Unit IV

PROFESSIONAL STANDARDS IN NURSING PRACTICE

Unit V

PSYCHOSOCIAL BASIS FOR NURSING PRACTICE

Unit VI

SCIENTIFIC BASIS FOR NURSING PRACTICE

Unit VII

BASIC HUMAN NEEDS

Unit VIII

CLIENTS WITH SPECIAL NEEDS

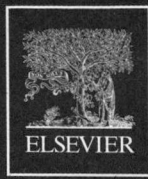

Fundamentals
of Nursing

Fundamentals *of* Nursing

Patricia A. Potter, RN, MSN, PhD, CMAC, FAAN
Research Scientist
Barnes-Jewish Hospital
St. Louis, Missouri

Anne Griffin Perry, RN, MSN, EdD, FAAN
Professor and Interim Director of Research
Saint Louis University School of Nursing
Saint Louis University Health Sciences Center
St. Louis, Missouri

ELSEVIER
MOSBY

6th Edition
With over 1100 illustrations

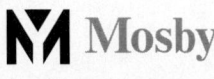

An Affiliate of Elsevier

11830 Westline Industrial Drive
St. Louis, Missouri 63146

NOTICE

Nursing is an ever-changing field. Standard safety precautions must be followed, but as new research and clinical experience broaden our knowledge, changes in treatment and drug therapy may become necessary or appropriate. Readers are advised to check the most current product information provided by the manufacturer of each drug to be administered to verify the recommended dose, the method and duration of administration, and contraindications. It is the responsibility of the licensed prescriber, relying on experience and knowledge of the patient, to determine dosages and the best treatment for each individual patient. Neither the publisher nor the authors assume any liability for any injury and/or damage to persons or property arising from this publication.

Previous editions copyrighted 1985, 1989, 1993, 1997, 2001
NCLEX is a registered trademark of the National Council of State Boards of Nursing, Inc.

International Standard Book Number: 0-323-02586-2

Executive Editor: Susan Epstein
Senior Developmental Editor: Maria Broeker
Publishing Services Manager: John Rogers
Senior Project Manager: Beth Hayes
Senior Designer: Kathi Gosche

Printed in the United States of America

Last digit is the print number: 9   8   7   6   5   4   3   2   1

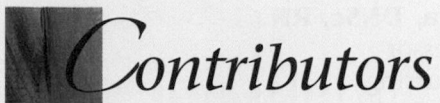

Contributors

Jeanette Adams, PhD, MSN, APRN, CRNI
Nursing Consultant
Coconut Grove, Florida

Myra. A. Aud, PhD, RN
Assistant Professor
Sinclair School of Nursing, University of Missouri–
   Columbia
Columbia, Missouri

Marjorie Baier, RN, PhD, APRN, BC
Associate Professor
School of Nursing, Southern Illinois University
   Edwardsville
Edwardsville, Illinois

Janice Boundy, RN, PhD
Professor, Director of Graduate Program
Saint Francis College of Nursing
Peoria, Illinois

Anna Brock, PhD, MSN, MEd, BSN
Professor
University of Southern Mississippi College
   of Nursing
Hattiesburg, Mississippi

Pamela L. Cherry, RN, BSN, MSN, DNSc
Associate Professor of Nursing
Humboldt State University
Arcata, California

Janice C. Colwell, RN, MS, CWOCN
Clinical Nurse Specialist, Wound, Ostomy & Skin
   Care
University of Chicago Hospitals
Chicago, Illinois

Eileen Costantinou, RN, MSN
Professional Practice Consultant
Barnes-Jewish Hospital
St. Louis, Missouri

Christine Durbin, RN, MSN, JD, PhDc
Instructor, School of Nursing
Southern Illinois University–Edwardsville
Edwardsville, Illinois

Margaret Ecker, RN, MS, PNP
Director of Education
Saint John's Health Center
Santa Monica, California

Martha Keene Elkin, RN, MS, IBCLC
Nursing Educator for Associate Degree Nursing
Private Practice Lactation Consultant
Mother Care of Maine
Sumner, Maine

**Susan Jane Fetzer, RN, BA, BSN, MSN, MBA,
   PhD**
Associate Professor
University of New Hampshire
Durham, New Hampshire

Victoria N. Folse, PhD, APRN, CS, LCPC
Assistant Professor
Illinois Wesleyan University
Bloomington, Illinois

Leah W. Frederick, MS, RN CIC
Infection Control Consultant
Infection Control Consultants
Scottsdale, Arizona

Amy Hall, RN, BSN, MS, PhD
Associate Professor
Saint Francis Medical Center College of Nursing
Peoria, Illinois

Mimi Hirshberg, RN, MSN
Clinical Assistant Professor
Barnes College of Nursing and Health Studies
University of Missouri–St. Louis
St. Louis, Missouri
IV Therapist
Vascular Access Service
Barnes-Jewish Hospital
St. Louis, Missouri

Steve Kilkus, RN, MSN
Nursing Faculty
Edgewood College
Madison, Wisconsin

Judith Ann Kilpatrick, RN, DNSc
Assistant Professor
Widener University School of Nursing
Chester, Pennsylvania

Kristine M. L'Ecuyer, RN, MSN, CCNS
Adjunct Assistant Professor
Saint Louis University School of Nursing
St. Louis, Missouri

Joyce Larson, PhD, MS, RN
President, Founder Culture and Counts
Adjunct Hillsborough Community College
Tampa, Florida

Ruth Ludwick, BSN, MSN, PhD, RNC
Professor
Kent State University, College of Nursing
Kent, Ohio

Annette G. Lueckenotte, MS, RN, BC, GNP GCNS
Gerontologic Nurse Practitioner and Educator
Barnes-Jewish West County Hospital
St. Louis, Missouri

Elaine K. Neel, BSN, MSN
Nursing Instructor
Graham Hospital School of Nursing
Canton, Illinois

Dula Pacquiao, BSN, MA, EdD
Professor, Director of Transcultural Nursing
 Institute and Coordinator of Graduate Program
Kean University
Union, New Jersey

Nancy C. Panthofer, RN, MSN
Lecturer
Kent State University College of Nursing
Kent, Ohio

Elaine U. Polan, RNC, BSN, MS
Nursing Program Supervisor
Vocational Education and Extension Board
 Practical Nursing Program
Uniondale, New York

Patsy L. Ruchala, DNSc, RN
Director and Professor
Orvis School of Nursing
University of Nevada–Reno
Reno, Nevada

Debbie Sanazaro, RN, MSN, GNP
Assistant Professor
Saint Louis University School of Nursing
St. Louis, Missouri

Marilyn Schallom, RN, MSN, CCRN, CCNS
Surgical Critical Care Clinical Nurse Specialist
Barnes-Jewish Hospital
St. Louis, Missouri

Patricia A. Stockert, RN, BSN, MS PhD
Associate Professor, Coordinator
Saint Francis Medical Center College of Nursing
Peoria, Illinois

Marshelle Thobaben, RN, MS, PHN, APNP, FNP
Chair and Professor
Humboldt State University
Arcata, California

Pamela Becker Weilitz, RN, MSN(R), BC, ANP, M-SCNS
Adult Nurse Practitioner
Private Practice
St. Louis, Missouri

Joan Domigan Wentz, BSN, MSN
Assistant Professor
Jewish Hospital College of Nursing and Allied
 Health
St. Louis, Missouri

Rita Wunderlich, BSN, MSN(r), PhD
Assistant Professor
Saint Louis University
School of Nursing
St. Louis, Missouri

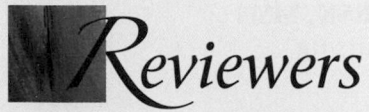

Reviewers

Pamela Adamshick, MSN, APRN, BC
Assistant Professor of Nursing
St. Luke's School of Nursing at Moravian College
Bethlehem, Pennsylvania

Sylvia K. Baird, RN, MM
Manager Patient Safety
Spectrum Health
Grand Rapids, Michigan

Martha C. Baker, RN, PhD, CCRN, CS
Director of BSN Program
Southwest Baptist University
Springfield, Missouri

Doris Bartlett, RN, MSN
Adjunct Facility
Bethel College
Mishawaka, Indiana

Julie Baylor, RN, MSN, PhDc
Assistant Professor
Bradley University
Peoria, Illinois

Margaret W. Bellak, RN, MN
Associate Professor
Indiana University of Pennsylvania
Indiana, Pennsylvania

Julie Bliss, EdD, RN
Associate Professor and Chairperson
Department of Nursing
William Paterson University of New Jersey
Wayne, New Jersey

Therese M. Bower, EdD, MSN, CNS, BSN, RN
Nursing Educator
Firelands Regional Medical Center School of
  Nursing
Sandusky, Ohio

Daya Breckinridge, RN, BSN, MSN, FNP
Clinical Faculty
Duke University School of Nursing
Durham, North Caroline

Anna Brock, PhD, MSN, MEd, BSN
Professor of Nursing
University of Southern Mississippi
Hattiesburg, Mississippi

Jacqueline Rosenjack Burchum, DNS, MSN, APRN, BC
Assistant Professor
The University of Memphis
Memphis, Tennessee

Susan Burkett, RN, MSN, CPNP, CPN
Chief Officer
TC Thompson Children's Hospital
Chattanooga, Tennessee

Darlene Nebel Cantu, MSN, RNC
Director
Baptist Health System
School of Professional Nursing
San Antonio, Texas
Faculty
San Antonio College
San Antonio, Texas

Kathlyn Carlson, BSN, MA, CPAN
Staff Nurse
Abbott Northwestern Hospital
Minneapolis, Minnesota

Patricia A. Castaldi, MSN, RN
Director
Practical Nursing Program
Union County College
Plainfield, New Jersey

Barbara Caton, RN, MSN
Assistant Professor
Southwest Missouri State University–West Plains
West Plains, Missouri

D. Sue Clarren, ND, RNC
Assistant Professor
University of Nevada Las Vegas
Las Vegas, Nevada

Barbara P. Daniel, CRNP, Med, MS
Professor of Nursing
Cecil Community College
North East, Maryland

Ken W. Edmisson, ND, EdD, RNC, FNP
Associate Professor
Middle Tennessee State University
Murfreesboro, Tennessee

Anne Falsone-Vaughan, MSN, RN
Clinical Instructor
Bellarmine University, Lansing School of Nursing
Louisville, Kentucky

Elizabeth Follis, BA, BSN, MS
Nursing Instructor
Northeastern Oklahoma A&M College
Miami, Oklahoma

Margaret S. Freel, RN, MSN, CNRN, APN/CS
Clinical Instructor and Clinical Simulation Lab
  Coordinator
Niehoff School of Nursing
Loyola University Chicago
Chicago, Illinois

Carrol Gold, PhD, RN
Case Manager
Palliative Care Center and Hospice of the North
  Shore
Evanston, Illinois

Linda C. Haynes, PhD, RN
Assistant Professor
Baylor University
Louise Herrington School of Nursing
Dallas, Texas

Adrienne Hentemann, RN, BSN, MS
Administrative Associate
Spectrum Health
Grand Rapids, Michigan

Monica Hentemann, RN, BSN
Staff Nurse and Preceptor
Spectrum Health
Grand Rapids, Michigan

Dorothy G. Herron, PhD, MS, MS, BS, RN
Assistant Professor
University of Maryland, School of Nursing
Baltimore, Maryland

Janice J. Hoffman, BSN, CCRN, MSN
SPRING Program Director
The Johns Hopkins Hospital
Baltimore, Maryland

Beth Hogan-Quigley, BSN, RN, MSN, CRNP
Clinical Lecturer
University of Pennsylvania School of Nursing
Philadelphia, Pennsylvania

Linda L. Kerby, BSN, RNC, MA, BA
Educational Consultant
Leawood, Kansas

Virginia Lester, RN, BSN, MSN
Assistant Professor of Nursing
Angelo State University
San Angelo, Texas

Rosemary Macy, RN, MSN
Assistant Professor
Boise State University
Boise, Idaho

Merry McBryde-Foster, PhD, CCM, RN
Assistant Professor
Baylor University
Louise Herrington School of Nursing
Dallas, Texas

Claudia Louth Mitchell, RN, BS, MS
Professor of Nursing
Santa Barbara City College
Santa Barbara, California

Teri A. Murray, PhD, MSN, MEd, BSN, RN
Director, Undergraduate Nursing Program
Barnes College of Nursing
University of Missouri–St. Louis
St. Louis, Missouri

Kathleen Ahem Nieubuurt, RN, MS
Nursing Instructor
Chemeketa Community College
Salem, Oregon

Ruth Novitt-Schumacher, BSN, MSN
Instructor
University of Illinois
Chicago, Illinois

Lynn Painter, DNSc, RN
Assistant Professor
Bloomsburg University
Bloomsburg, Pennsylvania

Marsha L. Ray, RN, BSN, MSN
Instructor of Nursing
Shasta College
Redding, California

Marisue Rayno, MSN, ACLS, BLS
Nursing Instructor
Luzerne County Community College
Nanticoke, Pennsylvania

Anita K. Reed, MSN, RN
Instructor of Nursing
St. Elizabeth School of Nursing
Lafayette, Indiana

Olive Santavenere, BSN, MSN, PhD, CNA
Associate Professor
Department of Nursing, Southern Connecticut
  State University
New Haven, Connecticut

Susan Parnell Scholtz, BSN, MN, DNSc
Associate Professor of Nursing
St. Luke's School of Nursing at Moravian College
Bethlehem, Pennsylvania

Susan R. Seager, MSN, EdD, RN
Associate Professor
Director Associate of Applied Science Nursing
  Program
Tennessee State University
Nashville, Tennessee

Ellen Shannon, RN, MSN, PhD(c)
Senior Clinical Quality Assurance Coordinator
  for North America
Aventis Pastur
Swiftwater, Pennsylvania

Julie Snyder, MSN, RN, C
Adjunct Faculty, School of Nursing
Old Dominion University
Norfolk, Virginia

Marilyn Teeter, MSN, RN
Associate Professor and Coordinator of Nursing
  Program
The Gettysburg Campus of the Harrisburg Area
  Community College
Gettysburg, Pennsylvania

Susanne M. Tracy, RN, MN, MA, PhD(c)
Associate Professor of Nursing
Rivier College
Nashua, New Hampshire

Kathleen Upham, BSN, MSN, ONC
Associate Professor of Nursing
Coastal Georgia Community College
Brunswick, Georgia

Debra J. Walden, BSN, MNSC, RNP
Assistant Professor of Nursing
Arkansas State University
State University, Arkansas

Katherine H. West, BSN, MSEd, CIC
Infection Control Consultant
Infection Control/Emerging Concepts, Inc.
Manassas, Virginia

Eileen Bagatti Whitwam, ARNP, MSN
Associate Professor of Nursing
Daytona Beach Community College
Daytona Beach, Florida

Rosemary H. Wittstadt, EdD, RN
Assistant Professor, Nursing
Towson University
Towson, Maryland

Thomas Worms, MSN, RN
Professor of Nursing
Truman College
Chicago, Illinois

Valerie Yancey, PhD, RN
Professor
Jewish Hospital College of Nursing and Allied
  Health
St. Louis, Missouri

Contributors to Previous Edition

Cynthia Hoppe Allen, BSN, MN, MPH
School of Nursing
Southeastern Louisiana University
Hammond, Louisiana

Charlene A. Allred, RN, PhD
Assistant Professor
College of Nursing
Medical University of South Carolina
Charleston, South Carolina

Denis E. Antle, BSN, MSN, RN, CCRN
CV/Critical Care Clinical Nurse Specialist
Genesis Medical Center
Davenport, Iowa

Della Aridge, RN, MSN
Clinical Nurse Specialist, General Surgery Division
Saint Louis University Hospital
St. Louis, Missouri

Elizabeth Ayello, PhD, MS, BSN, RN, CS, CWOCN
Clinical Assistant Professor
New York University, Division of Nursing
New York, New York

Genevieve Bahrt, RN, MN
Lecturer
School of Nursing
University of California–Los Angeles
Los Angeles, California

Karen Bailey, RN, MSN
Instructor of School Nursing
University of California–Los Angeles
Los Angeles, California

Julie K. Baylor, MSN, RN
Assistant Professor of Nursing
Bradley University
Peoria, Illinois

Billie J. Bodo, RN, MSN
Assistant Professor
Lakeland Community College
Mentor, Ohio

Peggy Breckinridge, MSN, FNP
Associate Professor
College of Health Sciences
Roanoke, Virginia

Penny S. Brooke, RN, BSN, MS, JD
Assistant Dean, Student-Affairs–Associate Professor
University of Utah College of Nursing
Salt Lake City, Utah

Judith C. Brostron, RN BA, JD, LLM
Attorney
Lashly and Baer
St. Louis, Missouri

Eleanor Lee Brown, RNC, MSN
Assistant Professor
Department of Nursing
Macon College
Macon, Georgia

Victoria Brown, RN, PhD
Associate Professor
School of Nursing
Georgia College
Milledgeville, Georgia

Kathryn Ann Caudell, PhD, RN, AOCN
Clinical Research and Education Manager
Amgen, Inc.
Thousand Oaks, California

Judith A. Chaney, RN, BSN, MS, PhD, AAMFT
Private Practice
Highland, Illinois

Mary F. Clarke, BSN, MA, RN
Informatics Nurse Specialists
Genesis Medical Center
Davenport, Iowa

Susan Cole, RN, MSN, CCRN
Clinical Resource Nurse, Department of Surgery
Saint Francis Medical Center
Cape Girardeau, Missouri

Judith A. Collins, MA, BSN, ARNP, CS
Psychiatric Liaison Clinical Nurse Specialist
Genesis Medical Center
Davenport, Iowa

Mary Coppola, RN, MSN
Assistant Professor
Salem State College
Salem, Massachusetts

Dorothy McDonnell Cooke, RN, PhD
Associate Professor, School of Nursing
Saint Louis University
St. Louis, Missouri

Sharon H. Cox, RN, MSN, CNAA
Principal Consultant, Founder
Cox and Associates
Brentwood, Tennessee

Rick Daniels, RN, BSN, MSN, PhD
Associate Professor of Nursing
Oregon Health Sciences University at Southern
Ashland, Oregon

Ruth Davidhizar, RN, BSN, MSN, DNS, CS, FAAN
Dean of Nursing
Bethel College
Mishawaka, Indiana

Lynne Dearing, RN, BSN, MSN, MA
Instructor in Nursing
Grays Harbor College
Aberdeen, Washington

Jana L. Weindel Dees, RN, BSN, MSN
Staff Nurse/Unit Based Educator
Barnes-Jewish Hospital
St. Louis, Missouri

Amy Deutschendorf, RN, MSN
Clinical Nurse Specialist
Sinai Hospital of Baltimore
Faculty Associate
University of Maryland
Baltimore, Maryland

Susan Dicke, BSN, BA, MS
School of Nursing
Mansfield General Hospital
Mansfield, Ohio

Catherine Doerrer, RN, MSN
Director of Medicine
Barnes Hospital
St. Louis, Missouri

Carole Edelman, RN, MS, CS
Director of Nursing, Waverly Care Center
New Canaan, Connecticut
Adjunct Faculty, Columbia University
New York, New York

Sally M. Featherstone, RN, BA, BSN, MN, CS, CGC, CDE
Director of Psychiatry
Dartmouth Hitchcock Medical Center
Lebanon, New Hampshire

Cathy Franklin, RN, BSN, MA
Professor of Nursing
Researcher
Director of Weekend Evening Program
Caldwell Community College
Hudson, North Carolina

Joyce Newman Giger, EdD, RN, CS, FAAN
Professor, Graduate Studies
School of Nursing, University of Alabama at
    Birmingham
Birmingham, Alabama

Brenda Goodner, RN, MSN, CS
Psychotherapist
Santa Teresa, New Mexico

Cynthia S. Goodwin, MSN, RN
Instructor, School of Nursing and Health
    Professions
University of Southern Indiana
Evansville, Indiana

Lois C. Hamel, MS, RN, CS, PhD(c)
Adult Nurse Practitioner/Adjunct Assistant
    Professor
University of New England/University of Vermont
    Medical School
Portland, Maine

Joyce J. Hamlin, RNC, BSN, MSN, CNS
Learning Resources Nurse Educator
Helene Fuld School of Nursing
Trenton, New Jersey

Renee Harrison, RN, MSN
Assistant Professor
Tulsa Junior College
Tulsa Oklahoma

Susan A. Hauser Jeffers, RN, BA, BSN, MS
Instructor, School of Nursing
Mansfield General Hospital
Mansfield, Ohio

Susan Herman, RN, MSN
Assistant Professor of Nursing
Chaffey College
Alta Loma, California

Lois K. Hess, RN, JD
Assistant In-House Counsel
Jewish Hospital Healthcare Systems, Inc.
Louisville, Kentucky

Wendy F. Higden, BN
Teacher and Clinical Instructor
Nursing Department
Vanier College
St. Laurent, Quebec, Canada

Karen Hill, RN, MN
Assistant Professor
School of Nursing
Southeastern Louisiana University
Hammond, Louisiana

Judith Hupcey, CRNP, EdD
Assistant Professor
School of Nursing
Pennsylvania State University
Hershey, Pennsylvania

Nancy C. Jackson, RN, BSN, MSN, CCRN
Pulmonary Clinical Nurse Specialist
St. Mary's Health Center
St. Louis, Missouri

Susan S. Johnson, RN, MSN
Lead Instructor
Nursing Education Options Program
Guilford Tech Community College
Jamestown, North Carolina

Marina K. Jones, RN, BSN, MSN(r)
Instructor of Nursing
Southern Illinois University–Edwardsville
Edwardsville, Illinois

Donna M. Kauffman, RN, MSN
Associate Professor
School of Nursing
Purdue University
West Lafayette, Indiana

Patricia T. Ketcham, RN, MSN, PhDc
Assistant Professor
Undergraduate Program Director
Oakland University
Rochester, Michigan

Carl A. Kirton, RN, BSN, MA, ACRN, ANP-CS
Clinical Assistant Professor of Nursing
New York University
New York, New York

Marjorie Knox, RN, MA, MPA
Professor of Nursing
Community College of Rhode Island
Warwick, Rhode Island

†Sister Kathleen Krekeler, RN, PhD
Professor of Nursing, School of Nursing
Saint Louis University
St. Louis, Missouri

Mary Ann Lavin, RN, BSN, MS, MSN, DSc, FAAN, ANP
Associate Professor of Nursing
Saint Louis University
St. Louis, Missouri

Jan L. Lee, CS, RN, PhD
Assistant Professor
Medical-Surgical/Physiological Section
School of Nursing
University of California–Los Angeles
Los Angeles, California

Pamela A. Lesser, RN, MS
Women's Services Coordinator
Women and Infants Service
Barnes Hospital
St. Louis, Missouri

Virginia Lester, RN, BSN, MSN, CNS
Assistant Professor
Angelo State University
San Angelo, Texas

Anne R. Lewis, BSN, MSN
Neuroscience Clinical Nurse Specialist
Genesis Medical Center
Davenport, Iowa

Gail B. Lewis, RN, MSN
Associate Professor
Barnes College
St. Louis, Missouri

Martha Long, RN, MSN, CIC
Infection Control Practitioner
University of Alabama Hospital
Birmingham, Alabama

Mary Kay Knight Macheca, RN, BSN, MSN(r) CDE
Nurse Practitioner
St. Louis, Missouri

---

† Deceased.

Jeffrey C. McManemy, RN, BSN, MSN, CS
Coordinator, Nursing Education, Clinical
  Instructor
Saint Louis University Health Sciences Center
St. Louis, Missouri

Sharon L. Merritt, RN, BSN, MSN, EdD
Associate Professor/Director, Center for Narcolepsy
  Research
University of Illinois at Chicago
Chicago, Illinois

Mary Dee Miller, RN, BSN, MS, CIC
Nurse Epidemiologist
Mercy Hospitals, Hamilton/Fairfield
Hamilton, Ohio

Janet Morgan, RN, MS
Associate Professor of Nursing
Tompkins-Cortland Community College
Dryden, New York

Kathleen Mulryan, BSN, MSN
Professor of Nursing
LaGuardia Community College
Long Island City, New York

Kathleen Nuwayhid, RN, BSN, MN
Instructor of Nursing
Vanier College
St. Laurent, Quebec, Canada

Susan Opas, RNC, MSN, CNS, CHES
Lecturer
School of Nursing
University of California–Los Angeles
Los Angeles, California

Marsha Evans Orr, RN, MS, CS
Regional Clinical Manger
Apria Healthcare
Phoenix, Arizona

Veronica (Ronnie) Peterson, RN, BA, BSN, MS
Nursing Supervisor
University of Wisconsin Hospital and Clinics
Madison, Wisconsin

Shelley-Rae Pheler, MSN, BSN, RN
Maternal Child/Pediatric Clinical Nurse Specialist
Genesis Medical Center
Davenport, Iowa

Victoria L. Poole, RN, DSN
Assistant Professor
School of Nursing
University of Alabama at Birmingham
Birmingham, Alabama

Ann M. Popkess, RN, BSN
Manager, Barnes Home Health Services
St. Louis, Missouri

Cheryl A. Prandoni, RN, MSN
Director of Learning Resources
School of Nursing
Catholic University of America
Washington, D.C.

Caroline Pritchard, RN, MSN, ND
Instructor and Clinical Director
BSN Program
Case Western Reserve University
Cleveland, Ohio

Peg Reiter, RN, MS
Assistant Professor
Galveston College
Galveston, Texas

Janet Robuck, MS, RD
Associate Professor of Nutrition
School of Nursing
University of Alabama
Birmingham, Alabama

Judith Roos, RN, BSN, MSN
Associate Professor of Nursing
Jewish Hospital College
St. Louis, Missouri

Janice Rumfelt, RNC, MSN, EdD
Assistant Professor of Nursing
Southern Illinois University–Edwardsville
Edwardsville, Illinois

Susan Schaffer, RN, MS, CFNP
Assistant Professor of Nursing
Old Dominion University
Norfolk, Virginia

Patti Pond Scott, RN, BS
Instructor Kilgore College
Longview, Texas

Nancy Semenza, RN, BSN, MS, PhD(c)
Nursing Faculty Adjunct
MacMurray College
Jacksonville, Illinois

Bobbi Shatto, BSN, MSN
Adjunct Instructor
Saint Louis University School of Nursing
St. Louis, Missouri

Thomas J. Smith, RN, BSN, MN, PhD
Associate Professor of Nursing
Nicholls State University
Thibodaux, Louisana

Margaret Souders, RNC, MSN
Instructor
Department of Nursing
Phoenix College
Phoenix, Arizona

Sharon Souter, RN, BSN, MSN
Nursing Program Director
New Mexico State University at Carlsbad
Carlsbad, New Mexico

Elizabeth Speakman, RN, MEd
Associate Professor of Nursing/Doctoral Candidate,
  Columbia University
Community College of Philadelphia
Philadelphia, Pennsylvania

**Rachel E. Spector, RN, BS, MS, PhD, CTN,
  FAAN**
Associate Professor of Nursing
Boston College School of Nursing
Chestnut Hill, Massachusetts

Martha Spies, RN, MSN
Assistant Professor
Deaconess College of Nursing
St. Louis, Missouri

Ruth Stephens, RN, PhD
Professor of Nursing
Florida Community College at Jacksonville
Jacksonville, Florida

**Ann Bernadette Tritak, RN, BS, MS, PhD,
  CTN, FAAN**
Associate Professor of Nursing
Fairleigh Dickinson University
Teaneck, New Jersey

Jean Urick, RN, MN
Assistant Professor
School of Nursing
Southeastern Louisiana University
Hammond, Louisiana

JoEtta A. Vernon, RN, MS, PhD
Research Consultant
Omaha, Nebraska

Mary E. Walker, RN, BSN, MA
Psychiatric Clinical Nurse Specialist
Veterans Administration Medical Center
Knoxville, Iowa

Flora Weirich, RN, MSN, CEN
Instructor
School of Nursing
Pennsylvania State University
University Park, Pennsylvania

Joyce Williams, RN, MSN
Assistant Professor
School of Nursing
George Mason University

Diane M. Wink, RN, MSN, MA, EdD
Assistant Professor
University of Central Florida
Orlando, Florida

Toni Wortham, RNC, MSN
Associate Professor
Nursing Program
Madisonville Community College
Madisonville, Kentucky

Valerie J. Yancey, PhD, RN
Professor
Jewish Hospital College of Nursing and Allied
  Health
St. Louis, Missouri

Susan SCHAFER, RN, MS, CCRN
Assistant Professor of Nursing
Old Dominion University
Norfolk, Virginia

Patti Pond Scott, RN, BS
Instructor in Nursing
... College
Bloomington, ...

Nancy Steffen..., RN, BSN, MS, PhD(c)
Nursing Faculty Adjunct
MacMurray College
Jacksonville, Illinois

Isabel Shatto, BSN, MSN
Adjunct Instructor
Saint Louis University ...
St. Louis, Missouri

Thomas J. Smith, RN, BSN, MN, PhD
Associate Professor of Nursing
Nicholls State University
Thibodaux, Louisiana

Margaret Soukup, RNC, MSN
Instructor
Department of Nursing
Phoenix College
Phoenix, Arizona

Ruth Stephens, RN, PhD
Professor of Nursing
Florida Community College at Jacksonville
Jacksonville, Florida

Ann Bernadette Irish, RN, BS, MS, PhD, RN, FAAN
Associate Professor of Nursing
Fairleigh Dickinson University
Teaneck, New Jersey

Jean Ulrich, RN, MN
Assistant Professor
School of Nursing
Southeastern Louisiana University
Hammond, Louisiana

Mary E. Walker, RN, BSN, MA
Psychiatric Clinical Nurse Specialist
Veterans Administration Medical Center
Knoxville, Iowa

This sixth edition is dedicated to
Ruth, Jim, Bess, and Anne,
uncommon friends who
bring joy and fulfillment to life.

Patricia A. Potter

This book is dedicated to the memory of my parents,
Florence Bowmaster Griffin and Cecil Howard Griffin,
for their love, support, compassion, and
commitment to lifelong learning.

Anne Griffin Perry

Student Preface

Learning **Objectives** begin each chapter to help you focus on the key information that follows.

Chapters end with **Key Concepts** to help you review.

Critical Thinking Exercises help you apply essential content.

Review Questions at the end of each chapter help you review and evaluate what you have learned. Answers and rationales are provided at the back of the book.

Key Terms are listed at the end of each chapter and are boldfaced and defined in the text. Page numbers help you quickly find where each term is defined.

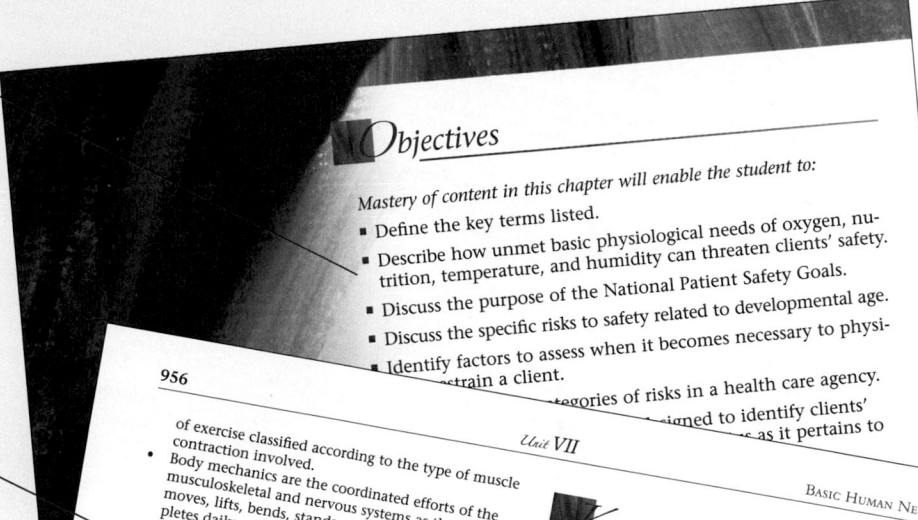

Objectives

Mastery of content in this chapter will enable the student to:

- Define the key terms listed.
- Describe how unmet basic physiological needs of oxygen, nutrition, temperature, and humidity can threaten clients' safety.
- Discuss the purpose of the National Patient Safety Goals.
- Discuss the specific risks to safety related to developmental age.
- Identify factors to assess when it becomes necessary to physically restrain a client.
- ... categories of risks in a health care agency.
- ... signed to identify clients' ... es as it pertains to

- of exercise classified according to the type of muscle contraction involved.
- Body mechanics are the coordinated efforts of the musculoskeletal and nervous systems as the person moves, lifts, bends, stands, sits, lies down, and completes daily activities.
- Coordinated body movement requires integrated functioning of the skeletal system, skeletal muscles, and nervous system.
- The skeleton provides bony support structure for movement, attachment of ligaments and muscles, protection of vital organs, some of the regulation of calcium, and production of red blood cells.
- Muscles primarily associated with movement are located near the skeletal region, where movement results from leverage, which is characteristic of movements of the upper extremities.
- Coordination and regulation of muscle groups depend on muscle tone and activity of antagonistic, synergistic, and antigravity muscles.
- Balance is assisted through nervous system control in the cerebellum and inner ear function.
- Body balance is achieved when there is a wide base of support, the center of gravity falls within the base of support, and a vertical line falls from the center of gravity through the base of support.
- Developmental changes, behavioral aspects, environmental issues, cultural and ethnic origin, and family and social support influence the client's perception and motivation to engage in physical activity and exercise.
- Ability to engage in normal physical activity and exercise depends on intact and functioning nervous and musculoskeletal systems.
- The nurse uses the nursing process to provide care for clients who are experiencing or are at risk for activity intolerance and impaired physical mobility.
- After identifying nursing diagnoses, the nurse plans and implements interventions to increase activity and exercise in collaboration with the client when possible.
- Range-of-motion exercises incorporated into daily activities can include one or all of the body joints.
- Mechanical devices to promote walking include canes, walkers, and crutches.

Key Terms

Activities of daily living (ADLs), *p. 931*
Activity tolerance, *p. 932*
Antagonistic muscles, *p. 933*
Antigravity muscles, *p. 933*
Body mechanics, *p. 930*
Cartilage, *p. 932*
Cartilaginous joints, *p. 932*
Center of gravity, *p. 931*
Crutch gait, *p. 950*
Exercise, *p. 930*
Fibrous joints, *p. 932*
Footboard, *p. 932*

Friction, *p. 931*
Gait, *p. 937*
Hemiparesis, *p. 937*
Hemiplegia, *p. 934*
Immobility, *p. 948*
Isometric contraction, *p. 932*
Isotonic contraction, *p. 932*
Joint, *p. 932*
Ligaments, *p. 932*
Mobility, *p. 937*
Muscle tone, *p. 931*
Posture, *p. 931*

Key Terms—cont'd

Proprioception, *p. 933*
Range of motion (ROM), *p. 937*

Synergistic muscles, *p. 933*
Synovial joints, *p. 932*
Tendons, *p. 932*

Critical Thinking Exercises

1. Ms. Moushey is an 52-year-old woman. She sustained a fracture of the left femur and must use crutches for 1 week until her follow-up visit at the orthopedic clinic. Her physician has ordered no weight bearing on the left leg. You are conducting the first home visit after her discharge from the hospital. What is the appropriate crutch gait for Ms. Moushey? List several teaching strategies that focus on crutch safety.

2. Mr. Neel has just undergone extensive abdominal surgery. What assessment parameters need to be considered before ambulation of this client? What precautions should you take before ambulating him for the first time?

3. The family of Mrs. Parks made the decision to care for her at home. She is a quadriplegic, weighs 72 kg, and requires total care. You are her nurse and responsible for instructing her family on several aspects of her care. Develop a list of basic principles describing body mechanics to protect Mrs. Parks's family members from injury.

Review Questions

1. Antagonistic muscles bring about movement at the:
   1. Muscle.
   1. Joint.
   1. Ligaments.
   1. Bones.

2. Proprioception is:
   1. Awareness of the position of the body.
   2. Needed for antigravity.
   3. Located within the semicircular canals.
   4. An uncommon metabolic disease.

3. Balance is controlled by the nervous system, specifically by the:
   1. Cerebrum and pons.
   2. Cerebellum and inner ear.
   3. Eye and ear.
   4. Cerebral cortex and gyrus.

4. A client with a right-sided cerebral hemorrhage may have:
   1. Left-sided hemiplegia.
   2. Right-sided hemiplegia.
   3. Bilateral hemiplegia.
   4. Degenerative hemiplegia.

The five-step **Nursing Process** provides a consistent framework for presentation of content in clinical chapters.

The unique **Critical Thinking Model** clearly shows how nursing process and critical thinking come together to help you provide the best care for your clients.

Unit VII   BASIC HUMAN NEEDS

968

Safety and the Nursing Process

NP Assessment

To conduct a thorough client assessment, the nurse considers possible threats to the client's safety, including the client's immediate environment, as well as any individual risk factors.

Nursing History. A nursing history will include data about the client's level of wellness to determine if any underlying conditions exist that pose threats to safety. For example, the nurse will give special attention to as-

sessing the client's gait, muscle strength and coordination, balance, and vision. A review of the client's developmental status must be considered as assessment information is analyzed. The nurse will also review if the client is taking any medications or undergoing any procedures that pose risks. For example, use of diuretics increases the frequency of voiding and may result in the client having to use toilet facilities more often. Falls often occur with clients who must get out of bed quickly because of urinary urgency.

Client's Home Environment. When caring for a client in the home, a home hazard assessment is necessary (Box 37-2). The nurse should walk through the home with the

---

Box 37-2 Home Hazard Assessment

Home Exterior
Are sidewalks uneven?
Are steps in good repair?
Is ice and snow removal adequate?
Do steps have securely fastened handrails?
Is there adequate lighting?
Is outdoor furniture sturdy?

Home Interior
Do al... ...airways, and halls have adequate, nonglare
... ...w nonslip floor

Bathroom
Are hand-washing facilities available?
Are there skidproof strips or surfaces in the tub or shower?
Are bath mats secured?
Does the client need grab bars near the bathtub and toilet?
Does the client need an elevated toilet seat?
Is the medicine cabinet well lighted?
Are medications in their original containers?
Are medication containers child resistant if children live in the home or visit?
Is ipecac syrup available in households with small children?
Have outdated medications been discarded?

Bedroom
Are beds of adequate height to allow getting on and off easily?
Is day and night lighting adequate?
Are floor coverings nonskid?
Does the client have a telephone nearby?
...e emergency numbers visible near the telephone?

... and Fire Hazards
...nonoxide detectors installed?
...tors tested every month and
...checked for proper
...priately?

Chapter 37   CLIENT SAFETY   967

KNOWLEDGE
• Basic human needs
• Potential risks to client safety from physical hazards, lifestyle, risks associated with health care environment, and environmental risks
• Influence of developmental stage on safety needs
• Influence of illness/medications on client safety

EXPERIENCE
• Caring for clients whose mobility or sensory impairments increase threats to safety
• Personal experience in caring for younger siblings or children

Assessment
• Identify actual and potential threats to the client's safety
• Determine impact of the underlying illness on the client's safety
• Identify the presence of risks for the client's developmental stage and client's environment

STANDARDS
• Apply intellectual standards such as accuracy, significance, and completeness when assessing for threats to the client's safety
• Apply ANA standards for nursing practice; JCAHO standards for health care settings
• Apply agency practice standards (e.g., fall prevention or restraint protocols)

ATTITUDES
• Demonstrate perseverance when necessary to identify all safety threats
• Be responsible for collecting unbiased, accurate data regarding threats to the client's safety
• Show discipline in conducting a thorough review of the client's home environment

FIGURE 37-5 Critical thinking model for safety assessment.

perience as he or she conducts a detailed assessment of a specific client. For example, while assessing a specific client's home environment, the nurse will consider knowledge regarding typical locations within the home where dangers commonly exist. If a client has a visual im-

pairment, the nurse will apply previous experiences in caring for clients with visual changes to anticipate how to thoroughly assess the client's needs. Critical thinking directs the nurse to anticipate what needs to be assessed and how to make conclusions about available data.

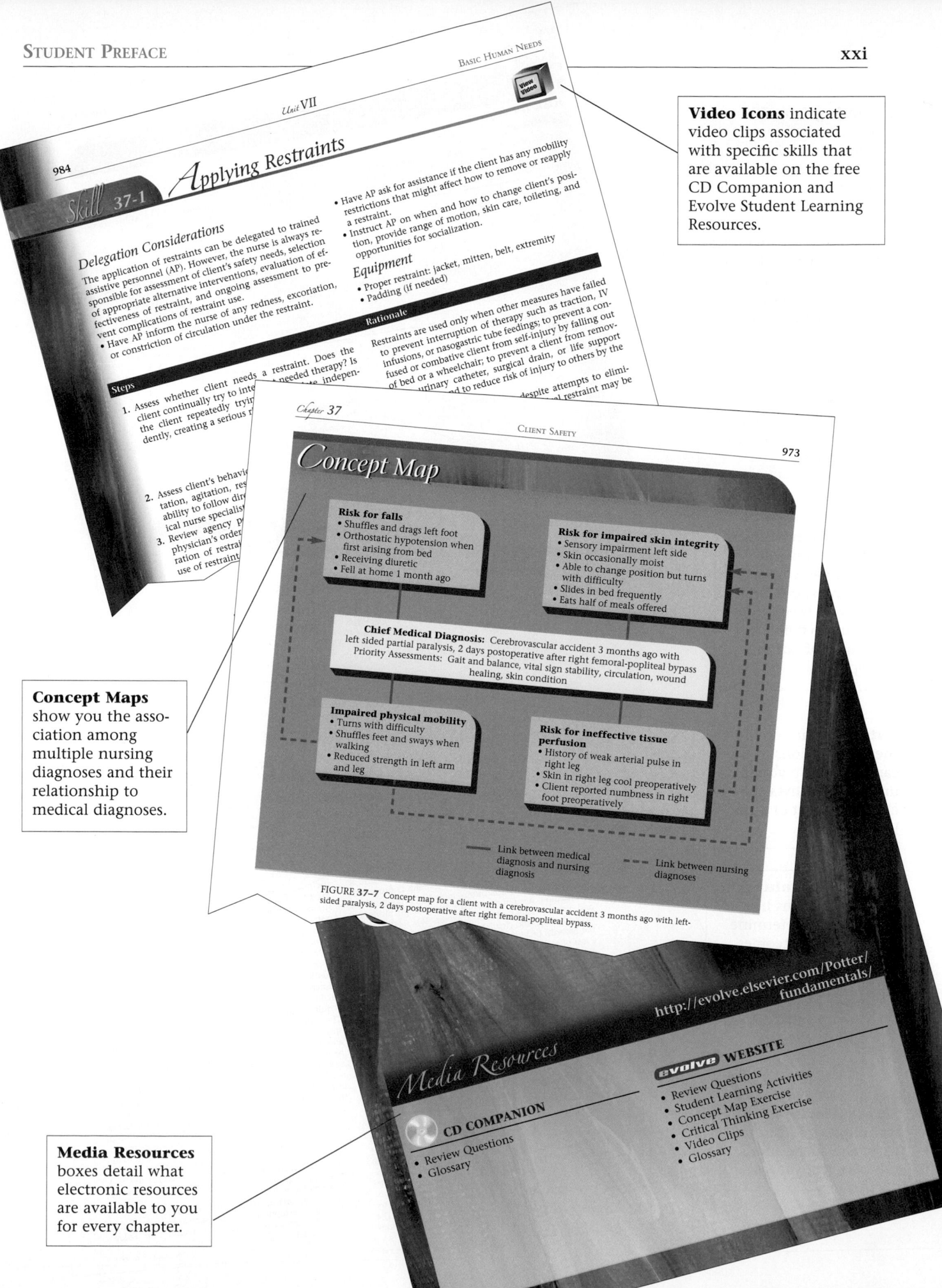

984

Skill 37-1

Applying Restraints

Delegation Considerations

The application of restraints can be delegated to trained assistive personnel (AP). However, the nurse is always responsible for assessment of client's safety needs, selection of appropriate alternative interventions, evaluation of effectiveness of restraint, and ongoing assessment to prevent complications of restraint use.

• Have AP inform the nurse of any redness, excoriation, or constriction of circulation under the restraint.

• Have AP ask for assistance if the client has any mobility restrictions that might affect how to remove or reapply a restraint.

• Instruct AP on when and how to change client's position, provide range of motion, skin care, toileting, and opportunities for socialization.

Equipment

• Proper restraint: jacket, mitten, belt, extremity
• Padding (if needed)

Rationale

Restraints are used only when other measures have failed to prevent interruption of therapy such as traction, IV infusions, or nasogastric tube feedings; to prevent a confused or combative client from self-injury by falling out of bed or a wheelchair; to prevent a client from removing urinary catheter, surgical drain, or life support and to reduce risk of injury to others by the

Steps

1. Assess whether client needs a restraint. Does the client continually try to inte... needed therapy? Is the client repeatedly tryi... ...te independently, creating a serious r...

2. Assess client's behavi... ...tation, agitation, res... ability to follow dir... ical nurse specialis...

3. Review agency p... physician's order... ration of restrai... use of restraint...

despite attempts to elimi... ...l restraint may be

Video Icons indicate video clips associated with specific skills that are available on the free CD Companion and Evolve Student Learning Resources.

Chapter 37

CLIENT SAFETY

973

Concept Map

Risk for falls
• Shuffles and drags left foot
• Orthostatic hypotension when first arising from bed
• Receiving diuretic
• Fell at home 1 month ago

Risk for impaired skin integrity
• Sensory impairment left side
• Skin occasionally moist
• Able to change position but turns with difficulty
• Slides in bed frequently
• Eats half of meals offered

Chief Medical Diagnosis: Cerebrovascular accident 3 months ago with left sided partial paralysis, 2 days postoperative after right femoral-popliteal bypass
Priority Assessments: Gait and balance, vital sign stability, circulation, wound healing, skin condition

Impaired physical mobility
• Turns with difficulty
• Shuffles feet and sways when walking
• Reduced strength in left arm and leg

Risk for ineffective tissue perfusion
• History of weak arterial pulse in right leg
• Skin in right leg cool preoperatively
• Client reported numbness in right foot preoperatively

——— Link between medical diagnosis and nursing diagnosis

- - - - Link between nursing diagnoses

FIGURE **37-7** Concept map for a client with a cerebrovascular accident 3 months ago with left-sided paralysis, 2 days postoperative after right femoral-popliteal bypass.

Concept Maps show you the association among multiple nursing diagnoses and their relationship to medical diagnoses.

http://evolve.elsevier.com/Potter/fundamentals/

Media Resources

evolve WEBSITE

CD COMPANION
• Review Questions
• Glossary

• Review Questions
• Student Learning Activities
• Concept Map Exercise
• Critical Thinking Exercise
• Video Clips
• Glossary

Media Resources boxes detail what electronic resources are available to you for every chapter.

Nursing Care Plans feature a revised format that helps you understand the process of assessment, the association of assessment findings with defining characteristics of nursing diagnoses, the identification of goals and outcomes, selection of interventions, and the process for evaluating care.

Assessment section tells you how to gather data instead of just listing findings.

Nursing Intervention Classification and **Nursing Outcome Classification** terminologies are used in the care plans to build your knowledge of nursing concepts.

Rationales for each of the interventions in the care plans help you to understand why a specific step or set of steps is performed.

Expanded Evaluation section explains how to evaluate and determine whether the outcomes have been achieved.

Safety Alerts indicate techniques you can use to ensure client and nurse safety.

Nursing Care Plan

Risk for Injury

Assessment

Mr. Key, a visiting nurse, is seeing Ms. Cohen, an 85-year-old woman, at her home. The client has been recovering from a mild stroke affecting her left side. Ms. Cohen lives alone but receives regular assistance from her daughter and son, who both live within 10 miles. Mr. Key's assessment included a discussion of Ms. Cohen's health problem and how the stroke has affected her, as well as a pertinent physical examination.

Assessment Activities

Ask Ms. Cohen how the stroke has affected her mobility.

Conduct a home hazard assessment.

Observe Ms. Cohen's gait and posture.

Assess Ms. Cohen's muscle strength.
Assess visual acuity with corrective lenses.

Findings/Defining Characteristics

She responds, "I bump into things, and I'm afraid I'm going to fall."
Cabinets in kitchen are in disarray and full of breakable items that could fall out. Throw rugs are on floors; lighting is poor (40-watt bulbs); bathroom lighting bars; home cluttered with furniture and small objects.
Ms. Cohen has kyphosis and has a hesitant, uncoordinated gait. She frequently holds walls for support.
Left arm and leg weaker than right.
Ms. Cohen has trouble reading and seeing familiar objects at a distance while wearing current glasses.

Nursing Diagnosis: Risk for injury related to impaired mobility, decreased visual acuity, and physical environmental hazards.

Planning

Goal

Home will be free of hazards within 1 month.

Client and family will be knowledgeable of potential hazards for Ms. Cohen's age-group within 1 week.

Ms. Cohen will

Expected Outcomes*
Risk Control
Modifiable hazards in kitchen and hallway will be the home within 1 week. Revisions to in 1 month.

Knowled

Nursing Care Plan

Risk for Injury—cont'd

Interventions†—cont'd

Fall Prevention
• Encourage daughter to schedule vision testing for new prescription within 2 to 4 weeks.
• Refer to a physical therapist to assess need for assistive devices for kyphosis, left-sided weakness, and gait.

Rationale

Improved visual acuity reduces incidence of falls (Ebersole and Hess, 2001).
Exercise often improves gait, balance, and flexibility.
Modifying gait problems by increasing lower extremity strength reduces fall risk (Schoenfelder, 2000).

†Intervention classification labels from Dochterman JM, Bulechek GM: *Nursing interventions classification (NIC)*, ed 4, St. Louis, 2004, Mosby.

Evaluation

Nursing Actions
Ask client and family to identify risks.

Observe environment for elimination of hazards.

Reassess Ms. Cohen's visual acuity.

Ms. Cohen's gait and posture.

Client Response/Finding
Ms. Cohen and daughter able to identify risks during a walk through the home and expressed a greater sense of safety as a result of changes made.
Throw rugs have been removed.
Lighting has increased to 75 watts except in bathroom and bedroom.
Ms. Cohen has new glasses and says she can read better, as well as see distant objects more clearly.
Ms. Cohen's gait remains hesitant and uncoordinated; she reports that her daughter has not had time to take her

Achievement of Outcome
Client and daughter are more knowledgeable of potential hazards.

Environmental hazards have been partially reduced.

Ms. Cohen's vision has improved, enabling her to ambulate more safely.

Outcome of safe ambulation has not been totally achieved; continue to encourage Ms. Cohen and daughter to go to physical therapy appointment.

---

comes necessary for a nurse to apply a vest restraint, it must be done safely. The use of any restraint is also associated with serious complications, including pressure ulcers, constipation, pneumonia, urinary and fecal incontinence, and urinary retention (see Chapter 46). Contractures, nerve damage, and circulatory impairment are also potential hazards. In addition, restrained clients can experience a loss of self-esteem, humiliation, fear, and anger.

Safety Alert. Routine assessment of a client in restraint is critical to prevent injury. Because of the risk of injury from restraints, regulatory agencies such as the JCAHO and the Centers for Medicaid and Medicare Services (CMS) enforce standards for the safe use of restraints and define clients' rights and choices regarding their use. Under these guidelines, reasons for use of a physical restraint are to be clearly stated. The use of restraints must be part of the client's medical treatment, all less restrictive interventions must be tried first, other disciplines must be consulted, and supporting documentation must be provided (CMS, 2001).

The impetus is for health care organizations to move to a restraint-free environment. Restraints do not prevent falls or injury. In fact, it has been shown that clients incur less severe injuries if left unrestrained (Capezuti and others, 1998; Strumpf and others, 1998). Research has shown that a multidisciplinary approach that conducts individualized assessments and develops structured treatment plans can reduce the number of restraints used. It is imperative that nurses try alternative measures instead of restraints (Box 37-8). The University of Iowa Gerontological Nursing Interventions

the family members and clients by explaining their purpose, expected care while the client is restrained, precautions taken to avoid injury, and that the restraint is temporary and protective. Informed consent from family members may also be required before using restraints, as is the case in long-term care settings.

For legal purposes, the nurse must know agency-specific policy and procedures for appropriate use and monitoring of restraints. The use of a restraint must be clinically justified and be a part of the client's prescribed medical treatment and plan of care. A physician's order is required, based on a face-to-face assessment of the client. The order must state the type of restraint, location, and specific client behaviors for which restraints are to be used and must have a limited time frame. These orders should be renewed within a specific time frame according to the agency's policy. Restraints are not to be ordered prn (as needed). Assessment of clients who are restrained is ongoing. Proper documentation, including the behaviors that necessitated the application of restraints, the procedure used in restraining, the condition of the body part restrained (e.g., circulation to hand), and the evaluation of the client response, is essential. Restraints must be periodically removed, and the nurse must assess the client to determine if the restraints continue to be needed.

Skill 37-1 includes guidelines for the proper use and application of restraints. Use of restraints must meet the following objectives:
• Reduce the risk of client injury from falls.
• Prevent interruption of therapy such as traction, IV infusions, nasogastric (NG) tube feeding, or Foley catheterization.

Text continued on p. 990

Procedural Guidelines provide streamlined, step-by-step instructions for performing basic skills.

Client Teaching boxes tell you what and how to teach clients and how to evaluate learning.

Chapter 37

Procedural Guidelines

Box 37-11

Interventions in Accidental Poisoning

1. Assess for airway patency, breathing, and circulation (ABCs) in all clients in whom accidental poisoning is suspected.
2. Remove any visible materials from areas such as the mouth and eyes to terminate exposure.
3. Identify the type and amount of substance ingested, if possible. This may help to determine the antidote.
4. Call the Poison Control Center before attempting any interventions. The universal phone number for poison control is (800) 222-1222.
5. If directed by a physician, give oral fluids to assist vomiting.
6. If directed, save vomitus for laboratory analysis, which may assist with further treatment.
7. Position the victim with the head to the side to prevent aspiration of vomitus, and assist in keeping the airway open.
8. Never induce vomiting in an unconscious victim or in a client experiencing convulsions, because aspiration may occur.
9. Never induce vomiting if any of the following substances have been ingested: lye, household cleaners, hair care products, grease or petroleum products, or furniture polish. Vomiting may increase internal burns.
10. If instructed to take the victim to the emergency department, call an ambulance. Emergency equipment may be needed en route.
11. In the case of convulsions, cessation of breathing or unconsciousness, call 911.
12. Do not administer syrup of ipecac to induce vomiting. It has not been proven effective in preventing poisoning (AAP, 2004).

American Academy of Pediatrics: News release—don't treat swallowed poison with syrup of ipecac, www.aap.org/advocacy/releases/novpoison.htm. Accessed Feb 27, 2004.

39). If the client has a pulse and remains alert and oriented, the nurse should quickly obtain vital signs and assess the skin for signs of thermal injury. The client's physician must be notified. If an electrical shock occurs in the home, the nurse follows the same procedure and then has the client go to the emergency department and then notifies the client's physician.

Seizures. Clients who have experienced some form of neurological injury or metabolic disturbance are at risk for a seizure. A seizure involves a hyperexcitation of neurons in the brain leading to a sudden, violent, involuntary series of contractions of a group of muscles. The client often loses consciousness. **Seizure precautions** encompass all nursing interventions to protect the client from traumatic injury, positioning for adequate ventilation and drainage of oral secretions, and providing privacy and support following the seizure (Skill 37-2).

During a seizure a client's jaw muscles can become tense. It has been found that significant injury to the client's oral cavity is rare, even during the most severe seizures. Injury may instead occur from a caregiver placing an object into the client's mouth and forcing biting down on a hard object. Soft objects, placed in the mouth during a seizure and be aspirated. For the Epilepsy Foundation of America, in its standard instructions for seizure first aid, includes avoiding the use of objects into the mouth (Seizure Recognition and Observation, 1992). The exception to this is with **status epilepticus,** a medical emergency in which a person has continual seizures with no recovery and adequate airway is maintained. Clients experiencing a seizure at home should be placed on seizure precautions and they should be protected from traumatic injury.

Chapter 37

Focus on Older Adults

Box 37-6

CLIENT SAFETY

- The older adult experiences alterations in vision and hearing. The nurse should encourage yearly vision and hearing examinations and frequent cleansing of glasses and hearing aids as a means of preventing falls and burns.
- Older adults may have slowed reaction time. Teach clients safety tips for avoiding automobile accidents. Driving may need to be restricted to daylight hours or suspended.
- Range of motion, flexibility, and strength are decreased. The nurse should encourage supervised exercise classes for older adults and teach them to seek assistance with household tasks as needed. Safety features, such as grab bars in the bathroom, may be needed.
- Reflexes are slowed, and the ability to respond to multiple stimuli is reduced. The nurse should provide adequate, meaningful stimuli but prevent sensory overload.
- Nocturia and incontinence are more frequent in older adults. The nurse should institute a regular toileting schedule for the client. A recommended frequency is every 3 hours. Diuretics should be given in the morning. Assistance should be provided, along with adequate lighting, to clients who need to go to the bathroom at night.
- Memory may be impaired. Clients should use medication organizers, which can be purchased at any drugstore at a very reasonable cost. These dispensers can be filled once a week with the proper medications to be taken at a specific time during the day.
- The family plays a significant role in the care of older adults. It is estimated that more than 8 million older adults living at home need and get some form of help from family and friends (Ebersole and Hess, 2001). Encourage the family to allow the older adult to remain as independent as possible and provide help only for those things that are especially stressful or depleted.
- The high prevalence of chronic conditions in older adults results in the use of a high number of prescription and over-the-counter medications. Coupled with age-related changes in pharmacokinetics, there is a greater risk of serious adverse effects. Medications typically prescribed for older adults include anticholinergics, diuretics, anxiolytic and hypnotic agents, antidepressants, antihypertensives, vasodilators, analgesics, and laxatives, all of which may themselves pose risks or may interact to increase the risk for falls. The nurse should review the client's drug profile to ensure that any of the above noted drugs are used cautiously and assess the client regularly for any adverse effects that may increase fall risk.

Client Teaching

Box 37-12

Prevention of Electrical Hazards

Objective

- Client will recognize electrical hazards in the home and eliminate them.

Teaching Strategies

- Discuss grounding appliances and other equipment.
- Provide examples of common hazards: frayed cords, damaged equipment, and overloaded outlets.
- Discuss guidelines to prevent electrical shocks; and use electrical tape to secure the cord to the floor where it will not be stepped on.
- Do not run wires under carpeting.
- Pull the plug, not the cord, when unplugging items.
- Keep appliances away from water.
- Know how to operate equipment.

involved in a crime. For example, some useful tips include always parking the car near a bright light or busy public area, carrying a whistle attached to the car keys, keeping car doors locked while driving, and always paying attention while driving to notice if anyone starts to follow the car.

To prevent the transmission of pathogens, nurses can teach aseptic practices. Medical asepsis, which includes hand hygiene and environmental cleanliness, reduces the transfer of organisms (see Chapter 33). Clients and family members need to learn thorough hand hygiene (hand washing or use of hand rub) and when to use it (e.g., before and after caring for a family member, before food preparation, before preparing a medication for a family member, and after contacting any body fluids). When clients require dressing changes or the use of syringes and needles, families should be shown how to properly dispose of contaminated items in the home. Most communities have regulations for the disposal of biohazardous waste.

Acute Care. There are a number of specific safety measures applicable to clients in the acute care environment. The nurse takes measures to help clients avoid falls, injuries from use of restraints and side rails, fires, poisoning, and electrical hazards. Special precautions are necessary to prevent injury in clients susceptible to having seizures. Radiation injuries are also a specific safety concern. Finally, the nurse must be prepared to respond to the emergency of a bioterrorist attack.

Falls. Modifications in the home and health care environment can easily reduce the risk of falls (Table 37-3). A heavy or debilitated client in a bed or wheelchair or on a toilet should be properly supported and secured. Side rails may be necessary unless a client is able to freely and easily ambulate independently. Safety bars on toilets, locks on beds and wheelchairs, and call lights are additional safety features found in health care settings (Figures 37-10 and 37-11). Excess furniture and equipment should be removed, and a weakened client should wear rubber-soled shoes or slippers for walking or transferring. When clients use assistive aids such as canes, crutches, or walkers, it is important to routinely check the condition of rubber tips and the integrity of the aid. To reduce the risk of injury in the home, all obstacles should be removed from halls and other heavily traveled areas. Necessary objects such as clocks, glasses, tissues, or medications should remain on bedside tables out of the reach of...

Focus on Older Adults boxes prepare you to address the special needs of older adults.

1368

2002). These exercises have demonstrated effectiveness in treating stress incontinence, overactive bladders, and mixed cause of urinary incontinence (Sampselle, 2003). A client begins these exercises during voiding to learn the technique. They are then practiced at nonvoiding times. Improvement is usually gradual. Clients should be alert and motivated to perform the exercises. The client must continue to use these exercises to maintain effectiveness (see Box 44-5, p. 1347). These exercises are noninvasive and carry a low risk of adverse effects.

Bladder Retraining. The goal of bladder retraining is to gradually increase the interval between voidings to decrease voiding frequency during both waking and sleeping hours (Sampselle, 2003). Ultimately the overall goal of this retraining is to restore a normal pattern of voiding. For bladder retraining to be successful, clients must be alert and physically able to follow a training program. The program includes education, scheduled voiding, and positive reinforcement.

The nurse first assesses the client's current pattern of urination. This information allows the nurse to plan a program that often takes 2 weeks or more to learn. Although the program may be started in the hospital or rehabilitation unit, it may need to be continued in an extended care facility or at home. If the client has an underlying UTI, this should be treated at the same time. The following measures may help the incontinent client gain control over urination and are part of restorative and rehabilitative care:

- Learning exercises to strengthen the pelvic floor
- Initiating a toileting schedule on awakening, at least every 2 hours during the day and evening, at least [getting into bed], and every 4 hours [... individ-]izing time frame as needed)
- Using methods to initiate void[ing ...] and stroking the inner thigh[...] [...] methods to [...]

Evidence-Based Practice Guideline Box 44-11

Prompted Voiding for Persons With Urinary Incontinence

- Apply prompted voiding protocol (Lyons, Specht, 2001).
- Approach person at scheduled prompted voiding times.
  - Wait 5 seconds for individual to self-initiate request (SIR) to toilet.
- Ask person if he or she is wet or dry.
  - Physically assess person to determine continence status.
  - Provide feedback. Praise if client is dry, no comment if client is wet.
- Prompt individual to toilet.
  - Offer assistance with toileting.
- Provide feedback.
- Inform individual of next scheduled prompted voiding session.
- Encourage individual to self-initiate requests to toilet.
- Record result of prompted voiding session.

Modified from Lyons S.S., Specht J.K.P. (1999). *Evidence-based protocol: Prompted voiding for persons with urinary incontinence.* In M.G. Titler (Series Ed.), Series on Evidence-Based Practice for Older Adults. Iowa City, IA, The University of Iowa College of Nursing Gerontological Nursing Interventions Research Center, Research Dissemination Co[re ... infor-]mation, http://www.nursing.uiowa.edu/cent[...]

Evidence-Based Practice Guideline boxes provide examples of recent state-of-the-science guidelines for nursing practice.

976

Cultural Aspects of Care Box 37-5

Cultural phenomena affecting health and safety include personal space, social organizations, communication, and environmental control. While conducting a home assessment for risks to safety, nurses must realize that they have entered the client's territory and that the client's attitude toward his or her residence and belongings must be appreciated. For example, clients from Western Europe and the British Isles are considered aloof and distant in terms of space. It may be very difficult for them to have an outsider in their home who is suggesting changes with regard to their personal belongings to reduce physical hazards. It is particularly difficult to determine a client's attitude toward his or her home environment when another language is spoken.

Another culturally sensitive issue is the client's sense of environmental control. The nurse must be aware of health beliefs and practices that will affect the outcome of interventions. For example, reliance on family and religious organizations, as opposed to community resources, may affect the client's compliance with nursing interventions and referrals.

Nurses and health care providers need to learn to ask questions sensitively and show respect for different cultural beliefs. Adapting to different cultural beliefs and practices requires flexibility and a respect for others' viewpoints. Respect for the belief systems of others and the effects of those beliefs on the client's well-being are critically important to competent care. Nurses must have the ability and knowledge to communicate and to understand health behaviors influenced by culture.

Implications for Practice

- Resistance to change long-standing habits can interfere with a cultural group's acceptance of injury prevention practices. Include family members who have a strong influence, such as a dominant male or older woman, when providing safety education.
- Evaluate the use of traditional ethnic remedies or foods that contain lead because they can increase a client's risk for lead poisoning.
- Living in rural areas and in manufactured housing places the client at greater risk for fire-related injuries and death. Stress the importance of having working smoke detectors and a multipurpose fire extinguisher.
- Assess the client's smoking and drinking habits. Residential fire deaths can be attributed to the use of cigarettes and alcohol.
- Clients who live in poverty and have low educational levels are at greater risk for injury and disease. Assist the client and family in identifying community resources such as the local health office or clinic.
- Be aware of family patterns and how the client and family interact with each other. Family disruption and weak intergenerational ties can increase a client's risk for injury due to violent behavior.

Cultural Aspects of Care boxes prepare you to care for clients of diverse populations by identifying actions needed to meet different cultural needs and preferences.

[Pouch external urinary device.]

[...]ent from **pelvic floor** [...] (PFEs).** Pelvic floor exercises, also known as Kegel exercises, improve the strength of pelvic floor muscles and consist of repetitive contractions of muscle groups (Thompson and Smith,

[... team may ben-]

Research Highlight Box 44-10

Cognitive Measures for Bladder Control

Research Focus

Alterations in urine elimination often include urinary leakage and/or frequency that cause discomfort for clients. Skin breakdown is a common condition resulting from consistent exposure of the skin to urine. Falls may occur secondary to clients' need to use toilet facilities. Because these urinary problems are often manageable by cognitive strategies, research has been done to determine the best methods to use.

Research Abstract

The purpose of this study was to determine if the introduction of an audiotape with reinforcing cognitive strategies would be successful in enhancing the comfort and quality of life for clients with urinary incontinence and/or frequency. Dowd and others investigated the use of cognitive strategies with two groups of adults with a history of incontinence and/or frequency. Thirty-one women and nine men entered into the study and were randomly assigned to the treatment group or the control group. Both groups received education about bladder health and recorded incontinence and/or frequency episodes in the voiding diary, but only the treatment group listened to an audiotape that contained relaxation, music, and cognitive strategies. The verbal side of the tape contained instructions for relaxation followed by cognitive strategy statements. These statements focused on concepts of self and on specific aspects of bladder management. Statements such as, "I am not alone; many other men and women have loss of urine and are okay" were designed to enhance social comfort. The statements ". . . being physically fit is important" and "I often tighten and relax the muscles that control my urine flow"

were designed to enhance physical comfort. Other statements reinforced concepts such as the effect of fluids on output and how to manage urge to void. Music was on the second side of the tape. Comfort was measured at four intervals during the study using the Urinary Incontinence and Frequency Comfort Questionnaire. The results demonstrated that self-report of increased comfort and decreased urinary episodes were significant, with the treatment group having better results. In addition, after the control group was given the audiotape treatment their levels of comfort and episodes of incontinence and/or frequency approximated the levels of the original treatment group.

Evidence-Based Practice

- Incontinence and/or frequency are experienced by adults of all ages, educational levels, economic status, and health status.
- Many adults wrongly believe that urinary incontinence and/or frequency are an expected part of the aging process.
- Clients who take an active part in their management of bladder control have improved self-esteem and decreased physical complications such as skin breakdown.
- Nurses can support the use of this inexpensive nonpharmacological intervention to enhance comfort in community-based and selected institutionalized older adults.

Reference

Dowd T, Kolcaba K, Steiner R: Using cognitive strategies to enhance bladder control and comfort. Holist Nurs Pract 14(2):91, 2000.

Research Highlight boxes provide abstracts of current nursing research studies and explain the implications for your daily practice.

Nursing Skills are presented in a clear, two-column format that includes Steps and Rationales to help you learn *how* and *why* a skill is performed.

Delegation Considerations guide you in delegating tasks to assistive personnel.

Critical Decision Points alert you to critical steps within a skill to ensure safe and effective client care.

Clear, close-up **photos** and **illustrations** show you how to perform important techniques.

Unit VII

BASIC HUMAN NEEDS

984

Skill 37-1

Applying Restraints

Delegation Considerations

The application of restraints can be delegated to trained assistive personnel (AP). However, the nurse is always responsible for assessment of client's safety needs, selection of appropriate alternative interventions, evaluation of effectiveness of restraint, and ongoing assessment to prevent complications of restraint use.

• Have AP inform the nurse of any redness, excoriation, or constriction of circulation under the restraint.

• Have AP ask for assistance if the client has any mobility restrictions that might affect how to remove or reapply a restraint.

• Instruct AP on when and how to change client's position, provide range of motion, skin care, toileting, and opportunities for socialization.

Equipment

• Proper restraint: jacket, mitten, belt, extremity
• Padding (if needed)

Steps	Rationale
1. Assess whether client needs a restraint. Does the client continually try to interrupt needed therapy? Is the client repeatedly trying to ambulate independently, creating a serious risk of injury?	Restraints are used only when other measures have failed to prevent interruption of therapy such as traction, IV infusions, or nasogastric tube feedings; to prevent a confused or combative client from self-injury by falling out of bed or a wheelchair; to prevent a client from removing a urinary catheter, surgical drain, or life support equipment; and to reduce risk of injury to others by the client.
2. Assess client's behavior, such as confusion, disorientation, agitation, restlessness, combativeness, or inability to follow directions. Consult with [...] ical nurse specialist if available.	If client's behavior continues despite attempts to eliminate cause of behavior, use of physical restraint may be necessary.
3. Review agency policies regarding res[...] physician's order for purpose, type, lo[...] ration of restraint. Determine if si[...] use of restraint is needed.	A physician's order is necessary to apply restraints. The [...] restrictive type of restraint should be ordered. [...] restraints limit the client's ability to move [...] e must make clinical judgments appro[...] condition and agency policy. If the [...] an emergency situation be[...] havior that presents an [...] sician assessment [...] ed for
4. Review manufacturer's ins[...] client's room. Determine [...] restraint.	
5. Perform hand hygiene, [...]	
6. Introduce self to clie[...] ings about restraint [...] porary and designe[...]	
7. Inspect area whe[...] condition of ski[...] to be applied.	
8. Approach clie[...] what you pla[...]	
9. Adjust bed[...] side of [...]	
10. Provide [...] in prope[...]	
11. Pad s[...] app[...]	

Chapter 37

CLIENT SAFETY

985

Steps	Rationale
12. Apply appropriate size restraint, making sure it is not over an IV line or other device (e.g., dialysis shunt).	IV lines and other therapeutic devices may become occluded.
A. **Jacket (vest or Posey) restraint:** Front and back of garment should be labeled as such. Apply over clothing or hospital gown (see illustration). Place client's hands through armholes or sleeves, and secure according to manufacturer's directions. Place straps at client's hips.	Restrains client while lying or reclining in bed and while sitting in chair or wheelchair. Proper application prevents suffocation or choking. Clothing or gown prevents friction against skin.

Critical Decision Point: Check agency policy. Some health care facilities have failed straints because they have been known to cause death due to strangulation.

| B. **Belt restraint:** Device that secures client to bed or stretcher. Apply over clothes or gown. Remove wrinkles from front and back of restraint while placing it around client's waist. Bring ties through slots in belt. Avoid placing belt across the chest or too tightly across the abdomen (see illustration). | Restrains center of gravity and prevents client from rolling off stretcher or sitting up while on stretcher or from falling out of bed. Tight application may interfere with ventilation. |

Warning: When a patient is in a restrictive (restraint or self-release) product in bed or on a stretcher or gurney, all side rails MUST be in the UP position. Side rail covers and/or gap protectors must be used when necessary to keep the patient's entire body on the mattress and to eliminate entrapment hazards.

STEP **12A** Vest restraint securely attached to bed frame. (Courtesy JT Posey Co, Arcadia, Calif.)

STEP **12B** Belt restraint tied to the bed frame and to an area that does not cause the restraint to tighten when the side rail is raised or lowered. (From Sorrentino SA: Mosby's textbook for nursing assistants, ed 5, St. Louis, 2000, Mosby.)

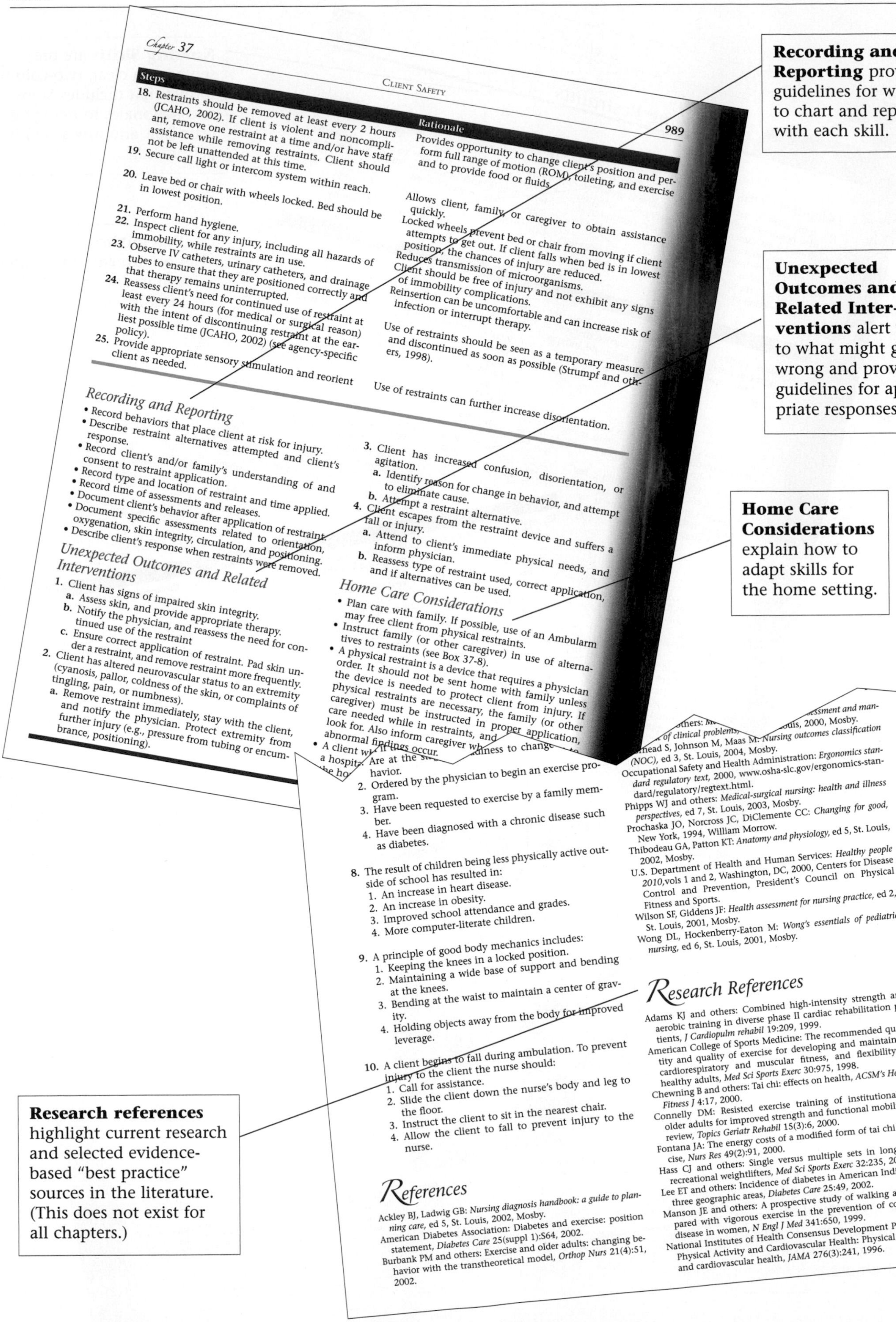

Chapter 37

Steps

CLIENT SAFETY

989

18. Restraints should be removed at least every 2 hours (JCAHO, 2002). If client is violent and noncompliant, remove one restraint at a time and/or have staff assistance while removing restraints. Client should not be left unattended at this time.
19. Secure call light or intercom system within reach.
20. Leave bed or chair with wheels locked. Bed should be in lowest position.
21. Perform hand hygiene.
22. Inspect client for any injury, including all hazards of immobility, while restraints are in use.
23. Observe IV catheters, urinary catheters, and drainage tubes to ensure that they are positioned correctly and that therapy remains uninterrupted.
24. Reassess client's need for continued use of restraint at least every 24 hours (for medical or surgical reason) with the intent of discontinuing restraint at the earliest possible time (JCAHO, 2002) (see agency-specific policy).
25. Provide appropriate sensory stimulation and reorient client as needed.

Rationale

Provides opportunity to change client's position and perform full range of motion (ROM), toileting, and exercise and to provide food or fluids.

Allows client, family or caregiver to obtain assistance quickly.
Locked wheels prevent bed or chair from moving if client attempts to get out. If client falls when bed is in lowest position, the chances of injury are reduced.
Reduces transmission of microorganisms.
Client should be free of injury and not exhibit any signs of immobility complications.
Reinsertion can be uncomfortable and can increase risk of infection or interrupt therapy.

Use of restraints should be seen as a temporary measure and discontinued as soon as possible (Strumpf and others, 1998).

Use of restraints can further increase disorientation.

Recording and Reporting

• Record behaviors that place client at risk for injury.
• Describe restraint alternatives attempted and client's response.
• Record client's and/or family's understanding of and consent to restraint application.
• Record type and location of restraint and time applied.
• Record time of assessments and releases.
• Document client's behavior after application of restraint.
• Document specific assessments related to orientation, oxygenation, skin integrity, circulation, and positioning.
• Describe client's response when restraints were removed.

Unexpected Outcomes and Related Interventions

1. Client has signs of impaired skin integrity.
   a. Assess skin, and provide appropriate therapy.
   b. Notify the physician, and reassess the need for continued use of the restraint
   c. Ensure correct application of restraint. Pad skin under a restraint, and remove restraint more frequently.
2. Client has altered neurovascular status to an extremity (cyanosis, pallor, coldness of the skin, or complaints of tingling, pain, or numbness).
   a. Remove restraint immediately, stay with the client, and notify the physician. Protect extremity from further injury (e.g., pressure from tubing or encumbrance, positioning).

3. Client has increased confusion, disorientation, or agitation.
   a. Identify reason for change in behavior, and attempt to eliminate cause.
   b. Attempt a restraint alternative.
4. Client escapes from the restraint device and suffers a fall or injury.
   a. Attend to client's immediate physical needs, and inform physician.
   b. Reassess type of restraint used, correct application, and if alternatives can be used.

Home Care Considerations

• Plan care with family. If possible, use of an Ambularm may free client from physical restraints.
• Instruct family (or other caregiver) in use of alternatives to restraints (see Box 37-8).
• A physical restraint is a device that requires a physician order. It should not be sent home with family unless the device is needed to protect client from injury. If physical restraints are necessary, the family (or other caregiver) must be instructed in proper application, care needed while in restraints, and what abnormal findings to look for. Also inform caregiver what to look for. Also inform caregiver of readiness to change behavior.

[overlapping lower page fragment:]
A client with ... a hospit... Are at the s... the ho... havior.
2. Ordered by the physician to begin an exercise program.
3. Have been requested to exercise by a family member.
4. Have been diagnosed with a chronic disease such as diabetes.

8. The result of children being less physically active outside of school has resulted in:
   1. An increase in heart disease.
   2. An increase in obesity.
   3. Improved school attendance and grades.
   4. More computer-literate children.

9. A principle of good body mechanics includes:
   1. Keeping the knees in a locked position.
   2. Maintaining a wide base of support and bending at the knees.
   3. Bending at the waist to maintain a center of gravity.
   4. Holding objects away from the body for improved leverage.

10. A client begins to fall during ambulation. To prevent injury to the client the nurse should:
    1. Call for assistance.
    2. Slide the client down the nurse's body and leg to the floor.
    3. Instruct the client to sit in the nearest chair.
    4. Allow the client to fall to prevent injury to the nurse.

References

Ackley BJ, Ladwig GB: Nursing diagnosis handbook: a guide to planning care, ed 5, St. Louis, 2002, Mosby.
American Diabetes Association: Diabetes and exercise: position statement, Diabetes Care 25(suppl 1):S64, 2002.
Burbank PM and others: Exercise and older adults: changing behavior with the transtheoretical model, Orthop Nurs 21(4):51, 2002.

[overlapping right page fragment:]
... others: M... ...essment and management
... of clinical problem... ...ouis, 2000, Mosby.
...head S, Johnson M, Maas M: Nursing outcomes classification (NOC), ed 3, St. Louis, 2004, Mosby.
Occupational Safety and Health Administration: Ergonomics standard regulatory text, 2000, www.osha-slc.gov/ergonomics-standard/regulatory/regtext.html.
Phipps WJ and others: Medical-surgical nursing: health and illness perspectives, ed 7, St. Louis, 2003, Mosby.
Prochaska JO, Norcross JC, DiClemente CC: Changing for good, New York, 1994, William Morrow.
Thibodeau GA, Patton KT: Anatomy and physiology, ed 5, St. Louis, 2002, Mosby.
U.S. Department of Health and Human Services: Healthy people 2010, vols 1 and 2, Washington, DC, 2000, Centers for Disease Control and Prevention, President's Council on Physical Fitness and Sports.
Wilson SF, Giddens JF: Health assessment for nursing practice, ed 2, St. Louis, 2001, Mosby.
Wong DL, Hockenberry-Eaton M: Wong's essentials of pediatric nursing, ed 6, St. Louis, 2001, Mosby.

Research References

Adams KJ and others: Combined high-intensity strength and aerobic training in diverse phase II cardiac rehabilitation patients, J Cardiopulm rehabil 19:209, 1999.
American College of Sports Medicine: The recommended quantity and quality of exercise for developing and maintaining cardiorespiratory and muscular fitness, and flexibility in healthy adults, Med Sci Sports Exerc 30:975, 1998.
Chewning B and others: Tai chi: effects on health, ACSM's Health Fitness J 4:17, 2000.
Connelly DM: Resisted exercise training of institutionalized older adults for improved strength and functional mobility: a review, Topics Geriatr Rehabil 15(3):6, 2000.
Fontana JA: The energy costs of a modified form of tai chi exercise, Nurs Res 49(2):91, 2000.
Hass CJ and others: Single versus multiple sets in long-term recreational weightlifters, Med Sci Sports Exerc 32:235, 2000.
Lee ET and others: Incidence of diabetes in American Indians of three geographic areas, Diabetes Care 25:49, 2002.
Manson JE and others: A prospective study of walking as compared with vigorous exercise in the prevention of coronary disease in women, N Engl J Med 341:650, 1999.
National Institutes of Health Consensus Development Panel on Physical Activity and Cardiovascular Health: Physical activity and cardiovascular health, JAMA 276(3):241, 1996.

[callout boxes:]

Recording and Reporting provides guidelines for what to chart and report with each skill.

Unexpected Outcomes and Related Interventions alert you to what might go wrong and provide guidelines for appropriate responses.

Home Care Considerations explain how to adapt skills for the home setting.

Research references highlight current research and selected evidence-based "best practice" sources in the literature. (This does not exist for all chapters.)

Preface to the Instructor

The future of nursing promises dynamic change and continual challenges. Nurses of tomorrow need a broad knowledge base from which to provide care. The role of the nurse includes assuming the lead in preserving nursing practice and demonstrating its contribution to the health care of our nation. Nurses of tomorrow need to become critical thinkers, client advocates, clinical decision makers, and client educators within a broad spectrum of care services.

The sixth edition of *Fundamentals of Nursing* has been revised to prepare today's students for the challenges of tomorrow. This textbook is designed for beginning students in all types of professional nursing programs. The comprehensive coverage provides fundamental nursing concepts, skills, and techniques of nursing practice and a firm foundation for more advanced areas of study.

Fundamentals of Nursing provides a contemporary approach to nursing practice, discussing the entire scope of primary, acute, and restorative care. This revision introduces 18 Concept Maps that visually demonstrate the relationship between multiple nursing diagnoses for associated medical diagnoses. Nursing Skills and Nursing Care Plans have been expanded. A new chapter on Nursing Today addresses emerging practice issues, including the nursing shortage. The increased focus on evidence-based practice in skills and care plans helps students understand how the latest research findings should guide their clinical decision making. We are indebted to the many educators and students who have shared their thoughts, visions, and ideas with us, and we credit each of them as valuable collaborators for this revision.

Patricia A. Potter
Anne Griffin Perry

Features

We have carefully developed this sixth edition with the student in mind. We have designed this text to welcome the new student to nursing, communicate our own love for the profession, and promote learning and understanding. Key features of the text include the following:

Classic Features
- **Comprehensive** coverage and readability of all fundamental nursing content.
- **Full-color** text to enhance visual appeal and instructional value.
- **Nursing process** provides a consistent organizational framework.
- Important nursing **skills** are presented in a clear, two-column format with rationales for all steps; whenever possible, rationales are based on research.
- Covers **health promotion, acute and tertiary care,** and **restorative care** to address today's practice in various settings.

- **Cultural diversity** is presented in Chapter 8, stressed in clinical examples throughout the text, and highlighted in special boxes.
- **Nursing research** principles and concepts are presented in Chapter 5. **Research Highlight** boxes integrated throughout the text provide current nursing research studies and explains the implications for your daily practice.
- **Client education** is presented in Chapter 24 and stressed in boxes that list teaching objectives, strategies, and evaluation for clinical topics throughout the text.
- **Gerontological nursing** principles are addressed in Chapter 13, as well as in special **Focus on Older Adults** boxes throughout the text.
- **Diverse clinical settings** are discussed, including clinics, extended care facilities, and the home, as well as acute care settings.
- A series of **Nursing Process** boxes in clinical chapters demonstrate how to apply the five-step process to client care.
- Critical thinking in clinical chapters is presented through a dimensional **critical thinking model** that visually demonstrates the ongoing assimilation of knowledge, critical thinking attitudes, intellectual and professional standards, and experience in relationship to clinical decision making and the nursing process.
- **NIC** and **NOC classifications** are included in sample nursing care plans.
- Real **Critical pathways** from progressive health care agencies across the country address collaborative care in the home, as well as acute care.
- **Procedural Guidelines** boxes provide streamlined, step-by-step instructions for performing very basic skills.
- A **health promotion/wellness** thread is used consistently throughout the text.

New Features
- **New chapter and expanded content:**
  - Nursing Today chapter
  - HIPAA regulations
  - Complementary and Alternative Therapies
  - Palliative care
  - Infection control—hand hygiene
  - Bioterrorism
  - Nursing assessment
  - Nursing diagnosis
  - Planning nursing care
  - Implementing nursing care
- **Concept Maps** show the association between multiple nursing diagnoses and their relationship to medical diagnoses.
- **Nursing Care Plans** feature a revised format that offers more detail to students on how to conduct an as-

sessment and consider the defining characteristics that indicate nursing diagnoses. In addition, the plans have incorporated NIC and NOC classifications to familiarize students with this important nomenclature. The evaluation section of the plans show students how to evaluate and then determine the outcomes of care.

- **Unexpected Outcomes and Related Interventions** are highlighted within nursing skills.
- **Evidence-Based Practice Guideline** boxes provide examples of recent state-of-the-science guidelines for nursing practice.
- **Research references** highlight evidence-based "best practice" sources in the literature.
- **Safety Alerts** indicate techniques students can use to ensure client and nurse safety.
- **Media Resources** boxes detail what electronic resources are available for the student in every chapter.
- **Video Icons** indicate video clips associated with specific skills that are available on the free CD Companion and Evolve Student Learning Resources.
- **Review Questions** at the end of each chapter help students review and evaluate what they have learned.
- **Free CD Companion** in each text has been enhanced to include **Test-Taking Skills** and **Review Questions** in addition to Butterfield's **Fluids and Electrolytes** program, and **Glossary.**

Ancillaries

- **Study Guide** provides an ideal supplement to help students understand and apply the content of the text. Each chapter includes multiple sections:
  - Preliminary Reading includes a chapter assignment from the text.
  - Comprehensive Understanding identifies topics and main ideas from the text in outline format. By com-

pleting the outline, students learn to extract key information from the chapter. Once completed, these outlines serve as ideal review tools for exams.
- Review Questions are NCLEX®-style multiple-choice questions that require students to provide a rationale for their answers.
- Clinical chapters include an Application of Critical Thinking Synthesis Model that expands the case study from the chapter's sample care plan and asks students to develop a step in the synthesis model based on the nurse and client in the scenario. This helps students learn to apply both content learned and the critical thinking synthesis model.
- Procedure Performance Checklists are included so that students can evaluate skill competency.
- **Instructor's Manual With Test Bank.**
- **Instructor's Resource CD** includes Instructor's Resource Manual, Computerized Test Bank, Electronic Image Collection, PowerPoint Slides, and Procedure Checklists.
- **evolve Online Courseware** includes WebLinks, Instructor's Manual, Computerized Test Bank, Electronic Image Collection, PowerPoint Slides, and Procedure Checklists.

We are pleased to note the growing number of men currently involved in the practice of nursing, and we acknowledge their dedication, skill, and professionalism. We have therefore made every effort to eliminate any gender-specific pronouns. In a very few instances, we have used "she" to refer to the nurse and "he" to refer to the client in order to clearly communicate to the reader.

The development of this textbook resulted from the combined efforts of many talented professionals committed to excellence. We appreciate their dedication and enthusiasm. Throughout the text we have attempted to acknowledge the contributions of our professional nurse colleagues who make a difference in the lives of their clients and the communities they serve. We are very proud to be associated with such fine individuals.

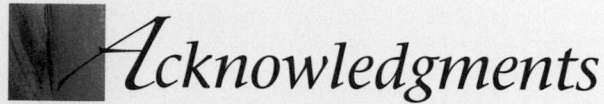

Acknowledgments

We wish to acknowledge and recognize the editorial, production, and design teams who have helped to make this textbook a reality.

Suzi Epstein, Executive Editor, Maria Broeker, Senior Developmental Editor, and Shari Malchow, Developmental Editor, for their support, expertise, guidance, and good humor. This is the editorial team whose creativity and commitment to excellence ensured a high-quality textbook with innovations in design and ancillary materials to assist both faculty and students in their use of the text.

Beth Hayes, Senior Project Manager, for her coordination of the manuscript, illustrations, and photographs through the production phases of the text.

Kathi Gosche, Senior Designer, whose innovative design and use of color makes the book both visually attractive and easy to use.

Rick Brady, Annapolis, Maryland, and Mike Defillipo, St. Louis, Missouri, for their photographs.

St. Luke's Hospital and Barnes-Jewish Hospital College of Nursing and Allied Health Professions, St. Louis, Missouri; Anne Arundel Medical Center, Annapolis, Maryland—our thanks for their assistance in making their facilities available for the photographs that make the text realistic and engaging.

The production teams at Graphic World, for the computer expertise that provides clear, detailed illustrations to enhance and complement the textbook.

Our contributors, whose expertise enables us to provide a state-of-the-art textbook that includes the most current practice and research. Our reviewers, whose painstaking critique of content and design ensures a high-quality textbook. The demands for accuracy from our contributors and reviewers have helped to set the standard for a comprehensive and accurate textbook.

To the professional managers and nursing staff at Barnes-Jewish Hospital, St. Luke's Hospital, the faculty and students at Jewish Hospital College of Nursing and Allied Health, the nursing faculty and students of Saint Louis University School of Nursing, and the nursing staff of Saint Louis University Hospital.

As always the creation of this textbook is no small feat. We continue to be grateful for our colleagues and their students who use this text. We are thankful to our family and friends who provide a tremendous amount of support in this endeavor. Last, we cherish the friendship and partnership that we have forged over the years. The rewards and blessings of this friendship are too numerous to count, but it is a once-in-a-lifetime experience. We hope to continue to challenge ourselves to meet the standards of excellences that you, our readers, expect.

Patricia A. Potter
Anne Griffin Perry

Contents

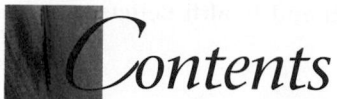

Unit V

Psychosocial Basis for Nursing Practice

26   Self-Concept, 500

27   Sexuality, 522

28   Spiritual Health, 543

29   The Experience of Loss, Death, and Grief, 567

33 *Infection Control, 772*

34 *Medication Administration, 821*

45 Bowel Elimination, 1373

Unit VIII

Clients With Special Needs

46 Mobility and Immobility, 1420

47 Skin Integrity and Wound Care, 1482

48 Sensory Alterations, 1565

$\mathcal{N}$ursing Today

1

Media Resources

http://evolve.elsevier.com/Potter/
fundamentals/

CD COMPANION

- Review Questions
- Glossary

evolve WEBSITE

- Review Questions
- Student Learning Activities
- Glossary

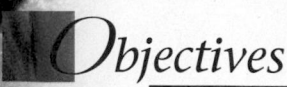

Mastery of content in this chapter will enable the student to:

- Define the key terms listed.
- Discuss the historical development of professional nursing roles.
- Describe educational programs available for professional registered nurse education.
- Describe the roles and career opportunities for nurses.
- List the five characteristics of a profession and discuss how nursing demonstrates these characteristics.
- Discuss the influence of social and economic changes on nursing practices.

Nursing is an art and a science. This means that a professional nurse learns to deliver care artfully with compassion, caring, and a respect for each client's dignity and personhood. As a science, nursing is based upon a body of knowledge that is always changing with new discoveries and innovations. When nurses integrate the science and art of nursing into their practice, the quality of care provided to clients is at a level of excellence that benefits clients in innumerable ways.

It is an exciting time to become a nurse. The opportunities for a nursing career are limitless. A new professional may choose any number of careers, including clinical practice, education, research, management, administration, and even entrepreneurship. There are many excellent health care facilities and educational institutions in this country to prepare nurses with the very best skills and knowledge. As a student beginning his or her career, it is important to understand the scope of nursing practice and how nursing influences the lives of the clients we care for.

At the center of a nurse's practice is the client, which includes the individual, family, and/or community. Clients enter a health care facility with a wide variety of health care problems, experiences, vulnerabilities, and expectations. But that is what makes nursing both challenging and rewarding. Making a difference in a client's life can be very fulfilling: helping a dying client find relief from pain, helping a young child and her parents learn to adjust to a disability, finding ways for an older adult to remain in the home to manage his or her own daily care. Nursing offers personal and professional rewards every day. This chapter presents a contemporary approach to the evolution of nursing and nursing practice. This approach presents to the reader elements of the historical, practical, social, and political influences on the discipline of nursing.

When giving care, a professional registered nurse provides a specified service according to standards of practice and follows a code of ethics. The foundation for professional practice arises from theories of nursing, scientific knowledge, relevance to basic social values, professional autonomy, a sense of commitment, a sense of community, and a code of ethics (Bernhard and Walsh, 1995). Nursing has many different philosophies and definitions. The following definition was developed by the **American Nurses Association (ANA):**

> **Nursing** is the protection, promotion, and optimization of health and abilities, prevention of illness and injury, alleviation of suffering through the diagnosis and treatment of human response, and advocacy in the care of individuals, families, communities, and populations (ANA, 2003).

This definition asserts the prominence and importance nursing holds in providing health care to people of our global community.

Expert clinical nursing practice is a result of a commitment to the application of knowledge and clinical experience. The expertise required to interpret clinical situations and make complex decisions is the essence of nursing care and is the basis for the advancement of nursing practice and the development of nursing science (Benner, 1984; Carnevali and Thomas, 1998). Critical thinking skills are essential to nursing (see Chapter 14). When providing nursing care, the nurse makes clinical judgments about the care needed for clients based on fact, experience, and standards of care (Alfaro-LeFevre, 1995). Knowledge, expertise, and lifelong learning are gained through the continual process of critical thinking.

Historical Perspective Highlights

Nursing has responded to and always will continue to respond to the needs of its clients. In times of war, nursing has responded by meeting needs of the wounded in the combat zones and in military hospitals in the United States and abroad. When communities face health care crises, such as those that occur from infectious diseases or a lack of health care resources, nursing is there to establish community-based immunization and screening programs, treatment clinics, and health promotion activities.

Our clients are most vulnerable when they are injured, sick, or dying. Historically nursing has been there and will continue to be there not only to meet the needs of the client, but also to assist in meeting the needs of the client's friends and families.

Nurses are active in social policy and political arenas. Nurses and their professional organizations lobby for health care legislation to meet the needs of clients, particularly the medically underserved. For example, nurses in communities provide home visits to newborns of high-risk mothers (e.g., adolescent, poorly educated mothers, or medically underserved). The results of these visits document fewer emergency department visits, fewer newborn infections, and reduced infant mortality. Changes in health care legislation allow these services to be paid by public and private insurance. Nurses are active in local government planning to ensure that health care resources are available in all clients' communities.

Throughout the nursing profession's history, nurses have studied and tested new and better ways to help their clients, their families, and their communities. Nurses have been leaders in expanding knowledge in nursing and other health care disciplines through health care research. Early in nursing's history during the Crimean War, Florence Nightingale studied and implemented methods to improve battlefield sanitation, which ultimately reduced illness, infection, and mortality. Today nurses are active in determining the best practices for skin care management, pain control, nutritional management, and care of older adults, to cite just a few examples.

Nursing continuously responds and adapts to new challenges as they arise. However, for nurses to understand and prepare for the future direction of nursing, the past shows how nursing evolved to meet the needs of the service community. The evolution of nursing has brought the profession to one of the most challenging and exciting times in history.

The historical roots of nursing enable both students and practicing professionals to prepare for the health care needs of the twenty-first century. Nursing is a combination of knowledge from the physical sciences, humanities, and social sciences, along with clinical competencies needed to meet the individual needs of clients and their families. Knowledge of the profession's history increases the nurse's awareness and promotes an understanding of the social and intellectual origins of the discipline (Keeling and Ramos, 1995) (Box 1-1). Although it is not feasible to describe all of the historical aspects of professional nursing, some of the more significant milestones are described below.

Florence Nightingale

The founder of modern nursing, Florence Nightingale, established the first nursing philosophy based on health maintenance and restoration in *Notes on Nursing: What It Is and What It Is Not* (Nightingale, 1860). Her views on nursing were derived from a spiritual philosophy, developed in her adolescence and adulthood (Macrae, 1995), and reflected the changing needs of society. She saw the role of nursing as having "charge of somebody's health" based on the knowledge of "how to put the body in such a state to be free of disease or to recover from disease" (Nightingale, 1860). During the same year, she developed the first organized program for training nurses, the Nightingale Training School for Nurses at St. Thomas' Hospital in London.

Nightingale was the first practicing nurse epidemiologist (Cohen, 1984). Her statistical analyses connected poor sanitation with cholera and dysentery. She viewed nursing as a search for truth in finding answers to health care questions or discovering and using God's laws of healing in nursing practice (Macrae, 1995). In 1853 Nightingale went to Paris to study with the Sisters of Charity and was later appointed superintendent of the English General Hospitals in Turkey. During this period she brought about major reforms in hygiene, sanitation, and nursing practice and reduced the mortality rate at the Barracks Hospital in Scutari, Turkey, from 42.7% to 2.2% in 6 months (Woodham-Smith, 1983; Donahue, 1996).

The Civil War to the Beginning of the Twentieth Century

The Civil War (1860 to 1865) stimulated the growth of nursing in the United States. Clara Barton, founder of the American Red Cross, tended soldiers on the battlefields, cleansing their wounds, meeting their basic needs, and comforting them in death. The U.S. Congress ratified the American Red Cross in 1882 after 10 years of lobbying by Barton. Dorothea Lynde Dix, Mary Ann Ball (Mother Bickerdyke), and Harriet Tubman also influenced nursing during the Civil War (Donahue, 1996). As superintendent

| Box 1-1 | Milestones in Nursing History |

300 AD	Entry of women into nursing.
1100-1200	Formation of charitable institutions to care for the aged, sick, and poor. These included the Hospital Brothers of St. Anthony's, Brothers of Misericordia (Italy), and the Alexian Brothers.
1633	Sisters of Charity founded by Louise de Marillac. Established the first educational program to be affiliated with a religious nursing order.
1809	Mother Elizabeth Seton introduced the Sisters of Charity into America, later known as the Daughters of Charity.
1836	Deaconess Institute of Kaiserwerth, Germany, founded. This is the institute where Florence Nightingale received her initial education in nursing.
1846	Florence Nightingale received the *Yearbook of the Institution of Deaconess at Kaiserwerth.*
1860	Establishment of the Nightingale Training School for Nurses at St. Thomas' Hospital in London, England. This was the first organized program for training nurses.
1860	Florence Nightingale published *Notes on Nursing: What It Is and What It Is Not.* This was the first nursing philosophy based on health maintenance and restoration of health.
1860-1865	Dorthea Lynde Dix served as superintendent of the Union Army female nurses; Mary Ann Ball (Mother Bickerdyke) organized ambulance services, searched for wounded, and supervised nurses; Harriett Tubman tended to soldiers and led over 300 slaves to freedom through the Underground Railroad movement.
1874	First nurses training school in Canada founded: St. Catherine's, Ontario.
1882	United States ratified the American Red Cross, founded by Clara Barton.
1884	Mary Agnes Snively assumed directorship of Toronto General Hospital and began to form the Canadian National Association of Trained Nurses, which was to become the Canadian Nurses Association (CNA).
1890	Establishment of the Nurses' Associated Alumni of the United States and Canada (NAAUSC). This group was an initial nursing professional group. It later became the American Nurses Association.
1893	First community health service for the poor: Henry Street Settlement opened by Lillian Wald and Harriet Brewster.
1894	Isabel Hampton Robb, RN, was the first superintendent of the Johns Hopkins Training School in Baltimore, Maryland.
1897	Initial discussion of nursing code of ethics.
1901	First university-affiliated nursing program.

1901	The Army Nurse Corps was established.
1902	Sigma Theta Tau, National Honor Society of Nursing, was formed by six student nurses from Indiana University.
1907	First professor of nursing, Mary Adelaide Nutting.
1908	Navy Nurse Corps established; Canadian National Association of Trained Nurses (later changed to the Canadian Nurses Association, 1924) founded.
1911	NAAUSC became the American Nurses Association (ANA).
1920	Graduate nurse-midwifery programs were established.
1923	Goldmark Report: Rockefeller Foundation–funded survey identified need for increased financial support to university-based schools of nursing.
1926	ANA Code of Ethics proposed.
1948	Brown Report: Dr. Esther Lucille Brown concluded that all nursing education programs should be affiliated with universities and have their own budgets. She recommended a broad academic education within a university and 2 years of nursing education focused on technical skills.
1949	Association of Operating Room Nurses formed.
1952	Dr. Mildred Montag established the first associate degree nursing program.
	Nursing Research, a journal reporting on the scientific investigations of nursing, was established.
1953	National League for Nursing (NLN), in collaboration with universities, developed graduate nursing education.
1960	Yale University School of Nursing defined nursing as a profession, interaction, and relationship between two human beings.
1965	Jerome Lysaught directed the National Commission on Nursing and Nursing Education Report, which recommended that nursing roles and responsibilities be clarified in relation to other health care professionals and that increased financial support and career opportunities were needed to attract and retain nurses; ANA position paper defined nursing.
1969	American Association of Critical Care Nurses formed.
1975	Oncology Nursing Society formed.
	NLN required theory-based curriculum for accreditation.
1985	ANA published *Code for Nurses With Interpretive Statements.*
1994	Health care reform.
1996	The Pew Report: Looking at future nursing needs and shortages.
	Institute of Medicine (IOM) Report. Parallel to the Pew Report.

Data from Donahue MP: *Nursing: the finest art—an illustrated history,* ed 2, St. Louis, 1996, Mosby.

of the female nurses of the Union Army, Dix organized hospitals, appointed nurses, and oversaw and regulated supplies to the troops. Mother Bickerdyke organized ambulance services, supervised nurses, and walked abandoned battlefields at night, looking for wounded soldiers. Harriet Tubman was active in the Underground Railroad

movement and assisted in leading over 300 slaves to freedom (Donahue, 1996).

The first African-American professional nurse was Mary Mahoney, RN. She was concerned with relationships between cultures and races, and as a noted nursing leader, she brought forth an awareness of cultural diversity and respect for the individual, regardless of background, race, color, or religion.

Isabel Hampton Robb, a graduate of St. Catherine's in Ontario, was the first superintendent of the Johns Hopkins Training School in Baltimore, Maryland, in 1894. As one of her many contributions to nursing, she helped found the Nurses' Associated Alumnae of the United States and Canada in 1896. This organization became the American Nurses Association (ANA) in 1911. She authored many nursing textbooks, including *Nursing: Its Principles and Practice for Hospital and Private Use* (1894), *Nursing Ethics* (1900), and *Educational Standards for Nurses* (1907), and was one of the original founders of the *American Journal of Nursing* (AJN) (Donahue, 1996). Today, the AJN continues to present current insights into nursing practice and professional issues.

Nursing in hospitals expanded in the late nineteenth century. However, nursing in the community did not increase significantly until 1893, when Lillian Wald and Mary Brewster opened the Henry Street Settlement, which focused on the health needs of poor people who lived in tenements in New York City (Donahue, 1996). Nurses working in this settlement were some of the first to demonstrate autonomy in practice because they frequently encountered situations that required quick and innovative problem solving and critical thinking without the supervision or direction of a physician. The poor people also needed nursing therapies aimed at maintaining wellness through proper nutrition, hygiene, and shelter. Wald described her activities with the Henry Street Settlement in the textbooks *The House on Henry Street* (1915) and *Windows on Henry Street* (1934).

Twentieth Century

In the early twentieth century a movement toward a scientific, research-based defined body of nursing knowledge and practice was evolving. Nurses began to assume expanded and advanced practice roles. Mary Adelaide Nutting, a member of the first graduating class at Johns Hopkins Hospital and successor to Isabel Hampton Robb as superintendent of the Johns Hopkins Training School, was instrumental in the affiliation of nursing education with universities. She became the first professor of nursing at Columbia University Teachers College in 1907 (Donahue, 1996). In addition, a landmark report, the Goldmark Report, concluded that nursing education needed increased financial support and suggested that the money be given to university schools of nursing.

As nursing education developed, nursing practice also expanded. In 1901 the Army Nurse Corps was established, followed in 1908 by the Navy Nurse Corps. By the 1920s nursing specialization was developing. Graduate nurse-midwifery programs were initiated, and in the late 1940s and early 1950s specialty nursing organizations, such as the Association of Operating Room Nurses, American Association of Critical Care Nurses, and Oncology Nursing Society, were formed.

Twenty-first Century

Nursing practice and education must continue to evolve to meet the needs of society. In 1990 the American Nurses Association established the Center for Ethics and Human Rights. The Center provides a forum to address the complex ethical and human rights issues confronting nurses and designs activities and programs to increase ethical competence in nurses (ANA, 2001). Nursing's code of ethics was revised in 2001 to reflect current ethical issues affecting health care and nursing practice (see Chapter 21).

Today the profession is faced with multiple challenges. Nurses and nurse educators are revising nursing practice and school curricula to meet the ever-changing needs of society, including bioterrorism, emerging infections, and disaster management. Advances in technology, the rising acuity of hospitalized clients, and early discharge from health care institutions require nurses in all settings to have a strong and current knowledge base from which to practice. In addition, nursing along with the Robert Wood Johnson Foundation, through the *Last Acts Campaign*, is taking a leadership role in developing standards and policies for end-of-life care (see Chapter 29). The End-of-Life Nursing Education Consortium (ELNEC) offered collaboratively by the American Association of Colleges of Nursing (AACN) and the City of Hope Medical Center has brought end-of-life care and practices into the nursing curricula (ANA, 2002d).

Nursing practice can now be found in multiple care settings, including health care institutions and foundations, the community, and the home. In addition, nurses are active in political and lobbying groups, social and not-for-profit agencies, and work on establishing social health care policies. These activities increase nursing's public viability and, at the same time, increase the public's awareness of professional nursing. The challenge now is to prepare professional nurses to deliver complex, multifaceted care in the client's home.

Societal Influences on Nursing

There are many external forces that affect nursing. These include demographic changes of the population, human rights, increasing numbers of medically underserved, and the threat of bioterrorism.

Demographic Changes

Demographic changes affect the population as a whole. Changes that have influenced health care in recent decades include the population shift from rural areas to urban centers; the increasing life span; the higher incidence of chronic, long-term illness; and the increased incidence of diseases such as alcoholism and lung cancer. Nursing as a profession responds to such changes by exploring new methods for providing care, by changing educational emphases, and by establishing practice standards in new areas.

Women's Health Care Issues

The women's movement has brought about many changes in society as women have increasingly sought economic, political, occupational, and educational equality. As a result, there is greater sensitivity to the health care needs of women and the role of women in health care research. There are and continue to be emerging health care specialties dealing with the needs of women.

These new specialties expand on the traditional obstetrical specialty. These new specialties address issues ranging from well women's examinations, to oncological subspecialties, and management of menopause. In addition, health care researchers acknowledge the prior lack of female subjects in biomedical research, and now the federal government mandates that women must be routinely included in research, unless specific exception criteria are met. For example, research focusing on management of prostatic cancer is such an exception.

Nursing is responding in two ways to women's health care issues and the women's movement. Because most nurses are women, they are increasingly asserting their equal rights as human beings, employees, and health care professionals. The women's movement has encouraged nurses to seek greater autonomy and responsibility in providing care. The women's movement has caused female clients to seek more responsibility for and control for their bodies, health, and lives in general. As women become more aware of their own unique needs and qualities, they seek health care that can help them meet those needs and reach their full potential.

Human Rights Movement

The human rights movement is changing the way society views the rights of all of its members, including minorities, clients with terminal illness, pregnant women, and older adults. Many groups have special health care needs, and nursing has responded by respecting all clients as individuals with a right to quality care and by supporting basic human rights. Nurses advocate the rights of all clients, but they have also recognized the special needs of some groups and thus have created bills of rights for dying, hospitalized, and pregnant clients, as well as other groups, to ensure that quality care is provided without sacrificing these rights.

Medically Underserved

The rising rates of unemployment, homelessness, and health care costs all contribute to an increase in the medically underserved population. The medically underserved population may be poor and on Medicaid or may be part of the working poor in that they cannot afford their own insurance but make too much money to qualify for Medicaid. In addition, there is an increase in the mentally ill population who have little or no access to health care. Nurses work in many rural, neighborhood, and community-based settings providing health promotion and disease management (Masson, 2001). Frequently these nurses have advanced preparation and function as advanced practice nurses, giving them the capability to provide direct health care. This area of nursing is rapidly expanding as more nurses are seeking to work with this population in need.

Threat of Bioterrorism

The world is a changing place; the treats of bioterrorism are no longer fictitious. Many health care agencies and communities have educational programs for nurses to prepare them in the event of nuclear, chemical, or biological attack. Nurses are active in disaster preparedness. For example, nurses work in conjunction with community disaster preparedness groups and hospitals to determine what specific nursing activities are needed before the disaster. This activity may range from participating in vaccine research, decontamination in the event of biological attack, triage for mass casualty, to crisis response units. It should also be remembered that if a disaster were to occur nurses would also be essential in evaluating the strengths and weaknesses of any disaster plan that was implemented. (See Chapter 37.)

Needs of the Consumer

The consumers' movement is a heightened public awareness of the value and costs of products and services. It has influenced health care by calling for new kinds of health care agencies, such as health maintenance organizations, demanding culturally sensitive care, creating new forms of health insurance, and voicing concern about the rising costs of health care (see Chapter 2). Consumers are also more knowledgeable about health and illness and are becoming more vocal in their desire for high-quality care. Because nurses generally interact with clients more than other health care professionals do, they must often answer questions about the quality and costs of health care.

Cultural Diversity

As the people of the world move about, nurses are confronted with caring for clients of many cultures different from their own. The nurse must now have an awareness of how different cultures view health and illness (see Chapter 8). Nurses are challenged to be culturally aware and competent. Care that is not culturally competent may be more costly and may be ineffective (Sullivan, 1999). *Healthy People 2010,* a federal document that outlines health care goals for the public, is one example of meeting the health of multiple cultures by defining goals and objectives for health (U.S. Department of Health and Human Services [USDHHS], 2002).

Health Promotion and Wellness

Today there is a great emphasis on health promotion, health maintenance, and illness prevention (see Chapter 6). Exercise, nutrition, and healthy lifestyles are subjects that interest many people. Nursing has responded to this greater concern for health promotion by providing programs in the community such as health fairs and wellness programs; educational programs for specific diseases; and client and family teaching activities in hospitals, clinics, primary care facilities, and other health care settings. Health promotion activities are an important part of the role of a nurse (see Chapter 6).

Influence of Today's Health Care Delivery System

Today's health care delivery system is a complex and highly regulated system (see Chapter 2). Nurses working in the system must be aware of their roles in containing health care costs, providing the best evidenced-based practice, and participating in nursing and biomedical research. In addition, today's health care system is further challenged by the nursing shortage.

Rising Health Care Costs

Skyrocketing health care costs present challenges to the nursing profession, consumer, and the health care delivery system as well (see Chapter 2). Nursing's responsibility is to provide the consumer with the best-quality care in an efficient and economically sound manner. Nurses are challenged to use health care and client resources wisely. For example, clients may be taught to perform procedures in the home with clean versus sterile equipment. This does not compromise care because clients are in their home environments, which are cleaner and without the risks of nosocomial infections. However, nurses need to clinically evaluate each client to determine which clients can perform procedures safely using clean technique. Nurses also play a role in managing health care costs by participating in product evaluation. Most health care institutions invite nurses to participate in product review committees to select the most clinically effective, reasonable-cost items for clinical use.

Evidenced-Based Practice

Consumers of health care are more informed than ever, and with the Internet consumers have access to more health care and treatment information. As a result, consumers expect and should receive the most current, effective, state-of-the-art care in a rapidly changing health care system. As providers of health care, nurses are faced with the challenge of providing safe, effective care. One way to achieve this goal is to provide evidence-based practice. Evidence-based practice is defined as "the integration of best research evidence with clinical expertise and patient values" (Sackett and others, 2000). Evidence-based nursing practice involves accurate and thoughtful decision making about health care delivery for clients (see Chapters 2 and 5).

Nursing and Biomedical Research

Nursing knowledge, scientific knowledge, and research findings have rapidly expanded over the last few years. Nurses share a "commitment to the advancement of nursing science and the ethical conduct of nursing science" (ANA, 1997). The scientific knowledge base for professional practice is developed through scholarly inquiry of nursing and biomedical research literature, utilization of research findings, and conducting research (see Chapter 5). Through nursing research, nurses base their care on scientific findings, rather than tradition. The beneficiary of this care is the client. Through research, nursing practice changes to provide the highest-quality state-of-the-art nursing care.

Nursing Shortage

Although there is much in the professional and public media about the nursing shortage, this shortage also represents challenges and opportunities for the profession. Vast health care dollars are being invested in strategies aimed at recruiting a well-educated, critically thinking, motivated, and dedicated nursing work force (Boychuk, 2001). Research documents the direct link between nursing care and positive client outcomes, reduced complication rate, and a more rapid return of the client to the preillness state (Romig, 2001; Blendon and others, 2002; Consumer Reports, 2003).

Like it or not, the nursing shortage affects the needs of the consumer (Romig, 2001; Consumer Reports, 2003). With fewer nurses in the workplace, nurses must use their client contact time efficiently and professionally. Time management, therapeutic communication, client education, and compassionate implementation of psychomotor skills are just a few of the essential skills needed for the provision of quality nursing care. For example, using a well-organized approach to prepare a client to self-administer blood pressure medication at home results in a scenario in which the client adheres to medication, blood pressure remains within the target range, and most importantly the client leaves the health care setting with a positive image of nursing and a feeling that quality care was provided. The client should never feel rushed or that he or she was one of many clients or tasks for the nurse. If a certain aspect of client care requires 15 minutes of contact, it will take the same time to deliver the care in an organized manner as it would in a rushed, harried manner. However, the impression left with the client will be far different. As nurses we all have the opportunities and obligation to present our profession and practice in the best possible manner.

Nursing as a Profession

Nursing is not simply a collection of specific skills, and the nurse is not simply a person trained to perform specific tasks. Nursing is a profession. No one factor absolutely differentiates a job from a profession, but the difference is important in terms of how nurses practice. When we say a person acts "professionally," for example, we imply that the person is conscientious in actions, knowledgeable in the subject, and responsible to self and others. Professions possess the following primary characteristics:

- A profession requires an extended education of its members, as well as a basic liberal foundation.
- A profession has a theoretical body of knowledge leading to defined skills, abilities, and norms.
- A profession provides a specific service.
- Members of a profession have autonomy in decision making and practice.
- The profession as a whole has a code of ethics for practice.

The practice of professional nursing and nursing knowledge has been developed over time through development of nursing theories and research. Theoretical models serve as frameworks for nursing curricula and clinical practice (see Chapter 4). Nursing research increases the scientific basis of nursing practice through the systematic inquiry into health care problems and issues.

Standards of Professional Performance

The ANA Standards of Professional Performance (Table 1-1) describes a competent level of behavior in the professional role, including activities related to quality of care, perfor-

Table 1-1	ANA Standards of Professional Performance	
Standard	Definition	Measurement Criteria
VII: Quality of practice	The registered nurse systematically enhances the quality and effectiveness of nursing practice.	The registered nurse: • Demonstrates quality by documenting the application of the nursing process in a responsible, accountable, and ethical manner. • Uses the results of quality improvement activities to initiate changes in nursing practice and in the health care delivery system. • Uses creativity and innovation in nursing practice to improve care delivery. • Incorporates new knowledge to initiate changes in nursing practice if desired outcomes are not achieved. • Participates in quality improvement activities. Such activities may include: identifying aspects of practice important for quality monitoring such as: Using indicators developed to monitor quality and effectiveness of nursing practice Collecting data to monitor quality and effectiveness of nursing practice. Analyzing quality data to identify opportunities for improving nursing practice Formulating recommendations to improve nursing practice or outcomes Implementing activities to enhance the quality of nursing practice Developing, implementing, and evaluating policies, procedures and/or guidelines to improve the quality of practice Participating on interdisciplinary teams to evaluate clinical care or health services Participating in efforts to minimize costs and unnecessary duplication Analyzing factors related to safety, satisfaction, effectiveness, and cost/benefit options Analyzing organizational systems for barriers Implementing processes to remove or decrease barriers within organizational systems *Additional Measurement Criteria for the Advanced Practice Registered Nurse:* The advanced practice registered nurse: • Obtains and maintains professional certification if available in the area of expertise. • Designs quality improvement initiatives. • Implements initiatives to evaluate the need for change. • Evaluates the practice environment and quality of nursing care rendered in relation to existing evidence, identifying opportunities for the generation and use of research. *Additional Measurement Criteria for the Nursing Role Specialty:* The registered nurse in a nursing role specialty: • Obtains and maintains professional certification if available in the area of expertise. • Designs quality improvement initiatives. • Implements initiatives to evaluate the need for change. • Evaluates the practice environment in relation to existing evidence, identifying opportunities for the generation and use of research.
VIII: Education	The registered nurse attains knowledge and competency that reflects current nursing practice.	The registered nurse: • Participates in ongoing educational activities related to appropriate knowledge bases and professional issues. • Demonstrates a commitment to lifelong learning through self-reflection and inquiry to identify learning needs. • Seeks experiences that reflect current practice in order to maintain skills and competence in clinical practice or role performance. • Acquires knowledge and skills appropriate to the specialty area, practice setting, role, or situation. • Maintains professional records that provide evidence of competency and lifelong learning. • Seeks experiences and formal and independent learning activities to maintain and develop clinical and professional skills and knowledge.

Excerpted from American Nurses Association: *Nursing: scope and standards of practice,* Washington, DC, 2004, The Association.

Table 1-1	ANA Standards of Professional Performance—cont'd	
Standard	**Definition**	**Measurement Criteria**
VIII: Education— cont'd		*Additional Measurement Criteria for the Advanced Practice Registered Nurse:* The advanced practice registered nurse: • Uses current healthcare research findings and other evidence to expand clinical knowledge, enhance role performance, and increase knowledge of professional issues. *Additional Measurement Criteria for the Nursing Role Specialty:* The registered nurse in a nursing role specialty: • Uses current research findings and other evidence to expand knowledge, enhance role performance, and increase knowledge of professional issues.
IX: Professional practice evaluation	The registered nurse evaluates one's own nursing practice in relation to professional practice standards and guidelines, relevant statutes, rules, and regulations.	The registered nurse: • The registered nurse's practice reflects the application of knowledge of current practice standards, guidelines, statutes, rules, and regulations. The registered nurse: • Provides age-appropriate care in a culturally and ethnically sensitive manner. • Engages in self-evaluation of practice on a regular basis, identifying areas of strength as well as areas in which professional development would be beneficial. • Obtains informal feedback regarding one's own practice from patients, peers, professional colleagues, and others. • Participates in systematic peer review as appropriate. • Takes action to achieve goals identified during the evaluation process. • Provides rationales for practice beliefs, decisions, and actions as part of the informal and formal evaluation processes. *Additional Measurement Criteria for the Advanced Practice Registered Nurse:* • The advanced practice registered nurse engages in a formal process seeking feedback regarding one's own practice from patients, peers, professional colleagues, and others. *Additional Measurement Criteria for the Nursing Role Specialty:* • The registered nurse in a nursing role specialty engages in a formal process seeking feedback regarding role performance from individuals, professional colleagues, representatives and administrators of corporate entities, and others.
X: Collegiality	The registered nurse interacts with and contributes to the professional development of peers and colleagues.	The registered nurse: • Shares knowledge and skills with peers and colleagues as evidenced by such activities as patient care conferences or presentations at formal or informal meetings. • Provides peers with feedback regarding their practice and/or role performance. • Interacts with peers and colleagues to enhance one's own professional nursing practice and/or role performance. • Maintains compassionate and caring relationships with peers and colleagues. • Contributes to an environment that is conducive to the education of health care professionals. • Contributes to a supportive and healthy work environment. *Additional Measurement Criteria for the Advanced Practice Registered Nurse:* The advanced practice registered nurse: • Models expert practice to interdisciplinary team members and health care consumers. • Mentors other registered nurses and colleagues as appropriate. • Participates with interdisciplinary teams that contribute to role development and advanced nursing practice and health care. *Additional Measurement Criteria for the Nursing Role Specialty:* The registered nurse in a nursing role specialty: • Participates on multiprofessional teams that contribute to role development and, directly or indirectly, advance nursing practice and health services. • Mentors other registered nurses and colleagues as appropriate.

Continued

Table 1-1	ANA Standards of Professional Performance—cont'd	
Standard	**Definition**	**Measurement Criteria**
XI: Collaboration	The registered nurse collaborates with patient, family, and others in the conduct of nursing practice.	The registered nurse: • Communicates with patient, family, and health care providers regarding patient care and the nurse's role in the provision of that care. • Collaborates in creating a documented plan focused on outcomes and decisions related to care and delivery of services that indicates communication with patients, families, and others. • Partners with others to effect change and generate positive outcomes through knowledge of the patient or situation. • Documents referrals, including provisions for continuity of care. *Additional Measurement Criteria for the Advanced Practice Registered Nurse:* The advanced practice registered nurse: • Partners with other disciplines to enhance patient care through interdisciplinary activities, such as education, consultation, management, technological development, or research opportunities. • Facilitates an interdisciplinary process with other members of the health care team. • Documents plan of care communications, rationales for plan of care changes, and collaborative discussions to improve patient care. *Additional Measurement Criteria for Nursing Role Specialty:* The registered nurse in a nursing role specialty: • Partners with others to enhance health care, and ultimately patient care, through interdisciplinary activities such as education, consultation, management, technological development, or research opportunities. • Documents plans, communications, rationales for plan changes, and collaborative discussions.
XII: Ethics	The registered nurse integrates ethical provisions in all areas of practice.	The registered nurse: • Uses the *Code of Ethics for Nurses With Interpretive Statements* (ANA, 2001) to guide practice. • Delivers care in a manner that preserves and protects patient autonomy, dignity, and rights. • Maintains patient confidentiality within legal and regulatory parameters. • Serves as a patient advocate assisting patients in developing skills for self-advocacy. • Maintains a therapeutic and professional patient-nurse relationship with appropriate professional role boundaries. • Demonstrates a commitment to practicing self-care, managing stress, and connecting with self and others. • Contributes to resolving ethical issues of patients, colleagues, or systems as evidenced in such activities as participating on ethics committees. • Reports illegal, incompetent, or impaired practices. *Additional Measurement Criteria for the Advanced Practice Registered Nurse:* The advanced practice registered nurse: • Informs the patient of the risks, benefits, and outcomes of health care regimens. • Participates in interdisciplinary teams that address ethical risks, benefits, and outcomes. *Additional Measurement Criteria for the Nursing Role Specialty:* The registered nurse in a nursing role specialty: • Participates on multidisciplinary and interdisciplinary teams that address ethical risks, benefits, and outcomes. • Informs administrators or others of the risks, benefits, and outcomes of programs and decisions that affect health care delivery.

Excerpted from American Nurses Association: *Nursing: scope and standards of practice,* Washington, DC, 2004, The Association.

Table 1-1	ANA Standards of Professional Performance—cont'd	
Standard	**Definition**	**Measurement Criteria**

XIII: Research	The registered nurse integrates research findings into practice.	The registered nurse:
		• Utilizes the best available evidence, including research findings, to guide practice decisions.
		• Actively participates in research activities at various levels appropriate to the nurse's level of education and position. Such activities may include:
		    Identifying clinical problems specific to nursing research (patient care and nursing practice).
		    Participating in data collection (surveys, pilot projects, formal studies).
		    Participating in a formal committee or program.
		    Sharing research activities and/or findings with peers and others.
		    Conducting research.
		    Critically analyzing and interpreting research for application to practice.
		    Using research findings in the development of policies, procedures, and standards of practice in patient care.
		    Incorporating research as a basis for learning.
		Additional Measurement Criteria for the Advanced Practice Registered Nurse:
		The advanced practice registered nurse:
		• Contributes to nursing knowledge by conducting or synthesizing research that discovers, examines, and evaluates knowledge, theories, criteria, and creative approaches to improve health care practice.
		• Formally disseminates research findings through activities such as presentations, publications, consultation, and journal clubs.
		Additional Measurement Criteria for the Nursing Role Specialty:
		The registered nurse in a nursing role specialty:
		• Contributes to nursing knowledge by conducting or synthesizing research that discovers, examines, and evaluates knowledge, theories, criteria, and creative approaches to improve health care.
		• Formally disseminates research findings through activities such as presentations, publications, consultation, and journal clubs.

XIV: Resource utilization	The registered nurse considers factors related to safety, effectiveness, cost, and impact on practice in the planning and delivery of nursing services.	The registered nurse: • Evaluates factors such as safety, effectiveness, availability, cost and benefits, efficiencies, and impact on practice when choosing practice options that would result in the same expected outcome. • Assists the patient and family in identifying and securing appropriate and available services to address health-related needs. • Assigns or delegates tasks, based on the needs and condition of the patient, potential for harm, stability of the patient's condition, complexity of the task, and predictability of the outcome. • Assists the patient and family in becoming informed consumers about the options, costs, risks, and benefits of treatment and care. *Additional Measurement Criteria for the Advanced Practice Registered Nurse:* The advanced practice registered nurse: • Utilizes organizational and community resources to formulate multidisciplinary or interdisciplinary plans of care. • Develops innovative solutions for patient care problems that address effective resource utilization and maintenance of quality. • Develops evaluation strategies to demonstrate cost effectiveness, cost benefit, and efficiency factors associated with nursing practice. *Additional Measurement Criteria for the Nursing Role Specialty:* The registered nurse in a nursing role specialty: • Develops innovative solutions and applies strategies to obtain appropriate resources for nursing initiatives. • Secures organizational resources to ensure a work environment conducive to completing the identified plan and outcomes. • Develops evaluation methods to measure safety and effectiveness for interventions and outcomes. • Promotes activities that assist others, as appropriate, in becoming informed about costs, risks, and benefits of care or the plan and solution.

Continued

Table 1-1	ANA Standards of Professional Performance—cont'd	
Standard	**Definition**	**Measurement Criteria**
XV: Leadership	The registered nurse provides leadership in the professional practice setting and the profession.	The registered nurse: • Engages in teamwork as a team player and a team builder. • Works to create and maintain healthy work environments in local, regional, national, or international communities. • Displays the ability to define a clear vision, the associated goals, and a plan to implement and measure progress. • Demonstrates a commitment to continuous, lifelong learning for self and others. • Teaches others to succeed by mentoring and other strategies. • Exhibits creativity and flexibility through times of change. • Demonstrates energy, excitement, and a passion for quality work. • Willingly accepts mistakes by self and others, thereby creating a culture in which risk-taking is not only safe, but expected. • Inspires loyalty through valuing of people as the most precious asset in an organization. • Directs the coordination of care across settings and among caregivers, including oversight of licensed and unlicensed personnel in any assigned or delegated tasks. • Serves in key roles in the work setting by participating on committees, councils, and administrative teams. • Promotes advancement of the profession through participation in professional organizations. *Additional Measurement Criteria for the Advanced Practice Registered Nurse:* The advanced practice registered nurse: • Works to influence decision-making bodies to improve patient care. • Provides direction to enhance the effectiveness of the health care team. • Initiates and revises protocols or guidelines to reflect evidence-based practice, to reflect accepted changes in care management, or to address emerging problems. • Promotes communication of information and advancement of the profession through writing, publishing, and presentations for professional or lay audiences. • Designs innovations to effect change in practice and improve health outcomes. *Additional Measurement Criteria for the Nursing Role Specialty:* The registered nurse in a nursing role specialty: • Works to influence decision-making bodies to improve patient care, health services, and policies. • Promotes communication of information and advancement of the profession through writing, publishing, and presentations for professional or lay audiences. • Designs innovations to effect change in practice and outcomes. • Provides direction to enhance the effectiveness of the multidisciplinary or interdisciplinary team.

Excerpted from American Nurses Association: *Nursing: scope and standards of practice,* Washington, DC, 2004, The Association.

mance appraisal, education, collegiality, ethics, collaboration, research, and resource utilization. This document serves as objective guidelines for nurses to be accountable for their actions, their patients, and their peers (ANA, 1998). The standards provide a method to assure clients that they are receiving high-quality care, that the nurses know exactly what is necessary to provide nursing care, and that measures are in place to determine whether the care meets the standards.

Standards of Care

The Standards of Care in the ANA *Nursing: Scopes and Standards of Practice* (2004) describe a competent level of nursing care (Table 1-2). The levels of care are demonstrated through the nursing process: assessment, diagnosis, outcome identification and planning, implementation, and evaluation. The nursing process is the foundation of clinical decision making and includes all significant actions taken by nurses in providing care to clients. Within these

Table 1-2 ANA Standards of Nursing Practice

Standard	Measurement Criteria
1: Assessment The registered nurse collects comprehensive data pertinent to the patient's health or the situation.	The registered nurse: • Collects data in a systematic and ongoing process. • Involves the patient, family, other healthcare providers, and environment, as appropriate, in holistic data collection. • Prioritizes data collection activities based on the patient's immediate condition, or anticipated needs of the patient or situation. • Uses appropriate evidence-based assessment techniques and instruments in collecting pertinent data. • Uses analytical models and problem-solving tools. • Synthesizes available data, information, and knowledge relevant to the situation to identify patterns and variances. • Documents relevant data in a retrievable format. *Additional Measurement Criteria for the Advanced Practice Registered Nurse:* • The advanced practice registered nurse initiates and interprets diagnostic tests and procedures relevant to the patient's current status.
2: Diagnosis The registered nurse analyzes the assessment data to determine the diagnoses or issues.	The registered nurse: • Derives the diagnoses or issues based on assessment data. • Validates the diagnoses or issues with the patient, family, and other health care providers when possible and appropriate. • Documents diagnoses or issues in a manner that facilitates the determination of the expected outcomes and plan. *Additional Measurement Criteria for the Advanced Practice Registered Nurse:* The advanced practice registered nurse: • Systematically compares and contrasts clinical findings with normal and abnormal variations and developmental events in formulating a differential diagnosis. • Utilizes complex data and information obtained during interview, examination, and diagnostic procedures in identifying diagnoses. • Assists staff in developing and maintaining competency in the diagnostic process.
3: Outcomes Identification The registered nurse identifies expected outcomes for a plan individualized to the patient or the situation.	The registered nurse: • Involves the patient, family, and other health care providers in formulating expected outcomes when possible and appropriate. • Derives culturally appropriate expected outcomes from the diagnoses. • Considers associated risks, benefits, costs, current scientific evidence, and clinical expertise when formulating expected outcomes. • Defines expected outcomes in terms of the patient, patient values, ethical considerations, environment, or situation with such consideration as associated risks, benefits and costs, and current scientific evidence. • Includes a time estimate for attainment of expected outcomes. • Develops expected outcomes that provide direction for continuity of care. • Modifies expected outcomes based on changes in the status of the patient or evaluation of the situation. • Documents expected outcomes as measurable goals. *Additional Measurement Criteria for the Advanced Practice Registered Nurse:* The advanced practice registered nurse: • Identifies expected outcomes that incorporate scientific evidence and are achievable through implementation of evidence-based practices. • Identifies expected outcomes that incorporate cost and clinical effectiveness, patient satisfaction, and continuity and consistency among providers. • Supports the use of clinical guidelines linked to positive patient outcomes.
4: Planning The registered nurse develops a plan that prescribes strategies and alternatives to attain expected outcomes.	The registered nurse: • Develops an individualized plan considering patient characteristics or the situation (e.g., age and culturally appropriate, environmentally sensitive). • Develops the plan in conjunction with the patient, family, and others, as appropriate.

Excerpted from American Nurses Association: *Nursing: scope and standards of practice,* Washington, DC, 2004, The Association.

Continued

Table 1-2	ANA Standards of Nursing Practice—cont'd
Standard	**Measurement Criteria**

4: Planning—cont'd

- Includes strategies within the plan that address each of the identified diagnoses or issues, which may include strategies for promotion and restoration of health and prevention of illness, injury, and disease.
- Provides for continuity within the plan.
- Incorporates an implementation pathway or timeline within the plan.
- Establishes the plan priorities with the patient, family, and others as appropriate.
- Utilizes the plan to provide direction to other members of the health care team.
- Defines the plan to reflect current statutes, rules and regulations, and standards.
- Integrates current trends and research affecting care in the planning process.
- Considers the economic impact of the plan.
- Uses standardized language or recognized terminology to document the plan.

Additional Measurement Criteria for the Advanced Practice Registered Nurse:
The advanced practice registered nurse:
- Identifies assessment, diagnostic strategies, and therapeutic interventions within the plan that reflect current evidence, including data, research, literature, and expert clinical knowledge.
- Selects or designs strategies to meet the multifaceted needs of complex patients.
- Includes the synthesis of patients' values and beliefs regarding nursing and medical therapies within the plan.

Additional Measurement Criteria for the Nursing Role Specialty:
The registered nurse in a nursing role specialty:
- Participates in the design and development of multidisciplinary and interdisciplinary processes to address the situation or issue.
- Contributes to the development and continuous improvement of organizational systems that support the planning process.
- Supports the integration of clinical, human, and financial resources to enhance and complete the decision-making processes.

5: Implementation

The registered nurse implements the identified plan.

The registered nurse:
- Implements the plan in a safe and timely manner.
- Documents implementation and any modifications, including changes to or omissions of the identified plan.
- Utilizes evidence-based interventions and treatments specific to the diagnosis or problem.
- Utilizes community resources and systems to implement the plan.
- Collaborates with nursing colleagues and others to implement the plan.

Additional Measurement Criteria for the Advanced Practice Registered Nurse:
The advanced practice registered nurse:
- Facilitates utilization of systems and community resources to implement the plan.
- Supports collaboration with nursing colleagues and other disciplines to implement the plan.
- Incorporates new knowledge and strategies to initiate change in nursing care practices if desired outcomes are not achieved.

Additional Measurement Criteria for the Nursing Role Specialty:
The registered nurse in a nursing role specialty:
- Implements the plan using principles and concepts of project or systems management.
- Fosters organizational systems that support implementation of the plan.

5A: Coordination of Care

The registered nurse coordinates care delivery.

The registered nurse:
- Coordinates implementation of the plan.
- Documents the coordination of the care.

Measurement Criteria for the Advanced Practice Registered Nurse:
The advanced practice registered nurse:
- Provides leadership in the coordination of multidisciplinary health care for integrated delivery of patient care services.
- Synthesizes data and information to prescribe necessary system and community support measures, including environmental modifications.
- Coordinates system and community resources that enhance delivery of care across continuums.

Excerpted from American Nurses Association: *Nursing: scope and standards of practice,* Washington, DC, 2004, The Association.

Table 1-2	ANA Standards of Nursing Practice—cont'd
Standard	**Measurement Criteria**
5B: Health Teaching and Health Promotion	The registered nurse: • Provides health teaching that addresses such topics as healthy lifestyles, risk-reducing behaviors, developmental needs, activities of daily living, and preventive self-care. • Uses health promotion and health teaching methods appropriate to the situation and the patient's developmental level, learning needs, readiness, ability to learn, language preference, and culture. • Seeks opportunities for feedback and evaluation of the effectiveness of the strategies used. *Additional Measurement Criteria for the Advanced Practice Registered Nurse:* The advanced practice registered nurse: • Synthesizes empirical evidence on risk behaviors, learning theories, behavioral change theories, motivational theories, epidemiology, and other related theories and frameworks when designing health information and patient education. • Designs health information and patient education appropriate to the patient's developmental level, learning needs, readiness to learn, and cultural values and beliefs. • Evaluates health information resources, such as the Internet, within the area of practice for accuracy, readability, and comprehensibility to help patients access quality health information.
5C: Consultation The advanced practice registered nurse and the nursing role specialist provide consultation to influence the identified plan, enhance the abilities of others and effect change. NOTE: Advanced practice and nursing role specialty only.	*Measurement Criteria for the Advanced Practice Registered Nurse:* The advanced practice registered nurse: • Synthesizes clinical data, theoretical frameworks, and evidence when providing consultation. • Facilitates the effectiveness of a consultation by involving the patient in decision-making and negotiating role responsibilities. • Communicates consultation recommendations that facilitate change. *Measurement Criteria for the Nursing Role Specialty:* The registered nurse in a nursing role specialty: • Synthesizes data, information, theoretical frameworks and evidence when providing consultation. • Facilitates the effectiveness of a consultation by involving the stakeholders in the decision-making process. • Communicates consultation recommendations that influence the identified plan, facilitate understanding by involved stakeholders, enhance the work of others, and effect change.
5D: Prescriptive Authority and Treatment The advanced practice registered nurse uses prescriptive authority, procedures, referrals, treatments, and therapies in accordance with state and federal laws and regulations. NOTE: Advanced practice nurse only.	*Measurement Criteria for the Advanced Practice Registered Nurse:* The advanced practice registered nurse: • Prescribes evidence-based treatments, therapies, and procedures considering the patient's comprehensive health care needs. • Prescribes pharmacological agents based on a current knowledge of pharmacology and physiology. • Prescribes specific pharmacological agents and/or treatments based on clinical indicators, the patient's status and needs, and the results of diagnostic and laboratory tests. • Evaluates therapeutic and potential adverse effects of pharmacological and nonpharmacological treatments. • Provides patients with information about intended effects and potential adverse effects of proposed prescriptive therapies. • Provides information about costs, alternative treatments and procedures, as appropriate.
6: Evaluation The registered nurse evaluates progress towards attainment of outcomes.	The registered nurse: • Conducts a systematic, ongoing, and criterion-based evaluation of the outcomes in relation to the structures and processes prescribed by the plan and the indicated timeline. • Includes the patient and others involved in the care or situation in the evaluative process. • Evaluates the effectiveness of the planned strategies in relation to patient responses and the attainment of the expected outcomes.

Continued

Table 1-2	ANA Standards of Nursing Practice—cont'd
Standard	**Measurement Criteria**
6: Evaluation—cont'd	• Documents the results of the evaluation. • Uses ongoing assessment data to revise the diagnoses, outcomes, the plan, and the implementation as needed. • Disseminates the results to the patient and others involved in the care or situation, as appropriate, in accordance with state and federal laws and regulations. *Additional Measurement Criteria for the Advanced Practice Registered Nurse:* The advanced practice registered nurse: • Evaluates the accuracy of the diagnosis and effectiveness of the interventions in relationship to the patient's attainment of expected outcomes. • Synthesizes the results of the evaluation analyses to determine the impact of the plan on the affected patients, families, groups, communities, and institutions. • Uses the results of the evaluation analyses to make or recommend process or structural changes including policy, procedure, or protocol documentation, as appropriate. *Additional Measurement Criteria for the Nursing Role Specialty:* The registered nurse in a nursing role specialty: • Uses the results of the evaluation analyses to make or recommend process or structural changes including policy, procedure, or protocol documentation, as appropriate. • Synthesizes the results of the evaluation analyses to determine the impact of the plan on the affected patients, families, groups, and communities, and on institutions, networks, and organizations.

Excerpted from American Nurses Association: *Nursing: scope and standards of practice,* Washington, DC, 2004, The Association.

standards are the nursing responsibilities for diversity, safety, education, health promotion, treatment, self-care, and planning for the continuity of care (ANA, 1998). Standards of care are important if a legal dispute arises over whether a nurse practiced appropriately in a particular case (see Chapter 22).

Code of Ethics. Nursing has a **code of ethics** that defines the principles by which nurses provide care to their clients. In addition, nurses incorporate their own values and ethics into practice. The ANA has a number of publications that address ethics and human rights in nursing. The *Code of Ethics for Nurses With Interpretive Statements* provides a guide for carrying out nursing responsibilities that provide quality nursing care and provides for the ethical obligations of the profession (ANA, 2001). In addition, the ANA established The Center for Ethics and Human Rights to address the complex and ethical human rights issues confronting nursing (ANA, 2002d). Chapter 21 gives several examples of specific statements of nursing's code of ethics and how nurses apply ethics in their everyday practice.

Nursing Education

As a profession, nursing requires that its members possess a significant amount of education. The issue of standardization of nursing education and entry into practice remains a major controversy. In 1965 the ANA published a position paper on nursing education that emphasizes the role of education in the profession (Box 1-2). Most nurses agree that nursing education is important to practice and that it must respond to changes in health care created by scientific and technological advances. There are various education preparations for the registered nurse. In addi-

tion, there is graduate nurse education and continuing and in-service education for the practicing nurse.

Professional Registered Nurse Education
There are various educational routes for becoming a professional **registered nurse (RN).** Initially, hospital schools of nursing were developed to educate nurses to work within those institutions. As nursing increasingly defined its own body of knowledge, formalized educational processes developed to ensure a consistent level of education in institutions. Such consistency was also necessary for RN licensure.

Currently in the United States the most frequent route an individual can choose to become an RN is through completion of an associate degree or baccalaureate degree program. Graduates of both programs are eligible to take the National Council Licensure Examination for Registered Nurses (NCLEX-RN) to become registered nurses in the state in which they will practice.

The associate degree program in the United States is a 2-year program that is usually offered by a university or junior college. This program focuses on the basic sciences and theoretical and clinical courses related to the practice of nursing. Graduates of this type of program take the state board examination for RN licensure.

The baccalaureate degree program usually encompasses 4 years of study in a college or university. The program focuses on the basic sciences and on theoretical and clinical courses, as well as courses in the social sciences, arts, and humanities to support nursing theory. In Canada the degree of Bachelor of Science in Nursing (BScN) or Bachelor in Nursing (BN) is equivalent to the degree of Bachelor of Science in Nursing (BSN) in the United States. The AACN published the *Essentials of Baccalaureate Education for Professional Nursing: A Final Report* (1998). This document

Box 1-2	**Premises for ANA's First Position Paper on Education for Nursing**

Nursing is a helping profession and, as such, provides services which contribute to the health and well-being of people.

Nursing is of vital consequence to the individual receiving services; it fills needs which cannot be met by the person, by the family, or by other persons in the community.

The demand for services of nurses will continue to increase.

The professional practitioner is responsible for the nature and quality of all nursing care that clients receive.

The services of professional practitioners of nursing will continue to be supplemented and complemented by the services of nurse practitioners who will be licensed.

Education for those in the health professions must increase in depth and breadth as scientific knowledge expands.

In addition to those licensed as nurses, the health care of the public, in the amount and to the extent needed and demanded, requires the services of large numbers of health occupation workers to function as assistants to nurses. These workers are presently designated: nurses' aides, orderlies, assistants, attendants, etc.

The professional association must concern itself with the nature of nursing practice, the means for improving nursing practice, the education necessary for practice, and the standards for membership in the professional association.

From American Nurses Association: *A position paper: educational preparation for nurse practitioners and assistants to nurses,* Kansas City, Mo, 1965, The Association.

delineated essential knowledge, practice and values, attitudes, personal qualities, and professional behavior for the baccalaureate-prepared nurse and guides faculty on the structure and evaluation of the curriculum and the performance of the graduate (American Association of Colleges of Nursing, 1998).

Graduate Education

Master's Education. After obtaining a baccalaureate degree in nursing, a nurse can pursue further education in any number of graduate fields, including nursing. A nurse completing a graduate program can receive the degree of Master of Arts (MA) in nursing, Master in Nursing (MN), or Master of Science in Nursing (MSN). The graduate degree provides the advanced clinician with strong skills in nursing science and theory with emphasis in the basic sciences and research-based clinical practice. A master's degree in nursing can be valuable for nurses seeking roles of nurse educator, clinical nurse specialist, nurse administrator, or nurse practitioner. These roles are described later in this chapter.

Doctoral Preparation. Professional doctoral programs in nursing (DSN or DNSc) emphasize the application of research findings to clinical nursing. Other programs emphasize more basic research and theory and award the degree of Doctor of Philosophy (PhD) in nursing. The need for nurses with doctorate degrees is rising. Expanding clinical roles, new areas of nursing such as nursing informatics, and rapidly advancing technology are just a few reasons for increasing the number of doctorally prepared nurses. It is important to continue to do research in areas such as nursing theory, basic science, and clinical practice to expand nursing knowledge. Doctorally prepared nurses are needed to educate the beginning nurse and those seeking advanced academic and clinical preparation.

Continuing and In-Service Education

Because nursing is a dynamic profession, continuing education programs help nurses remain current in nursing skills, knowledge, and theory. **Continuing education**

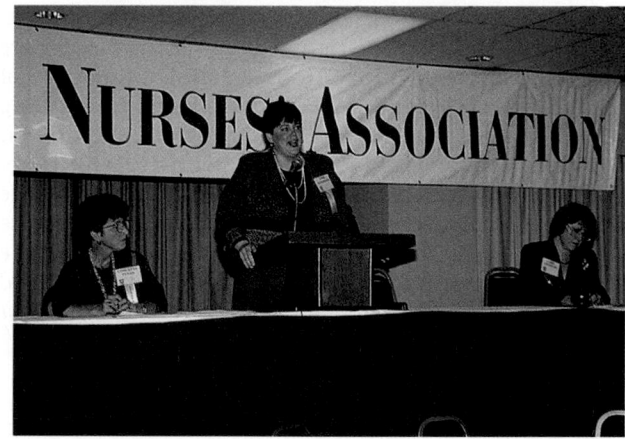

FIGURE **1-1** Participating at State Nurses Association meetings provides continuing education and networking opportunities.

involves formal, organized, and educational programs offered by State Nurses Associations (Figure 1-1) and educational and health care institutions. For example, a State Nurses' Association might offer a class on caring for older adults with dementia. As expressed by the ANA (1994), the goals of continuing education in nursing are to improve and maintain nursing practice, promote and exercise leadership in effecting change in health care delivery systems, and fulfill professional learning needs. Other goals include helping nurses become specialized in a particular area of practice and teaching nurses new skills and techniques.

An **in-service education** program is instruction or training provided by a health care agency or institution. An in-service program is held in the institution and is designed to increase the knowledge, skills, and competencies of nurses and other health care professionals employed by the institution. For example, a hospital might offer an in-service program to inform nurses about primary nursing before it is implemented at the hospital or a program on the newest safety syringes for administering parenteral medications.

Continuing and in-service education continues to be important after the nurse begins practice, whether the practice setting focuses on the adult or child, the chronically or acutely ill, or the home or hospital. Nursing encompasses an ever-widening range of roles. Multiple career paths and goals are open to new and experienced practitioners.

Nursing Practice

Nurses practice in a variety of settings, in many roles within those settings, and with other caregivers in the allied health professions. Administrators in hospitals and other health care agencies and institutions guide the practice of nursing only in part. State and provincial Nurse Practice Acts establish specific legal regulations for practice, and professional organizations establish standards of practice as criteria for nursing care

The Congress of Nursing Practice is the part of the ANA concerned with legal aspects of nursing practice, public recognition of the significance of nursing practice to health care, and implications for nursing practice of trends in health care. In 1980 the Congress for Nursing Practice defined nursing as the diagnosis and treatment of human responses to actual or potential health problems (ANA, 1980, 1995). This definition illustrates the consistent orientation of nurses to the provision of care to promote the well-being of their clients. Today the nursing profession remains committed to the care and nurturing of both healthy and ill people, individually or in groups and communities (ANA, 1995).

Nurse Practice Acts
In all states in the United States, Nurse Practice Acts regulate the licensure and practice of nursing. Each state or province defines for itself the scope of nursing practice, but most have similar practice acts. The definition of nursing practice published by the ANA is in some ways representative of the scope of nursing practice as defined in most states. In the last decade, however, many states have revised their Nurse Practice Acts to reflect nursing's growing autonomy and the expanded roles of nurses in practice.

Licensure and Certification
Licensure. In the United States, RN candidates must pass the NCLEX-RN, which is administered by the individual State Boards of Nursing. Regardless of educational preparation, the examination for RN licensure is exactly the same in every state in the United States. This provides a standardized minimum knowledge base for the client population nurses serve.

Certification. Beyond the NCLEX-RN, the nurse may choose to work toward certification in a specific area of nursing practice. Minimum practice requirements are set, based on the certification the nurse is seeking. National nursing organizations, such as the ANA, have many types of certification that the nurse can work toward. After passing the initial examination, the nurse maintains cer-

tification by ongoing continuing education and clinical or administrative practice.

Science and Art of Nursing Practice
Nursing is a multidimensional profession. Nursing reflects the needs and values of society, implements the standards of professional performance and the standards of care, meets the needs of each client, and integrates current research and evidence-based findings to provide the highest level of care. Although nursing has a specific body of knowledge, socialization into the profession and practice are essentials components of the discipline. Clinical expertise takes time and commitment. According to Benner (1984), an expert nurse passes through five levels of proficiency when acquiring and developing generalist or specialized nursing skills (Box 1-3).

Nurses use the competencies of critical thinking to integrate information from the scientific and nursing knowledge bases, derive knowledge from past and present experiences, apply critical thinking attitudes to a clinical situation, and implement intellectual and professional standards (see Chapter 14). Providing well thought out care with the compassion and caring attributes of the

---

Box 1-3   Benner: From Novice to Expert

Novice—Beginning nursing student, or any nurse entering a situation in which there is no previous level of experience, for example, an experienced operating room nurse chooses to now practice in home health. The learner learns via a specific set of rules or procedures, which are usually stepwise and linear.

Advanced Beginner—A nurse who has had some level of experience with the situation. This experience may only be observational in nature, but the nurse is able to identify meaningful aspects or principles of nursing care.

Competent—A nurse who has been in the same clinical position for 2-3 years. This nurse understands the organization and the specific care required by the type of clients, e.g., surgical, oncology, or orthopedic clients. This nurse is a competent practitioner who is able to anticipate nursing care and establish long-range goals. In this phase, the nurse has usually had experience with all types of psychomotor skills required by this specific group of clients.

Proficient—A nurse with greater than 2-3 years of experience in the same clinical position. This nurse perceives a client's clinical situation as a whole, is able to assess an entire situation, and can readily transfer knowledge gained from multiple previous experiences to a situation. This nurse focuses on managing care as opposed to managing and performing skills.

Expert—A nurse with diverse experience who has an intuitive grasp of an existing or potential clinical problem. This nurse is able to zero in on the problem and focus on multiple dimensions of the situation. This nurse is skilled at identifying client-centered problems, as well as problems related to the health care system or perhaps the needs of the novice nurse.

Data from Benner P: *From novice to expert: excellence and power in clinical nursing practice*, Menlo Park, Calif, 1984, Addison-Wesley.

profession enables nurses to provide each client the best of the science and art of nursing care (see Chapter 7).

Professional Responsibilities and Roles

Contemporary nursing requires that the nurse possess knowledge and skills for a variety of professional roles and responsibilities. In the past, the principal role of nurses was to provide care and comfort as they carried out specific nursing functions. However, changes in nursing have expanded the role to include increased emphasis on health promotion and illness prevention, as well as concern for the client as a whole.

Autonomy and Accountability

Autonomy is an essential element of professional nursing. Autonomy means that a person is reasonably independent and self-governing in decision making and practice. In the case of nursing, there are independent nursing measures a nurse can initiate without medical orders. A professional nurse also actively collaborates with health professionals to pursue the best treatment plan for a client. Nurses attain increased autonomy through higher levels of education. In the changing health care system, advanced practice nurses are increasingly taking on independent roles in nurse-run clinics, collaborative practice, and advanced nurse practice settings.

With increased autonomy come greater responsibility and accountability. Accountability means that the nurse is responsible, professionally and legally, for the type and quality of nursing care provided. The nurse is accountable for keeping current and competent in technical skills and informed of the knowledge needed to perform nursing care. The nursing profession itself regulates accountability through nursing audits and standards of practice.

Caregiver

As **caregiver,** the nurse helps the client regain health through the healing process. Healing is more than just curing a specific disease, although treatment skills that promote physical healing are important to caregivers. The nurse addresses the holistic health care needs of the client, including measures to restore emotional, spiritual, and social well-being. The caregiver helps the client and families set goals and meet those goals with a minimal cost of time and energy.

Advocate

In the role of **client advocate,** the nurse protects the client's human and legal rights and provides assistance in asserting those rights if the need arises. The nurse advocates for the client, keeping in mind the client's religion and culture. For example, the nurse may provide additional information for a client who is trying to decide whether or not to accept a treatment, or the nurse may assist with communication within the family. The nurse may also defend clients' rights in a general way by speaking out against policies or actions that might endanger their well-being or conflict with their rights.

Educator

As an educator, the nurse explains to clients concepts and facts about health, demonstrates procedures such as self-care activities, determines that the client fully understands, reinforces learning or client behavior, and evaluates the client's progress in learning. Some client teaching can be unplanned and informal, such as when a nurse responds to a question about a health issue in casual conversation. Other teaching activities may be planned and more formal, such as when the nurse teaches a client with diabetes to self-administer insulin injections. The nurse uses teaching methods that match the client's capabilities and needs and incorporates other resources, such as the family, in teaching plans (see Chapter 24).

Communicator

The role of communicator is central to all nursing roles and activities. Nursing involves communication with clients and families, other nurses and health care professionals, resource persons, and the community. Without clear communication, it is impossible to give care effectively, make decisions with clients and families, protect clients from threats to well-being, coordinate and manage client care, assist the client in rehabilitation, offer comfort, or teach. The quality of communication is a critical factor in meeting the needs of individuals, families, and communities (see Chapter 23).

Manager

As a manager, the nurse coordinates the activities of other members of the health care team, such as nutritionists and physical therapists, when managing care for a group of clients. To effectively manage a single client or group of clients the nurse implements solid clinical decision-making skills. As a **clinical decision maker,** the nurse uses critical thinking skills throughout the nursing process to provide effective care. Before undertaking any nursing action, whether it is assessing the client's condition, giving care, or evaluating the results of care, the nurse plans the action by deciding the best approach for each client (see Unit 3). The nurse makes these decisions alone or in collaboration with the client and family (Figure 1-2). In each of these situations, the nurse collaborates and consults with other health care professionals (Keeling and Ramos, 1995).

Career Development

Innovations in health care, expanding health care systems and practice settings, and the increasing needs of clients have been a stimulus for new nursing roles. Today nurses need to commit to lifelong learning and career development in order to provide clients with the state-of-the-art care they need (Table 1-3).

Career roles are specific employment positions or paths. Because of increasing educational opportunities for nurses, the growth of nursing as a profession, and a greater concern for job enrichment, the nursing profession offers expanded roles and different kinds of career opportunities. A

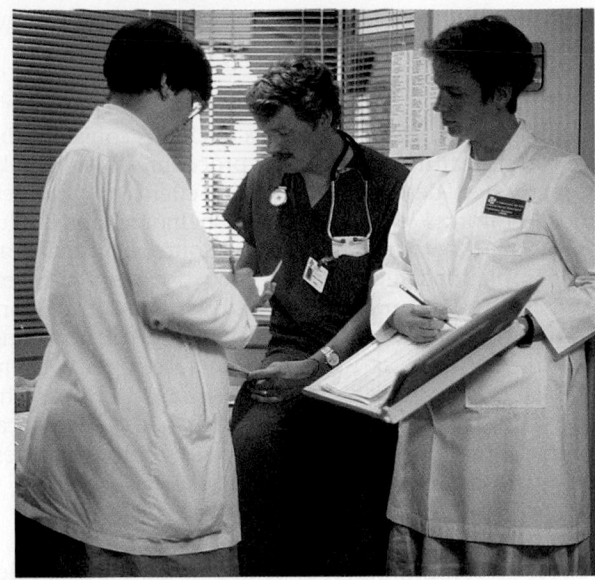

FIGURE **1-2** Decision making is at the core of nursing practice.

Table 1-3	Demographics for Today's Registered Nurses	
		United States*
Licensed nurses		2,239,816 million
Employed nurses		1,853,024 million
Gender		
Female		95.7%
Male		4.3%
Race		
White/Caucasian		90%
African-American		4%
Asian/Pacific Islanders		3.4%
Hispanics		1.4%
American Indian/Alaska Natives		0.4%
Age		
<30 years		11%
30-49 years		>60%
Education		
Diploma program		<15%
Associate degree		59%
Bachelor's degree		31%
Master's degree		7.5%
Doctorate		0.5%
Site of Employment		
Hospitals		66%
Nursing homes/extended care		7%
Community/public health		10%
Ambulatory care		8%
Other (physician office, nursing education)		10%

*Data from American Nurses Association: Nursing facts: today's registered nurse—number and demographics. From *National sample survey of registered nurses, 1996,* U.S. Department of Health and Human Services, Public Health Service, Division of Nursing, Health Resources and Services Administration, 2002, http://nursingworld.org/readroom/fsdemogr/htm.

nurse's career path can be limitless. Examples of career roles include nurse educators, advanced practice nurses, nurse managers and administrators, nurse researchers, nurse risk managers, quality improvement nurses, consultants, and even business owners.

Clinician. Most nurses enter the profession with the goal of providing direct client care. The nurse providing direct client care accounts for the majority of practicing nurses. Until recently, this has been in the acute care hospital setting. As health care returns to the home care setting, there are increased opportunities for nurses to provide direct care in the client's home. The clinical nurse provides direct care to the client, using the nursing process and critical thinking skills. The focus is restorative and curative. The clinical nurse provides education to the client and family to promote health maintenance and self-care. In collaboration with other health care team members, the clinician focuses on returning the client to his or her home and usual state of health.

In the hospital, nurses may choose to practice in a medical-surgical setting or concentrate on a specific area of practice, such as critical care or emergency care. Most specialty care areas require some experience as a medical-surgical nurse and additional continuing or in-service education. Many intensive care unit (ICU) and emergency department nurses are required to have training in advanced cardiac life support and certification in critical care, emergency nursing, or trauma nursing. Hospital-based nurses may also choose to practice in specialty areas such as transplantation, rehabilitation, or oncology. Larger medical centers offer more opportunity to concentrate practice in a single area.

Advanced Practice Nurses. The **advanced practice nurse (APN)** is generally the most independent functioning nurse. An APN has a master's degree in nursing,

advanced education in pharmacology and physical assessment, and certification and expertise in a specialized area of practice (ANA, 1996). The APN may work in primary, acute, or restorative care settings. The APN functions as a clinician, educator, case manager, consultant, and researcher within his or her area of practice, to plan or improve the quality of nursing care for the client and family. For example, a nurse practitioner in a community clinic will manage the health care of a group of clients by monitoring their chronic health problems and diagnosing and treating any new developing problems. The term *advanced practice nurse* is an umbrella term for an advanced clinical nurse that includes nurse practitioners, clinical nurse specialists, certified registered nurse anesthetists, and nurse-midwives.

Clinical Nurse Specialist. The **clinical nurse specialist (CNS)** is an APN with nursing expertise in a specialized area of practice and may work in any practice setting. Traditionally, the CNS has practiced most often in the hospital setting. The CNS may specialize in a specific disease, such as diabetes mellitus, cancer, or cardiac problems, or in a specific field, such as pediatrics or gerontology. The CNS

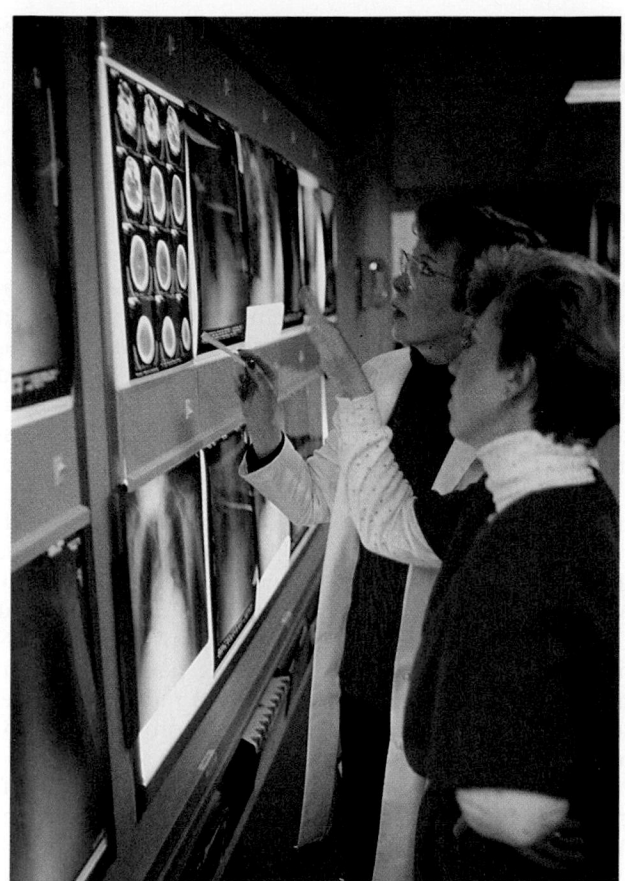

FIGURE **1–3**   Nurse specialist consults on a difficult client case.

functions as an expert clinician, educator, case manager, consultant, and researcher to plan or improve the quality of care provided to the client and family (Figure 1-3).

Nurse Practitioner. The **nurse practitioner** provides health care to clients, usually in an outpatient, ambulatory care, or community-based setting. Nurse practitioners provide care for clients with complex problems and provide a more holistic approach, attending to symptoms of nonpathological conditions, comfort, and comprehensiveness of care. A significant percentage of primary care visits by clients extend beyond the boundaries of medicine and demand the expertise of the nurse. The nurse practitioner is able to establish a collaborative provider-client relationship. A nurse practitioner may work with a specific group of clients or with clients of all ages and health care needs. The major nurse practitioner categories are adult, family, pediatric, obstetrics-gynecology, and geriatric. A nurse practitioner has the knowledge and skills necessary to detect and manage self-limiting acute and chronic stable conditions.

An adult nurse practitioner (ANP) provides primary, ambulatory care to adults with a nonemergent acute or chronic illness and in some settings tertiary care. ANPs work collaboratively with one or more primary care physicians; for example, in a five-physician primary care practice, a nurse practitioner may exclusively manage all diabetic clients who have a foot ulcer. In this example,

the nurse practitioner is working collaboratively with all physicians. A family nurse practitioner (FNP) provides primary ambulatory care for families, usually in collaboration with a family care physician. The FNP meets the family's general health care needs, manages some illnesses by providing direct care, and guides or counsels the family as needed.

A pediatric nurse practitioner (PNP) provides health care to infants and children. PNPs practice in hospital, ambulatory care, emergency care, and physicians' offices. A women's health nurse practitioner (WHNP) provides primary ambulatory care to women seeking obstetrical or gynecological health care.

An **acute care nurse practitioner** functions in collaboration with a physician or house staff physician in an acute care setting, such as a hospital or specialty clinic. The acute care nurse practitioner is a generalist, usually based in internal medicine, focusing on the care of the hospitalized patient.

The **geriatric nurse practitioner (GNP)** is an ANP with specialization in care of the older adult. GNPs are trained in the special needs of the aging adult, with emphasis on health promotion, health maintenance, and functional status. The GNP works with the client and family to manage existing health problems so as to promote independence and self-care. The client population is usually age 65 and older.

Certified Nurse-Midwife. A **certified nurse-midwife (CNM)** is an RN who is also educated in midwifery and is certified by the American College of Nurse-Midwives. The practice of nurse-midwifery involves providing independent care for women during normal pregnancy, labor, and delivery, as well as care for the newborn. It may include some gynecological services such as routine Papanicolaou (Pap) smears, family planning, and treatment for minor vaginal infections. A CNM practices with a health care agency that provides medical consultation, collaborative management, and referral.

Certified Registered Nurse Anesthetist. A **certified registered nurse anesthetist (CRNA)** is an RN who has received advanced training in an accredited program in anesthesiology. Nurse anesthetists provide surgical anesthesia under the guidance and supervision of an anesthesiologist, who is a physician with advanced knowledge of surgical anesthesia.

Nurse Educator. A **nurse educator** works primarily in schools of nursing, staff development departments of health care agencies, and client education departments. Nursing educators need experience in clinical practice to provide them with practical skills and theoretical knowledge. A faculty member in a school of nursing educates students to become professional nurses. Nursing faculty members are responsible for teaching current nursing practice, trends, theory, and necessary skills in laboratories and clinical settings. Nurse educators in nursing schools are usually required to have graduate degrees in nursing and additional education in the educational process. Many hold doctorate or advanced degrees in nursing, education, or administration, such as a master's degree in business administration

(MBA). Generally they have a specific clinical, administrative, or research specialty and advanced clinical experience.

Nurse educators in staff development departments of health care institutions provide educational programs for nurses within their institution. These programs include orientation of new personnel, critical care nursing courses, assisting with clinical skill competency, safety training, and instruction about new equipment or procedures. These nursing educators often participate in the development of nursing policies and procedures.

The primary focus of the nurse educator in an agency's department of client education is to teach ill or disabled clients and their families how to provide care in the home. These nurse educators may be specialized and certified, such as a certified diabetic educator (CDE) or an ostomy care nurse, and see only a discrete population of clients. In most health care agencies, however, the budget does not permit a separate client education department. Therefore the responsibility usually falls to the staff nurse to plan and provide client and family education.

Nursing Administrator. A **nurse administrator** manages client care and the delivery of specific nursing services within a health care agency. Nursing administration begins with positions such as the charge nurse or assistant nurse manager. Experience and additional education may lead to a middle-management position, such as nurse manager of a specific patient care area(s) or house supervisor, or to an upper-management position, such as assistant or associate director or director of nursing services.

Nurse manager's positions usually require at least a baccalaureate degree in nursing, and director and nurse executive positions generally require a master's degree. Chief nurse executive and vice president positions in large health care organizations often require preparation at the doctorate level. Nurses may have advanced degrees such as a master's degree in business administration (MBA), hospital administration (MHA), or public health (MPH).

In today's health care organizations, directors may have responsibility for more than nursing personnel. Responsibilities may include a particular service or product line, such as medicine or cardiology, and include supportive functions and personnel such as medicine clinics, cardiac diagnostics, or outpatient services such as cardiac catheterization. In addition, the director may be responsible for ancillary personnel such as cardiology technicians, respiratory therapists, social workers, and dietitians.

Vice presidents of nursing or chief nurse executives often have responsibilities for all clinical functions within the hospital. This may include all ancillary personnel who provide and support patient care services. The nursing administrator needs to be skilled in business and management, as well as understand all aspects of nursing and client care. Functions of administrators include budgeting, staffing, strategic planning of programs and services, employee evaluation, and employee development (Douglas, 1996).

Nurse Researcher. The **nurse researcher** investigates problems to improve nursing care and to further define and expand the scope of nursing practice (see Chapter 5). The nurse researcher may be employed in an academic setting, hospital, or independent professional or community service agency. The minimum educational requirement is a doctoral degree, with at least a master's degree in nursing.

Professional Nursing Organizations

A **professional organization** is created to deal with issues of concern to those practicing in the profession. In North America the major professional nursing organizations are the **National League for Nursing (NLN)** and American Nurses Association (ANA). The NLN is concerned with the improvement of nursing education, nursing service, and health care delivery in the United States.

ANA was formed in the late nineteenth century to improve standards of health and the availability of health care, to foster high standards for nursing, and to promote the professional development and general and economic welfare of nurses. The ANA is part of the **International Council of Nursing (ICN)**. The objectives of the ICN parallel those of the ANA: promoting national associations of nurses, improving standards of nursing practice, seeking a higher status for nurses, and providing an international power base for nurses.

The ANA is active in political, professional, and financial issues affecting health care and the nursing profession. ANA is a strong lobbyist in professional practice issues, such as limits of overtime hours. In this example, ANA extensively lobbied state legislatures to restrict the length of overtime any one nurse's shift can be extended. This was due to the safety risk of 12 to 16 hours on client and nurse safety. There is an increased risk of treatment errors and nurse injury when the nurse's workday is extended.

Nursing students take part in organizations such as the National Student Nurses Association (NSNA) in the United States and the Canadian Student Nurses Association (CSNA) in Canada. These organizations consider issues of importance to nursing students, such as career development and preparation for licensing. NSNA often cooperates in activities and programs with the professional organizations.

Some professional organizations focus on specific areas such as critical care, nursing administration or research, or nurse-midwifery. These organizations seek to improve the standards of practice, expand nursing roles, and foster the welfare of nurses within the specialty areas. In addition, professional organizations present education programs and publish journals.

Future Trends in Nursing

This chapter has emphasized that nursing is not a static, unchanging profession but is continuously growing and evolving as society changes, as health care emphases and methods change, as lifestyles change—and as nurses themselves change. To speak of nursing at all is to speak of nursing as it is at a given time, and in this sense, this chapter is about trends in nursing.

The current philosophies and definitions of nursing demonstrate the holistic trend in nursing—to address the whole person in all dimensions, in health and illness, and in interaction with the family and community. Nursing continues to draw on the social sciences and other fields as the focus of nursing care expands.

Expansion of Employment Opportunities

Nursing practice trends include a growing variety of employment settings in which nurses have greater independence, autonomy, and respect as members of the health care team. Nursing roles continue to expand and develop, broadening the focus of nursing care and providing a more holistic and all-encompassing domain. Nursing therapies are not only drawing from traditional nursing and medicine, spiritual, and emotional realms, but also expanding into alternative therapies such as healing touch, massage therapy, and use of natural herbs and vitamins (see Chapter 35).

Nursing's Public Perception

Any member of society who has been ill, hospitalized, or visited an emergency department has experienced nursing care; as an ANA campaign noted, "Everybody needs a *Nurse.*" The Johnson and Johnson Foundation has developed a compelling, attention-getting media campaign on the nursing profession. These media clips show nursing practice, and the nurses featured in the advertisements describe their satisfaction with the profession.

Nursing is a pivotal health care profession; as frontline health care providers, nurses practice in all health care settings and constitute the largest number of professionals. Nurses are essential to provide skilled, specialized, knowledgeable care; to improve the health status of the public; and to ensure safe, effective quality care (ANA, 2002c). In addition, the American public rated nurses high in honesty and ethics in their professional role (Gallup Organization, 1999-2001).

Nursing's Impact on Politics and Health Policy

The ability to influence or persuade an individual holding a government office to exert the power of that office to affect a desired outcome is known as political power or influence. Nurses' involvement in politics is receiving greater emphasis in nursing curricula, professional organizations, and health care settings. Professional nursing organizations have employed lobbyists to urge state legislatures and the U.S. Congress to improve the quality of health care.

The ANA works for the improvement of health standards and the availability of health care services for all people, fosters high standards of nursing, stimulates and promotes the professional development of nurses, and advances their economic and general welfare. The purposes are unrestricted by considerations of nationality, race, creed, lifestyle, color, sex, or age. The ANA employs RNs as lobbyists at the federal level, and state nursing organizations also hire lobbyists and legislative specialists to work on state nursing issues and assist with federal efforts. Finally, lobbyists working on behalf of nursing are employed in Washington, D.C., by professional organizations such as the American Federation of Teachers,

NLN, American College of Nurse-Midwives, American Public Health Association, and AACN. These groups aim to remove financial barriers to health care, increase the quality of nursing care available, increase economic rewards to nurses, and expand professional nursing roles.

In addition, individual nurses can influence policy decisions at all governmental levels, and organized nursing's unified efforts, such as with *Nursing's Agenda for Health Care Reform* (ANA, 1991) and *Nursing's Agenda for the Future: A Call to the Nation* (ANA, 2002c), will be critical to exert nurses' influence early in the political process. If nurses become serious students of social needs, activists in influencing policy to meet those needs, and generous contributors of time and money to nursing and their organizations and to candidates working for universal good health care, then the future is bright indeed.

Nurses are becoming more involved in health care reform. Nursing's Agenda for Health Care Reform supports the creation of a health care system that ensures access, quality, and services at affordable costs. The plan for reform focuses on primary health care services and the promotion, restoration, and maintenance of health (ANA, 1991, 2002c).

Healthy People 2010 (USDHHS, 2002) is a document for public health policy for the new millennium (see Chapter 6). It outlines goals for vulnerable populations, such as low-income groups, minorities, and persons with disabilities (Lancaster, 1999).

Political activism and commitment are a part of professionalism, however, and politics are an important aspect of the delivery of health care. Therefore nurses should view politics as a reality that includes the arts of influence, compromise, and social interaction. Nurses have been involved in a different sort of politics in schools of nursing and in health care settings when seeking additional resources, more self-direction, and accountability with authority. The skills gained in such experiences can be transferred to the politics of health care policy making.

As long as nurses maintain involvement in health care policy and practice, misinformed outsiders cannot attempt to impose their will on nursing and nursing practice. Nonnursing groups, often led by other health care providers, have made attempts to impose institutional licensure, mandatory continuing education, curtailment of advanced nursing practice, and other constraints on the nursing profession. Nursing should have its own voice in decisions made in these and numerous other areas affecting the practice and quality of nursing care. Although nurses have often successfully prevented infringement on the profession's self-governance, the future of nursing requires that nurses individually and collectively seek a greater influence on health care policies affecting nursing practice.

Key Concepts

- Nursing has responded to the health care needs of society, which were influenced by economic, social, and cultural variables of a specific era.
- Changes in society, such as increased technology, new demographic patterns, consumerism, health

promotion, and the women's and human rights movements, have led to changes in nursing.
- Nursing education became affiliated with universities early in the twentieth century.
- Expansion of nursing into the military occurred in the early twentieth century, and the development of specialty nursing organizations began in the 1950s and has continued to the present.
- Nursing definitions reflect changes in the practice of nursing and help bring about changes by identifying the domain of nursing practice and guiding research, practice, and education.
- Nursing standards provide the guidelines for implementing and evaluating nursing care.
- The multiple roles and functions of the nurse include caregiver, client advocate, manager, communicator, and educator.
- Specific career roles include nurse educator, advanced practice nurse, nurse practitioner, certified nurse-midwife, nurse anesthetist, administrator, and researcher.
- Nursing is a profession encompassing educational preparation for the nurse, nursing theory, a provided service, autonomy, and a code of ethics.
- Professional nursing organizations deal with issues of concern to specialist groups within the nursing profession.
- Nurses are becoming more politically sophisticated and, as a result, are able to increase nursing's influence on health care policy and practice.

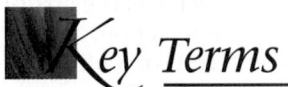

Key Terms

Acute care nurse practitioner (ACNP), *p. 21*	Continuing education, *p. 17*
Advanced practice nurse (APN), *p. 20*	Geriatric nurse practitioner (GNP), *p. 21*
American Nurses Association (ANA), *p. 5*	In-service education, *p. 17*
Caregiver, *p. 19*	International Council of Nurses (ICN), *p. 2*
Certified nurse-midwife (CNM), *p. 21*	National League for Nursing (NLN), *p. 22*
Certified registered nurse anesthetist (CRNA), *p. 21*	Nurse administrator, *p. 22*
Client advocate, *p. 19*	Nurse educator, *p. 21*
Clinical decision maker, *p. 19*	Nurse practitioner, *p. 21*
Clinical nurse specialist (CNS), *p. 20*	Nurse researcher, *p. 22* Nursing, *p. 2*
Code of ethics, *p. 16*	Professional organization, *p. 22*
	Registered nurse (RN), *p. 16*

Critical Thinking Exercises

1. Observe various levels of nursing practice, such as a staff nurse, advanced practice nurse, and nurse educator. Identify similarities and differences in their roles and educational preparation.

2. Outline some career objectives for yourself over the next 5 years. Obviously the first would be to complete your nursing program. But decide what you want to do as a professional nurse, and then outline strategies to achieve these goals.

3. Part of your education includes experiences in different types of health care settings. How would your role in the primary care setting be different from your role in the acute care setting?

Review Questions

1. Nursing has a code of ethics that professional registered nurses follow and:
   1. Defines the principles by which nurses' provide care to their clients.
   2. Ensures identical care to all clients.
   3. Protects the client from harm.
   4. Improves self-health care.

2. The founder of modern nursing is:
   1. Dorthea Dix.
   2. Florence Nightingale.
   3. Clara Barton.
   4. Harriet Tubman.

3. The founder of the American Red Cross is:
   1. Florence Nightingale.
   2. Dorthea Dix.
   3. Clara Barton.
   4. Mary Mahoney.

4. Evidence-based practice is defined as:
   1. The integration of best research evidence with clinical expertise and patient values.
   2. Scholarly inquiry of nursing and biomedical research literature.
   3. Nursing care based on tradition.
   4. Quality nursing care provided in an efficient and economically sound manner.

5. The Standards of Care described in the *ANA Standards of Clinical Practice,* second edition, include:
   1. The nursing process: assessment, diagnosis, outcome identification and planning, implementation, and evaluation.
   2. Administration of medications, personal hygiene, and grooming.
   3. Care of vulnerable populations.
   4. Care of persons in financial crisis.

6. Regardless of educational preparation, the examination for RN licensure is exactly the same in every state in the United States. This:
   1. Provides a standardized minimum knowledge base for the client population nurses serve.
   2. Guarantees safe care for all clients.
   3. Ensures identical care for all clients.
   4. Ensures an honest caregiver.

7. Contemporary nursing requires that the nurse possess knowledge and skills for a variety of professional roles and responsibilities. Examples include:
   1. Autonomy and accountability.
   2. Following physician orders.
   3. Providing bedside care.
   4. Increased emphasis on health promotion and illness prevention.

8. Advanced practice nurses generally:
   1. Work in the university setting.
   2. Function independently.
   3. Work in acute care settings.
   4. Function as unit directors.

9. In North America the major professional nursing organization(s) is (are):
   1. The National Institute of Health and Critical Care Nurses.
   2. National League for Nursing and the American Nurses Association.
   3. National Council Licensure Examination.
   4. The American Medical Association.

10. As long as nurses maintain involvement in health care policy and practice:
    1. Nurses will have significant increases in salaries.
    2. Outsiders will not impose their will on nursing and nursing practice.
    3. Major health problems will subside.
    4. Physicians will have more control over nursing and nursing functions.

*R*eferences

Alfaro-LeFevre R: *Critical thinking in nursing: a practical approach,* Philadelphia, 1995, WB Saunders.

American Association of Colleges of Nursing: *Essentials of baccalaureate education for professional nursing: a final report,* Washington, DC, 1998, The Association.

American Nurses Association: *A position paper: educational preparation for nurse practitioners and assistants to nurses,* Kansas City, Mo, 1965, The Association.

American Nurses Association: *Nursing and social policy statement,* Kansas City, Mo, 1980, The Association.

American Nurses Association: *Nursing's agenda for health care reform,* Washington, DC, 1991, The Association.

American Nurses Association: *Standards for nursing professional development: continuing education and staff development,* ANA Pub No. COE-17, Washington, DC, 1994, American Nurses Publishing.

American Nurses Association: *Nursing and social policy statement,* Washington, DC, 1995, American Nurses Publishing.

American Nurses Association: *Scope and standards of advanced practice registered nursing,* Pub No. ADV-1, Washington, DC, 1996, American Nurses Publishing.

American Nurses Association: *Position statement: educational preparation for participation in nursing research,* Washington, DC, 1997, The Association.

American Nurses Association: *Code for of ethics for nurses with interpretive statements,* Washington, DC, 2001, The Association.

American Nurses Association: Advanced practice nursing: a new age in health care, 2002a, http://nursingworld.org/readroom/fsadvprac.htm.

American Nurses Association: Nursing facts: today's registered nurse—number and demographics. From *National sample survey of registered nurses, 1996,* U.S. Department of Health and Human Services, Public Health Service, Division of Nursing, Health Resources and Services Administration, 2002b, http://nursingworld.org/readroom/fsdemogr/htm.

American Nurses Association: *Nursing's agenda for the future: a call to the nation,* Washington, DC, 2002c, The Association.

American Nurses Association: 2002d, The Center for Ethics and Human Rights, http://nursingworld. org/ethics.

American Nurses Association: *Standards of nursing practice,* ed 3, Washington, DC, 2003, The Association.

American Nurses Association: *Nursing: scopes and standards of practice,* Washington, DC, The Association.

Benner P: *From novice to expert: excellence and power in clinical nursing practice,* Menlo Park, Calif, 1984, Addison-Wesley.

Bernhard LA, Walsh M: *Leadership: the key to the professionalization of nursing,* ed 3, St. Louis, 1995, Mosby.

Carnevali DL, Thomas MD: *Diagnostic reasoning and treatment decision making in nursing,* Philadelphia, 1998, JB Lippincott.

Cohen IB: Florence Nightingale, *Sci Am* 250(128):137, 1984.

Donahue MP: *Nursing: the finest art—an illustrated history,* ed 2, St. Louis, 1996, Mosby.

Douglas LM: *The effective nurse: leader and manager,* ed 5, St. Louis, 1996, Mosby.

International Council of Nurses: ICN definition of nursing, 2002, http://icn.ch/definition.htm.

Keeling AW, Ramos MC: The role of nursing history in preparing nursing for the future, *Nurs Health Care* 16:30, 1995.

Lancaster J: *Nursing issues in leading and managing change,* St. Louis, 1999, Mosby.

Macrae J: Nightingale's spiritual philosophy and its significance for modern nursing, *Image J Nurs Sch* 27:8, 1995.

Masson V: The underserved: just who do we think they are, *Am J Nurs* 101(7):25, 2001.

Nightingale F: *Notes on nursing: what it is and what it is not,* London, 1860, Harrison & Sons.

Romig C: The nursing shortage demands action now—state and federal legislation passes, *AORN J* 74(5):733, 2001.

Sackett DL and others: *Evidence-based medicine: how to practice and teach EBM,* London, 2000, Churchill Livingstone.

Sullivan EJ: *Creating nursing's future: issues, opportunities, and challenges,* St. Louis, 1999, Mosby.

U.S. Department of Health and Human Services, Public Health Service. *Healthy People 2010: a systematic approach to health improvement,* Washingtion, DC, 2000b, U.S. Government Printing Office, www.health.gov/healthypeople/document/HTML.

Woodham-Smith C: *Florence Nightingale,* New York, 1983, McGraw-Hill.

*R*esearch References

Blendon RJ and others: Views of practicing physicians and the public on medical errors, *N Engl J Med* 347:1933, 2002.

Boychuk JE: Out in the real world: newly graduated nurses in acute-care speak out, *J Nurs Adm* 31(9):426, 2001.

Consumer Reports: How safe is your hospital, *Consumer Reports,* p 1, January 2003, www.consumerreports.org/main.

The Gallup Organization: *Honesty and ethics poll,* Princeton, NJ, 1999-2001, The Gallup Organization.

*H*ealth Care Delivery System

Media Resources

http://evolve.elsevier.com/Potter/
fundamentals/

CD COMPANION

- Review Questions
- Glossary

evolve WEBSITE

- Review Questions
- Student Learning Activities
- Glossary

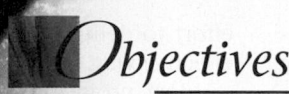

Objectives

Mastery of content in this chapter will enable the student to:

- Define the key terms listed.
- Discuss the effects that managed health care has had on health care services.
- Explain the rationale for regulatory and competitive approaches used to control health care costs.
- Explain the concept of prospective reimbursement.
- Describe the six levels of health care.
- Describe the types of services found within each level of health care.
- Explain the relationship between levels of health care and levels of prevention.
- Discuss the role of nurses in different health care delivery settings.
- Discuss the health care issues that have implications for the nursing profession.
- Differentiate evidence-based practice from research-based practice.
- Explain the role nursing has in promoting client satisfaction.

*T*he U.S. health care system is very complex. Although a broad variety of services are offered to the public by health professionals from varied disciplines, gaining access to services can be very difficult for those with limited or no health care insurance. There are few small independent hospitals remaining, with most having merged with large health care systems. Many of these systems continue to struggle to seamlessly integrate all levels of care to their clients. With the arrival of managed care, the organizations that pay for health care have the capacity to dramatically influence who provides care, how the care is furnished, and who receives compensation (Levi, 2000).

Clients are now limited as to who they can choose as their primary health care provider. Generally certain criteria must be met before a client can be referred to a health care specialist. Continuity of health care does not exist in all institutions. As a client moves from one physician or service to another, oftentimes little information is passed on about the client's needs or planned treatment. Many clients who would have been hospitalized for their condition 10 years ago are now treated in outpatient facilities or in the home, in part to reduce the costs resulting from lengthy hospitalization. Clients who are hospitalized truly do require acute care; they are sicker and their treatment involves a higher level of technological management. Clients are discharged from hospitals sooner, often leaving families with the burden of providing care in the home. The question being asked is, how can health care in the United States be financed so that health care services are produced efficiently, costs are effectively controlled, and quality is maintained or improved?

Nursing finds itself in the middle of the health care dilemma. As a caring discipline, nursing is rooted in helping individuals to regain, maintain, or improve their health, prevent illness, find comfort, and retain their individuality and dignity. The health care system of the new millennium has become less service oriented and significantly more business oriented in light of cost-saving initiatives. As a result, the practice of nursing is changing. In the face of rapid change, nursing must lead the way and retain its values for client care while meeting the challenges of new roles and new responsibilities in the health care environment. To become leaders in health care, nurses must understand the health care system and the issues that affect how care is provided to clients and their families.

Health Care Regulation and Competition

During most of the twentieth century there were few incentives for controlling health care costs existed. If a client needed to be in the hospital a few extra days for a wound to heal or to have time to complete rehabilitation, there were few obstacles. Insurers (third-party payers) paid for whatever a physician chose to order for a client's care and treatment. However, total health expenditures grew from $41.9 billion in 1965 to $425 billion in 1985 (Grace, 1997). As health care costs continued to rise out of control, regulatory and competitive approaches were created to control health care spending. Regulatory approaches included **professional standards review organizations (PSROs)** that functioned to review the quality, quantity, and cost of hospital care provided through Medicare (Garg and others, 1997). The PSROs largely reviewed the clinical care provided by physicians to determine if the best diagnostic and treatment approaches were utilized. Medicare-qualified hospitals have been required to have physician-supervised **utilization review (UR)** committees to review admissions, diagnostic testing, and treatments provided by physicians to clients. The intent was to identify and eliminate overuse of diagnostic and treatment services. In order to meet Medicare and other payer guidelines, many hospitals have added nurse case coordinators, whose functions are to monitor utilization of resources by clients, track their progress in the hospital, determine their financial resources, and assist in expediting discharge planning.

One of the most significant factors to influence how health care was paid for and to affect cost control and competition was the **prospective payment system** (PPS), established by Congress in 1983. The PPS eliminated cost-based reimbursement. Hospitals serving Medicare clients were no longer paid for all costs incurred to deliver care to a client. Instead, inpatient hospital services for Medicare clients were bundled into 468 **diagnosis-related groups (DRGs)**. Each group has a fixed reimbursement amount with adjustments for the severity of a case, rural/urban/regional labor costs, and teaching costs (of medical staff). Under the DRG system hospitals are reimbursed a set dollar amount for each DRG, regardless of the client's length of stay or use of services in the hospital. This system has provided a strong incentive for hospitals to better monitor the care of clients and to reduce length of stay of all clients. Because of prospective payment, hospitals within a given community compete in an effort to deliver the most efficient care in the most cost-effective way.

Most providers of health care (e.g., health care networks or managed care organizations) now receive capitated payments for their services. **Capitation** is the payment mechanism in which providers receive a fixed amount per client or enrollee of a health care plan (Appleby, 1996). The aim of capitation is to build a payment plan for select diagnoses or surgical procedures that includes the best standards of care, including essential diagnostic and treatment procedures at the lowest cost.

Capitation and prospective payment have influenced the way health care is delivered in all types of health care settings. DRGs are used in the rehabilitation setting, and **resource utilization groups (RUGs)** are used in long-term care. In all settings, efforts are made to manage costs so that the organization can remain profitable. For example, when clients are hospitalized for lengthy periods, hospitals absorb the portion of costs not reimbursed. This simply adds more pressure to ensure that clients are managed effectively and discharged as soon as is reasonably possible. As a result, the health care team within hospitals begins discharge planning activities as soon as clients are admitted. Staff will evaluate if outpatient rehabilitation, extended care facilities, and home care services are appropriate resources when planning the client's discharge. Most clients' third-party payers will only pay for a select number of home care visits. This places considerable burden on families, considering that home care services now include complex technological care, including infusion therapy, mechanical ventilation, and dialysis.

The term **managed care** describes health care systems in which there is administrative control over primary health care services for a defined client population. The managed care organization (MCO) or health care system receives a predetermined capitated payment for each client enrolled in the program. In this case the MCO bears financial risk in addition to providing client care. A client who belongs to an MCO must use only those primary care physicians approved by the organization. Referral to a medical specialist must be approved by the MCO. The MCO contract determines what treatments and procedures are reimbursed. In an effort to control costs, the organization's focus of care shifts from individual illness care to concern for the health of its covered population.

In theory, if people stay healthy, the cost of medical care declines. Managed care, properly managed, offers potential for the public's health, especially for populations who have traditionally had poor access to health care (Levi, 2000). For example, managed care organizations that are responsible for the coverage of **Medicaid** beneficiaries must ensure access to services, not just coverage. Debate exists about the scope and quality of such services; however, managed care implemented correctly can increase access to care for certain populations. Unfortunately, the influence of managed care has not reduced health care costs nationally. The Centers for Medicare and Medicaid Services (CMS) (2002), formerly the Health Care Financing Administration, reports that although health care spending seemed to even out during the late 1990s, total health care expenditures grew from $888 billion in 1993 to $1,299 trillion in the year 2000. Increase in spending is related to rising health care wages, legislation that increased **Medicare** spending, increasing insurance premiums, technology, and consumer demand for less restrictive insurance plans (CMS, 2002).

Nursing Implications

Nurses need not become health care financing experts. However, it is important for nurses to understand the basics of health care financing to recognize the effects on employers and clients (Table 2-1). Health care organizations are influenced daily by both regulatory and competitive approaches to control costs and maintain quality health care services. These pressures alter the amount and

the way that organizations are paid for producing health care services, directly affecting employers' demand for nurses and transforming the economic environment in which nurses work (Buerhaus, 1997). Nursing has been vulnerable, because it typically makes up a large percentage of a health care institution's labor budget. It is easy for an organization to change the nursing care delivery model, hire fewer nurses, and instead hire less-educated technical staff with the idea that costs will be reduced with minimal sacrifice to quality. However, recent research has shown that when the proportion of hours of care delivered on a patient care unit by professional registered nurses (RNs) is reduced, there are adverse client outcomes (Blegen and others, 1998; Needleman and others, 2001). Nursing units with a lower proportion of hours

Table 2-1   Health Care Plans

Type	Definition	Characteristics
Managed care organization (MCO)	Provides comprehensive, preventive, and treatment services to a specific group of voluntarily enrolled persons. Structures include a variety of models: *Staff model:* Physicians are salaried employees of the MCO. *Group model:* MCO contracts with single group practice. *Network model:* MCO contracts with multiple group practices and/or integrated organizations. *Independent practice association (IPA):* MCO contracts with physicians who usually are not members of groups and whose practices include fee-for-service and capitated clients.	Focus on health maintenance, primary care. All care provided by a primary care physician. Referral needed for access to specialists and hospitalization.
Medicare MCO	Program same as MCO but designed to cover health care costs of senior citizens.	Premium generally less than supplemental plans.
Preferred provider organization (PPO)	One that limits an enrollee's choice to a list of "preferred" hospitals, physicians, and providers. An enrollee pays more out-of-pocket expenses for using a provider not on the list.	Contractual agreement exists between a set of providers and one or more purchasers (self-insured employers or insurance plans). Comprehensive health services at a discount to companies under contract. Focus on health maintenance.
Exclusive provider organization (EPO)	One that limits an enrollee's choice to providers belonging to one organization. May or may not be able to use outside providers at additional expense.	Limited contractual agreement. Less access to select specialists.
Medicare	Federally funded national health insurance program in the United States for people over age 65. Part A provides basic protection for medical, surgical, and psychiatric care costs based on diagnosis-related groups (DRGs). Part B is a voluntary medical insurance; covers physician and certain outpatient services.	Payment for plan deducted from monthly individual Social Security check. Covers services of nurse practitioners (varies by state). Does not pay full cost of certain services. Supplemental insurance is encouraged.
Medicaid	Federally funded, state-operated program of medical assistance to people with low incomes. Individual states determine eligibility and benefits.	Finances a large portion of maternal and child care for the poor. Reimburses for nurse midwifery and other advanced practice nurses (varies by state). Reimburses nursing home funding.
Private insurance	Traditional fee-for-service plan. Payment computed after services are provided on basis of number of services used.	Policies typically expensive. Most policies have deductibles that clients must meet before insurance pays.
Long-term care insurance	Supplemental insurance for coverage of long-term care services. Policies provide a set amount of dollars for an unlimited time or for as little as 2 years.	Very expensive. Good policy has a minimum waiting period for eligibility, payment for skilled nursing, intermediate or custodial care, and home care.

of care delivered by RNs saw greater negative outcomes (e.g., medication errors, pressure sore rates, and client complaints). In the study by Needleman and others a greater number of RN hours of care per day was associated with a shorter average length of hospital stay and lower rates of urinary tract infections, pneumonia, and cardiac arrest.

Despite the threats posed to nursing, the profession has the talent, knowledge, and initiative to make a significant difference in health care. In the eyes of a health care employer, the most valuable employees will be those who contribute the most to the organization's ability to survive in a competitive and rapidly changing financial environment (Buerhaus, 1997).

*L*evels of Health Care

The health care industry is moving toward health care practices that emphasize managing health rather than managing illness. The premise is that in the long term, health promotion reduces health care costs. A wellness perspective focuses on the health of populations and the communities in which they live rather than just on finding a cure for an individual's disease. Larger health care systems have attempted to develop **integrated delivery networks (IDNs).** An IDN is a set of providers and services organized to deliver a coordinated continuum of care to the population of clients served at a capitated cost. An integrated system should, in theory, reduce duplication of services, coordinate care across settings, and ensure that clients receive care in the most appropriate and cost-effective settings (Curran, 1997).

The health care system provides six levels of care (Figure 2-1): preventive, primary, secondary, tertiary, restorative, and continuing care. Levels of care describe the scope of services and settings where health care is offered to clients in all stages of health and illness. For example, the secondary level of care is the traditional acute care setting where clients who present signs and symptoms of disease are diagnosed and treated. The restorative care level includes those settings and services where clients who are recovering from illness or disability receive rehabilitation and supportive care. Levels of care are not the same as levels of prevention (see Chapter 6). Levels of prevention instead describe the focus of health-related activities: avoiding disease (health promotion and disease prevention [primary prevention]), curing disease (secondary prevention), and diminishing complications (tertiary prevention). At any level of care, nurses and other health care providers might offer a variety of levels of prevention. The nurse working in an acute care hospital setting, for example, might monitor the recovery of a client following open heart surgery, while also providing health promotion information to the family concerning diet and exercise.

It is important to understand how levels of care are organized and delivered. Each level creates different requirements and opportunities for the nurse. In addition, changes unique to each level of care have developed as a result of health care reform. There is greater emphasis being placed on the importance of wellness and primary

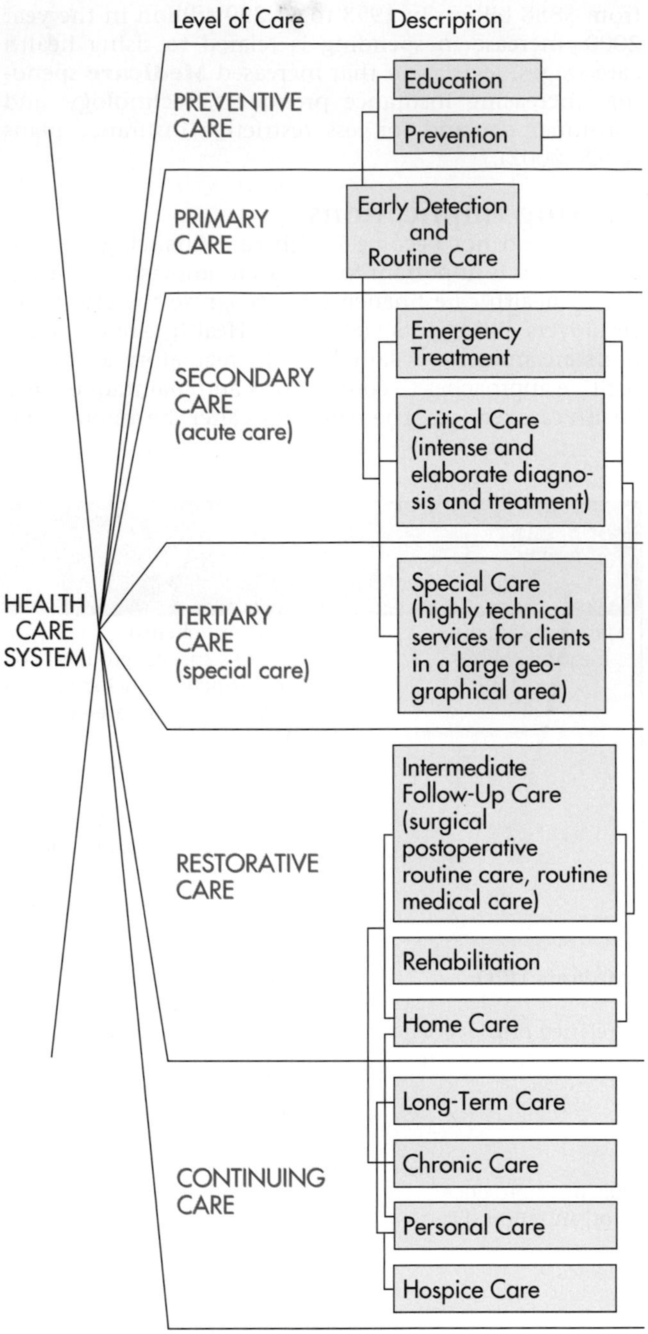

FIGURE 2–1 Spectrum of health services delivery. (Modified from Cambridge Research Institute: *Trends affecting the U.S. health care system,* 262, Health Planning Information Series, Human Resources Administration, Public Health Service, Department of Health, Education, and Welfare, Washington, DC, 1976, revised and updated 1992, U.S. Government Printing Office.)

and preventive care. More resources are being dedicated to these levels of care, particularly health promotion. Nursing has the chance to provide leadership to communities and health care systems that are aligning resources to better serve their populations. For example, nurses play a role in developing immunization programs, school health, and breast cancer screening. Critical to the suc-

Box 2-1 Examples of Health Care Services

Health Promotion

Prenatal care
Well-baby care
Nutrition counseling
Exercise classes
Family planning

Illness Prevention

Blood pressure and cancer screening
Immunizations
Poison control information
Community legislation (seat belts, air bags)
Mental health counseling and crisis prevention

Acute and Tertiary Care

Radiological procedures
Serum testing
Surgical outpatient and inpatient services
Emergency care

Restorative Care

Cardiovascular and pulmonary rehabilitation
Sports medicine
Spinal cord injury programs

Continuing Care

Assisted living
Psychiatric day care

---

cess of improving health care delivery will be the ability to find the type of services (Box 2-1) that better address client needs at all levels of care.

Preventive and Primary Health Care Services

Primary care has been defined by the Institute of Medicine (1994) as the "provision of integrated, accessible health care services by clinicians who are accountable for addressing a large majority of personal health care needs, developing a sustained partnership with clients, and practicing in the context of family and community." The emphasis is on personal health services. The Institute of medicine describes six core attributes of primary care:

1. Excellent primary care is grounded in both the biomedical and social sciences.
2. Clinical decision making in primary care differs from that in specialty care.
3. Primary care has as its core a sustained relationship between clinical care and clients.
4. Primary care does not consider mental health separately from physical health.

5. Important opportunities to promote health and prevent disease are intrinsic to primary care.
6. Primary care is information intensive.

In the settings where preventive and primary care are delivered, health promotion is a major theme. Successful health promotion programs are designed to help clients acquire healthier lifestyles and achieve a decent standard of living (see Chapter 6). The focus of health promotion is to keep people healthy through personal hygiene, good nutrition, clean living environments, regular exercise, rest, and the adoption of positive health attitudes. Health promotion programs can lower the overall costs of health care by reducing the incidence of disease, minimizing complications, and thus reducing the need to use more expensive health care resources. In contrast, preventive care is more disease oriented and focused on reducing and controlling risk factors for disease through activities such as immunization and occupational health programs.

School Health Services. Approximately 50,000 licensed professional school nurses provide health services to children and youth in the school setting (NASN, 2002). School nursing is a specialized practice of professional nursing that facilitates the well-being, academic success, and lifelong achievement of students. School health services have the goal of supporting educational success by enhancing health. Effective school health services are comprehensive programs that integrate health promotion principles throughout a school's curriculum. A school nurse develops programs that foster children's growth, positive life skills for successful coping, and acquisition of knowledge and skills for self-care, and that reinforce positive health attitudes (Pender, 1996). Specific nursing interventions in the school setting include health education, parent programming and counseling, communicable disease control, physical assessment, crisis intervention, environmental safety, nutrition planning, and emergency care. The school nurse role is rewarding when one is able to contribute to the overall process of education within a school.

To remove barriers to access to primary care, school-based health centers (SBHCs) were developed. The staff of SBHCs work along with school nurses. The centers make available age-appropriate primary services such as health, dental, mental health, and social services as well as health education (NASN, 2002). Services are available to those students who enroll to receive care in the centers.

Occupational Health Services. Recently, occupational health in the work setting has gained importance as employers seek to reduce the costs of health insurance benefits for injured or ill workers. Occupational health is a national concern, affecting individuals, families, and communities. A comprehensive occupational health program geared to health promotion and accident or illness prevention can increase worker productivity, decrease absenteeism, reduce use of expensive medical care, and lower disability claims (Pender, 1996). An occupational health program increases the health-enhancing potential of social and physical environments.

The foundation of occupational health nursing is epidemiology, worker advocacy, occupational health risk assessment, critical thinking, and educational principles

(OOHN, 2002). Occupational health nurses conduct environmental surveillance (e.g., investigating hazardous equipment, injuries occurring in the workplace, and potential stressors), direct nursing care (e.g., physical assessment, screening, and emergencies), health education, communicable disease control, counseling, administration, and research (Clemen-Stone, McGuire, and Eigsti, 1998). Recurring issues that nurses face in the work site are drug testing, right-to-know issues, concerns related to acquired immunodeficiency syndrome (AIDS), and exposure to environmental hazards. One of the nurse's roles is to help ensure that workers who have been injured are recovered and able to return to the work site safely. Some businesses try to reintroduce employees back into the workforce as soon as possible following illness or injury, even if an employee assumes a different job temporarily. The nurse can help to optimize the work experience by creating programs that involve workers in health promotion and in creating a safe work environment.

Physicians' Offices. Physicians' offices have traditionally provided primary care for most of the population. Physicians in office practices tend to focus on the diagnosis and treatment of specific illnesses rather than on health promotion. However, this trend is changing. More health care plans are requiring enrollees to have regular physical examinations with their primary care physician. During these visits physicians and nurse practitioners screen for possible health problems, identify clients' health promotion practices, and make recommendations to minimize or control risk factors. The addition of advanced practice nurses to physicians' offices looks beyond diagnosis and treatment to the holistic needs of clients. The advanced practitioner's time spent with a client addresses education, counseling, and community referrals (see Chapter 1).

RNs are often employed in physicians' offices in the role of office or practice manager. This includes supervision of secretarial and medical assistant staff and medical record personnel. The office manager is a problem solver who helps with referral questions, managing the flow of clients through the office, and dealing with physician concerns. The nurse can also be an important bridge to the physician in becoming closely familiar with their population of clients, in identifying trends in the types of problems clients present, and in recognizing opportunities to increase health promotion activities.

Clinics. Clinics that assess and treat ambulatory clients on an outpatient basis are often called ambulatory health services. A clinic may be affiliated with a hospital, medical school, group practice, MCO, church, or community organization (Clemen-Stone, McGuire, and Eigsti, 1998). The nature of the clinic affiliation often determines the type of services the clinic provides. For example, hospital clinics offer diagnostic and treatment services. A clinic in a community organization may offer primary care such as screening services for high blood pressure, tuberculosis, and glaucoma testing. There are also clinics that offer comprehensive care to specific client populations (e.g., well-baby, mental health, and allergy clinics). Hospital emergency departments often serve as ambulatory clinics for neighborhoods or towns with no formal outpatient clinic facility or primary care physicians. Emergency departments can also serve as "fast track" clinics to refer clients to primary care providers who accept new clients. This ensures that clients develop relationships with a stable and consistent physician rather than relying on episodic emergency care.

Community health nurses plan and provide clinic health care services. A comprehensive assessment of community needs is critical to ensure that clinic programs address the health status, lifestyle patterns, and cultural diversity of its clients. Often a neighborhood clinic becomes a focal point for a community. The successful clinic recognizes the work and lifestyle patterns of its clients and establishes a strong network of relationships with churches, schools, and businesses. Those networks become important for clients' continued care following hospitalization.

Nursing Centers. Nurse-managed clinics, or community nursing centers, provide high-quality nursing services with a focus on health promotion and health education, disease prevention, chronic disease management, and support for self-care and caregivers (Riesch, 1992; Barger and Rosenfeld, 1993). Many centers are academically sponsored and managed to educate advanced practice nurses in how to deliver cost-effective and community responsive care (Pohl and others, 2001). Typically, nursing centers serve vulnerable populations such as minority and ethnic groups of low-income status, older adults, and the disabled. Riesch (1992) identified three criteria for nursing centers: direct access by the client to the nurse, a nursing model of care, and holistic reimbursed services. Nurse practitioners and clinical nurse specialists typically manage a nursing center. However, public health nurses are also actively involved. The public health nurse's chief concern is the health of the community. Community health problems related to family dysfunction, illegal drug use, violent crimes, and poverty have a direct effect on clients using a nursing center.

The services offered in a nurse-managed clinic are varied (Box 2-2). It is how the services are delivered that makes a nurse-managed clinic unique. The nurse in an

---

Box 2-2 Nurse-Managed Clinic Services

Day care
Recreation
Physical and developmental assessment
Health risk appraisal
Wellness counseling
Health education
Youth and family support services
Employment readiness
Psychosocial counseling
Care and prevention of common diseases
Acute and chronic care management
Home care services

advanced practice role combines nursing and medical knowledge within a perspective of client-centered care. The advanced practice nurse stresses education and self-care. Clients with chronic illness are taught to partner with family members or friends to do the work of managing their illness. The public health nurse works to improve the conditions within the home and the community. A nurse-managed clinic designs services to help people assume more responsibility for their health and to acquire necessary coping skills.

Block and Parish Nursing. Two nontraditional settings where preventive and primary care can be found are in block and parish nursing. Both fill in gaps of the formal health care system, usually with older clients or those unable to leave the home or who are underserved (Clemen-Stone, McGuire, and Eigsti, 1998). **Block nursing** happens where the nurse lives, and services are available based on need rather than on the availability of reimbursement (Jamieson, 1990). Nurses who live within a neighborhood, through networks of friends, church groups, Girl Scouts, or Boy Scouts, collaborate to offer services to people in the community. These services might include running errands to the grocery store or pharmacy, transporting clients to a physician's office, providing respite care to family members, and being homemaker aides. **Parish nursing** is the same as block nursing, except churches and synagogues offer the site and support system for the program's activities. In a study by Wallace and others (2002), members of a southeastern Appalachian area served by parish nurses found that having a parish nurse was positive and beneficial for individ-

uals, their congregation, and the community. Important themes of clients' perceptions of parish nursing included being available, helping clients to help themselves, and integrating spirituality and health.

Primary Health Care in the Community. Primary care focuses on personal health services. In contrast, **primary health care** is an approach for building interventions that lead to improved health outcomes for an entire population (Shoultz and Hatcher, 1997). The primary health care model (Figure 2-2) focuses on collaboration of health professionals, community members, and others working in multiple sectors, emphasizing health promotion, development of health policies, and prevention of diseases for all individuals. A closer look at each sector finds that they are all linked and that events within each sector have an impact, either positive or negative, on each other and on the outcome of the population's health (Hatcher and others, 1994). For example, the health problems that commonly affect members of a lower socioeconomic level can often be traced to poor community services (e.g., water treatment, waste disposal, air quality, and transportation services). A primary health care approach requires a multisectoral approach by addressing many of the determinants of health (Shoultz and Hatcher, 1997). Primary care is a key component of the primary health care model. However, primary health care looks beyond primary care, with essential elements that include health education, proper nutrition, maternal/child health care, family planning, immunizations, and control of locally endemic diseases. Chapter 3 provides a more comprehensive discussion of primary health care in the community.

Secondary and Tertiary Care

Diagnostic and treatment services are generally the most commonly used services of the health care delivery system. With the arrival of managed care, these services are being delivered in primary care settings. For example, more physicians than ever before are performing simple surgeries in office surgical suites. However, once a client develops a more complicated problem and the primary care provider is not able to care for a particular condition, a medical specialist is needed. This often requires hospitalization of the client.

Hospitals. Hospital emergency departments and urgent care centers, critical care units, and inpatient medical-surgical units are the sites where secondary and tertiary levels of care are provided. In these settings nurses work closely with all members of the health care team to plan, coordinate, and deliver care for clients who are seriously ill. Nurses participate in constantly monitoring and evaluating whether care is effective and how it can be improved. Nurses must also recognize that in a busy, stress-filled location such as an inpatient nursing unit, client satisfaction is a priority. Clients are more informed than ever before and have higher expectations of services in a competitive environment. Acute care nurses must respond to client needs and expectations so as to form effective care partnerships. Customer service has become the philosophy of successful acute care organizations.

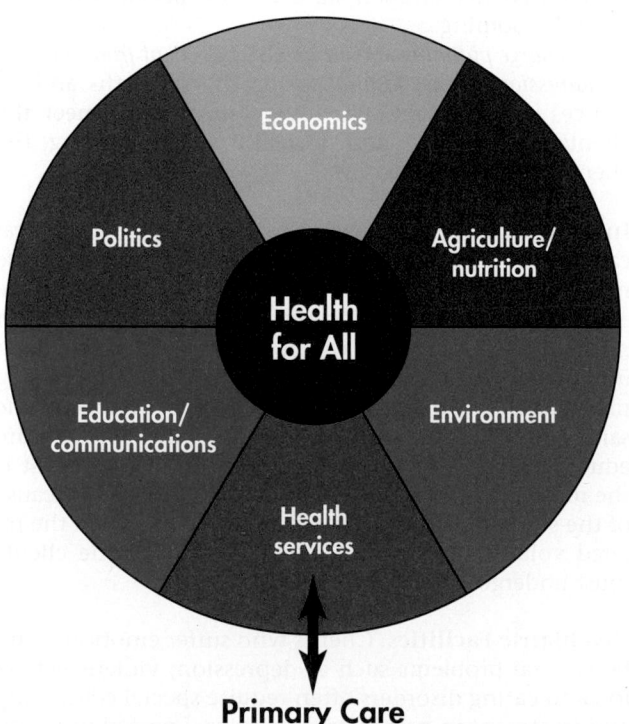

FIGURE 2–2 Primary health care model: a multisectoral or intersectoral approach. (© 1996 by P. Hatcher, J. Shoultz, W. Patrick; From *Nurs Outlook* 45(1):24, Jan-Feb, 1997.)

With the arrival of managed care, a hospitalized client with a given medical diagnosis or who undergoes surgery is expected to be cared for and discharged within a projected time period. Emphasis is on efficiency and the use of only those resources that are necessary to adequately care for the client until discharge. In some hospitals, nursing case managers have the primary responsibility to coordinate the efforts of all disciplines to achieve the most efficient and appropriate plan of care for the client. In a **case management** model of care, the case manager advises nursing staff on specific nursing care issues, coordinates the referral of clients to services provided by other disciplines, ensures that client education has been implemented, and monitors the client's progress through discharge (see Chapter 1). A multidisciplinary team, including physicians, nurses, social workers, and therapists, works closely with the client and family to ensure that the client has a well-designed discharge plan. In many settings a case manager continues caring for clients after discharge from acute care facilities.

When a hospital does not have a case manager, the staff nurse frequently plays the pivotal role in **discharge planning.** In the busy environment of an acute care hospital, continuity of care is important. To achieve continuity of care, the staff nurse must anticipate and identify clients' continuing needs, based on nursing assessments and medical plans of care. Once a client's needs are identified, the nurse works with all members of the multidisciplinary team to develop a plan that transfers the client's care from the hospital to another environment (e.g., hospital to home, hospital to extended care, or hospital to nursing home).

One tool that staff may use to coordinate care is a critical pathway. A **critical pathway** is a multidisciplinary treatment plan that sequences clinical interventions over a projected length of stay or a projected time frame for specific case types. For example, a pathway can be developed to sequence care for a normal vaginal delivery, cardiac surgery, or management of a client undergoing testing for cancer. Members of all disciplines that normally care for a particular client type develop a critical pathway. Pathways typically outline standard clinical assessments, treatments and procedures, activity and exercise therapies, client education, and referral activities required to ensure a smooth and uneventful discharge. When a client is placed on a pathway, staff collaborate more effectively because everyone understands what care should be given and when.

Because clients leave hospitals as soon as their physical conditions allow, they often have continuing health care needs when they go home or to another facility. This creates significant physical, psychological, and economic stress on clients and their families. Clients and family members typically worry about how they will care for the client's needs and manage his or her illness over the long term. The nurse often partners with social workers in understanding the client's concerns, determining the client's resources (e.g., financial and personal), and knowing the available health care resources in the client's community. Effective discharge planning often requires referrals to other health care disciplines. In many agencies a physician's order is needed for a referral. It is best to have clients and families participate in the referral process so that they are involved early in decision making. Some tips on making the referral process successful include the following:

- Initiate a referral as soon as possible
- Inform the care provider receiving the referral of as much information about the client as possible. This avoids duplication of effort and exclusion of important information.
- Involve the client and family in the referral process, including selecting the necessary referral. Explain the service to be provided, the reason for the referral, and what to expect from the referral's services.
- Determine what the referral discipline recommends for the client's care and incorporate into the nursing plan of care as soon as possible.

Good discharge planning depends on comprehensive client and family education (see Chapter 24). Clients need to know what to do when they get home, how to do it, and what to observe for when problems develop. The Joint Commission on Accreditation of Healthcare organizations (JCAHO) (2002) requires the following instruction before clients leave health care facilities:

- Safe and effective use of medications and medical equipment
- Instruction in potential food-drug interactions and counseling on nutrition and modified diets
- Rehabilitation techniques to support adaptation to and/or functional independence in the environment
- Access to available community resources (as needed)
- When and how to obtain further treatment
- The client's and family's responsibilities in the client's ongoing health care needs and the knowledge and skills needed to carry out those responsibilities
- Maintenance of good standards for personal hygiene and grooming

Discharge planning should involve the client from the time of admission to the hospital, using the strengths and resources of the client, providing resources to meet the client's limitations, and focusing on improving the client's long-term outcomes.

Intensive Care. An intensive care unit (ICU) or critical care unit is a hospital unit in which clients receive close monitoring and intensive medical care. The units are equipped with the most advanced technologies. Although many of the technologies can be found on regular nursing units, the clients hospitalized within ICUs are being monitored and maintained on multiple devices at the same time. Nursing and medical staff within an ICU are educated in critical care principles and techniques. It is the most expensive delivery site for medical care because of the staffing pattern required to deliver care and the related volume of treatments and procedures the clients must undergo.

Psychiatric Facilities. Clients who suffer emotional and behavioral problems such as depression, violent behavior, and eating disorders often require special counseling and treatment in psychiatric facilities. Located in hospitals, independent outpatient clinics, or private mental health hospitals, psychiatric facilities offer inpatient and outpatient services, depending on the seriousness of the problem. Clients may enter these facilities voluntarily or involuntarily. Hospitalization involves relatively short stays with the purpose of stabilizing clients before transfer to outpatient treatment centers. Psychiatric clients receive a comprehensive multidisciplinary treatment plan involving them and their families. All disciplines collaborate to develop a plan of care that will enable clients to return to functional states within the community. At discharge from inpatient facilities, clients are usually referred for follow-up care at clinics or with counselors.

Rural Hospitals. Access to health care in rural areas has been a serious problem. Most rural hospitals have had a severe shortage of primary care providers. Many have been forced to close because of economic failure. In 1989 the Omnibus Budget Reconciliation Act (OBRA) directed the Department of Health and Human Services to create a new health care entity, the rural primary care hospital (RPCH). An RPCH provides 24-hour emergency care, with no more than six inpatient beds for providing temporary care for 72 hours or less to clients needing stabilization before transfer to a larger hospital. Physicians, nurse practitioners, or physician assistants staff the RPCH. The RPCH can provide inpatient care to acutely ill or injured persons before they are transferred to better-equipped facilities. Basic radiological and laboratory services are also available.

With health care reform, more big-city health care systems are branching out and establishing affiliations or mergers with rural hospitals. The rural hospitals provide a referral base to the larger tertiary care medical centers. Nurse practitioners who work in rural hospitals or clinics often function independently in the absence of a physician. Nurse practitioners use medical protocols or work under collaborative agreements with staff physicians.

Restorative Care

Clients recovering from acute illnesses or who have chronic illnesses or disabilities usually require services designed to restore the client's level of health. Care is necessary until clients return to their previous level of function or they reach a new level of function limited by their illness or disability. The goal of **restorative care** is to assist an individual in regaining maximal functional status, thereby enhancing the individual's quality of life while promoting client independence and self-care. With the emphasis on early discharge from hospitals, there are few clients who do not require some level of restorative care. For example, surgical clients will require ongoing wound care, activity and exercise management, and sometimes diet interventions until they have recovered to a point where they can independently resume normal activities of daily living.

The intensity of care has increased in restorative care settings, because clients leave hospitals earlier. It is not uncommon to have clients in a home or rehabilitation setting still receiving infusion therapy (see Chapter 40), enteral nutrition (see Chapter 43), and oxygen therapy (see Chapter 39). The restorative health care team is an interdisciplinary group of health professionals that includes the client and family or significant others. In restorative settings, nurses recognize early that success is dependent on effective partnering with clients and their families. Clients and families require a clear understanding of goals for physical recovery, the rationale for any physical limitations, and the purpose and potential risks associated with therapies. The more clients and families are involved in restorative care, the more likely it is that they will be motivated to follow treatment plans and clients will be able to achieve optimal functioning.

Home care. **Home care** is the provision of medically related professional and paraprofessional services and equipment to clients and families in their homes for health maintenance, education, illness prevention, diagnosis and treatment of disease, palliation, and rehabilitation. It is the component of a continuum of comprehensive health care whereby health services are provided to individuals and families in their home to promote, maintain, or restore health, or to maximize the level of independence while minimizing the effects of disability and illness (Stanhope, 2000). Home care is unique, with health care providers practicing in the client's environment. For this reason, family dynamics (see Chapter 9), cultural practices (see Chapter 8), spiritual values (see Chapter 28), and communication principles (see Chapter 23) are just some of the knowledge areas that nurses must apply in making critical decisions regarding client and family care. Services are planned, coordinated, and made available by providers organized for the delivery of home care through the use of employed staff, contractual arrangements, or a combination of both. Nursing is the primary service offered under Medicare; however, home care might also include medical services; physical, occupational, speech, and respiratory therapy; and nutritional therapy. Home care equipment or durable medical equipment (DME) is any medically related product adapted for home use.

For the purpose of this chapter, home care is discussed under the category of restorative care, because a good percentage of home care services occur following hospitalization. However, all levels of care can occur within the home setting. Stanhope (2000) notes that home care involves a primary preventive focus (community health), as well as secondary and tertiary prevention (care of individuals). Figure 2-3 shows that home nursing is a synthesis of community-based nursing practice (see Chapter 3) and selected knowledge and skills from other nursing specialties.

The nurse who works in an acute care setting should be able to recognize the client characteristics that suggest evaluation for a home care referral (Box 2-3). These characteristics alone do not warrant the need for home care, but in combination with one another or with a new diagnosis that requires monitoring, they offer a guideline to determine the need for services (Lueckenotte, 2000). The assessment for these characteristics should be part of a nurse's ongoing assessment either at a prehospitalization screening, at the time of admission to the hospital, after a client's condition has changed, or as a client is being discharged. Ideally an assessment is conducted at the time of admission to ensure continuity of care. A uniform approach to assessment of adult home care clients,

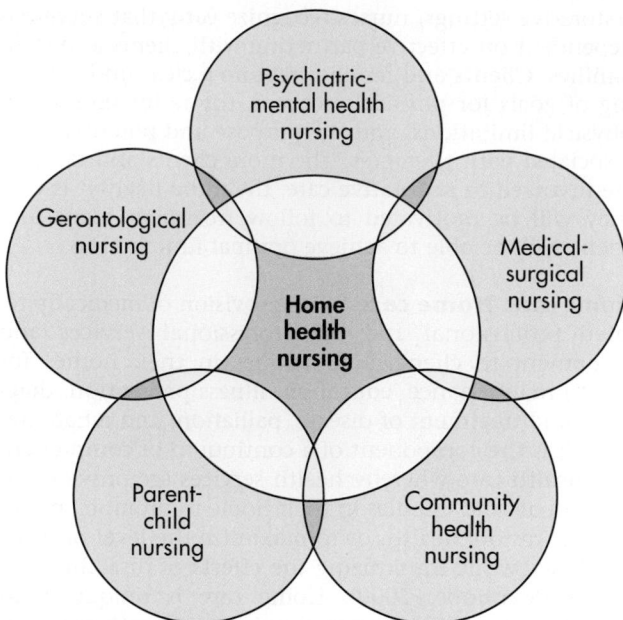

FIGURE **2-3** Home care nursing synthesizes community health nursing and other nursing specialties.

- Unexpected readmission to a hospital within 15 to 30 days
- Frequent hospital readmissions
- Alteration of health care problem or management
- Changes in client's mental status
- Noncompliant behavior before or during hospitalization
- Terminal or preterminal condition
- Received physical, occupational, or speech therapy in hospital
- Postamputation
- Post–hip replacement or post–knee replacement
- New assistive devices (e.g., cane, walker, brace)
- Foley catheter, urinary or bowel diversion, and/or incontinence
- Complex health management regimen
- Enteral or parenteral feedings
- Tubes of any kind
- Draining wounds
- Postwound debridement or irrigation and debridement for decubiti
- Pain management
- Intravenous antibiotics or chemotherapy
- Peripherally inserted central catheter (PICC)
- Multiple medications or a major medication change
- Ventilator dependent
- Low–air loss bed or other complex medical equipment

Modified from Lueckenotte A: *Gerontologic nursing,* ed 2, St. Louis, 2000, Mosby.

known as the Outcome and Assessment Information Set (OASIS), is being tested in a number of locations across the country (Lueckenotte, 2000). The tool aims to provide a set of essential data items necessary for measuring client outcomes that have utility for such purposes as outcome monitoring, clinical assessment, and care planning. It is likely that CMS will issue rules relating to home care agencies using OASIS data.

Home care agencies provide skilled and intermittent professional services and home care aide services (e.g., infusion therapy, home dialysis, home birthing, wound care, respiratory care, and ostomy management). These services usually are delivered once or twice a day, up to 7 days a week. Approved home care agencies usually receive reimbursement for services from the government (such as Medicare and Medicaid in the United States), private insurance, and private pay. The government has strict regulations governing reimbursement for home care services. An agency cannot simply charge for a service and expect to receive full reimbursement. Most professional services are reimbursed at the costs for providing the service by government programs.

Rehabilitation. Rehabilitation is the restoration of a person to the fullest physical, mental, social, vocational, and economic usefulness possible (Clemen-Stone, McGuire, and Eigsti, 1998). Clients require rehabilitation after a physical or mental illness, injury, or chemical addiction. Rehabilitation was once available primarily for clients with illnesses or injury to the nervous system and/or musculoskeletal system, but the health care delivery system has expanded its scope of such services. Today, specialized rehabilitation services, such as cardiovascular and pulmonary rehabilitation programs, help clients and families adjust to necessary changes in lifestyle and learn to function with the limitations of their disease. Drug re-

habilitation centers help the client become free from drug dependence and return to the community.

Rehabilitation services include physical, occupational, and speech therapy and social services. Ideally rehabilitation begins the moment a client enters a health care setting for treatment. For example, some orthopedic programs now have clients undergo physical therapy exercises before major joint repair so as to enhance their recovery postoperatively. Initially rehabilitation may focus on the prevention of complications related to the illness or injury. As the condition stabilizes, rehabilitation is directed at maximizing the client's functioning and level of independence.

Rehabilitation occurs in many health care settings, including rehabilitation institutions, outpatient settings, and the home. Frequently clients needing long-term rehabilitation (e.g., stroke and spinal injury clients) have severe disabilities affecting their ability to carry out activities of daily living. When rehabilitation services are provided in outpatient settings, clients receive treatment at specified times during the week but remain at home the rest of the time. Specific rehabilitation strategies are applied to the home environment so that maximal levels of function and independence can be achieved. Nurses and other members of the health care team visit homes and help clients and families learn to adapt to illness or injury.

Extended Care Facilities. An **extended care facility** provides intermediate medical, nursing, or custodial care for clients recovering from acute or chronic illnesses or disabilities. Extended care facilities include intermediate care and skilled nursing facilities. Some include long-term care and assisted living facilities (see later discussion of continuing care). At one time, extended care facilities cared primarily for older adults. However, as hospitals manage clients toward early discharge, there is a greater need for intermediate care settings for clients of all ages. For example, a young client who has experienced a traumatic accident may be transferred to an extended care facility for rehabilitative or supportive care until discharge to the home becomes a safe option. The growth of extended care facilities will increase as the number of older adults grows.

An intermediate care facility, or **skilled nursing facility (SNF),** offers skilled care from a licensed nursing staff. This may include administration of intravenous (IV) fluids, wound care, long-term ventilator management, and physical rehabilitation. Medicare covers stays at SNFs for 100 days but at a decreasing dollar amount after the first 20 days. The client's diagnosis must be appropriate for the therapy received (Lueckenotte, 2000). Extensive supportive care is provided until clients can move back into the community or into residential care. All extended care facilities provide around-the-clock nursing coverage. Nurses employed in such setting have expertise similar to that of nurses working in acute care inpatient settings. In addition, the nurse should have a background in gerontological nursing principles.

Continuing Care

Clients across the life span who have long-term health care needs are the chronically ill and disabled. Continuing care describes a collection of health, personal, and social services provided over a prolonged period to persons who are disabled, who never were functionally independent, or who suffer a terminal disease. The need for continuing health care services is growing in the United States. People are living longer, and many of those with continuing health care needs have no immediate family members to care for them. A decline in the number of children families choose to have, the aging of care providers, and the increasing rates of divorce and remarriage complicate this problem. Continuing care is available within institutional settings (e.g., nursing centers or nursing homes, group homes, and retirement communities), communities (e.g., adult day care and senior centers), or the home (e.g., home care, home-delivered meals, and hospice) (Lueckenotte, 2000).

Area Agencies on Aging. The Older Americans Act (OAA) of 1965 established a national network of federal, state, and area agencies on aging (AAAs), which are responsible for providing a range of community services for older adults (Lueckenotte, 2000). States are divided into areas for planning and service administration. Each AAA must designate community "focal points" as places where anyone in the community can receive information, services, and access to all of a community's resources for older adults. Multipurpose senior citizen centers, churches, community centers, hospitals, and town halls may serve as focal points. The types of services provided through the OAA and AAAs include information and referral for medical and legal advice; psychological counseling; preretirement and postretirement planning; programs to prevent abuse, neglect, and exploitation; programs to enrich life through educational and social activities; health screening and wellness promotion; and nutrition services.

Nursing Centers or Facilities. The language of continuing, or long-term, care can be confusing. The nursing home has been the dominant setting for long-term care (Lueckenotte, 2000). With OBRA 1987 the term *nursing facility* became the term for nursing homes and other skilled nursing facilities where long-term care is provided. Now, *nursing center* is the most appropriate term. A **nursing center** typically provides 24-hour intermediate and custodial care such as nursing, rehabilitation, dietary, recreational, social, and religious services for residents of any age with chronic or debilitating illnesses. The majority of persons living in nursing centers are older adults. A nursing center is a resident's temporary or permanent home with surroundings made to be as homelike as possible (Sorrentino, 2000). In a long-term care setting, the philosophy of care is to provide a planned, systematic, and interdisciplinary approach that helps residents reach and maintain their highest level of function, taking into account their feelings, thoughts, lifestyle, and physical condition (Resnick and Fleishell, 2002). Residents are encouraged to help themselves by establishing short-term, attainable goals that focus on a resident's potential and not on a diagnosis or the resident's limitations.

As life expectancy increases, the size of the older adult population grows. The number of people in the United States who will live in nursing centers is expected to increase, although the increased availability of home care services and alternative housing options such as assisted living may moderate any increase (Lueckenotte, 2000). Nursing centers have been under attack for years because of claims regarding inadequate care and abuse. Many of the claims have been justified. However, the nursing center industry has become one of the most highly regulated industries in the United States. These regulations have raised the standard of services provided. One regulatory area that deserves special mention is that of resident rights. OBRA's resident bill of rights states that a nursing center must promote the exercise of rights such as the right to select a personal attending physician, to receive complete information about one's care, to have privacy with regard to accommodations, treatment, and communication, and to participate in resident and family groups and social, religious, and community activities. Nursing facilities must recognize residents as active participants and decision makers in their care and life in institutional settings (Lueckenotte, 2000). This also means that family members are active partners in the planning of residents' care. Box 2-4 summarizes the types of standards currently established for nursing centers.

Interdisciplinary functional assessment of residents is the cornerstone of clinical practice within nursing centers (Lueckenotte, 2000). Government regulations require that each resident be comprehensively assessed, with care planning decisions made within a prescribed time period. A client's functional ability and long-term physical and psychosocial well-being are the focus. The Resident

Box 2-4 **The Major Regulatory Level A Requirements Defined by OBRA 1987**

Resident rights	Dietary services
Admission, transfer, and discharge rights	Physician services
	Specialized rehabilitative services
Resident behavior and facility practices	Dental services
Quality of life	Pharmacy services
Resident assessment	Infection control
Quality of care	Physical environment
Nursing services	Administration

From Lueckenotte A: *Gerontologic nursing,* ed 2, St. Louis, 2000, Mosby.

Box 2-5 **Minimum Data Set and Examples of Resident Assessment Protocols**

Minimum Data Set

Resident's background
Customary routines including usual cycle of daily events, eating patterns, and functional ability
Cognitive, communication/hearing, and vision patterns
Physical functioning and structural problems
Mood, behavior, and activity pursuit patterns
Psychosocial well-being
Physical functioning and structural problems
Bowel and bladder continence in last 14 days
Health conditions
Disease diagnoses
Oral/nutritional and dental status
Skin condition
Activity pursuit patterns
Medication use
Special treatments and procedures
Discharge potential

Resident Assessment Protocols (Examples)

Delirium
Falls
Pressure ulcers
Psychotropic drug use

Data from Briggs Corporation: *Minimum data set (MDS)—version 2.0 for nursing home resident assessment and care screening,* Form 1728HH, Des Moines, 1997, Briggs Corporation.

Assessment Instrument (RAI) must be completed on all residents. The RAI consists of the Minimum Data Set (MDS) (Box 2-5), Resident Assessment Protocols (RAPs), and utilization guidelines of each state. The RAI ultimately can provide a national database for nursing facilities to improve the quality of long-term care and to help policy makers understand the health care needs of the long-term care population.

Assisted Living. **Assisted living** is one of the fastest-growing industries within the United States. There are approximately 32,000 assisted living facilities in the United States according to the National Center for Assisted Living (Chicago Tribune, 2001). Assisted living offers an attractive long-term care setting with a homier environment and greater resident autonomy. Clients are generally in need of some assistance with activities of daily living but remain relatively independent within a partially protective setting. A group of residents live together, but each resident has his or her own room and shares dining and social activity areas. Usually people keep all personal possessions in their residences. Facilities range from hotel-like buildings with hundreds of units to modest group homes that house a handful of seniors. Services within an assisted living facility might include meals, social and recreational programs, personal laundry and housekeeping, transportation, 24-hour oversight, an emergency call system, and health checks (Sorrentino, 2000). Some facilities provide assistance with medication administration. Nursing care services are not directly provided, although a home care nurse can visit an assisted living facility after a client is discharged home.

The greatest limitation to assisted living is that most residents pay privately (Meyer, 1998). There are no government fee caps and little regulation. This severely limits the choices in long-term care for those individuals with limited financial resources.

Respite Care. The need to care for family members within the home creates great physical and emotional burdens for adult caregivers. The caregiver is usually an adult who not only has the responsibility for providing care to a loved one (e.g., spouse, parent, or sibling), but often must also maintain a full-time job and manage the routines of daily living. **Respite care** is a service that provides short-term relief or time off for persons providing home care to the ill or disabled (e.g., children, psychiatric clients, or frail older adults). Adult day care is one form of respite care. However, respite care can also be provided within the home by health professionals and trained volunteers. The caregiver is able to leave the home for errands or for just some social time while a responsible person stays in the home to care for the loved one.

Adult Day Care Centers. **Adult day care centers** provide a variety of health and social services to specific client populations who live alone or with family in the community. Services offered during the day allow family members to maintain their lifestyles and employment and still provide home care for their relatives (Lueckenotte, 2000). Day care centers may be associated with a hospital or nursing facility or exist as independent centers. Frequently the clients of such centers do not require hospitalization but need continuous health care services while their families or support persons work. These clients include older adults needing daily physical rehabilitation, individuals with emotional illnesses needing daily counseling or supervision, and individuals with chemical dependence problems who are involved in rehabilitation programs. The centers usually operate 5 days per week during typical business hours and usually charge on a per diem basis. Adult day care centers allow clients to retain more independence by living at home, thus potentially reducing the costs of health care by avoiding or delaying an older adult's admission to a nursing center.

Services offered in day care settings include transportation to and from the facility, assistance with personal care, nursing and therapeutic services (e.g., counseling and rehabilitation), meals, and recreational activities (Lueckenotte, 2000). Nurses working in day care centers provide continuity between care delivered in the home and in the center. For instance, nurses can ensure that the client continues to take prescribed medication and administer specific treatments. Knowledge of community needs and resources is essential in providing adequate support of clients who often spend only a few hours a week in the day care setting (Ebersole and Hess, 1998).

Hospice. A **hospice** is a system of family-centered care designed to allow clients to live and remain at home with comfort, independence, and dignity while alleviating the strains caused by terminal illness. The focus of hospice care is palliative care, not curative treatments (see Chapter 29). Hospice can benefit a client in the terminal phases of any disease, such as multiple sclerosis, AIDS, and cancer. A client entering a hospice has reached the terminal phase of illness (generally, the final 6 months or less), and the client, family, and physician have agreed that no further treatment could reverse the disease process. An attempt is made to provide care that ensures death with dignity in the client's home.

Occasionally a client must be admitted to a hospice unit within a hospital or independent location. The client and family must accept the fact that the hospice will not use emergency measures such as cardiopulmonary resuscitation to prolong life. Instead, the hospice uses a multidisciplinary approach to provide pain control and comfort measures. Hospice nurses work in institutional and community settings. They are committed to the philosophy and objectives of the facilities for which they work. They provide care and support for the client and the family during the terminal phase and at the time of death, and they continue to offer bereavement counseling and follow-up to the family following the client's death. Many hospice programs provide respite care, which is important in maintaining the health of the primary caregiver and family.

Issues in Health Care Delivery

The climate in health care today is influencing health care professionals, as well as consumers. In the midst of an evolving health care system, nurses must be prepared to participate fully and effectively within a managed care environment. Berwick (1994) has noted that "only those who provide care can in the end change care." As nurses struggle with issues of how to maintain health care quality while reducing costs, they need to acquire the knowledge, skills, and values that will allow them to practice competently and effectively as professionals. It is also important for nurses to collaborate with health care colleagues in designing new approaches for client care delivery.

Box 2-6 **Pew Health Professions Commission Twenty-one Competencies for the Twenty-first Century**

1. Embrace a personal ethic of social responsibility and service.
2. Exhibit ethical behavior in all professional activities.
3. Provide evidence-based, clinically competent care.
4. Incorporate the multiple determinants of health in clinical care.
5. Apply knowledge of the new sciences.
6. Demonstrate critical thinking, reflection, and problem-solving skills.
7. Understand the role of primary care.
8. Rigorously practice preventive health care.
9. Integrate population-based care and services into practice.
10. Improve access to health care for those with unmet health needs.
11. Practice relationship-centered care with individuals and families.
12. Provide culturally sensitive care to a diverse society.
13. Partner with communities in health care decisions.
14. Use communication and information technology effectively and appropriately.
15. Work in interdisciplinary teams.
16. Ensure care that balances individual, professional, system, and societal needs.
17. Practice leadership.
18. Take responsibility for quality of care and health outcomes at all levels.
19. Contribute to continuous improvement of the health care system.
20. Advocate for public policy that promotes and protects the health of the public.
21. Continue to learn and help others learn.

From the Pew Health Professions Commission, The Fourth Report of the Pew Health Professions Commission: *Recreating Health Professional Practice for a New Century,* 1998, The Commission.

Competency

The Pew Health Professions Commission was created in 1989 to focus on the health care workforce. The Commission is a national and interdisciplinary group of health care leaders that aims to help policy makers and educators produce health care professionals who meet the changing needs of the American health care system. The report *Recreating Health Professional Practice for a New Century* (1998) identifies 21 competencies for the twenty-first century. The competencies emphasize the importance of public service, caring for the community's health, and development of ethically responsible behaviors (Box 2-6). The Pew Commission's recommendations clearly show a prioritization for health care professionals to become more competent in health promotion efforts. The competencies offer an excellent yardstick for determining how well nurses practice and the type of professionals they become. A consumer of health care should expect that the standards of nursing care and practice in a health care setting are appropriate, safe, and efficacious. Ongoing competency is a nurse's responsibility. Health care organizations ensure quality care by establishing policies, procedures, and protocols that are scientifically sound and follow national accrediting standards. A nurse is responsible for following policies and procedures and knowing the most current evidence-based practice standards. As a nurse, it is important to obtain necessary continued education and to earn certifications when choosing to practice in specialty areas. In addition, a professional nurse should always pursue knowledge, whether it involves reading the nursing literature, consulting with peers on practice trends, or critiquing information from quality improvement reports, to improve and strengthen his or her level of practice.

Evidence-Based Practice

Each nurse is challenged to stay familiar with new information in order to provide the highest quality of client care. Nursing practice is dynamic and always changing because of new information originating from research, practice trends, technological development, and social issues affecting clients. It is important that all nurses have a link to new knowledge and expertise in using that knowledge to make sound, informed, client-care decisions (Barnsteiner and Prevost, 2002).

Evidence-based practice is defined as "the integration of best research evidence with clinical expertise and patient values" (Sacket and others, 2000). Evidence-based practice, research-based practice, and best practice are terms often used interchangeably. However, research-based practice refers to the use of knowledge based on systematic research studies, whereas evidence-based practice also takes into account a nurse's clinical experience, practice trends, and even individual client preferences (Barnsteiner and Prevost, 2002). Box 2-7 provides one researcher's views on this important concept.

Nurses in all client care settings must pursue knowledge by taking the time to review research and practice findings, critique research studies, and discuss with colleagues the implications when new knowledge is not integrated into practice. There are many reliable web-based resources that provide clinicians with links to evidence-based education and practice information. The University of York Centre for Evidence-based Nursing is an example of a website that provides links to evidence-based education and practice information (http://www.york.ac.uk/healthsciences/). The Cochran Collaboration provides systematic reviews of the literature related to specific clinical topics (http://www.cochrane.org). Reviews from the Cochrane database are constantly updated as new research becomes available. The Agency for Healthcare Research and Quality (AHRQ) provides evidence-based information on health care outcomes, quality, and cost (http://www.AHRQ.gov/clinic/epcix.htm). Finally, the National Guidelines Clearinghouse is a U.S. government database for evidence-based clinical practice guidelines and related documents (http://www.guideline.gov/index.asp). Chapter 5 discusses the use of evidence-based findings in practice in more detail.

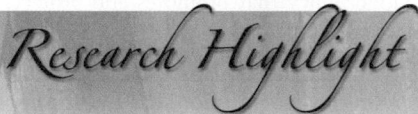

Box 2-7

Clarifying Evidence-Based Practice and Best Practice

Research Focus

The terms *evidence-based practice* and *best practice* are often used interchangeably and thus create issues in understanding and implementing evidence to improve nursing care processes and in achieving desired client outcomes. The purpose of this research article was to develop a working definition of evidence-based practice that can serve as a foundation for defining the concept of best nursing practice.

Research Abstract

Evidence on which nursing practice is based is derived from the synthesis of knowledge from research, data analyzed from the medical record, quality improvement, risk management data, infection control data, national and local standards, pathophysiology, client preferences, and clinical expertise. Evidence-based nursing practice involves accurate and thoughtful decision making about health care delivery for individuals or groups of clients based on the consensus of the most relevant and supported evidence derived from research and data-based information to respond to clients' preferences and societal expectations.

Best practice is more often the concept of choice and describes an organization's use of evidence to improve practice. In the clinical setting, best practice often refers to the use of clinical guidelines, is associated with disease management, and serves as a way of targeting interventions to reach desired client outcomes. Evidence should be the core to accomplishing the goals desired in implementing best practices. A best practice is a service, function, or process that is best from the context of an organization—best for an organization's clients or community, or an organization's mission and strategies.

Evidence-Based Practice

An organization benefits when evidence-based practice is successfully and meaningfully translated into nursing practice. Best practice built on a foundation of evidence-based practice can bridge the gap of practice and research and provide a basis for nurses to translate research into quality care.

There are six characteristics of quality health care that reinforce critical aspects of evidence-based and best practices:
- Client centered
- Scientifically based
- Population outcomes based
- Refined through quality improvement and benchmarking
- Individualized to each client
- Compatible with system policies and resources

Reference

Driever MJ: Are evidenced-based practice and best practice the same? *West J Nurs Res* 24(5):591, 2002.

Knowing Clients

The phenomenon of "knowing clients" is a measure of a nurse's experience and maturity. Knowing clients is a new concept of therapeutic decision making that comprises a nurse's understanding of a specific client and the nurse's subsequent selection of interventions (Radwin, 1996). Knowing develops as a result of a nurse's experience in a specific clinical area, the time the nurse has been in practice, and the quality of relationships the nurse has formed with clients. It means that a nurse gets a grasp of a client, understands the client's situation in context of an illness, and recognizes the nuances in behavior and responses that reflect the client's state of health. Knowing clients builds each time a nurse takes care of a new client. A nurse gradually develops a knowledge base that allows him or her to recognize the clinical conditions of clients in his or her area of specialty and to therefore anticipate clinical needs and problems. Tanner and others describe five aspects of knowing clients: (1) responses to therapeutic measures (e.g., medications and exercise), (2) routines and habits, (3) coping resources, (4) physical capacities and endurance, and (5) body typology and characteristics. Knowing is critical to nurses being able to understand a client's clinical condition, anticipate needs and clinical changes, make appropriate and timely decisions, and to take action.

The current health care environment within hospitals can make it difficult for nurses to know clients. Registered nurses care for more clients than ever before, and clients are more acutely ill, reducing the time spent with any one client. The work of client care can be stressful, fragmented because of the many procedures to be performed, and oftentimes interrupted by the constant inquiries and requests made by clients and other health care professionals. This fragmentation and interruption prevents nurses from focusing on the priorities of each client. In many settings, RNs work with assistive personnel (AP) to deliver care. Unless RNs and AP have good working relationships and RNs display good delegation skills (see Chapter 20), care can become even more fragmented and task focused rather than client focused. Finally, in areas where there are few senior nurses, new nurses do not have the mentors needed to demonstrate how knowing clients improves nursing practice.

Each time a nurse cares for a client, there must be some quality time for the nurse to assess and understand the client's needs and to know what illness or disability means to the client. Regardless of the setting or time available, quality client interaction is critical. Student nurses can begin to develop work habits that will foster knowing clients and ultimately help them to become better decision makers and critical thinkers:

- Before caring for a client in a clinical area, thoroughly review his or her medical record and the information that is available from other health care professionals who cared for the client.
- Plan your first interaction with a client. Learn to ask questions that will allow you to know what illness or disability means to the client, how it has affected his or her life, and what expectations the client has for his or her care. Never assume how a client feels. Apply principles of communication (see Chapter 23) in developing strong therapeutic relationships.

- Be observant and thoughtful. When you conduct an assessment, reflect on your findings and compare them with what is expected for the client's condition. Ask what your findings mean, and consider how the client might respond to any treatments you might administer.
- Use any time you have with a client to assess his or her condition and ongoing needs: assess during all routine care visits, during meals, when administering medications or other treatments, when responding to requests.
- Do not be afraid of the family. Family members are important resources who oftentimes know the client very well. Learn to take time to establish relationships with family members and recognize that they often require care, as well as the client.
- When working on a client care unit, make rounds regularly to determine the client's most current status and whether changes in therapy are needed.
- Talk with colleagues who also know your client. Learn what information they have been able to gain from their caregiving experience.

Assistive Personnel

Professional nurses in hospitals and skilled care facilities are finding themselves in situations where more support is needed to do the daily, repetitive tasks of client care. Many institutions have fewer RNs to care for hospitalized clients who are acutely ill. The RN is expected to coordinate care delivery for groups of clients, perform assessments, make professional judgments and clinical decisions, deliver and change therapies as needed, and provide client counseling and education. At the same time, clients still require basic supportive care activities (e.g., daily hygiene, ambulatory activities, and nutritional support). A professional nurse simply cannot do all of the work necessary to care for a group of clients. An issue that concerns many hospital nurses is that they have more to do and less time to do it in, and they are worried that quality of care and client safety might suffer.

More institutions are hiring **assistive personnel (AP)** to provide support to RNs and licensed practical nurses (LPNs) in the health care setting. AP might include certified nurse assistants, trained technicians, or staff who transfer from non–client care areas (e.g., dietary or housekeeping) to clinical areas. One problem with AP personnel is the inconsistency in training. Certified nurse assistants receive excellent preparation for basic client care responsibilities, but often their focus is in long-term care. There are many AP who receive only in-house training and minimal clinical preparation for their roles. AP must become competent and demonstrate consistent performance in the nursing care skills delegated by RNs and LPNs. Then and only then can the RN or LPN have a level of trust in assistive personnel so that they can team together and deliver client care safely and effectively.

Good working relationships are critical between RNs and AP. When AP show initiative and good ongoing communication to keep RNs informed and when RNs demonstrate trust in AP and acknowledge their contributions, very positive working relationships can develop (Potter and Grant, 2002). A key to success is RNs and AP working one-on-one so that each can understand the role of the other and RNs can mentor AP in important basic care skills. Another important factor in good working relationships is effective delegation. When delegating responsibilities to a competent individual, the RN still remains accountable for the overall nursing care of the client (Parkman, 1996). However, **delegation** is designed to make the work of client care more efficient. An RN must use good judgment in deciding what aspects of client care can be delegated and in what situations so that ultimately all clients are cared for effectively and efficiently. Delegation is not assigning a task without considering the specific client and whether it is appropriate for an AP to perform a task. Delegation is also not assigning a task without explaining to AP possible variations based on client status. Delegation must be driven by the RN's assessment of a client. The RN then decides what tasks or aspects of care are appropriate for the AP to perform for that client. Ultimately it allows the RN and AP to work as an effective team. Chapter 20 covers specific guidelines for safe and appropriate delegation.

Quality Health Care

Quality health care is difficult to define. What clients define as quality health care may not be the same as what health professionals define as quality. Unless health care providers can define quality, the purchasers of health care will buy ser-

vices based on price alone. The health care system that can deliver a given service (e.g., delivery of a baby and mother-infant care) for the cheapest price will become the primary provider of that service. Health care providers are now defining and measuring quality in terms of outcomes. An outcome is a measure of what actually does or does not happen as a result of a process of care; it is the end result (desirable or undesirable) of care delivered (Donabedian, 1966; Bernstein and Hilborne, 1993). Examples of outcomes are the readmission rates for surgical clients, the functional health status of clients following discharge (e.g., ability and time frame for returning to work), the successful relief of a client's pain, and the ability of clients to assume new self-care skills. Health plans throughout the United States are now relying on the Health Plan Employer Data and Information Set (HEDIS) as a quality measure (Greene, 1998). Participating health plans provide vital statistics on more than 70 quality indicators, allowing employers to check on the performance of different health plans. HEDIS is the database of choice for CMS, which requires the information from Medicare MCOs. One of the most common outcome measures is client satisfaction. The JCAHO (2002) requires health care organizations to deter-

---

Box 2-8   The Dimensions of Client-Centered Care

Respect for Clients' Values, Preferences, and Expressed Needs

Clients expect to be treated with dignity and respect.
Clients want to be informed and involved in decisions about their care.
Clients' perception of needs should not be completely different from those identified by a care provider.

Coordination and Integration of Care

Clients' feelings of powerlessness can be reduced by a competent and caring staff.
Clients look for someone to be in charge of care and to communicate clearly with other health team members.
Clients look to have services and procedures well coordinated.
Clients need to know at all times whom to call for help.

Information, Communication, and Education

Clients expect to receive accurate and timely information about their clinical status, progress, or prognosis.
Clients and families need to be informed of major changes in therapies or status.
Tests and procedures must be explained clearly in language clients understand.
Clients and family members want to know how to manage care on their own to the extent they desire or are able.

Physical Comfort

Physical care that comforts clients is one of the most elemental services caregivers can provide.

Nurses should respond in a timely and effective way to any request for pain medication, explain the extent of pain clients can expect, and offer alternatives for pain management.
Clients expect privacy and to have their cultural values respected.
The health care setting environment should be clean and comfortable.

Emotional Support and Relief of Fear and Anxiety

Clients look to care providers to share their fears and concerns.
Clients need to understand the impact illness will have on their ability to care for themselves and their family.
Clients worry about the ability to pay for their medical care. Are there staff who can help with those worries?

Involvement of Family and Friends

Care providers must recognize and respect the family and friends on whom clients rely for support.
Clients have the right to determine if family members are to be involved in decisions about their care.
Clients expect those family or friends who will provide physical support and care after discharge to be properly informed.

Transition and Continuity

Clients want information about medications to take, dietary or treatment plans to follow, and danger signals to look for after hospitalization or treatment.
Clients expect to have their continuing health care needs met after discharge with well-coordinated services.
Clients and family members expect access to any necessary health care resources after discharge.

Data from Gerteis M and others: *Through the patient's eyes,* San Francisco, 1993, Jossey-Bass.

mine how well an organization meets client needs and expectations. Organizations are using outcomes such as client satisfaction as a basis to redesign how care is managed and delivered in hopes of improving quality in the long term.

Client Satisfaction. Almost every major health care organization measures certain aspects of client satisfaction. The Picker/Commonwealth Program for Patient-Centered Care has identified seven dimensions of client-centered care (Box 2-8) that most affect clients' experiences with health care (Gerteis and others, 1993). The seven dimensions cover much of what is the scope of nursing practice. This should be no surprise because nurses are involved in almost every aspect of a client's care in a hospital. A close look shows that most of the dimensions that can be reflected in client satisfaction can be applied to almost any health care setting.

The Picker/Commonwealth program has a survey tool that measures client satisfaction along the seven dimensions. The survey looks globally at client perceptions of care in an attempt to understand how all hospital departments influence client satisfaction. The survey is conducted through telephone interviews after the client is discharged from the health care setting. Many other companies have developed similar client satisfaction surveys that are distributed in the mail to clients. Staff involved in client care receive the satisfaction scores as feedback regarding their success in meeting client expectations. It is the responsibility of staff to identify the unique issues that influence client satisfaction for their area. Client satisfaction findings become the basis for many quality improvement studies (see Chapter 19).

It is important for nurses to recognize the need to identify client expectations. The seven dimensions of care provide a useful guide. By learning early what a client expects in regard to information, comfort, and availability of family and friends, the nurse can better plan client care. When should the nurse ask about a client's expectations? It should become a routine question when the client first enters a health care setting and episodically as care continues. For example, many clients receive analgesics for pain relief on a prn, or as-needed, basis. The nurse may wish to say, "The medication is here when you need it," and then ask, "Would you like me to offer it when it is available, or would you prefer to ask for it?" Client expectations are an important measure of the evaluation of nursing care.

The Future of Health Care

This discussion on the health care delivery system began with the issues of complexity and change. Both issues are threatening but also create opportunities for improvement. At issue is the health and welfare of our population. Health care in the United States is not perfect. However, many health care organizations are striving to find ways to redesign their services, reduce unnecessary costs, improve access to services, and guarantee high-quality client care. Professional nursing is an important player in the future of health care delivery. The solutions necessary to improve the quality of health care will likely not be found without nursing's active participation.

Key Concepts

- Under managed care, the organizations that pay for health care have the capacity to dramatically influence who provides care, how the care is furnished, and who receives compensation.
- Regulatory approaches review the quality, quantity, and cost of hospital care provided through Medicare.
- Prospective reimbursement does not pay for all hospital costs incurred to deliver care to a client. Instead, inpatient hospital services for Medicare clients are paid a fixed amount based on diagnosis or condition.
- The aim of capitation is to build a payment plan for select diagnoses or surgical procedures that includes the best standards of care, including essential diagnostic and treatment procedures at the lowest cost.
- A managed care organization bears financial risk in addition to providing client care. The organization's focus of care shifts from individual illness care to concern for the health of its covered population.
- Research has shown that when the proportion of hours of care delivered by RNs on a patient care hospital unit is reduced, there are adverse client outcomes.
- Levels of care describe the scope of services and settings where health care is offered to clients in all stages of health and illness.
- At any level of care, nurses and other health care providers might offer a variety of levels of prevention.
- Successful health promotion programs, such as those found in nursing centers, schools, and community clinics, are designed to help clients acquire healthier lifestyles and achieve a decent standard of living.
- To achieve continuity of care when a client is discharged from a hospital, the staff nurse must anticipate and identify the client's continuing needs and then work with all members of the multidisciplinary team to develop a plan that transfers the client's care from the hospital to another environment.
- The intensity of care has increased in restorative care settings (e.g., home care, extended care) because clients leave hospitals earlier.
- Home care is unique, with health care providers practicing in the client's environment.
- Continuing care describes a collection of health, personal, and social services provided over a prolonged period to persons who are disabled, who never were functionally independent, or who suffer a terminal disease.
- It is important that all nurses have a link to new knowledge and expertise in using that knowledge to make sound, informed, client-care decisions.
- Knowing clients develops as a result of a nurse's experience in a specific clinical area, the time the nurse has been in practice, and the quality of relationships the nurse has formed with clients.
- Characteristics of good working relationships between RNs and AP include initiative, ongoing communication, trust, and acknowledging one another's contributions.

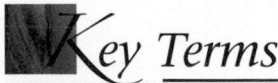

Key Terms

Adult day care centers,
  p. 38
Assisted living, *p. 38*
Assistive personnel (AP),
  p. 41
Block nursing, *p. 33*
Capitation, *p. 28*
Case management, *p. 34*
Critical pathway, *p. 34*
Delegation, *p. 42*
Diagnosis-related groups
  (DRGs), *p. 28*
Discharge planning, *p. 34*
Evidence-based practice,
  p. 40
Extended care facility, *p. 36*
Home care, *p. 35*
Hospice, *p. 39*
Integrated delivery net-
  works (IDNs), *p. 30*
Managed care, *p. 28*

Medicaid, *p. 28*
Medicare, *p. 29*
Nursing center, *p. 37*
Parish nursing, *p. 33*
Primary care, *p. 31*
Primary health care, *p. 33*
Professional standards
  review organizations
  (PSROs), *p. 28*
Prospective payment
  system (PPS), *p. 28*
Rehabilitation, *p. 36*
Respite care, *p. 38*
Resource utilization groups
  (RUGs), *p. 28*
Restorative care, *p. 35*
Skilled nursing facility
  (SNF), *p. 37*
Utilization review (UR),
  p. 28

Critical Thinking Exercises

1. Mr. Giesler is an 82-year-old man who underwent surgery for a total knee replacement. He is alert and oriented and has been able to give good feedback when asked to explain activity restrictions at home. He will be taking a pain medication for his knee along with his regular antihypertensive medication and vitamins. Mr. Giesler will continue to go to rehabilitation even after discharge. His doctor has recommended use of a walker and gait training and muscle strengthening. What health care service might you refer Mr. Giesler to, and what is your rationale?

2. When entering Mrs. Saguchi's room, the nurse notices that the client seems anxious to speak. Mrs. Saguchi explains, "I am worried about going home. My doctor wants me to go home today. My daughter is coming in from out of town but will not be here until three days from now. I live by myself, and I would like to stay here at least until my daughter arrives. The hospital is making money off of my surgery. Can't I stay one more day?" Is Mrs. Saguchi's request reasonable? What would be your response as the nurse?

3. Spend time observing a nurse who works on one of the clinical areas on which you are assigned. Ask if you can follow him or her during client rounds. Then ask the nurse what he or she knows about one of his or her clients. Ask the nurse to explain how this knowledge will affect how he or she plans care for that client.

Review Questions

1. The professional standards review organizations (PSROs) function to:
   1. Review the quality, quantity, and cost of hospital care provided through Medicare.
   2. Review admissions, diagnostic testing, and treatments provided by physicians to clients.
   3. Find incentives for controlling health care costs.
   4. Identify and eliminate overuse of diagnostic and treatment services.

2. This payment mechanism is one in which health care networks or managed care organizations receive a fixed amount per client or enrollee of a health care plan.
   1. Prospective payment system.
   2. Diagnosis-related groups (DRGs).
   3. Capitation.
   4. Managed care.

3. In this type of managed care organization (MCO), the physicians are salaried employees of the MCO.
   1. Group model.
   2. Network model.
   3. Independent practice association.
   4. Staff model.

4. The nurse organizes a blood pressure screening program. This is an example of which health care service?
   1. Health promotion.
   2. Illness prevention.
   3. Restorative care.
   4. Continuing care.

5. Recurring issues that nurses face in the this type of nursing are drug testing, right-to-know issues, concerns related to acquired immunodeficiency syndrome (AIDS), and exposure to environmental hazards.
   1. Occupational health nursing.
   2. School health nursing.
   3. Office nursing.
   4. Hospital nursing.

6. This type of nursing has a nontraditional setting in which preventive and primary care can be found.
   1. Community health nursing.
   2. Office nursing.
   3. Occupational nursing.
   4. Parish nursing.

7. This site provides provide secondary and tertiary health care.
   1. Home care organization.
   2. Rehabilitation facility.
   3. Extended care facility.
   4. Hospital.

8. Medicare covers stays at this type of facility for 100 days but at a decreasing dollar amount after the first 20 days.
   1. Extended care facility.
   2. Skilled nursing facility.
   3. Rehabilitation faculty.
   4. Hospital.

9. The following develops as a result of a nurse's experience in a specific clinical area, the time the nurse has been in practice, and the quality of relationships the nurse has formed with clients.
   1. Ability to delegate care.
   2. Personal ethics.
   3. "Knowing clients."
   4. Leadership.

References

Appleby C: Managed care's true values, *Hosp Health Netw* 70(8):20, 1996.

Barger S, Rosenfeld P: Models in community health care, *Nurs Health Care* 14(8):426, 1993.

Barnsteiner J, Prevost S: How to implement evidence-based practice: some tried and true pointers, *Reflections on Nursing Leadership* 28(2):18, 2002.

Bernstein SJ, Hilborne LH: Clinical indicators: the road to quality care? *Jt Comm J Qual Improv* 19(11):501, 1993.

Berwick DM: Eleven worthy aims for clinical leadership of health system reform, *JAMA* 272:797, 1994.

Blegen M and others: Nurse staffing and patient outcomes, *Nurs Res* 47(1):43, 1998.

Briggs Corporation: *Minimum data set (MDS)—version 2.0 for nursing home resident assessment and care screening,* Form 1728HH, Des Moines, 1995.

Buerhaus PI: How changes in payment systems are affecting nurses. In McCloskey JC, Grace HK, editors: *Current issues in nursing,* ed 5, St. Louis, 1997, Mosby.

Cambridge Research Institute: *Trends affecting the U.S. health care system,* 262, Health Planning Information Series, Human Resources Administration, Public Health Service, Department of Health, Education, and Welfare, Washington, DC, 1976, revised and updated 1992, U.S. Government Printing Office.

Centers for Medicare and Medicaid Services: National health expenditures and human services, 2002, http://www.cms.hhs.gov/stats.

Clemen-Stone S, McGuire SL, Eigsti DG: *Comprehensive community health nursing,* ed 5, St. Louis, 1998, Mosby.

Curran C: The future of academic health centers in a cost-driven market. In McCloskey JC, Grace HK, editors: *Current issues in nursing,* ed 5, St. Louis, 1997, Mosby.

Donabedian A: Evaluating the quality of medical care, *Milbank Mem Fund Q* 44:166, 1966.

Driever MJ: Are evidence-based practice and best practice the same? *West J Nurs Res* 24(5)591, 2003.

Ebersole P, Hess P: *Toward healthy aging,* ed 5, St. Louis, 1998, Mosby.

Garg ML and others: Controlling health care costs: regulation versus competition. In McCloskey JC, Grace HK, editors: *Current issues in nursing,* ed 5, St. Louis, 1997, Mosby.

Gerteis M and others: *Through the patient's eyes,* San Francisco, 1993, Jossey-Bass.

Grace HK: From a medical care system for a few to a comprehensive health care system for all. In McCloskey JC, Grace HK, editors: *Current issues in nursing,* ed 5, St. Louis, 1997, Mosby.

Greene J: Blue skies or black eyes? *Hosp Health Netw* 72(8):27, 1998.

Hatcher PA and others: Impacts: a primary health care game to develop global health consciousness, *J Fam Community Health* 17(2):74, 1994.

Institute of Medicine: *Defining primary care: an interim report,* Washington, DC, 1994, National Academy Press.

Jamieson MK: Block nursing: practicing autonomous professional nursing in the community, *Nurs Health Care* 11(5):250, 1990.

Joint Commission on Accreditation of Healthcare Organizations: *Manual of hospital accreditation: 2002 standards,* Chicago, 2002, The Commission.

Levi J: Managed care and public health, *Am J Public Health* 90(12):1823, 2000.

Lueckenotte A: *Gerontologic nursing,* ed 2, St. Louis, 2000, Mosby.

Meyer H: The bottom line on assisted living, *Hosp Health Netw* 72(14):22, 1998.

National Association of School Nurses (NASN): The role of the school nurse in school based health centers, 2002, http://www.nasn.org/positions/schoolbased.htm.

National Center for Assisted Living 2001, *Chicago Tribune.*

Office of Occupational Health Nursing (OOHN), 2002, www.osha.gov/dts/oohn.

Parkman CA: Delegation: are you doing it right? *Am J Nurs* 96(9):43, 1996.

Pender NJ: *Health promotion in nursing practice,* ed 3, St. Louis, 1996, Mosby.

Pew Health Professions Commission, The Fourth Report of the Pew Health Professions Commission: *Recreating Health Professional Practice for a New Century,* 1998, The Commission.

Pohl JM and others: Development of an academic consortium for nurse-managed primary care, *Nurs Health Care Perspect* 22(6):308, 2001.

Potter P, Grant E: A qualitative investigation of registered nurse and unlicensed assistive personnel working relationships, Unpublished manuscript, 2002.

Resnick B, Fleishell A: Developing a restorative care program: a five step approach that involves the resident, *Am J Nurs* 102(7):95, 2002.

Riesch SK: Nursing centers: state of the art survey results. In *Nursing centers: meeting the demand for quality health care,* NLN Pub No. 21-2311, New York, 1992, National League for Nursing.

Sackett DL and others: Evidence-based medicine: how to practice and teach EBM, London, 2000, Churchill Livingstone.

Shoultz J, Hatcher PA: Looking beyond primary care to primary health care: an approach to community-based action, *Nurs Outlook* 45(1):23, 1997.

Sorrentino S: *Mosby's textbook for nursing assistants,* ed 5, St. Louis, 2000, Mosby.

Stanhope M: Community health nurse in home health and hospice care. In Stanhope M, Lancaster J, editors: *Community health nursing: process and practice for promoting health,* ed 5, St. Louis, 2000, Mosby.

Research References

Driever MJ: Are evidenced-based practice and best practice the same? *West J Nurs Res* 24(5):591, 2002.

Needleman J and others: Nurse staffing and patient outcomes in hospitals: executive summary, February 28, 2001, U.S. Department of Health and Human Services, HRSA.

Radwin LE: "Knowing the patient": a review of research on an emerging concept, *J Adv Nurs* 23:1142, 1996.

Wallace DC and others: Client perceptions of parish nursing, *Public Health Nurs* 19(2):128, 2002.

3

Community-Based Nursing Practice

Media Resources

http://evolve.elsevier.com/Potter/
fundamentals/

CD COMPANION

- Review Questions
- Glossary

evolve WEBSITE

- Review Questions
- Student Learning Activities
- Glossary

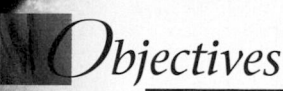

Objectives

Mastery of content in this chapter will enable the student to:

- Define the key terms listed.
- Explain the relationship between public health and community health nursing.
- Differentiate community health nursing from community-based nursing.
- Discuss the role of the community health nurse.
- Discuss the role of the nurse in community-based practice.
- Explain the characteristics of clients from vulnerable populations that influence a nurse's approach to care.
- Describe the competencies important for success in community-based nursing practice.
- Describe elements of a community assessment.

The rapid pace of today's health care climate usually results in the client moving from acute care, hospital-based settings to community-based care that may focus on health promotion, disease prevention, or restorative care. There is a growing need to organize health care delivery services where people live, work, and learn. One way to achieve this goal is through a community-based health care model (Flynn, 1998). Community-based health care organizations frequently spend resources on keeping individuals healthy and well, provide illness care in the client's home environment, and contain costs (U.S. Department of Health and Human Services [USDHHS], 2000a). With this new focus, nursing is in a particularly advantageous position to play an important role in health care delivery. The focus of keeping individuals healthy and well has always been appropriate to the holistic practice of professional nursing.

Nursing's history documents the roles of nurses in establishing and meeting the public health goals of their clients. Within the community health settings, nursing is developing a role as a leader in assessing, implementing, and evaluating the types of public and community health services needed by their clients. Community health nursing and community-based nursing are components of health care delivery necessary to improve the health of the general public.

Community-Based Health Care

It is important for nurses to gain an understanding of community-based health care. Historically, government-funded agencies have supported community health programs that improve the safety and adequacy of food supplies and provide a safe water supply and adequate sewage disposal. Public health policy has largely been responsible for the dramatic gain in life expectancy for Americans during the last century (Stanhope and Lancaster, 2004).

Today, the challenges in community-based health care are many. Social lifestyles, political policy, and economic initiatives have all influenced some of the major public health problems, including the following: an increase in sexually transmitted diseases, environmental pollution, underimmunization of infants and children, and the appearance of new life-threatening diseases (e.g., acquired immunodeficiency syndrome [AIDS] and other emerging infections). More than ever before, a commitment is needed to reform the health care system and bring attention to the health care needs of all communities.

Achieving Healthy Populations and Communities

The U.S. Department of Health and Human Services Public Health Service designed a program to improve the overall health status of people living in this country (see Chapter 6). The *Healthy People Initiative* was initially created to establish health care goals for the year 2000. These goals are continually revised; for example, *Healthy People 2010's* overall goals are to increase the life expectancy and quality of life and to eliminate health disparities (USDHHS, 2000b).

The current revision, *Healthy People 2010,* is designed to improve the delivery of health care services to the general public. This can be achieved through the assessment of health care needs of individuals, families, or communities; development and implementation of public health policies; and improved access to care. For example, assessment may include systematic data collection on the population, monitoring of the population's health status, and accessing available information about the health of the community (Stanhope and Lancaster, 2004). Examples of assessment can include, but are not limited to, gathering information on **incident rates** for certain cancers, identification and reporting of emerging infections, determining adolescent pregnancy rates, and reporting the number of motor vehicle accidents by teenage drivers. Public policy development and implementation refers to health professionals providing leadership in developing policies that support the population's health. An example is using research-based findings in developing policies such as the use of immunization and seat belts to reduce prevalence of disease or disability due to motor vehicle accidents or initiating new driving restrictions for the new teenage driver. Improved access to care refers to the role of public health in making sure that essential community-wide health services are available and accessible (Stanhope and Lancaster, 2004). Examples of assurance include the provision of prenatal care to the uninsured and establishing educational programs to ensure the competency of public health professionals. Population-based public health programs focus on disease prevention, health protection, and health promotion. This focus provides the foundation for health care services at all levels (see Chapter 2).

The five-level health services pyramid is an example of how to provide community-based services within existing health care services within a community (Figure 3-1). For example, a rural community may have a hospital to meet the acute care needs of their clients. However, community assessment notes that there are minimal services to meet the needs of expectant mothers, reduce teenage smoking, or provide nutritional support for older adults. Community-based programs to provide these three services are effective in improving health of the specific populations and the population of the community. When the lower level services are accessible and effective, there

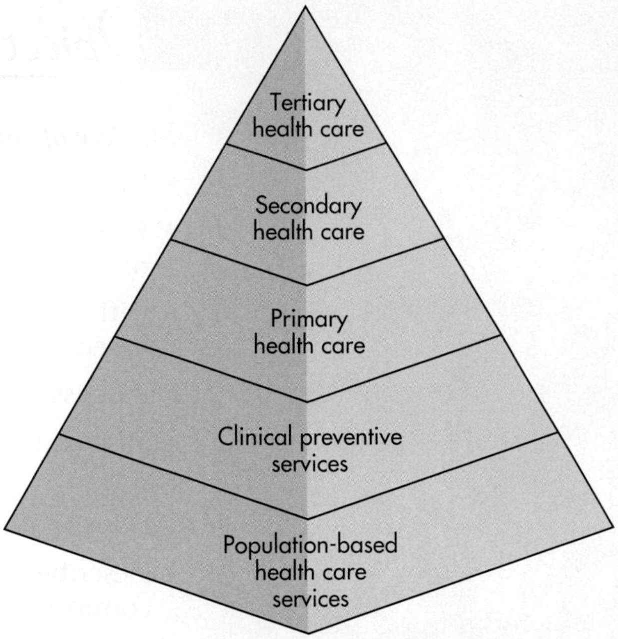

FIGURE **3–1**   Health services pyramid. (From Stanhope M, Lancaster J: *Community health nursing: a process and practice for promoting health,* ed 5, St. Louis, 2000, Mosby.)

is a greater likelihood that the higher tiers will contribute to the total health of the community (U.S. Public Health Service, 1995). For example, if there is inadequate mosquito control in a community, it becomes more difficult to enforce health promotion efforts and to prevent the occurrence of mosquito-borne diseases. On the other hand, when a community has the resources for providing childhood immunizations, primary preventive care services can focus on child developmental problems and child safety. The principles of public health practice aim at achieving a healthy environment for all individuals to live in. These principles can be applied with individuals, families, and the communities in which they live. Nursing plays a role in all levels of the health services pyramid. By using public health principles, the nurse is able to better understand the types of environments in which clients live and the types of interventions necessary to help keep clients healthy.

Community Health Nursing

Frequently the terms *community health nursing* and *public health nursing* are used interchangeably. There are similarities. A **public health nursing** focus requires understanding the needs of a **population,** or a collection of individuals who have in common one or more personal or environmental characteristics (Stanhope and Lancaster, 2004). Examples of populations might include high-risk infants, older adults, or a cultural group such as Native Americans. A public health nursing professional must understand factors that influence health promotion and health maintenance of groups, the trends and patterns influencing the incidence of disease within populations, environmental factors contributing to health and illness, and the political processes used to affect public policy. A public health nurse requires preparation at the basic entry level and may require a baccalaureate degree in nursing that includes educational preparation and clinical practice in public health nursing. A specialist in public health is prepared at the graduate level with a focus in the public health sciences (American Nurses Association [ANA], 1999).

Community health nursing is a nursing approach that merges knowledge from the public health sciences with professional nursing theories to safeguard and improve the health of populations in the community (ANA, 1986; Ayers, Bruno, and Langford, 1999). The focus of such nursing care is somewhat broader than that of public health, with an emphasis on the health of a community. In addition to considering the needs of populations, the community health nurse is prepared to provide direct care services to subpopulations within a community. These subpopulations may be a clinical focus in which the nurse has gained expertise (e.g., a case manager who follows older adults recovering from stroke and sees the need for community rehabilitation services, or a nurse practitioner who gives immunizations to clients with the objective of managing communicable disease within the community). By focusing on subpopulations, the community health nurse cares for the community as a whole and considers the individual or family to be only one member of a group at risk. Competence as a community health nurse requires the ability to use interventions that take into account the broad social and political context in which community problems occur and are resolved (Stanhope and Lancaster, 2004). The educational requirements for entry-level nurses practicing in community health nursing roles are not as clear-cut as those for public health nurses. An advanced degree may not be required by a hiring agency. However, nurses with a graduate degree in nursing who practice in community settings are considered community health nurse specialists, regardless of their public health experience (Stanhope and Lancaster, 2004).

Nursing Practice in Community Health

Community-focused nursing practice requires a unique set of skills and knowledge. In the health care delivery system, nurses who become expert in community health practice may have advanced nursing degrees, yet the baccalaureate-prepared generalist can also become quite competent in formulating and applying population-focused assessments and interventions (Diekemper, SmithBattle, and Drake, 1999). The expert community health nurse comes to understand the needs of a population or community through experience with individual families and working through their social and health care issues. Critical thinking becomes important for the nurse who applies knowledge of public health principles, community health nursing, family theory, and communication in finding the best approaches in partnering with families. Diekemper, SmithBattle, and Drake (1999) interviewed community health nurses to hear their stories and to understand what population-focused practice involves. Often community health nurses see their practice evolve "naturally" as they serve families and communities. This is best supported when the working environment does not restrict the nurse's ability to work closely with members of the community.

A successful community health nursing practice involves building relationships with the community and being responsive to changes within the community (Diekemper, SmithBattle, and Drake, 1999). For example, when there is an increase in the incidence of grandparents assuming child care responsibilities, establishing an instructional program in cooperation with local schools can begin to assist and support grandparents in this caregiving role. The community health nurse is responsive by becoming an active part of a community; knowing the community's members, needs, and resources, and then working to establish effective health promotion and disease prevention programs. This may require working with highly resistant systems (e.g., welfare system) and trying to encourage them to be more responsive to the needs of a population. Skills of client advocacy, communicating people's concerns, and designing new systems in cooperation with existing systems help to make community nursing practice effective.

Community-Based Nursing

Community-based nursing involves the acute and chronic care of individuals and families that enhances their capacity for self-care and promotes autonomy in decision making (Ayers, Bruno, and Langford, 1999). Care takes place in community settings such as the home or a clinic; however, the focus is nursing care of the individual or family. The nurse's competence is based on critical thinking and decision making at the level of the individual client—assessing health status, selecting nursing interventions, and evaluating outcomes of care. Because direct care services are provided where clients live, work, and play, it is important for community-based nursing to remain individual and family oriented and to appreciate the values of a community (Zotti, Brown, and Stotts, 1996).

The philosophical foundation for community-based nursing is the human ecological model, which conceptualizes human systems as open and interactive with the environment (Chalmers and others, 1998). In an ecological model the individual is viewed within the larger systems of family, community, culture, and society. The social interaction units seen in Figure 3-2 depict four circles: the inner circle of the client and the immediate family, the second circle of people and settings that have frequent contact with the client and family, the third circle of the local community and its values and policies, and the outer circle of larger social systems such as government and church (Ayers, Bruno, and Langford, 1999). A nurse in a community-based practice must understand the interaction of all of the units while caring for the client and family in their natural environment. The nurse will typically become involved in the domain of the first three circles when providing health care. For example, a home health nurse working with a newly diagnosed diabetic client will work closely with the client and family to establish a comprehensive plan for the client's health. The nurse may become involved in knowing the habits or lifestyle patterns when the client is with friends and co-

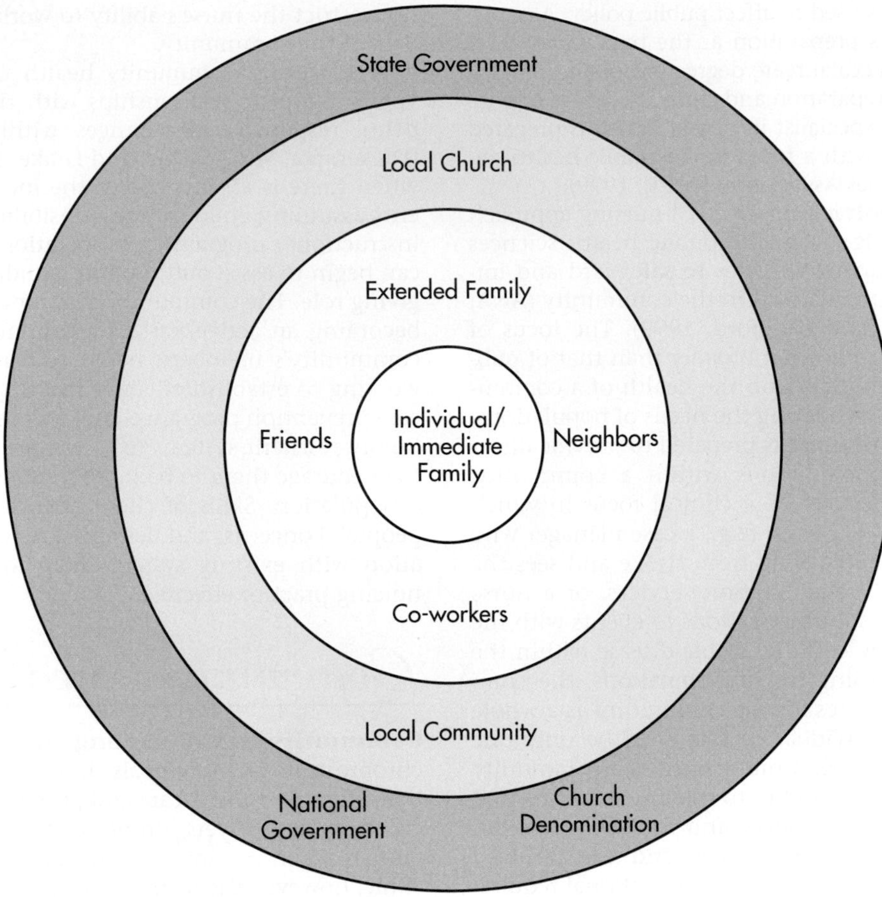

FIGURE **3–2**   These concentric circles represent the social interaction units of the human ecology model. (From Ayers M, Bruno AA, Langford RW: *Community-based nursing care: making the transition*, St. Louis, 1999, Mosby.)

workers to anticipate ways to plan the client's exercise schedule and meal routines. Knowing the resources available in the community (e.g., medical supply shops for glucose monitoring supplies and local diabetes association support groups) enables the nurse to provide comprehensive support for the client's needs.

With the individual and family as the clients, the context of community-based nursing is family-centered care within the community (Ayers, Bruno, and Langford, 1999). This focus requires the nurse to have a strong knowledge base in family theory (see Chapter 9), principles of communication (see Chapter 23), group dynamics, and cultural diversity (see Chapter 8). The nurse learns to partner with clients and families so that ultimately the client and family assume responsibility for their health care decisions. The family becomes involved in planning, decision making, implementation, and evaluation of health care approaches.

Vulnerable Populations

Community-based nurses care for clients from diverse cultures and backgrounds, and with various health conditions. However, changes in the health care delivery system have made high-risk groups the nurse's principal clients. Home health nurses, for example, are not likely to visit low-risk mothers and babies. Instead, adolescent mothers or mothers with drug addiction are more likely to receive home care services. **Vulnerable populations** of clients are those who are more likely to develop health problems as a result of excess risks, who have limits in access to health care services, or who are dependent on others for care. Individuals living in poverty, older adults, homeless persons, individuals in abusive relationships, substance abusers, severely mentally ill persons, and new immigrants are examples of vulnerable populations (Hwang, 2000). Vulnerable individuals and their families often belong to more than one of these groups. In addition, health care vulnerability affects all age-groups (Corrarino and others, 2000). Vulnerable individuals may also be a specific population with a unique health care problem. For example, the older adult who has received heart transplantation presents unique health care needs (Baas and other, 2002).

Frequently, vulnerable clients come from varied cultures, have different beliefs and values, face language barriers, and may have few sources of social support (Chalmers and others, 1998). Their special needs form the backdrop for the challenges nurses face in caring for increasingly complex acute and chronic health conditions.

To become competent in the care of vulnerable populations, it is especially important for nurses in community-based practice to provide culturally appropriate care.

Box 3-1   Guidelines for Assessing Members of Vulnerable Population Groups

Setting the Stage

Create a comfortable, nonthreatening environment.

Learn as much as you can about the culture of the clients you work with so that you will understand cultural practices and values that may influence their health care practices.

Provide culturally competent assessment by understanding the meaning of language and nonverbal behavior in the client's culture.

Be sensitive to the fact that the individual or family you are assessing may have other priorities that are more important to them. These might include financial or legal problems. You may need to give them some tangible help with their most pressing priority before you will be able to address issues that are more traditionally thought of as health concerns.

Collaborate with others as appropriate; you should not provide financial or legal advice. However, you should make sure to connect your client with someone who can and will help them.

Nursing History of an Individual or Family

You may have only one opportunity to work with a vulnerable person or family. Try to complete a history that will provide all the essential information you need to help the individual or family on that day. This means that you will have to organize in your mind exactly what you need to ask, and no more, and why the data are necessary.

It will help to use a comprehensive assessment form that has been modified to focus on the special needs of the vulnerable population group with whom you work. However, be flexible. With some clients, it will be both impractical and

unethical to cover all questions on a comprehensive form. If you know that you are likely to see the client again, ask the less pressing questions at the next visit.

Be sure to include questions about social support, economic status, resources for health care, developmental issues, current health problems, medication, and how the person or family manages their health status. Your goal is to obtain information that will enable you to provide family-centered care.

Does the individual have any condition that compromises his or her immune status, such as AIDS, or is the individual undergoing therapy that would result in immunodeficiency, such as cancer chemotherapy?

Physical Examination or Home Assessment

Again, complete as thorough a physical examination (on an individual) or home assessment as you can. Keep in mind that you should collect only data for which you have a use.

Be alert for indications of physical abuse, substance use (e.g., underweight, being inadequately clothed).

You can assess a family's living environment using good observational skills. Does the family live in an insect- or rat-infested environment? Do they have running water, functioning plumbing, electricity, and a telephone? Is perishable food (e.g., mayonnaise) left sitting out on tables and countertops? Are bed linens reasonably clean? Is paint peeling on the walls and ceilings? Is ventilation adequate? Is the temperature of the home adequate? Is the family exposed to raw sewage or animal waste? Is the home adjacent to a busy highway, possibly exposing the family to high noise levels and automobile exhaust?

From Stanhope M, Lancaster J: *Community health nursing: process and practice for promoting health,* ed 6, St. Louis, 2004, Mosby.

Chapter 8 addresses factors influencing individual differences within cultural groups and the nurse's role in providing culturally appropriate care. To be culturally competent, the nurse must be more than just sensitive to a client's cultural uniqueness. The nurse must be able to appraise and understand a client and family's cultural beliefs, values, and practices to determine their specific needs and the interventions that will most likely be successful in improving their state of health. The nurse cannot judge or evaluate a client's beliefs and values about health in terms of the nurse's own culture. Communication and caring practices become critical in learning a client's perceptions of his or her problems and then planning health care strategies that will be meaningful, culturally appropriate, and successful.

Vulnerable populations typically experience poorer outcomes than those clients with ready access to resources and health care services. Dramatically shorter life spans and higher morbidity rates pose real threats to members of ethnically and racially diverse minority groups (Barr and others, 2002; Hwang, 2000). Members of vulnerable groups frequently have cumulative risks or combinations of risk factors that make them more sensitive to the adverse effects of individual risk factors that others might overcome (Rew and others, 2001). It be-

comes essential for the community-based nurse to assess members of vulnerable populations by taking into account the multiple stressors that affect their clients' lives. It is also important to learn the clients' strengths and resources for coping with stressors. Box 3-1 summarizes guidelines to follow when assessing members of vulnerable population groups.

Poor and Homeless Persons. People who live in poverty are more likely to live in hazardous environments, work at high-risk jobs, eat less nutritious diets, and have multiple stressors in their life. When the life expectancies of European Americans and African-Americans have been compared, the causes of the differences have been found to be related to low socioeconomic status rather than race (Barr and others, 2002; Hwang, 2000). Clients with low income not only lack financial resources, but also are forced to live in poor living environments and face practical problems such as poor or unavailable transportation. Homeless clients have even fewer resources than the poor (Box 3-2). They do not have the advantage of shelter and must cope with finding a place to sleep at night and finding food. Exacerbations of chronic health problems are common because the homeless have no place to store medications if they can afford them and cannot obtain

Research Highlight

Box 3-2

Health Risks for Homeless Adolescents

Research Focus

Homeless adolescents have increased social, behavioral, physical, and health risks. Community-based nurses are frequently the first and only health care provider available to these youth. Early identification and intervention of risks can assist homeless youth in reaching higher levels of health and wellness.

Research Abstract

The purposes of this study were first, to describe reasons for homelessness and identify physical, behavioral, and health risks of homeless youth; and second, to determine relationships between resilience and risk and protective factors, and to determine best predictors of resilience and reduction of risk. Fifty-nine homeless adolescents who sought health care in a community-based clinic were asked to complete three surveys, which were valid measures of resilience, hopelessness, and social connectedness for a homeless adolescent population. These youth were also asked to complete a death-related attitude schedule. Of the sample, 36% were self-identified as gay, lesbian, or bisexual. Over half of the samples were thrown out of their homes by their parents, 37% left home because parents disapproved of their substance abuse, and one third left home because they were sexually abused by at least one parent. In addition, 47% of the sample reported a history of sexual abuse.

Lack of resilience was related to hopelessness, loneliness, life-threatening behaviors, and connectedness, but not to gender or sexual orientation. Youth who perceived themselves as resilient were less lonely, less hopeless, and engaged in fewer life-threatening behaviors. These youth survived by adapting to street life and by becoming overly self-reliant.

Evidence-Based Practice

- Interventions directed toward preventing life-threatening behaviors (including suicide prevention) are aided by increasing social connectedness and reducing loneliness.
- Interventions directed to reducing and eliminating substance abuse increase youth's perception of resilience and reduction in life-threatening behaviors.
- Because these youth lack the usual social resources and connection to family, they lack the perception of feeling cared about.
- Educating youth about available social programs may increase their feelings of being cared for, as well as reducing hopelessness and loneliness.

Reference

Rew L and others: Correlates of resilience in homeless adolescents, *J Nurs Scholarsh* 33(1):33, 2001.

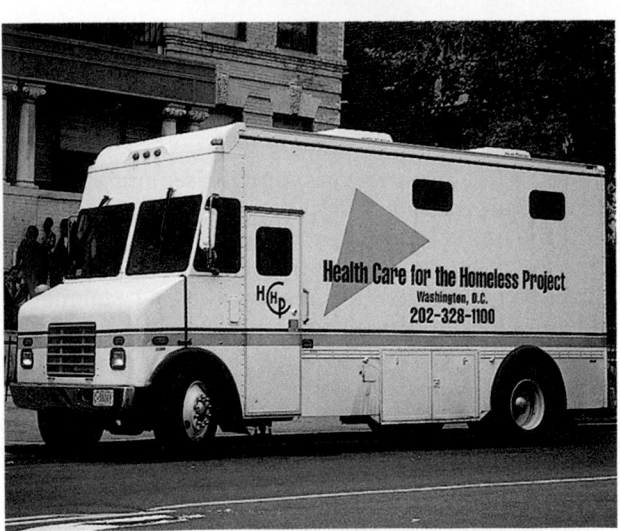

FIGURE **3–3**   The homeless population has unique health care needs.

nutritious meals. In addition, they lack a healthy balance of rest and activity because of the necessity to walk throughout the day to meet basic needs and because of vagrancy laws that prohibit loitering (Hwang and Bugeja, 2000). There is a high incidence of mental illness, personality disorder, and substance abuse among the homeless population. The nurse must help homeless people identify the resources they may have (e.g., mobile health care unit, Figure 3-3), their eligibility for assistance, and the interventions that may promote an increased ability to improve their health status (Table 3-1).

Abused Clients. Physical, emotional, and sexual abuse, as well as neglect, are major public health problems affecting older adults, women, and children (Rew and others, 2001; Sebastian, 1996). Risk factors for abusive relationships may include mental health problems, substance abuse, socioeconomic stressors, and dysfunctional family relationships. There may not be any risk factors present as well. When dealing with clients at risk for or who may have suffered abuse it is important to provide protection. The nurse must interview clients at a time when their privacy is ensured and the individual suspected of being the abuser is not present. Clients who have been abused fear retribution if they discuss their problems with a health care provider. Most states have abuse hot lines that must be notified when an individual has been identified as being at risk.

Substance Abusers. Substance abuse is a blanket term used to describe more than the use of illegal drugs. This term also includes the abuse of alcohol and prescribed medications such as antianxiety agents and opioid analgesics. A client with substance abuse has health and socioeconomic problems. The socioeconomic problems result from the financial strain of the cost of drugs, criminal convictions from illegal activities used to obtain drugs, communicable disease from sharing drug paraphernalia,

Table 3-1	Nursing Interventions for Care of the Homeless	
Level of Prevention		
Primary Intervention	**Secondary Intervention**	**Tertiary Intervention**
Stage 1: Prevent or Reduce Frequency of Homeless Experiences		
Improvement of physical environment (community, home)	Health screening	Control of spread of disease
Provision of adequate housing	Referral programs	Treatment of tuberculosis and acquired immunodeficiency syndrome (AIDS)
Health education	Case management	
Sex education	Case finding	Drug and alcohol treatment programs
Drug and alcohol education	Screening for iron, tuberculosis, human immunodeficiency virus (HIV), hemoglobin, substance use	Treatment of mental illnesses
Good nutrition		Strengthening of support systems
Pregnancy and nutrition	Diagnostic services	
Advocacy	Treatment of acute illnesses	
Support of legislation that helps the poor Increased minimum wage	Treatment of potentially life-threatening illnesses (e.g., rehydration of young children)	
Child day care		
Access to health care		
Stage 2: Assist Homeless in Reducing Factors That Keep Them Homeless and in Gaining Skills to Move Into Higher Level of Functioning		
Teaching regarding effective coping behaviors	Screening for chronic illnesses	Treatment for major mental illnesses Treatment for major illnesses and injuries
Teaching regarding avoidance of potentially violent situations	Leg ulcers	
	Drug abuse	
Advocacy	Trauma	Detoxification programs
Health education	Hypertension	Management of chronic illnesses
Interpersonal skills training	Cancer	Management of AIDS symptoms
Development of interrelationships with service providers	Immunizations	
	Monitoring of psychiatric status and compliance with medical regimen	
Recommendations regarding food and handling and exposure to infectious diseases	Monitoring for status of infectious diseases	
Teaching regarding importance of good nutrition	Provision of on-site care in shelters and service centers	
Referrals for legal assistance		
Stage 3: Increase Amount of Interaction With Service Providers and Acceptance of Resources		
Advocacy	Case management	Protection from violence
Outreach program	Mobile treatment programs	Promotion of wet and dry detoxification
Promotion of legislation regarding homeless mentally ill	Monitoring for changes in health status	
Promotion of legislation for care to homeless	Provision of access to basic nutritional needs	Treatment for major illnesses
		Help for persons in getting into mental health programs
Location of homeless through outreach programs		Supervised housing
Multiservice programs in service sites		Promotion of increased independence

Data from Scholler-Jaquish A: Homelessness in America. In Smith CM, Maurer FA, editors: *Community health nursing: theory and practice*, Philadelphia, 1995, WB Saunders; Hwang SW: Mortality among men using homeless shelters in Toronto, Ontario, *JAMA*, 283(16):2152, 2000; Hwang SW, Bugeja AL: Barriers to appropriate diabetes management among homeless people in Toronto, *Can Med Assoc J* 163(2):161, 2000; and Rew L and others: Correlates of resilience in homeless adolescents, *J Nurs Scholarsh* 33(1):33, 2001.

and family breakdown. For example, health problems for cocaine users can include nasal and sinus disorders and cardiac alterations that can be fatal (Sebastian, 1996). Health care providers who objectively assess substance use in terms of the amount, frequency, and type of use will gain useful information to assist the substance abuser. Frequently these clients may avoid health care for fear of judgmental attitudes by health care providers and concern over being turned in to criminal authorities.

Severely Mentally Ill Persons. When a client has a severe mental illness such as schizophrenia or severe personality disorders such as bipolar disorder, there are mul-

tiple health and socioeconomic problems that must be explored. Many clients with pervasive mental illnesses are homeless or marginally housed. Others lack the ability to maintain employment or to even care for themselves on a daily basis. Clients suffering from pervasive mental illness require medication therapy, counseling, housing, and vocational assistance. In addition, mentally ill clients are at greater risk of abuse and assault (Eckert, Sugar, and Fine, 2002).

The mentally ill are no longer routinely hospitalized in long-term psychiatric institutions. Instead, the goal is to offer community resources within their community; however, comprehensive service networks have not de-

Table 3-2	Major Health Problems in Older Adults and Community Health Nursing Roles and Interventions
Problem	**Community Health Nursing Roles and Interventions**
Hypertension	Monitor blood pressure and weight; educate about nutrition and antihypertensive drugs; teach stress management techniques; promote an optimal balance between rest and activity; establish blood pressure screening programs; assess client's current lifestyle and promote lifestyle changes; promote dietary modifications by using techniques such as a diet diary.
Cancer	Obtain health history; promote monthly breast self-examinations and yearly Pap smears and mammograms for older women; promote regular physical examinations; encourage smokers to stop smoking; correct misconceptions about processes of aging; provide emotional support and quality of care during diagnostic and treatment procedures.
Arthritis	Help adult avoid the false hope and expense of arthritis quackery; educate adult about management of activities, correct body mechanics, availability of mechanical appliances, and adequate rest; promote stress management; counsel and assist the family in improving communication, role negotiation, and use of community resources.
Visual impairment (e.g., loss of visual acuity, eyelid disorders, opacity of the lens)	Provide support in a well-lighted, glare-free environment; use printed aids with large, well-spaced letters; assist adult with cleaning eyeglasses; help make arrangements for vision examinations and obtain necessary prostheses; teach adult to be cautious of fraudulent advertisements.
Hearing impairment (e.g., presbycusis)	Speak with clarity at a moderate volume and pace, and face audience when performing health teaching; help make arrangements for hearing examination and obtain necessary prostheses; teach adult to be cautious of fraudulent advertisements.
Confusional states	Provide complete assessment; correct underlying causes of disease (if possible); provide for a protective environment; promote activities that reinforce reality; assist with adequate personal hygiene, nutrition, and hydration; provide emotional support to the family; recommend applicable community resources such as adult day care, home health aides, and homemaker services.
Alzheimer's disease	Maintain optimal functioning, protection, and safety; foster human dignity; demonstrate to the primary family caregiver techniques to dress, feed, and toilet adult; provide frequent encouragement and emotional support to caregiver; act as an advocate for client when dealing with respite care and support groups; ensure that clients' rights are protected; provide support to maintain family members' physical and mental health; maintain family stability; recommend financial services if needed.
Dental problems	Perform oral assessment and refer as necessary; emphasize regular brushing and flossing, proper nutrition, and dental examinations; encourage clients with dentures to wear and take care of them; allay fears about dentist; help provide access to financial services (if necessary) and access to dental care facilities.
Drug use and abuse	Obtain drug history; educate adult about safe storage, risks of drug-drug, and drug-food interactions, and general information about drug (e.g., drug name, purpose, side effects, dosage); instruct adult about presorting techniques (using small containers with one dose of drug that are labeled with specific administration times).
Substance abuse	Arrange and monitor detoxification if appropriate; counsel adults about substance abuse; promote stress management to avoid need for drugs or alcohol; encourage adult to use self-help groups such as Alcoholics Anonymous and Al-Anon; educate public about dangers of substance abuse.

Data from Stanhope M, Lancaster J: *Community health nursing: process and practice for promoting health,* ed 4, St. Louis, 1996, Mosby; Baas LD and others: The challenge of managing the care of older heart transplant recipients, *AACN Clin Issues* 13(1):114, 2002; Hwang SW: Mortality among men using homeless shelters in Toronto, Ontario, *JAMA* 283(16):2152, 2000; and Hwang SW, Bugeja AL: Barriers to appropriate diabetes management among homeless people in Toronto, *Can Med Assoc J* 163(2):161, 2000.

veloped in every community (Stanhope and Lancaster, 2004). Many clients are left with fewer and more fragmented services, with little skill in surviving and functioning within the community. There are more young mentally ill persons who have had only episodic hospital care. Collaboration with multiple community resources is a key to helping the pervasively mentally ill to obtain adequate health care.

Older Adults. With the increase in the older adult population, there is a simultaneous increase in the number of clients suffering from chronic disease and a greater demand for health care services. Health promotion and prevention of disease are infrequently associated with older adults because of the image of aging and its association with poor health and disease (Barr and others, 2002). However, it is important for the nurse to view health promotion from a broad context. This begins with the understanding of what health means to older adults and the steps they can take to maintain their own health (Zahn and others, 1998). When individuals feel empowered to control their own health, disability from chronic disease can be reduced (Baas and others, 2002). There is an opportunity to improve the lifestyle of older adults and their quality of life. Table 3-2 describes the major health problems encountered by older adults and the role of community health nurses.

Competency in Community-Based Nursing

A nurse in community-based practice must have a variety of skills and talents to be successful in assisting clients with their health care needs and in developing relationships within the community. The Pew Health Professions Commission, in response to the *Healthy People 2010* initiative (see Chapter 2), recommended competencies for health care professionals that included the practice of prevention and caring for the community's health (Dower, O'Neil, and Hough, 2001). Being able to apply the nursing process (see Unit III) in a critical thinking approach ensures good, individualized nursing care for specific clients and their families. Additional competencies reviewed here enable the nurse to deliver care within the context of the client's community so that long-term success is more likely.

Case Manager
Chapter 2 describes briefly the case management model for care delivery. In community-based practice, case management is an important competency. It is the ability to establish an appropriate plan of care based on assessment of clients and families and to coordinate needed resources and services for the client's well-being across a continuum of care. Generally, a community-based nurse will assume responsibility for the case management of multiple clients. This usually involves clients who are at greatest risk for needing extensive coordination of health care services (e.g., clients with neurological disease, trauma victims, psychiatric clients, and clients with complex med-

ical conditions). The greatest challenge is coordinating the activities of multiple providers and payers, in different settings, throughout a client's continuum of care. Although the nurse may be employed and located in one setting, the nurse will influence the selection and monitoring of care provided in other settings by formal and informal caregivers (Stanhope and Lancaster, 2004). An effective case manager eventually learns the roadblocks, deficits, and even the opportunities that exist within the community that influence the ability to find solutions for clients' health care needs. Case management with individual clients and families reveals the big picture of health services and the health status of a community.

Collaborator
A nurse who practices community-based nursing must be competent in working not only with individuals and their families, but also with other related health care disciplines. Collaboration, or working in a combined effort with all those involved in care delivery, is required for a mutually acceptable plan to be obtained that will achieve common goals (Ayers, Bruno, and Langford, 1999). For example, when a client is discharged home with terminal cancer, the home care nurse must be able to collaborate with hospice staff, social workers, and pastoral care to initiate a plan to support the client and family. For collaboration to be effective, there must be mutual trust and respect for each professional's abilities and contributions. Similarly, clients must share trust in the health care providers. Teamwork is central to being able to explore client issues, knowing the contributions each professional can offer, clarifying roles, and developing a plan of care that client and health care providers can accept and support.

Educator
Community-based nurses must also demonstrate competency in client education. The nurse will have the opportunity to work with single individuals and groups of clients. A nurse who is competent in establishing relationships with community service organizations can offer educational support to a wide range of client groups. Perinatal classes, infant care, child safety, and cancer screening are just some of the health education programs in which a nurse in community practice may participate (Corrarino and others, 2000).

With the goal of helping clients assume responsibility for their own health care, the role of educator takes on greater importance in community-based nursing than in episodic care (Ayers, Bruno, and Langford, 1999). Clients and families are expected to gain the skills and knowledge needed to learn how to give care themselves (see Chapter 24). In community-based practice the nurse must assess a client's learning needs and readiness to learn within the context of the individual, the systems the individual interacts with (e.g., family, business, and school), and the resources available for support. Teaching skills likewise must be adapted so that the nurse can instruct within the home setting and make the learning process meaningful. The nurse in community-based practice has the opportunity to follow clients over time. Planning for return demonstration of skills, use of follow-up phone calls, and referral to community support and self-help groups give the nurse the opportunity to provide continuity in instruction and to reinforce important instructional topics. Evaluation of client learning occurs over time, requiring the nurse's patience and commitment.

Counselor

A counselor assists clients in identifying and clarifying health problems and in choosing appropriate courses of action to solve those problems (Ayers, Bruno, and Langford, 1999). For example, a community-based nurse may work in employee assistance programs or women's shelters. In this setting a major amount of nurse-client interaction is through counseling. A counselor is responsible for providing information, listening objectively, and being supportive, caring, and trustworthy. Counselors do not make decisions; they help clients reach decisions that best suit them (Stanhope and Lancaster, 2004). The nurse in community-based practice will face many situations where counseling is an important skill. Clients and families often require assistance in first identifying and clarifying health problems. For example, a client who repeatedly reports a problem in following a prescribed diet may actually have the problem of being unable to afford nutritious foods or have family members who do not support good eating habits. The nurse may discuss with the client factors that block or aid problem resolution, identify a range of solutions, and then discuss which solutions are most likely to be successful. The nurse encourages the client to make decisions and fosters confidence in the choice that is made.

An important factor in the nurse's ability to be an effective counselor is knowing what a community can offer clients. Frequently clients must go outside their own family to obtain the support that is necessary to improve their health status. Directing clients to appropriate resources requires the nurse to know those resources well; what services do agencies provide, which staff members can be accessed quickly, what reimbursement limitations affect access, and is there coordination between agencies within the community?

Client Advocate

Client advocacy perhaps is even more important today in community-based practice because of the confusion surrounding access to health care services. Clients often need someone to help them walk through the system, identifying where to go for services, how to reach the individuals with the appropriate authority, what services to request, and how to follow through with the information they received. The community-based nurse may be the one who presents the client's point of view so that appropriate resources can be obtained. The nurse will provide the information necessary for clients to make informed decisions in utilizing and choosing services appropriately. Then the nurse supports clients in defending those decisions. There are similar principles used in both counseling and advocacy.

Change Agent

A community-based nurse also must be competent as a change agent. This involves seeking to implement new and more effective approaches to problems (Ayers, Bruno,

---

> **Box 3-3** **Success Factors in Adopting Change**
>
> The innovation or change must be perceived as more advantageous than other alternatives. The nature of the innovation determines what specific type of relative advantage (e.g., social, economic, community good) is important to those who adopt the change.
>
> The innovation or change must be compatible with existing values, past experiences, and needs of potential adopters. A change agent will determine needs of clients and recommend changes that fulfill those needs.
>
> The innovation or change must be tried on a limited basis. New ideas that can be experimented with are usually adopted more quickly. Clients trying out a new technology can find out how it works in their own situation.
>
> Simple innovations or changes are more readily adopted than those that are complex. An innovation must be easy to understand and use.
>
> An innovation is more quickly adopted when its results are clearly communicated and visible to others.

Data from Rogers EM: *Diffusion of innovations*, ed 4, New York, 1995, Free Press.

---

and Langford, 1999). The nurse may act as a change agent within a family system or intercede with problems that reside within the client's community. The nurse might identify any number of problems (e.g., quality of community child care services, availability of older adult day care services, or the status of neighborhood violence). The nurse may act to empower individuals and their families to creatively solve problems or become instrumental in creating change within a health care agency. As a change agent, the nurse gathers and analyzes facts and implements programs. This requires the nurse to be very familiar with the community itself. Many communities are resistant to change, preferring to provide services in an established manner as they always have. Before the nurse can analyze necessary facts, it is necessary to manage conflict between the health care providers involved in the client's care, clarify their roles, and clearly identify the needs of the clients. If the community has a history of poor problem solving, the nurse may have to focus on developing problem-solving capabilities (Stanhope and Lancaster, 2004). Box 3-3 describes the factors that increase the likelihood of change being accepted and adopted. Each factor should be considered as having potential in helping the nurse successfully bring about change. For example, if a nurse is trying to improve a client's adherence to routine health care visits, it may be useful to offer an alternative site, such as a nursing clinic, that is closer and has more convenient hours for the client to visit.

Community Assessment

When a nurse practices within a community setting, it is important to learn how to assess the community at large. This is the environment where the nurse's clients live and work. Without an adequate understanding of that envi-

Box 3-4	**Community Assessment**

Structure

Name of community or
  neighborhood
Geographical boundaries
Environment
Water and sanitation
Housing
Economy

Population

Age distribution
Sex distribution
Growth trends

Density
Education level
Predominant cultural groups
Predominant religious
  groups

Social System

Education system
Government
Communication system
Transportation system
Welfare system
Volunteer programs
Health system

ronment, any effort to promote the client's health and to institute necessary change is unlikely to be successful. The community can be viewed as having three components: structure or locale, the people, and the social systems. A complete assessment involves a careful look at each component to begin to identify needs for health policy, health program development, and service provision (Box 3-4). When assessing the structure or locale, the nurse should travel around the neighborhood or community and observe its design, the location of services, and the locations where residents congregate. An assessment of the demographics of the population may be facilitated by accessing statistics on the community from a local public health department or public library. Information about existing social systems, such as schools or health care facilities, are frequently acquired by visiting various sites and learning about their services.

Once the nurse has a good understanding of the community, any individual client assessment is then performed against that background. For example, consider the situation of the nurse assessing a client's home for safety. Does the client have secure locks on doors? Are windows secure and intact? Is lighting along walkways and entryways operational? The nurse will conduct the assessment, knowing at the same time the level of community violence and the resources that are available to the client when help is necessary. No individual client assessment should occur in isolation from the environment and conditions of the client's community.

Changing Clients' Health

The nurse in community-based practice will care for clients from diverse backgrounds and in diverse settings. It is relatively easy over time to become familiar with the resources that are available within a particular community practice setting. Likewise, with practice a nurse is able to learn how to identify the unique needs of individual clients. However, the challenge is how to promote and protect a client's health within the context of the community. Can a client with lung disease, for example, have the quality of life necessary when a community has a se-

rious environmental pollution problem? Similarly, the nurse brings together the resources necessary to improve the continuity of care that clients receive. The nurse can be a key figure in reducing the duplication of health care services and locating the best services for a client's needs.

Perhaps the most important theme to consider to be an effective community-based nurse is to understand clients' lives. This begins by being able to establish strong, caring relationships with clients and their families (see Chapter 7). This becomes more difficult as the amount of time that professional nurses have to spend with clients continues to decline. However, the expert nurse becomes able to advise, counsel, and teach effectively after being accepted into the client's family and by understanding what truly makes the client unique. The day-to-day activities of family life are the variables that influence how the nurse must adapt nursing interventions. The time of day a client goes to work, the availability of the spouse and client's parents to provide child care, and the family values that shape views about health are just a few examples of the many factors nurses must consider in community-based practice. Once the nurse acquires a picture of a client's life, interventions designed to promote health and prevent disease can be introduced so that the picture becomes enhanced.

Key Concepts

- The principles of public health nursing practice aim at assisting individuals in acquiring a healthy environment in which to live.
- Essential public health functions include assessment, policy development, and access to resources.
- When population-based health care services are effective, there is a greater likelihood of the higher tiers of services contributing efficiently to health improvement of the population.
- The community health nurse cares for the community as a whole and considers the individual or family to be only one member of a group at risk.
- A successful community health nursing practice involves building relationships with the community and being responsive to changes within the community.
- The community-based nurse's competence is based on decision making at the level of the individual client.
- Within the ecological model of community-based nursing, the individual is viewed within the larger systems of family, community, culture, and society.
- Vulnerable individuals and their families often belong to more than one vulnerable group.
- The special needs of vulnerable populations form the backdrop for the challenges nurses face in caring for these clients' increasingly complex acute and chronic health conditions.
- Exacerbations of chronic health problems are common among the homeless because they have few resources.
- An important principle in dealing with clients at risk or who may have suffered abuse is protection of the client.

- Clients who are substance abusers may often avoid health care for fear of being turned in to criminal authorities.
- In community-based practice it is important to understand what health means to older adults and the steps they can take to maintain their own health.
- A community-based nurse must be competent as a collaborator, educator, counselor, change agent, and client advocate.
- The likelihood of a change being accepted and adopted is increased if the change is more advantageous, it is compatible, it is realistic, and it is easily adopted.
- Assessment of a community includes three elements: structure or locale, the people, and the social systems.

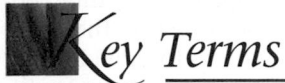

Key Terms

Community-based nursing, *p. 49*
Community health nursing, *p. 49*
Incident rates, *p. 48*

Population, *p. 48*
Public health nursing, *p. 48*
Vulnerable populations, *p. 50*

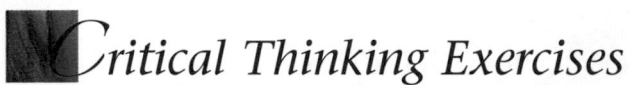

Critical Thinking Exercises

1. As a nurse managing a severely disabled child, you learn that there is an absence of respite services to provide parental support and limited educational resources in your community. What role of the community-based nurse would be important to establish a special education day care service, operated by volunteer educators?
2. Mr. Crowder is a 42-year-old man with diabetes mellitus and visual impairment. Your assessment reveals that he is homeless and that he currently spends nights in a shelter two blocks away. He has been unable to acquire medications or proper diet to control his blood sugar. What factors might you consider in attempting to improve Mr. Crowder's adherence to medication administration?
3. Conduct a community assessment of an area that you have visited infrequently. Observe the community locale by driving through the more populated area. Look for the following services: hospital, clinic, drugstore, grocery, schools, park or playground, and police and fire departments.

Review Questions

1. *Healthy People 2010's* overall goals are to:
   1. Increase the life expectancy and quality of life and to eliminate health disparities.
   2. Gather information on incident rates of certain diseases and social problems.
   3. Assess the health care needs of individuals, families, or communities.
   4. Develop and implement public health policies and improve access to care.

2. Community health nursing is a nursing approach that merges knowledge from professional nursing theories and the:
   1. Population sciences.
   2. Public health sciences.
   3. Environmental sciences.
   4. Mental health sciences.

3. Community-based nursing involves the acute and chronic care of individuals and families that enhance their capacity for:
   1. Nursing care that promotes autonomy in decision-making.
   2. Improving their health care and self-care.
   3. Self-care and promotes autonomy in decision making.
   4. Learning about their illnesses.

4. Vulnerable populations of clients are those who are more likely to develop health problems as a result of:
   1. Chronic diseases, homelessness, and poverty.
   2. Lack of transportation, dependent on other for care, and homelessness.
   3. Poverty and limits in access to health care services.
   4. Excess risks, limits in access to health care services, and dependency on others for care.

5. Major public health problems affecting older adults, women, and children are:
   1. Prescribed medication abuse, poverty, sexual abuse.
   2. Physical, emotional, and sexual abuse, as well as neglect.
   3. Acute illnesses, neglect, abandonment.
   4. Financial strain, poverty, physical abuse.

6. Control of spread of disease is an example of which level of prevention?
   1. Primary intervention.
   2. Secondary intervention.
   3. Tertiary intervention.
   4. Nursing intervention.

7. Teaching classes about infant care, child safety, and cancer screening are examples of a nurse in the role of a(n):
   1. Case manager.
   2. Collaborator.
   3. Educator.
   4. Counselor.

8. A community-based nurse working in employee assistance programs is an example of a nurse in the role of a(n):
   1. Educator.
   2. Collaborator.
   3. Case manager.
   4. Counselor.

9. The nurse has his client try a new technology that the client finds works for her. The nurse is using the following change factor that increases the likelihood that she will accept and adopt her situation.
   1. The innovation or change must be perceived as more advantageous that other alternatives.
   2. The innovation or change must be compatible with existing values, past experiences, and needs of potential adopters.
   3. The innovation or change must be tried on a limited basis.
   4. Simple innovations or changes are more readily adopted than those that are complex.

10. Assessment of a community includes three elements, which are:
    1. Structure or locale, the people, and the social systems.
    2. People, neighborhoods, and social systems.
    3. Health care systems, geographic boundaries, and the people.
    4. Environment, families, and social systems.

References

American Nurses Association: *Standards of community health nursing practice,* Washington, DC, 1986, The Association.

American Nurses Association: *Standards of public health nursing practice,* Washington, DC, 1999, The Association.

Ayers M, Bruno AA, Langford RW: *Community-based nursing care: making the transition,* St. Louis, 1999, Mosby.

Baas LD and others: The challenge of managing the care of older heart transplant recipients, *AACN Clin Issues* 13(1):114, 2002.

Chalmers KI and others: The changing environment of community health practice and education: perceptions of staff nurses, administrators, and educators, *J Nurs Educ* 37:109, 1998.

Diekemper M, SmithBattle L, Drake MA: Bringing the population into focus: a natural development in community health nursing practice, part I, *Public Health Nurs* 16:3, 1999.

Dower C, O'Neil E, Hough H: *Profiling the professions: a model for evaluating emerging health professions,* San Francisco, 2001, Center for Health Professions, University of California, San Francisco.

Flynn BC: Communicating with the public: community-based nursing research and practice, *Public Health Nurs* 15(3):165, 1998.

Hwang SW: Mortality among men using homeless shelters in Toronto, Ontario, *JAMA* 283(16):2152, 2000.

Hwang SW, Bugeja AL: Barriers to appropriate diabetes management among homeless people in Toronto, *Can Med Assoc J* 163(2):161, 2000.

Rew L and others: Correlates of resilience in homelss adolescents, *J Nurs Scholarsh* 33(1):33, 2001.

Rogers EM: *Diffusion of innovations,* ed 4, New York, 1995, Free Press.

Scholler-Jaquish A: Homelessness in America. In Smith CM, Maurer FA, editors: *Community health nursing: theory and practice,* Philadelphia, 1995, WB Saunders.

Sebastian JG: Vulnerability and vulnerable populations: an introduction. In Stanhope M, Lancaster J, editors: *Community health nursing: process and practice for promoting health,* ed 4, St. Louis, 1996, Mosby.

Stanhope M, Lancaster J: *Community health nursing: process and practice for promoting health,* ed 4, St. Louis, 1996, Mosby.

Stanhope M, Lancaster J: *Community health nursing: process and practice for promoting health,* ed 6, St. Louis, 2004, Mosby.

U.S. Department of Health and Human Services, Public Health Service: *Healthy People 2010,* vol 1 (ed 2), Part A Focus area 7, Educational and community-based programs, Washington, DC, 2000a, U.S. Government Printing Office, www.health.gov/healthypeople/document/HTML/VolumeI.

U.S. Department of Health and Human Services, Public Health Service. *Healthy People 2010: A systematic approach to health improvement,* Washington, DC, 2000b, U.S. Government Printing Office, www.health.gov/healthypeople/document/HTML.

U.S. Public Health Service: *A time for partnership: prevention report,* Rockville, Md, December 1994/January 1995, Office of Disease Prevention and Health Promotion.

Zhan L and others: Promoting health: perspectives from ethnic elderly women, *J Community Health Nurs* 15:31, 1998.

Zotti ME, Brown P, Stotts RC: Community-based nursing versus community health nursing: what does it all mean? *Nurs Outlook* 44(5):211, 1996.

Research References

Barr RG and others: The national asthma education and prevention program (NAEPP), *Arch Internal Med* 162(15):1761, 2002.

Corrarino JE and others: The Cool Kids Coalition: a community effort to reduce scald burn risk in children, *MCN Am J Maternal Child Nurs* 25(1):10, 2000.

Eckert LO, Sugar N, Fine D: Characteristics of sexual assault in women with a major psychiatric diagnosis, *Am J Obstet Gynecol* 186(96):1284, 2002.

Hwang SW: Mortality among men using homeless shelters in Toronto, Ontario, *JAMA* 283(16):2152, 2000.

Hwang SW, Bugeja AL: Barriers to appropriate diabetes management among homeless people in Toronto, *Can Med Assoc J* 163(2):161, 2000.

Rew L and others: Correlates of resilience in homeless adolescents, *J Nurs Scholorsh* 33(1):33, 2001.

4

*T*heoretical Foundations of Nursing Practice

Media Resources

http://evolve.elsevier.com/Potter/fundamentals/

CD COMPANION

- Review Questions
- Glossary

evolve WEBSITE

- Review Questions
- Student Learning Activities
- Glossary

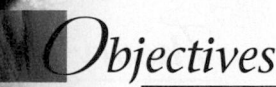

Objectives

Mastery of content in this chapter will enable the student to:

- Define the key terms listed.
- Define nursing theory.
- Describe types of nursing theories.
- Describe the relationship between theory, the nursing process, and client needs.
- Describe the historical development of nursing theory.
- Discuss selected theories from other disciplines.
- Discuss the value of nursing theory in nursing practice.
- Discuss selected nursing theories.
- Describe the relationship between theory and knowledge development in nursing.

*M*odern nursing involves the application of knowledge from nursing science, basic social sciences, physical sciences, biobehavioral sciences, ethics, and contemporary issues. This broad knowledge base applies to nursing because it is a unique profession, addressing the many responses individuals and families experience with their health problems. One form of knowledge that can be very useful to nurses as they design and implement nursing interventions to meet the needs of their clients is nursing theory. For many beginning students, nursing theory can be difficult to understand or appreciate. However, nursing theories serve to describe, explain, predict, and/or prescribe nursing care measures. The scientific work involved in developing theories is such that once one is found to be relevant for a science such as nursing, a theory offers a well-grounded rationale or reason for how and why nurses perform specific interventions.

Expertise in nursing is a result of knowledge and clinical experience. The expertise required to interpret clinical situations and make clinical judgments is the essence of nursing care and is the basis for the advancement of nursing practice and the development of nursing science (Benner and Tanner, 1987; Carnevali and Thomas, 1993). Nurses learn from experience. They also learn and grow professionally by becoming familiar with nursing theory and finding ways to apply theory in their practice. Well-developed theories can become an important basis for the nurse's approach to client care.

The Domain of Nursing

Any science has a **domain,** which is the view or perspective of the discipline. The domain contains the subject, central concepts, values and beliefs, phenomena of interest, and the central problems of the discipline. The domain of medicine is the diagnosis and treatment of disease. Nursing's domain is the identification and treatment of clients' health care needs at all levels of health and in all health care settings. Because the domain of a science can comprise many variables, it is helpful to have a model for conceptual understanding. Nursing has a model or **paradigm** that explains the linkages of science, philosophy, and theory accepted and applied by the discipline (Alligood and Marriner-Tomey, 2002). The elements of **nursing's paradigm** direct the ac-

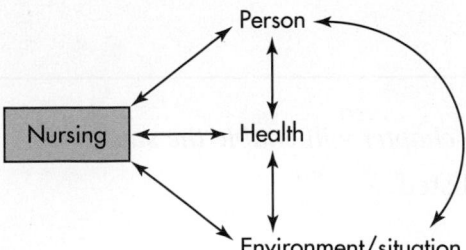

FIGURE **4–1** Nursing's paradigm.

tivity of the nursing profession, including knowledge development, philosophy, theory, educational experience, research, practice, and literature identified with the profession (Alligood and Marriner-Tomey, 2002). Nursing identified its domain in a paradigm that includes four linkages: the person, health, environment/situation, and nursing (Figure 4-1).

Person refers to the recipient of nursing care, including individual clients, families, and the community. The person is central to the care being provided. Because the person's needs are multidimensional, it is important that nursing provides care that is individualized to the client's needs.

Health is defined in different ways by the client, the clinical setting, and the health care profession (see Chapter 6). It is the goal of nursing care. The American Nurses Association (ANA) (1995) defines health as "a dynamic state of being in which the developmental and behavioral potential of the individual is realized to the fullest extent possible." Health is dynamic and continuously changing. The nurse is challenged to provide care based on the client's individualized level of health and health care needs at the time of care delivery.

Environment/situation includes all possible conditions affecting the client and the setting in which health care needs occur. For example, a client's level of health and health care needs can be influenced by factors in the home, school, workplace, or community. An adolescent girl with immune-mediated (or type 1) diabetes may need to adapt her care regimen to physical activities of school, to the demands of a part-time job, and to the timing of social events, such as her prom. There is continuous interaction between the client and the environment. This interaction can have positive and negative effects on the person's level of health and health care needs. Nursing has a unique focus in helping clients within all situations achieve a stable or improved level of health.

Nursing is the "diagnosis and treatment of human responses to actual or potential health problems" (ANA, 1995). For example, a nurse does not medically diagnose the client's heart condition but instead assesses the client's response to the disease and develops nursing diagnoses of fatigue, change in body image, and altered coping. From these nursing diagnoses, the nurse creates an individualized plan of care (see Unit 3). Nurses use critical thinking skills to integrate knowledge, experience, attitudes, and standards into the individualized plan of care for each client.

Theory

A **theory** is a set of concepts, definitions, relationships, and assumptions that project a systematic view of phenomena. For example, Orem's self-care deficit theory defines nursing as a helping service, a creative effort to help people (Fawcett, 1995). In addition, Orem's theory suggests that the goal of nursing is to help people to meet their own therapeutic self-care demands. From this theoretical view, nursing assists clients by acting for, doing, or guiding physical and/or psychological support. Orem's theory contains a detailed framework of self-care concepts that are linked in such a way as to explain, describe, or predict the type of nursing care that will assist clients to achieve a better level of health. A theory is a way of seeing through a "set of relatively concrete and specific concepts and the propositions that describe or link the concepts" (Fawcett, 1999).

A **nursing theory** is a conceptualization of some aspect of nursing communicated for the purpose of describing, explaining, predicting, and/or prescribing nursing care (Meleis, 1997). For example, Orem's theory (2001) explains the factors within a clients' living situation that support or interfere with the client's self-care ability. It is important to note that this theory has value in helping nursing design nursing interventions to promote the client's self-care in managing an illness such as diabetes or arthritis.

Theories constitute much of the knowledge of a discipline, and theory and inquiry are vital linkages to each other (Fawcett and others, 2001). Nursing theories provide nurses with a perspective to view client situations, a way to organize data, and a method to analyze and interpret information. When a nurse uses Orem's theory in practice, the nurse assesses and interprets the data to determine the client's self-care needs, self-care deficits, and self-care abilities in the management of a disease. The theory then guides the nurse to design individualized nursing interventions. Application of nursing theory in practice depends on the nurse's knowledge of nursing and other theoretical models, how these models relate to each other, and the use of these models in designing nursing interventions.

Nursing is a learned profession, a science, and an art (Rogers, 1990). Nurses need a theoretical base to exemplify the science and art of the profession when they promote health and wellness for their clients, whether the client is an individual, a family, or a community.

Components of a Theory

As previously stated, a theory is a set of concepts, definitions, and assumptions or propositions to explain a phenomenon (Figure 4-2). The theory explains how these elements are uniquely related in the phenomenon. It is developed after extensive research, which allows the researcher to see a clear perspective of all components of a phenomenon. For example, Kristin Swanson studied the phenomenon of caring by conducting extensive interviews with clients and their professional caregivers (Swanson, 1991). Swanson's theory of caring defines five components of caring: knowing, being with, doing for,

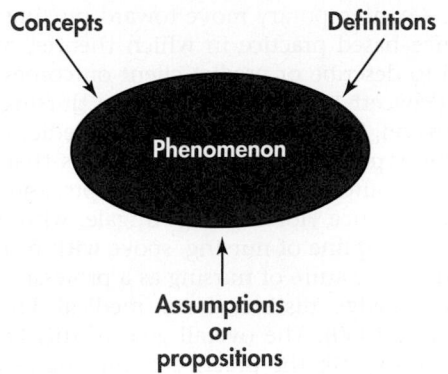

FIGURE **4–2** Components of a nursing theory.

enabling, and maintaining belief (see Chapter 7). These components provide a foundation of knowledge for the direction and delivery of caring nursing practice. Swanson's theory provides a basis for identifying nurse caring behaviors, which can then be tested, to determine if caring can improve client health outcomes.

Concepts. A theory consists of interrelated concepts. **Concepts** are mental formulations of an object or event that come from individual perceptual experience (Alligood and Marriner-Tomey, 2002). They are ideas, mental images. Concepts help to describe or label phenomena (Alligood and Marriner-Tomey, 2002). Using Neuman Systems Model (1972) as an example, there are concepts that affect the client system. Some of these concepts are physiological, psychological, sociocultural, and environmental or related to health and wellness, prevention, stressors, and defense mechanisms (Meleis, 1997).

Definitions. The definitions within the description of a theory convey the general meaning of the concepts in a manner that fits the theory. These definitions also describe the activity necessary to measure the constructs, relationships, or variables within a theory (Chinn and Kramer, 2004; Marriner-Tomey and Alligood, 2002). For example, Neuman Systems Model defines clients as people who are anticipating stress or who are dealing with stress. Thus nurses who use Neuman's theory in practice focus their care on client responses that could be labeled as stressful (Meleis, 1997). These responses are within the domain of nursing (Meleis, 1997).

Assumptions. **Assumptions** are statements that describe concepts or connect two concepts that are factual. Assumptions are the "taken for granted" statements that determine the nature of the concepts, definitions, purpose, relationships, and structure of the theory (Meleis, 1997; Chinn and Kramer, 2004). The assumptions in Neuman Systems Model are that clients are dynamic; the relationships between the theory's concepts influence a client's protective mechanisms and determine a client's response; clients have a normal range of responses; stressors attack flexible lines of defense followed by the normal lines of defense; and nurse's actions are focused on primary, secondary, and tertiary prevention (Neuman, 1972).

Phenomenon. Nursing theories focus on the phenomena of nursing and nursing care. A **phenomenon** is an aspect of reality that can be consciously sensed or experienced (Meleis, 1997). Examples of phenomena of nursing include caring, self-care, and client responses to stress. In Neuman Systems Model (1972), phenomena include all client responses, environmental factors, and nursing actions. Within a specific discipline, phenomena are part of the domain of the discipline. In nursing, phenomena reflect the domain of nursing practice.

Types of Theory

The general purpose of a theory is important because it specifies the context and situation in which the theory applies (Chinn and Kramer, 1999). Theories have different purposes and may be classified by levels of abstraction (grand theories versus middle-range theories) or the goals of the theory (descriptive or prescriptive). Theories may describe, predict, or prescribe activities for the phenomena of interest (Box 4-1).

Grand theories are broad in scope and complex and therefore require further specification through research before they can be fully tested (Chinn and Kramer, 1999). A grand theory is not intended to provide guidance for specific nursing interventions, but to provide the structural framework for broad, abstract ideas about nursing (Fawcett, 1995).

Theories that have more limited scope, less abstraction, address specific phenomena or concepts and reflect practice (administration, clinical, or teaching) are considered **middle-range theories.** The phenomena or concepts tend to cross different nursing fields and reflect a wide variety of nursing care situations, such as uncertainty, incontinence, social support, quality of life, and caring (Meleis, 1997). For example, Mishel's theory of uncertainty in illness (1988, 1990) focuses on the experience of clients with cancer while living with continual uncertainty. The theory provides a basis for nurses to assist clients in appraising and adapting to the uncertainty and the illness response.

Descriptive theories are the first level of theory development. They describe phenomena, speculate on why phenomena occur, and describe the consequences of phenomena. They have the ability to explain, relate, and in some situations predict nursing phenomena (Meleis, 1997). For example, theories of growth and development describe the maturation processes of an individual at various ages (see Chapter 10). Descriptive theories do not direct specific nursing activities, but may help to explain client assessments.

Prescriptive theories address nursing interventions and predict the consequence of a specific nursing intervention. In nursing, a prescriptive theory should designate the prescription (i.e., nursing interventions), the conditions under which the prescription should occur, and the consequences (Meleis, 1997). Prescriptive theories are action oriented, which tests the validity and predictability of a nursing intervention. These theories guide nursing research to develop and test specific nursing interventions (Fawcett, 1999). For example, Mishel's theory of uncertainty predicts that increasing the coping skills of clients with gynecological cancer assists their ability to deal with the uncertainty of the cancer diagnosis and treatment (Mishel and Sorenson, 1991; Mishel, 1997). Thus the theory provides a framework to design interventions that support and bolster clients' coping resources.

Theoretical Models

A **theoretical model** refers to global ideas about the individuals, groups, situations, or events of interest to a specific discipline from the view of the theorist. Theories focus more specifically on the events and phenomena of the discipline and are specific enough to contribute to a sound basis for nursing practice (Chinn and Kramer, 1999; Fawcett, 1999). Development of theory enhances nursing science, which involves the generation of knowledge. Although this knowledge can be used with knowledge from other disciplines, it is designed to advance and support nursing practice and health care (Chinn and Kramer, 1999).

There are multiple nursing theories, some of which are presented in this and other chapters in the text. It is important to understand the influence of theories from other disciplines and their effects on nurses' clinical practice and client care and to use them in developing innovative nursing interventions.

*R*elationship of Theory to the Nursing Process and Client Needs

Historically, nursing theories were studied in an isolated academic environment independent of nursing practice (Table 4-1). Many nurses argued that theories were not relevant to what occurs in clinical practice. There is,

however, a contemporary move toward nursing science– or evidence–based practice in which theories are tested and used to describe or predict client outcomes of nursing care (Fawcett and others, 2001). For nursing to grow as a profession, knowledge is needed to predict with confidence the types of nursing interventions that will improve client outcomes. Nursing concepts and theories have evolved since Florence Nightingale, who, in establishing the discipline of nursing, spoke with firm conviction about the "nature of nursing as a profession that required knowledge distinct from medical knowledge" (Nightingale, 1860). The overall goal of this knowledge has been to explain the practice of nursing as different and distinct from the practice of medicine, psychology, and social work (Chinn and Kramer, 2004).

Theory generates nursing knowledge for use in practice. The integration of theory into nursing practice is the basis for professional nursing (Torres, 1986). Nurses use the nursing process as a means to determine the individual needs of clients. The nursing process is central to the domain of nursing (Meleis, 1997). However, the nursing process is not a theory. It provides the process for the delivery of nursing care, not the knowledge component of the discipline. The process is a systematic approach for nursing care that allows a nurse to apply theory. For example, a theory of caring influences what to assess, how to determine client needs, how to plan care, how to select individualized nursing interventions, and how to evaluate client outcomes. Useful theories are adaptable to different clients and all care settings (see Unit III).

*I*nterdisciplinary Theories

To practice in today's health care systems, nurses need a strong scientific knowledge base from nursing and other disciplines, such as the physical, social, and behavioral sciences. Knowledge from these other disciplines includes relevant theories that explain phenomena. An **interdisciplinary theory** explains a systematic view of a phenomenon specific to the discipline of inquiry, such as Erickson's development theory (see Chapter 11).

Systems Theory

A system is made up of separate components. The parts rely on one another, are interrelated, share a common purpose, and together form a whole. A system has a specific purpose or goal and uses a process to achieve that goal. The content is the product and information obtained from the system.

Input is the information that enters the system. **Output** is the end product of a system. **Feedback** is the process through which the output is returned to the system. Systems can either be open or closed. An open system interacts with its environment, exchanging information between the system and the environment. Factors that change the environment can also have an impact on the system. A closed system is one that does not interact with the environment. An example of a closed system is a chemical reaction occurring under specific conditions.

One example of an open system is the nursing process (Figure 4-3). The purpose of the nursing process is to provide systematic and individualized client care. The process is the five components: assessment, nursing diagnosis, planning, implementation, and evaluation. The content is the information obtained and used from each component. The nursing process is an open system because the nurse applies the process to interact with the client care environment. The nursing process continually changes as the client's nursing needs change. Input to the system comes from the client's assessment data (e.g., how the client interacts with the environment). The output is returned as feedback to the system (e.g., the client's response to nursing interventions designed to assist the

Table 4-1	Chronology of Conceptual Models in Nursing (1952-1989)	
Year of First Major Publication	**Theorist**	**Key Emphasis**
1952	Hildegard E. Peplau	Interpersonal process is maturing force for personality.
1960	Faye G. Abdellah Irene L. Beland Almeda Martin Ruth V. Matheney	Client's problems determine nursing care.
1961	Ida Jean Orlando	Interpersonal process alleviates distress.
1964	Ernestine Weidenbach	Helping process meets needs through art of individualizing care.
1966	Lydia E. Hall	Nursing care is person directed toward self-love.
1966	Joyce Travelbee	Meaning in illness determines how people respond.
1967	Myra E. Levine	Holism is maintained by conserving integrity.
1970	Martha E. Rogers	Person-environment are energy fields that evolve negentropically.
1971	Dorothea E. Orem	Self-care maintains wholeness.
1971	Imogene M. King	Transactions provide a frame of reference toward goal setting.
1974	Sr. Callista Roy	Stimuli disrupt an adaptive system.
1976	Josephine G. Paterson Loretta T. Zderad	Nursing is an existential experience of nurturing.
1978	Madeleine M. Leininger	Caring is universal and varies transculturally.
1979	Jean Watson	Caring is moral ideal: mind-body-soul engagement with another.
1979	Margaret A. Newman	Disease is a clue to preexisting life patterns.
1980	Dorothy E. Johnson	Subsystems exist in dynamic stability.
1981	Rosemarie Rizzo Parse	Indivisible beings and environment co-create health.
1989	Patricia Benner and Judith Wrubel	Caring is central to the essence of nursing. It sets up what matters, enabling connection and concern. It creates possibility for mutual helpfulness.

Used with permission from Chinn PL, Kramer ML: *Integrated knowledge development in nursing,* ed 6, St. Louis, 1999, Mosby, p 42.

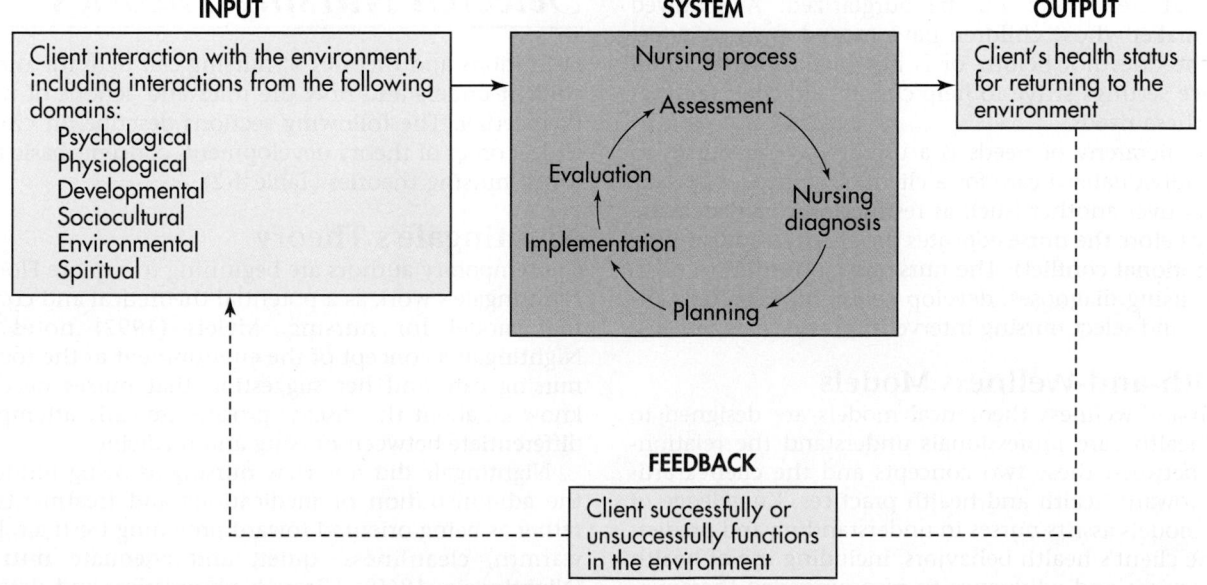

FIGURE **4-3** Nursing process as a system.

client to successfully or unsuccessfully function in the environment).

Nursing theories may have a systems model as the theoretical base. For example, Neuman (1972, 1995) defines a total-person model of wholism and an open-systems approach. As an open system, the person interacts with the environment. The environment is both external and internal, and the person interacts with stressors from the environment that affect the system.

Basic Human Needs

Maslow's hierarchy of needs is an interdisciplinary theory that is useful for designating priorities of care. The hierarchy of basic human needs includes five levels of priority. The most basic, or first, level includes physiological needs, such as air, water, and food. The second level includes safety and security needs, which involve physical and psychological security. The third level contains love and belonging needs, including friendship, social relationships, and sexual love. The fourth level encompasses esteem and self-esteem needs, which involve self-confidence, usefulness, achievement, and self-worth. The final level is the need for self-actualization, the state of fully achieving potential and having the ability to solve problems and cope realistically with life's situations. Maslow's hierarchy is extremely useful to nurses who must continually prioritize a client's nursing care needs. Basic physiological and safety needs are usually the first priority, especially when a client is severely dependent physically. However, the nurse may encounter situations in which a client has no emergent physical or safety needs. Instead, high priority is given to the psychological, sociocultural, developmental, or spiritual needs of the client.

Clients entering the health care system generally have unmet needs. For example, a person brought to an emergency department experiencing acute pneumonia has an unmet need for oxygen, the most basic physiological need. An older woman in a high-crime area may be concerned about physical safety and, while hospitalized, have a need for psychological security because of fear that her home will be burglarized. A widowed homemaker whose children have moved away may feel that she does not belong or is not loved. Nurses in all practice settings strive to help clients and their families meet these needs.

The hierarchy of needs is a useful way for nurses to plan individualized care for a client. One need may take priority over another (such as restoration of an adequate airway before the nurse educates the client in adjusting to an emotional conflict). The nurse uses priorities to organize nursing diagnoses, develop goals and expected outcomes, and select nursing interventions (see Chapter 17).

Health-and-Wellness Models

Health-and-wellness theoretical models are designed to help health care professionals understand the relationships between these two concepts and the client's attitudes toward health and health practices. Knowledge of these models assists nurses in understanding and predicting the client's health behaviors, including use of health care services and adherence to recommended therapies. Chapter 6 includes a variety of models that explain and predict client behavior related to health promotion activities. An understanding of these models is important when meeting the health promotion and disease prevention needs of the client.

Stress and Adaptation

Stress and adaptation are universal and dynamic. Everyone experiences stress and attempts to adapt to life stressors. Stressors and stress responses are physiological and behavioral. As a result, the models that explain the stress response are usually biobehavioral and provide the framework for care of clients experiencing stress. Chapter 30 explains the more prominent theories and demonstrates how these models are used in nursing practice.

Developmental Theories

Human growth and development is an orderly predictive process that begins with conception and continues through death. There are a variety of well-tested theoretical models that describe and predict behavior and development at various phases of the life continuum. Chapter 10 details these theories, and Chapters 11 through 13 demonstrate changes in growth and development in various age-groups.

Psychosocial Theories

Nursing is an eclectic discipline that strives to meet the holistic needs of clients in their physiological, psychological, sociocultural, developmental, and spiritual domains. There are theoretical models that explain and/or predict client responses in each of these domains. For example, Chapter 8 discusses models for understanding cultural diversity and implementing care to meet the diverse needs of the client. Chapter 9 describes family theory and how to meet the needs of the family when the family is the client or when the family is the caregiver. Chapter 29 discusses several models of grieving and demonstrates how to assist the clients through loss, death, and grief.

Selected Nursing Theories

Definitions and theories of nursing can help the nursing student understand how the roles and actions of nurses fit together. The following sections describe, in chronological order of theory development, concepts basic to selected nursing theories (Table 4-2).

Nightingale's Theory

Contemporary authors are beginning to explore Florence Nightingale's work as a potential theoretical and conceptual model for nursing. Meleis (1997) notes that Nightingale's concept of the environment as the focus of nursing care and her suggestion that nurses need not know all about the disease process are early attempts to differentiate between nursing and medicine.

Nightingale did not view nursing as being limited to the administration of medications and treatments but rather as being oriented toward providing fresh air, light, warmth, cleanliness, quiet, and adequate nutrition (Nightingale, 1860). Through observation and data collection, she linked the client's health status with envi-

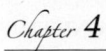

Table 4-2	Summary of Nursing Theories	
Theorist	**Goal of Nursing**	**Framework for Practice**
Nightingale—1860	To facilitate "the body's reparative processes" by manipulating client's environment	Client's environment is manipulated to include appropriate noise, nutrition, hygiene, light, comfort, socialization, and hope.
Peplau—1952	To develop interaction between nurse and client (Peplau, 1952)	Nursing is a significant, therapeutic, interpersonal process (Peplau, 1952). Nurses participate in structuring health care systems to facilitate natural ongoing tendency of humans to develop interpersonal relationships (Marriner-Tomey and Alligood, 2002).
Henderson—1955	To work independently with other health care workers (Marriner-Tomey and Alligood, 2002), assisting client in gaining independence as quickly as possible (Henderson, 1966); to help client gain lacking strength	Nurses help client to perform Henderson's 14 basic needs (Henderson, 1966).
Abdellah—1960	To provide service to individuals, families, and society; to be kind and caring but also intelligent, competent, and technically well prepared to provide this service (Marriner-Tomey and Alligood, 2002)	This theory involves Abdellah's 21 nursing problems (Abdellah and others, 1960).
Rogers—1970	To maintain and promote health, prevent illness, and care for and rehabilitate ill and disabled client through "humanistic science of nursing" (Rogers, 1970)	"Unitary man" evolves along life process. Client continuously changes and coexists with environment.
Orem—1971	To care for and help client attain total self-care	This is self-care deficit theory. Nursing care becomes necessary when client is unable to fulfill biological, psychological, developmental, or social needs (Orem, 2001).
King—1971	To use communication to help client reestablish positive adaptation to environment	Nursing process is defined as dynamic interpersonal process between nurse, client, and health care system (King, 1981).
Neuman—1972	To assist individuals, families, and groups in attaining and maintaining maximal level of total wellness by purposeful interventions	Stress reduction is goal of systems model of nursing practice. Nursing actions are in primary, secondary, or tertiary level of prevention (Neuman, 1972).
Leininger—1978	To provide care consistent with nursing's emerging science and knowledge with caring as central focus (Chinn and Kramer, 2004)	With this transcultural care theory, caring is the central and unifying domain for nursing knowledge and practice.
Roy—1979	To identify types of demands placed on client, assess adaptation to demands, and help client adapt	This adaptation model is based on the physiological, psychological, sociological, and dependence-independence adaptive modes (Roy, 1980).
Watson—1979	To promote health, restore client to health, and prevent illness (Marriner-Tomey and Alligood, 2002)	This theory involves philosophy and science of caring; caring is interpersonal process comprising interventions that result in meeting human needs (Watson, 1979, 1985).
Brenner and Wrubel—1989	To focus on client's need for caring as a means of coping with stressors of illness (Chinn and Kramer, 2004)	Caring is central to the essence of nursing. Caring creates the possibilities for coping and enables possibilities for connecting with and concern for others (Benner and Wrubel, 1989).

Modified from Chinn PL, Kramer ML: *Integrated knowledge development in nursing,* ed 6, St. Louis, 2004, Mosby.

ronmental factors and initiated improved hygiene and sanitary conditions during the Crimean War.

Nightingale provided basic concepts and propositions that could be supported and used for practice in nursing. Nightingale's "descriptive theory" provides nurses with a way to think about nursing with a frame of reference that focuses on clients and the environment. Nightingale's letters and writings direct the nurse to act on behalf of the client. Her principles were visionary and encompassed the areas of practice, research, and education. Most important, her concepts and principles shaped and delineated nursing practice (Alligood and Marriner-Tomey, 2002). Nightingale taught and used the nursing process, noting that "vital observation [assessment] . . . is not for the sake of piling up miscellaneous information or curious facts, but for the sake of saving life and increasing health and comfort."

Peplau's Theory

Hildegard Peplau's theory (1952) focuses on the individual, the nurse, and the interactive process; the result is the nurse-client relationship (Yamashita, 1997). According to this theory, the client is an individual with a felt need, and nursing is an interpersonal and therapeutic process.

Nursing's goal is to educate the client and family and to help the client reach mature personality development (Chinn and Kramer, 2004). The nurse strives to develop a nurse-client relationship in which the nurse serves as a resource person, counselor, and surrogate.

For example, when the client seeks help, the nurse and client first discuss the nature of the problem and the nurse explains the services available. As the nurse-client relationship develops, the nurse and client mutually define the problem and potential solutions. The client gains from this relationship by using available services to meet needs, and the nurse assists the client in reducing anxiety related to the health care problem. Peplau's theory is unique in that the collaborative nurse-client relationship creates a "maturing force" through which interpersonal effectiveness meets the client's needs. When the client's original needs have been resolved, new needs may emerge. The nurse-client interpersonal relationship is characterized by the following overlapping phases: orientation, identification, explanation, and resolution (Chinn and Kramer, 1999).

Henderson's Theory

Virginia Henderson defines nursing as "assisting the individual, sick or well, in the performance of those activities that will contribute to health, recovery, or a peaceful death and that the individual would perform unaided if he or she had the necessary strength, will, or knowledge" (Harmer and Henderson, 1955; Henderson, 1966). The process of nursing strives to do this as rapidly as possible, and the goal is independence. Henderson organized the theory into 14 basic needs of the whole person and includes phenomena from the following domains of the client: physiological, psychological, sociocultural, spiritual, and developmental. Together the nurse and client work in unison to meet these needs and attain client-centered goals.

Abdellah's Theory

The nursing theory developed by Faye Abdellah and others (1960) emphasizes delivering nursing care for the whole person to meet the physical, emotional, intellectual, social, and spiritual needs of the client and family. When using this approach, the nurse needs knowledge and skills in interpersonal relations, psychology, growth and development, communication, and sociology, as well as a knowledge of the basic sciences and specific nursing skills. The nurse is a problem solver and decision maker. The nurse formulates an individualized view of the client's needs, which may occur in the following four areas:
1. Comfort, hygiene, and safety
2. Physiological balance
3. Psychological and social factors
4. Sociological and community factors

Johnson's Theory

Dorothy Johnson's theory of nursing (1968) focuses on how the client adapts to illness and how actual or potential stress can affect the ability to adapt. The goal of nursing is to reduce stress so that the client can move more easily through recovery. According to Johnson, the nurse assesses the client's needs in behavioral subsystems.

Under normal conditions the client functions effectively in the environment. When stress disrupts normal adaptation, however, behavior becomes erratic and less purposeful. The nurse identifies this inability to adapt and provides nursing care to resolve problems in meeting the client's needs.

Rogers' Theory

Martha Rogers (1970) considered the individual (unitary human being) as an energy field coexisting within the universe. The individual is in continuous interaction with the environment and is a unified whole, possessing personal integrity and manifesting characteristics that are more than the sum of the parts (Rogers, 1970). The unitary human being is a "four dimensional energy field identified by pattern and manifesting characteristics that are specific to the whole and which cannot be predicted from the knowledge of parts" (Alligood and Marriner-Tomey, 2002). The four dimensions used in Rogers' theory—energy fields, openness, pattern and organization, and dimensionality—are used to derive principles related to human development.

Orem's Theory

Dorothea Orem (1971) developed a definition of nursing that emphasizes the client's self-care needs. Orem defines self-care as a learned, goal-oriented activity directed toward the self in the interest of maintaining life, health, development, and well-being. The goal of Orem's theory is to help the client perform self-care. According to Orem, nursing care is necessary when the client is unable to fulfill biological, psychological, developmental, or social needs. The nurse determines why a client is unable to meet these needs, what must be done to enable the client to meet them, and how much self-care the client is able to perform. The goal of nursing is to increase the client's ability to independently meet these needs (Orem, 2001).

Neuman's Theory

Betty Neuman's theory (1995) defines a total-person model for nursing, incorporating a wholistic concept and an open-systems approach (Alligood and Marriner-Tomey, 2002). Neuman believes that nursing is concerned with the whole person. The goal of nursing is to assist individuals, families, and groups in attaining and maintaining a maximal level of total wellness (Neuman and Young, 1972). The nurse assesses, manages, and evaluates client systems. Nursing focuses on the variables affecting the client's response to the stressor (Chinn and Kramer, 2004). Nursing actions include the primary, secondary, and tertiary levels of prevention. Primary prevention focuses on strengthening a line of defense through the identification of actual or potential risk factors associated with stressors. Secondary prevention strengthens internal defenses and resources by establishing priorities and treatment plans for identified symptoms, and tertiary prevention focuses on readaptation. The principal goal in tertiary prevention is to strengthen resistance to stressors through client education and to assist in preventing a recurrence of the stress response (Chinn and Kramer, 2004; Alligood and Marriner-Tomey, 2002).

Leininger's Theory

Leininger's cultural care diversity and universality theory (1991) states that care is the essence of nursing and the dominant, distinctive, and unifying feature of nursing. Human caring varies among cultures in its expressions, processes, and patterns. To provide care to clients of unique cultures the nurse selects interventions from one of the following:

- Culture care preservation and maintenance
- Culture care accommodation, negotiation, or both
- Culture care restructuring and repatterning

King's Theory

Imogene King's goal attainment theory (1997) focuses on three dynamic interacting systems: personal, interpersonal, and social. A personal relationship forms between client and nurse. The nurse-client relationship is the vehicle for the delivery of nursing care, which King (1971, 1981) defines as a dynamic interpersonal process in which the nurse and client are affected by each other's behavior, as well as by the health care system. The nurse's goal is to use communication to assist the client in reestablishing or maintaining a positive adaptation to the environment.

Roy's Theory

Sister Callista Roy's adaptation theory (Roy and Obloy, 1979; Roy, 1980, 1989) views the client as an adaptive system. According to Roy's model, the goal of nursing is to help the person adapt to changes in physiological needs, self-concept, role function, and interdependent relations during health and illness (Alligood and Marriner-Tomey, 2002). The need for nursing care arises when the client cannot adapt to internal and external environmental demands. All individuals must adapt to the following demands:

1. Meeting basic physiological needs
2. Developing a positive self-concept
3. Performing social roles
4. Achieving a balance between dependence and independence

The nurse determines what demands are causing problems for a client and assesses how well the client is adapting to them. Nursing care is then directed at helping the client adapt. For example, a postoperative client who has a significant blood loss and now has a low hematocrit value needs nursing interventions designed to assist the client in adapting to the associated fatigue. The nurse may design interventions to allow sufficient rest.

Watson's Theory

Jean Watson's philosophy of transpersonal caring (1979, 1985, 1988) defines the outcome of nursing activity in regard to the humanistic aspects of life (Alligood and Marriner-Tomey, 2002). The action of nursing is directed at understanding the interrelationship between health, illness, and human behavior. Nursing is concerned with promoting and restoring health and preventing illness.

Watson's model is designed around the caring process, assisting clients in attaining or maintaining health or in dying peacefully. This caring process requires that the nurse be knowledgeable about human behavior and human responses to actual or potential health problems, individual needs, how to respond to others, and strengths and limitations of the client and family, as well as those of the nurse. In addition, the nurse comforts and offers compassion and empathy to clients and their families. Caring represents all of the factors the nurse uses to deliver health care to the client (Watson, 1987).

Benner and Wrubel's Theory

The primacy of caring is a model proposed by Patricia Benner and Judith Wrubel (1989). In this model, caring is central. Caring creates possibilities for coping, enables possibilities for connecting with and concern for others, and allows for the giving and receiving of help (Chinn and Kramer, 1999). As defined in this theory, caring means that persons, events, projects, and things matter to people. Caring itself presents a connection (Edwards, 2001). Caring represents a wide range of involvement (e.g., caring about one's family, caring about one's friendships, and caring about one's clients). Benner and Wrubel see the personal concern as an inherent feature of nursing practice. In caring for one's clients, nurses help clients recover by noticing those interventions that are successful and that can guide future caregiving (Edwards, 2001). Chapter 7 describes this theory and other theoretical perspectives on caring within the nursing context.

•••

Application of nursing theory in practice depends on nurses having knowledge of the theories, as well as an understanding of how the theories relate to one another. Theories are the organizing frameworks for the science of nursing and the substantive approaches for nursing care. They provide critical thinking structures to guide clinical reasoning and problem solving.

The Link Between Theory and Knowledge Development in Nursing

Nursing has its own body of knowledge that is both theoretical and practical. Theoretical knowledge includes and "reflects on the basic values, guiding principles, elements, and phases of a conception of nursing" (Meleis, 1997). The goals of theoretical knowledge stimulate thinking and create a broad understanding of the "science" and practices of the nursing discipline.

Practical knowledge is not organized in the same manner as theoretical knowledge. Practical knowledge or the "art" of nursing is based on nurses' experience in providing care to clients. It is achieved through personal knowing gained through reflection on care experiences, synthesis, and integration of the art and science of nursing.

An earlier discussion in this chapter described the types of nursing theories and indicated that theories provided direction to nursing research. The relationships of components in a theory help to drive the research ques-

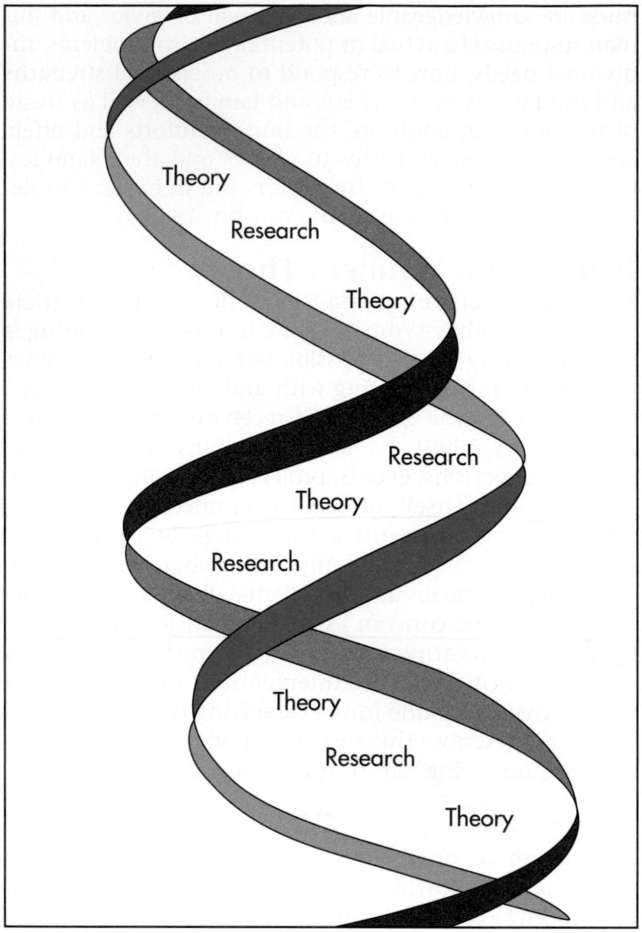

FIGURE **4-4**   Theory-research spiral of knowledge. (Chinn PL, Kramer MK: *Theory and nursing: integrated knowledge development,* ed 5, St. Louis, 1999, Mosby.)

tions for understanding nursing phenomena. For example, the relationship of components within Orem's self-care deficit theory has led nurse researchers to test approaches for their efficacy in improving self-care. The relationship between nursing theory and nursing research helps to build the discipline's knowledge base. As more research is conducted, the discipline learns to what extent a given theory can be useful in providing knowledge that improves client care.

Chinn and Kramer (2004) note that one view of the relationship between research and theory is a spiral (Figure 4-4). This spiral represents the interaction between theory and research and an underlying assumption that research increases nursing's knowledge base. Research is linked to theory in two ways: generation of theory and testing of theory (Fawcett, 1993; Chinn and Kramer, 2004).

Theory-generating research is designed to discover and describe relationships of phenomena without imposing preconceived notions (e.g., hypotheses) of what the phenomena under study mean (Chinn and Kramer, 2004). In theory-generating research, the investigator makes observations with an open mind in order to view a phenomenon in a new way. For example, a researcher may want to understand end-of-life surrogate decision making. In this example, the researcher interviews surrogate decision makers. From these interviews, the researcher would make objective

observations about the surrogate decision-making process, resulting in an initial theory of surrogate decision making.

Theory-testing research is used to determine how accurately a theory describes a nursing phenomenon. The investigator has some preconceived notions as to how the phenomenon is described and generates research questions or hypotheses to test the assumptions of the theory. Using the previous example of surrogate decision making, the researcher may test elements of the theory. For example, interviews of decision makers indicated that more knowledge about end-of-life care expectations was needed. The researcher may then initially test an educational program on end-of-life care for groups of surrogate caregivers. No one study can test all components of a theory; the theory is tested through a variety of research activities.

The result of theory-generating or theory-testing research is to increase nursing's knowledge base. As a result, nurses are able to incorporate research-based interventions into the practice of the discipline (King and Fawcett, 1997). As these research activities continue, not only does the knowledge and science of nursing increase, but also clients are the recipients of best evidence–based nursing practice (see Chapter 5).

As an art, nursing relies on knowledge gained from practice and reflection of past experiences. As a science, nursing draws on scientifically tested knowledge that is applied in the practice setting (Kikuchi, Simmons, and Romyn, 1996). But it is the "expert nurse" who transports the art and science of nursing into the scientific realm of creative caring.

Key Concepts

- Theoretical nursing models provide knowledge to improve practice, guide research and nursing curricula, and identify the domain and goals of nursing practice.
- A theory is a set of concepts, definitions, and assumptions that project a systematic view of a phenomenon by designing specific interrelationships among concepts for the purposes of describing, explaining, predicting, and/or prescribing.
- A nursing theory is a conceptualization of some aspect of nursing communicated for the purpose of describing, explaining, predicting, and/or prescribing nursing care.
- Theories may be classified by levels of abstraction or the goals of the theory.
- Grand theories are the complex structural framework for broad, abstract ideas.
- Middle-range theories are more limited in scope and less abstract. These theories address specific phenomena or concepts and reflect practice.
- A theoretical model refers to global ideas about the individuals, groups, situations, or events of interest to a specific discipline.
- Nursing's paradigm identifies four linkages of interest to the profession: the person, health, environment/situation, and nursing. Nurse theorists agree that these four components are integral to the development of theory.

- Theory is the generation of nursing knowledge used for practice. Process is the method for applying the theory or knowledge. The integration of theory and process is the basis for professional nursing.
- Theories from nursing and other disciplines help the nursing student understand how the roles and actions of nurses fit together in nursing.
- Nursing is an applied discipline with its own body of knowledge that can be theoretical and practical.
- Practical knowledge is achieved through personal knowing, which is achieved through practice, reflection on experiences, synthesis of knowledge, and integration of the art, science, and practice of nursing.
- Theory-generating research is designed to discover and describe relationships without imposing preconceived notions (e.g., hypotheses) of what the phenomenon under study means.
- Theory-testing research is used to determine how accurately a theory describes nursing phenomena.

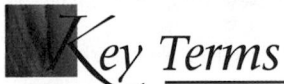 **ey Terms**

Assumptions, *p. 63*	Middle-range theory, *p. 63*
Concepts, *p. 63*	Nursing, *p. 62*
Descriptive theory, *p. 64*	Nursing theory, *p. 62*
Domain, *p. 61*	Nursing's paradigm, *p. 61*
Environment/situation, *p. 62*	Output, *p. 64*
	Paradigm, *p. 61*
Feedback, *p. 64*	Person, *p. 62*
Grand theory, *p. 63*	Phenomenon, *p. 63*
Health, *p. 62*	Prescriptive theory, *p. 64*
Input, *p. 64*	Theoretical model, *p. 64*
Interdisciplinary theory, *p. 64*	Theory, *p. 62*

Critical Thinking Exercises

1. Part of your education includes experiences in different types of health care settings. Take a theory and explain how it might apply in different health care settings.
2. What differences would you expect between the application of the theory in a hospital, skilled care facility, and community-based facility? Would you expect any commonalities?
3. From the following identify those questions you think are theory-generating or theory-testing research. Would you expect that some of these are related to one another, and, if so, how?
    a. Do clients who receive a prescribed exercise program wean quicker from the mechanical ventilator?
    b. What are the perspectives of family members in making end-of-life care decisions for a loved one?
    c. How does a family of divorce perceive their family hardiness?
    d. Do family members who know their loved ones' advance directives have an easier time with end-of-life care?

e. What are the perceptions of clients who wean from mechanical ventilation?
f. How does a family member in a divorced family measure his or her own level of hardiness?
g. Do family members who know their loved ones' advance directives implement these directives during end-of-life care?

Review Questions

1. Nursing identifies its domain in a paradigm that includes:
    1. The person, health, environment/situation, and nursing.
    2. Concepts, theory, health, and environment.
    3. Health, person, environment, and theory.
    4. Nurses, physicians, models, and client needs.

2. Prescriptive theories:
    1. Provide a structural framework for broad abstract ideas.
    2. Describe phenomena.
    3. Reflect practice and address specific phenomena.
    4. Have the ability to explain, relate, and in some situations predict nursing phenomena.

3. A theory is a set of concepts, definitions, relationships, and assumptions that:
    1. Explain a phenomenon.
    2. Formulate legislation.
    3. Measure nursing functions.
    4. Reflect the domain of nursing practice.

4. There is a contemporary move toward nursing science—or evidenced-based practice. This suggests:
    1. Scientists will decide nursing decisions.
    2. Theories are tested and used to describe or predict client outcomes of nursing care.
    3. Nursing will base client care on the practice of medicine, psychology, social work, and other sciences.
    4. One theory will guide nursing practice.

5. To practice in today's health care systems, nurses need a strong scientific knowledge base from nursing and other disciplines, such as the physical, social, and behavioral sciences. This is an example of which of these:
    1. Developmental theories.
    2. Health and wellness models.
    3. Systems theories.
    4. Interdisciplinary theories.

6. Knowledge of these assist nurses in understanding and predicting the client's health behaviors, including use of health care services and adherence to recommended therapies:
    1. Systems theories.
    2. Interdisciplinary theories.
    3. Stress and adaptation models.
    4. Health-and-wellness models.

7. These theories begin with conception and continue through death in an orderly process:
   1. Stress and adaptation theories.
   2. Systems theories.
   3. Developmental theories.
   4. Interdisciplinary theories.

8. Maslow's hierarchy of needs is useful to nurses who continually prioritize a client's nursing care needs. The most basic or first-level needs include:
   1. Esteem and self esteem needs.
   2. Self-actualization.
   3. Love and belonging.
   4. Air, water, and food.

9. Leininger's theory of cultural care diversity and universality specifically addresses:
   1. Caring for clients from unique cultures.
   2. Caring for client's who cannot adapt to internal and external environmental demands.
   3. Understanding of the humanistic aspects of life.
   4. Variables affecting a client's response to a stressor.

10. As an art, nursing relies on knowledge gained from practice and reflection of past experiences. As a science, nursing draws on:
    1. Scientifically tested knowledge that is applied in the practice setting.
    2. Physician generated research.
    3. Experimental research.
    4. Nonexperimental research.

*R*eferences

Abdellah FG and others: *Patient-centered approaches to nursing,* New York, 1960, Macmillan.

Alligood MR, Marriner-Tomy A: *Nursing theory: utilization and practice,* ed 2, St. Louis, 2002, Mosby.

American Nurses Association: *Nursing's social policy statement,* Washington, DC, 1995, The Association.

Benner P, Tanner C: How expert nurses use intuition, *Am J Nurs* 87(1):23, 1987.

Benner P, Wrubel J: *The primacy of caring: stress and coping in health and illness,* Menlo Park, Calif, 1989, Addison-Wesley.

Carnevali DL, Thomas MD: *Diagnostic reasoning and treatment decision making in nursing,* Philadelphia, 1993, JB Lippincott.

Chinn PL, Kramer MK: *Integrated knowledge development in nursing,* ed 6, St. Louis, 2004, Mosby.

Edwards S: Benner and Wrubel on caring in nursing, *J Adv Nurs* 33(2):167, 2001.

Fawcett J: *Analysis and evaluation of conceptual models of nursing,* ed 3, Philadelphia, 1995, FA Davis.

Fawcett J: *The relationship of theory and research,* ed 3, Philadelphia, 1999, FA Davis.

Fawcett J and others: On nursing theories and evidence, *J Nurs Scholarsh* 33(2):115, 2001.

Harmer D, Henderson V: *Textbook of the principles and practice of nursing,* ed 5, Riverside, NJ, 1955, Macmillan.

Henderson V: *The nature of nursing,* New York, 1966, Macmillan.

Johnson DE: Theory in nursing: borrowed and unique, *Nurs Res* 11:206, 1968.

Kikuchi JF, Simmons H, Romyn D: *Truth in nursing inquiry,* Thousand Oaks, Calif, 1996, Sage Publications.

King IM: *Toward a theory for nursing,* New York, 1971, John Wiley & Sons.

King IM: *Toward a theory for nursing: systems, concepts, process,* New York, 1981, John Wiley & Sons.

King IM: King's theory of goal attainment in practice, *Nurs Sci Q* 10(4):180, 1997.

King IM, Fawcett J: *The language of nursing theory and metatheory,* Sigma Theta Tau International, Indianapolis, 1997, Center Nursing Press.

Leininger MM: *Culture care diversity and universality: a theory of nursing,* Pub No. 15-2402, New York, 1991, National League for Nursing Press.

Marriner-Tomey A, Alligood MR: *Nursing theorists and their work,* ed 5, St Louis, 2002, Mosby.

Meleis AI: *Theoretical nursing: development and progress,* ed 3, Philadelphia, 1997, JB Lippincott.

Neuman B: *The Neuman systems model,* ed 3, Norwalk, Conn, 1995, Appleton & Lange.

Neuman BM, Young RJ: A model for teaching total person approach to patient problems, *Nurs Res* 21:264, 1972.

Nightingale F: *Notes on nursing: what it is and what it is not,* London, 1860, Harrison & Sons.

Orem DE: *Nursing: concepts of practice,* New York, 1971, McGraw-Hill.

Orem DE: *Nursing: concepts of practice,* ed 6, New York, 2001, McGraw-Hill.

Peplau HE: *Interpersonal relations in nursing,* New York, 1952, GP Putnam's Sons.

Rogers ME: *An introduction to the theoretical basis of nursing,* Philadelphia, 1970, FA Davis.

Rogers ME: Nursing: science of unitary, irreducible, human beings: update 1990. In Barrett EAM, editor: *Visions of Rogers's science-based nursing,* Pub No. 15-2285, New York, 1990, National League for Nursing.

Roy C: The Roy adaptation model. In Riehl JP, Roy C, editors: *Conceptual models for nursing practice,* New York, 1980, Appleton-Century-Crofts.

Roy C: The Roy adaptation model. In Riehl JP, Roy C, editors: *Conceptual models for nursing practice,* ed 3, New York, 1989, Appleton-Century-Crofts.

Torres G: *Theoretical foundations of nursing,* Norwalk, Conn, 1986, Appleton-Century-Crofts.

Watson J: *Nursing: the philosophy and science of caring,* Boston, 1979, Little, Brown.

Watson J: *Nursing: human science and human care,* Norwalk, Conn, 1985, Appleton-Century-Crofts.

Watson J: *Nursing: human science, human care: a theory of nursing,* Pub No. 15-2236, New York, 1988, National League for Nursing.

*R*esearch References

Mishel MH: Uncertainty in illness, *Image J Nurs Sch* 20(4):225, 1988.

Mishel MH: Reconceptualization of the uncertainty in illness theory, *Image J Nurs Sch* 22(4):256, 1990.

Mishel MH: Uncertainty in acute care, *Annu Rev Nurs Res* 15:57, 1997.

Mishel MH; Sorenson DS. Uncertainty in gynecological cancer: a test of the mediating functions of mastery and coping, *Nurs Res* 40(3):167, 1991.

Roy C, Obloy SM: The practitioner movement: toward a science of nursing, *Am J Nurs* 79:1698, 1979.

Swanson K: Empirical development of a middle-range theory of caring, *Nurs Res* 40(3):161, 1991.

Watson J: Nursing on the caring edge: metaphorical vignettes, *ANS Adv Nurs Sci* 10(1):10, 1987.

Yamashita M: Family caregiving: application of Neuman's and Peplau's theories, *J Psychiatr Ment Health Nurs* 4(6):401, 1997.

5

Nursing Research as a Basis for Practice

http://evolve.elsevier.com/Potter/fundamentals/

Media Resources

CD COMPANION

- Review Questions
- Glossary

evolve WEBSITE

- Review Questions
- Student Learning Activities
- Glossary

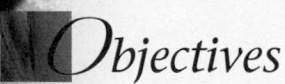

Objectives

Mastery of content in this chapter will enable the student to:

- Define the key terms listed.
- Compare the various ways to acquire knowledge.
- List the characteristics of scientific investigation.
- Define nursing research.
- Explain how nursing research can improve nursing practice.
- Discuss the steps of the research process.
- Discuss priorities for nursing research.
- Explain how the rights of human research subjects are protected.
- Discuss methods of locating research reports in nursing and related areas.
- Explain how to organize information from a research report.
- Describe the process of research utilization.

*H*ealth care is continually changing in the way nurses organize and deliver care to clients. For this reason, nursing knowledge must continuously grow and expand to keep nursing care approaches relevant, current, and appropriate. Without new knowledge, nursing cannot improve techniques for therapies such as infant care, pain management, grief counseling, or client education. One important source of new knowledge is research. Research provides a solid foundation on which nurses base their practice. The scientific knowledge base for professional nursing practice is developed through scholarly inquiry of the research literature, use of existing research findings, and the actual conduct of research.

Research means to search again or to examine carefully (Langford, 2001). Through the use of a systematic process that asks and answers questions that generate knowledge, the research process provides a scientific basis for nursing practice and validates the effectiveness of nursing interventions.

The International Council of Nurses (ICN) (1986) supports the need for nursing research as a means for improving the health and welfare of people. **Nursing research** is a way to identify new knowledge, improve professional education and practice, and use resources effectively. The National Center for Nursing Research (NCNR) and the ICN periodically update the broad priorities for nursing research. These priorities promote an in-depth knowledge base for nursing practice, recognize nursing research as an integral aspect of nursing practice and education, facilitate cross-cultural research, and encourage nursing associations to establish ethical research standards (NCNR/ICN, 1990). Research-based practice is essential if the nursing profession is to meet the needs of society for safe, effective, and efficient care (American Nurses Association, 1997).

Historical Perspective

Nursing leaders and organizations have made considerable efforts to increase nurses' awareness of the importance of nursing research as a foundation for practice. The conduct of nursing research has its roots with Florence Nightingale, who observed in detail the effects of nursing actions, such as the impact of nutrition and hygiene, during the Crimean War (Polit and Beck, 2004). Her work was the first to study the clinical care of clients. In the 1920s, nurse researchers conducted educational research to understand the preparation of educators, administrators, and public health nurses and the clinical experiences of nursing students. The results were published in the Goldmark report, which identified gaps in nursing education. As a result, more university-based nursing curricula were implemented.

In the 1950s, there was an increase in the number of nurses with advanced degrees, and the journal *Nursing Research* was initiated. This was the first journal dedicated to nursing research, and it was written for a broad nursing audience. In the 1960s several professional nursing organizations initiated development of nursing research priorities. The Lysaught report recommended increases in research toward nursing practice and nursing education. During the 1970s nursing studies tended to focus on the roles and characteristics of nurses rather than on problems in delivering professional care to clients. During this time more nurses were receiving doctoral preparation and initiating their own research, and more nursing research journals were published.

In 1981 the American Nurses Association (ANA) published recommendations for studying research at the different nursing education levels, which have since been updated and refined (ANA, 1997). In 1993 the National Institute of Nursing Research (NINR) was established. The NINR (2000) supports:

> Clinical and basic research to establish a scientific basis for the care of individuals across the life span—from management of clients during illness and recovery to the reduction of risks for disease and disability, the promotion of healthy lifestyles, promoting quality of life in those with chronic illness, and care for individuals at the end of life. This research may also include families within a community context. According to its broad mandate, the Institute seeks to understand and ease the symptoms of acute and chronic illness, to prevent or delay the onset of disease or disability or slow its progression, to find effective approaches to achieving and sustaining good health, and to improve the clinical settings in which care is provided. Nursing research involves clinical care in a variety of settings, including the community and home in addition to more traditional health care sites. The NINR's research extends to problems encountered by clients, families, and caregivers. It also focuses on the special needs of at-risk and underserved populations, with an emphasis on health disparities.

Nurse researchers meet to develop research priorities for the NINR. The current research priorities of the NINR are listed in Box 5-1.

An ongoing trend for nursing research is outcomes research. Outcomes research in nursing is research designed to assess and document the effectiveness of health care services (Polit and Beck, 2004). For example, studying the effects of an outpatient education program on the ability of older adult clients to follow a nutrition and exercise program is an outcome study. This type of research represents a response of the health care industry to the increased demand from policy makers, insurers, and the public to justify care practices and systems in terms of im-

---

Box 5-1   Examples of National Institute of Nursing Research Priorities

Chronic Illnesses or Conditions

Chronic illness self-management and quality of life

Behavioral Changes and Interventions

Decreasing low-birth-weight infants among minority populations
Enhancing health promotion among minority men

Responding to Compelling Public Health Concerns

End of life: bridging life and death
Nursing research training and centers

Data from National Institute of Nursing Research: *National Institute of Nursing Research, 2004 areas of research opportunity,* Bethesda, Md, 1997, National Institutes of Health, http://www.nih.gov/ninr/research/dea/2004AoRo.html.

---

proved client outcomes and costs (Hinshaw, Feetham, and Shaver, 1999; Polit and Beck, 2004).

Nursing research also has the support of professional and specialty organizations. In 2003, the ANA (2003) revised the *Standards of Nursing Practice*. Within this document are the Standards of Professional Performance (see Chapter 1). Standard XIII recommends that the professional nurse use research findings in practice (ANA, 2003). In addition to the ANA, nursing specialty organizations recommend that nurses incorporate research findings into clinical practice to restore health, prevent illness, manage symptoms, and minimize the effects of acute and chronic disease and disability (ANA, 2003).

Scientific Research in Nursing

Acquisition and application of new knowledge is essential in contributing to nursing practice. The expansion of technology, changes in the health care delivery system, and aging of the population all require nurses to apply research findings to identify and solve clinical nursing problems and issues.

Knowledge Acquisition

One hallmark of a mature discipline is the development of multiple research methods designed to develop a knowledge base unique to the discipline (Barrett, 1998). Although acquired in many ways, knowledge is information, and discovery is the creative process of obtaining new knowledge. A person continuously takes in information, and, through the process of critical thinking, evaluates numerous pieces of information to understand experiences.

Tradition. One way of acquiring knowledge is by tradition. One generation of nurses passes knowledge to the next. In nursing, certain traditional methods of practice, such as the change-of-shift report, methods for securing an intravenous (IV) dressing, and other daily hospital work practices, are passed from one practitioner to the next. Tradition is an efficient way of learning, although it can also limit the ability to seek new ways of doing things. If tradition becomes so ingrained that a person does not question the practice, other, more appropriate or research-based approaches may be overlooked.

Information Seeking. Knowledge is also acquired by seeking information from experts in a particular field. Experts are often asked to solve problems or answer questions. For example, nursing students often seek the advice of instructors and practicing nurses when assessing and caring for clients. Expert nurses are able to share their personal knowledge and experiences in caring for clients with a wide range of clinical problems. Authority, like tradition, is not infallible, although it is commonly treated as absolute truth.

Another method of seeking information is by investigating knowledge from other disciplines, such as physiology. For example, by using Selye's model of general adaptation, the nurse is able to use knowledge and apply it to clinical situations in which the client is experiencing stress. As a result, nursing interventions are designed to assist the client in reducing the stress response (see Chapter 30).

Experience. Knowledge is also based on experience. Without experience-based knowledge a person would have to relearn a procedure every time it was performed or how to establish a nurse-client relationship. Practice leads to the development of routines that help build skills. For example, a student nurse taking a blood pressure measurement for the first time may feel awkward and unsure of hearing the sounds, but with practice the student's confidence, technique, and interpretation of findings improve. Although experience is an important way of learning, it has limitations. A person may continue to do something simply because it was learned that way and may overlook improved or other ways of doing the same thing.

Problem Solving. Learning by problem solving is yet another way of gaining knowledge. Trying various ways of resolving clients' health care needs, developing new staffing patterns, or evaluating health care products are examples of problem solving. This method of learning is practical, but it is unsystematic and often a haphazard way of learning. In nursing, because clients' health status depends on nursing actions, the problem-solving method may lead toward specific research questions.

Critical Thinking. The nurse uses the skills of critical thinking to analyze information acquired through traditional learning, information seeking, experiential learning, investigating ideas from other disciplines, and problem solving to determine a course of nursing action (see Chapter 14). In addition, the nurse can use the skills of critical thinking to identify and investigate a clinical, professional, or educational issue.

Scientific Method

The **scientific method** is the foundation of research. Scientific research is the most reliable and objective of all methods of gaining knowledge. This method is an advanced, objective means of acquiring and testing knowledge. It guides the nurse in the utilization of research findings in practice as well as in conducting research.

When using research findings to add to or change practice, the nurse must understand the process the researcher used to guide the research. For example, when a nurse considers whether to change how to insert a feeding tube it is important to know if a newly recommended procedure was tested on similar clients and what were the beneficial results. The scientific method is a systematic step-by-step process. As the nurse reviews research articles, the article must include a clear description of the problem, research method, and research findings.

The researcher uses the scientific method to understand, explain, predict, or control a nursing phenomenon (Polit and Beck, 2004). The method is characterized by systematic, orderly procedures that, although not without fault, seek to limit the possibility for error. In addition, the scientific method minimizes the likelihood that any bias or opinion by the researcher might influence the results of research and thus the knowledge gained. Polit and Beck (2004) describe the characteristics of scientific research as follows:

- The problem area or what needs to be studied is identified.
- The steps of planning and conducting an investigation are undertaken in a systematic, orderly fashion.
- Researchers attempt to control external factors that are not under direct investigation but that can influence a relationship between phenomena they are studying. For example, if a nurse were studying the relationship between diet and heart disease, other characteristics such as stress or smoking history would have to be controlled for contributing factors to this disease.
- Evidence that is part of experience (**empirical data**) is gathered directly or indirectly through use of observations and assessments and is the basis for discovering new knowledge.
- The goal is to understand phenomena in such a way that the knowledge gained can be applied generally, not just to isolated cases or circumstances.

Nursing and the Scientific Approach

Nurses in all client care settings must pursue knowledge by taking the time to review research and practice findings, critique research studies, and discuss with colleagues the implications when new knowledge is not used in practice. The scientific method is a systematic approach to generate questions and test knowledge.

Compared with other ways of acquiring knowledge, the scientific method is more orderly and objective in its approach. In the past, much of the information used in nursing practice was borrowed from other disciplines such as biology, physiology, psychology, and sociology. Often this information was applied to nursing without testing or comparing ways of caring for clients. For example, nurses use several methods to help clients sleep. Interventions such as giving a client a back rub, making sure that the bed is clean and comfortable, preparing the environment by dimming the lights, and talking to a worried or anxious client are frequently used nursing measures and, in general, are logical, commonsense approaches. However, when these measures are considered in greater depth, questions may arise about their applications. For example, are they the best methods to promote sleep? Do different clients in different situations require other interventions to promote sleep?

Research provides a way for nursing questions and problems to be studied in greater depth within the context of nursing. Frequently nurses rely on personal experience or the statements of nursing experts. If an intervention works for most clients, the nurse may be satisfied with this success without questioning whether there might be a better way. If the intervention is not successful, the nurse might use an approach practiced by a colleague or try a different sequence of accepted measures. Even if an intervention discovered with this approach is effective for one or more clients, it may not be appropriate for other clients in other settings. Nursing interventions must be tested through nursing research to determine the measures that work best with specific clients.

Nursing Research

Nursing research addresses issues that are important to the discipline of nursing. For example, some of these issues relate to the profession itself, education of nurses, client and family needs, and issues within the health care delivery system. Once research is completed it is important to disseminate or communicate the findings. One method of dissemination is through publication of the findings in professional journals.

When reading the results of research studies, nurses should not interpret results in terms of cause and effect because there is a difference between cause-and-effect and other kinds of relationships. For example, as people get older, they tend to lose their hair, and their skin becomes wrinkled. These factors are related to each other as part of the aging process, but neither causes the other. In contrast, research studies on the side effects of chemotherapeutic agents have shown that a majority of these agents do cause hair loss and some skin changes. Researchers often study such relationships without being able to determine why or how these changes take place.

Nurses are interested in acquiring knowledge about a wide range of human needs and responses to health problems. Nursing research uses many methods to study clinical problems (Box 5-2). There are two broad approaches to research: quantitative and qualitative methods (Table 5-1).

Quantitative Research. **Quantitative nursing research** is the investigation of nursing phenomena that lend themselves to precise measurement and quantification. For example, pain severity, rate of wound healing, and body temperature changes can be quantitatively measured. Quantitative research is the rigorous, systematic,

---

| Box 5-2 | Types of Research |

Historical Research

Systematic studies designed to establish facts and relationships concerning past events (Polit and Beck, 2004)

Exploratory Research

Initial study designed to develop or refine the dimensions of phenomena or to develop or refine a hypothesis about the relationships among phenomena (Polit and Beck, 2004)

Evaluation Research

Study that tests how well a program, practice, or policy is working

Descriptive Research

Study in which the objective is to accurately portray characteristics of persons, situations, or groups and the frequency with which certain events or characteristics occur

Experimental Research

Study in which the investigator controls the study variable and randomly assigns subjects to different conditions

Correlational Research

Study that explores the interrelationships among variables of interest without any active intervention by the researcher

---

objective examination of specific concepts. Quantitative research focuses on numerical data, statistical analysis, and controls to eliminate bias in findings (Knapp, 1998; Polit and Beck, 2004). Although there are many quantitative methods, the following sections briefly describe experimental, survey, and evaluation research.

Experimental Research. The hallmark of scientific research is the experiment. In a true **experimental study,** the conditions under which a treatment or measure is investigated are tightly controlled. Experimental approaches to studying a problem require that the information about human subjects be collected and quantified in a prescribed manner. For example, a nurse wants to study the relationship between postoperative anxiety and preoperative teaching. In this example, the problem under study is postoperative anxiety and the treatment is preoperative teaching.

The study usually includes a control or comparison group, which does not receive the treatment being investigated. The results for this group are compared with those of the study or experimental group—the group that receives some form of treatment. The **subjects**—persons selected for the comparison and experimental groups—are chosen at random from among those eligible for the study. Random selection of subjects gives all eligible subjects the same chance to be in the control or experimental (treatment) group and eliminates sampling bias. Using the pre-

Table 5-1	Comparison of Quantitative and Qualitative Research	
Concept	**Quantitative Term**	**Qualitative Term**
Focus	Focus on a small number of clearly identified problems	Attempts to understand a phenomenon or experience
Person contributing information	Subject	—
	Study participant	Study participant
	Respondent	Informant, key informant
Area of investigation	—	Phenomena
	Concepts	Concepts
	Constructs	—
	Variables	—
System of organizing concepts	Theory, theoretical framework	Theory
	Conceptual framework, conceptual model	Conceptual framework
Information gathered	Data (numerical value)	Data (narrative descriptions)
Connection between concepts	Relationships—cause and effect, functional	Patterns of association
Quality of the evidence	Reliability	Dependability
	Validity	Credibility
	Generalizability	Transferability
	Objectivity	Confirmability

Data from Polit DF, Beck CT: *Nursing research: principles and methods,* ed 7, Philadelphia, 2004, JB Lippincott.

viously cited example, the subjects under study are clients undergoing surgery. The control group will be clients who do not receive preoperative teaching, and the treatment group includes clients who do receive the teaching. Each subject will be randomized into one of the two groups. Therefore each subject has a 50-50 chance of being in the treatment group.

Designing an experiment to study physical causes of disease is less difficult than designing an experiment that also includes psychological or social aspects of health. There are generally too many variables to consider in psychosocial studies. For example, in the study to examine the relationship between postoperative anxiety and preoperative teaching, the researcher can control one psychological factor by using only subjects having surgery for the first time. However, the researcher cannot control all of the other experiences that the clients may have had, such as hearing a friend's "horror" stories about surgery or reading about surgical experiences in the newspapers. These psychological factors, which cannot be controlled, may influence the subject's level of anxiety.

Surveys. Surveys are commonly used in quantitative research. **Surveys** are designed to obtain information from populations regarding the prevalence, distribution, and interrelation of variables within the study population (Polit and Beck, 2004). An example is a survey designed for a descriptive study to measure nurses' perceptions of physicians' willingness to collaborate in practice. Surveys may be conducted for the general purposes of obtaining information about practices, opinions, attitudes, and other characteristics of people (Knapp, 1998). For example, the most basic function of a survey is description. Surveys can gather a large amount of data to describe the population being studied, as well as the topic of study. It is important in survey research that the population sampled is large enough to keep sampling error at a minimum. The survey items used in questionnaires and interviews must be constructed carefully and pretested to determine correctness in style, ease of use, and appropriateness for the research question.

Evaluation Research. **Evaluation research** is a form of quantitative research that involves finding out how well a program, practice, procedure, or policy is working (Polit and Beck, 2004). Ultimately, the purpose of evaluation research is to determine the success of a program.

For example, a health center in a rural community develops a 5-year health initiative program to improve dental care of its preschool and school-age residents (ages 3 to 14). The dental program includes educational programs in the elementary schools, well-baby clinics, and prenatal clinics. In addition, each child receives two dental examinations each year. These examinations include dental cleaning, x-ray films, and follow-up treatment for tooth decay. Some of the overall outcomes of this study may include (1) improved overall oral hygiene practices, as evidenced by decreases in plaque and tarter, (2) reduced amount of tooth decay, and (3) reduced number of "missed" appointments to the dental clinic for oral hygiene and treatment.

Evaluation research can determine specifically why a program or some components of the program were successful or unsuccessful. When programs are unsuccessful, evaluation research can assist in identifying problems with the program and opportunities for change, why it was not successful, or even barriers to implementation of programs.

•••

Nursing studies use many quantitative methods for investigating clinical problems; some may be similar to the experimental approach. Other research methods may be similar to those used in the social sciences, such as anthropology and sociology. The amount of knowledge about the problem and the type of problem being investigated are factors that determine the methods used. Nursing is a practice discipline that deals with unique physical, emotional, and social problems that people experience in regaining, maintaining, and promoting health.

Qualitative Research. Qualitative nursing research is the investigation of phenomena that are not easily quantified or categorized. This method is used to describe information obtained in a nonnumeric form (e.g., data in the form of written transcripts from a series of interviews). Qualitative research involves inductive reasoning used to develop generalizations or theories from specific observations or interviews (Morse and Field, 1995; Polit and Beck, 2004). Qualitative research involves the discovery and understanding of important characteristics and the ways that they might be related. For example, a qualitative research study might involve an interview measuring clients' perceptions of mechanical ventilation (Wunderlich and others, 1999).

When qualitative methods are used, the investigator can use one of several design strategies. Ethnography involves the description and interpretation of cultural behavior (Polit and Beck, 2004). For example, a researcher will study the behaviors of residents suffering Alzheimer's disease within a nursing home. This type of research is closely associated with the field of anthropology, which focuses on the culture of a study population.

Phenomenology is a research method with roots in philosophy (Polit and Beck, 2004) with a focus on what people experience in regard to daily practices or experiences and how they interpret those experiences. For example, an investigator may want to study the impact of surrogate decision making regarding end-of-life decisions (Jeffers, 1998).

Grounded theory is a method of collecting and analyzing qualitative data with the aim of developing theories and theoretical propositions that are grounded in real-world observations (Polit and Beck, 2004). For example, in studying weaning from mechanical ventilation, Wunderlich and others (1999) interviewed clients who were successfully weaned from mechanical ventilation. As a result of these interview data, the investigators noted that social support was the most important factor that assisted clients in being weaned from mechanical ventilation.

Research Process

The **research process** consists of an orderly series of phases or steps that allow the researcher to move from asking the research question to finding the answer (Figure 5-1) (Langford, 2001). Usually the answer to the initial research question suggests new questions and areas of further study. The research process is used to gain knowledge that can be used in other, similar situations. Nurses may want to gain knowledge about the reason why a particular event happens or the best way to provide care for clients with a certain health problem. The research process is used to gain knowledge that can be repeatedly applied to a whole group or class of clients.

The research process usually consists of the following: problem identification, study design, conducting the study, data analysis, and use of the findings (Table 5-2). Initially the researcher identifies an area of inquiry (identifying a problem), which may result from clinical practice. For example, a nurse notices that many clients seem to have a difficult time sleeping the night before discharge following open-heart surgery. Based on work with these clients, the nurse determines that most of them have concerns about their activity tolerance and pain in the home care setting. The nurse reviews the relevant literature to determine what is known about postoperative activity level and pain immediately following open-heart surgery. After reviewing the literature, the researcher notes that many clients report poor activity tolerance and pain control. However, there is limited research on nursing interventions to improve these areas.

Following identification of the problem and review of the literature, the researcher will design the study protocol. In this example, the nurse might design a research study in which some of the clients receive the standard discharge planning and others receive an additional discharge planning intervention for activity tolerance and pain control. In this study the sample will include all first-time open-heart surgical patients who are having an aortic valve repair. The subjects in this study cannot be on preoperative pain medication for arthritis, cancer, or other chronic painful conditions. Each subject will be randomized to one of the two groups. The control group will receive standard discharge planning, whereas the experimental or treatment group will receive the standard discharge planning plus the additional intervention for activity tolerance and pain control. Each subject will have a 50-50 chance of being in each group. The researcher will also select appropriate instruments to measure postoperative pain and activity tolerance. In the study design the researcher has noted that all subjects will be followed in the same manner with regard to postoperative home care, follow-up appointments, and physical examinations.

The researcher will then conduct the study. Before conducting any study with human subjects, appropriate approvals must be obtained from the agency's human subject committee. Additional approvals from the agency in which the study is to be conducted may also be needed. The researcher will consistently collect all data from the subjects as indicated in the study design protocol. Each subject will receive the designated (e.g., control or treatment) discharge planning and all other postoperative care.

The researcher analyzes the results after collecting all information from the two groups studied. The results of both groups are compared to determine whether clients who received the new discharge interventions had improved activity levels and pain control when compared with clients receiving only standard discharge planning. If the clients receiving the new care slept better, had better pain control, and reported adequate activity toler-

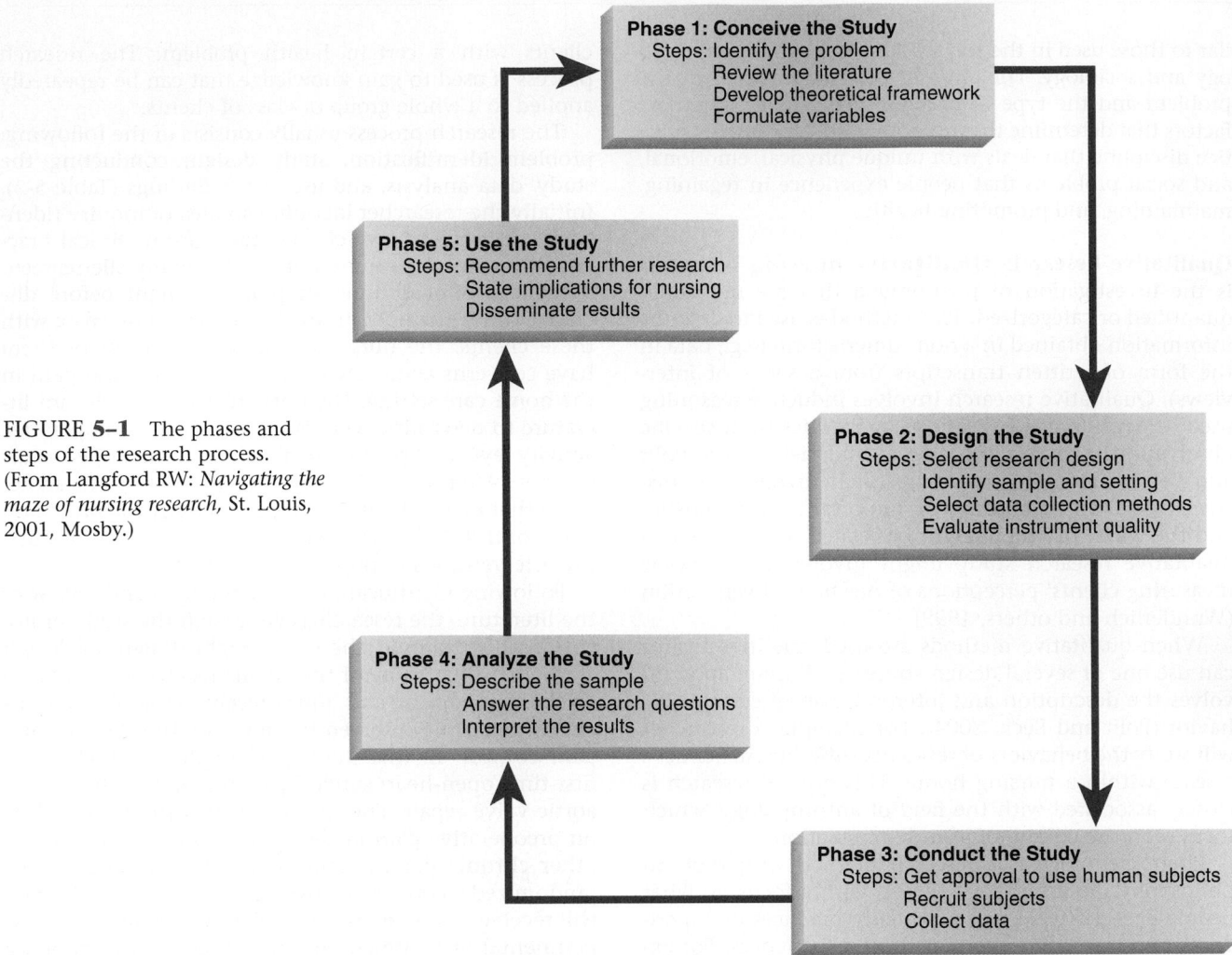

FIGURE **5-1** The phases and steps of the research process. (From Langford RW: *Navigating the maze of nursing research,* St. Louis, 2001, Mosby.)

Phase 1: Conceive the Study
Steps: Identify the problem
Review the literature
Develop theoretical framework
Formulate variables

Phase 2: Design the Study
Steps: Select research design
Identify sample and setting
Select data collection methods
Evaluate instrument quality

Phase 3: Conduct the Study
Steps: Get approval to use human subjects
Recruit subjects
Collect data

Phase 4: Analyze the Study
Steps: Describe the sample
Answer the research questions
Interpret the results

Phase 5: Use the Study
Steps: Recommend further research
State implications for nursing
Disseminate results

Table 5-2	Research Process
Nursing Process	**Research Process**
Problem identification	Identify area of interest or clinical problem: • Review the literature. • Formulate the theoretical framework. • Identify study variables. • Devise research question(s)/hypotheses.
Study design	Design the study protocol: • Select research design/methodology. • Identify sample population: number, recruitment, assignment to groups. • Select data collection methods. • Select instrumentation: questionnaires, physiological measures, interviews, treatments. • Formulate proposed analysis: statistical methods to answer the research questions/hypotheses.
Conducting the study	Obtain necessary approvals. Recruit subjects. Implement the study protocol/collect data: • Pilot study may be done initially. • Continually assess study methodology. Is study consistently carried out? Are all investigators following the study protocol?
Data analysis	Analyze the results of the study: • Interpret demographics of study population. • Analyze each research questions/hypothesis. • Interpret the results, including conclusions, limitations.
Use of the findings	Formulate recommendations for further research. Determine implications for nursing. Disseminate the findings: presentations, publications, research utilization.

ance, the nurse has acquired new knowledge about how generally to help first-time postoperative open-heart clients with an aortic valve repair.

However, this may be a first-time study and the results are not ready for use for all clients discharged after an aortic valve repair. The researcher must address limitations of the study. For example, was the sample size adequate, were there any subjects who did not complete the research? Were there large differences in the client's ages, home caregivers and family, or postoperative medications?

The implications for nursing practice are also important. In this study, the nurses may determine that all open-heart clients should receive the expanded discharge planning instruction. They will then do follow-up phone calls with these clients to determine their levels of postoperative activity tolerance and pain control.

Conducting Nursing Research

In 1997 the ANA published a position statement on the educational preparation for participation in nursing research. In this document, the ANA (1997) noted that all nurses share a "commitment to the advancement of nursing science and the ethical conduct of nursing science."

Nurses conduct research in a variety of settings. Student nurses and clinicians may be asked to participate in studies that investigate client outcomes and the effectiveness of nursing care. These types of research projects are commonly called quality assurance or improvement studies (see Chapter 19). Data are collected on clinical problems or care processes in a particular clinical setting. Because the results of such research are usually applicable only in a specific setting, this is not scientific research as discussed earlier. However, such research is important to the institution because the nursing department can use it to demonstrate the contributions made by nurses to client care.

Clinical nursing research should be undertaken by nurses educated to conduct scientific investigations (Figure 5-2). An experienced researcher is usually more qualified than a beginning researcher to undertake a complex, long-term project. Nurses new to research may, however, make important contributions by assisting with data collection, conducting replicated studies (studies

previously performed elsewhere), or conducting less complex studies.

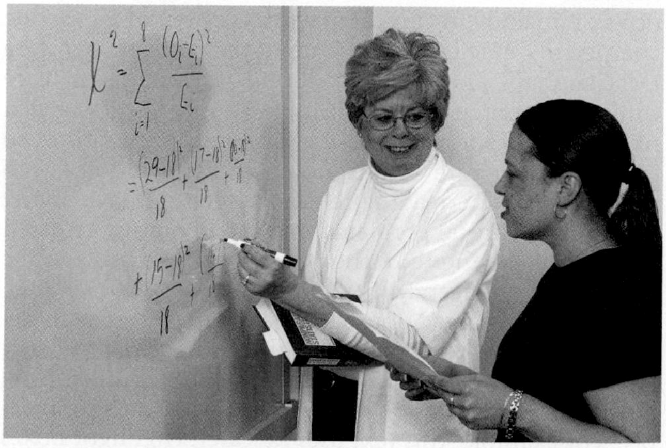

Research Preparation. The preparation of nurse scientists, who have primary responsibility for the conduct of research, is begun at the master's level and is concentrated at the doctoral and postdoctoral levels. However, the ANA's position paper (1997), which describes the participation of nurses in research according to their academic preparation, does include research activities for nurses with various levels of academic preparation.

Associate Degree in Nursing. Nurses with an associate degree are prepared to participate in research activities (1) through identification of clinical problems in nursing practice; (2) by assisting with organized data collection; and (3) in conjunction with nurses holding more advanced credentials, appropriately using research findings in clinical practice.

Baccalaureate Degree in Nursing. Nurses with a baccalaureate degree are prepared to read research critically and use existing standards to determine the readiness of the findings for clinical practice. In addition, nurses with this preparation participate in research activities (1) through identification of clinical problems in nursing practice, (2) by assisting experienced investigators in gaining access to clinical sites, (3) by influencing the selection of appropriate methods of data collection, and (4) by collecting data and implementing nursing research findings.

Master's Degree in Nursing. Nurses with a master's degree are prepared to be active members of a research team. This level of preparation allows nurses to assume the role of clinical expert and be able to create a climate in which research-based change can be implemented into practice. Master's-prepared nurses assume leadership roles in creating an environment for nursing research and integrating the findings into clinical practice.

Doctoral Education. Nurses are prepared to contribute to nursing knowledge through the conduct of research aimed at advancing the scientific basis of nursing practice. Doctorally prepared nurses are prepared to design studies independently, as well as collaborate with other clinicians and researchers in conducting studies. Doctorally prepared nurses are responsible for acquiring funding for research from public and private sources.

Ethical Issues in Research

The conduct of research must meet ethical standards in which the rights of human subjects are protected. In addition, other research participants (e.g., health care professionals, teachers, and students) also have rights as research participants.

Rights of Human Subjects

To refine existing knowledge and develop new knowledge, clinical research is sometimes directed at trying new

FIGURE **5–2** Nurses collaborating on research.

procedures whose outcomes are doubtful or unknown (e.g., a new wound treatment or a new approach in counseling pregnant adolescents) (ANA, 1995). This kind of research may conflict with the purpose of nursing practice, which is to meet specific clients' needs. In such cases the researcher is responsible for structuring the investigation to avoid or minimize harm to the subjects. Although it is not always possible to anticipate all potential undesirable effects, researchers are obligated to inform everyone involved about the known potential risks.

Informed Consent. Informed consent means that research subjects (1) are given full and complete information about the purpose of the study, procedures, data collection, potential harm and benefits, and alternative methods of treatment; (2) are capable of fully understanding the research and the implications of participation; (3) have the power of free choice to voluntarily consent or decline participation in the research; and (4) understand how confidentiality or anonymity is maintained.

Confidentiality guarantees that any information provided by the subject will not be reported in any manner that identifies the subject and will not be made accessible to people outside the research team (Polit and Beck, 2004). **Anonymity** occurs when even the researcher cannot link the subject to the data (Polit and Beck, 2004). The subject is assured of voluntary participation in giving consent, including the right to withdraw from the study at any time (Polit and Beck, 2004). Procedures for obtaining informed consent must be outlined in the study protocol.

Within the consent document, the investigator must outline in lay language the purpose of the study, the role of the subjects, types of data that are to be obtained, how the data are obtained, the duration of the study, subject selection, procedures, risks to the subject (including financial risks), potential benefits (including the possibility of no benefit), alternatives to participation, and contact information concerning the principal investigator and local institutional review board. This consenting process is done to provide subjects with complete information regarding the study's risks, benefits, and costs.

The Health Information Portability and Accountability Act (HIPAA). HIPAA went into effect in April of 2003. The federal law provides the first comprehensive federal protection for the privacy of health information (HIPAA Advisory, 2003). The privacy rule requires health care institutions to take reasonable steps to limit the use or disclosure of protected health information to the minimum necessary to protect clients. In the case of research, institutions now have HIPAA regulations that identify how protected health information of potential research subjects is to be managed. For example, if a study involves collection of research subjects' names, medical histories, and demographic data, the researcher will have to acquire authorization from the subjects to use that information. In addition, the researcher must be able to ensure that the data will be protected and used only by the researcher.

Box 5-3   Requirements Governing Institutional Review Board Decisions

Risks to participants are minimized.

Risks to participants are reasonable in relation to anticipated benefits.

Listing of potential benefits to subjects, acknowledging the possibility of no benefit, is provided in the consent form.

Selection of participants is equitable.

Informed consent will be sought, as required.

Informed consent will be appropriately documented.

Adequate provision is made for monitoring the research to ensure the safety of participants.

Appropriate provisions are made to protect the privacy of participants and the confidentiality of data.

When vulnerable subjects are involved, appropriate additional safeguards are included to protect their rights and welfare.

Data from Code of Federal Regulations: *Protection of human subjects,* 45CFR46 (1983, revised as of March 1993), Washington, DC, 1993, U.S. Department of Health and Human Services.

HIPAA has broad implications for how research studies will be designed and the steps needed to acquire subject consent.

Institutional Review Board. Federal regulations (Code of Federal Regulations, 1993) require that institutions receiving any federal funding or conducting drug or medical device research regulated by the Food and Drug Administration establish institutional review boards (IRBs). Such groups review all studies conducted in the institution to ensure that ethical principles (see Chapter 21) are observed. A major responsibility of an IRB is to determine the risk status of all research projects (Box 5-3).

Applying Research to Nursing Practice

Research evidence as a basis for scholarly, professional decision making in clinical practice is essential to provide competent, efficient, and state-of-the art nursing care (McCaughan and others, 2002). Advances in care through research are meaningless unless they reach nurses at the point of care. Linking research findings to direct nursing care results from scholarly inquiry into practices through reading relevant literature, identifying appropriate clinical problems, and incorporating research utilization activities into the nursing practice of a specific nursing unit or agency (Dufault, 2001).

Nurses must read journals that contain research reports, as well as textbooks and other sources, in nursing and related fields. Within these resources, findings from research studies may be suitable for use in nursing practice. For example, this text uses Research Highlight boxes

Research Highlight   Box 5-4

End of Life and Advance Directives

Research Focus

In recent years, there has been an increased focus on end-of-life decisions and the use of medical technology. It is not well documented in the literature whether or not and to what extent clients' advance directives are used for directing resuscitative efforts.

Research Abstract

The purpose of this descriptive study was to determine how useful clients' advance directives were to members of the health care team in determining treatment and end-of-life decisions among clients who received cardiopulmonary resuscitation (CPR) efforts. In addition, the researchers wanted to know what percentage of clients who experienced a cardiopulmonary arrest had meaningful and clear advance directives and what interventions occurred during CPR that were or were not addressed in the client's advance directive. This descriptive study was conducted in a large tertiary care medical center. A retrospective chart review of 135 adult clients who had undergone CPR efforts within the previous year was conducted to determine if and to what extent advance directives were useful in directing end-of-life care and treatment decisions. Only 35 of these clients had advance directives. Three categories for advance directives emerged: those that were "independently directive," clear directives as to what the client wanted and did not want done; those that were "vague and required further clarification," either from the family or friend; last, those that were "nondirective." Information from this study may be used to clarify treatment options for end-of-life care and to determine if and what further interventions are required to ensure that advance directives can be executed as meaningful documents.

Evidence-Based Practice

- Discussion of advance directives not only increases opportunities for the client and family to discuss issues, but more importantly provides an opportunity for the client to communicate his or her wishes.
- Nurses are active advocates for clients making decisions for advance directives.
- Nurses provide empathetic advocacy and support to family members who carry out their loved one's advance directives.
- The total health care team is responsible for implementing a client's advance directives.
- The total health care team can support one another and family caregivers when implementing a client's advance directives.

Reference

Gilbert M and others: Determining the relationship between end-of-life decisions expressed in advanced directives and resuscitation efforts during cardiopulmonary resuscitation, *Outcomes Manag Nurs Pract* 5(2):87, 2001.

---

to illustrate how research can progress from the phase of clinical problem investigation to application in day-to-day client care situations. To use findings in clinical practice, the nurse must be aware of the problems already studied, be able to identify and understand relevant research studies, and be able to determine which findings are applicable to his or her client's needs.

Biomedical research is concerned primarily with discovering the causes and treatments of disease. In contrast, nursing research focuses on the full range of human responses in health and illness and is directed toward helping well people improve their health status and stay healthy, as well as assisting clients who are sick or disabled in maintaining or improving their health. For example, the effect of preoperative teaching on postoperative recovery is an area that has been studied extensively. Some studies have examined the effect of preoperative teaching on positive postoperative outcomes (Meeker, 1994; Planchock and Wiggins, 1994). Timmons and Bower (1993) examined the effect of preoperative teaching on clients' understanding of patient-controlled analgesia and their management of postoperative pain. The group receiving preoperative education managed their pain significantly better. Teaching clients what they can expect on the day of surgery and in the immediate postoperative period is now a widely accepted and implemented nursing measure.

Research Report Versus Clinical Article

When reading health care literature, the nurse must distinguish a research report or article from other types of writing. This may not be as simple as it seems. Even if the title has the word *research* in it, the article does not necessarily report the results of a research study. The nurse can determine whether an article reports a research study only by examining its contents. Sometimes, however, an article's title can give a clue to its contents. Phrases such as "a study of" or "comparison of" suggest a research report. The abstract and the introductory paragraphs of an article can also indicate whether the article is based on research.

An **abstract** is a short summary of the purpose of a study, the subjects included in the research, the way the study was conducted, and the results obtained in the investigation (Box 5-4). An abstract is often quite brief and does not contain all of the essential information in the article. The first few paragraphs of the article should provide further clues about whether it describes a research study. Phrases such as "the purpose of this study was" and "this research was carried out to determine" are indications that the article is a research report. If the article describes only the author's experience with a particular aspect of nursing care, it probably is not a research article. In addition to the abstract, a typical research report has the following parts:

- *Introduction section:* An introductory section presenting the purpose, a summary of literature used to formulate the study, the hypotheses tested, or the research questions posed
- *Methods section:* Description of the methods used to conduct the study, including the sample (what or who was studied), type of data collected, including the device or instrument used to measure empirical information
- *Results section:* Description of the results obtained in the study, including appropriate statistical tests used to analyze data
- *Discussion section:* Presentation of the author's interpretation of the results, including conclusions and implications that can be drawn from the study
- *Reference list:* Articles used to support the study

If the report is written by one of the researchers in the study, it is a **primary source.** Any other article about the study is considered a **secondary source** (e.g., an article in which the author was not directly involved in conducting the study but collected the information from a primary or another secondary source). Most nursing textbooks are secondary sources of information. Authors of these texts incorporate knowledge and information gathered from nursing and related literature, including research written by original investigators.

The fact that a report is a primary source does not guarantee its accuracy, which depends on the ability of researchers to be scientific, impersonal, and impartial in conducting studies. However, a primary source does report firsthand knowledge, whereas a secondary source may include another person's interpretation of the original work.

Locating Research Studies

Nurses often need to find research articles on subjects that interest them. In the health care field a number of resources are useful when searching the literature for research articles.

To locate primary research sources related to a particular subject, the first source is the journals where original research reports are usually published. The most efficient way to locate research articles is to consult a computerized database or an index of journal articles, such as the *Cumulative Index to Nursing and Allied Health Literature (CINAHL), International Nursing Index, MEDLINE,* or *PubMed.*

Major nursing journals publish research studies or research reports. Some journals, such as *Nursing Research,* are devoted solely to research; other nursing journals, such as the *American Journal of Critical Care,* also publish original reports of research studies. Specialty practice journals publish research articles devoted to the particular specialty.

Identifying Clinical Nursing Problems

Diers (1979) defined a **clinical nursing problem** as "a difference between two states of affairs, a discrepancy between the way things are and the way they ought to be, or between what one knows and what one needs to know to eliminate the problem." The following questions are raised by this definition:

- Given the nursing interventions recommended for clients with a particular health care problem, how might the suggested care be improved so that the results or outcomes of care are better?

- Given the knowledge about how to provide nursing care, what additional information would be needed to plan new interventions for clients with a particular health care problem?

Unanswered questions and the desire to improve nursing practice can provide the stimulus for conducting a research study.

Experience can make it possible to identify a researchable clinical nursing problem, but a nurse does not need to have years of clinical practice to identify a nursing problem. Sometimes a person who is relatively new in a situation can more easily see how things could be improved than those who have more experience and who take present conditions for granted. The nurse also considers whether the problem frequently occurs in a particular client group, whether it can be consistently and accurately measured, and whether a possible nursing solution might change the way care is delivered.

Sometimes nursing students or practicing nurses think that their ideas about nursing problems for study are not worthwhile unless they are certain that the proposed clinical study would make a radical change in client care. However, research efforts also may have to refine ideas about a clinical problem before the investigator can test alternative nursing interventions. In fact, some nurse researchers think that more investigative work needs to be conducted to describe the client response before research is designed to test an alternative intervention. In addition, the researcher may have to devise correct ways for measuring results before the study can proceed. All of these factors may discourage a nurse from undertaking a nursing research project. On the other hand, such projects can be viewed as stimulating challenges because much information has yet to be scientifically tested for its relevance to nursing practice.

Research Utilization

Not all research related to clinical nursing problems can or should be applied in practice. The nurse must judge the scientific worth of a study before considering its use in practice. This chapter can provide only a foundation for judging the worth of a research study. Other aspects that should be considered follow (Stetler, 1994, 2001; Stetler and DiMaggio, 1991):

- The amount of supportive evidence provided by other scientific studies that have obtained similar results
- Determination of whether the subjects and environment in the study are similar to the clients for whom the nurse provides care in the particular practice setting
- The theoretical basis for present nursing care and the effectiveness of current theory in solving clinical nursing problems
- The feasibility of applying findings, including ethical and legal limitations; institutional policy; changes in the organization of nursing services that might be required; and potential costs in time, money, and equipment

The nurse must take specific steps to make judgments that involve validating the scientific soundness of a study, comparatively evaluating whether any use can be made of the findings, and deciding the type of application that would be appropriate (Box 5-5).

Box 5-5	**Steps for Successful Research Utilization**

1. *Relevance*—Topic/problem needs to be relevant to the nursing and administrative staff participating in the utilization project.
   a. Identify and gather research studies appropriate to the clinical problem.
   b. Critique the research studies.
   c. Determine the merit of each study in terms of applicability to clinical practice.
   d. Develop a specific practice innovation based on research findings of studies critiqued.
   e. Apply the practice innovation to a defined clinical population.
   f. Determine outcomes of the innovation.
   g. Evaluate outcomes of the innovation for widespread use.
2. *Education*—Prepare method to educate and inform staff about the research utilization process.
3. *Support*—Determine necessary support resources (e.g., librarian, university faculty, doctorally prepared researchers) to streamline and assist in the process.
4. *Expectation*—Create a climate that utilization of research findings in a practice setting is expected.
5. *Alignment*—Set goals for research utilization, implementation of change, and the educational process.
6. *Reward*—Acknowledge the work of others in utilizing research findings; build activities into career building.
7. *Caring*—Emphasize state-of-the-art nursing care, the impact on the client and family, and acknowledge impact on the total care provided by the staff, not just the people active in the research utilization project.
8. Continue to incorporate the innovation into daily client care routine.

Data from Maljanian R: Supporting nurses in their quest for evidence-based practice: research utilization and conduct, *Outcomes Manag Nurs Pract* 4(4):155, 2000; and Feldman HR: Strategies for teaching nursing research: teaching baccalaureate nursing students, *West J Nurs Res* 18:479, 1996.

Box 5-6	**Barriers to Research Utilization in a Health Care Organization**

- Lack of time to investigate research findings
- Lack of support from administration to implement new practices
- Existing nursing culture (e.g., ritualistic care, no authority to change practice, lack of incentive to change practice, and reluctance of staff to change practice)
- Poor team-building and team-working skills
- Financial constraints
- Shortage in professional nursing staff
- Rising acuity rates
- Limited interest in utilization of research findings
- Perception that research is an intimidating process

Data from Maljanian R: Supporting nurses in their quest for evidence-based practice: research utilization and conduct, *Outcomes Manage Nurs Pract* 4(4):155, 2000; Walsh M: Barriers to research utilization and evidence based practice in A & E nursing, *Emerg Nurse* 5(2):24, 1997; and Carroll DL and others: Barriers and facilitators to the utilization of nursing research, *Clin Nurse Spec* 11(5):207, 1997.

When implementing **research utilization** in practice, it must be remembered that the problem area chosen must have an established research base in the literature, be relevant to practice, and be reliably evaluated by nurses in clinical settings. When selecting the problem area, the nurse first determines whether a solid research base exists for changing practice, the scientific merit of the studies that constitute the research base, and the potential risk to the client in implementing the practice change. The final phases include developing a clinical protocol that can be used to implement the change and clinically evaluating the outcomes of the new nursing care to determine its effectiveness.

Nurses should not change from accepted to unproven ways of providing client care without careful deliberation and consultation with colleagues. Experimenting with new nursing measures is inappropriate, especially if an increased risk to clients' health is possible.

Evidence-based practice (EBP) incorporates critical thinking and research utilization competencies (Stetler and others, 1998). The research utilization skills enable the nurse to systematically transfer or translate research-based knowledge into the clinical practice setting (Kajermo and others, 2001). EBP recognizes that the best evidence available may not be research based. But it is important to acknowledge the evidence of clinical experts in the field. Integration of evidence-based practice is essential to provide competent, safe nursing care.

Evidence-based practice and *research-based* practice are terms often used interchangeably (see Chapter 2). However, research-based practice refers to the use of knowledge based on systematic research studies, while evidence-based practice also takes into account a nurse's clinical experience, practice trends, and even individual client preferences (Stevens, 2001; Barnsteiner and Prevost, 2002).

Evidence-based nursing practice demphasizes ritual, isolated and unsystematic clinical experiences, ungrounded opinion, and tradition as a basis for nursing practice. It stresses the use of research findings, and as appropriate, quality improvement data, other evaluation data, and the consensus of recognized experts and affirmed experience to support a specific practice (Stetler and others 1998).

Barriers to Research Utilization. Nursing has long been urged to base care on research findings rather than tradition and ritual. The rapid growth of doctorally prepared nurse researchers has enabled the scientific base for nursing practice to grow. There are, however, barriers to utilization of research in clinical settings. Sitzia (2001) and Funk, Tournquist, and Champagne (1995), among others, have tried to identify some of these barriers. Barriers such as those listed in Box 5-6 limit the potential of identifying clinical outcomes of nursing care. However, recognizing and acknowledging the existence of these barriers enable nurses to implement change in practice in a timelier manner.

•••

Nursing research improves the practice of nursing and raises the standards for the profession. Involvement in nursing research takes place in many ways: designing studies, being part of a research team, collecting data, using research findings to change clinical practice, improving client outcomes, and maintaining the cost of health care (Titler and others, 1994). Promoting research and research utilization in practice increases the scientific knowledge base for nursing practice. The recipients of these improvements to practice are the consumers of nursing care.

Key Concepts

- Knowledge is acquired through tradition, from authorities in a field, through experience, through problem solving and critical thinking, and through application of the scientific method.
- The research process is an orderly, planned, and controlled way of studying a problem in clinical practice, nursing education, or nursing administration.
- Nursing research is conducted to study the physical or psychosocial responses of people of all ages in health and illness.
- An experimental research study controls factors that could influence the results, includes comparison and experimental treatment groups of subjects, and uses random means for selecting study subjects.
- A qualitative study organizes information in narrative format so that phenomena can be described and patterns of relationships can be discovered.
- Participation of human subjects in research studies requires the researcher to obtain informed consent of study subjects, to maintain the confidentiality of subjects, and to protect subjects from undue risk or injury.
- When summarizing data reported in a research study, the nurse should note when, how, where, and by whom the investigation was conducted and who and what were studied.
- A researchable clinical nursing problem is one that is not satisfactorily resolved by present nursing interventions, occurs frequently in a particular group, can be consistently and accurately measured, and has a possible solution within the realm of nursing practice.
- To determine whether research findings can be used as a basis for nursing practice, the nurse should consider the scientific worth of the study, the substantiating evidence provided in other studies, the similarity of the research setting to the nurse's own clinical practice setting, the status of current nursing theory, and factors affecting the feasibility of application.

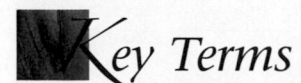

Key Terms

Abstract, *p. 83*	Nursing research, *p. 74*
Anonymity, *p. 82*	Primary source, *p. 84*
Biomedical research, *p. 83*	Qualitative nursing
Clinical nursing problem,	research, *p. 77*
p. 84	Quantitative nursing
Confidentiality, *p. 82*	research, *p. 79*
Empirical data, *p. 76*	Research process, *p. 79*
Evaluation research, *p. 78*	Research utilization, *p. 85*
Evidence-based practice,	Scientific method, *p. 76*
p. 85	Secondary source, *p. 84*
Experimental study, *p. 77*	Subjects, *p. 77*
Informed consent, *p. 82*	Surveys, *p. 78*

Critical Thinking Exercises

1. The nurse is concerned about learning to properly clean a pressure ulcer. Explain the benefits to the client if the nurse learns how to clean the sore by the scientific method versus trial and error.
2. If you wished to determine the best method for cleaning a pressure ulcer, how would you approach this problem?
3. You have noticed an increase in client falls. What method would you use to determine the exact number of falls in a specific time period? How would you determine which clients are falling? How could you use nursing research to implement an intervention for fall prevention? How would you determine the success or failure of the intervention?

Review Questions

1. The conduct of nursing research has its roots with:
    1. Florence Nightingale.
    2. The American Nurses Association.
    3. The National Institute of Nursing Research.
    4. The Goldmark report.

2. The first journal dedicated to nursing research is:
    1. Standards of Clinical Nursing Practice.
    2. Nursing Research.
    3. Goldmark report.
    4. The National Institute of Nursing Research.

3. Tradition is an efficient way of learning, although it also can limit the ability to seek new ways of doing things when:
    1. A person does not question the practice.
    2. A client is experiencing stress.
    3. It is treated as absolute truth.
    4. A client is disinterested in learning new things.

4. The foundation of research is based on:
   1. Experience.
   2. Problem solving.
   3. Critical thinking.
   4. Scientific method.

5. The hallmark of scientific research is the:
   1. Experiment.
   2. Survey.
   3. Evaluation.
   4. Literature review.

6. Persons selected for comparison and experimental research groups are known as the:
   1. Subjects.
   2. Control group.
   3. Researchers.
   4. Experimental group.

7. Nursing studies use many research methods. The method chosen depends on:
   1. The preference of the researcher.
   2. The amount of knowledge known about the problem.
   3. The latest healthcare issue.
   4. The availability of other research studies.

8. Qualitative nursing research is the investigation of phenomena that are:
   1. Not easily quantified.
   2. Easily categorized.
   3. Obtained in a numerical form.
   4. Developed through deductive reasoning.

9. The preparation of nurse scientists, who have primary responsibility for the conducting of research, is begun at the master's level and is concentrated at the doctoral and postdoctoral levels. However:
   1. Only doctorally prepared nurses identify a problem to be studied.
   2. Only doctorally prepared nurses conduct the study.
   3. Only master's prepared nurses apply research findings to practice.
   4. ANA's position paper (1997) describes and includes research activities for nurses.

10. Although it is not always possible to anticipate all potential undesirable effects, researchers are obligated to inform everyone involved about the known potential risks. This is an example of:
   1. Confidentiality.
   2. Anonymity.
   3. Informed consent.
   4. Autonomy.

References

American Nurses Association: *Standards of nursing practice,* ed 3, Washington DC, 2003, The Association.

American Nurses Association: *Position statement: educational preparation for participation in nursing research,* Washington, DC, 1997, The Association.

American Nurses Association: *Ethical guidelines in the conduct, dissemination, and implementation of nursing research,* Washington, DC, 1995, The Association.

Barnsteiner J, Prevost S: How to interpret evidence-based practice: some tried and true pointers, *Reflect Nurs Leadersh* 28(2):18, 2002.

Carroll DL and others: Barriers and facilitators to the utilization of nursing research, *Clin Nurse Spec* 11(5):207, 1997.

Code of Federal Regulations: *Protection of human subjects,* 45CFR46 (1983, revised as of March 1993), Washington, DC, 1993, U.S. Department of Health and Human Services.

Diers D: *Research in nursing practice,* Philadelphia, 1979, JB Lippincott.

Feldman HR: Strategies for teaching nursing research: teaching baccalaureate nursing students, *West J Nurs Res* 18:479, 1996.

Gilbert M and others: Determining the relationship between end-of-life decisions expressed in advanced directives and resuscitation efforts during cardiopulmonary resuscitation, *Outcomes Manag Nurs Pract* 5(2):87, 2001.

Hinshaw AS, Feetham SL, Shaver JL: *Handbook of clinical nursing research,* Thousand Oaks, Calif, 1999, Sage Publications.

HIPPA Advisory: *General overview of standards for privacy of individually identifiable health information,* http://www.hipaadvisory.com/regs/finalprivacymod/goverview.htm.

International Council of Nurses: *Nursing research: ICN position statement,* Geneva, 1986, The Council.

Knapp TR: *Quantitative nursing research,* Thousand Oaks, Calif, 1998, Sage Publications.

Langford, RW: *Navigating the maze of nursing research,* St. Louis, 2001, Mosby.

Maljanian R: Supporting nurses in their quest for evidence-based practice: research utilization and conduct, *Outcomes Manag Nurs Pract* 4(4):155, 2000.

McCaughan D and others: Acute care nurses' perceptions of barriers to using research information in clinical decision making, *J Adv Nurs* 39(1):46, 2002.

Morse JM, Field PA: *Qualitative research methods for health professionals,* ed 2, Thousand Oaks, Calif, 1995, Sage Publications.

National Center for Nursing Research/International Council of Nurses: *Nursing research worldwide: report of the Task Force on International Nursing Research,* Geneva, Switzerland, 1990, The Association.

National Institute of Nursing Research: *National Institute of Nursing Research, 2003 areas of research opportunity,* Bethesda, Md, 1997, National Institutes of Health, http://www.nih.gov/ninr/research/dea/2003AoRo.html.

National Institute of Nursing Research: *National Institute of Nursing Research mission statement,* Bethesda, Md, 2000, National Institutes of Health, http://www.nih.gov/ninr/research/diversity/mission.html.

Polit DF, Beck CT: *Nursing research: principles and methods,* ed 7, Philadelphia, 2004, JB Lippincott.

Sitzia J: Barriers to research utilization: the clinical setting and nurses themselves, *Eur J Oncol Nurs* 5(3):154, 2001.

Stetler CB: Refinement of the Stetler/Marram model for application of research findings to practice, *Nurs Outlook* 42(1):15, 1994.

Stetler CB: Updating the Stetler model of research utilization to facilitate evidence-based practice, *Nurs Outlook* 49(6):272, 2001.

Stetler CB, DiMaggio G: Research utilization among clinical nurse specialists, *Clin Nurs Spec* 5(3):151, 1991.

Stetler CB and others: Evidence-based practice and the role of nursing leadership, *J Nurs Adm* 28(7/8):45, 1998.

Stevens K: Systematic reviews: the heart of evidence-based practice, *AACN Clin Issues* 12(4):29, 2001.

Titler MG and others: Infusing research into practice to promote quality care, *Nurs Res* 43(50):307, 1994.

Walsh M: Barriers to research utilization and evidence based practice in A & E nursing, *Emerg Nurse* 5(2):24, 1997.

*R*esearch *References*

Barrett EAM: Unique nursing research methods: the diversity chant of pioneers, *Nurs Sci Q* 11(3):94, 1998.

Dufault MA: A program of research evaluating the effects of collaborative research utilization model, *Online J Knowl Synth Nurs* 8(3):7, 2001.

Feldman HR: Strategies for teaching nursing research: teaching baccalaureate nursing students, *West J Nurs Res* 18:479, 1996.

Funk SG, Tournquist EM, Champagne MT: Barriers and facilitators of research utilization: an integrative review, *Nurs Clin North Am* 30(3):395, 1995.

Gilbert M and others: Determining the relationship between end-of-life decisions expressed in advance directives and resuscitation efforts during cardiopulmonary resuscitation, *Outcomes Manag Nurs Pract* 5(2):87, 2001.

Jeffers BR: Research for practice: the surrogate's experience during treatment decision making, *Medsurg Nurs* 7(6):357, 1998.

Kajermo KN and others: Nurses' experiences of research utilization within the framework of an educational programme, *J Clin Nurs* 10(5):671, 2001.

Maljanian R: Supporting nurses in their quest for evidence-based practice: research utilization and conduct, *Outcomes Manag Nurs Pract* 4(4):155, 2000.

Meeker BJ: Preoperative education: evaluating postoperative patient outcomes, *Patient Educ Couns* 23(1):41, 1994.

Planchock NY, Wiggins MV: Preoperative assessment and teaching: physiological and psychological preparation, *Semin Perioper Nurs* 3(2):61, 1994.

Timmons ME, Bower FL: The effect of structured preoperative teaching on patients' use of patient-controlled analgesia (PCA) and their management of pain, *Orthop Nurs* 12(1):23, 1993.

Wunderlich R and others: Patients' perceptions of uncertainty and stress during weaning from mechanical ventilation, *Dimens Crit Care Nurs* 18(1):2, 1999.

Health and Wellness

Media Resources

http://evolve.elsevier.com/Potter/
fundamentals/

 CD COMPANION

- Review Questions
- Glossary

evolve WEBSITE

- Review Questions
- Student Learning Activities
- Glossary

Objectives

Mastery of content in this chapter will enable the student to:

- Define the key terms listed.
- List the two general *Healthy People 2010* public health goals for Americans.
- Discuss the definition of health.
- Discuss the health belief, health promotion, basic human needs, and holistic health models to understand the relationship between the client's attitudes toward health and health practices.
- Describe variables influencing health beliefs and practices.
- Describe health promotion, wellness, and illness prevention activities.
- Discuss the three levels of preventive care.
- Describe four types of risk factors.
- Discuss risk factor modification and changing health behaviors.
- Describe variables influencing illness behavior.
- Describe the impact of illness on the client and family.
- Discuss the nurse's role in health and illness.

In the past, most individuals and societies viewed good health, or wellness, as the opposite or absence of disease. This simple attitude ignores states of health between disease and good health. Health is a multidimensional concept and must be viewed from a broader perspective. An assessment of the client's state of health is an important aspect of nursing.

Models of health offer a perspective to understand the relationships between the concepts of health, wellness, and illness. Nurses are in a unique position to assist clients in achieving and maintaining optimal levels of health. Nurses understand the challenges of today's health care system and embrace the opportunity to use wellness activities to promote health and wellness and prevent illness. In an era of cost containment and advanced technology, nurses can be a vital link to the improved health of individuals and society. Nurses can identify actual and potential risk factors that predispose a person or a group to illness. In addition, the nurse may use risk factor modification strategies to promote health and wellness and prevent illness.

When illness does occur, different attitudes about illness cause people to react in different ways to illness or the illness of a family member. Medical sociologists call the reaction to illness, **illness behavior.** Nurses who understand how clients react to illness can minimize the effects of illness and assist clients and their families in maintaining or returning to the highest level of functioning.

Healthy People Documents

In 1979 an influential document, *Healthy People: The Surgeon General's Report on Health Promotion and Disease Prevention,* was published. This report introduced national goals for improving the health of Americans by 1990. It outlined priority objectives for preventive services, health protection, and health promotion that addressed improvements in health status, risk reduction, public and professional awareness of prevention, health services and protective measures, and surveillance and evaluation. The report served as a framework for the 1990s as the United States began to focus more on health promotion and disease prevention instead of illness care. The strategy announced by the Secretary of Health and Human Services required a cooperative effort by government, voluntary and professional organizations, businesses, and individuals. Widely cited by popular media, in professional journals, and at health conferences, it has inspired health promotion programs throughout the country.

The next document, published in 1990, *Healthy People 2000: National Health Promotion and Disease Prevention Objectives,* identified health improvement goals and objectives to be reached by the year 2000 (U.S. Department of Health and Human Services [USDHHS], 1990). Research has shown dramatic progress in improving the nation's health (Burggraf and Barry, 2000). For example, since the 2000 initiatives, infant mortality has declined, childhood vaccinations have risen to an all time high, and the death rate from coronary heart disease and stroke have declined.

Healthy People 2010 is the latest document and is designed to serve as a road map for improving the health of all people in the United States for the first decade of the twenty-first century (USDHHS, 1998). This newest edition emphasizes the link between individual health and community health and the premise that the health of communities determines overall health status of the nation. The two overarching goals for *Healthy People 2010* are (1) to increase quality and years of healthy life and (2) to eliminate health disparities (USDHHS, 1998). The 2010 document includes 28 focus areas with 467 objectives (www.health.gov/healthypeople). The document is divided into four areas: (1) promoting healthy behaviors, (2) promoting healthy and safe communities, (3) improving systems for personal and public health, and (4) preventing and reducing diseases and disorders.

Definition of Health

Defining health is difficult. The World Health Organization (WHO) defines **health** as a "state of complete physical, mental and social well-being, not merely the absence of disease or infirmity" (WHO, 1947). Many other aspects of health need to be considered. Health is a state of being that people define in relation to their own values, personality, and lifestyle. Each person has a personal concept of health. Pender, Murdaugh, and Parsons (2002) define health as the actualization of inherent and acquired human potential through goal-directed behavior, competent self-care, and satisfying relationships with others, while adjustments are made as needed to maintain structural integrity and harmony with the environment.

Individuals' views of health can vary among different age-groups, gender, race, and culture (Pender, 1996; Pender, Murdaugh, and Parsons, 2002). Pender (1996) explains that "all people free of disease are not equally healthy." Pender, Murdaugh, and Parsons (2002) note that views of health have broadened to include mental, social, and spiritual well-being, as well as a focus on health at the family and community levels.

To help clients identify and reach health goals, the nurse must discover and use information about their concepts of health. Pender, Murdaugh, and Parsons (2002) suggest that for many people, conditions of life rather than pathological states are what define health. Life conditions can have positive or negative effects on health long before an illness is evident (Pender, Murdaugh, and Parsons, 2002). Life conditions may include socioeconomic variables such as environment, diet, and lifestyle practices or choices, as well as many other physiological and psychological variables.

Health and illness must be defined in terms of the individual. Health can include conditions previously considered to be illness. For example, a person with epilepsy who has learned to control seizures with medication and who functions at home and at work may no longer consider himself or herself ill. Nurses' attitudes toward health and illness should consider the total person, as well as the environment in which the person lives, to individualize nursing care and enhance meaningfulness of the client's future health status.

Models of Health and Illness

A model is a theoretical way of understanding a concept or idea. Models represent different ways of approaching complex issues. Because health and illness are complex concepts, models are used to understand the relationships between these concepts and the client's attitudes toward health and **health behaviors.**

Health beliefs are a person's ideas, convictions, and attitudes about health and illness. They may be based on factual information or misinformation, common sense or myths, or reality or false expectations. Because health beliefs usually influence health behavior, they can positively or negatively affect a client's level of health. Positive health behaviors are activities related to maintaining, attaining, or regaining good health and preventing illness. Common positive health behaviors include immunizations, proper sleep patterns, adequate exercise, and nutrition. Negative health behaviors include practices actually or potentially harmful to health, such as smoking, drug or alcohol abuse, poor diet, and refusal to take necessary medications.

Nurses have developed the following health models to understand clients' attitudes and values about health and illness so that effective health care can be provided. These nursing models allow nurses to understand and predict clients' health behavior, including how they use health services and adhere to recommended therapy.

Health Belief Model

Rosenstoch's (1974) and Becker and Maiman's (1975) **health belief model** (Figure 6-1) addresses the relationship between a person's beliefs and behaviors. It provides a way of understanding and predicting how clients will behave in relation to their health and how they will comply with health care therapies.

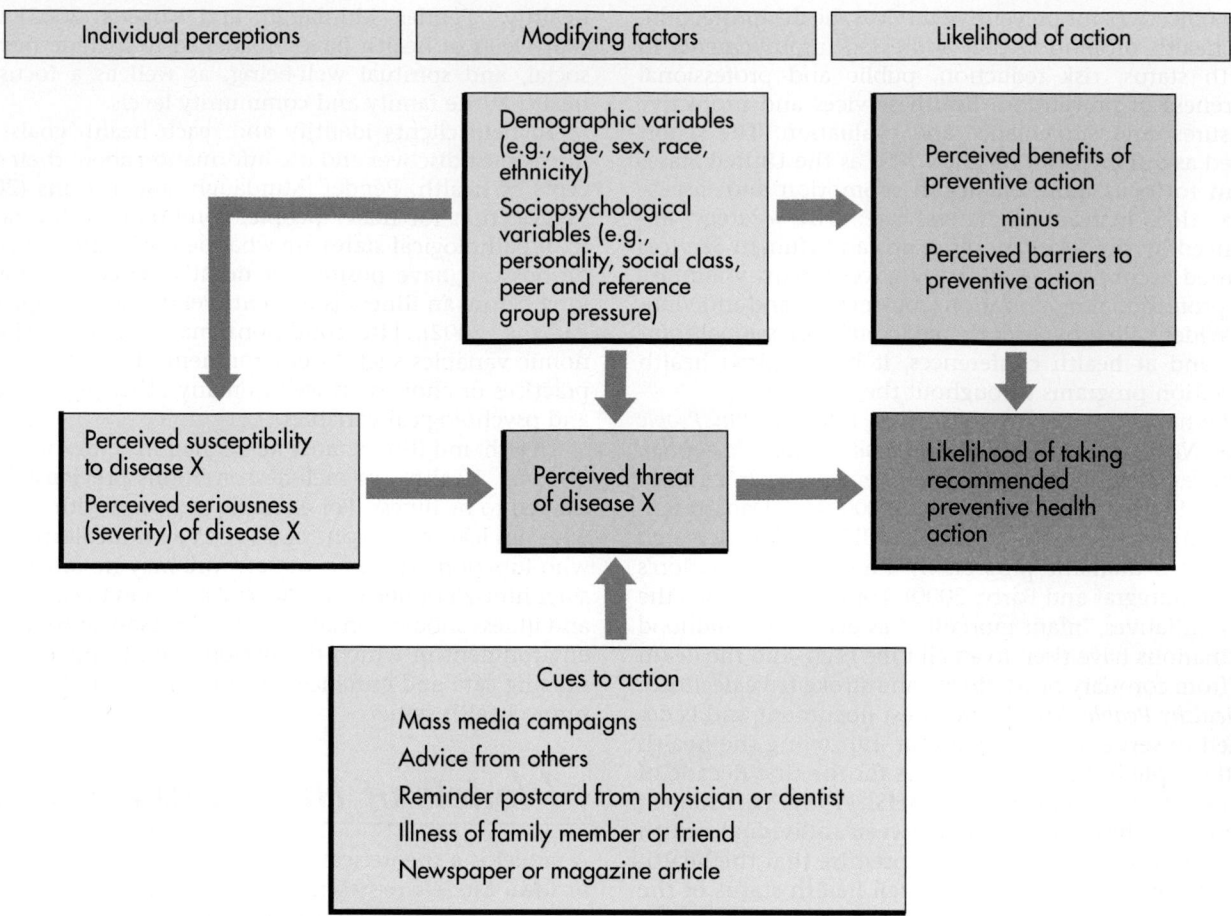

| Individual perceptions | Modifying factors | Likelihood of action |

FIGURE **6–1**   Health belief model. (Data from Becker M, Maiman L: Sociobehavioral determinants of compliance with health and medical care recommendations, *Med Care* 13(1):10, 1975.)

The first component of this model involves the individual's perception of susceptibility to an illness. For example, a client needs to recognize the familial link for coronary artery disease. After this link is recognized, particularly when one parent and two siblings have died in their fourth decade from myocardial infarction, the client may perceive the personal risk of heart disease.

The second component is the individual's perception of the seriousness of the illness. This perception is influenced and modified by demographic and sociopsychological variables, perceived threats of the illness, and cues to action (e.g., mass media campaigns and advice from family, friends, and medical professionals). For example, a client may not perceive his heart disease as serious, which may affect the way he takes care of himself.

The third component—the likelihood that a person will take preventive action—results from the person's perception of the benefits of and barriers to taking action. Preventive action may include lifestyle changes, increased adherence to medical therapies, or a search for medical advice or treatment. A client's perception of susceptibility to disease, as well as his or her perception of the serious of an illness, helps to determine the likelihood that the client will or will not partake in healthy behaviors.

The health belief model helps nurses understand factors influencing clients' perceptions, beliefs, and behavior

in order to plan care that will most effectively assist clients in maintaining or restoring health and preventing illness.

Health Promotion Model

The health promotion model (HPM) proposed by Pender (1982; revised, 1996) was designed to be a "complementary counterpart to models of health protection" (Figure 6-2). It defines health as a positive, dynamic state, not merely the absence of disease (Pender, Murdaugh, and Parsons, 2002). Health promotion is directed at increasing a client's level of well-being. The health promotion model describes the multidimensional nature of persons as they interact within their environment to pursue health (Pender, 1993, 1996; Pender, Murdaugh, and Parsons, 2002). The model focuses on the following three areas: (1) individual characteristics and experiences, (2) behavior-specific knowledge and affect, and (3) behavioral outcomes. The HPM notes that each person has unique personal characteristics and experiences that affect subsequent actions. The set of variables for behavioral-specific knowledge and affect have important motivational significance. These variables can be modified through nursing actions. Health-promoting behavior is the desired behavioral outcome and is the end point in the HPM. Health-promoting behaviors should result in improved health, enhanced functional

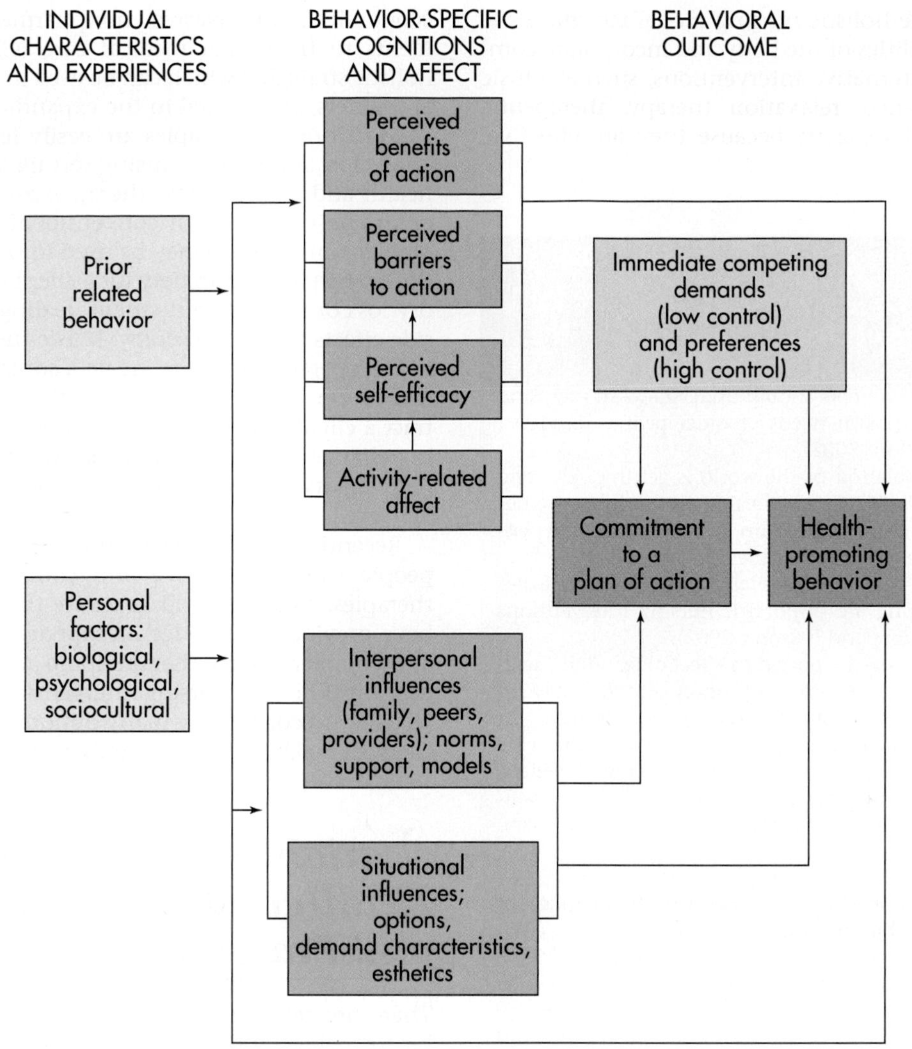

FIGURE **6–2**   Health promotion model (revised). (Redrawn from Pender NJ, Murdaugh CL, Parsons MA: *Health promotion in nursing practice,* ed 4, Upper Saddle River, NJ, 2002, Prentice Hall.)

ability, and better quality of life at all stages of development (Pender, Murdaugh, and Parsons, 2002) (Box 6-1).

Basic Human Needs Model

Basic human needs are elements that are necessary for human survival and health (e.g., food, water, safety, and love). Although each person has other unique needs, all people share the basic human needs, and the extent to which basic needs are met is a major factor in determining a person's level of health.

Maslow's hierarchy of needs is a model that nurses can use to understand the interrelationships of basic human needs (Figure 6-3). According to this model, certain human needs are more basic than others; that is, some needs must be met before other needs (e.g., fulfilling the physiological needs before the needs of love and belonging).

This model can provide a basis for nursing clients of all ages in all health settings. However, when the model is applied, the focus of care should be on the client's needs rather than on strict adherence to the hierarchy. In all cases an emergent physiological need takes precedence over a higher-level need. In other situations a psychological or physical safety need takes priority. For example, in a house fire, fear of death and injury take priority over self-esteem issues. It is unrealistic to always expect a client's basic needs to occur in the fixed hierarchical order. To provide the most effective care, the nurse needs to understand the relationships of different needs and the factors that determine the priorities for each client individually.

Holistic Health Models

Health care has begun to take a more holistic view of health by considering emotional and spiritual well-being, as well as other dimensions of an individual, as important aspects of physical wellness. The **holistic health model** of nursing attempts to create conditions that promote optimal health. In this model, nurses using the nursing process consider clients the ultimate experts regarding their own health and respect clients' subjective experience as relevant in maintaining health or assisting in healing. In the holistic health model, clients are involved in their healing process, thereby assuming some responsibility for health maintenance (Edelman and Mandle, 2002).

Nurses using the holistic nursing model recognize the natural healing abilities of the body and incorporate complementary and alternative interventions, such as music therapy, reminiscence, relaxation therapy, therapeutic touch, and guided imagery, because they are effective,

economical, noninvasive, nonpharmacological complements to traditional medical care (Chapter 35). These holistic strategies, which can be used in all stages of health and illness, are integral in the expanding role of nursing.

Most holistic therapies are easily learned and can be applied to almost any nursing setting and in all stages of health and illness. These therapies are used either alone or in conjunction with conventional medicine. For example, reminiscence may be used in the geriatric population to help relieve anxiety for a client dealing with memory loss or for a cancer patient dealing with the difficult side effects of chemotherapy. Music therapy may be used in the operating room to create a soothing environment. Relaxation therapy may be useful in any setting to distract a client during a painful procedure, such as a dressing change. Breathing exercises are commonly taught to help clients deal with the pain associated with labor and delivery.

Recently there has been an increase in the number of people using alternative and complementary medical therapies. Nurses should be aware that their clients may have previous knowledge or experience with alternative and complementary therapies and may therefore be accepting of holistic nursing interventions. Nurses can help all clients recognize the many options available and assist them in making choices to enhance health.

Variables Influencing Health and Health Beliefs and Practices

There are many variables that can influence a client's health beliefs and practices. Internal and external variables can influence how a person thinks and acts. As previously stated, health beliefs usually influence health behavior, or health practices, and likewise can positively or negatively affect a client's level of health. Therefore un-

FIGURE **6–3**   Maslow's hierarchy of needs. (Redrawn from Maslow AH: *Motivation and personality,* Upper Saddle River, NJ, 1970, Prentice Hall.)

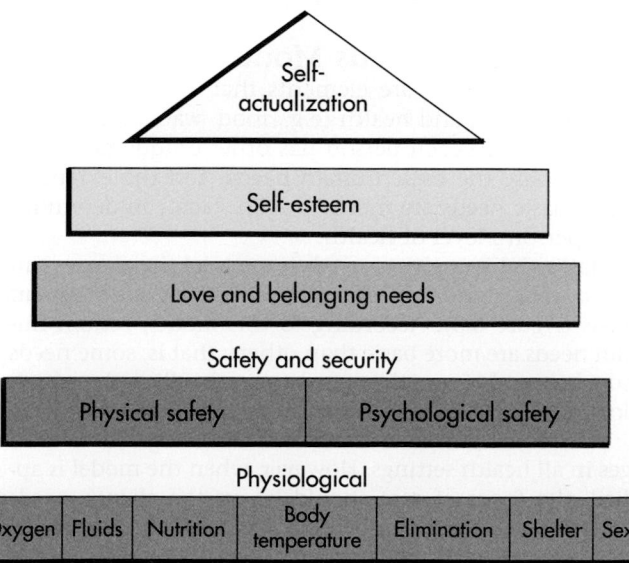

derstanding the effects of these variables allows the nurse to plan and deliver individualized care.

Internal Variables

Internal variables include a person's developmental stage, intellectual background, perception of functioning, and emotional and spiritual factors.

Developmental Stage. A person's thought and behavior patterns change throughout life. The nurse must consider the client's level of growth and development when using his or her health beliefs and practices as a basis for planning care. The study of development involves finding patterns or general principles that apply to most people most of the time (Murray and Zentner, 2000). The concept of illness for a child, adolescent, or adult is dependent on the individual's developmental stage. Fear and anxiety are common among ill children, especially if thoughts about illness, hospitalization, or procedures are based on lack of information or lack of clarity of information. Emotional development may also influence personal beliefs about health-related matters. For example, the nurse uses different techniques for teaching about contraception to an adolescent than would be used for an adult. Knowledge of the stages of growth and development helps the nurse predict the client's response to the present illness or the threat of future illness. The planning of nursing care is then adapted to these expectations, as well as to the client's abilities to participate in self-care.

Intellectual Background. A person's beliefs about health are shaped in part by the person's knowledge, lack of knowledge, or incorrect information about body functions and illnesses, educational background, and past experiences. These variables influence how a client thinks about health. In addition, cognitive abilities shape the *way* a person thinks, including the ability to understand factors involved in illness and to apply knowledge of health and illness to personal health practices. Cognitive abilities also relate to a person's developmental stage. A nurse considers intellectual background so that these variables can be incorporated into nursing care (Edelman and Mandle, 2002).

Perception of Functioning. The way people perceive their physical functioning affects health beliefs and practices. When nurses assess a client's level of health, they gather subjective data about the way the client perceives physical functioning, such as level of fatigue, shortness of breath, or pain. They also obtain objective data about actual functioning, such as blood pressure, height measurements, and lung sound assessment. This information allows nurses to more successfully plan and implement individualized care.

Emotional Factors. The client's degree of stress, depression, or fear, for example, can influence health beliefs and practices. The manner in which a person handles stress throughout each phase of life will influence the way the person reacts to illness. A person who generally is very calm may have little emotional response during illness, whereas an individual unable to cope emotionally with the threat of illness may either overreact to illness and assume it is life threatening or deny the presence of symptoms and not take therapeutic action (see Chapter 30).

Spiritual Factors. Spirituality is reflected in how a person lives his or her life, including the values and beliefs exercised, the relationships established with family and friends, and the ability to find hope and meaning in life. Spirituality serves as an integrating theme in people's lives (see Chapter 28). Religious practices are one way that people exercise spirituality. There are some religions that restrict the use of certain forms of medical treatment. Nurses must understand clients' spiritual dimensions to involve them effectively in nursing care.

External Variables

External variables influencing a person's health beliefs and practices include family practices, socioeconomic factors, and cultural background.

Family Practices. The way that clients' families use health care services generally affects their health practices. Their perceptions of the seriousness of diseases and their history of preventive care behaviors (or lack of them) can influence how clients will think about health. For example, if a young woman's mother never had annual gynecological examinations or Pap smears, it is unlikely the daughter will follow such practices.

Socioeconomic Factors. Social and psychosocial factors can increase the risk for illness and influence the way that a person defines and reacts to illness. Psychosocial variables include the stability of the person's marital or intimate relationship, lifestyle habits, and occupational environment. A person generally seeks approval and support from social networks (neighbors, peers, and co-workers), and this desire for approval and support affects health beliefs and practices.

Social variables partly determine how the health care system provides medical care. Because the health care system is organized in certain ways, it determines how clients can obtain care, the treatment method, the economic cost to the client, and potential reimbursement to the health care agency or client.

Like social variables, economic variables may affect a client's level of health by increasing the risk for disease and influencing how or at what point the client enters the health care system. A person's compliance with the treatment that is designed to maintain or improve health is also affected by economic status. A person who has high utility bills, a large family, and a low income tends to give a higher priority to food and shelter than to costly drugs or treatment or expensive foods for special diets.

Cultural Background. Cultural background influences beliefs, values, and customs. It influences the approach to the health care system, personal health practices, and the nurse-client relationship. Cultural background may also influence an individual's beliefs about causes of illness, as well as remedies or practices to restore health (Box 6-2).

Kundhal KK: Cultural diversity: an evolving challenge to physician-patient communication, *JAMA* 289(1):94, 2003; McEvoy M: Culture and spirituality as an integrated concept in pediatric care, *MCN Am J Matern Child Nurs* 28(1):39, 2003; and Crawley L and others: Strategies for culturally effective end-of-life care, *Ann Intern Med* 136(9):673, 2002.

Box 6-2 — Cultural Aspects of Care

The cultural and ethnic backgrounds of clients can shape their views of health, wellness, and illness. Cultural understanding of illness may affect the way a client reports symptoms. For example, because clinical depression is stigmatized in some cultures, a client with depression may report only physical symptoms such as fatigue and weight loss. Culture can also affect client's perceptions of illness causation and treatment. For example, some cultures have been found to attribute breast cancer to "sinful" behaviors, and other cultures have been found to believe that surgical treatment of breast cancer would cause it to metastasize. Differences in beliefs, values, and traditional health care practices are also relevant when planning end-of-life care. In addition, many cultures incorporate spiritual practices, and therefore spirituality overlaps with culture. When exploring information about culture, nurses should consider beliefs, values, daily practices, spirituality, and their implications for the way a client understands illness, perceives treatment plans, and makes health care decisions.

Implications for Practice

- Nurses should be aware of the impact of culture on a client's view and understanding of illness.
- When teaching clients about their illness and treatment regimens, it is important for nurses to understand that unique cultural perceptions exist regarding the cause of an illness and its treatment.
- Nurses should focus on understanding the client's traditions, values, and beliefs and how these dimensions may affect health, wellness, and illness.

If nurses are not aware of their own and other cultural patterns of behavior and language, they may not be able to recognize and understand a client's behavior and beliefs and may have difficulty interacting with the client. As with family and socioeconomic variables, cultural variables must be incorporated into a client's care plan (see Chapter 8).

Health Promotion, Wellness, and Illness Prevention

Health care has become increasingly focused on health promotion, wellness, and illness prevention. The rapid rise of health care costs has motivated people to seek ways of decreasing the incidence and minimizing the results of illness or disability.

The concepts of health promotion, wellness, and illness prevention are closely related and, in practice, overlap to some extent. All are focused on the future; the difference between them involves motivations and goals. **Health promotion** activities such as routine exercise and good nutrition, help clients maintain or enhance their present levels of health. Health promotion activities motivate people to act positively to reach more stable levels of health. **Wellness** education teaches people how to care for themselves in a healthy way and includes topics such as physical awareness, stress management, and self-responsibility. Wellness strategies are designed to help persons achieve new understanding and control of their lives. **Illness prevention** activities such as immunization programs protect clients from actual or potential threats to health. Illness prevention activities motivate people to avoid declines in health or functional levels.

Nurses emphasize health promotion, wellness-enhancing strategies, and illness prevention activities as important forms of health care because they assist clients in maintaining and improving health. The goal of a total health program is to improve a client's level of well-being in all dimensions, not just physical health. Total health programs are based on the belief that many factors can affect a person's level of health.

The following categories are identified as important determinants of health status (Edelman and Mandle, 2002): tobacco use, nutrition, alcohol use, habituating drug use, driving, exercise, sexuality and contraceptive or barrier use, family relationships, risk factor modification, coping and adaptation.

Health can be influenced by individual practices, such as poor eating habits and little or no exercise. It can also be affected by physical stressors, such as a poor living environment, exposure to air pollutants, and an unsafe environment. Hereditary and psychological stressors, such as emotional, intellectual, social, developmental, and spiritual factors, can also influence one's level of health. Total health programs are directed at individuals changing their lifestyle by developing habits that can improve their level of health.

Other programs are aimed at specific health care problems. For example, support groups exist to help people with human immunodeficiency virus (HIV) infection. Exercise programs encourage participants to exercise regularly to reduce their risk of cardiac disease. Stress reduction programs teach participants to cope with stressors and reduce their risks for multiple illnesses, such as infections, gastrointestinal disease, and cardiac disease.

Some health promotion, wellness education, and illness prevention programs are operated by health care agencies; others are independently operated. Many corporations have developed on-site health promotion activities for employees. Likewise, colleges and community centers offer health promotion and illness prevention programs. Nurses may be actively involved in these programs or may be consultants or give referrals. The goal of these activities is to improve the client's level of health through preventive health services, environmental protection, and health education.

Health care professionals who work in the field of health promotion use proactive attempts to prevent illness or disease. Health promotion activities can be passive or active. With **passive strategies of health promotion,** individuals gain from the activities of others without acting themselves. The fluoridation of municipal drinking water and the fortification of homogenized milk with vitamin D are examples of passive health promotion strategies. With **active strategies of health promotion,** individuals are motivated to adopt specific health programs. Weight reduction and smoking cessation programs require clients to be actively involved in measures to improve their present and future levels of wellness while decreasing the risk of disease.

Health promotion, as outlined in the *American Journal of Health Promotion,* is the science and art of helping people change their lifestyle to move toward a state of optimal health. This definition suggests that health and illness are affected by choices made by individuals (Raphael, 2002). An individual takes responsibility for health and wellness by making appropriate lifestyle choices. Lifestyle choices are important in that they affect a person's quality of life. Positive lifestyle choices and the avoidance of negative lifestyle choices may also play a role in the prevention of illness. Prevention of illness has an economic impact in that it decreases health care costs.

Levels of Preventive Care

Nursing care oriented to health promotion, wellness, and illness prevention can be understood in terms of health activities on primary, secondary, and tertiary levels (Figure 6-4).

Primary Prevention. **Primary prevention** is true prevention; it precedes disease or dysfunction and is applied to clients considered physically and emotionally healthy. Primary prevention aimed at health promotion includes health education programs, immunization, and physical and nutritional fitness activities. It can be provided to an individual or to a general population, or it can focus on individuals at risk for developing specific diseases. Wellness activities (Edelman and Mandle, 2002) are synonymous with the activities identified for primary prevention by Leavell and Clark (1965) in Figure 6-4. Primary prevention includes all health promotion efforts, as well as wellness activities that focus on maintaining or improving the general health of individuals, families, and communities (Edelman and Mandle, 2002).

Secondary Prevention. **Secondary prevention** focuses on individuals who are experiencing health problems or illnesses and who are at risk for developing complications or worsening conditions. Activities are directed at diagnosis and prompt intervention, thereby reducing severity and enabling the client to return to a normal level of health as early as possible (Edelman and Mandle, 2002; Pender, 1993). A large portion of nursing care related to secondary prevention is delivered in homes, hospitals, or skilled nursing facilities. It includes screening techniques and treating early stages of disease to limit disability by averting or delaying the consequences of advanced disease.

Tertiary Prevention. **Tertiary prevention** occurs when a defect or disability is permanent and irreversible. It involves minimizing the effects of long-term disease or disability by interventions directed at preventing compli-

cations and deterioration (Edelman and Mandle, 2002). Activities are directed at rehabilitation rather than diagnosis and treatment. Care at this level aims to help clients achieve as high a level of functioning as possible, despite the limitations caused by illness or impairment. This level of care is called preventive care because it involves preventing further disability or reduced functioning.

Risk Factors

A **risk factor** is any situation, habit, social or environmental condition, physiological or psychological condition, developmental or intellectual condition, or spiritual or other variable that increases the vulnerability of an individual or group to an illness or accident. An understanding of risk factors, behavior, risk factor modification, and behavior modification are integral components of health promotion, wellness, and illness prevention activities. Nurses in all areas of practice often have opportunities to assist clients in adopting activities to promote health and decrease risks of illness.

The presence of risk factors does not mean that a disease will develop, but risk factors increase the chances that the individual will experience a particular disease or dysfunction. Nurses and other health care professionals are concerned with risk factors, sometimes called health hazards, for several reasons. Risk factors play a major role in how a nurse identifies a client's health status. They can also influence health beliefs and practices if a person is aware of their presence. Risk factors can be placed in the following interrelated categories: genetic and physiological factors, age, physical environment, and lifestyle.

Genetic and Physiological Factors

Physiological risk factors involve the physical functioning of the body. Certain physical conditions, such as being pregnant or overweight, place increased stress on physiological systems (e.g., the circulatory system), increasing susceptibility to illness in these areas. Heredity, or genetic predisposition to specific illness, is a major physical risk factor. For example, a person with a family history of diabetes mellitus is at risk for developing the disease later in life. Other documented genetic risk factors include family histories of cancer, heart disease, kidney disease, or mental illness.

Age

Age increases or decreases susceptibility to certain illnesses. For example, an infant born prematurely and all neonates are more susceptible to infections. The risk of heart disease increases with age for both sexes. Also, many kinds of cancer pose a greater risk for persons over age 45 than for younger persons. Age risk factors are often closely associated with other risk factors such as family history and personal habits. Nurses need to educate their clients about the importance of regularly scheduled checkups for their age-group. U.S. authorities have identified a schedule of recommendations for health screenings, immunizations, and counseling. Access to scientific evidence, recommendations on clinical prevention ser-

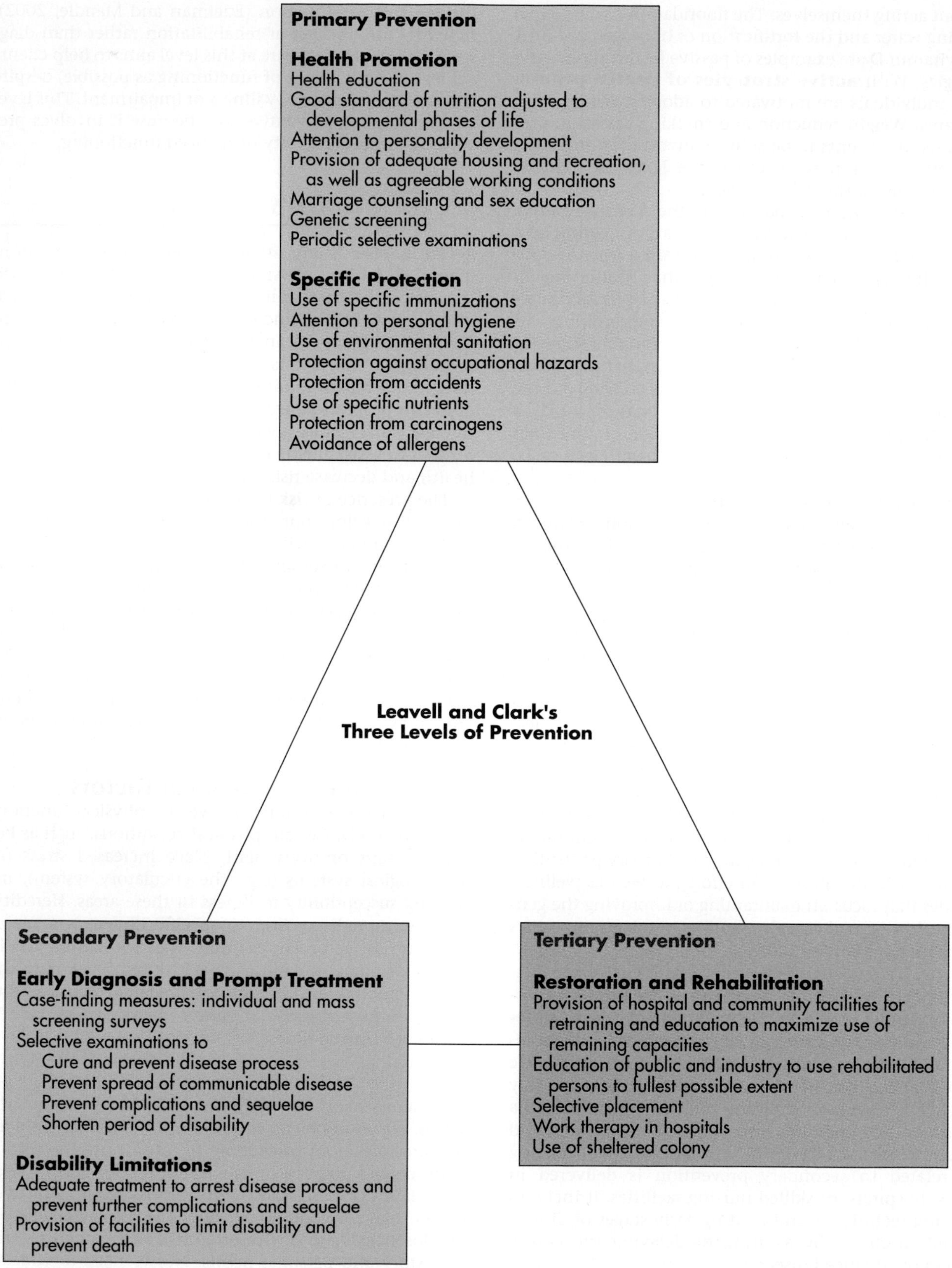

Primary Prevention

Health Promotion
Health education
Good standard of nutrition adjusted to
    developmental phases of life
Attention to personality development
Provision of adequate housing and recreation,
    as well as agreeable working conditions
Marriage counseling and sex education
Genetic screening
Periodic selective examinations

Specific Protection
Use of specific immunizations
Attention to personal hygiene
Use of environmental sanitation
Protection against occupational hazards
Protection from accidents
Use of specific nutrients
Protection from carcinogens
Avoidance of allergens

**Leavell and Clark's
Three Levels of Prevention**

Secondary Prevention

Early Diagnosis and Prompt Treatment
Case-finding measures: individual and mass
    screening surveys
Selective examinations to
    Cure and prevent disease process
    Prevent spread of communicable disease
    Prevent complications and sequelae
    Shorten period of disability

Disability Limitations
Adequate treatment to arrest disease process and
    prevent further complications and sequelae
Provision of facilities to limit disability and
    prevent death

Tertiary Prevention

Restoration and Rehabilitation
Provision of hospital and community facilities for
    retraining and education to maximize use of
    remaining capacities
Education of public and industry to use rehabilitated
    persons to fullest possible extent
Selective placement
Work therapy in hospitals
Use of sheltered colony

FIGURE **6–4**   The three levels of prevention developed by Leavell and Clark. (Data from Leavell H, Clark AE: *Preventive medicine for doctors in the community,* ed 3, New York, 1965, McGraw-Hill; and modified from Edelman CL, Mandle CL: *Health promotion throughout the lifespan,* ed 5, St. Louis, 2002, Mosby.)

vices and information on how to implement recommended preventative services into practice can be found at www.ahrq.gov/clinic/prevenix.htm.

Environment

Where we live and the condition of that area (its air, water, and soil) determine how we live, what we eat, the disease agents to which we are exposed, our state of health, and our ability to adapt (Murray and Zentner, 2000). The physical environment in which a person works or lives can increase the likelihood that certain illnesses will occur. For example, some kinds of cancer and other diseases are more likely to develop when industrial workers are exposed to certain chemicals or when people live near toxic waste disposal sites. Nursing assessments extend from the individual to the family and the community in which they live (Murray and Zentner, 2000).

Lifestyle

Many activities, habits, and practices involve risk factors. Lifestyle practices and behaviors can have positive or negative effects on health. Practices with potential negative effects are risk factors; these include sedentary lifestyle, overeating or poor nutrition, insufficient rest and sleep, and poor personal hygiene. Other habits that put a person at risk for illness include tobacco use, alcohol or drug abuse, unsafe sex, multiple sex partners, and activities involving a threat of injury, such as skydiving or mountain climbing. Some habits are risk factors for specific diseases. For example, excessive sunbathing increases the risk of skin cancer, and being overweight increases the risk of cardiovascular disease. These lifestyle risk factors have gained increased attention because it is known that many of the leading causes of death in the United States are related to lifestyle patterns or habits. This also represents a huge impact on the economics of the health care system. Therefore it is important to understand the impact of lifestyle behaviors on health status. Nurses can educate their clients and the public on wellness-promoting lifestyle behaviors.

Care must be taken however, not to blame clients for their illnesses. Gunderman (2000) discusses the phenomenon of assigning moral blame for illness and states that although it is sometimes appropriate to warn clients that their habits jeopardize their health, blaming clients who are ill is failing to offer care when it is needed most. Blaming clients may also discourage them from seeking care.

Stress can be a lifestyle risk factor if it is severe or prolonged, or if the person is unable to cope with life events adequately. Stress can threaten mental health (emotional stress), as well as physical well-being (physiological stress). Both may play a part in the development of an illness and affect the ability to adapt to potential changes associated with an illness, as well as the ability to survive a life-threatening illness. Stress may also interfere with health promotion activities and the ability to implement needed lifestyle modifications. Emotional stressors may result from life events such as divorce, pregnancy, death of a spouse or family member, and financial instabilities. Job-related stressors, for example, may overtax a person's cognitive skills and decision-making ability, leading to

"mental overload" or "burnout" (see Chapter 30). Stress can also threaten physical well-being and has been associated with illnesses such as heart disease, cancer, and gastrointestinal disorders (Pender, Murdaugh, and Parsons, 2002). Life stressors should be reviewed as part of a comprehensive risk factor analysis.

The goal of risk factor identification is to merely assist clients in visualizing those areas in their life that can be modified or even eliminated to promote wellness and prevent illness. More comprehensive health risk appraisals, using a variety of available health risk appraisal forms, can be done to estimate a person's specific health threats based on the presence of various risk factors (Edelman and Mandle, 2002). It is important to understand that implementation of a health risk appraisal must be linked with educational programs and other community resources in order to result in necessary lifestyle changes and in risk reduction (Pender, Murdaugh, and Parsons, 2002).

Risk Factor Modification and Changing Health Behaviors

Identifying risk factors is the first step in health promotion, wellness education, and illness prevention activities. Health hazards should be discussed with the client following a comprehensive nursing assessment; then the client can decide if he or she wants to maintain or improve his or her health status by taking risk reduction actions (Edelman and Mandle, 2002). Risk factor modification, health promotion or illness prevention activities, or any program that attempts to change unhealthy lifestyle behaviors can be considered a wellness strategy. Wellness strategies that teach clients to care for themselves in a healthier way need to be emphasized because they have the ability to increase the quality of life, as well as decrease the potential high costs of unmanaged health problems.

Attempts to change may be aimed at the cessation of a health-damaging behavior (tobacco use, alcohol misuse) or at the adoption of a healthy behavior (healthy diet, exercise) (Pender, Murdaugh, and Parsons, 2002). Changing health behavior is difficult, especially those behaviors that are ingrained in lifestyle patterns. The role of nurses using a health promotion model for identification of risky behaviors and implementation of the change process cannot be overemphasized, because it is the nurse who spends the greatest amount of time in direct contact with clients. In addition, leading causes of death continue to relate to health behaviors that require a change, and nurses are challenged to motivate and facilitate health behavior change in working with individuals, families, and communities (Shinitzky and Kub, 2001).

An understanding of the process of changing behaviors can help nurses support difficult **health behavior change** in their clients. It is believed that change involves movement through a series of stages. The stages of change are described by DiClemente and Prochaska (1998) in the transtheoretical model of change (Table 6-1). These stages range from no intention to change (precontemplation),

Table 6-1	**Stages of Health Behavior Change**	
Stage	**Definition**	**Nursing Implications**
Precontemplation	Not intending to make changes within the next 6 months.	Client will not be interested in information about the behavior and may be defensive when confronted with the information.
Contemplation	Considering a change within the next 6 months.	Ambivalence may be present, but clients will more likely accept information as they are developing more belief in the value of change.
Preparation	Making small changes in preparation for a change in the next month.	Client believes advantages outweigh disadvantages of behavior change. May need assistance in planning for the change.
Action	Actively engaged in strategies to change behavior. This stage may last up to 6 months.	Be aware of previous habits that may prevent action on new behaviors. Identify barriers and facilitators of change.
Maintenance stage	Sustained change over time. This stage begins 6 months after action has started and continues indefinitely.	Changes need to be integrated into the client's lifestyle.

Data from Prochaska JO, DiClemente CC: Stages of change in the modification of problem behaviors, *Prog Behav Modif* 28:184, 1992; and Conn VS: A staged-based approach to helping people change health behaviors, *Clin Nurs Spec* 8(4):187, 1994.

Client Teaching Box 6-3

Lifestyle Changes

Objective

- Health risks related to poor lifestyle habits (e.g., high-fat diet, sedentary lifestyle) will be reduced through behavior change.

Teaching Strategies

- Begin with determining what information client has regarding health risks related to poor lifestyle.
- Assist client in establishing goals for change.
- In collaboration with client, establish time lines for modification of eating and exercise lifestyle habits.
- Reinforce the process of change with client.
- Use therapeutic discussions in a respectful manner with the intention of motivating a change within a client (motivational interviewing) and helping motivated clients to be successful in making and maintaining behavioral change (cognitive-behavioral therapy) (Saarmann, Daugherty, and Riegel, 2000).
- Identify or build resources in the community and family that are needed to support the change.

Evaluation

- Have client maintain exercise and eating calendar to track adherence.
- Ask client to discuss success with lifestyle changes.
- Have client identify community resources used in making change.

considering a change within the next 6 months (contemplation), making small changes (preparation), actively engaging in strategies to change behavior (action), to maintaining a changed behavior (maintenance stage). As individuals attempt a change in behavior, relapse followed by recycling through the stages occurs frequently. When relapse occurs, the person will return to the contemplation or precontemplation stage before attempting the change again. Relapse can be viewed as a learning process, and what is learned from relapse can be applied to the next attempt to change. It is important to understand what occurs at the various stages of the change process in order to time the implementation of interventions (wellness strategies) adequately and to provide appropriate care at each stage.

Once a stage of change has been identified, the processes of change facilitate movement through the stages. The processes of change, or nursing interventions, should be appropriately chosen to match the stage of change (DiClemente and Prochaska, 1998). Most behavior change programs are designed (and have a chance of success) for those people who are ready to take action regarding their health behavior problems. Only a minority of people are actually in this action stage (Prochaska, 1991). Further work needs to be done to design interventions and wellness strategies for people in all stages of health behavior change. Changes will be maintained over time only if they are integrated into an individual's overall lifestyle (Box 6-3). Maintenance of healthy lifestyles can prevent hospitalizations and potentially lower the cost of health care.

Illness

Illness is a state in which a person's physical, emotional, intellectual, social, developmental, or spiritual functioning is diminished or impaired compared with previous experience. Cancer is a disease process, but one client with leukemia who is responding to treatment may continue to function as usual, whereas another client with breast cancer who is preparing for surgery may be affected in dimensions other than the physical.

Illness, therefore, is not synonymous with disease. Although nurses must be familiar with different kinds of diseases and their treatments, they are concerned more with illness, which may include disease but also includes the effects on functioning and well-being in all dimensions.

Acute Illness and Chronic Illness

Acute illness and chronic illness are two general classifications of illness used in this chapter. Both acute and chronic illnesses have the potential to be life threatening. An **acute illness** usually has a short duration and is severe. The symptoms appear abruptly, are intense, and often subside after a relatively short period. An acute illness may affect functioning in any dimension. A **chronic illness** persists, usually longer than 6 months, and can also affect functioning in any dimension. The client may fluctuate between maximal functioning and serious health relapses that may be life threatening. A person with a chronic illness is similar to a person with a disability in that both have limitations (of varying degrees) in function resulting from either a pathological process or an injury. Mechanic (1995) notes that "a chronic disabling disease interferes with ongoing life adaptations by making the performance of routine tasks more challenging." In addition, the social surroundings and physical environment in which the individual lives can affect the abilities, motivation, and psychological maintenance of the disabled person.

Chronic illnesses and disabilities remain a leading health problem in North America for older adults and children. Issues of coping and living with a chronic illness can be complex and overwhelming. A major role for nursing is to provide client education aimed at helping clients manage their illness or disability. The goal of managing a chronic illness is to reduce the occurrence of symptoms or to improve the tolerance of symptoms. By enhancing wellness, nurses may help improve the quality of life for clients living with chronic illnesses or disabilities.

It is important to understand that clients with chronic diseases and families of children with chronic diseases are faced with a process called normalization, in which they adapt to the disease. Studies of families facing illness challenges have found that over time, family members come to view both the child and their life as normal (Knafl and Deatrick, 2002). There is a relationship between family members' beliefs about their illness experiences and their illness management behaviors that affects the process of normalization (Knafl and Deatrick, 2002).

Illness Behavior

People who are ill generally act in a way that medical sociologists call illness behavior. It involves how people monitor their bodies, define and interpret their symptoms, take remedial actions, and use the health care system (Mechanic, 1982) (Box 6-4). Personal history, social situations, social norms, and the opportunities and constraints of community institutions can all affect illness behavior (Mechanic, 1995). Although there is a large variability in the way people react to an illness, illness behavior displayed in sickness can be used to manage life adversities (Mechanic, 1995). In other words, if people perceive themselves to be ill, illness behaviors can be coping mechanisms. For example, illness behavior can result in clients being released from roles, social expectations, or responsibilities. For a homemaker, for example, the "flu" may be viewed as an added stressor, or it may be a temporary release from child care and household responsibilities.

Variables Influencing Illness and Illness Behavior

Just as health and health behavior are affected by internal and external variables, so are illness and illness behavior. The influences of these variables, as well as the stage of illness behavior the client is in, may affect the likelihood of

---

Research Highlight **Box 6-4**

Impact of Chronic Illness on Level of Health

Research Focus

The lifestyle changes required to manage diabetes and its treatment can be extremely demanding for clients. In addition, 20% of clients with type 1 diabetes also have renal disease. As clients adapt to these diseases, constraints on their lifestyle can lead to feelings of depression and a reduced quality of life.

Research Abstract

The purpose of this study was to examine the clients' experiences in adapting to diabetic renal disease, a common chronic health disease. In-depth interviews were done with 20 adults with diabetic renal disease. Interviews covered participants' histories of diabetes before the diagnosis of their disease, the impact of renal disease on their lives, their involvement with the medical system, and their hopes and fears for the future. Participants told their own stories of their experiences with diabetic renal disease. Findings indicate variations in experiences but also some common themes. Clients' experiences can be found in four major themes: immediate reactions of diagnosis; participant explanations of renal disease; living with renal disease; and hopes, fears, and expectations for the future.

Evidence-Based Practice

- Nurses need to understand that clients respond differently to chronic illnesses.
- Chronically ill people have to find ways of adapting to illness.
- Coping is how people think about themselves and also how people present themselves in relation to their illness.
- Some ways people present themselves are control seeking, denial, optimism, defeatism, and stoicism.
- In attempt to adapt to uncertainty, clients may develop stoicism rather than express themselves emotionally.

Reference

King N and others: You can't cure it so you have to endure it: the experience of adaptation to diabetic renal disease, *Qual Health Res* 12(3):329, 2002.

seeking health care, compliance with therapy, and therefore health outcomes. Based on an understanding of these variables and behaviors, nurses can plan individualized care to assist clients in coping with their illness at various stages of illness. The goal of nursing is to promote optimal functioning in all dimensions throughout an illness.

Internal Variables. Internal variables influencing the way clients behave when they are ill are their perceptions of symptoms and the nature of the illness. If clients believe that the symptoms of their illnesses disrupt their normal routine, they are more likely to seek health care assistance than if they do not perceive the symptoms to be disruptive. If clients believe that the symptoms are serious or perhaps life threatening, they are also more likely to seek assistance. Persons awakened by crushing chest pains in the middle of the night generally view this symptom as potentially serious and life threatening, and they will probably be motivated to seek assistance. However, such a perception can also have the opposite effect. Individuals may fear serious illness, react by denying it, and not seek medical assistance.

The nature of the illness, either acute or chronic, can also affect a client's illness behavior. Clients with acute illnesses are likely to seek health care and comply readily with therapy. On the other hand, a client with a chronic illness, in which the symptoms may not be cured, but only partially relieved, may not be motivated to comply with the therapy plan. Chronically ill clients may become less actively involved in their care, may experience greater frustration, and may comply less readily with care. Because nurses generally spend more time than other health care professionals with chronically ill clients, they are in the unique position of being able to assist these clients in overcoming problems related to illness behavior. A client's coping skills, as well as his or her locus of control, are other internal variables that affect the way the client behaves when ill (see Chapter 30).

External Variables. External variables influencing a client's illness behavior include the visibility of symptoms, social group, cultural background, economic variables, accessibility of the health care system, and social support. The visibility of the symptoms of an illness can affect body image and illness behavior. A client with a visible symptom may be more likely to seek assistance than a client without such a visible symptom.

Clients' social groups may assist them in recognizing the threat of illness or support the denial of potential illness. Families, friends, and co-workers all may influence clients' illness behavior. Clients often react positively to social support while practicing positive health behaviors. A person's cultural and ethnic background teaches the person how to be healthy, how to recognize illness, and how to be ill. The effects of disease and its interpretation vary according to cultural circumstances. Ethnic differences can influence decisions about health care and the use of diagnostic and health care services (Murray and Zentner, 2000). Dietary practices among ethnic groups, occupations held by certain cultural groups, and cultural beliefs are other factors that contribute to illness and the distribution of disease (Murray and Zentner, 2000).

Economic variables influence the way a client reacts to illness. Because of economic constraints, a client may delay treatment and in many cases may continue to carry out daily activities. Clients' access to the health care system is closely related to economic factors. The health care system is a socioeconomic system that clients must enter, interact within, and exit. For many clients, entry into the system is complex or confusing, and some clients may seek nonemergency medical care in an emergency department because they do not know how otherwise to obtain health services. The physical proximity of clients to a health care agency often influences how soon they enter the system after deciding to seek care.

Impact of Illness on the Client and Family

Illness is never an isolated life event. The client and family must deal with changes resulting from illness and treatment. Each client responds uniquely to illness, and therefore nursing interventions must be individualized. The client and family commonly experience behavioral and emotional changes, as well as changes in roles, body image and self-concept, and family dynamics.

Behavioral and Emotional Changes

People react differently to illness or the threat of illness. Individual behavioral and emotional reactions depend on the nature of the illness, the client's attitude toward it, the reaction of others to it, and the variables of illness behavior.

Short-term, non–life-threatening illnesses evoke few behavioral changes in the functioning of the client or family. A husband and father who has a cold, for example, may lack the energy and patience to spend time in family activities and may be irritable and prefer not to interact with his family. This is a behavioral change, but the change is subtle and does not last long. Some may even consider such a change a normal response to illness.

Severe illness, particularly one that is life threatening, can lead to more extensive emotional and behavioral changes, such as anxiety, shock, denial, anger, and withdrawal. These are common responses to the stress of illness. The nurse can develop interventions to assist the client and the family in coping with and adapting to this stress because the stressor itself cannot usually be changed.

Impact on Body Image

Body image is the subjective concept of physical appearance (see Chapter 26). Some illnesses result in changes in physical appearance, and clients and families react differently to these changes. Reactions of clients and families to changes in body image depend on the type of changes (e.g., loss of a limb or an organ), their adaptive capacity, the rate at which changes takes place, and the support services available.

When a change in body image occurs, such as results from a leg amputation, the client generally adjusts in the following phases: shock, withdrawal, acknowledgment, acceptance, and rehabilitation. Initially the client may be shocked by the change or impending change and may de-personalize it and talk about it as though it were happening to someone else. As the client and family recognize the reality of the change, they become anxious and may withdraw, refusing to discuss it. Withdrawal is an adaptive coping mechanism that can assist the client in making the adjustment. As the client and family acknowledge the change, they move through a period of grieving. At the end of the acknowledgment phase, they accept the loss. During rehabilitation the client is ready to learn how to adapt to the change in body image through use of a prosthesis or changing lifestyles and goals.

Impact on Self-Concept

Self-concept is a mental self-image of strengths and weaknesses in all aspects of personality. Self-concept depends in part on body image and roles but also includes other aspects of psychology and spirituality (see Chapters 26 and 28). The impact of illness on the self-concepts of clients and family members may be more complex and less readily observed than role changes.

Self-concept is important in relationships with other family members. A client whose self-concept changes because of illness may no longer meet family expectations, leading to tension or conflict. As a result, family members may change their interactions with the client. In the course of providing care, a nurse is able to observe changes in the client's self-concept (or in the self-concepts of family members) and develop a care plan to help them adjust to the changes resulting from the illness.

Impact on Family Roles

People have many roles in life, such as wage earner, decision maker, professional, child, sibling, or parent. When an illness occurs, parents and children try to adapt to major changes resulting from a family member's illness. Role reversal is common (see Chapter 9). If a parent of an adult becomes ill and cannot carry out usual activities, the adult child often assumes many of the parent's responsibilities and in essence becomes a parent to the parent. Such a reversal of the usual situation can lead to stress, conflicting responsibilities for the adult child, or direct conflict over decision making.

Such a change may be subtle and short term or drastic and long term. An individual and family generally adjust more easily to subtle, short-term changes. In most cases they know that the role change is only temporary and will not require prolonged adjustment phases. Long-term changes, however, require an adjustment process similar to the grief process (see Chapter 29). The client and family often require specific counseling and guidance to assist them in coping with the role changes.

Impact on Family Dynamics

Because of the effects of illness on the client and family, family dynamics often change. Family dynamics is the process by which the family functions, makes decisions, gives support to individual members, and copes with everyday changes and challenges. If a parent in a family becomes ill, family activities and decision making often come to a halt as the other family members wait for the illness to pass, or they delay action because they are reluctant to assume the ill person's roles or responsibilities. Because of the effects of illness, family dynamics often change. The nurse must view the whole family as a client under stress, planning care to help the family regain the maximal level of functioning and well-being (see Chapter 9).

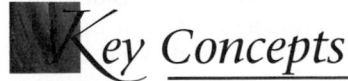 **ey** *Concepts*

- Health and wellness are not merely the absence of disease and illness.
- A person's state of health, wellness, or illness depends on individual values, personality, and lifestyle.
- The health belief model considers the relationship between a person's health beliefs and health behaviors.
- The health promotion model highlights factors that increase individual well-being and self-actualization.
- Holistic health models of nursing promote optimal health by incorporating active participation of clients in improving their health state.
- Health beliefs and practices are influenced by internal and external variables and should be considered when planning care.
- Health promotion activities help maintain or enhance health.
- Wellness education teaches clients how to care for themselves.
- Illness prevention activities protect against health threats and thus maintain an optimal level of health.
- Nursing incorporates health promotion, wellness, and illness prevention activities rather than simply treating illness.
- The three levels of preventive care are primary, secondary, and tertiary.
- Risk factors threaten health, influence health practices, and are important considerations in illness prevention activities.
- Improvement in health may involve a change in health behaviors.
- Illness behavior, like health practices, is influenced by many variables and must be considered by the nurse when planning care.
- Illness can have many effects on the client and family, including changes in behavior and emotions, family roles and dynamics, body image, and self-concept.

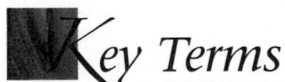 **ey** *Terms*

Critical Thinking Exercises

1. Identify two people you know—one whom you consider "healthy," the other whom you consider "unhealthy." What are the differences between these individuals? What characteristics did you use to determine health status?

2. How would you describe your current state of health: excellent, good, fair, or poor? What definition of health did you use to make this judgment? List the current health promotion, wellness, and illness prevention activities that you regularly engage in. Are there any areas that need to be improved or changed? What will influence your ability to adopt any needed changes?

3. Assess the lifestyle patterns of someone you know. Identify risk factors that increase this person's vulnerability to illness or susceptibility to disease. Are there risk factors present that could be modified?

4. With this same individual, how could you approach the subject of risk factor modification? What influences exist that will assist the individual in making a change? What barriers exist that may prevent maintenance of a change in health behavior? What resources are available to you and to this individual that may assist in the change process?

5. Have you witnessed illness behavior of yourself or someone you know? Did you (or they) respond differently to an acute versus a chronic illness? Evaluate the different responses you remember. Explore how the various internal and external variables influenced your reactions and behaviors. Was there an impact on the individual's self-concept or on family roles and dynamics?

Review Questions

1. When illness does occur, different attitudes about illness cause people to react in different ways. Medical sociologists call the reaction to illness:
   1. Illness behavior.
   2. Health belief.
   3. Health promotion.
   4. Illness prevention.

2. Defining health is difficult. The World Health Organization (WHO) defines health as:
   1. The absence of disease.
   2. A personal concept of health.
   3. Reaching full potential.
   4. A state of complete physical, mental, and social well-being, not merely the absence of disease or infirmity.

3. The health belief model addresses the relationship between a person's belief and behaviors, thus:
   1. A person who smokes does not practice the model.
   2. A person who does not take necessary medications does not practice the model.
   3. It provides a way of understanding and predicting how clients will behave in relation to their health and how they will comply with health care therapies.
   4. This model provides a basis for caring for clients of all ages.

4. Nurses using the holistic nursing model:
   1. Utilize only complementary interventions.
   2. Recognize the natural healing abilities of the body and incorporate complementary and alternative interventions.
   3. Consider only the mind and the body in providing care.
   4. Consider only the spiritual aspect in providing care.

5. Internal and external variables can influence how a person thinks and acts. Internal variables include:
   1. Temperature, blood pressure, and respirations.
   2. Anxiety, fever, respirations, blood pressure, and temperature.
   3. Developmental stage, intellectual background, perception of functioning, and emotional and spiritual factors.
   4. Bladder, heart, liver and gallbladder functioning.

6. A person's beliefs about health are shaped in part by the person's:
   1. Confidence in a healthcare provider.
   2. Knowledge of disease progression.
   3. Knowledge, lack of knowledge, or incorrect information about illness.
   4. Confidence in the healthcare system.

7. Health promotion activities can include:
   1. Exercise and good nutrition.
   2. Smoking and drinking excessive alcohol.
   3. Unsafe sex.
   4. Exposure to air pollutants.

8. Primary prevention aimed at health promotion includes:
   1. Rehabilitation and prevention of complications.
   2. Screening techniques and treating of early stages of disease.
   3. Health education programs, immunization, and physical and nutritional fitness activities.
   4. Care for a diabetic client using insulin.

9. This level of prevention would be directed at minimizing complications of disease:
   1. Primary prevention.
   2. Secondary prevention.
   3. Tertiary prevention.
   4. Illness prevention.

10. Acute illness and chronic illness are two general classifications of illness. Acute illness refers to an illness that:
   1. Is longer than 6 months, and can also affect functioning in any dimension.
   2. Has a short duration and is severe.
   3. Causes an irreversible condition.
   4. Is synonymous with disease.

References

Becker M, Maiman L: Sociobehavioral determinants of compliance with health and medical care recommendations, *Med Care* 13(1):10, 1975.

Conn VS: A staged-based approach to helping people change health behaviors, *Clin Nurs Spec* 8(4):187, 1994.

Crawley L and others: Strategies for culturally effective end-of-life care, *Ann Intern Med* 136(9): 673, 2002.

DiClemente C, Prochaska J: Toward a comprehensive thransthe-oretical model of change. In Miller WR, Healther N, editors: *Treating addictive behaviors,* New York, 1998, Plenum Press.

Edelman CL, Mandle CL: *Health promotion throughout the life span,* ed 5, St. Louis, 2002, Mosby.

Gunderman R: Illness as failure: blaming patients, *Hastings Cent Rep* 30(4):7, 2000.

King N and others: You can't cure it so you have to endure it: the experience of adaptation to diabetic renal diseases, *Qual Health Res* 12(3):329, 2002.

Kundhal KK: Cultural diversity: an evolving challenge to physician-patient communication, *JAMA* 289(1):94, 2003.

Leavell H, Clark A: *Preventive medicine for the doctor in his community,* ed 3, New York, 1965, McGraw-Hill.

Maslow AH: *Motivation and personality,* Upper Saddle River, NJ, 1970, Prentice Hall.

McEvoy M: Culture and spirituality as an integrated concept in pediatric care, *MCN Am J Matern Child Nurs* 28(1):39, 2003.

Mechanic D: The epidemiology of illness behavior and its relationship to physical and psychological distress. In Mechanic D: *Symptoms, illness behavior, and help seeking,* New York, 1982, Prodist.

Mechanic D: Sociological dimensions of illness behavior, *Soc Sci Med* 41(9):1207, 1995.

Murray RB, Zentner JP: *Health promotion strategies throughout the lifespan,* ed 7, Upper Saddle River, NJ, 2000, Prentice Hall.

Pender NJ: *Health promotion and nursing practice,* Norwalk, Conn, 1982, Appleton-Century-Crofts.

Pender NJ: Health promotion and illness prevention. In Werley HH, Fitzpatrick JJ, editors: *Annual review of nursing research,* New York, 1993, Springer.

Pender NJ: *Health promotion and nursing practice,* ed 3, Stamford, Conn, 1996, Appleton & Lange.

Pender NJ, Murdaugh CL, Parsons MA: *Health promotion in nursing practice,* ed 4, Upper Saddle River, NJ, 2002, Prentice Hall.

Prochaska JO: Assessing how people change, *Cancer* 67(3, suppl):805, 1991.

Raphael D: Models of illness, models of health, models of society, *Health Promotion: Global Perspective* 5(1):2, 2002.

Rosenstoch I: Historical origin of the health belief model, *Health Educ Monogr* 2:334, 1974.

Saarmann L, Daugherty J, Riegel B: Patient teaching to promote behavioral change, *Nurs Outlook* 48(6):281, 2000.

Shinitzky HE, Kub J: The art of motivating behavior change: the use of motivational interviewing to promote health, *Pub Health Nurs* 18(3):178, 2001.

U.S. Department of Health and Human Services, Public Health Service: *Healthy people 2000: national health promotion and disease prevention objectives,* Washington, DC, 1990, U.S. Government Printing Office.

U.S. Department of Health and Human Services, Public Health Service: *Healthy people 2010 objectives: draft for public comment,* Washington, DC, 1998, Office of Disease Prevention and Health Promotion.

World Health Organization Interim Commission: *Chronicle of WHO,* Geneva, 1947, The Organization.

Research References

Burggraf V, Barry RJ: Healthy people 2010: Protecting the health of older individuals, *J Gerontol Nurs* 26(12):16, 2000.

King N and others: You can't cure it so you have to endure it: the experience of adaptation to diabetic renal disease, *Qual Health Res* 12(3):329, 2002.

Knafl KA, Deatrick JA: The challenge of normalization for families of children with chronic conditions, *Pediatr Nurs* 28(1):49, 2002.

Leenerts MH, Teel CS, Pendelton MK: Building a model of self-care for health promotion in aging, *J Nurs Scholarsh* 34(4):355, 2002.

Prochaska JO, DiClemente CC: Stages of change in the modification of problem behaviors, *Prog Behav Modif* 28:184, 1992.

Resnick B: Health promotion practices of older adults: testing an individualized approach, *J Clin Nurs* 12(1):46, 2003.

7

$\mathscr{C}$aring in Nursing Practice

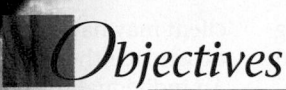

Objectives

Mastery of content in this chapter will enable the student to:

- Define the key terms listed.
- Discuss the role that caring plays in building a nurse-client relationship.
- Compare and contrast theories on the concept of caring.
- Discuss the potential implications when nurses' and clients' perceptions of caring might differ.
- Explain how an ethic of care influences nurses' decision making.
- Describe ways to convey caring through presence and touch.
- Describe the therapeutic benefit of listening to clients.
- Explain the relationship between knowing a client and clinical decision making.

Caring is central to nursing practice, but perhaps it has never been more important because of today's hectic health care environment. The pressure and time constraints on health care workers in most health care settings can result in nurses and other health professionals becoming cold and indifferent to client needs. The use of technological advances for rapid diagnosis and treatment often causes nurses and other health care providers to perceive the client relationship as less important. Benner and Wrubel (1989) warn that technological advances can be dangerous without a context of skillful and compassionate care. It is time to value and embrace the caring practices and expert knowledge that are the heart of nursing practice. A nurse who is able to engage clients in a caring and compassionate manner and recognizes the therapeutic gain in caring will make enormous contributions to the health and well-being of those clients.

Have you ever been ill or experienced a problem requiring health care intervention? Think about that experience for a moment. Then consider the following two scenarios and select the situation that you believe most successfully conveys a sense of caring (Box 7-1).

Case Study

Box 7-1

A nurse enters a client's room, greets the client warmly while touching the client lightly on the shoulder, makes eye contact, sits down for a few minutes and asks about the client's thoughts and concerns, listens to the client's story, looks at the intravenous (IV) solution hanging in the room, briefly examines the client, and then checks the vital sign summary on the bedside computer screen before departing the room.

A second nurse enters the client's room, looks at the IV solution hanging in the room, checks the vital sign summary sheet on the bedside computer screen, and acknowledges the client but never sits down or touches the client. Eye contact with the client is from the nurse's lofty vertical position to the client's vulnerable horizontal position. The nurse asks a few brief questions about the client's symptoms and then departs.

There is little doubt that the first scenario presents the nurse in specific acts of caring. The nurse's calm presence, parallel eye contact, attention to the client's concerns, and physical closeness all convey a person-centered, comforting approach. In contrast, the second scenario conveys a sense of indifference and interest only in the tasks of nursing care. During times of illness or when a person seeks the professional guidance of a nurse, caring is essential in helping the individual reach positive outcomes.

Theoretical Views on Caring

Caring is a universal phenomenon that influences the ways in which people think, feel, and behave in relation to one another. Caring in nursing has been studied from a variety of philosophical and ethical perspectives since the time of Florence Nightingale. A number of nursing scholars have developed theories on caring because of its importance to the practice of nursing as well as the existence of humankind. This chapter does not detail all of the theoretical positions on caring, but it should help beginning nurses understand that caring is at the heart of a nurse's ability to work with people in a respectful and therapeutic way.

Caring Is Primary
The works of Patricia Benner (1984) and Benner and Wrubel (1989) offers nurses a rich, holistic understanding of nursing practice and caring through the interpretation of expert nurses' stories. After listening to nurses' stories and analyzing their meaning, Benner is able to describe the essence of excellent nursing practice, which is caring. The nurses' stories revealed to Benner the nurses' behaviors and decisions that express caring. Caring means that persons, events, projects, and things matter to people (Benner and Wrubel, 1989). It is a word for being connected. Because caring determines what matters to a person, it describes a wide range of involvements, from parental love to friendship, from caring for one's work to caring for one's pet, to caring for and about one's clients. Benner and Wrubel (1989) note: "Caring creates possibility." Personal concern for another person, an event, or thing provides motivation and direction for people to care. Caring is an inherent feature of nursing practice, whereby nurses help clients to recover in the face of illness, to give meaning to that illness, and to maintain or reestablish connection. Caring makes nurses notice which interventions are successful, and this concern then guides future caregiving.

Clients are not all the same. Each individual brings a different background of experiences, values, and cultural perspectives to a health care encounter. Caring is always specific and relational for each nurse-client encounter. As nurses acquire more experience, they typically learn that caring helps them to focus on the clients for whom they care. Caring facilitates a nurse's ability to know a client, allowing the nurse to recognize a client's problems and to find and implement individualized solutions.

In addition to their work in understanding caring, Benner and Wrubel (1989) describe the relationship between health, illness, and disease. Health is not the absence of illness, nor is illness identical with disease (Chapter 6). Health is a state of being that people define in relation to their own values, personality, and lifestyle. Health exists along a continuum. Illness is the experience of loss or dysfunction, whereas disease is the manifestation of an abnormality at the cellular, tissue, or organ level. A client may have a disease (e.g., arthritis or diabetes) but not experience the sense of being ill or decrease in function. An individual may not seek health care until there is a disruption, loss, or concern. For example, a client may have had diabetes for a number of years but not sense being ill until the disease begins to cause serious visual impairment, threatening the ability to work. Illness therefore has meaning only within the context of the person's life.

Because illness is the human experience of loss or dysfunction, any treatment or intervention given without consideration of its meaning to an individual is likely to be worthless. Expert nurses understand the difference between health, illness, and disease. Through caring relationships, nurses learn to listen to clients' stories about their illness so that an understanding of the meaning of illness can be obtained. With this understanding, therapeutic, client-centered care can be provided.

The Essence of Nursing and Health
From a **transcultural** perspective, Madeleine Leininger (1978) describes the concept of care as the essence and central, unifying, and dominant domain that distinguishes nursing from other health disciplines. Care is also an essential human need, necessary for the health and survival of all individuals. Care, unlike cure, is oriented to assisting an individual or group in improving a human condition. Acts of caring refer to the nurturant and skillful activities, processes, and decisions that assist people in ways that are empathetic, compassionate, and supportive. An act of caring is dependent on the needs, problems, and values of the individual being assisted. Leininger's studies of numerous cultures around the world have found that care helps protect, develop, nurture, and provide survival to people. Care is vital to recovery from illness and to the maintenance of healthy life practices in all cultures.

Leininger (1988) stresses the importance of nurses' understanding both universal and nonuniversal folk and professional caring behaviors to be effective in the care of clients. Even though human caring is a universal phenomenon, the expressions, processes, and patterns of caring vary among cultures. Caring is very personal, and thus expression of caring will differ for each client. For caring to achieve cure, nurses must learn those culturally specific behaviors and words that reflect human caring in different cultures to identify and meet the needs of all clients (see Chapter 8).

Transpersonal Caring
Clients and their families should be able to expect a high quality of human interaction from nurses. Unfortunately, many of the conversations that occur between clients and their nurses are very brief and oftentimes disconnected. Jean Watson's theory of caring (1979, 1988) is a holistic model for nursing that suggests that a conscious intention to care potentiates healing and wholeness (Hoover, 2002). It does not discard conventional science or modern nursing practices, but is complementary to it. The theory of caring describes a consciousness that allows nurses to raise new questions about what it means to be a nurse, to be ill, and to be caring and healing. Watson's transpersonal caring theory (1988) rejects the disease orientation to health care and places care before cure. The

practitioner looks beyond the external disease and its treatment by conventional means. Transpersonal caring looks for deeper sources of inner healing to protect, enhance, and preserve a person's dignity, humanity, wholeness, and inner harmony.

In Watson's view, caring becomes almost spiritual. A nurse communicates caring-healing to the client through the consciousness of the nurse. This takes place during a single caring moment between nurse and client. An interconnectedness forms between the one cared for and the one caring. The model is **transformative,** as both the nurse and the client are influenced by the relationship, for better or for worse (Hoover, 2002). The caring-healing consciousness can promote healing. Application of Watson's caring model in practice can enhance nurses' caring practices. Box 7-2 summarizes a research study that successfully improved nursing students' awareness of caring practices.

Swanson's Theory of Caring

Kristen Swanson (1991) has conducted research with clients and professional caregivers in an effort to develop a theory of caring that applies to nursing practice. Swanson conducted interviews with three different groups: women who had miscarried, parents and health care professionals in a newborn intensive care unit, and socially at-risk mothers who had received long-term, public health intervention. All groups were in a perinatal (before, during, or after the birth of a child) setting or context and had experienced the phenomenon of caring.

Each group was asked questions regarding how caring was experienced or expressed in their situation. After analyzing the stories and descriptions of the three research groups, Swanson was able to develop a theory of caring. The theory describes caring as consisting of five categories or processes (Table 7-1). Swanson (1991) defines caring as a nurturing way of relating to a valued other, toward whom one feels a personal sense of commitment and responsibility. This theory supports the claim that caring is a central nursing phenomenon but not necessarily unique to nursing practice.

The contributions by Swanson (1991) are valuable in providing direction for how to develop useful and effective caring strategies. Each of the caring processes has definitions and subdimensions that can serve as the basis for nursing interventions. Thus the research findings used to develop the theory can be used in clinical nursing practice. For example, Swanson (1999) tested the effects of caring-based counseling on women's emotional well-being in the first year after miscarrying. Results from the study showed that caring-based counseling had significant benefit in reducing women's depression and anger, particularly for women in the first 4 months following miscarriage. Future research is needed to determine if Swanson's caring theory applies to other populations of clients.

Summary of Theoretical Views

There are common themes in nursing caring theories. Caring is highly relational. The nurse and the client enter into a relationship that is much more than one person

---

Research Highlight

Box 7-2

Enhancing Caring Practices

Research Focus

Caring has been shown to facilitate healing in clients and to improve client satisfaction with nursing care. A question to ask is, can human caring be influenced by the instructional process? Can educators of nurses present instructional methods that will improve students' caring practices?

Research Abstract

Hoover implemented an innovative 15-week module on nursing as human caring for a group of undergraduate nurses. The aim of the study was to improve students' understanding of caring practices and to thus make them more caring practitioners. The researcher interviewed students before and after completing the module to understand the impact of this module on their caring practices. For example, to gain a fuller understanding of the students' practices, they were asked what factors facilitated and impeded them caring in practice.

The students reported an increased self-awareness in regard to (1) connecting in relationships with self and others, (2) finding purpose and meaning in life, and (3) clarifying values. Several students spoke of becoming more tolerant of others, recognizing persons' uniqueness and appreciating their perspectives. By recognizing themselves as caring persons, the students

gained meaning in their lives. Many were able to relate a great deal of satisfaction in recognizing that they were caring persons and how nursing allowed them to express that. Finally, students also expressed an enhanced appreciation of what they valued.

Evidence-Based Practice

- When students acquire an increased knowledge and understanding of caring, they are able to understand a client's lifeworld and to change their approach to care delivery.
- Students who use caring in their practice also use a more holistic approach to care delivery. They recognize the importance of getting to know clients in order to elicit and therefore better meet their needs.
- The caring model involves a closeness, commitment, and involvement in the nurse-client relationship. This can be stressful for both nurse and client. The students who participated in the caring module were able to work through the emotional issues and practical constraints, which allowed them to grow spiritually and connect with clients at a deeper level.

Reference

Hoover J: The personal and professional impact of undertaking an educational module on human caring, *J Adv Nurs* 37(1):79, 2002.

Table 7-1	Swanson's Theory of Caring	
Caring Process	**Definitions**	**Subdimensions**
Knowing	Striving to understand an event as it has meaning in the life of the other	Avoiding assumptions Centering on the one cared for Assessing thoroughly Seeking cues Engaging the self or both
Being with	Being emotionally present to the other	Being there Conveying ability Sharing feelings Not burdening
Doing for	Doing for the other as he or she would do for the self if it were at all possible	Comforting Anticipating Performing skillfully Protecting Preserving dignity
Enabling	Facilitating the other's passage through life transitions (e.g., birth, death) and unfamiliar events	Informing/explaining Supporting/allowing Focusing Generating alternatives Validating/giving feedback
Maintaining belief	Sustaining faith in the other's capacity to get through an event or transition and face a future with meaning	Believing in/holding in esteem Maintaining a hope-filled attitude Offering realistic optimism "Going the distance"

From Swanson K: Empirical development of a middle-range theory of caring, *Nurs Res* 40(3):161, 1991.

simply "doing tasks for" another. There is a mutual give-and-take that develops as nurse and client begin to know and care for one another. Frank (1998) described a personal situation when he was suffering from cancer: "What I wanted when I was ill, was a mutual relationship of *persons* who were also clinician and client." It was important for Frank to be seen as one of two fellow human beings, not the dependent client being cared for by the expert technical clinician.

Caring may seem highly invisible at times, when a nurse and client enter a relationship of respect, concern, and support. The nurse's empathy and compassion become a natural part of every client encounter. However, when caring is absent, it becomes very obvious. For example, if the nurse shows disinterest or chooses to avoid a client's request for help, the nurse's inaction will quickly convey an uncaring attitude. Benner and Wrubel (1989) relate the story of a clinical nurse specialist who learned from a client what caring is all about: "I felt that I was teaching him a lot, but actually he taught me. One day he said to me (probably after I had delivered some well-meaning technical information about his disease), 'You are doing an OK job, but I can tell that every time you walk in that door you are walking out.'" The client perceived that the nurse was simply going through the motion of teaching and showed little caring toward the client.

Clients quickly know when nurses fail to relate to them. In contrast, when caring is practiced, the client senses a commitment on the part of the nurse and is willing to enter into a relationship that allows the nurse to gain an understanding of the client's experience of illness. In a study of oncology clients, one client described a

nurse's caring as "putting the heart in it" and "having an investment" that makes "clients feel that you are with them" (Radwin, 2000). This allows the nurse to become a coach and partner rather than a detached provider of care.

Another theme is understanding the context of the person's life and illness. It is difficult to show caring to another individual without gaining an understanding of who they are and their perception of their illness. Exploring the following questions with a client can assist the nurse in understanding a client's perception of illness: How was the illness first recognized? How does the client feel? What does the client think is the cause? How does the illness affect the client's daily life practices? Knowing the context of a client's illness helps the professional nurse to choose and individualize interventions that will actually help the client. This approach is more successful than simply selecting interventions on the basis of the client's symptoms or disease process.

Clients' Perceptions of Caring

Swanson's theory of caring (1991) provides an excellent beginning to understanding the behaviors and processes that characterize caring. Other researchers have also studied caring from clients' perceptions (Table 7-2). The identification of behaviors that clients perceive as caring helps to emphasize what clients expect from their caregivers. Clients have always valued nurses' effectiveness in performing tasks, but, clearly, clients also value the affective dimension of nursing care (Williams, 1997). Establishing a reassuring presence, recognizing an individual as unique, and keeping a close, attentive eye on the client are recur-

Table 7-2	A Comparison of Research Studies Exploring Nurse Caring Behavior (as Perceived by Clients)		
Riemen (1986)		Attree (2001)	Mayer (1986)
Perceptions of Female Clients	Perceptions of Male Clients	General Medical Patients' and Families' Perceptions	Perceptions of Cancer Clients
Responding to client's uniqueness	Being physically present so client feels valued	Checking up on clients	Knowing how to give injections and manage equipment
Being perceptive and supportive of client's concerns	Returning voluntarily without being called	Being compassionate and patient	Being cheerful
Being physically present	Making client feel comfortable, relaxed, and secure	Demonstrating sensitivity and sympathy	Encouraging clients to call if they have problems
Having attitudes and displaying behaviors that make client feel valued as a human being	Attending to comfort and needs of client before doing tasks	Using a calm, gentle, and kind approach	Putting clients first
Returning to client voluntarily without being asked	Using a kind, soft, pleasant, gentle voice and attitude		Anticipating that first experiences are the hardest
Showing concern that is comforting and relaxing			
Using a soft, gentle voice			
Invoking feelings of security			
Invoking feelings in client of wanting to reciprocate			

rent caring behaviors that researchers have identified. All clients are unique; however, understanding common behaviors that clients associate with caring will help the beginning student learn to express caring in practice.

The study of clients' perceptions is important because health care is placing greater emphasis on client satisfaction (see Chapter 2). What clients experience in their interactions with institutional services and health care professionals, and what they think of that experience, can determine how clients use the health care system and how they can benefit from it (Gerteis and others, 1993). When clients sense that health care providers are interested in them as people, clients will be more willing to follow recommendations and therapeutic plans. Williams (1997) studied the relationship between clients' perceptions of four dimensions of caring and their satisfaction with nursing care. Clients in the study indicated that they were more satisfied when they perceived nurses to be caring. Radwin (2000) found that oncology clients associated excellent nursing care with attentiveness, partnership, individualization, rapport, and caring. As institutions look to ways of improving client satisfaction, creating an environment of caring is a necessary and worthwhile goal. Clients' satisfaction with nursing care is an important factor in their decision to return to a hospital.

As a nurse begins clinical practice, it is important to consider how clients perceive caring and what are the best approaches to providing care. The behaviors that researchers have associated with caring offer an excellent starting point. It is also important to determine an individual client's perceptions and unique expectations. Researchers have learned that frequently clients and nurses differ in their perceptions of caring (Mayer, 1987).

For that reason, nurses must focus on building a relationship that allows them to learn what is important to their clients. A client who is fearful of having an intravenous catheter inserted may benefit more from the novice nurse's acquiring assistance from a staff member who can quickly and skillfully insert the catheter than from the novice nurse's attempt to relieve anxiety through a lengthy description of the procedure. Knowing who clients are helps the nurse to select those caring approaches that are most appropriate to the clients' needs.

Ethic of Care

Caring is interpreted by many as being a moral imperative. Through caring for other human beings, ultimately human dignity is protected, enhanced, and preserved. Watson (1988) suggests that caring, as a moral ideal, provides the stance from which one intervenes as a nurse. This stance is critical for ensuring that nurses practice ethical standards for good conduct, character, and motives. Chapter 21 explores the importance of ethics in professional nursing. The term *ethics* refers to the ideals of right and wrong behavior. In any client encounter, a nurse must know what behavior is ethically appropriate. An ethic of care is unique so that professional nurses do not make professional decisions based solely on intellectual or analytical principles. Instead, an ethic of care places caring at the center of decision making. Should an indigent client be cared for? Is it caring to place a disabled relative in a long-term care facility?

An **ethic of care** is concerned with relationships between people and with a nurse's character and attitude toward others. Nurses who function from an ethic of care are sensitive to unequal relationships that can lead to an abuse of one person's power over another—intentional or otherwise. In health care settings clients and families are often on unequal footing with professionals because of the client's illness, lack of information, regression caused by pain and suffering, and unfamiliar circumstances. An ethic of care places the nurse as the client's advocate, solving ethical dilemmas by attending to relationships and by giving priority to each client's unique personhood.

Caring in Nursing Practice

It is impossible to prescribe ways that will guarantee whether or when a nurse becomes a caring professional. Scholars disagree as to whether caring can be taught or is more fundamentally a way of being in the world. For those who find caring a normal part of their life, caring is a product of their culture, values, experiences, and relationships with others. Persons who do not experience care in their lives often find it difficult to act in caring ways. As nurses deal with health and illness in their practice, they grow in the ability to care. Nursing behaviors that have been shown to be related to caring include providing presence, a caring touch, and listening. Nurses who are able to demonstrate caring use a caring approach in each encounter with clients.

Providing Presence

To provide **presence** is to have a person-to-person encounter that conveys a closeness and a sense of caring. Fredriksson (1999) explains that presence involves "being there" and "being with." "Being there" is not only a physical presence, but also communication and understanding. The interpersonal relationship of "being there" seems to depend on the fact that a nurse is attentive to the client (Cohen and others, 1994). This type of presence is something the nurse offers to the client with the purpose of achieving some goal, such as support, comfort, or encouragement, to diminish the intensity of unwanted feelings or for reassurance (Pederson, 1993; Fareed, 1996).

"Being with" is also interpersonal. The nurse gives himself or herself, which is understood as being available and at a client's disposal (Pederson, 1993). If clients accept the nurse, they will invite him or her to see, share, and touch their vulnerability and suffering. The nurse then enters the client's world. In this presence, the client is able to put words to feelings and to understand himself or herself in a way that leads to identifying solutions, seeing new directions, and making choices (Gilje, 1997).

When a nurse establishes presence, eye contact, body language, voice tone, listening, and having a positive and encouraging attitude act together to create an openness and understanding. The message conveyed is that the other's experience matters to the one caring (Swanson, 1991). Being able to establish presence with a client also enhances the nurse's ability to learn from the client. As a result, the nurse's ability to provide adequate and appropriate nursing care is strengthened.

It is especially important to establish presence when clients are experiencing stressful events or situations. Awaiting a doctor's report of test results, preparing for an unfamiliar procedure, and planning for a return home after serious illness are just a few examples of events in the course of a person's illness that can create unpredictability and dependency on care providers. The nurse's presence can help to allay anxiety and fear related to stress. Giving reassurance and thorough explanations about a procedure, remaining at the client's side, and coaching the client through the experience all convey a presence that is invaluable to the client's well-being.

Touch

Clients face situations that can be embarrassing, frightening, and painful. Whatever the feeling or symptom, clients look to nurses to provide comfort. The use of touch is one **comforting** approach whereby the nurse reaches out to clients to communicate concern and support.

Touch is a form of relating that leads to a connection between nurse and client. Touch involves contact and noncontact touch (Fredriksson, 1999). Contact touch involves obvious skin-to-skin contact, whereas noncontact touch refers to eye contact. It is difficult to separate the two. Both in turn are described within three categories: task-orientated touch, caring touch, and protective touch (Fredriksson, 1999).

A nurse uses task-orientated touch when performing a task or procedure. The skillful and gentle performance of a nursing procedure conveys security and a sense of competence in the nurse. An expert nurse learns that any procedure is more effective when it is administered carefully and in consideration of any client concern. For example, if a client is anxious about having a procedure, such as the insertion of a nasogastric tube, the nurse affords comfort through a full explanation of how the procedure will be done and what the client will feel. The nurse then conveys the sense that the procedure will be performed safely, skillfully, and successfully in the way the nurse prepares supplies, positions the client, and gently manipulates and inserts the nasogastric tube. Throughout a procedure the nurse talks quietly with the client to provide reassurance and support.

Caring touch is a form of nonverbal communication that can successfully influence a client's comfort and security, enhance self-esteem, and improve reality orientation (Boyek and Watson, 1994). It may be expressed in the way a nurse holds a client's hand, gives a back massage, gently positions a client, or participates in a conversation. When using a caring touch, the nurse is making a connection with the client and showing acceptance of the individual (Tommasini, 1990).

Protective touch is a form of touch used to protect the nurse and/or client (Fredriksson, 1999). It can be viewed by the client either positively or negatively. The most obvious form of protective touch is that used to prevent an accident, for example, holding and bracing the client to avoid a fall. Protective touch is also a kind of touch that protects the nurse emotionally. A nurse might withdraw or distance herself or himself from a client when the nurse cannot tolerate suffering or needs to escape from a

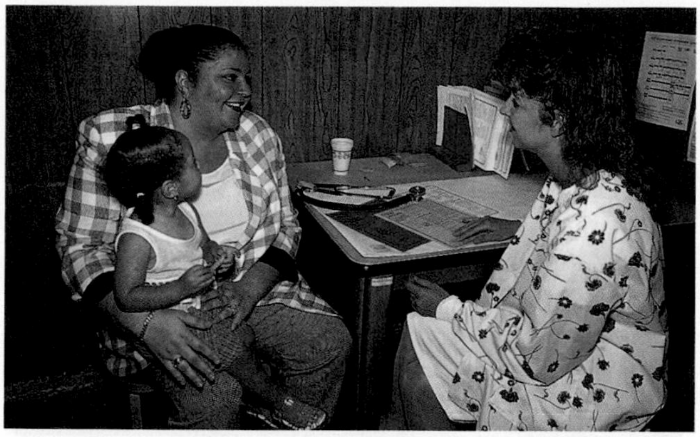

FIGURE **7-1** Nurse listening to client.

situation that is causing tension. When used in this way, protective touch can elicit negative feelings in a client (Fredriksson, 1999).

Because touch can convey many messages, it must be used with discretion. Task-orientated touch is generally sanctioned by the client, as most individuals give nurses and doctors a license to enter their personal space to provide care. However, exceptions can exist because of clients' cultural backgrounds. A nurse should understand if clients are accepting of touch and how they interpret the nurse's intentions.

Listening

Caring involves an interpersonal interaction that is much more than two persons simply talking back and forth. In a caring relationship the nurse establishes trust, opens lines of communication, and listens to what the client has to say (Figure 7-1). Listening is key, because it can convey the nurse's full attention and interest. Listening not only is "taking in" what a client says, but also includes interpretation and understanding of what is said and giving back that understanding to the person talking (Kemper, 1992). Listening to the meaning of what a client says helps create a mutual relationship.

When an individual becomes ill, he or she usually has a story to tell about the meaning of the illness. Any critical or chronic illness affects all of a client's life choices and decisions, sometimes affecting the individual's identity. Being able to tell that story helps the client break the distress of illness. Thus a story needs a listener. Frank (1998) described his own feelings during his experience with cancer: "I needed a [health care professional's] gift of listening in order to make my suffering a relationship between *us,* instead of an iron cage around *me.*" He needed to be able to express what he needed when he was ill. The personal concerns that are part of a client's illness story determine what is at stake for the client. Caring through listening enables the nurse to be a participant in the client's life.

To be able to listen, listeners needs to silence themselves to listen with openness (Fredriksson, 1999). Fredriksson describes silencing one's mouth and also the mind. It is important to remain intentionally silent and to concentrate on what the client has to say. A nurse

must be able to give clients his or her full, focused attention as their stories are told.

When an ill person chooses to tell his or her story, it involves reaching out to another human being. Telling the story implies a relationship that can develop only if the clinician exchanges his or her stories as well. Frank (1998) argues that professionals do not routinely take seriously their own need to be known as part of a clinical relationship. Yet, unless the professional acknowledges this need, there is no reciprocal relationship, only an interaction (Campo, 1997). There is pressure on the clinician to know as much as possible about the client, but it isolates the clinician from the client. By contrast, knowing and being known each supports the other (Frank, 1998).

Learning to listen to a client is sometimes difficult. It is easy to become distracted by tasks at hand, colleagues shouting instructions, or other clients waiting to have their needs attended to. However, the time one takes to listen (and listen effectively) is worthwhile both in the information gained and in the strengthening of the nurse-client relationship. Listening involves paying attention to the individual's words and tone of voice and entering his or her frame of reference. By observing the expressions and body language of the client, the nurse can find cues to help assist the client in exploring ways to achieve greater peace, take action, or do whatever a situation requires (Hungelmann and others, 1996). Chapter 23 discusses additional listening techniques.

Knowing the Client

One of the five caring processes described by Swanson (1991) is knowing the client. The concept comprises both the nurse's understanding of a specific client and the nurse's subsequent selection of interventions (Radwin, 1995). Knowing develops over time as a nurse learns the array of clinical conditions within a specialty and the behaviors and physiological responses of clients. To know a client means that the nurse avoids assumptions, focuses on the client, and engages in a caring relationship with the client that reveals information and cues that facilitate critical thinking and clinical judgments (see Chapter 14). Knowing the client is at the core of the process by which nurses make clinical decisions. By establishing a caring relationship, the mutuality that develops helps the nurse to better know the client as a unique individual and to then choose the most appropriate and efficacious nursing therapies.

The caring relationships that a nurse develops over time, coupled with the nurse's growing knowledge and experience, provide a rich source of meaning when changes in a client's clinical status occur. Expert nurses develop the ability to detect changes in clients' conditions almost effortlessly. Clinical decision making, perhaps the most important responsibility of the professional nurse, involves various aspects of knowing the client: responses to therapies, routines and habits, coping resources, physical capacities and endurance, and body typology and characteristics (Tanner and others, 1993). The experienced nurse knows additional facts about his or her clients such as their experiences, behaviors, feelings, and perceptions (Radwin, 1995). When clinical decisions are made accurately in the context of knowing a client well, improved client outcomes will result. Swanson-Kaufman (1986) notes that when care is based on knowing the client, it is perceived by clients as personalized, comforting, supportive, and healing.

The most important thing for a beginning nurse to recognize is that knowing a client is much more than simply gathering data about the client's clinical signs and condition. Of course, this information must be gathered. But success in knowing the client lies in the relationship that is established. To know a client is to enter into a caring, social process that results in a "bonding" whereby the client comes to feel known by the nurse (Lamb and Stempel, 1994). The bonding then sets the stage for the relationship to evolve into "working" and "changing" phases so that the nurse can help the client become involved in his or her care and accept help when needed.

Spiritual Caring

Spiritual health is achieved when a person finds a balance between his or her own life values, goals, and belief systems and those of others. Research has shown a link between spirit, mind, and body. An individual's beliefs and expectations can and do have effects on the person's physical well-being (Coe, 1997).

Establishing a caring relationship with a client involves an interconnectedness between the nurse and the client. This interconnectedness is why Watson (1979) describes the caring relationship in a spiritual sense. Spirituality offers a sense of connectedness as well, intrapersonally (connected with oneself), interpersonally (connected with others and the environment), and transpersonally (connected with the unseen, God, or a higher power). When a caring relationship is established, the client and the nurse come to know one another so that both move toward a healing relationship by:

- Mobilizing hope for the client and for the nurse
- Finding an interpretation or understanding of illness, symptoms, or emotions that is acceptable to the client
- Assisting the client in using social, emotional, or spiritual resources

Chapter 28 describes in detail the significance that spirituality plays in an individual's health.

Family Care

People live in their worlds in an involved way. Each individual experiences life through relationships with others. Caring for an individual thus cannot occur in isolation from that person's family. As a nurse, it is important to know the family almost as thoroughly as one knows a client (Figure 7-2). The family is an important resource. Success with nursing interventions often depends on the family's willingness to share information about the client, their acceptance and understanding of therapies, whether the interventions fit with the family's daily practices, and whether the family can support and deliver the therapies recommended.

Mayer (1986) identified 10 nurse caring behaviors that were perceived as most helpful by families of clients with cancer (Box 7-3). Ensuring the client's well-being and helping the family to become active participants are crit-

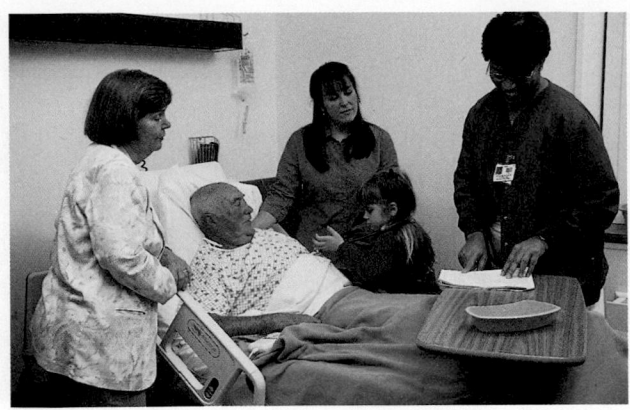

FIGURE 7–2   Nurse discusses client's health care needs with the family.

Box **7-3**	**Nurse Caring Behaviors as Perceived by Families**

Being honest
Giving clear explanations
Keeping family members informed
Trying to make the client comfortable
Showing interest in answering questions
Providing necessary emergency care
Assuring the client that nursing services will be available
Answering family members' questions honestly, openly, and willingly
Allowing clients to do as much for themselves as possible
Teaching the family how to keep the relative physically comfortable

Data from Mayer DK: Cancer patients' and families' perceptions of nurse caring behaviors, *Top Clin Nurs* 8(2):63, 1986.

ical for family members. Although specific to families of clients with cancer, the behaviors offer useful guidelines for developing a caring relationship with all families. The nurse begins a relationship by learning who makes up the client's family and what their roles are in the client's life. Showing the family care and concern for the client creates an openness that then enables a relationship to form with the family. Caring for the family takes into consideration the context of the client's illness and the stress it imposes on all members (see Chapter 9).

The Challenge of Caring

For many nurses, being able to assist individuals during a time of need is the reason for entering the profession. Hoover (2002) found that when nurses are able to affirm themselves as caring individuals, they achieve a meaning and purpose to their lives. The profession of nursing, unlike medicine, can care for and assist people without medical diagnoses or new technologies and treatments. Caring is a motivating force for people to become nurses and it becomes the source of satisfaction when nurses know they have made a difference in their clients' lives.

It is becoming more of a challenge to care in today's health care system. Being a part of the helping professions is difficult and demanding. Nurses are given less time to spend with clients, making it much harder to know who they are. A reliance on technology and cost-effective health care strategies and efforts to standardize and refine work processes all undermine the nature of caring. Too often clients become just a number, with their real needs either overlooked or ignored.

Recently the Tri-Council for Nursing (2001), an organization representing an alliance of the American Nurses Association (ANA), National League for Nursing (NLN), American Organization of Nurse Executives (AONE), and American Association of Colleges of Nursing (AACN), has recommended strategies to reverse the current nursing shortage. A number of the strategies have potential for creating work environments that enable nurses to demonstrate more caring behaviors. The strategies include introducing greater flexibility into the work environment structure, rewarding experienced nurse mentors, improving nurse staffing, and providing nurses with autonomy over their practice.

Human beings cannot be treated like machines or robots if health care is to make a positive difference in their lives. Instead, health care must become more humanizing. As professionals, nurses play an important role in making care an integral part of health care delivery. This begins by nurses' making caring a part of the philosophy and environment in the workplace. Incorporating care concepts into standards of nursing care establishes the guidelines for professional conduct. Finally, during the day-to-day practice with clients and families, nurses must be committed to caring and be willing to establish the relationships necessary for personal, compassionate, and meaningful nursing care to be delivered.

Key Concepts

- Caring is at the heart of a nurse's ability to work with people in a respectful and therapeutic way.
- Caring is always specific and relational for each nurse-client encounter.
- For caring to achieve cure, nurses must learn those culturally specific behaviors and words that reflect human caring in different cultures.
- Since illness is the human experience of loss or dysfunction, any treatment or intervention given without consideration of its meaning to the individual is likely to be worthless.
- Swanson's theory of caring includes five caring processes: knowing, being with, doing for, enabling, and maintaining belief.
- Caring involves a mutual give and take that develops as nurse and client begin to know and care for one another.
- It is difficult to show caring to another individual without gaining an understanding of who they are and their perception of their illness.

- Presence involves a person-to-person encounter that conveys a closeness and a sense of caring that involves "being there" and "being with" clients.
- Research has shown that touch, both contact and noncontact, includes task-orientated touch, caring touch, and protective touch.
- The skillful and gentle performance of a nursing procedure conveys security and a sense of competence in the nurse.
- Listening is not only "taking in" what a client says, it also includes interpretation and understanding of what is said and giving back that understanding to the person talking.
- Knowing the client is at the core of the process by which nurses make clinical decisions.
- A nurse demonstrates caring by helping family members become active participants in a client's care.

Key Terms

Caring, *p. 108*
Comforting, *p. 112*
Ethic of care, *p. 111*

Presence, *p. 112*
Transcultural, *p. 108*
Transformative, *p. 109*

Critical Thinking Exercises

1. Lindsey is a senior nursing student assigned to care for Mrs. Lowe, a 62-year-old client being treated for lymphoma (cancer of the lymph nodes). Mrs. Lowe is to receive an injection for her pain. In what way can Lindsay show caring in the way she administers the injection to Mrs. Lowe?
2. Mr. Leonard is a 42-year-old man who is married and has two teenage daughters. He underwent surgery this morning for an angioplasty to correct obstruction of his coronary arteries. The recovery room nurse calls the nursing division and tells you that Mr. Leonard has arrived, is stable, and will likely be there for 2 to 3 hours. His doctor will be up to the division shortly. What can you do to demonstrate caring for Mr. Leonard?
3. During your next clinical practicum, select a client to talk with for at least 15 to 20 minutes. Ask the client to tell you about his or her illness. Review the skills of listening in this chapter and in Chapter 23. Immediately after your discussion, reflect on the discussion with the client and answer the following questions:
   a. What do you believe the client was trying to tell you about his or her illness?
   b. Why was it important for the client to share his or her story?
   c. What did you do that made it easy or difficult for the client to talk with you?
   d. Would you rate yourself a good listener? If not, why not? If so, explain.
   e. The next time you are assigned to a clinical agency, ask to read their philosophy and standards of care documents. Does the language in the documents represent a caring ethic?

Review Questions

1. A nurse hears a colleague tell a student nurse she never touches the clients unless she is performing a procedure or doing an assessment. The nurse tells the colleague that:
   1. She does not touch the clients either.
   2. Touch is a verbal communication.
   3. Touch is a form of relating that leads to a connection between nurse and client.
   4. There is never a problem with using touch.

2. One of the five caring processes is "knowing" the client. This concept is best described as:
   1. Gathering task-oriented information.
   2. Knowing reasons for the client's physician preference.
   3. Knowing the client's personal business information.
   4. Avoiding assumptions and focusing on the client.

3. A nurse is overheard saying there is no place in nursing for spiritual caring. A nursing colleague replies:
   1. You are correct. Religion is a personal decision.
   2. Nurses should not force their religious beliefs on clients.
   3. Spiritual care should be left to a professional.
   4. There is a link between spirit, mind, and body that can have a direct effect on a client's health.

4. A nurse is overheard complaining about a client's family being "too involved" in the client's care. A colleague replies:
   1. The family is an important resource.
   2. "You are right, the family should just stay out of nursing matters!"
   3. "The client doesn't like her family anyway."
   4. "The family will not follow through with care when she goes home."

5. A number of strategies have potential for creating work environments that enable nurses to demonstrate more caring behaviors. Some of these include:
   1. Increases in monetary gain.
   2. Increasing working hours.
   3. Flexibility, autonomy, and improved staffing.
   4. Increased imput concerning nursing functions from physicians.

6. As professionals, nurses play an important role in making care an integral part of health care delivery. This begins by nurses:
   1. Making caring a part of the philosophy and environment in the workplace.
   2. Incorporating personal views in the workplace.
   3. Disregarding the family's views of care.
   4. Making all decisions in the care of the clients.

7. A nurse can demonstrate caring by helping family members:
   1. Make health care decisions for the client.
   2. Provide activities of daily living (ADLS).
   3. Become active participants in care.
   4. Remove themselves from any form of personal care.

8. Listening is not only "taking in" what a client says, it also includes:
   1. Interpreting and understanding of what is said and giving back that understanding to the person talking.
   2. Injecting the nurse's personal views and statements.
   3. Correcting any errors in the client's understanding.
   4. Incorporating the views of the physician.

9. Presence involves a person-to-person encounter that:
   1. Provides personal care to a client.
   2. Conveys a closeness and a sense of caring.
   3. Describes being in close contact with a client.
   4. Enables clients to care for self.

10. The study of clients' perceptions is important because health care is:
    1. Placing greater emphasis on client satisfaction.
    2. Always in the best interest of the client.
    3. Carefully watched by the federal government.
    4. Under investigation for misappropriation of funds.

References

Attree M: Patients' and relatives' experiences and perspectives of "good" and "not so good" quality care, *J Adv Nurs* 33(4):456, 2001.

Benner P: *From novice to expert,* Menlo Park, Calif, 1984, Addison-Wesley.

Benner P, Wrubel J: *The primacy of caring: stress and coping in health and illness,* Menlo Park, Calif, 1989, Addison Wesley.

Campo R: *The poetry of healing: a doctor's education in empathy, identification, and desire,* New York, 1997, WW Norton.

Coe RM: The magic of science and the science of magic: an essay on the process of healing, *J Health Soc Behav* 38(3):1, 1997.

Cohen MZ and others: Knowledge and presence: accountability as described by nurses and surgical patients, *J Prof Nurs* 3:177, 1994.

Fareed A: The experience of reassurance: patients' perspectives, *J Adv Nurs* 23:272, 1996.

Frank AW: Just listening: narrative and deep illness, *Fam Syst Health* 16(3):197, 1998.

Gerteis M and others: What patients really want, *Health Manage Q* 15:2, 1993.

Hoover J: The personal and professional impact of undertaking an educational module on human caring, *J Adv Nurs* 37(1):79, 2002.

Hungelmann J and others: Focus on spiritual well-being: harmonious interconnectedness of mind-body-spirit—use of the JAREL spiritual well-being scale, *Geriatr Nurs* 17(6):262, 1996.

Lamb G, Stempel G: Nursing case management from the client's view: growing as insider-expert, *Nurs Outlook* 42(7):7, 1994.

Leininger M: *Transcultural nursing: concepts, theories and practices,* New York, 1978, John Wiley & Sons.

Leininger M: *Care: the essence of nursing and health,* Detroit, 1988, Wayne State University Press.

Mayer DK: Cancer patients' and families' perceptions of nurse caring behaviors, *Top Clin Nurs* 8(2):63, 1986.

Mayer DK: Oncology nurses' versus cancer patients' perceptions of nurse caring behaviors: a replication study, *Oncol Nurs Forum* 14(3):48, 1987.

Swanson K: Empirical development of a middle-range theory of caring, *Nurs Res* 40(3):161, 1991.

Swanson-Kauffman K: Caring in the instance of unexpected early pregnancy loss, *Top Clin Nurs* 8(2):37, 1986.

Tri-Council for Nursing: Tri-Council for Nursing policy statement, January 31, 2001, NLNupdate@nln.org.

Watson MJ: *Nursing: the philosophy and science of caring,* Boston, 1979, Little, Brown.

Watson MJ: New dimensions of human caring theory, *Nurs Sci Q* 1:175, 1988.

*R*esearch References

Boyek K, Watson R: A touching story, *Elderly Care* 3:20, 1994.

Fredriksson L: Modes of relating in a caring conversation: a research synthesis on presence, touch, and listening, *J Adv Nurs* 30(5):1167, 1999.

Gilje F: Presence: Us-Norway nursing research perspectives. In Hummelvoll JK, Lindstrom UA, editors: *Nordiska Perspektiv Psykiatrisk Omvudnad,* Lund, 1997, Studentlitteratur.

Hoover J: The personal and professional impact of undertaking an educational module on human caring, *J Adv Nurs* 37(1):79, 2002.

Kemper BJ: Therapeutic listening: developing the concept, *J Psychosoc Nurs* 7:21, 1992.

Pederson C: Presence as a nursing intervention with hospitalized children, *Matern Child Nurs J* 3:75, 1993.

Radwin L: Knowing the patient: a process model for individualized interventions, *Nurs Res* 44:364, 1995.

Radwin L: Oncology patients' perceptions of quality nursing care, *Res Nurs Health* 23(3):179, 2000.

Riemen DJ: The essential structure of a caring interaction: doing phenomenology. In Munhall PL, Oiler CJ: *Nursing research: a qualitative perspective,* Norwalk, Conn, 1986, Appleton-Century-Crofts.

Swanson KM: Empirical development of a middle-range theory of caring, *Nurs Res* 40(3):161, 1991.

Swanson, KM: Effects of caring, measurement, and time on miscarriage impact and women's well-being, *Nurs Res* 48(6):288, 1999.

Tanner C and others: The phenomenology of knowing the patient, *Image J Nurs Sch* 25:273, 1993.

Tommasini NR: The use of touch with the hospitalized psychiatric patient, *Arch Psychiatr Nurs* 4:213, 1990.

Williams SA: The relationship of patients' perceptions of holistic nurse caring to satisfaction with nursing care, *J Nurs Care Qual* 11(5):15, 1997.

8

Culture and Ethnicity

Media Resources

http://evolve.elsevier.com/Potter/
fundamentals/

 CD COMPANION

- Review Questions
- Glossary

evolve WEBSITE

- Review Questions
- Student Learning Activities
- Glossary

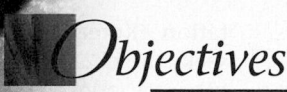

Objectives

Mastery of content in this chapter will enable the student to:

- Define key concepts relevant to cultural diversity in nursing and health care.

- Describe social and cultural influences in health, illness, and caring patterns.

- Differentiate culturally congruent from culturally competent care.

- Describe steps toward developing cultural competence.

- Identify major components of cultural assessment.

- Use cultural assessment to identify significant values, beliefs, and practices critical to nursing care of individuals through life transitions.

- Demonstrate nursing interventions to achieve culturally congruent care.

- Analyze outcomes of culturally congruent care.

- Apply research findings in culturally congruent care.

Population Diversity

The demographic profile of the United States is changing dramatically as a result of immigration patterns and significant increases in culturally diverse populations already residing in the country. Population projections beyond 2000 show Hispanics/Latinos, Asian-Americans, and African-Americans outpacing the growth of white, European-descended groups. In the state of California, Hispanics/Latinos constitute the majority of the total population (http://factfinder.census.gov.servlet). In 2020 the population of African-Americans is predicted to double and that of Asian-Americans and Hispanics/Latinos to triple. Linguistic diversity is also proliferating with over 300 languages spoken in 2000 (www.census.gov/population/www/estimates/popest.html).

Health Disparities

Elimination of longstanding disparities in access to health services and the health status of people from diverse racial, ethnic, and cultural backgrounds (*Healthy People 2010*) have resulted in many initiatives at the local and national level (U.S. Department of Health and Human Services, 1998). Title VI of the Civil Rights Act mandates that no person in the United States, regardless of race, color, or national origin, should be excluded from participation, denied benefits, or be subjected to discrimination under any program receiving federal funding. In compliance with these mandates, legislative, regulatory, and accreditation agencies have set standards in support of cultural and linguistic competence in health care.

Understanding Cultural Concepts

Culture consists of the totality of socially transmitted knowledge of values, beliefs, norms, and lifeways of a particular group that guides their thoughts and behaviors (Purnell and Paulanka, 1998; Leininger, 2002a). Culture evolves as a way of life by a group of people who deal with similar issues of survival over a period of time in their environment. People who live in an environment with distinct seasonal changes such as fall, winter, spring, and summer tend to plan for the future in order to survive the changes and hardships imposed by different weather conditions. Preoccupation with distinct future time is not characteristic of cultures that live in geographical areas with stable temperatures and abundant sunlight and rain. Social organization is also shaped by human-environmental interaction. In the harsh, difficult environment of the Kalahari Desert, group reliance and communal sharing of food and game facilitate survival. Concepts of personal property and territory are foreign to the **Kalahari bushmen,** whose kinship unit is a tribe comprised of several families governed by a council of elder males.

Culture has both **visible** (easily seen) and **invisible** (less observable) components. It is important to understand that the invisible value-belief system of a particular culture is the major driving force behind visible practices. Although a **Sikh** man can be easily identified by the visible artifacts that he wears (uncut hair with wooden comb, beard, turban, cotton underwear, steel bracelet, and short sword), the meanings and beliefs associated with these artifacts are not easily appreciated without further assessment. These artifacts symbolize a devotee's allegiance to the pillars of Sikhism, and removal of these artifacts without expressed consent of the individual or his family is considered sacrilegious and violates the ethnoreligious identity of the person (Singh, 2000).

In any society, there is a dominant culture that exists along with other variant cultural patterns (Kluckhohn, 1976). These variant patterns may be referred to as diverse cultures, subcultures, or minority cultures. Although subcultures may have similarities with the dominant culture, they maintain their unique life patterns, values, and norms. In the United States, the dominant culture is Anglo-American with origins from Western Europe. **Subcultures** such as the Appalachian and Missouri Ozark cultures represent various ethnic, religious, and other groups with distinct characteristics from the dominant culture. **Ethnicity** refers to a shared identity related to social and cultural heritage such as values, language, geographical space, and racial characteristics. Members of an ethnic group feel a common sense of identity. Individuals may declare their ethnic identity as Irish, Vietnamese, or Brazilian. A term that is usually contrasted from ethnicity is race, which is limited to the common biological attributes shared by a group such as skin color (Spector, 2000; Leininger and McFarland, 2002). Examples of racial classifications include blacks and whites.

In any intercultural encounter, there is an insider or native perspective **(emic worldview)** and an outsider's perspective **(etic worldview).** A nurse is baffled by a Korean female's request for seaweed soup for her first meal after giving birth. Although the nurse has an emic view of professional postpartal care, as an outsider to the Korean culture, she is not aware of the significance of the practice to the client. Conversely, the Korean client who has an etic view of American professional care assumes that seaweed soup should be available in the hospital because it cleanses the blood and promotes healing and lac-

tation (Korean health beliefs, 2003). Unless the nurse seeks the client's emic view, he or she is likely to suggest other varieties of soups available from the dietary department, disregarding the cultural meaning of the practice to the client.

The processes of enculturation and acculturation facilitate cultural learning. Socialization into one's primary culture as a child is known as **enculturation.** The process of adapting to and adopting a new culture is **acculturation** (Padilla, Wagatsuma, and Lindholm, 1984). Acculturation outcomes may result in varying degrees of affiliation with the dominant culture. **Assimilation** results when an individual gives up his or her ethnic identity in favor of the dominant culture (Spector, 2000). **Biculturalism** (sometimes known as multiculturalism) occurs when an individual identifies equally with two or more cultures (Purnell and Paulanka, 1998). Filipino nurses who migrate to seek better economic opportunities in the United States have been enculturated to the mainstream culture of the Philippines and are motivated to acculturate to the new American culture. Rather than assimilating to the American culture, many are choosing to be bicultural and acculturate their American-born children to the Filipino culture through their own ethnic community.

Cultural backlash (Leininger and McFarland, 2002) may occur as a countercultural effect when experience with the new or different culture is extremely negative and the culture is then rejected. The devaluation of education as a pathway to success in mainstream society has been observed among poor, inner-city African-American youths. Because of varying degrees of affiliation with new cultures, nurses must avoid stereotypes or unwarranted generalizations about any particular group that prevents further assessment of the individual's unique characteristics. Nurses should determine the degree to which an individual's life patterns are consistent with his or her heritage (Spector, 2002). Previous knowledge about a culture is maintained as *holding* knowledge (Leininger, 2002a), which persists until an accurate assessment of the individual's emic stance about his or her life is obtained.

Culturally Congruent Care

Leininger (1991, 2002a) has defined **transcultural nursing** as a comparative study of cultures to understand similarities (culture universal) and differences (culture-specific) across human groups. The goal of transcultural nursing is **culturally congruent care**—care that fits the people's valued life patterns and set of meanings—which is generated from the people themselves, rather than based on predetermined criteria. Culturally congruent care may be distinct from the values and meanings of the professional health care system. Discovering clients' culture care values, meanings, beliefs, and practices as they relate to nursing and health care requires nurses to assume the role of learners of clients' culture and copartners with clients and families in defining the characteristics of meaningful and beneficial care (Leininger, 2002b).

Culturally competent care requires specific knowledge, skills, and attitudes in the delivery of culturally congruent care. Pacquiao (2003) identifies three distinct levels of cultural competence at the practitioner, organizational, and societal levels. Culturally competent care is the ability of the practitioner to bridge cultural gaps in caring, work with cultural differences, and enable clients and families to achieve meaningful and supportive caring. Cultural competence is the synthesis of all three levels. Although practitioners constitute organizations, they need systemwide support to implement culturally congruent care. Culturally competent communities and societies are knowledgeable and skilled in using health care services and articulating their rights, as well as needs, to practitioners and organizations. For example, an individual practitioner, who is aware of Gypsy culture and skilled in dealing with Gypsy families, may not be able to provide for their need to be present in groups near the bedside of a hospitalized family member. The practitioner also needs organizational support in adapting space resources to accommodate the volume of visitors who tend to remain within the premises for long periods. Communities of Gypsies need to inform, negotiate, and demand accommodations for their caring patterns from hospital administration and staff. Box 8-1 lists the federally mandated guidelines for cultural competence in health care services delivery. These guidelines target systems and organizations engaged in providing health services.

Campinha-Bacote (2002) defines cultural competence as a process of development with five interlocking components: cultural awareness, knowledge, skill, encounters, and desire, as shown in Figure 8-1. Cultural awareness is an in-depth self-examination of one's own background, recognizing biases and prejudices and assumptions about other people. Cultural knowledge is obtaining sufficient comparative knowledge of diverse groups, including their indigenous values, health beliefs, care practices, worldview, and biocultural ecology. Cultural skills includes assessment of social, cultural, and biophysical factors influencing treatment and care of clients. Cultural encounters involve the engagement in cross-cultural interactions that can provide learning of other cultures and opportunities for effective intercultural communication development. Cultural desire is the motivation and commitment to caring that moves an individual to learn from others, accept the role as learner, be open and accepting of cultural differences, and build upon cultural similarities. Cultural competence is the process of acquiring specific knowledge, skills, and attitudes that ensure delivery of culturally congruent care. For example, a nurse assigned to a female Egyptian client decides to seek information about the Egyptian culture. Upon learning that female modesty and gender-congruent care are valued in the culture, the nurse encourages female relatives to provide for the client's hygienic needs. The nurse's cultural encounter allows her to understand nonverbal cues of the client's discomfort with lack of privacy. The nurse also notes that the client's male relatives are more assertive in their interactions.

Box *8-1*   Office of Minority Health Standards for Culturally and Linguistically Appropriate Health Care by Health Care Organizations

- Promote and support attitudes, behaviors, knowledge, and skills necessary for staff to work respectfully and effectively with patients and each other in a culturally diverse work environment.
- Have a comprehensive management strategy, including strategic goals, plans, policies, procedures, and designated staff responsible for implementation.
- Utilize formal mechanisms of community and consumer involvement in the development and execution of service delivery.
- Develop and implement a strategy to recruit, retain, and promote qualified diverse and culturally competent administrative, clinical, and support staff who are trained to address the needs of racial and ethnic communities.
- Require and arrange for ongoing education and training for administrative, clinical, and support staff in culturally and linguistically competent delivery of service.
- Provide all clients having limited English proficiency with access to bilingual interpretation services.
- Provide oral and written notices, including translated signage at key points of entry, to clients in their primary language, informing them of their right to receive interpreter services.
- Translate and make available signage and commonly used written patient educational materials in the predominant language(s) in the service area.

- Ensure that interpreters and bilingual staff can demonstrate bilingual proficiency and receive training that includes the skills and ethics of interpreting.
- Ensure that the clients' primary spoken language and self-identified race/ethnicity are included in the health care organization's information system.
- Use a variety of methods to collect and utilize accurate demographic, cultural, epidemiological, and clinical outcome data for racial and ethnic groups and become informed about the ethnic/cultural needs, resources, and assets of the surrounding community.
- Undertake ongoing organizational self-assessment of cultural and linguistic competence and measures for access, satisfaction, quality, and outcome using internal audits and performance improvement programs.
- Develop structures and procedures to address cross-cultural ethical and legal issues in health care delivery and complaints or grievances by patients and staff about unfair, culturally insensitive, or discriminatory treatment, or difficulty in accessing services, or denial of services.
- Prepare an annual progress report documenting progress in implementing these standards, including information on programs, staffing, and resources.

Office of Minority Health: Assuring cultural competence in health care: recommendations for national students and an outcomes-focused research agenda, Washington, DC, 1999, Department of Health and Human Services, U.S. Public Health Service, www.omhre.gov/clas/ds/htm.

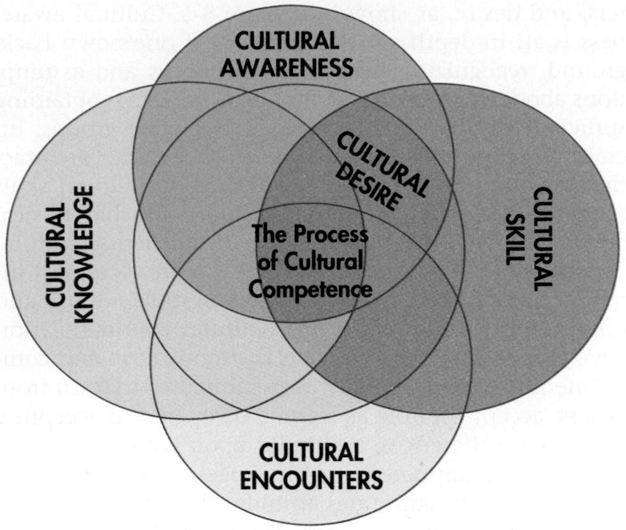

FIGURE **8–1** The process of cultural competence in delivery of health care services. (From Campinha-Bacote: 1999. The process of cultural competence in the delivery of health care services: a model of care, *J Transcult Nurs* 13(3):181, 2002. Printed with permission from Transcultural C.A.R.E. Associates, Cincinnati, Ohio.)

Cultural Conflicts

Culture provides the context for valuing, evaluating, and categorizing our life experiences. Cultural groups transmit their values, morals, and norms from one generation to another, which predisposes members to **ethnocentrism,** a tendency to hold one's own way of life as superior to others. Ethnocentrism is the root of biases and prejudices comprising beliefs and attitudes associating negative permanent characteristics with people who are perceived to be different from the valued group. When action is taken on one's prejudices, discrimination occurs. This is exemplified by a nurse who refuses to give the prescribed pain medication to a young African male with sickle cell anemia because of his or her belief (stereotyped bias) that young male Africans are likely to be drug abusers. Health care practitioners who have cultural ignorance or cultural blindness about differences generally resort to **cultural imposition** and use their own values and lifeways as the absolute guide in dealing with clients and interpreting their behaviors. Hence, a nurse who believes that pain is to be borne quietly as a demonstration of strong moral character will be annoyed by a client's insistence to have pain medication and may try to deny the client's discomfort.

Cultural Context of Health and Caring

Health, illness, and caring are phenomena embedded in a culture (Kleinman, 1979; Leininger, 2002a). Culture is the context in which groups of people interpret and define their experiences relevant to life transitions such as birthing, illness, and dying. It is the system of meanings by which people make sense of their experiences. Culture is

the framework used in defining social phenomena such as when a person is healthy or requires intervention. For example, in most African groups, a robust body is considered a sign of health in the same way that a plump baby is viewed as healthy in some Hispanic cultures (Loustaunau and Sobo, 1997; Higgins, 2000). In Jamaican culture, pregnancy is not viewed as a medical condition but rather as a normal life transition, hence a pregnant woman need not go to a doctor unless she has a problem (Sobo, 1993).

Table 8-1 provides a comparison of cultural contexts of health and illness in Western and non-Western cultures. Attributed causes of illness are highly influenced by cultural beliefs. Among the Hmong refugees (group of people who originated from the mountainous regions of Laos) in California, epilepsy or seizure disorder is believed to be caused by wandering of the soul, hence treatment includes intervention by a **shaman** who can perform the ritual to retrieve the client's soul (Fadiman, 1997). Their belief is distinct from the scientifically determined neurological abnormality causing seizures. The biomedical orientation of Western cultures emphasizing scientific investigation and reducing the human body into distinct parts is in conflict with the holistic conceptualization of health and illness in non-Western cultures. Holism is evident in the belief in continuity between humans and nature, and between human events and metaphysical and magico-religious phenomena. Hence, epilepsy as conceived by the Hmong people is caused by loss of one's spirit to the magical and supernatural forces in nature. Establishing a diagnosis of epilepsy in Western cultures requires scientifically proven techniques and confirmed criteria for the abnormality. Such medical criteria are meaningless to the **Hmong,** who believe in the global causation of the illness that goes beyond the mind and body of the person to forces in nature. The choice of healers or health care practitioners is conditioned by the attributed cause. Whereas a Hmong will seek a shaman, a Westerner will seek a neurologist who meets universalistic criteria for practice. A shaman, on the other hand, has an established reputation in the Hmong community, whose qualifications for healing are neither determined by published standardized criteria nor confined to specific bodily systems. A shaman uses rituals symbolizing the supernatural, spiritual, and naturalistic modalities of prayers, herbs, and incense burning.

The dominant value orientation in North American society is individualism and self-reliance in achieving and maintaining health. Caring approaches generally promote the client's independence and ability for self-care. In collectivistic cultures that value group reliance and interdependence such as traditional Asians, Hispanics, and Africans, caring behaviors are manifested by actively providing physical and psychosocial support for kin members. An adult client is not expected to be solely responsible for his or her care and well-being; rather, family and kin are relied upon to make decisions and provide for his or her care (Pacquiao, 2001). A traditional Chinese older adult woman's refusal to independently perform rehabilitation exercises after hip surgery until her daughter is present to assist her may be misconstrued by Western practitioners as lack of self-responsibility and motivation

Table 8-1	Comparative Cultural Contexts of Health and Illness	
	Western Cultures	**Non-Western Cultures**
Cause of illness	Biomedical causes	Imbalance between humans and nature Supernatural Magico-religious
Method of diagnosis	Scientific, high-tech Specialty focused Organ-specific manifestations	Naturalistic, magico-religious Holistic Mixed Global, nonspecific symptomatology
Treatment	Specialty specific Pharmacological Surgery	Holistic Mixed (magico-religious, supernatural herbal, biomedical, etc.)
Practitioners/Healers	Uniform standards and qualifications for practice	May be learned through apprenticeship Criteria for practice not uniform Reputation established in community
Caring pattern	Self-care Self-determination	Caring provided by others Group reliance and interdependence

Data from Foster G: Disease etiologies in non-Western medical systems, *Am Anthropol* 78:773,1976; Kleinman A: *Patients and healers in the context of culture*, Berkeley, 1979, University of California Press; and Leininger M, McFarland M: *Transcultural nursing: concepts, theories, research and practice*, ed 3, New York, 2002, McGraw-Hill.

for her care. In contrast, the client may interpret the nurse's insistence on self-care as uncaring behavior.

Cultural Healing Modalities and Healers

Health care systems have evolved into externalizing or internalizing systems (Young, 1976). **Externalizing systems** connect health and illness to social and cosmological factors. For instance, human immunodeficiency virus (HIV)/acquired immunodeficiency syndrome (AIDS) may be seen as punishment from God for one's evil deeds (cosmological) or transgression of social taboos (dishonoring one's elders). **Internalizing systems** are observed in modern societies with highly scientific and technological capacity to examine internal structural and biological causes of health and illness. An example is the Western biomedical system, which has been criticized for being specialty driven and having a tendency to minimize effects of social and cultural factors on health and illness.

Disparities in health outcomes between the rich and poor illustrate the influence of socioeconomic factors in morbidity and mortality. Social factors such as poverty and lack of universal medical insurance compromise the health status of the poor and unemployed. Cultural practices may pose advantages and health risks to members of a particular society. Sedentary lifestyle and high caloric intake have increased risks to cardiovascular disorders among Americans who value a convenient and efficient way of life. This value is translated in fast-foods, cars, and obsession with technology to perform many of the physical tasks of daily life.

Foster (1976) has identified two distinct categories of healers cross-culturally. **Naturalistic practitioners** attribute illness to natural, impersonal, and biological forces that cause alteration in the equilibrium of the human body. Healing emphasizes naturalistic modalities using herbs, chemicals, heat, cold, massage, and surgery. In contrast, **personalistic practitioners** believe that health

and illness can be caused by active influence of an external agent, which can be human (i.e., sorcerer) or nonhuman (e.g., ghosts, evil, or deity). Personalistic beliefs emphasize the importance of humans' relationship with others, both living and deceased, and with their deities. For example, a voodoo priest uses modalities that combine supernatural, magical, and religious beliefs through the active facilitation of an external agent or personalistic practitioner. A Haitian woman who believes in voodoo attributes her illness to a curse placed by someone and seeks the services of a voodoo priest to remove the cause. Personalistic approaches also include naturalistic modalities such as massage, aromatherapy, and herbs (see Chapter 35). A combination of modalities is used by some clients who seek both types of practitioners to achieve health and treat illness. Table 8-2 is a list of cultural healers commonly used by different groups in the United States.

Because of coexisting and simultaneous use of both healing systems, nurses must avoid making rash judgments about clients' practices. Nurses need to gain knowledge and understanding of folk remedies used by clients to prevent cultural imposition. Many Southeast Asian cultures practice folk remedies such as coining, cupping, pinching, and burning to relieve aches and pains and remove bad wind or noxious elements that cause illness. It should be noted that other groups, including Eastern Europeans, also use cupping as an acceptable treatment for respiratory ailments. These remedies leave peculiar visible markings on the skin in the form of ecchymosis, superficial burns, strap marks, or local tenderness. Cultural ignorance may precipitate a practitioner to call authorities for suspicion of abuse. Different groups commonly use herbal therapy with some distinct differences from each other. Instead of dismissing the practice as dangerous and incompatible with Western medicine, practitioners need to investigate further whether the practice needs changing. Consultation and collaboration with herbalists and

Table 8-2	Cultural Healers	
Cultural Group	**Healer**	**Nature of Practice**
Chinese and Southeast Asians	Herbalist	Combination of plant, animal, and mineral products in restoring balance based on yin/yang concepts
	Acupuncturist	Yin treatment using needles to restore balance and flow of *qi*; yang treatment using moxibustion or heat with acupuncture may be indicated to restore yin/yang balance
	Fortune teller	Consultation to foretell outcomes of plans and seek spiritual advice to enhance good fortune and deal with misfortune
	Shaman	Combination of prayers, chanting, and herbs to treat illnesses caused by supernatural, psychological, and physical factors
Asian Indians	Ayurvedic practitioner	Combination of dietary, herbal, and other naturalistic therapies to prevent and treat illness
Native American	Shaman	Combination of prayers, chanting, and herbs to treat illnesses caused by supernatural, psychological, and physical factors
African-American	Old lady "granny midwife"	Consultation in diagnosing and treating common illnesses and care of women in childbirth and children
	Spiritualist	Spiritual advisement, counseling, and prayers to treat illness or cope with personal and psychosocial problems
	Voodoo practitioners *Hougan* (male) *Mambo* (female)	Combination of herbs, drumming, and symbolic offerings to cure illness, remove curses, and protect a person
Hispanic	*Curandero/a*	Combination of prayers, herbs, and other rituals to treat traditional illnesses, especially in children
	Parteras Lay midwives	Assistance for women in childbirth and newborn care
	Yerbero Herbalist	Consultation for herbal treatment of traditional illnesses
	Sabador Bonesetters	Massage and manipulation of bones and joints used to treat a variety of ailments, including musculoskeletal conditions
	Espiritista Spiritualist	Foretelling of future and interpretation of dreams; combination of prayers, herbs, potions, amulets, and prayers for curing illnesses, including witchcraft
	Santero/a	Combination of prayers, symbolic offerings, herbs, potions, and amulets against witchcraft and curses

Data from Hautman MA: Folk health and illness beliefs, *Nurse Practitioner* 4(4):23, 1976; Loustaunau MO, Sobo EJ: *The cultural context of health, illness and medicine,* Westport, Conn, 1997, Bergin & Garvey; and Spector RE: *Cultural diversity in health and illness,* Englewood Cliffs, NJ, 2000, Prentice Hall.

other naturalistic practitioners can prevent unwarranted distress for the client.

Culture-Bound Syndrome

Kleinman (1980) has identified that human groups create their own interpretation and descriptions of biological and psychological malfunctions within their unique social and cultural context. **Culture-bound syndromes** are illnesses constituted by the personal, social, and cultural explanations and reactions of a given society to perceived dysfunctions or abnormalities in its members. ***Hwa-Byung*** is a Korean culture-bound syndrome observed among middle-age, low-income women who are overwhelmed and frustrated by the burden of caregiving for their in-laws, husbands, and children. Symptoms are generally somatic manifestations consisting of insomnia, fatigue, anorexia, indigestion, feelings of an epigastric mass, palpitations, heat, panic, feelings of impending doom, dyspnea, and others. Women unconsciously avoid expressions of symptoms that counter the cultural ideal of females as the caretaker of elders, husbands, and children. Symptoms reflect the cultural definition of illness as

imbalance between heat (yang) and cold (yin) (Park and others, 2001). In the United States, these symptoms are defined as depression related to anger and treated differently (American Psychological Association, 1994).

Culture and Life Transitions

Transitions to different phases of life are generally marked by rituals that symbolize cultural values and meanings attached to these life passages. Van Gennep (1960) originated the concept of **rites of passage** as significant social markers of changes in a person's life. Examining the practices surrounding these life events provides a glimpse of the cultural meanings and expressions relevant to these transitions. Sending flowers and get-well greetings to a sick person is a ritual denoting love and caring for the client in the Western world. In collectivistic groups such as the Hispanic culture, physical presence of loved ones with the client demonstrates caring. Whereas Americans value individual privacy, most Hispanics value group interdependence.

Pregnancy

Reproduction is valued across cultures because it promotes continuity of the family and community. Infertility in a woman is considered grounds for divorce and rejection among Arabs (AbuGharbeih, 1998). Pregnancy that occurs outside of accepted societal norms is generally considered taboo. Among traditional Muslims, pregnancy out of wedlock may result in severe sanctions meted out by the family against the female member (Moazam, 2000).

Pregnancy is generally associated with caring practices that symbolize the significance of this life transition in women. Some Asian, African, and Hispanic cultures believe that a mother's activities and predispositions also affect the fetus. Many cultures believe that if a pregnant woman's food craving is not met, negative consequences to the baby will occur. Among traditional Koreans, the family protects the pregnant woman from emotional and physical stress lest the baby will also be stressed. She is prevented from viewing the dead or being burdened by news of someone's illness. Pregnant Korean women avoid eating chicken, crab, eggs, duck, rabbit, and blemished fruits as these may harm the baby's appearance (Reardon, 1996).

Some cultures that subscribe to hot and cold theory of illness, such as the Hindus, view pregnancy as a hot state, so cold foods such as milk and milk products, yogurt, sour foods, and vegetables are encouraged. Hot foods such as chilies, ginger, and animal products are believed to cause miscarriage and fetal abnormality (Turrell, 1985). Although heat and cold theory is shared by many cultures, there is no agreement on what foods and beverages are classified as hot or cold. These classifications are made distinct by their unique ecological and ethnohistorical attributes. Because lactose intolerance is common among Asians, milk and milk products are generally avoided. Pregnant women are encouraged to have vegetables, and nourishing soups are generally part of everyday meals.

Modesty is a strong value among Afghan (Lipson and others, 1995) and Arab women (Meleis, 1996; Meleis and Sorrell, 1981), who may avoid prenatal visits because of embarrassment and may demand to be examined by a female practitioner. Religious beliefs may interfere with prenatal testing, as in the case of a Filipino couple refusing amniocentesis because they believe that the outcome of pregnancy is God's will. Supernatural beliefs associated with pregnancy are evident in the belief among some Hispanics that baby showers early in pregnancy bring bad luck or **mal de ojo** (evil eye) (Spector, 2000). Orthodox Jews avoid baby showers and do not announce the baby's name before the naming ceremony for the same reason (Lewis, 2003).

Childbirth

The manner by which pain is expressed and the expectation about how one's suffering is treated vary cross-culturally. Puerto Rican and Mexican women are verbally expressive of their pain during labor. **Parteras** or lay midwives commonly advise a screaming woman in labor to close her mouth as an open mouth will cause the uterus to rise (Purnell, 1998). Middle Eastern mothers are observed to be verbally expressive, crying and screaming aloud, yet may refuse pain medication (Meleis and Sorrell, 1981).

Fear of drug addiction and the belief that pain is a form of spiritual atonement for one's past deeds motivate most Filipino mothers to tolerate pain without much complaining or asking for medication (Pacquiao, 2001). Southeast Asian women believe that crying and screaming are shameful and consider labor pains as expected and to be endured (Lee and Essoka, 1998).

Religious beliefs may prohibit the presence of males, including husbands, from the delivery room. This may be observed among devout Muslims, Hindus, and Orthodox Jews. Husbands generally leave the room with the appearance of the bloody show (Lewis, 2003; Meleis and Sorrell, 1981; Callister, Semenic and Foster, 1999). As soon as the child is born, a Muslim father or mother whispers the Islamic call to prayer in the newborn's ear, welcoming the baby into the life of the world where the responsibility to Allah's call is the greatest (Emerick, 2002).

Practitioners other than medical doctors attend childbirth in some groups, such as *parteras* among Mexicans, granny midwives among Appalachian and southern African-Americans, and **hilots** among Filipinos (Barry and Boyle, 1996; Frankel, 1977; Miranda, McBride and Spangler, 1998). Known in their communities, these practitioners are affordable and accessible in remote areas. They use a combination of naturalistic, religious, and supernatural modalities combining herbs, massage, and prayers.

A growing number of cultural groups in the United States are now asking to take home the placenta after delivery (Box 8-2). Some Native Americans and Hispanics bury or dispose of the placenta congruent with gender-differentiated attributes for the child. For females, whose primary task is to take care of the family, the placenta is buried close to home. For males, who are expected to be adventurous and become the family breadwinner, the placenta is buried far from home. Ashes from the ceremonial burning of the placenta may be kept for future medicinal purposes in some Asian cultures.

Newborn

The age of the newborn may vary in some cultures. Among traditional Vietnamese and Koreans, a newborn is considered a year old at birth. Once acculturated to the U.S. culture, they assume a bicultural view, deducting 1 year from the age of the child when speaking to an outsider. In the Yoruba tribes in Nigeria, the baby is named at the official naming ceremony that occurs 8 days after birth and coincides with circumcision. Birth of a son is greatly celebrated in many cultures around the world, including Chinese, Asian Indians, Islamic groups, and **Igbos** in West Africa.

The name of the child reflects cultural values of the group. It is typical for a Hispanic baby to have several first names followed by the surnames of the father and mother (Maria Kristina Lourdes Lopez Vega). The bilineal tracing of descent from both the mother's and father's side in the Hispanic group is in stark contrast to the patrilineal system, where the last name of the father precedes the child's first name. In the Chinese culture, descent is traced only from the paternal side. Hence the name Chen Lu means that Lu is the daughter of Mr. Chen.

Box 8-2

Research Highlight

Afterbirths in the Afterlife: Cultural Meaning of Placental Disposal in a Hmong-American Community

Research Focus

Culturally congruent care is increasingly expected by clients and families in the hospital setting. Cultural knowledge of beliefs and practices of clients enables nurses to provide culturally competent care during life transitions such as birthing and dying as illustrated by the study of Hmong refugees in California.

Abstract

The Hmong are mostly Buddhists and animists who originated from the mountainous regions of Laos. They assisted the Americans during the Vietnam War and were granted refugee status after the fall of South Vietnam. The study involved interviews of 94 older Hmong adults living in California regarding their cultural beliefs and practices. The study findings revealed that the Hmong maintain their cultural belief in burying the placenta at home after birth. Informants reported that they were hesitant to ask their health care practitioners for their babies' afterbirths. They believe that upon death a person's soul travels into the spirit world to rejoin deceased ancestors. Because the home is the burial place of afterbirths, one's spirit is unable to unite with one's ancestors if one's placenta is not brought home and given proper burial. Because men are expected to be the center of the family hierarchy, a baby boy's afterbirth is buried at the center of the home. Women are expected to join and support their husbands, so a girl's afterbirth is buried near the home.

Evidence-Based Practice

- Clients may have difficulty communicating their cultural care values and practices to outsiders such as nurses and other health care practitioners. Failure of Hmong clients to ask for afterbirths does not mean the practice no longer exists.
- Inability to practice valued traditions has enormous impact on clients and families. For the Hmong, inability to practice placental burial at home has implications for the person's life in the present and beyond.
- Cultural knowledge and assessment is significant in understanding cultural care meanings, beliefs, and practices of clients.
- The goal of cultural assessment is to discover the emic meanings of care that enables nurses to act in ways that clients themselves recognize as beneficial and enabling.
- Culturally congruent care allows for meaningful, supportive, and facilitative care respectful of diverse values and practices of people.

Reference

Helsel DG, Mochel M: Afterbirths in the afterlife: cultural meaning of placental disposal in a Hmong-American community, *J Transcult Nurs* 13(4):282, 2002.

Newborns and young children are considered vulnerable cross-culturally, and many societies use a variety of ways to prevent the evil eye by using amulets, religious medals, herbs, or spices. Among the mostly Catholic Filipinos, the newborn is kept inside the home until after the baptism to ensure the baby's health and protection. The practice of using a cotton binder or **fajita** on the baby's abdomen to prevent gas and umbilical hernia may be evident among Filipinos and Hispanic groups (Miranda, McBride, and Spangler, 1998). Filipinos may rub warm oil on the baby's belly to prevent and relieve gas. Babies are believed to be vulnerable to cold and wind; hence they are not bathed for a number of days among traditional Iranians. They remain indoors with their mothers for a period of 30 to 40 days (Lipson and Hafizi, 1998).

Some cultures do not regard the colostrum (initial cloudy breast secretion following delivery) as healthy for the baby. For some Hindus and Muslims, the colostrum is dirty and not fit to be given to a newborn. Breast-feeding is postponed until regular milk appears. Alternative measures should be instituted to promote expulsion of meconium (thick secretion in the fetus's gastrointestinal tract) and lactation in the meantime (Jambunathan, 1998; Lipson and Hafizi, 1998). Higginbottom's study (2000) of mothers of African ancestry who migrated to the United Kingdom found that their attitudes toward breast-feeding are influenced by the social structure of their new environment. Lacking their traditional support systems and faced with a societal norm that does not encourage or provide facilities for breast-feeding at work or in public places, these women decide not to breast-feed. Nurses need to investigate the reasons for refusal to breast-feed rather than assume that once informed of the advantages, mothers should comply. Attempt should be made to address the barriers first before any mother can be expected to implement the teaching.

Postpartum Period

In many non-Western cultures the postpartum period is associated with vulnerability of the mother to cold. To restore balance, mothers may refuse a shower and prefer a sponge bath. Mothers may refuse sitz baths but may agree to heat lamp treatments to promote perineal healing. Special dietary practices are observed by some groups to give food and beverages classified as hot to restore balance. Cultural groups have preferences in terms of what types of foods are considered appropriate to restore balance in women after birth. Soups, eggs, and tea may be preferred by Chinese mothers, whereas rural Iranian families may provide pistachio nuts and eggs (Lipson and Hafizi, 1998; Matocha 1998). The length of the postpartum period is generally much longer (30 to 40 days) in non-Western cultures to provide much attention and support for the mother and her baby. This is one of the reasons given for the rarity of postpartum depression in these cultures when compared to the United States

(Stewart and Jambunathan, 1996). Hispanic women may go into a 40-day period of **la cuarantena** and may be placed on a regimen of dietary **(la dieta)** and restricted physical activity (Horn, 1981). This cultural belief that the mother needs much rest and relaxation after delivery may conflict with the Western belief in early ambulation.

Use of an abdominal binder to prevent air from entering the woman's uterus and promote healing is practiced among Filipino, Mexicans, and Pacific Islanders (Miranda, McBride, and Spangler, 1998; Purnell, 1998). Among Orthodox Jewish, Islamic, and Hindu cultures, bleeding is associated with pollution. A woman goes into a ritual bath after bleeding stops before she can resume relations with her husband (Lewis, 2003; Lipson and Hafizi, 1998). In some African cultures, such as in Ghana and Sierra Leone, some women will not resume sexual relations with their husbands until the baby is weaned.

Grief and Loss

Dying and death bring a resurgence of traditions that have been meaningful to groups of people most of their lives (see Chapter 29). When traditional medical measures fail, cultural beliefs and practices that are religious and spiritual take center stage. Societies assign different meanings to death of a child, a young person, and an older adult. In Western cultures with strong future time orientation and where a child is expected to survive his or her parents, death of a young person is devastating. In cultures, however, where infant mortality is very high, the emotional distress over a child's death is tempered by the reality of the commonly observed risks of growing up. Hence, untimely death of an adult may be mourned more deeply.

Societies that believe in the concept of reincarnation, such as devout Hindus and Buddhists, may view death as a step toward rebirth. Care of the dying is focused in supporting the client's preparation for a good death. The family will pray and read religious scriptures to the client to improve his or her chances in the next cycle. Buddhists generally believe that life is suffering and suffering is mitigated when a person moves beyond the earthly desires and atones for past misdeeds. A dying Hindu male prepares for a good death by refusing nourishment and medications, concentrating all his energies on the spiritual aspects of the journey to the next cycle (Pacquiao, 2002). Belief in afterlife allows some Jewish Americans to let go and accept death (Bonura and others, 2001).

Culture strongly influences pain expression and need for pain medication. Whereas a typical American believes in individual freedom and autonomy as synonymous with freedom from pain and suffering, other groups accept suffering. Nurses need not assume that pain relief is equally valued across groups. **Cultural pain** may be suffered by a client whose valued way of life is disregarded by practitioners (Leininger and McFarland, 2002). Inability of Orthodox Jews to pray in groups at the bedside with the dying client because of limitations in the number of visitors allowed can cause cultural pain in the client and family. Working with the family and their religious/spiritual leader will facilitate culturally congruent care (Pacquiao, 2003).

Regulatory mandates and organizational policies intended to benefit clients should be implemented with sensitivity and understanding of their cultural life patterns. The dominant value in American society of individual autonomy and self-determination may be in direct conflict with diverse groups. Advance directives, informed consent, and consent for hospice are examples of mandates that may violate clients' values. Informed consent and advance directives protect the right of the individual to know and make decisions insuring continuity of these rights even to the time when the individual is incapacitated. However, other cultures are organized so that the group assumes decision making for a family member in these situations and is trusted to make the rightful decision for the individual. Indeed, some groups such as African-Americans, Asian-Americans, and Hispanics expect their family to make decisions for them, and family members prefer to protect the individual from unnecessary suffering by knowing the reality of imminent death. These cultures value group interdependence and view individual autonomy as an unnecessary burden for a loved one who is ill (Pacquiao, 2002, 2003).

In the case of cultures that share the religious belief that events in their life are God's will, prognostication is not an acceptable human act. Hence, devout Muslims may object to a diagnosis of terminal illness or cancer. This belief may hinder their ability to get into hospice programs unless organizational policies are flexibly applied to accommodate their values and beliefs (Pacquiao, 2002, 2003). Cultural knowledge and skills are needed to enable nurses to provide culturally congruent care for dying clients and work with their families and religious leaders.

Rituals associated with dying and death are highly conditioned by culture. Orthodox Jews rally behind members of their congregation and provide care for the dying, as well as assistance to the family. They may come in groups of about 10 and pray together with the client and the family at the bedside (Bonura and others, 2001). Among Orthodox Jews and Muslims a special group knowledgeable in the religious rituals is called to perform postmortem care. Gender-congruent care and provision of privacy are strictly observed as a show of respect for the dead person. Immediate burial is generally scheduled; hence preparations should be planned with the family beforehand. Among Orthodox Jews the dead person is generally buried before sundown (Bonura and others, 2001). Some Buddhists may refuse to move the dead body after death because of their belief that the spirit of the dead takes some time to leave the body. They define death as the absence of consciousness and loss of body warmth. Indeed, many other groups do not agree with using brain death as a criterion of death (Lin, 1995).

The dominant practice of bringing a stillborn fetus to the mother immediately after birth to promote healthy grieving is not viewed as positive in some cultures. Some Asian Indians regard this practice as adding to the mother's and family's suffering. Hindus and Buddhists believe that it is the soul that lives on and the body is only a shell. A dead body without the soul is but an empty shell (Vatuk, 1996).

The meaning and expressions of grief are culturally constituted. The color black is not always a symbol of grief. Hindu mourners wear white. Among the usually stoic East

Asians, the extent to which mourners publicly express grief reflects the social position and status of the deceased. Korean families may hire people to lead the open grieving. Loud crying and screaming is to be expected.

Religious beliefs also affect attitudes toward cremation, organ donation, and the treatment of body parts. Devout Muslims may refuse an autopsy or organ donation for fear of desecrating the dead and because of their belief that one has to be whole to appear in front of the creator. Burial is preferred over cremation (Geissler, 1998). A Muslim client who is having a leg amputated may request a blessing of the leg from a priest **(Imam)** before surgery (Pacquiao, 2003).

Cultural Assessment

Cultural assessment is a systematic and comprehensive examination of the cultural care values, beliefs, and practices of individuals, families, and communities. The goal of cultural assessment is to generate from the clients themselves significant information and understanding that will enable the nurse to implement culturally congruent care (Leininger and McFarland, 2002). There are several models for cultural assessment, each involving different levels of skill and knowledge. Leininger's Sunrise Model (2002a) in Figure 8-2 demonstrates the inclusive-

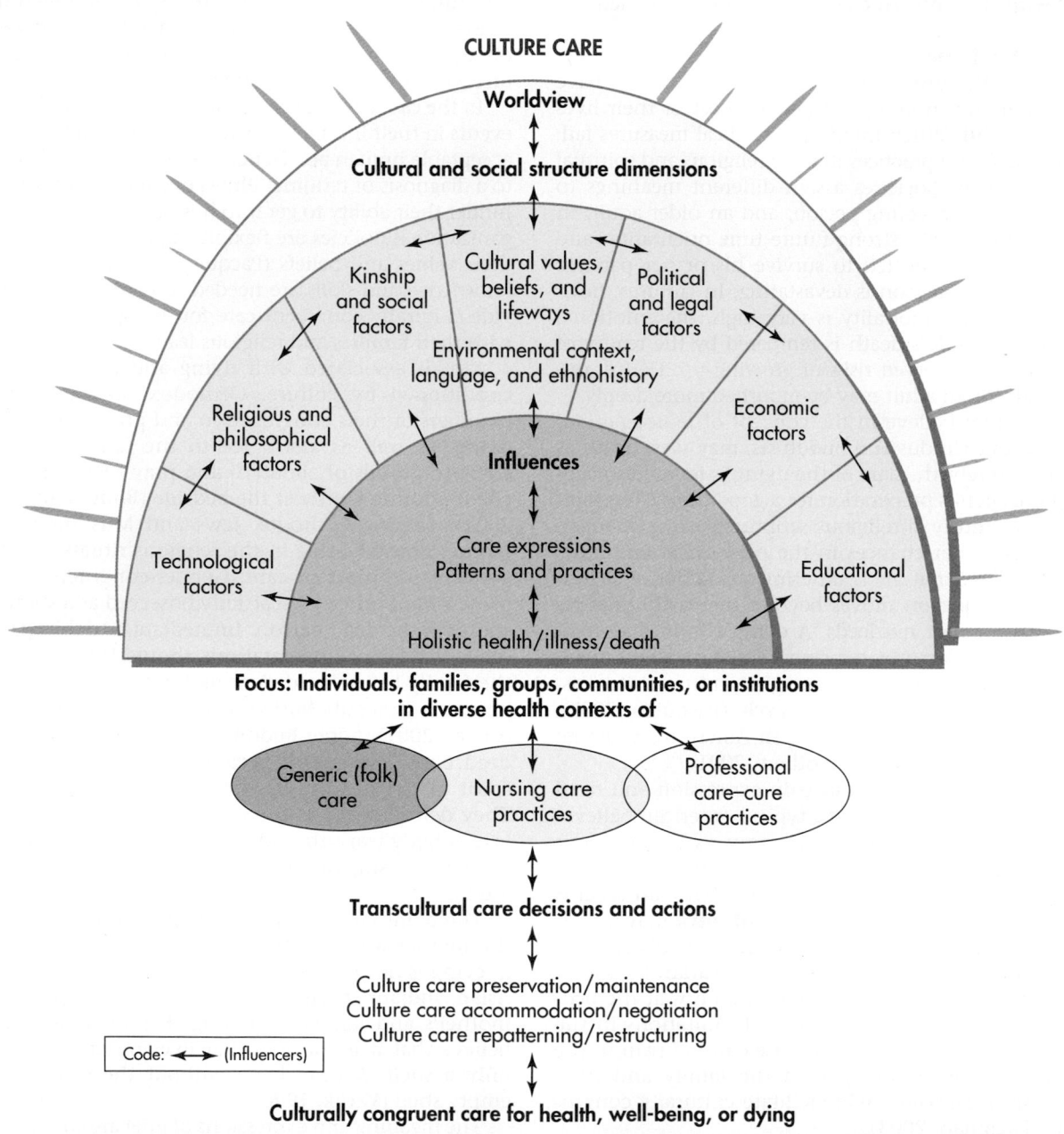

FIGURE **8–2**   Leininger's culture care theory and Sunrise Model. (Reprinted with permission from Leininger MM, McFarland MR: *Transcultural nursing: concepts, theories, research and practice,* ed 3, New York, 2002, McGraw-Hill.)

ness of culture in everyday life and helps to explain why cultural assessment must be comprehensive. The model assumes that cultural care values, beliefs, and practices are embedded in the cultural and social structural dimensions of society, which include environmental contexts, language, and ethnohistory. **Ethnohistory** refers to significant historical experiences of a particular group. For example, the experience with the Great Depression of older Americans has resulted in their tendency to be frugal and to save everything. Clients' caring patterns and expressions as conditioned by their cultural and social dimensions need to be assessed from a contextual and holistic integration of these dimensions. In other words, a nurse needs to have clients share stories about their lives that will reveal the broad picture of who they are and the cultural lifestyle they embrace. Leininger's model differentiates folk care, which is caring as defined by the people, from the health care professions, which is based on the scientific, biomedical caring system. Culturally congruent care is achieved by using the three action modes (discussed later in this chapter) individually or simultaneously to fit those patterns of care that the clients identify as meaningful and supportive to them.

Census Data

A nurse begins cultural assessment by knowing population demographic changes in the community setting of practice. Nurses should anticipate the client populations that use their services and gain some knowledge about their cultures before they come to the setting. Having a background knowledge of a culture assists the nurse in conducting a focused assessment when time is limited. Demographics can be gathered from the local and regional census data, as well as from the demographic breakdown of clients who come to the setting. Population demographics might include the distribution of ethnic groups, education, occupations, and incidence of the most common illnesses. Comprehensive cultural assessment requires skill and time; hence preparation and anticipation of need are important.

Asking Questions

One problem in cultural assessment is the lack of ability to assess the insider or emic perspective of the clients and interpret the information during the assessment. It helps to use open-ended, focused, and contrast questions (Spradley, 1979). The aim is to encourage clients to describe those values, beliefs, and practices that are significant to their care that may be taken for granted unless otherwise uncovered. Culturally oriented questions are by nature broad and require a lot of descriptions. Nurses need to have a set of questions to elicit the clients' descriptions. The following interaction shows these three types of questions. Table 8-3 provides a list of guiding questions relevant to each social and cultural dimension.

Open-ended: What do you think caused your illness?
Focused: Did you have this problem before?
Contrast: How different is this problem from the one you had previously?
Open-ended: How do you want us to help you with your problem?

Contrast: What is the difference between what we are doing from what you think we should be doing for you?
Focused: Is there someone you want us to talk to about your care?

Establishing Relationship

In contrast to other types of interviews, cultural assessment is intrusive and time consuming and requires a trusting relationship between participants. Miscommunication commonly occurs in intercultural interactions. This is due to language and communication differences between and among participants, as well as different contextual frames for interpreting each other's behaviors and communication. Skill in impression management is essential for nurses. It is based on one's ability to interpret the other's behavior within his or her own context of meanings and to behave in a culturally congruent way. In a sense, it is managing the impression one makes on the other to achieve desired outcomes of communication (Pacquiao, 2000). Impression management requires linguistic skills, culturally congruent interpretation of behaviors of others, and listening and observation skills. In cultural assessment, the goal is to generate knowledge about the client's values, beliefs, and practices about nursing and health care. If the nurse's behavior is offensive to the client, he or she will not likely participate in the interaction. Box 8-3 provides the general rules of impression management with specific recommendations for working with interpreters.

Effectiveness of interpreters is facilitated by their knowledge of the dialect spoken by the client. For example, among the Chinese, although the same words are used, the meanings are differentiated by the accentuation that is unique to the dialect spoken in a specific region of China (Purnell and Paulanka, 1998). Language(s) spoken and written by a client should be assessed on admission. Client need for an interpreter must also be established on admission. Federal mandates for culturally competent health care delivery include accommodation for language differences (see Box 8-1, p. 121). Nurses should know their organization's policies and procedures regarding these mandates. Working with interpreters and clients with little or no fluency in English requires skill development. Nurses should attend training programs and practice applications of principles of impression management before an actual client encounter. In hospital settings an interpreter must be used for communicating to the client information about his or her medical condition. It is not acceptable for family members to translate health care information, but they can assists with ongoing interaction during the client's care.

The content to be discussed with a client is another factor to be considered in selecting an interpreter. In some Hispanic and Asian groups, a woman's private parts are not generally discussed with members of the opposite sex, including male members of one's family. In societies where adults occupy higher status than the young, a child interpreter may be regarded as disrespectful. With immigrant groups, children learn the English language faster than their parents because of their schooling experience in the new culture when they immigrate at a young age. However, assuming that children are ideal in-

Table 8-3	Cultural Assessment Guide
	Suggested Questions
Cultural identity/ancestry/ heritage	Where were you born?
	Where were your parents born?
Ethnohistory	How long have you/your parents resided in this country?
	What is your ethnic background or ancestry?
	How strongly are you influenced by your culture?
	Why did you leave your homeland?
Social organization	Who lives with you?
	Who do you consider members of your family?
	Where do you live?
	Where do other members of your family live?
	How do you contact them?
	How often do you have contact with your family members?
	Who makes the decisions for you or your family?
	Who do you go to outside of your family for support?
	What do you expect your family members to do for you?
	How different are your expectations of them from other times?
	What expectations do you have of your family members who are males, females, old, or young?
Socioeconomic status	What do you do for a living?
	What did you do back in your homeland?
	Where did you go to school?
	What did you finish in school?
	How different is your life here from back home?
	Do you have medical insurance?
	Do you have a primary health care provider?
	What other care providers have you seen?
Biocultural ecology and health risks	What is your purpose for coming here?
	What caused your problem?
	Have you had this problem before?
	How does this problem affect or has affected your life and your family?
	Are there other members of your family with this kind of problem?
	How do you treat this problem at home?
	Who do you go to for this kind of problem?
	What other plans do you have for dealing with this problem?
	What do you think we should do for you?
	What other problems do you have?
	Have these problems occurred to any other member of your family?
Language and communication	What language(s) do you speak at home?
	What language(s) are you most comfortable speaking?
	In what language(s) can you read and write?
	How do you want us to talk to you?
	How should we address or call you?
	What kinds of communication upset or offend you?
	What words would you use to describe how you feel?
	Do you need an interpreter?
	Would you prefer a female or male interpreter?
Religion/spirituality	What is your religion?
	Who is your religious or spiritual leader?
	Do you want to be in touch with your religious leader?
	How do we contact your spiritual leader?
	What are some of the things we need to do within your religion?
	How do you practice your religion?
	Are there specific dietary practices you follow?
Caring beliefs and practices	What do you do to keep yourself well?
	What do you do to show someone you care?
	How does your family or you take care of sick family members?
	Which caregivers do you seek when you are sick?
	How do you decide when to go and which one to go to?
	How different is what we do from what your family does for you when you are sick?
	Are we doing what you think we should be doing for you?
	How should we give you care?
Experience with professional health care	Since you came to this country, have you had contact with doctors or hospitals?
	How do you compare your past experience with now?
	What were some of the problems that you encountered?
	How were they resolved?
	What were the positive experiences you have?
	What type of care provider do you prefer? Why?
	If you have a choice, what changes do you wish to see?

Box 8-3 **Rules of Impression Management**

1. Greet the client and the family in their own language if you know it.
2. Introduce yourself. Tell clients what to call you.
3. Request each one to introduce himself or herself and how she or he is related to client.
4. Welcome the family, and thank them for coming to visit.
5. Request to talk with client, and offer to accompany the family to the waiting room.
6. Inform the family that you will get them when you are done with the client.
7. Tell client your purpose.
8. Clarify if client wants a family member to be present.
9. Avoid asking client questions in front of family or spouse that can put him or her at risk with this group.
10. Ask client who is the person who needs to be consulted for major decisions and how to contact this person.
11. Observe nonverbal behavior, and match degree of distance exhibited by client.
12. If client needs an interpreter:
    a. Introduce yourself to the interpreter.
    b. Determine qualifications of interpreter.
       (1) Make sure that interpreter can speak the dialect of the client.
       (2) Ensure gender, age, and ethnic compatibility of interpreter with client's preference and topic to be discussed.
       (3) Watch for differences in educational and socioeconomic status between client and interpreter.
       (4) Orient interpreter to your purpose and expectation (e.g., assessment of the client's level of pain, intent to explain procedure to client).
    c. Clarify your questions about the interpreter's training, compatibility with the client, and interpreter understanding of your expectations beforehand.
    d. Introduce the interpreter to the client.
    e. Pace your speech slowly, and allow time for back translation.
    f. Direct your questions to the client.
    g. Request interpreter to ask client for feedback and clarification at regular intervals.
    h. Observe client's nonverbal and verbal behaviors.
    i. Thank both client and interpreter.

terpreters for their parents may in fact be an affront to the authority of the elder who has to take directions from a child.

Compatibility between the ethnic backgrounds of the interpreter and client is another consideration to facilitate trust. An Israeli interpreter may precipitate much anxiety and distrust in a Palestinian immigrant who experienced violent clashes between these groups in the home country. Socioeconomic and educational differences between interpreters and clients can become barriers to effective interpretation. Interpreters need training not only in interpretation but also in knowing their role to repeat back what was said without making judgment about the content. Any personal and subjective reactions to the conversation should be communicated to the practitioner.

Selected Components of Cultural Assessment

Cultural assessment is important to the total care of any client. A nurse will learn over time various skills needed to gather an accurate and comprehensive assessment. The following components of cultural assessment provide insight into the type of information that can be useful in planning and delivering nursing care.

Ethnic Heritage and Ethnohistory

Knowledge of a client's country of origin and its history and ecological contexts are significant to health care. For example, Haitian immigrants have linguistic and communication patterns distinct from those of Jamaicans though they both come from the Caribbean and have a common history of slavery. Differences can be traced back to their colonial history and intermingling with the local indigenous people. Hindu immigrants from Jamaica have different cultural characteristics from those originating from India because of the cultural contexts of the different regions. Their nutritional, communication, and health patterns may be more similar to African Jamaicans than South Asian Hindus. In giving care for an Indian Hindu who grew up in Jamaica, the nurse can expect that the client will interact more like a Jamaican although he or she looks south Indian.

People emigrate to another country for various reasons and have different motivations for acculturating to the new country. Refugees are relocated without any choice in their initial residence, in contrast to immigrants, who have options as to where they go. Refugees experience greater dislocation and deprivation than immigrants who enter the United States with specialized skills and education and have the option to return to their homeland. Age of immigration may determine the level of acculturation, with younger immigrants acculturating faster than their older counterparts. Similarities shared by an immigrant group with the dominant culture in society are strong predictors of assimilation. Experiences of white European immigrants contrast with those of nonwhite immigrants from Europe and other continents. Although acculturation and length of residence in the new culture are related, the outcome may be differentiated by other factors such as education, racial characteristics, and familiarity with the language and religion. A nurse asks clients what was the condition or situation that brought them to the United States and how they feel they are adjusting. Any problems (such as becoming comfortable with the language or the routines used to set medical appointments) need to be understood by the nurse so that reasonable and appropriate adjustments can be made.

Socioeconomic status in the new society may not be comparable to one's previous status in the country of origin. New immigrants begin with meager existence but retain those values and aspirations congruent with their previous status. It is important for a nurse to explore the background of the client such as preimmigration and postimmigration status, available resources for medical coverage, health risks in the new environment, and availability of support systems.

Biocultural History

Identification of clients' health risks related to sociocultural and biological history can be assessed on admission. Distinct health risks can be attributed to the ecological context of the culture. For example, immigrants originating from the region near the Nile River are generally predisposed to parasitic infestations endemic to the region. Immigrants from the Third World with poor sanitary conditions and water supply succumb to infections such as hepatitis. Certain genetic disorders are also linked with specific ethnic groups, such as Tay-Sachs among Ashkenazi Jews and malignant hypertension among African-Americans. Lactose intolerance is frequently observed among Asians, Africans, and Hispanics. Aboriginal Canadians descended from Native North American Indians and living on reservations have a higher incidence of tuberculosis than their nonaboriginal counterparts. Mortality from diabetes mellitus is 3 to 4 times higher among Utes, Pimas, and Papago Indians (Overfield, 1995; U.S. Department of Health and Human Services, 1998; Health Canada, 1999).

Social Organization

Cultural groups consist of units of organization delineated by kinship, status hierarchy, and appropriate roles for their members. In the dominant American society the most common unit of social organization is the nuclear family where married children and adults are expected to establish separate residences from their parents. Although different configurations of a family may exist, the most common is the nuclear household comprising parents and their young children (see Chapter 9). In collectivistic cultures, family composition may be extended to distant blood relatives across three generations and **fictive** or nonblood kin. Kinship maybe extended to both the father's and mother's side of the family **(bilineal)** or limited to the side of either father **(patrilineal)** or mother **(matrilineal).** Patrilineally extended families are observed among Chinese and Hindus, where a woman is expected to move into her husband's clan after marriage and kinship ties with her family of orientation (her own parents and siblings) are minimized. The nurse must consider all options when determining a client's next of kin. This is especially relevant to new immigrants and refugees, who may not have relocated with intact families. Collectivistic groups may regard members of their ethnic group as closest kin and would want to consult them for health care decisions, as well as permit them to speak on their behalf.

A client's status within the social hierarchy is generally linked with qualities such as age and gender, as well as achieved status such as education and position. The dominant culture in the United States emphasizes achievement as the determinant of status, whereas most collectivistic cultures give higher priority to age and gender. The eldest male is next to his father in terms of authority in many Asian and African cultures. A Korean mother is subject to the authority of her oldest son in the absence of her husband. An adult Hispanic client may not sign her surgical consent without consulting her husband, oldest son, or brothers. Older adults generally occupy higher status in some societies such that grandparents may impose their decisions over their married children regarding the care of the grandchildren. Nurses determine who has authority for making decisions within the family and how to communicate with the proper individuals.

Expected roles of members are defined by culture. Certain behaviors are accepted in children and not tolerated among adults. Role expectations may also be differentiated by gender. In Islamic and Arabic cultures, females perform the task of caregiving whereas males are expected to be the providers and major decision makers. Thus nurses should expect a woman's insistence on staying at the bedside of her child, in-laws, or husband. To assume, however, that as the primary caregiver she can be relied upon to make decisions independently is unrealistic. An Orthodox Jewish husband may respond to questions posed to his wife, which can annoy nurses operating from a context of individual autonomy. The family social hierarchy needs to be determined as soon as possible to prevent offending clients and their families. Working with established family hierarchy prevents delays and achieves outcomes in nursing care.

Religious and Spiritual Beliefs

Religious and spiritual beliefs are major influences in the client's worldview about health and illness, pain and suffering, and life and death. The distinction between religion and spirituality is often blurred. It is advisable for a nurse to understand the emic perspective of the client. Many cultures do not separate religion and spirituality, whereas many have a totally distinct concept of spirituality. To a Hmong animist, spirits could be those of dead ancestors or forces external to the person. To an Anglo-American, spirituality may mean an inner, personal relationship with God. Although discussion of religious and spiritual philosophies is difficult in a hospital setting, nurses must assess what is important to the spiritual well-being of clients and learn as much as possible about clients' spiritual and religious practices (see Chapter 28).

Devout Muslims pray five times daily and undergo an obligatory ritual cleansing of some parts of their body before praying. Nurses need to anticipate the ritual cleansing needs of the client and provide privacy for praying. Diagnostic procedures may be rescheduled so that Buddhist clients can participate in the festivities of their New Year. Anticipating the needs of Jewish clients during **Sabbath,** when they refrain from using electrical appliances requires creative accommodations by the staff such as placing articles of care near the client so he or she need not use the call light or telephone to get assistance. Consent for emergency surgeries can be sent by facsimile to the **rabbi,** who can contact the client's next of kin unreachable by telephone during Sabbath.

Religious beliefs are evident in clients' dietary practices. Devout Hindus avoid beef, and many are vegetarians. Many Buddhists are vegetarians. **Halal** foods, which include meat, fish, fresh fruit, vegetables, eggs, milk, and cheese, are permissible for Muslims. Halal meat comes from animals that have been slaughtered during a prayer ritual. Prohibited, or **Haram,** foods include non-Halal meat, animals with fangs, pork products, gelatin products and alcohol (Akhtar, 2002). Fasting during daylight is required during the 28 days of **Ramadan,** observed during the ninth lunar month. Although children and sick and frail individuals are exempt from fasting, nurses must not assume that these individuals will eat regular meals during Ramadan. Rescheduling of treatments and medications may be required to prevent complications such as hypoglycemia.

Jewish clients who follow a **Kosher** diet will avoid meat from carnivores, pork products, and fish without scales or fins. Kosher meat comes from permissible animals that are slaughtered with the least amount of suffering. Kosher foods must not be contaminated by non-Kosher foods. Hence meat is served separately from dairy, and dishes used for serving and eating these products are also kept separate among strict adherents (Selekman, 1998).

Background information should be available to the nursing staff about major holy days and practices for commonly encountered religions. Such information prevents scheduling nonemergency treatments and procedures on major holy days such as the Jewish Yom Kippur, Rosh Hashanah, or Passover. Religious mandates followed by Jehovah's Witnesses require followers to have bloodless surgery and to avoid blood transfusions. Nurses should identify and contact clients' religious and spiritual leaders before problems arise. These leaders can be called upon to act as cultural brokers in times of crises. On admission, nurses should obtain this information from the client or his or her family. Spiritual leaders may also be regarded as cultural healers, such as the voodoo priest, spiritualists, or ministers.

Life transitions are often manifested in religious and spiritual beliefs. Several examples follow. Male circumcision is practiced among Jewish and Islamic groups. Female circumcision is practiced among some African and Muslim groups. Annointing of the sick is a sacrament observed among Roman Catholics. Hospitalized Catholic clients may request daily communion. The family of a critically ill Jewish client will turn his or her head eastward or to the right side. The family of a dying Hindu remains at the bedside so they can place a drop of the holy water from the River Ganges on the client's lips immediately after death to facilitate transcendence of his or her soul to the next life. A dying Hispanic client will not be left alone so that his or her wishes can be conveyed to a close kin so that his or her soul can leave in peace.

Communication Patterns

Distinct linguistic and communication patterns are associated with different cultural groups. These patterns reflect core cultural values of a society. In the dominant American culture that upholds individualism, assertive communication is valued because it manifests the ideal of individual autonomy and self-determination. The individual is less encumbered by the context of relationships and is expected to say what he or she means and to mean what he or she says. In collectivistic cultures, communication is shaped by the context of relationships among participants. Promoting group harmony is given priority, so participants interact based on their expected positions and relationships within the social hierarchy. Individuals are more likely to remain respectful and show deference to older adults or family leaders, even though they may disagree on an issue. Differences in status and position, age, gender, and outsider versus insider determine the content and process of communication. Among Asian cultures, face-saving communication promotes harmony by indirect, ambiguous communication and conflict avoidance. Messages spoken may have little to do with their meanings. Saying "no" to a superior or older person may not be permitted, hence a subordinate's affirmative response may only mean "I heard you" rather than full agreement. This is likely to happen when a doctor or perceived authority speaks to some Asian, African, or Hispanic clients. Observing a client's behavior and clarifying messages heard from a trusted insider can prevent misinterpretation.

In cultural groups with distinct linear hierarchy, negotiation of conflict occurs between persons within the same level of position or authority. Identifying and working with established family hierarchy can prevent miscommunication. In cultures with highly differentiated gender roles, some clients may place more value on the advice of a male physician than a female nurse. By recognizing and working within this cultural context, the nurse can become more effective in achieving outcomes.

Nonverbal communication is also shaped by culture. Distance between participants in an interaction is embedded in the degree of eye contact, extent of touching, and degree to which private information is shared. Less distance is observed when speaking to trusted insiders, and persons of the same age, gender, and position in the social hierarchy. Many ethnic groups tend to speak their own dialect with insiders for ease and privacy and as a marker of insider status. To minimize this distance when communicating with clients, nurses need to establish rapport and behave in a culturally congruent manner through impression management.

Time Orientation

All cultures have past, present, and future time dimensions. It is important for a nurse to understand a client's time orientation. This information can be useful in planning a day of care, setting up appointments for procedures, and helping a client plan self-care activities in the home. Differences exist in the dimensions of time that cultures emphasize and the manner of expressing time. Time orientation is reflected in communication patterns. Future time orientation minimizes present time, so communication tends to be direct and focused on task achievement. Business time is separate and distinct from social time. This is the norm in the dominant American culture. In contrast, collectivistic cultures emphasize past and present times to preserve social hierarchy and promote group harmony. Communication may be circular and indirect to avoid risks of offending and disrespecting others. Social time is often emphasized and mixed with business time. Rushed, hurried, and businesslike communication may be perceived as uncaring or disrespectful. This is true with Mexican-Americans, who tend to trust **(confianza)** caregivers who interact with them in a personalistic **(personalismo)**, warm, friendly **(simpatia)**, and respectful **(respeto)** manner (Zoucha, 1998).

Present time orientation is in conflict with the dominant organizational norm in health care that emphasizes punctuality and adherence to appointments. This should be expected, and adjustments need to be made when dealing with ethnic groups. Improving a client's access to health services mandates culturally congruent time schedules that accommodate his or her cultural patterns. When making appointments and referrals, anticipated barriers to time adherence should be explored and managed with the client. For organizational accommodation to occur, nurses must seek clients' input and advocate for clients in recommending changes.

Caring Beliefs and Practices

It can be very helpful for nurses to draw from clients and families their own concepts of meaningful and supportive caring. Caring expressions integrate the central values of a culture. In collectivistic cultures, caring means active involvement of the group, emphasizing mutual and reciprocal obligations of members to care for each other. This caring norm is in conflict with the individualism and self-care ideology of the dominant American culture (Leininger, 1992). Nurses need to adopt their caring practices, learn to work with client's families as a group, using their social hierarchy, and assume a copartnership role with them.

Religious and spiritual beliefs are integrated in caring practices. The critical role of African-American churches in caring for their community members is an example. Gender-congruent care is a strong value among Islamic, Orthodox Jews, Hindus, and many other groups emphasizing female modesty. Caring roles of males and females are differentiated by culture. In many cultures, caretaking tasks are the primary responsibility of women, whereas men provide financial support and are called upon to make major decisions. Caring roles and responsibilities are also influenced by age and position in the social hierarchy. In some cultures, older women are the first group consulted during illness of family members and in the care of women and children.

Information about folk remedies and cultural healers used by the client should be obtained. Data can yield information about the client's beliefs about the illness and the meaning of the signs and symptoms. Assessment should focus on the emic perspective of the client. Allowing the client to describe the meanings of care and identify caring behaviors is fundamental to culturally congruent care. Studies conducted with approximately 100 Western and non-Western cultures identified several recurrent caring constructs, which are presented below in priority of dominant rankings in meanings and actions of care (Leininger and McFarland, 2002):

1. Respect for and about
2. Concern for and about
3. Attention to details/in anticipation of
4. Helping/assisting or facilitative acts
5. Active listening
6. Presence (being physically there)
7. Understanding (beliefs, values, lifeways, and environmental context)
8. Connectedness
9. Protection (gender related)
10. Touching
11. Comfort measures

This list represents major care meanings and expressions as defined by the people studied. Further discussion on many of these topics can be found in Chapter 7. Nurses can use this list to guide their behaviors when caring for clients from different cultures.

Experience With Professional Health Care

Understanding the emic perspective of the client about professional health care is valuable in correcting misconceptions and preventing culturally offensive actions. Previous encounters with professional caregivers have enormous implications for adherence to therapies and continuing access of services by clients. Assessing this information needs a trusting relationship between nurses and clients. Partnership between professionals and the community provides proactive and authentic feedback from culturally diverse client groups. Use of comparative

Case Study   Box 8-4

A young Mexican mother remains at the bedside of her 3-year-old daughter who has been diagnosed with croup and is inside a croupette. Early in the morning the attending physician, Dr. Lopez, who is also Mexican, calls the nurses' station to tell the mother to keep the baby in the croupette because her oxygen saturation level is dropping. The nurse informs the mother of the doctor's instructions and tells her to give plenty of clear liquids to her daughter. Each time the nurse gives her a bottle of jello or juice for the baby, the mother immediately goes to the bathroom to heat the bottle under running hot water. She later communicates to another nurse, who speaks Spanish, that the cold croupette is bad for the child's lungs.

Her belief in the heat and cold theory is evident in her distress over putting her daughter inside a cold tent when the respiratory illness of croup is classified as a cold condition. By giving warm fluids to her baby she is attempting to restore balance. Dr. Lopez suspects that at night she takes her daughter out of the croupette. It is clear that her cultural beliefs cannot be preserved or maintained without aggravating the child's condition. Cultural care accommodation or negotiation can be implemented by heating the bottle in the microwave before giving it to the mother. Since the child is afebrile, the nurse can allay her fear by allowing her to dress the child in the same way as when she takes her out in the cold weather. These accommodations do not alter the benefit of the croupette, which is to deliver cool humidity to her respiratory tract. The nurse could periodically inform her of signs of effectiveness of the treatment. Cultural repatterning may not achieve quick changes despite repeated instructions because cultural beliefs are deeply embedded in people's lives. This should be done along with accommodations of her cultural beliefs and caring patterns. Positive outcomes from the treatment and positive experience with the providers in the hospital are the best strategies for repatterning. Sensitive and respectful mediation by a Spanish-speaking practitioner may help allay the mother's fears and minimize her guilt in leaving her baby inside the tent. In order to use any of these action modes, the nurse has to first repattern his or her own thinking. Repatterning requires acceptance of one's role as a learner of the mother's cultural beliefs and practices, understanding their meanings to the mother, and allowing her to be a copartner in making decisions about the care of her daughter.

assessment questions will generate insight into clients' comparative perceptions and reactions to different aspects of the health care system. This is an essential step in outcomes evaluation.

Nursing Decisions

Leininger (1991) identified three nursing decision and action modes to achieve culturally congruent care. All three modes of professional decisions and actions are aimed to assist, support, facilitate, or enable people of particular cultures.

1. **Cultural care preservation** or **maintenance—** Retain and/or preserve relevant care values so that clients can maintain their well-being, recover from illness, or face handicaps and/or death.
2. **Cultural care accommodation** or **negotiation—**Adapt or negotiate with others for a beneficial or satisfying health outcome.
3. **Cultural care repatterning or restructuring—**Reorder, change, or greatly modify clients' lifeways for a new, different, and beneficial health care pattern.

Nurses can use any or all of these action modes simultaneously. These actions require that nurses have knowledge of clients' culture and have the willingness, commitment, and skills to copartner with clients and families in decision making. The intended outcome of these actions and decisions is meaningful, supportive, and facilitative care as judged by the client. The example in Box 8-4 illustrates application of the three modes.

Key Concepts

- Culture is the context for interpreting human experiences such as health and illness and provides direction to decisions and actions.
- Culturally congruent care is meaningful, supportive, and facilitative because it fits valued life patterns of clients. It is achieved through cultural assessment and the application of cultural preservation, accommodation, and repatterning.
- Culturally competent care requires knowledge, attitudes, and skills supportive of implementation of culturally congruent care.
- Cultural assessment requires a comprehensive and thorough investigation of a client's cultural values, beliefs, and practices.
- Transcultural nursing is a comparative study and understanding of cultures to identify culture-specific and culture-universal caring constructs across cultures.
- Impression management facilitates culturally congruent communication and intercultural relationships.

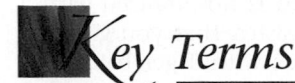

Key Terms

Acculturation, *p. 120*
Assimilation, *p. 120*
Biculturalism, *p. 120*
Bilineal, *p. 132*
Confianza, p. 133
Cultural backlash, *p. 120*
Cultural care accommodation or negotiation, *p. 135*
Cultural care preservation or maintenance, *p. 135*
Cultural care repatterning or restructuring, *p. 135*
Cultural imposition, *p. 122*
Cultural pain, *p. 127*
Culturally congruent care, *p. 120*
Culture, *p. 119*
Culture-bound syndrome, *p. 124*
Emic worldview, *p. 120*
Enculturation, *p. 120*
Ethnicity, *p. 120*
Ethnocentrism, *p. 122*
Ethnohistory, *p. 129*
Etic worldview, *p. 120*
Externalizing system, *p. 123*
Fajita, p. 126
Fictive, *p. 132*
Halal, p. 132
Haram, p. 132
Hilots, p. 125

Hmong, *p. 122*
Hwa-Byung, p. 124
Igbos, *p. 125*
Imam, *p. 128*
Internalizing system, *p. 123*
Invisible culture, *p. 120*
Kalahari bushmen, *p. 120*
Kosher, *p. 133*
La cuarantena, p. 127
La dieta, p. 127
Mal de ojo, p. 125
Matrilineal, *p. 132*
Naturalistic practitioners, *p. 123*
Parteras, p. 125
Patrilineal, *p. 132*
Personalismo, p. 133
Personalistic practitioners, *p. 123*
Rabbi, *p. 132*
Ramadan, *p. 133*
Respeto, p. 133
Rites of passage, *p. 124*
Sabbath, *p. 132*
Shaman, *p. 122*
Sikh/Sikhism, *p. 120*
Simpatia, p. 133
Subcultures, *p. 120*
Transcultural nursing, *p. 120*
Visible culture, *p. 120*

Critical Thinking Exercises

1. You were about to begin giving a male Arabic Muslim his morning care when he stated, "I don't want a bath now." He got annoyed when you tried explaining that you have to do it at this time. Before you left the room, he asked you to leave a basin of water and towel by his bedside. He also asked you to get his small rug from his closet.

   a. How would you respond to the client?

   b. What might be the reasons for his refusal and annoyance?

2. A 50-year-old Chinese woman is hospitalized with a respiratory condition. She insisted that you give her warm water and rub her back with Tiger balm liniment. When her lunch came, consisting of a turkey sandwich, tossed salad, and milk, she asked that you take it back.
   a. How would you respond to the client's requests?
   b. What is the significance of her requests?
   c. Why did she refuse her lunch?

3. You are assigned to a 60-year-old Indian Hindu widow who is admitted with chest pain and shortness of breath. The client recently arrived from India to visit her son and pregnant daughter-in-law. She can speak only Gujarati and understands very little English. She is accompanied by her son.
   a. What areas would you include in your focused cultural assessment?
   b. How would you communicate with the client?
   c. Identify ways to preserve and/or accommodate the client's culture.
   d. What aspects of the client's life way may need repatterning?

Review Questions

1. Socialization into one's primary culture as a child is known as:
   1. Enculturation.
   2. Acculturation.
   3. Assimilation.
   4. Biculturalism.

2. Assimilation results when an individual:
   1. Has an experience with the new or different culture that is extremely negative.
   2. Gives up his/her ethnic identity in favor of the dominant culture.
   3. Adapts to and adopts a new culture.
   4. Chooses to be bicultural.

3. Cultural awareness is an in-depth self-examination of one's:
   1. Background, recognizing biases and prejudices.
   2. Social, cultural, and biophysical factors.
   3. Engagement in cross-cultural interactions.
   4. Motivation and commitment to caring.

4. Cultural competence is the process of:
   1. Learning about vast cultures.
   2. Acquiring specific knowledge, skills, and attitudes.
   3. Influencing treatment and care of clients.
   4. Motivation and commitment to caring.

5. Ethnocentrism is the root of:
   1. Biases and prejudices.
   2. Meanings by which people make sense of their experiences.
   3. Cultural beliefs.
   4. Individualism and self-reliance in achieving and maintaining health.

6. When action is taken on one's prejudices:
   1. Discrimination occurs.
   2. Sufficient comparative knowledge of diverse groups is obtained.
   3. Delivery of culturally congruent care is ensured.
   4. Effective intercultural communication develops.

7. The dominant value orientation in North American society is:
   1. Use of rituals symbolizing the supernatural.
   2. Group reliance and interdependence.
   3. Healing emphasizing naturalistic modalities.
   4. Individualism and self-reliance in achieving and maintaining health.

8. Disparities in health outcomes between the rich and poor illustrates: a (an)
   1. Illness attributed to natural, impersonal, and biological forces.
   2. Creation of own interpretation and descriptions of biological and psychological malfunctions.
   3. Influence of socioeconomic factors in morbidity and mortality.
   4. Combination of naturalistic, religious, and supernatural modalities.

9. Culture strongly influences pain expression and need for pain medication. However, cultural pain:
   1. May be suffered by a client whose valued way of life is disregarded by practitioners.
   2. Is more intense, thus necessitating more mediation.
   3. Is not expressed verbally or physically.
   4. Is expressed only to others of like culture.

10. The dominant values in American society on individual autonomy and self-determination:
    1. Rarely have an effect on other cultures.
    2. Do not have an effect on healthcare.
    3. May hinder ability to get into hospice programs.
    4. May be in direct conflict with diverse groups.

References

AbuGharbeih P: Arab-Americans. In Purnell LD, Paulanka BJ: *Transcultural healthcare: a culturally competent approach*, Philadelphia, 1998, FA Davis.

Akhtar S: Nursing with dignity. VII. Islam, *Nurs Times* 98(16):40, 2002.

American Psychological Association: *Diagnostic and statistical manual of mental disorders (DSM IV),* ed 4, Washington, DC, 1994, The Association.

Campinha-Bacote J: The process of cultural competence in the delivery of healthcare services: a model of care, *J Transcult Nurs* 13(3):181, 2002.

Emerick Y: *The complete idiot's guide to understanding Islam,* Indianapolis, 2002, Pearson Education.

Fadiman A: *The spirit catches you and you fall down,* New York, 1997, Farrar, Straus & Giroux.

Foster G: Disease etiologies in non-western medical systems, *Am Anthropol* 78:773, 1976.

Frankel B: *Childbirth in the ghetto: folk beliefs of Negro women in a north Philadelphia hospital ward,* San Francisco, 1977, R&R Research Associates.

Geissler E: *Mosby's pocket guide series of cultural assessment,* ed 2, St. Louis, 1998, Mosby.

Hautman MA: Folk health and illness beliefs, *Nurse Pract* 4(4):23, 1976.

Health Canada: *Toward a healthy future: second report on the health of Canadians,* Ottawa, 1999, Health Canada.

Helsel DG, Mochel M: Afterbirths in the afterlife: cultural meaning of placental disposal in a Hmong-American community, *J Transcult Nurs* 13(4):282, 2002.

Higgins B: Puerto Rican cultural beliefs: Influence on infant feeding practices in western NY, *J Transcult Nurs* 11(1):12, 2000.

Jambunathan J: Hindu-Americans. In Purnell LD, Paulanka BJ: *Transcultural healthcare: a culturally competent approach,* Philadelphia, 1998, FA Davis (CD-ROM).

Kleinman A: *Patients and healers in the context of culture,* Berkeley, 1979, University of California Press.

Kleinman A: *Patients and healers in the context of cultures,* Berkeley, 1980, University of California Press.

Kluckhohn F: Dominant and variant value orientations. In Brink P, editor: *Transcultural nursing: a book of readings,* Englewood Cliffs, NJ, 1976, Prentice Hall.

Korean health beliefs, 2003, http://web.hawcc.hawaii.edu/nursing/RNKorean00.htm.

Leininger MM, editor: *Culture care diversity and universality: a theory of nursing,* New York, 1991, NLN Press.

Leininger MM: Self-care ideology and cultural incongruities: some critical issues, *J Transcult Nurs* 4(1):2, 1992 (editorial).

Leininger MM: Essential transcultural nursing care concepts, principles, examples and policy statements. In Leininger MM, McFarland MR: *Transcultural nursing: concepts, theories, research and practice,* ed 3, New York, 2002a, McGraw-Hill.

Leininger MM: Culture care theory: a major contribution to advance transcultural nursing knowledge and practices, *J Transcult Nurs* 13(3):189, 2002b.

Leininger MM, McFarland MR: *Transcultural nursing: concepts, theories, research and practice,* ed 3, New York, 2002, McGraw-Hill.

Lewis JA: Jewish perspectives on pregnancy and childbearing, *Am J Maternal Child Nurs* 28(5):306.

Lin Y: Crossing the gate of death in Chinese Buddhist culture, Buddhist Yogi C.M. Chen's Homepage, 2002, http://www.yourdictionary.com/ahd/p/p0576600.html.

Lipson JG, Hafizi H: Iranians. In Purnell LD, Paulanka BJ: *Transcultural healthcare: a culturally competent approach,* Philadelphia, 1998, FA Davis.

Loustaunau MO, Sobo EJ: *The cultural context of health, illness and medicine,* Westport, Conn, 1997, Bergin & Garvey.

Matocha LK: Chinese-Americans. In Purnell LD, Paulanka BJ: *Transcultural healthcare: a culturally competent approach,* Philadelphia, 1998, FA Davis.

Meleis AI: Arab-Americans. In Lipson JG, Dibble SL, Minarik PA, editors: *Culture and nursing care: a pocket guide,* San Francisco, Calif, 1996, UCSF Nursing Press.

Miranda BF, McBride MR, Spangler Z: Filipino-Americans. In Purnell LD, Paulanka BJ: *Transcultural healthcare: a culturally competent approach,* Philadelphia, 1998, FA Davis.

Moazam F: Families, patients and physicians in medical decision making: a Pakistani perspective, *Hastings Cent Rep* 30(6):28, 2000.

Office of Minority Health: *Assuring cultural competence in health care: recommendations for national standards and an outcomes-focused research agenda,* Washington, DC, 1999, Department of Health and Human Services, U.S. Public Health Service, www.omhre.gov/clas/ds.htm.

Overfield T: *Biologic variation in health and illness: race, age and sex differences,* New York, 1995, CRC Press.

Pacquiao DF: Impression management: an alternative to assertiveness in intercultural communication, *J Transcult Nurs* 11(1):5, 2000.

Pacquiao DF: Cultural incongruities of advance directives, *Bioethics Forum* 17(1):27, 2001.

Pacquiao DF: Ethics and cultural diversity: a framework for decision-making, *Bioethics Forum* 17(3-4):12, 2002.

Pacquiao DF: Cultural competence in ethical-decision-making. In Andrews MM, Boyle JS: *Transcultural concepts in nursing care,* Philadelphia, 2003, Lippincott Williams & Wilkins.

Purnell LD: Mexican-Americans. In Purnell LD, Paulanka BJ: *Transcultural healthcare: a culturally competent approach,* Philadelphia, 1998, FA Davis.

Purnell LD, Paulanka BJ: *Transcultural healthcare: a culturally competent approach,* Philadelphia, 1998, FA Davis.

Reardon T: Koreans. In Lipson JG, Dibble SL, Minarik PA, editors: *Culture and nursing care: a pocket guide,* San Francisco, Calif, 1996, UCSF Nursing Press.

Selekman J: Jewish-Americans. In Purnell LD, Paulanka BJ: *Transcultural healthcare: a culturally competent approach,* Philadelphia, 1998, FA Davis.

Singh P: *The Sikhs,* New York, 2000, Random House.

Sobo E: *One blood: the Jamaican body,* Albany, 1993, SUNY Press.

Sobo EJ: The cultural context of health, illness and medicine, Westport, Conn, 1997, Bergin & Garvey.

Spector RE: *Cultural diversity in health and illness,* Englewood Cliffs, NJ, 2000, Prentice Hall.

Spector RE: Cultural diversity in health and illness, *J Transcult Nurs* 13:(3), 197, 2002.

Spradley J: *The ethnographic interview,* New York, 1979, Harcourt Brace.

Stewarts S, Jambunathan J: Hmong women and postpartum depression, *Health Care Women Int* 17(4):319, 1996.

Turrell S: Asians' expectations: customs surrounding pregnancy and childbirth, *Nurs Times* 81(18):44, 1985.

U.S. Department of Commerce, Bureau of the Census: *Population profile of the United States.* Washington, DC, 2001, U.S. Department of Commerce. (www.census.com).

U.S. Department of Health and Human Services: *Racial and ethnic disparities in health,* 1998, http://www.raceandhealth.hhs.gov.

U.S. Department of Health and Human Services: *Healthy People 2010,* Washington, DC, 2000.

Van Gennep A: *The rites of passage,* Chicago, 1960, University of Chicago Press (Translated by MB Vizedom and GL Caffee).

Vatuk S: The art of dying in Hindu India. In Spiro HM, McCrea Curnen MG, Wandel IP, editors: *Facing death,* New Haven, Conn, 1996, Yale University Press.

Young A: Internalizing and externalizing medical systems: an Ethiopian example. In Currer C, Stacey M, editors: *Concepts of health, illness and disease: a comparative perspective,* Oxford, England, 1976, Berg Publishers.

Research References

Barry D, Boyle JS: An ethnohistory of a granny midwife, *J Transcult Nurs* 8(1):13, 1996.

Bonura D and others: Culturally-congruent end-of-life care for Jewish patients and their families, *J Transcult Nurs* 12(3):211, 2001.

Callister LC, Semenic S, Foster JC: Cultural and spiritual meanings of childbirth: Orthodox Jewish and Mormon women, *J Holistic Nurs* 17(3):280, 1999.

Helsel DG, Mochel M: Afterbirths in the afterlife: cultural meaning of placental disposal in a Hmong-American community, *J Transcult Nurs* 13(4):282, 2002.

Higginbottom GM: Breast-feeding experiences of women of African heritage in the United Kingdom, *J Transcult Nurs* 11(2):55, 2000.

Horn BM: Cultural concepts and postpartal care, *Nurs Health Care* 2(9):516, 1981.

Lee M, Essoka G: Continuing education: patients' perception of pain—comparison between Korean-American and Euro-American obstetric patients, *J Cult Divers* 5(1):29, 1998.

Lipson JG and others: Health issues among Afghan in California, *Health Care Women Int* 16(4):279, 1995.

Meleis AI, Sorell L: Bridging cultures: Arab American women and their birth experiences, *MCN Am J Matern Child Nurs* 6:171, 1981.

Padilla AM, Wagatsuma Y, Lindholm KJ: Acculturation and personality as predictors of stress in Japanese and Japanese-Americans, *J Soc Psychol* 125(3):295, 1984.

Park Y-J and others: A survey of Hwa-Byung in middle-aged Korean women, *J Transcult Nurs* 12(2):115, 2001.

Zoucha R: The experience of Mexican Americans receiving professional nursing care: an ethnonursing study, *J Transcult Nurs* 9(3):34, 1998.

Caring for Families

Media Resources

http://evolve.elsevier.com/Potter/
fundamentals/

CD COMPANION

- Review Questions
- Glossary

evolve WEBSITE

- Review Questions
- Student Learning Activities
- Glossary

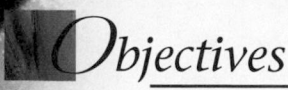

Objectives

Mastery of content in this chapter will enable the student to:

- Define the key terms listed.
- Discuss how the term *family* can be defined to reflect family diversity.
- Examine current trends in the American family.
- Describe two theoretical approaches to the study of families.
- Explain how the relationship between family structure and patterns of functioning affect the health of individuals within the family and the family as a whole.
- Discuss the way family members influence one another's health.
- Discuss the role of families and family members as caregivers.
- Interpret external and internal factors that promote family health.
- Compare family as context to family as client and explain the way that these perspectives influence nursing practice.
- Use the nursing process to provide for the health care needs of the family.

The Family

The family continues to be a central institution in American society. The concept, structure, and functioning of the family unit continue to change over time. Although the family is in transition and may look very different from the families of the 1950s, the family unit is here to stay. Families face many challenges, including the impact of health and illness, childbearing and child rearing, changes in family structure and dynamics, and caring for an older parent. However, family characteristics or attributes, such as durability, resiliency, and diversity, can assist in adapting to these challenges.

Family durability is the term for the intrafamilial system of support and structure that may extend beyond the walls of the household. The players may change, the parents may remarry, and the children may or may not leave home as adults, but the "family" is considered to transcend long periods and inevitable lifestyle changes.

Family resiliency is the ability to cope with expected and unexpected stressors. The family's ability to adapt to role changes, developmental milestones, and crises shows resilience. The goal of the family is not only to survive "the challenge," but also to thrive and to grow as a result of the newly gained knowledge.

Family diversity is the attention to uniqueness. Some families will be experiencing marriage for the first time and having children in later life, when others are grandparents at the same age. Every person within a family unit has specific needs, strengths, and important developmental considerations.

Nurses are responsible for first understanding the makeup (configuration), structure, function, and coping capacity of the family and then building on the

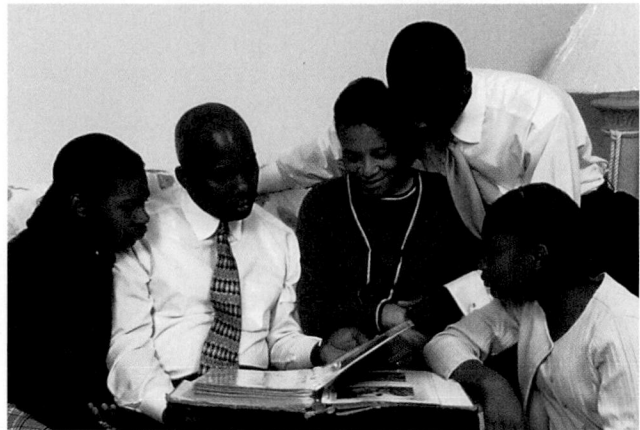

FIGURE **9–1**   Family celebrations and traditions strengthen the role of the family.

family's relative strengths and resources (Feeley and Gottlieb, 2000). The goal of family-centered nursing care is to promote, support, and provide for the well-being and health of the family and individual family members (Astedt-Kurki and others, 2002).

Concept of Family

For some the term *family* may evoke a visual image of adults and children living together in a satisfying, harmonious manner. Or this term may have an exact opposite image for other people. Families represent more than a set of individuals, and a family is more than a sum of its individual members (Astedt-Kurki and others, 2001). Families are as diverse as the individuals that compose them, and clients may have deeply ingrained values about their families that deserve respect. Thus the nurse must think of family as defined by each individual. In other words, the nurse can think of the **family** as a set of relationships that the client identifies as family or as a network of individuals who influence each other's lives whether or not there are actual biological or legal ties.

Definition: What Is a Family?

Defining family may initially appear to be a simple undertaking. However, different definitions have resulted in heated debates among social scientists and legislators. The definition of family can have a significant impact on who is included on health insurance policies, who has access to children's school records, who can file joint tax returns, and who has eligibility for sick-leave benefits or public assistance programs. The family can be defined biologically, legally, or as a social network with personally constructed ties and ideologies. To some clients, family may include only persons related by marriage, birth, or adoption. To others, aunts, uncles, close friends, cohabitating persons, and even pets are considered family. The nurse's personal beliefs do not have to coincide with those of the client. To provide individualized care, the nurse understands that families take many forms and have diverse cultural and ethnic orientations. In addition, no two families are alike, each has its own strengths, weaknesses, resources, and challenges (Bell and others,

Box 9-1   Family Forms

Nuclear Family

The nuclear family consists of husband and wife (and perhaps one or more children).

Extended Family

The extended family includes relatives (aunts, uncles, grandparents, and cousins) in addition to the nuclear family.

Single-Parent Family

The single-parent family is formed when one parent leaves the nuclear family because of death, divorce, or desertion, or when a single person decides to have or adopt a child.

Blended Family

The blended family is formed when parents bring unrelated children from prior or foster parenting relationships into a new, joint living situation.

Alternate Patterns of Relationships

These relationships include multiadult households, "skip-generation" families (grandparents caring for grandchildren), communal groups with children, "nonfamilies" (adults living alone), cohabitating partners, and homosexual couples.

2001). In other words, the nurse can think of the family as a set of relationships that the client identifies as family or as a network of individuals who influence each other's lives (Figure 9-1).

Current Trends and New Family Forms

Family forms are patterns of people considered by family members to be included in the family. Although all families have some things in common, each family form has unique problems and strengths. The nurse needs to have an open mind about what constitutes a family so that potential resources and concerns are not overlooked. Several family forms are displayed in Box 9-1.

Although the institution of the family remains strong, the family itself is changing. The "typical" family (two biological parents and children) is no longer the norm. People are marrying later, women are delaying childbirth, and couples are choosing to have fewer children or none at all. The number of people living alone is expanding rapidly and represents approximately 26% of all households. Divorce rates have tripled since the 1950s, and although the rate appears to have stabilized, it is now estimated that 55% of marriages will end in divorce (U.S. Bureau of the Census, 2001). About 90% of young Americans are likely to marry, and between 66% and 75% of those who divorce remarry. The median interval between divorce and remarriage is about 3 years. Men are more likely to remarry than women, younger persons are more likely to remarry than older persons, and divorcees are more likely to remarry than widows or widowers. Remarriage often results in a blended family with a complex set of relationships among stepparents, stepchildren, half brothers and sisters, and extended family members.

Marital roles are also more complex as families increasingly comprise two wage earners. The majority of women work outside the home, and about 62% of mothers are in the workforce (U.S. Bureau of the Census, 2001). Balancing employment and family life creates a variety of challenges in terms of child care and household work. Concerns that maternal employment is detrimental for children are unsubstantiated (Nichols, 1994; Harvey, 1999). However, finding quality substitute child care is a major issue for parents. Managing household tasks can also be a major challenge. Research demonstrates that although equal division of labor receives verbal approval, the majority of household tasks remain "women's work." There is some evidence that the fathering role is changing. Fathers are now expected to participate more fully in day-to-day parenting responsibilities. Twenty-four percent of children (ages 0 to 4), as reported by the U.S. Bureau of the Census in 2001, have their fathers as caretakers whether or not the fathers are employed.

The number of single-parent families doubled from the 1970s to the 1990s but now appears to be stabilizing at about 26% of all families with children. Although 83% of single-parent families are headed by mothers, father-only families are on the rise. Forty-one percent of children are living with mothers who have never married; many of these children are a result of an adolescent pregnancy (U.S. Bureau of the Census, 2001).

Adolescent pregnancy is an ever-increasing concern. The majority of these adolescents continue to live with their families. A teenage pregnancy tends to have long-term consequences for the mother and often severely stresses family relationships and resources. In addition, there is an increased risk for continued poverty for these families (SmithBattle, 2000). Teenage fathers also have stressors placed on them when their partner becomes pregnant. These young men have poorer support systems and fewer resources to teach them how to parent (James-Childs, 2000). As a result, both of these adolescents are often struggling with the normal tasks of development and identity but now are also forced to accept a responsibility that they may not be ready for physically, emotionally, socially, and/or financially.

Although unable to marry by law, many homosexual couples define their relationship in family terms. Approximately half of all gay male couples live together, compared with three fourths of lesbian couples. These couples have become more open about their sexual preferences and more vocal about their legal rights. Some homosexual families include children, either through adoption or artificial insemination, or from prior relationships.

The fastest-growing age-group in America is 65 years of age and over. For the first time in history the average American has more living parents than children, and children are more likely to have living grandparents and even great-grandparents. This "graying" of America has

---

Box 9-2

Focus on Older Adults

- The nurse must consider caregiver strain; caregivers are usually either spouses, who may also be an older adult and may have declining physical stamina, or middle-age children, who often have other responsibilities.
- Later-life families have a different social network than younger families because friends and same-generation family members may have died or been ill themselves. The nurse may need to look for social support within the community and church affiliation.
- Greater physical health impairment increases the risk of the older adult's depression.
- As in the other stages of life, members of later-life families need to be working on developmental tasks (see Chapter 13).
- Abuse of older adults in families occurs across all social classes. Spouses are the most frequent abusers. Unexplained bruises and skin trauma should not be ignored but should be reported by nurses to state protective agencies.

---

had an impact on the family life cycle that has perhaps been most significant for the middle generation. These individuals are finding that they must balance their own needs with those of their offspring and the needs of their aging parents. This balance often occurs at the expense of their own well-being and resources. In addition, many of these caregivers report that support received from professional health professionals is often lacking (Isaksen, Thuen, and Hanestad, 2003). The majority (75%) of these caregivers are women and frequently provide an average of 18 hours of care per week (Farran, Thuen, and Hanestad, 2002). Caring for a frail or chronically ill relative is a primary concern for a growing number of families, and it is not uncommon for people in their 60s and 70s to be the major caregivers of each other predominantly, as well as of their own elderly parents. Box 9-2 provides a list of family nursing gerontological concerns.

Grandparents are also increasingly being called on to raise their grandchildren (U.S. Bureau of the Census, 2001). This parenting responsibility is due to a number of societal factors: the increase in the divorce rate, dual-income families, and single parenthood. Most often it is a consequence of legal intervention when parents are deemed unfit or renounce their parental obligations.

Families face many challenges, including changing structures and roles in the changing economic status of society. Here we observe the lack of parental supervision, role modeling, and positive interaction with caring adults because more single parents or dual-income families are spending so much time on the job. In addition to family challenges related to divorce, changing structures and roles, and the aging of its older members, there are four further trends that social scientists identify as threats or concerns facing the family: (1) changing economic status (e.g., declining family income and lack of access to health care), (2) homelessness, (3) family violence, and (4) the presence of acute or chronic illnesses.

Changing Economic Status

Making ends meet is a daily concern because of the declining economic status of families. Although two-income families have become the norm, real family income has not increased since 1973. Families at the lower end of the income scale have been particularly affected, and single-parent families are especially vulnerable. According to the Children's Defense Fund, the number of American children living below the poverty line fell to 11.6 million in 2000, which was the lowest in 20 years. However, child poverty rose in full-time working families; this number rose to 4.1 million in 2000, up from 3.8 million in 1999 (Children's Defense Fund [CDF], 2003a).

The Children's Health Insurance Program (CHIP) was initiated in 1997. CHIP was designed to provide assistance to help children in working families with incomes too high to qualify for Medicaid but too low to afford private family coverage. This is an essential service to provide health promotion, vaccines, well child, and illness coverage. Currently 90% of uninsured children have at least one parent who works but is unable to afford insurance (CDF, 2003b).

Homelessness

Homelessness is a major public health issue. According to public health organizations, "absolute homelessness" describes people without physical shelter who sleep outdoors, in vehicles, abandoned buildings, or other places not intended for human habitation. "Relative homelessness" describes those who have a physical shelter, but one that does not meet the standards of health and safety (Hwang, 2001).

The fastest growing segment of the homeless population is families with children; this includes complete nuclear families and single-parent families. In 2000, families with children accounted for 36% of the homeless population (National Coalition for the Homeless, 2001). Poverty and lack of affordable housing are primary causes. Homelessness severely affects the functioning, health, and well-being of the family and its members. Children of homeless families are often in fair or poor health and have higher rates of asthma, ear infections, stomach problems, and mental illness. As a result, usually the only access to health care for these children is through the emergency department (Kushel and others, 2002).

In addition, these children face barriers, such as meeting residency requirements for public schools, inability to obtain previous enrollment records, enrolling in and attending school. As a result, these children are more likely to drop out of school and become unemployable (Shinn and others, 1998). Homeless families and their children are at serious risk for developing long-term health, psychological, and socioeconomic problems, thus posing a major challenge for our entire society (Kushel and others, 2002; Shinn and others, 1998).

Family Violence

The statistics regarding family violence are even more disturbing. Clemen-Stone, McGuire, and Eigsti (1998) state that 2.7 million children were reported as being abused or neglected in the period from 1991 to 1995, up from 1.1 million in the preceding 11 years, and in the 4 years between 1986 and 1990 the need for foster care increased by almost 50%. Emotional, physical, and sexual abuse occurs toward spouses, children, and older adults and across all social classes. Research spanning two decades has demonstrated that the cause of family violence is complex and multidimensional. Factors associated with violence include stress, poverty, social isolation, psychopathology, and learned family behavior. In addition, other factors such as alcohol and drug abuse, pregnancy, sexual orientation, and mental illness may increase the incidence of abuse within a family (Robrecht, 1998). Although abuse may end when one leaves a specific family environment, negative long-term physical and emotional consequences are often evident. One of these consequences includes moving from one abusive situation to another (Richardson and others, 2002). For example, a child may see marriage as a way to leave an abusive home and in turn may marry a person who will continue the abuse within the marriage (Wathen and MacMillan, 2003).

Human Immunodeficiency Virus

During the mid to late 1990s advances in human immunodeficiency virus (HIV) treatment led to declines in acquired immunodeficiency syndrome (AIDS) deaths and slowed the progression from HIV to AIDS. However, in recent years the rate of decline for both new cases and deaths began to slow, and in 1999 the annual number of AIDS cases appeared to be leveling, with a decline in death rate slowing (Centers for Disease Control and Prevention [CDC], 2003). AIDS-related mortality is down, indicating that people with HIV are living longer and better lives. While the epidemic has slowed, high-risk behaviors, such as unprotected sex, continue to rise (CDC, 1998a; Hwang, 2001). The characteristics of HIV are changing over time, although the rates of incidence have not changed much since about 1992 (CDC, 1998b). The rates appear highest in African-Americans and Hispanics, and a fifth of the persons with AIDS are women. The increasing incidences are now seen with intravenous (IV) drug use and heterosexual transmission. Finding that one is HIV positive is devastating, not only for the individual, but for the family and friends as well. As with all serious illnesses, caring for a family member who develops active HIV infection is emotionally and financially devastating. As with any chronic illness, when a family member is diagnosed with HIV, the entire family and individual family members are affected.

Theoretical Approaches: An Overview

Although there are a number of different perspectives that can be applied when working with or studying families, it is important that the beginning student understand some of the broader perspectives for family nursing. The family health system (FHS) and developmental theories are two perspectives most fully incorporated in this chapter and can assist a nurse in providing nursing care to the family as a whole and the individuals within the family structure.

Box 9-3 **Five Realms of Family Life: Family Health System—Family Assessment Plan**

Interactive Processes

Family relationships
Family communication
Family nurturing
Intimacy expression
Social support
Conflict resolution
Roles (instrumental and expressive)
Family leisure life

Developmental Processes

Current family transitions
Family stage task completion or progression
Individual developmental issues that affect family development
Development of health issue and family impact

Coping Processes

Problem solving
Use of resources
Family life stressors and daily hassles
Family coping strategies and effectiveness
Past experiences with handling crises
Family resistance resources

Integrity Processes

Family values
Family beliefs
Family meaning
Family identify
Family rituals
Family spirituality
Family culture and practices

Health Processes

Family health beliefs and beliefs about health concern or
    problem
Health behaviors of the family
Health patterns and health management activities
Family caretaking responsibilities
Disease conditions, treatments and consequences for the family
Family illness stressors
Relationship with health care providers and health system
    access

From Anderson KH: The family health system approach to family systems nursing, *J Fam Nurs* 6(2):103, 2000.

These theoretical perspectives and their concepts provide the foundation for family assessment.

Family Health System

The FHS offers a holistic perspective for nurses to examine, assess, and care for families (Anderson, 2000). In this system there are five realms or processes of family life: interactive, developmental, coping, integrity, and health (Box 9-3). The FHS approach uses family assessment to determine the areas of concern and strengths according to the realms of family life, and, as a result, the nurse develops a nursing care plan documenting family outcomes and family nursing interventions. The family is an open social system that exists in and interacts with the larger systems of the community (e.g., political, religious, school, and health care systems). As with all systems, the family system has both implicit and explicit goals, which vary according to the stage in the family life cycle, family values, and individual concerns of the family members. The goals of the FHS include improved family health or well-being, family management of illness conditions or transitions, and achievement of health outcomes related to the family areas of concern (Anderson, 2000).

Developmental Stages

Families, like individuals, change and grow over time. Although families are far from identical to one another, they tend to go through certain stages. Each developmental stage has its own challenges, needs, and resources and includes tasks that need to be completed before the

family can successfully move on to the next stage. Societal changes and an aging population have precipitated changes in the stages and transitions in the family life cycle. For example, adult children are not leaving the nest as predictably or as early as in the past, and many are returning home. In addition, more people are living into their 80s and 90s. Sixty-five is now considered the "backside of middle-age," and the length of the midlife stage in the family life cycle has increased, as has the later stage in family life.

McGoldrick and Carter's classic model of family life stages (1985) is based on expansion, contraction, and realignment of family relationships that support the entry, exit, and development of the members. This model describes the emotional aspects of lifestyle transition and the changes and tasks necessary for the family to proceed developmentally (Table 9-1). Thus the nurse can use this model to promote behaviors to achieve essential tasks and help families prepare for later transitions. It should be noted that this model does not address diverse family forms, such as blended families, single-parent families, or cohabitating partners.

Attributes of Families

Structure

Families also have a structure and a way of functioning. Structure and function are closely related and continually interact with one another. Structure is based on the ongoing membership of the family and the pattern of rela-

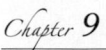

Table 9-1	Stages of the Family Life Cycle	
Family Life Cycle Stage	**Emotional Process of Transition: Key Principles**	**Changes in Family Status Required to Proceed Developmentally**
Between families: unattached young adult	Accepting parent-offspring separation	a. Differentiation of self in relation to family of origin b. Development of intimate peer relationships c. Establishment of self in work
Joining of families through marriage: newly married couple	Commitment to new system	a. Formation of marital system b. Realignment of relationships with extended families and friends to include spouse
Family with young children	Accepting new generation of members into system	a. Adjusting marital system to make space for children b. Taking on parental roles c. Realignment of relationships with extended family to include parenting and grandparenting roles
Family with adolescents	Increasing flexibility of family boundaries to include children's independence	a. Shifting of parent-child relationships to permit adolescents to move into and out of system b. Refocus on midlife material and career issues c. Beginning shift toward concerns for older generation
Launching children and moving on	Accepting multitude of exits from and entries into family system	a. Renegotiation of marital system as dyad b. Development of adult-to-adult relationships between grown children and their parents c. Realignment of relationships to include in-laws and grandchildren d. Dealing with disabilities and death of parents (grandparents)
Family in later life	Accepting shifting of generational roles	a. Maintaining own or couple functioning and interests in the face of physiological decline; exploration of new familial and social role options b. Support for more central role for middle generation c. Making room in system for wisdom and experience of older adults; supporting older generations without overfunctioning for them d. Dealing with loss of spouse, siblings, and other peers, and preparation for own death; life review and integration

Reprinted from McGoldrick M, Carter E: The stages of the family life cycle. In Walsh F: *Normal family processes,* New York, 1982, Guilford Press.

tionships. Relationships can be numerous and complex. For example, a woman's relationships may include wife-husband, mother-son, mother-daughter, employee-boss, and colleague-colleague, each with different demands, roles, and expectations. Patterns of relationships form power and role structures within the family. These structures can be determined by observing family behavior and interactions.

Structure may enhance or detract from the family's ability to respond to stressors. Very rigid or very flexible structures can impair functioning. A rigid structure specifically dictates who is permitted to accomplish a task, and it may also limit the number of persons outside the immediate family who are allowed to assume these tasks. For example, the mother might be considered the only acceptable person to provide emotional support for the children, or the husband might be considered the only one to provide financial support. A change in the health status of the person responsible for a task places a burden on the family because no other person is available or considered acceptable to assume that task.

An extremely open structure can also present problems for the family. Consistent patterns of behavior that lead to automatic action do not exist, and enactment of roles is overly flexible. A common example is an incon-

sistent parenting role. The parent sometimes is a strict authoritarian figure and at other times treats the child as a "best friend and confidant." This type of conduct can cause family members to become confused about what behavior is appropriate and who can be relied on for support. A general feeling of instability is created. During a crisis or rapid change, family members do not have a defined structure to "fall back on," and family disintegration can be a result.

Function

Friedman (1992) describes functioning as what the family does. Family functioning focuses on the processes used by the family to achieve its goals. These processes include communication among family members, goal setting, conflict resolution, caregiving, nurturing, and use of internal and external resources. The reproductive, sexual, economic, and educational goals that were once considered universal family goals no longer apply to all families. Although many families pursue these goals at various times during their development, they provide psychological support to their members throughout the life span. When the psychological needs of family members are not met, symptoms of family dysfunction are the usual consequence.

Box 9-4

Research Highlight

Well-Being of Parents of Young Children With Asthma

Research Focus

This study investigated the impact of caring for children with asthma on the parents' well-being, their level of health, perceived quality of life, recreation, and social relationships.

Research Abstract

Researchers explored the relationship between caring for a young child with asthma and family demands, caregiving demands, family hardiness, and parents' perception of their well-being. The researchers wanted to objectively identify if there was an impact or change in family life and dynamics when caring for a child with asthma. In addition, the researchers wanted to know how the family changed when the child was well as compared to when the child was experiencing an asthmatic attack. Asthma is one of the most common chronic diseases in children, and 10% of children under 6 years of age are believed to have asthma. Because the children are so young, primary symptom and disease management is the responsibility of the parents.

In this study investigators not only noted changes in family dynamics, but also noted that when the child was ill more than 80% of the major caregiving responsibility fell to the mother, who also needed to miss work. When the child was stable, fathers were more active in disease and symptom management, but 55% of the mothers still shared the bulk of this responsibility. When the child was ill, fathers perceived the family as hardy and able to cope. Mothers, on the other hand, had an opposite view of the family and noted changes in their own health status as well.

Evidence-Based Practice

- Mothers of children with asthma are at great risk for missing workdays due to caregiving responsibilities.
- Fathers can learn to assist in illness and disease management.
- Communication between parents may increase sharing of workload and decrease perception of one parent feeling overwhelmed.
- Mothers of children with asthma are more likely to feel overwhelmed with care of the child.
- Mothers are at greater risk of having health problems that may be timed with their child's exacerbation of asthma.

Reference

Svarvarsdottir EK, McCubbin MA, Kane JH: Well-being of parents of young children with asthma, *Res Nurs Health* 23:346, 2000.

Family goals are more easily achieved when communication is clear and direct. Clear communication enhances problem solving and conflict resolution, and it can facilitate coping with life-threatening stressors (Box 9-4). Another family process, facilitating goal achievement, includes the ability to nurture and promote growth. Families must have available, and must be able to use, internal and external resources. A social network is useful as an external resource. Social relationships, such as friends or churches, within the community act as buffers, particularly during times of stress, and reduce a family's vulnerability.

The Family and Health

The health of the family is influenced by many factors (e.g., its relative position in society, economic resources, and geographical boundaries). Although American families exist within the same culture, they live in very different ways. The structure, function, and health of any family are a reflection and result of many variables. These variables include social class, economic resources, and racial and ethnic background. For some minority groups and the poor, patterned differences in family living are consequences of inequalities deeply rooted in society. Class and ethnicity can produce differences in the access of families to society's resources and rewards, and this access creates differences in family life, most significantly in different life chances for its members.

Distribution of wealth greatly affects the capacity to maintain health. Low educational preparation, poverty, and decreased amounts of support compound one another, magnifying each other's impact *on* sickness in the family, and magnifying the amount of sickness *in* the family. Economic stability increases a family's access to adequate health care, creates more opportunity for education, increases sound nutrition, and decreases stress.

The family is the primary social context in which health promotion and disease prevention take place. The family's beliefs, values, and practices strongly influence health-promoting behaviors of its members (Hartrick, 2000). In turn, the health status of each individual influences how the family unit functions and its ability to achieve goals. When the family satisfactorily functions to meet its goals, its members tend to feel positive about themselves and their family. Conversely, when they do not meet goals, families view themselves as ineffective.

Good health may not be highly valued; in fact, detrimental practices may be accepted. In some cases a family member may provide mixed messages about health. For example, a parent may continue to smoke while telling children that smoking is bad for them. Family environment is crucial because health behavior reinforced in early life has a strong influence on later health practices. In addition, the family environment can be a crucial factor in an individual's adjustment to a crisis. Although relationships can be strained when confronted with illness, research indicates that family members have the potential to be a primary force for coping.

Attributes of Healthy Families. Ruebin Hill's classic work (1958) noted that it is possible to explain the reactions of crisis-proof and crisis-prone families. The crisis-proof, or effective, family is able to integrate the need for stability with the need for growth and change. This family has a flexible structure that allows adaptable performance of tasks and acceptance of help from outside the family system. The structure is flexible enough to allow adaptability but not so flexible that the family lacks cohesiveness and a sense of stability. The effective family has control over the environment and exerts influence on the immediate environment of home, neighborhood, and school. The ineffective, or crisis-prone, family may lack or believe it lacks control over these environments.

Recently health promotion research has started to focus on the stress-moderating effect of **hardiness** and **resiliency** as factors that contribute to long-term health. Family hardiness has been defined as the internal strengths and durability of the family unit and is characterized by a sense of control over the outcome of life, a view of change as beneficial and growth producing, and an active rather than passive orientation in adapting to stressful events (McCubbin, McCubbin, and Thompson, 1996). Resiliency helps to evaluate healthy responses when individuals and families are experiencing stressful events. Resources and techniques a family or individuals within the family use to maintain a balance or level of health can assist in understanding a family's level of resiliency (Svarvarsdottir, McCubbin, and Kane, 2000).

Family Nursing

To begin working with families, nurses must have a scientific knowledge base in family theory, as well as an adequate knowledge base in family nursing. Although the past and present health care systems tend to emphasize the individual, family focus is now needed in order to be able to safely discharge clients back to the family or community settings. The aging population now finds adult children as primary caregivers of their aging parents (Carruth, 1996). This emerging group of family caregivers has unique nursing and caregiving needs. To provide care for a family member, this group frequently must make major adjustments to integrate the challenges and time commitments of caring for a family member with their own lives (Hunt, 2003).

Family nursing is based on the assumption that all people regardless of age are a member of some type of family form. This family form may be the traditional nuclear family, a single-parent family, extended family, or alternate family forms previously described. The goal of family nursing is to help the family and its individual members reach and maintain maximum health throughout and beyond the illness experience. Family nursing is the focus of the future across all practice settings and is emphasized in all health care environments.

There are different approaches for family nursing practice. Friedman (1992) suggests three focuses: (1) the individual with family as context, (2) relationships within the family (relational), and (3) processes within the family (transactional). A very similar approach is a focus on (1) the individual within the context of the family, (2) the family with the individual as context, and (3) the whole family as the unit of care. The perspective that a nurse uses is related to the clinical setting, the clinical problem, and realistic and practical considerations. Dealing with

very complex family system problems often requires an interdisciplinary approach. The nurse must always be aware of the limits of nursing practice and make referrals when appropriate.

For the purposes of this chapter, family nursing practice is conceptualized as having three levels of approaches: (1) **family as context**, (2) **family as client**, and (3) the newest model, called **family as system**, which includes both relational and transactional concepts. If only one family member is receptive to nursing care, it is realistic and practical to view the family as context. When all family members are involved in the day-to-day care of one another, nursing intervention with one individual necessitates some change in the activities of the others, suggesting that family as client would be the best approach. Both family as context and family as client are approaches that can be useful in providing effective nursing care.

Family as Context
When the nurse views the family as context, the primary focus is on the health and development of an individual member existing within a specific environment (i.e., the client's family). Although the nurse focuses the nursing process on the individual's health status, the nurse also assesses the extent to which the family provides the individual's basic needs. These needs vary, depending on the individual's developmental level and situation. Because families provide more than just material essentials, their ability to help the client meet psychological needs must also be considered. Family members may need direct interventions themselves.

Family as Client
When the family as client is the approach, family processes and relationships (e.g., parenting or family caregiving) are the primary focuses of nursing care. The focus of nursing assessment is usually on family patterns versus individual characteristics. The nursing process concentrates on the extent to which these patterns and processes are consistent with reaching and maintaining family and individual health.

Family as System
It is important to understand that although theoretical and practical distinctions can be made between the family as context and the family as client, they are not necessarily mutually exclusive, and both are often used simultaneously, such as with the perspective of the family as system. The following clinical scenario illustrates the differences:

> *If the family is viewed as context, the nurse (Susan) focuses on the client (Patrick) as an individual. Susan assesses Patrick's knowledge of high-sodium foods, strategies for reducing the number of high-sodium foods in his diet, realistic opportunities to reduce the number and extent of perceived stressors in Patrick's work and family environment, and Patrick's knowledge and skill in stress management, such as relaxation or biofeedback techniques.*
>
> *If the family is viewed as client, Susan assesses Patrick's family's current dietary patterns and their desire and resources for changing the patterns as a result of Patrick's hy-*

pertension. The nurse determines the demands placed on Patrick and the family. The family's capabilities to support Patrick's efforts at changing eating patterns and use of stress management techniques are also assessed.

Using the family as system, elements of both of the above perspectives are used. The decision and application is very individualized, based on the nursing assessment and clinical judgment. For instance, Susan decides, based on her assessment, that the cultural impact of diet on the family is great. The decision is made by the family for all members to adjust their diet to incorporate Patrick's needs, but Patrick decides that he is the only one who needs to join the gym to work on exercise and stress management. This combination of decisions is based on several factors: (1) Patrick wants time away alone to "unwind," (2) the family's financial priorities are to place their income toward living expenses and college savings, and (3) the family's schedules do not allow easy access to the gym. They will, however, all decide to exercise as a family on the weekends, once per day for at least 45 minutes (walking, jogging, bicycling, or roller blading).

Nursing Process for the Family

Nurses interact with families in a variety of community-based and clinical settings. The nurse uses the nursing process to care for an individual within a family (e.g., the family as context) or the entire family (e.g., the family as client). When initiating the care of families, there are three factors that organize the family approach to the nursing process:

1. That all individuals must be viewed within their family context
2. That families have an impact on individuals
3. That individuals have an impact on families

Assessing the Needs of the Family

Family assessment is essential to providing adequate family care and support. To ensure nurses have a pivotal role in helping families adjust to acute and chronic illness, they first need to understand the family unit, what the illness means to the family members, what the illness means to family functioning, how the family structure and function have been affected by the illness, and the support the family requires (Neabel, Fothergill-Bourbonnais, and Dunning, 2000). Although the family as a whole differs from individual members, the measure of family health is more than a summation of the health of all members. Assessment realms unique to family assessment are the form, structure, function, and health of the family and the five realms of family life noted in Box 9-3.

In caring for the family, the nurse must incorporate knowledge of the client's illness and assess the primary client as well as the family (Neabel, Fothergill-Bourbonnais, and Dunning, 2000). When focusing on the family, the nurse begins the family assessment by determining the client's definition of and attitude toward family and the extent to which the family can be incorporated into nursing care. To determine family form and membership, the nurse can ask who the client considers family or with whom the

client shares strong emotional feelings. If the client is unable to express a concept of family, the nurse asks with whom the client lives, spends time, and shares confidences and then ask whether the client considers them to be family or like family. To further assess the family structure, the nurse asks questions that determine the power structure and patterning of roles and tasks (e.g., "Who decides where to go on vacation?" "How are tasks divided in your family?" "Who mows the lawn?" "Who usually prepares the meals?").

The nurse assesses family functions such as the ability to provide emotional support for members, the ability to cope with its current health problem or situation, and the appropriateness of its goal setting and progress toward achievement of developmental tasks (Figure 9-2). The nurse also assesses whether the family is able to provide and allocate sufficient economic resources and whether its social network is extensive enough to provide support.

A family's cultural background (see Chapter 8) is an important variable when assessing the family because race and ethnicity can affect structure, function, health beliefs, values, and the way events are perceived (Box 9-5). The United States is increasingly more diverse. A large number of immigrants enter the country daily, adding to both the number and the variety of the many ethnic groups that make up the population. American health care institutions tend to operate from a white, middle-class perspective, and immigrant populations may have particular difficulty understanding and "fitting into" the system. Cultural assessment educators encourage the use of a "culturagram," which assesses and empowers culturally diverse families and encourages ethnic-sensitive practice. This tool assesses a variety of factors such as language spoken in the home, impact of crisis events, and values regarding family, education, and work.

Drawing conclusions based on cultural backgrounds requires critical thinking and careful consideration. It is imperative to remember that categorical generalizations can be misleading (e.g., all Asian-Americans are good at math). As many caution, overgeneralizations in terms of racial and ethnic group characteristics do not lead to greater understanding of the culturally diverse family. Culturally different families can vary in meaningful and significant ways; however, neglecting to examine similar-

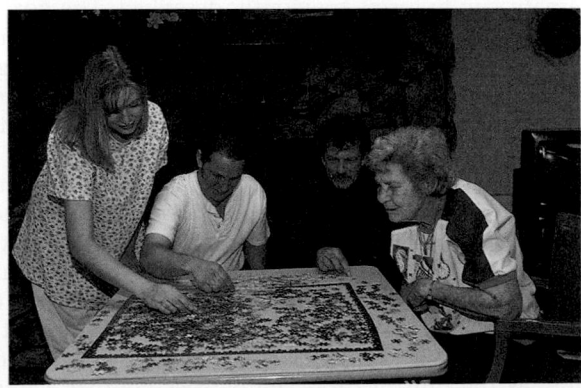

FIGURE **9-2** Observing family interactions assists in understanding family functioning.

ities can lead to inaccurate assumptions and stereotyping. Some studies reveal a lack of cultural differences in certain family processes. For example, more similarities than differences exist in parenting behaviors among white, African-American, Hispanic, and Asian-American parents. In addition, Asian-American families may use alternative therapies. Other cultures, such as Latino may prefer to stay with their family members during illness (see Chapter 8).

A comprehensive, culturally sensitive family assessment is critical to forming an understanding of family life, current changes in family life, and overall goals and expectations. These data provide the foundation for future family-centered nursing care (Anderson, 2000).

Cultural Aspects of Care
Box 9-5

Families have their unique perspectives and characteristics. Family have differences in values, beliefs, and philosophies. They range from traditional nuclear families, to single-parent families, to extended families. The cultural heritage of the family or member of the family can affect, for example, religious practices, child-rearing practices, recreational activities, and nutrition. Nurses need to have cultural competence and sensitivity when caring for multicultural clients. Incorporating cultural preferences into the plan of care can increase clients' adherence to therapy and assist in transition from hospital to home.

Implications for Practice

- Perception of certain events can vary across cultural groups and have particular impact on families. For example, the death of a grandparent may take on greater significance in families whose culture emphasizes veneration of older family members. Stressors such as rape may have an especially devastating effect on Hispanic women and their families, because great importance is placed on female virginity.
- Intergenerational support and patterns of living arrangements can be related to cultural background. For example, older Chinese, African-American, Japanese, and Hispanic persons are more likely to live in extended family households than are their white counterparts.
- Caregiving values and practices vary across cultures. In some cultures it is considered a sign of elder disrespect to place older adults in nursing homes, even those older adults with severe dementia.
- Health beliefs differ among various cultures, which may affect the decision of a family and its members about when and where to seek help. For example, Asians rarely consider symptoms as psychological and are not likely to go to mental health clinics.

Cox C, Monk A: Strain among caregivers: comparing the experiences of African-American and Hispanic caregivers of Alzheimer's relatives, *Int J Aging Hum Dev* 43(2):93, 1996; Kamo Y, Zhou M: Living arrangements of elderly Chinese and Japanese in the United States, *J Marriage Fam* 56(3):544, 1994; and Feeley N, Gottlieb LN: Nursing approaches for working with family strengths and resources, *J Fam Nurs* 6(1):9, 2000.

Family-Focused Care

Nursing practice is enhanced by a family-focused approach. When the nurse has established a relationship with a family, it is important to identify potential and external resources so that effective nursing care approaches can be implemented. The assessment provides this information. Any plan for nursing care must be clearly understood by the family and mutually agreed on by all members. Whatever goals the nurse sets in caring for the family must be concrete and realistic, compatible with the family's developmental stage, and acceptable to family members. The nurse collaborates closely with all appropriate family members when determining what they hope to achieve with regard to the family's health.

Collaboration with family members is essential, whether the family is the client or the context of care (Figure 9-3). A positive collaborative relationship is based on mutual respect and trust. The nurse's ability to care facilitates the building of trust. The family must feel "in control" as much as possible. By offering alternative actions and asking family members for their own ideas and suggestions, the nurse can help to reduce the family's feelings of powerlessness. For example, offering options for how to prepare a low-fat diet or how to rearrange the furnishings of a room to accommodate a family member's disability gives the family an opportunity to express their preferences, make choices, and ultimately feel as though they have contributed. Collaborating with other disciplines increases the likelihood of a comprehensive approach to the family's health care needs, and it ensures better continuity of care. Using other disciplines is particularly important when discharge planning from a health care facility to home or an extended care facility is necessary (Neabel, Fothergill-Bourbonnais, and Dunning, 2000).

When the family is viewed as the client, the nurse will aim to support communication among all family members. This ensures that the family remains informed as to the nurse's intent and progress in providing health care. Often the nurse must support conflict resolution between family members so that each member can confront and resolve problems in a healthy way. The nurse also helps family members use the external and internal resources that are necessary. Ultimately, the nurse's aim is to help the family reach a point of optimal function,

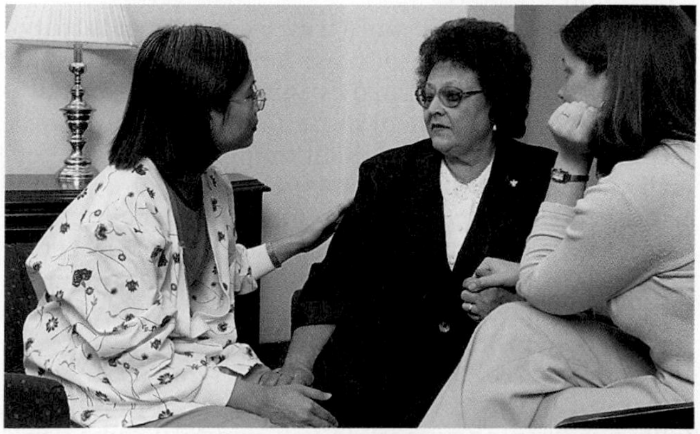

FIGURE **9–3** Nurse and family members.

given the family's resources, capacities, and desire to become healthier.

Challenges for Family Nursing

Delegation in the management of nursing care activities can become a challenge in family nursing. Often nurses are trying to make an impact on family health by delegating duties to family members or to other members of the health care team. For example, the nurse helps family members learn how to provide certain types of procedures to care for an ill family member. With earlier discharge and more complex family needs at the time of discharge, planning for discharge begins with the initiation of care by the registered nurse.

Discharge planning with a family involves an accurate assessment of what will be needed for care at the time of discharge, along with any shortcomings in the home setting. For example, if a postoperative client will be discharged to home and the older adult husband does not feel comfortable with the dressing changes required, the nurse first finds out if there is anyone else in the family or neighborhood who would or could do this. If not, the nurse arranges for a home care service referral. If the client also needs exercises and strength training, then perhaps a physical therapy referral is required.

Cultural sensitivity (see Chapter 8) in family nursing requires recognizing not only the diverse ethnic, cultural, and religious backgrounds of clients, but also the differences and similarities within the same family. In family-centered care, nurses learn how to integrate cultural practices, religious ceremonies, and rituals into family-centered care. Using effective and respectful communication techniques enables the nurse to determine the family's cultural practices and collaborate with the family to determine how best to integrate these beliefs and practices within the prescribed health care regimen.

Implementing Family-Centered Care

Whether caring for a client with the family as context or directing care to the family as client, nursing interventions aim to increase family members' abilities in certain areas, to remove barriers to health care, and to do things that the family cannot do for itself. The nurse guides the family in problem solving, provides practical services, and conveys a sense of acceptance and caring by listening carefully to family members' concerns and suggestions.

One of the roles the nurse will need to adopt is that of educator (Box 9-6). Health education is a process by which information is shared by nurse and client in a two-way fashion. Family/client needs for information may be recognized through direct questioning, but they are generally far more subtle. The nurse may recognize that the father is fearful of cleaning the newborn's umbilical cord or that an older adult woman is not using her cane or walker safely. Respectful communication is required. Often the subtle needs for information can be approached by saying, "I notice you are trying to not touch the umbilical cord; I see that a lot." Or "You use the cane the way I did before I was shown a way to keep from falling or tripping over it; do you mind if I show you?" When the nurse assumes a humble position instead of

---

Client Teaching **Box 9-6**

Family Caregiving: Newborn Cord Care

Objectives

- Client/family will be able to explain the purpose of cord care for the newborn.
- Client/family will be able to perform cord care correctly by return demonstration.
- Client/family will know who/when/where/why/how to call if problems develop.

Teaching Strategies

- Explain the following to the parents/grandparents/mature children:
  1. The umbilical cord does not have nerve endings, and if the baby cries, it is because of the cold alcohol near its skin and because of being exposed to the cooler air.
  2. The cord needs to be kept dry to promote its "falling off" without risk of infection.
  3. Tub baths will have to wait until the cord falls off.
  4. Diapers will need to be rolled down so that the cord stays dry (and the penis needs to be pointed down for boys).
  5. The cord will fall off at around 2 weeks of age.
  6. Signs and symptoms of infection include a red ring around the umbilical area, foul smell, moist oozing cord, drainage at the site, and either a high or very low core temperature in the newborn.
- Allow them to watch the nurse perform cord care correctly, and ask them to repeat for return demonstration.
- Offer them the opportunity to ask questions and repeat the skill as often as necessary for their comfort.

Evaluation

- Ask the client and family to explain the reasons and strategies used to care for the cord.
- Review with the family and provide feedback during their demonstrations. Frame it positively, and provide gentle encouragement.
- Remind them that the hospital nursing staff is available 24 hours a day, 365 days a year, for questions. They will refer the client/family to their own physician if there are problems or complications that are in need of medical evaluation.

---

coming across as an authority on the subject, this often decreases the client's defenses and makes the client more willing to listen without feeling embarrassed.

However, the nurse must also determine the best time to provide health care information. The nurse must be knowledgeable and able to provide accurate health information about diagnosis, necessary self-care activities, and the projected course of the condition. Such information helps the family caregiver to interpret behavior correctly and not to "blame" the client. Caregivers are not born with the knowledge of how to be caregivers, and older adults are not born with the knowledge of how to accept dependency (Hartrick, 2000).

Health Promotion. Although the family is the basic social context in which health behaviors are learned, the primary focus on health promotion has traditionally been on individuals. When implementing family nursing, health promotion interventions are needed to improve or maintain the physical, social, emotional, and spiritual well-being of the family unit and its members (Ford-Gilboe, 2002). Individual members and the total family are encouraged to reach their optimal levels of wellness. Identifying attributes that contribute to healthy, resilient families has been a focus of ongoing research for at least three decades. "Strong" families that adapt to expected transitions and unexpected crises and change tend to be characterized by clear communication among members, good problem-solving skills, a commitment to each other and to the family unit, and a sense of cohesiveness and spirituality (Svarvarsdottir, McCubbin, and Kane, 2000). Health promotion programs aimed at enhancing these attributes are available for families and children in many communities. The nurse must be aware of family-oriented offerings so that families can be referred as needed. Health promotion behaviors that the nurse needs to encourage are often tied to the developmental stage of the family (e.g., adequate prenatal care for the childbearing family and effective parenting and adherence to immunization schedules for the child-rearing family).

One approach for meeting goals and promoting health is the use of family strengths. Families do not look at their own system as one that has inherent, positive components. The nurse can help the family become aware of its own unique strengths, thereby increasing its potential and capabilities. Family strengths include clear communication, adaptability, healthy child-rearing practices, support and nurturing among family members, and the use of crisis for growth. The nurse can help the family focus on these strengths instead of its problems and weaknesses. For example, the nurse can point out that a couple's 10-year marriage must have endured many crises and transitions. Therefore they are likely to have the capabilities to adapt to this latest challenge.

Acute Care. Because family is becoming more of the focus, nursing will need to take more of a role in emphasizing family and client needs within the context of health care delivery in a managed care environment. Nurses need to be ever mindful of the early discharge states, paired with the increasing numbers of people within the household now being employed outside the home. These factors are challenges to the nurse to prepare family members to assist with health care or to locate appropriate community resources. Often when family members assume the role of caregiver, they may lose support from significant others. The nurse must be sure that families are willing to assume care responsibilities.

Family nursing requires a holistic view not only of the client but of the family as well. Nursing care in the acute environment can become very complex, making it a challenge for the client to feel cared for and to keep family members involved. A helpful tool is an independent journal in which clients and family members can communicate their thoughts, ideas, and reactions. The client or family members can use the journal as an open communication tool, updating entries based on their needs and observations of the acute care experience. It may also be helpful for a family member to use the journal as a record of care activities. The journal can be used to record data about when the client was turned, who visited, when the last pain medication was administered, and any special client requests. This information helps clients and families who are trying to "keep up" with what is happening in the acute care environment.

Restorative Care. In restorative care settings the challenge in family nursing is in trying to maintain clients' functional abilities within the context of the family. This includes having home care nurses help clients remain in their homes following acute injuries or illnesses, surgery, or exacerbation of a chronic illness. It may also entail finding ways to better the lives of chronically ill and disabled individuals and their families.

Family Caregiving. One way the nurse can best provide family care is through support of family caregivers. Family caregiving involves the routine provision of services and personal care activities for a family member by spouses, siblings, or parents. Caregiving activities might include personal care (bathing, feeding, or grooming), monitoring for complications or side effects of medications, instrumental activities of daily living (shopping or housekeeping), and the ongoing emotional support and decision making that is necessary. Whenever an individual becomes dependent on another family member for care and assistance, there is significant stress affecting both the caregiver and the care recipient. In addition, the caregiver must continue to meet the demands of his or her normal lifestyle (e.g., raising children, working full time, or dealing with personal problems or illness). In many cases older adult children are caring for their parents or older relatives. Without adequate preparation and support from health care providers, caregiving can predispose the family to serious problems, including a decline in the health of the caregiver and that of the care receiver, dysfunctional relationships, and even abusive relationships.

Despite its demands, caregiving can be a positive and rewarding experience (Picot, Youngblut, and Zeller, 1997). Caregiving is more than simply a series of tasks and often occurs within the context of a family. Whether it is a wife caring for a husband or a daughter caring for a mother, caregiving is an interactional process. The interpersonal dynamics between family members influence the ultimate quality of caregiving. Thus the nurse can play a key role in helping family members develop better communication and problem-solving skills to build the relationships needed for caregiving to be successful.

Researchers have identified variables, such as caregiver and care recipient expectations of one another, influencing caregiving quality. Carruth (1996) has studied the concept of **reciprocity**, acknowledging the importance of the capability of care recipients to share exchanges that contribute to a caregiver's perception of self-worth. When the caregiver knows that the care recipient appreciates his or her efforts and values the assistance provided, a healthier and more satisfying caregiving relationship will exist. When caregiver and client solve problems together, overprotection or oversolicitous behavior can be avoided. Clients feel in control of their care and responsible for care decisions. The caregiver also feels very positive and enjoys the caregiving experience (Isaksen, Thuen, and Hanestad, 2003).

Providing care and support for family caregivers often involves using available family and community resources. Establishing a caregiving schedule enabling all family members to participate, having extended family members share any financial burdens posed by caregiving, and having distant relatives send cards and letters communicating their support can be very useful. However, it is imperative for the nurse to understand the relationship between potential caregivers and care recipients. If the relationship is not a supportive one, community services may be a resource for both the client and family.

Use of community resources might include locating a service required by the family or providing respite care so that the family caregiver has time away from the care recipient. Examples of services that may be beneficial to families include caregiver support groups, housing and transportation services, food and nutrition services, housecleaning, legal and financial services, home care, hospice, and mental health resources. Before referring a family to a community resource, it is critical that the nurse understands the family's dynamics and knows whether support is desired or welcomed. Often a family caregiver will resist help, feeling obligated to be the sole source of support to the care recipient. The nurse must be sensitive to family relationships and help caregivers understand the normalcy of caregiving demands. Given the appropriate resources, caregivers can acquire the skills and knowledge necessary to effectively care for the loved ones within the context of the home while maintaining rich and rewarding personal relationships.

Key Concepts

- The family structure and functions influence the lives of its individual members.
- Family members influence one another's health beliefs, practices, and status.
- The concept of family is highly individual; thus the nurse should base care on the client's attitude toward the family rather than on an inflexible definition of family.
- The family's structure, functioning, and relative position in society significantly influence its health and ability to respond to health problems.
- Two theories that help nurses assess families are the family health system (FHS) and the developmental stages perspectives.
- The family can be viewed as an important context for the individual family member, the family unit can be viewed as the client, or the family unit can be viewed as a system (simultaneously viewing the family as both client and family in context).
- Measures of family health involve more than a summation of individual members' health.

- Its social class, economic stability, and racial and ethnic background influence the family's health.
- Family members as caregivers are often spouses who may be either older adults themselves or adult children trying to work full time, care for aging parents, and launch teenagers successfully.
- Health promotion through health education is an important tool in family nursing practice.
- Cultural sensitivity is paramount to family nursing. Members may subscribe to differing beliefs, traditions, and restrictions even within the same generation.
- Family nursing requires that nurses continually examine the current trends in the American family and its health care implications.
- Family caregiving is an interactional process that occurs within the context of the relationships among its members.

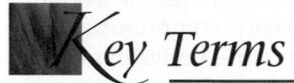

Key Terms

Family, *p. 141*

Family forms, *p. 141*

Family as client, *p. 147*

Family as context, *p. 147*

Family as system, *p. 147*

Hardiness, *p. 147*

Reciprocity, *p. 151*

Resiliency, *p. 147*

Critical Thinking Exercises

1. Kathy is a parish nurse and is working with a family in her church. This is a family of four: Carol, a 45-year-old single mother; her two adolescent sons, Matt and Kent; and Sara, her 76-year-old mother, who is in the last stages of terminal breast cancer. This family has lived together for 10 years, and Sara was a great support to Carol when her husband died 11 years ago. She helped Carol parent Matt and Kent. This family has decided to care for Sara in the home until the end. Kathy is going to help the family achieve this goal.
   a. What assessments are important?
   b. How will Kathy help the family achieve this goal?
   c. How will Kathy help the family determine their strengths, weaknesses, and resources?
2. Dan has been divorced from Kim for 7 years. Neither has remarried, and they have three girls: Annie, Angela, and Abby, ages 10 to 14. At the time of the divorce Dan was HIV positive. He has had active disease for 5 years and has not responded to therapy and is in the end stages of the disease. Kim has had repeated tests and remains HIV negative. They have shared all parenting responsibilities and maintain a friendly relationship. Dan and Kim have decided that it might be easier for this family of five to live together again. This decision is so Dan can be active in his girls' lives without placing caregiver demands on Kim when the family visits Dan overnight. Kim also wants to care for her former husband.
   a. What challenges will this family face as they reunite?

b. How will the nurse determine what support services are needed by the family?

3. Mr. and Mrs. Baillargeron, both in their early 50s, are the youngest members of large Catholic French Canadian families. They are employed full time and have two teenage children of their own. Both sets of their parents are in their 80s and have chronic health problems. All of their brothers and sisters are geographically farther away. How can you assist Mr. and Mrs. Baillargeron in developing extended resources to aid in caring for their parents and at the same time maintain the responsibilities of their own family unit?

Review Questions

1. The players may change, the parents may remarry, and the children may or may not leave home as adults, but the "family" is considered to transcend long periods and inevitable lifestyle changes. This is an example of family:
1. Diversity.
2. Resiliency.
3. Durability.
4. Configuration.

2. These family forms—"skip-generation" families (grandparents caring for grandchildren), "nonfamilies" (adults living alone), and homosexual couples— are considered:
1. Alternative patterns of relationships.
2. Blended families.
3. Extended families.
4. Diverse families.

3. The client is remarried, and her two children from a previous marriage live in the same household. Her husband's children visit on the weekend. This is an example of a (an):
1. Nuclear family
2. Blended family.
3. Extended family.
4. Alternative family.

4. The most common reason grandparents are called on to raise their grandchildren is due to:
1. The increase in divorce rate.
2. Dual-income families.
3. Single parenthood.
4. Legal interventions due to unfit parents.

5. The Family Health System (FHS) has five realms used to examine, assess, and care for families. An example of the interactive processes realm is:
1. Family relationships
2. Current family transitions
3. Family life stresses
4. Family values.

6. Communication among family members is an example of family:
1. Structure.
2. Function.
3. Goals.
4. Development.

7. A family's access to adequate health care, opportunity for education, sound nutrition, and decrease stress is increased by:
1. Economic stability.
2. Family structure.
3. Family function.
4. Development.

8. The primary social context in which health promotion and disease prevention take place is:
1. At educational institutions.
2. From friends and colleagues.
3. From doctors and nurses.
4. The family.

9. When nurses view the family as client, their primary focus is on the:
1. Health and development of an individual member existing within a specific environment.
2. Family process and relationships.
3. Family relational and transactional concepts.
4. Family within a system.

10. This type of nursing approach often decreases the clients' defenses and makes the client more willing to listen without feel embarrassed.
1. Authoritarian.
2. Problem solver.
3. Humble position.
4. Subtle.

References

Anderson KH: The family health system approach to family systems nursing, *J Fam Nurs* 6(2):103, 2000.

Bell JM and others: Learning to nurse the family, *J Fam Nurs* 7(2):117, 2001 (editorial).

Centers for Disease Control and Prevention: Combating complacency in HIV prevention, Atlanta, 1998a, Division of HIV/AIDS Prevention, www.cdc.gov/hiv/pubs/facts/combat. htm.

Centers for Disease Control and Prevention, U.S. Public Health Service: *HIV/AIDS surveillance reports* 10(2), 1998b.

Centers for Disease Control and Prevention: HIV/AIDS update: a glance at the HIV epidemic, 2003, www.cdc.gov/hiv/pubs/facts.htm.

Children's Defense Fund: Issues: fair start—child poverty, Washington, DC, 2003a, Children's Defense Fund, www.childrensdefense.org/fs_chpov.

Children's Defense Fund: What's CHIP? An introduction to the Children's Health Insurance Program, Washington, DC, 2003b, Children's Defense Fund, www.childrensdefense.org/hs_chipmain.php.

Clemen-Stone S, McGuire SL, Eigsti DG: *Comprehensive community health nursing*, St. Louis, 1998, Mosby.

Cox C, Monk A: Strain among caregivers: comparing the experiences of African-American and Hispanic caregivers of Alzheimer's relatives, *Int J Aging Hum Dev* 43(2):93, 1996.

Farran CJ: Family caregivers: a critical resource in today's changing healthcare climate, *Chart* 99(4):4, 2002.

Feeley N, Gottlieb LN: Nursing approaches for working with family strengths and resources, *J Fam Nurs* 6(1):9, 2000.

Friedman M: *Family nursing: theory and assessment,* ed 3, New York, 1992, Appleton-Century-Crofts.

Kamo Y, Zhou M: Living arrangements of elderly Chinese and Japanese in the United States, *J Marriage Fam* 56(3):544, 1994.

McGoldrick M, Carter E: The stages of the family life cycle. In Walsh F, editor: *Normal family processes,* New York, 1982, Guilford Press.

National Coalition for the Homeless: Homeless families with children: NCH fact sheet No. 7, Washington, DC, 2001, The Association, www.nationalhomeless.org/families.html.

Nichols SY: Work and family stress. In McHenry PC, Price SJ, editors: *Families and change: coping with stressful events,* London, 1994, Sage Publications.

Svarvarsdottir EK, McCubbin MA, Kane JH: Well-being of parents of young children with asthma, *Res Nurse Health* 23:346, 2000.

U.S. Bureau of the Census: *Population profile of the United States: 2000 (Internet release),* Washington, DC, 2001, The Bureau, http//: www.census.gov.

Walsh F: *Normal family processes,* New York, 1982, Guilford Press.

*R*esearch References

Anderson KH: The family health system approach to family systems nursing, *J Fam Nurs* 6(2):103, 2000.

Astedt-Kurki P and others: Methodological issues in interviewing families in family nursing research *J Adv Nurs* 35(2):288, 2001.

Astedt-Kurki P and others: Development and testing of a family nursing scale, *West J Nurs Res* 24(5):567, 2002.

Carruth AK: Development and testing of the caregiver reciprocity scale, *Nurs Res* 45:92, 1996.

Cox C, Monk A: Strain among caregivers: comparing the experiences of African-American and Hispanic caregivers of Alzheimer's relatives, *Int J Aging Hum Dev* 43(2):93, 1996.

Feeley N, Gottlieb LN: Nursing approaches for working with family strengths and resources, *J Fam Nurs* 6(1):9, 2000.

Ford-Gilboe M: Developing knowledge about family health promotion by testing the developmental model of health and nursing, *J Fam Nurs* 8:140, 2002.

Hartrick G: Developing health-promoting practice with families: one pedagogical experience, *J Adv Nurs* 3:27, 2000.

Harvey E: Short-term and long-term effects of early parental employment on children: the National Longitudinal Survey of Youth, *Dev Psychol* 35(2):445, 1999.

Hill R: Generic features of families under stress, *Soc Casework* 39:145, 1958.

Hunt CK: Concepts in caregiver research, *J Nurs Scholarsh* 35:27, 2003.

Hwang SW: Homelessness and health, *CMAJ-JAMC (Canadian Medical Association)* 164:229, 2001.

Isaksen AS, Thuen F, Hanestad B: Patients with cancer and their close relatives: experiences with treatment, care, and support, *Cancer Nurs* 26(1):68, 2003.

James-Childs EY: Adolescent and young adult male parenting: the forgotten half, doctoral dissertation, 2000, University of Colorado Health Sciences Center.

Kamo Y, Zhou M: Living arrangements of elderly Chinese and Japanese in the United States, *J Marriage Fam* 56(3):544, 1994.

Kushel M and others: Emergency department use among the homeless and marginally housed: results from a community-based study, *Am J Public Health* 92:778, 2002.

McCubbin MA, McCubbin HI, Thompson AI: Family Hardiness Index (FHI). In McCubbin HI, Thompson AI, McCubbin MS, editors. *Family assessment: resiliency, coping, and adaptation, inventories for research and practice,* Madison, 1996, University of Wisconsin Press.

Neabel B, Fothergill-Bourbonnais F, Dunning J: Family assessment tools: a review of the literature from 1978-1997, *Heart Lung* 29:196, 2000.

Picot SJF, Youngblut J, Zeller R: Development and testing of a measure of perceived caregiver rewards in adults, *J Nurs Meas* 5:33, 1997.

Richardson J and others: Identifying domestic violence: cross sectional study in primary care, *Br Med J* 324:274, 2002.

Robrecht LC: Interpersonal violence and the pregnant homeless woman, *J Obstet Gynecol Neonatal Nurs* 27:684, 1998.

Shinn M and others: Predictors of homelessness among families in New York City: from shelter request to housing stability, *Am J Public Health* 88:1651, 1998.

SmithBattle L: The vulnerabilities of teenage mothers: challenging prevailing assumptions, *ANS Adv Nurs Sci* 23(1):29, 2000.

Svarvarsdottir EK, McCubbin MA, Kane JH: Well-being of parents of young children with asthma, *Res Nurs Health* 23:346, 2000.

Wathen CN, MacMillan HL: Interventions for violence against women: scientific review, *JAMA* 289:589, 2003.

Developmental Theories

Media Resources

http://evolve.elsevier.com/Potter/
fundamentals/

CD COMPANION

- Review Questions
- Glossary

evolve WEBSITE

- Review Questions
- Student Learning Activities
- Glossary

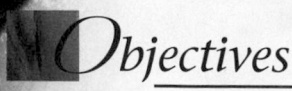

Objectives

Mastery of content in this chapter will enable the student to:

- Define the key terms listed.

- Identify basic principles of growth and development.

- Discuss factors influencing growth and development.

- Describe biophysical developmental theories under the categories of genetic theory, nongenetic cellular theories, and the physiological theories of aging.

- Describe and compare the psychoanalytic/psychosocial theories proposed by Freud, Erikson, and Havighurst.

- Describe Piaget's theory of cognitive development.

- Discuss how Kohlberg built upon Piaget's stages of moral development.

- Discuss Gilligan's criticism of Kohlberg's moral developmental stage theory.

- Apply developmental theories when planning interventions in the care of clients.

- Discuss nursing implications for the application of developmental principles to client care.

Growth and Development

Understanding normal growth and development helps nurses predict, prevent, and detect any deviations from clients' normal expected patterns. Growth refers to the changes that can be measured and compared to norms, for example, taking the height and weight of a pediatric client and comparing the measurements to the standardized growth charts. Development implies a progressive and continuous process of change leading to a state of organized and specialized functional capacity; for example, a child's progressions from rolling over to crawling to walking are developmental changes. Individuals have unique patterns of growth and development within broad limits. Knowledge of these patterns assists each person in reaching their full potential (Behrman and Kliegman, 2000).

Human growth and development are orderly, predictable processes beginning with conception and continuing until death. All persons progress through definite phases of growth and development, from the simple to the complex, and at a highly individualized rate. Children learn to walk before they can run, but one child may walk at 10 months, and another may not walk until 15 months of age.

The ability to progress through each developmental phase influences the holistic health of the individual. The success or failure experienced within a phase may affect the ability to complete subsequent phases. If individuals experience repeated developmental failures, inadequacies may result. However, when the individual experiences repeated successes, health is promoted. A child not learning to walk by 20 months, for example, demonstrates delayed gross motor ability that slows exploration and manipulation of the environment. A child walking by 10 months is able to explore and find stimulation in the environment, thereby enhancing learning.

Accurate assessment of patterns of growth and development helps set the stage for future patterns of adjustment to life (Edelman and Mandle, 2002). A clear understanding of these patterns assists the nurse in planning questions for health screening and health history and in health teaching for clients of all ages.

Major Factors Influencing Growth and Development

The human being is a complex, open system influenced by natural forces from within and from the environment (Table 10-1). Interaction between these forces affects development. The nurse applies knowledge of these factors in selecting therapies to promote normal growth and developmental progression. It is important, for example, that the nurse considers a female client's genetic endowment as well as her preconception state of health as part of planning for a healthy, positive pregnancy experience.

Definitions. Growth and development are synchronous processes that are interdependent in the healthy individual. Growth, development, maturation, and differentiation depend on a sequence of endocrine, genetic, constitutional, environmental, and nutritional influences (Edelman and Mandle, 2002).

Physical Growth. Physical growth is the measurable aspect of an individual's increase in physical measurements. Measurable growth indicators include changes in height, weight, teeth, skeletal structures, and sexual characteristics. For example, children generally double their birth weight by 5 months of age and their birth height by 36 months.

Development. Development occurs gradually and refers to changes in skill and capacity to function. These changes are qualitative in nature and difficult to measure in exact units. These are certain predictable charac-

---

Table 10-1 Major Factors Influencing Growth and Development

Factors	
Forces of Nature	
Heredity	Genetic endowment determines sex, race, hair and eye color, physical growth, stature, and to some extent psychological uniqueness.
Temperament	Temperament is characteristic psychological mood with which the child is born and includes behavioral styles of easy, slow-to-warm, and difficult. It influences interactions between the individual and environment.
External Forces	
Family	Family purpose is to protect and nurture its members.
	Family functions include means for survival, security, assistance with emotional and social development, assistance with maintenance of relationships, instruction about society and world, and assistance in learning roles and behaviors.
	Family influences through its values, beliefs, customs, and specific patterns of interaction and communication.
	Ordinal position and sex influence individual's interaction and communication in family.
Peer group	Peer group provides new and different learning environment.
	Peer group provides different patterns and structures of interaction and communication, necessitating different style of behavior.
	Functions of peer group include allowing individual to learn about success and failure; to validate and challenge thoughts, feelings, and concepts; to receive acceptance, support, and rejection as unique persons apart from family; and to achieve group purposes by meeting demands, pressures, and expectations.
Life experiences	Life experiences and learning processes allow individual to develop by applying what has been learned to what needs to be learned.
	Learning process involves series of steps: recognition of need to know task; mastery of skills to perform task; mastery of task; expertise in performing task, which expands capabilities; integration into whole functioning; and use of accumulated skills and experiences to develop repertoire of effective behavior.
Health environment	Level of health affects individual's responsiveness to environment and responsiveness of others to the individual.
Prenatal health	Preconception (e.g., genetic and chromosomal factors, maternal age, health) and postconception (e.g., nutrition, weight gain, use of tobacco and alcohol, medical problems, use of prenatal services) factors affect fetal growth and development.
Nutrition	Growth is regulated by dietary factors. Adequacy of nutrients influences whether and how physiological needs, as well as subsequent growth and development needs, are met.
Rest, sleep, and exercise	Balance between rest or sleep and exercise is essential to rejuvenating body. Disturbances diminish growth, whereas equilibrium reinforces physiological and psychological health.
State of health	Illness or injury potentially hampers growth and development. Nature and duration of health problem influences its impact. Prolonged injury or illness may cause inability to cope and respond to demands and tasks of developmental stages.
Living environment	Factors affecting growth and development include season, climate, home life, and socioeconomic status.

teristics, such as development proceeds from simple to complex, from general to specific, from head to toe **(cephalocaudal),** and from the trunk to the extremities **(proximodistal).**

Maturation. Maturation is the process of aging. The individual begins to adapt and show competence in new situations. Maturation involves an individual's biological ability, physiological condition, and desire to learn more mature behavior. To mature, the individual may have to give up previous behavior and learning, integrate new patterns into existing behavior, or both. Maturation influences the sequence and timing of the changes associated with growth and development. For example, the infant relinquishes crawling for walking because walking permits more extensive investigation of the environment and more learning. However, the infant cannot walk until the biological ability and structures to perform the action (i.e., increased muscle cells and tone) have developed.

Differentiation. **Differentiation** is the process by which cells and structures become modified and develop more refined characteristics. It is a simple-to-complex development of activities and functions. Embryonal cells begin as vague and undifferentiated and develop into complex, highly diversified cells, tissues, and organs.

Developmental Theories

A theory is an organized, often observable, and logical set of statements about a subject. Human developmental theories are models intended to account for how and why people become as they are (Thomas, 1997). Useful theories explain behavior, as well as predict behavior that can be tested and observed. By testing and observing behavior, caregivers can develop programs that can further enhance the development of children (Berk, 2003; Bukatko and Daehler, 2001; Edelman and Mandle, 2002). For example, knowledge of Erikson's psychosocial theory of development helps caregivers understand the importance of supporting the development of basic trust in the infancy stage. Trust establishes the foundation for all of one's future relationships. Developmental theories are also important in helping nurses assess and treat a person's response to an illness. Understanding the specific task or need of each developmental stage guides caregivers in planning appropriate individualized care for clients.

Four Areas of Theory Development

To help the reader understand the number of developmental theories, this chapter has been grouped into four main areas of theory development: biophysical, psychoanalytic/psychosocial, cognitive, and moral development. The areas of learning theory and spiritual development are covered in Chapters 24 and 28, respectively.

Biophysical development attempts to describe the way our physical bodies grow and change. These changes are quantified and can be compared against established norms. Biophysical developmental theory is defined as the process of biological maturation. Biological influences on development include many factors such as ge-

netics, exposure to teratogens (infections, maternal diseases, drugs, substance abuse, environmental chemicals or other hazardous substances). All theories give some credence to the role of nature and nurture; however, the theories differ sharply on how much influence they have on development (Berk, 2003).

Psychoanalytic/Psychosocial development attempts to describe the development of the human personality, behavior, and emotions. This development is thought to occur with varying degrees of influence from internal biological forces and external societal/cultural forces. These theories each have stages that children go through while attempting to resolve conflicts between biological drives and social forces (Berk, 2003).

Cognitive development is focused on reasoning and thinking processes, including the changes in how people come to perform intellectual operations. These operations are related to the ways persons learn to understand the world in which they live. Mental processes, including perceiving, reasoning, remembering, and believing, permit certain types of emotional behavior. The young child will, for example, have a different emotional reaction to the death of a grandparent as compared to an older sibling or a parent.

Moral development focuses on the description of moral reasoning. Moral reasoning is how people think about the rules of ethical or moral conduct but does not predict what a person would actually do in a given situation. Moral development is the ability of an individual to distinguish right from wrong and to develop ethical values on which to base his or her actions (Berk, 2003).

Biophysical Developmental Theories

Biophysical development is how our physical bodies grow and change. The changes that occur as a newborn infant grows into adulthood can be quantified and compared against established norms. How does the physical body age? What are the triggers that move the body from the physical characteristics of childhood, through adolescence, to the physical changes of adulthood? Biophysical developmental theory is defined as the process of biological maturation. Biophysical development was described by Gesell, who developed a theory based on his observations of children as related to their physical growth. The aging theories covered in Chapter 13 are named by how they define the aging process; they are not linked to any one person but instead are being studied by a number of different scientists.

Gesell's Theory of Development

Arnold Gesell (1880-1961) was a psychologist who also obtained his medical degree to help him explain the physiological processes he was observing in the behavior of children. Through extensive observations in the 1940s, he developed behavior norms that still serve as a primary source of information for childhood development today.

Fundamental to Gesell's theory of development is that although each child's pattern of growth (development) is unique, this pattern is directed by the activity of the genes.

Environmental factors can support, change, and modify the pattern, but they do not generate the progressions of development (Gesell, 1948). Gesell found the pattern of maturation as a fixed developmental sequence in all humans. Sequential development is seen in fetuses, where there is a specified order of development of the various organ systems (Crain, 1992). After birth, children grow according to their genetic blueprint and gain skills in an orderly fashion, but at each individual's own pace. For example, most children will learn first how to hold a cup with digital grasp at around 15 months of age and handle a cup well, lifting, drinking, and replacing, at 21 months of age. Gesell was clear that not every child develops those skills at exactly the same time. Gesell pointed out that the environment does play a part in the development of the child, but it does not have any part in the sequence of development. Gesell believed that a child could not be pushed to develop faster than that child's own unique timetable. Although Gesell felt genes controlled the person's development, he did not know the process by which the genes programmed development in an individual.

The biophysical theories all attempt to describe the processes of why our bodies age. Gesell went as far as to propose that it is our biological body that determines our behavioral development. The psychoanalytic/psychosocial theories look at the process of development from a very different perspective.

Psychoanalytic/Psychosocial Theory

The psychoanalytic/psychosocial theories describe human development from the perspective of personality, thinking, and behavior (Table 10-2). Human behavior is extremely complex and therefore difficult to capture within one theory. Many theorists have devoted their entire lifetime to the development of a consistent understanding of how we become successful human beings.

Sigmund Freud

The first person to provide a formal, structured theory of personality development was Sigmund Freud (1856-1939). His theory is grounded in the belief that two internal biological forces essentially drive psychological change in the child: sexual (**libido**) and aggressive energies. Motivation for behavior is to achieve pleasure and avoid pain created by these forces. These forces come into conflict with the reality of the world as maturational changes occur.

Freud's psychoanalytic model of personality development has five psychosexual developmental stages associated with different pleasurable zones serving as the focus for gratification and bodily pleasure (Behrman and Kliegman, 2000).

Stage 1: Oral (Birth to 12 to 18 Months). Initially, sucking and oral satisfaction is not only vital to life, but also extremely pleasurable in its own right. Late in this stage, the infant begins to realize that the mother/parent is something separate from self. Disruption in the physical or emotional availability of the parent (e.g., inadequate bonding or chronic illness) could have an impact on the infant's development.

Stage 2: Anal (12 to 18 months to 3 Years). The focus of pleasure changes to the anal zone. Children become increasingly aware of the pleasurable sensations of this body region with interest in the products of their effort. Through the toilet-training process the child is asked to delay gratification in order to meet parental and societal expectations.

Table 10-2	Comparison of Major Developmental Theories			
Developmental Stage/Age	Freud (Psychosexual Development)	Erikson (Psychosocial Development)	Piaget (Cognitive/ Moral Development)	Kohlberg (Development of Moral Reasoning)
Infancy (Birth to 18 months)	Oral stage	Trust versus mistrust Ability to trust others	Sensorimotor period Progress from reflex activity to simple repetitive actions	
Early childhood/ toddler (18 months to 3 years)	Anal stage	Autonomy versus shame and doubt Self-control and independence	Preoperational period— thinking using symbols; egocentric	Preconventional level Punishment-obedience orientation
Preschool (3-5 years)	Phallic stage	Initiative versus guilt Highly imaginative	Use of symbols; egocentric	Preconventional level Premoral Instrumental orientation
Middle childhood (6-12 years)	Latent stage	Industry versus inferiority Engaged in tasks and activities	Concrete operations period Logical thinking	Conventional level Good–boy, nice–girl orientation
Adolescence (12-19 years)	Genital stage	Identity versus role confusion Sexual maturity, "Who am I?"	Formal operations period Abstract thinking	Postconventional level Social contract orientation

Stage 3: Phallic or Oedipal (3 to 6 Years). It is during this stage that the genital organs become the focus of pleasure. According to Freud, the boy becomes interested in the penis; the girl becomes aware of the absence of the penis known as penis envy. This is the time of exploration and imagination as the child fantasizes about the parent of the opposite sex as his or her first love interest, known as the Oedipal or Electra complex. By the end of this stage, the child attempts to reduce this conflict by identifying with the parent of the same sex in a way to win recognition and acceptance.

Stage 4: Latency (6 to 12 Years). This is a stage in which Freud believed that sexual urges, from the earlier Oedipal stage, are repressed and channeled into productive activities that are socially acceptable. Within the educational and social worlds of the child, there is much to learn and accomplish. This is where the child places energy and effort.

Stage 5: Genital (Puberty Through Adulthood). This is Freud's final stage. This is a time of turbulence when earlier sexual urges reawaken and are directed to an individual outside the family circle. Unresolved prior conflicts surface during adolescence. Once conflicts are resolved, the individual is then capable of having a mature adult sexual relationship.

Components of the human personality develop through Freud's developmental stages. Freud believed that the functions of these components regulate behavior. These components are the id, the ego, and the superego. The id, basic instinctual impulses driven to achieve pleasure, is the most primitive part of the personality and originates in the infant. The ego represents the reality component mediating conflicts between the environment and the forces of the id. The ego helps us judge reality accurately, regulate impulses, and make good decisions. The third component, the superego, performs regulating, restraining, and prohibiting actions. Often referred to as the conscience, the superego is influenced by the standards of outside social forces (parent, teacher).

The goal was the development of balance between pleasure-seeking drives and societal pressures. The mature adult should have a strong sense of conscience that allows for the experience of pleasure within the boundaries of society. Although Freud's theory has been soundly criticized for gender and cultural biases, it is clear that he gave other theorists a basis for observation of emotion and behavior. Some of Freud's critics contend that people are more influenced by their life experiences than by their sexual energies. Other critics feel that Freud's basic assumptions such as the Oedipal complex are not applicable across different cultures.

Erik Erikson

Freud had a strong influence on his psychoanalytic followers, including Carl Jung, Erik Erikson, and others who continued to develop and refine his theory. Erikson expanded Freud's psychoanalytic stages into a psychosocial model that covered the whole life span (Erikson, 1963, 1997; Behrman and Kliegman 2000).

According to **Erikson's eight stages of life,** individuals need to accomplish a particular task before suc-

cessfully completing the stage. Each task is framed with opposing conflicts, such as the adolescent's need to develop a sense of personal identity challenged by many confusing choices. These tasks are triggered by life forces.

Each stage builds upon the successful resolution of the previous developmental conflict. Readiness for the task is necessary for success. Tasks once mastered are challenged and tested during new situations or at times of conflict (Hockenberry and others, 2003). For example, the infant's trust is built through consistent, reliable caregiving; yet the concept of trust is tested when an infant is hospitalized or after the birth of a new baby. Erickson's eight stages of life are described below:

Trust Versus Mistrust (Birth to 1 Year). Starting with oral satisfaction, the infant learns to trust the caregiver as well as self. Trust is achieved when the infant will let the caregiver out of sight without undo distress. Key to this stage is consistent caregiving. The parent's struggle with building the sense of competence can be assisted by the nurse's use of anticipatory guidance and other educative interventions. The parent may need to have guidance to understand the importance of a safe environment when meeting the child's need to explore through creeping and crawling before walking.

Autonomy Versus Sense of Shame and Doubt (1 to 3 Years). The growing child is now becoming accomplished in some basic self-care activities, including walking, feeding, and toileting. This newfound independence is the result of maturation and imitation. The toddler develops his or her autonomy by making choices. Choices typical for the toddler age-group include activities related to relationships, desires, and playthings. There is also opportunity to learn that parents and society have expectations about these choices. The nurse can model empathetic guidance that offers support for and understanding of the challenges of this stage. Limiting choices and or harsh punishment can lead to feelings of shame and doubt.

Initiative Versus Guilt (3 to 6 Years). Children like to pretend and try out new roles. Fantasy and imagination allow children to further explore their environment. Also at this time children are developing their superego, or conscience. Conflicts often arise between the child's desire to explore and the limits placed on his or her behavior. These conflicts may lead to feelings of frustration and guilt. Guilt may also occur if the caregiver's responses are too punitive. Teaching impulse control and cooperative behaviors to the child can help the family avoid the risks of altered growth and development.

Industry Versus Inferiority (6 to 11 Years). School-age children are eager to apply themselves to learning socially productive skills and tools. They learn to work and play with their peers. School-age children thrive on their accomplishments and praise. Without proper support for learning of new skills or if skills are too difficult, children may then develop a sense of inadequacy and inferiority. Erikson believed that the adult's attitudes toward work can be traced to successful achievement of this task (Erikson, 1963).

Identity Versus Role Confusion (Puberty). Dramatic physiological changes associated with sexual maturation mark this stage. There is a marked preoccupation with appearance and body image. This stage in which identity development begins with the goal of achieving some perspective or direction answers the question, "Who am I?" Acquiring a sense of identity is essential for making adult decisions such as choice of vocation or marriage partner. Each adolescent moves in his or her unique way into society as an interdependent member. There are also new social demands, opportunities, and conflicts that relate to the emergent identity and separation from family. The nurse can provide education and anticipatory guidance for the parent about the changes and challenges to the adolescent. Nurses can also assist hospitalized adolescents in dealing with their illness by giving them enough information to allow them to make decisions about their treatment plan.

Intimacy Versus Isolation (Young Adult). Young adults, having developed a sense of identity, deepen their capacity to love others and care for them. This is the time to become fully participative in the community, enjoying adult freedom and responsibility. If young persons have not achieved a sense of personal identity, they may experience feelings of isolation from others and the inability to form meaningful attachments. The nurse should understand that during hospitalization young adults may benefit from the support of their partner or significant other because this strengthens their need for intimacy.

Generativity Versus Self-Absorption and Stagnation (Middle Age). Following the successful development of an intimate relationship, the adult can focus on supporting future generations. The ability to expand one's personal and social involvement is critical to this stage of development. Middle-age adults should be able to see beyond their needs and accomplishments to the needs of society. Dissatisfaction with one's place and achievements often leads to self-absorption and stagnation. Nurses can assist physically ill adults in choosing creative ways to foster social development. Middle-age persons may find a sense of fulfillment by volunteering some time in a local school, hospital, or church.

Integrity Versus Despair (Old Age). As the aging process creates physical and social losses, the adult may also suffer loss of status and function, such as through retirement or illness. These external struggles are also met with internal struggles, such as the search for meaning in life. Meeting these challenges creates the potential for growth and wisdom (Figure 10-1). Many older adults review their lives with a sense of satisfaction even with their inevitable mistakes, whereas others see themselves as failures with their lives marked by despair and regret. Research pertaining to the losses experienced by older adults is presented in Box 10-1.

Nurses are in positions of influence within their communities and can contribute to the valuing of persons at all ages and stages. Persons at all ages and stages need to feel valued, appreciated, and needed. Erikson stated, "Healthy children will not fear life, if their parents have

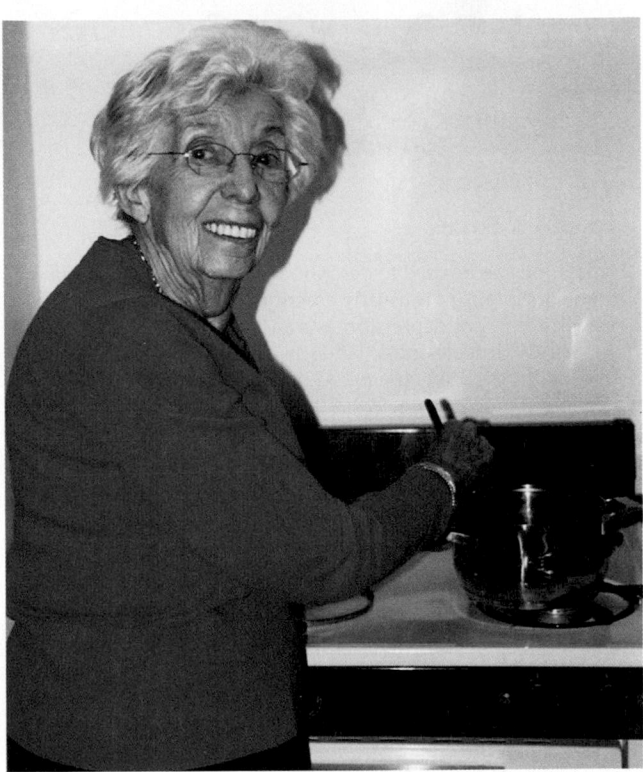

FIGURE 10–1 Maintaining independence is important to one's self-esteem.

integrity enough not to fear death" (Erikson, 1963). Erikson did significant research during his academic career with varied cultural traditions and gender groups. He believed his theory to be widely applicable.

Robert Havighurst

Robert Havighurst (1900-1991) was influenced by Erikson's work and observations of the developmental tasks critical to healthy development. Havighurst defined a series of essential tasks that arise from predictable internal and external pressures (Ashburn, 1978). These pressures include increasing physical maturity, cultural pressure of society, and the individual's personal goals and aspirations.

Looking at **Havighurst's developmental tasks,** it is clear that several sources of pressure may be present at the same time. Increasing physical maturity would be associated with the development of skills such as walking, talking, or eating. Cultural pressure creates the conditions necessary to learn social behaviors and ethical norms. Although the adolescent girl may be physically able to accomplish the task of having a child, the preparation and timing for the onset of parenthood can also be considered from a perspective of cultural pressure from both the youth and adult cultures. The desire to have a child might also grow out of the individual's personal goal or aspiration to be a parent.

Havighurst believed that there are critical periods when the individual is most receptive to the learning necessary to achieve success in performing these tasks. Effective learning and achievement of tasks during one

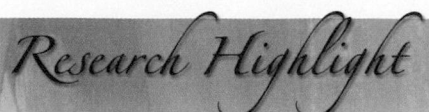

Box 10-1

Older Adult Women's Explanation of Depression

Research Focus

Depression can be used to describe a mood, a symptom, or a syndrome. Its intensity is usually described as mild, moderate, or severe. Examples of depression as a mood include the expression of sadness, hopelessness, and disappointment. The grieving process also expresses the mood of depression. Symptoms of depression appear in three spheres: cognitive (thinking), affective (feeling tone), and psychomotor (action) behaviors. It is not uncommon to see symptoms of depression during chronic illness or as a side effect of many medications. Depression is a common psychiatric condition affecting individuals of all ages. It is important that nurses understand what impact depression and other emotional states have on a person's perceptions about his or her health condition and treatment. As the older adult population increases, the rate of age-related disabilities, chronic illness, and depression will also increase.

Research Abstract

This research uses the Kleinman explanatory model to describe an individual's interpretation of an illness. This model is determined by the individual's general beliefs about health and illness. It provides personal and social meaning to the illness experience. Using this model, clients are permitted to construct from their beliefs an explanation of the illness and plan their course of treatment. Using the explanatory model, nurses should ask questions designed to gain the client's perspective of his or her illness with relationship to its etiology, symptoms, and treatment options.

Using the Kleinman explanatory model, 30 older adult women with depression were interviewed. Hand-recorded interviews focused on the person's perception of the cause and contributing factors for the start of her illness. The participants identified their perceptions of the severity, duration, and expected results of treatment.

The results showed that most of the women believed that their depression was a result of changes in their health. Some identified loss of function (poor eyesight, pain) as contributing factors. The second most common reason cited for the onset of depression was due to a death of a family member. The women believe that these deaths contributed to their loneliness. Thoughts of suicide were not commonly described; however, somatic symptoms such as generalized aches and pains were frequently expressed.

Evidenced-Based Practice

- Understanding the older person's concept of depression assists nurses in explaining complementary and alternative treatment measures.
- Further public education is needed to prepare for the growing numbers of older persons.
- Treatment centers should be extended to churches, synagogues, and other social or civic centers.
- Further studies are needed to look at the cultural display of depression.

Reference

Ugarriza DN: Elderly women's explanation of depression, *J Gerontol Nurs* 28(5):22, 2002.

---

period lead to happiness and success with later tasks. Failure leads to unhappiness, disapproval by society, and difficulty with later tasks. An example might be the struggle that adolescents might experience in preparing for a work career after having failed to develop fundamental skills in reading and calculating.

As an educator, Havighurst believed that schools have considerable responsibility in helping a child attain success necessary to lead to achievement of later adult development. His theory is a structure of both nonrecurrent tasks specific to a stage of development, such as learning to walk, and recurrent tasks that reemerge in new ways, such as learning to get along with age-mates. Havighurst's theory is limited in its cultural application according to critics who believe that it describes developmental milestones from the perspective of middle-class norms within the American culture. It would be difficult to fit all cultural or ethnic mores within this theoretical framework.

Roger Gould

Psychiatrist Roger Gould reviewed the work of other theorists and found that a lack of understanding of the adult years contributed to the maturing and changing of personality (Table 10-3) (Gould, 1972). He conducted extensive research that supported a set of development themes within stages of adult development. Gould found that over the adult years, persons dismantle the protective thinking developed during childhood. Over a period of years beliefs are shed, marking a shift from childhood into adult consciousness.

Gould's development themes start when individuals are in their 20s with "I have to get away from my parents." This is challenged in minor ways before the end of high school but culminates as young persons begin to live away from home. The move away from parental influence is gradual as young adults establish themselves as adults.

The second theme occurs during the early 30s and asks, "Is what I am the only way for me to be?" This question occurs when young adults experience the consequences of the decisions of their independence. Everything does not work out magically as might have been expected. There are failures to be overcome. Acceptance for who they are is essential. So is acceptance of their own growing children as being unique and separate.

The third theme occurs in the mid to late 30s and asks, "Have I done the right thing? Is there time to change?" These questions recognize the complexities of adult decisions. The impact of a growing family and aging parents influences this theme. There is a beginning sense of time left to effect wanted results.

Table **10-3** Adult Developmental Theorists			
Adult Stages (Approximate Ages)	**Erickson**	**Havighurst**	**Gould**
Early-early adult (12-22 years) Middle-early adult (22-28 years)	Intimacy versus isolation Ability to form intimate relationships	Early adulthood stage Selecting a mate Learning to live with a marriage partner Starting a family Rearing children Getting started in an occupation Taking on civic responsibilities Finding a congenial social group	Theme: "I have to get away from my parents." Gradually establishing control of self as an adult
Late-early adult (28-34 years)			Theme: "Is what I am the only way for me to be?" Demonstrating independent competence while overcoming failures
Middle adult (34-45 years)	Generativity versus self absorption and stagnation Ability to expand personal and social involvement	Middle age Assisting teenage children to become responsible adults Achieving adult social and civic responsibility Reaching and maintaining satisfactory performance in one's occupation Developing adult leisure-time activities Relating to one's spouse as a person Accepting and adjusting to the physiological changes of middle age Adjusting to aging of parents	Theme: "Have I done the right thing?" Learning to live with ambivalence without need to prove self Beginning sense of time to effect wanted results
Middle adult (continued) (40-50 years) Middle adult (continued) (50-60 years)			Theme: "The die is cast." Believing that possibilities are limited Seeing time as having an end point Decreased negativism Increased feelings of self-satisfaction Realizing mortality and concern for health
Late adult/old age (60-85 years)	Integrity versus despair, disgust Ability to adapt to changes in lifestyle, functional level, and family structure	Later maturity Adjusting to decreasing physical strength and health Adjusting to retirement and reduced income Adjusting to death of a spouse Establishing an affiliation with one's age-group Adopting and adapting social roles in a flexible way Satisfactory physical living space	

The fourth theme, identified in the 40s, "The die is cast," is indicative of resignation and the belief that possibilities are limited. The personality is set. Changes in career are believed to be less likely to be successful. Parents are blamed for their lack of choices. Regret is faced for mistakes made with children.

During the 50s a decrease in negativism occurs. Gould finds a realization of mortality with a concern for one's state of health. There is less responsibility for the welfare of the children and more attachment to the spouse, as might be expected.

Gould believes his research describes a sequential process that takes place between the internal life (personality) of adults and their outer world (culture, lifestyle). For example, Gould would look at the timing and sequencing of an event, as well as the individual's adjustment and transition into a particular stage. It seemed clear to Gould that events of adulthood may be similar in adults; however, the timing and sequencing will affect the adjustment and consequences in different individuals. Marriage, for example, may occur before or after pregnancy, the time between the birth of the first and second child may differ, and retirement may occur in one's 50s or 60s. Gould's theoretical work can focus the nurse's appreciation on life issues affecting the adult client. Nurses may help adults realistically appreciate their accomplishments and foster their continued development.

Stella Chess and Alexander Thomas

Psychiatrists Stella Chess and Alexander Thomas conducted a 20-year longitudinal study. It included children from a wide range of populations, including normal children of middle-class parents born in the United States and Puerto Rican and American working-class parents with mentally challenged children. The breadth of the data allowed them to look at the behavior of persons from childhood to early adulthood as they interacted with their environment. Their work defined the concept of temperament (Chess and Thomas, 1986).

Temperament is a behavioral style that affects the child's interactions with others (Hockenberry and others, 2003). It is the way a child deals with life. The individual differences children display in responding to their environment significantly influence the way others respond to them and their needs. Knowledge of temperament helps parents to have a clearer perspective of their child and enables health caregivers to guide them appropriately (Hockenberry and others, 2003). Chess and Thomas (1983) described three common categories of temperament but explain that there are wide ranges of the behavior and approximately 30% of children do not appear in any of these groups:

- **The easy child**—easygoing and even-tempered. Regular and predictable in his or her habits. An easy child is open and adaptable to change and displays a mild to moderately intense mood that is typically positive.
- **The difficult child**—highly active, irritable, and irregular in habits. Negative withdrawal towards others is typical, and the child requires a more structured environment. A difficult child adapts slowly to new routines, people, or situations. Mood expressions are usually intense and primarily negative.
- **The slow-to-warm-up child**—typically reacts negatively and with mild intensity to new stimuli. The child adapts slowly with repeated contact unless pressured and responds with mild but passive resistance to novelty or changes in routine.

Cognitive Developmental Theory

Jean Piaget's Theory of Cognitive Development

Jean Piaget (1896-1980), a Swiss biologist and philosopher, was most interested in the development of children's intellectual organization, how they think, reason, and perceive the world. **Piaget's theory of cognitive development** includes four periods and recognizes that children move through these specific periods at different rates but in the same sequence or order (Berk, 2003; Crain, 1992; Maier, 1965). His theory was built on years

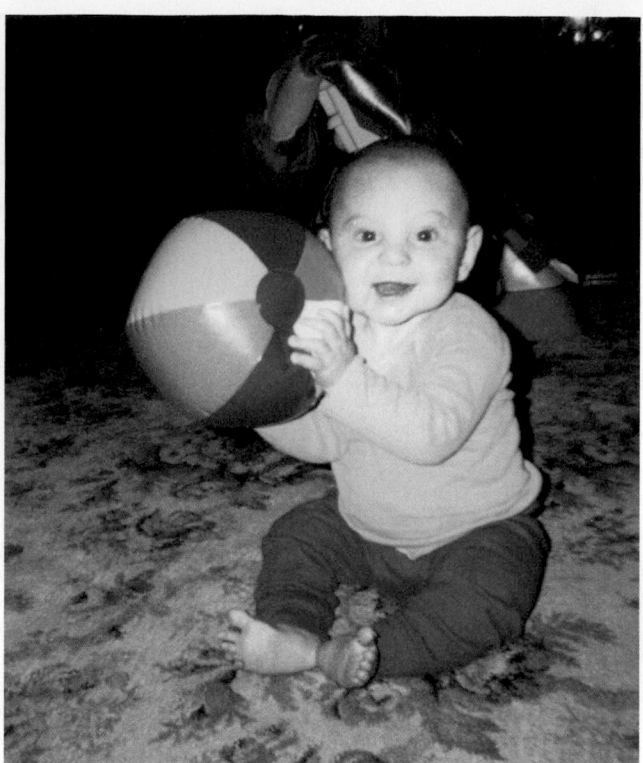

FIGURE **10–2**   Successful achievement of action patterns such as grasping leads to learning and more exploration.

of observing children as they explored, manipulated, and tried to make sense out of the world in which they lived. In Piaget's theory external or internal forces did not shape thinking, although he acknowledged their presence in the process. Piaget's theory includes four general periods of development with a number of stages within each (see Table 10-2).

Period I: Sensorimotor (Birth to 2 Years). During a time of unparalleled changes, the infant develops the schema or action pattern for dealing with the environment (Berk, 2003; Singer and Revenson, 1996). These schemas may include hitting, looking, grasping, or kicking (Figure 10-2). Schemas become self-initiated activities; for example, the infant learning that sucking achieves a pleasing result generalizes the action to suck fingers, blanket, or clothing. Successful achievement leads to greater exploration.

Toward the end of this stage, infants are able to form primitive mental images as they acquire object permanence. Before this they do not realize that objects out of sight exist. When a 6-month-old is shown a toy before it is hidden, he or she will not search for it. At 18 months the child can understand that even if it cannot be seen it still exists and will search for it.

Period II: Preoperational (2 to 7 Years). This is a time when children learn to think with the use of symbols and mental images. Still egocentric, the child sees objects and persons from only one point of view, the child's own. Play is the initial method of nonlanguage use of symbols

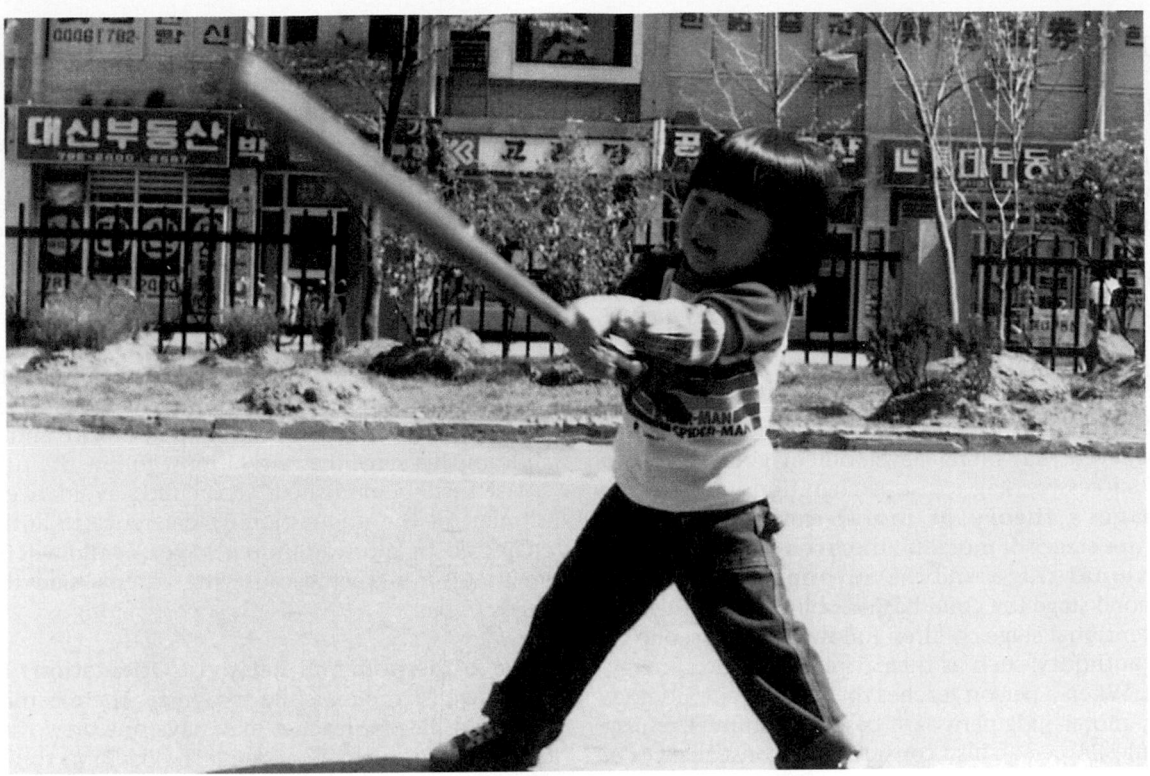

FIGURE **10–3**   Play is important to a child's development.

(Figure 10-3). This is a time of parallel play. Parallel play can be observed as children engage in activities side-by-side without a common goal. Imitation and make-believe play are ways to represent experience (Berk, 2003; Singer and Revenson, 1996). Nursing interventions during this period will recognize the use of play as the way the child understands the events taking place. Parents can be assisted in the use of play materials such as thermometers, blood pressure equipment, and play needles that will allow children to communicate feelings about health care procedures they experience.

Later, language develops and broadens possibilities for thinking about the past or the future. Children can now communicate about events with others. As the language fits into a logical form, it mirrors the thinking process at the time.

Period III: Concrete Operations (7 to 11 Years). Children now achieve the ability to perform mental operations. For example, the child can now think about an action that before was performed physically. At the earlier stage the child could count to 10 but now he or she can count and understand what each number represents. Children can now describe a process without actually performing it. At this time they are able to coordinate two concrete perspectives in social as well as scientific thinking. In other words, they can appreciate the difference between their perspective and that of a friend. Reversibility is the primary characteristic of concrete operational thought. Children can mentally reverse the direction of their thoughts. Children can

now mentally classify objects according to their quantitative dimensions, known as seriation. Another major accomplishment of this stage is conservation, or the ability to see objects or quantities as remaining the same despite a change in their physical appearance (Berk, 2003; Singer and Revenson, 1996). Children can begin to cooperate and share with new information about the acts they perform. Parents will be able to adjust their approaches to guide the child into helpful activities within the home, such as bargaining about chores in exchange for wishes for privileges (TV time, play with friends).

Period IV: Formal Operations (11 Years to Adulthood). During this stage the individual's thinking moves to abstract and theoretical subjects. Thinking can venture into such subjects as achieving world peace, finding justice, and seeking meaning in life. Adolescents can organize their thoughts in their minds. They have the capacity to reason with respect to possibilities. New cognitive powers allow the adolescent to do more far-reaching problem solving, including their futures and that of others. This thinking matures, and the depth of understanding increases with experience.

Piaget believed that the sequencing of these stages occurs for all children but that the rate of achievement may vary. He also theorized that this would be true in all cultures. He acknowledged that biological maturation plays a role in this developmental theory but believed that rates of development depend upon the intellectual stimulation and challenge in the environment of the child.

Moral Developmental Theory

Moral developmental theories try to explain "how individuals acquire moral values and how such values help guide the way persons treat other people" (Thomas, 1997). Although various psychosocial and cognitive theorists have addressed moral development within their respective theories, Piaget and Kohlberg are the two who have done the most to propose a theory of moral development (see Table 10-2).

Jean Piaget's Moral Developmental Theory

Piaget believed that moral development goes through a series of successive stages just as cognition and learning does. **Piaget's theory of moral development** presented three stages of morality: the **premoral stage**, the **conventional stage**, and the **autonomous stage.** In the premoral stage the child has no obligation to rules. In the conventional stage children follow the rules set up by those in authority, such as their parents, teachers, clergy, or police. When a person reaches the stage of autonomous morality, moral judgments are based on mutual respect for the rules. A person also considers the consequences of a moral decision. The person at this stage starts to consider information related to the subjective intent in making moral judgments that involve others (Berk, 2003).

Piaget first saw the child following the rules without understanding the rules. Children see these rules as fixed and handed down by adults or by God, so they cannot change them. Young children base their moral decisions on the extent of the consequences to the action, not necessarily on the action itself. For example, a young child will not eat a cookie before supper not because the mother said not to, but because the child is afraid of the punishment that would result if he or she did.

Around 10 or 11 years of age, children's cognitive ability matures and the rules children follow are understood within the context of community life, the interaction with those around them. Children understand that the rules can be modified "by legal channels" if everyone agrees to change the rules (Singer and Revenson, 1996). Moral maturity is the internalization of the principles, the desire to weigh all the relationships and circumstances before making a decision.

Lawrence Kohlberg's Moral Developmental Theory

Kohlberg expanded on Piaget's moral developmental theory. Kohlberg initially interviewed boys at ages 10, 13, and 16. Kohlberg felt that Piaget did not go far enough in the development of his stages. From a series of moral dilemmas, he identified six stages of moral development under three levels (Kohlberg, 1981). Kohlberg found a link between moral development and Piaget's cognitive development. A child's moral development did not advance if the child's cognitive development did not also mature. In this way, **Kohlberg's theory of moral development** follows Piaget's cognitive developmental theories (see Table 10-2).

Level I: Preconventional Level. At Level I the person reflects on moral reasoning based on personal gain. This closely correlates with Piaget's first stage, in that the person's moral reason for acting, the "why," relates to the consequences the person believes will occur. These consequences can come in the form of punishment or reward. It is at this level that children may view illness as a punishment for fighting with their siblings or disobeying their parents. The nurse must be aware of this thinking and reinforce teaching that the child cannot become ill because of wrongdoing.

Stage 1: Punishment and Obedience Orientation. In this first stage, the child's response to a moral dilemma is in terms of absolute obedience to authority and rules. A child in this stage reasons, "I must follow the rules; otherwise I will be punished." The child's avoidance of punishment or the unquestioning deference to authority is characteristic motivation to behave. A child will be home on time for supper because the parents said the child needs to be.

Stage 2: Instrumental Relativist Orientation. This second stage is where a child recognizes there is more than one right view; a teacher may have one view that is different than the child's parent. The decision to do something morally right is based on satisfying one's own needs, and occasionally the needs of others. Punishment is perceived not as proof of the child being wrong (as in Stage 1), but as something that one wants to avoid (Taffell, 2002). Children at this stage will follow their parent's rule about being home in time for supper because they do not want to be confined to their room for the rest of the evening if they do not get home on time.

Level II: Conventional Level. At level II, the person sees moral reasoning based on his or her own personal internalization of societal and others' expectations. A person wants to fulfill the expectations of the family, group, or nation and also develop a loyalty to and actively maintain, support, and justify the order. Moral decision making at this level moves from "What's in it for me?" to "How will it affect my relationships with others?" Nurses may observe this when family members make end-of-life decisions for their loved ones. Individual members often struggle with this type of moral dilemma. Grief support will involve an understanding of the level of moral decision making of each family member (see Chapter 29).

Stage 3: Good Boy–Nice Girl Orientation. Stage 3 correlates with Piaget's second stage of moral development. The individual wants to win approval and maintain the expectations of one's immediate group. "Being good" means having good motives, showing concern for others, and keeping mutual relationships through trust, loyalty, respect, and gratitude. One earns approval by "being nice." A person in this stage may stay after school and do odd jobs to win the teacher's approval.

Stage 4: Society-Maintaining Orientation. Individuals expand their focus from a relationship with others to societal concerns during Stage 4. Moral decisions take into account societal perspectives. Right behavior is doing one's duty, showing respect for authority, and maintaining the social order. Adolescents may choose not to attend a party where they know beer will be served, not because they are afraid of getting caught, but because they know that it is not right.

Level III: Postconventional Level. The person finds a balance between basic human rights and obligations and societal rules and regulations in this level. Individuals move away from moral decisions based on authority or conformity to groups to define their own moral values and principles. Individuals at this stage start to look at what an ideal society would be like.

Stage 5: Social Contract Orientation. Having reached Stage 5, an individual may follow the societal law but recognizes the possibility of changing the law to improve society. The individual also recognizes that different social groups may have different values but believes that all rational people would agree on basic rights, such as liberty and life. Individuals at this stage make more of an independent effort to think out what society ought to value, not related to what the society as a group would value, as would occur in Stage 4. The United States Constitution is based on this morality. An individual at this stage recognizes laws as social contracts that the citizens have agreed to uphold but believes that there must be a mechanism to change unfair laws by democratic means (Crain, 1992).

Stage 6: Universal Ethical Principle Orientation. Stage 6 defines "right" by the decision of conscience in accord with self-chosen ethical principles. These principles are abstract, like the Golden Rule, and appeal to logical comprehensiveness, universality, and consistency (Kohlberg, 1981). For example, the principles of justice would require the individual to treat everyone in an impartial manner, respecting the basic dignity of all people, and would guide the individual to base decisions on an equal respect for all (Figure 10-4). Stage 5 emphasizes the basic rights and the democratic process, whereas Stage 6 defines the principles by which agreements will be most just.

Further research on the part of Kohlberg made him question Stage 6 because he found that very few subjects consistently reasoned at this stage. He concluded that his research method of using moral dilemmas did not draw out difference between Stages 5 and 6. He termed Stage 6 a "theoretical stage" and no longer scored individuals as achieving this stage in his research.

Nurses need to know their moral reasoning level. Recognizing one's own moral developmental level is essential in separating one's own beliefs from others when helping clients with their moral decision-making process. Nurses should recognize the level of moral reasoning used by members of the health care team and its influence on the client's care plan. Ideally all members of the health care team will be on the same level, creating a unified outcome. This can be exemplified in the following scenario: The nurse is caring for a homeless person and believes that all clients deserve the same level of care. The case manager, being responsible for resource allocation, complains about the client's length of stay and the amount of resources being expended on this one client.

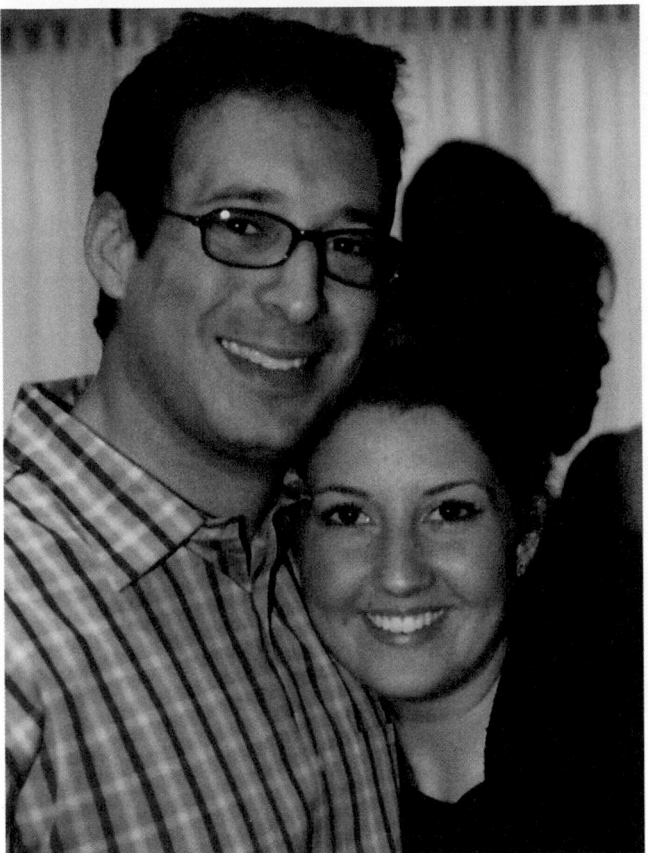

FIGURE **10–4**   Adults need meaningful, close, respectful relationships.

The nurse and the case manager are in conflict because of their different levels of moral decision making within their practices.

Kohlberg's Critics. Kohlberg constructed a systemized way of looking at moral development. He has been recognized as a leader in moral developmental theory. However, critics of his work raise questions about his choice of research subjects. Most of Kohlberg's subjects were males of the Western philosophical traditions.

Research attempting to support Kohlberg's theory with individuals raised in the Eastern philosophies has found that those study participants never rose above Stages 3 or 4 of Kohlberg's model. Does that mean that they have not reached higher levels of moral development, as most of the adults raised in the Western traditions? Or is it that Kohlberg's research design did not allow a way to measure those raised within a different culture?

Kohlberg has also been criticized for age and gender bias. Carol Gilligan, an associate, has criticized Kohlberg for his gender biases (Berk, 2003). Gilligan's research looked at moral development and concentrated on the differences that may be related to gender. According to Gilligan, all developmental theories are subject to gender bias, and it has only been recently that our society has researched and recognized the differences between men and women, in the way they think and how they have been raised to make decisions (Kail, 2001).

Carol Gilligan

Gilligan proposes that Kohlberg's theory is biased in favor of men. She believes there may be parallel ways that men and women develop, with one not being superior to the other. Basic to Gilligan's argument is the developmental difference in relationships and issues of dependency between women and men (Berk, 2003; Crain, 1992; Gilligan, 1982; Schroeder, 1992). **Separation** and **individuation** are critically tied to male development. Separation refers to the child's recognition of biological distinctness and is based on his emergence from a dependent relationship with his mother. This separation from the mother is essential for the boy in his development of masculinity. Girls do not need to separate from their mothers to achieve feminine identity; it is through this attachment to their mother that their identity is formed. Most developmental theories use achievement of increasing separation as a developmental norm. When women are measured against this norm as it relates to their need to maintain relationships, they are seen as failures or less evolved developmentally. Individuation is based on the child's awareness of differences in will, viewpoint, and needs. This process permits the individual to gradually assume a more independent role and identity.

Male moral development may focus on logic, justice, and social organization, whereas female moral development focuses on interpersonal relationships. Interestingly, studies using Gilligan's critique as the research design have been inconclusive. As a result, Gilligan's position remains controversial (Cavanaugh, 1993).

Conclusion

Developmental theories help nurses to use critical thinking skills when asking how and why people respond as they do. From the diverse set of theories included in this chapter, it is clear how complex human behavior is. No one theory successfully describes human growth and development in all of its complexity. Theorists themselves demonstrate their own values and beliefs in their focus and the subjects chosen for their work. They work within a cultural and historical perspective. As nurses apply the theories, it is important to keep this in mind.

A nurse's assessment of a client requires a thorough analysis and interpretation of data to form accurate conclusions about a client's developmental needs. Accurate identification of nursing diagnoses relies on the nurse's ability to consider developmental theory in data analysis. A nurse compares normal developmental behaviors with those projected by developmental theory. Examples of nursing diagnoses applicable to clients with developmental problems include *risk for delayed development, delayed growth and development,* and *risk for disproportionate growth.* Further detail regarding these diagnoses can be found in Chapter 11.

Growth and development is not a linear process, as most theories tend to be, but multidimensional. The theories included are meant to be the basis for a meaningful observation of an individual's pattern of growth and development. All theories require validation through research to become fact. They are important guidelines for understanding important human processes that can allow nurses to begin to predict human responses and recognize deviations from the norm.

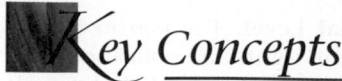 **ey** *Concepts*

- Nurses administer care for individuals at various developmental stages. Developmental theory provides a basis for nurses to assess and understand the responses seen in their clients.
- Humans continue to develop throughout their lives. Development does not end at adolescence; persons grow and develop throughout their life span.
- Theory is a way to account for how and why people grow up as they do. Theories provide a framework and a way to clarify and organize existing observations to explain and try to predict human behavior.
- Growth refers to the quantitative changes that can be measured and compared to norms.
- Development implies a progressive and continuous process of change leading to a state of organized and specialized functional capacity. These changes can be measured quantitatively but are more distinctly measured in qualitative changes.
- Biophysical development explores theories of why individuals age from a biological standpoint.
- Cognitive development focuses on the rational-thinking processes that include the changes in how children and adolescents perform intellectual operations.
- Developmental tasks are age-related achievements, the success of which leads to happiness, whereas failure may lead to unhappiness, disapproval, and difficulty in achieving later tasks.
- Developmental crisis is when a person is having great difficulty in meeting tasks of the current developmental period.
- Socialization is the outside influence a person receives from family, peers, and society.
- Psychosocial theories attempt to describe the development of the human personality with varying degrees of influence from the internal biological forces and the external societal/cultural forces.
- Temperament is a behavioral pattern that affects the child's interactions with others.
- Moral development attempts to define how moral reasoning matures for an individual.

ey *Terms*

Autonomous stage, *p. 166*

Biophysical development, *p. 158*

Cephalocaudal, *p. 158*

Cognitive development, *p. 158*

Conventional stage, *p. 166*

Differentiation, *p. 158*

Erikson's eight stages of life, *p. 160*

Freud's psychoanalytic model of personality development, *p. 159*

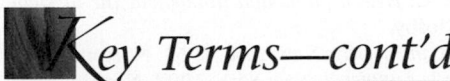

Key Terms—cont'd

Gould's development themes, *p. 162*
Havighurst's developmental tasks, *p. 161*
Individuation, *p. 168*
Kohlberg's theory of moral development, *p. 166*
Libido, *p. 159*
Moral development, *p. 158*

Piaget's theory of cognitive development, *p. 164*
Piaget's theory of moral development, *p. 166*
Premoral stage, *p. 166*
Proximodistal, *p. 158*
Psychoanalytic/ psychosocial development, *p. 158*
Separation, *p. 168*

Critical Thinking Exercises

1. A 76-year-old woman has just been diagnosed with breast cancer. She also has severe cardiovascular disease that limits her choices of treatment. Her oncologist has recommended a series of chemotherapy that her cardiologist believes would be fatal. Her family is urging her to do all that is recommended. The client, who is in good spirits despite her diagnosis, chooses palliative care. Based on her developmental stage, how can you help the family adjust to her choice?

2. A 50-year-old woman expresses dismay that her children ages 20 and 23 are no longer living at home. Her husband is still working full-time but looking to retire in a couple of years. She is concerned that she is not needed and is bored with her life. Identify the developmental task of Erickson's theory that best fits this woman's situation. How will the nurse assist this client in changing her lifestyle while understanding her developmental tasks?

3. Parents of an 18-month-old toddler describe to the nurse during their routine visit to the pediatrician that their child is walking and getting into everything. Using your knowledge of Erikson's developmental theories, what stage is this child at, and what approach would be helpful for these parents?

4. Two 11-year-old girls are spending the day together at the mall. They exit one store, and one of the girls shows her friend a small purse that she stole from the store. Her friend is upset and wonders how she should respond. What moral advice would you want to discuss with this young girl?

Review Questions

1. Children generally double their birth weight by 5 months of age. This is an example of:
   1. Development.
   2. Heredity.
   3. State of health.
   4. Physical growth.

2. _____ development is the ability of an individual to distinguish right from wrong and to develop ethical values on which to base his or her actions.
   1. Moral.
   2. Cognitive.
   3. Pyschosocial.
   4. Psychoanalytic.

3. Freud's _____ developmental stage is a time of turbulence when earlier sexual urges reawaken and are directed to an individual outside the family circle.
   1. Anal.
   2. Phallic or oedipal.
   3. Latency.
   4. Genital.

4. The nurse teaches parents how to have their children learn impulse control and cooperative behaviors. This would be during Erickson's stage of development:
   1. Trust Versus Mistrust.
   2. Autonomy Versus Sense of Shame and Doubt.
   3. Initiative Versus Guilt.
   4. Industry Versus Inferiority.

5. A 47-year-old woman expresses dismay to the nurse that her young adult children are unemployed. Her husband is working and near retirement. She is not working, and feels bored with her life and unneeded. She is experiencing Erickson's _____ stage of development.
   1. Integrity Versus Despair.
   2. Intimacy Versus Isolation.
   3. Identity Versus Confusion.
   4. Generativity Versus Self-Absorption and Stagnation.

6. The developmental theorist who believes his research describes a sequential process that takes place between the internal life (personality) of adults and their outer world (culture, lifestyle) is:
   1. Erickson.
   2. Gould.
   3. Freud.
   4. Thomas.

7. "The die is cast" is consistent with Gould's theme for the:
   1. 30s.
   2. 40s.
   3. 50s.
   4. 70s.

8. During this stage the individual's thinking moves to abstract and theoretical subjects. Thinking can venture into such subjects as achieving world peace, finding justice, and seeking meaning in life.
   1. Formal operations.
   2. Concrete operations.
   3. Sensorimotor.
   4. Preoperational.

9. In this level of Kohlberg's moral developmental theory the person reflects on moral reasoning based on personal gain.
   1. Instrumental Relativist Orientation.
   2. Conventional.
   3. Preconventional.
   4. Conventional.

10. The theorist who believes that girls do not need to separate from their mothers to achieve feminine identity is:
   1. Gilligan.
   2. Kohlberg.
   3. Gould.
   4. Freud.

References

Ashburn SS: Selected theories of development. In *The process of human development: a holistic approach,* Boston, 1978, Little, Brown.

Behrman R, Kliegman R: *Nelson Textbook of Pediatrics,* ed 16, Philadelphia, 2000, WB Saunders.

Berk L: *Child Development,* ed 6, Boston, 2003, Allyn & Bacon.

Bukatko D, Daehler M.: *Child development: a thematic approach,* ed 4, Boston, 2001, Houghton Mifflin.

Cavanaugh JC: *Adult development and aging,* ed 2, Pacific Grove, Calif, 1993, Brooks/Cole.

Chess S, Thomas A: *Temperament in clinical practice,* New York, 1986, Guilford Press.

Crain W: *Theories of development: concepts and applications,* ed 3, Englewood Cliffs, NJ, 1992, Prentice Hall.

Edelman C, Mandle C: *Health promotion throughout the lifespan,* St. Louis, 2002, Mosby.

Erikson E: *Childhood and society,* New York, 1963, Norton.

Erikson E: *The lifecycle completed,* New York, 1997, Norton.

Gesell A: *Studies in child development,* New York, 1948, Harper.

Gilligan C: *In a different voice: psychological theory and women's development,* Cambridge, Mass, 1982, Harvard University Press.

Hockenberry MJ and others: *Wong's nursing care of infants and children,* ed 7, St. Louis, 2003, Mosby.

Kail R: Development change in proactive interference, *Child Dev* 73(5):1392, 2002.

Kohlberg L. *The philosophy of moral development: moral stages and the idea of justice,* San Francisco, 1981, Harper & Row.

Maier HW: *Three theories of child development,* New York, 1965, Harper & Row.

Schroeder BA: *Human growth and development,* St. Paul, Minn, 1992, West Publishing.

Singer DG, Revenson TA: *A Piaget primer: how a child thinks,* New York, 1996, Penguin Books.

Taffell R: Values you teach your child by age five, *Parents,* p 118, December 2002.

Research References

Chess S, Thomas A: Individuality: dynamics of individual behavioral development. In Levine MD and others, editors: *Developmental-behavioral pediatrics,* Philadelphia, 1983, WB Saunders.

Gould RL: The phases of adult life: a study in developmental psychology, *Am J Psychiatry* 129:5, November 1972.

Thomas RM: Moral development theories: secular and religious—a comparative study, Westport, Conn, 1997, Greenwood Press.

Ugarriza DN: Elderly women's explanation of depression, *J Gerontol Nurs* 28(5):22,2002.

Conception Through Adolescence

Media Resources

http://evolve.elsevier.com/Potter/
fundamentals/

CD COMPANION

- Review Questions
- Glossary

evolve WEBSITE

- Review Questions
- Student Learning Activities
- Glossary

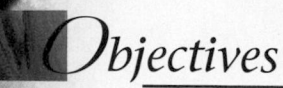

Objectives

Mastery of content in this chapter will enable the student to:

- Define the key terms listed.
- Discuss physiological and psychosocial health concerns during the transition of the child from intrauterine to extrauterine life.
- Describe characteristics of physical growth of the unborn child and from birth to adolescence.
- Describe cognitive and psychosocial development from birth to adolescence.
- Describe the interactions that occur between parent and child.
- Describe variables influencing how children learn about and perceive their health status.
- Explain the role of play in the development of the child.
- Identify factors that contribute to self-esteem in youth.
- Describe the influence of the school environment on the development of the child.
- Plan culturally appropriate health promotion activities for children of all backgrounds.
- Discuss ways in which the nurse can help parents meet their children's developmental needs.

Stages of Growth and Development

*H*uman growth and development are continuous and intricate, complex processes that are often divided into stages organized by age-groups, such as from conception to adolescence. Although this chronological division is arbitrary, it is based on the timing and sequence of developmental tasks that the child must accomplish to progress to another stage (Box 11-1). Major factors affecting growth and development can be found in Chapter 10. This chapter focuses on the various physical, psychosocial, and cognitive changes, as well as the health risks and concerns, during the different stages of growth and development.

Selecting a Developmental Framework for Nursing

Providing developmentally appropriate nursing care is easier when planning is based on a theoretical framework (see Chapter 10). An organized, systematic approach ensures that the child's needs are assessed and met by the plan of care. If nursing care is delivered only as a series of isolated actions, some of the child's developmental needs may be overlooked. A developmental approach encourages organized care directed at the child's current level of functioning to

---

Box 11-1   Developmental Age Periods

Prenatal Period: Conception to Birth

Germinal: Conception to approximately 2 weeks
Embryonic: 2 to 8 weeks
Fetal: 8 to 40 weeks (birth)

A rapid growth rate and total dependency make this one of the most crucial periods in the developmental process. The relationship between maternal health and certain manifestations in the newborn emphasizes the importance of adequate prenatal care to the health and well-being of the infant.

Infancy Period: Birth to 12 or 18 Months

Neonatal: Birth to 28 days
Infancy: 1 to approximately 12 months

The infancy period is one of rapid motor, cognitive, and social development. Through mutuality with the caregiver (parent), the infant establishes a basic trust in the world and the foundation for future interpersonal relationships. The critical first month of life, although part of the infancy period, is often differentiated from the remainder because of the major physical adjustments to extrauterine existence and the psychologic adjustment of the parent.

Early Childhood: 1 to 6 Years

Toddler: 1 to 3 years
Preschool: 3 to 6 years

This period, which extends from the time the children attain upright locomotion until they enter school, is characterized by intense activity and discovery. It is a time of marked physical and personality development. Motor development advances steadily. Children at this age acquire language and wider social relationships, learn role standards, gain self-control and mastery, develop increasing awareness of dependence and independence, and begin to develop a self-concept.

Middle Childhood: 6 to 11 or 12 Years

Frequently referred to as the school age, this period of development is one in which the child is directed away from the family group and is centered around the wider world of peer relationships. There is steady advancement in physical, mental, and social development with emphasis on developing skill competencies. Social cooperation and early moral development take on more importance with relevance for later life stages. This is a critical period in the development of a self-concept.

Later Childhood: 11 to 19 Years

Prepubertal: 10 to 13 years
Adolescence: 13 to approximately 18 years

The period of rapid maturation and change known as adolescence is considered to be a transitional period that begins at the onset of puberty and extends to the point of entry into the adult world—usually high school graduation. Biologic and personality maturation are accompanied by physical and emotional turmoil, and there is redefining of the self-concept. In the late adolescent period the child begins to internalize all previously learned values and to focus on an individual, rather than a group, identity.

From Hockenberry MJ and others: *Wong's nursing care of infants and children,* ed 7, St. Louis, 2003, Mosby.

---

motivate self-direction and health promotion. For example, nurses might encourage toddlers to feed themselves to advance their developing independence and thus promote their sense of autonomy. Or understanding an adolescent's need to be independent should prompt the nurse to establish a contract about the care plan and its implementation.

Conception

From the moment of conception, human development proceeds at a predictive and rapid rate. During gestation or the prenatal period, the embryo grows from a single cell to a complex, physiological being. All major organ systems develop in utero, with some functioning before birth. The psychosocial being also begins to emerge during gestation.

Intrauterine Life

Intrauterine life that reaches full term lasts 10 lunar or 9 calendar months, 40 weeks, or 280 days. The length of pregnancy is computed using **Nagele's rule,** which counts back 3 months from the first day of the last menstrual period (LMP) and then adds 7 days. **Fertilization** occurs when one sperm penetrates the ovum. Fertilization of the ovum takes place in the outer one third of the fallopian tube and occurs within 24 hours of the ovum's release. Once fertilization takes place, the material from both cell nuclei unites. The newly formed organism, known as a **zygote,** has its full genetic complement (one pair of sex chromosomes and 22 pairs of autosomal chromosomes). The ovum and the sperm each contribute one chromosome to each pair. It is through this mechanism that genetically programmed diseases (such as Down syndrome) and genetically determined characteristics (such as eye color) are transmitted from parent to child.

The zygote moves through the fallopian tube to the uterus within 3 to 4 days. During this time the zygote continues to divide. Within 3 days a solid ball of cells, the **morula,** has formed. The morula continues to develop and forms a central cavity, or **blastocyst.** Even at this early stage of development, cells begin to differentiate in structure and function. Cells at one end of the blastocyst develop into the **embryo,** and those at the opposite end will begin to form the **placenta.** Between days 6 and 10, enzymes are secreted that allow the blastocyst to burrow into the endometrium and become completely covered. This portion of the process is known as **implantation.** Chorionic villi, fingerlike projections, develop to obtain oxygen and nutrition from the maternal blood supply and dispose of carbon dioxide and waste products.

The placenta produces essential hormones that help maintain the pregnancy. Because the placenta is extremely porous, noxious materials such as viruses and drugs can also pass from mother to child. The effect of noxious agents on the unborn child depends on the developmental stage in which exposure takes place, with the embryonic stage being the most crucial. The embryonic stage covers from 2 to 8 weeks after conception. This is a crucial stage in the development of organ systems and the main external features. The period of gestation is divided equally into three periods called trimesters.

First Trimester

Physical Changes. During the first trimester, the first 3 calendar months, the uterus continues to be a pelvic organ. After implantation, fetal cells continue to differentiate and develop into essential organ systems. These processes of cellular change (differentiation) and staged organ change (development) occur at different rates and times, and each organ is extremely vulnerable to conditions in the environment. Interference with growth can cause the congenital absence of an organ system or extensive structural or functional alterations. Because several organ systems develop at the same time, disruption of one system often occurs with disruption of others. Toward the end of the first trimester, it is possible to detect fetal heart tones (FHTs) by fetoscope or ultrasound.

Health Promotion. Three risk factors have been cited as having a possible effect on prenatal development: nutrition, stress, and mother's age (Kail, 2001). The diet of a woman both before and during pregnancy has a significant effect on the development of the unborn. It has been repeatedly demonstrated that mothers who eat well have fewer complications of pregnancy and childbirth and bear healthier babies than those with inferior nutritional intake (Hilton, 2002; Kail, 2001). An adequate folic acid intake is encouraged for any woman before and during pregnancy (Box 11-2). Folic acid intake is believed to be responsible for decreasing the incidence of neural tube defects (Hilton, 2002). An average weight gain during pregnancy is between 25 and 30 pounds. Some women experience morning sickness, or transient nausea usually in the morning. By eating dry crackers upon awakening, not drinking fluids with meals, and avoiding greasy fried foods, one can prevent morning sickness. Excessive nausea and vomiting is not normal and should be reported to the physician.

Many woman today are overly concerned about their weight and dieting. As a result, many have diets that are inadequate in nutrients with many skipping meals. The age of the pregnant woman may or may not play a role in the health of the unborn and the overall pregnancy. Studies have indicated that often pregnant adolescents seek out less prenatal care than women in their 20s and 30s do. Older women may be at risk for chromosomal defects but show no other prenatal difficulties (Berk, 2003).

Agents capable of producing functional or structural damage to the developing fetus are called **teratogens.** The nurse educates the mother about avoiding exposure to teratogenic agents. One such teratogen is the rubella or German measles virus, which can cause spontaneous

---

Client Teaching Box 11-2

Folic Acid for Women Contemplating Pregnancy

Objective

- Client will consume 0.4 mg of folic acid (vitamin B_9) every day.

Teaching Strategies

- Educate females of childbearing age about the benefits of folic acid to a developing fetus.
- Discuss the need for women to have an adequate daily intake of folic acid because the moment of conception is not always known. Folic acid is a water-soluble vitamin and is readily excreted in the urine.
- Encourage consumption of 0.4 mg of folic acid daily. This amount may be consumed in food sources; however, adolescents are usually deficient. Deficiency is not related to socioeconomic status.
- Discuss foods rich in folic acid, such as green leafy vegetables, liver, kidney, and asparagus. More limited amounts may be found in milk, poultry, and eggs.
- Assist clients in developing menus with folic acid–rich foods.
- Encourage clients to take a daily multivitamin to supplement dietary intake.

Evaluation

- Have client identify dietary sources of folic acid.
- Review client's 3-day diet intake diary.

---

abortion, stillbirth, or birth defects of the eyes, ears, and heart, primarily when exposure is in the first trimester.

Many drugs are teratogenic during rapid organ growth (**organogenesis**) in the first trimester. Past and present use of home remedies, herbs, and prescription, over-the-counter, and illegal drugs must be carefully assessed. Barbiturates, anticoagulants, antimicrobials, alcohol, cancer chemotherapeutics, and anticonvulsants are only a few of the chemical agents associated with fetal abnormalities, and many other agents are still under investigation. Benefits of any drug needed to maintain the mother's health must be weighed against potential harm to the fetus. Abuse of drugs such as cocaine and LSD may result in preterm labor and chromosomal breakage, respectively. Smoking has been shown to reduce birth weight and increase the incidence of fetal and neonatal death (Kail, 2001; Pletsch and Morgan, 2002). Infants exposed prenatally to alcohol can develop fetal alcohol syndrome (FAS), fetal alcohol effect (FAE), or an alcohol-related birth defect (ARBD) (Kail, 2001). Although the effect on the fetus of maternal caffeine use is controversial, the safest policy is to avoid caffeine. With this knowledge, the nurse can explore lifestyle changes that can help a pregnant woman protect the health of her **fetus.**

Second Trimester

Physical Changes. During the second trimester, the end of month 3 through month 6, the uterus becomes an abdominal organ. Measurement of the height of the uterus above the symphysis pubis is one indicator of fetal growth. The height of the uterus can also indicate approximate gestational age and high-risk situations. Between 16 and 20 weeks, the mother begins to feel fetal movement. This feeling of life is referred to as **quickening.**

Some organ systems continue basic development while the functional capabilities of others are refined. By the end of the sixth month, most organ systems are complete and can function. The fetus is therefore considered viable, or capable of life outside the uterus, if given intensive environmental support. Fingers and toes are differentiated, rudimentary kidneys function, and the sex of the fetus can be determined. The fetus is covered with **vernix caseosa,** a cheeselike substance coating the skin. **Lanugo,** or fine hair, covers most of the body. These substances protect the thin, fragile skin and decrease in amount as the pregnancy nears its completion; thus infants born before 38 weeks' gestation have more of these protective coverings than full-term infants.

Health Promotion. In the second trimester the fetal heartbeat becomes audible to stethoscope auscultation, and the mother becomes aware of fetal movement. Both events are highly significant to the parents because they provide tangible evidence of the pregnancy and reassure them that the fetus is alive. Therefore the nurse should focus on these events during prenatal care.

Changes in maternal behavior during this period include planning for the birth, concern for personal safety, and preoccupation with health and appearance. The nurse can help the woman adapt to these changes and plan for the impending birth. This is often a good time for education about gestational events and appropriate maternal rest, nutrition, dental care, physical activity, posture, employment, and infant feeding options.

Due to dramatic changes occurring in the renal system, it is possible for a mother to have an asymptomatic urinary tract infection. Urinary tract infections greatly increase the risk of preterm labor. Proper voiding habits should be discussed with the mother during this time.

The mother should be educated to recognize potential complications and preterm labor, as well as the appropriate actions to take with each. With advances in modern technology, it is possible for 500-g babies of 24 to 26 weeks' gestation to survive; however, there may be significant risk of morbidity. **Prematurity** is identified as any infant between 20 and 37 weeks' gestation. Causes for prematurity are poorly understood and may be the result of maternal, fetal, or placental problems. Maternal risk factors include physiological stresses such as renal and cardiovascular disease, diabetes mellitus, or uterine and cervical abnormalities. Research has also demonstrated an increased risk among mothers living in poverty, smokers, and mothers receiving poor prenatal care (Berk, 2003). Multiple pregnancies and fetal infections are two of the potential fetal factors for prematurity. Placental factors include abruptio placentae and placenta previa. Several measures are instituted to stop labor when labor occurs before 37 weeks. Interventions can include medications, intravenous (IV) fluids, and bed rest. The primary goal is to allow for further fetal development by prolonging the onset of labor until closer to term.

Third Trimester

Physical Changes. During the last 3 months of intrauterine life the fetus grows to approximately 50 cm (19 to 20 inches) in length. Subcutaneous fat is stored, and weight increases to between 3.2 and 3.4 kg (7 to 7½ pounds). The skin thickens, lanugo begins to disappear, and the fetal body becomes rounder and fuller.

A tremendous spurt in brain growth begins during this trimester and lasts well into the first few years of life. The central nervous system has established its total number of neurons and connections between neurons, and myelination of nerve fibers progresses at a rapid rate.

At the end of the third trimester the normal fetus is physically able to make the transition from intrauterine to extrauterine life. The cardiac system can change its circulation to end bypassing of the lungs. The lungs are capable of maintaining the inflated state for gas exchange. The primitive temperature maintenance systems, reflexes, and sensory organs are ready for use.

Health Promotion. Thoughts of delivering a healthy infant are foremost in the mother's mind as she focuses on preparing her mind and body for the delivery. Parents often seek information regarding the childbirth process and breast-feeding.

Birth-setting choices should also be discussed at this time. Hospitals have been the more traditional setting for childbirth for the past 60 years. Many hospitals have taken a family-centered approach to childbirth. The majority of births in this country take place in the hospital because it is homelike and emergency backup is available in case of difficulties.

In some areas of the country, freestanding birthing centers are available for those who do not prefer the hospital setting. Women delivering in this setting are required to attend childbirth and parenting classes, and the pregnancy must be considered low risk. Physicians and midwives with hospital privileges may attend births in this facility. Mothers must understand that there is always a possibility of transfer to a hospital if the conditions warrant.

A small percentage of mothers choose to deliver at home. Home birth has been popular in Sweden and the Netherlands but has a limited following in this country. Control over the birth process seems to be the most attractive factor for mothers who do not believe they will have choices in a hospital setting. Another advantage is that the entire family or other persons close to the family can be part of the event. Providing support and reassurance about the pregnancy's progression and the decisions that need to be made are appropriate nursing actions at this stage.

Nurses can make a significant difference in supporting the functions of young families. Following an assessment of the couple's strengths and weaknesses, nurses can direct parents to available services to enhance their coping skills (Knauth, 2001).

Cognitive Changes. Relationships between prenatal events and cognitive development are difficult to establish. However, periods of diminished oxygen (anoxia) during fetal life are known to cause deficits in later cognitive functioning, and inadequate prenatal nutrition has been associated with lower brain weight (Behrman, Kliegman, and Jenson, 2000). The large volume of research on developmental outcomes in low-birth-weight (LBW) and very low-birth-weight (VLBW) infants indicates these infants have an increased risk for learning disorders, school failures, **temperament** problems, neurological and motor impairment, and developmental delays. The implication of this research is that families of LBW infants must be assessed for need of nursing interventions that may facilitate a supportive home environment for optimal cognitive outcomes.

Psychosocial Changes. Little information is available about the relationship between prenatal factors and the child's psychosocial development. Some authorities believe that nutritional deficiencies of the fetus can significantly influence later psychosocial development.

Transition From Intrauterine to Extrauterine Life

The transition from intrauterine to extrauterine life requires rapid changes in the newborn. The nurse assesses the newborn's ability to make these changes and plans for appropriate nursing interventions (Askin, 2002). Circulatory, pulmonary, and thermal changes all contribute to the infant's adaptation to neonatal life. Gestational age and development, exposure to depressant drugs before or during labor, and the newborn's own behavioral style also influence the adjustment to the external environment. Therefore initial assessment encompasses a variety of physical and psychosocial elements. The nurse also provides opportunities for the parents and child to develop close emotional bonds.

Physical Changes

An immediate assessment of the newborn's condition is performed to determine the physiological functioning of the major organ systems. The most extreme physiological change occurs when the newborn leaves the in utero circulation and develops independent respiratory functioning. Nursing care is directed at maintaining an open airway, stabilizing and maintaining body temperature, and protecting the newborn from infection. The most widely used assessment tool is the **Apgar score.** Heart rate, respiratory effort, muscle tone, reflex irritability, and color are rated to determine overall status. The Apgar assessment is generally conducted at 1 and 5 minutes after birth and may be repeated until the newborn's condition stabilizes. Table 11-1 outlines the scoring criteria of physiological functioning. A total score of 0 to 3 signifies severe distress, a score of 4 to 6 represents moderate difficulty, and a score of 7 to 10 indicates little difficulty in adjusting to extrauterine life. The nurse can use the Apgar score to determine areas requiring further assessment and careful observation. In addition, the nurse monitors the newborn's body temperature and other vital signs until they stabilize.

Psychosocial Changes

After immediate physical evaluation and application of identification bracelets, the nurse promotes the parents and newborn's need for close physical contact. Early parent-child interaction encourages parent-child attachment. Physical factors (e.g., fatigue, hunger, and health) and emotional factors (e.g., happiness and needs for affection and touch) are assessed.

Merely placing the family together does not promote closeness. The parents and newborn must be capable and desirous of exploring and responding to each other. Most healthy newborns are awake and alert for the first half-hour after birth. This is a good time for parent-child interaction to begin. Close body contact, often including breast-feeding, is a satisfying way for most families to start. If immediate contact is not possible, the nurse incorporates it into the care plan as early as possible, which may mean bringing the newborn to an ill parent or bringing the parents to an ill or premature child.

Bonding occurs when parents and newborn elicit reciprocal and complementary behavior. Parental bonding behaviors include attentiveness and physical contact. Newborn bonding behavior involves maintenance of contact with the parent. Preterm, ill newborns and ill mothers have more difficulty forming this bond if separation is prolonged. The bonding process is further complicated if parents are unable to care for the usual infant needs. The nurse should give the parents support throughout the early attachment process, particularly if the newborn or mother is ill or if the newborn is separated from the parents.

Table 11-1	**Apgar Scoring**		
Sign	**Score 0**	**Score 1**	**Score 2**
Heart rate	Absent	Slow (below 100)	Over 100
Respiratory effort	Absent	Slow, irregular, hypoventilation	Good, crying lustily
Muscle tone	Flaccid	Some flexion of extremities	Active motion, well flexed
Reflex irritability	No response	Crying, some motion	Vigorous cry
Color	Blue, pale	Pink body, blue hands and feet	Completely pink

Modified from Hockenberry MJ and others: *Wong's nursing care of infants and children,* ed 7, St. Louis, 2003, Mosby.

Health Risks

The removal of nasopharyngeal and oropharyngeal secretions with suction or a bulb syringe ensures airway patency. Newborns are susceptible to heat loss and cold stress (Askin, 2002). Because hypothermia increases oxygen needs, the newborn's body temperature must be stabilized and maintained. The newborn may be placed directly on the mother's abdomen and covered in warm blankets; be dried and wrapped in warm blankets, being sure to keep the head well covered; or placed unclothed in an infant warmer with a temperature probe in place. For newborns unable to sustain adequate body temperature, isolettes and incubators, which supply radiant heat, are preferred. Box 11-3 outlines measures to prevent cold stress.

Prevention of infection is a major concern in the care of the newborn, whose immune system is immature. Good hand-washing technique is the most important factor in protecting the newborn and nurse from infection. Cover gowns do not need to be worn while providing care for the healthy newborn once the blood and amniotic fluid have been removed from the infant's skin (Hockenberry and others, 2003). Other precautions include wearing gloves when touching mucous membranes or nonintact skin such as in a new wound (i.e., fresh circumcision) and when drawing blood (e.g., heel stick) (Garner, 1996).

The most commonly used prophylactic treatment against ophthalmic conjunctivitis is erythromycin (0.5%) because it prevents *Neisseria gonorrhoeae* and other infections, which can be transmitted during passage through an infected vaginal canal. Application should occur during the newborn's initial assessment.

Vitamin K is administered as a single intramuscular injection shortly after birth. Vitamin K is important for the synthesis of prothrombin necessary for clotting. Normally vitamin K is synthesized by the intestinal flora. On about the third day the infant will begin to have enough intestinal flora to start to synthesize its vitamin K.

The stump of the moist umbilical cord is an excellent medium for bacterial growth. The cord should be cleansed by application of 70% alcohol at each diaper change. Until the cord dries and falls off, the diaper should be folded below the umbilicus to prevent accumulation of moisture.

Box *11-3*	Measures to Prevent Cold Stress
Mechanism of Heat Loss	**Nursing Intervention**
Evaporation	Immediately dry newborn after delivery. Wrap in blanket. Delay first bath until temperature and other vital signs are stable.
Conduction	Warm objects that have direct contact with newborn. Cover newborn's head.
Convection	Prevent unnecessary exposure to cold.
Radiation	Use radiant warmer until temperature stabilizes. Avoid cold drafts.

Newborn

The **neonatal period** is the first month of life. During this stage the newborn's physical functioning is mostly reflexive, and stabilization of major organ systems is the body's primary task. Behavior greatly influences interaction between the newborn and the environment and caregivers. For example, the average 2-week-old smiles spontaneously and is able to regard the mother's face. The impact of these reflexive behaviors is generally a surge of maternal feelings of love that prompt the mother to cuddle the baby.

Nurses can apply their knowledge of this stage of growth and development to promote newborn and parental health. If the nurse understands, for example, that the newborn's cry is generally a reflexive response to an unmet need (such as hunger), parents can be assisted in identifying ways to meet those needs, such as counseling the parents to feed their baby on demand rather than on a rigid schedule.

Physical Changes

A comprehensive nursing assessment is performed as soon as the newborn's physiological functioning is stable, generally within a few hours after birth. At this time the nurse measures height, weight, head circumference, temperature, pulse, and respirations and observes general appearance, body functions, sensory capabilities, reflexes, and responsiveness.

The average newborn weighs 3400 g (7 pounds, 8 ounces), is 50 cm (20 inches) in length, and has a head circumference of 35 cm (14 inches). Up to 10% of birth weight is lost in the first few days of life, primarily through fluid losses by respiration, urination, defecation, and low fluid intake. Birth weight is usually regained by the second week of life, and a gradual pattern of increase in weight, height, and head circumference is evident. During the first month, these increases average 4 to 8 ounces in weight per week, 0.6 to 2.5 cm (¼ to 1 inch) in length, and 2 cm in head circumference.

The newborn's heart rate ranges from 120 to 160 beats per minute. The average blood pressure is 74/46 mm Hg. The newborn's respiratory movements are primarily abdominal and vary in rate and rhythm, with an average rate of 30 to 50 breaths per minute. The axillary temperature ranges from 36° to 37.5° C (96.8° to 99.5° F) and generally stabilizes within 24 hours after birth.

Normal physical characteristics include the continued presence of lanugo on the skin of the back; cyanosis of the hands and feet for the first 24 hours; and a soft, protuberant abdomen. Skin color varies according to racial and genetic heritage and gradually changes during infancy. **Molding,** or overlapping of the soft skull bones, allows the fetal head to adjust to various diameters of the maternal pelvis and is a common occurrence with vaginal births. The bones readjust within a few days, producing a rounded appearance. The sutures and **fontanels** are usually palpable at birth. The diamond shape of the anterior fontanel and the triangular shape of the posterior fontanel between the unfused bones of the skull are shown in Figure 11-1.

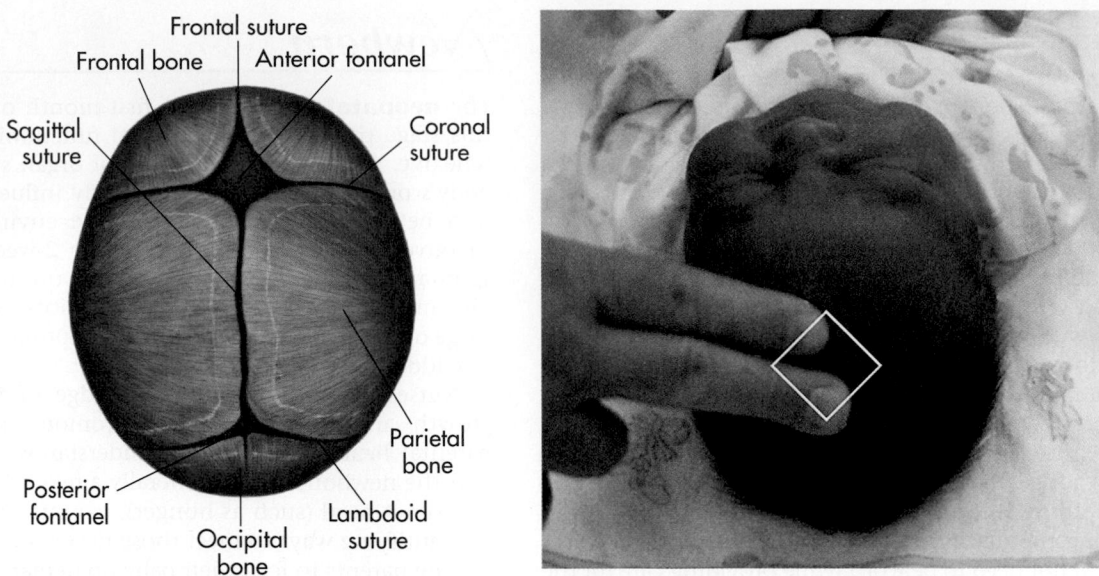

FIGURE **11–1**   Fontanels and suture lines. (From Hockenberry MJ and others: *Wong's nursing care of infants and children,* ed 7, St. Louis, 2003, Mosby.)

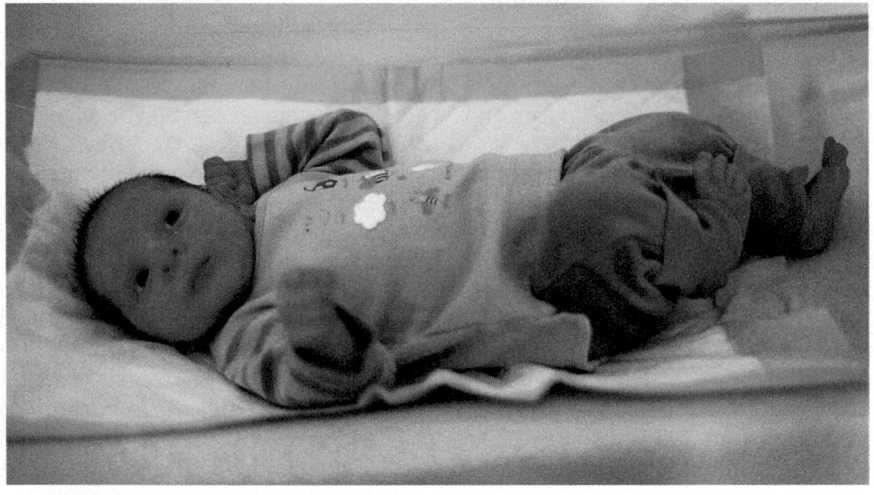

FIGURE **11–2**   Tonic neck reflex. Newborns assume this position while supine. (Courtesy Elaine Polan, RNC, BSN, MS.)

Neurological function is assessed by observing the newborn's level of activity, alertness, irritability, responsiveness to stimuli, and the presence and strength of reflexes. Normal reflexes include blinking in response to bright lights, startling in response to sudden, loud noises, and sucking, rooting, grasping, yawning, coughing, sneezing, and hiccoughing. An absence of any of these or other reflexes indicates prematurity, possible trauma, or central nervous system complications. Assessment of these reflexes is vital because the newborn depends largely on reflexes for survival and in response to its en-

vironment. Figure 11-2 shows the tonic neck reflex in the newborn.

Normal behavioral characteristics of the newborn include periods of sucking, crying, sleeping, and activity. Movements are generally sporadic, but they are symmetrical and involve all four extremities. The relatively flexed fetal position of intrauterine life continues as the newborn attempts to maintain an enclosed, secure feeling. Newborns normally watch the caregiver's face, reflexively smile, and respond to sensory stimuli, particularly the primary caregiver's face, voice, and touch.

The first hour of the newborn's life is spent in a primarily quiet alert state with wide-open eyes and vigorous sucking activity. Then infants sleep almost continuously for the next 2 to 3 days to recover from the exhausting birth process. Thereafter sleep periods vary from 20 minutes to 6 hours with little day-night differentiation. Infant behavior is characterized by five distinct states that are highly influenced by environmental stimuli. It is important for parents to understand these states and their implications for parental interaction.

In accordance with the recommendations of the American Academy of Pediatrics (AAP) infants who are put down for sleep should be positioned on their side or back to decrease the risk of sudden infant death syndrome (SIDS) (Behrman, Kliegman, and Jenson, 2000). Co-sleeping or bed sharing has also been reported to be possibly associated with an increased risk for SIDS (Behrman, Kliegman, and Jenson, 2000). Safeguards include proper positioning; removing stuffed animals, soft bedding, and pillows; and avoiding overheating of the infant. Smoking should be avoided during pregnancy and around the infant as it may place the infant at greater risk for SIDS (U.S. Department of Health and Human Services [USDHHS], 2000). Premature birth and intrauterine growth restriction have been linked to maternal smoking. Neonates and young children who are exposed to secondhand smoke are at further risk for developing respiratory conditions such as asthma or dying from sudden infant death syndrome (Pletsch and Morgan, 2002). *Healthy People 2010* targeted a 30% reduction of smoking for all pregnant women. In 1991 only 12% of pregnant women quit smoking during their first trimester (USDHHS, 2000). Creating smoke-free educational programs for pregnant women and their families continues to be a challenge for all health providers.

Cognitive Changes

Early cognitive development begins with innate behavior, reflexes, and sensory functions. Newborns initiate reflex activities, learn behaviors, and learn their desires. For example, newborns learn to turn to the nipple and learn that crying results in parent response of feeding, diapering, and cuddling.

Sensory functions contribute to cognitive development in the newborn. At birth, children can focus on objects about 8 to 10 inches from their faces and can perceive forms. A preference for the human face is apparent. Auditory and vestibular systems function from birth. These sensory capabilities allow newborns to elicit stimuli rather than simply receive them. Parents should be taught the importance of providing sensory stimulation, such as talking to their babies and holding them to see their faces. This allows infants to seek or take in stimuli, thereby enhancing learning and promoting cognitive development.

It is debatable whether infant crying is the precursor of refined language. However, crying elicits a response, and caregivers discriminate cry patterns. Crying therefore has significance to newborns and parents. For newborns, crying is a means of communication to provide cues to parents. Some babies cry because their diapers are wet or

they are hungry or want to be held. Others cry just to make noise or because they need a change in position or activity. Their crying may frustrate the parents if they cannot see an apparent cause. With the nurse's help, parents can learn to recognize infants' cry patterns and take appropriate action when necessary.

Psychosocial Changes

During the first month of life, parents and newborns normally develop a strong bond that grows into a deep attachment. Interactions during routine care enhance or detract from the attachment process. Feeding, hygiene, and comfort measures consume much of infants' waking time. These interactive experiences provide a foundation for the formation of deep attachments. Early on, older siblings should have opportunity to be involved in the newborn's care. Family involvement helps support growth and development and promotes nurturing (Figure 11-3).

If parents or children experience health complications after birth, attachment and bonding may be compromised. Infants' behavioral cues may be weak or absent, and caregiving may be less mutually satisfying. Tired, ill parents have difficulty interpreting and responding to their infants. Children who have congenital anomalies are often too weak to be responsive to parental cues and require special supportive nursing care. For example, infants born with heart defects may tire easily during feedings. They may rest frequently after several bursts of sucking and fall asleep after taking 1 to 1½ ounces of milk. Infants may awaken after 1½ hours, crying because they are hungry again. Mothers, not understanding that the crying is a physiologically dictated sequence of events, may think that the infants are being fussy or that they are inadequate. Both infants and mothers derive decreasing pleasure from feeding experiences. In this case, however, bonding is not enhanced and may even be reduced unless nursing intervention breaks the sequence of events.

Health Risks

Hyperbilirubinemia refers to an excessive amount of accumulated bilirubin in the blood and is characterized by a yellow coloring of the skin, or jaundice. The accumulation occurs when the infant's body is unable to balance the destruction of red blood cells (RBCs) and the use or excretion of by-products. The balance can be upset by prematurity, breast-feeding, excess production of bilirubin, certain disease states, or a disturbance in the liver. Bilirubin at high levels is highly toxic to neurons and places newborns at risk for brain damage. Phototherapy is used to help break down the bilirubin for easier excretion. Special care must be given to properly shielding the infant's eyes to protect exposure to the light. Because excretion of the extra bilirubin can cause watery stools, adequate fluid balance in the infant must be maintained.

Health Concerns

Screening. The nurse coordinates screening tests and other laboratory tests as indicated by the newborn's state of health. Blood tests can be used to determine **inborn**

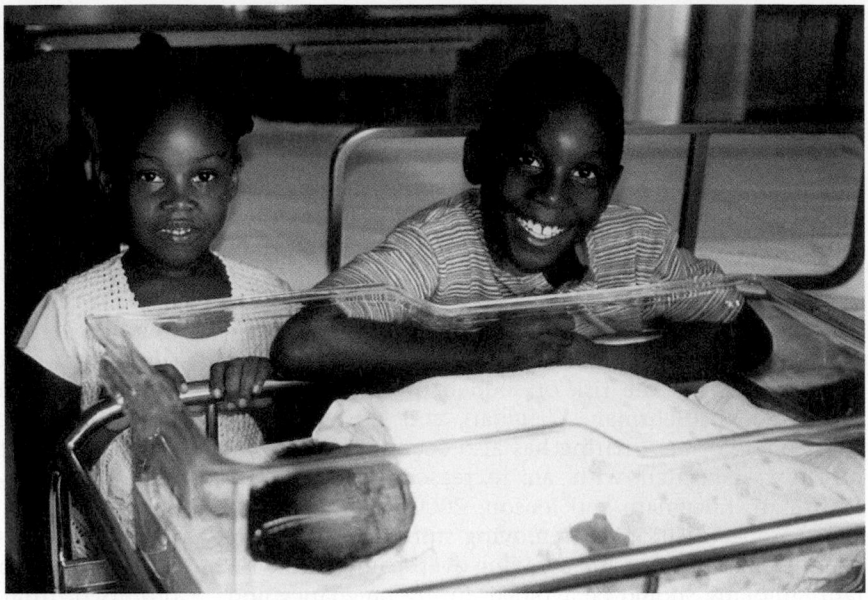

FIGURE **11–3** Siblings should be involved in newborn care. (Courtesy Elaine Polan, RNC, BSN, MS.)

errors of metabolism (IEMs). This term applies to genetic disorders caused by the absence or deficiency of a substance, usually an enzyme, essential to cellular metabolism that results in abnormal protein, carbohydrate, or fat metabolism. Although IEMs are rare, they account for a significant proportion of health problems in children. Neonatal screening can detect phenylketonuria (PKU), hypothyroidism, and galactosemia and thus allow appropriate treatment that can prevent permanent mental retardation and other health problems. This testing is mandatory in most of the United States.

Circumcision. Circumcision is a common and controversial procedure in this country. The controversy surrounds the risks and benefits, especially with respect to pain control. Risks have been identified as hemorrhage, infection, adhesions, and meatal stenosis. Benefits include prevention of penile cancer and urinary tract infections, and preservation of male body image to be consistent with peers (Hockenberry and others, 2003). Parents should give informed consent before the procedure. Because of the newborn's unstable physiological state during the first day, circumcision is not recommended to take place during this time. Care of the site depends on the type of method used for the procedure. The newborn should be checked frequently for evidence of swelling or oozing and the ability to void.

Infant

Infancy, the period from 1 month to 1 year of age, is characterized by rapid physical growth and change. This is the only period marked by such dramatic physical changes and marked development. Psychosocial development advances, aided by the progression from reflexive to more purposeful behavior. Interaction between infants and the environment is greater and more meaningful. Infants who giggle and roll over in response to tickling

are interacting more with their social environments and are displaying a greater response than when they merely smile in response to a hug. During this first year of life the nurse can easily observe the adaptive potential of infants because qualitative and quantitative changes in growth and development occur so rapidly.

Physical Changes

Steady and proportional growth of the infant is more important than absolute growth values. Charts of normal age- and gender-related growth measurements enable the nurse to compare growth with norms for a child's age. Using growth charts, the nurse can also evaluate an individual infant's growth patterns by recording measurements of weight, length, and head circumference at selected intervals. Measurements recorded over time are the best way to monitor growth and identify problems. An infant with a growth problem may be generally below the expected norms at all intervals or may experience an acute, brief interference with growth. An infant with a feeding problem may be below the expected norm for weight.

Size increases rapidly during the first year of life; birth weight doubles in approximately 5 months and triples by 12 months. An average weight gain is 1½ pounds the first 5 months and ¾ pound for months 7 to 12. Height increases an average of 1 inch during each of the first 6 months and ½ inch the next 6 months. This 50% increase in birth height occurs primarily in the trunk, with the chest diameter approximating that of the head by the first birthday (Hockenberry and others, 2003). The fontanels become smaller; the posterior fontanel closes at about 2 months; the anterior at about 12 to 18 months.

Physiological functioning stabilizes, and by the end of the first year the heart rate is 80 to 150 beats per minute, the blood pressure averages 90/50 mm Hg, and the respiratory rate is 30 to 35 breaths per minute. Patterns of body function also stabilize, as evidenced by predictable sleep, elimination, and feeding routines. Motor development proceeds steadily in a cephalocaudal (from the head

Table 11-2	Milestones in Infant Motor Development			
Month 3	**Month 6**	**Month 9**	**Month 12**	**Month 15**
Gross Motor				
Lifts head 90 degrees when prone Sits with support	Lifts head 90 degrees when prone Good head control in sitting position Crawls on abdomen with arms	Attains sitting position independently Creeps on all four extremities Pulls self to standing position	Walks holding onto walls and furniture (cruising) Stands alone Takes 1 to 2 steps	Walks alone
Fine Motor				
Grasps and briefly holds objects and takes them to mouth	Uses palm grasp with fingers encircling object Transfers cube from hand to hand	Crude thumb-finger pincer grasp Bangs hand-held cubes together	Places tiny object, such as raisin, into container Makes marks with crayon	Scribbles with crayon Builds tower of two cubes

Modified from Frankenburg WK and others: The Denver II: a major revision and restandardization of the Denver Developmental Screening Test, *Pediatrics* 89(1):93, 1992.

toward the feet) direction. Table 11-2 identifies milestones in gross motor and fine motor development.

Cognitive Changes

The infant learns by experiencing and manipulating the environment. Developing motor skills and increasing mobility expand an infant's environment and, with developing visual and auditory skills, enhance cognitive development. For these reasons Piaget (1952) named his first stage of cognitive development, which extends until around the third birthday, the sensorimotor period. The characteristics of each of the three subphases of this period that occur during the first year of life are described in Chapter 10.

Before the acquisition of language the extraordinary development of the mind occurs through the child's developing senses and motor abilities. For example, a 1-month-old can follow the path of a moving object. Improved visual acuity and eye-hand coordination allow grasping and exploration of objects. In addition, rudimentary color vision begins by 2 months and improves throughout the first year, making the environment more interesting to see and explore. The infant's hearing also progresses, allowing localization and discrimination of sounds.

Infants need opportunities to develop and use their senses. Nurses must evaluate the appropriateness and adequacy of these opportunities. For example, ill or hospitalized infants may lack the energy to interact with their environments, thereby slowing their cognitive development. Infants need to be stimulated according to their temperament, energy, and age. The nurse uses stimulation strategies that maximize the development of infants while conserving their energy and orientation. An example of this is the nurse talking to and encouraging an infant to suck on a pacifier while administering the infant's tube feeding.

Language. Speech is an important aspect of cognition that develops during the first year. Infants proceed from crying, cooing, and laughing to imitating sounds, comprehending the meaning of simple commands, and repeating words with knowledge of their meaning. By 1 year, infants not only recognize their own names but also have two- or three-word vocabularies including *Da-Da*, *Ma-Ma*, and *no*. The nurse can promote language development by encouraging mothers to name objects on which their infants' attention is focused.

Psychosocial Changes

Separation. During their first year, infants begin to differentiate themselves from others as separate beings capable of acting on their own. Initially, infants are unaware of the boundaries of self, but through repeated experiences with the environment, they learn where the self ends and the external world begins. As infants determine their physical boundaries, they begin to respond to others. Fathers should get involved in infant care from the onset (Figure 11-4).

Two- and 3-month-old infants begin to smile responsively rather than reflexively. Similarly, they can recognize differences in people when their sensory and cognitive capabilities improve. By 8 months, most infants can differentiate a stranger from a familiar person and respond differently to the two. Close attachment to the primary caregivers, most often parents, is usually established by this age. Infants seek out these persons for support and comfort during times of stress. The ability to distinguish self from others allows infants to interact and socialize more within their environments. By 9 months, for example, infants play simple social games such as patty-cake and peekaboo. More complex interactive games such as hide-and-seek involving objects are possible by age 1. Erikson (1963) describes the psychosocial developmental crisis for the infant as trust versus mistrust. He explains that the quality of parent-infant interactions determines development of trust or mistrust (see Chapter 10).

The nurse assesses the availability and appropriateness of experiences contributing to psychosocial development.

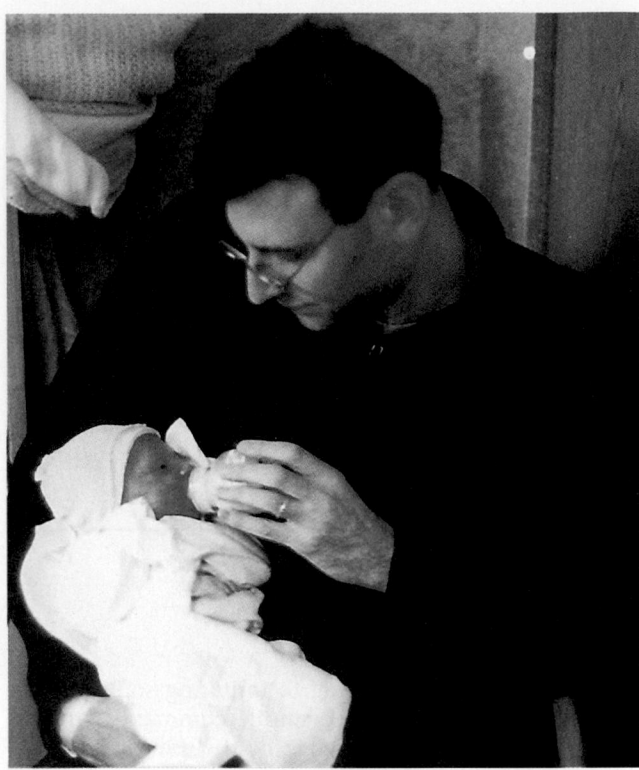

FIGURE **11–4** Smiling at and talking to an infant encourages bonding. (Courtesy Elaine Polan, RNC, BSN, MS.)

Hospitalized infants may have difficulty establishing physical boundaries because of repeated bodily intrusions and painful sensations. Limiting these negative experiences and providing pleasurable sensations are interventions that support early psychosocial development. Extended separations from parents complicate the attachment process and increase the number of caregivers with whom the infant must interact. Ideally, the parents should provide the majority of care during hospitalization. When parents are not present, an attempt should be made to limit the number of caregivers who have contact with the infant and to follow the parents' directions for care. These interventions will foster the infant's continuing development of trust.

Play. Play is a meaningful set of activities through which individuals interact with their environment and relate to others. Play provides opportunities for the infant to develop many motor skills. Much of infant play is exploratory as they use their senses to observe and examine their own bodies and objects of interest in their surroundings. Activities such as the infants' placement of their toes in their mouths provide them with pleasure, information about their own body, and help form their early self-concept. Play becomes manipulative as the child learns control of the hands. Adults can facilitate infant learning by planning activities that promote the development of milestones and by providing toys that are safe for the infant to explore with the mouth and manipulate with the hands, such as rattles, wooden blocks, plas-

tic stacking rings, squeezable stuffed animals, and busy boxes. Infants most frequently engage in solitary (one-sided) play but do enjoy watching others, particularly the antics of their siblings. Infants need to be played with and stimulated through interactions with others. They delight in activities such as peekaboo and patty-cake.

Health Risks

Injury Prevention. Injury is a major cause of death in children 6 to 12 months old. An understanding of the major developmental accomplishments during this time period will allow for injury prevention planning. Box 11-4 lists the main types of injuries occurring in this age-group and possible prevention strategies based on major developmental accomplishments.

Automobile injuries are a leading cause of death in children under 1 year of age. Many of these deaths occur when the child is not properly restrained. All infants must be restrained in a U.S. federally approved car seat restraint. Infant restraints may also convert into a toddler type of restraint (Figure 11-5).

The infant should always be placed in a restraint that is rear facing in the backseat of the vehicle. Placing an infant in a rear-facing restraint in the front seat of a vehicle is extremely dangerous in any vehicle with a passenger-side air bag.

Child Maltreatment. Child maltreatment includes intentional physical abuse or neglect, emotional abuse or neglect, and sexual abuse (Hockenberry and others, 2003). More children suffer from neglect than any other type of maltreatment. Many suffer from more than one type of maltreatment. The Child Protective Services agencies reported that of the 1 million children suffering from maltreatment, half suffered from some type of neglect, one quarter from physical abuse, and 13% from sexual abuse. More than half, 56%, were under the age of 4 years (USDHHS, 2000). All 50 states have a mandatory reporting law for all health professionals to report suspected abuse. No one profile fits a victim of maltreatment. Although signs and symptoms vary, Box 11-5 includes possible findings of child maltreatment.

A combination of signs and symptoms or a pattern of injury should arouse suspicion. It is important for the health care provider to be aware of certain disease processes and cultural practices. Lack of awareness of normal variants such as mongolian spots or cultural practices such as coining will cause the health care provider to arouse undue suspicion of abuse.

Health Concerns

Health Perception. The foundation for children's perceptions of their health status is laid early in life. Internal body sensations and experiences with the outside world affect self-perceptions. The nature of this influence and the value of nursing interventions to alter later perceptions are unknown. It is known, however, that parents tend to label children who are ill in early life as more vulnerable than their siblings and that this labeling may affect the children's perceptions of their own health. In addition, because infants and children depend on others for their health care, their experiences

---

Box 11-4   **Injury Prevention During Infancy**

Age: Birth-4 Months

Major Developmental Accomplishments
Involuntary reflexes, such as the crawling reflex, may propel infant forward or backward, and the startle reflex may cause the body to jerk

May roll over

Increasing eye-hand coordination and voluntary grasp reflex

Injury Prevention
Aspiration
Not as great a danger to this age-group, but should begin practicing safeguarding early (see under Age: 4-7 Months)

Never shake baby powder directly on infant; place powder in hand and then on infant's skin; store container closed and out of infant's reach

Hold infant for feeding; do not prop bottle

Know emergency procedures for choking*

Use pacifier with one-piece construction and loop handle

Suffocation/Drowning
Keep all plastic bags stored out of infant's reach; discard large plastic garment bags after tying in a knot

Do not cover mattress with plastic

Use a firm mattress and loose blankets; no pillows

Make sure crib design follows federal regulations and mattress fits snugly—crib slats 2⅜ in (6 cm) apart

Position crib away from other furniture and away from radiators

Do not tie pacifier on a string around infant's neck

Remove bibs at bedtime

Never leave infant alone in bath

Do not leave infant under 12 months alone on adult or youth mattress

Falls
Always raise crib rails

Never leave infant on a raised, unguarded surface

When in doubt as to where to place child, use the floor

Injury Prevention—cont'd
Falls—cont'd
Restrain child in infant seat and never leave child unattended while the seat is resting on a raised surface

Avoid using a high chair until child can sit well with support

Poisoning
Not as great a danger to this age-group, but should begin practicing safeguards early (see under Age: 4-7 Months)

Burns
Install smoke detectors in home

Use caution when warming formula in microwave oven; always check temperature of liquid before feeding

Check bathwater

Do not pour hot liquids when infant is close by, such as sitting on lap

Beware of cigarette ashes that may fall on infant

Do not leave infant in the sun for more than a few minutes; keep exposed areas covered

Wash flame-retardant clothes according to label directions

Use cool-mist vaporizers

Do not leave child in parked car

Check surface heat of car restraint before placing child in seat

Motor Vehicles
Transport infant in federally approved, rear-facing car seat,* preferably in backseat

Do not place infant on the seat or in lap

Do not place child in a carriage or stroller behind a parked car

Do not place infant or child in front passenger seat with an air bag

Bodily Damage
Avoid sharp, jagged objects

Keep diaper pins closed and away from infant

Age: 4-7 Months

Major Developmental Accomplishments
Rolls over

Sits momentarily

Grasps and manipulates small objects

Resecures a dropped object

Has well-developed eye-hand coordination

Can focus on and locate very small objects

Mouthing is very prominent

Can push up on hands and knees

Crawls backward

Injury Prevention
Aspiration
Keep buttons, beads, syringe caps, and other small objects out of infant's reach

Keep floor free of any small objects

Injury Prevention—cont'd
Aspiration—cont'd
Do not feed infant hard candy, nuts, food with pits or seeds, or whole or circular pieces of hot dog

Exercise caution when giving teething biscuits, because large chunks may be broken off and aspirated

Do not feed infant while child is lying down

Inspect toys for removable parts

Keep baby powder, if used, out of reach

Avoid storing large quantities of cleaning fluid, paints, pesticides, and other toxic substances

Discard used containers of poisonous substances

Do not store toxic substances in food containers

Discard used button-sized batteries; store new batteries in safe area

Know telephone number of local poison control center (usually listed in front of telephone directory)

From Hockenberry MJ and others: *Wong's nursing care of infants and children*, ed 7, St. Louis, 2003, Mosby.

*Information available from U.S. Consumer Product Safety Commission; (800) 638-CPSC.

Continued

Box 11-4   **Injury Prevention During Infancy—cont'd**

Age: 4-7 Month—cont'd

Injury Prevention—cont'd

Suffocation

Keep all latex balloons out of reach

Remove all crib toys that are strung across crib or playpen when child begins to push up on hands or knees or is 5 months old

Falls

Restrain in a high chair

Keep crib rails raised to full height

Poisoning

Make sure that paint for furniture or toys does not contain lead

Place toxic substances on a high shelf or in locked cabinet

Hang plants or place on high surface rather than on floor

Burns

Keep faucets out of reach

Place hot objects (cigarettes, candles, incense) on high surface

Limit exposure to sun; apply sunscreen

Motor Vehicles

See under Age: Birth-4 Months

Bodily Damage

Give toys that are smooth and rounded, preferably made of wood or plastic

Avoid long, pointed objects as toys

Avoid toys that are excessively loud

Keep sharp objects out of infant's reach

Age: 8-12 Months

Major Developmental Accomplishments

Crawls/creeps

Stands, holding onto furniture

Stands alone

Cruises around furniture

Walks

Climbs

Pulls on objects

Throws objects

Is able to pick up small objects; has pincer grasp

Explores by putting objects in mouth

Dislikes being restrained

Explores away from parent

Injury Prevention

Aspiration

Keep lint and small objects off floor, furniture, and out of reach of children

Take care in feeding solid table food to ensure that very small pieces are given

Do not use beanbag toys or allow child to play with dried beans

See also under Age: 4-7 Months

Suffocation/Drowning

Keep doors of ovens, dishwashers, refrigerators, coolers, and front-loading clothes washers and dryers closed at all times

If storing an unused appliance, such as a refrigerator, remove the door

Supervise contact with inflated balloons; immediately discard popped balloons and keep uninflated balloons out of reach

Fence swimming pools

Always supervise when near any source of water, such as cleaning buckets, drainage areas, toilets

Keep bathroom doors closed

Eliminate unnecessary pools of water

Keep one hand on child at all times when in tub

Injury Prevention—cont'd

Falls

Fence stairways at top and bottom if child has access to either end*

Dress infant in safe shoes and clothing (soles that do not "catch" on floor, tied shoelaces, pant legs that do not touch floor)

Avoid walkers, especially near stairs

Ensure that furniture is sturdy enough for child to pull self to standing position and cruise

Poisoning

Administer medications as a drug, not as a candy

Do not administer medications unless so prescribed by a practitioner

Replace medications and poisons immediately after use; replace caps properly if a child-protector cap is used

Burns

Place guards in front of or around any heating appliance, fireplace, or furnace

Keep electrical wires hidden or out of reach

Place plastic guards over electrical outlets; place furniture in front of outlets

Keep hanging tablecloths out of reach (child may pull down hot liquids or heavy or sharp objects)

From Hockenberry MJ and others: *Wong's nursing care of infants and children,* ed 7, St. Louis, 2003, Mosby.
*Information available from U.S. Consumer Product Safety Commission; (800) 638-CPSC.

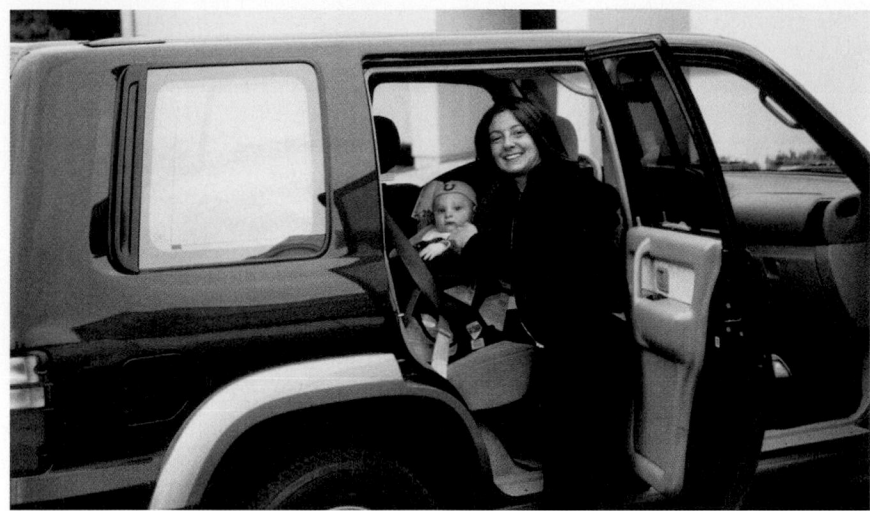

FIGURE **11–5**   Federally approved infant car restraint. Note that the seat is rear facing in the backseat. (Courtesy Elaine Polan, RNC, BSN, MS.)

with caregivers influence their health attitudes and behavior. The nurse has a responsibility to educate parents and other caregivers about health promotion behavior that will positively affect perception of health and self.

Nutrition. The quality and quantity of nutrition influence the infant's growth and development. The nurse helps parents select and provide a nutritionally adequate diet for their infant. The nurse must understand that nutrition is influenced by many variables (e.g., family culture, food preferences, slow eating, or food allergies) and that no diet is effective for all children or for one age-group.

Feeding Alternatives. Supplying essential nutrients to the infant is both the nurse's and parents' goal. The nurse should support the parents' choice of feeding methods and facilitate a successful feeding process (Gill, 2001). Breast-feeding is recommended for infants because breast milk contains the essential nutrients of protein, fats, carbohydrates, and immunoglobulins that bolster the ability to resist infection and it is considered the most complete nutritional source until 6 months of age (Box 11-6). Breast-feeding has been associated with a decreased frequency of gastroenteritis, otitis media, and food allergies (Behrman and others, 2000; USDHHS, 2000; Hockenberry and others, 2003).

However, if breast-feeding is not possible or not desired by the parent, an acceptable alternative is iron-fortified commercially prepared formula. Commercially prepared formulas are popular because they are convenient, contain standard ingredients, and are fortified with vitamins and minerals. All types of cow's milk—skim, 2%, or whole—or imitation milks are not recommended in the first year because of the infant's decreased ability to digest the contained fat. Cow's milk also contains more sodium and protein and less iron (Hockenberry and others, 2003). Because cow's milk is low in iron and high in calcium and phosphorus, absorption of iron may be decreased, causing anemia.

The average 1-month-old infant takes approximately 18 to 21 ounces of breast milk or formula per day. This amount increases slightly during the first 6 months and decreases when solid foods are introduced. The amount of formula per feeding and the number of feedings vary among infants. The addition of solid foods is not recommended before the age of 6 months because the gastrointestinal tract is not sufficiently mature to handle these complex nutrients and infants are exposed to food antigens that may produce food protein allergies. Developmentally, infants are not ready for solid food before 6 months. The extrusion (protrusion) reflex causes food to be pushed out of the mouth. The introduction of cereals, fruits, vegetables, and meats during the second 6 months of life provides iron and additional sources of vitamins. These become especially important when children are taken off breast milk or formula and begun on whole cow's milk after the first birthday. Well-cooked table foods are also tolerated by 1 year. The amount and frequency of feedings vary among infants, so the nurse should discuss differing feeding patterns with parents.

Honey has been used to sweeten water and coat pacifiers. Honey should not be used in infants less than 1 year because of the potential for infant botulism poisoning (Behrman, Kliegman, and Jenson, 2000).

Supplementation. The need for dietary vitamin and mineral supplements depends on the infant's diet. Full-term infants are born with some iron stores. The breast-fed infant absorbs adequate iron from breast milk during the first 4 to 6 months of life. After 6 months, iron-fortified cereal is generally considered an adequate supplemental source. Because iron in formula is less readily absorbed than that in breast milk, formula-fed infants should receive iron-fortified formula throughout the first year.

Adequate concentrations of fluoride to protect against dental caries are not available in human milk, and therefore fluoridated water or supplemental fluoride is generally recommended. The presence of fluoride in formula depends on the type of formula and the source of water used in preparing the concentrated forms. Fluoride supplementation may be necessary.

Box 11-5   Clinical Manifestations of Potential Child Maltreatment

Physical Neglect

Suggestive Physical Findings
Failure to thrive, signs of malnutrition, evidence of poor health care
Poor personal hygiene, especially of teeth, unclean and/or inappropriate dress
Frequent injuries from lack of supervision

Suggestive Behaviors
Dull and inactive
Self-stimulatory behaviors, such as finger-sucking or rocking
Begging or stealing food, vandalism or shoplifting
Absenteeism from school
Drug or alcohol addiction

Emotional Abuse and Neglect

Suggestive Physical Findings
Failure to thrive
Feeding disorders, such as rumination
Enuresis
Sleep disorders

Suggestive Behaviors
Self-stimulatory behaviors such as biting, rocking, sucking
During infancy, lack of social smile and stranger anxiety
Withdrawal, unusual fearfulness
Antisocial behavior, such as destructiveness, stealing, cruelty
Extremes of behavior, such as overcompliant, passive, aggressive, or demanding
Lags in emotional and intellectual development, especially language
Suicide attempts

Physical Abuse

Suggestive Physical Findings
Bruises and welts on face, lips, mouth, back, buttocks, thighs, or areas of torso
Regular patterns descriptive of object used, such as belt buckle, hand, wire hanger, chain, wooden spoon, squeeze or pinch marks
Burns, injuries, fractures, lacerations or bruises in various stages of healing on soles of feet, palms of hands, back, or buttocks
Patterns descriptive of object used, such as round cigar or cigarette burns, "glovelike" sharply demarcated areas from immersion in scalding water, rope burns on wrists or ankles from being bound, burns in the shape of an iron, radiator, or electric stove burner
Absence of "splash" marks and presence of symmetric burns
Whiplash from shaking the child
Unusual symptoms, such as abdominal swelling, pain, and vomiting from punching
Descriptive marks such as from human bites or pulling out of hair
Unexplained repeated poisoning or unexplained sudden illness

Physical Abuse—cont'd

Suggestive Behaviors
Wariness of physical contact with adults
Apparent fear of parents or of going home
Lying very still while surveying environment, lack of reaction to frightening events
Inappropriate reaction to injury, such as failure to cry from pain
Apprehensiveness when hearing other children cry
Indiscriminate friendliness and displays of affection, superficial relationships
Acting-out behavior, attention-seeking behaviors
Withdrawn behavior

Sexual Abuse

Suggestive Physical Findings
Bruises, bleeding, lacerations or irritation of external genitalia, anus, mouth, or throat
Torn, stained, or bloody underclothing
Pain on urination or pain, swelling, and itching of genital area, penile discharge, unusual odor in the genital area
Sexually transmitted disease, nonspecific vaginitis, or venereal warts or presence of sperm
Difficulty in walking or sitting
Recurrent urinary tract infections
Pregnancy in young adolescent

Suggestive Behaviors
Sudden emergence of sexually related problems, including excessive or public masturbation, age-inappropriate sexual play, promiscuity, or overtly seductive behavior
Withdrawn behavior, excessive daydreaming, preoccupation with fantasies, especially in play
Poor relationships with peers
Sudden changes, such as anxiety, loss or gain of weight, clinging behavior
In incestuous relationships, excessive anger at mother for not protecting daughter
Regressive behavior, such as bed-wetting or thumb-sucking
Sudden onset of phobias or fears, particularly fears of the dark, men, strangers, or particular settings or situations (e.g., undue fear of leaving the house or staying at the day care center or the baby-sitter's house)
Running away from home
Substance abuse, particularly of alcohol or mood-elevating drugs
Profound and rapid personality changes, especially extreme depression, hostility, and aggression (often accompanied by social withdrawal)
Rapidly declining school performance
Suicidal attempts or ideation

From Hockenberry MJ and others: *Wong's nursing care of infants and children,* ed 7, St. Louis, 2003, Mosby.

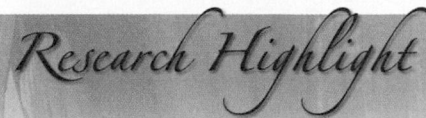

Box 11-6

Breast Feeding

Research Focus

Success in breast-feeding largely depends on the information and support a woman receives during the postpartum period. Nurses can play an important role in assisting mothers in their attempts to breast-feed. This article addresses how a group of mothers perceived the support that they received from their postpartum nurses.

Research Abstract

The purpose of this study was to describe how maternal-child nurses facilitated mothers' breast-feeding attempts during their hospital stay. Also investigated were the mother's perceptions of support by their nurses. Earlier research indicated that a mother's choice to breast-feed is influenced by several factors, including age, education, ethnicity, and income. Those who have difficulties initiating or continuing breast-feeding often have feelings of failing, which may further undermine their confidence in parenting. Different forms of support have been identified as informational support, tangible support, emotional or interpersonal support, and appraisal support. Informational support provides the mother with information verbally, nonverbally, or in writing. Tangible support utilizes physical assistance and or money. Appraisal support encourages and evaluates one's progress. Using a research approach known as ethnography, in-

formation was obtained from the subjects by interview and observation. Some of the postpartum nurses were reported to be well informed and knowledgeable about breast-feeding and willing to offer support. For the most part, the mothers interviewed reported that they were disappointed and did not feel supported. They were left feeling very frustrated and discouraged. Mothers expressed a need for the nurses to stay with them during their feeding attempts. They felt that the written instructions were not supportive enough for them to feel satisfied.

Evidence-Based Practice

- Maternal-child nurses must provide education and support to breast-feeding mothers.
- Nurses must try to anticipate mother's needs rather than wait for them to be asked for assistance.
- In order to best facilitate breast-feeding, all nurses should use consistent approaches.
- Nurses should provide breast-feeding mothers with verbal support, as well as written information.
- Nurses should assess mothers' support system's knowledge of breast-feeding.

Reference

Gill S: The little things: perceptions of breastfeeding support, *J Obstet Gynecol Neonatal Nurs* 30(4):401, 2001.

Cultural Aspects of Care

Box 11-7

Cultural practices and beliefs have a significant influence on the choice of infant feeding methods. Although cultural norms exist, application of the norms may not be appropriate for all individuals.

Implications for Practice

- Immigrants to the United States from poorer countries may choose to bottle-feed their infants because it is believed to be better and more modern. Others may choose bottle-feeding because of a desire to adapt to American culture.
- Many cultures choose not to give the infants colostrum. Filipinos, Mexican-Americans, Vietnamese, Hmong, Koreans,

Nigerians, and Indians are a few of the 50 known cultures that delay breast-feeding until the milk has "come in." Other cultures may begin breast-feeding immediately after delivery and offer the breast each time the infant cries.
- Cultural attitudes regarding breast-feeding, modesty, and dietary beliefs are important considerations for the nurse.
- The balance between energy forces may be the basis for food selections. "Hot" foods in some cultures are considered to be the best. "Hot" does not refer to the temperature of the foods. Chicken and broccoli are considered "hot." "Cold" foods include fresh fruits and vegetables.
- Families may bring desired foods into the health care setting.

Data from Edelman C, Mandle C: *Health promotion throughout the life span,* ed 5, St. Louis, 2002, Mosby; and Gill S: The little things: perceptions of breastfeeding support, *J Obstet Gynecol Neonatal Nurs* 30(4):401, 2001.

Overfeeding. The association between overfeeding, infant obesity, and later adult obesity is still controversial. However, early feeding experiences can influence later eating habits. The nurse should therefore emphasize balanced nutrition and good dietary habits through feeding experiences mutually satisfying for the parents and infant. Eating habits are frequently affected by the sociocultural background of the family. Certain cultures regard "a fat baby as a healthy baby." Because some cultures con-

sider a fat baby to be a sign of good mothering, any suggestion to limit intake or slow weight gain may be seen as a threat. It is important for the nurse to develop an understanding of the cultural influences to develop effective nursing interventions (Box 11-7).

Dentition. The average age for the first tooth to erupt is 7 months, but there is considerable variation among infants because of their genetic endowment. An occasional infant is born with a tooth whereas others remain toothless at 1 year. The order of tooth eruption is fairly predictable with the lower central incisors being first to appear, closely followed by the upper central incisors. Most 1-year-olds have six teeth.

Teething may result in considerable discomfort for some infants and little or none for others. The inflammation of the gums as the tooth prepares to emerge may result in a low-grade fever and irritability. Some have increased drooling, biting, or finger sucking. The use of a frozen teething ring or ice cube wrapped in a washcloth is soothing. Over-the-counter teething medications to rub on the inflamed gums and appropriate doses of acetaminophen are helpful when the infant is irritable and has difficulty eating or sleeping.

Most dentists recommend that parents cleanse their infant's teeth after each feeding. This can be accomplished very simply and quickly with a wet washcloth

Table 11-3	Selected Sleep Disturbances During Infancy and Early Childhood
Disorder/Description	**Management**
Nighttime Feeding	
Colic, irritability Prolonged need for night bottle or breast-feeding Child goes to sleep at the breast or with a bottle Irregular sleep patterns Child returns to sleep after feeding; other comfort measures (e.g., rocking or holding) are usually ineffective	Soothe, rock for brief periods, offer pacifier Gradually increase daytime feeding intervals to 4 hours or more Offer last feeding as late as possible at night Gradually increase amount of fluid during day Offer no bottles in bed Put to bed *awake* When child is crying, check at progressively longer intervals each night; reassure child but do not hold, rock, take to parent's bed, or give bottle or pacifier
Developmental Night Crying	
Child age 6-12 months with undisturbed nighttime sleep now awakes abruptly; may be accompanied by nightmares	Reassure parents that this phase is temporary Enter room immediately to check on child but keep reassurances *brief* Avoid feeding, rocking, taking to parent's bed, or any other routine that may initiate trained night crying
Trained Night Crying (Inappropriate Sleep Associations)	
Child typically falls asleep in place other than own bed (e.g., rocking chair or parent's bed) and is brought to own bed while asleep; on awakening, cries until usual routine is instituted (e.g., rocking)	Put child in own bed when *awake* If possible, arrange sleeping area separate from other family members Check crying child at progressively longer intervals each night; reassure child but do not resume usual routine
Refusal to Go to Sleep	
Child resists bedtime and comes out of room repeatedly Nighttime sleep may be continuous, but frequent awakenings and refusal to return to sleep may occur and become a problem if parent allows child to deviate from usual sleep pattern	Evaluate if hour of sleep is too early (child may resist sleep if not tired) Assist parents with consistent bedtime routine If child persists in leaving bedroom, close door for progressively longer periods Reinforce positive behavior
Nighttime Fears	
Child resists going to bed or wakes during the night because of fears Child seeks parent's physical presence and falls asleep easily with parent nearby. Overwhelming fears	Evaluate if hour of sleep is too early (child may fantasize when nothing to do but think in dark room) Calmly reassure the frightened child; keeping a night-light on may be helpful Use reward system with child to provide motivation to deal with fears Avoid patterns that can lead to additional problems (e.g., sleeping with child or taking child to parent's room) If child's fear is overwhelming, consider desensitization (e.g., progressively spending longer periods of time alone; consult professional help for protracted fears) Distinguish between nightmares and sleep terrors (confused partial arousals)

and the parent's finger. Dietary considerations should also be addressed with the parents. Prolonged breast- or bottle-feeding, especially bottle propping when the infant is likely to fall asleep and leave milk in the mouth to surround the teeth, should be discouraged due to the risk of developing dental caries (Behrman and others, 2000).

Immunizations. The widespread use of immunizations has resulted in the dramatic decline of infectious diseases over the past 50 years and is therefore a most important factor in health promotion during childhood. Although most immunizations can be given to persons of any age, it is recommended that the administration of the primary series begin soon after birth and be completed during early childhood. Vaccines are among the safest and most reliable drugs used. Minor side effects may occur; however, serious reactions are rare. Parents should receive instructions regarding the potential side effects of immunizations. High fever and extreme irritability should be reported to their health care provider.

Complacency and fear regarding the side effects of certain vaccines, especially diphtheria and tetanus toxoids and pertussis vaccine (DTP), have resulted in large numbers of children not receiving appropriate immunizations during recent years. General contraindications to vaccination include moderate illness, allergic response to a previous dose of a particular vaccine, immunosuppression, and persons receiving high doses of corticosteroids. Live virus vaccines are generally not recommended for pregnant women (Behrman, Kliegman, and Jenson, 2000).

Sleep. Sleep patterns vary among infants, with many having their days and nights mixed up until 3 to 4 months of age. By this time, most infants are nocturnal and sleep between 9 and 11 hours. Total daily sleep averages 15 hours. Most infants take one or two naps a day by the end of the first year. Sleep disturbances with a physiological basis are rare, with the possible exception of colic. More common sleep disturbances are described in Table 11-3.

Toddler

Toddlerhood ranges from the time when children begin to walk independently until they walk and run with ease, which is from 12 to 36 months. The toddler is characterized by increasing independence bolstered by greater physical mobility and cognitive abilities. Toddlers are increasingly aware of their abilities to control and are pleased with successful efforts with this new skill. This success leads them to repeated attempts to control their environments. Unsuccessful attempts at control may result in negative behavior and temper tantrums. These behaviors are most common when parents thwart the initial independent action. Parents cite these as the most problematic behaviors during the toddler years and at times express frustration with trying to set consistent and firm limits while simultaneously encouraging independence.

Physical Changes

The rapid development of motor skills allows the child to participate in self-care activities such as feeding, dressing, and toileting. In the beginning the toddler walks in an upright position with a broad-stance and gait, protuberant abdomen, and arms out to the sides for balance. Soon the child begins to navigate stairs, using a rail or the wall to maintain balance while progressing upward, placing both feet on the same step before continuing. Success provides courage to attempt the upright mode for descending the stairs in the same manner. Locomotion skills soon include running, jumping, standing on one foot for several seconds, and kicking a ball. Most toddlers can ride tricycles, climb ladders, and run well by their third birthday.

Fine motor capabilities move from scribbling spontaneously to drawing circles and crosses accurately. By 3 years the child draws simple stick people and can usually stack a tower of small blocks. Increased locomotion skills, the ability to undress, and development of sphincter control allow toilet training if the toddler has developed the necessary language and cognitive abilities. Parents often consult nurses for an assessment of readiness for toilet training. Recognizing the urge to urinate and or defecate is crucial in determining the child's mental readiness. At this stage children usually show a willingness to please parents and take pride in their accomplishments (Kinservik and Friedhoff, 2000). The nurse needs to remind parents that patience, consistency, and a nonjudgmental attitude, in addition to the child's readiness, are essential to successful toilet training.

The cardiopulmonary system becomes stable in the toddler years. The heart and respiratory rates slow to an average of 110 beats and 25 breaths per minute, respectively, and the blood pressure varies slightly from infancy. The average blood pressure for a toddler is 90/50 mm Hg.

The anterior fontanel closes between 12 and 18 months of age, ending the period of most rapid growth of the skull and brain. Routine measurement of head circumference should be done until 3 years of age.

The rate of increase in weight and length slows. By $2\frac{1}{2}$ years the child weighs 4 times the birth weight. Height during toddlerhood increases by approximately 3 inches a year, mainly as a result of increases in leg length. The average height of 2-year-olds is 34 inches. Slowed growth rates are accompanied by decreased caloric need, and smaller food intake leads some parents to worry about the adequacy of dietary intake. Parents need encouragement to offer the child appropriate servings of food from the food pyramid and to avoid force feeding or allowing the child to fill up on foods that are high in fat and sugar. The nurse can reassure parents that the child's nutrition is adequate by demonstrating the child's satisfactory status on a growth grid.

Cognitive Changes

Toddlers' completion of the development of **object permanence,** their ability to remember events, and their beginning ability to put thoughts into words at about 2 years of age signal their transition from Piaget's sensorimotor stage of cognitive development to the **preoperational thought** stage (Piaget, 1952). Toddlers recognize that they are separate beings from their mothers, but they are unable to assume the view of another. They use symbols to represent objects, places, and persons.

This function is demonstrated when children imitate the behavior of another that they viewed earlier (e.g., pretend to shave like daddy), pretend one object is another (use a finger as a gun), and use language to stand for absent objects (e.g., request bottle).

Language. The 18-month-old child uses approximately 10 words. The 24-month-old child has a vocabulary of up to 300 words and is generally able to speak in two-word sentences (Deering and Cody, 2002). "Who's that?" and "What's that?" typify questions asked during this period. Verbal expressions such as "me do it" and "that's mine" demonstrate the 2-year-old child's use of pronouns and desire for independence and control. Despite the expanded vocabulary of an older toddler, most parents comment that their child's favorite word is *no* until well into the third year. Offering choices to the toddler helps reduce their sense of frustration and builds their sense of independence (Deering and Cody, 2002).

Because children's moral development is closely associated with their cognitive abilities, the moral development of toddlers is only beginning and is also egocentric. Toddlers do not understand concepts of right and wrong. However, they do grasp the fact that some behaviors bring pleasant results (positive reinforcement) and others elicit unpleasant results (negative reinforcement). Therefore until toddlers achieve a higher level of cognitive function, they behave simply to avoid the unpleasant and seek out the pleasant (Hockenberry and others, 2003).

Psychosocial Changes

According to Erikson (1963), a sense of autonomy emerges during toddlerhood. Children strive for independence by using their developing muscles to do everything for themselves and become the master of their bodily functions. Their strong wills are frequently exhibited in negative behavior when caregivers attempt to direct their actions. Temper tantrums may result when toddlers are frustrated by parental restrictions. Parents need to provide toddlers with graded independence, allowing them to do things that do not result in harm to themselves or others. This prevents them from doubting their ability to do things that they are capable of learning or feeling a sense of shame for those things that they have done. Firm consistent limits, patience, and support allow toddlers to develop socially acceptable behavior and cope with the frustration of learning self-control (Kinservik and Friedhoff, 2000). Young toddlers who want to learn to hold their own cups may benefit from two-handled cups with spouts and plastic bibs with pockets to collect the milk that spills during the learning process.

Socially, toddlers remain strongly attached to their parents and fear separation from them. In their presence they feel safe, and their curiosity is evident in their exploration of the environment. Mothers of toddlers are rarely allowed any bathroom privacy because closing of the door results in incessant crying until the door is opened.

The child continues to engage in solitary play during toddlerhood but also begins to participate in parallel play, which is playing beside rather than with another child. Toddlers who are just learning what belongs to them are

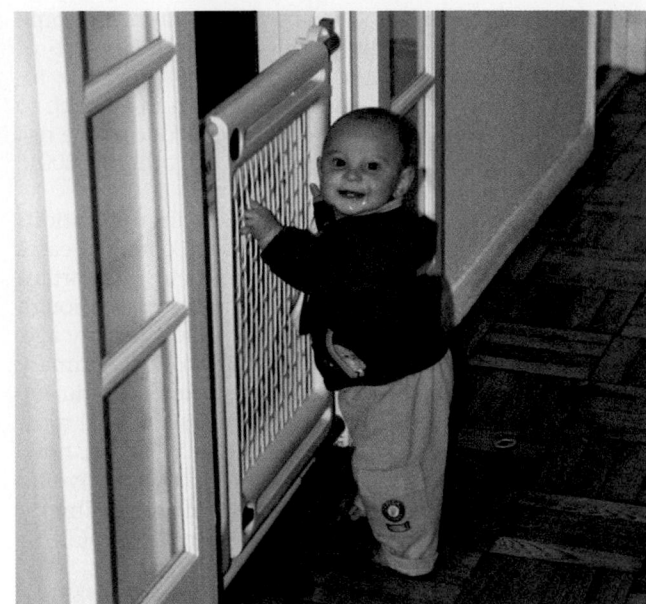

FIGURE 11–6 Safety precautions should be provided for toddlers. (Courtesy Elaine Polan, RNC, BSN, MS.)

often possessive of their toys. They learn the joy of sharing when they offer parents toys to hold and the parents express pleasure.

Health Risks

The newly developed locomotion abilities and insatiable curiosity of toddlers make them at risk for injury. Toddlers need close supervision at all times and particularly when in environments that have not been childproofed (Figure 11-6).

Poisonings occur frequently because children near 2 years of age are interested in placing any object or substance in their mouths to learn about it. The wise parent removes or locks up all possible poisons, including plants, cleaning materials, and medications. These parental actions create a safer environment for exploratory behavior. Lead poisoning continues to be a serious health hazard in the United States (Cohen, 2001). Health care providers need to educate families living in older homes about the risks, screening, and treatment of lead poisoning. The toddlers' lack of awareness regarding the danger of water and their newly developed walking skills make drowning a major cause of accidental death in this age-group. Limit setting is extremely important for toddlers' safety. Automobile safety requires toddlers to remain in car seats (Kamerling, 2002). Studies have shown that it is significantly safer to secure the child seat in the rear seat of the vehicle. Children often learn to release the car restraints, and parents must be firm in their resolve not to drive unless the children are securely restrained. Toddlers completely depend on their parents for physical safety. Health care workers have a moral and professional obligation to educate parents on the proper use of child passenger restraint use. Table 11-4 identifies developmental abilities acquired during this age period and injury prevention strategies.

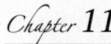
Table 11-4   Injury Prevention During Early Childhood

Developmental Abilities Related to Risk of Injury	Injury Prevention
	Motor Vehicles
Walks, runs, and climbs Able to open doors and gates Can ride tricycle Can throw ball and other objects	Use federally approved car restraint; if restraint is not available, use lap belt Supervise child while playing outside to avoid entering street Do not allow child to play on curb or behind a parked car Do not permit child to play in pile of leaves, snow, or large cardboard container in trafficked area Supervise tricycle riding Lock fences and doors if not directly supervising children Teach child to obey pedestrian safety rules Obey traffic regulations; walk only at crosswalks and when traffic signal indicates it is safe to cross Stand back a step from curb until it is time to cross Look left, right, and left again and check for turning cars before crossing street Use sidewalks; when there is no sidewalk, walk on left, facing traffic Wear light colors at night, and attach fluorescent material to clothing
	Drowning
Able to explore if left unsupervised Has great curiosity Helpless in water, unaware of its danger; depth of water has no significance	Supervise closely when near any source of water, including buckets Keep bathroom doors and lid on toilet closed Have fence around swimming pool and lock gate Teach swimming and water safety (not a substitute for protection)
	Burns
Able to reach heights by climbing, stretching, standing on toes, and using objects as a ladder Pulls objects Explores any holes or opening Can open drawers and closets Unaware of potential sources of heat or fire Plays with mechanical objects	Turn pot handles toward back of stove Place electric appliances, such as coffeemaker, frying pan, and popcorn popper, toward back of counter Place guardrails in front of radiators, fireplaces, or other heating elements Store matches and cigarette lighters in locked or inaccessible area; discard carefully Place burning candles, incense, hot foods, ashes, embers, and cigarettes out of reach Do not let tablecloth hang within child's reach Do not let electric cord from iron or other appliance hang within child's reach Cover electrical outlets with protective devices Keep electrical wires hidden or out of reach Do not allow child to play with electrical appliance, wires, or lighters Stress danger of open flames; teach what "hot" means Always check bathwater temperature; adjust hot-water heater temperature to 48.9° C (120° F) or lower; do not allow children to play with faucets Apply a sunscreen with SPF 15 or higher when child is exposed to sunlight
	Poisoning
Explores by putting objects in mouth Can open drawers, closets, and most containers Climbs Cannot read warning labels Does not know safe dose or amount	Place all potentially toxic agents (including plants) in a locked cabinet or out of reach Replace medications and poisons immediately; replace child-resistant caps properly Refer to medications as drugs, not as candy Do not store large surplus of toxic agents Promptly discard empty poison containers; never reuse to store a food item or other poison Teach child not to play in trash containers Never remove labels from containers of toxic substances Know number and location of nearest poison control center (usually listed in front of telephone directory)

From Hockenberry MJ and others: *Wong's nursing care of infants and children,* ed 7, St. Louis, 2003, Mosby.   *Continued*

Table 11-4	Injury Prevention During Early Childhood—cont'd

Developmental Abilities Related to Risk of Injury	Injury Prevention
Falls	
Able to open doors and some windows	Keep screen in window, nail securely, and use guardrail
Goes up and down stairs	Place gates at top and bottom of stairs
Depth perception unrefined	Keep doors locked or use child-resistant doorknob covers at entry to stairs, high porch, or other elevated area, such as laundry chute
	Remove unsecured or scatter rugs
	Apply nonskid mat in bathtub or shower
	Keep crib rails fully raised and mattress at lowest level
	Place carpeting under crib and in bathroom
	Keep large toys and bumper pads out of crib or playpen (child can use these as "stairs" to climb out), then move to youth bed when child is able to crawl out of crib
	Avoid using walkers, especially near stairs
	Dress in safe clothing (soles that do not "catch" on floor, tied shoelaces, pant legs that do not hang on floor)
	Keep child restrained in vehicles; never leave unattended in shopping cart or stroller
	Supervise at playgrounds; select play areas with soft ground cover and safe equipment
Choking and Suffocation	
Puts things in mouth	Avoid large, round chunks of meat, such as whole hot dogs (slice lengthwise into short pieces)
May swallow hard or nonedible pieces of food	Avoid fruit with pits, fish with bones, dried beans, hard candy, chewing gum, nuts, popcorn, grapes, marshmallows
	Choose large, sturdy toys without sharp edges or small removable parts
	Discard old refrigerators, ovens, and so on; if storing old appliance, remove doors
	Keep automatic garage door transmitter in inaccessible place
	Select safe toy boxes or chests without heavy, hinged lids
	Keep venetian blind strings out of child's reach
	Remove drawstrings from clothing
Bodily damage	
Still clumsy in many skills	Avoid giving sharp or pointed objects—such as knives, scissors, or toothpicks—especially when walking or running
Easily distracted from tasks	Do not allow lollipops or similar objects in mouth when walking or running
Unaware of potential danger from strangers or other people	Teach safety precautions (e.g., to carry fork or scissors with pointed end away from face)
	Store all dangerous tools, garden equipment, and firearms in locked cabinet
	Be alert to danger of animals, including household pets
	Use safety glass and decals on large glassed areas, such as sliding glass doors
	Teach personal safety
	Teach name, address, and phone number and to ask for help from appropriate people (cashier, security guard, policeman) if lost; have identification on child (sewn in clothes, inside shoe)
	Avoid personalized clothing in public places
	Teach child to never go with a stranger
	Teach child to tell parents if anyone makes child feel uncomfortable in any way
	Always listen to child's concerns regarding others' behavior
	Teach child to say "no" when confronted with uncomfortable situations

From Hockenberry MJ and others: *Wong's nursing care of infants and children*, ed 7, St. Louis, 2003, Mosby.

Health Concerns

Health Perceptions. Toddlers' perceptions of their own health are limited by their cognitive capabilities. Children increasingly recognize internal body sensations but have difficulty pinpointing their location. Therefore children often associate generalized responses with illness. Children who deviate radically from their usual patterns of eating, sleeping, or playing require assessment to determine whether these alterations result from illness. During this stage, children begin to internalize the labels that parents or health care professionals give to the somatic states. That is, if the parents label particular sensations, such as abdominal discomfort, an "illness," children begin to label related sensations similarly. At the same time, children observe and mimic parents' health care practices. Health beliefs and practices are therefore being significantly shaped, even in these early years.

Nutrition. Most toddlers change from breast milk or formula to cow's milk, consuming three to four 8-ounce servings per day. Nutritional requirements are increasingly met by solid foods from the food pyramid. Because the consumption of more than a quart of milk per day usually decreases the child's appetite for these essential solid foods and results in inadequate iron intake, the nurse should advise parents to limit milk intake to 2 to 3 cups per day. Children are usually not offered low fat or skim milk until age 2 because they need the fat for satisfactory physical and intellectual growth. The healthy toddler requires a balanced daily intake of bread and grains, vegetables, fruit, dairy products, and proteins. Because parents frequently overestimate the size of a normal serving for their child, the nurse can reduce their anxiety about inadequate intake by pointing out the normal serving size.

Children who are ill, are undergoing surgery, or have diseases involving ingestion, absorption, or use of nutrients require special dietary considerations. Alterations in the type of foods and caloric requirements may be necessary. Children on strict vegetarian diets also require careful planning to ensure adequate, balanced protein intake. Regardless of children's health status, several basic principles of nutrition apply. Mealtime has psychosocial and physical significance. If the parents struggle to control toddlers' dietary intake, problem behavior and conflicts may result. Toddlers often develop "food jags," or the desire to eat one food repeatedly. Rather than becoming disturbed by this behavior, parents should be encouraged by the nurse to offer a variety of nutritious foods at meals and to provide only nutritious snacks between meals. Serving finger foods to toddlers allows them to eat by themselves and to satisfy their need for independence and control. Small, reasonable servings allow toddlers to eat all of their meals.

Preschooler

The **preschool period** refers to those years between 3 and 5. Children refine the mastery of their bodies and eagerly await the beginning of formal education. Many people consider these the most intriguing years of parenting because children are less negative, can more accurately share their thoughts, and can more effectively interact and communicate. Physical development occurs at a slower pace than cognitive and psychosocial development.

Physical Changes

Several aspects of physical development continue to stabilize in the preschool years. Heart and respiratory rates range from 60 to 100 beats and 23 to 25 breaths per minute, respectively. Blood pressure rises slightly to an average of 92/56 mm Hg. Children gain about 5 pounds per year; the average weight at 3 years is 32 pounds, at 4 years is 37 pounds, and at 5 years is about 41 pounds. Preschoolers grow 2½ to 3 inches per year, double their birth length around 4 years, and stand an average of 43 inches tall by their fifth birthday. The elongation of the legs results in more slender appearing children. Little difference exists between the sexes, although boys are slightly larger with more muscle and less fatty tissue.

Large and fine muscle coordination improves. Preschoolers run well, walk up and down steps with ease, and learn to hop. By 5 years they can usually skip on alternate feet, jump rope, and begin to skate and swim. Improving fine motor skills allows intricate manipulations. They learn to copy crosses and squares. Triangles and diamonds are usually mastered between ages 5 and 6. Scribbling and drawing help to develop fine muscle skills and eye-hand coordination needed for the printing of letters and numbers.

Children need opportunities to learn and practice new physical skills. Nursing care of healthy and ill children includes an assessment of the availability of these opportunities. Although children with acute illnesses benefit from rest and exclusion from usual daily activities, children who have chronic conditions or who have been hospitalized for long periods need ongoing exposure to developmental opportunities. The parents and nurse weave these opportunities into the children's daily experiences, depending on their abilities, needs, and energy level.

Cognitive Changes

Preschoolers continue to master the preoperational stage of cognition. The first phase of this period, known as preconceptual thought (2 to 4 years), is characterized by perceptual-bound thinking, in which children judge persons, objects, and events by their outward appearance or what seems to be (Piaget, 1952). For example, children may determine that an 8-ounce glass full of fluid contains more than a 10-ounce glass that also contains 8 ounces of fluid because they center their thoughts on the fullness of the glass. Even if they watch the 8 ounces of fluid from the full glass being poured into the 10-ounce glass and the 8-ounce glass refilled, they will still assert that the full 8-ounce glass contains more because they cannot attend to the transfer. Thinking is hindered by their limited attention and attending skills. **Artificialism,** the misconception that everything in the world has been created by humanity, may result in children asking questions such as who built the mountains. Another misconception of preschool thinking, **animism,** the attribution of life to inanimate objects, often results in statements such as "Trees cry when their branches are broken." A third misconception is a type of reasoning called **immanent justice,** the notion that the world is equipped with a built-in code of law and order. It may result in children's beliefs that matches burned them because they were not supposed to handle them.

Around the age of 4 years, the intuitive phase of preoperational thought develops. Children's ability to think more complexly is demonstrated by their ability to classify objects according to size or color and by questions such as "Why do they call it the thirty-first day of the month instead of the thirty last?" Egocentricity persists, but during these 3 years, it begins to be replaced with social interaction, as is illustrated by the 5-year-old child who offers a bandage to a child with a cut finger. Children become aware of cause-and-effect relationships, as illustrated by the statement "The sun sets because people want to go to bed." Early causal thinking is also evident in preschoolers' transductive thoughts (reasoning occurs from one particular to another). If two events are related in time or space, children link them in a causal fashion. The hospitalized child, for example, may reason, "I cried last night, and that's why the nurse gave me the shot." As children near age 5, they begin to use or can be taught to use rules to understand causation. They then begin to reason from the general to the particular. This forms the basis for more formal logical thought. The child can now reason, "I get a shot twice a day, and that's why I got one last night."

Preschoolers' knowledge of the world remains closely linked to concrete (perceived by the senses) experiences. Even their rich fantasy life is grounded in the perception of reality. The mixing of the two aspects can lead to many childhood fears and may be misinterpreted by adults as lying when children are actually presenting reality from their perspective.

The greatest fear of this age-group appears to be that of bodily harm, and it can be seen in children's fear of the dark, animals, thunderstorms, and medical personnel. This fear often interferes with their willingness to allow nursing interventions such as measurement of vital signs. Preschoolers may cooperate if they are allowed to help the nurse measure the blood pressure of a parent or if they are allowed to manipulate the nurse's equipment.

The preschooler's moral development expands to include a beginning understanding of behaviors considered socially right or wrong. The child continues to be motivated, however, by the wish to avoid punishment or the desire to obtain a reward. The primary difference between this stage of moral development and that of a toddler is that a preschooler is better able to identify behaviors that elicit rewards or punishment and begins to label these behaviors as right or wrong.

Language. Preschoolers' vocabularies continue to increase rapidly, and by the age of 6 children have more than 10,000 words that they can use to define familiar objects, identify colors, and express their desires and frustrations (Deering and Cody, 2002). Language is more social, and questions expand to "Why?" and "How come?" in the quest for information. Phonetically similar words such as *die* and *dye* or *wood* and *would* may cause confusion in preschool children. The nurse avoids such words when preparing children for procedures and assesses comprehension of explanations.

Psychosocial Changes
The world of preschoolers expands beyond the family into the neighborhood where children meet other children and adults. Their curiosity and developing initiative lead to the active exploration of the environment, the development of new skills, and the making of new friends. Preschoolers have a surplus of energy that permits them to plan and attempt many activities that may be beyond their capabilities, such as pouring milk from a gallon container into their cereal bowls. Guilt arises within children when they overstep the limits of their abilities and feel they have not behaved correctly. Children who in anger have wished their sibling were dead experience guilt if

that sibling becomes ill. Children need to be taught that "wishing" for something to happen does not make it occur. Erikson (1963) recommends that parents help their children strike a healthy balance between initiative and guilt by allowing them to do things on their own while setting firm limits and providing guidance.

During times of stress or illness, preschoolers may revert to bed-wetting or thumb sucking and want the parents to feed, dress, and hold them. Box 11-8 lists potential sources of stress in the preschooler. These dependent behaviors are often confusing and embarrassing to parents, who can benefit from the nurse's reassurance that they are the child's normal coping behaviors. The nurse should provide experiences that these children can master. Such successes help children return to their prior level of independent functioning. As language skills develop, children should be encouraged to talk about their feelings. Play is also an excellent way for preschoolers to vent frustration or anger and is a socially acceptable way to deal with stress.

Play. The play of preschool children becomes more social after the third birthday as it shifts from parallel to associative play. Children playing together engage in similar if not identical activity; however, there is no division of labor, or rigid organization or rules. Most 3-year-old children are able to play with one other child in a cooperative manner in which they make something or play designated roles such as mother and baby. By age 4, children play in groups of two or three, and by 5 years the group has a temporary leader for each activity.

In many play activities, preschoolers display awareness of social context. Sex-role identification is strengthening, and children most often assume roles of persons of their own sex. Children frequently mimic or repeat social experiences. This tendency is especially significant for the nurse working with hospitalized children. Through play, children may express questions, fears, anger, and misunderstanding about their illnesses and care. The nurse should be alert to such clues and ensure that children can play within energy limits. Play can provide a healthy outlet for frustration when children have been subjected to painful or restrictive experiences against their will.

Pretend play involving imaginary situations depends on children's ability to retain images of things they have seen or heard. This sociodramatic play involving other children occupies about a third of 5-year-old children's playtime. Pretending allows children to learn to understand other's points of view, develop skills in solving social problems, and become more creative. Some children have imaginary playmates. These playmates serve many purposes—friends when they are lonely, they can accomplish what the child is still attempting and can experience what the child wants to forget or remember. Imaginary playmates are a sign of health and allow the child to distinguish between reality and fantasy.

Health Risks
As fine and gross motor skills develop and the child becomes more coordinated with better balance, falls become much less of a problem. Guidelines for injury prevention in the toddler also apply to the preschooler. The

Box 11-8   Sources of Stress in Preschoolers

Three-Year-Old

Infantile behavior—Reverts to babyish ways; can't completely let go of babyhood

Stubbornness—Although is developing an interest in social relationships and a concept of "we," may lapse into uncooperative behavior

Possessiveness—Guards belongings and may be bossy about them

Jealousy—Particularly when it comes to parents' love

Separation anxiety

Stranger anxiety

Confusion—Cannot always discriminate between fantasy and reality

White lies—May result from wishful thinking, fantasy, and desire to please or impress

Imaginary playmate—Often blamed for misdeeds

Fears—May be precipitated by imagination, may also fear dogs or other animals

Speech—May stutter or stumble over words

Activity level—Seems to be in perpetual motion; may exhaust himself or herself

Eating—May forget to eat or lose interest in food

Nap or bedtime—May fear bad dreams, the dark, or missing out on some fun while asleep

Destructiveness—May damage or destroy objects

Questions—Continually asks "why," and is upset if trusted adults do not respond or do not know the answer

Four-Year-Old

Insecurity—May develop nervous habits such as nail biting, facial tics, thumb sucking, genital manipulation, eye blinking, or nose picking; may insist on bringing a familiar item from house to preschool

Four-Year-Old—cont'd

Exaggerations—May attempt to boost self-image with boasts

Companionship—Enjoys interacting with friends, although there may be many quarrels

Silliness—Tends to engage in silly play; likes words and is fascinated by rhyming syllables or foul language; is disciplined for lack of control

Property rights—Protects belongings; may become bossy

Sex—Interested in the human body; may engage in exhibitionism

Activity level—Enjoys running, jumping, and slamming doors; may be punished for disruptive behavior

Fears—Picks up fears from adults; may fear dark room, snakes and lizards, or anything perceived as "creepy"

Attention—Likes to talk and is frustrated if ignored or put off; whines to get own way

Five-Year-Old

Approval—Parents' love and acceptance are vital; seeks praise

School—May have difficulty adjusting to kindergarten

Separation anxiety—Particularly fears loss of mother

Infantile behavior—May occasionally lapse into babyish behavior as a result of realizing that babyhood has ended

Worrying—May develop irrational fears, take information out of context, or fret over a misinterpreted, overheard conversation

Masturbation—Is concerned about being "bad"

Belongings—Protects possessions

Showing off—Performs in order to gain praise

Procrastination—May dillydally now and then

Name-calling—Insults others to boost self-image but is upset when she or he is the victim of mockery

Modified from Kuczen B: *Childhood stress: don't let your child be a victim,* New York, 1982, Delacorte Press.

nurse should alert parents of children in this age-group to the risks of poisoning and pedestrian–motor vehicle accidents. The leading cause of death in U.S. children remains due to unintentional injury (Hall-Long, Schell, and Corrigan, 2001). Most of these injuries are preventable. Children should be taught about safety in the home and reinforced early in elementary school. Educating children and their families will help facilitate the *Healthy People 2010* objectives (USDHHS, 2000).

Health Concerns

Little research has explored preschoolers' perceptions of their own health. Parental beliefs about health, children's bodily sensations, and their ability to perform usual daily activities help children develop attitudes about their health. Preschoolers are usually quite independent in washing, dressing, and feeding. Alterations in this independence can influence their feelings about their own health.

Nutrition. Nutrition requirements for the preschooler vary little from those of the toddler. The average daily in-

take is 1800 calories. Parents may still worry about the amount of food their child is consuming. The quality of the food is more important than quantity in most situations. Preschoolers consume about half of the average adult portions. Finicky eating habits are characteristic of the 4-year-old; however, the 5-year-old is more interested in trying new foods.

Sleep. Preschoolers average 12 hours of sleep a night and take infrequent naps. Sleep disturbances are not uncommon during these years. Disturbances may range from trouble getting to sleep to nightmares to prolonging bedtime with extensive rituals. Frequently, the child has had an overabundance of activity and stimulation. Helping them to slow down before bedtime usually results in better sleeping habits.

Vision. Preschoolers should routinely be screened for vision problems. One of the common problems in the preschool period is amblyopia. Early detection and treatment can improve vision for most children (Berry and others, 2001).

School-Age Children and Adolescents

School-age children and adolescents lead demanding, challenging lives. The developmental changes between ages 6 and 18 are diverse and span all areas of growth and development. Physical, psychosocial, cognitive, and moral skills are developed, expanded, refined, and synchronized so that the individual may become an accepted and productive member of society. The environment in which the individual develops skills also expands and diversifies. Instead of the boundaries of family and close friends, the environment now may include the school, community, and church. Because of expectations for development, increasing skill and knowledge base, and environmental expansion, the individual experiences new difficulties and dilemmas. With age-specific assessment, the nurse must review the appropriate developmental expectations for each age-group. For example, before assessing risk-taking behaviors, the nurse recognizes that adolescents normally strive to achieve a sense of identity while developing a moral code compatible with society.

The nurse needs to direct school-age children and adolescents toward normal developmental behaviors, assisting them in maximizing their abilities and using them to cope. By helping children and adolescents achieve a necessary developmental balance, the nurse promotes health. Table 11-5 provides an overview of developmental behavior typical of school-age children and adolescents. The nurse must also increasingly involve the child or adolescent in charting a developmental course. Because preadolescents have increased cognitive and social skills, they are better able to plan developmental activities. Not only can they describe their feelings about the changes, but they can also think through these changes. Problem solving becomes more purposeful and sophisticated and results in the achievement of the outcomes that they desire. This paced, active participation may initiate a style of involvement in lifelong self-care.

School-age children and adolescents must cope with changes involving other areas of development. For example, 6-year-old children are confronted with new authority figures, teachers, as well as new rules and restrictions. They need to cooperatively work and play with a large group of children of various cultural backgrounds. School-age children must meet the challenge of developing cognitive skills that enhance their reasoning and allow them to learn to read, write, and manipulate numbers. Because of the stress of these changes, a child may develop physical and psychosocial health problems (e.g., increased susceptibility to upper respiratory infections, school maladjustment, inadequate peer relationships, or learning disorders). The nurse designs health promotion interventions that are based on the child's developmental stage.

Table 11-5	Developmental Behaviors of School-Age Children and Adolescents
School-Age Children	**Adolescents**
Relationships With Parents	
Children gradually learn that parents are less than perfect; they can be disillusioned with them and wish that friends' parents were their own. Sometimes they believe that they must be adopted. They rely on parents for unconditional love, security, guidance, and nurturing.	Adolescents' desire for increasing independence and autonomy and continuing need for some dependence and limit setting by parents place strain on their relationship. Effective communication and democratic parenting are best tools for meeting this challenge.
Relationships With Siblings	
Seem to be at odds with one another at home; yet they are each others' best defenders away from home. Younger children often idolize older siblings, and this frequently leads to competition. Older children may envy attention that younger siblings require and be quite bossy and somewhat abusive.	Younger siblings rarely understand their adolescent siblings' need for privacy to think, dream, and talk with peers. Adolescents often enjoy interacting with and guiding younger brothers and sisters when timing is convenient for them and they can remain in control.
Relationships With Peers	
During primary grades (6-7 years), children of both sexes play together, depending on who is available and interested. Around age 8, social groupings of same-sex peers form. These "gangs" allow children to declare their independence from parental rules and establish their own secret codes or languages and rules of membership and behavior. This period is often referred to as *secret society* of childhood. Preadolescent (10-12 years) friendships are characterized by having best friend of same sex. These relationships may be transient, but they are intense and allow discussion of all areas of life. Some interest in heterosexual relationships develops but they usually are not reciprocal.	Peer group is factor of critical influence to adolescents, who have increasing need for recognition and acceptance. Companionship offered by peer groups provides secure environment for individuals to try out new ideas and share similar feelings and attitudes. Adolescents often form cliques with peers from same socioeconomic group with similar interests. Cliques, which are highly exclusive, help their members, who have strong emotional bonds, develop their identities. The crowd, which is more impersonal than the clique, offers opportunities for heterosexual interaction and social activities. The crowd also maintains rigid membership requirements; clique membership is usually a prerequisite for crowd membership.

Table 11-5 **Developmental Behaviors of School-Age Children and Adolescents—cont'd**	
School-Age Children	**Adolescents**

Self-Concept

Children's feelings of competence regarding mastery of tasks are key elements in forming self-esteem. Children need to receive positive feedback from teachers and parents regarding their efforts. It is important for children to develop skills in at least one area such as reading, music, or swimming. Pets that require children's care and attention reward them with unconditional love and promote feelings of self-worth.

Formal and informal peer groups are primary force in shaping self-concept of group members. Popularity and recognition within peer group enhance self-esteem and reinforce self-concept. Total immersion in peer group may make it appear that adolescents have no original thoughts and are incapable of making decisions. Adolescents who withdraw from peers into isolation struggle with developing identity.

Fears

There is decline in fears related to body safety such as storms, dogs, darkness, noises, scrapes, and scratches. Fears of supernatural such as ghosts and witches persist and decline slowly. New fears related to school and family occur. They fear ridicule from teachers and friends and disapproval and rejection of parents. They also become frightened about death and items that they hear on news such as war and destruction of environment.

Fears in this age-group center around peer group acceptance, body changes, loss of self-control, and emerging sexual urges. Adolescents constantly examine their bodies for changes and signs of imperfection. Any defect, real or imagined, is cause of endless worry. Adolescents' developing awareness of economic and political problems may result in fear of going to war with its resulting death and destruction.

Coping Patterns

To deal with stress, school-agers use problem solving and defense mechanisms such as denial and aggression. Several categories of coping behaviors of hospitalized school-agers include inactivity (total silence, lack of activity, and apathy), orientation or precoping (looking and listening, walking around and exploring, and asking questions), cooperation (compliance with care), resistance (attempt to get away from the situation by turning away or making physical or verbal attacks), and controlling (assuming responsibility for self-care and suggesting how things could be done).

Coping behaviors expand with experiences adolescents have gained from life and from developing cognitive maturity. By age 15, most use full range of defense mechanisms, including rationalization and intellectualization. Adolescents' problem-solving abilities have matured, and they can reason through philosophical discussions and complex situations that require abstract thinking and proposition of hypotheses. Some adolescents use avoidance coping strategies in which the problem is denied or repressed and an attempt is made to reduce tension by engaging in substance abuse or avoiding people.

Morals

Children learn rules from parents, but their understanding of rules or reasons for them is limited until about 10 years. Before that, they are concerned with own needs first and may cheat to win. After 10, justice is based on "eye for an eye," and punishment should correct situation (e.g., if children break something, they should pay to have it fixed).

According to Kohlberg (1964), as youths approach adolescence they reach conventional level, where internalization of expectations of their family and society begins. Initially there is considerable conformity to rules to win praise or approval from others and to avoid social disapproval or rejection; later, they seek to avoid criticism from persons of authority in institutions.

Diversional Activity

School-agers play cooperatively in group activities such as jumping rope, hopscotch, soccer, and baseball. Play becomes competitive, and children often have difficulty learning to lose. Teasing, insults, dares, superstitions, and increased sensitivity are characteristics of this age.

Many teenagers develop special interests in certain sports and concentrate on developing maximal skills therein. Recreational activities are often determined by what is popular with peers and what can provide independence from parents (e.g., computers, cars).

Nutrition

Children have definite likes and dislikes. Few nutritional deficiencies occur in this age-group. Children have voracious appetites after school and need quality snacks such as fruit and sandwiches to avoid empty calorie foods such as chips and candy.

Total nutritional needs become greater during adolescence. Girls' caloric needs decrease, and their need for protein increases slightly. Iron needed by adolescents is almost twice that of adult men, and growth spurt increases calcium demand.

School-Age Child

During these "middle years" of childhood, the foundation for adult roles in work, recreation, and social interaction is laid. In industrialized countries this school-age period begins when the child starts elementary school around the age of 6 years. Puberty, around 12 years of age, signals the end of middle childhood. Great developmental strides are made during these years when children develop competencies in physical, cognitive, and psychosocial skills. During these years children become "better" at things; for example, they can run faster and farther as proficiency and endurance develop.

The school or educational experience expands the child's world and is a transition from a life of relatively free play to a life of structured play, learning, and work. The school and home influence growth and development, requiring adjustment by the parents and child. The child must learn to cope with rules and expectations presented by the school and peers. Parents must learn to allow their child to make decisions, accept responsibility, and learn from life's experiences.

Physical Changes

The rate of growth during these early school years is slower than any time since birth but continues steadily. A particular child may not follow the pattern precisely. The school-age child appears slimmer than the preschooler, as a result of changes in fat distribution and thickness (Edelman and Mandle, 2002). Growth accelerates at different times for different children. The average increase in height is 2 inches per year, and weight, which is more variable, increases by 4 to 7 pounds per year. An average 6-year-old is 45 inches tall and weighs 46 pounds; the average 12-year-old is 59 inches tall and weighs 88 pounds. Many children double their weight during these middle childhood years (Hockenberry and others, 2003).

School provides children with the opportunity to compare themselves with large numbers of children of the same age. The physical examination usually required for entrance to formal school is an excellent opportunity for the nurse to discuss with the child and parents the influences of genetic endowment, nutrition, and exercise on height and weight. Annual measurement of height and weight may reveal alterations in growth that are symptoms of the onset of a variety of childhood diseases.

Boys are slightly taller and heavier than girls during these early school years. Approximately 2 years before puberty, children experience a rapid acceleration in skeletal growth. Girls, who reach puberty first, begin to surpass boys in height and weight, which causes embarrassment to both sexes. These changes may begin as early as 9 years in girls but do not usually occur in boys before 12 years of age.

Cardiovascular functioning is refined and stabilized during the school-age years. The heart rate averages 70 to 90 beats per minute, the blood pressure normalizes to approximately 110/70 mm Hg, and the respiratory rate stabilizes to 19 to 21 breaths per minute. Lung growth is minimal, and respirations become slower, deeper, and more regular. However, by the end of this period the heart is 6 times the size it was at birth and has generally reached its adult size.

School-age children become more graceful during the school years because their large muscle coordination improves and their strength doubles. Most children practice the basic gross motor skills of running, jumping, balancing, throwing, and catching during play, resulting in refinement of neuromuscular function and skills. Individual differences in the rate of mastering skills and ultimate skill achievement become apparent during their participation in their many activities and games. Fine motor skills improve and as control is gained over fingers and wrists, children become proficient in a wide range of activities.

Most 6-year-old children can hold a pencil adeptly and print letters and words, but by age 12 the child can make detailed drawings and write sentences in script. Painting, drawing, playing computer games, and modeling allow children to practice and improve newly refined skills. Nurses should encourage children and have parents encourage them to pursue these activities. Table 11-6 describes specific gross motor and fine motor skills and their use in self-care activities.

The improved fine motor capabilities of youngsters in middle childhood allow them to become very independent in bathing, dressing, and taking care of other personal needs. They develop strong personal preferences in the way these needs are met. Illness and hospitalization threaten children's control in these areas. Therefore it is important to allow them to participate in care and maintain as much independence as possible. Children whose care demands restriction of fluids cannot be allowed to decide the amount of fluids they will drink in 24 hours, but they can help decide the type of fluids and can help keep a record of intake.

Assessment of neurological development is often based on fine motor coordination. This assessment may include penmanship, stacking ability, and performance of sequential, rapid, alternating movements such as touching the finger to the nose and then to the examiner's finger (smooth movement without tremors is the normal response). Fine motor coordination is critical to success in the typical American school, where children must be able to hold pencils and crayons and use scissors and rulers. The opportunity to practice these skills through schoolwork and play is essential to the acquisition of coordinated, complex behaviors.

Other physical changes take place during the school-age years. Steady skeletal growth in the trunk and extremities occurs, and small- and long-bone ossification is present but not complete by age 12. Dental growth is prominent during the school-age years. The first permanent or secondary teeth erupt at approximately 6 years of age. Development of the permanent teeth has been occurring for some time prior to eruption. The root is absorbed, leaving the crown, which causes the tooth to become loose and fall out. This makes room for the new permanent teeth. Eruption usually begins with the 6-year molar and follows the same order as with the primary teeth. By 12 years, all primary teeth have been shed, and the majority of permanent teeth have erupted. Infrequent or inadequate dental care remains a persistent problem for many American children.

Table 11-6   Motor Development in the School-Age Child

6-7 Years	8-10 Years	11-12 Years
Fine Motor Skills		
Uses knife to butter bread and learns to cut tender meat	Uses knife and fork simultaneously	Learns to peel apples and potatoes
Cuts, folds, and pastes paper	Learns to thread needle and tie knot	Sews simple garments on machine
Prints with pencil	Uses hammer, saw, and screwdriver	Builds simple objects like birdhouse
Draws man with 12-16 details	Becomes proficient at writing cursive	Enjoys using decorative script
Copies triangle at 6 years and diamond by 7 years	Uses symbols in drawing (e.g., bird, star)	Begins to use creative and artistic talents
Colors within lines of picture	Builds simple models of cars and planes and does simple handcrafts	Builds complex models of cars and planes and does complex handcrafts
Needs assistance to clean teeth thoroughly	Learns to play jacks and marbles	Learns to play musical instrument
	Can learn to floss teeth effectively and be independent in tooth care	Becomes proficient in caring for teeth with braces and other appliances
Gross Motor Skills		
Remains in constant motion	Can catch, throw (70 feet), and hit baseball	Can do standing broad jump of 5 feet
Moves more cautiously at 7 years than at 6 years	Engages in alternate rhythmic hopping in 2-2, 2-3, or 3-3 pattern	Can do standing high jump of 3 feet
Hops and jumps into small squares	Engages in complex styles of skipping rope accompanied by verbal jingles	Plays games involving simultaneous use of two or more complex motor skills such as roller skating, ice hockey, or dance skating
Learns to roller skate, skip rope, ride bicycle, and swim		
Self-Care		
Takes bath without supervision	Learns to clean bathroom after bath	Dusts, vacuums, and straightens own room
Often returns to finger feeding	Enjoys fixing own snacks and sack lunch	Learns to cook simply prepared foods
Learns to brush and comb hair in acceptable fashion without help	Learns to part hair and insert hair ribbons and barrettes	Washes, dries, and fixes own hair in braids, curls, and ponytails
Puts on most clothes but may need assistance with shirttails, sashes, and final adjustments	Dresses self completely and can help younger siblings with clothes	Learns to sort, wash, dry, and press own clothing
	Can make own bed	Learns to care for fingernails and toenails

As skeletal growth progresses, body appearance and posture change. Earlier posture, which was characterized by a stoop-shouldered, slight lordosis and prominent abdomen, changes to a more erect posture. It is essential that children, especially girls after the age of 12 years, be evaluated for scoliosis, the lateral curvature of the spine.

Eye shape alters because of skeletal growth. This improves visual acuity, and normal adult 20/20 vision is achievable. Screening for vision and hearing problems is easier, and results are more reliable because school-age children can more fully understand and cooperate with the test directions. The school nurse typically assesses the dental, visual, and auditory status of school-age children and refers those with possible deviations to a health care provider, such as their family practitioner or pediatrician.

Cognitive Changes

Cognitive changes provide the school-age child with the ability to think in a logical manner about the here and now and to understand the relationship between things and ideas (Hockenberry and others, 2003). The thoughts of school-age children are no longer dominated by their perceptions, and thus their ability to understand the world greatly expands. Around 7 years of age, children enter Piaget's third stage of cognitive development, known as **concrete operations,** in which they are able to use symbols to carry out operations (mental activities) in thought rather than in action. They begin to use logical thought processes with concrete materials (objects, people, and events they can touch and see).

Children in the concrete operational stage are considerably less egocentric than younger children and develop the ability to concentrate on more than one aspect of a situation. School-age children now have the ability to recognize that the amount or quantity of a substance remains the same even when its shape or appearance changes. For instance, two balls of clay of equal size remain the same amount of clay even when one is flattened and the other remains in ball shape.

The mental process of **classification** becomes more complex during the school years. The young child can separate objects into groups according to shape or color, whereas the school-age child understands that the same element can exist in two classes at the same time. School-age children have the ability to place objects in order according to their increasing or decreasing size, which develops by age 7 or 8. The school-age child is becoming a "thinker" and is less egocentric and capable of understanding another's views and feelings (Bukatko and Daehler, 2001).

Middle childhood youngsters can use their newly developed cognitive skills to solve problems. Some individuals are better than others at problem solving because of native intelligence, education, and experience, but all children can improve these skills. Middle school-age children who are good problem solvers demonstrate the following characteristics: a positive attitude that the problem can be solved with persistence, a concern for accuracy, the ability to divide the problem into parts for study, and the ability to avoid guessing while searching for facts. Techniques that adults can use to help children improve their problem-solving strategies include helping them define the problem and its nature, plan and then evaluate their solution. Nurses can use these strategies to help school-age children understand their illness and assume responsibility for their general health.

Language Development. Language growth is so rapid during middle childhood that it is no longer possible to match age with language achievements. Children improve their use of language and expand their structural knowledge. They become more aware of the rules of syntax, the rules for linking words into phrases and sentences. They can also identify generalizations and exceptions to rules. They accept language as a means for representing the world in a subjective manner and realize that words have arbitrary, rather than absolute, meanings. They can use different words for the same object or concept, and they understand that a single word may have many meanings. Similar to younger children, school-age children watch parents and other adults to gain clues about how to understand events (Deering and Cody, 2002). Many school-age children use "bad language" to gain peer status and to shock adults. It often begins with bathroom language and progresses to sexual or genital words. Children begin to think about language, which enables them to appreciate jokes and riddles. Language acquisition is nurtured by social interactions with their parents and caretakers (Bukatko and Daehler, 2001).

Psychosocial Changes

Erikson (1963) identifies the developmental task for school-age children as industry versus inferiority. During this time, children strive to acquire competence and skills necessary for them to function as adults. School-age children who are positively recognized for success feel a sense of worth. Those faced with failure can feel a sense of mediocrity or unworthiness, which may result in withdrawal from school and peers.

Moral Development. The need for a moral code and social rules becomes more evident as school-age children's cognitive abilities and social experiences increase. For example, 12-year-old children are able to consider what society would be like without rules because of their ability to reason logically and their experiences with group play. They view rules as necessary principles of life, not just dictates from authorities. In the early school years, children strictly interpret and adhere to rules. As they develop, they make more flexible judgments and evaluate

rules for applicability to a given situation. School-age children consider motivations and the actual behavior when making judgments about the way that their behaviors affect themselves and others. The ability to be flexible when applying rules and to take the perspective of others is essential in developing moral judgments. These abilities are present at times in earlier years but are more consistently displayed in later school years.

Peer Relationships. Group and personal achievements become important to the school-age child. Success is important in physical and cognitive activities. Play involves peers and the pursuit of group goals. Although solitary activities are not eliminated, they are overshadowed by group play. Learning to contribute, collaborate, and work cooperatively toward a common goal becomes a measure of success (Figure 11-7).

The school-age child prefers same-sex peers to opposite-sex peers. In general, girls and boys view the opposite sex negatively. Peer influence becomes quite diverse during this stage of development. Conformity is evidenced in mannerisms, clothing styles, and speech patterns, which are reinforced and influenced by contact with peers. During this time period, clubs and peer groups become prominent. Group identity increases as the school-age child approaches adolescence.

Sexual Identity. Freud described middle childhood as the latency period because he felt that children of this period had little interest in their sexuality. Today many researchers believe that school-age children have a great deal of curiosity about their sexuality. Some may experiment, but this play is usually transitory. Children's curiosity about adult magazines or meanings of sexually explicit words is also an example of their sexual interest.

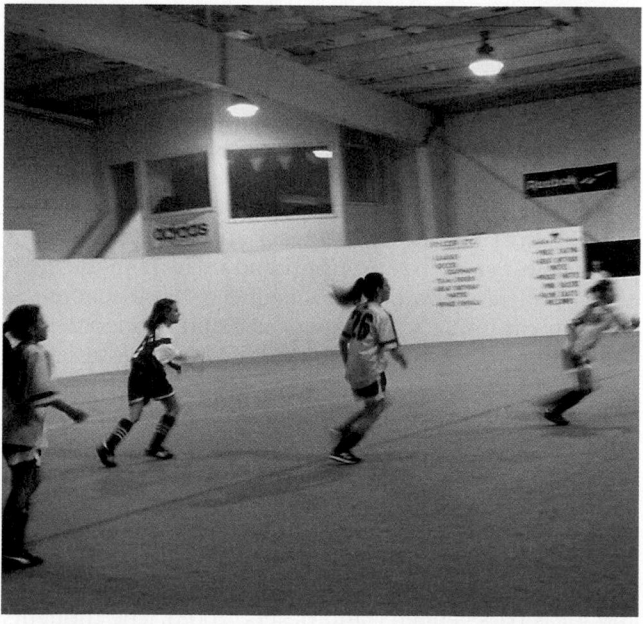

FIGURE **11-7** School-age children gain a sense of achievement working and playing with peers. (Courtesy Elaine Polan, RNC, BSN, MS.)

This is the time for children to have exposure to sex education, including sexual maturation, reproduction, and relationships (Edelman and Mandle, 2002).

While the child goes through the adjustments in this stage, the nurse assists in promoting health. This is done by helping the parents and child to identify potential stressors and by designing interventions to minimize stress and the child's stress response. Interventions must include parent, child, and teacher for maximal success. Box 11-9 provides an overview of stressors commonly encountered by school-age children and appropriate nursing interventions.

Health Risks

Accidents and injuries are a major health problem affecting school-age children. Motor vehicle accidents and accidents related to recreational activities or equipment are the leading causes of death or injury from age 1 to adulthood (Edelman and Mandle, 2002). These unintentional injuries account for nearly half of all childhood deaths (Table 11-7).

Box 11-9   Potential Sources of Stress in Middle Childhood*

Sources of Stress for the 6-Year-Old

Expectations—Parents, teachers, and other adults begin to demand more

School—First grade introduces the child to the more formal academic setting

Activity level—May find it difficult to sit still for long periods of time; may have frequent accidents, such as spilling milk

Competition—The child wants to be "first" or best

Shyness—May initially be shy in a new situation but usually recovers quickly

Aggression—May become hostile or aggressive; temper tantrums peak

Sensitivity—Begins to read body language or facial expressions and becomes upset when disapproval is sensed

Teasing—Engages in teasing, but becomes upset when on the receiving end

Decisions—Has difficulty coping with increasing independence

Jealousy—Sibling rivalry is common

Fears—Usually center around newly found independence and might include fear of getting lost or fear of making an embarrassing social blunder

Sources of Stress for the 7-Year-Old

Moodiness —Is often moody, unhappy, or pensive

Approval—Continues to need praise and approval from peer group and parents

Modesty—Demands privacy when in the bathroom or dressing

Organization—Is comfortable with rules, regulations, routines, and order; becomes upset when they are disrupted

Interruptions—Hates to be disturbed when intensely involved in an activity

Idols—Has a desire to be more like an admired idol

Friendship—Becomes more selective about playmates

Sources of Stress for the 8-Year-Old

Self-criticism—Is very critical of personal ability and performance

Parental authority—Is beginning to resent parental authority

Loneliness—Likes frequent interaction with friends; may hate to miss school

Praise—Continues to seek approval but can identify when praise is not genuine

Independence—Many begin to stay alone for brief periods of time while parents run errands, with resulting feelings of uneasiness

Sources of Stress for the 9-Year-Old

Rebelliousness—Occasionally tests independence by rebelling

Opposite sex—Engages in sex-segregated play, expresses an aversion to the opposite sex

Fair play—Has a keen sense of what is fair and is vehement in demanding personal rights when a situation is perceived as unfair

Interruptions—Continues to dislike interruptions but will usually resume an activity after an interruption

Propriety—Has a sense of propriety and will often be upset if siblings or parents offend the child's notion of decorum or dignity

Sources of Stress for the 10- to 12-Year-Old

Sexual maturation—Girls, in particular, may become self-conscious regarding obvious signs of development

Social issues—A new level of awareness can generate concern regarding pressing societal problems

Size—Both boys and girls may be upset by the fact that the girls are taller; the extremely small or extremely large child may be concerned about his or her size

Shyness—If the child already has a problem in this area, it is likely to become more pronounced at this stage

Opposite sex—May become interested, yet shy, around members of the opposite sex

Confusion—Too much freedom can cause the child to flounder

Health—It is not uncommon for a child to become a hypochondriac during this period of development

Money—Child is anxious to earn and handle money, but often uses poor judgment

Competition—Continues to be highly competitive and looks to peer group for prestige

Burnout—Child may become vigorously involved in so many activities that he or she finally becomes exhausted

Self-concept—May engage in teasing, scapegoating, or vicious attacks to temporarily boost his or her self-image; guilt often ensues; may be self-conscious about attempting a new skill

Parents—Often becomes highly critical or intolerant of parents

Idols—Continues hero worshipping

Fair play—Continues to have a highly developed sense of fair play

Drugs and sex—May be tempted to experiment with drugs or sex because "everyone" is doing it

Peer pressure—Becomes a powerful motivating force

Self-criticism—Child may be highly critical of personal performance

From Kuczen B: *Childhood stress: don't let your child be a victim,* New York, 1982, Delacorte Press.
*Violence is a universal stress at all ages.

Table 11-7 Injury Prevention During School-Age Years

Developmental Abilities Related to Risk of Injury	Injury Prevention
Motor Vehicles	
Is increasingly involved in activities away from home Is excited by speed and motion Can be reasoned with Does not always perceive injury risk Is easily distracted by environment	Educate child regarding proper use of seat belts while a passenger in a vehicle Maintain discipline while a passenger in a vehicle (e.g., keep arms inside, do not lean against doors or interfere with driver) Remind parents and children that no one should ride in the bed of a pickup truck Emphasize safe pedestrian behavior Insist on wearing safety apparel (e.g., helmet) where applicable, such as when riding a bicycle, motorcycle, moped, or all-terrain vehicle
Drowning	
Is apt to overdo May work hard to perfect a skill Is cautious, but not fearful	Teach child to swim Teach basic rules of water safety Select safe and supervised places to swim Check sufficient water depth for diving Swim with a companion Use an approved flotation device in water or boat Advocate for legislation requiring fencing around pools Learn CPR
Burns	
Has increasing independence Enjoys trying new things	Make sure smoke detectors are in homes Set hot water temperatures (120°-130° F) to avoid scald burns Instruct child in behavior in areas involving contact with potential burn hazards (e.g., gasoline, matches, bonfires or barbecues, lighter fluid, firecrackers, cigarette lighters, cooking utensils, chemistry sets); avoid climbing or flying kites around high-tension wires Instruct child in proper behavior in the event of fire (e.g., fire drills at home and school) Teach child safe cooking (use low heat, avoid any frying, be careful of steam burns, scalds, or exploding foods, especially from microwaving)
Substance Abuse and Poisoning	
May be easily influenced by peers Has strong allegiance to friends	Educate child regarding hazards of taking nonprescription drugs and chemicals, including aspirin and alcohol Teach child to say "no" if offered illegal or dangerous drugs or alcohol Keep potentially dangerous products in properly labeled receptacles—preferably locked and out of reach
Bodily Damage	
Has increased physical skills Needs strenuous physical activity Is interested in acquiring new skills and perfecting attained skills Is daring and adventurous, especially with peers Frequently plays in hazardous places Confidence often exceeds physical capacity Desires group loyalty and has strong need for friends' approval Attempts hazardous feats Accompanies friends to potentially hazardous facilities Delights in physical activity Is likely to overdo Growth in height exceeds muscular growth and coordination	Help provide facilities for supervised activities Encourage playing in safe places Keep firearms safely locked up except during adult supervision Teach proper care of, use of, and respect for devices with potential danger (e.g., power tools, firecrackers) Teach children not to tease or surprise dogs, invade their territory, take dogs' toys, or interfere with dogs' feeding Stress eye, ear, or mouth protection when using potentially hazardous objects or devices or when engaged in potentially hazardous sports (e.g., baseball) Teach safety regarding use of corrective devices (glasses); if child wears contact lenses, monitor duration of wear to prevent corneal damage Stress careful selection, use, and maintenance of sports and recreation equipment such as skateboards and in-line skates Emphasize proper conditioning, safe practices, and use of safety equipment for sports or recreational activities Caution against engaging in hazardous sports, such as those involving trampolines Use safety glass and decals on large glassed areas, such as sliding glass doors Use window guards to prevent falls Teach name, address, and phone number and to ask for help from appropriate people (cashier, security guard, policeman) if lost; have identification on child (sewn in clothes, inside shoe) Teach stranger safety: Avoid personalized clothing in public places Caution child to never go with a stranger Have child tell parents if anyone makes child feel uncomfortable in any way Always listen to child's concerns regarding others' behavior Teach child to say "no" when confronted with uncomfortable situations

From Hockenberry MJ and others: *Wong's nursing care of infants and children*, ed 7, St. Louis, 2003, Mosby.

Although falls account for a major portion of pediatric hospital admissions, they account for less than 5% of pediatric deaths resulting from injury. More children die from automobile accidents than from all major preventable childhood diseases. The rates of injury and death have begun to decrease with the institution of automobile child restraint laws.

School-age children are also significantly affected by cancer, birth defects, homicide, and heart disease (Hockenberry and others, 2003). In this age-group, these problems have a relatively low mortality rate but a high morbidity rate compared to accidents. Cancers are the second leading cause of death in children 1 to 14 years of age (Hockenberry and others, 2003). Leukemia is the most frequent type, with brain tumors and lymphoma second and third, respectively.

Infections account for the majority of all childhood illnesses; respiratory infections are the most prevalent. The common cold remains the chief illness of childhood. Certain groups of children are more prone to disease and disability, often as a result of barriers to health care. Mental retardation, learning disorders, sensory impairments, and malnutrition are far more prevalent among children living in poverty (USDHHS, 2000).

Poverty and the prevalence of illness are highly correlated. Access to care is often very limited and health promotion and preventative health care activities are minimal. Infant mortality, dental problems, poor nutrition, and lack of immunizations continue to be major health concerns for uninsured or impoverished families. Education, social and health care reform, and environmental change are necessary if the nurse wants to positively influence the health of children. Children's developing cognitive and psychomotor skills make it possible for them to become more involved in health promotion and the management of chronic illness.

Health Concerns

Perceptions. During the school-age years, identity and self-concept become stronger and more individualized. Perception of wellness is based on readily observable facts such as presence or absence of illness and adequacy of eating or sleeping. Functional ability is the standard by which personal health and the health of others are judged.

Six-year-olds are aware of their body and modest and sensitive about being exposed. Nurses should provide for privacy and offer explanations of common procedures. This helps foster children's self-esteem and lessen their fear of pain and intrusion (Popovich, 2000).

Health Education. The school-age period is a crucial period for the acquisition of behaviors and health practices for a healthy adult life. Because cognition is advancing during the period, effective health education must be developmentally appropriate. Promotion of good health practices is a nursing responsibility. Programs directed at health education are frequently organized and conducted in the school. Edelman and Mandle (2002) identify the critical aspects of school-based health promotion programs (Box 11-10).

During these programs, the nurse focuses on the development of behaviors that positively affect children's

---

> **Box 11-10   Critical Functions of School-Based Health Promotion Program**
>
> Promote health teaching appropriate to cognitive level of functioning.
> Assess child's understanding of cause of illness.
> Reinforce health promotion and illness prevention measures.
> Foster parental education on health issues.
> Facilitate growth and self-actualization.
> Emphasize positive health attitudes.
> Foster positive life skills that enhance successful coping.

---

health status. School-age children should receive age-appropriate human immunodeficiency virus (HIV) education that begins before the onset of sexual activity (Behrman, Kliegman, and Jenson, 2000). Other topic areas for elementary health education curricula that are consistent with *Healthy People 2010* include the promotion of adequate nutrition, oral hygiene, and regular health supervision. School-age children should also be exposed to programs that highlight tobacco and alcohol use prevention (USDHHS, 2000).

Nurses also instruct parents regarding health promotion appropriate for the school-age child. Parents need to recognize the importance of annual health maintenance visits for immunizations, screenings, and dental care. When their school-age child reaches 10 years of age, parents need to begin discussions in preparation for upcoming pubertal changes. Topics should include introductory information regarding menstruation, sexual intercourse, and reproduction. Nurses should provide age-appropriate written materials to aid parents in their efforts. The settings where health promotion activities can occur are varied. These include the classroom, school nurse's office, school-based clinic, community-based clinic, or in the community itself.

Examples of topics that encourage positive behaviors by children are dental health and illness prevention. Table 11-8 presents a comprehensive list of health promotion topics.

Safety. Because accidents are the leading cause of death and injury in the school-age period, safety is a priority health teaching consideration. Nurses can contribute to the general health of children by educating them about safety measures to prevent accidents. At this age, children should be encouraged to take responsibility for their own safety.

Nutrition. Nurses can contribute to meeting national policy goals by promoting healthy lifestyle habits, including nutrition. School-age children should participate in educational programs that enable them to plan, select, and prepare healthy meals and snacks. These foods should be consistent with the U.S. Department of Agriculture food guide pyramid nutritional guidelines limiting intake of total and saturated fats and increasing the intake of complex carbohydrates, fruits, and vegeta-

Table 11-8 — Health Promotion in the School-Age Period

School-Age Health Concerns	Health Promotion Interventions
Nutrition	Provide nutrition education that promotes healthy lifestyle: food guide pyramid; limiting fat intake to 30% of calories, saturated fat to 10% of calories.
Oral hygiene	Provide examples of low cariogenic snacks.
	Review mechanics of dental hygiene: brushing, flossing.
	Stress importance of biannual dental checkups.
Infections	Provide immunization information and follow-up.
	Teach infection prevention practices (hand washing, care of minor skin injuries).
	Teach concepts of viral and bacterial illness.
Tobacco, alcohol, and drug use	Provide tobacco use prevention programs.
	Provide information regarding the hazards of drug use.
Human sexuality	Provide information about sexual maturation and reproduction in age-appropriate manner.
	Encourage parents to view their child's sexual curiosity as part of the developmental process.
	Discuss with parents the learning needs of their child regarding sexuality.
	Provide age-appropriate HIV education.

Box 11-11 — School-Based Interventions to Promote Nutrition Education

Have young children collect pictures of healthy foods and make a poster for display in the school cafeteria.

Make healthy foods (fruits, vegetables, whole grains, low-fat snacks) available in school vending machines and at school sporting events.

Discourage the use of high-fat foods (candy bars) as part of school fund-raising projects.

Avoid the use of food as rewards for behavior; use verbal praise and token gifts to reinforce healthy eating and physical activity.

Have teachers and school personnel model healthy eating habits.

Ask children to select foods from a fast-food restaurant menu and to identify those foods high in fat, cholesterol, and sodium.

Ask each child to keep a diary of foods eaten in 1 day; using the food guide pyramid, evaluate these foods.

Incorporate nutrition education into other classes (such as using a computer to analyze the nutritional content of foods).

Have students keep a diary to identify cues for their eating behavior (e.g., hunger, stress, other people, social situations).

Teach students how to read and discuss the nutrition labels on foods.

Ask students to examine television commercials, magazine advertisements, and billboards to identify social influences on eating and physical activities.

Use role-playing to help students learn to cope with social and peer pressures to eat specific foods.

Have students identify environmental barriers to healthy eating.

Have students prepare nutritious foods, plan menus, and develop a recipe book of healthy foods.

Involve parents in nutrition education through homework assignments or by inviting parents to attend student-led nutrition fairs.

Modified from Center for Communicable Diseases: Guidelines for school programs to promote lifelong healthy eating, *J Sch Health* 67:9, 1996.

bles. Box 11-11 outlines several learning activities appropriate for this age-group. In addition, nurses need to promote an increase in the number of children involved in daily physical activity.

Growth may slow down during the school-age period as compared to infancy and adolescence. Obesity is believed to begin during infancy and childhood (Edelman and Mandle, 2002). Obesity places the child at increased risk for hypertension, diabetes, and coronary heart disease. Emotionally the obese child is at risk for problems caused by low self-esteem (Jerum and Melnyk, 2001). Obesity may occur because children often rush into the home after school or play and eat the most easily obtainable and appealing foods. Unfortunately, these foods are often high in calories and low in nutrition. Providing nutritious snacks is often the best way for a parent to ensure good nutritional intake. Caregivers should provide ready access to fresh fruit, raw vegetables, cheese, popcorn, and high-protein snacks such as skim-milk pudding and hot chocolate. Children should be praised when making healthy food choices (Jerum and Melnyk, 2001). Nurses must consider cultural, economic, and social issues when planning successful interventions (Edelman and Mandle, 2002).

Nurses can help families and children prevent obesity through proper nutrition and exercise. Today's families may often eat in fast-food restaurants where the food is high in fat, calories, and salt. Nurses need to encourage healthy food choices in these situations. Selections should include meats that are not breaded and are broiled, shakes that are made with low-fat yogurt or skim milk, and fruits and vegetables that are fresh or prepared in a low-calorie manner.

Preadolescent

Preadolescence or early adolescence, also known as **puberty,** is a transitional period between childhood and adolescence. The onset of preadolescence or puberty is varied and influenced by heredity (Berk, 2003). There will be changes in body size as well as other physical changes.

The primary sexual characteristic involving the reproductive organs mature. The visible secondary sexual characteristic changes such as the development of pubic hair and female breasts begin. These physical changes often begin about 2 years earlier in girls than boys. In addition, children become much more social, and their behavioral patterns become much less predictable. Cultural variations exist in rapidity of growth. For example, African-American youths obtain a greater proportion of their adult stature earlier (Behrman, Kliegman, and Jenson, 2000). This preparatory period often includes experimentation with makeup by girls and an interest in music and performers that are popular among older adolescents. Both sexes usually develop "best friends" with whom they share intimate feelings. New interest in the opposite sex develops. Youths of both sexes often develop a friendship with adults other than their parents (ego ideal), which allows them to acquire information about grown-ups.

Adolescent

Adolescence is the period of development during which the individual makes the transition from childhood to adulthood, usually between 13 and 20 years. The term *adolescent* usually refers to psychological maturation of the individual, whereas *puberty* refers to the point at which reproduction becomes possible. The hormonal changes of puberty result in changes in the appearance of the young person, and mental development results in the ability to hypothesize and deal with abstractions. Adjustments and adaptations are needed to cope with these simultaneous changes and the attempt to establish a mature sense of identity. In the past, many have referred to adolescence as a stormy and stressful period filled with inner turmoil, but today it is recognized that most teenagers successfully meet the challenges of this period. These challenges may cause the adolescent to be moody and difficult. Within adolescence, three subphases exist: early (pre) adolescence (11 to 14 years), middle adolescence (15 to 17 years), and late adolescence (18 to 20 years). Opportunities, challenges, changes, skills, pressures, and physical, cognitive, and psychosocial development vary widely between the subphases (Table 11-9).

The nurse's understanding of development provides a unique perspective for helping teenagers and parents anticipate and cope with the stresses of adolescence. Nursing activities, particularly education, can promote healthy development. These activities occur in a variety of settings and can be directed at the adolescent, parents, or both. For example, the nurse can conduct seminars in a high school to provide practical suggestions for solving problems of concern to a large group of students, such as treating acne or making responsible decisions about drugs or alcohol use. Similarly, a group education program for parents about how to cope with teenagers would promote parental understanding of adolescent development. These programs can be held in the school, clinic, private office, or community center. To learn more about specific topics or problems, the nurse must identify teenagers' needs and desires. Involvement produces more active, interested learners.

Physical Changes

Physical changes occur rapidly in adolescence. Sexual maturation occurs with the development of primary and secondary sexual characteristics. Four main focuses of the physical changes are:
1. Increased growth rate of skeleton, muscle, and viscera
2. Sex-specific changes, such as changes in shoulder and hip width
3. Alteration in distribution of muscle and fat
4. Development of the reproductive system and secondary sex characteristics

Wide variation exists in the timing of physical changes associated with puberty between sexes and within the same sex. Girls tend to begin their physical changes earlier than boys. Variations are more pronounced in boys (Behrman, Kliegman, and Jenson, 2000). The sequence of pubertal growth changes is the same in most individuals (Table 11-10).

Changes are created by hormonal changes within the body when the hypothalamus begins to produce gonadotropin-releasing hormones. This sends the pituitary a signal to secrete gonadotropic hormones. Gonadotropic hormones stimulate ovarian cells to produce **estrogen** and testicular cells to produce **testosterone.** These hormones contribute to the development of secondary sex characteristics such as hair growth and voice changes and play an essential role in reproduction. The changing concentrations of these hormones are also linked to acne and body odor. Understanding these hormonal changes enables the nurse to reassure adolescents and educate them about body care needs.

Boys who mature early have been shown by some researchers to be more poised, relaxed, good-natured, skilled in athletic activities, and more likely to be school leaders than boys who mature late. In contrast, girls who mature early have been found to be less sociable and more shy and introverted, perhaps from feeling so conspicuous (Edelman and Mandle, 2002).

The ranges of normal are stressed. As with increases in height and weight, the pattern of sexual changes is more significant than their time of onset. Large deviations from normal frames require investigation. Being like peers is extremely important for adolescents (Figure 11-8).

Any deviation in the timing of the physical changes can be extremely difficult for adolescents to accept. The nurse should therefore provide emotional support for those undergoing early or delayed puberty. Even adolescents whose physical changes are occurring at the normal times may seek confirmation of and reassurance about their normalcy.

Height and weight increases usually occur during the prepubertal growth spurt. The growth spurt for girls generally begins between 8 and 14 years of age. Height increases 2 to 8 inches, and weight increases by 15 to 55 pounds. The male growth spurt usually takes place between 10 and 16 years of age. Height increases approximately 4 to 12 inches, and weight increases by 15 to 65 pounds. The final 20% to 25% of adult height and 50% of adult weight is gained during this time period (Hockenberry and others, 2003).

Girls attain 90% to 95% of their adult height by **menarche** (the onset of menstruation) and reach their

Table 11-9   Growth and Development During Adolescence

Early Adolescence (11-14 years)	Middle Adolescence (14-17 years)	Late Adolescence (17-20 years)
Growth		
Rapidly accelerating growth reaches peak velocity Secondary sex characteristics appear	Growth decelerating in girls Stature reaches 95% of adult height Secondary sex characteristics well-advanced	Physically mature Structure and reproductive growth almost complete
Cognition		
Explores newfound ability for limited abstract thought Clumsy groping for new values and energies Comparison of "normality" with peers of same sex	Developing capacity for abstract thinking Enjoys intellectual powers, often in idealistic terms Concern with philosophic, political, and social problems	Establishes abstract thought Can perceive and act on long-range operations Able to view problems comprehensively Intellectual and functional identity established
Identity		
Preoccupied with rapid body changes Tries out various roles Measurement of attractiveness by acceptance or rejection of peers Conformity to group norms	Modifies body image Very self-centered; increased narcissism Tendency toward inner experience and self-discovery Has a rich fantasy life Idealistic Able to perceive future implications of current behavior and decisions; variable application	Body image and gender-role definition nearly secured Mature sexual identity Phase of consolidation of identity Stability of self-esteem Comfortable with physical growth Social roles defined and articulated
Relationships With Parents		
Defining independence-dependence boundaries Strong desire to remain dependent on parents while trying to detach No major conflicts over parental control	Major conflicts over independence and control Low point in parent-child relationship Greatest push for emancipation; disengagement Final and irreversible emotional detachment from parents; mourning	Emotional and physical separation from parents completed Independence from family with less conflict Emancipation nearly secured
Relationships With Peers		
Seeks peer affiliations to counter instability generated by rapid change Upsurge of close, idealized friendships with members of the same sex Struggle for mastery takes place within peer group	Strong need for identity to affirm self-image Behavioral standards set by peer group Acceptance by peers extremely important—fear of rejection Exploration of ability to attract the opposite sex	Peer group recedes in importance in favor of individual friendship Testing of male-female relationships against possibility of permanent alliance Relationships characterized by giving and sharing
Sexuality		
Self-exploration and evaluation Limited dating, usually socializes with a group Limited intimacy	Multiple plural relationships Decisive turn toward heterosexuality (if is homosexual, knows by this time) Exploration of "self-appeal" Feeling of "being in love" Tentative establishment of relationships	Forms stable relationships and attachment to another Growing capacity for mutuality and reciprocity Dating as a male-female pair Intimacy involves commitment rather than exploration and romanticism
Psychological Health		
Wide mood swings Intense daydreaming Anger outwardly expressed with moodiness, temper outbursts, and verbal insults and name-calling	Tendency toward inner experiences; more introspective Tendency to withdraw when upset or feelings are hurt Vacillation of emotions in time and range Feelings of inadequacy common; difficulty in asking for help	More constancy of emotion Anger more apt to be concealed

From Hockenberry MJ and others: *Wong's nursing care of infants and children*, ed 7, St. Louis, 2003, Mosby.

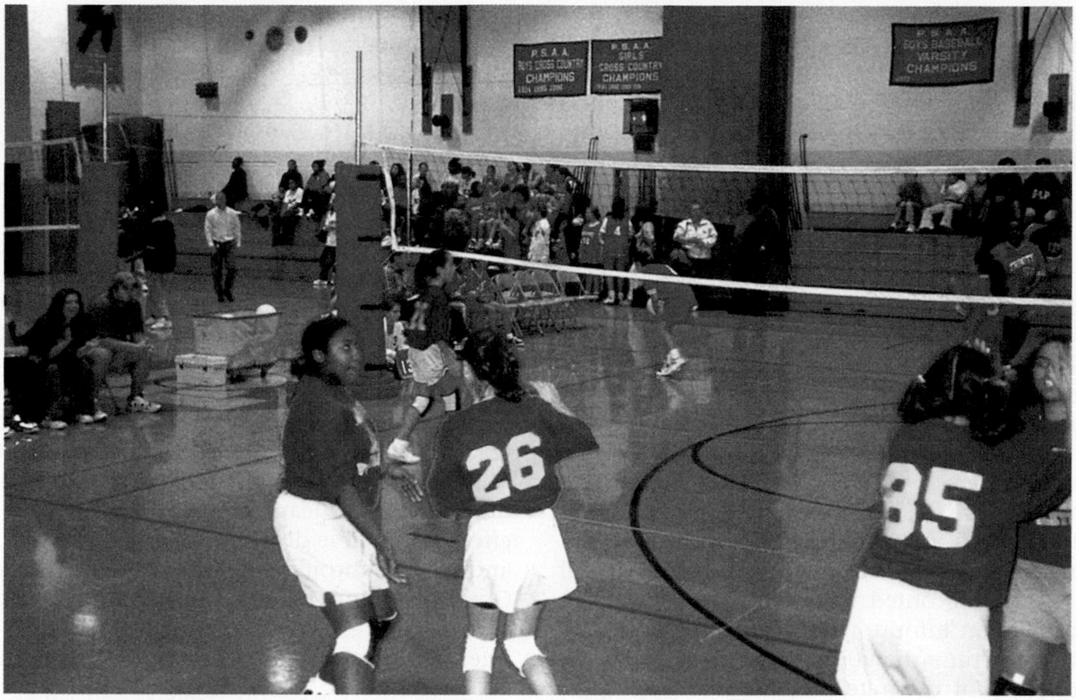

FIGURE **11-8** Peer interactions help increase self-esteem during puberty. (Courtesy Elaine Polan, RNC, BSN, MS.)

Table 11-10	Average Sequences of Physiological Changes in Adolescence	
Characteristics	**Girls***	**Boys***
Beginning of skeletal growth spurt	8-14½ (peak: 12)	10½-16 (peak: 14)
Beginning of breast development	8-13	
Enlargement of testes and scrotal sac		10-13½
Appearance of straight, pigmented pubic hair, which gradually becomes curly	8-14	10-15
Early voice changes (cracks)		11-14½
Enlargement of penis and prostate gland		11-14½
Menarche	10-18 (average: 12¼)	
Spermatogenesis (ejaculation of sperm)		11-17 (average: 13½)
Ovulation and completion of breast development	14-18 (average: 15½)	
Appearance of downy facial hair		12-17
Appearance of axillary (underarm) hair and increased output of oil and sweat-producing glands, which may lead to acne	10-16	12-17
Widening and deepening of female pelvis, with deposition of subcutaneous fat that gives rounded appearance to body	10-18	
Increase in shoulder width		11-21
Deepening of voice in males, with appearance of coarse and pigmented facial hair and appearance of chest hair		16-21

*Age range is in years.

full height by 16 to 17 years of age, whereas boys continue to grow taller until 18 to 20 years of age. Fat is redistributed into adult proportions as height and weight increase, and gradually the adolescent torso takes on an adult appearance. Although there are individual and sex differences, growth follows a similar pattern for both sexes. Growth in the length of the extremities occurs earliest, making the hands and feet appear very large and the legs very long; the individual often appears awkward and clumsy. At the same time the lower jaw and nose become

longer and the forehead higher and wider as the baby face of childhood disappears. Next the thighs widen; then the shoulders broaden, and growth of the trunk proceeds. Widening of the female hips and broadening of the male shoulders continue throughout adolescence.

Personal growth curves help the nurse assess physical development. The individual's sustained progression along the curve, however, is more important than a comparison to the norm. The nurse charts growth measurements during routine health assessments to evaluate changes.

Adolescents are sensitive about physical changes that make them different from peers. For this reason they are generally interested in the normal pattern of growth and their personal growth curves. Consequently, the nurse should share this information to reassure adolescents that their own patterns are normal.

Cognitive Changes

According to Piaget, the changes that occur within the mind and the widening social environment of the adolescent result in the highest level of intellectual development, known as formal operations. Without an appropriate educational environment, young persons who possess sufficient neurological development to reach this stage may not attain it, and those who are guided toward rational thinking may reach this stage early.

The adolescent develops the ability to determine possibilities, rank possibilities, solve problems, and make decisions through logical operations. The teenager can think abstractly and deal effectively with hypothetical problems. When confronted with a problem, the teenager can consider an infinite variety of causes and solutions. For the first time the young person can move beyond the physical or concrete properties of a situation and use reasoning powers to understand the abstract. School-age individuals think about what is, whereas adolescents can imagine what might be. These newly developed abilities allow the individual to have more insight and skill in playing games such as video games, computer games, and board games that require abstract thinking and deductive reasoning about many possible strategies. A teenager can even solve problems requiring simultaneous manipulation of several abstract concepts. Development of this ability is important in the pursuit of an identity. For example, newly acquired cognitive skills allow the teenager to define appropriate, effective, and comfortable sex-role behaviors and to consider their impact on peers, family, and society. The ability to think logically about these behaviors and their outcomes encourages the adolescent to develop personal thoughts and means of expressing sexual identity. In addition, a higher level of cognitive functioning makes the adolescent receptive to more detailed and diverse information about sexuality and sexual behaviors. For example, sex education can include an explanation of physiological sexual changes and birth control measures.

By midadolescence there is an introspective quality emerging with regard to cognition. At this time adolescents believe that they are unique and the exception, giving rise to their risk-taking behaviors. They often express that they "can drive fast and not get into an accident." Other typical adolescent behaviors includes self-consciousness and the desire for privacy.

The complex development of thought during this period leads adolescents to question society and its values. Although adolescents have the capability to think as well as an adult, they do not have experiences on which to build. It is common for teenagers to consider their parents too narrow minded or too materialistic. This can result in conflicts between teens and their parents. Cognitive abilities and performance vary greatly among adolescents. In fact, an adolescent may perform at different levels in different situations based on past experiences, formal education, and motivation in the use of logic and effective deductive reasoning.

Language Skills. Language development is fairly complete by adolescence, although vocabulary continues to expand. The primary focus becomes communication skills that can be used effectively in various situations. Adolescents need to communicate thoughts, feelings, and facts to peers, parents, teachers, and other persons of authority. The skills used in these diverse communication situations are varied. Adolescents must select the person with whom to communicate, decide on the exact message, and choose the way to transmit the message. For example, the way teenagers tell parents about failing grades is not the same as the way that they tell friends. Adolescents develop different skills and styles of communication and learn how and when to use them most effectively. These diverse communication skills are used and refined throughout life (Deering and Cody, 2002). Good communication skills are critical for adolescents in overcoming peer pressure and unhealthy behaviors. The following are some hints for communicating with adolescents:

- Do not avoid discussing sensitive issues. Asking questions about sex, drugs, and school opens the channels for further discussion.
- Ask open-ended questions.
- Look for the meaning behind their words or actions.
- Be alert to clues to their emotional state.
- Involve other individuals and resources when necessary.

Psychosocial Changes

The search for personal identity is the major task of adolescent psychosocial development. Teenagers must establish close peer relationships or remain socially isolated. Erikson (1963) sees identity (or role) confusion as the prime danger of this stage and suggests that the cliquishness and intolerance of differences seen in adolescent behavior are defenses against identity confusion (Erikson, 1968). Adolescents work at becoming emotionally independent from their parents, while retaining family ties. In addition, they need to develop their own ethical systems based on personal values. Choices about vocation, future education, and lifestyle must be made. The various components of total identity evolve from these tasks and compose adult personal identity that is unique to the individual. Indecisiveness and the inability to make an occupational choice are behaviors indicating negative resolution of the developmental task.

Sexual Identity. Achievement of sexual identity is enhanced by the physical changes of puberty. According to Freud these physiological changes of puberty stimulate the libido, the energy source that fuels the sex drive. This is evidenced by the teenager's interest in heterosexual relationships, as well as their practice of masturbation. The physical evidence of maturity encourages the development of masculine and feminine behaviors. If these physical changes involve deviations, the person has more difficulty developing a comfortable sexual identity. Adolescents de-

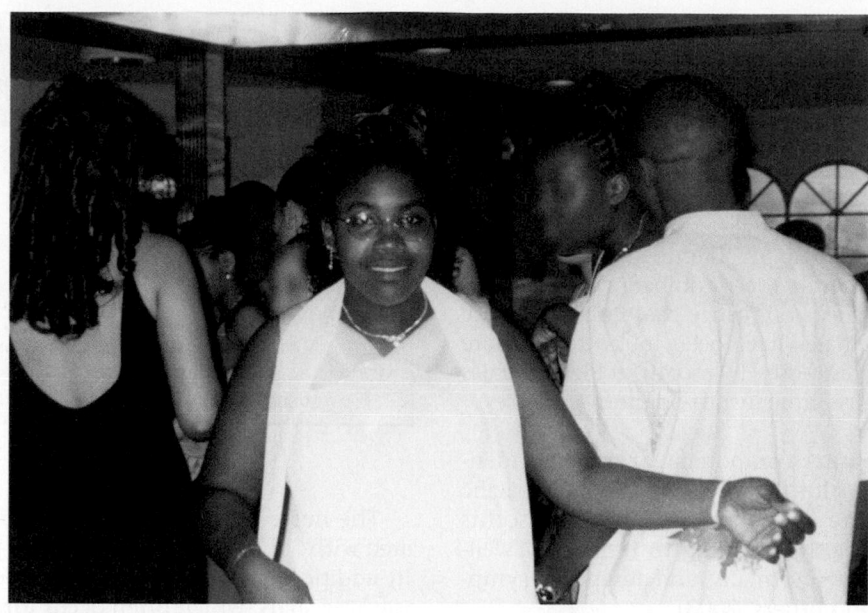

FIGURE **11–9**   Social interactions strengthen a teen's sexual identity. (Courtesy Elaine Polan, RNC, BSN, MS.)

pend on these physical clues because they want assurance of maleness or femaleness and because they do not wish to be different from peers.

Without these physical characteristics, achieving sexual identity is difficult. Other influences are cultural attitudes and expectations of sex-role behavior and available role models (Katz, 2003). The masculine and feminine behaviors that teenagers see affect the way that they express sexuality.

Group Identity. Adolescents seek a group identity because they need esteem and acceptance (Figure 11-9). Similarity in dress or speech is common in teenage groups. Popularity is a major concern for teens. Peer groups provide the adolescent with a sense of belonging, approval, and the opportunity to learn acceptable behavior. Popularity with opposite-sex and same-sex peers is important. The strong need for group identity seems to conflict at times with the search for personal identity. It is as though adolescents require close bonds with peers so that they can later achieve a sense of individuality.

Family Identity. The movement toward stronger peer relationships is contrasted with adolescents' movements away from parents. Although financial independence for adolescents is not the norm in American society, many adolescents work part time, using their income to bolster independence. When adolescents cannot have a part-time job because of studies, school-related activities, and other factors, parents can provide allowances for clothing and incidentals, which encourage adolescents to develop decision-making and budgeting skills.

Some adolescents and families have more difficulty during these years than others. Adolescents need to make choices, act independently, and experience the consequences of actions. This testing, however, is best done against a firm, supportive, family foundation. The family

needs to allow independence while providing a haven in which adolescents can contemplate actions. Families unable to provide this support complicate movement toward identity formation. Support to the family and adolescent may be essential to their success.

Nurses can assist families in considering ways that are appropriate for them to foster the independence of their adolescent while maintaining family structure. Many of these discussions often involve curfews, jobs, and participation in family chores. Emancipation from the immediate family is most successful when accomplished gradually and results in a balance between independence and family ties.

Vocational Identity. The selection of an occupation or a vocational direction in life provides a goal for adolescents. Because of society's changing needs, adolescents must be future oriented when making these choices. However, adolescents do not know which jobs will be available or which jobs will be rewarding 10 or 20 years in the future, so selecting a career is a complicated task. The nurse should provide emotional support during this process and should help adolescent clients select courses of action that promote self-satisfaction, identity, and continued opportunity for growth.

Moral Identity. The development of moral judgment depends heavily on cognitive and communication skills and peer interaction. Although moral development begins in early childhood, it is consolidated in adolescence because of the presence of certain skills. Adolescents learn to understand that rules are cooperative agreements that can be modified to fit the situation, rather than absolutes. Regarding rules, adolescents learn to use their own judgment rather than use the rules to avoid punishment as in earlier years. Kohlberg (1964) explains moral development in terms of stages (see Chapter 10). At the highest level, morality is derived from individual principles of conscience. Adolescents judge themselves by internalized ideals, which often leads to conflict between personal and group values. Group values become less significant in later adolescence.

Not all adolescents attain the same level of moral development. There is, however, a general forward movement through the stages of moral development, and the sequence of the stages is similar for all individuals even when their time of achievement varies. Kohlberg's moral development (1964) has a focus on justice based on reciprocity and equal respect. Females have been found to be more likely to give caring responses to moral problems. Males have been found to give more justice-oriented responses.

Health Identity. Another component of personal identity is perception of health. This component is of specific interest to health care providers. Healthy adolescents evaluate their own health according to feelings of well-being, ability to function normally, and absence of symptoms (Hockenberry and others, 2003).

Interventions to improve health perception might, therefore, concentrate on the adolescent period. The rapid changes during this period make health promotion programs especially crucial. Adolescents try new roles, begin to stabilize their identity, and acquire values and behaviors from which their adult lifestyle will evolve.

Health Risks

Accidents. Accidents remain the leading cause of death in adolescence. Motor vehicle accidents, which are the most common cause of death, resulted in almost half of the fatalities among 16- to 19-year-olds (Edelman and Mandle, 2002). Such accidents are often associated with alcohol intoxication or drug abuse. Bicycling fatalities were 4 to 7 times more likely to occur in males than females. Other frequent causes of accidental death in teenagers are drowning and firearms. Feelings of being indestructible lead to risk-taking behavior. Many injuries are preceded by the use of alcohol (USDHHS, 2000). Youths continue to be both the victims and perpetrators of violence.

Homicide. Homicide is the second leading cause of death in the 15- to 24-year-old age-group. Males and African-Americans have shown the greatest increases. Individuals 12 years of age and older are most likely to be killed by an acquaintance or gang member and most frequently with a firearm. Firearm homicides are 6 times greater in urban than nonurban areas. Firearm injuries are the second leading cause of death in young people 10 to 20 years of age (Ahmann, 2001; Behrman, Kliegman, and Jenson, 2000). American children spend an enormous amount of time watching television, listening to music, and playing video/computer games (Box 11-12). Much of what they encounter contains content that is violent or encourages antisocial behavior (Muscari, 2002).

Suicide. Suicide is the third leading cause of death in adolescents between 15 and 24 years of age (Edelman and Mandle, 2002). Depression and social isolation commonly precede a suicide attempt, but suicide probably results from a combination of several factors (Box 11-13).

Box *11-12*   **Parental Guidelines for Media Use**
Parents should do the following:
Set-up computer in family room
Use blocking software
Recognize that children can bypass some parental controls
Limit time children spend online
Supervise computer use
Communicate issues of concern
Reinforce concept of *stranger guidelines* on or off the computer
Monitor and track e-mail and chat room activity
Review ratings listed on video games, movies, and music CDs

The nurse must be able to identify the factors associated with adolescent suicide risk and precipitating events. In addition, the nurse should be alert to the following warning signs, which often occur for at least a month before suicide is attempted:

- Decrease in school performance
- Withdrawal
- Loss of initiative
- Loneliness, sadness, and crying
- Appetite and sleep disturbances
- Verbalization of suicidal thought

Immediate referrals to mental health professionals need to be made when assessment suggests that adolescents may be considering suicide. Guidance can help them focus on the positive aspects of life and strengthen coping abilities.

Substance Abuse. Substance abuse is in fact a concern to those who work with adolescents. Adolescents may believe that mood-altering substances create a sense of well-being or improve level of performance. All adolescents are at risk for experimental or recreational substance use, but those who have dysfunctional families are more at risk for chronic use and physical dependency. Some adolescents believe that substance use makes them more mature. They further believe that they will look and feel better with drug usage. The majority of adolescents experiment with marijuana. Other substances frequently abused by teens include steroids used to enhance their athletic performances. It is believed that the use of these products may increase the likelihood of using other illicit drugs (USDHHS, 2000).

Tobacco use continues to be a problem among adolescents. It is estimated that more than 3,000 young persons become regular smokers every day with over 1 million each year. The average age at which a teen begins to smoke is between 10 and 12, and the average age by which these teens become addicted is 14.5 years (LaSala and Todd, 2000). An attempt to decrease availability to those under 18 years of age resulted in a law that requires proof of age to purchase cigarettes. However, enforcement is far from being met (USDHHS, 2000).

Eating Disorders. The number of eating disorders is on the rise in adolescent girls, and knowledge of growth pro-

---

Box 11-13   Suicide Risk Assessment

History

Previous suicide attempt
Family member or friend has attempted suicide
History of child abuse or neglect
Past psychiatric hospitalization
Death of a parent when child was young

Individual Factors

Hopelessness
Marked, persistent depression
Alcohol or drug abuse
Impulsive
Difficulty tolerating frustration
Feelings of self-hatred or excessive guilt, feelings of humiliation
Thinking disorder (wishes to join a deceased person, hears voices telling to kill self)
Physical/body image problems (delayed puberty, chronic illness, disability, attention deficit hyperactivity disorder, learning disorders)
Gender identity concerns; gay or lesbian in an unsupportive environment
Sees self as totally helpless—a victim of fate
A need to do things perfectly

Family Factors

Difficult home situation—long, bitter parent-child conflict
Hostile parents
Overt rejection by one or both parents
Divorce or separation of parents
Recent or impending move
Family breakup or parental loss
Exposure to unrealistically high parental expectations
Parental indifference with very low expectations

Social/Environmental Factors

Firearms in the home
Incarceration
Lack of effective social support system
Isolation
Exposure to suicide of another
Few social, vocational, educational opportunities

From Hockenberry MJ and others: *Wong's nursing care of infants and children,* ed 7, St. Louis, 2003, Mosby.

---

gression may be a way to discourage radical weight reduction activities. If an adolescent deviates radically from the usual pattern, further assessment is necessary to identify the cause. Areas to include in the assessment are past and present diet history, food records, eating habits, attitudes, health beliefs, and socioeconomic and psychosocial factors (Hockenberry and others, 2003; Kail, 2001). Weight extremes resulting from excessive or inadequate caloric intake are common during the adolescent years. Allowing the adolescent to see when and how the weight curve changed can be a first step in identifying the problem and implementing dietary changes.

Although anorexia nervosa and bulimia are classified as separate disorders, there is significant overlap between the two eating disorders (Kail, 2001). Anorexia nervosa is considered a clinical syndrome with both physical and psychosocial components. The majority of clients are adolescents and young women. Attending a highly competitive high school and being from a professional, upper middle-class family increases the risk for this disorder. Persons with anorexia nervosa have an intense fear of gaining weight and refuse to maintain body weight at the minimal normal weight for their age and height.

Bulimia nervosa is most identified with binge eating and behaviors to prevent weight gain. Behaviors include self-induced vomiting, misuse of laxatives and other medications, and excessive exercise (Kail, 2001). Because adolescents rarely volunteer information about behaviors to prevent weight gain, it is important to take a thorough dietary history. Bulimia is considered a biopsychosocial illness. Society's expectations for thinness may have a strong influence on the development of these eating disorders.

Sexual Experimentation. Sexual experimentation is common among adolescents. Peer pressure, physiological and emotional changes, and societal expectations contribute to early heterosexual and homosexual relations. According to the Centers for Disease Control and Prevention (1999), 54% of adolescents between grades 9 and 12 have admitted to having sexual intercourse at least once. Two prominent consequences of adolescent sexual activity are sexually transmitted disease and pregnancy (Bukatko and Daehler, 2001).

Sexually Transmitted Disease. Sexually transmitted disease (STD) annually afflicts around 10 million persons under the age of 25 years. This high degree of incidence makes it imperative that sexually active adolescents be screened for STDs, even when they have no symptoms. The annual physical examination of a sexually active adolescent should include a thorough sexual history and a careful examination of the genitalia so that condylomata acuminata (genital warts), herpes, *Phthirus pubis* (crab lice), primary syphilitic chancres, and other STDs are not missed. Recommended tests for women include Papanicolaou (Pap) smears, cervical cultures for gonorrhea and *Chlamydia* species, and syphilis tests; for men, urethral cultures for gonorrhea and *Chlamydia* species and syphilis tests are recommended. If men have participated in homosexual activities, rectal and pharyngeal cultures also need to be taken to check for gonorrhea. The health care provider can be proactive by using the interview process to identify risk factors in the adolescent (Berk, 2003). Once identified, the risk factors should lead to strategies for prevention.

Human immunodeficiency virus, which causes acquired immunodeficiency syndrome (AIDS), is transmitted through unprotected sexual intercourse, the use of shared needles, and through infected blood products. Therefore the risk-taking behaviors of adolescent sexual activity and drug use make adolescents vulnerable to the threat of AIDS. Approximately 30,000 HIV-infected adolescents live in the United States today; AIDS is the sixth leading cause of death among individuals between 15 and 24 years of age (USDHHS, 2000). Adolescents who have placed themselves at risk for AIDS should be tested for HIV.

Pregnancy. Adolescent pregnancy continues to be a major social challenge for our nation. The United States has the highest rate of teenage pregnancy yearly as compared to other developed nations (Hockenberry and others, 2003; Spear, 2001). *Healthy People 2010* set as its objectives: (a) reduce teen pregnancy, (b) decrease infant mortality, and (c) encourage prenatal care (USDHHS, 2000). Adolescent pregnancy occurs across socioeconomic classes, in public and private schools, among all ethnic and religious backgrounds, and in all parts of the country. Teenage pregnancy with early prenatal supervision is considered less harmful to both mother and child than earlier believed. Pregnant teens need special attention to nutrition, as well as health supervision and psychological support.

Health Concerns

Perceptions. One area of concern is the formation of healthy habits of daily living. Emphasis on exercise, sleep, nutrition, and stress reduction habits is increasing. The nurse must recognize the importance of these habits and identify ways to adapt them to each adolescent. To do this the nurse must assess the individual's positive and negative habits and attitudes about health. Extensive and long-term follow-up is required if individualized interventions are to succeed. The nurse needs to be aware of the prevalence of health problems and make assessments accordingly.

Health Education. Community and school-based health programs for adolescents are focused on health promotion and illness prevention. Nurses are involved in community health through screening and teaching programs (Table 11-11).

Through their efforts in the school and community, nurses can make a contribution in meeting the *Healthy People 2010* objectives (USDHHS, 2000). Discussions with adolescents must be private and confidential. Deering and Cody (2002) found that for adolescents to reveal intimate information about their risk-taking behaviors, they must first feel comfortable and respected as individuals. Large numbers of school-based clinics have been developed and implemented to respond to adolescents' needs. Helping adolescents make decisions about their health care strengthens their autonomy and promotes healthy behaviors (Dickey and Deatrick, 2000; McGahee, Kemp, and Tingen, 2000).

Nurses can play an important role in preventing injuries and accidental deaths. Injury prevention activities and support of organizations that promote responsible behavior, including Mothers Against Drunk Driving (MADD) and Drug Abuse Resistance Education (DARE), and encouraging students to participate in Students Against Drunk Driving (SADD) are types of important activities. Stimulating adolescents to discuss alternatives to driving when under the influence of drugs or alcohol prepares them to consider alternatives when such an occasion arises. The nurse must identify those adolescents at risk for abuse, provide education to prevent accidents related to substance abuse, and provide counseling to those in rehabilitation.

Nurses can play a strategic role in an antismoking movement. Smoke prevention programs can be initiated in schools. Communities can also play a role in creating tobacco control policies at the local level (Dickey and Deatrick, 2000).

The nurse must provide sex education and counseling. Nurses play a key role in counseling teenagers on ways to avoid pregnancies. After pregnancy has occurred, the nurse can assist them in obtaining medical care and developing skills that will enhance their infants' development.

Extensive educational efforts to prevent the spread of AIDS and other STDs in this age-group are a nursing

Table 11-11	Health Promotion During the Adolescent Period
Adolescent Health Concerns	**Health Promotion Intervention**
Unintentional injuries	Advise adolescent to take driver's education course and to wear seat belts.
	Inform the adolescent of risk associated with drinking and driving, use of drugs.
	Promote helmet use by adolescent bicyclists and motorcyclists.
	Ensure adolescent receives proper orientation to the use of all sports equipment.
	Encourage adolescent to swim with a "buddy."
Firearm use and violence	Teach conflict resolution skills.
Tobacco, alcohol, and drug use	Screen for tobacco (including smokeless), alcohol, and drug use and inform of the risks of use.
Suicide	Offer suicide prevention information.
	Teach methods to deal with a suicidal peer.
	Promote suicide alternatives.
Sexually transmitted diseases	Provide adolescent with information regarding disease, mode of transmission, and related symptoms.
	Encourage abstinence from sexual activity; or if sexually active, the use of condoms.
	Provide accurate information about the consequences of sexual activity.

responsibility. Education may occur in the school or community and be formal, informal, one-on-one, or in a group setting. Speakers and organizations can be used to help in the educational process.

Rural Adolescents. Fifty percent of adolescents live in the rural South, 27% live in the rural Midwest, and the remaining adolescents are fairly evenly distributed among the two remaining regions of the United States. Areas of concern for these adolescents include limited access to health care, limited health care insurance, limited privacy, lack of transportation to health care, poverty, and farming accidents.

Nurses can play an important role in improving the health of the adolescent. Decreasing barriers to care, health promotion education, development of coping strategies, and assessment of health beliefs are important areas for the nurse to address.

Minority Adolescents. By the next century it is expected that minorities as a group will become the majority. Minority adolescents have been identified as experiencing a greater percentage of health problems and barriers to health care.

Issues of concern for these adolescents living in a high-risk environment include learning or emotional difficulties, death related to violence, unintentional injuries, increased rate for adolescent pregnancy, STDs, and AIDS. Poverty is a major factor negatively affecting the lives of minority adolescents. Limited access to health services is common. Nurses can make a significant contribution to improving access to appropriate health care for adolescents. Health promotion initiatives must be based on topics of concern for these adolescents.

Nurses working in the community must adopt culturally sensitive interventions to meet the needs of minority adolescents and their families (Hockenberry and others, 2003). They must be able to communicate in another language by speaking it or using an interpreter. Teaching materials need to be written in the appropriate language. Information regarding health beliefs and healing practices must be assessed. With knowledge about various cultures and the means to care for minority adolescents, the nurse acts as an advocate to ensure accessibility of appropriate services.

Key Concepts

- A developmental perspective helps the nurse understand commonalities and variations in each stage and the impact they have on the client's health.
- During critical periods of development, a multitude of factors can foster or hinder optimal physical, cognitive, and psychosocial development.
- Growth and development are influenced by inner forces of heredity and temperament and by the outer forces of family, peers, life experiences, and environmental elements.
- During the intrauterine period, while embryo and fetus grow and develop, genetic factors and environ-

mental factors (teratogens) may cause impairments in any body system.

- Physiological, cognitive, and psychosocial development continue from conception through adolescence, and the nurse must be familiar with normal parameters to determine potential problems and promote normal development.
- Physical growth during the school years is slow and steady until the skeletal growth spurt just before puberty.
- The major psychosocial developmental task of the school-age child is the development of a sense of industry.
- Cognitively, the young school-age child develops the ability to think in a logical manner.
- The prepubertal growth spurt usually occurs 2 years earlier in girls than in boys; during this time, development of secondary sexual changes begins.
- Preadolescents move forward to the last stage of cognitive development, formal operations, in which they begin to think in an abstract manner, reflect on thought processes, and plan for the future.
- Adolescence begins with puberty, when primary sexual characteristics begin to develop and secondary sexual characteristics complete development.
- Adolescents are able to solve complex mental problems which includes use of deductive reasoning.
- The adolescent's rapid change in physical appearance heightens self-consciousness and concerns regarding body image.
- Accidents are the major cause of death in all age-groups.
- Motor vehicle accidents are the major cause of accidental death in adolescence.
- Sexually transmitted diseases are the most common communicable diseases among adolescents.
- Adolescents begin the long process of emancipation from their parents and need parental support to accomplish this in a timely manner.

Key Terms

Adolescence, *p. 205*
Animism, *p. 193*
Apgar score, *p. 176*
Artificialism, *p. 193*
Blastocyst, *p. 173*
Bonding, *p. 176*
Classification, *p. 199*
Concrete operations, *p. 199*
Embryo, *p. 173*
Estrogen, *p. 205*
Fertilization, *p. 173*
Fetus, *p. 174*
Fontanels, *p. 177*
Hyperbilirubinemia, *p. 179*
Immanent justice, *p. 193*
Implantation, *p. 173*
Inborn errors of metabolism, *p. 179*

Infancy, *p. 180*
Lanugo, *p. 175*
Menarche, *p. 205*
Molding, *p. 177*
Morula, *p. 173*
Nagele's rule, *p. 173*
Neonatal period, *p. 177*
Object permanence, *p. 189*
Organogenesis, *p. 174*
Placenta, *p. 173*
Preadolescence, *p. 204*
Prematurity, *p. 175*
Preoperational thought, *p. 189*
Preschool period, *p. 193*
Puberty, *p. 204*
Quickening, *p. 175*
School-age, *p. 196*

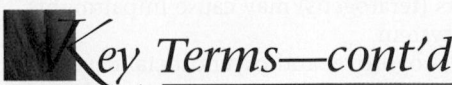

Key Terms—cont'd

Sexually transmitted disease (STD), *p. 211*	Testosterone, *p. 205*
Temperament, *p. 176*	Toddlerhood, *p. 189*
Teratogens, *p. 174*	Vernix caseosa, *p. 175*
	Zygote, *p. 173*

Critical Thinking Exercises

1. Mrs. Yeigh is attending the antepartum clinic for the first visit. A major area for focus is health promotion. What other topics should the nurse present at this time? Mrs. Yeigh asks whether it is better to breast-feed or bottle-feed.
2. The parents of 2-year-old Tyrese are concerned because he cries and fusses when his parents leave him at the day care center and go to work. Identify nursing measures that will minimize separation anxiety for Tyrese.
3. What measure can parents and teacher use to help the school-age child accomplish Erikson's task for this stage of development?
4. Twelve-year-old Elizabeth is brought to the pediatric clinic for a physical examination. She is concerned about her lack of physical development compared to her peers. Discuss ways to educate Elizabeth about puberty and the variations that occur.
5. Seventeen-year-old Ricardo wants very much to belong and be accepted by his peers. He expresses concern when his peers begin to plan a party with alcohol and girls. What should be discussed to help support his feelings and need to belong?

Review Questions

1. In an interview with her pregnant client, the nurse discussed the three risk factors that have been cited as having a possible effect on prenatal development. They are:
   1. Prematurity, stress, and mother's age.
   2. Nutrition, stress, and mother's age.
   3. Fetal infections, prematurity, placenta previa.
   4. Nutrition, mother's age, fetal infections.

2. The most extreme physiological change occurs when the newborn leaves the in utero circulation and develops:
   1. Respiratory functioning.
   2. Cardiac functioning.
   3. Reflex irritability.
   4. Temperature control.

3. The leading cause of death in children older than 1 year is:
   1. Falling.
   2. Maltreatment injuries.
   3. Automobile injuries.
   4. Malnutrition.

4. A child who is a toddler pretends to shave after watching his father shave. This is an example of Piaget's:
   1. Sensorimotor stage.
   2. Intuitive phase of preoperational thought stage.
   3. Autonomy stage.
   4. Preoperative thought stage.

5. By this age children are able to play with others in a cooperative manner and have a temporary leader for each activity.
   1. 3 years of age.
   2. 4 years of age.
   3. 5 years of age.
   4. 6 years of age.

6. The nurse counsels the parent that a preschooler sleeps an average of:
   1. 8 hours a night and takes frequent naps.
   2. 12 hours a night and takes infrequent naps.
   3. 10 hours a night and takes frequent naps.
   4. 6 hours a night and takes frequent naps.

7. The nurse can counsel a parent that her child can his floss teeth effectively and be independent in tooth care by the age of:
   1. 8 to 10 years.
   2. 6 to 7 years.
   3. 11 to 12 years.
   4. 7 to 8 years.

8. The chief illness of childhood is:
   1. Flu.
   2. Common cold.
   3. Measles.
   4. Ear infections.

9. When nurses are communicating with adolescents, they should:
   1. Avoid discussing sensitive issues, such as asking questions about sex and drugs.
   2. Ask closed-ended questions to get straight answers.
   3. Be alert to clues to their emotional state.
   2. Avoid looking for meaning behind adolescents' words or actions.

10. The leading cause of death in adolescence is:
    1. Homicide.
    2. Substance abuse.
    3. Accidents.
    4. Eating disorders.

References

Ahmann E: Guns in the home: nurse's roles, *Pediatr Nurs* 27(6):587, 2001.

Behrman R, Kliegman R, Jenson H: *Nelson textbook of pediatrics*, Philadelphia, 2000, WB Saunders.

Berk L: *Child development*, ed 6, Boston, 2003, Allyn & Bacon.

Bukatko D, Daehler M: *Child development a thematic approach,* ed 4, Boston, 2001, Houghton Mifflin.

Center for Communicable Diseases: Guidelines for school programs to promote lifelong healthy eating, *J Sch Health* 67:9, 1996.

Centers for Disease Control and Prevention: Trends in HIV related sexual risk behaviors among high school students— selected U.S. cities, *MMWR Morbid Mortal Wkly Rep* 48(21): 400, 1999.

Deering C, Cody D: Communicating with children and adolescents, *Am J Nurs* 102(3):34, 2002.

Edelman C, Mandle C: *Health promotion throughout the life span,* ed 5, St. Louis, 2002, Mosby.

Erikson EH: *Childhood and society,* ed 2, New York, 1963, Norton.

Erikson EH: *Identity: youth and crises,* New York, 1968, Norton.

Garner J: Guidelines for isolation precautions in hospitals, *Infect Control Hosp Epidemiol* 17(1):54, 1996.

Frankenburg WK and others: The Denver II: a major revision and restandardization of the Denver Development Screening Test, *Pediatrics* 89(1):91, 1992.

Hockenberry MJ and others: *Wong's nursing care of infants and children,* ed 7, St. Louis, 2003, Mosby.

Kail R: *Children and their development,* ed 2, Upper Saddle River, NJ, 2001, Prentice Hall.

Kamerling S: Airbags and children: making correct choices in child passenger restraints, *MCN Am J Matern Child Nurs* 27(5):264, 2002.

Katz A: "Where I come from we don't talk about that": exploring sexuality and culture among Blacks, Asians and Hispanics, *AWHONN Lifelines* 6(6):533, 2003.

Kinservik M, Friedhoff M: Control issues in toilet training, *Pediatr Nurs* 26(3):267, 2000.

Knauth D: Maternal Change during the transition to parenthood, *Pediatr Nurs* 27(2):169, 2001.

Kohlberg L: Development of moral character and moral ideology. In Hoffman ML, Hoffman LNW, editors: *Review of child development research,* vol 1, New York, 1964, Russell Sage Foundation.

Kuczen B: *Childhood stress: don't let your child be a victim,* New York, 1982, Delacorte Press.

LaSala K, Todd S: Preventing youth use of tobacco products: the role of nursing, *Pediatr Nurs* 26(2):143, 2000.

Muscari M: Media violence: advice for parents, *Pediatr Nurs* 28(6):585, 2002.

Piaget J: *The origins of intelligence in children,* New York, 1952, International Universities Press.

Spear H: Teenage pregnancy: "having a baby won't affect me that much," *Pediatr Nurs* 27(6):574, 2001.

U.S. Department of Health and Human Services: *Healthy People 2010,* Washington, DC, 2000.

*R*esearch *References*

Askin D: Complication in the transition from fetal to neonatal life, *J Obstet Gynecol Neonatal Nurs* 31(3):318, 2002.

Berry B and others: Preschool vision screening using the MTI-Photo screener, *Pediatr Nurs* 27(1):27, 2001.

Cohen S: Lead poisoning: a summary of treatment and prevention, *Pediatr Nurs* 27(2):125, 2001.

Dickey S, Deatrick J: Autonomy and decision making for health promotions in adolescence, *Pediatr Nurs* 26(5):461, 2000.

Gill S.: The little things: perceptions of breastfeeding support, *J Obstet Gynecol Neonatal Nurs* 30(4):401, 2001.

Hall-Long B, Schell K, Corrigan V: Youth safety education and injury prevention program, *Pediatr Nurs* 27(2):141, 2001.

Hilton J: Folic acid intake of young women, *J Obstet Gynecol Neonatal Nurs* 31(2):172, 2002.

Jerum A, Melnyk B: Effectiveness of intervention to prevent obesity and obesity-related complications in children, adolescents, *Pediatr Nurs* 27(6):606, 2001.

McGahee T, Kemp V, Tingen M: A theoretical model for smoking prevention studies in preteen children, *Pediatr Nurs* 26(2):135, 2000.

Pletsch P, Morgan S: Smoke-free families: a tobacco control program for pregnant women and their families, *J Obstet Gynecol Neonatal Nurs* 31(1):39, 2002.

Popovich D: Sexuality in early childhood: pediatric nurses' attitudes, knowledge, and clinical practice, *Pediatr Nurs* 26(5):484, 2000.

12

Young to Middle Adult

Media Resources

http://evolve.elsevier.com/Potter/
fundamentals/

CD COMPANION

- Review Questions
- Glossary

evolve WEBSITE

- Review Questions
- Student Learning Activities
- Glossary

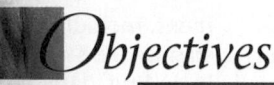

Objectives

Mastery of content in this chapter will enable the student to:

- Define the key terms listed.
- Discuss developmental theories of young and middle adults.
- List and discuss major life events of young and middle adults and the childbearing family.
- Describe developmental tasks of the young adult, the childbearing family, and the middle adult.
- Discuss the significance of family in the life of the adult.
- Describe normal physiological changes in young and middle adulthood and in pregnancy.
- Discuss cognitive and psychosocial changes occurring during the adult years.
- Describe health concerns of the young adult, the childbearing family, and the middle adult.
- Apply the nursing process to administer care to young and middle adults.

*Y*oung and middle adulthood is a period of challenges, rewards, and crises. Challenges may include the demands of working and raising families, although adults can also be rewarded by successes in their career endeavors and in their personal lives. Adults also face crises such as caring for their aging parents, the possibility of job loss in a changing economic environment, and dealing with their own developmental needs as well as those of their family members.

Adult developmental changes are based on earlier characteristics that help shape subsequent behavior and characteristics. Each person's development, however, is a unique process (Stuart and Laraia, 2001). Young adulthood is the period between the late teens and the mid to late 30s (Edelman and Mandle, 2002), and young adults constitute approximately 27% of the population (U.S. Department of Commerce, 2000). During young adulthood, individuals increasingly move away from their families of origin, establish career goals, and decide whether to marry and begin families or remain single. Young adults are active and must adapt to new experiences and newly acquired independence.

Middle age occurs between the mid to late 30s and the mid 60s. The transition into middle age occurs when young persons become aware of changes in reproductive and physical abilities that signify the beginning of another stage in life. This is a time of continuing transitions when individuals may reassess their life goals and add new goals. In 2000, almost 39% of the U.S. population was middle-age adults between the ages of 35 and 64, an increase of approximately 5% from the year 1990 (U.S. Department of Commerce, 2000).

Classic works by such developmental theorists as Levinson and others (1978), Diekelmann (1976), Erikson (1963, 1982), and Havighurst (1972) have attempted to describe the phases of young and middle adulthood and related developmental tasks (see Chapter 10 for an in-depth discussion of developmental theories). It has been proposed that intellectual and moral development differ between men and women. According to Gilligan (1993), women struggle with the issues of care and responsibility, and in turn their relationships progress toward a maturity of interdependence. As women progress toward adulthood, the moral dilemma changes from how to exercise their rights without interfering in the rights of others to "how to lead a moral life," which includes obligations to themselves and their families and people in general (Gilligan, 1993).

In many cultures familial authority has historically been associated with the male. Men have traditionally assumed the overwhelming majority of positions of power. Traditional masculine roles include providing and protecting. Recently, however, men have been characterized as moving into greater disequilibrium. Faced with a societal structure that differs greatly from the norms of 20 or 30 years ago, many men are challenged with determining what it means to be a man and how to feel good about it in today's society (Sheehy, 1995). As a provider, for example, a man is traditionally viewed as the primary supporter of the family. However, more women have been successful in entering the workforce and pursuing careers. In 1999, 60% of women age 16 and over in the United States were in the labor force. Women contribute significantly to their families' incomes, and families with the wife in the paid labor force have the highest median income of all family types. In 1998, women who were single heads of households maintained 13 million (18%) of the 71 million families in the U.S. (U.S. Department of Labor, 2000).

Developmental theories provide nurses with a basis for understanding the life events and developmental tasks of the young and middle adult. Clients may present challenges to nurses who themselves may be young or middle adults coping with the demands of their respective developmental period. Nurses must be careful to recognize the needs of their clients even if they are not experiencing the same challenges and events.

Young Adult

Physical Changes

The young adult has usually completed physical growth by the age of 20. An exception to this is the pregnant or lactating woman. The physical, cognitive, and psychosocial changes and the health concerns of the pregnant woman and the childbearing family are extensive.

Young adults are usually quite active, experience severe illnesses less commonly than older age-groups, tend to ignore physical symptoms, and often postpone seeking health care. Physical characteristics of young adults begin to change as middle age approaches. Unless clients have illnesses, assessment findings are generally within normal limits.

Nonetheless, clients in this developmental stage may benefit from a personal lifestyle assessment (see Chapter 6). A personal lifestyle assessment can help nurses and clients identify habits that increase the risk for cardiac, malignant, pulmonary, renal, or other chronic diseases. A personal lifestyle assessment of the young adult includes assessment of general life satisfaction; hobbies and interests; habits such as diet, sleeping, exercise, sexual habits, and use of caffeine, alcohol, and illicit drugs; home conditions, including housing, economic condition, type of health insurance, and pets; and occupational environ-

ment, including type of work, exposure to hazardous substances, and physical or mental strain. Military records, including dates and geographical area of assignments, may also be useful in assessing the young adult for risk factors.

Cognitive Changes

Critical thinking habits increase steadily through the young and middle adult years. Formal and informal educational experiences, general life experiences, and occupational opportunities dramatically increase the individual's conceptual, problem-solving, and motor skills.

Identifying preferred occupational areas is a major task of young adults. When people know their skills, talents, and personality characteristics, educational preparation and occupational choices are easier and more satisfying. Many young adults, however, either lack the resources or the support systems to facilitate further education or the development of skills necessary for many positions in the workplace. As a result, some young adults may have limited occupational choices.

An understanding of how adults learn assists the nurse in developing teaching plans (see Chapter 24). Adults enter the teaching-learning situation with a background of unique life experiences, including illness. Therefore the nurse always views adults as individuals. Their compliance with regimens such as medications, treatments, or lifestyle changes such as smoking cessation, involves decision-making processes. When determining the amount of information that the individual needs to make decisions about the prescribed course of therapy, the nurse should consider those factors that may affect the individual's compliance with the regimen, including educational level, socioeconomic factors, and motivation and desire to learn.

Because young adults are continually evolving and adjusting to changes in the home, workplace, and personal lives, their decision-making processes should be flexible. The more secure young adults are in their roles, the more flexible and open they are to change. Insecure persons tend to be more rigid in making decisions.

Psychosocial Changes

The emotional health of the young adult is related to the individual's ability to address and resolve personal and social tasks. The young adult is usually caught between wanting to prolong the irresponsibility of adolescence and wanting to assume adult commitments. Certain patterns or trends, however, are relatively predictable. Between the ages of 23 and 28, the person refines self-perception and ability for intimacy. From 29 to 34 the person directs enormous energy toward achievement and mastery of the surrounding world. The years from 35 to 43 are a time of vigorous examination of life goals and relationships. Alterations are made in personal, social, and occupational lives. Often the stresses of this reexamination may result in a "midlife crisis" in which marital partner, lifestyle, and occupation may change.

During the young adult years, people generally give more attention to occupational and social pursuits. During this period individuals attempt to improve their socioeconomic status. Upward mobility is sought through career choices. Recent trends toward corporate downsizing, however, are leading to fewer high-level positions. Subsequently, many young adults are facing the added stress of greater competition in the workplace for fewer positions. For many young adults, a dual-income family is also needed to achieve and maintain middle-class status. Career and personal counseling can help individuals identify career choices and set realistic goals.

Ethnic and gender factors have a sociological and psychological influence in an adult's life, and these factors can pose a distinct challenge for nursing care. Each person holds culture-bound definitions of health and illness. Nurses and other health professionals bring with them distinct practices for the prevention and treatment of illness. Knowing too little about a client's self-perception or beliefs regarding health and illness may create conflict between the nurse and the client. Changes in the traditional role expectations of both men and women in young and middle adulthood have also led to greater challenges for nursing care. Women often continue to work during the child-rearing years, and many women struggle with the enormity of balancing three careers: wife, mother, and employee. This is a potential source of stress for the adult working woman. Men are more aware of parental and household responsibilities and find themselves having more responsibilities at home while achieving their own career goals (Stuart and Laraia, 2001). An understanding of ethnicity, race, and gender differences enables the nurse to provide individualized care (see Chapter 8).

Support from the nurse, access to information, and appropriate referrals provide opportunities for achievement of a client's potential. Because health is not merely the absence of disease but involves wellness in all human dimensions, the holistic, humanistic nurse acknowledges the importance of the young adult's psychosocial needs and needs in other dimensions.

The young adult must make decisions concerning career, marriage, and parenthood. Although each person makes these decisions based on individual factors, the nurse should understand the general principles involved in these aspects of psychosocial development while assessing the young adult's psychosocial status.

Lifestyle. Family history of cardiovascular, renal, endocrine, or neoplastic disease increases the risk of illness as well. The nurse's role in health promotion is to identify modifiable factors that increase the young adult's risk for health problems and to provide client education and support to reduce unhealthy lifestyle behaviors.

Those lifestyle habits that activate the stress response (see Chapter 30) increase the risk of illness. Smoking is a well-documented risk factor for pulmonary, cardiac, and vascular diseases in smokers and the individuals who receive secondhand smoke. Inhaled cigarette pollutants increase the risk of lung cancer, emphysema, and chronic bronchitis. The nicotine in tobacco is a vasoconstrictor that acts on the coronary arteries, increasing the risk of angina, myocardial infarction, and coronary artery disease. Nicotine also causes peripheral vasoconstriction and may lead to vascular problems.

Lifestyle habits such as diet, smoking, stress, substance abuse, lack of exercise, and poor personal hygiene increase the risk of future illness. Prolonged stress increases wear and tear on the body's adaptive capacities. Stress-related diseases such as ulcers, emotional disorders, and infections can occur (see Chapter 30).

Career. Young men and women hope to have careers that will enable them to realize the occupational dreams of their childhood. They may formulate short- and long-term goals in traditional or nontraditional careers. A successful vocational adjustment is important in the lives of most men and women. Successful employment not only ensures economic security but also leads to friendships, social activities, support, and respect from co-workers.

Two-career marriages are increasing. The two-career marriage has benefits and liabilities. In addition to increasing the family's financial base, the person who works outside the home is able to expand friendships, activities, and interests. However, stress may occur in a two-career family. These stressors can result from a transfer to a new city; increased expenditures of physical, mental, or emotional energy; child care demands; or household needs. To avoid stress in a two- career family, neither partner can assume all responsibilities. For some families a solution may be to limit recreational expenses and instead hire someone to do routine housework. Others may set up an equal division of household, shopping, and cooking duties.

Sexuality. The development of secondary sexual characteristics occurs during the adolescent years (see Chapter 11). Physical development is accompanied by the ability to perform sexual acts. The young adult usually has emotional maturity to complement the physical ability and is therefore able to develop mature sexual relationships and establish intimacy. Young adults who have failed to achieve the developmental task of personal integration may develop relationships that are superficial and stereotyped (Stuart and Laraia, 2001).

Masters and Johnson (1970) have contributed important information about the physiological characteristics of the adult sexual response (see Chapter 27). The psychodynamic aspect of sexual activity is as important as the type or frequency of sexual intercourse to young adults. Psychological beliefs and expectations give feelings of pleasure and satisfaction to adults. To maintain total wellness, adults should be encouraged to explore various aspects of their sexuality and be aware that their sexual needs and concerns evolve. As the rate of early initiation of sexual intercourse continues to increase, young adults are at risk for sexually transmitted diseases. Consequently, there is an increase in the need for education regarding the mode of transmission, prevention, and symptom recognition and management for sexually transmitted diseases.

Childbearing Cycle. Conception, pregnancy, birth, and the puerperium are major phases of the childbearing cycle. The changes during these phases are complex. Education such as Lamaze classes can prepare pregnant women, their partners, and other support persons to participate in the birthing process (Figure 12-1). Social support has a positive impact on pregnant women and their families (Box 12-1). A current trend in some health care

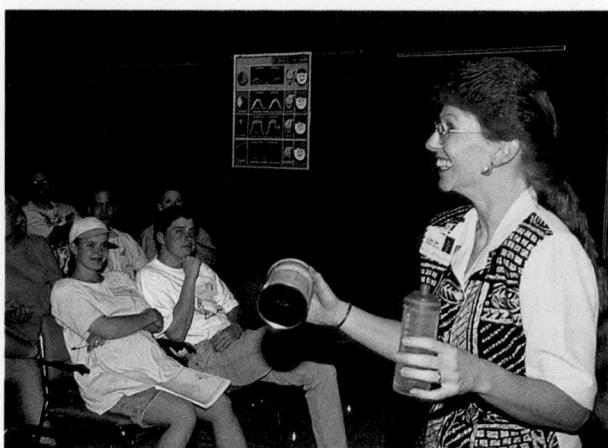

FIGURE **12–1**   Nurse providing Lamaze class for expectant young adults.

agencies is to provide a lay **doula** or support person to be present during labor to assist women who have no other source of support.

Lactation, or the process of breast-feeding, offers many advantages to both the new mother and baby. For the inexperienced mother, breast-feeding may also be a source of anxiety and frustration. Women who have had no contact with other mothers who breast-feed and who have had little or no contact with newborns require assistance to breast-feed successfully. The nurse must be alert for signs that the mother needs information and assistance. Direct observation of the breast-feeding mother-infant pair alerts the nurse to such problems as proper positioning of either the mother and infant or ineffective sucking by the infant (Lawrence and Lawrence, 1999).

The personal and social changes occurring in the lives of a couple after the birth of a baby cannot be underestimated (Figure 12-2). The nursing assessment of the couple's response to the birthing experience and parent-child bonding are discussed in a later section of this chapter.

Types of Families. During young adulthood most individuals experience singlehood and the opportunity to be on their own. Those who eventually marry experience several changes as they take on new responsibilities. For example, many married couples choose to become parents. There are also young adults who choose alternative lifestyles. Chapter 9 reviews forms of families.

Singlehood. Social pressure to get married is not as great as it once was, and many young adults do not expect to be married until their late 20s or early 30s, or not at all (Sheehy, 1995). For young adults who remain single, parents and siblings become the nucleus for a family, although the single young adult maintains independence from parental controls. Close friends and associates of the single young adult may also be viewed as the individual's "family."

One cause for the increased single population is the expanding career opportunities for women. Women enter the job market with greater career potential and have

Research Highlight
Box 12-1

Culture and Social Support in Pregnancy

Research Focus

Although Mexican-Americans have lower levels of prenatal care than non-Hispanic whites, they have relatively the same or better infant mortality rates and favorable birth-weight distributions, despite relatively low socioeconomic status. Questions arose regarding the reasons for this unusual "contemporary health enigma."

Research Abstract

The purpose of this study was to describe the experience of social support in Hispanic families during pregnancy. Verbatim interviews with Hispanic mothers, family members, and health care providers, along with field notes from participant observation, historical data of the region, and area demographics constituted the data for this qualitative study. Findings indicated that pregnancy outcomes were positive because of a socialization process that helped pregnant Hispanic women and family members adapt and change to support the pregnancy. The aspects of mutual adaptation helped reinforce the family structure, integrate cultural beliefs, define roles for both mother and family members, define the nature of mother-child and family-child relationships, and facilitate a positive process through a supportive orientation.

Evidence-Based Practice

- Recognizing the importance of cultural and social contexts in which pregnancies occur is an important aspect of nursing care and intervention.
- Family support of pregnant women is a major factor in the well-being of pregnant women and their unborn children.
- Health care practices and policy focused on increasing social support of pregnant women could improve birth outcomes.

Reference

Domian E: Cultural practices and social support of pregnant women in a northern New Mexico community, *J Nurs Scholarsh* 33(4):331, 2001.

greater opportunities for financial independence. More single individuals are choosing to live together outside of marriage, as well as to become parents either biologically or through adoption. Similarly, many married couples choose to separate or divorce if they find their marital situation unsatisfactory.

Marriage. Every couple's relationship is unique. Although no rules guarantee a successful marriage, some guidelines are useful for building a happy marriage. Before marriage the couple ideally should complete five tasks. First, the partners should make certain that their emotions are based on love rather than physical or sexual attraction. Second, both partners should explore their motivation for

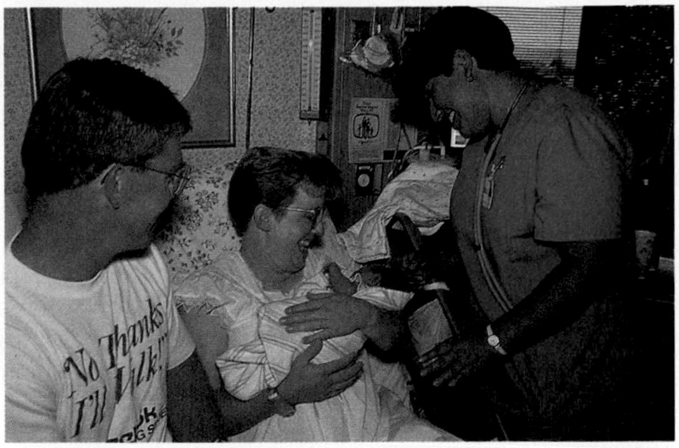

FIGURE **12–2** Parent-child nurturing is important in adapting to a newborn. (Modified from Stanhope M, Lancaster J: *Community and public health nursing,* ed 5, St. Louis, 2001, Mosby.)

Box 12-2   Ten Hallmarks of Emotional Health

A sense of meaning and direction in life
Successful negotiation through transitions
Absence of feelings of being cheated or disappointed by life
Attainment of several long-term goals
Satisfaction with personal growth and development
When married, feelings of mutual love for partner; when single, satisfaction with social interactions
Satisfaction with friendships
Generally cheerful attitude
No sensitivity to criticism
No unrealistic fears

wanting to marry. Third, they should focus on developing clear communication. Fourth, they should understand that any annoying behavior patterns and habits are unlikely to change after marriage. Last, they should determine their compatibility in important beliefs and values.

When establishing a household and family, the married couple must begin to work as a team. The major tasks of adults, establishing an intimate relationship; deciding on and working toward mutual goals; establishing guidelines for power and decision-making issues; setting standards for extrafamily interactions; finding companionship with other people for a social life; and choosing morals, values, and ideologies acceptable to both require considerable maturity and self-esteem. When accomplished, however, they provide the foundation for a stable relationship.

A marital relationship involves different developmental stages. The establishment stage begins at the wedding and continues as the couple attempts to function as a dyad. The couple learns patterns of sexual expression and ways to live intimately with each other. They must learn styles of conflict resolution, decision making, and role patterns. In addition, each partner may experience a sense of loss of individuality and self in the transition from *me* to *we*.

The family orientation stage is directed at childbearing and child-rearing activities. Parenting roles must be defined and practiced. Nurturing and socialization needs of the children can put pressure on the couple's intimate relationship. In addition, parents' images of the "perfect parent" conflict with reality.

Parenthood. The availability of contraception makes it easier for today's couples to decide when and if to start a family. One factor influencing this decision is the reason for wanting a child. Social pressures may encourage a couple to have a child or may influence them to limit the number of children they have. Economic considerations frequently enter into the decision-making process because having and bringing up children are expensive. General health status and age are also considerations in decisions about parenthood because couples are getting married later and are postponing pregnancies.

Alternative Family Structures and Parenting. Changing norms and values about family life in the United States reveal basic shifts in attitudes in our society. The trend toward greater acceptance of cohabitation without marriage has been a factor in the greater numbers of infants being born to unmarried women. Also, approximately 1.5 million parents are gay or lesbian, and up to one third of lesbians are mothers. Many times parents from alternative family structures feel a lack of support and even bias from the health care system (Coll, Surrey, and Weingarten, 1998). In recognizing the needs of gay and lesbian parents and their children, the American Academy of Pediatrics (2002) published a policy statement supporting adoption of children and the parenting role by same-sex parents.

Hallmarks of Emotional Health. Most young adults have the physical and emotional resources and support systems to meet the many challenges, tasks, and responsibilities they face. During psychosocial assessment of young adults, the nurse can assess for 10 hallmarks of emotional health (Box 12-2) that indicate successful maturation in this developmental stage.

Health Risks

Risk Factors. Health risk factors for a young adult originate in the community, lifestyle patterns, and family history.

Family History. A family history of a disease may put a young adult at risk for developing it in the middle or older adult years. For example, a young man whose father and paternal grandfather had myocardial infarctions (heart attacks) in their 50s has a risk for a future myocardial infarction. The presence of certain chronic illnesses in the family increases the family member's risk of developing a disease. This family risk is distinct from hereditary disease.

Personal Hygiene Habits. As in all age-groups, personal hygiene habits in the young adult can be risk factors. Sharing eating utensils with a person who has a contagious illness increases the risk of illness. Poor dental hygiene increases the risk of periodontal disease. Gingivitis (inflammation of the gums) and periodontitis (loss of tooth support) can be avoided through oral hygiene (see Chapter 38).

Violent Death and Injury. Violence is the greatest cause of mortality and morbidity in the young adult population. Factors that may predispose to violence, with subsequent injury or death, include poverty, family breakdown, child abuse and neglect, repeated exposure to violence, and ready access to guns. It is important that the nurse perform a thorough psychosocial assessment, including such factors as behavior patterns, history of physical abuse and substance abuse, education, work history, and social support systems, to detect personal and environmental risk factors for violence. Death and injury can occur from physical assaults, motor vehicle or other accidents, and suicide attempts. In 1999 the death rate (per 100,000 population) for 25- to 34-year-olds in the United States due to homicide was 11.2; the death rate due to accidents was 31.3; and the death rate due to suicide was 13.5 (U.S. Department of Health and Human Services [USDHHS], 2001).

Substance Abuse. Substance abuse directly or indirectly contributes to mortality and morbidity in young adults. Intoxicated young adults may be severely injured in motor vehicle accidents that may result in death or permanent disability to other young adults as well.

Dependence on stimulant or depressant drugs can result in death. Overdose of a stimulant drug ("upper") can stress the cardiovascular and nervous systems to the extent that death occurs. The use of depressants ("downers") can lead to an accidental or intentional overdose and death.

Caffeine is a naturally occurring legal stimulant that is readily available in carbonated beverages, chocolate-containing foods, coffee and tea, and over-the-counter medications, such as cold tablets, allergy and analgesic preparations, and appetite suppressants. It is the most widely ingested stimulant in North America. Caffeine can stimulate catecholamine release, which, in turn, stimulates the central nervous system; increases gastric acid secretion, heart rate, and basal metabolic rate; alters blood pressure; increases diuresis; and relaxes smooth muscle. Consumption of large amounts of caffeine can result in restlessness, anxiety, irritability, agitation, muscle tremor, sensory disturbances, heart palpitations, nausea or vomiting, and diarrhea in some individuals.

Substance abuse is not always diagnosable, particularly in its early stages. Nonjudgmental questions about use of legal drugs (prescribed drugs, tobacco, and alcohol), use of soft drugs (marijuana), and use of more problematic drugs (cocaine or heroin) should be a routine part of any physical assessment. Important information may be obtained by making specific inquiries about past medical problems, changes in food intake or sleep patterns, or problems of emotional lability. Reports of arrests because of driving while intoxicated, wife or child abuse, or disorderly conduct should alert the health care provider to probe the possibility of drug abuse more carefully.

Unplanned Pregnancies. Unplanned pregnancies, although more common among adolescents, account for 49% of pregnancies in young and middle adult women (USDHHS, 1999). Unplanned pregnancies are a contin-

ued source of stress that can result in adverse health outcomes for the mother, infant, and family. Often young adults have educational and career goals that take precedence over family development. Interference with these goals can affect future relationships and affects later parent-child relationships.

Determination of situational factors that may affect the progress and outcome of an unplanned pregnancy is important. Exploration of problems such as financial, career, and living accommodations; family support systems; potential parenting disorders; depression; and coping mechanisms is important in assessing the woman with an unplanned pregnancy.

Sexually Transmitted Diseases. Sexually transmitted diseases (STDs) are a major health problem in young adults. STDs include syphilis, chlamydia, gonorrhea, genital herpes, and acquired immunodeficiency syndrome (AIDS). Sexually transmitted diseases have immediate physical effects such as discharge, discomfort, and infection. They may also lead to chronic disorders, which can result from genital herpes; infertility, which can result from gonorrhea; or even death, which results from AIDS. These diseases may occur in sexually active persons, and it is estimated that there are 4 million new infections of chlamydia each year, 3 million new infections of gonorrhea, and 100,000 new infections of syphilis (Ament and Whalen, 1996).

Environmental or Occupational Factors. A common environmental or occupational risk factor is exposure to work-related hazards or agents, which may cause diseases and cancer (Table 12-1). Such lung diseases include silicosis from inhalation of talcum and silicon dust and emphysema from inhalation of smoke. Cancers resulting from occupational exposures may involve the lung, liver, brain, blood, or skin. Questions regarding occupational exposure to hazardous materials should be a routine part of the nurse's assessment.

Health Concerns

Health Promotion. Young adults are generally active and have a minimum of major health problems. However, their lifestyles (e.g., use of tobacco or alcohol) may put them at risk for illnesses or disabilities during their middle or older adult years. Young adults may also be genetically susceptible to certain chronic diseases such as diabetes mellitus and familial hypercholesterolemia (McCance and Huether, 1998). Crohn's disease, a chronic inflammatory disease of the small intestine, most commonly occurs between 15 and 35 years of age. Many young adults have misconceptions regarding transmission and treatment of STDs. Partners are encouraged to know one another's sexual history and sexual practices. The nurse should be alert for STDs when clients come to clinics with complaints of urological or gynecological problems (see Chapter 32). Young adults should be assessed for their knowledge and use of safe-sex practices and genital self-examinations.

Infertility. The term **infertility** refers to a prolonged time to conceive. An estimated 10% to 15% of reproductive couples are infertile, and many are young adults. However, about half of the couples evaluated and treated

Table 12-1	Occupational Hazards/Exposures Associated With Diseases and Cancers	
Job Category	**Occupational Hazard/Exposure**	**Work-Related Condition/Cancer**
Agricultural workers	Pesticides, infectious agents, gases, sunlight	Pesticide poisoning, "farmer's lung," skin cancer
Anesthetists	Anesthetic gases	Reproductive effects, cancer
Automobile workers	Asbestos, plastics, lead, solvents	Asbestosis, dermatitis
Carpenters	Wood dust, wood preservatives, adhesives	Nasopharyngeal cancer, dermatitis
Cement workers	Cement dust, metals	Dermatitis, bronchitis
Dry cleaners	Solvents	Liver disease, dermatitis
Dye workers	Dyestuffs, metals, solvents	Bladder cancer, dermatitis
Glass workers	Heat, solvents, metal powders	Cataracts
Hospital workers	Infectious agents, cleansers, latex gloves, radiation	Infections, latex allergies, unintentional injuries
Insulators	Asbestos, fibrous glass	Asbestosis, lung cancer, mesothelioma
Jackhammer operators	Vibration	Raynaud's phenomenon
Lathe operators	Metal dusts, cutting oils	Lung disease, cancer
Office computer workers	Repetitive wrist motion on computers and eye strain	Tendonitis, carpal tunnel syndrome, tenosynovitis

From Stanhope M, Lancaster J: *Community and public health nursing,* ed 6, St. Louis, 2001, Mosby.

in infertility clinics become pregnant. In about 15% of infertile couples the cause is unknown. Female factors such as ovulatory dysfunction or a pelvic factor is responsible for infertility in 50% of couples, and infertility in 35% of couples is due to a male factor such as sperm and semen abnormalities. For some infertile couples the nurse may be the first resource identified. Nursing assessment of the infertile couple should include comprehensive histories of both the male and female partners to determine factors that may have affected fertility as well as pertinent physical findings (Lowdermilk and Perry, 2003).

Exercise. Exercise patterns can affect health status. Exercise that produces a sustained increase in the pulse rate for 15 to 20 minutes 3 times a week improves cardiopulmonary function by decreasing blood pressure and heart rate. In addition, exercise decreases fatigability, insomnia, tension, and irritability. The nurse should conduct a thorough musculoskeletal assessment, including joint mobility and muscle tone, and psychosocial assessment for improved tolerance to stress to determine the effects of exercise.

Routine Health Screening. Poor adherence to routine screening examinations can put the client at risk for severe illnesses because of failed early detection. Clients should be encouraged to perform monthly skin, breast (BSE), or male genital self-examination (see Chapter 32). The nurse's role is extremely important in educating female clients about BSE and the current breast screening recommendations because breast cancer is the most common major cancer among women in the United States with a steadily increasing incidence. Routine assessment of the skin for recent changes in color or presence of lesions and changes in their appearance should be encouraged. Prolonged exposure to ultraviolet rays of the sun by the adolescent and young adult can increase the risk for development of skin cancer later in life.

Psychosocial Health. The psychosocial health concerns of the young adult are often related to stress, such as job

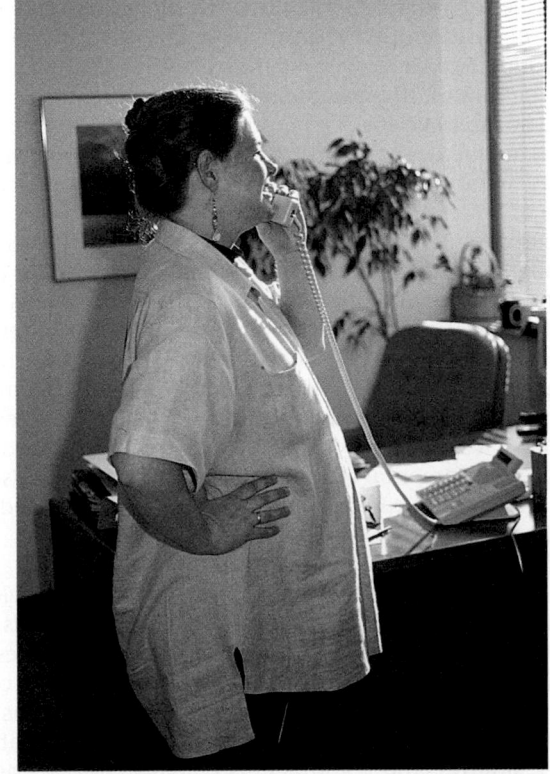

FIGURE **12–3** The ability to handle day-to-day challenges at work minimizes stress.

or family stress. As noted in Chapter 30, stress can be valuable because it motivates a client to change. However, if the stress is prolonged and the client is unable to adapt to the stressor, health problems can develop.

Job Stress. Job stress can occur every day or from time to time. Most young adults are able to handle day-to-day crises (Figure 12-3). Situational job stress may occur when a new boss enters the workplace, a deadline is approaching, or the worker is given new or greater numbers of responsibilities. A recent trend in today's business world and risk factor for job stress is corporate downsizing, leading to increased responsibilities for employees with fewer positions within the corporate structure. Job stress also occurs when a person becomes dissatisfied with a job or the associated responsibilities. Because individuals perceive jobs differently, the types of job stressors vary from client to client. The nurse's assessment of the young adult should include a description of the usual work performed and present work if different. Job assessment also includes conditions and hours, duration of employment, changes in sleep or eating habits, and evidence of increased irritability or nervousness.

Family Stress. Family stressors can occur at any time in family life (see Chapter 9). Family life has peaks, when everyone in the family works together, and valleys, when everyone appears to pull apart. Situational stressors occur during events such as births, deaths, illnesses, marriages, and job losses. Because of the multiplicity of changing relationships and structures in the emerging young adult family, stress is frequently high. Stress may be related to a number of variables, including the work trajectories of both husband and wife, and may lead to dysfunction in the young adult family. This may be reflected in the fact that the highest divorce rate occurs during the first 3 to 5 years of marriage for young adults under the age of 30. When a client seeks health care and presents stress-related symptoms, the nurse should assess for the occurrence of a life change event.

Each family has certain predictable roles or jobs for members. These roles enable the family to function and be an effective part of society. One necessary role is the family leader. In most families one parent is the leader, or both parents act as co-leaders. In single-parent families the parent or occasionally a member of the extended family is the family leader. When this changes as a result of illness, a situational crisis may occur. The nurse should assess environmental and familial factors, including support systems and coping mechanisms commonly used by family members.

Pregnant Woman and Childbearing Family. A developmental task for most young adult couples is the decision to begin a family. Although the physiological changes of pregnancy and childbirth occur only in the woman, cognitive and psychosocial changes and health concerns affect the entire childbearing family, including the baby's father, siblings, and grandparents (Diemer, 1997). Single-parent families and young single mothers tend to be particularly vulnerable both economically and socially.

Health Practices. Women who are anticipating pregnancy benefit from good health practices before conception; these include a balanced diet, exercise, dental checkups, avoidance of alcohol, and cessation of smoking. Women trying to become pregnant should not try weight-reduction diets.

Prenatal Care. **Prenatal care** is the routine examination of the pregnant woman by an obstetrician, nurse practitioner, or certified nurse-midwife. Health promotion interventions are important during the prenatal period and can improve the well-being of the woman and fetus. Prenatal care includes a thorough physical assessment of the pregnant woman during regularly scheduled intervals; provision of information regarding sexually transmitted diseases, other vaginal infections, and urinary infections that could adversely affect the fetus; and counseling about exercise patterns, diet, and child care. Regular prenatal care can address health concerns that arise during the pregnancy.

Physiological Changes. The physiological changes and needs of the pregnant woman vary with each trimester (Table 12-2). The nurse must be familiar with these physiological changes, their causes, and helpful interventions. All women experience some physiological changes in the first trimester, but some changes affect only certain women. During the second trimester, growth of the uterus and fetus results in some of the physical signs of pregnancy. If this is the woman's first pregnancy, she may be able to see and feel the enlarged uterus. However, it is common for her abdomen to stay relatively flat. In subsequent pregnancies she may "show" as early as the beginning of the second trimester. During the third trimester increases in **Braxton Hicks contractions** (irregular, short contractions), fatigue, and urinary frequency occur. Close to the onset of labor, the woman may experience a burst of energy during which she cleans house and prepares for the baby by shopping for baby supplies. This period is called **nesting.** Many experts in obstetrics and seasoned veterans of pregnancy believe that nesting indicates a rapidly approaching time of delivery.

Puerperium. The **puerperium** is a period of approximately 6 weeks after delivery. During this time the woman's body reverts to its prepregnant physical status. The nurse should assess the woman's knowledge of and ability to care for both herself and for her newborn baby. Assessment of parenting skills and maternal-infant interactions is particularly important.

Cognitive Changes. Cognitive changes during pregnancy, primarily involving sensory perception and needs for education, affect both parents and may occur gradually or quickly.

Sensory Perception. The pregnant woman generally experiences changes in sensory perception. Temporary changes occur in visual and hearing acuity, taste, and smell. Many pregnant women frequently stroke the abdomen, possibly because of a change in the sensation of touch or other sensory need. The woman may be using the sensation of touch to initiate bonding with her child.

Needs for Education. The entire childbearing family needs education about pregnancy, labor, delivery, breastfeeding, and integration of the newborn into the family structure. Traditionally, childbirth classes help parents plan for the birth of the child and focus on the normal physiological changes of pregnancy, the processes of labor and delivery, methods of pain control, symptoms of impending labor, and care of the newborn. Many health care centers also have sibling and grandparent preparation

Table 12-2	Major Physiological Changes During Pregnancy
Signs and Symptoms	**Causes**
First Trimester	
Amenorrhea	Fertilization and implantation of egg
	Increases in hormone levels
Morning sickness	Increased serum hormone levels
Breast changes	Increased estrogen levels
Enlargement	
Tenderness	
Darkened and enlarged nipples	
Urinary frequency	Pressure of uterus on bladder
Fatigue	Increases in hormone levels
	Increased nutritional demands
	Decreased nutritional intake resulting from morning sickness
Second Trimester	
Integumentary changes	Increased levels of melanocyte-stimulating hormone
Pigmented nipple and breast	
Hyperpigmentation of abdominal line (linea nigra)	
Mottling of cheeks or forehead (chloasma or "mask of pregnancy")	
Local or generalized pruritus	
Hypertrophy of gums causing gingival swelling and bleeding	Proliferation of interdental papillary blood vessels, resulting in local inflammation and hyperplasia
Increasing size of uterine fundus	Growth of fetus
Sensation of movement or gaslike movements (quickening)	Fetal movement
Braxton Hicks contractions	Expanding uterus and preparation of uterus for labor
Third Trimester	
Increased colostrum	Hormonal influence; preparation of breasts for lactation
Increased urinary frequency	Pressure on bladder from enlarged fetus

Data from Lowdermilk D, Perry S: *Maternity nursing,* ed 6, St. Louis, 2003, Mosby; and Dickason E, Silverman B, Kaplan J: *Maternal-infant nursing care,* St. Louis, 1998, Mosby.

classes. Not all pregnant women, however, attend childbirth classes for a variety of reasons.

Psychosocial Changes. Like the physiological changes of pregnancy, psychosocial changes may occur at various times during the 9 months of pregnancy and in the puerperium. Table 12-3 summarizes the major categories of psychosocial changes and implications for nursing intervention.

Health Concerns. The pregnant woman and her partner have many health questions. For example, they may wonder whether the pregnancy and baby will be normal. The majority of the health needs related to pregnancy can be met with proper prenatal care.

Acute Care. The young adult years are generally a time of good physical and emotional health. Potential health hazards may be related to lifestyle. Acute care for young adults is frequently related to accidents, substance abuse, exposure to environmental and occupational hazards, stress-related illnesses, respiratory infections, gastroenteritis, influenza, urinary tract infections, and minor surgery. An acute minor illness can cause a disruption in life activities of the young adult and increase stress in an already hectic lifestyle. Dependency and limitations posed by treatment regimens can also increase frustration for the young adult. To give young adults a sense of maintaining control of their health care choices, it is important to keep them informed about their health status and involve them in health care decisions.

Restorative and Continuing Care. Chronic conditions are not common in young adulthood, but they can occur. Chronic illnesses such as hypertension, coronary artery disease, and diabetes may have their onset in young adulthood without being known to the young adult until later in life. Causes of chronic illness and disability in the young adult can include accidents, multiple sclerosis, rheumatoid arthritis, AIDS, and cancer. Chronic illness and disability can affect the accomplishment of important developmental tasks in young adulthood. The threat to the young adult's independence that is caused by chronic illness or disability can result in the need to change personal, family, and career goals. Nursing interventions for the young adult faced with chronic illness or disability should include potential developmental problems related to sense of identity, the establishment of independence, reorganization of intimate relationships and family structure, and launching of a chosen career (Lewis, Heitkemper, and Dirksen, 2000).

Table 12-3	Major Psychosocial Changes During Pregnancy
Category	**Implications for Nursing**
Body image	Morning sickness and fatigue may contribute to poor body image
	Client may feel big, awkward, and unattractive during third trimester when fetus is growing more rapidly
	Increase in breast size may make the woman feel more feminine and sexually appealing
	May take extra time with hygiene and grooming, trying new hairstyles and makeup
	Begins to "show" during the second trimester and starts to plan maternity wardrobe
	General feeling of well-being when woman can feel the baby move and hear the heartbeat
Role changes	Both partners think about and can have feelings of uncertainty about impending role changes
	May have feelings of ambivalence about becoming parents and concern about ability to be parents
Sexuality	Need reassurance that sexual activity will not harm fetus
	Desire for sexual activity may be influenced by body image
	May desire cuddling and holding rather than sexual intercourse
Coping mechanisms	Need reassurance that childbirth and child rearing are natural and positive experiences, but can also be stressful
	Often unable to cope with particular stressors such as finding new housing, preparing the nursery, or participating in childbirth classes
Stresses during puerperium	May return home from hospital fatigued and unfamiliar with infant care
	May experience physical discomfort or feelings of anxiety or depression
	May be necessary for woman to return to work soon after delivery with subsequent feelings of guilt, anxiety, or, possibly, sense of freedom or relief

Middle Adult

In middle adulthood, the individual makes lasting contributions through involvement with others. Generally the middle adult years begin around the early to mid 30s and last through the late 60s, corresponding to Levinson's developmental phases of "settling down" and the "payoff years." During this period, personal and career achievements have often already been experienced. Many middle adults find particular joy in assisting their children and other young people to become productive and responsible adults (Figure 12-4). They may also begin to help aging parents while being responsible for their own children, placing them in the "sandwich generation." Using leisure time in satisfying and creative ways is a challenge that, if met satisfactorily, enables middle adults to prepare for retirement.

Although most middle adults have achieved socioeconomic stability, recent trends in corporate downsizing have left many middle adults either jobless or forced to accept lower-paying jobs. Economists at the Agency for Health Care Policy and Research have revealed that in 1996, 75% of U.S. workers were offered health insurance by their employers, an increase from 72% in 1987. However, the number of workers who turned down employer-offered health insurance coverage has more than doubled over the past decade, from 2.6 million in 1987 to 6 million in 1996. During that same time period, health insurance premiums rose by 90%, and fewer employers have shared the cost of health insurance plans that include coverage for dependents (Cooper and Schone, 1997). As a result, a greater proportion of the population is currently unable to afford adequate health insurance coverage (Scanlon, Chernew, and Lave, 1997).

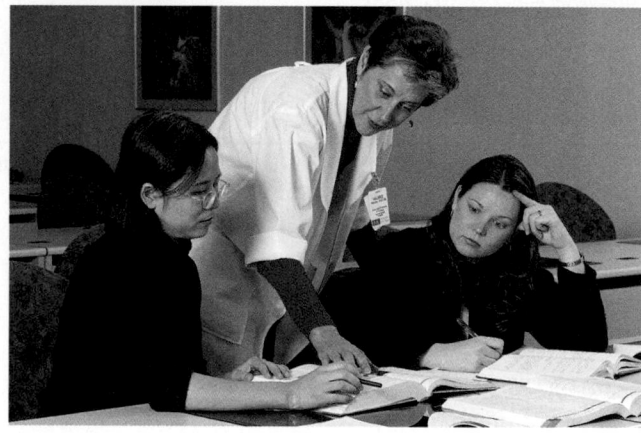

FIGURE **12–4** Ongoing prenatal care reduces complications of pregnancy.

Men and women must adjust to inevitable biological changes. As in adolescence, middle adults use considerable energy to adapt self-concept and body image to physiological realities and changes in physical appearance. High self-esteem, a favorable body image, and a positive attitude toward physiological changes are fostered when adults engage in physical exercise, balanced diets, adequate sleep, and good hygiene practices that promote vigorous, healthy bodies.

Physical Changes

Major physiological changes occur between 40 and 65 years of age. Table 12-4 summarizes these normal developmental changes that the nurse considers when con-

Table 12-4	Physical Assessment Findings in the Middle Adult
Body System	**Findings**
Integument	Intact condition
	Appropriate distribution of pigmentation
	Slow, progressive decrease in skin turgor
	Graying and loss of hair (Baldness patterns in males are established by age 55; hair loss after this time might have other causes.)
Head and neck	Symmetry of scalp, skull, and face
	Normal accessory organs of vision
Eyes	Visual acuity by Snellen chart that is less than 20/50
	Pupillary reaction to light and accommodation
	Normal visual fields and extraocular movements
	Normal retinal structures
Ears	Normal auditory structures and acuity
Nose, sinuses, and throat	Patent nares and intact sinuses, mouth, and pharynx
	Location of trachea at midline
	Nonpalpable lateral thyroid lobes
Thorax and lungs	Increased anteroposterior diameter
	Respiratory rate 16-20 breaths per minute and regular
	Ratio of respiratory rate to heart rate: 1:4
	Normal tactile fremitus, resonance, and breath sounds
Heart and vascular system	Normal heart sounds
	Systole: S_1 less than S_2 at base
	Diastole: S_1 greater than S_2 at apex
	Point of maximal impulse: at fifth intercostal space in midclavicular line and 2 cm or less in diameter
	Vital signs
	Temperature: 36.1°-37.6° C (97°-99.6° F)
	Pulse: 60-100 bpm (conditioned athlete <50)
	Blood pressure:
	<130 mm Hg systolic
	<85 mm Hg diastolic
	Respirations: 12-20 breaths per minute
	All pulses palpable
Breasts	Decreased size resulting from decreased muscle mass
	Normal nipples
Abdomen	No tenderness or organomegaly
	Decreased strength of abdominal muscles
Female reproductive system	Change in menstrual cycle and in duration and quality of menstrual flow to cessation of menses
	"Hot flashes"
	Change in cervical mucosa
Male reproductive system	Normal penis and scrotum
	Prostatic enlargement in some individuals
Musculoskeletal system	Decreased muscle mass
	Decreased range of joint motion
Neurological system	Appropriate affect, appearance, and behavior
	Lucidity and appropriate level of cognitive ability
	Intact cranial nerves
	Adequate motor responses
	Responsive sensory system

ducting a physical examination. The most visible changes are graying of the hair, wrinkling of the skin, and thickening of the waist. Decreases in hearing and visual acuity are often noted during this period. Often these physiological changes have an impact on self-concept and body image. The most significant physiological changes during middle age are menopause in women and the climacteric in men.

Perimenopause and Menopause. Menstruation and ovulation occur in a cyclical rhythm in the woman from adolescence into middle adulthood. Perimenopause is the period during which ovarian function declines, resulting in a diminishing number of ova and irregular menstrual cycles. **Menopause** is the disruption of this cycle, primarily because of the inability of the neurohormonal system to maintain its periodic stimulation of the endocrine system. The ovaries no longer produce estrogen and progesterone, and the blood levels of these hormones drop markedly. Menopause typically occurs between 45 and 60 years of age (see Chapter 27). Approximately 10% of women have no symptoms of menopause other than cessation of menstruation, 70% to 80% are aware of other changes but have no problems, and approximately 10% experience changes severe enough to interfere with activities of daily living.

Climacteric. The **climacteric** occurs in men in their late 40s or early 50s (see Chapter 27). It is caused by decreased levels of androgens. Throughout this period and thereafter, a man is still capable of producing fertile sperm and fathering a child. However, penile erection is less firm, ejaculation is less frequent, and the refractory period is longer.

Cognitive Changes

Changes in the cognitive function of middle adults are rare except with illness or trauma. The middle adult can learn new skills and information. Some middle adults enter educational or vocational programs to prepare themselves for entering the job market or changing jobs.

Psychosocial Changes

The psychosocial changes in the middle adult may involve expected events, such as children moving away from home, or unexpected events, such as a marital separation or the death of a close friend. Many middle adults may find themselves in the **"sandwich generation,"** having the responsibility of raising their own children while caring for aging parents. These changes may result in stress that can affect the middle adult's overall level of health.

Nurses should assess the major life changes occurring in the middle adult and the impact that the changes have on that person's state of health. Nursing assessment should also include individual psychosocial factors such as coping mechanisms and sources of social support.

In the middle adult years, as children depart from the household, the family enters the postparental family stage. Time and financial demands on the parents decrease, and the couple faces the task of redefining their own relationship. As grandchildren arrive, grandparenting styles must be chosen. It is during this period that many middle adults begin to take on a healthier lifestyle. Although not advisable to wait until this stage in life to think about health promotion, "better late than never" does apply. Assessment of health promotion needs for the middle adult include adequate rest, leisure activities, regular exercise, good nutrition, reduction or cessation in the use of tobacco or alcohol, and regular screening examinations. Assessment of the middle adult's social environment is also important, including relationship concerns; communication and relationships with children, grandchildren, and aging parents; and caregiver concerns with their own aging or disabled parents.

According to Erikson's developmental theory, the primary developmental task of the middle years is to achieve generativity (Erikson, 1968, 1982). Generativity is the willingness to care for and guide others. Middle adults can achieve generativity with their own children or the children of close friends or through guidance in social interactions with the next generation. If middle adults fail to achieve generativity, stagnation occurs. This is shown by excessive concern with themselves or destructive behavior toward their children and the community.

Career Transition. Career changes may occur by choice or as a result of changes in the workplace or society. In recent decades, middle adults more often change occupations for a variety of reasons, including limited upward mobility, decreasing availability of jobs, and seeking an occupation that is more challenging to the individual. In some cases technological advances or other changes force middle adults to seek new jobs. Such changes, particularly when unanticipated, may result in stress that can affect health, family relationships, self-concept, and other dimensions.

Sexuality. After the departure of their last child from the home, many couples recultivate their relationships and find increased marital and sexual satisfaction during middle age. The onset of menopause and the climacteric can affect the sexual health of the middle adult. A woman may desire increased sexual activity because pregnancy is no longer possible. Menopausal women may also experience vaginal dryness and dyspareunia or pain during sexual intercourse (see Chapter 27).

During middle age a man may notice changes in the strength of his erection and a decrease in his ability to experience repeated orgasm. Other factors influencing sexuality during this period include work stress, diminished health of one or both partners, and the use of prescription medications, for example, antihypertensive agents, with side effects that may influence sexual desire or functioning. Both partners may experience stresses related to sexual changes or a conflict between their sexual needs and self-perceptions and social attitudes or expectations (see Chapter 27).

Family Types. Psychosocial factors involving the family may include the stresses of singlehood, marital changes, transition of the family as children leave home, and the care of aging parents.

Singlehood. Many adults over 35 years of age in the United States have never been married. Many of those are college-educated people who have embraced the philosophy of choice and freedom, have delayed marriage, and have delayed parenthood. Some middle adults who have chosen to remain single, however, have also opted to become parents either biologically or through adoption. Many single middle adults may have no relatives but share a family type of relationship with close friends or work associates. Consequently, some single middle adults may feel isolated during traditional "family" holidays such as Thanksgiving or Christmas. In times of illness, middle adults who have chosen to remain single and childless may have to rely on other relatives or friends, increasing caregiving demands of those family members who may also have other caregiving responsibilities. Nursing assessment of single middle adults should include a thorough assessment of psychosocial factors, including the individual's definition of family and available support systems.

Marital Changes. Marital changes that may occur during middle age include death of a spouse, separation, divorce, and the choice of remarrying or remaining single.

A widowed, separated, or divorced client goes through a period of grief and loss in which it is necessary to adapt to the change in marital status. Normal grieving progresses through a series of phases, and resolution of grief may take a year or more. The nurse should assess effective coping of the middle adult to the grief and loss associated with certain life changes (Chapter 29).

If a single middle adult decides to marry, the stressors of marriage are similar to those for the young adult. In addition, the couple may have to cope with the social expectations and pressures related to marriage.

Family Transitions. The departure of the last child from the home may be a stressor. Many parents welcome freedom from child-rearing responsibilities, whereas others feel lonely or without direction because of this change. Eventually parents must reassess their marriage and try to resolve conflicts and plan for the future. Occasionally this readjustment phase may lead to marital conflicts, separation, and divorce.

Care of Aging Parents. Increasing life spans in the United States and Canada have led to increased numbers of older adults in the population. Therefore greater numbers of middle adults must address the personal and social issues confronting their aging parents. Many middle adults find themselves in the "sandwich generation" caught between the responsibilities of caring for dependent children and those of caring for aging and ailing parents. The needs of the caregivers is an area that continues to grow.

Housing, employment, health, and economic realities have changed the traditional social expectations between generations in families. The middle adult and the older adult parent may have conflicting priorities related to their relationship while the older adult strives to remain independent. Negotiations and compromises help in defining and resolving problems. Nurses deal with middle and older adults in the community, long-term care facilities, and hospitals. The nurse can help identify the health needs of both groups and can assist the multigenerational family in determining the health and community resources available to them as they make decisions and plans. The nurse should also assess family relationships to determine family members' perceptions of responsibility and loyalty in relation to caring for older adult members. Assessment of environmental resources (e.g., number of rooms in the house or stairwells) in relation to the complexity of health care demands for the older adult is also important.

Health Concerns

Health Promotion. Physiological concerns for the middle adult include stress, level of wellness, obesity, and the formation of positive health habits.

Stress and Stress Reduction. Because middle adults are experiencing physiological changes and face certain health realities, their perceptions of health and health behaviors are often important factors in maintaining health. Today's complex world makes individuals more prone to stress-related illnesses such as heart attacks, hypertension, migraine headaches, ulcers, colitis, autoimmune disease, backache, arthritis, and cancer.

When adults seek health care, the nurse's focus on the goal of wellness can guide clients to evaluate health behaviors, lifestyle, and environment. Attention to risk factors that can be altered to improve the client's health, such as stress, obesity, use of tobacco, excessive alcohol consumption, poor nutrition, and unsafe sexual practices, can increase the quality of life and add years to it.

Throughout life, people are exposed to many stressors (see Chapter 30). After these stressors are identified, the client and nurse can work together to intervene and modify the stress response. Specific interventions for stress reduction can fall into three categories. First, the frequency of stress-producing situations is minimized. Together the nurse and client identify approaches to prevent stressful situations, such as habituation, change avoidance, time blocking, time management, and environmental modification. The second category is psychophysiological preparation to increase stress resistance, such as increasing self-esteem, improving assertiveness, redirecting goal alternatives, and reorienting cognitive appraisal. Last, the physiological response to stress is avoided. The nurse uses relaxation techniques, imagery, and biofeedback to recondition the client's response to stress. Chapter 35 explains these general interventions in greater detail.

Levels of Wellness. The nurse must be able to assess the health status of the middle adult client. Such assessment offers direction for planning nursing care and is useful in evaluating the effectiveness of nursing interventions. Table 12-4, which shows the physical changes of the middle adult, can be used with other standard assessment techniques as a guide for physical assessment (see Chapter 32).

Obesity. Obesity is a growing health concern for middle adults. The prevalence of obesity, defined as having a body mass index (BMI) of 30 or more, among U.S. adults was 19.8% in 2000, reflecting a 61% increase since 1991 (National Center for Chronic Disease Prevention and Health Promotion, 2002). Health consequences of obesity include such ailments as high blood pressure, high blood cholesterol, Type 2 (non–insulin dependent) diabetes, coronary heart disease, osteoarthritis, and obstructive sleep apnea. Continued focus on the goal of wellness can assist clients in evaluating health behaviors and lifestyle that contribute to obesity during the middle adult years. Counseling related to physical activity and nutrition is an important component of the plan of care for overweight and obese clients.

Forming Positive Health Habits. A habit is a person's usual practice or manner of behavior. This behavior pattern is reinforced by frequent repetition until it becomes the individual's customary way of behaving. Some habits support health, such as exercise and brushing and flossing the teeth each day. Other habits involve risk factors to health, such as smoking or eating foods with little or no nutritional value.

During assessment the nurse frequently obtains data indicating positive and negative health behaviors by the client. Examples of positive health behaviors include regular exercise, adherence to good dietary habits, avoidance of excess consumption of alcohol, participation in routine screening and diagnostic tests (laboratory work for serum cholesterol, mammography) for disease prevention and health promotion, and lifestyle changes to reduce stress. In the planning, implementation, and evaluation phases, the nurse helps the client maintain habits that protect health and offers healthier alternatives to poor habits.

Health teaching and health counseling are often directed at improving health habits (Box 12-3). The more fully the nurse understands the dynamics of behavior and habits, the more likely interventions will help the client to achieve or reinforce health-promoting behaviors.

To help clients form positive health habits the nurse becomes a teacher and facilitator. By providing information about how the body functions and how habits are formed and changed, the nurse raises clients' levels of knowledge regarding the potential impact of behavior on health. A nurse cannot change clients' habits. Clients have control of and are responsible for their own behaviors. The nurse can explain psychological principles of changing habits and offer information about health risks. The nurse can also offer positive reinforcement (such as praise and rewards) for health-directed behaviors and decisions. Such reinforcement increases the likelihood that the behavior will be repeated. Ultimately, however, the client decides which behaviors will become habits of daily living.

The nurse may assist young and middle adults in considering factors such as prevention of STDs, substance abuse, and accident prevention in relation to decreasing health risks. For example, clients should be provided with factual information on sexually transmitted disease causes, symptoms, and transmission. The nurse should discuss methods of protection during sexual activity with the client in an open and nonjudgmental manner and reinforce the importance of practicing "safe sex" (see Chapter 27). The nurse can provide counseling and support for clients seeking treatment for substance abuse. The nurse can assist clients in recognizing and altering unsafe habits and potential health hazards (see Chapter 37). The nurse should also encourage clients to express their feelings to promote problem solving and recognition of risk factors by clients themselves. Barriers to change do exist (Box 12-4). Unless these barriers are minimized or eliminated, it is futile to encourage the client to take actions that are going to be blocked.

Psychosocial Concerns. Two common psychosocial health concerns of the middle adult are anxiety and depression.

Anxiety. Anxiety is a critical maturational phenomenon related to change, conflict, and perceived control of the environment (Stuart and Laraia, 2001)). Adults often experience anxiety in response to the physiological and psychosocial changes of middle age. Such anxiety can motivate the adult to rethink life goals and can stimulate productivity. For some adults, however, this anxiety precipitates psychosomatic illness and preoccupation with death. In this case the middle adult views life as being half or more over and thinks in terms of the time left to live.

Box 12-3

Client Teaching

Positive Health Habits

Objective

- Client will increase exercise patterns to include three 1-mile walks per week to assist in weight loss and improve cardiopulmonary functions.

Teaching Strategies

- Review with client the daily work schedule and identify potential times for exercise.
- Inform client about the effect of exercise on weight control and improved cardiac function.
- Demonstrate how to calculate target heart rate and assess pulse correctly.
- Provide warm-up and cool-down exercises and demonstrate how to do them.
- Instruct client about support shoes for walking exercises.

Evaluation

- Have client keep log of exercise periods.
- Have client demonstrate pulse measurement.
- Have client demonstrate warm-up and cool-down exercises.
- Inspect client's feet for blisters or sores.

Clearly, a life-threatening illness, marital transition, or job stressor increases the anxiety of the client and family. The nurse may need to use crisis intervention or stress management techniques to help the client adapt to the changes of the middle adult years (see Chapter 30).

Depression. Depression is a mood disorder that manifests itself in many ways. Although the most frequent age of onset is between ages 25 and 44, it is common among adults in the middle years and may have many causes (Stuart and Laraia, 2001). The risk factors for depression include being female; disappointments or losses at work, school, or in family relationships; departure of the last child from the home; and family history. In fact, the incidence of depression in women is twice that of men. Persons experiencing mild depression describe themselves as feeling sad, blue, downcast, down in the dumps, and tearful. Other symptoms include alterations in sleep patterns such as difficulty in sleeping (insomnia) or sleeping too much (hypersomnia), irritability, feelings of social disinterest, and decreased alertness. Physical changes such as weight loss or weight gain, headaches, or feelings of fatigue regardless of the amount of rest may also be depressive symptoms. Depression that occurs during the middle years is commonly characterized by moderate-to-high anxiety and physical complaints. Mood changes and depression are common phenomena during menopause. Depression may be worsened by the abuse of alcohol or other substances. Nursing assessment of the depressed middle adult includes focused data collection regarding individual and family history of depression, mood changes, cognitive changes, behavioral and social

Box 12-4　Barriers to Change

External Barriers	Internal Barriers
Lack of facilities	Lack of knowledge
Lack of materials	Lack of motivation
Lack of social supports	Insufficient skills to effect change in health habits
	Undefined short- and long-term goals

changes, and physical changes. Assessment data should be collected from both the client and the client's family, because family data may be particularly important, depending on the level of depression being experienced by the middle adult.

Community Health Programs. Community health programs for young and middle adults are designed to prevent illness, promote health, and detect disease in the early stages. Nurses can make valuable contributions to the community's health by taking an active part in the planning of screening and teaching programs and support groups for middle adults.

Family planning, birthing, and parenting skills are program topics in which adults might be interested. Health screening for diabetes, hypertension, eye disease, and cancer is a good opportunity for the nurse to perform assessment and provide health teaching and health counseling.

Health education programs can promote changes in behavior and lifestyle. The nurse as health teacher offers information that enables the client to make decisions about health practices within the context of health promotion for young to middle adults. The nurse must be sure that educational programs are culturally appropriate (Box 12-5). Changes to more positive health practices during young and middle adulthood may lead to fewer or less complicated health problems as an older adult. During health counseling the nurse and client design a plan of action that addresses the client's health and well-being. Through objective problem solving, the nurse helps the client grow and change.

Acute Care. Acute illnesses and conditions experienced in middle adulthood are similar to those of young adulthood. Injuries and acute illnesses in middle adulthood, however, may take a longer recovery period because of the slowing of recuperative processes. In addition, acute illnesses and injuries experienced in middle adulthood are more likely to become chronic conditions. For those middle adults who are in the "sandwich generation," stress levels may also increase as the middle adult tries to balance responsibilities related to employment, family life, care of children, and care of aging parents while recovering from an injury or acute illness.

Restorative and Continuing Care. Chronic illnesses such as diabetes mellitus, hypertension, rheumatoid arthritis, chronic obstructive pulmonary disease, or multiple sclero-

Cultural Aspects of Care
Box 12-5

Breast cancer is the most common cancer among American women and accounts for one of every three cancer diagnoses. Five-year survival has increased significantly over the past 25 years; however, survival rates differ among various cultural groups. Investigators have found that cultural beliefs and the actual experience of breast cancer screening may influence womens' decisions to not engage in regularly scheduled breast cancer screening and thus result often in late-stage diagnosis.

Implications for Practice

- Be aware of cultural influences that may affect the performance of monthly breast self-examinations (BSEs) or obtaining mammograms.
- Review BSE teaching, and encourage clients to report any findings that they think may be abnormal.
- Emphasize the importance of breast cancer screening for all women.
- Send reminders for annual physical examinations and mammograms.

Phillips JM and others: African American women's experiences with breast cancer screening, *J Nurs Scholarsh* 33(2):135, 2001.

sis may affect the roles and responsibilities assumed by the middle adult. Strained family relationships, modifications in family activities, increased health care tasks, increased financial stress, the need for housing adaptation, social isolation, medical concerns, and grieving may all result from chronic illness. The degree of disability and the client's perception of both the illness and the disability determine the extent to which lifestyle changes will occur. A few examples of the problems experienced by clients who develop debilitating chronic illness during adulthood include role reversal, changes in sexual behavior, and alterations in self-image. Along with the current health status of the chronically ill middle adult, the nurse must assess the knowledge base of both the client and family. This assessment should include the medical course of the illness and the prognosis for the client. In addition, the nurse determines the coping mechanisms of the client and family, adherence to treatment and rehabilitation regimens, and the need for community and social services, along with appropriate referrals.

Key Concepts

- Adult development involves orderly and sequential changes in characteristics and attitudes that adults experience over time.
- Many changes experienced by the young adult are related to the natural process of maturation and socialization.
- Young adults are in a stable period of physical development, except for changes related to pregnancy.

- Cognitive development continues throughout the young and middle adult years.
- Emotional health of young adults is correlated with the ability to address and resolve personal and social problems.
- Young adults must choose a career and decide whether to remain single or marry and begin a family.
- Pregnant women need to understand physiological changes occurring in each trimester.
- Psychosocial changes and health concerns during pregnancy and the puerperium affect the parents, the siblings, and often the extended family.
- Prenatal care reduces maternal and fetal mortality and morbidity.
- Midlife transition begins when a person becomes aware that physiological and psychosocial changes signify passage to another stage in life.
- Two significant physiological changes of the middle years are menopause in women and the climacteric in men.
- Cognitive changes are rare in middle age except in cases of illness or physical trauma.
- Psychosocial changes for middle adults may be related to career transition, sexuality, marital changes, family transition, and care of aging parents.
- Health concerns of middle adults commonly involve stress-related illnesses, health assessment, and adoption of positive health habits.

Key Terms

Braxton Hicks
  contractions, *p. 224*
Climacteric, *p. 228*
Doula, *p. 220*
Infertility, *p. 222*
Lactation, *p. 220*

Menopause, *p. 227*
Nesting, *p. 224*
Prenatal care, *p. 224*
Puerperium, *p. 224*
Sandwich generation, *p. 228*

Critical Thinking Exercises
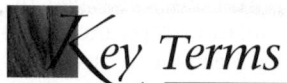

1. Joan K. is a 24-year-old woman who smokes two packs of cigarettes per day. She began smoking when she was 14 years old. Joan complains to the nurse at the clinic, "I just can't seem to kick the habit no matter how hard I try." What information does the nurse need to know to assist Joan in quitting smoking?
2. James D., age 48, married, and the father of 13- and 16-year-old sons, has recently had to assume the responsibility of caring for his 78-year-old mother after she suffered a stroke. Describe the nurse's role in assisting James in caring for his mother.

Review Questions

1. With the exception of pregnant or lactating women, the young adult has usually completed physical growth by the age of:
   1. 18.
   2. 20.
   3. 25.
   4. 30.

2. When assessing young adults, the nurse will find this population usually has a high level of wellness. However, it is important to direct health care education toward activities related to:
   1. Health promotion.
   2. Primary prevention.
   3. Secondary prevention.
   4. Tertiary prevention.

3. When determining the amount of information that the individual needs to make decisions about the prescribed course of therapy, the nurse should consider those factors that may affect the individual's compliance with the regimen, including educational level, socioeconomic factors, and:
   1. Sexuality.
   2. Lifestyle.
   3. Gender.
   4. Motivation.

4. A support person who is present during labor to assist women who have no other source of support is called a (an):
   1. Assistant.
   2. Nurse.
   3. Lay doula.
   4. Midwife.

5. The process of breast-feeding is known as:
   1. Lactation.
   2. Sucking.
   3. Nesting.
   4. Bottle feeding.

6. Close friends and associates of the single young adult may also be viewed as the individual's:
   1. Siblings.
   2. "Family."
   3. Alternative family structure.
   4. Substitute parents.

7. A young man's father and paternal grandfather had myocardial infarctions (heart attacks) in their 50s. He has a risk for a future myocardial infarction. The young man faces what type of health risk:
   1. Lifestyle.
   2. Personal hygiene habit.
   3. Family history.
   4. Community.

8. Sharing eating utensils with a person who has a contagious illness increases the risk of illness. This type of health risk is:
   1. Lifestyle.
   2. Personal hygiene habit.
   3. Family history.
   4. Community.

9. To improve an adult's health habits, the nurse uses often uses health counseling and:
   1. Medications.
   2. Referrals.
   3. Health teaching.
   4. Stress management techniques.

10. To help the client adapt to the changes of the middle adult years, the nurse may need to use crisis intervention or:
    1. Medications.
    2. Referrals.
    3. Health promotion.
    4. Stress management techniques.

References

American Academy of Pediatrics: Technical report: coparent or second-parent adoption by same-sex parents, *Pediatrics* 109(2):341, 2002, http://www.aap.org/policy/020008t.html.

Coll C, Surrey J, Weingarten K: *Mothering against the odds,* New York, 1998, The Guilford Press.

Cooper P, Schone B: More offers, fewer takers for employment-based health insurance: 1987 and 1996, *Health Aff* 16(6):142, 1997.

Dickason E, Silverman B, Kaplan J: *Maternal-infant nursing care,* St. Louis, 1998, Mosby.

Diekelmann J: The young adult: the choice is health or illness, *Am J Nurs* 76:1276, 1976.

Edelman C, Mandle C: *Health promotion throughout the lifespan,* ed 5, St. Louis, 2002, Mosby.

Erikson E: *Childhood and society,* ed 2, New York, 1963, WW Norton.

Erikson E: *Identity: youth and crisis,* New York, 1968, WW Norton.

Erikson E: *The life cycle completed: a review,* New York, 1982, WW Norton.

Gilligan C: *In a different voice,* Cambridge, Mass, 1993, Harvard University Press.

Havighurst R: Successful aging. In Williams RH, Tibbits C, Donahue W, editors: *Process of aging,* vol 1, New York, 1972, Atherton.

Lawrence R, Lawrence R: *Breastfeeding: a guide for the medical profession,* ed 5, St. Louis, 1999, Mosby.

Levinson D and others: *The seasons of a man's life,* New York, 1978, Knopf.

Lewis S, Heitkemper M, Dirksen S: *Medical-surgical nursing,* ed 4, St. Louis, 2000, Mosby.

Lowdermilk D, Perry S: *Maternity nursing,* ed 6, St. Louis, 2003, Mosby.

Masters W, Johnson V: *Human sexual response,* Boston, 1970, Little, Brown.

McCance K, Huether S: *Pathophysiology: the biologic basis for disease in adults and children,* ed 3, St. Louis, 1998, Mosby.

National Center for Chronic Disease Prevention and Health Promotion: *Overweight and obesity,* 2002, http://www.cdc.gov/nccdphp/dnpa/obesity.

Scanlon D, Chernew M, Lave J: Consumer health plan choice: current knowledge and future directions, *Annu Rev Public Health* 18:507, 1997.

Sheehy G: *New passages: mapping your life across time,* New York, 1995, Random House.

Stanhope M, Lancaster J: *Community and public health nursing,* ed 5, St. Louis, 2001, Mosby.

Stanhope M, Lancaster J: *Community and public health nursing,* ed 6, St. Louis, 2004, Mosby.

Stuart G, Laraia M: *Principles and practice of psychiatric nursing,* ed 7, St. Louis, 2001, Mosby.

U.S. Department of Commerce, Census Bureau: *Resident population estimates of the United States by age and sex,* 2000, http://eire.census.gov/popest/archives/national/nation2/intfile2-1.txt.

U.S. Department of Health and Human Services, Public Health Service: *Mortality & morbidity weekly report: insurance coverage of unintended pregnancies resulting in live-born infants,* 48(5) Hyattsville, Md, 1999, Centers for Disease Control and Prevention, National Center for Health Statistics, http://cdc.gov/nccdphp/drh/pdf/mm4805.pdf.

U.S. Department of Health and Human Services, Public Health Service: *National vital statistics report: deaths—leading causes for 1999,* 49(11), Hyattsville, Md, 2001, Centers for Disease Control and Prevention, National Center for Health Statistics, http://www.cdc.gov/nchs/data/nvsr/nvsr49/nvsr49_11.pdf.

U.S. Department of Labor: *20 facts on women workers,* 2000, http://permanent.access.gpo.gov/lps5581/20fact00.htm.

Research References

Ament L, Whalen E: Sexually transmitted diseases in pregnancy: diagnosis, impact, and intervention, *J Obstet Gynecol Neonatal Nurs* 25(8):657, 1996.

Diemer G: Expectant fathers: influence of perinatal education on stress, coping, and spousal relations, *Res Nurs Health* 20(4):281, 1997.

Domian E: Cultural practices and social support of pregnant women in a northern New Mexico community, *J Nurs Scholarsh* 33(4):331, 2001.

Phillips JM and others: African American women's experiences with breast cancer screening. *J Nurs Scholarsh* 33(2):135, 2001.

13

$\mathcal{O}$lder Adult

Media Resources

http://evolve.elsevier.com/Potter/
fundamentals/

CD COMPANION

- Review Questions
- Glossary

evolve WEBSITE

- Review Questions
- Student Learning Activities
- Glossary

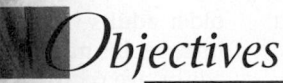

Objectives

Mastery of content in this chapter will enable the student to:

- Discuss demographic trends related to older adults in the United States.
- Identify common myths and stereotypes about older adults.
- List the types of community-based and institutional health care services available to older adults.
- Identify selected biological and psychosocial theories of aging.
- Discuss common developmental tasks of older adults.
- Describe common physiological changes of aging.
- Differentiate among delirium, dementia, and depression.
- Discuss issues related to psychosocial changes of aging.
- Describe selected health concerns of older adults.
- Identify nursing interventions related to the physiological, cognitive, and psychosocial changes of aging.

*T*he identification of age 65 as the start of older adulthood dates back to social reform in Germany in the nineteenth century. Age 65 continues to be used as the lower boundary for "old age" in demographics and social policy although many older adults consider themselves to be "middle-aged" well into their seventh decade. Chronological age may have little relation to the reality of aging for an older adult. Each of us ages in our own ways according to our own schedules and life histories. Every older adult is unique and must be approached as a unique individual by the nurse even though in this chapter generalizations will be made about the aging process and its effect on individuals.

The number of older adults in the United States is growing, both absolutely and as a proportion of the total population. In 2000 there were 35 million adults over age 65 in the United States, representing 12.4% of the population (Administration on Aging [AOA], 2002). This represented an increase of 3.7 million since 1990. Among those 35 million older adults in 2000, 18.4 million were between ages 65 and 74, 12.4 million were between ages 75 and 85, and 4.2 million were over age 85. The number of older adults is expected to increase to 70 million by 2030. Part of that increase is due to extension of the average life span. If you were age 65 in 2000, you could expect to live another 17.9 years if you are a woman or another 16.3 years if you are a man.

Two other factors that contribute to the projected increase in the number of older adults are the aging of the baby boom generation and the growth of the population segment over age 85. The baby boomers are the large cohort of adults born between 1946 and 1964. The first baby boomers will reach age 65 in 2011. As the baby boomers swell the numbers of older adults, it will be necessary for social and health care programs for older adults to expand to meet the aging baby boomers' needs while meeting the needs of the over age 85 group. The 4.2 million older adults currently over age 85, who are sometimes called the frail elderly, are projected to increase to 8.9 million by 2030. Furthermore, the centenarians, those age 100 and over, increased from 37,306 in 1990 to 50,545 in 2000 and are expected to continue to increase in number.

The diversity of the over age 65 group is also projected to increase (AOA, 2002). In 2000, minorities (African-Americans, Hispanics, American Indians/Eskimos/Aleuts, Asian/Pacific Islanders) constituted 16.4% of the over age 65 group. The percentages of older adults from minorities in 2000 were as follows: African-Americans, 8%; Hispanics, 5.6%; American Indians/Eskimos/Aleuts, less than 1%; Asian/Pacific Islanders, 2.4%. By 2030 the older adults from these minority groups are expected to account for 25.4% of the total over age 65 group. The degree of increase will vary for each minority group. According to population predictions for 2030, Hispanics over age 65 will experience the most dramatic increase over the statistics from 2000 (an estimated increase of 328%). The other minority groups will also increase: Asian/Pacific Islanders (an estimated increase of 285%), American Indians/Eskimos/Aleuts (an estimated increase of 147%), and African-Americans (an estimated increase of 131%).

Nurses must take the cultural, ethnic, and racial diversity represented by these numbers into account as they care for older adults from these groups. Examples of culturally sensitive nursing approaches to older adults include respect for preferences in food, music, and religion; attentive listening; use of physical assessment norms appropriate for the ethnic group; and asking about personal health practices, family customs, lifestyle preferences, and spiritual resources (Ebersole and Hess, 2001). Chapter 8 provides further information on cultural care.

Variability Among Older Adults

The nursing care of older adults poses special challenges because of great variation in their physiological, cognitive, and psychosocial health. Older adults also vary widely in their levels of functional ability. The majority of older adults are active and involved members of their communities. A smaller number have lost the ability to care for themselves, are confused or withdrawn, and/or are unable to make decisions concerning their needs. Most older adults live in noninstitutional settings. In 2000 55% of older adults in noninstitutional settings lived with a spouse (41% of older women, 73% of older men) (AOA, 2002). However, 30% lived alone (40% of older women, 17% of older men), and 15% had other noninstitutional living arrangements such as living with a family member (19% of older women, 10% of older men). Only 4.5% of all older adults resided in institutions such as nursing homes. Age influenced living arrangements: the proportion of older adults living with a spouse decreased with age, the proportion living alone increased with age, and the proportion living in an institution increased with age.

Aging does not inevitably lead to disability and dependence. Most older people remain functionally independent despite the increasing prevalence of chronic disease. Nursing assessment, a complex and challenging process, can provide valuable clues to the effect of a disease or illness on a client's functional status. Chronic conditions add to the complexity of assessment and care of the older adult. Approximately 70% of older adults have multiple chronic conditions with arthritis, hypertension, heart disease, vision impairment, and diabetes mellitus as the most common in noninstitutionalized

older adults (Adelman, 2001). These chronic conditions impose limitations on activities, with 28.8% of older adults age 65 to 74 and 50.6% of older adults age 75 and over reporting some limitations (AOA, 2002).

The physical and psychosocial aspects of aging are closely related. For the older person, a reduced ability to respond to stress, the experience of multiple losses, and the physical changes associated with normal aging may combine to place the person at high risk for illness and functional deterioration. Although the interaction of these physical and psychosocial factors can be serious, the nurse should not assume that all older adults have signs, symptoms, or behaviors representing disease and decline or that these are the only items to be assessed. The older adult's strengths and abilities must also be identified during the assessment.

Terminology

As the number of older adults increases, the specialty of gerontological nursing is gaining in importance. Several terms are used, at times interchangeably, to describe this specialty (Lueckenotte, 2000).

- **Geriatrics** the branch of medicine dealing with the physiological and psychological aspects of aging and with diagnosis and treatment of diseases affecting older adults.
- **Gerontology** is the study of all aspects of the aging process and its consequences.
- **Gerontological nursing** is concerned with assessment of the health and functional status of older adults; diagnosis, planning, and implementing health care and services to meet the identified needs; and evaluating the effectiveness of such care. This is the term most often used by nurses specializing in this field.
- **Gerontic nursing,** a seldom-used term, considers the nursing care of older adults to be the art and practice of nurturing, caring, and comforting rather than merely the treatment of disease.

Myths and Stereotypes

Despite ongoing research in the field of gerontology, false beliefs, or myths, about older adults persist. These stereotypes include beliefs about the physical and psychosocial characteristics and the lifestyles of older adults. Stereotypes, both positive and negative, may be held by younger and older adults but do not automatically imply age-based prejudice (Chasteen, Schwarz, and Park, 2002). However, when health care providers holding negative stereotypes about aging care for older adults, those stereotypes may adversely affect the quality of the care provided. Nurses, while personally susceptible to the myths and stereotypes held by society, have the responsibility to dispel the myths and replace the stereotypes with accurate information.

Older adults are sometimes stereotyped as ill, disabled, and physically unattractive. However, although many experience chronic conditions or have at least one disability that limits their performance of activities of daily living (ADLs), only 26.2% of older adults describe their health as poor or fair (AOA, 2002). Other common misconceptions hold that older adults are not interested in sex and that any interest in sexual activities is abnormal and should be discouraged. Yet older adults report continued enjoyment of sexual relationships.

Some people believe that older adults are forgetful, confused, rigid, bored, and unfriendly and that they are unable to understand and learn new information. Yet centenarians, the oldest of the old, are described as having an optimistic outlook on life, good memories, broad social contacts and interests, and tolerance for others (Ebersole and Hess, 1998). Although the process of learning may be affected by age-related changes in vision or hearing or by reduced energy and endurance, older adults are lifelong learners. The nurse should use teaching techniques that compensate for sensory changes, provide additional time for remembering and responding, and present concrete rather than abstract material to facilitate learning by older adults. Other effective teaching techniques draw on the older adult's past experiences and correspond to the identified interests of the older adult rather than to the content areas believed important by the health care professional. Box 13-1 presents additional teaching strategies that the nurse can use to address the special learning needs of older adults.

Stereotypes about lifestyles include mistaken notions about living arrangements and finances. Most older adults live in noninstitutional settings, either with family members or alone. Only 4.5% live in institutions such as nursing homes (AOA, 2002). Misconceptions about the financial status of older adults range from beliefs that many are affluent to beliefs that many are poor. According to the Administration on Aging (2002), 10.2% of persons over age 65 have incomes below the poverty level with another 6.7% classified as near poor. Most (90%) of older adults receive Social Security benefits. In the aggregated income of all older adults Social Security benefits accounted for only 38%, with earnings (21%), assets (20%), and pensions (19%) constituting the remainder of the aggregate income.

In a society that values attractiveness, energy, and youth these myths and stereotypes lead to the undervaluing of older adults. Some people believe that older adults become worthless after they leave the workforce. Others consider the knowledge and experience of older adults to be too old-fashioned to have any current value. These notions underlie the concept of **ageism,** which is discrimination against people because of increasing age, just as people who are racists and sexists discriminate because of skin color and gender. Ageism, unopposed, has the potential to undermine the self-confidence of older adults, limit their access to care, and distort caregivers' understanding of the uniqueness of each older adult (Cutillo-Schmitter, 1996).

Today there are laws banning discrimination on the grounds of age. The economic and political power of older adults also acts against ageism. Older adults are a significant proportion of the consumer economy. As voters and activists in various issues, they influence the formation of

---

Box 13-1 Older Adult Client's Special Learning Needs

Teaching Strategies

- Make sure the client is ready to learn before trying to teach. Watch for clues that would indicate that the client is preoccupied or too anxious to comprehend the material.
- Sit facing the client so that he or she can watch your lip movements and facial expressions.
- Speak slowly.
- Keep your tone of voice low; older adults can hear low sounds better than high-frequency sounds.
- Present one idea at a time.
- Emphasize concrete rather than abstract material.
- Give the client enough time in which to respond because older adults' reaction times are longer than those of younger persons.
- Focus on a single topic to help the client concentrate.
- Keep environmental distractions to a minimum.
- Defer teaching if the client becomes distracted or tired or cannot concentrate for other reasons.
- Invite another member of the household to join the discussion.
- Use audio, visual, and tactile cues to enhance learning and help the client remember information.
- Ask for feedback to ensure that the information has been understood.
- Use past experience; connect new learning to that already learned.
- Compensate for physical discomfort and sensory decrements.
- Support a positive self-image in the learner.
- Use creative teaching strategies.
- Respond to identified interests of learners.
- Emphasize and integrate emotional and personal values in the acquisition of skills and ideas.

Modified from Ebersole P, Hess P: *Geriatric nursing and healthy aging,* St. Louis, 2001, Mosby. (Original source: Fielo S, Rizzolo M: Handle with caring: meeting elderly clients' special learning needs, *Nurs Health Care* 9[4]:193, 1988.)

---

public policy. Their participation adds a unique perspective on social, economic, and technological issues because they have experienced almost 100 years of developments. In the past 100 years, we have gone from riding in horse-drawn carriages to observing space shuttle flights. Gaslights and steam power have given way to electricity and nuclear power. Typewriters and carbon paper have been replaced by computers and copier machines. Older adults have lived through the Great Depression. Older adults have also experienced two world wars and wars in Korea, Vietnam, and the Persian Gulf. Older adults have seen changes in health care as the era of the family doctor gave way to the age of specialization. After witnessing the government initiatives that established the Social Security system, Medicare, and Medicaid, older adults are currently living with the changes imposed by health care reform. Having lived through all of these events and changes, older adults have stories and examples of coping with change to share.

Nurses' Attitudes Toward Older Adults

It is important for nurses to assess their attitudes toward older adults, their own aging, and the aging of their family, friends, and clients. The attitudes of the nurse toward older adults comes in part from personal experiences with older adults, education, employment experiences, and attitudes of co-workers and employing institutions. The nurse's own age, either as a factor contributing to the amount of experience or as a factor reflecting the nurse's own aging, also contributes to the nurse's attitude toward older adults. Given the increasing number of older adults in health care settings, cultivation of positive attitudes toward older adults and specialized knowledge about aging and the health care needs of older adults are priorities for nurses.

Positive attitudes are based in part on a realistic portrayal of the characteristics and health care needs of older adults. In the past, negative attitudes about aging and older adults have contributed to the persistence of stereotypes of older adults as dependent and less attractive than younger clients. Nursing care, under the influence of these attitudes, has often ignored the opportunity to respect older adults and actively involve them in care decisions and activities. At times institutional settings such as hospitals and nursing homes have treated older adults as objects to be acted upon rather than independent, dignified adults. What older adults perceive as important in promoting their independence may differ from what nurses and other caregivers may assume to be important (Mastrian, 2001) (Box 13-2).

Theories of Aging

Various theorists have attempted to describe the complex biopsychosocial process of aging. Although many theories have been developed, there is no single universally accepted theory that predicts and explains the complexities of the aging process. The nurse must be aware of the scientific attempts to explain the aging process and the concepts included in the theories. Although the theories are in various stages of development and have limitations, nurses can use them to increase understanding of the phenomena affecting the health and well-being of older adults.

The biological theories of aging are categorized as either **stochastic theories** or **nonstochastic theories.** Stochastic theories view aging as the result of random cellular damage that occurs over time. The accumulated damage leads to the physical changes that we recognize as characteristic of the aging process. According to the nonstochastic theories, genetically programmed physiological

---

Research Highlight

Box 13-2

Staying Independent

Research Focus

Staying independent is a goal for older adults. This study explored the opinions of older adults, nurses, and nonnurses about skills necessary to stay independent and diseases or symptoms that interfered with staying independent.

Research Abstract

Older adults, nurses, and nonnurses (young and middle-age adults) were asked to indicate the relative importance of 18 skills for independent living and the amount of interference in independent living posed by nine diseases and symptoms. Examples from the list of 18 skills include bathing, using a telephone, ability to make decisions, managing medications, and using a toilet. The nine diseases and symptoms were Alzheimer's disease, hypertension, diabetes, forgetfulness, fractures, dialysis, paralysis, stroke, and night wandering.

There was considerable agreement among the participants about the diseases/symptoms that interfere with independent living. The participants agreed that Alzheimer's disease, paralysis, and night wandering were the three diseases/symptoms with the greatest impact on independent living.

There were significant differences among the groups in the choices of skills deemed necessary for independent living. The nurses selected managing medications as the most important skill and ranked using a telephone, using a toilet, being able to lock/unlock doors, having family willing to help, and being able to see in descending order of importance. For their first choice the young (age 19 to 29) and middle-age (age 30 to 60) nonnurses agreed with the nurses by selecting managing medications as the most important skill for independent living. However, the older adults selected balance as the most important skill for remaining independent. Other skills selected by the older adults were, in descending order of importance, being able to see, being able to lock/unlock doors, using a toilet, and managing medications.

Evidence-Based Practice

- Because older adults had different opinions than nurses and younger nonnurses, it is important to ask older adults about their needs rather than assuming what they may be.
- Although medication management was important to all participants in this study, older adults rated balance (a skill necessary to prevent falls) as the skill most necessary for staying independent.
- Nursing interventions to improve balance and reduce the risk of falling may promote older adults' efforts to stay independent.

Reference

Mastrian K: Differing perceptions in defining safe independent living for elders, *Nurs Outlook* 49:213, 2001.

mechanisms within the body control the process of aging. In another approach to the explanation of the biological changes of the aging process, Sloane (1992) suggests a "rule of thirds" in which functional decline due to disease, inactivity or disuse, and aging itself each contribute one third to the complex process we call aging.

The psychosocial theories of aging attempt to explain changes in behavior, roles, and relationships that come with aging. As with biological theories of aging, there is no single theory that is universally accepted. The theories also reflect the values held by the theorist and society at the time the theory was first articulated. The three classic psychosocial theories of aging are disengagement theory, activity theory, and continuity theory (Ebersole and Hess, 1998). Disengagement theory, the oldest psychosocial theory, states that aging individuals withdraw from customary roles and engage in more introspective, self-focused activities (Cummings and Henry, 1961). The activity theory, unlike the disengagement theory, considers the continuation of activities performed during middle age as necessary for successful aging (Lemon, Bengston, and Peterson, 1972). Continuity theory or developmental theory (Neugarten, 1964) states that personality remains the same and behavior becomes more predictable as people age. The personality and behavior patterns developed during a lifetime determine the degree of engagement and activity in older adulthood.

Critics suggest that all three psychosocial theories either fail in some measure to consider the many factors that affect an individual's response to the aging process or address those factors in a too simplistic fashion. Although we may generalize about aging, biologically and psychosocially each individual ages uniquely.

*D*evelopmental Tasks for Older Adults

Theories of aging are closely linked to the concept of developmental tasks appropriate for distinct stages of life. Although no two individuals age in the same way, either biologically or psychosocially, frameworks outlining tasks appropriate developmentally for older adults have been developed. Seven developmental tasks for older adults are listed in Box 13-3.

These developmental tasks are common to many older adults and are associated with varying degrees of change and loss. The more common losses are of health, significant others, a sense of being useful, socialization, income, and independent living. The ways that older adults adjust to the changes of aging are highly individualized. For some, adaptation and adjustment are relatively easy. For others, coping with aging changes may require the assistance of family, friends, and health care professionals. The nurse must be sensitive to the effect of such losses on older adults and their families and be prepared to offer support.

Older adults face the necessity of adjustment to the physical changes that accompany aging. The extent and timing of these changes vary from individual to individual, but as body systems age, changes in appearance and functioning occur. These changes are not associated with

a disease but are normal changes. The presence of disease may alter the timing of the changes or their impact on daily life. Structural and functional changes associated with aging are described in the section on physiological development.

Some older adults find it difficult to accept themselves as aging. This is seen in benign behaviors as some older adults, both men and women, understate their ages when asked, adopt younger styles of clothing, or attempt to conceal physical evidence of aging with cosmetics. But other older adults deny their own aging in ways that are potentially problematic. For example, some older adults may deny functional declines and refuse to ask for assistance with tasks that place their safety at great risk. Others avoid activities designed to benefit older adults, such as senior citizens' centers and senior health promotion activities and thus do not receive these benefits. Acceptance of personal aging does not mean retirement into inactivity, but it does require a realistic review of strengths and limitations.

Older adults retired from employment outside the home are challenged to cope with the loss of that work role. Older adults who worked at home and the spouses of those who worked outside the home also face role changes as they age. Because retirement is usually anticipated, persons can plan ahead to make financial plans and to consider replacement activities. Many older adults welcome retirement as a time to pursue new interests and hobbies, to participate in volunteer activities, to continue their education, or to start a new business career. Retirement plans for some older adults include changes of residence such as moving to a different city or state or moving to a different type of housing within the same area.

Reasons other than retirement may also lead to changes of residence. For example, physical impairments may require relocation to a smaller, single-level home. Severe health problems may require the older adult to live with relatives or friends. A change in living arrangements for the older adult may require an extended period of adjustment during which assistance and support from health care professionals, friends, and family members are needed.

The majority of older adults are faced with the deaths of spouses. In 2000 almost half (45%) of all older women were widows, and 14% of older men were widowers (AOA, 2002). Some older adults must cope with the death of adult children and grandchildren. All experience the deaths of friends. These deaths represent both losses and

---

Box 13-3   **Developmental Tasks of the Older Adult**

Adjusting to decreasing health and physical strength
Adjusting to retirement and reduced or fixed income
Adjusting to death of a spouse
Accepting self as aging person
Maintaining satisfactory living arrangements
Redefining relationships with adult children
Finding ways to maintain quality of life

reminders of personal mortality. Coming to terms with these deaths is often difficult. By assisting older adults through the grieving process, the nurse can help them resolve the issues posed by these deaths.

The redefining of relationships with children that occurred as those children grew up and left home continues as older adults experience the challenges of aging. A variety of issues may arise, including, but not limited to, role reversal, control of decision making, dependence, conflict, guilt, and loss. How these issues surface in situations and how they are resolved depends in part on the past relationship between the older adult and the adult children. All the involved parties bring past experiences and powerful emotions to the table. When adult children assist the older adults of their family, they must find ways to balance the demands of their own children and their careers. Adult children also debate over how much assistance to provide and how much decision-making authority to assume. As adult children and aging parents negotiate the parameters of the changed roles, nurses may act as counselors to both the parents and the children. Nurses can assist adult children by listening and by helping them distinguish between changes and behaviors related to illness, normal aging changes, and their parents' lifelong preferences and patterns of behavior.

In the face of the changes that come with aging, older adults must find ways to maintain their quality of life. What defines quality of life varies from person to person. Nurses must listen to what the older adult considers to be most important rather than making assumptions about that individual's priorities. Together the nurse and the older adult may set objectives that lead to the maintenance of quality of life. Whether quality of life is defined as maintenance of social relationships, continuing to live alone, or continuing activities such as driving or gardening, older adults look to the nurse for assistance.

Community-Based and Institutional Health Care Services

Nurses encounter older adult clients in a wide variety of community-based and institutional health care settings. Outside of the acute care hospital setting, nurses care for older adults in private homes and apartments, retirement communities, adult day care centers, assisted living facilities, and nursing centers or facilities (extended care facilities, intermediate care facilities, skilled nursing facilities). Chapter 2 describes these settings and the services provided in detail.

Nurses can also assist older adults and their families by providing information and answering questions as they make choices among care options. The assistance of the nurse is especially valuable when older adults and their families are making decisions about moving to a nursing center. Family caregivers may consider nursing center placement when in-home care becomes increasingly difficult or when convalescence from hospitalization requires more assistance than can be provided out-

---

Box 13-4

Focus on Older Adults

Selection of a Nursing Home: Six Aspects of Quality to Consider

An important step in the process of selecting a nursing home is to visit the nursing home. While looking around the nursing home, consider these aspects of quality.

- **Home:** The nursing home should not feel like a hospital. It is a home, a place where people live. Residents should be encouraged to personalize their rooms. Privacy is to be respected.
- **Care:** In addition to assistance with basic activities of daily living such as bathing, dressing, eating, oral hygiene, and toileting, staff should assist residents with social and recreational activities. Residents should be out of bed and dressed according to their preferences. Visitors should be able to see the staff actively assisting and interacting socially with residents.
- **Family involvement:** Families should be welcomed by the staff when they visit the facility. Whether families wish to provide information, ask questions, participate in care planning, or assist with social activities or physical care, staff should encourage family involvement.
- **Environment:** Residents, their clothing, their belongings, and their surroundings should be clean. The staff should be clean and well-groomed. There should be no pervasive odors in the facility. Ample nonglare lighting, minimal noise, plants, comfortable furniture, and pets contribute to a homelike environment.
- **Communication:** Good communication among residents, families, and staff is necessary for quality care. Good communication is respectful and considerate.
- **Staff:** Members of the nursing home staff are observed to be attentive to resident requests and actively involved with assisting the residents. They focus on the person, not on the task. The assistance that they provide to residents includes assistance with social or recreational activities, as well as the performance of nursing duties.

Modified from Rantz M, Popejoy L, Zwygart-Stauffacher M: *The new nursing homes: a 20-minute way to find great long-term care,* Minneapolis, 2001, Fairview Press.

---

side of a skilled nursing facility. However, the decision to enter a nursing center should come only after the older adult and the family have considered the full range of long-term care choices. Although the decision to enter a nursing center is never final and a nursing center resident may be discharged to home or another less-institutional facility, many older adults view the nursing home as their final residence. During the decision-making period, the actual move to the nursing center, and the time after admission, the nurse's role is to support the older adult and the family and to provide information about the selection of a good nursing center. Although results of state and federal inspections of nursing homes are available to the public at the nursing homes and at the inspectors' offices, the best way to evaluate the quality of a nursing home is to visit that facility and inspect it personally (Rantz, Popejoy, and Zwygart-Stauffacher, 2001). Suggestions related to the selection of a good nursing center are listed in Box 13-4.

Assessing the Needs of Older Adults

Gerontological nursing offers creative approaches for maximizing the potential of older adults. With comprehensive assessment information regarding the older adult's strengths, resources, and limitations, the nurse and the older adult identify needs and problems and select interventions that maintain the older adult's physical abilities and create an environment for psychosocial and spiritual well-being. A thorough assessment requires the nurse to actively engage the older adult and provide the older adult enough time to share important information about his or her health. The nurse assesses for changes in physiology, cognition, and psychosocial behavior.

Nursing assessment must take into account five key points to ensure an age-specific approach: (1) the interrelation between physical and psychosocial aspects of aging, (2) the effects of disease and disability on functional status, (3) the decreased efficiency of homeostatic mechanisms, (4) the lack of standards for health and illness norms, and (5) altered presentation and response to specific disease (Lueckenotte, 2000). Obtaining a comprehensive assessment of an older adult will take more time than the assessment of a younger adult because of the longer life and medical history and the potential complexity of that history. By planning to spend extra time with the assessment, the nurse and the older adult are less likely to feel rushed. During the physical examination, the nurse may find it necessary to allow rest periods or to conduct the assessment in several sessions because of the reduced energy and limited endurance experienced by some frail older adults.

Sensory changes may also affect data gathering. The nurse's choices of communication techniques will be influenced by any visual or hearing impairments experienced by the older adult. If older adults are unable to understand the nurse's visual or auditory cues, assessment data may be inaccurate or misleading. For example, if older adults have difficulty hearing the nurse's questions, inappropriate responses may lead the nurse to believe that they are confused. Communication techniques for the nurse to use when older adults have visual impairments include the following:

- Sit or stand in front of the client in full view.
- Face the older adult while speaking; do not cover your mouth.
- Provide diffuse, bright, nonglare lighting.
- Encourage the older adult to use his or her familiar assistive devices such as glasses or magnifiers.

Techniques for the nurse to use when older adults are hearing-impaired include the following:
- Speak directly to the client; do not cover your mouth.
- Speak in clear, low-pitched tones at a moderate rate and volume.
- Reduce background noises; move to a quiet, private room.
- Ask if there is a "good ear," and speak toward that ear.
- Encourage the older adult to use assistive devices such as hearing aids or "microphone plus earphones" devices.

- Make sure the hearing aid is working properly (check the battery, check that the hearing aid is turned on, adjust volume controls).
- Check the ear canal for cerumen impaction.

Memory deficits, if present, will affect the accuracy and completeness of the data collected. Information contributed by a family member or other caregiver may be necessary to supplement the older adult's recollection of past medical events and information such as allergies and immunizations. Tact must be used when involving another person in the assessment interview with the older adult. The additional person supplements the answers of the older adult with the consent of the older adult, but the older adult remains the focus of the interview.

During assessment, caution should be exercised in the interpretation of the signs and symptoms of diseases and the interpretation of laboratory values. Typically, younger populations were used to establish the classic signs and symptoms of diseases and the norms for laboratory values. However, the classic signs and symptoms of diseases may be absent, blunted, or atypical in older adults (Lueckenotte, 2000). This may be due to age-related changes in organ systems and homeostatic mechanisms, progressive loss of physiological and functional reserves, or coexisting acute or chronic conditions (Emmett, 1998). As a result, the older adult with a urinary tract infection may present with confusion, loss of appetite, weakness, dizziness, or fatigue instead of fever, dysuria, frequency, or urgency. The older adult with pneumonia may have tachycardia, tachypnea, and confusion without the more common symptoms of fever and productive cough. Instead of substernal chest pain and diaphoresis, the older adult with a myocardial infarction may experience no pain, epigastric discomfort, referred pain, restlessness, hypotension, or confusion. Variations from the usual norms for laboratory values may be due to age-related changes in cardiac, pulmonary, renal, and metabolic function (Beers and Berkow, 2000). Examples of laboratory values that may be increased by the aging process include, but are not limited to, alkaline phosphatase, serum cholesterol, triglycerides, serum glucose (postprandial), and serum uric acid. Examples of laboratory values that may be decreased by the aging process include, but are not limited to, serum calcium, serum creatine kinase, and creatinine clearance.

Physiological Changes

Perception of well-being can define quality of life. Understanding the older adult's perceptions about health status is essential for accurate assessment and development of clinically relevant interventions. Older adults' concepts of health generally depend on personal perceptions of functional ability. Therefore older adults engaged in activities of daily living usually consider themselves healthy, whereas those whose activities are limited by physical, emotional, or social impairments may perceive themselves as ill.

There are frequently observed physiological changes in older adults that are called normal. Finding these "normal" changes during an assessment is not unexpected. These physiological changes are not always pathological processes in themselves, but they may make older adults more vulnerable to some common clinical conditions and diseases. Some older adults experience all

Table 13-1	**Common Physiological Changes With Aging**
System	**Common Changes**
Integument	Loss of skin elasticity (wrinkles, sagging, dryness, easily tears), pigmentation changes, glandular atrophy (oil, moisture, sweat glands), thinning hair (facial hair: decreased in men, increased in women), slower nail growth, atrophy of epidermal arterioles
Respiratory	Decreased cough reflex; decreased removal of mucus, dust, irritants from airways (decreased cilia); decreased vital capacity (increased anterior-posterior chest diameter); increased chest wall rigidity; fewer alveoli, increased airway resistance; increased risk of respiratory infections
Cardiovascular	Thickening of blood vessel walls; narrowing of vessel lumen; loss of vessel elasticity; lower cardiac output; decreased number of heart muscle fibers; decreased elasticity and calcification of heart valves; decreased baroreceptor sensitivity; decreased efficiency of venous valves; increased pulmonary vascular tension; increased systolic blood pressure; decreased peripheral circulation
Gastrointestinal	Periodontal disease; loss of teeth; decrease in saliva, gastric secretions, and pancreatic enzymes; smooth muscle changes with decreased esophageal peristalsis and small intestinal motility
Musculoskeletal	Decreased muscle mass and strength, decalcification of bones, degenerative joint changes, dehydration of intervertebral disks (decreased height)
Neurological	Degeneration of nerve cells, decrease in neurotransmitters, decrease in rate of conduction of impulses
Sensory	
Eyes	Decreased accommodation to near/far (presbyopia), difficulty adjusting to changes from light to dark, yellowing of the lens, altered color perception, increased sensitivity to glare, smaller pupils
Ears	Loss of acuity for high-frequency tones (presbycusis), thickening of tympanic membrane, sclerosis of inner ear, may have buildup of earwax (cerumen)
Taste	Often diminished, may have fewer taste buds
Smell	Often diminished
Touch	Decreased skin receptors
Proprioception	Decreased awareness of body positioning in space
Genitourinary	Fewer nephrons, decreased renal blood flow, decreased bladder capacity
Men	Enlargement of prostate
Women	Reduced sphincter tone
Reproductive	
Female	Decreased estrogen production, degeneration of ovaries, atrophy of vagina, uterus, breasts
Male	Sperm count diminishes, smaller testes, erections less firm and slow to develop
Endocrine	
General	Alteration in hormone production with decreased ability to respond to stress
Thyroid	Decreased secretion
Thymus	Involution of thymus gland
Cortisols, glucocorticoids	Increased antiinflammatory hormone
Pancreas	Increased fibrosis, decreased secretion of enzymes and hormones

Modified from Ebersole P, Hess P: *Geriatric nursing and healthy aging,* St. Louis, 2001, Mosby.

of these physiological changes, and others experience only a few. The body changes continuously with age, and specific effects on particular older adults depend on health, lifestyle, stressors, and environmental conditions. The nurse should know about these normal, or more commonly experienced, changes in order to provide appropriate care for older adults and to assist with adaptation to the changes. Common physiological changes are summarized in Table 13-1.

General Survey. The general survey begins during the initial nurse-client encounter and includes a quick, but careful, head-to-toe scan of the older adult that the nurse writes in a concise description. An initial inspection of an older adult might reveal eye contact and facial expression appropriate to the situation, as well as common aging changes such as facial wrinkles, gray hair, loss of body mass in the extremities, and an increase of body mass in the trunk.

Integumentary System. With aging, the skin loses resilience and moisture. The epithelial layer thins, and elas-

tic collagen fibers shrink and become rigid. Wrinkles of the face and neck reflect lifelong patterns of muscle activity and facial expressions, the pull of gravity on tissue, and diminished elasticity.

Spots and lesions may also be present on the skin. Smooth, brown, irregularly shaped spots (age spots, or senile lentigo) initially appear on the backs of the hands and on forearms. Small, round, red or brown cherry angiomas may be found on the trunk. Seborrheic lesions or keratoses may appear as irregular, round or oval, brown, watery lesions. Years of sun exposure contribute to the aging of the skin and may lead to premalignant and malignant lesions. Examination of skin lesions must rule out three malignancies related to sun exposure: melanoma, basal cell carcinoma, and squamous cell carcinoma (Beers and Berkow, 2000) (see Chapter 32).

Head and Neck. The facial features of the older adult become more pronounced from loss of subcutaneous fat and skin elasticity. Facial features may appear asymmetrical because of missing teeth or improperly fitting dentures. In addition, common vocal changes include a rise in pitch and a loss of power and range.

Visual acuity declines with age. This may be the result of retinal damage, reduced pupil size, development of opacities in the lens, or loss of lens elasticity. Presbyopia, a progressive decline in the ability of the eyes to accommodate for close, detailed work, is common. There is a reduced ability to see in darkness and to adapt to abrupt changes from dark areas to light areas (and the reverse). More ambient light is needed for tasks such as reading, as well as for other activities of daily living. However, older adults also have increased sensitivity to the effects of glare, and interventions to increase ambient light should not increase glare. Changes in color vision and discoloration of the lens make it difficult to distinguish between blues and greens and among pastel shades.

Auditory changes are often subtle. The earliest losses of hearing acuity may be ignored until friends and family members comment on compensatory attempts such as turning up the volume on televisions and radios. A common age-related change in auditory acuity is called presbycusis. Presbycusis affects the ability to hear high-pitched sounds and sibilant consonants such as *s, sh,* and *ch.* Before the nurse assumes presbycusis it is necessary to inspect the external auditory canal for the presence of cerumen. Impacted cerumen is an easily treated cause of diminished hearing acuity.

Taste buds atrophy and lose sensitivity. The older adult is less able to discern among salty, sweet, sour, and bitter tastes. The sense of smell is also decreased, further reducing taste. Salivary secretion is reduced.

Thorax and Lungs. Because of changes in the musculoskeletal system, the configuration of the thorax sometimes changes. After age 55 respiratory muscle strength begins to decrease (Beers and Berkow, 2000). The anteroposterior diameter of the thorax increases. Vertebral changes due to osteoporosis lead to dorsal kyphosis, the curvature of the thoracic spine sometimes called "dowager's hump" because of the increased incidence in older women. Calcification of the costal cartilage can cause decreased mobility of the ribs. The chest wall gradually becomes stiffer. Lung expansion decreases. If kyphosis or chronic obstructive lung disease is present, breath sounds are distant.

Heart and Vascular System. Decreased contractile strength of the myocardium results in a decreased cardiac output. The decrease is significant when the older adult is stressed by anxiety, excitement, illness, or strenuous activity. The body tries to compensate for decreased cardiac output by increasing the heart rate during exercise. However, after exercise, it takes longer for the older adult's rate to return to baseline.

Systolic and/or diastolic blood pressures may be abnormally elevated. More than 50% of older adults have systolic or diastolic hypertension (systolic pressure >140 mm Hg, diastolic pressure >90 mm Hg) (Beers and Berkow, 2000). Although a common chronic condition, hypertension is not a normal aging change and predisposes older adults to heart failure, stroke, renal failure, coronary heart disease, and peripheral vascular disease.

Peripheral pulses are frequently weaker, although still palpable, in the lower extremities. Older adults may complain that their lower extremities are cold, particularly at night. Changes in the peripheral pulses in the upper extremities are less common.

Breasts. Decreased muscle mass, tone, and elasticity result in smaller breasts in older women. In addition, the breasts sag. Atrophy of glandular tissue, coupled with more fat deposits, results in a slightly smaller, less dense, and less nodular breast. Gynecomastia, enlarged breasts in men, may be due to medication side effects, hormonal changes, or obesity. Both older men and women are at risk of breast cancer.

Gastrointestinal System and Abdomen. Aging leads to an increase in the amount of fatty tissue in the trunk. As a result, the abdomen increases in size. Because muscle tone and elasticity decrease, it also becomes more protuberant. Gastrointestinal function changes include a slowing of peristalsis and alterations in secretions. The older adult may experience these changes as the development of intolerance to certain foods and discomfort due to delayed gastric emptying. Alterations in the lower gastrointestinal tract may lead to constipation, flatulence, or diarrhea.

Reproductive System. Changes in the structure and function of the reproductive system occur as the result of hormonal alterations. Female menopause is related to a reduced responsiveness of the ovaries to pituitary hormones and a resultant decrease in estrogen and progesterone levels. In men, there is no definite cessation of fertility associated with aging. Spermatogenesis begins to decline during the fourth decade but continues into the ninth. The changes in reproductive structure and function, however, do not affect libido. Less frequent sexual activity can result from illness, death of a sexual partner, decreased socialization, or loss of sexual interest.

Urinary System. Hypertrophy of the prostate gland may develop in older men. This hypertrophy enlarges the gland, and pressure is displaced to the neck of the bladder. As a result, urinary retention, frequency, incontinence, and urinary tract infections may occur. In addition, prostatic hypertrophy can result in difficulty initiating voiding and maintaining a urinary stream. Benign prostatic hypertrophy must be distinguished from cancer of the prostate. Cancer of the prostate is the second most common cause of cancer death in men over age 50, and 75% of prostate cancers are diagnosed in men over age 65 (Gambert, 2001).

Urinary incontinence is an abnormal condition for older women, although for women over age 60 the prevalence of any urine loss is estimated to be 40% and of daily incontinence 7% to 17% (Luft and Vriheas-Nichols, 1998). Older women, particularly those who have had children, can experience stress incontinence, an involuntary release of urine that occurs when they cough, sneeze, or lift an object. This is a result of a weakening of the perineal and bladder muscles. Other types of urinary incontinence are urge, overflow, functional, and mixed incontinence. The risk factors for urinary incontinence include age, menopause, diabetes, hysterectomy, stroke, and obesity.

Musculoskeletal System. With aging, muscle fibers are reduced in size. Muscle strength diminishes in proportion to the decline in muscle mass. Bone mass also declines. Older adults who exercise regularly do not lose as much bone and muscle mass or muscle tone as those who are inactive. Postmenopausal women have a greater rate of bone demineralization than older men, but men are 20% of the 25 million individuals in the United States with osteoporosis (Thorndyke, 2001). Women who maintain calcium intake throughout life and into menopause have less bone demineralization than women with low calcium intake. Older men with poor nutrition and decreased mobility are also at risk for bone demineralization.

Neurological System. The decrease in the number of neurons in the nervous system that begins in the middle of the second decade can lead to changes such as those affecting the special senses described earlier. In addition, the older adult may experience a decreased sense of balance or uncoordinated motor responses. Older adults frequently report alterations in the quality and the quantity of sleep (see Chapter 41). Reports include difficulty falling asleep, difficulty staying asleep, difficulty falling asleep again after waking during the night, waking too early in the morning, and excessive daytime napping.

Cognitive Changes

A common misconception about aging is that cognitive impairments are widespread among older adults. Because of this misconception, older adults fear that they are, or soon will be, cognitively impaired. Younger adults often assume that older adults are confused and no longer able to handle their affairs. Structural and physiological changes within the brain, such as reduction in the number of cells, deposition of lipofuscin and amyloid in cells, and change in neurotransmitter levels, that have been linked with cognitive impairment are seen in older adults with cognitive impairment and without cognitive impairment. Symptoms of cognitive impairment such as disorientation, loss of language skills, loss of the ability to calculate, and poor judgment are not normal aging changes. When the nurse identifies these changes during the assessment, further investigation of the underlying causes is indicated.

The three common conditions affecting cognition are **delirium, dementia,** and **depression** (Table 13-2). Distinguishing among these three conditions is challenging, but essential (Foreman and others, 1996). The nurse should be able to distinguish among these three conditions to select appropriate nursing interventions. Appropriate nursing interventions are specific to the cause of the cognitive impairment. The use of techniques such as reality orientation, validation therapy, and reminiscence also depends on the nature of the cognitive impairment.

Delirium. Delirium, or acute confusional state, is a potentially reversible cognitive impairment that is often due to a physiological cause. Physiological causes of delirium include, but are not limited to, electrolyte imbalances, cerebral anoxia, hypoglycemia, medications, drug effects, tumors, subdural hematomas, and cerebrovascular infection, infarction, or hemorrhage. Delirium in older adults sometimes accompanies systemic infections and may be the presenting symptom for pneumonia or urinary tract infection. Delirium may also be due to environmental factors such as sensory deprivation or unfamiliar surroundings or psychosocial factors such as emotional distress or pain. Although delirium may occur in any setting, an older adult in the acute care setting is especially at risk because of predisposing factors (physiological, psychosocial, and environmental) in combination with the medical condition that led to the hospital admission.

Delirium is characterized by fluctuations in cognition, mood, attention, arousal, and self-awareness. Other signs may be hallucinations, occasional incoherent speech, disturbed sleep-wake cycle, and disorientation. The onset of delirium is typically sudden, and there are rapid fluctuations in symptoms and severity. The presence of delirium requires prompt assessment and intervention. The cognitive impairment secondary to delirium is usually reversed once the cause of delirium is identified and treatment started unless there has been permanent brain damage.

Dementia. Dementia is a generalized impairment of intellectual functioning that interferes with social and occupational functioning. Cognitive function deterioration leads to a decline in the ability to perform basic and instrumental activities of daily living. Unlike delirium, dementia is characterized by a gradual, progressive, irreversible cerebral dysfunction. Because of the close resemblance between delirium and dementia, the presence of delirium must be ruled out whenever dementia is suspected. Bolla and Fille (2000) describe four major types of dementia: Alzheimer's disease (50%), diffuse Lewy body disease (DLBD) (15%), frontotemporal dementia (15%), and vascular dementia (10%). Other causes of dementia, such as infection or trauma, account for another 10% of cases.

The most common form of dementia is **Alzheimer's disease.** The cause of the disease is not known, and although several theories are being studied, none are definitive. Cholinesterase-inhibiting medications (donepezil, rivastigmine, galantamine) are currently prescribed to slow the progression of symptoms. These medications prevent the breakdown of the neurotransmitter acetylcholine by the enzyme cholinesterase (Conn, 2001). It is hypothesized by increasing the amount of acetylcholine available to transmit impulses among neurons, cognition in some older adults with Alzheimer's disease will improve. The characteristic progressive symptoms of Alzheimer's disease are loss of memory (amnesia), loss of the ability to recognize objects and persons (agnosia), loss of the ability to perform familiar tasks (apraxia), and loss of language skills (aphasia). As Alzheimer's disease progresses, the older adult becomes more dependent on caregivers for assistance with activities of daily living. Safety issues must be addressed as the disease progresses and the ability to judge risks diminishes.

The features of DLBD include dementia, fluctuating cognition, visual and/or auditory hallucinations, and the

Table 13-2	A Comparison of the Clinical Features of Delirium, Dementia, and Depression		
Clinical Feature	**Delirium**	**Dementia**	**Depression**
Onset	Acute/subacute, depends on cause, often at twilight or in darkness	Chronic, generally insidious, depends on cause	Chronic, generally insidious, depends on cause
Course	Short, diurnal fluctuations in symptoms, worse at night, in darkness, and on awakening	Long, no diurnal effects, symptoms progressive yet relatively stable over time	Diurnal effects, typically worse in the morning, situational fluctuations, but less than with delirium
Progression	Abrupt	Slow but uneven	Variable, rapid or slow but even
Duration	Hours to less than 1 month, seldom longer	Months to years	At least 6 weeks, can be several months to years
Awareness	Reduced	Clear	Clear
Alertness	Fluctuates, lethargic or hypervigilant	Generally normal	Normal
Attention	Impaired, fluctuates	Generally normal	Minimal impairment, but is easily distracted
Orientation	Generally impaired, severity varies	Generally normal	Selective disorientation
Memory	Recent and immediate impaired	Recent and remote impaired	Selective or "patchy" impairment, "islands" of intact memory
Thinking	Disorganized, distorted, fragmented, incoherent speech, either slow or accelerated	Difficulty with abstraction, thoughts impoverished, judgment impaired, words difficult to find	Intact but with themes of hopelessness, helplessness, or self-deprecation
Perception	Distorted perception, illusions, delusions, and hallucinations, difficulty distinguishing between reality and misperceptions	Misperceptions usually absent	Intact, delusions and hallucinations absent except in severe cases
Psychomotor behavior	Variable, hypokinetic, hyperkinetic, and mixed	Normal, may have apraxia	Variable, psychomotor retardation or agitation
Sleep/wake cycle	Disturbed, cycle reversed	Fragmented	Disturbed, usually early morning awakening
Associated features	Variable affective changes, symptoms of autonomic hyperarousal, exaggeration of personality type, associated with acute physical illness	Affect tends to be superficial, inappropriate, and labile, attempts to conceal deficits in intellect, personality changes, aphasia, agnosia may be present, lacks insight	Affect depressed, dysphoric mood, exaggerated and detailed complaints, preoccupied with personal thoughts, insight present, verbal elaboration
Assessment	Distracted from task, numerous errors	Failings highlighted by family, frequent "near miss" answers, struggles with test, great effort to find an appropriate reply, frequent requests for feedback on performance	Failings highlighted by individual, frequently answers "don't know," little effort, frequently gives up, indifferent toward test, does not care or attempt to find answer

Data from Foreman M: A comparison of the clinical features of delirium, dementia, and depression. In Foreman M and others: Assessing cognitive function, *Geriatr Nurs* 17(5):228, 1996.

motor features of parkinsonism. Like Alzheimer's disease, DLBD is progressive. However, whereas features of parkinsonism may accompany Alzheimer's disease in its later stages, they appear early in DLBD. Another difference is in sensitivity to neuroleptic medications such as haloperidol. Neuroleptics are used in Alzheimer's disease to modify behaviors but should be avoided in DLBD because DLBD clients are extremely sensitive to neuroleptics and may respond to their use with exaggerated parkinsonian features (Bolla and Fille, 2000).

Frontal-temporal dementia has an insidious onset and progresses slowly. Early symptoms include poor hygiene, lack of social tact, hyper-orality, and sexual disinhibition. Incontinence is an early symptom in frontal-temporal dementia, although it is a late symptom in the more com-

mon Alzheimer's disease. Repetitive behaviors (wandering, clapping, singing, picking up objects) are frequently observed. Safety and behavior managements are major concerns for caregivers.

The cause of vascular dementia is interruption of blood supply to areas of the brain by thromboembolism, hemorrhage, or ischemia (Bolla and Fille, 2000). Symptoms of vascular dementia vary with the areas of the brain affected. Progression of vascular dementia may be either stepwise with repeated episodes of damage to the brain over time or steadily progressive. Management of vascular dementia parallels the recommendations for cerebrovascular disease (i.e., reduction of risk factors by treatment of hypertension, hyperlipidemia, carotid disease, arrhythmias, diabetes mellitus, and polycythemia vera). Because the use of nicotine-containing tobacco products has been linked with vascular disease, older adults with vascular dementia should stop or reduce their use of these products. If the older adult has a cardiac arrhythmia such as atrial fibrillation, anticoagulant therapy may be indicated to reduce the risk of thromboembolism.

Nursing management of older adults with any form of dementia must consider the needs of the older adult with dementia and the needs of the family. Those needs change as the progressive nature of dementia leads to increased cognitive deterioration. In addition to the physical needs of the older adult, safety needs and psychosocial needs must be considered. The older adult's family needs information and support. To meet the needs of the older adult with dementia, nursing care objectives are individualized and promote the use of remaining functional abilities.

Depression. Late-life depression may be experienced by 20% of older adults (Butler and Lewis, 1995). Depression reduces happiness and well-being, contributes to physical and social limitations, complicates the treatment of concomitant medical conditions, and increases the risk of suicide. From 20% to 25% of older adults with dementia of the Alzheimer's type also experience depression (Butler and Lewis, 1995; Tueth, 1995). When dementia and depression occur together, the distress of the older adult and the family is increased.

Delirium and depression, both reversible disorders, are often mistaken for irreversible dementia in the older adult because cerebral dysfunction and cognitive impairment occur with these conditions, as well as with dementia. Careful and thorough assessment of older adults with cognitive impairment is essential in order to distinguish among delirium, dementia, and depression. The beginning nurse may choose to consult with a clinical nurse specialist in gerontology. Accurate assessment is necessary to select appropriate nursing interventions.

Psychosocial Changes

The psychosocial changes that occur with aging involve changes in roles and relationships. Roles and relationships within the family change as parents become grandparents, adult children become caregivers for aging parents, or spouses become widows or widowers. Group membership roles and relationships change as the older adult retires from work, moves from a familiar neighborhood, or stops attending social activities because of declining health status.

The nurse assesses both the nature of the psychosocial changes facing an older adult and the adaptation of the older adult to those changes. In the assessment the nurse asks how the older adult feels about self, self in relation to others, and self as aging. Areas to be addressed during the assessment include the family, intimate relationships, past and present occupation, finances, housing, social networks, activities, and spirituality. Specific topics related to these areas include retirement, housing and environment, social isolation, sexuality, and death.

Retirement. Retirement is often mistakenly associated with passivity and seclusion. In actuality, it is a stage of life characterized by transitions and role changes. The psy-chosocial stresses of retirement may be related to role changes with spouse or within the family and to loss of role. There may also be problems related to social isolation and finances. The age of retirement varies. Retirement, which may be mandatory or voluntary, occurs at a variety of ages. But whether it occurs at age 55, age 65, or age 75, retirement is one of the major turning points in life.

Preretirement planning is an important advisable task for middle-age individuals. People who plan in advance for retirement generally have a smoother transition into retirement. Preretirement planning is more than financial planning, although financial planning is important. Planning begins with consideration of the "style" of retirement desired and includes an inventory of interests, current skills, and general health. Meaningful retirement planning is critical because retirement can last for 30 or more years.

Retirement has an impact on more individuals than the retired person. Spouses, adult children, and grandchildren are all affected. When the spouse is still working, the retired person faces time alone. For example, the working spouse may have new ideas about the amount of participation in housework expected of the retired person. Friction may develop when the plans of the retired person conflict with the work responsibilities of the working spouse. The working spouse may also have expectations of the retired person that need clarification. For couples the adjustment to retirement is affected by the quality of their communication with each other, their process of decision making about issues such as money or activities, their adherence to either traditional or shared role orientations, and their level of affection and intimacy (Ebersole and Hess, 1998). Adult children may expect the retired person to become an automatic baby-sitter for the grandchildren.

Loss of the work role has a major impact on some retired persons. When so much of life has revolved around work and the personal relationships at work, the loss of the work role may be devastating. Personal identity may be rooted in the work role, and with retirement a new identity must be constructed. The structure imposed on daily life by a work schedule is also lost with retirement. Also lost are the social exchanges and interpersonal support that occur in the workplace. In the adjustment to retirement the older adult is challenged to develop a personally meaningful schedule and a supportive social network.

The most powerful factors that influence the retired person's satisfaction with life are health status, the option to continue working, and sufficient income (Ebersole and Hess, 1998). Positive preretirement expectations also contribute to satisfaction in retirement. The nurse can help the older adult and family prepare for retirement by discussing with them several key areas, including relations with spouse and children, meaningful activities to replace the work role, adjusting or rebuilding social networks, issues related to income and health promotion and maintenance, and long-range planning, including wills and advance directives.

Social Isolation. Many older adults experience social isolation, and the degree of isolation experienced may increase with age. There are two forms of isolation.

Isolation may be a choice, the result of a desire not to interact with others. Isolation may also be a response to conditions that inhibit the ability or the opportunity to interact with others (Ebersole and Hess, 1998). Although some older adults may choose to be isolated or to continue a lifelong pattern of reduced interaction with others, other older adults do not choose isolation but are vulnerable to its consequences.

The vulnerability of older adults to isolation is increased in the absence of the support of other adults as may occur with loss of the work role or relocation to unfamiliar surroundings. Impaired hearing, diminished vision, and reduced mobility (e.g., impaired ambulation, inability to use assistive devices independently, or loss of ability to drive) all contribute to reduced interaction with others and isolation. The loss of the ability to drive may limit older adults' ability to live independently, as well as contributing to isolation.

Some older adults withdraw from social interaction because of feelings of rejection (Ebersole and Hess, 1998). Societal attitudes about aging as unattractive lead to feelings of rejection for some older adults. These older adults see themselves as unattractive and rejected because of changes in their personal appearance due to normal aging changes or because of body image changes following illness or surgery. Society, including health care professionals, also considers some behaviors and situations to be unacceptable. Older adults who are confused or incontinent, who are unable to communicate, who are institutionalized, or who are poor or homeless are examples of older adults who may be isolated by society. The societal trend toward the geographic dispersion of families leads to decreased opportunities for interaction among family members. Some older adults consider this to be rejection by their families.

The nurse can assist lonely older adults to rebuild social networks and reverse patterns of isolation (Ebersole and Hess, 1998). Many communities have outreach programs designed to make contact with isolated older adults. Outreach programs may meet nutritional needs, such as Meals on Wheels; socialization needs, such as daily telephone calls by volunteers; or need for activities, such as outings. Social service agencies in most communities welcome older adults as volunteers and provide the opportunity to serve as well as being served. Other organizations within communities such as churches, colleges, unions, and libraries offer a variety of programs for older adults that increase the opportunity to meet people with similar activities, interests, and needs.

Sexuality. Sexuality is increasingly recognized as an important factor in the care of older adults. All older adults, whether healthy or frail, need to express sexual feelings. Sexuality involves love, warmth, sharing, and touching, not just the act of intercourse. Sexuality is linked with identity and validates the belief that people can give to others and have the gift appreciated.

Maintaining sexual health requires integration of somatic, emotional, intellectual, and social aspects of the sexual being. To help the older adult achieve or maintain sexual health, the nurse needs to understand the physical changes in sexual response (see Chapter 27). The nurse should provide privacy for any discussion of sexuality and should maintain a nonjudgmental attitude. Open-ended questions inviting the older adult to explain sexual activities or concerns may elicit more information than a list of closed-ended questions about specific activities or symptoms. Older adults may appreciate information about the typical age-related changes in sexuality. Information about the prevention of sexually transmitted diseases should be included when appropriate.

The older adult's libido does not decrease, although frequency of sexual activity may decline. An older woman who does not understand physical changes affecting sexual activity may be concerned that her sex life is nearly over with the onset of menopause. The older man may feel the same when he discovers a change in the firmness of his erection, a decreased need for ejaculation with each orgasm, or a longer recovery period between episodes of intercourse.

In addition to the physical changes that affect sexual functioning, many older adults use prescription medications that depress sexual activity such as antihypertensives, antidepressants, sedatives, or hypnotics. Some drugs increase libido in older adults. For example, phenothiazines increase sexual desire in women, and levodopa has a similar effect in men.

While considering the older adult's need for sexual expression, the nurse must not ignore the important need to touch and be touched. Touch is an overt expression with many meanings and is an important part of sexuality. Touch can complement traditional sexual methods or serve as an alternative sexual expression when physical intercourse is not desired or possible and thus can serve as an important method of achieving intimacy (Wallace, 1996). The nursing student needs to recognize that knowledge of older adults' sexual and intimacy needs will increase with professional growth. Experience in caring for older adults combined with the ability to establish therapeutic connection allows the nurse to learn how to explore clients' sexual concerns. Knowing an older adult's sexual needs allows the nurse to incorporate this information into the nursing care plan.

The sexual preferences of older adults are as diverse as those of the younger population. Not all older adults are heterosexual. Older gay men and lesbians make up approximately 10% of the population over age 65 (Ebersole and Hess, 1998). Little information is available regarding older adult homosexuals and their health care needs, although Wojciechowski (1998) described the health care needs of older lesbian women and older heterosexual women as similar. To be effective caregivers for older homosexuals, nurses need to be aware of their own beliefs about sexuality and the potential impact of those beliefs on their ability to provide care.

Nurses may find that they are called on to help other health care professionals understand the sexual needs of older adults, as well as advising older adults. Not all nurses feel comfortable counseling older adults about sexual health and need not feel obligated to do so. But all nurses should be prepared to refer older adults to appropriate professional counselors.

Housing and Environment. The extent of the older adult's ability to live independently strongly determines housing choices. Changes in social roles, family responsibilities, and health status influence older adults' living arrangements. Some choose to live with family members. Others prefer their own homes or apartments near their families. Leisure or retirement communities provide older people with living and social opportunities in a one-generation setting. Federally subsidized housing, where available, offers apartments with communal, social, and, in some cases, food service arrangements.

When assisting older adults with housing needs, the nurse should assess their activity level, financial status, access to public transportation and community activities, environmental hazards, and support systems. Housing choices should also look to the future needs of the older adults in so far as these can be anticipated. A housing unit with only one floor and without exterior steps may be a prudent choice for the older adult with severe arthritis who has already had some lower extremity joint replacement surgeries and anticipates the need for future surgeries.

Housing and environment have a major impact on the health of older adults. The environment can support or hinder physical and social functioning, enhance or drain energy, and complement or tax existing physical changes such as vision and hearing. For example, the colors red, orange, and yellow are easiest for older adults to see. In contrast, older adults have difficulty distinguishing between green and blue and among pastel shades. To help older adults in health care settings find their rooms, pictures or other decorations near their doors have been used as landmarks. Door frames and baseboards in a color that contrasts with the color of the wall improve perception of the boundaries of halls and rooms. Glare from highly polished floors, metallic fixtures, and windows is poorly tolerated.

Furniture should be comfortable and designed for the musculoskeletal changes of older adults. Older adults should examine furniture carefully for size, comfort, and function before purchasing it. Furniture should be easy to get into and out of and should provide back support. Dining room chairs should be tested for comfort during meals and for height in relation to the table. Older adults may prefer transferring out of a wheelchair to another chair for meals because some styles of wheelchairs do not let older adults sit close enough to the table to eat comfortably. Raising the table to clear the wheelchair arms may bring the table closer to the older adult but may make it too high for comfortable use. To make getting out of bed easier and safer, the height of the bed should allow the older adult's feet to be flat on the floor when the older adult is sitting on the side of the bed.

The goal of nursing assessment of the environment is the promotion of independence and functional ability (Fielo and Warren, 2001). Assessment of safety, a major component of the older adult's environmental, includes risks within the environment and the older adult's ability to recognize and respond to the risks. Risks include factors leading to injury within the home, such as water heaters set at excessively hot temperatures or throw rugs that could cause a fall, and factors outside of the home, such as deteriorating sidewalks and steps or a high incidence of street crime.

Death. Part of the life history of an older adult is the experience of the death of family members and friends (see Chapter 29). This includes the experience of the loss of the older generations of their families and sometimes, sadly, the loss of a child. By age 75, 63% of women have experienced the death of a husband and 20% of men, the death of a wife (Ebersole and Hess, 1998). As the older adult ages, friends are gradually lost to death as those friends grow older. In spite of these experiences, it would be wrong to assume that the older adult is comfortable with the idea of death.

Fear of death in old age is a multidimensional concept. Religiosity and external locus of control have a direct impact on fear of death (Ciricelli, 1999). Ethnicity and gender indirectly affect fear of death by influencing religiosity. Age and socioeconomic status affect fear of death by influencing a person's external locus of control. The stereotype that the death of an older adult is a blessing and the culmination of a full life will not apply to every older adult. Even as death approaches, many older adults still have unfinished business and are not prepared to die. Families and friends may not be ready to let go of the older adult. The nurse may be the person to whom the older adult and family members or friends turn to for assistance in coping with death and loss.

Addressing the Health Concerns of Older Adults

The three most common causes of death in older adults are heart disease, cancer, and stroke. Other frequently reported causes of death are lung disease, accidents/falls, diabetes, kidney disease, and liver disease. All of these causes of death have preventive measures that could potentially reduce the frequency of these conditions and delay disability and/or death (Rubenstein and Nahas, 1998). The national initiative *Healthy People 2010* lists seven essential elements of health promotion programs for older adults (U.S. Department of Health and Human Services, Public Health Service, 2000):

- Addressing causes of death
- Addressing chronic conditions
- Addressing risk factors
- Enabling access to medical care
- Providing participation in the health care system
- Providing equal opportunities by gender
- Providing equal opportunities to racially and ethnically diverse people

Nurses participate in activities such as health screenings and fairs that can identify older adults at risk and advise them about preventive measures (Davidhizar, Eshlernan, and Moody, 2002). Nurses in acute care and long-term care settings also assess the health status of older adults, intervene in acute situations, and, with the older adults, plan strategies to reduce risk and manage chronic conditions. Each contact with an older adult, regardless of setting, offers opportunities to teach and counsel.

Nursing interventions for older adults are directed toward improving or maintaining the older adult's health needs and concerns. Although various interventions cross all three levels of care, health promotion, acute care, and restorative care, there are approaches unique to each level. When planning interventions it is important to incorporate the older adult's routines or rituals when possible because the older adult feels more secure when routines are continued. The interventions generally are aimed at promoting independence and supporting self-care abilities.

Health Promotion and Maintenance: Physiological Concerns

Older adults believe that activity is important for staying fit and remaining independent and that their own positive actions contribute to wellness and quality of life (Clark, 1998). The factors that lead to wellness in advanced age have not been fully identified, but four important factors seem to be genetics, good luck, good health habits, and preventive measures (Rubenstein and Nahas, 1998). The nurse is unable to do anything about an older adult's genetic heritage or luck, but the nurse is in a unique position to establish health maintenance programs that promote older adults' wellness and to recommend preventive measures. Senior citizens' centers, churches, schools, shopping malls, libraries, and hospital lobbies can be used as settings to conduct screening tests and present information on health topics. Using creative approaches, the nurse can include health promotion activities for older adults in all health care settings.

Approximately 90% of adults over 65 have at least one chronic health condition, and chronic conditions are more than 4 times more common among older adults than in other age-groups (Eliopoulos, 1999). The effect of chronic conditions on the lives of older adults varies widely, but, in general, chronic conditions diminish the well-being and threaten the independence of older adults. Nursing interventions are often directed at the management of these conditions, but interventions can also focus on prevention (Rubenstein and Nahas, 1998). General preventive measures that nurses can recommend to older adults include the following:

- Regular exercise
- Weight reduction if overweight
- Management of hypertension
- Smoking cessation
- Immunization for influenza, pneumococcal pneumonia, and tetanus

Approximately 95% of the estimated 20,000 to 40,000 deaths per year in the United States from influenza occur among adults age 65 and older (Regan and Fowler, 2002). Annual immunization for influenza of all older adults is strongly recommended with special emphasis on the immunization for influenza of residents of nursing centers and clients of any age with chronic cardiovascular, pulmonary, and metabolic disorders (Gomolin and Kathpalia, 2002). Receipt of the pneumococcal pneumonia vaccine is recommended for all adults over age 65. Unlike influenza vaccine, pneumococcal pneumonia vaccine is given only once, although revaccination 6 to 8 years after the initial vaccination is recommended by some authorities (Beers and Berkow, 2000). For tetanus immunization, booster

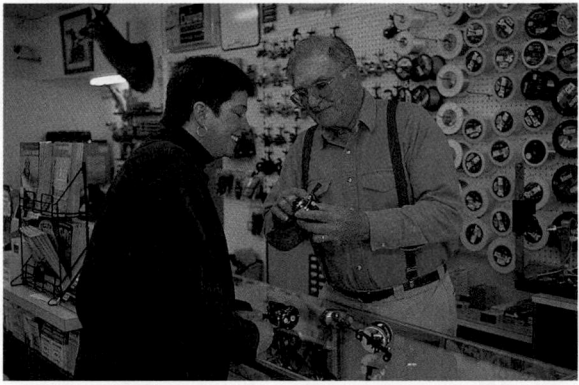

FIGURE **13–1** This older adult works part time at a sporting goods store.

injections every 10 years are recommended for adults who have had the primary series for tetanus immunization. However, not all older adults are current with their booster injections and some never received the primary series of injections. Nurses should ask older adults about the current status of all three types of immunizations, provide information about the immunizations, and make arrangements for the older adult to receive the immunizations as needed. Nurses should also refer older adults for screening for the early detection of cancer and depression.

Most older adults are interested in their health and are capable of taking charge of their lives. They want to remain independent and to prevent disability (Figure 13-1). Initial screenings establish baseline data that can be used to determine wellness, identify health needs, and design health maintenance programs. Following initial screening sessions, nurses can share with older adults information on nutrition, exercise, medications, and safety precautions. Information on specific conditions such as hypertension or arthritis or on self-care procedures such as foot and skin care may also be provided. By providing information about health promotion and self-care, nurses can significantly improve the health and well-being of older adults.

Heart Disease. Heart disease is the leading cause of death in older adults. Common cardiovascular disorders are hypertension and coronary artery disease. Hypertension is diagnosed when repeated blood pressure measurements of 90 mm Hg or greater diastolic and 140 mm Hg or greater systolic are present. Although over 50% of Americans have elevated diastolic and/or systolic pressures, the fact that hypertension is common does not make it normal or harmless. Systolic pressures higher than 160 mm Hg are associated with increased risk of stroke, increased risk of cardiovascular mortality, and increased risk of overall mortality (Beers and Berkow, 2000). In coronary artery disease, partial or complete blockage of one or more coronary arteries leads to myocardial ischemia and myocardial infarction. The risk factors for both hypertension and coronary artery disease include smoking, obesity, lack of exercise, and stress. Additional risk factors for coronary artery disease include hypertension, hyperlipidemia, and diabetes mellitus.

Nursing interventions for hypertension and coronary artery disease address weight reduction, exercise, dietary changes limiting salt and fat, stress management, and smoking cessation. Client teaching includes information about medications, blood pressure monitoring, nutrition, stress reduction techniques, and the symptoms indicating the need for emergency care.

Cancer. Malignant neoplasms are the second most common cause of death among older adults. Nurses participate in programs to educate older adults about early detection, treatment, and risk factors. Examples include smoking cessation, teaching breast self-examination (see Chapter 32), and encouraging all older adults to have annual screening for fecal occult blood. It is also important to educate older adults about the signs of cancer and encourage prompt reporting of nonhealing skin lesions, unexpected bleeding, change in bowel habits, and unexplained weight loss (Rubenstein and Nahas, 1998). Detection is complicated when cancer symptoms are mistakenly identified as part of the normal aging process, and the nurse must carefully distinguish between normal aging and pathological conditions.

Stroke (Cerebrovascular Accident). Cerebrovascular accidents, the third leading cause of death in the United States, occur as brain ischemia or brain hemorrhage (Beers and Berkow, 2000). In brain ischemia there is an inadequate supply of blood to areas of the brain due to blockage of blood vessels or general circulatory failure. Brain hemorrhage, either subarachnoid hemorrhage or intracerebral hemorrhage, is less common than brain ischemia. Risk factors for cerebrovascular accidents include hypertension, hyperlipidemia, diabetes mellitus, history of transient ischemic attacks, and family history of cardiovascular disease. Treatment usually includes hospitalization for days or months, depending on the degree of brain damage. Cerebrovascular accidents may impair the functional abilities of older adults and limit their ability to live independently. The scope of nursing interventions ranges from teaching older adults about risk reduction strategies to care of the older adult after a cerebrovascular accident and during recovery and rehabilitation.

Smoking. Cigarette smoking has been recognized as a risk factor in the four most common causes of death for older adults: heart disease, cancer, stroke, and lung disease. Smoking cessation is a health promotion strategy for older adults just as it is for younger adults. Older smokers can still benefit from smoking cessation (Boyd, 1996). In addition to reducing risk, smoking cessation may stabilize existing conditions such as chronic obstructive pulmonary disease (COPD). Smoking cessation may even contribute to the extension of life or of independent functioning.

There are four sequential approaches that nurses may use to encourage smoking cessation (Boyd, 1996). First, the nurse asks the older adult about smoking, including the type of tobacco product used, the frequency of smoking, and the number of years smoking. Then, the nurse provides information about the ill effects of smoking and the benefits of quitting. Finally, the nurse recommends quitting. If smoking cessation is rejected, the nurse should suggest a reduction in smoking. Assistance in developing a plan for quitting is offered, and various strategies such as the use of gum containing nicotine or nicotine patches and asking family members to reduce smoking are discussed. Lastly, the nurse, on subsequent visits with the older adult, offers encouragement and assistance in modifying the plan as necessary. Although some mistakenly believe that older adults do not want to quit smoking or are unable to quit, some older adults do choose to quit smoking and do succeed.

Alcohol Abuse. It is estimated that up to 15% of community-dwelling older adults are heavy drinkers (Gambert, 1997). Studies of alcohol abuse in older adults report two patterns: a lifelong pattern of heavy drinking that continues and a late-onset pattern when heavy drinking begins late in life. Frequently cited causes of excessive alcohol use are depression, loneliness, and lack of social support.

Abuse of alcohol may be underidentified in older adults. The clues to create suspicion of alcohol abuse are subtle, and the assessment may be complicated by coexisting dementia or depression. Suspicion of alcohol abuse increases when there is a history of repeated falls and accidents, a change in behavior or personality, social isolation, recurring episodes of memory loss and confusion, a history of skipping meals or medications, and difficulty managing household tasks and finances (Zimberg, 1996). When abuse of alcohol is suspected, treatment includes age-specific approaches that acknowledge the stresses experienced by the older adult and encourage involvement in activities that match the older adult's interests and boost feelings of self-worth. The identification and treatment of coexisting depression is also important.

Nutrition. How older adults meet their needs for good nutrition is influenced by lifelong eating habits and situational factors. Lifelong eating habits based in tradition, ethnicity, and religion influence choices of what foods are eaten and how those foods are prepared. Situational factors affecting nutrition include access to food stores, adequate finances, the physical and cognitive capability for food preparation, and a place to store food and prepare meals.

The nutritional needs of older adults are affected by their levels of activity and by clinical conditions. Level of activity has implications for the total amount of calories, with more sedentary older adults usually needing fewer calories than more active older adults. However, caloric requirements are not determined solely by activity. Additional calories may be required in clinical situations such as recovery from surgery, whereas calories may be restricted when the older adult is diabetic or overweight. Beyond caloric requirements, therapeutic diets may restrict fat, sodium, or simple sugars or may increase fiber or foods high in calcium, iron, vitamin A, or vitamin C.

Good nutrition for older adults includes appropriate caloric intake and limited intake of fat, salt, refined sugars, and alcohol. Although the nutritional guidelines displayed in the food guide pyramid (see Chapter 43) are the basic recommendations for older adult nutrition, some older adults do not follow these guidelines. Protein intake may be lower than recommended if older adults have reduced financial resources or limited access to grocery stores. Difficulty chewing meat may also limit protein intake. Fat intake may be higher than recommended because of the substitution of fast-food restaurant meals for meals prepared at home or because of methods of cooking featuring fried foods and sauces using butter and cream. Extra salt and sugar may be used while cooking or at the table to compensate for a diminished sense of taste. Vitamin intake may be reduced if shopping for fresh fruits and vegetables is difficult.

Older adults with dementia have special nutritional needs. As their memory and their functional skills decline with the progression of dementia, they lose the ability to remember when to eat, how to prepare food, and, eventually, how to feed themselves. At the same time their caloric needs may increase because of the energy expended in pacing and wandering activities. Nurses and other caregivers of older adults with dementia should routinely monitor weight and food intake, serve food that is easy to eat, provide assistance with eating, and offer food supplements as needed to maintain weight (Yen, 1997). Mealtime interventions for older adults with dementia also provide opportunities for socialization and practice with functional skills.

Dental Problems. Dental problems are common in older adults and include problems with natural teeth and dentures. Dental caries, gingivitis, broken or missing teeth, and ill-fitting or missing dentures may affect nutritional adequacy, cause pain, and lead to infection. The nurse can help prevent dental and gum disease through education about routine dental care (see Chapter 38). The nurse can also help older adults find dental services that offer reduced rates and that are accessible to those with impaired mobility.

Exercise. Older adults should be encouraged to maintain physical exercise and activity. The primary benefits of exercise include maintaining and strengthening functional ability and promoting a sense of enhanced well-being. An exercise such as walking builds endurance, increases muscle tone, improves joint flexibility, strengthens bones, reduces stress, and contributes to weight loss (Butler, 1998). Other benefits of a program of exercise include improvement of cardiovascular function, improved plasma lipoprotein profiles, increased metabolic rate, increased gastrointestinal transit time, and improved sleep quality (Butler and others, 1998). Frail older adults who exercise may experience improved mobility, gait, and balance plus less difficulty getting up from a chair or climbing stairs. Exercise may also have a positive effect on anxiety and depression (Gunnarsson and Judge, 1997).

The nurse should plan an exercise program that meets physical needs while allowing for physical impairments and encourage the older adult to persevere with the exercise program. Willingness to participate in and persevere with an exercise program is influenced by general beliefs about exercise, specific benefits from exercise, past experiences with exercise, personal goals, personality, and any unpleasant sensations associated with exercise (Resnick and Spellbring, 2000).

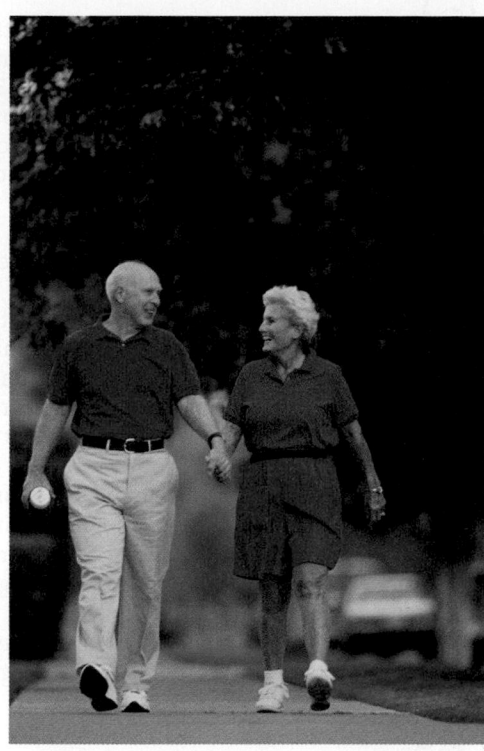

FIGURE **13–2**   This couple enjoys walking together.

Walking is the preferred exercise of many older adults (Figure 13-2). Walking and other low-impact exercises such as riding an exercise (stationary) bicycle or water exercises in a swimming pool protect the musculoskeletal system and joints (Ellingson and Conn, 2000). Other exercises can be incorporated into the older adult's activities of daily living. For example, arm and leg circles can be performed while watching television. But before beginning an exercise program, the older adult should have a physical examination. Exercise programs for sedentary older adults who have not been exercising regularly should begin conservatively and progress slowly. Safety considerations include wearing shoes and clothing appropriate to the exercise, drinking water before and after exercising, avoiding outdoor exercise when the weather is very warm or very cold, and exercising with a partner. Nurses should instruct the older adult to stop exercising and seek help if chest pain or tightness, shortness of breath, dizziness or light-headedness, or palpitations are experienced during exercise (Gunnarsson and Judge, 1997).

Arthritis. Arthritis is a common condition in older adults, especially in women. The degree to which the mobility of older adults is impaired depends on the extent of the disease and joints affected. The impact of arthritis on the lives of older adults is a combination of the changes in joint range of motion and stability and the amount of pain experienced. Arthritis has no cure, but recently developed pharmacological agents can decrease pain and swelling and therefore increase joint motion. Nursing interventions are aimed at promoting comfort, functional ability, and safety. Education about self-care techniques, joint protection, and exercises for flexibility and strength is also important.

Falls. Falls are a safety concern of many older adults. Falls may lead to fear of additional falls, withdrawal from usual activities, and loss of independence (see Chapters 37 and 46). Hospitalization and placement in a nursing home for rehabilitation or long-term placement may be required. Approximately 30% of older adults who live independently in their own homes will fall at least once a year (Tibbitts, 1996). A fracture will be sustained in 5% of those falls. Falls are more frequent and more serious for older adults over age 85.

The risk factors leading to falls are a combination of health-related issues and environmental hazards (Tideiksaar, 1996). Health-related issues include impaired vision; cardiovascular conditions such as postural hypotension or syncope; conditions affecting mobility such as arthritis, muscle weakness, and foot problems; conditions affecting balance; alterations in bladder function such as frequency or incontinence; cognitive impairment; and adverse medication reactions. Environmental hazards include, but are not limited to, poor lighting, slippery or wet floors, stairs or sidewalks in poor repair, shoes in poor repair or with slippery soles, and household items that could be tripped over, such as throw rugs, foot stools, and electric extension cords.

Nursing interventions are directed toward the management of health-related conditions and the reduction of environmental hazards. Older adults taking medications with adverse effects such as postural hypotension, dizziness, or sedation can be instructed to be aware of these potential effects and to take precautions such as changing position slowly or holding onto sturdy furniture if unsteady. Simple interventions in the home such as rearranging furniture to provide a clear pathway to the bathroom and providing a night-light in the bathroom can reduce falls related to nighttime trips to the toilet. Picking up throw rugs and other items on the floor reduces slipping and tripping. Nurses can also instruct older adults in the safe use of assistive devices such as canes, walkers, and wheelchairs.

Sensory Impairments. The older adult usually has changes in vision, hearing, taste, and smell that are a result of normal aging. Chapter 48 describes in detail the nursing interventions used to maintain and improve sensory function.

Pain. Between 25% and 50% of older adults living in the community and between 45% and 80% of older adults in nursing homes experience pain (Gloth, 2000). The causes of pain in older adults include acute and chronic conditions (e.g., trauma, infection, and neuropathies). Many factors influence the management of pain, including cultural influences on the meaning and expression of pain for older adults, fears related to the use of analgesic medications, and the problem of pain assessment with cognitively impaired older adults. Nurses caring for older adults are challenged to advocate for appropriate and effective pain management and to use standardized pain tools in their assessments (see Chapter 42).

Medication Use. Approximately two thirds of older adults use prescription and nonprescription drugs with one third of all prescriptions being written for older adults (Beers and Berkow, 2000). Most older adults use at least one drug daily; many use several drugs daily. The most commonly used medications are cardiovascular drugs, antihypertensives, analgesics, antiarthritic agents, sedatives, tranquilizers, laxatives, and antacids (Eliopoulos, 1999). **Polypharmacy,** the concurrent use of many medications, increases the risk for adverse reactions. Although polypharmacy may reflect inappropriate prescribing, the concurrent use of multiple medications may be necessary in situations where an older adult has multiple acute and chronic conditions. However, periodic and thorough review of all medications being used is important to restrict the number of medications used to the fewest necessary. The nurse's role with an older adult undergoing drug therapy is to ensure the greatest therapeutic benefit with the least amount of harm.

Older adults are at risk for adverse reactions because of age-related changes in the absorption, distribution, metabolism, and excretion of drugs (Table 13-3). Medications may interact with one another, adding or negating the effect of another drug. Medications may also cause confusion; affect balance and mobility; cause dizziness, nausea, and vomiting; or lead to constipation, urinary frequency, or incontinence. Because of these effects, some older adults are unwilling to take medications.

Managing medications is a very important component of maintaining and promoting good health in old age. For some older adults on large numbers of medications, safely managing medications can be a complex activity that can easily become overwhelming. Complicating the assessment of medication effects and side effects, some older adults, perhaps as many as 50%, take their medications incorrectly because they do not understand the instructions about their medications (Hayes, 1998). Nurses can provide valuable assistance to their older adult clients as they carry out this important self-care activity.

The nurse works collaboratively with the older adult to ensure safe and appropriate use of all medications, both prescribed and over-the-counter medications. The older adult should be taught the names of all drugs being taken, when and how to take them, and the desirable and undesirable effects of the drugs. The nurse also teaches how to avoid adverse effects and/or interactions of drugs and how to establish and follow an appropriate self-administration pattern. Strategies for reducing the risk for an adverse medication reaction in the older adult include reviewing the medications with the older adult at each visit, examining for potential interactions with food or other drugs, simplifying and individualizing the drug regimen, taking every opportunity to inform the older adult and family about all aspects of medication use, and encouraging the older adult to question the physician, advanced practice nurse, and/or pharmacist about all prescribed drugs and all over-the-counter drugs.

When drugs are used in the management of confusion, special care is necessary. The sedatives and tranquilizers sometimes prescribed for acutely confused older adults may themselves cause or exacerbate confusion. Drugs used to manage confused behaviors should be carefully administered, taking into account age-related changes in body systems that can affect the pharmacokinetic activity. When confusion has a physiological cause (such as an in-

Table 13-3   **Age-Related Changes Affecting Drug Therapy in Older Adults**

Change	Effect	Nursing Measures
Drier mucous membrane of oral cavity	Tablets and capsules may stick to roof or sides of mouth and not be swallowed, or dissolve in and irritate mouth.	Offer fluids before drug administration to moisten mouth and ample fluids during administration. Inspect client's mouth or advise client to inspect mouth for any tablet or capsule that may not have been swallowed (dentures and reduced oral sensations may cause client to be unaware of presence of medication). Unless contraindicated, break large tablets to facilitate swallowing.
Decreased circulation to lower bowel and vagina; lower body temperatures	Suppositories require more time to melt and can be expelled undissolved.	Explore possibility of using alternative route. Allow more time for suppository to melt. Check client or advise to check that the suppository has melted before getting out of bed to resume activities.
Decreased tissue elasticity; reduced muscle mass and activity	Poor seal of tissues after injection and oozing or poor absorption may result.	Use Z-track injection technique for injections to facilitate sealing.
Decreased pain sensation	Infection or other problem at injection site may not be detected.	Cleanse any medication that has oozed onto skin. Check injection sites regularly.
Decreased cardiac efficiency	Greater risk exists for circulatory overload during intravenous administration of medications.	Monitor intravenous drip closely. Observe for signs of circulatory overload, such as rise in blood pressure, rapid respirations, coughing, or shortness of breath.
Less gastric acid	Slower absorption of drugs that require low gastric pH may result.	Ensure that gastric acid is not further reduced by other drugs such as antacids.
Increase in adipose tissue compared with lean body mass; decreased cardiac output	Drugs stored in adipose tissue (lipid-soluble drugs) have increased tissue concentrations and decreased plasma concentrations and accumulate and remain in body longer. Plasma levels of drugs can increase while less is deposited in reservoirs (particularly true of water-soluble drugs).	Ensure that dosages are adjusted for age. Become familiar with adverse effects of drugs being administered and observe for these effects.
Reduced serum albumin levels	The administration of protein-bound drugs together can result in drugs competing for the same protein molecules. Some drugs may not effectively bind and may be less effective.	Advise physician of other protein-bound drugs client is taking when new protein-bound drug is prescribed. Highly protein-bound drugs include acetazolamide, amitriptyline, cefazolin, chlordiazepoxide, chlorpromazine, cloxacillin, digitoxin, furosemide, hydralazine, nortriptyline, phenylbutazone, phenytoin, propranolol, rifampin, salicylates, spironolactone, sulfisoxazole, and warfarin. Ensure that serum albumin level is evaluated along with blood level of drug. (If serum albumin level is low, client is at greater risk for toxicity despite normal or low blood levels of drug.)
Reduced number of functioning nephrons; decreased glomerular filtration rate; reduced blood flow	Biological half-life is extended, and drugs take longer to be filtered from body; risk of adverse reactions is increased.	Ensure that age-adjusted dosages are prescribed for drugs excreted through renal system.

From Eliopoulos C: *Manual of gerontologic nursing,* ed 2, St. Louis, 1999, Mosby.

fection), that cause, rather than the confused behavior, should be specifically treated. When confusion varies by time of day or is related to environmental factors, the nurse can use creative, nonpharmacological measures such as making the environment more meaningful, providing adequate light, encouraging use of assistive devices (glasses, hearing aids), or even making telephone calls to friends or family members to let older adults hear reassuring voices.

Health Promotion and Maintenance: Psychosocial Health Concerns

Interventions supporting the psychosocial health of older adults resemble those for other age-groups. However, some interventions are more crucial for older adults experiencing social isolation, cognitive impairment, or stresses related to retirement, relocation, or approaching death. These interventions include therapeutic communication, touch, reality orientation, validation therapy, reminiscence, and interventions to improve body image.

Therapeutic Communication. With therapeutic communication the nurse perceives and respects the older adult's uniqueness and meets the older adult's expectations. Older adults expect nurses to be attentive, caring, and knowledgeable (Santo-Novak, 1997). Attentive nurses provide care in a timely fashion, meeting client's expressed or unexpressed needs. A caring nurse expresses attitudes of concern, kindness, and compassion. Knowledgeable nurses not only demonstrate procedural competence but are adept at recognizing needs and relaying information. Older adult clients also expect nurses to respect their individuality (Marini, 1999). The nurse who meets these expectations and communicates effectively will be accepted as one who has a genuine concern for the older adult's welfare. However, the nurse cannot simply enter an older adult's environment and immediately establish a therapeutic relationship but must first be knowledgeable and skilled in communication techniques (see Chapter 23).

Touch. Throughout life, touch tells us about our environment and the people around us. Gentle touch conveys affection and friendliness. A firm handclasp may convey security. Touch is a therapeutic tool that nurses can use to help comfort the older adult. It can provide sensory stimulation, induce relaxation, provide physical and emotional comfort, orient the person to reality, convey warmth, and communicate interest. It is a powerful physical expression of a relationship.

Older adults may be deprived of touching when separated from family or friends. An older adult who is isolated, dependent, or ill; who fears death; or who lacks self-esteem has a greater need for touch. The nurse may recognize touch deprivation by behaviors as simple as an older adult reaching for the nurse's hand or standing close to the nurse. Unfortunately, older men are sometimes wrongly accused of sexual advances when they reach out to touch others. When nurses use touch, they must be aware of cultural variations as well as individual preferences (see Chapter 8). Touch should convey respect and sensitivity. Touch should not be used in a condescending way such as patting an older adult on the head. The nurse who reaches out to an older adult should not be surprised if the older adult reciprocates.

Reality Orientation. Reality orientation is a communication technique used to make an older adult more aware of time, place, and person. The purposes of reality orientation include restoring a sense of reality, improving the level of awareness, promoting socialization, elevating independent functioning, and minimizing confusion, disorientation, and physical regression.

Although the nurse can use reality orientation techniques in any health care setting, they may be especially useful in the acute care setting. The older adult experiencing a change in environment, surgery, illness, or emotional stress is at risk for becoming disoriented. Environmental changes, such as the bright lights, unfamiliar noises, and lack of windows in specialized units of a hospital, often lead to disorientation and confusion. Absence of familiar caregivers is also disorienting. When anesthesia, sedatives, tranquilizers, analgesics, and physical restraints are used, disorientation is increased. The nurse should anticipate and monitor for disorientation and confusion as possible consequences of hospitalization, relocation, surgery, loss, or illness and should incorporate interventions based on reality orientation into the care plan.

Once used as a therapy with disoriented individuals and groups of cognitively impaired individuals, the principles of reality orientation offer useful guidelines for communicating with acutely confused individuals. The key elements of reality orientation include frequent reminders of person, time, and place; the use of environmental aids such as clocks, calendars, and personal belongings; and stability of environment, routine, and staff (Eliopoulos, 1999). Communication is always respectful, patient, and calm. The nurse answers questions from the older adult simply and honestly with sensitivity and a caring attitude.

Validation Therapy. Validation therapy is an alternative approach to communication with a confused older adult. Where reality orientation insists that the confused older adult agree with our statements of time, place, and person, validation therapy accepts the description of time and place as stated by the confused older adult. Older adults with dementia are less likely to benefit and more likely to become agitated by the caregiver's insistence on the "correct" time, place, and person.

In validation therapy, statements and behaviors of the confused older adult are not challenged or disputed. The statements and behaviors are believed to represent an inner need or feeling. The appropriate nursing intervention is to recognize and address that inner need or feeling. Validation does not involve reinforcing the confused older adult's misperceptions, but reflects a sensitivity to hidden meanings in statements and behaviors. By listening with sensitivity and validating what is expressed, the nurse conveys respect, reassurance, and understanding. Validating or respecting confused older adults' feelings in the time and place that is real to them is more important than insisting on the literally correct time and place (Day, 1997).

Reminiscence. Reminiscence is recalling the past. Many older adults find enjoyment in sharing past experiences. As a therapy, reminiscence uses the recollection of the past to bring meaning and understanding to the present and to resolve current conflicts (Eliopoulos, 1999). Looking back to positive resolutions to problems reminds the older adult of coping strategies used successfully in the past. Reminiscing is also a way to express personal identity. Reflection on past achievements supports self-esteem. For some older adults the process of looking back on past events uncovers new meanings for those events.

During the assessment process, the nurse may use reminiscence to assess self-esteem, cognitive function, emotional stability, unresolved conflicts, coping ability, and expectations for the future (Eliopoulos, 1999). Reminiscence also occurs during direct care activities. Taking time to ask questions about past experiences and listening attentively conveys to an older adult the nurse's attitudes of respect and concern (Puentes, 1998).

Although reminiscence is often used in a one-on-one situation of nurse and older adult, reminiscence can also be a group therapy for cognitively impaired or depressed older adults. The nurse organizes the group and selects strategies to start a conversation. For example, the nurse might ask the group to discuss families or childhood memories. The group's size, structure, process, goals, and activities are adapted to meet its members' needs.

Body-Image Interventions. The way that older adults present themselves influences body image and feelings of isolation. Some physical characteristics of older adulthood are socially desirable, such as distinguished-looking gray hair. Other features are also impressive, such as a lined face that displays character or wrinkled hands that convey a lifetime of hard work. Too often, however, society sees older people as incapacitated, deaf, obese, or shrunken in stature. Consequences of illness and aging that threaten the older adult's body image include invasive diagnostic procedures, pain, surgery, loss of sensation in a body part, skin changes, loss of scalp hair, and incontinence. Body image is also affected by the use of devices such as dentures, hearing aids, artificial limbs, indwelling catheters, ostomy devices, and enteral feeding tubes.

The importance to the older adult of presenting a socially acceptable image must be considered. When older adults have acute or chronic illnesses, the related physical dependence makes it difficult for them to maintain body image. The nurse influences the older adult's appearance by assisting with grooming and hygiene. It takes little effort to assist the older adult with combing hair, cleaning dentures, shaving, or changing clothing. The older adult does not choose to have an objectionable appearance. The nurse should also be sensitive to odors in the environment. Odors created by urine and some illnesses are often present. By controlling odors, the nurse may prevent visitors from shortening their stay or not coming at all.

Older Adults and the Acute Care Setting

Older adults in the acute care setting need special attention to help them adjust to the acute care environment and to meet their basic needs for comfort, safety, nutrition/hydration, and skin integrity. The acute care setting poses increased risk for adverse events such as delirium, dehydration, malnutrition, nosocomial infections, urinary incontinence, and falls.

The risk for delirium is increased when hospitalized older adults experience immobilization, infection, dehydration, pain, and hypoxia. Multiple medications and multiple medical diagnoses are also risk factors for delirium (Simon, Jewell, and Brokel, 1997). Nonmedical causes of delirium include placement in unfamiliar surroundings, separation from supportive family members, and stress. Impaired vision or hearing contributes to confusion and interferes with attempts to reorient the older adult. When the prevention of delirium fails, interventions begin with treatment of the cause. Supportive interventions include encouraging family visits, providing memory cues (clocks, calendars, name tags), and compensating for sensory deficits. Reality orientation techniques may be useful.

Older adults are at greater risk for dehydration and malnutrition during hospitalization because of standard procedures such as limiting food and fluids in preparation for diagnostic tests (Sullivan, Sun, and Walls, 1999). The risk for dehydration and malnutrition is also increased when older adults are unable to reach beverages or to feed themselves while in bed or connected to medical equipment. Interventions include getting the client out of bed, providing beverages and snacks frequently, and including favorite foods and beverages in the diet plan.

The increased risk for nosocomial infections in older adults is related to age-related reductions in immune system response. The use of indwelling urinary catheters accounts for 80% of nosocomial urinary tract infections (Lee and Burnett, 1998). Other nosocomial infections include surgical site infection, pneumonia, and bloodstream infections (Russell, 1999). Prevention begins with hand hygiene and measures to minimize the risk of infection from procedures (see Chapter 33). Prevention also includes measures to increase the older adult's resistance to infection.

Older adults in acute care settings are also at risk for becoming incontinent of urine (transient incontinence). Causes of transient urinary incontinence include delirium, untreated urinary tract infection, excessive urine production, medications, restricted mobility, and constipation or impaction (Bradway, Hernly, and the NICHE faculty, 1998). Interventions for transient urinary incontinence are geared to correcting contributing factors. The interventions may include an individualized plan to provide voiding opportunities and modification of the environment to improve access to the toilet. Indwelling urinary catheters should be avoided if possible. Measures to prevent skin breakdown should be used.

The increased risk for skin breakdown and the development of pressure ulcers is related to changes in aging skin and to situations that arise in the acute care setting such as immobility, incontinence, and malnutrition. The key points in the prevention of skin breakdown are avoiding pressure, reducing shear forces and friction, providing skin care and moisture management, and providing nutritional support (Maklebust, 1997).

Older adults in the acute care setting are at risk for falling and sustaining injuries. Many of the falls occur as the older adult gets out of bed without assistance. Sedating medications may increase unsteadiness. Medications causing orthostatic hypotension may also increase the risk for falls because of the blood pressure drop when the older adult gets out of a bed or chair. The increase in urine output from diuretics increases the risk for falling by increasing the number of attempts to get out of bed to void. Attempts to get out of bed when physically restrained may lead to injury when the older adult becomes entangled in the restraint. Equipment such as wires from monitors, intravenous tubing, urinary catheters, and other medical devices become obstacles to safe ambulation. Impaired vision may prevent the older adult from seeing tripping hazards such as trash cans.

Confused older adults who may try to get out of bed although weak, unsteady, or drowsy may benefit from reality orientation or the presence of family members and friends. Interventions to reduce the risk for falling include assistance with ambulation, strengthening exercises, medication monitoring, assistance with toileting, and removal of tripping hazards (see Chapter 37).

Older Adults and Restorative Care

Restorative care refers to two types of ongoing care. The first type of restorative care continues the convalescence from acute illness or surgery that began in the acute care setting. The second type of restorative care addresses chronic conditions that affect day-to-day functioning. Both types of restorative care take place in private homes and in long-term care settings.

Interventions during convalescence from acute illness or surgery are directed toward regaining or improving the prior level of independence in ADLs. Interventions that began in the acute care setting should be continued and later modified as convalescence progresses. To achieve this continuation, the acute care setting's discharge information should include information on the ongoing interventions (e.g., exercise routines, wound care routines, medication schedules, vital sign monitoring, and blood glucose monitoring). Interventions should also address the restoration of interpersonal relationships and activities at either their previous level or at the level desired by the older adult.

When restorative care addresses chronic conditions, the goals of care include stabilizing the chronic condition, promoting health, and promoting independence in activities of daily living. Interventions to stabilize the chronic condition may focus on regulation or prevention. An example of a regulatory intervention is the monitoring of blood glucose levels in diabetes. An example of prevention is a smoking cessation program for the older adult with chronic obstructive pulmonary disease.

Health promotion for older adults, as addressed in this chapter, applies to all older adults. Health promotion interventions should occur in all health care settings. For example, nurse-directed programs in long-term care have improved ambulation, reversed urinary incontinence, and reduced confusion.

Interventions to promote independence in ADLs address physical ability, cognitive ability, and safety. The physical ability to perform ADLs requires strength, flexibility, and balance. Accommodation must be made for impairments of vision, hearing, and touch. The cognitive ability to perform ADLs requires the ability to recognize, judge, and remember. Cognitive impairments, such as Alzheimer's disease, may interfere with safe performance of ADLs, although the older adult is still physically capable of the activities. Interventions to promote independence in ADLs adapt these requirements to the needs and lifestyle of the older adult. Safety is always considered because it is not enough to be able to perform any of the ADLs. The older adult should be able to perform the ADLs with only an amount of risk that is acceptable to the older adult.

Beyond the basic activities of daily living, the older adult's ability to perform instrumental activities of daily living (IADLs) must be assessed and appropriate interventions implemented. Instrumental activities of daily living are tasks such as using a telephone, preparing meals, shopping, doing laundry, cleaning the home or apartment, and driving an automobile. To remain living independently at home or in an apartment, older adults must be able to perform IADLs, be able to purchase services by outside workers, or have a supportive network of family and friends who assist with these tasks.

Restorative care measures focus on activities to prevent, improve, reduce, or eliminate problems. Priorities of care are established, client goals and expected outcomes are determined, and appropriate interventions are selected. This is done with the older adult's participation so that the interventions are understood and conflicts in approaches or priorities can be avoided. Consideration by the nurse of the older adult's lifetime experiences, as well as the values and sociocultural patterns developed, serves as the basis for planning individual care. When the older adult's cognitive status prevents participation in health care decisions, the family must be included. Family and friends are rich sources of data because they knew the older adult before the impairment. Frequently, they can provide explanations for the older adult's behaviors and suggest methods of management. Thoughtful assessment and planning leads to goals of care that consider the influence of normal aging changes, facilitate an optimal level of comfort and coping, and promote independence in self-care activities.

Key Concepts

- The number of older adults, especially the number of older adults over age 85, is increasing.
- Because nurses' attitudes toward older adults influence the quality of care, those attitudes should be based on accurate information about older adults, rather than myths and stereotypes.
- The biological and psychosocial theories of aging offer possible explanations for the changes seen in aging, but every older adult is a unique individual who ages in a unique way.
- The physical changes that accompany aging are considered to be normal, not pathological, although they may predispose the older adult to disease.
- Cognitive impairment is not normal in older adults and requires assessment and intervention.
- Areas affected by psychosocial changes of aging include retirement, social isolation, change in housing, death, and sexuality.
- Cognitive impairment includes acute, potentially reversible disorders and chronic, irreversible, progressive disorders.
- Nursing interventions for psychosocial concerns include therapeutic communication, touch, reality orientation, validation therapy, reminiscence, and interventions to improve body image.

- The leading causes of death in the older population are heart disease, cancer, stroke, lung disease, accidents/falls, diabetes, kidney disease, and liver disease.
- Health promotion recommendations for older adults include good nutrition, regular exercise, smoking cessation, measures to reduce the risk for falls, and measures to reduce adverse medication reactions.
- Acute care settings place older adults at risk for delirium, dehydration, malnutrition, nosocomial infections, urinary incontinence, and falls.
- Restorative nursing interventions, whether accomplished in the older adult's home or in long-term care institutions, stabilize chronic conditions, promote health, and promote independence in basic and instrumental activities of daily living.

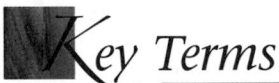

Key Terms

Ageism, *p. 237*	Gerontology, *p. 236*
Alzheimer's disease, *p. 244*	Nonstochastic theories,
Delirium, *p. 244*	*p. 238*
Dementia, *p. 244*	Polypharmacy, *p. 252*
Depression, *p. 244*	Reality orientation, *p. 254*
Geriatrics, *p. 236*	Reminiscence, *p. 254*
Gerontic nursing, *p. 236*	Stochastic theories, *p. 238*
Gerontological nursing,	Validation therapy, *p. 254*
p. 236	

Critical Thinking Exercises

1. Mr. Brown, age 73, has come to the clinic for a routine check of his blood pressure. It is normal (130/80 mm Hg). He tells you that he wants to do everything he can to stay healthy. What advice can you give him on health promotion and disease prevention?
2. Mrs. Shephard's daughter has come with her to the clinic. She is concerned about her mother's memory. She tells you that although her mother's memory is usually excellent with only occasional forgetting of names or the location of keys, this has suddenly changed. Two days ago Mrs. Shephard phoned her daughter 6 times in 2 hours asking where her husband (the late Mr. Shephard) was and when told of his death 4 years ago denied this fact. When her daughter arrived at her house to check on her, she found that Mrs. Shephard had emptied the contents of all the closets onto the floor and accused her daughter of theft. Mrs. Shephard has spent the last two nights at her daughter's house because her daughter is concerned about her safety. From Mrs. Shephard's daughter's report you suspect delirium (acute confusional state). What questions should you ask and what areas should you assess to identify the possible causes of Mrs. Shepard's confusion?
3. You and your colleague Jane Doe, RN, are having lunch together. She tells you that she does not know very much about assessing older adults and asks for some pointers on how to do a good, thorough assess-

ment. What advice can you give her on the process of geriatric assessment?

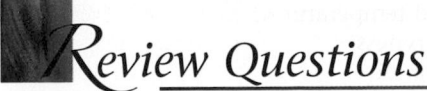

Review Questions

1. Two factors contribute to the projected increase in the number of older adults; they are:
   1. Financial success and improved environment.
   2. Greater acceptance of elderly and medical problems.
   3. Improved medication plan and increase in Medicare funding.
   4. The aging of the "baby boom" generation and the growth of the population segment over age 85.

2. Which of the following is true about the theories of aging?
   1. Genetic changes are solely responsible.
   2. Environment is the main factor.
   3. There is no single theory that explains aging.
   4. Disease causes a decline in function.

3. The three common conditions affecting cognition in the elderly are:
   1. Stroke, heart attack, and cancer of the brain.
   2. Cancer, Alzheimer's disease, stroke.
   3. Delirium, depression, and dementia.
   4. Blindness, hearing loss, and stroke.

4. Sexuality is recognized as a factor in the care of older adults, thus:
   1. Any expression of sexuality should be discouraged.
   2. All older adults, whether healthy or frail, need to express sexual feelings.
   3. A decrease in an older adult's libido does occur.
   4. The need to touch and be touched is decreased.

5. The older adult's libido does not decrease; however:
   1. Frequency of sexual activity may decline.
   2. Physical changes usually will not affect sexual functioning.
   3. The need to touch and be touched is decreased.
   4. The sexual preferences of older adults are not as diverse.

6. Visual acuity declines with age. Presbyopia, is a progressive decline in:
   1. Distinguishing between blues and greens and among pastel shades.
   2. Ability to see in darkness.
   3. The ability of the eyes to accommodate for close, detailed work.
   4. Adaptation to abrupt changes from dark areas to light areas.

7. A common age-related change in auditory acuity is called:
   1. Presbycusis.
   2. Presbyopia.
   3. Calcification.
   4. Hypertrophy.

8. Taste buds atrophy and lose sensitivity. The older adult is less able to discern:
    1. Salty, sweets, sour, and bitter tastes.
    2. Hot and cold temperatures.
    3. Moist and dryness.
    4. Spice and bland.

9. Changes in the musculoskeletal system lead to changes in the configuration of the thorax. This is known as:
    1. Hypertrophy.
    2. Calcification.
    3. Presbycusis.
    4. Kyphosis.

10. Frontal-temporal dementia has an insidious onset and progresses slowly. Early symptoms include:
    1. Poor hygiene, lack of social tact, and sexual disinhibition.
    2. More involvement in surroundings and social situations.
    3. Fluctuating cognition, visual and/or auditory hallucinations.
    4. Motor features of parkinsonism.

References

Adelman A: Managing chronic illness. In Adelman A, Daly M, editors: *20 common problems in geriatrics*, New York, 2001, McGraw-Hill.

Administration on Aging: *A profile of older Americans: 2001*, Washington, DC, 2002, U.S. Department of Health and Human Services, http://research.aarp.org/general/profile.

Beers M, Berkow R: *The Merck manual of geriatrics*, ed 3, Whitehouse Station, NJ, 2000, Merck.

Bolla L, Fille C, Palmer R: Office diagnosis of the four major types of dementia, *Geriatrics* 55(1):34, 2000.

Boyd N: Smoking cessation: a four-step plan to help older patients quit, *Geriatrics* 51(11):53, 1996.

Bradway C, Hernly S, the NICHE faculty: Urinary incontinence in older adults admitted to acute care, *Geriatr Nurs* 19:98, 1998.

Butler R: Tell your patients to take a walk, *Geriatrics* 53(5):15, 1998.

Butler R, Lewis M: Late-life depression: when and how to intervene, *Geriatrics* 50(8):44, 1995.

Butler R and others: Physical fitness: benefits of exercise for the older patient, *Geriatrics* 53(10):46, 1998.

Conn D: Cholinesterase inhibitors: comparing the options for mild-to-moderate dementia, *Geriatrics* 56(9):56, 2001.

Cummings E, Henry W: *Growing old: the process of disengagement*, New York, 1961, Basic Books.

Cutillo-Schmitter T: Aging: broaden our view for improved nursing care, *J Gerontol Nurs* 22(7):31, 1996.

Davidhizar R, Eshlernan J, Moody M: Health promotion for aging adults, *Geriatr Nurs* 23(1):28, 2002.

Day C: Validation therapy: a review of the literature, *J Gerontol Nurs* 23(4):29, 1997.

Ebersole P, Hess P: *Toward healthy aging: human needs and nursing response*, ed 5, St. Louis, 1998, Mosby.

Ebersole P, Hess P: *Geriatric nursing and healthy aging*, St. Louis, 2001, Mosby.

Eliopoulos C: *Manual of gerontologic nursing*, ed 2, St. Louis, 1999, Mosby.

Emmett K: Nonspecific and atypical presentation of disease in the older patient, *Geriatrics* 53(2):50, 1998.

Fielo S, Rizzolo M: Handle with caring: meeting elderly clients' special learning needs, *Nurs Health Care* 9(4):193, 1988.

Fielo S, Warren S: Home adaptation: helping older people age in place, *Geriatr Nurs* 22(5):239, 2001.

Foreman M and others: Assessing cognitive function, *Geriatr Nurs* 17(5):228, 1996.

Gambert S: Alcohol abuse: medical effects of heavy drinking in late life, *Geriatrics* 52(6):30, 1997.

Gambert S: Prostate cancer: when to offer screening in the primary care setting, *Geriatrics* 56(1):22, 2001.

Gloth FM III: Factors that limit pain relief and increase complications, *Geriatrics* 55(10):46, 2000.

Gomolin I, Kathpalia R: Influenza: how to prevent and control nursing home outbreaks, *Geriatrics* 57(1):28, 2002.

Gunnarsson O, Judge J: Exercise at midlife: how and why to prescribe it for sedentary patients, *Geriatrics* 52(5):71, 1997.

Lee V, Burnett E: A case report: special needs of hospitalized elders, *Geriatr Nurs* 19:185, 1998.

Lemon B, Bengston V, Peterson J: An exploration of the activity theory of aging: activity types and life satisfaction among in-movers to a retirement community, *J Gerontol* 27:516, 1972.

Lueckenotte A: Gerontologic assessment. In Lueckenotte A, editor: *Gerontologic nursing*, ed 2, St. Louis, 2000, Mosby.

Luft J, Vriheas-Nichols A: Identifying the risk factors for developing incontinence: can we modify individual risk? *Geriatr Nurs* 19(2):66, 1998.

Maklebust J: Pressure ulcers: decreasing the risk for older adults, *Geriatr Nurs* 18(6):250, 1997.

Neugarten B: *Personality in middle and late life*, New York, 1964, Atherton.

Puentes W: Incorporating simple reminiscence techniques into acute care nursing practice, *J Gerontol Nurs* 24(2):15, 1998.

Rantz M, Popejoy L, Zwygart-Stauffacher M: *The new nursing homes: a 20-minute way to find great long-term care*, Minneapolis, 2001, Fairview Press.

Regan S, Fowler C: Influenza: past, present, and future, *J Gerontol Nurs* 28(11):31, 2002.

Rubenstein I, Nahas R: Primary and secondary prevention strategies in the older adult, *Geriatr Nurs* 19(1):11, 1998.

Russell B: Nosocomial infections, *Am J Nurs* 99(6):24J, 1999.

Simon L, Jewell N, Brokel J: Management of acute delirium in hospitalized elderly: a process improvement project, *Geriatr Nurs* 18:150, 1997.

Sloane P: Normal aging. In Ham R, Sloane P, editors: *Primary care geriatrics: a case based approach*, ed 2, St. Louis, 1992, Mosby.

Sullivan D, Sun S, Walls R: Protein-energy undernutrition among elderly hospitalized patients, *JAMA* 281:2013, 1999.

Thorndyke L: Osteoporosis. In Adelman A, Daly M, editors: *20 common problems in geriatrics*. New York, 2001, McGraw-Hill.

Tibbitts G: Patients who fall: how to predict and prevent injuries, *Geriatrics* 51(9):24, 1996.

Tideiksaar R: Preventing falls: how to identify risk factors, reduce complications, *Geriatrics* 61(2):43, 1996.

Tueth M: How to manage depression and psychosis in Alzheimer's disease, *Geriatrics* 50(1):43, 1995.

U.S. Department of Health and Human Services, Public Health Service: *Healthy people 2010: national health promotion and disease prevention objectives*, Washington, DC, 2000, U.S. Government Printing Office.

Wallace M: Touch and intimacy. In Lueckenotte A, editor: *Gerontologic nursing*, St. Louis, 1996, Mosby.

Wojciechowski C: Issues in caring for older lesbians, *J Gerontol Nurs* 24(7):28, 1998.

Yen P: Weight loss resulting from Alzheimer's disease, *Geriatr Nurs* 18(3):132, 1997.

Zimberg S: Treating alcoholism: an age-specific intervention that works for older patients, *Geriatrics* 51(10):45, 1996.

Research References

Chasteen A, Schwarz N, Park D: The activation of aging stereotypes in younger and older adults, *J Gerontol B Psychol Sci Soc Sci* 57B:P540, 2002.

Ciricelli V: Personality and demographic factors in older adults' fear of death, *Gerontologist* 39:569, 1999.

Clark C: Wellness self-care by healthy older adults, *Image J Nurs Sch* 30:351, 1998.

Ellingson T, Conn V: Exercise and quality of life in elderly individuals, *J Gerontol Nurs* 26(3):17, 2000.

Hayes K: Randomized trial of geragogy-based medication instruction in the emergency department, *Nurs Res* 47:211, 1998.

Marini B: Institutionalized older adults' perceptions of nurse caring behaviors, *J Gerontol Nurs* 25(5):11, 1999.

Mastrian K: Differing perceptions in defining safe independent living for elders, *Nurs Outlook* 49:213, 2001.

Resnick B, Spellbring A: Understanding what motivates older adults to exercise, *J Gerontol Nurs* 26(3):34, 2000.

Santo-Novak D: Older adults' descriptions of their role expectations of nursing, *J Gerontol Nurs* 23(1):32, 1997.

14

Critical Thinking in Nursing Practice

Media Resources

http://evolve.elsevier.com/Potter/
fundamentals/

CD COMPANION

- Review Questions
- Glossary

evolve WEBSITE

- Review Questions
- Student Learning Activities
- Glossary

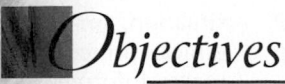

Mastery of content in this chapter will enable the student to:

- Define the key terms listed.
- Discuss the nurse's responsibility in making clinical decisions.
- Discuss how reflection can improve a nurse's practice.
- Describe how intuition affects clinical decisions.
- Compare and contrast critical thinking competencies.
- Describe the components of a critical thinking model for clinical decision making.
- Discuss critical thinking skills used in nursing practice.
- Explain the relationship between clinical experience and critical thinking.
- Discuss the critical thinking attitudes used in clinical decision making.
- Explain how professional standards influence a nurse's clinical decisions.
- Discuss the relationship of the nursing process to critical thinking.

Nurses face an endless variety of situations involving clients, family members, health care staff, and peers. Each situation poses new experiences and problems involving clients' care, different approaches to resolving problems, and different results as to whether approaches were successful. In every clinical situation it is important for a nurse to think critically and make sound judgments so that clients ultimately receive the very best nursing care. Critical thinking is not a simple step-by-step, linear process that can be learned overnight. It is a process acquired only through hard work, commitment, and an active curiosity toward learning. Ideally, critical thinking becomes a habit of mind, a part of each nurse's character (Facione and Facione, 1996).

Clinical Decisions in Nursing Practice

Nurses are responsible for making accurate and appropriate clinical decisions. Clinical decision making separates professional nurses from technical or ancillary personnel. It is the professional nurse, for example, who takes immediate action when a client's clinical condition deteriorates, who decides if a client is experiencing complications that warrant notification of the physician, or who determines if a teaching plan for a client is ineffective and must be revised. A nurse must be able to think critically, solve problems, and find the best solution for clients' needs to assist clients in maintaining, regaining, or improving their health. However, most clients have health care problems for which there are no clear textbook solutions. Each client's problem is unique, a product of many factors, including the client's physical health, lifestyle, culture, relationship with family and friends, living environment, and experiences. Thus a nurse does not always have a clear picture of the client's needs and the appropriate actions to take when first meeting a client. Instead, the nurse must learn to question, to wonder, and then to be self-directed in exploring different perspectives and interpretations and find a solution that can best help the client (Whiteside, 1997).

Because no two clients have identical types of health problems, a nurse is always challenged to observe each client closely, search for and examine ideas and inferences about client problems, consider scientific principles relating to the problems, recognize the problems, and develop an approach to nursing care. A nurse learns to creatively seek new knowledge as needed, act quickly when events change, and make sound decisions that promote the client's well-being. The challenges of clinical decision making make nursing a rewarding and fulfilling profession. Over time, a nurse gains the expertise to test and refine nursing approaches, to learn from successes and failures, and to apply new knowledge (e.g., nursing research findings). The ability to think critically through the application of knowledge and experience, problem solving, and decision making is central to professional nursing practice.

Critical Thinking Defined

Thinking and learning are interrelated, lifelong processes (Chaffee, 1994). Over time, a nurse's knowledge and experience in clinical practice help broaden the ability to make thoughtful observations, judgments, and choices. **Critical thinking** is an active, organized, cognitive process used to carefully examine one's thinking and the thinking of others (Chaffee, 1994). It involves use of the mind in forming conclusions, making decisions, drawing inferences, and reflecting (Gordon, 1995). It means taking nothing for granted. A critical thinker identifies and challenges assumptions, considers what is important in a

situation, imagines and explores alternatives, considers ethical principles, applies reason and logic, and thus makes informed decisions. As a new nurse caring for a client, critical thinking begins by asking these questions: What do I really know about this nursing care situation? How do I know it? What options are available to me? (Paul and Heaslip, 1995). For example, What do I really know about a client's pain? How do I know the client is in pain? What options are available to relieve the pain? Unless such questions are asked, a nurse can easily form inaccurate or inappropriate conclusions and take actions that are not beneficial to a client.

Critical thinking presupposes a certain basic level of intellectual humility (e.g., acknowledging one's own ignorance) and a commitment to thinking and reasoning, that is, to the clear, precise, and accurate assessment of a situation and to acting on the basis of genuine knowledge that comes from the situation and from nursing science.

Critical thinking requires not only cognitive skills but a person's habit to ask questions, to remain well informed, to be honest in facing personal biases, and always to be willing to reconsider and think clearly about issues (Facione, 1990). There are core critical thinking skills that, when applied to nursing, are useful in showing the complex nature of clinical decision making (Table 14-1). Being able to apply all of these skills takes practice, a sound knowledge base, and the thoughtful consideration of the knowledge gained in the clinical care of clients.

Nurses who apply critical thinking in their work focus on options for solving problems and making decisions, rather than hastily and carelessly forming quick, single solutions (Kataoka-Yahiro and Saylor, 1994). Indeed, nurses who work in crisis situations such as the emergency department or intensive care must often act quickly when client problems develop. However, even these nurses exer-

Table 14-1	Critical Thinking Skills Proposed by the American Philosophical Association	
Skill	**Description**	**Nursing Practice Applications**
Interpretation	Categorization Clarifying meaning	Be systematic in data collection. Look for patterns to categorize data (e.g., nursing diagnoses [see Chapter 16]). Clarify any data you are uncertain about.
Analysis	Examining ideas Analyzing arguments	Be open minded as you look at information about a client. Do not make careless assumptions. Do the data reveal what you believe is true, or are there other options?
Evaluation	Assessing results Assessing arguments	Look at all situations objectively. Use criteria (e.g., expected outcomes, pain characteristics, learning objectives) to determine results of nursing actions. Reflect on your own behavior.
Inference	Examining evidence Speculating or conjecturing alternatives Making conclusions	Look at the meaning and significance of findings. Are there relationships between findings? Does the data about the client help you determine that a problem exists?
Explanation	Stating results Justifying procedures Presenting arguments	Support your findings and conclusions. Use knowledge to select strategies you use in the care of clients.
Self-regulation	Self-examination Self-correction	Reflect on your experiences. Identify in what way you can improve your own performance. What will make you feel that you have been successful?

Modified from Facione P: *Critical thinking: a statement of expert consensus for purposes of educational assessment and instruction. The Delphi report: research findings and recommendations prepared for the American Philosophical Association,* ERIC Doc No. ED 315-423, Washington, DC, 1990, ERIC.

cise discipline in decision making so as to avoid premature and inappropriate decisions. Learning to think critically helps a nurse to care for clients as their advocate and to make better-informed choices about their care. Critical thinking is more than just problem solving. It is an attempt to continually improve how to apply oneself when faced with problems in client care. Each clinical experience helps a nurse pursue learning opportunities focused on excellence in practice. Three important aspects of critical thinking—reflection, language, and intuition—enable a nurse to excel in critical thinking.

Reflection

An important aspect of critical thinking is **reflection,** the process of purposefully thinking back or recalling a situation to discover its purpose or meaning (Miller and Babcock, 1996). As a nurse it helps to think back on a client situation, to make sense of the experience, and to thus gain insight as to the meaning of the situation. For example, after caring for a client who is recovering from heart surgery, one might reflect on how the client reacted when discussing diet restrictions and exercise guidelines. What did it mean when the client said, "I don't know what my family will think about this new diet" or "Exercise has never been something I enjoy doing"? Reflection provides new insight (Smith and Johnston, 2002). Reflection is like the playback function on a videotape. It involves playing back a situation in one's head and taking time to honestly review everything one can remember about the situation. Reflection requires adequate knowledge and is necessary for self-evaluation, to review one's successes or opportunities for improvement. O'Neill and Dluhy (1997) caution new clinicians to not question every judgment they make. An emphasis on reflection can deter thinking in a clinical situation because of the second-guessing it can create.

With reflection a nurse seeks to understand the relationships between concepts learned in the classroom and real-life clinical situations. In the example above, the client's response to new diet and exercise guidelines may be a result of fear, denial, or concern over family support. Reflection allows the nurse to consider all possibilities, refer to knowledge learned in class, and to then return to assess the client, identify relevant problems, and clarify any concerns. Reflection allows a nurse to judge personal performance while also judging whether standards of nursing practice were followed. It is a process that helps make sense out of an experience so that the next time a similar experience arises, a nurse can use approaches that were successful or revise a previous approach to achieve better client outcomes. For example, a nurse who uses reflection will not only consider the heart client's comments about diet and exercise but also his or her own responses to the client's comments. Did I respond so the client could express his views openly? Did I listen? Did I form unfounded conclusions without sufficient information?

Engaging in reflection is very individualized (Miller and Babcock, 1996). Learning to be reflective takes practice (Box 14-1). When a nurse reflects on a clinical experience, it is important to remain open to new information and be able to look at both the client's and nurse's perspectives. Paget (2001) suggests that reflective practice has

the potential for improving a nurse's clinical practice and for influencing a nurse's self-awareness and the manner in which he or she interacts with clients (Box 14-2). Paget also argues that the routine use of reflective practice has the potential to affect client outcomes in a favorable way.

Language

Another important aspect of critical thinking is the use of language. The ability to use language is closely associated with the ability to think meaningfully (Miller and Babcock, 1996). To think critically, a nurse must be able to use language precisely and clearly. When language is vague and inaccurate, it reflects sloppy thinking.

It is important to communicate clearly with clients, families, and health care professionals. When a nurse uses incorrect terminology, jargon, or vague descriptions, communication is ineffective. This may become obvious if the

---

Box *14-1* Tips on Facilitating Reflection

- As you care for a client, stop and think about what is going on with your client and what your assessment findings mean. What physical or psychological changes are occurring? How does this compare to normal functioning? When you chart or report on your client, what is the meaning of his or her symptoms and associated treatment? Always ask what could be happening (Fowler, 1998).
- Reflect carefully on any critical incidents (e.g., safety episodes, cardiac arrests, pivotal events in the progression of a client's disease) (Bittner and Tobin, 1998). What occurred? What actions were taken? How did the client respond? Were there other actions you might have taken?
- At the end of each day when you care for a client, take time to reflect. Ask yourself whether you achieved your original plan of care. If you did, what made it successful? If you did not, what were the barriers or factors requiring changes? What would you do differently or the same?
- Keep a journal or summative description of your experiences with clients. Be sure to include the following elements: identification, description, significance, and implications (Baker, 1996). Telling a story and drawing a picture are two ways to identify the situation or experience. Describe in detail what you felt, thought, and did. Analyze the significance of the experience by considering feelings, thoughts, and possible meanings. Describe the implications of the experience in terms of your own clinical practice or self-perceptions as a learner. Refer to the journal often when you care for clients in similar situations. The journal can become a rich resource for you to revisit important experiences and gain insight into the thoughts and actions that make up clinical practice.
- Talk with a close friend who works with you and has observed your clinical work. Ask if the friend's observations are the same as yours.
- Keep all of your written care plans or clinical papers. Use them frequently as a resource for future clients. Also maintain a logical filing system.
- Make time for reflection, both after having cared for a client and before caring for new clients with similar conditions. How is your current client similar to or different from previous clients?

Research Highlight   Box 14-2

Reflective Practice Improves Nursing Practice

Research Focus

Reflective practice, the use of reflection to help nurses expand and develop their clinical knowledge, is considered a useful method for developing nurses' practice. Techniques for developing reflective practice are being used in academic settings. The question is, does reflective practice influence a nurse's practice and client outcomes?

Research Abstract

This was an evaluative study to determine whether student nurses who had participated in a reflective practice course or course module perceived any change in their clinical practice. The study involved both undergraduate and graduate nurses. The research used a combination of focus groups (small groups of students sharing views together), questionnaires, and individual phone interviews. The majority of students found reflective practice useful, particularly when a group approach was used. In groups, students are able to discuss clinical events with individuals from similar backgrounds and experiences. The process of learning to reflect was perceived to improve students' self-awareness, their attitudes toward clients, and their insight into the clinical environment. Most students also felt that reflective practice changed their clinical practice in a way that benefited clients. Once learned, the skill of reflecting can be a medium for constant reviewing of professional practice. For a few students, reflective practice helped them learn to apply research findings to a specific area of clinical practice.

Evidence-Based Practice

The benefits of reflective practice should be considered for any student wishing to use reflection on a regular basis. Reflective practice was found to:
- Provide students with new insight
- Enhance communication skills
- Encourage use of research findings
- Increase a student's ability to reflect *in* actual practice
- Improve students' ability to deal with others more honestly and openly

Reference

Paget T: Reflective practice and clinical outcomes: practitioners' views on how reflective practice has influenced their clinical practice, *J Clin Nurs* 10(2):204, 2001.

It is an inner sensing that something is so. In other words, intuition occurs when an experienced nurse walks into a client's room, looks at the client's appearance without the benefit of a thorough assessment, and senses that the client is about to deteriorate physically. It is a common experience that many people have when interacting with their environments. Intuition in nursing develops as one's clinical experience increases. Intuition appears to act as a trigger, sparking an analytical process that leads nurses in a conscious search to acquire data that confirms their sense of change in a client's status (King and Clark, 2002). For example, when first entering the room to check on a client, an experienced surgical nurse may suspect that something is wrong. The nurse senses by looking at the client that something is out of place and the client is likely experiencing a surgical complication. The nurse will then act on intuition and begin an assessment of vital signs, the client's wound, the intravenous (IV) line status, and an analysis of how the client feels to gather information and verify whether the intuition was correct and a problem really exists.

It is important to remember that the quality of nursing practice depends on the nurse's ability to use all types of cognitive and emotional cues associated with a situation to trigger critical thinking and to then select effective nursing interventions. A nurse cannot safely act on intuition alone. Just as it is critical to know what knowledge we have, it is even more critical to know what we do not know. A nurse should trust his or her intuition as a red flag that something is not quite right, but should not take intuition as an automatic truth. As soon as intuition strikes, a nurse should probe further to assess a client's situation (Fowler, 1998). If nurses do not recognize what they do not know about their clients, there is a risk clients will receive improper care. Each clinical situation requires careful and thoughtful analysis for accurate and sound clinical decisions to be made.

Thinking and Learning

Learning is a lifelong process. Our intellectual and emotional growth involve acquiring new knowledge and refining the ability to think, problem solve, and make judgments. To learn, one must be flexible and always open to new information. The science of nursing is growing rapidly, and there will always be new information for nurses to apply in practice. Over time, as nurses have new experiences and apply the knowledge gained, they become better able to form assumptions, present ideas, and make valid conclusions.

A professional nurse must learn to think about a client's status and to anticipate nursing needs. This involves looking ahead and asking, What is a client's status? How might it change? and How can nursing knowledge be applied to improve the client's condition? A nurse cannot allow thinking to become routine or standardized. Instead, a nurse learns to look beyond the obvious in any clinical situation, explore the client's unique responses to health alterations, and recognize what actions are necessary to benefit the client's well-being. This does not mean that the nurse knows nothing about a

client is unable to cooperate with nursing therapies or if members of the nursing team do not follow through on the nurse's recommendations. Critical thinking requires a framing of one's thoughts so that the focus and resultant message are clear. It helps to reflect on one's language and to consider whether one communicates and expresses an idea, position, or judgment precisely and clearly.

Intuition

Intuition is the direct understanding of particulars in a situation without conscious deliberation (Benner, 1999).

client until having met him or her. A nurse's experience with other clients aids in recognizing patterns of behavior, seeing commonalities in signs and symptoms, and anticipating reactions to therapies. Thinking about those experiences enables the nurse to better anticipate client needs and recognize problems when they develop.

Nursing practice is always changing. As new knowledge becomes available, professional nurses must challenge traditional ways of doing things and discover those interventions that are most effective, have scientific relevance, and result in better client outcomes. For example, for many years nurses were taught to massage a client's reddened skin to improve circulation. Nursing research has shown that massaging a reddened pressure area causes capillary injury and promotes skin breakdown. Massage of reddened skin is no longer practiced, but the use of alternating air-flow mattresses is the new accepted therapy for pressure ulcer care. With knowledge a nurse is able to think critically and positively influence nursing practice.

*L*evels of Critical Thinking in Nursing

The ability to critically think expands as a nurse gains new knowledge and experience and matures into a competent professional. Kataoka-Yahiro and Saylor (1994) developed a critical thinking model that incorporates three levels of critical thinking in nursing: basic, complex, and commitment.

Basic Critical Thinking
At the basic level of critical thinking a learner trusts that experts have the right answers for every problem. Thinking is concrete and based on a set of rules or principles. For example, a nurse uses an institution's procedure manual to confirm how to insert a Foley catheter. The student nurse follows the procedure step-by-step without adjusting the procedure to meet a client's unique needs (e.g., positioning to accommodate the client's pain or mobility restrictions). For basic critical thinkers, answers to complex problems are either right or wrong (e.g., there is too much or insufficient air in the Foley catheter balloon), and one right answer usually exists for each problem. This is an early step in the development of reasoning ability (Kataoka-Yahiro and Saylor, 1994), revealing that the individual has had limited critical thinking experience. Despite the tendency to be governed by others, a person learns to accept the diverse opinions and values of experts (e.g., instructors and staff nurse role models). However, inexperience, weak competencies, and inflexible attitudes can restrict a person's ability to move to the next level of critical thinking.

Complex Critical Thinking
A person begins to detach from authorities and analyze and examine alternatives more independently at the complex level of critical thinking. Kataoka-Yahiro and Saylor (1994) note that the nurse's best answer to a problem at this level is "It depends." The person's thinking abilities and initiative to look beyond expert opinion begin to change. A nurse realizes that alternative, and perhaps conflicting, solutions do exist. Consider the case of Mr. Rosen, a 36-year-old man who underwent hip surgery. The client is having pain but refusing his ordered analgesic. His physician is concerned that the client will not progress as planned, delaying rehabilitation. While discussing the importance of rehabilitation with Mr. Rosen, the nurse realizes the client's conviction to avoid taking pain medication. The nurse learns that the client practices meditation at home and decides to discuss this with the client as a pain control option.

In complex critical thinking each solution has benefits and risks that the nurse weighs before making a final decision. There are options. Thinking can become more creative and innovative. There is a willingness to consider deviations from standard protocols or policies when complex situations develop. Nurses learn a variety of different approaches for the same therapy.

Commitment
The third level of critical thinking is commitment (Kataoka-Yahiro and Saylor, 1994). The individual anticipates the need to make choices without assistance from others and then assumes accountability for them. At this level the nurse does more than just consider the complex alternatives a problem poses. At the commitment level, the nurse chooses an action or belief based on the alternatives available and stands by it. Sometimes an action may be no action, or the nurse may choose to delay an action until a later time but does so as a result of experience and knowledge. Because the nurse assumes accountability for the decision, attention is given to the results of the decision and a determination of whether it was appropriate.

*C*ritical Thinking Competencies

Critical thinking competencies are the cognitive processes a nurse uses to make judgments. These include general critical thinking, specific critical thinking in clinical situations, and specific critical thinking in nursing (Kataoka-Yahiro and Saylor, 1994). General critical thinking processes include the scientific method, problem solving, and decision making. Specific critical thinking competencies in clinical situations include diagnostic reasoning, clinical inference, and clinical decision making.

General critical thinking competencies are not unique to nursing. They are used in other disciplines and in nonclinical, everyday situations. Physicians, nurses, and other health care professionals use critical thinking competencies in deciding about the clinical care and support of clients. The use of diagnostic reasoning and clinical decision making as parts of the nursing process makes the nursing process the specific critical thinking competency used in nursing practice.

Scientific Method
The scientific method is one approach to reasoning that is used in nursing, medicine, and a variety of other disci-

Table 14-2	Steps of the Scientific Method
Step	**Example in Practice**
Identify the problem to be investigated.	Family members have difficulty communicating with a dying loved one.
Collect data about the problem.	Review previous studies about grieving families. Review literature on methods for improving communication. Talk with dying clients about feelings they think are important to communicate.
Formulate a hypothesis or research question to explain or examine the problem.	Family members who receive instruction on ways to communicate with dying loved ones will be perceived as more supportive by the dying family member.
Test the hypothesis or questions.	Include family members in a group session on communication approaches. Have the family members use the new approaches when communicating with their dying loved ones.
Evaluate the results of the study to determine if the hypothesis was proved or disproved or to answer the research question.	Interview the clients to determine if they perceive family members to be more supportive.

plines. It is an approach to seeking the truth or verifying that a set of facts agrees with reality. Nurse researchers use the **scientific method** when testing research questions in nursing practice situations (Table 14-2). For example, a nurse researcher might observe that clients in a hospice program often have difficulty communicating their feelings to family members. The nurse learns more about what causes this problem and considers the possibility that family members might have ineffective communication skills. The nurse asks the question, "Can family members who receive instruction in communication principles provide support to loved ones with a terminal illness?" The nurse might design a study that involves formal instruction in communication skills and uses a support group to help family members practice and apply the skills. Once the instruction and application are complete, the nurse may ask clients to evaluate their feelings about communication with loved ones. The nurse hopes that results from the study will give other nurses working in hospice settings useful approaches for improving family communication. The scientific method is one formal way to approach a problem, plan a solution, test the solution, and come to a conclusion (see Chapter 5).

Problem Solving

We all face problems every day, such as a computer program that does not function properly or a kitchen cabinet that fails to close completely. When a problem arises, we obtain information and then use the information plus what we already know to find a solution. Clients routinely present problems in nursing practice. For example, consider the situation when a nurse visits a client at her home and learns that she has had difficulty taking her medications regularly. The nurse knows the client was discharged from the hospital and had five medications ordered. The nurse sits down with the client and finds that she has two over-the-counter medications she takes regularly as well. When the nurse asks the client to show the medications she takes in the morning, the nurse notices that the client has difficulty reading the medication labels. The client is able to describe the medications she is to take but is uncertain about the times of administration. The nurse recommends having the client's pharmacy relabel the medications in larger lettering. In addi-

tion, the nurse shows her some examples of pill organizers that can allow her to sort her medications by time of day for a period of 7 days.

Effective **problem solving** also involves evaluating the solution over time to be sure that it is still effective. It may become necessary to try different options if a problem recurs. From the example above, during a follow-up visit, the nurse finds that the client has organized her medications correctly and can read the labels without difficulty. The nurse obtained information that correctly clarified the cause of the client's problem and tested a solution that proved successful. Having solved a problem in one situation adds to a nurse's experience in practice and allows the nurse to apply that knowledge in future client situations.

Decision Making

When a person faces a problem or situation and must choose a course of action from several options, the person is engaged in decision making. **Decision making** is an end point of critical thinking that hopefully leads to problem resolution. For example, decision making occurs when a person decides on the choice of a physician. To make a decision, an individual must recognize and define the problem or situation (need for a certain type of physician to provide medical care), assess all options (consider recommended physicians or choose one whose office is close to home), weigh each option against a set of criteria (experience, friendliness, reputation), test possible options (talk directly with the physicians), consider the consequences of the decision (examine pros and cons of selecting one physician over another), and then make a final decision. Although the set of criteria follows a sequence of steps, decision making also involves moving back and forth among certain steps in order to consider all criteria. Using such a process leads to a conclusion that is informed and supported by evidence and reason (Bandman and Bandman, 1995). Examples of decision making in the clinical area include deciding on a choice of dressings for a client with a surgical wound or selecting the best approach for teaching a family how to assist a stroke client who is returning home. The nurse learns to make sound decisions by approaching each clinical situation thoughtfully and by applying each component of the decision-making process mentioned above.

Diagnostic Reasoning and Inference

As soon as a nurse receives information about a client in a particular clinical situation, **diagnostic reasoning** begins. It is a process of determining a client's health status after the nurse assigns meaning to the behaviors, physical signs, and symptoms presented by the client (O'Neill and Dluhy, 1997). Part of diagnostic reasoning is **inference,** that is, the process of drawing conclusions from related pieces of evidence (Smith Higuchi and Donald, 2002). An example of diagnostic reasoning is forming a nursing diagnosis (see Chapter 16). Diagnostic reasoning is a process of using the data gathered to logically explain a clinical judgment. For example, when a client presents symptoms of restlessness, guarded posturing, moaning, and abdominal discomfort, the nurse must retrieve knowledge regarding pain in the abdomen and then reason in a direct and precise way to determine the specific nature of the client's pain. The nurse collects as much information as possible to be sure a nursing diagnosis is accurate. Nurses do not make medical diagnoses, but they do assess and monitor clients closely and compare the clients' signs and symptoms with those that are common to a medical diagnosis. This type of diagnostic reasoning assists in making clinical inferences or judgments about a client's progress. When certain symptoms present themselves, the nurse considers all variables influencing the client, including what is known about the client's pathological condition, to infer if the client is doing better or worse.

Consider this clinical example. Mrs. Spellman had a myocardial infarction (heart attack) just 10 months ago. She must periodically be monitored for signs and symptoms of recurrent cardiac problems, such as chest pain, shortness of breath, and/or irregularity of vital signs. If Mrs. Spellman has a regular heart rate, denies discomfort, and is breathing without difficulty, the nurse may infer that the client's cardiac status is currently stable. The nurse must critically analyze changing clinical situations so that a client's status can immediately be determined. Careful analysis of the client's condition allows the nurse to initiate appropriate therapies, for example, activity restriction, so that the client's condition does not worsen. In addition, any diagnostic conclusions made by the nurse will help the physician pinpoint the nature of a problem more quickly and select proper medical therapies.

Clinical Decision Making

When a nurse approaches a clinical problem, such as a client who has developed a pressure ulcer or who is anxious about having surgery; the nurse collaborates with the client to make a decision that identifies the problem and then chooses those nursing interventions that will meet the mutually established goals of care. Nurses make clinical decisions all the time in an attempt to improve a client's health or to maintain ongoing wellness. This may mean minimizing the severity of the problem, or it might mean resolving the problem completely. The **clinical decision-making process** requires careful reasoning so that the options for the best client outcomes are chosen on the basis of the client's condition and the priority of the problem.

When making clinical decisions, the nurse first asks why a decision is necessary. For example, Mrs. Little is an 87-year-old client who lives alone. Her daughter, Marie, lives just a few minutes away and is Mrs. Little's primary caregiver. During a recent clinic visit the nurse, Ruth, observes a bruised area of the skin over Mrs. Little's right hip. Mrs. Little describes it as a scrape that she received when she slipped and fell on the edge of her bathtub. Knowing the client's age and the physiological changes that occur with aging, Ruth knows a decision is needed about whether Mrs. Little is living in a safe environment. In order for Ruth to make a decision about what actions are needed to promote healing and prevent further injury, she must collect facts and then select the information that is relevant to confirm the client's problems (Smith Higuchi and Donald, 2002). Before a decision can be made, Ruth must take into account Mrs. Little's actual physical condition (e.g., strengths and limitations), her home environment, and whether repeated injuries have been part of the client's history.

Strader (1992) has identified decision-making criteria to assist nurses in making appropriate choices:
- What needs to be achieved? (healing of the skin, a safe home environment)
- What needs to be preserved? (mobility, nutrition, comfort, and safety)
- What needs to be avoided? (further tissue injury or infection and further falls)

The answers to these questions help the nurse make clinical decisions and then set priorities as they relate to the client's situation (see Chapter 16). Because different clients bring different variables to a situation, an activity may be more of a priority in one situation and less of a priority in another. For example, if a client is physically dependent, unable to eat, and incontinent of urine, the nurse recognizes skin integrity as a greater priority than if the client were immobile but continent of urine and able to eat a normal diet. The nurse must not assume that certain health situations produce automatic priorities. For example, a client who has surgery is anticipated to experience a certain level of postoperative pain, which often becomes a priority of nursing care. However, if the client is experiencing severe anxiety that heightens pain perception, it may become necessary for the nurse to focus on ways to relieve the anxiety before pain relief measures can be effective.

After determining a client's nursing care priorities, a nurse selects therapies most likely to relieve each problem. A wide range of choices may be available from nurse-administered to client self-care strategies. The nurse collaborates with the client and then selects, tests, and evaluates the chosen approaches. The nurse tries to anticipate what might go wrong and considers alternative approaches to minimize or prevent problems. For example, Ruth will talk with Mrs. Little's daughter, Marie, about having someone check the condition of Mrs. Little's bathroom to see if there are any obstacles creating a risk for falls. A complete home safety assessment would be most helpful. Based on the findings, Ruth makes recommendations to Marie about ways to minimize hazards or obstacles so that further injury is less likely.

Nurses make decisions about individual clients and about groups of clients. A nurse who works on a busy hospital unit is likely to care for several clients. The nurse uses criteria such as the clinical condition of the client, Maslow's hierarchy of needs (see Chapter 6), risks involved in treatment delays, and clients' expectations of care to determine which clients have the greatest priorities for care. For example, a client who is having a sudden drop in blood pressure along with a change in consciousness requires the nurse's attention immediately as opposed to the client who needs to be assisted for a walk down the hallway. The nurse visits the client who has had no visitors and has recently been given a diagnosis of cancer before checking on the recovering surgical client whose family has just arrived. For nurses to be able to

---

Box 14-3   **Clinical Decision Making for Groups of Clients**

Identify the nursing and collaborative problems of each client.

Analyze clients' problems, and decide which problems are most urgent on the basis of basic needs, the clients' changing or unstable status, and problem complexity.

Consider the time it will take to care for clients whose problems are of high priority.

Consider the resources you have to manage each problem, other staff willing to assist, clients' family members.

Consider how to involve the clients as decision makers and participants in care.

Decide how to combine activities to resolve more than one client problem at a time.

Decide what if any nursing care procedures can be delegated to assistive personnel so that you can devote your time to activities requiring professional nursing knowledge.

---

manage the wide variety of problems associated with groups of clients, skillful, prioritized decision making is critical (Box 14-3).

Nursing Process as a Competency

Nurses apply the **nursing process** as a competency when delivering client care (Kataoka-Yahiro and Saylor, 1994). The nursing process consists of five steps: assessment, diagnosis, planning, implementation, and evaluation. The purpose of the nursing process is to diagnose and treat human responses to actual or potential health problems (American Nurses Association, 1980, 1995, 2003). Use of the process ultimately allows nurses to help clients meet agreed-upon outcomes for better health (Figure 14-1). The process provides a systematic approach for gathering client data, critically examining and analyzing the data, identifying the client's response to a health problem, determining priorities, establishing goals and expected outcomes of care, taking appropriate action, and then evaluating whether the action is effective. The process incorporates general and specific critical thinking competencies, described earlier, in a manner that focuses on a particular client's unique needs. The format for the nursing process is unique to the discipline of nursing and provides a common language and process for nurses to "think through" clients' clinical problems (Kataoka-Yahiro and Saylor, 1994). The nursing process is described in Unit III.

Creativity, or the use of innovation, is characteristic of the nursing process. The process is designed to be responsive to the continually changing needs of a client. For example, after a nurse has evaluated the results of nursing care and finds that the client has not improved, the nurse can reassess a client's condition to update data,

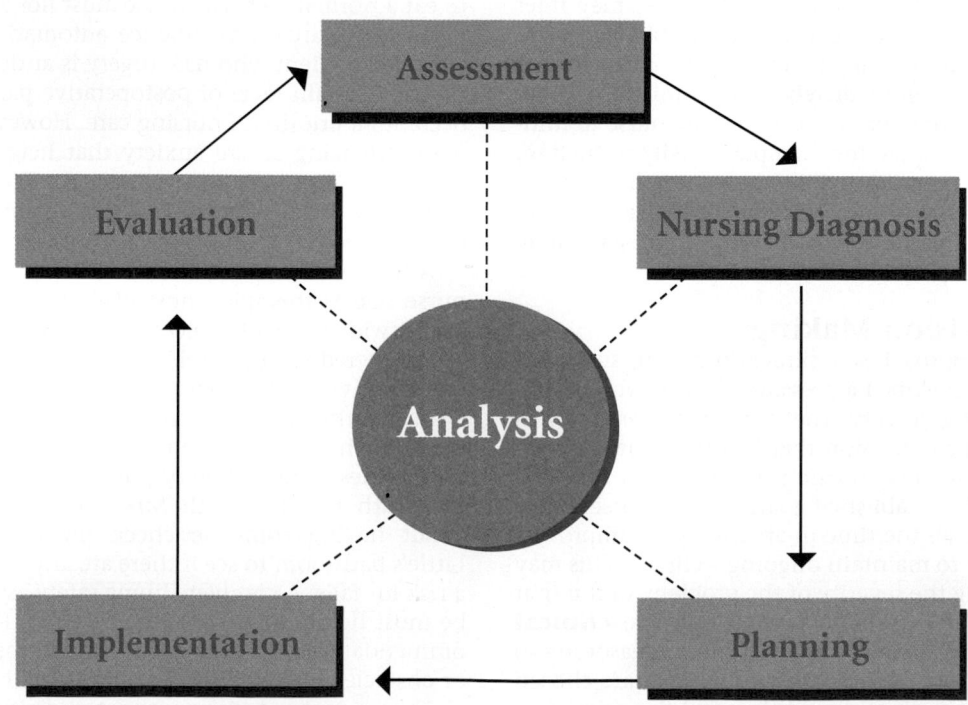

FIGURE **14–1**   Five-step nursing process model.

redefine problems, and select new interventions. The nursing process is not linear. In clinical practice, a nurse will move back and forth using steps of the nursing process that are most appropriate to a client's presenting situation.

The nursing process is a blueprint for care. It provides a creative, organized structure and framework for the delivery of nursing care, yet it is flexible enough to be used in all settings. At any time in the care of a client, a nurse may move back and forth from one step of the process to another should new data emerge. The nurse must always be thinking and recognizing what step of the process is being used. Chapters 15 to 19 of this unit describe each step of the nursing process.

Critical Thinking Model

Models help to explain concepts. Because critical thinking in nursing is complex, a model can help to explain all of the factors involved in making decisions and judgments about clients. Kataoka-Yahiro and Saylor (1994) have developed a model of critical thinking for nursing judgment based in part on previous work by Paul (1993), Glaser (1941), Perry (1979) and Miller and Malcolm (1990) (Figure 14-2). The model defines the outcome of critical thinking: nursing judgment that is relevant to nursing problems in a variety of settings. According to this model, there are five components of critical thinking: knowledge base, experience, competence, attitudes, standards, and the critical thinking competency of the nursing process. The elements of the model combine to explain how nurses make clinical judgments that are necessary for safe, effective, nursing care (Box 14-4).

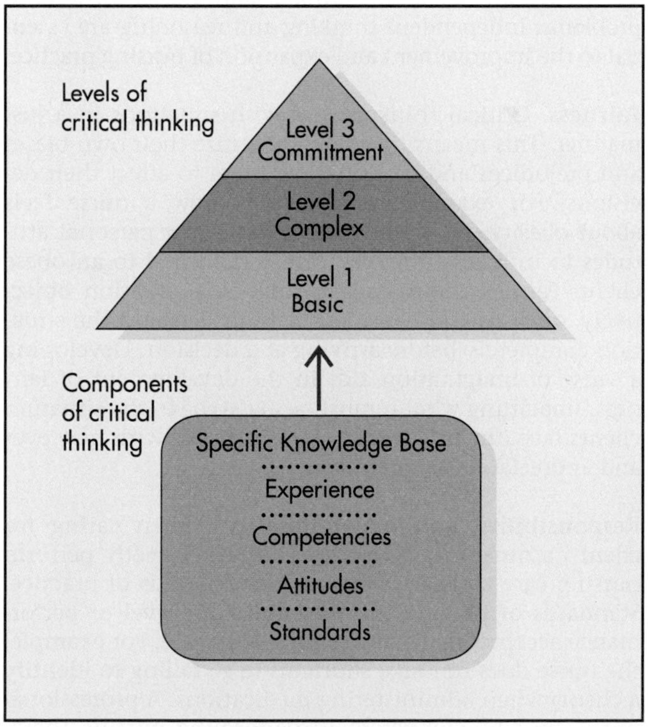

Specific Knowledge Base

The first component of critical thinking is a nurse's specific knowledge base. This varies according to a nurse's educational experience, including basic nursing education, continuing education courses, and additional college degrees. In addition, it includes the initiative a nurse shows in reading the nursing literature so as to remain current in nursing science. A nurse's knowledge base includes information and theory from the basic sciences, humanities, behavioral sciences, and nursing. Nurses use their knowledge base in a different way from other health care disciplines in regard to how they think about client problems. For example, a nurse's broad knowledge base gives the nurse a more holistic view of clients and their health care needs. The depth and extent of knowledge influence the nurse's ability to think critically about nursing problems.

FIGURE **14–2**   Critical thinking model for nursing judgment. (Redrawn from Kataoka-Yahiro M, Saylor C: A critical thinking model for nursing judgment, *J Nurs Educ* 33(8):351, 1994. Modified from Glaser, 1941; Miller and Malcolm, 1990; Paul, 1993; and Perry, 1979.)

Box **14-4**   **Components of Critical Thinking in Nursing**

I.   Specific knowledge base in nursing
II. Experience in nursing
III. Critical thinking competencies
   A.   General critical thinking competencies
   B.   Specific critical thinking competencies in clinical situations
   C.   Specific critical thinking competency in nursing
IV. Attitudes for critical thinking
   A.   Confidence   G.   Perseverance
   B.   Independence   H.   Creativity
   C.   Fairness   I.   Curiosity
   D.   Responsibility   J.   Integrity
   E.   Risk taking   K.   Humility
   F.   Discipline
V.   Standards for critical thinking
   A.   Intellectual standards
      1.   Clear   8.   Logical
      2.   Precise   9.   Deep
      3.   Specific   10. Broad
      4.   Accurate   11. Complete
      5.   Relevant   12. Significant
      6.   Plausible   13. Adequate (for purpose)
      7.   Consistent   14. Fair
   B.   Professional standards
      1.   Ethical criteria for nursing judgment
      2.   Criteria for evaluation
      3.   Professional responsibility

Modified from Kataoka-Yahiro M, Saylor C: A critical thinking model for nursing judgment, *J Nurs Educ* 33(8):351, 1994. Data from Paul RW: The art of redesigning instruction. In Willsen J, Blinker AJA, editors: *Critical thinking: how to prepare students for a rapidly changing world*, Santa Rosa, Calif, 1993, Foundation for Critical Thinking.

Consider this scenario: Robert Perez previously earned a bachelor's degree in education and taught high school for 1 year. He is starting his third year of study in his nursing program. He has successfully completed his required courses in the sciences, health ethics, introduction to nursing concepts, and communication principles. His first clinical course is on health promotion with a clinical assignment on a general medicine clinic. Although still a novice to nursing, his experiences as a teacher and his preparation and knowledge base in nursing will help him know how to interview clients and begin to make clinical decisions about clients' health promotion practices.

Experience

The second component of the critical thinking model is experience in nursing. Unless a nurse has the opportunity to practice and make decisions about client care, critical thinking in clinical decision making will not develop. In clinical situations, the nurse learns from observing, sensing, talking with clients and families, and then reflecting actively on all experiences. Clinical experience is the laboratory for testing nursing knowledge. The nurse will learn that "textbook" approaches lay important groundwork for practice, but safe adaptations or revisions in approaches must often be made to accommodate the setting, the unique qualities of the client, and the experience the nurse has gained from using the approaches for previous clients. With experience, the nurse begins to understand clinical situations, recognize cues of clients' health patterns, and interpret cues as relevant or irrelevant. Perhaps the best lesson to be learned by a new nursing student is to value all client experiences, which become stepping-stones for building new knowledge and stimulating innovative thinking.

During the previous summer, Robert worked as a nurse assistant in a nursing home. This experience provided him with valuable time spent in interacting with older adult clients and in giving basic nursing care. As Robert thinks about his clinical experience at the clinic, he recognizes he still has a lot to learn. However, each client has provided him valuable learning experiences. Specifically, he has been able to develop good interviewing skills and understand the importance of the family in an individual's health, and he has learned the role nurses play as advocates for clients. His time in the physical assessment laboratory and the time he worked in the nursing home have helped him begin to be a watchful observer. Robert also knows that his previous experience as a teacher will help him apply educational principles in his nursing role.

Attitudes for Critical Thinking

The fourth component of the critical thinking model is attitudes. Paul (1993) has identified 11 attitudes that are central features of a critical thinker (see Box 14-4, p. 269). These attitudes define how a person approaches a problem in order to be a successful critical thinker. For example, when a client complains of anxiety before undergoing a diagnostic procedure, the nurse will be curious and explore possible reasons for the client's concerns. The nurse will also show discipline in gathering a thorough assessment. Attitudes of inquiry involve an ability to recognize that problems exist and to accept the general need for evidence in support of what is asserted to be true (Watson and Glaser, 1980). Critical thinking attitudes offer guidelines for how to approach a problem or decision-making situation. An important part of critical thinking is interpreting, evaluating, and making judgments about the adequacy of various arguments and available data. Knowing when more information is needed, knowing when information is misleading, and recognizing one's own knowledge limits are examples of how critical thinking attitudes play a key role in decision making. Table 14-3 summarizes how critical thinking attitudes apply to nursing practice.

Confidence. To be confident is to feel certain in one's ability to accomplish a task or goal. Confidence grows with experience and the maturity to recognize one's strengths and limitations. Confidence is not arrogance or the feeling of superiority. Instead, confident critical thinkers remain aware of the balance between what they know and what they do not know. When a nurse shows confidence, clients recognize it in the manner in which the nurse communicates and performs nursing care. Confidence builds trust between the nurse and client and is often instrumental in achieving client outcomes.

Thinking Independently. As persons mature and gain new knowledge, they learn to consider a wide range of ideas and concepts before forming an opinion or making a judgment. This does not mean they ignore other people's ideas. All sides of a given situation should be considered. However, a critical thinker does not customarily accept another person's ideas without question. To think independently, one questions others' ways of interpreting knowledge and looks for rational and logical answers to problems. Independent thinking and reasoning are essential to the improvement and expansion of nursing practice.

Fairness. Critical thinkers deal with situations in a just manner. This means that they recognize their own biases and prejudices and do not allow them to affect their decisions. For example, regardless of how a nurse feels about obesity, he or she should not allow personal attitudes to influence the way care is delivered to an obese client. Fairness helps one to look at a situation objectively, analyzing all viewpoints, to understand the situation completely before arriving at a decision. Developing a sense of imagination aids in the development of fairness. Imagining what it must be like to be in the situation clients face can help a nurse see situations with new eyes and appreciate their complexity.

Responsibility and Accountability. When caring for clients, a nurse has a responsibility to correctly perform nursing care activities based upon standards of practice. Standards of practice are the minimum level of performance accepted to ensure high-quality care. For example, the nurse does not take shortcuts (e.g., failing to identify a client) when administering medications. A professional nurse must be competent in performing nursing therapies and in making clinical decisions about clients. The nurse who intervenes for a client must be answerable or accountable for the outcomes of any nursing actions. An accountable nurse is reliable and willing to recognize when nursing care is ineffective. Ultimately, the nurse as-

Table 14-3	Critical Thinking Attitudes and Applications in Nursing Practice
Critical Thinking Attitude	**Application in Practice**
Confidence	Learn how to introduce yourself to a client. Speak with conviction when you begin a treatment or procedure. Do not lead a client to think that you are uncertain of being able to perform care safely. Always be prepared before performing a nursing activity.
Thinking independently	Read the nursing literature, especially when there are different views on the same subject. Talk with colleagues and share ideas about nursing interventions.
Fairness	Listen to both sides in any discussion. If a client or family member complains about a colleague, listen to the story and then speak with the colleague as well. Weigh all facts.
Responsibility and authority	Ask for help if you are uncertain about an aspect of client care. Report any problems immediately. Follow standards of practice in your care.
Risk taking	If your knowledge causes you to question a physician's order, do so. Be willing to recommend alternative approaches to nursing care when colleagues are having little success with clients.
Discipline	Be thorough in whatever you do. Use known scientific and practice-based criteria for activities such as assessment and evaluation. Take time to be thorough, and manage your time effectively.
Perseverance	Be wary of an easy answer. If colleagues give you information about a client, and some fact seems to be missing, go clarify information or talk to the client directly. If problems of the same type continue to occur on a nursing division, bring colleagues together, look for a pattern, and find a solution.
Creativity	Look for different approaches if interventions are not working. A client may need a different positioning technique or a different instructional approach that will suit his or her unique needs.
Curiosity	Always ask why. A clinical sign or symptom can indicate a variety of problems. Explore and learn more about the client so as to make appropriate clinical judgments.
Integrity	Recognize when your opinions may conflict with those of a client; review your position, and decide how best to proceed to reach mutually beneficial outcomes. Do not compromise nursing standards or honesty in delivering nursing care.
Humility	Recognize when you need more information to make a decision. When you are newly assigned to a clinical division and you are unfamiliar with the clients, ask to be oriented to the area. Ask RNs regularly assigned to the area for assistance. Read the professional journals regularly to keep updated on new approaches to care.

sumes accountability for whatever decisions and resultant actions are made on the client's behalf.

Risk Taking. When a person takes a risk in acting or decision making, it often is perceived that a potential loss may be at stake. Driving 30 miles an hour over the speed limit is a risk that might result in injury to the driver and an unlucky pedestrian. But risk taking does not have to cause injury. Without intellectual risk taking, knowledge cannot advance. A critical thinker is willing to take risks in trying different approaches to solving problems. Willing to be wrong, willing to take a stance on an issue, willing to form close therapeutic relationships with clients in order to learn their concerns are ways critical thinkers discover client care innovations. The willingness to take risks often comes from experience with similar problems. Nurses in the past have taken risks in trying different approaches to skin and wound care, pulmonary hygiene, and pain management, to name a few. When taking a risk, the nurse considers all options, analyzes any potential danger to a client, and then acts in a well-reasoned, logical, and thoughtful manner.

Discipline. A disciplined thinker misses few details and follows an orderly approach when making decisions or taking action. Disciplined thinking ensures that decisions are made systematically and in a comprehensive manner. For example, assessment of a client's pain includes more than just the location. The nurse also assesses the severity of pain, its duration, factors that aggravate or relieve the pain, and the manner in which pain affects the client's lifestyle (see Chapter 42). An in-depth, disciplined assessment of the client's pain ensures correct identification of the nature of pain and the selection of the most appropriate nursing interventions.

Perseverance. A critical thinker will take on a problem with determination and diligence in spite of any opposition. Perseverance helps critical thinkers find effective solutions to client care problems. This is especially important when problems remain unresolved or when they reoccur. The nurse learns as much as possible about a problem, tries various approaches to care, and continues to seek additional resources until a successful approach is found. For example, a client who is unable to speak following throat surgery often poses challenges for the nurse to be able to communicate effectively. Perseverance leads the nurse to try different communication approaches (e.g., message boards or alarm bells) until a method that the client can easily use is found. A critical thinker who perseveres is not satisfied with minimal effort, but works to achieve the highest level of quality care.

Creativity. Creativity involves the use of imaginative and innovative skills in problem solving. This means finding new or innovative solutions to client problems while upholding standards of practice. Creativity is a great motivator that enables one to generate options and alternative approaches and to see the future (Miller and Babcock, 1996). Often clients pose problems that require unique approaches. A client's clinical problems, social support systems, and living environment are just a few examples of factors that can make the simplest nursing procedure more complicated if the nurse does not consider a creative approach for the client's situation. For example, a home health nurse must find a way to help an older client with arthritis gain greater mobility in the home. The client has difficulty lowering and raising herself in a chair because of pain and limited range of motion in her knees. The nurse uses wooden blocks to elevate the chair legs so that the client can easily sit and stand with minimal discomfort.

Curiosity. A critical thinker always has the desire to know or to seek knowledge. Curiosity is what drives a critical thinker to ask the question, Why? In any clinical situation, a nurse learns a great deal of information about a client. As the nurse analyzes client information, data patterns emerge that are not always clear. Having a sense of curiosity motivates the nurse to inquire further and to investigate a clinical situation so that all the information needed to make a decision is obtained.

Integrity. A person of integrity acts on the basis of a sound moral and ethical position. Personal integrity builds trust from peers and subordinates. Nurses face many dilemmas in day-to-day clinical practice, and few nurses do not make mistakes. A nurse of integrity is honest and willing to admit to any mistakes or inconsistencies in his or her own behavior, ideas, and beliefs. In addition, the professional nurse strives to adhere to high standards of practice even in the face of adversity. Critical thinkers question and test personal knowledge and beliefs as rigorously as they test the knowledge and beliefs of others.

Humility. It is important to be humble and admit to one's own limitations in knowledge and skills. Critical thinkers admit what they do not know and try to acquire the knowledge needed to make proper decisions. A client's safety and welfare may be at risk if the nurse is unable to admit to his or her inability to deal with a practice problem. The nurse must rethink a situation, acquire additional knowledge, and then use the new information to form opinions, draw conclusions, and take action.

Standards for Critical Thinking

The fifth component of the critical thinking model includes intellectual and professional standards (Kataoka-Yahiro and Saylor, 1994).

Intellectual Standards. Paul (1993) identified 14 intellectual standards (see Box 14-4, p. 269) universal for critical thinking. These standards are commonly applied when a nurse conducts the nursing process. When a nurse considers a client problem, it is important to apply intellectual standards such as preciseness, accuracy, and consistency to ensure that all data is available for making sound clinical decisions.

> *For example, Mrs. Lamar is an 82-year-old client who is transferred from intensive care to a general medicine nursing unit. During his assessment of Mrs. Lamar, the nurse, Robert, finds an ulcer on the client's left foot. A quick check of the client's medical record reveals a description of the ulcer by one of the intensive care unit (ICU) nurses from 2 days earlier. The client is receiving a topical medication for the ulcer. To be consistent in his assessment, Robert uses the same assessment criteria applied during the last examination. He methodically inspects the affected area of the skin, asks if the client is experiencing discomfort, measures the size of the ulcer, and notes the appearance of any drainage. The wound location and appearance are described in Mrs. Lamar's medical record using specific anatomical terms. Robert examines Mrs. Lamar further to ensure that his findings are accurate and to determine if any other ulcers are present. He adds an assessment of the client's ability to ambulate, knowing that the ulcer could impair function. By applying appropriate intellectual standards, Robert is able to determine that the ulcer is healing and has improved since the last assessment.*

A rigorous use of intellectual standards in clinical practice ensures that critical thinking is not done haphazardly.

Professional Standards. Professional standards for critical thinking refer to ethical criteria for nursing judgments, scientific and practice-based criteria used for evaluation, and criteria for professional responsibility (Paul, 1993). Application of professional standards requires that nurses use critical thinking for the good of individuals or groups (Kataoka-Yahiro and Saylor, 1994). Professional standards ensure that the highest level of quality nursing care is promoted.

Excellent nursing practice is a reflection of sound ethical standards. Client care requires more than just the application of scientific knowledge. Being able to focus on a client's values and beliefs helps a nurse to make clinical decisions that are just, faithful to the client's choices, and beneficial to the client's well-being. Critical thinkers maintain a sense of self-awareness through conscious awareness of their beliefs, values, feelings, and the multiple perspectives that clients, family members, staff, and peers present in clinical situations (Ludwick and Sedlak, 1998). Chapter 21 summarizes ethical standards used when clients face ethical dilemmas.

Critical thinking also requires the use of scientifically based and practiced-based criteria for making clinical judgments. These criteria may be scientifically based on research findings (see Chapter 5) or practice based on standards developed by clinical experts and quality improvement initiatives. An example is the clinical practice guidelines developed by individual clinical agencies and national organizations such as the Agency for Healthcare Research and Quality (AHRQ). A clinical practice guideline includes standards for the treatment of select clinical conditions. Another example is clinical criteria used to categorize clinical conditions, such as the criteria used to stage pressure ulcers (see Chapter 47). Scientific and practice-based evaluation criteria set the minimum requirements necessary to ensure appropriate and high-quality care.

Nurses routinely use scientific and practice-based criteria to assess clients' conditions and to determine the efficacy of nursing interventions. For example, accurate assessment of symptoms such as pain or shortness of breath includes use of assessment criteria such as the duration, severity, location, aggravating or relieving factors, and effects on daily lifestyle (see Chapter 32). In this case, assessment criteria allow a nurse to accurately determine the nature of a client's symptom, select appropriate therapies, and then evaluate if the therapies are effective. Another example is the determination of the stage of a pressure ulcer based on scientific criteria, including skin temperature, tissue consistency, and depth of wound (see Chapter 47). The criteria allow a nurse to select the stage of a pressure ulcer and to track the rate of healing.

The standards of professional responsibility that a nurse strives to achieve are those standards cited in nurse practice acts, institutional practice guidelines, and professional organizations' standards of practice. The American Nurses Association Standards of Care (see Chapter 1) is an example. These standards "raise the bar" for the responsibilities and accountabilities that a nurse must assume in guaranteeing quality health care to the public.

The Nursing Process Competency

The nurse applies each step of the nursing process by using critical thinking. Throughout the clinical chapters of this text, the relationship of critical thinking to the nursing process will be emphasized.

Critical Thinking Synthesis

Critical thinking is a reasoning process by which individuals reflect on and analyze their own thoughts, actions, and knowledge. To be a good critical thinker requires dedication and a desire to grow intellectually. A nurse learns that for each client cared for, there is a large source of scientific knowledge and practice-based information to consider. The depth of nursing knowledge coupled with knowledge of each client's unique clinical situation makes it challenging to provide the most appropriate plan of care for a client. As a beginning nurse, it is important to learn the steps of the nursing process and to incorporate the elements of critical thinking. For example, while assessing a client's pain, a nurse must consider all symptoms, analyze his or her interpretation of the source of pain, consider knowledge about the potential source, analyze the relevance of the pain to the client's clinical situation, choose interventions, and evaluate the consequences of treatment choices. Critical thinking is ongoing with information being analyzed from many sources.

If one places the nursing process within the context of the critical thinking model, one is able to see two processes occurring together (Figure 14-3). As the nurse engages in the nursing process for the care of a client, he or she is also synthesizing critical thinking knowledge, experience, standards, and attitudes. The nurse who is assessing a client's pain does not focus only on what the client reports about the pain and what the nurse is able to observe and measure. The nurse also reflects on prior experience with clients who have had similar pain so as to compare and the contrast this new client's response. The nurse refers to information in scientific texts about how the pain might be

relieved. The nurse also displays intellectual standards in being sure the pain assessment is accurate and objective. Finally, the nurse exercises the attitudes necessary for the client to be cared for fairly and responsibly.

The nursing process and critical thinking are synthesized, meaning the two come together in a manner that allows a student to become a competent professional. This text provides a model that reinforces the importance of critical thinking in practice. Throughout the clinical chapters of this text, the components of critical thinking are summarized to help readers better understand its relationship to the nursing process.

Key Concepts

- To assist persons in maintaining, regaining, or improving their health, a nurse must be able to think critically, problem solve, and find the best solution for a client's problems.
- The nurse who is a good critical thinker faces problems without forming a quick, single solution and instead is focused on the value of all available options.
- As a nurse it is helpful to reflect or think back on a client situation, to make sense of the experience, and to thus gain insight as to the meaning of the situation.
- Reflection is a form of self-evaluation that helps the nurse judge personal performance.
- To become a critical thinker, the nurse must be able to use language precisely and clearly.
- Intuition acts as a trigger, sparking an analytical process that leads nurses in a conscious search to acquire data that confirms their sense of change in a client's status.
- The three levels of critical thinking in nursing are basic, complex, and commitment.
- To make a decision, an individual must recognize and define the problem or situation, assess all options, weigh each option against a set of criteria, test possible options, consider the consequences of the decision, and then make a final decision
- Diagnostic reasoning involves the nurse in assigning meaning to the behaviors, physical signs, and reported client symptoms that arise in a clinical situation.
- A nurses makes clinical decisions by identifying client problems and then choosing the best nursing interventions that will reach mutually established goals.
- The model of critical thinking for nursing judgment consists of five elements: knowledge, experience, critical thinking competencies (e.g., nursing process), attitudes, and standards.
- With experience a nurse learns to understand clinical situations, recognize cues of clients' health patterns, and interpret cues as relevant or irrelevant.
- Critical thinking attitudes help a nurse to know when more information is needed, when information is misleading, and to recognize the nurse's own knowledge limits.
- The use of intellectual standards during assessment ensures a complete database of information.

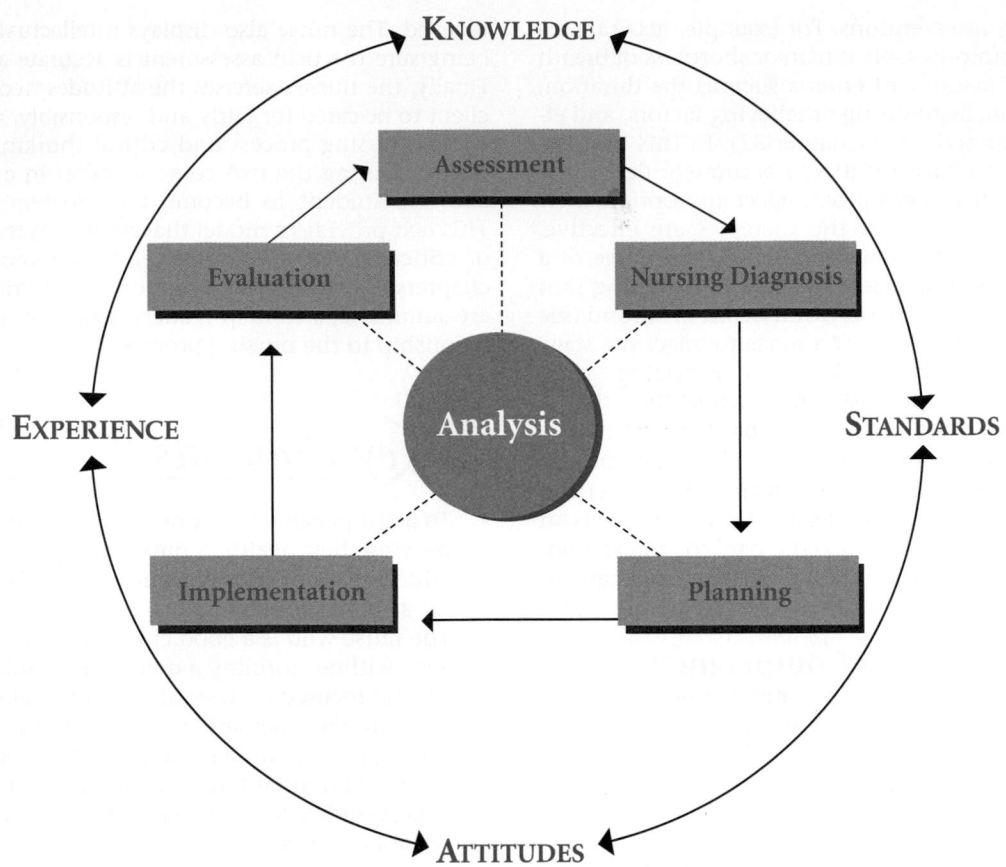

FIGURE **14–3**   Synthesis of critical thinking with the nursing process competency.

- Professional standards for critical thinking refer to ethical criteria for nursing judgments, scientific and practice criteria to be used for evaluation, and criteria for professional responsibility.
- As the nurse engages in the nursing process for the care of a specific client, the nurse is also synthesizing critical thinking knowledge, experience, standards, and attitudes.

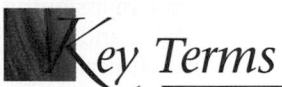**ey Terms**

Critical decision making process, *p. 267*
Critical thinking, *p. 262*
Decision making, *p. 266*
Diagnostic reasoning, *p. 267*
Inference, *p. 267*

Intuition, *p. 264*
Nursing process, *p. 268*
Problem solving, *p. 266*
Reflection, *p. 263*
Scientific method, *p. 266*

Critical Thinking Exercises

1. Select a day and write a journal entry describing any one of the following experiences *that stimulated your thinking:* an interaction you had with a client, an interaction you had with your spouse or one of your children, or an interaction you had with someone you

were trying to help. For the entry, discuss each of the following:
a. Describe, as thoroughly as you can, what you thought and what you did.
b. Describe your decision-making process.
c. Describe what you would do differently when a similar incident occurs.
d. Describe your strengths and weaknesses in dealing with the situation. Identify your thoughts, perceptions, and feelings.
2. The following nurse's note was entered for Mrs. Simmons, a client who visited the general medicine clinic.

Mrs. Simmons visited the general medicine clinic presenting with a 7-day bout of blurred vision and dizziness. Client reports vision is blurred or distorted, preventing her from performing routine activities such as preparing meals, writing checks, and some mornings performing her own hygiene and grooming. She has the most difficulty seeing close objects, although her distant vision is also blurred. Blurring is present with and without use of glasses. On examination pupils are equal and reactive to light and accommodation. Visual fields are normal. She was unable to read newsprint in the newspaper or read the instructions on the nutrition information chart on the wall. She is active in her local church activities, but this has declined recently. Mrs. Simmons denies having a headache but has also noticed some dizziness. She is currently taking estrogen, a calcium supplement, and Inderal.

Evaluate the nurse's note with regard to the use of intellectual standards. What is complete and significant in the note versus superficial or trivial? What is relevant versus irrelevant? What is clear versus unclear?

3. Consider the following statements, and describe which is an example of an inference, problem solving, or clinical decision making. Support your answer with a rationale.

   a. As the nurse enters a client's room, she observes the intravenous line is not infusing at the ordered rate. The nurse checks the flow regulator on the tubing, looks to see if the client is laying on the tubing, checks the point of connection between the tubing and the IV catheter, and then checks the condition of the site where the intravenous catheter enters the client's skin.

   b. The client is turning frequently in bed, holds his abdomen with his left hand, and tells the nurse, "My stomach is killing me." The nurse examines the client's abdomen, inspects the incision made during surgery 24 hours ago, and asks the client to rate the discomfort on a scale of 0 to 10. The client rates the pain a 9, compared to a 4 just 3 hours ago. The nurse concludes the pain is related to incisional trauma and administers a prescribed analgesic. The nurse checks the client 30 minutes later and finds that the client is more relaxed and the pain is at a 5.

   c. The nurse reviews a client's medical record and finds that the client has ingested only 600 ml of fluids over the last 24 hours. The client also has a low urinary output. The nurse conducts an assessment and finds the client to have poor skin turgor and difficulty concentrating when asked questions about his medical history. The nurse exits the client's room and tells the physician that the client is likely becoming dehydrated.

4. Mr. Spicer is a terminally ill client. His wife and son are asking you about the type of pain control he is receiving. Mrs. Spicer is asking that the physician increase her husband's medication, even if it means he will not be responsive. She does not want her husband to suffer. The son is vehemently opposed to too much narcotic, feeling that his father is still able to make decisions for himself. Mr. Spicer remains alert much of the time and is able to talk with you about his feelings regarding death. He seems to appreciate your availability in talking with him. How might you apply the critical thinking attitudes of fairness, responsibility, and creativity in this case study?

Review Questions

1. This process involves use of the mind in forming conclusions, making decisions, drawing inferences, and reflecting:
   1. Assessment.
   2. Critical thinking.
   3. Thinking independently.
   4. Intellectual humility.

2. The nurse identifies ways he can improve his own performance. He reflects on his nursing experiences. This is an example of the core critical thinking skill:
   1. Inference.
   2. Explanation.
   3. Analysis.
   4. Self-regulation.

3. During the day the nurse spends time instructing a client in how to self-administer insulin. After discussing the techniques and demonstrating an injection, the nurse has the client try it. After two attempts the client obviously does not understand how to prepare the correct dose. When the nurse returns to the medication room, he discusses the situation with the charge nurse, reviewing his approach with the client and asking for her suggestions on his technique. This is an example of:
   1. Reflection.
   2. Risk taking.
   3. Client assessment.
   4. Care plan evaluation.

4. An experienced surgical nurse enters a surgical client's room and suspects that the client is experiencing a surgical complication. The nurse begins an assessment of vital signs, the client's wound, and the intravenous (IV) line status and an analysis of how the client feels to gather information and verify whether the _____ was correct and a problem really exists.
   1. Knowledge.
   2. Intuition.
   3. Reflection.
   4. Risk taking.

5. A nurse uses an institution's procedure manual to confirm how to insert a Foley catheter. The level of critical thinking the nurse is using is:
   1. Commitment.
   2. Complex critical thinking.
   3. Scientific method.
   4. Basic critical thinking.

6. A client has a nursing diagnosis of anxiety and deficient knowledge concerning his impending surgery. The nurse decides that the client's anxiety must be addressed first in order for the client to be receptive to any formal instruction about surgery. This decision is considered a part of:
   1. Assessment.
   2. Planning.
   3. Intervention.
   4. Evaluation.

7. A client had hip surgery 24 hours ago. When the nurse begins the nursing shift, the nurse refers to the written plan of care, noting that the client has a drainage device collecting wound drainage. The physician's order requires that the physician be notified when drainage in the device exceeds 100 ml for the day. When the nurse enters the room, the nurse looks at the device

and carefully notes the amount of drainage currently in the device. This is an example of:
1. Assessment.
2. Planning.
3. Intervention
4. Evaluation.

8. The nurse asks a client how she feels about her impending surgery for breast cancer. Before the discussion the nurse reviewed the description in his textbook of loss and grief in addition to therapeutic communication principles. The critical thinking component involved in the nurse's review of the literature is:
   1. Experience.
   2. Problem solving.
   3. Knowledge application.
   4. Clinical decision making.

9. A 72-year-old woman has been a client on the medical unit for about 4 days. When she was first admitted, she was alert and oriented. For the last 24 hours she become acutely confused and repeatedly attempted to get out of bed. The nursing staff has discussed the possibility of using restraints; however, one nurse insists that use of orientation and meaningful diversion should be tried. This is an example of the critical thinking attitude:
   1. Integrity.
   2. Risk taking.
   3. Thinking independently.
   4. Responsibility and authority.

10. The nurse does not take shortcuts (e.g., failing to identify a client) when administering medications. This is an example of the critical thinking attitude:
    1. Responsibility and accountability.
    2. Thinking independently.
    3. Fairness.
    4. Discipline.

*R*eferences

American Nurses Association: *Nursing's social policy statement*, Kansas City, Mo, 1980, The Association.

American Nurses Association: *Nursing's social policy statement*, Washington, DC, 1995, The Association.

American Nurses Association: *Nursing's social policy statement*, Washington, DC, 2003, The Association.

Baker CR: Reflective learning: a teaching strategy for critical thinking, *J Nurs Educ* 35(1):19, 1996.

Bandman EL, Bandman B: *Critical thinking in nursing*, ed 2, Norwalk, Conn, 1995, Appleton & Lange.

Benner P and others: *Clinical wisdom and interventions in critical care*, Philadelphia, 1999, WB Saunders.

Bittner NP, Tobin E: Critical thinking: strategies for clinical practice, *J Nurs Staff Dev* 14(6):267, 1998.

Chaffee J: *Thinking critically*, ed 3, Boston, 1994, Houghton Mifflin.

Facione N, Facione P: Externalizing the critical thinking in knowledge development and clinical judgment, *Nurs Outlook* 44:129, 1996.

Fowler LP: Improving critical thinking in nursing practice, *J Nurs Staff Dev* 14(4):183, 1998.

Glaser E: *An experiment in the development of critical thinking*, New York, 1941, Bureau of Publications, Teachers College, Columbia University.

Gordon M: *Nursing diagnosis: process and application*, ed 3, St. Louis, 1995, Mosby.

Kataoka-Yahiro M, Saylor C: A critical thinking model for nursing judgment, *J Nurs Educ* 33(8):351, 1994.

Ludwick R, Sedlak CA: Ethical issues and critical thinking: students' stories, *Nursingconnections* 11(3):12, 1998.

Miller M, Malcolm N: Critical thinking in the nursing curriculum, *Nurs Health Care* 11:67, 1990.

Miller MA, Babcock DE: *Critical thinking applied to nursing*, St. Louis, 1996, Mosby.

O'Neill ES, Dluhy NM: A longitudinal framework for fostering critical thinking and diagnostic reasoning, *J Adv Nurs* 26:825, 1997.

Paul RW: The art of redesigning instruction. In Willsen J, Blinker AJA, editors: *Critical thinking: how to prepare students for a rapidly changing world*, Santa Rosa, Calif, 1993, Foundation for Critical Thinking.

Paul RW, Heaslip P: Critical thinking and intuitive nursing practice, *J Adv Nurs* 22:40, 1995.

Perry W: *Forms of intellectual and ethical development in the college years: a scheme*, New York, 1979, Holt, Rinehart, & Winston.

Smith B, Johnston Y: Using structured clinical preparation to stimulate reflection and foster critical thinking, *J Nurs Ed* 41(4):182, 2002.

Strader M: Critical thinking. In Sullivan EJ, Decker PJ, editors: *Effective management in nursing*, ed 3, Redwood City, Calif, 1992, Addison Wesley Nursing.

Watson G, Glaser E: *Watson-Glaser critical thinking appraisal manual*, New York, 1980, MacMillan.

Whiteside C: A model for teaching critical thinking in the clinical setting, *Dimens Crit Care Nurs* 16(3):152, 1997.

*R*esearch References

Facione P: *Critical thinking: a statement of expert consensus for purposes of educational assessment and instruction. The Delphi report: research findings and recommendations prepared for the American Philosophical Association*, ERIC Doc No. ED 315-423, Washington, DC, 1990, ERIC.

King L, Clark JM: Intuition and the development of expertise in surgical ward and intensive care nurses, *J Adv Nurs* 37(4):322, 2002.

Paget T: Reflective practice and clinical outcomes: practitioners' views on how reflective practice has influenced their clinical practice, *J Clin Nurs* 10(2):204, 2001.

Smith Higuchi KA, Donald JG: Thinking processes used by nurses in clinical decision making, *J Nurs Ed* 41(4):145, 2002.

15

Nursing Assessment

Media Resources

http://evolve.elsevier.com/Potter/
fundamentals/

CD COMPANION

- Review Questions
- Glossary

evolve WEBSITE

- Review Questions
- Student Learning Activities
- Glossary

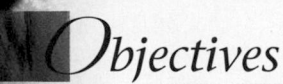

Objectives

Mastery of content in this chapter will enable the student to:

- Define the key terms listed.
- Discuss the purpose of nursing assessment.
- Explain the relationship of critical thinking to assessment.
- Discuss the steps that constitute nursing assessment.
- Describe the relationship between data collection and data analysis.
- Explain the difference between a comprehensive, problem-oriented, and focused assessment.
- Explain why client expectations are important to include in assessment.
- Discuss the purposes of a client interview.
- Explain the types of data that can be revealed from various interviewing techniques.
- Differentiate between objective and subjective data.
- State the sources of data for a nursing assessment.
- State the purpose of a nursing history.
- State the purpose of a physical examination.
- Explain the relationship between data interpretation, validation, and clustering.
- Conduct a nursing assessment.

*C*onsider the following scenario:

Lisa, an RN on a general nursing unit, enters Mrs. Devine's room for the first time. Mrs. Devine looks up and states, "I'm so glad you are here. I have had this pain in my back, and I cannot get comfortable." Lisa responds, "Mrs. Devine, I am Lisa, your RN. Let me take a look at your back." Lisa examines Mrs. Devine's back and then asks a series of questions: How long have you had the pain? Show me where the pain is located. Is there anything that relieves or worsens the pain? As Mrs. Devine responds to the questions, Lisa is analyzing the data and considering other relevant information, such as the client's medical diagnosis (ruptured lumbar disk) and knowledge of the alterations the condition typically causes (e.g., sciatic pain and change in sensation of the lower extremities). Lisa decides that Mrs. Devine has pain related to pressure on the spinal nerves. Lisa explains to Mrs. Devine the nursing interventions that can help relieve the discomfort. She then proceeds to administer the interventions, including administering an analgesic, repositioning Mrs. Devine, and discussing how Mrs. Devine can practice relaxation exercises. Forty-five minutes later Lisa returns to Mrs. Devine's room to determine if the pain is relieved and whether she would like to learn how to perform relaxation.

Lisa has just performed the nursing process while caring for Mrs. Devine. Each time a nurse meets a client, the nurse applies the nursing process to provide appropriate and effective nursing care. The process begins with an assessment or gathering and analysis of information about the client's health status. The nurse then makes clinical judgments about the client's response to health problems, defined as nursing diagnoses. Once the nurse defines appropriate nursing diagnoses, a plan of care is developed. The plan includes interventions individualized to each of the client's nursing diagnoses. The nurse performs all planned interventions in an effort to improve or maintain the client's health. After administering interventions, the nurse evaluates the client's response and whether the interventions were effective.

Nursing Process Overview

A nurse follows the **nursing process** to organize and deliver nursing care. Use of the process allows the nurse to integrate elements of critical thinking to make judgments and take actions based on reason. The nursing process is used to identify, diagnose, and treat human responses to health and illness (American Nurses Association [ANA],

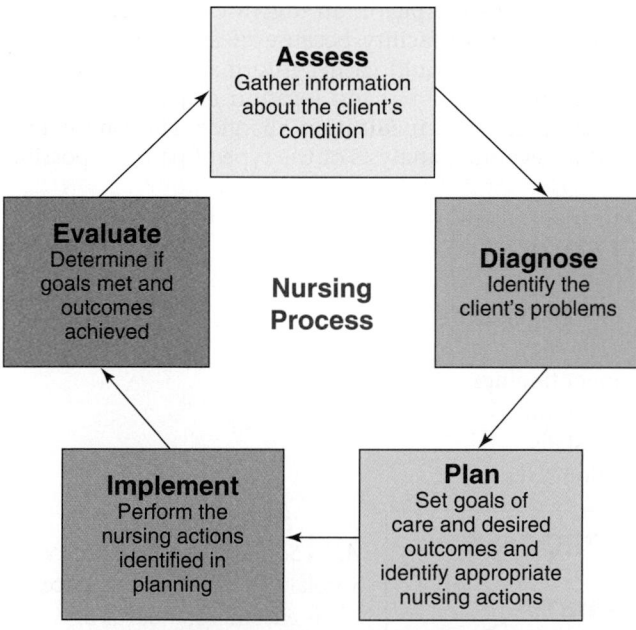

FIGURE 15–1　　Five-step nursing process.

2003). The process includes five steps: assessment, nursing diagnosis, planning, implementation, and evaluation (Figure 15-1). It is a dynamic continuous process, which allows a nurse to modify care as the client's needs change. Clients often have multiple needs, so the nurse will simultaneously apply the process to each of those needs. The use of the nursing process promotes individualized nursing care and assists the nurse in responding to client needs in a timely and reasonable manner.

The nursing process is a variation of scientific reasoning that allows nurses to organize and systematize nursing practice (Table 15-1). The nurse makes inferences about the meaning of a client's response to a health problem or generalizes about the client's functional state of health. A pattern will begin to form. For example, if the client is having acute back pain, the data allow the nurse to infer that the client's mobility will likely be limited. The nurse continues to gather more information (e.g., noting how the client moves and whether the client is able to walk, stand, and sit normally) until an accurate classification of the client's problem is determined, such as the following nursing diagnosis: *impaired physical mobility related to acute back pain*. The clear definition of the client's problem provides the basis for nursing interventions and evaluation of outcomes. In this example, the nurse's interventions are designed to relieve the pain so as to improve the client's mobility.

The nursing process applies to the care of all client systems, including individuals, families, groups, or communities. Use of the process allows nurses to differentiate their practice from that of physicians and other health care professionals. When nurses think critically, the client becomes an active participant and the ultimate outcome is a comprehensive, individualized approach to care.

A Critical Thinking Approach to Assessment

Assessment is the deliberate and systematic collection of data to determine a client's current and past health status and functional status and to determine the client's present and past coping patterns (Carpenito, 2000). Nursing **assessment** includes two steps. The first step involves the collection and verification of data from a primary source

Table 15-1	Comparison of Steps in Problem Solving, the Scientific Method, and the Nursing Process	
Problem Solving	**Copi and Cohen's Seven-Step Scientific Method***	**Nursing Process**
Encountering problem	The problem	Assessing
	Preliminary hypothesis	
Collecting data	Collecting additional facts	
Identifying exact nature of problem	Formulating hypotheses	Forming a nursing diagnosis
Determining plan of action	Deducing further consequences	Planning (outcome identification)
Carrying out plan	Testing consequences	Implementing
Evaluating plan in new situation	Application	Evaluating
Plan of action		

*Copi IM, Cohen C: *Introduction to logic*, ed 9, New York, 1994, Macmillan.

secondary sources (e.g., family, health pro-
medical record). The second step involves
all data as a basis for developing nursing di-
individualized plan of care for the client.
f the assessment is to establish a **database**
nt's perceived needs, health problems, and
responses to these problems. In addition, the data reveal
related experiences, health practices, goals, values, and expectations held about the health care system.

The nurse applies principles of critical thinking when
conducting a client assessment (see Chapter 14). Critical
thinking is the active, organized, cognitive process used to
carefully examine one's thinking, in this case the clinical
decision making of assessment. Critical thinking allows a
nurse to see the big picture when attempting to form conclusions or make decisions about a client's health condition. While gathering data about a client, the nurse synthesizes relevant knowledge, clinical experiences, critical
thinking standards and attitudes, and standards of practice simultaneously (Figure 15-2). Critical thinking thus
helps the nurse to direct the assessment in a meaningful
and purposeful way. The nurse brings knowledge from the
physical, biological, and social sciences to the assessment.
This knowledge enables the nurse to ask relevant questions and collect relevant history and physical assessment
data related to the client's presenting health care needs.
For example, by knowing that a client has a history of a
ruptured lumbar disk, the nurse knows to ask if the client
has sciatic pain (pain that radiates from the buttocks

down the leg) and to question how the discomfort affects
the client's ability to walk or sit, because these are common symptoms of disk disease. The use of good communication skills and critical thinking intellectual standards
enable the nurse to collect complete, accurate, and relevant data.

Prior clinical experience contributes to the skills of assessment. For example, if the nurse has cared for a client
with back pain in the past, the nurse knows the pain can
be very disabling and limits the client's normal motion.
Thus the nurse assesses thoroughly the extent to which
the pain affects the client's ability to walk normally and to
perform daily living activities. Validation of abnormal assessment findings and personal observation of assessments performed by skilled professionals enable a new
nurse to gain competency in the assessment process. The
nurse also applies standards of practice and accepted standards of "normal" for physical assessment data when assessing clients. The nurse brings attitudes such as curiosity, perseverance, risk taking, and confidence to the
nurse-client relationship so that a complete assessment
database is obtained.

An assessment must be relevant to a particular health
problem. For example, in an urgent care setting, when a
client enters the facility because of a possible ruptured
disk, the nurse would gather information regarding the
injury, intensity, type, and location of pain, initial first
aid measures, and medication allergies. The data is relevant for eventual analysis of the type of pain, its possible

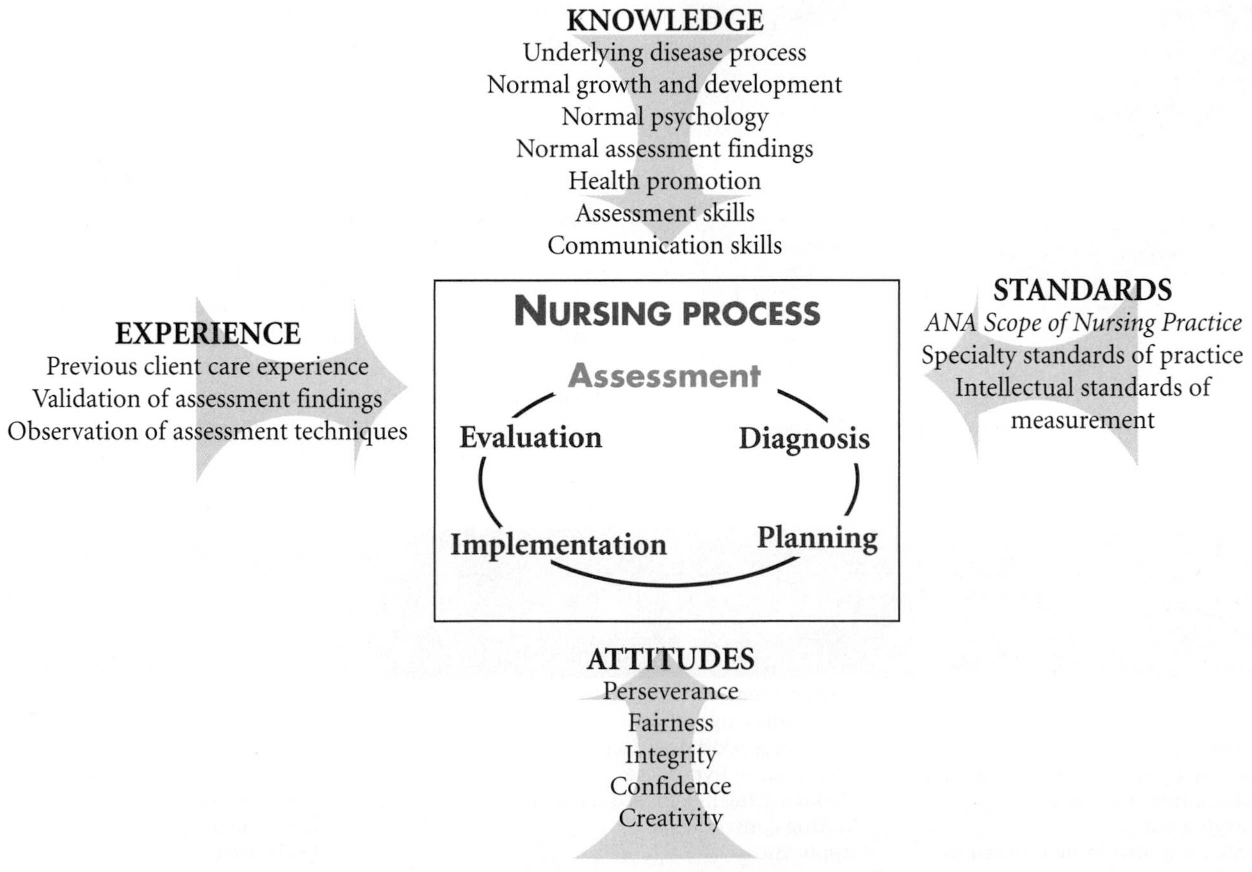

KNOWLEDGE
Underlying disease process
Normal growth and development
Normal psychology
Normal assessment findings
Health promotion
Assessment skills
Communication skills

EXPERIENCE
Previous client care experience
Validation of assessment findings
Observation of assessment techniques

NURSING PROCESS

Assessment

Evaluation   Diagnosis

Implementation   Planning

STANDARDS
ANA Scope of Nursing Practice
Specialty standards of practice
Intellectual standards of
measurement

ATTITUDES
Perseverance
Fairness
Integrity
Confidence
Creativity

FIGURE **15–2**   Critical thinking and the assessment process.

source, and the likely approaches that will relieve the pain. In settings such as an acute care hospital, the nurse collects assessment data on a standardized nursing assessment form, which is designed to collect targeted relevant data in a timely, efficient manner. In a community-based setting, where clients often present with less acute problems, the assessment focuses on the client's illness, circle of family and friends, and resources within the community (Bryans and McIntosh, 1996).

A nurse critically thinks when applying clinical knowledge and experience in judging the type of questions or measurements to make in an assessment. This level of judgment develops and matures over time. When first meeting a client, the nurse must decide whether an assessment can be a quick overview or a detailed examination of the client's case. An overview is usually based on the client's presenting priorities, the nurse's specialty of practice, or the treatment situation. For example, an emergency department nurse uses the A-B-C (airway-breathing-circulation) approach, because clients are usually experiencing acute injuries or conditions that threaten their survival. A psychiatric nurse may have more time to gather data and chooses to focus on the client's reality, anxiety level, and potential for violence (Carnevali and Thomas, 1993). The nurse must be able to differentiate important data from the data mass. A **cue** is information that the nurse acquires through use of the five senses. It is possible that the nurse will miss important cues with an intense focused assessment. However, the nurse tries to interpret cues from the client to know how in-depth an assessment should be. Assessment is dynamic; it should allow the nurse to freely explore relevant problems as they appear.

After an initial assessment, a nurse begins to focus on the client's potential problem areas by conducting a more comprehensive assessment. Two approaches may be used. One approach is the use of a structured database format, based upon an accepted theoretical framework or practice standard, such as Gordon's 11 **Functional Health Patterns** (1994), Pender's health promotion model (1996), or the Agency for Healthcare Research and Quality's (AHRQ's) standards for acute and chronic pain assessment (1992). The theory or practice standard provides categories of information for the nurse to assess. The premise is that the theoretical categories or standards provide for a comprehensive assessment of the client's health care problems.

The nurse's assessment moves from the general to the specific. For example, a nurse may assess all of Gordon's 11 functional health patterns and then determines if patterns or problems are revealed. More focused questions can be asked about those health patterns that suggest a problem exists. The nurse organizes patterns of behavior and physiological responses that pertain to a functional health category. The nurse then compares assessment data with the client's baseline (e.g., usual blood pressure, weight, and nutritional intake); established **norms** based on age, gender, height and weight; cultural, social, or other norms, such as religious practices, ethnic dietary guidelines, and health care practices. The complete assessment of the 11 functional health patterns represents the interaction of the client and the environment, which Gordon calls biopsychosocial integration. No one health pattern can be understood without knowledge of the

other patterns (Gordon, 1991). Ultimately the nurse's assessment identifies functional patterns (client strengths) and dysfunctional patterns (nursing diagnoses), which assist in developing the nursing care plan.

The second approach for conducting a comprehensive assessment is the problem-oriented approach. The nurse focuses on the client's presenting situation. For example, the nurse's assessment might begin with problem areas such as grieving and spread out to relevant areas of the client's life. The nurse will review with the client the nature of his or her loss and then broaden to categories such as the influence of loss on lifestyle, family relationships, and work habits (see Chapter 29). Once completed, the problems of loss and grief will be thoroughly analyzed so that a comprehensive approach can be used to plan interventions directed toward grief resolution.

Whatever approach is used to collect data, the nurse begins to cluster cues of assessment data and identifies emerging patterns and potential problems. To do this well, a nurse critically anticipates. In other words, the nurse always tries to stay a step ahead of the assessment. Once a question is asked of a client or an observation is made, the information often branches to an additional series of questions or observations (Figure 15-3). The risk the nurse takes in not anticipating assessment questions is to fail to recognize problems or to dismiss relevant problems (Hurst and others, 1991). Knowing how to frame questions is a basic skill, refined over time. The nurse decides which questions are relevant to the situation while at the same time being sure the assessment is complete. The nurse's thoughts about the client proceed from something given in the form of cues or data, to a conclusion. The extent of a nurse's ability to grasp the meaning of all the data being collected and analyzed is related to the nurse's knowledge and experience.

Assessment is part of a nurse's collaborative role. The nurse makes clinical observations of a client, reports the client's situation relative to a medical problem, and then follows delegated medical activities prescribed by the physician. In the independent role of a health care provider, the nurse assesses a client's response to health problems and institutes nursing interventions to maintain or improve the client's health. Accurate assessment is crucial to ensure client needs are properly identified and the right course of action is implemented.

Organization of Data Gathering

When beginning an assessment, it is helpful for the nurse to organize the assessment process and determine which data must be collected. The faculty of The Ohio State University developed one methodology for teaching nursing students problem-solving techniques (Ryan-Wenger, 1990). The approach emphasizes how assessment requires a level of detail to ensure accuracy (Table 15-2). Steps in the assessment phase are outlined to provide clearer direction for how nurses make client care decisions.

It is important for a nurse to have focus when initiating the nurse-client interaction during assessment. Why has the client sought health care? What is the purpose of any nurse-client interaction? Who will be involved? What knowledge does the nurse have about the situation that brings the nurse and client together? These factors

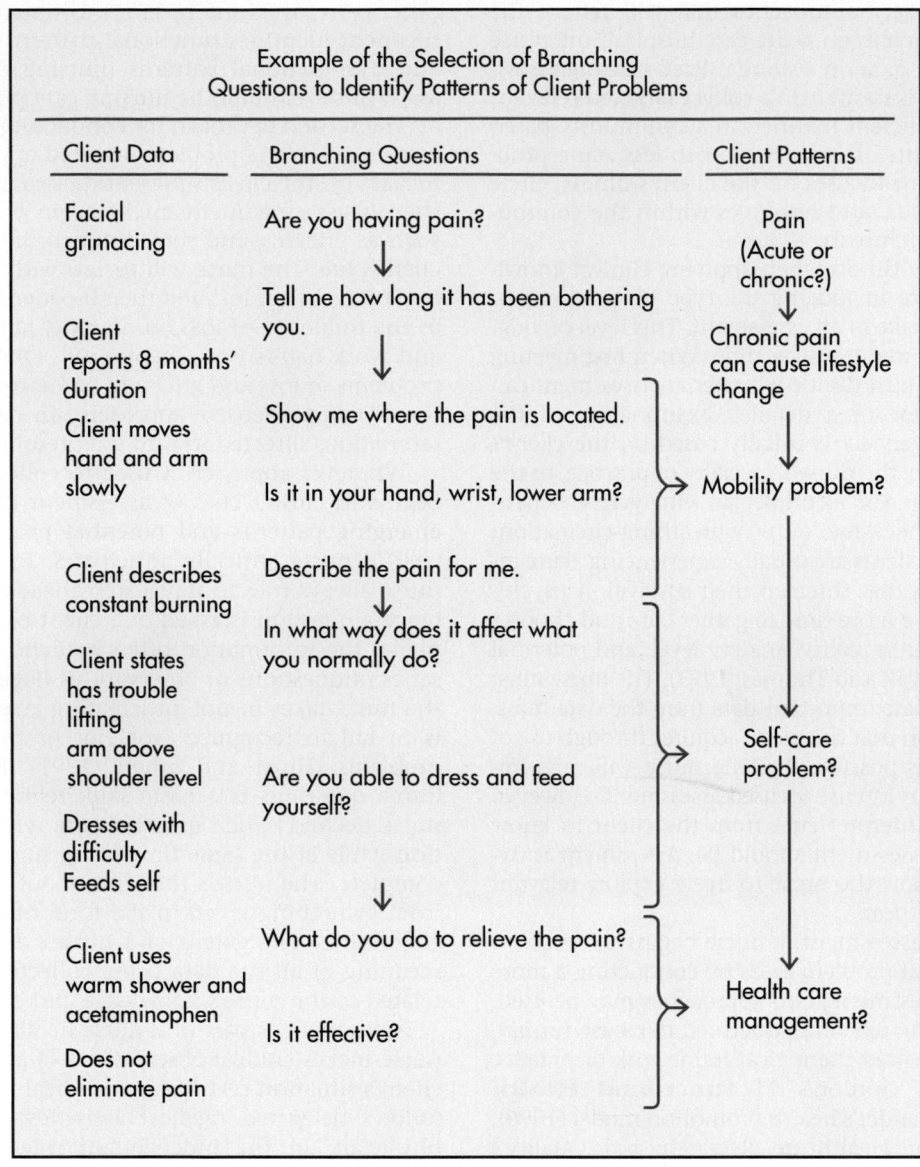

FIGURE **15–3**   Example of branching logic for selecting assessment questions.

influence the nurse's success in developing a relationship with the client that leads to a directed, purposeful, and comprehensive assessment.

During every nurse-client interaction, the nurse continually processes data (Carpenito, 1995). As a nurse conducts an assessment, there are considerable interactions (verbal and nonverbal) between the nurse and client. In addition, the client presents physiological responses such as posturing, breathing patterns, and body movement that relay information to the nurse. The nurse must use all senses to accurately assess client behavior.

Our senses collect experiences that we classify and judge (Bandman and Bandman, 1995). For example, when a nurse observes a client having difficulty breathing, sense impressions are formed that the client is in trouble. These sense impressions are sources of knowledge and often are reliable clues that lead the nurse to a more deliberate assessment. The skills of physical exami-

nation (see Chapter 32) enable the nurse to explore physical findings accurately and in detail, such as measurement of respiratory rate, rhythm, and depth. When making judgments, the nurse connects sense experiences to nursing knowledge to ensure accurate reasoning.

As a client and nurse interact, the nurse asks relevant questions to gather more data. If the nurse prematurely stops asking questions, the database can be incomplete and the resultant conclusions, made in the form of nursing diagnoses, can be inaccurate. Any **inferences** about the client or about the nurse's own behavior toward the client are separated from actual data.

Data Collection

Assessment data must be descriptive, concise, and complete. An assessment should not include inferences or interpretative statements that are unsupported with data. The nurse applies intellectual standards of critical think-

Table 15-2	A Methodology for Nursing Assessment
Element	**Nursing Activity**
Nurse-client interaction	Identify purpose of the nurse-client interaction (e.g., to provide hygiene care, administer a tube feeding, interact with an anxious client).
	Identify the system of study along with important subsystems (e.g., the client, nurse-client, group of clients, community).
	Recognize relationships between client and the environment that influence client's behavior and/or nurse-client interaction.
	Know the purpose of each nursing experience and type of client to prepare for the interaction. For example, practice hygiene skills before giving hygiene care.
Recording nurse and client behavior	Nurse and client are affected by each other's behavior and characteristics. Observe own verbal and nonverbal behavior to assess effect on client.
	Use all senses to accurately observe and record client's verbal/nonverbal behavior.
	Use tools and instruments (stethoscope, thermometer, height/weight chart) to accurately measure behavior and physiological signs.
Questions and inferences	Ask relevant questions to gather more data. *Do not be satisfied with simple answers.* For example:
	Nurse: Are you feeling nauseated?
	Client: Yes.
	Nurse: Tell me when it began; are you having other symptoms?
	Be aware of inferences about your own behavior: "My nervousness is showing"; "The client and I are not communicating well." *Keep inferences separate from data.* Use appropriate follow-up questions to clarify.
	The client responds to questions asked, and other data are collected to support or refute inferences.
Identifying patterns	Based on knowledge and data, identify patterns of nurse and client behavior. A pattern is similar to a nursing diagnosis and is defined as a particular behavior occurring over time (e.g., client walks 4 miles a day—has a pattern of regular exercise), or a pattern may be a cluster of behavior (e.g., client has shortness of breath, increased heart rate, rapid respirations following routine exercise—indicating poor activity tolerance).
	Identify positive and negative patterns. A positive pattern might be a client's spiritual strengths; a negative pattern might be poor eating habits. It is important to recognize and maintain positive health patterns as well as to decrease effects of negative health patterns.
	Identify interaction patterns based on observation of nurse-client interaction. For example, nurse asks questions and client responds in one-word phrases with no eye contact.
Apply theories and concepts	Concepts and theories help to support, refute, or give meaning to observed patterns. For example, while administering medication a student identifies a pattern of grief over a client's loss of a spouse and supports the finding by documenting that expression of guilt, crying, and poor eating habits are signs of dysfunctional grieving.
	Previously identified patterns are assessed for their potential or real effect on a client. Patterns with a negative effect on health (e.g., poor compliance in taking medication) are noted. Patterns that positively affect health (e.g., getting regular sufficient sleep) are reviewed.
	Also consider patterns of nurse behavior or client-nurse interaction that have positive or negative effects.
Validation	Document interpretation of patterns of data with reliable sources (e.g., literature, other nurses, family, health care professionals).

From Ryan-Wenger NM: A nursing process methodology, *Nurs Outlook* 38(4):190, 1990.

ing (see Chapter 14) to collect the level of detail necessary to fully understand a client's problems or needs. For example, when a client tells a nurse about difficulty sleeping, the nurse will be specific, "Do you have trouble falling asleep, staying asleep, or both?" or accurate, "Tell me how many hours of sleep you typically average."

A client's database originates with the client's perception of a symptom or health problem and then additional data originate from the perceptions and observations of the family, the nurse's observations, or reports from other members of the health care team. It is important to en-

courage clients to tell *their* story about their illness or health care problem. For example, a nurse might begin an assessment by saying, "Tell me what brings you to the clinic" or "In what way has your fatigue affected your daily way of life?" Open-ended questions allow a client to tell his or her story in detail and to relate what is important. This usually allows a nurse to focus on the client's priorities very quickly.

As a client begins to reveal data, the nurse immediately begins to anticipate the need for other questions and considers what the existing data means. For example, a client may describe pain as a "sharp, throbbing pain in the back." The nurse's observation may be, "The client lies on the right side with knees flexed. Facial grimacing is present. The client is unable to turn without assistance." The nurse then conducts a focused examination and records only observations (e.g., tenderness over L4 and L5) and avoids interpreting behavior (e.g., "The client tolerates pain poorly"). Concise data briefly describe the information obtained. The information is summarized in a short format using correct medical terms (e.g., "Client describes a constant, sharp, throbbing pain in the lower lumbar area of the back. Turning is limited. Pain began 48 hours ago after the client experienced a fall from his ladder"). Complete data collection results from obtaining all information relevant to the actual or potential health problem. To confirm that complete data have been collected, the nurse might ask, "Is there anything else? "Would you like to tell me more about your problem?" The nurse wants to have the information that answers the question, When, where, and what are the duration and influencing factors for the client's problems?

The collection of inaccurate, incomplete, or inappropriate data may lead to incorrect identification of the client's health care needs and subsequent inaccurate, incomplete, or inappropriate nursing diagnoses. Inaccurate data result if the nurse fails to collect information relevant to a specific area or if the nurse is disorganized or unskilled in assessment techniques. Data are incomplete if the nurse neglects to obtain all information about a specific area, jumps to conclusions about a potential problem, or makes assumptions without validation. Inappropriate data are unrelated to the area being assessed.

Types of Data

Data collection includes the gathering of subjective and objective data from or about a client. **Subjective data** are clients' perceptions about their health problems. Only clients can provide this kind of information. For example, a client's report of feeling fearful about impending surgery is a subjective finding. Other examples of subjective data include feelings of anxiety, pain, or mental stress. Although only clients can provide subjective data relevant to their feelings, the nurse must be aware that these problems can result in physiological changes, which are identified through objective data collection.

Objective data are observations or measurements made by the data collector. Assessment of a client's wound, a description of client behavior, and identification of the size of a localized body rash are examples of observed objective data. The measurement of objective data is based on an accepted **standard,** such as the Fahrenheit or Celsius measure on a thermometer, centimeters on a measuring tape, or known characteristics or definitions of behaviors. Body temperature and blood pressure are other examples of measured objective data.

Sources of Data

Subjective data are obtained from the client, family, significant others, health care team members, and health records. Objective data are obtained though physical examination, results of diagnostic and laboratory tests, and pertinent nursing and medical literature. The nurse's own past experiences with similar types of clients serves as a resource in validating accuracy of data. Each source of data provides information about the client's level of wellness, anticipated prognosis, risk factors, health practices and goals, and patterns of health and illness, as well as information relevant to the client's health care needs.

Client
A client is usually the best source of information. The client who is oriented and answers questions appropriately can provide the most accurate information about health care needs, lifestyle patterns, present and past illnesses, perception of symptoms, and changes in activities of daily living. It is important, however, to consider the setting where the nurse interacts with a client. A client experiencing acute symptoms in an emergency department will not be able to offer the same depth of information as one who comes to a primary care clinic for a routine checkup. It is also important for the nurse to always attend to a client. Clients are less likely to fully reveal the nature of their health care problems when health care providers show little interest or are easily distracted by activities around them. The nurse shows full attention and interest to a client to gather a detailed database.

Family and Significant Others
Family members and significant others can be interviewed as primary sources of information about infants or children and critically ill, mentally handicapped, disoriented, or unconscious clients. In cases of severe illness or emergency situations, families may be the only available sources of data about a client's health-illness patterns, current medications, allergies, onset of illness, and other information needed by nurses and physicians.

The family and significant others are also important secondary sources of information. They can confirm findings provided by a client. It is important to include them in assessment of the client when appropriate. Often spouses or close friends will sit in during an assessment and provide their view of the client's health problems or needs. Not only can they supply information about the client's current health status, but also they often are able to indicate when changes in the client's status occurred and how the client's functioning was affected. Family members are frequently very well informed, because they have had numerous experiences living with the client and observing how health problems affect the client's daily activities. Finally, family and friends can make pertinent observations about the client's needs that can affect the way care is delivered (e.g., how a client swallows or eats a meal, how a client makes choices, or how a client reacts to pain). The family is an invaluable resource for information about a client.

Health Care Team Members
For assessment to be comprehensive, the nurse must communicate with other health care team members, including physicians, physical therapists, social workers, other nurses, community health workers, and pastoral care staff, whenever possible. In the acute care setting the

change of shift report is often the vehicle for nurses from one shift to convey information to nurses on the oncoming shift (see Chapter 25). The health care team provides information about the way the client interacts within the health care environment; the client's reaction to information, diagnostic procedures, nursing and medical therapies; and how the client responds to visitors. Every member of the health care team is a potential source of information, and the team can identify and communicate data and verify information from other sources.

Medical Records

The medical record provides pertinent data about the client's medical history, laboratory tests and diagnostic study results, and the physician's proposed treatment plan. Data in the record are baseline information about the client's response to illness and information about the effects of later treatment measures. The Health Insurance Portability and Accountability Act (HIPAA) of 1996 has a privacy rule that came into effect on April 14, 2003, to set standards for the protection of health information (HIPAAdvisory, 2003). Information in a client's record is confidential. Each health care agency has policies governing how the information can be shared between health care providers. For example, hospitals may implement policies that permit nurses, physicians, and others involved in client treatment to have access to the entire medical record as necessary. Thus a nurse can review a client's medical record for the purpose of assessment but must be aware of agency policies governing how that information can be shared with other staff. The medical record is a valuable tool for checking the consistency and congruency of personal observations.

Other Records

Other records such as educational, military, and employment records may contain pertinent health care information (e.g., immunizations and prior illnesses). If the client received services at a community health center or day care clinic, the nurse should obtain data from these records but must first obtain written permission from the client or guardian to see them. New regulations from HIPAA (2003) dictate the manner in which an information release must be obtained. Consult agency policies. Any information obtained is confidential and is treated as part of the client's legal medical record (see Chapter 22).

Literature Review

Reviewing nursing, medical, and pharmacological literature about a client's illness helps the nurse complete the assessment database. The review increases the nurse's knowledge about the expected symptoms, treatment, and prognosis of specific illnesses, and established standards of therapeutic practice. The knowledgeable nurse is able to obtain pertinent, accurate, and complete information for the assessment database.

Nurse's Experience

Benner (1989) notes that through experience a nurse learns to ask the right questions, choosing those that yield the most useful information. A nurse's expertise develops after testing and refining propositions, questions, and principle- or standard-based expectations. For example, after a nurse has cared for a client with back pain there are lessons learned. The nurse more quickly recognizes the behavior the client showed while in acute pain. The nurse notes the extent to which positioning techniques help the client to relax and have less discomfort. The principle of administering a pain medication regularly rather than when the client requests it, to achieve better pain control, has been tested. Critical thinking is strengthened by practical experience and the opportunity to make decisions. A nurse's ability to assess clients improves from applying past experience, relevant knowledge, and focusing on data collection that avoids wasteful consideration of unnecessary information.

Methods of Data Collection

The nurse uses the interview, the nursing health history, the physical examination, and results of laboratory and diagnostic tests to establish the assessment database.

Interview

The first step in establishing the database is to collect subjective information by interviewing the client. An **interview** is an organized conversation with the client to obtain the client's health history and information about the current illness. During an interview nurses have the opportunity to:

- Be introduced to the client, explain their role, and the role of others during care
- Establish a sense of caring for the client as an individual
- Establish a therapeutic relationship with the client
- Gain insight about the client's concerns and worries
- Determine the client's goals and expectations of the health care system
- Obtain cues about which parts of the data collection phase require further in-depth investigation

Perhaps most important, the interview should help clients relate their own interpretation and understanding of their condition. This means the nurse and client must be partners during the interview rather than the nurse controlling the interview. This begins by establishing a therapeutic relationship with the client, where the nurse and client share a mutual concern, the client's well-being. This relationship builds a professional interpersonal closeness that develops and aids in the investigation and discussion of the client's responses to health and illness. A therapeutic relationship encourages the sharing of information, ideas, and emotions and enables the nurse to express a level of caring for the client.

Phases of the Interview. An interview with a client includes three phases, similar to that of a therapeutic relationship (see Chapter 23): orientation, working, and termination. A successful interview requires preparation on the part of the nurse by collecting any available information about the client and then creating an environment conducive to an interview. For example, an interview with a hospitalized client should be scheduled for a time when interruptions by other staff or visiting family members are minimal. An environment in which the client is comfortable and relaxed is conducive to a good interview.

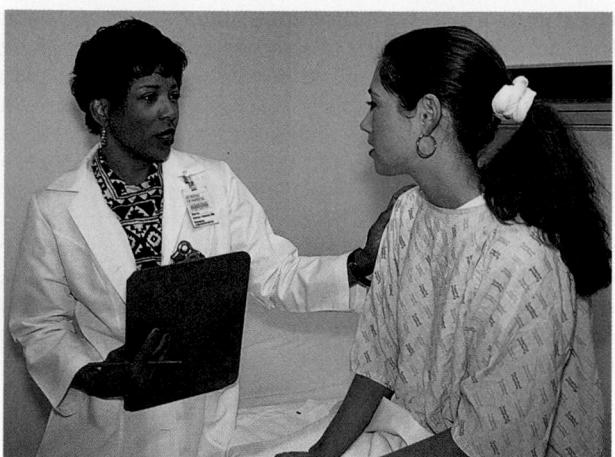

FIGURE **15–4**   Nurse explains the purpose of the interview.

A client interviewed at home may prefer that the interview take place in a bedroom away from other family members or in the living room with a spouse present. Remember to let a client decide whether to involve the family. Finally, the nurse selects a place private enough to allow the client to be comfortable when providing personal information.

Orientation Phase. The orientation phase begins with the nurse's introduction to the client, which includes the nurse's name, position, and an explanation of the purpose of the interview (Figure 15-4). It is important to explain to the client why the data are being collected (e.g., for a nursing history or for a focused assessment) and to assure the client that any information obtained will remain confidential and will be used by health care professionals in his or her care. HIPAA regulations require clients to sign an authorization before personal health data can be collected (HIPAAdvisory, 2003). This usually occurs in admitting and screening areas before the nurse sees the client. However, it is recommended that nurses refer to hospital policy for the authorization process.

The orientation phase is important in establishing trust and confidence with a client. While conducting the interview, the nurse remains aware that the client is forming an impression about nursing. For some clients, being interviewed by a nurse is a new experience. An important goal for the initial interview is to lay the groundwork for the nurse to understand the client's needs and to begin a relationship that allows the client to become an active partner in decisions about care.

As the orientation phase proceeds, a client should begin to feel more comfortable speaking with the nurse. This is important, because once the working phase begins, the nurse must gather information of a more personal and focused nature. The nurse consciously communicates a sense of trust and confidentiality to clients. Illnesses that cause people to seek help are often accompanied by anxiety, fear, helplessness, disruption of family relationships, and changes in self-image. Frequently clients are asked to provide very personal information about themselves and their families. Generally people share such information only with close friends, and there

Box 15-1

Focus on Older Adults

Nonverbal Behaviors Conducive to the Nurse-Client Relationship

Nonverbal communication includes all forms of communication that do not involve the spoken word. When older adults have limited hearing or visual deficits, it becomes more important for a nurse to use nonverbal communication when establishing nurse-client relationships.

- *Client-directed eye gaze*—Allows the nurse or client who is speaking to check whether information is understood. It is a signal for readiness to initiate interaction with a client. Eye contact conveys a sense of interest in a person with whom one is communicating.
- *Affirmative head nodding*—Has an important social function. It helps to regulate an interaction (especially when people change turns in speaking), it supports spoken language, and it allows for comment upon the interaction concerning the rapport and content of the communication.
- *Smiling*—Smiling is positively judged by others and is considered as a sign of good humor, warmth, and immediacy. It may be most important when a nurse wishes to establish good rapport with clients.
- *Forward leaning*—Shows awareness, attention, and immediacy. During an interaction it also clearly suggests interest in that person.
- *Touch*—Important in building rapport and a relationship with a client. If used appropriately it can also convey affection, care, and comfort.

Modified from Caris-Verhallen WMC and others: Non-verbal behaviour in nurse-elderly patient communication, *J Adv Nurs* 29(4):808, 1999.

is a certain amount of trust that this information will not be shared with others. The nurse assures clients that interviews are confidential before asking them to share personal information.

The **nurse-client relationship** is enhanced by the professionalism and competence conveyed by the nurse. The nurse's attitude, professional manner, and appearance encourage a supportive therapeutic relationship with the client. Box 15-1 outlines behaviors important in establishing good relationships, particularly with older adults. Open communication between nurse and client ensures the ongoing identification of the client's health care needs. The nurse is involved with the client and family and becomes an advocate for the client.

Box 15-2 is an introduction to a case study that will be used in subsequent chapters to demonstrate the nursing process. To begin, the nurse, Mr. Coffey, spends a few minutes becoming acquainted with the client, Mr. Brown. After introducing his role to Mr. Brown, Mr. Coffey reviews the interview process and its objectives, confidentiality, and length. The nurse and client agree mutually on an interview time. Before beginning the interview, Mr. Coffey asks his client if he has any questions. Clarifying Mr. Brown's concerns about his oxygen minimizes distractions during the interview. Mr.

Case Study   **Box 15-2**

Mr. Coffey is the nurse case manager assigned to Mr. Brown. Mr. Coffey is preparing an admission history on Mr. Brown, a 51-year-old man hospitalized for the first time. Mr. Brown is presenting with a history of diarrhea for 3 weeks. He also has a number of other physical problems including a history of emphysema, which requires a complete nursing assessment. Mr. Brown is married and has a 30-year-old son who has 2 children of his own.

Mr. Coffey: Good afternoon, Mr. Brown. I'm Joe Coffey, and I'm the nurse who will be managing your care during your hospital stay and through discharge to your home.

Mr. Brown: Hi, Joe. Please call me Bill. What do you mean by managing my care?

Mr. Coffey: That means I'm responsible for coordinating your nursing care with the rest of the nurses while you're hospitalized. I will work with them to plan for your discharge back to your home. Although other nurses will sometimes take care of you when I'm off, I'm the nurse who plans your care. Once you're discharged, I'll call you at home to see how you are doing and if you have any questions.

Mr. Brown: I guess that's a lot like being a coach. You may not play the game, but you're responsible for winning or losing.

Mr. Coffey: I suppose that's one way of looking at it. To better plan your care I will be asking some questions about your health. We call this a health interview. Any information you give me is confidential. The total interview should take about 20 to 30 minutes. Is it okay if I begin the interview in a few minutes?

Mr. Brown: How about giving me a half hour? My wife is about to leave. She needs to go pick up the grandkids at day care. That way we can have some time together. I'll be ready after that.

Mr. Coffey: That's fine. Because you're in a private room, I will do the health interview here. (Mr. Brown nods.)

Thirty minutes later, Mr. Coffey returns to the room.

Mr. Coffey: Okay. Before I get started, do you have any questions for me?

Mr. Brown: Yes. Why is there an outlet for oxygen on the wall above my bed? Does that mean that I'm really sick—did they put me in a special room?

Mr. Coffey: No, that's not it. Every bed in this hospital has an oxygen outlet located on the wall above the head of the bed. The reason is that this hospital has a central oxygen delivery system, and when a patient needs oxygen, we're able to supply it quickly, easily, and safely.

Mr. Brown: Okay. I wasn't actually worried. I was basically just curious. That was the only piece of equipment I couldn't explain.

Mr. Coffey: (pause) Mr. Brown, you mentioned that you and your wife have a son and grandchildren. Tell me a bit about your family.

Coffey's use of an open-ended question encourages Mr. Brown to begin the interview in a direction in which he feels comfortable.

Working Phase. During the working phase of the interview the nurse gathers information about the client's health status. The nurse may choose to use a health history form at this time or instead use an open-ended interview technique that allows the client to direct the conversation based upon the problems identified. Throughout the work-

ing phase, the nurse uses interview techniques to gather as comprehensive and complete a database as possible. In addition, the nurse uses a variety of communication strategies such as listening, paraphrasing, focusing, summarizing, and clarifying to facilitate communication and ensure that nurse and client clearly understand each other (see Chapter 23). The nurse's critical thinking also directs the interview so that sufficient detail can be gathered to understand the client's clinical condition. An example of Mr. Coffey's interview techniques follow:

Mr. Coffey: Tell me, Mr. Brown, about your difficulty breathing.

Mr. Brown: I can't get my breath after I do even the simplest activities.

Mr. Coffey: Can you give me an example?

Mr. Brown: After I get up in the morning, shower, and dress myself, I just can't catch my breath. I already feel worn out before I even start my day. I am beginning to feel helpless.

Mr. Coffey: (silence to encourage Mr. Brown to say more)

Mr. Brown: This problem with my heart is not something I ever expected.

The initial interview is normally the most extensive of all interviews. Major topics to be covered include biographical data, progress of current illness, the client's perceptions and beliefs about the illness, and the health history. Ongoing interviews, which occur each time a nurse interacts with a client, do not need to be as extensive. They update the client's status and are more focused toward changes in previously identified ongoing and new problems.

Termination Phase. As in the other phases of the interview, termination requires skill on the part of the interviewer. Ideally the client should be given a clue that the interview is coming to an end. For example, the nurse may say, "There are just two more questions," or "We'll be finished in 5 to 6 minutes." This helps the client remain attentive without being distracted by wondering when the interview will end. This approach also gives the client an opportunity to ask questions.

When concluding an interview, the nurse summarizes the important points and asks the client whether the summary was accurate. The interview is terminated in a friendly manner, with the nurse indicating specifically when there will be additional contact. For example, an appropriate way for Mr. Coffey to end his interview would be, "Thank you for your help, Mr. Brown. You have given me a good picture of your health and how you have been affected. You have indicated that you would like to know more about the procedures scheduled for your treatment. You also hope to be able to breathe more easily with less discomfort. Is that correct? This information will be helpful in planning your care. Another nurse will be caring for you this evening, but I'll be back on duty tomorrow morning. Do you have any other questions? Is there anything I can do for you now?"

A skillful interviewer is able to adapt interview strategies based on the client's responses. Pertinent health data are obtained when the nurse is prepared for the interview and is able to carry out each interview phase with minimal interruption.

Interview Techniques. The manner in which the interview is conducted is just as important as the questions asked. Attention to the environment, client comfort, and good communication techniques usually ensures a successful interview. During the interview the nurse directs the flow of the discussion so that adequate information is obtained and the client has the opportunity to contribute freely.

An interview may be focused, or it can be comprehensive. As the nurse listens and considers the information shared, the client may be directed to give more detail or discuss a topic that seems to reveal a possible problem. Because the client's report will include subjective information, the nurse uses data from the interview to later validate with objective data. For example, if the client reports difficulty in breathing, the nurse will later assess the client's respiratory rate and auscultate lung sounds.

During the interview the nurse obtains information about a client's physical, developmental, emotional, intellectual, social, and spiritual dimensions. Physical and developmental information reflects normal functioning and reveals any pathological changes induced by illness, trauma, or developmental crisis. Emotional information includes the client's behavioral responses to changes in health and pattern of living. Relevant emotional information includes mood, perceptions, body image, self-concept, and attitudes about sexuality. Intellectual information includes intellectual performance, problem-solving ability, educational level, communication patterns, and attention span. Social information involves environmental, cultural, ethnic, or social patterns that can affect the present or future level of wellness (e.g., values about health care and attitudes about family support). The nurse also collects information about life goals and values and religious practices, which are part of the spiritual dimension (see Chapter 28).

The interview allows the nurse to observe the client during interactions between the client and family and between the client and the health care environment. The nurse also observes the use of eye contact, nonverbal communication, and other body language. While observing this behavior, appearance, and interaction with the environment, the nurse determines whether the data obtained by observation are consistent with those obtained by verbal communication. For example, if the client states no concern about an upcoming diagnostic test but appears anxious and irritable, the data conflict. Observations during an interview lead the nurse to gather additional objective information to form accurate conclusions.

Clients also obtain information during the interview. If a positive nurse-client relationship has been established, the client will feel comfortable asking the nurse questions about the health care environment, planned treatments, diagnostic testing, and available resources. The client needs this information to make decisions about goals and the plan of care. It is important for the nurse to ask the client about his or her expectations of health care providers. In addition, the interview is a first step toward helping a client obtain education or counseling. For example, the interview allows a nurse to determine a client's readiness and ability to learn so that appropriate educational interventions can be used.

Types of Techniques. To interview a client successfully, a nurse needs experience and skills in initiating the nurse-client relationship, using correct interview techniques, and moving from one phase of the interview to the next. The nurse always remembers that the client's personality and health care needs and the health care setting affect the interview process.

An emergency situation may require a nurse to ask focused questions pertaining to the client's physical status. This approach moves quickly in an effort to problem solve and identify what factors or conditions are causing alterations in the client's health. A client entering an extended care facility with a chronic illness requires an interview approach that includes more elaboration and description of data. In this case the nurse collects a full picture of the client's health, living habits, familial and social resources, and the client's expectations for health care.

The interview in an emergent setting usually centers on the present illness or trauma, precipitating factors, medications, and allergies. In contrast, an interview with a client undergoing extensive rehabilitation may focus on past and present illnesses, coping strategies, family and community resources, daily living activities, and present limitations and goals for rehabilitation. The nurse uses the interview technique that elicits the necessary information from the client or another source.

When the interview involves collection of a complete nursing history, it is helpful to begin by trying to find out, in the client's own words, what the health problem is and what is likely causing it. Remember, clients are the best resource in most cases in being able to relate their health history. The nurse begins by asking the client a question to elicit the client's story. For example, the nurse may begin by asking, "So, tell me what brings you to the clinic today" or "Tell me about the problems you are having."

The use of **open-ended questions** prompts clients to describe a situation in more than one or two words (Box 15-3). This technique leads to a discussion in which

---

Box 15-3   Examples of Open- and Closed-Ended Questions

Open-Ended Questions

Tell me how you are feeling.
Your discomfort affects your ability to get around in what way?
Share with me the concerns you have about the x-ray test.
Describe how your wife has been helping you.
Give me an example of how you get relief from your pain at home.

Closed-Ended Questions

Do you feel like the medication is helping you?
Who is the person who helps you at home?
Do you understand why you are having the x-ray?
Has the warm compress given you relief from your back pain?
Are you having pain now?
How often do you awaken at night?
On a scale of 1 to 10, how would you rate your pain?

clients actively describe their health status. Open-ended questions give clients the chance to tell their stories and what is important to them. In contrast, closed-ended questions make it easy for clients to offer little detail while answering questions in only one or two words. The use of open-ended questions strengthens the nurse-client relationship because it shows that the nurse wants to invest time in hearing the client's thoughts. The nurse will encourage and let the client tell the story all the way through. The nurse's intent is reinforced through the use of good eye contact and listening skills. In addition, the nurse may use **back channeling,** which includes active listening techniques such as "all right," "go on," or "uh-huh," which indicate the nurse has heard what the client says and encourages even further elaboration.

As the client tells his or her story, the nurse encourages a full description without trying to control the direction the story takes. This may require the nurse to probe with further open-ended statements such as, "Is there anything else you can tell me?" or "What else is bothering you?" The nurse probes to exhaustion until the client has nothing else to say. It can also be very helpful to end the client's story by asking the client what might be causing his or her problem. This is described as the client's "explanatory model" (Lipkin and others, 1995). A physician is interested in a causal explanation so as to zone in on possible symptoms and their physical causes. In contrast, a nurse is interested in a causal explanation to understand the client's perceptions and response to a health problem and the meaning the problem has for the client. The client's sense of the cause of the problem will help to direct the nurse's subsequent focused assessment.

Once a client has told his or her story, the nurse uses a **problem-seeking interview** technique. This approach takes the information provided in the client's story to more fully describe and identify the client's specific problems. For example, a client may report experiencing indigestion over the course of several days and acknowledge having some diarrhea and loss of appetite. The client's explanation for the cause relates to a recent travel schedule that might have changed the client's eating habits. The nurse will focus on the symptoms the client identifies, as well as the general indigestion problem, by asking **closed-ended questions** that limit the client's answers to one or two words such as "yes" or "no" or a number or frequency of a symptom (see Box 15-3). For example, the nurse might ask, "How often does the diarrhea occur?" or "Do you have pain or cramping?" Closed-ended questions require concise answers and are used to clarify previous information or provide additional information. The questions do not encourage the client to volunteer more information than is directly requested. This type of questioning helps the nurse to acquire specific information about health problems such as symptoms, precipitating factors, or relief measures. As closed-ended questions reveal more information, the nurse may need to have the client elaborate more historical information. For example, after the client explains the cause of the indigestion, the nurse might ask the client to describe a normal day's food intake.

A good interviewer leaves with a complete story that contains enough details for understanding the client's perceptions of his or her problem, as well as the information needed to select appropriate nursing diagnoses for guiding the selection of nursing interventions.

Nursing Health History

The **nursing health history** is data collected about the client's current level of wellness, including a review of body systems, family and health history, sociocultural history, spiritual health, and mental and emotional reactions to illness. The history is obtained during an interview, and it is a major component of assessment. The objective is to identify patterns of health and illness, risk factors for physical and behavioral health problems, deviations from normal, and available resources for adaptation. Although many health history forms are structured, the nurse learns to use the questions as starting points. A good assessor learns to refine and broaden questions as needed so that the client's unique needs are correctly assessed. Time and client priorities determine how complete a history will be. Patterns of a client's health and illness are identified by collecting data about all health dimensions (Figure 15-5). Incorporating data from all dimensions enables the nurse to develop a complete plan of care. Although many formats for the nursing health history have been given in the literature, all contain similar basic components.

Biographical Information. Biographical information is factual demographic data about the client. The client's age, address, occupation and working status, marital status, source of health care, and types of insurance should be included.

Reason for Seeking Health Care. The nurse asks why the client is seeking health care, because the information contained on the initial admission form may differ from the client's subjective reason for seeking health care. For example, "Tell me, Mr. Lynn, why you have come to the clinic today." The nurse records the client's response in quotations to indicate the subjective response. The client's statement is not diagnostic; instead it is the client's perception of reasons for seeking health care. Clarification of the client's perception identifies potential needs for education, counseling, or referral to community resources.

Client Expectations. The assessment of client expectations is not the same as the reason for seeking medical care, although they are often related. It is important for nurses to acknowledge what is important to the client who is seeking health care. Failure to identify a client's expectations of health care providers and a health care institution can result in poor client satisfaction. Client satisfaction is a standard measure of quality for all hospitals throughout the country (see Chapter 2). Clients typically have expectations about information for making decisions regarding treatments and a plan of care for returning home, the likely outcome of treatment, cleanliness of the environment, relief of pain and other symptoms, and caring expressed by health care providers.

During the initial interview, the client's expresses expectations when entering the health care setting. Later, as

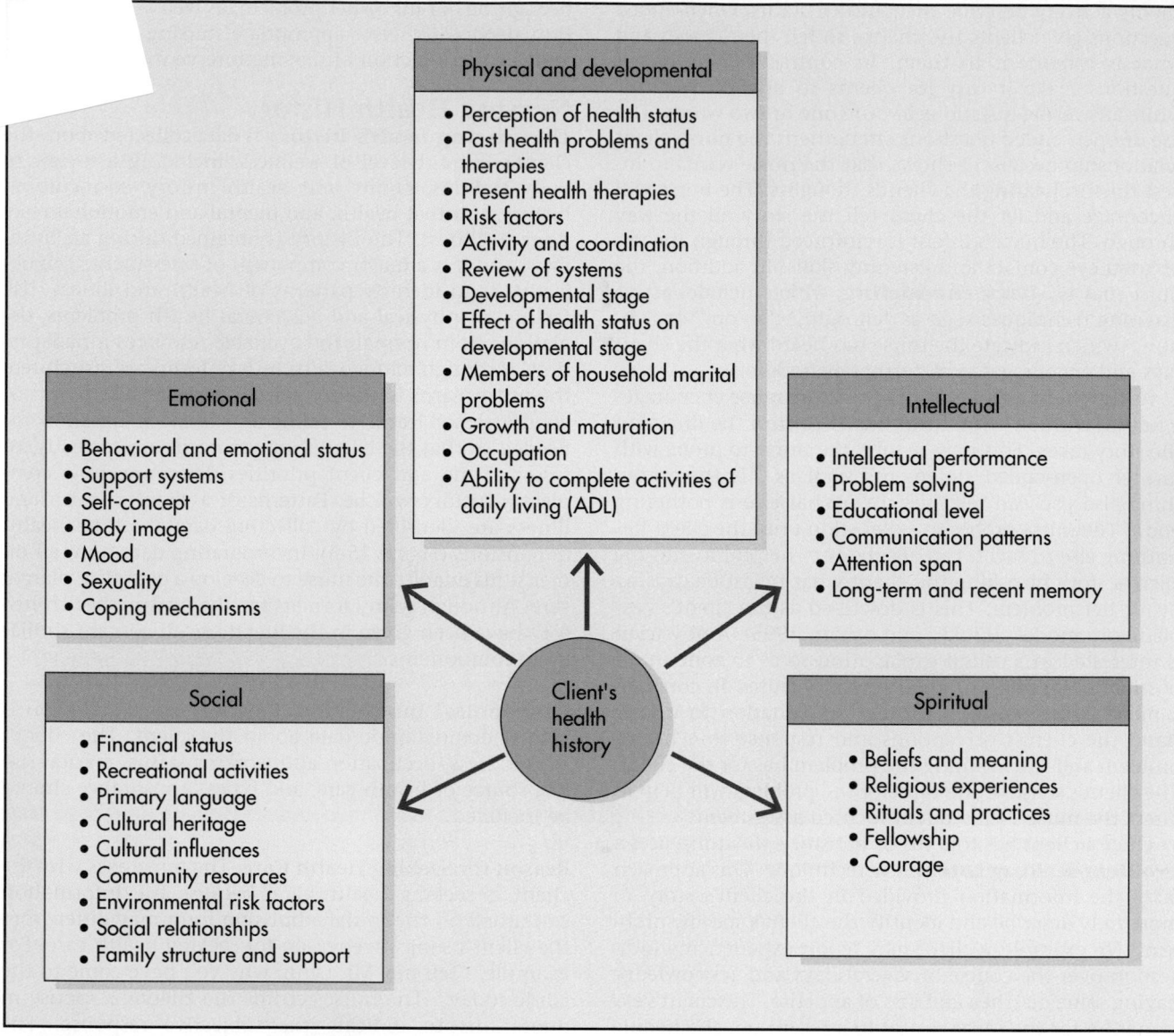

Physical and developmental

- Perception of health status
- Past health problems and therapies
- Present health therapies
- Risk factors
- Activity and coordination
- Review of systems
- Developmental stage
- Effect of health status on developmental stage
- Members of household marital problems
- Growth and maturation
- Occupation
- Ability to complete activities of daily living (ADL)

Emotional

- Behavioral and emotional status
- Support systems
- Self-concept
- Body image
- Mood
- Sexuality
- Coping mechanisms

Intellectual

- Intellectual performance
- Problem solving
- Educational level
- Communication patterns
- Attention span
- Long-term and recent memory

Social

- Financial status
- Recreational activities
- Primary language
- Cultural heritage
- Cultural influences
- Community resources
- Environmental risk factors
- Social relationships
- Family structure and support

Spiritual

- Beliefs and meaning
- Religious experiences
- Rituals and practices
- Fellowship
- Courage

Client's health history

FIGURE **15–5**   Dimensions for gathering data for a health history.

the client has had interactions with health care providers, it is valuable to assess if the client's expectations have changed or been met.

Present Illness or Health Concerns. If an illness is present, nurses gather essential and relevant data about the nature and onset of symptoms. The nurse determines when the symptoms began, whether they began suddenly or gradually, and whether they are always present or come and go. The nurse also asks about the duration of symptoms (most recently and over time). The nurse records information on the location, intensity, and quality of each symptom. For example, when the client describes the presence of pain, the nurse asks the client to point to or outline the area of the body affected and asks the client to rate the intensity on a scale of 0 to 10 (see Chapter 42). The nurse also assesses whether any action precipitates the symptoms, makes them worse, or provides relief.

Health History. The information collected about a client's health history provides data on the client's health care experiences and current health habits. The nurse assesses whether the client has ever been hospitalized or injured or has undergone surgery. A complete medication history (including herbal and over-the-counter drugs) is also included. Also essential are descriptions of allergies, including allergic reactions to food, latex, drugs, or contact agents (e.g., soap). For example, asking clients if they have had any problems with medications or food can help to clarify the type and amount of agent, the specific reaction, and whether the client has required treatment. If an allergy is present, the specific reaction and treatment are noted on the assessment form.

The nurse also identifies habits and lifestyle patterns. Assessing for the use of alcohol, tobacco, caffeine, or recreational drugs determines the client's risk for diseases involving the liver, lungs, heart, or nervous system. Noting the type of habit, as well as the frequency and duration of use, provides essential data.

Assessing patterns of sleep (see Chapter 41), exercise (see Chapter 36), and nutrition (see Chapter 43) is important when planning nursing care. The plan of care within a health care setting should match a client's lifestyle patterns as much as possible. Frequently, variations in sleep, activity, and nutritional patterns can be accommodated.

Family History. The purpose of the family history is to obtain data about immediate and blood relatives. The objectives are to determine whether the client is at risk for illnesses of a genetic or familial nature and to identify areas of health promotion and illness prevention (see Chapter 6). The family history also provides information about family structure, interaction, and function that may be useful in planning care (see Chapter 9). For example, a cohesive, supportive family can help a client adjust to an illness or disability and should be incorporated into the plan of care. On the other hand, if the client's family is not supportive, it may be better to not involve them in care. Stressful family relationships can be a significant barrier when a nurse tries to help clients with problems involving loss, self-concept, spiritual health, and personal relationships.

Environmental History. The environmental history provides data about clients' home and working environments with an emphasis on determining the client's safety. Information pertaining to the home environment may include function of utilities, layout of rooms in the house, and the presence of any barriers or risks for client injury. In addition, the environmental history identifies exposure to pollutants in the workplace, existence of high crime that prevents clients from walking around their neighborhoods, and available resources that can assist clients in returning to the community.

Psychosocial History. A complete psychosocial history reveals the client's support system, which may include spouse, children, other family members, and close friends. The psychosocial history includes information about ways that the client and family typically cope with stress (see Chapter 30). The same behavior, such as taking a walk, reading, or talking with a friend, can be used as a nursing intervention if the client experiences stress while receiving health care. The nurse also learns if the client has experienced any recent losses that create a sense of grief (see Chapter 29).

Spiritual Health. Life experiences and events are shaped by one's spirituality. The spiritual dimension represents the totality of one's being and is difficult to assess quickly (see Chapter 28). A nurse reviews with clients their beliefs about life, their source for guidance in acting on beliefs, and the relationship they have with family in exercising their faith. Rituals and religious practices as a way to express spirituality are also assessed.

Review of Systems. The **review of systems (ROS)** is a systematic method for collecting data on all body systems (Box 15-4). It is probable that all of the questions in each system will not be covered every time the nurse collects a history (Seidel, 2003). Nevertheless, some questions about each system should be included in the nursing history, particularly when a client mentions a symptom or sign. The systems that are assessed depend on the client's condition and the urgency in initiating care. During the ROS, the nurse asks the client about the normal functioning of each body system and any noted changes. Such changes are usually subjective data because they are described as perceived by the client. Findings from the ROS help the nurse to direct assessment during the physical examination.

Documentation of History Findings

As the nurse conducts the nursing health history, assessment data are recorded in a clear, concise manner using appropriate terminology. Standardized forms make it easy to enter data as the client responds to questions. A clear, concise record is necessary for use by other health care professionals (see Chapter 25). For example, when Gordon's Functional Health Patterns are the organizing framework for a nursing history form, data are collected for each of the 11 Functional Health Patterns in addition to the client's perception, evaluation, and explanation of any particular problems. The 11 patterns establish the nursing database. The historical and current information about all health patterns are used as baseline criteria against which any future changes are evaluated (Gordon, 1991, 1994). Assessments of functional health patterns and biomedical systems are easily integrated and aid in completing the client's physical and behavioral assessment database.

Physical Examination

During the **physical examination,** vital signs and other objective measurements are taken, and all body systems are examined. The nurse uses the techniques of inspection, palpation, percussion, auscultation, and olfaction to observe for abnormalities that may yield information about past, present, and future health problems. The physical examination is conducted after the nursing health history so that historical data can be verified. In addition, new data (e.g., appearance of the client's skin and muscle strength) are obtained during the examination.

Before conducting the physical examination, the nurse prepares the client, environment, and necessary equipment. The nurse informs the client about the process of the physical examination, specifically its purposes, the nurse's role, the client's role, and the approximate duration.

Order of Examination. The physical examination is performed systematically in a manner similar to the ROS in the health history. This component of assessment usually begins with the client's height, weight, and vital

---

Box 15-4   Review of Systems

- **General presentation of symptoms:** Fever, chills, malaise, pain, sleep patterns, fatigability
- **Diet:** Appetite, likes and dislikes, restrictions, written diary of food intake
- **Skin, hair, and nails:** Rash or eruption, itching, color or texture change, excessive sweating, abnormal nail or hair growth
- **Musculoskeletal:** Joint stiffness, pain, restricted motion, swelling, redness, heat, deformity
- **Head and neck:**
  - *Eyes:* Visual acuity, blurring, diplopia, photophobia, pain, recent change in vision
  - *Ears:* Hearing loss, pain, discharge, tinnitus, vertigo
  - *Nose:* Sense of smell, frequency of colds, obstruction, epistaxis, sinus pain, or postnasal discharge
  - *Throat and mouth:* Hoarseness or change in voice, frequent sore throat, bleeding or swelling of gums, recent tooth abscesses or extractions, soreness of tongue or mucosa
- **Endocrine and genital/reproductive:** Thyroid enlargement or tenderness, heat or cold intolerance, unexplained weight change, polyuria, polydipsia, changes in distribution of facial hair; *Males*—Puberty onset, difficulty with erections, emissions, testicular pain, libido, infertility;

Females—Menses (onset, regularity, duration, and amount), dysmenorrhea, last menstrual period, date of last Pap smear, frequency of intercourse, age at menopause, pregnancies (number, miscarriages, abortions), type of delivery, complications, use of contraceptives; breasts (pain, tenderness, discharge, lumps)
- **Chest and lungs:** Pain related to respiration, dyspnea, cyanosis, wheezing, cough, sputum (character and quantity), exposure to tuberculosis (TB), last chest x-ray
- **Heart and blood vessels:** Chest pain or distress, precipitating causes, timing and duration, relieving factors, dyspnea, orthopnea, edema, hypertension, exercise tolerance
- **Gastrointestinal:** Appetite, digestion, food intolerance, dysphagia, heartburn, nausea or vomiting, bowel regularity, change in stool color or contents, constipation or diarrhea, flatulence, hemorrhoids
- **Genitourinary:** Dysuria, flank or suprapubic pain, urgency, frequency, nocturia, hematuria, polyuria, hesitancy, loss in force of stream, edema, sexually transmitted disease
- **Neurological:** Syncope, seizures, weakness or paralysis, abnormalities of sensation or coordination, tremors, loss of memory
- **Psychiatric:** Depression, mood changes, difficulty concentrating, nervousness, tension, suicidal thoughts, irritability

Modified from Seidel HM and others: *Mosby's guide to physical examination*, ed 5, St. Louis, Mosby, 2003.

---

signs. Next the examiner writes a general statement about the client's appearance, behavior, and perceptions about health. This statement, called the general survey, includes information about mental status, signs of distress, body type, nutritional status, sex and race, chronological versus apparent age, behavior, appearance, grooming, and speech. Last is a head-to-toe physical examination of all body systems. The examiner describes and records objective data obtained, using clear, concise, and appropriate language. Throughout an examination the nurse works closely with a client to minimize any anxiety or discomfort. Chapter 32 describes the physical examination process.

Diagnostic and Laboratory Data

The results of diagnostic and laboratory tests can identify or verify alterations questioned or identified during the nursing health history and physical examination. For example, during the history the client indicates recurrent upper respiratory tract infections and at present has a productive cough with brown sputum. The nurse noted during examination an elevated body temperature, increased respirations, and decreased breath sounds in the right lower lobe. The nurse reviews results of a complete blood count (CBC) to look for an elevated white blood cell (WBC) count, indicative of an infection. In addition, the nurse would check the results of a chest x-ray examination to determine if there is right lung congestion. Together the findings suggest the client may have pneumonia. Laboratory data are compared with the established norms for a particular test, age group, and sex. The

nurse identifies variations from normal and interprets findings according to the disease process and treatments. In addition, the nurse uses laboratory data to evaluate the success or failure of nursing and medical interventions (e.g., review of WBC count following introduction of antibiotic therapy). Specific laboratory tests and the nursing responsibilities associated with them are detailed in the clinical chapters in Units VII and VIII.

Formulating Nursing Judgments

The successful interpretation of assessment data requires critical thinking. When nurses correctly collect and analyze data, they are able to make necessary clinical decisions in their clients' care. Useful and appropriate assessment data must refer to the intended purpose of nursing and relate to the client's health problems (Bandman and Bandman, 1995). These interrelated concepts are the basis for nursing judgments. The nurse critically chooses the type of information to collect about a client, interprets the information to determine abnormalities, conducts further observations to clarify information, and then names the client's problem(s) in the form of nursing diagnoses (see Chapter 16).

Data Validation and Interpretation

After gathering assessment data, the nurse validates the collected information to ensure its accuracy. Validation of

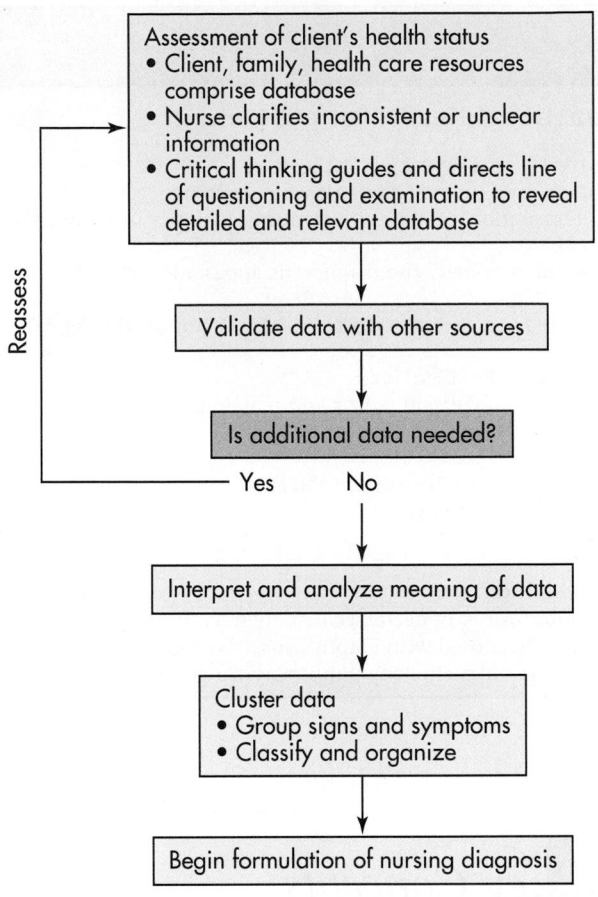

Assessment of client's health status
- Client, family, health care resources comprise database
- Nurse clarifies inconsistent or unclear information
- Critical thinking guides and directs line of questioning and examination to reveal detailed and relevant database

Reassess

Validate data with other sources

Is additional data needed?

Yes   No

Interpret and analyze meaning of data

Cluster data
- Group signs and symptoms
- Classify and organize

Begin formulation of nursing diagnosis

FIGURE **15–6**   Assessment and clinical nursing judgment.

assessment data involves comparing the data with another source (Figure 15-6). The nurse may ask a client or family member to validate information obtained during the interview and health history. Any additions or corrections are noted and added to the database. Findings concerning physical examination and observation of client behavior can be validated by comparing client data in the medical record or by consulting with other members of the health care team.

When a nurse validates data with both the client and family, it opens the door for gathering new information. It may become necessary for the nurse to reassess previously covered areas of the nursing history or gather more information in a physical examination. The nurse is continually analyzing and thinking about a client's database to make concise, accurate, and meaningful interpretations.

After the nurse collects extensive information about a client, it then becomes necessary to interpret the data. Through a process of inferential reasoning and judgment the nurse interprets data to decide what information has meaning in relation to the client's health status (Gordon, 1994). Inferential reasoning involves the process of attaching new meaning to known clinical data. For example, consider the following situation: When entering the client's room at 6 AM the nurse notices the client is out of

bed in the chair and the bed linen is pulled down to the end of the bed and twisted in a lump, with the blanket on the floor. (Inference: the bed linen is in disarray.) Closer inspection finds the client sitting up in the chair, holding his incision firmly, breathing slowly, and stating, "I didn't get much sleep last night." (Inference: the client received inadequate sleep.) A pattern of clinical data takes shape. In this example of inference in practice, one nurse will infer inadequate sleep and then assess further the nature of the problem. In this case, assessment of the client's comfort level may reveal important additional cues. Another nurse may not make the second inference, and simply tidy up the bed and leave the room. Interpretation of data summarizes the data and provides a focus for attention (Gordon, 1994). Critical thinking in client assessment enables a nurse to fully understand a client's problems, judge the extent of the problems more carefully, and discover possible relationships between problems.

Data Clustering

After validating and interpreting assessment data, the nurse organizes the information into meaningful clusters, keeping in mind the client's response to illness. A cluster is a set of signs or symptoms that are grouped together in a logical order. During data clustering, the nurse organizes data and focuses attention on client functions needing support and assistance for recovery. Focused data clustering using a systems approach or functional health pattern approach assists the nurse in correctly classifying and organizing data. For example, a client who has recently been diagnosed with diabetes, has had no opportunity to talk with a physician, and is asking questions about insulin obviously has a problem related to inadequate knowledge. As the nurse clusters cues, such as the client asking questions and reporting no previous experience with insulin use, a pattern of meaning forms. Clustering of data helps to focus on identification of the correct problem.

During data clustering, certain cues alert the nurse's thinking processes more than others. These cues help to generate nursing diagnoses (see Chapter 16). The nurse becomes experienced in recognizing features of health problems, such as pain, anxiety, or immobility. Over time the nurse stores knowledge from previous experiences so that more complicated clustering becomes recognizable. This explains the difference in the skill of a beginning nurse and a more expert nurse. Box 15-5 demonstrates focused data clustering using the system-oriented assessment and functional health pattern assessment completed on Mr. Brown. Sometimes cues for more than one nursing diagnosis overlap. For example, anger is a cue for the diagnoses of *anxiety, fear, ineffective coping,* and *caregiver role strain.* In this case the nurse must go back and gather and confirm additional data to be sure the correct diagnosis is made.

Data Documentation

Data documentation is the last part of a complete assessment. A thorough, concise, and accurate documentation

---

Box 15-5   **Focused Data Clustering for Mr. Brown**

System-Oriented Format

Integumentary System
Intact, flushed skin that is hot and dry to touch
Dry oral mucosa, coated tongue, and cracked lips

Gastrointestinal System
Distended, firm abdomen that is tender to palpation in lower quadrants
Hyperactive bowel sounds in all quadrants
History of diarrhea and cramping for 3 weeks
Poor nutritional intake over last week

Medical Record
Laboratory tests indicating elevated while blood cell (WBC) count and hematocrit level: hypernatremia
Abdominal x-ray examination showing gas-filled loops of bowel
Admitting diagnosis of gastroenteritis

Functional Health Pattern Format

Activity and Exercise Pattern
Statement of increased fatigue when walking
Demonstration of ability to perform activities of daily living (ADLs)
Fatigued, dyspneic, and diaphoretic appearance when performing ADLs
Increased pulse from 90 to 126 beats per minute during ADLs

Sleep and Rest Pattern
Report of difficulty in falling and remaining asleep
Denial of use of sleeping aids

Coping–Stress Tolerance Pattern
Anxiety about illness
Pain

Medical Record
Previous history of decreased activity tolerance and poor sleeping. Diagnosed with emphysema 1 year ago.
Chest x-ray film showing pulmonary congestion

---

of facts is necessary when recording client data (Figure 15-7). If an item is not recorded, it is lost and unavailable to anyone else caring for the client. If specific information is not given, the reader is left with only general impressions. Observation and recording of client status is a legal and professional responsibility. The nurse practice acts in all states and the American Nurses Association Policy Statement (2003) and Standards of Clinical Nursing Practice (1998) mandate accurate data collection and recording as independent functions essential to the role of the professional nurse.

Being factual is easy after it becomes a habit. The basic rule is to record all observations. When recording data, a nurse should pay attention to facts and should make an effort to be as descriptive as possible. Anything heard, seen, felt, or smelled should be reported exactly. Objective information must be recorded in accurate terminology (e.g., weighs 170 kg, abdomen is soft and nontender to palpation). Subjective information from a client should be recorded in quotation marks. When entering data, a nurse avoids generalizing or forming judgments through written communication. Conclusions about such data become nursing diagnoses and thus must be accurate. As a nurse gains experience and becomes familiar with patterns of signs and symptoms, he or she may correctly conclude the existence of that problem.

Concise information is also crucial. Documentation of ongoing assessments need not include repetitive data such as the client's age, diagnosis, or social-family history, if it has already been documented in the chart. Thorough documentation ensures that information is available to those caring for the client's needs. A general rule of thumb is that if it was assessed, it should be recorded.

Key Concepts

- The nursing process employs critical thinking to identify, diagnose, and treat human responses to health and illness.
- Nursing assessment involves the collection and verification of data and the analysis of all data to establish a database about a client's needs, health problems, and responses to those problems.
- Good assessment requires the nurse to apply knowledge and experience in making the necessary observations and measurements to gather data about clients.
- An assessment must be relevant to a client's problems and focused so that a comprehensive database, moving from general to specific, can be gathered.
- A nurse critically anticipates and uses an appropriate branching set of questions or observations to collect data and cluster cues of assessment information to identify emerging patterns and problems.
- Written data statements should be descriptive, concise, and complete and should not include inferences or interpretative statements.
- Collection of inaccurate, incomplete, or inappropriate data may result in incorrect identification of the client's health care needs.
- Subjective data are the client's perceptions.
- Family members and members of the health care team are important sources of information about the client's health status.
- When beginning an assessment, it is important to encourage clients to tell their stories about their illnesses or health care problems.

BARNES HOSPITAL ST. LOUIS, MISSOURI	Brown, William 4823 Independence Dr. Yorktown, MO

Person to Contact: Hannah (wife)	Emergency Phone:	555-4821

Why you came to the hospital? "To find out why I've had diarrhea for 3 weeks"

Allergies (food, drugs, latex, environment)?
Penicillin

Items brought in from home? ☐ Medications ☐ Dentures ☐ Contacts ☑ Glasses ☐ Hearing Aid	Did you bring: ☐ Money ☐ Jewelry ☐ Credit Cards ☐ Checkbook/Checks ☐ Other _____ *(These need to be locked up with security or sent home. Hospital will not be responsible* *for valuables left in room)* All sent home c̄ Hannah Brown

	MEDICINE NAMES	Dose & How Often Taken	Reason You Take Medicine	Time of Last Dose
	immodium	2 tabs	diarrhea	2° ago
Prescribed by a Doctor				
	acetaminophen		headaches	2 wks ago
Non-Prescription				

Do you have any problems with your medicines?

No – "but it isn't working"

Do you smoke? ☑ Yes ☐ No Do you chew tobacco? ☐ Yes ☑ No	Do you use "street" drugs? ☐ Yes ☑ No How much alcohol do you drink? _____	How much caffeine do you drink or eat? 4 cups coffee

Medical History:
☐ Heart Disease	☐ Epilepsy	☐ Cancer	☐ Chicken Pox/Shingles	☐ Menstrual Disease
☐ Lung Disease	☐ Stroke	☐ Hepatitis	☐ Fainting/Dizzy Spells	☐ Circulation Problems
☐ Liver Disease	☐ Diabetes	☐ High Blood Pressure	☐ Stomach Problems	☐ Swelling
☐ Immune Disorders	☐ TB	☐ Rheumatic Disease	☐ Bladder Problems	☐ Bleeding
☐ Other _____		☐ Sexually Transmitted Disease: _____		

HISTORY COMMENTS:

Could you be pregnant?   ☐ Yes   ☐ No   N/A   When was you last Period? _____

What surgeries or procedures have you had? (Date)

Family Health History: ☐ Hypertension   ☐ Diabetes   ☑ Heart Disease   ☐ Stroke   ☑ Cancer   ☐ Other _____

Which of the following have you had in the past 12 months?
☐ Self Breast Exam	☐ Prostate Check	☑ Glaucoma Check	☑ Rectal Check (over 40)	☑ Dental Exam
☐ Mammogram (over 40)	☑ Testicular Check	☐ Pelvic Exam	☐ Hearing Check	☑ Vision Check

Are your immunizations current?   ☑ Yes   ☐ No   ☐ Unknown
(Call ID Specialist)

FIGURE **15–7**   Admission nursing history for Mr. Brown.   *Continued*

Are you on a special diet? "no - but diarrhea occurs after all meals"	How is your appetite? poor last week
Any foods you can't eat and why? "everything causes diarrhea"	Any difficulty eating or swallow- no
Nutritional supplements/or diet substitutions (e.g., vitamins, artificial sweeteners salt, substitutes)	Weight loss/gain (amount) in the last 12 months? 15 lb. weight loss in last 3 weeks

How often do you have a BM? diarrhea
Do you have any difficulty having a bowel movement?
☐ use laxatives   ☐ hemorrhoids
☐ use stool softeners   ☐ black/tarry

Do you tire easily?   ☑ Yes   ☐ No

Have you fallen recently?   ☐ Yes   ☑ No

Do you have any difficulty urinating? no
☐ burning   ☐ blood   ☐ leaking   ☐ frequency

Do you get regular exercise?   ☐ Yes   ☐ No
What kind? _____   How often? _____
Usually walk ½ mile/day - hasn't done this for 1 mo.

What activities do you need help with?
☐ Feeding/eating   ☐ Meal preparation   ☐ Walking on level surfaces
☐ Dressing   ☐ Transportation   ☑ Walking on stairs
☐ Grooming/bathing   ☐ Housework   ☐ Paying for Medicines
☐ Taking medications   ☐ Handling finances
☐ Toileting   ☐ Grocery shopping
☐ Moving/positioning

(RN consider appropriate consults)

Aides used at home:
☑ Eye glasses   ☐ Contact lenses
☐ Hearing aid   ☐ Cane
☐ Walker   ☐ Wheelchair
☐ Prosthesis: _____
DENTURES: ☐ Upper   ☐ Lower
PARTIALS: ☐ Upper   ☐ Lower

Is it difficult for you to carry out prescribed health care regimens (Diet, Activity, Medications)?   ☐ Yes   ☐ No
If YES, explain: During last week, increased fatigue, increased abdominal pain

How much sleep do you normally get? 8 hrs.

What helps you fall asleep? nothing

Who do you live with?	☐ Alone	☐ Spouse only	☑ Family	☐ Friends	☐ Nursing Home
Who helps you at home?	☑ Spouse	☐ Family	☐ Friends	☐ Home Health	☐ Visiting Nurse

Do you have concerns about your family while you are in the hospital? no

What major changes have you had in your life in the past 12 months? none

Do you feel you deal successfully with stress?   ☑ Yes   ☐ No
"Afraid that I have cancer"

Would you like additional resources?   ☑ Yes   ☐ No

Do you have concerns that your illness/hospitalization will affect:
☐ appearance   ☐ job   ☐ male/female roles   ☐ how you feel about yourself

Is religion important in your life?   ☐ Yes   ☐ No
yes - Methodist

Will this illness/hospitalization interfere with any religious beliefs/practices?   ☐ Yes   ☑ No

What do you expect from us while in the hospital?
"To stop my diarrhea + pain" and "to tell me I don't have cancer"

Do you have a Living Will?   ☑ Yes   ☐ No
Do you have a copy with you?   ☑ Yes   ☐ No

Do you have a Power of Attorney?   ☑ Yes   ☐ No

Patient/Significant Other Signature: Relationship: William Brown	Date 7/3	Staff Signature: Title: Gary Jones, RN	Date 7/3

☐ REVIEWED BY REGISTERED NURSE   SIGNATURE: Gary Jones, RN   DATE: 7/3

TO BE COMPLETED BY STAFF ONLY

Patient provided: ☑ Admit kit   ☑ ID band   ☑ Sensitivity/Allergy band on patient   ☑ Allergy sticker on chart
Patient instructed: ☑ Valuables policy   ☑ Waiver signed   ☑ Smoking   ☑ Visitation
☑ Nursing call/Emergency   ☑ TV/phone   ☐ Fall precautions/band on wrist
☑ Patient's Rights/responsibilities   ☑ Received copy of Personal Directions for My Healthcare

Time patient arrived on Division: 0850   SIGNATURE: Gary Coffey

FIGURE **15–7, cont'd**   Admission nursing history for Mr. Brown.

- The interview is an organized conversation with a client that begins by establishing a therapeutic relationship with the client and that aids in the investigation and discussion of the client's health care needs.
- An interview includes an orientation, working, and termination phase.
- During an interview, clients obtain information about the health care environment, treatments, testing, and available resources.
- The nursing health history involves data about level of wellness, past medical history, family history, environmental history, psychosocial and cultural history, and a review of the body systems.
- To form a nursing judgment, the nurse critically assesses a client, validates the data, interprets the information gathered, looks for diagnostic cues, and identifies the client's problems.

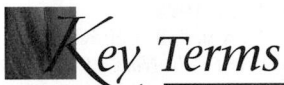ey Terms

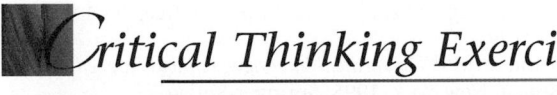ritical Thinking Exercises

1. Consider the following scenario:

   "Mr. Williams, I am your nurse, Sarah Mason. I am going to be asking some questions about your health so that we can do a good job planning your nursing care. Before we begin, do you have any questions?" (Patient has none.) "Ok, let's begin by my asking you, What has brought you to the hospital?" (Patient has had recurrent chest pain for 3 days.) "Is the pain sharp? Dull? Tell me what causes you to have the pain." (Pain begins with exercise.) "Is there anything else that causes you to have pain?"

   Critique this scenario by answering the following questions:

   a. During the interaction what questions did Sara use that were open ended?

   b. Did Sarah probe to exhaustion? If so, what was the purpose?

   c. Critique Sarah's introduction.

   d. What is the advantage of open-ended questions over closed-ended questions?

2. Mrs. Lewis comes to the well-baby clinic for her infant's 1-month examination. She tells her nurse, Ethan, that the baby has not been sleeping well during the night. In addition, Mrs. Lewis has noted a rash on the baby's abdomen. Write three questions that Ethan might ask to assess the two potential problems Mrs. Lewis has presented. What assessment technique might the nurse apply to assess the rash that would not be used to assess the baby's sleep pattern?

3. Dallas Hanson is waiting to have surgery this morning for a cancerous tumor of the larynx. He tells the nurse, "I am afraid I will not be able to speak again." The nurse asks, "What has your physician explained about the possible outcomes of surgery?" Mr. Hanson states, "He thinks he can save my voice but will not know until he gets inside and sees the tumor." The nurse asks, "Are you having any discomfort right now?" "No," replies Mr. Hanson. The nurse takes a set of vital signs while preparing Mr. Hanson for transport to the operating room. The nurse also examines Mr. Hanson's intravenous site, looking for any inflammation around the insertion area. She notes the site is clear, without inflammation or tenderness.

   Describe the subjective and objective data gathered in this scenario.

Review Questions

1. The purpose of assessment is to:
   1. Establish a database concerning the client.
   2. Teach the client about his or her health.
   3. Implement nursing care.
   4. Delegate nursing responsibility.

2. Critical thinking is the active, organized, cognitive process used to carefully examine one's thinking. Utilizing critical thinking during assessment allows the nurse to:
   1. Review the assessment with other healthcare providers.
   2. Determine the nursing care was delivered.
   3. Identify the anticipated client response to care.
   4. Direct the assessment in a meaningful and purposeful way.

3. Assessment data must be descriptive, concise, and complete. An assessment should not include:
   1. Inferences or interpretative statements that are unsupported with data.
   2. A detailed physical examination.
   3. The use of interpersonal and cognitive skills.
   4. Subjective data from the client.

4. Data collection includes the gathering of subjective and objective data from or about a client. Subjective data are:
   1. Observations made by the data collector.
   2. Ancillary reports from other services.
   3. Client's perceptions about their health problems.
   4. Obtained from the physician history and physical form.

5. One of the most important skills needed to obtain accurate information from your client is (are):
   1. Teaching and assessment.
   2. Cognitive and teaching.
   3. Good communication and critical thinking.
   4. Psychomotor.

6. The first step in establishing the database is to collect subjective information by interviewing the client. An interview is:
   1. An organized conversation with the client.
   2. Implementation of physician orders.
   3. Determining specific nursing actions.
   4. Delegating personnel responsible for care.

7. An interview with a client includes three phases, similar to those of a therapeutic relationship. These phases include:
   1. Orientation, working, and termination.
   2. Orientation, assessment, and delegation.
   3. Planning, evaluation, and assessment.
   4. Trust, planning, and honesty.

8. During data clustering the nurse:
   1. Implements the nursing process.
   2. Provides documentation of nursing care.
   3. Organizes data and focuses attention on client functions.
   4. Reviews the data with other healthcare providers.

9. A nurse might ask, "Do you have pain or cramping?" This is an example of:
   1. Problem seeking questioning.
   2. Open-ended questioning.
   3. Closed-ended questioning.
   4. Active listening.

10. A technique that allows for discussion is the use of:
    1. Use of closed-ended questions.
    2. Use of open-ended questions.
    3. Back channeling.
    4. Problem seeking.

References

Agency for Health Care Policy and Research, Acute Pain Management Guideline Panel: *Acute pain management: operative or medical procedures and trauma,* Clinical Practice Guideline, AHCPR Pub No. 92-0032, Rockville, Md, 1992, Agency for Health Care Policy and Research, Public Health Service, U.S. Department of Health and Human Services.

American Nurses Association: *Nursing's social policy statement,* ed 2, Washington, DC, 2003, The Association.

American Nurses Association: *Standards of clinical nursing practice,* American Nurses Association, ed 2, Washington, DC, 1998, American Nurses Publishing.

Bandman EL, Bandman B: *Critical thinking in nursing,* ed 2, Norwalk, Conn, 1995, Appleton & Lange.

Benner P, Wrubel J: *The primacy of caring,* Menlo Park, Calif, 1989, Addison-Wesley.

Bryans A, McIntosh J: Decision making in community nursing: an analysis of the stages of decision making as they relate to community nursing, *J Adv Nurs* 24(1):24, 1996.

Caris-Verhallen WMC and others: Non-verbal behaviour in nurse-elderly patient communication, *J Adv Nurs* 29(4):808, 1999.

Carnevali DL, Thomas MD: *Diagnostic reasoning and treatment decision making in nursing,* Philadelphia, 1993, JB Lippincott.

Carpenito LJ: *Nursing diagnosis: application to clinical practice,* ed 6, Philadelphia, 1995, JB Lippincott.

Carpenito LJ: *Nursing diagnosis: application to clinical practice,* ed 7, Philadelphia, 2000, JB Lippincott.

Copi IM, Cohen C: *Introduction to logic,* ed 9, New York, 1994, Macmillan.

Gordon M: *Manual of nursing diagnoses: 1991–1992,* St. Louis, 1991, Mosby.

Gordon M: *Nursing diagnosis: process and application,* ed 3, St. Louis, 1994, Mosby.

HIPAAdvisory, OCR guidance explaining significant aspects of the privacy rule, http://www.hipaadvisory.com/regs/finalprivacymod/guidance.htm.

Hurst K and others: The recognition and non-recognition of problem-solving stages in nursing practice, *J Adv Nurs* 16:1444, 1991.

Lipkin M and others: *The medical interview: clinical care, education, and research,* New York, 1995, Springer-Verlag.

Pender NJ: *Health promotion and nursing practice,* ed 3, Stamford, Conn, 1996, Appleton & Lange.

Ryan-Wenger NM: A nursing process methodology, *Nurs Outlook* 38(4):190, 1990.

Seidel HM and others: *Mosby's guide to physical examination,* ed 5, St. Louis, 2003, Mosby.

16

$\mathcal{N}$ursing Diagnosis

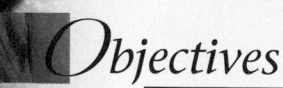

Objectives

Mastery of content in this chapter will enable the student to:

- Define the key terms listed.
- Differentiate between a nursing diagnosis and a medical diagnosis.
- Discuss the relationship of critical thinking to the nursing diagnostic process.
- List and discuss the steps of the nursing diagnostic process.
- Explain the relationship of defining characteristics to assessment cues.
- Explain the importance of the related factor in a nursing diagnosis.
- Explain what makes a nursing diagnosis correct.
- Discuss the limitations of nursing diagnoses.
- Formulate nursing diagnoses from a nursing assessment.

When physicians refer to commonly accepted medical diagnoses, such as myocardial infarction, diabetes mellitus, or osteoarthritis, they all know the meaning of the diagnoses and the standard approaches used for treatment. A **medical diagnosis** is the identification of a disease condition based on a specific evaluation of physical signs, symptoms, the client's medical history, and the results of diagnostic tests and procedures. Physicians are licensed to treat diseases or pathological processes described in medical diagnostic statements.

Nursing has a similar diagnostic language. Nursing diagnosis, the second step of the nursing process, is a term used to classify health problems within the domain of nursing. Diagnosis means "to distinguish" or "to know." A **nursing diagnosis** is a clinical judgment about individual, family, or community responses to actual and potential health problems or life processes (NANDA International, 2003). It is a statement that describes the client's actual or potential response to a health problem that the nurse is licensed and competent to treat. *Impaired skin integrity, risk for infection,* and *deficient knowledge* are examples of nursing diagnoses. Just as a medical diagnosis of diabetes mellitus provides the basis for selection of medical therapies such as insulin administration, an 1800-calorie diet, and a moderate exercise program, the nursing diagnosis of *impaired skin integrity* provides the basis for selection of nursing therapies such as application of pressure relief devices, regular turning schedules, and skin care. Nursing diagnoses provide the basis for selection of nursing interventions to achieve outcomes for which the nurse is accountable (NANDA International, 2003). The accurate selection of nursing diagnoses requires a nurse to use critical thinking and good clinical judgment. The statement of a nursing diagnosis is the result of a diagnostic process during which the nurse critically analyzes physical, developmental, intellectual, emotional, social, and spiritual assessment data (see Chapter 15).

Evolution of Nursing Diagnosis

When nursing schools were initially established, school curricula were organized around disease entities or medical models as frameworks for describing the role of the nurse in providing nursing care. However, in the mid 1950s and early 1960s, nursing leaders and educators started to revise curricula around **client-centered problems** (Carpenito, 1997). Nursing diagnosis was first introduced in the nursing literature in 1950 (McFarland and McFarlane, 1989). Fry (1953) proposed that nursing could be more creative by the formulation of nursing diagnoses and an individualized nursing care plan. This emphasized the nurse's independent practice (e.g., education and symptom relief) compared with the dependent practice driven by physicians' orders (e.g., medication administration and wound treatment). Initially, nursing diagnoses were not supported by professional nursing, and in 1955 the *Model Nurse Practice Act* of the American Nurses Association (ANA) excluded diagnosis or prescriptive therapies (ANA, 1955). As a result, nurses hesitated to use nursing diagnoses in their practice.

However, nursing theorists encouraged defining nursing in terms of client problems. Early theorists, by defining nursing intervention in terms of client-centered problems, were partly responsible for the interest and eventual use of nursing diagnosis in contemporary nursing education, practice, administration, and research (see Chapter 4).

In 1973 the first national conference for the classification of nursing diagnosis was held to identify nursing functions and establish a classification system. "A classification system for nursing defines the body of knowledge for which nursing is held accountable" (Carpenito, 1995). Over the years, participants of these conferences have developed the accepted nursing diagnoses (Box 16-1). In 1982 a professional association, the North American Nursing Diagnosis Association (NANDA), was established. The purpose of NANDA was "to develop, refine, and promote a taxonomy of nursing diagnostic terminology of general use for professional nurses" (Kim, McFarland, and McLean, 1984). Recently NANDA changed its name to **NANDA International** (NANDA International, 2003) to better reflect the international utility of nursing diagnosis for the global health community. NANDA International's work provides a common language for the health problems nurses deal with. The organization is the leader in nursing diagnosis classification and is endorsed by the ANA as having the responsibility to do so.

Nursing diagnosis was first incorporated into the ANA *Standards of Nursing Practice* (1973) in 1971, and it remains in the current *Standards of Clinical Nursing Practice* (ANA, 2003). In 1987 the definition of nursing diagnosis was strengthened in the refined definition of nursing in ANA's paper *Scope of Nursing Practice,* which defines nursing as the diagnosis and treatment of human responses to health and illness (ANA, 1987). The ANA included diagnosis as a separate activity in its publication *Nursing: A Social Policy Statement* (ANA, 1980). As a result, most state

---

Box 16-1   NANDA Nursing Diagnoses

Activity intolerance	Perceived **Constipation**
Risk for **Activity** intolerance	Risk for **Constipation**
Impaired **Adjustment**	**Coping**
Ineffective **Airway** clearance	Ineffective **Coping**
Latex **Allergy** response	Ineffective community **Coping**
Risk for latex **Allergy** response	Readiness for enhanced community **Coping**
Anxiety	Defensive **Coping**
Death **Anxiety**	Compromised family **Coping**
Risk for **Aspiration**	Disabled family **Coping**
Risk for impaired parent/infant/child **Attachment**	Readiness for enhanced family **Coping**
Autonomic dysreflexia	Ineffective **Denial**
Risk for **Autonomic** dysreflexia	Impaired **Dentition**
Disturbed **Body** image	Risk for delayed **Development**
Risk for imbalanced **Body** temperature	**Diarrhea**
Bowel incontinence	Risk for **Disuse** syndrome
Effective **Breastfeeding**	Deficient **Diversional** activity
Ineffective **Breastfeeding**	Disturbed **Energy** field
Interrupted **Breastfeeding**	Impaired **Environmental** interpretation syndrome
Ineffective **Breathing** pattern	Adult **Failure** to thrive
Decreased **Cardiac** output	Risk for **Falls**
Caregiver role strain	Dysfunctional **Family** processes: alcoholism
Risk for **Caregiver** role strain	**Family** processes
Impaired **Comfort**	Interrupted **Family** processes
Impaired verbal **Communication**	**Fatigue**
Readiness for enhanced **Communication**	**Fear**
Decisional **Conflict**	**Fluid** balance
Parental role **Conflict**	Deficient **Fluid** volume
Acute **Confusion**	Excess **Fluid** volume
Chronic **Confusion**	Risk for deficient **Fluid** volume
Constipation	Risk for imbalanced **Fluid** volume

Used with permission from NANDA International: *NANDA nursing diagnoses: definitions and classification 2003-2004,* Philadelphia, 2003, NANDA International.

Continued

Box 16-1   NANDA Nursing Diagnoses—cont'd

Impaired **Gas** exchange	**Rape-trauma** syndrome: compound reaction
Grieving	**Rape-trauma** syndrome: silent reaction
Anticipatory **Grieving**	**Relocation** stress syndrome
Dysfunctional **Grieving**	Risk for **Relocation** stress syndrome
Delayed **Growth** and development	Ineffective **Role** performance
Risk for disproportionate **Growth**	Bathing/hygiene **Self-care** deficit
Ineffective **Health** maintenance	Dressing/grooming **Self-care** deficit
Health-seeking behaviors	Feeding **Self-care** deficit
Impaired **Home** maintenance	Toileting **Self-care** deficit
Hopelessness	**Self-concept**
Hyperthermia	Chronic low **Self-esteem**
Hypothermia	Situational low **Self-esteem**
Disturbed personal **Identity**	Risk for situational low **Self-esteem**
Functional urinary **Incontinence**	**Self-mutilation**
Reflex urinary **Incontinence**	Risk for **Self-mutilation**
Stress urinary **Incontinence**	Disturbed **Sensory** perception
Total urinary **Incontinence**	**Sexual** dysfunction
Urge urinary **Incontinence**	Ineffective **Sexuality** patterns
Risk for urge urinary **Incontinence**	Impaired **Skin** integrity
Disorganized **Infant** behavior	Risk for impaired **Skin** integrity
Risk for disorganized **Infant** behavior	**Sleep**
Readiness for enhanced organized **Infant** behavior	**Sleep** deprivation
Ineffective **Infant** feeding pattern	Disturbed **Sleep** pattern
Risk for **Infection**	Impaired **Social** interaction
Risk for **Injury**	**Social** isolation
Risk for perioperative-positioning **Injury**	Chronic **Sorrow**
Decreased **Intracranial** adaptive capacity	**Spiritual** distress
Deficient **Knowledge**	Risk for **Spiritual** distress
Knowledge (specify)	Readiness for enhanced **Spiritual** well-being
Risk for **Loneliness**	Risk for **Sudden Infant Death Syndrome**
Impaired **Memory**	Risk for **Suffocation**
Impaired bed **Mobility**	Risk for **Suicide**
Impaired physical **Mobility**	Delayed **Surgical** recovery
Impaired wheelchair **Mobility**	Impaired **Swallowing**
Nausea	Effective **Therapeutic** regimen management
Unilateral **Neglect**	Ineffective **Therapeutic** regimen management
Noncompliance	Ineffective community **Therapeutic** regimen management
Imbalanced **Nutrition:** less than body requirements	Ineffective family **Therapeutic** regimen management
Imbalanced **Nutrition:** more than body requirements	Management of **Therapeutic** regimen
Nutrition	Ineffective **Thermoregulation**
Risk for imbalanced **Nutrition:** more than body requirements	Disturbed **Thought** processes
Impaired **Oral** mucous membrane	Impaired **Tissue** integrity
Acute **Pain**	Ineffective **Tissue** perfusion
Chronic **Pain**	Impaired **Transfer** ability
Impaired **Parenting**	Risk for **Trauma**
Parenting	Impaired **Urinary** elimination
Risk for impaired **Parenting**	**Urinary** elimination
Risk for **Peripheral** neurovascular dysfunction	**Urinary** retention
Risk for **Poisoning**	Impaired spontaneous **Ventilation**
Post-trauma syndrome	Dysfunctional **Ventilatory** weaning response
Risk for **Post-trauma** syndrome	Risk for other-directed **Violence**
Powerlessness	Risk for self-directed **Violence**
Risk for **Powerlessness**	Impaired **Walking**
Ineffective **Protection**	**Wandering**
Rape-trauma syndrome	

Used with permission from NANDA International: *NANDA nursing diagnoses: definitions and classification 2003-2004,* Philadelphia, 2003, NANDA International.

nurse practice acts include nursing diagnosis as part of the domain of nursing practice.

Recently work has been under way to create a unifying structure that links NANDA International nursing diagnoses and the nursing intervention (NIC) and nursing outcome (NOC) classifications developed by the Center for Nursing Classification and Clinical Effectiveness at the University of Iowa College of Nursing (Dochterman and Jones, 2003). The goal is to advance the development, testing, and refinement of a common nursing language. Nurses assist clients in improving their health outcomes through assessment, diagnosis, planning, intervention, and evaluation. A standardized nursing language incorporating NANDA, NIC, and NOC (NNN) represents a pooled nursing knowledge base for use in the nursing process (Dochterman and Jones, 2003).

Research in the field of nursing diagnosis continues to grow. As a result, new diagnostic labels are continually developed and added to the NANDA International listing (see Box 16-1, p. 301). The use of standard formal nursing diagnostic statements serves several purposes:

- Nursing diagnoses offer a language to promote understanding between nurses about clients' health problems so as to facilitate communication and care planning.
- Nursing diagnoses distinguish the nurse's role from that of the physician.
- Nursing diagnoses help nurses to focus on the role of nursing in client care.

The use of nursing diagnosis continues to draw interest because of its nature as a nursing vocabulary. With the development of a common language in nursing, there can be improvement in the documentation of care, a greater ability to link nursing contributions to quality outcomes, and the ability to cost out nursing care services (Jones, 2001).

Critical Thinking and the Nursing Diagnostic Process

Critical thinking is an active, organized, cognitive process used to carefully examine one's thinking and the thinking of others (Chaffee, 1994). The process is applicable to the formation of nursing diagnoses (Figure 16-1). A nurse integrates what is known from previous experience and scientific and practical knowledge bases, applies critical thinking attitudes and intellectual standards, and refers to standards of practice in making well reasoned, accurate, and relevant nursing diagnoses. The critical thinking process (see Chapter 14) is required in diagnostic reasoning and judgment.

Diagnostic Process

Diagnostic reasoning is a process of using the data gathered about a client to logically explain a clinical judgment, in this case making a nursing diagnosis. The **diagnostic process** includes decision-making steps, including gathering the assessment database, validating data, analyzing and interpreting data, identifying client needs, and

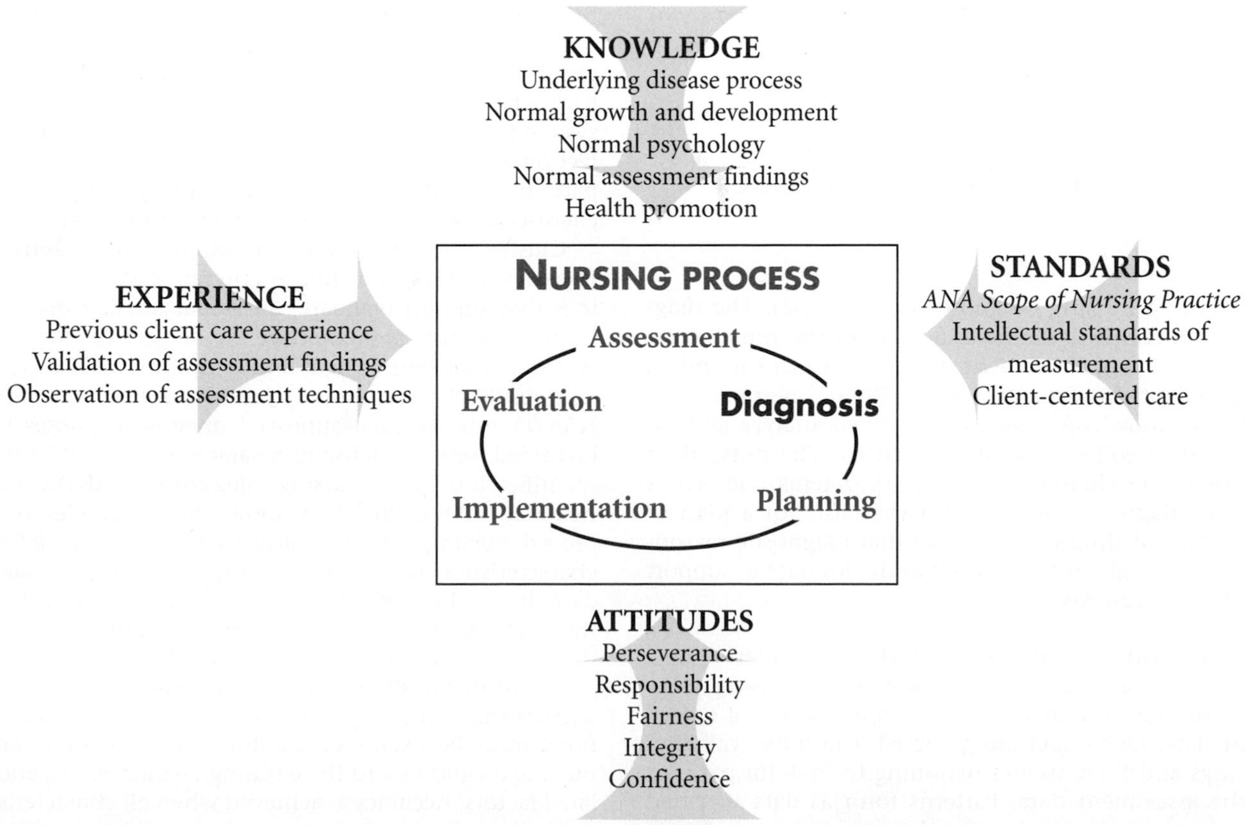

KNOWLEDGE
Underlying disease process
Normal growth and development
Normal psychology
Normal assessment findings
Health promotion

EXPERIENCE
Previous client care experience
Validation of assessment findings
Observation of assessment techniques

NURSING PROCESS
Assessment
Evaluation   **Diagnosis**
Implementation   Planning

STANDARDS
ANA Scope of Nursing Practice
Intellectual standards of measurement
Client-centered care

ATTITUDES
Perseverance
Responsibility
Fairness
Integrity
Confidence

FIGURE **16–1**   Critical thinking and the nursing diagnostic process.

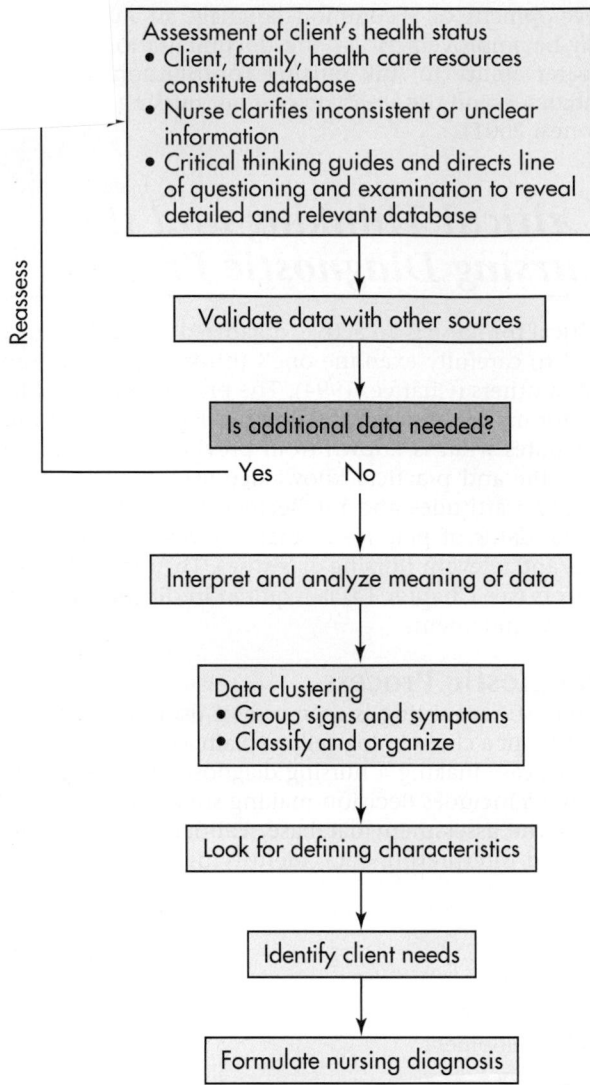

FIGURE **16–2**   Nursing diagnostic process.

formulating nursing diagnoses (Figure 16-2). The diagnostic process is dynamic and requires the nurse to reflect on existing assessment data and health care needs of the client (Da Cruz and Acuri, 1998). The nurse uses scientific knowledge and experience to analyze and interpret data collected about the client. The nurse then identifies the client's health care problems and writes nursing diagnoses, which form the basis for a plan of care. Clinical situations demand that diagnostic reasoning be thorough and rigorous in order for data to support a nursing diagnosis.

Analysis and Interpretation of Data. Chapter 15 discusses in detail the steps for formalizing nursing judgment through the analysis and interpretation of assessment data. Once data are gathered, the nurse validates findings and then applies reasoning to look for patterns in the assessment data. Patterns form as data is sorted into clusters or categories. The database is continually revised when additional information is needed to include

changes in the client's physical and emotional status and the results of laboratory and diagnostic tests.

Data analysis involves recognizing patterns or trends, comparing them with standards, and coming to a reasoned conclusion about the client's response to a health problem (Box 16-2). When looking for a pattern or trend, the nurse examines clusters of data that are a set of signs or symptoms grouped together in a logical order. Alone these signs or symptoms tell the nurse little, and no diagnostic conclusion can be made. However, when these signs are placed or clustered together as a group, the nurse sees a relationship between and among these assessment findings. The client Mr. Brown was introduced in Chapter 15. Box 16-3 includes a summary of relevant data collected by Mr. Coffey (the RN case manager) from Mr. Brown's assessment. Singly these symptoms could be related to multiple nursing diagnoses, but analyzing these together the nurse begins to think about functional health patterns (e.g., client's elimination pattern) or body system function (e.g., oxygenation), and the potential effect on Mr. Brown's health. When the nurse recognizes a pattern and identifies a relationship among patterns, client-centered needs begin to emerge (Box 16-4).

Clusters and patterns of data often contain **defining characteristics,** the clinical criteria or assessment findings that support (validate) an actual nursing diagnosis. Clinical criteria are objective or subjective signs and symptoms, clusters of signs and symptoms, or risk factors. As a result of research and clinical practice observation, NANDA International–approved nursing diagnoses have identified sets of defining characteristics that support identification of a nursing diagnosis (NANDA International, 2003). Box 16-5 shows two examples of approved nursing diagnoses and their associated defining characteristics and related factors. As a nurse analyzes data, he or she may begin to consider various diagnoses that might apply to the client. It is important to recognize that the absence of defining characteristics suggest that a proposed diagnosis should be rejected. Defining characteristics that either support or eliminate a particular diagnosis must be examined carefully. A nurse must know nursing diagnoses and the defining characteristics and related factors. Accuracy is achieved when all characteristics are evaluated, nonrelevant ones are eliminated, and relevant ones are confirmed (Collier and others, 1996).

Box 16-3 **Summary of Relevant Data From Mr. Brown's Complete Assessment**

Physical and Developmental

Diarrhea for 3 weeks
Productive cough upon rising each morning
Occasional rales in lung bases
15-pound weight loss 3 weeks before hospitalization
Hemoglobin 12 g/100 ml
Slight change of emphysema shown on chest roentgenogram
Distended abdomen
Squamous cell cancer
Biopsy obtained during outpatient colonoscopy June 24
Smoked for 15 years, 2 packs a day (30 pack-years)
Family history of stomach cancer
Family history of heart attack
Married 40 years
Self-employed for 20 years
One adult son, 30 years old
Two sisters, 50 and 48, with no major health problems
Anemia, hemoglobin level of 12 g/100 ml
Crackles auscultated in lung fields

Intellectual

Talkative
Frequently asks nurses if he has cancer and "Can it be treated?"
Good attention span

Emotional

Anxious
Withdrawn after biopsy report of squamous cell cancer
Awaiting colon resection and temporary colostomy

Social

Walks with neighbor
Active in his neighborhood
Married with a son and grandchildren

Spiritual

Methodist
Attends church weekly
Reads Bible daily

Box 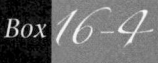 16-4 **Example of Data Analysis: Mr. William Brown**

Recognize Pattern (Cluster of Defining Characteristics)

Diarrhea for 3 weeks
Ribbon-shaped or watery stools
Distended abdomen
Cramping before and during each bowel movement

Compare With Normal Standards

Soft, formed stool daily
Abdomen soft, nondistended
Defecation nonpainful

Make a Reasoned Conclusion

Bowel elimination problem

While focusing on patterns of defining characteristics, the nurse also compares a client's pattern of data with data that are consistent with normal, healthful patterns. The nurse uses widely accepted norms, such as normal laboratory and diagnostic test values, and professional standards and knowledge as the basis for comparison and judgment. When comparing patterns, the nurse judges whether the grouped signs and symptoms are normal for the client and whether they are within the range of healthful responses. Defining characteristics that are not within healthy norms are isolated and form the basis for problem identification.

Identification of Client Needs. Before finalizing a nursing diagnosis, the nurse identifies the client's general health care needs or problems. For example, after reviewing clusters of data, such as dyspnea, increased respiratory rate, and cough, the nurse recognizes that the client has a general respiratory problem. However, before a nurse can effectively give care, the problem must be more specifically defined. NANDA International has a variety of nursing diagnoses that can apply to a respiratory problem (e.g., *ineffective breathing pattern, impaired gas exchange,* or *ineffective airway clearance*). It is critical for the nurse to eventually arrive at the correct diagnostic label for the client's need (Collier and others, 1996). When identifying the client's general problem, the nurse considers all assessment data and focuses on pertinent, relevant, and abnormal data (Gordon, 1994). It may help the inexperienced nurse to think of the problem identification phase as the general health care problem and the formulation of the nursing diagnosis as the specific health care problem. The nurse moves from general to specific.

It is important to review the assessment data to identify client needs and to not focus solely on the client's illness or medical diagnosis. For example, a client with a diagnosis of *social isolation related to relocation into extended care* has experienced the debilitating disease of Parkinson's syndrome. However, his greatest need is to increase friends, social supports, and familiarity with his new surroundings. Working with the client to resolve this nursing diagnosis will require the nurse to focus on social support rather than the physical symptoms of Parkinson's syndrome. Eventually the nurse will be able to improve the client's independence and level of wellness and help the client avoid future health problems.

Examples of NANDA International–Approved Nursing Diagnoses With Defining Characteristics and Related Factors

Diagnosis: Diarrhea
Definition: Passage of loose, unformed stool

Defining Characteristics:

- At least three loose, liquid stools a day
- Hyperactive bowel sounds
- Urgency
- Abdominal pain
- Cramping

Related Factors:

- *Psychological:* High stress and anxiety
- *Situational:* Alcohol abuse, toxins, laxative abuse, travel, radiation, tube feedings, adverse medication effects, contaminants
- *Physiological:* Inflammation, malabsorption, irritation, infectious processes, parasites

Diagnosis: Hopelessness
Definition: Subjective state in which individual sees limited or no alternatives or personal choices available and is unable to mobilize energy on own behalf.

Defining Characteristics:

- Passivity, decreased verbalization
- Decreased affect
- Verbal cues
- Closing eyes
- Decreased appetite
- Decreased response to stimuli
- Increased/decreased sleep

Related Factors:

- Lack of initiative
- Lack of involvement in care
- Shrugging in response to speaker
- Turning away from speaker
- Abandonment, prolonged activity restriction creating isolation, lost belief in transcendent values/God, long-term stress, failing or deteriorating physiological condition.

From NANDA International: *NANDA nursing diagnoses: definitions and classification, 2003-2004,* Philadelphia, 2003, NANDA International.

Formulation of the Nursing Diagnosis

Once patterns and clusters of data containing defining characteristics are sorted and client needs or problems are identified, the nurse is ready to formulate nursing diagnoses. NANDA International has identified three types of nursing diagnoses: actual diagnoses, at risk diagnoses, and wellness diagnoses (NANDA International, 2003).

An **actual nursing diagnosis** describes human responses to health conditions/life processes that exist in an individual, family, or community. It is a judgment that is supported by defining characteristics (manifestations, signs, and symptoms) that cluster in patterns of related cues or inferences (NANDA International, 2003). The presence of such a diagnosis indicates that sufficient assessment data are available to establish the nursing diagnosis (Collier and others, 1996).

A **risk nursing diagnosis** describes human responses to health conditions/life processes that may develop in a vulnerable individual, family, or community (NANDA International, 2003). For example, a client with a spinal cord injury that limits mobility is at *risk for impaired skin integrity.* The key assessment for this type of diagnosis is the presence of data revealing risk factors that support the client's vulnerability. Such data include physiological, psychosocial, familial, lifestyle, and environmental factors that increase the client's vulnerability to, or likelihood of developing, the condition.

A **wellness nursing diagnosis** describes human responses to levels of wellness in an individual, family, or community that have a readiness for enhancement (NANDA International, 2003). It is a clinical judgment about an individual, group, or community in transition from a specific level of wellness to a higher level of wellness. This type of diagnosis is used when the client wishes to or has achieved an optimal level of health, for example, *family coping: potential for growth related to unexpected birth of twins.* The nurse and the family unit work together to adapt to the stressors associated with twins and identify the family's strengths and resources, as well as their needs. In doing so, the nurse incorporates the client's strength into a plan of care, with the outcome directed at an enhanced level of coping.

Components of a Nursing Diagnosis

The nursing diagnosis flows from the assessment and diagnostic process. Throughout this text, nursing diagnoses are stated in a two-part format: the diagnostic label followed by a statement of a related factor (Table 16-1). It is this two-part format that provides a diagnosis meaning and relevance for a particular client. In addition, all NANDA International–approved diagnoses have a definition. Risk factors are a component of all risk nursing diagnoses.

Diagnostic Label

The diagnostic label is the name of the nursing diagnosis as approved by NANDA International (see Box 16-1,

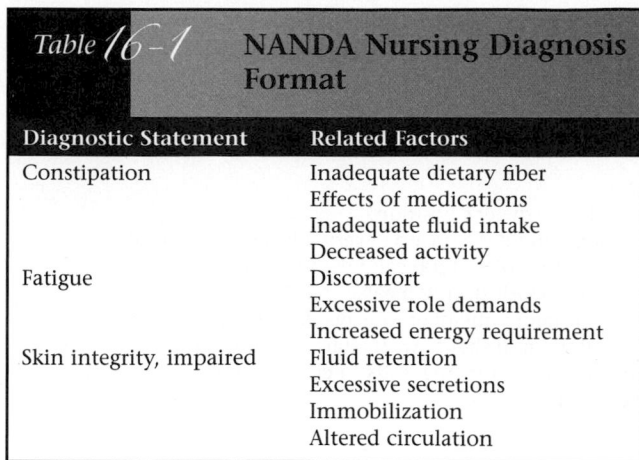

Table 16-1   NANDA Nursing Diagnosis Format

Diagnostic Statement	Related Factors
Constipation	Inadequate dietary fiber
	Effects of medications
	Inadequate fluid intake
	Decreased activity
Fatigue	Discomfort
	Excessive role demands
	Increased energy requirement
Skin integrity, impaired	Fluid retention
	Excessive secretions
	Immobilization
	Altered circulation

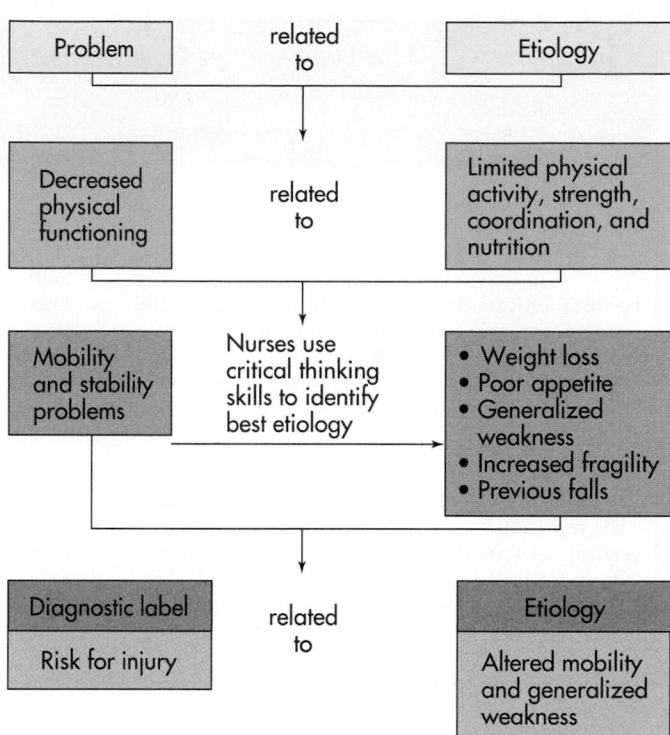

FIGURE 16-3 Relationship between a diagnostic label and etiology (related factor). (Redrawn from Hickey P: *Nursing process handbook,* St. Louis, 1990, Mosby.)

p. 301). It describes the essence of a client's response to health conditions in as few words as possible. Diagnostic labels include descriptors used to give additional meaning to the diagnosis. For example, the diagnosis *impaired physical mobility* includes the descriptor *impaired* to describe the nature or change in mobility that best describes the client's response. Examples of other descriptors include compromised, decreased, deficient, delayed, effective, imbalanced, impaired, and increased.

Related Factors

Related factors are causative or other contributing factors that have influenced the client's actual or potential response to the health problem and can be changed by nursing interventions. For example, the nursing diagnostic statement includes the diagnostic label (e.g., *impaired physical mobility*) and the related factor (e.g., *related to limited range of motion*). Related factors include four categories: pathophysiological (biological or psychological), treatment-related, situational (environmental or personal), and maturational (Carpenito, 1995).

The "related to" phrase identifies the etiology or cause of the client's response to health conditions/life processes. This is not a cause-and-effect statement; rather, it indicates that the etiology contributes to or is associated with the client's diagnosis (Figure 16-3). The inclusion of the "related to" phrase requires a nurse to use critical thinking skills to individualize the diagnosis to ensure appropriate interventions are chosen (Table 16-2).

The **etiology** or cause of the nursing diagnosis must be within the domain of nursing practice and a condition that responds to nursing interventions. Sometimes medical diagnoses are recorded as the etiology of the nursing diagnosis. This is incorrect. Nursing interventions cannot change a medical diagnosis. However, nursing interventions can be directed at behavior or conditions that a nurse can treat or manage. For example, the nursing diagnosis acute pain related to breast cancer is incorrect. Nursing actions cannot affect the medical diagnosis of breast cancer. Rewording the diagnosis to read *acute pain related to impaired skin integrity secondary to mastectomy incision* results in nursing interventions directed at reducing stress on the suture line and improving the client's comfort.

Definition

NANDA approves a definition for each diagnosis following clinical use and testing. The definition describes the characteristics of the human response identified. For example, the definition of the diagnostic label *impaired physical mobility* is the "limitation in independent, purposeful physical movement of the body or of one or more extremities" (NANDA International, 2003).

Risk Factors

Risk factors are environmental, physiological, psychological, genetic, or chemical elements that increase the vulnerability of an individual, family, or community to an unhealthful event (NANDA International, 2003). They serve as cues to indicate a risk nursing diagnosis is applicable to a client's condition. Examples of risk factors for the nursing diagnosis *risk for infection* include invasive procedures, trauma, malnutrition, immunosuppression, and insufficient knowledge to avoid exposure to pathogens. The risk factors help in selecting the correct risk diagnosis, similar to the manner in which defining characteristics help in the formulation of actual nursing diagnoses.

Support of the Diagnostic Statement

Nursing assessment data must support the diagnostic label, and the related factors must support the etiology. To collect complete, relevant, and correct assessment data it may help to identify assessment activities that produce specific kinds of data. For example, asking the client about the quality and perception of pain results in subjective data. However, palpating an area, which may

Table 16-2   **Comparison of Interventions for Nursing Diagnoses With Different Etiologies**

Nursing Diagnoses	Interventions
Client A	
Ineffective airway clearance related to obesity	Place client in high-Fowler's position.
	Have client cough and deep breathe every 2 hours while awake.
	Start weight-reduction diet (1200 calories) to decrease obesity.
Feeding self-care deficit related to inability to bend arms secondary to bilateral arm casts	Encourage family to visit during meals.
	Be certain staff or family members are available to feed client.
	Provide high-calorie milkshakes with straw at 3 and 8 PM.
Anxiety related to social isolation secondary to protective isolation	Plan staffing patterns to include visits to client's room 4 times a day.
	Provide diversional activities.
Client B	
Ineffective airway clearance related to poor coughing technique	Teach client deep breathing and coughing.
	Splint client's abdominal incision during coughing.
Feeding self-care deficit related to inability to grasp feeding utensils	Provide large-handled eating utensils.
	Offer finger foods cut in large pieces for between-meal snacks: 10-2-8.
Social isolation related to unfamiliarity with neighborhood	Provide client with phone numbers and location of local senior citizens' center.
	Draw client a map of neighborhood stores, restaurants, and libraries.

Table 16-3   **Formulation of Nursing Diagnoses for Mr. Brown**

Clustering Data	Identification of Client Need	Nursing Diagnosis
Diarrhea for 3 weeks	Alteration of elimination patterns	Diarrhea related to irritation
Distended abdomen		
Family history of stomach cancer		
Weight loss: 15 pounds	Excessive weight loss	Altered nutrition: less than body requirements related to inability to absorb nutrients because of chronic diarrhea for 3 weeks
Anemia, hemoglobin level of 12 g/100 ml	Risk for postoperative respiratory complications	Risk for ineffective airway clearance after surgery related to incisional pain
30 pack-year history of smoking		
Slight change of emphysema shown on chest x-ray film		
Crackles auscultated in lung fields		
Productive cough on rising each morning		
Temporary colostomy	Possible change in body image	Risk for situational low self-esteem related to change in body image
Scheduled surgery:		
Abdominal incision		
Client verbalization of fear of stomach cancer	Changes in interpersonal interactions	Ineffective individual coping related to fear about unknown prognosis
Client withdrawal after biopsy report		
Anxiety		

elicit a painful grimace, provides objective information. Likewise, asking a client to describe the perception of an irregular heartbeat elicits subjective information, and using auscultation to obtain a pulse produces an objective measurement of heart rate and rhythm. Box 16-3 summarizes the relevant preoperative assessment data for Mr. Brown that may lead to the identification of an actual or potential health care problem. Table 16-3

demonstrates data clustering, identification of client need, and formulation of nursing diagnoses from Mr. Brown's assessment data.

Table 16-4 uses the two nursing diagnoses, *ineffective airway clearance* and risk for *situational low self-esteem,* to demonstrate how defining characteristics and probable related factors assist in the development of the total diagnostic label.

Table 16-4   Defining Characteristics and Etiologies to Support Nursing Diagnoses

Assessment Activities	Defining Characteristics	Nursing Diagnoses	Etiologies ("Related to")
Auscultate lungs.	Abnormal breath sounds	Ineffective airway clearance	Decreased energy or fatigue
Observe respiration.	Changes in rate or depth of respiration		Tracheobronchial infection, obstruction, or secretion
Observe cough.	Cough		Pain
Inspect skin color.	Cyanosis		
Ask client about shortness of breath and observe for it.	Dyspnea		
Ask client about smoking.	Smoking history		
Observe client's grooming.	Verbal or nonverbal response to actual or perceived change in structure or function	Situational low self-esteem	Biophysical factors (e.g., amputation or loss of function of extremity)
Observe client's willingness to participate in rehabilitation.	Missing or impaired body part, not looking at or touching body or body part		Cognitive or perceptual factors (e.g., expressions of worthlessness and sorrow)
Review history of trauma injury.	Trauma to body Refusal to acknowledge change		Psychosocial factors (e.g., withdrawal behavior or excessive crying)

Defining characteristics and relevant etiologies are from Kim MJ, McFarland GK, McLean AM: *Pocket guide to nursing diagnoses,* ed 7, St. Louis, 1997, Mosby and are derived from the NANDA classification.

Mind Mapping Nursing Diagnosis

When caring for a client or groups of clients, a nurse must critically think about client needs and how to prevent problems from developing. The challenge of thinking about all client needs and problems is heightened by a nurse's holistic view of a client. Few clients have single problems. Often a nurse cares for a client with multiple nursing diagnoses. Therefore a picture of each client usually consists of a myriad of interconnections between sets of data all associated with identified client problems (Mueller, Johnston, and Bligh, 2002). Mind mapping is one way to graphically represent the connections between concepts and ideas that are related to a central subject (e.g., the client's health problems).

The benefit of mind mapping is to allow a student nurse to plot out associated thoughts, link together lines of reasoning, and see the relationship of one problem or diagnosis with another. A mind map provides a whole picture of a client's health situation with all of its interrelationships seen spatially. As a student develops a mind map for nursing diagnoses, eventually it expands and develops into a plan of care (see Chapter 17). The mind map shown in Figure 16-4 demonstrates a surgical client's three nursing diagnoses (*acute pain related to incisional trauma, ineffective airway clearance related to restrained coughing,* and *deficient knowledge regarding postoperative recovery related to inexperience*). The defining characteristics used to identify each diagnosis are drawn in octagons. The student draws connecting arrows between diagnoses and defining characteristics to show relationships between diagnoses. For example, the client's difficulty in performing postoperative exercises, a defining characteristic for *deficient knowledge,* could affect the client's ability to cough and clear the airway. The mind map helps the student to see the total picture and the way each of the diagnoses are related. Ultimately the nurse selects nursing interventions on the basis of each nursing diagnosis.

The advantage of a mind map is its central focus on the client rather than the client's disease or health alteration. This encourages students of nursing to concentrate on clients' specific health problems and nursing diagnoses (Mueller, Johnston, and Bligh, 2002). This focus promotes client participation with the eventual plan of care.

Sources of Diagnostic Errors

Errors can occur in the nursing diagnostic process during data collection, clustering, interpretation, and statement of the diagnosis (Box 16-6). This demonstrates the methodical level of critical thinking required for an accurate nursing diagnostic process.

Errors in Data Collection
A nurse must be knowledgeable and skilled in interviewing, observation, and physical examination to gather a complete and comprehensive database. If data are incomplete, omitted, or inaccurate, nursing diagnoses may be missed or incorrect. If data collection is disorganized, the diagnostic process is scattered. The following practices are essential to avoid data collection errors:
- Before assessment the nurse critically reviews his or her level of comfort and competence with interview and physical assessment skills.
- New students should approach assessment in steps. For example, the first experience may be completing an interview of a family member or collecting physical assessment data on one body system. The learner then moves on to more complex assessments.

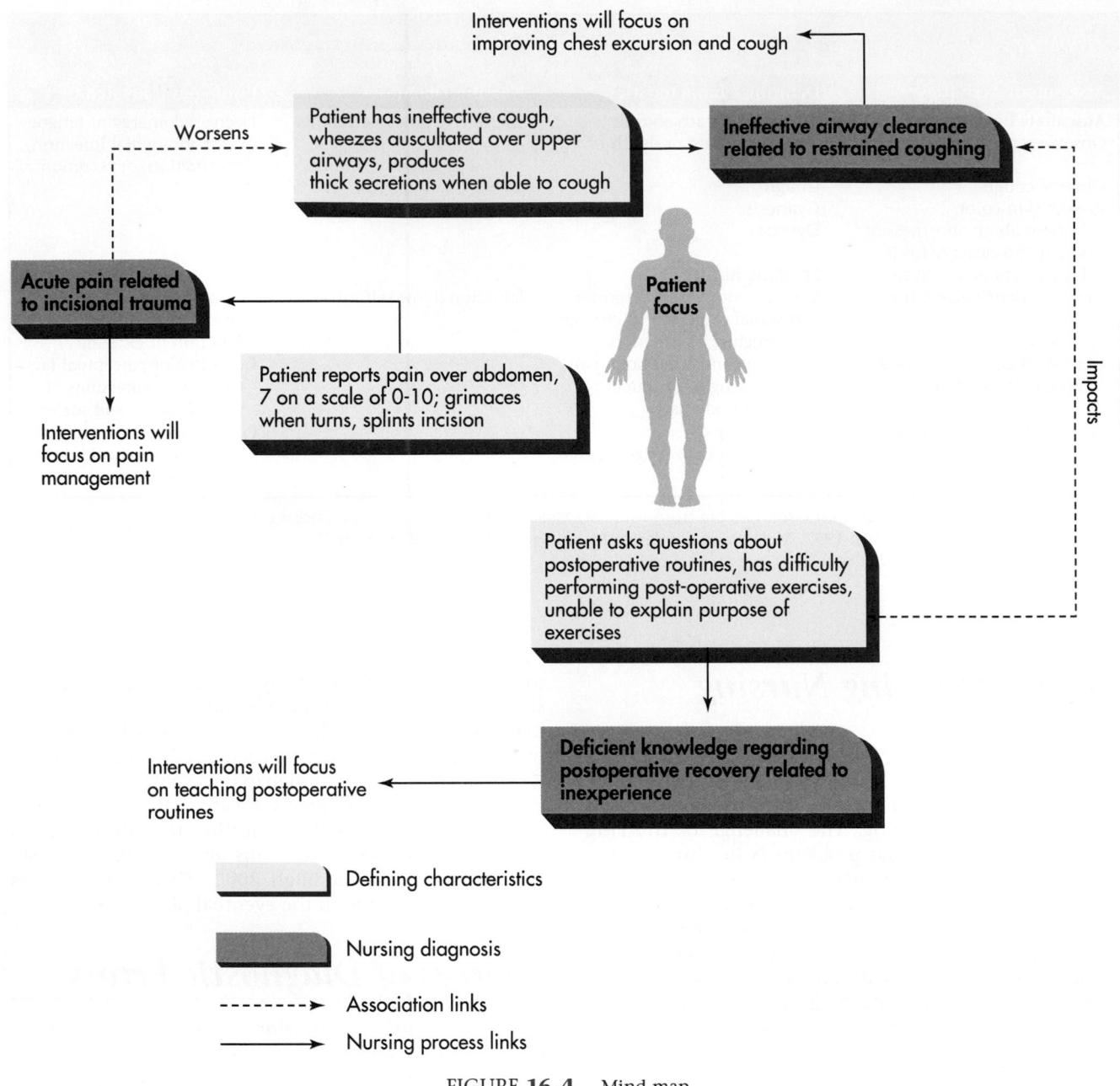

Interventions will focus on
improving chest excursion and cough

Worsens

Patient has ineffective cough,
wheezes auscultated over upper
airways, produces
thick secretions when able to cough

Ineffective airway clearance
related to restrained coughing

Patient
focus

Acute pain related
to incisional trauma

Patient reports pain over abdomen,
7 on a scale of 0-10; grimaces
when turns, splints incision

Interventions will
focus on pain
management

Impacts

Patient asks questions about
postoperative routines, has difficulty
performing post-operative exercises,
unable to explain purpose of
exercises

Interventions will focus
on teaching postoperative
routines

Deficient knowledge regarding
postoperative recovery related to
inexperience

Defining characteristics

Nursing diagnosis

- - - - - - - - ▶   Association links

————————▶   Nursing process links

FIGURE **16–4**   Mind map.

- The nurse determines the accuracy of data collected. For example, the nurse who auscultates abnormal lung sounds for the first time may be unsure of what is being heard through the stethoscope. Inaccurate assessment data means that data from clients are misinterpreted, inappropriate interventions may be selected, and the quality of care is jeopardized (Lunney, 1998). To minimize the risk of inaccuracy, the nurse must have a more experienced colleague validate findings or explain why they are incorrect.

- When developing assessment skills, the nurse needs to check completeness of assessment data. Reviewing client assessments in clinical or classroom settings provides the nurse with a constructive learning opportunity to determine when assessments are complete or when further revisions are needed.

- Errors in data collection are reduced when an organized approach is used for the assessment. Prior to assessment the nurse should have the appropriate forms and examination equipment. It is easier for the nurse

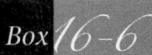

Box 16-6   Sources of Diagnostic Error

Collecting

Lack of knowledge or skill
Inaccurate data
Missing data
Disorganization

Interpreting

Inaccurate interpretation of cues
Failure to consider conflicting cues
Using an insufficient number of cues
Using unreliable or invalid cues
Failure to consider cultural influences or developmental stage

Clustering

Insufficient cluster of cues
Premature or early closure
Incorrect clustering

Labeling

Wrong diagnostic label selected
Evidence exists that another diagnosis is more likely
Condition is a collaborative problem
Failure to validate nursing diagnosis with client
Failure to seek guidance

to achieve an organized assessment if the environment is private, quiet, and comfortable for the client.

Errors in Interpretation and Analysis of Data

Following data collection the nurse reviews the database to determine if it is accurate and complete. The nurse reviews the data to validate that subjective data are supported by measurable objective physical findings when necessary. For example, when a client reports "difficulty breathing" the nurse also listens to lung sounds, assesses respiratory rate, and measures the client's chest excursion. When data are not appropriately validated, there may be an inaccurate match between the clinical cues and the diagnosis (Lunney, 1998). The nurse may also review supportive literature to ensure an adequate knowledge base to form a correct nursing diagnosis. Last, the nurse begins to identify and organize relevant assessment patterns to support the presence of client problems.

Errors in Data Clustering

Errors in data clustering occur when data are clustered prematurely, incorrectly, or not at all (Gordon, 1994). Premature closure of clustering occurs when the nurse makes the nursing diagnosis before all data have been grouped. For example, a nurse may learn that a client has had urinary incontinence and complains of urgency and nocturia. The nurse may cluster data and consider that *impaired urinary elimination* is a probable diagnosis.

However, incorrect clustering occurs when the nu to make the nursing diagnosis fit the signs and syn obtained. In this example, further assessment reve client has bladder distention and dribbling, and th ...,pe of incontinence is likely overflow incontinence. As a result of these findings a more accurate diagnosis, *urinary retention,* is made. The nursing diagnosis should be derived from the data, not the reverse. An incorrect nursing diagnosis affects quality of client care.

Errors in the Diagnostic Statement

The correct selection of a diagnostic statement is more likely to result in the appropriate selection of nursing interventions and outcomes (Dochterman and Jones, 2003). There are some common guidelines for reducing errors in the diagnostic statement. The statement should be worded in appropriate, concise, and precise language, which involves using correct terminology reflecting the client's response to the illness or condition. Use of standardized nursing language such as NANDA International diagnoses helps to ensure accuracy. A diagnostic statement such as "unhappy and worried about health" is not a scientifically based diagnosis, and it can lead to errors. The language needs to be more precise and appropriate, such as *ineffective individual coping related to fear of medical diagnosis.* Also, the problem and etiology portions must be within the scope of nursing to diagnose and treat.

Avoiding and Correcting Errors. Nursing diagnoses are easy to write when the nurse remembers that the problem portion of the statement is concerned with a client's response to the illness or condition and that the etiology portion must be within the scope of nursing practice. The following suggestions should help the nurse to avoid the most common errors in formulating nursing diagnoses accurately:

1. Identify the client's response, not the medical diagnosis (Carpenito, 2000). Because the medical diagnosis requires medical interventions, it is legally inadvisable to include it in the nursing diagnosis. The diagnosis, pain related to myocardial infarction, should be changed to *acute pain related to physical exertion.*

2. Identify a NANDA International diagnostic statement rather than the symptom. Nursing diagnoses are derived from a cluster of defining characteristics; one symptom is insufficient for problem identification. For example, shortness of breath, pain on inspiration, and productive cough with thick secretions should cue the nurse to *ineffective breathing pattern related to increased airway secretions.*

3. Identify a treatable etiology rather than a clinical sign or chronic problem. Nursing interventions are directed toward correcting the etiology of the problem. A diagnostic test or a chronic dysfunction is not an etiology that can be treated by a nursing intervention. A client with pneumonia may present restlessness, hypoxia, abnormal blood gas levels, and dyspnea. Impaired gas exchange related to altered blood gases is an incorrect diagnostic statement. *Impaired gas exchange related to alveolar capillary membrane changes* is a correct statement.

4. Identify the problem caused by the treatment or diagnostic study rather than the treatment or study itself. Clients experience many responses to diagnostic tests and medical treatment. These responses are the area of nursing concern. The diagnosis cardiac catheterization related to angina should be restated to read *anxiety related to lack of knowledge about cardiac catheterization.*

5. Identify the client response to the equipment rather than the equipment itself. Clients are often unfamiliar with medical technology. The diagnosis anxiety related to cardiac monitor can be changed to *deficient knowledge regarding the need for cardiac monitoring.*

6. Identify the client's problems rather than the nurse's problems. Nursing diagnoses are always client centered and form the basis for goal-directed care. Potential complications related to poor vascular access indicates a nursing problem in initiating and maintaining intravenous therapy. The diagnosis *risk for infection related to presence of invasive lines* properly centers attention on client needs.

7. Identify the client problem rather than the nursing intervention. Nursing interventions are planned to alleviate client problems and are not part of the diagnostic statement. Failure to state a diagnostic label results in an inability to evaluate problem resolution. The statement offer bedpan frequently because of altered elimination patterns should be changed to identify the problem and etiology. *Diarrhea related to food intolerance* corrects the misstatement and allows proper implementation of the nursing process.

8. Identify the client problem rather than the goal. Goals are based upon accurate identification of a client's problems The goals then serve as a basis to determine if problem resolution is achieved. If the problem is not first identified, goal selection and evaluation of problem resolution is difficult. Client needs high-protein diet related to potential alteration in nutrition should be changed to *imbalanced nutrition: less than body requirements related to inadequate protein intake* to allow for planning to correct the etiology.

9. Make professional rather than prejudicial judgments. Nursing diagnoses are based on subjective and objective client data and should not include the nurse's personal beliefs and values. The nurse's judgment can be removed from risk for impaired skin integrity related to poor hygiene habits by changing the diagnosis to read *risk for impaired skin integrity related to knowledge about perineal care.*

10. Avoid legally inadvisable statements (Carpenito, 2000). Statements that imply blame, negligence, or malpractice can result in litigation. The diagnosis recurrent angina related to insufficient medication implies inadequate prescription by the physician. Correct problem identification might read *chronic pain related to improper use of medications.*

11. Identify the problem and etiology. Be careful to avoid a circular statement. Such statements are vague and give no direction to nursing care. Alteration in comfort related to pain can be changed to identify the client problem and the cause: *ineffective breathing pattern related to incisional pain.*

12. Identify only one client problem in the diagnostic statement. Every problem has different specific expected outcomes. Confusion during the planning step occurs when multiple problems are included in a nursing diagnosis. Pain and anxiety related to difficulty in ambulating should be restated as two nursing diagnoses, such as *impaired physical mobility related to pain in right knee* and *anxiety related to difficulty in ambulating.* It is permissible to include multiple etiologies contributing to one client problem, for example, *dysfunctional grieving related to diagnosed terminal illness and change in family role* would be an acceptable diagnostic statement.

Diagnostic errors often shift the focus of the diagnostic statement from nursing to medicine or shift the focus from the cause to the intervention. As expertise with the diagnostic process is gained, the likelihood of errors is reduced, and the nurse is able to develop nursing diagnoses based on the actual or potential nursing needs of the client. Errors in the diagnostic process result in the development of an incomplete or inappropriate nursing care plan.

Nursing Diagnosis and Other Health Care Problems

A nursing diagnosis focuses on a client's needs or responses to health care alterations. A diagnosis reflects the client's level of health or response to a disease or pathological process, an emotional state, a sociocultural phenomenon, or a developmental stage. A medical diagnosis identifies a specific disease or pathological condition of organs or body systems. Medical diagnoses provide information about the signs and symptoms of a disease process and a means to communicate treatment requirements.

Medical and nursing diagnoses are developed using assessment databases. The nursing database is global and includes an in-depth assessment of the physiological, psychological, sociocultural, developmental, and spiritual dimensions of the client. Medicine's database includes the physiological systems and the personal and social systems. The personal and social systems may be limited to a family medical history and the economic and insurance history of the client (Gordon, 1994).

The goals and objectives of a nursing diagnosis differ from those of a medical diagnosis. The goal of a nursing diagnosis is to direct an individualized plan of care to assist clients and their families in adapting to their illness and resolving health care problems. The goals of a medical diagnosis are to identify and to design a treatment plan for curing the disease or the pathological process. For example, a 20-year-old college student is admitted with right lower quadrant abdominal pain. The physician makes a medical diagnosis of appendicitis, and the client undergoes an emergency appendectomy to remove the infected appendix. After the appendectomy the nurse develops several nursing diagnoses, one of which is *impaired physical mobility related to pain secondary to an abdominal incision.* The nursing care will be directed at gradually increasing the client's mobility to preoperative levels.

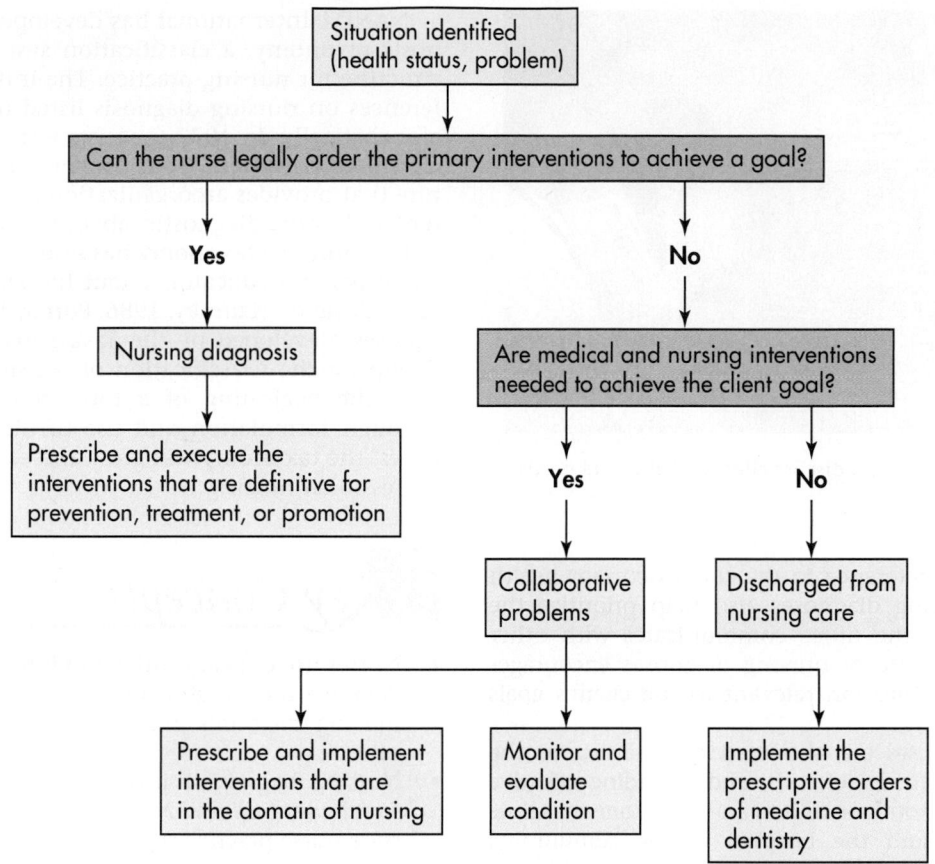

FIGURE **16–5**   Differentiating nursing diagnoses from collaborative problems. (© 1990, 1988, 1985 Lynda Juall Carpenito. Redrawn from Carpenito LJ: *Nursing diagnosis: application to clinical practice*, ed 6, Philadelphia, 1995, JB Lippincott.)

Collaborative problems are actual or potential physiological complications that can result from disease, trauma, treatment, or diagnostic studies for which nurses intervene in collaboration with personnel of other health care disciplines (Carpenito, 2000). Examples include wound infection and respiratory insufficiency. It is important to clarify collaborative problems from nursing diagnoses. If a nurse can prevent the onset of a complication or provide primary treatment, then the problem is a nursing diagnosis. For example, nurses can prevent pressure ulcers, so an appropriate nursing diagnosis might be *risk for impaired skin integrity*. Collaborative problems represent situations that are the primary responsibility of nurses, who often diagnose the onset of the problem and manage any changes in status. Consider a client who presents with clinical signs and symptoms of pneumonia. The client will have the collaborative problem of respiratory insufficiency, and an associated nursing diagnosis of *ineffective airway clearance related to tracheobronchial secretions*. The nurse will select independent interventions for both the collaborative problem and nursing diagnosis. However, for the nursing diagnosis the nurse will prescribe the definitive treatment to achieve desired outcomes, whereas the physician and nurse both prescribe treatments for respiratory insufficiency (Carpenito, 2002). Figure 16-5 provides a comparison of nursing diagnoses and collaborative problems.

Nursing Diagnoses: Application to Care Planning

The use of nursing diagnoses is a mechanism for identifying the domain of nursing. The formulated nursing diagnoses provide direction for the planning process and the selection of nursing interventions to achieve the desired outcomes. Unifying the languages of NANDA, NIC, and NOC will facilitate the process of matching nursing diagnoses with accurate and appropriate interventions and outcomes (Dochterman and Jones, 2003). The care plan (see Chapter 17) is a map for nursing care and demonstrates accountability for client care (Carpenito, 1997). In addition, the nursing diagnoses and subsequent care plan assist in communicating to other professionals the client-centered problems through the nursing care plan, consultations, discharge planning, and client care conferences (Figure 16-6).

Advantages of Nursing Diagnoses
Nursing diagnoses are advantageous for both nurses and clients. They facilitate communication among nurses about a client's level of wellness and assist in discharge planning. Nursing diagnoses facilitate communication in several ways. The initial list of nursing diagnoses is an

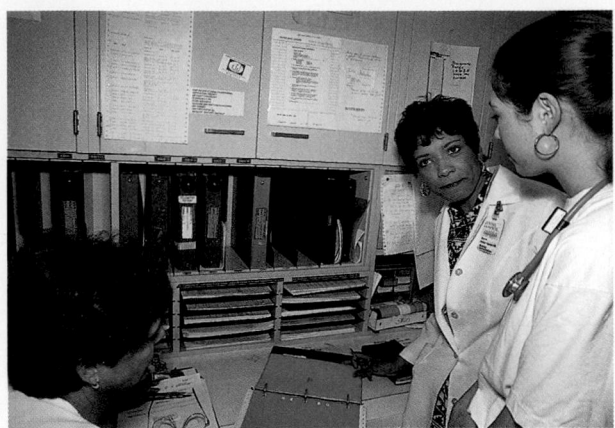

FIGURE 16–6   Nurses discuss clients' health care needs.

easily obtainable reference to the client's current health care needs. Nursing diagnoses also help prioritize the client's needs. As the nurse communicates with other professionals, the use of nursing diagnoses encourages organized communication relevant to the client's goals and priorities.

Nursing diagnoses are also used for charting in the progress notes, writing referrals, and providing effective transition of care from one unit to another, from one clinic to another, or from the hospital to the community. Discharge planning is the set of decisions and activities designed to give continuity and coordination to nursing care (see Chapter 2). Discharge planning is necessary when a client is discharged from one hospital to another or from the hospital to a community-based agency. In discharge planning, nursing diagnoses are a mechanism for communicating and delineating care the client still requires.

Nursing diagnoses can also serve as a focus for quality improvement (Gordon, 1994). Quality improvement is the monitoring and evaluation of process and outcomes to identify opportunities for improvement (see Chapter 20). When a quality improvement team focuses on practice issues pertaining to a nursing diagnosis, there is the opportunity to improve standards of practice and quality of care to clients. For example, when examining the practices in caring for clients with the diagnosis of *deficient knowledge,* nursing staff can identify ways to improve teaching interventions to reach better learning outcomes for clients.

Limitations of Nursing Diagnoses

Nursing diagnoses have limitations primarily with respect to what a diagnosis communicates. Because of the continuous evolution of the terms and use of nursing diagnoses, the language can occasionally be verbose and contain jargon. This may limit the use of nursing diagnoses to only nursing professionals and result in confusion among other members of the health care team (Seahill, 1991; Carpenito, 1997).

Imprecise language of the diagnosis may incorrectly "label" a client. One such diagnostic label is noncompliance. Unless based upon an accurate assessment, the term can be value laden and incomplete (Stantis and Ryan, 1982).

NANDA International has developed a nursing diagnosis taxonomy, a classification system, to provide a structure for nursing practice. The initial national conferences on nursing diagnosis listed nursing diagnoses alphabetically. In 1977 theorists were asked to create a classification system. Today there is a taxonomic structure that provides an organizational framework for current and future diagnostic labels. However, terminology in the form of a taxonomy has resulted in confusion for clinicians and educators about the language of the diagnostic labels (Lunney, 1986; Porter, 1986). Nursing diagnoses, developed by the Task Force of the National Group for the Classification of Nursing Diagnoses, are only the beginning of a total classification system. Through formulation and use of other nursing diagnoses, the taxonomy will grow and expand the focus of professional nursing.

Key Concepts

- Nurses use critical thinking to interpret assessment data in a meaningful and relevant way to identify nursing diagnoses and provide direction for nursing care.
- Nursing diagnosis is incorporated into the ANA's *Standards of Clinical Nursing Practice,* as well as most state nurse practice acts.
- Nursing diagnoses give all members of the health care team a clear understanding of client needs and distinguish the nurse's role from that of the physician.
- NANDA International has developed a common language for the health problems nurses manage.
- The diagnostic process includes critical analysis and interpretation of data that reveal a client's response to health care problems, identification of client needs, and formulation of nursing diagnoses.
- The analysis and interpretation of data requires the nurse to validate data, recognize patterns or trends, compare data with healthful standards, and then form diagnostic conclusions.
- Absence of defining characteristics suggests that a proposed diagnosis should be rejected.
- Nursing diagnoses state the actual or potential problems of the client's health status.
- Nursing diagnoses are written for the physical, developmental, intellectual, emotional, social, and spiritual dimensions of the client.
- There are three types of nursing diagnoses: actual diagnoses, at risk diagnoses, and wellness diagnoses.
- Nursing diagnoses are necessary to develop a plan of care that will help the client and family adapt to changes resulting from an illness or change in lifestyle.
- The "related to" factor of the diagnostic statement assists the nurse in individualizing a client's nursing diagnoses and provides direction for the selection of appropriate interventions.
- Mind mapping is a technique that allows a student to see the relationship of one problem or nursing diagnosis to another.

- Nursing diagnostic errors can occur by errors in data collection, interpretation and analysis of data, clustering of data, or in the diagnostic statement.
- Nursing diagnoses improve communication between nurses and other health professionals.

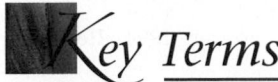

Key Terms

Actual nursing diagnosis, *p. 306*

Client-centered problems, *p. 301*

Collaborative problems, *p. 313*

Defining characteristics, *p. 304*

Diagnostic process, *p. 303*

Etiology, *p. 307*

Medical diagnosis, *p. 300*

NANDA International, *p. 301*

Nursing diagnosis, *p. 300*

Risk nursing diagnosis, *p. 306*

Wellness nursing diagnosis, *p. 306*

Critical Thinking Exercises

1. Mrs. Spezio has a pressure ulcer over the coccyx that is 5 cm in diameter and approximately 1 cm deep. The tissue surrounding the ulcer is inflamed and tender to touch. Mrs. Spezio is a transfer from a nursing home where she had resided for 6 months following a massive stroke. She is unable to move independently in bed and does not sense pressure or discomfort over her coccyx or hips. Given this clinical situation, identify the defining characteristics and related factors for the nursing diagnosis *impaired skin integrity.*
2. Examine the following two sets of data. Identify normal standards with which to compare the data, and then make a reasoned conclusion about the client need or problem the data tend to support.

Data Set I
Poor oral intake
Low white blood cell (WBC) count
Has a surgical wound

Data Set II
Awakens 2 to 3 times during night
Takes about 1 hour to fall asleep
Reports becoming tired easily at work
Worried about job security

3. Identify nursing diagnoses that might apply to the data sets in question 2.
4. Review the following nursing diagnoses and identify those that are stated correctly and those that are stated incorrectly:
   Anxiety related to fear of dying
   Self-care deficit: toileting related to incontinence
   Fatigue related to chronic emphysema
   Need for mouth care related to inflamed mucosa

Review Questions

1. A nursing diagnosis is:
   1. A clinical judgment about individual, family, or community responses to actual and potential health problems or life processes.
   2. The identification of a disease condition based on a specific evaluation of physical signs, symptoms, the client's medical history, and the results of diagnostic tests and procedures.
   3. The diagnosis and treatment of human responses to health and illness.
   4. The advancement of the development, testing, and refinement of a common nursing language.

2. This organization is the leader in nursing diagnosis classification:
   1. ANA (American Nurses Association).
   2. AMA (American Medical Association).
   3. NANDA (North American Nursing Association International).
   4. American Nurses Diagnostic Society.

3. One of the purposes of the use of standard formal nursing diagnostic statements is to:
   1. Gather information on patient data.
   2. Help nurses to focus on the role of nursing in client care.
   3. Facilitate understanding among nurses and health care providers.
   4. Evaluate nursing care.

4. Critical thinking is:
   1. A language to promote understanding among nurses about clients' health problems so as to facilitate communication and care planning.
   2. A process to help nurses to focus on the role of nursing in client care.
   3. A process to link nursing contributions to quality outcomes and the ability to cost out nursing care services.
   4. An active, organized, cognitive process used to carefully examine one's thinking and the thinking of others.

5. The nursing diagnosis: *Family coping: potential for growth related to unexpected birth of twins* is an example of a:
   1. Wellness nursing diagnosis.
   2. Risk nursing diagnosis.
   3. Potential nursing diagnosis.
   4. Diagnostic nursing diagnosis.

6. The nursing diagnosis: *Risk for impaired skin integrity* is an example of a:
   1. Wellness nursing diagnosis.
   2. Risk nursing diagnosis.
   3. Potential nursing diagnosis.
   4. Diagnostic nursing diagnosis.

7. The word *impaired* in the diagnosis *Impaired physical mobility* is an example of a:
   1. Related factor.
   2. Nursing diagnosis.
   3. Risk factor.
   4. Descriptor.

8. The nurse using auscultation to obtain a pulse. This is an example of a (an):
   1. Subjective measurement.
   2. Related factor.
   3. Objective measurement.
   4. Risk nursing diagnosis.

9. A practice to avoid data collection errors is:
   1. The nurse who auscultates abnormal lung sounds is unsure of what is being heard through the stethoscope so she asks her co-worker to listen to her client's lungs.
   2. After doing an assessment the nurse critically reviews his or her level of comfort and competence with interview and physical assessment skills.
   3. The nurse's client assessments vary depending on which part of the assessment she remembers to do first.
   4. The nurse asks her colleague to chart her assessment data.

10. "Unhappy and worried about health" is not a scientifically based diagnosis, and it can lead to error in:
    1. Data collection.
    2. Diagnostic statement.
    3. Medical diagnosis.
    4. Date clustering.

*R*eferences

American Nurses Association: *Model nurse practice act,* Washington, DC, 1955, The Association.

American Nurses Association: *Standards of nursing practice,* Washington, DC, 1973, The Association.

American Nurses Association: *Nursing: a social policy statement,* Washington, DC, 1980, The Association.

American Nurses Association: *Scope of nursing practice,* Washington, DC, 1987, The Association.

American Nurses Association: *Nursing: a social policy statement,* ed 2, Washington, DC, 2003, The Association.

American Nurses Association: *Standards of clinical nursing practice,* American Nurses Association, ed 2, Washington, DC, 1998, American Nurses Publishing.

Carpenito LJ: *Nursing diagnoses: application to clinical practice,* ed 6, Philadelphia, 1995, JB Lippincott.

Carpenito LJ: *Nursing diagnoses: application to clinical practice,* ed 7, Philadelphia, 1997, JB Lippincott.

Carpenito LJ: *Nursing diagnoses: application to clinical practice,* ed 8, Philadelphia, 2000, JB Lippincott

Carpenito LJ: *Nursing diagnoses: application to clinical practice,* ed 9, Philadelphia, 2002, JB Lippincott.

Chaffee J: *Thinking critically,* ed 3, Boston, 1994, Houghton Mifflin.

Collier IC and others: *Writing nursing diagnoses: a critical thinking approach,* St. Louis, 1996, Mosby.

Dochterman JM, Jones, DA: Unifying nursing languages: the harmonization of NANDA, NIC, NOC, Washington, DC, 2003, American Nurses Association.

Fry VS: The creative approach to nursing, *Am J Nurs* 53:301, 1953.

Gordon M: *Nursing diagnosis: process and application,* ed 3, St. Louis, 1994, Mosby.

Hickey P: *Nursing process handbook,* St. Louis, 1990, Mosby.

Jones D: Linking nursing language and knowledge development. In Chaska NL, editor: *The nursing profession: tomorrow and beyond,* Thousand Oaks, Calif, 2001, Sage Publications.

Kim MJ, McFarland GK, McLean AM, editors: *Classification of nursing diagnoses: proceedings of the fifth conference (NANDA),* St. Louis, 1984, Mosby.

Kim MJ, McFarland GK, McLean AM: *Pocket guide to nursing diagnoses,* ed 7, St. Louis, 1997, Mosby.

Lunney M: Nursing diagnoses: refining the system, *Am J Nurs* 82:456, 1986.

Lunney M: Accuracy of nurses' diagnoses: foundation of NANDA, NIC, and NOC, *Nurs Diagn* 9(2):83, 1998.

McFarland GK, McFarlane EA: *Nursing diagnosis and intervention: planning for patient care,* St. Louis, 1989, Mosby.

Mueller A, Johnston M, Bligh D: Joining mind mapping and care planning to enhance student critical thinking and achieve holistic nursing care, *Nurs Diagn* 13(1):24, 2002.

NANDA International: *NANDA nursing diagnoses: definitions and classifications, 2003-2004,* Philadelphia, 2003, NANDA International.

Porter EJ: Critical analysis of NANDA nursing diagnoses taxonomy, part I, *Image J Nurs Sch* 18:137, 1986.

Seahill L: Nursing diagnosis vs goal-oriented treatment planning in child psychiatry, *Image J Nurs Sch* 23:95, 1991.

Stantis MA, Ryan J: Noncompliance, an unacceptable diagnosis, *Am J Nurs* 82:941, 1982.

*R*esearch Reference

Da Cruz DALM, Acuri EAM: The influence of nursing diagnosis on information processing on undergraduate students, *Nurs Diagn* 9(3):93, 1998.

17

$\mathcal{P}$lanning Nursing Care

Media Resources

http://evolve.elsevier.com/Potter/
fundamentals/

CD COMPANION

- Review Questions
- Glossary

evolve WEBSITE

- Review Questions
- Student Learning Activities
- Glossary

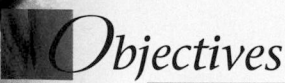

Objectives

Mastery of content in this chapter will enable the student to:

- Define the key terms listed.
- Explain the relationship of planning to assessment and nursing diagnosis.
- Discuss the process of priority setting.
- Describe goal setting.
- Discuss the difference between a goal and an expected outcome.
- List the seven guidelines for writing an outcome statement.
- Discuss the process of selecting nursing interventions.
- Discuss the differences between nurse-initiated, physician-initiated, and collaborative interventions.
- Describe the purposes of a written nursing care plan.
- Describe the elements of a concept map.
- Describe the consultation process.
- Develop a care plan from a nursing assessment.
- Develop a concept map from a nursing assessment.

*O*nce a nurse assesses a client's condition and identifies appropriate nursing diagnoses, a plan is developed for the client's nursing care. **Planning** is a category of nursing behaviors in which client-centered goals and expected outcomes are established and nursing interventions are selected. The interventions are specifically chosen to resolve the client's problem and achieve the goals and outcomes. Planning requires a nurse to use deliberate decision-making and problem-solving skills to design care for each client (Liukkonen, 1992). During planning, priorities are set because a client often has more than one nursing diagnosis and a variety of proposed interventions. In addition to collaborating with the client and family, the nurse consults with other members of the health care team and reviews pertinent literature during the planning process, A plan of care is dynamic and will change as the clients needs are met or as new needs are identified.

Establishing Priorities

Priority setting involves ranking nursing diagnoses in order of importance. The process helps a nurse attend to the client's most important needs and assists the nurse in organizing ongoing care activities. Priorities are established to help the nurse anticipate and sequence nursing interventions when a client has multiple problems or alterations (Carpenito, 1997). Because clients have multiple nursing diagnoses, the nurse and client select mutually agreed-on priorities based on the urgency of the problem, the client's safety and desires, the nature of the treatment indicated, and the relationship among the diagnoses. Establishing priorities is not merely a matter of numbering the nursing diagnoses on the basis of severity or physiological importance.

Priorities are classified as high, intermediate, or low (Table 17-1). The nurse considers those nursing diagnoses that, if untreated, could result in harm to the client. For example, *risk for other-directed violence, impaired gas exchange,* and *acute pain* are high-priority nursing diagnoses that drive the priorities of safety, maintaining adequate oxygenation, and providing comfort. In many cases, priorities that protect clients' basic needs of safety, adequate oxygenation, and comfort are always considered high priorities. However, it is always important to consider each client's unique case. Consider Mr. Brown who was introduced in Chapter 15. He has now successfully undergone surgery for a colon resection. Among Mr. Brown's nursing diagnoses are *acute pain, risk for ineffective airway clearance, deficient knowledge,* and *ineffective peripheral tissue perfusion.* Mr. Brown's high priorities are pain control postoperatively and maintaining a patent airway. Pain control is the highest priority because unless it is managed, Mr. Brown will be unable to cough effectively to remove secretions for a clear airway. High priorities can occur in both the psychological and physiological dimensions, and the nurse should avoid classifying only physiological nursing diagnoses as high priority. For example, lowering anxiety may become a priority over teaching a client information about impending surgery. If the client is too anxious to learn, then the nurse is unable to address a knowledge deficit at that time. Anxiety becomes the initial priority.

Intermediate priority nursing diagnoses involve the nonemergent, non–life threatening needs of the client. In Mr. Brown's case the intermediate priority pertains to the nursing diagnosis of *ineffective peripheral tissue perfusion.* Mr. Brown has no immediate impairment in circulation but is at risk for postoperative venous stasis. Aggressive preventive care is a part of Mr. Brown's routine postoperative care. Thus, maintaining normal circulation to the lower extremities becomes the nurse's immediate priority.

Low-priority nursing diagnoses are client needs that may not be directly related to a specific illness or prognosis but may affect the client's future well-being. Many low-priority diagnoses focus on the client's long-term health care needs. For example, Mr. Brown eventually will be discharged following surgery and will be required to manage his wound and nutritional needs in the home. *Deficient knowledge* is an important diagnosis that the nurse must attend to, but teaching the client is a low priority, especially if pain management and a patent airway have not been achieved. The nurse will begin teaching Mr. Brown as soon as the client becomes receptive and able to learn.

The order of priorities changes as a client's condition changes, sometimes within a matter of minutes. Each time a nurse begins a sequence of care such as at the beginning of a hospital shift or a client's clinic visit, it is important to reorder priorities. This requires the nurse to monitor assessment data to be sure that nursing diagnoses have been identified or that existing diagnoses have been resolved. For example, once Mr. Brown's pain is under control and the client is breathing without congestion or difficulty, *deficient knowledge* will become a higher priority. The appropriate ordering of priorities will ensure that client's needs are met in a timely and efficacious way.

Clients entering the health care system will have different types of priority needs. For example, a person brought to an emergency department experiencing acute

---

Table 17-1   Priority Setting for Mr. Brown

Mr. Brown has returned to the postoperative nursing unit following surgery for a colon resection. His condition presents numerous nursing diagnoses. The nurse sets priorities as follows:

Nursing Diagnoses	Rationale
High Priority	
Risk for ineffective airway clearance related to abdominal incisional pain	Client is at risk for postoperative pulmonary complications such as atelectasis and pneumonia, unless he is able to cough and deep breathe. Nurse will institute aggressive pulmonary hygiene.
Acute pain related to tissue trauma of surgical incision	Client is experiencing typical acute incisional pain. If the pain is not controlled or managed to a level the client can tolerate, it will be difficult for the client to participate in pulmonary hygiene.
Intermediate Priority	
Ineffective peripheral tissue perfusion related to postoperative venous status and risk for thrombophlebitis	All clients are at risk for altered peripheral tissue perfusion following major abdominal surgery. Mr. Brown does not currently show signs of thrombophlebitis; however, preventive measures such as frequent turning, leg exercises, and early ambulation will be essential.
Low Priority	
Deficient knowledge regarding postoperative home care related to inexperience	Mr. Brown will require instruction on wound care, infection prevention, and nutrition. The nurse will plan to begin teaching once pain control is achieved and the client is receptive to learning.
Risk for infection related to history of smoking for 20 years	This diagnosis reflects the client's long-term needs. The client will have to have a desire and willingness to change behavior and stop smoking. Postdischarge referral to a stop smoking class may be appropriate.

pneumonia has an unmet need for oxygen, the most basic physiological need. An older woman living in a high-crime area may be concerned about physical safety and, while hospitalized, may have a need for psychological security from fear that her home will be burglarized. A widowed homemaker whose children have moved away may feel that she does not belong or is not loved. Nursing care includes helping clients, and often the family, meet their needs.

Whenever possible, the client should be involved in priority setting. In some situations the client and the nurse assign different priority rankings to nursing diagnoses. If both place different values on health care needs and treatments, these differences can be resolved though open communication. However, when the client's physiological and emotional needs are at stake, the nurse needs to assume primary responsibility for setting priorities.

Critical Thinking in Establishing Goals and Expected Outcomes

Once a nursing diagnosis is identified for a client, the nurse must ask what is the best approach to address and resolve the problem. Goals and expected outcomes are specific statements of client behavior or physiological responses that a nurse sets to achieve problem resolution. The goals and outcomes provide a clear focus for the type of interventions necessary to care for the client. When goals and outcomes are met, a client's health problems are resolved. For example, when a client has a diagnosis of *impaired physical mobility related to acute pain,* there are two associated health problems: reduced mobility and pain. Appropriate goals would include "Client will achieve normal mobility" and "Client will achieve pain control." Both goals are necessary because the nurse must attend to both the client's mobility and comfort needs. In order for the nurse to monitor progress toward the ultimate goals, outcomes or measurable criteria to evaluate goal achievement are necessary. Outcomes for the goal of "Client will achieve normal mobility" include "Client will initiate turning and repositioning in bed" and "Client will sit and stand by first postoperative evening." Outcomes for the goal of "Client will achieve pain control" include "Client will report pain severity below 4 on a scale of 0 to 10" and "Client will report ability to sleep during the night without discomfort." The nurse's interventions will include exercise therapy (ambulation and turning), analgesic administration, and nonpharmacological pain management (relaxation exercises). In summary, the purposes for writing goals and expected outcomes are twofold: to provide direction for the selection and use of nursing interventions and to provide focus for evaluation of the effectiveness of the interventions.

Planning nursing care requires critical thinking (Figure 17-1). The nurse critically evaluates the preestablished nursing diagnoses, the urgency of the problems, and the resources of the client and the health care delivery system (Bandman and Bandman, 1995). The nurse applies knowledge from the medical, sociobehavioral, and nursing sciences to plan care. Goals, expected outcomes, and interventions are selected by considering previous experience with similar client problems, as well as any established standards for clinical problem management. The goals and outcomes must meet intellectual standards by being relevant to client needs, specific, singular, observable, measurable, and time-limited. The nurse uses critical thinking attitudes in selecting interventions with the greatest likelihood of success. For example, the nurse creatively selects comfort measures the client practices at home in choosing a plan for managing the client's chronic pain. Figure 17-2 graphically illustrates the relationships between nursing diagnoses, goals, expected outcomes, and nursing interventions.

Goals of Care

A **client-centered goal** is a specific and measurable behavior or response that reflects a client's highest possible level of wellness and independence in function. Examples include "Client will perform self-care hygiene independently," "Client will remain free of infection," and "Client will accept body image alteration." A goal contains singular behaviors or responses. The example of "Client will communicate needs and adhere to treatment plan" is written incorrectly because the statement includes two different behaviors, communicate and adhere. A goal must also be observable and measurable. A nurse is able to observe the condition of a surgical wound and measure the amount of drainage or appearance of the incision for the goal "Client will remain free of infection." The specific criteria used to measure success of a goal are written in the form of outcome statements (see statements below). Each goal and outcome must be time-limited so that the health care team has a common time frame for problem resolution. The time frame depends on the nature of the problem, etiology, overall condition of the client, and treatment setting. For example, a client with acute pain following surgery will likely have a shorter time frame for achievement of goals than a client with chronic recurrent pain. The statements "Client will achieve pain control within 48 hours" and "Client will remain free of infection by discharge home" are correctly written goals.

Role of the Client in Goal Setting. It is desirable for the nurse to partner with clients when setting goals. Mutual goal setting is an activity that includes the client and family (when appropriate) in prioritizing the goals of care and in developing a plan of action to achieve those goals (McCloskey and Bulechek, 1994). Unless goals are mutually set and there is a clear plan for action, clients may fail to adhere to the plan of care. Clients must understand and see the value of nursing therapies, even though they are oftentimes totally dependent on the nurse. Once a client shares the nurse's goals, there is a greater likelihood of client participation in the plan of care.

Goals should be realistic and based on client needs and resources. For clients to participate in goal setting, they should be alert and have some degree of independence in completing activities of daily living, problem solving, and decision making. This is important because the nurse and client partner together in the client's care.

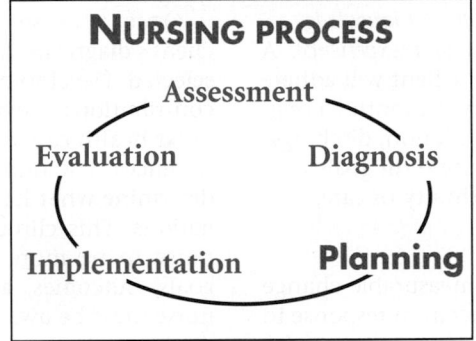

KNOWLEDGE
Client's database and selected nursing diagnoses
Anatomy and physiology
Pathophysiology
Normal growth and development
Evidence-based nursing interventions
Role of other health care disciplines
Community resources
Family dynamics
Teaching/learning process
Delegation principles

EXPERIENCE
Previous client care experience

NURSING PROCESS

Assessment

Evaluation   Diagnosis

Implementation   **Planning**

STANDARDS
ANA Scope of Nursing Practice
Specialty standards of practice
Client-centered goals and outcomes
Intellectual standards

ATTITUDES
Creativity
Responsibility
Perseverance

FIGURE **17–1**   Critical thinking and the process of planning care.

If clients' cognitive and physical impairments are so severe that they cannot actively participate in goal setting, the nursing team acts in their behalf to develop client-centered goals. When developing goals, the nurse acts as an advocate for the client to develop nursing interventions to promote the client's return to health or to prevent further deterioration in the client's level of wellness or cognitive and physical functioning (Carpenito, 1997).

Goals should not only meet the immediate needs of the client but should also strive toward prevention and rehabilitation. Two types of goals, short-term goals and long-term goals, are developed for the client depending upon the nature of the client's need or problems and the nature of the nursing services provided.

Short-Term Goals. A **short-term goal** is an objective that is expected to be achieved within a short time frame, usually less than a week (Carpenito, 1997). With the present health care system and shorter hospital stays, short-term goals are the direction for the immediate care plan. In the case of Mr. Brown, the client has the nursing diagnosis of *acute pain related to the tissue trauma of a surgical incision.* A short-term goal for Mr. Brown would be "Client will achieve comfort within 24 hours postoperatively."

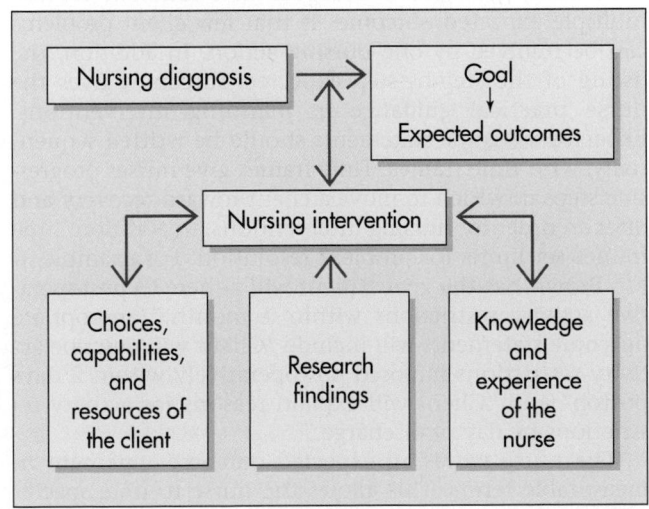

FIGURE **17–2**   From diagnosis to outcome. (Revised and redrawn from Gordon M: *Nursing diagnosis: process and application,* ed 3, St. Louis, 1994, Mosby.)

The goal is realistic because of the importance placed on aggressively managing clients' postoperative pain.

Long-Term Goals. A **long-term goal** is an objective that is expected to be achieved over a longer time frame, usually over weeks or months. Long-term goals may be more appropriate for problem resolution after discharge, especially from acute care settings (Carpenito, 1997). Long-term goals are appropriate for clients in home care settings and those adapting to chronic illnesses who reside in long-term care facilities and for some clients in rehabilitation, mental health, ambulatory care, and community nursing settings (Carpenito, 1997). For example, Mr. Brown has the nursing diagnosis of *deficient knowledge regarding postoperative home care related to inexperience.* A long-term goal for Mr. Brown may be "Client will adhere to postoperative activity restrictions for 1 month." Long-term goals focus on prevention, rehabilitation, discharge, and health education. Failure to set long-term goals may prevent the client from receiving continuity of care.

Expected Outcomes

An **expected outcome** is a specific measurable change in a client's status that is expected to occur in response to nursing care. An outcome is an objective criterion for measuring goal achievement. Client outcomes are the ultimate definition of effectiveness and efficiency by identifying and measuring the desired results of nursing interventions and practice (Deaton, 1998). Outcomes provide a focus for nursing care because they are the desired responses of a client's condition in the physiological, social, emotional, developmental, or spiritual dimensions. The expected outcomes determine when a specific, client-centered goal has been met and evaluate the response to nursing care and the resolution of the etiology of a nursing diagnosis.

Several expected outcomes are usually developed for each nursing diagnosis and goal. The rationale for the multiple expected outcomes is that few client problems can be resolved by one nursing action. In addition, the listing of the step-by-step expected outcomes gives the nurse practical guidance in planning interventions. Expected outcome statements should be written sequentially, with time frames. Time frames give nurses progressive steps in which to move a client toward recovery and offer an order for nursing interventions. In addition, time frames set limits for problem resolution. For example, if Mr. Brown has the goal "Client will adhere to postoperative activity restrictions within 1 month," appropriate outcome statements will include "Client will describe activity restrictions imposed postoperatively within 2 days postop" and "Client will explain reasons for activity restrictions by day of discharge."

The nurse writes an expected outcome statement in measurable terms. This allows the nurse to note specifically the behavior or physiological response expected for resolution of the client's problem. For example "Client will have less pain" is an inaccurate outcome statement because the phrase "less pain" is nonspecific. The statement "Client will report pain acuity less than 4 on a scale of 0 to 10" is accurate.

There is much attention in the current health care environment to measuring outcomes of nursing interventions. The Iowa Intervention Project has published a classification of nursing outcomes and has linked the outcomes to nursing diagnoses (Moorhead, Johnson, and Maas, 2004). These nursing outcomes are dependent on the delivery-of-care setting. For example, outcomes in a critical care setting are not necessarily appropriate for a community-based setting or a rehabilitation facility. Outcomes are also dependent on the acute or chronic disease state of the client (Chase, 1998). It is important to reflect on the goals and expected outcomes of care to ensure that they are specific to the client, care delivery setting, the discipline delivering the care, and the underlying medical diagnosis.

Once a nurse develops goals and outcomes for a client's diagnosis, the interventions in the plan of care are selected. Developing a plan of care must incorporate the contributions of evidence-based research (see Chapter 5), other health care disciplines, the family, and community resources. The nurse also applies previous experiences to determine what has worked or not worked in similar situations. This clinical testing of interventions helps the nurse to be more therapeutic for each new client. As goals, outcomes, and interventions are developed, the nurse must be aware of and committed to accepted standards of practice from nursing and other disciplines in designing safe and relevant client-centered care. In the planning of care the nurse displays attitudes such as creativity, perseverance, and humility to develop a plan of care that is individualized to the client/family needs.

Combining Goal and Outcome Statements

It is important to clarify that many schools of nursing and health care institutions use a format for stating goals and outcomes as one statement. Often the terms *goals* and *outcomes* are used interchangeably in health care settings. This is acceptable as long as the criteria for writing goals and outcomes are met. For example, the statement "Client will achieve pain control as evidenced by reporting pain acuity less than 4 on a scale of 0 to 10 within 48 hours" is an acceptable statement. The goal portion of the statement provides a broad description of the desired client status (achieve pain control), and the outcome portion of the statement contains the observable criterion (4 on a pain scale) needed to measure success. The format for the many documentation forms found within health care settings dictates how goals and outcomes are written.

●●●

It is now 1 day after Mr. Brown had surgery for a bowel resection. He was found to have colon cancer. His operative course has some complications. His blood loss was greater than anticipated, and his hemoglobin level is now 8.5 g/100 ml. He has developed fatigue, and his tolerance of routine postoperative leg exercises and ambulation is poor. He therefore has a new nursing diagnosis of "*activity intolerance.*" Although he is receiving around-the-clock (ATC) pain medications, he still periodically reports pain at a level above 5 on the pain scale. It is important for the nurse to continue to emphasize the need for pulmonary hygiene. Because of his current fatigue and level of pain, teaching Mr. Brown is not a priority at this time. Table

Table 17-2	The Relationship of Nursing Diagnoses, Goals, and Outcomes Application of the Case Study for Mr. Brown	
Nursing Diagnoses	**Goals**	**Expected Outcomes**
Risk for ineffective airway clearance related to abdominal incisional pain	Client will maintain patent airway through postoperative period to discharge.	Lungs will be clear to auscultation within 48 hours postoperatively. Client achieves incentive spirometer goal of 90% every 2 hours.
Acute pain related to tissue trauma of surgical incision	Client will achieve pain control within 48 hours.	Client will report pain severity below 4 on a scale of 0-10 by 24 hours. Client will report ability to sleep during night without discomfort within 48 hours.
Activity intolerance related to reduced oxygenation from blood loss	Client will increase ambulation progressively during postoperative period.	Client will walk 5 minutes without verbal report of fatigue by postoperative day 2. Client will sit up in chair 20 minutes without abnormal heart rate by day 2.
Ineffective peripheral tissue perfusion related to postoperative venous stasis	Client will maintain adequate peripheral tissue perfusion by discharge.	Client's toes remain warm, dry, with capillary refill of 2 seconds. Client remains negative for Homan's sign.

17-2 shows the relationship between nursing diagnoses, goals, and expected outcomes for Mr. Brown.

Guidelines for Writing Goals and Expected Outcomes

It is important to write goals and outcomes clearly so that all members of the nursing team understand a client's plan of care and are able to collaborate on achieving the same goals and outcomes. Several of the guidelines for writing goals and expected outcomes have been mentioned earlier. There are seven guidelines: client-centered, singular, observable, measurable, time-limited, mutual, and realistic.

Client-Centered. Outcomes and goals should reflect the client behavior and responses expected as a result of nursing interventions. A common error occurs when the goals are written to reflect the nurse's goals or outcomes. A correct outcome statement is "Client will ambulate in the hall 3 times a day." A common error is to write "Ambulate client in the hall 3 times a day."

Singular Goal or Outcome. Each goal and expected outcome statement should address only one behavior or response. This ensures a precise method to evaluate the client's response to a nursing intervention. If an outcome statement reads, "Client's lungs will be clear to auscultation, and respiratory rate will be 20 breaths per minute by 8/22," but the nurse evaluates the client after suctioning and finds the lungs to be clear with the respiratory rate at 28 per minute, it will be difficult to determine whether the expected outcome was achieved. By splitting the outcome into two parts, "Lungs will be clear to auscultation by 8/22" and "Respiratory rate will be 20 breaths per minute by 8/22," the nurse can determine specifically the outcome that has been achieved. In addition, singularity assists the nurse in determining if modification of the care plan is necessary.

Observable. The nurse must be able to determine through observation if change has taken place. Observable changes

can occur in physiological findings, the client's level of knowledge, perceptions or expressed feelings, and behavior. The results can be obtained by directly asking the client about the condition or can be observed using assessment skills. For example, the goal "Client will be able to self-administer insulin" is observed through the outcomes "Client prepares insulin dosage correctly by 8/30" and "Client performs subcutaneous injection correctly by 8/31." The outcome statement "Client will appear less anxious" is not a correct statement because there is no specific behavior observable for "will appear."

Measurable. Goals and expected outcomes are written to give the nurse a standard against which to measure the client's response to nursing care. Examples are "Body temperature will remain 98.6," and "Apical pulse will remain between 60 and 100 beats per minute." A goal or an outcome that is stated in measurable terms allows the nurse to objectively quantify changes in the client's status. Common mistakes are made when the nurse uses vague qualifiers such as *normal, stable, acceptable,* or *sufficient* in the expected outcome statement. Vague terms result in guesswork in determining the client's response to care. Terms specifically describing quality, quantity, frequency, length, or weight allow the nurse to evaluate whether outcomes are achieved.

Time-Limited. The time frame for each goal and expected outcome indicates when the expected response should occur. Time frames assist the nurse and client in determining that progress is being made at a reasonable rate. When the date of evaluation arrives, the nurse assesses the client to determine whether that particular expected outcome has been reached. If the outcome is unmet, but it is still appropriate for the client's care, another future evaluation date is set. Time frames promote accountability in the delivery of nursing care.

Mutual Factors. Mutually set goals and expected outcomes ensure that the client and nurse agree on the direction and time limits of care. Mutual goal setting can increase the client's motivation and cooperation. The nurse does not impose personal values on the client. However, the nurse must be aware of standards of practice, client safety, and basic human needs. The nurse may need to direct some of the goals and expected outcomes to keep the client physically and emotionally stable and safe.

Realistic. The nurse sets goals and expected outcomes that can be achieved. This provides clients with a sense of accomplishment. In turn, this sense of accomplishment can increase the client's motivation and cooperation. When establishing realistic goals, the nurse, through assessment, must know the resources of the health care facility, family, and client; the client's physiological, emotional, cognitive, and sociocultural potential; and the economic cost and resources available to reach expected outcomes in a timely manner.

Critical Thinking in Designing Nursing Interventions

Nursing interventions are any treatment or action, based upon clinical judgment and knowledge, that nurses perform to enhance clients' outcomes (Dochterman and Bulechek, 2004). Nursing interventions are designed to assist the client in moving from the present level of health to that which is described in the goal and measured by the expected outcomes (Gordon and others, 1994). Implementation of these interventions occurs during the implementation phase of the nursing process (see Chapter 18).

Choosing suitable nursing interventions involves decision making. The nurse uses critical thinking by applying knowledge pertinent to the client's situation, experience from caring for similar clients, critical thinking attitudes, and standards to select interventions that will successfully meet established goals and expected outcomes for each diagnostic statement. In addition, to initiate the intervention the nurse must be competent in three areas: (1) knowing the scientific rationale for the intervention, (2) possessing the necessary psychomotor and interpersonal skills, and (3) being able to function within a particular setting to use the available health care resources effectively (Dochterman and Bulechek, 2004).

Types of Interventions

Generally there are three categories of nursing interventions: nurse-initiated or independent, physician-initiated or dependent, and collaborative interventions. Category selection is based on client needs. One client may require all three categories, whereas another client may need only nurse- and physician-initiated interventions.

Nurse-Initiated Interventions. Nurse-initiated interventions are the independent response of the nurse to the client's health care needs and nursing diagnoses. A nurse is able to act within his or her own scope of practice to intervene on a client's behalf. Nurse-initiated interventions are autonomous actions based on scientific rationale that is expected to benefit the client in a predicted way related to the nursing diagnosis and client-centered goals (Dochterman and Bulechek, 2004). Nurse-initiated interventions involve aspects of professional nursing practice encompassed by licensure and law. These interventions require no supervision or direction from others. For example, instructing clients in ways to manage their nutrition or activities of daily living or positioning clients to minimize the effects of pressure on bony prominences are independent nursing actions.

Nurse-initiated interventions do not require a physician's or an independent care provider's (e.g., nurse practitioner) order or an order from another health professional. Physicians frequently include in their written orders the specifics of independent nursing interventions. However, according to the nurse practice acts in a majority of states, nursing actions pertaining to activities of daily living, health education, health promotion, and counseling are in the domain of nursing practice. Nurse practice acts delineate the legal scope of nursing practice within the geographical boundaries of each state's jurisdiction (see Chapter 22).

Physician-Initiated Interventions. Physician-initiated interventions are based on a physician's response to treat or manage a medical diagnosis. Nurse practitioners working under collaborative agreements with physicians or who are licensed independently by state practice acts are also able to write such interventions. The nurse intervenes by carrying out the independent provider's written orders. This may be in the form of an individual written order, a signed treatment protocol, or standing orders. Administering a medication, implementing an invasive procedure, changing a dressing, and preparing a client for diagnostic tests are examples of physician-initiated interventions. It is not always within the legal practice of nursing for the nurse to prescribe and order these treatments independently, but it is within the practice of nursing for the nurse to complete such orders and to individualize approaches to their administration. For example, a physician may order a dressing change twice a day and a bone scan for a client. The nurse incorporates each of these orders into the client's plan of care so that they are safely and efficiently completed.

Each physician-initiated intervention requires specific nursing responsibilities and technical nursing knowledge. For example, when administering medications, the nurse is responsible for knowing the classification of the drug, its physiological action, normal dosage, side effects, and nursing interventions related to its action or side effects (see Chapter 34). With an invasive procedure the nurse is responsible for knowing when the procedure is necessary, the clinical skills necessary to complete it, and its expected outcome and possible side effects. The nurse is also responsible for adequate preparation of the client and proper communication of the results. When a specific diagnostic or laboratory test is ordered by a physician or nurse practitioner, the nurse is responsible for scheduling the test, preparing the client, and knowing the normal findings and nursing implications associated with it.

Collaborative Interventions. Collaborative interventions are therapies that require the knowledge, skill, and expertise of multiple health care professionals. For example, Mr. Joseph is a 68-year-old man who is a hemiplegic from a recent cerebrovascular accident (stroke) and also has a long-term history of dementia. His cognitive functions are limited, he is at risk for problems related to impaired sensation and mobility, and he is unable to independently complete activities of daily living. In order for Mr. Joseph to maintain his present level of health, he requires multiple interventions, including nursing interventions to prevent pressure ulcers, physical therapy interventions to prevent musculoskeletal changes from immobility, and occupational therapy interventions for eating and hygiene needs. The care for this client requires the coordination of collaborative interventions from multiple health care professionals, all directed toward the long-term goal of maintaining Mr. Joseph's present level of health.

•••

Nurse-initiated, physician-initiated, and collaborative interventions require critical thinking and decision making. When encountering physician-initiated or collaborative interventions, the nurse does not automatically implement the therapy but must determine whether it is appropriate for the client. Every nurse faces an inappropriate or incorrect order at some time. The nurse with a strong knowledge base recognizes the error and seeks to correct it. The ability to recognize incorrect therapies is particularly important when administering medications or implementing procedures. An error can occur in writing the order or transcribing it to a documentation form or computer screen. Clarifying an order is competent nursing practice, and it protects the client and members of the health care team. The nurse carrying out an incorrect or inappropriate intervention is as much in error as the person who wrote or transcribed the original order and is liable for any complications resulting from the error. Chapter 22 explains legal issues affecting nursing practice.

Selection of Interventions

A nurse does not select interventions haphazardly. Clients who have the diagnosis of *Anxiety;* for example, are not cared for in the same way with the same interventions. *Anxiety* related to the uncertainty of an impending diagnostic test will be treated very differently than *anxiety* related to a threat to loss of family role function. When choosing interventions, a nurse deliberates about six important factors: (1) characteristics of the nursing diagnosis, (2) expected outcomes, (3) research base (nursing knowledge) for the interventions, (4) feasibility of the intervention, (5) acceptability to the client, and (6) competencies of the nurse (McCloskey and Bulechek, 1998; Dochterman and Bulechek, 2004) (Box 17-1). During deliberation the nurse may review available

---

Box 17-1 Choosing Nursing Interventions

Characteristics of the Nursing Diagnosis

- Interventions must be directed toward altering the etiological (related to) factors associated with the diagnosis.
- When an etiological factor cannot change, the interventions must be directed toward treating the signs and symptoms (e.g., NANDA defining characteristics).
- For potential or high-risk diagnoses, interventions must be aimed at altering or eliminating the risk factors for the diagnosis.

Expected Outcomes

- Client outcomes must be specified before selecting an intervention.
- Because an outcome is stated in terms used to evaluate the effectiveness of an intervention, this language can assist in selecting the intervention.
- Nursing Interventions Classification (NIC) is designed to show the link to Nursing Outcomes Classification (NOC) (Moorehead, Johnson, and Maas, 2004).

Research Base

- Research in support of a nursing intervention will indicate the effectiveness of using the intervention with certain types of clients.
- Refer to research articles or evidence-based practice protocols that describe the utilization of research findings in similar clinical situations and settings.
- When research is not available, use scientific principles (e.g., infection control) or consult a clinical expert about your client population.

Feasibility

- A specific intervention may have the potential for interacting with other interventions chosen by the nurse or other health care providers.
- The nurse must be knowledgeable of the total plan of care.
- Consider cost: Is the intervention clinically effective and cost efficient?
- Consider time: Are time and personnel resources available?

Acceptability to the Client

- An intervention must be acceptable to the client and family and congruent with the client's goals, health care values, and culture.
- To facilitate informed choice, a client must know how he or she is expected to participate and the anticipated effect of the intervention.

Capability of the Nurse

- The nurse must be able to carry out the intervention.
- The nurse must be knowledgeable of the scientific rationale for the intervention.
- The nurse must possess the necessary psychosocial and psychomotor skills to complete the intervention.
- The nurse must be able to function within the particular setting to effectively use health care resources.

Modified from Dochterman JM, Bulechek GM: *Nursing interventions classification (NIC)*, ed 4, Mosby, St. Louis, 2004.

Table 17-3	Nursing Interventions Classification (NIC) Taxonomy	
Domain 1	**Domain 2**	**Domain 3**

Level 1 Domains

1. **Physiological: Basic**
   Care that supports physical functioning

2. **Physiological: Complex**
   Care that supports homeostatic regulation

3. **Behavioral**
   Care that supports psychosocial functioning and facilitates lifestyle changes

Level 2 Classes

A *Activity and Exercise Management:* Interventions to organize or assist with physical activity and energy conservation and expenditure	G *Electrolyte and Acid-Base Management:* Interventions to regulate electrolyte/acid-base balance and prevent complications	O *Behavior Therapy:* Interventions to reinforce or promote desirable behaviors or alter undesirable behaviors
B *Elimination Management:* Interventions to establish and maintain regular bowel and urinary elimination patterns and manage complications due to altered patterns	H *Drug Management:* Interventions to facilitate desired effects of pharmacological agents	P *Cognitive Therapy:* Interventions to reinforce or promote desirable cognitive functioning or alter undesirable cognitive functioning
C *Immobility Management:* Interventions to manage restricted body movement and the sequelae	I *Neurologic Management:* Interventions to optimize neurologic functions	Q *Communication Enhancement:* Interventions to facilitate delivering and receiving verbal and nonverbal messages
D *Nutrition Support:* Interventions to modify or maintain nutritional status	J *Perioperative Care:* Interventions to provide care before, during, and immediately after surgery	R *Coping Assistance:* Interventions to assist another to build on own strengths, to adapt to a change in function, or to achieve a higher level of function
E *Physical Comfort Promotion:* Interventions to promote comfort using physical techniques	K *Respiratory Management:* Interventions to promote airway patency and gas exchange	S *Patient Education:* Interventions to facilitate learning
F *Self-Care Facilitation:* Interventions to provide or assist with routine activities of daily living	L *Skin/Wound Management:* Interventions to maintain or restore tissue integrity	T *Psychological Comfort Promotion:* Interventions to promote comfort using psychological techniques
	M *Thermoregulation:* Interventions to maintain body temperature within a normal range	
	N *Tissue Perfusion Management:* Interventions to optimize circulation of blood and fluids to the tissue	

From Dochterman JM, Bulechek GM: *Nursing interventions classification (NIC)*, ed 4, St. Louis, 2004, Mosby.

resources such as standardized care plans, the Nursing Interventions Classification (NIC), critical pathways, policy or procedure manuals, textbooks, and nursing literature. Collaboration is also useful. Through **collaboration** the nurse taps the best resources to individualize nursing interventions. During collaboration, the nurse includes the client, family, and members of the health team. In addition, the nurse also reviews previous clinical experiences and priorities to select nursing interventions that have the best potential for achieving the expected outcomes. With experience, the deliberation process becomes more efficient and experience based (Benner, 1984).

Nursing Interventions Classification. The Iowa Intervention Project has developed a taxonomy of nursing interventions that provides a level of standardization to enhance communication of nursing care across settings and to compare outcomes (Iowa Intervention Project, 1993; Dochterman and Bulechek, 2004). Extensive nursing research, expert review, and clinical judgment have merged to form the NIC taxonomy: 486 interventions are grouped into 30 classes and 7 domains for ease of use

(Table 17-3). Each class includes interventions that will enhance the condition of a client who has an alteration within the class (Box 17-2). Each intervention then has a variety of nursing activities from which the nurse chooses to perform (Box 17-3). In addition, NIC interventions have been linked with NANDA International nursing diagnoses (Dochterman and Jones, 2003; NANDA International, 2003). For example, if a client has a problem in the area of activity and exercise management, specifically the diagnosis of *activity intolerance,* there are a variety of interventions from which to choose (e.g., body mechanics promotion or exercise promotion). NIC is a valuable resource to assist nurses in the selection of appropriate interventions. NIC is evolving and is practice oriented; it is designed to enable nurses in all practice settings to have a standard classification system for documenting nursing care. The classification is designed to be comprehensive, including independent and collaborative interventions that cover all specialty areas (Carter and others, 1995). However, it still remains the individual nurse's decision to determine which interventions are most appropriate for the client's needs and situation.

Table *17-3*	Nursing Interventions Classification (NIC) Taxonomy—cont'd		
Domain 4	**Domain 5**	**Domain 6**	**Domain 7**
4. Safety Care that supports protection against harm	**5. Family** Care that supports the family unit	**6. Health System** Care that supports effective use of the health care delivery system	**7. Community** Care that supports the health of the community
U Crisis Management: Interventions to provide immediate short-term help in both psychological and physiological crises *V Risk Management:* Interventions to initiate risk-reduction activities and continue monitoring risks over time	*W Childbearing Care:* Interventions to assist in understanding and coping with the psychological and physiological changes during the childbearing period *Z Childrearing Care:* Interventions to assist in rearing children *X Lifespan Care:* Interventions to facilitate family unit functioning and promote the health and welfare of family members throughout the lifespan	*Y Health System Mediation:* Interventions to facilitate the interface between patient/family and the health care system *a Health System Management:* Interventions to provide and enhance support services for the delivery of care *b Information Management:* Interventions to facilitate communication among health care providers	*c Community Health Promotion:* Interventions that promote the health of the whole community *d Community Risk Management:* Interventions that assist in detecting or preventing health risks to the whole community

From Dochterman JM, Bulechek GM: *Nursing interventions classification (NIC)*, ed 4, St. Louis, 2004, Mosby.

*P*lanning Nursing Care

When planning care, a nurse will usually have more interventions than are necessary to meet a client's expected outcomes. Some are discarded as inappropriate, and others are adapted to the client's needs and abilities. As a result, the list of possible interventions is narrowed down to those suitable to the client (Redman, 1997). These interventions are then written on the nursing care plan.

A **nursing care plan** is a guide for clinical care. It also serves as a document that communicates a client's nursing care to all members of the health care team. It is made available to the team as a ready reference for nursing care interventions. There are different forms of care plans. This chapter will describe student care plans, institutional care plans, and concept maps.

Purpose of Care Plans

A written care plan is designed to direct clinical care and to decrease the risk of incomplete, incorrect, or inaccurate care. The plan is organized so that any nurse can quickly identify the client's nursing diagnoses, goals, and outcomes and nursing interventions to be delivered. In hospitals and outpatient and community-based settings, the client often receives care from more than one nurse, physician, or allied health professional. A written nursing care plan makes possible the coordination of nursing care, subspecialty consultations, and scheduling of diagnostic tests.

The care plan can identify and coordinate resources used to deliver nursing care. The listing of specific equipment and supplies necessary for nursing actions is an economically efficient mechanism for selecting equipment. If all equipment and supplies are included in the care plan, the nurse's time is used more effectively in providing care.

The nursing care plan enhances the continuity of nursing care by listing specific nursing actions necessary to achieve the goals and outcomes of care. These nursing actions can be carried out daily. A correctly formulated written care plan facilitates the continuity of care from one nurse to another. As a result, all nurses have the opportunity to deliver high-quality, consistent care.

Written nursing care plans organize information exchanged by nurses in change-of-shift reports (see Chapter

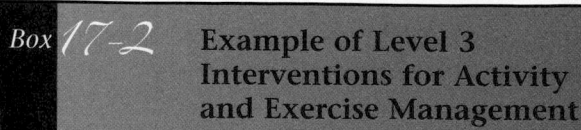

Box 17-2   Example of Level 3 Interventions for Activity and Exercise Management

A. Activity and Exercise Management

Interventions to organize or assist with physical activity and energy conservation and expenditure.

Level 3 Interventions
Body Mechanics Promotion
Energy Management
Exercise Promotion
Exercise Promotion: Strength Training
Exercise Promotion: Stretching
Exercise Therapy: Ambulation
Exercise Therapy: Balance
Exercise Therapy: Joint Mobility
Exercise Therapy: Muscle Control
Teaching Prescribed Activity/Exercise

Examples of Linked Nursing Diagnoses:
Activity Intolerance
Fatigue
Mobility, Impaired Physical

From Dochterman JM, Bulechek GM: *Nursing interventions classification (NIC)*, ed 4, St. Louis, 2004, Mosby.

Box 17-3   Example of Level 3 Interventions and Associated Nursing Activities

Body Mechanics Promotion

Examples of Activities:
Determine client's commitment to learning and using correct posture
Collaborate with physical therapy in developing a body mechanics promotion plan
Determine client's understanding of body mechanics and exercises
Instruct client on structure and function of spine and optimal posture for moving and using the body
Instruct client need for correct posture to prevent fatigue, strain, or injury
Instruct client how to use posture and body mechanics while performing any physical activities
Determine client awareness of own musculoskeletal abnormalities and potential effects of posture and muscle tissue
Instruct to use firm mattress/chair or pillow as appropriate
Instruct to avoid sleeping prone
Assist to demonstrate appropriate sleeping positions
Assist to avoid sitting in the same position for prolonged periods
Demonstrate how to shift weight from one foot to another while standing

From Dochterman JM, Bulechek GM: *Nursing interventions classification (NIC)*, ed 4, St. Louis, 2004, Mosby.

25). Nurses focus their reports on nursing care and treatments and client outcomes as delineated in care plans. At the end of shifts, nurses discuss care plans and the client's overall progress with the next caregivers. Thus all nurses are able to discuss current and pertinent information about the client's plan of care.

The written care plan also includes the long-term needs of the client. Incorporating the goals of the care plan into discharge planning is particularly important for a client who will be undergoing long-term rehabilitation in the community or who will require ongoing home care. A complete care plan enhances the continuity of nursing care between nurses in the hospital and community.

When developing an individualized care plan, the nurse involves the family and client. The family is a resource to help the client meet health goals. In addition, meeting some of the family's needs can improve the client's level of wellness.

Most written plans include expected outcome criteria used in the evaluation of care. Proper listing of the criteria provides the nurse with objective statements that help determine whether the goals of care have been achieved. The complete care plan is the blueprint for nursing action. It provides direction for implementation of the plan and a framework for evaluation of the client's response to nursing actions.

Student Care Plans

Nursing students learn to write and use a nursing care plan as part of their education. The student care plan is essential for learning the problem-solving technique, the nursing process, skills of written communication, and organizational skills needed for nursing care. Most important, by using the nursing care plan students can apply the knowledge gained from nursing and medical literature and the classroom to a practice situation.

Students typically write care plans for each of a client's nursing diagnoses before they actually provide clinical care for a client. The most common format used in writing student nursing care plans is a columnar plan that includes assessment, goals, nursing interventions, supporting scientific rationales, and outcome criteria (Table 17-4).

The nursing diagnosis with the highest priority is the beginning point for the nursing care plan and is followed by other nursing diagnoses in order of assigned priority. The example in Table 17-4 uses a six-column format. In the assessment column (column 1), the nurse includes all assessment data relevant to the corresponding nursing diagnosis. The nurse then includes the goals (column 2) and outcomes (column 3) identified for the client. At this point, the nurse begins to translate the goals and outcomes into an action plan that includes appropriate nursing interventions and ensures a coordinated approach to nursing care. The nurse writes the action plan in the implementation column (column 4) of the care plan. Each nursing action is written to include information necessary to implement nursing care. It may help the beginning nurse to ask whether the stated interventions answer the following questions:
What is the intervention?
When should each intervention be implemented?

Table 17-4		Example of Student Care Plan			
Nursing Diagnosis: Risk for impaired skin integrity related to physical immobility secondary to impaired consciousness					
Assessment	**Goals**	**Expected Outcomes**	**Interventions**	**Rationale**	**Evaluation**
Fever >102° F for 48 hr Diaphroresis Changes position on own infrequently Incontinent of urine Decreased skin turgor Braden scale = 10 No skin breakdown noted, 2-cm area of redness over left shoulder lasting 15 min	Skin will remain intact through discharge. Client will achieve fluid intake > output within 24 hr.	Skin color returns to normal in 48 hr. Client is afebrile in 24 hr Skin remains dry and without breakdown through discharge. Skin turgor returns to normal in 48 hr.	Turn client every 1½ hr as follows: 8 AM supine 9:30 AM 30-degree left lateral position 11 AM 30-degree right lateral position 12:30 PM supine Continue cycle as above. Keep head of bed below 30-degree elevation. Apply air fluidized bed until body fluids are contained. Apply condom urinary catheter. Administer IV fluids as ordered.	Turning interval should be based on standard 2-hr turning minus hypoxia time (skin redness usually persists half of time hypoxia occurs) (AHCPR, 1994). Head of bed below 30-degree angle reduces shear (Bryant and others, 2000). When excess moisture on intact skin is potential source of skin maceration, an air flow support surface dries skin and prevents pressure ulcers (AHCPR, 1994). Provides urinary drainage when clients have spontaneous and complete bladder emptying.	*Student* enters notes to evaluate success of plan in this column.

How should the intervention be performed for this specific client?

Who should be involved in each aspect of intervention?

The nurse enters a scientific rationale (column 5) for a specific intervention. A **scientific rationale** is the reason that, based on supporting literature, a specific nursing action was chosen. Each rationale should include a reference, whenever possible, to document the source from the scientific literature. This reinforces the importance of evidence-based nursing practice. It is important that each intervention be specific and unique to a client's situation. Nonspecific nursing interventions result in incomplete or inaccurate nursing care, lack of continuity among caregivers, and poor use of resources. Common omissions in writing nursing interventions include action, frequency, quantity, method, or person to perform them. These errors can occur if the nurse is unfamiliar with the planning process. Table 17-5 illustrates these types of errors by showing incorrect and correct statements of nursing interventions. Column 6 of the care plan includes a section for the student nurse to evaluate

the plan of care: was each outcome fully met or only partially met? The student can use the evaluation column to document whether the plan requires revision. The student can also enter when outcomes are met, thus indicating when a particular nursing diagnosis is no longer relevant to the client's plan of care.

The student care plan is more elaborate than a care plan in a hospital or community health care agency because its purpose is to teach the process of planning care. Student care plans vary from one educational program to another and between beginning and more advanced students. Some educational institutions model the student care plan on the care plan used in the affiliated health care agency.

Institutional Care Plans

Institutional care plans are concise documents that become part of the client's medical record. Many hospitals use the Kardex nursing care plan. **Kardex** is a trade name for a card-filing system that allows quick reference to the particular needs of the client for certain aspects of nurs-

Table 17-5	Frequent Errors in Writing Nursing Interventions	
Type of Error	**Incorrectly Stated Nursing Intervention**	**Correctly Stated Nursing Intervention**
Failure to precisely or completely indicate nursing actions	Turn client every 2 hours.	Turn client every 2 hours, using the following schedule: 8 AM—supine, 10 AM—left side, Noon—prone, 2 PM—right side. Repeat at 4 PM and 2 AM
Failure to indicate frequency	Perform blood glucose measurements.	Measure blood glucose before each meal: 7 AM—11 AM—5 PM.
Failure to indicate quantity	Irrigate wound once a shift: 6 AM — 2 PM—8 PM.	Irrigate wound with 100 ml normal saline unil clear: 6 AM—2 PM—8 PM
Failure to indicate method	Change client's dressing once a shift: 6 AM—2 PM—10 PM.	Replace client's dressing with Neosporin ointment to wound and two dry 4 × 4 dressings secured with hypoallergenic tape, once a shift: 2 PM—10 PM—6 AM.

ing care. Information about medications, activity levels, level of self-care, diet, treatments, and procedures is usually included on the outside of the card. The nursing care plan is commonly placed on the inside (Figure 17-3). Each institution has its own format for the Kardex, but the basic information contained on it is universal. The care plan section of the Kardex also has institutional variations. One institution might use a three-column nursing care plan, which includes the problem, goal or outcome, and nursing action. Another institution may incorporate a four-column nursing care plan, which includes the nursing diagnosis, goal or outcome, nursing action, and evaluation. Although the format of the care plan varies from setting to setting, its overall purpose is to provide a written guideline for care so that the health care needs of the client and subsequent therapies are communicated among the health care team. One feature of an institutional care plan, different from that of student care plans, is the omission of scientific rationale. In practice, it is assumed that professional nurses know the rationales for the interventions selected for clients.

The focus of a nursing care plan will differ by setting and the evolving client situation. For example, the nursing care plan developed for the client returning home is usually based solely on long-term health needs. The plan includes interventions to involve the client, family, and significant others in assuming more responsibility for care because the client is to receive nursing care in the home. Same-day surgeries usually have plans focused on clients' short-term needs, (e.g., immediate recovery from surgery and instructions for assuming self-care following discharge). A long-term care facility will have a plan of care focused on the client's long-term rehabilitation needs.

Computerized Care Plans. The use of computers and the need to efficiently organize the nurse's time have resulted in standardized care plans, which are prewritten plans created for a specific nursing diagnosis or clinical problem (e.g., immobility, abdominal surgery, or postpartum care). After completing a nursing assessment, the nurse determines whether a standardized care plan should be used for that particular client. Even if the care plan is generally appropriate for a client, the nurse must add or

delete information on the standardized form to individualize it for the client's needs. Failure to do so can result in incomplete and inaccurate care. For example, the nurse selects a nursing diagnosis and then individualizes the standard care plan by making selections from menus. Each care plan lists generalized nursing diagnoses, goals, outcome criteria, and interventions for specific clients (Figure 17-4).

Computerized/standardized nursing care plans are a method to streamline and augment care planning, and provide documentation for third-party reimbursement (Hirtzel-Trexler, 1994). They are designed to incorporate current evidence-based practice guidelines to achieve the desired client outcomes for a specific group of clients. In addition, these plans encourage the nurse to incorporate individual client care needs into the plan of care.

Care Plans for Community-Based Settings. Planning care for clients in community-based settings, for example, clinics, community centers, or client's homes, involves using the same principles of nursing practice. However, in these settings the nurse must complete a more comprehensive community, home, and family assessment. In this setting, the client/family unit is in equal partnership with health care professionals (Bond, Phillips, and Rollins, 1994). Ultimately the client/family must be able to independently provide the majority of health care. The nurse designs a plan (1) to educate the client/family about the necessary care techniques, (2) to teach the client/family how to integrate care within family activities, and (3) to allow the client/family to assume a greater percentage of care in graduated increments (Bond, Phillips, and Rollins, 1994; Lund, 1994). Last, the plan is designed to include nurses' and the client's/family's evaluation of expected outcomes.

Critical Pathways. **Critical pathways** allow staff from all disciplines, such as medicine, nursing, pharmacy, and social work, to develop integrated care plans for a projected length of stay or number of visits for clients with a specific case type (Zander and McGill, 1994). For example, a pathway for a surgical procedure such as a colon resection will recommend on a day-by-day basis the client's activities, consults, procedures, and discharge planning activities, and

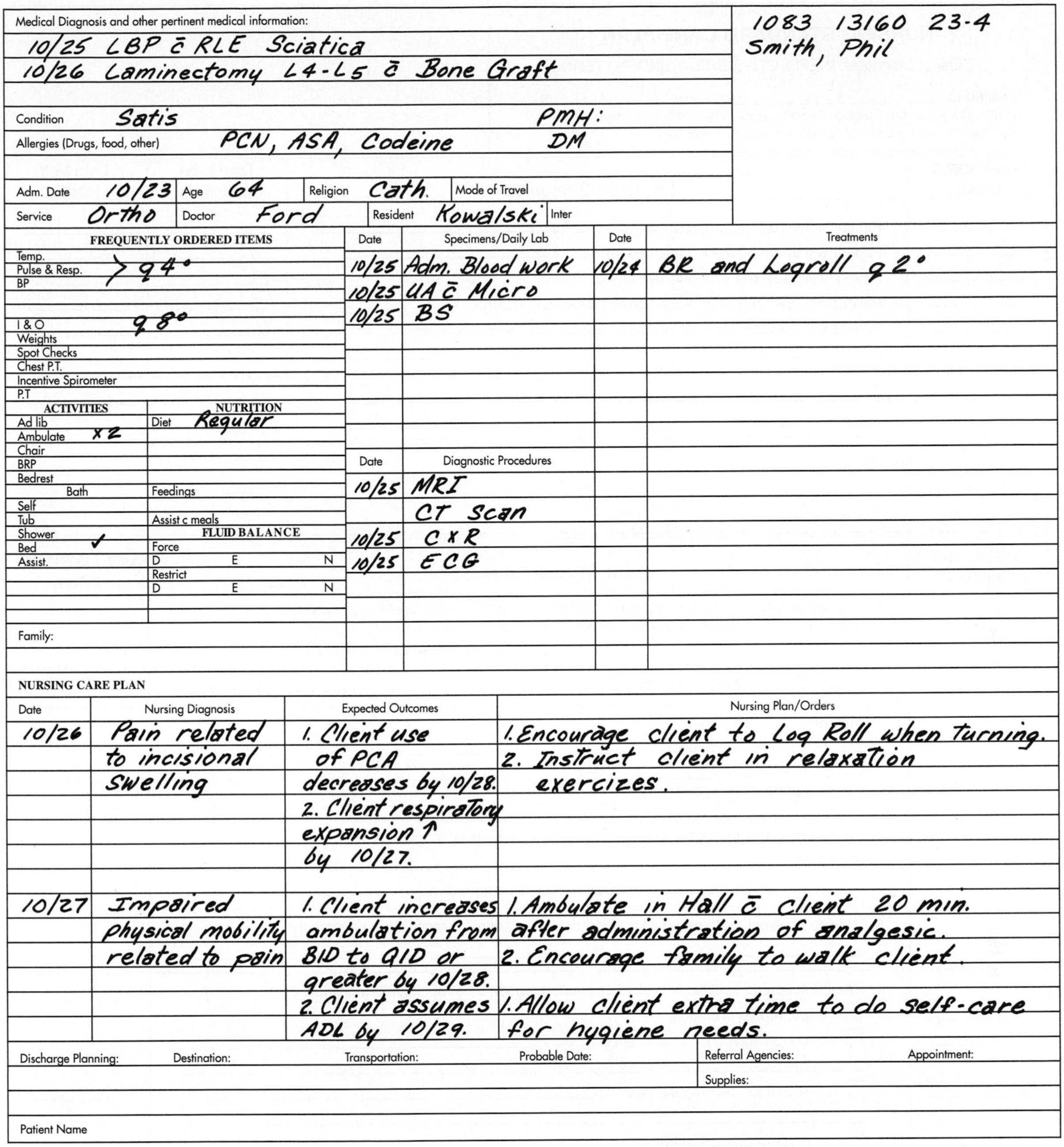

Medical Diagnosis and other pertinent medical information:			1083 13160 23-4 Smith, Phil

10/25 LBP c̄ RLE Sciatica
10/26 Laminectomy L4-L5 c̄ Bone Graft

Condition	Satis		PMH:
Allergies (Drugs, food, other)	PCN, ASA, Codeine		DM

Adm. Date 10/23	Age 64	Religion Cath.	Mode of Travel
Service Ortho	Doctor Ford	Resident Kowalski	Inter

FREQUENTLY ORDERED ITEMS		Date	Specimens/Daily Lab	Date	Treatments
Temp. Pulse & Resp. BP	> q4°	10/25	Adm. Blood work	10/24	BR and Logroll q2°
		10/25	UA c̄ Micro		
		10/25	BS		
I & O	q8°				
Weights					
Spot Checks					
Chest P.T.					
Incentive Spirometer					
P.T					

ACTIVITIES		NUTRITION		Date	Diagnostic Procedures	
Ad lib		Diet	Regular			
Ambulate	X2					
Chair						
BRP				10/25	MRI	
Bedrest					CT Scan	
Bath		Feedings				
Self				10/25	CXR	
Tub		Assist c̄ meals		10/25	ECG	
Shower	✓	FLUID BALANCE				
Bed		Force				
Assist.		D E N				
		Restrict				
		D E N				

Family:

NURSING CARE PLAN

Date	Nursing Diagnosis	Expected Outcomes	Nursing Plan/Orders
10/26	Pain related to incisional Swelling	1. Client use of PCA decreases by 10/28. 2. Client respiratory expansion ↑ by 10/27.	1. Encourage client to Log Roll when turning. 2. Instruct client in relaxation exercizes.
10/27	Impaired physical mobility related to pain	1. Client increases ambulation from BID to QID or greater by 10/28. 2. Client assumes ADL by 10/29.	1. Ambulate in Hall c̄ client 20 min. after administration of analgesic. 2. Encourage family to walk client. 1. Allow client extra time to do self-care for hygiene needs.

Discharge Planning:	Destination:	Transportation:	Probable Date:	Referral Agencies:	Appointment:
				Supplies:	

Patient Name

FIGURE 17–3 Nursing care plan on a nursing Kardex.

educational topics expected for client's progression to discharge. A critical pathway ensures better continuity of care because it maps out clearly the responsibility of each health care discipline. When well developed, pathways incorporate evidence-based protocols typically used in the care of the specific case type. The nurse and other health team members use the pathway to monitor a client's progress and as a documentation tool. Due to managed care (see Chapter 2), documentation tools that integrate the standards of care for multiple disciplines are necessary. Critical pathways help all members of the health care team to meet this need, and charting by exception is frequently the method of choice (see Chapter 25).

Initially, critical pathways were developed to manage clients in acute care settings. However, these pathways are now integrated into community-based settings (e.g., home care, restorative care settings, and same-day surgery) (Leininger and Laux, 1998). When using critical pathways to plan care, many other forms (e.g., the nursing care plan, flow sheets, and nurses' notes) are eliminated because all the pertinent components are included on the pathway format.

Concept Maps

Students care for clients who present with multiple health problems and related nursing diagnoses. It is

NURSING STANDARD CARE PLAN

Nursing Diagnosis: INEFFECTIVE BREATHING PATTERN

Related to: _____
(respiratory muscle fatigue, anxiety, pain, impaired respiratory
mechanics such as chest tubes, incisions, anatomy)

Date Initiated/ Initials	Expected Outcomes	Date to be Met/Initials	Date Met/ Initials
_____	Patient will verbalize understanding of _____ .	_____	_____
_____	Patient will demonstrate ability to perform _____ .	_____	_____
_____	Patient will pace and schedule activities.	_____	_____
_____	Patient will use relaxation techniques for breathing control.	_____	_____
_____	Patient will maintain respiratory rate of _____ with PaCO2 of _____ .	_____	_____
_____	Other: _____	_____	_____

Relevant baseline data: _____
_____

Referrals: (date contacted)

☐ Nurse Specialist: _____ ☐ Home Care: _____ ☐ Social Work: _____
☐ Other: _____ ☐ Other: _____

Date Initiated/ Initials	Nursing Interventions	Date Inactivated/ Initials

	1. Assess respiratory function for rapid, shallow, irregular, or slow breathing, dyspnea,
	   use of accessory muscles, breath sounds, restlessness, confusion, and cyanosis
	   every _____ .	

	2. Monitor patient's mental status/LOC every _____ .	

_____
_____
_____
	3. Maintain adequate airway by:
	   ☐ a. cough/splinting every _____
	   ☐ b. suction every _____
	   ☐ c. incentive spirometry every _____
		_____
		_____
		_____

	4. Pace and schedule activity to avoid dyspnea resulting from fatigue. Schedule is _____	
	5. Provide physical and emotional support during episodes of respiratory distress by: _____	

_____
_____
_____
_____
_____
	6. Provide teaching specific to patient or support person's needs. Initiate individual plan:
	   ☐ a. pursed lip breathing
	   ☐ b. coughing/splinting techniques (specify) _____
	   ☐ c. relaxation techniques (specify) _____
	   ☐ d. diaphragmatic breathing _____
	   ☐ e. other: _____
		_____
		_____
		_____
		_____
		_____

_____
_____
_____
_____
	7. Other interventionsl specific to patient:
	   a. _____
	   b. _____
	   c. _____
	   d. _____	

	Signature/Initials: _____	

☐ **PLAN OF CARE MUTUALLY SET WITH PATIENT AND/OR FAMILY**

FIGURE **17–4** Standardized nursing care plan. (Courtesy Barnes-Jewish Hospital, St. Louis, Mo.)

often not realistic to have a written columnar plan developed for each nursing diagnosis. Plus, the columnar plans do not contain a means to show the association between different nursing diagnoses and different nursing interventions. A **concept map** is a tool that assists learners in developing a self-appraisal of their own individual thinking processes (Daley and others, 1999). Basically, it is a diagram of client problems and interventions that shows their relationships to one another (Schuster 2002). When used as a plan of care, a concept map fosters a careful consideration of evidence from clinical practice. Students learn to consider the context of nursing practice in their conceptualization of nursing problems (Daley and others, 1999). The use of a concept map promotes critical thinking and helps student nurses to organize complex client data, process complex relationships, and achieve a holistic view of a client's situation (Baugh and Mellott, 1998).

There are different approaches to writing concept maps. Schuster (2000) suggests some simple steps in preparing for concept mapping and in developing a clinical plan of care:

1. Before caring for an assigned client, gather the clinical assessment database from the client's medical record, including health history, physical assessment data, laboratory and diagnostic data, medication history, and treatment plan.
2. Review information on the client's health problems, treatments, and medications in course textbooks, pharmacology texts, and other related resources.
3. Review on the nursing unit any standardized nursing care plans, clinical pathways, clinical protocols, or

client education materials appropriate for client care preparation.

4. Prepare the map by first developing a skeleton diagram of the client's health problems. Write the client's major medical diagnoses in the middle of the map, then add associated nursing care needs like spokes on a wheel (Figure 17-5). Often students initially have difficulty labeling nursing diagnoses correctly. It is important for you to recognize the major nursing care focus for the client. Later appropriate diagnostic labels can be added to the map.
5. Identify and group clinical assessment data, treatments, medications, and medical history data related to the nursing diagnoses (Figure 17-6). These include assessments you must complete during your first contact with the client. Remember, sometimes symptoms apply to more than one nursing diagnosis. Repeat symptoms under different categories when appropriate; for example, lethargy and fatigue would be appropriate under "activity intolerance," and "altered nutrition."
6. Next, analyze relationships among the nursing diagnoses. Draw lines between nursing diagnoses to indicate relationships (Figure 17-7). It is important for you to make meaningful associations between one concept and another concept. The links must be accurate, meaningful, and complete. You must be able to explain why nursing diagnoses are related.
7. Finally, on a separate sheet of paper or on the map itself, list nursing interventions to attain the outcomes for each nursing diagnosis (Box 17-4). This

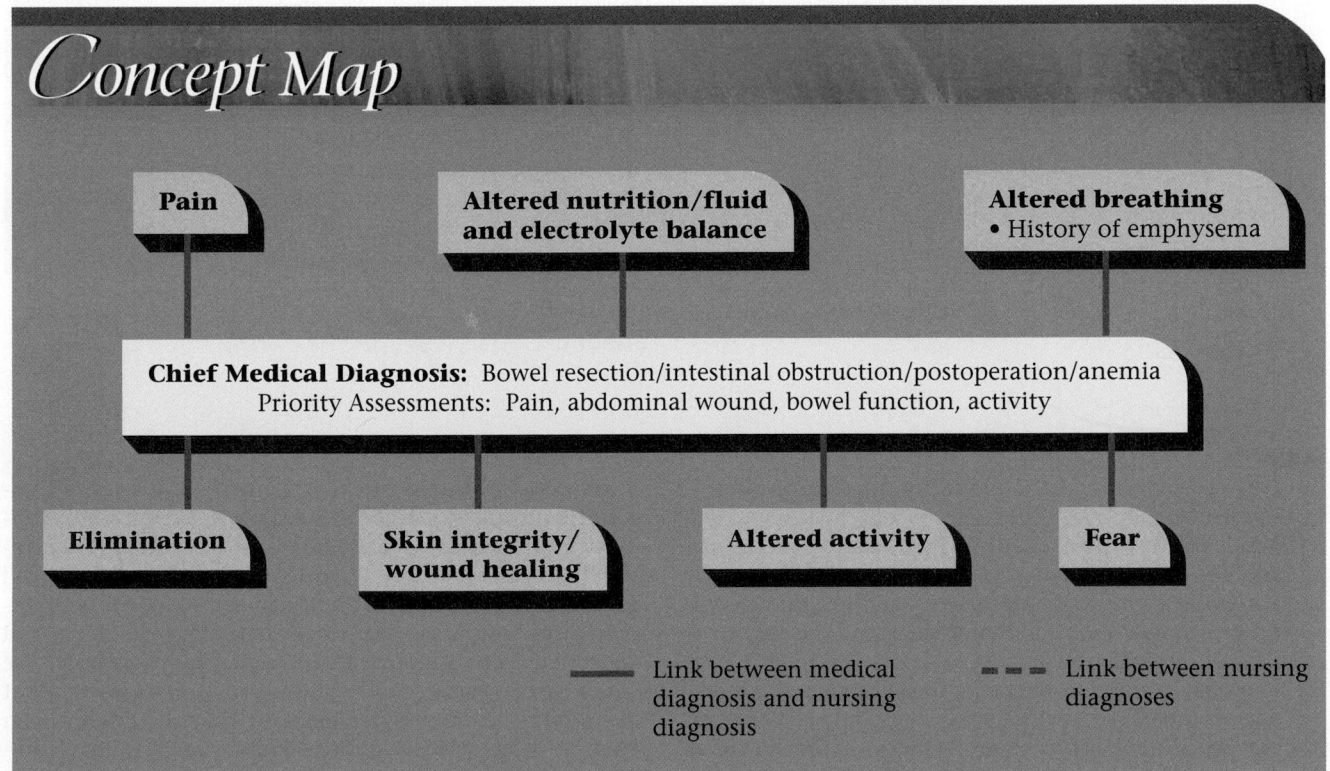

FIGURE **17–5** Concept map with nursing and medical diagnoses.

Concept Map

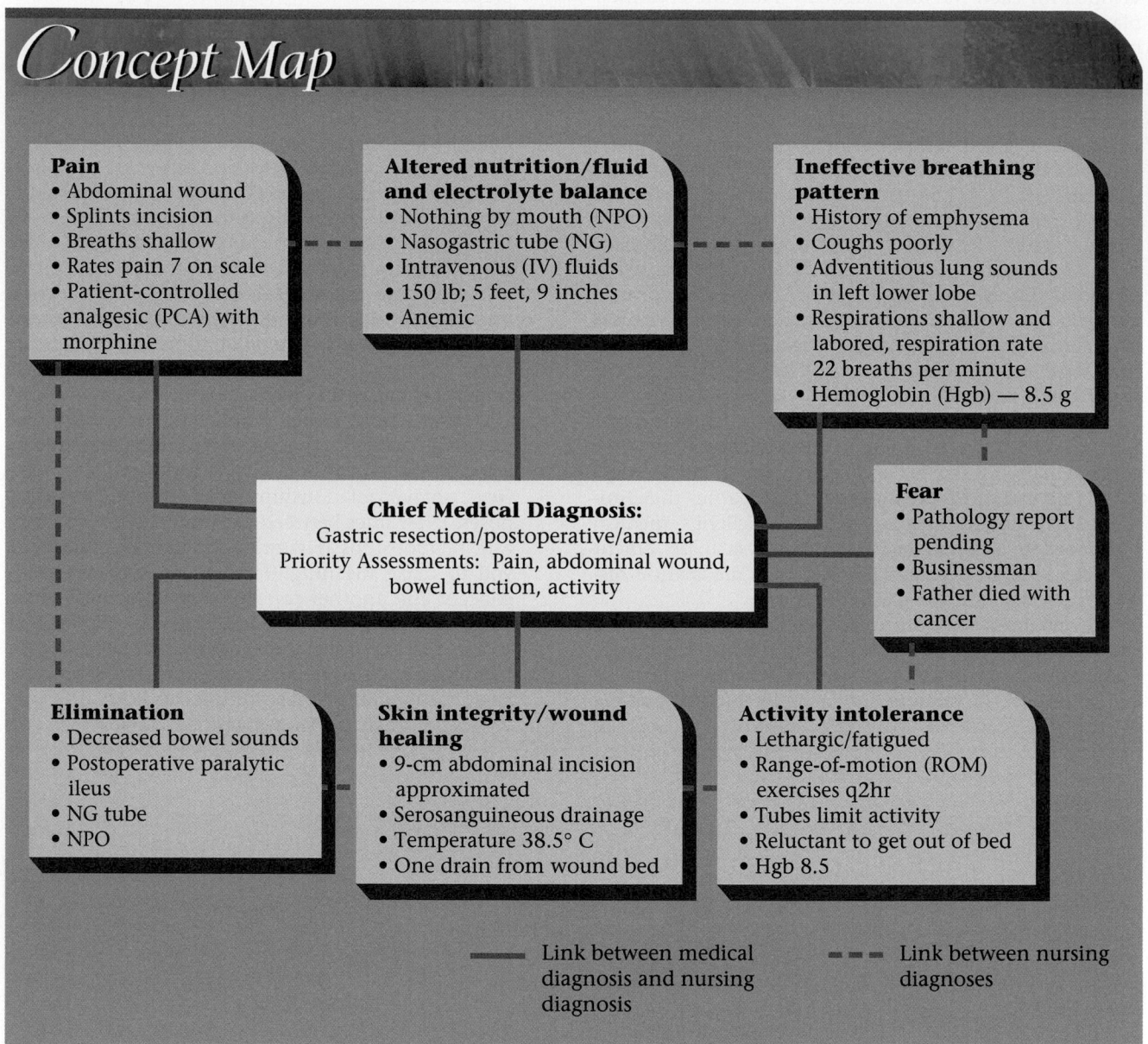

Pain
- Abdominal wound
- Splints incision
- Breaths shallow
- Rates pain 7 on scale
- Patient-controlled analgesic (PCA) with morphine

Altered nutrition/fluid and electrolyte balance
- Nothing by mouth (NPO)
- Nasogastric tube (NG)
- Intravenous (IV) fluids
- 150 lb; 5 feet, 9 inches
- Anemic

Ineffective breathing pattern
- History of emphysema
- Coughs poorly
- Adventitious lung sounds in left lower lobe
- Respirations shallow and labored, respiration rate 22 breaths per minute
- Hemoglobin (Hgb) — 8.5 g

Chief Medical Diagnosis:
Gastric resection/postoperative/anemia
Priority Assessments: Pain, abdominal wound, bowel function, activity

Fear
- Pathology report pending
- Businessman
- Father died with cancer

Elimination
- Decreased bowel sounds
- Postoperative paralytic ileus
- NG tube
- NPO

Skin integrity/wound healing
- 9-cm abdominal incision approximated
- Serosanguineous drainage
- Temperature 38.5° C
- One drain from wound bed

Activity intolerance
- Lethargic/fatigued
- Range-of-motion (ROM) exercises q2hr
- Tubes limit activity
- Reluctant to get out of bed
- Hgb 8.5

—— Link between medical diagnosis and nursing diagnosis

- - - Link between nursing diagnoses

FIGURE **17–6** Concept map data to support nursing diagnoses.

step corresponds to the planning phase of the nursing process.

8. While caring for the client, write down the client's responses to each nursing activity. Also write your clinical impressions and inferences regarding the client's progress toward expected outcomes and the effectiveness of interventions.

9. Keep the care map with you throughout the clinical day. As the plan is revised, take notes and add or delete nursing interventions. Use the information recorded on the map for your documentation of client care.

Critical thinkers learn by organizing and relating cognitive concepts. Concept maps help learners to link concepts such as nursing diagnoses and to assimilate the interrelationships so as to create a unique meaning and organization of information. A concept map will help students link important ideas between client problems and treatments for those problems. A map helps to build the structure of what a student knows, as well as reveal what a student does not understand, so that the student can learn to ask questions and discover what to learn to provide quality client care.

Concept Map

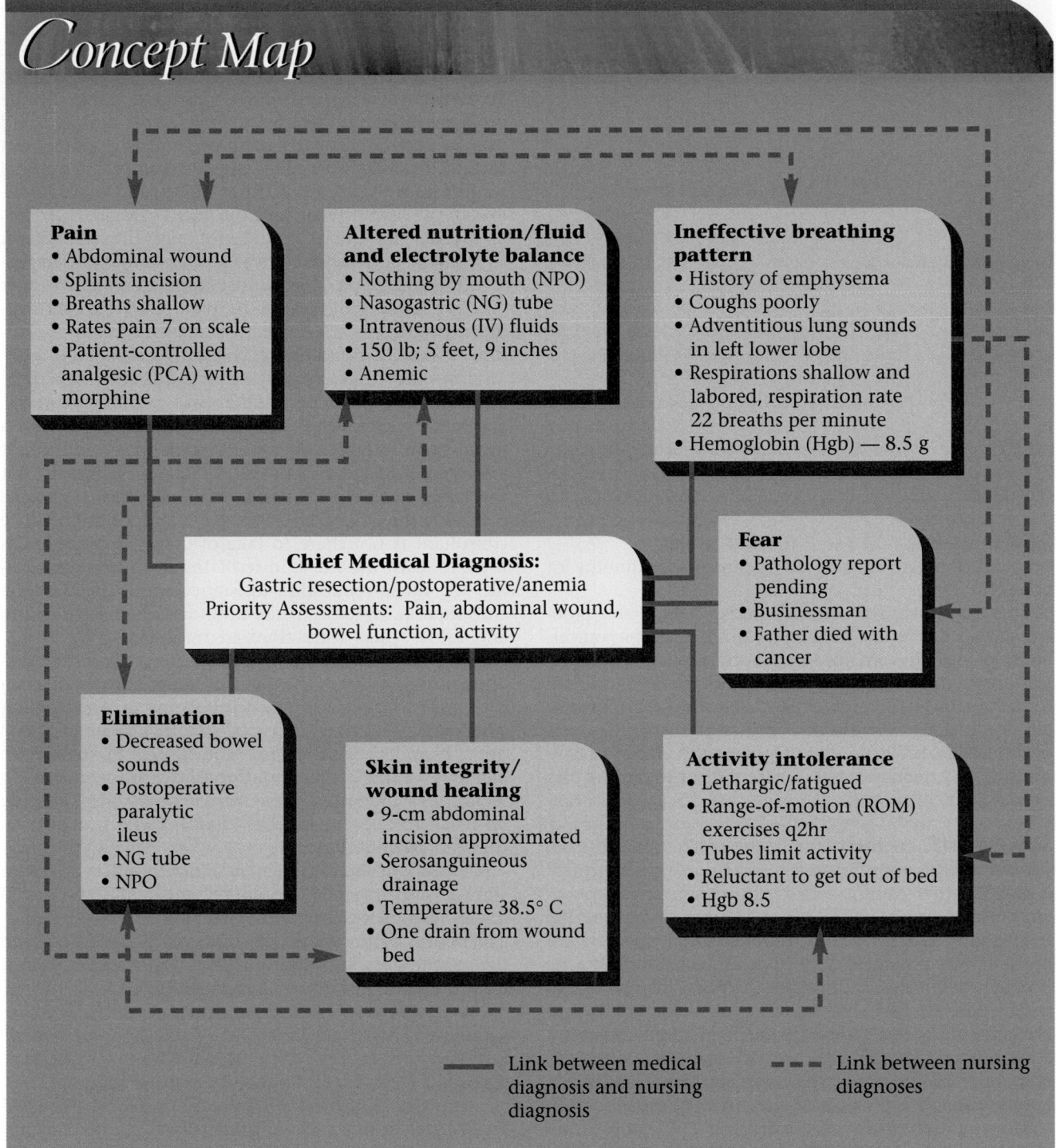

Pain
- Abdominal wound
- Splints incision
- Breaths shallow
- Rates pain 7 on scale
- Patient-controlled analgesic (PCA) with morphine

Altered nutrition/fluid and electrolyte balance
- Nothing by mouth (NPO)
- Nasogastric (NG) tube
- Intravenous (IV) fluids
- 150 lb; 5 feet, 9 inches
- Anemic

Ineffective breathing pattern
- History of emphysema
- Coughs poorly
- Adventitious lung sounds in left lower lobe
- Respirations shallow and labored, respiration rate 22 breaths per minute
- Hemoglobin (Hgb) — 8.5 g

Chief Medical Diagnosis:
Gastric resection/postoperative/anemia
Priority Assessments: Pain, abdominal wound, bowel function, activity

Fear
- Pathology report pending
- Businessman
- Father died with cancer

Elimination
- Decreased bowel sounds
- Postoperative paralytic ileus
- NG tube
- NPO

Skin integrity/wound healing
- 9-cm abdominal incision approximated
- Serosanguineous drainage
- Temperature 38.5° C
- One drain from wound bed

Activity intolerance
- Lethargic/fatigued
- Range-of-motion (ROM) exercises q2hr
- Tubes limit activity
- Reluctant to get out of bed
- Hgb 8.5

——— Link between medical diagnosis and nursing diagnosis

– – – Link between nursing diagnoses

FIGURE **17–7** Concept map relationships among nursing diagnoses.

Consulting Other Health Care Professionals

Planning nursing care involves consultation with other members of the health care team. **Consultation** may occur at any step in the nursing process, but it is needed most often during planning and implementation, when the nurse is more likely to identify a problem requiring additional knowledge, skills, or resources (Lund, 1994). Consultation is a process in which the expertise of a specialist is sought to identify ways to handle problems in client management or the planning and implementation of therapies. Consultation is based on the problem-

---

Box 17-4   **Example of Nursing Interventions for Nursing Diagnoses on Concept Map**

Pain

Reinforce appropriate use of patient-controlled analgesia (PCA) device.
Splint abdomen.
Position for comfort.
Use distraction or guided imagery.

Ineffective Breathing Pattern

Support incisional area during cough/deep breathing exercises.
Administer incentive spirometer every hours.
Turn every 2 hours.
Monitor respiratory rate, chest excursion.
Auscultate breath sounds.
Monitor hemoglobin level.
Position semi-Fowler's, Fowler's if tolerated.

---

solving approach, and the consultant is the stimulus for change.

In clinical nursing, consultation is used to solve problems in the delivery of nursing care or the use of resources. Nurse consultants are most frequently approached for advice about difficult clinical problems. Nurses are consulted for their clinical expertise, client education skills, or staff education skills. Nurses also consult with other members of the health care team, such as physical therapists, nutritionists, and social workers. Again, the consultant focuses on problems in providing nursing care.

When to Consult

Consultation is appropriate when the nurse has identified a problem that cannot be solved using personal knowledge, skills, and resources. Consultation increases the nurse's knowledge about the problem and helps in learning skills and obtaining the resources needed to solve the problem. After the consultation, the nurse may be able to resolve similar problems in the future. For example, a nurse caring for a client with diabetes might request a consultation from a diabetes educator to determine the best approach to instruct the client and the teaching materials available on insulin administration.

Consultation is also used when the exact problem remains unclear. A consultant objectively entering a situation can more clearly assess and identify the exact nature of the problem, whether it is client, personnel, or equipment oriented. An unbiased consultant can often objectively identify the problem and outline a method for resolving it.

How to Consult

The nurse will have a general understanding of a client's clinical problems. When making a consult, the first step is identification of the general problem area, which will give the consultant a starting point for identifying the specific problem. Second, the consultation should be di-

rected to the appropriate professional, who may be another nurse or another member of the health care team.

Third, the nurse provides the consultant with pertinent assessment information and resources about the problem area. This includes a brief assessment of the problem, interventions used to manage the problem, and the outcome of those interventions. Other resources can include the client's complete nursing history and medical record, information from other nurses and other members of the health team, and the client's family.

Fourth, the nurse should not bias the consultant. Consultants are in the clinical setting to identify and resolve a nursing problem, and biasing them can hinder problem resolution. Bias can be avoided by not overloading consultants with subjective and emotional conclusions about the client and problem.

Fifth, the nurse requesting consultation should be available to discuss the findings and recommendations. When a consultation is requested, the nurse provides a private, comfortable atmosphere in which the consultant and client can meet. However, this does not mean that the nurse leaves the client care unit. A common mistake is turning the whole problem over to the consultant. The consultant is not there to take over the problem but is there to assist the nurse in resolving it. Whenever possible, the nurse requesting assistance should request the consultation for a day when both are scheduled to work and a time when distractions are minimal.

Finally, the nurse incorporates the consultant's recommendations into the plan of care. The changes in care must be communicated in writing on the nursing care plan or Kardex and verbally to all nursing and other health care providers. The success of the advice depends on the implementation of the problem-solving techniques suggested. The nurse should also provide feedback to the consultant regarding the outcome of the recommendations.

Consultants are a valuable adjunct to nursing care. In clinical nursing practice, competent and experienced nurses encounter problems beyond their knowledge or experience. Professional and competent nurses recognize their limitations, seek appropriate consultation, and learn from the findings and recommendations.

Key Concepts

- During planning, client goals are determined and prioritized, expected outcomes of nursing care are developed, and a nursing care plan is written.
- Priority setting helps a nurse anticipate and sequence nursing interventions when a client has multiple problems.
- A nurse writes goals and expected outcomes to direct selection and use of nursing interventions and to provide focus for evaluation of client care.
- A client-centered goal is specific, measurable, time limited, and mutually set with a client when possible.
- An expected outcome is an objective criteria for goal achievement.
- To initiate an intervention the nurse must know the

scientific rationale for the intervention, possess necessary psychomotor and interpersonal skills, and function effectively within the health care setting.

- Nurse-initiated interventions require no supervision or direction from others.
- Physician-initiated interventions require specific nursing responsibilities and technical nursing knowledge.
- Critical pathways are multidisciplinary treatment plans that predict the interventions and outcomes to be met for selected clients over a projected length of stay.
- Care plans and critical pathways increase communication among nurses and facilitate the continuity of care from one nurse to another and from one health care setting to another.
- A concept map provides a graphic way to show the relationship between clients' nursing diagnoses and interventions.
- The Nursing Interventions Classification taxonomy provides a standardization to assist nurses in selecting suitable interventions for clients' problems.
- Correctly written nursing interventions include actions, frequency, quantity, method, and the person to perform them.
- Consultation increases the nurse's knowledge about the problem and helps in learning skills and obtaining the resources needed to solve the problem.

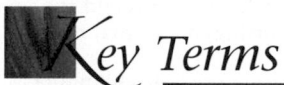

Key Terms

Client-centered goal, *p. 320*	Long-term goal, *p. 322*
Collaboration, *p. 326*	Nurse-initiated
Collaborative	interventions, *p. 324*
interventions, *p. 324*	Nursing care plan, *p. 327*
Concept map, *p. 333*	Physician-initiated
Consultation, *p. 335*	interventions, *p. 324*
Critical pathways, *p. 330*	Planning, *p. 318*
Expected outcome, *p. 322*	Scientific rationale, *p. 329*
Goals, *p. 320*	Short-term goal, *p. 321*
Kardex, *p. 329*	

Critical Thinking Exercises

1. Write a goal and expected outcome for each of the following clinical scenarios:
   a. Mr. Jacko has recently been diagnosed with asthma and is to be discharged tomorrow. His physician has ordered a metered dose inhaler for Mr. Jacko to use daily. The client has not used an inhaler before. He asks the nurse, "What do I do at home if I have trouble using this thing?" The nursing diagnosis for Mr. Jacko is *deficient knowledge regarding use of a metered dose inhaler related to inexperience.*
   b. Ms. Snow has been suffering from a high fever for several days. She is diaphoretic and very fatigued. She has difficulty turning herself in bed because she has little energy and she is overweight. The skin over her bony prominences is intact at this time, with some redness appearing over the coccyx area. Reddened area blanches with fingertip pressure. The nursing diagnosis for Ms. Snow is *risk for impaired skin integrity related to moisture and impaired mobility.*

2. Mrs. Drew is a 68-year-old woman with a diagnosis of congestive heart failure. Her heart does not have the strength to contract as strongly as normal and thus is unable to efficiently pump blood through the circulation. As a result, she is experiencing fatigue, shortness of breath especially following light exertion, edema of the lower extremities, cough, and occasional palpitations. She complains of feeling weak and tired when ambulating down the hall. She tends to have more palpitations after walking only about 10 to 20 feet. Mrs. Drew lives alone, and she expresses concerns as to how she will care for herself. When asked if her neighbors can assist, she says she would rather not have to depend on them. The nurse talks with her at length and finds that Mrs. Drew has difficulty problem solving ways she can minimize her exertion when performing routine activities at home.

   Identify three nursing diagnoses for Mrs. Drew, and order those diagnoses by high, intermediate, or low priority.

3. Which of the following are errors in writing a nursing intervention?
   a. Suction client nasotracheally.
   b. Assigned RN will assist client with active ROM exercises 0800, 1200, 1600, 1900.
   c. Assigned RN will instruct client in medication administration 11/10 and 11/11.

Review Questions

1. Once a nurse assesses a client's condition and identifies appropriate nursing diagnoses, a:
   1. Plan is developed for nursing care.
   2. Physical assessment begins.
   3. List of priorities is determined.
   4. Review of the assessment is conducted with other team members.

2. Planning is a category of nursing behaviors in which:
   1. The nurse determines the health care needed for the client.
   2. The physician determines the plan of care for the client.
   3. Client-centered goals and expected outcomes are established.
   4. The client determines the care needed.

3. Priorities are established to help the nurse anticipate and sequence nursing interventions when a client has multiple problems or alterations. Priorities are determined by the client's:
   1. Physician.
   2. Nonemergent, non–life threatening needs.
   3. Future well-being.
   4. Urgency of problems.

4. A client-centered goal is a specific and measurable behavior or response that reflects a client's:
   1. Desire for specified health care interventions.
   2. Highest possible level of wellness and independence in function.
   3. Physician's goal for the specific client.
   4. Response when compared to another client with a like problem.

5. For clients to participate in goal setting, they should be:
   1. Alert and have some degree of independence.
   2. Ambulatory and mobile.
   3. Able to speak and write.
   4. Able to read and write.

6. The nurse writes an expected outcome statement in measurable terms. An example is:
   1. Client will have less pain.
   2. Client will be pain free.
   3. Client will report pain acuity less than 4 on a scale of 0 to 10.
   4. Client will take pain medication every 4 hours.

7. As goals, outcomes, and interventions are developed, the nurse must:
   1. Be in charge of all care and planning for the client.
   2. Be aware of and committed to accepted standards of practice from nursing and other disciplines.
   3. Not change the plan of care for the client.
   4. Be in control of all interventions for the client.

8. When establishing realistic goals, the nurse:
   1. Bases the goals on the nurse's personal knowledge.
   2. Knows the resources of the health care facility, family, and client.
   3. Must have a client who is physically and emotionally stable.
   4. Must have the client's cooperation.

9. To initiate an intervention the nurse must be competent in three areas, which include:
   1. Knowledge, function, and specific skills.
   2. Experience, advanced education, and skills.
   3. Skills, finances, and leadership.
   4. Leadership, autonomy, and skills.

10. Collaborative interventions are therapies that require:
    1. Physician and nurse intervention.
    2. Nurse and client intervention.
    3. Client and physician intervention.
    4. Multiple health care professionals.

*R*eferences

Bandman EL, Bandman B: *Critical thinking in nursing,* ed 2, Norwalk, Conn, 1995, Appleton & Lange.

Baugh NG, Mellott KG: Clinical concept mapping as preparation for student nurses' clinical experiences, *J Nurs Educ* 37(6):253, 1998.

Benner P: *From novice to expert: excellence and power in clinical nursing practice,* Menlo Park, Calif, 1984, Addison-Wesley.

Bond N, Phillips P, Rollins JA: Family-centered care at home for families with children who are technology dependent, *Pediatr Nurs* 20:123, 1994.

Bryant RA: *Acute and chronic wounds,* ed 2, St. Louis, 2000, Mosby.

Carpenito LJ: *Nursing diagnoses: application to clinical practice,* ed 7, Philadelphia, 1997, JB Lippincott.

Carter J and others: Using the nursing interventions classification to implement Agency for Health Care Policy and Research guidelines, *J Nurs Care Qual* 9(2):166, 1995.

Chase S: Teaching baccalaureate nursing students to project outcomes to nursing interventions, *Nurs Diagn* 9(2):62, 1998.

Deaton C: Outcomes measurement, *J Cardiovasc Nurs* 12(4):49, 1998.

Dochterman JM, Bulechek GM: *Nursing interventions classification (NIC),* ed 4, St. Louis, 2004, Mosby.

Dochterman JM, Jones DA: *Unifying nursing: the harmonization of NANDA,* NIC, NOC, Washington, DC, 2003, American Nurses Association.

Gordon M: *Nursing diagnosis: process and application,* ed 3, St. Louis, 1994, Mosby.

Gordon M and others: Clinical judgment: an integrated model, *Adv Nurs Sci* 16:55, 1994.

Hirtzel-Trexler BJ: Commentary on practice guidelines: a standard whose time has come, *AONE's Leadership Perspectives* 2(2):22, 1994.

Iowa Intervention Project: the NIC taxonomy structure, *Image J Nurs Sch* 25:1816, 1993.

Leininger SM, Laux LH: The continuum of health care: highlights of orthopaedic and general medical pathways, *Home Health Care Management and Practice* 10(4):1, 1998.

Liukkonen A: The nurse's decision-making process and the implementation of psychogeriatric nursing in a mental hospital, *J Adv Nurs* 17(3):356, 1992.

Lund SM: Family-centered nurse coordinator-early childhood intervention: development and implementation of the CNS role, *Clin Nurse Spec* 8:109, 1994.

McCloskey JC, Bulechek GM: Standardizing the language for nursing treatments: an overview of the issues, *Nurs Outlook* 42:56, 1994.

McCloskey JC, Bulechek GM: Nursing interventions core to specialty practice, *Nurs Outlook* 46(2):67, 1998.

Moorhead S, Johnson M, Maas M: *Nursing outcomes classification,* ed. 3, St. Louis, Mo, 2004, Mosby.

NANDA International: *NANDA nursing diagnosis: definitions and classifications 2003-2004,* Philadelphia, 2003, NANDA International.

Redman BK: *The practice of patient education,* ed 8, St. Louis, 1997, Mosby.

Schuster PM: Concept mapping: Reducing clinical care plan paperwork and increasing learning, *Nurse Educ* 25(2):76, 2000.

Schuster PM: *Concept mapping: a critical-thinking approach to care planning,* St. Louis, 2002, Mosby.

Zander K, McGill R: Critical and anticipated recovery paths: only the beginning, *Nurs Manage* 25(8):34, 1994.

*R*esearch References

Agency for Health Care Policy and Research, Panel for treatment of pressure ulcers, Clinical practice guideline, No 15, ANCPR Pub No. 95-0653, Rockville, Md, 1994.

Daley BJ and others: Concept maps: a strategy to teach and evaluate critical thinking, *J Nurs Educ* 38(1):42, 1999.

18

*I*mplementing Nursing Care

Media Resources

http://evolve.elsevier.com/Potter/
fundamentals/

CD COMPANION

- Review Questions
- Glossary

evolve WEBSITE

- Review Questions
- Student Learning Activities
- Glossary

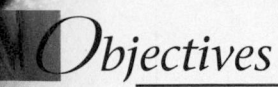

Mastery of content in this chapter will enable the student to:

- Define the key terms listed.
- Explain the relationship of implementation to the diagnostic process.
- Discuss the differences between protocols and standing orders.
- Describe the association between critical thinking and selecting nursing interventions.
- Identify preparatory activities the nurse uses before implementation.
- Explain when it may become necessary to revise a plan of care before implementation is performed.
- Discuss the relationship between the three implementation skills.
- Describe both direct and indirect implementation methods.
- Select appropriate implementation methods for an assigned client.

*I*mplementation, the fourth step of the nursing process, begins after the care plan has been developed. With the care plan based on clear and relevant nursing diagnoses, the nurse then selects and initiates interventions that are most likely to support or improve the client's health status. In theory, implementation of the nursing care plan follows the planning component of the nursing process. However, in many health care settings implementation may begin directly after assessment. For example, immediate implementation is necessary when the nurse identifies urgent needs of the client in situations such as cardiac arrest or sudden death of a loved one.

Implementation is the step of the nursing process where nurses provide care to patients. The nurse initiates and completes actions or interventions necessary for achieving the goals and expected outcomes of nursing care. A **nursing intervention** is any treatment, based upon clinical judgment and knowledge, that a nurse performs to enhance client outcomes (Dochterman and Bulechek, 2004). Interventions include both direct and indirect care; those aimed at individuals, families, and the community. **Direct care** interventions are treatments performed through interaction with the client. For example, a client may require direct intervention in the form of medication administration, insertion of an intravenous infusion to support circulatory function, or the provision of psychosocial counseling during a client's time of grief. **Indirect care** interventions are treatments performed away from the client but on behalf of the client or group of clients (Dochterman and Bulechek, 2004). Examples of indirect care include actions aimed at managing the client's environment (e.g., safety and infection control), documentation, and interdisciplinary collaboration.

Implementation is a continuous process that interacts with all steps of the nursing process. As the nurse carries out interventions, the client's condition can change, requiring further assessment, or the client may respond to the interventions as expected based on evaluation (Table 18-1). For implementation to be effective, the nurse must be knowledgeable about the implementation

Table 18-1	Sample Nursing Care Plan

CASE STUDY: A nursing care plan has been developed for Mrs. Coyle, a 32-year-old woman who had a normal vaginal delivery of an 8-pound, 6-ounce newborn. The nursing diagnosis of *impaired urinary elimination related to perineal swelling after vaginal delivery* provides the focus for the plan. Just before inserting the straight catheter, the nurse reassesses Mrs. Coyle to determine if she has voided spontaneously. Spontaneous voiding of 150 ml of urine would indicate that the straight catheterization procedure was no longer appropriate. However, Mrs. Coyle has not voided and the straight catheterization is still indicated.

NURSING DIAGNOSIS: Impaired urinary elimination related to perineal swelling after vaginal delivery.

DEFINITION: Impaired urinary elimination is the state in which an individual experiences a disturbance in urine elimination.*

Assessment	Goals/*Outcomes*	Implementation	Evaluation (Outcomes)
Client has not voided in 8 hours.	Achieve emptying of bladder (8/17) as evidenced by: *Urine output greater than 240 ml during single voiding.*	Insert straight catheter, using sterile technique, if client has not voided in 8 hours and bladder is palpable.	1000 ml of clear yellow urine is returned via straight catheter (8/16).
Fluid intake for last 8 hours is 2400 ml.			Bladder is not palpable (8/16).
Client states that she "feels the urge" to void and experiences bladder discomfort.	*Verbalizes no urge to void and no bladder discomfort.*		Client no longer has urge to void (8/17).
Bladder is palpable to 2 cm below umbilicus.	*Bladder is not palpable.*		Client no longer complains of bladder discomfort (8/17).

*Data from NANDA International: *Nursing diagnoses: definitions and classification 2003-2004,* Philadelphia, 2003, NANDA International.

process, implementation skills, and specific direct and indirect care interventions.

Types of Nursing Interventions

Direct and indirect care interventions include those that are nurse-initiated, physician-initiated, and collaborative (see Chapter 17). Nurse-initiated interventions are the independent response of the nurse to the client's health care needs and nursing diagnoses. These are autonomous actions based on scientific rationale that is executed to benefit the client in a predicted way in relation to the nursing diagnoses and client-centered goals (Bulechek and McCloskey, 1990). Physician-initiated interventions are based on a physician's response to treat or manage a medical diagnosis. It is not always within the legal practice of nursing for the nurse to prescribe and order these treatments independently, but it is within the practice of nursing for the nurse to complete such orders and to individualize approaches to their administration. Collaborative interventions are therapies that require the knowledge, skill, and expertise of multiple health care professionals. Each member of the team has a responsibility for his or her discipline's contribution to the client's care.

At times, nursing interventions are developed, communicated, and organized on the basis of protocols or preprinted (standing) orders. An understanding of these clinical guidelines is necessary for safe nursing practice.

Protocols and Standing Orders

A **protocol** is a written plan specifying the procedures to be followed during care of clients with a select clinical condition or situation, such as the care of postoperative clients. A protocol provides a standard of care or clinical guideline, which can still be individualized for a specific client, depending on how an institution recommends protocol implementation. Nurses who provide primary care for clients in an outpatient setting frequently follow diagnostic and treatment protocols. In such a setting, nurses assess the client and identify abnormalities. The protocol delineates the conditions that nurses are permitted to treat, such as controlled hypertension, and the types of treatment they are permitted to administer, such as antihypertensive medications.

A protocol can also be strictly within the framework of independent nursing interventions, such as a protocol for admission and discharge, pain management, or initiating cardiopulmonary resuscitation (CPR). Protocols are also used in interdisciplinary settings for diagnostic testing and physical, occupational, and speech therapies.

A **standing order** is a preprinted document containing orders for the conduct of routine therapies, monitoring guidelines, and/or diagnostic procedures for specific clients with identified clinical problems. The orders direct the conduct of client care in various clinical settings. Standing orders must be approved and signed by the licensed, prescribing physician or health care provider in charge of care before their implementation. Often they are implemented at the time a client is admitted to a health care setting. Standing orders are commonly found in critical care settings, where client's needs can change rapidly and require immediate attention. Such a standing order might specify certain medications, such as lidocaine or propranolol, for an irregular heart rhythm. After assessing the client and identifying the irregular rhythm, the critical care nurse gives the specified medication without first notifying the physician. The physician's initial order covers the nurse's action. Standing orders are also common in the community health setting, in which the nurse encounters situations that do not permit immediate contact with a physician. Thus standing orders and protocols give the nurse legal protection to intervene appropriately in the client's best interest.

•••

Before implementing any intervention, the nurse must use sound judgment in determining whether the intervention is correct and appropriate. Second, the nurse has the responsibility to have the correct theoretical knowledge and develop the clinical competency necessary to perform the intervention. Nursing responsibility is equally great for all types of interventions.

*C*ritical Thinking in Implementation

When nurses use the nursing process, they make two types of decisions. During the diagnostic process, the nurse forms conclusions, makes decisions, and draws inferences about the client's assessment data and health care needs (Miller and Babcock, 1996). Next, the nurse uses a methodical, systematic, research-based approach to plan and select appropriate nursing interventions (Gordon, 1994). The selection of nursing interventions for a specific client is part of the clinical decision making of the nurse (Dochterman and Bulechek, 2004). Six factors should be considered when choosing interventions:

1. *Desired or expected client outcome*—Outcomes are the criteria against which to judge the success of a nursing intervention. The nurse identifies for each client the outcomes that can be reasonably expected and attained as a result of nursing intervention (see Chapter 17).
2. *Characteristics of the nursing diagnosis*—An intervention should be directed toward altering the etiological or related factor of a client's nursing diagnosis. An intervention will alter the related factor or treat the client's signs and symptoms. For a risk nursing diagnosis, interventions are aimed at altering or eliminating risk factors for the diagnosis.
3. *Evidence base for the intervention*—A nurse should know the evidence base for an intervention. An evidence base includes the research or proven practice guidelines that indicate the effectiveness of using an intervention with certain types of clients (Dochterman and Bulechek, 2004). Sometimes choosing among nurse-initiated interventions can be difficult because research is not available to support all nursing interventions (Snyder, Egan, and Nojima, 1996). Some interventions have been widely tested for specific populations. Examples are interventions in patient education and pain management. Other interventions are still in the development phase, with scant evidence of their efficacy. Nurses should stay informed of the evidence base for their practice. When

evidence is not available, the nurse uses scientific principles and/or consults with clinical experts.

4. *Feasibility for performing an intervention*—A single intervention can interact with other interventions delivered by the nurse or members of the health care team. The nurse must consider how a proposed intervention will affect other planned interventions. For example, a nurse should consider how educating a client about adjusting lifestyle so as to follow a diabetic diet will affect the information a dietitian covers during diet instruction. In addition, the cost and time it takes to deliver an intervention must also be considered when determining if an intervention is feasible.
5. *Acceptability to the client*—An intervention must be acceptable to a client and family (Dochterman and Bulechek, 2004). When choosing interventions, the nurse explains how the client is to participate, what the intervention involves, and how the client might be affected. This type of summary is necessary for clients to make informed decisions about their care. It is also important to consider the client's values, beliefs, and culture when selecting interventions.
6. *Capability of the nurse*—A nurse must be competent to perform the intervention. The nurse must have knowledge of the scientific rationale for the intervention, possess necessary psychomotor and interpersonal skills, and function within the setting to effectively use all resources. No one nurse is expert in all interventions. Consultation with other nurses and disciplines is critical.

The critical thinking model discussed in Chapter 14 provides a framework for how to make decisions for implementing nursing care (Figure 18-1). The nurse implements the care plan using the knowledge bases necessary for care planning (see Chapter 17) and for then completing the planned interventions most effectively. An important knowledge base is the Nursing Interventions Classification (NIC) taxonomy developed by the University of Iowa. The interventions help to differentiate nursing practice from the practice of other health care professionals (Box 18-1). In addition to knowledge, the nurse applies prior clinical experiences in performing specific interventions. The nurse considers what interventions have worked and what have not worked in certain clinical situations. The nurse also learns to adapt interventions on the basis of different client needs and situations. To intervene effectively, the nurse must be aware of both professional and agency standards of practice. The standards of practice offer guidelines for the selection of interventions, their frequency, and the determination of whether the procedures may be delegated. When performing interventions, the nurse applies intellectual standards. For example, any client instruction should be relevant, clear, logical, and complete to promote client learning. All critical thinking attitudes apply to implementation. For example, the confidence a nurse shows in performing a procedure builds trust with a client. Creativity and self-discipline will guide the nurse in reviewing, modifying, and implementing interventions. A critical thinker shows integrity by questioning personal knowledge. A beginning student or

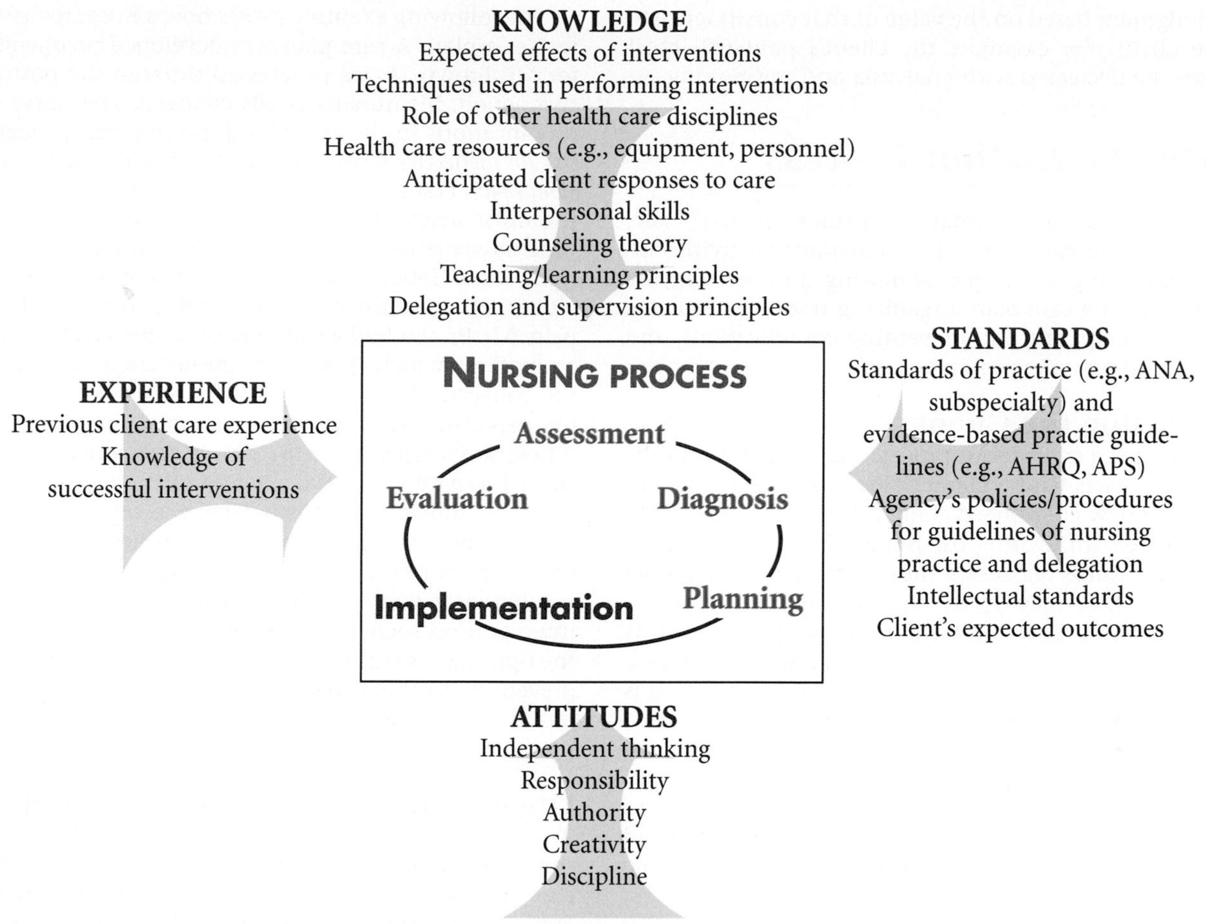

KNOWLEDGE
Expected effects of interventions
Techniques used in performing interventions
Role of other health care disciplines
Health care resources (e.g., equipment, personnel)
Anticipated client responses to care
Interpersonal skills
Counseling theory
Teaching/learning principles
Delegation and supervision principles

EXPERIENCE
Previous client care experience
Knowledge of
successful interventions

NURSING PROCESS
Assessment
Evaluation   Diagnosis
Implementation   Planning

STANDARDS
Standards of practice (e.g., ANA,
subspecialty) and
evidence-based practie guidelines (e.g., AHRQ, APS)
Agency's policies/procedures
for guidelines of nursing
practice and delegation
Intellectual standards
Client's expected outcomes

ATTITUDES
Independent thinking
Responsibility
Authority
Creativity
Discipline

FIGURE **18–1** Critical thinking and the process of implementing care.

Box 18–1   **Purposes of the Nursing Interventions Classification (NIC) Project**

1. Standardization of the nomenclature (e.g., labeling, describing) of nursing interventions. Needed to standardize the language nurses use to describe specific actions used to deliver nursing care.
2. Expansion of nursing knowledge about connections between nursing diagnoses, treatments, and outcomes. These connections will be determined through the study of actual client care using a database that the classification will generate.
3. Development of nursing and health care information systems. Information systems will standardize a system for describing the interventions that nurses perform.
4. Teaching decision making to nursing students. Defining and classifying nursing interventions will help in teaching beginning nurses how to determine a client's need for care and respond appropriately. In addition, a classification of nursing interventions will make it easier to identify nursing interventions requiring higher knowledge and skill levels.
5. Determination of the cost of services provided by nurses.
6. Planning for resources needed in all types of nursing practice settings.
7. Language to communicate the unique functions of nursing.
8. Articulate with the classification systems of other health care providers.

From Dochterman JM, Bulechek GM: *Nursing interventions classification (NIC),* ed 4, St. Louis, 2004, Mosby.

---

practitioner still needs supervision from an instructor or experienced nurse to guide the decision-making process for implementation.

When making decisions about implementing care, the nurse may want to consider the following (Snyder, 1985):
• The set of all possible nursing actions (e.g., pain-control measures, including analgesia, relaxation, and positioning).

• A listing of all possible consequences associated with each possible nursing action, such as relief of pain, no relief of pain, and an adverse reaction to analgesia.
• The determination of the probability that each of the consequences will occur. For example, the client's pain decreased with previous analgesia and positioning; therefore adverse reactions are unlikely.

- A judgment based on the value of that consequence to the client. For example, the client's pain will most likely be decreased with analgesia and positioning.

Implementation Process

Preparation for implementation ensures efficient, safe, and effective nursing care. Five preparatory activities include reassessing the client, reviewing and revising the existing nursing care plan, organizing resources and care delivery, anticipating and preventing complications, and implementing nursing interventions.

Reassessing the Client

Assessment is a continuous process that occurs each time a nurse interacts with a client. When new data are gathered and a new client need is identified, the nurse modifies the care plan. During the initial phase of implementation, the nurse reassesses the client. This is a partial assessment that may focus on one dimension of the client, such as level of comfort, or on one system, such as the cardiovascular system. The reassessment provides a way to determine whether the proposed nursing action is still appropriate for the client's level of wellness. For example, the nurse plans to ambulate a client following lunch; however, a reassessment reveals shortness of breath and increased fatigue, which requires the nurse to return the client to bed. When new data are obtained and a new client need is identified, the nurse modifies the nursing care plan.

Reviewing and Revising the Existing Nursing Care Plan

After reassessing a client, the nurse reviews the care plan, compares assessment data to validate the stated nursing diagnoses, and determines whether the nursing interventions remain the most appropriate for the clinical situation. If the client's status has changed and the nursing diagnosis and related nursing interventions are no longer appropriate, the nursing care plan needs to be modified. An out-of-date or incorrect care plan compromises the quality of nursing care, whereas review and modification enable the nurse to provide timely nursing interventions to best meet the client's needs. Modification of the existing written care plan includes four steps:

1. Data in the assessment column are revised to reflect the client's current status. New data entered in the care plan should be dated to inform other members of the health care team of the time that the change occurred.
2. Nursing diagnoses are revised. Nursing diagnoses that are no longer relevant are deleted, related factors are revised, and new nursing diagnoses are added and dated. In addition, the client's priorities, goals, and expected outcomes also must be revised. The revisions are also dated on the care plan.
3. Specific interventions are revised to correspond to the new nursing diagnoses and client goals. This revision reflects the client's present status.
4. The nurse determines what methods of evaluation will be used to determine if outcomes are achieved.

The following example shows how a nurse reviews and revises a plan. A care plan was developed preoperatively for Mr. Brown. As he progressed through the postoperative period, his nursing needs changed. The nurse made modifications in the care plan for one nursing diagnosis: *risk for ineffective airway clearance related to abdominal incisional pain* (Table 18-2). On the second postoperative day the nurse assessed the client and noted decreased chest wall movements, crackles that were auscultated in the right lower lobes, and an elevated temperature (39° C [102.2° F]). Mr. Brown also reported increased abdominal pain. Mr. Brown had a standing order for a chest x-ray examination, which was taken immediately and revealed the collapse of alveoli in the right lower lobe. The nursing diagnosis was revised to an actual diagnosis with a different etiology, *ineffective airway clearance related to decreased inspiratory effort secondary to abdominal incisional pain.* The nursing diagnostic label was revised because of the presence of right lower lobe crackles and decreased chest wall movement. The goal of Mr. Brown's airway becoming clear was still appropriate. Specific new nursing interventions such as the use of incentive spirometry and the optional use of suctioning were developed to assist in preventing further alveolar collapse. Finally, the nurse determined the method of evaluation for the new clinical problem.

Organizing Resources and Care Delivery

A facility's resources include equipment and skilled personnel. Organization of equipment and personnel makes efficient, skilled client care possible (see Chapter 20). Before delivering an intervention, the nurse prepares the necessary supplies and decides on the time and provider of care. Preparation for care delivery also involves preparing the environment and client for nursing intervention.

Equipment. Most nursing procedures, from bed making to client teaching, require some equipment or supplies. The nurse determines needed items and their availability. Equipment should be in working order to ensure safe use. All necessary supplies should be gathered and put in a convenient location, usually where they will be used. Extra supplies should be available in case of mishaps. By having extra sterile gloves, for example, the nurse anticipates the possibility of a break in sterile technique. However, extra supplies should not be opened unless they are needed; this controls health care costs. The nurse also arranges the supplies in the order in which they will be used. Following the procedure the nurse appropriately returns any unopened supplies.

Personnel. Nursing care delivery systems vary among facilities and must be considered when deploying nursing staff. The system by which nursing is organized determines the way in which personnel are designated for client care delivery. For example, an RN's accountabilities differ in a team nursing model compared with a primary nursing model. A primary nurse is accountable for the nursing care a client receives during his or her length of stay. A team nurse is accountable for the care a client receives for a specific shift in which the nurse works. Chapter 20 summarizes the various care delivery models.

Table 18-2	Modified Nursing Care Plan for Mr. Brown

NURSING DIAGNOSIS: Risk for ineffective airway clearance related to abdominal incisional pain.
Modified Nursing Diagnosis: Ineffective airway clearance related to decreased inspiratory effort secondary to abdominal incisional pain.
DEFINITION: Ineffective airway clearance is the state in which an individual is unable to clear secretions or obstructions from the respiratory tract to maintain a clear airway.*

Assessment	Goals/*Outcomes*	Implementation	Evaluation
Smoked two packs/day for 20 years; chest x-ray film showing slight change of emphysema; crackles auscultated in RLL; scheduled for abdominal surgery	Airway will remain clear (11/8) as evidenced by: *Lungs clear to auscultation* *Client coughs productively*	**Airway management†** Demonstrate turn, cough, and deep breathing exercise to client. Have client perform exercises every 2 hours while awake.	Productive cough produced. Airway clear to auscultation.

Modified 24 Hours After Surgery

Assessment	Goals/*Outcomes*	Implementation	Evaluation
Decreased chest wall movements; crackles bilaterally in base that do not clear with coughing; elevated temperature (39° C [102.2° F]); reports incisional pain 6 on scale of 0 to 10	Airway will remain clear (11/8) as evidenced by: *Lungs clear to auscultation* *Temperature <100° F* *Pain intensity will be less than client's baseline*	**Airway management†** Administer chest physiotherapy to all lobes of the lung: 8-12-4-8-12-4. Have Mr. Brown perform incentive spirometry every 2 hours around the clock. Teach client to splint incision with pillow before and during coughing. Administer analgesics as ordered for incisional pain. **Airway suctioning** Suction nasotracheally every 2 hours if client is unable to cough productively.	Lung fields are clear on auscultation. Client becomes afebrile. Chest x-ray film demonstrates atelectasis resolving. Client does not report increased pain during coughing.

*Data from NANDA International: *Nursing diagnoses: definitions and classification 2003-2004,* Philadelphia, 2003, NANDA International.
†Intervention categories supported by NIC. From Dochterman JM, Bulechek GM: *Nursing interventions classification (NIC),* ed 4, St. Louis, 2004, Mosby.

It is the nurse's responsibility to determine whether to perform an intervention or to delegate it to another member of the nursing team. The nurse's assessment of the client should direct the decision about delegating an intervention, not the intervention alone. For example, assistive personnel (AP) are trained to competently ambulate clients. However, if a nurse learns that a client experienced cardiac irregularities the previous shift, the nurse may decide to personally assist the client with ambulation and evaluate the client's cardiac status. The assistive personnel can be then be asked to perform an intervention for a different client.

Nursing staff work together when client needs demand it. If a client makes a request, such as use of a bedpan, the RN should position the client on the pan if she or he has time rather than trying to find the technician who is in a different room. When interventions are complex or physically difficult, an RN may need assistance. For example, an RN and a technician can more effectively change a dressing in a large gaping wound, with the nurse performing the procedure and the technician assisting with client positioning and handing off of supplies.

Environment. Environmental factors influence the delivery and reception of care. The surroundings in which nursing activities occur should be safe and conducive to

the implementation of the therapy. Client safety is always the first concern. If the client has sensory deficits, physical disability, or an alteration in level of consciousness, the environment must be arranged to prevent injury. Using special rooms, providing assistive devices (e.g., walkers, eyeglasses), rearranging furniture and equipment, and making rooms free of clutter are examples of creating safe surroundings.

The client benefits most from nursing interventions when surroundings are compatible with activities. Privacy promotes relaxation when body parts are exposed. Reducing distractions enhances a client's learning opportunities. Provision of adequate space and lighting provides for efficiency when procedures are performed.

Client. Before beginning to perform interventions, the nurse should make the client as physically and psychologically comfortable as possible. Symptoms such as nausea, dizziness, or pain, for example, frequently interfere with a client's full concentration and cooperation. Administering comfort measures before initiating interventions enables the client to participate more fully. In the case of analgesic administration, for example, if client alertness is needed, the dose of pain medication should be sufficient to relieve discomfort but not impair mental faculties.

Even if symptoms are not a factor, the client should be made physically comfortable during interventions. Controlling environmental factors, positioning, and taking care of other physical needs (e.g., elimination) should precede initiation of interventions. The nurse should also consider the client's level of endurance and plan only the amount of activity that the client can comfortably tolerate.

Awareness of the client's psychosocial needs helps the nurse to create a favorable emotional climate. Some clients feel reassured by having a significant other present to lend encouragement and moral support. Other strategies include planning sufficient time or multiple opportunities for the client to work through and ventilate feelings and anxieties. Adequate preparation allows the client to obtain maximal benefit from each intervention.

Anticipating and Preventing Complications

Risks to the client arise from both illness and treatment. The nurse must identify these risks, evaluate the relative benefit of the treatment versus the risk, and initiate risk prevention measures. Many client conditions place the client at risk for additional complications. For example, the client with preexisting left-sided paralysis following a stroke 2 years earlier is at risk for developing a pressure ulcer following orthopedic surgery, which requires traction and bed rest. The nurse's knowledge of pathophysiology helps in identifying the risk of complications that can occur. Scientific rationales for how certain interventions (e.g., pressure relief devices and turning and repositioning) can prevent or minimize complications help the nurse to evaluate the usefulness of preventive measures. If the client's postoperative pain is not controlled, the risk for pressure ulcer development increases because the client may be unwilling or unable to change position frequently, because of pain. The nurse anticipates when the client's pain will be aggravated, administers ordered analgesics, and then positions the client to remove pressure on the skin and underlying tissues.

Identifying Areas of Assistance. Some nursing situations require the nurse to acquire assistance by seeking additional personnel, knowledge, and/or nursing skills. Before implementing care, the nurse reviews the plan to determine the need for assistance and the type required. Situations requiring additional personnel vary. Assistance may be needed in performing a procedure, comforting a client, or preparing the client for a procedure. For example, a nurse assigned to care for an overweight, immobilized client may need additional personnel to help turn, transfer, and position the client. The nurse needs to determine the number of additional personnel and when they are needed. The nurse then explains the type of assistance needed, when it is needed, and how the client has responded in the past when more than one caregiver is needed to perform the intervention.

Some nursing situations require additional knowledge and skills, as well as additional personnel. A nurse needs additional knowledge when administering a new medication or implementing a new procedure. Such information can be obtained from a hospital's formulary or procedure book. If the nurse still is uncertain about the new medication or procedure, other members of the health care team can be consulted.

Because of the continual growth of health care professions and related technology, a nurse may lack the skills to perform a new procedure. When this occurs, information about the procedure is obtained from the literature and the agency's procedure book. Next, all equipment necessary for the procedure is collected. Finally, another nurse who has completed the procedure correctly and safely provides assistance and guidance. The assistance can come from another staff nurse, a supervisor, an educator, or a nurse specialist. Requesting assistance occurs frequently in all types of nursing practice and is a learning process that continues throughout educational experiences and into professional development.

Implementation Skills

Nursing practice includes cognitive, interpersonal, and psychomotor (technical) skills. Each type of skill is needed to implement direct and indirect nursing interventions. The nurse is responsible for knowing when one type of implementation skill is preferred over another and for having the necessary knowledge and skill to perform each.

Cognitive Skills. Cognitive skills involve the application of nursing knowledge. To perform any intervention, the nurse should use good judgment and make sound clinical decisions. This ensures that no nursing intervention is automatic. The nurse must continually think and anticipate so that client care is well designed, individualized, and appropriate. The nurse must know the rationale for therapeutic interventions, understand normal and abnormal physiological and psychological responses, know nursing science, be able to identify client learning and discharge needs, and recognize the client's health promotion and illness prevention needs.

Interpersonal Skills. Interpersonal skills are essential for effective nursing action. The nurse develops a trusting relationship, expresses a level of caring, and communicates clearly with the client and family (see Chapter 23) Good interpersonal communication is critical for keeping clients informed, providing individualized client teaching, and effectively supporting clients with challenging emotional needs. Proper use of interpersonal skills also enables the nurse to be perceptive of the client's verbal and nonverbal communication. As a member of the health care team, the nurse communicates client problems and needs clearly, intelligently, and in a timely manner.

Psychomotor Skills. Psychomotor skills involve the integration of cognitive and motor activities. For example, knowing the angle of insertion and the function of syringe parts, a nurse uses good coordination and precision to administer an injection correctly. With time and practice the nurse learns to perform skills correctly, smoothly, and confidently. This ensures safe performance and conveys that the nurse is competent. The nurse has a professional responsibility to acquire necessary psychomotor skills. In the case of a new skill, nurses assess their level of competency and obtain the necessary resources to ensure that the client receives the treatment safely.

Direct Care

Nurses provide a wide variety of **direct care** measures. Because interaction with the client is involved, the nurse must always be sensitive to the client's clinical condition, values and beliefs, expectations, and cultural views. This ensures an individualized approach. All direct care measures require competent and therefore safe practice. When administering direct care, the nurse learns to avoid or compensate for clients' adverse reactions to therapy and takes action to ensure preventive care.

Activities of Daily Living

Activities of daily living (ADLs) are activities usually performed in the course of a normal day; they include ambulating, eating, dressing, bathing, brushing the teeth, and grooming (see Chapter 38). Conditions resulting in the need for assistance with ADLs can be acute or chronic. An acute disease is characterized by symptoms that are usually severe and are present for a relatively short time, usually less than 6 months. An episode of acute disease results in recovery to a state of health and activity comparable to the state before the disease, passage into a chronic phase of the disease, or death. An example is the postoperative client who because of lingering sedation and pain is often unable to independently complete all ADLs. While progressing through the postoperative period, the client gradually depends less on nurses for completing ADLs.

A chronic disease persists longer. Although the symptoms are usually less severe than those of the acute phase of the same disease, chronic disease may result in complete or partial disability. An example is a client with partial paralysis after a cerebrovascular accident (stroke). The client will be unable to use the affected extremity or extremities and generally will require long-term assistance with ADLs.

The client's need for assistance with ADLs may be temporary, permanent, or rehabilitative. In the case of temporary assistance with ADLs, the client needs assistance during a limited period of time. A client with impaired mobility because of bilateral arm casts has a temporary need for assistance. After the casts are removed, the client will gradually regain the strength and range of motion needed to perform ADLs. However, a client with a total self-care deficit related to an irreversible injury high in the cervical spinal cord has a permanent need for assistance. It is unrealistic for the nurse to plan a rehabilitation program with the goal that this client will be able to independently complete all ADLs. However, through restorative care, the client will learn new ways to perform ADLs, thus becoming more independent.

As is the case with any intervention, assessment verifies a client's need for assistance with ADLs. Clients whose assessment data reveal fatigue, limitations in mobility, confusion, and pain, for example, often need assistance with ADLs. A client who experiences severe shortness of breath may avoid eating because of the associated fatigue. The nurse will assist the client with feeding and plan for more frequent, small meals to maintain the client's nutrition. Assistance with ADLs can range from partial assistance to complete care. In clients with chronic conditions, assistance with ADLs can change from day to day.

When assisting with ADLs, the nurse must also assess client preferences. For example, a client whose activities are limited because of mobility restrictions may prefer to have assistance with partial hygiene but maintain independence in feeding and grooming activities. Another client may wish to have assistance with ADLs spaced throughout the day and maintain independence in all ADLs. Involving the client in planning the timing and types of interventions aimed at meeting individualized ADLs can be a significant boost to the client's self-esteem and willingness to become more independent in some aspects of care.

Instrumental Activities of Daily Living

Illness or disability can alter clients' ability to be independent in society. **Instrumental activities of daily living (IADLs)** include such skills as shopping, preparing meals, writing checks, and taking medications. Nurses within the home care and community health setting have an excellent opportunity to assist clients in adapting to ways to perform IADLs. Often family and friends can serve as excellent resources to assist clients. In the acute care setting, it is important for a nurse to anticipate how a client's illness might affect the ability to perform IADLs so that appropriate referrals can be made to support the client following discharge.

Physical Care Techniques

The nurse will deliver a wide array of physical care techniques when caring for clients. Just a few examples include turning and positioning clients, performing invasive procedures, administering medications, and providing comfort measures. Physical techniques involve the safe and competent administration of nursing skills or procedures (e.g., urinary catheter insertion, range-of-motion exercises, and administration of injections). The specific knowledge and skills needed to carry out these nursing procedures are detailed in subsequent clinical chapters in this text. However, there are common methods to use to ensure physical care techniques are administered appropriately. These methods include protecting the nurse and client from injury, using proper infection-control practices, using an organized approach, and positioning clients correctly. When these methods are integrated within a procedure, the ultimate outcome is safe and effective nursing care.

To carry out a procedure, the nurse must be knowledgeable about the procedure itself, the standard frequency, the steps, and the expected outcomes. In a hospital the nurse completes many procedures each day. Some of these procedures might be new, so before conducting a new procedure the nurse assesses personal competencies and determines the need for assistance, new knowledge, or new skills.

Lifesaving Measures. A **lifesaving measure** is implemented when a client's physiological or psychological state is threatened (see Chapter 39). The purpose of the lifesaving measure is to restore physiological or psychological equilibrium. Such measures include administering emergency medications, instituting cardiopulmonary resuscitation, intervening to protect a confused or violent client, and obtaining immediate counseling from a crisis center for a severely anxious client. As with any procedure, the nurse must be knowledgeable about the lifesaving procedure itself, steps, and expected outcomes. If an inexperienced nurse faces a situation requiring emergency measures, the proper nursing action may be to get an experienced professional.

Counseling

Counseling is a direct care method that helps the client use a problem-solving process to recognize and manage stress and to facilitate interpersonal relationships among the client, family, and health care team. Nurses provide counseling to help the client accept actual or impending changes resulting from stress. Counseling involves emotional, intellectual, spiritual, and psychological support. A client and family who need nursing counseling have normal adjustment difficulties and are upset or frustrated, but they are not necessarily psychologically disabled. For example, more families are now taking care of their older adult relatives who have physical disabilities following surgery, stroke, or chronic illnesses. These families need assistance in adjusting to the demands placed on the caregiver. Likewise, the recipient of care also needs assistance in adjusting to the disability. Clients with psychiatric diagnoses require therapy by nurses specializing in psychiatric nursing or by social workers, psychiatrists, or psychologists.

Many counseling techniques are used to foster cognitive, behavioral, developmental, experiential, and emotional growth in clients. Most of the techniques listed in Box 18-2 require additional knowledge beyond the scope of this text. Counseling encourages individuals to examine available alternatives and decide which choices are useful and appropriate. When clients are able to examine alternatives, they can develop a sense of control and are able to better manage stress. To assist clients in need of counseling techniques, the nurse must be able to identify the need for counseling and possess communication skills to develop a therapeutic relationship (Sundeen and others, 1998).

Clients or families needing counseling include persons who must adjust lifestyle patterns, as in smoking cessation, weight reduction, or increasing activity. Clients coping with chronic or disabling diseases require counseling to help them adapt to changes in lifestyle or body image as the disease progresses. During life-threatening illnesses, clients and families need counseling to cope with the possibility of death.

Teaching

Counseling is closely aligned with teaching. Both involve using communication skills to effect a change in the client. However, with counseling the change results in the development of new attitudes and feelings, whereas in teaching the focus of change is intellectual growth or the acquisition of new knowledge or psychomotor skills (Redman, 2001).

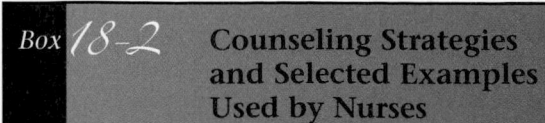

| Box *18-2* | **Counseling Strategies and Selected Examples Used by Nurses** |

Behavior Modification

Client changes from smoking to meditating to cope with stress
Client uses exercise as a health promotion activity

Bereavement Counseling

Nurse assists client in productive reminiscing of loved one
Nurse supports client in removing loved one's belongings from home

Biofeedback

Regulation of stress
Meditation

Relaxation Exercises

Progressive muscle relaxation exercises
Meditation

Crisis Intervention

Therapy designed to assist in coping with crisis
Anticipatory guidance to recognize and avoid modifiable crises

Play Therapy

Assist children through play to cope with loss and grief
Assist children in coping with chronic illness
Assist children in becoming competent in self-care activities

Teaching is an implementation method used to present correct principles, procedures, and techniques of health care to clients and to inform clients about their health status (see Chapter 24). As a nursing responsibility, teaching is implemented in all health care settings (Figure 18-2). The nurse is responsible for assessing the learning needs and readiness of clients and is accountable for the quality of education delivered. The teaching-learning process is an interaction between the teacher and the learner in which specific learning objectives are presented (Redman, 2001). This process provides the organizational structure and framework for client education. The teaching-learning process is much like the basic nursing process.

During assessment the nurse determines the client's learning needs and readiness to learn. The nurse then interprets the data to formulate nursing diagnoses reflecting the identified needs. During planning the nurse and client establish goals and outcomes for learning, with consideration of the skills and knowledge clients will require in their self-care. Implementation is the initiation of the teaching strategies designed to achieve the learning goals. Finally, evaluation measures the learning that has occurred. The purpose of the teaching-learning process is to develop and implement a teaching plan in-

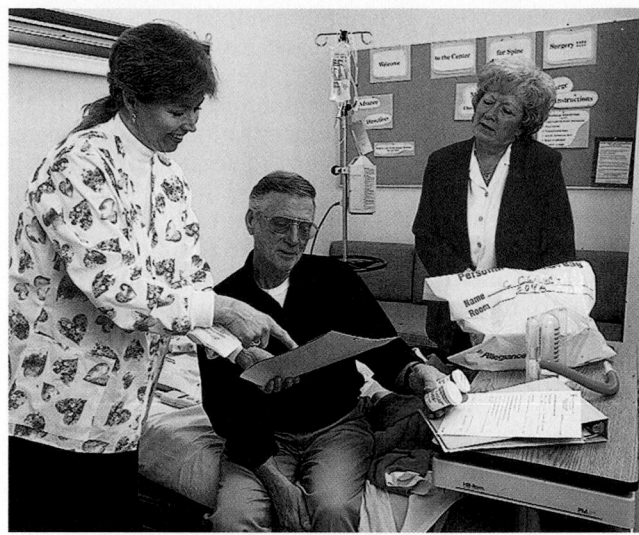

FIGURE **18-2** Teaching client discharge instructions.

dividualized for the client's needs, level of knowledge, and learning resources. The goal is to give clients the knowledge and skills necessary to assume health-related behaviors.

Controlling for Adverse Reactions

An **adverse reaction** is a harmful or unintended effect of a medication, diagnostic test, or therapeutic intervention. Adverse reactions can follow any nursing interventions, so the nurse learns to anticipate and know the adverse reactions to expect. For instance, the client receiving feedings through a nasogastric tube is at risk for aspiration. The nurse should elevate the head of the bed and have pharyngeal suction equipment at the bedside before initiating the feedings.

Nursing actions that control for adverse reactions reduce or counteract the reaction. For example, when applying a moist heat compress, the nurse assesses the area requiring the compress. Following application of the compress, the nurse evaluates the area every 5 minutes for any adverse reaction, such as excessive reddening of the skin from the heat or skin maceration from the moisture of the compress. When completing a physician-directed intervention, such as medication administration, the nurse understands the known and potential side effects of the drug. After administration of the medication, the nurse evaluates the client for any adverse effects. The nurse should be aware of drugs that can counteract the side effects. For example, a client may have an unknown hypersensitivity to penicillin and may develop hives after three doses. The nurse records the reaction and stops further administration of the drug. The nurse also consults the physician's orders and, for example, may administer diphenhydramine (Benadryl), an antihistamine and antipruritic medication, to reduce the allergic response and to relieve the itching.

When caring for a client who is undergoing a particular diagnostic test, the nurse must understand the test and any potential adverse effects. For example, a client

has not had a bowel movement in 24 hours after a barium enema. Because bowel impaction is a potential side effect of a barium enema, the nurse increases fluid intake and instructs the client to let the nursing personnel know when a bowel movement occurs.

Although adverse effects are not common, they do occur. Ultimately, the nurse wants to prevent any adverse effects. It is imperative that the nurse recognizes the signs and symptoms of an adverse reaction and intervenes in a timely manner.

Preventive Measures

Preventive nursing actions promote health and prevent illness to avoid the need for acute or rehabilitative health care. Prevention includes assessment and promotion of the client's health potential, application of prescribed measures (e.g., immunizations), health teaching, and identification of risk factors for illness and/or trauma.

Consider, for example, the case of Mrs. Schmidt, who is providing in-home care to an older parent, maintaining a career, and caring for two school-age children as a single parent. Mrs. Schmidt and the nurse agree that the client is experiencing a great deal of stress. The nurse can implement preventive measures to assist the client in controlling some of the stress. The nurse initiates stress-reducing interventions, such as relaxation therapy, for Mrs. Schmidt. In addition, the nurse assists Mrs. Schmidt in identifying community agencies and resources, such as respite care (see Chapter 2). The nurse teaches Mrs. Schmidt how to provide hygiene, nutrition, and medications. Together, the nurse and Mrs. Schmidt identify signs and symptoms that indicate whether her parent's health status is changing and what actions should be taken.

Preventive nursing interventions aimed at promoting health and preventing illness are needed in all types of care settings and with all age-groups. As changes in the health care system continue, there is and will be greater emphasis on health promotion and illness prevention.

Indirect Care

Indirect care measures are actions that support the effectiveness of direct care interventions (Dochterman and Bulechek, 2004). Many of the measures are managerial in nature, such as emergency cart checking, environmental management, and supply management (Box 18-3). A good percentage of a nurse's time is spent in indirect and unit management activities. Communication of information about clients (e.g., change of shift report and consultation) is critical to ensuring that direct care activities are planned, coordinated, and ultimately performed with the proper resources. Delegation of care to AP is another indirect care activity. When performed correctly, delegation ensures that the right tasks are performed by the right care providers so that the RN and AP work most efficiently for the client's benefit.

Communicating Nursing Interventions

Nursing interventions are written and/or communicated orally. Written interventions are part of the nursing care plan and client's permanent medical record. In many in-

Box *18-3*   **Examples of Indirect Care Activities**

Documentation
Delegation
Order transcription
Environmental management (e.g., make client rooms safe, strategically making client room assignments)
Computer entry
Telephone consultation
Shift report
Specimen management
Visitation facilitation
Transport
Product evaluation

From Dochterman JM, Bulechek GM: *Nursing interventions classification (NIC)*, ed 4, St. Louis, Mosby, 2004.

stitutions, **interdisciplinary care plans** are developed. These plans represent the contributions of all disciplines caring for a client. For example, a client recovering from total hip surgery will have a care plan for the problem of impaired mobility that includes interventions from nursing, the surgeon, and physical therapy. Any client care plan reflects proposed nursing interventions. After the interventions are completed, the client's response to the treatment is recorded on the appropriate record (see Chapter 25). The record entry usually includes a brief description of pertinent assessment findings, the specific procedure, and the client's response. This information validates the need for the specific nursing intervention. Writing the time and the details of the intervention documents that the procedure was completed.

Nursing interventions are also communicated orally from one nurse to another or to other health care professionals. Unless communication is timely and accurate, caregivers can be uninformed, interventions may be needlessly duplicated, procedures may be delayed, or tasks may be left undone (Gerteis and others, 1993). Clients can quickly tell when members of the health care team communicate inconsistent messages, indicating that no one is in charge. Nurses commonly communicate orally when conferring with colleagues, changing shifts, transferring a client to another unit, or discharging a client to another health care agency. Whether the nursing intervention is written or communicated orally, the language should be clear, concise, and to the point.

Delegating, Supervising, and Evaluating the Work of Other Staff Members

Depending on the system of health care delivery, the nurse who develops the care plan frequently does not perform all of the nursing interventions. Some activities may be delegated to other members of the health care team and coordinated by the nurse. Repetitive, noninvasive interventions such as skin care, range-of-motion ex-

ercises, ambulation, grooming, and hygiene measures are typically delegated to AP such as certified nurse assistants. A licensed practical nurse (LPN) can perform these measures in addition to medication administration and certain invasive tasks (e.g., catheterization, dressing care, and suctioning). When a nurse delegates aspects of a client's care to another staff member, the nurse assigning tasks is responsible for ensuring that each task is appropriately assigned and is completed according to the standard of care and that the direct care interventions are delegated to those personnel competent to provide the specific type of care (McCloskey and others, 1996). Chapter 20 covers guidelines for effective delegation.

*A*chieving Client Goals

Regardless of the type of interventions, the nurse implements care to meet client goals and outcomes. Goals can be achieved by providing an environment conducive to meeting such goals; adjusting care in accordance with the client's expressed or implied needs; stimulating and motivating clients, thereby enabling them to achieve self-care and independence; and encouraging clients to accept care or adhere to the treatment regimen.

Nurses can help create a health care environment conducive to achieving clients' goals. An early step in establishing an appropriate environment is to orient clients and families to the health care agency. If it is a hospital, clients need to be oriented to their rooms, the health care team, and other clients. Clients in clinics should be oriented to clinic policies and procedures, the location of restrooms and cafeterias, and the health care team. When clients receive care in the home, the nurse should take time to acquaint clients and their families with the purposes and expectations of the home visits.

Ideally, the nurse provides clients with adequate privacy for meeting basic needs and for allowing them to feel safe and free to interact with the health care team. This includes closing privacy curtains or room doors, selecting appropriate room placement, and using private meeting rooms when appropriate. Obviously, clients need privacy to carry out activities of hygiene, grooming, and elimination. In addition, they need privacy to talk with family, friends, or members of the health care team. In an environment of privacy, clients may feel free to share concerns, ask questions about their diagnosis and treatment, and resolve personal problems.

As a further aid in the attainment of health care goals, the nursing care plan should be flexible so that the client is not placed in a fixed routine. Obviously, the degree of flexibility depends on the nature of the need, the severity of the client's disability or illness, and the client's dependence on nursing care. However, even the smallest degree of flexibility, giving the client an opportunity to have some choice about the type or timing of nursing care, is valuable.

Clients with severe and chronic diseases should be encouraged to increase their levels of self-care and independence. To avoid discouraging clients, it is best to attempt to achieve this nursing goal gradually. The care plan is

Case Study

Box 18-4

Mr. Porter is a 50-year-old executive, husband, and father of three teenagers. He is recovering from a severe myocardial infarction (heart attack) and cardiac arrest. For the past 3 days, all of Mr. Porter's hygiene and grooming needs have been met by the nursing staff. Mr. Porter has expressed doubts about ever getting his energy back and being able to care for himself. Mr. Martin, a student nurse, assesses Mr. Porter and develops a nursing care plan. One of the goals is complete self-care by Mr. Porter within 1 week. With the help of his instructor, Mr. Martin implements the following plan, which is designed to achieve the overall goal of independence in various phases:

Day 1: Wash face, shave, and comb hair

Day 2: Feed himself meals, wash face, shave, and comb hair

Day 4: Perform grooming activities and feed himself

Day 6: Shower

implemented so that clients successfully achieve one level of independence before attempting the next (Box 18-4). In the case study, each day includes achievable tasks for Mr. Porter. Placing the tasks in sequential order has been done for the following reasons: (1) each task was developed with the knowledge that Mr. Porter could indeed successfully complete the activity, (2) a sequence of successes will motivate Mr. Porter to continue with the plan, and (3) the sequence was designed to gradually increase Mr. Porter's activity tolerance.

Clients with chronic diseases may need to adhere to many treatment modalities. **Client adherence** means that clients and families invest time in carrying out the required home treatments. For example, a client with chronic obstructive pulmonary disease (COPD) may need to spend several hours a day performing respiratory therapies designed to keep the airway open and maintain an acceptable level of wellness.

Some treatment plans include the need for the client and family to adjust to functional changes as a result of medications. For example, a client with high blood pressure being treated with atenolol (Tenormin) occasionally feels increasingly fatigued during the early stages of treatment. Another client with cancer who is undergoing chemotherapy may have changes in energy level and body image as a result of the medication.

Finally, adherence to treatment plans can require an increased financial investment by the client and family. For example, for a client who has cardiac disease, a two-story house may no longer be suitable because the client is unable to climb stairs without feeling short of breath. Thus the client and family may need to invest in a new house or have their present home modified.

Investments of time, money, and personal resources for a long period can be discouraging. The discouraged client may neglect the treatment regimen. After the client begins to reduce adherence to treatment, levels of wellness may decline.

Nurses intervene to assist clients in adhering to their treatment plan. Adequate discharge planning and educa-

tion of the client and family help promote a smooth transition from one health care setting to another or to the home. They also help increase the client's level of knowledge about the treatment plan. Counseling helps the client and family adapt to change resulting from the disease process or treatment. Continuity of care also provides a supportive professional who is familiar with the client's pattern of living, pattern of wellness, and treatment. In addition, reinforcing successes with the treatment plan encourages the client to adhere to the regimen.

Key Concepts

- Implementation is the step of the nursing process where nurses provide direct and indirect nursing care interventions to clients.
- Standing orders and protocols give the nurse legal protection to intervene appropriately in the client's best interest.
- Six factors to consider when choosing nursing interventions include desired or expected client outcome, characteristics of the nursing diagnosis, research base for the intervention, feasibility of the intervention, acceptability to the client, and capability of the nurse.
- During the initial phase of implementation, the nurse reassesses the client to determine whether the proposed nursing action is still appropriate for the client's level of wellness.
- The implementation of nursing care may require additional knowledge, nursing skills, and personnel resources.
- Before beginning to perform interventions, the nurse should make the client as physically and psychologically comfortable as possible.
- To anticipate and preventing complications, a nurse identifies risks to the client, evaluates the relative benefit of a treatment versus the risk, and initiates risk prevention measures.
- Successful implementation of nursing interventions requires the nurse to use appropriate cognitive, interpersonal, and psychomotor skills.
- The methods used to ensure physical care techniques are administered appropriately include protecting the nurse and client from injury, using proper infection-control practices, using an organized approach, and positioning clients correctly.
- Counseling is a direct care method that helps the client use a problem-solving process to recognize and manage stress and to facilitate interpersonal relationships among the client, family, and health care team.
- Preventive nursing actions include assessment and promotion of the client's health potential, application of prescribed measures (e.g., immunizations), health teaching, and identification of risk factors for illness and/or trauma.
- To complete any nursing procedure, the nurse must know the procedure, its frequency, the steps, and the expected outcomes.

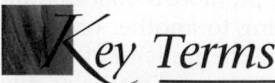

Key Terms

Activities of daily living
(ADLs), *p. 347*
Adverse reaction, *p. 349*
Client adherence, *p. 351*
Counseling, *p. 348*
Direct care, *p. 340*
Implementation, *p. 340*
Indirect care, *p. 340*
Instrumental activities of
daily living (IADLs), *p. 347*

Interdisciplinary care
plans, *p. 350*
Lifesaving measure, *p. 347*
Nursing intervention,
p. 340
Preventive nursing
actions, *p. 349*
Protocol, *p. 341*
Standing order, *p. 341*

Critical Thinking Exercises

1. Sue is a junior nursing student. She is to care for Mr. Nelson, a 56-year-old client who underwent a total knee replacement yesterday. Sue was able to talk with Mr. Nelson briefly after surgery and reviewed his complete medical record. In preparing for clinical today (postoperative day 1) Sue has identified *acute pain* and *impaired physical immobility* as his primary nursing diagnoses. Sue has developed a plan of care with interventions to relive pain and promote mobility; including use of patient-controlled analgesia (PCA), safe positioning techniques, use of guided imagery, and support of the use of range-of-motion exercises on a continuous passive motion (CPM) machine. As Sue prepares to implement her plan of care, what should she specifically do initially? What complications might she anticipate and prevent?

2. Brad is assigned to care for Ms. Reznick, who has been diagnosed to have Crohn's disease, an inflammatory condition of the bowel. Ms. Reznick has had considerable abdominal pain, accompanied by cramping and frequent diarrheal stools. Her nursing history shows that she has lost 15 pounds over the last 2 months. Her appetite has been poor. One of the many nursing diagnoses for Ms. Reznick is *imbalanced nutrition: less than body requirements related to decreased nutrient intake and increased nutrient loss through diarrhea.* What factors should Brad consider in selecting interventions for Ms. Reznick?

3. You are assigned to ambulate Mr. Clay, who had abdominal surgery 24 hours ago. Mr. Clay weighs 270 pounds and is 6 feet tall. He has a PCA system for pain control. His intravenous (IV) fluids are running at 100 ml/hr, and he has two IV antibiotics scheduled to run every 6 hours. What questions do you need to answer before you attempt to ambulate this client?

Review Questions

1. Implementation begins when in the nursing process?
   1. During the assessment phase.
   2. Immediately, in some critical situations.
   3. After there is mutual goal setting between nurse and client.
   4. After the care plan has been developed.

2. An example of the difference between direct care and indirect care is that during indirect care:
   1. Actions are aimed at managing environment and documentation.
   2. Medication administration is performed.
   3. Psychological counseling is provided.
   4. Intravenous infusion is begun.

3. A standing order is a:
   1. Protocol followed during care of clients with select clinical conditions.
   2. Physician order documented on each client's chart.
   3. Preprinted document directing the conduct of client care in certain settings.
   4. Document written and signed by an advanced practice nurse.

4. Some nursing activities may be delegated to other health care team members. The nurse must remember that:
   1. Delegation may reduce the client's cost of care.
   2. The delegated personnel are responsible for the care.
   3. The nurse has the primary responsibility for the quality of client care.
   4. Delegation occurs only upon a physician's order.

5. Interdisciplinary care plans represent:
   1. Contributions of all disciplines caring for the client.
   2. All nursing personnel having input in the care plan.
   3. The client's expressed wishes and advanced directives.
   4. Physicians and nurses working together to develop a plan of care.

6. Reassessment of a client is:
   1. Utilized when needed.
   2. A continuous process.
   3. Utilized when a new medical problem is identified.
   4. Utilized only in emergency situations.

7. Environmental factors heavily affect a client's care. The first environmental client concern is always:
   1. Safety.
   2. Food and fluids.
   3. Adequate pain relief.
   4. Location of fire exits.

8. An out-of-date care plan:
   1. Reflects a discharge of the client.
   2. Compromises the quality of care.
   3. Ensures the nursing care was delivered.
   4. Identifies the client response was successful.

9. Goals can be achieved by providing an environment that is:
   1. Stimulating and motivating.
   2. Encouraging dependence.
   3. Goal directed by the nursing staff.
   4. Rigid and nonflexible.

10. When a new procedure is needed the nurse may obtain information from the agency's:
    1. Procedure manual.
    2. Infection control department.
    3. Inservice director.
    4. Nursing supervisor.

*R*eferences

Bulecheck GM, McCloskey JC: Nursing interventions taxonomy development. In McCloskey JC, Grace HK, editors: *Current issues in nursing,* ed 3, St. Louis, 1990, Mosby.

Dochterman JM, Bulechek GM: *Nursing interventions classification (NIC),* ed 4, St. Louis, 2004, Mosby.

Gerteis M and others, editors: *Through the patient's eyes,* San Francisco, 1993, Jossey-Bass Health Series.

Gordon M: *Nursing diagnosis: process and application,* ed 3, St. Louis, 1994, Mosby.

McCloskey JC and Bulechek GM: Nurses' use and delegation of indirect care interventions, *Nurs Econ* 14(1):22, 1996.

Miller MA, Babcock DE: *Critical thinking applied to nursing,* St. Louis, 1996, Mosby.

NANDA International: *Nursing diagnoses: definitions and classification 2003-2004,* Philadelphia, 2003, NANDA International.

Redman BK: *The practice of patient education,* ed 9, St. Louis, 2001, Mosby.

Snyder M: *Independent nursing interventions,* New York, 1985, John Wiley & Sons.

Snyder M, Egan EC, Nojima Y: Defining nursing interventions, *Image J Nurs Sch* 28(2):137, 1996.

Sundeen SJ and others: *Nurse-client interaction: implementing the nursing process,* ed 6, St. Louis, 1998, Mosby.

Evaluation

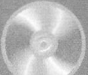

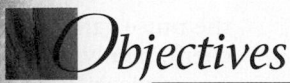

Objectives

Mastery of content in this chapter will enable the student to:

- Define the key terms listed.
- Discuss the relationship between critical thinking and evaluation.
- Identify the five elements of the evaluation process.
- Explain the relationship between goals of care, expected outcomes, and evaluative measures when evaluating nursing care.
- Give examples of evaluation measures used to determine a client's progress toward outcomes.
- Evaluate a set of nursing actions selected for a client.
- Describe how evaluation leads to discontinuation, revision, or modification of a plan of care.
- Explain the association between evaluation and quality improvement (QI).
- Discuss how outcomes management can assist an organization in improving the quality of care it delivers.

*W*hen a repairman comes to a home to fix a leaking faucet, he turns the faucet on to determine the problem, changes or adjusts parts to the faucet, and then turns the faucet on once again to determine if the leak is fixed. After a client diagnosed with pneumonia has completed a 5-day dose pack of antibiotics, the physician may have the client return to the office to have a chest x-ray examination to determine if the pneumonia has cleared. When a nurse delivers an intervention such as applying a warm compress to a wound, several steps are involved. The nurse assesses the appearance of the wound, determines the severity of the wound, applies the appropriate form of compress, and then returns to determine if the condition of the wound has improved. These three scenarios depict what ultimately occurs during the process of evaluation. The repairman rechecks the faucet, the physician orders a chest x-ray film, and the nurse reinspects the client's wound. Evaluation involves two components: an examination of a condition or situation and then a judgment as to whether change has occurred. Ideally, after an intervention takes place, evaluation should reveal an improvement.

The nursing process is a series of nursing actions based on and supported by clinical judgments. The previous chapters describe how the nurse uses critical thinking skills to gather client data, form nursing diagnoses, develop a plan of care, and implement the care plan. **Evaluation,** the final step of the nursing process, is crucial to determine whether, after application of the nursing process, the client's condition or well-being improves. The nurse applies all that is known about a client and the client's condition, as well as experience with previous clients, to evaluate whether nursing care was effective. The nurse conducts evaluation measures to determine if expected outcomes are met, not the nursing interventions. The expected outcomes are the standards against which the nurse judges if goals have been met and thus if care is successful.

Critical Thinking and Evaluation

Evaluation is one of the most critical phases of the nursing process because it determines the usefulness and effectiveness of nursing practice (Lin, 1996). During evaluation the nurse decides if the previous steps of the nursing process were effective by examining the client's responses and comparing them with the behaviors or physical indicators stated in the expected outcomes. For example, a client may have a diagnosis of *impaired oral mucous membrane related to effects of chemotherapy*. The nurse administers oral care and adjusts the client's food intake with the intent of meeting the outcome of "Client's mucosa will be well hydrated and client will deny oral pain." Evaluation will involve inspection of the oral mucosa and questioning the client about pain. Evaluation is not simply recording that oral care was performed. Evaluation informs the nurse of the need to change or revise the plan of care when interventions are ineffective or less effective than anticipated. Effective evaluation requires the use of critical thinking skills (Figure 19-1).

Evaluation is ongoing whenever the nurse has contact with the client. Once an intervention has been delivered, the nurse gathers objective and subjective data from the client, family, and health care team members. The nurse also reviews knowledge regarding the client's current condition, treatment, resources available for recovery, and the anticipated outcomes. By referring to previous experiences caring for similar clients, the nurse is in a better position to know how to evaluate the client. Finally, the nurse applies critical thinking attitudes and standards to determine whether outcomes of care are achieved. If outcomes are met, the overall goals for the client are also met. The nurse compares client behavior and responses assessed before nursing intervention with behaviors and responses reassessed after administering nursing care. Critical thinking directs the nurse to analyze evaluation findings. What do I know about the client's health problem, and has it improved? For example, has the skin's appearance returned to normal after administering pressure relief therapies? Is pain relieved following the use of guided imagery and distraction? Is the client expressing less anxiety following instruction and the opportunity to ask questions about his diagnosis?

During evaluation, the nurse makes clinical decisions and redirects nursing care to best meet client needs. For example, when evaluating a client for a change in vital signs, the nurse applies knowledge of the disease process, physiological responses to interventions, and the correct

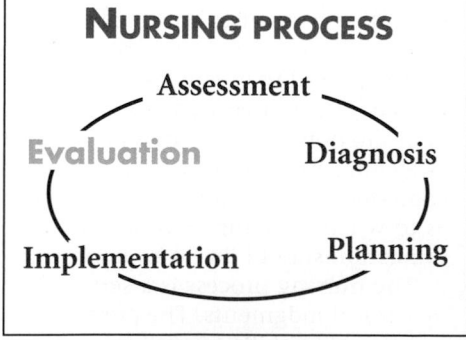

KNOWLEDGE
Characteristics of improved phsyiological, psychological, spiritual, and sociocultural status
Expected outcomes of pharmacological, medical, nutritional, and other therapies
Unexpected outcomes of pharmacological, medical, nutritional, and other therapies
Characteristics of improved family and group dynamics
Community resources

EXPERIENCE
Previous client care experience

NURSING PROCESS
Assessment
Evaluation   Diagnosis
Implementation   Planning

STANDARDS
Expected outcomes of care
Specialty standards of practice
(e.g., American Pain Society;
University of Iowa Evidence
Based Protocols)
Intellectual standards

ATTITUDES
Creativity
Responsibility
Perseverance
Humility

FIGURE **19–1**   Critical thinking and evaluation.

procedure for vital sign measurement to interpret whether a change has occurred and whether the change is desirable. A client experiencing deficient fluid volume following blood loss from surgery may have an increased heart rate and reduced blood pressure. The nurse knows this is the expected physiological response to an isotonic fluid loss (see Chapter 40). The nurse knows the client has a history free of complications and rules out other factors that may cause an increased heart rate or drop in blood pressure. After administering intravenous (IV) fluids and making the client comfortable so as to reduce stressors, the nurse returns to evaluate if vital signs have returned either to a more acceptable level or to the client's baseline before surgery. Evaluative findings determine the nurse's next course of action.

Positive evaluations occur when desired results are met and lead the nurse to conclude that nursing interventions are effective. For example, in the example above, a return to normal vital signs indicates the client achieves the goal of a normal fluid balance. Negative evaluations or undesired results, such as the continuation of an elevated or irregular heart rate, indicate that interventions are not effective in minimizing or resolving the actual problem or avoiding an at-risk problem. A negative evaluation reveals the client's inability to meet the expected outcomes. As a result, the nurse changes the plan of care by trying different therapies or changing the frequency or approach of existing therapies.

This sequence of critically evaluating and revising therapies continues until clients' problems, as defined by nursing diagnoses, are appropriately resolved. The nurse must realize that evaluation is dynamic and ever changing, depending on the client's nursing diagnoses and condition. As problems change, so too may expected outcomes. A client whose health status continuously changes requires more frequent evaluation. In addition, priority diagnoses are usually evaluated first. For example, a nurse evaluates a client's *acute pain* before evaluating the status of *deficient knowledge*.

The Evaluation Process

The purpose of nursing care is to assist the client in resolving actual health problems, preventing the occurrence of potential problems, and maintaining a healthy state. The evaluation process, which determines the effectiveness of nursing care, includes five elements: (1) identifying evaluative criteria and standards, (2) collecting data to determine whether the criteria or standards are met, (3) interpreting and summarizing findings, (4) documenting findings and any clinical judgment, and (5) terminating, continuing, or revising the care plan.

Identifying Criteria and Standards

A nurse evaluates care by knowing what to look for. With clearly defined goals and expected outcomes the nurse has objective criteria from which to judge the client's response to care.

Goals. A goal specifies the expected behavior or response that indicates resolution of a nursing diagnosis or maintenance of a healthy state. It is a summary statement of what is to be accomplished when all expected outcomes have been met. In the case of Mr. Brown, who is 2 days postoperative, the nursing diagnosis of *ineffective airway clearance related to decreased inspiratory effort secondary to abdominal incisional pain* remains his primary health problem. The nurse selected the goal of "Client's airway will become clear in 48 hours." Successful achievement of this goal depends on the success of rigorous pulmonary hygiene (Table 19-1). The nurse compares evaluative findings with all expected outcomes to determine if the goal is achieved. For example, the nurse auscultates the client's lungs to determine if crackles have decreased and lung sounds are clear. When a goal has been accomplished, the nurse knows that interventions were successful toward improving the client's well-being. If a goal remains unmet, either the plan must continue or revi-

Table 19-1	Evaluation of Mr. Brown's Plan of Care			
Assessment	**Goals**	**Expected Outcomes**	**Evaluative Measures**	**Evaluation Statement**
Decreased chest wall movements	Airway will become clear in 48 hours.	Chest excursion will increase by 2.5 cm.	Auscultate lung fields bilaterally.	Lung sounds reveal crackles in bases with clearing on left during coughing.
Crackles bilaterally in bases do not clear with coughing		Lungs will be clear to auscultation within 48 hours.	Observe and record volume of air inspired by client using spirometry.	Client is achieving 60% of incentive spirometry goal.
Chest x-ray film reveals right lower lobe infiltrate present		Client will achieve 90% of incentive spirometry goal in 24 hours.		
Elevated temperature (39° C [102.2° F])		Temperature will be <100° F in 48 hours.	Measure client's oral temperature.	Temperature is 101° F.
Reports incisional pain 5-6 on scale of 0-10		Pain intensity will be less than client's baseline in 24 hours.	Administer pain scale.	Client rates pain at level of 6.
				Client continues to have difficulty clearing airway due to ongoing abdominal pain.

sions may be necessary. In Mr. Brown's case revisions are likely needed.

Goals often are based on standards of care or guidelines established for minimal safe practice. For example, the infusion nurses society (INS) has standards of care for prevention of the IV complication phlebitis. When a nurse cares for a client with a peripheral intravenous line, the goal of "The IV site will remain free of phlebitis" is established on the basis of sound practice standards. The INS has developed a scale containing physical criteria for determining phlebitis (Chapter 40).

Expected Outcomes. Expected outcomes are the expected measurable results of the goal-oriented nursing process. A nurse-sensitive client outcome is a measurable client or family state, behavior, or perception, largely influenced by and sensitive to nursing interventions (Moorhead, Johnson, and Maas, 2004). Outcomes are statements of progressive, step-by-step responses or behaviors that the client needs to accomplish to achieve the goals of care. An outcome defines the effectiveness, efficiency, and measurement of the results of nursing interventions (Deaton, 1998). When outcomes are achieved, the related factors for a nursing diagnosis no longer exist. For example, for Mr. Brown's nursing diagnosis of *ineffective airway clearance related to decreased inspiratory effort secondary to abdominal incisional pain,* the client must achieve the goal of the airway remaining clear. This will be accomplished by meeting the outcomes of "The client's lungs will become clear to auscultation within 48 hours," "Client will achieve 90% of incentive spirometry goal," and "Oral temperature will return to normal within 48 hours." If the outcomes are met, the nurse has successfully promoted mucus clearance and the maintenance of a patent airway.

It is important for a beginning nurse to understand that evaluation is not a description of the achievement of an intervention. Evaluation of Mr. Brown *does not* involve observation of his ability to use the incentive spirometer. Evaluation *does* involve the actual incentive spirometry volume achieved by the client compared with the desired outcome of 90%.

During the planning phase of the nursing process (see Chapter 17) it is imperative for nurses to select an observable client state, behavior, or self-reported perception that will reflect goal achievement. One valuable resource is the Nursing Outcomes Classification (NOC), which provides a classification system of nurse-sensitive outcomes. NOC is designed to provide the language for the evaluation step of the nursing process. The purposes of NOC are (1) to identify, label, validate, and classify nursing-sensitive client outcomes; (2) to field test and validate the classification; and (3) to define and test measurement procedures for the outcomes and indicators using clinical data (Johnson, Mass, and Moorhead, 2004). The NOC project complements the work of the North American Nursing Diagnosis Association (NANDA) and the Nursing Interventions Classification (NIC) project. The NOC classification offers nurse-sensitive outcomes for NANDA nursing diagnoses (Table 19-2). For each outcome there are specific recommended evaluation indicators.

If a critical pathway or CareMap is used to direct client care (see Chapter 17), the nurse and team members clearly know what client outcomes are to be met for a given day (Figure 19-2). The CareMap as a documentation tool includes expected outcomes that the care team predicts will be met during the client's projected length of stay. The nurse and other team members refer to the outcomes on the CareMap on an ongoing basis. If there is variance (unexpected outcomes or outcomes occurring at a different time than expected), the nurse reports these responses and revises the plan of care as needed. By having outcomes

Table 19-2	**Linkages Between Nursing Outcomes Classification and Nursing Diagnoses**	
Nursing Diagnosis	**Suggested Outcomes**	**Indicators (examples)**
Pain	Comfort level	Reported physical well-being
		Reported satisfaction with symptom control
		Expressed satisfaction with pain control
	Pain control	Recognizes pain onset
		Uses analgesics appropriately
		Reports pain controlled
	Pain: disruptive effects	Difficulty eating
		Impaired mood
	Pain level	Reported pain level
		Frequency of pain
		Muscle tension
Ineffective airway clearance	Aspiration control	Avoids risk factors
		Positions self upright for eating
	Respiratory status: airway patency	Moves sputum out of airway
		Free of adventitious lungsounds
	Respiratory status: gas exchange	Ease of breathing
		PaO$_2$ and PaCO$_2$ within normal limits (WNL)
	Respiratory status: ventilation	Respiratory rate in expected range
		Chest expansion symmetrical
		Shortness of breath not present

Modified from Moorhead S, Johnson M, Maas M: *Nursing outcomes classification (NOC),* ed 3, St. Louis, 2004, Mosby.

Norman Regional Hospital CareMap®
(Heart Catheterization)

Check (✓) Precautions

☐ Falls   ☐ Skin   ☐ DNR

Page 1

Admitting Physician:	Primary Care Physician:	Consulting Physician(s):	Expected LOS 23 hours	M&R LOS

Allergy/Reaction   Secondary Diagnosis

Prob.	Patient Problem	Expected Discharge Outcome (Responsible Discipline)	Outcome	Date	Signature
#1	★ Hematoma	-Hematoma present (significant swelling > 5 cm²) at arterial puncture site? (RN) -If **yes**, check intervention required. (RN) ☐ Delayed ambulation ☐ Surgical repair of laceration ☐ Blood transfusion ☐ CT r/t retroperitoneal hematoma ☐ other:	☐ YES ☐ <u>NO</u>		
#2	Knowledge deficit of Patient and Family	-Verbally demonstrates understanding of procedure (pre/post) and the disease process? (RN)	☐ YES ☐ <u>NO</u>		
#3	★ Procedural priority	-Cardiac catheterization performed as an elective procedure, (patient admitted for procedure)? (RN)	☐ YES ☐ <u>NO</u>		
#4	★ Procedural complications	-Discharged home in less than 23 hours? (RN) - If no, why? ☐ PTCA ☐ Heart surgery ☐ Anticoagulant therapy ☐ MI this admission ☐ Other ___	☐ YES ☐ <u>NO</u>		
			Patient removed from Heart Catheterization CareMap r/t: ☐ PTCA ☐ Heart surgery ☐ Other ___		
	★ = Key Exception __ = Documentaion Required	Copyright© 1999 Norman Regional Hospital		**Patient Sticker**	

Statement of Intent:
The CareMap® serves as an optional guideline for patient care and is subject to alteration based on the individual needs of the patient.
(CareMap® used with permission of the Center for Case Management.)

Authors: Dr. M. Anwar, Dr. J. Crook, Dr. M. Salim, Dr. M. Sellers, Dr. A. Sohail, J. Eisen, L. Rickner, B. McTasney, K. Calbone, L. Velez.

Date: 10/1/99   Form CMAP#111   Revised: 4/24/01

Continued

FIGURE 19–2 Sample CareMap. (From Norman Regional Hospital CareMap®, Heart Catheterization, Copyright 1999, Norman Regional Hospital. Used with the permission of Norman Regional Hospital, Norman, Okla.)

Page 2

Norman Regional Hospital CareMap® (Heart Catheterization) CareMap® Summary

PATIENT STICKER

Time Admitted:		Pre-procedure Date:	Peri-procedural Date:	Post-procedure Date:
Assessments/Monitoring		-Nursing Assessment -Complete Permits -VS q 4° or per unit policy -I & O q shift -Assess pulses	-Nursing Assessment -Review lab results, permits, IV site -Assess and mark pulses -Confirm patient identity -Check for H&P on chart	-Nurse Assessment -VS, pulses & procedure site as ordered -CM/Tele monitoring, if ordered -I & O q shift
Consults				-Cardiac Rehab Phase II if ordered.
Procedures/Tests		-CBC, BMP, PTT, PT (if not done in last 24 hours) -FSBS (if diabetic)	-ACT as ordered	-If diabetic, check FSBS upon arrival to recovery area
Treatments		-Have patient void prior to Cath Lab transfer. -Foley cath prn	-Assist with procedure site prep -Remove sheath once ACT <180 sec	-In & out straight cath prn if unable to void
Medications/IV		-Continue home meds except insulin. -Pre-medicate for Iodine allergies -Initiate Pre-op meds -Start IV 1/2 NS	-Medications as ordered	-Resume pre-procedure meds -Initiate post-procedure meds -DC IV at discharge
Nutrition		-HHD, if diabetic, 1800 cal ADA -NPO 6 hours prior to procedure	-NPO	-HHD, if diabetic, 1800 cal ADA -Encourage po fluids -HHD instructions
Activity/Safety		-Up with assistance. -Bedrails up after pre-op med	-Patient flat and supine	-Bedrest 4-6 hrs as ordered -HOB ↑ 30° -Immobilize affected extremity -Ambulate following bedrest
Patient/Family Education		-Initiate Heart Cath Patient/Family CareMap® -Show Heart Cath Video	-Reinforce procedure instructions -Orient to room and equipment -Discuss sensations and communication	-Reinforce lifestyle changes -Final Review Patient/Family CareMap®
Discharge Planning		-Assess discharge needs -Notify Social Services if indicated		
Psychosocial/Emotional/Spiritual		-Encourage questions/discussion of procedure with patient/family	-Give patient/family frequent status reports	-Encourage family visitation and participation in pt. care
CMAP #111				

Additional Daily Treatments/Other

Isolation Precautions:

Special Procedures/Surgeries:

Additional Daily Lab: CareMap® entered into the computer (US/RN) initial: _____

Diabetic? □ Yes □ No

Pharmacy notified: □ Yes □ No □ N/A

Other Pertinent Information:

Family Spokesperson:

Emergency Phone #:

FIGURE 19–2, cont'd   Sample CareMap. (From Norman Regional Hospital CareMap®, Heart Catheterization, Copyright 1999, Norman Regional Hospital. Used with the permission of Norman Regional Hospital, Norman, Okla.)

clearly documented on either a CareMap or other documentation form, the nurse and other health care providers clearly know what to evaluate. All members of the health care team should monitor a client's progress. Each nurse summarizes data on an ongoing basis to ensure that the client is progressing to an optimal level of health.

Collecting Evaluative Measures

When nurses provide care to clients, two aspects of care must be evaluated. First, what is the client's response to nursing care? Was the therapy effective in improving the client's physical or emotional heath? Did the client benefit? It is important to evaluate whether each client reaches a level of wellness or recovery that the health care team and client established in the goals of care. Second, have the client's expectations of care been met? The nurse asks clients about their perceptions of care, such as "Did you receive the type of pain relief you expected?" "Did you receive enough information to care for your baby at home?" This level of evaluation is important to determine the client's satisfaction with care and to strengthen the partnering between nurse and client. The nurse selects appropriate evaluative measures to evaluate client response and expectations.

Evaluating a client's response to nursing care requires the use of evaluative measures, which are simply the assessment skills and techniques used to collect data for evaluation (e.g., auscultation of lung sounds, observation of a client's skill performance, discussion of the client's feelings, and inspection of the skin) (Figure 19-3). In fact, evaluative measures are the same as assessment measures but are performed at the point of care when decisions are made about the client's status and progress. The intent of assessment is to identify what if any problems exist. The intent of evaluation is to determine if the known problems have remained the same, improved, worsened, or otherwise changed. In Mr. Brown's situation, the nurse uses evaluative measures that include auscultation of lung sounds, measurement of the inhaled volume on the incentive spirometer, and measurement of the client's oral temperature (see Table 19-1, p. 357).

In many clinical situations it is important to collect evaluative measures over a period of time to determine if

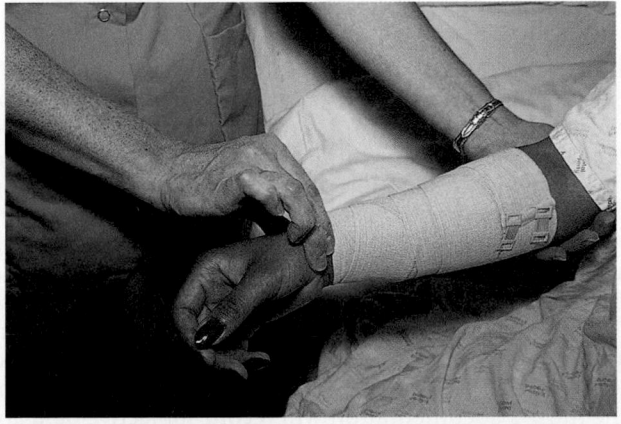

FIGURE **19–3**   Nurse evaluates circulation following application of elastic wrap bandage.

a pattern of improvement or change exists. A one-time observation of a pressure ulcer is insufficient to determine that the ulcer is healing. It is important to note a consistency in change. For example, over a period of 2 days is the pressure ulcer gradually decreasing in size, is the amount of drainage declining, is the redness of inflammation resolving? Recognizing a pattern of improvement or deterioration allows the nurse to reason and decide whether the client's problems are resolved.

The primary source of data for evaluation is the client. However, the nurse also uses the family and other caregivers. For example, the nurse might ask a family member to report on the amount of food the client eats during a meal or how well a client prepared medications in the home. A nurse might consult with a colleague about how the client responded to pain medication on a previous shift.

Interpreting and Summarizing Findings

Expert nurses engage in an ongoing dialogue with a situation (Benner, Hooper-Kyriakidis, and Stannard, 1999). They are able to read a clinical situation and then provide an appropriate response. An expert nurse recognizes relevant evidence, even evidence that sometimes does not match clinical expectations, and makes judgments about a client's condition. To develop clinical judgment, a new nurse learns to match a clinical situation with expected outcomes and clinical goals to determine if a client's status is improving or not. When interpreting findings, the nurse compares the client's behavioral responses and physiological signs and symptoms expected to be seen with those actually seen from the evaluative database. Comparing expected and actual findings allows the nurse to interpret and judge the client's condition and whether predicted changes have occurred (Table 19-3). To objectively evaluate the degree of success in achieving a goal, the nurse should use the following steps:

1. Examine the goal statement to identify the exact desired client behavior or response.
2. Assess the client for the presence of that behavior or response.
3. Compare the established outcome criteria with the behavior or response.
4. Judge the degree of agreement between outcome criteria and the behavior or response.
5. If there is no agreement (or only partial agreement) between the outcome criteria and the behavior or response, what is/are the barriers? Why did they not agree?

Evaluation is easier to perform after a nurse cares for a client over a long period. The nurse is then able to make subtle comparisons of client responses and behaviors. When a nurse has not had the opportunity to care for a client over an extended time, evaluation is enhanced by referring to previous experience and by asking colleagues, familiar with the client, to confirm evaluation findings. The accuracy of any evaluation improves when the nurse is familiar with the client's behavior and physiological status or has cared for more than one client with a similar problem.

Evaluation of each expected outcome and its place in the sequence of care is essential. Failure to evaluate each

Table 19-3	Evaluation Measures to Determine the Success of Goals and Expected Outcomes	
Goals	**Evaluative Measures**	**Expected Outcomes**
Client's pressure ulcer will heal within 7 days.	Inspect color, condition, and location of pressure ulcer. Measure diameter of ulcer daily. Note odor and color of drainage from ulcer.	Erythema will be reduced in 2 days. Diameter of ulcer will decrease in 5 days. Ulcer will have no drainage in 2 days. Skin overlying ulcer will be closed in 7 days.
Client will tolerate ambulation to end of hall by 11/20.	Palpate client's radial pulse before exercise. Palpate client's radial pulse 10 minutes after exercise. Assess respiratory rate during exercise. Observe client for dyspnea or breathlessness during exercise.	Pulse will remain below 110 beats per minute during exercise. Pulse rate will return to resting baseline within 10 minutes after exercise. Respiratory rate will remain within two breaths of client's baseline rate. Client will deny feeling of breathlessness.
Client will have improved grief resolution by 1/15.	Ask client about frequency of periods of crying, sadness. Review client's sleeping log. Review client's dietary intake.	Client reports decreased frequency of crying, sadness in 2 months. Client has periods of 6-7 hours of sleep without interruption within 10 days. Client has no weight loss in 1 month.

Table 19-4	Examples of Objective Evaluation of Goal Achievement		
Goals	**Outcome Criteria**	**Client Response**	**Evaluation Findings**
Client will self-administer insulin by 12/18.	Client prepares insulin dosage in syringe by 12/17. Client demonstrates self-injection by 12/18.	Client prepared accurate dosage in syringe on 12/17. Client administered morning insulin dosage; self-injection was correctly performed on 12/18.	Client has progressed and achieved desired behavior.
Client's lungs will be free of secretions by 11/30.	Coughing will be nonproductive by 11/29. Lungs will be clear to auscultation by 11/30. Respirations will be 20 per minute by 11/30.	Client coughed frequently and productively on 11/29. Lungs were clear to auscultation on 11/30. Respirations were 18 per minute on 11/29.	Client will require continued therapy. Condition is improving.
Client will be able to perform self-care measures without discomfort in 2 days.	Client will rate pain as 3 on a scale of 0-10 within 2 days. Client will initiate bathing within 2 days.	Client rates severe right-sided abdominal pain as 5 on a scale of 0-10 while attempting bathing on day 2.	Client's condition still indicates a problem. Continued therapy with possibly new care measures is required.

expected outcome results in an inability to determine the place in which the sequence faltered. In other words, the nurse is not able to revise and redirect the plan of care at the most appropriate time. If the client achieves the expected outcomes, the nurse either continues the care plan or discontinues interventions because the goal of care is met. If evaluation determines that the expected outcomes were not met or only partially met, the nurse begins reassessment and revision of the care plan.

There are different degrees of goal achievement. If the client's response matches or exceeds the outcome criteria, the goal is met. If the client's behavior begins to show changes but does not yet meet criteria set, the goal is partially met. If there is no progress, the goal is not met (Table 19-4). A clearly defined goal with specific outcomes is easily measured (see Chapter 17).

Documenting Findings

Documentation and reporting are an important part of the evaluation process. Accurate information must be present in a client's medical record in order for nurses to make ongoing evaluation decisions. When documenting the client's response to interventions, the nurse always includes the same evaluative measures gathered during assessment. The nurse presents a clear argument from the data whether a client is progressing or not. All objective data should be documented using precise measurements and thorough detail (see Chapter 25). If a client is asked to explain or describe a situation as part of evaluation, the nurse's documentation will record subjective data appropriately, for example, "Client reports that nausea has subsided." Written nursing progress notes, assessment flow sheets, and information shared among nurses during change-of-shift reports should communicate a client's progress toward meeting expected outcomes and goals for the nursing plan of care.

Care Plan Revision and Critical Thinking

As goals are evaluated, the nurse makes adjustments to the care plan as indicated. If a goal was successfully met, that portion of the care plan is discontinued. Unmet and partially met goals require the nurse to continue intervention. After a nurse reassesses a client, nursing diagnoses may be modified or added with appropriate goals and expected outcomes, and interventions are established. The nurse also redefines priorities. This is an important step in critical thinking—knowing how the client is progressing and how problems either resolve or worsen. In the case of Mr. Brown, his pain continues to be a problem. The nurse on days recognized that Mr. Brown was not using his patient-controlled analgesia (PCA) device routinely. Mr. Brown consistently was reporting pain at a level of 6 on a scale of 0 to 10. The nurse revises the plan of care to place more emphasis on pain control (Box 19-1). The nurse reviews the care plan developed immediately following surgery for the nursing diagnosis of *acute pain* (see Chapter 17). In addition, the nursing diagnosis of *ineffective airway clearance* has already been revised to include poor pain control as the related factor. The nurse revises the *acute pain* care plan's expected outcomes and interventions for managing Mr. Brown's abdominal pain. The nurse's logic in revising the plan is to focus attention on pain management and to administer pain relief therapies so that the client can then breathe more deeply, cough with minimal discomfort, and eventually achieve airway clearance.

The nurse's careful monitoring and early detection of problems are a client's first line of defense (Benner, Stannard, and Hooper, 1996). Benner, Stannard, and Hooper describe the importance of nurses' learning how to anticipate the client's future course. Clinical judgments are based on the nurse's observations of what is occurring with a specific client and not merely what may happen to clients in general. Frequently changes are very subtle. Evaluation must be client specific, based on a close familiarity with each client's behavior, physical status, and reaction to caregivers. Critical thinking skills promote accurate evaluation, which leads to the appropriate revision of ineffective care plans and discontinuation of therapy that has successfully resolved a problem.

Discontinuing a Care Plan

After determining that expected outcomes and goals have been achieved, the nurse confirms this evaluation with the client when possible. If the nurse and client agree that the expected outcomes have been met, the nurse discontinues that care plan. For example, a client has the nursing diagnosis of *deficient knowledge regarding self-administration of insulin related to inexperience.* To achieve the goal of accurate client administration of insulin, the nurse establishes outcomes, including "Client will describe the purpose of insulin by 9/20," "Client will cor-

rectly prepare insulin in syringe by 9/20," and "Client will administer insulin injection independently by 9/22." The nurse asks the client to describe the purpose of insulin and observes as the client prepares the dosage and administers the injection. When outcomes are met successfully, it becomes unnecessary to teach additional information about insulin administration. The care plan can be documented as discontinued. This ensures that other nurses will not unnecessarily continue the care plan. Continuity of care assumes that care provided is relevant to client needs. Significant time is wasted when achieved goals are not communicated.

Modifying a Care Plan

When goals are not met, the nurse identifies the variables or factors that interfere with goal achievement. Usually a change in the client's condition, needs, or abilities makes alteration of the care plan necessary. For example, when teaching self-administration of insulin, the nurse discovers that the client has developed a new problem, a tremor associated with a side effect of a medication. The client is unable to draw medication from a syringe or inject the needle safely. As a result, the original outcomes of "Client will correctly prepare insulin in a syringe" and "Client will administer insulin injection independently" cannot be met. The nurse introduces new interventions (instructing wife in insulin preparation and administration) and revises outcomes to meet the goal of care.

Lack of goal achievement may also result from an error in nursing judgment or failure to follow each step of the nursing process. Clients frequently have multiple and complex problems. The nurse should always remember the possibility of overlooking or misjudging something. When there is failure to achieve a goal, no matter what the reason, the entire nursing process sequence for that nursing diagnosis is repeated to discover changes that need to be made to promote, maintain, or restore the client's health.

Reassessment. A complete reassessment of all client factors relating to the nursing diagnosis and etiology is necessary when modifying a plan. Reassessment requires critical thinking when the nurse compares new data about the client's condition with previously assessed information. Often a nurse applies knowledge from experiences with other clients to direct the reassessment process. Encounters over time with clients and families who have similar health problems give nurses a strong background of knowledge to use for anticipating client needs and planning care. For example, consider Mr. Brown, who has the nursing diagnosis of *acute pain related to surgical trauma of incision.* Two days following surgery, the client continues to have a poor appetite despite the fact that there are no obvious surgical complications. If the client continues to have pain, the nurse may automatically associate loss of appetite with discomfort. However, the experienced nurse may recall a previous client who became almost depressed following surgery. After exploring the problem further, the nurse learns that Mr. Brown's family has not been visiting, the client is fearful of his cancer diagnosis, and in addition to experiencing loss of appetite, the client is not sleeping well. Although the client continues to have pain, a new priority diagnosis may be

Box 19-1   Modification of Nursing Care Plan for Mr. Brown

Mr. Brown is continuing to have difficulty with abdominal incision pain. As a result, Mr. Brown has resisted pulmonary hygiene implemented by the nursing staff. The nurse on the evening shift returns to Mr. Brown's room to reassess the client's condition.

Assessment Activities
Auscultate client's lung sounds.
Observe client use incentive spirometer and observe volume of air inspired.
Observe client's ability to turn, cough, and deep breathe.

Observe client's technique with splinting incision during coughing.
Measure oral temperature.
Monitor use of patient-controlled analgesia (PCA) device and ask client to rate pain on a scale of 0 to 10.

Findings/Defining Characteristics
Crackles present in both lower lobes
Achieves only 60% to 70% of incentive spirometry goal

Reluctant to turn, cough, and deep breathe; states that pain is "too much"
Does not splint abdominal incision

Oral temperature of 39.8° C (103.6° F)
Infrequent, irregular use of PCA
Rates incisional pain as 6 on a scale of 0 to 10

Nursing Diagnosis: Acute Pain Related to Surgical Trauma of Incision

Planning

Goal

Client's pain will be reduced in 24 hours.

Expected Outcomes*
Pain Control
Client will use PCA more frequently, receiving 6 mg morphine every hour for next 24 hours.
Client's level of pain decreases to level below baseline within 36 hours.
Client will splint incision before each cough and deep breathing exercise.

Interventions†
Pain Management
Instruct client in proper use of PCA and rationale for regular use of medication.

Have client administer a single PCA dose 10 minutes before performing incentive spirometry.
Demonstrate correct splinting procedure. Allow for return demonstration by client.
Assist client in performing splinting during coughing and deep breathing and during turning and repositioning.
When pain is under control, instruct client in relaxation exercises.

Rationale

PCA is a drug delivery system that allows clients to self-administer opioids with minimal risk of overdose On-demand doses typically add 1 mg morphine every 6 minutes, with a total hourly limit of 6 mg (American Pain Society, 1999).
Provides level of pain relief before incentive spirometer exercise that will cause expansion of thoracic and abdominal muscles.
Splinting provides support to underlying tissues disrupted by surgical incision, preventing stimulation of pain fibers.

Relaxation techniques provide individuals with self-control when discomfort or pain occurs, reversing the physical and emotional stress of pain.

Evaluation

Nursing Actions	Client Response/Finding	Achievement of Outcome
Ask client to rate severity of pain on scale of 0 to 10 after coughing or activities such as routine hygiene.	Client rates pain at level of 5 after coughing. Is able to perform hygiene activities with pain at level of 3 to 4.	Pain control is improving. Continue reinforcement of splinting and use of PCA.
Observe regularity of client splinting incision during turning, coughing and deep breathing.	Client uses splinting technique about 75% of the time. May forget to splint when coughing develops without warning. Turns without splinting.	Reinforce use of splinting during turning.
Check dosage delivered on PCA pump for 24-hour period.	Client receiving average of 4 to 6 mg morphine per hour.	Client using PCA more regularly, receiving safe dosage of medication.

*Outcome label from Moorhead S, Johnson M, Maas M: *Nursing outcomes classification (NOC)*, ed 3, St. Louis, 2004, Mosby.
†Intervention Classification label from Dochterman JM, Bulechek GM: *Nursing interventions classification (NIC)*, ed 4, St. Louis, 2004, Mosby.

anticipatory grieving related to losses associated with illness. Focusing on this diagnosis may improve the client's appetite more than the original plan. As in the original assessment, data are collected from all sources. Depending on the nurse's findings, it often becomes necessary to assess variables that were not covered on the initial assessment.

Reassessment ensures that the database is accurate and current. It may also reveal the missing link (i.e., a critical piece of new information that was overlooked and thus interfered with goal achievement). All new data are sorted, validated, and clustered to analyze and interpret differences from the original database. The nurse documents reassessment data to alert other nursing staff to the client's status.

Nursing Diagnoses. After reassessment the nurse determines what nursing diagnoses are accurate for the situation. The nurse asks whether the correct diagnosis was selected and whether it and the etiological factor are current. The problem list should then be revised to reflect the client's changed status. A new diagnosis may be made. If a previous diagnosis no longer accurately reflects the problem, it should be discontinued. For example, after finding that the client with diabetes is unable to self-administer insulin, the nurse decides a family member is available as a resource. To develop a plan designed to educate an alternate caregiver about the administration of insulin, the nurse then establishes a new diagnosis: *ineffective health maintenance related to impaired dexterity.*

A nurse's care is based on an accurate list of nursing diagnoses. Accuracy is more important than the number of diagnoses selected. As the client's condition changes, the diagnoses do as well.

Goals and Expected Outcomes. When care plans are revised, the nurse reviews goals and expected outcomes for needed changes. Even the goals for unchanged nursing diagnoses should be examined for appropriateness, because a change in one problem may affect others. Determining that each goal and expected outcome is realistic for the problem, etiology, and time frame is particularly important. Unrealistic expected outcomes and time frames make goal achievement difficult.

The nurse clearly documents goals and expected outcomes for new or revised nursing diagnoses so that all team members are aware of the revised care plan. When the goal is still appropriate but has not yet been met, the nurse may change the evaluation date to allow more time. All goals and expected outcomes should be client centered, with realistic expectations for client achievement.

Interventions. The evaluation of interventions examines two factors: the appropriateness of the interventions selected and the correct application of the intervention. The appropriateness of an intervention may be based on the standard of care for a client's health problem. A **standard of care** is the minimum level of care accepted to ensure high quality of care to clients. Standards of care define the types of therapies typically administered to clients with defined problems or needs. If the client who is postoperative for abdominal surgery has a specific nursing diagnosis, such as *ineffective airway clearance,* the stan-

dard of care established by a nursing department for this problem may include pain-control measures with coughing or deep breathing exercises to help the client breathe more easily with a clear airway. The nurse reviews the standard of care to determine whether the right interventions have been chosen or whether additional ones are required.

Increasing or decreasing the frequency of interventions is one approach to ensure appropriate application of the intervention. The nurse adjusts interventions on the basis of the client's actual response to therapy, as well as previous experience with similar clients. For example, if a client continues to have congested lung sounds, the nurse increases the frequency of coughing and deep breathing exercises to remove secretions.

During evaluation the nurse may find that some planned interventions are designed for an inappropriate level of nursing care. If the level of care needs to be changed, a different action verb, such as *assist* in place of *provide,* may be substituted. Sometimes the level of care is appropriate but the interventions are unsuitable because of a change in the expected outcome. In this case the interventions should be discontinued and new ones planned.

Changes in implementation should be guided by the nature of the client's unfavorable response. Consulting with other nurses may yield suggestions for improving the approach to care delivery. Senior nurses are often excellent resources because of their experience. Simply changing the care plan is not enough. The nurse must implement the new plan and reevaluate the client's response to the nursing actions.

Occasionally during evaluation the nurse may discover unmet client needs. This should be anticipated. The nursing process is designed to be a systematic, problem-solving approach to individualized client care, but there is a wide array of variables for each client with a health care problem. Clients with the same health care problem are not treated the same way. As a result, the nurse sometimes makes errors in judgment. The systematic use of evaluation provides a way for nurses to catch these errors in judgment. The nurse consistently incorporates evaluation into practice to minimize errors and ensure that the client's plan of care is appropriate and relevant.

Quality Improvement

Quality of care is defined in many ways. The Institute of Medicine (2002) defines quality as the "degree to which health services for individuals and populations increase the likelihood of desired health outcomes and are consistent with current professional knowledge." Just as each individual health care professional is responsible for evaluating the care he or she provides to a client, health care organizations must be responsible and accountable for evaluating and improving the quality of client care services being provided to all clients. This requires health professionals at all levels to critically evaluate their practices, to incorporate the latest scientific findings into client care, and to measure the success of meeting client outcomes on an ongoing basis (see Chapter 20).

Quality improvement (QI) and performance improvement are terms used to describe an approach to the continuous study and improvement of the processes of providing health care services to meet the needs of clients and others (Joint Commission on the Accreditation of Healthcare Organizations, 2003). Among the processes that most directly influence clients are those that constitute nursing practice, such as medication administration, diet management, wound care, and discharge planning (see Chapter 20).

Outcomes Management

Outcomes management is a term that encompasses managing the individual clinical outcomes of clients as a result of prescribed treatments. In outcomes management, a hospital, clinic, or physician's office, for exmaple, conducts formal measurement of system level performance and effectiveness (Pelletier, 1998). An outcome is the condition to be achieved as a result of care delivery or prescribed treatment. An **outcome** reveals whether interventions are effective, whether clients progress, how well standards of care are being met, and whether changes in therapy or delivery of care are necessary. In health care today, outcomes management programs can be found on the individual nursing unit or point of care level to the level of a health care system or managed care program. The move toward outcomes management was the result of several national initiatives: reduction of unnecessary health care costs, identification and use of best practices, and health risk appraisal. Outcomes management has become a priority for all health care organizations because quality is one way to differentiate good and poor performers.

When professional nurses think in terms of outcomes management, their actions become much more purpose-ful and focused on improving the condition of their clients' health. The purpose of quality improvement is not to identify problems after the fact, but to identify opportunities prospectively to improve the quality of care or service (Patton and Stanley, 1993). Two types of outcomes, professional and client, are important to differentiate (Peters, 1995).

Professional outcomes: Measures of the professional caregiver's performance. For example, the RN is responsible for the ongoing assessment of clients' status and will communicate changes in a client's condition to appropriate health team members.

Client outcomes: Measures of clients' status after receiving care. For example, following the implementation of a fall prevention program, there will be a reduction in the number of client falls on the nursing unit.

A well-organized QI program focuses on processes of care or systems that significantly contribute to client outcomes. A systematic approach with everyone in an organization participating creates a culture where all staff understand their responsibility toward maintaining and improving quality. Quality improvement is concerned with exceeding the standard of care, examining ways to be more efficient, improving client satisfaction, and focusing on service (Bower, 2002).

As a member of the nursing team, each nurse participates in recognizing trends in nursing practice, identifying when recurrent problems develop, and initiating opportunities to improve the quality of care. For example, after reviewing clients who have undergone hip surgery, nursing staff might ask, "Are our clients regaining functional mobility without severe pain?" "Are the best practices being applied in the choice and administration of analgesics?" "Is rehabilitation delayed unnecessarily?"

Table 19-5	Quality Accreditation and Advocacy Organizations	
Organization	**Initiative**	**Description**
ANA (American Nurses Association) Voluntary http://www.nursingworld.org	ANCC magnet recognition	Provides national recognition to health care organizations that demonstrate sustained excellence in nursing care. The program is based on quality indicators and standards of nursing practice as defined by the ANA.
	Nursing report card for acute care settings	Provides indicators and measurement tools for evaluating quality of nursing care in acute care settings. Outcome indicators include educational information, nosocomial infection rates, patient injury (e.g., falls), pain management, and patient satisfaction.
JCAHO (Joint Commission on Accreditation of Healthcare Organizations) Accreditation (private) http://www.jcaho.org	ORYX	Integrates outcomes and performance measures into accreditation process; requires accredited hospitals and long-term care agencies to identify clinical measures population. Percentage to be adjusted annually.
NCQA (National Committee for Quality Assurance) Nonprofit, accreditation for managed care http://www.ncqa.org	HEDIS (Health plan Employer Data and Information Set)	HEDIS targets effectiveness of care, access and availability of care, patient satisfaction, health plan stability, use of services, costs, and health plan descriptive information.
URAC (American Accreditation Healthcare Commission) Nonprofit, charitable, accreditation for managed care		Promotes continuous improvement through the establishment of standards, programs of education and communication, and a process of accreditation.

The QI process begins at the staff level, where problems are more readily defined. Nursing staff collaborate with all appropriate disciplines (e.g., physicians, pharmacists, and physical therapists) to define appropriate standards of care (e.g., appropriate analgesic selection and use of nonpharmacological therapies) and to then determine whether those standards and good client outcomes are being met. If desired outcomes are unmet, the staff will then devise approaches to ensure appropriate standards are practiced.

The challenge of maintaining quality care is imposing. A number of accrediting, professional, and governmental agencies provide quality criteria for organizations to use in developing and maintaining quality improvement efforts (Table 19-5). Quality improvement has become a routine part of every professional nurse's responsibility. Chapter 20 provides detail on how quality improvement programs are conducted and managed on individual nursing units.

•••

Providing health care in a timely, competent, and cost-effective manner is complex and challenging. This chapter on the evaluation process has discussed multiple methods to determine the effectiveness of care, make necessary modifications, and to continuously ensure favorable client outcomes. Evaluation of care is a professional responsibility, and it is a crucial component of nursing care. Evaluation can focus on a single client's plan of care, or it can focus on the delivery of care provided by an agency or a specific nursing division within an agency. Through the continuous evaluation of care, nurses play a key role in the ongoing improvement of client care.

Key Concepts

- Evaluation involves two components: an examination of a condition or situation and a judgment as to whether change has occurred.
- Evaluation is a step of the nursing process that allows a nurse to determine whether nursing interventions are successful in improving a client's condition or well-being.
- During evaluation the nurse applies critical thinking to make clinical decisions and redirect nursing care to best meet client needs.
- The nurse compares the client's actual response (e.g., behaviors and physiological signs and symptoms) to nursing interventions with expected outcomes established during planning to determine if goals of care are met.
- A nurse interprets evaluative findings to judge the client's condition and to know whether predicted changes have occurred.
- Evaluation measures are assessment skills used to collect data for evaluation.
- Documentation of evaluative findings allows all members of the health team to know whether a client is progressing or not.
- As a result of evaluation, a client's nursing diagnoses, priorities, and interventions may change.

- Health care organizations are responsible for evaluating and improving the quality of client care services they provide.
- The processes of health care that most directly influence clients are those that constitute nursing practice.
- When professional nurses think in terms of outcomes management, their actions become more purposeful and focused on improving the condition of their client's health.

Key Terms

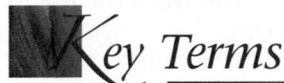

Evaluation, *p. 355*	Quality improvement (QI),
Outcome, *p. 366*	*p. 366*
Outcomes management,	Standard of care, *p. 365*
p. 366	

Critical Thinking Exercises

1. Mr. Vicar has been visiting the clinic for more than a month. He visits weekly for follow-up care for a chronic venous stasis ulcer of the left leg. The nurse's note at the time of his first visit contained the following information: "Ulcer with irregular margins, 4 cm wide by 5 cm long, approximately 0.5 cm deep, draining foul-smelling purulent yellowish drainage. Only subcutaneous tissue visible. Skin around ulcer, brownish rust in color. Zinc oxide and calamine gauze applied to ulcer; elastic wrap bandage applied to gauze. Client instructed to return in 1 week." As the nurse who is caring for the client on the follow-up visit, what expected outcomes would you anticipate for the goal of "Wound will demonstrate healing within 4 weeks"? What evaluative measures would you use to determine if the wound was healing?

2. The nursing staff on the general medicine unit are discussing a number of issues during their monthly staff meeting. Two additional RNs have been hired to work the night shift. Staff nurses have not been conducting routine reviews of clients' discharge plans. The nurse manager has announced that discharge planning conferences will be held at 1:30 PM each weekday. A new safety syringe is being introduced that will require staff to attend in-service training sessions. Over the last 3 months there has been a 10% incidence rate for pressure ulcers. That is an increase when compared to the last 6 months. The wound care nurse specialist will be consulting on the floor.

   a. Of all the nursing unit issues, which one would you identify as a professional outcome?

   b. Which one would you identify as a client outcome?

3. Mr. Becker is a 78-year-old man who has been diagnosed with terminal lung cancer. He reports a loss of appetite and a 6-pound weight loss over the last month (152 pounds down to 146 pounds). He is able to chew and swallow food without difficulty. Mr. Becker denies feeling nauseated but states, "I just have no interest in food." His wife reports that he eats only

a portion of what is served, "He gets full so quickly." Mrs. Becker also reports that her husband is less active around the house, sleeps poorly, and is unable to talk about his diagnosis. The nurse develops a nursing diagnosis of *imbalanced nutrition, less than body requirements related to a decline in food intake.*
   a. What would be an appropriate goal for Mr. Becker's plan of care?
   b. Identify expected outcomes to use in measuring success of the care plan.
   c. What evaluative measures would the nurse use to determine Mr. Becker's progress?
4. Mr. Becker returns to the physician's office 2 weeks later. Mrs. Becker has been serving smaller and more frequent meals as recommended by the nurse. She has also worked hard to select a menu that is appealing to Mr. Becker. He continues to deny feeling nauseated. Mrs. Becker reports, "Some days he seems to eat better, but other days he just won't eat much. I think the smaller portions help." Mr. Becker's weight is now 145 pounds. His food diary shows that there are meals where he has eaten most of his food, but other meals where intake is minimal. He tells the nurse, "I know I should try to eat more, but what is the use?"
   a. How would you interpret Mr. Becker's progress?
   b. How would you revise the plan of care?

Review Questions

1. Evaluation is an important part of nursing care. During this process you determine the effectiveness of a specific nursing action by:
   1. Reassessing the client for new problems.
   2. Determining that the specific nursing action was completed.
   3. Comparing the client's response to the nursing action with other clients receiving the same nursing action.
   4. Comparing the client's response with expected outcomes established during the planning phase.

2. Evaluation is one of the most critical phases of the nursing process because it determines the usefulness and effectiveness of nursing practice and is:
   1. Client driven and client centered.
   2. Nurse driven and client centered.
   3. Physician and nurse centered.
   4. Client and nurse driven.

3. Evaluation is ongoing whenever the nurse has contact:
   1. With the client.
   2. With the family.
   3. With the physician.
   4. With the physician and family.

4. The nurse must realize that evaluation is
   1. The second step in nursing care.
   2. Dynamic and ever changing.
   3. The reassessment of the client for new problems.
   4. At the direction of the physician's orders.

5. The evaluation process, which determines the effectiveness of nursing care, includes five elements; these are:
   1. Implementing, evaluating, documenting, revising, and continuing.
   2. Planning, diagnosing, interpreting, evaluating, and revising.
   3. Identifying, collecting, interpreting, documenting, and terminating, continuing, or revising the care plan.
   4. Assessing, diagnosing, planning, implementing, and evaluating.

6. A goal specifies the expected behavior or response that indicates:
   1. Resolution of a nursing diagnosis or maintenance of a healthy state.
   2. The nurse has made the correct nursing diagnoses.
   3. The validation of the nurse's physical assessment.
   4. The specific nursing action was completed.

7. Expected outcomes are the expected measurable results of the:
   1. Physician's orders.
   2. Goal-oriented nursing process.
   3. Nurse-initiated goals.
   4. Need for additional health care personnel.

8. Evaluating a client's response to nursing care requires the use of evaluative measures, which are:
   1. Computer generated.
   2. Provided by ancillary staff.
   3. Determined by the physician.
   4. Assessment skills and techniques used to collect data for evaluation.

9. The primary source of data for evaluation is the
   1. Physician.
   2. Client.
   3. Family.
   4. Nurse.

10. Unmet and partially met goals require the nurse to:
   1. Compare the client's response with that of another client.
   2. Relinquish care of the client to another nurse.
   3. Continue intervention.
   4. Begin new interventions.

References

American Pain Society: *Principles of analgesic use in the treatment of acute and cancer pain,* ed 4, Glenview, Ill, 1999, American Pain Society.

Benner P, Hooper-Kyriakidis P, Stannard D: Clinical wisdom and interventions in critical care, Philadelphia, 1999, WB Saunders.

Benner P, Stannard D, Hooper PL: A "thinking-in-action" approach to teaching clinical judgment: a classroom innovation for acute care advanced practice nurses, *Adv Pract Nurs Q* 1(4):70, 1996.

Bower JO: Designing and implementing a patient safety program for the OR, *AORN J,* 76(3):452, 2002.

Deaton C: Outcomes measurement, *J Cardiovasc Nurs* 12(4):49, 1998.

Dochterman JM, Bulechek GM: *Nursing interventions classification (NIC),* ed 4, St. Louis, 2004, Mosby.

Institute of Medicine, Definition of quality of care, 2002, www.iom.edu/iom.

Joint Commission on Accreditation of Healthcare Organizations: *2003 Accreditation manual for hospitals,* vol 1, Standards, Chicago, 2003, The Commission.

Lin C: Patient satisfaction with nursing care as an outcome variable: dilemmas for nursing evaluation researchers, *J Prof Nurs* 1294:207, 1996.

Moorhead S, Johnson M, Maas M: *Nursing outcomes classification (NOC),* ed 3, St. Louis, 2004, Mosby.

Patton S, Stanley J: Bridging quality assurance and continuous quality improvement, *J Nurs Care Qual* 7(2):15, 1993.

Pelletier LR: Implementing outcomes management, *J Nurs Care Qual* 13(1):vii, 1998 (editorial).

Peters DA: Outcomes: the mainstay of a framework for quality care, *J Nurs Care Qual,* 10(1):61, 1995.

20

Managing Client Care

Media Resources

http://evolve.elsevier.com/Potter/
fundamentals/

CD COMPANION

- Review Questions
- Glossary

evolve WEBSITE

- Review Questions
- Student Learning Activities
- Glossary

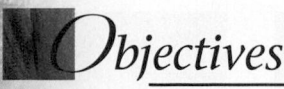

Objectives

Mastery of content in this chapter will enable the student to:

- Define the key terms listed.
- Differentiate among the types of nursing care delivery models.
- Describe the elements of decentralized decision making.
- Discuss the ways in which a nurse manager can support staff involvement in a decentralized decision-making model.
- Discuss ways to apply clinical care coordination skills in nursing practice.
- Discuss principles to follow in the appropriate delegation of client care activities.
- Differentiate total quality management and quality improvement.
- Discuss the elements of the Joint Commission on Accreditation of Healthcare Organizations' (JCAHO's) standards for improving organization performance.
- Describe an example of a quality improvement project on a nursing unit.

As a student nurse, it is important for you to acquire the necessary knowledge and competencies that ultimately allow you to practice as an entry-level staff nurse (Box 20-1). Regardless of the type of setting you eventually choose to work in as a staff nurse, you will be responsible for using organizational resources, participating in organizational routines while providing direct client care, using time productively, collaborating with all members of the health care team, and using certain leadership characteristics to manage others on the nursing team (Wywialowski, 1997). The delivery of nursing care within the health care system is a challenge because of the changes that are influencing health professionals, clients, and health care organizations (see Chapter 2). However, change offers opportunities. As you develop the knowledge and skills to become a staff nurse you will learn what it takes to effectively manage the clients you care for and to take the initiative in becoming a leader among your professional colleagues.

Building a Nursing Team

Nurses are self-directed and, with proper leadership and motivation, can solve most complex problems. A nurse's education and commitment in practicing within established standards and guidelines will ensure a rewarding professional career. It is also important for a nurse to work as a member of a cohesive and strong nursing team. An empowering work environment is one that brings out the best in a professional, concentrating on effective delivery of client care (e.g., client assessment, referral mechanisms, and physician-nurse collaboration), supporting risk taking and innovation, focusing on results and rewards, and offering professional opportunities for growth and advancement.

Building an empowered nursing team begins with the nurse executive. The nurse executive often holds the title of vice president or director of nursing.

Box 20-1   Entry-Level Staff Nurse Competencies

Identify organization resources (people, equipment, services), and determine when they are needed.
Work within various nursing care delivery models.
Use position descriptions to establish the scope and limitations of one's own and other nursing team members' practices.
Manage time purposefully and productively.
Prioritize client needs and related care.
Exhibit flexibility in providing care within available time constraints.
Show initiative and creativity as leadership qualities.
Use decision-making skills.
Defend one's own decisions.
Work with other health team members.
Resolve conflicts within the health team.
Delegate care activities appropriately.

Modified from Wywialowski EF: *Managing client care,* ed 2, St. Louis, 1997, Mosby.

Box 20-2   Developing a Vision for a Nursing Unit

What Is the Nursing Unit's Purpose or Mission?

Why do we exist?
Who are our customers (internal and external)?
What makes us unique?
What is unique about our clients?
How do we accomplish organizational goals or vision?

How Will Staff Work With Clients and Families?

Placing client and family needs first with a client-focused approach
Involving clients and families in all aspects of care
Making communication a priority

What Are the Standards of the Work Unit?

All staff will be competent.
Each staff member is accountable for the care delivered to clients.
Staff will work collaboratively with all members of the health care team.

Key Values

Creating an environment of caring
Being self-motivated and self-managed
Supporting a learning environment

The executive's position within an organization is critical in uniting the strategic direction of an organization with the philosophical values and goals of nursing. The nurse executive is both a clinical and business leader in the organization who is concerned with maximizing quality of care and cost-effectiveness while maintaining relationships and professional satisfaction of the staff (Pinkerton, 2001). Perhaps the most important responsibility of the nurse executive is to establish a vision for nursing that lays the groundwork that enables managers and staff to provide quality nursing care.

It takes an excellent nurse manager and an excellent nursing staff to achieve an empowering work environment. Together a manager and the nursing staff must share a vision and philosophy of care for their work unit. A philosophy of care incorporates the professional nursing staff's values and concerns for the way in which clients should be viewed and cared for. For example, a philosophy should address the nursing unit's purpose, how staff will work with clients and families, and the standards of care for the work unit (Box 20-2). A philosophy is a vision for how nursing is to be practiced. It should inspire the soul and be something about which all staff members can be proud (Hansten and Washburn, 1999). Integral to the philosophy of care is the selection of a nursing care delivery model and a management structure that support professional nursing practice.

Nursing Care Delivery Models

Since the time of Florence Nightingale there have been a variety of nursing care delivery models, methods by which nursing care is provided for clients. Ideally, the vision and philosophy nurses establish for the quality care of clients should drive the selection of a care delivery model (Coughlin, 2000). However, too often the scarcity of nursing resources and business initiatives from the health care organization influence the final decision. Care delivery must be effective in helping nurses achieve

desirable outcomes for their clients. Key factors contributing to success are decision-making authority for nurses who provide direct care, autonomy, collaborative practice, and effective methods of communicating with colleagues, physicians, and other health care providers (Coughlin, 2000; Ritter-Teitel, 2002).

Functional Nursing. Functional nursing was popular during World War II during a nursing shortage. This model of care is task focused, not client focused. In this model, tasks are divided, with one nurse assuming responsibility for specific tasks, for example, hygiene and dressing changes, whereas another nurse may assume responsibility for medication administration. Typically a lead nurse responsible for a specific shift assigns available nursing staff members according to their qualifications, their particular abilities, and tasks to be completed. Nurses become highly competent with the tasks that are repeatedly assigned to them.

The major disadvantages of functional nursing are problems with continuity of care, absence of a holistic view of clients, and the possibility that care will become mechanical (Dadich, 2003). In other words, a task-focused approach does not ensure that client care needs are met shift to shift. Communication is not always clear, because a single nurse is not responsible for the overall care of the client. The task-focused approach and ineffective communication lead to fragmented care and client dissatisfaction (Dadich, 2003).

Team Nursing. **Team nursing** developed as a care delivery model in response to the severe nursing shortage following World War II (Ritter-Teitel, 2002). In team nursing a registered nurse (RN) leads a team that is composed of other RNs, licensed practical nurses (LPNs) or licensed vocational nurses (LVNs), and nurse assistants or technicians. The team members provide direct client care to groups of clients, under the direction of the RN team leader. In this model, nurse assistants are given client assignments rather than being assigned particular nursing tasks.

The team leader develops client care plans, coordinates care delivered by the nursing team, provides care requiring complex nursing skills, problem solves with physicians and members of other disciplines, and assists the team in evaluating the effectiveness of their care (Wywialowski, 1997).

Limitations to the model include the lack of time the team leader spends with clients. Depending on the mix of staff members, this may mean that clients see an RN infrequently. Risks exist if an RN is unable to make necessary client assessments and be involved in important clinical decision making. The task orientation of the model and the fact that nurses may not be assigned to the same clients each day potentially may cause lack of continuity of care.

An advantage of team nursing is the collaborative style that encourages each member of the team to help the other members. This model has a high level of autonomy for the team leader and is an example of decision making occurring at a clinical level (Ritter-Teitel, 2002).

Total Patient Care. **Total patient care** delivery was the original care delivery model developed during Florence Nightingale's time. An RN is responsible for all aspects of care for one or more clients. The model became popular during the 1970s and 1980s, when the number of RNs were on the increase. The RN may delegate aspects of care to an LPN or unlicensed staff, but retains accountability for care of all assigned clients. The nurse works directly with the client, family, physician, and health care team members. The model typically has a shift-based focus. The same nurse does not necessarily care for the same client over time. Continuity of care from shift to shift or day to day can be a problem if staff members do not clearly communicate client needs to one another.

Primary Nursing. The **primary nursing** model of care delivery was developed with the aim of placing RNs at the bedside and improving nursing's accountability for client outcomes and the professional relationships among staff members (Ritter-Teitel, 2002). The model became more popular in the 1970s and early 1980s as hospitals began to employ more RNs. Primary nursing supports a philosophy regarding nurse and client relationships.

Primary nursing is a model of care delivery whereby an RN assumes responsibility for a caseload of clients over time. Typically the RN selects the clients for his or her caseload and cares for the same clients during their hospitalization or stay in the health care setting. The RN assesses client needs, develops a care plan, and ensures that appropriate nursing interventions are delivered to the client.

Primary nursing maintains continuity of care across shifts, days, or visits. It can be applied in any health care setting. When a primary nurse is off-duty, associate nurses, including LPNs or other RNs follow through with the developed plan of care. If there are differences in opinion as to client needs, associates and primary nurses collaborate to redefine the plan as needed.

Although primary nursing may require the presence of more professional staff members, this does not mean that the model is more costly. Care consistently managed by a single professional can minimize delays in therapies, improve collaboration with other professionals, and enhance the client-nurse relationship. In this model, the RN has a high level of clinical autonomy and authority that enhances collaboration with physicians (Ritter-Teitel, 2002).

Case Management. **Case management** is a care management approach that coordinates and links health care services to clients and their families while streamlining costs and maintaining quality (Dadich, 2003) (see Chapter 2). The Case Management Society of America (2003) defines case management as "a collaborative process which assesses, plans, implements, coordinates, monitors, and evaluates the options and services required to meet an individual's health needs, using communications and available resources to promote quality, cost-effective outcomes." What is unique about case management is that clinicians, either as individuals or as part of a collaborative group, oversee the management of clients with specific case types (e.g., clients with specific diagnoses presenting complex nursing and medical problems) and are usually held accountable for some standard of cost management and quality.

A case manager coordinates a client's acute care in the hospital, for example, and then follows up with the client after discharge home. Case managers may not provide direct care but instead they collaborate with and supervise the care delivered by other staff members and actively coordinate client discharge planning. The case manager frequently oversees a caseload of clients with complex nursing and medical problems.

Many organizations use critical pathways or CareMaps in a case management delivery system (see Chapter 17). These are multidisciplinary treatment plans that are designed for clients of a specific case type. The case manager, along with members of the health care team, uses the critical pathways or CareMaps to implement timely interventions in a coordinated plan of care. The plans eliminate the guesswork in client care by having all members of the health care team working from the same plan.

Decentralized Decision Making

With a vision for nursing established, it is the manager who directs and supports staff in the realization of that vision. The nurse executive supports managers by establishing a management structure that will help to achieve organizational goals and provide appropriate support to care delivery staff (Table 20-1). It takes a committed nurse executive, an excellent manager, and empowered nursing staff to create an enriching work environment where nursing practice thrives.

Table 20-1	Examples of Management Structures
Structural Approach	**Characteristics**
Centralized management	Single administrator leads organization, with directors overseeing departmental responsibilities. Typically, decisions are made by virtue of a person's position in an organization. Decisions are made from top down, with minimal input from staff. Managers tend to have minimal responsibility or accountability for 24-hour operation of nursing unit.
Decentralized management	Structure may appear similar to that of centralized organization. Often there are fewer directors. Those staff members who are best informed about a problem or issue make decisions on basis of knowledge. Managers often have 24-hour accountability and responsibility for staff, budget, and day-to-day management of work unit.
Matrix	Traditional hospital departments become reorganized into business units. Staff may report to more than one manager.

Decentralized management, in which decision making is moved down to the level of staff, is very common within health care organizations. This type of management structure has the advantage of creating an environment where managers and staff become more actively involved in shaping a health care organization's identity and determining success. Decentralized management requires workers to be empowered to accept greater responsibility for the quality of client care provided (Maddox, 1999). Working in a decentralized structure has the potential for greater collaborative effort, increased competency of staff, and ultimately a greater sense of professional accomplishment and satisfaction.

It is clear that progressive organizations achieve more when employees at all levels are actively involved. As a result, the role of a nurse manager has become critical in the management of effective nursing units or groups. The diverse responsibilities assumed by nursing managers are highlighted in Box 20-3. To make decentralized decision-making work, managers must know how to move decision making down to the lowest level possible. On a nursing unit, it is important for all nursing staff members (RNs, LPNs, LVNs), nurse assistants, and unit secretaries to become involved. This means that they must be kept well informed and given the opportunity by managers to participate in problem-solving activities. This includes opportunities in direct client care, as well as unit activities such as committee participation. Key elements to the decision-making process are responsibility, autonomy, authority, and accountability (Cox, 1995; Ritter-Teitel, 2002).

Responsibility refers to the duties and activities that an individual is employed to perform. A professional nurse's responsibilities in a given role are outlined in a position description describing the nurse's duties in client care and in participating as a member of the nursing unit.

Responsibility reflects ownership. The individual who oversees the employee must allocate it, and the employee must accept it. Managers must be sure that staff clearly understand their responsibilities, particularly in the face of change. For example, when hospitals participate in work redesign, client care delivery models can change significantly. It is the manager's responsibility to clearly define the RN's role within the new care delivery model. If decentralized decision making is in place, professional staff have a voice in identifying the new RN role. Each RN

Box 20-3	Responsibilities of the Nurse Manager

Assist staff in establishing annual goals for the unit and systems needed to accomplish goals.
Monitor professional nursing standards of practice on the unit.
Develop an ongoing staff development plan, including one for new employees.
Recruit new employees (interview and hire).
Conduct routine staff evaluations.
Establish self as a role model for positive customer service (customers include clients, families, and other health care team members).
Submit staffing schedules for the unit.
Conduct regular client rounds and problem solve client or family complaints.
Establish and implement a unit quality improvement plan.
Review and recommend new equipment for the unit.
Conduct regular staff meetings.
Conduct rounds with physicians.
Establish and support staff and interdisciplinary committees.

on the work team is responsible for knowing his or her role and how it is to be implemented on the busy nursing unit. For example, a primary nurse is responsible for completing a nursing assessment of all assigned clients and for developing a plan of care that addresses each of the client's nursing diagnoses (see Unit III). As the plan of care is delivered, the primary nurse is responsible for evaluating whether the plan is successful. This responsibility becomes a work ethic for the nurse in delivering excellent client care.

Autonomy is the freedom to decide and act (Hicks, 2003). Autonomy consistent with the scope of professional nursing practice will maximize the effectiveness of the nurse (Hicks, 2003). With autonomy, a professional nurse can make an independent decision about client care. The nurse plans care for the client within the scope of professional nursing practice, and provides the client independent nursing interventions without physician permission (Chapter 17) (Ritter-Teitel, 2002). Autonomy is not an absolute, but occurs in degrees. Innovation by nurses, increased productivity, higher nurse retention, and greater client satisfaction are results of autonomy in nursing practice (Hicks, 2003). For example, a nurse has the autonomy to develop and implement a discharge teaching plan based on specific client needs for any client who has been hospitalized. The nurse is providing nursing care that complements the prescribed medical therapy.

Authority refers to the right to act in areas where an individual has been given and accepts responsibility (Cox, 1995). Fox example, a primary nurse, managing a caseload of clients, may discover that members of the nursing team did not follow through on a discharge teaching plan for an assigned client. The primary nurse has the authority to consult other nurses to learn why recommendations on the plan of care were not followed and to choose appropriate teaching strategies for the client that all members of the team will follow. The primary nurse has the final authority in selecting the best course of action for the client's care.

Accountability refers to individuals being answerable for their actions. It involves follow-up and a reflective analysis of one's decisions to evaluate their effectiveness (Cox, 1995). A primary nurse is accountable for his or her clients' outcomes. In the example above, the primary nurse is accountable for ensuring that the client learns the information necessary to improve self-care. The nurse demonstrates accountability in checking on the client and family after discharge and in reviewing with the nursing team whether continuity in teaching occurred.

A successful decentralized nursing unit exercises on an ongoing basis the four elements of decision making: responsibility, autonomy, authority, and accountability. An effective manager sets the same expectations for the staff in how decisions are made. Staff must routinely meet to discuss and negotiate how to maintain an equality and balance in the elements. Staff members must feel comfortable in expressing differences of opinion and in challenging ways in which the team functions, while recognizing their own responsibility, autonomy, authority, and accountability. Ultimately, decentralized decision making is the vehicle for realizing the unit's vision of what professional nursing care should be.

Staff Involvement. When decentralized decision making exists on a nursing unit, all staff members actively participate in unit activities (Figure 20-1). Because the work environment promotes participation, all staff members benefit from the knowledge and skills of the entire work group. If the staff learns to value knowledge and the contributions of colleagues, better client care becomes an outcome. The nursing manager supports staff involvement through a variety of approaches:

1. *Establishment of nursing practice or problem-solving committees or professional **shared governance** councils.* Chaired by senior clinical staff, these groups are empowered to establish and maintain care standards for nursing practice on their work unit. The committees review and establish standards of care, develop policy and procedures, resolve client satisfaction issues, or develop new documentation tools. It is important for the committees to focus on client outcomes rather than only work issues in order to ensure quality care is delivered on the unit (Hansten and Washburn, 1999). Mechanisms are established to ensure that all staff have

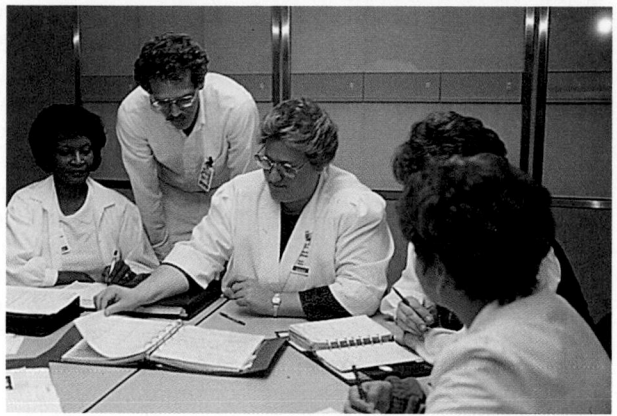

FIGURE **20-1**   Staff collaborating on practice issues.

input on practice issues. Managers might not sit on the committee, but they receive regular reports of committee progress. The nature of work on the nursing unit determines committee membership. At times, members of other disciplines, for example, pharmacy, respiratory therapy, or clinical nutrition, might participate in practice committees or shared governance councils.

2. *Nurse/physician collaborative practice.* The nursing unit's care delivery model influences how nurse and physician collaboration can best be fostered. If the unit practices team nursing, it is important for team leaders to regularly participate in physician rounds. If the unit practices primary nursing, the physician should communicate either with each primary nurse or the associate nurse who is assuming care for the client on that day. In a home care or extended care setting, the staff should be able to contact physicians with minimal delay and be able to work together on decisions regarding client care. The manager avoids taking care of problems for the staff. Instead, staff members learn to keep physicians informed on what is important regarding their clients. Open communication is critical. Physicians are invited to attend practice committees when clinical problems are addressed and to present timely in-service programs on new medical procedures or research findings.

3. *Interdisciplinary collaboration.* The emphasis on efficiency in health care delivery brings all members of the health care team together. Whenever systems or programs are redesigned, interdisciplinary involvement is crucial because most health care processes involve more than one discipline. At the client care level, the staff must recognize the importance of prompt referrals and timely communication with other health professionals. Including representatives of the various disciplines together in practice projects, in-service programs, conferences, and staff meetings fosters interdisciplinary collaboration.

4. *Staff communication.* Perhaps one of the manager's greatest challenges, especially if a work group is large, is communication with staff. It is difficult to ensure that all staff receive the same message: the correct message. In the present health care environment, staff quickly become uneasy and distrusting if they

fail to hear about planned changes on their work unit. However, a manager cannot assume total responsibility for all communication. Instead, the manager can use a variety of approaches to ensure that information is communicated quickly and accurately to all staff. For example, many managers distribute biweekly or monthly newsletters of ongoing unit or health care agency activities. Minutes of committee meetings should be posted in an accessible location for all staff to read. When vital issues regarding the operations of the unit or the organization are to be discussed, the manager should conduct staff meetings. When the unit has practice or quality improvement committees, each member should be assigned responsibility to communicate directly to a select number of staff. In that way, all staff are contacted and given the opportunity for input.

5. *Staff education.* A professional nursing staff should always grow in knowledge. It is impossible to remain knowledgeable of current medical and nursing practice trends without ongoing education. The nurse manager is responsible for making learning opportunities available so that staff remain competent in their practice. This involves planning in-service programs, sending staff to continuing education classes and professional conferences, and having staff present case studies or practice issues during staff meetings. Staff members are responsible for pursuing educational opportunities when they know that their competencies are lacking.

*L*eadership Skills for Nursing Students

As nursing students become involved in clinical assignments with clients, it is important that they prepare themselves for leadership roles. This does not mean that they have to quickly learn how to lead a team of nursing staff. Instead, they first learn to become dependable and competent providers of client care. Just as is the case with the staff nurse, the nursing student has a responsibility for the care given to his or her clients and must assume accountability for that care. Even though the student has limited authority and consults with instructors and staff regarding decisions, the student must not avoid making decisions in client care. The student can learn to become a leader by making good clinical decisions, learning from mistakes and seeking guidance, collaborating closely with professional nurses, and striving to improve his or her performance during each client interaction. There are certain leadership skills that the nursing student can learn to use, including clinical care coordination, team communication, delegation, and knowledge building.

Clinical Care Coordination

A student must acquire the skills necessary so that client care can be delivered in a timely and effective manner. In the beginning, this might involve only one client but eventually will involve groups of clients. Clinical care coordination includes clinical decision making, priority setting, use of organizational skills and resources, time management, and evaluation.

Clinical Decisions. When a nurse begins an assignment with a client, the first activity involves a focused but complete assessment of the client's condition that enables the nurse to make an accurate clinical decision as to the client's needs and required nursing therapies. This initial contact is also an important first step in developing a caring relationship with a client. The nurse uses a critical thinking approach, applying previous knowledge and experience to the decision-making process (see Chapter 14).

The nursing process is the framework used by the nurse in determining the level of care required, implementing the plan of care, and evaluating its results (see Unit III). If the nurse fails to make accurate clinical judgments about a client, there can be undesirable outcomes. The client's condition might worsen or remain the same when the potential for improvement has been lost. An important lesson in organizational skills is to be thorough. The nurse must learn to attend and listen to the client, look for any cues (obvious or subtle) that point to a pattern of findings, and direct the assessment to explore the pattern further. Accurate clinical decision making keeps the nurse focused on the proper course of action. A student nurse should never hesitate to ask for assistance when a client's assessment reveals a changing clinical condition.

Priority Setting. After forming a picture of the client's total needs, the nurse must then decide on what client needs or problems need to be cared for first. If a client is experiencing serious physiological or psychological problems, the nurse's priority becomes clear. It becomes essential to act immediately to stabilize the client's condition. If the client is in no acute distress, priority setting might be based on the client's basic needs. Wywialowski (1997) describes categories of priority nursing needs of individual clients:

- *First-order priority needs*—An immediate threat to a client's survival or safety, such as a physiological episode of obstructed airway, loss of consciousness, or a psychological episode of an anxiety attack
- *Second-order priority needs*—Actual problems for which the client or family has requested immediate help, such as comfort measures, nausea, or a full bladder or bowel
- *Third-order priority needs*—Relatively urgent actual or potential problems that the client or family does not recognize, such as monitoring for postoperative complications or anticipating teaching needs of a client who may be unaware of side effects of a drug
- *Fourth-order priority needs*—Actual or potential problems with which the client or family may need help in the future, such as teaching for self-care in the home

Many clients can have all four types of priorities, requiring a nurse to make careful judgments in choosing a course of action. Obviously first-order priority needs demand a nurse's immediate attention. When a client has diverse priority needs, sometimes it helps to focus on the client's basic needs. For example, a client who is immobilized in traction might report being uncomfortable from being in the same position. The dietary assistant arrives in the room to deliver a meal tray. Instead of immediately assisting the client with the meal, the nurse repositions the client and offers basic hygiene measures. The client will likely become more interested in eating after being made to feel comfortable. The client will also then be more receptive to any instruction the nurse wishes to provide.

Over time the nurse will also be required to meet the priority needs of a group of clients. This requires the nurse to know the priority needs of each client within the group, assessing each client's needs as soon as possible while addressing first- and second-priority needs in a timely manner (Wywialowski, 1997). To identify which clients require assessment first, the nurse relies on information from the change-of-shift report, the agency's classification system that identifies client acuity, and information from the medical record. Over time the nurse learns to spontaneously rank clients' needs by priority or urgency. It is important to think about the resources available, to be flexible in recognizing that priority needs can change, and to consider how time can be used wisely.

Priorities must also be made on the basis of client expectations. A nurse might have an excellent plan of care established, but if the client is resistant to certain therapies or disagrees with the approach, little success will be gained. Working closely with the client and showing a caring attitude is important. A nurse shares the priorities defined with the client to establish a level of agreement and cooperation.

Organizational Skills. Implementing a plan of care requires the nurse to be effective and efficient. Effective use of time entails doing the right things, whereas efficient use of time entails doing things right (Wywialowski, 1997). A nurse learns to become efficient by combining various nursing activities—in other words, doing more than one thing at a time. For example, during medication administration or while obtaining a specimen, the nurse combines therapeutic communication skills, teaching interventions, and assessment and evaluation. The nurse always tries to establish and strengthen relationships with clients and uses any client contact as an opportunity to convey important information. Client interaction also provides the nurse the opportunity to convey caring and interest in the client. The nurse always attends to the client's behaviors and responses to therapies to assess if any new problems are developing and to evaluate responses to interventions.

A well-organized nurse approaches any planned procedures by having all of the necessary equipment available and making sure the client is prepared. Being sure the client is comfortable and well informed will increase the likelihood of the procedure going smoothly. Sometimes the nurse requires the assistance of colleagues to perform or complete a procedure. It is always wise to have the work area organized and preliminary steps completed before asking colleagues for assistance.

As the nurse begins to deliver care based on established priorities, events may occur within the health care setting that can interfere with plans. For example, just as a nurse begins to provide morning hygiene for a hospitalized client, an x-ray technician may enter to take a chest film. Once the x-ray film is completed, a phlebotomist may arrive to draw a sample of blood. In such a case the nurse's priorities may seem to conflict with the priorities of other health care personnel. It is important

to always keep the client's needs as the center of attention. The client may have experienced symptoms earlier that required a chest film and laboratory work. In such a case it is important to be sure that the diagnostic tests are completed. In another example, a client may be waiting to visit family, and a chest film may be a routine order from 2 days earlier. The client's condition may have since stabilized, and the x-ray technician may be willing to return later to shoot the film. In this situation attending to the client's hygiene and comfort so that family can visit is more of a priority at this time.

Use of Resources. Another important aspect of clinical care coordination is appropriate use of resources. Resources in this case include members of the health care team. In any setting the administration of client care occurs more smoothly when staff members work together. Students should never hesitate to have staff assist them, especially when there is an opportunity to make a procedure or activity more comfortable and safer for the client. For example, assistance in turning, positioning, and ambulating clients is frequently necessary when clients experience impaired mobility. Having a staff member assist with handling equipment and supplies during more complicated procedures such as catheter insertion or dressing change can help make procedures more efficient. This is an excellent way for students to learn how to work with assistive personnel. There are also times when the student must recognize personal limitations and use professional resources for assistance. For example, the student may assess a client and find relevant clinical signs and symptoms but be unfamiliar with the underlying physical condition. Consulting with an RN leads to confirmation of findings and assurance that the proper course of action will be taken for the client. Throughout a nurse's professional career there are always new experiences. A leader knows his or her limitations and seeks professional colleagues for guidance and support.

Time Management. Nurses can experience stress on the clinical unit while trying to meet the multiple needs of assigned clients. One way to manage this stress is through the use of time management skills. These skills involve learning how, where, and when to use your time. Because the nurse has a limited amount of time with clients, it is essential to remain goal oriented and to use time wisely. The nurse learns early the importance of using client goals as a way to identify priorities. However, the nurse must also learn how to establish personal goals and time frames. For example, a nurse may be caring for two clients on a busy surgical nursing unit, one of whom underwent surgery the day before and the other of whom is anticipating discharge the next day. Clearly, the first client's goals center on restoring physiological function impaired as a result of the stress of surgery. The second client's goals center on adequate preparation to assume self-care at home. The nurse, in reviewing the therapies required for both clients, must learn how to organize his or her time so that the activities of care, as well as client goals, can be achieved. The nurse must anticipate when care will be interrupted for medication administration, any diagnostic testing, and when is the best time for planned therapies such as dressing changes, client education, and client ambulation.

One useful time management skill involves keeping a to-do list. When a nurse first begins working with a client or clients, it helps to make a list that sequences the nursing activities to be performed. The change-of-shift report may help in sequencing activities based on what the nurse learns about the client's condition and the care provided before the nurse's arrival to the unit. It is helpful to consider activities that have specific time limits in terms of addressing client needs, such as administering a pain medication before a scheduled procedure or instructing clients before their discharge home. The nurse also analyzes the items on the list that are scheduled by agency policies or routines (e.g., medications or intravenous [IV] tubing changes). A nurse notes which activities need to be done on time and which activities can be done on discretion (Wywialowski, 1997). The administration of medications must be performed within a specific schedule, but a nurse can also perform other activities while in the client's room. Finally, estimate the amount of time needed to complete the various activities. Activities requiring the assistance of other staff members usually take longer because the nurse must plan around their schedule.

Good time management also involves completing one task before starting another. A nurse completes the activities started with one client before moving on to the next if possible. Care will then become less fragmented, and the nurse can better focus on what he or she is doing for each client. As a result, it is less likely that errors will be made. Time management requires an ability to anticipate the day's activities, to combine activities when possible, and to not be interrupted by nonessential activities. Box 20-4 summarizes principles of time management.

Box 20-4 Principles of Time Management

Goal setting: Review the client's goals of care for the day and any goals you have for activities, such as completing documentation, attending a client care conference, giving a staff report, or preparing medications for administration.

Time analysis: Reflect on how you use your time. While working on a clinical area, keep track of how you use your time in different activities. This may provide valuable information to reveal how well organized you really are.

Priority setting: Set the priorities that you have established for clients within set time frames. Determine when is the best time, for example, to conduct teaching sessions, plan ambulation, and provide rest periods, based on what you know about the client's condition. For example, if a client is nauseated or in pain, it is not a good time for a teaching session.

Interruption control: Everyone needs time to socialize or to discuss issues with colleagues. However, do not let this interrupt important client care activities such as medication administration. Use time during report, mealtime, or team meetings to the best of your advantage. Also, plan time to assist fellow colleagues so that it complements your client care schedule.

Evaluation: At the end of each day, take time to think about how effectively time was used. If you are having difficulties, discuss them with an instructor or a more experienced staff member.

Evaluation. One of the most important aspects of clinical care coordination is evaluation (see Chapter 19). It is a mistake to think that evaluation occurs at the end of an activity. Evaluation is an ongoing process. Once a nurse assesses a client's needs and begins therapies directed at a specific problem area, the nurse should immediately evaluate if therapies are effective and the client's response. The process of evaluation compares actual client outcomes with those that are expected. For example, a clinic nurse may assess the condition of a diabetic client's foot ulcer to determine if healing has progressed since the last clinical visit. When expected outcomes are not being met, evaluation reveals the need to continue current therapies for a longer period, revise approaches to care, or introduce new therapies. Throughout the day as a nurse cares for a client it is important to anticipate when to return to the bedside to evaluate care, for example, 30 minutes after a medication was administered, 15 minutes after an IV line has begun infusing, or 60 minutes after discussing discharge instructions with the client and family.

Keeping a focus on evaluation of the client's progress lessens the chance of becoming distracted by the tasks of care. It is common to assume that staying focused on planned activities ensures that care is performed appropriately. However, task orientation does not ensure good client outcomes. The competent nurse learns that at the heart of good organizational skills is the constant inquiry into the client's condition and progress toward an improved level of health.

Team Communication. As a part of a nursing team, each nurse is responsible for open, professional communication. Regardless of the setting, nurses learn that an enriching, professional environment is one in which staff members respect one another's ideas, share information, and keep one another informed. On a busy hospital unit this means keeping colleagues informed about clients with emerging problems, physicians who have been called for consultation, and unique approaches that solved a complex nursing problem. In a clinic setting it may mean sharing unusual diagnostic findings or conveying important information regarding a client's source of family support. One way of fostering good team communication is by setting expectations of one another. A nurse always treats colleagues with respect, listens to the ideas of other staff members without interruption, is honest and direct in what is said, and is responsible for professional actions without displacing anger or frustration on co-workers (Kreitzer and others, 1997). An efficient team knows it can count on all members when needs arise. Sharing expectations of what, when, and how to communicate is a step toward establishing a strong work team.

Delegation. The art of effective delegation is a skill nursing students need to observe and practice to improve their own management skills. The American Nurses Association (1995) defines **delegation** as transferring responsibility for the performance of an activity or task while retaining accountability for the outcome. One purpose of delegation is to improve efficiency. Asking a staff member to obtain an ordered specimen while the nurse attends to a client's pain medication request effectively prevents a delay in the client gaining pain relief. Delegation can also provide job enrichment. A nurse shows trust in colleagues by delegating tasks to them and showing staff members that they are important players in the delivery of care. A nurse never delegates a task that he or she dislikes doing or would not do independently because this can create negative feelings and poor working relationships. For example, if a nurse is in the room when a client asks to be placed on a bedpan, the nurse should assist the client rather than leave the room to find the nurse assistant. Remember that even though the delegation of a task transfers the responsibility and authority to another person, the nurse who is delegating retains accountability for the delegated task.

It is important to recognize that in regard to delegation to assistive personnel, tasks are delegated, not clients. Leah Curtin (1994), a distinguished nursing leader and past editor of the journal *Nursing Management,* wrote that assistive personnel should not be at the bedside, but at the nurse's side. This means that assistive personnel should not be assigned sole responsibility for the care of clients. Instead, it is the professional nurse in charge of client care who decides what activities assistive personnel may perform independently and what activities must be performed by the RN and assistant in partnership. One way to accomplish this is to have the RN and technician or nurse assistant conduct rounds together. The nurse can assess each client as the technician helps to attend to basic client needs. The nurse then delegates care based upon assessment findings and priority setting. An RN will always be responsible for the assessment of a client's ongoing status, but if a client is stable, the RN may delegate vital sign monitoring to the assistive personnel. The RN is the one in most settings who makes judgments during client care as to when delegation is appropriate. The LPN directs care in many long-term care facilities. The National Council of State Boards of Nursing (1995) has provided some guidelines for delegation of tasks in accordance with an RN's legal scope of practice (Box 20-5). As the leader of the health care team, the RN must know how to give clear instructions, effectively prioritize client needs and therapies, and be able to give staff members timely and meaningful feedback. Assistive personnel respond positively when they are included as part of the nursing team.

A nurse cannot simply assign assistive personnel to tasks without considering the implications. The nurse assesses a client and determines a plan of care before identifying which tasks someone else can perform. When directing assistive personnel, the RN must determine the degree of supervision that may be required. Is it the first time a staff member performed the task? Does the client present a complicating factor whereby the RN's assistance is necessary? Does the staff member have prior experience with a particular type of client in addition to having received training on skill performance? The RN's final responsibility is to evaluate whether assistive personnel performed a task properly and whether desired outcomes were realized.

Appropriate delegation begins with knowing what skills can be delegated. This requires the RN to be familiar with the state's nurse practice act, institutional policies and procedures, and the institution's job description

for assistive personnel. These standards help to define the necessary level of competency of assistive personnel.

An institution's policies and procedures and job description for assistive personnel provide specific guidelines in regard to what tasks or activities can be delegated. The job description should specify any required education and the types of tasks assistive personnel can perform, either independently or with RN direct supervision. Institutional policy helps in defining the amount of training required of assistive personnel while employed. Procedures specify who is qualified to perform a given nursing procedure, whether supervision is necessary, and the type of reporting required. Nurses should have a means to easily access policies or have supervisory staff who can inform them as to assistive personnel's job duties.

Efficient delegation requires constant communication—sending clear messages and listening so that all participants understand expectations regarding client care. An RN should provide clear instructions when delegating tasks. These instructions may initially focus on the procedure itself, as well as on the unique needs of a given client. As the RN becomes more familiar with a staff member's competency, trust builds and fewer instructions may be needed, but clarification of clients' specific needs will always be necessary.

Box 20-5   The Five Rights of Delegation

Right Task

The right task in one that is delegable for a specific client, such as tasks that are repetitive, require little supervision, and are relatively noninvasive.

Right Circumstances

The appropriate client setting, available resources, and other relevant factors are considered. In an acute care setting, clients' conditions can change quickly. Good clinical decision making is needed to determine what to delegate.

Right Person

The right person is delegating the right tasks to the right person to be performed on the right person.

Right Direction/Communication

A clear, concise description of the task, including its objective, limits, and expectations, is given. Communication must be ongoing between RN and assistive personnel during a shift of care.

Right Supervision

Appropriate monitoring, evaluation, intervention as needed, and feedback are provided. Assistive personnel should feel comfortable to ask questions and seek assistance.

Modified from National Council of State Boards of Nursing: *Delegation: concepts and decision-making process,* Chicago, 1995, The Council.

Another important step in delegation is evaluation of the staff member's performance and the client's outcomes. When assistive personnel do a good job, it is important to provide praise and recognition. If the staff member's performance is not satisfactory, the RN must give constructive and appropriate feedback. The RN should always give specific feedback in regard to any mistakes that were made, explaining how the mistakes could have been avoided. Giving feedback in private is the professional way and preserves the staff member's dignity. Frequently when the performance of assistive personnel does not meet expectations, the cause is due to inadequate training or assignment to too many tasks. The RN may discover the need to review a procedure with staff and offer demonstration or even recommend that additional training be scheduled with the education department. If too many tasks are being delegated, this might be a nursing practice issue. All staff should discuss the appropriateness of delegation on their unit. Some assistive personnel may need help in learning how to prioritize. In some cases RNs may need to learn that they are overdelegating.

Here are a few tips on appropriate delegation (Keeling and others, 2000):

- *Assess the knowledge and skills of the delegate:* Determine what assistive personnel know and what they can do by asking open-ended questions that will elicit conversation and details on what the person knows; for example, "How do you usually put the cuff on when you measure a blood pressure?" or "Tell me how you prepare the tubing before you give an enema."

- *Match tasks to the delegate's skills:* Know what skills are included in the training program for assistive personnel at your facility. Determine if personnel have learned critical thinking skills, such as knowing when a client may be in harm or knowing the difference between normal clinical findings and changes to report.

- *Communicate clearly:* Always provide unambiguous and clear directions by describing a task, the desired outcome, and the time period within which the task should be completed. Never give instructions through another staff member. Make the person feel as though he or she is part of the team. For example, "I'd like you to help me by getting Mr. Floyd up to ambulate before lunch. Be sure to check his blood pressure before he stands and write your finding on the graphic sheet. OK?"

- *Listen attentively:* Listen to the response of assistive personnel after you provide directions. Do they feel comfortable in asking questions or requesting clarification? If you encourage a response, listen to what the person has to say. Be especially attentive if the staff member has been given a deadline to meet by another nurse. Help sort out priorities.

- *Provide feedback:* Always give assistive personnel feedback regarding performance, regardless of outcome. Let them know of a job well done. If an outcome is undesirable, find a private place to discuss what occurred, any miscommunication, and how to achieve a better outcome in the future.

Knowledge Building. All professional nurses recognize the importance of pursuing knowledge to remain competent. A leader recognizes that there is always something new to learn. Opportunities for learning occur with each client interaction, each encounter with a professional colleague, and each meeting or class session where health care professionals gather to discuss clinical care issues. There is always someone who has had different experiences and knowledge. In-service programs, workshops, and collegiate courses offer innovative and current information on the rapidly changing world of health care. To become a leader, a nurse actively pursues learning opportunities, both formal and informal, and learns to share knowledge with the professional colleagues he or she encounters.

Quality Management

Within a health care environment where business initiatives and client care activities create constant demands on all levels of staff, it is sometimes difficult to reflect and take the time to consider how improvements can be made in the way work is done. If you would ask a busy staff nurse who just completed caring for six clients, "How can you improve what you just did," you likely might get a skeptical look. It would be easy for the nurse to say that he or she is just too busy to take the time to think about how changes can be made. This is the case unless the nurse works for an organization where **total quality management (TQM)** is a well-integrated philosophy.

Quality and value were major health care issues that came to the forefront in the 1990s. Quality management recognizes that the client or customer defines quality (Wendt and Vale, 2003). Value is a function of balance between excellent care and services, good outcomes, and cost (JCAHO, 2002). Health care organizations cannot ignore the need for quality, value, and improvement. Quality improvement is a must for customer satisfaction and business success and survival. TQM has become the philosophy for change within many business organizations. It is a philosophy that influences every single department and thus every single employee of an organization. TQM requires employees to think differently and therefore to act differently from what may be their usual habit (Marriner-Tomey, 2000; Triolo and others, 1997). An organization that accepts TQM as a work principle acknowledges that perfection is never reached, recognizes that an attempt to improve is not a condemnation of the past, and accepts that change is a continuous process. Table 20-2 summarizes principles and conditions for TQM.

In a well-established TQM program, customer service is a priority. Customers are more interested today in the quality of health care because of rising costs and because they are more informed. They want easy access to services, timely and safe delivery of services, coordinated care, and effective services that result in desired outcomes. In a TQM philosophy the term *customer* is not intended to devalue how health care providers perceive their client relationships (Triolo and others, 1997). Instead, it is intended to broaden each staff member's concept of relationships with others in doing work. In addition to clients, customers may include families, physicians, other health care professionals, and even product suppliers. To make improvements in how health care is provided, each em-

Table 20-2	Principles and Conditions for Total Quality Management
Principles	**Conditions in the Work Environment**
Continuous quality improvement	Employee involvement
Knowledge of customer expectations, needs	Empowerment
Processes of customer-supplier relationships	An environment that supports risk taking
Belief in people	Teamwork
Statistical analysis	Data collection and analysis skills
Costs of poor quality	Group interaction skills
	Structure and management to enable improvement
	Tools to facilitate the improvement

ployee of a health care organization must be willing to work with others.

Another important principle of TQM is that work towards improvement is accomplished through a focus on processes and systems (Wendt and Vale, 2003). For improvement of client outcomes, organizations must systematically monitor, analyze, and improve its processes (JCAHO, 2002). Typically, many individuals are involved in a single process. For example, medication delivery might seem to be simply the concern and responsibility of the nurse. But consider that physicians prescribe the medications, the pharmacy must prepare the medications, secretaries communicate orders and changes, transporters often deliver medications to work areas, and the nurse finally administers the medications. With so many individuals involved in most work processes, strong leadership, employee empowerment, good collaboration, effective communication, and support of staff's ideas are essential factors for TQM to be successful. TQM begins with executive leaders and then is integrated through the work of managers and staff. The following section explores the influence a TQM philosophy can have on nursing practice and the involvement of staff nurses.

Quality in Nursing Practice

The JCAHO (2002) defines **quality improvement (QI)** as a method for continuously studying and improving the processes related to the provision of health care services to meet the needs of clients and others. Quality improvement focuses on improving organization performance related to processes. JCAHO (2002) identifies performance as what is done and how well it is done to provide health care (Box 20-6). Among the processes that most directly influence clients are those that constitute nursing practice. The quality of nursing practice is a principal responsibility of nursing managers and their staff. Each professional nurse must learn to evaluate his or her success in delivering appropriate and effective client care. Does the nurse perform competently? Is appropriate care delivered? What outcomes does the client experience? These questions drive any QI effort.

The outcomes of care are a measure of the performance of the entire health care team. Managing quality ultimately is a multidisciplinary effort. With all disciplines contributing to client care, the nurse manager and staff assume the critical role in recognizing trends in nursing practice, identifying when recurrent problems

Box 20-6	Dimensions of Performance

Doing the Right Thing

The *efficacy* of the procedure or treatment in relation to the client's condition

The *appropriateness* of a specific test, procedure, or service to meet the client's clinical needs

Doing the Right Thing Well

The *availability* of a needed test, procedure, treatment, or service to the client who needs it

The *timeliness* with which a needed test, procedure, treatment, or service is provided to the client

The *effectiveness* with which tests, procedures, treatments, and services are provided

The *continuity* of the services provided to the client with respect to other services, practitioners, and providers and over time

The *safety* of the client and others to whom the services are provided

The *efficiency* with which care and services are provided

The *respect and caring* with which care and services are provided

Modified from Joint Commission on Accreditation of Healthcare Organizations: *Comprehensive accreditation manual for hospitals: the official handbook,* Chicago, 2002, The Commission.

develop, and initiating opportunities to improve the quality of care. For example, after reviewing clients who have undergone hip surgery, the nurse manager asks, "Do clients regain functional mobility without severe pain?" "Is rehabilitation delayed?" and "Are there complications of wound infection?" An effective nurse manager will enforce a work ethic that has nursing staff continually improving on how care is administered. The first step is to define quality of nursing practice.

Quality Defined. Before the nurse manager and staff can measure trends in nursing practice, they first must know the standards or guidelines that define quality. In other words, to judge if clients with hip surgery have functional mobility impaired by pain, there must be an agreement as to how functional clients should become after surgery and how pain is assessed. Similarly, to judge if rehabilitation has been delayed, there must be a standard for when

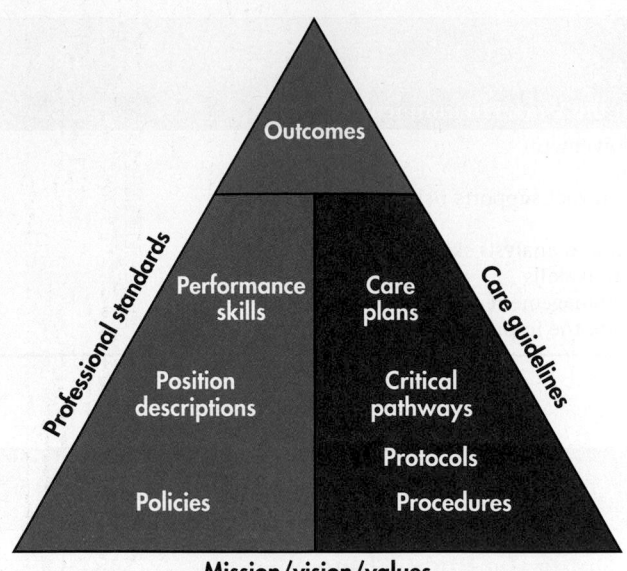

FIGURE **20–2**   Framework for quality. (Data from Peters: Outcomes: the mainstay of a framework for quality care, *J Nurs Care Qual* 10(1):61, 1995.)

clients begin rehabilitation. Quality of care and nursing practice is not something arbitrarily defined. The process is ongoing, involving all members of a nursing department. It therefore occurs at an administration level and at a work unit level. A definition of quality begins with the mission, vision, and philosophy of the nursing department. These statements lay the foundation of values that define how all nurses within an organization are to perform and the services that are to be made available to clients. A well-written set of values for a nursing department then provides direction for professional standards and care guidelines that when administered should guarantee excellent client outcomes. Figure 20-2 provides a framework for quality nursing care.

Professional Standards. Professional standards are authoritative statements used by the profession in describing the responsibilities for which its practitioners are accountable (Peters, 1995). Included are the policies and position descriptions that identify the performance skills within an institution. Standards are an organization's interpretation of the professional's competency. Whenever a work unit such as a nursing staff attempts to define quality, professional performance is a critical element. When the process is done well, the staff will be able to recognize evidence of quality standards in all aspects of their work. The adherence to professional standards is measured through professional outcomes.

Care Guidelines. Care guidelines are systematically developed statements to assist in determining how diseases, disorders, and other health conditions can be most effectively and appropriately prevented, diagnosed, treated, and clinically managed. Guidelines may be developed by single disciplines or be multidisciplinary in focus. There may be care guidelines jointly developed by nurses from

similar clinical areas or from a single, unique clinical unit. An example of a nursing clinical protocol is one used for instructing clients newly diagnosed with diabetes. The effectiveness of clinical guidelines is measured through client outcomes.

Care guidelines include procedures, care plans (see Chapter 17), protocols and critical pathways (see Chapter 17). Procedures are step-by-step descriptions of how to perform a psychomotor skill. An example is the nursing skill for changing a sterile dressing. Depending on complexity, skills include cognitive abilities (e.g., assessment steps) and manual dexterity. Clinical protocols outline steps to be taken in treating a certain condition (Peters, 1995). A specific course of action is usually prescribed in specific terms under specific conditions. In the example of treatment for pressure ulcers, a protocol will establish the course of action to take in treating the condition, depending on the stage of the ulcer.

Outcomes. Outcomes are the conditions to be achieved as a result of care delivery (see Chapter 17). Analysis of outcomes is a key component of quality improvement (Moorhead, Johnson, and Maas, 2004; Titler, 2001). An **outcome** tells whether interventions are effective, whether clients progress, how well standards are being met, and whether changes are necessary. When a nursing staff is able to think in terms of outcomes, their actions become much more purposeful and focused on improving the condition of their clients' health. There are two types of outcomes important to differentiate (Peters, 1995):

1. *Professional outcomes:* A measure of the professional caregiver's performance. Professional standards of care, institutional policies, and job descriptions set expectations for how care is to be delivered and the professional nurse's responsibility in care delivery. These discipline-specific outcomes are also important in evaluating the quality of practice (Moorhead and others, 2000). *Example:* The RN is responsible for the ongoing assessment of clients' status and will communicate changes in a client's condition to appropriate health team members.
2. *Client outcomes:* A measure of the client's status after receiving care. All clients have outcomes reflected in their nursing plan of care (see Chapter 17). Client outcomes are also defined in other clinical guidelines, such as critical pathways and clinical protocols. This type of outcome is generally organization specific and is stated as an expected goal (Moorhead and others, 2004). *Example:* Following use of reminiscent therapy, a client will be able to discuss concerns regarding the client's terminal illness.

Developing Quality Improvement Teams. It makes sense for health care providers who are most familiar with client care activities to collaborate on QI efforts. For example, if a team of nursing staff identifies an opportunity to improve the timeliness and efficiency of the admission process to their unit, it makes sense to include admitting, transporters, pharmacy, and physicians in the improvement effort. In many health care organizations there are organization-wide and unit-based QI teams or committees. The organization-wide teams are composed of staff

Table 20-3	Models for Process Improvement		
PRIDE	**FOCUS-PDCA**	**FADE**
Process—select one to improve	**F**ind process to improve	**F**ocus on a problem
Relevant dimensions of performance measurement	**O**rganize team that knows process	**A**nalyze the problem
Interpret data and evaluate variance	**C**larify current knowledge of process	**D**evelop a plan
Design or redesign the process	**U**nderstand causes of process variation	**E**xecute the plan
Execute the plan	**S**elect process improvement	
Improve—validate by remeasuring	**PDCA: P**lan, **D**o, **C**heck, **A**ct	

Modified from Keill P, Johnson T: Optimizing performance through process improvement, *J Nurs Car Qual* 9(1):1, 1994.

Box 20-7 — Standards for Improving Organization Performance

The leaders establish a planned, systematic, organization-wide approach to process design and performance measurement, analysis, and improvement.

New or modified processes are designed well.

Data are collected to monitor the stability of existing processes, identify opportunities for improvement, identify changes that will lead to improvement, and sustain improvement.

Data are systematically combined and analyzed on an ongoing basis.

Improved performance is achieved and sustained.

Modified from Joint Commission on Accreditation of Healthcare Organizations: *Comprehensive accreditation manual for hospitals: the official handbook,* Chicago, 2002, The Commission.

---

from all departments within a hospital. The problems these teams seek to solve usually affect processes that occur on all units within an organization. For example, the redesign of a client documentation system requires participation by all disciplines who enter information in the medical record. These organizational QI teams are given the responsibility to create innovations to make work more efficient and to improve the quality of care provided. In contrast, unit-based QI teams identify clinical priorities for a work unit. Client understanding of discharge instructions and the associated education process is an example of a unit-based QI project for a nursing unit. Unit-based teams are ideally participative, decentralizing decision making and accountability for practice and placing them at the staff level. An effective QI program leads to improved clinical practice, better participation by professional staff members, and increased sophistication of evaluation. It also achieves better client outcomes.

Components of a QI Program. A well-organized QI program focuses on processes or systems that significantly contribute to outcomes. To identify the greatest opportunity for improving quality, an organization considers those activities that are high volume, high risk, and/or problem areas (JCAHO, 2002). A systematic approach is needed organizationally to ensure that everyone speaks the same language with regard to QI projects. The JCAHO's Standards for Improving Organization Performance (Box 20-7) are incorporated within many health care organizations' programs. In addition to the JCAHO's model, there are numerous process improvement models to be found across the country (Table 20-3). The models have similar elements, such as process or problem identification, establishment of a target to guide the process, collection and analysis of data, interpretation of results and implementation of the improvements followed by evaluation of the improvement effectiveness (Wendt and Vale, 2003). An organization may use the JCAHO's standards to organize their QI program but use a QI model such as FOCUS-PDCA (see Table 20-3) to structure problem analysis and resolution.

Responsibility for a QI Program. Leadership and planning are essential components of quality improvement (JCAHO, 2002). Organizational leadership must create a work culture that supports continuous quality improvement (CQI) beliefs and practice. This work culture is a nonthreatening environment that shows belief in people; a promotion of teamwork; treatment of everyone in the workplace with respect, dignity, and trust; open communication; and work toward a win-win situation for all involved in the process (Wendt and Vale, 2003; Werner, 1999). Most organizations have a director responsible for TQM or system CQI activities. In nursing care areas, home care sections, or clinics, a nurse manager is responsible for supporting a unit-based program. Individual staffs are responsible for monitoring practice, making decisions about ways to improve practice, and evaluating results.

Scope of Service. Each nursing care area involved in the care of a select group of clients provides a well-defined set of services. A unit's scope of service includes the types of clients who receive nursing care and the types of processes involved in delivering care. An example might be a general medicine unit in a hospital that cares for middle-age and older adult clients who have diabetes, heart disease, and gastrointestinal disorders. Such a unit would be involved in processes that include intravenous administration, diabetes education, referrals for cardiac diagnostic testing, and endoscopy. An understanding of the scope of service allows staff to focus on quality issues related to typical client groups. Unit-based committees review activities or services considered most important in providing quality service to clients. It is a way of prioritizing activities within the unit's scope of service.

Developing Quality Indicators. A **quality indicator** is a quantitative measure of an important aspect of service that determines whether the service conforms to established standards or requirements. The quality indicator is the focus for a QI project, with the staff monitoring criteria that will show whether indicator standards have been met. There are three types of indicators: structure, process, and outcome.

Structure indicators evaluate the structure or systems for delivering care; an example is adherence in checking if emergency carts are adequately stocked or if forms documenting restraint use are completed correctly. Process indicators evaluate the manner in which care is delivered (e.g., the process of pain assessment, recovery of clients from sedation, and clients' referral to community services). Outcome indicators, as described earlier, evaluate the end result of care delivered (e.g., incidence of nosocomial infection and adherence to medication therapy). Outcomes are the most important indicators in any QI program, but structural and process indicators cannot be ignored.

Processes of care are obviously closely related to outcomes and the structure in which a process of care occurs, enhances, or hinders the effectiveness of care (Titler, 2001). When a unit-based team selects a QI indicator, it is important that the indicator be relevant. It is often appropriate to measure a process, as well as the expected outcome, to know if standards of care are being met. In the example of the medicine unit, staff may choose to measure their success in implementing the process of diabetes instruction early while also measuring the outcome of whether clients learn to administer insulin correctly. When a unit-based team sits together to select quality indicators for a QI project, it helps to ask what processes and related outcomes are in need of improvement and are most likely to make a significant contribution to how nursing care is being practiced. Processes to improve may include the following:

- A weak process that is causing problems (e.g., poor pain management for clients with sickle cell anemia)
- A stable process that is adequate, but that can benefit from improvement (e.g., waiting time for ambulatory surgery clients)
- A process linked to negative outcomes (e.g., care of intravenous access sites with the occurrence of phlebitis)

Establishing Thresholds for Evaluation. After selecting a quality indicator, staff members must determine ways to quantitatively measure the indicator. The occurrence of an indicator, or the percentage of times the indicator is observed (e.g., the number of clients having surgery who can successfully explain their discharge instructions) is a common measure. A threshold is a standard for determining whether a problem exists. A measurement that falls below the threshold indicates a problem. For example, a staff may set a threshold that states that 95% of older adult clients over age 65 who visit a clinic will receive flu shots. If monitoring of records shows that only 90% of clients scheduled visits to have flu shots, the threshold is not being met. Staff will

then thoroughly review the factors interfering with successful client education and adherence. When QI is an ongoing process, staff continuously work to improve outcomes or performance by raising thresholds.

It is important to understand that almost all processes have variation. For example, consider the process of diabetic instruction and the associated outcome of clients' administering insulin. Possible variations in the process might include the time when teaching begins, materials used in instruction, and learner motivation. Outcome variations might include accuracy in injection site selection and proficiency in preparing the insulin in a syringe. Setting specific thresholds may not always be achievable. The intent in any QI program is to seek ways to continuously improve. This includes defining the acceptable level of performance and allowing for normal variability.

Data Collection and Analysis. The process of data collection and analysis can be simple or complex. The importance, however, is in obtaining accurate results that help in making appropriate decisions regarding quality care issues. Many organizations have made QI so important that formal research studies are conducted (see Chapter 25). In this case the process of data collection and analysis is very formal and well designed. Statistical techniques are used to determine if problems that have been identified are significant. Similarly, if a QI project involves introduction of a new practice or procedure, statistics can show whether the improvement made a significant difference in outcomes.

When formal research is not conducted, staff may become involved in simple evaluation studies involving the collection of data on frequencies and percentages for a predetermined number of clients or cases. Evaluation studies offer valuable information on practice trends and whether problems are evident. What is important in data collection is to collect data on the right criteria and to then have adequate data from which to make decisions. QI teams usually have access to resources within their organization that can help determine how much information is needed for QI analysis. In the example of diabetic instruction and insulin administration, staff might monitor criteria that include use of recommended teaching materials, staff's compliance with teaching standards, and each client's score on a return demonstration test. When sufficient data have been collected, the QI team can determine whether problems exist and analyze their possible causes. For example, if diabetic clients perform poorly on their test, staff can analyze whether standards are inconsistently met or if teaching is unnecessarily delayed.

Evaluation of Care. Monitoring of quality indicators evaluates whether a specifically defined process reaches desired outcomes. If results exceed or meet a threshold, or if performance is within controls set for a process, no problem has been identified and the process is performing well. When thresholds for satisfactory care are not met or when performance is below the control limits set, staff must try to find the cause of problems. For example, if diabetic clients score an average of only 70% on a return demonstration test, staff must determine the reasons. This step requires nurses and colleagues to honestly review practice activities and look for opportunities to reinforce nursing care standards or improve practice.

When a process is not working well, one of the models for QI (e.g., FOCUS-PDCA) may be used. This allows staff to find the aspect of the process to improve, organize an expert team that knows the process, clarify knowledge about the process, understand any sources of variation, and select an improvement or solution. The process may take several team meetings before the group can agree on the actions to take. In the case of diabetic instruction, it would be important to have staff nurses, dietitians, diabetes nurse specialists, and pharmacists involved as part of the QI team. Many of these staff members might have been on the original QI committee. However, once a problem is identified, additional team members may be needed. The team collaborates to discover what factors are associated with a practice problem. Eventually the team recommends approaches for improving the process with the goal of achieving desired outcomes.

Resolution of Problems. After evaluating quality problems, staff develop action plans to improve the process and outcomes. It is important to establish actions that will be successful. For example, the action of merely notifying staff that a problem exists is unlikely to change practice or improve outcomes. An action plan should be more direct. In FOCUS-PDCA, staff *P*lan the action or improvement to make, *D*o or implement the change, *C*heck or analyze results of the change, and then *A*ct on the findings. For example, the QI team may discover that clients are not administering insulin correctly because they do not have all of the necessary information. (Staff are not beginning teaching as soon as clients learn that insulin will be a form of therapy. Staff are also found to have trouble acquiring necessary teaching materials for instruction.) In this case the team may recommend having the pharmacy send instructional materials when insulin is sent to the unit and having a clinical pharmacist assist with instruction on insulin therapy. The staff nurses and nurse specialist may develop a practice protocol that outlines specific content to teach until the client learns to administer injections. Collectively, the team may develop an innovative approach that is designed to get appropriate information to clients more quickly and efficiently so that learning can take place.

Evaluation of Improvement. After implementing an action plan, the staff must reevaluate its success. In the example, staff members may repeat monitoring of the teaching process and the results of client testing to see if improvement has been made. The change may be positive or negative. For example, if client test scores improve, the team has successfully improved outcomes. Similarly, if test scores show no improvement or even worsen, a new plan of action is needed. The QI process is similar to the nursing process (see Unit III) in that when desired outcomes are not met, the staff reinstitutes the QI process.

Communication of Results. The results of QI activities must be communicated to staff in all appropriate organizational departments. If findings and results are not communicated, practice changes will likely not occur. Regular discussions of QI activities through staff meetings, newsletters, and memos are examples of communication strategies. Often a QI study reveals information requiring organization-wide change. In this case the organization must be responsible for responding to the problem with the resources needed to make changes. Revision of policies and procedures, modification of standards of care, and implementation of system changes are examples of ways that an organization may respond.

•••

The incorporation of a QI program within a health care setting benefits the client, the professional staff, and the institution. With a focus on client and professional outcomes, QI activities lead to a selection of interventions that result in improved client care. Professional staff members learn from their own practice, identify opportunities to change practice, and gain greater satisfaction from improved client outcomes. An institution benefits from an improved level of care delivery that reduces excessive or unnecessary use of resources and improves client satisfaction.

Key Concepts

- A manager must set a vision or philosophy for a work unit, ensure appropriate staffing, mobilize staff and institutional resources to achieve objectives, motivate staff members to carry out their work, set standards of performance, and make the right decisions to achieve objectives.
- Consideration conveys mutual trust, respect, and rapport between the manager and staff members.
- Empowering staff members brings out the best in a manager and allows him or her to concentrate on effective client care systems, to support risk taking and innovation, and to focus on results and rewards.
- An empowered nursing staff has decision-making authority to change how they practice.
- Nursing care delivery models vary by the responsibility of the RN in coordinating care delivery and the roles other staff members play in assisting with care.
- Continuity of nursing care can be compromised in total patient care delivery, functional nursing, and team nursing.
- Critical to the success of decentralized decision making is making staff members aware that they have the responsibility, authority, autonomy, and accountability for the care they give and the decisions they make.
- A nurse manager can foster decentralized decision making by establishing nursing practice committees, supporting nurse-physician and interdisciplinary collaboration, setting and implementing quality improvement plans, and maintaining timely staff communication.
- Clinical care coordination involves accurate clinical decision making, establishing priorities, efficient organizational skills, appropriate use of resources and time management skills, and an ongoing evaluation of care activities.

- To promote an enriching professional environment, each member of a nursing work team is responsible for open, professional communication.
- Delegation involves transferring responsibility for performing an activity while retaining accountability for the outcome.
- When done correctly, delegation can improve job efficiency and job enrichment.
- An important responsibility for the nurse who delegates nursing care is evaluation of the staff member's performance and client outcomes.
- In a total quality management environment, every staff member becomes involved in finding ways to improve or change work processes so as to promote client or customer satisfaction.
- A well-organized quality improvement program focuses on processes or systems that significantly contribute to improvement of outcomes.

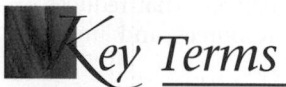

Key Terms

Accountability, *p. 375*
Authority, *p. 375*
Autonomy, *p. 374*
Case management, *p. 373*
Decentralized management, *p. 374*
Delegation, *p. 378*
Functional nursing, *p. 372*
Outcome, *p. 382*
Primary nursing, *p. 373*

Quality improvement, *p. 381*
Quality indicator, *p. 384*
Responsibility, *p. 374*
Shared governance, *p. 375*
Team nursing, *p. 373*
Total patient care, *p. 373*
Total quality management (TQM), *p. 380*

Critical Thinking Exercises

1. John, an RN, is working with Tammy, a nursing assistant, to manage care for five clients. John has completed morning assessments and rounds on the assigned clients and is giving Tammy directions for what she needs to do in the next hour. John says to Tammy, "Why don't you go to room 415 and see what Mr. Thomas needs and go to room 418 to check if Mrs. Landry is doing all right." Based on what you know about delegation, were these appropriate or inappropriate directions for the nursing assistant? Provide a rationale for your answer.
2. The unit you are working has identified a problem: clients are receiving initial doses of newly ordered medications 6 to 8 hours after the order is written. Your manager asks you to be the head of a quality improvement team to investigate this problem. Who would you want to be on your team? What would your first priority be? What data would you want to collect related to this problem?
3. You have just received morning shift report on your clients. You have been assigned the following clients:
   - A 52-year-old man who was admitted yesterday with a diagnosis of angina. He is scheduled for a cardiac stress test at 9:00 AM.
   - A 60-year-old woman who was transferred out of intensive care at 6:30 AM today. She had uncomplicated coronary bypass surgery yesterday.
   - A 45-year-old man who experienced a myocardial infarction 3 days ago and is complaining of pain rated as 5 on a scale of 0 to 10.
   - A 76-year-old woman who had a permanent pacemaker inserted yesterday and is complaining of incision pain rated as a 7 on a scale of 0 to 10.
   Which one these clients do you need to see first? Explain your answer.

Review Questions

1. The nursing model of client care in which tasks are divided, with one nurse assuming responsibility for specific tasks, for example, hygiene and dressing changes, whereas another nurse may assume responsibility for medication administration, is:
   1. Team nursing.
   2. Total patient care.
   3. Functional nursing.
   4. Primary nursing

2. The model of nursing care delivery that was developed with the aim of placing RNs at the bedside and improving nursing's accountability for client outcomes and the professional relationships among staff members is:
   1. Team nursing.
   2. Total patient care.
   3. Functional nursing.
   4. Primary nursing.

3. The type of care management approach that coordinates and links health care services to clients and their families while streamlining costs and maintaining quality is:
   1. Case management.
   2. Total patient care.
   3. Functional nursing.
   4. Primary nursing.

4. The type of management structure in which there is the potential for greater collaborative effort, increased competency of staff, and ultimately a greater sense of professional accomplishment and satisfaction is:
   1. Case management.
   2. Primary nursing.
   3. Total patient care.
   4. Decentralized.

5. While administering medications, the nurse realizes she has given the wrong dose of medication to a client. The nurse acts by completing an incident report and notifying the client's physician. The nurse is exercising:
   1. Authority.
   2. Responsibility.
   3. Accountability.
   4. Decision making.

6. Many managers distribute biweekly newsletters of ongoing unit or health care agency activities and post minutes of committee meetings in an accessible location for all staff to read. This is an example of:
   1. Problem-solving committees.
   2. Nurse/physician collaborative practice.
   3. Interdisciplinary collaboration.
   4. Staff communication.

7. During the morning rounds a nurse assesses the client's condition. He had major heart surgery 2 days ago. His vital signs are stable and his incision is clean and healing well. He complains of pain in his lower leg where the vein graft was removed. The nurse finds that the IV infusion is running on time but only 100 ml remains before the infusion runs out. An order exists for the IV infusion to continue. A second order of priority is:
   1. The need to replace the IV bag with a new one.
   2. The need to have an analgesic administered to the client for his leg pain.
   3. The need to instruct the client on complications of wound health.
   4. The need for the nurse to determine if the pharmacy has delivered IV solutions ordered for the day.

8. A client is experiencing an anxiety attack. This is which priority nursing need for this client:
   1. First-order priority.
   2. Second-order priority.
   3. Third-order priority.
   4. Fourth-order priority.

9. The nurse checks on her client who was admitted to the hospital with pneumonia. He has been coughing profusely and has required nasotracheal suctioning. He has an IV infusion of antibiotics. He is febrile. The client asks the nurse if he can have a bath because he has been perspiring profusely. The nurse delegates to the nursing assistant working with her today the task of:
   1. Assessing vital signs.
   2. Changing IV dressing.
   3. Nasotracheal suctioning.
   4. Administering a bed bath.

10. An example of a quality improvement (QI) outcome indicator is the:
    1. Rate of postoperative wound infection.
    2. Percentage of time it takes to count narcotics by nursing staff every shift.
    3. Number of patients receiving postoperative education on possible surgical complications.
    4. Time it takes for a client to be transported from the emergency department to an inpatient nursing unit.

References

American Nurses Association: Position statement on registered nurse utilization of assistive personnel, *Am Nurse* 25(2):7, 1995.

Case Management Society of America: Membership information, http: www.cmsa.org/meminfo/mem-main.html, 2003.

Coughlin C: Is now the time to design new care delivery models? *J Nurs Adm* 30(9):403, 2000.

Cox S: Managing the workplace 2000. Seminar conducted at Barnes-Jewish Hospital, St. Louis, 1995.

Curtin L: The heart of patient care, *Nurs Manage* 25(5):7, 1994.

Dadich KA: Care delivery strategies. In Yoder-Wise PS, editor: *Leading and managing in nursing,* ed 3, St. Louis, 2003, Mosby.

Hansten R, Washburn M: Seven steps to shift from tasks to outcomes, *Nurs Manage* 30(7):25, 1999.

Hicks F: Collective action. In Yoder-Wise PS, editor: *Leading and managing in nursing,* ed 3, St. Louis, 2003, Mosby.

Joint Commission on Accreditation of Healthcare Organizations: *Comprehensive accreditation manual for hospitals: the official handbook,* 2002, The Commission.

Keeling B and others: Appropriate delegation, *Am J Nurs* 100(12): 24, 2000.

Keill P, Johnson, T: Optimizing performance through process improvement, *J Nurs Car Qual* 9(1):1, 1994.

Kreitzer MJ and others: Creating a healthy work environment in the midst of organizational change and transition, *J Nurs Adm* 27(6):35, 1997.

Maddox PJ: Quality management in nursing practice. In Lancaster J, editor: *Nursing issues in leading and managing change,* St. Louis, 1999, Mosby.

Marriner-Tomey A: *Guide to nursing management and leadership,* ed 6, St. Louis, 2000, Mosby.

Moorhead S, Johnson M, Maas M: *Nursing outcomes classification (NOC),* ed 3, St. Louis, 2004, Mosby.

National Council of State Boards of Nursing: *Delegation: concepts and decision-making process,* Chicago, 1995, The Council.

Peters DA: Outcomes: the mainstay of a framework for quality care, *J Nurs Care Qual* 10(1):61, 1995.

Pinkerton SE: Nurses executives: Who are they; what do they do; and what challenges do they face? In McCloskey JC, Grace HK, editors: *Current issues in nursing,* ed 6, St. Louis, 2001, Mosby.

Ritter-Teitel J: The impact of restructuring on professional nursing practice. *J Nurs Adm* 32(1):31, 2002.

Titler MG: Outcomes management for quality improvement. In McCloskey JC, Grace HK, editors: *Current issues in nursing,* ed 6, St. Louis, 2001, Mosby.

Triolo PK and others: Total quality management, redesign, reengineering, what's the difference? In McCloskey JC, Grace HK, editors: *Current issues in nursing practice,* ed 5, St. Louis, 1997, Mosby.

Wendt DA, Vale DJ: Managing quality and risk. In Yoder-Wise PS, editor: *Leading and managing in nursing,* ed 3, St. Louis, 2003, Mosby.

Werner KM: Nursing's role in improving the quality of health care. In Chery B, Jacob SR, editors: *Contemporary nursing: issues, trends and management,* St. Louis, 1999, Mosby.

Wywialowski E: *Managing client care,* ed 2, St. Louis, 1997, Mosby.

21

$\mathcal{E}$thics and Values

Media Resources

http://evolve.elsevier.com/Potter/
fundamentals/

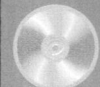 **CD COMPANION**

- Review Questions
- Glossary

evolve WEBSITE

- Review Questions
- Student Learning Activities
- Glossary

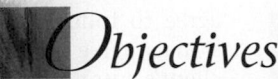

Mastery of content in this chapter will enable the student to:

- Define the key terms listed.
- Explain the relationship between ethics and professional practice.
- Discuss the role of values in the study of ethics.
- Examine and clarify personal values.
- Discuss how values influence client care.
- Describe some basic philosophies of bioethics.
- Describe a nursing perspective in ethics.
- Apply a method of ethical analysis to a clinical situation.
- Identify contemporary ethical issues with nursing implications.

The term **ethics** refers to the study of philosophical ideals of right and wrong behavior. In professional practices such as nursing, a **code of ethics** provides guidelines for safe and compassionate care. Nurses' commitment to a code of ethics guarantees the public that nurses adhere to professional practice standards. This chapter reviews professional nursing ethics.

The study of **bioethics** has developed in the past several decades. Built on the foundation of professional ethics in health care, the field of bioethics guides discourse about difficult issues that arise in health care. Advances in management of disease can create concerns about the implementation of new technologies. Principles of bioethics guide difficult negotiations that can characterize decisions about health care. This chapter also reviews the development of bioethics and reviews the vital role that nurses play.

Discussion and resolution of ethical issues requires critical thinking skills. Unlike the resolution of clinical problems, however, the resolution of ethical issues involves the negotiation of closely held personal values and philosophies, not facts or measurable clinical data. Resolution of ethical issues incorporates not only the nurse's personal values, but also the interpretation of the client's personal values, based on the unique perspective of nurses. The ethical process works best in a climate where skills of values clarification and critical thinking are protected and nurtured.

*E*thics

Ethics is the study of good conduct, character, and motives. It is concerned with determining what is good or valuable for all people. Acts that are ethical often reflect a commitment to standards beyond personal preferences—standards on which individuals, professions, and societies agree.

Basic Terms

To discuss ethics, it is helpful to establish a basic vocabulary. Although the terms may have a certain meaning in a larger context, they provide specific meanings within the context of ethics that further the understanding and discussion about ethical matters. These basic terms include *autonomy, beneficence, nonmaleficence, justice,* and *fidelity.*

In his essay "Autonomy Under Duress," Leonard Harris (1992) challenges the notion that respect for autonomy guarantees respect for all persons. Most researchers investigating the concept of autonomy focus on appreciating culture differences. For example, investigators on a Navajo reservation identified a cultural tradition where thought and language are considered to have the power to shape reality (Carrese and Rhodes, 1995). As a result, the discussion of a poor prognosis, often considered a duty out of respect for autonomy, can have a devastating effect for a client who is from a Navajo tradition.

Harris is also concerned that the definition of autonomy is influenced by the culture of the people using the term. His concerns, however, led him to conclude that there can be limits in other more subtle ways to the value of respect for autonomy. His argument is based on his experience as an African-American. "If race-targeted advertising such as cigarette and alcohol advertising elicits less social consternation than we might hope, one reason may be that the target is not invested by physicians and society in general with ties of affection, compassion, . . . and value among those empowered to create change." Society may claim respect for autonomy, and health care providers specifically commit to this respect in their professional practices. Nonetheless, Harris argues, certain groups of poor or historically underserved peoples may not enjoy equal respect for autonomy. The respect they enjoy is lessened as a result of racial prejudice. Respect for autonomy applied in this way promotes harm. Harris does not argue to abandon the concept of autonomy. He does warn, however, that an honest appraisal of its use is critical.

Implications for Practice

Harris recommends a thorough self-examination to ensure that when the term *autonomy* is applied, it is applied with respect, compassion, and value, as though no differences existed between classes or races of people.

References

Carrese J, Rhodes L: Western bioethics on the Navajo reservation: benefit or harm?, *JAMA* 274(10):826, 1995.

Harris L: Autonomy under duress. In Flack HE, Pellegrino ED, editors: *African-American perspectives on biomedical ethics,* Washington, DC, 1992, Georgetown University Press.

Autonomy. **Autonomy** refers to a person's independence. As a standard in ethics, autonomy represents an agreement to respect another's right to determine a course of action. Respect for another's autonomy is fundamental to the practice of health care. It serves to justify the inclusion of clients in all aspects of decision making regarding their health care. The agreement to respect autonomy involves the recognition that clients are "in charge of their own destiny in matters of health and illness" (O'Neil, 1995). For example, the purpose of the preoperative consent that clients must read and sign before surgery is the assurance in writing that the health care team respects the client's independence by obtaining permission to proceed.

The consent process implies that a client may refuse treatment, and in most cases the health care team must agree to follow the client's wishes. Health care professionals agree to abide by a standard of respect for the client's autonomy (Box 21-1).

Beneficence. **Beneficence** refers to taking positive actions to help others. The practice of beneficence encourages the urge to do good for others. Commitment to beneficence helps to guide difficult decisions wherein the benefits of a treatment may be challenged by risks to the client's well-being or dignity. A child's immunization may cause discomfort during administration, but the benefits of protection from disease, both for the individual and for society, outweigh the temporary discomforts. The agreement to act with beneficence also requires that the best interests of the client remain more important than self-interest. For example, a nurse will not simply follow medical orders but will act thoughtfully to understand client needs and then work actively to help meet those needs.

Nonmaleficence. Maleficence refers to harm or hurt; thus **nonmaleficence** is the avoidance of harm or hurt. In health care ethics it is important to remember that ethical practice involves not only the will to do good, but also the equal commitment to do no harm. The health care professional tries to balance the risks and benefits of a plan of care while striving to do the least harm possible. This principle is often helpful in guiding discussions about new or controversial technologies. For example, a new bone marrow transplant procedure may promise a chance at cure. The procedure, however, may require long periods of pain and suffering. These discomforts should be considered in light of the suffering that the disease itself might cause, and in light of the suffering that other treatments might cause. The commitment to provide least harmful interventions illustrates the term *nonmaleficence*. The standard of nonmaleficence promotes a continuing effort to consider the potential for harm even when it may be necessary to promote health.

Justice. **Justice** refers to fairness. Health care providers agree to strive for justice in health care. The term often is used during discussions about resources. What constitutes a fair distribution of resources may not always be clear. In these cases national discussion about just distribution of resources often helps to clarify methods for achieving fairness. For example, in the United States the number of candidates awaiting liver transplants is approximately 3 times larger than the number of available organs for transplantation. Decisions about who should receive available organs are always difficult. Criteria set by a national multidisciplinary committee strive for justice by ranking recipients according to need. These criteria are preferable to resorting to selling organs for profit, which would favor recipients with the most money, and preferable to distributing them by lottery, which would result in random distribution without regard to justice.

Fidelity. **Fidelity** refers to the agreement to keep promises. A commitment to fidelity explains the reluctance to abandon clients, even when disagreement arises about decisions that a client may make. The standard of fidelity also includes an obligation to follow through with care offered to clients. For example, if a nurse assesses a client for pain and then offers a plan to manage the pain, the standard of fidelity encourages the nurse to monitor the client's response to the plan. Professional behavior by the nurse includes revision of the plan as necessary to try to keep the promise to reduce pain.

Professional Nursing

Code of Ethics. A code of ethics is a set of ethical principles that are accepted by all members of a profession. A profession's ethical code is a collective statement about the group's expectations and standards of behavior. Codes serve as guidelines to assist nurses and other professional groups when questions arise about correct practice or behavior. The nursing code of ethics, as in other professions, sets forth ideals of conduct. The American Nurses Association (ANA) and the International Council of Nurses (ICN) have established widely accepted codes that professional nurses attempt to follow. These codes differ somewhat in specific emphasis, but they reflect the same basic principles, including responsibility, accountability, advocacy, confidentiality, and veracity (Boxes 21-2 and 21-3). Nurses agree to responsibility for specific actions and accountability for the consequences. To practice responsibly, professional nurses also agree to maintain competence in their practice and to use competence in the application of judgment.

Accountability. **Accountability** refers to the ability to answer for one's own actions. The nurse balances accountability to the client, the profession, the employer, and society. For example, a nurse may know that a client who will be discharged soon remains confused about how to administer insulin. The action that a nurse takes in response to this situation will be guided by the sense of accountability. The client, the institution, and society rely on the good judgment of the nurse and trust that the nurse will take action in response to this situation. The nurse may request more hospitalization to provide further teaching or arrange home care to continue teaching at home. The goal is the prevention of injury to the client. The nurse's sense of accountability guides actions that achieve this goal (Box 21-4).

To remain accountable to society, nursing professionals agree to evaluate practices and actions and to take action to preserve nursing excellence. The Joint Commission on Accreditation of Healthcare Organizations (JCAHO), a national accreditation association, recommends standards for the delivery of nursing care. These standards provide a basic structure against which nursing care is objectively measured. Accountability is best ensured and measured when quality of care has been defined. National organizations such as the JCAHO and ANA provide these definitions and offer standards of practice to achieve quality, as well as a structure for evaluation of continuing practice (JCAHO, 2002). The following activities serve to support standards of the JCAHO and ANA in the nursing professions:

- Evaluation of new professional practices and reassessment of existing ones
- Maintenance of standards of health care
- Facilitation of personal reflection, ethical thought, and personal growth
- Provision of a basis for ethical decision making

Box 21-2   **American Nurses Association Code of Ethics**

The nurse, in all professional relationships, practices with compassion and respect for the inherent dignity, worth and uniqueness of every individual, unrestricted by considerations of social or economic status, personal attributes, or the nature of health problems.

The nurse's primary commitment is to the patient, whether an individual, family, group, or community.

The nurse promotes, advocates for, and strives to protect the health, safety, and rights of the patient.

The nurse is responsible and accountable for individual nursing practice and determines the appropriate delegation of tasks consistent with the nurse's obligation to provide optimum patient care.

The nurse owes the same duties to self as to others, including the responsibility to preserve integrity and safety, to maintain competence, and to continue personal and professional growth.

The nurse participates in establishing, maintaining, and improving health care environments and conditions of employment conducive to the provision of quality health care and consistent with the values of the profession through individual and collective action.

The nurse participates in the advancement of the profession through contributions to practice, education, administration, and knowledge development.

The nurse collaborates with other health professionals and the public in promoting community, national, and international efforts to meet health needs.

The profession of nursing, as represented by associations and their members, is responsible for articulating nursing values, for maintaining the integrity of the profession and its practice, and for shaping social policy.

From American Nurses Association: *Code of ethics for nurses with interpretive statements*, Washington, DC, 2001, American Nurses Publishing.

Responsibility. The term **responsibility** refers to the characteristics of reliability and dependability. The term implies an ability to distinguish between right and wrong. In professional nursing, responsibility includes a duty to perform actions well and thoughtfully. When administering a medication, for example, a nurse is responsible for assessing the client's need for the drug, for giving it safely and correctly, and for evaluating the response to it. By agreeing to act responsibly, the nurse gains trust from clients, colleagues, and society.

Confidentiality. The concept of **confidentiality** in health care enjoys widespread acceptance in the United States. Federal legislation known as HIPAA (Health Insurance Portability and Accountability Act of 1996) requires it. The legislation defines the rights and privileges of clients for protection of privacy without diminishing access to quality care. In addition to a requirement for education of all employees in health care about the HIPAA protections, the legislation establishes fines for infractions (HHS fact sheet, 2002). Medical records may not be copied or forwarded without a client's consent. Health care information, including laboratory results, diagnosis, and prognosis, is not shared with others without specific

---

Box 21-3   International Council of Nurses Code of Ethics for Nurses

Nurses have four fundamental responsibilities: to promote health, to prevent illness, to restore health, and to alleviate suffering. The need for nursing is universal.

Inherent in nursing is respect for human rights, including the right to life, to dignity and to be treated with respect. Nursing care is unrestricted by considerations of age, colour, creed, culture, disability or illness, gender, nationality, politics or social status.

Nurses render health services to the individual, the family, and the community and coordinate their services with those of related groups.

Nurses and People

The nurse's primary responsibility is to those people requiring nursing care.

In providing care, the nurse promotes an environment in which the human rights, values, customs, and spiritual beliefs of the individual, family, and community are respected.

The nurse ensures that the individual receives sufficient information on which to base consent for care and related information.

The nurse holds in confidence personal information and uses judgment in sharing this information.

The nurse shares with society the responsibility for initiating and supporting action to meet the health and social needs of the public, in particular those of vulnerable populations.

The nurse also shares responsibility to sustain and protect the natural environment from depletion, pollution, degradation and destruction.

Nurses and Practice

The nurse carries personal responsibility and accountability for nursing practice and for maintaining competence by continual learning.

The nurse maintains a standard of personal health such that the ability to provide care is not compromised.

The nurse uses judgment regarding individual competence when accepting and delegating responsibility.

The nurse at all times maintains standards of personal conduct which reflect well on the profession and enhance public confidence.

Nurses and the Profession

The nurse assumes the major role in determining and implementing acceptable standards of critical nursing practice, management, research, and education.

The nurse is active in developing a core of research-based professional knowledge.

The nurse, acting through the professional organization, participates in creating and maintaining equitable social and economic working conditions in nursing.

Nurses and Co-workers

The nurse sustains a cooperative relationship with co-workers in nursing and other fields.

The nurse takes appropriate action to safeguard individuals when their care is endangered by a co-worker or any other person.

From International Council of Nurses: *ICN code of ethics for nurses,* Geneva, 2000, The Council.

Focus on Older Adults   Box 21-4

- Older people may not be as familiar with the concept of autonomy as people from younger generations. As a result, older adults may be uncomfortable disagreeing with doctors or nurses. They may view assertiveness as a violation of trust.

- As people age, they may develop clinical conditions that affect the communication process: hearing deficits, memory impairments, chronic illness, isolation. Clients may become incapacitated by stroke or disease. Most older adults take multiple medications, some of which may affect cognitive skills in subtle ways. It is important to evaluate the competence of a client to make decisions, and to provide assistance where necessary, especially when treatment choices, consent, or ethical issues arise.

- Consensus about medical goals for clients in the geriatric population can be hard to achieve. When is a person so diminished by old age that a treatment plan not only prolongs life, it also prolongs suffering? Working to ensure dignity and comfort can be as important as achieving medical success.

Modified from Burke MM, Laramie JA: *Primary care of the older adult: a multidisciplinary approach,* St. Louis, 2000, Mosby.

---

client consent. This practice even includes preventing other family members or friends of the client from acquiring health care information. Conflicting obligations may arise when a client wants to keep information from insurance companies to preserve coverage or from employers to preserve a job. The commitment to confidentiality is particularly challenged as medical records become computerized. Preservation of confidentiality is often in competition with the need to facilitate access to information. In the case of computer access, health care institutions work to protect confidentiality by using special access codes that limit what certain employees can find on a computer system.

Veracity. A part of the ANA code of conduct addresses the issue of veracity, another aspect of reliability. **Veracity** in general means accuracy or conformity to truth. As a part of the nursing code of ethics, veracity guides nurses to practice truthfulness. Although in most circumstances veracity is an obvious asset, the practice of truthfulness may be challenged during the delivery of health care. A nurse may have to balance competing interests in certain cases. For example, a spouse may make an urgent plea that a client not be given news of a poor prognosis. In this case, principles generally in effect that may take precedence over the spouse's wishes include respect for the client's autonomy and the principle of veracity. In some instances it may be tempting to tell a child that a medicine tastes good when it does not or that a procedure will not hurt when it probably will, to achieve a level of compliance. Professional codes of ethics guide the nurse to tell the truth, however, and it is a rare circumstance where other principles would support another behavior.

Values

Nursing is essentially a work of intimacy. The tasks of nursing require the nurse to be in close contact with clients, physically and emotionally. This kind of contact is usually not acceptable in public relationships. As a result, the work of nursing involves the negotiation of values, whether those values be of the client, the physician, the employer, or other groups. To negotiate values, it is important to have clarity about one's own values: what they are, where they came from, and how they stand in relationship to others' values and to society's values.

A **value** is a personal belief about the worth of a given idea, attitude, custom, or object that sets standards that influence behavior (Maslow, 1959; Rokeach, 1973). The values that an individual holds reflect cultural and social influences, relationships, and personal needs. Values vary among people and develop and change over time. Understanding one's own value system and assessing the value systems of others helps to facilitate decision making while ensuring respect for client autonomy.

Value Formation

People acquire values in many ways. An understanding of values begins in earliest childhood and is influenced by the way a child is raised. Children develop through different stages of cognitive and emotional growth. Basically, as children become more complex cognitively, they become more capable of complex emotional behavior. Because a fundamental part of value formation involves the ability to identify strong feelings and to act on them, the acquiring of values depends in large part on experiences within the family.

The character of parenting influences what children come to value as adults. In some cultures children may be prized and indulged until they reach school age and then must face more rigorous discipline as they enter school and the world outside the family. In other cultures children may be raised according to strict gender expectations. For example, girls assume household duties early in their lives and boys acquire more physical or labor-related skills. In still other cultures children are raised quite separately from adult activities, in communal settings with less exposure to adult socialization or patterning opportunities. These variations in child rearing result in variations in values and variations in adult behavior. The fundamental urge to love and nurture children takes on many different expressions and produces many different kinds of value systems with which we must contend, as individuals and as professionals.

Once children begin to experience life outside the family, they experience a broad range of influences on value formation. Religious institutions are often charged with the primary responsibility for teaching and enforc-

ing values. Schools, governments, and other social institutions also play a role. The nature of the role depends to a large degree on the nature of the institution. Religions with a strict code of behavior might teach the value of obedience, whereas religions with a focus on helping the poor might focus on the value of charity. A young person who begins to learn about other religions might experience conflict over these differences. Institutional lessons may undergo change from one generation to another. A basic task of the young adult is the identification of values within the context of the community. Over time, an individual acquires values by choosing some that are strongly held in the community and perhaps discarding or transforming others.

Finally, individual experience influences what we come to value. A person who suffers much loss early in life, of a parent or sibling, may grow to value certain things very differently than someone whose life has been free of suffering. A person whose employment has been menial may form certain values that reflect experience of a lack of dignity in the workplace. An appreciation of the source of these differences may promote respectful and effective communication. Within health care, nurses and other providers agree to respect the wide variety of value systems that clients may hold and to try to understand how these differences affect client health and wellness.

Values Clarification

To better articulate one's point of view, it will be helpful to clarify one's own values. One's values constitute an important part of the way one sees the world, and they influence how a person interprets confusing or conflicting information. As individuals mature and experience new situations, their values change. It would be unusual if any one value remained the primary motivating factor throughout a person's life. Value changes may involve a reordering of values or the replacement of old values with new ones. As a result of changing values, a person may modify attitudes and behavior. The willingness to change shows a healthy attitude toward life and the ability to adapt to new experiences.

To adopt new values, a person must first be aware of existing values and how those values affect behavior. To achieve awareness of personal values, it may be helpful to practice the process of **values clarification.** This is a process of self-discovery that helps a person gain insight into values. It is not a set of rules designed to interfere with conscientious decision making, and it does not suggest that a specific set of values should be accepted by all persons. If persons hold a particular value, they have personally chosen, interpreted, justified, and preferred that value over others. Louis Raths (1979) pioneered values clarification as an approach to individual appraisal of values (Box 21-5). A person clarifying values learns to make choices when alternatives are presented and determines whether choices are carefully made. The result of values clarification is greater self-awareness and personal insight. Critical thinking skills are invaluable during the process of values clarification, especially an understanding of attitudes and standards (see Chapter 14).

Cultural values are those adopted as a result of the social setting in which a person lives. Cultural values vary

Three Steps of Values Clarification

Choosing One's Beliefs and Behaviors

Choosing from alternatives
Choosing freely
Considering all consequences

Prizing One's Beliefs and Behaviors

Prizing and cherishing the choice
Publicly affirming the choice

Acting on One's Beliefs

Making the choice part of one's behavior
Acting with a pattern of consistency and repetition

A Values Clarification Exercise

1. Consider a choice that you make about a fundamental value. For example, how do you feel about the separation of church and state? Or what do you consider your obligation to be regarding your contributions to society? Think through all the possible choices you could make and the consequences of each possibility.
2. Describe how the evidence of your choice might be made to your friends and family, and to your colleagues in school or at work. How would people you know understand your cherishing this particular value?
3. List three or four activities in which you might participate where your behavior reflects consistent commitment to this specific value.

Modified from Raths LE, Harmin M, Simon SB: *Values and teaching,* ed 2, Columbus, Ohio, 1979, Merrill Publishing.

according to the community and the needs of the community. **Ethnocentrism** refers to the belief that one's own culture is superior. As Kirkpatrick and Deloughery (1995) explain, the nurse who holds this belief "may assess and plan intervention for the client, as well as evaluate the effectiveness of what was done, based on personal perceptions and values, without taking into account the perceptions and beliefs of the client." The exercise in Box 21-6 illustrates the wide variety of cultural values that affect perception of health care issues.

By understanding one's own point of view, the nurse will become better prepared to understand a client's values, as well as the values of other members of the health care team. The ultimate test of a value system lies in its ability to guide individuals through dissent or confusion. The technologies of contemporary medicine often cause ethical dilemmas wherein competing points of view leave members of the health care team or the team and the client in conflict. Values clarification plays a significant role in the resolution of these dilemmas. In addition, nurses strengthen their ability to advocate for a client when nurses are able to identify personal values and then accurately identify the values of the client.

Once the nurse has mastered the skill of clarifying personal values, it will be possible to turn to the client and apply similar practices that improve the nurse's ability to implement health care interventions. Values clarification can help clients gain an awareness of personal priorities, identify ambiguities in values, and resolve major conflicts between values and behavior. The goal of values clarification with a client is effective nurse-client communication. As the client becomes more willing to express problems and feelings, the nurse can better establish an individualized plan of care.

A useful method for values clarification with a client is structured communication. Simple strategies that promote the process of sharing feelings can be quite effective. For example, responding to a client by repeating the client's sentence as a question ("You wish you could be at home?") will encourage the client to elaborate. Avoiding questions that can be answered with a yes or no encourage the client to answer in greater detail. Rather than asking, "Do you want to live at home with your daughter?" the nurse might say, "Tell me how you feel about living at home with your daughter."

The character of a nurse's response to a client can motivate the client to examine personal thoughts and actions. When the nurse makes a clarifying response, it should be brief and nonjudgmental. For example, when talking with a client who says he exercises rarely, the nurse might say, "I see. So, what is your understanding of the purpose of exercise?" An effective clarifying response encourages the client to think about personal values after the exchange is over without imposing one's own values onto the client's. In this way, the nurse respects the client and avoids introducing personal values into the conversation.

Values clarification plays an important role in communication. Especially when the topic concerns issues of personal health, private habits, and quality of life, participants in a discussion will benefit from a clarity of values. The nurse who appreciates values will accurately identify differences between personal opinion and the values that others embrace. The respect demonstrated for the client and the skill used in helping the client clarify values promote a nurse's ability to teach and to heal.

Bioethics

Just as health care and society itself have changed radically in the past two decades, so, too, has the practice of ethical consideration of health care issues. Perhaps the most striking change in the philosophy of health care delivery is the change in the relationship between health care provider and health care recipient. Half a century ago, a sick person would seek a physician's care and advice and then usually follow the advice without question. The assumption was that the physician knew everything about sickness and the client knew very little. Issues of client consent and concepts of shared knowledge did not begin until relatively recently.

In an infamous research project conducted in this century, a population of African-American men with syphilis were observed but not treated for many years so that more could be learned about the progress of syphilis, even though treatment modalities were available, and even though the transmission of syphilis was well under-

---

Box 21-6   Cultural Values Exercise

If persons from a variety of cultures were given this questionnaire, some would strongly agree with the beliefs listed on the left and others would strongly agree with the opposite viewpoint listed on the right. Circle 1 if you strongly agree or 2 if you moderately agree with the statement on the left. Circle 3 if you moderately agree or 4 if you strongly agree with the statement on the right.

1.	Preparing for the future is an important activity and reflects maturity.	1 2 3 4	Life has a predestined course. The individual should follow that course.
2.	Vague answers are dishonest and confusing.	1 2 3 4	Vague answers are sometimes preferred because they avoid embarrassment and confrontation.
3.	Punctuality and efficiency are characteristics of a person who is both intelligent and concerned.	1 2 3 4	Punctuality is not as important as maintaining a relaxed atmosphere, enjoying the moment, and being with family and friends.
4.	When in severe pain, it is important to remain strong and not to complain too much.	1 2 3 4	When in severe pain, it is better to talk about the discomfort and express frustration.
5.	It is self-centered and unwise to accept a gift from someone you do not know well.	1 2 3 4	It is an insult to refuse a gift when it is offered.
6.	Addressing someone by their first name shows friendliness.	1 2 3 4	Addressing someone by their first name is disrespectful.
7.	Direct questions are usually the best way to gain information.	1 2 3 4	Direct questioning is rude and could cause embarrassment.
8.	Direct eye contact shows interest.	1 2 3 4	Direct eye contact is intrusive.
9.	Ultimately, the independence of the individual must come before the needs of the family.	1 2 3 4	The needs of the individual are always less important than the needs of the family.

Modified from Renwick GW, Rhinesmith SH: *An exercise in cultural analysis for managers,* Chicago, 1995, Intercultural Press.

---

stood. Studies such as this one eventually came under criticism as the concept of consent gained recognition (Twenty Years After, 1992). In many ways, the notion of autonomy was developed to explain and define a society's growing desire to protect clients from scientific endeavors. The notion of client autonomy reflects a change in society's definition of power and knowledge.

Philosophical Constructions

Philosophical discussion about health care issues has progressed over time, just as developments in health care and society itself have progressed. The philosophical constructions that shape the discussions have also changed. Ethics began as a standard reference point for the determination of right action. It has now grown into a field of study that is filled with differences of opinion, competing systems of values, and deeply meaningful efforts to understand human interaction with new technologies. The following discussion introduces the reader to a variety of contemporary ethical systems. The list is neither exclusive nor comprehensive.

Deontology. A traditional ethical theory, **deontology** proposes a system of ethics that is perhaps most familiar to practitioners in health care. Its foundations are often associated with the work of the eighteenth-century philosopher Immanuel Kant (1724-1804). Deontology defines actions as right or wrong based on their "right-making characteristics such as fidelity to promises, truthfulness, and justice" (Beauchamp and Childress, 2001). It locates the essence of right or wrong within these principles. Deontology specifically does not look to consequences of actions to determine rightness or wrongness. Instead, it critically examines a situation for the existence of essential rightness or wrongness. Ethical terms such as justice, au-

tonomy, and beneficence serve to define right or wrong. If an act is just, respects autonomy, and provides good, then the act will be ethical. The process depends on a mutual understanding and acceptance of these principles.

Difficulty arises when a person must choose between conflicting principles, which is often the case in health care ethical dilemmas. For example, how to apply the principle of respect for autonomy can be confusing when dealing with the health care of children. The health care team may recommend a certain course of treatment, but the parent may disagree or even refuse the recommendation. In discussion of the dilemma, participants may refer to a guiding principle such as respect for autonomy. But questions will remain. Whose autonomy should receive the respect? The parent's? Who should speak for the child's best interest? Society often struggles to understand who should be ultimately responsible for the well-being of children. A commitment to respect autonomy does not guarantee that controversy can be avoided.

Utilitarianism. A utilitarian system of ethics proposes that the value of something is determined by its usefulness. This philosophy may also be known as **consequentialism,** because its main emphasis is on the outcome or consequence of action. A third term associated with this philosophy is **teleology,** from the Greek word *telos,* meaning "end," or the study of ends or final causes. Its philosophical foundations were first proposed by John Stuart Mill (1806-1873), a British philosopher and social commentator. The greatest good for the greatest number of people is the guiding principle for determining right action in this system. As with deontology, this theory relies on the application of a certain principle, namely, measures of "good" and "greatest" (Beauchamp and Childress, 2001). The difference between utilitarianism and deontology is in the focus on consequences or outcomes. Utilitarianism measures the effect that an act will have; deontology looks to the presence of principle regardless of outcome.

Individuals or groups of individuals may have conflicting definitions of "greatest good." For example, research suggests that education regarding safe sex practices may reduce the spread of human immunodeficiency virus (HIV). But some argue that education about sex should be provided in the family and that sex education in public schools diminishes the role and the value of family. For some, the greater good is defined as educating the greatest number of people in the most effective way possible. For others, the greater good is the preservation of family values and the protection of individual choices regarding sex education of children. The concepts of utilitarianism provide guidance, but they do not invariably provide for universal agreement.

Feminist Ethics. A newer philosophy focuses on feminism and bioethics. Feminist ethicists consider their work a critique of conventional ethics, as well as a critique of social values. Their work focuses on inequalities between people (Holmes and Purdy, 1992; Wolf, 1996). They look to the nature of relationships between people for guidance in the processing of ethical dilemmas. Writers with a feminist perspective concentrate more on practical solutions than on ethical theory.

Changes in the regard of women reflect changes in women's relationship to family, to work, to science, and to society (Sherwin, 1993). For example, until the early 1980s moral development was thought to reach highest stages more often in men than in women. According to this theory, moral development occurred in predictable stages. The most complex stage involved a sense of justice, and young girls did not reach this sense as often as young boys (Kohlberg, 1981). Research from the early 1980s disputed these findings. Carol Gilligan (1993) proposed that Kohlberg's tools to measure moral development were **gender biased.** Gilligan went on to build a revised theory of moral development based on her findings. She attempted to accommodate gender differences. Specifically, she concluded that young girls tend to pay attention to community and to individual circumstances and that young boys tend to process dilemmas through ideals or principles determined abstractly.

Feminist ethics builds on the idea that principles may distract participants from dealing with larger issues of community. Feminist ethicists value the role of relationships and the stories about relationships. They emphasize the importance of stories and the role of community over an attention to universal principles. In fact, they argue that it is impossible to be unbiased or not influenced by relationships to people. They even propose that the natural human urge to be influenced by relationships is a positive value (Wolf, 1996).

This system of ethics also addresses issues of gender inequality. Feminists propose that an inequality of attention to women can be remedied by routinely asking, in the midst of any ethical dilemma, how decisions will affect women (Sherwin, 1993). For example, in a discussion regarding the ethics of fetal surgery (surgical intervention before birth of the child), feminist ethics would propose that questions about the effects of the intervention on the mother are at least as important as questions about the effects on the fetus. In a discussion about a proposal to ration services to the very old so that younger people would have better resources, feminists might ask how such a proposal would affect women. In the United States, older women outnumber older men. Older women also tend to be poorer and more often live alone. Bell (1992) concludes, "If age becomes a standard for limiting the provision of health care, the limits that will be set will affect women more drastically than they affect men." Gender-based investigations in ethical discussion would ensure that social facts about women, and men, are addressed.

Critics of feminist ethics argue that feminist ethics favors social relevance, at the sacrifice of moral content. In this argument, the critics agree that feminists are concerned about inequities that occur in society, but they argue that a feminist reluctance to endorse universal principles decreases their moral strength.

Ethic of Care. The ethic of care and feminist ethics are closely related. Many theorists who developed ideas about the ethic of care are nurses. The ethic of care explores the notion of care as a central activity of human behavior. Those who write about **ethic of care** maintain that ethical theory based on principles is a male-biased theory. They advocate a more female-biased theory that is based on understanding relationships, especially personal narratives.

Nel Noddings (1984), an early proponent of the ethic of care, uses the term "the one-caring" to identify the individual who provides care, and "the cared-for" to refer to the client or patient. In adopting this language, Noddings hopes to emphasize the role of feelings but not at the expense of conventional principles such as autonomy and beneficence. Edmund Pellegrino (1985), a physician, writes about the moral obligation of physicians and nurses to incorporate notions of care into a definition of professional behavior. His definition of care includes the obligation to appreciate, understand, and even share the pain or condition of a client.

Some nurse authors propose a nursing ethics that distinguishes the work of nurses from the work of physicians (Boyer and Nelson, 1990; Fry, 1989; Leininger, 1988; Watson, 1994). As Leininger (1988) writes, care has been the "central and unifying domain for the body of knowledge and practices in nursing." These writers propose that dilemmas can be solved by attention to relationships and by attention to clients' stories. A focus on the individual client narratives will lead to clarity about decisions, because individual values and moral preferences are often revealed within clients' personal histories. Chapter 7 describes in further detail an ethic of care in caring relationships with clients.

Consensus in Bioethics

Each of the above philosophical constructions could be used to justify a stand on an issue. None of them guarantees a solution to an ethical dilemma, however. Bringing different points of view to consensus requires skill and patience. The understanding of group process, how to incorporate principles and social values into the process of resolving a dilemma represents elements of consensus building. Those who study consensus turn to academic fields for help in understanding and refining the process, including sociology and psychology, as well as philosophy, medicine, and nursing.

The process of bioethics consensus diminishes dissent by encouraging respect for unusual points of view while still striving to come to agreement between all participants (Moreno, 1995). Bioethics consensus proposes equal regard for different points of view. As a strategy for solving dilemmas, consensus promotes respect and agreement, rather than a philosophy or moral system itself. Critics of consensus are concerned that the insistence on agreement will decrease efforts to identify social, religious, or personal values (Callahan, 1993).

Nursing Point of View

Professional nurses play a vital role in the management of health care in both outpatient and inpatient settings. All clients interact with a nurse at some point in the health care system.

When ethical dilemmas arise, the nurse's point of view is unique and critical. The nurse usually interacts with clients over longer time intervals than do other disciplines. Because nurses may be involved in intimate physical acts such as bathing, feeding, and special procedures, clients and families reveal information not generally shared with physicians or others. Details about family life, information about coping styles, personal preferences, and details about fears and insecurities are likely to come out during nursing interventions (Shannon, 1997).

On the other hand, it is important for nurses to remember that care of any one client has become multidisciplinary and often fragmented. The nursing point of view is part of a larger picture that is best built by all members of the health care team, including the client and family. Managers and administrators from many different professional backgrounds may also contribute to ethical discourse with their knowledge of systems, allocation of resources, financial possibilities, or constraints (Figure 21-1).

How to Process an Ethical Dilemma

Ethical problems can cause distress and confusion for both clients and caregivers. Controversy is the very nature of ethical problems, and few people like conflict. To overcome controversy and determine a course of action, ethical issues are processed carefully and deliberately. Participants refrain from making decisions solely on an emotional level, but at the same time, the process promotes the free expression of feelings. As discussed previously, however, an ethical outcome is not obtained by considering only what people want and feel.

Resolving an ethical dilemma is in many ways similar to the nursing process. It requires deliberate, systematic thinking (Miller and Babcock, 1996). Processing an ethical dilemma differs from the nursing process, on the other hand, because it requires negotiation of differences, incorporation of conflicting ideas, and an effort to respect differences of opinion. The process of negotiating ethical dilemmas may in part be the process of understanding ambiguities.

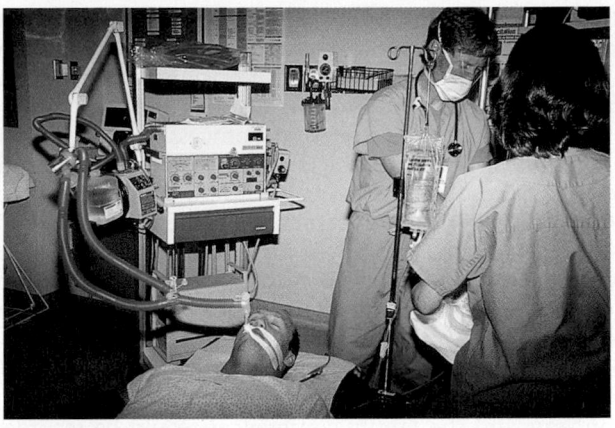

FIGURE **21-1** Nurses collaborate with other professionals in making ethical decisions.

Each step in processing an ethical dilemma resembles steps in critical thinking (see Chapter 14). The nurse begins by gathering information and moves through assessment, identification of the problem, planning, implementation, and evaluation. The first step guides the nurse in determining whether the problem is an ethical one. Not all problems are ethical in nature. The nurse learns to distinguish ethical problems from questions of procedure, legality, or medical diagnosis. To distinguish an ethical problem from other problems, Curtin and Flaherty (1982) recommend that the nurse decide whether the problem has one or more of the following characteristics:

- It cannot be resolved solely through a review of scientific data. To make this determination, it will be necessary to gather detailed information about the situation. This information may come from medical records, health care literature, consultation with colleagues, or with the client and the client's family. What at first appears to be a dilemma may resolve on the nurse's learning, for example, that a review of a diagnostic procedure reveals a different prognosis.
- It is perplexing. One cannot easily think logically or make a decision about the problem. Or, the nurse may disagree with a decision that others are making, and the difference of opinion is perplexing.
- The answer to the problem will have a profound relevance for several areas of human concern.

A part of gathering information includes an examination of one's own values as they relate to the issues. The distinction between personal opinion and the facts of the case, or the opinions of others, is essential for resolution to proceed. To clarify the true ethical issues in any situation, a nurse needs to be aware of personal responses. People come to different conclusions about the same situation with no malice intended toward other people. Remembering this will help the nurse arbitrate conversations.

After reviewing relevant information and personal values, a clear statement of the ethical problem becomes the groundwork to begin negotiation. Discussions are more likely to remain focused and constructive when all parties agree on the statement of the dilemma. These discussions are next facilitated by listing possible courses of action as they occur to the group. Possibilities may occur at any time during deliberations. After alternatives are considered, persons in an ethical conflict come to a point of resolution or agreement, and action is taken. Decisions are made that can be evaluated in an ongoing manner (Box 21-7).

Documentation of the ethical process can take a variety of forms. Whenever the process involves a family conference or results in a change in the management plan, the process should be documented in the medical record. Some institutions may use a formal consultation format whenever a request for discussion comes to the ethics committee. If the ethical dilemma does not directly affect client care, however, documentation may occur by means of minutes from a meeting or in a memorandum to affected parties. In the following case study, the nursing concerns and the family conferences would be recorded in the medical record and in nursing flow sheets.

On your unit, a young 35-year-old woman has been hospitalized in the final stages of a struggle with brain cancer. She is a single mother with two young children at home. Although she has been treated by conventional, as well as some experimental treatments, the tumor continues to grow, and the medical team has agreed that further treatment would be futile. You have cared for this client during past admissions, and during an especially open discussion, she expressed wishes to explore "do not resuscitate" (DNR) orders. During the current admission, her primary physician is out of town. The attending physician does not know the client personally, but he has spent time with her. He has reviewed the clinical data and agrees that the client is entering the terminal stage of her disease. In his opinion,

however, the client is not ready to discuss end-of-life issues. In fact, he states that on offering the option to discuss DNR, the client declined. You have asked him to convene a family conference to discuss DNR orders, but he refuses to do so, because in his opinion the client is not ready to participate.

Step 1. Is this an ethical dilemma? What may at first appear to be a question of ethics may be resolved by clarifying one's knowledge base about clinical facts. A review of policy and procedure, or of standards of care, may explain legal obligations that determine a course of action, regardless of personal opinion. If the question remains perplexing, and the answer will have profound relevance for several areas of human concern, then an ethical dilemma may exist.

The single mother's situation meets the criteria for an ethical dilemma. Further review of scientific data will probably not contribute to a resolution of the dilemma, but it is important to review the data carefully to make this determination. The disagreement does not revolve around whether the client is in a terminally ill state, so further clinical information will not change the basic question: Should the client have an opportunity to discuss DNR orders at this time? The question is perplexing. Basically, two professional team members disagree on an assessment of a client's readiness to confront the very difficult issues related to dying. The answer to the question "Is this client ready to discuss end of life?" has important human implications. If she is not ready, then raising the issues may cause anguish and fear in the client and her family. If she is ready and the team avoids discussion, she may suffer unnecessarily in silence. If she is very close to death, then the lack of a DNR order will necessitate the application of cardiopulmonary resuscitation (CPR) in a futile situation. As a nurse, you know that CPR can cause pain. If applied in a situation where further life is unlikely, then CPR could prolong suffering and reduce dignity.

Step 2. Gather as much information as possible that is relevant to the case. Because resolution to dilemmas may arise from unlikely sources, it is helpful to incorporate as much knowledge as possible at every step of the process. At this point, the information could include looking at laboratory and test results, the clinical state of the client in question, and perhaps current literature about the diagnosis or condition of the client. It may include careful investigation into the psychosocial concerns of the client, as well as those of the client's significant others. A client's religious, cultural, and family orientation are part of the nurse's assessment.

You obtain all of the clinical information that is pertinent to the question. It may be helpful in this case to determine if the client retains most cognitive functions, even though her brain tumor is aggressive. You review the chart and discuss this aspect with the physician, and you agree that the client is fully competent, but definitely afraid, and overwhelmed by the prognosis. Because the dilemma exists because two professionals do not agree on a client's state of mind, it may be helpful to reassess the client, or even to request that an independent person assess the client's readiness to discuss end-of-life issues. Sometimes family members or significant others in the client's life will hold important clues to a client's psychological state of mind.

Box 21-7 **How to Process an Ethical Dilemma**

Step 1. Is this an ethical dilemma? If a review of scientific data does not resolve the question, the question is perplexing, and the answer will have profound relevance for several areas of human concern, then an ethical dilemma may exist.

Step 2. Gather all of the information relevant to the case. To be sure it is a true dilemma, it will be important to review all pertinent information. Occasionally an overlooked fact may provide quick resolution. At this point, client, family, institutional, and social perspectives are important sources of relevant information.

Step 3. Examine and determine your own values on the issues. Values clarification provides a foundation for clarity and for confidence during discussions that will be necessary for resolution of a dilemma.

Step 4. Verbalize the problem. A clear, simple statement of the dilemma may not always be easy, but it is essential for the next step to take place.

Step 5. Consider possible courses of action. To respect all sides of an issue, it is helpful to list potential actions, especially when the list will reflect opinions that conflict.

Step 6. Negotiate the outcome. Sometimes courses of action that seem unlikely at the beginning of the process take on new possibility as they are put to rational and respectful consideration. Negotiation requires a confidence in one's own point of view and a deep respect for the opinions of others.

Step 7. Evaluate the action.

Step 3. Examine and determine your own values on the issues. This step is important for all participants in the discussion. It is at this stage that the nurse, and others, will practice values clarification and try to differentiate between their own values and the values of the client and other team members. Part of the goal is the accurate formation of one's own opinion. An equally essential part of the goal is the establishment of respect for others' opinions.

At this point, you stop to reflect on your own values. You realize that your own religious practices would not prohibit you from deciding to forego further treatment if you were in the client's condition. You also realize that you do not yet have family members who rely on you, such as children or elderly parents. This client's religious practices are perhaps more strictly constructed than your own. Her religion discourages actions that diminish life in any way, and you realize that she may have come to see a DNR order as giving up, or as "acting like God." In addition, you understand that the attending physician has not had time to know this client as her own physician has or as you have. You continue to believe that the client would be capable of a discussion, in spite of her statements to the physician. In fact, you believe that she would benefit from a discussion, because perhaps the combination of an unfamiliar caretaker and declining physical health have silenced her even though her fears and concerns persist.

Step 4. Verbalize the problem. Once all of the relevant information has been gathered, then accurate definition of the problem may proceed. It is helpful to try to state the problem in a few sentences. By agreeing to a statement of the problem, the group can proceed with discussion in a focused way.

Here, the problem seems to be this: Should this client discuss DNR at this time? What are the benefits and what constitute risks of a DNR order at this time? An important question also seems to be on the table regarding the client's current state of mind: Is she afraid to speak? Is she feeling cut off from her normal network (a primary physician)? Are these feelings contributing to confusion about DNR decisions?

Step 5. Consider possible courses of action. What options are available within the context of the situation and the client's values?

Once you have asked the basic question, other questions and possible courses of action arise. Should you initiate a discussion with the client independently of the physician? Would you be outside your professional domain if you facilitated a DNR order? What if your assessment were incorrect? Would you contribute not to the dignity but to the distress of the client? The answers to these questions may be elusive, because they depend on an understanding of client feelings and values that are not necessarily obvious. Even if legally the nurse cannot actually write a DNR order, this fact does not relieve the nurse of troubling questions, because the ability to influence a physician's or client's decision regarding DNR remains.

Step 6. Negotiate the outcome. This step represents the most important and delicate part of the process. These negotiations may happen informally at the bedside or in the charting room. Or a formal ethics meeting may

be necessary. Wherever negotiations occur, the nurse has an obligation to speak for the nursing point of view. The nurse's point of view, by definition, represents a unique contribution to the discussion.

If an ethics committee meeting is convened, then the discussion will usually be multidisciplinary by definition. A facilitator or chairperson will ensure that all points of view are examined and that all pertinent issues are identified. A decision or recommendation is the usual outcome of discussion. In the best of circumstances, participants discover a course of action that meets criteria for acceptance by all. Occasionally, however, participants may leave the discussion disappointed or even opposed to the decision. But in a successful discussion, all members will have agreed on an action or decision that can be implemented.

The discussion focuses on the disagreement between your assessment and the physician's regarding the client's readiness to discuss end-of-life issues. The principles involved during the discussion include beneficence and nonmaleficence: Which plan would provide the most good for this client, a DNR order or no order? A separate question addresses the client's point of view: Would a discussion with the client promote well-being or promote anguish? The principle of autonomy reveals that a troublesome question remains: Does the client want something different from what she is expressing?

With several members of the health care team present, the discussion proceeds. You present your point of view. You continue to sense that the client is ready to discuss DNR orders, but that she may be reluctant to trust the circumstances of this admission. But you also respect the attending physician and his analysis and continue to have concerns that the client may have experienced a change of mind between the last admission and this one. In the end, the team proposes the following: a formal meeting with the client, where you, the attending physician, and a supportive family member, are all present. You support this proposal because you sense that it will maximize the support of the client's existing network. In addition, you recognize that in a trusting environment, the client is most likely to express her fears, insecurities, and wishes most accurately. Team members agree to keep the discussion open ended and exploratory. You suggest that rather than asking if the client wants a DNR order, perhaps the team could wait for her to bring up the issue. In this way, the team could be assured of her consent and willingness to participate in the discussion.

Step 7. Evaluate the action.

At the meeting the client in fact opens up. She expresses relief at the chance to explore her options and feelings. Pain management issues are clarified. She wants to discuss a DNR order but requests a visit from her priest before making a final decision.

Institutional Resources

Most health care institutions have established ethics committees to support the processing of ethical dilemmas. Ethics committees are usually multidisciplinary. They can be a valuable resource for the nurse who identifies an ethical conflict or dilemma.

Ethics committees serve several purposes: education, policy recommendation, and case consultation or review. Any involved person, including nurses, physicians, clients, and families of clients may request access to an ethics committee.

Ethical issues may also be processed in settings other than in a committee, however. Nurses provide insight about ethical problems at family conferences, staff meetings, or even in meetings one-to-one. Many ethical problems begin when people feel misled or are not aware of their options and do not know when to speak up about their concerns. Such concerns may be addressed in a variety of constructive settings. Ethics committees serve to complement relationships and offer a valuable resource for strengthening them.

*I*ssues in Bioethics

Nurses will deal with ethical issues in a variety of ways, throughout all settings and throughout their careers (Box 21-8). Issues change as society and as technologies change. Several current issues are described below.

Quality of Life
For each individual, quality of life is something that is intensely personal and particular. In health care, researchers try to develop quality-of-life measures to help determine the benefits of medical intervention. Discussions about quality of life abound. Some social scientists have proposed formulas or other objective measuring devices that can be applied to individual situations (Fallowfield, 1990; Levine and Ganz, 2002). These formulas take into account the age of the client, the client's ability to live independently, and the client's ability to contribute to society in a gainful way. A quality-of-life measure could help a client and family decide on the merits of a certain risky intervention, such as an organ transplant or experimental drug management. The question of quality of life is central to discussions about futile care, physician-assisted suicide, and DNR discussions.

The definition of quality has been especially challenged by the population of disabled persons in the past few decades. The national movement to pay respect to the abilities of the "disabled" has raised the visibility of quality-of-life issues and forced a reconsideration of the definition of quality. Many school districts, for example, no longer separate physically or mentally challenged children but now integrate these children into "mainstream" classrooms. Public places are accessible to people who use wheelchairs (Figure 21-2). Economic security has been enhanced by laws that protect people who are physically or otherwise challenged from discrimination. These changes have greatly increased the integration of disabled persons into general society. They remind society in general and health care workers specifically that definitions of quality begin as an individual's definition. Society as a whole benefits from these lessons.

Genetic Screening
Genetic testing may alert a client to a condition that is not yet evident, but that is certain to develop in the future. What are the risks and what are the benefits to learning about the presence of disease that has not yet caused symp-

Research Highlight   Box 21-8

When Clients Request Assisted Suicide

Research Focus

Oregon legislators passed the Death With Dignity Act in 1997, legalizing physician-assisted suicide for the first time in the United States. Nearly 80% of clients who have requested physician-assisted suicide in Oregon were enrolled in a hospice program. Researchers were interested in the experiences of the hospice workers—nurses and social workers—who manage hospice clients who request assisted suicide.

Research Abstract

Researchers constructed a questionnaire and mailed it to all Oregon hospice nurses and social workers. Seventy three percent of workers returned the questionnaire. About half of these had cared for a client who requested assistance with suicide.

The nurses and social workers were asked to rate the importance that different reasons played in the client's decision to ask for this option. Workers based their responses on information that they gathered from patient care conferences and in individual interviews with clients.

A consensus among the workers was that a very important reason for assisted suicide was a wish to control the circumstances of death, including a desire to die at home. A readiness for death was also listed as an important reason. Far less important, according to the workers, were reasons of depression, lack of social support, or fear of being a financial burden on loved ones.

According to Ganzini, lead author of the study, the findings suggest that enrollment in hospice programs can act as safeguards for physician-assisted suicide "by increasing opportunities to find alternatives, and ensuring that clients have adequate decision-making capacity, aren't depressed, and aren't acting impulsively."

Evidence-Based Practice

- Hospice nurses can provide client safeguards for physician-assisted suicide.
- Nurses play a key role in the assessment and management of end-of-life care.
- A client's request for suicide assistance may be more influenced by a sense of a loss of control than by depression or concerns for the burden of the client's illness on family members.

Reference

Ganzini L and others: Experiences of Oregon nurses and social workers with hospice patients who requested assistance with suicide, *N Engl J Med* 347(8):582, 2002.

toms? An ethical dilemma could arise for clients or for providers while trying to make a decision whether or not to have the test done. The gene that indicates the presence of Huntington's disease, for example, is detectable upon genetic screen. Huntington's disease is an inherited degenerative neurological disease, incurable at this time. The disease affects cognitive and emotional function as well as physical function. Symptoms usually do not appear until the third or fourth decade of life. If a parent or grandparent

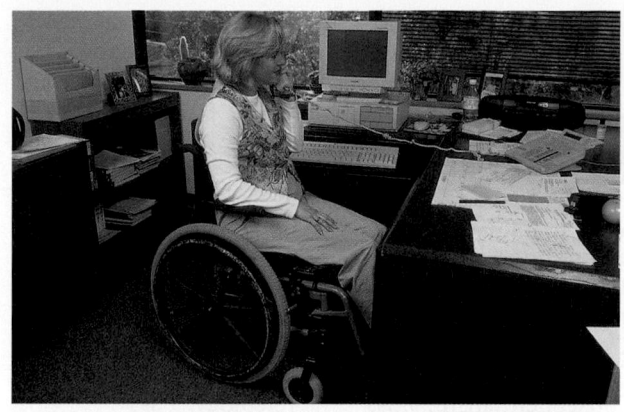

FIGURE **21–2** Measures can be made to provide accessibility in the work environment.

has the disease, offspring are at risk for developing the disease. Some clients might be eager to learn if they will develop the disease so that they can make decisions about childbearing, career, and retirement planning. Others might be reluctant to face the knowledge before symptoms begin, preferring to live life with the uncertainties. As one person whose mother died of Huntington's disease explained, "Cheerful predictions that people could use a positive diagnosis to make rational life choices mystify me . . . I doubt if I'd have the confidence to continue. To think that my brain was slowly dying, never to know if thoughts or feelings were artifacts of a diseased brain—how to live with that and keep on working?" (Wexler, 1995).

Futile Care

The dictionary defines futile as something that is "useless; vain; hopeless; lacking vigor or purpose." In discussions about health care, the term usually refers to interventions unlikely to produce benefit for the client. In practice, however, the term can be slippery. Predictions about medical outcomes can never be 100% guaranteed. Even when an outcome can be predicted with some certainty, people's opinions about the value or worth of the outcome can differ.

Hypothetically, a client might request gall bladder surgery before experiencing any symptoms of gall bladder disease, thinking he could prevent future suffering. Physicians would be reluctant to provide this intervention. They would argue that the intervention is futile: unlikely to produce benefit that outweighs risks. In another situation, a physician might want to provide an arduous intervention where the outcome is uncertain, for example, a liver transplant for a client whose underlying disease is aggressive. In this case, the client might have the opinion that the transplant is futile, unlikely to produce benefit that outweighs the suffering. Agreement on what is and is not futile is often hard to pin down.

If the client is dying, in a condition with little or no hope of recovery, then almost any intervention beyond pain management and comfort measures might be deemed futile. In this situation, an agreement to label an intervention as futile helps providers, families, and clients to refrain from prolonging the dying. In other circumstances, the decision may be reasonably and respectfully made to use certain interventions, such as dialysis for renal failure even though a cancer has metastasized and is unresponsive to any treatment. This use of an intervention, although technically futile clinically, may be justified as a way to provide loved ones time to prepare final farewells, allow distant relatives to arrive at the bedside, resolve important personal legal issues such as a will or other financial matters. In this case, the intervention may be useless clinically, but it produces benefit in other ways.

Allocation of Scarce Resources: Medical Technologies

The concept of scarce resources once was used primarily to assist with discussion of organ transplantation. The term *scarce resource* usually referred to the difficult but common situation wherein far more recipients existed than organs available for transplantation. However, the term has grown to have greater implication as society in the United States is faced with the unequal availability of all health care resources. More than 14% of people living in the United States have no health insurance, and many of those people are women and children. Furthermore, the national costs of health care grow astronomically. The growth of managed care reflects a national and economic effort to control these spiraling costs, but the successes are few, and they generally raise controversy as providers and clients alike struggle with a sense of chaos and lost control.

Although this issue is often larger than a nurse's individual relationship with a client, the application of ethical process or discussion is still applicable. The discussion about allocation of scarce resources easily accommodates the language of ethical principles: respect for autonomy requires that a client not only be able to make an informed choice, but that the treatment chosen be available. Issues of justice apply when certain treatments are available only to certain populations. Processing these thoughts in a way that suggests a clear plan of action, however, is challenging. The individual nurse is still left to ponder personal thoughts. Should resources be focused on research for treatment of devastating disease or on prevention? Which activity is more valuable, research or delivery of care? If public funds are made available for a very expensive intervention, will other populations suffer a diminished level of basic care?

Allocation of Scarce Resources: The Nursing Shortage

The nursing shortage in the United States is a real and a growing problem. The factors that contribute to the shortage are complex and numerous. The statistics about the shortage are startling. According to the federal Bureau of Health Professions, for example, the demand for nurses in 2000 was 2 million, and the supply was at 1.89 million, a 6% shortfall. When predictions about the shortfall were originally forecast, a gap this large was not expected until 2007 (Bureau of Health Professions, 2000). The nursing shortage produces difficult working conditions and affects client outcomes (Needleman and others, 2001). The Institute of Medicine's report on the magnitude of medication errors includes discussion on the role of the nurse, and the role of inadequate staffing as a source of medication error (Kohn, Corrigan, and Donaldson, 2000).

The shortage can also be seen in terms of ethical concerns. How does a nurse decide what is the best course to take when the client care assignment feels too large to be safe? California is the first state in the United States to pass mandated staffing ratios. The number of clients in an assignment will be limited by law. Some hospitals in California have up to 25% of their nursing positions unfilled, however. The law stipulates that if a hospital does not have enough nurses to staff by the law, then the hospital will "close beds." Clients will be turned away.

Professional issues of advocacy and client abandonment compete with ethical concerns about beneficence, maleficence, and justice. An obligation to participate in political solutions may play as important a role as the negotiation of personal concerns.

•••

The courage and intelligence to act, both as an advocate for clients and as a professional member of the health care team, comes only after a committed effort to learn and to understand ethical principles. The professional nurse has a unique point of view regarding clients, the health care system that supports clients, and the institutions that make up the health care system. The nurse has both a duty and the privilege to articulate that point of view. Learning the language of ethical discourse is a part of the skill necessary to exercise this duty and privilege. In addition, review and consideration of various ethical principles assists nurses in forming personal points of view, a necessary ingredient in the negotiation of difficult ethical situations.

Key Concepts

- Ethics refers to the study of philosophical ideals of right and wrong behavior.
- Bioethics refers specifically to ethical issues that affect health and the delivery of health care.
- A code of ethics provides a foundation for professional nursing.
- Professional nursing promotes accountability, responsibility, and advocacy.
- Basic standards of ethics in health care include autonomy, beneficence, nonmaleficence, justice, and fidelity.
- Personal ethics grow from personal values.
- Feelings and beliefs play an important role in the resolution of ethical problems.
- The process of values clarification helps a nurse to explore personal values and feelings and to decide how to act on personal beliefs.
- Ethical problems arise from differences in values, changing professional roles, technological advances, and social issues that influence quality of life.
- A standard process for thinking through ethical dilemmas helps providers resolve conflict or uncertainty about right actions.
- Critical thinking is an important part of processing ethical dilemmas.

- The nurse's point of view provides a unique and valuable voice in the resolution of ethical dilemmas.

Key Terms
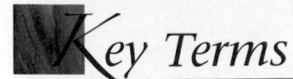

Accountability, *p. 391*	Ethnocentrism, *p. 394*
Autonomy, *p. 390*	Fidelity, *p. 390*
Beneficence, *p. 390*	Gender biased, *p. 396*
Bioethics, *p. 389*	Justice, *p. 390*
Code of ethics, *p. 389*	Nonmaleficence, *p. 390*
Confidentiality, *p. 391*	Responsibility, *p. 391*
Consequentialism, *p. 395*	Teleology, *p. 395*
Cultural values, *p. 393*	Value, *p. 393*
Deontology, *p. 395*	Values clarification, *p. 393*
Ethic of care, *p. 396*	Veracity, *p. 392*
Ethics, *p. 389*	

Critical Thinking Exercises

1. Complete the "cultural values" exercise (see Box 21-6, p. 395) with your classmates or with members of another class of professionals. Compare the answers and discuss the differences.

2. You are caring for a 17-year-old client who has been admitted for treatment of sickle cell crisis. She needs fluid management and comfort management. Even though she is receiving narcotics around the clock, she continues to complain of pain. She also complains about her roommate, the food, and the intravenous line. She comes from a community far from the hospital, and her mother cannot visit every day. She has an older brother who has been convicted of possession of illegal drugs. Discuss your approach to this client. Rank her needs. What is your priority action, based on what you know so far? Examine and describe your opinions about pain, pain management, and addiction.

3. You are a clinic nurse in an small community clinic. A 45-year-old male client has been coming to the clinic for several years for treatment and support of his acquired immunodeficiency syndrome (AIDS). During recent months he has lost his long-term companion to AIDS. In addition, both his parents died many years ago. His clinical condition has deteriorated. His vision is failing, his nutritional status is difficult to maintain, and he has been hospitalized 3 times in the past 3 months for pneumonia. He asks for your help in planning his suicide. Discuss your response to his request. Begin by an examination of your personal feelings about suicide. Include a discussion about your understanding of AIDS: Where does it come from? Who gets the disease? Why? What are your feelings and opinions about people with AIDS? Construct your response, keeping in mind the ethical principles of fidelity, autonomy, beneficence, and nonmaleficence. Because all of these principles collide in this example, it will be important to identify each and recognize personal responses to the role that each plays in this narrative. Just as important is the role that one imagines they play for the client, especially as they differ from

one's own. For the sake of this discussion, it is illegal in your state for nurses to prescribe medicines. What are your possible courses of action?

4. You have been assigned the care of a 98-year-old woman who was recently admitted from home with a diagnosis of pneumonia. She has a history of cardiac disease and takes a number of medications. She had been fairly active until the past few days, when her cough worsened and she developed a fever. You note that her pulse has become weak and thready and that her respirations are increasingly labored. The client is now too weak to respond to you. When you mention to the family that you may need to call the physician and even "call a code," the son and the daughter become distraught, saying that they do not want their mother to be kept alive on "machines." They report that they have discussed this situation with their mother. You find that documentation of these wishes is not in the chart. The family members have not discussed this situation with their doctor. What actions would you consider taking at this moment? Take into account the ethical principles of autonomy and beneficence. What are your personal values about interventions at the end of life?

Review Questions

1. In the United States, access to health care usually depends on a client's ability to pay for health care, either through insurance or by paying cash. The client the nurse is caring for needs a liver transplant to survive. This client has been out of work for several months and does not have insurance or enough cash. A discussion about the ethics of this situation would involve predominately the principle of:
   1. Accountability, because you as the nurse are accountable for the well-being of this clients.
   2. Respect for autonomy, because this client's autonomy will be violated if he does not receive the liver transplant.
   3. Ethics of care, because the caring thing that a nurse could provide this patient is resources for a liver transplant.
   4. Justice, because the first and greatest question in this situation is how to determine the just distribution of resources.

2. It may seem redundant that health care providers, including professional nurses, agree to "do no harm" to their clients. The point of this agreement is to reassure the public that in all ways the health care team will not only work to heal patients, they agree to do this in the least painful and harmful way possible. The principle that describes this agreement is called:
   1. Beneficence.
   2. Accountability.
   3. Nonmaleficence.
   4. Respect for autonomy.

3. A child's immunization may cause discomfort during administration, but the benefits of protection from disease, both for the individual and for society, outweigh the temporary discomforts. This involves the principle of:
   1. Beneficence.
   2. Fidelity.
   3. Nonmaleficence.
   4. Respect for autonomy.

4. If a nurse assesses a client for pain and then offers a plan to manage the pain, the principle that encourages the nurse to monitor the client's response to the plan is:
   1. Beneficence.
   2. Fidelity.
   3. Nonmaleficence.
   4. Respect for autonomy.

5. The code of ethics for nurses is composed and published by:
   1. The National League for Nursing.
   2. The American Nurses Association.
   3. The American Medical Association.
   4. The National Institutes of Health, Nursing Division.

6. Nurses agree to be advocates for their patients. Practice of advocacy calls for the nurse to:
   1. Seek out the nursing supervisor in conflicting situations.
   2. Work to understand the law as it applies to the client's clinical condition.
   3. Assess the client's point of view and prepare to articulate this point of view.
   4. Document all clinical changes in the medical record in a timely manner.

7. Successful ethical discussion depends on people who have a clear sense of personal values. When many people share the same values it may be possible to identify a philosophy of utilitarianism, which proposes that:
   1. The value of people is determined solely by leaders in the Unitarian Church.
   2. The decision to perform a liver transplant depends on a measure of the moral life that the client has led so far.
   3. The best way to determine the solution to an ethical dilemma is to refer the case to the attending physician.
   4. The value of something is determined by its usefulness to society.

8. The philosophy sometimes called the ethics of care suggests that ethical dilemmas can best be solved by attention to:
   1. Relationships.
   2. Ethical principles.
   3. Clients.
   4. Code of ethics for nurses.

9. In most ethical dilemmas, the solution to the dilemma requires negotiation among members of the health care team. The nurse's point of view is valuable because:
   1. Nurses have a legal license that encourages their presence during ethical discussions.
   2. The principle of autonomy guides all participants to respect their own self-worth.
   3. Nurses develop a relationship to the client that is unique among all professional health care providers.
   4. The nurse's code of ethics recommends that a nurse be present at any ethical discussion about client care.

10. Ethical dilemmas often arise over a conflict of opinion. Once the nurse has determined that the dilemma is ethical, a critical first step in negotiating the difference of opinion would be to:
   1. Consult a professional ethicist to ensure that the steps of the process occur in full.
   2. Gather all relevant information regarding the clinical, social, and spiritual aspects of the dilemma.
   3. List the ethical principles that inform the dilemma so that negotiations agree on the language of the discussion.
   4. Ensure that the attending physician has written an order for an ethics consultation to support the ethics process.

*R*eferences

American Nurses Association: *Code for nurses with interpretive statements,* Washington, DC, 2001, American Nurses Publishing, http://nursingworld.org/ethics/code/ethicscode150.htm.

Beauchamp T, Childress J: *Principles of biomedical ethics,* ed 4, New York, 2001, Oxford University Press.

Bell NK: If age becomes a standard for rationing health care. In Holmes HB, Purdy LM, editors: *Feminist perspectives in medical ethics,* Bloomington, 1992, Indiana University Press.

Boyer JR, Nelson JL: A comment on Fry's "The Role of Caring in a Theory of Nursing Ethics," *Hypatia* 5(3): 153, 1990.

Bureau of Health Professions: *Projected supply, demand, and shortages of registered nurses: 2000-2020,* 2000, http://bhpr.hrsa.gov/healthworkforce/rnproject/default.htm.

Burke MM, Laramie JA: *Primary care of the older adult: a multidisciplinary approach,* St. Louis, 2000, Mosby.

Callahan D: Why America accepted bioethics, *Hastings Cent Rep* 23(6 suppl): 58, 1993.

Canadian Nurses Association: *Code of ethics for registered nurses,* Ottowa, Ontario, September 2002, The Association, www.cna-nurses.ca/pages/ethics/ethics.htm.

Curtin L, Flaherty MJ: *Nursing ethics: theories and pragmatics,* Bowie, Md, 1982, Brady.

Deloughery G: *Issues and trends in nursing,* ed 3, St. Louis, 1998, Mosby.

Fallowfield L: *The quality of life: the missing measurement in health care,* London, 1990, Souvenir Press.

Fry ST: The role of caring in a theory of nursing ethics, *Hypatia* 4(2): 89, 1989.

Gilligan C: *In a different voice,* Cambridge, Mass, 1993, Harvard University Press.

Harris L: Autonomy under duress. In Flack HE, Pellegrino ED, editors: *African-American perspectives on biomedical ethics,* Washington, DC, 1992, Georgetown University Press.

HHS Fact Sheet: Modifications to the standards for privacy of individually identifiable health information—final rule, August 9, 2002, U.S. Department of Health and Human Services, www.hhs.gov/news/press/2002pres/20020809.html.

Holmes HB, Purdy LM, editors: *Feminist perspectives in medical ethics,* Bloomington, 1992, Indiana University Press.

International Council of Nurses: *The ICN code of ethics for nurses,* The Council, Geneva, 2000, www.icn.ch/ethics.htm.

Joint Commission on Accreditation of Healthcare Organizations: *2003 accreditation manual for hospitals,* vol 1, Standards, Chicago, 2002, The Commission.

Kirkpatrick SM, Deloughery GL: Cultural influences on nursing. In Deloughery GL, editor: *Issues and trends in nursing,* ed 2, St. Louis, 1995, Mosby.

Kohlberg L: *Essays on moral development,* vols 1-3, San Francisco, 1981, Harper & Row.

Kohn LT, Corrigan JM, Donaldson MS, editors: *To err is human,* Washington, DC, 2000, National Academy Press.

Leininger M: *Caring: an essential human need,* Detroit, 1988, Wayne State University Press.

Levine M, Ganz P: Beyond the development of quality-of-life instruments: where do we go from here? *J Clin Oncol* 20(9):2215, 2002.

Maslow A: *New knowledge in human values,* New York, 1959, Harper & Row.

Miller MA, Babcock, DE: *Critical thinking applied to nursing,* St. Louis, 1996, Mosby.

Moreno J: *Deciding together: bioethics and moral consensus,* New York, 1995, Oxford University Press.

Noddings N: *Caring: a feminist approach to ethics and moral education,* Berkeley, 1984, University of California Press.

O'Neil J: Ethical decision making and the role of nursing. In Deloughery GL, editor: *Issues and trends in nursing,* ed 2, St. Louis, 1995, Mosby.

Pellegrino ED: The caring ethic: the relation of physician to patient. In Bishop AH, Scudder JR, editors: *Caring, curing, coping: nurse, physician, and patient relations,* Birmingham, 1985, University of Alabama Press.

Raths LE, Harmin M, Simon SB: *Values and teaching,* ed 2, Columbus, Ohio, 1979, Merrill Publishing.

Renwick GW, Rhinesmith SH: *An exercise in cultural analysis for managers,* Chicago, 1995, Intercultural Press.

Rokeach M: *The nature of human values,* New York, 1973, Free Press.

Shannon SE: The roots of interdisciplinary conflict around ethical issues, *Crit Care Nurs Clin North Am* 9(1):13, 1997.

Sherwin S: *No longer patient: feminist ethics and health care,* Philadelphia, 1993, Temple University Press.

Twenty years after: the legacy of the Tuskegee syphilis study, *Hastings Cent Rep* 22 (6):29 November–December 1992.

Watson J, editor: *Applying art and science of human caring,* New York, 1994, National League of Nursing Press.

Wexler A: *Mapping fate: a memoir of family, risk, and genetic research,* New York, 1995, Times Books.

Wolf SM, editor: *Feminism and bioethics,* New York, 1996, Oxford University Press.

*R*esearch References

Carrese J, Rhodes L: Western bioethics on the Navajo reservation: benefit or harm? *JAMA* 274(10):826, 1995.

Ganzini L and others: Experiences of Oregon nurses and social workers with hospice patients who requested assistance with suicide, *N Engl J Med* 347(8):582, 2002.

Needleman J and others: *Nurse staffing and patient outcomes in hospitals: executive summary,* Boston, February 2001, Harvard School of Public Health, http://bhpr.hrsa.gov/nursing/staffstudy.htm.

Legal Implications in Nursing Practice

Media Resources

CD COMPANION

- Review Questions
- Glossary

evolve WEBSITE

- Review Questions
- Student Learning Activities
- Glossary

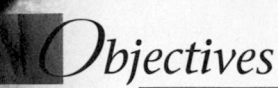

Objectives

Mastery of content in this chapter will enable the student to:

- Define the key terms listed.
- Explain the legal concepts of standard of care and informed consent.
- Describe the legal responsibilities and obligations of nurses regarding the following federal statutes: Americans With Disabilities Act (ADA), Emergency Medical Treatment and Active Labor Act (EMTALA), Health Insurance Portability and Accountability Act of 1996 (HIPAA), and the Patient Self-Determination Act (PSDA).
- List sources for standards of care for nurses.
- Describe the nurse's role regarding a "do not resuscitate" (DNR) order.
- Define legal aspects of nurse-client, nurse-physician, nurse-nurse, and nurse-employer relationships.
- List the elements needed to prove negligence.
- Describe the nursing implications associated with legal issues that arise in nursing practice.

*S*afe nursing practice includes an understanding of the legal boundaries within which nurses must function. As with all aspects of nursing today, an understanding of the implications of the law supports critical thinking on the nurse's part. Nurses must understand the law to protect themselves from liability and to protect their clients' rights. Nurses need not fear the law but rather should view the information that follows as the foundation for understanding what is expected by our society from professional nursing care providers. The laws in our society are fluid and constantly changing to meet the needs of the persons the laws are intended to protect. As technology has expanded the role of the nurse, the ethical dilemmas associated with client care have increased and often become legal issues as well. The public is better informed than in the past about their rights to health care. As health care evolves in our society, so, too, the legal implications for health care evolve. Frequently, nurses function under several sources and jurisdictions of health law simultaneously. Nurses' familiarity with the laws enhances their ability to be client advocates.

Legal Limits of Nursing

Professional nurses must understand the legal limits influencing their daily practice. This, coupled with good judgment and sound decision making, ensures safe and appropriate nursing care.

Sources of Law

The legal guidelines that nurses must follow are derived from statutory law, regulatory law, and common law. **Statutory law** is created by elected legislative bodies such as state legislatures and the U.S. Congress. An example of state statutes are the Nurse Practice Acts found in all 50 states. These **Nurse**

Practice Acts describe and define the legal boundaries of nursing practice within each state. An example of a federal statute enacted by the U.S. Congress is the Americans with Disabilities Act (ADA) (1995). This statute protects the rights of handicapped individuals in the workplace, in educational institutions, and throughout our society. **Regulatory law,** or **administrative law,** is created by administrative bodies such as State Boards of Nursing when they pass rules and regulations. An example of regulatory law is the duty to report incompetent or unethical nursing conduct to the State Board of Nursing. **Common law** is created by judicial decisions made in courts when individual legal cases are decided. An example of common law is informed consent and the client's right to refuse treatment.

Statutory law is either civil or criminal. **Criminal laws** prevent harm to society and provide punishment for crimes (Black, 1999). There are two classifications of **crimes.** A **felony** is a crime of a serious nature that has a penalty of imprisonment for greater than 1 year or even death. A **misdemeanor** is a less serious crime that has a penalty of a fine or imprisonment for less than 1 year. An example of criminal conduct for nurses would be misuse of a controlled substance.

Civil laws protect the rights of individual persons within our society and encourage fair and equitable treatment among people (Black, 1999). Generally, violations of civil laws cause harm to an individual or property. The damages for civil laws involve the payment of money, unlike criminal laws, which are punished by imprisonment. However, under many federal and state laws, sanctions for violations may include both civil and criminal penalties.

Standards of Care

Standards of care are the legal guidelines for nursing practice. Nursing standards of care are defined in the Nurse Practice Acts and by the State Board of Nursing of each state, by the federal and state laws regulating hospitals and other health care institutions, by the professional and specialty nursing organizations, and by the written policies and procedures of employing institutions (Illinois Nursing Practice Act, 1997). In a malpractice lawsuit, nursing standards of care are used to measure nursing conduct and to determine whether the nurse acted as any reasonably prudent nurse would act under the same or similar circumstances. A breach of the nursing standard of care is one element that must be proven in the tort of nursing negligence or malpractice.

The law defines the standards of care that nurses must follow. All state legislatures have passed Nurse Practice Acts that define the scope of nursing practice. Since assistive personnel (e.g., nurse assistants) have been employed, some State Boards of Nursing have defined the registered nurse's responsibilities specifically and developed position statements and guidelines to help licensed nurses delegate safely (Sheehan, 2001). Nurse Practice Acts establish educational requirements for nurses, distinguish between nursing and medical practice, and generally define the scope of nursing practice. The rules and regulations enacted by the State Board of Nursing define the practice of nursing more specifically. For example, a state board may develop a rule regarding intravenous therapy. All nurses are responsible for knowing the provisions of the Nurse Practice Act for the state in which they work, as well as the rules and regulations enacted by the State Board of Nursing and other regulatory administrative bodies.

Professional organizations are another source for defining standards of care. The American Nurses Association (ANA) has developed standards for nursing practice, policy statements, and similar resolutions. The standards delineate the scope, function, and role of the nurse in practice. For example, the standards for community health nursing practice include guidelines for data collection, diagnosis, planning, treatment, and evaluation. Nursing specialty organizations also have standards of practice defined for certifying nurses who work in specialty areas such as the operating room (OR) or critical care. These same standards also serve as practice guidelines for defining safe and appropriate nursing care in specialty areas.

The Joint Commission on Accreditation of Healthcare Organizations (JCAHO) (2003) requires that accredited hospitals have written nursing policies and procedures. The written policies and procedures of the employing institution detail how nurses are to perform their duties. These internal standards of care are quite specific and should be accessible on all nursing units. For example, a policy/procedure outlining the steps that should be taken when changing a dressing or administering medication provides specific information about how nurses are to perform these tasks. Some hospitals are also now using commercially published procedural textbooks to reference the institution's general policies and procedures. Nurses must know the policies and procedures of their employing institution because the same standard of care should be used by all nurses in the health care institution (*Quijano v United States*, 2003). Institutional policies and procedures must conform to state and federal laws, as well as community standards, and cannot conflict with legal guidelines that define acceptable standards of care (*Quijano v United States*, 2003).

In a lawsuit for malpractice or nursing negligence, a nursing expert is called to testify to the jury about the standards of nursing care as applied to the facts of the case (Box 22-1). The standards of care are used by the jury to determine whether the nurse acted appropriately. Nurse experts must base their opinions on existing standards of practice established by Nurse Practice Acts, professional organizations, institutional policies and procedures, federal and state hospital licensing laws, standards of the JCAHO, job descriptions, and current nursing research literature (Manson, 2002).

Usually, general duty nurses are responsible for meeting the same standards as other general duty nurses in similar settings. However, specialized nurses such as nurse anesthetists, OR nurses, intensive care nurses, or certified nurse-midwives are held to standards of care and skill exercised by those in the same specialty as defined by applicable standards. All nurses should know the standards of care that they are expected to meet within their specific specialty and work setting. Ignorance of the law or of standards of care is not a defense against malpractice. However, at the time of trial, the standard of care is

---

Box 22-1   Anatomy of a Lawsuit

Petition—elements of the claim: The plaintiff outlines what the defendant nurse did wrong and how as a result of that alleged negligence the plaintiff was injured.

Answer: The nurse admits or denies each allegation in the petition. Anything that is not admitted must be proved.

Discovery

Interrogatories: Written questions requiring answers under oath. Usual questions concern witnesses, insurance experts, and which health care providers the plaintiff has seen before and after the incident.

Medical records: The defendant obtains all of the plaintiff's relevant medical records for treatment before and after the incident.

Witnesses' depositions: Questions are posed to the witness under oath to obtain all relevant, nonprivileged information about the case.

Parties' depositions: The plaintiff and defendants (doctor, nurse, hospital personnel) are almost always deposed.

Other witnesses: Factual witnesses, both neutral and biased, are deposed to obtain information and their version of the case. This may include family members on the plaintiff's side and other medical personnel (e.g., nurses) on the defendant's side.

Treating physicians' depositions: Before subsequent treating, physicians' depositions may be taken to establish issues such as those concerning preexisting conditions, causation, the nature and extent of injuries, and permanency.

Experts: The plaintiff selects experts to establish the essential legal elements of the case against the defendant. The defendant selects experts to establish the appropriateness of the nursing care.

Trial: Usually occurs at least 2 to 3 years, and sometimes as long as 6 to 8 years, after the filing of the petition. (Only about 5% of cases are tried. Most are dismissed or settled. Settlement means that money has been paid for the case to be dismissed, usually without any admission of liability.)

Proof of Negligence

The nurse owed a duty to the client.

The nurse did not carry out the duty or breached the duty (failure to use that degree of skill and learning ordinarily used under the same or similar circumstances by members of his or her profession).

The client was injured:
    Medical bills, lost wages
    Pain and suffering
    Perinatal damages
    Wrongful death damages

The client's injury was caused by the nurse's failure to carry out that duty ("but for" the breach of duty the client would not have been injured).

---

what the nurse experts testify that standard to be and ultimately what the jury believes (Manson, 2002).

One of the first and most important cases to discuss a nurse's liability was *Darling v Charleston Community Memorial Hospital.* This 1966 Illinois Supreme Court case has been adopted in almost every state. It involved an 18-year-old man with a fractured leg. The emergency department physician applied a cast with insufficient padding. The man's toes became swollen and discolored, and he developed decreased sensation. He complained to the nursing staff many times. Although the nurses recognized the symptoms as signs of impaired circulation, they failed to tell their supervisor that the physician did not respond to their calls or the client's needs. Gangrene developed, and the man's leg had to be amputated. Although the physician was held liable for incorrectly applying the cast, the nursing staff was also held liable for failing to adhere to the standards of care for monitoring and reporting the client's symptoms. Even though the nurses attempted to contact the physician, this case holds that when the physician fails to respond, the nurse must go over the physician's head to make sure that the client is appropriately treated.

The nurse is obligated to seek appropriate treatment for the client not only ethically but legally. The nurse bears a fiduciary relationship to the client. A fiduciary relationship is one in which a professional, the nurse, provides services which by their nature cause the recipient, the client, to trust in the specialized knowledge, the integrity, and the fidelity of the professional (5 CFR §2636.305 (b) (2)). The nurse is obligated in the fiduciary relationship to provide knowledgeable, safe care to the client. The nurse

is obligated to behave honestly and truthfully with regard to the client. Last, the nurse must be faithful to provide care in the best interests of the client.

The best way for nurses to keep up with the current legal issues affecting nursing practice is to read the nursing literature in their practice area. Current nursing literature deals with the changing obligations and standards of care for nurses, explains pertinent state and federal laws, and keeps the nurse up to date on any new rules or regulations and case law (Laughlin, 2002).

Federal Statutory Issues in Nursing Practice

Americans With Disabilities Act

The Americans with Disabilities Act (ADA) (1995) is a very broad-reaching civil rights statute. It protects the rights of disabled people. It is also the most extensive law on how employers must treat health care workers and clients infected with the human immunodeficiency virus (HIV). The Supreme Court ruled in 1998 in *Bragdon v Abbott* that even asymptomatic HIV constitutes a disability within the meaning of the ADA. This means that the HIV-positive individual who does not have acquired immunodeficiency syndrome (AIDS) is still protected by the ADA. The ADA regulations protect the privacy of infected people by giving individuals the opportunity to decide whether to disclose their disability. However, several cases have held that the health care provider may be obligated to disclose the fact that he or she is infected with HIV. Despite these rulings, health care workers with disabilities, such as HIV infection, are protected in the workplace under the ADA. Likewise, health care workers may not discriminate against HIV-positive clients (Vernaglia, 2002).

Emergency Medical Treatment and Active Labor Act

As a result of clients being transferred from private hospitals to public hospitals without appropriate screening and stabilization (referred to as "patient dumping"), Congress enacted the Emergency Medical Treatment and Active Labor Act (EMTALA) (1986). This act provides that when a client comes to the emergency department or the hospital, an appropriate medical screening must be done within the hospital's capacity. If an emergency condition exists, the client may not be discharged or transferred until the condition is stabilized. The client can be discharged or transferred before he is stable. For example, if the client requests in writing to be transferred or discharged after being informed of the benefits and risks, or if a physician certifies that the benefits of transfer outweigh the risks, the client may be transferred without an EMTALA violation. The transfer must always be appropriate, which means (1) that the receiving facility agrees to the transfer, has space for the client, and has qualified personnel to receive the client; (2) the medical records must be forwarded to the receiving hospital; and (3) the client must be transported by qualified personnel and transportation equipment.

Mental Health Parity Act

Health insurance plans are free to eliminate coverage for certain specialties and can impose limits on the amount of coverage that they will pay for certain illnesses. However, if mental health benefits are provided, a recent federal statute regulates restrictions on mental health benefits. The Mental Health Parity Act of 1996 forbids health plans from placing lifetime or annual limits on mental health coverage that are less generous than those placed on medical or surgical benefits.

A client can be admitted to a psychiatric unit involuntarily or on a voluntary basis. A petition for involuntary detention must be filed with the court within 96 hours of the client's initial detention. A hearing must be conducted within 2 days of the filing of the involuntary petition. If the judge determines that the client is a danger to self or others, the judge will grant the involuntary detention, and the client can be detained for 21 more days for psychiatric treatment.

Potentially suicidal clients are admitted to psychiatric units. If the client's history and medical records indicate suicidal tendencies, the client must be kept under supervision. Lawsuits result from clients' attempts at suicide within the hospital. The allegations in the lawsuits are that the health care provider failed to provide adequate supervision and failed to safeguard the facilities. Documentation of precautions against suicide is essential.

Advance Directives

There are two basic advance directives: living wills and durable powers of attorney for health care (Scanlon, 2003). Many clients have living wills or have signed a durable power of attorney for health care. The Patient Self-Determination Act (PSDA) (1991) requires health care institutions to provide written information to clients concerning the clients' rights under state law to make decisions, including the right to refuse treatment and formulate advance directives. Under the act, it must be documented in the client's record whether the client has signed an advance directive. The hospital is also required to ensure that state law is followed and provide education for the staff and the public concerning living wills and durable powers of attorney. It is especially important to understand clients' cultural beliefs when explaining advance directives. Regulatory mandates to benefit the public are based on the dominant value in American society of self-determination. This may be in conflict with a client's cultural heritage (see Chapter 8). In order for living wills or durable powers of attorney for health care to be enforceable, the client must be legally incompetent or lack decisional capacity to make decisions regarding health care treatment (Furrow and others, 1991). The determination of legal competency is made by a judge, and the determination of decisional capacity is usually made by the physician and family. Therefore the implementation of the advance directive is done within the context of the health care team and the health care institution. The nurse should be familiar with the institution's policies complying with the act.

Living Wills. **Living wills** are written documents that direct treatment in accordance with a client's wishes in the event of a terminal illness or condition (Lueckenotte, 2000). Living wills may be difficult to interpret and not clinically specific in unforeseen circumstances. Each state providing for living wills has its own requirements for executing them. Generally, two witnesses, neither of whom can be a relative or physician, are needed when the client signs the document. If health care workers follow the directions of the living will, they are immune from liability.

A durable power of attorney for health care designates an agent, surrogate, or proxy to make health care decisions if and when the client is no longer able to make decisions on his or her own behalf. This agent is appointed to make health care treatment decisions based on the client's wishes (Scanlon, 2003).

In addition to federal statutes, the ethical doctrine of autonomy ensures the client the right to refuse medical treatment. This right to refuse medical treatment was upheld in the *Bouvia v Superior Court* case in 1986. That case allowed the discontinuation of the client's tube feedings at her request. The courts have also upheld the right of a legally competent client to refuse medical treatment for religious reasons. Christian Scientists refuse medical treatment based on religious beliefs, and Jehovah's Witnesses accept medical treatment but refuse blood transfusions for religious beliefs. In the absence of a truly compelling reason otherwise, the right to make those choices are protected. The U.S. Supreme Court stated in the *Cruzan v Director Missouri Department of Health* case in 1990 that "we assume that the U.S. Constitution would grant a constitutionally protected competent person the right to refuse lifesaving hydration and nutrition." In cases involving the client's right to refuse or withdraw medical treatment, the courts balance the client's interest with the state's interest in protecting life, preserving medical ethics, preventing suicide, and protecting innocent third parties. Children are generally considered innocent third parties. Although the courts will not force adults to undergo treatment that is refused for religious reasons, they will grant an order allowing hospitals and doctors to treat children of Christian Scientists or Jehovah's Witnesses who have denied consent for treatment of their minor children.

Where clients are legally incompetent and are unable to make health care decisions, the courts balance the state's interest with what the client would have wanted. The courts attempt to substitute their judgment as to what the client would have chosen if the client were competent. The Supreme Court held in the Cruzan case that states had the right to require "clear and convincing evidence" of a legally incompetent client's prior wishes when making determinations to discontinue life-sustaining treatment. In that case nutrition and hydration were recognized as life-sustaining medical treatment that could be withdrawn.

Every state now requires "clear and convincing" evidence of the client's choice, but individual states differ as to what standard satisfies the amount of evidence required. If there is no evidence of the client's prior choice, most states allow treatment to be stopped based on other factors, including the best interest of the client balanced with the state's interest.

In addition to client refusals of treatment, the nurse will frequently encounter the DNR order. DNR means "do not resuscitate" or "no code." The DNR order was first developed in 1976 and marks an important change in health care because it was the first order to withhold treatment instead of deliver treatment (Burns and others, 2003). A DNR order should be written, not given verbally. The physician should routinely review DNR orders in case the client's condition warrants a change. "Slow codes" or "partial" codes may be defined differently by various institutions and may be interpreted as not performing resuscitative procedures as a competent person would. If resuscitative procedures are performed more slowly than recommended by the American Heart Association, they may be interpreted as being below the standard of care and therefore become the basis for a lawsuit.

Cardiopulmonary resuscitation (CPR) is an emergency treatment that is provided without client consent. It is a procedure that is performed on an appropriate client unless a DNR order is written in the client's chart. Since 1988, when New York first adopted legislation regarding DNR orders, over 20 states have drafted similar statutes (New York DNR Statute, 1988). The statutes assume that all clients will be resuscitated unless there is a written DNR order in the chart. Legally competent adult clients may consent to a DNR order verbally or in writing after being given the appropriate information by the physician. A verbal consent requires two witnesses, one of whom must be a physician affiliated with the hospital. A written consent requires two adult witnesses. If the client lacks the decisional capacity to give consent, a surrogate may give consent for the client if two physicians say that within reasonable medical certainty the client has a terminal condition, the client is terminally unconscious, resuscitation would be medically futile, or resuscitation would impose extraordinary burden on the client in light of the client's medical condition and the expected outcome of resuscitation. If no surrogate is available to give consent, the DNR order can still be written but only if the physician is reasonably medically certain that the resuscitation would be futile. The statutes provide that the attending physician must review the DNR orders every 3 days for hospitalized clients or every 60 days for clients in residential health facilities.

Uniform Anatomical Gift Act

An individual who is at least 18 years of age may make an anatomical gift or organ donation (defined as a "donation of all or part of a human body to take effect upon or after death"). The gift must be made in writing and signed by the donor. If the donor cannot sign, the document must be signed by another individual and two witnesses. In many states adults may sign the back of their driver's license, indicating consent to organ donation. Pursuant to the Uniform Anatomical Gift Act of 1987, which has been adopted in nearly 20 states, unless the gift is revoked by the donor before death, no further consent is required after the donor's death.

In most states Required Request laws mandate that at the time of admission to a hospital, a qualified health care provider must ask each client over 18 whether they are an organ or tissue donor. If the answer is affirmative, a copy of the document should be obtained. If the answer is negative and the attending physician consents, the option to make or refuse an anatomical gift should be discussed. Documentation should be placed in the client's medical record. Required Request laws came about because of the shortage of suitable organs for transplantation. Required Request laws are also part of the Uniform Anatomical Gift Act (1987), which addresses many issues involving organ donation, including the rights and duties at death. The physician who certifies death shall not be involved in the removal or transplantation of organs (see Chapter 29).

The National Organ Transplant Act of 1984 prohibits the purchase or sale of organs. The act also provides civil and criminal immunity to the hospital and physician who acts in accordance with the act. The act also protects the donor's estate from liability for injury or damage that may result from the use of the gift. Organ transplantation is extremely expensive. Clients in end-stage renal disease are eligible for Medicare coverage for a kidney transplant, but other transplants have to be paid for by private insurance. The United Network for Organ Sharing has a contract with the federal government and sets policies and guidelines for the procurement of organs. Most clients who require organ transplantation have to be placed on a waiting list for an organ in their geographical area. Recently, the geographical system has changed to give priority to clients who demonstrate the greatest need. Nurses must be familiar with their employing institution's policies and procedures regarding organ donation.

Health Insurance Portability and Accountability Act

The Health Insurance Portability and Accountability Act of 1996 (HIPAA) limits the extent to which health plans may impose preexisting condition limitations and prohibits discrimination in health plans against individual participants and beneficiaries based on health status. One of the ways that insurance companies keep costs down is by not insuring certain preexisting conditions that clients have when they obtain group health insurance coverage. For example, if a client has heart disease, an insurer may agree to provide health insurance for the client for all medical problems except heart disease. HIPAA requires insurers to only limit coverage for a preexisting condition for 12 months in most cases. This means that if an employee has group health insurance coverage with his job for at least 12 months and then changes jobs, the second employer cannot impose preexisting condition exclusion on the individual. The advantages of HIPAA are that employees can change jobs without losing coverage as a result of preexisting coverage exclusion as long as they have had 12 months of continuous group health insurance coverage.

HIPAA also contains a section that sets standards regarding the electronic exchange of private and sensitive health information. Known as the Privacy Standards (Rosati, 2002), these rules create client rights to consent to use and disclose protected health information, to inspect and copy one's medical record, and to amend mistaken or incomplete information. In addition, the standards require all hospitals and health agencies to have specific policies and procedures in place to ensure compliance with the standards. These policies and procedures must provide reasonable safeguards to protect written and verbal communications about clients. Student nurses who visit patient care units before caring for clients usually prepare by reading clients' charts. However, no part of the chart can be copied. Although HIPAA will not require such measures as soundproof rooms in hospitals, it does mean that nurses and all health care providers should avoid discussing clients in public hallways and should provide reasonable levels of privacy in communicating with and about clients in any manner. Message boards used in clients' hospital rooms to post daily nursing care information can no longer contain information revealing the client's medical condition. HIPAA violations have civil and criminal sanctions. All nurses must understand the HIPAA policies of their organization.

Restraints

The Resident's Rights section of the Medicaid Statute (1988) regulates the use of physical or chemical restraints in nursing facilities. In addition, the FDA has set forth guidelines for the use of restraints (U.S. Department of Health and Human Services, 1992). The statutes provide that restraints may be imposed (1) only to ensure the physical safety of the resident or other residents and (2) only on the written order of a physician that specifies the duration (usually 24 hours) and circumstances under which the restraints are to be used (except in emergency circumstances until such an order could reasonably be obtained). The most frequent indications for restraints are as follows: (1) unanticipated risk of injury to self (falls) or others, (2) interference with treatment, and (3) clinically disruptive or disturbing behavior (Martin, 2002). The nurse must know when and how to use restraints correctly. After a client is restrained, the nurse is required to make frequent client assessments and to periodically release restraints (see Chapter 37). Liability for improper or unlawful restraint, as well as liability for client injury from unprotected falls, lies with the nurse and the health care institution.

State Statutory Issues in Nursing Practice

Licensure

All registered nurses are licensed by the State Board of Nursing of the state in which they practice. The requirements for licensure vary among states, but most states have minimum education requirements and require a licensure examination. All states use the National Council Licensure Examinations (NCLEX® examination) for registered nurse and licensed practical nurse examinations. Licensure permits persons to offer special skills to the public, but it also provides legal guidelines for protection of the public.

A license can be suspended or revoked by the State Board of Nursing if a nurse's conduct violates provisions in the licensing statute based on administrative law rules that implement and enforce the statute. For example, nurses who perform illegal acts such as selling or taking controlled substances jeopardize their license status. Because a license is viewed as a property right, due process must be followed before a license can be suspended or revoked. Due process means that nurses must be notified of the charges brought against them and that the nurses have an opportunity to defend against the charges in a hearing. Hearings for suspension or revocation of a license do not occur in court but are usually conducted by a hearing panel of professionals. Some states provide administrative and judicial review of such cases after nurses have exhausted all other forms of appeal.

Good Samaritan Laws

Nurses may act as Good Samaritans by providing emergency assistance at an accident scene. Good Samaritan laws have been enacted in almost every state to encourage health care professionals to assist in emergency situations (Good Samaritan Law, 1998). These laws limit liability and offer legal immunity for nurses who help at the scene of an accident. They also provide that a nurse can assist a minor in an emergency at the scene of an accident or competitive sports event before obtaining the parent's consent. If a nurse stops at the scene of an automobile accident and gives appropriate emergency care, such as applying pressure to stop hemorrhage, the nurse is acting within accepted standards, even though proper equipment was not available. If the client subsequently develops complications as a result of the nurse's actions, the nurse is immune from liability as long as he or she acted without gross negligence. Nurses should check their own state's Good Samaritan statute, because some states (e.g., Minnesota and Vermont) require nurses to stop and help in an emergency.

Public Health Laws

It is important that nurses, especially those employed in community health settings, understand the public health laws. State legislatures enact statutes under the health code, which describes the reporting laws for communicable diseases, school immunizations, and laws intended to promote health and reduce health risks in communities. The Centers for Disease Control and Prevention (CDC) (http://www.CDC.gov, 2003) and the Occupational Health and Safety Act (OHSA) (http://www.osha.gov, 2003) also provide guidelines on a national level for safe and healthy communities and work environments. The purposes of public health laws are protection of the public's health, advocating for the rights of people, regulating health care and health care financing, and ensuring professional accountability for the care provided. Community health nurses have the legal responsibility to enforce the laws enacted to protect the public's health. These laws may include reporting suspected abuse and neglect, such as child abuse, elder abuse, or domestic violence, reporting communicable diseases, ensuring that required immunizations have been received by clients in the community, and reporting of other health-related issues enacted to protect the public's health.

Every state with child abuse legislation requires that suspected child abuse or neglect must be reported. Health care professionals such as nurses are mandated to report suspected cases. To encourage reports of suspected cases, states provide legal immunity for the reporter if the report is made in good faith. Health care professionals who do not report suspected child abuse or neglect may be held liable for civil or criminal legal action.

As in all areas of nursing practice, negligence involving pediatric clients is possible, and the nurse is responsible for preventing a child in his or her care from accidentally coming to harm. Cribs, which sometimes have a restraining device over the top, are designed to keep infants and toddlers from climbing out of bed and injuring themselves. All poisonous substances and sharp objects should be kept out of the reach of small children. When possible, small children should be kept under constant watch to minimize opportunities for accidental harm.

The Uniform Determination of Death Act

Many legal issues surround the event of death, including a basic definition of the actual point at which a person is considered dead. There are essentially two standards for the determination of death. The cardiopulmonary standard requires irreversible cessation of circulatory and respiratory functions. The whole-brain standard requires irreversible cessation of all functions of the entire brain, including the brain stem. The reason for the development of different definitions is to facilitate recovery of organs for transplantation. Even though the client may be legally

"brain dead," the client's organs may be healthy for donation to other clients. The Uniform Determination of Death Act (1980) has been adopted in most states and provides that either the cardiopulmonary definition or the whole-brain definition may be used to determine death. Nurses must be aware of legal definitions of death because they must document all events that occur when the client is in their care. Nurses have a specific legal obligation to treat the deceased person's remains with dignity (see Chapter 29). Wrongful handling of a deceased person's remains could cause emotional harm to the surviving family.

Consent for an autopsy must have been given previously by the decedent before death or may be given by a close family member at the time of death. In many states there is an order of priority for the giving of consent for autopsies, such as (1) decedent, in writing; (2) durable power of attorney; (3) surviving spouse; and (4) surviving child, parent, brother, or sister in the order named (Autopsy Consent, 1998). It is important to know a client's cultural heritage. In some cultures, the accepted family social hierarchy may differ from what is expected by law (see Chapter 8). Nurses must help clients understand the law and what, if any, options are available. Death is to be reported and investigated by the coroner when there are reasonable grounds to believe that the person died as a result of violence, homicide, suicide, accident, or death occurring in any unusual or suspicious manner. The coroner should be also be contacted if a client's death is unforeseen and sudden and the client has not been seen by a physician in over 36 hours.

Physician-Assisted Suicide

In 1994 the State of Oregon passed the Oregon Death with Dignity Act, which was the first statute that permitted physician-assisted suicide. The statute provided that a competent individual with a terminal disease defined as an "incurable and irreversible disease that has been medically confirmed and will, within reasonable medical judgment, produce death within 6 months" could make an oral and written request for medication to end his or her life in a humane and dignified manner. The written request had to be signed and witnessed by two individuals. The attending physician had to refer the individual to a consulting physician and refer the individual for counseling, if appropriate. The attending physician also had to have the individual notify his or her next of kin and provide information regarding the medication so that an informed decision could be made. There was a 15-day waiting period between the initial oral request and the writing of the prescription and no less than a 48-hour waiting period between the written request and the writing of the prescription. The individual had a right to rescind the request at any time and had to be able to self-administer the medication. Despite efforts by the Oregon state legislature and the U.S. attorney general, the Oregon Death With Dignity Act went into effect in November 1997. However, it remains the object of several challenges in federal court.

In *Compassion in Dying v Washington* (1996) and *Quill v Vacco* (1996), challenges to state statutes that made assisting in suicide a criminal act in Washington and New York, respectively, were filed with the courts. The lower courts both held that the criminal statutes were unconstitutional. The cases were heard by the Supreme Court, and on June 26, 1997, the Supreme Court held in *Washington v Glucksberg* that there is no fundamental constitutional right to assisted suicide. In making its ruling, the Supreme Court did not preclude the states from passing legislation legalizing assisted suicide. The Supreme Court also relied on the fact that there are no legal barriers to obtaining pain medication and that dying persons in Washington and New York could "obtain palliative care, even when doing so would hasten their deaths."

Other states have proposed similar legislation. Legally, nurses must know their State Nurse Practice Act and their state laws regarding physician-assisted suicide. The American Nurses Association has stated that nurses should not participate in assisted suicide because it is an act that violates the Code for Nurses and the ethical traditions of the profession (Coughennower, 2003).

Civil and Common Law Issues in Nursing Practice

Torts

A **tort** is a civil wrong made against a person or property. Torts may be classified as unintentional or intentional. An example of an unintentional tort is negligence or malpractice. **Malpractice** is negligence committed by a professional such as a nurse or physician. **Intentional torts** are willful acts that violate another's rights. Examples are assault, battery, invasion of privacy, and defamation of character.

Intentional Torts

Assault. Assault is any intentional threat to bring about harmful or offensive contact. No actual contact is necessary. The law protects clients who are afraid of harmful contact. It is an assault for a nurse to threaten to give a client an injection or to threaten to restrain a client for an x-ray procedure when the client has refused consent. The key issue is the client's consent. In a lawsuit wherein assault is alleged, the client's consent would bar the claim of assault against a nurse.

Battery. Battery is any intentional touching without consent. The contact can be harmful to the client and cause an injury, or it can be merely offensive to the client's personal dignity. A battery always includes an assault, which is why the terms *assault* and *battery* are commonly combined. In the example of a nurse threatening to give a client an injection without the client's consent, if the nurse actually gives the injection, it is considered battery. Battery can also result if the health care provider performs a procedure that exceeds the client's consent. For example, if the client gives consent for an appendectomy and the physician performs a tonsillectomy, battery has occurred. Once again, the key issue is the client's consent.

In some situations consent is implied. For example, if a client gets into a wheelchair or transfers to a stretcher after being advised that it is time to be taken for an x-ray

procedure, the client has given implied consent to the procedure. If the client learns that an x-ray film of the head instead of the foot is to be taken and the client refuses to have the x-ray film taken, the consent has been revoked or withdrawn.

Invasion of Privacy. The tort of invasion of privacy protects the client's right to be free from unwanted intrusion into his or her private affairs. The four types of invasion of privacy torts are intrusion on seclusion, appropriation of name or likeness, publication of private or embarrassing facts, and publicity placing one in a false light (Prosser and Keeton, 1988).

Clients are entitled to confidential health care. For example, in a classic case, reporters published photographs of a female client in her hospital room without her consent. A claim for invasion of privacy was upheld. This case is an example of intrusion on seclusion or publication of private, embarrassing facts (*Barber v Time Magazine*, 1942).

Another form of invasion of privacy is the release of a client's medical information to an unauthorized person, such as a member of the press or the client's employer. The information that is contained in a client's medical record is a confidential communication. It should be shared with health care providers for the purpose of medical treatment only.

A client's medical record is confidential. The nurse should not disclose the client's confidential medical information without the client's consent. For example, a nurse should respect a wish not to inform the client's family of a terminal illness. Similarly, a nurse should not assume that a client's spouse or family members know all of the client's history, particularly with respect to private issues such as mental illness, medications, pregnancy, abortion, birth control, or sexually transmitted diseases.

An individual's right to privacy may conflict with the public's right to know. In one case a married couple was filmed by a television crew while attending a hospital program in which they participated. The couple had previously told no one but their immediate family that they were involved in the in vitro fertilization program and had been assured that there would be no publicity or public exposure. After the newscast they were subjected to phone calls and embarrassing questions. The couple filed a lawsuit. The court held that the husband and wife stated a claim for invasion of privacy and that even though the in vitro fertilization program may have been of public interest, the identity of the plaintiffs was a private matter (*YG v Jewish Hospital*, 1990).

Many states, through their respective public health departments, require that certain infectious or communicable diseases be reported. Sometimes the client is a public figure whose physical condition is considered newsworthy (Prosser and Keeton, 1988). There are also cases in which information is given out about a scientific discovery or a major medical breakthrough, as with the first heart transplant case or the first artificial heart recipient. If an event falls into any of these categories, information should be channeled through the public relations department of the institution to ensure that invasion of privacy does not occur. The nurse should not independently attempt to decide the legality of disclosing information.

Nursing standards for what constitutes confidential information are based on professional ethics (see Chapter 21) and the common law. The ideals of privacy and sensitivity to the needs and rights of clients who may not choose to have nurses intrude on their lives, but who depend on nurses for their care, guide the nurse's judgment. The nurse's fiduciary duty requires that confidential information not be shared with others.

Defamation of Character. **Defamation of character** is the publication of false statements that result in damage to a person's reputation. The statements must be published with malice in the case of a public official or public figure. **Malice** means that the person publishing the information knows it is false and publishes it anyway or that it is published with reckless disregard as to the truth or falsity of the statement. If the statement is presented orally, it is called **slander.** If the statement is made in writing, it is called **libel.** For example, if a nurse tells people erroneously that a client has venereal disease and the disclosure affects the client's business, the nurse could be held liable for slander.

Unintentional Torts

Negligence. **Negligence** is conduct that falls below the standard of care. The standard of care is established by law for the protection of others against an unreasonably great risk of harm (Black, 1999). For example, if a driver of a car acts unreasonably in failing to stop at a stop sign, it is negligence. In general, courts define negligence in car accident cases and other negligence cases as that degree of care that an ordinarily careful and prudent person would use under the same or similar circumstances (Missouri Approved Instructions, §11.02).

Malpractice. Malpractice is one type of negligence; it is referred to as professional negligence. Nursing malpractice results when nursing care falls below the standard of care. Nurses can be found liable for malpractice if the following criteria are established: (1) the nurse (defendant) owed a duty to the client (plaintiff); (2) the nurse did not carry out that duty; (3) the client was injured; and (4) the nurse's failure to carry out the duty caused the injury. Even though nurses do not intend to injure clients, if nurses give care that does not meet the appropriate standards, they may be held liable for negligence. Negligence may involve failing to check a client's arm band and then administering medication to the wrong client. Negligence may also involve administering a medication to a client even though it has been documented that the client has an allergy to that medication. In general, courts define nursing negligence as the failure to use that degree of skill or learning ordinarily used under the same or similar circumstances by members of the nursing profession (Missouri Approved Instructions, §11.06) (Box 22-2).

The best way for nurses to avoid being liable for negligence is to follow standards of care, give competent health care, communicate with other health care providers, develop a caring rapport with the client, and document assessments, interventions, and evaluations fully. If a nurse is brought into a lawsuit, careful, complete, and thorough documentation is one of the best de-

---

Box 22-2	**Common Negligent Acts**

Medication errors that result in injury to clients
Intravenous therapy errors resulting in infiltrations or phlebitis
Burns to clients caused by equipment, bathing, or spills of hot liquids and foods
Falls resulting in injury to clients
Failure to use aseptic technique where required
Errors in sponge, instrument, or needle counts in surgical cases
Failure to give a report, or giving an incomplete report, to an oncoming shift
Failure to adequately monitor a client's condition
Failure to notify a physician of a significant change in a client's status

---

fenses. Nurses should also know the current nursing literature in their areas of practice. They should know and follow the policies and procedures of the institution in which they work. Nurses should be sensitive to common sources of client injury, such as falls and medication errors. Finally, nurses must communicate with the client, explain the tests and treatment to be performed, document that specific explanations were provided to the client, and listen to the client's concerns about the treatment. Any significant changes in the client's condition must be reported to the physician and documented in the chart (see Chapter 25). Timely and truthful documentation is important to provide the communication necessary among the health care team members. Good documentation also keeps other health care providers up-to-date on the most recent treatments received by the client so that ongoing care can be safely provided. Nurses must be certain that documentation is legible and signed.

A number of courts have stated that when a health care provider negligently alters or loses medical records relevant to a malpractice claim, the health care provider must demonstrate why these events occurred. An institution has a duty to maintain nursing records. These duties are established by statutes and accreditation regulations. Nursing notes contain substantial evidence needed to understand the care received by a client. If records are lost or incomplete, there is a presumption that the care was negligent and therefore the cause of the client's injuries. In addition, incomplete or illegible records undermine the credibility or believability of the health care provider.

Consent

A signed consent form is required for all routine treatment, hazardous procedures such as surgery, some treatment programs such as chemotherapy, and research involving clients (JCAHO, 2003). A client signs general consent forms when admitted to the hospital or other health care facility (Figure 22-1). Separate special consent or treatment forms must be signed by the client or a representative before specialized procedures or treatments are performed.

State statutes provide the designation of individuals who are legally able to give consent to medical treatment (Consent to Surgical or Medical Treatment, 1998). Nurses

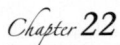

BARNES JEWISH Hospital
BJC HealthCare™

Washington University in St.Louis
SCHOOL OF MEDICINE

AUTHORIZATION FOR MEDICAL TREATMENT AND FINANCIAL RESPONSIBILITY

ADDRESSOGRAPH

1. CONSENT

I authorize my physician and other physicians who may attend me, their associates and assistants, including those employed by the Washington University School of Medicine (hereinafter referred to as "WU"), and Barnes-Jewish Hospital (hereinafter referred to as "Hospital"), its house staff, employees, and students to provide the medical care, tests, procedures, drugs, blood or blood products, services and supplies considered advisable by my physician. These services may include pathology, radiology, emergency services and other special services ordered by my physician(s). In consenting to treatment, I have not relied on any statements as to results. I further authorize my physician or Hospital staff to examine, use, store, and/or dispose of in any manner (except for organ donation and/or transplantation) any bones, organs, tissue, fluids or parts removed from my body.

In the event that any personnel assisting in the provision of care and treatment suffer inadvertent exposure to any of my blood and/or other bodily substances, that are capable of transmitting disease, and I am unable to consult timely with my physician prior to testing, I consent to limited testing to determine the presence, if any, of antibodies to hepatitis A, B, and C and HIV.

2. STORAGE AND RELEASE OF INFORMATION

I consent to the electronic storage and transmission of patient health information. I hereby authorize my treating physician, WU and Hospital and its affiliates, to release by electronic means or otherwise any medical and/or billing information concerning my care, including copies of my medical records, to the following:

   a. Any governmental or other entity as required by law for purposes of reporting, or for purposes of determining eligibility in goverment sponsored benefit programs.

   b. The supplier of any blood or blood products which may be administered to me for the purposes of quality control and recipient monitoring.

   c. Any continuing care, residential, or long-term care facility, or home health agency for the purpose of providing services for my care.

3. PERSONAL VALUABLES

The Hospital provides facilities that may be used for the safekeeping of money, valuables or other personal effects. If I choose not to use those facilities, I understand that I assume all responsibility for the loss of, damage to, any money, valuables or other personal effects during my stay. For the safety of its patients, the Hospital does not permit patients to use personal electrical appliances, battery chargers or converters for battery operated appliances during hospitalization. Battery operated personal appliances may be used. I understand that I assume all responsibility for any injuries or losses which may occur as a result of the unauthorized use of personal electrical appliances, battery chargers or converters for battery operated appliances.

4. IN PATIENT ROOM TELEVISION SERVICE

Standard network TV programming is available free of charge in all patient rooms. Premium Cable Channels are available for a daily fee. By choosing the cable TV service on my TV, I hereby release my name, address and telephone number to an authorized CCTV (Healthcare Cable Systems, Inc.) billing agent who will bill me for the cable service I used.

5. MEDICARE/TRICARE INSURANCE BENEFITS

I certify that the information given by me in applying for payment under Title XVIII of the Social Security Act is correct. I authorize the release of medical or other information to the Medicare Program or its Intermediaries or carriers concerning this or a related claim filed by the Hospital or WU. I request that payment of authorized benefits be made on my behalf. I understand that I am responsible for the Part A and Part B deductible for each year and/or visit, the remaining co-insurance and any other non-covered personal charges. I hereby acknowledge receipt of the Medicare/Tricare letter entitled "An Important Message from Medicare/Tricare" which is included in my Patient Binder.

I (or my representative) certify(ies) that I or he/she has read (or if the patient/representative is unable to read has had the form read to him/her) and understand(s), accept(s) the above and further certify(ies) that I am the patient, or am duly authorized on behalf of the patient to execute such an agreement.

6. PHOTOGRAPHS, FILM OR VIDEO TAPE

I hereby authorize Hospital or WU to photograph, film, and/or video tape me and to use such photographs, films or video tapes for treatment and/or instructional purposes.

7. GUARANTEE FOR PAYMENT

In accordance with the above terms and in consideration of the services provided to the above-named patient by WU and/or the Hospital, the undersigned agrees, whether he/she signs as patient or guarantor, to pay WU, physicians and the Hospital for all services ordered by the attending physician, or requested by the patient and the patient's family. If the requirements for referral, second opinion or pre-certification of care, as outlined by my insurer, benefit plan or other payer, have not been followed, the patient and/or guarantor may in some instances be personally responsible for all charges incurred.

8. ASSIGNMENT OF INSURANCE BENEFITS

In consideration of any and all medical services, care, drugs, supplies, equipment and facilities furnished by WU, all attending physicians and the Hospital, I authorize direct payment to WU and/or the Hospital of all insurance benefits applicable to these medical services, which are now or which shall become due and payable to me. In addition, I hereby authorize payment to the Hospital of all applicable insurance benefits for medical and/or surgical services rendered by physicians for whom the Hospital is authorized to bill and collect.

   HIPAA - NOTICE OF PRIVACY PRACTICES ACKNOWLEDGEMENT

     I acknowledge that I have received or I have been provided the opportunity to receive a copy of the "Notice of Privacy Practices" that explains when, where, and why my confidential health information may be used or shared. I acknowledge that Hospital, WU, the physicians, the nurses and other Hospital and WU staff may use and share my confidential health information with others in order to treat me, in order to arrange for payment of my bill and for issues that concern Hospital or WU operations and responsibilities.

     Initials of patient or person authorized to sign for patient. ☐

Signature of patient or person authorized to consent	Date	Patient's relationship to person
Signature of Guarantor	Date	Patient's Relationship to Guarantor
Signature of Witness	Date	

2120-02 V5 (03/03) Page 1 of 1 TAB: MANAGEMENT   **DO NOT WRITE BELOW THIS LINE**

2120-02

FIGURE 22–1   Sample consent form for admission to the hospital. (Courtesy Barnes-Jewish Hospital, St. Louis, Mo.)

should know the law in their own states and be familiar with the policies and procedures of their employing institution regarding consent (Box 22-3).

If a client is deaf, illiterate, or speaks a foreign language, an official interpreter must be available to explain the terms of consent. A family member or acquaintance that is able to speak a client's language should not be used to interpret health information. A client under the effects of a sedative is not able to clearly understand the implications of an invasive procedure. Every effort should be made to assist the client in making an informed choice.

Nurses must be sensitive to the cultural issues of consent. The nurse must understand the way in which clients and their families communicate and make important de-

---

Box 22-3   Statutory Guidelines for Legal Consent for Medical Treatment

Those who may consent to medical treatment are governed by state law but generally include the following:

I. Adults
  A. Any competent individual 18 years of age or older for himself or herself
  B. Any parent for his or her unemancipated minor
  C. Any guardian for his or her ward
  D. Any adult for the treatment of his or her minor brother or sister (if an emergency and parents are not present)
  E. Any grandparent for a minor grandchild (if an emergency and parents are not present)

II. Minors
  A. For his or her child and any child in his or her legal custody
  B. For himself or herself in the following situations:
    1. Lawfully married or a parent (emancipated)
    2. Pregnancy (excluding abortions)
    3. Venereal disease
    4. Drug or substance abuse
  C. Unemancipated minors may not consent to abortions without one of the following:
    1. Consent of one parent
    2. Self-consent being granted by court order
    3. Consent specifically given by a court

---

cisions. It is essential for nurses to understand the various cultures with which they interact. The cultural beliefs and values of the client may be very different from those of the nurse. It is important for nurses not to impose their own cultural values on the client. Insensitivity toward and stereotyping of different ethnic groups are of equal concern. A conscious awareness of the different values and beliefs held by various cultures is essential for sensitive nursing care (see Chapter 8).

Informed Consent. Informed consent is a person's agreement to allow something to happen, such as surgery or an invasive diagnostic procedure, based on a full disclosure of risks, benefits, alternatives, and consequences of refusal (Black, 1999). Informed consent creates a legal duty for the physician and/or health care provider to disclose material facts in terms the client can reasonably understand to make an informed choice (Guido, 2001). The explanation should also describe treatment alternatives, as well as the risks involved in all treatment options. Failure to obtain consent in situations other than emergencies may result in a claim of battery. Without informed consent, a client may bring a lawsuit against the health care provider for negligence. Informed consent requires providing adequate information for the client to form a decision and documenting that decision.

The following factors are required for informed consent (Guido, 2001):

1. A brief, complete explanation of the procedure or treatment must be given.

2. Names and qualifications of persons performing and assisting in the procedure should be provided.

3. A description of the serious harm, including death, which may occur as a result of the procedure, as well as anticipated pain and/or discomfort, should be provided.

4. An explanation of alternative therapies to the proposed procedure/treatment should be provided, as well as the risks of doing nothing.

5. The client needs to be informed of his or her right to refuse the procedure/treatment without discontinuing other supportive care.

6. The client may refuse the procedure/treatment even after the procedure has begun.

Informed consent is part of the physician-client relationship. Because nurses do not perform surgery or direct medical procedures, in most situations, obtaining clients' informed consent does not fall within the nursing duty. Even though the nurse assumes the responsibility for witnessing the client's signature on the consent form, the nurse does not legally assume the duty of obtaining informed consent (Figure 22-2). The nurse's signature witnessing the consent means that the client voluntarily gave consent, that the client's signature is authentic, and that the client appears to be competent to give consent (Sullivan, 1998). When nurses provide consent forms for clients to sign, the clients should be asked if they understand the procedures for which consent is being given. If clients deny understanding or the nurse suspects they do not understand, the nurse must notify the physician or nursing supervisor and must make certain that clients are informed before signing. Some consent forms also have a line for the physician to sign after explaining the risks and alternatives to a client. Such a form is helpful in a court case when a client alleges that consent was not informed. A client refusing surgery or other medical treatment must be informed about any harmful consequences of refusal. If the client persists in refusing the treatment, this rejection should be written, signed, and witnessed.

If a client participates in an experimental treatment program or submits to use of experimental drugs or treatments, an even more detailed and stringently regulated informed consent form is used. The Food and Drug Administration (FDA) and an organization's institutional review board (IRB) review the information in the consent form for research involving human subjects. The client may withdraw from the experiment at any time (see Chapter 25).

Parents are usually the legal guardians of pediatric clients, and therefore they are the persons who must sign consent forms for treatment. If the parents are divorced, the parent with legal custody must give consent. Occasionally a parent or guardian refuses treatment for a child. In those cases the court may intervene on the child's behalf.

In some instances obtaining informed consent is difficult. If, for example, the client is unconscious, consent must be obtained from a person legally authorized to give consent on the client's behalf. Other surrogate decision makers may have legally been delegated this authority through special process of attorney documents or through court guardianship procedures. In emergency

---

INFORMED CONSENT FOR AMNIOCENTESIS

I.   I hereby request and authorize Doctor _____ to perform a
     diagnostic amniocentesis (pass a needle through the abdominal wall and withdraw
     some of the amniotic fluid). I further request that an attempt be made to perform the
     following test(s) on my unborn child:

          A. Chromosome analysis _____ (Initial)
          B. Alpha-fetoprotein _____ (Initial)
          C. Acetylcholinesterase _____ (Initial)
             (if indicated)
          D. _____ (Initial)

II. I consent to the performance of an ultrasound examination for the purpose of dating
     the pregnancy, locating the placenta and selecting a site for placement of the needle.

III. I understand that:

          A. the procedure of amniocentesis involves a small risk to both mother and fetus
          and that these risks include; discomfort at the site where the needle was inserted,
          cramping, bloody spotting, leakage of amniotic fluid, intrauterine infection and
          miscarriage.

          B. there is a possibility that growing the fetal cells may not be successful and that
          repeat amniocentesis would then be required.

          C. although the likelihood of an error is considered to be extremely small, a
          complete and correct diagnosis of the condition of the fetus based on the test(s)
          performed cannot be guaranteed.

          D. the results provided of normal chromosomes or normal biochemical status of
          the fetus does not eliminate the possibility that the child may have birth defects
          and/or mental retardation because of other disorders.

          E. in the case of twins, the results may apply to only one of the pair.

          F. in some Rh negative mothers Rh sensitization has occurred following amnio-
          centesis.

IV. I have had my questions answered and understand and accept the risks and limitations
     of this test.

Signed: _____ (Patient)

          _____ (Spouse)

          _____ (Witness)

          Date: _____

FIGURE **22–2**   Sample consent form for a special procedure.

situations, if it is impossible to obtain consent from the client or an authorized person, the procedure required to benefit the client or save a life may be undertaken without liability for failure to obtain consent. In such cases the law assumes that the client would wish to be treated.

Psychiatric clients must also give consent. They retain the right to refuse treatment until a court has legally determined that they are incompetent to decide for themselves.

Abortion Issues

In 1973 in the case of *Roe v Wade*, the U.S. Supreme Court ruled that there is a fundamental right to privacy, which includes a woman's decision to have an abortion. The court ruled that during the first trimester a woman could end her pregnancy without state regulation because the risk of natural mortality from abortion is less than with normal childbirth. During the second trimester the state has an interest in protecting maternal health, and the state may enforce regulations regarding the person performing the abortion and the abortion facility. By the third trimester, when the fetus becomes viable, the state's interest is to protect the fetus, so the state can therefore prohibit abortion except when necessary to save the mother.

In 1989 in the case of *Webster v Reproductive Health Services*, the court substantially narrowed the *Roe v Wade* case. States may require viability tests before conducting abortions if the fetus is thought to be over 28 weeks' gestational age. States may also require a minor's parental consent or a judicial decision that the minor is mature and can self-consent.

In the case of *Planned Parenthood of Southeastern Pennsylvania v Casey* (1992), informed consent was upheld in that the physician must present the woman with a description of the nature of the abortion procedure, the health risk related to abortion and childbirth, the probable gestational age of the fetus, and the availability of state-published material about medical assistance, adoption agencies, and child support from the father. The court also upheld a mandatory 24-hour waiting period between when the materials are provided to the client and when the abortion is performed. An emancipated minor must get informed consent of one parent or a judicial determination that the minor is mature and can give her own informed consent.

Student Nurses

Student nurses are liable if their actions cause harm to clients. If a client is harmed as a direct result of a nursing student's actions or lack of action, the liability for the incorrect action is generally shared by the student, instructor, hospital or health care facility, and university or educational institution. Student nurses should never be assigned to perform tasks for which they are unprepared, and they should be carefully supervised by instructors as they learn new skills. Although student nurses may not be considered employees of the hospital, the institution has a responsibility to monitor the acts of student nurses. Student nurses are expected to perform as professional nurses would in providing safe client care. Faculty members are usually responsible for instructing and observing students, but in some situations staff nurses serving as preceptors may share these responsibilities. Every nursing school should provide clear definitions of preceptor and faculty responsibility.

When students are employed as nursing assistants or nurses' aides when not attending classes, they should not perform tasks that do not appear in a job description for a nurses' aide or assistant. For example, even if a student has learned to administer intramuscular medications in class, this task may not be performed by a nurse's aide. If a staff nurse overseeing the nursing assistant or aide knowingly assigns work without regard for the person's ability to safely conduct the task defined in the job description, the staff nurse will also be liable. If students employed as nurse's aides are requested to perform tasks that they are not prepared to safely complete, this information should be brought to the supervisor's attention so that the needed help can be obtained.

Malpractice Insurance

Malpractice or professional liability insurance is a contract between the nurse and the insurance company. Malpractice insurance provides for a defense when a nurse is sued for professional negligence or medical malpractice. As part of the insurance contract, the insurance company pays for any judgment or settlement of the case and also pays for the attorney's fees generated in the representation of the nurse. Nurses employed by health care institutions generally are covered by that institution's insurance and do not need to purchase any supplemental insurance unless the nurse plans to practice nursing outside of the employing institution. The employing institution's insurance, however, only covers nurses while they are working within the scope of their employment. Because nurses are professionals and it is often difficult to separate their private lives from their professional skills, they should consider purchasing individual professional liability insurance, even if the employing institution has coverage. A nurse who is called on by neighbors and friends to provide nursing care on a volunteer basis would not be covered by the hospital's policy if the neighbor or friend filed suit.

Nurses should consult their lawyers on what types of policies to purchase and what rights or duties, if any, exist under the policy. If the employing institution and the nurse are sued in a professional liability case, even though the nurse has insurance with the hospital, the nurse should notify his or her private insurance carrier of the lawsuit. If both the hospital policy and the private policy are considered primary and the hospital loses as a result of the nurse's acts, theoretically the hospital could sue the nurse's private insurer to recover its losses. Most private insurance policies for nurses, however, are considered excess policies and only begin covering the nurse after all of the primary (hospital) insurance coverage has been exhausted. Because the hospital insurance coverage is generally much greater than the private insurance coverage, hospitals very rarely sue nurses' private insurers.

Abandonment and Assignment Issues

Short Staffing. During nursing shortages or staff downsizing periods, the issue of inadequate staffing may arise. The JCAHO (2003) requires institutions to have guidelines for determining the number (staffing ratios) of nurses required to give care to a specific number of clients. Legal problems may arise if there are not enough nurses to provide competent care. If nurses are assigned to care for more clients than is reasonable, they should bring this information to the attention of the nursing supervisor. If nurses are required to accept assignments, they should make written protests to nursing administrators. Although these protests may not relieve nurses of responsibility if a client suffers an injury because of inattention, it would show that the nurses were attempting to act reasonably. Whenever a written protest is made, nurses should keep a copy of this document in their own personal file. Most administrators recognize that knowledge of a potential problem shifts some of the responsibility to the institution. Nurses should not walk out when staffing is inadequate, because charges of abandonment could be made. A nurse who refuses to accept an assignment may be considered insubordinate and clients will not benefit from having even less staff available. It is important to know the institution's policies and procedures on how to handle such reports before the situation arises (Mrayyan, 2003).

Floating. Nurses are sometimes required to "float" from the area in which they normally practice to other nursing units. In one case a nurse in obstetrics was assigned to an emergency department. A client entered the emergency department and complained of chest pain. The client was given an incorrect dosage of lidocaine by the obstetrical nurse and died after suffering irreversible brain damage and cardiac arrest. The nurse lost the malpractice lawsuit. Nurses who float should inform the supervisor of any lack of experience in caring for the type of clients on the nursing unit. They should also request and be given orientation to the unit. A supervisor can be held liable if a staff nurse is given an assignment he or she cannot safely handle. In the case of *Winkelman v Beloit Memorial Hospital* (1992), the court remarked that if an employer wishes to rotate nurses to areas outside of their usual area of expertise, the employer should provide the training and education to prepare nurses to work in an area outside of their normal assignment. Before accepting employment, nurses should find out the institution's policies regarding floating and have an understanding as to what is expected. For example, nurses should not be floated to areas where they have not been adequately cross-trained.

Physicians' Orders. The physician is responsible for directing medical treatment. Nurses are obligated to follow physicians' orders unless they believe the orders are in error or would harm clients. Therefore all orders must be assessed, and if one is found to be erroneous or harmful, further clarification from the physician is necessary. If the physician confirms the order and the nurse still believes it is inappropriate, the supervising nurse should be informed. A nurse should not proceed to perform a physician's order if it is foreseeable that harm will come to the client. The nursing supervisor should be informed and given a written memorandum detailing the events in chronological order; the reasons for refusing to carry out the order should also be written to protect the nurse from disciplinary action. The supervising nurse should help resolve the questionable order. A medical consultant may be called in to help clarify the appropriateness or inappropriateness of the order. A nurse carrying out an inaccurate or inappropriate order may be legally responsible for any harm suffered by the client.

In a malpractice lawsuit against a physician and a hospital, one of the most frequently litigated issues is whether the nurse kept the physician informed of the client's condition. To inform a physician properly, nurses must perform a competent nursing assessment of the client to determine the signs and symptoms that are significant in relation to the attending physician's tasks of diagnosis and treatment. Nurses must be certain to document that the physician was notified and document his or her response, the nurse's follow-up, and the client's response.

The physician should write all orders, and the nurse must make sure that they are transcribed correctly. Verbal orders are not recommended because they increase the possibilities for error. If a verbal order is necessary (e.g., during an emergency), it should be written and signed by the physician as soon as possible, usually within 24 hours. The nurse should be familiar with the institution's policy and procedures regarding verbal orders.

Risk Management

Risk management is a system of ensuring appropriate nursing care that attempts to identify potential hazards and eliminate them before harm occurs (Guido, 2001). The steps involved in risk management include identifying possible risks, analyzing them, acting to reduce the risks, and evaluating the steps taken. One tool used in risk management is the **incident report** or **occurrence report.**

Risk management also requires good documentation. The nurse's documentation can be the evidence of what actually was done for a client and can serve as proof that the nurse acted reasonably and safely. Documentation should be thorough, accurate, and performed in a timely manner (see Chapter 25). To protect the nurse and the client, the nurse should document the care given and the details associated with it (Guido, 2001). Charting the statement "physician notified" may be insufficient if at the time the nurse is being questioned about the lawsuit, he or she does not recall which physician and what specific facts were told to the physician. When a lawsuit is filed, very often the nurse's notes are the first thing reviewed by an attorney. The nurse's assessments and the reporting of significant changes in the assessments are very important factors in defending a lawsuit. Therefore the nurse should identify the physician contacted, the information communicated to the physician, and the physician's response.

For nurses in practice, the underlying rationale for quality improvement and risk management programs is the highest possible quality of care. Some insurance companies, medical and nursing organizations, and the JCAHO require the use of quality improvement and risk management procedures (JCAHO, 2003).

One area of potential risk is associated with the use of electronic monitoring devices. No monitor is totally reliable, and the nurse must not completely depend on it. Therefore the nurse's continual assessment of a client is necessary to help document the accuracy of electronic monitoring. There may also be electrical hazards to the nurse and the client. The equipment should be checked routinely by biomedical engineers to ensure that it is in proper working order and to make sure that a client will not receive an electrical shock.

In the operating room, sponge, needle, and instrument counts are routine surgical standards to prevent client injury and lawsuits. Even though it is the physician who inserts sponges and instruments into the surgical wound, the physician relies on the nurse's counts at the end of the procedure. Generally, when the chart records a correct sponge count and the client suffers an injury because of a retained sponge, the hospital is liable because the nurse charted a correct count when it was not correct.

Every piece of equipment must be carefully used to prevent injury to the client. There can also be liability for nurses because of incorrect positioning or insufficient padding placed when positioning the client. All nurses need to be risk managers.

Professional Involvement

Nurses must be involved in their professional organizations and on committees that define the standards of care for nursing practice. If current laws, rules and regulations, or policies under which nurses must practice do not reflect reality, nurses must become involved as advocates to see that the scope of nursing practice is accurately defined. Nurses must be willing to represent nursing and the client's perspective in the community as well. The voice of nursing can be powerful and effective when the organizing focus is the protection and welfare of the public entrusted to their care.

Key Concepts

- Registered nurses and licensed practical nurses are licensed by the state in which they practice; licensing is based on educational requirements, the passing of an examination, and other criteria.
- The civil law system is concerned with the protection of a person's private rights, and the criminal law system deals with the rights of individuals and society as defined by legislative statutes.
- A nurse can be found liable for malpractice if the following criteria are established: the nurse (defendant) owed a duty to the client (plaintiff), the nurse did not carry out that duty, the client was injured, and the nurse's failure to carry out the duty caused the client's injury.
- All clients are entitled to confidential health care and freedom from unauthorized release of information.
- Under the law, practicing nurses must follow standards of care, which originate in Nurse Practice Acts, the guidelines of professional organizations, and the written policies and procedures of employing institutions.
- Nurses are responsible for confirming that informed consent has been given for any surgery or other medical procedure before the procedure is performed.
- Nurses are responsible for performing all procedures correctly and exercising professional judgment as they carry out physicians' orders.
- Nurses are obligated to follow physicians' orders unless they believe the orders are in error or could be detrimental to clients.
- Staffing standards determine the ratio of nurses to clients, and if the nurse is required to care for more clients than is reasonable, a formal protest should be made to the nursing administration.
- Legal issues involving death include documenting all events surrounding the death, treating a deceased person with dignity, and obtaining consent for an autopsy from the decedent (before death) or a close family member (after death).
- A competent adult can legally give consent to donate specific organs, and nurses may serve as witnesses to this decision.
- All nurses should know the laws that apply to their area of practice.
- Depending on state laws, nurses are required to report possible criminal activities such as child abuse, as well as certain communicable diseases.
- Nurses are client advocates and ensure quality of care through risk management and lobbying for safe nursing practice standards.
- Nurses must file incident/occurrence reports in all situations when someone could or did get hurt.

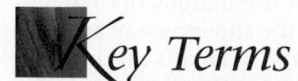

Key Terms

Administrative law, *p. 407*	Living wills, *p. 409*
Assault, *p. 413*	Malice, *p. 414*
Battery, *p. 413*	Malpractice, *p. 413*
Civil laws, *p. 407*	Misdemeanor, *p. 407*
Common law, *p. 407*	Negligence, *p. 414*
Crimes, *p. 407*	Nurse Practice Acts, *p. 406*
Criminal laws, *p. 407*	Occurrence report, *p. 419*
Defamation of character,	Regulatory law, *p. 407*
p. 414	Risk management, *p. 419*
Felony, *p. 407*	Slander, *p. 414*
Incident report, *p. 419*	Standards of care, *p. 407*
Informed consent, *p. 416*	Statutory law, *p. 406*
Intentional torts, *p. 413*	Tort, *p. 413*
Libel, *p. 414*	

Critical Thinking Exercises

1. Nurse Smith and Nurse Jones are getting on an elevator to go down to the cafeteria. There are several visitors present in the elevator, as well as hospital personnel. Nurse Smith and Nurse Jones are talking about a client who is in the intensive care unit who has just tested positive for HIV. They identify the client as the man in Room 14B. One of the visitors on the elevator who overhears this information is a woman who is engaged to the client in Room 14B.
   a. Have Nurse Smith and Nurse Jones breached a client's right to confidential health care?
   b. Will the client in Room 14B have any legal cause of action against the nurses?
   c. Even though the client's fiancée may have a right to know the HIV status of her future husband, is there any duty on the part of the nurses to disclose confidential information to the fiancée?
2. While transporting a client down the hall on a stretcher, Nurse Black stops to chat with an orderly. The side rails on the stretcher are down, and while Nurse Black has her back to the stretcher, the client rolls over, falls off the stretcher, and fractures his hip. In a lawsuit by the client against Nurse Black, what must the client establish to prove negligence against the nurse?
3. Sally Green, a 16-year-old girl, is the mother of a newborn baby. While driving in her car, without having her newborn baby in an appropriate infant car seat, Sally Green has a car accident. Her newborn baby suffers a head injury. Physicians tell Sally Green that her baby has suffered severe brain damage and that she cannot be maintained without life support. They request her consent to have the baby's organs donated for transplant.
   a. Because Sally Green is a minor, is she able to give consent?
   b. Does the hospital have any duty to report Sally Green to the Division of Family Services for failure to have her child in a protective seat?

c. If Baby Green should suffer a cardiac arrest, can the nurses and doctors perform CPR on the baby without consent?

Review Questions

1. The Nurse Practice Acts are an example of:
   1. Statutory law.
   2. Common law.
   3. Civil law.
   4. Criminal law.

2. The scope of nursing practice, the established educational requirements for nurses, and the distinction between nursing and medical practice is defined by:
   1. Statutory law.
   2. Common law.
   3. Civil laws.
   4. Nurse practice acts.

3. The client's right to refuse treatment is an example of:
   1. Statutory law.
   2. Common law.
   3. Civil laws.
   4. Nurse practice acts.

4. The most common sources of client injury are:
   1. Decubitus ulcers.
   2. Burns from hot liquids.
   3. Transfer from bed to cart.
   4. Medication errors and falls.

5. This act allows an individual who is at least 18 years of age to may make an anatomical gift or organ donation.
   1. Mental Health Parity Act.
   2. Advances directives.
   3. Uniform Anatomical Gift Act.
   4. Living wills.

6. When the nurse stops to help in an emergency at the scene of an accident, if the injured party files suit and the nurse's employing institution's insurance does not cover the nurse, the nurse would probably be covered by:
   1. The nurse's automobile insurance.
   2. The nurse's homeowner's insurance.
   3. The Patient Care Partnership, which may grant immunity from suit if the injured party consents.
   4. The Good Samaritan laws, which grant immunity from suit if there is no gross negligence.

7. The legal definition of death that facilitates organ donation is cessation of:
   1. Pulse.
   2. Respirations.
   3. Functions of entire brain.
   4. Circulatory and respiratory functions.

8. Even though the nurse may obtain the client's signature on a form, obtaining informed consent is the responsibility of the:
   1. Client.
   2. Physician.
   3. Student nurse.
   4. Supervising nurse.

9. The nurse's malpractice insurance covers the nurse for incidents that occur:
   1. At the nurse's home.
   2. While the nurse is driving to work.
   3. When the nursing is driving home from work.
   4. While the nurse is working within the scope of his employment.

10. The nurse is obligated to follow a physician's order unless:
    1. The order is a verbal order.
    2. The physician's order is illegible.
    3. The order has not been transcribed.
    4. The order is in error, violates hospital policy, or would be detrimental to the client.

References

Black HC: *Black's law dictionary,* ed 7, St. Paul, Minnesota, 1999, West Publishing.

Burns J and others: Do-not-resuscitate order after 25 years, *Crit Care Med* 31(5):1543, 2003.

Coughennower M: Physician-assisted suicide, *Gastroenterol Nurs* 26(2):55, 2003.

Furrow B and others: *Health law cases, materials and problems,* ed 2, St. Paul, 1991, West Publishing.

Guido G: *Legal and ethical issues in nursing,* ed 3, Upper Saddle River, NJ, 2001, Prentice Hall.

Joint Commission on Accreditation of Healthcare Organizations: *Hospital accreditation standards,* Oakbrook Terrace, Ill, 2003, The Commission.

Laughlin S: Nurse immunity from liability, protection under the ADA, *J Nurs Law* 8(3):39, 2002.

Lueckenotte A: *Gerontologic nursing,* ed 2, St. Louis, 2000, Mosby.

Manson P: Nurse is expert on victim behavior, 2002, *Chicago Daily Law Bulletin,* http://web.lexis-nexis.com/universe/docu.

Martin B: Restraint use in acute and critical care settings: changing practice, *AACN Clin Issues,* 13(2):294, 2002.

Missouri Approved Instructions: *Definition: negligence of adult,* §11.02.

Missouri Approved Instructions: *Definition: negligence of health care providers,* §11.06.

Mrayyan M, Huber D: The nurse's role in changing health policy related to patient safety, *JONAS Healthc Law Ethics Regul* 5(1):13, 2003.

Prosser W, Keeton W: *Prosser and Keeton on the law of torts,* ed 5, St. Paul, 1988, West Publishing.

Rosati K: HIPAA privacy: the compliance challenges ahead, *J Health Law* 35(1):45, 2002.

Scanlon C: Ethical concerns in end-of-life care: when questions about advance directives and the withdrawal of life-sustaining interventions arise, how should decisions be made? *Am J Nurs* 103(1):48, 2003.

Sheehan J: Delegating to UAPs: a practical guide, *RN* 64(11):65, 2001.

Sullivan G: Getting informed consent: role of nurses in obtaining informed consent from patients, *RN* 61(4):59, 1998.

U.S. Department of Health and Human Services, Food and Drug Administration: *Safety alert,* Rockville, Md, 1992, The Department.

Vernaglia L: Responses to questions commonly asked about health law, *JONA'S Healthcare Law Ethics Reg* 4(1):6, 2002.

Statutes

Americans With Disabilities Act (ADA), 42 USC §§121.010-12213 (1995).

Autopsy Consent, Mo Rev Stat §194.115 (1998).

Consent to Surgical or Medical Treatment, Mo Rev Stat §431.061 (1998).

Emergency Medical Treatment and Active Labor Act (EMTALA), 42 USC §1395 (dd) (1986).

Good Samaritan Law, Mo Rev Stat §537.037 (1998).

Health Insurance Portability and Accountability Act of 1996 (HIPAA), Public Law No. 104 (1996).

Illinois Nursing Practice Act (1997).

Mental Health Parity Act of 1996, 29 USC §1885 (1996).

National Organ Transplant Act, Public Law 98–507 (1984).

New York DNR Statute, NY Public Health Laws §2962 (1988).

Occupational Health and Safety Act (2003).

Oregon Death With Dignity Act, Ore Rev Stat §§127.800–127.897 (1994).

Patient Self-Determination Act, 42 CFR 417 (1991).

Resident's Rights, Medicaid Statute, 42 USCA §1396R (1988).

Uniform Anatomical Gift Act (1987).

Uniform Determination of Death Act (1980).

Cases

Barber v Time Magazine, 159 SW2d 291 (1942).

Bouvia v Superior Court, 225 Cal Rptr 297 (1986).

Bragdon v Abbott, 524 U.S. 624 (1998).

Compassion in Dying v Washington, 79 F3d 790 (9th Cir 1996).

Cruzan v Director Missouri Department of Health, 497 U.S. 261 (1990).

Darling v Charleston Community Memorial Hospital, 33 Ill 2d 326 (Ill 1966).

Planned Parenthood of Southeastern Pennsylvania v Casey, 505 U.S. 883 (1992).

Quijano v. United States, No. 02-50095 (5th Cir 2003).

Quill v Vacco, 80 F3d 716 (2nd Cir 1996).

Roe v Wade, 410 U.S. 113 (1973).

Washington v Glucksberg, 521 U.S. 702 (1997).

Webster v Reproductive Health Services, 492 U.S. 490 (1989).

Winkelman v Beloit Memorial Hospital, 484 NW2d 211 (W 1992).

YG v Jewish Hospital, 795 SW2d 488 (Mo App 1990).

23

Communication

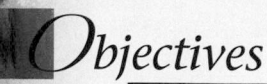

Objectives

Mastery of content in this chapter will enable the student to:

- Define the key terms listed.
- Describe aspects of critical thinking that are important to the communication process.
- Describe the five levels of communication and their uses in nursing.
- Describe the basic elements of the communication process.
- Identify significant features and therapeutic outcomes of nurse-client helping relationships.
- List nursing focus areas within the four phases of a nurse-client helping relationship.
- Identify significant features and desired outcomes of nurse–health team member relationships.
- Describe qualities, behaviors, and communication techniques that affect professional communication.
- Discuss effective communication techniques for clients at various developmental levels.
- Identify client health states that contribute to impaired communication.
- Discuss nursing care measures for clients with special communication needs.

Communication and Nursing Practice

Communication is a lifelong learning process for the nurse. Nurses make the intimate journey with clients and their families from the miracle of birth to the mystery of death. It is necessary to build therapeutic communications for this journey. Nurses communicate with people under stress: clients, families, and colleagues. Nurses function as client advocates and as members of interdisciplinary teams who may have different ideas about priorities for care. In addition, nurses must be assertive to ask the right questions and make their voices heard. Being assertive to communicate one's own needs ensures balance in a nurse's life. Without such balance, the high-stress environment may contribute to burnout and diminish the nurse's effectiveness (Balzer Riley, 2000).

Despite the complexity of technology and the multiple demands on nurses' time, it is the intimate moment of connection that makes all the difference in the quality of care and meaning for the client and the nurse. As nurses refine their communication skills and increase their confidence, they can progress professionally to become experts (Balzer Riley, 2000).

Nurses interact with many persons in the course of their profession. Competency in communication helps the nurse maintain effective relationships within the entire sphere of professional practice and helps meet legal, ethical, and clinical standards of care. Failure to effectively communicate causes serious difficulty, increases liability, and threatens professional credibility.

The qualities, behaviors, and therapeutic communication techniques described in this chapter characterize professionalism in helping relationships. Although the term *client* is often used, the same principles can be applied when communicating with any person, in any nursing situation.

Communication and Interpersonal Relationships

At the core of nursing are caring relationships formed between the nurse and those affected by the nurse's practice (see Chapter 7). Communication is the means to establish these helping-healing relationships. All behavior communicates, and all communication influences behavior. Communication is essential to the nurse-client relationship for the following reasons:

- It is the vehicle for establishing a therapeutic relationship.
- It is the means by which an individual influences the behavior of another, which leads to the successful outcome of nursing interventions.

Nurses with expertise in communication express caring by becoming sensitive to self and others, promoting and accepting the expression of positive and negative feelings, and developing helping-trust relationships. Caring is also demonstrated by instilling faith and hope, promoting interpersonal teaching and learning, providing a supportive environment, assisting with gratification of human needs, and allowing for spiritual expression (Watson, 1995).

The nurse's ability to relate to others is a very important aspect of interpersonal communication. This includes the nurse's ability to take initiative in establishing and maintaining communication, to be authentic (one's self), and to respond appropriately to the other person. Good interpersonal communication also requires the nurse to develop a sense of mutuality, a belief that the nurse-client relationship is a partnership and that both are equal participants. Nurses must honor the fact that people can be very complex and ambiguous. There is often more communicated than first meets the eye, and client responses are not always what the nurse might expect. It is very helpful for the nurse to purposefully focus on positive intentions for the other person and to use the technique of reimagining a possible future (Hartrick, 1997) so that a vision of hope and better health can be shared. For example, a client who's had a heart attack can be encouraged to set the intention for improved health through choosing healthy behaviors such as stress-reducing activities, an exercise regimen, and improved dietary habits.

A new perspective of human relationships suggests energy fields that permeate and connect everything to each other. Although the idea of using energy for healing has recently reemerged in the West, it has long been present in Eastern cultures. Healers in Eastern and primitive cultures treated their clients holistically and focused on the concept of a vital energy within each human being that must be maintained in balance to maintain health (Minor, 2001). Considering these principles, it is not sur-

prising that nurses often perceive the strong sense of connection to others that occurs within a helping relationship. Nurses know that attitudes and emotions are easily transmitted. Most nurses embrace the profession's view of the holistic nature of people and have experienced synergy in human interaction when client and nurse together accomplish much more than either can alone.

Accepting that humans are energy-based beings means that nurses of the twenty-first century must look at communication in new ways. All communication contains stimuli with the potential to influence others (Curtis, Floyd, and Winsor, 1997). Like any powerful therapeutic agent, the nurse's communication can result in both harm and good. Every nuance of posture, every small expression and gesture, every word chosen, every attitude held—all have the potential to hurt or heal, affecting others through the transmission of human energy. Knowing that intention and behavior directly influence human energy fields, and therefore health, gives nurses tremendous ethical responsibility to do no harm to those entrusted to their care. Communication must be respected for its potential power and not carelessly misused to hurt, manipulate, or coerce others. Good communication empowers others and enables people to know themselves and make their own choices, an essential aspect of the healing process. Nurses have wonderful opportunities to bring about good things for themselves, their clients, and their colleagues through this kind of therapeutic communication.

Developing Communication Skills

Gaining expertise in communication, as in any aspect of nursing, requires both an understanding of the communication process and reflection about one's communication experiences as a nurse. Nurses who have developed good critical thinking skills make the best communicators. They are able to draw upon theoretical knowledge about communication and integrate this knowledge with what has been learned through personal experience. They can interpret messages received from others, analyze their content, make inferences about their meaning, evaluate their effect, explain rationale for communication techniques used, and self-examine personal communication skills (Creasia and Parker, 2001).

Other qualities of good critical thinking are also important to the communication process. Critical thinking attitudes offer guidelines for how to approach a problem. These attitudes include being curious. Curiosity motivates the nurse to communicate and know more about a person. Clients are more likely to communicate with nurses who express an interest in them. Perseverance and creativity are also attitudes that are conducive to communication because they motivate the nurse to communicate and identify innovative solutions. A self-confident attitude is important because the nurse who conveys confidence and comfort while communicating can more readily establish interpersonal helping-trust relationships and convey competence in the professional role. Also, an independent attitude encourages the nurse to communicate with colleagues and share ideas about nursing interventions. Such an attitude sometimes involves risk taking because colleagues may question the suggested nursing interventions.

At the same time, an attitude of fairness goes a long way in the ability to listen to both sides in any discussion. An additional critical thinking attitude, integrity, allows nurses to recognize when their opinions may conflict with those of the client, review positions, and decide how to communicate to reach mutually beneficial decisions. It is also very important for the nurse to communicate responsibly and ask for help if uncertain about an aspect of client care. Furthermore, an attitude of humility is necessary to recognize and communicate the need for more information before a decision can be made (Paul, 1993).

The application of intellectual standards that are universal for critical thinking also promote effective communication. When a nurse considers a client problem, it is important to apply standards such as preciseness, accuracy, and consistency to ensure that communication and clinical decisions are sound (Paul, 1993).

It is challenging to understand human communication within interpersonal relationships. Each individual's **perceptions** are based on information received through the five senses of sight, hearing, taste, touch, and smell (Stuart and Laraia, 2001). An individual's culture and education also influence perception. Critical thinking can help the nurse overcome **perceptual biases,** human tendencies that interfere with accurately perceiving and interpreting messages from others. People often assume that others would think, feel, act, react, and behave as they would in similar circumstances. They tend to distort or ignore information that goes against their expectations, preconceptions, or stereotypes (Beebe, Beebe, and Redmond, 1999). By thinking critically about personal communication habits, the nurse can learn to control these tendencies and become more effective in interpersonal relationships.

As communication skills develop, the nurse's competence in the nursing process will also grow. Communication skills must be integrated throughout the nursing process as nurses collaborate with clients and health team members to achieve goals (Box 23-1). Nurses use communication skills to gather, analyze, and transmit information and to accomplish the work of each step of the process. Assessment, diagnosis, planning, implementation, and evaluation all depend on effective communication among nurse, client, family, and others on the health care team. Although the nursing process is a reliable framework for client care, it will not work well unless the nurse masters the art of effective interpersonal communication.

The nature of the communication process requires that nurses constantly make decisions about what, when, where, why, and how to convey messages to others. The nurse's decision making is always contextual—the unique features of any situation influence the nature of the decisions made. For example, the explanation of the importance of following a prescribed diet to a client with a newly diagnosed medical condition will differ from the explanation to a client who has repeatedly chosen not to follow diet restrictions. Effective communication techniques can be easily learned, but their application is more difficult. Deciding which techniques best fit each unique nursing situation is challenging.

Throughout this chapter, brief clinical examples guide students in the use of effective communication tech-

---

Box 23-1   Communication Throughout the Nursing Process

Assessment

Verbal interviewing and history taking
Visual and intuitive observation of nonverbal behavior
Visual, tactile, and auditory data gathering during physical examination
Written medial records, diagnostic tests, and literature review

Nursing Diagnosis

Intrapersonal analysis of assessment findings
Validation of health care needs and priorities via verbal discussion with client
Handwritten or computer-mediated documentation of nursing diagnosis

Planning

Interpersonal or small-group health team planning sessions
Interpersonal collaboration with client and family to determine implementation methods
Written documentation of expected outcomes
Written or verbal referral to health team members

Implementation

Delegation and verbal discussion with health care team
Verbal, visual, auditory, and tactile health teaching activities
Provision of support via therapeutic communication techniques
Contact with other health resources
Written documentation of client's progress in medical record

Evaluation

Acquisition of verbal and nonverbal feedback
Comparison of actual and expected outcomes
Identification of factors affecting outcomes
Modification and update of care plan
Verbal and/or written explanation of revisions of care plan to client

---

niques. Situations that challenge the nurse's decision-making skills and call for careful use of therapeutic techniques often involve the types of persons described in Box 23-2. Since the best way to acquire skill is through practice, it is useful for students to discuss and role play these scenarios before experiencing them in the clinical setting. Consider that clients, family, nurse colleagues, assistive personnel, physicians, or other health team members might be involved and decide which communication techniques might be most effective.

Levels of Communication

Nurses use different levels of communication in their professional role. The nurse's communication skills need to include techniques that reflect competence in each level.

Box 23-2   **Challenging Communication Situations**

Silent, withdrawn persons who do not express any feelings or needs

Sad, depressed persons who have slow mental and motor responses

Angry, hostile persons who do not listen to explanations

Sullen, uncooperative persons who resent being asked to do something

Talkative, lonely persons who want someone with them all the time

Demanding persons who want someone to wait on them or meet their requests

Ranting and raving persons who blame nursing staff unfairly

Sensory impaired persons who cannot hear or see well

Verbally impaired persons who cannot articulate words

Gossiping, catty persons who violate confidentiality and cause friction

Mentally handicapped persons who are frightened and distrustful

Confused, disoriented persons who are bewildered and uncooperative

Foreign-born persons who speak very little English

Anxious, nervous persons who cannot cope with what is happening

Grieving, crying persons who have had a major loss

Screaming, kicking toddlers who want their mother

Unresponsive, comatose persons who cannot communicate at all

Flirtatious, sexually inappropriate persons

Loud, obscene persons causing a disturbance or violating a rule

---

Intrapersonal Communication

Intrapersonal communication is a powerful form of communication that occurs within an individual. This level of communication is also called self-talk, self-verbalization and inner thought (Balzer Riley, 2000). People's thoughts strongly influence perceptions, feelings, behavior, and self-concept. Intrapersonal communication creates a set of conditions through which life is experienced. Nurses should be aware of the nature and content of their own thinking and try to replace negative, self-defeating thoughts with positive assertions. Positive self-talk can be used as a tool to improve the nurse's or client's health and self-esteem. For example, guided imagery, can be used to enhance coping and reduce stress (see Chapter 35). Self-instruction can provide a mental rehearsal for difficult tasks or situations so individuals can deal with them more effectively. Nurses and clients can use intrapersonal communication to develop self-awareness and a positive self-concept that will enhance appropriate self-expression.

Interpersonal Communication

Interpersonal communication is one-to-one interaction between the nurse and another person that often occurs face to face. It is the level most frequently used in nursing situations and lies at the heart of nursing practice. It takes place within a social context and includes all the symbols and cues used to give and receive meaning.

Because meaning resides in persons and not in words, messages received may be different from messages intended. Nurses work with people who have different opinions, experiences, values, and belief systems, so meaning must be validated or mutually negotiated between participants. Meaningful interpersonal communication results in exchange of ideas, problem solving, expression of feelings, decision making, goal accomplishment, team building, and personal growth.

Transpersonal Communication

Transpersonal communication is interaction that occurs within a person's spiritual domain. It has been predicted that our greatest advances in the next decade will come from our deeper understanding of what it means to be a human, spiritual being (Krebs, 2001). Many persons use prayer, meditation, guided reflection, religious rituals, or other means to communicate with their "higher power." Nurses who value the importance of human spirituality often use this form of communication with clients and for themselves.

Small-Group Communication

Small-group communication is interaction that occurs when a small number of persons meet together. This type of communication is usually goal directed and requires an understanding of group dynamics. When nurses work on committees, lead client support groups, form research teams, or participate in client care conferences, a small-group communication process is used. Small groups are more effective when they are a workable size, have an appropriate meeting place, suitable seating arrangements, and cohesiveness and commitment among group members (Hybels and Weaver, 1998). Furthermore, Darley (2002) suggests that there are two main principles that are important to ensure effective communication and working relationships between people in any group. The first is to respect people as partners; the second, listen actively to the other people in the group.

Public Communication

Public communication is interaction with an audience. Nurses have opportunities to speak with groups of consumers about health-related topics, present scholarly work to colleagues at conferences, or lead classroom discussions with peers or students. Public communication requires special adaptations in eye contact, gestures, voice inflection, and use of media materials to communicate messages effectively. Effective public communication increases audience knowledge about health-related topics, health issues, and other issues important to the nursing profession.

Basic Elements of the Communication Process

Communication is an ongoing, dynamic, and multidimensional process. Its basic elements are shown in Figure 23-1 and described below. This simple linear model underrepresents a very complex process but helps the

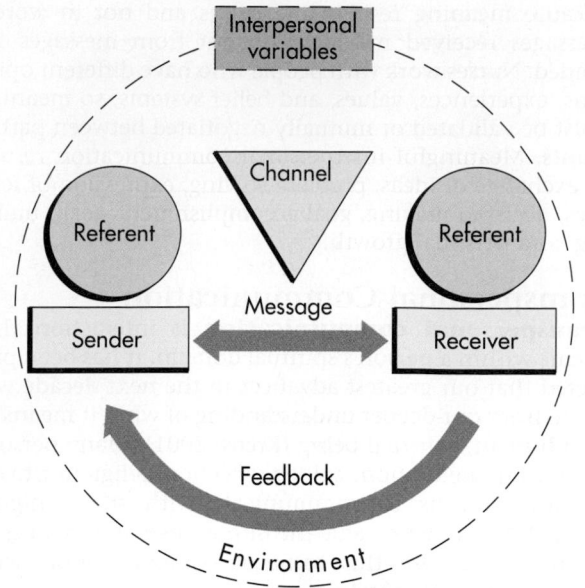

FIGURE **23–1**   Communication as active process between sender and receiver.

nurse identify its essential components. Nursing situations have many unique aspects that influence the nature of communication and interpersonal relationships. In the professional role, the nurse must use critical thinking to focus on each aspect of communication so interactions can be purposeful and effective.

Referent

The **referent** motivates one person to communicate with another. In a health care setting, sights, sounds, odors, time schedules, messages, objects, emotions, sensations, perceptions, ideas, and other cues initiate communication. The nurse who knows what stimulus initiated communication can develop and organize messages more efficiently and better perceive meaning in another's message. A client request for help prompted by difficulty breathing brings a different nursing response than a request prompted by boredom.

Sender and Receiver

The **sender** is the person who encodes and delivers the message, and the **receiver** is the person who receives and decodes the message. The sender puts ideas or feelings into a form that can be transmitted and is responsible for the accuracy of its content and emotional tone. The sender's message acts as a referent for the receiver, who is responsible for attending to, translating, and responding to the sender's message. Sender and receiver roles are fluid and change back and forth as two persons interact; sending and receiving may even occur simultaneously. The more the sender and receiver have in common and the closer the relationship, the more likely they will accurately perceive one another's meaning and respond accordingly.

Messages

The **message** is the content of the communication. It may contain verbal, nonverbal, and symbolic language. Mes-

sages are interpreted by those who receive them through personal perceptions that may or may not distort the meaning intended by the sender. Two nurses can provide the same information yet convey very different messages according to their personal communication styles. One nurse can send the same message to two persons and be understood differently by each. Nurses can send effective messages by expressing themselves clearly, directly, and in a manner familiar to the receiver. Watching the listener for nonverbal cues that suggest confusion or misunderstanding helps the nurse know whether the message needs to be clarified. Communication can be difficult when participants have different levels of education and experience. "Your incision is well approximated without purulent drainage" means the same as "Your wound edges are together, and there are no signs of infection," but a client more easily understands the latter. The nurse must be sure clients can read before sending messages in writing.

Channels

Channels are means of conveying and receiving messages through visual, auditory, and tactile senses. Facial expressions send visual messages, spoken words travel through auditory channels, and touch uses tactile channels. The more channels the sender uses to convey a message, the more clearly it is usually understood. For example, when teaching about insulin self-injection, the nurse talks about and demonstrates the technique, gives the client printed information, and encourages hands-on practice with the vial and syringe. Nurses use verbal, nonverbal, and mediated (technological) communication channels. They send and receive information in person, by informal or formal writing, over the telephone or pager, by audiotape and videotape, through fax and electronic mail, and through computer interactive and information sites.

Feedback

Feedback is the message returned by the receiver. It indicates whether the meaning of the sender's message was understood. Senders need to seek verbal and nonverbal feedback to ensure that good communication has occurred. To be effective, the sender and receiver must be sensitive and open to each other's messages, clarify the messages, and modify behavior accordingly. In a social relationship, both persons assume equal responsibility for seeking openness and clarification, but the nurse assumes primary responsibility in the nurse-client relationship.

Interpersonal Variables

Interpersonal variables are factors within both the sender and receiver that influence communication. Perception is one such variable that provides a uniquely personal view of reality formed by one's expectations and experiences. Each person senses, interprets, and understands events differently. A nurse might say, "You have been very quiet since your family left. Is there something on your mind?" One client might perceive the nurse's question as caring and concerned; another might perceive the nurse as invading privacy and be less willing to talk. Other interpersonal variables include educational and developmental levels, sociocultural backgrounds, values and beliefs, emotions, gender, physical health status, and roles and relationships. Variables associated with illness, such as pain, anxiety, and medication effects, can also affect nurse-client communication.

Environment

The **environment** is the setting for sender-receiver interaction. For effective communication, the environment should meet participant needs for physical and emotional comfort and safety. Noise, temperature extremes, distractions, and lack of privacy or space may create confusion, tension, and discomfort. Environmental distractions are common in health care settings and can interfere with messages sent between people, so nurses must try to control the environment as much as possible to create favorable conditions for effective communication.

Forms of Communication

Messages are conveyed verbally and nonverbally, concretely and symbolically. As people communicate, they express themselves through words, movements, voice inflection, facial expressions, and use of space. These elements can work in harmony to enhance a message or conflict with one another to contradict and confuse it.

Verbal Communication

Verbal communication uses spoken or written words. Verbal language is a code that conveys specific meaning as words are combined. The most important aspects of verbal communication are discussed below.

Vocabulary. Communication is unsuccessful if senders and receivers cannot translate each other's words and phrases. When a nurse cares for a client who speaks another language, an interpreter may be necessary. Even those who speak the same language use subcultural variations of certain words: *dinner* may mean a noon meal to one person and the last meal of the day to another. Medical jargon (technical terminology used by health care providers) may sound like a foreign language to clients unfamiliar with the health care setting and should be used only with other health team members. Children have a more limited vocabulary than adults. They may use special words to describe bodily functions or a favorite blanket or toy. Teenagers often use words in unique ways that are unfamiliar to adults.

Denotative and Connotative Meaning. A single word can have several meanings. Individuals who use a common language share the denotative meaning: *baseball* has the same meaning for everyone who speaks English, but *code* denotes cardiac arrest primarily to health care providers. The connotative meaning is the shade or interpretation of a word's meaning influenced by the thoughts, feelings, or ideas people have about the word. Families who are told a loved one is in serious condition may believe that death is near, but to nurses *serious* may simply describe the nature of the illness. Nurses should carefully select words that cannot be easily misinterpreted, especially when explaining a client's medical con-

dition or therapy. Even a much-used phrase such as "I'm going to take your vital signs" can be unfamiliar to an adult or frightening to a child.

Pacing. Conversation is more successful at an appropriate speed or pace. Nurses should speak slowly enough to enunciate clearly. Talking rapidly, using awkward pauses, or speaking slowly and deliberately can convey an unintended message. Long pauses and rapid shifts to another subject may give the impression that the nurse is hiding the truth. Pacing is improved by thinking before speaking and by developing awareness of the cadence of one's speech.

Intonation. Tone of voice dramatically affects a message's meaning. Depending on intonation, even a simple question or statement can express enthusiasm, anger, concern, or indifference. The nurse must be aware of voice tone to avoid sending unintended messages. For example, clients may interpret a nurse's patronizing tone of voice as condescending, and further communication may be inhibited. A client's voice tone often provides information about his or her emotional state or energy level.

Clarity and Brevity. Effective communication is simple, brief, and direct. Fewer words result in less confusion. Clarity is achieved by speaking slowly, enunciating clearly, and using examples to make explanations easier to understand. Repeating important parts of a message also clarifies communication. Phrases such as "you know" or "OK?" at the end of every sentence detract from clarity. Brevity is achieved by using short sentences and words that express an idea simply and directly. "Where is your pain?" is much better than "I would like you to describe for me the location of your discomfort."

Timing and Relevance. Timing is critical in communication. Even though a message is clear, poor timing can prevent it from being effective. For example, the nurse should not begin routine teaching when a client is in severe pain or emotional distress. Often the best time for interaction is when a client expresses an interest in communicating. If messages are relevant or important to the situation at hand, they are more effective. When a client is facing emergency surgery, discussing the risks of smoking is less relevant than explaining perioperative procedures.

Nonverbal Communication

Nonverbal communication includes all of the five senses and everything that does not involve the spoken or written word. It has been estimated that approximately 7 percent of meaning is transmitted by words, 38 percent is transmitted by vocal cues, and 55 percent is transmitted by body cues. It is common that nonverbal communication is unconsciously motivated and may more accurately indicate a person's intended meaning than the spoken words (Stuart and Laraia, 2001). When there is incongruity between verbal and nonverbal communication, the receiver usually "hears" the nonverbal message as the true message.

All kinds of nonverbal communication are important, but interpreting them can be problematic. Sociocultural background is a major influence on the meaning of non-verbal behavior. In the United States, with its diverse cultural communities, nonverbal messages between people of different cultures can easily be misinterpreted. Because the meaning attached to nonverbal behavior is so subjective, it is imperative that the nurse check its meaning (Stuart and Laraia, 2001). There are many kinds of nonverbal behavior.

Personal Appearance. Personal appearance includes physical characteristics, facial expression, manner of dress and grooming, and adornments. These factors help communicate physical well-being, personality, social status, occupation, religion, culture, and self-concept. First impressions are largely based on appearance. Nurses learn to develop a general impression of client health and emotional status through appearance, and clients develop a general impression of the nurse's professionalism and caring in the same way.

Posture and Gait. Posture and gait are forms of self-expression. The way people sit, stand, and move reflect attitudes, emotions, self-concept, and health status. For example, an erect posture and a quick, purposeful gait communicate a sense of well-being and confidence. Leaning forward conveys attention. A slumped posture and slow shuffling gait may indicate depression, illness, or fatigue.

Facial Expression. The face is the most expressive part of the body. Facial expressions convey emotions such as surprise, fear, anger, happiness, and sadness. Some persons have an expressionless face, or flat affect, which reveals little about what they are thinking or feeling. An inappropriate affect is a facial expression that does not match the content of a verbal message, for example, smiling when describing a sad situation. People can be unaware of the messages their expressions convey. For example, a nurse may frown in concentration while doing a procedure and the client may interpret this as anger or disapproval. Clients often closely observe nurses. Consider the impact a nurse's facial expression might have on a person who asks, "Am I going to die?" The slightest change in the eyes, lips, or facial muscles can reveal the nurse's feelings. Although it is hard to control all facial expression, the nurse should try to avoid showing shock, disgust, dismay, or other distressing reactions in the client's presence.

Eye Contact. People signal readiness to communicate through eye contact. Maintaining eye contact during conversation shows respect and willingness to listen. Eye contact also allows people to closely observe one another. Lack of eye contact may indicate anxiety, defensiveness, discomfort, or lack of confidence in communicating. However, persons from Asian cultures may consider eye contact intrusive, threatening, or harmful and minimize or avoid its use. Eye movements communicate feelings and emotions. Looking down on a person establishes authority, whereas interacting at the same eye level indicates equality in the relationship. Rising to the same eye level of an angry person helps establish one's autonomy.

Gestures. Gestures emphasize, punctuate, and clarify the spoken word. Gestures alone carry specific meanings, or they may create messages with other communication cues. A finger pointed toward a person may communicate several meanings, but when accompanied by a frown and stern voice, the gesture becomes an accusation or threat. Pointing to an area of pain may be more accurate than describing the pain's location.

Sounds. Sounds such as sighs, moans, groans, or sobs also communicate feelings and thoughts. Combined with other nonverbal communication, sounds help send clear messages. Sounds can be interpreted in several ways: moaning can convey pleasure or suffering, and crying can communicate happiness, sadness, or anger. The nurse must validate such nonverbal messages with the client to interpret them accurately.

Territoriality and Personal Space. Territoriality is the need to gain, maintain, and defend one's right to space. Territory is important because it provides people with a sense of identity, security, and control. Territory can be separated and made visible to others, such as a fence around a yard or a bed in a hospital room. Personal space is invisible, individual, and travels with the person. During interpersonal interaction, people maintain vary-

---

Box 23-3   Zones of Personal Space and Touch

Zones of Personal Space

Intimate zone (0 to 18 inches)
Holding a crying infant
Performing physical assessment
Bathing, grooming, dressing, feeding, and toileting a client
Changing a client's dressing
Personal zone (18 inches to 4 feet)
Sitting at a client's bedside
Taking the client's nursing history
Teaching an individual client
Exchanging information at change of shift
Social zone (4 to 12 feet)
Making rounds with a physician
Sitting at the head of a conference table
Teaching a class for clients with diabetes
Conducting a family support group
Public zone (12 feet and greater)
Speaking at a community forum
Testifying at a legislative hearing
Lecturing to a class of students

Zones of Touch

Social zone (permission not needed)
Hands, arms, shoulders, back
Consent zone (permission needed)
Mouth, wrists, feet
Vulnerable zone (special care needed)
Face, neck, front of body
Intimate zone (great sensitivity needed)
Genitalia, rectum

ing distances between each other depending on their culture, the nature of their relationship, and the situation. When personal space becomes threatened, people respond defensively and communicate less effectively. Situations dictate whether the interpersonal distance between nurse and client is appropriate. Examples of nursing actions within zones of personal space are listed in Box 23-3, along with zones of touch. Nurses frequently move into clients' territory and personal space due to the nature of caregiving. The nurse must convey confidence, gentleness, and respect for privacy, especially when actions require intimate contacts or involve a client's vulnerable zone.

Symbolic Communication

Good communication requires awareness of **symbolic communication,** the verbal and nonverbal symbolism used by others to convey meaning. Art and music are forms of symbolic communication that may be used by the nurse to enhance understanding and promote healing. Dreams, drawings, metaphorical language, a child's play, and even the symptoms of illness are all symbolic forms of self-expression that have rich messages for health care providers (Seigel, 1989).

Metacommunication

Metacommunication is important to effective interpersonal interaction. It is "communication about communication" so that the deeper "message within a message" can be uncovered and understood (Wood, 1999). Metacommunication can help people better understand what they have communicated. For example, the nurse observes a young client holding his body rigidly erect and his voice is sharp as he says, "Going to surgery is no big deal." The nurse replies, "You say having surgery doesn't bother you, but you look and sound tense. I'd like to help." This is metacommunication, and it may result in further exploration of the client's feelings and concerns.

Professional Nursing Relationships

Professional relationships are created through the nurse's application of knowledge, understanding of human behavior and communication, and commitment to ethical behavior. Having a philosophy based on caring and respect for others will help the nurse be more successful in establishing relationships of this nature.

Nurse-Client Helping Relationships

Helping relationships are the foundation of clinical nursing practice. In such relationships, the nurse assumes the role of professional helper and comes to know the client as an individual who has unique health needs, human responses, and patterns of living. The relationship is therapeutic, promoting a psychological climate that facilitates positive change and growth. The nurse's therapeutic use of communication is the mechanism by which clients can achieve successful outcomes for the problems cur-

rently preventing them from achieving optimum health (Fortinash and Holoday-Worret, 2000). There is an explicit time frame, a goal-directed approach, and a high expectation of confidentiality. The nurse establishes, directs, and takes responsibility for the interaction, and the client's needs take priority over the nurse's needs. The relationship is also characterized by the nurse's nonjudgmental acceptance of the client. Acceptance conveys a willingness to hear a message or to acknowledge feelings. It does not mean the nurse must always agree with the other person or approve of the client's decisions or actions. A helping relationship between nurse and client does not just happen—it is created with care and skill and is built on the client's trust in the nurse.

The nurse-client relationship is characterized by a natural progression of four goal-directed phases that often begin before the nurse meets the client and continue until the caregiving relationship ends (Box 23-4). Even a brief interaction uses an abbreviated version of the same preinteraction, orientation, working, and termination phases. For example, the student nurse may gather client information to prepare in advance for caregiving, meet the client and establish trust, accomplish health-related goals through use of the nursing process, and say goodbye at the end of the day.

Socializing is an important initial component of interpersonal communication. It helps people get to know one another and relax. It is easy, superficial, and not deeply personal, whereas therapeutic interactions are often more intense, difficult, and uncomfortable. A nurse often uses social conversation to lay a foundation for a closer relationship: "Hi, Mr. Simpson, I hear it's your birthday today. How old are you?" A friendly, informal, and warm communication style helps establish trust, but nurses must get beyond social conversation to talk about issues or concerns affecting the client's health. During social conversation, clients may ask personal questions about the nurse's family, place of residence, and so forth. Students often wonder whether it is appropriate to reveal such information. The skillful nurse uses judgment about what to share and provides minimal information or deflects such questions with gentle humor and refocuses conversation back to the client.

Creating a therapeutic environment depends on the nurse's ability to communicate, to comfort, and to help clients meet their needs. Comfort has been acknowledged as a critical value inherent in the practice of nursing. Hawley (2000) identified comforting strategies from the perspective of emergency department clients. Participants described nurses' comforting strategies under the following categories: competent and immediate technical/physical care, positive talk, vigilance, attention to physical discomforts, and attending to family. The comforting strategies used by nurses resulted in the clients feeling safe, secure, cared about, more relaxed, and better able to cope with pain and the unknown.

In a therapeutic relationship, nurses often encourage clients to share personal stories, which is called narrative interaction. Through narrative interactions, nurses begin to understand the context of others' lives and learn what is meaningful for them from their perspective (Canales, 1997). For example, a nurse asked a client to tell about a

Box 23-4   Phases of the Helping Relationship

Preinteraction Phase

Before meeting the client, the nurse:

Reviews available data, including the medical and nursing history

Talks to other caregivers who may have information about the client

Anticipates health concerns or issues that may arise

Identifies a location and setting that will foster comfortable, private interaction

Plans enough time for the initial interaction

Orientation Phase

When the nurse and client meet and get to know one another, the nurse:

Sets the tone for the relationship by adopting a warm, empathetic, caring manner

Recognizes that the initial relationship may be superficial, uncertain, and tentative

Expects the client to test the nurse's competence and commitment

Closely observes the client and expects to be closely observed by the client

Begins to make inferences and form judgments about client messages and behaviors

Assesses the client's health status

Prioritizes the client's problems and identifies the client's goals

Clarifies the client's and nurse's roles

Forms contracts with the client that specify who will do what

Lets the client know when to expect the relationship to be terminated

Working Phase

When the nurse and client work together to solve problems and accomplish goals, the nurse:

Encourages and helps the client to express feelings about his or her health

Encourages and helps the client with self-exploration

Provides information needed to understand and change behavior

Encourages and helps the client to set goals

Takes actions to meet the goals set with the client

Uses therapeutic communication skills to facilitate successful interactions

Uses appropriate self-disclosure and confrontation

Termination Phase

During the ending of the relationship, the nurse:

Reminds the client that termination is near

Evaluates goal achievement with the client

Reminisces about the relationship with the client

Separates from the client by relinquishing responsibility for his or her care

Achieves a smooth transition for the client to other caregivers as needed

---

time in his life when he had to make a hard decision. He related the following story:

> When I was a young man, I worked on the family farm. An uncle died and left me some money. All of a sudden I could afford to go to college, but Dad didn't want me to go because he needed me there. I had to decide whether to stay or go, and it was real hard, because at first I just wanted to get away. I talked to our preacher, and he said it was up to me, to pray about it and do what my heart told me to. So I stayed. Oh, I've thought from time to time what I might have made of myself, but I never regretted it. I had a good life in farming.

From this brief story, the nurse understood that it was important to the client to put his family's needs above his personal desires and that seeking spiritual guidance was an important component of his decision making. This same information may not have been revealed had the nurse used a standard history form that usually only elicits short answers.

The nurse and client work as a team in a helping relationship. The nurse offers clients the opportunity to make choices, even as simple as choosing a bath time or whether to take a prn (as needed) medication. The nurse also acts as an advocate to keep the client informed of health care alternatives and give support in decision making.

A good way to encourage autonomy is to collaborate with others. For example, the nurse can ask clients and family members for input and suggestions about goals, interventions, and evaluation of the plan of care. This type of mutuality (give-and-take) has been shown to balance power and respect and to promote productive provider-client communication (Henson, 1997). It gives the client a greater sense of purpose and direction, encourages personal responsibility for health, helps establish priorities for care, gives the opportunity for self-expression, and strengthens the client's problem-solving ability. Research has shown that successful collaboration requires an active and committed involvement by both client and nurse and a joint effort toward problem solving. Such a relationship will enhance the client's well-being and the nurse's feeling of success (Paavilainen and Astedt-Kurki, 1997).

Nurse-Family Relationships

Many nursing situations, especially those in community and home care settings, require the nurse to form helping relationships with entire families. The same principles that guide one-to-one helping relationships also apply when the client is a family unit, although communication within families requires additional understanding of the complexities of family dynamics, needs, and relationships (see Chapter 9).

Nurse–Health Team Relationships

Nurses function in roles that require interaction with multiple health team members. Many elements of the nurse-client helping relationship are also applied in these collegial relationships, which are focused on accomplishing the work and goals of the clinical setting. Communication in such relationships may be geared toward team building, facilitating group process, collaboration, consultation, delegation, supervision, leadership, and management (see Chapter 20). A variety of communication skills are needed, including presentational speaking, persuasion, group problem solving, providing performance reviews, and writing business reports.

Both social and therapeutic interactions are needed between the nurse and health team members to build morale and strengthen relationships within the work setting. Everyone has interpersonal needs for acceptance, inclusion, identity, privacy, power and control, and affection (Stewart and Logan, 1998). Nurses need friendship, support, guidance, and encouragement from one another to cope with the many stressors imposed by the nursing role and must extend the same caring communication used with clients to build positive relationships with colleagues and co-workers.

Nurse-Community Relationships

Many nurses form relationships with community groups by participating in local organizations, volunteering for community service, or becoming politically active. Nurses in a community-based practice must be able to establish relationships with their community to be effective change agents (see Chapter 3). Understanding the importance of community-oriented, population-focused nursing practice and developing the skills to practice it are critical in attaining a leadership role in health care regardless of the practice setting (Stanhope and Lancaster, 2000). Communication within the community occurs through channels such as neighborhood newsletters, public bulletin boards, newspapers, radio, television, and electronic information sites. Nurses can use these forms of communication to share information and discuss issues important to community health.

Elements of Professional Communication

Professional appearance, demeanor, and behavior are important in establishing the nurse's trustworthiness and competence. They communicate that the nurse has assumed the professional helping role, is clinically skilled, and is focused on the client. Nothing harms nursing's professional image like an individual nurse's inappropriate appearance or behavior.

A professional is expected to be clean, neat, well groomed, conservatively dressed, and scent- and odor-free. Professional behavior should reflect warmth, friendliness, confidence, and competence. Professionals speak in a clear well-modulated voice, use good grammar, listen to others, help and support colleagues, and communicate effectively. Being on time, organized, well prepared, and equipped for the responsibilities of the nursing role also communicate one's professionalism.

Courtesy

Common courtesy is part of professional communication. To practice courtesy, the nurse says hello and goodbye, knocks on doors before entering, and uses self-introduction. The nurse also states his or her purpose, addresses people by name, says please and thank you to team members, and apologizes for inadvertently making an error or causing someone distress. Being discourteous causes the nurse to be perceived as rude or insensitive. It sets up barriers between nurse and client and causes friction among team members.

Use of Names

Self-introduction is important. The nurse's failure to give a name, indicate status (e.g., registered nurse or licensed practical nurse) or acknowledge the client can create uncertainty about the interaction and convey an impersonal lack of commitment or caring. Making eye contact and smiling at others gives them recognition. Addressing others by name conveys respect for human dignity and uniqueness. Because using last names is respectful in most cultures, nurses usually use the client's last name in the initial interaction, then use the first name if it is requested by the client. The nurse should ask others how they would like to be addressed and let them know personal preference. Using first names is appropriate for infants, young children, confused or unconscious clients, and close team members. Avoid terms of endearment such as "honey," "dear," "Grandma," or "sweetheart." Avoid referring to clients by diagnosis, room number, or other attribute, which is demeaning and sends the message that the nurse does not care enough to know the person as an individual.

Privacy and Confidentiality

Maintaining confidentiality is an important aspect of professional behavior. It is essential that the nurse safeguard the client's right to privacy by carefully protecting information of a sensitive, private nature (see Chapter 22). Sharing personal information or gossiping about others violates nursing ethical codes and practice standards. It sends the message that the nurse cannot be trusted and damages interpersonal relationships. Team members directly involved in the client's care should be given only relevant information about the client's status. Respect for clients is demonstrated when the nurse treats others with dignity and maintains their physical and emotional privacy.

Trustworthiness

Trust is relying on someone without doubt or question. Being trustworthy means helping others without hesitation when help is needed. To foster trust, the nurse communicates warmth and demonstrates consistency, reliability, honesty, and competence. Sometimes it is not easy for a client to ask for help. Trusting another person involves risk and vulnerability, but it also fosters open, therapeutic communication and enhances the expression of feelings, thoughts, and needs. Without trust, a nurse-client relationship rarely progresses beyond social interaction and superficial care. Avoid dishonesty at all costs. Knowingly withholding key information, lying, or distorting the truth violates both legal and ethical standards of practice.

Autonomy and Responsibility

Autonomy is the ability to be self-directed and independent in accomplishing goals and advocating for others. Professional nurses make choices and accept responsibility for the outcomes of their actions (Townsend, 2003). They take initiative in problem solving and communicate in a manner that reflects what they really need and want (Burden, 1997). Autonomy can be beneficial to the client because people who seek health care are often concerned about losing control of decisions that influence how they live.

Assertiveness

According to Darley (2002) assertiveness comprises respect for others, respect for yourself, self-awareness, and effective, clear, and consistent communication. **Assertiveness** conveys a sense of self-assurance while also communicating respect for the other person (Stuart and Laraia, 2001). The advantages of assertive behavior include the following (Balzer Riley, 2000):

- It is more likely you will get what you want when you ask for it.
- People respect clear, open, honest communication.
- You stand up for your own rights and experience self-respect.
- You avoid the invitation of aggression when the rights of others are violated.
- You are more independent.
- You become a decision maker.
- You feel more peaceful and comfortable with yourself.

Nurses can teach assertiveness skills to others as a means for promoting personal health. Assertive people express feelings and emotions confidently, spontaneously, and honestly. They make decisions and control their lives more effectively than nonassertive individuals. They can better deal with criticism and manipulation by others and learn to say no, set limits, and resist intentionally imposed guilt.

Assertive responses are characterized by feelings of security, competence, power, optimism, and professionalism. They are good tools for dealing with criticism, change, negative conditions in personal or professional life, and conflict or stress in relationships. Assertive responses often contain "I" messages, such as "I want," "I need," "I think," or "I feel."

Communication Within the Nursing Process

In the following section the focus of the nursing process is on providing care for clients who need special assistance with communication. However, the nursing intervention section contains examples of therapeutic communication techniques that are appropriate strategies for use in any interpersonal nursing situation.

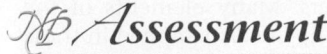 *Assessment*

Assessment of a client's ability to communicate includes gathering data about the many contextual factors that influence communication. The word *context* refers to all the parts of something that help determine its meaning. A context is the situation that influences the nature of communication, interpersonal relationships, and client needs (Beebe, Beebe, and Redmond, 1999). This includes the participants' internal factors and characteristics, the nature of their relationship, the situation prompting communication, the environment, and the sociocultural elements present. Box 23-5 lists the contextual factors that influence communication. Assessing these contextual factors helps the nurse make sound decisions during the communication process.

Physical and Emotional Factors. It is especially important to assess the psychophysiological factors that influence communication. There are many altered health states and human responses that limit communication. Persons with hearing or visual impairments have fewer channels through which to receive messages (see Chapter 48). Facial trauma, laryngeal cancer, or endotracheal intubation may prevent movement of air past vocal cords or mobility of the tongue, resulting in inability to articulate words. An extremely breathless person must use oxygen to breathe rather than speak. Persons with aphasia after a stroke or in late-stage Alzheimer's disease often cannot understand or form words. Certain mental illnesses such as psychoses or depression may cause clients to demonstrate flight of ideas, constant verbalization of the same words or phrases, a loose association of ideas, or slowed speech pattern. Persons with high anxiety may be unable to perceive environmental stimuli or hear explanations. Finally, unresponsive or heavily sedated persons cannot send or respond to verbal messages.

Review of the client's medical record helps provide relevant information about the client's ability to communicate. The medical history and physical examination may document physical barriers to speech, neurological deficits, and pathophysiology affecting hearing or vision. Reviewing the client's medication record is also important. For example, opiates, antidepressants, neuroleptics, hypnotics, or sedatives may cause a client to slur words or use incomplete sentences. The nursing progress notes may reveal other factors that contribute to communication difficulties, such as the absence of family members who could provide more information about a confused client.

Assessment should include communicating directly with clients to provide information about their ability to attend to, interpret, and respond to stimuli. If clients have difficulty communicating, it is important to assess how they are affected by the problem. The client who cannot communicate effectively will often have difficulty expressing needs and responding appropriately to the environment. A client who is unable to speak can be at risk for injury unless an alternate communication method

Box 23-5   Contextual Factors Influencing Communication

Psychophysiological Context

The internal factors influencing communication:
Physiological status (e.g., pain, hunger, weakness, dyspnea)
Emotional status (e.g., anxiety, anger, hopelessness, euphoria)
Growth and development status (e.g., age, developmental tasks)
Unmet needs (e.g., safety/security, love/belonging)
Attitudes, values, and beliefs (e.g., meaning of illness experience)
Perceptions and personality (e.g., optimist/pessimist, introvert/extrovert)
Self-concept and self-esteem (e.g., positive or negative)

Relational Context

The nature of the relationship between the participants:
Social, helping, or working relationship
Level of trust between participants
Level of caring expressed
Level of self-disclosure between participants
Shared history of participants
Balance of power and control

Situational Context

The reason for the communication:
Information exchange
Goal achievement
Problem resolution
Expression of feelings

Environmental Context

The physical surroundings in which communication takes place:
Privacy level
Noise level
Comfort and safety level
Distraction level

Cultural Context

The sociocultural elements that affect the interaction:
Educational level of participants
Language and self-expression patterns
Customs and expectations

---

can be found. If there are barriers that make it difficult to communicate directly with the client, family or friends become important sources about the client's communication patterns and abilities.

Developmental Factors. Aspects of a client's growth and development also influence nurse-client interaction. For example, an infant's self-expression is limited to crying, body movement, and facial expression, whereas older children can express their needs more directly. The nurse adapts communication techniques to the special needs of infants and children. Communication with children and their parents requires special considerations. The nurse can include the parents, child, or both as sources of information about the child's health, depending on the child's age. A young child can be given toys or other distractions so the parent can give full attention to the nurse. Children are especially responsive to nonverbal messages, and sudden movements, loud noises, or threatening gestures can be frightening. Children often prefer to make the first move in interpersonal contacts and do not like adults to stare or look down at them. A child who has received little environmental stimulation may be behind in language development, thus making communication more challenging.

Age also influences communication. Age alone does not determine an adult's capacity for communication. However, approximately one fifth of the adults in the United States who are age 65 and older have a speech disorder that prevents them from expressing themselves, such as expressive aphasia, or limits their ability to understand others, such as receptive aphasia. Box 23-6 highlights communication needs and barriers of older adults. The nurse's awareness of these factors facilitates the communication process with those older adults who do experience communication problems.

Sociocultural Factors. Culture is a blueprint for thinking, feeling, behaving, and communicating. Nurses need to be aware of the typical patterns of interaction that characterize various cultures. For example, European Americans are more open and willing to discuss private family matters, whereas Hispanics, African-Americans, and Asian-Americans may be reluctant to reveal personal or family information to strangers. Hispanics and Asian-Americans value a quiet demeanor and self-restraint; to be open or argumentative is thought to reflect negatively on family honor. Native Americans also value silence and are comfortable with it.

Foreign-born persons may not speak or understand English. Those who speak English as a second language often experience difficulty with self-expression or language comprehension. To practice cultural sensitivity in communication, the nurse understands that persons of different cultures use different degrees of eye contact, personal space, gestures, loudness of voice, pace of speech, touch, silence, and meaning of language. The nurse makes a conscious effort not to interpret messages through his or her cultural perspective but to consider the communication within the context of the other individual's background. The nurse avoids stereotyping, patronizing, or making fun of other cultures.

Gender. Gender is another factor that influences how we think, act, feel, and communicate. Male and female communication patterns tend to differ, which can sometimes create barriers to effective communication (Beebe, Beebe, and Redmond, 1999).

Males communicate to achieve goals, establish individual status and authority, and compete for attention and power. They typically prefer to talk about topics that do not expose personal feelings. Men tend to speak di-

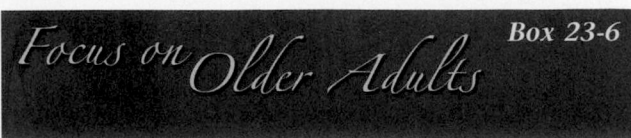

Tips for Improved Communication With Older Adults Who Have Communication Needs/Barriers

- Always start the communication process by checking for a hearing aid.
- Amplify your voice if necessary.
- Get the clients' attention before speaking. Face them so they can see your mouth.
- Structure the environment so it is conducive to good communication. Minimize visual and auditory distractions. Make sure there is adequate lighting.
- When caring for elderly clients with communication disorders, remember their deficit. Don't assume a communication breakdown is the result of the client being uncooperative.
- Don't expect to communicate the same way as you would with a nonimpaired person. Instead, act as a communication partner whose job is to facilitate the clients' self-expression and comprehension.
- Speak slowly and clearly while maintaining eye contact. Use short sentences with simple words.
- Supplement your words with visual gestures.
- Match your body language to your speech. For example, when reporting favorable test results, the message that the news is good should be evident in your expressions, posture, and tone of voice.
- Summarize the most important points of the conversation.
- Give clients plenty of time to ask and answer questions.
- Allow them to make errors. Don't constantly correct them. Suppress the desire to finish sentences.
- Be a good listener despite time constraints that make listening difficult.
- Stick to one topic at a time.
- Whenever possible have a family member or caregiver in the room with you. This person will usually be most familiar with the client's communication patterns and can assist in the communication process.

Used with permission: *Patient Care* 31(2):55-58, 1997. Copyright Medical Economics, Thomas Health Care.

rectly when giving criticism or orders. They use more banter, teasing, and playful put-downs. Men usually want others to know of their accomplishments.

Females communicate to build connections with others, include others, and cooperate with, respond to, show interest in, and support others. Women enjoy discussing feelings and personal issues and find closeness in dialogue. They tend to downplay their achievements. Women speak indirectly, couching criticism and commands in praise or vagueness to avoid causing offense or hurt feelings. A male nurse might say to his colleague, "Help me turn Jeremy." A female nurse might say, "Jeremy needs to be turned," expecting her colleague to understand the implied request for help. Research has shown there are differences in the way male and female nurses use silence, touch, and humor in their practice (Perry, 1996).

To practice gender sensitivity in communication, the nurse recognizes the differences in male and female pat-terns and does not misinterpret messages sent by someone of the opposite gender. The nurse avoids conversation with sexual overtones, gender-denigrating jokes, and male-female stereotyping.

Nursing Diagnosis

Most individuals experience difficulty with some aspect of communication. Persons who are free of illness or disability may lack skills in attending, listening, responding, and self-expression. Most often, the nurse's care is directed toward those individuals who experience more serious impairments in communication.

The primary nursing diagnostic label used to describe the client who has limited or no ability to communicate verbally is *impaired verbal communication*. This is the state in which an individual experiences a decreased or absent ability to receive, process, transmit, and use symbols (Johnson and others, 2001). A client will have defining characteristics such as the inability to articulate words, inappropriate verbalization, difficulty forming words, and difficulty in comprehending, which the nurse clusters together to form the diagnosis. This diagnosis is useful for a wide variety of clients with special problems and needs related to communication, such as impaired perception, reception, and articulation. Although a client's primary problem may be impaired verbal communication, the associated difficulty in self-expression or altered communication patterns may also contribute to other nursing diagnoses:

- Anxiety
- Social isolation
- Ineffective coping
- Compromised family coping
- Powerlessness
- Impaired social interaction

The related (contributing) factors for a nursing diagnosis focus on the causes of the communication disorder. In the case of impaired verbal communication, these can be physiological, mechanical, anatomical, psychological, cultural, or developmental in nature. Accuracy in the identification of related factors is necessary so that the nurse selects interventions that can effectively resolve the diagnostic problem. For example, the diagnosis of *impaired verbal communication related to cultural difference (Hispanic heritage)* would be managed very differently than the diagnosis of *impaired verbal communication related to deafness.*

Planning

Once the nurse has identified the nature of the client's communication dysfunction, several factors must be considered as the care plan is designed. Motivation is a factor in improving communication, and clients often require encouragement to try different approaches that involve significant change. It is especially important to involve the client and family in decisions about the plan of care to determine whether suggested methods are acceptable. The nurse needs to make sure basic comfort and safety needs are met before introducing new communication methods and techniques. Adequate time must be allowed for practice, and participants need to be patient with themselves and one another if effective communication is to be achieved. When the focus is on practicing communication, the nurse should arrange for a quiet, private place that is free of distractions such as television or visitors. Communication aids may be needed, such as a writing board for a client with a tracheostomy or a special call system for a client who is paralyzed.

Goals and Outcomes. In general, effective nursing interventions will have the goal of the client experiencing a sense of trust in the nurse and health team. Expected outcomes for the client with impaired communication are also important to identify. Outcomes are very specific and measurable and a way to determine if the broader goal is met. For example, outcomes for the client might include the following:

- Client initiates conversation about diagnosis or health care problem.
- Client is able to attend to appropriate stimuli.
- Client conveys clear and understandable messages with family members and health care team.
- Client will express increased satisfaction with the communication process.

At times nurses care for well clients whose difficulty in sending, receiving, and interpreting messages interferes with healthy interpersonal relationships. In this case, impaired communication may be a contributing factor to other nursing diagnoses such as *impaired social interaction* or *ineffective coping*. Nurses can plan interventions to help such clients improve their communication skills. For example, the nurse can model effective communication techniques and provide feedback regarding the client's communication. Role play can help clients rehearse situations in which they have difficulty communicating. Expected outcomes for a client in this situation might include demonstrating the ability to appropriately express needs, feelings and concerns; communicating thoughts and feelings more clearly; engaging in appropriate social conversation with peers and staff; and increasing feelings of autonomy and assertiveness.

Setting of Priorities. It is essential for the nurse to always maintain an open line of communication so that the client can express any emergent needs or problems. This may involve an intervention as simple as keeping a call light in reach for a client restricted to bed, or providing communication augmentative devices (e.g., message board, Braille computer). When the nurse plans to have lengthy interactions with a client, it is important that physical care priorities are addressed, so that the discussion can be uninterrupted. The nurse should make the client comfortable by ensuring that any symptoms are under control and that any elimination needs have been met.

Continuity of Care. To ensure an effective plan of care, the nurse may need to collaborate with other health team members who have expertise in communication strategies. Speech therapists can help clients with aphasia, interpreters may be needed for clients who speak a foreign language, and psychiatric nurse specialists might

help angry or highly anxious clients to communicate more effectively.

Implementation

In carrying out any plan of care, nurses need to use communication techniques that are appropriate for the client's individual needs. Before learning how to adapt communication methods to help clients with serious communication impairments, it is necessary to learn the communication techniques that serve as the foundation for professional communication. It is also important to understand those communication techniques that create barriers to effective interaction.

Therapeutic Communication Techniques. Therapeutic communication techniques are specific responses that encourage the expression of feelings and ideas and convey the nurse's acceptance and respect. Learning these techniques helps the student develop awareness of the variety of nursing responses available for use in different situations. Although some of the techniques may seem artificial at first, skill and comfort will increase with practice. Tremendous satisfaction will result as therapeutic relationships and outcomes are achieved.

Active Listening. **Active listening** means to be attentive to what the client is saying both verbally and nonverbally. Active listening facilitates client communication. Crouch (2002) suggests it is important to remember that we have two ears and one mouth; and, we should use them in that 2:1 ratio. With active listening, trust is enhanced because the nurse communicates acceptance and respect for the client. Several nonverbal skills have been identified as facilitative skills for attentive listening. They can be identified by the acronym SOLER (Townsend, 2003):

S—Sit facing the client. This posture gives the message that the nurse is there to listen and is interested in what the client is saying.

O—Observe an open posture (i.e., keep arms and legs uncrossed). This posture suggests that the nurse is "open" to what the client says. A "closed" position may convey a defensive stance, possibly invoking a similar response in the client.

L—Lean toward the client. This posture conveys that the nurse is involved and interested in the interaction.

E—Establish and maintain intermittent eye contact. This behavior conveys the nurse's involvement in and willingness to listen to what the client is saying. Absence of eye contact or shifting of the eyes gives the message that the nurse is not interested in what is being said.

R—Relax. It is important to communicate a sense of being relaxed and comfortable with the client. Restlessness communicates a lack of interest and may also convey a feeling of discomfort that may be transferred to the client.

Sharing Observations. Nurses make observations by commenting on how the other person looks, sounds, or acts. Stating observations often helps the client communicate without the need for extensive questioning, focusing, or clarification. This technique can help start a conversation with quiet or withdrawn persons. The nurse does not state observations that might embarrass or anger the client, such as telling someone "You look a mess!" Even if such an observation is made with humor, the client can become resentful.

Sharing observations differs from making assumptions, which means drawing unwarranted conclusions about the other person without validating them. Making assumptions puts the client in the position of having to contradict the nurse. Examples might include the nurse interpreting fatigue as depression or assuming that untouched food indicates lack of interest in meeting nutritional goals. Making observations is a gentler and safer technique: "You look tired . . . ," "You seem different today . . . ," or "I see you haven't eaten anything."

Sharing Empathy. **Empathy** is the ability to understand and accept another person's reality, to accurately perceive feelings, and to communicate this understanding to the other. Balzer Riley (2000) states: "When clients or colleagues are hurting, confused, troubled, anxious, alienated, terrified, doubtful of self-worth, or uncertain as to identity, then understanding is called for." To express empathy, the nurse reflects understanding of the importance of what has been communicated by the other person on a feeling level. Such empathic understanding requires the nurse to be both sensitive and imaginative, especially if the nurse has not had similar experiences. Although nurses are rarely empathetic in every situation, it is an important goal to work for, a key to unlocking concern and communicating support for others. Statements reflecting empathy are highly effective because they tell the person that the nurse heard the feeling content, as well as factual content, of the communication. Empathy statements are neutral and nonjudgmental. They can be used to establish trust in difficult situations. For example, the nurse might say to an angry client who has low mobility after a stroke: "It must be very frustrating to know what you want and not be able to do it."

Sharing Hope. Nurses recognize that hope is essential for healing and learn to communicate a "sense of possibility" to others. Appropriate encouragement and positive feedback are important in fostering hope and self-confidence and for helping people achieve their potential and reach their goals. The nurse can give hope by commenting on the positive aspects of the other person's behavior, performance, or response. Sharing a vision of the future and reminding others of their resources and strengths can also strengthen hope. Clients can be reassured that there are many kinds of hope and that meaning and personal growth can come from illness experiences. For example, the nurse might say to a client discouraged about a poor prognosis: "I believe you will find a way to face your situation, because I have seen your courage and creativity in the past."

Sharing Humor. Humor is an important but underused resource in nursing interactions. According to Astedt-Kurki and Isola (2001), humor has positive effects

on both a person's psyche and physiology. Laughter signifies positive events to people; it may contribute to feelings of togetherness, closeness, and friendliness. The use of humor is one indicator of mental well-being. Furthermore, humor tends to minimize the effect of negative factors and protects from difficulties.

When nurses were asked how they think humor works in health care, they replied that humor does the following:
- Shows you care
- Reduces tension and helps you get on with work
- Shows you your clients' personalities with their defenses down
- Makes us equals, because we all laugh at the same things
- Makes us more likely to be accepted (Balzer Riley, 2000).

Furthermore, Balzer Riley (2000) suggests that humor works to promote positive communication in the following three ways:
- *Prevention:* Using humor when a crisis occurs in a work environment makes staff more willing to work together when tension can be great.
- *Perception:* Injecting humor into a situation changes the perception that the situation is so terrible that it cannot be handled.
- *Perspective:* Humor assists us in keeping the big picture in view and not to take ourselves too seriously.

Smith (2000) notes that laughter loosens us up and facilitates open communication. Laughter is a "social lubricant." The goal in using humor as a health care provider is to bring hope and joy to the situation and to enhance the client's well-being and the therapeutic relationship. According to Stuart and Lararia (2001), humor serves several additional functions. It helps reduce stress and tension, provides social control, permits cognitive reframing, reflects social change, and expresses emotion.

Today it is common that nurses care for clients from different cultures. When the nurse interacts with clients who do not have a full grasp of the language, it is important to realize the jokes and statements meant to be humorous may not be understood or may be misinterpreted. It is also important to recognize that when either a nurse or client tries to speak in another language, mistakes may occur. The ability to laugh at oneself and with others serves to ease the anxiety that may be present in an intercultural situation (Geiger and Davidhizar, 1999).

A kind of dark, negative humor is sometimes used after difficult or traumatic situations as a way to deal with unbearable tension and stress. This coping humor has a high potential for being misinterpreted as uncaring by persons not involved in the situation. For example, student nurses are sometimes offended and wonder how staff can laugh and joke after unsuccessful resuscitation efforts. When nurses use coping humor within earshot of clients or their loved ones, great emotional distress can result.

Sharing Feelings. Emotions are subjective feelings that result from one's thought and perceptions. Feelings are not right, wrong, good, or bad, although they may be pleasant or unpleasant. If feelings are not expressed, stress and illness can worsen. Nurses can help clients express emotions by making observations, acknowledging feelings, encouraging communication, giving permission to express "negative" feelings, and modeling healthy emotional self-expression. At times, clients may direct anger or frustration prompted by their illness toward the nurse, who should not take such expressions personally. Acknowledging clients' feelings communicates that the nurse listened to and understood the emotional aspects of their illness situation.

When nurses care for clients they must be aware of their own emotions, because feelings are difficult to hide. Students may wonder whether it is helpful for the nurse to share feelings with clients. Sharing emotion makes nurses seem more human and can bring people closer. It is appropriate to share feelings of caring, or even cry with others, as long as the nurse is in control of how those feelings are expressed and does so in a way that does not burden the client or break confidentiality. Clients are perceptive and can sense a nurse's emotions. It is usually inappropriate to discuss negative personal emotions such as anger or sadness with clients. A social support system of colleagues is helpful, and employee assistance programs, peer group meetings, and the use of interdisciplinary teams such as social work and pastoral care provide other means for nurses to safely express feelings away from clients.

Using Touch. In today's fast-paced technical environments, nurses are required more than ever to bring the sense of caring and human connection to their clients (see Chapter 7). Touch is one of the nurse's most potent forms of communication. Nurses are privileged to experience more of this intimate form of personal contact than almost any other professional. Many messages, such as affection, emotional support, encouragement, tenderness, and personal attention, are conveyed through touch. Comfort touch, such as holding a hand, is especially important for vulnerable clients who are experiencing severe illness with its accompanying physical and emotional losses. Research has found that nurses use touch not connected with procedures to get a client's attention, arouse them from sleep, begin a nursing intervention, add emphasis to explanations, make requests, bring comfort, emphasize or point things out, tease, thank, and reprimand (Routasalo, 1996) (Figure 23-2).

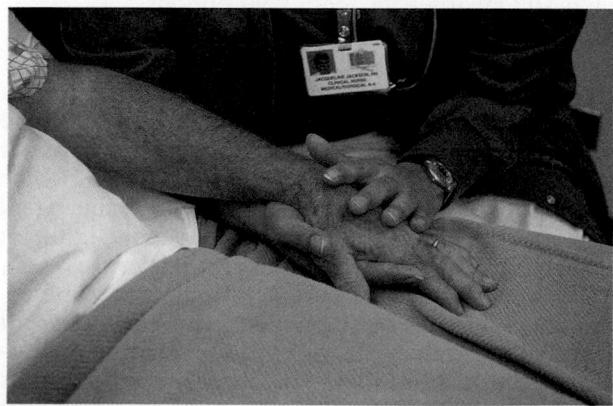

FIGURE **23–2** The nurse uses touch to communicate.

Seed (1995) found that students may initially find giving intimate care to be stressful, especially when caring for clients of the opposite gender, and that students learn to cope with intimate contact by changing their perception of the situation. Since much of what nurses do involves touching, nurses must learn to be sensitive to other's reactions to touch and use it wisely. Touch should be as gentle or as firm as needed and delivered in a comforting, nonthreatening manner. There are times when touch should be withheld; for example, highly suspicious or angry persons may respond negatively or even violently to the nurse's touch.

Using Silence. It takes time and experience to become comfortable with silence. Most people have a natural tendency to fill empty spaces with words, but sometimes what those spaces really need is time for the nurse and client to observe one another, sort out feelings, think how to say things, and consider what has been communicated. Silence can prompt people to talk. Silence allows the client to think and gain insight. In general, the nurse should allow the client to break the silence, particularly when the client has initiated it (Stuart and Laraia, 2001).

Silence is particularly useful when people are confronted with decisions that require much thought. For example, silence may help a client gain confidence needed to share the decision to refuse medical treatment. Silence also allows the nurse to pay particular attention to nonverbal messages such as worried expressions or loss of eye contact. Remaining silent demonstrates the nurse's patience and willingness to wait for a response when the other person is unable to reply quickly. Silence may be especially therapeutic during times of profound sadness or grief.

Providing Information. Providing relevant information tells other persons what they need or want to know so they can make decisions, experience less anxiety, and feel safe and secure. It is also an integral aspect of health teaching. It is usually not helpful to hide information from clients, particularly when they seek it. If a physician withholds information, the nurse needs to clarify the reason with the physician. Clients have a right to know about their health status and what is happening in their environment. Information of a distressing nature needs to be communicated with sensitivity, at a pace appropriate to what the client can absorb, and in general terms at first: "John, your heart sounds have changed from earlier today, and so has your blood pressure. I'll let your doctor know." The nurse provides information that enables others to understand what is happening and what to expect: "Mrs. Evans, John is getting an echocardiogram right now. This test uses painless sound waves to create a moving picture of his heart structures and valves and should tell us what is causing his murmur."

Clarifying. To check whether understanding is accurate, the nurse can restate an unclear or ambiguous message to clarify the sender's meaning. Instead of restating the message, the nurse can also ask the other person to rephrase it, explain further, or give an example of what the person means. Without clarification, the nurse may make invalid assumptions and miss valuable information. Despite efforts at paraphrasing, the nurse may not understand the client's message and should let the client know if this is the case: "I'm not sure I understand what you mean by 'sicker than usual.' What is different now?"

Focusing. Focusing is used to center on key elements or concepts of a message. If conversation is vague or rambling or clients begin to repeat themselves, focusing is a useful technique. The nurse does not use focusing if it interrupts clients while discussing an important issue. Rather, the nurse uses focusing to guide the direction of conversation to important areas: "We've talked a lot about your medications, but let's look more closely at the trouble you're having in taking them on time."

Paraphrasing. Paraphrasing is restating another's message more briefly using one's own words. Through paraphrasing, the nurse sends feedback that lets the client know that the nurse is actively involved in the search for understanding. Practice is required to paraphrase accurately. If the meaning of a message is changed or distorted through paraphrasing, communication may become ineffective. For example, a client may say, "I've been overweight all my life and never had any problems. I can't understand why I need to be on a diet." Paraphrasing this statement by saying, "You don't care if you're overweight or not," is incorrect. It would be more accurate to say, "You're not convinced you need a diet because you've stayed healthy."

Asking Relevant Questions. Nurses ask relevant questions to seek information needed for decision making. Nurses should ask only one question at a time and fully explore one topic before moving to another area. During client assessment, questions follow a logical sequence and usually proceed from general to more specific. Open-ended questions allow the client to take the conversational lead and introduce pertinent information about a topic. For example, "What's your biggest problem at the moment?" Focused questions are used when more specific information is needed in an area: "How has your pain affected your life at home?" The nurse should allow clients to fully respond to an open-ended question before asking more focused questions. Closed-ended questions elicit a yes, no, or one-word response: "How many times a day are you taking pain medication?" They are generally less useful during therapeutic exchanges, although they may be needed during assessment.

Asking too many questions can be dehumanizing, because seeking factual information does not allow the nurse or client to establish a more meaningful relationship or deal with important emotional issues. It may be a way for the nurse to ignore uncomfortable areas in favor of more comfortable, neutral topics. A useful exercise is to try conversing without asking the other person a single question. By giving general leads ("tell me about it . . ."), making observations, paraphrasing, focusing, providing information, and so forth, nurses can discover much of importance that would have remained hidden if questions alone were used during the communication process.

Summarizing. Summarizing is a concise review of key aspects of an interaction. Summarizing brings a sense of satisfaction and closure to an individual conversation and is especially helpful during the termination phase of a nurse-client relationship. By reviewing a conversation, participants focus on key issues and can add additional relevant information as needed. Beginning a new interaction by summarizing a previous one helps the client recall topics discussed and shows the client that the nurse has analyzed communication. Summarizing also clarifies expectations, as in this example of a nurse manager who has been working with a dissatisfied employee: "You've told me a lot of things about why you don't like this job and how unhappy you've been. We've also come up with some possible ways to make things better, and you've agreed to try some and let me know if any of them help."

Self-Disclosure. Self-disclosures are subjectively true, personal experiences about the self and are intentionally revealed to another person. This is not therapy for the nurse; rather, it shows clients that their experiences can be understood and are not unique. The nurse may choose to share experiences or feelings that are similar to those of the client and may emphasize both the similarities and differences. This kind of self-disclosure is indicative of the closeness of the nurse-client relationship and involves a particular kind of respect for the client. It is offered as an expression of genuineness and honesty by the nurse and is an aspect of empathy (Stuart and Laraia, 2001). Self-disclosures should be relevant and appropriate and made to benefit the client rather than the nurse. They are used sparingly so the client is the focus of the interaction: "That happened to me once, too. It was devastating, and I had to face some things about myself that I didn't like. I went for counseling, and it really helped. . . . What are your thoughts about seeing a counselor?"

Confrontation. To confront someone in a therapeutic way, the nurse helps the other person become more aware of inconsistencies in his or her feelings, attitudes, beliefs, and behaviors (Stuart and Laraia, 2001). This technique improves client self-awareness and helps the client recognize growth and deal with important issues. Confrontation should be used only after trust has been established, and it should be done gently, with sensitivity: "You say you've already decided what to do, yet you're still talking a lot about your options."

Nontherapeutic Communication Techniques. Certain communication techniques can hinder or damage professional relationships. These specific techniques are referred to as nontherapeutic or blocking and will often cause recipients to activate defenses to avoid being hurt or negatively affected. Nontherapeutic techniques tend to discourage further expression of feelings and ideas and may engender negative responses or behaviors in others.

Asking Personal Questions. "Why don't you and John get married?" Asking personal questions that are not relevant to the situation, simply to satisfy the nurse's curiosity, is not appropriate professional communication. Such questions are nosy, invasive, and unnecessary. If clients wish to share private information, they will. If the nurse needs to know more about the client's interpersonal roles and relationships, a question such as "How would you describe your relationship with John?" can be asked.

Giving Personal Opinions. "If I were you, I'd put your mother in a nursing home." When the nurse gives a personal opinion, it takes decision making away from the client. It inhibits spontaneity, stalls problem solving, and creates doubt. Personal opinions differ from professional advice. At times, clients need suggestions and help to make choices. Suggestions are presented to clients as options because the final decision rests with the client. Remember, the problem and its solution belong to the other person and not the nurse. A much better response would be, "Let's talk about what options are available for your mother's care."

Changing the Subject. "Let's not talk about your problems with the insurance company. It's time for your walk." Changing the subject when another person is trying to communicate something important is rude and shows a lack of empathy. It tends to block further communication, and the sender may then withhold important messages or fail to openly express feelings. Thoughts and spontaneity are interrupted, ideas become tangled, and information provided may be inadequate. In some instances, changing the subject can serve as a face-saving maneuver. If this happens, reassure the client you will return to his concerns: "After your walk, let's talk some more about what's going on with your insurance company."

Automatic Responses. "Older adults are always confused." "Administration doesn't care about the staff." Stereotypes are generalized beliefs held about people. Making stereotyped remarks about others reflects poor nursing judgment and can threaten nurse-client or team relationships. A cliché is a stereotyped comment such as "You can't win them all" that tends to belittle the other person's feelings and minimize the importance of his or her message. These automatic phrases communicate that the nurse is not taking concerns seriously or responding thoughtfully. Another kind of automatic response is parroting, repeating what the other person has said, word for word. Parroting is easily overused and is not as effective as paraphrasing. A simple "oh?" can give the nurse time to think if the other person says something that takes one by surprise.

A nurse who is task oriented automatically makes the task or procedure the entire focus of interaction with clients, missing opportunities to communicate with them as individuals and meet their needs. Task-oriented nurses are often perceived as cold, uncaring, and unapproachable. When students first perform technical skills, it is difficult to integrate therapeutic communication due to the need to focus on the procedure. In time, the nurse can learn to integrate communication with high-visibility tasks and accomplish several goals simultaneously.

False Reassurance. "Don't worry, everything will be all right." When a client is seriously ill or distressed, the nurse may be tempted to offer hope to the client with statements such as "You'll be fine" or "There's nothing to worry about." When a client is reaching for understanding, false reassurance from the nurse may discourage open communication. Offering reassurance not supported by facts or based in reality can do more harm than good. Although it might be intended kindly and have the secondary effect of helping the nurse avoid the other person's distress, it tends to block conversation and discourage further expression of feelings. A more facilitative nursing response would be "It must be difficult not to know what the surgeon will find. What can I do to help?"

Sympathy. "I'm so sorry about your mastectomy, it must be terrible to lose a breast." **Sympathy** is concern, sorrow, or pity felt for the client generated by the nurse's personal identification with the client's needs. Sympathy is a subjective look at another person's world that prevents a clear perspective of the issues confronting that person. Sympathy focuses on the nurse's feelings rather than the client's (Balzer Riley, 2000). Although sympathy is a compassionate response to another's situation, it is not as therapeutic as empathy. The nurse's own emotional issues can prevent effective problem solving and impair good judgment. A more empathetic approach would be "The loss of a breast is a major change. How do you think it will affect your life?"

Asking for Explanations. "Why are you so anxious?" A nurse may be tempted to ask the other person to explain why the person believes, feels, or has acted in a certain way. Clients frequently interpret "why" questions as accusations or think the nurse knows the reason and is simply testing them. Regardless of client perception of the nurse's motivation, "why" questions can cause resentment, insecurity, and mistrust. If additional information is needed, it is best to phrase a question to avoid using the word "why." "You seem upset. What's on your mind?" is more likely to help the anxious client to communicate.

Approval or Disapproval. "You shouldn't even think about assisted suicide, it's not right." Nurses must not impose their own attitudes, values, beliefs, and moral standards on others while in the professional helping role. Other people have the right to be themselves and make their own decisions. Judgmental responses by the nurse often contain terms such as *should, ought, good, bad, right,* or *wrong.* Agreeing or disagreeing sends the subtle message that nurses have the right to make value judgments about client decisions. Approving implies that the behavior being praised is the only acceptable one. Often the client shares a decision with the nurse, not in an effort to seek approval but to provide a means to discuss feelings. On the other hand, disapproving implies that the client must meet the nurse's expectations or standards. Instead, the nurse should help clients explore their own beliefs and decisions. The nursing response "I'm surprised you are considering assisted suicide. Tell me more about it . . ." gives the client a chance to express ideas or feelings without fear of being judged.

Defensive Responses. "No one here would intentionally lie to you." Becoming defensive in the face of criticism implies the other person has no right to an opinion. The sender's concerns may be ignored when the nurse focuses on the need for self-defense, defense of the health care team, or defense of others. When clients express criticism, nurses should listen to what they have to say. Listening does not imply agreement. To discover reasons for the client's anger or dissatisfaction, the nurse must listen uncritically. By avoiding defensiveness the nurse can defuse anger and uncover deeper concerns: "You believe people have been dishonest with you. It must be hard to trust anyone."

Passive or Aggressive Responses. "Things are bad, and there's nothing I can do about it." "Things are bad, and it's all your fault." Passive responses serve to avoid conflict or sidestep issues. They reflect feelings of sadness, depression, anxiety, powerlessness, and hopelessness. Aggressive responses provoke confrontation at the other person's expense. They reflect feelings of anger, frustration, resentment, and stress. Nurses who lack assertive skills may also use triangulation, complaining to a third party rather than confronting the problem or expressing concerns directly to the source. This lowers team morale and draws others into the conflict situation. Assertive communication is a far more professional approach for the nurse to take.

Arguing. "How can you say you didn't sleep a wink, when I heard you snoring all night long?" Challenging or arguing against perceptions denies that they are real and valid to the other person. They imply that the other person is lying, misinformed, or uneducated. The skillful nurse can give information or present reality in a way that avoids argument: "You feel like you didn't get any rest at all last night, even though I thought you slept well since I heard you snoring."

Adapting Communication Techniques for the Client With Special Needs. Interacting with those who have conditions that impair communication requires special thought and sensitivity. Such clients benefit greatly when the nurse adapts communication techniques to their unique circumstances or developmental level. For example, the nurse caring for a client with impaired verbal communication related to cultural differences may provide a table of simple words in the client's language. The nurse and client use the table to help communicate about basic needs such as food, water, toileting, pain relief, sleep, and so forth. Research findings suggest that many of the difficulties in communicating with clients with severe communication impairment can be viewed as a breakdown in understanding, arising from the lack of an understandable communication system that could be used by nurse and client (Box 23-7) (Hemsley and others, 2001).

The nurse's actions are directed at meeting the goals and expected outcomes identified in the plan of care, addressing both the communication impairment and its contributing factors. Box 23-8 lists many methods available to encourage, enhance, restore, or substitute for verbal communication. The nurse must be sure that the client is physically able to use the chosen method and

Research Highlight   Box 23-7

Difficulty in Communicating With Clients Unable to Speak

Research Focus

Effective communication with clients is critical to effective nursing practice. There is little information on nurses' experiences in caring for clients who are unable to speak. The focus of this descriptive study was to provide information about the nurses' experiences in communicating with clients who had severe communication impairment.

Research Abstract

The study was designed to include interviews with 20 nurses who cared for clients with severe communication impairment. The interview protocol explored positive and negative experiences of providing nursing care to clients with severe communication impairments as a result of cerebral palsy or traumatic brain injury. Frequency counts and descriptive analyses were conducted to identify the major themes emerging from the interviews.

The results suggest that nurse-client communication is difficult when the client has severe communication impairment, although some nurses discovered effective strategies to facilitate communication with such clients. Many of the difficulties could be viewed as a breakdown in understanding arising from the lack of a readily interpretable communication system that could be used by nurse and client.

Evidence-Based Practice

The results suggest a need for nurses to have the following:
- Training in the use of alternative modes of communication
- Access to a variety of simple augmentative communication devices for use with clients who are unable to speak
- Collaboration with speech pathologists on the development of preadmission information and bedside training for people who are admitted to the hospital with severe communication impairment

Reference

Hemsley B and others: Nursing the patient with severe communication impairment, *J Adv Nurs* 35(6):827, 2001.

that it does not cause frustration by being too complicated or difficult.

Box 23-9 provides general guidelines for communicating with persons at preadult developmental levels. Students may consult pediatric nursing textbooks for more detailed information about communication and establishing nurse-client relationships with children and their parents.

In helping older adults with impaired communication, the primary goal is to establish a reliable communication system that is easily understood by all health care team members, because nursing care of the older adult is ideally delivered through an interdisciplinary model. Effective communication involves adapting to any special needs resulting from sensory, motor, or cognitive impairments that may be present. Nurses can also encourage older adults to share life stories and reminisce about the

Box 23-8   Communicating With Clients Who Have Special Needs

Clients Who Cannot Speak Clearly (Aphasia, Dysarthria, Muteness)

Listen attentively, be patient, and do not interrupt.
Ask simple questions that require "yes" or "no" answers.
Allow time for understanding and response.
Use visual cues (e.g., words, pictures, and objects) when possible.
Allow only one person to speak at a time.
Do not shout or speak too loudly.
Encourage the client to converse.
Let client know if you have not understood him or her.
Collaborate with speech therapist as needed.
Use communication aids:
> Pad and felt-tipped pen or Magic Slate
> Communication board with commonly used words, letters, or pictures denoting basic needs
> Call bells or alarms
> Sign language
> Use of eye blinks or movement of fingers for simple responses ("yes" or "no")

Clients Who Are Cognitively Impaired

Reduce environmental distractions while conversing.
Get client's attention prior to speaking.
Use simple sentences and avoid long explanations.
Ask one question at a time.
Allow time for client to respond.
Be an attentive listener.
Include family and friends in conversations, especially in subjects known to client.

Clients Who Are Unresponsive

Call client by name during interactions.
Communicate both verbally and by touch.
Speak to client as though he or she could hear.
Explain all procedures and sensations.
Provide orientation to person, place, and time.
Avoid talking about client to others in his or her presence.
Avoid saying things client should not hear.

Clients Who Do Not Speak English

Speak to client in normal tone of voice (shouting may be interpreted as anger).
Establish method for client to signal desire to communicate (call light or bell).
Provide an interpreter (translator) as needed.
Avoid using family members, especially children, as interpreters.
Develop communication board, pictures, or cards.
Translate words from native language into English list for client to make basic requests.
Have dictionary (English/Spanish and so forth) available if client can read.

Box 23-9   Developmental Aspects of Communication

Communicating With Infants

Use firm touch and gentle physical contact such as cuddling, patting, or rocking.
Hold infant so he or she can see the parents.
Talk softly to the infant.

Communicating With Toddlers and Preschoolers

Interact with parents before communicating with child.
Assume a position that is at the child's eye level.
Allow children to touch and examine objects that will come in contact with them.
Offer a choice only if one exists.
Focus communication on the child, not on the experience of others.
Use simple words and short sentences.
Keep unfamiliar equipment out of view until it is needed.
Communicate through transition objects such as dolls, puppets, or stuffed animals before questioning a young child directly.

Communicating With Children

Allow time for the child to feel comfortable.
Avoid sudden or rapid advances, broad smiles, staring, or other threatening gestures.

Talk to the parent if the child is initially shy.
Give older children the opportunity to talk without the parents present.
Speak in a quiet, unhurried, and confident voice.
Give correct reason for why something is done or how equipment works.
State directions and suggestions specifically and positively.
Be honest and let the child know what to expect and how to participate.
Allow the child to express concerns and fears; allow time for questions.
Use a variety of communication techniques such as drawing or play.

Communicating With Adolescents

Give undivided attention.
Listen, listen, listen.
Be courteous, calm, and open-minded.
Avoid judging or criticizing.
Choose important issues when taking a stand.
Make expectations clear.
Respect their privacy and views.
Praise good points and tolerate differences.
Encourage expressions of ideas and feelings.

Modified from Wong D and others: *Whaley and Wong's nursing care of infants and children,* ed 6, St. Louis, 1999, Mosby.

Box **23-10**   **Sample Communication Analysis**

Nurse: "Good morning, Mr. Simpson."
(Smiles, approaches bed holding clipboard)
Acknowledging by name, social greeting to begin conversation

Client: "What's good about it?"
(Arms crossed over chest, frowning, direct stare)
Nonverbal signs of anger

Nurse: "You sound unhappy."
(Pulls up chair and sits at bedside)
Sharing observation, nonverbal communication of availability

Client: "You'd be unhappy, too, if nobody would answer your questions."
(Angry voice tone, challenging expression)
Further expression of feelings facilitated by nurse making accurate observation

Nurse: "Are you saying that you need some information you haven't been able to get?"
Clarifying what has been implied

Client: "Oh, I've tried to get it, all right. But nothing does any good."
Feeling powerless

Nurse: "I'd like to hear more about it."
(Leans forward slightly, lays clipboard in lap)
Offering self, removing barriers to active listening

Client: "You're probably just like all the rest of the incompetents in this hospital. Why should I talk to you?"
Testing and challenging nurse

Nurse: "This hospital has a fine staff, Mr. Simpson. I'm sure no one would intentionally keep information from you."
Feeling threatened and being defensive, a nontherapeutic technique

Client: "All right then: Why wouldn't that girl tell me what my blood sugar was?"

Nurse: "I'm not sure. If I were you, I'd forget about it and get a fresh start."
Giving advice and using cliché, which was nontherapeutic; would have been better to acknowledge that client had a right to know the information

Nurse: "I'm going to test your glucose in a minute, and I'll tell you the results." (does test) "Your blood sugar was 350."
Providing information, demonstrating trustworthiness

Client: "That's up pretty high, isn't it?"
(Worried facial expression)
Feeling very concerned about test results

Nurse: (Nods) . . . long pause . . .
Nonverbal affirmation, use of silence to allow client time to absorb information and gather thoughts

Client: "I'll never be normal again."
(Tears in eyes and voice)
Expressing feelings, which is therapeutic

Nurse: "This illness has changed a lot of things for you, hasn't it?"
Empathy statement, acknowledging implied feelings

Client: "I'm sorry, I shouldn't cry. I'm acting like a baby."
Embarrassed about showing his emotions

Nurse: "I don't think you're acting like a baby. I think being able to express your feelings is important and healthy."
(Hands him tissue box)
Sharing perception, giving professional opinion, meeting comfort needs

Client: "I'm so afraid complications will set in since my blood sugar is high."
(Stares out window)
Feels free to express deeper concerns, but they are hard to face

Nurse: "What kinds of things are you worried about?"
Open-ended question to seek information

Client: "I could lose a leg, like my mother did. Or go blind. Or have to live hooked up to a kidney machine for the rest of my life. I could go crazy!"

Nurse: "Go crazy? I'm not sure what you mean."
(Puzzled and faintly alarmed facial expression)
Concerned about meaning, trying to clarify

Client: "Go crazy from worrying, I guess."
(Both laugh)
Use of humor defuses tension

Nurse: "You've been thinking about all kinds of things that could go wrong, and it adds to your worry not to be told what your blood sugar is."
Summarizing to let client "hear" what he has communicated

Client: "I always think the worst."
(Shakes head in exasperation)
Expressing insight into his "inner dialogue"

Nurse: "I'll pass along to the tech that it's OK to tell you your glucose levels. And later this afternoon, I'd like us to talk more about some things you can do to help avoid these complications and set some goals for controlling your glucose."
(Stands up, keeps looking at client)
Providing information, encouraging collaboration and goal setting
Giving nonverbal cue that conversation is nearing end

Client: "OK, if you can stand an old pessimist like me."
(Smiles, appears relaxed)
Trust established, willing to work with nurse; anxiety lessened

Nurse: "Old pessimists are my biggest challenge! Seriously, I'm glad you let me know what was going on, and I'd like to help."
Humor, positive reinforcement for client's willingness to communicate

---

past, which has a therapeutic effect and increases their sense of well-being. The nurse should avoid sudden shifts from subject to subject. It is helpful to include the client's family and friends and to become familiar with the client's favorite topics for conversation.

NP Evaluation

The nurse and client determine whether the plan of care has been successful by evaluating the client communication outcomes. The nurse evaluates nursing interven-

tions to determine what strategies or interventions were effective and what client changes resulted because of the interventions. For example, if using a pen and paper proves frustrating for a nonverbal client whose handwriting is shaky, the care plan can be revised to include use of a picture board instead. If expected outcomes are not met or progress is not satisfactory, the nurse needs to determine what factors influenced the outcomes, then modify the plan of care.

Nurses can evaluate the effectiveness of their own communication by making process recordings, written records of their verbal and nonverbal interactions with clients.

Process recording analysis reveals how the nurse can improve personal communication techniques to make them more effective. Box 23-10 contains a sample communication analysis of such a record. Analysis of a process recording enables the nurse to evaluate the following:

- Determine whether he or she encouraged openness and allowed the client to "tell his story," expressing both thoughts and feelings
- Identify any missed verbal or nonverbal cues or conversational themes
- Examine whether nursing responses blocked or facilitated the client's efforts to communicate
- Determine whether nursing responses were positive and supportive or superficial and judgmental
- Examine the type and number of questions that were asked
- Determine the type and number of therapeutic communication techniques used
- Discover any missed opportunities to use humor, silence, or touch

Evaluation of the communication process will help nurses gain confidence and competence in interpersonal skills. Becoming an effective communicator greatly increases the nurse's professional satisfaction and success. There is no skill more basic, no tool more powerful.

Key Concepts

- Communication is a powerful therapeutic tool and an essential nursing skill used to influence others and achieve positive health outcomes.
- Communication involves the entire human being, including body, mind, emotions, and spirit.
- Critical thinking facilitates communication through creative inquiry, focused self-awareness and awareness of others, purposeful analysis, and control of perceptual biases.
- Nurses consider many contexts and factors influencing communication when making decisions about what, when, where, how, why, and with whom to communicate.
- Communication is most effective when the receiver and sender accurately perceive the meaning of one another's messages.
- Message transmission is influenced by the sender's and receiver's physical and developmental status, perceptions, values, emotions, knowledge, sociocultural background, roles, and environment.
- Effective verbal communication requires appropriate intonation, clear and concise phrasing, proper pacing of statements, and proper timing and relevance of a message.
- Effective nonverbal communication complements and strengthens the message conveyed by verbal communication so that the receiver is less likely to misinterpret the message.
- Nurses use intrapersonal, interpersonal, transpersonal, small-group, and public interaction to achieve positive change and health goals.
- Helping relationships are strengthened when the nurse demonstrates caring by establishing trust, empathy, autonomy, confidentiality, and professional competence.
- Effective communication techniques are facilitative and tend to encourage the other person to openly express ideas, feelings, or concerns.
- Ineffective communication techniques are inhibiting and tend to block the other person's willingness to openly express ideas, feelings, or concerns.
- The nurse must blend social and informational interactions with therapeutic communication techniques so that others can explore feelings and manage health issues.
- Methods that facilitate communication with children include sitting at eye level; interacting with parents; using simple, direct language; and incorporating play activities.
- Older-adult clients with sensory, motor, or cognitive impairments require the adaptation of communication techniques to compensate for their loss of function and special needs.
- Clients with impaired verbal communication require special consideration and alterations in communication techniques to facilitate the sending, receiving, and interpreting of messages.
- Desired outcomes for clients with impaired verbal communication include increased satisfaction with interpersonal interactions, the ability to send and receive clear messages, and attending to and accurately interpreting verbal and nonverbal cues.

Key Terms

Active listening, *p. 437*
Assertiveness, *p. 434*
Autonomy, *p. 434*
Channels, *p. 428*
Communication, *p. 424*
Empathy, *p. 438*
Environment, *p. 429*
Feedback, *p. 428*
Interpersonal communication, *p. 427*
Interpersonal variables, *p. 428*
Intrapersonal communication, *p. 427*
Message, *p. 428*
Metacommunication, *p. 431*
Nonverbal communication, *p. 429*

Perceptions, *p. 426*
Perceptual biases, *p. 426*
Public communication, *p. 427*
Receiver, *p. 428*
Referent, *p. 428*
Sender, *p. 428*
Small-group communication, *p. 427*
Symbolic communication, *p. 431*
Sympathy, *p. 441*
Therapeutic communication techniques, *p. 437*
Transpersonal communication, *p. 427*
Verbal communication, *p. 429*

Critical Thinking Exercises

1. Mrs. Maria Ramirez, an American of Puerto Rican descent, is faced with the difficult decision of whether of not to continue chemotherapy in the face of a rapidly spreading malignancy. What communication techniques could the nurse use to help her at this

point, and what traps must the nurse avoid in such a situation?

2. Jan, a nurse colleague, is having difficulty standing up to a physician who has an abrupt, intimidating communication style. She often ends up with a lot of unspoken anger, developing tension headaches and easily becoming tearful. What could the nurse do to help?

3. Mr. Hess, a client with Parkinson's disease living at an extended care facility, has a stiff, expressionless face. He sits slumped in a recliner chair all day and seems lost in his own world, rarely looking at or interacting with anyone. When he does talk, he mumbles in a soft voice and his words are difficult to understand. What kinds of things could the nurse do to establish a helping-healing relationship with Mr. Hess?

4. Jennifer Hughes, a new graduate, is very discouraged. In school, she had felt a great deal of anxiety about her own performance, and even now she find it difficult to be positive about herself or her job. What knowledge about communication could she us to help improve her situation?

5. Mrs. Esther Larson, a client who has been recently admitted to a hospice program, confides in the nurse that she feels overwhelmed with the number of things she must attend to now that she's facing the possibility of death. She says, "My thoughts are all over the place. I don't know where to start." What communication techniques, based on the critical thinking model, could the nurse use to help her at this point?

Review Questions

1. Communication is not the message that was intended but rather the message that was received. The statement that best helps explain this is:
   1. Clean communication can ensure the client will receive the message intended.
   2. Sincerity in communication is the responsibility of the sender and the receiver.
   3. Attention to personal space can minimize misinterpretation of communication.
   4. Contextual factors, such as attitudes, values, beliefs, and self-concept, influence communication.

2. The nurse demonstrates active listening by:
   1. Agreeing with the client.
   2. Repeating everything the client says to clarify.
   3. Assuming a relaxed posture and leaning toward the client.
   4. Smiling and nodding continuously throughout the interview.

3. The nurse builds helping, caring relationships by:
   1. Using touch for calming and comfort.
   2. Establishing trust and demonstrating empathy.
   3. Not asking the patient to do anything painful.
   4. Being sympathetic and protective of the client.

4. Gender influences how a person thinks, acts, feels, and communicates. In Western culture it is important for the nurse to remember when he is trying to be sensitive to gender in communicating that:
   1. Males communicate to achieve goals, establish individual status and authority, and compete for attention and power.
   2. Males use indirect communication to meet their needs, whereas females communicate directly.
   3. Males grow up using aggressive communication, whereas females use passive communication.
   4. Males and females should be treated equally; therefore it serves no purpose to distinguish between genders in communication.

5. The statement that best explains the role of collaboration with others for the client's plan of care is the professional nurse:
   1. Collaborates with colleagues and the client's family to provide combined expertise in planning care.
   2. Consults the physician for direction in establishing goals for clients.
   3. Depends on the latest literature to complete an excellent plan of care for clients.
   4. Works independently to plan and deliver care and does not depend on other staff for assistance.

6. "I'm not sure I understand what you mean by 'sicker than usual.' What is different now?" The nurse is using the therapeutic technique:
   1. Paraphrasing.
   2. Providing information.
   3. Clarifying.
   4. Focusing.

7. "We've talked a lot about your medications, but let's look more closely at the trouble you're having in taking them on time." The nurse is using the therapeutic technique:
   1. Paraphrasing.
   2. Providing information.
   3. Clarifying.
   4. Focusing.

8. "If I were you, I'd put your mother in a nursing home." The nurse is using the nontherapeutic technique:
   1. Asking personal questions.
   2. Changing the subject.
   3. Giving personal opinions.
   4. Automatic responses.

9. When working with an older adult, the nurse should remember to avoid:
   1. Touching the client.
   2. Shifting from subject to subject.
   3. Allowing the client to reminisce.
   4. Asking the client how he or she feels.

10. A nurse should consider zones of personal space and touch when caring for clients. If the nurse is taking the client's nursing history, she should:
1. Be 12 inches to 3 feet from the client.
2. Sit next to the client.
3. Be 4 to 12 feet from the client.
4. Be 18 inches to 4 feet from the client.

References

Balzer Riley J: *Communications in nursing,* ed 4, St. Louis, 2000, Mosby.

Beebe S, Beebe S, Redmond M: *Interpersonal communication: relating to others,* ed 2, Boston, 1999, Allyn & Bacon.

Burden N: Using self-responsibility to improve communication: one nurse's perspective, *J Perianesth Nurs* 12(1):25, 1997.

Canales M: Narrative interaction: creating a space for therapeutic communication, *Issues Ment Health Nurs* 18(5):477, 1997.

Creasia J, Parker P: *Conceptual foundations of professional nursing practice,* St. Louis, 2001, Mosby.

Crouch R: Communication is the key, *Emerg Nurse* 10(3):1, 2002.

Curtis D, Floyd J, Winsor J: *Business and professional communication,* ed 2, Dubuque, Iowa, 1997, Kendall/Hunt.

Darley M, editor: *Managing communication in health care,* New York, 2002, Baillere Tindall/Harcourt Publishers.

Fortinash K, Holoday-Worret P: *Psychiatric mental health nursing,* ed 2, St. Louis, 2000, Mosby.

Geiger J, Davidhizar R: *Transcultural nursing: assessment and intervention,* ed 3, St. Louis, 1999, Mosby.

Hartrick G: Relational capacity: the foundation for interpersonal nursing practice, *J Adv Nurs* 26(3):523, 1997.

Henson R: Analysis of the concept of mutuality, *Image J Nurs Sch* 29(1):77, 1997.

Hybels S, Weaver R: *Communicating effectively,* ed 5, Boston, 1998, McGraw-Hill.

Johnson M and others: *Nursing diagnoses, outcomes, and interventions,* St. Louis, 2001, Mosby.

Krebs K: The spiritual aspect of caring: an integral part of health and healing, *Nurs Adm Q* 25(3):55, 2001.

Mandel E, Shulman M, Begany T: Overcoming communication disorders in the elderly, *Patient Care* 31(2):55, 1997.

Minor A: Therapeutic touch, *Healthcare Rev* 14(3):4, 2001.

Paavilainen E, Astedt-Kurki P: The client-nurse relationship as experienced by public health nurses: toward better collaboration, *Public Health Nurs* 14(3):137, 1997.

Paul R: The art of redesigning instruction. In Willsen J, Blinker AJA, editors: *Critical thinking: how to prepare students for a rapidly changing world,* Santa Rosa, Calif, 1993, Foundation for Critical Thinking.

Perry B: Influence of nurse gender on the use of silence, touch, and humor, *Int J Palliat Nurs* 2(1):7, 1996.

Seigel B: *Peace, love and healing,* New York, 1989, Harper & Row.

Smith K: *Humor as a clinical skill: Are you joking?* Urol Nurs 20(16):382, 2000.

Stanhope M, Lancaster J: *Community and public health nursing,* ed 5, St. Louis, 2000, Mosby.

Stewart J, Logan C: *Together: communicating interpersonally,* ed 5, Boston, 1998, McGraw-Hill.

Stuart G, Laraia M: *Principles and practice of psychiatric nursing,* ed 7, St. Louis, 2001, Mosby.

Townsend M: *Psychiatric mental health nursing: Concepts of care,* ed 4, Philadelphia, 2003, FA Davis.

Watson J: *Nursing: human science and health care,* Norwalk, Conn, 1985, Appleton-Century-Crofts.

Wong D and others: *Whaley and Wong's nursing care of infants and children,* ed 6, St. Louis, 1999, Mosby.

Wood J: *Interpersonal communication,* ed 2, Cincinnati, 1999, Wadsworth.

Research References

Astedt-Kurki P, Isola A: Humour between nurse and patient, and among staff, *J Adv Nurs* 35(3):452, 2001.

Hawley M: Nurse comforting strategies, *Clin Nurs Res* 9(4):441, 2000.

Hemsley B and otehrs: Nursing the patient with severe communication impairment, *J Adv Nurs* 35(6):827, 2001.

Routasalo P: Non-necessary touch in the nursing care of elderly people, *J Adv Nurs* 23(5):904, 1996.

Seed A: Crossing the boundaries: experiences of neophyte nurses, *J Adv Nurs* 21(6):1136, 1995.

24

Client Education

Media Resources

http://evolve.elsevier.com/Potter/
fundamentals/

CD COMPANION

- Review Questions
- Glossary

evolve WEBSITE

- Review Questions
- Student Learning Activities
- Glossary

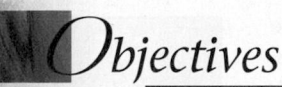

Objectives

Mastery of content in this chapter will enable the student to:

- Define the key terms listed.
- Identify appropriate topics for a client's health education needs.
- Describe the similarities and differences between teaching and learning.
- Identify the role of the nurse in client education.
- Identify the purposes of client education.
- Describe how to incorporate communication principles into client education.
- Describe the domains of learning.
- Identify basic learning principles.
- Differentiate factors that determine the readiness to learn from those that determine the ability to learn.
- Compare and contrast the nursing and teaching processes.
- Write learning objectives for a teaching plan.
- Describe characteristics of a good learning environment.
- Describe ways to incorporate teaching with routine nursing care.
- Identify methods for evaluating learning.

*C*lient education is one of the most important roles for a nurse in any health care setting. Teaching prenatal care to healthy mothers in a physician's office, instructing parents visiting a clinic about immunization of children, and teaching people who have had heart attacks about newly pre-scribed medications are all examples of client education. Clients and family members have the right to health education so that they are able to make in-telligent, informed decisions about their health and lifestyle. Client education is essential because many clients now receive treatments in their homes or in an outpatient setting. In addition, hospitalized clients are being discharged ear-lier. These situations require the nurse to provide adequate education to ensure the achievement of client outcomes. Furthermore, effective health education is essential to care for increasing numbers of clients in the community and to minimize the effects of preventable diseases.

Shorter hospital stays, increased demands on nurses' time, an increase in the number of chronically ill, and the need to give acutely ill clients concise, mean-ingful information as soon as possible emphasize the importance of quality client education. As nurses try to find the best way to educate clients, the gen-eral public has become more assertive in seeking knowledge and understand-ing of their health and the resources available within the health care system. Providing clients health care information is necessary to ensure continuity of care from the hospital to the home. A well-designed, comprehensive teaching plan that fits a client's learning needs can reduce health care costs, improve the quality of care, and help clients gain optimal wellness and increase indepen-dence (Cooper and others, 2001).

Client education is important because clients have the right to know and to be informed about their diagnoses, prognoses, and available treatments. Educational materials provided should be readily understandable. It is negligent to assume that clients will learn on their own. Accurate, timely teaching is needed for clients to make decisions about their health and improve their overall health status. More attention is being paid in courts of law as to whether clients are adequately informed about ways to manage their health. Competent professional nursing practice includes client education. The nurse can provide effective education only by identifying clients' learning needs and by using the most appropriate teaching strategies.

Standards for Client Education

Client education has long been a standard for professional nursing practice. Various accrediting agencies set guidelines for providing client education in health care institutions. These guidelines ensure that the client and family receive information necessary to maintain the client's optimal level of health. The Joint Commission on Accreditation of Healthcare Organizations (JCAHO) accredits health care institutions in the United States. According to the JCAHO (2003), the goal of client and family education is to promote healthy behaviors and encourage the client's involvement both in the delivery of health care and in health care decisions, to improve outcomes. Box 24-1 lists JCAHO's standards for client education. The successful accomplishment of these standards enhances client recovery and depends on participation of all health care professionals. Educational efforts must take into consideration the client's psychosocial, spiritual, and cultural values, as well as his or her desire to actively participate in the educational process (JCAHO, 2002). Evidence of successful client education must be documented in the client's medical record. Standards such as these help to direct nurses in client education.

Purposes of Client Education

The goal of educating others about their health is to assist individuals, families, or communities in achieving optimal levels of health (Edelman and Mandle, 2002). The American Nurses Association's *Position Statement on Promotion and Disease Prevention* (ANA) (1995) supports a focus on promoting health and preventing illness. Preventative health care is essential in reducing health care costs, as well as reducing hardships on individuals, families, and communities. Clients now know more about health and want to be involved in health maintenance. Nurses need to provide education about health and health care in places that are convenient and familiar to clients. Comprehensive client education includes three important purposes, each involving a separate phase of health care (Box 24-2).

> **Box 24-1**   **JCAHO Patient and Family Education and Responsibilities**
>
> **PF.1** The hospital plans for and supports the provision and coordination of patient education activities.
> **PF.1.1** The hospital identifies and provides the resources necessary for achieving educational objectives.
> **PF.2** The patient education process is coordinated among appropriate staff or disciplines who are providing care or services.
> **PF.3** The patient receives education and training specific to the patient's assessed needs, abilities, learning preferences, and readiness to learn as appropriate to the care and services provided by the hospital.
> **PF.3.1** Based on assessed needs, the patient is educated about how to safely and effectively use medications, according to law and regulation, and the hospital's scope of services, as appropriate.
> **PF.3.2** The patient is educated about nutrition interventions, modified diets, or oral health, when applicable.
> **PF.3.3** The hospital assures that the patient is educated about how to safely and effectively use medical equipment or supplies, as appropriate.
> **PF.3.4** Patients are educated about pain and managing pain as part of treatment, as appropriate.*
> **PF.3.5** Patients are educated about habilitation or rehabilitation techniques to help them be more functionally independent, as appropriate.
> **PF.3.6** The patient is educated about other available resources, and when necessary, how to obtain further care, services, or treatment to meet his or her identified needs.
> **PF.3.7** Education includes information about patient responsibilities in the patient's care.
> **PF.3.8** Education includes self-care activities, as appropriate.
> **PF.3.9** Discharge instructions are given to the patient and those responsible for providing continuing care.
> **PF.3.10** Academic education is provided to children and adolescents either directly by the hospital or through other arrangements, when appropriate.

From Joint Commission on Accreditation of Healthcare Organizations: *Accreditation manual of hospitals*, Oakbrook Terrace, Ill, 2003, The Commission.
*Effective January 1, 2001.

Maintenance and Promotion of Health and Illness Prevention

The nurse is a visible, competent resource for clients intent on improving physical and psychological well-being. In the school, home, clinic, or workplace, the nurse provides information and skills that allow clients to assume healthier behaviors (see Box 24-2). For example, in childbearing classes, nurses teach expectant parents about physical and psychological changes in the woman and about fetal development. After learning about normal childbearing, the mother is more likely to eat healthy foods, engage in physical exercise, and avoid substances that might harm the fetus. Promoting healthy behavior through education increases self-esteem by allowing clients to assume more responsibility for their health.

Box 24-2	Topics for Health Education

Health Maintenance and Promotion and Illness Prevention

First aid
Avoidance of risk factors (e.g., smoking, alcohol)
Stress management
Growth and development
Hygiene
Immunizations
Prenatal care and normal childbearing
Nutrition
Exercise
Safety (in home and health care setting)
Screening (e.g., blood pressure, vision, cholesterol level)
Behavior modification to change risk behaviors (e.g., smoking cessation, substance abuse treatment)

Restoration of Health

Client's disease or condition
Anatomy and physiology of body system affected
Cause of disease
Origin of symptoms
Expected effects on other body systems
Prognosis
Limitations on function
Rationale for treatment

Medications
Tests and therapies
Nursing measures
Surgical intervention
Expected duration of care
Hospital or clinic environment
Hospital or clinic staff
Long-term care
Methods for client participation in care
Limitations posed by disease or surgery

Coping With Impaired Functions

Home care
Medications
Intravenous therapy
Diet
Activity
Self-help devices
Rehabilitation of remaining function
Physical therapy
Occupational therapy
Speech therapy
Prevention of complications
Knowledge of risk factors
Implications of noncompliance with therapy
Environmental alterations

Greater knowledge can result in better health maintenance habits. When clients become more health conscious, they are more likely to seek early diagnosis of health problems (Redman, 2001).

Restoration of Health

Injured or ill clients need information and skills that will help them regain or maintain their levels of health (see Box 24-2. Clients recovering from illness or injury and adapting to the resultant changes often seek information about their conditions. For example, a woman recently having a hysterectomy asks about her pathology reports and expected length of recovery. However, clients who find it difficult to adapt to illness may become passive and uninterested in learning. The nurse learns to identify clients' willingness to learn and to help motivate interest in learning (Assessment, the Foundation of Good Teaching, 2002).

The family can be a vital part of a client's return to health and may need to know as much as the client. If the nurse excludes the family from a teaching plan, conflicts may arise. For example, if the family does not understand a client's need to regain independent function, their efforts may cause the client to become unnecessarily dependent and slow the client's recovery. The nurse should not assume that the family should be involved and must first assess the client-family relationship.

Coping With Impaired Functioning

Not all clients fully recover from illness or injury. Many must learn to cope with permanent health alterations.

New knowledge and skills are often necessary for clients to continue activities of daily living (see Box 24-2). For example, a client whose ability to speak is lost after surgery of the larynx must learn new ways of communicating. The client with severe heart disease learns to modify risk factors that might cause further heart damage.

In the case of serious disability, the client's family needs to understand and accept these changes. The family's ability to provide support can result from education, which begins as soon as the client's needs are identified and the family displays a willingness to help. The nurse teaches family members to assist the client with health care management (e.g., giving medications through gastric tubes and doing passive range-of-motion exercises). Families of clients with alterations such as alcoholism, mental retardation, or drug dependence also learn to adapt to the emotional effects of these chronic conditions.

A nurse learns to recognize the information to teach to clients at different levels of wellness by assessing clients' needs and abilities. Learning occurs when information is practical and useful to the learner (Redman, 2001). Comparing the desired level of health with the actual state enables the nurse to plan effective teaching programs.

Teaching and Learning

It is impossible to separate teaching from learning. **Teaching** is an interactive process that promotes learning. It consists of a conscious, deliberate set of actions that help individuals gain new knowledge, change attitudes, adopt new behaviors, or perform new skills (Bastable, 2003; Redman, 2001). A teacher provides information that prompts the learner to engage in activities that lead to a desired change.

Learning is the purposeful acquisition of new knowledge, attitudes, behaviors, and skills (Bastable, 2003). Complex patterns are required if the client is to learn new skills or change existing attitudes (Redman, 2001). A new mother exhibits learning when she demonstrates to the nurse how to bathe her newborn. Learning is also demonstrated when a client preparing for abdominal surgery demonstrates deep breathing and coughing while splinting the abdomen with a pillow. Generally, teaching and learning begin when a person identifies a need for knowing or acquiring an ability to do something. Teaching is most effective when it responds to the learner's needs. The teacher assesses these needs by asking questions and determining the learner's interests. Interpersonal communication is essential for successful teaching to occur (see Chapter 23).

Role of the Nurse in Teaching and Learning

Nurses have an ethical responsibility to teach their clients. In *The Patient Care Partnership,* formerly called *A Patient's Bill of Rights,* the American Hospital Association (2003) indicates that clients have the right to make informed decisions about their care. The information required to make informed decisions must be accurate, complete, and relevant to the client's needs. The nurse should anticipate clients' needs for information based on their physical conditions or treatment plans. The nurse's responsibility is to teach the information that clients and their families need. The nurse often clarifies information provided by physicians and other health care providers and may become the primary source of information needed for adjusting to health problems (Oermann, Harris, and Dammeyer, 2001).

Clients and their families often ask nurses for health information. For example, a client may request information about a new medication, or family members may

---

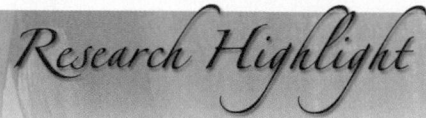

Box 24-3

Learning Preferences of Cancer Patients

Research Focus

Adult clients living with a diagnosis of cancer have unique learning needs. Information needs of these clients have been reported in many different publications. However, questions remain as to these clients' preferred learning methods.

Research Abstract

This study identified appropriate content to be included in a formal cancer education program for adults. The study also aimed to describe the learning and support preferences of adults with cancer. This study had three phases. In the first phase, a multidisciplinary cancer-care team identified key categories of information that should be included in an educational program. The key components included topics such as cancer diagnosis and treatment, coping, medication side effect management, sexuality, and pain control. The second phase included 100 structured interviews. Participants in this phase had been diagnosed with a variety of different cancer types, including breast cancer, lymphoma, colorectal cancer, prostate cancer, and lung cancer. The third phase of the study included the development of a 37-item survey. Items in the survey were based on information obtained during the interviews. The survey was mailed to 1310 adults who were receiving care in radiation oncology, medical oncology, and chemotherapy treatment outpatient areas. The survey asked clients to recall what they were taught about their cancer treatment and their preferences for the educational format. Respondents reported their most favored method for learning about all cancer topics was discussions with physicians, followed by personal communication with nurses. Adults over 60 years of age were less likely to indicate their preferences for learning, whereas those respondents with a postsecondary education endorsed a variety of learning preferences. Women were more likely to prefer speaking with a

nurse for all content areas, whereas men were more likely to discuss sexuality with their physicians. The majority of respondents did not attend support groups, and interest in computer-assisted learning (e.g., the Internet) was low. However, respondents did express an interest in using a toll-free number to enhance access to information and support.

Evidence-Based Practice

- Clients with cancer want clear, accurate information about their diagnosis and related treatment options.
- Adult clients with cancer prefer interactive, personal communication with physicians or nurses.
- Printed material that enhances knowledge was also preferred and should be distributed to clients with cancer.
- Assessing and adapting educational information and approaches to clients' needs and preferences enhances the success of educational efforts.
- Not all clients are comfortable in class settings or in support groups. Educational programs that use these methods should have other educational opportunities available to their clients.
- Computer-assisted learning (CAL) was not preferred by many of the participants in this study. As clients become more comfortable with computers, this preference may change. Nurses who use CAL in educational sessions need to assess the client's access and desire to use this learning technique.
- Nurses must remain creative and responsive to their clients when providing client education.

Reference

Chelf J and others: Learning and support preferences of adult patients with cancer at a comprehensive cancer center, *Oncol Nurs Forum* 29(5):863, 2002.

question the reason for their mother's pain. The leader of a support group for teenage mothers may ask the nurse to explain the importance of healthy food choices for children. Identification of the need for teaching is easy when clients request information. Often, however, a client's need for teaching may be less obvious.

To be an effective educator, the nurse must do more than just pass on facts. The nurse carefully determines what clients need to know and find the time when they are ready to learn. When nurses value client education and are able to implement it, clients are better prepared to assume health care responsibilities. Evaluating the positive impact of client education on client outcomes is an important nursing issue (Bastable, 2003; Redman, 2001) (Box 24-3).

Teaching as Communication

The teaching process closely parallels the communication process (see Chapter 23). Effective teaching depends in part on effective interpersonal communication. A teacher applies each element of the communication process while imparting information to learners. Thus the teacher and learner become involved together in a teaching process that increases the learner's knowledge and skills.

The steps of the teaching process can be compared with those of the communication process (Table 24-1). In teaching, the referent is the need to provide the client with information. The client may request information, or the nurse may perceive a need for information because of a client's health restrictions or the recent diagnosis of an illness. The nurse then identifies specific learning objectives. A **learning objective** describes what the learner will be able to do after successful instruction.

The nurse is the sender who wants to convey a message to the client. The nurse promotes learning by communicating in a language recognizable to the learner. Many intrapersonal variables influence the nurse's style and approach. The nurse's attitudes, values, emotions, and knowledge influence the way the information is delivered. Past experiences with teaching are also helpful as the nurse chooses the best way to present the necessary content.

The message or content to be taught is delivered clearly and precisely. The nurse organizes information to be taught in a logical sequence so that the client will more easily understand skills or ideas. Each lesson progresses from the simple to the more complex skills or ideas.

The nurse may use a variety of ways to present teaching content. All of the senses are channels for presenting information. The auditory channel is the simplest, as in a lecture or discussion. The learning process becomes more stimulating and effective, however, when several sensory channels are used together. For example, the nurse uses a

Table 24-1	Comparison of Terms Used in Teaching and Communication
Communication	**Teaching**
Referent	
Idea that initiates reason for communication	Perceived need to provide person with information; establishment of relevant learning objectives by teacher
Sender	
Person who conveys message to another	Teacher who performs activities aimed at helping other person to learn
Intrapersonal Variables (Sender)	
Knowledge, values, emotions, and sociocultural influences that affect sender's thoughts	Teacher's philosophy of education (based on learning theory); knowledge of teaching content; teaching approach; experiences in teaching; teacher's emotions and values
Message	
Information expressed or transmitted by sender	Content or information taught
Channels	
Methods used to transmit message (e.g., visual, auditory, touch)	Methods used to present content (e.g., visual and auditory materials, touch, taste, smell)
Receiver	
Person to whom message is transmitted	Learner
Intrapersonal Variables (Receiver)	
Knowledge, values, emotions, and sociocultural influences that affect receiver's thoughts	Willingness and ability to learn (e.g., physical and emotional health, education, experience, developmental level)
Feedback	
Information revealing that true meaning of message was received	Determination of whether learning objectives were achieved

tactile channel in helping a client with newly diagnosed heart disease learn how to measure a pulse by actually feeling the pulsation of the radial artery.

The receiver in the teaching-learning process is the learner. A number of intrapersonal variables affect motivation and ability to learn. Clients are ready to learn when they express a desire to do so and are more likely to receive the message when they understand the content. Attitudes, anxiety, and values influence the ability to understand a message. The ability to learn depends on factors such as emotional and physical health, education, the stage of development, and previous knowledge.

Effective communication involves feedback. An effective teacher provides a mechanism for evaluating the success of a teaching plan and then providing positive reinforcement (Bastable, 2003). Examples of ways to evaluate teaching sessions include having a client demonstrate a newly learned skill or asking the client to describe how the correct dosage schedule for a new medication will be incorporated into a daily routine. Feedback must show the success of the learner in achieving objectives; that is, the learner verbalizes information or provides a return demonstration of skills learned.

*D*omains of Learning

Learning occurs in three domains: cognitive (understanding), affective (attitudes), and psychomotor (motor skills) (Bloom, 1956). Any topic to be learned may involve one or all domains or any combination of the three. The nurse often works with clients who need to learn in each domain. For example, clients diagnosed with diabetes must learn how diabetes affects the body and how to control blood glucose levels for healthier lifestyles (cognitive domain). In addition, clients must learn to accept the chronic nature of diabetes by learning positive coping mechanisms (affective domain). Finally, many clients living with diabetes must learn to test their blood glucose levels at home. This requires learning how to use a glucose meter (psychomotor domain). The characteristics of learning within each domain affect the teaching and evaluation methods used. Understanding each learning domain prepares the nurse to select proper teaching techniques (Box 24-4). However, the nurse needs to also be able to apply the basic principles of learning to any teaching method.

Cognitive Learning

Cognitive learning includes all intellectual behaviors and requires thinking (Bastable, 2003). In the hierarchy of cognitive behaviors the simplest behavior is acquiring knowledge, whereas the most complex is evaluation.

Knowledge. Using knowledge is acquiring new facts or information and being able to recall them. For example, the client learns about a prescribed medication and is able to describe its purpose and potential side effects.

Comprehension. Comprehension is the ability to understand the meaning of learned material. For example, the

---

Box 24-4   Appropriate Teaching Methods Based on Domains of Learning

Cognitive

Discussion (one-on-one or group)
May involve nurse and one client or nurse with several clients
Promotes active participation and focuses on topics of interest to client
Allows peer support
Enhances application and analysis of new information
Lecture
Is more formal method of instruction because it is controlled by teacher
Helps learner acquire new knowledge and gain comprehension
Question-and-answer session
Designed specifically to address client's concerns
Assists client in applying knowledge
Role play, discovery
Allows client to actively apply knowledge in controlled situation
Promotes synthesis of information and problem solving
Independent project (computer-assisted instruction), field experience
Allows client to assume responsibility for completing learning activities at own pace
Promotes analysis, synthesis, and evaluation of new information and skills

Affective

Role play
Allows expression of values, feelings, and attitudes
Discussion (group)
Allows client to acquire support from others in group
Permits client to learn from others' experiences
Promotes responding, valuing, and organization
Discussion (one-on-one)
Allows discussion of personal, sensitive topics of interest or concern

Psychomotor

Demonstration
Provides presentation of procedures or skills by nurse
Permits client to incorporate modeling of nurse's behavior
Allows nurse to control questioning during demonstration
Practice
Gives client opportunity to perform skills using equipment in a controlled setting
Provides repetition
Return demonstration
Permits client to perform skill as nurse observes
Provides excellent source of feedback and reinforcement
Independent projects, games
Require teaching method that promotes adaptation and origination of psychomotor learning
Permit learner to use new skills

client is able to explain specifically how a new medication will improve a physical condition.

Application. Application involves using abstract, newly learned ideas in a concrete situation. For example, the client develops a medication schedule according to normal mealtimes to ensure optimal desired effects of the medication.

Analysis. Analysis involves breaking down information into organized parts. It allows a person to discriminate important from unimportant information. For example, the client is able to distinguish which side effects are more likely to be experienced from a medication and to compare them with the effects experienced by another person.

Synthesis. Synthesis is the ability to apply knowledge and skills to produce a new whole. For example, the client experiences side effects from a medication and is able to take preventive steps.

Evaluation. Evaluation is a judgment of the worth of a body of information for a given purpose. For example, the client is able to recognize the need for more information about a medication (e.g., insulin) to plan a safe exercise program.

Affective Learning

Affective learning deals with expression of feelings and acceptance of attitudes, opinions, or values. Values clarification (see Chapter 21) is an example of affective learning. The simplest behavior in the hierarchy is receiving, and the most complex is characterizing (Krathwohl and others, 1964).

Receiving. Receiving is being willing to attend to another person's words. For example, a woman shows a willingness to listen to a nurse explain the surgical procedure for removal of a breast by being attentive and maintaining eye contact while the nurse is talking.

Responding. Responding involves active participation through listening and reacting verbally and nonverbally. The person feels satisfied from the response. For example, the client asks the nurse about what the incision will look like after the surgery.

Valuing. Valuing means attaching worth to an object or behavior. This is shown through the learner's behavior. The person is motivated to act out the behavior. For example, the client who expresses concern about the appearance of a surgical incision before having a breast removed refuses to look at the incision and wears a gown with a high neck after the surgery.

Organizing. Organizing is developing a value system by identifying and organizing values and resolving conflicts. For example, the client learns to accept changes created by surgery and is willing to participate in social activities.

Characterizing. Characterizing involves acting and responding with a consistent value system. The person behaves consistently when values are tested or challenged. For example, the client assumes a normal lifestyle after having breast surgery and is able to discuss positive self-feelings with others.

Psychomotor Learning

Psychomotor learning involves acquiring skills that require the integration of mental and muscular activity, such as the ability to walk or to use an eating utensil. The simplest behavior in the hierarchy is perception, whereas the most complex is origination (Rankin and Stallings, 2001; Redman, 2001).

Perception. Perception is being aware of objects or qualities through the use of sense organs. A person associates a sensory cue with the task to perform. For example, a client who has had a stroke needs to learn to use a walker. While learning this skill, the client begins to recognize that changes in walking surfaces require an adjustment to placement of the walker.

Set. A set is a readiness to take a particular action. There are three sets: mental, physical, and emotional. For example, a person who has recently been injured in a motor vehicle accident uses judgment to determine the best way to get out of a wheelchair (mental readiness). Before getting out of the wheelchair, the person aligns and postures properly (physical readiness). The client makes a commitment (emotional set) to regularly perform strengthening exercises to facilitate recovery from the sustained injuries.

Guided Response. A guided response is the performance of an act under the guidance of an instructor. This involves imitation of a demonstrated act. For example, a client prepares an insulin injection after watching a nurse's demonstration. The nurse provides immediate reinforcement after the client correctly performs the self-injection.

Mechanism. A mechanism is a higher level of behavior by which a person gains confidence and skill in performing behavior. Usually the skill is more complex or involves several more steps than a guided response. For example, a client is able to fill the insulin syringe for different insulin doses.

Complex Overt Response. A complex overt response involves performing a motor skill involving a complex movement pattern. The person performs the skill smoothly and accurately without hesitation. For example, a client who is recently paralyzed from a spinal injury is able to perform self-catheterization and does not acquire a urinary tract infection.

Adaptation. Adaptation occurs when a person is able to change a motor response when unexpected problems arise. For example, a new mother who is breast-feeding and who plans to return to work learns how to collect breast milk, store it, and coordinate pumping times with her baby's feeding demands and her work schedule.

Origination. Origination is a highly complex motor act that involves creating new movement patterns. A person acts on the basis of existing psychomotor skills and abilities. For example, a client who has left-sided paralysis from a cerebrovascular accident must learn to eat, dress, and walk while on a rehabilitation unit.

Basic Learning Principles

To teach effectively and efficiently, the nurse must first understand how people learn. Learning depends on the learning environment and on the individual's motivation, learning preferences, and the ability to learn. An ideal learning environment allows a person to attend to instruction. Motivation addresses a person's desire or willingness to learn (Redman, 2001). The client's willingness to become involved in learning influences a nurse's teaching approach. Previous knowledge, attitudes, and sociocultural factors influence motivation.

A person's learning style affects preferences for learning. People process information in the following ways: by seeing and hearing, reflecting and acting, reasoning logically and intuitively, and analyzing and visualizing. Some people learn information gradually, whereas others learn more sporadically. Effective teaching plans include a combination of approaches that meet multiple learning styles (Felder, 2002).

The ability to learn depends on physical and cognitive attributes, developmental level, physical wellness, and intellectual thought processes. If a learning ability is impaired, such as with a client in pain, the nurse should postpone teaching activities or modify teaching strategies to better meet the needs of the learner.

Motivation to Learn

Attentional Set. An attentional set is the mental state that allows the learner to focus on and comprehend a learning activity. People often use mental pictures to visualize ideas. While a nurse explains how to give support to a dying client, the family members might envision grasping the fragile hand of their dying family member. Before learning anything, clients must give attention to, or concentrate on, the information to be learned.

Physical discomfort, anxiety, and environmental distractions can influence the ability to attend. Any physical condition that impairs the ability to concentrate (e.g., pain, fatigue, anxiety, or hunger) interferes with learning. Therefore the nurse determines the client's level of comfort and energy before beginning a teaching plan and ensures that the client is comfortable enough for discussion. Nonverbal cues can also reveal that a client is not ready to learn.

Anxiety may increase or decrease the ability of a person to pay attention. Anxiety is uneasiness or uncertainty resulting from anticipating a threat or danger. When faced with change or the need to act differently, a person feels anxious. Learning requires a change in behavior and thus produces anxiety. A mild level of anxiety may motivate learning. However, a high level of anxiety prevents learning from occurring. It incapacitates a person, creating an inability to attend to anything other than to relieve the anxiety.

Environmental distractions interfere with the ability to attend to a teacher and to learning activities.

Unplanned interruptions or an uncomfortable environment is not conducive to learning.

Motivation. **Motivation** is a force that acts on or within a person (e.g., an idea, emotion, or a physical need) that causes the person to behave in a particular way (Redman, 2001). If a person does not want to learn, it is unlikely that learning will occur. Motivation may result from a social, task, or physical motive.

Social motives are a need for connection, social approval, or self-esteem. People normally seek out others with whom they can compare opinions, abilities, and emotions. For example, new parents often seek validation of ideas and parenting techniques from others whom they have identified as role models in their social environment or health care workers with whom they have established a rapport.

Task mastery motives are based on needs such as achievement and competence. For example, a high school senior who has diabetes begins to test blood glucose levels and make decisions about insulin dosages in preparation for leaving home and establishing independence. The ability to successfully manage diabetes provides the motivation to master the task or skill. After a person succeeds at a task, the person is usually motivated to achieve more.

Often client motives are physical. A client can be motivated to return to a level of physical normalcy. For example, a client who has had a below-the-knee amputation is motivated to learn how to walk with assistive devices. Knowledge that is necessary for survival, problem recognition, and critical decision-making skills creates a stronger stimulus for learning than knowledge that merely promotes health (Rankin and Stallings, 2001). Teaching strategies reflect the relative importance of each kind of physical motive.

Not all persons are interested in maintaining health. Many people will not adopt new health behaviors or change unhealthy behaviors unless they perceive a disease as a threat, they overcome barriers to changing health practices, and they see the benefits to adopting a healthy behavior. For example, a client with lung disease may continue to smoke. An obese client may worsen a heart condition by refusing to follow a low-fat diet. No therapy will have an effect unless a person is motivated by the belief that health is important. The trend in health care is to treat clients in their homes after they recover from the acute phase of illness. Such treatment is successful only if clients follow caregiver's recommendations. **Compliance** is a client's adherence to the prescribed course of therapy. The nurse assesses the client's motivation to learn and what the client needs to know in order to adhere to the prescribed therapy. The nurse also determines interventions that will stimulate learning and positive behavior changes.

Use of Theory to Enhance Motivation and Learning. Health education often involves changing attitudes and values that are not altered by simple teaching of facts. Therefore nurses use various interventions, based on theory, when developing client education plans. The client's ideas, beliefs, and motivation must be thoroughly assessed in order for learning to occur.

Because of the complexity of the client education process, several theories and models have been used to guide client education (Bastable, 2003; Redman, 2001). Using a theory that matches the client's needs in practice helps the nurse provide effective client education. Social learning theory provides one of the most useful approaches to client education because it explains the characteristics of the learner and guides the educator in developing effective teaching interventions that result in enhanced learning and improved motivation (Bandura, 2001; Bastable, 2003; Saarmann, Daugherty, and Riegel, 2002).

According to social learning theory, people continuously attempt to control events that affect their lives. This allows people to attain desired outcomes and avoid undesired outcomes, resulting in improved motivation. **Self-efficacy,** a concept included in social learning theory, refers to a person's perceived ability to successfully complete a task. When people believe that they can execute a particular behavior, they are more likely to actually perform the behavior consistently and correctly (Bandura, 1997).

Self-efficacy beliefs arise from four sources: enactive mastery experiences, vicarious experiences, verbal persuasion, and physiological and affective states (Bandura, 1997). Understanding the four sources of self-efficacy allows nurses to develop interventions to help clients adopt healthy behaviors. For example, a nurse wishing to teach a child recently diagnosed with asthma to correctly use an inhaler expresses personal beliefs in the child's ability to use the inhaler (verbal persuasion). Then the nurse demonstrates how to use the inhaler (vicarious experience). Once the demonstration is complete, the child uses the inhaler (enactive mastery experience). As the child's wheezing and anxiety decrease after the correct use of the inhaler, the child experiences positive feedback, further enhancing the child's confidence to use the inhaler (physiological and affective states). Interventions such as these enhance perceived self-efficacy, which in turn improves the achievement of desired outcomes.

Psychosocial Adaptation to Illness. A temporary or permanent loss of health is difficult for clients to accept. Clients need to grieve, and the process of grieving gives clients time to adapt psychologically to the emotional and physical implications of illness. The stages of grieving (see Chapter 29) include a series of responses that clients experience during a loss such as illness. People experience these stages at different rates and sequences, depending on their self-concept before illness, the severity of the illness, and the changes in lifestyle that the illness creates. Effective, supportive care guides the client through the grieving process.

Readiness to learn is related to the stage of grieving (Table 24-2). Clients cannot learn when they are unwilling or unable to accept the reality of illness. However,

Table 24-2   **Relationship Between Psychosocial Adaptation to Illness and Learning**

Stage	Client's Behavior	Learning Implications	Rationale
Denial or disbelief	Client avoids discussion of illness ("There's nothing wrong with me"), withdraws from others, and disregards physical restrictions. Client suppresses and distorts information that has not been presented clearly.	Provide support, empathy, and careful explanations of all procedures while they are being done. Let client know you are available for discussion. Explain situation to family or significant other if appropriate. Teach in present tense (e.g., explain current therapy).	Client is not prepared to deal with problem. Any attempt to convince or tell client about illness will result in further anger or withdrawal. Provide only information client pursues or absolutely requires.
Anger	Client blames and complains and often directs anger toward nurse or others.	Do not argue with client but listen to concerns. Teach in present tense. Reassure family/significant other of client's normalcy.	Client needs opportunity to express feelings and anger; client is still not prepared to face future.
Bargaining	Client offers to live better life in exchange for promise of better health ("If God lets me live, I promise to manage my disease better").	Continue to introduce only reality. Teach only in present tense.	Client is still unwilling to accept limitations.
Resolution	Client begins to express emotions openly, realizes that illness has created changes, and begins to ask questions.	Encourage expression of feelings. Begin to share information needed for future, and set aside formal times for discussion.	Client begins to perceive need for assistance and is ready to accept responsibility for learning.
Acceptance	Client recognizes reality of condition, actively pursues information, and strives for independence.	Focus teaching on future skills and knowledge required. Continue to teach about present occurrences. Involve family/significant other in teaching information for discharge.	Client is more easily motivated to learn. Acceptance of illness reflects willingness to deal with its implications.

properly timed teaching can facilitate adjustment to illness or disability. The nurse identifies the client's stage of grieving on the basis of the client's behaviors. When the client enters the stage of acceptance, the stage compatible with learning, the nurse introduces a teaching plan. Continuous assessment of the client's behaviors determines the stages of grieving. Teaching continues as long as the client remains in a stage conducive to learning.

Active Participation. Learning is facilitated when the client is actively involved in the educational session (Edelman and Mandle, 2002). A client's involvement in learning implies an eagerness to acquire knowledge or skills. It also improves the opportunity for the client to make decisions during teaching sessions. For example, a nurse teaching car seat safety during a parenting class holds one teaching session in the parking lot where the participants park their cars. The nurse encourages active participation when the learners are provided with several different car seats for the participants to actually place in their cars. At the completion of this session, the parents are able to decide the types of car seats that fit in their cars and which are the easiest to use. This enables the participants to purchase the appropriate car seat.

Ability to Learn

Developmental Capability. Cognitive development influences the client's ability to learn. A nurse can be a competent teacher, but if the client's intellectual abilities are not considered, teaching will be unsuccessful. Sometimes a nurse has shared teaching booklets and brochures and then discovered that the client cannot read. Learning, like developmental growth, is an evolving process. The nurse must know the client's level of knowledge and intellectual skills before beginning a teaching plan. For example, measuring liquid or solid food portions requires the ability to perform mathematical calculations. Reading a medication label or discharge instructions requires reading and comprehension skills. Learning to regulate insulin dosages requires problem-solving skills. Following directions when performing self-care in accordance with limitations requires comprehension and application skills.

A requisite level of maturation and cognitive development must exist before an individual is capable of learning new information. It is wrong to assume that a client has a certain level of knowledge; instead, the nurse assesses the client's level of knowledge. Learning occurs more readily when new information complements existing knowledge.

Learning in Children. The capability for learning and the type of learning behaviors that can be acquired depend on the child's maturation. Without proper biological, motor, language, and personal-social development, many types of learning cannot take place. However, learning can occur in children of all ages. Intellectual growth moves from the concrete to the abstract as the child matures. Therefore information presented to children must be understandable, and the expected outcomes must be realistic, based on the child's developmental stage (Box 24-5). Teaching aids that are developmentally appropriate should also be used (Figure 24-1). Learning

occurs when behavior changes as a result of experience or growth (Wong and others, 2003).

Adult Learning. Teaching adults differs from teaching children. Because adults become independent and self-directed as they mature, they are often able to identify their own learning needs. These learning needs arise out of problems or tasks that result from real-life situations. Although adults may tend to be self-directed learners, they may become dependent in new learning situations. The amount of information that can be provided and learned and the amount of time that can be spent with the adult client varies depending on the client's personal situation and readiness to learn. An adult's readiness to learn is often associated with his or her developmental stage and what other events are occurring in his or her life. Needs or issues that are perceived as extremely important to the adult must be resolved before learning can occur.

Adults have a wide variety of personal and life experiences to draw on. Therefore adult learning is enhanced when they are encouraged to use these experiences to solve problems. Furthermore, educational topics and goals need to be developed in collaboration with the adult client. Adult clients are ultimately responsible for changing their own behavior. Assessing what the adult client currently knows, teaching what the client wants to know, and setting mutual goals will improve the outcomes of client education (Bastable, 2003).

Physical Capability. The ability to learn often depends on the client's level of physical development and overall physical health. To learn psychomotor skills, a client must possess the necessary level of strength, coordination, and sensory acuity. For example, it is useless to teach a client to transfer from a bed to a wheelchair if the client has insufficient upper body strength. An older client with poor eyesight or the inability to grasp objects tightly cannot learn to apply an elastic bandage. Therefore the nurse should not overestimate the client's physical development or status. The following physical attributes are required to learn psychomotor skills:

- Size (height and weight match the task to perform or the equipment to use [e.g., crutch walking])
- Strength (ability of the client to follow a strenuous exercise program)
- Coordination (dexterity needed for complicated motor skills, such as using utensils or changing a bandage)
- Sensory acuity (visual, auditory, tactile, gustatory, and olfactory; sensory resources needed to receive and respond to messages taught)

Any condition (e.g., pain) that depletes a person's energy will also impair the ability to learn. For example, a client who spends a morning undergoing rigorous diagnostic studies is unlikely to be capable of the effort needed for any learning discussion. When an illness becomes aggravated by complications, such as a high fever or respiratory difficulty, teaching should be postponed. After working with a client, the nurse assesses the client's energy level by noting the client's willingness to communicate, the amount of activity initiated, and the client's responsiveness toward questions. The nurse may halt teaching temporarily if the client needs rest. The nurse

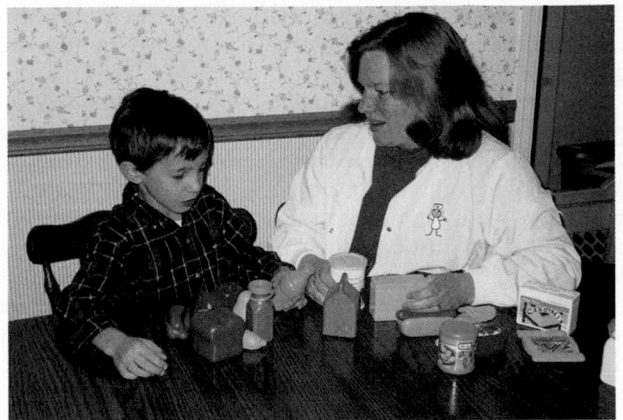

FIGURE **24-1** The nurse uses developmentally appropriate food models to teach healthy eating behaviors to the school-age child.

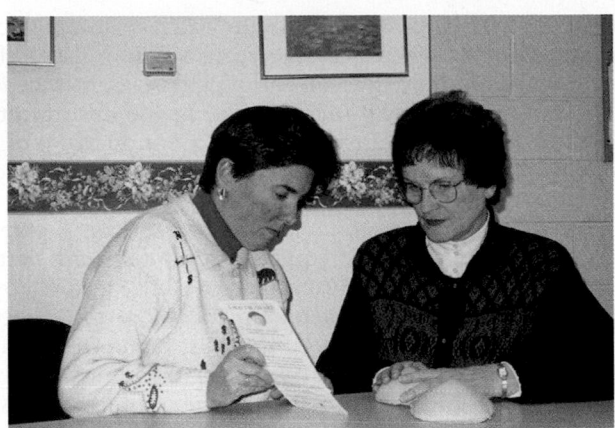

FIGURE **24-2** Choosing comfortable, pleasant environments enhances the learning experience. The nurse is explaining the breast self-examination procedure to the client.

Box 24-5   **Teaching Methods Based on Client's Developmental Capacity**

Infant

Keep routines (e.g., feeding, bathing) consistent.
Hold infant firmly while smiling and speaking softly to convey sense of trust.
Have infant touch different textures (e.g., soft fabric, hard plastic).

Toddler

Use play to teach procedure or activity (e.g., handling examination equipment, applying bandage to doll).
Offer picture books that describe story of children in hospital or clinic.
Use simple words such as *cut* instead of *laceration* to promote understanding.

Preschooler

Use role playing, imitation, and play to make it fun for preschoolers to learn.
Encourage questions and offer explanations. Use simple explanations and demonstrations.
Encourage children to learn together through pictures and short stories about how to perform hygiene.

School-Age Child

Teach psychomotor skills needed to maintain health. (Complicated skills, such as learning to use a syringe, may take considerable practice.)
Offer opportunities to discuss health problems and answer questions.

Adolescent

Help adolescent learn about feelings and need for self-expression.
Use teaching as collaborative activity.
Allow adolescents to make decisions about health and health promotion (safety, sex education, substance abuse).
Use problem solving to help adolescents make choices.

Young or Middle Adult

Encourage participation in teaching plan by setting mutual goals.
Encourage independent learning.
Offer information so that adult can understand effects of health problem.

Older Adult

Teach when client is alert and rested.
Involve adult in discussion or activity.
Focus on wellness and the person's strength.
Use approaches that enhance sensorially impaired client's reception of stimuli (see Chapter 48).
Keep teaching sessions short.

---

achieves greater teaching success when the client is an active participant in learning.

Learning Environment

Factors in the physical environment where teaching takes place make learning either a pleasant or a difficult experience. The ideal setting helps the client focus on the learning task. The number of persons being taught, the need for privacy, the room temperature, the room lighting, noise, the room ventilation, and the room furniture are important factors when choosing the setting. The ideal environment for learning is a room that is well lit and has good ventilation, appropriate furniture, and a comfortable temperature (Figure 24-2). A darkened room interferes with the client's ability to watch the nurse's actions, especially when demonstrating a skill or using visual aids such as posters or pamphlets. A room that is cold, hot, or stuffy will make the client too uncomfortable to attend to the nurse's activities. Comfortable furniture helps eliminate distractions, such as the need to change position or shift body weight.

It is also important to choose a quiet setting. A quiet setting offers privacy; infrequent interruptions are best. The nurse can provide privacy even in a busy hospital by closing cubicle curtains or taking the client to a quiet spot. In the home a bedroom might separate the client from household activities. If the client desires, family members or significant others may share in discussions. However, a client may be reluctant to discuss the nature of the illness when others, even close family members, are in the room.

Teaching a group of clients requires a room that allows everyone to be seated comfortably and within hearing distance of the teacher. The size of the room should not overwhelm the group, tempting participants to sit outside the group along the room's perimeter. Arranging the group to allow participants to observe one another further enhances learning. More effective communication occurs as learners observe others' verbal and nonverbal interactions.

Integrating the Nursing and Teaching Processes

A relationship exists between the nursing and teaching processes (Redman, 2001). During the assessment phase of the nursing process, the nurse determines the client's health care needs (see Unit III). At times assessment will reveal a client's need for health care information. The nursing diagnoses identified are individualized to the client's situation. The plan of care is established to meet desired goals and outcomes and to prescribe nursing interven-

tions for improving or maintaining the client's health. Evaluation determines the level of success in meeting goals of care.

While diagnosing a client's health care problems, the nurse may identify the need for education. When education becomes a part of the care plan, the teaching process begins. Like the nursing process, the teaching process requires assessment, in this case, analyzing the client's needs, motivation, and ability to learn. A diagnostic statement specifies the information or skills that the client requires. The nurse sets specific learning objectives and implements the teaching plan using teaching and learning principles to ensure that the client acquires knowledge and skills. Finally, the teaching process requires an evaluation of learning based on learning objectives.

The nursing and teaching processes are not the same. The nursing process requires assessment of all sources of data to determine a client's total health care needs. The teaching process focuses on the client's learning needs and willingness and capability to learn. Table 24-3 compares the teaching and nursing processes.

NP Assessment

Success in teaching a client requires the nurse to assess all factors influencing relevant content, the client's ability to learn, and the resources available for instruction. Learning needs, identified by both the client and the nurse, determine the choice of teaching content. An effective assessment is the basis on which instruction can be individualized to each client (Redman, 2001).

Expectations of Learning. Clients have the ability to identify their own learning needs based on the implications of living with their illness. To meet these learning needs, the nurse assesses what clients view as important information to know. For example, the nurse asks a young woman newly diagnosed with breast cancer what

Table 24-3	Comparison of the Nursing and Teaching Processes	
Basic Steps	**Nursing Process**	**Teaching Process**
Assessment	Collect data about client's physical, psychological, social, cultural, developmental, and spiritual needs from client, family, diagnostic tests, medical record, nursing history, and literature.	Gather data about client's learning needs, motivation, ability to learn, and teaching resources from client, family, learning environment, medical record, nursing history, and literature.
Nursing diagnosis	Identify appropriate nursing diagnoses based on assessment findings.	Identify client's learning needs on basis of three domains of learning.
Planning	Develop individualized care plan. Set diagnosis priorities based on client's immediate needs. Collaborate with client on care plan.	Establish learning objectives, stated in behavioral terms. Identify priorities regarding learning needs. Collaborate with client on teaching plan. Identify type of teaching method to use.
Implementation	Perform nursing care therapies. Include client as active participant in care. Involve family/significant other in care as appropriate.	Implement teaching methods. Actively involve client in learning activities. Include family/significant other participation as appropriate.
Evaluation	Identify success in meeting desired outcomes and goals of nursing care. Alter interventions as indicated when goals are not met.	Determine outcomes of teaching-learning process. Measure client's ability to achieve learning objectives. Reinforce information as needed.

she wants to know and listens to questions raised by the client or family about health issues. When a client feels a need to know something, the nurse recognizes that the client will likely be receptive to information presented.

Nurses also use assessment tools to determine the perceived learning needs of clients. For example, a short educational needs checklist was developed for clients diagnosed with coronary artery disease (Martinali and others, 2001). Clients who used this checklist to prepare for their visits to a cardiology clinic were better able to identify their educational needs and experienced less anxiety before their scheduled appointments.

Learning Needs. The nurse also determines the information that is critical for the client to learn. Learning needs change depending on the client's current health status. Because a client's health status is dynamic, assessment is an ongoing activity. The nurse assesses the following:

- Client's level of understanding of current health status, implications of illness, types of therapy, and prognosis to determine a client's perception of the threat of illness and its effect on lifestyle. For example, the nurse asks a client newly diagnosed with Type 1 diabetes, "Tell me what you know about diabetes and why you need to take insulin."
- Information or skills needed by the client to perform self-care and to understand the implications of a health problem. Health care team members anticipate learning needs related to specific health problems. For example, the nurse teaches a boy who has just entered high school to perform testicular self-examination.
- Client's experiences that influence the need to learn. For example, a woman who is pregnant for the third time is more likely to be familiar with the implications of pregnancy than a woman who is pregnant for the first time.
- Information that family members or significant others require to support the client's needs. The amount of information needed depends on the extent of the family's role in helping the client. For example, a nurse asks family members to describe their availability and how they plan to help the client.

Motivation to Learn. The nurse asks questions that define the client's motivation. These questions help to determine whether the client is prepared and willing to learn. Although a client may have a variety of learning needs, a lack of motivation seriously threatens the success of the teaching plan. The nurse assesses the following motivational factors:

- Client's behavior (e.g., attention span, tendency to ask questions, memory, and ability to concentrate during the teaching session).
- Client's health beliefs and perception of the severity and susceptibility of a health problem, and the benefits and barriers to treatment. For example, a nurse asks a client with coronary artery disease, "Explain how heart disease will affect you over time. What value is there in eating a low-fat diet?"
- Client's perceived ability to complete a required health behavior.
- Client's desire to learn.

- Client's attitudes about health care providers (e.g., role of client and nurse in making decisions). For example, a nurse caring for a client with Parkinson's disease asks, "Together we can choose the best way for you to learn about Parkinson's disease. In what way can I best help you?"
- Client's knowledge of information to be learned. The client must play an active role in seeking health-based information.
- Pain, fatigue, anxiety, or other physical symptoms that can interfere with the ability to maintain attention and participate. In acute care settings a client's physical condition can easily detract from learning.
- Client's sociocultural background. A client's beliefs and values about health and various therapies may be influenced by sociocultural norms or tradition (see Chapter 8 and Box 24-6).
- Client's learning style preference. Clients who learn better by seeing and hearing may benefit from a videotape. Clients who learn best by reasoning logically and intuitively may learn better if presented with a case study that requires careful analysis and discussion with others to arrive at conclusions.

Cultural Aspects of Care   **Box 24-6**

Assessing the preferred learning approaches and adapting educational efforts for clients enhances the attainment of educational outcomes. Sociocultural norms, values, and traditions often determine the importance of different health education topics and the preference of one learning approach over another. For example, one study determined that white women over 55 years of age preferred a one-on-one approach, whereas African-American and Hispanic women preferred the group approach. Another study found that health promotion teaching was perceived as being more important by African-Americans than whites and that client teaching and the availability of calling a nurse was more important to clients with lower incomes. Educational efforts can be especially challenging when clients and educators do not speak the same language.

Implications for Practice

- Sociocultural background influences a client's desire to learn, as well as what information is perceived as important to learn.
- Carefully assessing a client's preference for educational delivery method is vital to ensure successful learning.
- Nurses must have a wide variety of educational resources available to them to meet the needs of diverse populations.
- When the client and nurse do not speak the same language, accurate translators are necessary.

Data from Danigelis N and others: Two community outreach strategies to increase breast cancer screening among low-income women, *J Cancer Educ* 16(1):55, 2001; Edelman CL, Mandle CL: *Health promotion throughout the life*span, ed 5, St. Louis, 2002, Mosby; and Oermann M, Harris C, Dammeyer J: Teaching by the nurse: how important is it to patients? *Appl Nurs Res* 14(1):11, 2001.

Ability to Learn. The nurse determines the client's physical and cognitive ability to learn. Health care providers often underestimate the client's cognitive deficits. Many factors can impair the ability to learn, including body temperature, electrolyte levels, oxygenation status, and blood glucose level. In any health care setting, several of these factors may influence a client at one time. The nurse assesses the following factors related to the ability to learn:

- Physical strength, movement, dexterity, and coordination. The nurse determines the extent to which the client can perform skills. For example, the nurse encourages the client to manipulate equipment that will be used in self-care at home.
- Sensory deficits (see Chapter 48) that may affect the client's ability to understand or follow instruction.
- Client's reading level. This can be difficult to assess because a functionally illiterate client is often able to conceal it by using excuses such as not having the time or not being able to see. One way to assess a client's reading level and level of understanding is to ask the client to read instructions from a teaching brochure and then explain its meaning.
- Client's developmental level. This influences the approaches chosen by the nurse during teaching (see Box 24-5, p. 459).
- Client's cognitive function, including memory, knowledge, association, and judgment.

Teaching Environment. The environment for a teaching session must be conducive to learning. The nurse assesses the following factors when seeking a place to teach clients:

- Distractions or persistent noise. A quiet area should be set aside for teaching.
- Comfort of the room, including ventilation, temperature, lighting, and furniture.
- Room facilities and available equipment.

Resources for Learning. A client may require the support of family members or significant others. In this case the nurse assesses the readiness and ability of family and friends to learn the information necessary for the care of the client. The nurse also reviews resources within the home environment. Assessment of resources also includes a review of any teaching tools available. The nurse assesses the following:

- Client's willingness to have family members and significant others involved in the teaching plan and to provide health care. Information about the client's health care is confidential unless the client chooses to share it. Sometimes it is difficult for the client to accept the help of family members, especially when bodily functions are involved.
- Family members' perceptions and understanding of the client's illness and its implications. Family members' perceptions should match those of the client; otherwise, conflicts may arise in the teaching plan.
- Family's or significant other's willingness and ability to participate in care. If the client chooses to share information about his or her health status with family members, the family members must be responsible,

willing, or physically and cognitively able to assist in care activities, such as bathing or administering medications. Not all family members will fill this description. For example, the nurse asks, "Your husband may need some help in changing his colostomy bag. How do you feel about learning how to assist him?"

- Resources within the home. These include financial or material resources, such as obtaining health care equipment; and architectural resources, such as arrangement of rooms or stairways.
- Teaching tools, including brochures, audiovisual materials, or posters. Printed material should present current information that is written clearly and logically and that matches the client's reading level. Currently, printed educational materials often surpass clients' reading levels (Dreger and Trembeck, 2002).

Nursing Diagnosis

After assessing information related to the client's ability and need to learn, the nurse interprets data and clusters defining characteristics to form diagnoses that reflect the client's specific learning needs (Box 24-7). This ensures that teaching will be goal directed and individualized. If a client has several learning needs, the nursing diagnoses will guide priority setting. When the nursing diagnosis is *deficient knowledge,* the diagnostic statement should describe the specific type of learning need and its cause; for example, *deficient knowledge regarding psychomotor learning related to inexperience with medication self administration.* Classifying diagnoses by the three learning domains helps the nurse to focus specifically on subject matter and teaching methods. Clients may always require education to support resolution of their various health problems. Examples of additional nursing diagnoses that indicate a need for education include the following:

- Ineffective health maintenance
- Health-seeking behaviors
- Impaired home maintenance
- Deficient knowledge
- Ineffective therapeutic regimen management
- Ineffective community therapeutic regimen management
- Ineffective family therapeutic regimen management
- Noncompliance

When health care problems can be managed or eliminated through education, the related factor of the diagnostic statement is *deficient knowledge.* For example, an older adult client may have difficulty managing a medication regimen because of the number of medications that must be taken at different times of the day. In this case educating the client about the medications may improve the client's ability to schedule and take the medications as directed.

Some nursing diagnoses also indicate that teaching may be inappropriate. The nurse may identify conditions that cause barriers to effective learning (e.g., nursing diagnosis of *pain* or *activity intolerance*). In these cases the nurse delays teaching until the nursing diagnosis is resolved or the health problem is controlled.

Nursing Diagnostic Process

Box **24-7**

Assessment Activities	Defining Characteristics	Nursing Diagnosis
Have client describe how to walk with crutches. Have client demonstrate three-point crutch walking on level surfaces and up stairs.	States has not received information about use of crutches Asks questions about how to use crutches Uses crutches inappropriately Cannot go up or down stairs on crutches	Deficient knowledge (psychomotor) regarding use of crutches related to lack of exposure

Planning

After determining the nursing diagnoses that identify a client's learning needs, the nurse develops a teaching plan, determines goals and expected outcomes, and involves the client in selecting learning experiences (see care plan). Expected outcomes (or learning objectives) guide the choice of teaching strategies and approaches with a client. Client participation ensures a more relevant, meaningful plan.

Developing Learning Objectives. The first step in forming a teaching plan is developing learning objectives. A learning objective identifies the expected outcome of a planned learning experience and helps establish priorities for learning. Despite all planning, a particular instructional session often leads to unanticipated learning. It may be difficult to anticipate all objectives for a teaching session. However, by setting objectives a teacher can plan teaching sessions so that time is maximized and the best resources are available for learning.

Objectives are either short term or long term. Short-term objectives relate to the client's immediate learning needs, such as knowing the nature of gallbladder disease to understand an upcoming test. Long-term objectives relate to acquisition of the knowledge and skills that are needed to permanently adapt to a health problem (e.g., learning to plan a diet within restrictions caused by ulcerative colitis). Like a goal of care, a long-term objective is usually all encompassing. Short-term objectives can be compared with outcomes of care.

The objectives established by the nurse and client guide the teaching plan. Poorly determined objectives can create confusion throughout the teaching-learning process. Thus a learning objective includes the same criteria as outcomes in a nursing care plan (see Chapter 17):
- Singular behaviors
- Observable or measurable content
- Timing or conditions under which the objective is measured
- Goals mutually set between the nurse and client

Each objective is a statement of a singular behavior that identifies the learner's ability to do something after a learning experience. A behavioral objective contains an active verb, describing what the learner will do after the objective is met, such as *will empty* colostomy bag, or *will administer* an injection. The verb should have few interpretations (e.g., verbalize, demonstrate, identify, describe, or select) and be stated in terms of how the client is to demonstrate learning, rather than what or how the teacher is to teach (Bastable, 2003).

Behavioral objectives are measurable and observable and indicate how learning will be evidenced (e.g., "will perform *three-point crutch gait*"). The objective describes precise behaviors and content. An example of a vague or nonspecific objective might be "will be familiar with chronic renal failure." This example does not explain what the learner is to do, and it raises questions about how the behavior can be measured. If content is missing, the objective cannot guide teaching and learning. The precise behaviors and content set the standard for feedback that reflects learning and forms the basis for evaluation of the teaching plan.

An objective is more precise when it describes the conditions or timing under which the behavior occurs. Conditions or time frames should be realistic and designed for the learner's needs (e.g., "will identify the side effects of aspirin by discharge"). It also helps to consider conditions under which the client or family will typically perform the learning behavior (e.g., "will walk from bedroom to bathroom using crutches"). The criteria for acceptable performance set a standard by which achievement of objectives is measured. A teacher sets criteria on the basis of a desired level of accuracy, success, or satisfaction. For example, a client undergoing therapy for a fractured leg will walk on crutches *to the end of the hall within 3 days*. Criteria are more acceptable when the teacher and learner establish them mutually. However, the nurse serves as a resource in setting the minimum criteria for success. Criteria on which the client and nurse agree help define the expected behaviors and the quality of performance. The client also uses these criteria for self-evaluation, which is a powerful motivator of behavior.

After formulating objectives, the nurse and client establish a teaching plan. The nurse integrates basic teaching principles and develops a well-timed, organized teaching plan.

Setting Priorities. Priorities for teaching are based on the client's immediate needs, nursing diagnoses, and the learning objectives established for the client. Priorities also depend on what the client perceives to be most important, the client's anxiety level, and the amount of time available to teach. A client's learning needs must be set in order of priority to conserve the time and energy of

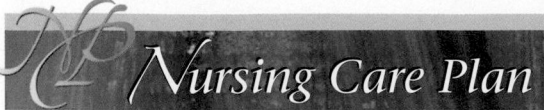

Nursing Care Plan

Learning Needs

Assessment

Connie, a nurse in a surgeon's office, is preparing Mr. Holland for a colon resection, which is scheduled in one week. Mr. Holland is 75 years old and has recently been diagnosed with colorectal cancer. Connie's assessment focuses on Mr. Holland's readiness to learn and factors that might affect his ability to understand the procedure and related postoperative care.

Assessment Activities	Findings/Defining Characteristics
Assess Mr. Holland's readiness to learn, and ask what the surgeon has already told him about the surgery.	Mr. Holland responds, "I can't remember what the doctor told me at my last appointment. But, I need to know how to take care of myself. My surgery is scheduled for next week."
Ask Mr. Holland to explain postoperative care, including performing a return demonstration of deep breathing and coughing.	Mr. Holland is unable to describe postoperative care or provide a return demonstration of deep breathing and coughing.
Assess Mr. Holland's visual acuity.	Mr. Holland states he has difficulty seeing small print.

Nursing Diagnosis: Deficient knowledge related to lack of recall and exposure to information.

Planning

Goal	Expected Outcomes* **Knowledge: Treatment Procedure**
Client will describe preoperative and postoperative care before surgery.	Mr. Holland will verbalize understanding of surgical procedure and related care on the day of surgery.
Client will participate in postoperative care during hospitalization.	Mr. Holland will demonstrate deep breathing and coughing and will advance his level of activity after his surgery.

*Outcome labels from Moorhead S, Johnson M, Maas M: *Nursing outcomes classification (NOC)*, ed 3, St. Louis, 2004, Mosby.

Interventions†

Learning Readiness Enhancement
Determine readiness to learn and what the client perceives as important to know.

Learning Facilitation
Give client large-print brochure describing preoperative and postoperative care during educational session.

Explain postoperative care, demonstrate deep breathing and coughing, and have client perform return demonstration.

Rationale

The adult client's learning is enhanced when the client is ready to learn and the information is perceived as important (Bastable, 2003).

Providing clients with educational methods that use multiple senses is effective in educating older adults. Large fonts with contrasting colors are easier to visualize for the older adult (Maas and others, 2001).

Improving self-efficacy by using role modeling and having the client perform behaviors enhances the successful adoption of healthy behaviors (Bandura, 1997).

†Intervention classification labels from Dochterman JM, Bulechek GM: *Nursing interventions classification (NIC)*, ed 4, St. Louis, 2004, Mosby.

Evaluation

Nursing Actions	Client Response/Finding	Achievement of Outcome
Ask Mr. Holland what he can expect before and after surgery.	Mr. Holland is able to state understanding of preoperative and postoperative care.	Mr. Holland's anxiety level has decreased, and he reports he is ready for surgery.
Observe client as he demonstrates deep breathing and coughing and advances his activity postoperatively.	Mr. Holland is able to deep breathe and cough postoperatively, but he is hesitant to advance his activity level after surgery.	Outcome of advancing activity postoperatively has not been totally achieved. Address and manage barriers inhibiting attainment of this outcome (e.g., pain), and continue to encourage and educate client.

the client and nurse. For example, a client recently diagnosed with coronary artery disease has deficient knowledge related to the illness and its implications. The client will benefit most by first learning about the correct way to take nitroglycerin and how long to wait before calling for help when chest pain occurs. Once these needs related to basic survival are met, then other topics, such as exercise and nutritional changes, can be discussed.

Timing. When is the right time to teach? Before a client enters a hospital? When a client first enters a clinic? At discharge? At home? Each may be appropriate because clients continue to have learning needs and opportunities as long as they stay in the health care system. The nurse should plan teaching activities for a time when the client is most attentive, receptive, and alert. The client's activities should be organized to provide time for rest and teaching-learning interactions.

Timing can be difficult because emphasis is placed on a client's early discharge from a hospital. For example, it may take several days after surgery for a client to become free of discomfort so that attention can be given to learning. By the time the client feels ready to learn, discharge may already be scheduled. Therefore nurses need to anticipate educational needs of clients before they occur. For example, the nurse educates a pregnant woman about care of the newborn 1 month before the expected delivery date, or a client scheduled to have a hip replacement receives information about what to expect during and after the surgery the week before admission. Anticipating a client's educational needs can improve the client's outcomes. For example, Donovan and Ward (2001) found that clients were better able to manage their pain after receiving structured education at an oncology clinic. Therefore, identifying clients with cancer at risk for experiencing pain and teaching them pain management strategies in a structured manner may help clients better manage pain as their disease progresses.

The duration of teaching sessions also influences learning ability. Prolonged sessions cause concentration and attentiveness to decrease. Frequent sessions lasting 20 minutes are more easily tolerated and retain the client's interest in the material. However, factors such as shorter hospital stays and lack of insurance reimbursement for outpatient education sessions may necessitate longer teaching sessions. The nurse assesses a client's loss of concentration by observing for nonverbal cues, such as poor eye contact or slumped posture. After loss of concentration is noted, the session should be stopped. However, teaching sessions should not be too brief. The client needs time to comprehend the information and to give feedback.

Teaching sessions should be held frequently enough to document the client's learning. The frequency of sessions depends on the learner's abilities and the complexity of the material. For example, a child newly diagnosed with diabetes will require more visits to an outpatient center than the older adult client who has had diabetes for 15 years and who lives in a nursing home. Intervals between teaching sessions should not be so long that the client might forget information. For a client discharged from a hospital, home care nurses must reinforce learning.

Organizing Teaching Material. A good teacher carefully considers the order of information to present. An outline of content helps organize information into a logical sequence. Material should progress from simple to complex ideas because a person must learn the simple facts and concepts before learning how to make associations or complex interpretations of ideas. For example, to teach a woman how to feed her husband who has a gastric tube, the nurse first teaches the wife how to measure the tube feeding and how to manipulate the equipment. Once this is accomplished, the process of administering the feeding occurs.

The nurse begins any instruction with essential content because clients are more likely to remember information that is taught early in the teaching session. For example, immediately after surgical removal of a malignant breast tumor, the client has many learning needs. The nurse starts with essential information such as how to monitor the incision site for signs of infection and how to deal with the emotional aspects of a cancer diagnosis and then completes the teaching session with informative but less critical content including the warning signs of cancer. Key points should be summarized. Repetition also reinforces learning. A concise summary of key topics helps the learner remember the most important information (Bastable, 2003).

Maintaining Learning Attention and Participation. Active participation is key to learning. Persons learn better when more than one of the body's senses are stimulated. Audiovisual aids and role playing are good teaching strategies. By actively experiencing a learning event, the person will be more likely to retain the knowledge gained.

A teacher's actions can also increase learner attention and interest. When conducting a discussion with a learner, the teacher should stay active by changing the tone and intensity of his or her voice, making eye contact, and using gestures that accentuate key points of discussion. An effective teacher often uses as much energy as the learner, talking and moving among a group rather than remaining stationary behind a lectern or table. A learner remains interested in a teacher who is actively enthusiastic about the subject under discussion.

Building on Existing Knowledge. A client learns best on the basis of preexisting cognitive abilities and knowledge. Thus a teacher is more effective by presenting information that builds on a learner's existing knowledge. A client quickly loses interest if a nurse begins with familiar information. For example, a client who has lived with multiple sclerosis for several years must begin a new medication that is given subcutaneously. Before teaching the client how to prepare the medication and give the injection, the nurse asks the client about previous experience with injections. On assessment, the nurse learns that the client's father had diabetes and that the client administered the insulin injections. The nurse individualizes the teaching plan by building on the client's previous knowledge and experience with insulin injections.

Selection of Teaching Methods. During planning, the nurse chooses appropriate teaching methods and encourages the client to offer suggestions. A teaching method is the way that the teacher delivers information, and it is based on the client's learning needs. For example, a client who learns best in the psychomotor domain will benefit from demonstrations and supervised practice. The client masters skills by manipulating equipment and practicing manual skills. Discussions, question-and-answer sessions, and formal lectures are effective methods for promoting cognitive learning. Clients with intellectual learning needs are given the opportunity to explore new ideas, recognize new relationships, and apply knowledge to their unique needs. A highly effective method for stimulating affective learning is group discussion. More than one method may be used for instruction.

Availability of Teaching Resources. The nurse is the primary member of the health care team responsible for ensuring that all client educational needs are met. However, sometimes client needs are highly complex. In these cases the nurse identifies appropriate health education resources within the health care system or the community during planning. Examples of resources for client education include diabetes education clinics, cardiac rehabilitation programs, prenatal classes, and support groups. When clients receive education and support from these types of resources, the nurse is responsible for obtaining a referral if necessary, encouraging clients to attend these resources, and reinforcing information taught. Resources that specialize in a particular health need are integral to successful client education.

Writing Teaching Plans. In all health care settings, nurses develop written teaching plans for use by colleagues. When one nurse, such as a primary nurse, is responsible for developing the initial teaching plan, all information about the client is incorporated appropriately. The teaching plan includes topics for instruction, resources (e.g., equipment, teaching booklets, and referrals to special educational programs), recommendations for involving family, and objectives of the teaching plan. A plan may be lengthy or in outline form.

The setting influences the complexity of any teaching plan. In an acute care setting, plans are concise and focused on the primary learning needs of the client because there is limited time for teaching. A home care teaching plan or outpatient clinic plan may be more comprehensive in scope because nurses often have more time to instruct clients and clients are often less anxious in outpatient settings.

A plan should provide continuity of instruction, particularly when several nurses are involved in caring for the client. The more specific the plan, the easier it is for nurses to follow through. To enhance communication among nurses and to avoid duplication, the nurse should know the point at which the last teaching session ended.

ℕℙ *Implementation*

The implementation of a teaching plan depends on the nurse's ability to critically analyze assessment data when identifying learning needs and developing the teaching plan (see care plan, p. 464). The nurse carefully evaluates the learning objectives and determines which teaching and learning principles will most effectively and efficiently assist the client in meeting expected goals and outcomes. Implementation involves believing that each interaction with a client is an opportunity to teach. The nurse uses a diversified approach to create an active learning environment (Box 24-8).

Box 24-8   **Example of Nursing Interventions Based on Client's Learning Needs**

Assessment Data

Mr. Kennedy is a 67-year-old man who has a 15-year history of type 2 diabetes. He is in the hospital because he has a foot ulcer that became infected and required frequent dressing changes. Mr. Kennedy used to take oral hypoglycemic agents to control his blood sugar levels. However, he now needs to start home insulin injections because of the infection and wound in his foot. He also needs to learn how to change his dressings. Mr. Kennedy is very anxious about his discharge and is requesting information about a local diabetes support group. The case manager indicates that Mr. Kennedy will be discharged soon.

Cognitive Interventions

- Ask Mr. Kennedy about what he believes he needs to know before his discharge.
- Encourage Mr. Kennedy to help establish learning outcomes and goals.
- Provide Mr. Kennedy with teaching materials regarding insulin preparation, administration, and how to recognize and manage hypoglycemia and hyperglycemia.
- During teaching sessions, give Mr. Kennedy examples of what problems he might experience at home and ask him how he would respond to the situations (e.g., if the wound's drainage increased and became purulent, what would he do?).

Affective Interventions

- Allow Mr. Kennedy to attend a support group meeting if possible to allow learning from others' experiences.
- Encourage Mr. Kennedy to verbalize his feelings and fears about this change in his health status.
- Have Mr. Kennedy role play how he will respond to his friends when they ask him about his health status.
- Provide Mr. Kennedy with feedback and positive reinforcement as he acquires new skills and behaviors.

Psychomotor Interventions

- Demonstrate insulin preparation and injection techniques.
- Demonstrate use of blood sugar meter and recording of blood sugar measurement results.
- Demonstrate dressing changes.
- Have Mr. Kennedy perform return demonstrations of insulin preparation and injection, blood sugar testing, and dressing changes.

Teaching Approaches. A nurse's approach in teaching is different from teaching methods. Some situations require a teacher to be directive. Others may require a nondirective approach. An effective teacher concentrates on the task and uses teaching approaches according to the learner's needs. A learner's needs and motives can change over time. Thus the teacher must always be aware of the need to modify teaching approaches.

Telling. The telling approach is useful when limited information must be taught (e.g., preparing a client for an emergent diagnostic procedure). If a client is highly anxious but it is vital for information to be given, telling can be effective. When using telling, the nurse outlines the task to be done by the client and gives explicit instructions. There is no opportunity for feedback with this method.

Selling. The selling approach uses two-way communication. The nurse paces instruction based on the client's response. Specific feedback is given to the client who shows success in learning. For example, the client learns a step-by-step procedure for changing a dressing. The nurse uses information from the client to adapt the teaching approach.

Participating. Participating involves the nurse and client setting objectives and becoming involved in the learning process together. The client helps decide content, and the nurse guides and counsels the client with pertinent information. In this method, there is opportunity for discussion, feedback, mutual goal setting, and revision of the teaching plan. For example, a parent caring for a child with leukemia and receiving chemotherapy must learn how to care for the child at home and how to recognize problems that need to be reported immediately. The parent and the nurse collaborate on developing an appropriate teaching plan that will facilitate the parent's learning and the child's discharge from the hospital. After each teaching session is completed, the parent and nurse review the objectives together, determine if the objectives were met, and plan what will be covered in the next session.

Entrusting. The entrusting approach provides the client the opportunity to manage self-care. Responsibilities are accepted, and the client performs tasks correctly and consistently. The nurse observes the client's progress and remains available to assist without introducing more new information. For example, a client has been managing diabetes well for 10 years. Because of the development of a complication of diabetes, the client must now walk instead of jog during exercise. The client understands how to adjust insulin when exercising to prevent hypoglycemia. The nurse instructs the client about the newly prescribed exercise therapy and allows the client to adjust insulin dosages independently.

Reinforcing. The principle of reinforcement applies to the process of learning; however, the teacher must often be the source of reinforcement. **Reinforcement** is using a stimulus that increases the probability for a response. A learner who receives reinforcement before or after a desired learning behavior is likely to repeat the behavior. Feedback is a common form of reinforcement.

Reinforcers are positive or negative. Positive reinforcement, such as a smile or spoken approval, produces desired responses. Although negative reinforcement, such as frowning or criticizing, can decrease an undesired response, people usually respond better to positive reinforcement (Bastable, 2003). The effects of negative reinforcement are less predictable and often undesirable.

Three types of reinforcers are social, material, and activity. When a nurse works with a client, most reinforcers are social ones (e.g., smiles, compliments, or words of encouragement), which are used to acknowledge a learned behavior. Examples of material reinforcers are food, toys, and music. These work best with young children. Activity reinforcers rely on the principle that a person is motivated to engage in an activity if he or she is promised that after its completion the opportunity to engage in more desirable activity will be available. For example, a client will more likely go to a mental health counseling session if he or she is given the chance to go outside for a walk with the nurse afterward.

Choosing an appropriate reinforcer involves giving careful thought and attention to individual preferences. Observing behavior often helps reveal the best reinforcer to use. Reinforcers should never be used as threats and are not always effective with every client. A young child responds more to social reinforcers than do older children or adults. An adult with whom the nurse has a good relationship is more effectively reinforced than an adult with whom the nurse has a poor relationship.

Incorporating Teaching With Nursing Care. Many nurses find that they can teach more effectively while delivering nursing care. This becomes easier as nurses gain confidence in their own clinical skills. For example, while hanging blood, the nurse explains why the blood is needed and the symptoms indicated with transfusion reactions that should be reported immediately. Another example is the nurse who explains a drug's side effects while administering the medication. An informal, unstructured style relies on the positive therapeutic relationship between nurse and client, which fosters spontaneity in the teaching-learning process. This does not suggest that teaching should occur without a formal plan. When the nurse follows a teaching plan informally, the client feels less pressure to perform and learning becomes more of a shared activity. Teaching during routine care is efficient and cost-effective (Figure 24-3).

Instructional Methods. A nurse's choice of instructional methods depends on the client's learning needs, the time available for teaching, the setting, the resources available, and the nurse's own comfort level with teaching. Skilled teachers are flexible in altering teaching methods according to the learner's responses. An experienced teacher uses a variety of techniques and teaching aids. A nurse cannot expect to be an expert educator when first entering nursing practice. Learning to become an effective educator takes time and practice.

When first starting to teach clients, it helps to remember that clients perceive the nurse as an expert. However,

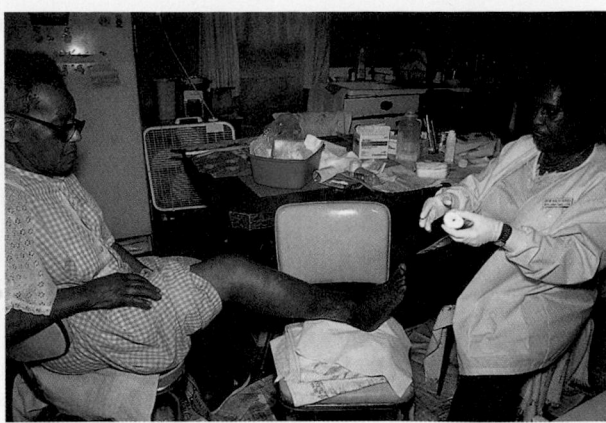

FIGURE 24–3 The nurse incorporates teaching about wound care during a home visit.

this does not mean that the nurse must have all of the answers. It simply means that clients expect that the nurse will keep them appropriately informed. The nurse can be effective by keeping the teaching plan simple and focused on clients' needs.

One-on-One Discussion. Perhaps the most common method of instruction is one-on-one discussion. When teaching a client at the bedside, in a physician's office, or in the home, the nurse directly shares information. Various teaching aids such as models or diagrams can be used during the discussion, depending on the client's learning needs. Information is usually given in an informal manner, allowing the client to ask questions or share concerns. The nurse uses unstructured and informal discussion when helping the client understand the implications of illness and ways to cope with health stressors.

Group Instruction. Nurses may choose to teach clients in groups because of the advantages associated with group teaching. Groups are an economical way to teach a number of clients at one time, and clients are able to interact with each other and learn from the experiences of others. Groups can also foster the development of positive attitudes that help clients meet learning objectives (Rankin and Stallings, 2001).

Group instruction often involves both lecture and discussion. Lectures are highly structured and are efficient in helping groups of clients learn standard content about a subject. For example, a nurse might teach groups of clients about the warning signs of breast cancer, the health risks of smoking, or the normal development of a fetus. A lecture does not ensure that learners are actively thinking about the material presented; thus discussion and practice sessions are essential (Rankin and Stallings, 2001). After a lecture, learners need the opportunity to share ideas and seek clarification. Group discussions allow clients and families to learn from each other as they review common experiences. A productive group discussion helps participants solve problems and arrive at solutions toward improving each member's health. To be an effective group leader, the nurse must be able to guide participation. Acknowledging a look of interest, asking questions, and summarizing key issues foster group involvement. However, not all clients benefit from group discussions, and sometimes the physical or emotional level of wellness may prohibit participation.

Preparatory Instruction. Clients frequently face unfamiliar tests or procedures that create significant anxiety. Providing information about procedures helps clients form realistic images of what to anticipate. This is a common expectation of clients in acute care settings because information helps to give them a sense of control. When the experience matches expectations, the client is more likely to attend to the nurse's future explanations. A nurse gains respect when preparatory explanations prove useful. The nurse uses the following guidelines for giving preparatory explanations:

- Physical sensations during the procedure are described but not evaluated. For example, when drawing a blood specimen, the nurse explains that the client will feel a sticking sensation as the needle punctures the skin.
- The cause of the sensation is described, preventing misinterpretation of the experience. For example, the nurse explains that a needle stick burns because the alcohol used to cleanse the skin enters the puncture site.
- Clients are prepared only for aspects of the experience that have commonly been noticed by other clients. For example, the nurse explains that it is normal for a tight tourniquet to cause a person's hand to tingle and feel numb.

The client finds comfort in knowing what to expect. When the nurse's descriptions accurately portray the actual experience, the client is able to cope more effectively with stress from procedures and therapies. The known is less threatening than the unknown.

Demonstrations. Demonstrations are useful methods for teaching psychomotor skills such as preparation of a syringe, bathing an infant, crutch walking, or measuring a pulse. The client is able to observe a skill before practicing it. Demonstrations are most effective when learners first observe the teacher and then during a **return demonstration** have the chance to practice the skill. Nurses commonly use demonstrations for teaching motor skills; however, motor skills are not learned separately from attitudes and factual knowledge (Redman, 2001). A demonstration should be combined with discussion to clarify concepts and feelings. An effective demonstration requires advanced planning:

1. Be sure the learner can easily see the demonstration. Position the learner to provide a clear view of the skill being performed.
2. Review the rationale and steps of the procedure.
3. Assemble and organize equipment. Be sure that all equipment works.
4. Perform each step in sequence while analyzing the knowledge and skills involved.
5. Determine when explanations are to be given, considering the client's learning needs.
6. Judge proper speed and timing of the demonstration, based on the client's cognitive abilities and anxiety level.

The nurse demonstrates a skill in the same order in which the client will perform it. The demonstration involves the following:

- Performing each step slowly and accurately
- Encouraging the client to ask questions so that each step is understood
- Explaining the rationale for each step
- Allowing the client to observe each step
- Avoiding a hurried approach
- Allowing the client to handle equipment and practice the skill under supervision

The client demonstrates the procedure to ensure that learning has occurred. The independent demonstration should occur under the same conditions that will be experienced at home or in the place where the skill is to be performed. For example, if a client is learning to walk with crutches, the nurse simulates the home environment. If short, narrow steps lead to the client's bedroom, the client should learn to climb similar stairs in the hospital.

Analogies. Learning occurs when a teacher translates complex language or ideas into words or concepts that the client understands. In addition, the client benefits by integrating new information into daily routines. **Analogies** supplement verbal instruction with familiar images that make complex information more real and understandable. For example, when explaining arterial blood pressure, an analogy would be the flow of water through a hose. To use analogies, the nurse uses the following general principles:

- Be familiar with the concept.
- Know the client's background, experience, and culture.
- Keep the analogy simple and clear.

Role Playing. A nurse uses role play for teaching ideas and attitudes. During role play, people are asked to play themselves or someone else. The technique involves rehearsing a desired behavior. For example, a nurse teaches a parent to respond to a child's behavior by pretending to be a child who is having a temper tantrum. This scenario allows the parent to practice responding in this situation. Afterward, the nurse evaluates the parent's response and determines whether an alternative approach would have been more appropriate. As a result of role play, clients are taught the skills required and feel more confident in being able to perform them independently.

Simulation. Simulation is a useful technique for teaching clients problem solving, application, and independent thinking. During individual or group discussion, a nurse poses a pertinent problem or situation for clients to solve. For example, clients with heart disease are asked to plan a meal that is low in cholesterol and fat. The clients in the group decide which foods would be appropriate. The nurse asks the group members to present their diet, providing an opportunity to identify mistakes and reinforce correct information.

Illiteracy and Other Disabilities. It is important to use words a client can understand. Medical jargon can be confusing. Clients understand fewer medical words than health care professionals predict. The problem of **functional illiteracy,** the inability to read above a fifth-grade level, is also real. The National Adult Literacy Survey (NALS), conducted in 1992, assessed the extent of literacy skills in Americans over the age of 16. Participants in this survey completed simulations of daily life experiences. Once the participants completed the survey, they were classified according to their literacy level, with level 1 representing the lowest level of literacy and level 5 being the highest level of literacy. Results from the NALS placed 21% to 23% (about 40 to 44 million) of Americans over the age of 16 in level 1. These people demonstrated only rudimentary reading and writing skills. About 8 million people were unable to perform even the simplest literacy tasks. Approximately 25% to 28% (about 50 million) of adults in America were placed in level 2. These adults had a limited ability to perform tasks that required integration or synthesis of information. Although illiteracy existed among all races, African-American, American Indian/Alaska Native, Hispanic, and Asian/Pacific Islander adults were more likely to be classified into the lowest two literacy levels when compared with Caucasian (white) adults (National Center for Education Statistics, 1996).

To compound the problem, the readability of printed health education material has been researched extensively and has been shown to range from elementary school level to college level. Researchers have found that printed client education material is consistently written above the reading levels of most clients. Unfortunately, the gap between the client's reading level and the readability of educational materials often goes undetected by health care professionals (Winslow, 2001).

In addition to illiteracy, some clients have learning disabilities that impede their ability to learn. For example, many self-care behaviors require an understanding of math, including computation and fractions. If a client's learning disability impairs the ability to effectively use math skills, teaching can be challenging, especially when trying to teach clients about complex medication dosages and frequencies. Another learning disability that can affect the client's ability to learn includes attention deficit and hyperactivity disorder (ADHD). Clients with ADHD may have difficulty recalling information and staying focused during educational sessions in addition to having a low threshold of frustration (Mennies, 2001).

Implications of illiteracy and learning disabilities include an impaired ability to analyze instructions or synthesize information and incorporate it into a behavior task. Also, many of these clients have not acquired the problem-solving skills of drawing conclusions and inferences from experience, and they will not ask questions to obtain or clarify information that has been presented. Nursing interventions that can be used when caring for clients who are illiterate or who have learning disabilities are summarized in Box 24-9.

Some clients have sensory deficits that affect how the nurse presents information (see Chapter 48). Clients, for example, who have hearing impairments may require a sign language interpreter. Not all people who are deaf can read lips. Therefore it is very important to ensure that clear written materials are provided. Written materials for the deaf population should be written at a fourth-grade

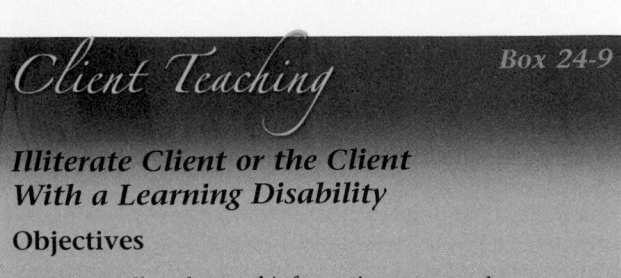

Client Teaching *Box 24-9*

Illiterate Client or the Client With a Learning Disability

Objectives

- Client will understand information presented.
- Client will perform desired behaviors accurately.

Teaching Strategies

- Establish trust with the client before beginning the teaching-learning session.
- Use simple terminology to enhance the client's understanding.
- Avoid medical jargon. If necessary, explain medical terms using basic one- or two-syllable words.
- Keep teaching sessions short and to the point and minimize distractions.
- Include the most important information at the beginning of the session.
- Relate practical information to personal experiences or real-life situations.
- Use visual cues and simple analogies when appropriate.
- Frequently ask the client for feedback to determine if the client comprehends information.
- Ask for return demonstrations (provides opportunity to clarify instructions and time to review procedures).
- Provide teaching materials that reflect the reading level of the client, with attention given to short words and sentences, large type, and simple format (generally, information written on a fifth-grade reading level is recommended for adult learners).
- Reinforce the most important information at the end of the session.
- Schedule teaching sessions at frequent intervals.
- Model appropriate behavior and use role playing to help client learn how to ask questions and ask for help effectively.

Evaluation

- Ask the client to verbalize understanding of information taught.
- Observe and evaluate the client's ability to perform desired behaviors.

Data from Bastable S: *Nurse as educator: principles of teaching and learning for nursing practice,* Sudbury, Mass, 2003, Jones & Bartlett; Mennies J: Teaching adult patients with learning disabilities, *Nurs Spec* 14(21):20, 2001; Osborne H: In other words . . . can they understand? *Testing patient education materials with intended readers,* 2001, http://www.healthliteracy.com/oncallnov2001.htm.

level (Bastable, 2003). Visual impairments can also impact the teaching strategy employed by the nurse. Many people who are blind have acquired acute listening skills. Nurses should be careful not to shout to these clients and should announce their presence to their clients before approaching them. If the client has partial vision, a careful assessment, including what colors the client can see, how large print must be in order for the client to see, and adequate lighting, is an important first step. Other helpful interventions may include audio taping teaching sessions and providing structured, well-organized instructions (Bastable, 2003).

Speaking the Client's Language. The nurse must have knowledge of the client's cultural background and beliefs, as well as the client's ability to understand instructions developed outside of his or her native language. The cultural diversity of clients poses a great challenge to the nurse trying to provide culturally sensitive care. When educating clients of different ethnic groups, the nurse must become aware of the distinctive aspects of each culture, being careful not to stereotype clients. Nurses must also collaborate with other nurses and educators to assist in dealing with cultural diversity and enlist the help of people in the cultural group to share values and beliefs. Ethnic nurses are excellent resources who can provide input through their experiences to improve the care provided to members of their own community. The nurse must especially assess cultural norms and values, as well as communication patterns and perceptions of time (Bastable, 2003).

Nurses also must assess for intergenerational conflict of values. This occurs when immigrant parents uphold their traditional values and their children, who are exposed to American values in social encounters, develop beliefs similar to those of their American peers. This conflict in values must be considered when providing information to families or groups that are composed of members from different generations.

To enhance client education in culturally diverse populations, nurses must know when and how to provide education so that cultural values are respected. Teaching regarding interventions or desired behaviors may need to be modified to mediate cultural differences. Effective educational strategies may require the nurse to use different patterns of communication.

Using Teaching Tools. Many teaching tools are available for nurses to use when instructing a client. Selection of the right tool depends on the instructional method chosen, the client's learning needs, and the client's ability to learn (Table 24-4). For example, a printed pamphlet may not be the best tool to use for a client with poor reading comprehension, and an audiotape may be the best choice for a client with visual impairment.

Special Needs of Children and Older Adults. Children, adults, and older adults learn differently. The nurse adapts teaching strategies to each learner. Children pass through several developmental stages (see Unit II). In each developmental stage, children acquire new cognitive and psychomotor abilities that respond to different types of teaching methods (Figure 24-4). For example, a nurse may teach school-age children of varying ages about dental hygiene, nutrition, safety measures, and sex education. Parental input is incorporated in planning health education for children.

Older adults experience numerous physical and psychological changes as they age (see Chapter 13). These changes not only increase the educational needs of older adults, they can also create barriers to learning unless adjustments are made in nursing interventions.

Table 24-4	Teaching Tools for Instruction
Description	**Learning Implications**

Printed Material

Written teaching tools available as pamphlets, booklets, brochures	Material must be easily readable for learner. Information must be accurate and current. Method is ideal for understanding complex concepts and relationships.

Programmed Instruction

Written sequential presentation of learning steps requiring that learners answer questions and that teachers tell them whether they are right or wrong	Instruction is primarily verbal, but teacher may use pictures or diagrams. Method requires active learning, giving immediate feedback, correcting wrong answers, and reinforcing right answers. Learner works at own pace.

Computer Instruction

Use of programmed instruction format in which computers store response patterns for learners and select further lessons on basis of these patterns (programs can be individualized)	Method requires reading comprehension, psychomotor skills, and familiarity with computer.

Nonprint Materials

Diagrams

Illustrations that show interrelationships by means of lines and symbols	Method demonstrates key ideas, summarizes, and clarifies key concept.

Graphs (Bar, Circle, or Line)

Visual presentations of numerical data	Graphs help learner to grasp information quickly about single concept.

Charts

Highly condensed visual summary of ideas and facts that may highlight series of ideas, steps, or events	Charts demonstrate relationship of several ideas or concepts. Method helps learners know what to do.

Pictures

Photographs or drawings used to teach concepts in which the third dimension of shape and space is not important	Photographs are more desirable than diagrams because they more accurately portray the details of the real item. Drawings are pertinent for removing the superfluous detail present in real objects.

Physical Objects

Use of actual equipment, objects, or models to teach concepts or skills	Models are useful when real objects are too small, large, or complicated or are unavailable. Learners can manipulate objects that are to be used later in skill.

Other Audiovisual Materials

Slides, audiotapes, television, and videotapes used with printed material or discussion	Materials are useful for clients with reading comprehension problems and visual deficits.

Sensory changes such as visual and hearing changes require teaching methods that enhance functioning. For example, the nurse faces the client with hearing problems and speaks in a low tone of voice during discussions. Older adult clients with visual problems can benefit from the use of printed materials containing large print. Older adults learn and remember effectively if the learning is paced properly and the material is relevant to the learner's needs and abilities. Although older adults may have slower cognitive function and reduced short-term memory, nurses can facilitate learning in several ways to support behaviors that maximize the individual's capacity for self-care (Box 24-10). When teaching older clients, short-term goals should be established. Family members who may be assuming partial care for the client must also be included. However, the nurse must be sensitive to the client's desire for assistance, because offering unwanted support may result in negative outcomes and may be perceived as nagging and interference. Furthermore, not all relationships between older adults and other family members are therapeutic. Because of the high incidence of abuse and neglect of older adults, the nurse needs to assess family dynamics before including family members in educational sessions.

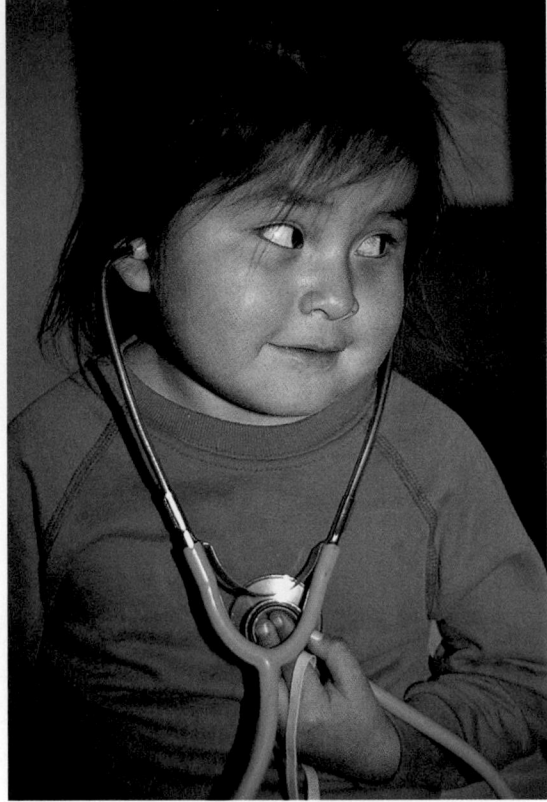

FIGURE 24–4 The preschool child learns not to be afraid of medical equipment by being allowed to handle the stethoscope and imitating its use.

Box 24-10

Focus on Older Adults

Nurses can facilitate learning by using the following interventions when providing client education to older adults:
- Begin and end each teaching session with the most important information.
- Present information slowly.
- Speak in a low tone of voice (lower tones are easier to hear than higher tones).
- Allow ample time for understanding of the material.
- Emphasize concrete material that applies to current situations.
- Present only crucial information to avoid overwhelming the learner.
- Provide specific information in frequent, small amounts.
- Repeat important information.
- Relate new material to previous life experiences.
- Build on existing knowledge.
- Allow clients to progress at their own pace (older adults are more cautious, so it may take longer to adopt a behavior change).
- Use group experiences if appropriate to enhance problem solving.
- If written material is used, assess the client's ability to read and use information that is printed in a large font size and in a color that contrasts highly with the background (e.g., black 14 point font print on buff-colored paper). Avoid blues and greens because they are more difficult to see.

Data from Edelman CL, Mandle CL: *Health promotion throughout the lifespan*, ed 5, St. Louis, 2002, Mosby; Maas M and others: *Nursing care of older adults: diagnoses, outcomes, and interventions*, St. Louis, 2001, Mosby; and Rankin SH, Stallings, KD: *Patient education: issues, principles, practices*, ed 4, Philadelphia, 2001, JB Lippincott.

Evaluation

Client education is not complete until the nurse evaluates outcomes of the teaching-learning process (see care plan). The nurse determines whether clients have learned the material. Evaluation reinforces correct behavior, helps learners realize how they should change incorrect behavior, and helps the teacher determine adequacy of teaching (Cronbach, 1977; Redman, 2001). The nurse evaluates success by observing the client's performance of each expected behavior. Success depends on the client's ability to meet the established outcome and goals. Rankin and Stallings (2001) developed a checklist for evaluating client education. This checklist includes the following:
- Were the objectives clearly stated in a way that allowed client behaviors to be observed?
- Were the client's goals or outcomes realistic?
- Were the learner's needs assessed thoroughly?
- Did the client perceive the education as important, and did the client state a willingness to change behavior?
- What obstacles or problems were encountered that provided barriers to change?
- Were educational goals set mutually between the nurse and the client?
- Were the interventions individualized to help the client meet the learning objectives?
- Was the client's behavioral change measured and documented accurately?

- Does the client continue to have a skill deficiency? If so, what changes in interventions should be made to enhance skill attainment?

Measurement methods. Direct observation of client behaviors is useful when determining how a person will act in the future. The client receives immediate feedback, and the nurse can collect accurate data (Rankin and Stallings, 2001). In direct observation, the nurse has the client demonstrate the behaviors described in the learning objectives. If the evaluation process indicates a knowledge or skill deficit, the nurse repeats or modifies the teaching plan. Watching a client demonstrate a skill helps the nurse to know whether the correct technique is being used. However, a client may choose to behave differently later. Therefore observation works best in real-life situations.

Oral and written questioning are other useful evaluation methods. When a nurse questions a client verbally, the client's success in cognitive learning about a specific topic can be measured. Questions measure behaviors that are not easily observed. The nurse should carefully phrase questions to ensure that the learner understands them and that objectives are truly measured.

Another form of evaluation includes self-reports (oral and written) and self-monitoring (written). This involves the client or family member providing information independently. An example might include a client's written log of the foods eaten during a specific week, matched against a newly prescribed diet. The nurse relies on the client's honesty and memory in self-reporting.

Client Expectations. Because of the increasing importance of client satisfaction (see Chapter 2), nurses should evaluate whether clients have the information they want. Have their expectations been met? A client may want specific information that he or she knows will be necessary to continue a normal lifestyle at home. For example, during teaching sessions, the nurse periodically asks clients if they understand what is being taught. At the end of the teaching session, the nurse asks clients to identify information that was not provided that should have been covered. Clients may also be asked to evaluate a teaching session or the nurse providing the information in writing. Questionnaires used in these situations ask clients to express their satisfaction with the education they received. At times, written evaluations may be more truthful than evaluations obtained in a face-to-face situation.

Evaluation may reveal new learning needs or the existence of new factors that may interfere with the client's ability to learn. Alternative teaching methods often help clarify information or skills that the client was unable to comprehend or perform originally. When a client has difficulty in an acute care setting, the nurse may make a referral to resources, such as home care or an outpatient clinic, for further education and evaluation. Like the nursing process, the teaching-learning process is continuous and ever changing.

Documentation of Client Teaching. Because client teaching often occurs informally between nurse and client, it is difficult to document it consistently. A nurse is legally responsible for providing accurate, timely client information that promotes continuity of care; therefore it is essential to document the outcomes of teaching. Documentation of client teaching also helps support quality improvement efforts, meet JCAHO standards, and promote third-party reimbursement. Many institutions have special forms that allow easy documentation. For instance, teaching flow sheets are excellent records that document the plan, implementation, and evaluation of learning. Rankin and Stallings (2001) suggest documenting the following regarding client education:

- *Assessment data and reassessment of learning needs.* Provides important information needed when developing the teaching plan.
- *Nursing diagnoses, client needs, and educational priorities.* Provides support for goals and outcomes that are established.
- *Interventions planned.* A specific plan, including the methods to be used in instruction, enhances continuity of care. When viewing the planned interventions, nurses can determine what information needs to be provided to the client.
- *Interventions provided.* Specifically describing subject matter enables other nurses to follow up and reinforce teaching (e.g., "Explained side effects of Inderal" or "Demonstrated umbilical cord care"). Note the date, time, and specific person or persons taught. Avoid

generalizations (e.g., "medications taught") that leave staff uninformed about what content has been taught. When resources such as pamphlets or audiovisual materials are used, the nurse documents this in the client's record.
- *Client's response and outcomes of care.* Documenting evidence of learning (e.g., a return demonstration or the ability to verbalize the purpose and side effects of a medication) informs staff about the client's progress and determines information that still must be taught.
- *Ability of client and/or family to manage needs after discharge.* A careful evaluation of educational needs that remain upon discharge will help identify the potential need for outpatient or home health follow-up after discharge. When the nurse makes appropriate referrals, the client and/or family are often able to successfully meet their needs and avoid unnecessary rehospitalizations.

Key Concepts

- The nurse ensures that clients, families, and communities receive information needed to maintain optimal health.
- Health education is aimed at the promotion, restoration, and maintenance of health.
- Teaching is most effective when it is responsive to the learner's needs.
- Teaching is a form of interpersonal communication, with the teacher and student actively involved in a process that increases the student's knowledge and skills.
- The ability to learn depends on a person's physical and cognitive attributes.
- The ability to attend to the learning process depends on physical comfort and anxiety levels and the presence of environmental distraction.
- A person's health beliefs influence the willingness to gain knowledge and skills necessary to maintain health.
- Teaching must be timed to coincide with the client's readiness to learn.
- Clients of different age-groups require different teaching strategies as a result of developmental capabilities.
- The client should be an active participant in a teaching plan, agreeing to the plan, helping choose instructional methods, and recommending times for instruction.
- Learning objectives describe what a person is to learn in behavioral terms.
- A combination of teaching methods improves the learner's attentiveness and involvement.
- A teacher is more effective when presenting information that builds on a learner's existing knowledge.
- A teacher who uses reinforcement for a behavior is increasing the probability of the behavior recurring.
- Older adults learn most effectively when information is slowly paced and presented in small amounts.
- A nurse evaluates a client's learning by observing performance of expected learning behaviors under desired conditions.

- Effective documentation describes the entire process of client education, promotes continuity of care, and demonstrates that educational standards have been met.

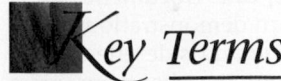

Key Terms

Affective learning, *p. 455*
Analogies, *p. 469*
Cognitive learning, *p. 454*
Compliance, *p. 456*
Functional illiteracy, *p. 469*
Learning, *p. 452*
Learning objective, *p. 453*
Motivation, *p. 456*

Psychomotor learning, *p. 455*
Reinforcement, *p. 467*
Return demonstrations, *p. 468*
Self-efficacy, *p. 457*
Teaching, *p. 451*

Critical Thinking Questions

1. Mrs. S has a 10-year history of hypertension and a 5-year history of diabetes. Recently her hypertension has become uncontrolled, and she has been diagnosed with depression. Her medications, which have recently been changed, include captopril (Capoten) 25 mg 3 times a day, diltiazem (Cardizem CD) 240 mg every morning, metformin (Glucophage XR) 1500 mg before the evening meal, and sertraline (Zoloft) 100 mg by mouth at bedtime. The nurse identifies the priority nursing diagnosis as *deficient knowledge related to change in medications*. The nurse wants to develop a plan of care that utilizes the three domains of learning. What are the client's teaching priorities? Which learning needs would require a cognitive method? Which needs would be more appropriate to satisfy through affective or psychomotor methods?
2. The nurse is caring for a client who is being discharged after an appendectomy. He is taking medication for the treatment of attention deficit and hyperactivity disorder (ADHD). Which teaching strategies should the nurse employ when providing discharge information to this client?
3. A 23-year-old man has recently sustained a spinal cord injury after being involved in a diving accident that has left him paralyzed from the waist down. He is verbally abusive to the staff and expresses anger toward his family and friends when they come to visit. He needs to begin learning transfer techniques. Which stage of grieving is this client experiencing? What approach should the nurse take in planning education for this client?
4. A 65-year-old woman is taking her 72-year-old husband home after a hip pinning. Which interventions should the nurse use in helping this couple transition to home smoothly?

Review Questions

1. A client must learn to use a walker. Acquisition of this skill will require learning in the:
   1. Cognitive domain.
   2. Affective domain.
   3. Psychomotor domain.
   4. Attentional domain.

2. The nurse should plan to teach a client about the importance of exercise:
   1. When there are visitors in the room.
   2. When the client's pain medications are working.
   3. Just before lunch, when the client is most awake and alert.
   4. When the client is talking about current stressors in his or her life.

3. A client newly diagnosed with cervical cancer is going home. The client is avoiding discussion of her illness and postoperative orders. In teaching the client about discharge instructions, the nurse should:
   1. Teach the client's spouse.
   2. Focus on knowledge the client will need in a few weeks.
   3. Provide only the information the client needs to go home.
   4. Convince the client that learning about her health is necessary.

4. The school nurse is about to teach a freshman-level health class about nutrition. To achieve the best learning outcomes, the nurse should:
   1. Provide information using a lecture.
   2. Use simple words to promote understanding.
   3. Complete an extensive literature search focusing on eating disorders.
   4. Develop topics for discussion that require problem solving.

5. A nurse is going to teach a client how to perform a breast self-examination. The behavioral objective that would best measure that the client's ability to perform the examination is:
   1. The client will verbalize the steps involved in breast self-examination within 1 week.
   2. The nurse will explain the importance of performing breast self-examination once a month.
   3. The client will perform breast self-examination correctly on herself before the end of the teaching session.
   4. The nurse will demonstrate breast self-examination on a breast model provided by the American Cancer Association.

6. A client who is having chest pain is going for an emergency cardiac catheterization. The most appropriate teaching approach in this situation is the:
   1. Telling approach.
   2. Selling approach.
   3. Entrusting approach.
   4. Participating approach.

7. The nurse is teaching a parenting class to a group of pregnant adolescents and has given the adolescents baby dolls to bathe and talk to. This is an example of:
   1. Discovery.
   2. An analogy.
   3. Role playing.
   4. A demonstration.

8. An older adult is being started on a new antihypertensive medication. In teaching the client about the medication, the nurse should:
   1. Allow the client time to express himself or herself and ask questions.
   2. Speak loudly.
   3. Present the information once.
   4. Expect the client to understand the information quickly.

9. A client must learn how to administer a subcutaneous injection. The nurse knows the client is ready to learn when the client:
   1. Has walked 400 feet.
   2. Expresses the importance of learning the skill.
   3. Can see and understand the markings on the syringe.
   4. Has the dexterity needed to prepare and inject the medication.

10. A client who is hospitalized has just been diagnosed with diabetes. He is going to need to learn how to give himself injections. The best teaching method would be:
    1. Demonstration.
    2. Group instruction.
    3. One-on-one discussion.
    4. Simulation.

*R*eferences

American Hospital Association: *The patient care partnership: understanding expectations, rights, and responsibilities,* http://www.hospitalconnect.com/aha/.

American Nurses Association: *Position statement on promotion and disease prevention,* 1995, http://www.nursingworld.org/readroom/position/social/scprmo.htm.

Assessment, the foundation of good teaching, *Patient Education Management* 9(4):40, 2002.

Bandura A: *Self-efficacy: the exercise of control,* New York, 1997, WH Freeman.

Bandura A: Social cognitive theory: an agentic perspective, *Annu Rev Psychol* 52:1, 2001.

Bastable S: *Nurse as educator: principles of teaching and learning for nursing practice,* Sudbury, Mass, 2003, Jones & Bartlett.

Bloom BS, editor: Taxonomy of educational objectives, *Cognitive domain,* vol 1, New York, 1956, Longman.

Cronbach LJ: *Educational psychology,* ed 3, New York, 1977, Harcourt Brace Jovanovich.

Dochterman JM, Bulechek GM: *Nursing interventions classification (NIC),* ed 4, St. Louis, 2004, Mosby.

Donovan H, Ward S: A representational approach to patient education, *J Nurs Scholarsh* 33(3):211, 2001.

Dreger V, Trembeck T: Optimize patient health by treating literacy and language barriers, *AORN J* 75(2):280, 2002.

Edelman CL, Mandle CL: *Health promotion throughout the lifespan,* ed 5, St. Louis, 2002, Mosby.

Felder R: *Learning styles,* http://www.ncsu.edu/felder-public/Learning_Styles.html.

Joint Commission on Accreditation of Healthcare Organizations: *Accreditation manual of hospitals,* Oakbrook Terrace, Ill, 2003, The Commission.

Krathwohl DR and others: *Taxonomy of educational objectives: the classification of educational goals, handbook II, affective domain,* New York, 1964, David McKay.

Maas M and others: *Nursing care of older adults: diagnoses, outcomes, & interventions,* St. Louis, 2001, Mosby.

Martinali J and others: A checklist to improve patient education in a cardiology outpatient setting, *Patient Educ Couns* 42(2001):231, 2001.

Mennies J: Teaching adult patients with learning disabilities, *Nurs Spec* 14(21):20, 2001.

Moorhead S, Johnson M, Maas M: *Nursing outcomes classification (NOC),* ed 3, St. Louis, 2004, Mosby.

National Center for Education Statistics: *1992 National adult literacy survey,* 1996, http://nces.ed.gov/naal.

Osborne H: In other words . . . can they understand? *Testing patient education materials with intended readers,* 2001, http://www.healthliteracy.com/oncallnov2001.htm.

Rankin SH, Stallings KD: *Patient education: issues, principles, practices,* ed 4, Philadelphia, 2001, JB Lippincott.

Redman BK: *The practice of patient education,* ed 9, St. Louis, 2001, Mosby.

Saarmann L, Daugherty J, Riegel B: Teaching staff a brief cognitive-behavioral intervention, *Medsurg Nurs* 11(3):144, 2002.

Winslow E: Patient education materials: can patients read them, or are they ending up in the trash? *Am J Nurs* 101(10):33, 2001.

Wong D and others: *Wong's nursing care of infants and children,* ed 7, St. Louis, 2003, Mosby.

*R*esearch References

Cooper H and others: Chronic disease patient education: lessons from meta-analyses, *Patient Educ Couns* 44:107, 2001.

Chelf J and others: Learning and support preferences of adult patients with cancer at a comprehensive cancer center, *Oncol Nurs Forum* 29(5):863, 2002.

Danigelis N and others: Two community outreach strategies to increase breast cancer screening among low-income women, *J Cancer Educ* 16(1):55, 2001.

Oermann M, Harris C, Dammeyer J: Teaching by the nurse: how important is it to patients? *Appl Nurs Res* 14(1):11, 2001.

25

Documentation

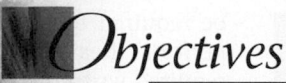
Objectives

Mastery of content in this chapter will enable the student to:

- Define the key terms listed.
- Describe multidisciplinary communication within the health care team.
- Identify purposes of a health care record.
- Discuss legal guidelines for documentation.
- Maintain confidentiality of records and reports.
- Describe five quality guidelines for documentation and reporting.
- Discuss the relationship between documentation and health care financial reimbursement.
- Describe the different methods used in record keeping.
- Discuss the advantages of standardized documentation forms.
- Identify elements to include when documenting a client's discharge plan.
- Describe the role of critical pathways in multidisciplinary documentation.
- Identify the important aspects of home care and long-term care documentation.
- Discuss issues related to computerization in documentation.
- Describe the purpose and content of a change-of-shift report.
- Explain how to verify telephone orders.

*D*ocumentation is anything written or printed that is relied on as record or proof for authorized persons. Documentation within a client medical record is a vital aspect of nursing practice. Nursing documentation must be accurate, comprehensive, and flexible enough to retrieve critical data, maintain continuity of care, track client outcomes, and reflect current standards of nursing practice. Information in the client record provides a detailed account of the level of quality of care delivered to clients. Effective documentation ensures continuity of care, saves time, and minimizes the risk of errors (Yocum, 2002). Today's health care environment creates many challenges for accurately documenting and recording care provided to clients.

Accreditation agencies such as the Joint Commission on Accreditation of Healthcare Organizations (JCAHO) specify guidelines for documentation. Under the prospective payment system, hospitals are reimbursed a set dollar amount by Medicare for each **diagnosis-related group (DRG)** (Box 25-1). Everything that is done for a client must be documented in the medical record for the health care institution to recover its costs.

As members of the health care team, nurses need to communicate information about clients accurately and in a timely, effective manner. The quality of client care depends on caregivers' ability to communicate with one another. All health care providers require the same information about clients so that they can plan an organized, comprehensive care plan. If the care plan is not com-

Box 25-1   Diagnosis-Related Groups

- A diagnosis-related group (DRG) is a series of decision trees designed to cluster groups of clients together by diagnosis, surgical procedures, complications, comorbidities (preexisting illness), and age.
- A hospital is reimbursed a fixed amount based on the hospital's specific rate of reimbursement.
- Each client with a particular diagnosis is reimbursed the same regardless of length of stay or cost of treatment.
- An assigned DRG may change on the basis of documentation.

municated to all members of the health care team, care can become fragmented, repetition of tasks occurs, and therapies may be delayed or omitted. Data recorded, reported, or communicated to other health care professionals are confidential and must be protected.

The health care environment creates many challenges for accurately documenting and reporting the care delivered to clients. The quality of care, the standards of regulatory agencies and nursing practice, the reimbursement structure in the health care system, and legal guidelines make documentation and reporting an extremely important responsibility of a nurse. Whether the transfer of client information occurs through verbal reports, written documents, or electronic transfer, there are principles that the nurse must follow to maintain confidentiality of information.

Confidentiality

Nurses are legally and ethically obligated to keep information about clients confidential. Nurses may not discuss a client's examination, observation, conversation, or treatment with other clients or staff not involved in the client's care. Only staff directly involved in a specific client's care have legitimate access to the records. Clients frequently request copies of their medical records, and they have the right to read those records. Each institution has policies for controlling the manner in which records are shared. In most situations, clients are required to give written permission for release of medical information.

Nurses are responsible for protecting records from all unauthorized readers. When nurses and other health care professionals have a legitimate reason to use records for data gathering, research, or continuing education, appropriate authorization must be obtained according to agency policy. Student nurses and faculty may be required to present identification indicating access to the record is authorized. The nurse should know the location of the record at all times. The record is stored by the health care agency after treatment ends.

Legislation to protect client privacy for health information, the Health Insurance Portability and Accountability Act (HIPAA), became a final rule in April 2001 and took effect in April 2003. This legislation governs all areas of information management, including reimbursement, coding, security, and client records. Health care providers (e.g., hospitals, physicians' offices, and pharmacies) will

be required to provide clients with greater control over personal health care information. Previously the rule required written consent for disclosure of all client information. Under new regulations, in order to eliminate barriers that could delay access to care, providers are required only to notify clients of their privacy policy and make a reasonable effort to get written acknowledgment of this notification (Frank-Stromborg and Gauschow, 2002).

HIPAA requires that disclosure or requests regarding health information are limited to the minimum necessary. This includes only the specific information required for a particular purpose. For example, if a client's home telephone number is needed to reschedule an appointment, access to the medical records will be limited solely to telephone information. According to the U.S. Department of Health and Human Services (USDHHS) (2001), clients will have significant new rights to understand and control how their health information is used.

- **Client education on privacy protections:** Providers and health plans will be required to give clients a clear written explanation of how the covered entity may use and disclose their health information.
- **Ensuring clients' access to their medical records:** Clients will be able to see and get copies of their records and request amendments. In addition, a history of nonroutine disclosures must be made accessible to clients.
- **Receiving client consent before information is released:** Health care providers who see clients will be required to obtain client consent before sharing their information for treatment, payment, and health care operations. In addition, separate client authorization must be obtained for nonroutine disclosures and most non–health care purposes. Clients will have the right to request restrictions on the uses and disclosures of their information.
- **Providing recourse if privacy protections are violated:** People will have the right to file a formal complaint with a covered provider or health plan, or with the USDHHS, about violations of the provisions of this rule or the policies and procedures of the covered entity.

Standards

Current JCAHO standards require that all clients who are admitted to a health care institution have an assessment of physical, psychosocial, environmental, self-care, client education, and discharge planning needs (JCAHO, 2003). The JCAHO requires documentation within the context of the nursing process, as well as evidence of client and family teaching and discharge planning.

The JCAHO also stresses the importance of evaluating client outcomes, including the client's response to treatments, teaching, or preventive care. If more than one discipline regularly cares for a client, the JCAHO also expects a multidisciplinary care plan. For example, the JCAHO standards recently incorporated a collaborative and interdisciplinary approach to pain management. This includes individualized pain control strategies involving frequent reassessment of pain, use of both pharmacological and nonpharmacological strategies and a formalized approach to the implementation and evaluation of pain management (see Chapter 42).

The nursing service department of each health care agency selects the method that is used to document client care. The method reflects the philosophy of the nursing department and incorporates the standards of care. For example, if a nursing department's standards of practice use nursing diagnosis or a framework such as Gordon's functional health patterns (Gordon, 2002), the documentation system uses nursing diagnoses and health patterns in care plans and other forms. Because the nursing process shapes a nurse's approach and direction of care, effective documentation reflects the nursing process.

Multidisciplinary Communication Within the Health Care Team

Client care requires effective communication among members of the health care team. Effective communication takes place along two approaches. A client's **record** or chart is a confidential, permanent legal documentation of information relevant to a client's health care. Information about the client's health care is recorded after each client contact. The record is a continuing account of the client's health care status and is available to all members of the health care team. All records basically contain the following information:

- Client identification and demographic data
- Informed consent for treatment and procedures
- Admission nursing history
- Nursing diagnoses or problems
- Nursing or multidisciplinary care plan
- Record of nursing care treatment and evaluation
- Medical history
- Medical diagnosis
- Therapeutic orders
- Medical and health discipline's progress notes
- Reports of physical examinations
- Reports of diagnostic studies
- Client education
- Summary of operative procedures
- Discharge plan and summary

Reports are oral, written, or audiotaped exchanges of information between caregivers (Figure 25-1). Common reports given by nurses include change-of-shift reports, telephone reports, transfer reports, and incident reports. A physician may call a nursing unit to receive a verbal report on a client's condition and progress. The laboratory submits a written report providing the results of diagnostic tests. Incident reports are documented on a record that is not part of the client medical record (see Chapter 22).

Information is also communicated through discussions or conferences among team members. For example, a discharge planning conference often involves members of all disciplines (e.g., nursing, social work, dietary, medicine, and physical therapy), who meet to discuss the client's progress toward established discharge goals.

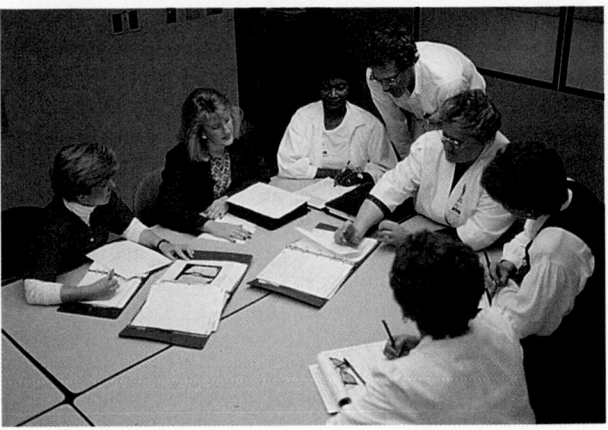

FIGURE **25-1**   Staff communicate information about their clients during a change-of-shift report.

Consultations are another form of discussion whereby one professional caregiver gives formal advice about the care of a client to another caregiver. For example, a nurse caring for a client with a chronic wound may need a consultation with a wound care specialist. **Referrals** (an arrangement for services by another care provider), consultations, and conferences must be documented in a client's permanent record so that all caregivers can plan care accordingly.

Purposes of Records

A record is a valuable source of data that is used by all members of the health care team. Its purposes include communication, legal documentation, financial billing, education, research, and auditing-monitoring.

Communication

The record is a means by which health care team members communicate client needs and progress, individual therapies, content of conferences, client education, and discharge planning. The plan of care needs to be clear to anyone reading the chart (see Unit III). The record should be the most current and accurate source of information about a client's health care status.

The manner in which the nursing process is conducted with a client is communicated in the record. The admitting nursing history and physical assessment is comprehensive and provides a baseline of the client's health status on admission to the facility. These data usually contains biographical data (e.g., age and marital status), method of admission, reason for admission, a brief past medical-surgical history (e.g., previous surgeries or illnesses), allergies, current medication (prescribed and over-the-counter), the client's perceptions about illness or hospitalization, and a review of health risk factors (see Chapter 15). A physical assessment of all body systems is either incorporated into the nursing history or included on a separate form (see Chapter 32).

The medical progress notes should complement nursing process information. The notes detail the physician's findings at the time of assessment. While caring for any client, the nurse refers to the medical record for relevant assessment findings. The nurse is able to enter a client's room, anticipate the status of the client, and then conduct an individualized assessment of the client.

The record provides data that nurses use to identify and support nursing diagnoses, establish expected outcomes of care, plan interventions for care, and evaluate the care according to clients' responses to the care provided. Information from the record adds to the nurse's observations and assessment. It is unnecessary for the nurse to collect information that is already available. If there is reason to believe that the information is inaccurate, information should be verified, and appropriate changes made to the client's record.

Legal Documentation

Accurate documentation is one of the best defenses for legal claims associated with nursing care (see Chapter 22). To limit nursing liability, nursing documentation must clearly indicate that individualized, goal-directed nursing care was provided to a client based on the nursing assessment. The record needs to describe exactly what happened to a client. This is best achieved when the nurse charts immediately after care was provided. Even though nursing care may have been excellent, in a court of law "care not documented is care not provided." Nurses need to indicate all assessments, interventions, client responses, instructions, and referrals in the medical record.

Four common issues in malpractice caused by inadequate documentation are (1) not charting the correct time when events occurred, (2) failing to record verbal orders or failing to have them signed, (3) charting actions in advance to save time, and (4) documenting incorrect data (Martin, 1994). Table 25-1 provides guidelines for legally sound documentation.

Financial Billing

Diagnosis-related groups (DRGs) have become the basis for establishing reimbursement for client care. DRGs are a prospective payment system. Hospitals are reimbursed a preestablished dollar amount by Medicare for each DRG. Detailed recording helps in establishing codable diagnoses that are used to determine a DRG. The nurse's contribution to documentation can help clarify the type of

Table 25-1　Legal Guidelines for Recording

Guidelines	Rationale	Correct Action
Do not erase, apply correction fluid, or scratch out errors made while recording.	Charting becomes illegible: it may appear as if you were attempting to hide information or deface record.	Draw single line through error, write word *error* above it and sign your name or initials. Then record note correctly.
Do not write retaliatory or critical comments about client or care by other health care professionals.	Statements can be used as evidence for nonprofessional behavior or poor quality of care.	Enter only objective descriptions of client's behavior; client comments should be quoted.
Correct all errors promptly.	Errors in recording can lead to errors in treatment.	Avoid rushing to complete charting; be sure information is accurate.
Record all facts.	Record must be accurate and reliable.	Be certain entry is factual; do not speculate or guess.
Do not leave blank spaces in nurse's notes.	Another person can add incorrect information in space.	Chart consecutively, line by line; if space is left, draw line horizontally through it and sign your name at end.
Record all entries legibly and in black ink.	Illegible entries can be misinterpreted, causing errors and lawsuits; ink cannot be erased; black ink is more legible when records are photocopied or transferred to microfilm.	Never erase entries or use correction fluid, and never use pencil.
If order is questioned, record that clarification was sought.	If you perform order known to be incorrect, you are just as liable for prosecution as the physician is.	Do not record "physician made error." Instead, chart that "Dr. Smith was called to clarify order for analgesic."
Chart only for yourself.	You are accountable for information you enter into chart.	Never chart for someone else (exception: if caregiver has left unit for day and calls with information that needs to be documented, include the name of the source of information in the entry and include that the information was provided via telephone).
Avoid using generalized, empty phrases such as "status unchanged" or "had good day."	Specific information about client's condition or case can be accidentally deleted if information is too generalized.	Use complete, concise descriptions of care.
Begin each entry with time, and end with your signature and title.	This guideline ensures that correct sequence of events is recorded; signature documents who is accountable for care delivered.	Do not wait until end of shift to record important changes that occurred several hours earlier; be sure to sign each entry.
For computer documentation keep your password to yourself.	Maintains security and confidentiality.	Once logged into the computer, do not leave the computer screen unattended.

treatment a client receives and help support the reimbursement to the health care agency.

Medical records are also audited to review financial charges used in the client's care. Private insurance carriers and auditors from federal agencies review records to determine the reimbursement that a client or a health care agency receives. Accurate documentation of supplies and equipment used assists in accurate and timely reimbursement.

Education
A client's record contains a variety of information, including diagnoses, signs and symptoms of disease, successful and unsuccessful therapies, diagnostic findings, and client behaviors. An effective way to learn the nature of an illness and the individual client's response to it is to read the client care record. No two clients have identical records, and patterns of information can be identified in records of clients who have similar health problems. With this information, students identify patterns for various health problems and can begin to anticipate the type of care required for a client.

Research
Statistical data relating to the frequency of clinical disorders, complications, use of specific medical and nursing therapies, recovery from illness, and deaths can be gathered from client records. For example, as a part of a quality improvement program for clients receiving intravenous therapy, a nurse manager may review clients' records to investigate the incidence of infection in clients with a specific type of intravenous catheter. A client record review indicates that the infection rate is increased, and the nurse manager and staff nurses design a new specific method for intravenous catheter care. Once this new intervention is implemented, the manager again reviews clients' records to determine if the infection rate decreases.

A nurse may use clients' records during a clinical research study to investigate a new nursing intervention. For example, a nurse wants to compare a new method of pain control with a standard pain protocol using two groups of clients. The client records provide data on the two types of interventions: the new method and the standard pain control. The nurse researcher collects data from the clients' records that describe the type and dose of analgesic medications used, objective assessment data, and clients' subjective reports of pain relief. The researcher then compares the findings to determine if the new method was more effective that the standard pain control protocol.

Some data collection activities may be part of the quality improvement practices at an agency, whereas other activities may be actual clinical research studies. There are different types of permissions that must be secured before reviewing client records for any type of research study or data analysis. It is the responsibility of the researcher to be sure the data collection and analysis adhere to federal and agency policies.

Auditing-Monitoring
The JCAHO requires hospitals to establish quality improvement programs for conducting objective, ongoing reviews of client care (JACHO, 2003). The JCAHO has established standards for the information to be found in the client's record, including indications that a plan of care is developed with the client as a participant and that discharge planning and client education have occurred. The JCAHO asks institutions to establish standards for quality care. Nurses monitor or review records throughout the year to determine the degree to which quality improvement standards are met (see Chapter 20). Deficiencies identified during monitoring are shared with all members of the nursing staff so that corrections in policy or practice can be made. Quality improvement programs keep nurses informed of standards of nursing practice to maintain excellence in nursing care (see Chapter 19).

Guidelines for Quality Documentation and Reporting

High-quality documentation and reporting are necessary to enhance efficient, individualized client care. Quality documentation and reporting have five important characteristics: they are factual, accurate, complete, current, and organized.

Factual
A record must contain descriptive, objective information about what a nurse sees, hears, feels, and smells. An objective description is the result of direct observation and measurement. The use of inferences without supporting factual data is not acceptable because it can be misunderstood.

The use of vague terms, such as *appears, seems,* or *apparently,* is not acceptable because these words suggest that the nurse is stating an opinion. For example, the description "the client seems anxious" does not accurately communicate facts and does not inform another caregiver of the details regarding the behaviors exhibited by the client that led to the use of the word *anxious.* The phrase *seems anxious* is a conclusion without supported facts. Objective documentation needs to include the nurse's observations of the client's behaviors. For example, objective signs of anxiety may include increased pulse rate, increased respiration, and increased restlessness.

A subjective description when recording subjective data, document the client's exact words within quotation marks whenever possible. For example, when a client exhibits anxiety the nurse may record, "Client states, 'I feel very nervous.'"

Accurate
The use of exact measurements establishes accuracy. For example, a description such as "Intake, 360 ml of water" is more accurate than "Client drank an adequate amount of fluid." These measurements can later be used as a means to determine whether a client's condition has changed. Charting that an abdominal wound is "5 cm in length without redness, drainage, or edema" is more descriptive than "large wound healing well."

Documentation of concise data is clear and easy to understand. It is essential to avoid the use of unnecessary words and irrelevant detail. For example, the fact that the client is watching TV is only necessary when this activity is significant to the client's status and plan of care.

Use of an institution's accepted abbreviations, symbols, and system of measures (e.g., metric) ensures that all staff members use the same language in their reports and records. A nurse should use abbreviations carefully to avoid misinterpretation. For example, od (every day) can be misinterpreted to mean O.D. (right eye). To minimize errors, abbreviations are spelled in their entirety when abbreviations become confusing.

Correct spelling demonstrates a level of competency and attention to detail. Many terms can easily be misinterpreted (e.g., *dysphagia* or *dysphasia* and *dram* or *gram*). Some spelling errors can also result in serious treatment errors; for example, the names of certain medications such as digitoxin and digoxin or morphine and Numorphan are similar and must be transcribed carefully to ensure that the client receives the correct medication.

JCAHO standards (2003) require that "all entries in medical records are dated and a method is established to identify the authors of entries." Therefore each entry in a client's record ends with the caregiver's full name or initials and status, such as "Julie Smith, RN." Each time initials are used, the full name and status must previously appear on the same page so the individual entering initials can be readily identified. A nursing student enters full name, student nurse abbreviation (e.g., SN or NS), and educational institution, such as "David Jones, SN (student nurse), CMTC (Central Maine Technical College)."

Records need to reflect accountability during the time frame of the entry, which is best accomplished when nurses chart only their own observations and actions. The signature holds that nurse accountable for information recorded. If information was inadvertently omitted from the record, it is acceptable for nurses to ask colleagues to chart information after they leave work. The entry needs to clearly show what was done and by whom (e.g., "At 11 AM Sam Turner, RN, called and reported that at 8 AM morphine sulfate 15 mg IM was administered to client for abdominal pain").

Complete

The information within a recorded entry or a report needs to be complete, containing appropriate and essential information. Criteria for thorough communication exist for certain health problems or nursing activities (Table 25-2). The nurse makes written entries in the client's medical record, describing nursing care that is administered and the client's response. An example of a thorough nurse's note follows:

> *1915 Client verbalizes sharp, throbbing pain localized along lateral side of right ankle, beginning approximately 15 minutes ago after twisting his foot on the stairs. Client rates pain as 8 on a scale of 0-10. Pain increased with movement, slightly relieved with elevation. Pedal pulses equal bilaterally. Right ankle circumference 1 cm larger than left. Ice applied. Percocet 2 tabs given for pain. Client states pain somewhat relieved with ice, rates pain as 6 on a scale of 0-10. Physician notified. Lee Turno, RN.*

Current

Timely entries are essential in the client's ongoing care (JCAHO, 2003). To increase accuracy and decrease unnecessary duplication, many health care agencies use records kept near the client's bedside, which facilitate immediate documentation of information as it is collected from a

Table 25-2	Examples of Criteria for Reporting and Recording
Topic	**Criteria to Report or Record**
Assessment	
Subjective data	Description of episode in quotation marks Onset, location, description of condition (severity, duration, frequency, precipitating, aggravating and relieving factors)
Client behavior (e.g., anxiety, confusion, hostility)	Onset, behaviors exhibited, precipitating factors
Objective data (e.g., rash, tenderness, breath sounds)	Onset, location, description of condition
Nursing Interventions and Evaluation	
Treatments (e.g., enema, bath, dressing change)	Time administered, equipment used (if appropriate), client's response (objective and subjective changes) compared to previous treatment; for example, "client denied pain during dressing change" or "client reported severe abdominal cramping during enema"
Medication administration	Immediately after administration, document: time medication given, preliminary assessment (e.g., pain level, vital signs), client response or effect of medication; for example, "1500 Pain reported at 6 (scale 0-10). Tylenol 500 mg given PO 1530: Client reports pain level 2 (scale 0-10)" or "Pruritus and hives developed over lower abdomen 1 hour after penicillin was given"
Client teaching	Information presented, method of instruction (e.g., discussion, demonstration, videotape, booklet), client response, including questions and evidence of understanding such as return demonstration or change in behavior
Discharge planning	Measurable client goals or expected outcomes, progress toward goals, need for referrals

client. Activities or findings to communicate at the time of occurrence include the following:

- Vital signs
- Administration of medications and treatments
- Preparation for diagnostic tests or surgery
- Change in client's status and who was notified, (e.g., physician, manager, client's family)
- Admission, transfer, discharge, or death of a client
- Treatment for a sudden change in client's status

This information is often included in flow sheets kept at the bedside. Nurses often keep notes on a worksheet when caring for several clients, making notes as the care occurs to ensure that entries recorded later in the record are accurate.

Most health care agencies use military time, a 24-hour system that avoids misinterpretation of AM and PM times (Figure 25-2). Instead of two 12-hour cycles in standard time, the military clock is one 24-hour time cycle. The military clock ends with midnight at 2400 and begins at 1 minute after midnight as 0001. For example, 10:22 AM is 1022 military time; 1:00 PM is 1300 military time.

Organized

The nurse communicates information in a logical order. For example, an organized note describes the client's pain, nurse's assessment and interventions, and the client's response. To write notes about complex situations in an organized fashion the nurse thinks about the situation and often makes notes of what is to be included before beginning to write in the permanent legal record.

Methods of Recording

There are several documentation systems for recording client data. These documentation systems are selected by the nursing service and reflect the philosophy of the department. The same documentation system is used throughout a specific agency and may be used throughout a health care system as well.

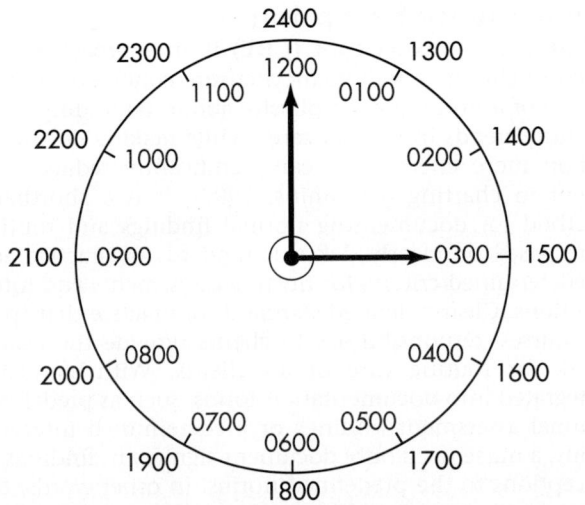

FIGURE 25-2   Military time clock.

Narrative Documentation

Narrative documentation is the traditional method for recording nursing care. It is simply the use of a storylike format to document information specific to client conditions and nursing care. Narrative charting, however, has many disadvantages, including the tendency to have repetitious information, to be time consuming, and to require the reader to sort through much information to locate desired data. There are several formats for recording health care information.

Problem-Oriented Medical Record

The **problem-oriented medical record (POMR)** is a method of documentation that places emphasis on the client's problems. Data are organized by problem or diagnosis. Ideally each member of the health care team contributes to a single list of identified client problems. This approach assists in coordinating a common plan of care. The POMR has the following major sections: database, problem list, care plan, and progress notes.

Database. The database section contains all available assessment information pertaining to the client (e.g., history and physical examination, the nurse's admission history and ongoing assessment, the dietitian's assessment, laboratory reports, and radiological test results). The database is the foundation for identifying client problems and planning care. As new data become available, the database is revised. It accompanies clients through successive hospitalizations or clinic visits.

Problem List. After data are analyzed, problems are identified and a single list is made. The problem list includes the client's physiological, psychological, social, cultural, spiritual, developmental, and environmental needs. The problems are listed in chronological order and filed in the front of the client's record to serve as an organizing guide for the client's care. New problems are added as they are identified. When a problem has been resolved, the date is recorded and it is highlighted or a line is drawn through the problem and its number.

Nursing Care Plan. A care plan is developed for each problem by the disciplines involved in the client's care (see Chapter 17). Nurses document the plan of care in a variety of formats. Generally these plans of care include nursing diagnoses, expected outcomes, and interventions.

Progress Notes. Health care team members monitor and record the progress of a client's problems (Box 25-2). The information can be expressed in various formats of structured notes. One method is the SOAP charting. **SOAP:** S—subjective data (verbalizations of the client), O—objective data (that which is measured and observed), A—assessment (diagnosis based on the data), P—plan (what the caregiver plans to do). An I and E are sometimes added (i.e., **SOAPIE**) in some institutions. The I stands for intervention, and the E represents evaluation. The logic for SOAPIE notes is similar to that of the nursing process. Collect data about the client's problems, draw conclusions, and develop a plan of care. The nurse numbers each SOAP note and titles it according to the problem on the list.

Box 25-2 **Examples of Progress Notes Written in Different Formats**

SOAP (Subjective—Objective—Assessment—Plan)

1/19/04 Knowledge deficit related to inexperience regarding surgery
4:30 PM
S—"I'm worried about what it will be like after surgery."
O—Client asking frequent questions about surgery. Has had no previous experience with surgery. Wife present, acts as a support person.
A—Knowledge deficit regarding surgery related to inexperience. Client also expressing anxiety.
P—Explain routine preoperative preparation. Demonstrate and explain rationale for turning, coughing, and deep breathing exercises. Provide explanation and teaching booklet on postoperative nursing care. S. Lazarus, RN

PIE (Problem—Intervention—Evaluation)

P—Knowledge deficit regarding surgery related to inexperience.
I—Explained to client normal preoperative preparations for surgery. Demonstrated TCDB exercises. Provided booklet to client on postoperative nursing care.
E—Client demonstrates TCDB exercises correctly. Needs review of postoperative nursing care. S. Lazarus, RN

Focus Charting (Data—Action—Response)

D—Client stating, "I'm worried about what it will be like after surgery." Client asking frequent questions about surgery. Has had no previous experience with surgery. Wife present, acts as a support person
A—Explained to client normal preoperative preparations for surgery. Demonstrated TCDB exercises. Provided booklet to client on postoperative nursing care.
R—Client demonstrates TCDB exercises correctly. Needs review of postoperative nursing care. S. Lazarus, RN
NOTE: Some agencies also add P (Plan).

A second progress note method is the **PIE** format. It is similar to SOAP charting in its problem-oriented nature. However, it differs from the SOAP method in that PIE charting has a nursing origin, whereas SOAP originated from medical records. The format simplifies documentation by unifying the care plan and progress notes. PIE differs from SOAP notes because the narrative does not include assessment information. A nurse's daily assessment data appear on flow sheets, preventing duplication of data. The narrative note includes P—problem, I—intervention, and E—evaluation. The PIE notes are numbered or labeled according to the client's problems. Resolved problems are dropped from daily documentation after the nurse's review. Continuing problems are documented daily.

A third narrative format is **focus charting**. It involves use of **DAR** notes, which include D—data (both subjective and objective), A—action or nursing intervention, and R—response of the client (i.e., evaluation of effectiveness). One distinction of focus charting is its movement away from charting only problems, which has a negative connotation. Instead the notes are structured according to client concerns: a sign or symptom, a condition, a nursing diagnosis, a behavior, a significant event, or a change in a client's condition. Documentation is written in accordance with the nursing process, nurses are encouraged to broaden their thinking to include any client concerns, not just problem areas, and critical thinking is encouraged. Focus charting is easily understood by caregivers and adaptable to most health care settings. Focus charting helps track the client's condition and progress (Smith, 2000).

Source Records

In a **source record** the client's chart is organized so that each discipline (e.g., nursing, medicine, social work, or respiratory therapy) has a separate section in which to record data. One advantage of a source record is that caregivers can easily locate the proper section of the record in which to make entries. Table 25-3 lists the components of a source record.

A disadvantage of the source record is that details about a specific problem may be distributed throughout the record. For example, the nurse describes the character of abdominal pain and use of relaxation therapy and analgesic medication in the nurses' notes. The physician's notes describe the progress of the client's bowel obstruction and the plan for surgery in a separate section of the record. The results of x-ray examinations that show the location of the bowel obstruction are in the test results section of the record. The method by which source records are organized does not show how information from the disciplines is related or how care is coordinated to meet all of the client's needs.

The notes section is where nurses enter a narrative description of nursing care and the client's response (Box 25-3). It is also a section for documenting care that is provided by the physician in the nurse's presence. The nurse may record key diagnostic test results from other sections of the record in the nurses' notes if they are of major importance in the care of the client.

Charting by Exception

Charting by exception (CBE) is an approach that is used to eliminate redundancy, ensure concise documentation of routine care, emphasize abnormal findings, and identify trends in clinical care. While making documentation more effective, it can significantly reduce time spent in charting (Cummins, 1999). It is a shorthand method for documenting normal findings and routine care based on clearly defined standards of practice and predetermined criteria for nursing assessments and interventions. Clearly defined standards of practice that specify nurses' responsibilities to clients provide the framework for routine care of all clients. With standards integrated into documentation forms, such as predefined normal assessment findings or predetermined interventions, a nurse need only document significant findings or exceptions to the predefined norms. In other words, the nurse writes a progress note only when the standardized

Table 25-3	Organization of Traditional Source Record
Sections	**Contents**
Admission sheet	Specific demographic data about client: legal name, identification number, sex, age, birth date, marital status, occupation and employer, health insurance, nearest relative to notify in an emergency, religious preference, name of attending physician, date and time of admission
Physician's order sheet	Record of physician's orders for treatment and medications, with date, time, and physician's signature
Nurse's admission assessment	Summary of nursing history and physical examination
Graphic sheet and flow sheet	Record of repeated observations and measurements such as vital signs, daily weights, and intake and output
Medical history and examination	Results of initial examination performed by physician, including findings, family history, confirmed diagnoses, and medical plan of care
Nurses' notes	Narrative record of nursing process: assessment, nursing diagnosis, planning, implementation, and evaluation of care
Medication records	Accurate documentation of all medications administered to client: date, time, dose, route, and nurse's signature
Physician's progress notes	Ongoing record of client's progress and response to medical therapy and review of disease process
Health care disciplines' records	Entries made into record by all health-related disciplines: radiology, social work, and laboratories
Discharge summary	Summary of client's condition, progress, prognosis, rehabilitation, and teaching needs at time of dismissal from hospital or health care agency

Box 25-3	Sample Narrative Note

8/6/04 1100
Client states, "I'm having a hard time catching my breath." Respirations, labored at 32/min; P, 120; BP, 112/70. Client using intercostal muscles during inhalation. Breath sounds auscultated, crackles and wheezes over both lower lobes. Chest excursion equal bilaterally. Elevated head of bed to Fowler's position. Obtained arterial blood gas analysis at 1045 and O_2 started at 2 L/min per mask as ordered. Remained at bedside to calm client. P. Haske, RN
1130 Results of ABGs reported to Dr Stein are pH, 7.34; P_{CO_2}, 44 mm Hg; P_{O_2}, 80 mm Hg. Client breathing less labored and now R, 28/min; P, 96; BP, 110/72. Crackles and wheezing still apparent. Client resting quietly. P. Haske, RN

statement on the form is not met. Assessments are standardized on forms so that all caregivers evaluate and document findings consistently (Figure 25-3).

Because the standard assessments are located in the chart, client data are already present on the permanent record, so nurses do not have to keep temporary notes for later transcription and caregivers have easy access to current data. The assumption with charting by exception is that all standards are met unless otherwise documented. When nurses see entries in the chart, they know that something out of the ordinary has been observed or has occurred. For that reason when changes in a client's condition have developed, it is easy to track them.

When clients' conditions change, thorough and precise descriptions of what happens to clients and the actions taken are essential. Charting by exception can pose

legal risks if nurses are not disciplined in documenting exceptions.

Case Management Plan and Critical Pathways

The **case management** model of delivering care (see Chapter 2) incorporates a multidisciplinary approach to documenting client care. In many organizations the standardized plan of care is summarized into critical pathways for a specific disease or condition. The **critical pathways** are multidisciplinary care plans that include client problems, key interventions, and expected outcomes within an established time frame (Figure 25-4). The use of a computerized charting system allows for integration of the chart by many disciplines. The nurse and other team members such as physicians, dietitians, social workers, physical therapists, and respiratory therapists use the same critical pathway to monitor the client's progress during each shift or in the case of home care, every visit. With the computerized record available at every computer terminal, each care provider can access it at any time.

Critical pathways promote integration of information so that each discipline has access to notes written by others. It also reduces duplication and the amount of charting (Braugh, 1998). Unexpected outcomes, unmet goals, and interventions not specified within the critical pathway time frame are called **variances.** A variance occurs when the activities on the critical pathway are not completed as predicted or the client does not meet the expected outcomes. An example of a variance is when a postoperative client develops pulmonary complications requiring oxygen therapy and monitoring with pulse oximetry. A positive variance occurs when a client pro-

BARNES-JEWISH HOSPITAL Nursing Shift Assessment C-6 Requested by: CAROL	789651458 X Collins, Joseph S.S. Dr. Unit: Bed:

Search Interval   From: 05-Dec-1999 at 07:00
                  To: 06-Dec-1999 at 14:51

Patient Assessment

		Monday 12/06 07:00
N/S	**NEUROSENSORY STANDARD** Alert and awake. If asleep awakens to name. Verbal appropriate, clear, and understandable. Swallows without coughing. Oriented to time, place, person and situation. Behavior is appropriate to situation. Moves all extremities well, ambulates with steady gait.	Within Normal Limits
RESP	**RESPIRATORY STANDARD** Respirations are even and unlabored. Nailbeds and mucous membranes are pink. Patent airway. Lung sounds clear to auscultation. No cough noted	Within Normal Limits
CARD	**CARDIOVASCULAR STANDARD** Regular palpable pulses. Skin pallor within patient's norm. Skin warm and dry. No edema.	Within Normal Limits
SKIN	**SKIN INTEGRITY STANDARD** Skin and mucous membranes intact without notable lesions or impaired integrity. Mucous membranes moist and pink. Braden Score greater than 17.	* Exception as noted below
	Braden Risk Assessment	Mobility: Slightly Limited (3) Sensory: Slightly Limited (3) Moisture: Occasionally Moist (3) Activity: Walks Occasionally (3) Nutrition: Adequate (3) Friction/Shear: Potential Problem (2) Total Score 17

	Casts, Splints, Braces
	  Type: Fiberglass Cast
	  Site: Right Lower Leg
		Maintains correct anatomical position No pressure areas noted Distal extremity pink warm to touch Palpable distal pulse Capillary Refill <3 seconds Sensation normal Able to move distal phalanges.

	VASCULAR ACCESS STANDARD IV SITE: Site free of redness, swelling, pain, bleeding, drainage, IV patent, dressing occlusive and intact.	
NUTR	**NUTRITION STANDARD** Tolerating prescribed diet without nausea and vomiting. Eating at least 75% of each meal without difficulty. Feeds self.	Within normal limits
	Diet Type	Regular
GI	**GASTROINTESTINAL STANDARD** Abdomen soft. Bowel sounds active all 4 quadrants. No pain with palpation. Having bowel movements within patient's normal pattern, consistency, and color.	Within Normal Limits
GU	**GENITOURINARY STANDARD** Continent of urine. Urine clear and yellow to amber color.	Within Normal Limits
PSYCH	**PSYCHOSOCIAL STANDARD** Accepts situation and facial expressions are appropriate. family support available and patient receives visitors. Able to communicate without assistance.	Within Normal Limits
EDU	Health Status Teaching	
	Tests/Procedures/Therapies	
	Medication Teaching	
	Nutrition Teaching	
	Medical Equipment Teaching	
HMGT	Equipment	
Charted By		cl

Signatures: cl   C. Logan, rn

Printed: 06-Dec-1999 at 14:51

FIGURE 25-3   Nursing care record. (Courtesy Barnes-Jewish Hospital, St. Louis, Mo.)

gresses more rapidly than expected (e.g., use of a Foley catheter may be discontinued a day early). A variance analysis is necessary to review the data for trends and for developing and implementing an action plan to respond to the identified client problems (Box 25-4). In addition, variances may result from changes in the client's health or may occur as a result of other health complications not associated with the primary reason for which the client requires care. The nurse's responsibility is to address the variance and to justify the actions taken to manage the critical pathway deviation (Iyer and Camp, 1999). Over time, the reoccurrence of similar variances may lead the health care team to revise a critical pathway.

Common Record-Keeping Forms

A variety of forms are available that are designed for the type of information nurses routinely document. The categories within a form are usually derived from institutional standards of practice or guidelines established by accrediting agencies.

Admission Nursing History Forms

A nursing history form is completed when a client is admitted to a nursing care unit. The history form guides the nurse through a complete assessment to identify relevant nursing diagnoses or problems (see Chapter 15). Data on history forms provide baseline data that can be compared with changes in the client's condition. Each institution designs a nursing history form differently, based on the standards of practice and philosophy of nursing care.

Flow Sheets and Graphic Records

Flow sheets are forms that allow nurses to quickly and easily enter assessment data about the client, including vital signs and routine repetitive care, such as hygiene measures, ambulation, meals, weights, and safety and re-straint checks. Flow sheets use a coding system for data entry (Figure 25-5). If an occurrence on the flow sheet is unusual or changes significantly, a focus note is needed. For example, if a client's blood pressure becomes dangerously high, the nurse completes a focus assessment and records this, as well as action taken, in the progress notes. Flow sheets provide a quick, easy reference for the health care team members in assessing a client's status. Critical care and acute care units commonly use flow sheets for all types of physiological data (Box 25-5).

Client Care Summary or Kardex

Many hospitals now have computerized systems that provide basic, summative information in the form of a client care summary. This is printed out for each client during each shift. This summary is continually updated and provides the nurse with a current detailed list of orders, treatment, and diagnostic testing. In some settings, a **Kardex,** a portable "flip-over" file or notebook, is kept at the nurses' station. Most Kardex forms have an activity and treatment section and a nursing care plan section that organize information for quick reference as nurses give change-of-shift reports or make walking rounds. An updated Kardex eliminates the need for repeated referral to the chart for routine information throughout the day. In many institutions Kardex entries are done in pencil because of the need for frequent revisions as the client's needs change. In settings in which the Kardex is a permanent part of the client's record, entries are made in ink.

Information commonly found on the client care summary or Kardex includes the following:
- Basic demographic data (e.g., age, religion)
- Physician's name
- Primary medical diagnosis
- Current physician's treatment orders to be carried out by the nurse (e.g., dressing changes, ambulation, glucose monitoring)
- Nursing care plan
- Nursing orders (e.g., education sessions, symptom relief measures, counseling)
- Scheduled tests and procedures
- Safety precautions to be used in the client's care
- Factors related to activities of daily living
- Nearest relative/guardian or person to contact in an emergency
- Emergency code status
- Allergies

Text continued on p. 492

Box 25-4   **Example of Variance Documentation**

A 56-year-old client is on a surgical unit 1 day after cholecystectomy. He is beginning to have an elevated temperature, his breath sounds are decreased bilaterally in the bases of both lobes of the lungs, and he is slightly confused. Ordinarily, 1 day after surgery the client should be afebrile with lungs clear. The following is an example of the variance documentation for this client.
9/23/05 1000
Breath sounds diminished bilaterally at the bases. T, 100.4; P, 92; R, 28/min; oxygen sat, 84%. Daughter states he is "confused" and did not recognize her when she arrived a few minutes ago. Oxygen started at 2 L per standing orders. Will monitor pulse oximetry and vital signs every 15 minutes. Physician notified of change in status. Daughter at bedside.

Box 25-5   **Benefits of Using a Flow Sheet**

Information is accessible to all members of the health care team.
Time spent on writing a narrative note is decreased.
Information is current.
Errors resulting from transfer of information are decreased.
Team members can quickly see trends over time.

Norman Regional Hospital CareMap®
Community Acquired Pneumonia

Check (✓) Precautions

☐ Falls   ☐ Skin   ☐ DNR

Page 1

Admitting Physician:	Consulting Physician(s):	Expected LOS	M&R LOS
Primary Care Physician:			
Allergy/Reaction		Secondary Diagnosis	

Prob	Patient Problem	Expected Outcome (Responsible Discipline)	Outcome	Date	Signature
#1 ★	Infection	Blood cultures obtained prior to start of antibiotics? (RN)	☐YES ☐NO		
#2	Activity Tolerance	Patient is at or above baseline activity (endurance) level? (RN)	☐YES ☐NO		
#3	Knowledge Deficit	Patient able to verbalize understanding of pneumonia signs and symptoms? (RN)	☐YES ☐NO		
#4 ★	Timeliness of Antibiotic Administration	First dose of antibiotic administered within 2 hours of order? (RN, RPh)	☐YES ☐NO		
#5 ★	Discharge Preparation	Patient switched from IV to oral antibiotic within 48hrs after delivery of 1st dose? (RN, RPh)	☐YES ☐NO		

★ = Key Exception
— = Documentation Required

Copyright©2000 Norman Regional Hospital

Statement of Intent:
The CareMap® serves as an optional guideline for patient care and is subject to alteration based on the individual needs of the patient.
(CareMap® used with permission of the Center for Case Management.)

Authors: Rosalie Lavon, M.D., Jerry Leu, M.D., John McCarter, M.D., Tom Merrill, M.D., Bruce Naylor, M.D., J. Kin Pirtle, M.D., Joe Riddle, M.D., Christian Sieck, M.D., Jackie Evans, Linda Fielder, Vicki Johnson, Wanda Maddox, Yvette Morrison, Wanda Morrow, Joyce Nolen, Barbara Poe, Michelle Rausch, Darin Smith, Brenda Wilson

Date: 7/00   Form# CMAP 114   Revised:

Patient Sticker

FIGURE 25–4   Example of a critical pathway for pneumonia. (From Norman Regional Hospital CareMap®, Community Acquired Pneumonia. Copyright 2000, Norman Regional Hospital. Used with the permission of Norman Regional Hospital, Norman, Okla.)

PATIENT STICKER	Norman Regional Hospital CareMap® Community Acquired Pneumonia CareMap® Summary	
Time Admitted: _____	Day #1 (ER/Floor) Date _____	Day #2 Date _____
Assessments/Monitoring	VS qshift (and Temp q4h if T>99.5) Nursing Assessment qshift Weight I&O Pain Assessment	VS qshift (and Temp q4h if T>99.5) Nursing Assessment qshift I&O Pain Assessment
Consults	Respiratory Therapy Assess need for Social Work Consult	
Procedures/Tests	CBC with diff, Basic Metabolic Panel, UA, Sputum gram stain + C&S Stat (induce if necessary), Blood cultures x2 (15 minutes apart), CXR (PA & Lateral)	CBC with diff
Treatments	Oxygen Therapy per protocol C&DB q2hr Suction prn Albuterol AN treatments/MDI per RT/RN if ordered Incentive Spirometry q2hr WA @ bedside if ordered	Continue oxygen therapy per protocol, evaluate for discontinuation of O2 RT to convert to MDI prn Incentive Spirometry q2hr WA @ bedside if ordered
Medications/IV	Initial Antibiotic STAT (to be administered within one hour of order) IV Fluids	Cont Abx-consider oral switch Evaluate and change to HL or DC IV if applicable
Nutrition	Diet as tolerated Encourage oral fluids if appropriate	Diet as tolerated Encourage oral fluids if appropriate Goal: 3-4 glasses H₂O if not fluid restricted
Activity/Safety	Activity as tolerated (Encourage up in chair for meals) Fall prevention program initiated if appropriate	Activity as tolerated (Encourage up in chair for meals) Goal: Ambulate 25-50ft x 2
Patient/Family Education	Assess knowledge level concerning disease process and medication Teach use of MDI if applicable	Reasses patient's ability to use MDI Reinforce med education, activity and follow-up
Discharge Planning	RN/SW initiates discharge planning	Interview patient/family re: discharge planning
Psychosocial/Emotional/ Spiritual	Explain procedures Encourage verbalization of feelings	Notify Chaplain to visit if requested
CMAP # 114		

Additional Daily Treatments/Other

Isolation Precautions

Special Procedures/Surgeries:

Additional Daily Lab:
Order for CareMap entered into computer:
initial (RN/US): _____

Other Pertinent Information:

Family Spokesperson:

Emergency Phone #: _____

Page 2

FIGURE 25-4 Example of a critical pathway for pneumonia. (From Norman Regional Hospital CareMap®, Community Acquired Pneumonia. Copyright 2000, Norman Regional Hospital. Used with the permission of Norman Regional Hospital, Norman, Okla.)

Oregon Health Sciences University
Hospitals and Clinics

ACUTE CARE
24 HOUR FLOW SHEET
4 YEARS TO ADULT

ACCOUNT NO. *8490*
MED. REC. NO. *8490821*
NAME *Kline, Richard*
BIRTHDATE *08/10/67*

DATE _*12/12*_ WEIGHT _*180 lb*_ YESTERDAY'S WEIGHT _*180 lb*_

ISOLATION _*0*_

TIME	0800	1300																						F	C
F C																									
103.1 39.5																								103.1	39.5
102.2 39.0																								102.2	39.0
101.3 38.5																								101.3	38.5
100.4 38.0	●																							100.4	38.0
99.5 37.5		●																						99.5	37.5
98.6 37.0																								98.6	37.0
97.7 36.5																								97.7	36.5
96.8 36.0																								96.8	36.0
95.9 35.6																								95.9	35.6
95.0 35.0																								95.0	35.0

PULSE RADIAL	88	84																**PAIN LEVEL**
APICAL																		
RESP.	16	16																0-NONE
B/P	120 / 80	110 / 78																10-SEVERE
PAIN	0	0																
SA O₂ O₂	90	90																

DAYS / INITIALS: RN: *PAF* CNA: *FP* | **EVENINGS / INITIALS:** RN: ___ CNA: ___ | **NIGHTS / INITIALS:** RN: ___ CNA: ___

HYGIENE
☐ BED BATH ☐ SHOWER ☐ ORAL CARE
☐ CATHETER CARE COMMENTS: _____
_____

HYGIENE
☐ BED BATH ☐ SHOWER ☐ ORAL CARE
☐ CATHETER CARE COMMENTS: _____

HYGIENE
☐ BED BATH ☐ SHOWER ☐ ORAL CARE
☐ CATHETER CARE COMMENTS: _____

ACTIVITY
☐ BED REST CHAIR: _____
AMBULATE: _✓_ SLEEP: ___ HRS
COMMENTS: *Ambulating in hall*
_____

ACTIVITY
☐ BED REST CHAIR: _____
AMBULATE: ___ SLEEP: ___ HRS
COMMENTS: _____

ACTIVITY
☐ BED REST CHAIR: _____
AMBULATE: ___ SLEEP: ___ HRS
COMMENTS: _____

SAFETY
☐ SAFETY POLICY
☐ RESTRAINTS TYPE: _____
☐ SITTER COMMENTS: _____

SAFETY
☐ SAFETY POLICY
☐ RESTRAINTS TYPE: _____
☐ SITTER COMMENTS: _____

SAFETY
☐ SAFETY POLICY
☐ RESTRAINTS TYPE: _____
☐ SITTER COMMENTS: _____

	BREAKFAST	LUNCH	DINNER
DIET *Reg*			
% TAKEN	80%	70%	
% SNACKS			
ASSIST S - SELF P-PARTIAL F - FEED	S	S	

RESOURCES/EQUIPMENT USED TO PROVIDE PATIENT CARE:
SCD ☐ K PAD ☐ TRAPEZE ☐ _____ ☐
NUMBER OF IV PUMPS SINGLE _____ DOUBLE ___ ✓
NUMBER OF SUCTION UNIITS _*0*_
SPECIAL BED _*0*_
OTHER _*0*_

8.1-4A (1) (10/94) 0748-1054

8.1-4A (1)

FIGURE 25–5 Twenty-four hour client care record (flow sheet). (Courtesy Oregon Health Sciences University Hospitals and Clinics, Portland, Ore.)

DATE: 12/12

START DATE/ TIME	STANDARDS AND INTERVENTIONS	✓ — ASSESSMENT STANDARD OR PROTOCOL MET. INTERVENTION CARRIED OUT		✳ — VARIANCE FROM STANDARDS OR ORDERED INTERVENTIONS. SEE NARRATIVE ENTRY.		→ — VARIANCES REMAIN. NO CHANGES FROM LAST NARRATIVE ENTRY.								
	RN INITIALS	PAF 0800	PAF 1200											
12/8 1400	*Neurological*	✓	✓											
12/8 1400	*Cardiovascular*	✓	✓											
12/8 1400	*Respiratory*	✓	✓											
12/8 1400	*Gastrointestinal*	✓	✓											
12/8 1400	*Integument*	✓	✓											
	TEACHING													

(Left margin: ASSESSMENT STANDARDS / PROTOCOLS / INTERVENTIONS)

ASSESSMENT STANDARDS: ADULTS AND PEDIATRIC PATIENTS ABOVE 4 YEARS. All normal assessments include patient without subjective

NORMAL NEUROLOGICAL ASSESSMENT:
- alert and oriented X3 (person place, time)
- behavior appropriate to situation
- PERL
- full range of motion with symmetry of strength
- no paresthesia
- verbalization clear and coherent
- swallows without coughing or choking on liquids or solids
- gait steady if patient ambulatory
- clear vision (corrective lenses allowable)
  PEDIATRIC:
- alert and oriented appropriately for developmental age
- verbalization/vocalization appropriate for developmental age
- tracks and recognizes objects appropriately for developmental age (if unable to assess clear vision)

NORMAL RESPIRATORY ASSESSMENT:
- rate appropriate for age while at rest
- respirations quiet, regular and unlabored
- equal and clear breath sounds over both lung fields
- nail beds and mucous membranes pink
- sputum and nasal drainage clear if present

NORMAL CARDIOVASCULAR ASSESSMENT:
- regular apical or radial pulse
- capillary refill less than 3 seconds
- no edema
- peripheral pulse palpable and of equal quality
- pink nail beds and mucous membranes

NORMAL GASTROINTESTINAL ASSESSMENT:
- abdomen soft and non-distended
- no pain with palpation
- bowel tones present
- tolerates prescribed diet without problem
- bowel movements appropriate in color, volume, and consistency for intake
- if NG present, drainage clear to light green in color, heme negative
- continent

NORMAL GENITOURINARY ASSESSMENT:
- able to empty bladder q shift without urgency, frequency, pain, or post-void feeling of fullness or distention
- urine clear yellow to amber without foul odor.
- absence of vaginal or penile drainage
- continent
- if catheter present, patent and draining freely.
  PEDIATRIC: urine output 1-3 cc/kg/hour

NORMAL NEUROVASCULAR (CMS) ASSESSMENT:
- pink nail beds
- warm
- full range of motion
- capillary refill less than 3 seconds
- palpable peripheral pulses
- no edema
- no paresthesia

NORMAL MUSCULOSKELETAL ASSESSMENT:
- absence of joint tenderness, swelling, redness, or increased temperature
- full range of motion all joints
- no muscle weakness

NORMAL INTEGUMENTARY ASSESSMENT:
- skin color consistent with race
- skin warm, dry, and intact
- mucous membranes moist and without lesions
- no rashes, petechiae, or purpura
- no signs of infestation

FIGURE 25-5, cont'd   Twenty-four hour client care record (flow sheet).

Acuity Records

Acuity records provide a method of determining the hours of care and staff required for a given group of clients. A client's acuity level is based on the type and number of nursing interventions required for providing care in a 24-hour period. The acuity level determined by the nursing care allows clients to be rated in comparison with one another. For example, an acuity system might rate bathing clients from 1 to 5 (1 is totally dependent, 5 is independent). A client returning from surgery requiring frequent monitoring and extensive care may be listed with an acuity level of 1. On the same continuum another client awaiting discharge after a successful recovery from surgery has an acuity level of 5. Accurate acuity ratings may also be used to justify overtime and the number and qualifications of staff needed to safely care for clients. The client-to-staff ratios established for a unit depend on a composite gathering of data for the 24-hour interventions that are necessary for each client receiving care.

Standardized Care Plans

Many institutions have attempted to make documentation easier for nurses with **standardized care plans.** The plans, based on the institution's standards of nursing practice, are preprinted, established guidelines that are used to care for clients who have similar health problems. After a nursing assessment is completed, the staff nurse identifies the standard care plans that are appropriate for the client. The care plans are placed in the client's medical record. Modifications can be made in ink to the standardized plans to individualize the therapies. Most standardized care plans also allow the nurse to write in specific goals or desired outcomes of care and the dates by which these outcomes should be achieved.

One advantage of standardized care plans is establishment of clinically sound standards of care for similar groups of clients. These standards can be useful when quality improvement audits are conducted. Another advantage is education. Nurses learn to recognize the accepted requirements of care for clients. The standardized care plans can also improve continuity of care among professional nurses.

The use of standardized care plans is controversial. The major disadvantage is the risk that the standardized plans inhibit nurses' identification of unique, individualized therapies for clients. When standardized care plans are used in a health care facility, the nurse remains responsible for an individualized approach to care. Standardized care plans cannot replace the nurse's professional judgment and decision making. In addition, care plans need to be updated on a regular basis to ensure that content is current and appropriate. There is the trend among many hospitals to computerize care plans. With such a system, daily computer-generated care plans are printed and incorporate several nursing diagnoses or problems in a single care plan. Such a system facilitates the process of revision and individualization of plans.

Discharge Summary Forms

Much emphasis is placed on preparing a client for an effective, timely discharge from a health care institution. A prospective payment system based on DRGs encourages health care institutions to be more efficient and to dis-

---

> **Box 25-6   Discharge Summary Information**
>
> - Use clear, concise descriptions in client's own language
> - Provide step-by-step description of how to perform a procedure (e.g., home medication administration). Reinforce explanation with printed instructions.
> - Identify precautions to follow when performing self-care or administering medications.
> - Review signs and symptoms of complications that should be reported to a physician.
> - List names and phone numbers of health care providers and community resources that the client can contact.
> - Identify any unresolved problem, including plans for follow-up and continuous treatment.
> - List actual time of discharge, mode of transportation, and who accompanied the client.

---

charge the client as soon as possible. The earlier a client is discharged, the more likely it is that a hospital will be fully reimbursed. However, it is important to ensure that a client's discharge results in desirable outcomes. Multidisciplinary involvement in discharge planning helps to ensure that a client leaves the hospital in a timely manner with the necessary resources (Box 25-6).

Ideally discharge planning begins at admission. Nurses revise the plan of care as the client's condition changes. There needs to be evidence of the involvement of the client and family members in the discharge planning process so that the client and family have the necessary information and resources to return home. The JCAHO (2003) has established standards for client education necessary for effective discharge planning:

- Instruction in potential food-drug interactions, nutrition intervention, and modified diets
- Rehabilitation techniques to support adaptation to and/or functional independence in the environment
- Access to available community resources
- Under what circumstances clients should obtain further treatment or follow-up care
- Methods of obtaining follow-up care
- The client's and family's responsibilities in the client's care
- Medication instructions, including when to take each medication and why, the dose, the route, precautions, and possible adverse reactions, and when and how to get prescriptions refilled.

In addition to the JCAHO standards, a common standard in nursing practice is to educate clients about the nature of their disease process, its likely progress, and the signs and symptoms of complications.

When a client is discharged from inpatient care, a discharge summary is prepared by the various members of the health care team. The summary is given to the client or family or to the home care, rehabilitation, or long-term care agency (JCAHO, 2003). Discharge summary forms (Figure 25-6) make the summary concise and instructive. A summary form emphasizes previous learning by the client and family and care that should be continued in any restorative care setting. When given directly to clients the form may be attached to pamphlets or teaching brochures.

Barnes Hospital

PATIENT DISCHARGE SUMMARY

C-16

Addressograph Plate

Date _10/17/--_   Time _1030_

MEANS: ☐ Ambulatory   ☒ Wheelchair   ☐ Stretcher

METHODS: ☒ M.D. order   ☐ AMA with release   ☐ AMA with release

Afebrile 24 hours? ☒ Yes ☐ No   TPR _36^8-72-16_   B/P _124/72_

☐ Physician notified of irregularities

DISCHARGED TO: ☐ Home ☐ Nursing Home ☒ Home with Home Health Care ☐ Other

If discharged to Nursing Home or other facility/service:

Name _____   Address/Phone _____

☐ Release of information form signed   ☐ Chart copied   ☐ Transfer form completed   ☐ Transportation Arranged

DISCHARGE CONSIDERATIONS:

☐ Valuables from cashier   ☐ PTA meds returned   ☐ Scripts given
☒ NA   ☒ NA   ☒ NA

DISCHARGE INSTRUCTIONS

FOR PROBLEMS OR FOLLOW-UP:

Physician _Dr. Stan Jones_   Phone _362-5000_   Appt. _10/24/91_

Other: _____

Activity: _To remain in bed with Ⓛ foot elevated on two pillows. May be up only to go to the bathroom._

Diet: _To follow 1800 calorie ADA diet as instructed by the dietitian. For questions about diet, call the dietitian (Sue Marlin) 362-3184._

Medications: _To take usual dosage of 30 units NPH insulin and 8 units of regular insulin every morning before breakfast._

Wound Care: _Change dressings to Ⓛ foot daily using moistened fine mesh gauze with dry 4x4 gauze and wrap dressings with 4 kling gauze._

Teaching Materials Given: _Copy of "Controlling Your Diabetes" and "Diabetic Menu Planning."_

Special Instructions: _Call doctor for increased pain, redness, swelling or drainage from Ⓛ foot wound. Barnes Home Health nurses will be visiting daily to change dressing to Ⓛ foot._

My discharge instructions have been explained and a copy has been given to me.

Patient/Significant Other _John Owens_   Relation _HUSBAND_

Nurse _B. Rand, RN_

FIGURE 25–6   Discharge summary form. (Courtesy Barnes-Jewish Hospital, St. Louis, Mo.)

The usual forms used to document home care include:
Client assessment
Referral source information/intake form
Discipline-specific care plans
Physician's plan of treatment
Medication sheet
Clinical progress notes
Miscellaneous (conference notes, verbal order forms, telephone calls)
Discharge summary
Reports to third-party payers

Modified from Iyer PW, Camp NH: *Nursing documentation: a nursing process approach*, St. Louis, 1999, Mosby.

Home Care Documentation

The home care business continues to grow with shorter hospitalizations and larger numbers of older adults requiring home care services. Medicare has specific guidelines for establishing eligibility for home care reimbursement. Documentation in the home care system has different implications than in other areas of nursing. One primary difference is that the majority of care is witnessed by the client and family rather than the nurse. Nurses must have astute assessment skills to gather the needed information about changes in the client's health care status. In addition, documentation systems need to provide the entire health care team with the necessary information to be able to work together effectively (Box 25-7). The documentation is both the quality control and the justification for reimbursement from Medicare, Medicaid, or private insurance companies. Nurses need to document all their services for payment (e.g., direct skilled care, client instructions, skilled observation, and evaluation visits) (JCAHO, 2003).

Some parts of the record are needed in the home with the client; other information is needed in an office setting. Thus duplication of documentation is necessary, or agency policies are needed regarding what forms nurses need to leave at their office versus what forms need to be taken into the homes. Computerized client records are evolving as one means of addressing these different needs. With the use of modems and laptop computers it is becoming possible for the records to be available in multiple locations, which allows greater access to the multidisciplinary needs that are often present in home care.

Long-Term Health Care Documentation

An increasing number of older adults require care in long-term health care facilities. Because many individuals will live in this setting for the rest of their lives, they are referred to as **residents** rather than clients. In the long-term care setting, nursing personnel face challenges much different from those in the acute care setting (Iyer and Camp, 1999).

In long-term care, governmental agencies are instrumental in determining the standards and policies for documentation. For example, the Omnibus Budget Reconciliation Act of 1987 included extremely significant Medicare and Medicaid legislation for long-term care documentation. Each resident is viewed holistically by using the Resident Assessment Instrument. This assessment must be gathered by a registered nurse who has clinical competence, observational skills, and assessment expertise. The overall goal is a system of clinical documentation that provides improved care for residents and increased reimbursement for that care (Boroughs, 1999).

In addition, the department of health in each state governs the frequency of written nursing records of the residents in long-term care facilities. Because residents are often stable, daily documentation is done using flow sheets. Assessments done several times a day in the acute care setting may be required only weekly or monthly in the long-term care setting.

Long-term care agencies also may have skilled care units where clients require increased levels of care in response to mandates for shorter hospital stays. Multidisciplinary communication among such health care providers as nurses, social workers, recreational therapists, and dietitians is essential in these settings as well. The fiscal support for long-term care residents hinges on the justification of nursing care as demonstrated in documentation of the services rendered.

Computerized Documentation

Nurses have been using computerized systems for supplies, equipment, stock medications, and diagnostic testing for some time. However, most larger hospitals have also been using computerized documentation systems. There is now a rapidly growing trend for computerized documentation even in smaller community hospitals. Computerized documentation systems are drastically changing. Many computerized systems have been developed in standardized formats with the ability to gain access to data across the continuum easily (regardless of setting) and the ability to capture useful information from both individual clients and population groups.

Increasingly, software programs allow nurses to quickly enter specific assessment data, fill in forms with typical entry choices, allow narrative for unique situations, have adequate computer memory for large amounts of data, and automatically transfer information to different reports. Computers also help generate nursing care plans and document all facets of client care.

Typical user interfaces (e.g., keyboard and monitor) require typing skills and can result in data entry errors. **Graphic user interfaces** (e.g., touch pads, mouse, and icons) are not well suited for nursing. Pen-based handwriting recognition or **automated speech-recognition (ASR)** or voice-recognition technology may eventually become extremely effective for nursing documentation

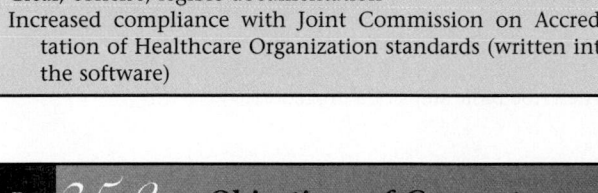

Box 25-8 Benefits of Automated Speech-Recognition (ASR) Technology

Comprehensive nursing documentation with minimal nursing effort
Decreased charting errors and omissions
Consistent documentation patterns
Increased interdisciplinary communication
Considerable time savings for the nurse
Clear, concise, legible documentation
Increased compliance with Joint Commission on Accreditation of Healthcare Organization standards (written into the software)

Box 25-9 Objectives of Computer-Based Patient Care Recording (CPCR)

Improved uniformity, accuracy, and retrievability of data about client care
Confidentiality of health care information ensured in the system
Access for authorized health care providers from any department
Ability to retrieve information selectively and choose various formats for examining it
Assistance with clinical application, including analysis tools, risk assessment, and clinical reminders
Support for data collection in a manner that adequately supports health care providers' direct entry and stores information according to a defined vocabulary
Easy access to client data, fast retrieval, and versatile data display that facilitates improved health care delivery
Availability of a lifelong record of health-related events incorporating records from various settings and time periods

Modified from National Coordination Office for Computing, Information, and Communications: *High performance computing and communications FY 1997 implementation plan,* Washington, DC, 1996, U.S. Government Printing Office, http://www.ccic.gov/pubs/imp97/136.html.

(Box 25-8). A notebook-sized computer is available, allowing nurses to document with ease and flexibility not possible in the current systems.

A complete **computer-based patient care record (CPCR)** is a comprehensive system that uses many components of data collection (Box 25-9). The CPCR permits the nurse to have an instrumental role in development of this form of documentation.

There are legal risks associated with computerized documentation. Any given person could theoretically access a computer station within a hospital and gain information on almost any client. Confidentiality of access to computerized records is a major issue. Security requires the use of a password to enter and sign off computer files. It is essential that the computer password is not under any circumstances shared with anyone other than the

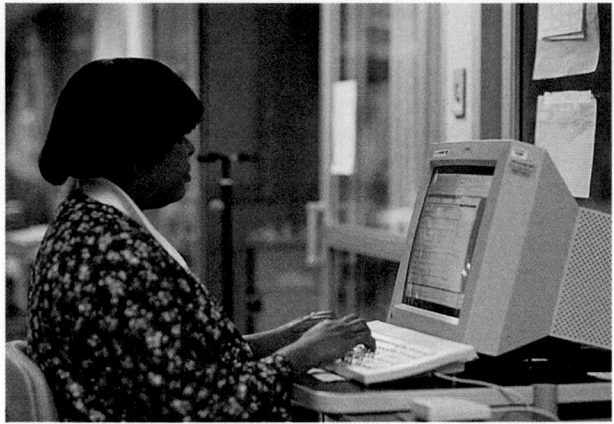

FIGURE **25-7**   Computerized documentation systems can improve uniformity, accuracy, and retrievability of data.

person to whom it was assigned. A good system requires periodic changes in personal passwords to prevent unauthorized persons from tampering with records. In addition, most staff have access only to clients in their work area. Select staff may be given authority to access all client records.

Nurses need to know how to correct charting errors on a computer. As with any documentation method, data that has been part of the record is not deleted. Incorrect entries must be corrected, indicating who made the correction and when.

One of the challenges of computerized documentation is inclusion of the nursing process (Ammenwerth and others, 2001). Those involved in this project suggest that there are important preconditions for the success of computer-based nursing process documentation, including a high acceptance of the nursing process, careful preparation of predefined care plans, organizational preparation, and inclusion of future users in the development process. It is also essential to have sufficient technical equipment with integration into the hospital information system.

The transition to computerized documentation presents both opportunities and challenges to nurses and nurse managers (Figure 25-7). The successful implementation of a computerized documentation system requires preparation, involvement, and commitment of the entire nursing staff. The transition from paper to computer presents challenges for nursing staff. Tools for transforming existing documents into interactive interdisciplinary computerized forms have been developed (Wenzel, 2002). Some studies, however, have shown that during the transition when charting must be done on both paper and the computer, the amount of time spent on documentation was not excessive (Korst, 2003).

Reporting

Nurses communicate information about clients so that all team members can make appropriate decisions about their care. It is important that any form of verbal report

Table 25-4	Comparison of Do's and Don'ts of Change-of-Shift Report
Do's	**Don'ts**
Provide only essential background information about client (i.e., name, sex, age, physician's diagnosis, and medical history).	Don't review all routine care procedures or tasks (e.g., bathing, scheduled changes).
Identify client's nursing diagnoses or health care problems and their related causes.	Don't review all biographical information already available in written form.
Describe objective measurements or observations about client's condition and response to health problem: emphasize recent changes.	Don't use critical comments about client's behavior, such as "Mrs. Wills is so demanding."
Share significant information about family members as it relates to client's problems.	Don't make assumptions about relationships between family members.
Continuously review ongoing discharge plan (e.g., need for resources, client's level of preparation to go home).	Don't engage in idle gossip.
Relay to staff significant changes in the way therapies are given (e.g., different position for pain relief, new medication).	Don't describe basic steps of a procedure.
Describe instructions given in teaching plan and client's response.	Don't explain detailed content unless staff members ask for clarification.
Evaluate results of nursing or medical care measures (e.g., effect of back rub or analgesic administration).	Don't simply describe results as "good" or "poor." Be specific.
Be clear about priorities to which oncoming staff must attend.	Don't force oncoming staff to guess what to do first.

be timely, accurate, and relevant. Four types of reports made by nurses are change-of-shift reports, telephone reports, transfer reports, and incident reports.

Change-of-Shift Reports

At the end of each shift nurses report information about their assigned clients to the nurses working on the next shift. The purpose of the report is to provide continuity of care among nurses who are caring for a client. For example, if one nurse finds a certain pain-relief measure effective for a client, it is important that the information be relayed to the next nurse caring for the client so that pain-control interventions can be continued.

A **change-of-shift report** may be given orally in person, by audiotape recording, or during "walking-planning" rounds at each client's bedside. Oral reports are given in conference rooms, with staff members from both shifts participating. An advantage of oral reports is that it allows staff members to ask questions or clarify explanations. When nurses make rounds, the client and family members also have the opportunity to participate in any decisions. The nurses can see the client together to perform needed assessments, evaluate progress, and discuss the interventions best suited to the client's needs. An audiotape report is given by the nurse who has completed care for the client and is left for the nurse on the next shift to review. Taped reports can improve efficiency by taping report before the end of the shift when time is available and by avoiding social conversations between peers. It is essential to schedule an opportunity for the oncoming nurses to ask questions for clarification after listening to the taped report.

Because of the many responsibilities nurses have to assume, it is important that a change-of-shift report be conducted quickly and efficiently (Table 25-4). An effective report describes each client's health status and lets staff on the next shift know what care the clients will require.

A change-of-shift report should *not* simply be reading documented information. Instead, significant information about clients are reviewed (e.g., the condition of wounds or episodes of chest pain) to provide a baseline for comparison during the next shift. Data about clients need to be objective, current, and concise.

An organized report follows a logical sequence. To prepare for the report, the nurse gathers information from work sheets, the client's records, and the client's care plan. A systematic approach such as using the nursing process can provide staff with critical information that is needed to continue care. The following is an example of a change-of-shift report:

Background information: *Cy Tolan in bed 4, a 32-year-old client of Dr. Lang, is scheduled for a colon resection this morning. He has had ulcerative colitis for 2 years with recent bouts of frank bleeding in stools. He was admitted last night with slight abdominal discomfort. This is his first experience with surgery. He knows he may require a colostomy. He has been NPO since midnight.*

Assessment: *Mr. Tolan expressed difficulty falling asleep last night. He had several questions about surgery. Early in the night he called for assistance several times.*

Nursing diagnosis: *His chief concerns are anxiety related to inexperience with surgery and risk for body image disturbance.*

Teaching plan: *He asks appropriate questions about surgery. Staff on evenings explained postoperative routines. I reinforced information with him early in the night. He stated that he feels less anxious now that he knows more what to expect.*

Treatments: *A cleansing enema was administered until clear at 9 PM; no blood was noted in the return. He complained of some abdominal cramping immediately afterward, and that subsided within an hour. He received Restoril 15 mg PO at 9:00 PM, and I gave him a back rub. When he awakened at 6:30 AM, he stated he slept OK.*

Family information: *His wife remained with him last evening until the end of visiting hours.*

She has returned and is in the room this morning.

Discharge plan: Mr. Tolan is a very active person at home. He participates in strenuous sports such as tennis, basketball, and swimming, and for this reason Mrs. Tolan is concerned about how he might react to a colostomy. I suggest making a referral to the enterostomal therapist early, if the colostomy is performed.

Priority needs: Right now, Mr. Tolan is relaxing in his room. The operative permit has been signed. All preoperative procedures have been completed except for his preop medications, due on call to the operating room.

A professional demeanor is essential when giving a report as the nurse discusses clients or family members. It is often necessary to describe the interactions among clients, nurses, and family members in behavioral terms. The nurse must avoid using judgmental language such as *uncooperative, difficult,* or *bad* when describing such behaviors.

In many settings assistive personnel are involved in the change-of-shift report. Assistive personnel are part of the team and can contribute more when they also know a client's condition and the nursing team's priorities in care. The registered professional nurse (RN) can use the report to emphasize to assistive personnel the tasks to be done.

Telephone Reports

Nurses inform physicians of changes in a client's condition and communicate information to nurses on other units about client transfer. The laboratory staff or a radiologist may report results of diagnostic tests. Persons involved with a telephone report also must provide clear, accurate, and concise information. In many cases information in a telephone report is documented when significant events or changes in a client's condition have occurred. To document a phone call, the nurse includes when the call was made, who made it (if other than the writer of the information), who was called, to whom information was given, what information was given, and what information was received, for example, "At 10:22 AM called Dr. Morgan's office; S. Thomas, RN, will inform Dr. Morgan that Mr. Rush's STAT potassium level drawn at 8:00 AM was 3.2. C. Towns, RN."

Telephone or Verbal Orders

A telephone order (TO) involves a physician stating a prescribed therapy over the phone to a registered nurse. A verbal order (VO) may be accepted when there is no opportunity for a physician to write the order, as in emergency situations. Clarifying for accuracy is important when a registered nurse accepts physician's orders over the telephone or verbally. The order needs to be verified by repeating it clearly and precisely. The registered nurse is responsible for writing the order on the physician's order sheet in the client's permanent record and signs it. An example follows: "1/16/2004: 7:20 PM acetaminophen 650 mg PO, 1 tab now and q4h prn. TO. Dr. Reiss/Carol Towns, RN." The physician later verifies the telephone order legally by signing it within a set time period (e.g., 24 hours). Telephone orders are frequently given at night or during an emergency and need to be used only when absolutely necessary. In some situations it may be prudent to have a second person listen to telephone orders. Check

> ### Box 25-10   Guidelines for Telephone Orders and Verbal Orders
>
> Clearly determine the client's name, room number, and diagnosis.
> Repeat any prescribed orders back to the physician.
> Use clarification questions to avoid misunderstandings.
> Write TO (telephone order) or VO (verbal order), including date and time, name of client, the complete order; and sign the name of the physician and nurse.
> Follow agency policies; some institutions require telephone (and verbal) orders to be reviewed and signed by two nurses.
> The physician must cosign the order within the time frame required by the institution (usually 24 hours).

agency policy. Box 25-10 provides some guidelines that can be used to prevent errors in receiving telephone and verbal orders.

Transfer Reports

Clients may transfer from one unit to another to receive different levels of care. For example, clients transfer from an intensive care unit or the recovery room to general nursing units when the client no longer requires such intense monitoring. To promote continuity of care, **transfer reports** may be given by phone or in person. When giving a transfer report, nurses include the following information:

1. Client's name, age, primary physician, and medical diagnosis
2. Summary of progress up to the time of transfer
3. Current health status (physical and psychosocial)
4. Allergies
5. Emergency code status
6. Family support
7. Current nursing diagnoses or problem and care plan
8. Any critical assessments or interventions to be completed shortly after transfer (helps receiving nurse to establish priorities of care)
9. Need for any special equipment, such as isolation equipment, suction equipment, or traction.

After completion of the transfer report, the receiving nurse needs an opportunity to ask questions about the client's status. In some cases written documentation must include a record of information reported.

Incident Reports

An incident is any event that is not consistent with the routine operation of a health care unit or routine care of a client. Examples of incidents include client falls, needlestick injuries, a visitor having symptoms of illness, medication administration errors, accidental omission of ordered therapies, and circumstances that led to injury or a risk for client injury. Analysis of incident reports helps with the identification of trends in systems and unit operations that provide justification for changes in policies and procedures or for in-service seminars. **Incident reports** are an important part of a unit's quality improvement program (see Chapter 22).

Key Concepts

- The medical record is a legal document and requires information describing the care that is delivered to a client.
- All information pertaining to a client's health care management that is gathered by examination, observation, conversation, or treatment is confidential.
- Multidisciplinary communication is essential within the health care team.
- Accurate record keeping requires an objective interpretation of data with precise measurements, correct spelling, and proper use of abbreviations.
- A nurse's signature on an entry in a record designates accountability for the contents of that entry.
- Any change in a client's condition warrants immediate documentation to keep a record accurate.
- The medical record is a financial record that serves as the basis for reimbursement.
- Problem-oriented medical records are organized by the client's health care problems.
- The intent of SOAP, SOAPIE, PIE, or DAR charting formats is to organize entries in the progress notes according to the nursing process.
- Critical pathways provide members of the health care team a way to document their contributions to the client's total plan of care.
- Medicare guidelines for establishing a client's home care cost reimbursement is the basis for documentation by home care nurses.
- Long-term care documentation is multidisciplinary and closely linked with fiscal requirements of outside agencies.
- Computerized information systems provide information about clients in an organized and easily accessible fashion.
- The major purpose of the change-of-shift report is to maintain continuity of care.
- Rounds allow nurses to perform needed assessments, evaluate clients' progress, and determine the best interventions for a client's needs.
- When information pertinent to care is communicated by telephone, the information needs to be verified.
- Incident reports objectively describe any event that is not consistent with the routine care of a client.

Key Terms

Key Terms—cont'd

Critical Thinking Exercises

1. Joseph Page is an 80-year-old man admitted with a diagnosis of possible pneumonia. He complains of general malaise and a frequent productive cough, worse at night. Vital signs are as follows: blood pressure, 150/90 mm Hg; pulse rate, 92 beats per minute; respirations, 22 breaths per minute; and temperature, 38.5° C (101.3° F). During your initial assessment he coughs violently for 40 to 45 seconds without expectorating. His lungs have wheezes and rhonchi in both bases and are otherwise clear. He states, "It hurts in my chest when I cough." Differentiate between objective and subjective data in this case example.

2. The nurse positions Mr. Page in a semi-Fowler's position, encourages increased fluid intake, and gives Tylenol 650 mg PO as ordered for fever. One hour later the client is resting in bed. Vital signs are as follows: blood pressure, 130/86 mm Hg; pulse rate, 86 beats per minute; respirations, 22 breaths per minute; and temperature, 37.7° C (99.8° F). He states he has been unable to sleep. His fluid intake has been 200 ml of water. Use the given information to write a nurse's progress note using the PIE format.

3. At the end of your shift you have identified *deficient fluid volume* as a nursing diagnosis for Mr. Page. Since his admission he has had fluid intake of about 600 ml, and his urine output was 300 ml of dark concentrated urine. His temperature is back up to 38.3° C (101° F), his mucous membranes are dry, and he states he feels very weak. Record significant data. List what should be included in the change-of-shift report.

4. Several days later, following treatment with intravenous antibiotics, Mr. Page is feeling much better and preparations are being made for discharge. He is to take Keflex 500 mg every 6 hours for the next 10 days, continue to drink extra fluids, and get extra rest. He lives alone. Although he is generally cooperative, he does not like drinking water or taking pills. He is to make an appointment with his physician for 1 week from today and should call the physician if he develops symptoms of recurrence. Write a discharge summary that is concise and instructive.

Review Questions

1. Accreditation agencies such as which of the following specify guidelines for documentation?
   1. Joint Commission on Accreditation of Healthcare Organizations (JCAHO).
   2. American Nurses Association.
   3. National League of Nursing.
   4. American Academy of Colleges of Nursing.

2. Under the prospective payment system, hospitals are reimbursed a set dollar amount by Medicare for each:
   1. Nursing diagnosis.
   2. JCAHO standard.
   3. Problem–oriented medical record.
   4. Diagnosis-related group (DRG).

3. A vital aspect of nursing practice is:
   1. Documentation.
   2. Evaluation.
   3. Implementation.
   4. Diagnosis.

4. Data recorded, reported, or communicated to other health care professionals are:
   1. Public knowledge.
   2. Available to all ancillary agencies.
   3. Confidential and must be protected.
   4. Available to all interested parties.

5. Clients frequently request copies of their medical records. The nurse understands:
   1. They have the right to read those records.
   2. They are not allowed to read those records.
   3. Only the healthcare workers have access to the records.
   4. Only the families may read the records.

6. Critical pathways are care plans that:
   1. Guide nursing care for all diseases.
   2. Are used only by nurses.
   3. Include key interventions and expected outcomes.
   4. Are written by the physician.

7. Acuity records are designed to:
   1. Guide all nursing care.
   2. Document the client admission.
   3. Determine hours of care needed.
   4. Establish guidelines for client care.

8. Ideally discharge planning begins:
   1. At the time they are preparing for discharge.
   2. At admission.
   3. After a diagnosis is made.
   4. After acuity has been determined.

9. In long-term care facilities the client is referred to as a (an):
   1. Resident.
   2. Occupant.
   3. Patient.
   4. Client.

10. A telephone order involves:
    1. A physician giving any health care worker an order via the phone.
    2. No liability on the part of the nurse taking a phone order.
    3. Use in only an acute emergency.
    4. Clarification, accuracy, and verification.

References

Ammenwerth E and others: Nursing process documentation systems in clinical routine—prerequisites and experiences, *Int J Med Inf* 64(2-3):187, 2000.

Boroughs DS: Documentation in the long-term care setting, *J Nurs Adm* 29(12):46, 1999.

Braugh LA: Automated Clinical Pathways in the patient record: legal implications, *Nurs Case Manag* 3(3), 1998.

Cummins KM: Charting by exception, a timely format for you? *Am J Nurs* 99(3):24G, 1999.

Frank-Stromborg JD, Ganschow JR: How HIPAA will change your practice, *Nursing* 32(9):54, 2002.

Gordon M: *Manual of nursing diagnosis,* ed 10, St. Louis, 2002, Mosby.

Iyer PW, Camp NH: *Nursing documentation: a nursing process approach,* St. Louis, 1999, Mosby.

Joint Commission on Accreditation of Healthcare Organizations: *Standards for the accreditation of home care,* Chicago, 2003, The Joint Commission.

Korst LM: Nursing documentation time during implementation of an electronic medical record, *J Nursing Adm* 33(1):24-30, 2003.

Martin F: Documentation tips: to help you stay out of court, *Nursing* 24(6):63, 1994.

National Coordination Office for Computing, Information, and Communications: *High performance computing and communications FY 1997 implementation plan,* Washington, DC, 1996, U.S. Government Printing Office, http://www.ccic.gov/pubs/imp97/136.html.

Smith LS: How to use focus charting, *Nursing* 30(5):76, 2000.

U.S. Department of Health and Human Services: HHS fact sheet: protecting the privacy of patients' health information, May 9, 2001, www.hhs.gov/news.

Wenzel, 2002.

Williams S: Computerized documentation of case management from diagnosis to outcomes: *Nurs Case Manag* 3(6), 1998.

Yocum RF: Documenting for quality patient care, *Nursing* 32(8):58, 2002.

$\mathcal{S}$elf-Concept

26

Media Resources

http://evolve.elsevier.com/Potter/
fundamentals/

CD COMPANION

- Review Questions
- Glossary

evolve WEBSITE

- Review Questions
- Student Learning Activities
- Glossary

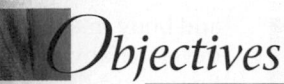# Objectives

Mastery of content in this chapter will enable the student to:

- Define key terms.
- Discuss factors that influence the following components of self-concept: identity, body image, and role performance.
- Identify stressors that affect self-concept and self-esteem.
- Describe the components of self-concept as related to psychosocial and cognitive developmental stages.
- Explore ways in which the nurse's self-concept and nursing actions can affect the client's self-concept and self-esteem.
- Incorporate research findings to promote evidence-based practice for identity confusion, disturbed body image, low self-esteem, and role conflict.
- Examine cultural considerations that affect self-concept.
- Apply the nursing process to promote a client's self-concept.

Self-concept is an individual's conceptualization about how one thinks about himself or herself. It is a subjective sense of the self and a complex mixture of unconscious and conscious thoughts, attitudes, and perceptions. Self-concept provides a frame of reference that affects the management of all situations and relationships with others. Self-concept, or how one thinks about himself or herself, directly affects one's self-esteem, or how one feels about himself or herself. Although these two terms are often used interchangeably, it is important to differentiate the two so that a nurse can correctly and completely assess the client and develop an individualized plan of care based on the client's needs.

Nurses care for clients who face a variety of health problems that can threaten their self-concept and self-esteem. The loss of bodily function, a decline in activity tolerance, and difficulty in managing a chronic illness, are just examples of situations that can change a client's self-concept. The nurse can play a key role in both helping clients to adjust to alterations in self-concept and to support components of self-concept that enable clients to cope with difficulties.

Scientific Knowledge Base

Despite inconsistencies in the literature that limit universal conclusions about self-concept and self-esteem, it is evident that development and maintenance of self-concept and self-esteem begin at a young age and continue across the life span. There is a tendency for men to report higher self-esteem than women. However, the exact magnitude of this gender difference and the way it varies across the life span remain unclear. The influence, parents and other primary caregivers have on the development of a child's self-concept and self-esteem has been established. In addition, cultural influences on self-concept and self-esteem are learned and internalized in childhood and adolescence. A significant amount of emphasis during the school years has been placed on fostering a child's academic identity. In general, young children tend to rate themselves higher than they rate other children, suggesting that their view of themselves is positively inflated. Adolescence is a particularly critical time when many

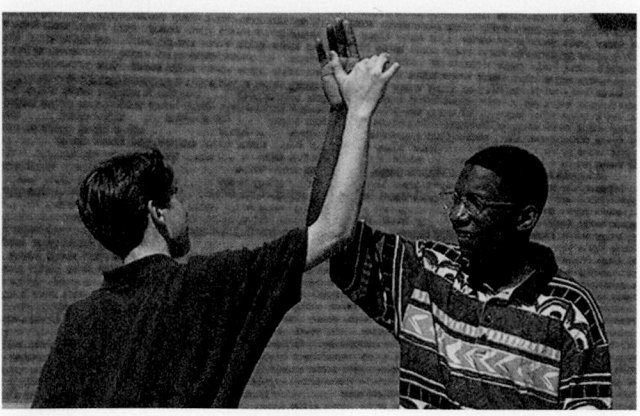

FIGURE **26–1**   Adolescents' participating in group activities can foster self-esteem. (From Birchenall J, Streight E: *Mosby's textbook for the home care aide,* ed 2, St. Louis, 2003, Mosby.)

variables affect the self-concept and self-esteem (Figure 26-1). The adolescent experience appear to adversely affect self-esteem, more strongly for girls than for boys. For example, adolescent girls may be more sensitive to their appearance and how others view them.

Job satisfaction and job performance in adulthood have been linked to self-esteem. When individuals are terminated or laid off from a job, their sense of self may be diminished, they may not be motivated to be active socially or may even become depressed. They lose their job identity, and as a result their self-perceptions are altered. The establishment of a sense of self that is stable and that transcends relationships and situations is a developmental goal of adulthood.

However, evidence exists that sense of self may be negatively affected in older adulthood because of the intensity of emotional and physical changes associated with aging (Robins and others, 2002). For example, when the older adult loses a partner or has a change in health, there may be a change in how that person makes decisions about his or her level of independent functioning, degree of social interaction, or even personal hygiene care.

Ethnic and cultural differences in self-concept and self-esteem have also been demonstrated across the life span, and recent findings may suggest that differences in the development of self-concept exist (Twenge and Crocker, 2002). Sensitivity to factors that affect self-concept and self-esteem in diverse cultures is essential to ensure an individualized approach to health care.

How individuals view themselves and their perception of their health are closely related. A client's belief in personal health can enhance his or her self-concept. Statements such as "I can get through anything" or "I've never been sick a day in my life" indicate that a person's thoughts about personal health are positive. Illness, hospitalization, and surgery can also affect self-concept. Chronic illness may affect the ability to provide financial support, thereby affecting an individual's self-esteem and perceived roles within the family. Negative perceptions regarding health status may be reflected in such statements as "It's not worth it anymore" or "I'm a burden to my family." Further, chronic illness can affect identity

and body image as reflected by verbalizations such as "I'll never get any better" or "I can't stand to look at this disfigurement."

What individuals think and how they feel about themselves affects the way in which they care for themselves physically and emotionally and the way in which they are able to care for others. Further, how one behaves is generally consistent with both self-concept and self-esteem. Individuals who have poor self-concepts often do not feel in control of situations and may not feel worthy of care, which can influence decisions regarding health care. Knowledge of variables that affect self-concept and self-esteem is critical for the nurse to provide effective treatment.

*N*ursing Knowledge Base

In providing evidence-based practice to clients, the nurse incorporates professional nursing knowledge developed from the humanities and sciences, nursing research, and clinical practice. The nurse's broad knowledge base allows for a holistic view of clients, thus promoting quality client care that can best meet the self-concept needs of each client and family.

Development of Self-Concept

The development of self-concept is a complex lifelong process that involves many factors. Erikson's psychosocial theory of development (1963) remains helpful in understanding key tasks that individuals face at various stages of development. Successful mastery of each stage can translate to a solid sense of self (Box 26-1).

A nurse learns to recognize an individual's failure in achieving an age-appropriate developmental stage or an individual's regression to an earlier stage in a period of crisis. This understanding allows a nurse to individualize care and determine appropriate nursing interventions. Self-concept is always changing and is based on the following:

- Sense of competency
- Perceived reactions of others to one's body
- Ongoing perceptions and interpretations of the thoughts and feelings of others
- Personal and professional relationships
- Academic and employment-related identity
- Spiritual identity
- Personality structure
- Perceptions of events that have an impact on the self
- Mastery of prior and new experiences
- Current feelings about the physical, emotional, and social self
- Self-expectations
- Racial identity

Global self-esteem levels are highest in childhood, drop during adolescence, rise gradually throughout adulthood, and decline sharply in old age (Robins and others, 2002). In general, this pattern holds true across gender, socioeconomic status, and ethnicity. Children may report high self-esteem because their sense of self is inflated by a variety of extremely positive sources, and the subsequent decline may be associated with a shift to more realistic in-

Box 26-1   Self-Concept: Developmental Tasks

0 to 1 Year

Develops trust from consistency in caregiving and nurturing interactions of parents and others
Distinguishes self from environment

1 to 3 Years

Begins to communicate likes and dislikes
Increasingly autonomous in thoughts and actions
Appreciates body appearance and function
Develops self through modeling, imitation, and socialization

3 to 6 Years

Takes initiative
Identifies with a gender
Gains an enhanced self-awareness
Increases language skills, including identification of feelings
Sensitive to family feedback

6 to 12 Years

Incorporates feedback from peers and teachers
Increases self-esteem with new skill mastery (e.g., reading, math, sports, music)
Sexual identity strengthens
Aware of strengths and limitations

12 to 20 Years

Accepts body changes/maturation
Examines attitudes, values, and beliefs; establishes goals for the future
Feels positive about expanded sense of self
Interacts with those whom he or she finds sexually attractive or intellectually stimulating

Mid-20s to Mid-40s

Has intimate relationships with family and significant others
Has stable, positive feelings about self
Experiences successful role transitions and increased responsibilities

Mid-40s to Mid-60s

Can accept changes in appearance and physical endurance
Reassesses life goals
Shows contentment with aging

Late 60s On

Feels positive about one's life and its meaning
Interested in providing a legacy for the next generation

---

formation about the self. Further, the adolescent decline in self-esteem could be partially understood in the context of maturational changes associated with puberty and increased expectations associated with the transition from grade school to junior high and high school.

> **Safety Alert.** An adolescent's decline in self-esteem may result in an increased need for attention. This need for attention may be demonstrated in unsafe behaviors, such as premature sexual activity, unprotected sex, or substance abuse. In addition, there is the increased risk of adolescents "showing off" when they begin to drive. These risks are a threat to the child's safety and have implications for health care interventions.

Erikson's emphasis on the generativity stage (1963) (see Chapter 10) may explain the rise in self-esteem and self-concept in adulthood. The individual is focused on being increasingly productive and creative at work, while at the same time promoting and guiding the next generation. Other than childhood, the mid-60s seem to represent the highest level of self-esteem across the life span. A sharp decline in self-esteem has been reported around age 70 (Robins and others, 2002). Again, based on Erikson's stages of development, a decline in self-concept at this age may reflect a diminished need for self-promotion and a shift in self-concept to a more modest and balanced view of the self. Identification of specific nursing interventions to address the unique needs of clients at various life stages is essential.

Components and Interrelated Terms of Self-Concept

A positive self-concept gives a sense of meaning, wholeness, and consistency to a person. A healthy self-concept has a high degree of stability and generates positive feelings toward the self. The components of self-concept frequently considered by nurses are identity, body image, and role performance. Self-esteem is traditionally viewed as a closely related concept.

Identity. Identity involves the internal sense of individuality, wholeness, and consistency of a person over time and in various circumstances. Identity implies being distinct and separate from others. Identity develops over time and ends in being a whole and unique self. Being "oneself" or living an authentic life is the core of identity. A child learns culturally accepted values, behaviors, and roles through identification and modeling. Identity is often gained from self-observations and from what individuals are told about themselves (Stuart and Laraia, 2001). An individual first identifies with parenting figures and later with teachers, peers, and role models. To form an identity, the child must be able to bring together learned behaviors and expectations into a coherent, consistent, and unique whole (Erikson, 1963).

The achievement of identity is necessary for intimate relationships because one's identity is expressed in relationships with others. Sexuality is a part of one's identity. Sexual identity is a person's conceptualization of the self as a man or as a woman and includes one's sexual orientation. This image and its meaning depend on culturally determined values that are affected by socialization (see Chapter 27).

Racial or cultural identity develops from identification and socialization within an established group, as well as through the experience of integrating the response of individuals outside the cultural or racial group into one's self-concept. Self-concept may be most influenced by the political, social, and cultural influences during childhood. In general, the more a person identifies with social groups, the greater is the person's self-esteem. In addition, when racial identity is central to self-concept and is positive, self-esteem tends to be high (Twenge and Crocker, 2002). An individual who experiences discrimination, prejudice, or environmental stressors such as low income or high-crime neighborhoods, may conceptualize himself or herself differently than an individual who has not had the same living conditions (Ruiz, Roosa, and Gonzales, 2002). Further, the opinion or approval of others may not constitute the basis for self-esteem in the same way for all racial and cultural groups. Cultural differences in self-concept exist and may also demonstrate some age-specific trends (Box 26-2).

Body Image. **Body image** involves attitudes related to the body, including physical appearance, structure, or function. Feelings about body image include those related to sexuality, femininity and masculinity, youthful-

ness, health, and strength. These mental images are not always consistent with a person's actual physical structure or appearance. Some body image distortions have deep psychological origins such as an eating disorder, for example anorexia. Other alterations occur as a result of situational events such as the loss or change in a body part. Nurses need to be aware that the majority of men and women experience some degree of body dissatisfaction, which can affect body image and overall self-concept. Disturbances in body image can be exaggerated when a change in health status occurs. The way others view a person's body and the feedback offered is also influential. For example, a controlling, violent husband might tell his wife that she is ugly and that no one else would want her. Over the years of marriage, this devaluation is incorporated into her self-concept.

Body image is affected by cognitive growth and physical development. Normal developmental changes such as puberty and aging have a more apparent effect on body image than on other aspects of self-concept. Hormonal changes during adolescence and menopause influence body image. The development of secondary sex characteristics and changes in body fat distribution have a tremendous impact on the self-concept of an adolescent. Changes associated with aging (i.e., wrinkles; graying hair; and decrease in visual acuity, hearing, and mobility) may also affect body image in an older adult.

Cultural and societal attitudes and values also influence body image. Culture and society dictate the accepted norms of body image and can influence one's attitudes (Figure 26-2). Values such as ideal body weight and shape, as well as attitudes toward body markings, piercing, and tattoos, are culturally based. In American society, youth, beauty, and wholeness are emphasized; this is apparent in television programs, movies, and advertisements. Western cultures have been socialized to dread the normal aging process, whereas in Eastern cultures aging is viewed very positively and the older adult is respected.

Body image depends only partly on the reality of the body. When physical changes occur, individuals may or may not incorporate these changes into their body image. For example, people who have experienced significant weight loss do not perceive themselves as thin and

---

Cultural Aspects of Care   Box 26-2

Racial and cultural identity are important components of a person's self-concept. Early in growth and development, an individual develops this identity within the context of family. As the individual grows, the cultural aspects of his or her self-concept may be reinforced through social, family, or cultural experiences. In addition, a person's self-concept may be strengthened or questioned through political, social, or cultural influences experienced in the school and workplace environments.

Implications for Practice

- Positive or negative role cultural modeling or past experiences can influence self-concept.
- Develop an open, nonrestrictive attitude for assessing for and encouraging cultural practices to improve a client's self-concept.
- Ask clients what they think are important to help them feel better or gain a stronger sense of self.
- Encourage cultural identity by individualizing hygiene practices and clothing to meet clients self-concept needs.

Data from Robins RW and others: Global self-esteem across the life span, *Psychol Aging* 17(3):423, 2002; Ruiz SY, Roosa MW, Gonzales NA: Predictors of self-esteem for Mexican American and European American youths: a reexamination of the influence of parenting, *J Fam Psychol* 16(1):70, 2002; Twenge JM, Crocker J: Race and self-esteem: meta-analyses comparing whites, blacks, Hispanics, Asians, and American Indians, *Psychol Bull* 128(3):371, 2002.

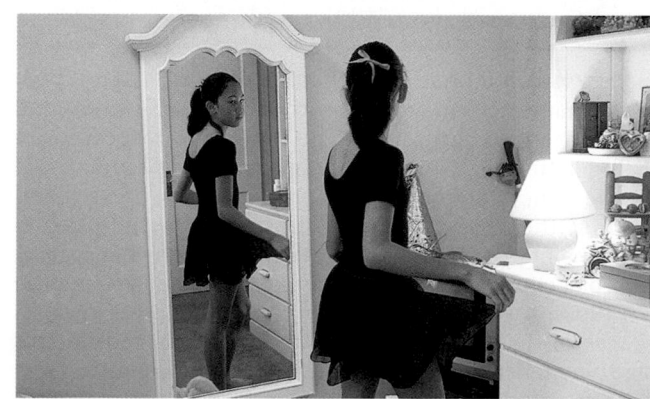

FIGURE **26–2**   An individual's appearance influences self-concept. (From Sorrentino SA: *Mosby's textbook for nursing assistants,* ed 6, St. Louis, 2004, Mosby.)

thus may present with a distorted body image. Body image issues are often associated with impaired self-concept and self-esteem and frequently focus on thinness for females and bigness and muscularity for males (Cohane and Pope, 2001).

Role Performance. **Role performance** is the way in which an individual perceives his or her ability to carry out significant roles. This includes roles such as parent, supervisor, or close friend. An individual's perception of competency in a role may or may not match the evaluation of others who relate to the person. Roles that individuals follow in given situations involve socialization to expectations or standards of behavior. The patterns are stable and change only minimally during adulthood. Behaviors that are approved by society are developed and maintained through the following processes:

- *Reinforcement-extinction:* Certain behaviors become common or are avoided, depending on whether they are approved and reinforced or discouraged and punished.
- *Inhibition:* An individual learns to refrain from behaviors, even when tempted to engage in them.
- *Substitution:* An individual replaces one behavior with another, which provides the same personal gratification.
- *Imitation:* An individual acquires knowledge, skills, or behaviors from members of the social or cultural group.
- *Identification:* An individual internalizes the beliefs, behavior, and values of role models into a personal, unique expression of self.

Ideal societal role behaviors are often hard to achieve in real life. Individuals have multiple roles and individual needs that may conflict. Successful adults learn to distinguish between ideal role expectations and realistic possibilities. To function effectively in multiple roles, a person must know the expected behavior and values, desire to conform to them, and be able to meet the role requirements. Common roles include mother or father, wife or husband, daughter or son, employee or employer, sister or brother, and friend. Each role involves meeting certain expectations. Fulfillment of these expectations leads to an enhanced sense of self. Difficulty or failure in meeting role expectations leads to deficits and often contributes to decreased self-esteem or altered self-concept.

Self-Esteem. **Self-Esteem** is an individual's overall sense of self-worth or the emotional appraisal of self-concept. It can be understood as the most fundamental core self-evaluation that an individual holds about himself or herself because it represents the overall judgment of personal worth or value (Judge and Bono, 2001). Self-esteem is positive when one feels capable, worthwhile, and competent (Rosenberg, 1965). According to Erikson (1963), young children begin to develop a sense of usefulness or industry by learning to act on their own initiative. A child's self-esteem is related to the child's evaluation of his or her effectiveness at school, within the family, and in social settings. The evaluation of others also is likely to have a profound influence on the child's self-esteem. Social support is positively related to self-esteem and well-being in early adolescence (Yarcheski,

Mahon, and Yarcheski, 2001). Once established, basic feelings about the self tend to be constant, even though there may be some fluctuation. A situational crisis may temporarily affect one's self-esteem.

Considering the relationship between a person's self-concept and his or her ideal self can enhance understanding self-esteem. The ideal self consists of the aspirations, goals, values, and standards of behavior that a person considers ideal and strives to attain. The ideal self originates in the preschool years and develops throughout life; it is influenced by societal norms and the expectations and demands of parents and significant others. In general, a person whose self-concept comes close to matching the ideal self has high self-esteem, whereas a person whose self-concept varies widely from the ideal self suffers from low self-esteem. A child who excels in school and who is liked by peers is more likely to have high academic self-esteem than a child who has difficulty in school and is not liked by peers.

Self-evaluation is an ongoing mental process. A positive sense of self-esteem is an important variable in determining how an individual functions in the world. A person's ability to contribute in a meaningful way to society often affects self-concept and self-esteem. Individuals who are sick and unable to be involved in society may feel a sense of worthlessness. The nurse's acceptance of a client as an individual with worth and dignity can be vital in maintaining and improving the client's self-esteem. It is important to recognize that a person's self-esteem stems from self-concept, and a person's self-esteem influences self-concept.

Stressors Affecting Self-Concept

A self-concept stressor is any real or perceived change that threatens identity, body image, or role performance (Figure 26-3). The individual's perception of the stressor is the most important factor in determining his or her response. The ability to reestablish balance is related to numerous factors, including the number of stressors, duration of the stressor, and health status (see Chapter 30). Stressors challenge a person's adaptive capacities. The normal process of maturation and development itself is a stressor. Changes that occur in physical, spiritual, emotional, sexual, familial, and sociocultural health can affect self-concept. Being able to adapt to stressors is likely to lead to a positive sense of self, whereas failure to adapt often leads to a negative sense of self.

Any change in health can be a stressor that potentially affects self-concept. A physical change in the body can lead to an altered body image affecting identity and self-esteem. Chronic illnesses often alter role performance, which may alter one's identity and self-esteem. Further, an essential process in the adjustment to loss is the development of a new self-concept. A loss of a partner, as an example, can lead to a loss of identity and a lower self-esteem (Van Baarsen, 2002). The case study in Box 26-3 illustrates the interrelationship of the components of self-concept.

A crisis occurs when a person cannot overcome obstacles with usual methods of problem solving and adaptation. Any crisis potentially threatens self-concept and self-esteem. Some crises, such as the case study in Box 26-3, directly affect all components of self-concept. The

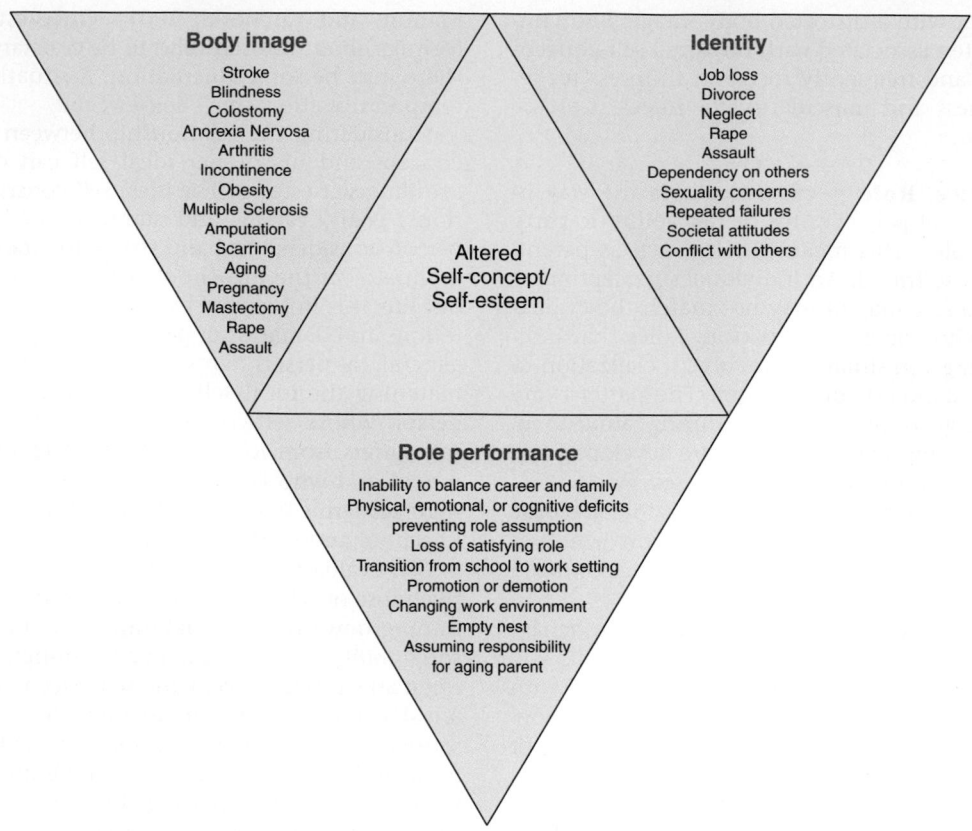

FIGURE **26–3** Common stressors that influence self-concept. (From Hockenberry M and others: *Nursing care of infants and children,* ed 7, St. Louis, 2003, Mosby.)

stressors created as a result of a crisis can also affect a person's health. If people are unable to adapt to such stressors, their health may be at risk. If the resulting identity confusion, disturbed body image, low self-esteem, role conflict, role strain, role ambiguity, or role overload is not relieved, illness may result. For example, the diagnosis of cancer places additional demands on a person's established living pattern. It changes the person's appraisal of and satisfaction with the current level of physical, emotional, and social functioning. Self-esteem, learned resourcefulness, and social support have been shown to predict health-related quality of life for long-term survivors of cancer, with self-esteem being the strongest predictor (Pedro, 2001). Health-related quality of life may increase with interventions such as nurse-led support groups aimed at supporting and improving self-esteem. During self-concept crises, supportive and educative resources can be valuable in helping a person learn new ways of coping with and responding to the stressful event or situation to maintain or enhance self-concept.

Identity Stressors. An individual's identity is affected by stressors throughout life but is particularly vulnerable during adolescence, which is a time of great change. Adolescents are trying to adjust to the physical, emotional, and mental changes of increasing maturity, which can result in insecurity and anxiety. It is also a time when the adolescent is developing psychosocial competence, including coping strategies (see Chapter 30).

An adult generally has a more stable identity and thus a more firmly developed self-concept. Cultural and social stressors, rather than personal stressors, may have more impact on an adult's identity. For example, an adult may have to balance career and family, or make choices regarding honoring religious traditions from one's family of origin. **Identity confusion** results when people do not maintain a clear, consistent, and continuous consciousness of personal identity. It may occur at any stage of life if a person is unable to adapt to identity stressors. Under extreme stress an individual may experience disturbed personal identity, a state in which the differences between the self and others cannot be determined.

Developmental markers such as the initiation of puberty, menopause, retirement, and decreasing physical abilities may affect identity. Identity, like body image, is closely related to appearance and abilities. Retirement may mean the loss of an important means of achievement and continued success. People at retirement may begin to reevaluate their identities and accomplishments. Loss of a significant other can lead the surviving individual to reexamine aspects of his or her identity.

Body Image Stressors. Changes in the appearance, structure, or function of a body part requires an adjustment in body image. An individual's perception of the change and the relative importance placed on body image will affect the significance of a loss of function or change in appearance. For example, if a woman's body image incor-

Case Study

Box 26-3

Paul, a 48-year-old man, suffers a stroke. The stroke is unexpected and sudden. He was not even aware that he had hypertension, because he had not been getting annual checkups. Paul awakens in the hospital bed to find that he cannot even move his right hand. He cannot care for himself and is unable to turn himself for days. With the nurse's constant encouragement, he is finally able to pull himself out of bed and into a chair. He wonders what lies ahead for him. Paul's body image has dramatically changed from that of a man of strength and endurance to that of a helpless individual. Paul worries about his family and what will happen. His daughter, the oldest child, is away at college, and his son is still in high school. Paul and his wife, Meredith, are terrified. Although Meredith works, they have not saved enough money to be able to meet monthly expenses or to educate their children without Paul's wages. Paul's role as primary financial provider for the family may be drastically changed if his condition does not improve.

Paul's self-esteem diminishes as his recovery and rehabilitation move slowly. His self-concept has changed from that of a strong laborer, one who did his own plumbing and car repairs, to a man who must rely on others. Although he is now at home in the rehabilitation process, Paul is not able to perform tasks for the family and must wait until his wife and son get home to help him with things that require strength. Paul's adaptation capabilities are stretched to the maximum, although his physician tells him that he is very fortunate to be alive. Paul's identity is not clear to him anymore, he has no clear role within the family, his body image has been drastically altered, and his self-esteem is spiraling lower and lower.

Paul continues in outpatient physical therapy. Significant time and energy are required even on simple tasks, but he begins to gain some strength. He is able to return to work, with a few modifications to ensure safety. He has some diminished mental quickness and some muscle weakening, but he is able to perform most aspects of his job. His self-esteem improves, and his body image is enhanced. Although he still feels somewhat altered, his physical capabilities closely resemble those before the stroke.

porates reproductive organs as the ideal, a hysterectomy secondary to uterine cancer may be a very significant alteration and may result in a perceived loss of femininity or wholeness. Changes in the appearance of the body, such as an amputation, facial disfigurement, or burns, are obvious stressors affecting body image. Mastectomy and colostomy are surgical procedures that alter the appearance and function of the body, although the changes may not be apparent to others when the individual is dressed. Although potentially undetected by others, these bodily changes have a significant impact on the individual. Even some elective changes such as breast augmentation or reduction may also affect body image. Chronic illnesses such as heart and renal disease involve a change in function, in which the body no longer functions at an optimal level. Anticipated body changes resulting from the developmental process can also affect body image. In addition, the effects of pregnancy, significant weight gain or loss, pharmacological management of illness, or radiation therapy change body image. Negative body image can lead to adverse health outcomes.

Many people associate success with a specific body part or function. For example, athletes may consider their bodies and physical activities to be the focus of personal success. If they can never again participate in athletics because of an accident or injury, their adaptation and rehabilitation may be affected. To a surgeon, use of the hands may be the foundation of his or her worth as a person; a traumatic amputation of a hand would significantly alter his or her self-concept. Body image changes necessitate the revision of long-accepted self-perceptions, as well as alterations in lifestyle. To regain a positive self-concept and self-esteem, each must adapt to his or her body image stressors.

Society's response to an individual's physical changes may be affected by the conditions surrounding the alteration. For example, paralysis resulting from an act of war or terrorism may result in the individual being treated as a hero and being praised for self-sacrifice. Donations from charitable organizations and governmental resources may be available for rehabilitation. However, people who drink and drive and who have an accident resulting in paralysis may receive a very different response from society.

Overall, positive social changes with regard to how the public responds to illness and altered body image have occurred. The media now frequently present positive stories about persons adjusting in a healthy manner following serious disabilities (e.g., Christopher Reeve's spinal cord injury) or adapting to a debilitating illness (e.g., Michael J. Fox's Parkinson's disease). These stories may change public perception of what constitutes a disability and certainly have provided positive role models for individuals undergoing self-concept stressors, as well as for their families, friends, and society as a whole.

Role Performance Stressors. Throughout life a person undergoes numerous role changes. Normal changes associated with growth and maturation result in developmental transitions. Situational transitions occur when parents, spouses, children, or close friends die or people move, marry, divorce, or change jobs. A health-illness transition is a movement from a state of health or well being to one of illness. It is important to recognize that a shift along the continuum from illness to wellness is as stressful as a shift from wellness to illness. Any of these transitions may lead to role conflict, role ambiguity, role strain, or role overload.

Role conflict results when a person is required to simultaneously assume two or more roles that are inconsistent, contradictory, or mutually exclusive. For example, when a middle-age woman with teenage children assumes responsibility for the care of her older parents, conflicts may arise in relation to being both a parent to her children and the child of her parents. Negotiating a balance of time and energy between her children and parents may create role conflicts. The perceived importance of each conflicting role influences the degree of conflict experienced. The **sick role** involves the expectations of others and society regarding how one should behave when sick. Role conflict may occur when general societal expectations (take care of yourself and you will get better) and the expectations of co-workers (need to get the job done) collide. The conflict of taking care of oneself while getting everything done can be a major challenge.

Role ambiguity involves unclear role expectations. When there are unclear expectations, people may be unsure about what to do or how to do it. Such a situation is often stressful and confusing. Role ambiguity is common in the adolescent years. Adolescents are pressured by parents, peers, and the media to assume adult-like roles, yet may lack the resources to move beyond the role of a dependent child. Role ambiguity is also common in employment situations. In complex, rapidly changing, or highly specialized organizations, employees often become unsure about job expectations.

Role strain blends role conflict and role ambiguity. Role strain may be expressed as a feeling of frustration when a person feels inadequate or feels unsuited to a role. Role strain is often associated with gender role stereotypes (Stuart and Laraia, 2001). Others may perceive women in positions typically held by men as less competent, less objective, or less knowledgeable than their male counterparts. Thus the women may feel that they must work harder and be better to compete. Men in typically female roles may also encounter gender bias, which, in turn, can unfortunately raise questions about their masculinity.

Role overload involves having more roles or responsibilities within a role than are manageable. It is frequently reflected in an individual who unsuccessfully attempts to meet the demands of work and family while carving out some personal time. Often during periods of illness or change, those involved, either as the one who is ill or as a significant other, find themselves in role overload.

Self-Esteem Stressors. Individuals with high self-esteem are generally more resilient and are better able to cope with demands and stressors than those with low self-esteem. Low self-worth can contribute to feeling unfulfilled and misunderstood and can result in depression and unremitting uneasiness or anxiety. Illness, surgery, or accidents that change life patterns may also influence feelings of self-worth. Chronic illnesses such as diabetes, arthritis, and cardiac dysfunction require changes in accepted and long-assumed behavioral patterns. The more the chronic illness interferes with the ability to engage in activities contributing to feelings of worth or success, the more it affects self-esteem.

Self-esteem stressors vary with developmental stages. Perceived inability to meet parental expectations, harsh criticism, inconsistent discipline, and unresolved sibling rivalry may reduce the level of self-worth of children. Some data suggest that the maximum difference in self-esteem between boys and girls occurs in junior high school and also indicate that a gender difference exists in early adolescent coping strategies (Bryne, 2000).

Negative thinking and low self-esteem in college-age women have been shown to be potential predictors for later development of depression (Pedan and others, 2000). Stressors affecting the self-esteem of an adult include failure in work and failures in relationships. Another developmental milestone, pregnancy, introduces unique self-concept stressors. Lowered self-esteem has emerged as one of the strongest predictors of postpartum depression. Additional risk factors include prenatal depression, child care stress, prenatal anxiety, life stress, marital relationship, history of previous depression, infant temperament, maternity blues, marital status, socioeconomic status, and unplanned/unwanted pregnancy (Beck, 2001). Self-concept stressors in older adults include health problems, declining socioeconomic status, spousal loss or bereavement, loss of social support, and decline in achievement experiences following retirement (Box 26-4).

Family Effect on Self-Concept Development

The family plays a key role in creating and maintaining the self-concepts of its members. Children develop a basic sense of who they are from their family caregivers. A child also gains accepted norms for how one should think, feel, and behave from family members. Negative self-concepts may be cultivated in children, even by well-meaning parents. Some literature suggests that parents are the most important influences on a child's development, yet variations in approach may be culturally determined. Specifically, a relationship exists between parents who respond in a firm, consistent, and warm manner and a child's positive self-esteem and school achievement (Ruiz, Roosa, and Gonzales, 2002). Parents who are harsh, inconsistent, or have low self-esteem themselves may behave in ways that foster negative self-concepts in their

---

Focus on **Older Adults**   Box 26-4

- Promoting a positive self-concept in all older adults is essential, but it is especially important for those experiencing disability or frailty.
- Conducting a life review or participating in a reminiscence group, recording an oral history, or arranging a photo scrapbook of meaningful life events are examples of activities the nurse can suggest to help older adults feel a sense of self-worth about the life lived, as well as provide a legacy for the younger family members (Eliopoulos, 2001).
- Potential threats to the self-esteem of older adults may arise from the institutional environments where they receive their care. These threats can include dependence, devaluation, depersonalization, functional impairments, and lack of control over one's environment. Nursing interventions directed toward reducing or eliminating these threats result in improved quality of life for the older adult (Miller, 1999).
- Self-concept may be negatively affected in older adulthood secondary to a number of life changes, including health problems, declining socioeconomic status, spousal loss or bereavement, loss of social support, and decline in achievement experiences following retirement (Stuart and Laraia, 2001).
- Be alert to the adults' preoccupation with physical complaints; assess thoroughly, and if no physical explanation exists, encourage older adult to verbalize needs (e.g., fear, insecurity, loneliness) (Robins and others, 2002).
- Convey that the older adult is worthwhile by actively listening to and accepting the person's feelings, being respectful, and praising health-seeking behaviors.

children. To reverse a client's negative self-concept, the nurse may first need to assess the family's style of relating (see Chapter 9). Negative health practices, such as cigarette smoking, may be influenced by family and cultural factors (Box 26-5). Self-concept change demands an evidence-based practice approach, supported by the entire health care team.

The Nurse's Effect on the Client's Self-Concept

A nurse's acceptance of a client with an altered self-concept helps promote positive change. When a client's physical appearance has changed, it is likely that both the client and the family will look to nurses and observe their verbal and nonverbal responses and reactions to the changed ap-

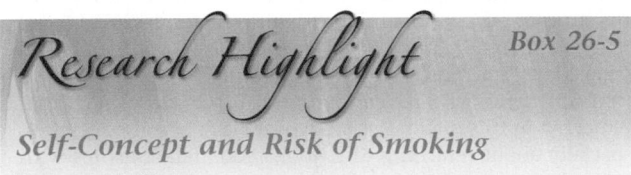

Box 26-5

Research Highlight

Self-Concept and Risk of Smoking

Research Focus

Cigarette smoking by young women is a growing health concern. The decision to smoke may be reflective of self-concept issues and may be culturally influenced. Awareness of risk factors is essential for implementation of preventative health care in a variety of nursing settings.

Research Abstract

The purpose of this 10-year study was to identify early predictors of daily smoking in young women. This study of 1,213 black and 1,166 white girls revealed that white girls were at higher risk of becoming daily smokers than black girls. Early predictors of daily smoking included parental education, single-family home, drinking alcohol at ages 11 to 12, higher drive for thinness at ages 11 to 12, lower behavioral conduct at ages 11 to 12, and a perceived increase in stress from ages 10 to 11 to ages 12 to 13.

Evidenced-Based Practice

- Body weight concerns, as well as family, social environment, and behavioral factors, are important issues to be addressed by the nurse during preadolescence.
- Effective, healthy, and realistic weight management methods for young adolescent girls must be implemented; techniques include promoting fun, family-oriented physical activity and the elimination of dieting.
- A priority nursing action is the assessment of child and adolescent coping strategies; appropriate techniques, including effective communication, conflict resolution, and stress management, must be taught to children.
- Identification of risk factors for early drug and alcohol use, including genetic predisposition and family environment, must be a priority for health care providers.

Reference

Voorhees CC and others: Early predictors of daily smoking in young women: the National Heart, Lung, and Blood Institute growth and health study, *Prev Med* 34:616, 2002.

pearance. Nurses need to remain aware of their own feelings, ideas, values, expectations, and judgments. Self-awareness is critical in initially understanding and accepting others. Nurses who are secure in their own identities more readily accept and thus reinforce clients' identities. It is critical for nurses to assess and clarify the following self-concept issues about themselves:

- Own thoughts and feelings about lifestyle, health, and illness
- Awareness of how own nonverbal communication may affect clients and families
- Personal values and expectations and how these affect clients
- Ability to convey a nonjudgmental attitude toward clients
- Preconceived attitudes toward cultural differences in self-concept and self-esteem

The client with a change in body appearance or function can be extremely sensitive to the verbal and nonverbal responses of the health care team. A positive and matter-of-fact approach to care can provide a model for the client and family to follow. Nurses can have a significant affect on clients by conveying genuine interest and acceptance. Recognizing and including self-concept issues in the planning and delivery of care can positively influence client outcomes. Building a trusting nurse-client relationship and appropriately involving the client and family in decision making can enhance self-concept. An individualized approach may highlight a client's unique needs, including the incorporation of alternative health care practices or methods of spiritual expression.

Nurses can also have a significant impact on their client's body image. For example, a nurse can influence the body image of a woman who has had a mastectomy in a positive way by showing acceptance of the mastectomy scar. On the other hand, a shocked or disgusted facial expression can contribute to the woman developing a negative body image. Clients closely watch the reactions of others to their wounds and scars. It is very important for the nurse to monitor responses toward the client. Statements such as "This wound is healing nicely" or "This looks healthy" can be very affirming for the body image of the client.

Inadvertently frowning or grimacing when performing procedures can have profound effects on the client. The nurse's nonverbal behaviors help to convey the level of caring that exists for a client and can affect self-esteem (Figure 26-4). For example, the self-concept of an incontinent client can be threatened by the perception that the caretakers find the situation unpleasant. Nurses should anticipate their own reactions, acknowledge them, and focus on the client instead of the unpleasant task or situation. If nurses can put themselves in the client's position, they can envision measures to ease embarrassment, frustration, anger, and denial.

Preventative measures, early identification, and appropriate treatment can minimize the intensity of self-esteem stressors and the potential effects for the client and family. The nurse learns to design specific self-concept interventions to fit a client's profile of risk factors. It is essential to assess the client's perception of a problem and to work collaboratively to resolve self-concept issues. For

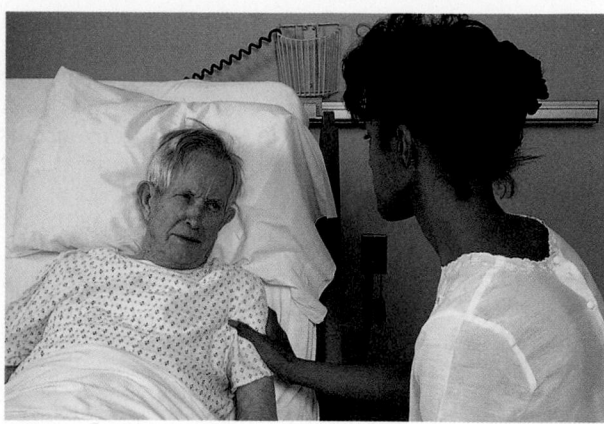

FIGURE **26-4**   Nurses can use touch and eye contact to enhance a client's self-esteem.

example, low-income women defined different barriers to returning to work than those that had been traditionally prioritized by professionals (Box 26-6). Thus the nurse must use a different set of interventions for this group of clients.

Critical Thinking

Successful critical thinking requires synthesis of knowledge, experience, information gathered from clients and families, critical thinking attitudes, and intellectual and professional standards. Solid clinical judgment requires the nurse to anticipate the information necessary, analyze the data, and make appropriate decisions regarding client care.

In the case of self-concept, the nurse must integrate knowledge from nursing and other disciplines, including self-concept theory, communication principles, and a consideration of cultural and developmental factors. Previous experience in caring for clients with self-concept alterations assists the nurse in individualizing care for each client. The nursing process is continuous until the client's self-concept is improved, restored, or maintained. Self-concept profoundly influences a person's response to illness. A critical thinking approach to care is essential.

Self-Concept and the Nursing Process

Assessment

In assessing self-concept and self-esteem, the nurse first focuses on each component of self-concept (identity, body image, and role performance). Assessment should also include behaviors suggestive of an altered self-concept (Box 26-7), actual and potential self-concept stressors (see Figure 26-3, p. 506), and coping patterns. Gathering comprehensive assessment data requires the nurse to critically synthesize information from multiple sources (Figure 26-5). In addition to direct questioning, much of the data

Research Highlight   Box 26-6

Promoting Self-Esteem and Self-Sufficiency

Research Focus

As low-income women struggle to become self-sufficient, they encounter many barriers. Inadequate child care and transportation were not identified as barriers by the women themselves but were viewed by the women as socially acceptable reasons for not working. Modifying the nursing approach to match the identified need of the women themselves is needed to ensure family health.

Research Abstract

A group of low-income women participated in in-depth interviews with nurse researchers. The women who were attending an occupational skills training center designed to assist low-income, unemployed or underemployed women in their transition to the workforce identified eight obstacles to self-sufficiency. Perceived barriers of self-sufficiency that emerged in this qualitative study were lack of self-esteem, especially about returning to school; "bad" relationships with men; lack of support from family and friends; limited life options; lack of training; lack of quality programs; criminal histories; and fear of success.

Evidence-Based Practice

- The promotion of empowerment, self-esteem building, and the development of self-efficacy are more important nursing interventions to promote behavioral change in low-income women than removing child care and transportation barriers.
- Nursing resources should be aimed at addressing fundamental self-concept deficits.
- Follow-up services, including home care and community health, are needed to promote family health.

Reference

Brown SG, Barbosa G: Nothing is going to stop me now: low-income women as they become self-sufficient, *Public Health Nurs* 18(5):364, 2001.

Box 26-7	Behaviors Suggestive of Altered Self-Concept
Avoidance of eye contact	Excessively dependent
Slumped posture	Hesitant to express views or opinions
Unkempt appearance	
Overly apologetic	Lack of interest in what is happening
Hesitant speech	
Overly critical or angry	Passive attitude
Frequent or inappropriate crying	Difficulty in making decisions
Negative self-evaluation	

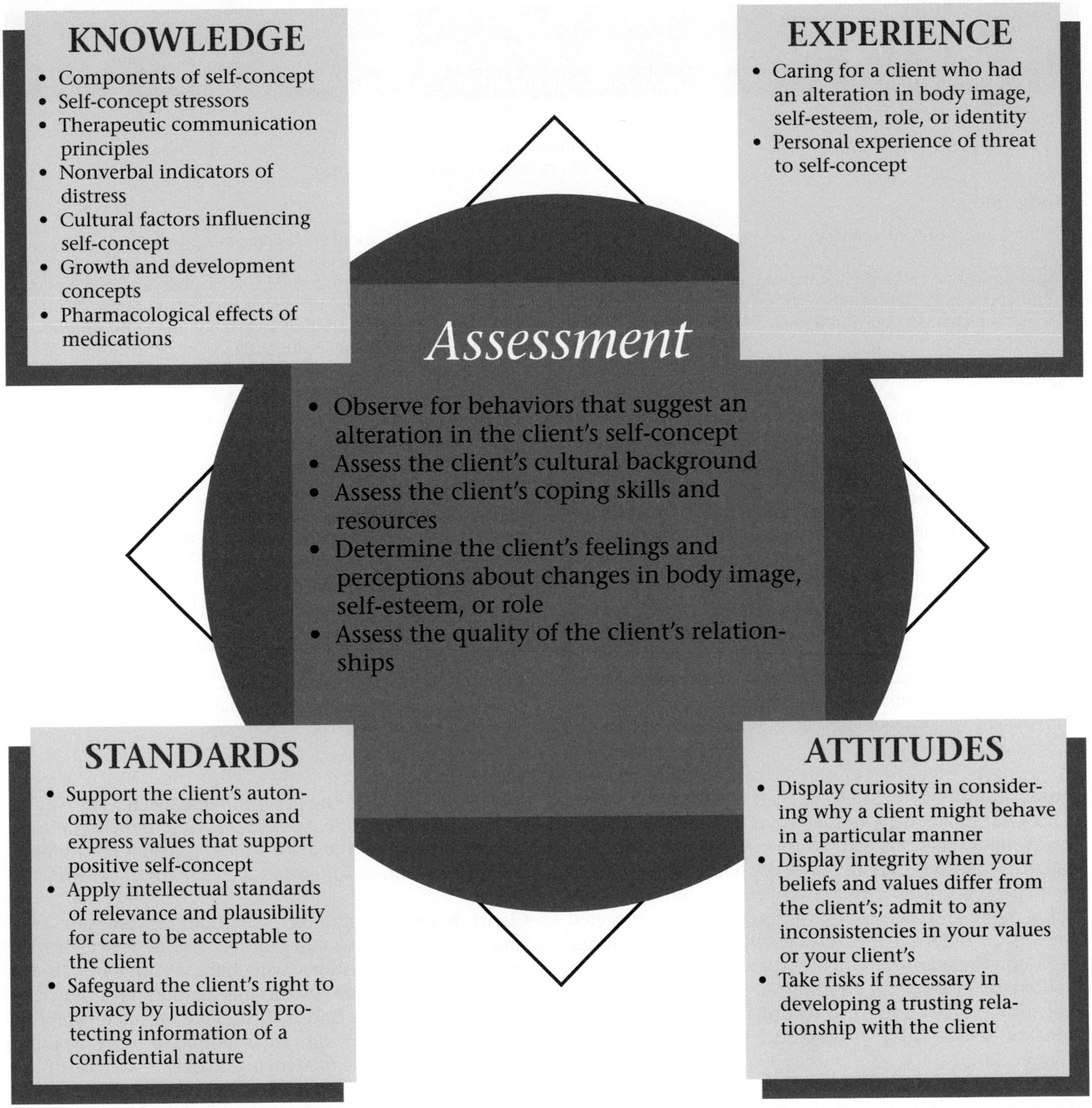

KNOWLEDGE

- Components of self-concept
- Self-concept stressors
- Therapeutic communication principles
- Nonverbal indicators of distress
- Cultural factors influencing self-concept
- Growth and development concepts
- Pharmacological effects of medications

EXPERIENCE

- Caring for a client who had an alteration in body image, self-esteem, role, or identity
- Personal experience of threat to self-concept

Assessment

- Observe for behaviors that suggest an alteration in the client's self-concept
- Assess the client's cultural background
- Assess the client's coping skills and resources
- Determine the client's feelings and perceptions about changes in body image, self-esteem, or role
- Assess the quality of the client's relationships

STANDARDS

- Support the client's autonomy to make choices and express values that support positive self-concept
- Apply intellectual standards of relevance and plausibility for care to be acceptable to the client
- Safeguard the client's right to privacy by judiciously protecting information of a confidential nature

ATTITUDES

- Display curiosity in considering why a client might behave in a particular manner
- Display integrity when your beliefs and values differ from the client's; admit to any inconsistencies in your values or your client's
- Take risks if necessary in developing a trusting relationship with the client

FIGURE 26–5   Critical thinking model for self-soncept assessment.

regarding self-concept is effectively gathered through observation of the client's nonverbal behavior and by paying attention to the content of the client's conversation. The nurse should take note of the manner in which clients talk about the people in their lives, because this can provide clues to both stressful and supportive relationships, as well as to key roles the client assumes. Using knowledge of developmental stages to determine what areas are likely to be important to the client, the nurse should inquire about these aspects of the person's life. For example, the nurse might ask a 65-year-old client about his or her life and what has been important to him or her. This is the stage of development in life in which individuals are examining their lives and considering the impact they have had in the world. The individual's conversation will likely provide data relating to role performance, identity, self-esteem, stressors, and coping patterns. At appropriate times, specific questions may be useful (Table 26-1).

Coping Behaviors. The nursing assessment should also include consideration of previous coping behaviors; the

Table 26-1   **Nursing Assessment of Client's Self-Concept**

Assessment Questions*	Responses Reflecting Difficulties With Self-Concept
Identity	
"How would you describe yourself?"	Derogatory answers (e.g., "I don't know; there's not too much worth mentioning") should raise the concern of the nurse.
Body Image	
"What aspects of your appearance do you like?" "Are there any aspects of your appearance that you would like to change? If yes, describe the changes you would make."	Most people can identify something about their appearance that they like (e.g., "People have always told me I have nice eyes"). If a person cannot identify any appreciated characteristic, this is suggestive of a negative body image and poor self-esteem. Most people have one or two areas that they would like to change (e.g., "My nose is too big" or "My hips are too large"), but a long list of problem areas should lead the nurse to consider difficulties with self-concept.
Self-Esteem	
"Tell me about the things you do that make you feel good about yourself." "How do you feel about yourself?"	Statements about not having any strengths or being able to do anything well should raise the concern of the nurse.
Role Performance	
"Tell me about your primary roles (e.g., partner, parent, friend, sister, professional role, volunteer). How effective are you at carrying out each of these roles?"	The nurse should listen for the number of primary roles identified. A large number of primary roles will put the client at risk for role conflicts and role overload. As with questions above, if the client indicates that he or she does not feel that these roles are adequately covered, the person may be experiencing alterations in self-concept. Although most people carry out many roles and often feel as though some of them are not adequately addressed, listen for the person's perception about his or her overall role competency.

*In addition to the verbal content of the client's answer, the nurse should note the client's nonverbal behaviors. Hesitant speech, poor eye contact, and hunched posture suggest alterations in self-concept.

nature, number, and intensity of the stressors; and the client's internal and external resources. Knowledge of how a client has dealt with stressors in the past can provide insight into the client's style of coping. Not all issues are addressed in the same way by clients, but often one uses a familiar coping pattern for newly encountered stressors. As the nurse identifies previous coping patterns, it is useful to determine whether these patterns have contributed to healthy functioning or created more problems. For example, the use of drugs or alcohol during times of stress often creates additional stressors (see Chapter 30).

Exploring resources and strengths, such as availability of significant others or prior use of community resources, can be important in formulating a realistic and effective plan. Also pertinent in assessment is determining how the client views the situation. For example, it may be that older women are more accustomed to changes in their health status because of the aging process in general, and experiencing heart disease may be one more aspect of growing older. On the other hand, a cardiac event occurring in middle age may be less expected and more problematic for women in terms of family and career responsibilities and thus elicit a more dramatic change in anxiety (Plach, Napholz, and Kelber, 2001).

Significant Others. Valuable data may also evolve out of conversations with family and significant others. Significant others may have insights into the person's way of dealing with stressors and may have knowledge about what is important to the person's self-concept. The way in which the person talks about the client and the significant others' nonverbal behaviors may provide information about what kind of support is available for the client.

Client Expectations. Also important in assessing self-concept is the person's expectations. Asking the client how he believes interventions will make a difference in his problem can provide useful information regarding the client's expectations and may provide an opportunity to discuss the client's goals. For example, a nurse working with a client who is experiencing anxiety related to an upcoming diagnostic study might ask the client about his expectations of the relaxation exercise that they have been practicing together. The client's response will provide the nurse with valuable information about the client's beliefs and attitudes regarding the efficacy of the interventions as well as the potential need to modify the nursing approach.

Nursing Diagnosis

Assessment data need careful consideration by the nurse to identify a client's actual or potential problem areas. The nurse will rely on knowledge and experience, apply appropriate professional standards, and look for clusters of defining characteristics that indicate a nursing diagnosis. Although there are multiple nursing diagnostic labels for altered self-concept, the following list provides examples of self-concept–related nursing diagnoses:

Nursing Diagnostic Process

Box 26-8

Assessment Activities

Observe client's behavior during conversation.

Empathically communicate, "Tell me how you are coping" or "Let's talk about what you are thinking and feeling about tomorrow's procedure."

Defining Characteristics

Client demonstrates restlessness, inability to maintain eye contact, facial tension, increased perspiration, and self-preoccupation.

Client replies, "I'm feeling really scared. You know there is a possibility they may amputate my leg tomorrow. I just don't know how I will manage if it comes to that. I just couldn't sleep last night. On top of the pain, I just kept thinking about all that is happening."

Nursing Diagnosis

Anxiety related to accidental injury, pain, uncertainty of outcome of upcoming surgery

---

- Impaired adjustment
- Anxiety
- Disturbed body image
- Caregiver role strain
- Decisional conflict
- Ineffective coping
- Ineffective denial
- Fear
- Hopelessness
- Disturbed personal identity
- Risk for loneliness
- Ineffective role performance
- Chronic low self-esteem
- Situational low self-esteem
- Ineffective sexuality patterns
- Impaired social interaction
- Spiritual distress
- Risk for self-directed violence

Making nursing diagnoses in the realm of self-concept is complex. Often, isolated data could be defining characteristics for more than one nursing diagnosis (Box 26-8). For example, a client might express feelings of uncertainty and inadequacy. These are defining characteristics for both *anxiety* and *situational low self-esteem*. The awareness that the client is demonstrating defining characteristics of more than one nursing diagnosis can guide the nurse in gathering specific data to validate and to differentiate the underlying problem. To further assess the possibility of *anxiety* as the nursing diagnosis, the nurse might consider whether the person has any of the following defining characteristics: Is the person experiencing increased muscle tension, shakiness, a sense of being "rattled," or restlessness? These symptoms would suggest *anxiety* as the more appropriate diagnosis. On the other hand, if the person expresses a predominantly negative self-appraisal, including inability to handle situations or events and difficulty making decisions, these characteristics would suggest that the more appropriate nursing diagnosis might be *situational low self-esteem*. To further aid the nurse in differentiating between the two demonstrated diagnoses, information regarding recent events in the person's life and how the person has viewed himself or herself in the past would provide insight into the most appropriate nursing diagnosis. As additional data are gathered, usually the priority nursing diagnosis becomes evident.

To validate critical thinking regarding a nursing diagnosis, the nurse can share observations with the client and allow the client to verify the nurse's perception. This approach often results in the client providing additional data, which further clarifies the situation. In the example above, if the nurse said to the client, "I notice you haven't eaten much of your breakfast or lunch today," the response to this observational statement coupled with the client's nonverbal communication could facilitate further discussion. An alternative approach may be to state, "I noticed that you jumped when I came up behind you. Are you feeling uneasy today?" This could allow the client to verify whether he or she is in fact anxious and to tell the nurse about his or her concerns.

Planning

During planning the nurse again synthesizes knowledge, experience, critical thinking attitudes, and standards (Figure 26-6). Critical thinking ensures that the client's plan of care integrates all that the nurse knows about the individual, as well as key critical thinking elements (see care plan). Professional standards are especially important to consider when the nurse develops a plan of care. These standards often establish ethical or evidence-based practice guidelines for selecting effective nursing interventions.

Another method to assist in planning care is a concept map (Figure 26-7). A concept map shows the relationship of a medical diagnosis, postoperative reconstruction of severe facial scars, with the four nursing diagnosis. The concept map also links the nursing diagnosis and shows how they are interrelated. In this example there is a relationship between disturbed body image and situational low self-esteem. As the client's facial scars improve and resolve she should begin to feel better about her appearance.

Goals and Outcomes. The nurse develops an individualized plan of care for each nursing diagnosis. The nurse and client set realistic expectations for care. Goals are to be individualized and realistic with measurable outcomes. In establishing goals, the nurse should consult with the client about whether the goals are perceived as realistic. Consultation with significant others, mental health clinicians, and community resources can result in

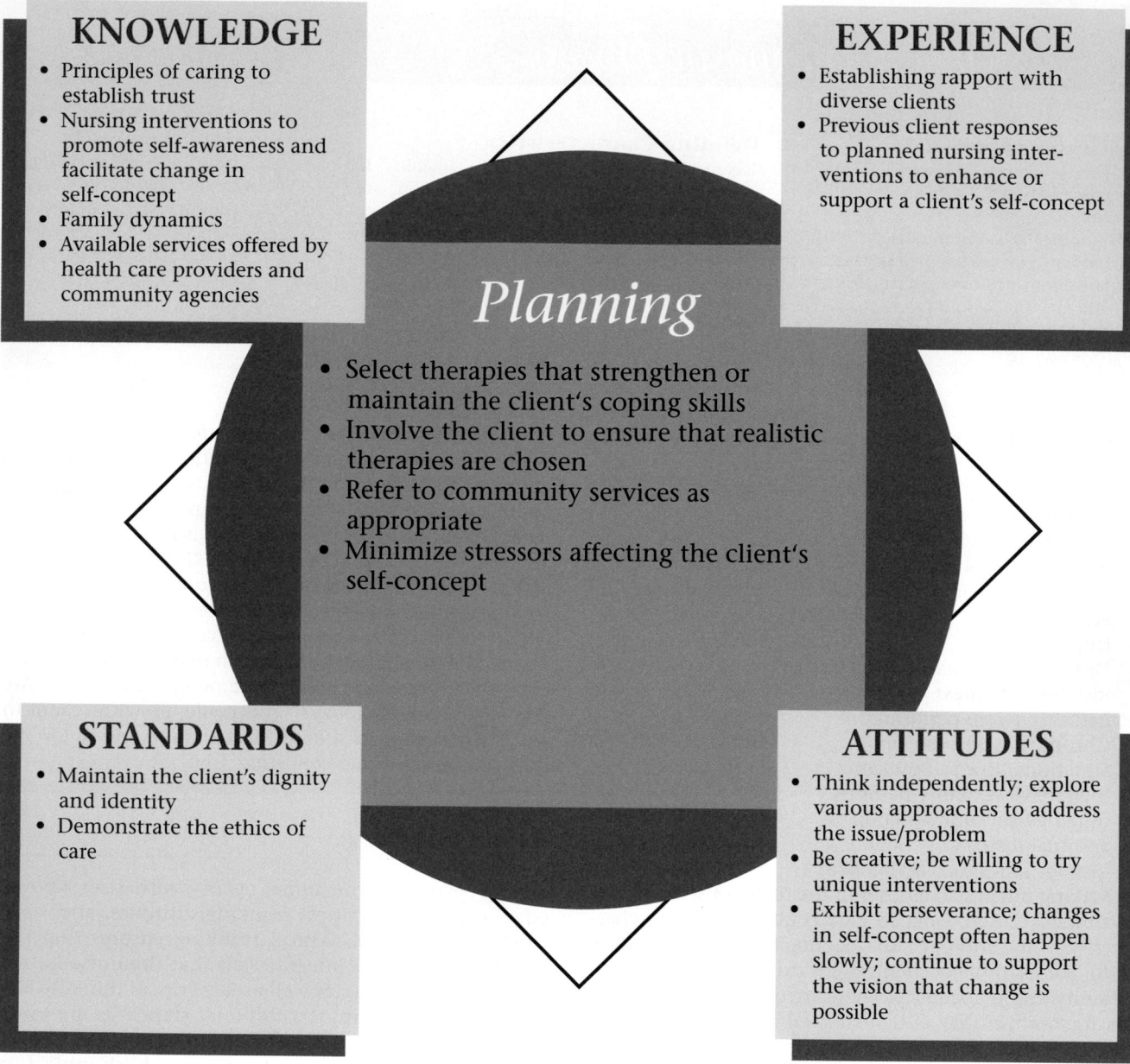

KNOWLEDGE
- Principles of caring to establish trust
- Nursing interventions to promote self-awareness and facilitate change in self-concept
- Family dynamics
- Available services offered by health care providers and community agencies

EXPERIENCE
- Establishing rapport with diverse clients
- Previous client responses to planned nursing interventions to enhance or support a client's self-concept

Planning
- Select therapies that strengthen or maintain the client's coping skills
- Involve the client to ensure that realistic therapies are chosen
- Refer to community services as appropriate
- Minimize stressors affecting the client's self-concept

STANDARDS
- Maintain the client's dignity and identity
- Demonstrate the ethics of care

ATTITUDES
- Think independently; explore various approaches to address the issue/problem
- Be creative; be willing to try unique interventions
- Exhibit perseverance; changes in self-concept often happen slowly; continue to support the vision that change is possible

FIGURE 26–6   Critical thinking model for self-concept planning.

a more comprehensive and workable plan. Once a goal has been formulated, the nurse should consider how the data that illustrated the problem would change if the problem were diminished. These changes should be reflected in the outcome criteria. For example, a client is diagnosed with *situational low self-esteem related to a recent job layoff.* The nurse and client establish a goal: "Client's self-esteem and self-concept should begin to improve in 2 weeks." Examples of expected outcomes directed toward that goal include the following:
- The client will discuss a minimum of three areas of her life where she is functioning well.
- The client will be able to voice the recognition that losing her job is not reflective of her worth as a person.
- The client attends a support group for out-of-work professionals.

Setting Priorities. The care plan presents the goals, expected outcomes, and interventions for a client with an alteration in self-concept. Interventions focus on helping the client adapt to the stressors that led to the self-concept disturbance and on supporting and reinforcing the development of coping methods.

Often a client perceives a situation as overwhelming and may feel hopeless about returning to the level of previous functioning. The client may need time to adapt to physical changes.

Establishing priorities may include therapeutic communication to address self-concept issues to ensure that the client's ability to address physical needs is maximized. The nurse should look for strengths in both the individual and the family and provide resources and education to turn limitations into strengths. Client teaching

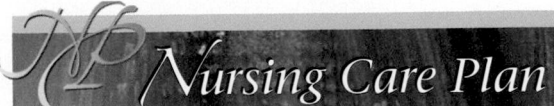

Nursing Care Plan

Alterations in Self-Concept

Assessment

Mrs. Johnson, a 45-year-old married woman who underwent a unilateral radical mastectomy due to malignancy, has been assigned to Miss Carr, a student nurse. Mrs. Johnson's physical assessment has been completed, and she has been adequately medicated for pain. Miss Carr sits down to engage in a discussion of how the mastectomy has affected Mrs. Johnson's self-concept.

Assessment Activities	Findings/Defining Characteristics
Assess identity concerns (e.g., sexual role, femininity). Ask Mrs. Johnson how the mastectomy is affecting her sense of self.	Mrs. Johnson looks away, shakes her head, and states, "I feel like less of a woman. My husband says I'm still sexy, but I don't believe him."
Observe Mrs. Johnson's mood and interactions with others, including family members.	Intermittent eye contact, frequent crying when alone, pulling hospital gown tightly across chest, superficial conversations with family members.
Determine Mrs. Johnson's participation in self-care activities.	Demonstrates avoidance of looking at self; refuses to bathe, comb hair, or apply typical makeup.

Nursing Diagnosis: Disturbed body image related to negative thoughts and feelings to actual change in body.

Planning

Goal	Expected Outcomes*
	Body Image
Mrs. Johnson will identify and express feelings verbally and nonverbally.	Mrs. Johnson will discuss disturbed body image with staff members and significant others within 3 days.
	Mrs. Johnson will consider exploring support groups by discharge.
	Acceptance; Health Status
Mrs. Johnson will participate in self-care related to mastectomy.	Mrs. Johnson will look at tissue surrounding surgery within 2 days.
	Mrs. Johnson will begin to attend to basic hygiene needs within 2 days.
	Social Involvement
Mrs. Johnson will identify and use resources outside the hospital.	Mrs. Johnson will verbalize commitment to participating in community resources (e.g., mastectomy support group) by discharge.
	By postoperative visit, Mrs. Johnson will determine if she wishes to attend support group.

*Outcome classification labels from: Moorhead S, Johnson M, and Maas M: *Nursing Outcomes Classification (NOC)*, ed 3, St. Louis, 2004, Mosby.

Interventions†	Rationale
Coping Enhancement	
Initially assign the same staff members to work with Mrs. Johnson.	Continuity in care will facilitate the establishment of a therapeutic relationship; familiarity and trust will enhance communication.
Approach Mrs. Johnson and initiate conversation; use silence and active listening to promote communication.	Mrs. Johnson's ability to initially find the words for what she is experiencing may be limited.
Remain aware of your own feelings regarding Mrs. Johnson's bodily changes and physical appearance.	Inadvertently communicating discomfort or reacting negatively will interfere with Mrs. Johnson's ability to openly communicate her own feelings.
Have Mrs. Johnson spend time alone and with supportive family members for crying, recording in her journal, and reflection on prayer.	Encourages expression of thoughts and feelings including depression, grief, resentment, and fear of rejection.
Facilitate evaluation of overall self-concept.	The impact on body image may influence other aspects of self-concept and self-esteem, including perception of identity and role performance.

Continued

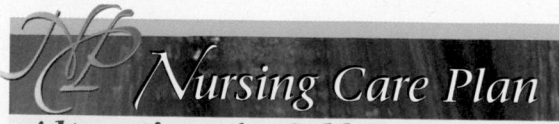

Nursing Care Plan

Alterations in Self-Concept—cont'd

Interventions†—cont'd

Coping Enhancement—cont'd

Involve Mrs. Johnson's husband in discussion of uncomfortable issues such as areas of sexual concerns.

Assist Mrs. Johnson to identify and use appropriate support systems outside the hospital including home health care.

Rationale

Family involvement is an essential element of comprehensive care. Sexuality is a basic need and concern for both men and women, yet can be one of the most difficult discussions for clients to initiate.

Support can assist the client in feeling normal again and in integrating a new body image into her self-concept.

†Intervention classification labels from Dochterman JM, Bulechek GM: *Nursing interventions classification (NIC)*, ed 4, St. Louis, 2004, Mosby.

Evaluation

Nursing Actions	Client Response/Finding	Achievement of Outcome
Ask Mrs. Johnson how effective she feels in her ability to identify and express feelings verbally and nonverbally.	Mrs. Johnson responds, "It's hard for me to talk about myself, but I have really made an effort to talk about what the loss of my breast means to me."	Mrs. Johnson reports improvement in communication skills and success with discussing disturbed body image with primary nurse and husband.
Observe Mrs. Johnson's participation in self-care related to mastectomy.	Mrs. Johnson assumed responsibility for basic hygiene immediately after establishing the goal and has used a mirror to examine her mastectomy scar.	Mrs. Johnson has increased her independence and has begun to integrate body image change into her self-concept.
Assist Mrs. Johnson in the identification of resources outside the hospital; secure a commitment to use resources.	Mrs. Johnson will verbalize commitment to participating in community resources (e.g., mastectomy support group).	Outcome has not been completely achieved; Mrs. Johnson has expressed hesitancy in attending a support group, but is receptive to home care. Home care nurse to ensure goal is reevaluated and addressed as appropriate.

creates understanding of the normalcy of certain situations (e.g., nature of a chronic disease, change in relationships, or effect of a loss). Often, once this is understood, the sense of hopelessness and helplessness can be lessened.

Continuity of Care. The perceptions of significant others are important to incorporate into the plan of care. Individuals who have experienced deficits in self-concept before the current episode of treatment may have established a system of support including mental health clinicians, clergy, and other community resources. Before involving the family, the nurse needs to consider the client's desires for their involvement and cultural norms regarding who most frequently makes decisions in the family.

Implementation

As with all the steps of the nursing process, a therapeutic nurse-client relationship is central to the implementation phase. Once the goals and outcome criteria have been developed, the nurse considers nursing interventions for promoting a healthy self-concept and helping the client move toward the goals. To develop effective nursing interventions, the nurse should consider the nursing diagnosis and broad interventions that address the diagnosis. These broad, standard interventions should be tailored to the individual client. Regardless of the health care setting, it is important that nurses work with clients and their families or significant others to promote a healthy self concept. For example, nursing interventions may include strategies to help clients regain or restore the elements that contribute to a strong and secure sense of self. The approaches that nurses choose will vary according to the level of care required.

Health Promotion. The nurse may work with clients to help them develop healthy lifestyle behaviors that contribute to a positive self-concept. Measures that support adaptation to stress, such as proper nutrition, regular exercise within the client's capabilities, measures that facilitate adequate sleep and rest, and stress-reducing practices may contribute to a healthy self-concept. Nurses are in a unique position to identify lifestyle practices that put a person's self-concept at risk or are suggestive of altered self-concepts. For example, a young teacher visits a clinic, with complaints of being unable to sleep and experiencing anxiety attacks. In gathering the nursing history, the nurse may learn of lifestyle practices such as too little rest, a large number of life changes occurring simultaneously, or excessive use of alcohol. These data, when taken together, can be suggestive of actual or potential self-concept disturbances. The nurse in this situation determines how the client views the various lifestyle elements, to facilitate the client's insight into behaviors, and to make appropriate referrals or provide needed health teaching.

Acute Care. In the acute care setting the nurse is likely to care for clients who are experiencing potential threats to their self-concept because of the nature of the treatment and diagnostic procedures. Threats to a person's self-concept can result in anxiety and/or fear. Numerous stressors, including unknown diagnoses, the need to make changes in lifestyle, and change in functioning, may be present and need to be addressed. In the acute care setting there is often more than one stressor, thus increasing the overall stress level for the client and family.

Nurses in the acute care setting also encounter clients who are faced with the need to adapt to an altered body image as a result of surgery or other physical change. Often a visit by someone who has experienced similar changes and adapted to them (e.g., someone who has had a laryngectomy) may be helpful. The timing of such a visit is important. Because addressing these needs may be difficult to do while in an acute care settings, appropriate follow-up and referrals, including home care, are essential. The nurse needs to be sensitive to the client's level of acceptance of the change. Forcing confrontation with the change before the client is ready could delay the person's acceptance. Signs that a person may be receptive to such a visit would include the client's asking questions related to how to manage a particular aspect of what has happened or looking at the changed area. As the client expresses readiness to integrate the body change into his or her self-concept, the nurse can either let the client know about groups that are available or ask the client if he or she would like the nurse to make the contact. Another way in which the nurse can facilitate adjustment to a change in physical appearance is through his or her own response to the wound or change. As the nurse responds with acceptance, this models acceptance for both the client and the family.

Restorative Care. It is often in a long-term nurse-client relationship in a home care environment that a nurse has the opportunity to work with a client to obtain the goal of attaining a more positive self-concept (Box 26-9). Interventions designed to help a client reach the goal of adapting to changes in self-concept or attaining a positive self-concept are based on the premise that the client first develops insight and self-awareness concerning problems and stressors and then acts to solve the problems and cope with the stressors. This approach, outlined by Stuart and Laraia (2001), can be incorporated into client teaching for alterations in self-concept, including situational low self-esteem, which might present in the home care setting.

Increasing the client's self-awareness is achieved through establishing a trusting relationship that allows the client to openly explore thoughts and feelings. A priority nursing intervention continues to be the expert use of communication skills to clarify the expectations of the client and family. Open exploration can make the situa-

---

Client Teaching   Box 26-9

Alterations in Self-Concept

Objective

- Risks for situational low self-esteem will be reduced in the home care setting.

Teaching Strategies

- Reinforce client's expression of thoughts and feelings; clarify meaning of verbal and nonverbal communication.
- Encourage opportunities for client to care for self.
- Elicit client's perceptions of strengths and weaknesses.
- Convey verbally and behaviorally that client is responsible for behavior.
- Identify relevant stressors with client and ask for appraisal of them.
- Explore client's adaptive and maladaptive coping responses to problems.
- Collaboratively identify alternative solutions; encourage alternatives not previously tried.
- Continue to reinforce strengths and successes.

Evaluation

- Confirm perception of and actual use of improved communication skills.
- Observe level of participation in decisions that affect care.
- Confirm with client and family that the increase in activities and tasks has been a positive experience.
- Observe the client's establishment of a simple routine.
- Observe client take necessary action to change maladaptive coping responses and maintain adaptive ones.
- Confirm with client and family how new coping resources can be applied to continued change.

Modified from Stuart GW, Laraia MT: *Principles and practice of psychiatric nursing*, ed 7, St. Louis, 2001, Mosby.

---

tion less threatening for the client and encourages behaviors that expand self-awareness.

Encouraging the client's self-exploration is achieved by accepting the client's thoughts and feelings, by helping the client to clarify interactions with others, and by being empathetic. The nurse encourages self-expression and stresses the client's self-responsibility.

Promoting the client's self-evaluation involves helping the client to define problems clearly and to identify positive and negative coping mechanisms. The nurse works closely with the client to help to analyze adaptive and maladaptive responses, contrast different alternatives, and discuss outcomes.

Collaborating with the client in establishing realistic goals involves helping the client to identify alternative solutions and develop realistic goals based on them. This facilitates real change and encourages further goal-setting behaviors. The nurse designs opportunities that result in success, reinforces the client's skills and strengths, and assists the client in getting needed assistance.

Assisting the client in becoming committed to decisions and actions to achieve goals involves teaching the client to move away from ineffective coping mechanisms and develop successful coping strategies. Supporting attempts that are health promoting is essential, because with each success another attempt can be made. Supporting adaptive, flexible coping is critical to intervening in self-concept alterations.

Clients who are experiencing threats to or alterations in self-concept often benefit from collaboration with mental health and community resources to promote increased awareness. Knowledge of available community resources allows the nurse to make appropriate referrals.

Establishing a therapeutic environment and a therapeutic relationship (see Chapter 23), and increasing self-awareness are critical to successfully intervening with clients who have alterations in self-concept, whether care is focused on health promotion, dealing with an acute process, or addressing restorative care. To support the development of a positive self-concept in a client, the nurse must convey genuine caring for the client (see Chapter

7). Then, and only then, can the nurse establish a partnership with the client to address underlying problems.

Evaluation

Client Care. Evaluating success in meeting each client goal and the established expected outcomes requires critical thinking (Figure 26-7). Frequent evaluation of client progress is recommended so that changes can be instituted if necessary. The nurse applies knowledge of behaviors and characteristics of a healthy self-concept when reviewing the actual behaviors clients display. This determines whether outcomes have been met.

Expected outcomes for a client with a self-concept disturbance may include nonverbal behaviors indicating a positive self-concept, statements of self-acceptance, and acceptance of change in appearance or function. Key indicators of a client's self-concept can be his or her nonverbal behaviors. For example a client who has had difficulty making eye contact may demonstrate a more

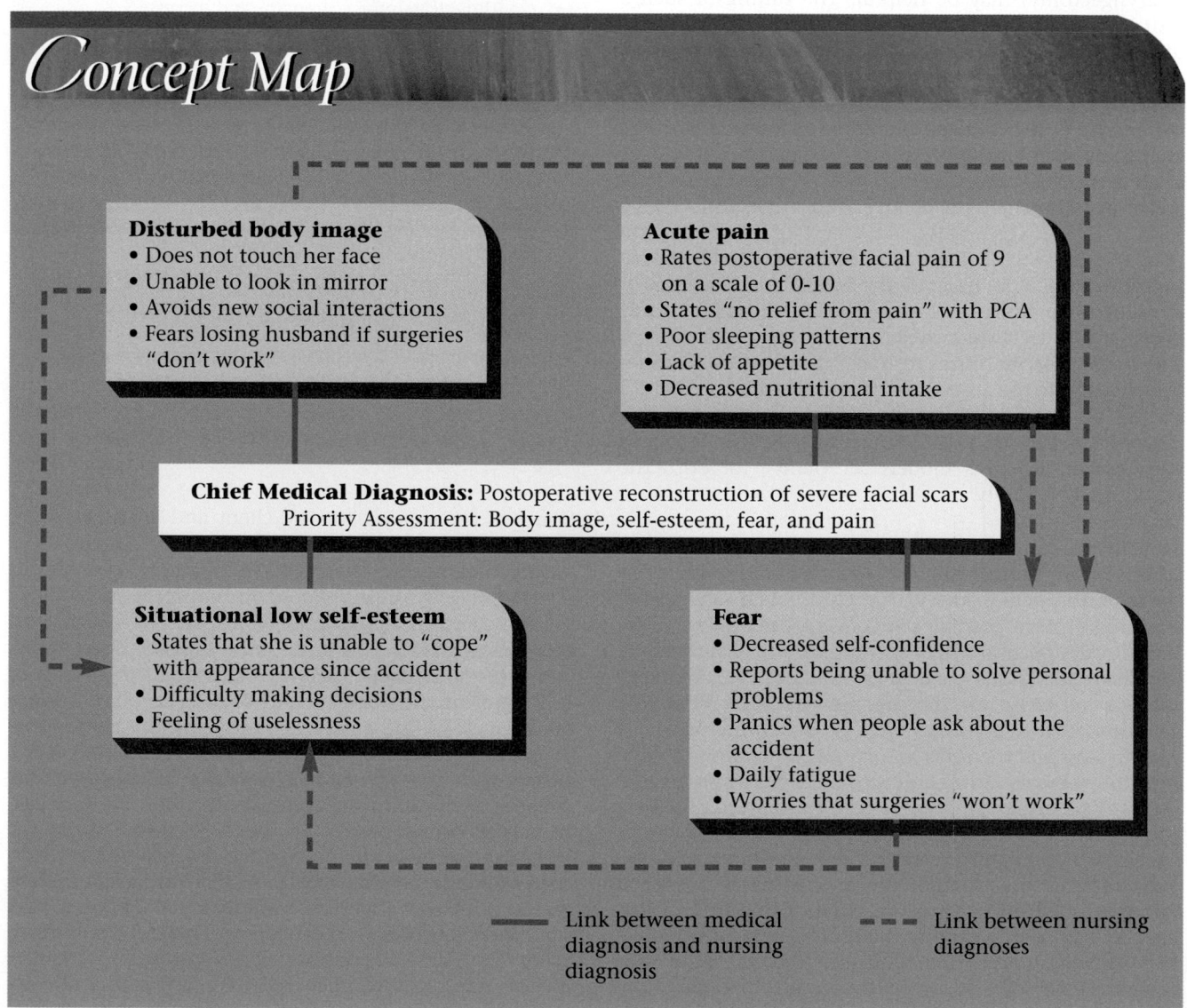

Concept Map

Disturbed body image
- Does not touch her face
- Unable to look in mirror
- Avoids new social interactions
- Fears losing husband if surgeries "don't work"

Acute pain
- Rates postoperative facial pain of 9 on a scale of 0-10
- States "no relief from pain" with PCA
- Poor sleeping patterns
- Lack of appetite
- Decreased nutritional intake

Chief Medical Diagnosis: Postoperative reconstruction of severe facial scars
Priority Assessment: Body image, self-esteem, fear, and pain

Situational low self-esteem
- States that she is unable to "cope" with appearance since accident
- Difficulty making decisions
- Feeling of uselessness

Fear
- Decreased self-confidence
- Reports being unable to solve personal problems
- Panics when people ask about the accident
- Daily fatigue
- Worries that surgeries "won't work"

——— Link between medical diagnosis and nursing diagnosis   - - - Link between nursing diagnoses

FIGURE **26-7**   Concept map for client who is postoperative for reconstruction of severe facial scars.

positive self-concept by making more frequent eye contact during conversation. Social interaction, adequate self-care, acceptance of the use of prosthetic devices, and statements indicating understanding of teaching all indicate progress. A positive attitude toward rehabilitation and increased movement toward independence facilitate a return to preexisting roles at work or at home. Patterns of interacting can also reflect changes in self-concept. For example, a client who has been hesitant to express his or her views may more readily offer opinions and ideas as self-esteem increases.

The goals of care may be unrealistic or inappropriate as the client's condition changes. The nurse may need to revise the plan, reflecting on successful experiences with other clients. Client adaptation to major changes may take a year or longer, but the fact that this period is long does not suggest problems with adaptation. The nurse should look for signs that the client has reduced some stressors and that some behaviors have become more adaptive. Changes in self-concept take time. Although change may be slow, care of the client with a self-concept disturbance can be rewarding.

Client Expectations. If the nurse has developed a good rapport with the client, the client may be able to share how things are going from his or her perspective. The nurse may be able to facilitate this sharing by initiating a review of what has happened over time. This offers the nurse the opportunity to share perceptions and encourages the client to consider and voice how he or she has conceptualized any changes.

Key Concepts

- Self-concept is an integrated set of conscious and unconscious attitudes and perceptions about the self.
- Components of self-concept are identity, body image, and role performance.
- Each developmental stage involves factors that are important to the development of a healthy, positive self-concept.
- Identity is particularly vulnerable during adolescence.

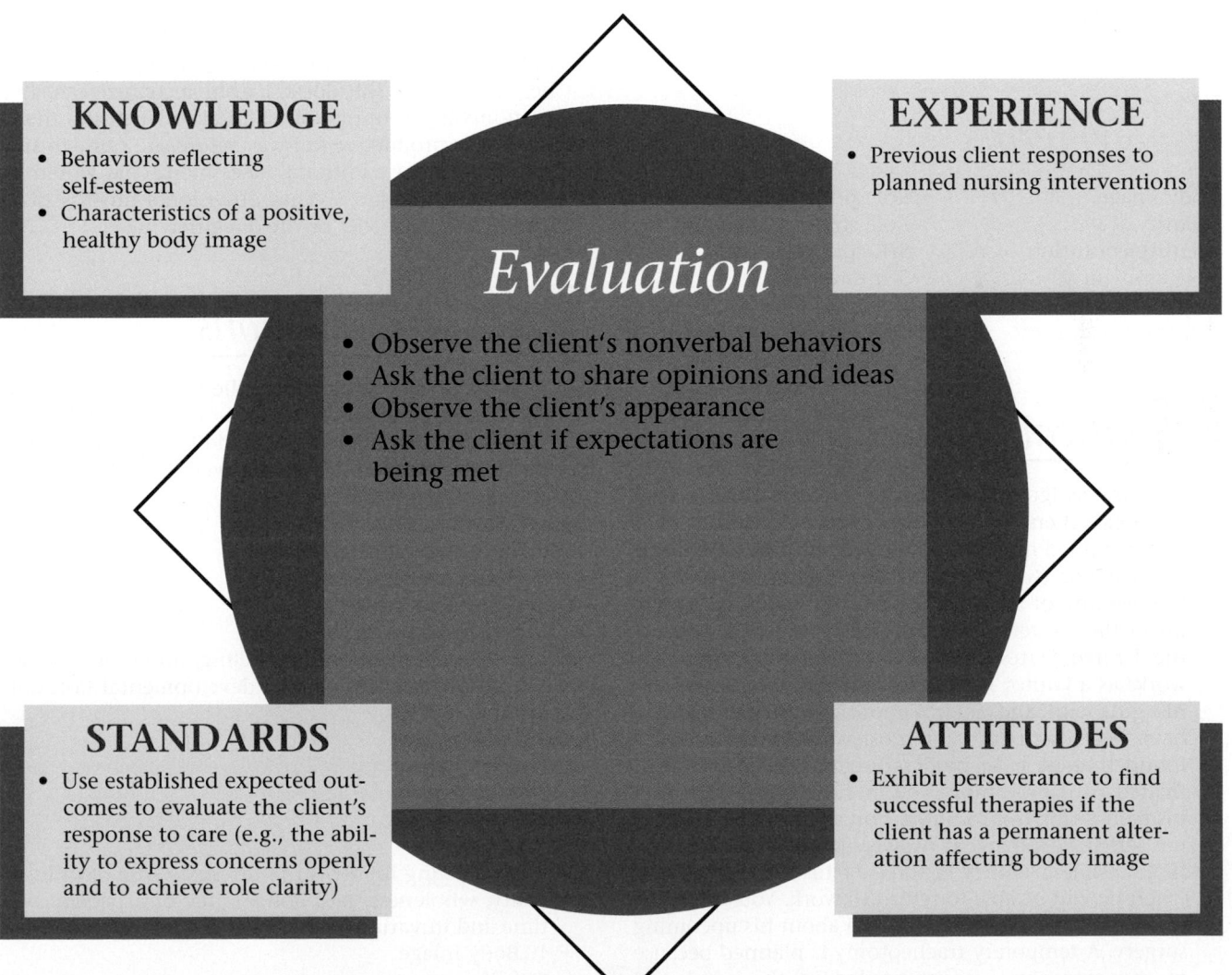

FIGURE **26–8**   Critical thinking model for self-concept evaluation.

- Body image is the mental picture of one's body and is not necessarily consistent with a person's actual body structure or appearance.
- Body image stressors include changes in physical appearance, structure, or functioning caused by normal developmental changes or illness.
- Self-esteem is the emotional appraisal of self-concept and reflects the overall sense of being capable, worthwhile, and competent.
- Self-esteem stressors include developmental and relationship changes, illness (particularly chronic illness involving changes in what were normal activities), surgery, accidents, and the responses of other individuals to changes resulting from these events.
- Role stressors, including role conflict, role ambiguity, and role strain, may originate in unclear or conflicting role expectations and may be aggravated by the effects of illness.
- The nurse's self-concept and nursing actions can have an effect on a client's self-concept.
- Planning and implementing nursing interventions for self-concept disturbance involve expanding the client's self-awareness, encouraging self-exploration, aiding in self-evaluation, helping formulate goals in regard to adaptation, and assisting the client in achieving those goals.

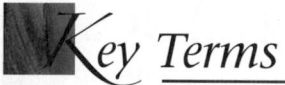

Key Terms

Body image, *p. 504*	Role performance, *p. 505*
Identity, *p. 503*	Role strain, *p. 508*
Identity confusion, *p. 506*	Self-concept, *p. 501*
Role ambiguity, *p. 508*	Self-esteem, *p. 505*
Role conflict, *p. 507*	Sick role, *p. 507*
Role overload, *p. 508*	

Critical Thinking Exercises

1. You are assigned to care for a 23-year-old Asian-American client who was in a motor vehicle accident and sustained multiple fractures to his face and a fractured femur (which was fixated through surgery on the evening of admission 4 days ago). He has grown up in the United States; he and his mother came to the United States when he was a young child. He works as a janitor for a local university. He lives with his girlfriend and their 7-month-old daughter. You have been with him for most of the morning and found that he is in moderate pain, which has been treated with morphine. The morphine has decreased his pain rating from a 6 to a 3 on a scale of 0 to 10 but has left him somewhat drowsy. During the morning he has shared with you some of his concerns about when he will be able to return to work. You are in the room when the surgeon tells him about his upcoming surgery. A temporary tracheotomy is planned because of the extensive surgery needed in the nasal and throat area. After the surgeon leaves, the client tells you that he does not want the tracheotomy. He indi-

cates that he is unclear about what it actually entails, even though the surgeon explained it in fairly simple terms. He says to you, "I just want to get back to my normal self." How would you address his comment regarding "get back to normal" and his lack of understanding regarding the tracheotomy?

2. A 16-year-old girl is preparing for discharge from the hospital after giving birth 2 days earlier. She is unmarried, not involved with the baby's father, and has minimal familial support to care for the child. Before admission, she arranged to terminate rights and give the baby up for adoption. She reaffirms this as a good decision because she will be able to return to school immediately and graduate, as scheduled, in 2 years. The client confides in you that her biggest concerns right now are how she feels about herself and how she looks. Taking into account developmental needs of this adolescent, how will you collaborate with her to establish priority interventions to address her self-concept deficits?

3. As a part of your community health experience, you are assigned to visit a 75-year-old woman who has gone to her daughter's home after being hospitalized for agitation and aggression secondary to Alzheimer's disease. When you go to the home, you find the 55-year-old daughter tearful. She says, "I just don't know if I can do this. She doesn't like anything I cook. She calls me two or three times during the night to sit with her; sometimes she doesn't even recognize me. I've been missing a lot of work, and even when I'm there, I'm not as productive as I was before she came to stay with us." What additional assessment data would be important to gather? What provisional nursing diagnosis could be made for the daughter?

Review Questions

1. When a nurse is caring for a client after mastectomy, interventions to promote physiological stability and pain control are necessary. In addition, the nurse also needs to design nursing interventions directed toward improving her:
   1. Mobility.
   2. Self-concept.
   3. Activity tolerance.
   4. Self-care activities.

2. Developing self though modeling, imitation, and socialization is a self-concept developmental task during the ages of:
   1. 0 to 1 year.
   2. 1 to 3 years.
   3. 3 to 6 years.
   4. 6 to 12 years.

3. The following involves the internal sense of individuality, wholeness, and consistency of a person over time and in various circumstances:
   1. Body image.
   2. Self-concept.
   3. Role performance.
   4. Identify.

4. Adolescents are at risk for body image disturbance. An accurate statement about body image is that:
   1. Body image is not influenced by the opinions of others.
   2. Body image refers to the external features of a person.
   3. Body image includes actual and perceived perceptions of one's body.
   4. Physical changes during adolescence are quickly incorporated into the person's body image.

5. Certain behaviors become common or are avoided, depending on whether they are approved and reinforced or discouraged and punished. This process is called:
   1. Reinforcement-extinction.
   2. Inhibition.
   3. Substitution.
   4. Identification.

6. When an individual internalizes the beliefs, behavior, and values of role models into a personal, unique expression of self, the process is called:
   1. Reinforcement-extinction.
   2. Inhibition.
   3. Substitution.
   4. Identification.

7. An individual's identity is affected by stressors throughout life, but the age-group that is particularly vulnerable to stressors because of it being a time of great change is:
   1. Infants.
   2. Children.
   3. Adolescents.
   4. Adults.

8. When a person does not maintain a clear, consistent, and continuous consciousness of personal identity, it results in:
   1. Identify confusion.
   2. Low self-esteem.
   3. Low self-concept.
   4. Body image difficulties.

9. The nurse asks the client, "How do you feel about yourself?" The nurse is assessing the client's:
   1. Identify.
   2. Body image.
   3. Self-esteem.
   4. Role performance.

10. Increasing a client's self-awareness is achieved:
    1. Though establishing a trusting relationship that allows the client to openly explore thoughts and feelings.
    2. By accepting the client's thoughts and feelings.
    3. By helping the client to define her problems clearly.
    4. Though having the client identify her positive and negative coping mechanisms.

*R*eferences

Eliopoulos C: *Gerontologic nursing,* ed 5, Philadelphia, 2001, Lippincott.

Erikson E: *Childhood and society,* ed 2, New York, 1963, WW Norton.

Fortinash KM, Holoday Worrett PA: *Psychiatric nursing care plans,* ed 4, St. Louis, 2003, Mosby.

McCloskey Dochterman JC, Bulechek GM: *Nursing interventions classification (NIC),* ed 3, St. Louis, 2000, Mosby.

Miller CA: *Nursing care of older adults: theory and practice,* ed 3, Philadelphia, 1999, Lippincott.

Moorhead S, Johnson M, and Maas M: *Nursing Outcomes Classification (NOC),* ed 3, St. Louis, 2004, Mosby.

Rosenberg M: *Society and the adolescent self-image,* Princeton, NJ, 1965, Princeton University Press.

Stuart GW, Laraia MT: *Principles and practice of psychiatric nursing,* ed 7, St. Louis, 2001, Mosby.

*R*esearch References

Beck CT: Predictors of postpartum depression, *Nurs Res* 50(5):275, 2001.

Brown SG, Barbosa G: Nothing is going to stop me now: low-income women as they become self-sufficient, *Public Health Nurs* 18(5):364, 2001.

Bryne B: Relationships between anxiety, fear, self-esteem, and coping strategies in adolescence, *Adolescence* 35(137):201, 2000.

Cohane GH, Pope HG: Body image in boys: a review of the literature, *Int J Eat Disord* 29:373, 2001.

Judge TA, Bono JE: Relationship of core self-evaluations traits—self-esteem, generalized self-efficacy, locus of control, and emotional stability—with job satisfaction and job performance: a meta-analysis, *J Appl Psychol* 86(1):80, 2001.

Pedan AR and others: Negative thinking mediates the effect of self-esteem on depressive symptoms in college women, *Nurs Res* 49(4):201, 2000.

Pedro LW: Quality of life for long-term survivors of cancer: influencing variables, *Cancer Nurs* 24(1):1, 2001.

Plach SK, Napholz L, Kelber ST: Differences in anxiety and role experiences between three age groups of women with heart disease, *Arch Psychiatr Nurs* 15(4):195, 2001.

Robins RW and others: Global self-esteem across the life span, *Psychol Aging* 17(3):423, 2002.

Ruiz SY, Roosa MW, Gonzales NA: Predictors of self-esteem for Mexican American and European American youths: a reexamination of the influence of parenting, *J Fam Psychol* 16(1):70, 2002.

Twenge JM, Crocker J: Race and self-esteem: meta-analyses comparing whites, blacks, Hispanics, Asians, and American Indians, *Psychol Bull* 128(3):371, 2002.

Van Baarsen B: Theories on coping with loss: the impact of social support and self-esteem on adjustment to emotional and social loneliness following a partner's death in later life, *J Gerontol* 57(1):S33, 2002.

Voorhees CC and others: Early predictors of daily smoking in young women: the National Heart, Lung, and Blood Institute growth and health study, *Prev Med* 34:616, 2002.

Yarcheski A, Mahon NE, Yarcheski TJ: Social support and well-being in early adolescents, *Clin Nurs Res* 10(2):163, 2001.

Sexuality

Media Resources

http://evolve.elsevier.com/Potter/
fundamentals/

CD COMPANION

- Review Questions
- Glossary

evolve WEBSITE

- Review Questions
- Student Learning Activities
- Glossary

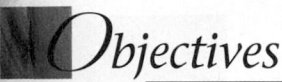

Objectives

Mastery of content in this chapter will enable the student to:

- Define the key terms listed.
- Identify personal attitudes, beliefs, and biases related to sexuality.
- Discuss the nurse's role in maintaining or enhancing a client's sexual health.
- Describe key concepts of sexual development across the life span.
- Describe the sexual response cycle.
- Identify potential causes of sexual dysfunction.
- Assess a client's sexuality.
- Define appropriate nursing diagnoses for clients with alterations in sexuality.
- Identify client risk factors in the area of sexual health.
- Identify and describe nursing interventions to promote sexual health.
- Evaluate a client's sexual health.
- Identify potential referral resources for clients' sexual concerns outside the nurse's level of expertise.
- Use critical thinking skills in assisting clients in meeting their sexual needs.

Sexuality is part of the person's personality and is important for overall health. Even though openness to sexual topics and discussion has increased over the years, many adults lack knowledge regarding **sexuality** and are reluctant to raise questions related to sexuality. For example, cardiac clients frequently have concerns about resumption of sexual **intercourse,** and anxiety over the effects new medications will have on sexual functioning. These clients are often hesitant to bring up these sexual concerns, yet when the nurse addresses sexuality in a relaxed, matter-of-fact manner, the client may feel it is safe to bring up his or her areas of concern. For the nurse to address sexuality in a relaxed, matter-of-fact manner, the nurse needs to have an adequate knowledge base regarding sexual functioning and sexual issues; well-developed communication skills; knowledge of areas to assess in regard to sexuality; personal comfort in discussing sexuality; and a caring, sensitive attitude. It is also critical that the nurse recognize that sexual issues are value laden. Religious teachings, culturally prescribed **gender roles,** beliefs about **sexual orientation,** and social and environmental climates all influence both the client's and the health care provider's value systems.

Sexuality is more than genital physical activity. Sexuality encompasses our whole being. It includes our sense of femaleness and maleness. Sexuality includes biological, sociological, psychological, spiritual, and cultural dimensions of each person's being. In addition, sexuality is influenced by values, attitudes, behaviors, relationships with others, and the need to establish emotional closeness with others (MacLaren, 1995). **Sexual health** can be described as a person's freedom from physical and psychological impairment, the awareness of open and positive attitudes toward sexual functioning, and accurate knowledge about sexuality (Heath and White, 2001).

Scientific Knowledge Base

A nurse assists a client in meeting his or her sexual needs, by having a sound scientific knowledge base regarding sexuality. A basic understanding of sexual development, sexual orientation, the **sexual response cycle, contraception,** abortion, and **sexually transmitted diseases (STDs)** is necessary.

Sexual Development

As a person grows and develops, so does his or her sexuality. Each stage of development brings changes in sexual functioning and the role of sexuality in relationships.

Infancy and Early Childhood. From birth on, children are treated differently according to their gender. The differential treatment results in shaping the behavior of the child. Freud's psychodynamic theory maintains that the first 3 years of life are crucial in the development of **gender identity.** It is during this time that the child identifies with the parent of the same sex and develops a complementary relationship with the parent of the opposite sex (Yarhouse, 2001).

The first step of gender identity development occurs as the child becomes aware of the differences of the sexes and perceives that he or she is male or female. Sexuality identity enables the child to interpret the behaviors of others as behavior appropriate for a female or a male.

School-Age Years. During the school years, children expand their horizons from parents and family. Parents, teachers, and the child's peer group serve as role models and teachers about how men and women act and relate with each other. School-age children generally have questions regarding the physical and emotional aspects of sex (Finan, 1997). They need accurate information from home and school about body and emotional changes during this period and what to expect as they move into puberty. Knowledge about normal emotional and physical changes associated with puberty may decrease the anxieties as these changes begin to happen. An uninformed child may be frightened by menstruation or nocturnal emission and view them as evidence of a dreadful disease.

Puberty/Adolescence. The emotional changes during puberty and adolescence are as dramatic as the physical ones. The adolescent functions within a powerful peer group, with the almost constant anxiety of "Am I normal?" and "Will I be accepted?" (Figure 27-1). Same-sex peers or friends remain influential in defining appropriate behavior, but the task of establishing a romantic relationship begins. Adolescence is a self-centered, egocentric stage. This introspection is necessary to establish a sense of self within the context of family, community, and emotional relationships. Assurance of normalcy in phys-

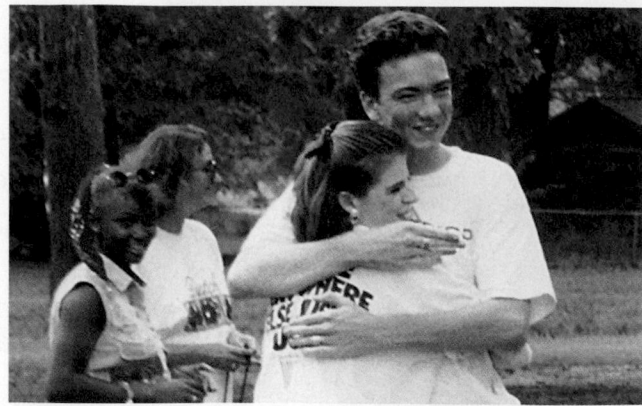

FIGURE **27–1**   Adolescents function within a powerful network of peers as they explore their sexual identity.

ical and emotional development should be given honestly and often.

The adolescent is faced with many decisions and needs accurate information on topics such as body changes, sexual activity, emotional responses within intimate sexual relationships, STDs, contraception, and pregnancy. In the United States 70% of adolescents have had sexual intercourse by the age of 18 (Kenney, Reinholtz, and Angelini, 1998). A substantial number of these teenagers do not protect themselves from pregnancy or STDs. The dynamics of sexual risk taking are not fully understood, but numerous studies have found correlations between drug/alcohol use, sexual abuse, and unsafe sex (Keller and others, 1996; Kenney, Reinholtz, and Angelini, 1998). Adolescents tend to have a sense of being invincible, believing that unwanted pregnancy, STDs, and other negative outcomes of sexual behavior are not likely to happen to them (Ross, Channon-Little, and Rosser, 2000).

Factual information regarding sexuality and sexual activity is important, but equally or perhaps more important is guidance in establishing a personal value or belief system to use as a framework for decision making. In healthy family networks much of this guidance will have been conveyed in the course of child rearing. Parents need to understand the importance of providing information, sharing their values, and promoting sound decision-making skills. Parents and significant others need to be counseled that even with the best guidance and information, adolescents will make their own decisions and must be held accountable for those decisions.

Adolescence is often a developmental phase during which an individual explores his or her primary sexual orientation. Many adolescents will have at least one **homosexual** experience with an individual or in a group (Stuart and Laraia, 1998). Adolescents may fear that this experience defines their total sexuality as homosexual. This is not true. Many individuals continue with a strictly **heterosexual** orientation after such experiences. However, some teenagers may recognize their preference as distinctly homosexual. This can be frightening and confusing for an adolescent. Support for the adolescent's sexual identity can be important during this time.

Support can come from a variety of sources, such as school counselors, clergy, family, or health professionals.

Young Adulthood. The adult has gained physical maturation but is continuing to explore and define emotional maturation in relationships. Intimacy and sexuality are issues for all adults whether they are in a sexual relationship, choose to abstain from sex, remain single by choice, are homosexual, or are widowed—whatever circumstances arise. People can be sexually healthy in numerous ways. Sexual activity is often defined as a basic need, but sexual desire can be channeled healthily into other forms of intimacy throughout a lifetime.

As sexually active adults develop intimate relationships, they need to learn techniques of stimulation that are satisfying to both themselves and their sexual partners. Some adults may need permission or affirmation that alternative ways of sexual expression other than penile-vaginal intercourse are normal. Other individuals may require significant education or therapy to achieve mutually satisfying sexual relationships.

Middle Adulthood. Later in the adult years, individuals may be adjusting to the social and emotional changes associated with children moving away from home. This can be a time of renewed intimacy between partners, or it may be a time when formerly intimate partners realize that they no longer care for each other or have common interests. In either case, children leaving home usually heralds a time of change in intimate relating.

Changing physical appearance related to aging may lead to concern about sexual attractiveness. In addition to concerns about changes in physical appearance, actual physical changes can affect sexual functioning. Decreasing levels of estrogen in the **perimenopausal** woman may lead to diminished vaginal lubrication and decreased vaginal elasticity. Both of these changes may lead to **dyspareunia** or the occurrence of pain during intercourse. Decreasing levels of estrogen can also result in a decreased desire for sexual activity. As men age, they are likely to experience an increase in the postejaculatory refractory period, delayed ejaculation, and other changes. Anticipatory guidance regarding these normal changes related to aging can ease concerns regarding functioning. Suggestions such as using vaginal lubrication and creating time for caressing and tenderness can help to ease adjustment to normal changes related to aging. Aging adults may also need to adjust to the impact of chronic illness, medications, aches, pains, and other health concerns on sexuality.

Older Adulthood. Studies of sexual behavior and interest of these behaviors among older adults have been limited and inconsistent in their findings. Many studies suggest that older adults retain an interest in sexual function and are sexually active. Other studies conclude that there is a decline of sexual interest and behavior among older adults (Box 27-1). Reported declines are largely the result of social, cultural, and psychological factors rather than biological or physical factors (Riley, 1999). Factors that determine sexual activity include present health status, past and present life satisfaction, and the status of mari-

---

Focus on Older Adults   **Box 27-1**

Changes Affecting Sexuality in Older Adults

- Sexuality and continued interest in sex throughout late life generally reflects life patterns (Lueckenotte, 2000).
- Pathological problems with the aging sexual response are often related to illnesses and medications. For example, impotence is often due to the use of tranquilizers, antidepressants, antihypertensives, or phenothiazines. Removal of causative agent generally results in resolution of the problem (Lueckenotte, 2000).
- In women vaginal tissue atrophies and lubrication is diminished or delayed over time.
- The nurse can demonstrate recognition, acceptance, and respect for an older adult's sexuality by displaying a willingness to openly discuss sex and sexuality-related concerns.
- Keeping abreast of current research in the filed of sexuality and aging and communicating these findings to nursing colleagues and older adult clients can promote a more realistic understanding of aging and sexuality (Eliopoulos, 2001).

---

tal or intimate relationships. For example, many older women are widowed or divorced and lack available sexual partners, which probably accounts for their decline in sexual activity. Nurses working with older adults need to be aware of the sexuality of their clients, assess interest and functioning, and plan accordingly.

Sexual Response Cycle

Kaplan (1979) identified three phases of the sexual response cycle: desire, arousal, and orgasm. These phases are a result of **vasocongestion** and **myotonia**, the basic physiological responses of sexual arousal. In women, this reaction leads to vaginal lubrication, swelling of the clitoris and the labia minora and majora, and engorgement of the outer third of the vagina (orgasmic platform). In men, vasocongestion leads to erection of the penis. Myotonia, or neuromuscular tension, gradually increases throughout the body during the excitement and plateau phases. Myotonia peaks during orgasm, resulting in involuntary contractions of the woman's vagina and the man's vas deferens and urethra. Women and men may experience contractions of the arm and leg muscles, facial muscles, and gluteal muscles. After orgasm, vasocongestion and myotonia return to prearousal levels. The phases described are not absolute. Male and female response patterns are similar.

Sexual Orientation

Sexual orientation describes the predominant gender preference of a person's sexual attraction over time. For about 10% of the population, the sexual preference is a member of the same sex. For another 20%, the sexual preference is a member of either sex (Ross, Channon-Little, and Rosser, 2000). Homosexuality among men and lesbianism among women is defined as the preference of a member of the same sex as a sexual partner. Bisexuality refers to an equal or almost equal preference for either sex.

Many stereotypical myths remain about homosexuals and **lesbians.** However, the nurse who is nonjudgmental and equipped with an appropriate knowledge base can help to dispel these myths and provide nursing care that includes attention to the person's sexual orientation.

Contraception

There are numerous contraceptive options available to sexually active couples today. The various methods provide varying levels of protection against unwanted pregnancies. Some methods do not require a prescription, whereas other methods do require intervention by a health care provider. Some methods, although effective for contraception, do not reduce the risk of STDs. For example, the pill and intrauterine device (IUD) are effective as birth control but not for protection from STDs.

Nonprescription Contraceptive Methods. Nonprescription methods for contraception include abstinence, various barrier methods, and timing of intercourse in regard to the menstrual cycle. Abstinence from sexual intercourse is 100% effective. But abstinence is often a difficult method for both men and women to use consistently. Any act of unprotected intercourse can result in pregnancy and exposure to STDs.

Barrier methods include over-the-counter spermicidal products (i.e., creams, jellies, foams, and sponges) that are put into the vagina before intercourse to create a spermicidal barrier between the uterus and ejaculated sperm. A **condom** is a thin rubber sheath that fits over the penis to prevent entrance of sperm into the vagina. Vaginal spermicides and condoms are most effective when instructions are carefully followed; their combined use has been found to be more effective in preventing pregnancy than the use of either one alone (Running and Berndt, 2003).

Effectiveness varies with each contraceptive method and the consistency of use. Two thirds of American females have at least one unplanned pregnancy and 40% of all pregnancies in the United States are unplanned. Unplanned pregnancies occur because contraceptives are not used, are used inconsistently, or are used improperly (Running and Berndt, 2003).

Nonprescription methods of contraception that are based on the physiological changes of the menstrual cycle include the rhythm, basal body temperature, cervical mucus, and fertility awareness methods. These methods require that the female client understand the reproductive cycle of her body and be aware of the subtle signs and signals her body gives during the cycle. These methods also require abstinence from sexual intercourse during designated fertile periods. The failure rate for these methods during the first year of use is 20% (Running and Berndt, 2003).

Methods That Require a Health Care Provider's Intervention. Contraceptive methods that require the intervention of a health care provider include hormonal contraception, IUDs, the **diaphragm,** the cervical cap, and **sterilization.** Hormonal contraception is available in several forms: oral contraceptive pills, intramuscular in-

jection, subdermal implant, transdermal skin patches, and IUDs. Hormonal contraception alters the hormonal environment to prevent ovulation and thicken cervical mucus.

An IUD is a plastic device inserted by a health care provider into the uterus through the cervical opening. IUDs vary in shape and may contain copper or may be impregnated with progesterone. The presence of the IUD results in the lining of the uterus being less favorable for the implantation of a fertilized ovum.

The diaphragm is a round, rubber dome that has a flexible spring around the edge. It must be used with a contraceptive cream or jelly and is inserted in the vagina so that it provides a contraceptive barrier over the cervical opening. The woman must be refitted after a significant weight gain/loss or pregnancy.

The cervical cap functions like the diaphragm; however, it covers only the cervix. It may be left in place longer and may be perceived as more comfortable than the diaphragm.

Effectiveness rates are reported as follows: oral contraceptives, 97% to 99.9%; IUDs, 98% to 99.9%; diaphragm, 82% to 97%; and cervical cap, 82% to 95% (Running and Berndt, 2003). The variation in rates for the diaphragm and cervical cap relates in part to the need for correct and consistent use during each act of intercourse for the method to be effective. Using a contraceptive method that requires specific action at the time of sexual excitement and activity can decrease the consistency of use.

Sterilization is the most effective contraception method other than abstinence. It should be considered permanent. Female sterilization, or **tubal ligation,** involves cutting, tying, or otherwise ligating the fallopian tubes. In male sterilization, or **vasectomy,** the vas deferens, which carries the sperm away from the testicles, is cut and tied. Both a tubal ligation and a vasectomy are considered minor surgical procedures, although a vasectomy is a less involved procedure and can be performed with the client under local anesthesia in a physician's office.

Sexually Transmitted Diseases

The incidence of STDs in the United States is increasing each year. The United States has the highest rate of STDs in the industrialized world (Centers for Disease Control and Prevention [CDC], 1999). The prevalence of STDs is a major health concern because treatment is costly and the incidence is high in minority populations of low socioeconomic status (CDC, 1999). Prevalent STDs include syphilis, gonorrhea, chlamydia, trichomoniasis, and infection with the human papillomavirus (HPV) and herpes simplex virus (HSV) type II (genital warts and genital herpes, respectively).

Safety Alert: Increasingly adolescents engage in oral sex, thinking there is less risk for acquiring STDs. Education about the risk must include parents and teachers as well as the adolescent.

As the name implies, STDs are transmitted from infected individuals to partners during intimate sexual contact. The site of transmission is usually genital, but it may also be oral-genital or anal-genital. Those persons most likely to be infected share one key characteristic: unprotected sex with multiple partners. Diseases that are caused by bacteria and that can usually be cured with antibiotics include gonorrhea, chlamydia, syphilis, and pelvic inflammatory disease. All clients need to understand that antibiotics need to be taken for the full course of treatment. An emerging concern, however, is that some of these bacterial infections (e.g., gonorrhea and syphilis) are now developing antibiotic-resistant strains. Two diseases—genital herpes and genital warts—are caused by viruses and cannot be cured.

A major problem in dealing with STDs is finding and treating the people who have them. Some people may not even know that they are infected, because symptoms are absent or go unnoticed. Because sexual behavior may include the whole body rather than just the genitalia, many parts of the body are potential sites for an STD. The ears, mouth, throat, tongue, nose, and eyelids can be used for sexual pleasure. The perineum, anus, and rectum are also frequently included in sexual activity. Furthermore, any contact with another person's body fluids around the head or an open lesion on the skin, anus, or genitalia can transmit an STD.

Sometimes people do not seek treatment because they are embarrassed to discuss sexual symptoms or concerns. They may also hesitate to talk about their sexual behavior if they believe that it is not "normal." Oral-genital sex, anal-genital sex, or any sexual behavior that embarrasses the client may hinder the detection of an STD.

The most valuable tool the nurse can develop for providing care in areas of sexuality involves communication skills and a nonjudgmental attitude. By questioning and talking with the client in a caring manner that evokes trust, the nurse can pick up valuable clues about an STD that the client may have missed. The nurse can also begin to assess the client's attitudes toward sexuality and adjust the intervention to make it acceptable to the client's sexual value system.

Human Immunodeficiency Virus Infection. Human immunodeficiency virus (HIV) infection or acquired immunodeficiency syndrome (AIDS) is also spread through sexual contact. Although HIV is present in the majority of body fluids, it is really a blood-borne pathogen. For transmission to occur, therefore, some exchange of body fluid, particularly blood, must occur. Primary routes of transmission include contaminated intravenous (IV) needles; anal intercourse, vaginal intercourse, and oral-genital sex; and transfusion of blood and blood products.

The Centers for Disease Control and Prevention (CDC) (2002) reported the percentage of AIDS cases by exposure category for adults and adolescents as follows: **gay** men (46%); IV drug users (25%); gay men and IV drug users (6%), and individuals with hemophilia (1%), and others who have received contaminated blood (1%). As with other STDs, heterosexual persons who have unprotected sex with multiple partners or who have a partner who has multiple other partners are also at risk. This category constituted 11% of the AIDS cases. For the pediatric exposure rates, 3% were related to hemophilia and 91% were related to a mother with HIV infection.

AIDS is the late stage of a continuum of symptoms that result from infection with HIV. AIDS is not the same as HIV infection, and not everyone infected with HIV develops AIDS. The time from initial HIV infection to development of AIDS ranges from 18 months to more than 10 years (CDC, 2000). The range differs among people, depending on the way in which HIV was acquired and a variety of personal factors (Department of Health, 2000).

AIDS is a serious, debilitating, and eventually fatal disease. The care of the person with AIDS can evoke complex personal issues for the nurse. There is fear of acquiring HIV and negative attitudes related to the client's lifestyle that contributed to the disease. Knowledge and practice of infection control procedures can reduce the nurse's fears about becoming infected through client care. Nurses must be willing to suspend judgment in order to provide competent, compassionate care to the person with AIDS.

> *Safety Alert.* The individual has an obligation not to infect others if infected, and if uninfected should take all possible steps to remain that way. These steps include avoidance of unsafe sex in which the transfer of body fluids may occur and not sharing needles during injecting drug use. Reduction of sexual partners to a minimum and use of condoms to reduce risk of infection should be advised.

*N*ursing Knowledge Base

As the nurse plans to assist the client in addressing his or her sexual needs, the nurse uses critical thinking skills and basic nursing knowledge. The nurse may draw from the following areas of nursing knowledge: sociocultural dimensions of sexuality; the impact of pregnancy and menstruation on sexuality; factors that influence discussion of sexual issues; factors that influence decisions regarding contraception, abortion, STD prevention, and abortion; **infertility;** sexual abuse; and **sexual dysfunction.**

Sociocultural Dimensions of Sexuality

Sexuality is influenced by cultural rules and norms that determine what is acceptable behavior within the culture. Global cultural diversity creates considerable variability in sexual norms and represents a wide spectrum of beliefs and values. Common areas of diversity include the meaning of dating and behavior allowed during dating, what is considered arousing, the types of sexual activity commonly practiced, sanctions and prohibitions concerning sexual behavior, whom one marries, and who is allowed to marry.

A definitive and comprehensive survey of sexual practices and beliefs in America confirmed that people are influenced by their social networks and tend to act out social scripts (Michael and others, 1994). Sexual behavior is very similar to any other social behavior (i.e., people behave the way they are rewarded for behaving). They tend to "play by the rules" when choosing someone to have sex with and when choosing someone to marry.

Society plays a powerful role in shaping sexual values and attitudes and in supporting specific expression of sexuality in its members. Each cultural and social group has its own set of rules and norms that guide the behavior of its members. These rules become an integral part of an individual's thinking and underlie sexual behavior, including, for example, how people find partners, who they choose as partners, how they relate to one another, how often they have sex, and what they do when they have sex.

Many factors affect a person's sexual health and his or her willingness to discuss this private part of life. Spanish-speaking clients and Native Americans tend to be hesitant to talk about sexual matters. People from these groups may talk more freely to a nurse or other health care provider of the same sex (Iannotta, 2002).

Cultural or religious background can also influence the individual's willingness to openly discuss sexual matters. Personal beliefs may enable certain practices and prohibit others (Box 27-2). For example, the teachings of the Roman Catholic Church prohibit the use of artificial contraception.

Impact of Pregnancy and Menstruation on Sexuality. Many cultures have taboos against sexual intercourse or even male-female contact during menstruation and pregnancy. For example, in the Hindu culture a woman must stay away from worship, cooking, and other members of the family during menstruation. Research has found no physiological contraindication to intercourse during men-

struation or during most pregnancies. Female sexual interest tends to fluctuate during pregnancy, with increased interest during the second trimester and often decreased interest during the first and third trimesters. There is often a decrease in libido during the first trimester because of nausea, fatigue, and breast tenderness. During the second trimester, there is an increased blood flow to the pelvic area to supply the placenta and sexual enjoyment and libido increases. During the third trimester the increased abdominal size may make finding a comfortable position difficult (Pillitteri, 1999). Emotional overtones (e.g., dealing with blood during menstruation or fear of injury to the fetus or mother during pregnancy) may need to be resolved to promote mutual sexual satisfaction.

Discussing Sexual Issues. Sexuality is a significant part of each person's being, yet sexual assessment and interventions are not always included in health care. The area of sexuality can be emotionally charged for nurses, as well as for clients. Discomfort with talking about sexual issues, lack of information, differences in values between the client and the nurse, and guilt may prevent the nurse from discussing issues regarding sexuality with clients. The most valuable tool that the nurse can develop for providing care in areas of sexuality involves communication skills. Nurses who have difficulty discussing topics related to sexuality should explore their discomfort and develop a plan for addressing their discomfort. If the nurse is uncomfortable with topics related to sexuality, the client is unlikely to share sexual concerns with the nurse.

Decisional Issues

There are numerous decisions individuals make about their sexuality. Some of those decisions that the nurse is likely to encounter and perhaps influence include decisions regarding contraception and abortion.

Contraception. The decisions that women and men make regarding contraception can have far-reaching effects on their lives. Pregnancy, whether planned or unplanned, significantly affects the life of the mother and father and often the larger support network. Effects are physical, interpersonal, social, financial, and societal. The choice to use contraception is multifaceted and is not completely understood. Robinson and colleagues (2000) report that two thirds of American females have at least one unplanned pregnancy and that 49% of all pregnancies in the United States are unplanned; 26.5% of all pregnancies end in elective abortion; 90% of pregnancies in adolescents age 15 to 19 years are unplanned. Effective contraception involves factors relating to the sexually active couple, the method of contraception, the couple's understanding of the contraceptive method, the consistency of use, and the compliance with the requirements of the chosen method. Personal characteristics that have been identified as positively influencing contraceptive use include motivation to avoid unplanned pregnancy, ability to plan, comfort with sexuality, and previous contraceptive use (Running and Berndt, 2003). Cultural and religious background may permit certain practices and prohibit others. For example, the teachings of the Roman Catholic Church prohibit the use of artificial contraception.

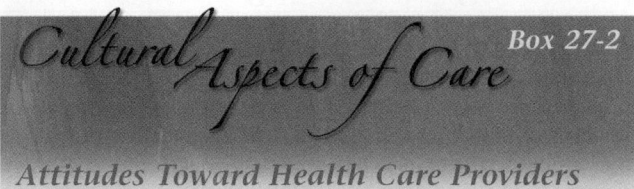

Cultural Aspects of Care   **Box 27-2**

Attitudes Toward Health Care Providers

Many Spanish-speaking clients are uncomfortable when treated by a physician. They often perceive the doctor's professional approach as being indifferent and impersonal. Spanish-speaking women may feel embarrassment and bashfulness in the presence of male health care professionals and may prefer to have a female conduct the interview or examination. A male would prefer not to be cared for by a female health provider. The impersonality of doctors and nurses and the infringement on one's modesty contribute to the anxiety and often reluctance of the client to cooperate.

Implications for Practice

- When possible, match the gender of a health care professional with gender of client when dealing with assessment of sexual needs, sex education, or individualized nursing interventions.
- Whenever possible, first establish a strong therapeutic relationship with client and family before discussing sexual health.
- Position yourself to maintain eye contact with client; avoid being separated from client by a desk or examination table.
- Continuously assess client's level of emotional, social, and psychological comfort with sexual health issues.

From Iannotta JG, editor: *Emerging issues in Hispanic health: summary of a workshop,* Washington, DC, 2002, The National Academies Press.

Abortion. Abortions have been performed since ancient times. The safety and availability of abortions in the United States improved after the 1973 Supreme Court decision *Roe v Wade*, which established the right of every woman to have an abortion legally. Abortions are safer and less costly when performed in the early weeks of pregnancy. This is possible with improved pregnancy testing and more accurate early diagnosis.

Abortion continues to be a hotly debated issue. Women and their partners who are faced with an unwanted pregnancy often consider abortion. The nurse can provide an environment in which the issue of abortion can be openly discussed, allowing exploration of various options with an unwanted pregnancy. The nurse should discuss religious, social, and personal issues in a nonjudgmental manner with clients. Reasons for choosing an abortion vary and may include terminating an unwanted pregnancy or aborting a fetus known to have birth defects. When abortion is chosen as a way of dealing with an unwanted pregnancy, the woman, and often her partner, may experience a sense of loss, grief, and/or guilt. Guilt may surface immediately or may be more covert and manifest as sexual dysfunction or altered perceptions.

Health care providers must sort out personal values related to abortion. The health care provider is entitled to personal views and should not be forced to participate in counseling or procedures contrary to beliefs and values. Nurses should choose specialties or places of employment where their personal values are not compromised and the care of a client in need of health care is not jeopardized.

STD Prevention. "Safe sex" is a term used to describe responsible sexual behavior aimed at preventing the spread of STDs, including AIDS. Responsible sexual behavior includes knowing one's sexual partner, being able to openly discuss sexual and drug-use history with the partner, not allowing one's decision to be influenced by drugs or alcohol, and using protective devices.

Alterations in Sexual Health

Infertility. A group with special health care needs is made up of individuals who want to conceive but cannot. Infertility is defined as the inability to conceive after 1 year of unprotected intercourse. A couple who want to conceive and cannot may experience a sense of failure and may feel that their bodies are somehow defective. A desire to become pregnant can grow until it permeates most waking moments. A woman or her partner may become preoccupied with creating just the right circumstances for conception. With advances in reproductive technology, infertile couples face many choices that involve religious and ethical values and financial constraints.

Choices for the infertile couple include pursuit of adoption, medical assistance with fertilization, or adapting to the probability of remaining childless. Organizations such as RESOLVE or international adoption groups can provide couples with support. RESOLVE, a national support group for couples with infertility, can be helpful in offering referral sources and support that a couple can use in planning.

Sexual Abuse. Sexual abuse is a widespread health problem in our society. Abuse crosses all gender, socioeconomic, age, and ethnic groups. Most often this abuse is at the hands of a former intimate partner or family member. Sexual abuse has far-ranging effects on physical and psychological functioning (Dickinson and others, 1999).

Evidence of sexual abuse in children may be uncovered during history taking or physical examination (see Chapter 32). Symptoms that should raise suspicion of the possibility of sexual abuse include a child showing an early, exaggerated awareness of sex or exhibiting seductive behavior toward adults; swelling or bruising of the external genitalia, anus, breasts, or buttocks; lacerations of or a foreign substance in the vagina or anus; and an STD in a child under 15 years of age.

Sexual abuse may begin, continue, or even intensify during pregnancy. The abuser may not fit any classic description. Cues that raise a question of possible sexual abuse include extreme jealousy and refusal to leave a woman's presence. The overall appearance may be of a very concerned and caring husband or boyfriend when the underlying dynamic is very different from this picture.

When abuse is recognized, support needs to be mobilized for the victim and the family. All family members may require therapy in situations of incest to promote healthy interactions and relationships. Rape victims may need to work through the crisis before feeling comfortable with intimate expressions of affection. The partner may need support in understanding this process and ways to assist the victim. Children who have been sexually molested need to understand that they are not at fault for the incident. The parents must understand that their response is critical to how the child reacts and adapts. The nurse may come in contact with clients confronting these stressors. Nurses are in an ideal position to assess occurrences of sexual violence and to educate individuals regarding community services. Nurses should be aware of resources for referral and support in the community.

Personal and Emotional Conflicts. Ideally, sex is a natural, spontaneous act that passes easily through a number of recognizable physiological stages and ends in one or more orgasms. In reality, this sequence of events is more the exception than the rule. Nurses encounter clients who have problems with one or more of the stages of sexual activity, including the feeling of wanting sex, the physiological processes and emotions of having sex, and the feelings experienced after sex. For example, some women who are taking antidepressants have noted that their ability to reach orgasm is negatively affected.

Sexual Dysfunction. Sexual dysfunction is common. Sexual dysfunction is defined as the absence of complete sexual functioning (Tables 27-1 and 27-2). A recent analysis of a large sample of U.S. men and women ages 18 to 59 found that 43% of women and 31% of men reported sexual dysfunction (Laumann and others, 1999). Sexual dysfunction is more prevalent in men and women with poor emotional and physical health. Sometimes the exact cause cannot be determined.

Running and Berndt (2003) report that erectile dysfunction (ED) affects about 30 million men in the United

Table 27-1	Types of Sexual Dysfunctions	
Category	**Type**	**Define**
Sexual desire disorders	Hypoactive sexual desire disorder	Persistent or recurrent deficiency or absence of sexual fantasies and desire for sexual activity.
	Sexual aversion disorder	Persistent or recurrent extreme aversion to, and avoidance of, all or almost all genital sexual contact with a sexual partner.
Sexual arousal disorders	Female sexual arousal disorder	Failure to attain or maintain the lubrication-swelling response or experience a subjective sense of sexual excitement and pleasure in a female during sexual activity.
	Male erectile disorder	Persistent or recurrent inability to attain, or maintain until completion of the sexual activity, an adequate erection.
Orgasmic disorders	Female orgasmic disorder (anorgasmia)	The recurrent and persistent inhibition of the female orgasm, as manifested by the absence or delay of orgasm following a period of sexual excitement judged adequate in intensity and duration to produce such a response.
	Male orgasmic disorder (retarded ejaculation)	Persistent or recurrent delay in, or absence of, orgasm following a normal sexual excitement phase during sexual activity that the clinician, taking into account the person's age, judges to be adequate in focus, intensity, and duration.
	Premature ejaculation	Persistent or recurrent ejaculation with minimal sexual stimulation or before, upon, or shortly after penetration and before the person wishes it.
Sexual pain disorders	Dyspareunia	Recurrent or persistent genital pain in either a male or female before, during, or after sexual intercourse that is not associated with vaginismus or with lack of lubrication.
	Vaginismus	An involuntary constriction of the outer one third of the vagina that prevents penile insertion and intercourse.
Sexual dysfunction due to drugs/diseases		With these disorders, the sexual dysfunction is judged to be caused by the direct physiological effects of a general medical condition or use of a substance.

Table 27-2	Predisposing Factors to Sexual Dysfunctions
Category	**Predisposing Factor**
Biological factors	Suggestive evidence exists of a relationship between serum testosterone and hypoactive sexual desire in men and increased libido in women.
	Certain medications, such as antihypertensives, antipsychotics, antidepressants, anxiolytics, and anticonvulsants may be linked to hypoactive sexual desire disorder.
	Erectile disorders in men may be affected by arteriosclerosis and diabetes.
	In women, consumption of alcohol, as well as certain medications, have been shown to affect ability to have orgasms.
	Various organic factors have also been associated with painful intercourse in both men and women.
Psychological factors	A number of psychological factors have been associated with sexual desire disorders, as well as with virtually all the sexual disorders. A few of these factors include religious orthodoxy, secret sexual deviations, fear of pregnancy, childhood sexual abuse, rape, fears, anxiety, and depression.
Transactional model of stress/adaptation	The etiology of sexual disorders is most likely influenced by multiple factors.

States and is often unreported. ED occurs more frequently in older men but can occur in younger men as well. Risk factors are similar to those for coronary artery disease (diabetes mellitus, hyperlipidemia, hypertension, hypothyroidism, chronic renal failure, smoking, obesity, alcohol abuse, and lack of exercise). The etiology of ED is often multifactorial. It can be caused by neurogenic problems, medications, or endocrine or psychogenic factors. An age-related decrease in testosterone may result in decreased tone of the erectile tissues.

Common issues of sexual dysfunction in women are vaginismus or orgasmic dysfunction. **Vaginismus** is a spastic contraction or tightening of the vagina during or before penetration for intercourse. Orgasmic dysfunction is the inability to achieve orgasm or difficulty attaining orgasm in certain situations. Physical causes such as infection, diabetes, neurological disease, drug or alcohol use, and aging changes are ruled out first. Unresolved anger, fear of pregnancy, and depression can cause a lack of desire and loss of interest in being sexual.

Critical Thinking

Successful critical thinking requires synthesis of knowledge, experience, information gathered from clients, critical thinking attitudes, and intellectual and professional standards. Clinical judgment requires the nurse to anticipate the information necessary, analyze the data, and make appropriate decisions regarding client care. Figure 27-2 demonstrates that the nurse must consider numerous critical thinking elements, as well as client assessment data, that contribute to appropriate nursing diagnoses.

In the case of sexuality the nurse integrates knowledge from nursing and other disciplines. The nurse must have a good understanding, for example, of the human sexual response, safe sex practices, and the risks and behaviors associated with sexual problems to anticipate how to assess a client and then how to interpret findings. Previous experience in caring for clients whose sexuality becomes threatened helps the nurse approach the next client in a more reflective and helpful way. Clients will have different customs and values from those of the nurse. Professional standards call for the nurse to respect each client as an individual. Critical thinking attitudes such as integrity require the nurse to recognize when his or her opinions and values are in conflict with those of the client and to consider how to proceed in a way that is mutually beneficial for the client and the nurse.

Sexuality and the Nursing Process

A person's sexuality has physical, psychological, social, and cultural elements. The nurse must assess all relevant elements to determine a client's sexual well-being. Many nurses find that they are uncomfortable talking about sexuality with clients. To increase comfort in discussing sexuality, the nurse should build a sound knowledge base and be willing to explore personal issues regarding sexuality. The nursing role in addressing sexual concerns can range from ongoing assessment to providing information to counseling to referral. Recognition that the nurse is not expected to have answers to all of the sexual issues and concerns identified can free the nurse to gather an appropriate sexual history database.

Assessment

Factors Affecting Sexuality. In gathering a sexual history, the nurse should consider physical, functional, relationship, lifestyle, and self-esteem factors that may influence sexual functioning. Sexual desire varies among individuals; some people want and enjoy sex every day, whereas others want sex only once a month, and still others have no sexual desire and are quite comfortable with that fact. Sexual desire becomes an issue if the person wants to feel sexual desire more often, if the person believes it is necessary to measure up to some cultural

norm, or if there is a discrepancy between the sexual desires of the partners in a relationship.

The nurse assesses for factors that typically can influence sexual desire. A person may experience a decrease in sexual desire for physical reasons, such as pain or discomfort during sexual activity. Even imagining that sex could hurt can lessen sexual desire. Minor illness, medications, and fatigue can also decrease sexual desire. Lifestyle factors, such as the use or abuse of alcohol, lack of sleep, lack of time, or the demands of caring for a new baby can also be influencing factors. Working parents, for example, may feel so overburdened that they perceive sexual advances from a partner as an additional demand on them. When the nurse identifies factors that can potentially affect sexual desire, he or she will confirm them with the client and then determine the extent to which sexual function is impaired.

Self-concept issues (see Chapter 26), including identity, body image, role performance, and self-esteem, affect a client's sexuality. Poor body image, particularly when magnified by feelings of rejection or by body-altering surgery, may result in diminished or absent sexual desire. A person's self-esteem can lead to conflicts involving sexuality. If a healthy sense of a sexual self and comfortable sexual behaviors have not been developed, sexuality may cause negative feelings or lead to the suppression of sexual feelings. Sexual self-esteem can be lowered in many ways. Low sexual self-esteem will negatively affect a person's self-concept. Rape, incest, and physical or emotional abuse leave deep scars. Low sexual self-esteem can also result from lack of adequate sex education, negative role models, and attempts to live up to unrealistic personal or cultural expectations.

Issues in a relationship can also affect sexual desire. After the initial glow of a new relationship has faded, couples may find that they are faced with major differences in their values or lifestyles. The degree to which they still feel close to each other and interact on an intimate level depends on their ability to negotiate and compromise. Thus communication between sexual partners plays a crucial role in sexual satisfaction within a relationship.

Sexual Health History. When taking a nursing history, the nurse should consider including a few questions related to sexual functioning to determine whether the client has any sexual concerns. These questions can be incorporated in the review of systems and addressed in a routine, matter-of-fact manner. The nurse needs to understand the reasons for the question and be able to provide them to the client on request. An opening statement such as "Sex is an important part of life and can be affected by our health status and vice versa. To better understand your health, it is useful to know . . ." is a possible introduction to these questions. Other questions for adults might include the following:

- How do you feel about the sexual aspects of your life?
- Have you noticed any changes in the way you feel about yourself (as a man, woman, husband, or wife)?
- How has your illness, medication, or surgery affected your sex life?
- It is not unusual for people with your condition to be experiencing some sexual changes. Have you noticed any changes, or do you have any concerns?

KNOWLEDGE

- Ways to phrase questions about sexuality
- Sexual development and human sexual response patterns
- Impact of self-concept on sexuality
- Sexual orientation
- Effective contraceptive methods
- STDs and associated risk factors
- Safe sex practices
- Behaviors suggestive of current or past sexual abuse
- Diseases and/or medications that affect sexual function
- Interpersonal relationship factors and sexual functioning

EXPERIENCE

- Communicating with clients and developing rapport
- Working with clients and exploring sexual concerns (e.g., working in OB-GYN setting)
- Personal sexual experience and response

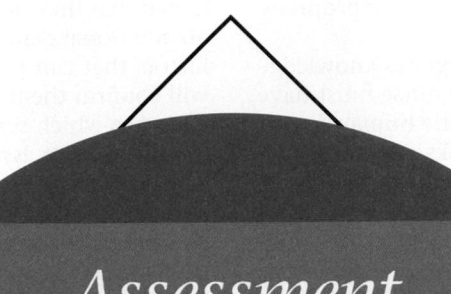

Assessment

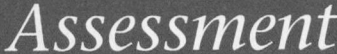

- Assess the client's developmental stage with regard to sexuality
- Perform physical assessment of urogenital area
- Determine the client's sexual concerns
- Assess the impact of high risk behaviors, safe sex practices, and use of contraception
- Assess medical conditions and medications that might affect sexual functioning

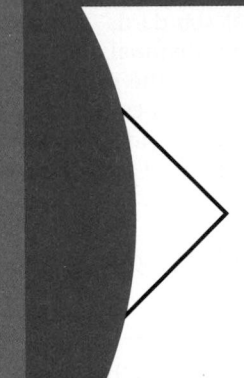

STANDARDS

- Apply intellectual standards of relevance and plausibility for care to be acceptable to the client
- Safeguard the client's right to privacy by judiciously protecting information of a confidential nature
- Apply ethic of care

ATTITUDES

- Display curiosity; consider why a client might behave or respond in a particular manner
- Display integrity; your beliefs and values may differ from client's; admit to any inconsistencies in your values and in the client's
- Take risks if necessary to explore both personal sexual issues and concerns and those of the client

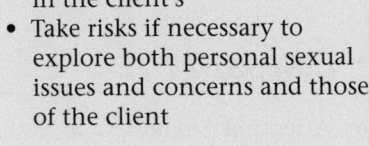

FIGURE **27–2** Critical thinking model for sexuality assessment.

When caring for older adults, the nurse may adjust his or her assessment approach. When the nurse gathers a sexual history from an older adult, it is important to keep in mind that the older adult may have difficulty discussing intimate details with health care providers. The nurse has the responsibility to help maintain the sexuality of older adults by offering the opportunity to discuss any concerns. Often, asking questions on the topic of sexuality in a comfortable, relaxed manner facilitates older adults' discussing their sexual needs.

Conducting a sexual assessment of children and adolescents provides special challenges for health care providers. Issues of language, of promoting normal development while not minimizing problems, of screening for sexual concerns while not unduly alarming them, are all common challenges. In addition, the sexual counseling of minors raises ethical and legal issues regarding the client's rights to health care and education on the one hand, and the parents' or guardian's right to supervise information on the other. Use of an open, positive, interested disposition when introducing sexual questions is helpful.

In light of the prevalence of domestic violence and sexual abuse, questions relating to abusive relationships can be important. Questions that address domestic violence or abuse should be addressed to the client in private. A question such as "Are you in a relationship in which someone is hurting you?" may open the door for a client to reveal present or previous abuse. An additional question such as "Has anyone ever forced you to have sex you did not wish to participate in?" may more specifically open the door for the client to discuss concerns. Recognizing both subjective and objective signs and symptoms of abuse can aid in recognition of this too common problem (Box 27-3).

It is also significant to explore, while gathering the sexual history for sexually active clients, the client's use of contraception and safe sex practices. Adolescents may respond to a comment that allows them to know that having questions related to sexuality is normal. A lead-in could be, "Many adolescents have questions about STDs or whether their bodies are developing at the right rate. Do you have any questions about sex or other things?"

Some individuals are too embarrassed or do not know how to ask sexual questions directly. The nurse may detect clues that a person has questions if the person expresses concern about how his or her partner may respond now or if the person makes a sexual comment or joke. Observing for and listening to concerns about sexuality takes practice. With experience the nurse develops skill in clarifying and paraphrasing to help individuals express sexual concerns. By including sexuality in the nursing history, the nurse acknowledges that sexuality is an important component of health and creates an opportunity for the person to discuss sexual concerns.

Sexual Dysfunction. Many illnesses, injuries, medications and aging changes can have a negative effect on sexual health. In some cases, sexual dysfunctions may result that can be temporary or permanent. The nurse applies a knowledge base of those conditions that may cause sexual dysfunction while assessing a client's risks. Awareness of the possible effects of physical problems, altered self-concept, medications, and the factors addressed thus far on sexual functioning assist the nurse in conducting a thorough assessment. A client may also bring up the topic of sexual dysfunction, or issues may become evident as the client answers other nursing history questions.

Physical Assessment. The physical examination is important in evaluating the cause of sexual concerns or problems and may be the best opportunity to teach an individual about sexuality. In examining a woman's breasts and the external and internal genitalia, the nurse has the opportunity to assess the woman's reaction, answer questions, and provide information about the examination of anatomical and physiological structures. A woman can learn to perform a breast self-examination during physical assessment (see Chapter 32). In addition, the nurse may choose to teach Kegel exercises (Box 27-4). These exercises strengthen the pubococcygeus muscle. Toning of this muscle often decreases as a result of stretching during childbirth and loss of general elasticity during aging. Maintaining good tone helps prevent bladder or rectal prolapse into the vagina (cystocele or rectocele), reduces problems with later urinary incontinence, and can enhance sexual enjoyment through and beyond menopause. During physical assessment of the genitalia, men can be taught to perform testicular self-examination (see Chapter 32). Knowledge of normal scrotal anatomical structures aids men in detecting signs of testicular cancer. The nurse can instruct both men and women on signs and symptoms of STDs during the examination when clients' histories suggest risks for STD.

Client Expectations. As in the case of any client assessment, it is important to understand the client's expectations regarding his or her care. Questions such as "What would you like to have happen in regard to [expressed concern]?" and "What initial steps might you take?" can help the person identify desired outcomes. It is important for the nurse to set aside personal views and not assume what a client's expectations might be.

Box **27-3**	**Signs and Symptoms That May Indicate Current Sexual Abuse or a History of Sexual Abuse**

Bruises	Premenstrual syndrome
Lacerations	Sleep pattern disturbances
Abrasions	Nightmares
Burns	Repetitive dreams
Frequent visits to health care providers	Insomnia
	Depression
Vague symptoms	Anxiety
Headaches	Fear
Gastrointestinal problems	Decreased self-esteem
Eating disorders	Difficulty developing trust
Abdominal pain	Difficulties with intimate relationships
Vaginal pain	
Dysmenorrhea	Substance abuse

Modified from Bohn D, Holz K: Sequelae of abuse: health effects of childhood sexual abuse, domestic battering, and rape, *J Nurse Midwifery* 41(6):442, 1996.

Kegel Exercises

Objective

- Client will demonstrate ability to tighten pubococcygeus muscle and will verbalize methods to assess correct procedures and increasing strength.

Teaching Strategies

- Explain method to identify proper muscle contraction: client sits on toilet with knees far apart and tightens muscles to stop the flow of urine.
- After muscle is identified, instruct client to contract muscle for a count of 3, hold and release for a count of 3, and

repeat this 10 times. Client should do this about 5 times a day.
- Explain that within first week of exercises, client should assess if proper muscle contraction is occurring by placing two fingers in vagina to identify if tightening can be felt or asking partner to identify during sexual intercourse when muscle is tightened.

Evaluation

- Ask client if she has identified pubococcygeus muscle via finger insertion or partner response.
- During vaginal bimanual examination, ask client to do exercises and assess muscle tone.

Assessment Activities	Defining Characteristics	Nursing Diagnosis
Observe readiness to discuss sex through verbalization (e.g., "When can I return to life as normal?" or "There goes my love life") or behavior (e.g., exhibitionism).	Client verbalizes concern that sexual activity may cause another myocardial infarction or death.	Ineffective sexuality patterns related to fear of recurrent myocardial infarction or death during intercourse.
Ask client and spouse about previous level and method of sexual expression (e.g., frequency, initiator).		
Observe for affectionate behavior (e.g., touching, hand holding, kissing).	Client's spouse exhibits reluctance to touch client.	
In privacy, ask spouse about perceptions of recovery and return to full functioning.	Spouse verbalizes concern that client will need continuous care, attention, and protection.	
Observe for anxiety (e.g., hand wringing).	Client maintains eye contact, shifts position frequently.	

Nursing Diagnosis

After completing an assessment and applying critical thought to the diagnostic process (Box 27-5), the nurse selects diagnoses applicable to the client's needs. Possible nursing diagnoses related to sexual functioning are listed below:

- Anxiety
- Ineffective coping
- Interrupted family processes
- Deficient knowledge (contraception/STDs)
- Sexual dysfunction
- Ineffective sexuality patterns
- Social isolation
- Risk for other-directed violence
- Risk for self-directed violence

Clues that may signal at-risk or an actual nursing diagnosis related to sexuality include history of surgery of reproductive organs, changes in appearance, past or current physical or sexual abuse, chronic illness, and developmental milestones such as puberty or menopause. When making nursing diagnoses related to sexual dysfunction, the nurse must have assessed anatomical, physiological, sociocultural, ethical, and situational issues thoroughly.

As with making any nursing diagnosis, the process in regard to sexuality is often one of clarification with the client to establish that the nursing diagnosis defining characteristics in fact exist and that the client perceives a problem or difficulty with regard to sexuality. Determining the etiological or contributing factors is important, to focus effective planning and to select appropriate nursing interventions. For example, the nursing interventions appropriate for the nursing diagnosis of *chronic low self-esteem* would be different for different etiological factors. *Self-esteem disturbance related to chronic, recurring herpes infection* would lead to counseling and education on how to maintain safe sexual practices. In contrast, *self-esteem disturbance related to sexual abuse* would require counseling

KNOWLEDGE

- PLISSIT model
- Community resources for sex education information
- Community resources for contraception and STD treatment and counseling

EXPERIENCE

- Establishing rapport with diverse clients
- Care of clients with HIV infection
- Care of clients with various sexual orientations

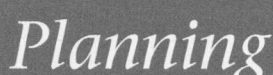

Planning

- Create an atmosphere in which the client can explore sexual concerns
- Refer to appropriate resources for exploration of sexual concerns
- Explore the client's understanding, beliefs, and attitudes regarding sexuality and sexual functioning

STANDARDS

- Maintain the client's dignity and identity
- Promote an environment in which the client's values, customs, and spiritual beliefs are respected
- Report STDs as required by law
- Report cases of suspected abuse as required by law

ATTITUDES

- Think independently; explore various approaches to address the issue/problem
- Be creative and try unique interventions
- Demonstrate perseverance—changes in self-concept often happen slowly; continue to support the vision that change is possible
- Take risks by asking about the client's concerns even when the topic is sensitive

FIGURE **27–3** Critical thinking model for sexuality planning.

and referral to community resources (e.g., crisis services or sexual abuse support group).

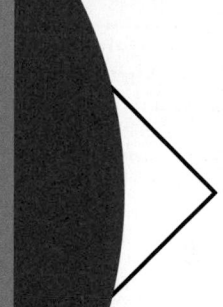 *Planning*

Goals and Outcomes. During planning the nurse again synthesizes information from multiple resources (Figure 27-3). Critical thinking ensures that the client's plan of care integrates all that the nurse knows about the individual, as well as critical thinking elements as they pertain to sexual-

ity. Professional standards are especially important to consider when the nurse develops a plan of care. Maintaining a client's dignity and identity is a significant consideration. For example, conveying respect for a client's gender preferences by including a lesbian or gay partner in the plan to the degree that the client wishes can assist the client in maintaining his or her identity and dignity.

The nurse develops an individualized plan of care for each nursing diagnosis (see care plan). The nurse and client together set realistic goals for care. Expected outcomes need to be individualized and realistic. For example,

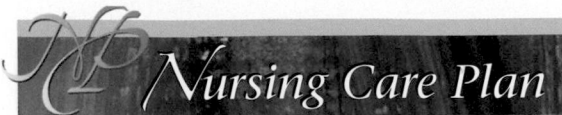

Sexual Dysfunction

Assessment

Mr. Clements is a 46-year-old black client who was last seen in the office 2 months ago, when he was found to have mild hypertension and was given a prescription for propranolol (Inderal). His blood pressure today is 122/82 mm Hg.

Jack Constant is a 25-year-old nursing student who goes in to talk with Mr. Clements after reading his records, which include the recent diagnosis of mild hypertension, the order for propranolol, and the current blood pressure reading of 122/82 mm Hg. The record also indicates that Mr. Clements is married and living with his wife.

In talking with Mr. Clements, Jack tells him of the improvement in his blood pressure since his last visit. He inquires if Mr. Clements is taking his medication regularly. Mr. Clements reports that he has been taking his medication regularly. He relates that it scared him when his blood pressure was up because both of his parents had died of strokes. Jack then inquires if he has noted any side effects from the medicine. Mr. Clements says not really, except he is maybe a little more tired than he use to be. Jack then asks the question he formulated, "Some people find that certain blood pressure medications affect their sexual performance. Have you noticed any changes in sexual functioning since you began your medication?" Mr. Clements replies that he finds he just is not very interested in sex any more and that this is becoming somewhat of a problem between him and his wife. Her interest does not seem to have waned at all, he tells Jack.

Assessment Activities	Findings/Defining Characteristics
Ascertain when Mr. Clements began noticing his decreased interest in sex.	He responds that it was at about the same time he started taking propranolol.
Ask Mr. Clements about his sexual relationship with his wife before taking propranolol.	He states they used to have intercourse 1 to 3 times per week.
Ask Mr. Clements if he has noticed any changes in his erect penis.	He states he sometimes has trouble having an erection.
Ask Mr. Clements if there have there been any changes to his lifestyle since the first of the year.	He denies any changes.

Nursing Diagnosis: Sexual dysfunction related to side effects of antihypertensive medication.

Planning

Goal	Expected Outcomes* **Sexual Functioning**
Client will express satisfaction with sexual relationship with wife within 1 month.	Client will report a renewed interest in sex within 1 month. Client will report resolution of problem with impotence.

*Outcome classification labels from Moorhead S, Johnson M, Maas M: *Nursing outcomes classification (NOC),* ed 3, St. Louis, 2004, Mosby.

Interventions†

Sexual Counseling
- Establish trust and respect with client. Offer privacy during conversations.
- Discuss possible effects of antihypertensive on sexual functioning, and encourage client to discuss sexual concerns with physician.
- Encourage client to discuss concerns with his wife. Role play so client can practice ways to approach concerns.

Anxiety Reduction
- Assure client that there are other blood pressure medications available that can maintain blood pressure control and that do not negatively affect sexual function.

Rationale

Conveys sense of caring, increasing likelihood of client's ability to express concerns fully (Ross and others, 2000).

Helps client to understand possible cause for sexual difficulties. Gives client important option to review with physician (Riley, 1999).

Many of the sexual problems in relationships involve poor communication (Finan, 1997).

Gives client sense of control knowing that there are options and that blood pressure can continue to be safely managed (Running and Berndt, 2003).

†Intervention classification labels from Dochterman JM, Bulechek GM: *Nursing interventions classification (NIC),* ed 4, St. Louis, 2004, Mosby.

Evaluation

Nursing Actions	Client Response/Finding	Achievement of Outcome
Ask Mr. Clements if his sexual relations with his wife has increased during return office visit.	He responds that since he has been on new medication his interest in sex is back to normal and he has no trouble now having an erection.	Mr. Clements reports sexual interest and function with the new medication.

while caring for a client with a nursing diagnosis of *sexual dysfunction related to dyspareunia or hypoactive sexual desire,* the nurse and client develop a goal to be free from pain or discomfort during sexual intercourse. Expected outcomes for this goal may include that the client will:

- Report decreased anxiety and greater satisfaction with sexual activity
- Consistently use a water-soluble lubricant before sexual intercourse
- Avoid the use of feminine hygiene products that destroy the natural flora and secretions of the vaginal walls

A concept map is another method that is useful in organizing client care (Figure 27-4). This concept map shows the relationship of a medical diagnosis (decreased libido and depression) with the four nursing diagnoses identified from the client assessment data. In addition, the map shows the links and relationship with the nursing diagnosis. For example, ineffective coping affects and contributes to social isolation; and as long as the client

has ineffective coping the social isolation continues or perhaps worsens.

Setting Priorities. A useful framework for guiding planning is the PLISSIT model developed by Annon (1976). In this model there are progressively more involved levels of intervention. The *P* stands for permission giving. During assessment the nurse's questions can bring up the topic of sexuality and can give the individual permission to talk about sexual concerns. *LI* stands for limited information, which involves providing basic information regarding sexuality and sexual functioning. An example would be discussing nocturnal emissions with a prepubescent boy to minimize fear that might develop if the boy did not know this was a normal part of development. *SS* stands for specific suggestions, whereby the nurse provides specific suggestions regarding a sexual concern or issue. For example, a postmenopausal woman might be concerned about her lack of vaginal lubrication. The nurse might

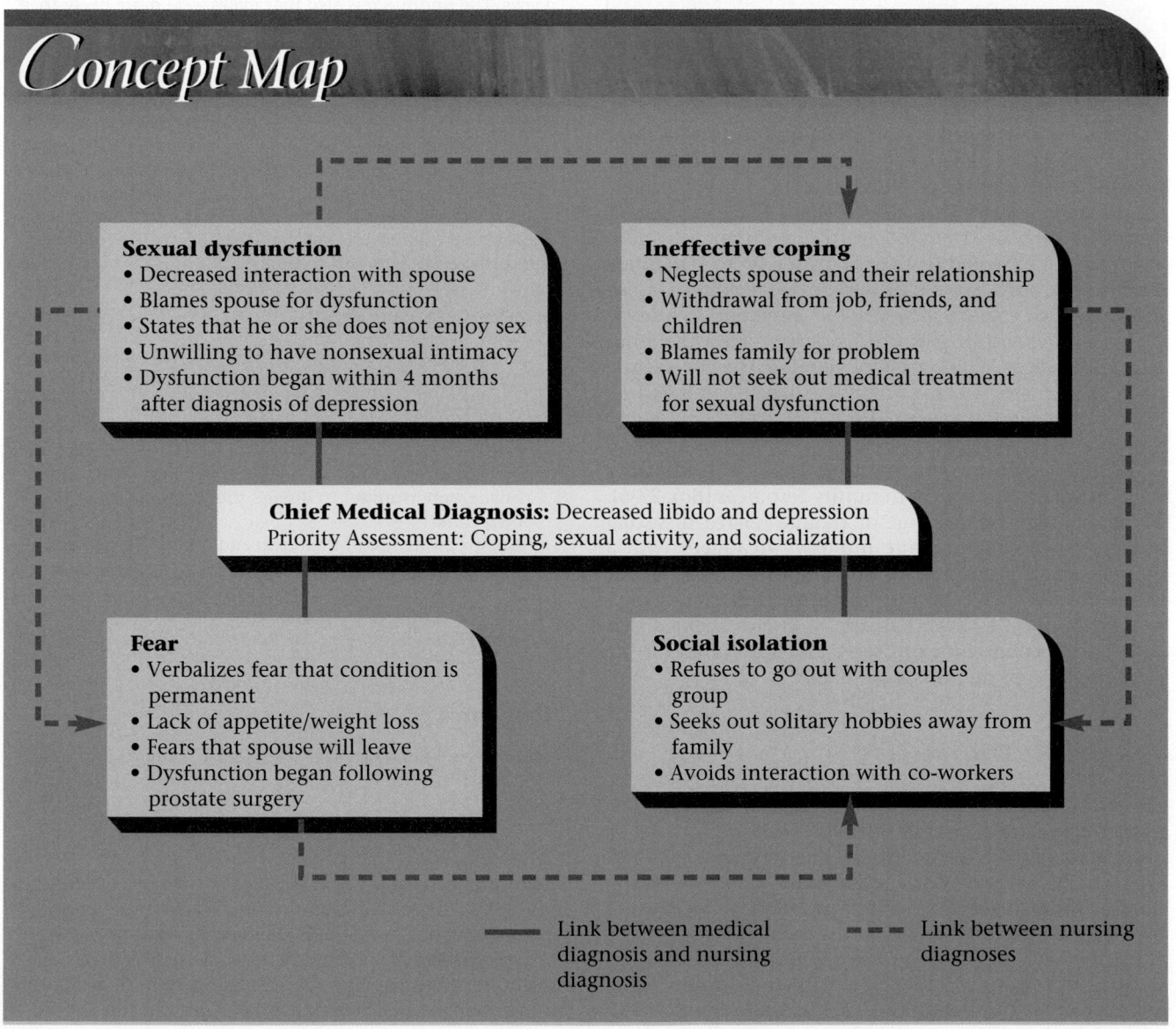

Concept Map

Sexual dysfunction
- Decreased interaction with spouse
- Blames spouse for dysfunction
- States that he or she does not enjoy sex
- Unwilling to have nonsexual intimacy
- Dysfunction began within 4 months after diagnosis of depression

Ineffective coping
- Neglects spouse and their relationship
- Withdrawal from job, friends, and children
- Blames family for problem
- Will not seek out medical treatment for sexual dysfunction

Chief Medical Diagnosis: Decreased libido and depression
Priority Assessment: Coping, sexual activity, and socialization

Fear
- Verbalizes fear that condition is permanent
- Lack of appetite/weight loss
- Fears that spouse will leave
- Dysfunction began following prostate surgery

Social isolation
- Refuses to go out with couples group
- Seeks out solitary hobbies away from family
- Avoids interaction with co-workers

—— Link between medical diagnosis and nursing diagnosis

– – – Link between nursing diagnoses

FIGURE **27–4** Concept map for client with decreased libido and depression.

Box 27-6   Community Resources Relating to Sexuality

Planned Parenthood
Sex therapists
Clinical psychologists
Social workers
Health department (often for both family planning and STDs)
Groups that provide education/services for those with partic-
ular conditions include:
    American Diabetes Association
    American Heart Association
    Muscular Dystrophy Association
    Muscular Sclerosis Society
Sexual abuse support groups
Women's shelters (for those who have been physically and/or
sexually abused)
Hot lines for help (will have lists of community support
resources)
Impotence Resource Center, www.impotence.org
Resolve Inc national office, www.resolve.org/international
North America Menopause Society, www.menopause.org

---

suggest use of a water-based lubricant during sexual intercourse, or the concern expressed might be one that the
nurse is not equipped to address. In this case the nurse
should refer to another health care provider. The *IT*
stands for intensive therapy. At this level of intervention,
the nurse's role would be to refer the client to a qualified
practitioner, such as a social worker or sex counselor, for
individualized therapy. The level of intervention a nurse
plans will depend in part on his or her own experience
and knowledge. When a client requires specific suggestions or intensive therapy, the nurse may recommend referral of the client to a specialist.

Continuity of Care. Planning in the area of sexuality
may include referrals to community resources (Box 27-6).
Sexual conflicts in marriage or trauma related to sexual
abuse or incest may require intensive treatment with a
mental health professional or certified sex therapist. For
the woman who is currently in an abusive relationship,
most communities have battered women's shelters that
can provide counseling and serve as a safe haven for the
woman while further plans are made.

Implementation

The nurse's role includes the promotion of sexual health
as a component of overall wellness. The nurse can promote sexual health by identifying clients at increased risk
(Box 27-7), by providing appropriate information, by
helping individuals gain insight into their problems, and
by exploring methods to deal with them effectively.

Health Promotion. Helping clients gain a healthy sexuality involves consideration of factors that influence sexual satisfaction. The nurse needs to educate clients about
sexual health, including measures for contraception and
prevention of STDs. Regular breast self-examinations,

Research Highlight   Box 27-7

The Effect of Social Stigma and Shame on STD-Isolated Care

Research Focus

At-risk clients who perceive that they will be judged adversely
because of STDs are less likely to seek appropriate care.

Research Abstract

The purpose of this study was to assess the relationship between social stigma and shame associated with seeking treatment for sexually transmitted diseases (STDs). Participants included 847 males and 1126 females (mean age was 24.9 years)
recruited from clinics, community-based organizations, and
through street intercept in seven cities throughout the
United States. The STD-related stigma and the STD-related
shame scales were administered during face-to-face interviews. The findings revealed that males were more likely than
females to have suspected gonorrhea in the past, but females
were more likely than males to have received a gonorrhea or
human immunodeficiency virus (HIV) test in the past year. A
significantly higher proportion of males were classified in the
"high shame" group. Gonorrhea testing was related to female
gender, younger age, enrollment from a health facility, health
service use in the past year, suspicion of gonorrhea, and low
levels of STD-related stigma. HIV testing was related to older
age, health service use, gonorrhea testing, and low levels of
STD-related stigma. STD-related shame was not related to
gonorrhea testing or HIV testing.

Evidence-Based Practice

- STD-related stigma, rather than shame, decreases the likelihood of a person being tested for gonorrhea or HIV.
- Nurses have the potential through education to promote
  community norms of healthy sexuality and STD-related
  care. They can act as advocates for STD-related care and
  prevention programs in high schools and colleges, organizing opportunities to discuss the issues of sexual at-risk
  behaviors.
- Nurses' awareness of their own and others' feelings and attitudes about STDs will enable them to respond more effectively to the needs of the client.
- Use of a caring, open, nonjudgmental manner with clients
  with STDs will increase the likelihood of a person seeking
  treatment.

Reference

Fortenberry M and others: Relationship of stigma and shame
to gonorrhea and HIV screening, *Am J Public Health* 92(3):378,
2002.

---

mammograms, and Papanicolaou (Pap) smear are important sexual health measures for women that should be
encouraged, as are testicular self-examinations for men.

   Exploring an individual's values, discussing levels of satisfaction, and providing sex education require good communication skills. The environment and timing should be
structured to provide privacy, comfort, and uninterrupted
time. For example, when discussing methods of contraception with a woman, the nurse should provide comfortable

chairs in a private area rather than discussing this in the examination room when the client is only partially clothed.

Topics of education vary, depending on the defining characteristics and related factors in the nursing diagnoses. Client education may provide guidelines for normal development; for example, the nurse might talk to a toddler's mother regarding a new baby, to a school-age child regarding appearance of pubic hair, or to a 60-year-old man regarding delayed ejaculation. Details of physiological changes should be provided as a part of general health care. Providing client education gives permission for clients to raise questions or concerns regarding personal functioning.

Discussions of healthy sex should include contraception when talking with both men and women of childbearing age. The discussion should include desire for children, usual sexual practices, and acceptable methods of contraception. Factors that need to be considered when discussing contraception include frequency of sexual activity, comfort with genital touching, comfort with sharing contraceptive responsibility with the partner, and comfort with interruption of sexual acts. Formulating questions related to sexuality can be uncomfortable for the nurse. The way in which questions are asked will depend on numerous factors, including the rapport between the client and the nurse, the comfort of both the client and the nurse when discussing sexually related topics, and the client's reason for the health care contact. The nurse might ask, "Are you using contraception with your partner now?" and then follow up, based on the client's answer. If the method of contraception is one that requires participation at the time of intercourse, such as condoms, foam, or a diaphragm, the nurse might ask, "What is it like for you to stop lovemaking to use contraception?" or "Some people find it difficult to use a method consistently that requires remembering or effort each time to actually use the method—has that been a problem for you?" or "How frequently do you have intercourse without protection?" The questions will need to flow from each situation. For clients who do not have a regular contraceptive method, who do not have a reliable contraceptive method, or who are not satisfied with their current method, the various methods of contraception should be reviewed to provide necessary information for an informed choice. The best method is the one that the person will use consistently.

Individuals having more than one sex partner or whose partner has other sexual experiences need to learn more about safe sex practices. Information should be provided regarding STD symptoms and transmission, use of condoms, and risky sexual activities (e.g., trauma from penile-anal sex). An area to consider in discussing sexual relating is the emotional risks within a relationship. Role play can be a useful educational tool in helping a person learn to say no or negotiate with a partner to use a condom.

Also significant in maintaining sexual health is regular health examinations. Often STDs, particularly chlamydia and gonorrhea in women and chlamydia in men, are asymptomatic and are only diagnosed during a physical examination with appropriate laboratory work. The annual health examination also provides an easy opportunity to discuss contraception and safe sex practices.

Acute Care. Nursing interventions that address alterations in sexuality generally are aimed at raising awareness, assisting in clarification of issues or concerns, and/or providing information. Nurses who have pursued specialized education in sexual functioning and counseling may provide more intensive sex therapy. Nurses should recognize when an individual's needs exceed their expertise and provide appropriate referral.

The initial intervention often includes exploring present sexual practices with the individual. The individual should be encouraged to investigate and acknowledge social and ethical values and consider the role of sexuality in his or her self-concept. When there is significant discrepancy between values and past or present practices, the person may need referral for more intensive counseling.

Major developmental crises (e.g., puberty, **climacteric,** or menopause) should prompt education about effects on sexuality. Situational crises such as a life change with pregnancy, illness, extreme financial stress, placement of a spouse in a nursing home, or loss and grief affect sexuality. Effects may last for days, months, or years and can generate performance anxieties that lead to continued sexual dysfunction. If an individual is prepared for possible changes in sexual functioning, performance anxieties may be minimized.

Illness and surgery are situational stressors that often affect a person's sexuality. During periods of illness, individuals may experience major physical changes, the effects of drugs or treatments, the emotional stress of a prognosis, concern about future functioning, and separation from significant others. Situational stressors could include survival of a heart attack (myocardial infarction); cancer diagnosis and treatment; or chronic disease such as diabetes, multiple sclerosis, or Parkinson's disease. The nurse should not assume that sexual functioning is not a concern because of an individual's age or severity of prognosis. When concerns are assessed and identified, they can be addressed in the context of the individual's value system.

In response to identified concerns, the nurse may initiate discussion in pertinent areas. It may be appropriate to discuss sexual practices such as oral-genital sex or mutual masturbation as methods of expressing intimate affection when penile-vaginal intercourse is contraindicated. A partner experiencing joint pain may appreciate a discussion of various positions for intercourse. Use of fantasy or a sense of playfulness may add new romance or stimulation to a long-term relationship. A couple may need confirmation or assurance that the thoughts and acting out of nonharmful fantasy is normal and healthy.

Restorative Care. In the home environment it is important to assist individuals in creating an environment that is comfortable for sexual activity. This may involve making recommendations for ways to arrange the bedroom to accommodate any limitations the individual may have. For example, wheelchair-bound individuals may prefer being able to move the chair close to the side of the bed at an angle that allows for more ease in touching and caressing. Suggestions regarding how to accommodate barriers such as Foley catheters or drainage tubes can contribute to sexual activity.

In the long-term care setting, facilities should make proper arrangements for privacy during residents' sexual experiences (Lueckenotte, 2000). The ideal situation is to set up a pleasant room that can be used for a variety of activities but may also be reserved for private visits with a spouse or partner. If this is not feasible, making arrangements for the roommate of a client to have another place to be can allow a couple time alone.

Evaluation

Client Care. The nurse will review client responses to interventions to determine if goals and outcome criteria have been met (Figure 27-5). Critical thinking ensures that the nurse applies what is known about sexuality and the client's unique situation.

Having follow-up discussions with the client or spouse will determine whether goals and outcomes have been achieved. Sexuality is felt more than observed, and sexual expression requires an intimacy that is not amenable to observation. Clients can be asked to relate risk factors, verbalize concerns, and share experiences and their level of satisfaction. The nurse can also observe behavioral cues, such as eye contact, posture, and extraneous hand movements, that indicate comfort or suggest continued

anxiety or concern as topics are addressed. As outcomes are evaluated, the individual, spouse, and nurse may need to modify expectations or establish more appropriate time frames in which to achieve the target goals. All involved may need to be reminded of the individual nature of sexual expression and the multiple factors that affect perceptions and responses. Sexual wellness is not an absolute. An individual must define what is acceptable and satisfying. The partner's level of sexual satisfaction must also be considered. Sexual performance is seldom the exclusive focus of sexual satisfaction. Open communication and positive self-esteem are essential factors in effectively resolving concerns.

Client Expectations. In evaluating the outcomes of interventions related to sexuality, the nurse must consult with the client. Resolution of sexual concerns must meet the client's perceptions of improvement. Sexuality is not an absolute. An individual must define what is acceptable and satisfying. In considering the status of sexual health, the client's partner's perceptions of sexual satisfaction are also significant.

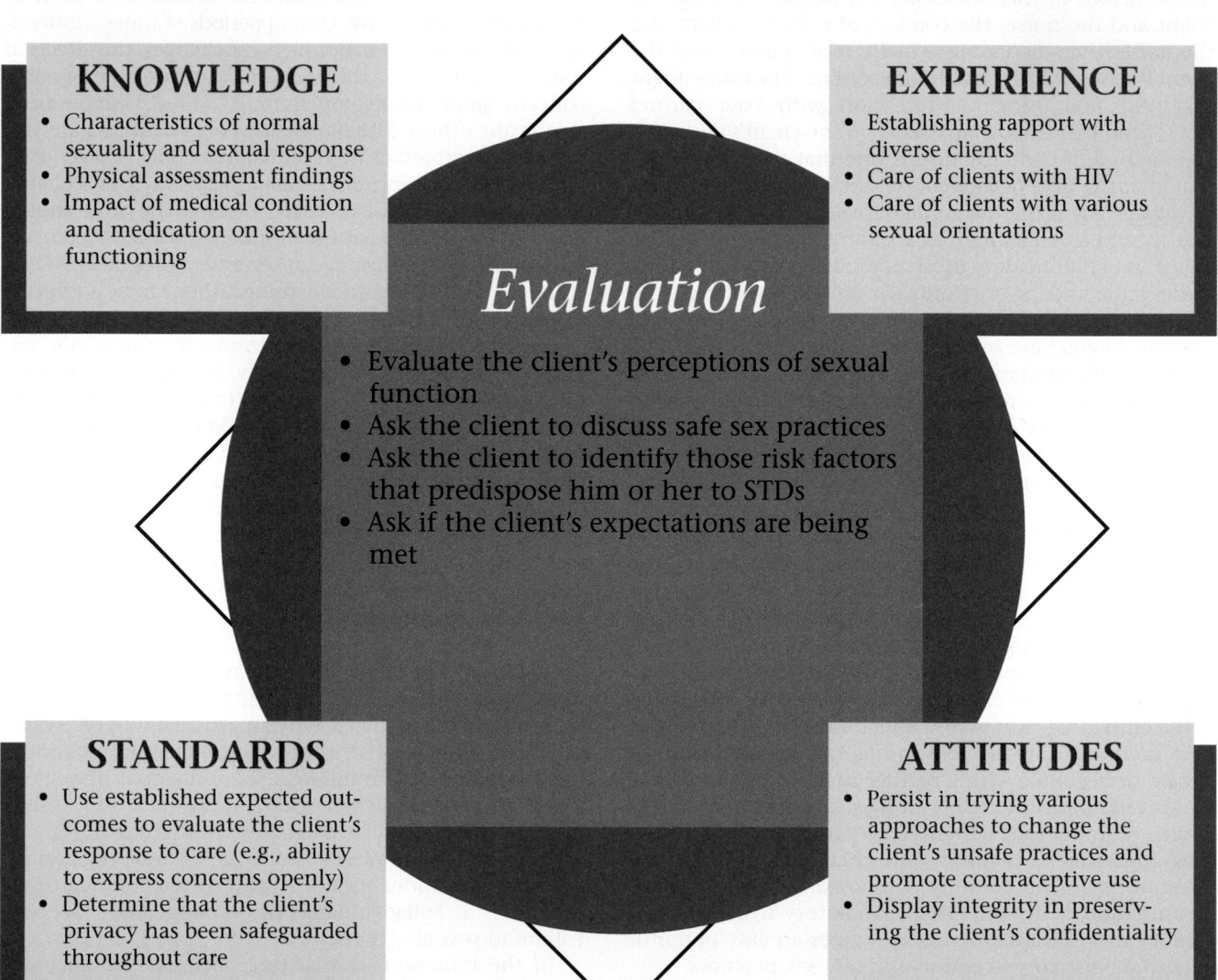

FIGURE 27–5 Critical thinking model for sexuality evaluation.

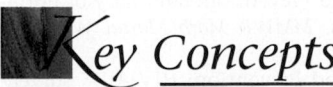

Key Concepts

- Sexuality is related to all dimensions of health; therefore sexual concerns or problems should be addressed as a part of nursing care.
- Sexuality is a part of each individual's identity and includes biological sex, gender identity, gender role, and sexual partner preference.
- Attitudes toward sexuality vary widely and are influenced by religious beliefs, society's values, the media, the family, and other factors.
- Nurses' attitudes toward sexuality also vary and may differ from those of clients; nurses should be sensitive to clients' sexual preferences and needs.
- Sexual response cycle includes three phases: desire, arousal, and orgasm.
- Sexual development is a process beginning in infancy and involves some level of sexual behavior or growth in all developmental stages.
- The physiological sexual response changes with aging, but aging does not lead to diminished sexuality.
- Sexual health involves physical and psychosocial aspects and contributes to an individual's sense of self-worth and positive interpersonal relationships.
- Sexual dysfunctions can result from an easily identified etiology or varied and complex etiologies.
- Interventions for sexual dysfunctions depend on the condition and the client; interventions may include giving information, teaching specific exercises, improving communication between partners, and referral to a knowledgeable professional.
- Choice and use of effective contraceptive methods are affected by sexual biases, comfort with touching genitalia, desire for future fertility, financial status, ability to plan sexual contact, and ability to communicate with the sex partner regarding sensitive issues.
- A brief review of sexuality should be included in every nursing assessment of a client's level of wellness.
- Most nursing interventions to enhance a client's sexual health involve providing information and education.
- Evaluation is formulated based on discussion with the individual and possibly his or her partner regarding satisfaction with sexual functioning and through observations of nonverbal behaviors that suggest anxiety.

Key Terms

Climacteric, *p. 538*
Condom, *p. 526*
Contraception, *p. 524*
Diaphragm, *p. 526*
Dyspareunia, *p. 525*
Gay, *p. 527*
Gender identity, *p. 524*
Gender roles, *p. 523*
Heterosexual, *p. 524*
Homosexual, *p. 524*
Infertility, *p. 527*
Intercourse, *p. 523*
Lesbian, *p. 526*
Myotonia, *p. 525*
Perimenopausal, *p. 525*
Sexual dysfunction, *p. 527*
Sexual health, *p. 523*
Sexual orientation, *p. 523*
Sexual response cycle, *p. 524*
Sexuality, *p. 523*

Sexually transmitted diseases (STDs), *p. 524*
Sterilization, *p. 526*
Tubal ligation, *p. 526*
Vaginismus, *p. 530*
Vasectomy, *p. 526*
Vasocongestion, *p. 525*

Critical Thinking Exercises

1. Your current clinical experience is in a community health care setting. You are conducting the initial interview with a 48-year-old man who started taking antihypertensives 2 weeks ago. You take his blood pressure and find it to be 136/74 mm Hg. You ask him how he has been doing since his last visit. He looks down at the floor and says, "Oh, OK I guess. Seems like I'm just getting old now." What kind of follow-up would be indicated based on this information?

2. You are assigned to care for a 15-year-old girl who was admitted after a motor vehicle accident. Yesterday she had an internal fixation of a fractured ankle. In gathering her nursing history, you explore sexuality and learn that she has just recently become sexually active with her boyfriend of 3 months. When you ask about safe sex and the use of birth control, she tells you that she knows she does not have to worry about STDs with him because he is just not one of those kind of boys. In regard to birth control, she says that her boyfriend has reassured her that because he is pulling out before ejaculation, there is no risk of her becoming pregnant. How would you proceed, given this assessment data?

3. You are working on a rehabilitation unit and caring for a 67-year-old man who had a stroke 3 weeks ago. He shares a room with another man who is recovering from a stroke. He has been progressing in his self-care skills and is now able to get around with a cane, feed himself, and do most of his bath. His wife is in fairly good health, and the plan is for him to return home within the next 1 to 2 weeks. As you work with him one morning, he says to you, "You know, one of the things that is hardest about being here is not being able to sleep in the same bed as Greta. I miss her so much. Even though she visits every day, it is just not the same." How would you explore his comment, and what planning would you consider?

Review Questions

1. Gender identity is the individual's:
   1. Sexual behavior.
   2. Sexual orientation.
   3. Sense of being feminine or masculine.
   4. Sense of preferring one sex over the other.

2. Sexual health refers to:
   1. Having no sexually transmitted diseases.
   2. Open and positive attitudes toward sexual functioning.
   3. Using contraception consistently.
   4. Sexual activity with multiple partners.

3. Inability or difficulty in sexual functioning caused by numerous factors is called:
   1. Sexual behavior.
   2. Sexual response.
   3. Sexual orientation.
   4. Sexual dysfunction.

4. Sexually transmitted diseases (STDs) in the industrialized world are increasing each year. The United States:
   1. Has the highest rate of STDs.
   2. Has the lowest rate of STDs.
   3. Is virtually unaffected by STDs.
   4. Considers STDs a minor health concern.

5. Methods of contraception requiring a health care provider intervention include:
   1. Diaphragm and sterilization.
   2. Condoms and hormones.
   3. Cervical caps and condoms.
   4. Sterilization and vaginal spermicidals.

6. Effectiveness rates for oral contraceptives are:
   1. 82% to 95%.
   2. 82% to 97%.
   3. 97% to 99.9%.
   4. 65% to 85%.

7. The most effective contraception method other than abstinence is:
   1. Sterilization.
   2. Oral contraceptives.
   3. Condoms.
   4. Barrier methods of contraception.

8. For transmission of human immunodeficiency virus (HIV) infection some exchange of body fluid must occur, particularly:
   1. Saliva.
   2. Blood.
   3. Semen.
   4. Urine.

9. When the nurse is gathering a sexual history form an older adult the nurse must keep in mind:
   1. Older adults do not usually participate in sexual activity.
   2. Older men lose fertility.
   3. Older adults may not reveal intimate details.
   4. Both male and female elders have sexual dysfunction.

10. A useful framework for the nurse in guiding planning and setting priorities regarding sexual activity for a client is the:
    1. PLISSIT model.
    2. NANDA International guidelines.
    3. NIC and NOC guidelines.
    4. The nurse's own theory of sexual behavior.

References

Annon JS: The PLISSIT model: a proposed conceptual scheme for the behavioral treatment of sexual problems, *J Sex Educ Ther* (2):1, 1976.

Centers for Disease Control and Prevention: Summary of notifiable diseases, United States, *MMWR Morb Mortal Wkly Rep* 47(53):1, 1999.

Centers for Disease Control and Prevention: HIV/AIDS surveillance report, *MMWR Morb Mortal Wkly Rep* 12(1):1, 2000.

Centers for Disease Control and Prevention: HIV/AIDS surveillance report, *MMWR Morb Mortal Wkly Rep* 13(2):1, 2002.

Department of Health: National sexual health and HIV strategy 2000, www.doh.gov.uk/nshs/background.htm.

Dochterman JM, Bulechek GM: *Nursing interventions classification (NIC)*, ed 4, St. Louis, 2004, Mosby.

Eliopoulos C: *Gerontological nursing*, ed 5, Philadelphia, 2001 Lippincott Williams & Wilkins.

Finan SF: Promoting healthy sexuality: guidelines for the school-age child and adolescent, *Nurse Pract* 22(11):62, 1997.

Heath H, White I: *Challenging sexuality in health care*, Oxford, 2001, Blackwell Science.

Iannotta JG, editor: *Emerging issues in Hispanic health: summary of a workshop*, Washington, DC, 2002, The National Academies Press.

Kaplan J: *Disorders of sexual desire*, New York, 1979, Simon & Schuster.

Laumann EO and others: Sexual dysfunction in the United States: prevalence and predictors, *JAMA* 281(6):537, 1999.

Leuckenotte AG: *Gerontologic nursing*, ed 2, St. Louis, 2000, Mosby.

MacLaren A: Primary care for women: comprehensive sexual health assessment, *J Nurse Midwifery* 40(2):104, 1995.

Michael RT and others: *Sex in America: a definitive survey*, New York, 1994, Little, Brown.

Moorhead S, Johnson M, Mass M: *Nursing outcomes classification (NOC)*, ed 4, St. Louis, 2004, Mosby.

Pillitteri A.: *Maternal and child health nursing: care of the childbearing and childrearing family*, ed 3, Philadelphia, 1999, Lippincott.

Robinson D, Dollins A, McConlogue-Shaughnessy M: Care of the woman before and after an elective abortion, *American Journal for Nurse Practitioners*, p 17, March 2000.

Ross MW, Channon-Little LD, Rosser BR: *Sexual health concerns: interviewing and history taking for health practitioners*, ed 2, Philadelphia, 2000, FA Davis.

Running A, Berndt A: *Management guidelines for nurse practitioners working in family practice*, Philadelphia, 2003, FA Davis.

Stuart GW, Laraia MT: *Principles and practice of psychiatric nursing*, ed 6, St. Louis, 1998, Mosby.

Yarhouse MA: Sexual identity development: the influence of valuative 3 frameworks on identity synthesis, *Psychotherapy: Theory, Research, Practice, Training* 38(3):331, 2001.

Research References

Bohn D, Holz K: Sequelae of abuse: health effects of childhood sexual abuse, domestic battering, and rape, *J Nurse Midwifery* 41(6):442, 1996.

Dickinson LM and others: Health-related quality of life and symptom profiles of female survivors of sexual abuse, *Arch Fam Med* 8(1):35, 1999.

Fortenberry M and others: Relationship of stigma and shame to gonorrhea and HIV screening, *Am J Public Health* 92(3):378, 2002.

Keller M and others: Adolescents' views of sexual decision-making, *Image J Nurs Sch* 28(2):125, 1996.

Kenney JW, Reinholtz CO, Angelini PO: Sexual abuse, sex before age 16, and high-risk behaviors of young females with sexually transmitted diseases, *J Obstet Gynecol Neonatal Nurs* 27(1): 54, 1998.

Riley A: Sex in old age: continuing pleasure or inevitable decline? *Geriatr Med* 29(3):25, 1999.

28

Spiritual Health

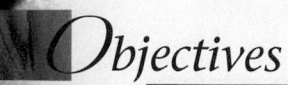

Objectives

Mastery of content in this chapter will enable the student to:

- Define the key terms listed.
- Discuss research findings that suggest spiritual practices influence clients' health status.
- Describe the relationship between faith, hope, and spiritual well-being.
- Explain the concepts of the Framework of Systemic Organization as it applies to spirituality.
- Compare and contrast the concepts of religion and spirituality.
- Perform an assessment of a client's spirituality.
- Explain how a nurse's caring relationship with clients affects their ability to gain spiritual insight.
- Discuss the risks and benefits of including spiritual intervention in nursing care.
- Discuss nursing interventions designed to promote spiritual health.
- Evaluate attainment of spiritual health.

The word **spirituality** derives from the Latin word *spiritus,* which refers to breath or wind. The spirit gives life to, or animates, a person. It signifies whatever is at the center of all aspects of a person's life (Dombeck, 1995). A person's health depends on a balance of physical, psychological, sociological, cultural, developmental, and spiritual factors. Friedemann, Mouch, and Racey (2002) define spirituality as the act of connecting to systems such as God, nature, or other people to find meaning through relationships. Spirituality can be the important factor that helps individuals achieve the balance needed to maintain health and well-being and to cope with illness.

There is debate over the danger of nurses applying a "one size fits all" concept of spirituality when administering care to clients (Draper and McSherry, 2002). There are studies that show most Americans claim to be religious (Gallop, 1985) and seek comfort through religion when they are seriously ill. However, there is also research showing that a significant proportion of people either do not know what is meant by the concept of spirituality or positively disagree with the suggestion that their lives have a spiritual dimension (McSherry and Ross, 2002).

Spirituality is a highly personal matter. Caring for a client's spiritual needs means caring for the whole person, accepting his or her beliefs and experiences, and helping the client with issues surrounding meaning and hope (Childe, 2002). Being able to determine the importance spirituality holds for clients depends on a nurse's ability to develop a caring relationship (see Chapter 7).

Nurses must therefore learn to recognize spirituality in their clients and likewise have an awareness of their own spirituality in order to provide appropriate and relevant spiritual care. Expert nursing care involves helping clients use their spiritual resources as they identify and explore what is meaningful in their lives and as they find ways to cope with the impact of illness and the ongoing stressors of life.

Scientific Knowledge Base

Health care research now shows the association between spirituality and health. There may be beneficial health outcomes when an individual is able to engage his or her beliefs in a higher power and sense a source of strength or support. The healing power of prayer may lower blood pressure (Koenig and others, 1997), reduce stress before surgery (Saudia and others, 1991), enhance cancer treatment (Lambe and others, 1996), or relieve depression and improve immune status in acquired immunodeficiency syndrome (AIDS) clients (Adair and others, 1991; Carson and Green, 1992). Prayer and meditation are frequently used as methods for coping and minimizing physical stressors. For example, meditation is successful in treating chronic pain, insomnia, anxiety, and depression (Culligan, 1996).

The relationship between spirituality and healing is not completely understood. However, it is the individual's intrinsic spirit that seems to be an important factor in healing. When clients are given a placebo (sugar pill) instead of a prescribed medication, often they improve, not because of the sugar pill but because of their faith in the physician who prescribed it. The placebo phenomenon shows that healing can take place because of believing.

There is a link between mind, body, and spirit. An individual's beliefs and expectations can and do have effects on the person's physical well-being (Coe, 1997). Many of these effects may be tied to hormonal and neurological function. Diabetic clients who did not attend religious services were more likely to have an elevated C-reactive protein (CRP) level than those clients who attended services (King, Mainous, and Pearson, 2002). CRP levels are believed to be associated with cardiovascular mortality. Laughter raises pain thresholds, boosts antibodies, reduces stress hormones, and elevates mood (Kellar, 2001). A person's inner beliefs and convictions can become powerful resources for healing. A nurse will be more successful in helping clients achieve desirable health outcomes after learning to support clients and families spiritually as well as mentally and physically.

Nursing Knowledge Base

Framework of Systemic Organization

Friedemann (1995) developed the Framework of Systemic Organization as a theoretical basis for family nursing. Use of such a theoretical model can be very helpful to a nurse in how to design and organize a client's assessment and to anticipate the types of interventions that will successfully support a client and family's spiritual well-being. The framework applies to various types of families and includes a model for the systemic life process that applies not only to families, but to individuals and larger social systems. It serves as an organizing structure through which nurses can engage in nurse-client relationships to explore their clients' diverse spiritual needs. Figure 28-1 pictures the relationships between the key concepts on the Framework of Systemic Organization.

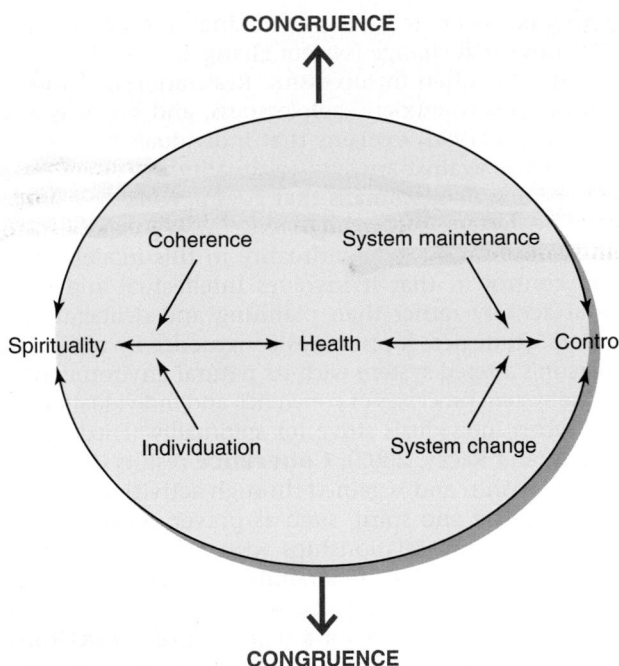

FIGURE **28–1**   Framework of Systemic Organization. (Redrawn from Friedemann M, Mouch J, Racey T: Nursing the spirit: the Framework of Systemic Organization, *J Adv Nurs* 39[4]:325, 2002.)

The ideal condition of all systems such as a family is **congruence,** a dynamic state in which a system's patterns and rhythms are in harmony with each other (Friedemann, 1995). For example, as individuals are subjected to ongoing changes and conflicting values, congruence is something continuously attempted but never reached. Tension created by incongruence leads to anxiety. Humans try to reduce the effect of tension in their life processes by balancing control in their lives with spirituality. The balance will differ from person to person, based on their culture, beliefs, and values.

Americans highly value control. **Control** is the process of changing what interferes with the individual's attempt to return to the status quo (homeostasis) or to effect a change that is least disruptive (Friedemann, 1995). Control protects individuals from vulnerability (e.g., feelings of powerlessness or loss of self-esteem) and provides a sense of security. To control something as threatening as a serious illness, individuals strive to reestablish preexisting conditions to whatever extent possible (Friedemann, Mouch, and Racey, 2002).

There are two processes to achieve control: system maintenance and system change (see Figure 28-1). An individual will practice system maintenance by using self-care to nurture the body and mind and meet his or her physical, psychological, and social needs. Patterns of system change include strategies used by the person to adapt to changes (Friedemann, 1995). Seeking medical care for a disease is one example of control as a client strives to battle a disease by taking medication or undergoing surgery. The client strives to maintain physical function through deliberate planning and acting (system maintenance) such as through activity or diet. At the same time the client channels energy, incorporating knowledge, and altering behaviors (e.g., stops smoking) in order to minimize unwanted change (system change).

Control is often unsuccessful. Realization of a loss of control leads to anxiety, helplessness, and hopelessness. Friedemann (1995) explains that individuals have a second defense against anxiety: spirituality. Spirituality is a practice unique to humans that goes beyond logical reasoning and promotes congruence through a sense of unity and inner peace. Spirituality in this model differs from control in that it involves intellectual and emotional activity rather than planning and deliberate behavioral strategies. It promotes congruence by realigning a person's altered system with its natural environment.

The system processes of coherence and individuation are used when individuals strive for spirituality (Friedemann, Mouch, and Racey, 2002). **Coherence** results in a sense of unity within and is gained through activities that nurture the mind and spirit, such as prayer, religious practices, meaningful relationships with others, and enjoying music and the arts. In a family, coherence represents togetherness with family members experiencing each other as connected parts of a whole. **Individuation** is human striving to connect and become a part of something outside of oneself, through integration of knowledge, adjustment of values, and alteration of behaviors. Individuation involves expanding one's consciousness and sharpening one's perceptions of the world. Friedemann, Mouch, and Racey (2002) give the example of a severely ill client, who may resort to spirituality by getting in touch with the inner self (coherence), connecting with family and friends for comfort (coherence), or experiencing a meaningful relationship with nature or God (individuation).

Spirituality is an active and positive way of dealing with problems. It is particularly useful and essential where problems do not seem solvable (Friedemann, 1995). Terminally ill clients who have given up their struggle to regain physical health exercise a level of spirituality that allows them to gain a sense of freedom from fear and anxiety.

According to Friedemann, Mouch, and Racey (2002) both control and spirituality are essential in each person's life. The interaction of both in a way that is true to the person's culture and values has the potential to promote congruence. The practice of a desired and individually defined blend of control and spirituality may signify health. Health is a lack of incapacitating anxiety and thus distinctly different from the absence of physical disease (Friedemann, Mouch, and Racey, 2002). Health is possible in the presence of disease. An older adult who is experiencing gradual decline in physical function, for example, is experiencing a natural occurrence and thus is in congruence with a healthy state.

Nurses will observe their clients struggle with illness by attempting to gain control. This can often be characterized by feelings of anxiety, anger, and resentment. Anxiety can destroy interpersonal relationships, often with friends and family members who could be the greatest source of comfort. By applying Friedemann's Framework of Systemic Organization, a nurse can assist individuals and their families in attempting to establish congruence. Spiritual care introduces interventions that promote coherence and individuation so that a client achieves a healthy state.

Traditional Concepts in Spiritual Health

A variety of concepts are used to describe spiritual health. To provide meaningful and supportive spiritual care, it is important for a nurse to understand the concepts of spirituality, faith, religion, and hope. Each concept offers direction in understanding the views individuals have of life and its value.

Spirituality. Spirituality is a concept that is unique to each individual, dependent upon a person's culture, development, life experiences, beliefs, and ideas about life. An individual's spirituality enables the person to love, have faith and hope, seek meaning in life, and to nurture relationships with others. Spirituality offers a sense of connectedness intrapersonally (connected within oneself), interpersonally (connected with others and the environment), and transpersonally (connected with the unseen, God, or a higher power). Elements of spirituality frequently found in the literature include spiritual well-being, spiritual needs, and spiritual awareness. Hungelmann and others (1996) describe **spiritual well-being** as a sense of harmonious interconnectedness between self, others/nature, and an ultimate other that exists throughout and beyond time and space. There are two important characteristics of spirituality agreed upon by most authors: (1) it is a unifying theme in people's lives, and (2) it is a state of being.

Spirituality begins as children learn about themselves and their relationships with others. Many adults experience spiritual growth by entering into lifelong relationships. An ability to care meaningfully for others and the self is evidence of a healthy spirituality. Older adults often turn to important relationships and the giving of themselves to others as spiritual tasks.

Establishing a connection with a supreme being, beings, or an important meaning or value is one way a person develops spiritually. Followers of Confucianism develop spirituality through their commitment to a code of ethics that emphasizes a hierarchy of society, worship of ancestors, and respect for age and custom (Giger and Davidhizar, 1995). In the Judeo-Christian context children often begin with a concept of a supreme being as presented to them by their home or religious community. Adolescents often reconsider their childlike concept of a spiritual power, and in the search for an identity, they may either question practices and values or find the spiritual power as the motivation to seek a clearer meaning to life.

As people mature, they often turn inward to enduring values and to a concept of a supreme being or a higher meaning that has been sustaining and meaningful. A healthy spirituality in older adults is one that gives peace and acceptance of the self and that is often based on a lifelong relationship with a supreme being. Illness and loss can threaten and challenge the spiritual developmental process. It thus becomes important for the nurse to understand the nature and status of a client's belief system and spiritual health.

There are individuals who either do not believe in the existence of God (**atheist**) or who believe that any ultimate reality is unknown **(agnostic).** Agnostics believe that the existence of a God or higher power cannot be proven or disproved. This does not mean that spirituality is not an important concept for the atheist or agnostic. Atheists search for meaning in life through their work and their relationships with other individuals (Burnard, 1988). Because atheists feel they are alone, they sense a strong responsibility for themselves. They also tend to believe in a joint responsibility for others. In acting for themselves, they feel they should also act for all of mankind (Burnard, 1988). It is important for agnostics to discover meaning in what they do or how they live. Burnard (1988) explains that since agnostics find no ultimate meaning for the way things are, they believe that we as people bring meaning to what we do.

Faith. The concept of faith has two uses described in the literature. In the first, faith is defined as a cultural or institutional religion, such as Judaism, Buddhism, Islam, or Christianity. Second, **faith** is a relationship with a divinity, higher power, authority, or spirit that incorporates a reasoning faith (belief) and a trusting faith (action) (Benner, 1985). Reasoning faith is an individual's belief and confidence in something for which there is no proof. Sometimes that involves a belief in a higher power, spirit guide, God, or Allah (Fryback, 1993). However, faith also might be the manner in which a person chooses to live life. Faith in this sense enables action. For example, a person might believe that having a positive outlook on life is the best way to achieve life's goals. The belief that comes with faith involves **transcendence,** or an awareness of that which one cannot see or know in ordinary physical ways (Reed, 1987). It gives purpose and meaning to an individual's life, allowing for action. For example, cancer clients who have faith in a positive outlook on life might pursue more knowledge about their disease and continue to pursue daily activities rather than resign themselves to the disease's symptoms. Hall (1998) studied clients diagnosed with human immunodeficiency virus (HIV) and found that spirituality frames individuals' lives. Individuals become open to discover their unique spiritual meaning after a crisis that threatens health. Their faith becomes strengthened, and they are better able to go on with life and engage in activities that fit the new definition of their selves.

Religion. Religion is associated with the "state of doing," or a specific system of practices associated with a particular denomination, sect, or form of worship. Emblen (1992) defines religion as a system of organized beliefs and worship that a person practices to outwardly express spirituality. Many persons practice a faith or belief in the doctrines and expressions of a specific religion or sect, such as the Lutheran church within Christianity or Orthodox Judaism. Religion influences how the person exercises a faith of belief and action. For example, a Buddhist believes in the Four Noble Truths taught by Buddha: life is suffering; suffering is caused by desire; suffering can be eliminated by eliminating desire; and to eliminate desire, one must follow an eightfold path (Giger and Davidhizar, 1995). The path includes right understanding, purpose, speech, conduct, vocation, effort,

thinking, and meditation. The Buddhist turns inward, valuing self-control, whereas a Christian looks to the love of God to provide enlightenment and direction in life.

When providing spiritual care to clients it is important to understand the differences between religion and spirituality. Many people tend to use the terms *spirituality* and *religion* interchangeably. Although closely associated, these terms are not synonymous. Religion provides a framework for beliefs and rituals (Peri, 1995). Spirituality is the umbrella under which religion is a part (Burgess, 1997). In other words, religious practice encompasses spirituality, but spirituality need not include religious practice. Religious care is seen as helping clients maintain their faithfulness to their belief systems and worship practices. Spiritual care is seen as helping people maintain personal relationships and a relationship to a higher being or life force, to identify meaning and purpose in life, and to hopefully look beyond the present (Alridge, 1993).

Hope. Spirituality is a key element in hope. When a person has the attitude of something to live for and look forward to, hope is present. **Hope** is a multidimensional concept that provides comfort while enduring life threats and personal challenges (Morse and Doberneck, 1995). Hope is also closely associated with faith. It is energizing, giving individuals a motivation to achieve and the resources to use toward that achievement. People express hope in all aspects of their lives to help them deal with life stressors. Hope is an invaluable personal resource whenever someone is faced with a loss (see Chapter 29) or a challenge that seems difficult to achieve. Morse and Doberneck (1995) conducted research with four different groups of clients: heart transplant recipients, spinal cord injured clients, breast cancer survivors, and breast-feeding mothers intending to continue nursing while employed. Their work identified seven concepts of hope, revealing how complex and unique hope can be for each individual (Box 28-1).

Spiritual Problems

When illness, loss, grief, or a major life change affects a person, spiritual resources either help a person move to recovery or spiritual needs and concerns develop. **Spiritual distress** is the disruption of an individual's

Box **28-1**	Conceptual Components of Hope

- A realistic initial assessment of threat or predicament
- The envisioning of options and setting of goals
- Bracing or preparing for negative outcomes
- A realistic assessment of personal resources and external conditions/resources
- The seeking out of mutually supportive relationships
- The continuous evaluation for signs that reinforce the selected goals
- A determination to endure

Modified from Morse JM, Doberneck B: Delineating the concept of hope, *Image J Nurs Sch* 27(4):277, 1995.

"life principle," which fills the person's entire being and transcends or exceeds one's biological and psychosocial nature (North American Nursing Diagnosis Association, 2003). A catastrophic illness, for example, can upset a person's spiritual well-being sufficiently to cause doubt and loss of faith. Spiritual distress may cause the person to feel alone or even abandoned by resources that at one time were very nurturing. Individuals may question their spiritual values, raising questions about their whole way of life, purpose for living, and source of meaning. Spiritual distress also occurs when there is conflict between a person's beliefs and prescribed health regimens or the inability to practice usual rituals.

Acute Illness. Sudden, unexpected illness that poses both an immediate and a long-term threat to a client's life, health, and/or well-being can create significant spiritual distress. For example, both the 50-year-old man who has a heart attack and the 20-year-old who is a victim of a motor vehicle accident face crises that may threaten their spiritual health. The illness or injury creates an unanticipated scramble to integrate and cope with new realities (e.g., disability). People look for ways to remain faithful to their beliefs and value systems. They may pray, attend religious services more often, or spend time reflecting on the positive aspects of their lives. Often conflicts can develop around a person's beliefs and the meaning of life. Anger is not uncommon, and clients may express it against God, their families, themselves, or the nurse. The strength of a client's spirituality influences how he or she copes with sudden illness and how quickly he or she can move to recovery. Yim and Vande Creek (1996) have developed a spiritual healing critical pathway for coronary artery bypass clients. Their research has shown that knowledge of a person's spiritual well-being can be used to maximize a client's recovery. Hope and the ability to speak about life values help the individual gain meaning from illness and influence the ability to recover from heart surgery. The pathway identifies where clients are in their spiritual recovery and recommends appropriate interventions that help clients find purpose and worth to move forward and recover.

Chronic Illness. Persons with chronic illness often suffer debilitating symptoms that change the ability to continue their lifestyles. A symptom is more than a signal for a persistent health problem or a clue for diagnosing a disease. A symptom can give a person permission to take needed rest, be a sign of impending disruption, or even raise feelings about the person's self-worth and strength (Benner and Wrubel, 1989). Symptoms are meaningful to the individual, and that meaning is shaped by the person's history and the current context of the illness.

With chronic illness independence can be threatened, causing fear, anxiety, and an overall dispiritedness. Dependence on others for routine self-care measures can create a feeling of powerlessness. A person may feel a loss of a sense of purpose in life that affects the inner strength needed to deal with alterations in functioning. A person's spirituality can be a significant factor in how he or she adapts to the changes resulting from chronic illness. Successful adaptation can strengthen a person spiritually. A reevaluation of life may occur. Those who are able to engage and use their spiritual resources will have a much better chance to reestablish a self-identity and live to their potential.

Terminal Illness. Terminal illness commonly causes fears of physical pain, isolation, the unknown, and dying (Turner and others, 1995). However, when people experience periods of disease remission, they may become asymptomatic for long periods of time and put off the idea of illness and any terminal outcome. Terminal illness creates an uncertainty about what death means and thus makes clients susceptible to spiritual distress. However, there are also clients who have a spiritual sense of peace that enables them to face death without fear. Hall (1998) interviewed 10 men and women in advanced-stage HIV disease who self-identified as having spiritual or religious experiences that had helped them cope with HIV disease. These individuals discovered a unique spiritual meaning after a crisis that threatened their health. Living with HIV required clearing one's life of the stressful existence, problematic relationships, and social memberships that did not work. Spirituality helped them find peace in themselves and their death.

Individuals experiencing a terminal illness will often find themselves reviewing their life and questioning its meaning. Common questions asked might include "Why is this happening to me?" or "What have I done?" Family and friends can be affected just as much as the client. Terminal illness causes members of the family to ask important questions about its meaning and how it will affect their relationship with the client (see Chapter 29).

Fryback (1993) conducted a study to learn how people with a terminal illness describe health. Clients in the study identified the following three domains of health: mental/emotional, spiritual, and physical (Figure 28-2). The spiritual domain was seen as being essential for health and included having a relationship with a higher power, recognizing mortality, and striving for self-actualization. Although many of the participants in the study either attended church or stated a desire to do so, others found that spirituality was not dependent on a religion or church. They associated health with belief in a higher power that gave them faith and the ability to love (Fryback, 1993). The study revealed that when terminally ill clients have a perception of being unhealthy, it is not due to the disease but to being unable to live their lives fully and do the things they desire.

Near-Death Experience. Nurses may care for clients who have had a near-death experience (NDE). An NDE is a psychological phenomenon of people who either have been close to clinical death or may have recovered after being declared dead. It is not associated with a mental disorder (Basford, 1990). Persons who experience an NDE after cardiopulmonary arrest, for example, often tell the same story of feeling themselves rising above their bodies and watching caregivers initiate lifesaving measures. Most individuals describe passing through a tunnel to a bright light, encountering people who had preceded them in death, and feeling an inner tranquility and peace. Instead of moving toward the light, they learn it is not time for them to die and they return to life.

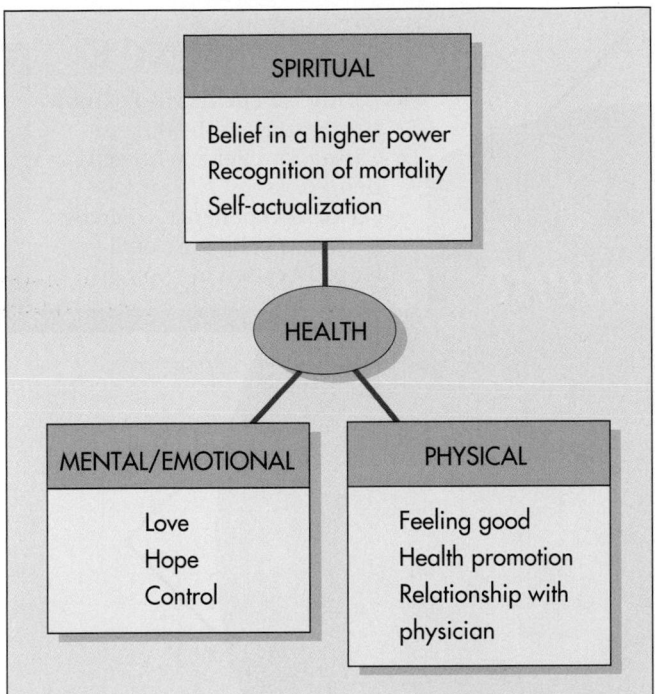

FIGURE **28–2**   Domains of health based on perceptions of terminally ill clients. (Modified from Fryback PB: Health for people with a terminal diagnosis, *Nurs Sci Q* 6[3]:147, 1993.)

Clients who have an NDE are often reluctant to discuss it, thinking family or caregivers will not understand. Isolation and depression can occur. However, individuals experiencing an NDE who can discuss it with family or caregivers find acceptance and meaning from this powerful experience. They consistently report positive aftereffects, including a positive attitude and spiritual development (Turner and others, 1995). After a client has survived cardiopulmonary arrest it is important for the nurse to remain open and give the client a chance to explore what happened.

Critical Thinking

The helping role is important in nursing practice (Benner, 1984). Clients look to nurses for a different kind of help than that sought from other health care professionals. Expert nurses acquire the ability to anticipate the personal issues affecting clients' abilities to receive and seek help, including their spiritual well-being. Critical thinking knowledge and skills help a nurse to enhance clients' spiritual well-being and health. While using the nursing process, the nurse applies knowledge, experience, attitudes, and standards in providing appropriate spiritual care (Figure 28–3).

Knowledge about spirituality begins with nurses' insight about their own spirituality. Friedemann, Mouch, and Racey (2002) believe it is important that nurses experience a self-exploration through reading, religious involvement, or activities such as meditation to understand their own beliefs and values. Applying knowledge of spir-

itual concepts, principles of caring (see Chapter 7), and therapeutic communication skills (see Chapter 23) positions a nurse to readily recognize and understand a client's spiritual needs. Personal experience in caring for clients in spiritual distress can be invaluable in helping each new client to examine coping options, test values, and try out new behaviors. A client's spirituality is unique, and thus a nurse must apply critical thinking attitudes in order to acquire the information needed to determine whether intervention is necessary and how to sensitively provide spiritual care. The application of intellectual standards helps the nurse to make accurate clinical decisions in helping clients find meaningful and logical ways to acquire spiritual healing. It is particularly important in giving spiritual care to apply sound ethical standards in practice. The standard or routine prescription of interventions such as relaxation exercises or meditation can be coercive and/or unethical, unless they are attuned to clients' needs and interests and based on a broad assessment of their life process (Friedemann, Mouch, and Racey, 2002). An ethic of caring (see Chapter 21) provides nurses with a framework for decision making. A client's spiritual beliefs may place the client on an unequal footing with professionals because of the influence those beliefs have on the client's choice of therapy. An ethic of care places the nurse as the client's advocate, solving ethical dilemmas by attending to relationships and honoring the client's personal choices.

Nursing Process

At the core of nursing is a commitment to caring and respect for an individual's uniqueness. In the case of spirituality, it is even more important to respect each client's personal systems of belief. There are fundamental differences in the ways in which people experience the world and find meaning in that experience (Martsolf and Mickley, 1998). There is a danger that any blanket application of a concept of spirituality will be equally disrespectful to the views of clients who embrace a broadly religious view of the world and to those who adopt a more secular (nonreligious) orientation.

Application of the nursing process from the perspective of a client's spiritual needs is not simple. It goes beyond assessing a client's religious practices. Understanding a client's spirituality and then appropriately identifying the level of support and resources needed requires a new, broader perspective. Heliker (1992) describes the importance of shared compassion and community. *Compassion* comes from the Latin words *pati* and *cum,* meaning "to suffer with." *Community* is derived from the Latin word meaning "fellowship." To be compassionate is to "enter into places of pain, to share in brokenness with other human beings" (Heliker, 1992). To practice compassion as a nurse requires awareness of the very human tie between clients and a healing community. This kind of work will generally consist of quiet conversations, effective listening, and communication through presence and touch (Draper and McSherry, 2002).

The nurse must remove from the assessment any personal biases or misconceptions and be willing to share

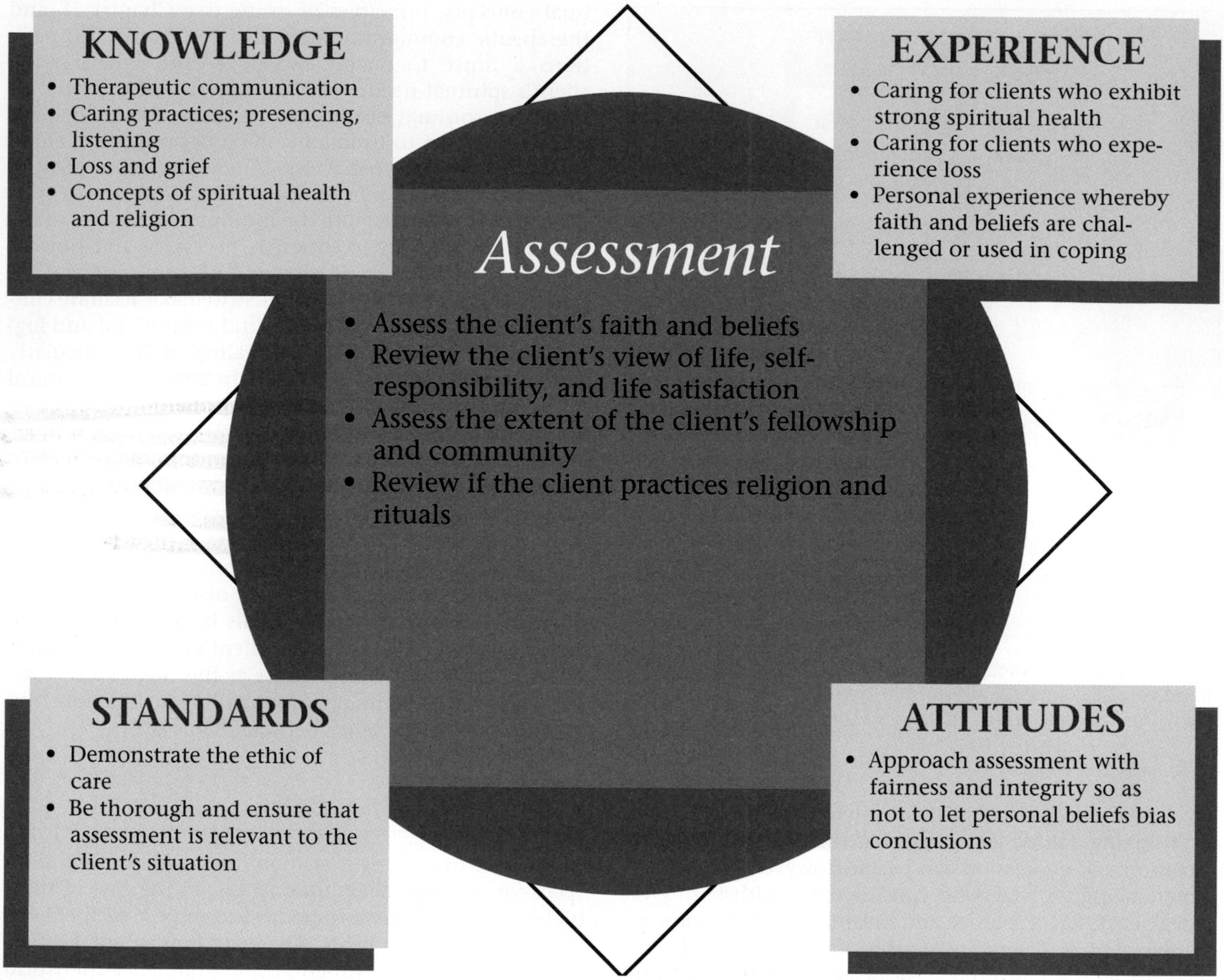

KNOWLEDGE
- Therapeutic communication
- Caring practices; presencing, listening
- Loss and grief
- Concepts of spiritual health and religion

EXPERIENCE
- Caring for clients who exhibit strong spiritual health
- Caring for clients who experience loss
- Personal experience whereby faith and beliefs are challenged or used in coping

Assessment
- Assess the client's faith and beliefs
- Review the client's view of life, self-responsibility, and life satisfaction
- Assess the extent of the client's fellowship and community
- Review if the client practices religion and rituals

STANDARDS
- Demonstrate the ethic of care
- Be thorough and ensure that assessment is relevant to the client's situation

ATTITUDES
- Approach assessment with fairness and integrity so as not to let personal beliefs bias conclusions

FIGURE **28–3**   Critical thinking model for spiritual health assessment.

and discover a client's meaning and purpose in life, sickness, and health. Typically one of the questions usually asked on a client's admission form is the client's "religion." Such a question leaves little doubt that the accepted position is that of a "believer" (Burnard, 1988). It is important for nurses to sort out value judgments about other people's belief systems. Working through values clarification exercises can be helpful (see Chapter 21). If the nurse is a believer, does he or she judge harshly the unbeliever? If the nurse is an agnostic or atheist, does he or she dismiss the believer? As nurses, it becomes important to accept and acknowledge others' beliefs and not spend work time trying to convert others to our personal beliefs. A nurse learns to look beyond a personal view when establishing a client relationship. This means identifying the common values that make us human and respecting the commitments and values that make humans unique. Love, trust, hope, forgiveness, meaning, and community are spiritual needs we all have. Learning to share these needs helps the nurse find a way to give clients spiritual care and support.

Another important aspect of spiritual care is recognizing that a client does not have to have a spiritual problem. Clients bring certain spiritual resources that the nurse can engage as resources to help them assume healthier lives, recover from illness, or face impending death. Supporting and recognizing the positive side of a client's spiritually will go a long way toward delivering effective, individualized nursing care.

Assessment

Because spirituality is deeply subjective, it can mean different things to different people (McSherry and Ross, 2002). There is considerable religious diversity in the United States, and there are many geographic regions that provide health care to multifaith users. Traditionally, the manner in which spirituality has been assessed in health care settings is an interpretation of Judeo-Christian spirituality. It is possible for clients of some faith traditions to be offended by such an approach.

DIRECTIONS: PLEASE CIRCLE THE CHOICE THAT **BEST** DESCRIBES HOW MUCH YOU AGREE WITH EACH STATEMENT.   CIRCLE ONLY **ONE** ANSWER FOR EACH STATEMENT.   THERE IS NO RIGHT OR WRONG ANSWER.

		Strongly Agree	Moderately Agree	Agree	Disagree	Moderately Disagree	Strongly Disagree
1.	Prayer is an important part of my life.	SA	MA	A	D	MD	SD
2.	I believe I have spiritual well-being.	SA	MA	A	D	MD	SD
3.	As I grow older, I find myself more tolerant of others' beliefs.	SA	MA	A	D	MD	SD
4.	I find meaning and purpose in my life.	SA	MA	A	D	MD	SD
5.	I feel there is a close relationship between my spiritual beliefs and what I do.	SA	MA	A	D	MD	SD
6.	I believe in an afterlife.	SA	MA	A	D	MD	SD
7.	When I am sick I have less spiritual well-being.	SA	MA	A	D	MD	SD
8.	I believe in a supreme power.	SA	MA	A	D	MD	SD
9.	I am able to receive and give love to others.	SA	MA	A	D	MD	SD
10.	I am satisfied with my life.	SA	MA	A	D	MD	SD
11.	I set goals for myself.	SA	MA	A	D	MD	SD
12.	God has little meaning in my life.	SA	MA	A	D	MD	SD
13.	I am satisfied with the way I am using my abilities.	SA	MA	A	D	MD	SD
14.	Prayer does not help me in making decisions.	SA	MA	A	D	MD	SD
15.	I am able to appreciate differences in others.	SA	MA	A	D	MD	SD
16.	I am pretty well put together.	SA	MA	A	D	MD	SD
17.	I prefer that others make decisions for me.	SA	MA	A	D	MD	SD
18.	I find it hard to forgive others.	SA	MA	A	D	MD	SD
19.	I accept my life situations.	SA	MA	A	D	MD	SD
20.	Belief in a supreme being has no part in my life.	SA	MA	A	D	MD	SD
21.	I cannot accept change in my life.	SA	MA	A	D	MD	SD

FIGURE **28–4**   JAREL spiritual well-being scale. (Copyright 1987 by J Hungelmann, E Kenkel-Rossi, L Klassen, R Stollenwerk, Marquette University College of Nursing, Milwaukee, Wisc.)

The purpose behind a spiritual assessment is fundamental in determining how such assessments are constructed and used in practice. Catterall and others (1998) suggest a two-stage approach to assessment. The first stage is commonly found in acute care settings where an initial assessment focuses only upon identifying a client's religious beliefs, affiliations, and practices. This information is important for making referrals to appropriate clergy and attempting to adapt clients' practices (e.g., diet preferences or rituals) into their care. The second stage is a more in-depth assessment for clients whom the nurse feels are experiencing or at risk for spiritual distress. With time pressures on nurses, it is often difficult to obtain an in-depth spiritual assessment. A key to success is to conduct an ongoing assessment over the course of the client's stay in the health care setting. The nurse must establish trust and rapport and have the opportunity to conduct meaningful discussions with clients.

Once a trusting relationship with a client is established, the nurse and client reach a point of learning together, and spiritual caring can occur. The nurse learns to consciously integrate an attitude of spiritual care into the nursing process. The assessment should focus on aspects of spirituality most likely to be influenced by life experiences, events, and questions in the case of illness and hospitalization. Even conducting an assessment can be therapeutic because it conveys a level of caring and support. Friedemann, Mouch, and Racey (2002) note, "An assessment done well is not simply a collection of data but becomes an intervention." The nurse who understands the overall approach to spiritual assessment can enter into thoughtful discussions with the client and gain a greater awareness of the personal resources an individual brings to a situation. These resources ought to be incorporated into an effective plan of care.

The JAREL spiritual well-being scale (Figure 28-4) provides nurses and other health care professionals with a simple tool for assessing a client's spiritual well-being (Hungelmann and others, 1996). The tool was developed for clients from Christian, non-Christian, and atheist belief systems. Items on the tool comprise three key dimensions: faith/belief, life/self-responsibility, and life-satisfaction/self-actualization. The tool is simple to use, requiring clients to rate their level of agreement with each item on a five-point scale (strongly agree to strongly disagree). For clients with visual or literacy problems, the nurse can read the items and record the client's response. If the client's score on any item, group of items, or particular dimension is low, it may indicate an area to explore further (Hungelmann and others, 1996).

The tool helps the nurse to explore with a client any perceptions or concerns he or she might have. For example, if a client disagrees about accepting life situations, the nurse will need to spend time understanding how an illness is being accepted and managed by the client. Whether a nurse uses a tool like the JAREL scale or directs an assessment with questions that are based on principles of spirituality, it is important to not impose personal value systems on the client. This is particularly true when the client's values and beliefs are similar to those of the nurse, as it can then become very easy to make false assumptions.

Faith/Belief. Each individual has some source of authority and guidance in his or her life. It is that inner voice or outer authority that leads persons to choose and act on their beliefs. The authority can be a supreme being, a code of conduct, a specific religious leader, family or friends, oneself, or a combination of sources. Faith in an authority provides a sense of confidence that guides a person in exercising beliefs and experiencing growth. Knowing a client's source of strength and faith can direct interaction with him or her. The nurse can assess a person's faith in an authority by asking, "To what or whom do you look as a source of strength or faith in life?" or "What is your personal source of strength or hope?"

The nurse determines if the client has a religious source of guidance that conflicts with medical treatment plans. This can seriously affect the options nurses and other health care providers can offer clients. For example, if a client looks to the Jehovah's Witnesses as a source of authority, blood products cannot be accepted as a form of treatment. Christian Scientists often refuse any medical intervention because they believe that their faith will heal them.

It is also important to understand a client's philosophy of life (Box 28-2). Asking the client, "Tell me what is most important in your life" or "Tell me what gives your life meaning," may help to assess what is the basis of the client's belief system regarding meaning and purpose in life. This information reveals the client's spiritual focus and may help to reflect the impact that illness, loss, or disability has on the person's life. Depending on a client's religious practices, views about health and the response to illness may influence how nurses provide support (Table 28-1).

Life and Self-Responsibility. Spiritual well-being includes life and self-responsibility (Hungelmann and others, 1996). Individuals who can accept change in life, make decisions about their lives, and are able to forgive others in times of difficulty have a higher level of spiritual well-being. During illness clients often are unable to

---

Research Highlight

Box 28-2

Spirituality in Thai Older Adults

Research Focus

In many cultures, spirituality is associated with health and what people value most in life. Little is known about the relationship between religion, spirituality, and health in the older Thai population. There is some evidence to suggest there is an association of the Buddhist religion with positive health behaviors of older Thai persons.

Research Abstract

The purpose of this study was to describe spirituality as perceived and experienced by older Thai persons living in an urban U.S. community. The researcher conducted interviews with 9 older Thai adults (5 women and 4 men) to describe how spirituality helped older Thai persons maintain health as they aged and to describe what older Thai persons valued most as they aged. The subjects ranged in age from 60 to 82 years. Examples of open-ended questions asked during the interviews included, "Describe how you keep healthy as you age" and "Describe what is most important to you in your life at this time." Five themes were identified: (1) connecting with spiritual resources, which provided comfort and peace, (2) finding harmony through a healthy mind and body, (3) living a valuable life, (4) valuing tranquil relationships with family and friends, and (5) experiencing meaning and confidence in death. Connecting with spiritual resources was a way the older Thai adult maintained spiritual health. This included activities such as going to the Buddhist temple, practicing devout rituals to achieve psychological harmony and reduce stress, and accumulating merit through activities such as meditation to ensure a peaceful life. Finding harmony included letting go of conflicts, problems, and worries; sustaining a body free of disease and disability; and continuing favorite activities. Living a valuable life involved making sense of life's struggles and successes through self-reflection. The older Thai adults found ways to contribute to their community and enjoyed sharing stories about events that made them feel valued. Valuing tranquil relationships represented the older adults' desires to achieve calm, healthy relationships with family and friends. Preserving family relationships was important. Finally, the older Thai adults thought about death and used their religious resources and faith to come to terms with it. Death was viewed as a normal part of life.

Evidence-Based Practice

- Thai people follow the rituals and teachings of Buddhism and perform spiritual activities to accumulate religious merit in their daily lives.
- Thai people choose to avoid conflict. Promoting harmonious and cooperative relationships is highly valued.
- Thai people receive high respect from friends and community members if they remain composed.
- Thai people are able to prepare for death and want to die peacefully without pain and discomfort.
- When a Thai person is seriously ill and near death, the family helps the person meditate on Buddha's teaching.

Reference

Pincharoen S, Congdon JG: Spirituality and health in older Thai persons in the United States, *West J Nurs Res* 25(1):93, 2003.

accept limitations or know what to do to regain a functional and meaningful life. Their sense of helplessness may reflect spiritual distress. However, if clients are able to adapt to changes and seek solutions for how to deal with any limitations, spiritual well-being reflects an important coping resource. The nurse assesses whether a client understands the limitations or threats posed by an illness and the manner in which the client has chosen to adjust to them. In addition, questions to ask might include "Tell me how you feel about the changes caused by this illness" and "How do these changes affect what you now need to do?"

Life Satisfaction. Spiritual well-being seems to be tied to a person's satisfaction with life and what he or she has accomplished (Hungelmann and others, 1996). When persons are satisfied with life and the manner in which they are using their abilities, more energy is available to deal with new difficulties and to resolve problems. Haase and colleagues (1992) have found satisfaction with someone or something to be associated with acceptance. Acceptance is the process of resolving issues within oneself or dealing with life experiences and is closely tied to hope and spirituality. A nurse can assess a client's life satisfaction by asking, "How happy or satisfied are you with your life?" or "Tell me to what extent you feel satisfied with what you have accomplished in life."

Culture. Spirituality is a personal experience within a cultural context (Pincharoen and Congdon, 2003). It is important to know a client's culture of origin and to assess what a client values in life. It is common in many cultures for individuals to feel that they have led a worthwhile and purposeful life (Box 28-3). Remaining connected with their cultural heritage often helps clients define their place in the world and to express their spirituality. Asking clients about their faith and belief systems (see above) is a good beginning for understanding the relationship between culture and spirituality.

Fellowship and Community. Fellowship is one kind of relationship an individual can have with other persons

Table 28-1	**Religious Beliefs About Health**	
Religious/Cultural Group	**Health Care Beliefs**	**Response to Illness**
Hinduism	Accepts modern medical science.	Illness is caused by past sins. Prolonging life is discouraged.
Sikhism	Accepts modern medical science.	Females to be examined by females. Removing undergarments causes great distress.
Buddhism	Accepts modern medical science. Believes in the Four Noble Truths taught by Buddha: life is suffering, suffering is caused by desire, suffering can be eliminated by eliminating desire, and to eliminate desire, one must follow an eightfold path of understanding, purpose, speech, conduct, vocation, effort, thinking, and meditation.	May refuse treatment on Holy Days. Dharma, the law of nature, teaches that life is impermanent and all persons have to age and die. May want a Buddhist priest. Usually accepts death as last stage of life and may permit withdrawal of life support. Does not practice euthanasia.
Islam	Must be able to practice the Five Pillars of Islam. May have a fatalistic view of health.	Uses faith healing. Family members are a comfort. Group prayer is strengthening. May permit withdrawal of life support. Does not practice euthanasia.
Judaism	Believes in the sanctity of life. God and medicine must have a balance. Observance of the Sabbath is important. May refuse treatments on the Sabbath.	Visiting the sick is an obligation. The sick are obligated to seek care. Euthanasia is forbidden.
Christianity	Accepts modern medical science. Many follow complementary alternative medicine (see Chapter 35)	Life supports are discouraged. Uses prayer, faith healing. Appreciates visits from clergy. Some will use laying on of hands. Holy Communion is commonly practiced.
Navajos	Concepts of health have a fundamental place in their concept of humans and their place in the universe.	Blessingway is a practice that attempts to remove ill health by means of stories, songs, rituals, prayers, symbols, and sand paintings (Sobralske, 1985).
Appalachians	External locus of control. Life and health are controlled by nature. Accept folk healers. Good Christian members of community are called as servants to minister to disabled (Giger and Davidhizar, 1995).	Dislike hospitals. Tend to be noncompliant in following medical regimens but expect to be helped directly when seeking episodic treatment.

Cultural Aspects of Care

Box 28-3

Spirituality should not be limited to a client's religious perspective, but rather include all of life. In caring for clients from different cultures it is important to determine what is important in their lives and what provides them with inner strength and meaning. Clients are usually attempting to find meaning in the changing circumstances of their health and illness. Often spirituality and health are closely associated. For example, Martinez (1999) found in a study of Hispanic older adults that spiritual aspects of life played a major role in their health. Health was seen as creating balance in life by living one's beliefs. The Hispanic older adults also fulfilled their obligations to self through fulfilling obligations to others, especially their family and community. Pincharoen and Congdon (2003) investigated how spirituality helped Thai older adults maintain health and found that finding harmony through a healthy mind and body was critical.

Implications for Practice

- Explore spirituality of clients from different cultures by assessing the meaning of health and how clients achieve balance, stability, peace, or comfort in their lives.
- Offer a universal and holistic approach to assessing clients' needs by demonstrating caring and using therapeutic communication techniques.
- Promote an environment during assessment in which human rights, values, customs, and spiritual beliefs are respected.
- Include appropriate pastoral care professionals in the assessment process.
- Avoid use of language that alienates or discriminates between different religions.

(Farran and others, 1989), including immediate family, close friends, associates at work or school, fellow members of a church, and neighbors. More specifically, this includes the extent of the community of shared faith between clients and their support networks. The nurse can ask, "With whom do you find the greatest source of support in times of difficulty?" or "When you have faced difficult times in the past, how has that resource been helpful?" The nurse explores the extent and nature of a person's support networks and their relationship with the client. It is unwise to assume that a given network offers the kind of support a client desires. For example, calling the client's clergy to request a visit might be inappropriate if the client finds little fellowship with that individual or their religious community. Does the client have one significant fellowship or several?

Ritual and Practice. One of the easiest areas to assess about a client's spirituality is the use of rituals and practices. Rituals include participation in a religious group or private worship, prayer, sacraments such as baptism or communion, fasting, singing, meditating, scripture reading, and making offerings or sacrifices. Different religions have established various rituals for certain life events. For example, Buddhists practice baptism later in life and find

burial or cremation acceptable at death. Muslims wash the body of a dead family member and wrap it in white cloth with the head turned toward the right shoulder. Orthodox and Conservative Jews circumcise their newborn sons 8 days after birth. The nurse assesses whether a client's usual rituals or practices have been interrupted as a result of illness or hospitalization. A ritual can provide the client with structure and support during difficult times (Table 28-2). If rituals are important to the client, the nurse uses them as part of nursing intervention.

Vocation. Individuals express their spirituality on a daily basis in life routines, work, play, and relationships (Farran and others, 1989). Spirituality can be used in their vocation in life and be part of their identity. The nurse determines if illness or hospitalization has altered the person's ability to express his or her spirituality. Expression of spirituality may include showing an appreciation for life in the variety of things people do, living in the moment and not worrying about tomorrow, appreciating nature, expressing love towards others, and being productive. Questions might include "Has your illness affected the way you live your life spiritually?" or "Has your illness affected your ability to express what's important in life for you?" When illness or loss prevents clients from expressing their spirituality, the nurse must understand the implications psychologically, socially, and spiritually and provide appropriate guidance and support.

Client Expectations. It is important to include in any client assessment a review of the client's expectations for his or her health care. This part of the assessment gives the nurse and the client the chance to share what is most important to the client in terms of what caregivers are expected to provide and what the client hopes to gain. The nurse should not try to anticipate a client's expectations. What a client needs from the perspective of the nurse may have nothing to do with what the client actually expects or wants. Assessing client expectations requires the nurse to ask questions such as "What do you hope we will be able to do for you?" or "Your expectations are important to us; how can we make your care most satisfactory?" During times of loss or crisis, the client might simply desire a trusting and open relationship with the nurse. It might also be important that the client perceive caregivers to be accepting of his or her religious rituals. Asking the client what expectations are held of caregivers and then following through in meeting those expectations can be very beneficial in establishing a strong nurse-client relationship.

Nursing Diagnosis

A spiritual assessment allows a nurse to learn a great deal about who a client is and the extent that spirituality plays in the client's life. Exploring the client's spirituality may reveal responses to health problems that require nursing intervention, or it may reveal existence of a strong set of resources that enable the client to cope effectively. As a nurse analyzes data to find patterns of defining characteristics, appropriate nursing diagnoses are selected (Box 28-4). In identifying diagnoses, it is important to recognize the sig-

Table 28-2   Religious Practices Related to Birth and Death

Religion	Birth Rituals	Death Rituals
Hinduism	No special rituals.	The dying may want to lie on the floor. A priest will tie a thread around the neck or wrist (do not remove) and pour water in the client's mouth. Family will wash the body before cremation.
Sikhism	Allow mother and child to remain together.	The deceased will need the five Ks: *Kesh,* uncut hair; *Kangra,* wooden comb; *Kara,* wrist band; *Kirpan,* sword; *Kach,* shorts.
Buddhism	No special rituals. Baptism later in childhood.	A priest should be called. Last rites and chanting at bedside are common. Burial or cremation is acceptable.
Shinto	No special rituals.	Remove all jewelry. The body is washed and dressed in a white kimono and straw shoes.
Islam	A prayer is said into the infant's ear.	The dying must confess their sins. The body is washed and wrapped in white cloth, and the head is turned toward the right shoulder. The body faces east, toward Mecca. A prayer called *Kalima* is said.
Judaism	Circumcision on day 8 for Orthodox and Conservative Jews.	Body is washed by burial society, and someone needs to remain with the body for Orthodox and Conservative Jews. Rituals vary among groups.
Christianity	Rituals vary. Many will baptize.	Many give last rites or communion. Prefers burial to cremation.
Church of Jesus Christ of Latter-Day Saints (Mormonism)	Baptism by immersion.	Many give last rites or communion. Prefers burial to cremation.
Navajos	After a child's delivery the umbilical cord is taken from the newborn, dried, and buried near a place that symbolizes what parents want for child's future.	Navajo medicine men and women conduct formal ceremonies.

Nursing Diagnostic Process

Box 28-4

Assessment Activities	Defining Characteristics	Nursing Diagnosis
Ask client to describe his or her source of faith. Have client describe level of satisfaction with life. Determine who provides the greatest source of strength and support to the client during times of difficulty.	Client expresses an inner strength and source of guidance. Life has purpose and meaning, provides community service as a volunteer. Person pursues interactions with friends and family.	Readiness for enhanced spiritual well-being

nificance that spirituality has for all types of health problems. Pain, fear, anxiety, and self-care deficit are just some examples of common nursing diagnoses that will require the nurse to incorporate spiritual care principles.

There are two nursing diagnoses, *readiness for enhanced spiritual well-being* and *spiritual distress*, accepted by the North American Nursing Diagnosis Association (2003) that pertain specifically to spirituality. *Readiness for enhanced spiritual well-being* is based on defining characteristics that show a person's ability to experience and inte-

grate meaning and purpose in life through connectedness with self and others. A client with this nursing diagnosis has potential resources to draw on when faced with illness or a threat to well-being. If the client does not know how to engage personal resources to cope with health problems, the nurse offers support in exploring options.

The nursing diagnosis of *spiritual distress* creates a different clinical picture. Defining characteristics from a nurse's assessment may find patterns that reflect a person's dispiritedness (e.g., expressing lack of hope, meaning, or purpose in life; refusing interaction with spiritual leaders, friends, or family; inability to express previous creativity; or inability to pray). A client with *spiritual distress* requires care that focuses on establishing or renewing faith and hope and offering resources that the client accepts.

Accurate selection of diagnoses requires critical thinking. The nurse reviews concrete data (e.g., religious rituals and sources of fellowship), an assessment of previous client experiences, the nurse's own spirituality, and the appraisal of the client's spiritual well-being. Defining characteristics must be validated and clarified with the client before a diagnosis and plan of care are made. Commonly clients will have multiple nursing diagnoses. The concept map in Figure 28-5 provides an example of how multiple diagnoses can be interrelated.

Each diagnosis must have an accurate related factor so that resulting interventions can be purposeful and goal directed. The following nursing diagnoses may apply to clients in need of spiritual care:

- Anxiety
- Compromised family coping
- Disabled family coping
- Readiness for enhanced family coping
- Ineffective coping
- Interrupted family processes
- Fear
- Dysfunctional grieving
- Hopelessness
- Powerlessness
- Chronic low self-esteem
- Readiness for enhanced spiritual well-being
- Spiritual distress
- Risk for spiritual distress

Planning

During the planning step of the nursing process, the nurse develops a plan of care for each of the client's nursing diagnoses. Critical thinking is again important because the nurse must reflect on previous experience and apply knowledge and critical thinking attitudes and standards

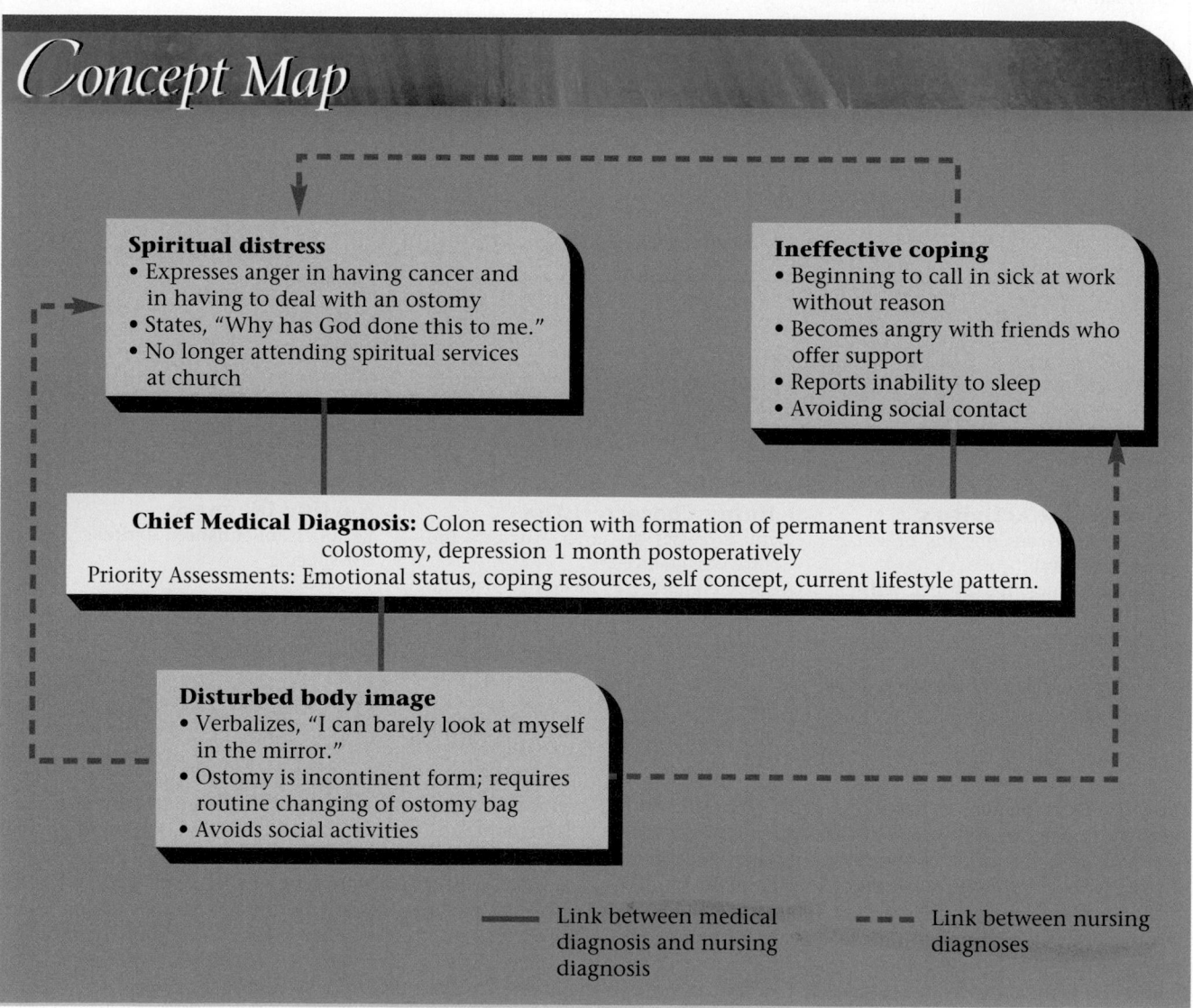

FIGURE **28–5**   Concept map for client with colon resection with formation of permanent transverse colostomy and depression 1 month postoperatively.

in selecting the most appropriate nursing interventions (Figure 28-6). Prior experience in selecting interventions that support clients' spiritual well-being is invaluable when the nurse considers the best options for clients with similar types of situations or problems. The nurse also integrates the knowledge gathered from assessment and knowledge relating to resources and therapies available for spiritual care to develop an individualized plan of care (see care plan). The nurse matches the client's needs with those interventions that are supported and recommended in the clinical and research literature. Confidence becomes an important critical thinking attitude as the nurse attempts to build a caring relationship with the client. Confidence works to build trust, enabling nurse and client to enter into a healing relationship together. Attempting to meet or support clients' spiritual needs is not simple, and often the new nurse will require humility in recognizing that additional resources may be needed. The

nurse's skills in helping clients interpret and understand the meaning of illness and loss, for example, may be limited. Because spiritual care is so personal, standards of autonomy and self-determination are critical in supporting the client's decisions about the plan of care.

Goals and Outcomes. A spiritual care plan must include realistic and individualized goals along with relevant outcomes. It is important for both nurse and client to collaborate closely in setting goals and choosing related interventions. Setting realistic goals will require the nurse to know the client well. In cases where spiritual care requires helping clients adjust to loss or stressful life situations, goals may be long-term oriented. However, short-term outcomes can be established so that the client progressively reaches a more spiritually healthy situation. In establishing a plan of care, an example of a goal and associated outcomes follows:

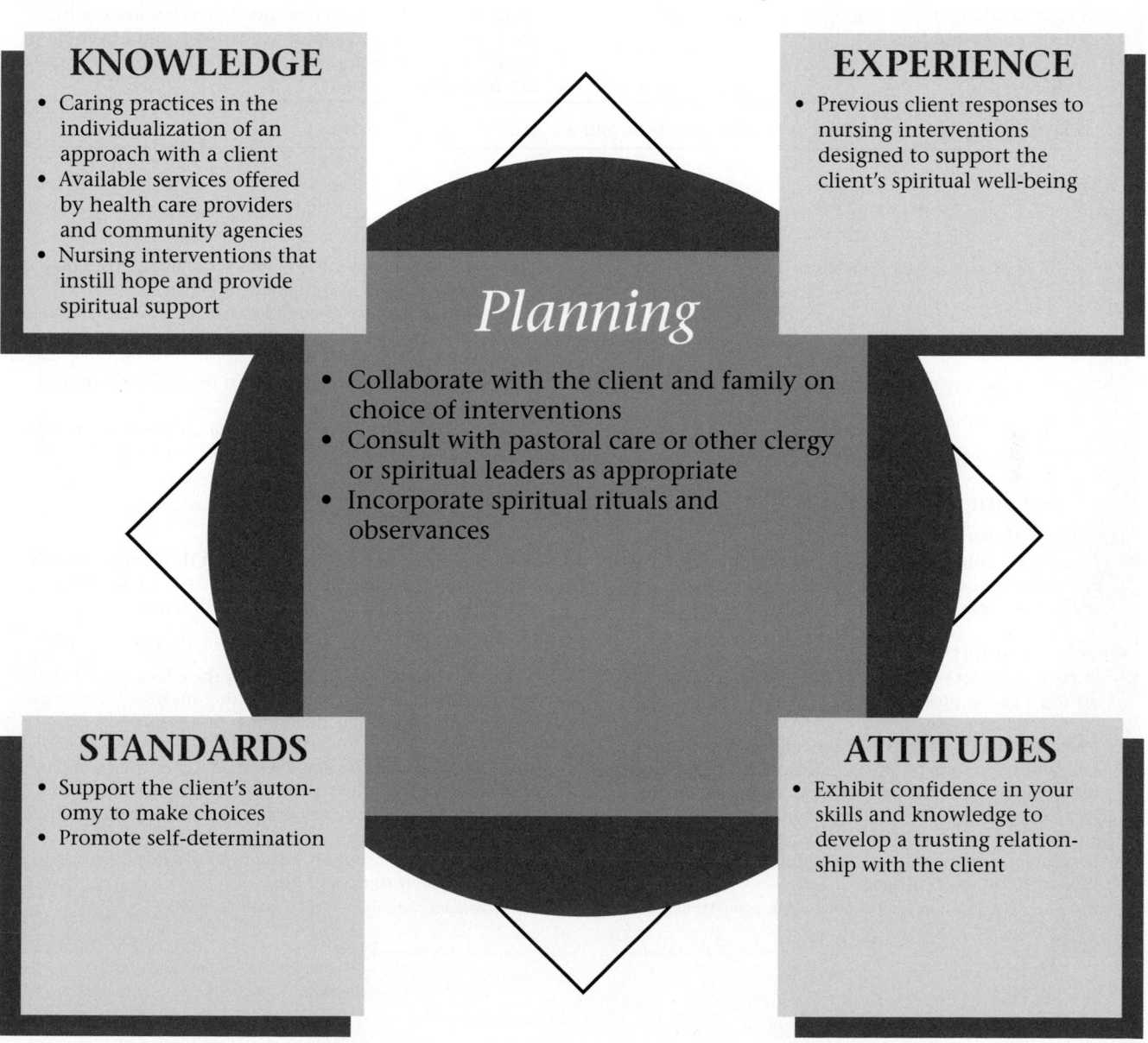

KNOWLEDGE
- Caring practices in the individualization of an approach with a client
- Available services offered by health care providers and community agencies
- Nursing interventions that instill hope and provide spiritual support

EXPERIENCE
- Previous client responses to nursing interventions designed to support the client's spiritual well-being

Planning
- Collaborate with the client and family on choice of interventions
- Consult with pastoral care or other clergy or spiritual leaders as appropriate
- Incorporate spiritual rituals and observances

STANDARDS
- Support the client's autonomy to make choices
- Promote self-determination

ATTITUDES
- Exhibit confidence in your skills and knowledge to develop a trusting relationship with the client

FIGURE **28–6**   Critical thinking model for spiritual health planning.

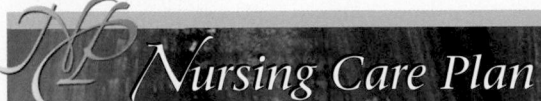

Nursing Care Plan

Spiritual Well-Being

Assessment

James is a 24-year-old who has recently been diagnosed with AIDS. The clinic nurse, Leah, has been talking with James during his last three visits. During that time James expresses a fear of dying. His partner, Will, visits James at home periodically but much less often than before the diagnosis. Leah now talks with James in a private conference area.

Assessment Activities	Findings/Defining Characteristics
Leah asks James, "How has your illness affected your own source of strength or hope?"	James responds, "I don't believe this is happening to me. How can God do this to me? There are moments when I just feel so angry. What is going to happen to me?"
Leah responds, "This is obviously a very difficult time. Who in your life provides you the greatest source of support?"	James begins to cry and admits, "I feel so alone. Will has just not been there when I need him. My family wants to help but they live out of town."
Leah clarifies, "You sound as though it would help to have someone to talk to."	James responds, "It would, but it is so hard to find someone who I can trust and who I feel will listen."
Leah questions, "You mentioned you could not understand why God has done this to you. How has this experience affected your faith and beliefs?"	James responds, "It has been hard. I have never been a religious person. My church does not accept homosexuality, but I always have had a faith in God. Will and I have attended a new ecumenical service at the local college. I have not been attending lately."

Nursing Diagnosis: Spiritual distress related to fear and uncertainty of terminal illness.

Planning

Goal	Expected Outcomes*
	Hope
Client will express a sense of purpose.	Client will discuss how the experience of having AIDS may have a positive influence in life within 1 month.
	Client expresses a sense of confidence in treatments available for AIDS in 2 weeks.
	Spiritual Well-being
Client establishes connection with significant others.	Client reports having more visits with partner, Will, in next 2 weeks.
	Client schedules attendance at AIDS support group in 1 month.

*Outcome classification labels from Moorhead S, Johnson M, Maas M: *Nursing outcomes classification (NOC)*, ed 3, St. Louis, 2004, Mosby.

Interventions†	Rationale
Hope Instillation	
• Plan instructional session to discuss typical course of AIDS, emphasizing the typical pattern of remissions with drug therapy. Review therapies available for treatment.	Knowledge about disease will help client think as a person living with AIDS rather than dying with AIDS (Hall, 1998). Reality of disease course will help instill hope.
Spiritual Support	
• Encourage client's expression of loneliness through establishing a caring presence.	Presencing reflects being in tune with the client and displays caring. It is an effective technique that makes a topic of discussion more approachable (Benner and Wrubel, 1989).
• Listen to client's feelings and concerns.	
• Use spiritual resources. Plan discussion session with client that includes Will, his partner. Have client discuss his ability to cope with AIDS and the meaning it has spiritually.	People question and become open to discover their unique spiritual meaning after a crisis that threatens health (Hall, 1998). Provides client a resource from client's community of faith to share concerns.
• Recommend client consider attending AIDS support group sponsored by local college.	Connections with a support system can provide meaning to illness and offer sources of hope.

†Intervention classification labels from Dochterman JM, Bulechek GM: *Nursing interventions classification (NIC)*, ed 4, St. Louis, 2004, Mosby.

Continued

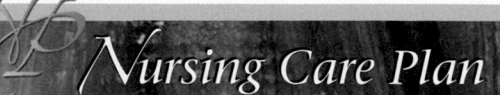

Nursing Care Plan
Spiritual Well-Being—cont'd

Evaluation

Nursing Actions	Client Response/Finding	Achievement of Outcome
Ask client how he currently feels about having AIDS.	"I am not quite as frightened as I was a few weeks ago. I believe the treatments will help me. I have been on the combination therapy for 2 weeks. I just hope it works."	James reports an improved outlook and confidence in treatment. May continue to have doubt about outcome.
Have client describe the session that included Will.	"It meant a great deal to tell Will how I feel. I know now he wants to help, but did not know how. Since then we have talked on the phone almost every day."	Successfully increased connection with significant other. May require support or guidance on how to discuss sensitive feelings with partner.
Ask client if he scheduled attendance at the support group.	"I have called the college. The support group meets next Tuesday evening. I plan to be there."	Client schedules attendance at support group.

The client will improve personal harmony and connections with members of his or her support system.
- The client will be able to express an acceptance of his or her illness.
- The client reports the ability to rely on family members for support.
- The client initiates social interactions with family and friends.

Setting Priorities. A client's spiritual health is closely tied to his or her physical and psychological well-being. When a client is in acute distress, the nurse focuses care on the relief of symptoms to provide the client a sense of control. Then the nurse supports the client's efforts to express the emotional and intellectual aspects of his or her spirituality. When a client suffers a chronic or terminal condition, the nurse's priorities may shift to helping the client deal with unresolved losses and to connect with the spiritual resources available. The nurse needs to reinforce the everyday life patterns that the client uses to maintain coherence and practice individuation.

Continuity of Care. Significant others, such as spouses, siblings, parents, and friends, need to be involved in the client's care, as appropriate. This means that the nurse learns from the assessment what individuals or groups have formed a relationship with the client. These individuals may become involved in all levels of the nurse's plan. The client's support network may assist in giving physical care, providing emotional comfort, and sharing spiritual support. In a hospital setting, one of the best resources to utilize in planning a client's spiritual care is the hospital's pastoral care department. A health care chaplain has special expertise in dealing with the spiritual problems confronted by clients. These professionals should be part of the health care team, lending insight about how and when to best support clients and families.

If the client participates in a formal religion, members of the clergy or members of the church, temple, mosque, or synagogue may need to be involved in the plan of care.

Depending on the client's health status and needs, part of the plan will involve a continuation of appropriate religious rituals. The nurse must make sure that any icons or religious materials such as scriptures or a prayer book are made available.

Implementation

Whether a nurse can provide spiritual care depends on the nurse's ability to establish a caring relationship with a client. Both the client and nurse must feel free to discover together the meaning illness or loss poses for the client and the impact it has on the meaning and purpose of life. Achieving this level of understanding with a client enables the nurse to deliver care in a sensitive, creative, and appropriate manner.

Health Promotion. Spiritual care should be a central theme in promoting an individual's overall well-being. Spirituality is one personal resource that affects the balance between health and illness. In settings where health promotion activities occur, clients are often in need of information, counseling, and guidance to make the necessary choices to remain healthy.

Establishing Presence. Clients have reported that the presence of nurses and their caregiving activities contributes to a sense of well-being and provides hope for recovery (Clark and others, 1991). Behaviors that establish the nurse's presence include giving attention, answering questions, listening, and having a positive and encouraging (but realistic) attitude. The ability to establish presence is part of the art of nursing. It is not simply being in the same room with a client while performing procedures or sharing technical information with a client, but presencing involves "being with" a client versus "doing for" a client (Benner, 1984). Presencing involves offering a closeness with the client, physically, psychologically, and spiritually (Box 28-5).

Case Study   **Box 28-5**

Miller Edmonds is a 51-year-old man who was diagnosed with bone cancer 3 months ago. His primary nursing care problem is that of pain control. Mr. Edmonds is receiving morphine infusions via an intravenous (IV) pump and has been receiving some relief. He has been experiencing a loss of appetite, and the nurses from the night shift reported that during the night Mr. Edmonds was frequently awake and crying. His family visits regularly but usually not until the early evening.

Diane Renthro is the nurse assigned to Mr. Edmonds on the day shift. When she enters Mr. Edmond's room during morning rounds, she finds the client sitting on the side of the bed, moving about restlessly. Diane asks Mr. Edmonds, "How can I help you this morning? Are you having pain?" Mr. Edmonds responds, "Yes, it is not as bad as it was, but I still have trouble really relaxing. I could not sleep at all last night." Diane places her hand on Mr. Edmond's shoulder and says, "Let me take a look at that IV in your arm. I want to be sure it is working properly." Diane silently checks the IV and realigns the tubing so that Mr. Edmonds has more freedom to move his arm. Diane asks, "Can you rate your pain for me on a scale of 0 to 10?" Mr. Edmonds responds, "Yes, they have been asking me that question, I guess it is about a 5." As Mr. Edmonds makes the gesture to lie down, Diane quietly but expertly helps him to his side in bed. She covers Mr. Edmonds with a light sheet and rearranges his pillow. She also tells Mr. Edmonds that she plans on checking with his physician to ensure the morphine dosage is adequate for his pain relief. Diane then places her hand on Mr. Edmonds arm and asks, "Tell me what is most important for us to do for you today." Mr. Edmonds thinks a moment and responds, "I would like to be able to enjoy my family's visit this afternoon. I haven't been a very good host when they visit." Diane takes a seat next to Mr. Edmonds bedside and says, "In what way would you enjoy your family's visit?" Mr. Edmonds begins to cry, "This is so hard for them, my illness and all." Diane uses good eye contact and encourages Mr. Edmonds to say more, "Go on, I want to know how you feel."

Diane's ability to exhibit a presence puts Mr. Edmonds at ease to describe his concerns about his family. He knows he has a terminal illness and has been unable to discuss his fears with his wife. Diane offers ideas for how Mr. Edmonds might share his feelings and then sets a plan with Mr. Edmonds to maximize pain control during the family's visit. As Diane leaves the room she notices Mr. Edmonds is more relaxed. Mr. Edmonds states, "Thanks for listening. You know, I think I might try to eat a little breakfast this morning."

When health promotion is the focus of care, the nurse's presence becomes important in instilling confidence in clients' abilities to take the steps necessary to remain healthy. A nurse can convey a caring presence by listening to clients' concerns over possible outcomes should their health become impaired, willingly involving family in discussions about clients' health, displaying self-confidence when health instruction is provided, and supporting clients' faith in the choices they make. Emblen and Halstead (1993) found in their research that nurses listening to clients was the option clients preferred when spiritual care was provided. The client who seeks health care may be fearful of experiencing an illness that would

threaten loss of control and looks for someone to offer competent direction. The nurse's encouraging words of support and the nurse's calm and decisive approach establish a presence that builds trust and well-being. Chapter 7 provides further details on how to establish presence.

Supporting a Healing Relationship. A nurse learns to look beyond isolated client problems and recognize the broader picture of a client's needs. For example, the nurse does not just look at a client's back pain as a problem to solve with quick remedies, but rather how the pain influences the client's ability to function and achieve goals established in life. A **holistic** view enables the nurse to establish a helping role and a healing relationship. Three factors are evident when a healing relationship develops between nurse and client:

1. Mobilizing hope for the nurse, as well as for the client
2. Finding an interpretation or understanding of the illness, pain, anxiety, or other stressful emotion that is acceptable to the client
3. Assisting the client in using social, emotional, and spiritual resources (Benner, 1984)

Central to a healing relationship is mobilizing the client's hope. Hope motivates people with strategies to face challenges in life. The nurse can help a client find things to hope for. For example, a newly diagnosed diabetic might hope to learn how to manage the disease so as to continue a productive and satisfying way of life. An adult daughter who has decided to become caregiver to her older adult parent might hope to be able to protect the parent from injury or worsening disability. Hope helps a client work toward recovery. To help clients achieve hope, the nurse and client work together to find an explanation of the situation that is acceptable to both. Then the nurse helps the client realistically exercise hope. This might include supporting a client's positive attitude toward life or a desire to be informed and to make decisions.

To further support a healing relationship the nurse must remain aware of the client's spiritual resources and needs. It is always important for a client to be able to express and exercise his or her beliefs and to find spiritual comfort. When life stressors or illness create confusion or uncertainty for the client, the nurse must recognize the possible effect this can have on a client's well-being. How can spiritual resources be used and strengthened? The nurse may begin by encouraging a client to discuss the effect illness has had on personal beliefs and faith. This gives the nurse the chance to clarify any misconceptions or inaccuracies in information. Having a clear sense of what illness may hold for an individual helps the person to apply all resources toward recovery.

Acute Care. Within acute care settings, clients experience multiple stressors that threaten their sense of control. Support and enhancement of a client's spiritual well-being can be a challenge when the focus of health care seems to be one of treatment and cure rather than care. The nurse works closely with the client and his or her support network in finding ways to make the client's spiritual resources become part of the therapeutic plan of care.

Table 28-3	Religious Dietary Regulations Affecting Health Care
Religion	**Dietary Practices**
Hinduism	Some sects are vegetarians. The belief is not to kill *any* living creature.
Buddhism	Some are vegetarians, and many will not use alcohol or tobacco and may hesitate to use drugs. Many will fast on Holy Days.
Islam	Prohibits consumption of pork and alcohol. Fasting is done during the month of Ramadan.
Judaism	Some observe the kosher dietary restrictions of avoiding pork and shellfish and not preparing and eating milk and meat at the same time.
Christianity	Some Baptists, Evangelicals, and Pentecostals discourage the use of alcohol, caffeine, and tobacco.
	Some Roman Catholics may fast during Lent, Ash Wednesday, Good Friday, and 1 hour before receiving Communion.
Jehovah's Witnesses	Members may avoid food prepared with or containing blood.
Mormonism	Members abstain from alcohol, caffeine, and tobacco.
Russian Orthodox Church	Followers must observe fast days as well as a "no meat" rule on Wednesdays and Fridays. During Lent all animal products, including dairy products and butter, are forbidden.
Native Americans	Food practices are influenced by individual tribal beliefs.

Support Systems. Use of support systems is of course important in any health care setting. Support systems provide clients with the greatest sense of well-being during hospitalization and serve as a human link connecting the client, the nurse, and the client's lifestyle before an illness (Clark and others, 1991). Part of the client's caregiving environment is the regular presence of family and friends viewed by the client as supportive. The nurse plans care with the client and the client's support network to promote the interpersonal bonding that is needed for recovery. The support system is a source of faith and hope, and it can be an important resource in conducting the religious rituals on which some clients rely.

When it is known that clients depend on family and friends for support, the nurse encourages them to visit the client regularly. The nurse's encouragement to family to be themselves during visits can facilitate the family's ability to provide the spiritual comfort that they are capable of sharing. Often illness and the treatment environment produce unknowns that intimidate family members and friends. The nurse helps family members to feel welcome and uses their support and presence to promote the client's healing. Including family members in prayer, for example, is a thoughtful gesture if it is appropriate to the client's religion and if family members are comfortable participating. Encouraging the family to bring meaningful religious symbols to the client's bedside can offer significant spiritual support.

Another important resource to clients are spiritual advisors and members of the clergy. Many hospitals have pastoral care departments that assist in notifying community clergy of their congregants' admission or who can provide trained clergy for support. Pastoral care professionals are expert at giving attention to both how an illness is influencing a person's beliefs and how the beliefs of the person can influence the actual illness and recovery experience. The nurse should ask if clients desire to have a member of the clergy visit during their hospitalization. All clergy should be made welcome on nursing units. When requested by clients or families, the nurse should keep clergy informed of any physical, psychoso-

cial, or spiritual concerns affecting the client. The nurse shows respect for clients' spiritual values and needs by willingly cooperating with others giving spiritual care and by facilitating the administration of sacraments, rites, and rituals.

Providing privacy for the client, family, and clergy is a thoughtful and sensitive gesture. The nurse determines the proper routine in a client's religion by asking the clergy, family, or client. Often a client within the hospital may want to discuss spiritual concerns in the evening or late at night, when support services such as clergy and social services are unavailable. The nurse can help to meet the client's needs through careful, skilled, and active listening.

Diet Therapies. Food and nutrition are important aspects of client care and often an important component of some religious observances (Table 28-3). Food and the rituals surrounding the preparation and serving of food can be important to a person's spirituality. The nurse can consult with the dietitian to integrate the client's dietary preferences into daily care. In the event that a hospital or other health care agency cannot prepare food in the preferred way, the family may be asked to bring meals fitting into any dietary restrictions posed by the client's condition.

Supporting Rituals. Nurses provide spiritual care by supporting clients' participation in spiritual rituals and activities. This is especially important for older adults, who typically perceive themselves as highly spiritual (Isaia, Parker, and Murrow, 1999) (Box 28-6). Personal care of the client should be planned to allow time for religious readings, spiritual visitations, or attendance at religious services. Some churches and synagogues offer audiotapes of their services for those members who cannot attend in person. Family members can plan a prayer session or an organized reading of scriptures on a regular basis. Arrangements may need to be made with pastoral care staff for the client and family to receive the sacraments. Clergy will routinely offer to make home visits for persons unable to attend religious services. Taped medi-

- Older adults become more aware of physical decline and inevitable losses, which allows them to find meaning to balance the developmental conflict of ego integrity versus despair (Carson, 1989).
- There is an association between an older adult's spirituality and ability to adjust or cope with illness.
- The very old are more likely to be interested in the nonorganizational aspects of religion than in active participation (Courtney and others, 1992).
- Consideration and a belief in the afterlife increase as adults grow older. Visits from clergy, social workers, lawyers, and even financial advisors can be made available so clients feel prepared. Leaving a legacy (e.g., oral histories, works of art, photographs) to loved ones prepares the older adult to leave the world with a sense of meaning (Ebersole and Hess, 1998).
- Higher levels of religiosity in older women may be related to the social structure in which women typically participate, including church activities, caregiving, and nurturing (Levin and others, 1994).
- Older adult caregivers, such as those caring for another with Alzheimer's dementia, often have a need to express spiritual needs in relation to decisions about the care of the care recipient. Feelings of guilt, hopelessness, fear, and the distresss of "playing God" are just some of those caregivers might express that could reflect spiritual distress (Miller, 1999).

Meditation Techniques
Objective

- The client will be able to achieve a state of relaxation and a transcendent state of being.

Teaching Strategies

- Instruct client to select a quiet room in the home where interruptions can be eliminated.
- Peaceful music or the quiet whirring of a fan may be useful in lessening distraction from the meditation exercise.
- Each meditation should involve about 20 minutes.
- Have client practice 2 or more times daily.
- To begin the exercise have the client assume a comfortable position with extremities unencumbered and supported.
- Coach the client in slow, rhythmic, deep breathing.
- Have the client focus on a sound, a thought, or an image.
- Chanting psalms, a poem, or a prayer repeatedly may assist in focusing.
- After meditation have the client think about what became the focus of meditation, what the client learned or felt about himself or herself.

Evaluation

- Have the client describe the meaning and feeling meditation provides.

---

tations, classical or religious music, and televised religious services provide other effective options. The nurse should be respectful of icons, medals, prayer rugs, or crosses that clients bring to a health setting to be sure they are not accidentally lost, damaged, or misplaced.

Restorative and Continuing Care. For clients who are recovering from a long-term illness or disability or who suffer chronic or terminal disease, spiritual care becomes especially important. Many of the nursing interventions applicable in health promotion and acute care apply to this level of health care as well.

Prayer. The act of prayer gives an individual the opportunity to renew personal faith and belief in a higher being in a specific, focused way that may be highly ritualized and formal or quite spontaneous and informal. Prayer has been shown to be an effective coping resource for physical as well as psychological symptoms. Clients may pray in private or pursue opportunities for group prayer with family, friends, or clergy. The nurse can be supportive of prayer by giving the client privacy if desired, learning if the client wishes to have the nurse participate, and by suggesting prayer when it is known to be a coping resource for the client. If prayer is not suitable for a client, an alternative may be to read from a book (e.g., the Bible or the Koran) selected by the client or from poetry or other inspirational texts.

Meditation. Meditation effectively creates a relaxation response that reduces daily stress. Chapter 35 reviews guided imagery, an approach nurses can use to help clients learn meditation. Individuals who regularly sit quietly in a comfortable position with their eyes closed and repeat a sound, phrase, or sacred word in rhythm with their breathing, gently disregarding intrusive thoughts as they do so, experience decreased metabolism and heart rate, easier breathing, and slower brain waves (Culligan, 1996). Meditation exercises give individuals relief from chronic pain, insomnia, anxiety, and depression and can help in coping with the side effects of therapies for cancer and AIDS. When clients use meditation in conjunction with their spiritual beliefs, often they report an increased spirituality that is described as experiencing the presence of a power, force, or energy, or what was perceived as God (Box 28-7).

Supporting Grief Work. Clients who experience terminal illness or who have suffered permanent loss in body function because of a disabling disease or an injury will require the nurse's support in grieving over and coping with their loss. Chapter 29 provides a variety of nursing interventions for support of clients' grief work. Supporting a client during times of grief can be strengthened by the nurse's ability to enter into a spiritual relationship with the client, whereby nurse and client come to know one another as individuals.

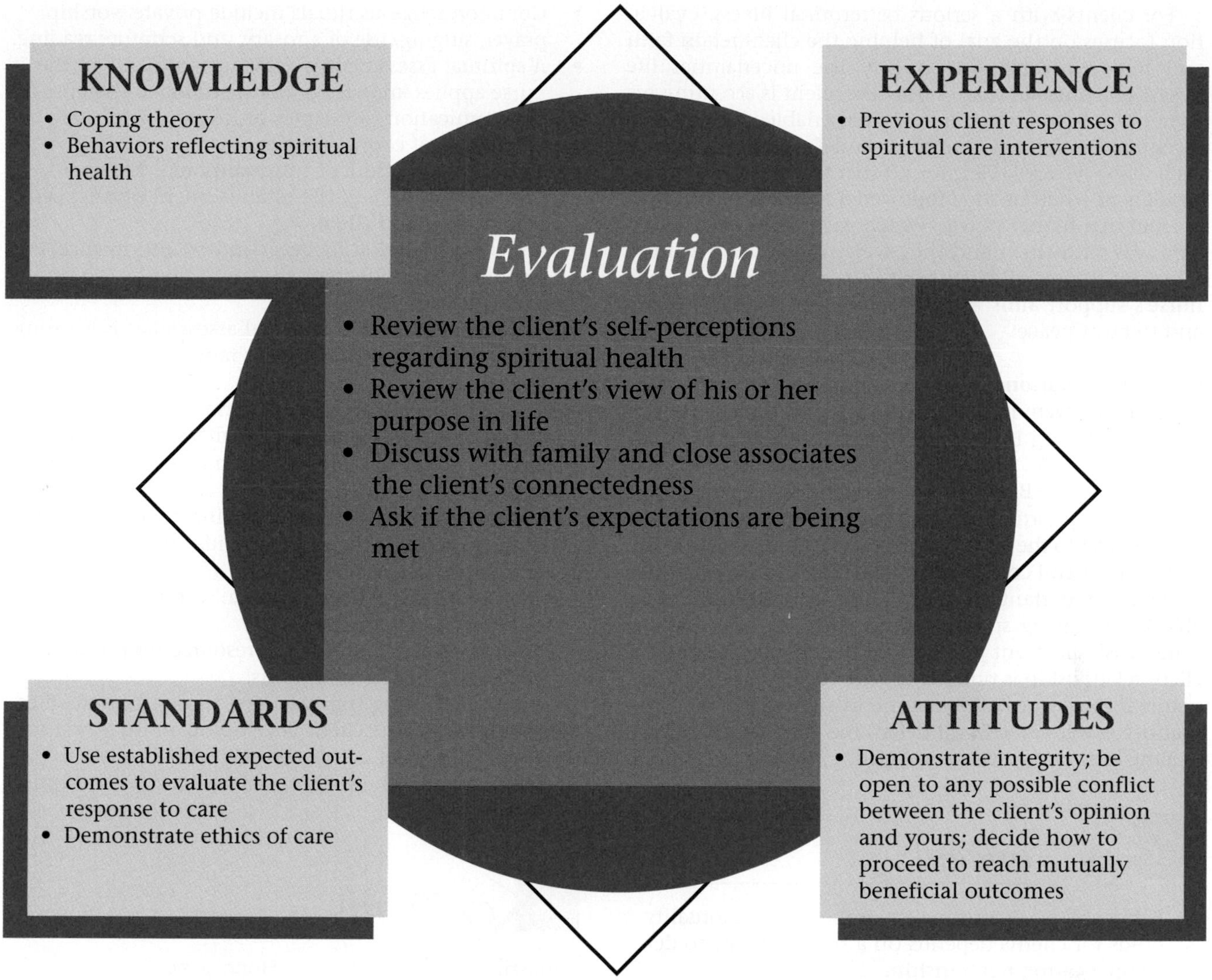

FIGURE 28–7   Critical thinking model for spiritual health evaluation.

Evaluation

The evaluation of a client's spiritual care requires the nurse to think critically in determining if efforts at restoring or maintaining the client's spiritual health were successful (Figure 28-7). The nurse will consider knowledge of spiritual concepts and coping theory (see Chapter 30) in evaluating whether the client has been able to adjust to those factors that threaten spiritual well-being. Outcomes established during the planning phase will serve as the standards to evaluate the client's progress. In addition, an ethic of caring ensures that the nurse evaluates any ethical concerns that may arise in the course of the client's spiritual care and support. Critical thinking attitudes are applied to ensure sound nursing judgments. The nurse's evaluation includes a review of the client's response to care and whether the client's expectations were achieved.

Client Care. Attainment of spiritual health is a lifelong goal. Clients will experience the need to clarify values (see Chapter 21), reshape philosophies, strengthen relationships, and live those experiences that help to shape one's purpose in life. The nurse provides spiritual care while always evaluating whether planned outcomes and goals were achieved. The nurse compares the client's level of spiritual health with the behaviors and perceptions noted in the nursing assessment. For example, if the nurse's assessment finds the client losing hope, the follow-up evaluation will involve a discussion with the client to determine if the client has regained an attitude of something to live for. Family and friends with whom the client seeks to have fellowship can be a useful source of evaluative information. Successful outcomes should reveal the client developing an increased or restored sense of connectedness with family; maintaining, renewing, or reforming a sense of purpose in life and, for some, a confidence and trust in a supreme being or power.

For clients with a serious or terminal illness, evaluation focuses on the goal of helping the client retain faith and hope or expressing openly the uncertainties life poses. The nurse evaluates how the client is accepting his or her illness and whether hope has enabled the client to recognize individual mortality and focus on living for each day. Fryback (1993) found that the terminally ill, regardless of whether they followed a formal religion, held a belief in a higher power, which gave them a sense that God was with them and they were not alone. The nurse must not assume all clients have such faith. However, the nurse's support aims to help clients accept their destiny and to be at peace.

Client Expectations. The nurse evaluates whether client expectations were met. In regard to spiritual care, this involves evaluating if the client's spiritual practices were respected and if the nurse-client relationship was one of caring and support. Both the client and family should be able to relate if opportunities were offered for religious rituals. With respect to the nurse-client relationship, does the client express trust and confidence in the nurse? Is the client able to discuss important issues or topics? Is the client comfortable in expressing spiritual needs with the nurse? Taking time to ask the client to reflect on the quality of the nurse-client relationship is time well spent. Asking the client, "Do you feel your expectations of me in supporting your spiritual needs were met?" will determine whether an effective healing relationship was developed.

Key Concepts

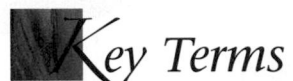

- Being able to determine the importance spirituality holds for clients depends on a nurse's ability to develop a caring relationship.
- There may be beneficial health outcomes when individuals are able to exercise their spiritual beliefs.
- The Framework of Systemic Organization is an organizing structure through which nurses can engage in nurse-client relationships to explore their clients' diverse spiritual needs.
- During times of illness and loss individuals seek control to protect themselves from vulnerability and provide a sense of security.
- When control is unsuccessful, individuals practice spirituality to promote congruence through a sense of unity and inner peace.
- Spirituality is highly personal and unique to each individual.
- Faith is a relationship with a higher power or authority that enables action and gives purpose and meaning to an individual's life.
- Religion is a system of organized beliefs and worship that a person practices to outwardly express spirituality.
- Hope provides comfort and a motivation to achieve when a person is faced with a loss.
- When clients experience acute or chronic illness or a terminal disease, spiritual resources either help a person move to recovery or spiritual distress develops.

- Common religious rituals include private worship, prayer, singing, use of a rosary, and scripture reading.
- A spiritual assessment is most successful when the nurse applies knowledge that pertains to therapeutic communication, principles of loss and grief, and knowledge of caring practices.
- The personal nature of spirituality requires open communication and the establishment of trust between nurse and client.
- If a client's religious beliefs conflict with medical treatment, options to nurses and other health care providers can be limited.
- An important part of spiritual assessment is learning who are the client's friends or family who share a community of faith.
- A hospital's pastoral care department is a valuable resource to use in planning a client's spiritual care.
- Central to a healing relationship is mobilizing the client's hope.
- Part of a client's caregiving environment can be the regular presence of family, friends, and spiritual advisors.
- Depending on a client's religion, certain foods may be restricted in the diet.
- Prayer is an effective coping resource for physical and psychological symptoms.
- When evaluating spiritual care, successful outcomes should reveal the client developing an increased or restored sense of connectedness with family and maintaining, renewing, or reforming a sense of purpose in life.

Key Terms

Critical Thinking Exercises

1. Mr. Jackson is a 40-year-old businessman who employs over 100 employees. A 12-hour-a-day work week is not unusual for him. Last evening he was admitted to the cardiac care unit with severe chest pain resulting from a myocardial infarction (heart attack). He is now stabilized but is making frequent requests of his nurses and doctors, asking about his diagnostic tests and what he needs to do to be able to go home. He tells his nurse, "My doctor tells me I will need surgery once I am more stable. I hope he can do that soon. I just can't believe this is happening. I worry about what will happen to my business while I am gone."
   a. Applying the Framework of Systemic Organization, what behaviors is Mr. Jackson demonstrating?

b. Identify three approaches you might use as his nurse to conduct a spiritual assessment with Mr. Jackson.

2. Celia is a new graduate nurse caring for Ms. Rosenbaum for the first time. Ms. Rosenbaum has been diagnosed with uterine cancer. Celia is helping Ms. Rosenbaum with her meal tray when she says, "I noticed that the information in your chart says you are Jewish. Would you like me to call a Rabbi to visit? Are there any diet considerations we should be making for you?" Are Celia's assessment and resultant interventions appropriate for this situation?

3. Critical thinking is an ongoing process. When you learn that you are assigned to Julio Gonsaga, you note that the Kardex information includes his religion, Catholic, and his place of birth, Cuba. A colleague tells you he can speak some English. The client is 80 years old and reportedly has a bit of a hearing deficit. What knowledge might you wish to reflect on critically before beginning a spiritual assessment of this client?

Review Questions

1. Caring for a client's spiritual needs means:
   1. The nurse must have the same beliefs as the client.
   2. Praying for the client.
   3. Accepting the client's beliefs and experiences.
   4. Calling for a religious leader if the nurse determines a need.

2. An individual who does not believe in the existence of God is an:
   1. Agnostic.
   2. Atheist.
   3. Anarchist.
   4. Agenic.

3. Hope is a concept related to spirituality that can be best described as:
   1. Satisfaction with someone or something.
   2. Having a bond with another person for ongoing support.
   3. Having confidence in something for which there is no proof.
   4. Knowing a threat exists and preparing for any undesired outcomes.

4. Hinduism discourages the prolonging of life and believes illness is:
   1. Caused by past sins.
   2. A blessing in disguise.
   3. A result of unhealthy personal habits.
   4. A personal experience.

5. Client's rituals and practice:
   1. Have no place in modern medicine.
   2. Have no place in the hospital.
   3. Can get in the way of nursing care.
   4. Provide structure and support for the client.

6. The ability to establish presence is part of the art of nursing. It is not simply being in the same room with a client but also:
   1. Involves offering a closeness with the client, physically, psychologically, and spiritually.
   2. Involves performing procedures.
   3. Involves sharing technical information with the client.
   4. Involves all team members.

7. For Hindus it is important to consider that:
   1. Some sects are vegetarian.
   2. Followers must observe fast days.
   3. Many individuals avoid meats containing blood.
   4. Members abstain from alcohol and caffeine.

8. Jehovah Witnesses may avoid:
   1. Caffeine and chocolate.
   2. Pork and shellfish.
   3. Dairy products and caffeine.
   4. Food prepared with or containing blood.

9. Members of the Mormon faith:
   1. Avoid pork and shellfish.
   2. Avoid alcohol, caffeine, and tobacco.
   3. Practice vegetarianism.
   4. Do not eat milk and meat at the same time.

10. Clients who experience terminal illness or who have suffered permanent loss in body function because of a disabling disease or an injury can benefit from:
    1. Grief work
    2. Prayer from the nurse.
    3. Acupuncture.
    4. Assisted suicide.

References

Adair MN and others: New behavioral strategies for enhancing immune function, *AIDS Patient Care* 5:297, 1991.

Aldridge D: Is there evidence for spiritual healing? *Adv J Mind-Body Health* 9(4):4, 1993.

Basford TK: *Near death experience: an annotated bibliography,* New York, 1990, Garland.

Benner DG: *Baker encyclopedia of psychology,* Grand Rapids, Mich, 1985, Baker Book House.

Benner P: *From novice to expert,* Menlo Park, Calif, 1984, Addison-Wesley.

Benner P, Wrubel J: *The primacy of caring,* Menlo Park, Calif, 1989, Addison-Wesley.

Burgess WA: *Psychiatric Nursing,* Stamford, Conn, 1997, Appleton & Lange.

Burnard P: The spiritual needs of atheists and agnostics, *Prof Nurse* 4(3):130, 1988.

Carson V: *Spiritual dimensions of nursing practice,* Philadelphia, 1989, WB Saunders.

Catterall RA and others: The assessment and audit of spiritual care, *Int J Palliat Nurs* 4:162, 1998.

Childe G: Spiritual healing, *Nurs Stand* 16(44):27, 2002.

Clark CC and others: Spirituality: integral to quality care, *Holist Nurs Pract* 5(3):67, 1991.

Coe RM: The magic of science and the science of magic: an essay on the process of healing, *J Health Soc Behav* 38(3):1, 1997.

Courtney BC and others: Religiosity and adaptation in the oldest-old. In Poon LW, editor: *The Georgia centenarian study,* Amityville, NY, 1992, Baywood.

Culligan K: Spirituality and healing in medicine, *America,* p 17, August 31, 1996.

Dombeck MB: Dream-telling: a means of spiritual awareness, *Holist Nurs Pract* 9(2):37, 1995.

Draper P, McSherry W: A critical view of spirituality and spiritual assessment, *J Adv Nurs* 39(1):1, 2002.

Ebersole P, Hess P: *Toward healthy aging,* ed 5, St. Louis, 1998, Mosby.

Emblen JD: Religion and spirituality defined according to current use in nursing literature, *J Prof Nurs* 8(1):41, 1992.

Emblen JD, Halstead L: Spiritual needs and interventions: comparing the views of patients, nurses, and chaplains, *Clin Nurs Spec* 7(4):175, 1993.

Farran CJ and others: Development of a model for spiritual assessment and intervention, *J Religion Health* 28(3):185, 1989.

Friedemann ML: *The framework of systemic organization: a conceptual approach to families and nursing,* Thousand Oaks, Calif, 1995, Sage.

Friedemann M, Mouch J, Racey T: Nursing the spirit: the Framework of Systemic Organization, *J Adv Nurs* 39(4):325, 2002.

Fryback PB: Health for people with a terminal diagnosis, *Nurs Sci Q* 6(3):147, 1993.

Gallop G: Religion in America: fifty years: 1935-1985—The Gallup Report, Princeton, NJ, 1985, Princeton Religious Research Center.

Giger JN, Davidhizar RE: *Transcultural nursing: assessment and intervention,* ed 2, St. Louis, 1995, Mosby.

Haase JE and others: Simultaneous concept analysis of spiritual perspective, hope, acceptance, and self-transcendence, *Image J Nurs Sch* 24(4):141, 1992.

Heliker D: Reevaluation of a nursing diagnosis: spiritual distress, *Nurs Forum* 27(4):15, 1992.

Hungelmann J and others: Focus on spiritual well-being: harmonious interconnectedness of mind-body-spirit—use of the JAREL spiritual well-being scale, *Geriatr Nurs* 17(6):262, 1996.

Kellar P: Mind-body medicine, *Midwest Pain Society Update,* p 3, July 2001.

Koenig HG and others: Attendance at religious services, interleukin-6, and other biological parameters of immune function in older adults, *Int J Psychiatry Med* 27:233, 1997.

Martsolf DS, Mickley JR: The concept of spirituality in nursing theories: differing world-views and extent of focus, *J Adv Nurs* 27:294, 1998.

McCloskey Dochterman JC, Bulechek GM: *Nursing interventions classification (NIC),* ed 4, St. Louis, 2004, Mosby.

McSherry W, Ross L: Dilemmas of spiritual assessment: considerations for nursing practice, *J Adv Nurs* 38(5):479, 2002.

Miller CA: Nursing care of older adults: theory and practice, ed 3, Philadelphia, 1999, Lippincott.

Morse JM, Doberneck B: Delineating the concept of hope, *Image J Nurs Sch* 27(4):277, 1995.

North American Nursing Diagnosis Association: *NANDA nursing diagnoses: definitions and classifications 2003-2004,* Philadelphia, 2003, The Association.

Peri TC: Promoting spirituality in persons with acquired immunodeficiency syndrome: a nursing intervention, *Holist Nurs Pract* 10(1):68, 1995.

Saudia TL and others: Health locus of control and helpfulness of prayer, *Heart Lung* 20:60, 1991. Sobralske M: Perceptions of health: Navajo Indians, *Top Clin Nurs* 7(3):32, 1985.

Turner RP and others: Religious or spiritual problem: a culturally sensitive diagnostic category in the DSM-IV, *J Nerv Ment Dis* 183(7):435, 1995.

Yim RJR, Vande Creek L: Unbinding grief and life's losses for thriving recovery after open heart surgery, *Caregiver J* 12(2):8, 1996.

*R*esearch References

Carson VB, Green H: Spiritual well-being: a predictor of hardiness in patients with acquired immunodeficiency syndrome, *J Prof Nurs* 8:209, 1992.

Hall BA: Patterns of spirituality in persons with advanced HIV disease, *Res Nurs Health* 21:143, 1998.

Isaia D, Parker V, Murrow E: Spiritual well-being among older adults, *J Gerontol Nurs* 26(8):15, 1999.

King DE, Mainous AG, Pearson WS: C-reactive protein, diabetes, and attendance at religious services, *Diabetes Care* 25(7):1172, 2002.

Lambe M and others: Malignant melanoma: reduced risk associated with early childbearing and multiparity, *Melanoma Res* 6:147, 1996.

Levin JS and others: Race and gender differences in religiosity among older adults: findings from four national surveys, *J Gerontology* 49:S137, 1994.

Martinez RJ: Close friends of God: an ethnographic study of health of older Hispanic adults, *J Multicult Nurs Health* 5(1):40, 1999.

Pincharoen S, Congdon JG: Spirituality and health in older Thai persons in the United States, *West J Nurs Res* 25(1):93, 2003.

Reed PG: Spirituality and well-being in terminally ill hospitalized adults, *Res Nurs Health* 10:335, 1987.

29

The Experience
of Loss, Death, and Grief

Media Resources

http://evolve.elsevier.com/Potter/
fundamentals/

 CD COMPANION

- Review Questions
- Glossary

evolve WEBSITE

- Review Questions
- Student Learning Activities
- Glossary

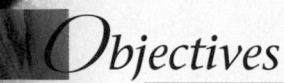

Objectives

Mastery of content in this chapter will enable the student to:

- Define key terms.
- Identify the nurse's role in assisting clients with problems related to loss, death, and grief.
- Describe and compare the phases of grieving from Kübler-Ross, Bowlby, and Worden.
- List and discuss the five categories of loss.
- Describe the types of grief.
- Describe characteristics of a person experiencing grief.
- Discuss variables that influence a person's response to grief.
- Develop a nursing care plan for a client or family experiencing loss and grief.
- Explain reasons for the need for improved end-of-life care for clients.
- Discuss principles of palliative care.
- Describe how to involve family members in palliative care.
- Describe the procedure for care of the body after death.
- Discuss the nurse's own loss experience when caring for dying clients.

*L*oss and grief are experiences that affect not only clients and their families but the nurses who care for them as well. America is a death-denying society (End-of-Life Nursing Education Consortium [ELNEC], 2000). This means that Americans often deny the need to express grief and to feel the pain associated with a loss, both of which are beneficial to healing. Grief affects survivors physically, psychologically, socially, and spiritually as a result of very real, concrete losses. Death of a client, for example, leaves family, friends, and caregivers feeling powerless. Most nurses enter the profession with the intent of helping clients recover from illness, adjust to illness-related changes in lifestyle, and move toward health restoration. It is frightening to learn that knowledge, skill, and technology cannot always come together to result in cure.

The nurse's role in facilitating the grief process includes assisting survivors to feel the loss, express the loss, and complete the tasks of the grief process (ELNEC, 2000). To be effective the nurse must have a thorough understanding of a client's loss, its significance and meaning to the client and family, and how it affects the client's and family's ability to carry on. Providing care for clients in crisis from loss or at the end of life requires knowledge and caring to help bring comfort to clients and families even when a hope for cure is gone.

Scientific Knowledge Base

Loss

Throughout our lives, from birth to death, we form attachments and suffer losses. We develop independence from our parents, start and leave school, change friends, begin careers, and form relationships. The growing-up process is natural and positive, yet as we move our lives forward, we suffer necessary losses (Hasler, 1996). **Necessary losses** are an integral part of each person's life. We expect our losses to be recovered and replaced by something different or better, but there are other losses that cause us to suffer an unbearable change in our safety and security (Hasler, 1996). Losses such as death of a loved one, divorce, or loss of independence are significant and can have long-term effects on our physical and psychological health.

Loss comes in many forms based on the values and priorities learned within a person's sphere of influence, including family, friends, society, and culture. A person experiences loss in the absence of an object, person, body part or function, emotion, or idea that was formerly present (Table 29-1). Losses may be actual or perceived. An **actual loss** is any loss of a person or object that can no longer be felt, heard, known, or experienced by the individual. Examples could include the loss of a body part, child, relationship, or role at work. Lost objects that have been valued by a client include any possession that is worn out, misplaced, stolen, or ruined by disaster. For example, a child may grieve over the loss of a favorite toy. A **perceived loss** is any loss that is uniquely defined by the grieving client. It may be less obvious to others. An example is the loss of confidence or prestige. Perceived losses are easily overlooked or misunderstood, yet the process of grief follows the same sequencing and progression as actual losses. Individual interpretation makes a difference in how the perceived loss is uniquely valued and the response that one will have during grieving.

Losses may also be maturational, situational, or both. A **maturational loss** includes any change in the developmental process that is normally expected during a lifetime. One example would be a mother's feeling of loss as a child goes to school for the first time. Events associated with maturational loss are part of normal life transitions, but the feelings of loss persist as grieving helps a person cope with the change. **Situational loss** includes any sudden, unpredictable external event. Often this type of loss includes multiple losses rather than a single loss, such as an automobile accident that leaves a driver paralyzed, unable to return to work, and grieving over the loss of the passenger in the accident.

The type of loss and the perception of the loss influence the depth and duration of grief a person experiences. Each individual responds to loss differently. It is incorrect to assume that the loss of an object does not generate the same level of stress as loss of a loved one. The value an individual places on the lost object (e.g., a family pet) determines the emotional response to the separation. A nurse must assess the special meaning that a loss has for a client and its effect on the client's health and well-being.

Hospitalization and chronic illness or disability are special circumstances that have multiple associated losses. When persons enter a hospital, they lose their privacy, control over body functions and their daily routines, their modesty, and any illusions that they may have about their personal indestructibility. A chronic illness or disability adds concern over financial security. Furthermore, long-term illness may require a job change, threaten independence, and force alterations in lifestyle. Even a brief illness or hospitalization requires temporary shifts in family role functioning. Chronic or debilitating illness may pose a major threat to the stability of relationships.

Death is the ultimate loss. Although death is part of the continuum of life and a universal and inevitable part of being human, it is also a mystical event that generates anxiety and fear. Death ends relationships that bind and unite families and individuals together, and it separates people from the physical presence of persons who influence their lives. Even in the presence of a strong spiritual grounding, facing death is often difficult for the dying person, as well as for the person's family, friends, and caregivers. A person's terminal illness reminds close friends and associates of their own mortality. A person with an advanced, progressive, ultimately fatal illness such as chronic renal failure, end-stage heart failure, amyotrophic lateral sclerosis, or metastatic cancer faces many levels of suffering. It is difficult to be sick, and many people dislike seeking help from others, yet nearly all want companionship in the face of death (Finucane, 2002).

Callahan (1995) suggests that talking about death has been banished from our society, our everyday lives, our language, and even our thinking. Feelings of guilt, anger, and fear arise when death must finally be faced. It may cause family members and caregivers to withdraw at a

Table 29-1	**Types of Loss**
Definition	**Implications of Loss**
Loss of external objects (e.g., loss, misplacement, deterioration, theft, destruction by natural causes)	Extent of grieving depends on object's value, sentiment attached to it, and its usefulness.
Loss of known environment (e.g., moving from a neighborhood, hospitalization, a new job, moving out of intensive care unit)	Loss occurs through maturational or situational events and through injury or illness. Loneliness or newness of unfamiliar setting threatens self-esteem and makes grieving difficult.
Loss of a significant other (e.g., being promoted, moving, or running away; loss of a family member, friend, trusted nurse, acquaintance, or animal companion)	Significant other typically fulfills another person's need for psychological safety, love and belonging, and self-esteem.
Loss of an aspect of self (e.g., body part, psychological or physiological function)	Illness, injury, or developmental changes result in loss of aspect of self that causes grief and permanent changes in body image and self-concept.
Loss of life (e.g., death of family members, friend, or acquaintance; own death)	Loss of life creates grief for those left behind. Person facing death often fears pain, loss of control, and dependency on others.

time when the dying person needs a trusted, unhurried companion, acting with gentle advocacy and humility. The way a person approaches dying will be influenced by personal fundamental beliefs and values, past experiences with death, culture, spirituality, and the quality of the human emotional support available.

Grief

Grief is the emotional response to a loss. It is manifested in a variety of ways that are unique to an individual and based on personal experiences, cultural expectations, and spiritual beliefs (Farber and others, 1999) (see Chapters 8 and 28). Coping with grief after a loss involves the process of mourning, the outward, social expression of a loss (ELNEC, 2000). It involves working through the grief until an individual accepts and adapts to his or her expectations to go on in life without that which was lost. **Bereavement** includes grief and mourning—the inner feelings and outward reactions of the survivor (ELNEC, 2000). Survivors go through a bereavement period that is not linear. It does not proceed in sequential stages that can be precisely predicted, which may imply passivity on the part of the bereaved. Rather an individual will move back and forth through a series of stages and/or tasks many times, possibly extending over a period of several years, before the process is completed. However, no one really "gets over" a loss, but the individual can heal and learn to live with a loss (ELNEC, 2000). There are several theorists who have developed stages of the grieving process and a series of tasks for survivors to work through their bereavement and adapt to life with a loss.

Theories of Grief

Kübler-Ross's Stages of Dying. The framework for Kübler-Ross's theory (1969) is behavior oriented and includes five stages (Table 29-2). During **denial** an individual acts as though nothing has happened and may refuse to believe or understand that a loss has occurred. In the **anger** stage the individual resists the loss and may strike out at everyone and everything. During **bargaining** the individual postpones awareness of the reality of the loss and may try to deal in a subtle or overt way as though the loss can be prevented. A person finally realizes the full impact and significance of the loss during the stage of **depression.** During depression the individual may feel overwhelmingly lonely and withdraw from interpersonal interaction. Finally, during the stage of **acceptance,** the individual accepts the loss and begins to look to the future.

Bowlby's Phases of Mourning. Bowlby's attachment theory (1980) is the foundation for his theory on mourning. Attachment is described as an instinctive behavior that leads to the development of affectional bonds between children and their primary caregiver. These bonds are present and active throughout the life cycle. Later the bonds are generalized to other persons with whom individuals form close relationships. Attachment behavior ensures our survival because it keeps us in close contact with persons who can offer us protection and support.

Bowlby describes four phases of mourning (see Table 29-2). As in the case of the other grief theories, a person can move back and forth between any two of the phases while responding to the loss. The phase of **numbing** may last from a few hours to a week or more and may be interrupted by periods of extremely intense emotion. It is the briefest phase of mourning. The grieving person may describe this phase as feeling "stunned" or "unreal." Numbing may serve to protect the body from the onslaught or consequence of the loss. The second phase of **yearning and searching** arouses emotional outbursts of tearful sobbing and acute distress in most persons. The phase is painful, but must be endured (Hasler, 1996). Parkes (1972) has explained that it is necessary for the bereaved person to experience the pain of grief in order to get the grief work done. Then, anything that continually allows the person to avoid or suppress the pain can be expected to prolong the course of mourning. Common physical symptoms include tightness in the chest and throat, a shortness of breath, a feeling of weakness and lethargy, and insomnia and loss of appetite. A person may also experience less openly an intense yearning for the object or individual who is lost. This phase may last for months or years. During the phase of **disorganization and despair** an individual may endlessly examine how and why the loss occurred. It is common for the person to express anger at anyone who might be responsible. Gradually, this examination gives way to an acceptance that the loss is permanent. During the final phase of **reorganization,** which may require as much as a year or more, the person begins to accept unaccustomed roles, acquire new skills, and build new relationships. Persons experiencing this phase must be encouraged to untie themselves from their old relationship, while not devaluing it or feeling that in doing so they are lessening its importance (Hasler, 1996).

Worden's Four Tasks of Mourning. Worden's four tasks of mourning (1982) imply that persons who mourn can be actively involved in helping themselves and can be assisted by outside intervention. Although time varies greatly in individuals, the tasks typically require a minimum of a full year to work through.

• *Task I: To accept the reality of the loss.* Even when a death has been expected, there is always some period of dis-

Table 29-2	The Grief Process	
Kübler-Ross's Five Stages of Dying	**Bowlby's Four Phases of Mourning**	**Worden's Four Tasks of Mourning**
Denial	Numbing	Accepting the reality of loss
Anger	Yearning and	Working through the
Bargaining	searching	pain of grief
Depression	Disorganization	Adjusting to the
Acceptance	and despair	environment without
	Reorganization	the deceased
		Emotionally relocating the deceased and moving on with life

belief and surprise that the event has really happened. This task involves the processes required to accept that the person or object is gone and will not return.

- *Task II: To work through the pain of grief.* Even though people respond to loss differently, it is impossible to experience a loss and work through grief without emotional pain. Individuals who deny or shut off the pain prolong their grief.
- *Task III: To adjust to the environment in which the deceased is missing.* According to Worden, a person does not realize the full impact of a loss for at least 3 months. At this point many friends and associates stop calling and the person is left to ponder the full impact of loneliness. People completing this task must take on roles formerly filled by the deceased, including some tasks that they never fully appreciated.
- *Task IV: To emotionally relocate the deceased and move on with life.* The goal of this task is not to forget the deceased or give up the relationship with the deceased but to have the deceased take a new, less prominent place in a person's emotional life. This is often the most difficult task to complete because people fear that if they make other attachments they will forget their loved one or become disloyal. A person completes this stage after realizing that it is possible to love other people without loving the deceased person less.

Types of Grief. A nurse's knowledge of the types of grief, which are based on characteristics or signs and symptoms of grief, allows for the implementation of appropriate bereavement therapies.

Normal Grief. Normal or uncomplicated grief consists of the normal feelings, behaviors, and reactions to a loss. These might include resentment, sorrow, anger, crying, loneliness, and temporary withdrawal from activities. Often the normal grief response to a loss can prove positive, helping one to mature and develop as a person. As people mature they develop ways of dealing with losses and learn to maintain and enhance their feelings of safety and security (Hasler, 1996).

Anticipatory Grief. The process of disengaging or "letting go" that occurs before an actual loss or death has occurred is called **anticipatory grief.** For example, once a person or family receives a terminal diagnosis, they begin the process of saying good-bye and completing life affairs. The process becomes more stressful when the client is unable to make decisions due to deterioration in health. Unless guided by a client's explicit decisions regarding end-of-life care, the family assumes the responsibility of deciding whether to continue life-sustaining measures. The family must weigh factors such as the client's values and choices, the medical facts and probabilities, the burden of treatment, the expected future quality of life for the client, and the limitations of their own emotional resources (Tilden and others 2001).

When the actual process of dying is extended for a long time, persons in the client's family may have few symptoms of grief once the death occurs. This seeming absence of grief symptoms may result because the family has engaged in the grief process over time. By the time the actual moment of death arrives, much of the shock, denial, and tearfulness have already been experienced.

There are risks in anticipatory grieving. Family members may withdraw emotionally from the client too soon, leaving the client with no emotional support as death approaches. There may also be complications if a person who was thought to be near death survives. Family members may then have difficulty reconnecting and may even be resentful that the person has lived past life expectancy.

Complicated Grief. When a person has difficulty progressing through the normal phases or stages of grieving, bereavement becomes complicated. In these cases bereavement appears to "go wrong" and loss never resolves. This can threaten a person's relationships with others. Complicated grief includes four types:

- *Chronic grief:* Active acute mourning that is characterized by normal grief reactions that do not subside and continue over very long periods of time (ELNEC, 2000). Persons verbalize an inability to "get past" the grief.
- *Delayed grief:* Characterized by normal grief reactions that are suppressed or postponed and the survivor consciously or unconsciously avoids the pain of the loss (ELNEC, 2000). Active grieving is held back, only to resurface later, usually in response to a trivial loss or upset. For example, a wife may only bereave a few weeks after the death of her spouse, only to become hysterical and sad a year later when she attends a family gathering. The extreme sadness is a delayed response to the death of her husband.
- *Exaggerated grief:* Persons become overwhelmed by grief, and they cannot function. This may be reflected in the form of severe phobias or self-destructive behavior such as alcoholism, substance abuse, or suicide.
- *Masked Grief:* Survivors are not aware that behaviors that interfere with normal functioning are a result of their loss (ELNEC, 2000). For example, a person who has lost a pet may develop alterations in eating or sleeping patterns.

Disenfranchised Grief. Persons experience grief when a loss is experienced and cannot be openly acknowledged, socially sanctioned, or publicly shared (ELNEC, 2000). An example includes the loss of a partner from human immunodeficiency virus (HIV) or acquired immunodeficiency syndrome (AIDS), children experiencing the death of a step-parent, or the mother whose child dies in utero or at birth.

Application of Grief Theory to Other Types of Loss. Although grief theories apply mainly to the way individuals cope with the death of a loved one, they also apply to other losses. The theories are relevant when describing the way persons respond to a loss of body function, as in the case of organ transplantation or heart attack, and disability such as amputation of a limb or a stroke. Grief theory applies to individuals who progress through stages of mourning for lost independence, body integrity, and a change in body image. These individuals experience emotional pain that is very real as they progress through the stages of grieving.

Nursing Knowledge Base

Nursing knowledge has traditionally focused on the acute care setting, where losses are more physical in nature. As nurses enter the home and community setting, the definitions of loss are more comprehensive, and in many ways different. Nurses face challenges to develop interventions when every client's situation is different. Nursing interventions for these challenges are being validated through nursing research and evidence-based practice.

Factors Influencing Loss and Grief

The way an individual perceives a loss and responds to it during bereavement is heavily influenced by many factors.

Human Development. Persons of differing ages and stages of development will display different and unique symptoms of grief. For example, toddlers are unable to understand loss or death, but they feel great anxiety over loss of objects and separation from parents. School-age children experience grief over the loss of a body part or function. They often associate misdeeds with causing death. Middle-age adults usually begin to reexamine life and are sensitive to their own physical changes. Older adults often experience anticipatory grief because of aging and the possible loss of self-care abilities. Aging is frequently associated with losses such as physical changes, loss of employment, loss of social respect, loss of relationships, and threat to a sense of fulfillment and contributions made in life. However, Lund (1989) found that older adults are often resilient in responding to grief despite it being a highly stressful process (Box 29-1).

Psychosocial Perspectives of Loss and Grief. Loss and death are universal life experiences that each person faces. Death is an overwhelming experience that affects everyone involved in the loss situation or in the death of the individual. According to psychologists, the valuing of individuals is a unique, learned response of a specific culture and society (Binstock and Spector, 1997). Concepts, perspectives, and definitions of "loss" are described within a cultural bias of a specific society (Witoszek, 1998). Age, gender, status, race, spirituality, religious beliefs, intellect, achievement, self-expression, and cultural opportunity are the basis for an individual to define and qualify the definition of life or death (Cressy, 1997). The nurse is a product of that same psychosocial environment and shares many of the biases or perspectives gained during sociological development. Norms for psychosocial patterns of loss and grief are reflected in caregivers as well as in clients.

An individual's expression of grief evolves as the person matures. Personal experiences shape the coping mechanisms that the individual uses to deal with stressors. As psychologists frequently explain, the coping mechanisms that were effective in the past are repeated as a first response to the pain of a loss. When older coping strategies are unsuccessful, new coping mechanisms are attempted (see Chapter 30). When faced with a loss, a client learns what is needed for his or her own coping through repetition that is based on the successes and failures of different coping mechanisms. Sometimes the number or depths of losses become overwhelming, and familiar coping styles are not successful. For example, in the case of disenfranchised grief, society has different expectations than the person experiencing the loss, and routine coping strategies become ineffective or unavailable. Professional assistance is often required to help the client and family understand and deal realistically with losses.

Socioeconomic Status. Socioeconomic status influences a person's ability to obtain options and use support mechanisms when coping with loss. Generally an individual feels greater burden from a loss when there is a lack of financial, educational, or occupational resources. For example, a client with limited finances may not be able to replace a home lost in a fire or may not be able to purchase necessary medications to manage a newly diagnosed disease. These clients require referral to community social service agencies that can provide needed resources.

Personal Relationships. When loss involves a loved one, the quality and meaning of the relationship are critical in understanding a person's grief experience. It has been said that to lose your parents is to lose your past, to lose your spouse is to lose your present, and to lose your child is to lose your future. When a relationship between two individuals has been very close and well connected, it can be very difficult for the one left behind to cope. The support that clients receive from family and friends is based in part on their relationships with members of their social network and the manner and circumstances of their loss. When clients do not receive supportive understanding and compassion from others, they become unable to handle grief and look to the future.

Nature of the Loss. The ability to resolve grief depends on the meaning of the loss and the situation surround-

---

Focus on Older Adults   **Box 29-1**

- Bereavement adjustments are multidimensional in that nearly every aspect of a person's life can be affected by a loss.
- The overall effect of bereavement on the physical and mental health of many older spouses is not as devastating as expected.
- Older bereaved spouses commonly experience both positive and negative feelings simultaneously.
- Loneliness and problems associated with the tasks of daily living are two of the most common and difficult adjustments for older bereaved spouses.
- There is a great deal of diversity in how older bereaved adults adjust to the deaths of spouses.

Data from Lund DA: Conclusions about bereavement in later life and implications for interventions and future research. In Lund DA, editor: *Older bereaved spouses: research with practical application,* New York, 1989, Hemisphere.

ing the loss. The ability to accept help from others influences whether the bereaved will be able to cope effectively. The visibility of a loss influences the support a person receives. For example, the total loss of one's home from a tornado will bring support from the community, whereas a private loss of an important possession may bring less support from others. The suddenness of a loss can often cause slower resolution from grief. For example, a sudden and unexpected death is generally more difficult for a family to accept than one following a long-term chronic disease.

Culture and Ethnicity. Interpretation of a loss and the expression of grief arise from cultural background and family practices (Box 29-2). When individuals lose control over aspects of their life due to illness, their basic core belief systems are critical components of culture that they can and often do hold on to (Thomas, 2001). Culture affects how clients and their support systems or families respond to loss (see Chapter 8). For example, in the Western hemisphere the grieving process is usually personal and private, with individuals showing restrained emotion. However, the ceremonies surrounding a person's death offer time for grief resolution and reminiscing. In Eastern nations, such as the Philippines or China, respect for the dead is shown by wailing and physical demonstration of grief for a specified period of time. Despite these trends, members of the same ethnocultural background may respond to loss and death differently. It is imperative for nurses to acquire an understanding and appreciation of each client's cultural values as they apply to the experience of loss, death, and grieving.

The conflict between core American cultural values of individualism and self-determination versus the emphasis on collectivity and family, clan, or tribal orientation can clash when end-of-life decisions mandate caregiver roles, treatment modalities, and service locations (Thomas, 2001). Nurses must be able to support and guide clients and families along the final life journey in a culturally informed and acceptable manner, and not solely within the context of Euro-American or Judeo-Christian belief systems (Kagawa-Singer, 1998). Culturally sensitive practices are needed to guide the development of effective nursing interventions.

Research has shown that ethnicity is strongly related to attitudes toward life-sustaining treatments during terminal illness (Blackhall and others, 1999). The challenge for the nurse dealing with these issues is to explore realistically and practically the desires of clients and their support systems to clearly identify concepts and approaches for effective guidance through the loss experience.

Spiritual Beliefs. Individuals' spirituality significantly influences their ability to cope with loss. A person's faith in a higher power or influence, the community of fellowship with friends, their sources of hope and meaning in life, and the use of religious rituals and practices are just some of the spiritual resources a client may depend upon during a loss. Loss can sometimes cause internal conflicts about spiritual values and the meaning of life. Clients who have a strong interconnectedness with a higher power or others are often very resilient and able to face

death with relatively minimal discomfort. Chapter 28 summarizes the role spirituality plays in dealing with loss.

Coping With Grief and Loss

In order for nurses to provide support for clients and families require during loss, it is necessary to understand how people normally cope with grief and loss. Nursing interventions will involve reinforcement of the client's successful coping mechanisms and introduction of new coping approaches. Chapter 30 summarizes the nursing care principles for assisting clients in coping with stressful situations.

Cultural Aspects of Care   Box 29-2

At the end of life, rituals, mourning practices, and specific expressions of grief of all cultures are necessary for participants to have a sense of acceptance and inner peace. There is controversy as to whether appropriate care at the end of life achieves a "good death" or an "acceptable death" for clients. Do clients achieve a sense of comfort and peace during the death experience? Most hospital policies and procedures support an "acceptable death" for the client who is dying. This means providing basic standard levels of care and support, which may or may not take into account a client's cultural beliefs and practices. The expectation is that death be nontheatrical, disciplined, and with minimal exchange of emotions. In contrast, Kagawa-Singer (1998) describes a "good death" as one that allows social adjustments and personal preparations for the transition that will occur. A good death allows time for the client and family to make both the private and public preparations that are needed to help the family begin the adjustment to a world without its loved one, and for the client to complete unfinished tasks. The disengagement that occurs between the person who is dying and loved ones takes many forms because of cultural differences:

- Hindus envision a circular pattern of life and death with multiple deaths and rebirths.
- Christians believe in a more linear trajectory as expressed in the construct of a heaven where all good people with gather after death and a hell where lost souls go for eternity.
- Some Native Americans envision the land of the dead as a parallel world, where the spirits of the dead can directly affect the lives of the living.
- For other cultures the disengagement can be abrupt and final even to the point of sanctions against speaking names of the deceased to avoid keeping them from leaving earth and gaining peace.

Implications for Practice

- A nurse's concept of social support must be broadened to include greater variation in the timing, form, and mode of support provided to grieving clients and families.
- Cultural beliefs influence who makes up a client's support network and what support is acceptable to both give and receive during death.
- Care provided at the end of life within the client and family's cultural context draws on the resources of their whole lives.

Data from Kagawa-Singer, M: The cultural context of death rituals and mourning practices, *Oncol Nurs Forum* 25(10):1752, 1998.

Hope. **Hope** is the anticipation of a continued good, an improvement or lessening of something unpleasant. It is a multidimensional concept that is energizing and provides comfort while enduring life threats and personal challenges (Bierman and others, 1998; Morse and Doberneck, 1995; Nowotny, 1991). Hope enhances coping skills and even influences a person's survival (Doka, 1993). A person often reveals hope through an expression of expectations for life, the present, and the future. Often in terminal illness a client focuses hope on milestones (e.g., a child's high school graduation or the completion of a project at work), significant events (e.g., an upcoming anniversary), or for the relief of pain or other disabling symptoms (Weissman and others, 1999). A person's spiritual distress is often based on his or her definition of hope or lack of hope. Persons may view hope as encouragement to work toward recovery. Others may view hope more negatively by not being able to see any future favorable outcomes.

Hope can be found in all aspects of life as a force that helps persons cope with life stressors. It has purpose and direction and gives reason for being (Post-White and others, 1996). The existence and maintenance of hope depend on a person having strong relationships and a sense of emotional connectedness to others. Nurses and other health care professionals may provide that personal connectedness essential to hope. Hope is often the basis in which clients find meaning in their illness. Hopefulness

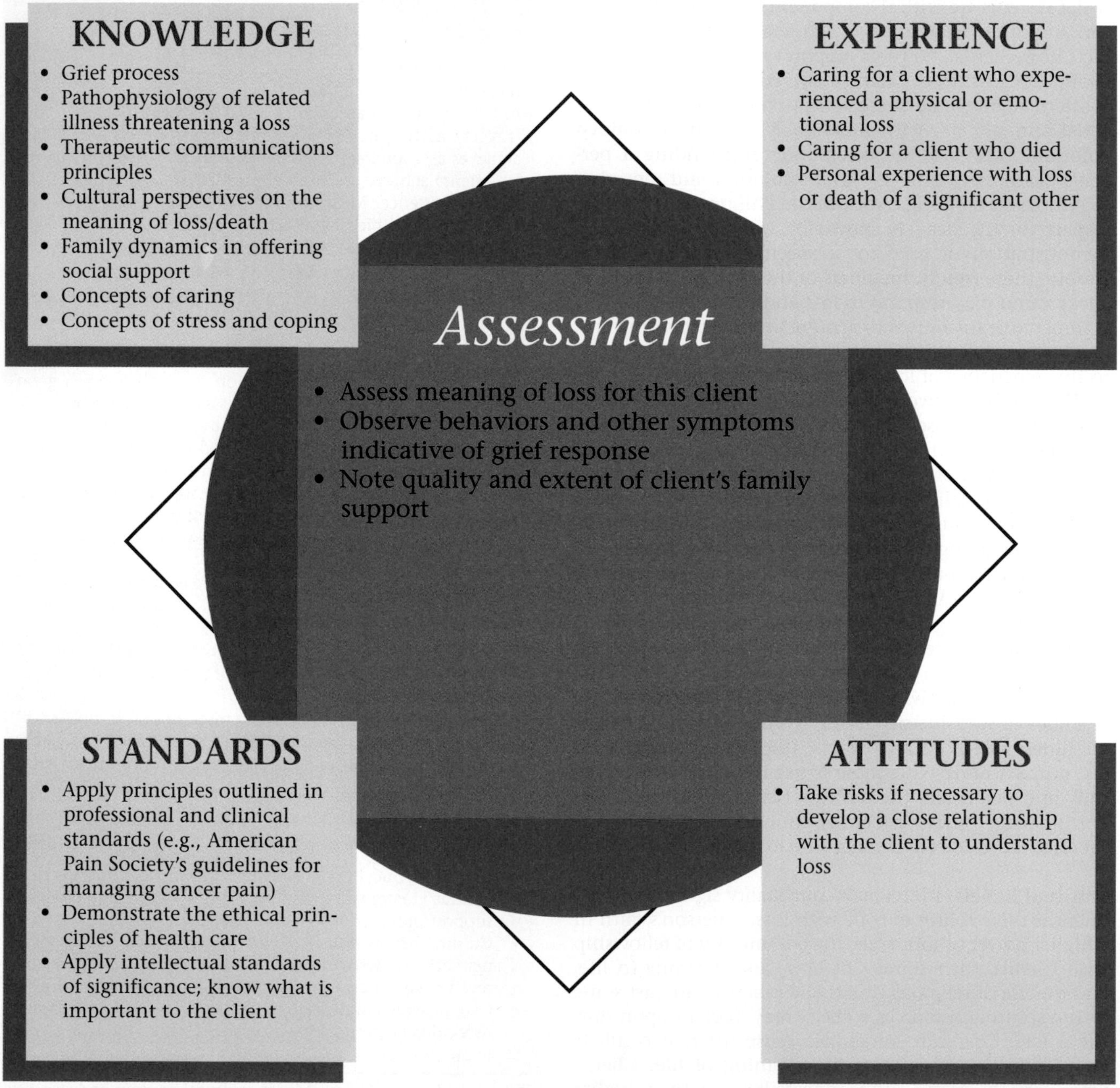

KNOWLEDGE

- Grief process
- Pathophysiology of related illness threatening a loss
- Therapeutic communications principles
- Cultural perspectives on the meaning of loss/death
- Family dynamics in offering social support
- Concepts of caring
- Concepts of stress and coping

EXPERIENCE

- Caring for a client who experienced a physical or emotional loss
- Caring for a client who died
- Personal experience with loss or death of a significant other

Assessment

- Assess meaning of loss for this client
- Observe behaviors and other symptoms indicative of grief response
- Note quality and extent of client's family support

STANDARDS

- Apply principles outlined in professional and clinical standards (e.g., American Pain Society's guidelines for managing cancer pain)
- Demonstrate the ethical principles of health care
- Apply intellectual standards of significance; know what is important to the client

ATTITUDES

- Take risks if necessary to develop a close relationship with the client to understand loss

FIGURE 29–1 Critical thinking model for loss, death, and grieving assessment.

offers an ability to see life as enduring or having sustained meaning or purpose (Chochinov, 2002). Chapter 28 discusses the conceptual components of hope and related nursing care implications.

Critical Thinking

When nurses care for clients who have experienced losses, successful critical thinking requires a synthesis of knowledge, previous experience with loss and grief, and information gathered from clients and families. In addition, the nurse must apply critical thinking attitudes and intellectual and professional standards to provide appropriate and responsive nursing care. Critical thinking applies to all steps of the nursing process.

During assessment the nurse must analyze all sources of information that lead to the selection of appropriate nursing diagnoses (Figure 29-1). To understand the process of grief and its effect on the client and family, the nurse integrates knowledge from nursing and other disciplines and previous experiences in caring for clients suffering loss. Knowledge of the stages of grief, for example, enables a nurse to better empathize with a client and family and to understand the behaviors exhibited by the client. Through identification of the various stages of grief, the nurse is able to direct assessment questions. The application of critical thinking attitudes and standards

---

Box 29-3   A Dying Person's Bill of Rights

I have the right to be in control.

I have the right to be treated as a living human being until I die.

I have the right to have a sense of purpose.

I have the right to be cared for by those who can maintain a sense of hopefulness.

I have the right to express my feelings and emotions about my approaching death in my own way.

I have the right to have a respected spirituality.

I have the right to participate in decisions about my care.

I have the right to expect continuing medical and nursing attention even though "cure" goals must be changed to "comfort" goals.

I have the right not to die alone.

I have the right to be comfortable.

I have the right to have my questions answered honestly.

I have the right not to be deceived.

I have the right to have help from and for my family in accepting my death.

I have the right to die in peace and dignity.

I have the right to laugh and to be angry and sad.

I have the right to retain my individuality and not be judged for my decisions that may be contrary to beliefs of others.

I have the right to be cared for by caring, sensitive, knowledgeable people who will try to understand my needs and will be able to gain some satisfaction in helping me face my death.

Modified from Barbus AJ: The dying person's bill of rights, *Am J Nurs* 75:99, 1975; and Hospice RN: Patient's bill of rights, 2003, http://www.geocities.com/HotSprings/5120/bill.htm.

---

then helps the nurse to apply this information in a relevant and therapeutic way for the client's benefit. For example, the critical thinking attitude of perseverance is needed to learn as much as possible about the type of grief a client is experiencing to ultimately select the most appropriate nursing interventions. The use of appropriate intellectual standards such as significance and relevance guide the nurse during assessment to ensure the information gathered is pertinent to the client's unique situation. Professional standards including those of bioethics, the dying person's bill of rights (Box 29-3), and clinical standards such as the American Pain Society's guidelines for managing cancer pain. All provide evidence-based guidelines for a thorough assessment and humane, compassionate nursing care.

The Nursing Process and Grief

Assessment

When a nurse cares for a client who has experienced or is facing a loss, assessment includes the client, family, and significant others. Grief assessment is ongoing throughout the course of an illness for the client and family and for the bereavement period after the death for the survivors (ELNEC, 2000). The nurse should not assume how or if the client or family experiences grief. The nurse should also avoid assuming that a particular behavior indicates grief; rather, the nurse should allow clients to share what is happening in their own way. An effective nurse encourages clients to tell their stories. This requires the nurse to establish trust with clients and to evoke a caring presence. It is helpful to have clients and families find a time and place to express their grief and describe their experiences (Figure 29-2). The nurse interviews clients and families separately unless a client requests having family members present. A thorough and comprehensive approach to the assessment of grief will result in a well-designed plan of care that will facilitate clients' abilities to work through grief.

A nurse begins by interviewing the client and family, using honest and open communication. Listening carefully and observing the client's responses and behaviors are important. The nurse assumes a neutral perspective and remains alert for nonverbal cues such as facial expressions, voice tones, and topics that are avoided. While gathering data, the nurse summarizes and validates any impressions formed with the client and family so that appropriate nursing diagnoses can be made. Information from other health care workers, such as physicians, social workers, and members of pastoral care will contribute to the database.

Type and Stage of Grief. It is important for the nurse to assess how a client *is* reacting rather than how the client *should be* reacting. The sequencing of stages or behaviors of grief may occur in order, they may be skipped, or they may reoccur. A single behavior can be representative of any number of types of grief. Therefore the identification of the type and stage of grief should be used only to guide the nurse's assessment and not to judge the outcomes of

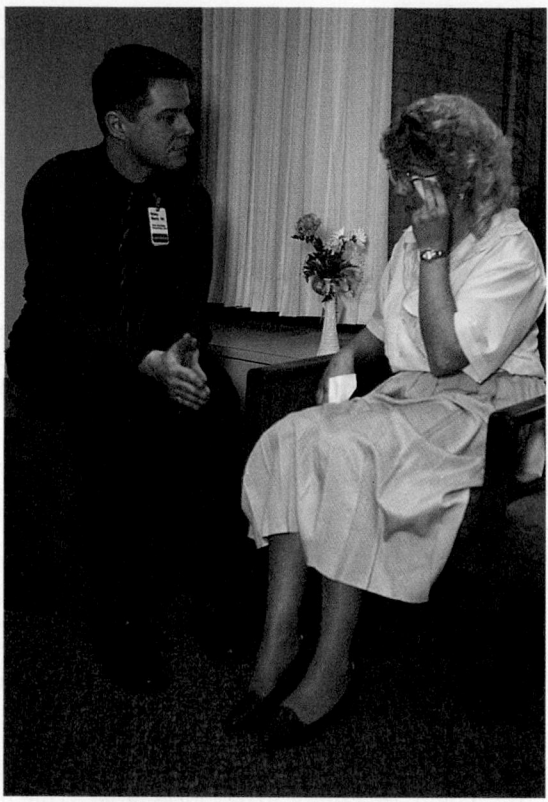

FIGURE **29–2**   Nurses assist family members in finding resources to help with the grieving process.

Box 29-4   Symptoms of Normal Grief

Feelings

Sadness
Anger
Guilt or self-reproach
Anxiety
Loneliness
Fatigue
Helplessness
Shock/numbness (lack of feeling)
Yearning
Emancipation/relief

Cognitions (Thought Patterns)

Disbelief
Confusion
Preoccupation about the deceased
Sense of the presence of the deceased
Hallucinations
Hopelessness ("I'll never be OK again")

Physical Sensations

Hollowness in the stomach
Tightness in the chest
Tightness in the throat
Oversensitivity to noise
Sense of depersonalization ("Nothing seems real")
Feeling short of breath
Muscle weakness
Lack of energy
Dry mouth

Behaviors

Sleep disturbances
Appetite disturbances
Absentminded behavior
Dreams of the deceased
Sighing
Crying
Carrying objects that belonged to the deceased

---

the grieving process. The application of a theorist's phase of grief aids the nurse in the accurate assessment of a situation. For example, if a client is complaining of loneliness and difficulty falling asleep, the nurse considers all factors surrounding the loss. When did the loss occur? What type of loss occurred? The client may be experiencing a normal grief reaction or if the loss occurred 2 years previously, chronic grief.

The nurse asks clients to describe their loss and how it has affected them. "Tell me how your diagnosis of heart disease makes you feel." The nurse can anticipate characteristics or responses during a phase of grieving but should allow clients to describe their feelings as thoroughly as possible. "How has this change in your life affected you day today?" "Tell me more." The nurse probes and validates feelings expressed in the client's emotions: "You seem angry, tell me more . . . ," "You seem sad, tell me . . . ," "What are your feelings about. . . ." The nurse continues assessment until the client has nothing more to share. The nurse avoids premature assumptions about the phase of grief a client might be experiencing so as to avoiding terminating assessment too early.

Grief Reactions. The nurse uses psychological and physical assessment skills to gather a complete database about the client and/or family. Although no two people grieve exactly the same way, most persons who grieve have at least some outward signs and symptoms (Box 29-4). Clinical reasoning is needed to analyze the data cues and to determine the appropriate related cause. For

example, a client who is experiencing dysfunctional grieving may have a changing affect, withdrawn activity level, somatic complaints such as headache, upset stomach, and alterations in concentration. The nurse might associate these symptoms with any number of problems such as anxiety, gastrointestinal disturbances, or even impaired memory. However, the focus is to assess the client's symptoms in context. What is the meaning and significance of loss, and how is it affecting the client in physical and psychological ways? What does the client associate the symptoms with? In what way are the symptoms related to one another when they occur? What symptoms are observed when the client openly expresses grief? Over what time period have the symptoms been present: before the loss, during the loss? Careful analysis refines the nurse's ability to make judgments about the client's condition.

A loss takes place in a social context. In the case of a family where the father is experiencing a terminal illness, the family begins to reorganize itself as soon as the client is no longer able to fulfill the same number and types of roles. When a person is disabled, both the client and family undergo similar reorganization, realigning roles and responsibilities to meet the demands. During this time clients and families can experience a variety of physical and psychological symptoms. The nurse assesses the entire family's response to loss, recognizing that family members may be dealing with different aspects of grief than the client. Good interviewing and physical assessment skills guide the nurse as caregiver and as an advocate of the client to ensure appropriate nursing care will be planned.

Table 29-3	Assessment of Factors Influencing Grieving
Factor	**Areas/Suggestions/Questions to Explore**
Nature of relationships	Functions of the family, community, and society *Examples:* How long have you known your friend? What role has your mother played in your family? What is your relationship? Will it change? How will family relationships change as a result of the loss?
Social support system	Availability of family, friends, health care workers *Examples:* Who is present? Absent? Supportive? Nonsupportive? What do family/friends do that is most meaningful? Are family/friends available when needed or do they just say, "Call me if you need me?" Are health care workers accepting and exploring ways to preserve the client's dignity and lifestyle?
Nature of loss	Actual versus perceived; death issues; impact on roles *Examples:* Tell me what the loss of your dog means in your own words. What factors help you to grieve? What factors interfere with grieving? What past experiences or outcomes have you had with loss?
Cultural and spiritual beliefs	Values, cultural norms, spirituality, customs, attitudes *Examples:* What is your belief about death? Meaning of life? What customs do you value at the time of death? How is this loss viewed by others of your culture or religious group? Do religious practices interfere with medical treatments? Who has the right to say "yes" or "no" to life-sustaining measures?
Loss of personal life goals	Actual or perceived individual losses affecting future decisions and options *Examples:* What is your goal in life for . . . ? How has this changed as a result of your diagnosis? How will your role change your personal goals? What planning have you and your family made for your own life?
Family's grief	Relationships, involvement with the dying process *Examples:* Observe client and family's level of grief, patterns of behavior, rank of leadership or power. What has helped family members deal with problems in the past? What was not helpful? What are the family's strengths and weaknesses?
Survivor risk factors	High risk, such as sudden death, violent death, loss of a child *Examples:* Describe your feelings at this time. Let's talk about why you think you could have prevented this. Are you feeling guilty because . . . ? What are unresolved issues or perceptions towards others?
Hope	Goals, worth, adaptation to future changes *Examples:* Tell me what you think about your treatment plan. What do you expect will happen to you? How does this illness affect your goals in life? What are you hoping for following your surgery?

Factors That Affect Grief. As was discussed previously, a number of factors influence loss and the grief response. It helps to discuss the meaning of loss to the client and family. This usually provides information that allows the nurse to explore a number of topics in detail, such as personal characteristics of the person experiencing loss, the nature of family relationships, support systems, and cultural and spiritual beliefs (Table 29-3). The nurse must then apply assessment skills from appropriate specialty areas (e.g., spiritual or family assessment; see Chapters 28 and 9, respectively) to acquire a thorough understanding of the client's loss.

End-of-Life Decisions. When a client is experiencing a terminal illness, family members must face end-of-life decisions. Families experience a very high level of stress when deciding whether to withdraw life-sustaining treatments (Tilden and others, 2001). Although some clients may have living wills, it is important for family members to know a client's wishes in regard to life-sustaining measures. The Study to Understand Prognoses and Preferences for Outcomes and Risks of Treatments (SUPPORT Principal Investigators, 1995) found that a larger proportion of clients received prolonged aggressive treatments even when clients and families had indicated preference for palliative care rather than life extension. Unfortunately, physicians and nurses often have difficulty helping clients to die with dignity. The Institute of Medicine (Field and Cassel, 1997) and other organizations (e.g., Robert Wood Johnson's Last Acts Coalition) have identified needed improvements in the areas of advance planning, respecting client and family preferences for location of death and amount of life-sustaining treatment, pain management, and supportive resources (Tolle and others, 2000).

One part of the country has attempted to create conditions for improving end-of-life care for its residents. The state of Oregon now permits physician-assisted suicide. Oregon also has a capitated health care plan that protects the uninsured and makes end-of-life care more accessible for its poorer citizens. Medicare data indicate that Oregon has one of the highest rates of hospice use in the country (Cushman, 1998). Tolle and others (2000) studied families of dying clients in Oregon to determine whether barriers to optimal care of the dying existed (Box 29-5).

A nurse must assess the client's and family's wishes for end-of-life care, including the preferred place for death, the use of and the level of life-sustaining measures, and expectations regarding pain control and symptom management. Does the client want to try all available treatments? Does the family or client insist on use of a feeding tube for continued nutritional support after the client stops eating? When life support requires use of a mechanical ventilator, is this something the client wants? Does the family feel comfortable in administering analgesics? Family members face complex decisions with unresolved burdens and guilt, limited knowledge, and an inability to conceptualize the dying trajectory or how a person's final days or weeks will be experienced (Forbes, Bern-Klug, and Gessert, 2000). The nurse must give the client and family time to discuss their preferences. Often it is necessary to return to a conversation on a subsequent day or visit. If the nurse feels uncomfortable in assessing a client's wishes, it is important to find a health care provider who is experienced with discussing end-of-life issues and can assist in communicating a client's preferences to the total health care team.

End-of-life care is one of the more significant topics a nurse will discuss with clients. A nurse cannot keep what is learned about a client's preferences private. Good interdisciplinary teamwork is essential to provide quality end-of-life care. Thus the nurse must communicate what is known about client preferences and decisions in change-of-shift reports, health team conferences, written care plans, and ongoing consultation with physicians and other health team members.

Nurse's Experience With Grief. When caring for clients experiencing grief, it is important for nurses to assess their own emotional well-being. Self-reflection, which is a part of critical thinking, becomes a valuable tool in asking whether one's personal sadness is related to caring for the client or to unresolved personal experiences

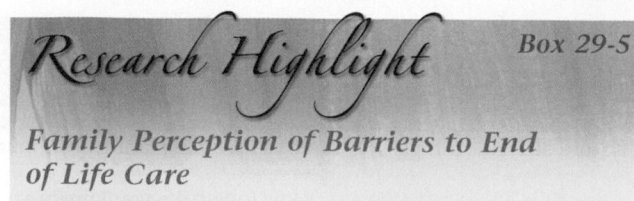

Research Highlight   Box 29-5

Family Perception of Barriers to End of Life Care

Research Focus

Family members are often involved in the decedent's care during the last month of life. Their perspectives of how a decedent's last days of life are spent provide valuable insight in the quality of end-of-life care and the potential barriers that might exist.

Research Abstract

This is a retrospective study of 1996-1997 decedents in Oregon and their families. Oregon provides data about family views of health services and clinicians' care during the last month of life. Researchers used this data in addition to conducting telephone surveys of family members using a 58-item survey. The survey obtained information about family members' perceptions of three aspects of end-of-life care: clinician respect for decedents' preferences for life-sustaining treatment, satisfaction with clinicians' support in the week before death, and barriers to pain management the week before death.

Findings suggest that a high rate of advance planning and a high level of clinician respect for client-family preferences existed. There was a low use of aggressive, life-sustaining treatments and greater frequency of decisions to forego aggressive treatments rather than to discontinue them once started. All clients who died at home preferred that location. However, almost half of hospital decedents preferred that setting. One third of the families indicated their family member experienced moderate to severe pain in the final week of life. Families had more complaints about the management of pain for decedents who died at home, even though they did not report higher levels of pain. Generally, there was a high level of satisfaction with clinicians' efforts to manage pain.

Evidence-Based Practice

- It is important to learn directly from clients and families their wishes regarding preferred location of the client's death.
- Families of dying clients may have low expectations of pain management; nonetheless more aggressive therapies are needed to help comfort dying clients.
- Nurses should recognize that family members are more aware of pain management problems and bear more responsibility for direct care of such needs.
- Nurses should provide guidance and support to help families administer necessary pain therapies.

Reference

Tolle S and others: Family reports of barriers to optimal care of the dying, *Nurs Res* 49(6):310, 2000.

from the past or a combination. It is normal to have personal feelings and emotions about certain illnesses and death. However, it is inappropriate to place personal family situations and values before those of the client. Talking with friends and close professional colleagues may offer a resource for the nurse to resolve any con-

Nursing Diagnostic Process

Box 29-6

Assessment Activities	Defining Characteristics	Nursing Diagnosis
Ask client to discuss future goals and plans.	Client sighs and says, "I have no future."	Hopelessness related to failing physical condition
Observe client's nonverbal behavior.	Client becomes passive with little affect and turns away from speaker.	
Offer client choices and observe responses.	Client shrugs and says, "What does it matter?"	
Assess activity level.	Client refuses to eat. Client sleeps all the time, keeping blinds pulled and lights out. Client refuses to participate in care.	

flicts about caring for dying clients. Sometimes a nurse must make the choice of working in a specialty area where the incidence of client deaths is low. Part of being a professional is knowing when to get away from a situation and take care of oneself.

Client Expectations. The nurse takes time to assess the client's and family's expectations for nursing care. The client's perceptions and expectations can influence how the nurse prioritizes nursing diagnoses. For example, if clients perceive that their level of pain and discomfort is severe, they will be less attentive to any attempts the nurse makes to discuss the significance and meaning of their loss. It will become a priority for the nurse to make a client comfortable before the nurse can institute meaningful discussion or counseling. The nurse should assess the client's expectations within the context of the loss by asking questions such as, "How can we help you cope with your loss?" and "What do you feel is necessary from us for you to be able to resolve the grief you feel?" "What is most important that we do for you while you are under our care?"

It is important to give family members the chance to explain how they perceive the nurse's role and what their goals are for the health care team. This part of the assessment helps the nurse to clarify any misunderstandings that might exist. For example, the family may have very unrealistic expectations regarding the type of treatment available to the client and the anticipated effects. The nurse should take time to assess what clients and families expect and desire from nursing care so as to ensure an individualized and comprehensive plan of care.

Nursing Diagnosis

Based on the nurse's conclusions during the assessment phase, the nurse identifies a nursing diagnosis that accurately reflects needs exhibited by the client or family experiencing the loss. Critical thinking skills are the tools used to apply concepts of assessment, clustering of cues, and drawing a conclusion of the actual or perceived needs of the client. The nurse will cluster defining characteristics and identify the nursing diagnosis applicable to the client's situation (Box 29-6). Clustering of client or

family behaviors, actual or potential losses, the client's attempts at coping, and data involving the nature and meaning of the loss will lead to individualized nursing diagnoses such as the following:

- Anxiety
- Caregiver role strain
- Compromised family coping
- Ineffective community coping
- Ineffective denial
- Fear
- Anticipatory grieving
- Dysfunctional grieving
- Hopelessness
- Powerlessness
- Social isolation
- Spiritual distress
- Readiness for enhanced spiritual well-being

The presence of one or two defining characteristics is usually insufficient to make an accurate diagnosis. The nurse must be vigilant by carefully reviewing the data to consider if competing diagnoses exist. For example, if a client who is dying manifests crying or tearfulness, displays anger, and reports nightmares, this could signal several possible nursing diagnoses because these characteristics are common to more than one diagnosis. Possibilities include *pain, ineffective coping,* and *spiritual distress.* The nurse examines all available data and inquires about the presence of other behaviors and symptoms until an accurate diagnosis can be identified.

Part of the diagnostic process is to identify the appropriate related factor for each diagnosis. For example, *dysfunctional grieving related to the loss of the ability to walk from paralysis* will require different interventions than *dysfunctional grieving related to the loss of a job.* Clarification of the related factor will ensure that appropriate interventions are selected for the client's care.

When identifying nursing diagnoses for the dying client, other problems are identified separately according to specific standards of care for the dying client. Other nursing diagnoses can include *disturbed body image, impaired physical mobility,* or *ineffective role performance.* More physical nursing diagnose are identified when the client begins to experience the physical changes accompanying death, including *impaired urinary elimination* and/or *bowel incontinence, acute pain, nausea, disturbed sensory perception,* and *ineffective breathing pattern*. Successful recovery is not always an expected outcome. The comfort of the dying, including pain control and the acceptance of the dying process by the family, are realistic expectations for the nurse to deal with in the dying situation. With terminal illness, physical assessment of the dying process is ongoing so the nurse can adapt or validate the actual nursing diagnoses with the changing condition of the client.

Planning

Grieving is the natural response to loss and thus has a therapeutic value. The focus in planning nursing care is to support the client physically, emotionally, developmentally and spiritually in the expression of grief. Figure 29-3 illustrates the interrelatedness of critical thinking factors during the planning phase of the nursing process. Application of critical thinking ensures a well-designed plan where the nurse supports the client's personhood, self-esteem, and autonomy by including the client in decisions about the plan of care. When caring for the dying client, it is important to devise a plan that helps a client to die with dignity and offers family members the assurance their loved one is cared for with care and compassion (see care plan, p. 582).

Goals and Outcomes. The nurse establishes realistic goals and expected outcomes based on the client's nursing diagnoses. Client resources such as physical energy and activity tolerance, supportive family members, spiritual faith, and methods for coping are integrated into the plan of care. For example, if a terminally ill client has the diagnosis of *powerlessness related to planned cancer therapy*, a goal of "Client will be able to discuss expected course of disease" will be realistic if the client is able to remain attentive and participate in educational discussions without becoming fatigued. In contrast, an expected outcome of "Client will participate in series of short planned teaching discussions about disease" accounts for the client's need to have short teaching sessions so as to avoid exhaustion.

Goals of care for a client dealing with loss might be long or short term, depending on the nature of the loss and the client's phase of grieving. Because a client may move back and forth between phases of grief, it may become necessary for the nurse to revise goals and outcomes to ensure they remain relevant. Having the client partner in deciding which goals are relevant is important. General nursing care goals for clients with a loss include accommodating grief, accepting the reality of a loss, and renewing regular relationships. When a client is suffering a terminal illness, pain and symptom control, maintaining autonomy, and achieving spiritual comfort are examples of important goals to achieve. For the goal of "achieving a sense of dignity" expected outcomes might include the following:

- Client will be able to continue parental responsibilities in care of toddler.
- Client will express hopefulness in cancer treatment ameliorating symptoms.
- Client will engage in playing chess with friends on a weekly basis.

Setting Priorities. When a client has multiple nursing diagnoses, it is not possible to address all of the problems simultaneously. On any given day or time when a nurse cares for a client, two or three problem areas will demand the nurse's attention. Figure 29-4 is an example of a concept map developed for a client diagnosed medically with depression, following the death of his wife 6 months ago. As a result of the client's medical condition, associated health problems include the nursing diagnoses of *dysfunctional grieving, disturbed sleep pattern*, and *imbalanced nutrition: less than body requirements*. In such a situation the nurse would determine which of the three diagnoses required greater attention. The continuing grief experienced by the client might be the focus. Until the client is able to accept the loss of his wife and begin resolving his grief, he may be unable to attend to those interventions that will improve his nutritional intake and sleep status.

Clients' conditions always change. Ongoing assessment of a client's condition can quickly focus the nurse's attention to a new problem. The nurse must always consider what are the client's most urgent physical or psychological needs requiring immediate intervention. The nurse considers the client's expectations and preferences in regard to the priorities of care. If the terminally ill client's priorities include pain control and promoting self-esteem, pain control will become a priority when analgesics become ineffective and the client experiences acute distress. If the client is progressing as desired, the nurse may refocus priorities to address unmet needs. For example, the client suffering depression has experienced the loss of a spouse and has problems of imbalanced nutrition and a disturbed sleep pattern. If the client reports an improved appetite and has shown weight stabilization since the last clinic visit, the nurse can focus more attention on the sleep pattern disturbance. The nurse must remember that the client's expectations, clinical condition, and preferences influence priorities. If a terminally ill client places more emphasis on spiritual support versus other priorities such as mobility or learning about planned treatments, the nurse must attend to the client's priorities. Meeting client priorities may allow the nurse to then address other needs more effectively with less effort.

Continuity of Care. Interdisciplinary teams help in identifying and meeting the needs of those who experience losses. Dietitians, clergy, physicians, social workers, physical therapists, psychologists, and other specialty health care workers can assist a client and family in their grief. A coordinated group approach to management of a client's needs ensures that little is left to chance and that the client's plan will be managed well. When a client dies, the loss experienced by the nurse and colleagues can be shared within the professional group. Support is needed to promote healing for all who worked with the dying client. Conflicts and differences can be openly discussed and solutions found in a healthy manner with the client as the primary focus. By working together, the sharing of experiences, feelings, alternatives, and solutions become the basis for dealing with future loss situations.

Often, terminally ill clients will return home and require continued intense nursing care. In that situation, home care nurses will collaborate closely with family

KNOWLEDGE

- Spirituality as a resource for dealing with loss
- Role other health professions play in helping clients deal with loss
- Services provided by community agencies
- Principles of providing comfort
- Principles of grief support

EXPERIENCE

- Previous client responses to planned nursing interventions for pain and symptom management or loss of a significant other

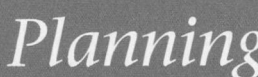

Planning

- Select communication strategies that assist the client/family in accepting and adapting to loss
- Select interventions designed to maintain the client's dignity and self-esteem
- Provide skills/knowledge for the family to manage and understand care for the dying client

STANDARDS

- Provide privacy for the client and family
- Apply ethical principles of autonomy in supporting the client's choice regarding treatment
- Individualize therapies for the client's self-esteem
- Apply appropriate professional standards for end-of-life care (e.g., American Pain Society's guidelines for managing cancer pain)

ATTITUDES

- Be responsible for delivering high-quality supportive care
- Demonstrate an openness to participate in experiencing the loss

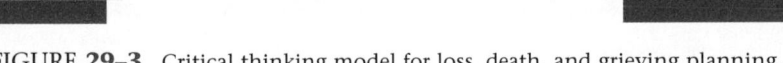

FIGURE **29–3** Critical thinking model for loss, death, and grieving planning.

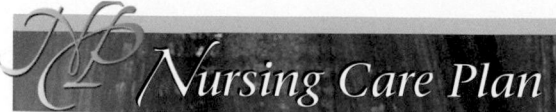

Nursing Care Plan

Grief and Loss

Assessment

Jan Runyon is the nurse who admits Mr. Miller, a 48-year-old man, from the emergency department to the intensive care unit (ICU) following massive head trauma incurred in a motor vehicle accident. Mr. Miller is a successful businessman who has a wife and two sons. The physician has explained to the family that Mr. Miller's prognosis is poor. Tests are under way to determine the extent of brain injury. The family is in the ICU waiting area, waiting on word about Mr. Miller.

Assessment Activities	Findings/Defining Characteristics
Jan asks the wife, "Tell me how you are feeling about your discussion with the physician."	"I know they are doing everything they can. He is going to be OK, I just know he is. He has never been sick a day in his life."
Jan observes Mrs. Miller's interaction with her children.	Mrs. Miller has difficulty problem solving. The family has posed several questions to her as to what she plans to say to the insurance company and Mr. Miller's employer. Mrs. Miller is unable to decide what to say at this time.
Jan overhears Mrs. Miller on the phone in the waiting area.	Mrs. Miller states over the phone, "Don't worry, he's having some tests right now. I know, Bill, he will be back in the office before you know it. Tell the staff everything will be OK."
Jan accompanies the transplant coordinator who asks Mrs. Miller if the family has ever discussed organ donation.	Mrs. Miller responds, "Bill will be fine, that's not important right now!"

Nursing Diagnosis: Ineffective coping related to husband's traumatic injury and uncertainty of prognosis.

Planning

Goal	Expected Outcomes*
	Grief Resolution
Wife will accept client's impending death within 48 hours.	Wife will verbalize to caregiver within the next 6 hours that husband's death is actually impending.
	Wife will inform children of their father's likely death within 24 hours.
	Wife will make a decision about organ donation within the next 12 hours.
	Wife will discuss immediate lifestyle changes that will occur as a result of husband's death over next 48 hours.
Wife will demonstrate effective expression of grief within next 48 hours.	Wife will discuss with children their concerns about what they need to do as a family to prepare for father's impending death within next 48 hours.
	Wife will discuss effects loss has on her personally with caregiver within next 48 hours.

*Outcome classification label from Moorhead S, Johnson M, Maas M: *Nursing outcomes classification (NOC)*, ed 3, Mosby, 2004, St. Louis.

Interventions†	Rationale
Presence	
• Display interest in wife's situation and accept her behaviors of denial.	Recognizing denial (based on Kübler-Ross's theory) gives the staff direction for planning unique interventions based on grief theory (Cressy, 1997).
• Establish trust and a positive regard by creating an atmosphere of sharing. Offer privacy and security.	Privacy offers a place of security to exhibit personal needs and to work through feelings (McLean, 1999). Anxiety about losing self-esteem when expressing grief will hinder an honest expression of feelings.

Continued

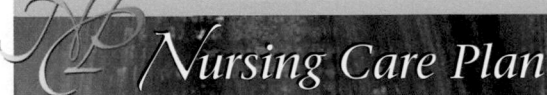

Nursing Care Plan

Grief and Loss—cont'd

Interventions†—cont'd

Grief Work Facilitation

- Offer wife encouragement to explore and verbalize feelings of grief.

- Identify personal coping strategies used in the past; assess effectiveness and promote when appropriate.

- Determine wife's acceptance of available community resources and initiate as appropriate: significant other (business partner), children, clergy (family is Methodist), or other health care workers.

Rationale

Encouragement refocuses on current needs and minimizes dysfunctional adaptation behaviors by facilitating resolution of grief through problem solving skills (Braza, 1993).

Previously successful coping strategies are the first to be used when one is under stress (Cressy, 1997). Discouraging maladaptive behaviors will minimize dysfunctional grieving (Lendhardt, 1997).

Professionals can use their expertise to direct the grieving process (Catalano, 1995). Trust in relationships already formed will speed the therapeutic communication process (Stocker, 1994).

†Intervention classification labels from Dochterman JM, Bulechek GM: *Nursing interventions classification (NIC),* ed 4, St. Louis, 2004, Mosby.

Evaluation

Nursing Actions	Client Response/Finding	Achievement of Outcome
Say to client, "This has been a difficult time. Your husband's injury has been so sudden."	Wife responds, "I still cannot believe it. The doctors do not believe he will live through the night."	Shows beginning acknowledgment of client's impending death.
Nurse asks, "Tell me how you are feeling now."	Wife explains, "I am worried about my kids. The boys are both close to their dad. I feel this unbelievable sadness."	Able to express normal grieving behaviors.
Observe wife's behavior when with children.	Wife discusses decisions that must be made because of impending death of husband. Allows children to express their sadness.	Wife is able to express grief with family; maintains role as supportive mother.

members to ensure the client's ongoing needs are met. Important interventions to include in planning are arranging for main-floor access, arranging appropriate medical equipment, and providing sufficient family respite support. When it is realistic for the client to remain independent, therapeutic strategies should bolster the client's sense of autonomy and the ability to function as independently as possible (Chochinov, 2002). For example, judicious application of orthotic devices, along with physical and occupational therapy, can often bolster a client's functional capacity.

Implementation

Health Promotion. Although a return to full function will not be an expected outcome for a terminally ill client or even a person who experiences significant disability, there is always the goal of enabling the client to return to optimal physical and emotional functioning. This does not mean the client and family will not experience sorrow, anger, or other disturbing emotions. However, the goal of nursing care is to help clients and families cope with the stressors in their lives and to move towards healthy grief resolution. Nurses will assist clients and families in learning to deal with loss, to make effective

decisions about the client's health care, and to adjust to any disappointment, frustration, and anxiety created by their loss.

Therapeutic Communication. Nursing care of the grieving client and family begins with establishing a caring presence and determining the significance of their loss. This is difficult if the client is unwilling or unable to express feelings or is experiencing numbing or denial. It is important for the nurse to use therapeutic communication strategies that enable clients to discuss their loss and work with them in finding ways to resolve it. The nurse uses open-ended questions, attentive listening, and presence to allow clients to freely share their thoughts and concerns. The use of closed-ended questions often results in the client discussing only what the nurse presumes is the problem. For example, asking the client, "Knowing you have cancer, does this make you fearful?" will not likely reveal as much useful information as, "Tell me how your diagnosis of cancer is making you feel." The nurse should acknowledge the client's grief and show support by demonstrating caring behaviors throughout the discussion (see Chapter 7). The nurse will gain the client's trust by showing a desire to become involved with the client at a level that fosters mutual understanding. Listening to the client's story can be very therapeutic

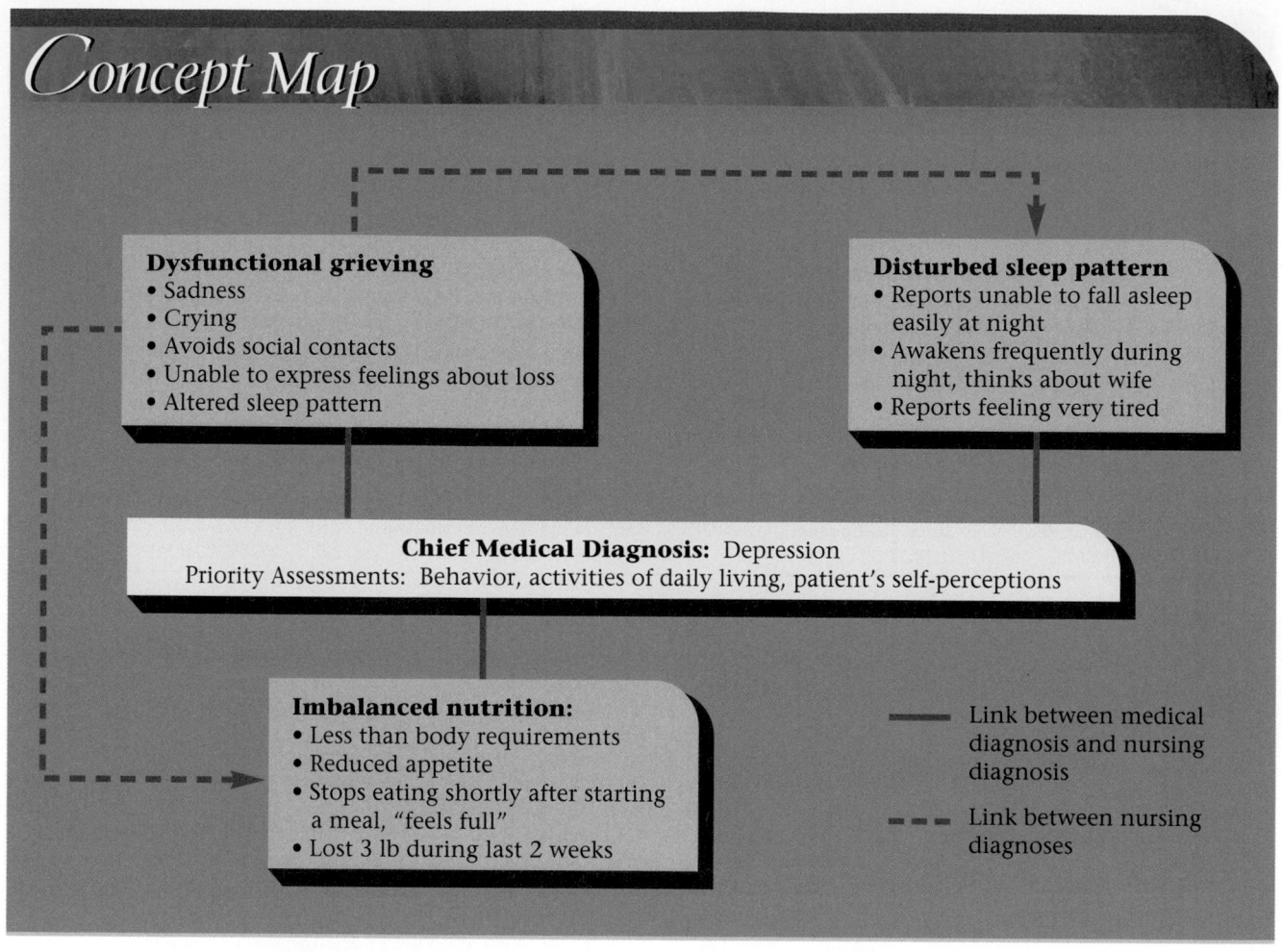

Concept Map

Dysfunctional grieving
- Sadness
- Crying
- Avoids social contacts
- Unable to express feelings about loss
- Altered sleep pattern

Disturbed sleep pattern
- Reports unable to fall asleep easily at night
- Awakens frequently during night, thinks about wife
- Reports feeling very tired

Chief Medical Diagnosis: Depression
Priority Assessments: Behavior, activities of daily living, patient's self-perceptions

Imbalanced nutrition:
- Less than body requirements
- Reduced appetite
- Stops eating shortly after starting a meal, "feels full"
- Lost 3 lb during last 2 weeks

——— Link between medical diagnosis and nursing diagnosis

- - - Link between nursing diagnoses

FIGURE **29–4**   Concept Map for a client with depression following death of spouse.

and will generally reveal details that enable the nurse to provide effective interventions.

If a client chooses not to share feelings or concerns, the nurse should convey a willingness to be available when needed. If the nurse is reassuring and respectful of the client's need for dignity and privacy, a therapeutic relationship will likely develop. Sometimes clients need to begin resolving their grief before they can discuss their loss.

It is important for the nurse to recognize that some clients will not discuss feelings about their loss. The nurse must be observant for expressions of anger, denial, depression, or guilt. It is also important for the nurse to know his or her own feelings before encouraging clients to express their anger. Individuals may retaliate against family, staff, or physicians. Clients can also become demanding and accusing. The nurse must remain supportive by letting clients and family members know that feelings such as anger are normal. For example, the nurse might say, "You are obviously upset, I just want you to know I am here to talk with you if you want." The nurse must always avoid barriers to communication such as denying the client's grief, providing false reassurance, or avoiding discussion of sensitive issues (see Chapter 23).

No topic that a dying client wishes to discuss should be avoided. When the nurse senses that clients desire to begin a discussion, it is important to find time to let them discuss their concerns. This can be very challenging for a nurse with limited experience with dying clients or who works in a busy acute care setting. The nurse responds to questions openly and honestly. The nurse also provides information that helps clients and their families to understand their condition, the trajectory or future course of their disease, the benefits and burdens of treatment, and clarification of values and goals (Forbes, Bern-Klug, and Gessert, 2000). In some cases it is appropriate for the nurse to recognize the need to consult with pastoral care or counseling services to help clients discuss these very difficult issues.

Promoting Hope. Hope can be an energizing resource for clients experiencing loss. For each dimension of hope, there are nursing strategies that promote hope.
- **Affective dimension.** Show empathic understanding of the client's strengths. Reinforce expressions of courage, positive thinking, and realistic goal setting. Encourage expression of both positive and negative feelings.
- **Cognitive dimension.** Offer information about the illness and correct any misunderstanding or misinformation. Clarify or modify the client's perceptions.

- **Behavioral dimension.** Assist the client in using personal resources and making use of external supports to balance need for independence with healthy interdependence and dependence.
- **Affiliative dimension.** Encourage clients to foster supportive relationships with others.
- **Temporal dimension.** Focus on short-term goals as life expectancy diminishes.
- **Contextual dimension.** Encourage development of achievable goals. Reminisce about achievements or positive moments in time so client can derive meaning from suffering.

Facilitating Mourning. There are nursing care strategies to help clients move through uncomplicated grief (Worden, 1982). The following guidelines are helpful for persons who are mourning a death, facing death, and grieving over an actual situational loss:

- **Help the client accept that loss is real.** Discuss how the loss or illness occurred or was discovered, when, under what circumstances, who told them about it, and other similar topics to help make the event real and to place it in perspective.
- **Support efforts to live without the deceased person or in the face of disability.** Using a problem-solving approach is often helpful. Have clients or family make a list of their problems, help them prioritize them, and then lead them step-by-step through a discussion of how they might tackle each one. Encourage them to make use of family members, community resources, or others who can help.
- **Encourage establishment of new relationships.** Many people will fear that in doing so they will be disloyal. They will need reassurance that new relationships do not mean that they are replacing the person who has died. Encourage the client to become involved in social relationships that are nonthreatening (e.g., religious gatherings or volunteer activities).
- **Allow time to grieve.** It is common to have "anniversary reactions" around the time of the loss in subsequent years. Some people worry that they are going crazy when sadness or other signs of grief recur after a period of relative calm. Encourage the client to reminisce.
- **Interpret "normal" behavior.** Being distractible, having difficulty sleeping or eating, and thinking they have heard the deceased's voice are common behaviors following loss. These symptoms do not mean an individual has an emotional problem or is becoming ill in some way. Reinforce that these behaviors are normal and will resolve over time.
- **Provide continuing support.** Clients and their families may need to talk and may look to the nurse for support for many months or years following a loss. If the nurse has occasion to see the client or family after an extended time, it is appropriate to ask about how they are coping or adjusting. This gives them the opportunity to talk if needed.
- **Be alert for signs of ineffective coping.** Be aware of coping mechanisms that may be harmful, such as alcohol or substance abuse, which can include excessive use of over-the-counter pain killers or sleep aids.

Acute Care

Palliative Care. People who face life-threatening illnesses have many medical and technological advances available to reverse the course of their disease or to prolong their lives. For clients with serious life-limiting illness, it becomes important for health care providers to find ways to help clients approach their end of life. Such is the goal of **palliative care,** the prevention, relief, reduction, or soothing of symptoms of disease or disorders without effecting a cure (Field and Cassel, 1997). Palliative care is for any age, any diagnosis, at any time, and not just during the last few months of life. Chochinov (2002) explains that when the preservation of dignity becomes the goal of palliation, care options encompass the physical, psychological, social, spiritual, and existential aspects of the client's illness. Palliative care thus allows clients to make more informed choices, achieve better alleviation of symptoms, and have more opportunity to work on issues of life closure. According to the World Health Organization (2003), when health care providers deliver palliative care, they do the following:

- Provide relief from pain and other distressing symptoms
- Affirm life and regard dying as a normal process
- Neither hasten nor postpone death
- Integrate psychological and spiritual aspects of client care
- Offer a support system to help clients live as actively as possible until death.
- Offer a support system to help families cope during the client's illness and their own bereavement
- Enhance the quality of life

Palliative care is a philosophy of total care. The approach to care usually involves an interdisciplinary team of physicians, nurses, social workers, pastoral care professionals, physical and occupational therapists, and pharmacists. Massage therapists or music/art therapists who provide alternative therapies might also be a part of the team (see Chapter 35). A palliative care approach ensures that a client experiences a "good death," free of avoidable pain and suffering, in accord with the client's and family's wishes, and reasonably consistent with clinical, cultural, and ethical standards (Tolle and others, 2000).

As a nurse, one of the most important skills in providing palliative care is establishing a caring relationship with both client and family. It also becomes very important for the nurse to provide appropriate symptom-control measures to maintain the client's dignity and self-esteem, to prevent abandonment or isolation, and to provide a comfortable and peaceful environment at the time of death.

Symptom Control. Comfort for a dying client requires management of symptoms of disease and therapies. For many clients, symptom distress is characteristic of the dying experience (Chochinov, 2002). Symptom distress is the experience of discomfort or anguish related to the progression of a disease. Clients experience anguish from not knowing or being unaware of aspects of their health status or treatment. Worry or fear are common in many clients and may heighten their perception of discomfort. The nurse assesses the character of the client's symptoms carefully in order to select appropriate therapies. Chapter 42 details the assessment of pain. Providing information about treatment options or the anticipated unfolding of an illness helps to conserve the dignity of clients and families plagued by not knowing what the future holds (Hinton, 1999).

One symptom common among the terminally ill is dyspnea, or air hunger. The sense of suffocation can cause great panic in the client and significant stress in the caregiver (Tarzian, 2000). As the client panics, unable to get a breath, the dyspnea simply worsens. Tarzian (2000) interviewed nurses who cared for the terminally ill and found that surrendering and sharing control help reduce pain and anxiety in these clients. For example, a client may choose to switch oxygen devices, even though they deliver the same concentration of oxygen. However, if the client believes there is a difference, it might be enough to relieve the dyspnea at least briefly. When there are options in respiratory therapy, it helps to give the client a choice.

Management of air hunger also involves the judicious administration of morphine and anxiolytics for relief of respiratory distress. Table 29-4 summarizes nursing care measures for additional symptoms of terminal disease.

Maintaining Dignity and Self-Esteem. The notion of dignity varies from client to client, and between one circumstance and the next (Chochinov, 2002). Dignity may revolve around a person's positive sense of self-regard, a feeling that the essence of who one is remains intact, along with an ability to invest in and gain strength from a rich spiritual life (Daaleman and VandeCreek, 2000). Dignity may also revolve around the extent to which a client feels valued and how he or she is treated by caregivers.

A nurse can promote a client's self-esteem and dignity by taking a therapeutic stance that conveys respect for the client as a whole person with feelings, accomplish-

Table 29-4	Promoting Comfort in the Terminally Ill Client	
Symptoms	**Characteristics or Causes**	**Nursing Implications**
Discomfort	Any source of physical irritation may worsen pain.	Provide thorough skin care including daily baths, lubrication of skin, and dry, clean bed linens to reduce irritants.
	As client approaches death, mouth remains open, tongue becomes dry and edematous, and lips become dry and cracked.	Provide oral care at least every 2 to 4 hours. Use soft toothbrushes or foam swabs for frequent mouth care. Apply a light film of petroleum jelly to lips and tongue (Chapter 28).
	Blinking reflexes diminish near death, causing drying of cornea.	Eye care removes crusts from eyelid margins. Artificial tears reduce corneal drying.
Fatigue	Metabolic demands of a cancerous tumor cause weakness and fatigue.	Help client to identify values or desired tasks; then help client to conserve energy for only those tasks. Promote frequent rest periods in a quiet environment.
	Exhaustion phase of the general adaptation syndrome causes energy depletion.	Time and pace nursing care activities.
Nausea	Nausea may occur as a side effect of medications and as a result of severe pain.	Administer antiemetics: provide oral care at least every 2 to 4 hours; offer clear liquid diet and ice chips; avoid liquids that increase stomach acidity such as coffee, milk, and citric acid juices.
Constipation	Narcotic medications and immobility slow peristalsis.	Give preventive care, which is most effective: increase fluid intake; include bran, whole grain products, and fresh vegetables in diet; encourage exercise (Chapter 45).
	Lack of bulk in diet or reduced fluid intake may occur with appetite changes.	
	Constipation can add to discomfort.	Administer prophylactic stool softeners. Assess for fecal impaction.
Diarrhea	Diarrhea results from disease process (e.g., colon cancer) and complications of treatment or medications.	Confer with physician to change medication if possible. Provide low-residue diet.
Urinary incontinence	Incontinence results from progressive disease (e.g., involvement of spinal cord, reduced level of consciousness.)	Protect skin from irritation or breakdown. Indwelling urinary catheter or condom catheters may be used (Chapter 44).
Inadequate nutrition	Nausea and vomitting can decrease appetite.	Serve smaller portions and bland foods, which may be more palatable.
	Depression from grieving may cause anorexia.	Allow home-cooked meals, which may be preferred by client and gives the family a chance to participate.
Dehydration	As disease progresses, client is less willing or able to maintain oral fluid intake.	Remove factors causing decreased intake; give antiemeticss, apply topical analgesics to oral lesions. Reduce discomfort from dehydration; give mouth care at least every 4 hours; offer ice chips or moist cloth to lips.
Ineffective breathing patterns, e.g. dyspnea, shortness of breath	Disease progression that involves lung tissue, e.g. progression of cancer, pneumonia, pulmonary edema	Treat or control underlying cause Maximize client's oxygenation, e.g. position client upright, provide supplemental oxygen, maintain a patent airway, reduce anxiety or fever
	Anemia which reduces oxygen carrying capacity	Administer medications such as bronchodilators, inhaled steroids, or narcotics to supress cough and ease breathing and apprehension.
	Anxiety which increases oxygen demand	
	Fever which increases oxygen demand	

ments, and passions independent of the illness experience (Chochinov, 2002). Giving importance to the things that a client holds dear acknowledges individual personhood, while also strengthening the empathic, therapeutic communication between the client, the client's family, and the nurse. Spending time to let clients share their life experiences, particularly what has been meaningful, enables the nurse to know clients better. Knowing clients then facilitates choice of therapies that promote client decision making and autonomy.

For many clients, preservation of dignity and self-esteem can be achieved by providing spiritual comfort. Facilitating connections to a spiritual practice or community and supporting the expression of culturally held beliefs is very important. Clients may also benefit by being assured that some aspect of their lives may transcend death. In other words, the client gains comfort from knowing that something of one's life will continue after death. Participating in a life project such as making an audiotape or videotape for the family, writing letters, or keeping a journal can offer clients the comfort of knowing that something of their essence will survive beyond death (Chochinov, 2000). Chapter 28 further discusses some of the spiritual practices and religious rituals that can support persons in need of spiritual comfort.

Basic to promoting a client's self-esteem and dignity is attending to the client's appearance and surroundings. Cleanliness, absence of body odors, attractive clothing, and personal grooming all contribute to a sense of worth. When caring for a client's bodily functions, the nurse always shows an attitude of respect, even when the client becomes dependent. It is important to keep the client's immediate surroundings pleasant by opening curtains and letting light change from the bright of day to the dark of night. The quick removal of liquid stool or vomitus will remove unpleasant odors.

Disabilities experienced by the client may threaten dignity, especially when caregivers take control of the client's life. The nurse allows the client to make nursing care decisions (e.g., how and when to administer personal hygiene, diet preferences, and timing of nursing therapies). The nurse keeps the client and family well informed about planned therapies, their purpose, and anticipated effects. It is also important to provide the client privacy during nursing care procedures and when the client and family need time together.

Preventing Abandonment and Isolation. A terminally ill client is often fearful of dying alone. Therefore it is important for the nurse to answer the call light quickly and to explain when staff will be giving care and performing assessments throughout the day and night. The nurse should establish presence and use appropriate touch when performing care measures. The nurse must be available to answer questions, even if there is no need for data, no further decisions to make, or no further curative interventions to offer (Finucane, 2002). Clients should not be placed in private rooms unless family members visit and plan to stay around the clock. Clients feel a sense of involvement when sharing a room and interacting with staff. Clients can share conversation and companionship with roommates and visitors.

If family members have difficulty accepting the client's impending death, they may avoid visitation. When family members do visit, it is important for the nurse to talk with them and keep them informed of the client's progress. It may be useful to give family members helpful hints about what to discuss with clients. For example, the nurse role models attentive listening and offering reassurance to improve the family members' communication skills. The nurse encourages the family to discuss activities other family members are involved in, to reminisce about enjoyable times, and to inquire about the client's concerns. It is also helpful to find simple and appropriate care activities for the family to perform, such as feeding the client, washing the client's face, combing hair, and filling out the client's menu. Older adults often become particularly lonely at night and may feel more secure if a family member stays at the bedside during the night. The nurse should allow visitors to remain with dying clients at any time if the client wants them. Also, the nurse must know how to contact family members at any time if the client requests a visit or if the client's condition worsens.

Providing a Comfortable and Peaceful Environment. The nurse keeps a client comfortable through frequent repositioning, keeping bed linens dry, and controlling extraneous environmental noise. Pictures, cherished objects, cards or letters from family members and friends, and plants and flowers create an environment that is more familiar and comforting. The nurse offers the client frequent back massage or guided imagery exercises and allows the client time to listen to preferred types of music. A comfortable, pleasant environment helps clients to relax, which promotes their ability to sleep and minimizes severity of symptoms.

Support for the Grieving Family. The family may be the primary caregivers when the client chooses to be at home during the last days of life. Family members require the nurse's support and benefit from being taught ways to care for their loved one (Box 29-7). Caring for a family member can be emotionally stressful and physically exhausting for the family caregiver. Not all families can manage care on their own. In the home setting, the nurse provides the opportunity for the family to be temporarily relieved of their duties so they can acquire needed rest and support. Respite care is a resource available through hospice programs. Families also need to be informed of home care, hospice, and community service options so that they can choose among the resources available. In some cases, families may need assistance and support in making the very difficult decision about nursing home placement.

The nurse keeps the family informed so that they can anticipate the type of symptoms the client will likely experience and the implications for care. The nurse encourages family members to express their grief openly with the client and to give the client opportunity to discuss any remaining concerns or requests. The family also needs personal time to share their concerns with the nurse and to ask questions about treatment options, course of the client's disease, and the meaning of the client's behaviors. It is wise for the nurse to communicate news of the client's impending death when the family is together, if possible. Family members can provide support for one another. The nurse conveys the news in a private area and remains willing to stay with the family as needed.

Preparing the Dying Client's Family
Objectives

- Family will be able to provide appropriate physical care for the dying client in the home.
- Family will be able to provide appropriate psychological support to the dying client.

Teaching Strategies

- Describe and demonstrate feeding techniques and selection of foods to facilitate ease of chewing and swallowing.
- Demonstrate bathing, mouth care, and other hygiene measures, and allow family to perform return demonstration.
- Show a video on simple transfer techniques to prevent injury to themselves and the client; help family to practice.
- Instruct family on need to enforce rest periods.
- Teach family to recognize signs and symptoms to expect as the client's condition worsens and provide information on whom to call in an emergency.
- Discuss ways to support the dying person and listen to needs and fears.
- Solicit questions from family and provide information as needed.

Evaluation

- Have the family members demonstrate physical care techniques (e.g., turning, feeding, mouth care).
- Ask the family members to describe how they vary approaches to care when the client has symptoms such as pain or fatigue.
- Ask the family to discuss how they feel about their ability to support the client.

In the hospital setting the nurse assists in planning a visitation schedule for family members to prevent the client and family from excessive fatigue. Young children should visit dying parents. At the time of the client's death, the nurse helps the family to stay in communication with the client through frequent visits, caring silence, attentive listening, touch, and telling the client of their love. After death the nurse assists the family with decision making such as notification of a mortician, transportation of family members, and collection of the client's belongings.

Hospice Care. **Hospice** care is an alternative care delivery model for the terminally ill. It is one phase of palliative care. Generally clients accepted into a hospice program have less than 6 months to live. Hospice is not a facility but a concept for family-centered care designed to assist the client in being comfortable and maintaining a satisfactory lifestyle until death. Hospice services are available in the home, hospital, and nursing home settings. Components of hospice care programs include the following:
- Client and family as the unit of care
- Coordinated home care with access to available inpatient and nursing home beds
- Control of symptoms (physical, sociological, psychological, and spiritual)

- Physician-directed services
- Provision of an interdisciplinary care team of physicians, nurses, spiritual advisers, social worker, and counselors
- Medical and nursing services available at all times
- Bereavement follow-up after a client's death
- Use of trained volunteers for frequent visitation and respite support
- Acceptance into the program on the basis of health care needs rather than the ability to pay

The nurse's role in hospice is to meet the primary wishes of the dying client and to be open to individual desires of each client. The nurse supports a client's choice in maintaining comfort and dignity. Whether the client ultimately dies at home or in a health care facility, the client's wishes are followed with the understanding that whatever choice is made, is made "for the good of all who are involved." When options are complicated by family needs, hospice will try to work with the clients' wishes. A hospice program emphasizes palliative care with the client and family as active participants. Client care goals are mutually set, and all participants fully understand the options and desires of the client. Efforts by the hospice team are made to meet the client's desires and to encourage the family to stay within those guidelines. Often a bereavement visit or visits will be made by the staff of the hospice team to the family even after the death of the client to help the family move through the grieving process successfully.

Many clients prefer to die at home in a familiar setting, whereas others choose not to burden their families and so prefer to die in a hospital or nursing home. It is important that the hospice team know the client's preference. Many clients suffer physical ailments that prevent them from being cared for at home despite the willingness of family and friends to care for the client. The health and welfare issues are viewed from a broader perspective than just the client's desires. The concern for family needs is also taken into consideration by the hospice team.

A client in hospice may become hospitalized, but the health care team will coordinate care between the home and inpatient setting. There must be a primary caregiver (e.g., family member or friend) in the home for a client to have hospice services. There is always the effort to keep clients at home for as long as possible. The family provides basic supportive care. However, if the family cannot meet all of the client's needs, a home care aide is available for hygienic needs and a nurse is available to coordinate and administer symptom management therapies. The interdisciplinary team has the goal of 24-hour accessibility as needed. As a client's death becomes imminent, members of the hospice team are there to give support to the client and family.

Care After Death. When a client dies in a hospital setting, the nurse is the one who provides **postmortem care.** It is important for the nurse to care for the client's body with dignity and sensitivity and in a manner consistent with the client's religious or cultural beliefs. After death the body undergoes many physical changes. For that reason, care must be provided as soon as possible to prevent tissue damage or disfigurement of body parts.

Federal and state legislation require hospitals to formulate policies and procedures based on current laws to validate death, identify potential organ or tissue donors, and to provide postmortem care. For transplantation of organs, the client must be maintained on ventilatory and circulatory support until vital organs are harvested. The family must clearly understand that the client is "brain dead," that the equipment (i.e., ventilator and vasopressor medications) is not keeping the client alive but keeping the physical body in a state so that the organs will not be damaged before harvesting.

The nurse can be very helpful in supporting families through the organ and tissue request process. It is important to provide a private area to discuss all issues with the family. The staff member designated to make a request, such as a formal transplant coordinator, a social worker, chaplain, or the nurse must offer the family clarification of what defines brain death because support systems must remain in place even after the client is pronounced "dead" for vital organ retrieval (i.e., heart, lungs, kidneys, and liver). The nurse reinforces explanations throughout the organ retrieval process. The family must know who legally can give final consent, what options there are for organ or tissue donation, whether there are associated costs, and how donation will affect burial or cremation. Nonvital tissues such as corneas, skin, long bones, and middle ear bones can be harvested when the client is proclaimed dead without artificially maintaining vital functions. Organ and tissue donation must be agreed on by the family if no specific documented requests were made by the client before death. Each nurse should review his or her state's organ retrieval laws and institutional policy and procedure regarding the formal consent process.

Another area that is difficult for the nurse and family concerns autopsy. According to Dracup and Brown (1998), getting permission through delicate questioning is difficult at best. Often the doctor will ask for permission for an autopsy, but it is the nurse's job to answer questions and support the family's choices. It is very difficult to approach a grieving family with such a request. Dracup and Brown (1998) suggest showing the value that an autopsy can have by improving knowledge in the field of medicine. To help the living, the autopsy can lead to new therapies or new understanding of diseases. The more reasons the nurse can think of to support organ donation or autopsy, the more the family will be helped to realize the good that can be accomplished by either donation or research autopsy.

Clients' and families' cultural beliefs become very important in postmortem care (see Chapter 8). Maintaining the integrity of rituals and mourning practices gives families a sense of acceptance of the client's death and an inner peace. Although there are individual variations within cultural groups, general preferences are described in Box 29-8. The ability of families to express their cultural values when a client dies becomes a tool to make predictable and controllable that which is unpredictable and inevitable (Kagawa-Singer, 1998). The ethical decisions that surround a client's death are based on the values of a culture. The U.S. health care system reflects Western, Judeo-Christian values. Difficulties arise when it is considered the "right way" compared to all others. For example, for many cultures the U.S. laws that govern who to approach for organ donation may not be acceptable. Many other cultures recognize the family as more than

Box **29-8**	**Cultural Considerations in Care of the Body After Death**

African Americans—Prefer having a member of the health care team to clean and prepare the loved one's body. Some consider organ donation a taboo but may agree to an autopsy.
Chinese Americans—Some families will prefer to bathe the client themselves. Often believe the body should remain intact; organ donation and autopsy are uncommon.
Filipino Americans—Some families may prefer to wash the body themselves and are likely to want time for all family members to say goodbye. May not permit organ donation or autopsy.
Hispanic or Latino Americans—Family members may help with care of the body and are likely to want time to say goodbye. Organ donation and autopsy are uncommon.

Modified from Mazanec P, Tyler MK: Cultural considerations in end-of-life care, *Am J Nurs* 103(3):50, 2003.

just the nuclear biological unit. Health care providers must determine the makeup of a family network and which members should be involved about decisions such as organ donation and end-of-life care.

The nurse is responsible for coordination of all aspects of care surrounding a client's death. Box 29-9 summarizes the nurse's and physician's responsibilities for care of the body after death. It is important for the nurse to be familiar with institutional policies and procedures that are established for postmortem care.

The family becomes the primary client when the actual death has occurred, and the shift of concern moves from the dead client to the living family. At this time it becomes important to appropriately use the resources that are available. For example, pastoral care staff can be a helpful resource to assist the family even before the actual death, if no bereavement team is available. However, it is important to know whether the family chooses to have spiritual counselors present. Some families prefer to grieve alone, whereas others may desire the support of others. Social workers and counselors can also offer assistance. If the family's expectations for support are unknown, the simple questions and suggestions for assistance can be offered by anyone who assists the family.

Documentation of all of the events surrounding a client's death is important to avoid misunderstandings and to clarify final event's in a client's life. There are legal guidelines that are supported by each facility's policies and procedures and that must be followed and accurately documented to avoid breaks in the law. Box 29-10 lists the content to be documented about end-of-life care. Documentation will validate the success of meeting the goals identified for the client or provide a justification for the failure to meet any goals. Complete and accurate documentation offers a summary of activities that can become the focus for risk management or legal investigations.

Some medical forms must be signed by a doctor or coroner, but most of the forms must be recorded by the registered nurse. Gathering of information for the forms may be delegated to assistive personnel, but the actual charting of data on the nurse's notes must be done by the

Box 29-9   *Procedural Guidelines*

Care of the Body After Death

Equipment: Bath towels, washcloths, wash basin, scissors, shroud kit with name tags, bed linen, room deodorizer, documentation forms.

Delegation: Care of the body after death can be delegated to assistive personnel (AP) except for requests of organ/tissue donation. Check agency policy for which staff member is to remove any invasive tubes or lines.

1. Physicians must certify the death—time pronounced, therapy used, actions taken.
2. Physicians may request an autopsy, especially for unusual circumstances.
3. Trained staff member provides an option for donation of organs or tissue—personal, religious, and cultural needs should be included during this process (see Chapter 28).
4. Nurses provide dignity and sensitivity to the client and the family.
   a. Check orders for any specimens or special orders needed by the physician.
   b. Make arrangements for staff, minister, or others to stay with the family while preparing the body for viewing; ask for special requests for viewing (e.g., shaving, a special gown, Bible in hand, rosary at the bedside).
   c. Before shaving of male client: Determine if the family wishes client to remain unshaven if it was his custom to wear a beard. Determine if client's religion or culture has a preference to facial hair.
   d. Remove all equipment, tubes, supplies, and dirty linens according to protocol (unless organ donation is to take place; in that case leave support systems in place).
   e. Cleanse the body thoroughly, apply clean sheets, and remove all trash from the room.
   f. Brush and comb client's hair. Apply any personal hairpiece.
   g. Position according to protocol—the eyes should be closed by gently holding them down a few minutes; dentures should be in the mouth to maintain facial alignment; packing should not be visible during viewing.
   h. Cover with a clean sheet up to the chin with arms outside covers if possible.
   i. Lower the lighting, and spray a deodorizer if possible to remove unpleasant odors.
   j. Give the family the option to view or not to view and go with them.
   k. Clarify that either option is acceptable.
   l. Encourage the family to say goodbye through both touch and talk.
   m. Do not rush this process. Once the family is more comfortable, *ask* if they would like to be left alone. Remind them that they can call you if needed.
   n. Clarify personal belongings that are to stay with the body or who has taken personal items; documentation will require both a descriptor of the objects and the name of who received them, with the time and date.
   o. Discard nothing if items are found after the family is gone—call the family and tell them what was found and ask who might pick it up—describing the articles will be helpful in the decision-making process for the client's family.
   p. Apply name tags according to protocol—such as at the wrist, right big toe, or outside a shroud.
   q. Complete documentation in the nursing notes (see Box 29-10).
   r. Remain sensitive to other hospitalized clients or visitors when transporting the body, such as covering the body with a clean sheet and watching to avoid visitors when moving the body to another part of the hospital or to the exit for the funeral home.
   s. Follow all protocol and policies to meet all legal requirements in caring for the body.

RN or LPN. A licensed professional should witness the signing of forms.

In cases of legal matters the family will expect a clear, concise description of what occurred in the care of the client at the time of death. Opinions must be avoided, and facts are stated in a nonjudgmental, objective fashion. Both state and federal guidelines will direct what type of information is charted and when it is to be charted. Reading of such a chart by family varies according to state laws, but if it is allowed, the family should be made aware of the documentation process. Copies of parts of the chart can be given to family members with a written request and the approval of the physician and hospital (see agency guidelines). The nurse must understand and uphold the legal guidelines of documentation at all times (see Chapter 25).

The Grieving Nurse. When a nurse has cared for a client for a period of time, it is possible to have deep personal feelings of loss and sadness when the client dies. McPhee and Markowitz (2002) describe an almost universal desire to hold on to the person who is dying, with the ability to "let go" becoming a fundamental challenge. When a nurse is able to "let go," there are four fundamental things to hold on to: faith, memory, love, and one another.

There are many ways in which a nurse can attempt to cope with the loss of a dying client. Attending the viewing at the mortuary or funeral is one way to say goodbye. Writing a letter of sympathy to the family can prove useful. It is natural for a nurse to go through the grieving process. When a nurse works in an area where there are multiple losses, it is easy for bereavement overload to develop unless there are ways to process grief. The nurse might feel frustration, anger, guilt, sadness, or anxiety. Often nurses seek out other nurses or health care workers to discuss their own grief (Figure 29-5). It is important for nurses to develop their own support systems that allow time away from the care setting and opportunities to share personal feelings. Stress management techniques (see Chapter 30) can help to

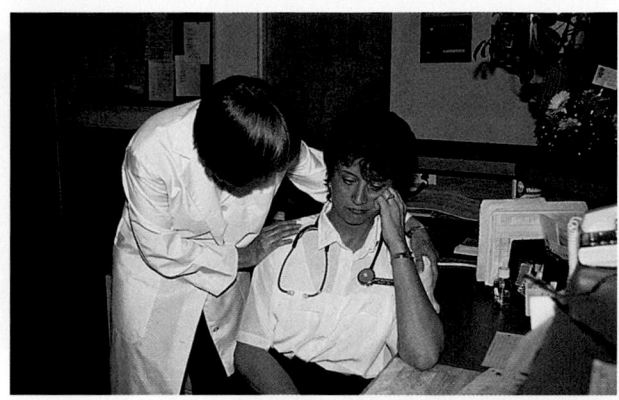

FIGURE 29–5   Nurses benefit from support of colleagues during their time of loss.

Box 29-10	Documentation of End-of-Life Care

Time of death and actions taken to prevent the death if applicable

Who pronounced the death of the client

Any special preparation and type of donation, including time, staff, and company

Who was called and who came to the hospital—donor organization, morgue, funeral home, chaplain, and individual family members making any decisions

Personal articles left on the body and taped to skin or tubes left in

Personal items given to the family—specific names and descriptors of items

Time of discharge and destination of the body

Location of name tags on the body

Special requests by the family

Any other personal statements that might be needed to clarify the situation

restore a nurse's energy and continued enjoyment in caring for clients. The nurse's self-care is critical to survival and recovery from loss, not only for his or her own sake, but also for the sake of future clients.

NP Evaluation

Client Care. A nurse will care for clients and families at every phase of the grief process. This requires the nurse to remain aware of signs and symptoms of grief, even when clients are not specifically seeking care directly related to a loss. These same signs and symptoms offer criteria to evaluate whether a client is able to deal with a loss and progress through the grief process. Critical thinking ensures that the evaluation process is thorough and relevant to the client's situation (Figure 29-6).

The nurse refers to the goals and expected outcomes established in the plan of care to determine the effectiveness of nursing interventions. By comparing actual client behaviors with expected outcomes the nurse evaluates the client's health status and whether there is a need to revise the plan of care. For example, if the goal is to have the client communicate a sense of hope with family members, the nurse evaluates the verbal and nonverbal communication process for cues related to hope. The client's responses will determine if new therapies are needed or if existing therapies should be revised. The nurse continues to evaluate the progress of the client, the effectiveness of the interventions and the interactions between the family and client. It is important for the client and family to share experiences and be active participants in the evaluation process.

Client Expectations. The client expects individualization of care, including relief of symptoms, preservation of dignity, and support of the family to maximize quality of life. The success of the evaluation depends partially on the bond formed with the client. Unless the client trusts the nurse, the sharing of personal expectations or desires is not likely to occur. It becomes important for the nurse to take the time to talk with the client and learn if expectations are being met. The following are examples of questions that will validate the achievement of client expectations:
- Am I helping you in the way you have hoped?
- Would you like me to assist you in a different way?
- Do you have a specific request that I have not been able to meet?
- What is most important for us to do for you at this time?
- Are we dealing with your problems in a timely manner?

Through communication and evaluation the nurse will continue to determine if outcome criteria were met to support the goals of care. Often the evaluation of the client's needs is easy, but the process is more complex as it relates to the family. Once a rapport is established, the nurse must be ever vigilant to avoid problems that threaten that rapport.

Key Concepts

- When caring for clients who have experienced a loss, the nurse facilitates the grief process by assisting survivors in feeling the loss, expressing the loss, and moving through the tasks of the grief process.
- Loss comes in many forms based on the values and priorities learned within a person's sphere of influence, including family, friends, society, and culture.
- The type of loss and the perception of the loss influence the degree of grief a person experiences.
- Death is difficult for the dying person, as well as for the person's family, friends, and caregivers.
- Survivors go through a bereavement period that is not linear; rather, an individual will move back and forth through a series of stages and/or tasks many times, possibly extending over a period of several years.
- Several theorists have developed stages of the grieving process and a series of tasks for survivors to successfully complete their bereavement and adapt to life with a loss.
- A nurse's knowledge of the types of grief allows for the implementation of appropriate bereavement interventions.

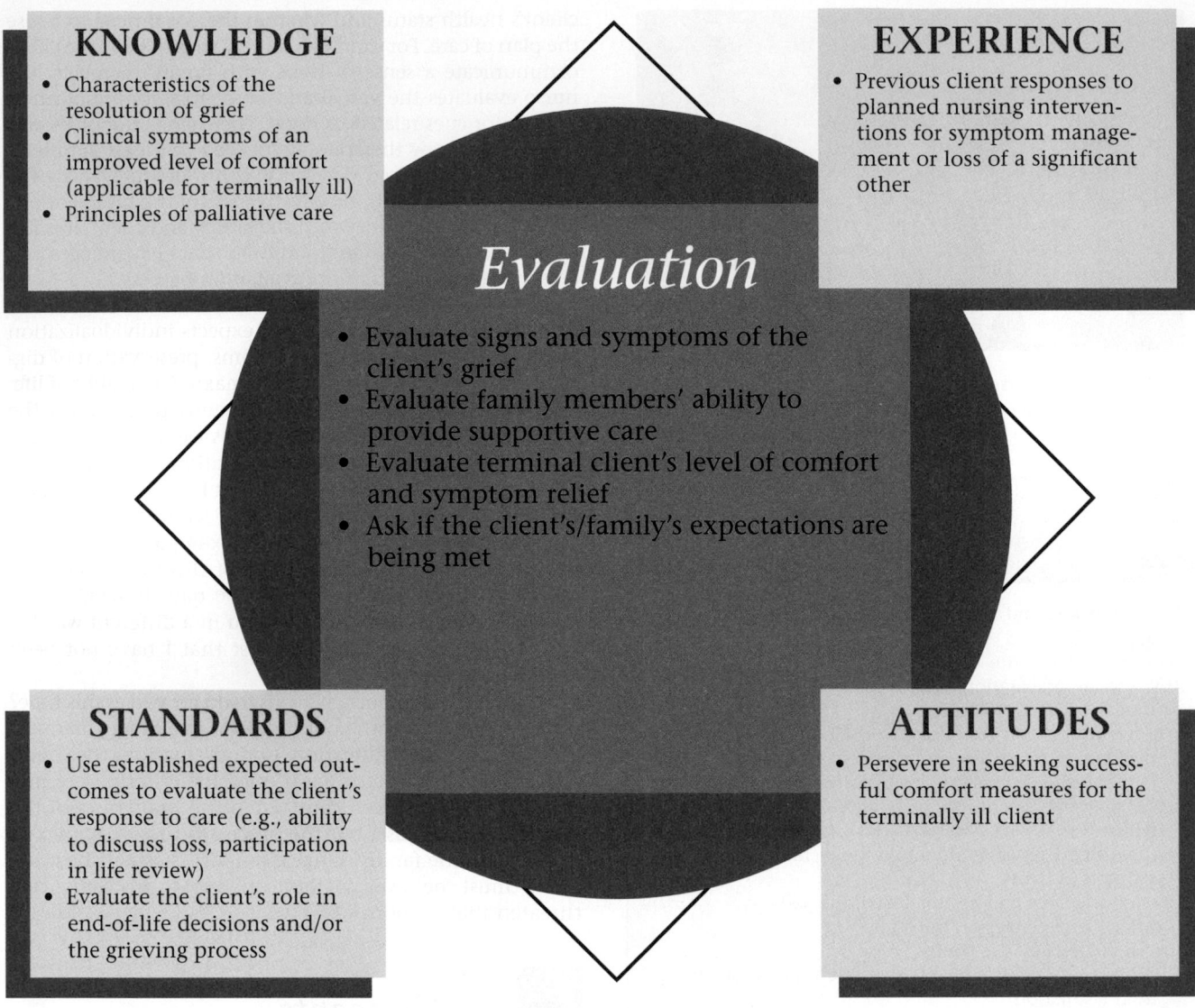

KNOWLEDGE
- Characteristics of the resolution of grief
- Clinical symptoms of an improved level of comfort (applicable for terminally ill)
- Principles of palliative care

EXPERIENCE
- Previous client responses to planned nursing interventions for symptom management or loss of a significant other

Evaluation
- Evaluate signs and symptoms of the client's grief
- Evaluate family members' ability to provide supportive care
- Evaluate terminal client's level of comfort and symptom relief
- Ask if the client's/family's expectations are being met

STANDARDS
- Use established expected outcomes to evaluate the client's response to care (e.g., ability to discuss loss, participation in life review)
- Evaluate the client's role in end-of-life decisions and/or the grieving process

ATTITUDES
- Persevere in seeking successful comfort measures for the terminally ill client

FIGURE 29–6 Critical thinking model for loss, death, and grieving evaluation.

- The way an individual perceives and responds to a loss is influenced by one's development, psychosocial perspectives, socioeconomic status, personal relationships, nature of loss, culture, and spiritual beliefs.
- Nursing interventions involve reinforcement of clients' successful coping mechanisms and introduction of new coping approaches such as the promotion of hope.
- When assessing clients in grief, the nurse does not assume how or if clients experience grief or that a particular behavior indicates grief; rather the nurse allows clients to share what is happening in their own way.
- A nurse must assess the terminally ill client's and family's wishes for end-of-life care, including the preferred place for death, the level of life-sustaining measures to employ, and expectations regarding pain and symptom management.

- The nurse develops a plan of care by integrating clients' resources such as physical energy and activity tolerance, supportive family members, spiritual faith, and methods for coping.
- The nurse establishes a caring presence and employs therapeutic communication strategies that enable clients to discuss their loss and find ways to resolve it.
- Palliative care allows clients to make more informed choices, achieve better alleviation of symptoms, and have more opportunity to work on issues of life closure.
- A nurse can promote a client's self-esteem and dignity by taking a therapeutic stance that conveys respect for the client as a whole person.
- Hospice is not a facility but a concept for family-centered care designed to assist the client in being comfortable and maintaining a satisfactory lifestyle until death.

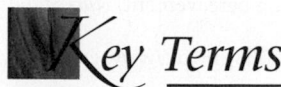

Key Terms

Acceptance, *p. 570*
Actual loss, *p. 569*
Anger, *p. 570*
Anticipatory grief, *p. 571*
Bargaining, *p. 570*
Bereavement, *p. 570*
Denial, *p. 570*
Depression, *p. 570*
Disorganization and
    despair, *p. 570*
Grief, *p. 570*
Hope, *p. 574*

Hospice, *p. 588*
Maturational loss, *p. 569*
Necessary loss, *p. 569*
Numbing, *p. 570*
Palliative care, *p. 585*
Perceived loss, *p. 569*
Postmortem care, *p. 588*
Reorganization, *p. 570*
Situational loss, *p. 569*
Yearning and searching,
    p. 570

Critical Thinking Exercises

1. Mr. Jamison visits the community health clinic and tells the nurse, "I do not know what is wrong with me. I lost my wife 6 months ago and I still get angry that God let her die. I still miss her so much. I have been going out with friends, but I just do not enjoy it that much. There are times when I wake up at night and I think my wife is still here. What is wrong with me? I thought I would be feeling better by now." As the nurse, how would you respond to Mr. Jamison?

2. You are assigned to care for two different clients. Mrs. Rouse has rheumatoid arthritis and is experiencing severe joint pain in both hands. Mrs. Nester has bone cancer and has experienced ongoing deep pain in the back and hips, with some discomfort also in the lower extremities. Refer to Chapter 42 on content about pain. Then discuss in what way management of pain will differ between the two patients.

3. A nursing colleague is discussing her client with you. She says, "My client is a 48-year-old man with a degenerative neurological disease. The disease is progressive. He is having trouble walking and taking care of his daily needs. The only thing I can do is assist him with bathing, feeding, and walking. He really is not a candidate yet for palliative care." What would be your response to your colleague?

Review Questions

1. A child is grieving over the loss of a favorite toy. This is an example of a (an):
   1. Actual loss.
   2. Perceived loss.
   3. Situational loss.
   4. Maturational loss.

2. A middle-age man comes to a community clinic for his annual flu examination. In the discussion with the nurse she learns that he still works at a local law firm. However, he has recently lost two important cases and his boss has been applying pressure on him "to turn it around." The client may be experiencing a (an):
   1. Actual loss.
   2. Perceived loss.
   3. Situational loss.
   4. Maturational loss.

3. The community health nurse's job is to provide grief counseling for the community residents where a major flood has occurred. The loss associated with flooding is best described as a (an):
   1. Actual loss.
   2. Perceived loss.
   3. Situational loss.
   4. Maturational loss.

4. The client has been diagnosed with terminal brain cancer. When the nurse visits him during rounds, he asks her whether the cancer could have been caused by something he ate or perhaps exposure to some chemical toxin. The client is likely experiencing:
   1. Bowlby's phase of numbing.
   2. Kübler-Ross's stage of acceptance.
   3. Worden's tasks of emotionally relocating.
   4. Bowlby's phase of disorganization and despair.

5. According to Kübler-Ross's *Stages of Dying*, during this phase the client may feel overwhelmingly lonely and withdraw from interpersonal interaction.
   1. Bowlby's phase of numbing.
   2. Kübler-Ross's stage of acceptance.
   3. Worden's tasks of emotionally relocating.
   4. Kübler-Ross's stage of depression.

6. Since the death of his wife, the client has assumed full responsibility for the care of his children. He has noticed over the last few weeks that friends are calling less often. He is most likely in the following phase of mourning:
   1. Anticipatory grieving.
   2. Worden's task III of mourning.
   3. Kübler Ross's phase of bargaining.
   4. Bowlby's disorganization and despair.

7. A factor that uniquely influences an older adult's grief response is:
   1. Cultural background.
   2. Socioeconomic resources.
   3. Sense of contributions in life.
   4. Support available from family and friends.

8. "Client will be able to discuss expected course of disease" is an example of a (an):
   1. Goal.
   2. Intervention.
   3. Plan.
   4. Expected outcome.

9. A sixteen-year-old client has been admitted to the intensive care unit after suffering a closed head injury. The physician and nurse are preparing to approach the family to consider donation of the heart and lungs. When working with families in this situation, it is important to explain that:
   1. The ventilator is being used to prevent brain death.
   2. The ventilator maintains organ perfusion until time for harvesting.
   3. Tissues such as corneas can be harvested only if the client remains ventilated.
   4. Organ donation can occur only if the client has made a request to donate organs in the past.

10. This type of care allows clients to make more informed choices, achieve better alleviation of symptoms, and have more opportunity to work on issues of life closure:
    1. Acute care.
    2. Mourning care.
    3. Palliative care.
    4. Terminal care.

References

Barbus AJ: The dying person's bill of rights, *Am J Nurs* 75:99, 1975.

Bierman E and others: Assessing access as a first step towards improving the quality of care for very old adults, *J Ambul Care Manage* 21(3):17, 1998.

Blackhall and others: Ethnicity and attitudes towards life-sustaining technology. *Social Service in Medicine,* 48: 1779, 1999.

Bowlby J: *Attachment and loss,* vol 3, Loss, sadness, and depression, New York, 1980, Basic Books.

Braza K: Families and the grief process, *ARCH Factsheet* 21, March 1993.

Callahan D: Terminating life-sustaining treatment of the demented, *Hastings Cent Rep* 25:25, 1995.

Catalano JT: *Ethical and legal aspects of nursing,* ed 2, Springhouse, Pa, 1995, Springhouse.

Chochinov, 2000.

Chochinov HM: Dignity-conserving care—a new model for palliative care: helping the patient feel valued, *JAMA* 287(17):2253, 2002.

Cressy D: *Birth, marriage, and death: ritual, religion, and the life-cycle in Tudor and Stuart England,* New York, 1997, Oxford University Press.

Cushman JD: *Hospice penetration: the use of public data to measure hospice performance.* Symposium conducted at the National Hospice Organization Senior Management and Leadership Conference in St. Louis, 1998.

Daaleman TP, VandeCreek L: Placing religion and spirituality in end-of-life care, *JAMA* 284:2514, 2000.

Doka KJ: *Living with life-threatening illness: a guide for patients, their families, and caregivers,* New York, 1993, Lexington.

Dracup K, Brown CW: Asking difficult questions, *Am J Crit Care* 7(6):399, 1998.

End-of-Life Nursing Education Consortium (ELNEC), American Association of Colleges of Nursing and City of Hope National Medical Center, 2000.

Farber SJ and others: Issues in end-of-life care: family practice faculty perceptions, *J Fam Pract* 48(7):525, 1999

Field MJ, Cassel CK: *Approaching death: improving care at the end of life,* Washington, DC, 1997, (Institute of Medicine Committee on Care at the End of Life), National Academy Press.

Finucane TE: Care of patients nearing death: another view, *J Am Geriatr Soc* 50(3):551, 2002.

Hasler K: Understanding and managing bereavement, *Nurs Stand* 10(24):51, 1996.

Hospice RN: Patient's bill of rights, 2003, http://www.geocities.com/HotSprings/5120/bill.htm.

Johnson M, Maas M, Moorhead S: *Nursing outcomes classification (NOC),* ed 2, St. Louis, 2000. Mosby.

Kagawa-Singer M: The cultural context of death rituals and mourning practices, *Oncol Nurs Forum* 25(10):1752, 1998.

Kübler-Ross E: *On death and dying,* New York, 1969, Macmillan.

Last Acts Palliative Care Task Force, 1997.

Lendhardt AMC: Grieving disenfranchised losses: background and strategies for counselors, *J Hum Educ Dev* 35(4):208, 1997.

Lund DA: Conclusions about bereavement in later life and implications for interventions and future research. In Lund DA, editor: *Older bereaved spouses: research with practical application,* New York, 1989, Hemisphere.

Mazanec P, Tyler MK: Cultural considerations in end-of-life care, *Am J Nurs* 103(3):50, 2003

McCloskey JC, Bulechek GM: *Nursing interventions classification (NIC),* ed 3, St. Louis, 2000, Mosby.

McLean S: The definition of death: contemporary controversies, *BMJ* 319:(7207):42A, 1999.

McPhee SJ, Markowitz AJ: Reflections at a palliative care unit, *JAMA* 288(10):1279, 2002.

Nowotny M: Every tomorrow a vision of hope, *J Psychosoc Oncol* 9(3):117, 1991.

Parkes CM: *Bereavement: studies of grief in adult life,* London, 1972, Tavistock.

Post-White J and others: Hope, spirituality, sense of coherence, and quality of life in patients with cancer, *Oncol Nurs Forum* 23(10):1571, 1996.

Stocker S: Beyond grief, *Prevention* 46(8):88, 1994.

Tarzian AJ: Caring for dying patients who have air hunger, *Image J Nurs Sch* 32:137, 2000.

Thomas ND: The importance of culture throughout all of life and beyond, *Holist Nurs Pract* 15(2):40, 2001.

Tolle S and others: Family reports of barriers to optimal care of the dying, *Nurs Res* 49(6):310, 2000.

Weissman DE and others: Pain assessment and management in the long-term care setting, *Theor Med Bioeth* 20(1):31, 1999.

Witoszek N: *Talking to the dead: a study of Irish funerary traditions,* Atlanta, 1998, Rodopi.

Worden JW: *Grief counseling and grief therapy,* New York, 1982, Springer.

World Health Organization: Palliative Care, 2003, http://www.who.int/hiv/topics/palliative/palliative care.

Research References

Binstock W, Spector W: Five priority areas for research on long term care, *Health Serv Res* 32(5):715, 1997.

Forbes S, Bern-Klug M, Gessert C: End-of-life decision making for nursing home residents with dementia, *J Nurs Scholarsh* 32(3):251, 2000.

Hinton J: The progress of awareness and acceptance of dying assessed in cancer patients and their caring relatives, *Palliat Med* 13:19, 1999.

Morse JM, Doberneck B: Delineating the concept of hope, *Image J Nurs Sch* 27(4):277, 1995.

SUPPORT Principal Investigators: A controlled trial to improve care for seriously ill hospitalized patients: The Study to Understand Prognoses and Preferences for Outcomes and Risks of Treatments (SUPPORT), *JAMA* 274:1591, 1995.

Tilden VP and others: Family decision-making to withdraw life-sustaining treatments from hospitalized patients, *Nurs Res* 50(2):105, 2001.

Tolle S and others: Family reports of barriers to optimal care of the dying, *Nurs Res* 49(6):310, 2000.

Stress and Coping

30

Media Resources

http://evolve.elsevier.com/Potter/
fundamentals/

CD COMPANION

- Review Questions
- Glossary

evolve WEBSITE

- Review Questions
- Student Learning Activities
- Glossary

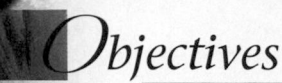

Objectives

Mastery of content in this chapter will enable the student to:

- Define key terms.
- Describe the three stages of the general adaptation syndrome.
- Differentiate acute stress disorder and posttraumatic stress disorder.
- Discuss the integration of stress theory with nursing theories.
- Formulate nursing diagnoses based on assessment data.
- Describe stress management techniques beneficial for coping with stress.
- Discuss the process of crisis intervention.
- Develop a care plan for clients experiencing stress.
- Discuss how stress in the workplace can affect the nurse.

Knowledge about stress in general is important so health care professionals can recognize stress in clients and families and intervene effectively. In addition, health care professionals are affected by stressful events that occur in the course of clinical practice. Nurses must recognize the signs and symptoms of stress and be knowledgeable about stress management techniques to aid personal coping, as well as to design stress management interventions for their clients and families.

People use the term **stress** in many ways. First, stress is an experience a person is exposed to, through a stimulus or stressor. **Stressors** are disruptive forces operating within or on any system (Neuman, 1995). Stress is also the appraisal, or perception, of a stressor. **Appraisal** is how people interpret the impact of the stressor on themselves, of what is happening and what they can do about it (Lazarus 1999). Finally, stress is a general term that links environmental demands and the person's capacity to meet those demands (Kasl 1992). Stress in this context refers to the consequences of the stressor, as well as to the person's appraisal of the stressor.

People experience stress as a consequence of daily life events and experiences. Stress can be helpful by stimulating thinking processes and helping people stay alert to their environment. Furthermore, stress can result in personal growth and facilitate development (Aguilera, 1998). How people react to stress depends on how they view and evaluate the impact of the stressor, its effect on their situation and support at the time of the stress, and their usual coping mechanisms. Stress is universal and is necessary for survival, affecting every person regardless of age, gender, race, economic condition, or educational level. Stress can provide stimulation and motivation, as well as cause discomfort and retreat. However, when stress overwhelms a person's existing coping mechanisms, disequilibrium occurs, and a **crisis** results (Aguilera, 1998). If symptoms of stress persist beyond the duration of the stressor, a person has experienced a **trauma** (Hyer and Sohnle 2001).

Scientific Knowledge Base

Over 60 years ago Walter Cannon proposed the **fight-or-flight response** to stress, which is arousal of the sympathetic nervous system (Aldwin, 2000). This reaction prepares a person for action by increasing heart rate; diverting blood

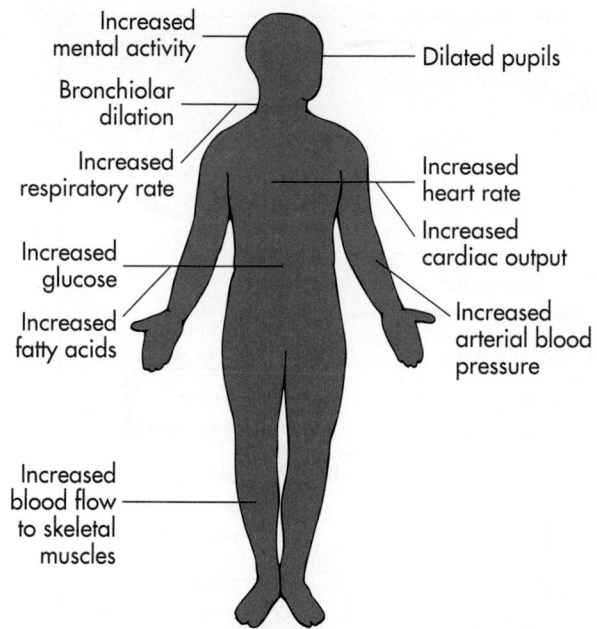

FIGURE **30–1**   Fight-or-flight response.

from the intestines to the brain and striated muscles; and increasing blood pressure, respiratory rate, and blood sugar levels (Figure 30-1).

Neurophysiological responses to stress function through negative feedback. This is a process by which the controlling mechanism senses an abnormal state, such as lowered body temperature, and makes an adaptive response, such as initiating shivering to generate body heat. Three of the major mechanisms of response to a stressor are controlled by the medulla oblongata, the reticular formation, and the pituitary gland.

Medulla Oblongata

The medulla oblongata controls vital functions necessary for survival. These include heart rate, blood pressure, and respiration. Impulses traveling to and from the medulla oblongata can increase or decrease these vital functions. For example, regulation of the heartbeat is the result of sympathetic or parasympathetic nervous system impulses traveling from the medulla oblongata to the heart. The heart rate increases in response to pulses from sympathetic fibers and decreases with impulses from parasympathetic fibers.

Reticular Formation

The reticular formation is a small cluster of neurons in the brain stem and spinal cord. It also controls vital functions and continuously monitors the physiological status of the body through connections with sensory and motor tracts. For example, certain cells within the reticular formation can cause a sleeping person to regain consciousness or increase the level of consciousness when a need arises.

Pituitary Gland

The pituitary gland, a small gland attached to the hypothalamus, supplies hormones that control vital functions. The pituitary gland produces hormones necessary for

adaptation to stress, such as the adrenocorticotropic hormone (ACTH), which in turn produces cortisol. In addition, the pituitary gland regulates the secretion of thyroid, gonadal, and parathyroid hormones. Hormone secretion, like other homeostatic mechanisms, is normally regulated by a feedback mechanism that continuously monitors hormone levels in the blood. When hormone levels drop, the pituitary gland receives a message to increase hormone secretion. When hormone levels rise, the pituitary gland decreases hormone production.

General Adaptation Syndrome

In the 1930s, 1940s, and 1950s Hans Selye enlarged on Cannon's fight-or-flight hypothesis to describe the **general adaptation syndrome (GAS),** a three-stage reaction to stress (Selye, 1991). The GAS describes how the body responds to stressors through the alarm reaction, the resistance stage, and the exhaustion stage. The GAS can be triggered either directly by a physical event or indirectly by a psychological event (Lazarus, 1999).

The GAS is an immediate physiological response of the body to stress and involves several body systems, especially the autonomic nervous system and the endocrine system (Figure 30-2). When a physical demand is made on the body, such as an injury, the GAS is initiated by the pituitary gland. The pituitary gland is closely linked to the hypothalamus, which secretes **endorphins.** Endorphins are hormones that act on the mind like morphine and opiates, producing a sense of well-being and reducing pain (Lazarus, 1999). In this way the GAS defends against stress both by activating the neuroendocrine system and by providing endorphins that decrease awareness of the pain.

During the **alarm reaction** rising hormone levels result in increased blood volume, blood glucose levels, epinephrine and norepinephrine amounts, heart rate, blood flow to muscles, oxygen intake, and mental alertness (Selye, 1991). In addition, the pupils of the eyes dilate to produce a greater visual field. This change in body systems prepares an individual for fight or flight and may last from 1 minute to many hours. If the stressor poses an extreme threat to life or remains for a long time, the person progresses to the second stage, resistance.

During the **resistance stage** the body stabilizes and responds in an opposite manner to the alarm reaction. Hormone levels, heart rate, blood pressure, and cardiac output return to normal, and the body repairs any damage that may have occurred. However, if the stressor remains, and there is no adaptation, the person enters the third stage, exhaustion.

The **exhaustion stage** occurs when the body can no longer resist the effects of the stressor and when the energy necessary to maintain adaptation is depleted. The physiological response is intensified, but the person's energy level is compromised, and adaptation to the stressor diminishes. The body is unable to defend itself against the impact of the event, physiological regulation diminishes, and, if the stress continues, death may result.

Physiological responses to stress also include immunological responses. The immune system differentiates between self and nonself, so that under normal conditions

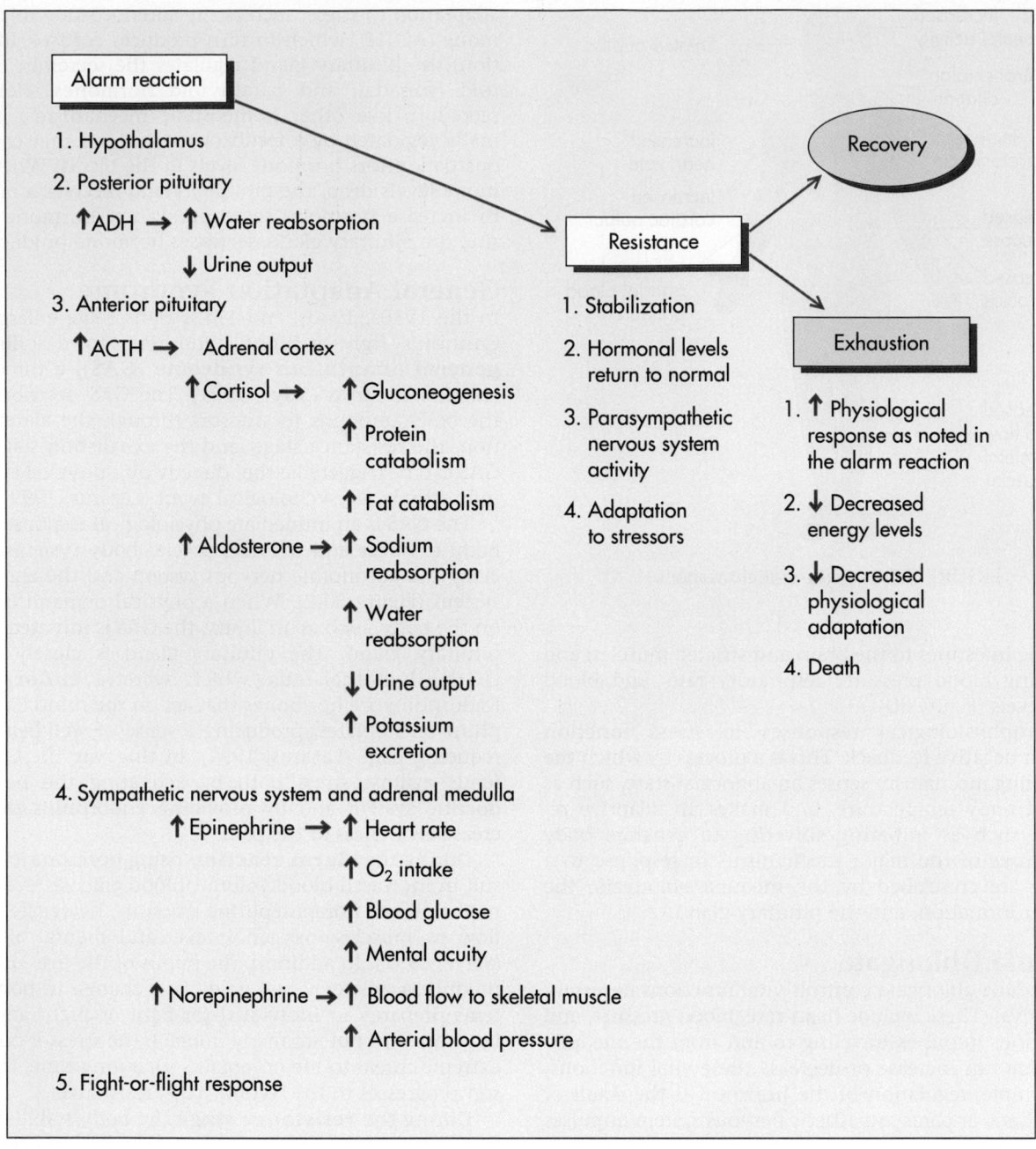

FIGURE **30–2** General adaptation syndrome (GAS).

one's own cells are not treated as threats, in the way that bacteria, viruses, parasites, or toxins are treated. Typically, the immune system recognizes bacteria, for example, as a threat and attacks them. An antigen on the surface of the bacteria cells identifies the bacteria as invaders. After being exposed to a particular antigen, the immune system remembers how to respond to that antigen and is prepared to respond with antibodies when the same antigen appears at a later time. However, a virus might create an antigen that is very similar to a naturally occurring protein and the immune system would attack it as if it were a threat. Problems occur when the immune system misinterprets antigens and makes a too vigorous response, leading to an autoimmune illness. The mechanisms through which stress affects the immune system are unclear (Aldwin, 2000).

Selye (1991) noted that a prolonged state of stress can cause disease. Stress can make people ill as a result of (1) increased levels of powerful hormones that change our bodily processes; (2) coping choices that are unhealthy, such as not getting enough rest or a proper diet or use of tobacco, alcohol, other substances, or caffeine; and (3) neglect of warning signs of illness or failure to adhere to prescribed medicines or treatments (Monat and Lazarus, 1991).

Reaction to Psychological Stress. The GAS is activated indirectly for psychological threats, which are different

---

Box 30-1   **Factors Influencing the Response to Stressors**

Aspects of a Stressor That Would Influence the Stress Response

Intensity
Scope
Duration
Number and nature of other stressors
Predictability

Characteristics of the Individual That Would Influence the Stress Response

Level of personal control
Availability of social supports
Feelings of competence
Cognitive appraisal

Box 30-2   **Examples of Ego-Defense Mechanisms**

- Compensation is making up for a deficiency in one aspect of self-image by strongly emphasizing a feature considered an asset. (Example: A person who is a poor communicator may rely on organizational skills.)
- Conversion is unconsciously repressing an anxiety-producing emotional conflict and transforming it into nonorganic symptoms (e.g., difficulty sleeping, loss of appetite).
- Denial is avoiding emotional conflicts by refusing to consciously acknowledge anything that might cause intolerable emotional pain. (Example: A person refuses to discuss or acknowledge a personal loss.)
- Displacement is transferring emotions, ideas, or wishes from a stressful situation to a less anxiety-producing substitute. (Example: A person transfers anger over an interpersonal conflict to a malfunctioning VCR.)
- Identification is patterning behavior after that of another person and assuming that person's qualities, characteristics, and actions.
- Dissociation is experiencing a subjective sense of numbing and a reduced awareness of one's surroundings.
- Regression is coping with a stressor through actions and behaviors associated with an earlier developmental period.

---

for each person and produce differing reactions (Box 30-1). Lazarus (1999) maintains that a person is under stress only if the person evaluates the event or circumstance as personally significant. Evaluating an event for its personal meaning is called **primary appraisal.** Appraisal of an event or circumstance is an ongoing perceptual process (Aguilera, 1998). If primary appraisal results in the person identifying the event or circumstance as a harm, loss, threat, or challenge, the person experiences stress. If stress is present, **secondary appraisal** focuses on possible coping strategies. Balancing factors contribute to restoring equilibrium. According to crisis theory (Aguilera, 1998), feedback cues lead to reappraisals of the original perception. Therefore coping behaviors constantly change as new information is perceived.

Coping is the person's effort to manage psychological stress (Lazarus, 1999). Effectiveness of coping strategies depends on the individual's needs. For this reason no single coping strategy works for everyone or for every stress. The same person may cope differently from one time to another. In stressful situations people may use a combination of problem-focused coping and emotion-focused coping strategies. In other words, when under stress, a person obtains information and takes action to change the situation, as well as regulating emotions tied to the stress. In some cases a person avoids thinking about the situation or changes the way he or she thinks about it, without changing the actual situation itself (Lazarus, 1999).

Lazarus (1999) suggests that not only does the type of stress make a difference, but that people's goals, their beliefs about themselves and the world, and personal resources determine how they cope with stress. "Resources include intelligence, money, social skills, supportive family and friends, physical attractiveness, health and energy, and ways of thinking, such as optimism" (Lazarus, 1999).

Psychological adaptive behaviors are also referred to as coping mechanisms. Such mechanisms can be task oriented, involving the use of direct problem-solving techniques to cope with the threats. They can also be **ego-defense mechanisms,** the purpose of which is to regulate emotional distress and thus give a person protection from anxiety and stress. Ego-defense mechanisms are indirect methods of coping with stress.

Ego-defense mechanisms, first described by Sigmund Freud, are unconscious behaviors that offer psychological protection from a stressful event. They are used by everyone and help protect against feelings of worthlessness and anxiety. Occasionally a defense mechanism can become distorted and is no longer able to assist the person in adapting to a stressor. There are many ego-defense mechanisms (Box 30-2). They are frequently activated by short-term stressors and usually do not result in psychiatric disorders.

Types of Stress

Selye identified two types of stress: **distress,** or damaging stress, and **eustress,** stress that protects health. Eustress is motivating energy, such as happiness, hopefulness, and purposeful movement (Varcarolis, 2002). However, the idea of healthy stress has become controversial because it is difficult to tell whether a person has benefited from stress or is coping by denying the stress in some way (Aldwin, 2000). There are several types of stress, including work stress, family stress, chronic stress, acute stress, daily hassles, trauma, and crisis. "Work and family stress interact, family being the background for work stress, and work the background for family stress" (Lazarus, 1999). One person may look at a stimulus and see it as a challenge, leading to mastery and growth. Another sees the same stimulus as a threat, leading to stagnation and loss. Lazarus suggests a spillover of stresses between work and home. The individual with family responsibilities and a full-time job outside the home may experience chronic stress. Chronic stress occurs in stable conditions and from stressful roles. Another example of chronic stress is living with a long-term illness. Conversely, acute stress is provoked by time-limited events that are threatening for a relatively brief period. Further complicating chronic or acute stress are daily hassles that are recurrent, such as commuting to work, maintaining a house, dealing with difficult people, and managing money.

When a trauma occurs, its effects may last well after the traumatizing event ends (Hyer and Sohnle, 2001). **Posttraumatic stress disorder (PTSD)** begins with an **acute stress disorder** (ASD) (Hyer and Sohnle, 2001). An acute stress disorder begins with the person experiencing, witnessing, or being confronted with a traumatic event and responding with intense fear, helplessness, or horror (American Psychiatric Association [APA], 2000). Other criteria of the acute stress disorder are that the person displays at least three acute dissociative symptoms, has at least one reexperiencing symptom, displays marked avoidance of stimuli that arouse memories of the trauma, shows marked hyperarousal, and has these symptoms between 2 days and 4 weeks after the trauma (Hyer and Sohnle, 2001). Examples of traumatic events that lead to ASD are motor vehicle crashes, natural disasters, violent personal assault, and military combat. Symptoms of PTSD may have a delayed onset longer than 4 weeks and persists longer than 1 month (APA, 2000). People with PTSD may experience **flashbacks,** or recurrent and intrusive recollections of the event. Traumatic events that can lead to PTSD include the same events that lead to ASD (Box 30-3).

Conversely, research is beginning to show that trauma can have positive effects. Benefits can enable the person to improve in coping skills and self-knowledge, social ties, and changes in values and perspectives (Hyer and Sohnle, 2001).

A crisis implies that a person is facing a turning point in life. That is, previous ways of coping are not effective and the person must change. Gerald Caplan, in 1964, described crisis intervention. Caplan distinguished two types of crises, those associated with changing developmental levels, or **developmental crises,** and **situational crises.** The frame of reference for a crisis is from the view of the person experiencing the crisis. Aguilera's crisis theory (1998) maintains that the vital question for a person in crisis is, "What does this mean to you; how is it going to affect your life?" What is extremely stressful for one person might not be at all stressful to another. The factors influencing the return of equilibrium or homeostasis are the perception of the event, situational supports, and coping mechanisms. A basic assumption of crisis theory is that a person can either advance or regress as a result of a crisis, depending upon how the crisis is managed (Lazarus, 1999).

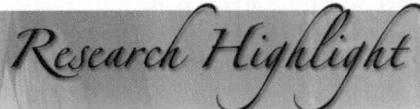

Box 30-3

Understanding Risks for Developing Psychological Distress

Research Focus

When caring for clients who have experienced trauma such as motor vehicle crashes, assaults, and industrial accidents, nurses focus first on life threatening effects of the trauma. However, other consequences of trauma, such as psychological distress, can be unnoticed. Nurses need to be aware of risk factors for anxiety, depression, and posttraumatic stress disorder following trauma.

Research Abstract

The purpose of this study was to describe the pretrauma characteristics of 152 people (87 women and 65 men) who experienced significant psychological distress shortly after physical injury. Individuals who had received treatment in the emergency department were contacted and asked to complete three questionnaires: the Posttraumatic Stress Disorder Scale, the Impact of Event Scale (IES), and the Hospital Anxiety and Depression Scale. A fourth questionnaire, the Abbreviated Injury Scale, was completed based upon a medical record review by the researchers. The presence of significant psychological distress among the 152 people identified from all the people receiving emergency treatment was documented. Overall, the people identified with distress reported very little functional impairment and a high level of contentment before the traumatic event. Most of their injuries were relatively minor and not life threatening. However, 141 (93%) of the subjects met the diagnostic criteria for posttraumatic stress disorder

(PTSD). The IES revealed that the subjects were experiencing high levels of trauma-related distress. The researchers examined the relationship between pretrauma variables and the total score on the IES. The pretrauma factors of being unemployed and having experienced previous trauma accounted for 10% of the variance in the total IES score. The researchers concluded that (a) trauma perceived as mild by medical personnel can result in severe stress, anxiety, and depression for the client; (b) high functioning before a traumatic event does not protect the client from developing PTSD; and (c) pretrauma unemployment can contribute to psychological distress after a traumatic injury.

Evidence-Based Practice

- Regardless of the severity of trauma or previous level of functioning, clients who have experienced a traumatic injury are at risk for developing PTSD.
- Nurses must monitor the client's perception of the meaning and impact of a traumatic injury, regardless of the apparent severity of the trauma.
- Two risk factors for developing PTSD after a traumatic injury are unemployment before the trauma and previous trauma.

Reference

Joy D and others: Posttraumatic stress reactions after injury, *J Trauma* 48(3):490, 2000.

Nursing Knowledge Base

Nurses have proposed theories related to stress and coping. Because stress plays a central role in vulnerability to disease, symptoms of stress often require nursing intervention.

Nursing Theory and the Role of Stress

Neuman Systems Model is based on the concepts of stress and reaction to stress. This nursing theory views nursing as being responsible for developing interventions to prevent or reduce stressors on the client or to make them more bearable for the client (Neuman, 1995). Because the Neuman model is a systems model, it is applied to not only understand clients' individual responses to stressors but families' and communities' responses as well. All systems experience multiple stressors, each of which has a differing potential to disturb the person's, family's, or community's balance. Examples of stress may include intrapersonal stressors, such as an illness or injury; interpersonal stressors, such as an argument or misunderstanding between two people, or extrapersonal stressors, such as financial concerns, that impinge on the person from life circumstances. Every person has developed a set of responses to stress that constitute the "normal line of defense" (Neuman, 1995). This line of defense helps to maintain health and wellness. However, when "physiological, psychological, sociocultural, developmental, or spiritual influences" are unable to buffer stress, the normal line of defense is broken, and disease can result. In this belief, Neuman Systems Model coincides with Selye's general adaptation syndrome.

Neuman Systems Model (1995) stresses the importance of accuracy in assessment and interventions that promote optimal wellness using primary, secondary, and tertiary prevention strategies. According to Neuman's theory, the goal of primary prevention is to promote client wellness by stress prevention and reduction of risk factors. Secondary prevention occurs after symptoms appear. The nurse determines the meaning of the illness and stress to the client and the client's needs and resources for meeting them. Tertiary prevention begins when the client system is becoming more stable and recovering. At the tertiary level of prevention the nurse supports rehabilitation processes involved in healing, moving the client back to wellness and the primary level of disease prevention. Neuman's model of nursing views the person, family, or community as constantly changing in response to the environment and stressors.

Pender's health promotion model proposes that health promotion is directed toward increasing the level of well-being of an individual or group (Pender, Murdaugh, and Parsons, 2002). Conversely, primary, secondary, and tertiary prevention (health protection) focus on avoiding negative events. Pender considers stress reduction strategies important to reduce threats to well-being, to help people fulfill their potential, and to shape and maintain health behaviors. To change behavior, the client must initiate the change and behave differently in interactions. People want to live in ways that enable them to be as healthy as possible and to be capable of assessing their own abilities and assets. Based on these assumptions of the capability and desire of people to be healthy, Pender suggests strategies for prevention and health promotion related to stress management.

Situational, Maturational, and Sociocultural Factors

Potential stressors and coping mechanisms vary across the life span. For example, adolescence, adulthood, and old age bring different stressors. Appraisal of stressors, amount and type of social support, and coping strategies are balancing factors when assessing stress, and all depend on previous life experiences (Aguilera, 1998). Furthermore, situational and social stressors place people who are vulnerable at higher risk for prolonged stress (Box 30-4).

Situational Factors. Situational stress can arise from job changes, either one's own or that of a family member, and relocation. Stressful job changes can include promotions, transfers, downsizing, restructuring, changes in supervisors, and additional responsibilities. Adjusting to chronic illness is another situational stress. Common diseases that provoke stress are obesity, hypertension, diabetes, depression, asthma, and coronary artery disease. Although being a family caregiver for someone with a chronic illness such as Alzheimer's disease is associated with stress, the source of the stress for caregivers is not necessarily the stress of caregiving, but other factors in the caregiver's life (Chiriboga 1992). More general stressors, such as work- or financial-related stressors, can affect caregivers adversely.

Maturational Factors. Stressors vary with life stage. Preadolescents experience stress related to self-esteem issues, changing family structure due to divorce or death of a parent, or hospitalizations. As adolescents search for their identity with peer groups and separate from their families, they undergo stress. In addition, they face questions about using mind-altering substances, sexuality, jobs, school, and career choices that cause stress. Stress for adults center around major changes in life circumstances (Aguilera, 1998). These include the many milestones of beginning a family and a career, losing parents, seeing children leave home, and accepting physical aging. In old age, stressors include the loss of autonomy and mastery due to general frailty or health problems that limit stamina and strength (Pearlin and Mullan, 1992) (Box 30-5).

Sociocultural Factors. Environmental and social stressors can lead to developmental problems. Potential stressors that could affect any age-group, but that are especially stressful for young people, include prolonged poverty, and physical handicap. Children are vulnerable when relationships with parents and caregivers are lost through divorce, imprisonment, or death or when parents have mental illness or substance abuse disorders. Furthermore, living under conditions of continuing violence, disintegrated neighborhoods, or homelessness is damaging for people of any age, but especially for young people (Pender, Murdaugh, and Parsons, 2002) (Box 30-6).

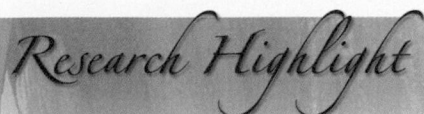

Box 30-4

Spousal Support for Psychological Distress

Research Focus

Holistic nursing care includes the client's family. Family members, especially the spouse, have an impact on the client's recovery from cardiac disease and surgery. More information is needed about stress experienced by spouses of clients in cardiac rehabilitation and interventions to help spouses cope with stress.

Research Abstract

The purposes of this study were (a) to describe the distress experienced by 213 spouses of men in cardiac rehabilitation, (b) to identify the most common heart disease stressors experienced by the women, (c) to compare distressed and nondistressed spouses in terms of demographic variables and coping strategies, and (d) to identify specific intervention needs for spouses of clients undergoing cardiac rehabilitation. Spouses were recruited by telephone at the time of the admission of the spouse into the cardiac rehabilitation program. Subjects agreed to participate in five spousal support group sessions and to complete five questionnaires that assessed psychological distress, coping, marital intimacy, family functioning, and heart disease hassles. The Brief Symptom Inventory measured psychological distress. Based upon this scale, 66 subjects were categorized as being psychologically distressed. Symptoms of distress were feeling tense, having trouble falling asleep, and feeling easily hurt. The group of spouses who were distressed was significantly younger than the group who were not dis-

tressed. The distressed spouses coped with the stress by disengagement strategies, such as avoidance, wishful thinking, self-criticism, and withdrawal. The Heart Disease Hassles Scale (HDHS) is a 75-item scale that identified common heart disease–related stressors. The five highest ranked stressors identified by spouses in this study were (a) worries about treatment, recovery, and prognosis; (b) moodiness of the client; (c) worries about the client returning to work and about money; (d) sexual concerns; and (e) helplessness or apathy on the part of the client and increased spousal responsibility.

Evidence-Based Practice

- Spouses of clients in cardiac rehabilitation could benefit from the following:
  - Stress-management techniques, such as relaxation training, assertiveness training, and self-care techniques
  - Training in problem-solving and cognitive-based coping strategies
  - Support groups for spouses
- Younger women need to be especially identified for supportive interventions when their husbands are in cardiac rehabilitation

Reference

O'Farrell P, Murray J, Hotz S: Psychologic distress among spouses of patients undergoing cardiac rehabilitation, *Heart Lung* 29(2):97, 2000.

Focus on Older Adults

Box 30-5

- There are very few age-related differences in coping strategies, and older adults are just as effective at coping as younger adults (Aldwin, 1992).
- Older adults are incorrectly presumed to be unique and more vulnerable to the effect of stressors; however, the effect of psychosocial factors on health status is not altered by age (Kasl, 1992).
- Losses in later life may be less stress provoking than generally assumed, partly because certain life transitions are anticipated and people prepare by coping in advance (Pearlin and Mullan, 1992).
- A study of stress and coping in old-old clients (ages 75 to 91) found them to be least likely to view their lives as having problems, and they expended less effort in coping (Aldwin and others, 1996). This may be due to the fact that the life experiences and perspectives of older adults may make most problems seem insignificant, and/or older adults have acquired appropriate stress management techniques.

- The timing of stress-inducing events can significantly influence older adults' ability to cope. The fact that older adults may have several stressful events (e.g., loss of a spouse and new medical diagnosis) occur with a short period of time can result in detrimental effects on coping ability.
- In people 85 and older there is a clear connection involving age, loss, and stress (Pearlin and Mullan, 1992). Stresses in this age-group are related to confronting one's own diminished autonomy and mastery (Pearlin and Mullan, 1992).
- Older adults effectively utilize religious coping in response to medical illness and disasters (Foster, 1997).
- Anxiety disorders are the most prevalent disorders in later life and are continuations of life-long illnesses (Hyer and Sohnle, 2001).

Aldwin CM: *Stress, coping and development: an integrative perspective*, New York, 2000, Guilford Press.

Cultural Aspects of Care　　Box 30-6

A client's culture defines what is stressful to the person and ways of coping with stress (Aldwin, 2000). Cultural context shapes the types of environmental stimuli that produce stress. For example, diverse cultures address developmental transitions and life's turning points differently. How a person leaves the parental home, experiences health crises or chronic illness, cares for the family or becomes disabled or dependent are all culturally bound. Furthermore, how a person appraises stress is also dependent upon the person's culture. What is perceived as a stressor in one culture might be viewed as a minor problem in another culture. A person's response to the stress of pain is an example of a culture-based response to stress, whether a person maintains personal control or becomes emotionally expressive. Coping strategies are also influenced by one's cultural background. According to Aldwin, cultures vary in their emotion-focused and problem-focused coping strategies. Related to emotion-focused coping, some cultures stress that emotions should be controlled whereas others believe in expressing emotions. Problem-focused coping refers to controlling or managing stress. Different cultures control stress in different ways. Finally, cultures provide different institutions for coping with stress. These include the legal system for conflict resolution, advice givers or support groups, and rituals.

Implications for Practice

- Realize that stressors and coping styles vary with different cultures.
- Use introspection to examine one's own perceptions of stress and coping in a cultural context.
- Assess the influence of culture on a client's appraisal of stress.
- Determine the institutions within a client's culture that may facilitate coping.

Critical Thinking

When caring for a client experiencing stress, the nurse uses skills of critical thinking to understand the stressor and the client's stress response. The nurse integrates knowledge from nursing and other disciplines, previous experiences, and information gathered from clients to understand stress and its impact on the client and family.

The nurse should know the neurophysiological changes that occur in the client experiencing the alarm reaction, resistance stage, and exhaustion stage of the general adaptation syndrome. In addition, knowledge of communication principles will contribute to assessing client's behaviors (see Chapter 23). Determining the client's perception of the situation and the ability of the client to cope with the stress is of utmost importance. If the client's usual coping skills are unsuccessful or support systems are inadequate, the nurse will need to use crisis intervention counseling.

The nurse's experience teaches the nurse to understand the client's unique perspective and to view every person as an individual, recognizing that no two people are exactly alike. Experience with clients will also help the nurse to recognize responses to stress. In addition, the nurse's own personal experiences with stress and coping will increase his or her ability to empathize with a client who is temporarily immobilized by stress.

The nurse is confident in the belief that stress can be effectively managed by the nurse, if necessary, and by the client. Clients who are overwhelmed and perceive events as being beyond their capacity to cope will rely on the nurse as an expert. Clients will respect the nurse's advice and counsel and gain confidence from his or her belief in their ability to move past the stressful event or illness. Clients overwhelmed by life events are often unable, at least initially, to act on their own behalf and require either direct intervention or guidance. Integrity is an essential attitude through which the nurse is reminded to respect the client's perception of or perspective about the stressor. Effort must be made to have clients explain their unique viewpoint and situation.

The nurse uses standards of practice to guide an accurate assessment of a client's stress, coping mechanisms, and support system before intervening. The nurse must be able to clearly and precisely understand a client's perception of the stress and focus on factors relevant to the client's well-being. In addition, the client will also have expectations of the nurse. Interacting with a client who is experiencing stress requires the nurse to have confidence and integrity in dealing with a client who may be temporarily vulnerable. The nurse must assess the client's situation accurately and be especially aware of the ethical responsibility in caring for someone who may have diminished autonomy due to stress.

Nursing Process

Assessment

Assessment of a client's stress level and coping resources requires that the nurse first establish a trusting nurse-client relationship because the nurse will be asking the client to share personal and sensitive information. The nurse learns from the client both by asking questions and by making observations of nonverbal behavior and the client's environment. The nurse synthesizes the information and adopts a critical thinking attitude while observing and analyzing client behaviors (Figure 30-3). Often the client has difficulty expressing exactly what is most bothersome about the situation until there is an opportunity to discuss it with someone who has time to listen.

Stress can occur to a family or a community, as well as to an individual. Stress to a family might be from a critically ill family member, the sudden loss of a job, a move, or becoming homeless. Stress to a community might be a natural disaster such as a major flood or the sudden, unexpected death of a beloved teacher or teen-

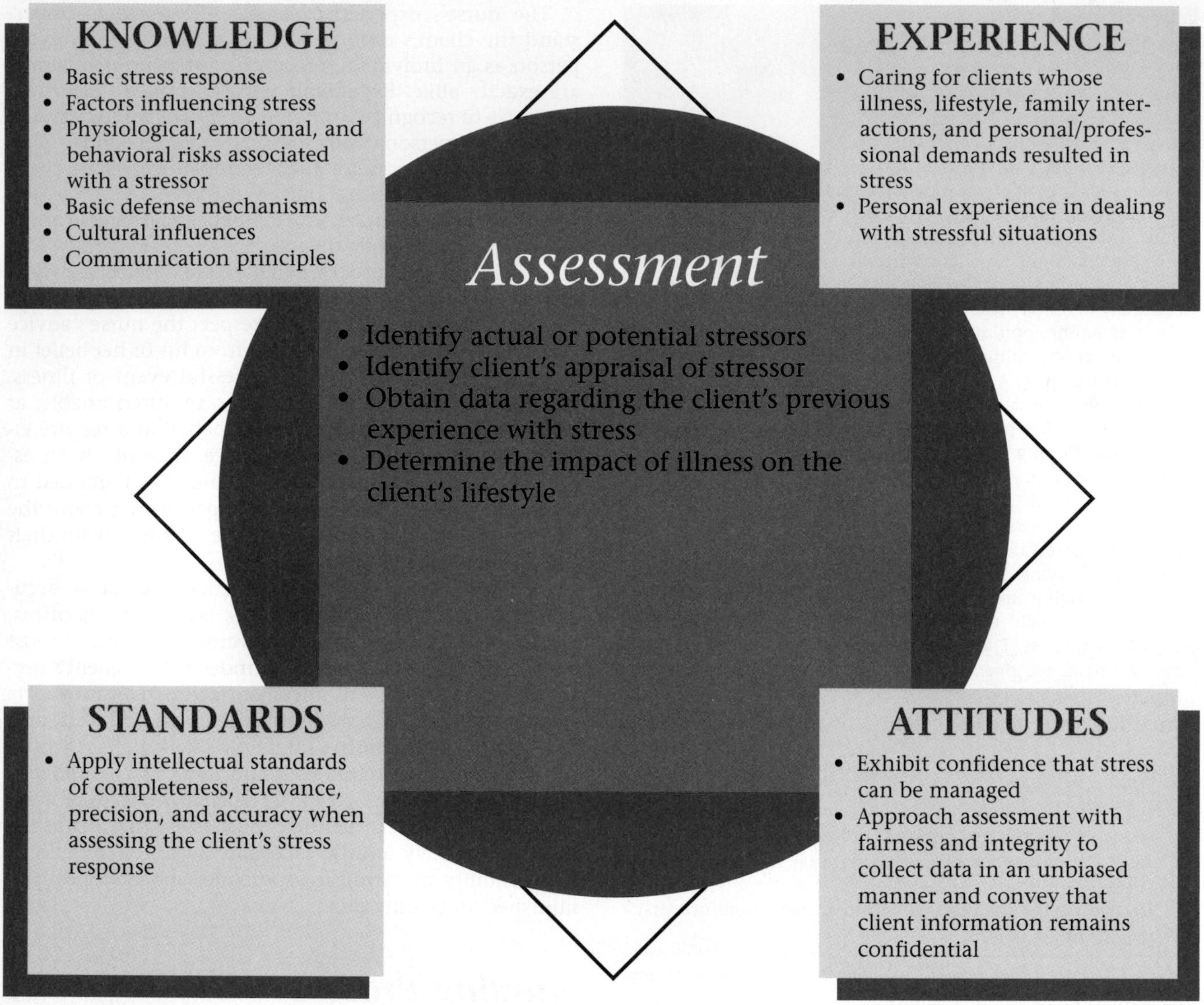

KNOWLEDGE

- Basic stress response
- Factors influencing stress
- Physiological, emotional, and behavioral risks associated with a stressor
- Basic defense mechanisms
- Cultural influences
- Communication principles

EXPERIENCE

- Caring for clients whose illness, lifestyle, family inter-actions, and personal/profes-sional demands resulted in stress
- Personal experience in dealing with stressful situations

Assessment

- Identify actual or potential stressors
- Identify client's appraisal of stressor
- Obtain data regarding the client's previous experience with stress
- Determine the impact of illness on the client's lifestyle

STANDARDS

- Apply intellectual standards of completeness, relevance, precision, and accuracy when assessing the client's stress response

ATTITUDES

- Exhibit confidence that stress can be managed
- Approach assessment with fairness and integrity to collect data in an unbiased manner and convey that client information remains confidential

FIGURE **30–3**   Critical thinking model for stress and coping assessment.

ager. Individuals experience stress and difficulty in coping while others are also experiencing the stress in their own ways.

Subjective Findings. When assessing a client's level of stress and coping resources, the nurse arranges a non-threatening physical environment, without a desk as a barrier, for the interaction (Varcarolis, 2002). The nurse assumes the same height as the client, arranging the inter-view environment so that eye contact can be comfortably maintained or avoided. This can be accomplished by plac-ing chairs at a 90-degree angle or side by side to reduce the intensity of the interaction (Varcarolis, 2002). The nurse gathers information about the health status of the client from the client's perspective and begins the process of de-veloping a trusting relationship with the client. The nurse uses the interview to determine the client's view of the stress, coping resources, any possible maladaptive coping, and adherence to prescribed medical recommendations,

such as medication or diet (Monat and Lazarus, 1991) (Table 30-1). If the client is using denial as a coping mech-anism, the nurse must be alert to whether the person is overlooking necessary information. As in all interactions with the client, the nurse must respect the confidentiality and sensitivity of the information shared.

Objective Findings. The nurse obtains objective findings related to stress and coping through observation of the appearance and nonverbal behavior of the client. The nurse observes grooming and hygiene, gait, characteris-tics of the client's handshake, actions of the client while sitting, quality of speech, eye contact, and the attitude of the client toward the nurse during the interview. Before the interview begins or at the end of the interview, de-pending upon the anxiety level of the client, the nurse takes basic vital signs to assess for physiological signs of stress such as elevated blood pressure, heart rate, or respi-ratory rate (Figure 30-4).

Table 30-1	Focused Assessment Interview	
Factors to Assess	**Questions and Approaches**	**Physical Assessment Strategies**
Perception of stressor	Ask the client what is of most concern at this time. Ask the client about problems sleeping, eating, working, and concentrating. Ask whether the client has had accidents in the home, in the car, or on the job.	Observe nonverbal behavior and expressions of feelings that indicate anxiety, fear, anger, irritability, or tension.
Available coping resources	Ask the client about current friendships and contacts with family members. Ask what the client has done in the past to cope with similar problems or stress. Ask how the client spends leisure time.	Observe whether the person is alone or with others. Observe grooming and hygiene. Observe the person's communication skills. Observe if the person is able to ask for help. Observe developmental level and sociocultural circumstances.
Maladaptive coping used	Ask about use of tobacco, alcohol, drugs, medications, and caffeine.	Observe for effects of smoking, alcohol, drugs, and caffeine.
Adherence to healthy practices	Ask if the client sees a physician or nurse practitioner regularly for checkups. Ask about nutritional habits, exercise, use of seat belts, helmets (if applicable), and safe sex.	Monitor pulse, blood pressure, weight. Observe nonverbal behavior.

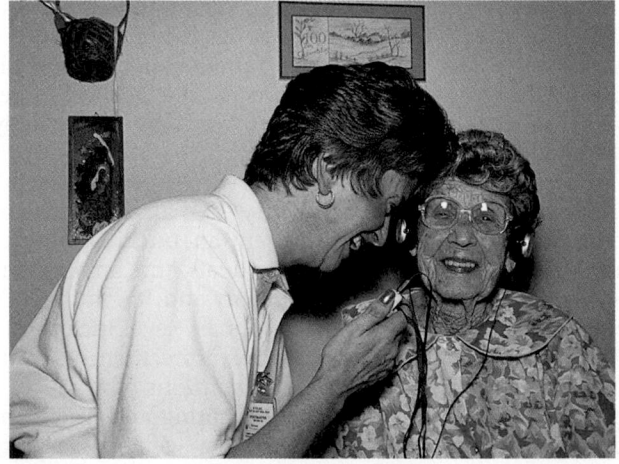

FIGURE 30–4   Sharing a joke or laughing with clients can assist in reducing stress and supporting a therapeutic relationship.

Safety Alert. Medical conditions such as hypoxia and thyroid dysfunction that are common in older adults can initially present symptoms that mimic the consequences of stress and anxiety. For this reason, a thorough physical assessment of an older adult appearing stressed or anxious is necessary to rule out potentially serious medical disorders (Kennedy, 1992). In addition, it is critical to differentiate signs of stress and crisis in older adults from dementia and from acute confusion, a condition that can be life threatening.

Client Expectations. A central point relating to stress is the importance of an understanding of the meaning of the precipitating event to the client and the ways in which stress is affecting the client's life. The nurse must allow time for the client to express priorities for coping with stress. For example, in the case of a woman who has just been told that a breast mass was identified on a routine mammogram, it would be important to know what the client wants and needs most from the nurse. Although some persons in this situation might identify their need for information about biopsy or mastectomy as their personal priority, other women might need guidance and support in discussing how to share the news with family members. In some cases, when nothing can be done to change or improve the situation, allowing the client to use denial as a coping mechanism can be helpful. Gaining an understanding of client expectations does not mean excluding certain types of care that are important simply because a client does not identify them as needs. However, by inquiring about client expectations and priorities, the nurse will be better able to ensure that *all* the client's needs will be addressed in some way.

Nursing Diagnosis

A review of assessment data leads the nurse to cluster data that may indicate a potential or actual stressor and the client's response. Clustering data, along with the application of the nurse's knowledge and experiences with clients in stress, leads to individualized nursing diagnoses (Box 30-7).

Nursing diagnoses for people experiencing stress generally focus on coping. Specifically, major defining characteristics of *ineffective coping* include verbalization of an inability to cope and an inability to ask for help. The nurse identifies defining characteristics when asking the client what is of most concern at the time of the interview and, importantly, when allowing the client sufficient time to answer. The nurse observes for nonverbal signs of anxiety,

Nursing Diagnostic Process

Box 30-7

Assessment Activities	Defining Characteristics	Nursing Diagnosis
Ask client about change in sleeping patterns.	Sleep disturbance; difficulty falling asleep at night	Ineffective coping
Ask client to complete a sleep diary for 2 weeks.	Sighing Excessive sleeping	
Observe client's behavior and response to questions during assessment.	Fatigue Inability to concentrate Inaccurate response to questions Inappropriate laugh or crying	
Observe client's appearance.	Poor grooming Self-harm	
Ask client about changes in eating patterns.	Weight gain or loss Lack of interest in food	

fear, anger, irritability, and tension in a client who is experiencing ineffective coping. Other defining characteristics include the presence of life stress, an inability to meet role expectations and basic needs, alteration in societal participation, self-destructive behavior, change in usual communication patterns, high rate of accidents, excessive food intake, drinking, smoking, and sleep disturbances. The nurse identifies these behaviors as part of the subjective and objective data collection. Stress can result in multiple nursing diagnoses. Examples of these diagnoses include but are not limited to the following:

- Anxiety
- Caregiver role strain
- Compromised family coping
- Ineffective coping
- Ineffective community coping
- Fear
- Chronic pain
- Post-trauma syndrome
- Powerlessness
- Relocation stress syndrome
- Situational low self-esteem
- Disturbed sleep pattern
- Impaired social interaction

Crisis differs from stress in the degree of severity, although there are also many similarities between stress and crisis. A client who perceives a situation as stressful, who is unable to cope in any ways that have worked before, and who has insufficient supports is experiencing a crisis. A crisis is devastating and requires use of all resources available (Aguilera, 1998). Unlike stress, which ends when the stressor is gone, the effects of a trauma can last for years (Hyer and Sohnle, 2001).

Planning

Goals and Outcomes. Desirable outcomes for persons experiencing stress are (1) effective coping, (2) family coping, (3) caregiver emotional health, and (4) psychosocial

adjustment: life change (Moorhead, Johnson and Maas, 2004). The nurse may select interventions for stress and improved coping such as coping enhancement and crisis intervention which are in the Nursing Interventions Classification (NIC) (Dochterman and Bulechek, 2004). In addition, the nurse selects individualized interventions after considering the nursing diagnosis, the resources available to the client, and the goals identified by the client and nurse (Figure 30-5).

Nursing interventions may be designed within the framework of primary, secondary, and tertiary prevention. At the primary level of prevention, nursing activities are directed to identifying individuals and populations who may be at risk for stress (Stuart and Wright, 1995). Nursing interventions at the secondary level include actions directed at symptoms, such as protecting the client from self-harm. Tertiary-level interventions have the purpose of assisting the client in readapting and might include relaxation training and time management training. According to Pender's health promotion model (Pender, Murdaugh, and Parsons, 2002), the nurse and the client assess the level and source of the existing stress and determine the appropriate points for intervention to reduce the stress (see Nursing Care Plan).

Another method of planning care is throught the use of a concept map (Figure 30-6). The nurse creates the map after identifying relevant nursing diagnoses from the assessment database. In this example, the nursing diagnoses are linked to the client's medical diagnosis of post-traumatic stress response. In addition, the concept map shows the relationships with the nursing diagnoses: *post-traumatic stress syndrome, ineffective coping, anxiety, and risk for other directed violence.* Using this approach uses critical thinking skills to organzie client data and assists in planning for client centered care.

Just as the nursing assessment of the client's stress and coping depends on the client's perception of the problem and coping resources, the interventions focus on a partnership with the client and support system, usually the family. In the case of a family or community stressor and

KNOWLEDGE

- Role of community resources in assisting client/family adaptation
- Role of health care professionals in stress management
- Impact of diet, exercise, medication, and other health promotion indicators on stress management
- Crisis intervention skills

EXPERIENCE

- Previous client responses to planned nursing interventions for improving client's adaptation to stress
- Previous experience in partnering with client in goal setting

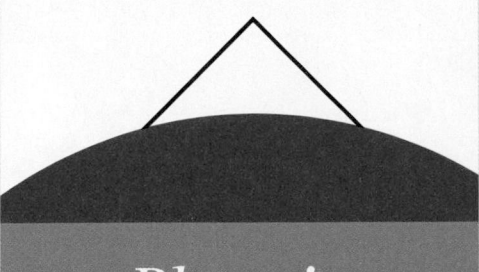
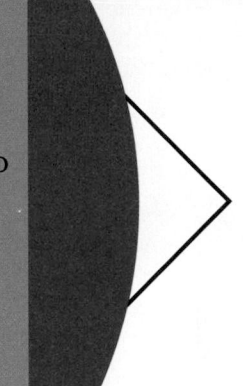
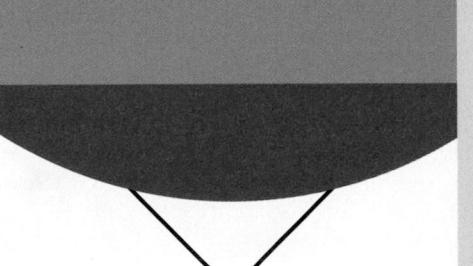

Planning

- Select nursing interventions to promote adaptation to stress
- Consult with mental health professionals
- Involve the client and family
- Identify community resources accessible to the client

STANDARDS

- Individualize interventions to meet the client's needs
- Apply ANA code of ethics by safeguarding the client's right to privacy and autonomy in the selection of interventions

ATTITUDES

- Display integrity when creating interventions for the client's lifestyle
- Act independently to seek out resources that could benefit the client
- Express confidence that stress can be managed

FIGURE **30–5**   Critical thinking model for stress and coping planning.

impaired family or community coping, the view of the situation and resources would be broader.

Setting Priorities. Prioritizing needs has special meaning for a person experiencing stress or crisis (see care plan). The first question to be answered is, "What is happening in your life that you needed to come today?" or "What happened in your life that is *different?*" This requires some focusing by the client. Next, assess the client's perception of the event, available situational supports, and what the person usually does when there is a problem the client cannot solve (Aguilera, 1998). As in all areas of nursing, safety of the client and others in the client's environment is the first priority.

Safety Alert. Determine if the person is suicidal or homicidal by asking directly. For example, the nurse might ask, "Are you thinking of killing yourself or someone else?" If so, determine in a caring and concerned manner if the person has a plan and determine how lethal the means are. If suicide or homicide is not an issue, examine other potential threats to the safety of vulnerable people who are under the care of the client. Provide for their temporary care or supervision if necessary. Determine the degree of disruption in the person's life with work, school, home, and family. When immediate assessment is completed and safety is ensured, begin the problem-solving process (Aguilera, 1998).

Concept Map

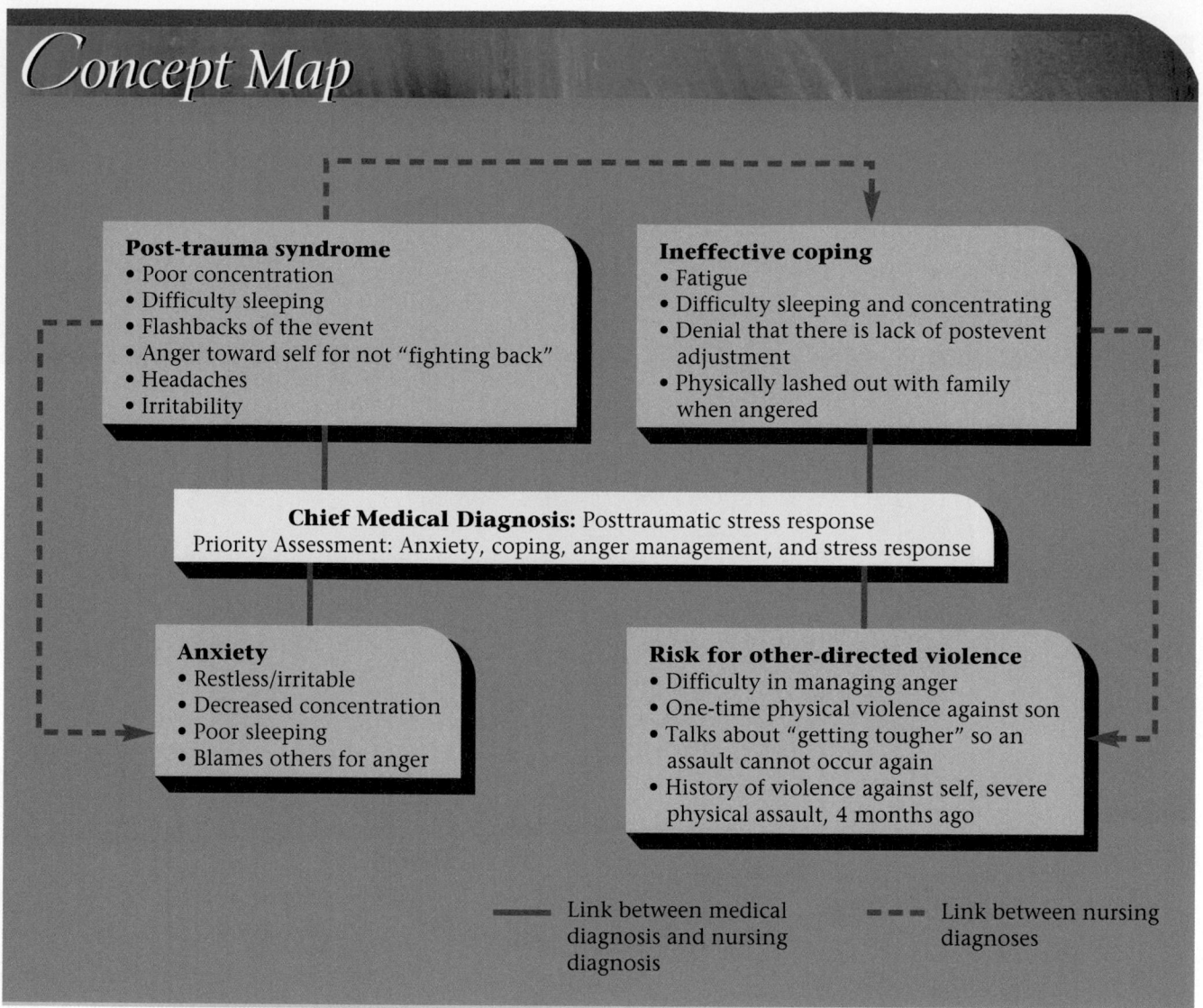

Post-trauma syndrome
• Poor concentration
• Difficulty sleeping
• Flashbacks of the event
• Anger toward self for not "fighting back"
• Headaches
• Irritability

Ineffective coping
• Fatigue
• Difficulty sleeping and concentrating
• Denial that there is lack of postevent adjustment
• Physically lashed out with family when angered

Chief Medical Diagnosis: Posttraumatic stress response
Priority Assessment: Anxiety, coping, anger management, and stress response

Anxiety
• Restless/irritable
• Decreased concentration
• Poor sleeping
• Blames others for anger

Risk for other-directed violence
• Difficulty in managing anger
• One-time physical violence against son
• Talks about "getting tougher" so an assault cannot occur again
• History of violence against self, severe physical assault, 4 months ago

——— Link between medical diagnosis and nursing diagnosis

– – – Link between nursing diagnoses

FIGURE 30–6 Concept map for client with posttraumatic stress response 4 months after a severe assault.

Continuity of Care. The nurse will collaborate with occupational therapists, dietitians, or pastoral care professionals. There will be times when the scope of nursing practice is insufficient to meet all of the client's needs. Clients experiencing stress from medical conditions or psychiatric disorders will present needs that will make it necessary for the nurse to consult with advanced practice mental health nurses, psychiatrists, psychologists, or psychiatric social workers. Such a multidisciplinary approach to care is often most effective in addressing the holistic needs of the client. The nurse's role is to recognize the need for collaboration and consultation, inform the client about potential resources, and make arrangements for interventions, such as consultations, group sessions, or therapy as needed.

Implementation

Health Promotion. Three primary modes of intervention for stress are to decrease stress-producing situations, in-

crease resistance to stress, and learn skills that reduce physiological response to stress (Pender, Murdaugh, and Parsons, 2002) (Box 30-8). The nurse is in a position to educate clients and families about the importance of health promotion.

Regular Exercise. A regular exercise program improves muscle tone and posture, controls weight, reduces tension, and promotes relaxation. In addition, exercise reduces the risk of cardiovascular disease and improves cardiopulmonary functioning. Clients who have a history of a chronic illness, who are at risk for developing an illness, or who are older than 35 years of age should begin a physical exercise program only after discussing the plan with a physician. In general, for a fitness program to have positive physical effects, a person should exercise daily for an hour (Figure 30-7).

Support Systems. A support system of family, friends, and colleagues who will listen, offer advice, and provide emotional support benefits a client experiencing stress.

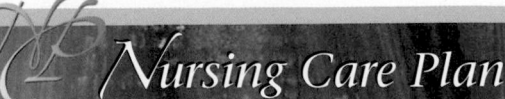

Nursing Care Plan

Caregiver Role Strain

Assessment

When Janet Rich first goes to Carl's house, she finds the home to be in slight disarray. The lawn is overgrown, there are dirty dishes in the sink, and an empty can of soup is sitting on the kitchen counter. Carl is standing in the living room folding clothes from a laundry basket, and Evelyn, Carl's wife, is sitting in a chair watching TV. Evelyn was recently diagnosed with Alzheimer's dementia.

Assessment Activities	Findings/Defining Characteristics
Ask Carl about his recent stressors and coping strategies.	He continues to fold clothes during the visit, stating, "There's so much to do that I don't even know where to begin."
	Carl describes being awakened 3 to 4 times per night to find Evelyn wandering in the house.
	He states that he has no outside activities and his children live in other states. He does have several close friends who live nearby but denies any knowledge of community resources.
Observe Carl's grooming and hygiene.	Carl is unshaven and appears disheveled.
Ask Carl about his sleep and nutrition patterns.	Carl states that he has lost 20 pounds in the past 6 months and that his appetite has been poor.
Assess Carl's mood and affect by asking how he is feeling.	Carl states, "I feel very tired. Everything feels overwhelming."
Assess Carl's suicide potential.	Carl denies being suicidal.
Assess health status and health care status.	Carl has not seen a nurse practitioner or physician for his own health in over a year.

Nursing Diagnosis: Caregiver role strain related to recent diagnosis of wife's Alzheimer's dementia.

Planning

Goal	Expected Outcomes*
	Caregiver Physical Health
Client will appear rested in 1 month.	• Client will report waking up less frequently during the night within 1 week.
	• Client will verbalize approaches used to involve others in wife's caregiving activities within 2 weeks.
Client will maintain a stable weight over next 4 weeks.	• Client will reestablish normal eating pattern within 1 week.
	• Client will report improved appetite.
	Caregiver Lifestyle Disruption
Client will state that he has resumed one outside activity within 1 month.	• Client will report a balanced routine that incorporates time for own rest or relaxation with 1 week.

*Outcome classification labels from Moorhead S, Johnson M, Maas M: *Nursing outcomes classification (NOC)*, ed 3, St. Louis, 2004, Mosby.

Interventions†	Rationale
Caregiver Support	
• Assist client in establishing a consistent care routine.	Routines can help tasks be simplified and more time efficient.
• Discuss ways that client agrees will simplify care routine such as hiring a teenage neighbor to mow the lawn, buying frozen meals, having groceries delivered, having a cleaning service twice a month.	Caregivers experience stress outside of their caregiving roles. Frequently, providing ways to assist the caregiver with home maintenance, meal planning, and shopping assists caregivers with stress management (Chiriboga 1992).
• Identify sources of respite care by encouraging client to identify available friends who can assist with caregiving.	Successful caregiving cannot normally occur with only one caregiver. Caregiver may be hesitant to ask for help because of past family conflict (Gulanick and others, 2003).
• Explore community resources such as home care, adult day care, and Meals on Wheels with client.	Feelings of burden have been found to be lower among caregivers with social supports (Solomon and Draine, 1995).
• Teach client stress management techniques.	Stress, especially long-term stress, can facilitate physical illness.
• Set up monthly health checks for client that include vital sign and weight checks.	Teaching the caregiver health maintenance strategies is important to sustain his own physical and mental health (McCloskey and Bulechek, 2000).

†Intervention classification labels from Dochterman JM, Bulechek GM: *Nursing interventions classification (NIC)*, ed 4, St. Louis, 2004, Mosby.

Continued

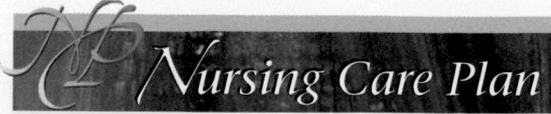

Nursing Care Plan

Caregiver Role Strain—cont'd

Evaluation

Nursing Actions	Client Response/Finding	Achievement of Outcome
Observe for signs of fatigue.	Carl states he feels more rested and less depressed.	Carl is able to sleep for 6 hours during night and takes a 30-minute nap in the afternoon.
Review new care routines. Ask client what other modifications may need to be made.	Carl buys frozen meals to use when he is busy with other caregiving.	Carl has reduced his personal expectation that he must cook every meal himself.
Ask client about how community and additional family support is helping to relieve stress.	Meals on Wheels delivers lunch 5 days per week.	Carl is mobilizing community resources.
Ask client to compare past and present energy levels.	A neighbor mows the lawn for Carl. Carl reports having more energy and smiles spontaneously.	Carl has improved balance in routine between Evelyn's and his own.
Weigh client regularly.	Carl reports gaining 5 pounds in 1 month.	Carl has resumed a normal eating pattern.
Ask client about recent food intake.	Carl reports having eaten lunch with Evelyn on the day of the visit.	

Client Teaching

Box 30-8

Stress Management

Objective

- Coping with daily hassles in the workplace will improve.

Teaching Strategies

- Instruct the client to participate in a committee that provides input to hospital administration about work assignments.
- Assist the client in analyzing new job possibilities if necessary.
- Instruct the client to avoid excessive change in lifestyle when other stress is present.
- Instruct the client in time management skills to become more organized and set priorities.
- Assist the client in creating an exercise plan that includes daily exercise.
- Assist the client in building a network of social support.
- Train the client in progressive muscle relaxation skills.

Evaluation

- Observe client for signs of stress.
- Ask client to keep a record of hours of sleep.
- Ask client to list participation in activities that are soothing or enjoyable.

Data from Pender NJ, Murdaugh C, Parsons MA: *Health promotion in nursing practice*, ed 4, Upper Saddle River, NJ, 2002, Howorth Press.

There are many support groups available to individuals, such as those sponsored by the American Heart Association, the American Cancer Society, local hospitals and churches, and mental health organizations.

Time Management. Time management techniques include developing lists of tasks to be performed in order of priority, for example, those tasks that require immediate attention, those that are important and can be delayed, and those tasks that are routine and can be accomplished when time becomes available. In many cases setting priorities helps individuals identify tasks that are not necessary or perhaps can even be delegated to someone else.

Guided Imagery and Visualization. Guided imagery is based on the belief that a person can significantly reduce stress with imagination. Guided imagery is a relaxed state in which a person actively uses imagination in a way that allows visualization of a soothing, peaceful setting. Typically the image created or suggested uses many sensory words to engage the mind and offer distraction and relaxation.

Progressive Muscle Relaxation. In the presence of anxiety-provoking thoughts and events, a common physiological symptom is muscle tension. Physiological tension will be diminished through a systematic approach to releasing tension in major muscle groups. Typically a relaxed state is achieved through deep chest breathing, and then the client is directed to alternately tighten and relax muscles in specific groupings.

Assertiveness Training. Assertiveness comprises skills for helping individuals communicate effectively regarding their needs and desires. The ability to resolve conflict

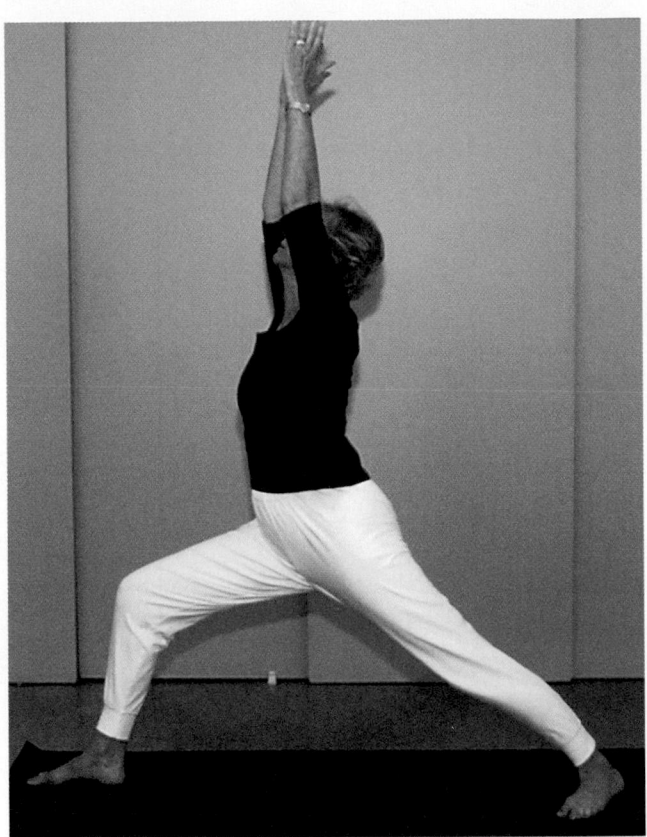

FIGURE 30-7 Regular exercise assists in coping with stress. (Lewis SM, Heitkemper MM, Dirksen SR: *Medical surgical nursing*, ed 6, St. Louis, 2004, Mosby.)

with others through assertiveness training is important for reducing stress. When assertiveness is taught in a group setting, benefits of the experience are increased.

Journal Writing. For many people, keeping a private, personal journal provides a therapeutic outlet for stress, and it is well within the realm of nursing to suggest journal keeping to clients experiencing difficult situations. In a private journal, clients can express a full range of emotion and vent their honest feelings without hurting anyone's feelings and without concern for how they might appear to others.

Stress Management in the Workplace. Rapid changes in health care technology, diversity in the workforce, organizational restructuring, and changing work systems can place stress on nurses (Manning and others, 1999). Additional causes of job stress include particular job assignments, difficult schedules, shift work, fear of failure, inadequate support services, and not knowing where you stand (Manning and others, 1999). **Burnout** occurs as a result of chronic stress. Burnout is "a syndrome of emotional exhaustion, depersonalization of others, and perceptions of reduced personal accomplishment, resulting from intense involvement with people in a care-giving environment" (Aguilera, 1998).

If you recognize feelings of burnout, you can make changes in your behavior to cope with workplace stress.

An important step is identifying the limits and scope of your responsibilities at work (Aguilera, 1998). Recognizing the areas over which you have control and can change and those that you do not have responsibility for is a vital insight. Making a clear separation between work and home life is crucial as well. Strengthening friendships outside of the workplace, arranging for temporary social isolation for personal "recharging" of emotional energy, and spending off-duty hours in interesting activities all help reduce burnout.

Acute Care

Crisis Intervention. When stress overwhelms a person's usual coping mechanisms and demands mobilization of all available resources, it becomes a crisis (Aguilera, 1998). A crisis creates a turning point in a person's life because it changes the direction of a person's life in some way. According to Aguilera (1998), the precipitating event usually occurs from 1 to 2 weeks before the individual seeks help, but it may have occurred within the past 24 hours. Generally a crisis is resolved in some way within approximately 6 weeks. Crisis intervention aims to return the person to a precrisis level of functioning and to promote growth (Figure 30-8).

Because an individual's or family's usual coping strategies are ineffective in managing the stress of the precipitating event, the use of new coping mechanisms is required. This experience, which forces the use of unfamiliar strategies, can result either in a heightened awareness of previously unrecognized strengths and resources or in deterioration in functioning. Thus a crisis is often referred to as a situation of both danger and opportunity. Some persons or families will emerge from a crisis state functioning more effectively, whereas others may find themselves weakened, and still others completely dysfunctional.

Crisis intervention is a specific type of brief psychotherapy with prescribed steps (Aguilera, 1998). Crisis intervention is more directive than traditional psychotherapy or counseling and can be used by any member of the health care team who has been trained in its techniques. The basic approach is problem solving and focuses only on the problem presented by the crisis.

When using a crisis intervention approach, the nurse helps the client make the mental connection between the stressful event and the client's reaction to it. This is crucial because the person may be unable to see the whole situation clearly. The nurse also helps the person become aware of present feelings, such as anger, grief, or guilt, to help the individual reduce feelings of tension. In addition, the nurse helps the client explore coping mechanisms, perhaps identifying ways of coping the client had not thought of. Finally, the nurse needs to help increase the scope of the person's social contacts if the person had been internally focused and isolated (Aguilera, 1998).

Restorative and Continuing Care. A person under stress recovers when the stress is removed or coping strategies are successful; however, a person who has experienced a crisis has changed, and the effects may last for years or for

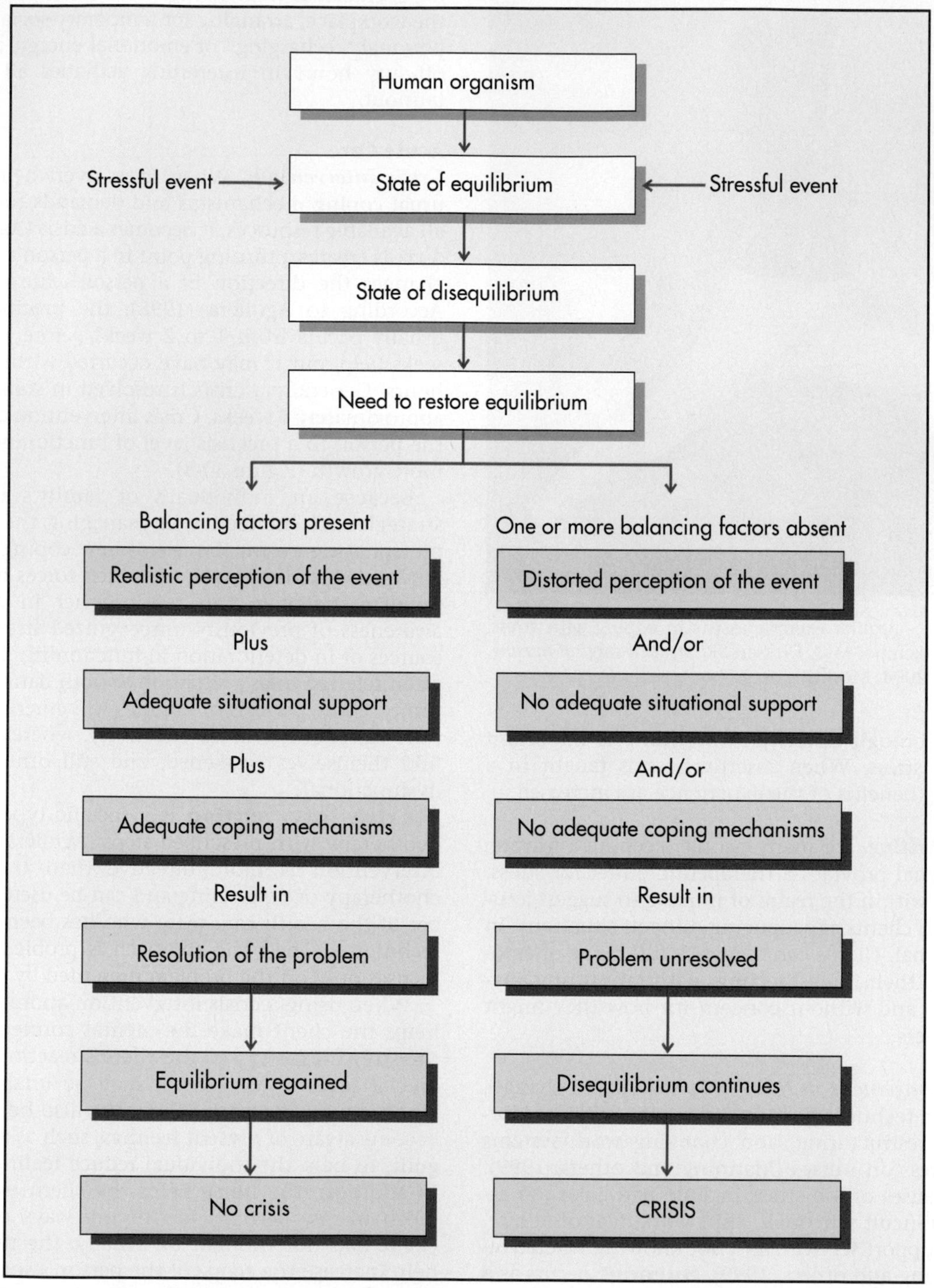

FIGURE **30–8** Crisis intervention model. (Redrawn from Aguilera DC: *Crisis intervention: theory and methodology,* ed 8, St. Louis, 1998, Mosby.)

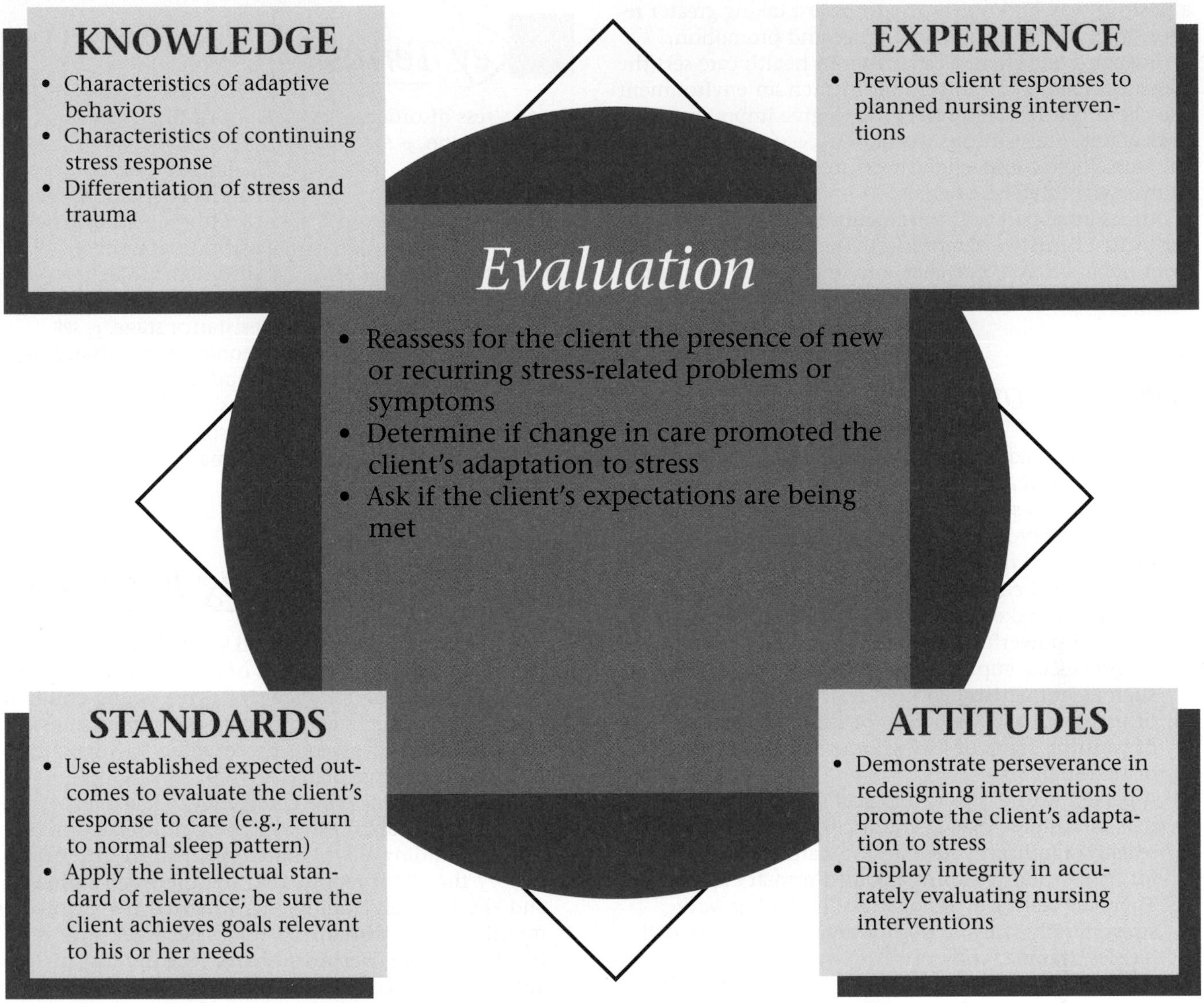

KNOWLEDGE

- Characteristics of adaptive behaviors
- Characteristics of continuing stress response
- Differentiation of stress and trauma

EXPERIENCE

- Previous client responses to planned nursing interventions

Evaluation

- Reassess for the client the presence of new or recurring stress-related problems or symptoms
- Determine if change in care promoted the client's adaptation to stress
- Ask if the client's expectations are being met

STANDARDS

- Use established expected outcomes to evaluate the client's response to care (e.g., return to normal sleep pattern)
- Apply the intellectual standard of relevance; be sure the client achieves goals relevant to his or her needs

ATTITUDES

- Demonstrate perseverance in redesigning interventions to promote the client's adaptation to stress
- Display integrity in accurately evaluating nursing interventions

FIGURE **30–9** Critical thinking model for stress and coping evaluation.

the rest of the person's life (Shontz, 1975). The final stage of adapting to a crisis is acknowledgment of the long-term implications of the crisis (Shontz, 1975). If a person has successfully coped with a crisis and its consequences, he or she becomes a more mature and healthy person. When a person has recovered from a stressful situation, the time is right for introducing stress management skills to reduce the number and intensity of stressful situations in the future.

Evaluation

Client Care. By evaluating the goals and expected outcomes of care, the nurse knows if the nursing interventions were effective and if the client is coping with the identified stress. The nurse reviews the measurable goals, and assesses whether or not the client has met the criteria for success as stated in the outcomes. If the nursing interventions have not been effective in helping the client

achieve targeted goals, the nurse must reevaluate the strategies implemented and revise the plan of care in light of the client's current health status (Figure 30-9).

To evaluate the client experiencing stress, observe client behaviors and talk with the client and family, if appropriate. Remember that coping with stress can take time. If contact with a client must end before resolution of goals has been achieved, it is important to refer clients to appropriate resources so that progress is not delayed or interrupted.

Client Expectations. It is crucial to maintain ongoing communication with clients regarding the plan of care. Clients under severe stress, or trauma, often experience feelings of powerlessness, vulnerability, and loss of control. The nurse can help to reduce these feelings by actively involving clients and families in the process of problem identification (assessment), prioritizing, and goal setting and evaluation. Involving clients in these processes gives them an opportunity to direct their energy in a positive way and moves them toward taking greater responsibility for health maintenance and promotion.

Engaging the client as a partner in health care sets the stage for open communication. In such an environment the client can feel more freedom to give important feedback about interventions that are successful and can help the nurse better understand why some interventions fail to meet the established goals.

An essential part of the evaluation process is collaborating with clients to determine if their own expectations from nursing have been met. Any revision in the plan of care must then include steps to address client expectations.

Key Concepts

- The general adaptation syndrome is an immediate physiological response of the whole body to stress and involves several body systems, especially the autonomic nervous system and the endocrine system. Physiological responses to stress also include immunological changes.
- Stress can make people ill as a result of increased levels of powerful hormones that change our bodily processes; coping choices that are unhealthy, such as not getting enough rest or a proper diet or use of tobacco, alcohol, or caffeine; and neglect of warning signs of illness or prescribed medicines or treatments.
- A person is under psychological stress only if the person evaluates the event or circumstance as personally significant. Such an evaluation of an event for its personal meaning is called primary appraisal.
- There are several types of stress, including work stress, family stress, chronic stress, acute stress, daily hassles, trauma, and crisis.
- Rapid changes in health care technology, diversity in the workforce, organizational redesign, and changing work systems can place stress on nurses.
- Potential stressors and coping mechanisms vary across the life span, from childhood through adolescence, adulthood, and old age.
- Coping means making an effort to manage psychological stress.
- Coping is a process that is constantly changing to manage demands on a person's resources.
- Three primary modes for stress intervention are to decrease stress-producing situations, increase resistance to stress, and learn skills that reduce physiological response to stress.
- A client whose stress is so severe that the person is unable to cope in any ways that have worked before is experiencing a crisis.
- A crisis is a turning point in life and can be developmental or situational.
- Generally a crisis is resolved in some way within approximately 6 weeks. Crisis intervention aims to return the person to a precrisis level of functioning and to promote growth.

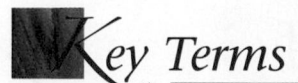

Key Terms

Acute stress disorder, *p. 600*
Alarm reaction, *p. 597*
Appraisal, *p. 596*
Burnout, *p. 611*
Coping, *p. 599*
Crisis, *p. 596*
Crisis intervention, *p. 611*
Developmental crises, *p. 600*
Distress, *p. 599*
Ego-defense mechanisms, *p. 599*
Endorphins, *p. 597*
Eustress, *p. 599*
Exhaustion stage, *p. 597*

Fight-or-flight response, *p. 596*
Flashback, *p. 600*
General adaptation syndrome (GAS), *p. 597*
Posttraumatic stress disorder (PTSD), *p. 600*
Primary appraisal, *p. 599*
Resistance stage, *p. 597*
Secondary appraisal, *p. 599*
Situational crises, *p. 600*
Stress, *p. 596*
Stressors, *p. 596*
Trauma, *p. 596*

Critical Thinking Exercises

1. You are caring for a 30-year-old single mother who has recently received a diagnosis of metastatic breast cancer. She is the sole provider for three young children (all under 7 years of age). Discuss the various stressors that will need to be considered when writing an appropriate discharge plan.

2. A client comes to the emergency department with complaints of dizziness, which are not related to any physical finding on examination. During the health history the client reports that her life is very stressful and she is barely coping. She finalized her divorce 3 months ago, is working 32 hours per week, and is attending college. Her ex-husband recently lost his job and can no longer pay child support. Finally, she tearfully confesses that she thinks she might be pregnant but does not want her ex-husband to know. Develop nursing diagnoses related to this situation.

3. An older adult woman is admitted to the hospital with a fractured hip. Before her injury she lived with her husband, who suffers from advancing Alzheimer's disease. While she is hospitalized, he is staying with a niece who lives 100 miles away, but this cannot be a permanent situation because her niece is also in frail health. The client has no children who can help her when she returns home. She is concerned not only about who will care for her after she is discharged but also about her husband. What approach would be the best to take in establishing goals for treatment?

Review Questions

1. The vital functions necessary for survival, which include heart rate, blood pressure, and respiration, are controlled by the:
   1. Medulla oblongata.
   2. Reticular formation.
   3. Pituitary gland.
   4. Brain.

2. While assessing a person for effects of the general adaptation syndrome, the nurse should be aware that:
   1. Heart rate increases in the resistance state.
   2. Blood volume increases in the exhaustion stage.
   3. Vital signs return to normal in the exhaustion stage.
   4. Blood glucose level increases during the alarm reaction stage.

3. A client avoids emotional conflict by refusing to consciously acknowledge anything that might cause intolerable emotional pain. The client is using the defense mechanism:
   1. Conversion.
   2. Denial.
   3. Dissociation.
   4. Displacement.

4. When doing an assessment of a young woman who was in an automobile accident 6 months before, the nurse learns that the woman has vivid images of the crash whenever she hears a loud, sudden noise. The nurse recognizes this as:
   1. Social phobia.
   2. Acute anxiety.
   3. Posttraumatic stress disorder.
   4. Borderline personality disorder.

5. A man is adjusting to chronic illness; this is an example of:
   1. A sociocultural factor.
   2. A maturational factor.
   3. A situational factor.
   4. Critical thinking.

6. A child who has been in a house fire comes to the emergency department with her parents. The child and parents are upset and tearful. During the nurse's first assessment for stress she should say:
   1. "Tell me whom I can call to help you."
   2. "Tell me what bothers you the most about this experience."
   3. "I will contact someone who can help get you temporary housing."
   4. "I will sit with you until other family members can come help you get settled."

7. The nurse is evaluating the coping success of a client experiencing stress from being newly diagnosed with multiple sclerosis and psychomotor impairment. The nurse realized that the client is coping successfully when the client says:
   1. "I am going to learn to drive a car so I can be more independent."
   2. "My sister says she feels better when she goes shopping, so I will go shopping."
   3. "I have always felt better when I go for a long walk. I will do that when I get home."
   4. "I am going to attend a support group to learn more about multiple sclerosis and what I will be able to do."

8. The nurse knows that the client is recovering from the stress of an emergency surgery when the client says:
   1. "I am going to change jobs."
   2. "I am learning progressive relaxation training."
   3. "I plan to have plastic surgery while I am here in the hospital."
   4. "I am planning to sell my house and move within the next 6 weeks."

9. A staff nurse is talking with her nursing supervisor about the stress she feels on the job: The supervising nurse recognizes that:
   1. Nurses who feel stress usually pass the stress along to their clients.
   2. A nurse who feels stress is ineffective as a nurse and should not be working.
   3. Nurses who talk about feeling stress are unprofessional and should calm down.
   4. Nurses frequently experience stress with the rapid changes in health care technology and organizational restructuring.

10. Generally a person's crisis is resolved in some way within approximately:
    1. 6 weeks.
    2. 1 month.
    3. 6 months.
    4. 2 weeks.

References

Aguilera DC: *Crisis intervention: theory and methodology*, ed 8, St. Louis, 1998, Mosby.

Aldwin C: Aging, coping, and efficacy: theoretical framework for examining coping in life-span developmental context. In Wykle M and others, editors: *Stress and health among the elderly*, New York, 1992, Springer.

Aldwin CM: *Stress, coping, and development: an integrative perspective*, New York, 2000, Guilford.

American Psychiatric Association: *Diagnostic and statistical manual of mental disorders*, ed 4, TR, Washington, DC, 2000, The Association.

Chiriboga DA: Paradise lost: stress in the modern age. In Wykle M and others, editors: *Stress and health among the elderly*, New York, 1992, Springer.

Dochterman JM, Bulechek G, editors: *Nursing interventions classification (NIC)*, ed 4, St. Louis, 2004, Mosby.

Gulanick M and others: *Nursing care plans: nursing diagnosis and intervention*, ed 5, St. Louis, 2003, Mosby.

Hyer LA, Sohnle SJ: *Trauma among older people,* Ann Arbor, Mich, 2001, Taylor & Francis.

Johnson M, Maas M, Moorhead S: *Nursing outcomes classification (NOC),* ed 2, St. Louis, 2000, Mosby.

Kasl SV: Stress and health among the elderly: an overview of issues. In Wykle M and others, editors: *Stress and health among the elderly,* New York, 1992, Springer.

Kennedy JS: Psychopharmacological management of stress in the elderly. In Wykle M and others, editors: *Stress and health among the elderly,* New York, 1992, Springer.

Lazarus R: *Stress and emotion: a new synthesis,* New York, 1999, Springer.

Manning G and others: *Stress: living and working in a changing world,* Duluth, Minn, 1999, Whole Person Associates.

Monat A, Lazarus R: *Stress and coping: an anthology,* New York, 1991, Columbia University Press.

Moorhead S, Johnson M, Mass M: *Nursing outcomes classification (NOC),* ed 3, St. Louis, 2004, Mosby.

Neuman B: *The Neuman systems model,* ed 3, Stamford, Conn, 1995, Appleton & Lange.

Pearlin LI, Mullan JT: Loss and stress in aging. In Wykle M and others, editors: *Stress and health among the elderly,* New York, 1992, Springer.

Pender NJ, Murdaugh C, Parsons MA: *Health promotion in nursing practice,* ed 4, Upper Saddle River, NJ, 2002, Howorth Press.

Selye H: History and present status of the stress concept. In Monat A, Lazarus R, editors: *Stress and coping: an anthology,* New York, 1991, Columbia University Press.

Shontz F: *The psychological aspects of physical illness and disability,* New York, 1975, Macmillan.

Stuart G, Wright L: Applying the Neuman systems model to psychiatric nursing practice. In Neuman B: *The Neuman Systems Model,* ed 3, Stanford Conn, 1995, Appleton & Lange.

Varcarolis EM: *Foundations of psychiatric mental health nursing: a clinical approach,* ed 4, St. Louis, 2002, Saunders.

Research References

Aldwin CM and others: Age differences in stress, coping, and appraisal: findings from the normative aging study, *J Gerontol B Psychol Sci Soc Sci* 51B(4):179, 1996.

Foster J: Successful coping, adaptation and resilience in the elderly: an interpretation of epidemiological data, *Psychiatr Q* 68(3)189, 1997.

Joy D and others: Posttraumatic stress reactions after injury, *J Trauma* 48(3):490, 2000.

O'Farrell P, Murray J, Hotz SB: Psychologic distress among spouses of patients undergoing cardiac rehabilitation, *Heart Lung* 29(2):97, 2000.

Soloman P, Draine J: Subjective burden among family members of mentally ill adults: relation to stress, coping, and adaptation, *Am J Orthopsychiatry* 65(3):419, 1995.

31

Vital Signs

Media Resources

http://evolve.elsevier.com/Potter/
fundamentals/

CD COMPANION

- Review Questions
- Animations
- Glossary

evolve WEBSITE

- Review Questions
- Student Learning Activities
- Animations
- Video Clips
- Glossary

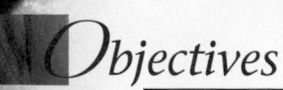

Objectives

Mastery of content in this chapter will enable the student to:

- Define the key terms listed.
- Explain the principles and mechanisms of thermoregulation.
- Describe nursing measures that promote heat loss and heat conservation.
- Discuss physiological changes associated with fever.
- Accurately assess tympanic, oral, rectal, and axillary temperatures.
- Accurately assess pulse, respirations, oxygen saturation, and blood pressure.
- Explain the physiology of normal regulation of blood pressure, pulse, oxygen saturation, and respirations.
- Describe factors that cause variations in body temperature, pulse, oxygen saturation, respirations, and blood pressure.
- Describe cultural and ethnic variations with blood pressure assessment.
- Identify ranges of acceptable vital sign values for an infant, a child, and an adult.
- Explain variations in technique used to assess an infant's, a child's, and an adult's vital signs.
- Describe the benefits and precautions involving self-measurement of blood pressure.
- Identify when vital signs should be taken.
- Accurately record and report vital sign measurements.
- Appropriately delegate vital sign measurement to assistive personnel.

The most frequent measurements obtained by health practitioners are those of temperature, pulse, blood pressure, respiratory rate, and oxygen saturation. As indicators of health status, these measures indicate the effectiveness of circulatory, respiratory, neural, and endocrine body functions. Because of their importance they are referred to as **vital signs.** Recently the Joint Commission on Accreditation of Healthcare Organizations and pain management experts have advocated for making pain the fifth vital sign to ensure routine screening for pain (Lynch, 2001). (Pain is covered in Chapter 42.) Measurement of vital signs provides data to determine a client's usual state of health (baseline data). Many factors, such as the temperature of the environment, the client's physical exertion, and the effects of illness, cause vital signs to change, sometimes outside an acceptable range. A change in vital signs can indicate a change in physiological function. Assessment of vital signs allows the nurse to identify nursing diagnoses, to implement planned interventions, and to evaluate success when vital signs have returned to acceptable values. An alteration in vital signs may signal the need for medical or nursing intervention.

Vital signs are a quick and efficient way of monitoring a client's condition or identifying problems and evaluating the client's response to intervention. When the nurse learns the physiological variables influencing vital signs and recognizes the relationship of vital sign changes to other physical assessment findings, precise determinations of the client's health problems can be made. The basic techniques of inspection, palpation, and auscultation are used to determine vital signs. These skills are simple but should not be taken for granted. Careful measurement techniques ensure accurate findings. Vital signs and other physiological measurements are the basis for clinical problem solving. Vital sign assessment is an essential ingredient when nurses and physicians collaborate to determine the client's health status.

Guidelines for Measuring Vital Signs

Vital signs are a part of the database that a nurse collects during assessment. Box 31-1 provides a reference for acceptable values in the adult client. Vital signs are included in a complete physical assessment (see Chapter 32) or obtained individually to assess a client's condition. Establishing a database of vital signs during a routine physical examination serves as a baseline for future assessments. The client's needs and condition determine when, where, how, and by whom vital signs are measured. The nurse must be able to measure vital signs correctly or delegate the measurement of vital signs appropriately to assistive personnel. When vital signs are obtained, the nurse must understand and interpret the values, communicate findings appropriately, and begin interventions as needed. The following guidelines assist the nurse in incorporating vital sign measurement into nursing practice:

- The nurse caring for the client is responsible for vital sign measurement. Measurement of selected vital signs (i.e., in stable clients) may be delegated to assistive personnel. However, the nurse must analyze the

---

vital signs to interpret their significance and make decisions about interventions.

- Equipment should be functional and appropriate for the size and the age of the client. Equipment used to measure vital signs (e.g., a thermometer) must work properly to ensure accurate findings.
- Equipment should be selected based on the client's condition and characteristics (e.g., an adult-size blood pressure cuff should not be used for a child).
- The nurse knows the client's usual range of vital signs. A client's usual values may differ from the acceptable range for that age or physical state. The client's usual values serve as a baseline for comparison with later findings. Thus a nurse can detect a change in condition over time.
- The nurse knows the client's medical history, therapies, and prescribed medications. Some illnesses or treatments cause predictable vital sign changes. Some medications affect one or more of the vital signs.
- The nurse controls or minimizes environmental factors that may affect vital signs. For example, assessing the client's temperature in a warm, humid room may yield a value that is not a true indicator of the client's condition.
- The nurse uses an organized, systematic approach when taking vital signs. Each procedure requires a step-by-step approach to ensure accuracy.
- The manner of approach to the client can alter the vital signs. The nurse approaches the client in a calm, caring manner while demonstrating proficiency in handling the supplies needed for vital sign measurement.
- Based on the client's condition, the nurse collaborates with the physician to decide the frequency of vital sign assessment. In the hospital, the physician orders a minimum frequency of vital sign measurements for each client. Following surgery or treatment intervention, vital signs are measured more frequently to detect complications. In a clinic or outpatient setting, vital signs are taken before the practitioner examines the client and after any invasive procedures. As a client's physical condition worsens, it may be necessary to monitor vital signs as often as every 5 to 15 minutes. The nurse is responsible for judging whether more frequent assessments are needed (Box 31-2).
- The nurse uses vital sign measurements to determine indications for medication administration. For example, the physician may order certain cardiac drugs to be given only within a range of pulse or blood pressure values. Antipyretics are often administered when temperature is elevated outside of the acceptable range for the client. The nurse does not administer these drugs if the vital sign assessment indicates the measurements are within the specified acceptable range.
- The nurse analyzes the results of vital sign measurement. The nurse is often in the best position to assess all clinical findings about a client. Vital signs are not interpreted in isolation. The nurse must also know related physical signs or symptoms and be aware of the client's ongoing health status.
- The nurse verifies and communicates significant changes in vital signs. Vital signs are documented and communicated to the nurse assuming care of the

---

| Box *31-1* | **Vital Signs: Acceptable Ranges for Adults** |

Temperature Range: 36° to 38° C (96.8° to 100.4° F)

Average oral/tympanic: 37° C (98.6° F)
Average rectal: 37.5° C (99.5° F)
Average axillary: 36.5° C (97.7° F)

Pulse

60 to 100 beats per minute

Respirations

12 to 16 breaths per minute

Blood Pressure

Average: 120/80 mm Hg
Pulse pressure: 30 to 50 mm Hg

Box 31-2 When to Take Vital Signs

When the client is admitted to a health care facility

In a hospital or care facility on a routine schedule according to the physician's order or the institution's standards of practice

Before and after a surgical procedure

Before and after an invasive diagnostic procedure

Before, during, and after the administration of medications that affect cardiovascular, respiratory, and temperature-control function

When the client's general physical condition changes (as with loss of consciousness or increased intensity of pain)

Before and after nursing interventions influencing a vital sign (e.g., before a client previously on bed rest ambulates or before a client performs range-of-motion exercises)

When the client reports nonspecific symptoms of physical distress (e.g., feeling "funny" or "different")

---

client. Baseline measurements allow a nurse to identify changes in vital signs. When vital signs appear abnormal, it may help to have another nurse or a physician repeat the measurement. The nurse informs the physician or nurse in charge of abnormal vital signs.

- The nurse develops a teaching plan to instruct the client or caregiver in vital sign assessment and the significance of findings.

Body Temperature

Physiology

The body temperature is the difference between the amount of heat produced by body processes and the amount of heat lost to the external environment.

Heat produced − Heat lost = Body temperature

Despite extremes in environmental conditions and physical activity, temperature-control mechanisms of human beings keep the body's **core temperature** (temperature of the deep tissues) relatively constant (Figure 31-1). However, surface temperature fluctuates depending on blood flow to the skin and the amount of heat lost to the external environment. Because of these surface temperature fluctuations, the acceptable temperature of human beings ranges from 36° to 38° C (96.8° to 100.4° F). The body's tissues and cells function best within the relatively narrow temperature range.

The site of temperature measurement (oral, rectal, axillary, tympanic membrane, esophageal, pulmonary artery, or even urinary bladder) is one factor that determines the client's temperature. For healthy young adults the average oral temperature is 37° C (98.6° F). In clinical practice, nurses learn the temperature range of individual clients. No single temperature is normal for all people.

The measurement of body temperature is aimed at obtaining a representative average temperature of core body tissues. Sites reflecting core temperatures are more reliable indicators of body temperature than sites reflecting

surface temperatures (Box 31-3). In addition, the temperature value obtained may differ depending on the measurement site.

Regulation. The balance between heat lost and heat produced, or **thermoregulation,** is precisely regulated by physiological and behavioral mechanisms. For the body temperature to stay constant and within an acceptable range, the relationship between heat production and heat loss must be maintained. This relationship is regulated by neurological and cardiovascular mechanisms. The nurse applies knowledge of temperature-control mechanisms to promote temperature regulation.

Neural and Vascular Control. The **hypothalamus,** located between the cerebral hemispheres, controls body temperature the same way a thermostat works in the home. A comfortable temperature is the "set point" at which a heating system operates. In the home a fall in environmental temperature activates the furnace, whereas a rise in temperature shuts the system down.

The hypothalamus senses minor changes in body temperature. The anterior hypothalamus controls heat loss, and the posterior hypothalamus controls heat production. When nerve cells in the anterior hypothalamus become heated beyond the set point, impulses are sent out to reduce body temperature. Mechanisms of heat loss include sweating, vasodilation (widening) of blood vessels, and inhibition of heat production. Blood is redistributed to surface vessels to promote heat loss.

If the posterior hypothalamus senses the body's temperature is lower than the set point, heat conservation mechanisms are instituted. Vasoconstriction (narrowing) of blood vessels reduces blood flow to the skin and extremities. Compensatory heat production is stimulated through voluntary muscle contraction and muscle shivering. When vasoconstriction is ineffective in preventing additional heat loss, shivering begins. Disease or trauma to the hypothalamus or to the spinal cord, which carries hypothalamic messages, can cause serious alterations in temperature control.

Heat Production. Thermoregulation depends on the normal function of heat production processes. Heat is produced in the body as a by-product of metabolism, which is the chemical reaction in all body cells. Food is the primary fuel source for metabolism. Activities requiring additional chemical reactions increase the metabolic rate. As metabolism increases, additional heat is produced. When metabolism decreases, less heat is produced. Heat production occurs during rest, voluntary movements, involuntary shivering, and nonshivering thermogenesis.

- Basal metabolism accounts for the heat produced by the body at absolute rest. The average **basal metabolic rate (BMR)** depends on the body surface area. Thyroid hormones also affect the BMR. By promoting the breakdown of body glucose and fat, thyroid hormones increase the rate of chemical reactions in almost all cells of the body. When large amounts of thyroid hormones are secreted, the BMR can increase 100% above normal. Absence of thyroid hormones can cut the BMR in half, causing a decrease in heat

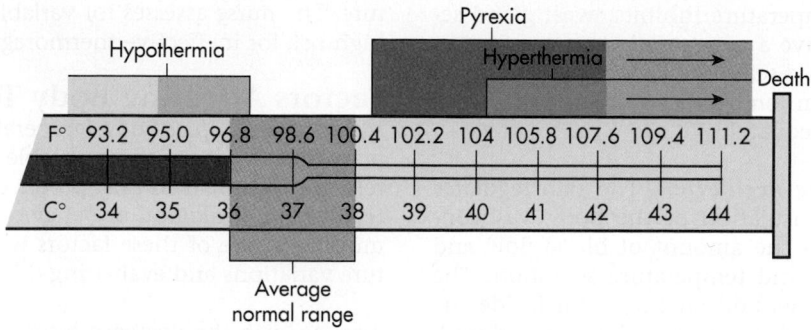

FIGURE **31–1** Ranges of normal temperature values and physiological consequences of abnormal body temperature.

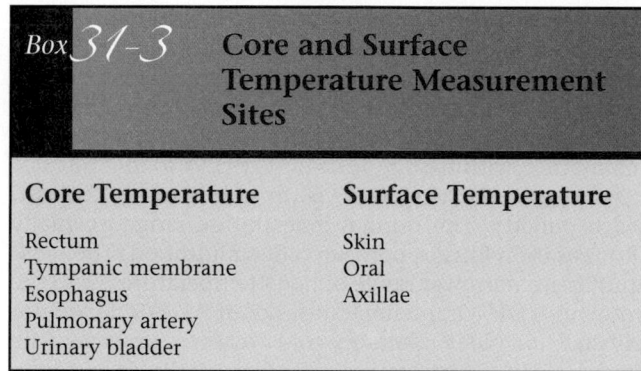

Box **31–3**	**Core and Surface Temperature Measurement Sites**
Core Temperature	**Surface Temperature**
Rectum	Skin
Tympanic membrane	Oral
Esophagus	Axillae
Pulmonary artery	
Urinary bladder	

production. The male sex hormone testosterone increases BMR. Men have a higher BMR than women.

- Voluntary movements such as muscular activity during exercise require additional energy. The metabolic rate can increase up to 2000 times normal during exercise. Heat production can increase up to 50 times normal.

- **Shivering** is an involuntary body response to temperature differences in the body. The skeletal muscle movement during shivering requires significant energy. In vulnerable clients shivering can seriously deplete energy sources, resulting in further physiological deterioration. Shivering can increase heat production 4 to 5 times greater than normal. The heat that is produced assists in equalizing the body temperature, and the shivering ceases.

- **Nonshivering thermogenesis** occurs primarily in neonates. Because neonates cannot shiver, a limited amount of vascular brown tissue, present at birth, is metabolized for heat production.

Heat Loss. Heat loss and heat production occur simultaneously. The skin's structure and exposure to the environment result in constant, normal heat loss through radiation, conduction, convection, and evaporation.

Radiation is the transfer of heat from the surface of one object to the surface of another without direct contact between the two. Up to 85% of the human body's surface area radiates heat to the environment. Peripheral vasodilation increases blood flow from the internal or-

gans to the skin to increase radiant heat loss. Peripheral vasoconstriction minimizes radiant heat loss. Radiation increases as the temperature difference between the objects increases. However, if the environment is warmer than the skin, the body absorbs heat through radiation.

The nurse increases heat loss through radiation by removing clothing or blankets. The client's position enhances radiation heat loss (e.g., standing exposes a greater radiating surface area and lying in a fetal position minimizes heat radiation). Covering the body with dark, closely woven clothing also reduces the amount of heat lost from radiation.

Conduction is the transfer of heat from one object to another with direct contact. Heat conducts through contact with solids, liquids, and gases. When the warm skin touches a cooler object, heat is lost. Conduction normally accounts for a small amount of heat loss. The nurse increases conductive heat loss when applying an ice pack or bathing a client with a cool cloth. Applying several layers of clothing reduces conductive loss. The body gains heat by conduction when contact is made with materials warmer than skin temperature (e.g., application of an aquathermia pad).

Convection is the transfer of heat away by air movement. A fan promotes heat loss through convection. Convective heat loss increases when moistened skin comes into contact with slightly moving air.

Evaporation is the transfer of heat energy when a liquid is changed to a gas. The body continuously loses heat by evaporation. About 600 to 900 ml a day evaporates from the skin and lungs, resulting in water and heat loss. By regulating perspiration or sweating, the body promotes additional evaporative heat loss. Millions of sweat glands located in the dermis of the skin secrete sweat through tiny ducts on the skin's surface. When body temperature rises, the anterior hypothalamus signals the sweat glands to release sweat. Sweat evaporates from the skin surface, resulting in heat loss. During exercise and emotional or mental stress, sweating is one way to lose excessive heat produced by the increased metabolic rate. **Diaphoresis** is visible perspiration primarily occurring on the forehead and upper thorax, though it can also be seen elsewhere on the body. Excessive evaporation can cause skin scaling and itching, as well as drying of the nares and pharynx.

A lowered body temperature inhibits sweat gland secretion. People who have a congenital absence of sweat glands or a serious skin disease that impairs sweating are unable to tolerate warm temperatures because they cannot cool themselves adequately.

Skin in Temperature Regulation. The skin regulates temperature through insulation of the body, vasoconstriction (which affects the amount of blood flow and heat loss to the skin), and temperature sensation. The skin, subcutaneous tissue, and fat keep heat inside the body. When blood flow between skin layers is reduced, the skin alone is an excellent insulator. Persons with more body fat have more natural insulation than do slim and muscular people.

The way that the skin controls body temperature is similar to the way that an automobile radiator controls engine temperature. The engine of an automobile generates a great deal of heat. Water is pumped through the engine's system to collect the heat and carry it to the radiator, where a fan transfers the heat from the water to the outside air. In the human body the internal organs produce heat, and during exercise or increased sympathetic stimulation, the amount of heat produced is greater than the usual core temperature. Blood flows from the internal organs, carrying heat to the body surface. The skin is well supplied with blood vessels, especially the areas of the hands, feet, and ears. Blood flow through these vascular areas of the skin may vary from minimal flow to as much as 30% of the blood ejected from the heart. Heat transfers from the blood, through vessel walls, to the skin's surface and is lost to the environment through the heat-loss mechanisms. The body's core temperature remains within safe limits.

The degree of vasoconstriction determines the amount of blood flow and heat loss to the skin. If the core temperature is too high, the hypothalamus inhibits vasoconstriction. As a result, blood vessels dilate, and more blood reaches the skin's surface. On a hot, humid day the blood vessels in the hands are dilated and easily visible. In contrast, if the core temperature becomes too low, the hypothalamus initiates vasoconstriction and blood flow to the skin lessens. Thus body heat is conserved.

Behavioral Control. Humans voluntarily act to maintain comfortable body temperature when exposed to temperature extremes. The ability of a person to control body temperature depends on (1) the degree of temperature extreme, (2) the person's ability to sense feeling comfortable or uncomfortable, (3) thought processes or emotions, and (4) the person's mobility or ability to remove or add clothes. Body temperature control is difficult if any of these abilities are absent or lost. Infants can sense uncomfortable warm conditions but need assistance in changing their environment. Older adults may need help in detecting cold environments and minimizing heat loss. Illness, a decreased level of consciousness, or impaired thought processes result in an inability to recognize the need to change behavior for temperature control. When temperatures become extremely hot or cold, health-promoting behaviors, such as removing or adding clothing, have a limited effect on controlling tempera-

ture. The nurse assesses for variables that place clients at high risk for ineffective thermoregulation.

Factors Affecting Body Temperature

Many factors affect body temperature. Changes in body temperature within an acceptable range occur when the relationship between heat production and heat loss is altered by physiological or behavioral variables. The nurse must be aware of these factors when assessing temperature variations and evaluating deviations from normal.

Age. At birth the newborn leaves a warm, relatively constant environment and enters one in which temperatures fluctuate widely. Temperature-control mechanisms are immature. An infant's temperature may respond drastically to changes in the environment. Extra care is needed to protect the newborn from environmental temperatures. Clothing must be adequate, and exposure to temperature extremes must be avoided. A newborn loses up to 30% of body heat through the head and therefore needs to wear a cap to prevent heat loss. When protected from environmental extremes, the newborn's body temperature is maintained within 35.5° to 37.5° C (95.9° to 99.5° F).

Temperature regulation is unstable until children reach puberty. The normal temperature range gradually drops as individuals approach older adulthood. The older adult has a narrower range of body temperatures than the younger adult. Oral temperatures of 35° C (95° F) are not unusual for older adults in cold weather. However, the average body temperature of older adults is approximately 36° C (96.8° F). Older adults are particularly sensitive to temperature extremes because of deterioration in control mechanisms, particularly poor vasomotor control (control of vasoconstriction and vasodilation), reduced amounts of subcutaneous tissue, reduced sweat gland activity, and reduced metabolism.

Exercise. Muscle activity requires an increased blood supply and an increased carbohydrate and fat breakdown. This increased metabolism causes an increase in heat production. Any form of exercise can increase heat production and thus body temperature. Prolonged strenuous exercise, such as long distance running, can temporarily raise body temperatures up to 41° C (105.8° F).

Hormone Level. Women generally experience greater fluctuations in body temperature than men. Hormonal variations during the menstrual cycle cause body temperature fluctuations. Progesterone levels rise and fall cyclically during the menstrual cycle. When progesterone levels are low, the body temperature is a few tenths of a degree below the baseline level. The lower temperature persists until ovulation occurs. During ovulation, greater amounts of progesterone enter the circulatory system and raise the body temperature to previous baseline levels or higher. These temperature variations can be used to predict a woman's most fertile time to achieve pregnancy.

Body temperature changes also occur in women during menopause (cessation of menstruation). Women who have stopped menstruating may experience periods of intense body heat and sweating lasting from 30 seconds to

5 minutes. There may be intermittent increases in skin temperature of up to 4° C (7.2° F) during these periods, referred to as hot flashes. This is due to the instability of the vasomotor controls for vasodilation and vasoconstriction.

Circadian Rhythm. Body temperature normally changes 0.5° to 1° C (0.9° to 1.8° F) during a 24-hour period. However, temperature is one of the most stable rhythms in humans. The temperature is usually lowest between 1:00 and 4:00 AM (Figure 31-2). During the day, body temperature rises steadily, until a maximum temperature value at about 6:00 PM, and then declines to early morning levels. Temperature patterns are not automatically reversed in people who work at night and sleep during the day. It takes 1 to 3 weeks for the cycle to reverse. In general, the circadian temperature rhythm does not change with age.

Stress. Physical and emotional stress increase body temperature through hormonal and neural stimulation. These physiological changes increase metabolism, which increases heat production. The client who is anxious about entering a hospital or a physician's office may register a higher normal temperature (see Chapter 30).

Environment. Environment influences body temperature. If body temperature is measured in a very warm room, a client may be unable to regulate body temperature by heat-loss mechanisms, and the body temperature will be elevated. If the client has just been outside in the cold without warm clothing, body temperature may be low because of extensive radiant and conductive heat loss. Infants and older adults are most likely to be affected by environmental temperatures because their temperature-regulating mechanisms are less efficient.

Temperature Alterations. Changes in body temperature outside the usual range affect the hypothalamic set point. These changes can be related to excess heat production, excessive heat loss, minimal heat production, minimal heat loss, or any combination of these alterations. The nature of the change affects the type of clinical problems a client experiences.

Fever. **Pyrexia,** or **fever,** occurs because heat-loss mechanisms are unable to keep pace with excess heat production, resulting in an abnormal rise in body temperature. A fever is usually not harmful if it stays below 39° C (102.2° F) and a single temperature reading may not indicate a fever. In addition to physical signs and symptoms of infection, a fever determination is based on several temperature readings at different times of the day compared with the usual value for that person at that time.

A true fever results from an alteration in the hypothalamic set point. **Pyrogens** such as bacteria and viruses cause a rise in body temperature. Pyrogens act as antigens, triggering immune system responses. The hypothalamus reacts to raise the set point, and the body responds by producing and conserving heat. Several hours may pass before the body temperature reaches the new set point. During this period the person experiences chills, shivers, and feels cold, even though the body temperature is rising (Figure 31-3). The chill phase resolves when the new set point, a higher temperature, is achieved. During the next phase, the plateau, the chills subside and the person feels warm and dry. If the new set point is "overshot," or the pyrogens are removed (e.g., destruction of bacteria by antibiotics), the third phase of a febrile episode occurs. The hypothalamus set point drops, initiating heat loss responses. The skin becomes warm and flushed because of vasodilation. Diaphoresis assists in evaporative heat loss. When the fever "breaks," the client becomes **afebrile.**

Fever is an important defense mechanism. Mild temperature elevations up to 39° C (102.2° F) enhance the body's immune system. During a febrile episode, white blood cell production is stimulated. Increased temperature reduces the concentration of iron in the blood plasma, suppressing the growth of bacteria. Fever also fights viral infections by stimulating interferon, the body's natural virus-fighting substance.

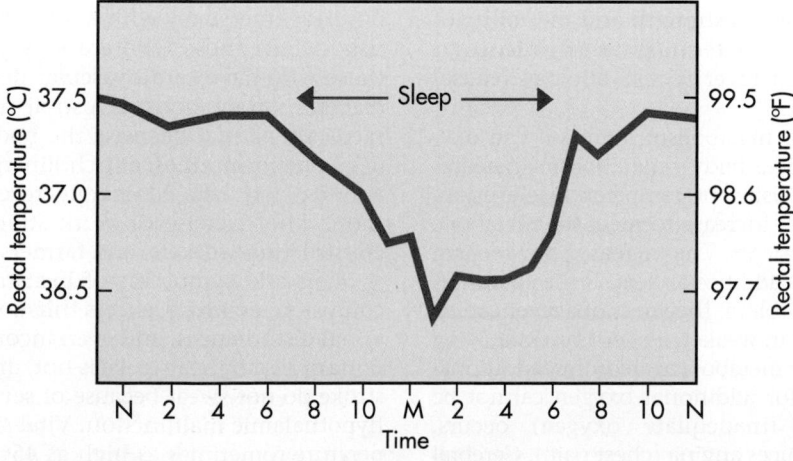

FIGURE **31–2** Temperature cycle for 24 hours.

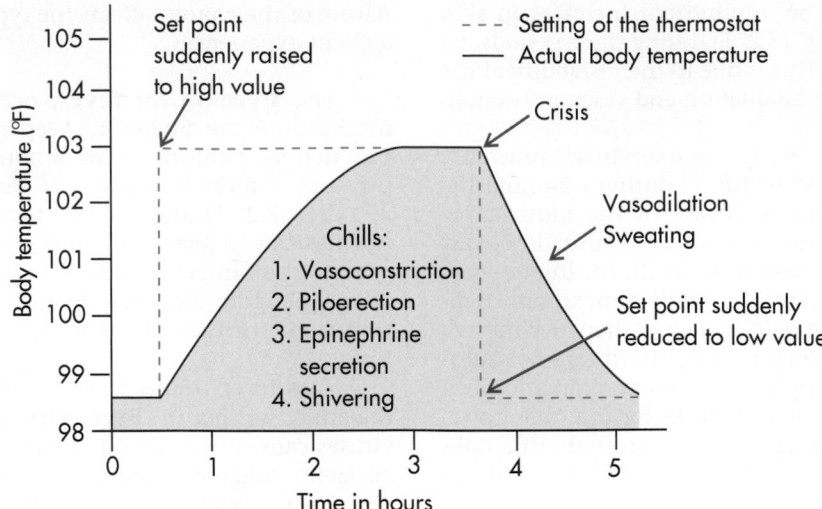

FIGURE **31-3** Effect of changing the set point of the hypothalamic temperature control during a fever. (Modified from Guyton AC, Hall JE: *Textbook of medical physiology,* ed 10, Philadelphia, 2000, WB Saunders.)

Box **31-4**   **Patterns of Fever**

Sustained—A constant body temperature continuously above 38° C (100.4° F) that demonstrates little fluctuation.
Intermittent—Fever spikes interspersed with usual temperature levels. Temperature returns to acceptable value at least once in 24 hours.
Remittent—Fever spikes and falls without a return to normal temperature levels.
Relapsing—Periods of febrile episodes interspersed with acceptable temperature values. Febrile episodes and periods of normothermia may be longer than 24 hours.

By analyzing the fever pattern, fevers can serve a diagnostic purpose. Fever patterns differ depending on the causative pyrogen (Box 31-4). The increase or decrease in pyrogen activity results in fever spikes and declines at different times of the day. The duration and degree of fever depend on the pyrogen's strength and the ability of the individual to respond. The term **fever of unknown origin (FUO)** refers to a fever whose etiology (cause) cannot be determined.

During a fever, cellular metabolism increases and oxygen consumption rises. The body's metabolism increases 13% for every degree Celsius of temperature elevation. Heart and respiratory rates increase to meet the metabolic needs of the body for nutrients. The increased metabolism uses energy that produces additional heat. If the client has a cardiac or respiratory problem, the stress of a fever can be great. A prolonged fever can weaken a client by exhausting energy stores. Increased metabolism requires additional oxygen. If the demand for additional oxygen cannot be met, cellular hypoxia (inadequate oxygen) occurs. Myocardial hypoxia produces angina (chest pain). Cerebral hypoxia produces confusion. Interventions during a fever may include oxygen therapy. Water loss through increased respiration and diaphoresis can be excessive, placing a client at risk for fluid volume deficit. Dehydration can be a serious problem for older adults and children with low body weight. Maintaining optimum fluid volume status is an important nursing action (see Chapter 40).

Hyperthermia. An elevated body temperature related to the body's inability to promote heat loss or reduce heat production is **hyperthermia.** Whereas fever is an upward shift in the set point, hyperthermia results from an overload of the body's thermoregulatory mechanisms. Any disease or trauma to the hypothalamus can impair heat-loss mechanisms. **Malignant hyperthermia** is a hereditary condition of uncontrolled heat production, occurring when susceptible persons receive certain anesthetic drugs.

Heatstroke. Prolonged exposure to the sun or high environmental temperatures can overwhelm the body's heat-loss mechanisms. Heat also depresses hypothalamic function. These conditions cause **heatstroke,** a dangerous heat emergency with a high mortality rate. Clients at risk include those who are very young or very old and those who have cardiovascular disease, hypothyroidism, diabetes, or alcoholism. Also at risk are those who take medications that decrease the body's ability to lose heat (e.g., phenothiazines, anticholinergics, diuretics, amphetamines, and beta-adrenergic receptor antagonists) and those who exercise or work strenuously (e.g., athletes, construction workers, and farmers).

Signs and symptoms of heatstroke include giddiness, confusion, delirium, excess thirst, nausea, muscle cramps, visual disturbances, and even incontinence. The most important sign of heatstroke is hot, dry skin. Victims of heatstroke do not sweat because of severe electrolyte loss and hypothalamic malfunction. Vital signs reveal a body temperature sometimes as high as 45° C (113° F) with an increase in heart rate and lowering of blood pressure. If the condition progresses, the client with heatstroke becomes

Table 31-1	Classification of Hypothermia	
	C	**F**
Mild	34°-36°	93.2°-96.8°
Moderate	30°-34°	86.0°-93.2°
Severe	<30°	<86.0°

unconscious with fixed, unreactive pupils. Permanent neurological damage occurs unless cooling measures are rapidly started.

Heat Exhaustion. **Heat exhaustion** occurs when profuse diaphoresis results in excess water and electrolyte loss. Caused by environmental heat exposure, the client exhibits signs and symptoms of fluid volume deficit (see Chapter 40). First aid includes transporting the client to a cooler environment and restoring fluid and electrolyte balance.

Hypothermia. Heat loss during prolonged exposure to cold overwhelms the body's ability to produce heat, causing hypothermia. **Hypothermia** is classified by core temperature measurements (Table 31-1). It can be unintentional, such as falling through the ice of a frozen lake. Hypothermia may be intentionally induced during surgical procedures to reduce metabolic demand and the body's need for oxygen.

Accidental hypothermia usually develops gradually and may go unnoticed for several hours. When skin temperature drops to 35° C (95° F), the client suffers uncontrolled shivering, loss of memory, depression, and poor judgment. As the body temperature falls below 34.4° C (94° F), heart rate, respiratory rate, and blood pressure fall. The skin becomes cyanotic. If hypothermia progresses, a client experiences cardiac dysrhythmias, loss of consciousness, and unresponsiveness to painful stimuli. In cases of severe hypothermia a person may demonstrate clinical signs similar to death (e.g., lack of response to stimuli and extremely slow respirations and pulse). The assessment of core temperature is critical when hypothermia is suspected. A special low reading thermometer may be required because standard devices do not register below 35° C (95° F).

Frostbite occurs when the body is exposed to subnormal temperatures. Ice crystals forming inside the cell can result in permanent circulatory and tissue damage. Areas particularly susceptible to frostbite are the earlobes, tip of the nose, and fingers and toes. The injured area becomes white, waxy, and firm to the touch. The client loses sensation in the affected area. Intervention includes gradual warming measures, analgesia, and protection of the injured tissue.

Nursing Process and Thermoregulation

Knowledge of the physiology of body temperature regulation helps the nurse to assess the client's response to temperature alterations and to intervene safely. Independent measures can be implemented to increase or minimize heat loss, to promote heat conservation, and to increase comfort. These measures complement the effects of medically ordered therapies during illness. Many measures can also be taught to family members, parents of children, or other caregivers.

Assessment

Sites. There are several sites for measuring core and surface body temperature. The core temperatures of the pulmonary artery, esophagus, and urinary bladder are used in intensive care settings. These measurements require the use of continuous invasive devices placed in body cavities or organs and continually display readings on an electronic monitor.

Intermittent temperature measurements are obtained from the routinely used invasive sites of the mouth, rectum, tympanic membrane, and axilla. Noninvasive chemically prepared thermometer patches can also be applied to the skin. Oral, rectal, axillary, and skin temperature sites rely on effective blood circulation at the measurement site. The heat of the blood is conducted to the thermometer probe. Tympanic temperature relies on the radiation of body heat to an infrared sensor. Because the tympanic membrane shares the same arterial blood supply as the hypothalamus, tympanic temperature is considered a core temperature.

To ensure accurate temperature readings, each site must be measured correctly (Skill 31-1). The temperature obtained varies, depending on the site used, but should be between 36.0° C (96.8° F) and 38.0° C (100.4° F). Rectal temperatures are usually 0.5° C (0.9° F) higher than oral temperatures, and axillary temperatures are usually 0.5° C (0.9° F) lower than oral temperatures. Each of the common temperature measurement sites has advantages and disadvantages (Box 31-5). The nurse chooses the safest and most accurate site for the client. When possible, the same site should be used when repeated measurements are necessary.

Thermometers. Two types of thermometers are commonly available for measuring body temperature: electronic and disposable. A third type, the mercury-in-glass thermometer, was once the standard device found in the clinical setting. However, most municipalities have prohibited the sale or use of mercury-containing medical devices because of the potential hazards.

Each device measures temperature using the **Celsius** or **Fahrenheit** scale. Electronic thermometers allow the nurse to convert scales by activating a switch. When it is necessary to convert temperature readings, the following formulas can be used:

1. To convert Fahrenheit to Celsius, subtract 32 from the Fahrenheit reading and multiply the result by 5/9

$$C = (F - 32°) \times 5/9$$
Example: $40° C = (104° F - 32° F) \times 5/9$

2. To convert Celsius to Fahrenheit, multiply the centigrade reading by 9/5 and add 32 to the product.

$$F = (9/5 \times C) + 32°$$
Example: $104° F = (9/5 \times 40° C) + 32°$

Electronic Thermometer. The electronic thermometer consists of a rechargeable battery-powered display unit, a thin wire cord, and a temperature-processing probe covered by a disposable plastic sheath (Figure 31-4). Separate unbreakable probes are available for oral and rectal use.

Text continued on p. 632

Skill 31-1 Measuring Body Temperature

Delegation Considerations

The skill of temperature measurement can be delegated to assistive personnel. The nurse is responsible for assessing the impact of changes in body temperature. It is important for the nurse to:

- Inform caregiver of appropriate route and device to measure temperature.
- Inform caregiver of specific factors related to client that can falsely raise or lower temperature.
- Inform caregiver of the frequency of temperature measurement for select client.
- Determine that caregiver is aware of the usual values for client.
- Inform caregiver of the abnormalities that should be reported and reconfirmed by the nurse.

Equipment

- Appropriate thermometer
- Soft tissue or wipe
- Lubricant (for rectal measurements only)
- Pen, pencil, vital sign flow sheet or record form
- Disposable gloves, plastic thermometer sleeve or disposable probe cover

Steps	Rationale
1. Assess for signs and symptoms of temperature alterations and for factors that influence body temperature.	Physical signs and symptoms may indicate abnormal temperature. Nurse can accurately assess nature of variations.
2. Determine any previous activity that would interfere with accuracy of temperature measurement. When taking oral temperature, wait 20 to 30 min before measuring temperature if client has smoked or ingested hot or cold liquids or foods.	Smoking or oral intake of food or fluids can cause false oral temperature readings.
3. Determine appropriate temperature site and device for client.	Chosen based on advantages and disadvantages of each site (see Box 31-5, p. 631). Disposable single-use thermometer is used for client who is on isolation precautions.
4. Explain route by which temperature will be taken and importance of maintaining proper position until reading is complete.	Clients are often curious about such measurements and should be cautioned against prematurely removing thermometer to read results.
5. Perform hand hygiene.	Reduces transmission of microorganisms.
6. Obtain temperature reading.	
A. Oral temperature measurement with electronic thermometer	
(1) Apply disposable gloves (optional).	Use of oral probe cover, which can be removed without physical contact, minimizes need to wear gloves.
(2) Remove thermometer pack from charging unit. Attach oral probe (blue tip) to thermometer unit. Grasp top of probe stem, being careful not to apply pressure on the ejection button.	Charging provides battery power. Ejection button releases plastic probe cover from tip.
(3) Slide disposable plastic probe cover over thermometer probe until cover locks in place (see illustration).	Soft plastic cover will not break in client's mouth and prevents transmission of microorganisms between clients.
(4) Have client sit or lie in bed. Ask client to open mouth; then gently place thermometer probe under tongue in posterior sublingual pocket lateral to center of lower jaw (see illustration).	Heat from superficial blood vessels in sublingual pocket produces temperature reading. With electronic thermometer, temperatures in right and left posterior sublingual pocket are significantly higher than in area under front of tongue.
(5) Ask client to hold thermometer probe with lips closed.	Maintains proper position of thermometer during recording.
(6) Leave thermometer probe in place until audible signal occurs and client's temperature appears on digital display; remove thermometer probe from under client's tongue.	Probe must stay in place until signal occurs to ensure accurate reading.
(7) Push ejection button on thermometer stem to discard plastic probe cover into appropriate receptacle.	Reduces transmission of microorganisms.

Steps	Rationale

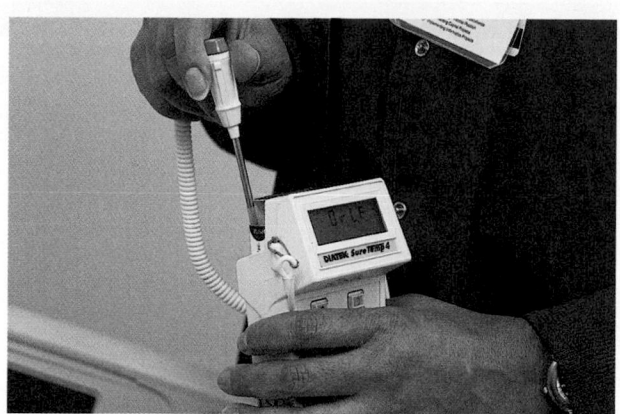

STEP **6A(3)** Inserting thermometer stem into plastic probe cover.

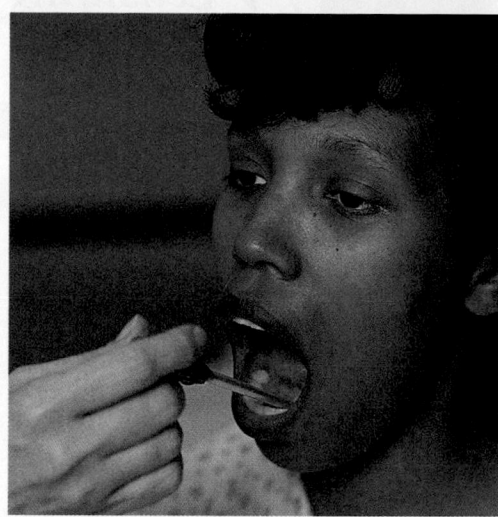

STEP **6A(4)** Probe under tongue in posterior sublingual pocket.

(8) Return thermometer stem to storage well of unit.	Protects probe from damage. Returning probe automatically causes digital reading to disappear.
(9) If gloves worn, remove and dispose in appropriate receptacle. Perform hand hygiene.	Reduces transmission of microorganisms.
(10) Return thermometer to charger.	Maintains battery charge.

B. **Rectal temperature measurement with electronic thermometer**

(1) Draw curtain around bed and/or close room door. Assist client to Sims' position with upper leg flexed. Move aside bed linen to expose only anal area. Keep client's upper body and lower extremities covered with sheet or blanket.	Maintains client's privacy, minimizes embarrassment, and promotes comfort. Exposes anal area for correct thermometer placement.
(2) Apply disposable gloves.	Maintains standard precautions when exposed to items soiled with body fluids (e.g., feces).
(3) Remove thermometer pack from charging unit. Attach rectal probe (red tip) to thermometer unit. Grasp top of probe stem, being careful not to apply pressure on the ejection button.	Charging provides battery power. Ejection button releases plastic probe cover from tip.
(4) Slide disposable plastic probe cover over thermometer probe until cover locks in place.	Probe cover prevents transmission of microorganisms between clients.
(5) Squeeze liberal portion of lubricant on tissue. Dip thermometer's blunt end into lubricant, covering 2.5 to 3.5 cm (1 to 1½ in) for adult.	Lubrication minimizes trauma to rectal mucosa during insertion. Tissue avoids contamination of remaining lubricant in container.
(6) With nondominant hand, separate client's buttocks to expose anus. Ask client to breathe slowly and relax.	Fully exposes anus for thermometer insertion. Relaxes anal sphincter for easier thermometer insertion.
(7) Gently insert thermometer into anus in direction of umbilicus 3.5 cm (1½ in) for adult. Do not force thermometer.	Ensures adequate exposure against blood vessels in rectal wall.
(8) If resistance is felt during insertion, withdraw thermometer immediately. Never force thermometer.	Prevents trauma to mucosa.

Critical Decision Point: If thermometer cannot be adequately inserted into rectum, remove thermometer and consider alternative method for obtaining temperature.

Skill 31-1   *Measuring Body Temperature—cont'd*

Steps	Rationale

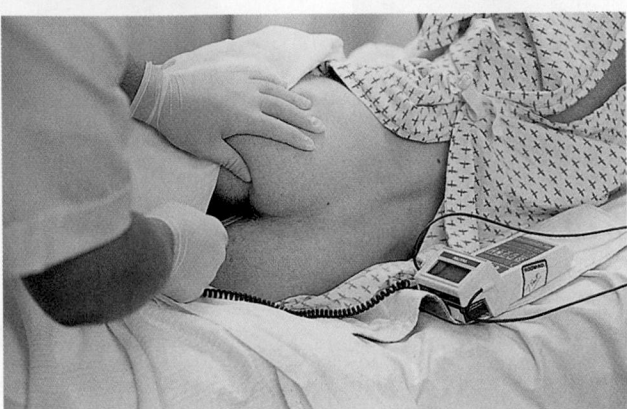

STEP **6B(9)**   Probe positioned in anus.

(9) Once positioned, leave thermometer probe in place (see illustration) until audible signal occurs and client's temperature appears on digital display; remove thermometer probe from anus.	Probe must stay in place until signal occurs to ensure accurate reading.
(10) Push ejection button on thermometer stem to discard plastic probe cover into appropriate receptacle. Wipe probe with alcohol swab, paying particular attention to ridges where probe cover connects to probe.	Reduces transmission of microorganisms.
(11) Return probe to storage position of thermometer unit.	Protects probe from damage. Returning probe automatically causes digital reading to disappear.
(12) Wipe client's anal area with soft tissue to remove lubricant or feces and discard tissue. Assist client in assuming a comfortable position.	Provides for comfort and hygiene.
(13) Remove and dispose of gloves in appropriate receptacle. Perform hand hygiene.	Reduces transmission of microorganisms.
(14) Return thermometer to charger. Verify that charger and probes are wiped with alcohol daily.	Maintains battery charge. Reduces transmission of microorganisms.

C. **Axillary temperature measurement with electronic thermometer**

(1) Draw curtain around bed and/or close door.	Maintains client's privacy, minimizes embarrassment.
(2) Assist client to a supine or sitting position.	Provides easy access to axilla.
(3) Move clothing or gown away from shoulder and arm.	Expose axilla for correct thermometer probe placement.
(4) Remove thermometer pack from charging unit. Be sure oral probe (blue tip) is attached to thermometer unit. Grasp top of probe stem, being careful not to apply pressure on the ejection button.	Charging provides battery power. Ejection button releases plastic cover from probe.
(5) Slide disposable plastic probe cover over thermometer probe until cover locks in place.	Soft plastic cover prevents transmission of microorganisms between clients.

Steps   **Rationale**

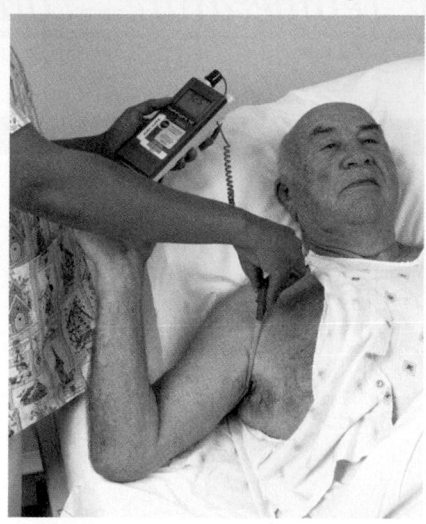 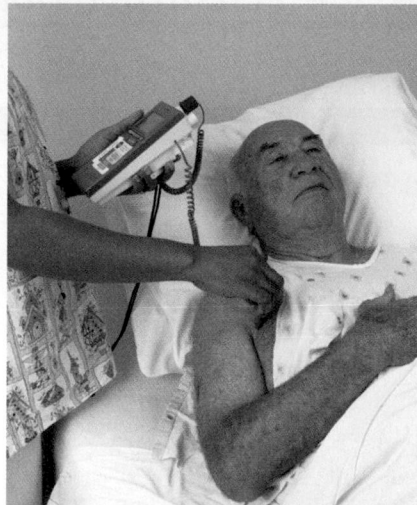

STEP **6C(7)** Thermometer tip in axilla.

(6) Raise client's arm away from torso; inspect for skin lesion and excessive perspiration. Insert probe into center of axilla, lower arm over probe, and place arm across client's chest (see illustration).	Maintains proper position of probe against blood vessels in axilla.

Critical Decision Point: Do not use axilla if skin lesions are present because local temperature may be altered and area may be painful to touch.

---

(7) Hold probe in place until audible signal occurs and temperature appears on digital display.	Probe must stay in place until signal occurs to ensure accurate reading.
(8) Remove probe from axilla.	
(9) Push ejection button on thermometer stem to discard plastic probe cover into appropriate receptacle.	Reduces transmission of microorganisms.
(10) Return thermometer stem to storage well of recording unit.	Protects probe from damage. Returning probe automatically causes digital reading to disappear.
(11) Assist client in assuming a comfortable position replacing linen or gown.	Restores comfort and promotes privacy.
(12) Perform hand hygiene.	Reduces transmission of microorganisms.
(13) Return thermometer unit to charger.	Maintains battery charge.

D. **Tympanic membrane temperature with electronic thermometer**

(1) Assist client in assuming comfortable position with head turned toward side, away from nurse. Right-handed persons should obtain temperature from client's right ear. Left-handed people should obtain temperature from client's left ear.	Ensures comfort and exposes auditory canal for accurate temperature measurement. The less acute the angle of approach, the better the probe seal.
(2) Note if there is obvious earwax in the client's ear canal.	To ensure clear optical pathway, lens cover of speculum must not be impeded by earwax. Switch to other ear or select alternative measurement site if needed.
(3) Remove thermometer handheld unit from charging base, being careful not to apply pressure on the ejection button.	Base provides battery power. Removal of handheld unit from base prepares it to measure temperature. Ejection button releases plastic probe cover from tip.

Skill 31-1   *Measuring Body Temperature—cont'd*

Steps	Rationale

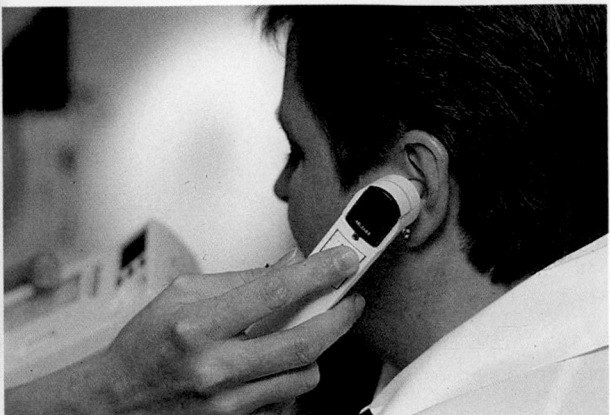

STEP **6D(5)c**   Tympanic thermometer with probe cover inserted into auditory canal.

Steps	Rationale
(4) Slide clean disposable speculum cover over otoscope-like lens tip until it locks into place, being careful not to touch lens cover.	Lens cover must be unimpeded by dust, fingerprints, or earwax to ensure clear optical pathway.
(5) Insert speculum into ear canal following manufacturer's instructions for tympanic probe positioning:	Correct positioning of the probe with respect to ear canal ensures accurate readings.
a. Pull ear pinna backward, up, and out for an adult.	The ear tug straightens the external auditory canal, allowing maximum exposure of the tympanic membrane.
b. Move thermometer in a figure-eight pattern.	Some manufacturers recommend movement of the speculum tip in a figure-eight pattern, which allows the sensor to detect maximum tympanic membrane heat radiation.
c. Fit otoscope probe snugly into canal and do not move (see illustration).	Gentle pressure seals ear canal from ambient temperature, which can alter readings as much as 2.7° C (5° F).
d. Point speculum tip toward nose.	
(6) As soon as probe is in place, depress scan button on handheld unit. Leave thermometer probe in place until audible signal occurs and client's temperature appears on digital display.	Depression of scan button causes infrared energy to be detected. Otoscope tip must stay in place until signal occurs to ensure accurate reading.
(7) Carefully remove speculum from auditory meatus.	
(8) Push ejection button on handheld unit to discard plastic probe cover into appropriate receptacle.	Reduces transmission of microorganisms. Automatically causes digital reading to disappear.
(9) If a second reading is necessary, replace probe lens cover and wait 2 to 3 min before inserting the probe tip.	Lens cover must be free of cerumen to maintain optical path. Time allows ear canal to regain usual temperature (Giuliano and others, 2000).
(10) Return handheld unit to charging base.	Protects sensory tip from damage.
(11) Assist client in assuming a comfortable position.	Restores comfort and sense of well-being.
(12) Perform hand hygiene.	Reduces transmission of microorganisms.
7. Discuss findings with client as needed.	Promotes participation in care and understanding of health status.
8. If temperature is assessed for the first time, establish temperature as baseline if it is within normal range.	Used to compare future temperature measurements.

Steps	Rationale
9. Compare temperature reading with client's previous baseline and acceptable temperature range for client's age-group.	Normal body temperature fluctuates within narrow range; comparison reveals presence of abnormality. Improper placement or movement of thermometer can cause inaccuracies. Second measurement confirms initial findings of abnormal body temperature.

Unexpected Outcomes and Related Interventions

- Temperature 1° C above usual range
  - Assess possible sites (e.g., central line catheter, wounds, etc.) for localized infection and for related data suggesting a systemic infection.
  - Follow interventions listed in Box 31-9, p. 636.
- Persistent fever
  - Notify physician and administer antipyretic and antibiotics as ordered.
- Temperature 1° C below usual range
  - Remove any drafts, wet clothing, or linen.
  - Apply extra blankets, and unless contraindicated offer warm liquids.

Recording and Reporting

- Record temperature in nurses' notes or vital sign flow sheet. Measurement of temperature after administration of specific therapies should be documented in narrative form in nurses' notes.
- Report abnormal findings to nurse in charge or physician.

Home Care Considerations

- Assess temperature and ventilation of client's environment to determine existence of any environmental condition that may influence outcome of client's temperature.
- In the home, clients may continue to use mercury-in-glass thermometers (see Box 31-6, p. 633). Assess safe storage of mercury-in-glass thermometers to protect from breakage and mercury spills. Educate client and caregiver about mercury hazards.

Box 31-5   **Advantages and Disadvantages of Select Temperature Measurement Sites**

Tympanic Membrane

Advantages

Easily accessible site
Minimal client repositioning required
Provides core reading
Very rapid measurement (2 to 5 seconds)
Can be obtained without disturbing or waking client
Eardrum close to hypothalamus; sensitive to core
Unaffected by oral intake of food, fluids, smoking
Can be used for tachypneic clients
Can be used in newborns to reduce infant handling and heat loss (Bailey and Rose, 2001)

Disadvantages

More variability of measurement than with other core temperature devices
Requires removal of hearing aids before measurement
Should not be used with clients who have had surgery of the ear or tympanic membrane
Requires disposable probe cover
Expensive
Does not accurately measure core temperature changes during and after exercise
Possible distortion of temperature readings for clients with otitis media
Cerumen impaction can lower readings (Giuliano and others, 2000)
Questions about measurement accuracy in newborns
Cannot obtain continuous measurement
Affected by ambient temperature devices such as incubators, radiant warmers, and facial fans (Giuliano and others, 2000)

Rectum

Advantages

Argued to be more reliable when oral temperature cannot be obtained

Disadvantages

May lag behind core temperature during rapid temperature changes (Giuliano and others, 2000)
Should not be used for children with diarrhea or clients who have had rectal surgery, a rectal disorder, or decreased platelets
Should not be used for routine vital signs in newborns
Requires positioning and may be source of client embarrassment and anxiety
Risk of body fluid exposure
Requires lubrication

Mouth

Advantages

Accessible-requires no position change
Comfortable for client
Provides accurate surface temperature reading
Reflects rapid change in core temperature
Acceptable route for clients with endotracheal tube in place (Fallis, 2000)

Continued

Box **31-5**   **Advantages and Disadvantages of Select Temperature Measurement Sites—cont'd**

Mouth—cont'd

Disadvantages

Affected by ingestion of fluids or foods, smoke, and oxygen delivery

Should not be used with clients who have had oral surgery, trauma, history of epilepsy, or shaking chills

Should not be used with infants, small children, or confused, unconscious, or uncooperative clients

Risk of body fluid exposure

Axilla

Advantages

Safe and noninvasive

Can be used with newborns and uncooperative clients

Disadvantages

Long measurement time

Requires continuous positioning by nurse

Lags behind core temperature during rapid temperature changes

Requires exposure of thorax

Not recommended to detect fever in infants and young children

Skin

Advantages

Inexpensive

Provides continuous reading

Safe and noninvasive

Does not require disturbing client

Can be used for neonates

Easy to read

Disadvantages

Lags behind other sites during temperature changes, especially during hyperthermia

Adhesion can be impaired by diaphoresis or sweat

Can be affected by environmental temperature

Unreliable during chill phase of fever

The oral probe can also be used for axillary temperature measurement. Within 20 to 50 seconds of insertion, a reading appears on the display unit. A sound signals when the peak temperature reading has been measured.

Another form of electronic thermometer is used exclusively for tympanic temperature. An otoscope-like speculum with an infrared sensor tip detects heat radiated from the tympanic membrane. Within 2 to 5 seconds of placement in the auditory canal, a reading appears on the display unit. A sound signals when the peak temperature reading has been measured.

The greatest advantages of electronic thermometers are that they can be inserted immediately, their readings appear within seconds, and they are easy to read. The plastic sheath is unbreakable and ideal for children. Their expense is a major disadvantage. Maintaining cleanliness of the probes is an important consideration. If not properly cleaned between clients, gastrointestinal contamination of the rectal probe can be a vector of disease transmission. The thermometer is wiped down daily with alcohol and the thermometer probe must be wiped down with an alcohol swab after each client. Particular attention is paid to the probe hub, which has ridges, where the probe cover is secured to the probe.

Disposable Thermometers. Disposable single-use thermometers are thin strips of plastic with a temperature sensor at one end. They are used for oral or axillary temperatures, particularly with children (Figure 31-5). They are useful when caring for clients on protective isolation (see Chapter 33) to avoid the need to take electronic instruments into client rooms. They are inserted the same way as an oral or axillary thermometer and used only once. Chemical dots on the thermometer change color to reflect the temperature reading. The thermometer is removed after 60 seconds and read after waiting about 10 seconds to ensure the temperature reading has stabilized. Research has shown that disposable single-use thermometers tend to overestimate or underestimate true temperature readings (Erickson and others, 1996). As a result the device is only recommended for screening purposes in adults. When an abnormal temperature is suspected, the temperature should be confirmed with an electronic thermometer.

Another form of disposable thermometer is a temperature-sensitive patch or tape. Applied to the forehead or abdomen, the patch changes color at different temperatures. These thermometers are also useful for screening clients, especially infants, for altered temperature. If an abnormal temperature is suspected, the temperature must be confirmed with an electronic temperature device. Disposable thermometers are not appropriate for monitoring temperature therapies.

Glass Thermometers. The mercury-in-glass thermometer is a glass tube sealed at one end, with a mercury-filled bulb at the other. Exposure of the bulb to heat causes the mercury to expand and rise in the enclosed tube. The length of the thermometer is marked with Fahrenheit or centigrade calibrations. Obtaining a temperature with a mercury-in-glass thermometer requires careful preparation of the device (Box 31-6). In addition to proper positioning of the thermometer using the oral, rectal, or axillary site, you must maintain this positions for the appropriate length of time to obtain an accurate reading. In addition to the time delay, the mercury-in-glass device is easily breakable and when broken, releases hazardous mercury. Although health care agencies no longer use

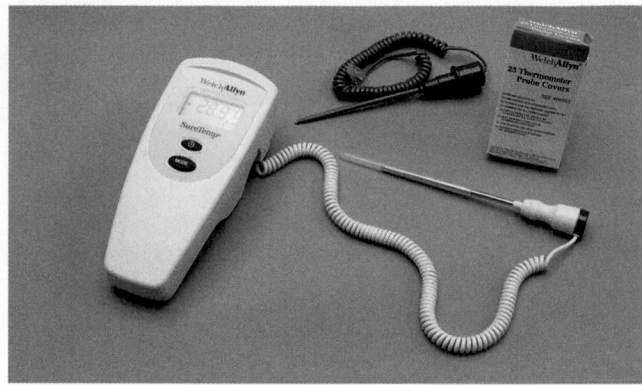

FIGURE 31-4 Electronic thermometer. Blue probe is for oral or axillary use. Red probe is for rectal use.

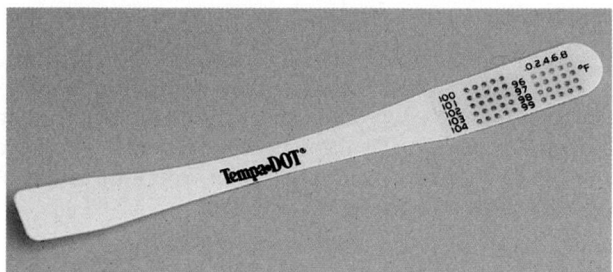

FIGURE 31-5 Disposable, single-use thermometer strip.

glass thermometers, many clients may have mercury-in-glass thermometers in their homes. If a thermometer is broken or a mercury spill is suspected, the nurse is required to take immediate action (Box 31-7). It is also important to teach clients and their families what to do in the event of breakage of a mercury-in-glass thermometer.

Nursing Diagnosis

The nurse identifies assessment findings and clusters defining characteristics to form a nursing diagnosis. Nursing diagnoses for clients with body temperature alterations include the following:

- Risk for imbalanced body temperature
- Hyperthermia
- Hypothermia
- Ineffective thermoregulation

For example, an increase in body temperature, flushed skin, skin warm to touch, and tachycardia indicate the diagnosis *hyperthermia*. The nursing diagnosis will be stated as either an at-risk or actual temperature alteration. If the client possesses risk factors for temperature alterations, the nurse minimizes or eliminates them.

Once a diagnosis is determined, the nurse must accurately select the related factor or etiology (Box 31-8). The related factor allows the nurse to select appropriate nursing interventions. In the example of hyperthermia, a related factor of vigorous activity will result in much different interventions than a related factor of decreased ability to perspire.

Box 31-6   Procedural Guidelines

Use of a Mercury-in-Glass Thermometer

Equipment: Mercury-in-glass thermometer (rectal or oral), plastic sleeve, lubricating jelly (rectal only), disposable gloves.

Delegation Considerations: The skill of measuring body temperature can be delegated to assistive personnel (see Skill 31-1, p. 626).

1. Perform hand hygiene. Apply disposable gloves to avoid contact with body fluids (e.g., saliva, stool).
2. Hold end (if color-coded, tip will be blue or red) of glass thermometer with fingertips to reduce contamination of bulb.
3. Read mercury level while gently rotating thermometer at eye level. If mercury is above desired level, grasp tip of thermometer securely, stand away from solid objects, and sharply flick wrist downward. Briskly shaking lowers mercury level in glass tube. Continue shaking until reading is below 35.6° C (96° F). Thermometer reading must be below client's actual temperature before use.
4. Insert thermometer into plastic sleeve cover to protect from body secretions (e.g., saliva, stool). Apply lubricant to cover 2.5 to 3.5 cm (1 to 1½ inches) on rectal thermometer.
5. Place thermometer using technique appropriate to oral, rectal, or axillary site (see Skill 31-1, p. 626).
6. Leave thermometer in place 3 minutes for oral or rectal temperature, 2 minutes for axillary temperature, or according to agency policy.
7. Remove the thermometer. Carefully discard the plastic sleeve. Wipe off secretions with clean tissue, moving toward the bulb.
8. Read thermometer at eye level, read findings, store thermometer in storage container. Remove gloves and perform hand hygiene.

Box 31-7   Steps to Take in the Event of a Mercury Spill

1. Do NOT touch spilled mercury droplets. If skin contact has occurred, immediately flush area with water for 15 minutes.
2. If possible, remove client from immediate contaminated environment.
3. Change any clothing or linen that has been contaminated with mercury. Perform hand hygiene thoroughly after changing. Wash clothing before reuse.
4. Notify the environmental services department or obtain a mercury spill kit if available.
5. Follow procedures for mercury removal as directed by Material Safety Data Sheet (MSDS). Spills are removed using special absorbent materials, filtered vacuum equipment, and protective clothing.
6. Promote exhaust ventilation to reduce concentration of mercury vapors.
7. Follow agency guideline for laundering clothing.
8. Complete occurrence report as directed by institution procedure.

Nursing Diagnostic Process

Box 31-8

Assessment Activities	Defining Characteristics Assessment	Nursing Diagnosis
Obtain vital signs, including temperature, pulse, respirations, SpO$_2$.	Increased body temperature above usual range Tachycardia Tachypnea Hypoxemia	Ineffective thermoregulation related to aging and inability to adapt to environmental temperature
Palpate skin. Observe client's appearance and behavior while talking and resting.	Warm, dry skin Restlessness Confusion Flushed appearance	
Review medical history.	Found in unventilated apartment during heat wave; 85 years old with history of dementia	

Planning

During planning, the nurse integrates the knowledge gathered from assessment and the client history to develop an individualized plan of care (see care plan). The nurse matches the client's needs with those interventions that are supported and recommended in the clinical research literature.

Goals and Outcomes. The plan of care for a client with alteration in temperature must include realistic and individualized goals along with relevant outcomes. This will require the nurse to collaborate closely with the client in setting goals and outcomes and ultimately choosing nursing interventions. Expected outcomes are established to gauge progress toward returning the body temperature to an acceptable range. In cases where the temperature alteration requires helping clients modify their environment, goals may be long term (e.g., obtaining appropriate clothing to wear in cold weather). Short-term goals, such as regaining normal range of body temperature, may be helpful in improving client health. Outcomes must relate to what the nurse learns about the client. For example, if a client has had excessive diaphoresis during a fever episode, an outcome for the goal of attaining fluid and electrolyte balance might be stated "Client intake and output will be equal for the next 24 hours."

Setting Priorities. Priorities of care must be set with regard to the extent the temperature alteration affects a client. The severity of a temperature alteration and its effects, together with the client's general health status, will influence the nurse's priorities in the care of a client. Safety is a top priority. Often, other medical problems complicate the care plan. For instance, alterations in body temperature affect the body's requirements for fluids. Clients with heart problems may have difficulty tolerating required fluid replacement therapy.

Continuity of Care. Clients at high risk for alterations in body temperature require an individualized care plan directed at maintaining normothermia and reducing risk factors. For example, the outcome that the client can explain appropriate actions to take during a heat wave is important to establish. The nurse teaches the client and caregiver the importance of thermoregulation and actions to take during excessive environmental heat. Education is particularly important for parents, who need to know how to take action at home when an infant or child develops a temperature alteration.

Implementation

Health Promotion. Health promotion for clients at risk for altered body temperature is directed toward promoting balance between heat production and heat loss. Client activity, temperature of the environment, and clothing are all considered. The nurse teaches clients to avoid strenuous exercise in hot, humid weather; to drink fluids such as water or clear fruity juices before, during, and after exercise; to wear light, loose-fitting, light-colored clothes; to avoid exercising in areas with poor ventilation; to wear a protective covering over the head when outdoors; and to expose themselves to hot climates gradually.

Prevention is the key for clients at risk for hypothermia. Prevention involves educating clients, family members, and friends. Clients most at risk include the very young and the very old and persons debilitated by trauma, stroke, diabetes, drug or alcohol intoxication, sepsis, and Raynaud's disease. Mentally ill or handicapped clients may fall victim to hypothermia because they are unaware of the dangers of cold conditions. Persons without adequate home heating, shelter, diet, or clothing are also at risk. Fatigue, skin color (African-Americans are more susceptible), malnutrition, and hypoxemia also contribute to the risk of frostbite.

Acute Care
Fever. When an elevated body temperature develops, the nurse initiates interventions to treat fever. The objective of therapy is to increase heat loss, reduce heat production, and prevent complications.

The procedures used to intervene and treat the temperature depend on the cause, any adverse effects, and the strength, intensity, and duration of the elevation. The nurse plays a key role in assessing and implementing temperature-reducing strategies (Box 31-9). The physi-

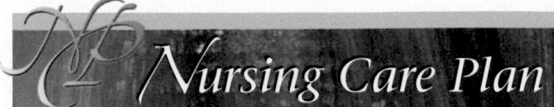

Nursing Care Plan

Elevated Body Temperature

Assessment

Mr. Coburn is a 45-year-old school teacher who arrives at the outpatient clinic with the complaint of malaise.

Assessment Activities	Findings/Defining Characteristics
Palpate skin.	Mr. Coburn's skin is warm and dry to touch.
Observe client's behavior while talking and resting.	Mr. Coburn appears to have labored breathing. His face is flushed.
Obtain vital signs.	Blood pressure right arm 116/62, left arm 114/64; right radial pulse 128, regular and bounding; respiratory rate 26; SpO$_2$ 98% on room air; oral temperature 39.2° C (102.6° F).
Review medical history.	He admits to smoking one pack of cigarettes per day and recently began expectorating yellow-green sputum. He has been tired for the past 3 days and upon rising in the morning has been dizzy.

Nursing Diagnosis: Hyperthermia related to infectious process.

Planning

Goals	Expected Outcomes*
	Thermoregulation
Client will regain normal range of body temperature within next 24 hours.	Body temperature will decline at least 1° C (1.8° F) within next 8 hours.
Client will attain sense of comfort and rest within next 48 hours.	Client will verbalize increased satisfaction with rest and sleep pattern.
	Client will report increase in energy level within next 3 days.
	Vital Signs
Fluid and electrolyte balance will be maintained during next 3 days.	Intake will equal output within next 24 hours.
	No evidence of postural hypotension during ambulation.

*Outcome classification labels from Moorhead S, Johnson M, Maas M: *Nursing outcomes classification (NOC)*, ed 4, St. Louis, 2004, Mosby.

Interventions†	Rationale
Fever Treatment	
• Instruct client to reduce external coverings and keep clothing and bed linen dry.	Promotes heat loss through conduction and convection.
• Instruct client to monitor temperature at home and administer acetaminophen every 4 hours as ordered for temperature over 39° C (102.2° F).	Antipyretics reduce set point.
• Instruct client to limit physical activity and increase frequency of rest periods over next 2 days.	Activity and stress increase metabolic rate, contributing to heat production.
• Instruct client to increase oral fluids of choice.	Fluids lost through insensible water loss require replacement.

†Intervention classification labels from Dochterman JM, Bulechek GM: *Nursing interventions classification (NIC)*, ed 4, St. Louis, 2004, Mosby.

Evaluation

Nursing Actions	Client Response/Finding	Achievement of Outcome
Obtain orthostatic blood pressure measurements.	Blood pressure measurements lying, sitting, and standing are within 5 mm Hg of each other	Fluid volume status adequate.
Review Mr. Coburn's fluid record.		
Ask Mr. Coburn if he has had any episodes of dizziness.	Mr. Coburn denies dizziness.	
Ask Mr. Coburn if his energy level has changed since the last visit.	He responds, "I am sleeping much better and have returned to work with a lot more energy."	Improved rest and sleep pattern and increased energy level.

Box 31-9   **Nursing Measures for Clients With a Fever**

Assessment

- Obtain core temperature during each phase of febrile episode.
- Assess for contributing factors such as dehydration, infection, or environmental temperature.
- Identify physiological response to temperature.
  - Obtain all vital signs.
  - Observe skin color.
  - Assess skin temperature.
  - Observe for shivering and diaphoresis.
  - Assess client comfort and well-being.
- Determine phase of fever: chill, plateau, fever break.

Intervention (Unless Contraindicated)

- Obtain blood cultures when ordered. Blood specimens are obtained to coincide with temperature spikes when the antigen-producing organism is most prevalent.
- Initiate therapies to minimize heat production.
  - Reduce the frequency of activities that increase oxygen demand such as excessive turning and ambulation.
  - Allow rest periods.
  - Limit physical activity.
- Initiate therapies to maximize heat loss.
  - Reduce external covering on client's body to promote heat loss through radiation and conduction. Do not induce shivering.
  - Keep clothing and bed linen dry to increase heat loss through conduction and convection.
- Initiate therapies to meet requirements for increased metabolic rate.
  - Provide supplemental oxygen therapy as ordered to improve oxygen delivery to body cells.
  - Provide measures to stimulate appetite and offer well-balanced meals.
  - Provide fluids (at least 3 L per day for client with normal cardiac and renal function) to replace fluids lost through insensible water loss and sweating.
- Initiate therapies to promote client comfort.
  - Encourage oral hygiene because oral mucous membranes dry easily from dehydration.
  - Control temperature of the environment without inducing shivering.
- Identify onset and duration of febrile episode phases.
- Examine previous temperature measurements for trends.
- Initiate health teaching as indicated.

---

cian may try to determine the cause of the elevated temperature by isolating the causative pyrogen. The nurse may be asked to obtain necessary culture specimens for laboratory analysis such as urine, blood, sputum, and wound sites (see Chapter 33). The physician will order antibiotic medications to be given after the cultures have been obtained. Administering antibiotics destroys pyrogenic bacteria and eliminates the body's stimulus for the elevated temperature.

Most fevers in children are of a viral origin, last only briefly, and have limited effects. However, children still have immature temperature-control mechanisms and temperatures can rise rapidly. Dehydration and febrile seizures occur during rising temperatures of children between 6 months and 3 years of age. Febrile seizures are unusual in children more than 5 years of age. The extent of the temperature, often exceeding 38.8° C (101.8° F), seems to be a more important factor than the rapidity of the temperature increase. Children are at particular risk for fluid volume deficit because they can quickly lose large amounts of fluids in proportion to their body weight. The nurse maintains accurate intake and output records and encourages fluids.

A fever may be a hypersensitivity response to a drug. Drug fevers can be accompanied by other allergy symptoms such as rash or pruritus (itching). Treatment involves withdrawing the medication.

Antipyretics are drugs that reduce fever. Nonsteroidal drugs such as acetaminophen, salicylates, indomethacin, and ketorolac reduce fever by increasing heat loss. Corticosteroids reduce heat production by interfering with the immune system and can mask signs of infection. Corticosteroids are not used to treat a fever. However, the nurse must be aware of their effect on sup-

pressing the ability of the client to develop a fever in response to a pyrogen.

Nonpharmacological therapy for fever uses methods that increase heat loss by evaporation, conduction, convection, or radiation. Traditionally nurses have used tepid sponge baths, bathing with alcohol water solutions, applying ice packs to axillae and groin areas, and cooling fans. These therapies should be avoided because they lead to shivering. There is no demonstrated advantage of these methods over antipyretic medications. Blankets cooled by circulating water delivered by motorized units increase conductive heat loss. The nurse must follow manufacturer's instructions for applying these hypothermia blankets because of the risk for skin breakdown and "freeze burns." Placing a bath blanket between the client and the hypothermia blanket and wrapping distal extremities (fingers, toes, and genitalia) is recommended to reduce the risk of injury to the skin and tissue from hypothermia therapy.

Nursing measures to enhance body cooling must avoid stimulating shivering. Shivering is counterproductive and can increase energy expenditure up to 400%. Wrapping the client's extremities has been recommended to reduce the incidence and intensity of shivering. A dependent nursing intervention for shivering may involve giving medications (e.g., meperidine or butorphanol) that can reduce shivering.

Heatstroke. Heatstroke is an emergency situation. First aid treatment for heatstroke includes moving the client to a cooler environment, reducing clothing covering the body, placing cool wet towels over the skin, and using oscillating fans to increase convective heat loss. Emergency medical treatment may include intravenous

(IV) fluids, irrigating the stomach and lower bowel with cool solutions, and hypothermia blankets.

Hypothermia. The priority treatment for hypothermia is to prevent a further decrease in body temperature. Removing wet clothes, replacing them with dry ones, and wrapping the client in blankets is a key nursing intervention. In emergencies away from a health care setting, the client lies under blankets next to a warm person. A conscious client benefits from drinking hot liquids such as soup, while avoiding alcohol and caffeinated fluids. Keeping the head covered, placing the client near a fire or in a warm room, or placing heating pads next to areas of the body (head and neck) that lose heat the quickest helps.

Restorative and Continuing Care. The nurse educates the client who has been febrile about the importance of taking and continuing any antibiotics as directed until the course of treatment is completed. Children and older adults are at risk for fluid volume deficit because they can quickly lose large amounts of fluids in proportion to their body weight. Identifying preferred fluids and encouraging oral fluid intake is an important ongoing nursing intervention.

Evaluation

All nursing interventions are evaluated by comparing the client's actual response to the expected outcomes of the care plan. This reveals whether goals of care have been met or if a revision to the plan is needed. After any intervention the nurse measures the client's temperature to evaluate for change. In addition, the nurse uses other evaluative measures such as palpation of the skin and assessment of pulse and respirations. If therapies are effective, body temperature will return to an acceptable range, other vital signs will stabilize, and the client will report a sense of comfort.

Pulse

The pulse is the palpable bounding of blood flow noted at various points on the body. Blood flows through the body in a continuous circuit. The pulse is an indicator of circulatory status.

Physiology and Regulation

Electrical impulses originating from the sinoatrial (SA) node travel through heart muscle to stimulate cardiac contraction. Approximately 60 to 70 ml of blood enters the aorta with each ventricular contraction **(stroke volume).** With each stroke volume ejection, the walls of the aorta distend, creating a pulse wave that travels rapidly toward the distal ends of the arteries. The pulse wave moves 15 times faster through the aorta and 100 times faster through the small arteries than the ejected volume of blood. When a pulse wave reaches a peripheral artery, it can be felt by palpating the artery lightly against underlying bone or muscle. The pulse is the palpable bounding of the blood flow in the peripheral artery. The number of pulsing sensations occurring in 1 minute is the pulse rate.

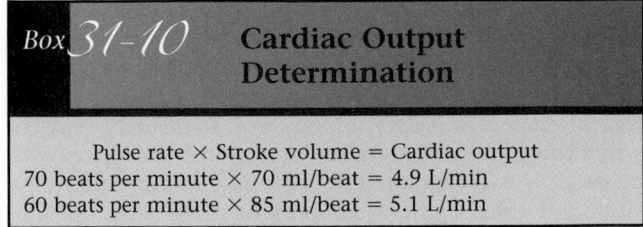

Box 31-10 **Cardiac Output Determination**

Pulse rate × Stroke volume = Cardiac output
70 beats per minute × 70 ml/beat = 4.9 L/min
60 beats per minute × 85 ml/beat = 5.1 L/min

The volume of blood pumped by the heart during 1 minute is the **cardiac output,** the product of heart rate and the ventricle's stroke volume. In an adult the heart normally pumps 5000 ml of blood per minute. A change in heart rate or stroke volume does not always change the heart's output or the amount of blood in the arteries. For example, if a person's heart rate is 70 beats per minute and the stroke volume is 70 ml, the cardiac output is 4900 ml per minute. What happens if the heart rate drops to 60 beats per minute and the stroke volume rises to 85 ml (Box 31-10)?

Mechanical, neural, and chemical factors regulate the strength of heart contractions and its stroke volume. But when mechanical, neural, or chemical factors are unable to alter stroke volume, a change in heart rate will result in a change in blood pressure. As heart rate increases, there is less time for the heart to fill. As heart rate increases without a change in stroke volume, blood pressure will decrease. As the heart rate slows, filling time is increased and blood pressure increases. The inability of blood pressure to respond to increases or decreases in heart rate may indicate a health deviation and is reported to the physician.

The cause of an abnormally slow, rapid, or irregular pulse may alter cardiac output. The nurse assesses the heart's ability to meet the demands of the body's tissue for nutrients by palpating a peripheral pulse or by using a stethoscope to listen to heart sounds (apical rate).

Assessment of Pulse

Any artery can be assessed for pulse rate, but the radial and carotid arteries are commonly used because they are easily palpated. When a client's condition suddenly worsens, the carotid site is recommended for quickly finding a pulse. The heart will continue delivering blood through the carotid artery to the brain as long as possible. When cardiac output declines significantly, peripheral pulses weaken and are difficult to palpate.

The radial and apical locations are the most common sites for pulse rate assessment. The radial pulse is used by persons learning to monitor their own heart rates (e.g., athletes, persons taking heart medications, and clients starting a prescribed exercise regimen). If the **radial pulse** at the wrist is abnormal or intermittent resulting from dysrhythmias, or if it is inaccessible because of a dressing or cast, the apical pulse is assessed. When a client takes medication that affects the heart rate, the apical pulse may provide a more accurate assessment of heart function. The brachial or apical pulse is the best site for assessing an infant's or young child's pulse because other peripheral pulses are deep and difficult to palpate accurately.

Assessment of other peripheral pulse sites such as the brachial or femoral artery is unnecessary when routinely obtaining vital signs. Other peripheral pulses are assessed when a complete physical is conducted, when surgery or treatment has impaired blood flow to a body part, or when there are clinical indications of impaired peripheral blood flow (see Chapter 32). Table 31-2 summarizes pulse sites and criteria for measurement. Skill 31-2 outlines pulse rate assessment.

Use of a Stethoscope. When assessing the apical rate, the nurse uses a stethoscope (Figure 31-6). The five major parts of the stethoscope are the earpieces, binaurals, tubing, bell chestpiece, and diaphragm chestpiece.

The plastic or rubber earpieces should fit snugly and comfortably in the nurse's ears. The binaurals should be angled and strong enough so the earpieces stay firmly in the ears without causing discomfort. To ensure the best reception of sound, the earpieces follow the contour of the ear canal pointing toward the face when the stethoscope is in place.

The polyvinyl tubing should be flexible and 30 to 40 cm (12 to 18 inches) in length. Longer tubing decreases the transmission of sound waves. The tubing should be thick walled and moderately rigid to eliminate transmission of environmental noise and to prevent the tubing from kinking, which distorts sound wave transmission. Stethoscopes can have single or dual tubes.

The chestpiece consists of a bell and a diaphragm that are rotated into position. The diaphragm or bell must be in proper position during use to hear sounds through the stethoscope. To test the position of the chestpiece, tap lightly on the diaphragm to determine which side is functioning. The diaphragm is the circular, flat portion of the chestpiece covered with a thin plastic disk. It transmits high-pitched sounds created by the high-velocity movement of air and blood. Bowel, lung, and heart sounds are auscultated using the diaphragm. The nurse positions the diaphragm to make a tight seal against the client's skin (Figure 31-7). Enough pressure is exerted to leave a temporary red ring on the client's skin when the diaphragm is removed.

The bell is the bowl-shaped chestpiece usually surrounded by a rubber ring. The ring avoids chilling the client with cold metal when placed on the skin. The bell transmits low-pitched sounds created by the low-velocity movement of blood. Heart and vascular sounds are auscultated using the bell. The nurse applies the bell lightly, resting the chestpiece on the skin (Figure 31-8). Compressing the bell against the skin reduces low-pitched sound amplification and creates a "diaphragm of skin." Some stethoscopes have one chestpiece that combines features of the bell and diaphragm. When the nurse uses light pressure, the chestpiece is a bell, whereas exerting more pressure converts the bell into a diaphragm.

The stethoscope is a delicate instrument and requires proper care for optimal function. The earpieces should be removed regularly and cleaned of cerumen (earwax). The bell and diaphragm are cleaned of dust, lint, and body oils. Clean the tubing with mild soap and water.

Character of the Pulse

Assessment of the radial pulse includes measurement of the rate, rhythm, strength, and equality. When auscultating an apical pulse, the nurse assesses rate and rhythm only.

Rate. Before measuring a pulse, the nurse reviews the client's baseline rate for comparison (Table 31-3). Some practitioners prefer to make baseline measurements of the pulse rate as the client assumes a sitting, standing, and lying position. Postural changes cause changes in pulse rate because of alterations in blood volume and sympathetic activity. The heart rate temporarily increases when a person changes from a lying to a sitting or standing position.

Text continued on p. 642

Table 31-2	**Pulse Sites**	
Site	**Location**	**Assessment Criteria**
Temporal	Over temporal bone of head, above and lateral to eye	Easily accessible site used to assess pulse in children
Carotid	Along medial edge of sternocleidomastoid muscle in neck	Easily accessible site used during physiological shock or cardiac arrest when other sites are not palpable
Apical	Fourth to fifth intercostal space at left midclavicular line	Site used to auscultate for apical pulse
Brachial	Groove between biceps and triceps muscles at antecubital fossa	Site used to assess status of circulation to lower arm Site used to auscultate blood pressure
Radial	Radial or thumb side of forearm at wrist	Common site used to assess character of pulse peripherally and assess status of circulation to hand
Ulnar	Ulnar side of forearm at wrist	Site used to assess status of circulation to hand; also used to perform an Allen's test
Femoral	Below inguinal ligament, midway between symphysis pubis and anterior superior iliac spine	Site used to assess character of pulse during physiological shock or cardiac arrest when other pulses are not palpable; used to assess status of circulation to leg
Popliteal	Behind knee in popliteal fossa	Site used to assess status of circulation to lower leg
Posterior tibial	Inner side of ankle, below medial malleolus	Site used to assess status of circulation to foot
Dorsalis pedis	Along top of foot, between extension tendons of great and first toe	Site used to assess status of circulation to foot

Skill 31-2 — *Assessing the Radial and Apical Pulses*

Delegation Considerations

The skill of pulse measurement can be delegated to assistive personnel. The nurse is responsible for assessing changes in pulse. It is important for the nurse to:
- Inform caregiver of client history or risk for irregular pulse.
- Inform caregiver of frequency of pulse measurement for select client.
- Determine that caregiver is aware of the usual values for the client.
- Inform caregiver of the abnormalities that should be reported and reconfirmed by the nurse.

Equipment
- Stethoscope (apical pulse only)
- Wristwatch with second hand or digital display
- Pen, pencil, vital sign flow sheet, or record form
- Alcohol swab

Steps	Rationale
1. Determine need to assess radial or apical pulse:	Nurse uses clinical judgment to determine need for assessment.
a. Note risk factors for alterations in apical pulse.	Certain conditions place clients at risk for pulse alterations. Heart rhythm can be affected by heart disease, cardiac dysrhythmias, onset of sudden chest pain or acute pain from any site, invasive cardiovascular diagnostic tests, surgery, sudden infusion of large volume of IV fluid, internal or external hemorrhage, and administration of medications that alter heart function.
b. Assess for signs and symptoms of altered stroke volume and cardiac output such as dyspnea, fatigue, chest pain, orthopnea, syncope, palpitations (person's unpleasant awareness of heartbeat), jugular venous distention, edema of dependent body parts, cyanosis or pallor of skin.	Physical signs and symptoms may indicate alteration in cardiac function.
2. Assess for factors that normally influence pulse rate and rhythm: age, exercise, position changes, fluid balance, medications, temperature, sympathetic stimulation.	Allows nurse to accurately assess presence and significance of pulse alterations.
3. Determine previous baseline apical rate (if available) from client's record. Otherwise note baseline radial rate.	Allows nurse to assess for change in condition. Provides comparison with future apical pulse measurements.
4. Explain that pulse or heart rate is to be assessed. Encourage client to relax and not speak.	Activity and anxiety can elevate heart rate. Client's voice interferes with nurse's ability to hear sound when apical pulse is measured.
5. Perform hand hygiene.	Reduces transmission of microorganisms.
6. If necessary, draw curtain around bed and/or close door.	Maintains privacy.
7. Obtain pulse measurement.	
A. **Radial pulse**	
(1) Assist client in assuming a supine or sitting position.	Provides easy access to pulse sites.
(2) If supine, place client's forearm straight alongside body or across lower chest or upper abdomen with wrist extended straight (see illustration). If sitting, bend client's elbow 90 degrees and support lower arm on chair or on nurse's arm. Slightly flex the wrist with palm down (see illustration).	Relaxed position of lower arm and slight flexion of wrist promotes exposure of artery to palpation without restriction.
(3) Place tips of first two fingers of hand over groove along radial or thumb side of client's inner wrist (see illustration).	Fingertips are most sensitive parts of hand to palpate arterial pulsation. Nurse's thumb has pulsation that may interfere with accuracy.
(4) Lightly compress against radius, obliterate pulse initially, and then relax pressure so pulse becomes easily palpable.	Pulse is more accurately assessed with moderate pressure. Too much pressure occludes pulse and impairs blood flow.

Skill **31-2**   *Assessing the Radial and Apical Pulses—cont'd*

Steps	Rationale

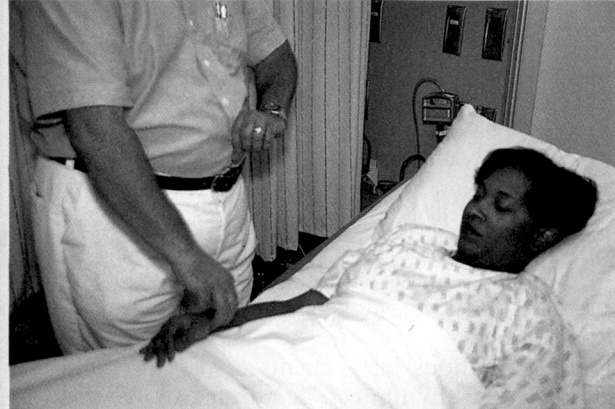

STEP 7A(2) Pulse check with client's forearm at side with wrist extended.

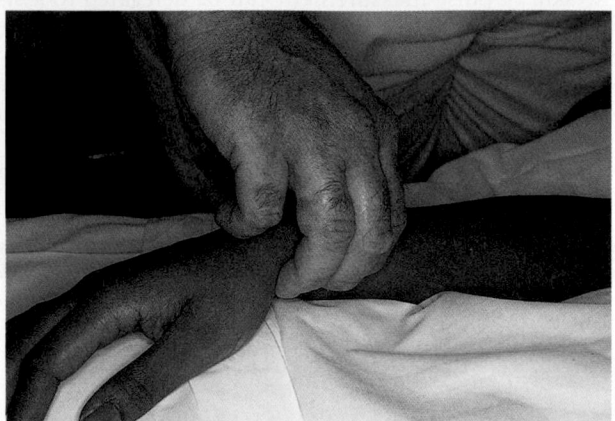

STEP 7A(3) Hand placement for pulse checks.

(5) Determine strength of pulse. Note whether thrust of vessel against fingertips is bounding, strong, weak, or thready.	Strength reflects volume of blood ejected against arterial wall with each heart contraction.
(6) After pulse can be felt regularly, look at watch's second hand and begin to count rate: when sweep hand hits number on dial, start counting with zero, then one, two, and so on.	Rate is determined accurately only after nurse is assured pulse can be palpated. Timing begins with zero. Count of one is first beat palpated after timing begins.
(7) If pulse is regular, count rate for 30 seconds and multiply total by 2.	A 30-second count is accurate for rapid, slow, or regular pulse rates.
(8) If pulse is irregular, count rate for 1 min (60 seconds). Assess frequency and pattern of irregularity.	Inefficient contraction of heart fails to transmit pulse wave, interfering with cardiac output, resulting in irregular pulse. Longer time ensures accurate count.

Critical Decision Point: If pulse is irregular, do an apical/radial pulse assessment to detect a pulse deficit. Count apical pulse while colleague counts radial pulse. Begin apical pulse count out loud to simultaneously assess pulses. If pulse count differs by more than 2, a pulse deficit exists.

B. Apical pulse

(1) Assist client to supine or sitting position. Move aside bed linen and gown to expose sternum and left side of chest.	Exposes portion of chest wall for selection of auscultatory site.
(2) Locate anatomical landmarks to identify the point of maximal impulse (PMI), also called the apical impulse (see illustrations A-D). Heart is located behind and to left of sternum with base at top and apex at bottom. Find angle of Louis just below suprasternal notch between sternal body and manubrium; can be felt as a bony prominence (illustration A). Slip fingers down each side of angle to find second intercostal space (ICS) (illustration B). Carefully move fingers down left side of sternum to fifth ICS (illustration C) and laterally to the left midclavicular line (MCL) (illustration D). A light tap felt within an area 1 to 2 cm (½ to 1 inch) of the PMI is reflected from the apex of the heart.	Use of anatomical landmarks allows correct placement of stethoscope over apex of heart, enhancing ability to hear heart sounds clearly. If unable to palpate the PMI, reposition client on left side. In the presence of serious heart disease, the PMI may be located to the left of the MCL or at the sixth ICS.

Steps	**Rationale**

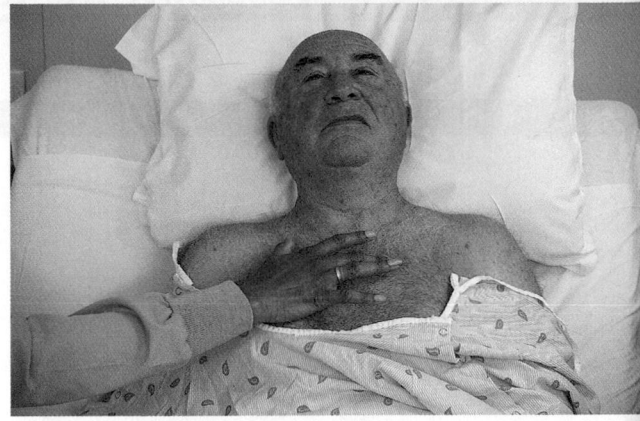

STEP **7B(2)a**   Locating the angle of Louis.

STEP **7B(2)b**   Locating the second intercostal space (ICS).

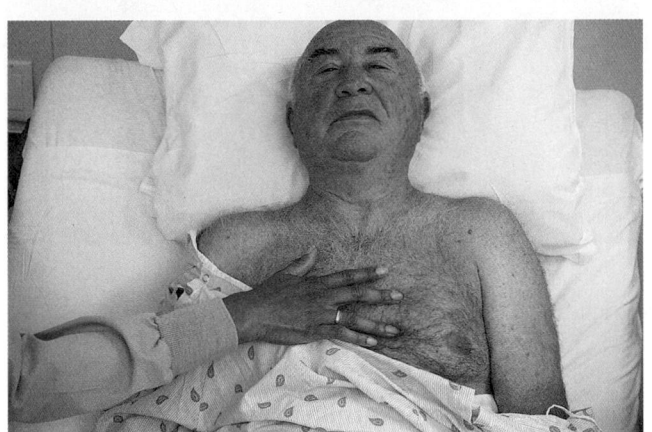

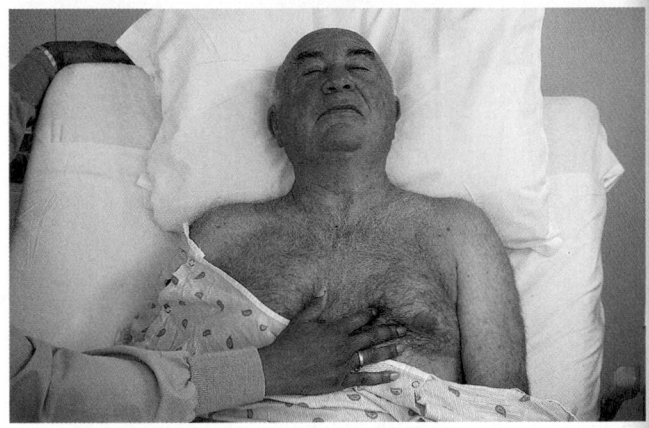

STEP **7B(2)c**   Locating the fifth ICS.

STEP **7B(2)d**   Identifying the midclavicular line (MCL).

Steps	Rationale
(3) Place diaphragm of stethoscope in palm of hand for 5 to 10 seconds.	Warming of metal or plastic diaphragm prevents client from being startled and promotes comfort.
(4) Place diaphragm of stethoscope over PMI at the fifth ICS, at left MCL, and auscultate for normal S_1 and S_2 heart sounds (heard as "lub-dub") (see illustrations).	Allow stethoscope tubing to extend straight without kinks that would distort sound transmission. Normal sounds S_1 and S_2 are high pitched and best heard with the diaphragm.
(5) When S_1 and S_2 are heard with regularity, use watch's second hand and begin to count rate: when sweep hand hits number on dial, start counting with zero, then one, two, and so on.	Apical rate is determined accurately only after nurse is able to auscultate sounds clearly. Timing begins with zero. Count of one is first sound auscultated after timing begins.
(6) If apical rate is regular, count for 30 seconds and multiply by 2.	Regular apical rate can be assessed within 30 seconds.
(7) If heart rate is irregular or client is receiving cardiovascular medication, count for 1 min (60 seconds).	Irregular rate is more accurately assessed when measured over longer interval.
(8) Note regularity of any dysrhythmia (S_1 and S_2 occurring early or later after previous sequence of sounds; for example, every third or every fourth beat is skipped).	Regular occurrence of dysrhythmia within 1 min may indicate inefficient contraction of heart and alteration in cardiac output.
(9) Replace client's gown and bed linen; assist client in returning to comfortable position.	Restores comfort and promotes sense of well-being.

Skill 31-2   *Assessing the Radial and Apical Pulses—cont'd*

Steps	Rationale

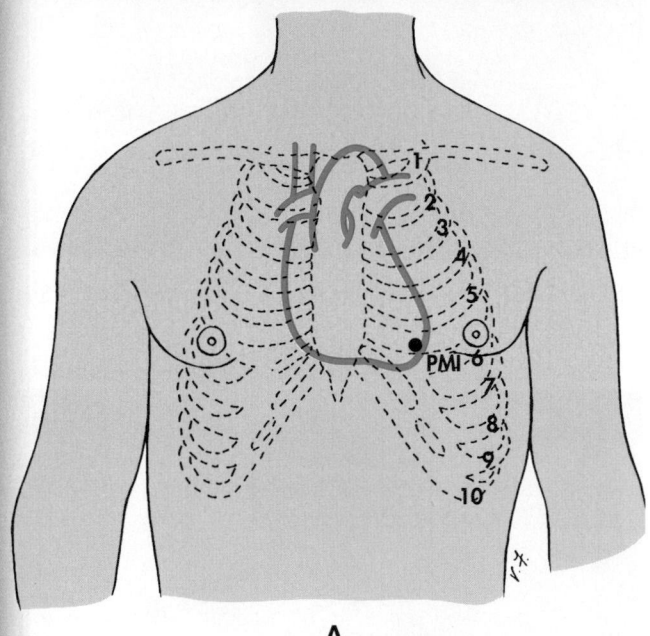

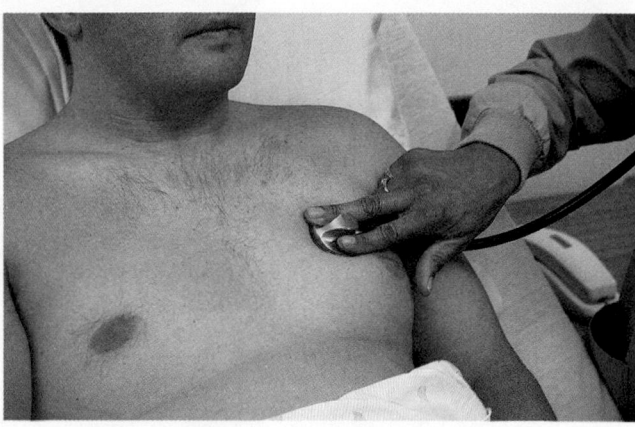

STEP **7B(4)**   **A,** Location of PMI in adult. **B,** Stethoscope over PMI.

(10) Clean earpieces and diaphragm of stethoscope with alcohol swab as needed (optional).	Controls transmission of microorganisms when nurses share stethoscope.
8. Perform hand hygiene.	Reduces transmission of microorganisms.
9. Discuss findings with client as needed.	Promotes participation in care and understanding of health status.
10. Compare readings with previous baseline and/or acceptable range of heart rate for client's age (see Table 31-3).	Evaluates for change in condition and alterations.
11. Compare peripheral pulse rate with apical rate and note discrepancy.	Differences between measurements indicate pulse deficit and may warn of cardiovascular compromise. Abnormalities may require therapy.
12. Compare radial pulse equality and note discrepancy.	Differences between radial arteries indicate compromised peripheral vascular system.
13. Correlate pulse rate with data obtained from blood pressure and related signs and symptoms (palpitations, dizziness).	Pulse rate and blood pressure are interrelated.

Unexpexcted Outcomes and Related Interventions

- Radial pulse is weak and thready.
  - Assess both radial pulses and compare findings. Local obstruction to one extremity (e.g., clot, edema) may decrease peripheral blood flow.
  - Perform complete assessment of all pulses (Chapter 32).
  - Observe for symptoms associated with decreased tissue perfusion (e.g., pallor and cool skin temperature of tissue distal to the weak pulse.
  - Measure apical and radial pulse simultaneously to determine presence of pulse deficit.
- Apical pulse is greater than 100 beats/min (tachycardia).
  - Assess for presence of fever, anxiety, pain, recent exercise, hypotension, decreased oxygenation, or dehydration, all of which can elevate pulse.

- Obtain complete vital signs.
- Assess for factors associated with decreased cardiac output (e.g., chest pain, dyspnea, dizziness).
- Apical pulse is less than 60 beats/min (bradycardia).
  - Assess for the presence of factors that may alter heart rate (e.g., digoxin or other cardiac medications). It may be necessary to withhold prescribed medications until the physician can evaluate the need to adjust dosage.
  - Assess for factors associated with decreased cardiac output.

Recording and Reporting

- Record pulse rate with assessment site in nurses' notes or vital signs flow sheet. Measurement of pulse rate after administration of specific therapies should be documented in narrative form in nurses' notes.
- Report abnormal findings to nurse in charge or physician.

Home Care Considerations

- Assess home environment to determine room that will afford quiet environment for auscultating apical rate.

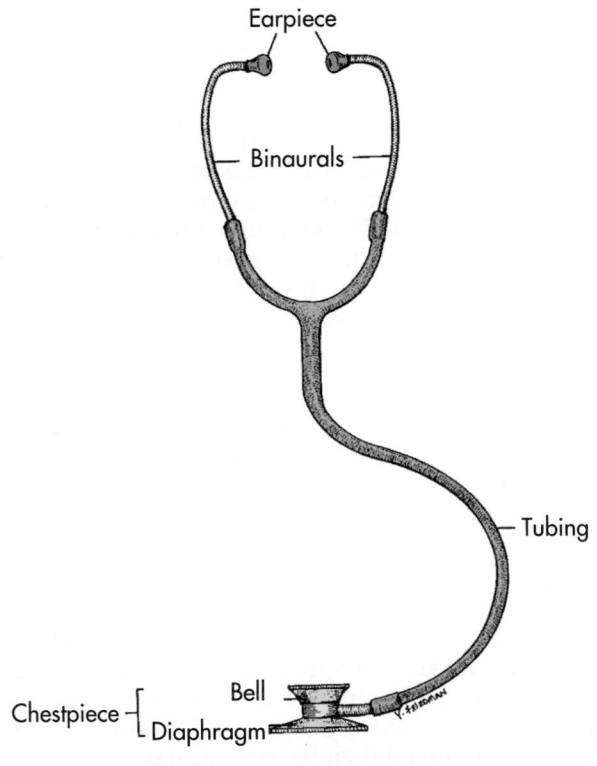

FIGURE **31–6** Parts of a stethoscope.

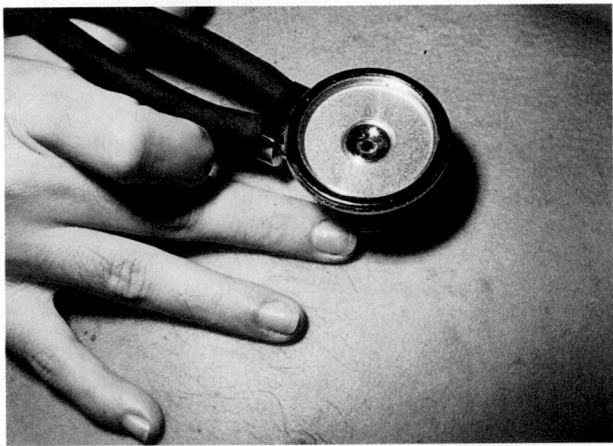

FIGURE **31–8** Positioning the bell of the stethoscope lightly on the skin to hear low-pitched heart sounds.

Table *31-3*	Acceptable Ranges of Heart Rate
Age	**Heart Rate (Beats per Minute)**
Infant	120-160
Toddler	90-140
Preschooler	80-110
School-ager	75-100
Adolescent	60-90
Adult	60-100

Data from Kinney MR and others: *AACN's clinical reference for critical care nursing*, ed 4, St. Louis, 1998, Mosby.

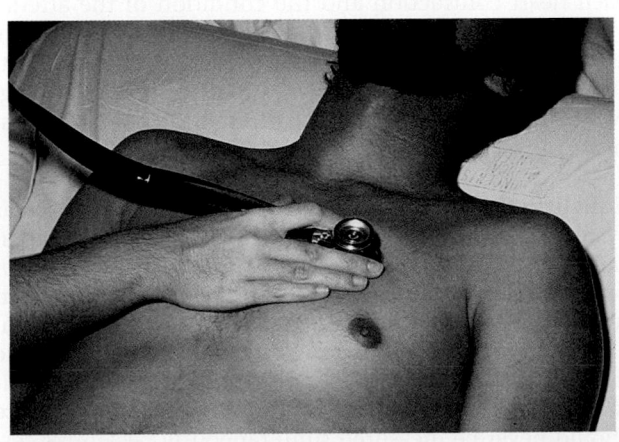

FIGURE **31–7** Positioning the diaphragm of the stethoscope firmly and securely when auscultating high-pitched heart sounds.

Table 31-4	Factors Influencing Pulse Rates	
Factor	**Increases Pulse Rate**	**Decreases Pulse Rate**
Exercise	Short-term exercise.	A conditioned athlete who participates in long-term exercise will have a lower heart rate at rest.
Temperature	Fever and heat.	Hypothermia.
Emotions	Acute pain and anxiety increase sympathetic stimulation, affecting heart rate.	Unrelieved severe pain increases parasympathetic stimulation, affecting heart rate; relaxation.
Drugs	Positive chronotropic drugs such as epinephrine.	Negative chronotropic drugs such as digitalis; beta and calcium blockers.
Hemorrhage	Loss of blood increases sympathetic stimulation.	
Postural changes	Standing or sitting.	Lying down.
Pulmonary conditions	Diseases causing poor oxygenation such as asthma, chronic obstructive pulmonary disease (COPD).	

When assessing the pulse, the nurse must consider the variety of factors influencing the pulse rate (Table 31-4). A single factor or a combination of these factors may cause significant changes. If the nurse detects an abnormal rate while palpating a peripheral pulse, the next step is to assess the apical rate. The apical rate requires auscultation of heart sounds, which provides a more accurate assessment of cardiac contraction.

The nurse assesses the apical rate by listening for heart sounds (see Chapter 32). The nurse tries to identify the first and second heart sounds (S_1 and S_2). At normal slow rates, S_1 is low pitched and dull, sounding like a "lub." S_2 is higher pitched and shorter, creating the sound "dub." Each set of "lub-dub" is counted as one heartbeat. Using the diaphragm or bell of the stethoscope, the nurse counts the number of lub-dubs occurring in 1 minute.

Peripheral and apical pulse rate assessment may reveal variations in heart rate. Two common abnormalities in pulse rate are tachycardia and bradycardia. **Tachycardia** is an abnormally elevated heart rate, above 100 beats per minute in adults. **Bradycardia** is a slow rate, below 60 beats per minute in adults.

An inefficient contraction of the heart that fails to transmit a pulse wave to the peripheral pulse site creates a **pulse deficit.** To assess a pulse deficit the nurse and a colleague assess radial and apical rates simultaneously and then compare rates. The difference between the apical and radial pulse rates is the pulse deficit. For example, an apical rate of 92 with a radial rate of 78 leaves a pulse deficit of 14 beats. Pulse deficits are frequently associated with abnormal rhythms.

Rhythm. Normally a regular interval occurs between each pulse or heartbeat. An interval interrupted by an early or late beat or a missed beat indicates an abnormal rhythm or **dysrhythmia.** A dysrhythmia threatens the heart's ability to provide adequate cardiac output, particularly if it occurs repetitively. The nurse identifies a dysrhythmia by palpating an interruption in successive pulse waves or auscultating an interruption between heart sounds. If a dysrhythmia is present, the regularity of its occurrence should be assessed and the apical rate is auscultated (see Chapter 32). Dysrhythmias may be described as regularly irregular or irregularly irregular.

To document a dysrhythmia, a physician may order an electrocardiogram, Holter monitor, or telemetry. An electrocardiogram records the electrical activity of the heart for a 12-second interval. This test requires placement of electrodes across the client's chest followed by recording of the heart rhythm. The Holter monitor records 24 hours of electrical activity in a small tape recorder that the client wears. Access to the information recorded is not available until after the 24 hours have passed and the data are printed for review. Cardiac telemetry provides continuous monitoring of the heart's electrical activity transmitted to a stationary monitor. Telemetry permits observation of heart rhythm during all of the client's daily activities and thus allows for immediate treatment if the rhythm becomes erratic or unstable.

Children often have a sinus dysrhythmia, which is an irregular heartbeat that speeds up with inspiration and slows down with expiration. This is a normal finding and can be verified by having the child hold his or her breath; the heart rate should then become regular.

Strength. The strength or amplitude of a pulse reflects the volume of blood ejected against the arterial wall with each heart contraction and the condition of the arterial vascular system leading to the pulse site. Normally the pulse strength remains the same with each heartbeat. Pulse strength may be graded or described as strong, weak, thready, or bounding. It is included during assessment of the vascular system (see Chapter 32).

Equality. Pulses on both sides of the peripheral vascular system should be assessed. The nurse assesses both radial pulses to compare the characteristics of each. A pulse in one extremity may be unequal in strength or absent in many disease states (e.g., thrombus [clot] formation, aberrant blood vessels, cervical rib syndrome, or aortic dissection). All symmetrical pulses can be assessed simultaneously except for the carotid pulse. The carotid pulse should never be measured simultaneously because excessive pressure may occlude blood supply to the brain.

Nursing Process and Pulse Determination

Pulse assessment determines the general state of cardiovascular health and the response to other system imbalances. Tachycardia, bradycardia, and dysrhythmias are defining characteristics of many nursing diagnoses including the following:

- Activity intolerance
- Anxiety
- Decreased cardiac uutput
- Fear
- Deficient/excess fluid volume
- Impaired gas exchange
- Hyperthermia
- Hypothermia
- Acute pain
- Ineffective tissue perfusion

The nursing care plan includes interventions based on the nursing diagnosis identified and the related factor. For example, the defining characteristics of an abnormal heart rate, exertional dyspnea, and a client's verbal report of fatigue lead to a diagnosis of *activity intolerance*. The nurse evaluates client outcomes by assessing the pulse rate, rhythm, strength, and equality following each intervention.

Respiration

Human survival depends on the ability of oxygen (O_2) to reach body cells and for carbon dioxide (CO_2) to be removed from the cells. Respiration is the mechanism the body uses to exchange gases between the atmosphere and the blood and the blood and the cells. Respiration involves **ventilation** (the movement of gases in and out of the lungs), **diffusion** (the movement of oxygen and carbon dioxide between the alveoli and the red blood cells), and **perfusion** (the distribution of red blood cells to and from the pulmonary capillaries). Analyzing respiratory efficiency requires integrating assessment data from all three processes. Ventilation is assessed by determining respiratory rate, respiratory depth, and respiratory rhythm. Diffusion and perfusion can be assessed by determining oxygen saturation.

Physiological Control

Breathing is generally a passive process. Normally a person thinks little about it. The respiratory center in the brain stem regulates the involuntary control of respirations. Adults normally breathe in a smooth, uninterrupted pattern, 12 to 16 times a minute.

Ventilation is regulated by levels of CO_2, O_2, and hydrogen ion concentration (pH) in the arterial blood. The most important factor in the control of ventilation is the level of CO_2 in the arterial blood. An elevation in the CO_2 level causes the respiratory control system in the brain to increase the rate and depth of breathing. The increased ventilatory effort removes excess CO_2 (hypercarbia) by increasing exhalation. However, clients with chronic lung disease have ongoing hypercarbia. For these clients chemoreceptors in the carotid artery and aorta become sensitive to **hypoxemia,** or low levels of arterial O_2. If ar-

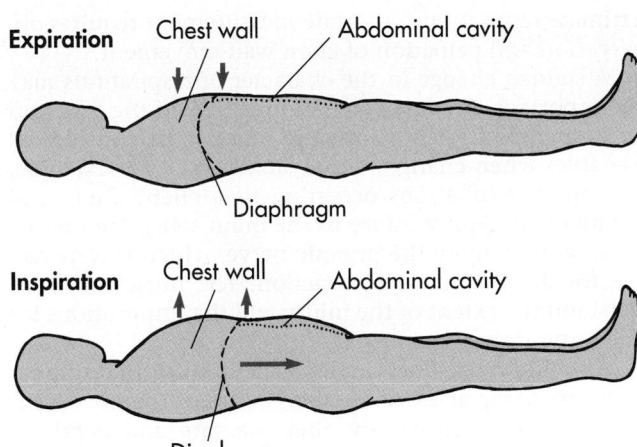

FIGURE 31–9   Illustration of diaphragmatic and chest wall movement during inspiration and expiration.

terial oxygen levels fall, these receptors signal the brain to increase the rate and depth of ventilation. Hypoxemia helps to control ventilation in clients with chronic lung disease. Because low levels of arterial O_2 provide the stimulus that allows the client to breathe, administration of high oxygen levels can be fatal for clients with chronic lung disease.

Mechanics of Breathing

Although breathing is normally passive, muscular work is involved in moving the lungs and chest wall. Inspiration is an active process. During inspiration the respiratory center sends impulses along the phrenic nerve, causing the diaphragm to contract. Abdominal organs move downward and forward, increasing the length of the chest cavity to move air into the lungs. The diaphragm moves approximately 1 cm ($\frac{4}{10}$ inch), and the ribs retract upward from the body's midline approximately 1.2 to 2.5 cm ($\frac{1}{2}$ to 1 inch). During a normal, relaxed breath, a person inhales 500 ml of air. This amount is referred to as the **tidal volume.** During expiration the diaphragm relaxes and the abdominal organs return to their original positions. The lung and chest wall return to a relaxed position (Figure 31-9). Expiration is a passive process. The normal rate and depth of ventilation, **eupnea,** is interrupted by sighing. The sigh, a prolonged deeper breath, is a protective physiological mechanism for expanding small airways and alveoli not ventilated during a normal breath.

The accurate assessment of respirations depends on the nurse's recognition of normal thoracic and abdominal movements. During quiet breathing the chest wall gently rises and falls. Contraction of the intercostal muscles between the ribs or contraction of the muscles in the neck and shoulders, the accessory muscles of breathing, is not visible. During normal quiet breathing, diaphragmatic movement causes the abdominal cavity to rise and fall slowly.

Assessment of Ventilation

Respirations are the easiest of all vital signs, but they are often the most haphazardly measured. A nurse must not estimate respirations. Accurate measurement requires observation and palpation of chest wall movement.

A sudden change in the character of respirations may be important. Because respiration is tied to the function of numerous body systems, the nurse must consider all variables when changes occur (Box 31-11). For example, a drop in respirations occurring in a client after head trauma may signify injury to the brain stem. Abdominal trauma may injure the phrenic nerve, which is responsible for diaphragmatic contraction. The nurse must understand the extent of the injury and the implications for the respiratory system.

A skillful nurse does not let a client know that respirations are being assessed. A client aware of the nurse's intentions may consciously alter the rate and depth of breathing. Measurement can best be done immediately after measuring pulse rate, with the nurse's hand still on the client's wrist as it rests over the chest or abdomen. When assessing a client's respirations, the nurse should keep in mind the client's usual ventilatory rate and pattern, the influence any disease or illness has on respiratory function, the relationship between respiratory and cardiovascular function, and the influence of therapies on respirations. The objective measurements of an assessment of respiratory status include the rate and depth of breathing and the rhythm of ventilatory movements (Skill 31-3).

Respiratory Rate. The nurse observes a full inspiration and expiration when counting ventilation or respiration rate. The respiratory rate varies with age (Table 31-5). The usual range of respiratory rate declines throughout life.

A respiratory monitoring device that aids the nurse's assessment is the apnea monitor. This device uses leads attached to the client's chest wall that sense movement. The absence of chest wall movement triggers the apnea alarm. Apnea monitoring is used frequently with infants in the hospital and at home to observe for prolonged apneic events.

Ventilatory Depth. The depth of respirations is assessed by observing the degree of excursion or movement in the chest wall. The nurse subjectively describes ventilatory movements as deep, normal, or shallow. A deep respiration involves a full expansion of the lungs with full exhalation. Respirations are shallow when only a small quantity of air passes through the lungs and ventilatory movement is difficult to see. More objective techniques are used if the nurse observes that chest excursion is unusually shallow (see Chapter 32). Table 31-6 summarizes types of breathing patterns.

Ventilatory Rhythm. Breathing pattern can be determined by observing the chest or the abdomen. Diaphragmatic breathing results from the contraction and relaxation of the diaphragm and is best observed by watching abdominal movements. Healthy men and children usually demonstrate diaphragmatic breathing. Women tend to use thoracic muscles to breathe; movements are observed in the upper chest. Labored respirations usually involve the accessory muscles of respiration visible in the neck. When something such as a foreign body interferes with the movement of air in and out of the lungs, the intercostal spaces retract during inspiration. A longer expiration

---

Box 31-11   Factors Influencing Character of Respirations

Exercise

Exercise increases rate and depth to meet the body's need for additional oxygen and to rid the body of CO_2.

Acute Pain

Pain alters rate and rhythm of respirations; breathing becomes shallow.
Client may inhibit or splint chest wall movement when pain is in area of chest or abdomen.

Anxiety

Anxiety increases rate and depth as a result of sympathetic stimulation.

Smoking

Chronic smoking changes the lung's airways, resulting in increased rate of respirations at rest when not smoking.

Body Position

A straight, erect posture promotes full chest expansion.
A stooped or slumped position impairs ventilatory movement.
Lying flat prevents full chest expansion.

Medications

Narcotic analgesics, general anesthetics, and sedative hypnotics depress rate and depth.
Amphetamines and cocaine may increase rate and depth.
Bronchodilators slow rate by causing airway dilation.

Neurological Injury

Injury to the brain stem impairs the respiratory center and inhibits respiratory rate and rhythm.

Hemoglobin Function

Decreased hemoglobin levels (anemia) reduce oxygen-carrying capacity of the blood, which increases respiratory rate.
Increased altitude lowers the amount of saturated hemoglobin, which increases respiratory rate and depth.
Abnormal blood cell function (e.g., sickle cell disease) reduces ability of hemoglobin to carry oxygen, which increases respiratory rate and depth.

Skill 31-3   Assessing Respirations

Delegation Considerations

The skill of respiration measurement can be delegated to assistive personnel. The nurse is responsible for assessing for change in respiration rate, rhythm, and depth. It is important for the nurse to:
- Inform caregiver of client history or risk for increased or decreased respiratory rate or irregular respirations.
- Inform caregiver of frequency of respirations measurement for specific client.

- Determine that caregiver is aware of the usual values for the client.
- Inform caregiver of the abnormalities that should be reported and reconfirmed by the nurse.

Equipment
- Wristwatch with second hand or digital display
- Pen, pencil, vital sign flow sheet or record form

Steps	Rationale
1. Determine need to assess client's respirations:	Nurse uses clinical judgment to determine need for assessment.
a. Note risk factors for respiratory alterations.	Certain conditions place client at risk for alterations in ventilation detected by changes in respiratory rate, depth, and rhythm. Fever, pain, anxiety, diseases of chest wall or muscles, constrictive chest or abdominal dressings, gastric distention, chronic pulmonary disease (emphysema, bronchitis, asthma), traumatic injury to chest wall with or without collapse of underlying lung tissue, presence of a chest tube, respiratory infection (pneumonia, acute bronchitis), pulmonary edema and emboli, head injury with damage to brain stem, and anemia can result in respiratory alteration.
b. Assess for signs and symptoms of respiratory alterations such as bluish or cyanotic appearance of nail beds, lips, mucous membranes, and skin; restlessness, irritability, confusion, reduced level of consciousness; pain during inspiration; labored or difficult breathing; adventitious breath sounds (see Chapter 32), inability to breathe spontaneously; thick, frothy, blood-tinged, or copious sputum produced on coughing.	Physical signs and symptoms may indicate alterations in respiratory status related to ventilation.
2. Assess pertinent laboratory values:	
A. **Arterial blood gases (ABGs):** Normal ABGs (values may vary slightly within institutions): pH 7.35-7.45 $PaCO_2$ 35-45 PaO_2 80-100 SaO_2 95%-100%	Arterial blood gases measure arterial blood pH, partial pressure of O_2 and CO_2, and arterial O_2 saturation, which reflects client's oxygenation status.
B. **Pulse oximetry (SpO_2):** Acceptable SpO_2 90%-100%; 85%-89% may be acceptable for certain chronic disease conditions; less than 85% is abnormal (see Skill 31-4, p. 651).	SpO_2 less than 85% is often accompanied by changes in respiratory rate, depth, and rhythm.
C. **Complete blood count (CBC):** Normal CBC for adults (values may vary within institutions): *Hemoglobin:* 14 to 18 g/100 ml, males; 12 to 16 g/100 ml, females *Hematocrit:* 40% to 54%, males; 38% to 47%, females *Red blood cell count:* 4.7 to 6.1 million/ml, males; 4.2 to 5.4 million/ml, females	Complete blood count measures red blood cell count, volume of red blood cells, and concentration of hemoglobin, which reflects client's capacity to carry O_2.
3. Determine previous baseline respiratory rate (if available) from client's record.	Allows nurse to assess for change in condition. Provides comparison with future respiratory measurements.

Skill 31-3   *Assessing Respirations*

Steps	Rationale
4. Perform hand hygiene. Draw curtain around bed and/or close door.	Prevents transmission of microorganisms. Maintains privacy.

Critical Decision Point: Clients with difficulty breathing (dyspnea) such as those with congestive heart failure or abdominal ascites or in late stages of pregnancy should be assessed in the position of greatest comfort. Repositioning may increase the work of breathing, which will increase respiratory rate.

---

5. Be sure client is in comfortable position, preferably sitting or lying with the head of the bed elevated 45 to 60 degrees. Be sure client's chest is visible. If necessary, move bed linen or gown.	Sitting erect promotes full ventilatory movement. Ensures clear view of chest wall and abdominal movements.
6. Place client's arm in relaxed position across the abdomen or lower chest, or place nurse's hand directly over client's upper abdomen (see illustration).	A similar position used during pulse assessment allows respiratory rate assessment to be inconspicuous. Client's hand or your hand rises and falls during respiratory cycle.
7. Observe complete respiratory cycle (one inspiration and one expiration).	Rate is accurately determined only after nurse has viewed respiratory cycle.
8. After cycle is observed, look at watch's second hand and begin to count rate: when sweep hand hits number on dial, begin time frame, counting one with first full respiratory cycle.	Timing begins with count of one. Respirations occur more slowly than pulse; thus timing does not begin with zero.
9. If rhythm is regular, count number of respirations in 30 seconds and multiply by 2. If rhythm is irregular, less than 12, or greater than 20, count for 1 full min.	Respiratory rate is equivalent to number of respirations per minute. Suspected irregularities require assessment for at least 1 min.

Critical Decision Point: Respiratory rate less than 12 or greater than 20 requires further assessment (see Chapter 32) and may require immediate intervention.

---

10. Note depth of respirations, subjectively assessed by observing degree of chest wall movement while counting rate. Nurse can also objectively assess depth by palpating chest wall excursion or auscultating the posterior thorax after rate has been counted (see Chapter 32). Depth is described as shallow, normal, or deep.	Character of ventilatory movement may reveal specific disease state restricting volume of air from moving into and out of the lungs.

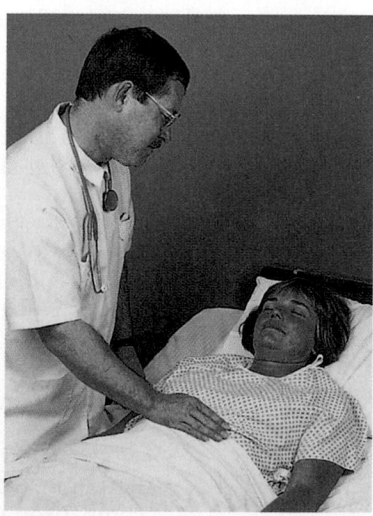

STEP **6**   Nurse's hand over client's abdomen to check respiration.

Steps	Rationale
11. Note rhythm of ventilatory cycle. Normal breathing is regular and uninterrupted. Sighing should not be confused with abnormal rhythm.	Character of ventilations can reveal specific types of alterations.

Critical Decision Point: Any irregular respiratory pattern or periods of apnea (the cessation of respiration for several seconds) are symptoms of underlying disease in the adult and must be reported to the physician or nurse in charge. Further assessment may be required (Chapter 32) and immediate intervention may be needed. An irregular respiratory rate and short apneic spells are normal for newborns.

Steps	Rationale
12. Replace bed linen and client's gown.	Restores comfort and promotes sense of well-being.
13. Perform hand hygiene.	Reduces transmission of microorganisms.
14. Discuss findings with client as needed.	Promotes participation in care and understanding of health status.
15. If respirations are assessed for the first time, establish rate, rhythm, and depth as baseline if within normal range.	Used to compare future respiratory assessment.
16. Compare respirations with client's previous baseline and normal rate, rhythm, and depth.	Allows nurse to assess for changes in client's condition and for presence of respiratory alterations.

Unexpexcted Outcomes and Related Interventions

- Client has abnormal respiratory rate, depth, or states a feeling of being short of breath.
  - Observe for related factors, including obstructed airway, abnormal breath sounds, productive cough, restlessness, irritability, anxiety, confusion.
  - Position client to a position to improve ventilation such as sitting position (semi- or high-Fowler's) unless contraindicated.
  - When possible, remove respiratory irritants from the environment, such as second-hand smoke, perfumes, etc.

Recording and Reporting

- Record respiratory rate and character in nurses' notes or vital sign flow sheet. Indicate type and amount of oxygen therapy if used by client during assessment. Measurement of respiratory rate after administration of specific therapies should be documented in narrative form in nurses' notes.
- Report abnormal findings to nurse in charge or physician.

Home Care Considerations

- Assess for environmental factors in the home that may influence client's respiratory rate such as secondhand smoke, poor ventilation, or gas fumes.

Table 31-5	Acceptable Range of Respiratory Rates for Age
Age	**Rate (Breaths per Minute)**
Newborn	30-60
Infant (6 months)	30-50
Toddler (2 years)	25-32
Child	20-30
Adolescent	16-19
Adult	12-20

phase is evident when the outward flow of air is obstructed (e.g., asthma).

With normal breathing a regular interval occurs after each respiratory cycle. Infants tend to breathe less regularly. The young child may breathe slowly for a few seconds and then suddenly breathe more rapidly. While assessing respirations, the nurse estimates the time interval after each respiratory cycle. Respiration is regular or irregular in rhythm.

Assessment of Diffusion and Perfusion

The respiratory processes of diffusion and perfusion can be evaluated by measuring the oxygen saturation of the blood. Blood flow through the pulmonary capillaries provides red blood cells for oxygen attachment. After oxygen diffuses from the alveoli into the pulmonary blood, most of the oxygen attaches to hemoglobin molecules in red blood cells. Red blood cells carry the oxygenated hemoglobin molecules through the left side of the heart and out to the peripheral capillaries, where the oxygen detaches, depending on the needs of the tissues.

The percent of hemoglobin that is bound with oxygen in the arteries is the percent of saturation of hemoglobin (or SaO_2). It is usually between 95% and 100%. SaO_2 is affected by factors that interfere with ventilation, perfusion, or diffusion (see Chapter 39). The saturation of venous blood (SvO_2) is lower because the tissues have removed some of the oxygen from the hemoglobin molecules. A normal value for SvO_2 is 70%. SvO_2 is affected by factors that interfere with or increase the tissue's need for oxygen.

Table 31-6	Alterations in Breathing Pattern
Alteration	**Description**
Bradypnea	Rate of breathing is regular but abnormally slow (less than 12 breaths per minute).
Tachypnea	Rate of breathing is regular but abnormally rapid (greater than 20 breaths per minute).
Hyperpnea	Respirations are labored, increased in depth, and increased in rate (greater than 20 breaths per minute). Occurs normally during exercise.
Apnea	Respirations cease for several seconds. Persistent cessation results in respiratory arrest.
Hyperventilation	Rate and depth of respirations increase. Hypocarbia may occur.
Hypoventilation	Respiratory rate is abnormally low, and depth of ventilation may be depressed. Hypercarbia may occur.
Cheyne-Stokes respiration	Respiratory rate and depth are irregular, characterized by alternating periods of apnea and hyperventilation. Respiratory cycle begins with slow, shallow breaths that gradually increase to abnormal rate and depth. The pattern reverses, breathing slows and becomes shallow, climaxing in apnea before respiration resumes.
Kussmaul's respiration	Respirations are abnormally deep, regular, and increased in rate.
Biot's respiration	Respirations are abnormally shallow for two to three breaths followed by irregular period of apnea.

Measurement of Arterial Oxygen Saturation. A pulse oximeter permits the indirect measurement of oxygen saturation (Skill 31-4). The pulse oximeter is a probe with a light-emitting diode (LED) and photo detector connected by cable to an oximeter (Figure 31-10). The LED emits light wavelengths that are absorbed differently by the oxygenated and deoxygenated hemoglobin molecules. The photo detector detects the light-absorbing differences, and the oximeter calculates the pulse saturation (SpO_2). SpO_2 is a reliable estimate of SaO_2 when the SaO_2 is over 70%. Values obtained with pulse oximetry are less accurate at saturations less than 70% (Grap, 2002).

The photo detector is contained within the oximeter probe. Selecting the appropriate probe is important to reduce measurement error. Digit probes are spring loaded and conform to various sizes. Earlobe probes have greater accuracy at lower saturations and are least affected by peripheral vasoconstriction (Grap, 2002). Disposable sensor pads can be applied to a variety of sites, even the bridge of an adult's nose or the sole of an infant's foot. The ability of the photo detector to measure SpO_2 is affected by factors that affect light transmission or peripheral arterial pulsations (Box 31-12). An awareness of these factors allows accurate interpretation of abnormal SpO_2 measurements.

Nursing Process and Respiratory Vital Signs

Vital sign measurement of respiratory rate, pattern, and depth, along with SpO_2, allows the nurse to assess ventilation, diffusion, and perfusion. The nurse may also conduct other assessments to measure respiratory status (see Chapter 32). Each measurement can provide clues in determining the nature of a client's problem. Respiratory assessment data are defining characteristics of many nursing diagnoses including the following:

- Activity intolerance
- Ineffective airway clearance
- Anxiety
- Ineffective breathing pattern
- Impaired gas exchange
- Acute pain

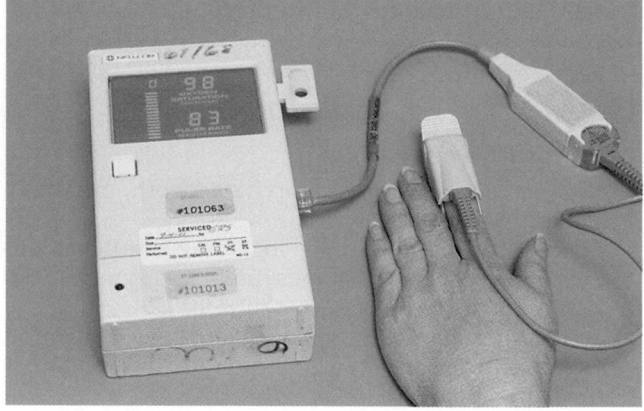

FIGURE **31–10**   Portable pulse oximeter with digit probe.

- Ineffective tissue perfusion
- Dysfunctional ventilatory weaning response

The nursing care plan includes interventions based on the nursing diagnosis identified and the related factor. For example, the defining characteristics of tachypnea, changes in depth of respirations, use of accessory muscles, cyanosis, and a decline in SpO_2 lead to a diagnosis of *impaired gas exchange*. Related factors may include postoperative lobectomy with chest tube placement, a history of chronic obstructive lung disease, and 30 pack-year history of smoking. The nurse evaluates client outcomes by assessing the respiratory rate, ventilatory depth, rhythm, and SpO_2 following each intervention.

Blood Pressure

Blood pressure is the force exerted on the walls of an artery by the pulsing blood under pressure from the heart. Blood flows throughout the circulatory system because of pressure changes. It moves from an area of high pressure to an area of low pressure. Systemic or arterial blood pressure, the blood pressure in the system of arteries in the body, is a good indicator of cardiovascular

Skill 31-4   *Measuring Oxygen Saturation (Pulse Oximetry)*

Delegation Considerations

The skill of oxygen saturation measurement can be delegated to assistive personnel. The nurse is responsible for assessing the impact of changes in oxygen saturation. It is important for the nurse to:

- Inform caregiver to notify nurse immediately of any reading lower than SpO_2 of 90%.
- Inform caregiver of appropriate sensor site and probe for measurement of oxygen saturation.
- Inform caregiver of frequency of oxygen saturation measurements for specific client.
- Determine that caregiver is aware of factors that can falsely lower SpO_2 (see Box 31-11, p. 646).

Equipment

- Oximeter
- Oximeter probe appropriate for client and recommended by manufacturer
- Acetone or nail polish remover
- Pen, pencil, vital sign flow sheet, or record form

Steps	Rationale
1. Determine need to measure client's oxygen saturation:	Nurse uses clinical judgment to determine need for assessment.
a. Note risk factors for alteration of oxygen saturation.	Certain conditions place clients at risk for decreased oxygen saturation: acute or chronic compromised respiratory function, recovery from general anesthesia or conscious sedation, or traumatic injury to chest wall with or without collapse of underlying lung tissue, ventilator dependence, changes in supplemental oxygen therapy.
b. Assess for signs and symptoms of alterations in oxygen saturation such as altered respiratory rate, depth, or rhythm; adventitious breath sounds (see Chapter 32); cyanotic appearance of nail beds, lips, mucous membranes, and skin; restlessness, irritability, confusion; reduced level of consciousness; labored or difficult breathing.	Physical signs and symptoms may indicate abnormal oxygen saturation.
2. Assess for factors that normally influence measurement of SpO_2 such as oxygen therapy, hemoglobin level, and temperature.	Allows nurse to accurately assess oxygen saturation variations. Peripheral vasoconstriction related to hypothermia can interfere with SpO_2 determination.
3. Review client's medical record for physician's order or consult agency policy or procedure manual for standard of care.	Medical order may be required to assess oxygen saturation.
4. Determine previous baseline SpO_2 (if available) from client's record.	Baseline information provides basis for comparison and assists in assessment of current status and evaluation of interventions.
5. Perform hand hygiene.	Reduces transmission of microorganisms.
6. Explain purpose of procedure to client and how oxygen saturation will be measured. Instruct client to breathe normally.	Promotes client cooperation and increases compliance. Prevents large fluctuations in minute ventilation and possible error in SpO_2 readings.
7. Assess site most appropriate for sensor probe placement (e.g., digit, earlobe). Site must have adequate local circulation and be free of moisture.	Peripheral vasoconstriction can interfere with SpO_2 determination. Dark nail polish and acrylic nails impede sensor detection of emitted light and produce falsely elevated SpO_2. Moisture impedes ability of sensor to detect SpO_2 levels.
8. Position client comfortably. If finger is chosen as monitoring site, support lower arm.	Ensures probe positioning and decreases motion artifact that interferes with SpO_2 determination.
9. Instruct client to breathe normally.	Prevents large fluctuations in respiratory rate and depth and possible changes in SpO_2.
10. If finger is to be used, remove any fingernail polish with acetone from digit to be assessed.	Ensures accurate readings. Opaque coatings decrease light transmission; nail polish containing blue pigment can absorb light emissions and falsely alter saturation.
11. Attach sensor probe to monitoring site. Instruct client that clip-on probe feels like a clothespin on the finger but will not hurt.	Pressure of sensor probe's spring tension on a peripheral digit or earlobe may be unexpected.

Skill 31-4   *M*easuring Oxygen Saturation (Pulse Oximetry)—cont'd

Steps	Rationale

Critical Decision Point: Do not attach probe to finger, ear, or bridge of nose if area is edematous or skin integrity is compromised. Do not attach probe to fingers that are hypothermic. Select ear or bridge of nose if adult client has history of peripheral vascular disease. Earlobe and bridge of nose sensors are not used for infants and toddlers because of skin fragility. Disposable adhesive probes contain latex and should not be used if client has latex allergy.

Steps	Rationale
12. Turn on oximeter by activating power. Observe pulse waveform/intensity display and audible beep. Correlate oximeter pulse rate with client's radial pulse. Differences require reevaluation of oximeter probe placement and may require reassessment of pulse rates.	Pulse waveform/intensity display enables detection of valid pulse or presence of interfering signal. Pitch of audible beep is proportional to SpO_2 value. Double-checking pulse rate ensures oximeter accuracy. Oximeter pulse rate, client's radial pulse, and apical pulse rate should be the same. Any difference requires reevaluation of oximeter sensor probe placement and reassessment of pulse rates. Reading may take 10 to 30 seconds, depending on site selected.
13. Leave probe in place until oximeter readout reaches constant value and pulse display reaches full strength during each cardiac cycle. Inform client that oximeter will alarm if the probe falls off or if client moves the probe. Read SpO_2 on digital display.	
14. If continuous SpO_2 monitoring is planned, verify SpO_2 alarm limits and alarm volume, which are preset by the manufacturer at a low of 85% and a high of 100%. You must determine limits for SpO_2 and pulse rate alarms based on each client's condition. Verify that alarms are on. Assess skin integrity under sensor probe and relocate sensor probe at least every 4 hr.	Alarms must be set at appropriate limits and volumes to avoid frightening clients and visitors. Spring tension of sensor probe or sensitivity to disposable sensor probe adhesive can cause skin irritation and lead to disruption of skin integrity.
15. Assist client in returning to comfortable position.	Restores comfort and promotes sense of well-being.
16. Perform hand hygiene.	Reduces transmission of microorganisms.
17. Discuss findings with client as needed.	Promotes participation in care and understanding of health status.
18. If intermittent or spot-checking SpO_2 measurements are planned, remove probe and turn oximeter power off. Store probe in appropriate location.	Batteries can be depleted if oximeter is left on. Sensor probes are expensive and vulnerable to damage.
19. Compare SpO_2 readings with client baseline and acceptable values.	Comparison reveals presence of abnormality.
21. Correlate SpO_2 with SaO_2 obtained from arterial blood gas measurements (see Chapter 40) if available.	Documents reliability of noninvasive assessment.
22. Correlate SpO_2 reading with data obtained from respiratory rate, depth, and rhythm assessment (see Skill 31-3, p. 647).	Measurements assessing ventilation, perfusion, and diffusion are interrelated.

Unexpexcted Outcomes and Related Interventions

- SpO_2 is less than 90%.
  - Verify that oximeter probe is intact and correctly positioned.
  - Obtain vital signs and notify physician if indicated.
  - Observe for signs associated with decreased oxygenation (e.g., anxiety, restlessness, tachycardia, cyanosis).
  - Verify that supplemental oxygen delivery system is delivered as ordered and is functioning properly.
  - Position client to promote optimal ventilation.

- Pulse rate indicated on the oximeter is less than client's radial or apical pulse.
  - Reposition sensor probe to an alternative site with increased blood flow.
  - Assess client for signs of altered cardiac output (e.g., decreased blood pressure, cool skin, confusion).

Recording and Reporting

- Record SpO_2 value on nurses' notes or vital sign flow sheet indicating type and amount of oxygen therapy used by client during assessment. Also record any signs and symptoms of oxygen desaturation in narrative form in nurses' notes. Report abnormal findings to nurse in charge or physician.

- Assessment of oxygen saturation after administration of specific therapies should be documented in narrative form in nurses' notes.
- Record in nurses' notes client's use of continuous or intermittent pulse oximetry. Documents use of equipment for third-party payers.

Home Care Considerations

- Pulse oximetry is used in home care to noninvasively monitor oxygen therapy or changes in oxygen therapy.
- Instruct caregivers to examine oximeter site prior to applying sensor.
- Instruct caregivers on procedure to implement when oxygen saturation not within acceptable values.

Box 31-12   Factors Affecting Determination of Pulse Oxygen Saturation (SpO$_2$)

Interference With Light Transmission

Outside light sources can interfere with the oximeter's ability to process reflected light.

Carbon monoxide (caused by smoke inhalation or poisoning) artificially elevates SpO$_2$ by absorbing light similar to oxygen.

Client motion can interfere with the oximeter's ability to process reflected light.

Jaundice may interfere with the oximeter's ability to process reflected light.

Intravascular dyes (methylene blue) absorb light similar to deoxyhemoglobin and artificially lower saturation.

Reduction of Arterial Pulsations

Peripheral vascular disease (atherosclerosis) can reduce pulse volume.

Hypothermia at assessment site decreases peripheral blood flow.

Pharmacological vasoconstrictors (epinephrine, phenylephrine, dopamine) will decrease peripheral pulse volume.

Low cardiac output and hypotension decrease blood flow to peripheral arteries.

Peripheral edema can obscure arterial pulsation.

Tight probe will record venous pulsations in the finger that compete with arterial pulsations.

---

health. The heart's contraction forces blood under high pressure into the aorta. The peak of maximum pressure when ejection occurs is the **systolic** blood pressure. When the ventricles relax, the blood remaining in the arteries exerts a minimum or **diastolic** pressure. Diastolic pressure is the minimal pressure exerted against the arterial walls at all times.

The standard unit for measuring blood pressure is millimeters of mercury (mm Hg). The measurement indicates the height to which the blood pressure can raise a column of mercury. Blood pressure is recorded with the systolic reading before the diastolic (e.g., 120/80). The difference between systolic and diastolic pressure is the **pulse pressure.** For a blood pressure of 120/80, the pulse pressure is 40.

Physiology of Arterial Blood Pressure

Blood pressure reflects the interrelationships of cardiac output, peripheral vascular resistance, blood volume, blood viscosity, and artery elasticity. A nurse's knowledge of these hemodynamic variables helps in the assessment of blood pressure alterations.

Cardiac Output. A person's cardiac output (CO) is the volume of blood pumped by the heart (stroke volume [SV]) during 1 minute (heart rate [HR]):

$$CO = HR \times SV$$

The blood pressure (BP) depends on the cardiac output and peripheral vascular resistance (R):

$$BP = CO \times R$$

When volume increases in an enclosed space, such as a blood vessel, the pressure in that space rises. Thus, as cardiac output increases, more blood is pumped against arterial walls, causing the blood pressure to rise. Cardiac output can increase as a result of an increase in heart rate, greater heart muscle contractility, or an increase in blood volume. Changes in heart rate can occur faster than changes in heart muscle contractility or blood volume. An increase in heart rate may decrease the heart's filling time. As a result there is a decrease in blood pressure.

Peripheral Resistance. Blood circulates through a network of arteries, arterioles, capillaries, venules, and veins. Arteries and arterioles are surrounded by smooth muscle that contracts or relaxes to change the size of the lumen. The size of arteries and arterioles changes to adjust blood flow to the needs of local tissues. For example, when more blood is needed by a major organ, the peripheral arteries constrict, decreasing their supply of blood. More blood becomes available to the major organ because of the resistance change in the periphery. Normally, arteries and arterioles remain partially constricted to maintain a constant flow of blood. Peripheral vascular resistance is the resistance to blood flow determined by the tone of vascular musculature and diameter of blood vessels. The smaller the lumen of a vessel, the greater peripheral vascular resistance to blood flow. As resistance rises, arterial blood pressure rises. As vessels dilate and resistance falls, blood pressure drops.

Blood Volume. The volume of blood circulating within the vascular system affects blood pressure. Most adults have a circulating blood volume of 5000 ml. Normally

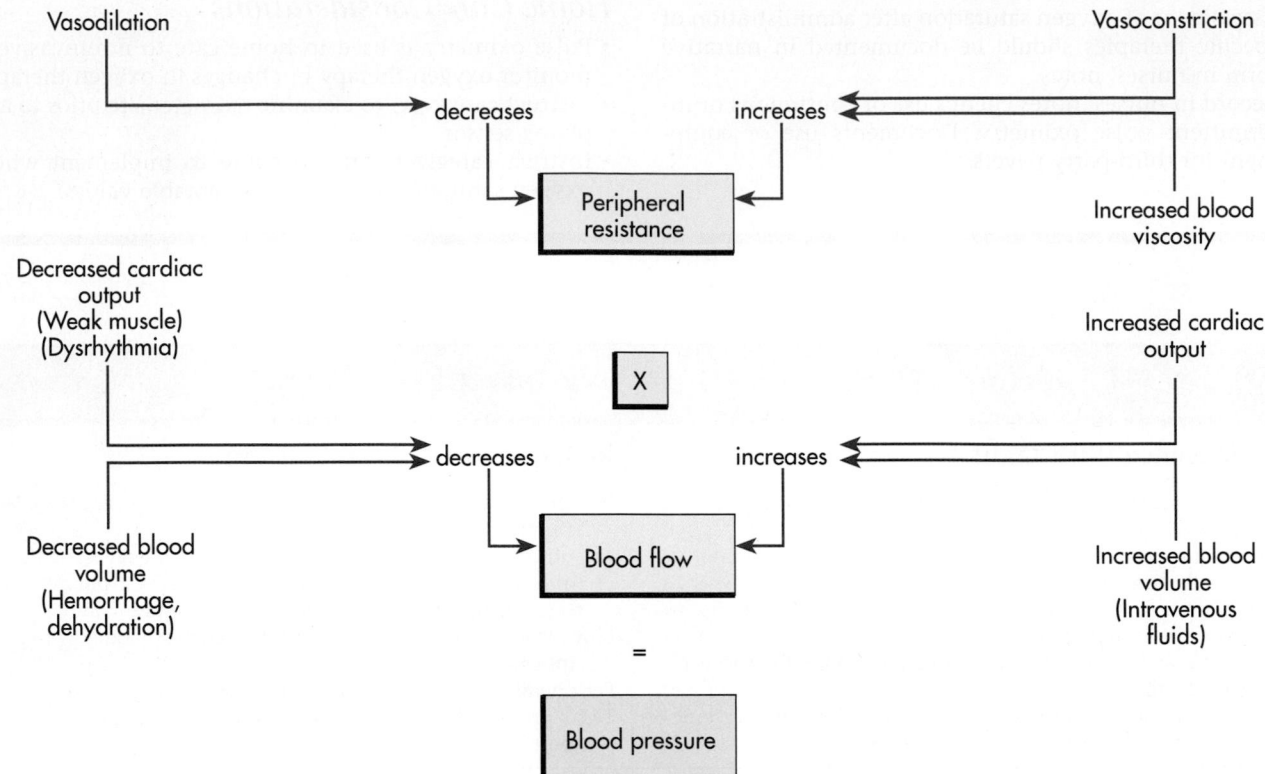

FIGURE **31–11** Hemodynamic factors that affect blood pressure.

the blood volume remains constant. However, if volume increases, more pressure is exerted against arterial walls. For example, the rapid, uncontrolled infusion of intravenous fluids elevates blood pressure. When circulating blood volume falls, as in the case of hemorrhage or dehydration, blood pressure falls.

Viscosity.   The thickness or viscosity of blood affects the ease with which blood flows through small vessels. The **hematocrit,** or percentage of red blood cells in the blood, determines blood viscosity. When the hematocrit rises and blood flow slows, arterial blood pressure increases. The heart must contract more forcefully to move the viscous blood through the circulatory system.

Elasticity.   Normally the walls of an artery are elastic and easily distensible. As pressure within the arteries increases, the diameter of vessel walls increases to accommodate the pressure change. Arterial distensibility prevents wide fluctuations in blood pressure. However, in certain diseases, such as arteriosclerosis, the vessel walls lose their elasticity and are replaced by fibrous tissue that cannot stretch well. With reduced elasticity there is greater resistance to blood flow. As a result, when the left ventricle ejects its stroke volume, the vessels no longer yield to pressure. Instead, a given volume of blood is forced through the rigid arterial walls, and the systemic pressure rises. Systolic pressure is more significantly elevated than diastolic pressure as a result of reduced arterial elasticity.

Each hemodynamic factor significantly affects the others. For example, as arterial elasticity declines, peripheral vascular resistance increases. The complex control of the cardiovascular system normally prevents any single factor from permanently changing the blood pressure. For example, if the blood volume falls, the body compensates with an increased vascular resistance. Figure 31-11 illustrates how hemodynamic variables can affect blood pressure.

Factors Influencing Blood Pressure

Blood pressure is not constant but is continually influenced by many factors. One blood pressure measurement cannot adequately reflect a client's blood pressure. Even under the best conditions, blood pressure changes from heartbeat to heartbeat. Blood pressure trends, not individual measurements, guide nursing interventions. Understanding these factors ensures a more accurate interpretation of blood pressure readings.

Age. Normal blood pressure levels vary throughout life (Table 31-7). They increase during childhood. The level of a child's or adolescent's blood pressure is assessed with respect to body size and age. An infant's blood pressure ranges from 65-115/42-80. The normal blood pressure for a 7-year-old is 87-117/48-64. Larger children (heavier and/or taller) have higher blood pressures than smaller children of the same age. During adolescence, blood pressure continues to vary according to body size.

An adult's blood pressure tends to increase with advancing age. The optimal blood pressure for a healthy,

Table 31-7	Average Optimal Blood Pressure for Age
Age	**Blood Pressure (mm Hg)**
Newborn (3000 g [6.6 lb])	40 (mean)
1 month	85/54
1 year	95/65
6 years*	105/65
10-13 years*	110/65
14-17 years*	120/75
>18	<120/80

From National High Blood Pressure Education Program (NHBPEP); National Heart, Lung, and Blood Institute; National Institutes of Health: The seventh report of the Joint National Committee on Detection, Evaluation, and Treatment of High Blood Pressure, *JAMA* 289(19):2560, 2003.
*In children and adolescents, hypertension is defined as BP that is, on repeated measurement, at the 95th percentile or greater adjusted for age, height, and gender (NHBPEP, 1997).

Table 31-8	Classification of Blood Pressure for Adults Ages 18 and Older		
Category	**Systolic (mm Hg)***		**Diastolic (mm Hg)***
Normal	<120		<80
Pre-hypertension†	120-139	or	80-89
Stage 1 Hypertension	140-159	or	90-99
Stage 2 Hypertension	>160	or	>100

Data from National High Blood Pressure Education Program (NHBPEP); National Heart, Lung, and Blood Institute; National Institutes of Health: The seventh report of the Joint National Committee on Detection, Evaluation, and Treatment of High Blood Pressure, *JAMA* 289(19):2560, 2003.
*Treatment based on highest category.
†Based on average of two or more readings.

middle-age adult is less than 120/80. Values of 120-139/80-89 are considered hypertensive (NHBPEP, 2003) (Table 31-8). Older adults may have a rise in systolic pressure related to a decreased vessel elasticity; however, blood pressure greater than 140/90 increases an older adult's risk for hypertension and other related illness.

Stress. Anxiety, fear, pain, and emotional stress result in sympathetic stimulation, which increases heart rate, cardiac output, and peripheral vascular resistance. The effects of sympathetic stimulation increase blood pressure.

Ethnicity. The incidence of hypertension (high blood pressure) is higher in African-Americans than in European-Americans. African-Americans tend to develop more severe hypertension at an earlier age and have twice the risk for complications such as stroke and heart attack. Genetic and environmental factors are believed to be contributing factors. Hypertension-related deaths are also higher among African-Americans.

Gender. There is no clinically significant difference in blood pressure levels between boys and girls. After puberty, males tend to have higher blood pressure readings. After menopause, women tend to have higher levels of blood pressure than men of similar age.

Diurnal Variation. Blood pressure levels vary over the course of a day. Blood pressure is typically lowest in the early morning, gradually rises during the morning and afternoon, and peaks in late afternoon or evening. No two persons have the same pattern or degree of variation. Students may find it interesting to have their blood pressure checked by a friend at intervals during 24 hours.

Medications. Some medications can directly or indirectly affect blood pressure. During blood pressure assessment, the nurse asks whether the client is receiving antihypertensive or other cardiac medications, which lower blood pressure (Table 31-9). Another class of medications affecting blood pressure is opioid analgesics, which can lower blood pressure.

Other. Blood pressure can be reduced for several hours after a period of exercise. Older adults often experience a 5- to 10-mm fall in blood pressure about 1 hour after eating.

Hypertension

The most common alteration in blood pressure is **hypertension.** Hypertension is an often asymptomatic disorder characterized by persistently elevated blood pressure. The diagnosis of pre-hypertension in adults is made when an average of two or more diastolic readings on at least two subsequent visits is between 80 and 89 mm Hg or when the average of multiple systolic blood pressures on two or more subsequent visits is between 120 and 139 mm Hg. Hypertension is noted with diastolic readings greater than 90 mm Hg and systolic readings greater than 140 mm Hg (NHBPEP, 2003). Categories of hypertension have been developed and determine medical intervention (see Table 31-8). One elevated blood pressure measurement does not qualify as a diagnosis of hypertension. However, if the nurse assesses a high reading during the first blood pressure measurement (e.g., 150/90 mm Hg), the client is encouraged to return for another checkup within 2 months.

Hypertension is associated with the thickening and loss of elasticity in the arterial walls. Peripheral vascular resistance increases within thick and inelastic vessels. The heart must continually pump against greater resistance. As a result, blood flow to vital organs such as the heart, brain, and kidney decreases.

Persons with a family history of hypertension are at significant risk. Obesity, cigarette smoking, heavy alcohol consumption, high sodium (salt) intake, sedentary lifestyle, and continued exposure to stress are also linked to hypertension. The incidence of hypertension is greater in diabetic clients, older adults, and African-Americans. It

Table 31-9	Antihypertension Medications	
Medication Type	Names	Action
Diuretics	Furosemide (Lasix), spironolactone (Aldactone), metolazone, polythiazide, benzthiazide	Lower blood pressure by reducing reabsorption of sodium and water by the kidneys, thus lowering circulating fluid volume
Beta-adrenergic blockers	Atenolol (Tenormin), nadolol (Corgard), timolol maleate (Blocadren), propranolol (Inderal)	Combine with beta-adrenergic receptors in the heart, arteries, and arterioles to block response to sympathetic nerve impulses; reduce heart rate and thus cardiac output
Vasodilators	Hydralazine hydrochloride (Apresoline), minoxidil (Loniten)	Act on arteriolar smooth muscle to cause relaxation and reduce peripheral vascular resistance
Calcium channel blockers	Diltiazem (Cardizem, Dilacor XR), verapamil hydrochloride (Calan SR), nifedipine (Procardia), nicardipine (Cardene)	Reduce peripheral vascular resistance by systemic vasodilation
Angiotensin-converting enzyme (ACE) inhibitors	Captopril (Capoten), enalapril (Vasotec), lisinopril (Prinivil, Zestril), benazepril (Lotensin)	Lower blood pressure by blocking the conversion of angiotensin I to angiotensin II, preventing vasoconstriction; reduce aldosterone production and fluid retention, lowering circulating fluid volume

is a major factor underlying deaths from strokes and is a contributing factor to myocardial infarctions (heart attacks). When clients are diagnosed with hypertension, the nurse helps to educate them about blood pressure values, long-term follow-up care and therapy, the usual lack of symptoms (the fact that it may not be "felt"), therapy's ability to control but not cure hypertension, and a consistently followed treatment plan that can ensure a relatively normal lifestyle (NHBPEP, 2003).

Hypotension

Hypotension is considered present when the systolic blood pressure falls to 90 mm Hg or below. Although some adults have a low blood pressure normally, for the majority of people, low blood pressure is an abnormal finding associated with illness.

Hypotension occurs because of the dilation of the arteries in the vascular bed, the loss of a substantial amount of blood volume (e.g., hemorrhage), or the failure of the heart muscle to pump adequately (e.g., myocardial infarction). Hypotension associated with pallor, skin mottling, clamminess, confusion, increased heart rate, or decreased urine output is life threatening and should be reported to a physician immediately.

Orthostatic hypotension, also referred to as **postural hypotension,** occurs when a normotensive person develops symptoms and low blood pressure when rising to an upright position. When a healthy individual changes from a lying, to sitting, to standing position, the peripheral blood vessels in the legs constrict. Constriction of the lower extremity vessels when standing prevents the pooling of blood in the legs due to gravity. Thus no symptoms are normally felt in standing. In contrast, when clients have a decreased blood volume, their blood vessels are already constricted. When a volume-depleted client stands, there is a significant drop in blood pressure with an increase in heart rate to compensate for the drop in cardiac output. Clients who are dehydrated, anemic, or have experienced prolonged bed rest or recent blood loss are at risk for orthostatic hypotension. Some medications

can cause orthostatic hypotension if misused, especially in older adults or young clients. Blood pressure should always be measured before administering such medications.

The nurse assesses for orthostatic hypotension during vital sign measurements by obtaining blood pressure and pulse with the client supine, sitting, and standing. When recording orthostatic blood pressure measurements, the nurse records the client's position in addition to the blood pressure measurement. For example: 140/80 supine, 132/72 sitting, 108/60 standing. The readings are obtained 1 to 3 minutes after the client changes position. In most cases, orthostatic hypotension is detected within a minute of standing. If orthostatic hypotension is assessed, the client is assisted to a lying position and the physician or nurse in charge is notified. While obtaining orthostatic measurements, the nurse observes for other symptoms of hypotension such as fainting, weakness, or light-headedness. Because the skill of orthostatic measurements requires critical thinking and ongoing nursing judgment, this procedure is not delegated to unlicensed assistive personnel.

Measurement of Blood Pressure

Arterial blood pressure may be measured either directly (invasively) or indirectly (noninvasively). The direct method requires the insertion of a thin catheter into an artery. Tubing connects the catheter with electronic monitoring equipment. The monitor displays a constant arterial pressure waveform and reading. Because of the risk of sudden blood loss from an artery, invasive blood pressure monitoring is used only in intensive care settings. The more common noninvasive method requires use of the sphygmomanometer and stethoscope. The nurse measures blood pressure indirectly by auscultation or palpation. Auscultation is the most widely used technique (Skill 31-5).

Blood Pressure Equipment. Before assessing blood pressure, the nurse must be comfortable using a sphygmomanometer and stethoscope. A **sphygmomanometer** includes a pressure manometer, an occlusive cloth or

Text continued on p. 661

Skill 31-5 *Measuring Blood Pressure*

Delegation Considerations

The skill of blood pressure measurement can be delegated to assistive personnel. The nurse is responsible for assessing changes in blood pressure. It is important for the nurse to:

- Inform caregiver if client has alterations affecting the appropriate limb for blood pressure measurement.
- Inform caregiver of appropriate-size blood pressure cuff for designated extremity.
- Inform caregiver if client is at risk for orthostatic hypotension.
- Inform caregiver of frequency of blood pressure measurement for select client.
- Determine that caregiver is aware of the usual values for the client.
- Inform caregiver of the abnormalities that should be reconfirmed by the nurse.

Equipment

- Aneroid sphygmomanometer
- Cloth or disposable vinyl pressure cuff of appropriate size for client's extremity
- Stethoscope
- Alcohol swab
- Pen, pencil, vital sign flow sheet or record form

Steps	Rationale
1. Determine need to assess client's BP:	Nurse uses clinical judgment to determine need for assessment.
a. Note risk factors for alteration in BP.	Certain conditions place clients at risk for BP alteration: history of cardiovascular disease, renal disease, diabetes, circulatory shock (hypovolemic, septic, cardiogenic, or neurogenic), acute or chronic pain, rapid intravenous infusion of fluids or blood products, increased intracranial pressure, postoperative conditions, toxemia of pregnancy.
b. Observe for signs and symptoms of BP alterations:	Physical signs and symptoms may indicate alterations in BP.
(1) Assess for symptoms of high blood pressure: headache (usually occipital), flushing of face, nosebleed, and fatigue in older adults.	High BP (hypertension) is often asymptomatic until pressure is very high.
(2) Assess for symptoms associated with low blood pressure: dizziness, mental confusion; restlessness; pale, dusky, or cyanotic skin and mucous membranes; cool, mottled skin over extremities.	
2. Determine best site for BP assessment. Avoid applying cuff to extremity when intravenous fluids are infusing; an arteriovenous shunt or fistula is present; breast or axillary surgery has been performed on that side; extremity has been traumatized, diseased, or requires a cast or bulky bandage. The lower extremities may be used when the brachial arteries are inaccessible.	Inappropriate site selection may result in poor amplification of sounds, causing inaccurate readings. Application of pressure from inflated bladder temporarily impairs blood flow and can further compromise circulation in extremity that already has impaired blood flow.
3. Select appropriate cuff size.	Improper cuff size results in inaccurate readings (see Table 31-10, p. 664). If cuff is too small, it tends to come loose as inflated or results in false high readings. If the cuff is too large, false low readings may be recorded. For the adult client the bladder, enclosed by the cuff, should encircle 80% of the arm (NHBPEP, 2003).
4. Determine previous baseline BP (if available) from client's record.	Allows nurse to assess for change in condition. Provides comparison with future BP measurements.
5. Identify factors likely to interfere with accuracy of blood pressure measurement: exercise, coffee (i.e., caffeine), smoking. Encourage client to avoid exercise, smoking, and ingestion of caffeine for 30 min before assessment of BP.	Exercise and smoking can cause false elevations in BP. Smoking increases BP immediately and lasts up to 15 min. The effects of coffee or caffeine increases BP for up to 3 hr (Pickering, 2001).

Skill **31-5**   *Measuring Blood Pressure—cont'd*

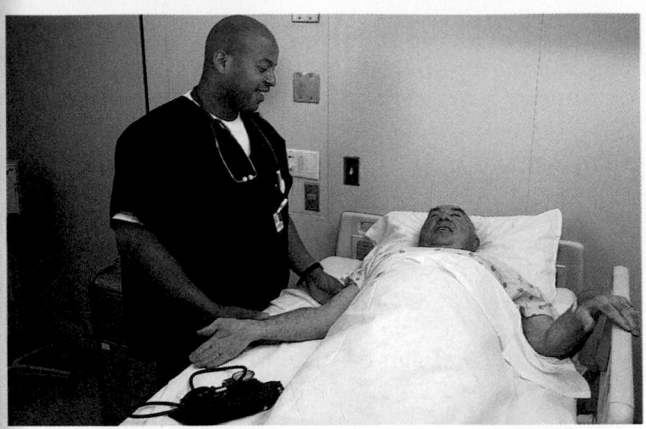

STEP **8**   Client's forearm supported in bed.

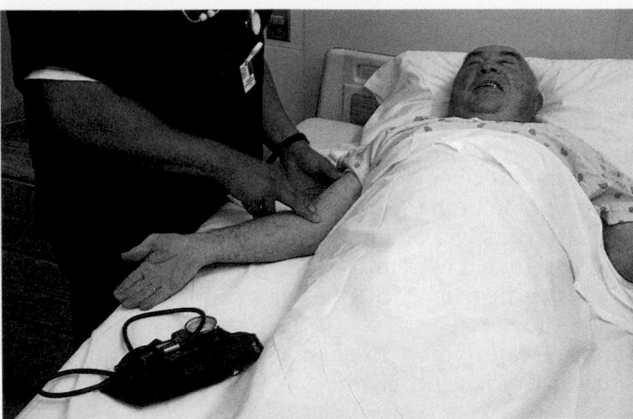

STEP **10**   Nurse palpating client's brachial artery.

6. Perform hand hygiene. Have client assume sitting or lying position. Be sure room is warm, quiet, and relaxing.	Reduces transmission of microorganisms. Maintains client's comfort during measurement. The client's perceptions that the physical or interpersonal environment is stressful affect the BP measurement.
7. Explain to client that BP is to be assessed and have client rest at least 5 min before measurement. When possible, client should be sitting in a chair (NHBPEP, 2003). Ask client not to speak when BP is being measured.	Allows client to relax and helps to avoid falsely elevate readings. Blood pressure readings taken at different times can be objectively compared when assessed with client at rest (NHBPEP, 2003). Talking to a client when the BP is being assessed may increase readings 10% to 40%.
8. With client sitting or lying, position client's forearm at heart level, position thigh flat (provide support as needed). For arm, turn palm up (see illustration); for thigh, position with knee slightly flexed.	If extremity is unsupported, client may perform isometric exercise that can increase diastolic blood pressure.
9. Expose extremity (arm or leg) fully by removing constricting clothing.	Ensures proper cuff application.

Critical Decision Point: Do not place blood pressure cuff over clothing.

---

10. Palpate brachial artery (arm) (see illustration) or popliteal artery (leg). Position cuff 2.5 cm (1 in) above site of pulsation (antecubital or popliteal space).	Inflating bladder directly over artery ensures proper pressure is applied during inflation.
11. Apply bladder of cuff above artery by centering arrows marked on cuff over artery. If no center arrows on cuff, estimate the center of the bladder and place this center over artery. With cuff fully deflated, wrap cuff evenly and snugly around extremity (see illustrations).	Loose-fitting cuff causes false high readings.
12. Measure blood pressure.	
A. Two-Step Method	
(1) Relocate brachial pulse. Palpate the artery distal to the cuff with fingertips of nondominant hand while inflating cuff rapidly to pressure 30 mm Hg above point at which pulse disappears. Slowly deflate cuff and note point when pulse reappears. Deflate cuff fully and wait 30 seconds.	Estimating prevents false low readings, which may result in the presence of an auscultatory gap. Maximal inflation point for accurate reading can be determined by palpation. If unable to palpate artery because of weakened pulse, an ultrasonic stethoscope can be used (see Chapter 32). Deflating cuff prevents venous congestion and false high readings.
(2) Place stethoscope earpieces in ears and be sure sounds are clear, not muffled.	Each earpiece should follow angle of ear canal to facilitate hearing.
(3) Relocate brachial or popliteal artery and place bell or diaphragm chestpiece of stethoscope over it. Do not allow chestpiece to touch cuff or clothing (see illustration).	Proper stethoscope placement ensures optimal sound reception. Stethoscope improperly positioned causes muffled sounds that often result in false low systolic and false high diastolic readings.

Steps	Rationale

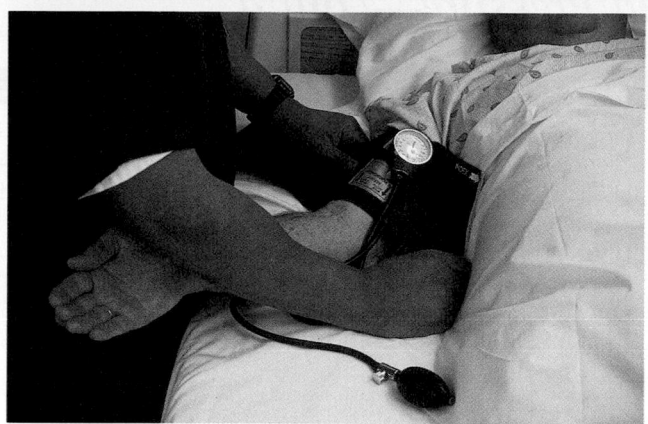

A

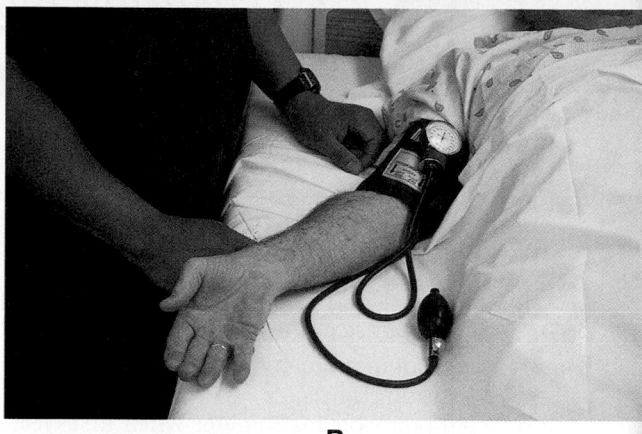

B

STEP **11** **A,** Center bladder of cuff above artery. **B,** Blood pressure cuff wrapped around upper arm.

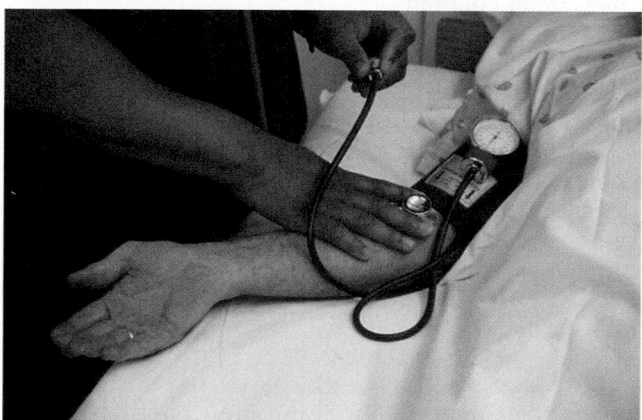

STEP **12A(3)**   Stethoscope over brachial artery to measure BP.

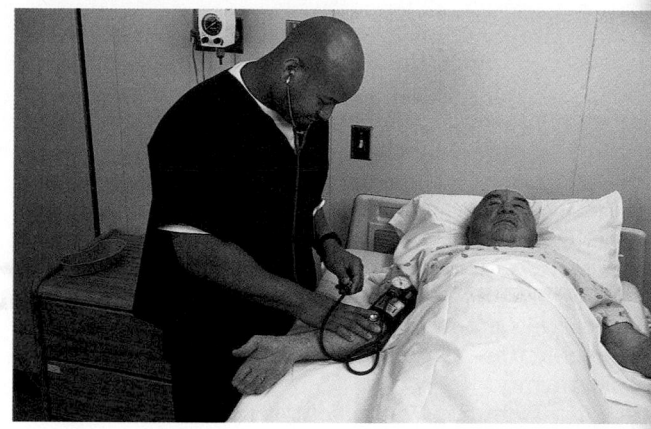

STEP **12A(4)**   Inflating BP cuff.

(4) Close valve of pressure bulb clockwise until tight. Quickly inflate cuff to 30 mm Hg above palpated systolic pressure (client's estimated systolic pressure) (see illustration).

Tightening of valve prevents air leak during inflation. Inflation ensures accurate measurement of systolic pressure.

(5) Slowly release pressure bulb valve and allow needle of manometer gauge to fall at rate of 2 to 3 mm Hg/sec.

Too rapid or slow a decline in pressure can cause inaccurate readings.

(6) Note point on manometer when first clear sound is heard. The sound will slowly increase in intensity.

First Korotkoff sound indicates systolic pressure.

(7) Continue to deflate cuff, noting point at which muffled or dampened sound appears.

Fourth Korotkoff sound involves distinct muffling of sounds and is recommended as indication of diastolic pressure in children.

(8) Continue to deflate cuff gradually, noting point at which sound disappears in adults. Listen for 10 to 20 mm Hg after the last sound, and then allow remaining air to escape quickly.

Beginning of the fifth Korotkoff sound is recommended by American Heart Association as indication of diastolic pressure in adults.
Continuous cuff inflation causes arterial occlusion, resulting in numbness and tingling of client's arm.

B. One-Step Method
(1) Place stethoscope earpieces in ears and be sure sounds are clear, not muffled.

Each earpiece should follow angle of ear canal to facilitate hearing.

Skill 31-5   *Measuring Blood Pressure—cont'd*

Steps	Rationale
(2) Relocate brachial or popliteal artery and place bell or diaphragm chestpiece of stethoscope over it. Do not allow chestpiece to touch cuff or clothing.	Proper stethoscope placement ensures optimal sound reception. Stethoscope improperly positioned causes muffled sounds that often result in false low systolic and false high diastolic readings.
(3) Close valve of pressure bulb clockwise until tight. Quickly inflate cuff to 30 mm Hg above palpated systolic pressure.	Tightening of valve prevents air leak during inflation. Inflation ensures accurate measurement of systolic pressure.
(4) Slowly release pressure bulb valve and allow needle of manometer gauge to fall at rate of 2 to 3 mm Hg/sec.	Too rapid or slow a decline in pressure can cause inaccurate readings.
(5) Note point on manometer when first clear sound is heard. The sound will slowly increase in intensity.	First Korotkoff sound indicates systolic pressure.
(6) Continue to deflate cuff, noting point at which muffled or dampened sound appears.	Fourth Korotkoff sound involves distinct muffling of sounds and is recommended as indication of diastolic pressure in children.
(7) Continue to deflate cuff gradually, noting point at which sound disappears in adults. Listen for 10 to 20 mm Hg after the last sound, and then allow remaining air to escape quickly.	Beginning of the fifth Korotkoff sound is recommended by American Heart Association as indication of diastolic pressure in adults. Continuous cuff inflation causes arterial occlusion, resulting in numbness and tingling of client's arm.
13. Remove cuff from extremity unless measurement must be repeated. The Joint National Commission (NHBPEP, 2003) recommends that two or more readings separated by 2 min should be averaged. If readings are different by more than 5 mm Hg, additional readings are necessary. If this is the first assessment of client, repeat blood pressure assessment on other extremity.	Comparison of BP in both extremities detects circulation problems. (Normal difference of 5 to 10 mm Hg exists between extremities.)
14. Discuss findings with client as needed.	Promotes participation in care and understanding of health status.
15. Perform hand hygiene.	Reduces transmission of microorganisms.
16. Assist client in returning to comfortable position and cover upper arm if previously clothed.	Restores comfort and promotes sense of well-being.
17. Compare reading with previous baseline and/or acceptable value of blood pressure for client's age.	Evaluates for change in condition and alterations.
18. Compare blood pressure in both arms or both legs.	If using upper extremities, the arm with the higher pressure should be used for subsequent assessments unless contraindicated.
19. Correlate blood pressure with data obtained from pulse assessment and related cardiovascular signs and symptoms.	Blood pressure and heart rate are interrelated.

Unexpexcted Outcomes and Related Interventions

- Unable to obtain BP reading
  - Assess for signs of decreased cardiac output (e.g., weak thready pulse, confusion, pallor, or cyanosis).
  - Palpate radial artery if strong, reposition BP cuff, and repeat measurement.
  - Use palpation method to obtain BP.
  - If BP is low or obtainable, place client in supine position.
  - Notify physician.

- BP is less than 90 mm Hg, systolic
  - Repeat BP measurement
  - If using automatic BP device, switch and use ascultation or palpation method to obtain client's BP.
  - Notify physician.
- BP is elevated above client's usual value
  - Repeat measurement in other arm.
  - Assess client for headache, confusion, fatigue.
  - Report elevated BP to physician.

Recording and Reporting

- Inform client of value and need for periodic reassessment.
- Record blood pressure in nurses' notes or vital sign flow sheet. Measurement of blood pressure after administration of specific therapies should be documented in narrative form in nurses' notes.
- Report abnormal findings to nurse in charge or physician.

Home Care Considerations

- Assess home noise level to determine room that will provide quietest environment for assessing BP.
- Consider electronic blood pressure cuff for home if client has hearing difficulties, if client has sufficient financial resources, and if client has adequate dexterity.

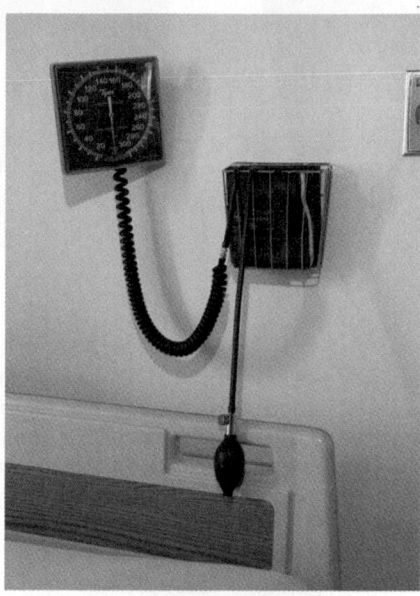

FIGURE **31–12** Wall-mounted aneroid sphygmomanometer.

vinyl cuff that encloses an inflatable rubber bladder, and a pressure bulb with a release valve that inflates the bladder. The two types of manometers are the aneroid and the mercury (Figure 31-12). Aneroid manometers have the advantages of being safe, lightweight, portable, and compact. The aneroid manometer has a glass-enclosed circular gauge containing a needle that registers millimeter calibrations. Before using the aneroid model, the nurse makes sure that the needle points to zero and that the manometer is correctly calibrated. Aneroid sphygmomanometers require biomedical calibration at routine intervals to verify their accuracy.

Mercury manometers, once the gold standard, are less common because they contain mercury, a hazardous substance. However, some agencies or specific units, for example, operating rooms or intensive care units, may still use the mercury manometer. Pressure created by the inflation of the compression cuff moves the column of mercury upward against the force of gravity. Millimeter calibrations mark the height of the mercury column. To ensure accurate readings, the mercury column should fall freely as pressure is released and should always be at zero when the cuff is deflated. Accurate readings are obtained by looking at the meniscus of the mercury at eye level. Looking up or down at the mercury results in distorted readings. Because most municipalities have prohibited the sale or use of mercury-containing devices because of

the potential hazards, fewer mercury manometers are available, but they still exist.

Cloth or disposable vinyl compression cuffs contain the inflatable bladder and come in several sizes. The size selected is proportional to the circumference of the limb being assessed (Figure 31-13). Ideally, the width of the cuff should be 40% of the circumference (or 20% wider than the diameter) of the midpoint of the limb on which the cuff is to be used. The bladder, enclosed by the cuff, should encircle at least 80% of the arm of an adult and the entire arm of a child (NHBPEP, 2003). In children the lower edge of the cuff should be above the antecubital fossa, allowing room for placement of the stethoscope bell or diaphragm. Blood pressure measurements will not be accurate unless the correct size blood pressure cuff is applied appropriately.

Before using a sphygmomanometer the nurse should inspect the parts of the release valve and the pressure bulb. The valve should be clean and freely moveable in either direction. If it sticks or becomes too tightly closed, the deflation of the pressure cuff will be hard to regulate. The pressure bulb is made of tough rubber and should be free of leaks.

Auscultation. The best environment for blood pressure measurement by auscultation is a quiet room at a comfortable temperature. Although the client may lie or stand, sitting is the preferred position (Box 31-13). In most cases blood pressure readings obtained with the client in the supine, sitting, and standing positions are similar.

The client's position during routine blood pressure determination should be the same during each measurement to permit a meaningful comparison of values. Before assessment the nurse should attempt to control factors responsible for artificially high readings, such as pain, anxiety, or exertion. The client's perceptions that the physical or interpersonal environment is more or less stressful will affect the blood pressure measurement. Blood pressure measurements taken at the client's place of employment or in a physician's office are higher than those taken at the client's home.

During the initial assessment the nurse should obtain and record the blood pressure in both arms. Normally there is a difference of 5 to 10 mm Hg between the arms. In subsequent assessments the blood pressure should be measured in the arm with the higher pressure. Pressure differences greater than 10 mm Hg indicate vascular problems and are reported to the physician or nurse in charge.

The nurse asks the client to state his or her usual blood pressure. If the client does not know, the nurse informs the client after measuring and recording the blood pres-

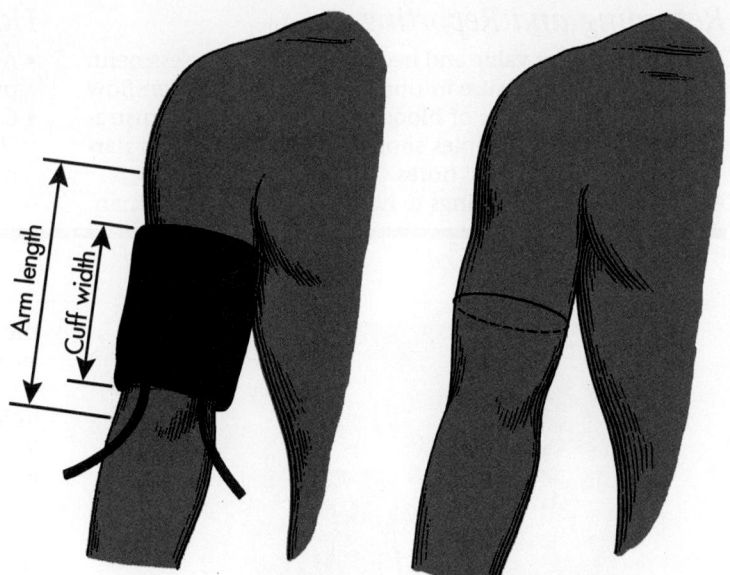

FIGURE **31–13** Guidelines for proper blood pressure cuff size. Cuff width 20% more than upper arm diameter, or 40% of circumference and two thirds of arm length.

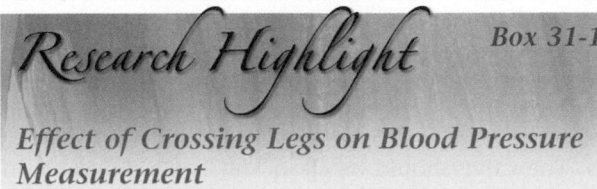

Research Highlight

Box 31-13

Effect of Crossing Legs on Blood Pressure Measurement

Research Focus

Blood pressure measurement is an important factor when determining the diagnosis of hypertension. Because hypertension can lead to serious complications, eliminating errors in measuring blood pressure is important.

Research Abstract

The purpose of this study was to determine if the client's position affects the measurement of blood pressure. One hundred and three senior citizens participated in a study to determine the influence of leg crossing. The blood pressure of male and female senior citizens with and without a diagnosis of hypertension was measured two times. Blood pressure was measured after 3 minutes of rest while sitting with feet flat on the floor. A second blood pressure was measured after the seniors had crossed one leg over the knee for 3 minutes. Results indicate that systolic and diastolic blood pressure were greater when legs were crossed for both groups of seniors.

Evidence-Based Practice

- Clients should be instructed to keep their feet flat on the floor during blood pressure measurement.
- A client's positions should be considered when comparing two different blood pressure measurements.

Reference

Keele-Smith R, Price-Daniel C: Effects of crossing legs on blood pressure measurement, *Clin Nurs Res* 10(2):202, 2001.

sure. This is a good opportunity to educate a client about optimal values of blood pressure, the risk factors for developing hypertension, and dangers of hypertension.

Indirect measurement of arterial blood pressure works on a basic principle of pressure. Blood flows freely through an artery until an inflated cuff applies pressure to tissues and causes the artery to collapse. After the cuff pressure is released, the point at which blood flow returns and sound appears through auscultation is the systolic pressure.

In 1905, Korotkoff, a Russian surgeon, first described the sounds heard over an artery distal to the blood pressure cuff. The first Korotkoff sound is a clear rhythmical tapping corresponding to the pulse rate that gradually increases in intensity. *Onset of the sound corresponds to the systolic pressure.* A murmur or swishing sound occurs as the cuff continues to deflate, resulting in the second Korotkoff sound. As the artery distends, there is a turbulence in blood flow. The third Korotkoff sound is a crisper and more intense tapping. The fourth Korotkoff sound becomes muffled and low pitched as the cuff is further deflated. At this point the cuff pressure has fallen below the pressure within the vessel walls; *this sound is the diastolic pressure in infants and children.* The fifth Korotkoff sound marks the disappearance of sound. *In adolescents and adults, the fifth sound corresponds with the diastolic pressure* (Figure 31-14). In some clients the sounds are clear and distinct. In other clients only the beginning and ending sounds are clear.

The American Heart Association (NHBPEP, 1997, 2003) recommends recording two numbers for a blood pressure measurement: the point on the manometer when the first sound is heard for systolic and the point on the manometer when the fifth sound is heard for diastolic. Some institutions recommend recording the point when the fourth sound is heard as well, especially for clients with hypertension. The numbers are divided by slashed lines (e.g., 120/80 or 120/100/80), and the arm used to measure the blood pressure is noted (e.g., right arm [RA] 130/70), and the client's position when the pressure is assessed (e.g., sitting).

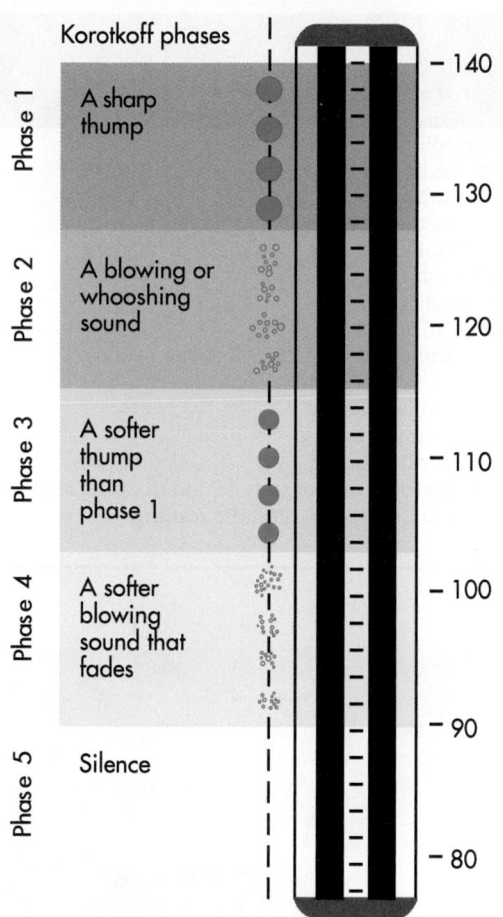

FIGURE 31–14 The sounds auscultated during blood pressure measurement can be differentiated into five Korotkoff phases. In this example blood pressure is 140/90.

Many medical decisions and nursing interventions about a client's health care are made on the basis of blood pressure findings. The importance of obtaining an accurate blood pressure cannot be overemphasized. There are several sources for error. Table 31-10 summarizes common mistakes in measurement. When a nurse is unsure of a reading, a colleague should reassess the blood pressure.

Assessment in Children. All children 3 years of age through adolescence should have blood pressure checked at least yearly. Blood pressure in children changes with growth and development. The nurse can help parents to understand the importance of this routine screening to detect children who may be at risk for hypertension. The measurement of blood pressure in infants and children is difficult for several reasons:

- Different arm size requires careful and appropriate cuff size selection. Do not choose a cuff based on the name of the cuff. An "infant" cuff may be too small for some infants.
- Readings are difficult to obtain in restless or anxious infants and children. A delay of at least 15 minutes to allow children to recover from recent activities and apprehension is recommended. Preparing the child for

the blood pressure cuff's unusual sensation can increase cooperation. Most children will understand the analogy of a "tight hug on your arm."

- Placing stethoscope too firmly on the antecubital fossa can cause errors in auscultation.
- Korotkoff sounds are difficult to hear in children because of low frequency and amplitude. A pediatric stethoscope bell can be helpful.

Ultrasonic Stethoscope. If a nurse is unable to auscultate sounds because of a weakened arterial pulse, an ultrasonic stethoscope can be used (see Chapter 32). This stethoscope allows the nurse to hear low-frequency systolic sounds and is commonly used when measuring the blood pressure of infants, children, and low blood pressure in adults.

Palpation. The indirect palpation technique is useful for clients whose arterial pulsations are too weak to create Korotkoff sounds. Severe blood loss and decreased heart contractility are examples of conditions that result in blood pressures too low to auscultate accurately. Only the systolic blood pressure can be assessed by palpation because the diastolic pressure is difficult to appreciate (Box 31-14). When the palpation technique is used, the systolic value and the manner in which it was measured are recorded (e.g., RA 90/−, palpated, supine).

The palpation technique is used along with auscultation in some instances. In some hypertensive clients, the sounds usually heard over the brachial artery when the cuff pressure is high disappear as pressure is reduced and then reappear at a lower level. This temporary disappearance of sound is the auscultatory gap. It typically occurs between the first and second Korotkoff sounds. The gap in sound may cover a range of 40 mm Hg and thus may cause an underestimation of systolic pressure or overestimation of diastolic pressure. The examiner must be certain to inflate the cuff high enough to hear the true systolic pressure before the auscultatory gap. Palpation of the radial artery helps to determine how high to inflate the cuff. The examiner inflates the cuff 30 mm Hg above the pressure at which the radial pulse was palpated. The range of pressures in which the auscultatory gap occurs is recorded (e.g., BP RA 180/94 with an **auscultatory gap** from 180 to 160, sitting).

Lower Extremity Blood Pressure. Dressings, casts, intravenous catheters, or arteriovenous fistulas or shunts, can make the upper extremities inaccessible for blood pressure measurement. Blood pressure must then be measured in the lower extremities. Comparing upper extremity blood pressure with that in the legs is also necessary for clients with certain peripheral vascular abnormalities. The popliteal artery, palpable behind the knee in the popliteal space, is the site for auscultation. The cuff must be wide and long enough to allow for the larger girth of the thigh. Placing the client in a prone position is best. If such a position is impossible, the client should be asked to flex the knee slightly for easier access to the artery. The cuff is positioned 2.5 cm (1 inch) above the popliteal artery with the bladder over the posterior aspect of the midthigh (Figure 31-15). The procedure is identical to brachial artery auscultation. Systolic pressure in the legs

Table 31-10   Common Mistakes in Blood Pressure Assessment

Error	Effect
Bladder or cuff too wide	False low reading
Bladder or cuff too narrow	False high reading
Cuff wrapped too loosely or unevenly	False high reading
Deflating cuff too slowly	False high diastolic reading
Deflating cuff too quickly	False low systolic and false high diastolic reading
Arm below heart level	False high reading
Arm above heart level	False low reading
Arm not supported	False high reading
Stethoscope that fits poorly or impairment of the examiner's hearing, causing sounds to be muffled	False low systolic and false high diastolic reading
Stethoscope applied too firmly against antecubital fossa	False low diastolic reading
Inflating too slowly	False high diastolic reading
Repeating assessments too quickly	False high systolic reading
Inaccurate inflation level	Inaccurate interpretation of systolic and diastolic readings
Multiple examiners using different Korotkoff sounds for diastolic readings	False high systolic and low diastolic reading

Box 31-14   Palpating the Systolic Blood Pressure

1. Apply blood pressure cuff to the upper arm in the same manner as the auscultation method.
2. Continually palpate the pulse of the brachial, radial, or popliteal artery with fingertips of one hand.
3. Inflate blood pressure cuff 30 mm Hg above the point at which the radial pulse is palpated.
4. Release valve and allow manometer needle mercury to fall 2 mm Hg per second.
5. As soon as the pulse is palpable, note the manometer reading, which will be the systolic blood pressure.
6. Deflate cuff rapidly and completely.
7. Remove cuff from extremity and discuss findings with client as needed. Record pressures systolic/−, palpated (e.g., BP 108/−, palpated).

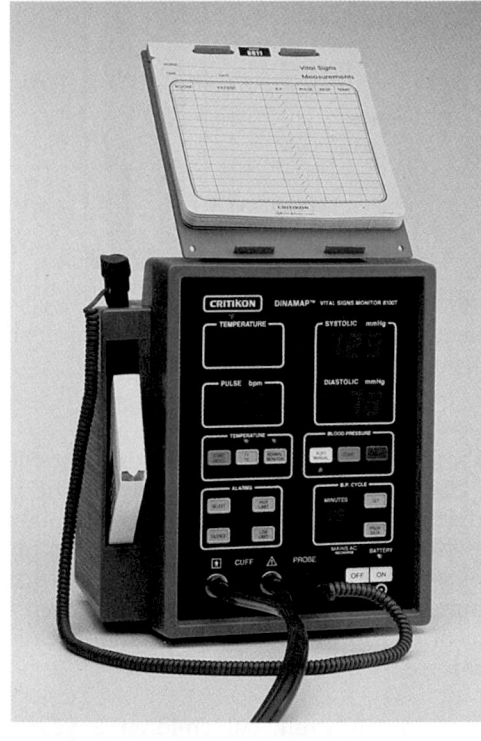

FIGURE 31–16   Automatic blood pressure monitor. (Dinamap Vital Signs Monitor is a trademark of Critikon, Inc. Photo courtesy Critikon, Inc., Tampa, Fla.)

is usually higher by 10 to 40 mm Hg than in the brachial artery, but the diastolic pressure is the same.

Automatic Blood Pressure Devices. Many electronic devices can determine blood pressure automatically (Figure 31-16). These devices are applied when frequent blood pressure assessment is required such as in the critically ill or potentially unstable client, during or after invasive procedures, or when therapies require frequent monitoring (e.g., intravenous heart and blood pressure medications).

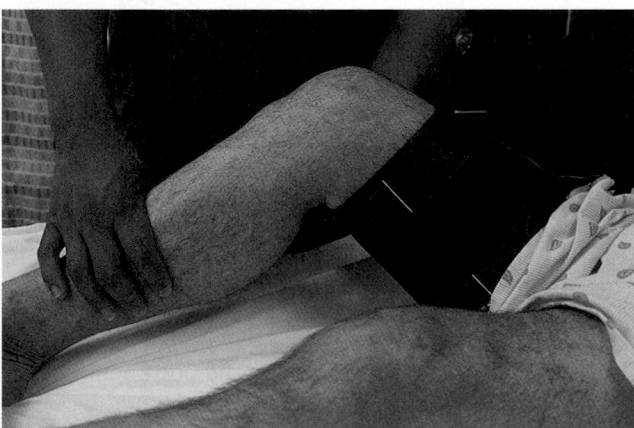

FIGURE 31–15   Lower extremity blood pressure cuff positioned above popliteal artery at midthigh with knee flexed.

> **Box 31-15**   **Client Conditions Not Appropriate for Electronic Blood Pressure Measurement**
>
> Irregular heart rate
> Peripheral vascular obstruction (e.g., clots, narrowed vessels)
> Shivering
> Seizures
> Excessive tremors
> Inability to cooperate
> Blood pressure less than 90 mm Hg systolic

However, some client conditions are not appropriate for automatic blood pressure devices (Box 31-15).

Whereas the auscultatory technique relies on the detection of Korotkoff sounds, some electronic devices rely on the principle of oscillometry. The system includes either a microphone or a pressure sensor built into the inflatable cuff. The microphone or acoustic system hears Korotkoff sounds and registers diastolic and systolic readings. The pressure sensor or ultrasonic system responds to the pressure waves generated by the movement of blood through the artery. The sensor determines the initial burst of oscillations and translates the information into a systolic pressure reading. The diastolic pressure is measured when the oscillations are lowest, just before they stop.

A baseline blood pressure should be obtained using the auscultatory method before applying automatic devices. A comparison assists in evaluation of a client's status and allows proper programming of the device. Once the blood pressure cuff is applied, the nurse can program the device to obtain and record blood pressure readings at preset intervals. Alarm limits can be programmed to alert the nurse if the blood pressure measurement is outside desired parameters.

The advantages of automatic devices are the ease of use and efficiency when repeated or when frequent measurements are indicated. The ability to use a stethoscope is not required. However, automatic devices are more sensitive to outside interference and are susceptible to error. The microphone or pressure sensor must be positioned directly over the artery for proper function. Client movements or vibration or outside noise can interfere with the microphone or sensor signal. Most automatic blood pressure devices are unable to process sounds or vibrations of low blood pressure. The range of device sophistication also can make blood pressure measurement comparisons difficult. The use of automatic blood pressure devices permits assessment of blood pressure during interpersonal interactions. However, the nurse should avoid speaking to the client for at least a minute before initiating a blood pressure recording. Talking to a client when the blood pressure is being assessed can increase readings 10% to 40% (Pickering, 2001).

Self-Measurement of Blood Pressure. More people measure their own blood pressures because of improved technology in home monitoring devices and a greater interest in health promotion. Two of the more common devices used by the general public include portable home sphygmomanometers and stationary automatic blood pressure machines.

The portable home devices include the aneroid sphygmomanometer and electronic digital readout devices that do not require use of a stethoscope. The electronic devices inflate and deflate cuffs with the push of a button. The electronic devices may be easier to manipulate but can easily become inaccurate and require recalibration more than once a year. Because of their sensitivity, improper cuff placement or movement of the arm can cause electronic devices to give incorrect readings.

Stationary automatic blood pressure devices can be found in public places such as grocery stores, fitness clubs, banks, airports, or work sites. Users simply rest their arms within the machine's inflatable cuff, which contains a pressure sensor. The cuff fits over clothing. A visual display tells users their blood pressure within 60 to 90 seconds. The reliability of the stationary machines is limited. Blood pressure values may vary by 5 to 10 mm Hg or more (for both systolic and diastolic values) compared with pressures taken with a manual sphygmomanometer.

Self-measurement of blood pressure has several benefits. Elevated blood pressure may be detected in persons previously unaware of a problem. Persons with high normal blood pressure can provide information about the pattern of blood pressure values. Clients with hypertension can benefit from participating actively in their treatment through self-monitoring, which may help compliance with treatment. The disadvantages of self-measurement include improper use of the device and risk of inaccurate readings. A client may be needlessly alarmed with one elevated reading. Clients with hypertension may become overly conscious of their blood pressures and make inappropriate self-adjustment of medications.

Consumers can learn to use self-measurement devices if they have the information needed to perform the procedure correctly and if they know when to seek medical attention. The nurse can advise clients of possible inaccuracies in the blood pressure devices, help clients understand the meaning and implications of readings, and teach them proper measurement techniques.

Nursing Process and Blood Pressure Determination

The assessment of blood pressure along with pulse assessment is used to evaluate the general state of cardiovascular health and responses to other system imbalances. Hypotension, hypertension, orthostatic hypotension, and narrow or wide pulse pressures are defining characteristics of certain nursing diagnoses including the following:

- Activity intolerance
- Anxiety
- Decreased cardiac output
- Deficient/excess fluid volume
- Risk for injury
- Acute pain
- Ineffective tissue perfusion

The nursing care plan includes interventions based on the nursing diagnosis identified and the related factor. For example, the defining characteristics of hypotension,

Client Teaching   Box 31-16

Health Promotion

Temperature

- Identify client's ability to initiate preventive health measures and recognize alteration in body temperature. Educate client and caregiver about measures to prevent body temperature alterations.
- Teach clients risk factors for hypothermia and frostbite: fatigue; malnutrition; hypoxemia; cold, wet clothing; alcohol intoxication.
- Teach clients risk factors for heat stroke: strenuous exercise in hot, humid weather; tight-fitting clothing in hot environments; exercising in poorly ventilated areas; sudden exposures to hot climates; poor fluid intake before, during, and after exercise.
- Teach clients the importance of taking and continuing antibiotics as directed until course of treatment is completed.

Pulse Rate

- Clients taking certain prescribed cardiac medications should learn to assess their own pulse rates to detect side effects of medications.
- Clients undergoing cardiac rehabilitation should learn to assess their own pulse rates to determine their response to exercise.

Blood Pressure

- Teach client risk factors for hypertension. Persons with family history of hypertension are at significant risk. Obesity, cigarette smoking, heavy alcohol consumption, high blood cholesterol and triglyceride levels, and continued exposure to stress are risk factors linked to hypertension.

- Clients with hypertension should learn about their BP values, long-term follow-up care and therapy, the usual lack of symptoms, therapy's ability to control but not cure, and benefits of a consistently followed treatment plan.
- Instruct clients on the importance of appropriate-size blood pressure cuff for home use.
- Instruct client or primary caregiver to take BP at same time each day and after client has had a brief rest. Take BP sitting or lying down, use same position and arm each time pressure is taken.
- Instruct client or primary caregiver that if it is difficult to hear the pressure, it may be that the cuff is too loose, not big enough, or too narrow; the stethoscope is not over arterial pulse; cuff was deflated too quickly or too slowly; or cuff was not pumped high enough for systolic readings.

Respirations

- Clients who demonstrate decreased ventilation may benefit from being taught deep breathing and coughing exercises (see Chapter 49).
- Instruct caregiver to contact home care nurse or physician if unusual fluctuations in respiratory rate occur.
- Teach client signs and symptoms of hypoxemia: headache, somnolence, confusion, dusky color, shortness of breath, dyspnea.
- Teach client effect of high-risk behaviors such as cigarette smoking on oxygen saturation.

dizziness, pulse deficit, and dysrhythmia lead to a diagnosis of *decreased cardiac output*. Related factors may include poor oral intake, excessive heat exposure, and a history of valvular heart disease. The related factor guides the choice of nursing interventions. The nurse evaluates client outcomes by assessing the blood pressure following each intervention.

Health Promotion and Vital Signs

The emphasis on health promotion and health maintenance, as well as early discharge from hospital settings, has resulted in an increase in the need for clients and their families to monitor vital signs in the home. Teaching considerations affect all vital sign measurements and should be incorporated within the client's plan of care (Box 31-16).

When considering how to teach clients and their families about vital sign measurements and their importance and significance, the client's age is an important factor. With the increased older adult population there is an in-

creased need for caregivers to be aware of changes that are unique to older adults. Box 31-17 identifies some of these variations unique to the older adult.

Recording Vital Signs

Special graphic flow sheets exist for recording vital signs (Figure 31-17). The nurse identifies the institution's procedure for documenting on the graphic or vital sign flow sheet. In addition to the actual vital sign values, the nurse records in the nurses' notes any accompanying or precipitating symptoms such as chest pain and dizziness with abnormal blood pressure, shortness of breath with abnormal respirations, cyanosis with hypoxemia, or flushing and diaphoresis with elevated temperature. The nurse documents any interventions initiated as a result of vital sign measurement such as administration of oxygen therapy or an antihypertensive medication.

Clients being managed on critical paths or CareMaps may have vital sign values listed as outcomes (see Chapter 19). If a vital sign value is above or below the anticipated outcomes, a variance note is written to explain

Focus on Older Adults

Temperature

- Normal body temperatures are lower in later life; mean body temperature ranges from 36° to 36.8° C (96.9° to 98.3° F) orally and 36.6° to 37.2° C (98° to 99° F) rectally (Eliopoulos, 2001).
- Know the older adult's baseline body temperature when making a determination about febrile status. In fact, document the actual temperature and its deviation from baseline, rather than using terminology such as "febrile" or "afebrile" (Miller, 1999).
- Manifestations of delayed or diminished febrile response to infection are subtle and variable in their presentation and very difficult to assess. In fact, do not assume that an infection in an older adult will cause an elevated temperature (Miller, 1999).
- The nurse needs to be especially attentive to subtle temperature changes and other manifestations of fever in this population, such as tachypnea, anorexia, falls, delirium, and overall functional decline (Lueckenotte, 1998).
- Increased age is associated with a reduced ability to respond to cold environments due to inefficient vasoconstriction, decreased cardiac output, diminished shivering, and reduced muscle mass and subcutaneous tissue.
- A reduced ability to respond to hot environments is due to impaired sweating mechanisms and decreased cardiac output (Eliopoulos, 2001).

Pulse Rate

- If it is difficult to palpate the pulse of an older adult or obese client, a Doppler device will provide a more accurate reading.
- The older adult has a decreased heart rate at rest (Ebersole and Hess, 2001).
- Once elevated, the pulse rate of an older adult takes longer to return to normal resting rate (Lueckenotte, 2000).
- When assessing older adult women with sagging breasts, the breast tissue is gently lifted and the stethoscope placed at the fifth intercostal space (ICS) or the lower edge of the breast.
- Heart sounds may be muffled or difficult to hear in older adults because of an increase in air space in the lungs.

Blood Pressure

- Older adults, especially those who are frail, have lost upper arm mass, requiring special attention to selection of BP cuff size.
- An older adult's blood pressure may elevate with age. However, such elevations should not be considered a normal aspect of aging and older adults need minor elevations monitored (NHBPEP, 2003).
- Older adults have an increase in systolic pressure related to decreased vessel elasticity. The diastolic pressure remains the same, resulting in a wider pulse pressure (Lueckenotte, 2000).
- Older adults are instructed to change position slowly and wait after each change to avoid postural hypotension and prevent injuries.

Respirations

- Aging causes ossification of costal cartilage and downward slant of ribs, resulting in a more rigid rib cage, which reduces chest wall expansion. Kyphosis and scoliosis that can occur in older adults may also restrict chest expansion and decrease tidal volume (Sheahan and Musialowski, 2001).
- Older adults may depend more on diaphragmatic and accessory abdominal muscles during respiration than on weakened thoracic muscles (Sheahan and Musialowski, 2001).
- Decreased efficiency of respiratory muscles results in breathlessness at low exercise levels.
- A change in lung function with aging results in respiratory rates that are generally higher in older adults with a normal of 16 to 25 breaths per minute (Lueckenotte, 2000).
- Responses to hypercapnia and hypoxia are reduced 50% in older adults as compared with the young, limiting the ability of older adults to respond to hypoxia with respiratory changes (Ebersole and Hess, 2001).
- Identifying an acceptable pulse oximeter probe site may be difficult on older adults because of the likelihood of peripheral vascular disease, decreased cardiac output, cold-induced vasoconstriction, and anemia.

---

the nature of the variance and the nurse's course of action. For example, a CareMap for a client who has undergone a thoracotomy may have an outcome during the postoperative period of "afebrile." If the client has a fever, the nurse's variance note may address possible sources of fever (e.g., retained pulmonary secretions) and nursing interventions (e.g., increased suctioning, postural drainage, or hydration).

Key Concepts

- Vital signs include the physiological measurement of temperature, pulse, blood pressure, respirations, and oxygen saturation.
- Vital signs are measured as part of a complete physical examination or in a review of a client's condition.
- The nurse assesses vital sign changes with other physical assessment findings, using clinical judgment to determine measurement frequency.
- Knowledge of the factors influencing vital signs assists the nurse in determining and evaluating abnormal values.
- Vital signs provide a basis for evaluating response to nursing interventions.
- Vital signs are best measured when the client is inactive and the environment is controlled for comfort.
- The nurse assists the client in maintaining body temperature by initiating interventions that promote heat loss, production, or conservation.
- A fever is one of the body's normal defense mechanisms.
- Rectal temperature measurements should not be performed on newborn infants or adults with rectal alterations.

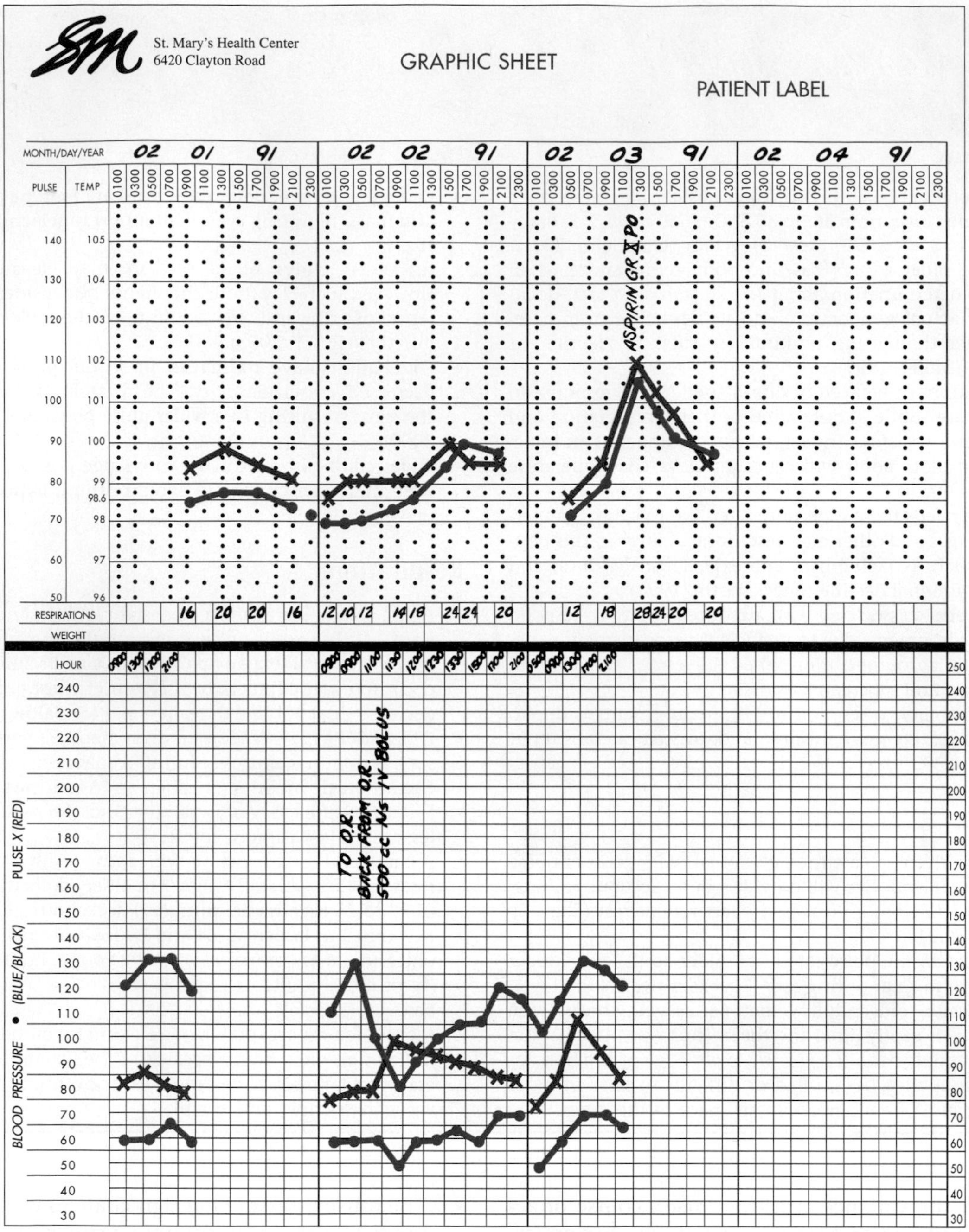

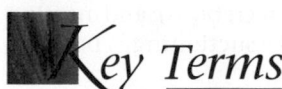

FIGURE **31–17**   Vital signs graphic flow sheet. (Courtesy St. Mary's Health Center, St. Louis, Mo.)

- Respiratory assessment includes measurement to determine the effectiveness of ventilation, perfusion, and diffusion.
- Several hemodynamic variables contribute to blood pressure determination.
- Hypertension is diagnosed only after an average of readings made during two or more subsequent visits reveals an elevated blood pressure.
- Errors in blood pressure measurement can be made by selecting and applying the cuff improperly.
- Changes in one vital sign can influence characteristics of the other vital signs.

Key Terms

Afebrile, *p. 623*

Antipyretics, *p. 636*

Auscultatory gap, *p. 663*

Basal metabolic rate (BMR), *p. 620*

Blood pressure, *p. 650*

Bradycardia, *p. 644*

Cardiac output, *p. 637*

Celsius, *p. 625*

Conduction, *p. 621*

Convection, *p. 621*

Core temperature, *p. 620*

Diaphoresis, *p. 621*

Diastolic, *p. 653*

Diffusion, *p. 645*

Dysrhythmia, *p. 644*

Eupnea, *p. 645*

Evaporation, *p. 621*

Key Terms—cont'd

Critical Thinking Exercises

1. A 47-year-old African-American man is coming to the health clinic for a physical examination by the nurse practitioner for a routine employment physical. The nursing assistant obtains the following routine vital signs: tympanic temperature, 36.9° C (98.4° F); right radial pulse rate of 96 beats per minute and irregular; BP, sitting, right arm 162/82 mm Hg, left arm 150/70 mm Hg; SpO$_2$, 95% on room air; respiratory rate, 22 breaths per minute.
   a. As the admitting nurse, what questions would you ask this client to evaluate his risk for hypertension?
   b. Based on these vital signs, what actions should you take?

2. A teenage mother brings her 3-year-old child to the walk-in health center. She notes that he has been fussy, has not had much of an appetite, and is not his active self. The boy is crying and struggling to get out of his mother's lap during your interview. You note that he is small for his age, but otherwise well developed.
   a. Describe the sequence you would use for obtaining vital signs.
   b. When selecting the appropriate equipment for obtaining the vital signs, what, if any, special considerations are needed?
   c. The nursing assistant reports she has obtained a temperature of 37.7° C (99.8° F). What additional information do you request from the assistant?

3. A 52-year-old woman is admitted to the medical unit for chronic dyspnea and discomfort in her left chest with deep breathing and coughing. She has been smoking for 35 years and has a 20-year history of emphysema. Over the past 4 months she has lost 10 pounds and currently weighs 110 pounds.

   a. When delegating the vital signs to assistive personnel what information and directions should you provide?
   b. The blood pressure and heart rate are within acceptable ranges. The temperature is 37.5° C (99.5° F) obtained with an oral electronic thermometer; the respiratory rate 32 breaths per minute and shallow; the SpO$_2$ is 89%. Based on these results, list your actions in priority.

4. An 82-year-old resident in your subacute extended care facility is being treated for pneumonia with antibiotics. She has been on bed rest for the past 2 days. She has a history of hypertension, treated with diuretics, but is otherwise healthy. She has been afebrile for the past 24 hours and is eager to walk to the activity room. She has activity orders "up ad lib."
   a. Should you delegate the ambulation assistance to a nursing assistant?
   b. What places this client at risk for fainting?
   c. Explain to this client the reason you are obtaining orthostatic measurements.

5. A 25-year-old Hispanic woman arrives at the prenatal clinic for her first visit. She is 8 months pregnant. The nursing assistant checks her vital signs and height and weight. The client weighs 230 pounds and is 5'3" tall; BP in right arm is 210/92 mm Hg; HR, 104 beats per minute; respiratory rate, 24 breaths per minute; tympanic temperature, 98.8° F. You are concerned with the client's blood pressure and repeat the measurement. You obtain 148/86 mm Hg in the right arm and 144/84 mm Hg in the left arm.
   a. What blood pressure measurement should be recorded? Provide some possible explanations for the difference in the measurements between you and the nursing assistant.
   b. How might you explain the abnormal vital signs to the client?
   c. What will be included in your discharge teaching?

Review Questions

1. During a nursing assessment an adult client is noted to have shallow respirations at a rate of 8 beats per minute. His heart rate is 46 beats per minute. His vital signs would be described as:
   1. Bradycardia and apnea.
   2. Tachycardia and apnea.
   3. Bradycardia and bradypnea.
   4. Tachycardia and bradypnea.

2. A pulse deficit provides information about the heart's ability to adequately perfuse the body. A pulse deficit is:
   1. The difference between the radial and apical pulse rates.
   2. The digital pressure felt when taking radial and ulnar pulses.
   3. The amount of pressure felt when taking radial and ulnar pulses.
   4. The difference between the systolic and diastolic blood pressure readings.

3. The nursing assistant reports to the nurse that a client is "feeling funny." The nurse's first action would be to:
   1. Obtain the vital signs herself.
   2. Instruct the nursing assistant to retake the vital signs.
   3. Instruct the nursing assistant to continue to assess the client and report any further complaints.
   4. Notify the physician.

4. If a blood pressure cuff is too narrow or wrapped too loosely the blood pressure reading will be:
   1. Falsely low.
   2. Falsely high.
   3. Difficult to hear because sounds will be muffled.
   4. Dependent on the examiner's hearing acuity.

5. Clients with apnea experience:
   1. Difficult respirations requiring more effort.
   2. Slowness of breathing followed by rapid breathing.
   3. Cessation of breathing that may be temporary.
   4. Lack of oxygen to body tissues and organs.

6. The nurse obtains a supine blood pressure reading of 130/64. One hour later the nurse obtains a supine blood pressure reading of 134/62 and a sitting blood pressure reading of 95/62. The nurse's immediate action is to:
   1. Assist the client to return to a supine position.
   2. Obtain a blood pressure in the other arm.
   3. Report the findings to the nurse in charge.
   4. Question the client about lightheadedness.

7. A nurse is taking vital signs and notes the client has a strong radial pulse that diminishes in intensity and has an interruption in rhythm about every four to six beats. The nurse's immediate action is to:
   1. Report the findings to a physician.
   2. Measure a 60-second apical pulse.
   3. Connect the client to a cardiac monitor.
   4. Obtain a 60-second apical-radial pulse.

8. Nursing interventions such as removing excess blankets from the client and applying cool cloths to the axilla act to decrease body temperature through:
   1. Conduction.
   2. Convection.
   3. Evaporation.
   4. Radiation.

9. Poor oxygenation of the blood ordinarily will affect the pulse rate and cause it to become:
   1. Bounding.
   2. Irregular.
   3. Faster than normal.
   4. Slower than normal.

10. The basic techniques of which of these are used to determine vital signs:
    1. Inspection, palpation, and auscultation.
    2. Inspection, blood work, and x-rays.
    3. Rhythm, rate, and open communication.
    4. Psychology, physiology, and nursing skills.

References

Dochterman JM, Bulechek GM: *Nursing interventions classification (NIC)*, ed 4, St. Louis, 2004, Mosby.

Ebersole P, Hess P: *Geriatric nursing and healthy aging*, St. Louis, 2001, Mosby.

Eliopoulos C: *Gerontologic nursing*, ed 5, Philadelphia, 2001, Lippincott.

Grap MJ: Pulse oximetry, *Crit Care Nurse* 22(3):69, 2002.

Guyton AC, Hall J: *Textbook of medical physiology*, ed 9, Philadelphia, 1995, WB Saunders.

Kinney MR and others: *AACN's clinical reference for critical care nursing*, ed 4, St. Louis, 1998, Mosby.

Lueckenotte AG: *Pocket guide to gerontologic assessment*, ed 3, St. Louis, 1998, Mosby.

Lueckenotte AG: *Gerontologic nursing*, ed 3, St. Louis, 2000, Mosby.

Lynch M: Pain as the fifth vital sign. *J Intraven Nurs* 24(2):85, 2001.

Mass ML and others: *Nursing care of older adults*, St. Louis, 2001, Mosby.

McCloskey JC, Bulecek GM: *Nursing interventions classification (NIC)*, ed 3, St. Louis, 2000, Mosby.

Miller CA: *Nursing care of older adults: theory and practice*, ed 3, Philadelphia, 1999, Lippincott.

Moorhead S, Johnson M, Maas M: *Nursing outcomes classification (NOC)*, ed 3, St. Louis, 2004, Mosby.

National High Blood Pressure Education Program (NHBPEP); National Heart, Lung, and Blood Institute; National Institutes of Health: The sixth report of the Joint National Committee on Detection, Evaluation, and Treatment of High Blood Pressure, *Arch Intern Med* 157:2413, 1997.

National High Blood Pressure Education Program (NHBPEP); National Heart, Lung, and Blood Institute; National Institutes of Health: The seventh report of the Joint National Committee on Detection, Evaluation, and Treatment of High Blood Pressure, *JAMA* 289(19):2560, 2003.

National Institutes of Health (NIH): *National Heart, Lung and Blood Institute update on the task force report (1987) on high blood pressure in children and adolescents*, Bethesda, Md, 1996, NIH.

Pickering TG: Self-monitoring of blood pressure. In White WB: *Blood pressure monitoring in cardiovascular medicine and therapeutics*, NJ, 2001, Humana Press.

Sheahan SL, Musialowski R: Clinical implications of respiratory system changes in aging, *J Gerontol Nurs* 27(5):26, 2001.

Thibodeau GA, Patton KT: *Anatomy and physiology*, ed 4, St. Louis, 1999, Mosby.

Research References

Bailey J, Rose P: Axillary and tympanic membrane temperature recording in the preterm neonate: A comparative study, *J Adv Nurs* 34(4):465-474, 2001.

Erickson, RS and others: Accuracy of chemical dot thermometers in critically ill adults and young children. *Image J Nurs Sch* 28:23, 1996.

Fallis WM: Oral measurement of temperature in orally intubated critical care patients: State of the science review, *Am J Crit Care* 9(5):334, 2000.

Futterman LG, Lemberg L: Hypertension in the aged population, *Am J Crit Care* 11(1):80, 2002.

Giuliano KK and others: Temperature measurement in critically ill adults: a comparison of tympanic and oral methods, *Am J Crit Care* 9(4):254, 2000.

Keele-Smith R, Price-Daniel C: Effects of crossing legs on blood pressure measurement, *Clin Nurs Res* 10(2):202, 2001.

Thomas SA, Dekeyser F: Blood pressure, *Annu Rev Nurs Res* 14:3, 1996.

Yucha CB: Ambulatory blood pressure monitoring: measurement implications for research, *J Nurs Meas* 9(1):49, 2001.

32

*H*ealth Assessment and Physical Examination

Media Resources

http://evolve.elsevier.com/Potter/
fundamentals/

CD COMPANION

- Review Questions
- Glossary

evolve WEBSITE

- Review Questions
- Student Learning Activities
- Animations
- Glossary

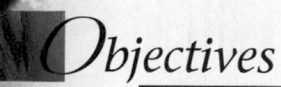# Objectives

Mastery of content in this chapter will enable the student to:

- Define the key terms listed.

- Discuss the purposes of physical assessment.

- Describe the techniques used with each physical assessment skill.

- Discuss the importance of understanding cultural diversity as it influences the approach to health assessment.

- List techniques used to prepare a client physically and psychologically before and during an examination.

- Describe interview techniques used to enhance communication during history taking.

- Make environmental preparations before an examination.

- Identify information to collect from the nursing history before an examination.

- Discuss normal physical findings in a young and middle-age adult compared with an older adult.

- Discuss ways to incorporate health teaching into the examination.

- Use physical assessment skills during routine nursing care.

- Describe physical measurements made in the assessment of each body system.

- Identify self-screening examinations commonly performed by clients.

- Identify preventive screenings and the appropriate age(s) for each screening to occur.

- Discuss factors to consider in documenting examination findings.

- Communicate abnormal findings to appropriate personnel.

Nurses are most often the first persons to detect changes in clients' conditions, regardless of the setting. For this reason, the ability to think critically and interpret the meaning of client behaviors and presenting physiological changes is very important. The skills of physical assessment and examination provide nurses with powerful tools to detect subtle, as well as obvious, changes in a client's health. Physical assessment enables the nurse to assess patterns reflecting health problems and to evaluate the client's progress following therapy.

The nurse works in a variety of settings, seeking information about clients' health status. The nurse conducts health assessments at health fairs, at screening clinics, in physicians' offices, in acute care agencies, and in the client's home. Health screenings involve measurement of specific physical functions such as blood pressure or diagnostic tests such as a tuberculosis (TB) skin test to detect persons with high probabilities of having a disease or condition. This information then determines the need for more comprehensive examinations.

A complete health assessment involves a more detailed review of a client's condition. The nurse collects a nursing history (see Chapter 15) and performs a behavioral and physical examination. The health history interview is an opportunity to establish a relationship with the client that promotes sharing of information. A physical examination is a head-to-toe review of each body system that offers objective information about the client and allows the nurse to make clinical judgments. The client's condition and response affect the extent of the examination. The accuracy of a physical assessment influences the choice of therapies a client receives and the determination of the response to those therapies. Continuity in health care improves when the nurse makes ongoing, objective, and comprehensive assessment.

Purposes of Physical Examination

An examination should be designed for the client's needs. If a client is acutely ill, the nurse recognizes the presenting symptoms and may choose to assess only the involved body systems. A more comprehensive examination is conducted when the client feels more at ease, and the nurse then learns about the client's total health status. A complete physical examination is performed for routine screening to promote wellness behaviors and preventive health care measures; to determine the client's eligibility for health insurance, military service, or a new job; or for the client's admission to a hospital or long-term care facility. The nurse uses physical assessment for the following reasons:

- To gather baseline data about the client's health
- To supplement, confirm, or refute data obtained in the nursing history
- To confirm and identify nursing diagnoses
- To make clinical judgments about a client's changing health status and management
- To evaluate the physiological outcomes of care

Gathering a Health History

The main objective of interacting with clients is to find out what is central to their concerns and to help find solutions. It is important for the nurse to pay attention to clients'

worries and to direct an interview and examination so that a clear picture is created of their condition. This means that collection of a health history and a physical examination require patience and a dedication to thoroughness and detail. There are some basic principles that can help in conducting a successful health history (see Chapter 15) and in laying the groundwork for a well-organized physical examination. The interview allows the nurse to form a partnership with the client so that the interview is oriented to the client, not to a disease. Knowing one's own idiosyncrasies (e.g., wanting to be liked, fear of harming the client, or catching a disease) can prevent resultant feelings from harming the relationship with the client.

Developing Nursing Diagnoses and a Care Plan

The nursing health history allows the nurse to gather a complete and detailed database about the client's health status. After collecting a history, the nurse conducts a physical assessment to refute, confirm, or supplement the existing database. The nurse critically thinks about the information provided by the client, applies knowledge from previous clinical care, and methodically conducts an examination to create a clear picture of the client's status. For example, a client may complain of back pain. The nurse asks several questions to clarify the nature of the pain. During the examination the nurse carefully looks for the source of the pain (e.g., discomfort when changing position or a bruise across the client's back) to rule out a variety of potential ailments.

One assessment finding cannot conclusively reveal the nature of an abnormality. A complete assessment is needed to form a definitive diagnosis. The nurse learns to group significant findings into patterns of data that reveal actual or "risk for" nursing diagnoses. In addition, each abnormal finding directs the nurse to gather additional information. Information gathered during an initial physical assessment provides a baseline of the client's functional abilities. The baseline is not necessarily the normal range of physical findings but rather the pattern of findings identified when the client was first assessed. This baseline serves as a comparison for future assessment findings. During a subsequent assessment the nurse can determine whether the client's condition has changed.

The accuracy of the database allows the nurse to develop individualized nursing diagnoses (Table 32-1).

Table 32-1	Development of Individualized Nursing Diagnoses		
Assessment Method	**Findings**	**Patterns**	**Nursing Diagnosis**
Inspection of skin	Skin along sacral area is intact. There is 3-cm area of redness around coccyx; skin blanches on palpation. No skin lesions are observed.	There is pressure area around coccyx.	Risk for impaired skin integrity.
Palpation of skin	Skin is moist from diaphoresis. There is tenderness to palpation around sacral area. There is elastic skin turgor.	Skin moisture promotes maceration.	
Historical data	Client suffered fractured left leg. Client is immobilized as a result of left leg traction.		

Physical assessment findings help determine the etiology of diagnoses so that the nurse can select the correct type of interventions for the care plan. Physical assessment is ongoing, and thus the care plan changes with the client's condition. The nurse monitors the client's progress and responses to therapies to review existing diagnoses and identify new problems.

Managing Client Problems

When caring for clients, the nurse makes many observations and performs a variety of therapies. Yet the nurse's success in giving care depends on the ability to recognize change in status and to modify therapies so that clients gain the most desirable outcome. Physical assessment skills allow the nurse to judge the status of the client's health and direct the management of care. For example, the nurse inspects the skin during a routine bath and finds it excessively dry. The nurse does not use soap and applies body lotion to the skin. The nurse revises the written care plan so that other nurses know the type of skin care to provide. Instruction is also given to the client about skin care. Performing the mechanics of physical assessment is relatively simple. The more difficult challenge lies in using findings to make decisions.

Evaluating Nursing Care

Nurses demonstrate accountability for their nursing care through evaluating the results of nursing interventions. Physical assessment skills enhance the evaluation of nursing measures through monitoring physiological and behavioral outcomes of care. The same physical assessment skills used to assess a condition (e.g., palpation of the client's pulse) can be used as an evaluation measure after care is administered (e.g., an evaluation of a client's tolerance to an exercise plan).

Nurses make accurate, detailed, objective measurements through physical assessment. The measurements determine whether the expected outcomes of care are met.

Cultural Sensitivity

As is the case with any other aspect of nursing, a physical examination must be performed with the nurse respecting the cultural differences of clients. How individuals behave as a result of their cultural heritage influences their willingness to assume responsibility for their health and their tendency to seek professional health care (see Chapter 8). This is important for the nurse to remember before attempting to conduct a physical examination. A client's health beliefs, use of alternative therapies, nutritional habits, relationships with family, and comfort with the nurse's physical closeness during an examination and history taking must be considered.

It is extremely important for nurses to remain culturally aware and to avoid stereotyping clients on the basis of gender or race. There is a sharp difference between distinguishing cultural characteristics and distinguishing physical characteristics. It is important for nurses to learn common disorders of those ethnic populations within the nurse's community. For example, Navajo Indians often have ear anomalies, Polynesians often suffer clubfoot, and many blacks experience sickle cell disease. Similarly, it is important to know variations in physical characteristics, such as in the skin and musculoskeletal system that are related to cultural variables. Recognition of cultural diversity helps the nurse to respect a client's uniqueness and to provide care of a higher quality (see Chapter 8).

Integration of Physical Assessment With Nursing Care

Whether a complete or partial physical assessment is performed, an examination should be integrated into routine care. For example, the nurse can assess the condition of the skin and other body parts during a bed bath. When a client undergoes oral hygiene, the nurse can carefully assess oral cavity structures. As a client ambulates down the hall, the nurse assesses the client's range of motion, balance, and gait. This practice makes more efficient use of time. The nurse also learns that physical assessment should become an automatic behavior when the nurse and client interact. Physical assessment skills enable the nurse to gather more comprehensive and relevant assessment findings.

Skills of Physical Assessment

Chapter 15 briefly describes the skills of inspection, palpation, percussion, and auscultation. This chapter provides a more detailed description of those skills and their application in the physical examination.

Inspection

Inspection is the process of observation. The nurse inspects body parts to detect normal characteristics or significant physical signs. An experienced nurse learns to make several observations, almost simultaneously, while becoming very perceptive of early warnings of abnormalities. The secret to inspection is to always pay attention to the client, watching all movements and looking very carefully at any body part or area being inspected.

It helps to know normal physical characteristics before trying to distinguish abnormal findings. It is especially important to know normal characteristics of clients of different ages. Dry, wrinkled, inelastic skin is normal in an older adult but not in a young adult. Experience is needed to recognize normal variations among clients, as well as ranges of normal in an individual. Inspection is a simple technique, but it is often underused. The quality of an inspection depends on the nurse's willingness to spend time doing a thorough job. To use inspection effectively, the nurse observes the following principles:

- Make sure good lighting is available.
- Position and expose body parts so that all surfaces can be viewed.
- Inspect each area for size, shape, color, symmetry, position, and abnormalities.
- If possible, compare each area inspected with the same area on the opposite side of the body.

Table 32-2	Examples of Characteristics Measured by Palpation	
Area Examined	**Criteria Measured**	**Portion of Hand to Use**
Skin	Temperature	Dorsum of hand/fingers
	Moisture	Palmar surface
	Texture	
	Turgor and elasticity	Grasping with fingertips
	Tenderness	
	Thickness	Palmar surface
Organs (e.g., liver and intestine)	Size	Entire palmar surface of hand or palmar surface of fingers
	Shape	
	Tenderness	
	Absence of masses	
Glands (e.g., thyroid and lymph)	Swelling	Pads of fingers
	Symmetry and mobility	
Blood vessels (e.g., carotid or femoral artery)	Pulse amplitude	Palmar surface/pads of finger tips
	Elasticity	
	Rate	
	Rhythm	
Thorax	Excursion	Palmar surface
	Tenderness	Finger pads/palmar surface fingers
	Fremitus	Palmar or ulnar surface of entire hand

- Use additional light (e.g., a penlight) to inspect body cavities.
- Do not hurry inspection. Pay attention to detail.

After inspection of a body part is completed, findings may indicate further examination. Palpation is often used with or after visual inspection.

Palpation

Further assessment of body parts is made through the sense of touch. Through palpation the hands can make delicate and sensitive measurements of specific physical signs, including resistance, resilience, roughness, texture, and mobility (Table 32-2). The nurse uses different parts of the hand when touching the skin to detect characteristics such as texture and temperature.

The client should be relaxed and positioned comfortably because muscle tension during palpation impairs its effectiveness. Asking the client to take slow, deep breaths enhances muscle relaxation. Placing the arms along the side of the body will decrease abdominal rigidity. *Tender areas are palpated last.* The nurse asks the client to point out the more sensitive areas and notes any nonverbal signs of discomfort.

Clients appreciate warm hands, short fingernails, and a gentle approach. Palpation may be either light or deep and is controlled by the amount of pressure applied with the fingers or hand. Light palpation always precedes deep palpation. The nurse applies tactile pressure slowly, gently, and deliberately. Light palpation of structures such as the abdomen determines areas of tenderness (Figure 32-1, *A*). The nurse's hand is placed on the part to be examined and depressed about 1 cm (½ inch). Tender areas are examined further for potentially serious abnormalities. The sensation of touch is best preserved with light, intermittent pressure. Heavy, prolonged pressure causes a loss of sensitivity in the nurse's hand.

After light palpation, deeper palpation is used to examine the condition of organs, such as those in the abdomen (Figure 32-1, *B*). The nurse depresses the area be-

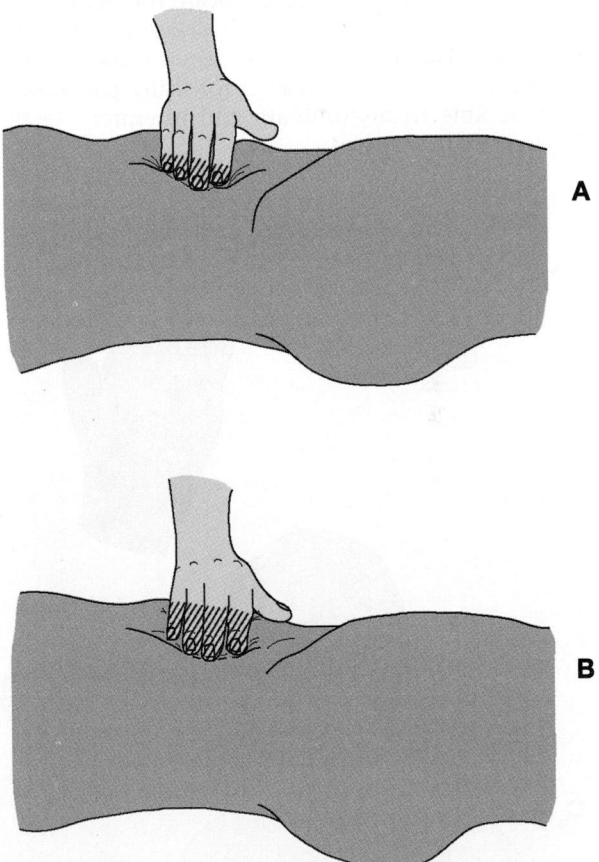

FIGURE 32-1 **A,** During light palpation, gentle pressure against underlying skin and tissues can detect areas of irregularity and tenderness. **B,** During deep palpation, the nurse depresses tissue to assess the condition of underlying organs.

ing examined approximately 2 to 4 cm (1 to 2 inches) (Seidel and others, 2003). Caution is the rule. A nursing student should not attempt deep palpation without clinical supervision to avoid injuring a client. Deep palpation may be applied with one hand or both hands (bimanually). When the nurse uses bimanual palpation, one hand (sensing hand) is relaxed and placed lightly over the client's skin. The other hand (active hand) applies pressure to the sensing hand. The lower hand does not exert pressure directly and thus retains the sensitivity needed to detect organ characteristics.

The most sensitive parts of the hand, the palmar surface of the fingers and finger pads, are used to assess position, texture, size, consistency, form of a mass, and pulsation (Figure 32-2, *A*). Temperature is best measured using the dorsum or back of the hand (Figure 32-2, *B*) and fingers, where the skin is thinnest. The palm or ulnar surface of the hand (Figure 32-2, *C*) is more sensitive to vibration. The nurse measures position, consistency, and turgor by lightly grasping the body part with the fingertips (Figure 32-2, *D*).

The nurse must not palpate without considering the client's condition. For example, if the client has a fractured rib, extra care is used to locate the painful area. A vital artery is not palpated with pressure that obstructs blood flow. The nurse also considers the body area being palpated, as well as the reason for using palpation, and must be able to discriminate and interpret the significance of what is sensed.

Percussion

Percussion involves tapping the body with the fingertips to evaluate the size, borders, and consistency of body organs and to discover fluid in body cavities. It requires considerable skill. It is perhaps the least-used assessment skill; however, it can help to confirm other assessment findings. Through percussion the location, size, and density of an underlying structure are determined. Percussion helps verify reported abnormalities. For example, if the nurse hears abnormal breath sounds when auscultating the lungs, percussion may rule out the presence of consolidated fluid or air in the pleural space.

Percussion involves striking one object against another, thus producing vibration and subsequent sound waves. When the examiner strikes the body's surface with a finger, vibration is transmitted through the body tissues. Sound waves are heard as percussion tones arising from vibrations 4 to 6 cm deep in body tissue (Seidel and others, 2003). The character of the sound depends on the density of the underlying tissue. For example, the normal lung transmits sounds with high intensity and low pitch, whereas the more solid liver transmits a high-pitched sound of soft intensity. By knowing the way that densities influence sound, the nurse can locate organs or masses, map their boundaries, and determine their size. An abnormal sound suggests a mass or substance such as air or fluid within an organ or body cavity.

The two methods of percussion are direct and indirect. The direct method involves striking the body surface di-

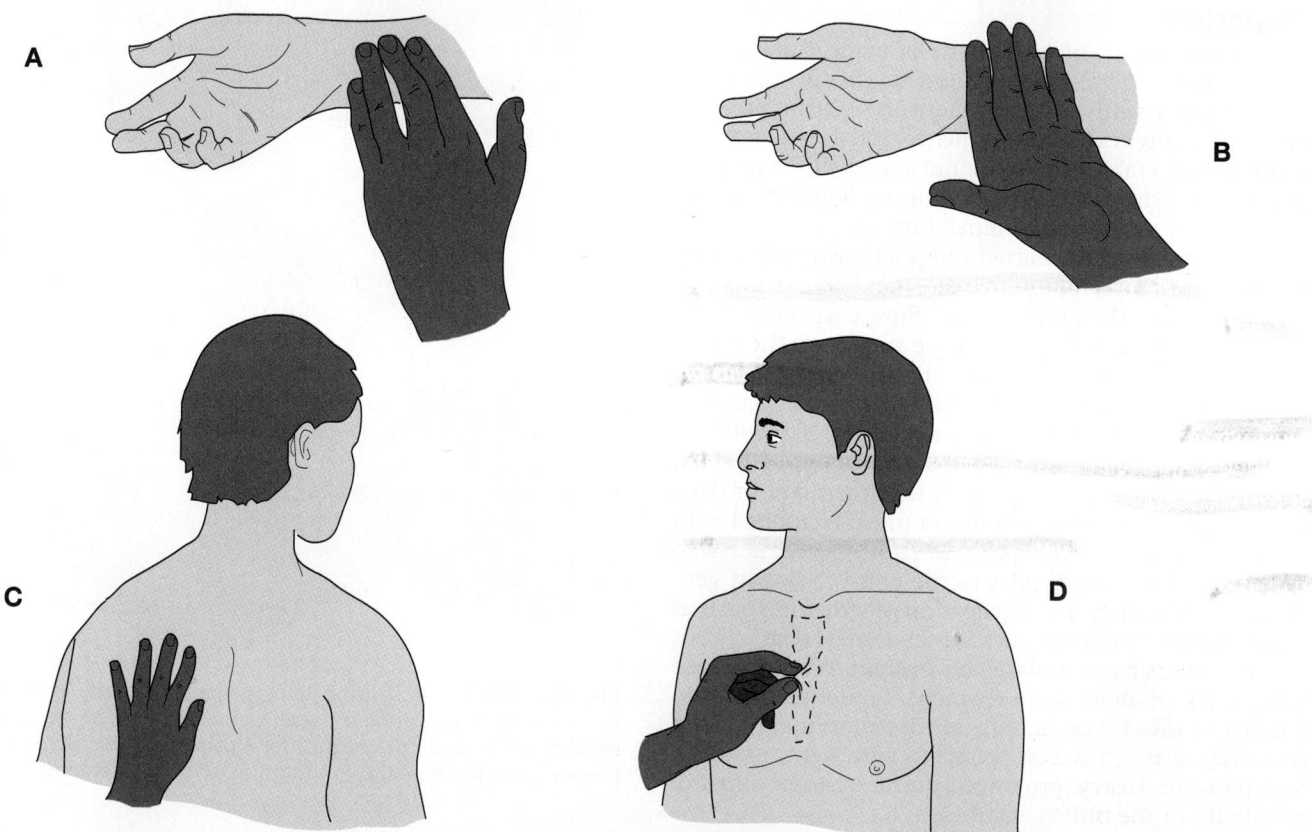

FIGURE 32–2   **A,** The radial pulse is detected with the pads of the fingertips, the most sensitive part of the hand. **B,** The dorsum of the hand allows the nurse to detect temperature variations in skin. **C,** The nurse uses the bony part of the palm at the base of the fingers to detect vibration. **D,** The nurse grasps the skin with the fingertips to assess turgor.

rectly with one or two fingers. The indirect technique is performed by placing the middle finger of the nondominant hand (called the pleximeter) firmly against the body surface, keeping the palm and remaining fingers off the skin. The tip of the middle finger of the dominant hand (called the plexor) strikes the base of the distal joint of the pleximeter (Figure 32-3). The examiner uses a quick, sharp stroke with the plexor finger, keeping the forearm stationary. The wrist remains relaxed to deliver the proper blow. If the blow is not sharp, if the pleximeter is held loosely, or if the palm rests on the body surface, the sound is dampened or softened, preventing transmission of sound to underlying structures. The same force must be applied to each area so that an accurate comparison of sounds can be made. A light, quick blow usually produces the clearest sound. Use of direct versus indirect percussion or firm versus light percussion can lead to different interpretations of results.

Percussion produces five types of sounds: tympany, resonance, hyperresonance, dullness, and flatness. Each sound is created by certain types of underlying tissues and is judged by its intensity of pitch, duration, and quality (Table 32-3).

Auscultation

Auscultation is listening to sounds produced by the body. This skill should be carried out last, except during the ab-

dominal examination, after the other techniques have provided information that will assist in interpreting what is heard. Some sounds can be heard with the unassisted ear, although most sounds can be heard only through a stethoscope. To auscultate correctly, the nurse should listen in a quiet environment, listening for the presence of sound, as well as its characteristics.

It is important to first learn the normal sounds created by the cardiovascular, respiratory, and gastrointestinal systems, such as the passage of blood through an artery. Abnormal sounds can be recognized only after normal variations are learned. The nurse becomes more successful in auscultation by knowing the types of sounds arising from each body structure and the location in which they can most easily be heard. Likewise, the nurse becomes familiar with the areas that normally do not emit sounds.

To auscultate correctly, the nurse needs good hearing acuity, a good stethoscope, and knowledge of how to use the stethoscope properly. Nurses with hearing disorders should purchase stethoscopes with greater sound amplification or ask colleagues to check findings through auscultation. The stethoscope should always be placed on naked skin, because clothing obscures sound. Chapter 31 describes the parts of the stethoscope and the general use of the bell and diaphragm. The bell is best for low-pitched sounds, such as vascular and certain heart sounds, and the diaphragm is best for high-pitched sounds, such as bowel and lung sounds.

A nurse must become familiar with the stethoscope before attempting to use it on a client. It helps to practice using it with a friend. By deliberately producing extraneous sounds, the nurse learns to recognize and disregard them during the actual examination (Box 32-1). Through auscultation the nurse notes the following characteristics of sounds:

- Frequency, or the number of oscillations generated per second by a vibrating object. The higher the frequency, the higher the pitch of a sound, and vice versa.
- Loudness, or the amplitude of a sound wave. Auscultated sounds are described as loud or soft.
- Quality, or sounds of similar frequency and loudness from different sources. Terms such as *blowing* or *gurgling* describe the quality of sound.
- Duration, or the length of time that sound vibrations last. The duration of sound is short, medium, or long. Layers of soft tissue dampen the duration of sounds from deep internal organs.

Auscultation requires concentration and practice. Closing your eyes may help to focus on a particular sound. Taking time to listen to a sound is important. The

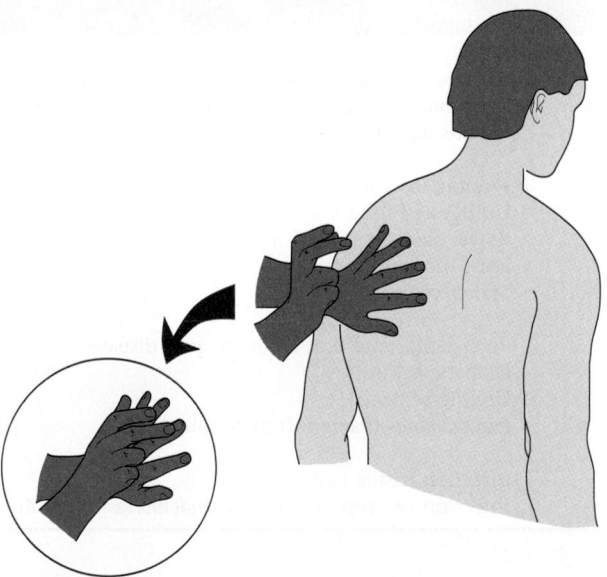

FIGURE 32–3 To perform indirect percussion, the nurse places the middle finger of the nondominant hand against the body's surface. The tip of the middle finger of the dominant hand strikes the top of the middle finger of the nondominant hand.

Table 32-3	Sounds Produced by Percussion				
Sound	**Intensity**	**Pitch**	**Duration**	**Quality**	**Common Location**
Tympany	Loud	High	Moderate	Drumlike	Enclosed, air-containing space; gastric air bubble; puffed-out cheek
Resonance	Moderate to loud	Low	Long	Hollow	Normal lung
Hyperresonance	Very loud	Very low	Longer than resonance	Booming	Emphysematous lung
Dullness	Soft to moderate	High	Moderate	Thudlike	Liver
Flatness	Soft	High	Short	Flat	Muscle

Box 32-1	Exercises to Increase Familiarity With the Stethoscope

Ensure that the earpiece follows the contour of the ear canal. Learn what fit is best for you by comparing amplification of sounds with the earpieces in both directions.

Place the earpieces in your ears with the tips of the earpieces turned toward the face. *Lightly* blow into the diaphragm. Again place the earpieces in your ears, this time with the ends turned toward the back of the head. *Lightly* blow into the diaphragm. You will find that clearer sounds are heard with the earpiece turned toward the face. After you have learned the right fit for the loudest amplification, wear the stethoscope the same way each time.

Put on the stethoscope and *lightly* blow into the diaphragm. If the sound is barely audible, *lightly* blow into the bell. Sound is carried through only one part of the chestpiece at a time. If the sound is greatly amplified through the diaphragm, the diaphragm is in position for use. If the sound is barely audible through the diaphragm, the bell is in position for use. Rotation of the diaphragm and bell places the chestpiece in the desired position. Leave the diaphragm in position for the next exercise.

Place the diaphragm over the anterior part of your chest. Ask a friend to speak in a normal conversational tone. Environmental noise seriously detracts from hearing the noise created by body organs. When a stethoscope is used, the client and the examiner should remain quiet.

Put the stethoscope on and gently tap the tubing. It is often difficult to avoid stretching or moving the stethoscope's tubing. The examiner should be in a position so that the tubing hangs free. Moving or touching the tubing creates extraneous sounds.

Care of the stethoscope: Earpieces should be removed regularly and cleaned of cerumen (earwax). The bell and diaphragm should be kept free of dust, lint, and body oils. The tubing should be kept away from nurse's body oils. Avoid draping the stethoscope around the neck next to the skin. The entire stethoscope (diaphragm, tubing, etc.) can be wiped clean with alcohol or soapy water. Be sure to dry all parts thoroughly. Please follow the manufacturer's recommendations.

Table 32-4	Assessment of Characteristic Odors	
Odor	**Site or Source**	**Potential Causes**
Alcohol	Oral cavity	Ingestion of alcohol, diabetes
Ammonia	Urine	Urinary tract infection
Body odor	Skin, particularly in areas where body parts rub together (e.g., underarms and under breasts)	Poor hygiene, excess perspiration (hyperhidrosis), foul-smelling perspiration (bromhidrosis)
	Wound site	Wound abscess
	Vomitus	Undigested food
Feces	Vomitus/oral cavity (fecal odor)	Bowel obstruction
	Rectal area	Fecal incontinence
Foul-smelling stools in infant	Stool	Malabsorption syndrome
Halitosis	Oral cavity	Poor dental and oral hygiene, gum disease
Sweet, fruity ketones	Oral cavity	Diabetic acidosis
Stale urine	Skin	Uremic acidosis
Sweet, heavy, thick odor	Draining wound	*Pseudomonas* (bacterial) infection
Musty odor	Casted body part	Infection inside cast
Fetid, sweet odor	Tracheostomy or mucus secretions	Infection of bronchial tree (*Pseudomonas* bacteria)

nurse must also consider the part of the body auscultated and the causes of the sounds. For example, the first heart sound is caused by closure of the mitral valve. The nurse learns where sounds can best be heard. The first heart sound is best auscultated at the fifth intercostal space along the midclavicular line. The nurse also learns the characteristics of normal sounds. The first heart sound has the quality of a loud "lub," whereas the second sound is a "dub." After the cause and character of normal auscultated sounds are understood, it becomes easier to recognize abnormal sounds and their origins.

Olfaction

While assessing a client, the nurse should be familiar with the nature and source of body odors (Table 32-4).

Olfaction helps the nurse detect abnormalities that cannot be recognized by any other means. For example, a client with a cast is expected to experience discomfort after an injury. However, the nurse who notes a strong odor will suspect that the discomfort may also be related to wound infection. The discomfort alone does not reveal the presence of infection. Findings from olfaction and other assessment skills allow the nurse to detect serious abnormalities.

Preparation for Examination

Proper preparation of the environment, equipment, and client ensures a smooth physical examination with few interruptions. A disorganized approach when preparing for a physical examination can cause errors and incomplete findings.

Infection Control

During an examination the nurse may find clients with open skin lesions or weeping wounds. Examination techniques cause the nurse to contact body fluids and discharge. Standard precautions should be used throughout the examination (see Chapter 33) as appropriate. At times, it becomes necessary to wear gloves during palpation and percussion to reduce contact with microorganisms. If a client has excessive drainage from a wound, the examiner may need to wear a gown. Before initiating and after completing a physical assessment or portions of an assessment the nurse should follow the agency's hand hygiene policies.

Environment

A physical examination requires privacy. A well-equipped examination room is preferable. However, in hospitals the examination usually occurs in the client's room, where it may be necessary to use room curtains or dividers around the bed. In the home the nurse may perform an examination in the client's bedroom.

Any examination room should be well equipped for all necessary procedures. Adequate lighting is needed for proper illumination of body parts. Primary lighting can be either daylight or artificial, as long as the light is direct enough to reveal skin characteristics without distortion from shadows. Ideally, an examination room is soundproofed so that clients feel comfortable discussing their conditions. The nurse eliminates sources of noise such as televisions or radios, takes steps to prevent interruptions from others, and makes sure the room is warm enough for the client's comfort.

Sometimes it is difficult to examine clients who are in beds or on stretchers. Special examination tables make clients easily accessible and help them assume special positions. The tables are high and narrow. The nurse must carefully assist clients so that they do not fall while getting on and off them. A confused, combative, or uncooperative client should not be left unsupervised on an examination table.

Examination tables are often hard and uncomfortable. When the client lies supine, the head of the table can be raised about 30 degrees. The client may also be given a small pillow. When examining a client in bed, the nurse can raise the bed to reach body parts more easily.

Equipment

Hand hygiene is completed before equipment preparation and before the examination. Hand hygiene reduces the transmission of microorganisms. The equipment needed for an examination should be clean, readily available, and arranged in order for easy use (Figure 32-4). It should be kept warm as appropriate. The diaphragm of the stethoscope may be briskly rubbed between the hands before it is applied to the skin. Warm water should be run over the vaginal speculum. All equipment must be checked to ensure that it functions properly. The ophthalmoscope and otoscope require good batteries and lightbulbs. Equipment typically used is listed in Box 32-2.

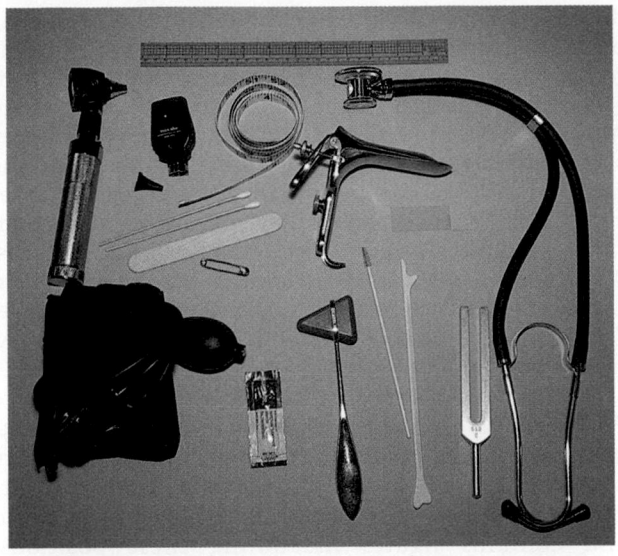

FIGURE 32-4   Equipment used during a physical examination.

Box 32-2   Equipment and Supplies for Physical Assessment

Cotton applicators
Cytobrush
Disposable pad
Drapes
Eye chart (e.g., Snellen chart)
Flashlight and spotlight
Forms (e.g., physical, laboratory)
Gloves (sterile or clean)
Gown for client
Water-soluble lubricant
Ophthalmoscope
Otoscope
Papanicolaou smear slides
Paper towels
Percussion hammer

Ruler
Scale with height measurement rod
Specimen containers and microscope slides
Sphygmomanometer and cuff
Stethoscope
Swabs or sponge forceps
Tape measure
Thermometer
Tissues
Tongue depressors
Tuning fork
Vaginal speculum
Wristwatch with second hand or digital display

Physical Preparation of the Client

The client's physical comfort is vital for a successful examination. Before starting, the nurse asks if the client needs to use the toilet. An empty bladder and bowel facilitate examination of the abdomen, genitalia, and rectum and provide the opportunity to collect urine or fecal specimens. The nurse explains the proper method for collecting specimens and ensures that each specimen is properly labeled. When obtaining specimens, infection-control practices are necessary (see Chapter 33).

Physical preparation involves being sure the client is dressed and draped properly. A client in the hospital will likely be wearing only a simple gown. In an outpatient setting the client is instructed to undress and apply a light cover gown. If the examination is limited to certain body systems, it may be unnecessary for the client to undress completely. The client should have privacy during undressing and plenty of time to finish. Walking into the room as the client undresses causes embarrassment. Drapes and gowns are made of linen or disposable paper. After clients have undressed and donned the gown, they should sit or lie down on the examination table with the drape over the lap or lower trunk. The examiner makes sure that the client stays warm by eliminating drafts, controlling room temperature, and providing warm blankets. A seriously ill client or older adult is more susceptible to chills. The nurse should ask if the client is comfortable. The client may become more relaxed if offered a pillow, sip of water, or tissue.

Positioning. During the examination the nurse asks clients to assume proper positions so that body parts are accessible and clients stay comfortable. Table 32-5 lists the preferred positions for each part of the examination and contains figures illustrating these positions. Clients' abilities to assume positions will depend on their physical strength, mobility, ease of breathing, age, and degree of wellness. The examiner explains the positions and assists clients in attaining them. The drapes are adjusted to be sure that the area to be examined is accessible and that no body part is unnecessarily exposed. More than one position can be assumed for the same part of an examination (e.g., supine and sitting for assessment of the anterior thorax), so the nurse first chooses the position that provides greater accessibility and accuracy in assessing body parts (sitting for assessment of the anterior thorax). However, if clients are too weak or are physically unable to assume a position, the nurse may choose an alternative position. The nurse uses extra care to position older adults so that they may avoid looking into the source of light, which can cause discomfort from glare.

Psychological Preparation of the Client

Clients are easily embarrassed when forced to answer sensitive questions about bodily functions or when body parts are exposed and examined. The possibility that the examiner will find something abnormal also creates anxiety, so reduction of this anxiety may be the nurse's highest priority before the examination. The nurse should convey an open, receptive, and professional approach. A stiff, formal demeanor may inhibit the client's ability to communicate, but a style that is too casual may fail to instill confidence (Seidel and others, 2003). A thorough explanation lets clients know what to expect and what to do so that they can cooperate. The nurse first explains the examination in general terms, and then a more detailed explanation is given as each system is examined.

The nurse uses simple terms when describing the steps of the examination. Complicated terminology confuses clients and adds to their fears. The nurse's manner should be professional, but the voice tone and facial expressions should be relaxed to put clients at ease. The nurse encourages clients to ask questions and mention any discomfort they feel during the assessment. When the client and nurse are of opposite gender, it may be necessary to have a third person of the client's gender in the room, especially when examination of the sexual organs is re-

quired. The presence of a third person assures the client that the examiner will behave ethically, and the third person acts as a witness to the examiner's proper conduct.

During the examination the nurse watches the client's emotional responses. The nurse observes whether the client's facial expression conveys fear or concern and whether body movements reveal anxiety, such as frequently pulling the drape around the body or tensing up as the examiner touches the body. The nurse must remain calm and clearly explain each step of the assessment. It may be necessary to stop the examination and ask whether the client feels anxious, afraid, or uncomfortable. The client should not be forced to continue. Postponing the examination until a later time may be advantageous because the findings may be more accurate when the client can cooperate and relax. If the fears result from misconceptions, the nurse clarifies the purpose of the examination and how it is to be performed.

Assessment of Age-Groups

The nurse uses different interview styles and approaches to physical examination for clients of different age-groups. When assessing children, the nurse must be sensitive and anticipate the child's reaction to the examination as a strange and unfamiliar experience. Routine pediatric examinations have a focus on health promotion and illness prevention. The focus of the examination is on growth and development, sensory screening, dental examination, and behavioral assessment. Children who are chronically ill or disabled, foster children, and foreign-born adopted children may require additional examination visits. These visits may be to evaluate required therapies or treatments, evaluate nutritional needs for proper growth and development, or to provide for additional immunizations. When examining children, the following tips assist in data collection:

- When obtaining histories on infants and children, gather all or part of the information from parents or guardians.
- Perform the examination in a nonthreatening area and provide time for play to become acquainted.
- Because parents may think they are being tested by the examiner, offer support during the examination and do not pass judgment.
- Call children by their first name, and address the parents as "Mr. and Mrs." rather than by their first names.
- Use open-ended questions to allow parents to share more information and describe more of the children's problems.
- Interview older children to allow observation of parent-child interactions. Also, older children can often provide details about their health history and severity of symptoms.
- Treat adolescents as adults and individuals because they tend to respond best when treated as such.
- Remember that adolescents have the right to confidentiality. After talking with parents about historical information, speak alone with adolescents.

A comprehensive health assessment and examination of older adults should include physical data, as well as a review of the client's cognitive, affective, and social level of functioning (Lueckenotte, 2000). An important aspect

Table 32-5   Positions for Examination

Position	Areas Assessed	Rationale	Limitations
Sitting	Head and neck, back, posterior thorax and lungs, anterior thorax and lungs, breasts, axillae, heart, vital signs, and upper extremities	Sitting upright provides full expansion of lungs and provides better visualization of symmetry of upper body parts.	Physically weakened client may be unable to sit. Examiner should use supine position with head of bed elevated instead.
Supine	Head and neck, anterior thorax and lungs, breasts, axillae, heart, abdomen, extremities, pulses	This is most normally relaxed position. It provides easy access to pulse sites.	If client becomes short of breath easily, examiner may need to raise head of bed.
Dorsal recumbent	Head and neck, anterior thorax and lungs, breasts, axillae, heart, abdomen	Position is used for abdominal assessment because it promotes relaxation of abdominal muscles.	Clients with painful disorders are more comfortable with knees flexed.
Lithotomy*	Female genitalia and genital tract	This position provides maximal exposure of genitalia and facilitates insertion of vaginal speculum.	Lithotomy position is embarrassing and uncomfortable, so examiner minimizes time that client spends in it. Client is kept well draped.
Sims'	Rectum and vagina	Flexion of hip and knee improves exposure of rectal area.	Joint deformities may hinder client's ability to bend hip and knee.
Prone	Musculoskeletal system	This position is used only to assess extension of hip joint.	This position is poorly tolerated in clients with respiratory difficulties.
Lateral recumbent	Heart	This position aids in detecting murmurs.	This position is poorly tolerated in clients with respiratory difficulties.
Knee-chest*	Rectum	This position provides maximal exposure of rectal area.	This position is embarrassing and uncomfortable.

*Clients with arthritis or other joint deformities may be unable to assume this position.

is to assess basic activities of daily living as well as complex instrumental activities of daily living.

Throughout an examination the nurse must recognize that with advancing age the body does not respond vigorously to injury or disease. Therefore older persons do not always exhibit the expected signs and symptoms (Lueckenotte, 2000). Characteristically, older adults present more blunted or atypical signs and symptoms.

Principles to follow during examination of an older adult include the following:

- Do not stereotype aging clients. Most are able to adapt to change and to learn about their health. Similarly, most are reliable historians.
- Recognize that sensory or physical limitations can affect how quickly you are able to interview older adults and conduct examinations. Plan for more than one examination session. Sometimes it helps to give clients an initial health questionnaire before they come to a clinic or office (Lueckenotte, 2000).
- Perform the examination with adequate space; this is especially important for clients with mobility aids such as a cane or walker.
- During the examination use patience, allow for pauses, and observe for details. Recognize normalities of later life that would be abnormal in a younger client.
- Older clients may find giving certain types of health information stressful. Illness is seen as a threat to independence and a step toward institutionalization.
- Perform the examination near bathroom facilities. The client may experience an urgent need to void.
- Be alert to signs of increasing fatigue, such as sighing, grimacing, irritability, leaning against objects for support, and drooping of the head and shoulders.

Organization of the Examination

Regardless of the age of a client, a basic physical examination follows a similar approach. A physical examination is composed of individual assessments for each body system. The extent of an examination depends on its purpose and the client's condition. A client who comes to a clinic with symptoms of a severe chest cold will not routinely require a neurological assessment. A client entering the emergency department with an acute illness requires assessment of the body systems most at risk for being abnormal. When a client is admitted to the hospital, a complete examination is usually performed. A client who is receiving a routine health promotion examination may undergo specific preventive screenings, depending on the client's age or health risk (Table 32-6). Clients with specific symptoms or needs often require only portions of an examination. The nurse's judgment is needed to ensure that an examination is relevant and includes the correct observations.

The performance of a complete health assessment follows the format of the nursing history (see Chapter 15). The nurse uses information from the history to focus attention on specific parts of the examination. Findings from the history generally reveal a pattern of related signs and symptoms. The physical examination supplements information from the history to confirm or refute the data.

The examination should be systematic and well organized so that important assessments are not omitted. A head-to-toe approach includes all body systems and helps the nurse anticipate each step. In an adult the nurse begins by assessing the head and neck area, progressing methodically down the body to incorporate all body systems. The following tips help the nurse keep an examination well organized:

- Compare both sides of the body for symmetry. A degree of asymmetry is normal (e.g., the biceps muscles in the dominant arm may be more developed than the same muscles in the nondominant arm).
- If a client is seriously ill, first assess the systems of the body more at risk for being abnormal. For example, a client with chest pain should undergo a cardiovascular assessment first.
- If a client becomes fatigued, offer rest periods between assessments.
- Perform painful procedures near the end of the examination.
- Record results of the examination in specific anatomical and scientific terms so that any professional can interpret the findings.
- Use common and accepted medical abbreviations to keep notes brief and concise.
- Record quick notes during the examination to avoid keeping the client waiting. Complete any observations at the end of the examination.
- A physical assessment form allows recording of information in the same sequence it is gathered.

General Survey

Assessment begins when the nurse first meets the client. The nurse determines the reason the client is seeking health care. Initial data from the general survey begins with a review of the client's primary health problems. The nurse makes mental notes of the client's behavior and appearance. The examination begins with a general survey that includes observation of general appearance and behavior, vital signs, and height and weight measurements. The survey provides information about characteristics of an illness, a client's hygiene and body image, emotional state, recent changes in weight, and developmental status. If abnormalities or problems are found, the affected body system is closely assessed later.

General Appearance and Behavior

Assessment of appearance and behavior begins while the nurse prepares the client for the examination. The review of general appearance and behavior includes the following:

- *Gender and race:* A person's gender affects the type of examination performed and the manner in which assessments are made. Different physical features are related to gender and race. Certain illnesses are more likely to affect a specific gender or race; for example, the incidence of skin cancer is 20 times higher in whites than

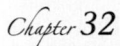

Table 32-6	**Recommended Preventive Screenings**	
Disease/Condition	**Age-Group**	**Screening Measures**
Breast cancer*	Ages 20 to 39	Monthly breast self-examination (BSE). Clinical breast examination by health care professional every 3 years.
	Ages 40 and up	Monthly BSE. Annual clinical breast examination by health care professional.
Colon/rectal cancer*	Ages 50 and up	Men and women should have one of the following: fecal occult blood test (FOBT) yearly, or flexible sigmoidoscopy every 5 years, or FOBT yearly and a flexible sigmoidoscopy every 5 years (ACS recommends this one) or double-contrast barium enema every 5 years or colonoscopy every 10 years. A digital rectal examination should be done at the same time as above. Earlier screening is needed if risk factors exist.
Ear disorders	All ages	Periodic hearing checks as needed.
	Over age 65	Regular hearing checks.
Eye disorders	Age 40 and under	Complete eye examination every 3 to 5 years (more if positive history).
	Ages 40 to 64	Complete eye examination every 2 years.
	Age 65 and up	Complete eye examination every year.
Heart/vascular disorders	Men age 45 to 65/ Women age 45 to 65	Regular measurement of total blood cholesterol levels and triglycerides; blood pressure screenings.
Obesity	All ages	Periodic height and weight measurements.
Oral cavity/ pharyngeal disorders/cancer	All ages (children, adults, older adults)	Regular dental examinations every 6 months.
Ovarian cancer*	Age 18 and up or on becoming sexually active	Annual pelvic examinations by health care professional.
Prostate cancer*	Ages 50 and up	Men who have at least a 10-year life expectancy should have a digital rectal examination and prostate-specific antigen (PSA) blood test annually. Men at high risk require earlier screening.
Skin cancer*	All ages	Regular skin self-examination.
	Ages 20 to 40	See specialist every 3 years.
	Over 40	Annual skin checkups with biopsy of suspicious lesions.
Testicular cancer*	Age 15 and up	Monthly testicular self-examination (TSE).
Uterine cancer*	Age 18 and up or on becoming sexually active	Annual pelvic examination by health care professional plus an annual Pap test.
Cervical cancer	Age 18 and up or on becoming sexually active	Annual pelvic examination by health care professional.
Endometrial cancer	Age 18 and up or on becoming sexually active	Endometrial biopsy at age 35 for high-risk clients. At menopause, women at average and high risk should be informed of high risks and signs and symptoms to report.

*Data from American Cancer Society: *Cancer prevention and early detection: Facts and figures 2003*, New York, 2003, The Society.
Web site for further information on preventative screenings: *Guide to clinical preventive services*, prepared by the U.S. Preventive Services Task Force, http://cpmcnet.columbia.edu/texts//gcps/gcpsoooo.html.

in blacks, the incidence of prostate cancer is higher in African-American than in white American men, and cancer of the bladder is more common in men (American Cancer Society [ACS], 2003).

- *Age:* Age influences normal physical characteristics. The ability to participate in some parts of the examination is also influenced by age.
- *Signs of distress:* There may be obvious signs or symptoms indicating pain, difficulty in breathing, or anxiety. These signs establish priorities regarding what to examine first.
- *Body type:* The nurse observes if a client appears trim and muscular, obese, or excessively thin. Body type can reflect the level of health, age, and lifestyle.
- *Posture:* Normal standing posture is an upright stance with parallel alignment of the hips and shoulders. Normal sitting posture involves some degree of rounding of the shoulders. Observe whether the client has a

slumped, erect, or bent posture. Posture may reflect mood or presence of pain. Many older adults assume a stooped, forward-bent posture, with the hips and knees somewhat flexed and the arms bent at the elbows, raising the level of the arms.

- *Gait:* Observe the client walk into the room or at the bedside (if the client is ambulatory). Note whether movements are coordinated or uncoordinated. A person normally walks with the arms swinging freely at the sides, with the head and face leading the body.
- *Body movements:* Observe whether movements are purposeful and note if there are any tremors involving the extremities. Determine if any body parts are immobile.
- *Hygiene and grooming:* The client's level of cleanliness is noted by observing the appearance of the hair, skin, and fingernails. Observe if the client's clothes are clean. Grooming may depend on the activities being performed just before the examination, as well as the

client's occupation. Also note the amount and type of cosmetics used.

- *Dress:* Culture, lifestyle, socioeconomic level, and personal preference affect the type of clothes worn. Note if the type of clothing worn is appropriate for the temperature and weather conditions. Depressed or mentally ill persons may be unable to choose proper clothing. An older adult tends to wear extra clothing because of the sensitivity to cold.
- *Body odor:* An unpleasant body odor may result from physical exercise, poor hygiene, or certain disease states. Poor oral hygiene or certain diseases may cause bad breath.
- *Affect and mood:* Affect is a person's feelings as they appear to others. A person's mood or emotional state is expressed verbally and nonverbally. Note if verbal expressions match nonverbal behavior and observe if

the client's mood is appropriate for the situation. For example, the mood is inappropriate if the client seems unusually happy after recently being diagnosed with cancer. Observe facial expressions as questions are asked.

- *Speech:* Normal speech is understandable and moderately paced and shows an association with the person's thoughts. Note if the client talks rapidly or slowly. An abnormal pace may be caused by emotions or neurological impairment. Also note if the client speaks in a normal tone with clear inflection of words.
- *Client abuse:* Abuse of children, women, and older adults is a growing and serious health problem. It may be suspected in clients who have suffered obvious physical injury or neglect (e.g., evidence of malnutrition or presence of bruising on the extremities or

---

Box 32-3   **Clinical Indicators of Abuse**

Physical Findings

Child Sexual Abuse

Vaginal or penile discharge
Blood on underclothing
Pain, itching, or unusual odor in genital area
Genital injuries
Difficulty sitting or walking
Pain while urinating; recurrent urinary tract infections
Foreign bodies in rectum, urethra, or vagina
Sexually transmitted diseases
Pregnancy in young adolescent

Behavioral Findings

Problem in sleeping or eating
Fear of certain people or places
Play activities recreate the abuse situation
Regressed behavior
Sexual acting out
Knowledge of explicit sexual matters
Preoccupation with other's or own genitals
Profound and rapid personality changes
Rapidly declining school performance
Poor relationship with peers

Domestic Abuse

Injuries and trauma are inconsistent with reported cause
Multiple injuries involving head, face, neck, breasts, abdomen, and genitalia (black eyes, orbital fractures, broken nose, fractured skull, lip lacerations, broken teeth, strangulation marks)
X-ray films show old and new fractures in different stages of healing
Abrasions, lacerations, bruises/welts
Burns
Human bites

Attempted suicide
Eating or sleeping disorders
Anxiety
Panic attacks
Pattern of substance abuse (follows physical abuse)
Low self-esteem
Depression
Sense of helplessness
Guilt
Increased forgetfulness
Stress-related complaints (headache, anxiety)

Older Adult Abuse

Injuries and trauma are inconsistent with reported cause (cigarette burn, scratch, bruise, or bite)
Hematomas
Bruises at various stages of resolution
Bruises, chafing, excoriation on wrist or legs (restraints)
Burns
Fractures inconsistent with cause described
Dried blood

Dependent on caregiver
Physically and/or cognitively impaired
Combative
Wandering
Verbally belligerent
Minimal social support
Prolonged interval between injury and medical treatment

Data from Gerard M: Domestic violence: how to screen and intervene, *RN* 63(12):52, 2000; Hoban S, Kearney K: Elder abuse and neglect, *Am J Nurs* 100(11):49, 2000; Kramer A: Domestic violence: how to ask and how to listen, *Nurs Clin North Am* 37(1):189, 2002; and Wong DL, Hockenberry-Eaton M: *Wong's essentials of pediatric nursing,* ed 6, St. Louis, 2001, Mosby.

trunk). Assess for the client's fear of the spouse or partner, caregiver, parent, or adult child. Note if the partner or caregiver has a history of violence, alcoholism, or drug abuse. Is the person unemployed, ill, or frustrated in caring for the client? Most states mandate a report to a social service center if abuse or neglect is suspected. When abuse is suspected, interview the client in private. It is difficult to detect abuse, because victims often will not complain or report that they are in an abusive situation (Kramer, 2002). Clients are much more likely to reveal any problems to a nurse when the suspected abuser is absent from the room (Hoban and Kearney, 2000). Clinical indicators for abuse are summarized in Box 32-3.

> **Safety Alert.** The risk for further abuse is high once the victim has reported the abuse or tries to leave the abusive situation. Provide counseling options for these individuals.

- *Substance abuse.* Health care providers' recognition of clients who abuse alcohol, prescribed medications, or illegal drugs is typically poor. The problem affects all socioeconomic groups, and a single visit to a clinic may not reveal the problem. Several visits often reveal behaviors that can be confirmed with a well-focused history and physical examination. The nurse must approach the client in a caring and nonjudgmental way, because issues of substance abuse involve both emo-

---

Box 32-4   **Red Flags for Suspicion of Substance Abuse**

Clients who frequently miss appointments

Clients who frequently request written excuses for work

Clients who have chief complaints of insomnia, "bad nerves," or pain that does not fit a particular pattern

Clients who often report lost prescriptions (e.g., tranquilizers or pain medications) or ask for frequent refills

Clients who make frequent emergency department visits

Clients who have a history of changing doctors or who bring in medication bottles prescribed by several different providers

Clients with a history of gastrointestinal bleeds, peptic ulcers, pancreatitis, cellulitis, or frequent pulmonary infections

Clients with frequent sexually transmitted diseases (STDs), complicated pregnancies, multiple abortions, or sexual dysfunction

Clients who complain of chest pains or palpitations or who have a history of admissions to rule out myocardial infarctions

Clients with a history of activities that place them at risk for human immunodeficiency virus (HIV) infections (multiple sexual partners, multiple rapes)

Clients with a family history of addiction; history of childhood sexual, physical, or emotional abuse; or social and financial or marital problems

Modified from Master S, Terpstra JK: Recognition and diagnosis. In Schnoll SH, Horvatich PK, Terpstra JK, editors: *Prescribing drugs with abuse liability,* Richmond, Va, 1992, DSAM, MCV-VCU; and Friedman L and others: *Source book of substance abuse and addiction,* Baltimore, 1996, Williams & Wilkins.

---

tional and lifestyle issues. Clients to suspect for substance abuse include those listed in Box 32-4. When substance abuse is suspected, it is recommended that the nurse or examiner ask the following CAGE questions: Have you ever felt the need to *Cut down* on your drinking or drug use? Have people *Annoyed* you by criticizing your drinking or drug use? Have you ever felt bad or *Guilty* about your drinking or drug use? Have you ever used or had a drink first thing in the morning as an *Eye-opener* to steady your nerves or feel normal? If answers to two or more of the CAGE (a mnemonic for the four questions) questions are positive, the nurse should strongly suspect abuse and consider how to motivate the client to seek treatment (Stuart and Laraia, 2001).

Vital Signs

Assessment of vital signs (see Chapter 31) should be the first part of the physical examination. Positioning or moving the client during the examination can interfere with obtaining accurate values. However, it is also appropriate for the nurse to measure specific vital signs during assessment of individual body systems. For example, the pulse can be assessed during examination of the peripheral pulses, and the heart and respirations can be assessed during examination of the thorax. Body temperature is always measured during the general survey.

Height, Weight, and Circumference

A person's general level of health can be reflected in the ratio of height to weight. Weight is a routine measure during health screenings and visits to physicians' offices or clinics. Both measures are routine when clients are admitted to a health care setting. A nurse measures infants' and children's height and weight to assess growth and development. In older adults, height and weight coupled with a nutritional assessment are important in determining the cause of and treatment for chronic disease and in assessing the older adult who has difficulty with feeding and other functional activities (Box 32-5). The nurse should look for overall trends in height and weight changes.

A client's weight will normally vary daily because of fluid loss or retention. Progressive weight gain is expected during pregnancy. A downward trend in a frail older adult may indicate serious reduction in nutritional reserves. The assessment screens for abnormal weight changes. The nursing history can help to focus on possible causes for a change in weight (Table 32-7). Before measurement the nurse asks clients their current height and weight. Standardized tables can help reveal the normal expected weight for a client at a given height (Table 32-8). A weight gain of 5 pounds (2.3 kg) in a day may indicate fluid retention problems. If the client has lost more than 5% of body weight in a month or 10% in 6 months, the loss is significant.

Clients should be weighed at the same time of day, on the same scale, and in the same clothes to allow an objective comparison of subsequent weights. Although measuring body weight may seem routine, care should be taken to be certain of accuracy, because medical and nursing decisions (e.g., drug dosage determinations, lift-

Box 32-5	Dietary History for Older Adults

Does the older adult need or have help in preparing meals? Are meals ever skipped?

Are the five primary food groups from the food guide pyramid represented in the daily diet (bread, cereal, rice and pasta group, 6 to 11 servings; fruit group, 2 to 4 servings; vegetable group, 3 to 5 servings; meat, poultry, fish, dry beans, eggs and nut group, 2 to 3 servings; and milk, yogurt and cheese group, 2 to 3 servings)? Refer to Chapter 43.

Does the older adult take nutritional supplements, such as multivitamins?

Does the older adult take any medication affecting appetite or absorption of nutrients?

Does the older adult have any religious or cultural beliefs and practices that influence diet?

Does the older adult have a special diet, or does the client's diet contain an unusual amount of alcohol, sweets, or fried food?

Does the older adult have temperomandibular joint (TMJ) dysfunction?

Data from Lueckenotte A: *Gerontologic nursing,* ed 2, St. Louis, 2000, Mosby; and Moore MC: *Pocket guide to nutritional care,* ed 4, St. Louis, 2001, Mosby.

Table 32-7	Nursing History for Weight Assessment

Assessment Category	Rationale
Ask about total weight lost or gained; compare with usual weight; note time period for loss (e.g., gradual, sudden, desired, or undesired).	Determines severity of problem and may reveal if related to disease process, change in eating pattern, or pregnancy.
If weight loss desired, ask about eating pattern, diet plan followed, usual daily calorie intake, and appetite.	Helps to determine appropriateness of diet plan followed.
If weight loss undesired, ask about anorexia, vomiting, diarrhea, thirst, frequent urination, and change in lifestyle or activity.	Focuses on problems that may cause weight loss (e.g., gastrointestinal problems).
Assess if client has noted changes in social aspects of eating: more meals in restaurants, rushing to eat meals, stress at work, or skipping meals.	Lifestyle changes can contribute to weight changes.
Assess if client takes chemotherapy, diuretics, insulin, psychotropics, steroids, nonprescription diet pills, or laxatives.	Weight gain or loss can be side effect of these medications.

Table 32-8	Height and Weight Table: Weights for Persons 25 to 59 Years According to Build*

Men				Women				
HEIGHT		Small Frame	Medium Frame	Large Frame	HEIGHT†		Small Frame	Medium Frame	Large Frame
Feet	Inches				Feet	Inches			
5	2	128-134	131-141	138-150	4	10	102-111	109-121	118-131
5	3	130-136	133-143	140-153	4	11	102-111	111-123	120-134
5	4	132-138	135-145	142-156	5	0	103-113	113-126	122-137
5	5	134-140	137-148	144-160	5	1	104-115	115-129	125-140
5	6	136-142	139-151	146-164	5	2	106-118	118-132	128-143
5	7	138-145	142-154	149-168	5	3	108-121	121-135	131-147
5	8	140-148	145-157	152-172	5	4	111-124	124-138	134-151
5	9	142-151	148-160	155-176	5	5	114-127	127-141	137-155
5	10	144-154	151-163	158-180	5	6	117-130	130-144	140-159
5	11	146-157	154-166	161-184	5	7	120-133	133-147	143-163
6	0	149-160	157-170	164-188	5	8	123-136	136-150	146-167
6	1	152-164	160-174	168-192	5	9	126-139	139-153	149-170
6	2	155-168	164-178	172-197	5	10	129-142	142-156	152-173
6	3	158-172	167-182	176-207	5	11	132-145	145-159	155-176
6	4	162-176	171-187	181-207	6	0	138-151	148-162	158-179

Courtesy Metropolitan Life Insurance Company: *Statistical bulletin,* New York, 2000, Metropolitan.
*Indoor clothing weighing 5 pounds for men and 3 pounds for women.
†Shoes with 1-inch heels.

ing, and positioning) may be based on weight changes. Clients capable of bearing their own weight use a standing scale. The nurse calibrates a standard platform scale by moving the large and small weights to zero. The balance beam should be made level and steady by adjusting the calibrating knob. Electronic scales are automatically calibrated each time they are used. The client stands on the scale platform and remains still. Electronic scales automatically display the weight within seconds. Stretcher and chair scales are available for clients unable to bear weight. After being transferred to the scale, the client is lifted above the bed by a hydraulic device and the weight is measured on a balance beam or digital display. Caution must be used when transferring clients to and from the scales.

Infants are weighed using an infant scale. The nurse removes clothing and weighs infants in dry, disposable diapers to ensure accurate readings. The weight can later be adjusted for the weight of the diaper. The room should be warm to prevent chills. A light cloth or paper placed on the scale's surface prevents cross infection from urine or feces. The scale is recalibrated to provide for weighing of clothes. Care should be used to prevent accidental falls. Weight is measured in ounces and grams.

Different techniques exist for measuring the height of weight-bearing and non–weight-bearing clients. Clients able to stand remove their shoes. A paper towel can be placed on the scale platform or floor so that the client's feet remain clean. A measuring stick or tape is attached vertically to the weight scales or wall. Have the client stand erect. On a standing scale a metal rod, which is attached to the back of the scale, swings out and over the crown of the head. A measuring stick or flat book can also be placed on the head when a scale is unavailable. With the rod or stick placed level horizontally at a 90-degree angle to the measuring stick, the nurse measures height in inches or centimeters.

A non–weight-bearing client (such as an infant) is positioned supine on a firm surface. There are portable devices available that provide a reliable means to measure height. The nurse places the infant on the device, having the parent hold the infant's head against the headboard. With the infant's legs straight at the knees, the footboard is placed against the bottom of the infant's feet (Figure 32-5). The infant's length is recorded to the nearest 0.5 cm or ¼ inch.

A more detailed assessment of infants and children requires measurement of the circumferences of the head and chest. The nurse records the infant's measurements at each health visit until 2 years of age and then measures the child's head circumference yearly until age 6 (Seidel and others, 2003).

Accurate head measurements require the nurse to wrap the paper measuring tape snugly around the child's head at the occipital protuberance and supraorbital prominence, the location of the largest circumference. The nurse records the measurement to the nearest 0.5 cm or ⅛ inch. Growth charts indicate the appropriate circumference for the child's age.

A chest circumference can be compared with the head circumference to rule out problems in head or chest size.

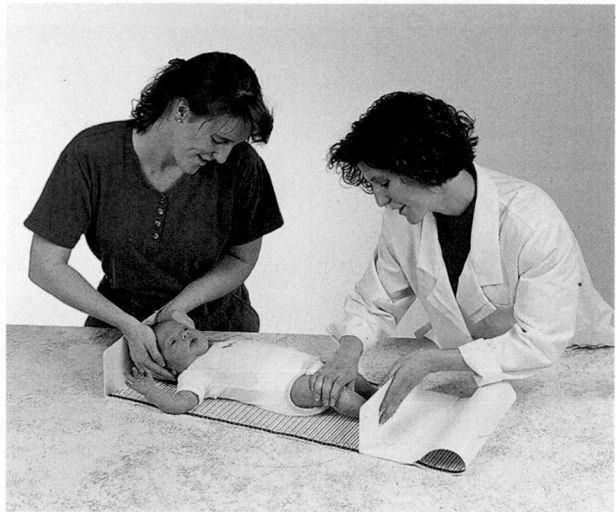

FIGURE **32–5**   Measurement of infant length. (From Seidel HM and others: *Mosby's guide to physical examination*, ed 5, St. Louis, 2003, Mosby.)

The measuring tape is firmly wrapped around the infant's chest at the nipple line without causing a skin indentation. Measurement is taken midway between inspiration and expiration and read to the nearest 0.5 cm or ¼ inch.

Skin, Hair, and Nails

The skin provides the body's external protection, regulates body temperature, and acts as a sensory organ for pain, temperature, and touch. Assessment of the **integument** includes the skin, hair, scalp, and nails. The nurse may initially inspect all skin surfaces or may assess the skin gradually while other body systems are examined. The physical assessment skills of inspection, palpation, and olfaction are used to assess the integument's function and integrity.

Skin

Assessment of the skin can reveal a variety of conditions, including changes in oxygenation, circulation, nutrition, local tissue damage, and hydration. In a hospital setting the majority of clients are older adults, debilitated clients, or young but seriously ill clients. As a result, there are significant risks for skin lesions resulting from trauma to the skin during administration of care, from exposure to pressure during immobilization, or from reaction to various medications used in treatment. Clients most at risk are neurologically impaired clients; chronically ill clients; orthopedic clients; and clients with diminished mental status, poor tissue oxygenation, low cardiac output, or inadequate nutrition. In nursing homes and extended care facilities, clients may be at risk for many of the same problems, depending on their level of mobility and the presence of chronic illness. Nurses must routinely assess the skin to look for primary or initial lesions that may develop. Without proper care, primary lesions can quickly

Client Teaching

Box 32-6

Skin Assessment

Objectives

- Client will perform a monthly self-examination of the skin.
- Client will identify factors that increase the risk of skin cancer.
- Client will follow hygiene practices aimed at maintaining skin integrity.

Teaching Strategies

- Instruct client to conduct a complete monthly self-examination of the skin, noting moles, blemishes, and birthmarks. Tell client to inspect all skin surfaces. Cancerous melanomas start as small, molelike growths that increase in size, change color, become ulcerated, and bleed. A simple ABCD rule (ACS, 2003) outlines warning signals:

  A   is for *A*symmetry.

  B   is for *B*order irregularity; edges are ragged, notched, or blurred.

  C   is for *C*olor; pigmentation is not uniform; variations in shading/multiple colors—blue, black, or variegated (Lapka, 2000).

  D   is for *D*iameter; greater than 6 mm.

- Tell client to report to a physician or health care provider any change in skin lesions or a sore that does not heal.
- Instruct client to prevent skin cancer by avoiding overexposure to the sun: wear wide-brimmed hats and long sleeves,

apply broad spectrum sunscreens with SPF of 15 or greater to protect against UVB and UVA rays approximately 15 minutes before going into the sun and after swimming or perspiring, avoid tanning under the direct sun at midday (10 AM to 4 PM), and do not use indoor sunlamps, tanning parlors, or tanning pills (ACS, 2003). Medications such as oral contraceptives, antibiotics, immunosuppressive agents, antiinflammatories, and antihypertensives can make the skin more sensitive to the sun (Lapka, 2000). Special care should be taken to protect children from the sun.

- Instruct client to report any lesion that bleeds or fails to heal to a physician. Especially instruct older adults, who tend to have delayed wound healing.
- To treat excessively dry skin, tell client to avoid hot water, harsh soaps, and drying agents such as rubbing alcohol. Use a superfatted (Dove) soap and pat rather than rub the skin after bathing.
- Apply moisturizers (mineral oil) to the skin regularly to reduce itching and drying, and wear cotton clothing (Hardy, 1996).

Evaluation

- Observe client perform skin assessment.
- Have client describe signs of skin cancer and measures to take to prevent skin cancer.
- Ask client to describe methods for keeping the skin lubricated and supple.

---

deteriorate to become secondary lesions that require more extensive nursing care. The development of a pressure ulcer, for example, can lengthen a hospital stay unless it is prevented or discovered early and treated properly (see Chapter 47).

There will be approximately 53,600 new cases of **melanoma,** an aggressive form of skin cancer, diagnosed in 2002 (ACS, 2003). In addition, one million new cases of the highly curable basal cell and squamous cell cancers will be seen (ACS, 2003). Cutaneous malignancies are the most common neoplasms seen in clients. The nurse must incorporate performing a thorough skin assessment on all clients with educating them about self-examination (Box 32-6).

The condition of the client's skin reveals the need for nursing intervention. The nurse uses assessment findings to determine the type of hygiene measures required to maintain integrity of the integument (see Chapter 38). Adequate nutrition and hydration become goals of therapy if the nurse identifies alterations in the integument's status (see Chapter 43).

Adequate illumination of the skin is required for accurate observations. The recommended choice is natural or halogen lighting (Bennett, 1998). For detecting skin changes in the dark-skinned client, sunlight is the best choice (Talbot and Curtis, 1996). Room temperature may also affect skin assessment. A room that is too warm may cause superficial vasodilation, resulting in an increased

redness of the skin. A cool environment may cause the sensitive client to develop cyanosis around the lips and nail beds (Talbot and Curtis, 1996).

Disposable gloves are required for palpation if open, moist, or draining lesions are present. Although the nurse observes each part of the body during an examination, it helps to make a brief but careful overall visual sweep of the entire body. This gives the nurse a good idea of the distribution and extent of any lesions, as well as the overall symmetry of skin color. Because the nurse inspects all skin surfaces, the client must assume several positions. The nursing history for skin assessment is outlined in Table 32-9. If abnormalities are seen during an examination, the nurse palpates the involved areas. Skin odors are usually noted in the folds of the skin, such as the axillae or under the female client's breasts. Figure 32-6 illustrates a normal cross section of the skin.

Color. Skin color varies from body part to body part and from person to person. Despite individual variations, skin color is usually uniform over the body. Table 32-10 lists common variations. Normal skin pigmentation ranges in tone from ivory or light pink to ruddy pink in light skin and from light to deep brown or olive in dark skin. **Basal cell carcinomas** are most commonly seen in sun-exposed areas and frequently occur in a background of sun-damaged skin. In older adults, **pigmentation** increases unevenly, causing discolored skin.

Table 32-9   **Nursing History for Skin Assessment**

Assessment Category	Rationale
Ask client about history of changes in the skin: dryness, pruritus, sores, rashes, lumps, color, texture, odor, lesion that does not heal.	Client is best source to recognize change. Skin cancer may first be noticed as a localized change in skin color.
Consider if the client has the following history: fair, freckled, ruddy complexion; light-colored hair or eyes; tendency to burn easily.	Characteristics are risk factors for skin cancer.
Determine whether client works or spends excessive time outside. If so, ask whether a sunscreen is worn and the level of protection.	Exposed areas such as face and arms will be more pigmented than rest of body. Use of sunscreen is recommended by the American Cancer Society (ACS, 2003).
Determine whether client has noted lesions or changes in skin.	Most skin changes do not develop suddenly. Change in character of lesion might indicate cancer. Bruising indicates trauma or bleeding disorder.
Question client about frequency of bathing and type of soap used.	Excessive bathing and use of harsh soaps can cause dry skin.
Ask if client has had recent trauma to skin.	Injury can cause bruising and changes in skin texture.
Determine whether client has history of allergies.	Skin rashes commonly occur from allergies.
Ask if client uses topical medications or home remedies on skin.	Incorrect use of topical agents may cause inflammation or irritation.
Ask if client goes to tanning parlors, uses sun lamps, or takes tanning pills.	Overexposure of skin to these irritants can cause skin cancer.
Ask if client has family history of serious skin disorders such as skin cancer or psoriasis.	Family history may reveal information about client's condition.
Determine if client works with creosote, coal, tar, petroleum products, arsenic compounds, or radium.	Exposure to these agents creates risk for skin cancer.

Table 32-10   **Skin Color Variations**

Color	Condition	Causes	Assessment Locations
Bluish (cyanosis)	Increased amount of deoxygenated hemoglobin (associated with hypoxia)	Heart or lung disease, cold environment	Nail beds, lips, mouth, skin (severe cases)
Pallor (decrease in color)	Reduced amount of oxyhemoglobin	Anemia	Face, conjunctivae, nail beds, palms of hands
	Reduced visibility of oxyhemoglobin resulting from decreased blood flow	Shock	Skin, nail beds, conjunctivae, lips
Loss of pigmentation	Vitiligo	Congenital or autoimmune condition causing lack of pigment	Patchy areas on skin over face, hands, arms
Yellow-orange (jaundice)	Increased deposit of bilirubin in tissues	Liver disease, destruction of red blood cells	Sclera, mucous membranes, skin
Red (erythema)	Increased visibility of oxyhemoglobin caused by dilation or increased blood flow	Fever, direct trauma, blushing, alcohol intake	Face, area of trauma, sacrum, shoulders, other common sites for pressure ulcers
Tan-brown	Increased amount of melanin	Suntan, pregnancy	Areas exposed to sun: face, arms, areolae, nipples

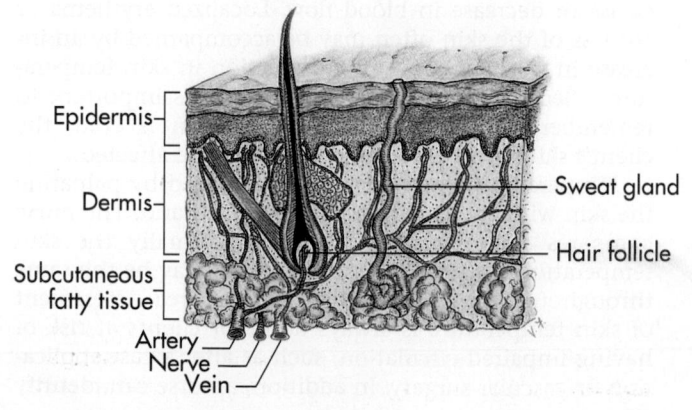

FIGURE **32–6**   A cross section of the skin reveals three layers: epidermis, dermis, and subcutaneous fatty tissues.

While inspecting the skin, the nurse must be aware that color may be masked by cosmetics or tanning agents. The assessment of color first involves areas of the skin not exposed to the sun, such as the palms of the hands. The nurse notes if the skin is unusually pale or dark. Areas exposed to the sun, such as the face and arms, will be darker. It is more difficult to note changes such as pallor or cyanosis in clients with dark skin. Usually color hues are best seen in the palms, soles of the feet, lips, tongue, and nail beds. Areas of increased color (hyperpigmentation) and decreased color (hypopigmentation) are common. Skin creases and folds are darker than the rest of the body in the dark-skinned client. The nurse inspects sites where abnormalities are more easily identified. For example, pallor is more easily seen in the face, buccal (mouth) mucosa, conjunctiva, and nail beds. **Cyanosis** (bluish discoloration) is best observed in the lips, nail beds, palpebral conjunctivae, and palms. In recognizing pallor in the dark-skinned client, the nurse would observe that normal brown skin appears to be yellow-brown and normal black skin appears to be ashen gray. The lips, nail beds, and mucous membranes should also be assessed for generalized pallor; if pallor is present, the mucous membranes will be ashen gray. Assessment of cyanosis in the dark-skinned client requires that the nurse observe areas where pigmentation occurs the least (conjunctiva, sclera, buccal mucosa, tongue, lips, nail beds, and palms and soles). In addition, the nurse should verify findings with clinical manifestations (Talbot and Curtis, 1996). The best site to inspect for **jaundice** (yellow-orange discoloration) is the client's sclera. Normal reactive hyperemia, or redness, is most often seen in regions exposed to pressure such as the sacrum, heels, and greater trochanter.

The nurse inspects for any patches or areas of skin color variation. Localized skin changes, such as pallor or **erythema** (red discoloration), may indicate circulatory changes. For example, an area of erythema may be due to localized vasodilation resulting from a sunburn or fever. In the dark-skinned client, erythema is not easily observed, so the nurse must palpate the area for heat and warmth to note the presence of skin inflammation (Talbot and Curtis, 1996). An area of an extremity that appears unusually pale may result from arterial occlusion or edema. It is important to ask if the client has noticed any changes in skin coloring. The client usually knows whether a change has occurred.

A pattern of findings that is becoming more common is that associated with clients who are chemically dependent and are intravenous (IV) drug abusers. A client who takes repeated IV injections may have edematous, reddened, and warm areas along the arms and legs. This pattern suggests recent injections. Evidence of old injection sites appears as hyperpigmented and shiny or scarred areas. Box 32-7 summarizes additional physical findings associated with substance abuse.

Moisture. The hydration of skin and mucous membranes helps to reveal body fluid imbalances, changes in the skin's environment, and regulation of body temperature. Moisture refers to wetness and oiliness. The skin is normally smooth and dry. Skin folds such as the axillae are

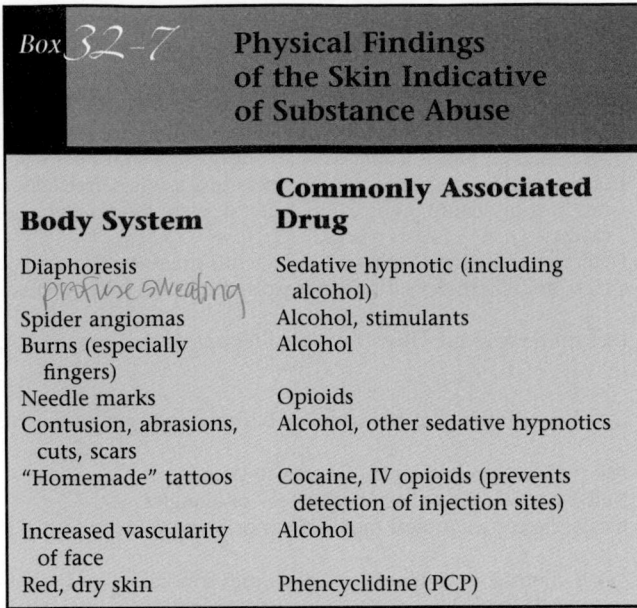

Box 32-7   Physical Findings of the Skin Indicative of Substance Abuse

Body System	Commonly Associated Drug
Diaphoresis *(profuse sweating)*	Sedative hypnotic (including alcohol)
Spider angiomas	Alcohol, stimulants
Burns (especially fingers)	Alcohol
Needle marks	Opioids
Contusion, abrasions, cuts, scars	Alcohol, other sedative hypnotics
"Homemade" tattoos	Cocaine, IV opioids (prevents detection of injection sites)
Increased vascularity of face	Alcohol
Red, dry skin	Phencyclidine (PCP)

Modified from Caulker-Burnett I: Primary care screening for substance abuse, *Nurse Pract* 19(6):42, 1994; and Friedman L and others: *Source book of substance abuse and addiction*, Baltimore, 1996, Williams & Wilkins.

normally moist. Minimal perspiration or oiliness should be present (Seidel and others, 2003). Increased perspiration may be associated with activity, warm environments, obesity, anxiety, or excitement. The nurse uses ungloved fingertips to palpate skin surfaces and observe for dullness, dryness, crusting, and flaking. Flaking is the appearance of flakes resembling dandruff when the skin surface is lightly rubbed. Scaling involves fishlike scales that are easily rubbed off the skin's surface. Both flaking and scaling are believed to indicate abnormally dry skin (Hardy, 1996). Excessively dry skin is common in older adults and persons who use excessive amounts of soap during bathing. Other factors causing dry skin include lack of humidity, exposure to sun, smoking, stress, excessive perspiration, and dehydration (Hardy, 1996). Excessive dryness can worsen existing skin conditions such as **eczema** and **dermatitis.**

Temperature. The temperature of the skin depends on the amount of blood circulating through the dermis. Increased or decreased skin temperature indicates an increase or decrease in blood flow. Localized erythema or redness of the skin often may be accompanied by an increase in skin temperature. A reduction in skin temperature reflects a decrease in blood flow. It is important to remember that if an examination room is cold, the client's skin temperature and color may be affected.

Temperature is more accurately assessed by palpating the skin with the dorsum or back of the hand. The nurse compares symmetrical body parts. Normally the skin temperature is warm. Skin temperature may be the same throughout the body or may vary in one area. Assessment of skin temperature is always done for clients at risk of having impaired circulation, such as after a cast application or vascular surgery. In addition, a nurse can identify a stage I pressure ulcer early when noting warmth and erythema on an area of the skin (see Chapter 47).

Texture. The character of the skin's surface and the feel of deeper portions are its texture. The nurse determines whether the client's skin is smooth or rough, thin or thick, tight or supple, and **indurated** (hardened) or soft by stroking it and palpating it lightly with the fingertips. The texture of the skin is normally smooth, soft, even, and flexible in children and adults. However, the texture is usually not uniform throughout. The palms of the hand and soles of the feet tend to be thicker. In older adults the skin becomes wrinkled and leathery because of a decrease in collagen, subcutaneous fat, and sweat glands.

Localized changes may result from trauma, surgical wounds, or lesions. When irregularities in texture such as scars or hardening are found, the nurse asks if the client has had a recent injury to the skin. Deeper palpation may reveal irregularities such as tenderness or localized areas of induration commonly caused by repeated intramuscular or subcutaneous injections. If the client has diabetes or receives vitamin B_{12} or iron injections, indurated areas may be seen.

Turgor. **Turgor** is the skin's elasticity, which can be diminished by edema or dehydration. Normally the skin loses its elasticity with age. To assess the skin turgor, a fold of skin on the back of the forearm or sternal area is grasped with the fingertips and released (Figure 32-7). Normally the skin lifts easily and snaps back immediately to its resting position. The back of the hand is not the best place to test for turgor, since the skin is normally loose and thin (Seidel and others, 2003). The skin stays pinched when turgor is poor. The nurse notes the ease with which the skin moves and the speed at which it returns to place. Failure of the skin to reassume its normal contour or shape indicates dehydration. The client with poor skin turgor does not have a resilience to the normal wear and tear on the skin. The skin tends to stay pinched or tented when turgor is poor. A decrease in turgor predisposes the client to skin breakdown.

Vascularity. The circulation of the skin affects the appearance of superficial blood vessels. With aging, capillaries become fragile. Localized pressure areas, found after a client has lain or sat in one position, appear reddened, pink, or pale (see Chapter 47). **Petechiae** are pinpoint-sized, red or purple spots on the skin caused by small hemorrhages in the skin layers. Petechiae may indicate serious blood-clotting disorders, drug reactions, or liver disease.

Edema. Areas of the skin become swollen or edematous from a buildup of fluid in the tissues. Direct trauma and impairment of venous return are two common causes of **edema.** Edematous areas should be inspected for location, color, and shape. For the client with dependent edema caused by poor venous return, typical sites of edema are the feet, ankles, and sacrum. The formation of edema separates the skin's surface from the pigmented and vascular layers, masking skin color. Edematous skin looks stretched and shiny. The nurse palpates areas of edema to determine mobility, consistency, and tenderness. When pressure

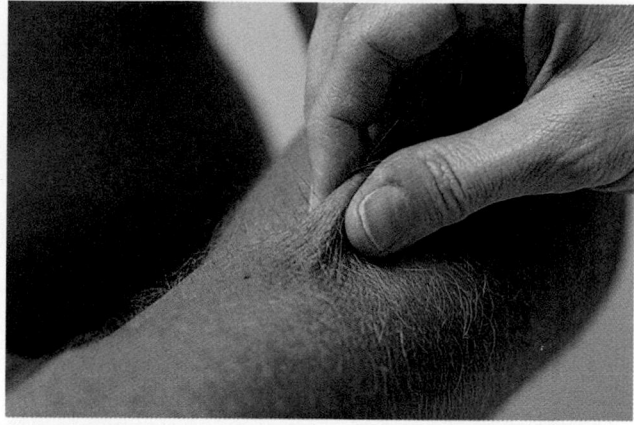

FIGURE **32–7** Assessment for skin turgor. (From Seidel HM and others: *Mosby's guide to physical examination,* ed, 5 St. Louis, 2003, Mosby.)

from the examiner's fingers leaves an indentation in the edematous area, it is called pitting edema. To check the degree of pitting edema, the nurse presses the edematous area firmly with the thumb for 5 seconds and releases. The depth of pitting, recorded in millimeters determines the degree of edema (Seidel and others, 2003). For example, 1+ edema equals a 2-mm depth, 2+ edema equals a 4-mm depth and so on.

Lesions. During palpation the nurse may locate skin lesions, which are any pathological skin changes (Seidel and others, 2003). The skin is normally free of lesions, except common freckles or age-related changes such as skin tags, **senile keratosis** (thickening of skin), **cherry angiomas** (ruby red papules), and atrophic warts. Lesions may be primary (occurring as initial spontaneous manifestations of a pathological process), such as the wheal of an insect bite, or secondary (resulting from later formation or trauma to a primary lesion), such as a pressure ulcer.

When a lesion is detected, it is inspected for color, location, texture, size, shape, type, grouping (clustered or linear), and distribution (localized or generalized). Any exudate is observed for color, odor, amount, and consistency. The size is best measured by using a small, clear, flexible ruler marked in centimeters. Comparing a lesion with a household measure, such as a coin or eraser, is not reliable (Seidel and others, 2003). Lesions should be measured in centimeters in all dimensions (height, width, and depth) when possible.

Palpation determines the lesion's mobility, contour (flat, raised, or depressed), and consistency (soft or indurated). Certain types of lesions present a characteristic pattern. For example, a tumor is usually an elevated, solid lesion larger than 2 cm. Primary lesions, such as macules and nodules, arise from some stimulus to the skin (Box 32-8). Secondary lesions, such as ulcers, occur as alterations in primary lesions. After it is identified, a lesion is closely inspected with good illumination. The lesion is palpated gently, covering its entire area. If the lesion is moist or draining fluid, gloves are worn during palpation.

It helps to ask clients if they have noticed any lesions, their causes, and any recent changes in their character.

Box 32-8 Types of Primary Skin Lesions

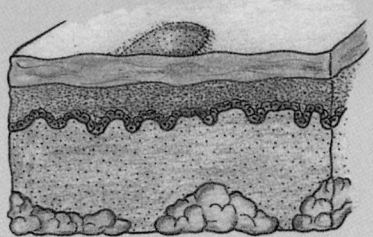

Macule: Flat, nonpalpable change in skin color, smaller than 1 cm (e.g., freckle, petechia)

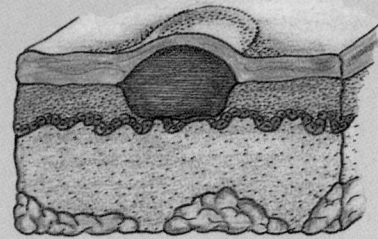

Papule: Palpable, circumscribed, solid elevation in skin, smaller than 0.5 cm (e.g., elevated nevus)

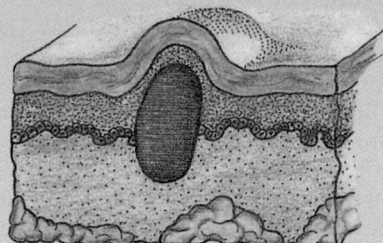

Nodule: Elevated solid mass, deeper and firmer than papule, 0.5-0.2 cm (e.g., wart)

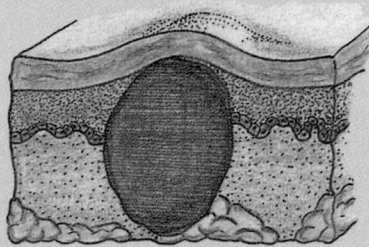

Tumor: Solid mass that may extend deep through subcutaneous tissue, larger than 1-2 cm (e.g., epithelioma)

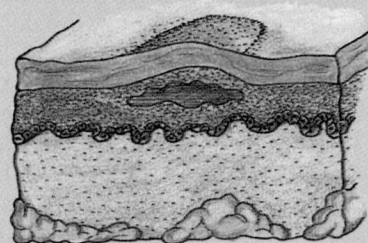

Wheal: Irregularly shaped, elevated area or superficial localized edema; varies in size (e.g., hive, mosquito bite)

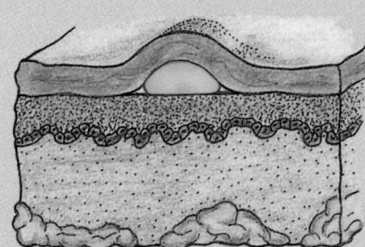

Vesicle: Circumscribed elevation of skin (filled with serous fluid, smaller than 0.5 cm (e.g., herpes simplex, chickenpox)

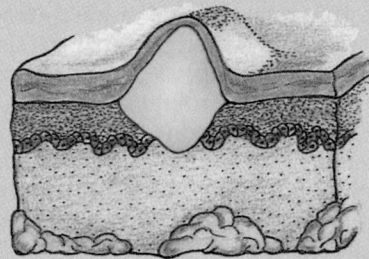

Pustule: Circumscribed elevation of skin similar to vesicle but filled with pus; varies in size (e.g., acne, staphylococcal infection)

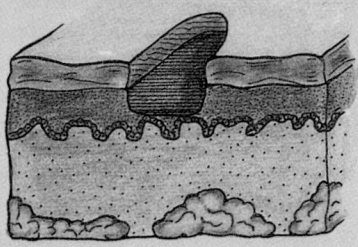

Ulcer: Deep loss of skin surface that may extend to dermis and frequently bleeds and scars; varies in size (e.g., venous stasis ulcer)

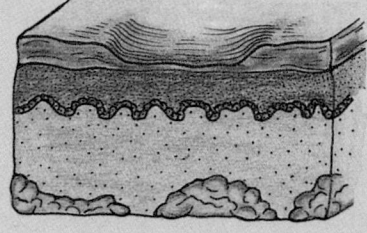

Atrophy: Thinning of skin with loss of normal skin furrow, with skin appearing shiny and translucent; varies in size (e.g., arterial insufficiency)

Further questioning as to how a lesion bothers a client and what has been done to care for it may reveal how a client feels about the disorder. Many clients react with fear and anxiety to rashes or other lesions. Cancerous lesions frequently undergo changes in color and size (Box 32-9). Abnormal lesions are reported to the physician because further examination may be required.

Safety Alert. Individuals exposed to the sun through sunbathing or artificial means increase their risk for development of skin cancer. Provide appropriate teaching to inform clients of ways to decrease their risk.

Hair and Scalp

The following types of hair cover the body: terminal hair (long, coarse, thick hair easily visible on the scalp, axillae, pubic areas, and in the beard in men) and vellus hair (small, soft, tiny hairs covering the whole body except for the palms and soles). Good lighting allows the nurse to inspect the condition and distribution of hair and the integrity of the scalp. Assessment of the hair occurs during all portions of the examination.

Inspection. Clients are sensitive about personal appearance. During inspection the nurse explains the need to separate parts of the hair to detect problems. If lesions or

---

Box *32-9*   **Skin Malignancies in the Older Adult**

Basal Cell Carcinoma

0.5- to 1.0-cm crusted lesion that may be flat or raised and may have a rolled, somewhat scaly border.

Frequently there are underlying, widely dilated blood vessels that can be seen clinically within the lesion.

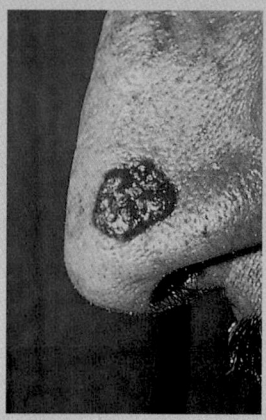

Squamous Cell Carcinoma

Occurs more often on mucosal surfaces and nonexposed areas of skin, compared with basal cell.

0.5- to 1.5-cm scaly lesion, may be ulcerated or crusted. Appears frequently and grows more rapidly than basal cell.

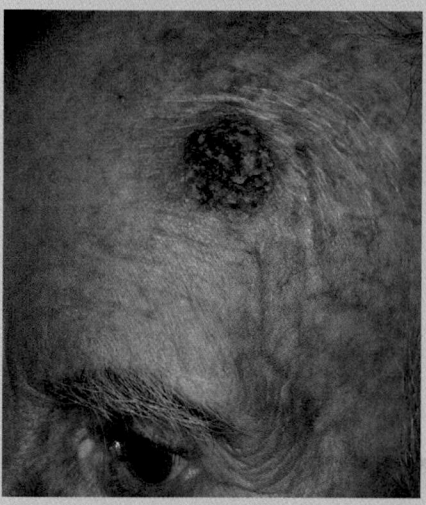

Melanoma

0.5- to 1.0-cm brown, flat lesion that may arise on sun-exposed or nonexposed skin. Variegated pigmentation, irregular borders, and indistinct margins.

Ulceration, recent growth, or recent change in long-standing mole are ominous signs.

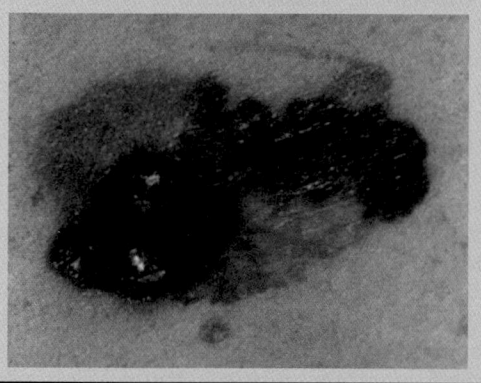

Illustrations from Belcher AE: *Cancer nursing,* St. Louis, 1992, Mosby; Habif TP: *Clinical dermatology: a color guide to diagnosis and therapy,* ed 3, St. Louis, 1996, Mosby; and Zitelli B, Davis H: *Atlas of pediatric physical diagnosis,* ed 2, St. Louis, 1991, Mosby.

---

lice are probable, the nurse wears disposable gloves to avoid infection. Table 32-11 describes the nursing history for assessment of the hair and scalp.

The nurse begins inspection by noting the color, distribution, quantity, thickness, texture, and lubrication of body hair. Scalp hair may be coarse or fine; may be curly or straight; and should be shiny, smooth, and pliant. While separating sections of scalp hair, the nurse observes characteristics of color and coarseness. Color varies from very light blond to black to gray and may show alterations

Table 32-11	Nursing History for Hair and Scalp Assessment	
Assessment Category	**Rationale**
Ask client if wig or hairpiece is being worn and request that it be removed.	Wigs or hairpieces interfere with inspection of hair and scalp. (Client may request to omit this part of examination.)
Determine if client has noted change in growth or loss of hair.	Change may occur slowly over time.
Identify type of shampoo, other hair care products, and curling irons used for grooming.	Excessive use of chemical agents and burning of hair causes drying and brittleness.
Determine if client has recently had chemotherapy (if hair loss noted) or taken a vasodilator (minoxidil) if hair growth noted.	Chemotherapeutic agents kill cells that rapidly multiply, such as tumor cells and normal hair cells. Minoxidil causes excessive hair growth.
Has client noted changes in diet or appetite?	Nutrition can influence condition of hair.

from rinses or dyes. In older adults the hair becomes dull gray, white, or yellow. It also thins over the scalp, axillae, and pubic areas. Older men lose facial hair, whereas older women may develop hair on the chin and upper lip.

Much of the information gathered about characteristics of hair growth comes from the client. The nurse needs to be aware of the normal distribution of hair growth in a man and a woman. At puberty a change in the amount and distribution of hair growth occurs. A client with hormone disorders may experience an unusual distribution and growth. A woman with **hirsutism** has hair growth on the upper lip, chin, and cheeks, with vellus hair becoming coarser over the body. A change in hair growth can negatively affect body image and emotional well-being.

Changes may occur in the thickness, texture, and lubrication of scalp hair. Disturbances such as a febrile illness or scalp disease can result in hair loss. Conditions such as thyroid disease can alter the condition of the hair, making it fine and brittle. Hair loss **(alopecia),** or thinning of the hair, is usually related to genetic tendencies and endocrine disorders such as diabetes, thyroiditis, and even menopause. Poor nutrition can cause stringy, dull, dry, and thin hair. The hair is lubricated from the oil of sebaceous glands. Excessively oily hair is associated with androgen hormone stimulation. Dry, brittle hair occurs with aging and with excessive use of shampoo or other chemical agents. The amount of hair covering the extremities may be reduced as a result of aging and arterial insufficiency and is most commonly seen over the lower extremities. In women, loss of hair should not be confused with shaven legs.

When inspecting the scalp, the nurse asks if the client has noticed anything unusual. The scalp is normally smooth and inelastic, with even coloration. By carefully separating strands of hair, the nurse can thoroughly examine the scalp for lesions, which can easily go unnoticed in thick hair. The nurse notes the characteristics of any scalp lesion. If lumps or bruises are found, the nurse asks if the client has experienced recent trauma to the head. Moles on the scalp are common. The nurse should warn the client that combing or brushing can cause a mole to bleed. Scaliness or dryness of the scalp is frequently caused by dandruff or psoriasis.

Careful inspection of hair follicles on the scalp and pubic areas may reveal lice or other parasites. The three

types of lice are *Pediculus humanus capitis* (head lice), *Pediculus humanus corporis* (body lice), and *Pediculus pubis* (crab lice). Head and crab lice attach their eggs to hair. The tiny eggs look like oval particles of dandruff. The lice themselves are difficult to see. Head and body lice are very small with grayish white bodies. Crab lice have red legs. The nurse looks for bites or pustular eruptions in the hair follicles and in areas where skin surfaces meet, such as behind the ears and in the groin. The discovery of lice requires immediate treatment (Box 32-10).

Nails

The condition of the nails can reflect an individual's general state of health, state of nutrition, occupation, and level of self-care. Even a person's psychological state may be revealed by evidence of nail biting. Before assessing the nails, the nurse gathers a brief history (Table 32-12). The most visible portion of the nails is the nail plate, the transparent layer of epithelial cells covering the nail bed (Figure 32-8). The vascularity of the nail bed creates the nail's underlying color. The semilunar, whitish area at the base of the nail bed is called the lunula, from which the nail plate develops.

Inspection and Palpation. The nurse inspects the nail bed for color, cleanliness, and length; the thickness and shape of the nail plate, the texture of the nail; the angle between the nail and the nail bed; and the condition of the lateral and proximal nail folds around the nail. The nurse also palpates the nail base. By inspecting the nails, the nurse can obtain a quick sense about the client's hygiene practices. The nails are normally transparent, smooth, well rounded, and convex, with a nail bed angle of about 160 degrees. The surrounding cuticles are smooth, intact, and without inflammation. If the nails are ragged, dirty, and poorly kept, there is a good indication that either the client practices infrequent nail care or is physically unable to perform care. However, the nurse must consider the client's profession, because some individuals may have dirty nails as part of their employment (e.g., mechanics, coal miners, and farmers) despite excellent nail care. Jagged, bitten, or broken nail edges or cuticles can predispose a client to localized infection. Abnormalities such as erythema or swelling should be reported.

Client Teaching

Box 32-10

Hair and Scalp Assessment

Objective

- Client will perform proper hygiene practices for care of the hair and scalp.

Teaching Strategies

- Instruct client about basic hygiene practices for care of the hair and scalp (see Chapter 38).
- Instruct clients who have head lice to shampoo thoroughly with appropriate medicated shampoo using cold water, to comb thoroughly with a fine-tooth comb (following product directions); and to discard the comb. Caution against use of products containing Lindine, a toxic ingredient known to cause adverse reactions.
- Repeat shampoo treatment 12 to 24 hours later.
- After combing, remove any detectable nits or nit cases with tweezers or between the fingernails. A dilute solution of vinegar and water may help loosen nits.
- Instruct clients and parents about ways to reduce transmission of lice:
  - Do not share personal care items with others.

- Vacuum all rugs, car seats, pillows, stuffed animals, mattresses, and upholstered furniture thoroughly. Discard the vacuum bag.
- Seal nonwashable items in plastic bags for 14 days if unable to dry-clean or vacuum.
- Use thorough hand hygiene practices.
- Launder all clothing, linen, and bedding in hot soap and water and dry in a hot dryer for at least 20 minutes. Dry-clean nonwashable items.
- Instruct client that his or her partner must be notified if lice were sexually transmitted.
- Avoid physical contact with infested individuals and their belongings, especially clothing and bedding.
- Soak combs, brushes, and hair accessories in lice-killing products for 1 hour or in boiling water for 10 minutes.

Evaluation

- Have client describe methods used to care for the hair and scalp.
- Have client explain steps taken to reduce lice transmission in the home.

Data from Benenson AS, editor: *Control of communicable diseases manual,* Washington, DC, 1995, American Public Health Association; National Pediculosis Association: Child care provider's guide to controlling head lice, www.headlice.org.

Table 32-12	Nursing History for Nail Assessment
Assessment Category	**Rationale**
Ask if client has experienced recent trauma or changes in nails (splitting, breaking, discoloration, thickening).	Trauma may change shape and growth of nail. Systemic conditions cause changes in color, growth, and shape.
Has the client had other symptoms of pain, swelling, presence of systemic disease with fever, or psychological or physical stress?	Alterations may occur slowly over time.
Question client's nail care practices.	Can help to indicate if change in nails is due to local or systemic problem.
Determine if client has risks for nail or foot problems (e.g., diabetes, older adulthood, obesity).	Chemical agents can cause drying of nails. Improper care may damage nails and cuticles.
	Vascular changes associated with diabetes reduce blood flow to peripheral tissues; foot lesions and thickened nails are common. Older adult may have trouble performing foot and nail care because of poor vision, uncoordination, or inability to bend over. Obese clients have difficulty bending over.

Safety Alert. Clients with impaired circulation are at greater risk for localized infection. It is important to observe the condition of hand and foot nails and nail beds to identify risks for and early signs of infection.

In whites the nail beds are pink with translucent white tips. In clients with dark skin, brown or black pigmentation is normally present in longitudinal streaks (Figure 32-9). Splinter hemorrhages can be caused by trauma, cirrhosis, diabetes mellitus, and hypertension. Vitamin, pro-

tein, and electrolyte changes can also cause lines or bands in the nail beds.

Nails normally grow at a constant rate, but direct injury or generalized disease can impair growth. With aging, the nails of the fingers and toes become harder and thicker. Longitudinal striations develop, and the rate of nail growth slows. Nails become more brittle, dull, and opaque and may turn yellow in older adults because of insufficient calcium. Also with age, the cuticle becomes less thick and wide. Inspection of the angle between the

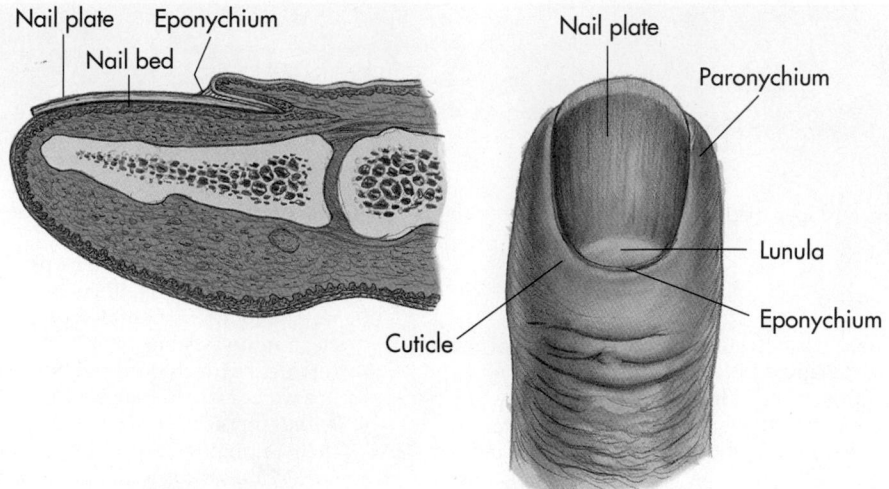

FIGURE **32–8**   Components of the nail unit. (Redrawn from Thompson JM and others: *Mosby's Clinical Nursing,* ed 4, St. Louis, 1997, Mosby.)

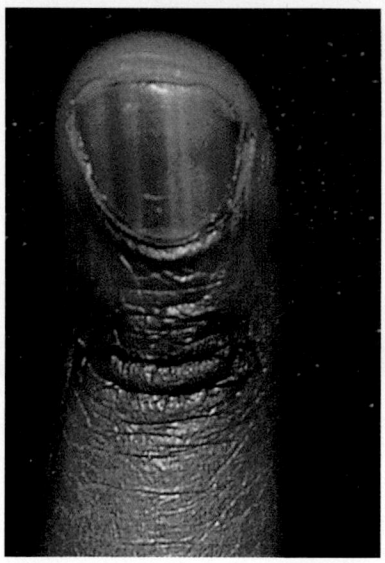

FIGURE **32–9**   Pigmented bands in nail of client with dark skin. (From Seidel HM and others: *Mosby's guide to physical examination,* ed 5, St. Louis, 2003, Mosby.)

nail and nail bed normally reveals an angle of 160 degrees (Box 32-11). A larger angle and softening of the nail bed can indicate chronic oxygenation problems. The nurse palpates the nail base to determine firmness and the condition of circulation. The nail base is normally firm.

To palpate, the nurse gently grasps the client's finger and observes the color of the nail bed. Next, gentle, firm, quick pressure is applied with the thumb to the nail bed and released. As the pressure is applied, the nail bed appears white or blanched; however, the pink color should return immediately on release of pressure. Failure of the pinkness to return promptly indicates circulatory insufficiency. An ongoing bluish or purplish cast to the nail bed

occurs with cyanosis. A white cast or pallor results from anemia.

Calluses and corns are commonly found on the toes or fingers. A callus is flat and painless. It results from a thickening of the epidermis. Corns are caused by friction and pressure from shoes and can usually be seen over a bony prominence. During the examination the nurse instructs clients about proper nail care (Box 32-12).

Head and Neck

An examination of the head and neck includes assessment of the head, eyes, ears, nose, mouth, pharynx, and neck (lymph nodes, carotid arteries, thyroid gland, and trachea). The carotid arteries can also be assessed during assessment of peripheral arteries. Assessment of the head and neck uses inspection, palpation, and auscultation, with inspection and palpation often used simultaneously.

Head

Inspection and Palpation. The nursing history will screen for intracranial injury and local or congenital deformities (Table 32-13). The nurse begins by inspecting the client's head position and facial features. The head is normally held upright and still. Holding the head tilted to one side may be an indication of unilateral hearing or visual loss.

The nurse also notes the client's facial features, looking at the eyelids, eyebrows, nasolabial folds, and mouth for shape and symmetry. It is normal for slight asymmetry to exist. If there is facial asymmetry, the nurse notes if all features on one side of the face are affected or if only a portion of the face is involved. Various neurological disorders (e.g., facial nerve paralysis) affect different nerves that innervate muscles of the face.

Examination continues with the nurse noting the size, shape, and contour of the skull. The skull is generally

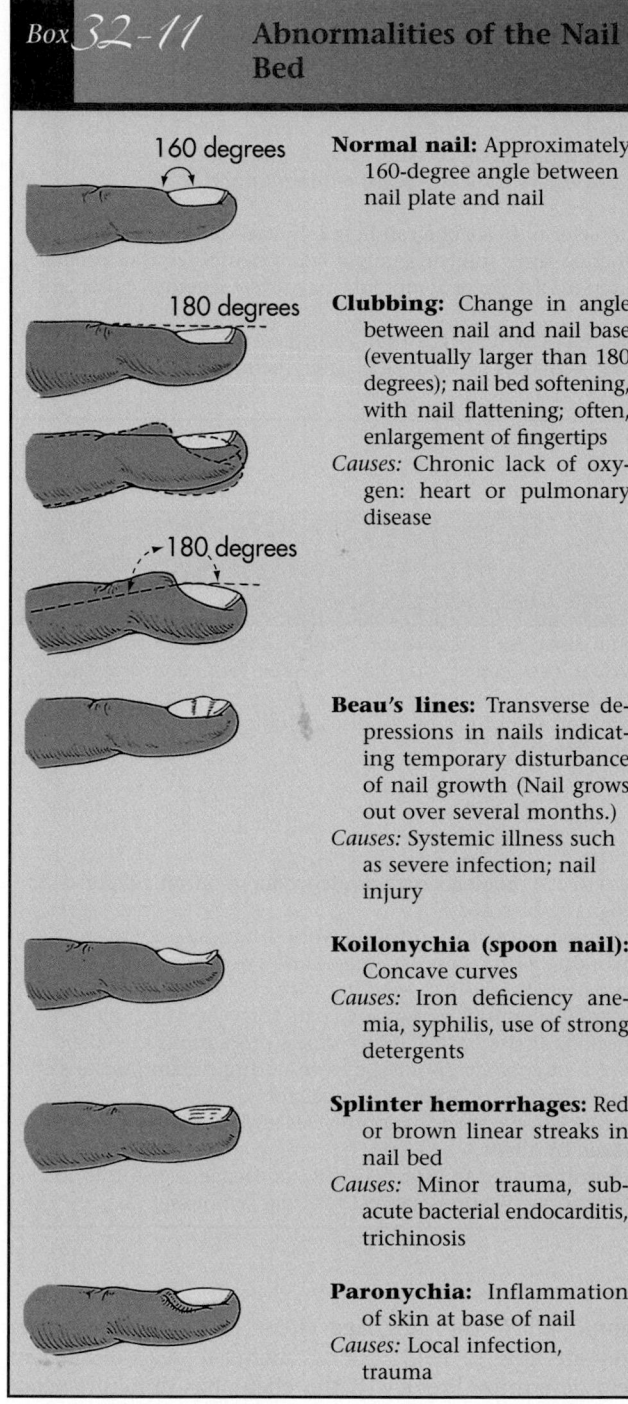

Box 32-11   **Abnormalities of the Nail Bed**

160 degrees

Normal nail: Approximately 160-degree angle between nail plate and nail

180 degrees

Clubbing: Change in angle between nail and nail base (eventually larger than 180 degrees); nail bed softening, with nail flattening; often, enlargement of fingertips
Causes: Chronic lack of oxygen: heart or pulmonary disease

180 degrees

Beau's lines: Transverse depressions in nails indicating temporary disturbance of nail growth (Nail grows out over several months.)
Causes: Systemic illness such as severe infection; nail injury

Koilonychia (spoon nail): Concave curves
Causes: Iron deficiency anemia, syphilis, use of strong detergents

Splinter hemorrhages: Red or brown linear streaks in nail bed
Causes: Minor trauma, subacute bacterial endocarditis, trichinosis

Paronychia: Inflammation of skin at base of nail
Causes: Local infection, trauma

Client Teaching   *Box 32-12*

Nail Assessment
Objective

- Client will be able to properly care for fingernails, feet, and toenails.

Teaching Strategies

- Instruct client to avoid use of over-the-counter preparations to treat corns, calluses, or ingrown toenails.
- Tell clients to cut nails straight across and even with the tops of the fingers or toes. If client has diabetes, tell client to file, not cut, nails (see Chapter 38).
- Instruct client to shape nails with a file or emery board.
- If client is diabetic:
  - Wash feet daily in warm water. Inspect feet each day in a place with good lighting, looking for dry places and cracks in the skin. Soften dry feet by applying a cream or lotion such as Nivea, Eucerin, or Alpha Keri.
  - Do not put lotion between the toes.
  - Caution client against using sharp objects to poke or dig under the toenail or around the cuticle.
  - Have client see a podiatrist for treatment of ingrown toenails and nails that are thick or tend to split.

Evaluation

- Inspect nails during the next home visit.
- Have client explain steps to take to avoid injury.

---

round with prominences in the frontal area anteriorly and the occipital area posteriorly. Local skull deformities are typically caused by trauma. In infants, large heads may result from congenital anomalies or the buildup of cerebrospinal fluid in the ventricles **(hydrocephalus).** Adults may have enlarged jaws and facial bones resulting from **acromegaly,** a disorder caused by excessive secretion of growth hormone. The nurse palpates the skull for nodules or masses. Gentle rotation of the fingertips down the midline of the scalp and then along the sides

of the head reveals abnormalities. The nurse then palpates the temporomandibular joint (TMJ) space bilaterally. The nurse places the fingertips just anterior to the tragus of each ear. The fingertips should slip into the joint space as the client's mouth opens, to gently palpate the joint spaces. Normally the movements should be smooth, although it is not unusual to hear or feel a clicking or snapping in the TMJ (Seidel and others, 2003).

Eyes
Examination of the eyes includes assessment of visual acuity, visual fields, extraocular movements, and external and internal eye structures. Figure 32-10 shows a cross section of the eye. The assessment detects visual alterations and determines the level of assistance that clients require when ambulating or performing self-care activities. Clients with visual problems may also need special aids for reading educational materials or instructions (e.g., medication labels). Table 32-14 reviews the nursing history for an eye examination. Box 32-13 describes common types of visual problems.

Visual Acuity. The assessment of visual acuity, the ability to see small details, tests central vision. The easiest way to assess near vision is to ask clients to read printed material under adequate lighting. If clients wear glasses, they should wear them during the examination. The nurse

Table 32-13	Nursing History for Head Assessment
Assessment Category	**Rationale**
Determine if client experienced recent trauma to the head. If so, assess state of consciousness after injury (immediately on return and 5 minutes later), duration of unconsciousness, and predisposing factors (e.g., seizure, poor vision, blackout).	Trauma is major cause for lumps, bumps, cuts, bruises, or deformities of scalp or skull. Loss of consciousness following head injury indicates possible brain injury.
Ask if client has history of headache; note onset, duration, character, pattern, and associated symptoms.	Character of headache can help to reveal causative factors such as sinus infection, migraine, or neurological disorders.
Determine length of time client has experienced neurological symptoms.	Duration of signs or symptoms may reveal severity of problem.
Review client's occupational history for use of safety helmets.	Nature of client's occupation can create a risk for head injury.
Ask if client participates in contact sports, cycling, roller blading, or skateboarding.	These activities require use of safety helmets.

Table 32-14	Nursing History for Eye Assessment
Assessment Category	**Rationale**
Determine if client has history of eye disease, eye trauma, diabetes, hypertension, or eye surgery.	Some diseases or trauma can cause risk for partial or complete visual loss. Surgery may have been performed for a visual disorder.
Determine problems that prompted client to seek health care. Ask client about eye pain, photophobia (sensitivity to light), burning, itching, excess tearing or crusting, diplopia (double vision), blurred vision, awareness of a "film" over field of vision, floaters (small, black spots that seem to float across field of vision), flashing lights, or halos around lights.	Common symptoms of eye disease indicate need for physician referral.
Determine whether there is family history of eye disorders or diseases.	Certain eye problems such as glaucoma or retinitis pigmentosa are inherited.
Assess client's occupational history and recreational hobbies; are safety glasses worn?	Performance of close, intricate work can cause eye fatigue. Working with computers may cause eye strain. Certain occupational tasks (e.g., working with chemicals) and recreational activity (e.g., fencing or motorcycle riding) place persons at risk for eye injury unless precautions are taken.
Ask client if glasses or contacts are worn; how often?	Glasses or contacts should be worn during certain portions of examination for accurate assessment.
Determine when client last visited ophthalmologist or optometrist.	Date of last eye examination reveals level of preventive care taken by client.
Assess medications client is taking, including eye drops or ointment.	Determines need to assess client's knowledge of medications. Certain medications can cause visual symptoms.

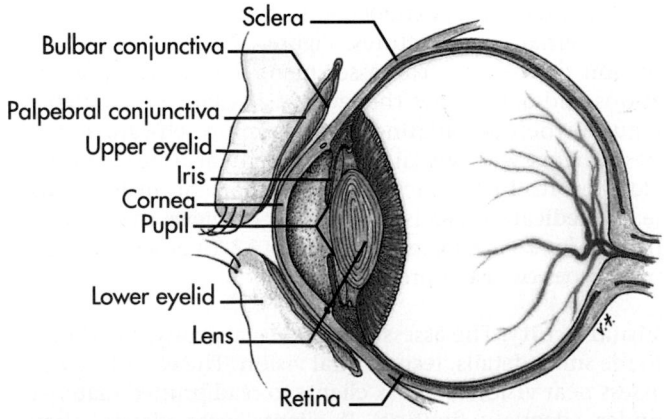

Sclera
Bulbar conjunctiva
Palpebral conjunctiva
Upper eyelid
Iris
Cornea
Pupil
Lower eyelid
Lens
Retina

FIGURE **32–10**   Cross section of the eye.

should know the language clients speak and whether they are able to read. Asking clients to read aloud can help determine literacy. If the client has difficulty reading, move to the next step.

Assessment of distant vision requires use of a Snellen chart (paper chart or projection screen). The chart should be well lighted. Vision is tested without corrective lenses first. The nurse has the client sit or stand 20 feet (6.1 m) away from the chart and try to read all of the letters beginning at any line with both eyes open and then with each eye separately (with the opposite eye covered by an index card or eye cover (Figure 32-11). The client should avoid applying pressure to the eye. The nurse notes the smallest line in which the client can read all of the letters correctly and records the visual acuity for that line. The test is repeated with the client

Box 32-13   Common Eye and Visual Problems

Hyperopia

Hyperopia is farsightedness, a refractive error in which rays of light enter the eye and focus behind the retina. Persons are able to clearly see distant objects but not close objects.

Myopia

Myopia is nearsightedness, a refractive error in which rays of light enter the eye and focus in front of the retina. Persons are able to clearly see close objects but not distant objects.

Presbyopia

Presbyopia is impaired near vision in middle-age and older adults, caused by loss of elasticity of the lens and associated with the aging process.

Astigmatism

Astigmatism is a condition in which parallel light rays do not focus on a single point on the retina. An uneven curvature of the cornea or lens causes light to be focused on different points.

Retinopathy

Retinopathy is a noninflammatory eye disorder resulting from changes in retinal blood vessels. It is a leading cause of blindness.

Strabismus

Strabismus is a congenital problem in which the eyes appear crossed. The muscles controlling movement of the eyes are not coordinated.

Cataracts

A cataract is an increased opacity of the lens, which blocks light rays from entering the eye. Cataracts may develop slowly and progressively after age 35 or suddenly after trauma. Cataracts are one of the most common eye disorders. By age 70, most older adults have some evidence of visual impairment from cataracts.

Glaucoma

Glaucoma is intraocular structural damage resulting from elevated intraocular pressure. It is caused by obstruction of the outflow of aqueous humor. Without treatment the disorder can cause blindness.

Macular Degeneration

Macular degeneration is blurred central vision often occurring suddenly, caused by a progressive degeneration of the center of the retina. It is the most common visual impairment of individuals over age 50 and the most common cause of blindness in older adults. There is no cure.

---

wearing corrective lenses. The nurse does the test rapidly enough that the client does not memorize the chart (Seidel and others, 2003).

If a client is unable to read, the nurse uses an *E* chart or one with pictures of familiar objects. Instead of reading letters, clients tell the nurse which direction each *E* is pointing or the name of the object. The visual acuity score is recorded for each eye and for both eyes.

The Snellen chart has standardized numbers at the end of each line of the chart. The numerator is the number 20, or the distance the client stands from the chart. The denominator is the distance from which the normal eye can read the chart. Normal vision is 20/20. The larger the denominator, the poorer the client's visual acuity. For example, a value of 20/40 means that the client, standing 20 feet away, can read a line that a person with normal vision can read from 40 feet away. The nurse records visual acuity as *sc* (without correction) or *cc* (with correction), depending on whether or not the client wears glasses or contact lenses.

If clients cannot read even the largest letters or figures of a Snellen chart, the nurse tests their ability to count upraised fingers or distinguish light. The nurse holds a hand 30 cm (1 foot) from the face and instructs clients to count the upraised fingers. To check light perception, the nurse shines a penlight into the eye and then turns the light off. If clients note when the light is turned on or off, light perception is intact.

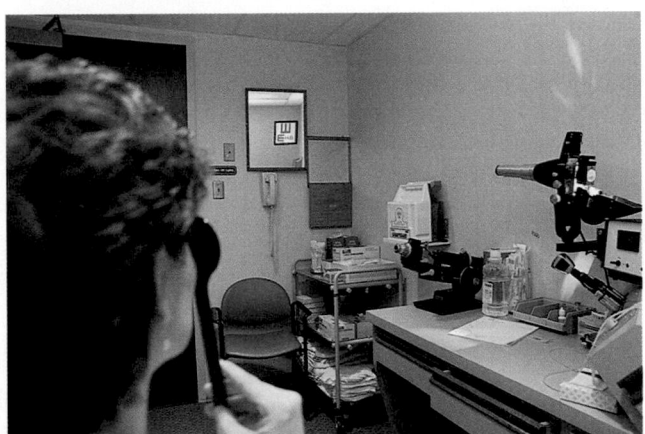

FIGURE 32–11 Assessment of visual acuity using a projection screen with an *E* chart.

Near vision can be assessed by asking the client to read a handheld card containing a vision screening chart. The client is instructed to hold the card a comfortable distance (5 to 6 cm, or about 12.5 to 14 inches) from the eyes. The client reads the smallest line possible.

Extraocular Movements. Six small muscles guide the movement of each eye. Both eyes move parallel to each other in each of the six directions of gaze (Figure 32-12). The client sits or stands 60 cm (2 feet) away, facing the nurse. The nurse holds a finger at a comfortable distance (15 to 30 cm, or 6 to 12 inches) from the client's eyes. The client keeps the head in a fixed position facing the nurse and follows the movement of the finger with the eyes only. The client looks to the right, to the left, and diagonally up and down to the left and right. The nurse's finger moves smoothly and slowly within the normal field of vision.

As the client gazes in each direction, the nurse observes for parallel eye movement, the position of the upper eyelid in relation to the iris, and the presence of abnormal movements. As the eyes move through each direction of gaze, the upper eyelid covers the iris only slightly. By periodically stopping movement of the finger, the nurse can assess **nystagmus,** an involuntary, rhythmical oscillation of the eyes. The nurse can also often initiate nystagmus in clients with normal eye movements by having them gaze to the far left or right. Disturbances in eye movement reflect local injury to eye muscles and supporting structures or a disorder of the cranial nerves innervating the muscles.

The nurse can also check the alignment of the eyes by assessing the corneal light reflex. A weakness or imbalance of the extraocular muscles can cause misalignment. The nurse shines a penlight onto the bridge of the client's nose from 60 to 90 cm (2 to 3 feet) away in a darkened room. The client looks straight ahead. Normally light reflects on the cornea in the same spot on both eyes. If an abnormality is present, the light shines on a different spot on each eye.

Visual Fields. As a person looks straight ahead, all objects in the periphery can normally be seen. To assess visual fields, the nurse has the client stand or sit 60 cm (2 feet) away, facing the nurse at eye level. The client gently closes or covers one eye (e.g., the left) and looks at the nurse's eye directly opposite. The nurse closes the opposite eye (in this case the right) so that the field of vision is superimposed on that of the client. The nurse moves a finger equidistant from the nurse and client outside the field of vision, then slowly brings it back into the visual field. The client is asked to tell when the nurse's finger is seen. If the nurse sees the finger before the client does, a portion of the client's visual field is reduced. To test temporal field vision, the object should be slightly behind the client. (NOTE: The nurse can see the finger.) The procedure is repeated for each field of vision for the other eye.

> ***Safety Alert.*** Clients with visual field problems may be at risk for injury because they cannot see all of the objects in front of them. Older adults commonly have loss of peripheral vision caused by changes in the lens.

External Eye Structures. To inspect external eye structures, the nurse stands directly in front of the client at eye level and asks the client to look at the nurse's face.

Position and Alignment. The nurse assesses the position of the eyes in relation to one another. The eyes are normally parallel to each other. Bulging **(exophthalmos)** is usually caused by hyperthyroidism when both eyes are involved. Crossing of eyes (strabismus) results from neuromuscular injury or inherited abnormalities. Tumors or inflammation of the orbit can cause abnormal eye protrusion.

Eyebrows. The eyebrows are normally symmetrical. The eyebrows are inspected for size, extension, texture of hair, alignment, and movement. A loss or absence of hair may indicate a hormonal disturbance or is a result of waxing or plucking. Aging causes loss of the lateral third of the eyebrows. The brows should raise and lower symmetrically. Paralysis of the facial nerve exists if a client cannot move the eyebrows.

Eyelids. The nurse inspects the eyelids for position, color, condition of the surface, condition and direction

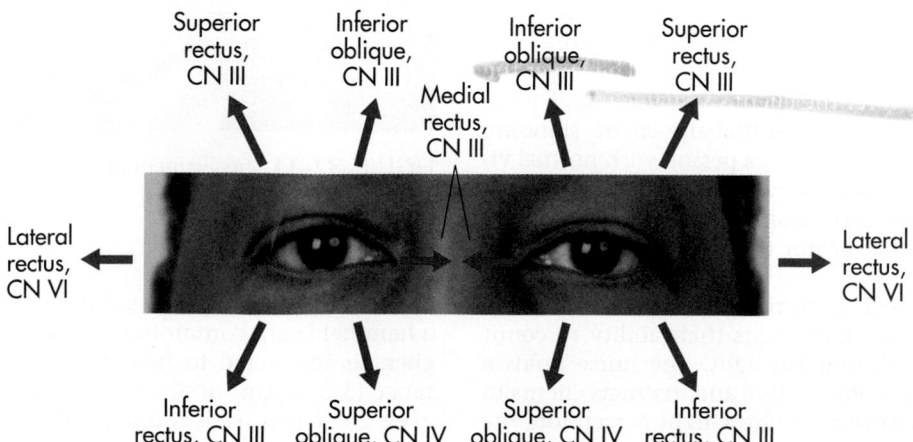

FIGURE 32–12 Six directions of gaze. The nurse directs the client to follow finger movement through each gaze. (From Seidel HM and others: *Mosby's guide to physical examination,* ed 5, St. Louis, 2003, Mosby.)

of the eyelashes, and the client's ability to open, close, and blink. When the eyes are open in a normal position, the lids do not cover the pupil and the sclera cannot be seen above the iris. The lids are also close to the eyeball. An abnormal drooping of the lid over the pupil is called **ptosis** (pronounced "toe-sis") and is caused by edema or impairment of the third cranial nerve. Defects in the position of the lid margins may also be observed. An older adult frequently has lid margins that turn out **(ectropion)** or in **(entropion).** An entropion may lead to the lid's lashes irritating the conjunctiva and cornea, increasing the risk of infection. The eyelashes are normally distributed evenly and curved outward away from the eye. An erythematous or yellow lump (hordeolum or sty) on the follicle of an eyelash indicates an acute suppurative inflammation.

To inspect the surface of the upper lids, the nurse first asks clients to close their eyes. The nurse then raises both eyebrows gently with the thumb and index finger to stretch the skin. The lids are normally smooth and the same color as the skin. Redness indicates inflammation or infection. Lid edema may be due to allergies or to heart or kidney failure. Edema of the eyelids prevents them from closing. Lesions are inspected for typical characteristics and discomfort or drainage. Gloves should be worn if drainage is present.

The lids normally close symmetrically. Failure of the lids to close exposes the cornea to drying. This condition is common in unconscious clients or in those with facial nerve paralysis.

The nurse asks the client to open the eyes for inspection of the lower lids. The same characteristics noted for the upper lids are assessed. Normally a person blinks involuntarily and bilaterally up to 20 times a minute. The blink reflex helps lubricate the cornea. The nurse reports absent or infrequent, rapid, or monocular (one-eyed) blinking.

Lacrimal Apparatus. The anterior surface of the eye, made up of the sensitive cornea and conjunctivae, is moistened or lubricated by tears secreted from the lacrimal gland (Figure 32-13). The gland is located in the upper outer wall of the anterior part of the orbit. Tears

flow from the gland across the eye's surface to the lacrimal duct, which is located in the nasal corner or inner canthus of the eye. The lacrimal gland can be the site of tumors or infections. The area of the gland is inspected for edema and redness, and it is palpated gently to detect tenderness. Normally the gland cannot be felt.

The nasolacrimal duct may become obstructed, blocking the flow of tears. If the client complains of excess tearing, the nurse looks for evidence of edema in the inner canthus. Mild palpation of the duct at the lower eyelid just inside the lower orbital rim, not on the side of the nose, may cause a regurgitation of tears.

Conjunctivae and Sclerae. The bulbar conjunctiva covers the exposed surface of the eyeball up to the outer edge of the cornea, and the palpebral conjunctiva is the delicate membrane lining the eyelids. Normally the conjunctiva is transparent, enabling the examiner to view the tiny underlying blood vessels that give it a light pink color. The sclera is seen under the bulbar conjunctiva and normally is the color of white porcelain in whites and light yellow in African-Americans. Sclerae may become pigmented and appear either yellow or green if liver disease is present.

Care must be taken when inspecting the conjunctivae. For adequate exposure of the bulbar conjunctiva, the eyelids must be retracted without placing pressure directly on the eyeball. Both lids are gently retracted, with the thumb and index finger pressed against the lower and upper bony orbits. The client is asked to look up, down, and from side to side. Many clients begin to blink, making the examination difficult. The nurse inspects for color, texture, and the presence of edema or lesions. Normally the conjunctivae are free of erythema. The presence of redness may indicate an allergic or infectious **conjunctivitis.** Bright red blood in a localized area surrounded by normal-appearing conjunctiva usually indicates subconjunctival hemorrhage.

To inspect the palpebral conjunctiva, the nurse must evert the lower eyelids. The lower lid is gently depressed with the thumb or index finger. Often the client can depress the eyelid to facilitate examination. A pale conjunctiva results from anemia, whereas a fiery red appearance is a result of inflammation (conjunctivitis). Conjunctivitis is a highly contagious infection. The crusty drainage that collects on eyelid margins can easily spread from one eye to the other. The nurse should wear gloves during the examination. Performing proper hand hygiene is necessary before and after the examination.

Corneas. The cornea is the transparent, colorless portion of the eye covering the pupil and iris. From a side view, the cornea looks like the crystal of a wristwatch. As the client looks straight ahead, the nurse inspects the cornea for clarity and texture while shining a penlight obliquely across the cornea's entire surface. The cornea is normally shiny, transparent, and smooth. However, in an older adult the cornea loses its luster. Any irregularity in the surface may indicate an abrasion or tear that warrants immediate examination by a physician. Both conditions are very painful. The color and details of the underlying iris should be easy to see. In an older adult the iris becomes

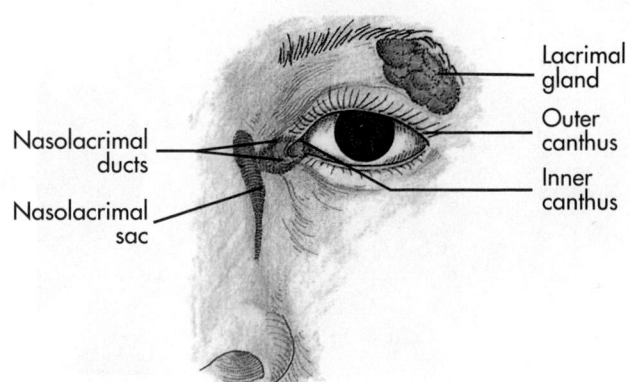

Nasolacrimal ducts

Nasolacrimal sac

Lacrimal gland

Outer canthus

Inner canthus

FIGURE **32–13** The lacrimal apparatus secretes and drains tears, which moisten and lubricate eye structures.

faded. A thin white ring along the margin of the iris, called an **arcus senilis,** is common with aging but is abnormal in anyone under age 40. To test for the corneal blink reflex, see the cranial nerve test section of this chapter.

Pupils and Irises. The nurse observes the pupils for size, shape, equality, accommodation, and reaction to light. The pupils are normally black, round, regular, and equal in size (3 to 7 mm in diameter) (Figure 32-14). The iris should be clearly visible.

Cloudy pupils indicate cataracts. Dilated pupils can result from glaucoma, trauma, neurological disorders, eye medications (e.g., atropine), or withdrawal from opioids. Constricted pupils may be caused by inflammation of the iris or use of drugs (e.g., pilocarpine, morphine, or cocaine). Pinpoint pupils are a common sign of opioid intoxication. When a beam of light is shined through the pupil and onto the retina, the third cranial nerve is stimulated and innervates the muscles of the iris to constrict. Any abnormality along the nerve pathways from the retina to the iris alters the ability of the pupils to react to light. Changes in intracranial pressure, lesions along the nerve pathways, locally applied ophthalmic medications, and direct trauma to the eye may alter pupillary reaction.

Pupillary reflexes (to light and accommodation) should be tested in a dimly lit room. As the client looks straight ahead, the nurse brings a penlight from the side of the client's face, directing the light onto the pupil (Figure 32-15). If the client looks at the light, there will be a false reaction to accommodation. A directly illuminated pupil constricts, and the opposite pupil constricts consensually. The nurse observes the quickness and equality of the reflex. The examination is repeated for the opposite eye.

To test for accommodation, the client is asked to gaze at a distant object (the far wall) and then at a test object (finger or pencil) held by the nurse approximately 10 cm (4 inches) from the bridge of the client's nose. The pupils normally converge and accommodate by constricting when looking at close objects. The pupillary responses are equal. Testing for accommodation is only important if the client has a defect in the pupillary response to light (Seidel and others 2003). If assessment of pupillary reaction is normal in all tests, the nurse records the abbreviation **PERRLA** (pupils equal, round, reactive to light, and accommodation).

Internal Eye Structures. The internal eye cannot be observed without an instrument to illuminate its structures. The **ophthalmoscope** is used to inspect the fundus, which includes the retina, choroid, optic nerve disc, macula, fovea centralis, and retinal vessels. Clients in greatest need of an examination are those with diabetes, hypertension, and intracranial disorders. The nurse should feel competent in using an ophthalmoscope before attempting this examination.

The ophthalmoscope has a battery tube light source, two dials or disks, and a keyhole viewer (Figure 32-16). The dial at the top of the battery tube changes the light image. Five lenses are available, but the large white light is used for general examination. The dial at the top of the viewer rotates clockwise for selection of the lens, which adjusts the focus for the examiner.

The nurse should practice holding the ophthalmoscope in each hand, using the index finger to rotate the lens dial. The nurse turns the white light on, rotates the lens dial to *0*, and looks through the keyhole, focusing on near objects, such as the palm of the hand. Reading the newspaper with the ophthalmoscope is useful practice. During an examination the nurse keeps both eyes open when looking through the keyhole.

The examination is done in a darkened room. The nurse and client stand or sit in comfortable positions facing each other with their eyes at the same height. The client removes eyeglasses, but contact lenses may be left

2 3 4 5 6 7 8 9

FIGURE **32–14** Chart depicting pupillary size in millimeters.

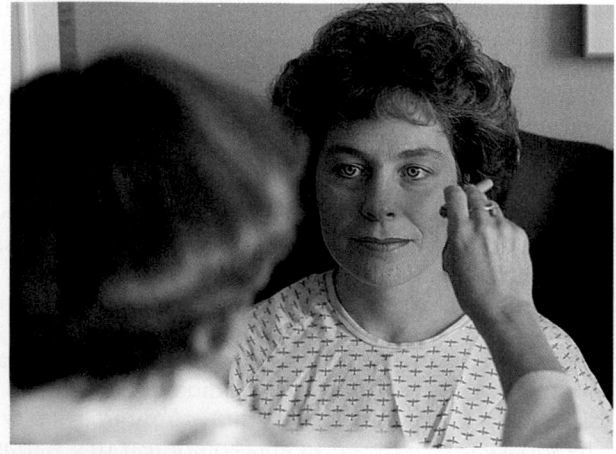 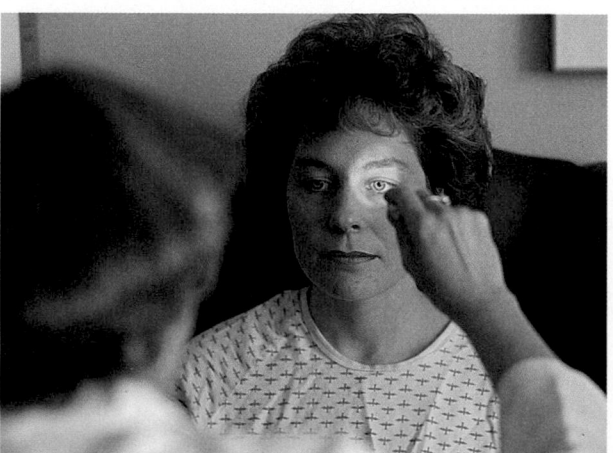

A B

FIGURE **32–15** **A,** To check pupillary reflexes, the nurse first holds the penlight to the side of the client's face. **B,** Illumination of the pupil causes pupillary constriction.

in place. The ophthalmoscope's light is switched on, and the lens is rotated to *0*. The index finger is kept on the lens dial to refocus the ophthalmoscope.

The examiner's right hand and eye are used to examine the client's right eye, and the left hand and eye are used to examine the client's left eye. The ophthalmoscope is held comfortably against the nurse's face. As the client gazes straight ahead with both eyes open, the examiner, at a distance of approximately 25 cm (10 inches) from the client and 25 degrees lateral to the client's central line of vision, shines the light on the pupil (Figure

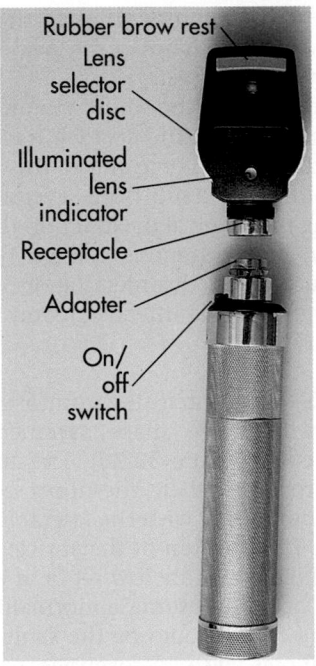

FIGURE **32–16**   Ophthalmoscope. (From Seidel HM and others: *Mosby's guide to physical examination*, ed 5, St. Louis, 2003, Mosby.)

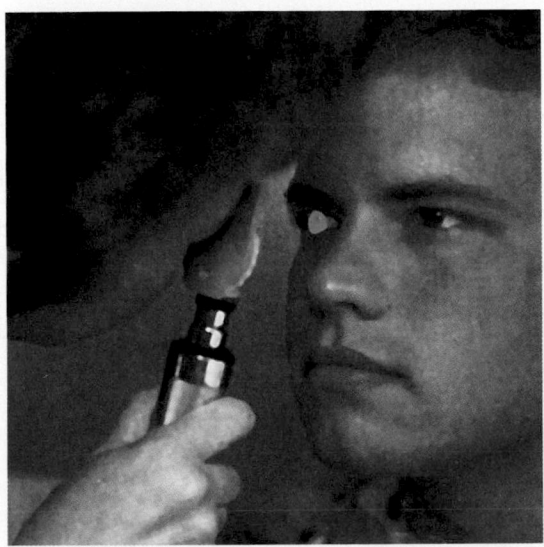

FIGURE **32–17**   To visualize internal eye structures, the nurse moves in toward the pupil with the ophthalmoscope's light focused on the red reflex.

32-17). A bright orange glow in the pupil, called the red reflex, can then normally be seen. The light from the ophthalmoscope causes the pupil to constrict. The light is slowly moved toward the pupil while the nurse keeps it focused on the red reflex. The nurse must relax and keep both eyes open. As the light approaches the pupil, the nurse begins to see structures of the fundus. Rotating the lens dial brings the internal structures into focus. The examiner inspects the size, color, and clarity of the disc; checks the integrity of the vessels; looks for the presence of retinal lesions; and assesses the appearance of the macula and fovea (Figure 32-18). Normally the following structures are observed:

- A clear, yellow optic nerve disc
- Reddish pink retina (whites) or darkened retina (African-Americans)
- Light red arteries and dark red veins
- A 3:2 vein-to-artery ratio in size proportion
- The avascular macula

If any abnormalities are observed, the client should be examined by an ophthalmologist (Box 32-14). The client's fundus should not be illuminated for extended periods. The bright light of the ophthalmoscope is very irritating and can cause discomfort and tearing. During the examination, the nurse assesses the client for discomfort.

Ears

The ears are easy to examine because of their accessibility. The three parts of the ear are the external, middle, and inner ear (Figure 32-19). The nurse inspects and palpates external ear structures, inspects middle ear structures with an otoscope, and tests the inner ear by measuring hearing acuity. External ear structures consist of the auricle, outer ear canal, and tympanic membrane (eardrum). The ear canal is normally curved and approximately 2.5 cm (1 inch) long in an adult. It is lined with skin containing fine hairs, nerve endings, and glands secreting cerumen. The middle ear is an air-filled cavity containing the three bony ossicles (malleus, incus, and stapes). The eustachian tube connects the middle ear to the nasopharynx. Pressure between the outer atmosphere and the middle ear is stabilized through the eustachian tube.

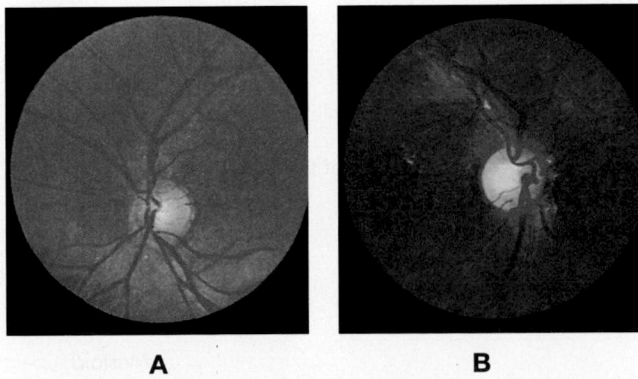

FIGURE **32–18**   Fundus of, **A,** white patient and, **B,** black patient. (Courtesy MEDCOM, Cypress, Calif.)

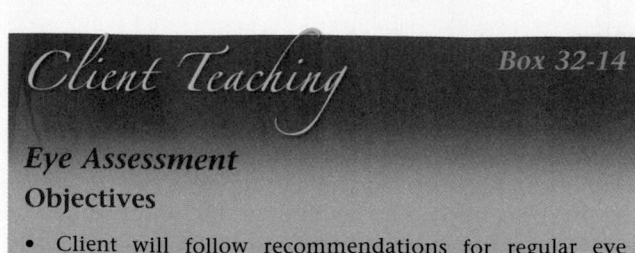

Client Teaching

Box 32-14

Eye Assessment

Objectives

- Client will follow recommendations for regular eye examinations.
- Client will be able to recognize warning signs and symptoms of eye disease.
- Client will take appropriate safety precautions for visual deficits.

Teaching Strategies

- Tell client that persons under age 40 should have a complete eye examination every 3 to 5 years (or more often if family histories reveal risks such as diabetes or hypertension).
- Tell client that persons over age 40 should have eye examinations every 2 years to screen for conditions that may develop without awareness (e.g., glaucoma).
- Tell client that persons over age 65 should have yearly eye examinations.
- Describe the typical symptoms of eye disease (see Box 32-13, p. 699).
- Instruct older adult to take the following precautions because of normal visual changes: avoid or use caution while driving at night, increase lighting in the home to reduce risk of falls, and paint the first and last steps of a staircase and the edge of each step in between a bright color to aid depth perception.

Evaluation

- Ask client or family member to report on client's most recent visit to an ophthalmologist.
- Have client describe when to have an eye examination.
- Ask client to describe common symptoms of eye disease.
- Observe the home environment of a client with visual deficits.

The inner ear contains the cochlea, vestibule, and semicircular canals. The nurse assesses the ears to determine the integrity of ear structures and the condition of hearing. Nursing history data (Table 32-15) aid in identifying risks for hearing disorders.

Understanding the mechanisms for sound transmission helps the nurse identify the nature of hearing disorders. Sound travels through the ear by air and bone conduction; the following explains the steps of hearing:

1. Sound waves in the air enter the external ear, passing through the outer ear canal.
2. The sound waves reach the tympanic membrane, causing it to vibrate.
3. Vibrations are transmitted through the middle ear by the bony ossicular chain to the oval window at the opening of the inner ear.
4. The cochlea receives the sound vibration.
5. Nerve impulses from the cochlea travel to the auditory (eighth cranial) nerve and to the cerebral cortex.

Disorders of the ear result from several types of problems, including mechanical dysfunction (blockage by ear wax or foreign body), trauma (foreign bodies or noise exposure), neurological disorders (auditory nerve damage), acute illnesses (viral infection), and toxic effects of medications.

Auricles. With the client sitting comfortably, the nurse inspects the auricle's size, shape, symmetry, landmarks, position, and color (Figure 32-20). The auricles are normally level with each other. The upper point of attachment is in a straight line with the lateral canthus, or corner of the eye. The position of the auricle should also be almost vertical. Ears that are low set or at an unusual angle are a sign of chromosome abnormality (e.g., Down syndrome). The color should be the same as that of the face, without moles, cysts, deformities, or nodules. Redness is a sign of inflammation or fever. Extreme pallor can indicate frostbite.

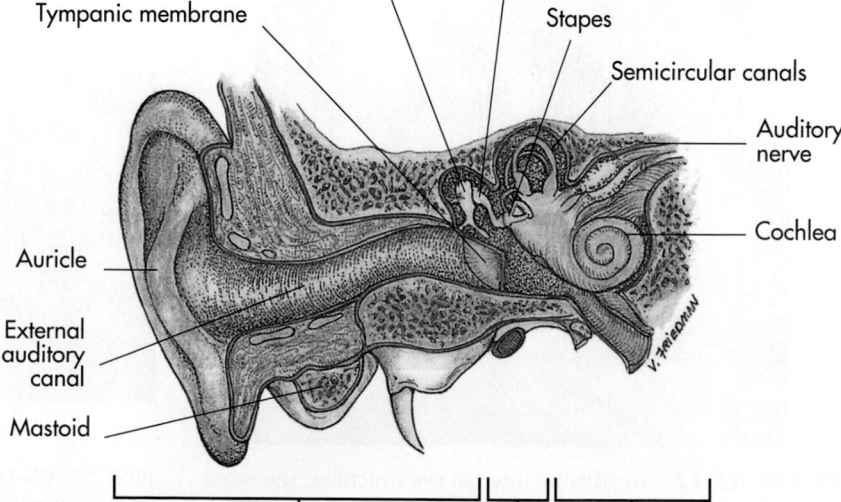

FIGURE **32–19** Structures of the external, middle, and inner ear.

The nurse palpates the auricles for texture, tenderness, and skin lesions. The auricle is normally smooth, without lesions. If the client complains of pain, the nurse gently pulls the auricle and presses on the tragus and palpates behind the ear over the mastoid process. If palpating the external ear increases the pain, an external ear infection is likely. If palpation of the auricle and tragus does not influence the pain, the client may have a middle ear infection. Tenderness in the mastoid area can indicate mastoiditis.

The nurse inspects the opening of the ear canal for size and discharge. Discharge may be accompanied by an odor. The meatus should not be swollen or occluded. A yellow, waxy substance called **cerumen** is common. Yellow or green, foul-smelling discharge may indicate infection or a foreign body.

Ear Canals and Eardrums. The deeper structures of the external and middle ear can be observed only with an **otoscope,** which is an ophthalmoscope with a special ear speculum attached to the battery tube. Speculums come in different sizes to conform to the different sizes of ear canals. For best visualization the largest speculum that fits comfortably into the ear canal should be used.

Before inserting the speculum, the examiner checks for foreign bodies in the opening of the auditory canal. Clients must not move their heads during the examination to avoid damage to the canal and tympanic membrane. Infants and young children often need to be restrained. Infants should lie supine with their heads turned to one side and their arms held securely at their sides. Young children can sit on their parents' laps with their legs held between the parents' knees.

The nurse turns on the otoscope by rotating the dial at the top of the battery tube. To insert the speculum prop-

erly, the nurse asks the client to tip the head slightly toward the opposite shoulder. The nurse holds the handle of the otoscope in the space between the thumb and index finger, supported on the middle finger. This leaves the ulnar side of the hand to rest against the client's head,

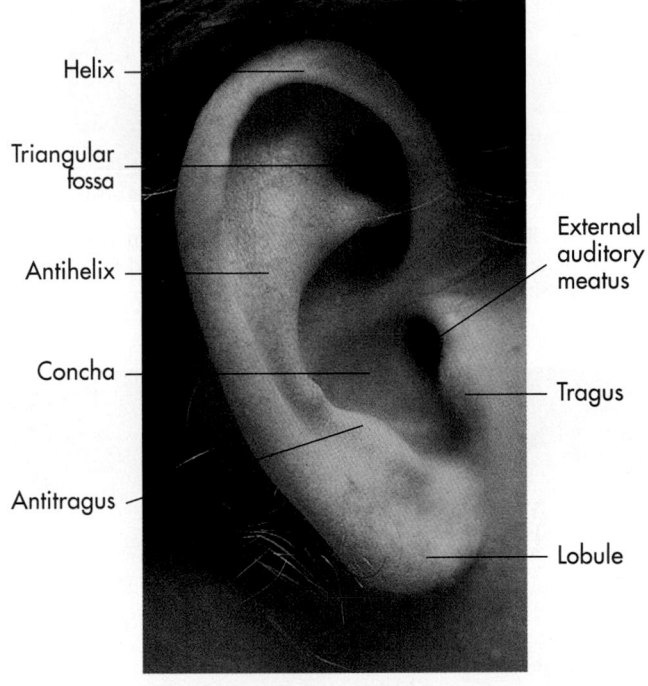

FIGURE 32–20 Anatomical structures of the auricle. (From Seidel HM and others: *Mosby's guide to physical examination,* ed 5, St. Louis, 2003, Mosby.)

Table 32-15 Nursing History for Ear Assessment

Assessment Category	Rationale
Ask if client has experienced ear pain, itching, discharge, vertigo, tinnitus (ringing in ears), or change in hearing.	These signs and symptoms indicate infection or hearing loss.
Assess risks for hearing problem.	Risk factors predispose client to permanent hearing loss. It may be difficult to assess infant's hearing status with examination only.
Infants/children: Hypoxia at birth, meningitis, birth weight less than 1500 g, family history of hearing loss, congenital anomalies of skull or face, nonbacterial intrauterine infections (rubella, herpes), maternal drug use, excessively high bilirubin, head trauma	
Adults: Exposure to industrial or recreational noise, genetic disease (Meniere's disease), neurodegenerative disorder	
Determine client's exposure to loud noises at work and availability of protective devices.	Prolonged noise exposure can cause temporary or permanent hearing loss.
Note behaviors indicative of hearing loss, such as failure to respond when spoken to, requests to repeat comments, leaning forward to hear, and child's inattentiveness or use of monotonous voice tone.	Persons with hearing loss cope with sensory deficit through a variety of behavioral cues.
Assess if client takes large doses of aspirin or other ototoxic drugs (e.g., aminoglycosides, furosemide, streptomycin, cisplatin, ethacrynic acid).	Medications have side effects of hearing loss.
Determine whether client uses hearing aid.	Determination allows nurse to assess ability to care for device and allows nurse to adjust voice tone to communicate.
If client had recent hearing problem, note onset, contributing factors, affected ear, and effect on activities for daily living.	Nature and severity of hearing problem are determined.
Determine whether client has repeated history of cerumen buildup in ear.	Cerumen impaction is common cause for conduction deafness.

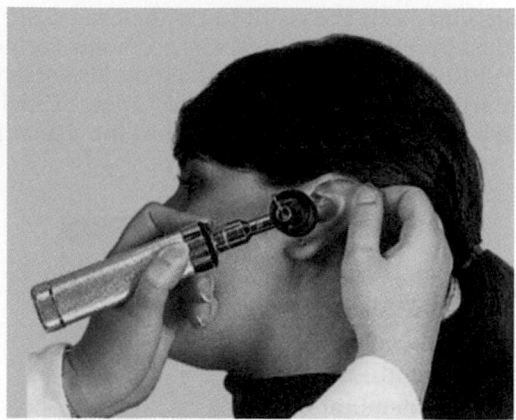

FIGURE **32–21** Otoscopic examination. (From Seidel HM and others: *Mosby's guide to physical examination,* ed 5, St. Louis, 2003, Mosby.)

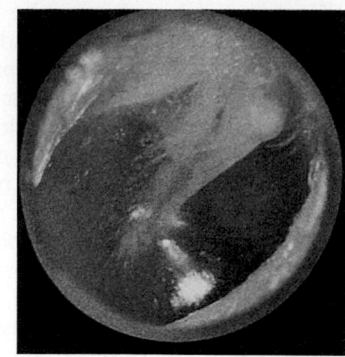

FIGURE **32–22** Normal right tympanic membrane. (Courtesy Dr. Richard A. Buckingham, Abraham Lincoln School of Medicine, University of Illinois, Chicago.)

Client Teaching

Box 32-15

Ear Assessment

Objectives

- Client will use proper technique for cleansing the ears.
- Client will follow preventive guidelines for screening of hearing loss.
- Client with hearing loss will communicate effectively.

Teaching Strategies

- Instruct client about the proper way to clean the outer ear (see Chapter 38), avoiding use of cotton-tipped applicators and sharp objects such as hairpins, which may cause impaction of cerumen deep in the ear canal.
- Tell client to avoid inserting pointed objects into the ear canal.
- Encourage clients over age 65 to have regular hearing checks. Explain that a reduction in hearing is a normal part of aging (see Chapter 48).
- Instruct family members of clients with hearing losses to avoid shouting, speaking instead in low tones, and to be sure the client can see the speaker's face.

Evaluation

- Ask client to explain the proper technique for cleansing the ears.
- In a follow-up visit, question client about frequency of hearing checks.
- Observe client with hearing loss interacting with family members.

stabilizing the otoscope as it is inserted into the canal (Seidel and others, 2003). Two grips on the otoscope may be used. In one grip, the nurse holds the battery tube along the client's face with the fingers against the face or neck. In the other grip, the inverted otoscope is lightly braced against the side of the client's head or cheek. This grip, used with children, prevents accidental movement

of the otoscope deeper into the ear canal. The nurse inserts the scope while pulling the auricle upward and backward in the adult and older child (Figure 32-21). Pulling the auricle gently up, back, and slightly out in the adult or older child straightens the ear canal. In infants the nurse pulls the auricle back and down.

The nurse inserts the speculum slightly down and forward 1 to 1.5 cm (½ inch) into the ear canal. Care is taken not to abrade the sensitive lining of the ear canal, because this can be painful. The skin has little subcutaneous fat between it and the underlying bone. The canal normally has little cerumen and is uniformly pink with tiny hairs in the outer third of the canal. The nurse observes for color, discharge, scaling, lesions, foreign bodies, and cerumen. Normally cerumen is dry (light brown to gray and flaky) or moist (dark yellow or brown) and sticky. Dry cerumen occurs in Asians and Native Americans about 85% of the time (Seidel and others, 2003). A reddened canal with discharge is a sign of inflammation or infection. In other adults, accumulated cerumen is a common problem. Buildup of cerumen can create a mild hearing loss. During the examination the examiner asks about methods that the client uses to clean the ear canal (Box 32-15).

The light from the otoscope allows visualization of the tympanic membrane. The nurse must be familiar with the common anatomical landmarks and their appearances (Figure 32-22). This takes practice. The otoscope is slowly moved so that the entire tympanic membrane and its periphery can be seen. Because the tympanic membrane is angled away from the ear canal, the light from the otoscope appears as a cone rather than a circle. A ring of fibrous cartilage surrounds the oval membrane. The umbo is near the center of the membrane, and the attachment of the malleus is behind it. A knoblike structure at the top of the tympanic membrane is created by the underlying short process of the malleus. The nurse should check carefully to make sure that there are no tears or breaks in the membrane. The normal tympanic membrane is translucent, shiny, and pearly gray. It is free from tears or breaks. A pink or red bulging membrane indicates inflammation. A white color reveals pus behind it. The membrane is taut, except for the small triangular pars flaccida near the top. If the tympanic membrane is blocked by cerumen, irrigation with warm water will safely remove the wax.

Hearing Acuity. Often the nurse can tell whether the client has a hearing loss from a response to conversation. The three types of hearing loss are conduction, sensorineural, and mixed. A conduction loss interrupts sound waves as they travel from the outer ear to the cochlea of the inner ear because the sound waves are not transmitted through the outer and middle ear structures. Examples of causes of a conduction loss are swelling of the auditory canal or tears in the tympanic membrane. A sensorineural loss involves the inner ear, auditory nerve, or hearing center of the brain. Sound is conducted through the outer and middle ear structures, but the continued transmission of sound becomes interrupted at some point beyond the bony ossicles. A mixed loss involves a combination of conduction and sensorineural loss.

> *Safety Alert.* Clients working or living around loud noises are at risk for hearing loss. In addition, adolescents may be at risk for premature hearing loss from continued exposure to loud music in their car or home or at concert events.

Older adults experience an inability to hear high-frequency sounds and consonants (e.g., *S, Z, T,* and *G*). Deterioration of the cochlea and a thickening of the tympanic membrane cause older adults to gradually lose hearing acuity. They are especially at risk for hearing loss due to **ototoxicity** (injury to auditory nerve) resulting from high maintenance doses of antibiotics (e.g., the aminoglycosides).

To begin a hearing assessment, the nurse has the client remove any hearing aid that is worn. The nurse notes the client's response to questions. Normally the client should respond without excessive requests to have the nurse repeat questions. If hearing loss is suspected, the nurse checks the client's response to the whispered voice. One ear is tested at a time while the client occludes the other ear with a finger. The nurse asks the client to gently move the finger up and down during the test. While standing 30 to 60 cm (1 to 2 feet) from the ear being tested, the nurse covers the mouth so that the client is unable to read lips. After exhaling fully, the nurse first whispers softly toward the unoccluded ear, reciting random numbers with equally accented syllables, such as *nine-four-ten.* If necessary, the nurse gradually increases voice intensity until the client correctly repeats the numbers. The other ear is then tested for comparison. Seidel and others (2003) report that clients normally hear numbers clearly when whispered, responding correctly at least 50% of the time.

If a hearing loss is present, there are tests that can be performed using a tuning fork or audiometry. A tuning fork of 256 to 512 hertz (Hz) is most commonly used. The tuning fork allows for comparison of hearing by bone conduction with that of air conduction. The nurse holds the base of the tuning fork with one hand without touching the tines. The fork should be lightly tapped against the palm of the other hand, setting the fork in vibration (Table 32-16).

Nose and Sinuses

The nurse uses inspection and palpation to assess the nose and sinuses. The client sits during the examination. A penlight allows for gross examination of each naris. A more detailed examination requires use of a nasal speculum to inspect the deeper nasal turbinates. A student should not use a speculum unless a qualified practitioner is present. Table 32-17 lists components of the nursing history.

Nose. When inspecting the external nose, the nurse observes for shape, size, skin, color, and the presence of deformity or inflammation. The nose is normally smooth and symmetric and the same color as the face. Recent trauma may have caused edema and discoloration. If swelling or deformities exist, the nurse gently palpates the ridge and soft tissue of the nose by placing one finger on each side of the nasal arch and gently moving the fingers from the nasal bridge to the tip. The nurse notes any tenderness, masses, or underlying deviations. Nasal structures are usually firm and stable.

Air normally passes freely through the nose as a person breathes. To assess patency of the nares, the nurse places a finger on the side of the client's nose and occludes one naris. The client is asked to breathe with the mouth closed. The examination is repeated for the other naris.

While illuminating the anterior nares, the nurse inspects the mucosa for color, lesions, discharge, swelling, and evidence of bleeding. If discharge is present, gloves should be worn. Normal mucosa is pink and moist without lesions. Pale mucosa with clear discharge indicates allergy. A mucoid discharge indicates rhinitis. A sinus infection results in yellowish or greenish discharge. Habitual use of intranasal cocaine and opioids can cause puffiness and increased vascularity of the nasal mucosa (Friedman and others, 1996). For the client with a nasogastric or nasopharyngeal tube, the nurse routinely checks for local skin breakdown (**excoriation**) of the naris, characterized by redness and sloughing of the skin.

To view the septum and turbinates, the client tips the head back slightly to give the nurse a clear view. The septum is inspected for alignment, perforation, or bleeding. Normally the septum is close to the midline, and thicker anteriorly than posteriorly. The turbinates are covered with mucous membranes that warm and moisten inspired air. The mucosa is pink and moist, with clear mucus. A deviated septum can obstruct breathing and interfere with passage of a nasogastric tube. Perforation of the septum can occur after repeated use of intranasal cocaine. The nurse notes any **polyps** (tumorlike growths) or purulent drainage.

Sinuses. Examination of the sinuses involves palpation. In cases of allergies or infection, the interior of the sinuses become inflamed and swollen. The most effective way to assess for tenderness is by externally palpating the frontal and maxillary facial areas (Figure 32-23). The frontal sinus is palpated by exerting pressure with the thumb up and under the client's eyebrow. Gentle, upward pressure elicits tenderness easily if sinus irritation is present and reveals the severity of sinus irritation. Pressure should not be

Table 32-16   Tuning Fork Tests

Tests and Steps	Rationale
Weber's Test (Lateralization of Sound) Hold fork at its base and tap it lightly against heel of palm. Place base of vibrating fork on midline vertex of client's head or middle of forehead (see illustration *A*). Ask client if the sound is heard equally in both ears or better in one ear.	Client with normal hearing hears sound equally in both ears or in midline of head. In conduction deafness, sound is heard best in impaired ear. In unilateral sensorineural hearing loss, sound is identified only in normal ear.
Rinne Test (Comparison of Air and Bone Conduction) Place stem of vibrating tuning fork against client's mastoid process (see illustration *B*). Begin counting the interval with your watch. Ask client to tell you when the sound is no longer heard; note number of seconds. Quickly place still-vibrating tines 1 to 2 cm (½ to 1 inch) from ear canal and ask client to tell you when the sound is no longer heard (see illustration *C*). Continue counting time the sound is heard by air conduction. Compare number of seconds the sound is heard by bone conduction versus air conduction.	Air-conducted sound should be heard twice as long as bone-conducted sound. In conduction deafness, bone-conducted sound can be heard longer. In sensorineural loss, sound is reduced and heard longer through air.

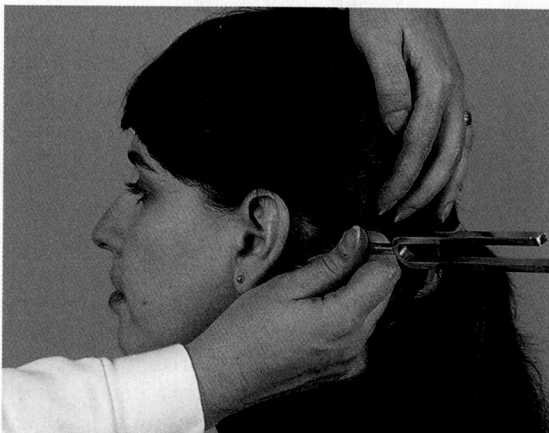

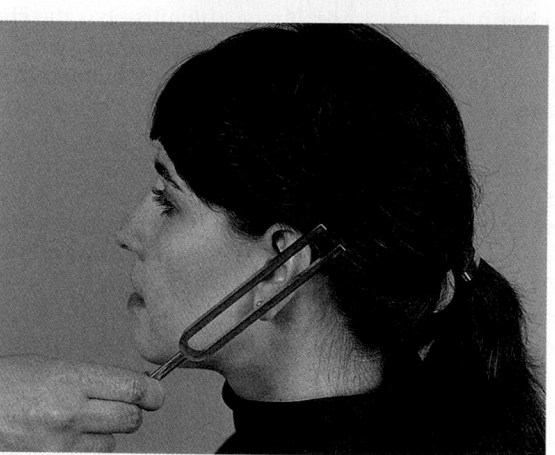

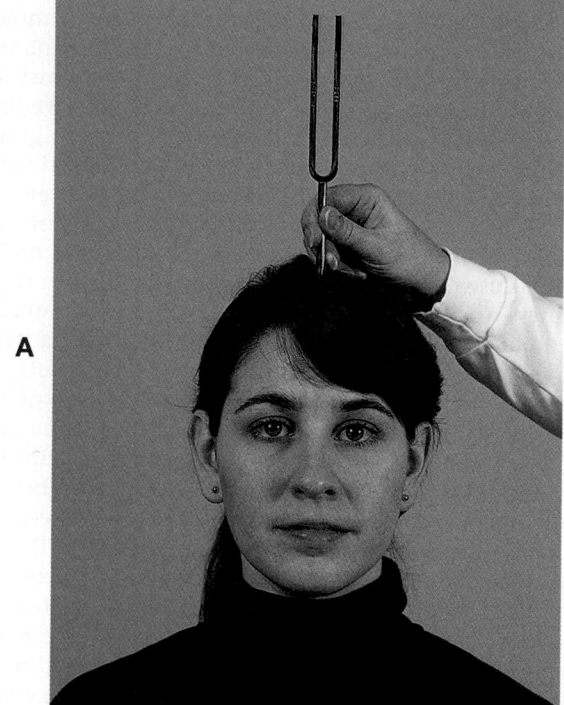

Illustrations from Seidel HM and others: *Mosby's guide to physical examination*, ed 5, St. Louis, 2003, Mosby.

Table 32-17	Nursing History for Nose and Sinus Assessment
Assessment Category	**Rationale**
Ask if client has had trauma to nose.	Trauma can cause septal deviation and asymmetry of external nose.
Ask if client has history of allergies, nasal discharge, epistaxis (nosebleeds), or postnasal drip.	History is useful in determining source or nature of nasal and sinus drainage.
If there is history of nasal discharge, assess color, amount, odor, duration, and associated symptoms (e.g., sneezing, nasal congestion, obstruction, or mouth breathing).	Can help to rule out presence of infection, allergy, or drug use.
Assess for history of nosebleed, including site, frequency, amount of bleeding, treatment, and difficulty stopping bleeding.	Characteristics may reveal trauma, medication use, or excessive dryness as causative factors.
Ask if client uses nasal spray or drops.	Overuse of over-the-counter nasal preparations can cause physical change in mucosa.
Ask if client snores at night or has difficulty breathing.	Difficulty with breathing or snoring may indicate septal deviation or obstruction.

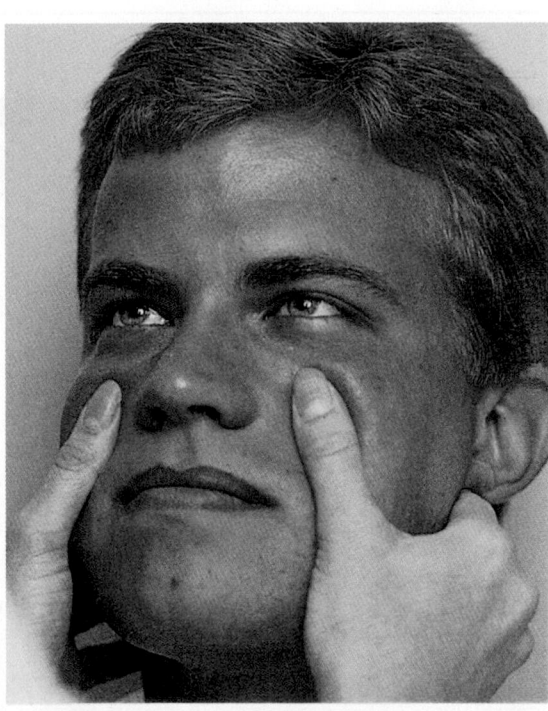

FIGURE **32–23** Palpation of maxillary sinuses.

applied to the eyes. Box 32-16 describes teaching guidelines during nose and sinus assessment.

Mouth and Pharynx

The nurse assesses the mouth and pharynx to detect signs of overall health, determine oral hygiene needs, and develop nursing therapies for clients with dehydration, restricted intake, oral trauma, or oral airway obstruction. To assess the oral cavity, the nurse uses a penlight and tongue depressor or a single gauze square. Gloves should be worn during the examination. The client may sit or lie during the examination. Assessment of the oral cavity can be made during administration of oral hygiene (see Chapter 38). Table 32-18 describes the nursing history for assessment of the mouth and pharynx.

Client Teaching   Box 32-16

Nose and Sinus Assessment

Objectives

- Client will safely use over-the-counter nasal sprays.
- Parents will take proper measures to stop a child's nosebleed.
- Older adult will take safety precautions with loss of olfaction.

Teaching Strategies

- Caution client against overuse of over-the-counter nasal sprays, which can lead to "rebound" effect, causing excess nasal congestion.
- Instruct parents on care of a child with nosebleeds: have child sit up and lean forward to avoid aspiration of blood, apply pressure to the anterior nose with the thumb and forefinger as the child breathes through the mouth, and apply ice or a cold cloth to the bridge of the nose if pressure fails to stop bleeding.
- Instruct older adults to install smoke detectors on each floor of their home.
- Instruct older adults to always check dated labels on food to ensure against spoilage.

Evaluation

- Have client explain proper use of over-the-counter nasal sprays.
- Have parents demonstrate and describe technique for stopping a nosebleed.
- Inspect client's home during visit and look for smoke detectors. Ask to check some food items in the refrigerator.

Lips. The lips are inspected for color, texture, hydration, contour, and lesions. With the client's mouth closed, the nurse views the lips from end to end. Normally they are pink, moist, symmetrical, and smooth (Figure 32-24). Female clients should remove their lipstick before the examination. Pallor of the lips can be caused by anemia, with cyanosis caused by respiratory or cardiovascular

Table 32-18   Nursing History for Mouth and Pharyngeal Assessment

Assessment Category	Rationale
Determine if client wears dentures or retainers and if they are comfortable.	Dentures must be removed to visualize and palpate gums. Ill-fitting dentures chronically irritate mucosa and gums.
Determine if client has had recent change in appetite or weight.	Symptoms may result from painful mouth conditions or poor hygiene.
Determine if client smokes or chews tobacco.	Tobacco users have greater risk for mouth and throat cancers than nonusers (ACS, 2003).
Review history for alcohol consumption.	Heavy drinkers appear to have greater risk for oral cancer. Effects of alcohol are independent of tobacco use.
Assess dental hygiene practices, including use of fluoride toothpaste, frequency of brushing and flossing, and frequency of dental visits.	Assessment reveals client's need for education and/or financial support. Periodontal disease has a higher prevalence in older adults who have history of high plaque buildup, use tobacco, and visit the dentist infrequently.
Ask if client has pain from chewing or eating. If so, ask if mouth lesions are present, including duration and associated symptoms.	May be associated with broken tooth, tooth grinding, or temporomandibular joint problems. Extra care needed during oral hygiene administration.

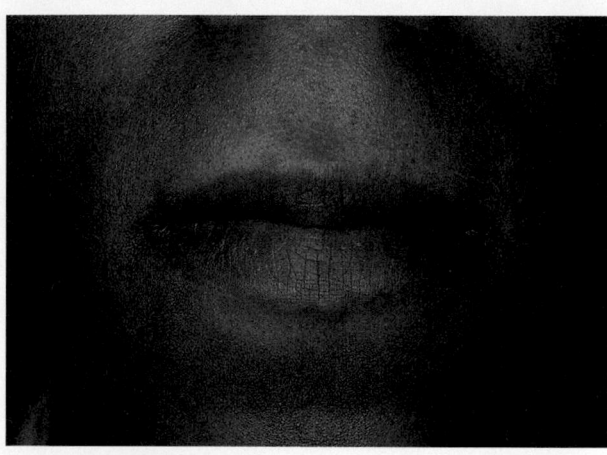

FIGURE **32-24** The lips are normally pink, symmetrical, smooth, and moist.

problems. Cherry-colored lips may indicate carbon monoxide poisoning. Any lesions such as nodules or ulcerations can be related to infection, irritation, or skin cancer.

Buccal Mucosa, Gums, and Teeth. The nurse begins inspection by having the client clench the teeth and smile. The maneuver allows assessment of teeth occlusion. The upper molars should rest directly on the lower molars with the upper incisors slightly overriding the lower incisors. A symmetrical smile reveals normal facial nerve function.

The quality of dental hygiene is easily determined by inspecting the teeth (Box 32-17). The position and alignment of the teeth are noted. To examine the posterior surface of the teeth, the nurse has the client open the mouth with the lips relaxed. A tongue depressor may be needed to retract the lips and cheeks, especially when viewing the molars. Tartar along the base of the teeth, dental **caries** (cavities), extraction sites, and tooth color should be

Client Teaching   Box 32-17

Mouth and Pharyngeal Assessment

Objectives

- Client will practice proper oral hygiene measures and dental care.
- Client will describe warning signs of oral cancer.
- Older adult will maintain normal solid food intake.

Teaching Strategies

- Discuss proper techniques for oral hygiene, including brushing and flossing (see Chapter 38).
- Explain the early warning signs of oral cancer, including a sore that bleeds easily and does not heal, a lump or thickening, and a red or white patch on the mucosa that persists.* Difficulty chewing or swallowing is a late symptom.
- Encourage regular dental examination every 6 months for children, adults, and older adults.
- Identify older clients who have difficulty in chewing and changes in the teeth. Teach clients to eat soft foods and cut food into small pieces.

Evaluation

- Ask client to demonstrate brushing.
- Have client identify when to have regular dental checkups.
- Have client identify the warning signs of oral cancer.
- Ask older adult to keep a diet record for 3 days.

*Data from American Cancer Society: *Cancer facts and figures 2003*, New York, 2003, The Society.

noted. Normal, healthy teeth are smooth, white, and shiny. A chalky white discoloration of the enamel is an early indication of caries formation. Brown or black discolorations indicate the formation of caries. In the older adult, loose or missing teeth are common because bone re-

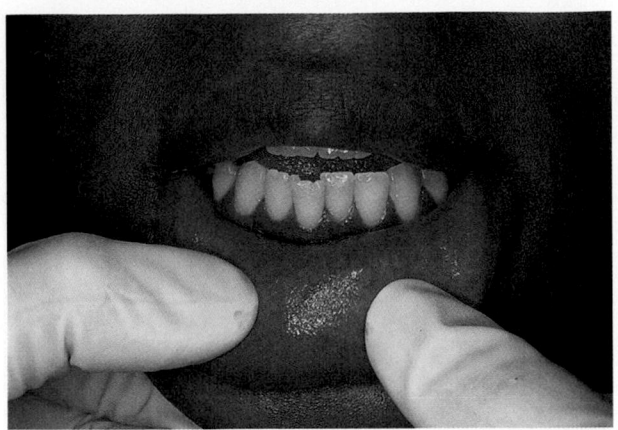

FIGURE 32–25   Inspection of inner oral mucosa of lower lip.

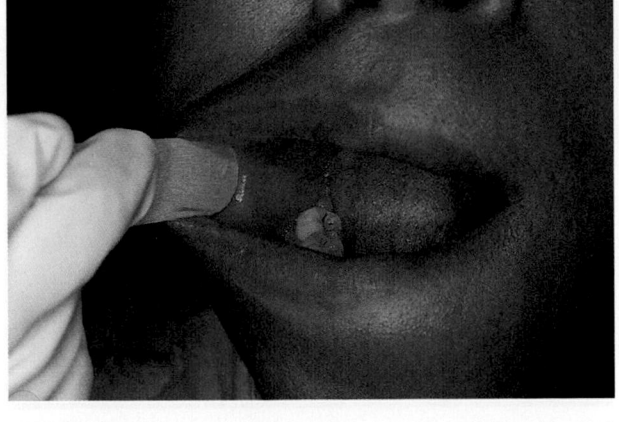

FIGURE 32–26   Retraction of the buccal mucosa allows for clear visualization.

sorption increases. An older adult's teeth often feel rough when tooth enamel calcifies. Yellow or darkened teeth are also common in the older adult because of the general wear and tear that exposes the darker, underlying dentin.

To view the mucosa and gums, the nurse asks the client to first remove any dental appliance. The nurse views the inner oral mucosa by having the client open and relax the mouth slightly and then gently retracts the client's lower lip away from the teeth (Figure 32-25). This process is repeated for the upper lip. The mucosa is inspected for color, hydration, texture, and lesions such as ulcers, abrasions, or cysts. Normal mucous membrane is pinkish red, smooth, and moist. Small, yellow-white raised lesions commonly seen on the buccal mucosa and lips are Fordyce spots, or ectopic sebaceous glands (Seidel and others, 2003). If lesions are present, the nurse palpates them gently with a gloved hand for tenderness, size, and consistency.

To visualize the buccal mucosa, the nurse asks the client to open the mouth and then gently retracts the cheeks with a tongue depressor or gloved finger covered with gauze (Figure 32-26). The surface of the mucosa must be viewed from right to left and top to bottom. A penlight illuminates the most posterior portion of the mucosa. Normal mucosa is glistening, pink, soft, moist, and smooth. An increase in color or hyperpigmentation is normal in 10% of whites after age 50 and in up to 90% of African-Americans by the same age. For clients with normal pigmentation, the buccal mucosa is a good site to inspect for jaundice and pallor. In older adults the mucosa is normally dry because of reduced salivation. Thick white patches **(leukoplakia)** can be seen in heavy smokers and alcoholics. Leukoplakia should be reported because it can also be a precancerous lesion. The nurse palpates the cheek with one finger along the inner mucosa and the thumb along the outside cheek to check for deep-seated lumps or ulcerations.

> *Safety Alert.* Clients who smoke cigarettes, cigars, or pipes and those who use chewing tobacco have an increased risk of oral cancer. These individuals may have leukoplakia or other lesions anywhere in their oral cavity (e.g., lips, gums, or tongue) at an early age.

While the nurse retracts the cheeks, the gums (gingivae) are inspected for color, edema, retraction, bleeding, and lesions. The gums around the back molars should be viewed because this is a difficult area to reach when cleaning teeth. Healthy gums are pink, smooth, and moist, with a tight margin at each tooth. African-Americans may have patchy pigmentation. In older adults the gums are usually pale. Using gloves, the nurse palpates the gums to assess for lesions, thickening, or masses. There should be no tenderness on palpation. Spongy gums that bleed easily indicate periodontal disease and vitamin C deficiency. If the client has loose or mobile teeth, swollen gums, or pockets containing debris at the tooth margins, periodontal disease or gingivitis can be suspected.

Tongue and Floor of Mouth. The tongue is carefully inspected on all sides, and the floor of the mouth is checked. The client first relaxes the mouth and sticks the tongue out halfway. The nurse notes any deviation, tremor, or limitation in movement. This tests hypoglossal nerve function. If the client protrudes the tongue too far, the gag reflex may be elicited. When the tongue protrudes, it lies midline. To test for tongue mobility, the nurse asks the client to raise the tongue up and move it from side to side. The tongue should move freely.

Using the penlight for illumination, the nurse examines the tongue for color, size, position, texture, and coatings or lesions. The tongue should be medium or dull red in color, moist, slightly rough on the top surface, and smooth along the lateral margins. The undersurface of the tongue and the floor of the mouth are highly vascular (Figure 32-27). Extra care is taken to inspect these areas, which are common sites for oral cancer lesions. The client lifts the tongue by placing its tip on the palate behind the upper incisors. The nurse looks for color, swelling, and lesions such as nodules or cysts. The ventral surface of the tongue is pink and smooth, with large veins between the frenulum folds. To palpate the tongue, the nurse explains the procedure and then asks the client to protrude the tongue. The nurse grasps the tip with a gauze square and gently pulls it to one side. With a gloved hand, the nurse palpates the full length of the

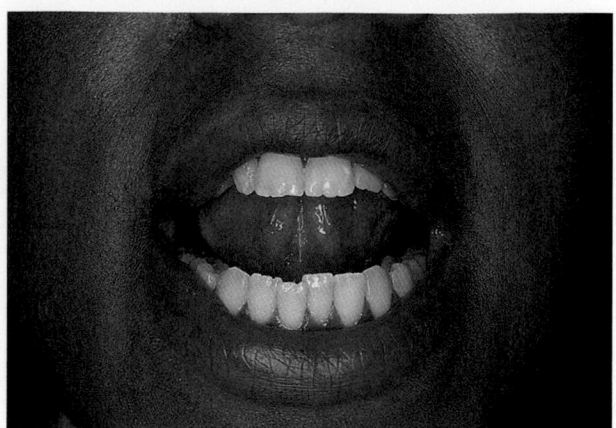

FIGURE **32–27** The undersurface of the tongue is highly vascular.

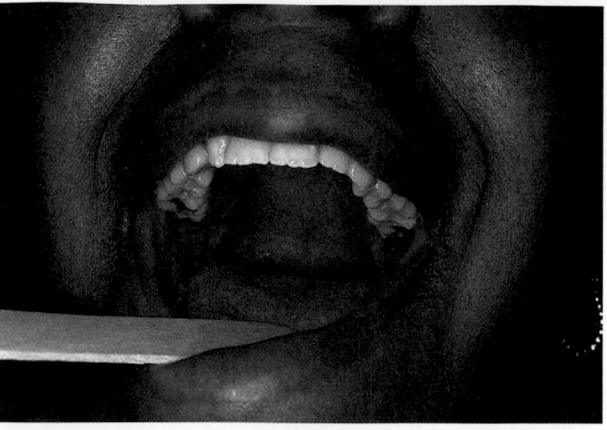

FIGURE **32–29** A penlight and tongue depressor allow the nurse to visualize the uvula and posterior soft palate.

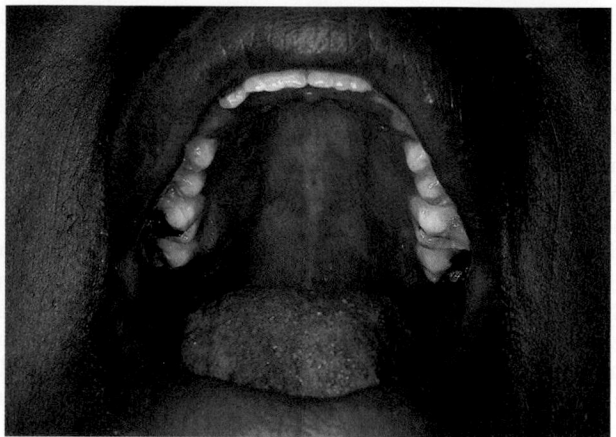

FIGURE **32–28** The hard palate is located anteriorly in the roof of the mouth.

pressor is placed too far anteriorly, the posterior part of the tongue mounds up, obstructing the view. The gag reflex is elicited when the tongue depressor touches the posterior tongue.

With a penlight, the nurse inspects the uvula and soft palate (Figure 32-29). Both structures, which are innervated by the tenth cranial (vagus) nerve, should rise centrally as the client says "ah." The nurse also inspects the arch formed by the anterior and posterior pillars, soft palate, and uvula. The tonsils can be viewed in the cavities between the anterior and posterior pillars and are oval, with infoldings of tissue. The posterior pharynx is behind the pillars. The pharyngeal tissues are normally pink and smooth. Edema, ulceration, or inflammation indicates infection or abnormal lesions. Clients with chronic sinus problems frequently exhibit a clear exudate that drains along the wall of the posterior pharynx. Yellow or green exudate indicates infection. A client with a typical sore throat has redness and swelling of the uvula, and tonsillar pillars, as well as the possible presence of yellow exudate.

Neck

The neck muscles, lymph nodes of the head and neck, carotid arteries, jugular veins, thyroid gland, and trachea are located within the neck (Figure 32-30). An examination of the jugular veins and carotid arteries can be deferred until assessment of the vascular system. The nurse inspects and palpates the neck to determine the integrity of the neck structures and to examine the lymphatic system. The lymphatic system is examined region by region during the assessment of other body systems (head and neck, breast, genitalia, and extremities). An abnormality of superficial lymph nodes may reveal an infection or malignancy. Examination of the thyroid gland and trachea also aids in ruling out malignancies. Examination is best performed with the client sitting. The areas of the neck are outlined by the sternocleidomastoid and trapezius muscles, which divide each side of the neck into two triangles. The anterior triangle contains the trachea, thyroid gland, carotid artery, and anterior cervical lymph nodes. The posterior triangle contains the posterior lymph nodes. Table 32-19 reviews the nursing history for the head and neck examination.

tongue and the base for any areas of hardening or ulceration. **Varicosities** (swollen, tortuous veins) may be seen. Varicosities rarely cause problems but are common in the older adult.

Palate. The client should extend the head backward, holding the mouth open so that the nurse can inspect the hard and soft palates for color, shape, texture, and extra bony prominences or defects (Figure 32-28). The hard palate, or roof of the mouth, is located anteriorly. It is whitish and should be dome shaped. The soft palate, best seen while depressing the tongue with a tongue blade, extends posteriorly toward the pharynx. It is normally light pink and smooth. A bony growth, or **exostosis,** between the two palates is common.

Pharynx. The pharynx can be a site for infection, inflammation, or lesions. Before examining the pharynx, the nurse explains the procedure to the client. The client tips the head back slightly, opens the mouth wide, and says "ah." The nurse places the tip of a tongue depressor on the middle third of the tongue, taking care not to press the lower lip against the teeth. If the tongue de-

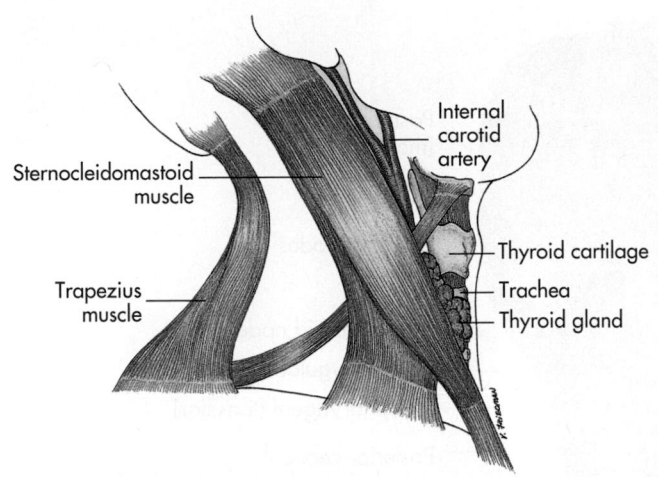

Sternocleidomastoid muscle

Trapezius muscle

Internal carotid artery

Thyroid cartilage

Trachea

Thyroid gland

FIGURE 32–30 Anatomical position of the major neck structures. Note the triangles formed by the sternocleidomastoid muscle, lower jaw, and anterior neck anteriorly and by the sternocleidomastoid muscle, trapezius muscle, and lower neck posteriorly.

Table 32-19   **Nursing History for Neck Assessment**

Assessment Category	Rationale
Assess for history of recent cold or infection or enlarged lymph nodes.	Colds or infections can cause temporary or permanent lymph node enlargement. Lymph nodes may also be enlarged in various diseases such as cancer.
If there is an enlarged lymph node, consider reviewing history of IV drug use, hemophilia, sexual contact with persons infected with HIV, history of blood transfusion, multiple and indiscriminate sexual contacts, or male with homosexual or bisexual activities.	These are risk factors for HIV infection.
Ask if client has had history of neck pain with restriction in movement.	May indicate muscle strain, head injury, local nerve injury, or enlarged or swollen lymph node.
Ask if client has had change in temperature preference (more or less clothing); swelling in neck; change in texture of hair, skin, or nails; or change in emotional stability.	Symptoms indicative of thyroid disease.
Ask if client has history of thyroid problem or takes thyroid medication.	Disease or medications may influence tissue growth of gland.
Review medical history of pneumothorax (collapsed lung) or bronchial tumor.	Conditions place client at risk for tracheal displacement or lateral deviation.

Neck Muscles. The nurse begins the examination by inspecting the neck in the usual anatomical position, in slight hyperextension. The nurse inspects for bilateral symmetry of the neck muscles. To test the function of the sternocleidomastoid muscle, the nurse asks the client to flex the neck with the chin to the chest. Then the client hyperextends the neck backward so that the nurse can check for trapezius muscle function. Movement of the head sideways so that the ear moves toward the shoulder further tests function of the sternocleidomastoid muscle. The neck should move freely without discomfort or dizziness. Other tests for muscle strength and function can be performed during assessment of the musculoskeletal system.

Lymph Nodes. An extensive system of lymph nodes collects lymph from the head, ears, nose, cheeks, and lips (Figure 32-31). The immune system protects the body from foreign antigens, removes damaged cells from the circulation, and provides a partial barrier to growth of malignant cells within the body. The nurse should be-

come particularly competent in assessing the lymph nodes when caring for clients with suspected immunoincompetence, which can be linked to allergies, human immunodeficiency virus (HIV) infection, autoimmune disease (e.g., lupus erythematosus), or serious infection.

With the client's chin raised and head tilted slightly, the nurse first inspects the area where lymph nodes are distributed and compares both sides. This position stretches the skin slightly over any possible enlarged nodes. Visible nodes are inspected for edema, erythema, or red streaks. Nodes are not normally visible.

A methodical approach is used to examine the lymph nodes to avoid overlooking any single node or chain. The client relaxes with the neck flexed slightly forward and, if needed, toward the nurse. This maneuver relaxes tissues and muscles. Both sides of the neck are inspected and palpated for comparison. During palpation the nurse faces or stands to the side of the client for easy access to all nodes. Using the pads of the middle three fingers of the hand, the nurse palpates gently in a rotary motion for superficial lymph nodes (Figure 32-32). Each node is

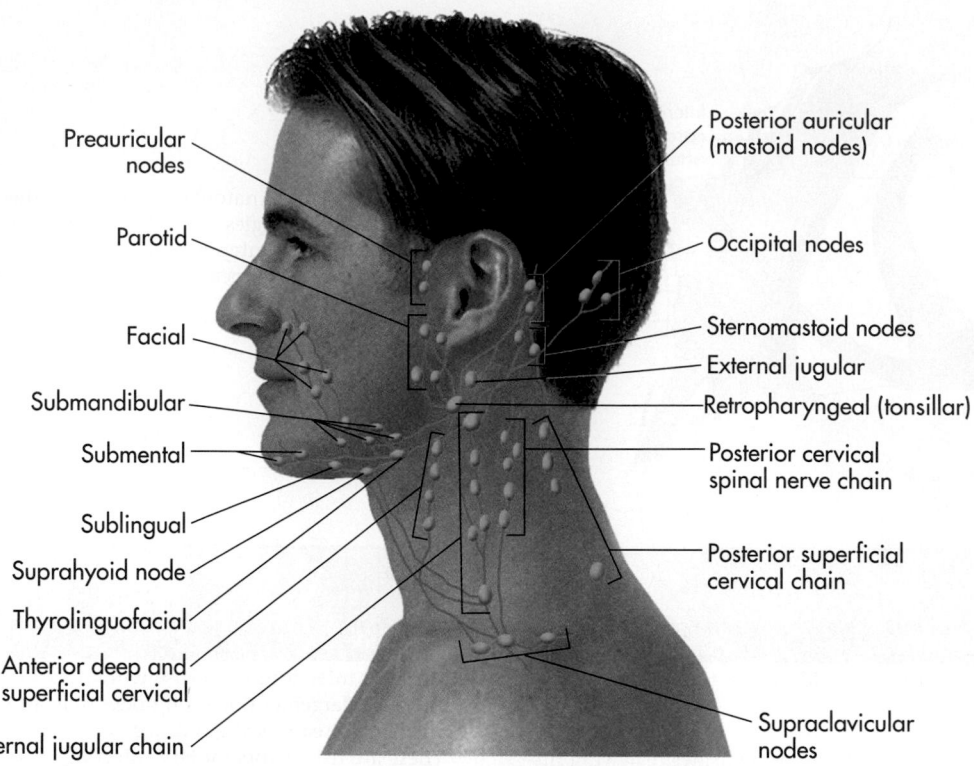

Preauricular nodes

Parotid

Facial

Submandibular

Submental

Sublingual

Suprahyoid node

Thyrolinguofacial

Anterior deep and superficial cervical

Internal jugular chain

Posterior auricular (mastoid nodes)

Occipital nodes

Sternomastoid nodes

External jugular

Retropharyngeal (tonsillar)

Posterior cervical spinal nerve chain

Posterior superficial cervical chain

Supraclavicular nodes

FIGURE **32–31** Lymphatic drainage system of the head and neck. If the group of nodes is often referred to by another name, the second name appears in parentheses. (From Seidel HM and others: *Mosby's guide to physical examination,* ed 5, St. Louis, 2003, Mosby.)

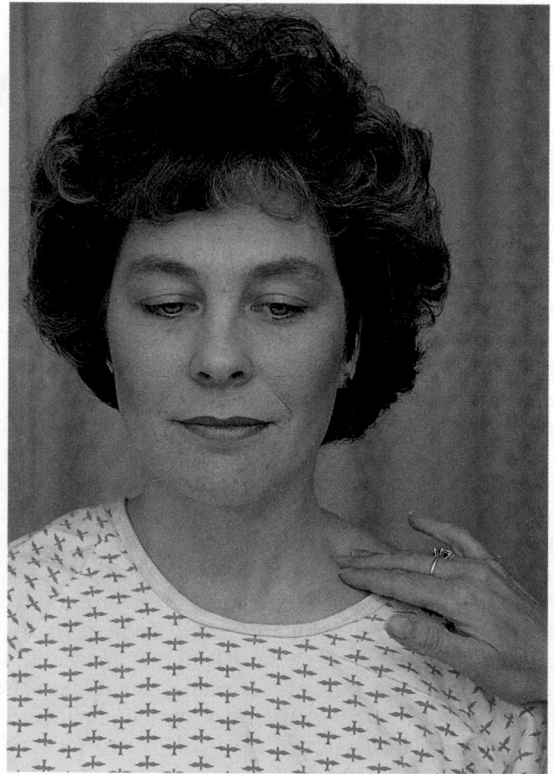

FIGURE **32–32** Palpation of cervical lymph nodes.

checked methodically in the following sequence: occipital nodes at the base of the skull, postauricular nodes over the mastoid, preauricular nodes just in front of the ear, retropharyngeal nodes at the angle of the mandible, submaxillary nodes, and submental nodes in the midline behind the mandibular tip. The nurse tries to detect enlargement and notes the location, size, shape, surface characteristics, consistency, mobility, tenderness, and warmth of the nodes. If the skin is mobile, the nurse moves the skin over the area of the nodes. It is important to press underlying tissue in each area and not simply move the fingers over the skin. However, if excessive pressure is applied, small nodes are missed and palpable nodes are obliterated.

To palpate supraclavicular nodes, the nurse asks the client to bend the head forward and relax the shoulders. The nurse may have to hook the index and third finger over the clavicle, lateral to the sternocleidomastoid muscle, to palpate these nodes. The deep cervical nodes can be palpated only with the nurse's fingers hooked around the sternocleidomastoid muscle.

Normally lymph nodes are not easily palpable. However, small, mobile, nontender nodes are common. Lymph nodes that are large, fixed, inflamed, or tender indicate a problem such as local infection, systemic disease, or neoplasm (Seidel and others, 2003) (Box 32-18). When enlarged nodes are found, the nurse explores adjacent areas and regions drained by the nodes for signs of infection or malignancy. Tenderness is usually a result of inflammation. Noting which nodes are enlarged may help

Client Teaching

Box 32-18

Neck Assessment

Objective

- Client will take proper preventive action if a mass is noted in the neck.

Teaching Strategies

- Stress importance of regular compliance with medication schedule to clients with thyroid disease.
- Instruct client about the lymph nodes and how infection can commonly cause node tenderness.
- Instruct client to call the physician when an enlarged lump or mass is noted in the neck.
- Teach client risk factors for HIV infection.

Evaluation

- Have client explain when to notify a physician about a neck mass.

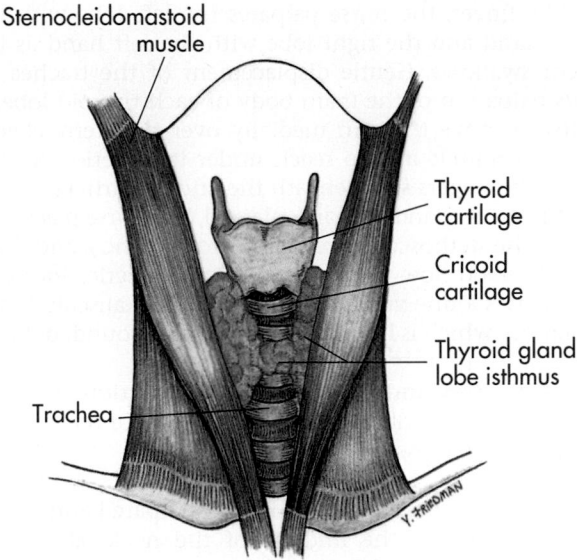

FIGURE 32–33 Anatomical position of the thyroid gland.

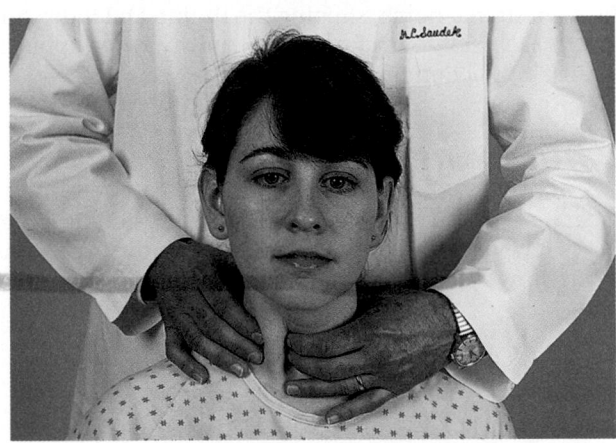

FIGURE 32–34 Palpation of the right thyroid lobe from behind the client. (From Seidel HM and others: *Mosby's guide to physical examination,* ed 5, St. Louis, 2003, Mosby.)

locate the site of an infection. For example, ear infections usually drain to the preauricular or deep cervical nodes. Malignancy is usually associated with nontender, hard, discrete nodes. After a serious infection a node may remain permanently enlarged but may not be tender.

Thyroid Gland. The thyroid gland lies in the anterior lower neck, in front of and to both sides of the trachea. The gland is fixed to the trachea with the isthmus overlying the trachea and connecting the two irregular, cone-shaped lobes (Figure 32-33). The nurse assesses the gland by inspection, palpation, and auscultation.

The nurse stands in front of the client and inspects the area of the lower neck overlying the thyroid gland for visible masses, symmetry, and any subtle fullness at the base of the neck. Asking the client to hyperextend the neck helps tighten the skin for better visualization. The nurse offers the client a glass of water and then has the client swallow while the nurse notes whether there is a bulging of the gland. Normally the thyroid cannot be visualized.

To palpate the gland, the examiner stands in front of or behind the client. Light, gentle palpation is needed to feel any abnormalities. Seidel and others (2003) recommend allowing the fingers to drift over the gland. For both the anterior and posterior approach, the client flexes the neck forward and laterally toward the side being examined to relax the neck muscles. The client holds a cup of water and takes a sip to swallow once instructed by the nurse.

For the posterior approach, the nurse has the client sit with the neck at a comfortable level. Both of the nurse's hands are placed around the neck, with two fingers of each hand on the sides of the trachea just beneath the cricoid cartilage. As the client swallows the nurse feels for movement of the thyroid isthmus. The thyroid should move beneath the fingers when the client swallows. Enlargement of the isthmus as it rises should be noted. To

examine each lobe, the nurse has the client swallow while the nurse displaces the trachea to the right or left. The nurse then palpates the main body of each lobe (Figure 32-34). During examination of the right lobe, for example, the nurse moves the fingers of the left hand between the trachea and the right sternocleidomastoid muscle. Then the nurse places the fingers of the right hand behind the right sternocleidomastoid muscle and gently presses the hands together to palpate the lobe as the client swallows. The approach is repeated for the left lobe with the hands in the reverse positions. Normally the thyroid gland is small, smooth, and free of nodules. However, in extremely thin individuals the thyroid is more easily palpable. Enlargement is a manifestation of thyroid dysfunction. Masses or nodules may be signs of malignant disease. However, not all nodules are malignant.

The anterior approach requires the client to sit as the nurse stands to the side. Using the pads of the index and middle finger, the nurse palpates the left lobe with the right hand and the right lobe with the left hand as the client swallows. Gentle displacement of the trachea allows palpation of the main body of each thyroid lobe. It helps to move the skin medially over the sternocleidomastoid muscle and to reach under its anterior borders while the fingers stay beneath the cricoid cartilage.

When the gland appears enlarged, the nurse places the bell of the stethoscope over the thyroid. If the gland is enlarged, blood flow through the thyroid arteries increases and causes a fine vibration. The nurse can auscultate the vibration, which is heard as a soft, rushing sound, or bruit.

Carotid Artery and Jugular Vein. This portion of the examination is described under examination of the vascular system (see later section).

Trachea. The trachea can be directly palpated and is normally located in the midline of the neck, above the suprasternal notch. Masses in the neck or mediastinum and pulmonary abnormalities can cause displacement laterally. The client may sit or lie down during palpation. The position of the trachea is determined by palpating at the suprasternal notch, slipping the thumb and index fingers to each side. Forceful pressure must not be applied, because this action may elicit a cough.

Thorax and Lungs

Accurate physical assessment of the thorax and lungs requires review of the ventilatory and respiratory functions of the lungs. If the lungs are affected by disease, other body systems will reflect alterations. For example, reduced oxygenation can cause changes in mental alertness because of the brain's sensitivity to lowered oxygen levels. The alert nurse uses the data from all body systems to determine the nature of pulmonary alterations.

Before assessing the thorax and lungs, the nurse must be familiar with the landmarks of the chest (Figure 32-35). These landmarks help the nurse locate findings and use assessment skills correctly. For example, by knowing the position of underlying organs in relation to the landmarks, the nurse can anticipate where to percuss or auscultate the chest wall. The client's nipples, angle of Louis, suprasternal notch, costal angle, clavicles, and vertebrae are key landmarks that provide a series of imaginary lines for sign identification. The lungs and thorax are assessed posteriorly, laterally (on both sides), and anteriorly, with the nurse using landmarks to record localized findings.

During the examination the nurse keeps a mental image of the location of the lobes of the lung and the position of each rib (Figure 32-36). Locating the position of each rib is critical to visualizing the lobe of the lung being assessed. To begin, the nurse locates the angle of Louis at the manubriosternal junction. The angle is a visible and palpable angulation of the sternum and is the point at which the second rib articulates with the sternum. The nurse counts the ribs and intercostal spaces (between the ribs) from this point. The number of each intercostal space corresponds with that of the rib just above it. The spinous process of the third thoracic vertebra and the fourth, fifth, and sixth ribs help to locate the lung's lobes laterally. The lower lobes project laterally and anteriorly (Figure 32-37). Posteriorly the tip or inferior margin of the scapula lies approximately at the level of the sev-

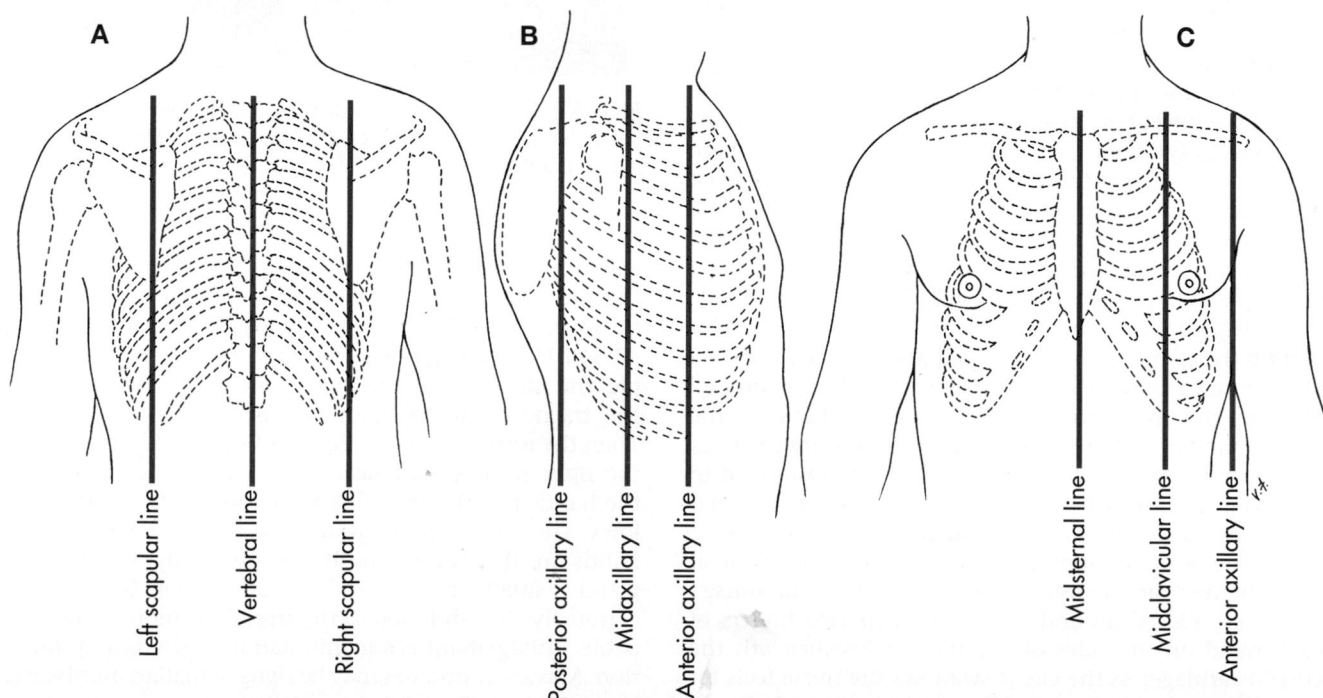

FIGURE 32–35 Anatomical chest wall landmarks. **A,** Posterior chest landmarks. **B,** Lateral chest landmarks. **C,** Anterior chest landmarks.

enth rib (Figure 32-38). After identifying the seventh rib, the examiner can count upward to locate the third thoracic vertebra and align it with the inner borders of the scapula to locate the posterior lobes.

Examination of the lungs and thorax requires the client to be undressed to the waist. Good lighting is essential. The nurse should assess clients at risk for pulmonary problems, such as the client confined to bed rest or the client with chest pain who cannot fully expand the lungs. The examination begins with the client sitting for assessment of the posterior and lateral chest. For assessment of the anterior chest, the client sits or lies. Table 32-20 reviews the nursing history for lung examination.

Posterior Thorax

The nurse first inspects the shape and symmetry of the client's chest from the back and front. The anteroposterior diameter is noted. The shape of the chest or the client's posture can significantly impair ventilatory movement. Normally the chest contour is symmetrical, with the anteroposterior diameter one third to one half of the transverse, or side-to-side, diameter. Aging and chronic lung disease are characterized by a barrel-shaped chest (anteroposterior diameter equals transverse diameter). Infants have an almost round shape. Abnormal contours are caused by congenital and postural alterations. A client may assume a posture such as leaning over a table or splinting the side of the chest as a result of a breathing problem. Splinting or holding the chest wall as a result of localized pain causes a client to bend toward the side affected. Such a posture impairs ventilatory movement.

Standing at a midline position behind the client, the nurse looks for deformities, the position of the spine, the slope of the ribs, retraction of the intercostal spaces during inspiration, and bulging of the intercostal spaces during expiration. The scapulae are normally symmetrical and closely attached to the thoracic wall. The normal spine is straight without lateral deviation. Posteriorly, the

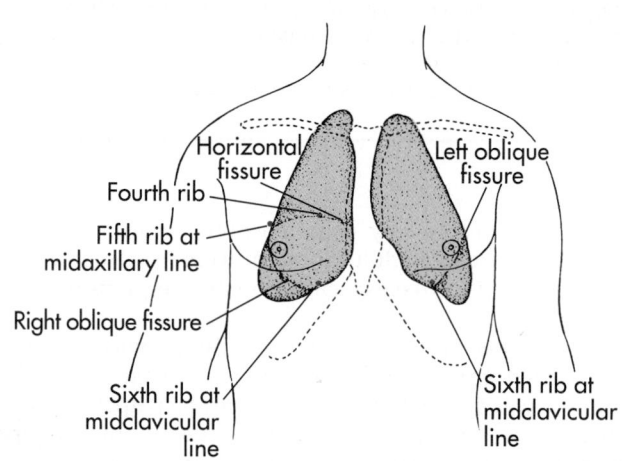

FIGURE 32–36 Anterior position of lung lobes in relation to anatomical landmarks.

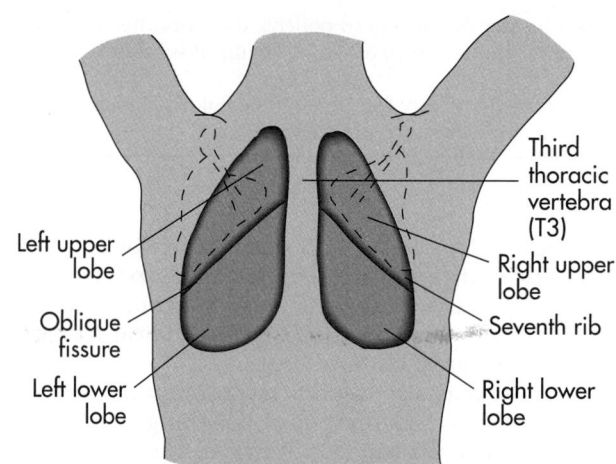

FIGURE 32–38 Posterior position of lung lobes in relation to anatomical landmarks.

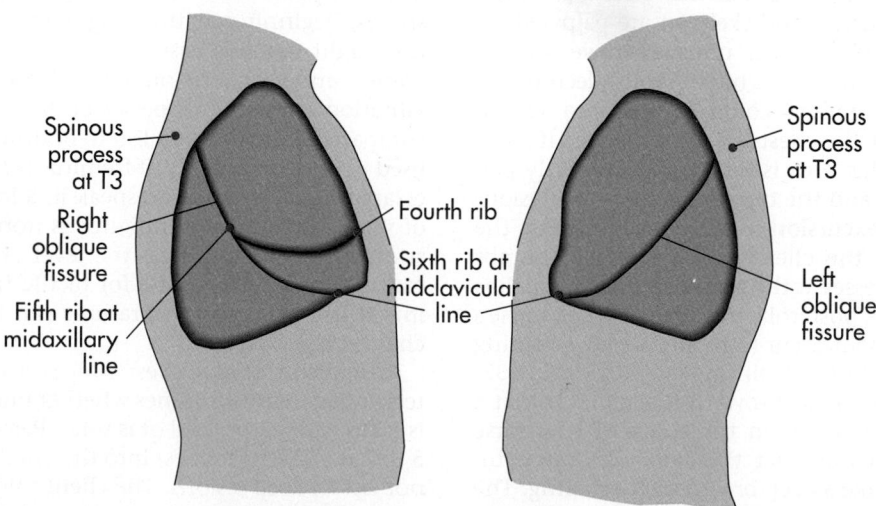

FIGURE 32–37 Lateral position of lung lobes in relation to anatomical landmarks.

Table 32-20	Nursing History for Lung Assessment	
Assessment Category	**Rationale**
Assess history of tobacco or marijuana use, including type of tobacco, duration and amount (pack-years = number of years smoking × number of packs per day), age started, and efforts to quit.	Smoking is a risk factor for lung cancer, heart disease, and emphysema or bronchitis. Cigarette smoking accounts for a significant percentage of all cancer deaths.
Ask if client has had a *persistent cough* (productive or nonproductive), *sputum production, chest pain,* shortness of breath, orthopnea, dyspnea during exertion or at rest, poor activity tolerance, or *recurrent attacks of pneumonia or bronchitis.*	Symptoms of respiratory alterations may help nurse localize objective physical findings. (Warning signals for lung cancer are in italic type.)
Determine if client works in environment containing pollutants (e.g., asbestos, arsenic, coal dust) or requiring exposure to radiation. Does client have exposure to sidestream cigarette smoke?	These risk factors increase chance for various lung diseases.
Review history for known or suspected HIV infection, substance abuse, low income, residence in nursing home, or recent immigration to United States.	These are risk factors for tuberculosis.
Ask if client has history of persistent cough, hemoptysis, unexplained weight loss, fatigue, night sweats, or fever.	These are risk factors for both tuberculosis and HIV infection.
Does client have history of chronic hoarseness?	Hoarseness may indicate laryngeal disorder or abuse of cocaine or opioids (sniffing).
Assess history of allergies to pollens, dust, or other airborne irritants and to foods, drugs, or chemical substances.	Symptoms such as choking feeling, bronchospasm with respiratory stridor, wheezes on auscultation, and dyspnea may be caused by allergic response.
Review family history for cancer, tuberculosis, allergies, or chronic obstructive pulmonary disease.	Conditions place client at risk for lung disease.

ribs tend to slope across and down. The ribs and intercostal spaces are easier to see in a thin person. Normally no bulging or active movement occurs within the intercostal spaces during breathing. Bulging indicates that the client is using great effort to breathe.

The nurse may also inspect the posterior thorax to determine the rate and rhythm of breathing (see Chapter 31). The thorax as a whole is observed. The entire thorax normally expands and relaxes regularly with equality of movement. In healthy adults the normal respiratory rates vary from 12 to 20 respirations per minute.

Palpation of the posterior thorax assesses further characteristics and confirms or supplements assessment findings. The thoracic muscles and skeleton are palpated for lumps, masses, pulsations, and unusual movement. If pain or tenderness is noted, the nurse avoids deep palpation. Fractured rib fragments could be displaced against vital organs. Normally the chest wall is not tender. If a suspicious mass or swollen area is detected, it is lightly palpated for size, shape, and the typical qualities of a lesion.

To measure chest excursion or depth of breathing, the nurse stands behind the client and places the thumbs along the spinal processes at the tenth rib, with the palms lightly contacting the posterolateral surfaces. The nurse's thumbs should be about 5 cm (2 inches) apart, pointing toward the spine and fingers pointing laterally (Figure 32-39, *A*). The hands are pressed toward the spine so that a small skinfold appears between the thumbs. The nurse does not slide the hands over the skin. The nurse instructs the client to take a deep breath after exhaling. The nurse notes movement of the thumbs (Figure 32-39, *B*). Chest excursion should be symmetrical, separating the thumbs 3 to 5 cm (1¼ to 2 inches). Reduced chest excursion may be caused by pain, postural deformity, or fatigue. In the older adult, chest movement declines because of costal cartilage calcification and respiratory muscle atrophy.

During speech the sound created by the vocal cords is transmitted through the lung to the chest wall. The sound waves create vibrations that can be palpated externally. These vibrations are called **vocal** or **tactile fremitus.** The accumulation of mucus, the collapse of lung tissue, or the presence of lung lesions can block the vibrations from reaching the chest wall.

To palpate for tactile fremitus, the nurse places the ball or lower palm of the hand over symmetrical intercostal spaces, beginning at the lung apex (Figure 32-40, *A*). A firm, light touch is best. The nurse asks the client to say "ninety-nine" or "one-one-one." Normally there is a faint vibration as the client speaks. Both sides of the thorax are compared, moving from top to bottom. Only one hand is used to ensure accuracy. If fremitus is faint, it may be necessary to ask the client to speak in a louder or lower tone of voice. Symmetry of fremitus is normal. Vibrations are strongest at the top, near the level of the tracheal bifurcation. It is easy to assess for tactile fremitus in a crying infant because strong vibrations can be felt through the chest wall.

Percussion of the chest wall is a difficult assessment technique that determines whether underlying lung tissue is filled with air or fluid or is solid. Percussion reaches only 5 to 7 cm (2 to 3 inches) into the chest wall and thus cannot detect deep lesions. The client folds the arms forward across the chest with the head bent forward. This position separates the scapulae further to expose more lung to assessment. Using the indirect technique, the nurse

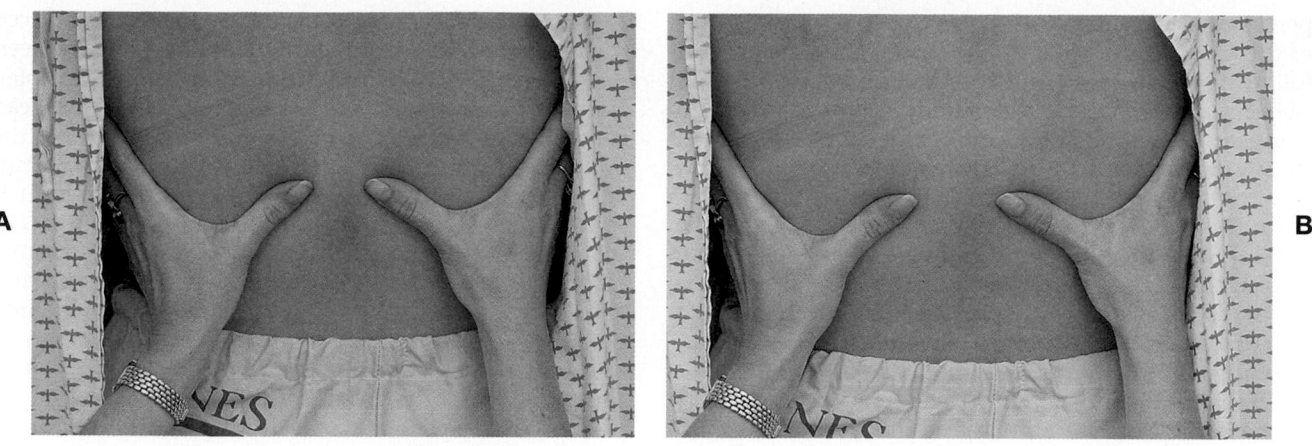

FIGURE **32–39** **A,** Position of nurse's hands for palpation of posterior thorax excursion. **B,** As the client inhales, the movement of chest excursion separates the nurse's thumbs.

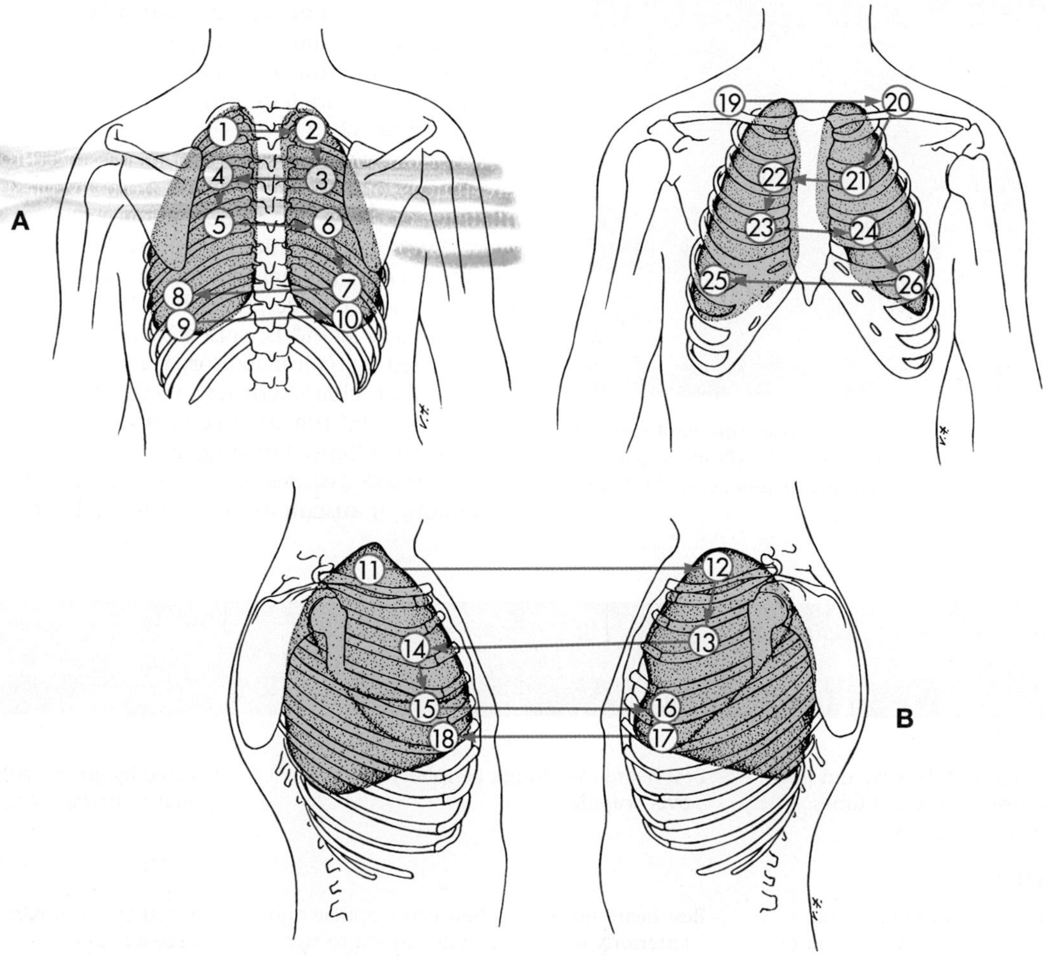

FIGURE **32–40** **A** to **C,** The nurse follows a systematic pattern (posterior-lateral-anterior) when comparing fremitus, percussion notes, and auscultation.

percusses in the intercostal spaces over symmetrical areas of the lungs moving side to side. Figure 32-40 shows how following a systematic pattern, starting posteriorly and then moving laterally and anteriorly, allows the nurse to compare percussion notes for all lung lobes. Resonance, the sound created by air-filled lungs, is normally heard over the posterior thorax. Percussion over the scapula, ribs, or spine is dull. The chest is normally more resonant in the child than in the adult. A lung mass causes a flat sound. Conditions such as emphysema, asthma, or pneumothorax produce a hyperresonant sound because of hyperinflation of lung tissue. A dull or flat sound may suggest atelectasis, pleural effusion, pneumothorax, or asthma.

Auscultation assesses the movement of air through the tracheobronchial tree and detects mucus or obstructed airways. Normally air flows through the airways in an unobstructed pattern. Recognizing the sounds created by normal airflow allows the nurse to detect sounds caused by obstruction.

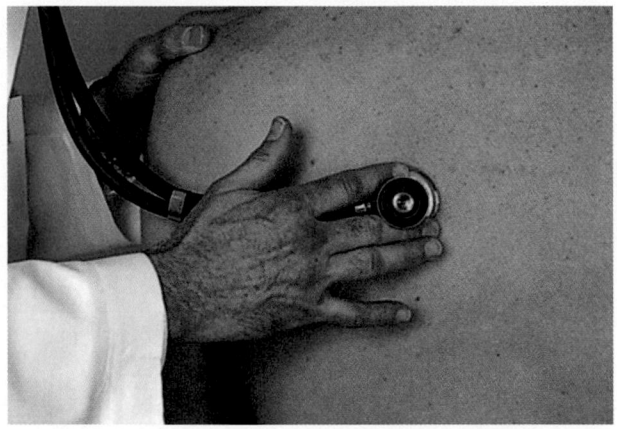

FIGURE **32–41** In an adult the nurse uses the diaphragm of the stethoscope to auscultate breath sounds. (From Seidel HM and others: *Mosby's guide to physical examination,* ed 5, St. Louis, 2003, Mosby.)

In an adult the diaphragm of the stethoscope is placed firmly on the skin, over the posterior chest wall between the ribs (Figure 32-41). The client sits upright (if possible), folds the arms in front of the chest, and keeps the head bent forward while taking slow, deep breaths with the mouth slightly open. It helps to demonstrate for the client. The nurse listens to an entire inspiration and expiration at each position of the stethoscope. If sounds are faint, as in the obese client, the client should be asked to breathe harder and faster. Breath sounds are much louder in children because of the thinness of the chest wall. In children the bell works best because of a child's small chest.

A systematic pattern throughout should be used when comparing the right and left sides (see Figure 32-40, *A*, p. 719). An inexperienced student may attempt to auscultate all of the left side and then return to the right side. This is incorrect. The examiner compares lung sounds in one region on one side of the body with sounds in the same region on the opposite side. It is impossible to remember the quality of all sounds noted on one side of the body and then compare them with sounds on the other side.

The nurse auscultates for normal breath sounds and abnormal or **adventitious sounds.** Normal breath sounds differ in character, depending on the area of the lungs being auscultated. Sounds normally heard over the posterior thorax include bronchovesicular and vesicular sounds (Table 32-21).

Abnormal sounds result from air passing through moisture, mucus, or narrowed airways; from alveoli suddenly reinflating; or from an inflammation between the lung's pleural linings. Adventitious or added sounds often occur superimposed over normal sounds. The four types of adventitious sounds are crackles, rhonchi, wheezes, and pleural friction rub. Each sound is caused by a specific entity and is characterized by typical auditory features (Table 32-22). The location and characteristics of the sounds should be noted, as should the absence of breath sounds (found in clients with collapsed or surgically removed lobes).

If the nurse assesses abnormalities in tactile fremitus, percussion, or auscultation, another test is performed for

Table 32-21	Normal Breath Sounds		
Description	**Location**		**Origin**
Vesicular			
Vesicular sounds are soft, breezy, and low pitched. Inspiratory phase is 3 times longer than expiratory phase.	Best heard over lung's periphery (except over scapula)		Created by air moving through smaller airways
Bronchovesicular			
Bronchovesicular sounds are blowing sounds that are medium pitched and of medium intensity. Inspiratory phase is equal to expiratory phase.	Best heard posteriorly between scapulae and anteriorly over bronchioles lateral to sternum at first and second intercostal spaces		Created by air moving through large airways
Bronchial			
Bronchial sounds are loud and high pitched with hollow quality. Expiration lasts longer than inspiration (3:2 ratio).	Best heard over trachea		Created by air moving through trachea close to chest wall

spoken and whispered voice sounds. With the stethoscope placed over the same locations used to assess breath sounds, the client says "ninety-nine" in a normal voice tone. Normally the sounds are muffled. If fluid is compressing the lung, vibrations from the client's voice are transmitted to the chest wall and the sounds become clear **(bronchophony).** The nurse then asks the client to whisper "ninety-nine." The whispered voice is usually faint and indistinct. Certain lung abnormalities may cause the whispered voice to become clear and distinct **(whispered pectoriloquy).**

Lateral Thorax

The client sits during examination of the lateral chest. Usually the nurse extends the assessment of the posterior thorax to the lateral sides of the chest. The client is asked to raise the arms, which improves access to lateral thoracic structures. The nurse uses all four assessment skills to methodically examine the lateral thorax (see Figure 32-40, *B*, p. 719). Excursion cannot be assessed laterally. Normally, percussion notes are resonant, and breath sounds are vesicular.

Anterior Thorax

The anterior thorax is inspected for the same features as the posterior thorax. The client sits or lies down with the head elevated. The nurse observes the accessory muscles of breathing: sternocleidomastoid, trapezius, and abdominal muscles. The accessory muscles move little with normal passive breathing. When a client requires effort to breathe

Table 32-22	**Adventitious Breath Sounds**		
Sound	**Site Auscultated**	**Cause**	**Character**
Crackles	Are most commonly heard in dependent lobes: right and left lung bases	Random, sudden reinflation of groups of alveoli; disruptive passage of air	Fine crackles are high-pitched fine, short, interrupted crackling sounds heard during end of inspiration, usually not cleared with coughing. Medium crackles are lower, more moist sounds heard during middle of inspiration; not cleared with coughing. Coarse crackles are loud, bubbly sounds heard during inspiration; not cleared with coughing.
Rhonchi (sonorous wheeze)	Are primarily heard over trachea and bronchi; if loud enough, can be heard over most lung fields	Muscular spasm, fluid, or mucus in larger airways, causing turbulence	Are loud, low-pitched, rumbling coarse sounds heard most often during inspiration or expiration; may be cleared by coughing.
Wheezes (sibilant wheeze)	Can be heard over all lung fields	High-velocity airflow through severely narrowed bronchus	Are high-pitched, continuous musical sounds like a squeak heard continuously during inspiration or expiration; usually louder on expiration.
Pleural friction rub	Is heard over anterior lateral lung field (if client is sitting upright)	Inflamed pleura, parietal pleura rubbing against visceral pleura	Has dry, grating quality heard best during inspiration; does not clear with coughing; heard loudest over lower lateral anterior surface.

Data from Siedel HM and others: *Mosby's guide to physical examination,* ed 5, St. Louis, 2003, Mosby.

Lung Assessment

Objectives

- Client will describe warning signs of lung disease.
- Older adult will receive influenza and pneumonia vaccines annually.
- Client with chronic obstructive pulmonary disease (COPD) will clear airways more effectively and report less shortness of breath.

Teaching Strategies

- Explain risk factors for chronic lung disease and lung cancer, including cigarette smoking, history of smoking for over 20 years, exposure to environmental pollution, and radiation exposure from occupational, medical, and environmental sources. Residential radon exposure may also increase risk especially in cigarette smokers. Exposure to sidestream cigarette smoke increases risk for nonsmokers (ACS, 2003).
- Share brochures on lung cancer from American Cancer Society (ACS) with client and family.
- Discuss warning signs of lung cancer, such as a persistent cough, sputum streaked with blood, chest pains, and recurrent attacks of pneumonia or bronchitis.
- Counsel older adult on benefits from receiving annual influenza and pneumonia vaccinations because of a greater susceptibility to respiratory infection.
- Instruct client with COPD in coughing and pursed-lip breathing exercises.
- Persons at risk for tuberculosis who visit clinics or health care centers should be referred for skin testing.

Evaluation

- Have client describe risk factors for lung disease and cancer.
- Ask client to identify any known risks for cancer.
- Ask client to name warning signs for cancer.
- In a follow-up visit, review client's immunization record.
- Observe client performing breathing exercises and coughing.

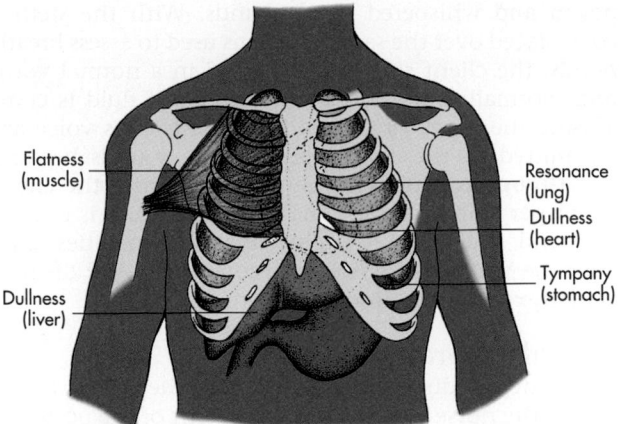

FIGURE 32–42　Variations in percussion notes in the normal thorax and upper abdomen.

angled along each costal margin. The thumbs are pushed toward the midline to create a fold of skin between the thumbs. As the client inhales deeply, the thumbs should normally separate approximately 2.5 to 5 cm (1 to 2 inches), with each side expanding equally.

Tactile fremitus is assessed over the chest wall. Anterior findings differ from posterior findings because of the heart and female breast tissue. Fremitus is best felt next to the sternum at the second intercostal space, at the level of the bronchial bifurcation. It is decreased over the heart, lower thorax, and breast tissue. The nurse will not be able to sense vibrations over breast tissue and thus must retract the breasts gently during palpation. If the breasts are large, this portion of the examination may be omitted.

Percussion of the anterior thorax follows a systematic pattern. The nurse must imagine the location of all internal organs anteriorly accessible to examination. The underlying liver, heart, and stomach create percussion notes characteristically different from those of the lung (Figure 32-42). Percussion may be conducted with the client in a sitting or lying position. However, the procedure is easier if the client lies down. The nurse starts above the clavicles and moves across and then down. The female breasts are displaced as needed. The normal lung is resonant. As the examiner proceeds downward, the areas of heart and liver dullness and the tympanic gastric air bubble will be detectable.

Auscultation of the anterior thorax follows the same pattern as percussion (see Figure 32-40, *C*, p. 719). The client should sit, if possible, to maximize chest expansion. Special attention should be paid to the lower lobes, where mucus commonly gathers. Bronchovesicular and vesicular sounds are heard above and below the clavicles and along the lung periphery. An additional normal breath sound, the bronchial sound, can be heard over the trachea. It is loud, high pitched, and hollow sounding, with expiration lasting longer than inspiration (3:2 ratio).

Heart

The assessment of heart function involves a review of signs and symptoms from the nursing history, pulse assessment,

as a result of strenuous exercise or disease (e.g., chronic obstructive pulmonary disease), the accessory muscles and abdominal muscles contract (Box 32-19). Some clients produce a grunting sound.

The nurse observes the width of the costal angle. It is usually larger than 90 degrees between the two costal margins. The nurse observes the breathing pattern. Normal breathing is quiet and barely audible near the open mouth. Respiratory rate and rhythm are more often assessed anteriorly (see Chapter 31). A man's respirations are usually diaphragmatic, whereas a woman's are more costal. Accurate assessment occurs as a client breathes passively.

The examiner palpates the anterior thoracic muscles and skeleton for lumps, masses, tenderness, or unusual movement. The sternum and xiphoid are relatively inflexible. To measure chest excursion anteriorly, the nurse uses a technique similar to that for assessing the posterior thorax.

The nurse places the hands over each lateral rib cage, with the thumbs approximately 2.5 cm (1 inch) apart and

Table 32-23	Nursing History for Heart Assessment
Assessment Category	**Rationale**
Determine history of smoking, alcohol intake, use of drugs, exercise habits, and dietary patterns and intake (including fat and sodium intake).	Smoking, alcohol ingestion, cocaine use, lack of regular exercise, and intake of foods high in carbohydrates, fats, and cholesterol are risk factors for cardiovascular disease.
Determine if client is taking medications for cardiovascular function (e.g., antidysrhythmics, antihypertensives) and if client knows their purpose, dosage, and side effects.	Knowledge allows nurse to assess compliance with drug therapies. Medications may affect vital sign values.
Assess for chest pain, palpitations, excess fatigue, cough, dyspnea, leg pain or cramps, edema of feet, cyanosis, fainting, and orthopnea. Ask if symptoms occur at rest or during exercise.	These are key symptoms of heart disease. Cardiovascular function may be adequate during rest but not during exercise.
If client reports chest pain, determine if it is cardiac in nature. Anginal pain is usually a deep pressure or ache that is substernal and diffuse, radiating to one or both arms, neck, or jaw.	Determines nature of pain and need to initiate care immediately.
Determine whether client has a stressful lifestyle. What physical demands or emotional stress exists?	Repeated exposure to stress may increase risk for heart disease.
Assess family history for heart disease, diabetes, high cholesterol levels, hypertension, stroke, or rheumatic heart disease.	Factors increase risk for heart disease.
Ask client about history of heart trouble (e.g., congestive heart failure, congenital heart disease, coronary artery disease, dysrhythmias, murmurs).	Knowledge reveals client's level of understanding of condition. Preexisting condition influences examination techniques used by nurse, as well as findings to expect.
Determine whether client has preexisting diabetes, lung disease, obesity, or hypertension.	These disorders may alter heart function.
Determine whether client drinks excessive amounts of coffee, tea, other caffeine-containing soft drinks, or chocolate.	Caffeine can cause heart dysrhythmias.

and direct examination of the heart. A client who has signs or symptoms of heart (cardiac) problems (e.g., chest pain and irregular heart rate) may be suffering a life-threatening condition requiring immediate attention. In this case the nurse acts quickly and decides on the portions of the examination that are absolutely necessary. When a client's condition is stable, a more thorough assessment can reveal baseline heart function and any risks for heart disease. Abnormal findings require a physician's attention. The nurse performing a cardiac assessment compares findings with those made in the vascular examination (see later section). The nursing history (Table 32-23) provides data that help the nurse interpret physical findings.

Assessment of cardiac function is performed through the anterior thorax. The nurse forms a mental image of the heart's exact location (Figure 32-43). In the adult it is in the center of the chest (precordium), behind and to the left of the sternum, with a small section of the right atrium extending to the sternum's right. The base of the heart is the upper portion, and the apex is the bottom tip. The surface of the right ventricle composes most of the heart's anterior surface. A section of the left ventricle shapes the left anterior side of the apex. The apex actually touches the anterior chest wall at approximately the fourth to fifth intercostal space just medial to the left midclavicular line. This location is known as the **apical impulse** or **point of maximal impulse (PMI).**

An infant's heart is positioned more horizontally and has a larger diameter compared with that of an adult. The apex of the heart in an infant is at the third or fourth intercostal space, just to the left of the midclavicular line. By the age of 7 a child's PMI is in the same location as the adult's.

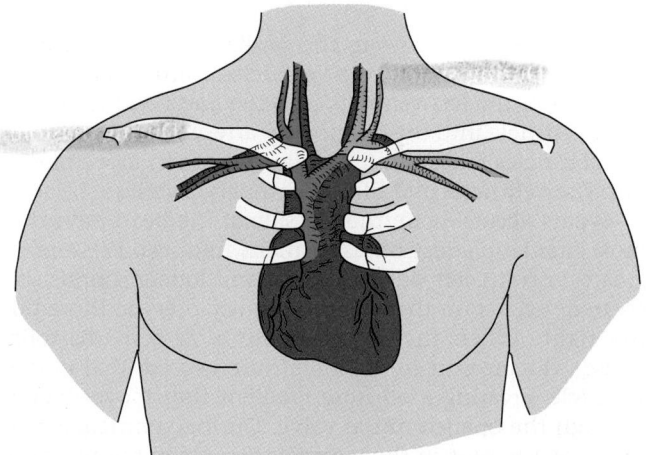

FIGURE **32-43** Anatomical position of the heart.

In tall, slender persons the heart hangs more vertically and is positioned more centrally. In persons who are stocky and short, the heart tends to lie more to the left and horizontally (Seidel and others, 2003).

To understand the significance of cardiac assessment findings, the nurse must first understand timing in relation to the cardiac cycle (Figure 32-44). The heart normally pumps blood through its four chambers in a methodical, even sequence. Events on the left side occur just before those on the right. As blood flows through each chamber, the valves open and close, the pressures within chambers rise and fall, and the chambers contract. Each event creates a physiological sign that can be detected by

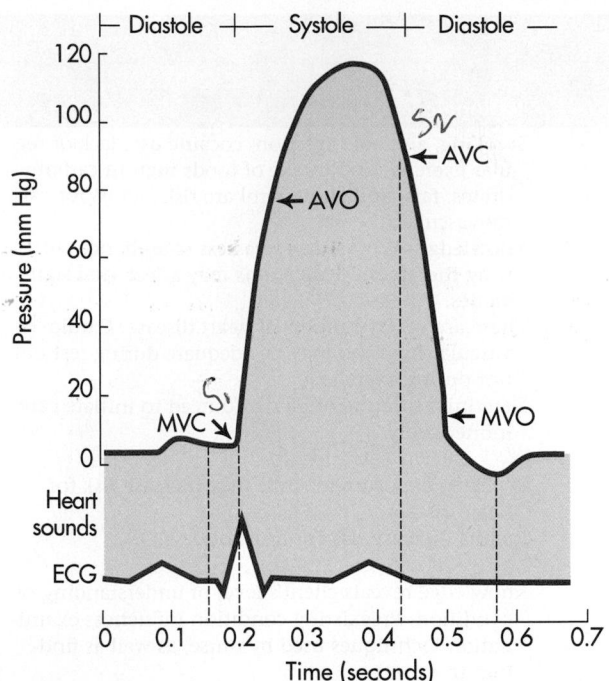

FIGURE 32–44 Cardiac cycle. *MVC,* Mitral valve closes; *AVO,* aortic valve opens; *AVC,* aortic valve closes; *MVO,* mitral valve opens.

an examiner. Both sides of the heart function in a coordinated fashion.

There are two phases to the cardiac cycle: systole and diastole. During systole the ventricles contract and eject blood from the left ventricle into the aorta and from the right ventricle into the pulmonary artery. During diastole the ventricles relax and the atria contract to move blood into the ventricles and fill the coronary arteries.

Events occurring on the left side of the heart have the most dramatic effect on assessment findings. Pressure is greatest on the left side, so longer and louder sounds are created. Events on the left side slightly precede those on the right. When the left ventricle is at rest (diastolic phase), the pressure in the left atrium exceeds that in the ventricle, creating a pressure gradient that moves blood through the opened mitral valve. During ventricular filling, pressure rises in the ventricle to exceed the pressure in the left atrium. Just before the ventricle contracts, the mitral valve closes to prevent regurgitation of blood into the atrium, creating the first heart sound (S_1), often described as "lub." Ventricular pressure builds, causing the aortic valve to open as the ventricle contracts (systolic phase). Blood flows into the aorta, elevating aortic pressure. When the ventricle empties, pressure within the chamber falls. To prevent regurgitation from the aorta into the left ventricle, the aortic valve closes, creating the second heart sound (S_2), described as "dub." As ventricular pressure continues to fall, it drops below that of the left atrium. The mitral valve reopens to again allow ventricular filling. The rapid filling of the ventricle may create a third heart sound (S_3), heard more often in children and young adults. An S_3 can also be heard as an abnormality in adults over 30 years of age. When the atria con-

tract to enhance ventricular filling, a fourth heart sound (S_4) is produced. The S_4 is not normally heard in adults but may be heard in healthy older adults, children, and athletes. Because it may also indicate an abnormal condition, it should be reported to a physician.

Inspection and Palpation

Before beginning the examination, the nurse ensures that the client is relaxed, comfortable, and explains the procedure to relieve the client's anxiety. An anxious or uncomfortable client can have mild tachycardia that may lead the nurse to misinterpret the findings. Findings from the examination of other body systems, such as signs of heart failure (rapid heart rate, tachypnea, and crackles in the lungs), influence judgments made during cardiovascular assessment. The nurse must be able not only to successfully examine the client, but also to integrate and interpret findings correctly.

The nurse uses inspection and palpation simultaneously. The examination begins with the client in the supine position or with the upper body elevated 45 degrees because clients with heart disease frequently suffer shortness of breath while lying flat. The nurse stands at the client's right side. The client must not talk, especially when the nurse auscultates heart sounds. Good lighting in the room is essential.

During inspection and palpation the nurse will methodically look for visible pulsations and exaggerated lifts and palpate for the apical impulse and any source of vibrations (thrills). It helps to follow an orderly sequence beginning with assessment of the base of the heart and moving toward the apex. First the nurse inspects the angle of Louis, which lies between the sternal body and manubrium and can be felt as a ridge in the sternum approximately 5 cm (2 inches) below the sternal notch. The nurse can slip the fingers along the angle on each side of the sternum to feel adjacent ribs. The intercostal spaces are just below each rib. The second intercostal space allows identification of the first two anatomical landmarks (Figure 32-45): the second right and left interspace. The third and fourth left interspaces can be found by progressing down along the left side of the sternum, palpating each intercostal space. This maneuver locates the second pulmonic and trucuspid areas. Deeper palpation is required to feel the spaces in obese clients or in those with well-developed chest muscles. To find the apical or mitral area, the nurse locates the fifth intercostal space just to the left of the sternum and moves the fingers laterally, just medial to the left midclavicular line. Some examiners are able to locate the apical area with the palm of the hand, but others use their fingertips. Normally at the apical impulse there is a light tap felt in an area 1 to 2 cm (½ inch) in diameter at the apex (Figure 32-46). Another landmark is the epigastric area at the tip of the sternum. It is typically used to palpate for aortic abnormalities.

As the nurse locates the six anatomical landmarks of the heart, each area is inspected and palpated. The nurse looks for the appearance of pulsations, viewing each area over the chest at an angle to the side. Normally no pulsations can be seen, except perhaps at the PMI in thin clients or at the epigastric area as a result of abdominal aorta pulsation.

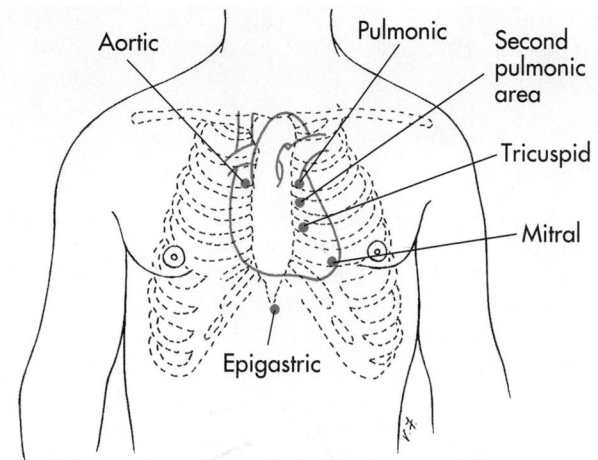

FIGURE 32–45 Anatomical sites for assessment of cardiac function.

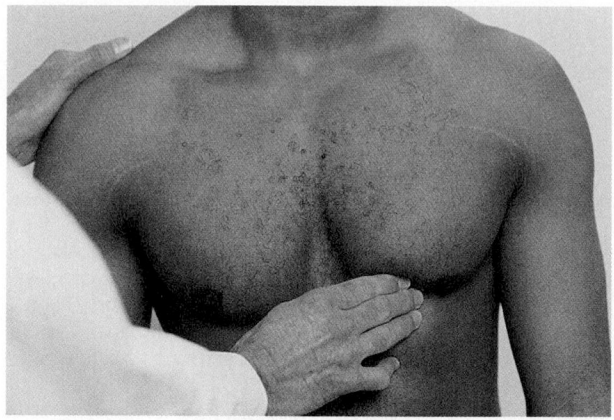

FIGURE 32–46 Palpation of apical pulse. (From Seidel HM and others: *Mosby's guide to physical examination,* ed 5, St. Louis, 2003, Mosby.)

Palpation for pulsations is best done using the proximal halves of the four fingers together and then alternating with the ball of the hand. The nurse touches the areas gently to allow movements to lift the hand. Normally no pulsations or vibrations can be felt in the second, third, or fourth intercostal spaces. A vibration is caused by loud murmurs. If pulsations or vibrations are palpated, the nurse times their occurrence in relation to systole or diastole by auscultating heart sounds simultaneously.

If the PMI cannot be found with the client in the supine position, the nurse asks the client to roll onto the left side, which moves the heart closer to the chest wall. The nurse estimates the heart's size by noting the diameter of the PMI and its position relative to the midclavicular line. In cases of serious heart disease, the cardiac muscle enlarges, with the PMI found to the left of the midclavicular line. The PMI may be difficult to find in the older adult because the chest deepens in its anteroposterior diameters. It may also be difficult to locate in a client who is very muscular or overweight. The PMI of an infant can usually be found near the third or fourth intercostal space. It is easy to palpate the child's PMI because of the thin chest wall.

Auscultation

Auscultation of the heart detects normal heart sounds, extra heart sounds, and murmurs. The nurse should first become skilled in detecting normal heart sounds. These low-intensity sounds created by the closing of the valves are often difficult to hear, especially if breath sounds are noisy. Concentration is needed when detecting heart sounds. To begin auscultation, the nurse eliminates all sources of room noise. The nurse follows a pattern during auscultation, starting at the second right interspace, moving systematically and inching the stethoscope across each of the anatomical sites (see Figure 32-45). It is important to hear heart sounds clearly at each location. Then the sequence is repeated using the bell of the stethoscope. The client may be asked to assume three different positions during the examination (Figure 32-47): sitting up and leaning forward (good position to hear all areas and to hear high-pitched murmurs), supine (good for all areas), and left lateral recumbent (good for all areas and best position to hear low-pitched sounds in diastole).

The nurse usually must lift the female client's left breast to listen better to the chest wall. The nurse learns to identify the first (S_1) and second (S_2) heart sounds. At normal rates, S_1 occurs after the long diastolic pause and preceding the short systolic pause. S_1 is high pitched, dull in quality, and heard best at the apex. If the nurse has difficulty hearing S_1, it can be timed in relation to the carotid pulse. It occurs just before the carotid pulsation. S_2 follows the short systolic pause and precedes the long diastolic pause. It is heard best at the aortic area.

The nurse auscultates for rate and rhythm after both sounds can be heard clearly. Each combination of S_1 and S_2 or "lub-dub" counts as one heartbeat. The nurse counts the rate for 1 minute, listening for the interval between S_1 and S_2, and then the time between S_2 and the next S_1. A regular rhythm involves regular intervals of time between each sequence of beats. There is a distinct silent pause between S_1 and S_2. Failure of the heart to beat at regular successive intervals is a **dysrhythmia.** Some dysrhythmias can be life threatening.

When the heart rhythm is irregular, the nurse compares apical and radial pulse rates simultaneously to determine if a pulse deficit exists. The apical pulse is auscultated first, and then the radial pulse is immediately palpated (one-examiner technique). When two examiners are available, the apical and radial rates are assessed at the same time. When a client has a **pulse deficit,** the radial pulse is slower than the apical pulse because ineffective contractions fail to send pulse waves to the periphery. A difference in pulse rates is reported to the physician immediately.

The nurse also learns to assess for extra heart sounds at each auscultatory site. Using the bell of the stethoscope, the nurse listens for low-pitched extra heart sounds such as S_3 and S_4 gallops, clicks, and rubs. The nurse auscultates over all anatomical areas. S_3, or a **ventricular gallop,** occurs just after S_2 at the end of ventricular diastole. It may be caused by a premature rush of blood into a ventricle that is stiff or dilated as a result of heart failure and hypertension. Some examiners describe the combination of S_1, S_2, and S_3 as sounding like "Ken-tuck'-y."

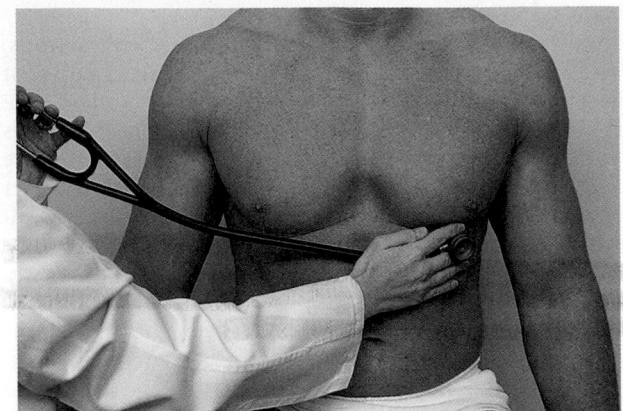

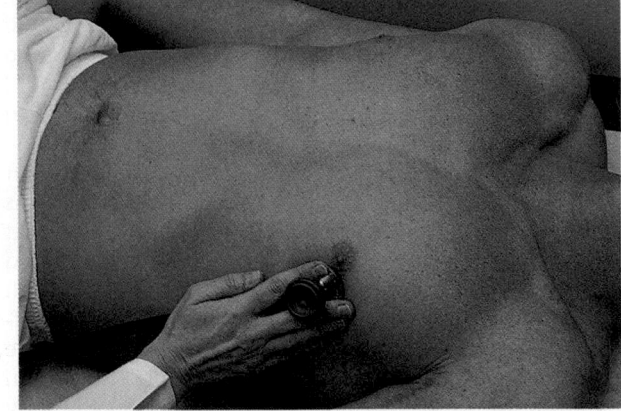

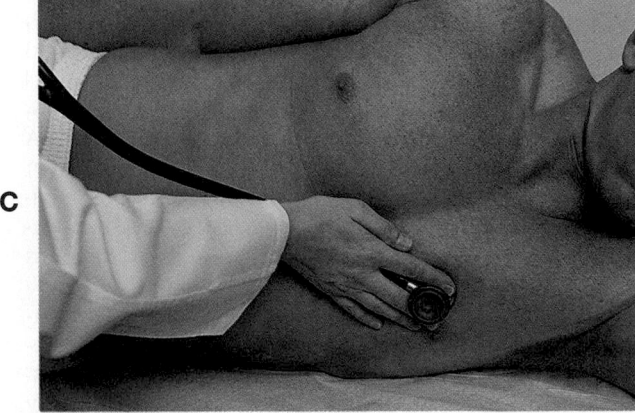

FIGURE **32–47**   Sequence of client positions for heart auscultation. **A,** Sitting, **B,** Supine, **C,** Left lateral recumbent. (From Seidel HM and others: *Mosby's guide to physical examination,* ed 5, St. Louis, 2003, Mosby.)

S₄, or an atrial gallop, occurs just before S_1 or ventricular systole. The sound of an S_4 is similar to that of "Ten'-es-see." Physiologically it may be due to an atrial contraction pushing against a ventricle that is not accepting blood because of heart failure or other alterations. One can often hear extra heart sounds more easily with the client lying on the left side and the stethoscope at the apical site.

The final portion of the examination includes assessment for heart murmurs. **Murmurs** are sustained swishing or blowing sounds heard at the beginning, middle, or end of the systolic or diastolic phase. They are caused by

increased blood flow through a normal valve, forward flow through a stenotic valve or into a dilated vessel or heart chamber, or backward flow through a valve that fails to close. A murmur can be asymptomatic or a sign of heart disease (Box 32-20). Murmurs are common in children. The nurse keeps the following factors in mind when auscultating to detect murmurs:

- When a murmur is detected, the nurse auscultates the mitral, tricuspid, aortic, and pulmonic valve areas for its place in the cardiac cycle (timing), the place it is heard best (location), radiation, loudness, pitch, and quality.
- If a murmur occurs between S_1 and S_2, it is a systolic murmur. If it occurs between S_2 and the next S_1, it is a diastolic murmur.

Table 32-24	Nursing History for Vascular Assessment
Assessment Category	**Rationale**
Determine if client experiences leg cramps, numbness or tingling in extremities, sensation of cold hands or feet, pain in legs, or swelling or cyanosis of feet, ankles, or hand.	These signs and symptoms indicate vascular disease.
If client experiences leg pain or cramping in lower extremities, ask if it is relieved or aggravated by walking or standing for long periods or during sleep.	Relationship of symptoms to exercise can clarify whether problem is vascular or musculoskeletal. Pain caused by vascular condition tends to increase with activity. Musculoskeletal pain is not usually relieved when exercise ends.
Ask women if they wear tight-fitting garters or hosiery and sit or lie in bed with legs crossed.	Tight hosiery around lower extremities and crossing legs can impair venous return.
Reconsider previous heart risk factors (e.g., smoking, exercise, nutritional problems).	These predispose client to vascular disease.
Assess medical history for heart disease, hypertension, phlebitis, diabetes, or varicose veins.	Circulatory and vascular disorders influence findings gathered during examination.

- The location of a murmur is not necessarily directly over the valves. With experience, a nurse can learn where each type of murmur is best heard. For example, mitral murmurs are heard best at the apex of the heart.
- To assess for radiation, the nurse listens for a murmur over areas besides where it is heard best. Murmurs can also sometimes be heard over the neck or back.
- Intensity or loudness is related to the rate of blood flow through the heart or the amount of blood regurgitated. In serious murmurs the nurse may feel a thrust or intermittent palpable sensation at the auscultation site. A **thrill** is a continuous palpable sensation like the purring of a cat. Intensity is recorded in the following grades:
  - *Grade 1* Barely audible
  - *Grade 2* Audible immediately but faint
  - *Grade 3* Loud, without thrust or thrill
  - *Grade 4* Loud, with thrust or thrill
  - *Grade 5* Very loud, with thrust or thrill; audible with stethoscope only partially applied
  - *Grade 6* Louder, may be heard without stethoscope
- A murmur may be low, medium, or high in pitch, depending on the velocity of blood flow through the valves. A low-pitched murmur is heard best with the bell of the stethoscope. If it is heard best with the diaphragm, a murmur is high pitched.

The quality of a murmur refers to its characteristic pattern and sound. A crescendo murmur starts softly and builds in loudness. A decrescendo murmur starts loudly and then becomes less intense.

Vascular System

Examination of the vascular system includes measurement of the blood pressure (see Chapter 31) and a thorough assessment of the integrity of the peripheral vascular system. Table 32-24 reviews the nursing history data collected before the examination. The nurse may perform portions of the vascular examination during assessment of other body systems. For example, the carotid pulse may be checked after palpation of cervical lymph nodes.

As the nurse inspects the skin, signs and symptoms of arterial and venous insufficiency are noted. An experienced nurse integrates vascular assessment with other portions of the examination if it is important to minimize time spent in the total examination.

Blood Pressure
When auscultating blood pressure, it is important to know that readings between the arms may vary by as much as 10 mm Hg and tend to be higher in the right arm (Seidel and others, 2003). The higher reading is always recorded. Systolic readings that differ by 15 mm Hg or more suggest atherosclerosis or disease of the aorta.

Carotid Arteries
When the left ventricle pumps blood into the aorta, pressure waves are transmitted through the arterial system. Pressure waves are manifested as pulses that are palpable in arteries close to the skin or that lie over bones. The carotid arteries reflect heart function better than peripheral arteries because they are positioned closest to the heart and thus their pressure correlates with that of the aorta.

The carotid arteries supply oxygenated blood to the head and neck (Figure 32-48) and are protected by the overlying sternocleidomastoid muscle. To examine the carotid arteries, the nurse has the client sit or lie supine with the head of the bed elevated 30 degrees. One carotid artery is examined at a time. If both arteries were occluded during palpation, the client could lose consciousness as a result of inadequate circulation to the brain. The carotids must not be vigorously palpated or massaged. The carotid sinus is located at the bifurcation of the common carotid arteries in the upper third of the neck. The sinus sends impulses along the vagus nerve. Its stimulation can cause a reflex drop in heart rate and blood pressure, which causes **syncope** or circulatory arrest. This can be a particular problem for older adults.

The neck is first inspected for obvious pulsation of the artery. The client turns the head slightly away from the artery being examined. Sometimes the wave of the pulse can be seen. The carotid is the only site for assessing the quality of a pulse wave. Only an experienced assessor can evaluate the quality of the wave in relation to

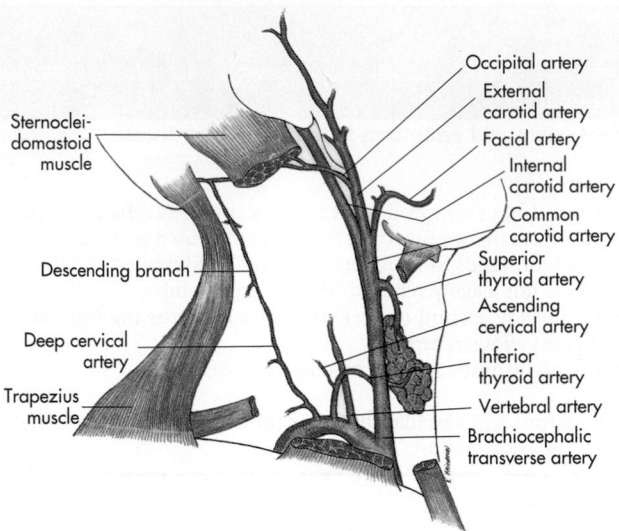

FIGURE **32–48**   Anatomical position of the carotid artery.

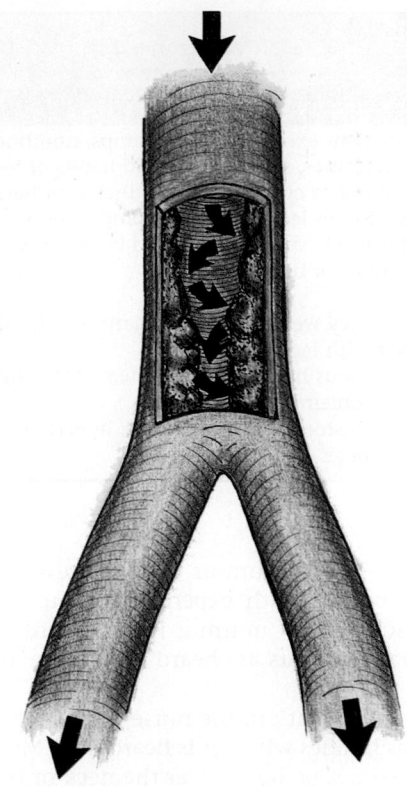

FIGURE **32–50**   Occlusion or narrowing of the carotid artery disrupts normal blood flow. The resultant turbulence creates a sound (bruit) that the nurse can auscultate.

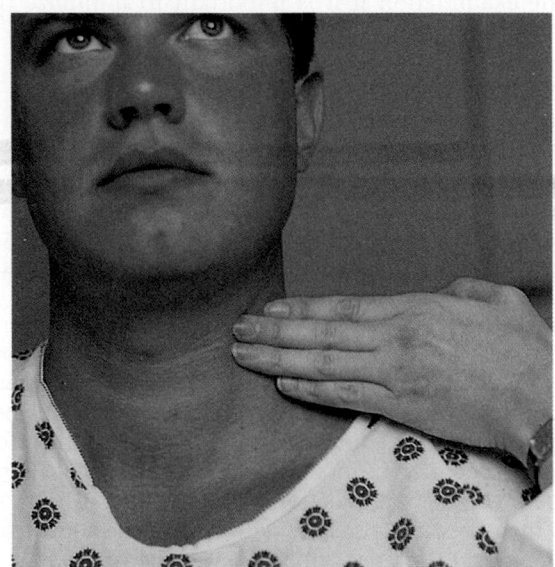

FIGURE **32–49**   Palpation of internal carotid artery along the margin of the sternocleidomastoid muscle.

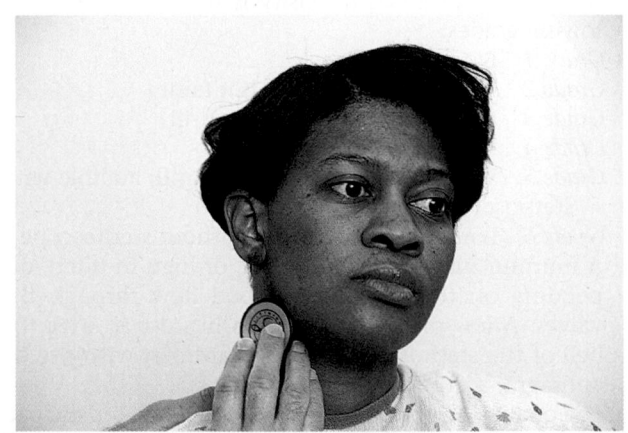

FIGURE **32–51**   Auscultation for carotid artery bruit. (From Seidel HM and others: *Mosby's guide to physical examination,* ed 5, St. Louis 2003, Mosby.)

systole and diastole of the cardiac cycle. An absent pulse wave can indicate arterial **occlusion** (blockage) or **stenosis** (narrowing).

For palpation of the pulse, the client turns the head slightly toward the side being examined. This maneuver relaxes the neck muscles for easier palpation. The nurse slides the tips of the index and middle fingers around the medial edge of the sternocleidomastoid muscle. Gentle palpation avoids occlusion of circulation (Figure 32-49).

The normal carotid pulse is localized rather than diffuse. A strong pulse, the carotid has a thrusting quality. As the client breathes, no change occurs during inspiration or expiration. Rotation of the neck or a shift from a sitting to a supine position does not change the carotid artery's quality. Both carotid arteries should be equal in

pulse rate, rhythm, and strength and should be equally elastic. Diminished or unequal carotid pulsations can indicate **atherosclerosis** or aortic arch disease.

The carotid is the most commonly auscultated pulse. (Others might include the jugular, temporal, femoral, renal, and abdominal arteries.) Auscultation is especially important for middle-age clients, older adults, or clients suspected of having cerebrovascular disease manifested by carotid artery obstruction. When the lumen of a blood ves-

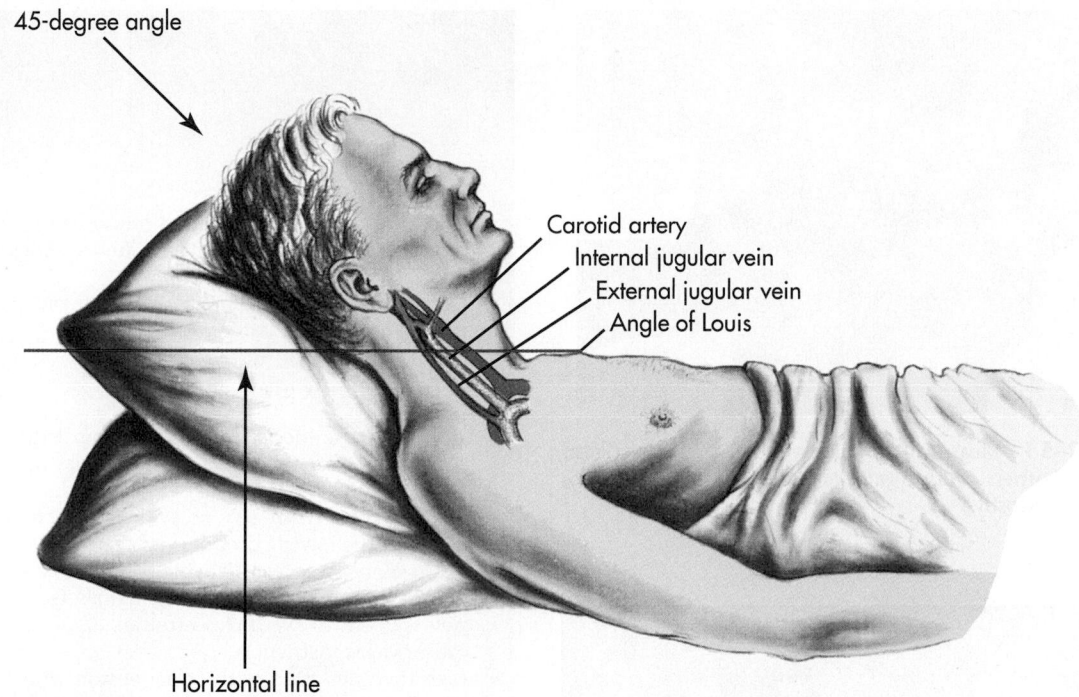

45-degree angle

Carotid artery
Internal jugular vein
External jugular vein
Angle of Louis

Horizontal line

FIGURE 32–52   Position of client to assess jugular vein distention. (From Thompson JM and others: *Mosby's manual of clinical nursing,* ed 4, St. Louis, 1997, Mosby.)

sel is narrowed, its blood flow is disturbed. As blood passes through the narrowed section, a turbulence is created, causing a blowing or swishing sound. The blowing sound is called a **bruit** (pronounced "brew-ee") (Figure 32-50).

The bell of the stethoscope is placed over the carotid artery at the lateral end of the clavicle and the posterior margin of the sternocleidomastoid muscle. The client turns the head slightly away from the side being examined (Figure 32-51). The nurse asks the client to hold the breath for a moment so that breath sounds do not obscure a bruit. Normally no sound is heard during carotid auscultation. If a bruit is heard, the nurse palpates the artery lightly for a thrill (palpable bruit).

Jugular Veins

The most accessible veins are the internal and external jugular veins in the neck. Both veins drain bilaterally from the head and neck into the superior vena cava. The external jugular vein lies superficially and can be seen just above the clavicle. The internal jugular vein lies deeper, along the carotid artery.

It is best to examine the right internal jugular vein because it follows a more direct anatomical path to the right atrium of the heart. The column of blood inside the internal jugular vein serves as a manometer, reflecting pressure in the right atrium. The higher the column, the greater the venous pressure. Raised venous pressure reflects right-sided heart failure.

Normally when a client lies in the supine position, the external jugular vein distends and becomes easily visible. In contrast, the jugular veins normally flatten when the client is in a sitting position. A client with heart disease, however, may have distended jugular veins when sitting.

The jugular veins are inspected to measure venous pressures, which are influenced by blood volume, the capacity of the right atrium to receive blood and send it to the right ventricle, and the ability of the right ventricle to contract and force blood into the pulmonary artery. Any factor resulting in greater blood volume within the venous system results in elevated venous pressure. The nurse assesses venous pressure by using the following steps:

1. Have the client lie supine with the head elevated 30 to 45 degrees (semi-Fowler's position).
2. Be sure the neck and upper thorax are exposed. Use a pillow to align the head. Avoid neck hyperextension or flexion to ensure that the vein is not stretched or kinked (Figure 32-52).
3. Usually pulsations are not evident with the client sitting up. As the client slowly leans back into a supine position, the level of venous pulsations begins to rise above the level of the manubrium as much as 1 or 2 cm as the client reaches a 45-degree angle. Measure venous pressure by measuring the vertical distance between the angle of Louis and the highest level of the visible point of the internal jugular vein pulsation.
4. Use two rulers. Line up the bottom edge of a regular ruler with the top of the area of pulsation in the jugular vein. Then take a centimeter ruler and align it perpendicular to the first ruler at the level of the sternal angle. Measure in centimeters the distance between the second ruler and the sternal angle (Figure 32-53).
5. Repeat the same measurement on the other side. Bilateral pressures higher than 2.5 cm (1 inch) are considered elevated and are a sign of right-sided heart failure. One-sided pressure elevation can be caused by obstruction.

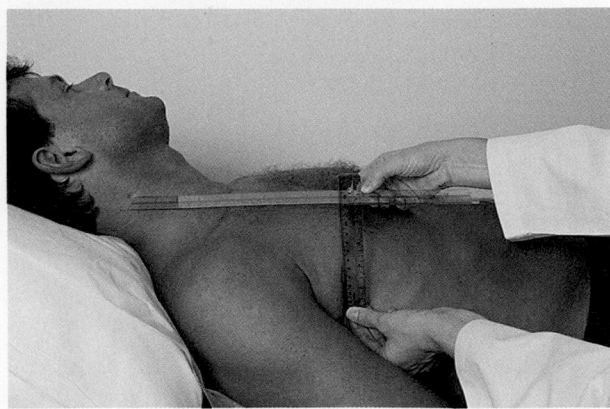

FIGURE **32–53** Measuring jugular venous pressure. (From Seidel HM and others: *Mosby's guide to physical examination*, ed 5, St. Louis, 2003, Mosby.)

Table 32-25	Indicators for Assessing Local Blood Flow
Indicator	**Rationale**
Systemic diseases (e.g., arteriosclerosis, atherosclerosis, diabetes)	Diseases result in changes in integrity of walls of arteries and smaller blood vessels.
Coagulation disorders (e.g., thrombosis, embolus)	Blood clot causes mechanical obstruction to blood flow.
Local trauma or surgery (e.g., contusion, fracture, vascular surgery)	Direct manipulation of vessels or localized edema impairs blood flow.
Application of constricting devices (e.g., casts, dressings, elastic bandages, restraints)	Constriction causes tourniquet effect, impairing blood flow to areas below site of constriction.

Peripheral Arteries and Veins

To examine the peripheral vascular system, the nurse first assesses the adequacy of blood flow to the extremities by measuring arterial pulses and inspecting the condition of the skin and nails. The integrity of the venous system is also assessed, with attention given to determining whether the client has abnormalities.

A number of factors can impair circulation to the extremities, including altered blood vessel integrity and overlying constriction on vessel walls (Table 32-25). The nurse should anticipate the risk for circulatory impairment (Box 32-21). Some clients, such as older adults and diabetic persons, suffer physical changes in blood vessel walls that increase the risk of perfusion problems.

Peripheral Arteries. The nurse examines each peripheral artery using the distal pads of the second and third fingers. The thumb may help anchor the brachial and femoral artery. The nurse applies firm pressure but avoids

Vascular Assessment

Objectives

- Client will know normal blood pressure range for age and compare it with own blood pressure readings to identify normalcy of blood pressure.
- Client with vascular insufficiency will avoid activities that worsen circulatory status.

Teaching Strategies

- Tell client the blood pressure reading. Explain the normal reading for the client's age. Discuss implications of abnormalities.
- Instruct client with risk or evidence of vascular insufficiency in the lower extremities to avoid tight clothing over the lower body or legs, to avoid sitting or standing for long periods, to walk regularly, and to elevate feet when sitting.
- Advise client to avoid cigarette smoking because nicotine causes vasoconstriction.
- Identify older adult with hypertension who may benefit from regular monitoring of blood pressure (daily, weekly, or monthly). Teach client how to use home monitoring kits (see Chapter 31).

Evaluation

- Ask client to identify if blood pressure reading is within normal limits for age.
- Have client with vascular insufficiency describe precautions to take to avoid further circulatory deficiency.
- Have older adult demonstrate self-monitoring of blood pressure.

occluding the pulse. When it is difficult to find a pulse, it is helpful to vary pressure and feel all around the pulse site. The nurse must be sure not to palpate his or her own pulse.

Routine vital signs usually include assessment of the rate and rhythm of the radial artery because it is easily accessible. The pulse is counted for either 30 seconds or a full minute, depending on the character of the pulse. With palpation the nurse normally feels the pulse wave at regular intervals. When an interval is interrupted by an early, late, or missed beat, the pulse rhythm is irregular. In emergencies the carotid artery is chosen because it is accessible and most useful in evaluating heart activity. To check local circulatory status of tissues, the nurse palpates peripheral arteries long enough to note that a pulse is present.

The nurse assesses each peripheral artery for elasticity of the vessel wall, strength, and equality. A systematic technique is useful, starting with the temporal arteries in the head and moving down to the arteries in the upper and lower extremities. The wall of an artery is normally elastic, making it easily palpable. After the artery is depressed, it will spring back to shape when pressure is released. An abnormal artery may be described as hard, inelastic, or calcified.

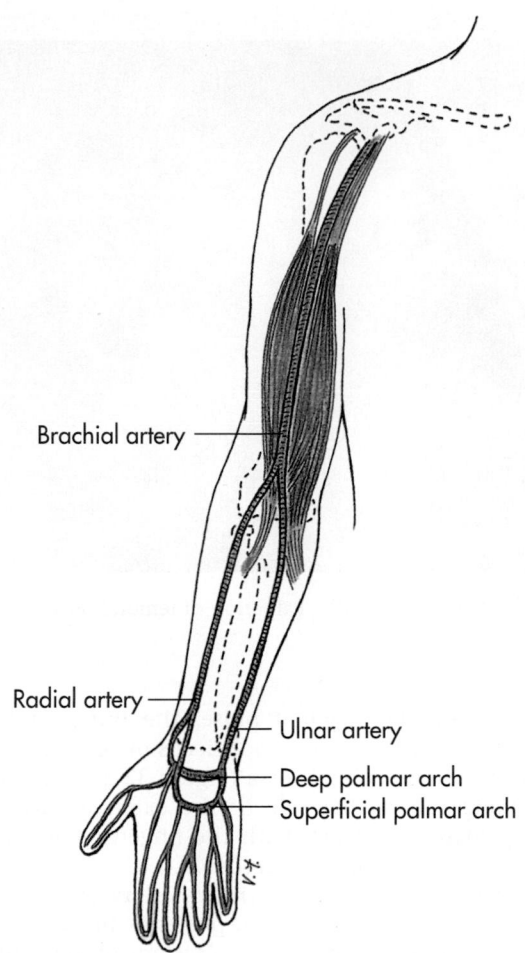

FIGURE **32–54**   Anatomical positions of brachial, radial, and ulnar arteries.

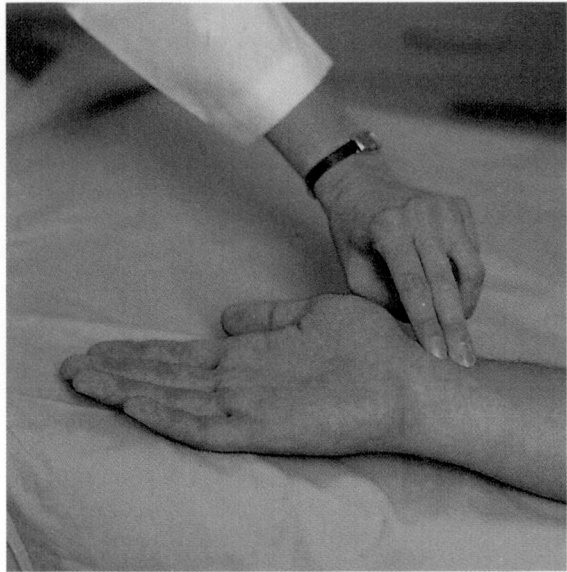

FIGURE **32–55**   Palpation of radial pulse.

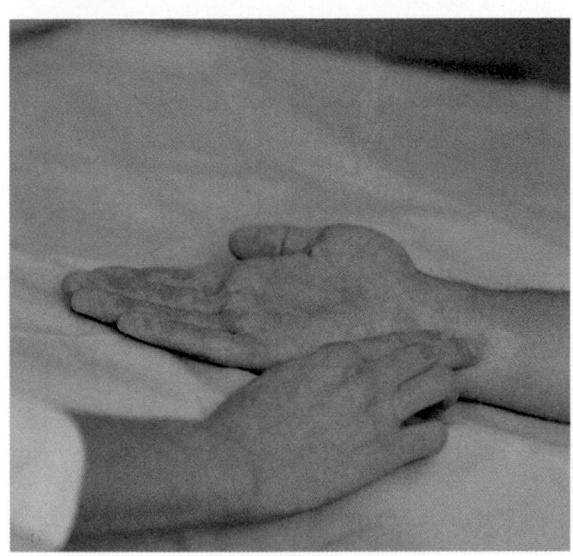

FIGURE **32–56**   Palpation of ulnar pulse.

The strength of a pulse is a measurement of the force at which blood is ejected against the arterial wall. Some examiners use a scale rating from 0 to 4+ for the strength of a pulse (Seidel and others, 2003):

0   Absent, not palpable
1+   Pulse diminished, barely palpable
2+   Easily palpable, normal pulse
3+   Full pulse, increased
4+   Strong, bounding pulse, cannot be obliterated

All peripheral pulses are measured for equality and symmetry. The left radial pulse is compared with that of the right, the left brachial pulse is compared with the left radial, and so on. An inequality may indicate localized obstruction or an abnormally positioned artery.

In the upper extremities the primary artery is the brachial artery, which channels blood to the radial and ulnar arteries of the forearm and hand. If circulation in this artery becomes blocked, the hands will not receive adequate blood flow. If circulation in the radial or ulnar arteries becomes impaired, the hand will still receive adequate perfusion. An interconnection between the radial and ulnar arteries guards against arterial occlusion (Figure 32-54).

The nurse should practice locating pulses on a friend. To locate pulses in the arm and hand, the nurse has the client sit or lie down. The radial pulse is found along the radial side of the forearm, at the wrist. In a thin individual a groove is formed lateral to the flexor tendon of the wrist. The radial pulse can be felt with light palpation in the groove (Figure 32-55). The ulnar pulse is on the opposite side of the wrist and tends to feel less prominent than the radial pulse (Figure 32-56). An examiner palpates the ulnar pulse only when arterial insufficiency to the hand is expected.

The **Allen's test** can be performed to assess collateral circulation. The client makes a fist as the ulnar and radial arteries are compressed simultaneously. The client then opens the hand, and the nurse releases the ulnar artery. The hand should quickly turn pink if the ulnar artery is patent. The test may be repeated by releasing only the radial artery.

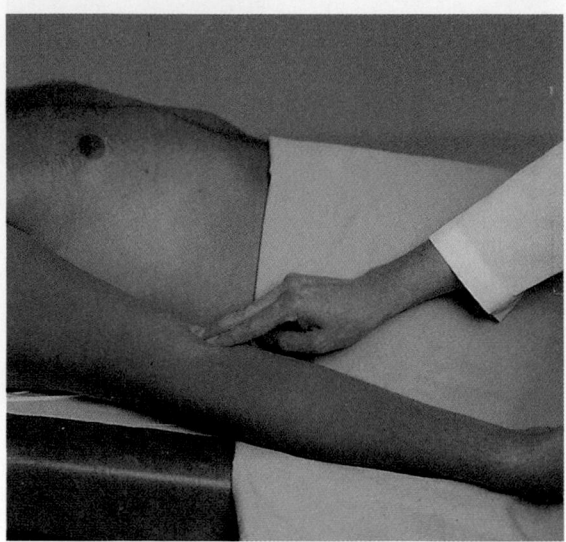

FIGURE 32–57   Palpation of brachial pulse.

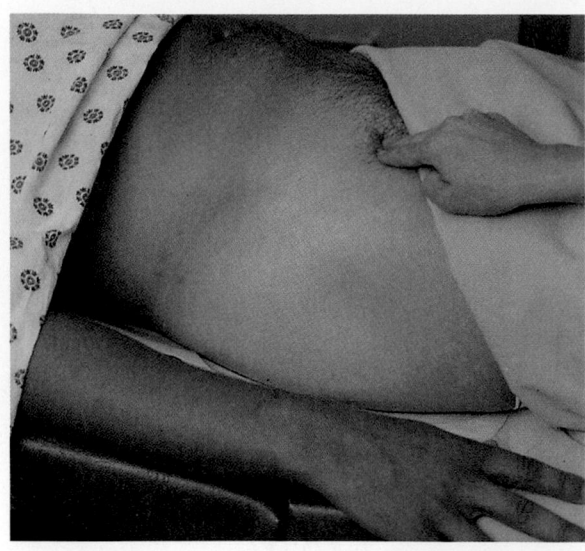

FIGURE 32–59   Palpation of femoral pulse.

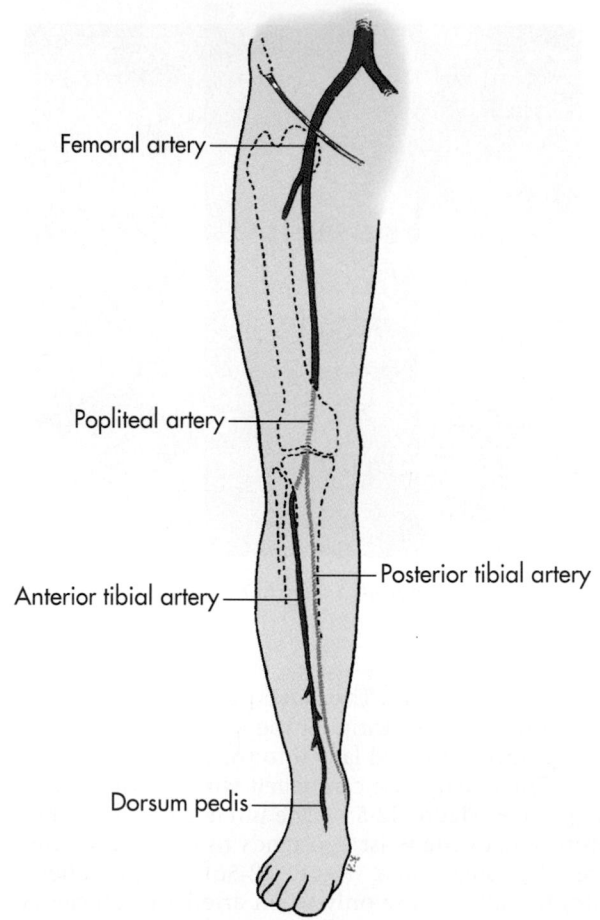

Femoral artery

Popliteal artery

Anterior tibial artery

Posterior tibial artery

Dorsum pedis

FIGURE 32–58   Anatomical position of femoral, popliteal, dorsum pedis, and posterior tibial arteries.

To palpate the brachial pulse, the nurse finds the groove between the biceps and triceps muscles above the elbow at the antecubital fossa (Figure 32-57). The artery runs along the medial side of the extended arm. The nurse palpates the artery with the fingertips of the first three fingers in the muscle groove.

The femoral artery is the primary artery in the leg, delivering blood to the popliteal, posterior tibial, and dorsalis pedis arteries (Figure 32-58). It is one of the strongest arteries in an infant or small child. An interconnection between the posterior tibial and dorsalis pedis arteries guards against local arterial occlusion.

The femoral pulse is found best with the client lying down with the inguinal area exposed (Figure 32-59). The femoral artery runs below the inguinal ligament, midway between the symphysis pubis and the anterosuperior iliac spine. Deep palpation may be required to feel the pulse. Bimanual palpation is effective in obese clients. This technique differs from the previous description of bimanual palpation. The nurse places the fingertips of both hands on opposite sides of the pulse site. A pulsatile sensation can be felt as the fingertips are pushed apart by arterial pulsation.

The popliteal pulse is found behind the knee. The client should slightly flex the knee, with the foot resting on the examination table, or assume a prone position with the knee slightly flexed (Figure 32-60). The client is instructed to keep leg muscles relaxed. The nurse palpates with the fingers of both hands deeply into the popliteal fossa, just lateral to the midline. The popliteal pulse is difficult to locate.

With the client's foot relaxed, the nurse locates the dorsalis pedis pulse. The artery runs along the top of the foot in line with the groove between the extensor tendons of the great toe and first toe (Figure 32-61). Often an examiner finds the pulse by placing the fingertips between the great and first toe and slowly inching up the foot. This pulse may be congenitally absent.

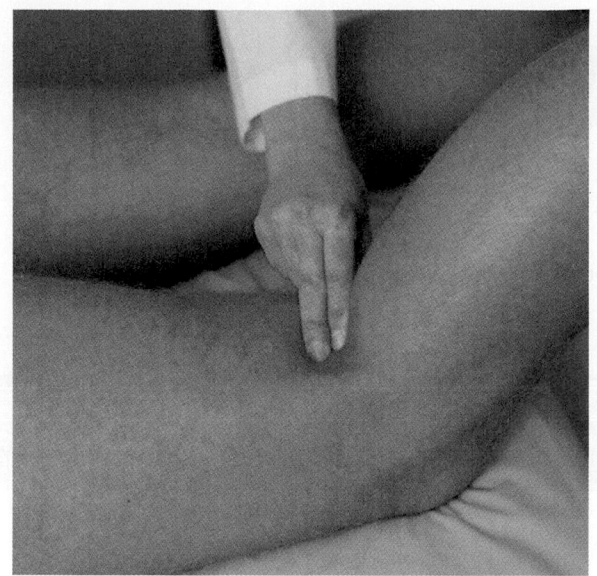

FIGURE **32–60**   Palpation of popliteal pulse.

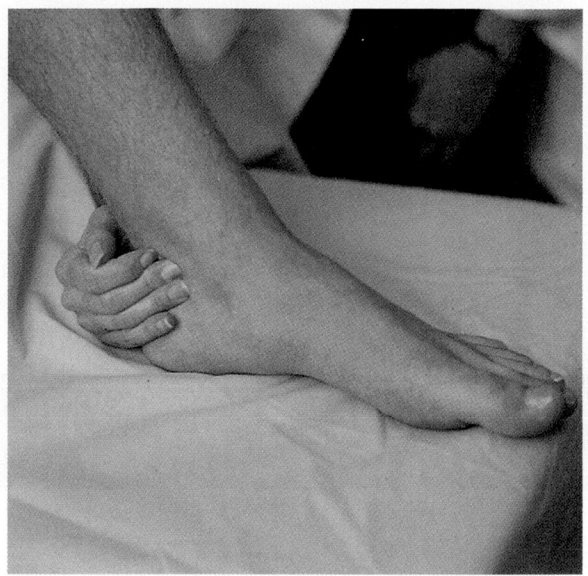

FIGURE **32–62**   Palpation of posterior tibial pulse.

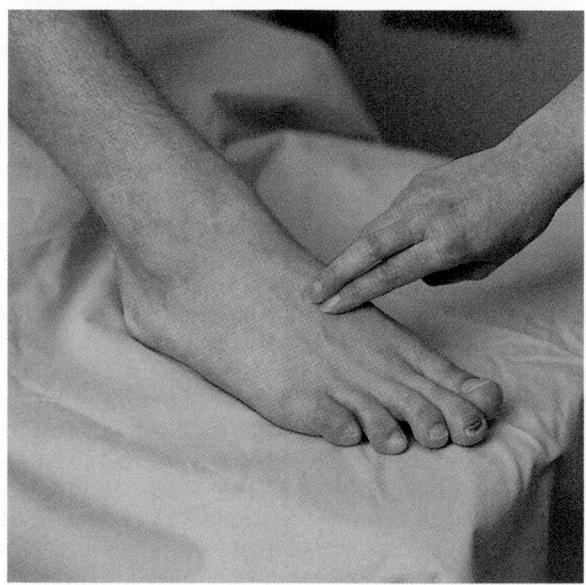

FIGURE **32–61**   Palpation of dorsalis pedis pulse.

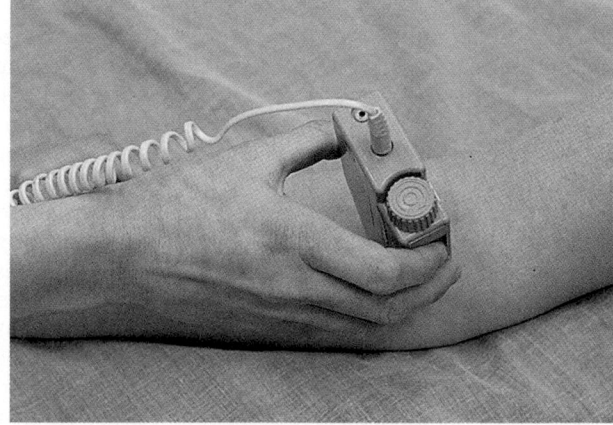

FIGURE **32–63**   Ultrasound stethoscope in position on brachial artery.

The posterior tibial pulse is found on the inner side of each ankle (Figure 32-62). The nurse places the fingers behind and below the medial malleolus (ankle bone). The artery is easily located with the foot relaxed and slightly extended.

Ultrasound Stethoscopes. If a nurse cannot palpate a pulse, an ultrasound stethoscope is a useful tool that amplifies the sounds of a pulse wave. Factors that may weaken a pulse or make palpation difficult include obesity, reduction in the heart's stroke volume, diminished blood volume, or arterial obstruction. A thin layer of transmission gel is first applied to the client's skin at the

pulse site or directly onto the transducer tip of the probe. The nurse then turns the volume control to "on" and places the tip of the probe at a 45- to 90-degree angle on the skin (Figure 32-63). The nurse moves the probe until a pulsating "whooshing" sound is heard, indicating that arterial blood flow is present.

Tissue Perfusion. The condition of the skin, mucosa, and nail beds offers useful data about the status of circulatory blood flow. The nurse first examines the face and upper extremities, looking at the color of the skin, mucosa, and nail beds. The presence of cyanosis requires special attention. Central cyanosis, which indicates poor arterial oxygenation, may be due to heart disease. It can be noted by a bluish discoloration of the lips, mouth, and conjunctivae. Peripheral cyanosis, which indicates peripheral vasoconstriction, is noted by blue lips, earlobes, and nail beds. When cyanosis is present, the nurse refers

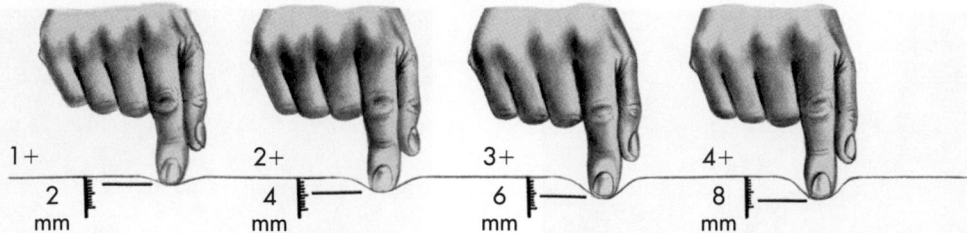

FIGURE **32–64** Assessing for pitting edema. (From Seidel HM and others: *Mosby's guide to physical examination,* ed 5, St. Louis, 2003, Mosby.)

Table 32-26	**Signs of Venous and Arterial Insufficiency**	
Assessment Criterion	**Venous**	**Arterial**
Color	Normal or cyanotic	Pale; worsened by elevation of extremity; dusky red when extremity is lowered
Temperature	Normal	Cool (blood flow blocked to extremity)
Pulse	Normal	Decreased or absent
Edema	Often marked	Absent or mild
Skin changes	Brown pigmentation around ankles	Thin, shiny skin; decreased hair growth; thickened nails

to available laboratory data on oxygen saturation to determine the severity of the problem. Examination of the nails involves inspection for clubbing, a bulging of the tissues at the nail base. **Clubbing** is due to insufficient oxygenation at the periphery resulting from conditions such as chronic emphysema and congenital heart disease.

The nurse inspects the lower extremities for changes in color, temperature, and condition of the skin indicating either arterial or venous alterations (Table 32-26). This is a good time to ask the client about any history of pain in the legs. If an arterial occlusion is present, the client has signs resulting from an absence of blood flow. Pain will be distal to the occlusion. The three *P's*—pain, pallor, and pulselessness—characterize an occlusion. Venous congestion causes tissue changes indicating an inadequate circulatory flow back to the heart.

During examination of the lower extremities, the nurse also inspects skin and nail texture; hair distribution on the lower legs, feet, and toes; the venous pattern; and scars, pigmentation, or ulcers. As the nurse palpates the feet, an assessment is made about their color and temperature. In addition the nurse should also assess **capillary refill.** Capillary refill is measured by blanching the nail bed with a substantial pressure of several seconds. The pressure is released, and the nurse observes the time elapsed before the nail regains its full color. An acceptable capillary refill time is less than 2 seconds (Seidel and others, 2003).

The absence of hair growth over the legs may indicate circulatory insufficiency. The nurse should not be misled by shaven lower legs. Also, many men have less hair around the calves from wearing tight-fitting dress socks. Chronic recurring ulcers of the feet or lower legs are a serious sign of circulatory insufficiency and require a physician's intervention.

Peripheral Veins. The nurse assesses the status of the peripheral veins by asking the client to assume sitting and standing positions. Assessment includes inspection and palpation for varicosities, peripheral edema, and phlebitis. Varicosities are superficial veins that become dilated, especially when the legs are in a dependent position. They are common in older adults because the veins normally fibrose, dilate, and stretch. They are also common in people who stand for prolonged periods. Varicosities in the anterior or medial part of the thigh and the posterolateral part of the calf are abnormal.

Dependent edema around the area of the feet and ankles can be a sign of venous insufficiency and right-sided heart failure. Dependent edema is common in older adults and persons who spend a lot of time standing (e.g., waitresses, security guards, or nurses). To assess for pitting edema, the nurse uses a thumb to press firmly for 5 seconds and then release over the medial malleolus or the shins. A depression left in the skin indicates edema. The severity of the edema is characterized by grading 1+ through 4+ (Figure 32-64).

Phlebitis is an inflammation of a vein that occurs commonly after trauma to the vessel wall, infection, prolonged immobilization, and prolonged insertion of IV catheters (see Chapter 40). Phlebitis promotes clot formation, a potentially dangerous situation because a clot within a deep vein of the leg can become dislodged and travel through the heart, causing a pulmonary embolus. To assess for phlebitis, the nurse inspects the calves for localized redness, tenderness, and swelling over vein sites. Gentle palpation of calf muscles reveals tenderness and firmness of the muscle. If the calf appears normal, the nurse may also check for Homans' sign by supporting the leg while flexing the foot upward. If phlebitis is present in the lower leg, forceful dorsiflexion of the foot often causes pain in the calf. Homans' sign is not always a reliable indicator of phlebitis and may be present in other conditions (Breen, 2000).

Lymphatic System

Assessment of the lymphatic drainage of the lower extremities is performed during examination of the vascular system. The nurse may also perform this examination

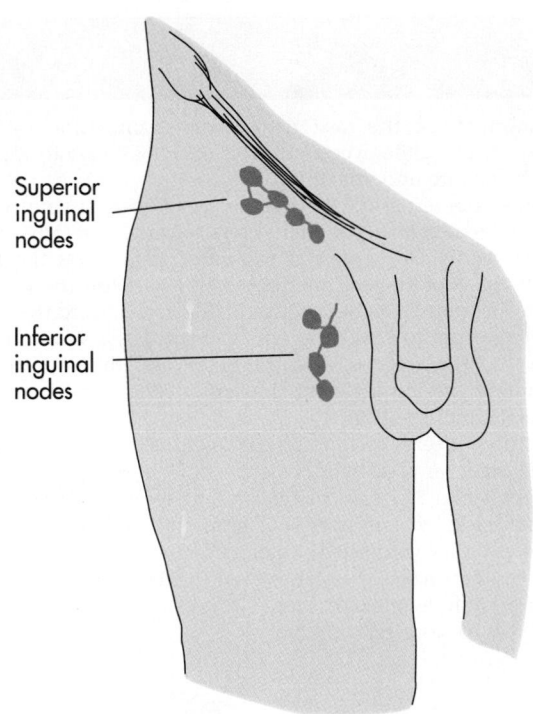

Superior inguinal nodes

Inferior inguinal nodes

FIGURE **32–65**   Inguinal lymph nodes.

just before the female or male genital examination. The legs are drained by superficial and deep nodes, but only the two groups of superficial nodes are palpable. The nurse palpates the area of the superficial inguinal nodes (Figure 32-65), beginning in the groin area and moving down toward the inner thigh. The vertical group of nodes lies close to the upper portion of the great saphenous vein. The horizontal group lies below the inguinal ligament. The nurse uses a firm but gentle pressure when palpating over each lymphatic chain. Multiple nodes are not normally palpable, although a few soft, nontender nodes are not unusual. Enlarged, hardened, tender nodes can reveal potential sites of infection or metastatic disease.

Breasts

It is important to examine the breasts of female and male clients. A small amount of glandular tissue, a potential site for the growth of cancer cells, is located in the male breast. In contrast, the majority of the female breast is glandular tissue.

Female Breasts

Breast cancer was projected to affect an estimated 192,200 women in the United States in 2002 (ACS, 2003). The disease is second to lung cancer as the leading cause of death in women with cancer. Early detection is the key to cure. A major responsibility for nurses is to teach clients health behavior such as breast self-examination (BSE). Studies suggest that a minority of women actually perform BSE. Nurses should know factors that increase the likelihood of a woman performing BSE. Incorporating these interventions into teaching strategies may improve

the likelihood of a client detecting breast cancer early. The American Cancer Society (ACS, 2003) recommends the following guidelines for the early detection of breast cancer:

- BSE should be performed monthly by women 20 years of age and older.
- An examination by a health care professional should be performed every 3 years from ages 20 to 40, and yearly for women over age 40.
- Women with a family history of breast cancer should have a yearly examination by a health care professional.
- Asymptomatic women should have a screening mammogram by age 40; women age 40 and over should have a mammogram annually.
- For women with a history of breast cancer, a yearly examination is recommended.

During an examination the nurse explains how to perform a BSE. While assessing the client's breasts, the nurse uses many of the same techniques the client will use in the home (Box 32-22).

If the client already performs BSE, the nurse can ask about the method she uses and times she does the examination in relation to her menstrual cycle. The best time for a BSE is 2 to 3 days after the menstrual period ends, when the breast is no longer swollen or tender from hormone elevations. If the woman has already experienced menopause, she should check her breasts the same time each month. The pregnant woman also must check her breasts monthly.

Older women may require special attention when reviewing the need for regular BSE. Many older women are limited by fixed incomes and thus fail to pursue regular clinical breast examination and mammography. Unfortunately, many older women ignore changes in their breasts, assuming that they are a part of aging. In addition, physiological factors can affect the ease with which older women can perform a BSE. Musculoskeletal limitations, diminished peripheral sensation, reduced eyesight, and changes in joint range of motion can limit palpation and inspection abilities. The nurse should find resources for older women, including free screening programs. Often family members can be taught to perform examinations.

The client's history (Table 32-27) should alert the nurse to any signs of breast disease and normal developmental changes. Because of its glandular structure, the breast undergoes changes during a woman's life. Knowledge of these changes (Box 32-23) helps the nurse complete an accurate assessment. Both men and women are encouraged to observe their breast for changes.

Inspection. The client removes the top gown or drape to allow simultaneous visualization of both breasts. The client may stand or sit with her arms hanging loosely at her sides. If possible, the nurse places a mirror in front of the client so that she can see what to look for when performing a BSE. To recognize abnormalities, the client must be familiar with the normal appearance of her breasts. The nurse describes observations or findings in relation to imaginary lines that divide the breast into four quadrants and a tail. The lines cross at the center of the nipple. Each tail extends outward from the upper outer quadrant (Figure 32-66).

Box 32-22   **Breast Self-Examination**

Breast self-examination (BSE) should be done once a month so that you become familiar with the usual appearance and feel of your breasts. Familiarity makes it easier to notice any changes in the breast from one month to another. Early discovery of a change from what is "normal" is the main idea behind BSE.

If you menstruate, the best time to do BSE is 2 or 3 days after your period ends, when your breasts are least likely to be tender or swollen. If you no longer menstruate, pick a day, such as the first day of the month, to remind yourself it is time to do BSE.

Here is how to do BSE:

1. Stand before a mirror. Inspect both breasts for anything unusual, such as any discharge from the nipples, puckering, dimpling, or scaling of the skin.

The next two steps are designed to emphasize any change in the shape or contour of your breasts. As you do them, you should be able to feel your chest muscles tighten.

2. Watching closely in the mirror, clasp hands behind your head and press hands forward.

3. Next, press hands firmly on hips and bow slightly toward your mirror as you pull your shoulders and elbows forward.

Some women do the next part of the examination in the shower. Fingers glide over soapy skin, making it easy to appreciate the texture underneath.

4. Raise your left arm. Use three or four fingers of your right hand to explore your left breast firmly, carefully, and thoroughly. Beginning at the outer edge, press the flat part of your fingers in small circles, moving the circles slowly around the breast. Gradually work toward the nipple. Be sure to cover the entire breast. Pay special attention to the area between the breast and the armpit, including the armpit itself. Feel for any unusual lump or mass under the skin.

5. Gently squeeze the nipple and look for a discharge. Repeat the exam on your right breast.

6. Steps 4 and 5 should be repeated lying down. Lie flat on your back, left arm over your head and a pillow or folded towel under your left shoulder. This position flattens the breast and makes it easier to examine. Use the same circular motion described earlier.

Repeat on your right breast.

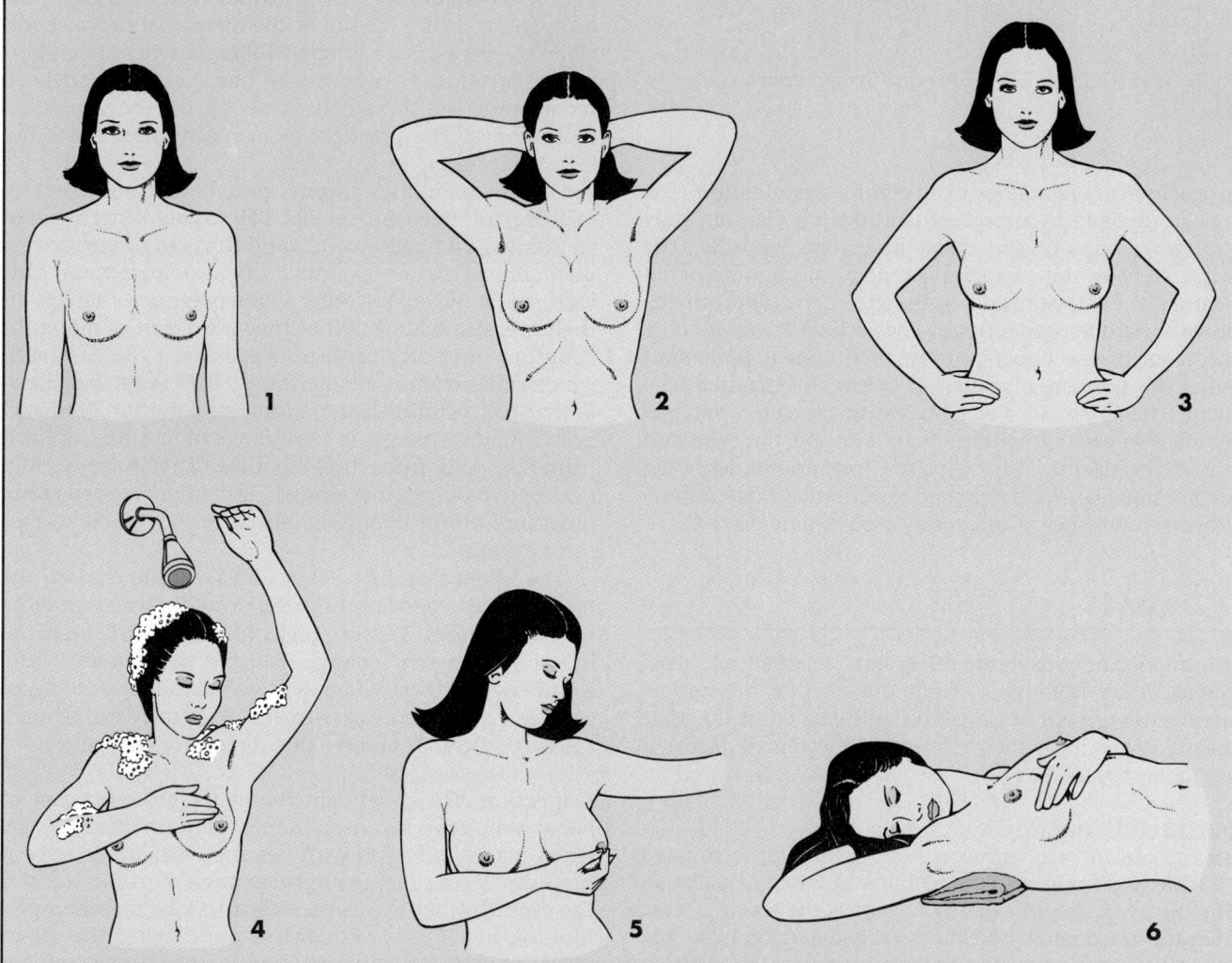

From Seidel HM and others: *Mosby's guide to physical examination*, ed 5, St. Louis, 2003, Mosby.

Table 32-27   **Nursing History for Breast Assessment**

Assessment Category	Rationale
Determine if woman is over age 40; has a personal or family history of breast cancer, early-onset menarche (before age 12), or late-age menopause (after age 50); has never had children or gave birth to first child after age 30; or has not breast-fed.	These are risk factors for breast cancer.
Ask if client (both sexes) has noticed lump, thickening, pain, or tenderness of breast; discharge, distortion, retraction, or scaling of nipple; or change in size of breast.	Potential signs and symptoms of breast cancer allow nurse to focus on specific areas of breast during assessment.
Determine if client is taking oral contraceptives, digitalis, diuretics, steroids, or estrogen hormones.	Medications may cause nipple discharge. Hormones and caffeine may cause fibrocystic changes in breast.
Determine client's caffeine intake and intake of foods high in fat.	Breast cancer incidence rates may correlate with intake high in total fat (Moore, 2001).
Ask if client performs monthly BSE. If so, determine time of month she performs examination in relation to menstrual cycle. Have client describe or demonstrate method used.	Nurse's role is to educate client about breast cancer and techniques for BSE.
If client reports a breast mass, ask about length of time since lump was first noted. Does lump come and go, or is it always present? Have there been changes in the lump (e.g., size, relationship to menses), and are there associated symptoms?	Helps to determine nature of mass.

Box 32-23   **Normal Changes in the Breast During a Woman's Life Span**

Puberty (8 to 20 Years)*

Breasts mature in five stages. One breast may grow more rapidly than the other. The ages at which changes occur and rate of developmental progression vary.

Stage 1 (Preadolescent)
- This stage involves elevation of the nipple only.

Stage 2
- The breast and nipple elevate as a small mound, and the areolar diameters enlarge.

Stage 3
- There is further enlargement and elevation of the breast and areola, with no separation of contour.

Stage 4
- The areola and nipple project into the secondary mound above the level of the breast (may not occur in all girls.)

Stage 5 (Mature Breast)
- Only the nipple projects, and the areola recedes (may vary in some women).

Young Adulthood (20 to 30 Years)

- Breasts reach full (nonpregnant) size. Shape is generally symmetrical. Breasts may be unequal in size.

Pregnancy

- Breast size gradually enlarges to 2 to 3 times the previous size. Nipples enlarge and may become erect. Areolae darken, and diameters increase. Superficial veins become prominent. A yellowish fluid (colostrum) may be expelled from the nipples.

Menopause

- Breasts shrink. Tissue becomes softer, sometimes flabby.

Older Adulthood†

- Breasts become elongated, pendulous, and flaccid as a result of glandular tissue atrophy. The skin of the breasts tends to wrinkle, appearing loose and flabby.
- Nipples become smaller, flatter and lose erectile ability. Nipples may invert because of shrinkage and fibrotic changes.

*Data from Wong DL and others: *Whaley and Wong's nursing care of infants and children*, ed 6, St. Louis, 1999, Mosby.
†Data from Ebersole P, Hess P: *Toward healthy aging*, ed 5, St. Louis, 1998, Mosby.

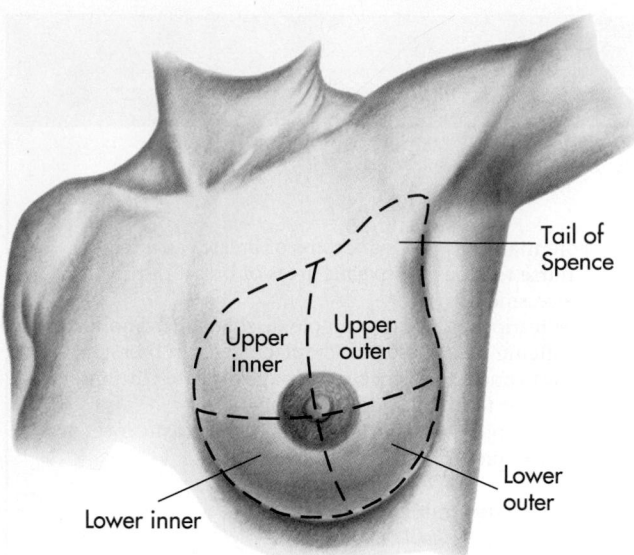

FIGURE 32–66   Quadrants of the left breast and axillary tail of Spence. (From Seidel HM and others: *Mosby's guide to physical examination,* ed 5, St. Louis, 2003, Mosby.)

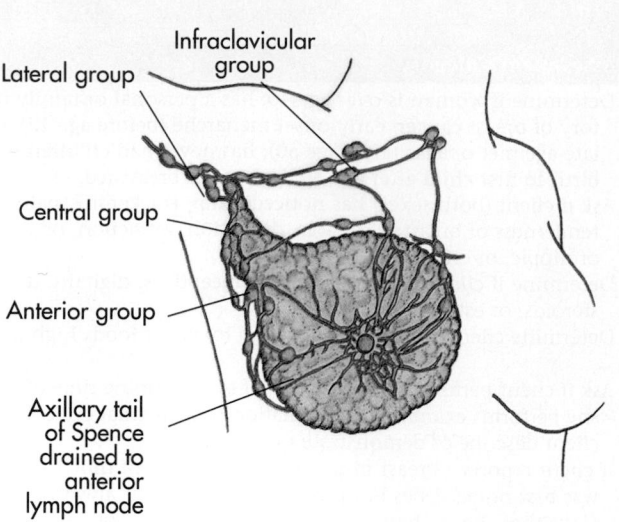

FIGURE 32–67   Anatomical position of axillary and clavicular lymph nodes.

The breasts are inspected for size and symmetry. The breasts usually extend from the third to the sixth ribs, with the nipple at the level of the fourth intercostal space. One breast is commonly larger than the other. However, a difference in size may be caused by inflammation or a mass. As the woman becomes older, the ligaments supporting the breast tissue weaken, causing the breasts to sag and the nipples to lower.

The nurse observes the contour or shape of the breasts and notes masses, flattening, retraction, or dimpling. Breasts vary in shape from convex to pendulous or conical. Retraction or dimpling results from invasion of underlying ligaments by tumors. The ligaments become fibrotic and pull the overlying skin inward toward the tumor. Edema also changes the breasts' contour. To bring out retraction or changes in the shape of breasts, the nurse asks the client to assume three positions: raise arms above the head, press hands against the hips, and extend arms straight ahead while sitting and leaning forward. Each maneuver causes a contraction of the pectoral muscles, which will accentuate retraction.

The overlying skin is carefully inspected for color and venous pattern. Venous patterns are more easily seen in thin clients or pregnant women. The presence of lesions, edema, or inflammation is also noted. The nurse lifts each breast when necessary to observe lower and lateral aspects for color and texture changes. The breasts are the color of neighboring skin, and venous patterns are the same bilaterally. For women with large breasts, the nurse should be sure to look carefully at the undersurface, a common site for redness and excoriation caused by rubbing of skin surfaces.

The nurse inspects the nipple and areola for size, color, shape, discharge, and the direction the nipples point. The normal areolae are round or oval and nearly equal bilaterally. Color ranges from pink to brown. In light-skinned women the areola turns brown during pregnancy and re-

mains dark. In dark-skinned women the areola is brown before pregnancy (Seidel and others, 2003). Normally the nipples point in symmetrical directions, they are everted, and there is no drainage. Their surface may be either smooth or wrinkled. If the nipples are inverted, the nurse asks if this has been a lifetime history. A recent inversion or inward turning of the nipple may indicate an underlying growth. Rashes or ulcerations are not normal on the breast or nipples. Bleeding or discharge from the nipple is noted. Clear yellow discharge 2 days after childbirth is common. While inspecting the breasts, the nurse explains the characteristics observed. The client must be taught the significance of abnormal signs or symptoms.

Palpation. Palpation allows the nurse to determine the condition of underlying breast tissue and lymph nodes. Breast tissue consists of glandular tissue, fibrous supportive ligaments, and fat. Glandular tissue is organized into lobes that end in ducts that open onto the nipple's surface. The largest portion of glandular tissue is in the upper outer quadrant and tail of each breast. Suspensory ligaments connect to skin and fascia underlying the breast to support the breast and maintain its upright position. Fatty tissue is located superficially and to the sides of the breast.

A large portion of lymph from the breasts drains into axillary lymph nodes. If cancerous lesions **metastasize** (spread), the nodes are commonly involved. The nurse learns the location of supraclavicular, infraclavicular, and axillary nodes (Figure 32-67). The axillary nodes drain lymph from the chest wall, breasts, arms, and hands. A tumor of one breast may involve nodes on the opposite side, as well as those on the same side.

The lymph nodes are best palpated when the client sits, although the examination can be performed with the client supine. Easy access is gained to the axillary nodes with the client's arms at her sides and the muscles relaxed. While facing the client and standing on the side

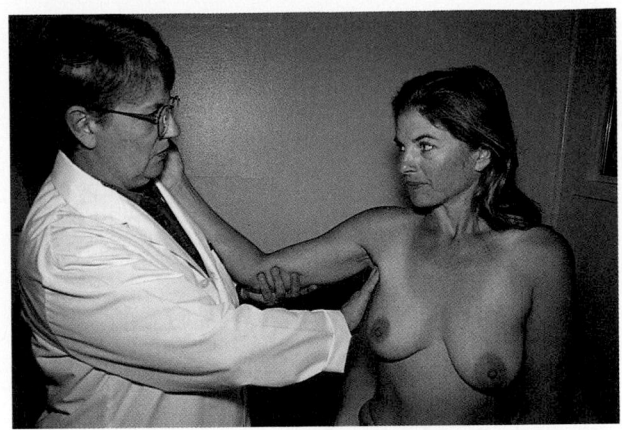

FIGURE **32–68**   The nurse supports the client's arm and palpates axillary lymph nodes.

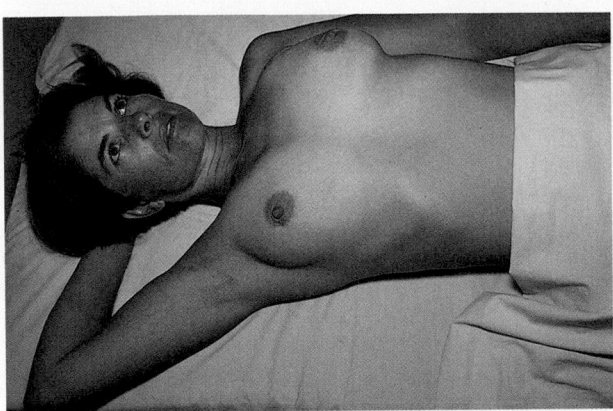

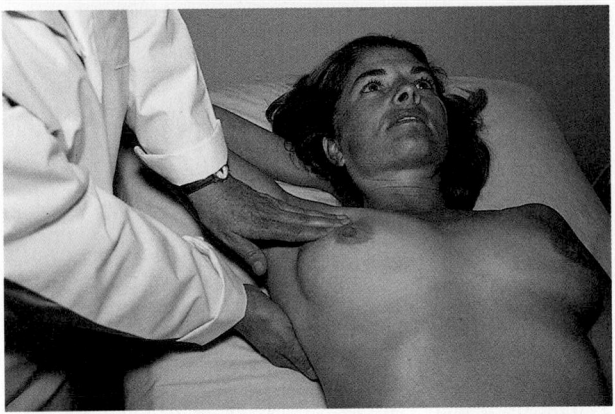

FIGURE **32–69**   **A,** The client lies flat with arm abducted and hand under head to help flatten breast tissue evenly over the chest wall. **B,** The nurse palpates each breast in systemic fashion.

being examined, the nurse supports the client's arm in a slightly flexed position and abducts the arm away from the chest wall. Then the nurse places the free hand against the client's chest wall and high in the axillary hollow. With the fingertips the nurse presses gently down over the surface of the ribs and muscles. The axillary nodes are palpated with the fingertips gently rolling soft tissue (Figure 32-68). Four areas of the axilla are palpated:

1. The edge of the pectoralis major muscle along the anterior axillary line
2. The chest wall in the midaxillary area
3. The upper part of the humerus
4. The anterior edge of the latissimus dorsi muscle along the posterior axillary line

Normally lymph nodes are not palpable. Each area must be assessed carefully because enlarged nodes are easily missed. The nurse notes their number, consistency, mobility, and size. One or two small, soft, nontender nodes may be normal. A palpable node feels like a small mass that may be hard, tender, and immobile. The nurse also palpates along the upper and lower clavicular ridges. The procedure is reversed for the other side.

It may be difficult for the client to learn to palpate for lymph nodes. Lying down with the arm abducted makes the area more accessible. The client is instructed to use her left hand for the right axillary and clavicular areas. The nurse can take the client's fingertips and move them in the proper circular fashion. The client then uses her right hand to palpate for nodes on the left side.

Palpation of breast tissue is best performed with the client lying supine with one arm behind the head (alternating with each breast). The supine position allows the breast tissue to flatten evenly against the chest wall. The client should raise her hand and place it behind the neck to further stretch and position breast tissue evenly (Figure 32-69, *A*). The examiner often places a small pillow or towel under the shoulder blade to further position breast tissue.

The consistency of normal breast tissue varies widely. The breasts of a young client are firm and elastic. In an older client the tissue may feel stringy and nodular. The client's familiarity with the texture of her own breasts is

very important. This familiarity is gained through monthly BSE (Box 32-24).

If the client complains of a mass, the nurse examines the opposite breast to ensure an objective comparison of normal and abnormal tissue. The nurse uses the pads of the first three fingers to compress breast tissue gently against the chest wall, noting tissue consistency (Figure 32-69, *B*). Palpation is performed systematically in one of three ways: (1) clockwise or counterclockwise, forming small circles with the fingers along each quadrant and the tail; (2) a back-and-forth technique with the fingers moving up and down each quadrant; or (3) palpating from the center of the breast in a radial fashion, returning to the areola to begin each spoke (Figure 32-70). Whatever approach is used, the nurse must be sure to cover the entire breast and tail, directing attention to any areas of tenderness.

When palpating large, pendulous breasts, the nurse uses a bimanual technique. The inferior portion of the breast is supported in one hand while the nurse uses the other hand to palpate breast tissue against the supporting hand.

During palpation the nurse notes the consistency of breast tissue. It normally feels dense, firm, and elastic. In fibrocystic disease, a common problem in women, tissue feels lumpy, but it is found bilaterally. With menopause, breast tissue shrinks and becomes softer. The lobular feel of glandular tissue is normal. The lower edge of each breast

Female Breast Assessment

Objectives

- Client will perform BSE (see Box 32-22, p. 736).
- Client will have screening mammography performed at recommended intervals, beginning at age 40.
- Client will identify signs and symptoms of breast cancer.
- Client will identify signs and symptoms of fibrocystic disease.
- Client will follow a low-fat diet.

Teaching Strategies

- Have client perform return demonstration of BSE and offer the opportunity to ask questions.
- Explain recommended frequency of mammography and assessment by a health care provider.
- Discuss signs and symptoms of breast cancer.
- Discuss signs and symptoms of fibrocystic disease.
- Inform a woman who is obese or who has a family history of breast cancer that she is at higher risk for the disease (ACS, 2003). Encourage dietary changes, including limiting meat consumption to well-trimmed, lean beef, pork, or lamb; removing skin from cooked chicken before eating it; selecting tuna and salmon packed in water and not oil; and using low-fat dairy products.
- Encourage client to reduce intake of caffeine and theophyllines. Although this approach is controversial, it may reduce symptoms of fibrocystic disease.

Evaluation

- Have client demonstrate BSE.
- During follow-up visit, determine whether client has had mammography performed.
- Ask client to explain frequency of mammography.
- Have client describe signs and symptoms of breast cancer compared with fibrocystic disease.

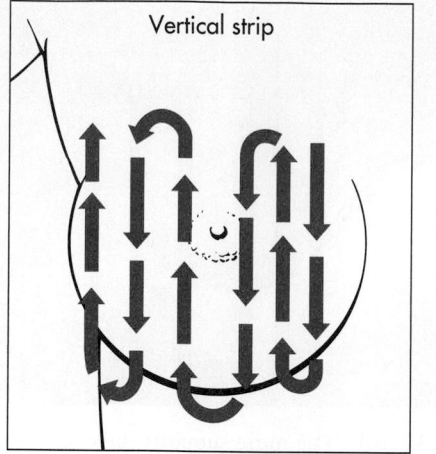

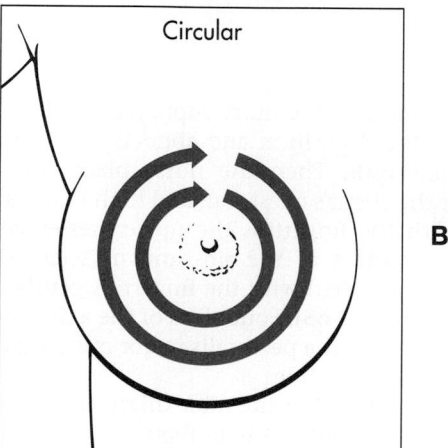

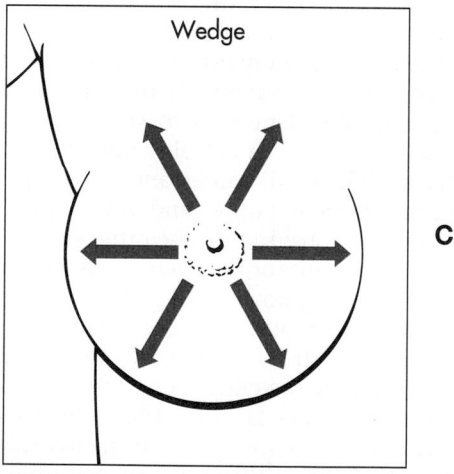

FIGURE 32–70 Various methods for palpation of the breast. **A,** Palpate from top to bottom in vertical strips. **B,** Palpate in concentric circles. **C,** Palpate out from the center in wedge sections. (From Seidel, HM and others: *Mosby's guide to physical examination,* ed 5, St. Louis, 2003, Mosby.)

may feel firm and hard. This is the normal inframammary ridge and not a tumor. It may be helpful to move the client's hand so that she can feel normal tissue variations. Abnormal masses are palpated to determine the following:

- Location in relation to quadrants
- Diameter in centimeters
- Shape (e.g., round or discoid)
- Consistency (soft, firm, or hard)
- Tenderness
- Mobility
- Discreteness (whether boundaries of mass are clear or unclear)

Cancerous lesions are hard, fixed, nontender, and irregular in shape. A common benign condition of the breast is **fibrocystic breast disease.** This condition is characterized by lumpy, painful breasts and sometimes nipple discharge. Symptoms are more apparent during the menstrual period. When palpated, the cysts (lumps) are soft, well differentiated, and movable. Deep cysts may feel hard.

Special attention is given to gently palpating the nipple and areola. The thumb and index finger compress the nipple gently, and the nurse notes any discharge. As the nurse examines the nipple and areola, the nipple may become erect with wrinkling of the areola. These changes are normal.

Table 32-28	Nursing History for Abdominal Assessment
Assessment Category	**Rationale**
If client has abdominal or low back pain, assess character of pain in detail (location, onset, frequency, precipitating factors, aggravating factors, type of pain, severity, course).	Pattern of characteristics of pain helps determine its source.
Carefully observe client's movement and position, including lying still with knees drawn up, moving restlessly to find comfortable position, and lying on one side or sitting with knees drawn to chest.	Positions assumed by client may reveal nature and source of pain, including peritonitis, renal stone, and pancreatitis.
Assess normal bowel habits and stool character; ask if client uses laxatives.	Data compared with physical findings can help identify cause and nature of elimination problems.
Determine if client has had abdominal surgery, trauma, or diagnostic tests of GI tract.	Surgical or traumatic alterations of abdominal organs may cause changes in expected findings (e.g., position of underlying organs). Diagnostic tests may change character of stool.
Assess if client has had recent weight changes or intolerance to diet (e.g., nausea, vomiting, cramping, especially in last 24 hours).	Data may indicate alterations in upper GI tract (stomach or gallbladder) or lower colon.
Assess for difficulty in swallowing, belching, flatulence, bloody emesis (hematemesis), black or tarry stools (melena), heartburn, diarrhea, or constipation.	These characteristic signs and symptoms indicate gastrointestinal alterations.
Ask if client takes antiinflammatory medication (e.g., aspirin, ibuprofen, or steroids) or antibiotics.	Pharmacological agents may cause GI upset or bleeding.
Ask client to locate tender areas.	Nurse assesses painful areas last to minimize discomfort and anxiety.
Inquire about family history of cancer, kidney disease, alcoholism, hypertension, or heart disease.	Data may reveal risk for alterations identifiable during examination.
Determine if female client is pregnant; note last menstrual period.	Pregnancy causes changes in abdominal shape and contour.
Assess client's usual intake of alcohol.	Chronic alcohol ingestion can cause gastrointestinal and liver problems.
Review client's history for the following factors: health care occupation, hemodialysis, IV drug user, household or sexual contact with hepatitis B virus (HBV) carrier, heterosexual person with more than one sex partner in previous 6 months, sexually active homosexual or bisexual male, international traveler in area of high HBV infection rate.	Risk factors for HBV exposure.

After the nurse completes the examination, the client can demonstrate self-palpation. Observing the client's technique helps the nurse emphasize the importance of a systematic approach. The client is urged to see her physician if she discovers an abnormal mass during routine monthly BSE. She should also know all of the signs and symptoms of breast cancer.

Male Breasts

Examination of the male breast is relatively easy. The nipple and areola are inspected for nodules, edema, and ulceration. An enlarged male breast may result from obesity or glandular enlargement. Breast enlargement in young males may be indicative of steroid use. Fatty tissue feels soft, whereas glandular tissue is firm. Any masses are palpated for the same characteristics as in the female breast. Because breast cancer in men is relatively rare, routine self-examinations are unnecessary.

Safety Alert. Men, especially men who have a first-degree relative (e.g., mother or sister) with breast cancer, are at risk for breast cancer and should palpate their breasts at regular intervals. In discussion with their health care provider these men may also be scheduled for routine mammograms.

Abdomen

The abdominal examination can be complex because of the organs located within and near the abdominal cavity. A thorough nursing history (Table 32-28) helps the nurse interpret physical signs. The examination includes an assessment of structures of the lower gastrointestinal (GI) tract in addition to the liver, stomach, uterus, ovaries, kidneys, and bladder. Abdominal pain is one of the most common symptoms that clients report when seeking medical care. An accurate assessment requires matching client history data with a careful assessment of the location of physical symptoms.

Landmarks help the nurse map out the abdominal region. The xiphoid process (tip of the sternum) marks the upper boundary of the abdominal region, and the symphysis pubis delineates the lower boundary. By dividing the abdomen into four imaginary quadrants (Figure 32-71, *A*) the nurse can refer to assessment findings and record them in relation to each quadrant. For example, the nurse may determine that the client is experiencing tenderness over the left lower quadrant (LLQ) with normal bowel sounds present. Posteriorly the kidneys, located from the T12 to L3 vertebrae, are protected by the lower ribs and heavy back muscles (Figure 32-71, *B*). The costovertebral

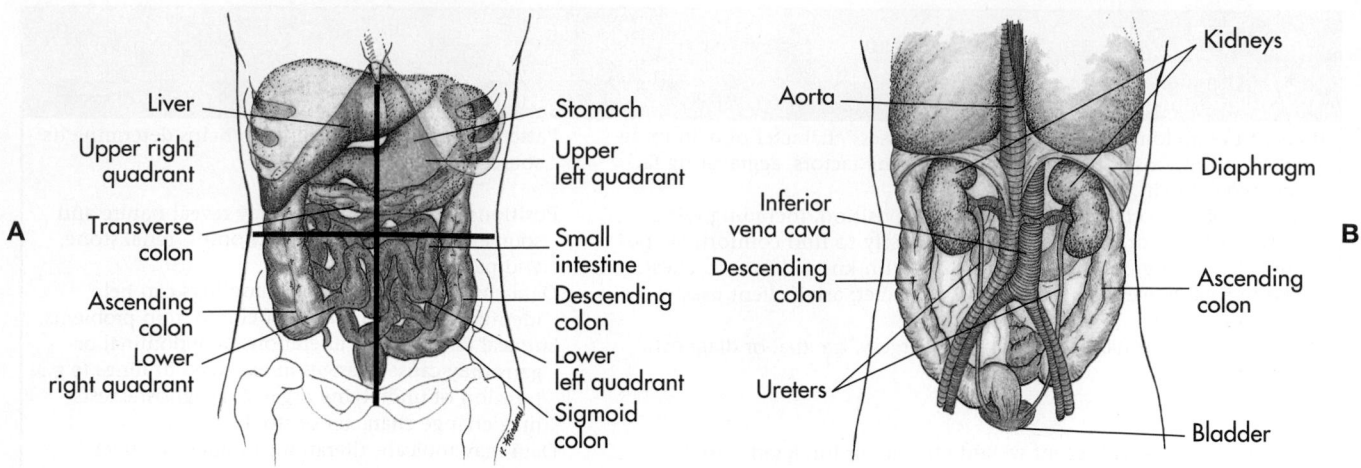

FIGURE 32–71 **A,** Anterior view of abdomen divided by quadrants. **B,** Posterior view of abdominal section.

angle formed by the last rib and vertebral column is a landmark used during kidney palpation.

Clients must be relaxed for abdominal examinations. A tightening of abdominal muscles hinders accuracy with palpation and auscultation. The nurse asks the client to void before beginning. The room should be warm, and the client's upper chest and legs should be draped. The client lies supine or in a dorsal recumbent position with the arms at the sides and knees slightly bent. Small pillows can be placed beneath the knees. If the client places the arms under the head, the abdominal muscles may tighten. The examiner proceeds calmly and slowly, making sure that there is adequate lighting. The abdomen is exposed from just above the xiphoid process down to the symphysis pubis. Warm hands and a warm stethoscope further promote relaxation. Maintaining conversation except during auscultation helps to distract clients. Clients should be asked to report pain and point out tender areas. Tender areas are assessed last.

The order of an abdominal examination differs slightly from previous assessments. The nurse begins with inspection and then follows with auscultation. It is important to auscultate before palpation and percussion because palpation and percussion may alter the frequency and character of bowel sounds. The nurse also needs a tape measure and marking pen.

Inspection

The nurse may be able to observe the client during routine care activities. The nurse notes the client's posture and looks for evidence of abdominal splinting: the client's lying with the knees drawn up or moving restlessly in bed. A client free from abdominal pain will not stoop or splint the abdomen. To inspect the abdomen for abnormal movement or shadows, the nurse stands on the client's right side and inspects from above the abdomen. By sitting down to look across the abdomen, the nurse assesses contour. The examination light is directed over the abdomen.

Skin. The nurse inspects the skin over the abdomen for color, scars, venous patterns, lesions, and **striae** (stretch

marks). The skin is subject to the same color variations as the rest of the body. Venous patterns are normally faint, except in thin clients. Striae result from stretching of tissue by obesity or pregnancy. An artificial opening may indicate a drainage site resulting from surgery (see Chapter 49) or an ostomy (see Chapters 44 and 45). Scars indicate past trauma or surgery that may have created permanent changes in underlying organ anatomy. Bruising may indicate accidental injury, physical abuse, or a type of bleeding disorder. The nurse should ask if the client self-administers injections (e.g., heparin or insulin). Unexpected findings include generalized color changes such as jaundice or cyanosis. A glistening, taut appearance indicates ascites.

Umbilicus. When examining the umbilicus, the position; shape; color; and signs of inflammation, discharge, or protruding masses are noted. Normally the umbilicus is a flat or concave hemisphere positioned midway between the xiphoid process and symphysis pubis. The color is the same as that of the surrounding skin. Underlying masses can cause displacement. An everted (pouched-out) umbilicus usually indicates distention. **Hernias** (protrusions of abdominal organs through the muscle wall) cause upward protrusion of the umbilicus. Normally no discharge is emitted from the umbilical area.

Contour and Symmetry. The nurse inspects for contour, symmetry, and surface motion of the abdomen, noting any masses, bulging, or distention. A flat abdomen forms a horizontal plane from the xiphoid process to the symphysis pubis. A round abdomen protrudes in a convex sphere from the horizontal plane. A concave abdomen appears to sink into the muscular wall. Each of these findings is normal if the abdomen's shape is symmetrical. In older adults there is often an overall increased distribution of adipose tissue. The presence of masses on only one side, or asymmetry, may indicate an underlying pathological condition.

Intestinal gas, a tumor, or fluid in the abdominal cavity may cause **distention** (swelling). When distention is generalized, the entire abdomen protrudes. The skin often appears taut, as if it were stretched over the abdomen. When gas causes distention, the flanks do not bulge. However, if fluid is the source of the problem, the flanks bulge. The client should be asked to roll onto one side. A protuberance forms on the dependent side if fluid is the cause of the distention. The nurse asks the client if the abdomen feels unusually tight. The nurse must be careful not to confuse distention with obesity. In obesity the abdomen is large, rolls of adipose tissue are often present along the flanks, and the client does not complain of tightness in the abdomen. If abdominal distention is expected, the nurse may choose to measure the abdomen's girth by placing a tape measure around the abdomen at the level of the umbilicus. Consecutive measurements will show any increase or decrease in distention. A marking pen is used to indicate where the tape measure was applied.

Enlarged Organs or Masses. While observing the abdominal contour, the nurse asks the client to take a deep breath and hold it. The contour should remain smooth and symmetrical. This maneuver forces the diaphragm downward and reduces the size of the abdominal cavity. Any enlarged organs in the upper abdominal cavity (e.g., liver or spleen) may descend below the rib cage to cause a bulge. Closer examination can be performed with palpation.

To evaluate the abdominal musculature, the nurse has clients raise their heads. This position causes superficial abdominal wall masses, hernias, and muscle separations to become more apparent.

Movement or Pulsations. The nurse should remember that a man breathes abdominally and a woman breathes more costally. If the client has severe pain, respiratory movement is diminished, and the client tightens abdominal muscles to guard against the pain. On closer inspection the nurse may see peristaltic movement and aortic pulsation by looking across the abdomen from the side to detect movement. It may take several minutes to see a peristaltic wave. In contrast, aortic pulsations occur with each beat of systole and appear in the midline above the umbilicus (epigastric area).

Auscultation

The nurse changes the usual sequence of assessment skills when auscultating the abdomen. Auscultation always precedes percussion and palpation during the abdominal assessment because manipulation of the abdomen may alter the frequency and intensity of bowel sounds. Clients are asked to not talk. If a client has a nasogastric or intestinal tube connected to intermittent suction, it should be momentarily turned off. Sound from the suction obscures bowel sounds.

Bowel Motility. Peristalsis, or intestinal motility, is a normal function of the small and large intestine. Bowel sounds are the audible passage of air and fluid created by peristalsis. The warmed diaphragm of the stethoscope is placed lightly over each of the four quadrants. Normally air and fluid move through the intestines, creating soft gurgling or clicking sounds that occur irregularly 5 to 35 times per minute (Seidel and others, 2003). Sounds may last ½ second to several seconds. It normally takes 5 to 20

seconds to hear a bowel sound. However, it may take 5 minutes of continuous listening before it can be determined that bowel sounds are absent (Seidel and others, 2003). All four quadrants are auscultated to make sure that no sounds are missed. The best time to auscultate is between meals. When the nurse auscultates just after meals or long after the client eats, bowel sounds tend to be increased. Sounds are generally described as normal, audible, absent, hyperactive, or hypoactive. Absent sounds indicate a cessation of gastrointestinal motility that may result from late-stage bowel obstruction, **paralytic ileus,** or **peritonitis.** Absent sounds are normal postoperatively following general anesthesia. Hyperactive sounds are loud, "growling" sounds called **borborygmi,** which indicate increased gastrointestinal motility. Inflammation of the bowel, anxiety, diarrhea, bleeding, excessive ingestion of laxatives, and reaction of the intestines to certain foods cause increased motility (Box 32-25).

Client Teaching   *Box 32-25*

Abdominal Assessment
Objectives

- Client will maintain normal bowel elimination.
- Client will achieve pain relief.
- Clients at high risk for hepatitis B virus (HBV) will receive immunization.
- Client will identify signs and symptoms of colon cancer.

Teaching Strategies

- Explain factors that promote bowel elimination, such as diet, regular exercise, limited use of over-the-counter drugs causing constipation, establishment of regular elimination schedule, and a good fluid intake (see Chapter 45). Stress importance for older adults.
- Caution clients about dangers of excessive use of laxatives or enemas.
- If client has acute pain, explain activities or positions to avoid.
- If client has chronic pain, explain measures used for pain relief (e.g., relaxation exercises, positioning) (see Chapter 42).
- If client is a health care worker or has contact with blood or fluids of affected person, encourage client to receive the series of three vaccine doses.
- Instruct client about warning signs of colon cancer, including bleeding from rectum, pain, black or tarry stools, blood in stool, and a change in bowel habits (constipation or diarrhea).

Evaluation

- Reassess client's bowel elimination pattern and stool character after therapies are started.
- Observe client using pain-relief measures and reassess character of pain.
- During follow-up clinic or office visit, check client's compliance with HBV vaccine schedule.
- Ask client to state signs and symptoms of colon cancer.

Vascular Sounds. The presence of bruits in the abdominal area can reveal aneurysms or stenotic vessels. The nurse uses the stethoscope's bell to auscultate in the epigastric region and each of the four quadrants. Normally there are no vascular sounds over the aorta (midline through the abdomen) or femoral arteries (lower quadrants). Renal artery bruits can be heard by placing the stethoscope over each upper quadrant anteriorly or over the costovertebral angle posteriorly (which can be done when the client sits). A bruit should be reported immediately to a physician.

Percussion

Percussion of the abdomen maps out underlying organs, bone, and masses and helps reveal the presence of air in the stomach and intestines. The beginning student uses this skill in a limited fashion. Practice is needed to ensure accuracy.

Organs and Masses. The nurse systematically percusses each quadrant to assess areas of tympany and dullness. Potentially painful areas are always percussed last. Tympany usually predominates because of air in the stomach and intestines. A dull percussion note is a medium- to high-pitched short sound heard over solid masses such as the liver, spleen, pancreas, kidneys, and distended bladder. In addition, a dull note may indicate a tumor. When dullness is noted, it may be useful to also use palpation to complete a detailed assessment.

Liver Size. Percussion allows the nurse to identify borders of the liver to detect organ enlargement. The nurse starts at the right iliac crest and percusses upward along the right midclavicular line. The percussion note changes from tympanic to dull at the liver's lower border, which is usually at the right costal margin. Extension beyond the right costal margin should be reported immediately. The nurse may mark the lower border on the client's abdomen with a water-soluble pencil. The upper border is found by percussing down from the clavicle along the intercostal spaces at the midclavicular line. This time, the note changes from resonant to dull (Figure 32-72). The liver's upper border is usually found in the fifth, sixth, or seventh intercostal space. The distance between the upper and lower liver borders should be 6 to 12 cm (2½ to 5 inches) at the right midclavicular line. Diseases such as **cirrhosis,** cancer, and **hepatitis** cause liver enlargement.

Kidney Tenderness. With the client sitting or standing erect, the nurse uses direct or indirect percussion to assess for kidney inflammation. With the ulnar surface of the partially closed fist, the nurse percusses posteriorly the costovertebral angle at the scapular line. If the kidneys are inflamed, the client feels tenderness during percussion.

Palpation

With palpation, beginning nurses are primarily concerned with detecting areas of abdominal tenderness and noting the quality of abnormal distentions or masses. As nurses become more skilled, they learn to palpate for specific organs such as the liver. Light and deep palpation are used.

After rubbing the hands together, the nurse uses light palpation over each quadrant. The nurse waits to palpate painful areas last. The nurse lays the palm of the hand with fingers extended and approximated lightly on the abdomen. The nurse keeps the palm and forearm horizontal (Figure 32-73). The pads of the fingertips depress approximately 1.3 cm (½ inch) in a gentle dipping mo-

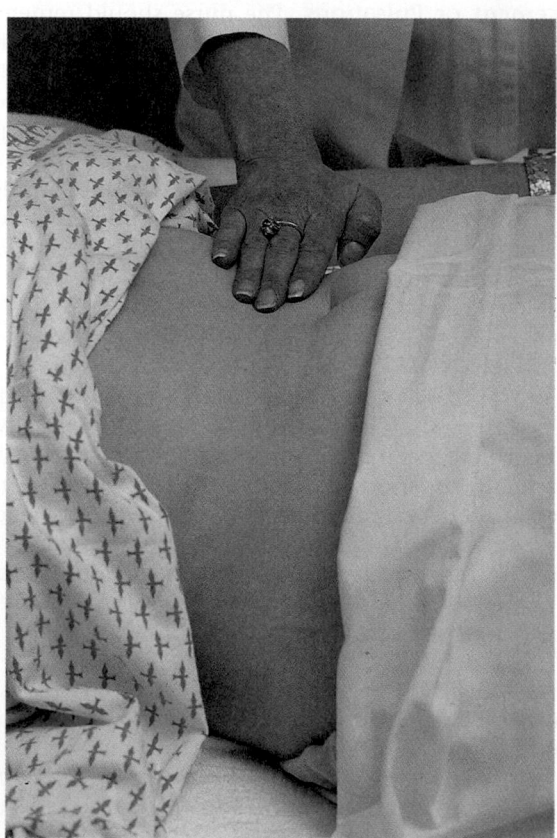

FIGURE **32–73**   Light palpation of abdomen.

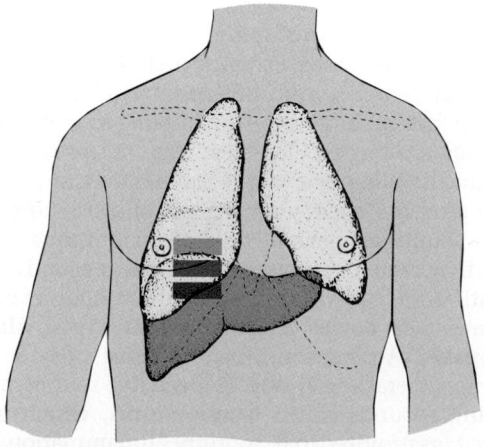

FIGURE **32–72**   To locate the liver's upper border, the nurse percusses downward, noting the change in sound from resonance (lung) to dullness (liver).

tion. The nurse avoids quick jabs and uses smooth, coordinated movements. If the client is ticklish, it may help to place the client's hand on the abdomen with the nurse's hand on the client's. This continues until the nurse can gradually remove the client's hand.

A systematic palpation of each quadrant assesses for muscular resistance, distention, tenderness, and superficial organs or masses. While palpating, the nurse observes the client's face for signs of discomfort. The abdomen is normally smooth with consistent softness and nontender without masses. The older adult often lacks abdominal tone. If the nurse palpates a sensitive area, guarding or muscle tenseness may occur. If tightening remains after the client is helped to relax, peritonitis, acute **cholecystitis,** or appendicitis may be the cause. A distended bladder is easy to detect with light palpation. Normally the bladder lies below the umbilicus and above the symphysis pubis. The nurse routinely checks for a distended bladder if a client has been unable to void (e.g., because of anesthesia or sedation) or has been incontinent, or if an indwelling urinary catheter is not draining well.

With experience the nurse can perform deep palpation to delineate abdominal organs and to detect less obvious masses. Short fingernails are needed. It is important for the client to be relaxed as the nurse's hands are depressed approximately 2.5 to 7.5 cm (1 to 3 inches) into the abdomen (Figure 32-74). Deep palpation is never used over a surgical incision or over extremely tender organs. It is also unwise to use palpation on abnormal masses. Deep pressure may cause tenderness in the healthy client over the cecum, sigmoid colon, aorta, and the midline near the xiphoid process (Seidel and others, 2003).

Each quadrant is surveyed systematically. Masses palpated are assessed for size, location, shape, consistency, tenderness, pulsation, and mobility. If tenderness is found, the examiner tests for rebound tenderness by pressing a hand slowly and deeply into the involved area and then letting go quickly. If pain is elicited with the release of the hand, the test is positive. Rebound tenderness occurs in clients with peritoneal irritation such as occurs in appendicitis; **pancreatitis;** or any peritoneal injury causing bile, blood, or enzymes to enter the peritoneal cavity.

Liver. The liver lies in the right upper quadrant under the rib cage. The nurse uses deep palpation to locate the liver's lower edge. This technique detects liver enlargement. To palpate the liver, the nurse places the left hand under the client's right posterior thorax at the eleventh and twelfth ribs and then applies upward pressure. This maneuver makes it easier to feel the liver anteriorly. With the fingers of the right hand pointing toward the right costal margin, the nurse places the hand on the right upper quadrant well below the liver's lower border. As the nurse presses gently in and up (Figure 32-75), the client takes a deep abdominal breath. As the client inhales, the nurse tries to palpate the liver's edge as it descends. A nor-

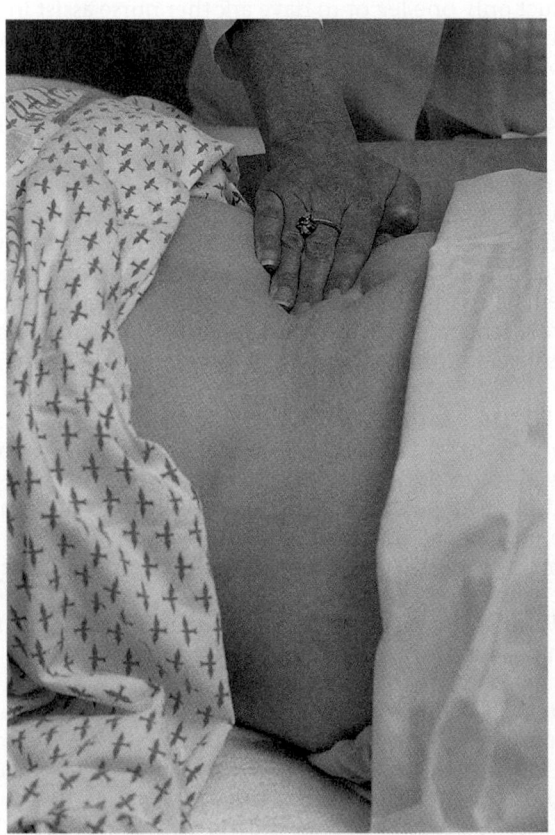

FIGURE **32–74**   Deep palpation of abdomen.

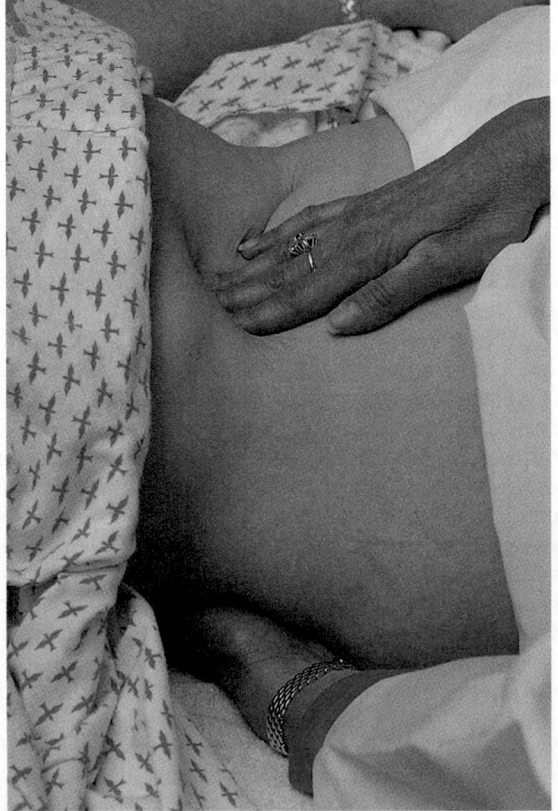

FIGURE **32–75**   The nurse's left hand is placed under the client's posterior thorax at the eleventh and twelfth ribs. The nurse's right hand palpates in and up to feel the liver's edge as the client inhales.

mal liver may not be palpable. However, it is nontender and has a firm, regular, and sharp edge. If the liver is palpable, the nurse traces its edge medially and laterally by repeating the maneuver.

Aortic Pulsation. To assess aortic pulsation, the nurse palpates with the thumb and forefinger of one hand deeply into the upper abdomen, just left of the midline. Normally a pulsation is transmitted forward. If there is enlargement of the aorta from an **aneurysm** (localized dilation of a vessel wall), the pulsation expands laterally. In obese clients it may be necessary to palpate with both hands, one on each side of the aorta.

> *Safety Alert.* When enlargement from an aneurysm is present, this area should only have light palpation. In addition, palpation of this area should only be performed by someone with advanced education and training.

Female Genitalia and Reproductive Tract

An examination of the female genitalia can be embarrassing for many women unless the nurse uses a calm and relaxed approach. The gynecological examination is one of the most difficult experiences for adolescents. Cultural background may further add to apprehension. For example, female Mexican-Americans have a strong social value that women do not expose their bodies to men or even to other women. Similarly, Chinese-Americans may believe that the examination of genitalia is offensive. The nurse must provide very thorough explanations as to the reason for the procedure used in the examination. The lithotomy position assumed during the examination is an added source of embarrassment. Comfort is established through correct positioning and draping. Each portion of the examination is explained in advance so that clients can anticipate the nurse's actions. Adolescents may choose to have parents present in the examination room.

The client may require a complete examination of the female reproductive organs, which includes assessment of the external genitalia and a vaginal examination. Most nurses do not perform a vaginal examination until they become nurse practitioners with extensive experience. However, it is important for the nurse to understand the procedure because a physician will require the nurse's assistance. An examination should be part of each woman's preventive health care because uterine cancers have a high incidence rate and ovarian cancer causes more deaths than any other cancer of the female reproductive system (ACS, 2003). Frequently a client will undergo an examination of external genitalia during routine hygiene measures or urinary catheter care.

Adolescents and young adults should be examined because of the growing incidence of sexually transmitted diseases (STDs). The average age of menarche among young girls has declined, and the majority of male and female teenagers are sexually active by age 19 (Hockenberry and others, 2003). As the nurse collects a history (Table 32-29), it is also important to assess the client's level of anxiety. The nurse should ask if the client has ever had a vaginal examination before. Rectal and anal assessment is easily combined with this examination because the client can assume a lithotomy or dorsal recumbent position.

Preparation of the Client

If a complete examination will be performed, the following special equipment will be needed: examination table with stirrups, vaginal speculum of correct size, adjustable light source, sink, clean disposable gloves, glass microscopic slides and coverslips, plastic spatula and/or cytobrush, and specimen bottles with fixative spray (hairspray).

Equipment must be ready before the examination begins. The client is asked to empty her bladder so that urine is not accidentally expelled during the examination. Often it is necessary to collect a urine specimen. The client is assisted in assuming the lithotomy position, in bed or on an examination table for an external genitalia assessment, and is assisted into stirrups if a speculum examination is to be performed. The woman stabilizes each foot in a stirrup and then slides her buttocks down to the edge of the examining table. The nurse places a hand at the edge of the table and instructs the client to move until touching the hand. The client's arms should be at her sides or folded across the chest to prevent tightening of abdominal muscles.

A woman suffering from pain or deformity of the joints may be unable to assume a lithotomy position. In this situation it may be necessary to have the client abduct only one leg or to have another nurse assist in separating the client's thighs. The side-lying position may also be used with the client on the left side with the right thigh and knee drawn up to her chest.

A square drape or sheet is given to the client. She holds one corner over her sternum, the adjacent corners fall over each knee, and the fourth corner covers the perineum. Once the examination begins, the drape over the perineum is lifted. The male examiner should always have a female attendant present during the examination. A female examiner may prefer to work alone but should have a female attendant if the client is particularly anxious or emotionally unstable.

External Genitalia

The perineal area must be well illuminated. The nurse gloves both hands to prevent contact with infectious organisms. The perineum is extremely sensitive and tender. The area is not touched suddenly without warning the client. It is best to touch the neighboring thigh first before advancing to the perineum.

To assess sexual maturity, the quantity and distribution of hair growth is noted. A preadolescent has no pubic hair except for fine body hair like that on the abdomen. During adolescence, hair grows along the labia, becoming darker, coarser, and curlier as it spreads over the pubic symphysis. Hair growth eventually forms a triangle over the female perineum and along the medial surfaces of the thighs. Hair growth should not spread up over the abdomen. Hair should be free of nits and lice. The underlying skin should be free of inflammation, irritation, or lesions.

Table 32-29	Nursing History for Female Genitalia and Reproductive Tract Assessment
Assessment Category	**Rationale**
Determine if client has had previous illness or surgery involving reproductive organs, including STD.	Illness or surgery can influence appearance and position of organs being examined.
Review menstrual history, including age at menarche, frequency and duration of menstrual cycle, character of flow (e.g., amount, presence of clots), presence of dysmenorrhea (painful menstruation), pelvic pain, dates of last two menstrual periods, and premenstrual symptoms.	This information helps to reveal level of reproductive health, including normalcy of menstrual cycle.
Ask client to describe obstetrical history, including each pregnancy and history of abortions or miscarriages.	Observed physical findings will vary, depending on woman's history of pregnancy.
Ask client to describe current and past contraceptive practices and problems encountered. Determine whether client uses safe sex practices. Discuss risk of STDs and HIV infection.	Use of certain types of contraceptives may influence reproductive health (e.g., sensitivity reaction to spermicidal jelly). Sexual history reveals risk for and understanding of STDs.
Assess if client has signs and symptoms of vaginal discharge, painful or swollen perianal tissues, or genital lesions.	These signs and symptoms indicate STD.
Determine if client has symptoms or history of genitourinary problems, including burning during urination, frequency, urgency, nocturia, hematuria, incontinence, or stress incontinence (see Chapter 44).	Urinary problems may be associated with gynecological disorders, including STDs.
Ask if client has had signs of bleeding outside of normal menstrual period or after menopause or has had unusual vaginal discharge.	These are warning signs for cervical and endometrial cancer.
Determine if client is between ages 40 and 50 and has history of condyloma acuminatum, herpes simplex, or cervical dysplasia; has multiple sex partners; smokes; has had multiple pregnancies; or was young at first intercourse.	These are risk factors for cervical cancer (ACS, 2003).
Determine if client is between ages 40 and 60 and has history of ovarian dysfunction, breast or endometrial cancer, irradiation of pelvic organs, or endometriosis; has family history of ovarian or breast cancer; or has history of infertility or nulliparity.	These are risk factors for ovarian cancer (ACS, 2003).
Determine if client is postmenopausal, obese, or infertile; had early menarche (before age 12); had late menopause (after age 50); has history of hypertension, diabetes, or gallbladder disease; has family history of endometrial, breast, or colon cancer; or has a history of estrogen-related exposure (ERT, tamoxifen use).	These are risk factors for endometrial cancer (ACS, 2003).

The nurse inspects surface characteristics of the labia majora. The skin of the perineum is smooth, clean, and slightly darker than other skin. The mucous membranes appear dark pink and moist. The labia majora may be gaping or closed and appear dry or moist. They are usually symmetrical. After childbirth the labia majora are separated, causing the labia minora to become more prominent. When a woman reaches menopause, the labia majora become thinned, and with advancing age, they become atrophied. The labia majora are normally without inflammation, edema, lesions, or lacerations.

To inspect the remaining external structures, the nurse gently places the thumb and index finger of the nondominant hand inside the labia minora and retracts the tissues outwardly (Figure 32-76). The nurse should have a firm hold to avoid repeated retraction against the sensitive tissues. The nurse uses the other hand to palpate the labia minora between the thumb and second finger. On inspection, the labia minora are normally thinner than the labia majora, and one side may be larger. The tissue should feel soft on palpation and without tenderness. The size of the clitoris is variable. However, it normally is about 2 cm (⅘ inch) or less in length and 0.5 cm (⅕ inch) in width. The nurse looks for atrophy, inflammation, or adhesions. If inflamed, the clitoris will be a bright cherry red. In young women it is a common site for syphilitic lesions, or **chancres,** which appear as small open ulcers that drain serous material. Older women may have malignant changes that result in dry, scaly, nodular lesions.

The urethral orifice is carefully observed for color and position. It is normally intact without inflammation. The urethral meatus is anterior to the vaginal orifice and is pink. At times it is difficult to locate. It may appear as a small slit or pinhole opening just above the vaginal canal. In women who have had several vaginal childbirths, the opening to the vaginal canal often extends upward, interfering with the view of the urethra. The nurse notes any discharge, polyps, or fistulas.

When inspecting the vaginal orifice (introitus), the nurse inspects for inflammation, edema, discoloration, discharge, and lesions. Normally the introitus is a thin, vertical slit or a large orifice. The tissue is moist. The hymen is just inside the introitus. In the virgin the hymen may restrict the opening of the vagina. Only remnants of the hymen remain after sexual intercourse.

With the labia still retracted, the nurse examines Skene's and Bartholin's glands. The client is told that the nurse is going to insert one finger into the client's vagina and that she will feel pressure. With the palm facing upward, the nurse inserts an index finger of the examining hand into the vagina as far as the second joint. Exerting upward pressure, the nurse milks Skene's glands by mov-

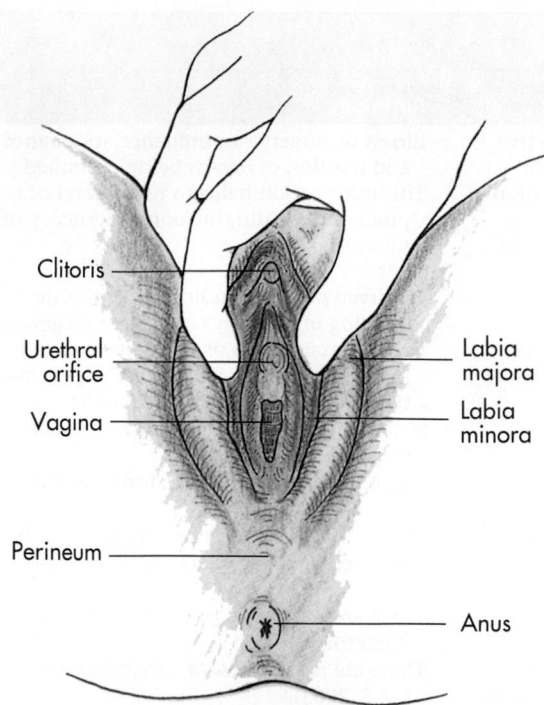

FIGURE 32–76   Female external genitalia.

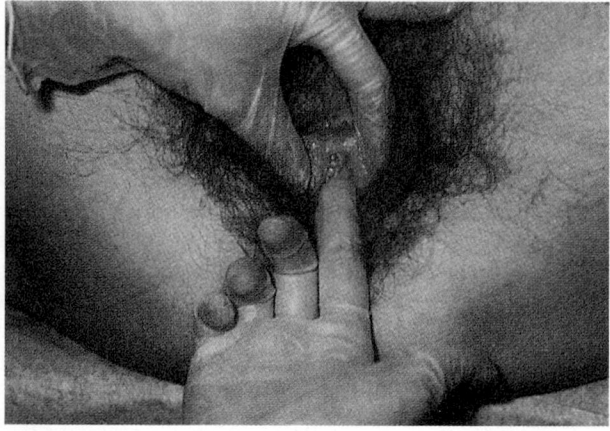

FIGURE 32–77   Milking the urethra and paraurethral glands.

ing the finger outward. Discharge and tenderness are abnormal. The examination is done on both sides of the urethra and then directly on the urethra (Figure 32-77). The technique may cause discharge to appear. If so, the nurse notes the color, odor, and consistency and obtains a culture. The nurse then changes into a new pair of gloves.

If inflammation and edema are found near the posterior end of the introitus, Bartholin's glands may be infected. The glands cannot normally be palpated. To attempt palpation, the nurse places a thumb and index finger between the labia majora and introitus and palpates one side at a time.

With the gloved index and middle fingers in the vaginal orifice, the nurse asks the client to strain downward as

if she were voiding. If the client lacks adequate muscular support, the vaginal walls bulge, blocking the introitus. A portion of the vaginal wall and bladder may prolapse or fall into the orifice anteriorly; this is a **cystocele.** Bulging of the posterior wall may be caused by prolapse of the rectum **(rectocele).** Normally when a client is asked to constrict or close the vaginal orifice, the nurse palpates tension in the muscles. A woman who has undergone vaginal childbirth has less muscle tone than one who has not.

The nurse may also inspect the anus at this time, looking for lesions and hemorrhoids (see section on rectal ex-

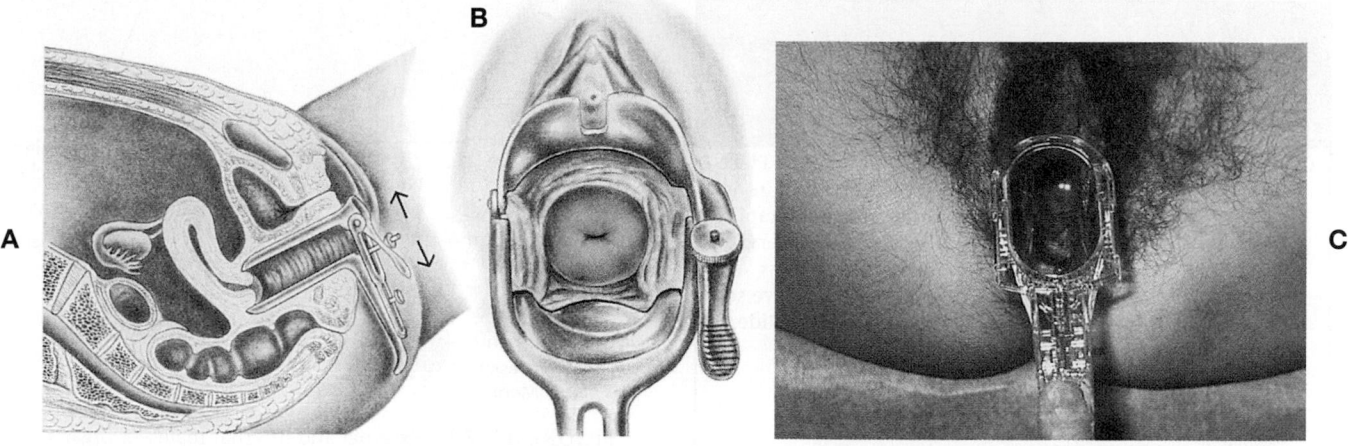

FIGURE 32–78 **A,** Angle of speculum insertion. **B,** View of cervix. **C,** Vaginal speculum in place with cervix in full view.

amination). If the nurse performs only the external examination, the examination gloves are disposed of at this time. The client is then offered perineal hygiene if the skin is soiled with secretions.

Clients who are at risk for contracting an STD should learn to perform a genital self-examination (GSE) (Box 32-26). The purpose is to detect any signs or symptoms of an STD. Many persons do not know they have an STD, and some STDs can remain undetected for years.

Speculum Examination of Internal Genitalia

An examination of the internal genitalia requires much skill and practice. Usually it is performed only by advanced nurse practitioners or nurse-midwives. Beginning students will probably only observe the procedure or assist the examiner.

The examination involves use of a plastic or metal speculum. Consisting of two blades and an adjustable thumbscrew, the speculum is inserted into the vagina to assess the internal genitalia for cancerous lesions and other abnormalities. During the examination a **Papanicolaou (Pap) smear** is collected to test for cervical and vaginal cancer.

To assist an examiner, the nurse makes sure that the client is comfortably positioned in the stirrups. A variety of speculum sizes (small, medium, large) should be available so that the examiner may select the appropriate size for the client. The smallest size will fit a virgin. If the woman is sexually active, a medium-sized speculum is best. For women who have had children vaginally, the examiner uses a medium-to-large speculum.

In addition, the nurse will have gloves, specimen slides, and a spatula and/or cytobrush close at hand. Water-soluble lubricant is used only when specimens are not being collected. Most examiners lubricate the speculum with warm water.

Cervix. The first portion of the examination involves careful insertion of the speculum until the examiner can fully visualize the cervix (Figure 32-78). The examiner sits on a

stool facing the client's perineum. The adjustable light is placed over the examiner's shoulder, directed at the examination site. The examiner holds the speculum in the dominant hand and explains the procedure to the client. If the woman has never been examined, two fingers are gently inserted into the vagina to explore for abnormalities. Then with two fingers the examiner presses down on the perineal body just inside the introitus. After checking to be sure that the speculum blades are closed, the examiner introduces the closed speculum obliquely (rotated 50 degrees counterclockwise from the vertical position) past the fingers. The speculum is inserted downward at a 45-degree angle toward the examination table to avoid trauma to the urethra (this maneuver corresponds with the normal downward slope of the vaginal canal). Care is taken to avoid pulling the pubic hair or pinching the labia.

After the wide portions of the blades have passed the introitus, the speculum is rotated so that the blades are horizontal. The blades are opened slowly after full insertion, and the speculum is moved to visualize the cervix. When the cervix is in full view, the blades are locked in the open position. The examiner inspects the cervix for color, appearance of the os or opening, position, size, surface characteristics, and discharge. The normal cervix is glistening pink, smooth, and round. Its diameter is 2.5 to 3 cm (about 1 inch) in a young woman and smaller in an older adult. The cervix should be midline and without lesions.

Papanicolaou Smear. The surface of the cervix at the cervical canal opening is lined with layers of vaginal squamous cells. The cells meet a different group of cells—columnar cells. The columnar cells secrete mucus and line the passageway that leads up into the central cavity of the uterus. The squamous cells have a protective role for the cervix, and the columnar cells have a reproductive role (helping sperm to enter the uterus for fertilization). A Pap smear is a painless screening test for cervical cancer. Specimens are taken from the endocervix and ectocervix (Table 32-30). The test is simple and has no side effects. It should be performed annually with a pelvic examination in women who are, or have been, sexually active, and in women who have reached the age of 18. After three or

Table 32-30	Methods for Obtaining Pap Smears
Location	**Technique**
Outer cervix 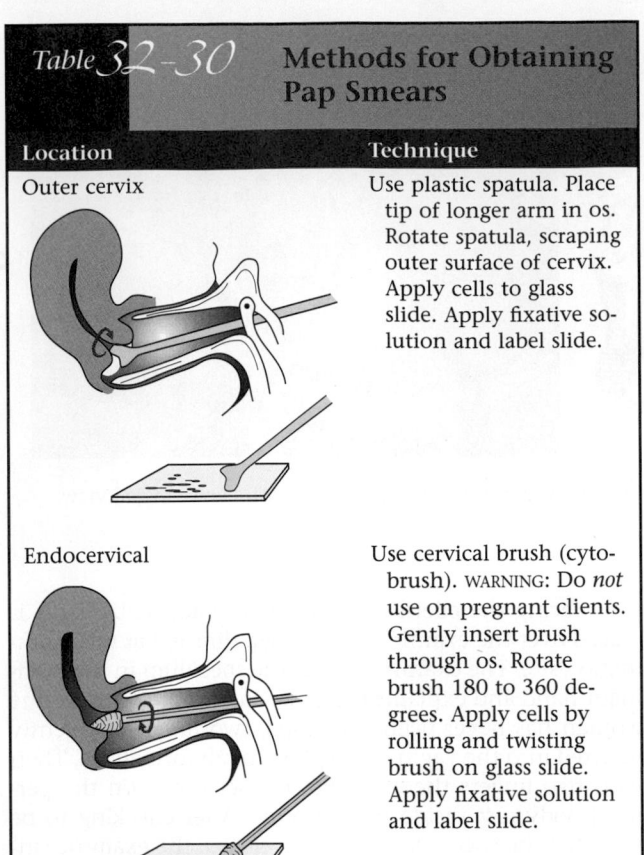	Use plastic spatula. Place tip of longer arm in os. Rotate spatula, scraping outer surface of cervix. Apply cells to glass slide. Apply fixative solution and label slide.
Endocervical	Use cervical brush (cytobrush). WARNING: Do *not* use on pregnant clients. Gently insert brush through os. Rotate brush 180 to 360 degrees. Apply cells by rolling and twisting brush on glass slide. Apply fixative solution and label slide.

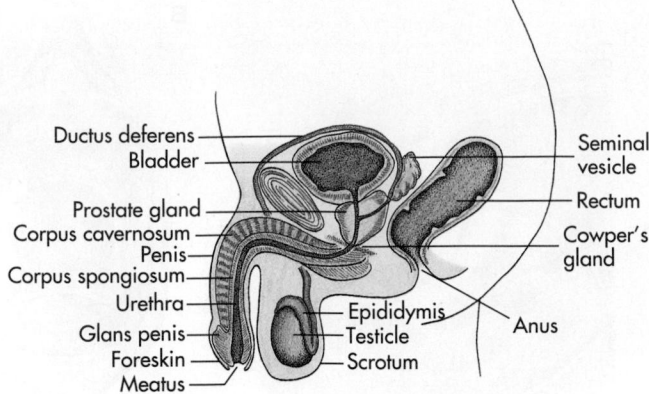

FIGURE **32–79** External and internal male sex organs.

more consecutive annual examinations with normal findings, the Pap test may be done less often at the discretion of the physician. Women at high risk for cervical cancer and those over 40 should have annual checkups.

The examiner first collects a sample of the outer cervix or ectocervix. A plastic spatula is rotated 360 degrees against the cervical surface. Once the spatula is withdrawn, the examiner spreads the specimen lightly over a glass slide. The nurse who is assisting sprays the specimen with cytological fixative and labels the slide. The examiner next uses a cytobrush to collect endocervical cells. The cytobrush is inserted into the cervical os and rotated one full turn. The specimen is then spread across the slide by rolling the brush with moderate pressure. The specimen is sprayed again, and the slide is labeled. At the end of the procedure the nurse warns the client that blood spotting is normal for a few hours.

There is also a paintbrush device (Cervex-brush) that can be used to collect both specimens at the same time. It uses flexible plastic bristles, which reportedly cause less blood spotting (Seidel and others, 2003).

Vagina. Once specimens are collected, the examiner views the vaginal walls as the speculum is slowly withdrawn. As the speculum leaves the cervix, the thumbscrew is loosened, but the blades are kept open with the thumb. During the withdrawal the examiner notes the color, surface characteristics, and secretions. The vaginal walls are normally pink throughout and free from discharge and lesions. The surface should be moist and smooth or rugated.

Normal secretions are thin, clear or cloudy, and odorless. Women commonly acquire yeast infections, causing a thick, white, patchy, malodorous, curdlike discharge.

After speculum withdrawal the nurse assists the client to a sitting position and allows the client to dress and perform hygiene. In a hospital setting the client may need assistance with perineal hygiene. The nurse makes sure the gloves, speculum, and other disposable equipment are appropriately discarded in a receptacle. The client is informed that Pap smear results will be available in 3 to 4 days (check agency policy).

*M*ale Genitalia

An examination of the male genitalia includes assessment of the external genitalia (Figure 32-79) and the inguinal ring and canal. Because the incidence of STDs in adolescents and young adults is high, an assessment of the genitalia should be a routine part of any health maintenance examination for this age-group (Box 32-27). The client may be lying or standing for this part of the examination. Inspection and palpation are used. The nurse applies disposable gloves to prevent the chance of cross infection from urethral discharge.

The nurse uses a calm and gentle approach to lessen the client's anxiety. Often adolescents and men are fearful of having an erection during the examination. Boys and adolescents may worry about their genitals being normal. The nurse should limit discussion of the client's sexual activity during the examination because the client might perceive this as evaluative or judgmental. The client's modesty must be preserved. It may help to provide teaching after the examination. Do not joke or use nonverbal expressions that may convey concern or worry. The genitalia are gently manipulated to avoid causing erection or discomfort. A thorough nursing history (Table 32-31) before the examination ensures that the assessment will be complete.

Sexual Maturity

The nurse begins by assessing the sexual maturity of the client, noting the size and shape of the penis and testes, the color and texture of the scrotal skin, and the character and distribution of pubic hair. The first sign of puberty, an

Male Genitalia Assessment

Objectives

- Client will describe methods to prevent transmission of STDs.
- Client will perform genital self-examination.
- Client with an STD will follow safe sex practices.

Teaching Strategies

- Counsel client with an STD about diagnosis and treatment.
- Teach measures to prevent STDs:
  - Use of condoms
  - Avoiding sex with partner who is infected
    - Restricting number of sexual partners
    - Avoiding sex with persons who have multiple partners
    - Using regular perineal hygiene
  - Tell clients with an STD that sexual partners must be informed of the need to have an examination.
  - Instruct client on how to perform genital self-examination (see Box 32-28, p. 752).

Evaluation

- Ask client to describe methods for treating and preventing STDs.
- During a follow-up visit, determine whether client with an STD has used safe sex practices.

Table **32-31** **Nursing History for Male Genitalia Assessment**

Assessment Category	Rationale
Review normal urinary elimination pattern, including frequency of voiding; history of nocturia; character and volume of urine; daily fluid intake; symptoms of burning, urgency, and frequency; difficulty starting stream; and hematuria (see Chapter 44).	Urinary problems can be directly associated with genitourinary problems because of anatomical structure of men's reproductive and urinary systems.
Assess client's sexual history and use of safe sex habits (multiple partners, infection in partners, failure to use condom).	Sexual history reveals risk for and understanding of STDs and HIV.
Determine if client has had previous surgery or illness involving urinary or reproductive organs, including STD.	Alterations resulting from disease or surgery may be responsible for symptoms or changes in organ structure or function.
Ask if client has noted penile pain or swelling, genital lesions, or urethral discharge.	These signs and symptoms indicate STD.
Determine if client has noticed heaviness or painless enlargement of testis or irregular lumps.	These signs and symptoms are early warning signs for testicular cancer.
If client reports an enlargement in inguinal area, assess if it is intermittent or constant, associated with straining or lifting, and painful, and whether pain is affected by coughing, lifting, or straining at stool.	Signs and symptoms reflect potential inguinal hernia.
Ask if client has difficulty achieving erection or ejaculation; also review whether client is taking diuretics, sedatives, antihypertensives, or tranquilizers.	These medications may influence sexual performance.

---

increase in genital and pubic hair development, is variable but generally does not start before 9½ years of age. During the preadolescent stage there is no pubic hair except for the fine body hair found on the abdomen. By puberty the pubic hair extends from the base of the penis over the symphysis pubis and becomes coarse and curly. The testes and penis develop, with the scrotal skin darkening and becoming thinner and more wrinkled in texture. The penis slowly lengthens, eventually reaching to the bottom of the scrotum (Figure 32-80). The nurse inspects the skin covering the genitalia for lice, rashes, excoriations, or lesions.

Penis

The nurse inspects the structures of the penis, including the shaft, corona, prepuce (foreskin), glans, and urethral meatus. The dorsal vein should be apparent on inspection. In uncircumcised males the foreskin is retracted to reveal

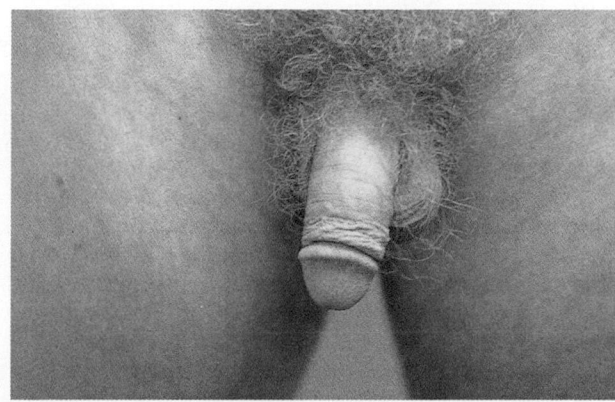

FIGURE **32-80** Normal male genitalia (circumcised). (From Seidel HM and others: *Mosby's guide to physical examination*, ed 5, St. Louis, 2003, Mosby.)

the glans and urethral meatus. The foreskin should retract easily. A small amount of thick, white secretion between the glans and foreskin is normal. If there is evidence of abnormal discharge, a culture is usually obtained. The urethral meatus is slitlike and should be positioned on the ventral surface just millimeters from the tip of the glans. In some congenital conditions the meatus is displaced along the penile shaft. Gentle compression of the glans between the nurse's thumb and index finger opens the urethral meatus to allow inspection for discharge. The opening should be glistening and pink. The meatus is also inspected for lesions, edema, and inflammation.

The glans is carefully checked around its entire circumference for lesions. The area between the foreskin and glans is a common site for venereal lesions. Any lesion is palpated gently to note tenderness, size, consistency, and shape.

The nurse continues to inspect the entire shaft of the penis, including the undersurface, looking for lesions, scars, and edema. The shaft is palpated between the thumb and first two fingers to detect any localized areas of hardness and tenderness. When inspection and palpation of the penis is completed, the foreskin is pulled down to its original position. It is important for any male client to learn to perform a genital self-examination to detect signs or symptoms of an STD. Many people who have an STD do not know it. A self-examination should be a routine part of self-care (Box 32-28).

Box 32-28   Male Genital Self-Examination

All men 15 years and older should perform this examination monthly using the following steps.

Genital Examination

Perform the examination after a warm bath or shower when the scrotal sac is relaxed.

Stand naked in front of a mirror and hold the penis in your hand and examine the head. Pull back the foreskin if uncircumcised.

Inspect and palpate the entire head of the penis in a clockwise motion, looking carefully for any bumps, sores, or blisters.

Look also for any bumpy warts (see illustration).

Look at the opening at the end of the penis for discharge.

Look along the entire shaft of the penis for the same signs.

Be sure to separate pubic hair at the base of the penis and carefully examine the skin underneath.

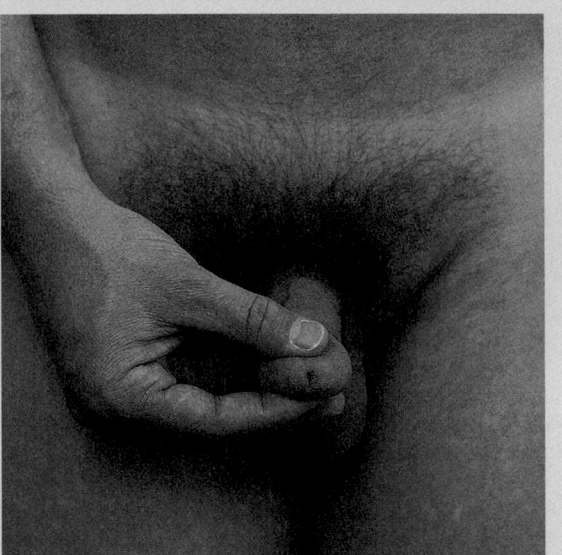

Testicular Self-Examination

Look for swelling or lumps in the skin of the scrotum while looking in the mirror.

Use both hands, placing the index and middle fingers under the testicles and the thumb on top (see illustration).

Gently roll the testicle, feeling for lumps, thickening, or a change in consistency (hardening).

Find the epididymis (a cordlike structure on the top and back of the testicle; it is not a lump).

Feel for small, pea-sized lumps on the front and side of the testicle. The lumps are usually painless and are abnormal.

Call your physician if you find a lump.

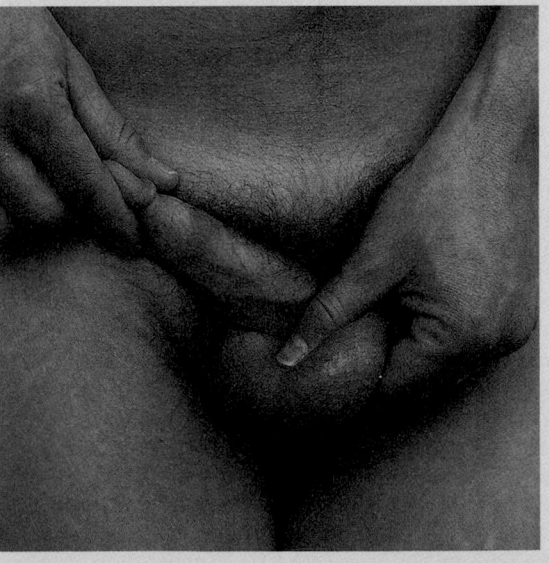

Illustrations from Seidel HM and others: *Mosby's guide to physical examination*, ed 5, St. Louis, 2003, Mosby.

Scrotum

The nurse must be particularly cautious when inspecting and palpating the scrotum because the structures lying within the scrotal sac are very sensitive. The scrotum is a saclike structure divided internally into two halves. Each half contains a testicle, epididymis, and the vas deferens, which travels upward into the inguinal ring. Normally the left testicle is lower than the right. The nurse inspects the scrotum's size, shape, and symmetry while observing for lesions or edema. The scrotum is usually more deeply pigmented than the body skin, and the surface is coarse. It is gently lifted to view the posterior surface. The scrotal skin is usually loose. A tightening of the skin may reveal edema. The scrotum's size normally changes with temperature variations as the dartos muscle contracts in cold and relaxes in warm temperatures.

Testicular cancer has become a common solid tumor among young men ages 18 to 34 years. Early detection is critical, and thus clients must learn to perform testicular self-examination (TSE) (see Box 32-28). The nurse can explain the technique while examining the client. The underlying testicles are normally ovoid and approximately 2 to 4 cm (⅘ to 1⅗ inches) in size. The testicles and epididymis are gently palpated between the nurse's thumb and first two fingers. They should be sensitive to gentle compression but not tender, and they should feel smooth, rubbery, and free of nodules. The most common symptoms of testicular cancer are a painless enlargement of one testis and the appearance of a palpable, small, hard lump, about the size of a pea, on the front or side of the testicle. The size, shape, and consistency of the organs are noted. In the older man the testicles decrease in size and are less firm during palpation. The client should be asked about any unusual tenderness. The nurse continues palpating the vas deferens separately as it forms the spermatic cord toward the inguinal ring, noting the presence of nodules or swelling. It normally feels smooth and discrete.

Inguinal Ring and Canal

The external inguinal ring provides the opening for the spermatic cord to pass into the inguinal canal. The canal forms a passage through the abdominal wall, a potential site for hernia formation. A hernia is a protrusion of a portion of intestine through the inguinal wall or canal. An intestinal loop may even enter the scrotum. The client stands during this portion of the examination.

During inspection the client is asked to strain or bear down. The maneuver helps make a hernia more visible. The nurse looks for obvious bulging. The nurse next palpates the inguinal ring and canal to be sure a hernia is not present. Standing on the right side of the client, the nurse places the index finger of the examining hand against the scrotal skin low on the right side. Gently the nurse moves the finger toward the inguinal canal with the folds of the scrotal tissue covering the finger. Carrying the index finger upward along the vas deferens into the inguinal canal, the nurse follows the spermatic cord. It is important not to force the finger into the canal. When the finger reaches the farthest point along the canal, the nurse asks the client to cough and strain down. The maneuver is repeated on the left side. As the client strains,

no bulging pressure will be felt. A tightening around the finger is normal.

The nurse completes the examination by palpating for inguinal lymph nodes. Small, nontender, mobile horizontal nodes may normally be found. Any abnormality may indicate local or systemic infection or malignant disease.

Rectum and Anus

A good time to perform the rectal examination is after the genital examination. Usually the examination is not performed in young children or adolescents. The examination can detect colorectal cancer in its early stages. In men the rectal examination can also detect prostatic tumors. The nurse collects a thorough history (Table 32-32) to detect the client's risk for bowel or rectal disease or prostatic disease.

The rectal examination can be uncomfortable and embarrassing, so the nurse uses a calm, slow-paced, gentle approach. Explanation of the steps of the procedure helps clients to relax and lessens discomfort during the digital examination. Women can be examined immediately after examination of the genitalia while they are still in a dorsal recumbent position. Otherwise the left lateral side-lying (Sims') position is preferred. Men are best examined by having the client bend over forward with his hips flexed and upper body resting across the examination table. A nonambulatory client can be examined in Sims' position. Clients are draped with only the anal area exposed. The nurse applies disposable gloves for the examination.

Inspection

The nurse begins by inspecting the perianal and sacrococcygeal areas. The skin should be smooth and uninterrupted. The nurse looks for lumps, rashes, inflammation, excoriation, and scars. Fungal infection can cause perianal irritation.

Using the nondominant hand, the nurse gently retracts the buttocks apart to inspect the anus. Anal tissues are normally moist and hairless compared with perianal skin. The tissue is coarser and more darkly pigmented. The anus is held closed by the voluntary external muscle sphincter. The nurse inspects anal tissue for skin lesions, external **hemorrhoids** (dilated veins that appear as reddened protrusions), fissures and fistulas, inflammation, rashes, or discoloration. Next, the nurse asks the client to bear down as though having a bowel movement. Any internal hemorrhoids, fistulas, fissures, or polyps will appear at this time. Normally the anal lining is intact.

Digital Palpation

Some institutions do not permit nurses to perform digital examinations. In institutions where it is permitted, the nursing student should have a qualified examiner present during the first examination.

The nurse lubricates the index finger of the gloved dominant hand. The procedure is explained, and then the client is asked to bear down gently as if having a bowel movement. As the anal sphincter relaxes, the nurse's fingertip is gently slipped into the anal canal in a

Table 32-32	Nursing History for Rectal and Anal Assessment
Assessment Category	**Rationale**
Determine whether client has experienced bleeding from rectum, black or tarry stools (melena), rectal pain, or change in bowel habits (constipation or diarrhea).	These are warning signs of colorectal cancer* or other gastrointestinal alterations.
Determine whether client has personal or strong family history of colorectal cancer, polyps, or chronic inflammatory bowel disease. Ask if client is over age 40.	These are risk factors for colorectal cancer.*
Assess dietary habits for high-fat intake or deficient fiber content.	Bowel cancer may be linked to dietary intake of fat or insufficient fiber intake.*
Determine whether client has undergone screening for colorectal cancer (digital examination, fecal occult blood test, flexible sigmoidoscopy, and colonoscopy).	Undergoing this screening reflects understanding and compliance with preventive health care measures.
Assess medication history for use of laxatives or cathartic medications.	Repeated use can cause diarrhea and eventual loss of intestinal muscle tone.
Assess for use of codeine or iron preparations.	Codeine causes constipation. Iron turns the color of feces black and tarry.
Ask male client if weak or interrupted urine flow, inability to urinate, difficulty in starting or stopping urine flow, polyuria, nocturia, hematuria, or dysuria has been experienced. Does client have continuing pain in lower back, pelvis, or upper thighs?	These are warning signs of prostatic cancer.* Symptoms also can suggest infection or prostate enlargement.

*Data from American Cancer Society: *Cancer facts and figures 2003,* New York, 2003, The Society.

Client Teaching

Box 32-29

Rectal and Anal Assessment

Objectives

- Client will have a regular digital examination performed appropriate to age.
- Client will be able to identify symptoms of colorectal and prostatic cancer.
- Client will follow a diet of increased fiber and reduced fat.

Teaching Strategies

- Discuss the ACS's guidelines (2003) for early detection of colorectal cancer:
  - Digital rectal examination yearly after age 50
  - Fecal occult blood test (FOBT) yearly after age 50
  - Flexible sigmoidoscopy (FSIG): visual inspection of the rectum and lower colon with a hollow, lighted tube, performed by a physician every 5 years after age 50 on the advice of a physician
  - Colonoscopy every 10 years
  - Individuals at increased risk should discuss options with their health care professional.
- Discuss warning signs of colorectal cancer (see Tables 32-6, p. 683 and 32-32).

- Discuss dietary planning to reduce fat and increase fiber content.
- Warn client against problems caused by overuse of laxatives, cathartic medications, codeine, or enemas.
- Discuss with male client the ACS's guidelines (2003) for early detection of prostatic cancer:
  - Digital rectal examination performed annually after age 50
  - Annual prostate-specific antigen (PSA) blood test for men age 50 and over
  - Prostate ultrasound testing if results of either digital rectal examination or PSA test are suspicious
  - African-American men or those with a first-degree relative diagnosed with prostate cancer should begin testing at age 45
  - Warning signs of prostatic cancer

Evaluation

- During follow-up visits, determine whether client has had a rectal examination performed.
- Have client explain warning signs of colorectal and prostatic cancer.
- Ask client to describe foods high in fiber and low in fat.

---

direction toward the umbilicus. Normally the client feels as though stool is being passed. The nurse never forces digital insertion, so mucosal tissues are not injured.

The anal canal is the distal portion of the gastrointestinal tract. The canal extends in a line toward the umbilicus before turning into the mucus-lined rectum. The anus contains a rich supply of sensory nerve fibers. Thus digital manipulation can be painful. At the junction of the anal

canal and rectum, the rectum balloons out and turns posteriorly into the hollow of the coccyx and sacrum.

Initially the nurse notes the tone of the anal sphincter as the muscle closes snugly around the finger. After asking the client to tighten the sphincter around the finger, the nurse notes sphincter tone. The sphincter should tighten evenly without discomfort. A weak sphincter may indicate a neurological problem. Acute rectal pain is not

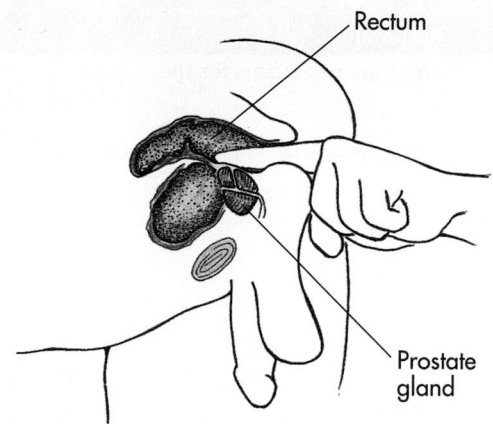

Rectum

Prostate
gland

FIGURE **32–81** Palpation of prostate gland during rectal examination.

normal. Irritation, fissures, inflamed hemorrhoids, or rock-hard constipation can be the source of discomfort.

Beyond the anal canal the nurse palpates each side of the rectal wall for tenderness, irregularities, polyps, masses, or nodules. The wall should feel even and smooth. After the finger is advanced fully, the client is asked to bear down again. High lesions within the rectum will descend against the fingertip (Box 32-29).

In men the nurse turns the hand so that the finger palpates the anterior rectal wall. The client should be warned that he may feel the urge to urinate, but that he will not. The prostate gland is palpable anteriorly as a rounded, heart-shaped structure about 2.5 to 4 cm (1 to 1½ inches) in diameter with less than 1 cm (½ in) protrusion into the rectum (Figure 32-81). A small medial groove separates the gland into two lateral lobes. The nurse palpates the size, shape, and consistency of the prostate. The gland normally is firm, without bogginess, tenderness, or nodules. Hardness or nodules may indicate the presence of a cancerous lesion. Prostate enlargement is classified by the amount of projection into the rectum: grade I is 1 to 2 cm protrusion; grade II, 2 to 3 cm; grade III, 3 to 4 cm; grade IV, more than 4 cm (Seidel and others, 2003).

In women it may be possible to palpate the cervix through the anterior rectal wall. It is common to mistake the cervix or an inserted tampon for a rectal tumor.

After palpation is completed, the nurse gently withdraws the finger and observes it for feces. Feces are normally brown. The presence of mucus; blood; or black, tarry stool should be reported. A sample of the feces is tested for occult blood (see Chapter 45). For women suspected of having an STD, a rectal culture may be taken to rule out cross infection from vaginal discharge. The nurse cleans the perianal area before continuing to the next part of the examination.

Musculoskeletal System

The nurse can learn to integrate portions of the musculoskeletal assessment when the client walks, moves in bed, or performs any type of physical activity. The assessment of musculoskeletal function focuses on determining range of joint motion, muscle strength and tone, and joint and muscle condition. Assessment of musculoskeletal integrity is especially important when the client reports pain or loss of function in a joint or muscle. Frequently, muscular disorders are manifestations of neurological disease. For this reason, a neurological assessment is often conducted simultaneously.

It is important to review the anatomy of bone and muscle placement and joint structure (see Chapter 46). Joints vary in their degree of mobility. Some, as in the knee, are freely movable. The spinal vertebrae are examples of slightly movable joints.

The examination uses inspection and palpation. The muscles and joints should be exposed and free to move. Depending on the muscle groups assessed, the client assumes a sitting, supine, prone, or standing position. Table 32-33 lists the information gathered in the nursing history.

General Inspection

The nurse observes the client's gait and the anterior, posterior, and lateral aspects of the client's posture as the client walks into and stands in the examination room. When the client is unaware of the nature of the observations, the gait is more natural. Later a more formal test involves having the client walk in a straight line away from the nurse and then return. The nurse looks for foot dragging, limping, shuffling, and the position of the trunk in relation to the legs. Normally the client walks with the arms swinging freely at the sides and the head and face leading the body. An older adult often walks with smaller steps and a wider base of support.

The normal standing posture is an upright stance with parallel alignment of the hips and shoulders (Figure 32-82). There should be an even contour of the shoulders, level scapulae and iliac crests, alignment of the head over the gluteal folds, and symmetry of extremities. Looking sideways at the client, the nurse notes the normal cervical, thoracic, and lumbar curves. The head is held erect. As the client sits, some degree of rounding of the shoulders is normal. Older adults tend to assume a stooped, forward-bent posture with the hips and knees somewhat flexed and arms bent at the elbows, raising the level of the arms.

Common postural abnormalities include lordosis, kyphosis, and scoliosis (Figure 32-83). **Kyphosis,** or hunchback, is an exaggeration of the posterior curvature of the thoracic spine. This postural abnormality is common in the older adult. **Lordosis,** or swayback, is an increased lumbar curvature. A lateral spinal curvature is called **scoliosis.** Loss of height is frequently the first clinical sign of **osteoporosis,** in which height loss occurs in the trunk as a result of vertebral fracture and collapse (Pachucki-Hyde, 2001). Osteoporosis is a metabolic bone disease that causes a decrease in quality and quantity of bone and affects over 20 million Americans (Wishnia, 2001). Kessenich (2000) reports that over 28 million Americans are at risk for development of this disease, with 20% of these individuals being men. Although a small amount of height loss is to be expected with aging, if the amount of loss is greater than expected, osteoporosis is likely (Box 32-30). As men and women age, they are more likely to have osteoporotic fractures of the wrists, hips, and vertebrae (Kessenich, 2000; Pachucki-Hyde, 2001).

Table **32-33**   **Nursing History for Musculoskeletal Assessment**

Assessment Category	Rationale
Determine if client is involved in competitive sports (particularly involving collision and contact), fails to warm up adequately, is in poor physical condition, or had had a rapid growth spurt (adolescents).	These are risk factors for sports injury.
Review client history for heavy alcohol use; cigarette smoking; constant dieting; calcium intake less than 500 mg daily; thin and light body frame; nulliparous status; menopause before age 45; postmenopause status; family history of osteoporosis; Caucasian, Asian, Native American, or northern European ancestry; excessive caffeine intake; advanced age; history of fractures/falls; inadequate calcium intake; sedentary lifestyle; chronic diseases (Cushing's hyperthyroidism and hypothyroidism, malabsorption/malnutrition disorders, neoplasms); long-term use of corticosteroids, methotrexate, phenytoin, heparin, aluminum-containing antacids (Peterson, 2001).	These are risk factors for osteoporosis.
Ask client to describe history of alteration in bone, muscle, or joint function (e.g., recent fall, trauma, lifting of heavy objects, history of bone or joint disease with sudden or gradual onset, location of alteration).	History assists in assessing nature of musculoskeletal problem.
Assess nature and extent of pain, including location, duration, severity, predisposing and aggravating factors, relieving factors, and type.	Alterations in bone, joints, or muscle are frequently accompanied by pain, which has implications for not only comfort but also ability to perform activities of daily living.
Assess client's normal activity pattern, including type of exercise routinely performed.	Provides baseline in assessment. Sedentary lifestyle and lack of appropriate exercise increases bone loss and risk of fractures (Peterson, 2001).
Determine how alteration influences ability to perform activities of daily living (e.g., bathing, feeding, dressing, toileting, and ambulating) and social functions (e.g., household chores, work, recreation, sexual activities).	Level of nursing care will be determined by extent to which client is able to perform self-care. Type and degree of restriction in continuing social activities influence topics for client education and ability of nurse to identify alternative ways to maintain function.
Assess height loss of woman over age 50 by subtracting current height from recall of maximum adult height.	Measurement may be useful screening tool to predict osteoporosis.

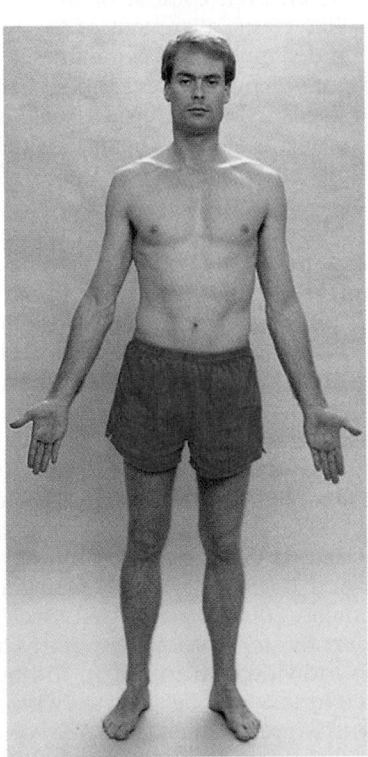 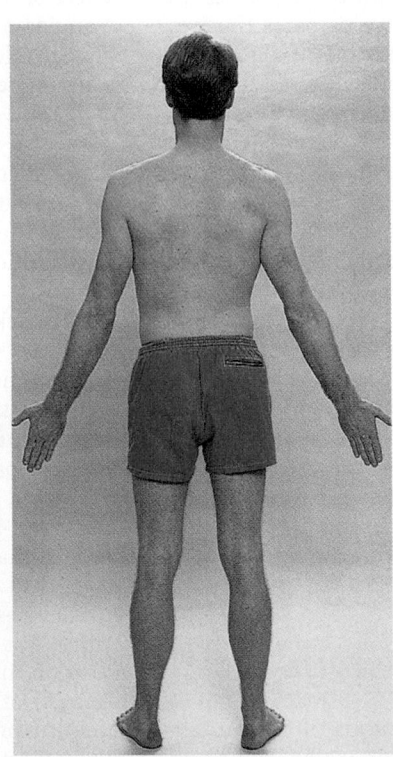 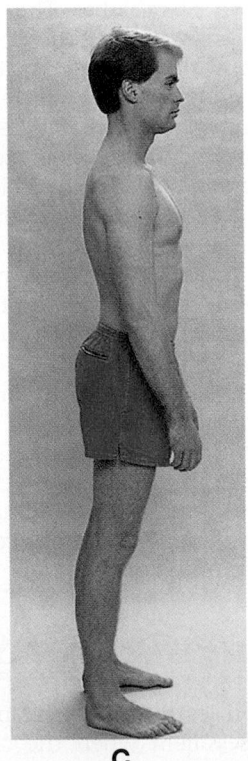

A   **B**   **C**

FIGURE **32–82**   Inspection of overall body posture. **A,** Anterior view. **B,** Posterior view. **C,** Lateral view. (From Seidel HM and others: *Mosby's guide to physical examination,* ed 5, St. Louis, 2003, Mosby.)

During general inspection the nurse looks at the extremities for overall size, gross deformity, bony enlargement, alignment, and symmetry. There should be bilateral symmetry in length, circumference, alignment, and position, and in the number of skin folds (Seidel and others, 2003). A general review pinpoints areas requiring specialized assessment.

Palpation

The nurse applies gentle palpation to all bones, joints, and surrounding muscles in a complete examination. In the case of a focused assessment, only an involved area needs to be examined. The nurse notes any heat, tenderness, edema, or resistance to pressure. The client should feel no discomfort when palpation is applied. Muscles should be firm.

Range of Joint Motion

The nurse asks the client to put each major joint through active and passive full range of motion (see Chapter 46). It is important to have plenty of room for the client to fully move each extremity. The nurse assesses range of motion passively by gently supporting and moving the extremities through their range of motion. The nurse must learn the correct terminology for the movements that the joints are capable of making (Table 32-34) and instruct the client on how to move through each range of motion. It also helps to demonstrate range of motion to the client when possible. The same body parts are compared for equality in movement. Figure 32-84 shows an example of range-of-motion positions for the hand and wrist.

When assessing range of motion, the nurse does not force a joint if there is pain or muscle spasm. The nurse must know the joint's normal range and the extent to which it can be moved. Range of motion should be equal between contralateral joints. Ideally, the normal range is assessed to determine a baseline for assessing later change.

A **goniometer,** frequently used by physical and occupational therapists, measures the precise degree of motion in a particular joint and is used mainly in clients who have a suspected reduction in joint movement. The instrument has two flexible arms with a 180-degree protractor in the center. The center of the protractor is positioned at the center of the joint being measured (Figure 32-85).

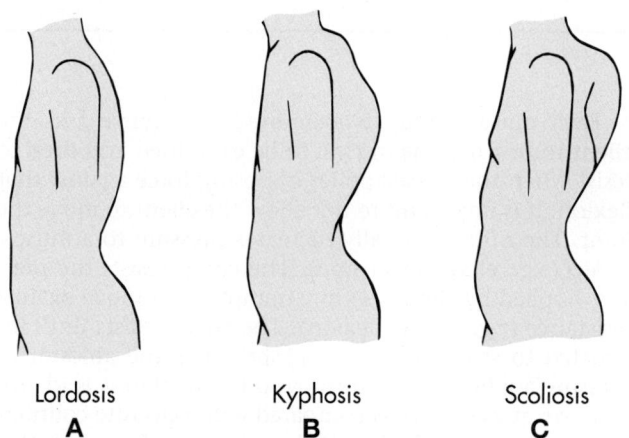

Lordosis	Kyphosis	Scoliosis
A	**B**	**C**

FIGURE **32–83**   Common postural abnormalities. **A,** Lordosis. **B,** Kyphosis. **C,** Scoliosis.

Client Teaching   Box 32-30

Musculoskeletal Assessment

Objectives

- Client will follow measures to prevent or minimize osteoporosis.
- Client will assume proper body posture.
- Client will be able to perform self-care measures.

Teaching Strategies

- Instruct client about correct postural alignment. Consult with physical therapist to provide client with exercises for improving posture.
- To reduce bone demineralization, instruct older adults about a proper exercise program (e.g., low-impact aerobics or vigorous water exercise) to be followed 3 or more times a week.
- Encourage intake of calcium to meet the recommended daily allowance. Increased vitamin D will aid calcium absorption. Recommendations for daily calcium supplements are as follows: Men and premenopausal women and postmenopausal women on estrogen—1000 mg; postmenopausal women on no estrogen—1500 mg; men and women over 65—1500 mg.
- Explain to clients with low back pain that they can benefit from modification of worker risk factors (e.g., lifting heavy weights, use of protective equipment), regular aerobic exercise, exercises that strengthen the back and increase trunk flexibility, and learning how to lift properly.
- Encourage clients who are employed in jobs that require lifting to wear a back support device.
- Instruct older adults and those with osteoporosis, on proper body mechanics, as well as range-of-motion and moderate weight-bearing exercises (e.g., swimming and walking) to minimize trauma and subsequent fracture of bones.
- When client is unable to perform self-care, instruct on use of assistive devices (e.g., zippers on clothing instead of buttons; elevation of chairs to minimize bending of knees and hips).
- Instruct older clients to pace activities to compensate for loss in muscle strength.

Evaluation

- Observe client's posture.
- Ask client to describe therapies for preventing osteoporosis.
- Observe client perform range-of-motion exercises.
- Have client keep log of regular weight-training exercises.
- Ask client or family members to describe client's use of self-care aids.

Table 32-34	Terminology for Normal Range-of-Motion Positions	
Term	**Range of Motion**	**Examples of Joints**
Flexion	Movement decreasing angle between two adjoining bones; bending of limb	Elbow, fingers, knee
Extension	Movement increasing angle between two adjoining bones	Elbow, knee, fingers
Hyperextension	Movement of body part beyond its normal resting extended position	Head
Pronation	Movement of body part so that front or ventral surface faces downward	Hand, forearm
Supination	Movement of body part so that the front or ventral surface faces upward	Hand, forearm
Abduction	Movement of extremity away from midline of body	Leg, arm, fingers
Adduction	Movement of extremity toward midline of body	Leg, arm, fingers
Internal rotation	Rotation of joint inward	Knee, hip
External rotation	Rotation of joint outward	Knee, hip
Eversion	Turning of body part away from midline	Foot
Inversion	Turning of body part toward midline	Foot
Dorsiflexion	Flexion of toes and foot upward	Foot
Plantar flexion	Bending of toes and foot downward	Foot

The arms extend along the body parts on each side of the protractor. A measurement is taken of the joint angle before moving the joint. After taking the joint through a full range of motion, the nurse measures the angle again to determine the degree of movement. The reading is compared with the normal degree of joint movement.

When putting each joint through its range of motion, the nurse makes a number of basic observations, noting pain, limited mobility, spastic movement, joint instability, stiffness, and contracture. Normal joints are nontender, without swelling, and move freely. In older adults, joints often become swollen and stiff with reduced range of motion resulting from cartilage erosion and fibrosis of synovial membranes (see Chapter 46). If a joint appears swollen and inflamed, the nurse palpates it for warmth.

Muscle Tone and Strength

The nurse may assess muscle strength and tone during measurement of range of motion. Findings are integrated with those from the neurological assessment. Tone is the slight muscular resistance felt by the examiner as the relaxed extremity is passively moved through its range of motion.

The client is asked to allow an extremity to relax or hang limp. This is often difficult, particularly if the client feels pain in the extremity. The extremity is supported, and each limb is grasped, moving it through the normal range of motion (Figure 32-86). Normal tone causes a mild, even resistance to movement through the entire range.

If a muscle has increased tone, or **hypertonicity,** any sudden passive movement of a joint is met with considerable resistance. Continued movement eventually causes the muscle to relax. A muscle that has little tone **(hypotonicity)** feels flabby. The involved extremity hangs loosely in a position determined by gravity.

For assessment of muscle strength, the client assumes a stable position. The client performs maneuvers demonstrating strength of major muscle groups (Table 32-35). Symmetrical muscle pairs are compared (Table 32-36). The arm on the dominant side is normally stronger than the arm on the nondominant side. In the older adult a loss of muscle mass causes bilateral weakness, but muscle strength remains greater in the dominant arm or leg.

Each muscle group is examined. The nurse asks the client to first flex the muscle to be examined and then to resist when the nurse applies opposing force against that flexion. It is important to not allow the client to move the joint. The nurse gradually increases pressure to a muscle group (e.g., elbow extension). The client resists the pressure applied by the nurse by attempting to move against resistance (e.g., elbow flexion). The client resists until instructed to stop. As the examiner varies the amount of pressure applied, the joint moves. If a weakness is identified, the muscle's size is compared with opposite counterpart by measuring the muscle body's circumference with a tape measure. A muscle that has **atrophied** (reduced in size) may feel soft and boggy when palpated.

*N*eurological System

The neurological system is responsible for many functions, including initiation and coordination of movement, reception and perception of sensory stimuli, organization of thought processes, control of speech, and storage of memory. A close integration exists between the neurological system and all other body systems. For example, urine production relies in part on the adequacy of blood flow to the kidneys, and the size of arterioles supplying the kidneys is under neural control.

An assessment of neurological function can be time consuming. An efficient nurse integrates neurological measurements with other parts of the physical examination. For example, cranial nerve function can be tested during the survey of the head and neck. Mental and emotional status is observed as the nursing history is collected.

Many variables must be considered when deciding the extent of the examination. A client's level of consciousness influences the ability to follow directions. A person's general physical status influences tolerance to assessment. For example, an inability to walk makes a detailed assessment of coordination difficult. The client's chief complaint also helps determine the need for a thorough neurological assessment. If the client complains of headache or a recent loss of function in an extremity, a complete neurological review is needed. Table 32-37 reviews the data collected in

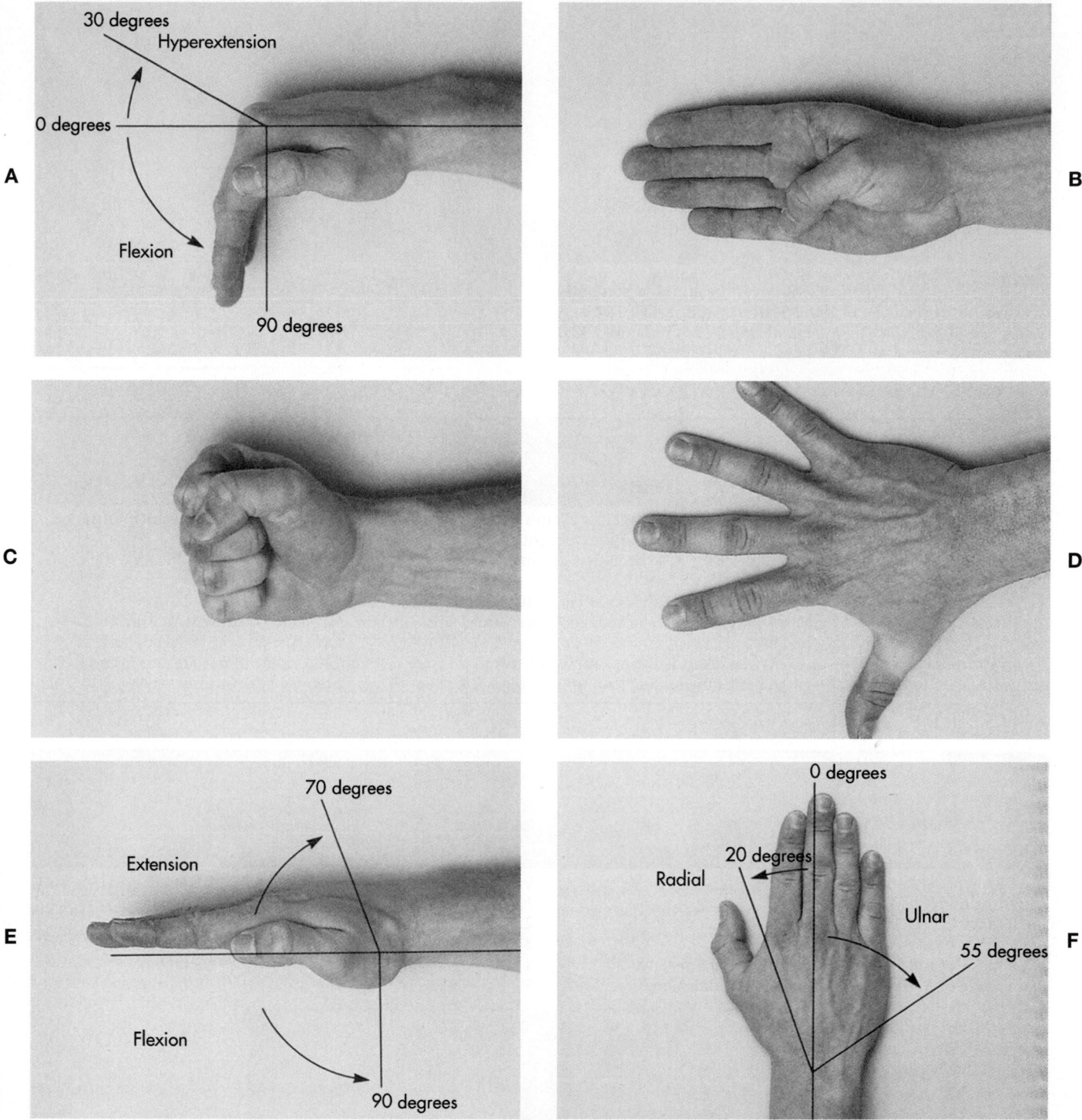

FIGURE 32–84 Range of motion of the hand and wrist. **A,** Metacarpophalangeal flexion and hyperextension. **B,** Finger flexion: thumb to each fingertip and to the base of the little finger. **C,** Finger flexion, first formation. **D,** Finger abduction. **E,** Wrist flexion and hyperextension. **F,** Wrist radial and ulnar movement. (From Seidel HM and others: *Mosby's guide to physical examination,* ed 5, St. Louis, 2003, Mosby.)

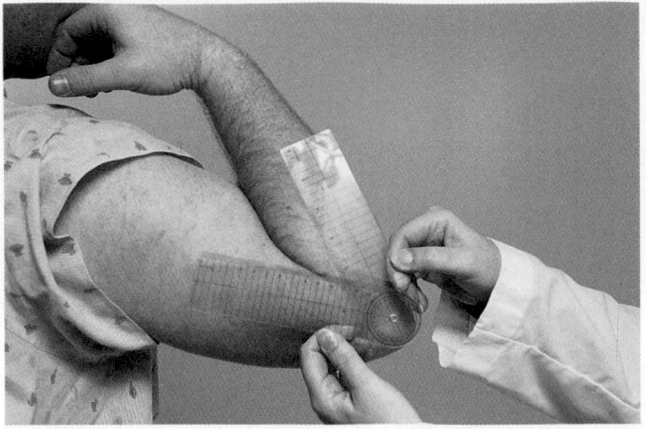

FIGURE **32–85** After the client flexes the arm, the goniometer measures the degree of joint flexion. (From Seidel HM and others: *Mosby's guide to physical examination,* ed 5, St. Louis, 2003, Mosby.)

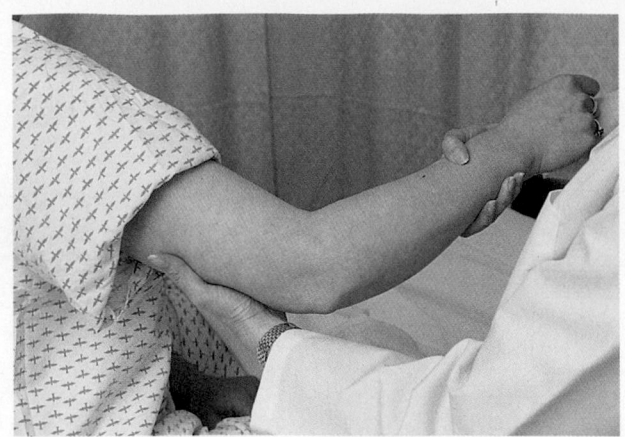

FIGURE **32–86** The nurse assesses muscle tone.

Table 32-35	Maneuvers to Assess Muscle Strength
Muscle Group	**Maneuver**
Neck (sternocleidomastoid)	Place hand firmly against client's upper jaw. Ask client to turn head laterally against resistance.
Shoulder (trapezius)	Place hand over midline of client's shoulder, exerting firm pressure. Have client raise shoulders against resistance.
Elbow	
Biceps	Pull down on forearm as client attempts to flex arm.
Triceps	As client's arm is flexed, apply pressure against forearm. Ask client to straighten arm.
Hip	
Quadriceps	When client is sitting, apply downward pressure to thigh. Ask client to raise leg up from table.
Gastrocnemius	Client sits, holding shin of flexed leg. Ask client to straighten leg against resistance.

Table 32-36	Muscle Strength			
		Scales		
Muscle Function Level	**Grade**	**% Normal**	**Lovett Scale**	
No evidence of contractility	0	0	0 (zero)	
Slight contractility, no movement	1	10	T (trace)	
Full range of motion, gravity eliminated*	2	25	P (poor)	
Full range of motion with gravity	3	50	F (fair)	
Full range of motion against gravity, some resistance	4	75	G (good)	
Full range of motion against gravity, full resistance	5	100	N (normal)	

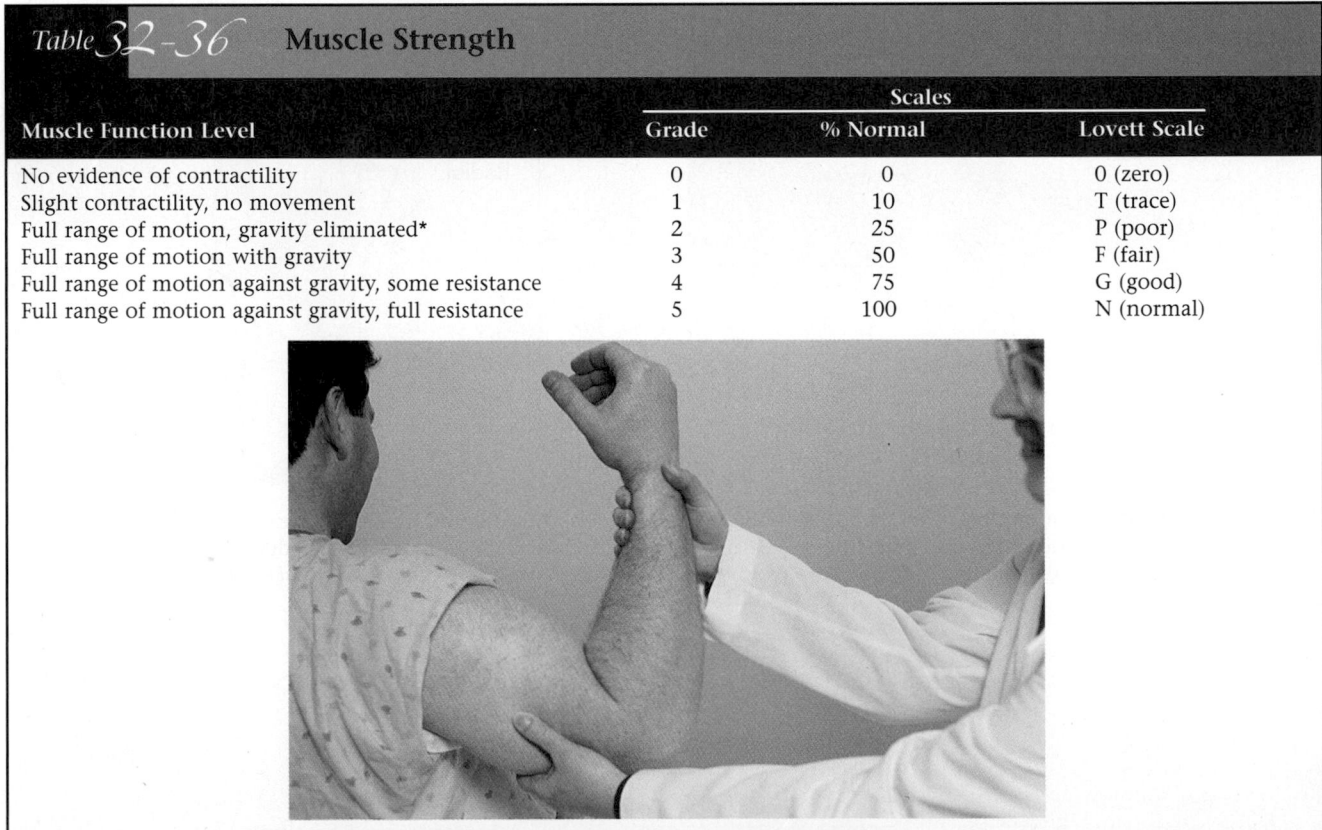

From Barkauskas VH and others: *Health and physical assessment,* ed 2, St. Louis, 1998, Mosby.
*Passive movement.

Table 32-37　　Nursing History for Neurological Assessment	
Assessment Category	**Rationale**
Determine if client is taking analgesics, antipsychotics, antidepressants, or nervous system stimulants.	These medications can alter level of consciousness or cause behavioral changes.
Assess client's use of alcohol, sedative-hypnotics, or recreational drugs.	Abuse can cause tremors, ataxia, and changes in peripheral nerve function.
Determine if client has recent history of seizures/convulsions: clarify sequence of events (aura, fall to ground, motor activity, loss of consciousness); character of any symptoms; and relationship of seizure to time of day, fatigue, or emotional stress.	Seizure activity often originates from central nervous system alteration. Characteristics of seizure help determine its origin.
Screen client for headache, tremors, dizziness, vertigo, numbness or tingling of body part, visual changes, weakness, pain, or changes in speech.	These symptoms frequently originate from alterations in central nervous system or peripheral nervous system function. Identification of specific patterns may aid in diagnosis of pathological condition.
Discuss with spouse, family members, or friends any recent changes in client's behavior (e.g., increased irritability, mood swings, memory loss, change in energy level).	Behavioral changes may result from intracranial pathological states.
Assess client for history of change in vision, hearing, smell, taste, or touch.	Major sensory nerves originate from brain stem. These symptoms may help to localize nature of problem.
If an older client displays sudden acute confusion (delirium), review history for drug toxicity (anticholinergics, diuretics, digoxin, cimetidine, sedatives, antihypertensives, antiarrhythmics), serious infections, metabolic disturbances, heart failure, and severe anemia.	This is one of the most common mental disorders in older persons. Condition is always potentially reversible (see Box 32-32, p. 762).
Review past history for head or spinal cord injury, hypertension, or psychiatric disorders.	Factors may cause neurological symptoms or behavioral changes to develop, focusing assessment on possible cause.

the nursing history. For a complete examination, the following special equipment will be needed:
- Reading material
- Vials containing aromatic substances (e.g., vanilla and coffee)
- Opposite tip of cotton swab or tongue blade broken in half
- Snellen eye chart
- Penlight
- Vials containing sugar or salt
- Tongue blade
- Two test tubes, one filled with hot water and the other with cold water
- Cotton balls or cotton-tipped applicators
- Tuning fork
- Reflex hammer

Mental and Emotional Status

A great deal can be learned about mental capacities and emotional state by simply interacting with a client. A nurse can ask questions throughout an examination to gather data and observe the appropriateness of emotions and ideas. There are special assessment tools designed to assess a client's mental status. Kahn and Goldfarb's mental status questionnaire (MSQ) (1960) is a 10-item instrument and a widely used tool (Kahn and others, 1960). Folstein, Folstein, and McHugh (1975) developed the Mini-Mental State (MMS) to measure orientation and cognitive function. The sample questions in Box 32-31 are only a portion of those found in the examination. A maximum score on the MMS is 30. Clients with scores of 21 or less generally reveal cognitive impairment requiring further evaluation.

To ensure an objective assessment, the nurse considers the client's cultural and educational background, values, beliefs, and previous experiences. Such factors influence the client's response to questions. An alteration in mental or emotional status may reflect a disturbance in cerebral functioning. The cerebral cortex controls and integrates intellectual and emotional functioning. Primary brain disorders, medication, and metabolic changes are examples of factors that may change cerebral function.

A common mental disorder affecting older adults is delirium. It is an acute mental disorder characterized by confusion, disorientation, and restlessness. The acute condition is often misdiagnosed as a form of dementia, a more progressive, organic mental disorder such as Alzheimer's disease. Thus the underlying cause of the condition is missed. When it occurs, many nurses and physicians think it is common older adult behavior. Delirium is often overlooked in older adults because of a failure to adequately assess mental status. The condition can fortunately be reversed when correctly assessed by treating the underlying cause (central nervous system [CNS], metabolic, and cardiopulmonary disorders; systemic illnesses; and sensory deprivation or overload) (Stuart and Laraia, 2001). Frequently clients who develop delirium are labeled with sundowner's syndrome because the delirium frequently worsens at night. Many practitioners mistake this as being common with old age. The nurse should obtain a good history of the client's behavior before delirium develops so as to recognize the condition early. Family members can usually be a good resource. Box 32-32 summarizes clinical criteria for delirium.

Box 32-31   **MMSE Sample Questions**

Orientation to time
   "What is the date?"
Registration
   "Listen carefully. I am going to say three words. You say them back after I stop.
   Ready? Here they are...
   HOUSE (pause), CAR (pause), LAKE (pause). Now repeat those words back to me."
   [Repeat up to 5 times, but score only the first trial.]
Naming
   What is this?" [Point to a pencil or pen.]
Reading
   "Please read this and do what it says." [Show examinee the words on the stimulus form.]
   CLOSE YOUR EYES

Reproduced by special permission of the Publisher, Psychological Assessment Resources, Inc., 16204 North Florida Avenue, Lutz, Florida 33549, from Mini-Mental State Examination, by Marshal Folstein and Susan Folstein, Copyright 1975, 1998, 2001 by Mini Mental, LLC, Inc. Published 2001 by Psychological Assessment Resources, Inc. Further reproduction is prohibited without permission of PAR, Inc. The MMSE can be purchased from PAR, Inc. by calling (800) 331-8378 or (813) 968-3003.

Box 32-32   **Clinical Criteria for Delirium**

Definition: An acute disturbance of consciousness that is accompanied by a change in cognition. It cannot be accounted for by a preexisting or evolving dementia. Delirium develops over a short period of time, usually hours to days, and tends to fluctuate during the course of the day. It is usually a direct physiological consequence of a general medical condition.
There is reduced clarity of awareness of the environment.
Ability to focus, sustain, or shift attention is impaired (questions must be repeated).
Person is easily distracted by irrelevant stimuli.
There is an accompanying change in cognition (memory impairment, disorientation, or language disturbance).
Recent memory is most commonly affected.
Disorientation is usually shown, with client disoriented to time or place.
Language disturbance may involve impaired ability to name objects or ability to write; speech may be rambling.
Perceptual disturbances may include misinterpretations, illusions, or hallucinations.

Modified from American Psychiatric Association: *Diagnostic and statistical manual of mental disorders*, ed 4, text revision, Washington, DC, 2000, The Association; and Stuart G, Laraia M: *Principles and practice of psychiatric nursing*, ed 7, St. Louis, 2001, Mosby.

Level of Consciousness. The level of consciousness exists along a continuum from full awakening, alertness, and cooperation to unresponsiveness to any form of external stimuli. A fully conscious client responds to questions spontaneously. As consciousness lowers, a client may show irritability, a shortened attention span, or an unwillingness to cooperate. To avoid ambiguity in the assessment of the level of consciousness, the Glasgow coma scale (GCS) measures consciousness by an objective numerical scale (Table 32-38). Caution is needed in using the scale with clients who have sensory losses (e.g., vision or hearing). As consciousness deteriorates, a client becomes disoriented to name, time, and place. The nurse asks short, to-the-point questions regarding information that the client knows (e.g., "Tell me your name," "What's the name of this place?" and "What day is this?"). The client's ability to understand and answer questions has a direct effect on the nurse's ability to perform a complete examination. The client must be aroused to full alertness before the assessment can be conducted.

A client may be unable to follow simple commands, such as "Squeeze my finger" or "Move your toes." At this lowered level of consciousness the client often is responsive only to painful stimuli. The nurse tests the client by applying firm pressure with the thumb over the root of the fingernail. The client should withdraw the hand from the painful stimulus. A client with serious neurological impairment exhibits abnormal posturing in response to pain. A flaccid response indicates the absence of muscle tone in the extremities and severe injury to brain tissue.

Table 32-38   **Glasgow Coma Scale**

Action	Response	Score
Eyes open	Spontaneously	4
	To speech	3
	To pain	2
	None	1
Best verbal response	Oriented	5
	Confused	4
	Inappropriate words	3
	Incomprehensible sounds	2
	None	1
Best motor response	Obeys commands	6
	Localized pain	5
	Flexion withdrawal	4
	Abnormal flexion	3
	Abnormal extension	2
	Flaccid	1
	TOTAL SCORE	15

The GCS allows the nurse to evaluate a client's neurological status over time. The higher the score, the more improved or normal the level of functioning.

Behavior and Appearance. Behavior, moods, hygiene, grooming, and choice of dress reveal pertinent information about mental status. The nurse must be perceptive of mannerisms and actions during the entire physical assessment. The nurse notes nonverbal, as well as verbal, behavior. Does the client respond appropriately to directions? Does the client's mood vary with no apparent cause? Does the client show concern about appearance? Is the client's hair clean and neatly groomed, and are the nails trim and clean? The client should behave in a manner expressing concern and interest in the examination. The client should make eye contact with the nurse and express appropriate feelings that correspond to the situation. Normally the client will show some degree of personal hygiene.

Choice and fit of clothing may reflect socioeconomic background or personal taste rather than deficiency in self-concept or self-care. The nurse avoids being judgmental and focuses assessment on the appropriateness of clothing for the weather. Older adults may neglect their appearance because of a lack of energy, finances, or reduced vision.

Language. The ability of an individual to understand spoken or written words and to express the self through writing, words, or gestures is a function of the cerebral cortex. The nurse assesses the client's voice inflection, tone, and manner of speech. The client's voice should have inflections, be clear and strong, and increase in volume appropriately. Speech should be fluent. When communication is clearly ineffective (e.g., omission or addition of letters and words, misuse of words, or hesitations), the nurse assesses for **aphasia.** An injury to the cerebral cortex may result in aphasia.

The two types of aphasia are sensory (or receptive) and motor (or expressive). With receptive aphasia a person cannot understand written or verbal speech. With expressive aphasia a person understands written and verbal speech but cannot write or speak appropriately when trying to communicate. A client may suffer a combination of receptive and expressive aphasia, depending on the portion of the cerebral cortex involved. The nurse assesses language capabilities when it is clear that communication with the client is ineffective. Some simple assessment techniques include the following:
- Asking the client to name a familiar object to which the nurse points
- Asking the client to respond to simple verbal and written commands, such as "Stand up" or "Sit down"
- Asking the client to read simple sentences out loud
Normally a client names objects correctly, follows commands, and reads sentences correctly.

Intellectual Function
Intellectual function includes memory (recent, immediate, and past), knowledge, abstract thinking, association, and judgment. Each aspect of intellectual function is tested through a specific technique. However, because cultural and educational background influence the ability to respond to test questions, the nurse should not ask questions related to concepts or ideas with which the client is unfamiliar.

Memory. The nurse assesses immediate recall and recent and remote memory. Often a problem with memory becomes apparent when the nurse takes the nursing history. To assess immediate recall, the nurse has the client repeat a series of numbers (e.g., *7, 4, 1*) in the order they are

presented or in reverse order. The nurse gradually increases the number of digits (e.g., *7, 4, 1, 8, 6*) until the client fails to repeat the digits correctly. Normally an individual is able to repeat a series of 5 to 8 digits forward and 4 to 6 digits backward.

The nurse asks if the client's memory can be tested. Then the nurse says clearly and slowly the name of three unrelated objects. After the nurse says all three, the client is asked to repeat each. This is continued until the client is successful. Then, later in the assessment, the nurse asks the client to repeat the three words again. The client should be able to identify the three words. Another test for recent memory involves asking the client to recall events occurring during the same day (e.g., what was eaten for breakfast). Information may need to be validated with a family member.

To assess past memory, the nurse can ask the client to recall his or her mother's maiden name, a birthday, or a special date in history. It is best to ask open-ended questions rather than simple yes/no questions. A client should have immediate recall of such information. With older adults a nurse should not interpret a hearing loss as confusion. Good communication techniques are necessary throughout the examination to ensure that the client clearly understands all directions and testing.

Knowledge. The nurse can assess knowledge by asking clients what they know about their illnesses or the reason for seeking health care. By assessing knowledge, the nurse determines clients' abilities to learn or understand. If an opportunity to teach exists, the nurse can test mental status by asking for feedback during a follow-up visit.

Abstract Thinking. Interpreting abstract ideas or concepts reflects the capacity for abstract thinking. A higher level of intellectual functioning is required for an individual to explain such phrases as "A stitch in time saves nine" or "Don't count your chickens before they're hatched." The nurse notes whether the client's explanations are relevant and concrete. The client with altered mentation will likely interpret the phrase literally or merely rephrase the words.

Association. Another higher level of intellectual functioning involves finding similarities or associations between concepts: a dog is to a beagle as a cat is to a Siamese. The nurse names related concepts and asks the client to identify their associations. Questions should be appropriate to the client's level of intelligence. It is sufficient to use simple concepts.

Judgment. Judgment requires a comparison and evaluation of facts and ideas to understand their relationships and to form appropriate conclusions. The nurse attempts to measure the ability to make logical decisions. By assessing judgment, the nurse also measures the ability to organize thought processes. The nurse may choose to ask clients why they decided to seek health care or how they plan to adjust to limitations after returning home. A simpler test would involve asking what clients would do if placed in a situation such as being locked out of their homes or suddenly becoming ill when alone at home.

Cranial Nerve Function

The nurse may assess all 12 cranial nerves or test a single nerve or related group of nerves. A test of the oculomotor nerve measures pupillary response. Assessment of the glossopharyngeal and vagus nerves reveals integrity of the gag reflex. Measurements used to assess the integrity of organs within the head and neck also assess cranial nerve function. For example, the cochlear branch of the eighth cranial nerve is tested during a hearing assessment. The function of the ninth and tenth nerves can be assessed during examination of the pharynx. A dysfunction in any nerve reflects an alteration at some point along the cranial nerve's distribution. Cranial nerve assessment is easy after the nurse is familiar with the nerve's normal functions. To remember the order of the 12 nerves, the nurse can use this simple phrase, "On old Olympus' towering tops, a Finn and German viewed some hops." The first letter of each word in the phrase is the same as the first letter of the names of the cranial nerves (Table 32-39).

Sensory Function

The sensory pathways of the central nervous system conduct sensations of pain, temperature, position, vibration, and crude and finely localized touch. Different nerve pathways relay the sensations. For most clients a quick screening of sensory function is sufficient unless there are symptoms of reduced sensation, motor impairment, or paralysis.

> **Safety Alert.** When a client has impaired sensation, the risk of skin breakdown is greater. When decreased sensation is assessed, it is important to do a complete skin and tissue assessment of the area affected by the sensory loss. In addition, these clients should also be taught to avoid pressure, thermal, and/or chemical trauma to the area.

Normally a client has sensory responses to all stimuli that are tested. Sensations along the body's surface are felt equally on both sides of the face, trunk, and extremities. A nurse can assess the major sensory nerves by knowing

Table 32-39 Cranial Nerve Function and Assessment

Number	Name	Type	Function	Method
I	Olfactory	Sensory	Sense of smell	Ask client to identify different nonirritating aromas such as coffee and vanilla.
II	Optic	Sensory	Visual acuity	Use Snellen chart or ask client to read printed material while wearing glasses.
III	Oculomotor	Motor	Extraocular eye movement	Assess directions of gaze.
			Pupil constriction and dilation	Measure pupillary reaction to light reflex and accommodation.
IV	Trochlear	Motor	Upward and downward movement of eyeball	Assess directions of gaze.
V	Trigeminal	Sensory and motor	Sensory nerve to skin of face	Lightly touch cornea with wisp of cotton. Assess corneal reflex. Measure sensation of light pain and touch across skin of face.
			Motor nerve to muscles of jaw	Palpate temples as client clenches teeth.
VI	Abducens	Motor	Lateral movement of eyeballs	Assess directions of gaze.
VII	Facial	Sensory and motor	Facial expression	As client smiles, frowns, puffs out cheeks, and raises and lowers eyebrows, look for asymmetry.
			Taste	Have client identify salty or sweet taste on front of tongue.
VIII	Auditory	Sensory	Hearing	Assess ability to hear spoken word.
IX	Glossopharyngeal	Sensory and motor	Taste	Ask client to identify sour or sweet taste on back of tongue.
			Ability to swallow	Use tongue blade to elicit gag reflex.
X	Vagus	Sensory and motor	Sensation of pharynx	Ask client to say "ah." Observe movement of palate and pharynx.
			Movement of vocal cords	Assess speech for hoarseness.
XI	Spinal accessory	Motor	Movement of head and shoulders	Ask client to shrug shoulders and turn head against passive resistance.
XII	Hypoglossal	Motor	Position of tongue	Ask client to stick out tongue to midline and move it from side to side.

the sensory dermatome zones (Figure 32-87). Some areas of the skin are innervated by specific dorsal root cutaneous nerves. For example, if the nurse notes reduced sensation when checking for light touch along an area of the skin (e.g., the lower neck), the nurse can determine, in general, where a neurological lesion may exist (e.g., fourth cervical spinal cord segment).

All sensory testing is performed with the client's eyes closed so that the client is unable to see when or where a stimulus strikes the skin (Table 32-40). Stimuli are applied in a random, unpredictable order to maintain the client's attention and prevent detection of a predictable pattern. The client is asked to tell the nurse when, what, and where each stimulus is felt. The nurse compares symmetrical areas of the body while applying stimuli to the client's arms, trunk, and legs.

Motor Function

An assessment of motor function includes the same measurements made during the musculoskeletal examination. In addition, cerebellar function is assessed. The cerebellum coordinates muscular activity by producing smooth, steady, and efficient movements of muscle groups. The maintenance of balance and equilibrium is also a function of the cerebellum. Sensory impulses from the vestibular portion of the inner ear travel to the cerebellum, where impulses are relayed to proper motor nerves to maintain body equilibrium. The cerebellum also controls posture.

Coordination. It is difficult for the nurse to explain the tests used to measure coordination. To avoid confusion, the nurse demonstrates each maneuver and then has clients repeat it after determining that their mobility is normal and they are physically able to make the necessary movements. The nurse observes the smoothness and balance of movements (Box 32-33). In older adults a slow reaction time may cause movements to be less rhythmical.

To assess fine motor function, the nurse has the client extend the arms out to the sides and touch each forefinger alternately to the nose (first with eyes open, then with eyes closed). Normally the client alternately touches the nose smoothly. Performing rapid, rhythmical, alternating movements demonstrates coordination in the upper extremities. While sitting, the client begins by patting the knees with both hands. Then the client alternately turns up the palm and back of the hands while continuously patting the knees. The maneuver should be done smoothly and regularly with increasing speed.

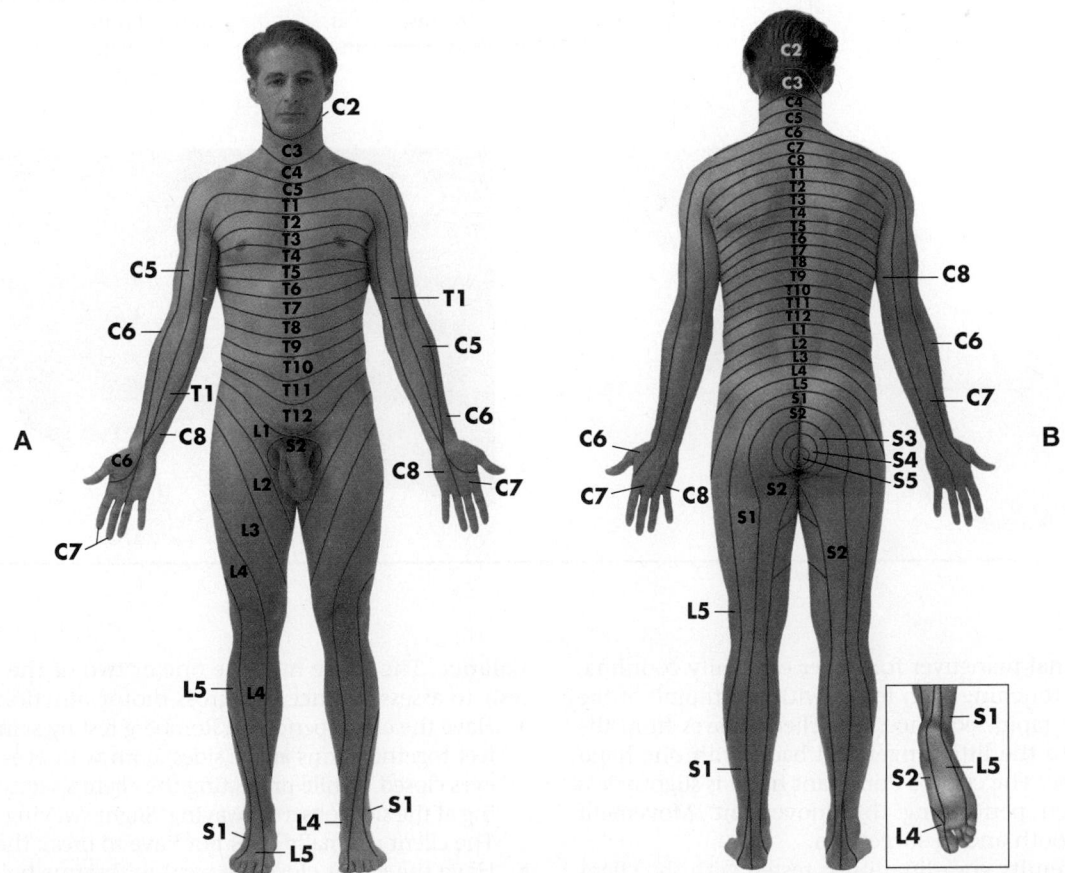

FIGURE 32–87   Dermatomes of the body, the body surface areas innervated by particular spinal nerves; C1 usually has no cutaneous distribution. **A,** Anterior view. **B,** Posterior view. It appears that there is a distinct separation of surface area controlled by each dermatome, but there is almost always overlap between spinal nerves. (From Seidel HM and others: *Mosby's guide to physical examination,* ed 5, St. Louis, 2003, Mosby.)

Table 32-40   Assessment of Sensory Nerve Function

Function	Equipment	Method	Precautions
Pain	Broken tongue blade or wooden end of cotton applicator	Ask client to voice when dull or sharp sensation is felt. Alternately apply sharp and blunt ends of tongue blade to skin's surface. Note areas of numbness or increased sensitivity.	Remember that areas where skin is thickened, such as heel or sole of foot, may be less sensitive to pain.
Temperature	Two test tubes, one filled with hot water and other with cold	Touch skin with tube. Ask client to identify hot or cold sensation.	Omit test if pain sensation is normal.
Light touch	Cotton ball or cotton-tip applicator	Apply light wisp of cotton to different points along skin's surface. Ask client to voice when sensation is felt.	Apply at areas where skin is thin or more sensitive (e.g., face, neck, inner aspect of arms, top of feet and hands).
Vibration	Tuning fork	Apply stem of vibrating fork to distal interphalangeal joint of fingers and interphalangeal joint of great toe, elbow, and wrist. Have client voice when and where vibration is felt.	Be sure client feels vibration and not merely pressure.
Position		Grasp finger or toe, holding it by its sides with thumb and index finger. Alternate moving finger or toe up and down. Ask client to state when finger is up or down. Repeat with toes.	Avoid rubbing adjacent appendages as finger or toe is moved. Do not move joint laterally; return to neutral position before moving again.
Two-point discrimination	Two broken tongue blades	Lightly apply one or both tongue blade tips simultaneously to the skin's surface. Ask client whether one or two pricks are felt. Find the distance at which client can no longer distinguish two points.	Apply blade tips to same anatomical site (e.g., fingertips, palm of hand, or upper arms). Minimum distance at which client can discriminate two points varies (2 to 8 mm on fingertips).

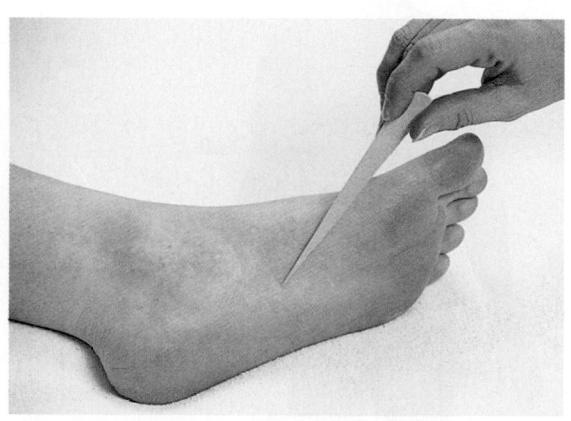
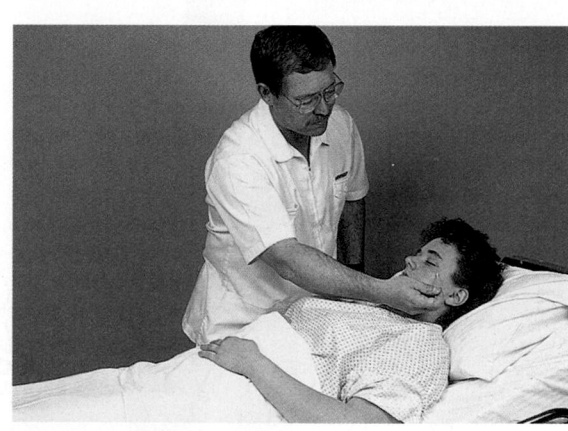

An additional maneuver for upper extremity coordination involves touching each finger with the thumb of the same hand in rapid sequence. The client moves from the index finger to the little finger and back, with one hand tested at a time. The client's dominant hand is slightly less awkward when performing this movement. Movement should be smooth and in succession.

Lower extremity coordination is tested with the client lying supine, legs extended. The nurse places a hand at the ball of the client's foot. The client taps the nurse's hand with the foot as quickly as possible. Each foot is tested for speed and smoothness. The feet do not move as rapidly or evenly as the hands.

Balance. The nurse may use one or two of the following tests to assess balance and gross motor function:
- Have the client perform a Romberg test by standing with feet together, arms at the sides, both with eyes open and eyes closed. While protecting the client's safety by standing at the side, observe swaying. Slight swaying is normal. The client normally does not have to break the stance.
- Have the client close the eyes, with arms held straight at the sides, and stand on one foot and then the other. Normally balance is maintained for 5 seconds with slight swaying.
- Ask the client to walk a straight line by placing the heel of one foot directly in front of the toes of the other foot.

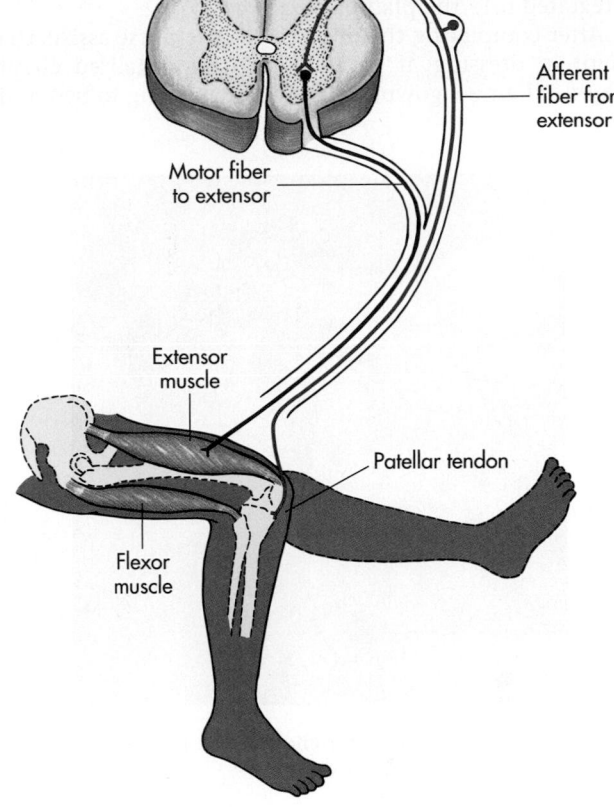

FIGURE 32–88   Pathway of the reflex arc.

Neurological Assessment

Objectives

- Client's family will understand relationship of client's behavioral and mental changes to physical status.
- Client with sensory or motor impairment will select safety measures for self-care.
- Older adult will routinely inspect skin for injuries.

Teaching Strategies

- Explain to family or friends the neurological implications of any behavioral or mental impairment shown by client.
- If client has sensory or motor impairments, explain measures to ensure safety (e.g., use of ambulation aids or safety bars in bathrooms or stairways).
- Teach older adult to plan enough time to complete tasks, because reaction time is slowed.
- Teach older adult to observe skin surfaces for areas of trauma, because perception of pain is reduced.

Evaluation

- Ask family to discuss client behaviors that result from neurological impairments.
- Have client explain safety measures used to avoid injury from sensory and motor limitations.
- Have older client explain reason for inspecting skin surface routinely.

Safety Alert When examining the older adult client's gait, be aware of the risk for falls. Older adult clients may need assistance with this portion of the examination.

Reflexes

Eliciting reflex reactions allows the nurse to assess the integrity of sensory and motor pathways of the reflex arc and specific spinal cord segments. Assessment of reflexes does not determine higher neural center functioning. Figure 32-88 traces the pathway of the reflex arc. Each muscle contains a small sensory unit called a muscle spindle, which controls muscle tone and detects changes in the length of muscle fibers. By tapping a tendon with a reflex hammer, the nurse stretches the muscle and tendon, lengthening the spindle. The spindle sends nerve impulses along afferent nerve pathways to the dorsal horn of the spinal cord segment. Within milliseconds the impulses reach the spinal cord and synapse to travel to the efferent motor neuron in the spinal cord. A motor nerve sends the impulses back to the muscle, causing the reflex response.

The two categories of normal reflexes are deep tendon reflexes, elicited by mildly stretching a muscle and tapping a tendon, and cutaneous reflexes, elicited by stimulating the skin superficially. Reflexes are graded as follows:

0 No response
1+ Low normal with slight muscle contraction

2+ Normal with visible muscle twitch and movement of the arm or leg
3+ Brisker than normal; may not indicate disease
4+ Hyperactive and very brisk; often associated with spinal cord disorders

When reflexes are being assessed, the client should relax as much as possible to avoid voluntary movement or tensing of muscles. The nurse positions the limbs to slightly stretch the muscle being tested. The reflex hammer is held loosely between the nurse's thumb and fingers so that it can swing freely and tap the tendon briskly (Figure 32-89). The nurse compares the symmetry of the reflex from one side of the body with that of the other side. In the older adult, reflexes are normally slowed. Reflexes can be hyperactive in clients with alcohol, cocaine, or opioid intoxication (Caulker-Burnett, 1994). Practitioners often use stick figures to record reflexes. Table 32-41 summarizes common deep tendon and cutaneous reflexes.

After the Examination

The nurse may choose to record findings from the physical assessment during the examination or at the end. Most institutions have special forms that make it easy to record examination data (see Chapter 25). The nurse reviews all findings before assisting the client with dressing, in case there is a need to recheck any information or gather additional data. Physical assessment findings are integrated into the plan of care.

After completing the assessment, the nurse assists the client in dressing, if necessary. The hospitalized client may need a new gown and help in returning to bed and

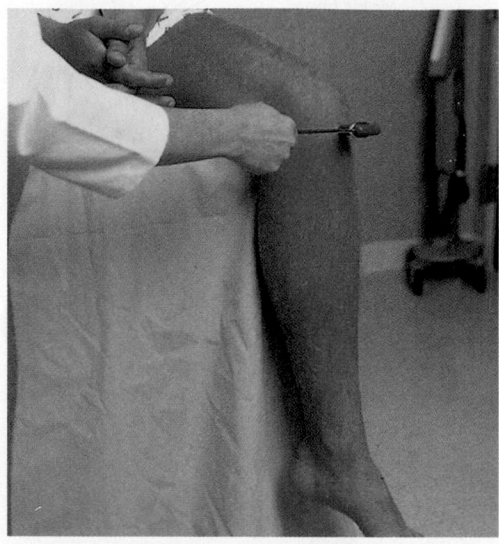

FIGURE **32–89**   Position for eliciting the patellar tendon reflex. The lower leg normally extends.

assuming a comfortable position. The client in the home may only need time to dress and join the nurse in the living room or kitchen. When the client is comfortable, it helps to share a summary of the assessment findings. If the findings have revealed serious abnormalities, such as a mass or highly irregular heart rate, the client's physician should be consulted before any findings are revealed. It is the physician's responsibility to make definitive medical diagnoses. The nurse can explain the type of abnormality found and the need for the physician to conduct an additional examination.

The nurse may delegate cleaning the examination area to assistive personnel. Infection-control practices are used in removing materials or instruments soiled with potentially infectious wastes. If the client's bedside was the examination site, the assistant clears away soiled items from the table and makes sure that the bed linen is dry and clean. The client may appreciate a clean gown and the opportunity to wash the face and hands. Afterward, the nurse performs hand hygiene.

The nurse checks to make sure that the recording of the assessment is complete. If entry of items into the assessment form was delayed, the nurse records them at this time to avoid forgetting any important information. If entries were made periodically during the examination, they are reviewed for accuracy and thoroughness. Significant findings are communicated to appropriate medical and nursing personnel, either verbally or in the written care plan.

Table 32–41	Assessment of Common Reflexes	
Type	**Procedure**	**Normal Reflex**
Deep Tendon Reflexes		
Biceps	Flex client's arm up to 45 degrees at elbow with palms down. Place your thumb in antecubital fossa at base of biceps tendon and your fingers over biceps muscle. Strike triceps tendon with reflex hammer.	Flexion of arm at elbow
Triceps	Flex client's arm at elbow, holding arm across chest, or hold upper arm horizontally and allow lower arm to go limp. Strike triceps tendon just above elbow.	Extension at elbow
Patellar	Have client sit with legs hanging freely over side of table or chair or have client lie supine and support knee in a flexed 90-degree position. Briskly tap patellar tendon just below patella.	Extension of lower leg
Achilles	Have client assume same position as for patellar reflex. Slightly dorsiflex client's ankle by grasping toes in palm of your hand. Strike Achilles tendon just above heel at ankle malleolus.	Plantar flexion of foot
Cutaneous Reflexes		
Plantar	Have client lie supine with legs straight and feet relaxed. Take handle end of reflex hammer and stroke lateral aspect of sole from heel to ball of foot, curving across ball of foot toward big toe.	Plantar flexion of all toes
Gluteal	Have client assume side-lying position. Spread buttocks apart and lightly stimulate perineal area with cotton applicator.	Contraction of anal sphincter
Abdominal	Have client stand or lie supine. Stroke abdominal skin with base of cotton applicator over lateral borders of rectus abdominus muscle toward midline. Repeat test in each abdominal quadrant.	Contraction of rectus abdominus muscle with pulling of umbilicus toward stimulated side

The client often needs a number of ancillary examinations, such as x-ray examinations, laboratory tests, or ultrasonography, after a physical examination. These tests provide additional screening information to rule out the presence of abnormalities and help in the diagnosis of specific abnormalities found during the examination. The nurse explains the purpose of these tests and the sensations that the client can expect.

Key Concepts

- Baseline assessment findings reflect the client's functional abilities when the nurse first assesses the client and serve as the basis for comparison with subsequent assessment findings.
- Assessment data are used to make nursing diagnoses, select appropriate nursing interventions, and evaluate the outcomes of nursing care.
- Physical assessment of varying age-groups requires the nurse to apply principles of growth and development and understand normal age-related changes.
- Client teaching should be integrated throughout the examination to help clients learn about health promotion and disease prevention.
- Inspection requires good lighting, full exposure of the body part, and a careful comparison of the part with its counterpart on the opposite side of the body.
- Palpation involves the use of parts of the hand to detect different types of physical characteristics.
- Percussion is the detection of differences in density of underlying tissues by listening to sounds produced while striking the body's surface.
- Through auscultation with a good stethoscope, the nurse assesses the character of sounds created in various body organs.
- A physical examination should be performed only after proper preparation of the environment and equipment and after preparing the client physically and psychologically.
- Throughout the examination the nurse should keep the client warm, comfortable, and informed of each step of the process.
- The nurse uses a systematic approach when conducting a physical assessment and learns to integrate the assessments of different body systems simultaneously.
- During assessments of the skin, breast, and genitalia, the nurse explains the techniques for self-examination.
- Assessment of musculoskeletal function can easily be conducted by observing the client ambulating or participating in other active movements.
- The nurse continually assesses the client's cognitive function throughout the examination.
- At the end of the examination the nurse provides for the client's comfort and then completes a detailed review of physical assessment findings.

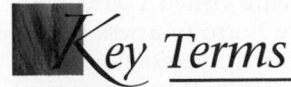

Key Terms

Acromegaly, *p. 697*	Hypotonicity, *p. 758*
Adventitious sounds, *p. 720*	Indurated, *p. 691*
Allen's test, *p. 721*	Integument, *p. 687*
Alopecia, *p. 694*	Jaundice, *p. 690*
Aneurysm, *p. 746*	Kyphosis, *p. 755*
Aphasia, *p. 763*	Leukoplakia, *p. 711*
Apical impulse, *p. 723*	Lordosis, *p. 755*
Arcus senilis, *p. 702*	Melanoma, *p. 688*
Atherosclerosis, *p. 728*	Metastasize, *p. 738*
Atrophied, *p. 758*	Murmurs, *p. 726*
Basal cell carcinoma, *p. 688*	Nystagmus, *p. 700*
Borborygmi, *p. 743*	Occlusion, *p. 728*
Bronchophony, *p. 721*	Ophthalmoscope, *p. 702*
Bruit, *p. 729*	Osteoporosis, *p. 755*
Capillary refill, *p. 734*	Otoscope, *p. 705*
Caries, *p. 710*	Ototoxicity, *p. 707*
Cerumen, *p. 705*	Pancreatitis, *p. 745*
Chancres, *p. 747*	Papanicolaou (Pap) smear, *p. 749*
Cherry angiomas, *p. 691*	Paralytic ileus, *p. 743*
Cholecystitis, *p. 745*	Peristalsis, *p. 743*
Cirrhosis, *p. 744*	Peritonitis, *p. 743*
Clubbing, *p. 734*	PERRLA, *p. 702*
Conjunctivitis, *p. 701*	Petechiae, *p. 691*
Cyanosis, *p. 690*	Phlebitis, *p. 734*
Cystocele, *p. 748*	Pigmentation, *p. 688*
Dermatitis, *p. 690*	Point of maximal impulse (PMI), *p. 723*
Distention, *p. 742*	Polyps, *p. 707*
Dysrhythmia, *p. 725*	Ptosis, *p. 701*
Ectropion, *p. 701*	Pulse deficit, *p. 725*
Eczema, *p. 690*	Rectocele, *p. 748*
Edema, *p. 691*	Scoliosis, *p. 755*
Entropion, *p. 701*	Senile keratosis, *p. 691*
Erythema, *p. 690*	Stenosis, *p. 728*
Excoriation, *p. 707*	Striae, *p. 742*
Exophthalmos, *p. 700*	Syncope, *p. 727*
Exostosis, *p. 712*	Tactile fremitus, *p. 718*
Fibrocystic breast disease, *p. 740*	Thrill, *p. 727*
Goniometer, *p. 757*	Turgor, *p. 691*
Hemorrhoids, *p. 753*	Varicosities, *p. 721*
Hepatitis, *p. 744*	Ventricular gallop, *p. 725*
Hernias, *p. 742*	Vocal fremitus, *p. 718*
Hirsutism, *p. 694*	Whispered pectoriloquy, *p. 721*
Hydrocephalus, *p. 697*	
Hypertonicity, *p. 758*	

Critical Thinking Exercises

1. A 32-year-old client entering a neighborhood clinic has the following symptoms: frequent productive cough, fatigue, decreased appetite, and persistent fever. What focused assessment should the nurse conduct?
2. The nurse is performing an abdominal assessment and observes a pulsating midline abdominal mass. What is the nurse's next line of action?

3. A 75-year-old black man is being visited 1 week post-operatively by the home care nurse to assess his peripheral vascular status following a femoral-popliteal bypass graft for arterial insufficiency. What assessment data need to be obtained by the nurse?

4. Develop a teaching plan for a female client (age 40) with a family history of breast cancer who acknowledges that she does not perform a monthly breast self-examination (BSE).

5. What physical examination techniques does the nurse use during assessment of the following clients?
   a. A client suspected of having a head injury
   b. A client with a cast on the lower leg
   c. A client reporting abdominal pain

6. A 55-year-old client is to be evaluated for osteoporosis. Which specific questions would the nurse ask to ascertain the client's risk? What physical examination techniques would the nurse employ?

Review Questions

1. The first technique the nurse employs when conducting a client's physical examination is:
   1. Palpation.
   2. Inspection.
   3. Percussion.
   4. Auscultation.

2. The main reason that auscultation proceeds palpation of the abdomen is to:
   1. Prevent distortion of vascular sounds.
   2. Prevent distortion of bowel sounds.
   3. Determine any areas of tenderness or pain.
   4. Allow the client to relax and be comfortable.

3. To correctly palpate the client's skin for temperature, the nurse will use the:
   1. Base of the hands
   2. Fingertips of the hands.
   3. Dorsal surface of the hands.
   4. Palmar surface of the hands.

4. To assess a client's superficial lymph nodes, the nurse would:
   1. Deeply palpate using the entire hand.
   2. Deeply palpate using a bimanual technique.
   3. Lightly palpate using a bimanual technique.
   4. Gently palpate using the pads of the index and middle fingers.

5. The nurse is teaching the client to inspect all skin surfaces and to report pigmented skin lesions that:
   1. Are symmetrical.
   2. Have irregular borders.
   3. Are uniform in color.
   4. Are less than 6 mm in diameter.

6. The client is being assessed for range-of-joint movement. You ask the client to move the arm away from the body, evaluating the movement of:
   1. Flexion.
   2. Extension.
   3. Abduction.
   4. Adduction.

7. When inspecting the adult client's thorax, the nurse observes for:
   1. Presence of fremitus.
   2. Presence of breath sounds.
   3. Movement of the diaphragm.
   4. Symmetry of chest excursion.

8. The nurse is auscultating the client's lung fields. The systematic pattern used for comparison is:
   1. Side to side.
   2. Top to bottom.
   3. Anterior to posterior.
   4. Interspace to interspace.

9. The nurse asks the client to interpret the saying "Don't count your chickens before they're hatched." The client's response reveals:
   1. Judgment.
   2. Knowledge.
   3. Association.
   4. Abstract reasoning.

10. The nurse is conducting a general survey on an adult client. The general survey includes:
    1. Appearance and behavior.
    2. Measurement of vital signs.
    3. Observing specific body systems.
    4. Conducting a detailed health history.

References

American Cancer Society: *Cancer facts and figures 2003,* New York, 2003a, The Society, www.cancer.org/docroot/STT/stt_0.asp.

American Cancer Society: *Cancer prevention and early detection: facts and figures 2003,* New York, 2003b, The Society, www.cancer.org/docroot/STT/stt_.asp.

American Psychiatric Association: *Diagnostic and statistical manual of mental disorders,* ed 4, text revision, Washington, DC, 2000, The Association.

Barkauskas VH and others: *Health and physical assessment,* ed 2, St. Louis, 1998, Mosby.

Belcher AE: *Cancer nursing,* St. Louis, 1992, Mosby.

Benenson AS, editor: *Control of communicable diseases manual,* Washington, DC, 1995, American Public Health Association.

Bennett MA: Report of the taskforce on the implications for darkly pigmented intact skin in the prediction and prevention of pressure ulcers, *Adv Wound Care* 8(6):34, 1998.

Breen P: DVT: what every nurse should know, *RN* 63(4): 58-62, 2000.

Caulker-Burnett I: Primary care screening for substance abuse, *Nurse Pract* 19(6):42, 1994.

Ebersole P, Hess P: *Toward healthy aging,* ed 5, St. Louis, 1998, Mosby.

Friedman L and others: *Source book of substance abuse and addiction,* Baltimore, 1996, Williams & Wilkins.

Gerard M: Domestic violence: how to screen and intervene, *RN* 63(12):52, 2000.

Habif TP: *Clinical dermatology: a color guide to diagnosis and therapy,* ed 3, St. Louis, 1996, Mosby.

Hardy MA: What can you do about your patient's dry skin, *J Gerontol Nurs* 22(5):10, 1996.

Hoban S, Kearney K: Elder abuse and neglect, *Am J Nurs* 100(11):49, 2000.

Hockenberry MJ and others: *Wong' nursing care of infants and children,* ed 7, St. Louis, 2003, Mosby.

Kessenich CR: Update on osteoporosis in elderly men, *Geriatr Nurs* 21(5):242, 2000.

Kramer A: Domestic violence: how to ask and how to listen, *Nurs Clin North Am* 37(1):189, 2002.

Lapka DV: Skin cancer, *RN* 63(7):32, 2000.

Lueckenotte A: *Gerontologic nursing,* ed 2, St. Louis, 2000, Mosby.

Master S, Terpstra JK: Recognition and diagnosis. In Schnoll SH, Horvatich PK, Terpstra JK, editors: *Prescribing drugs with abuse liability,* Richmond, Va, 1992, DSAM, MCV-VCU.

Metropolitan Life Insurance Company, *Statistical bulletin,* New York, 2000, Metropolitan.

Moore MC: *Pocket guide to nutritional care,* ed 4, St. Louis, 2001, Mosby.

National Pediculosis Association: Child care provider's guide to controlling head lice, www.headlice.org.

Pachucki-Hyde L: Assessment of risk factor for treatment and prevention of osteoporosis, *Nurs Clin North Am* 36(3):401, 2001.

Peterson JA: Osteoporosis overview, *Geriatr Nurs* 22(1):17, 2001.

Seidel HM and others: *Mosby's guide to physical examination,* ed 5, St. Louis, 2003, Mosby.

Stuart G, Laraia M: *Principles and practice of psychiatric nursing,* ed 7, St. Louis, 2001, Mosby.

Talbot L, Curtis L: The challenges of assessing skin indicators in people of color, *Home Health Nurse* 14(3), 1996.

U.S. Preventive Services Task Force: Guide to clinical preventive services, ed 2, Washington, DC, 1996, U.S. Department of Health and Human Services, Office of Disease Prevention and Health Promotion, http://cpmcnet.columbia.edu/texts/gcps/gcps0000.html.

Wishnia G: Challenges in the area of adults with osteoporosis, *Geriatr Nurs* 22(3):160, 2001.

Wong DL, Hockenberry-Eaton M: *Wong's essentials of pediatric nursing,* ed 6, St. Louis, 2001, Mosby.

Zitelli B, Davis H: *Atlas of pediatric physical diagnosis,* ed 2, St. Louis, 1991, Mosby.

*R*esearch References

Folstein MF, Folstein S, McHugh PR: Mini-mental state: a practical method for grading the cognitive state of patients for the clinician, *J Psychiatr Res* 12:82, 1975.

Kahn RL and others: Brief objective measures for the determination of mental status of the aged, *Am J Psychiatry* 117:326, 1960.

33

Infection Control

Media Resources

http://evolve.elsevier.com/Potter/
fundamentals/

CD COMPANION

- Review Questions
- Glossary

evolve WEBSITE

- Review Questions
- Student Learning Activities
- Animations
- Video Clips
- Glossary

Objectives

Mastery of content in this chapter will enable the student to:

- Define the key terms listed.
- Explain the relationship of the chain of infection to transmission of infection.
- Identify the body's normal defenses against infection.
- Discuss the events in the inflammatory response.
- Describe the signs/symptoms of a localized infection and those of a systemic infection.
- Identify clients most at risk for infection.
- Explain conditions that promote the transmission of nosocomial infection.
- Explain the difference between medical and surgical asepsis.
- Give an example for preventing infection for each element of the infection chain.
- Explain the rationale for standard precautions.
- Perform proper procedures for hand hygiene.
- Explain how infection-control measures may differ in the home versus the hospital.
- Properly don a surgical mask, sterile gown, and sterile gloves.

Good health depends in part on a safe environment. Practices or techniques that control or prevent transmission of infection help to protect clients and health care workers from disease. Clients in all health care settings are at risk for acquiring infections because of lower resistance to infectious **microorganisms,** increased exposure to numbers and types of disease-causing microorganisms, and **invasive** procedures. In acute care or ambulatory care facilities, clients can be exposed to pathogens, some of which may be resistant to most antibiotics. By practicing infection prevention and control techniques, the nurse can avoid spreading microorganisms to clients.

In all settings, clients and their families must be able to recognize sources of infections and be able to institute protective measures. Client teaching should include information concerning infections, modes of transmission, and methods of prevention.

Health care workers can protect themselves from contact with infectious material or exposure to a communicable disease by having knowledge of the infectious process and appropriate barrier protection. Diseases such as hepatitis B and C, acquired immunodeficiency syndrome (AIDS), and tuberculosis (TB) have resulted in a greater emphasis on infection-control techniques.

Nature of Infection

An infection is the entry and multiplication of an infectious agent in the tissues of a host. If the infectious agent **(pathogen)** fails to cause injury to cells or tissues, the pathogen is colonizing the cells or tissue without causing harm.

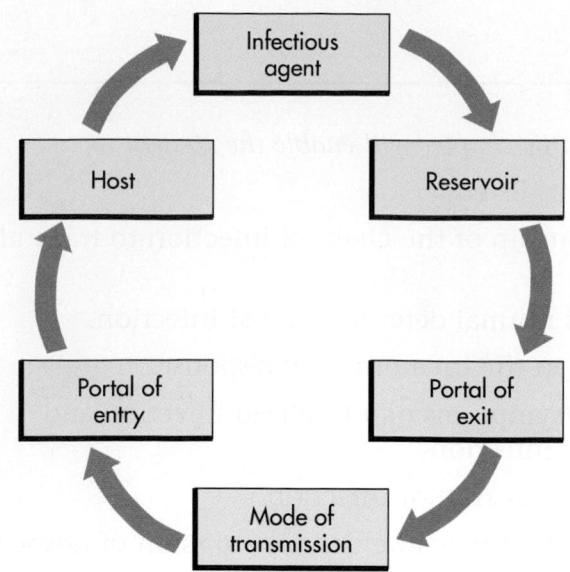

FIGURE **33–1** Chain of infection.

If the pathogens multiply and cause clinical signs and symptoms, the infection is symptomatic. If the infectious disease can be transmitted directly from one person to another, it is a **communicable,** or contagious, disease.

Chain of Infection

The presence of a pathogen does not mean that an infection will begin. Development of an infection occurs in a cycle that depends on the presence of all of the following elements:

• An infectious agent or pathogen
• A reservoir or source for pathogen growth
• A portal of exit from the reservoir
• A mode of transmission
• A portal of entry to a host
• A susceptible host

An infection will develop if this chain remains intact (Figure 33-1). Nurses follow infection prevention and control practices to break the chain so that infection will not develop.

Infectious Agent. Microorganisms include bacteria, viruses, fungi, and protozoa (Table 33-1). Microorganisms on the skin are called resident or transient flora. Resident organisms are considered permanent residents of the skin, where they survive and multiply without causing harm. Resident organisms are not easily removed by hand washing with plain soaps unless considerable friction is used. Resident microorganisms in deep skin layers are usually killed only by performing hand hygiene with products containing antimicrobial ingredients.

Transient microorganisms attach to the skin when a person has contact with another person or object during normal activities of living. For example, when a nurse touches a bedpan or a contaminated dressing, transient bacteria adhere to the nurse's skin. The organisms attach loosely to the skin in dirt and grease or under fingernails.

These organisms may be readily transmitted unless removed by hand washing (Larson, 1996).

The potential for microorganisms or parasites to cause disease depends on the following factors:

• Sufficient number of organisms
• **Virulence,** or ability to produce disease
• Ability to enter and survive in the host
• Susceptibility of the host

Some resident skin microorganisms are not virulent and may cause only minor skin infections. However, they can cause serious infection when surgery or other invasive procedures allow them to enter deep tissues or when a client is severely **immunocompromised** (impaired immune system).

Reservoir. A reservoir is a place where a pathogen can survive but may or may not multiply. For example, hepatitis A virus survives in shellfish but does not multiply; *Pseudomonas* organisms may survive and multiply in nebulizer reservoirs used in the care of clients with respiratory problems. The most common reservoir is the human body. A variety of microorganisms live on the skin and within the body cavities, fluids, and discharges. The presence of microorganisms does not always cause a person to be ill. **Carriers** are persons or animals who show no symptoms of illness but who have pathogens on or in their bodies that can be transferred to others. For example, a person can be a carrier of hepatitis B virus without having signs or symptoms of infection. Animals, food, water, insects, and inanimate objects can also be reservoirs for infectious organisms. *Clostridium botulinum* toxin survives in improperly processed foods (e.g., home-canned green beans) to cause botulism. The bacterium *Legionella pneumophila,* which causes Legionnaires' disease, lives in contaminated water and water systems. To thrive, organisms require a proper environment, including appropriate food, oxygen, water, temperature, pH, and light.

Food. Microorganisms require nourishment. Some, such as *Clostridium perfringens,* the microbe that causes gas gangrene, thrive on organic matter. Others, such as *Escherichia coli,* consume undigested foodstuff in the bowel. Carbon dioxide and inorganic material such as soil provide nourishment for other organisms.

Oxygen. **Aerobic** bacteria require oxygen for survival and for multiplication sufficient to cause disease. Aerobic organisms are more commonly the cause of infections in humans, as compared with **anaerobic** organisms. Examples of aerobic organisms are *Staphylococcus aureus* and strains of *Streptococcus organisms.*

Anaerobic bacteria thrive where little or no free oxygen is available. Infections deep within the pleural cavity, in a joint, or in a deep sinus tract are typically caused by anaerobes. Bacteria that cause tetanus, gas gangrene, and botulism are anaerobes.

Water. Most organisms require water or moisture for survival. For example, a favorite place of microorganisms is the moist drainage from a surgical wound. Some bacteria assume a form, called a spore, that is resistant to dry-

Table 33-1   Common Pathogens and Some Infections or Diseases They Produce

Organism	Major Reservoir(s)	Major Infections/Diseases
Bacteria		
Escherichia coli	Colon	Gastroenteritis, urinary tract infection
Staphylococcus aureus	Skin, hair, anterior nares	Wound infection, pneumonia, food poisoning, cellulitis
Streptococcus (beta-hemolytic group A) organisms	Oropharynx, skin, perianal area	"Strep throat," rheumatic fever, scarlet fever, impetigo, wound infection
Streptococcus (beta-hemolytic group B) organisms	Adult genitalia	Urinary tract infection, wound infection, post-partum sepsis, neonatal sepsis
Mycobacterium tuberculosis	Droplet nuclei from lungs	Tuberculosis
Neisseria gonorrhoeae	Genitourinary tract, rectum, mouth	Gonorrhea, pelvic inflammatory disease, infectious arthritis, conjunctivitis
Rickettsia rickettsii	Wood tick	Rocky Mountain spotted fever
Staphylococcus epidermidis	Skin	Wound infection, bacteremia
Viruses		
Hepatitis A virus	Feces	Hepatitis A
Hepatitis B virus	Blood and body fluids	Hepatitis B
Hepatitis C virus	Blood	Hepatitis C
Herpes simplex virus (type I)	Lesions of mouth or skin, saliva, genitalia	Cold sores, aseptic meningitis, sexually transmitted disease, herpetic whitlow
Human immunodeficiency virus (HIV)	Blood, semen, vaginal secretions (also isolated in saliva, tears, urine, and breast milk, but not proved to be sources of transmission)	Acquired immunodeficiency syndrome (AIDS)
Fungi		
Aspergillus organisms	Soil, dust, mouth, skin, colon, genital tract	Aspergillosis, pneumonia, sepsis
Candida albicans	Mouth, skin, colon, genital tract	Candidiasis, pneumonia, sepsis
Protozoa		
Plasmodium falciparum	Blood	Malaria

ing. These spore-forming bacteria, such as those that cause anthrax, botulism, and tetanus, can live without water.

Temperature. Microorganisms can live only in certain temperature ranges. The ideal temperature for most human pathogens is 35° C (95° F) (Keroack and Rosen-Kotilainen, 1996). However, some can survive temperature extremes that would be fatal to humans. Cold temperatures tend to prevent growth and reproduction of bacteria (**bacteriostasis**). A temperature that destroys bacteria is **bactericidal.**

pH. The acidity of an environment determines the viability of microorganisms. Most microorganisms prefer an environment within a pH range of 5 to 8. Bacteria in particular thrive in urine with an alkaline pH. Most organisms cannot survive the acid environment of the stomach. Acid-reducing medications (e.g., antacids and H_2 blockers) may cause an overgrowth of gastrointestinal organisms, which can contribute to nosocomial pneumonia in a client receiving these medications (Centers for Disease Control and Prevention [CDC], 2002).

Light. Microorganisms thrive in dark environments such as those under dressings and within body cavities.

Ultraviolet light may be effective in killing certain forms of bacteria (e.g., *Mycobacterium tuberculosis*).

Portal of Exit. After microorganisms find a site to grow and multiply, they must find a portal of exit if they are to enter another host and cause disease. Microorganisms can exit through a variety of sites, such as the skin and mucous membranes, respiratory tract, urinary tract, gastrointestinal tract, reproductive tract, and blood.

Skin and Mucous Membranes. The skin may be considered a portal of exit because any break in the integrity of the skin and mucous membranes may allow pathogens to exit the body. Often the body responds to a pathogenic organism with the creation of purulent drainage. For example, *S. aureus* causes a characteristic yellow, creamy drainage, whereas *Pseudomonas aeruginosa* causes a greenish, creamy drainage. This purulent drainage is a potential portal of exit.

Respiratory Tract. Pathogens that infect the respiratory tract, such as *M. tuberculosis,* can be released from the body when an infected person sneezes, coughs, talks, or even breathes. Microorganisms exit through the mouth and nose in normal clients. In clients with artificial airways such as tracheostomy or endotracheal tubes (see

Chapter 39), organisms easily exit the respiratory tract through these devices.

Urinary Tract. Normally urine is sterile. However, when a client has a urinary tract infection, microorganisms exit during urination or through urinary diversions such as ileostomies and suprapubic drains (see Chapter 44).

Gastrointestinal Tract. The mouth is one of the most bacterially contaminated sites of the body, although most of the organisms are normal flora—bacteria that normally reside within the body and defend against infection. However, organisms that are normal flora in one person can be pathogens in another. Organisms, for example, exit when a person expectorates saliva. Kissing can also provide a means of exit. Additional portals of exit include bowel elimination, drainage of bile via surgical wounds or drainage tubes, and escape of gastric contents during vomiting.

Reproductive Tract. Organisms such as *Neisseria gonorrhoeae* and human immunodeficiency virus (HIV) may exit through a man's urethral meatus or a woman's vaginal canal. In the man, semen may be the vehicle of pathogens. Discharge and vaginal fluid from the woman's vaginal canal may carry pathogens.

Blood. The blood is normally sterile, but in the case of infectious diseases such as hepatitis B or C, it becomes a reservoir for pathogens. A break in the skin allows pathogens to exit the body. Caregivers may become exposed during activities such as blood drawing, unless precautions are taken.

Modes of Transmission. There are many modes for transmission of microorganisms from the reservoir to the host. Table 33-2 summarizes common modes of transmission. Certain infectious diseases tend to be transmitted more commonly by specific modes. However, the same microorganisms may be transmitted by more than one route. For example, herpes zoster may be spread by the airborne route in droplet nuclei or by direct contact. Although the major mode of transmission of microorganisms is the hands of the health care worker, almost any object within the environment (e.g., a stethoscope or thermometer) can become a means of transmitting pathogens. All hospital personnel providing direct care (e.g., nurses, physical therapists, and physicians) or performing diagnostic and support services (e.g., laboratory technicians, respiratory therapists, and dietary workers) must follow practices to minimize the spread of infection. Each group follows procedures for handling equipment and supplies used by a client. For example, respiratory

Table 33-2   Modes of Transmission

Routes and Means	Examples of Organisms
Contact	**Contact**
Direct	
Person-to-person (fecal, oral) or physical contact between source and susceptible host (e.g., touching client)	Hepatitis A virus, *Shigella, Staphylococcus,* herpes simplex
Indirect	
Personal contact of susceptible host with contaminated inanimate object (e.g., needles or sharp objects, dressings)	Hepatitis B virus, hepatitis C virus, HIV, *Staphylococcus,* respiratory syncytial virus (RSV), *Pseudomonas*
Droplet	
Large particles that travel up to 3 feet and come in contact with susceptible host (e.g., coughing, sneezing, or talking)	Influenza virus, rubella virus
Air	**Air**
Droplet nuclei, or residue or evaporated droplets suspended in air (e.g., coughing, sneezing) or carried on dust particles	*Mycobacterium tuberculosis* (TB), varicella zoster virus (chickenpox), *Aspergillus,* measles virus
Vehicles	**Vehicles**
Contaminated items	*Vibrio cholerae*
Water	*Pseudomonas*
Drugs, solutions	*Pseudomonas*
Blood	Hepatitis B virus, hepatitis C virus, HIV, syphilis
Food (improperly handled, stored, or cooked, fresh or thawed meats)	*Salmonella, Escherichia coli, Clostridium botulinum*
Vector	**Vector**
External mechanical transfer (flies)	*Vibrio cholerae*
Internal transmission such as parasitic conditions between **vector** and host, such as:	
Mosquito	*Plasmodium falciparum* (malaria), West Nile virus
Louse	*Rickettsia typhi*
Flea	*Yersinia pestis* (plague)
Tick	*Borrelia burgdorferi* (Lyme disease)

therapists perform hand hygiene before working with each client and dispose of contaminated therapy equipment in a prescribed manner. Certain medical devices and diagnostic procedures provide avenues for the spread of pathogens. Invasive procedures such as cystoscopy (visualization of the bladder) facilitate diagnosis of problems but also increase the risk of transmitting infection. Because so many factors can promote the spread of infection to a client, all health care workers must be conscientious in using infection-control practices, such as proper hand washing and ensuring that equipment has been adequately disinfected or sterilized.

Portal of Entry. Organisms can enter the body through the same routes they use for exiting. For example, when a needle pierces a client's skin, organisms enter the body. More organisms enter the body as long as the device is in place. Any obstruction to the flow of urine from a urinary catheter allows organisms to travel up the urethra. Factors that reduce the body's defenses enhance the chances of pathogens entering the body.

Susceptible Host. Whether a person acquires an infection depends on susceptibility to an infectious agent. **Susceptibility** depends on the individual degree of resistance to a pathogen. Although everyone is constantly in contact with large numbers of microorganisms, an infection does not develop until an individual becomes susceptible to the strength and numbers of microorganisms capable of producing infection. The more virulent an organism, the greater the likelihood of a person's susceptibility. Organisms with resistance to antibiotics are becoming more common in acute care settings. This is believed to be associated with the frequent and sometimes inappropriate use of antibiotics. A person's resistance to an infectious agent is enhanced by vaccines or by actually contracting the disease.

The Infectious Process

By understanding the chain of infection, the nurse intervenes to prevent infections from developing. When the client acquires an infection, the nurse observes signs and symptoms of infection and takes appropriate actions to prevent its spread. Infections follow a progressive course (Box 33-1). The severity of the client's illness depends on the extent of the infection, the **pathogenicity** of the microorganisms, and the susceptibility of the host.

If infection is **localized** (e.g., a wound infection), proper care controls the spread and minimizes the illness. The client may experience localized symptoms such as pain and tenderness at the wound site. An infection that affects the entire body instead of just a single organ or part is **systemic** and can become fatal.

The course of an infection influences the level of nursing care provided. The nurse is responsible for properly administering antibiotics and monitoring the response to drug therapy (see Chapter 34). Supportive therapy includes providing adequate nutrition and rest to bolster defenses against the infectious process. The complexity of care further depends on body systems affected by the infection.

Regardless of whether infection is localized or systemic, the nurse plays a critical role in minimizing its spread. For example, the organism causing a simple wound infection can spread to involve an intravenous (IV) needle insertion site if the nurse uses improper technique during an IV dressing change. Nurses who have breaks in their own skin can also acquire infections from clients if their techniques for controlling infection transmission are inadequate.

Defenses Against Infection

The body has normal defenses against infection. Normal body flora that reside inside and outside of the body protect a person from several pathogens. Each organ system has defense mechanisms that defend against exposure to infectious microorganisms. The **inflammatory response** is a protective reaction that neutralizes pathogens and repairs body cells. Normal flora, body system defenses, and inflammation are all nonspecific defenses that protect against microorganisms regardless of prior exposure. The immune system is composed of separate cells and molecules that help the body resist disease. Certain responses of the immune system are nonspecific, whereas others are specific defenses against specific pathogens. If any of the body's defenses fail, an infection can quickly progress to a serious health problem.

Normal Flora. The body normally contains microorganisms that reside on the surface and deep layers of skin, in

---

Box 33-1   Course of Infection by Stage

Incubation Period

- Interval between entrance of pathogen into body and appearance of first symptoms (e.g., chickenpox, 2-3 weeks; common cold, 1-2 days; influenza, 1-3 days; mumps, 15-18 days)

Prodromal Stage

- Interval from onset of nonspecific signs and symptoms (malaise, low-grade fever, fatigue) to more specific symptoms (During this time, microorganisms grow and multiply, and client may be more capable of spreading disease to others.)

Illness Stage

- Interval when client manifests signs and symptoms specific to type of infection (e.g., common cold manifested by sore throat, sinus congestion, rhinitis; mumps manifested by earache, high fever, parotid and salivary gland swelling)

Convalescence

- Interval when acute symptoms of infection disappear (Length of recovery depends on severity of infection and client's general state of health; recovery may take several days to months.)

the saliva and oral mucosa, and in the gastrointestinal and genitourinary tracts. A person normally excretes trillions of microbes daily through the intestines. The skin also has a large population of resident flora. **Normal flora** do not usually cause disease when residing in their usual area of the body but instead participate in maintaining health.

Normal flora of the large intestine exist in large numbers without causing injury. Normal flora also secrete antibacterial substances within the intestine's walls. The skin's normal flora exert a protective action by inhibiting multiplication of organisms landing on the skin. The mouth and pharynx are also protected by flora that impair growth of invading microbes. The mass of normal flora maintains a sensitive balance with other microorganisms to prevent infection. Any factor that disrupts this balance places a person at increased risk for acquiring an infectious disease. For example, the use of **broad-spectrum antibiotics** for the treatment of infection can lead to **suprainfection.** A suprainfection develops when broad-spectrum antibiotics eliminate a wide range of microorganisms, not just those causing infection. Normal bacterial flora are eliminated, reducing the body's defenses and thus allowing disease-producing microorganisms to multiply.

Body System Defenses. A number of the body's organ systems have unique defenses against infection (Table 33-3). The skin, respiratory tract, and gastrointestinal tract are easily accessible to microorganisms. Pathogenic organisms easily adhere to the skin's surface, are inhaled into the lungs, or are ingested with food. Each organ system has defense mechanisms physiologically suited to its structure and function. For example, the lungs cannot completely control the entrance of microorganisms. However, the airways are lined with hairlike projections, or cilia, that rhythmically beat to move a blanket of mucus and adherent or trapped organisms up to the pharynx to be removed. Conditions that impair an organ's specialized defenses increase susceptibility to infection.

Inflammation. The body's cellular response to injury or infection is inflammation. Inflammation is a protective vascular reaction that delivers fluid, blood products, and nutrients to interstitial tissues in an area of injury. The process neutralizes and eliminates pathogens or dead **(necrotic)** tissues and establishes a means of repairing body cells and tissues. Signs of localized inflammation may include swelling, redness, heat, pain or tenderness, and loss of function in the affected body part. When inflammation becomes systemic, other signs and symptoms develop, including fever, leukocytosis, malaise, anorexia, nausea, vomiting, and lymph node enlargement.

The inflammatory response may be triggered by physical agents, chemical agents, or microorganisms. Mechanical trauma, temperature extremes, and radiation are examples of physical agents. Chemical agents include external and internal irritants such as harsh poisons or gastric acid. Microorganisms may trigger this response, as previously discussed.

After tissues are injured, a series of well-coordinated events occurs. The inflammatory response includes the following:
1. Vascular and cellular responses

2. Formation of inflammatory **exudates** (fluid and cells that are discharged from cells or blood vessels, e.g., pus or serum)
3. Tissue repair

Vascular and Cellular Responses. Acute inflammation is an immediate response to cellular injury. Arterioles supplying the infected or injured area dilate, allowing more blood into the local circulation. The increase in local blood flow causes the characteristic redness of inflammation. The symptom of localized warmth results from a greater volume of blood at the inflammatory site. Local vasodilation delivers blood and white blood cells (WBCs) to injured tissues. Injury causes tissue necrosis, and as a result the body releases histamine, bradykinin, prostaglandin, and serotonin. These chemical mediators increase the permeability of small blood vessels. Fluid, protein, and cells enter interstitial spaces. Accumulated fluid appears as localized swelling **(edema).**

Another sign of inflammation is pain. The swelling of inflamed tissues increases pressure on nerve endings, causing pain. Chemical substances such as histamine stimulate nerve endings. As a result of physiological changes occurring with inflammation, the involved body part usually undergoes a temporary loss of function. For example, a localized infection of the hand causes the fingers to become swollen, painful, and discolored. Joints may become stiff as a result of swelling, but function of the fingers returns when inflammation subsides.

The cellular response of inflammation involves WBCs arriving at the site. WBCs pass through blood vessels and into the tissues. Through the process of **phagocytosis,** specialized WBCs, called neutrophils and monocytes, ingest and destroy microorganisms or other small particles. As inflammation becomes systemic, other signs and symptoms develop. **Leukocytosis,** or an increase in the number of circulating WBCs, is the body's response to WBCs leaving blood vessels. A serum WBC count is normally 5000 to 10,000/mm^3 but may rise to 15,000 to 20,000/mm^3 and higher during inflammation. Fever is caused by phagocytic release of pyrogens from bacterial cells that cause a rise in the hypothalamic set point (see Chapter 31). Other systemic signs and symptoms include malaise, anorexia, and lymph node enlargement.

Inflammatory Exudate. Accumulation of fluid and dead tissue cells and WBCs forms an exudate at the site of inflammation. Exudate may be **serous** (clear, like plasma), **sanguineous** (containing red blood cells), or **purulent** (containing WBCs and bacteria). Eventually the exudate is cleared away through lymphatic drainage. Platelets and plasma proteins such as fibrinogen form a meshlike matrix at the site of inflammation to prevent its spread.

Tissue Repair. When there is injury to tissue cells, healing involves the defensive, reconstructive, and maturative stages (see Chapter 47). Damaged cells are eventually replaced with healthy new cells. The new cells undergo a gradual maturation until they take on the same structural characteristics and appearance as the previous cells. If inflammation is chronic, tissue defects may fill with fragile **granulation tissue.** Granulation tissue is not as strong as tissue collagen and assumes the form of scar tissue.

Table 33-3   Normal Defense Mechanisms Against Infection

Defense Mechanisms	Action	Factors That May Alter Defense
Skin		
Intact multilayered surface (body's first line of defense against infection)	Provides barrier to microorganisms and antibacterial activity	Cuts, abrasions, puncture wounds, areas of maceration
Shedding of outer layer of skin cells	Removes organisms that adhere to skin's outer layers	Failure to bathe regularly
Sebum	Contains fatty acid that kills some bacteria	Excessive bathing
Mouth		
Intact multilayered mucosa	Provides mechanical barrier to microorganisms	Lacerations, trauma, extracted teeth
Saliva	Washes away particles containing microorganisms	Poor oral hygiene, dehydration
	Contains microbial inhibitors (e.g., lysozyme)	
Eye		
Tearing and blinking	Provides mechanisms to reduce entry (blinking) or to assist in washing away (tearing) particles containing pathogens	Injury
Respiratory Tract		
Cilia lining upper airway, coated by mucus	Trap inhaled microbes and sweep them outward in mucus to be expectorated or swallowed	Smoking, high concentration of oxygen and carbon dioxide, decreased humidity, cold air
Macrophages	Engulf and destroy microorganisms that reach lung's alveoli	Smoking
Urinary Tract		
Flushing action of urine flow	Washes away microorganisms on lining of bladder and urethra	Obstruction to normal flow by urinary catheter placement, obstruction from growth or tumor, delayed micturition
Intact multilayered epithelium	Provides barrier to microorganisms	Introduction of urinary catheter, continual movement of catheter in urethra
Gastrointestinal Tract		
Acidity of gastric secretions	Administration of antacids	Administration of antacids
Rapid peristalsis in small intestine	Prevents retention of bacterial contents	Delayed motility resulting from impaction of fecal contents in large bowel or mechanical obstruction by masses
Vagina		
At puberty, normal flora causing vaginal secretions to achieve low pH	Inhibit growth of many microorganisms	Antibiotics and oral contraceptives disrupting normal flora

Nosocomial Infections

Clients in health care settings may have an increased risk of acquiring infections. **Nosocomial infections** result from delivery of health services in a health care facility. A hospital is one of the most likely places for acquiring an infection because it harbors a high population of virulent strains of microorganisms that may be resistant to antibiotics. Unfortunately, many nosocomial infections are transmitted by health care workers.

Iatrogenic infections are a type of nosocomial infection resulting from a diagnostic or therapeutic proce-

dure. A urinary tract infection that develops after catheter insertion is an example of an iatrogenic nosocomial infection. The incidence of nosocomial infections can be reduced if nurses use critical thinking when practicing aseptic techniques. The nurse should always consider the client's risks for infection and anticipate how the approach to care may increase or decrease the chances of infection transmission.

Nosocomial infections may be exogenous or endogenous. An **exogenous infection** arises from microorganisms external to the individual that do not exist as normal

Box 33-2 Sites for and Causes of Nosocomial Infections

Urinary Tract

Unsterile insertion of urinary catheter
Open drainage system
Catheter and tube becoming disconnected
Drainage bag port touching contaminated surface
Improper specimen collection technique
Obstruction or interference with urinary drainage
Urine in catheter or drainage tube being allowed to reenter bladder (reflux)
Repeated catheter irrigations
Improper hand hygiene

Surgical or Traumatic Wounds

Improper skin preparation (shaving and bathing) before surgery
Failure to cleanse skin surface properly
Failure to use aseptic technique during dressing changes
Use of contaminated antiseptic solutions
Improper hand hygiene

Respiratory Tract

Contaminated respiratory therapy equipment
Failure to use aseptic technique while suctioning airway
Improper disposal of secretions
Improper hand hygiene

Bloodstream

Contamination of IV fluids by tubing or needle changes
Insertion of drug additives to IV fluid
Addition of connecting tube or stopcocks to IV system
Improper care of needle insertion site
Contaminated needles or catheters
Failure to change IV access site when inflammation first appears
Improper technique during administration of multiple blood products
Improper care of peritoneal or hemodialysis shunts
Improper hand hygiene

Box 33-3 *Focus on Older Adults*

- An age-related decline in immune system function, termed immune senescence, increases the body's susceptibility to infection and lessens the strength of the overall immune response (Eliopoulos, 2001).
- The older adult's higher prevalence of chronic disease allows infectious agents to readily invade, and higher rates of hospitalization and institutionalization because of these chronic diseases increases their exposure to pathogens (Eliopoulos, 2001).
- Risks associated with the development of nosocomial infections in older clients include poor nutrition, unintentional weight loss, and low serum albumin levels (Lueckenotte, 2000).
- Age-related changes in immunity contribute to the increased risk of acquiring pneumonia and influenza in older adulthood, both of which have significant age-related increases in mortality rates (Miller, 1999).

Data from Eliopoulos C: *Gerontologic nursing,* ed 5, Philadelphia, 2001, Lippincott; Miller CA: *Nursing care of older adults: theory and practice,* ed 3, Philadelphia, 1999, Lippincott; and Lueckenotte AG: *Gerontologic nursing,* ed 2, St. Louis, 2000, Mosby.

wounds, urinary and respiratory tracts, and the bloodstream (Box 33-2).

Nosocomial infections significantly increase costs of health care. Older adults have increased susceptibility to these infections because of their affinity to chronic disease and the aging process itself (Box 33-3). Extended stays in health care institutions, increased disability, increased costs of antibiotics, and prolonged recovery times add to the expenses of the client, as well as the expenses of the health care institution and funding bodies (e.g., Medicare). Often, costs for nosocomial infections are not reimbursed; as a result, prevention has a beneficial financial impact and is an important part of managed care.

The Nursing Process in Infection Control

Assessment

The nurse assesses the client's defense mechanisms, susceptibility, and knowledge of infections. A review of disease history with the client and family may reveal an exposure to a communicable disease. A thorough review of the client's clinical condition may detect signs and symptoms of actual infection or risk for infection. An analysis of laboratory findings provides information about a client's defense against infection. By knowing the factors that increase susceptibility or risk for infection, the nurse is better able to plan preventive therapy that includes aseptic techniques. By recognizing early signs and symptoms of infection, the nurse can alert others on the health care team to the potential need for therapy and initiate supportive nursing measures.

flora; examples are *Salmonella* organisms and *Clostridium tetani*. An **endogenous infection** can occur when part of the client's flora becomes altered and an overgrowth results. Examples are infections caused by enterococci, yeasts, and streptococci. When sufficient numbers of microorganisms normally found in one body cavity or lining are transferred to another body site, an endogenous infection develops. For example, transmission of enterococci, normally found in fecal material, from the hands to the skin is a common cause of wound infections. The number of microorganisms needed to cause a nosocomial infection depends on the virulence of the organism, the host's susceptibility, and the site affected.

The number of health care employees having direct contact with a client, the type and number of invasive procedures, the therapy received, and the length of hospitalization influence the risk of infection. Major sites for nosocomial infection include surgical or traumatic

---

Box 33-4   **Risk Factors for Infection**

Inadequate Primary Defenses

Broken skin or mucosa
Traumatized tissue
Decreased ciliary action
Obstructed urine outflow
Altered peristalsis
Change in pH of secretions
Decreased mobility

Inadequate Secondary Defenses

Reduced hemoglobin level
Suppression of WBCs (drug or disease related)
Suppressed inflammatory response (drug or disease related)
Low WBC count (leukopenia)

Status of Defense Mechanisms. A review of physical assessment findings and the client's medical condition reveals the status of normal defense mechanisms against infection. For example, any break in the skin or mucosa is a potential site for infection. Similarly, a chronic smoker is at greater risk for acquiring a respiratory tract infection after general surgery because the cilia of the lung are less likely to propel retained mucus from the lung's airways. Any reduction in the body's primary or secondary defenses against infection places a client at risk (Box 33-4).

Client Susceptibility. Many factors influence susceptibility to infection. The nurse gathers information about each factor through the client's and family's history.

Age. Throughout the life span, susceptibility to infection changes. An infant has immature defenses against infection. Born with only the antibodies provided by the mother, the infant's immune system is incapable of producing the necessary immunoglobulins and WBCs to adequately fight some infections. However, breast-fed infants have greater immunity than bottle-fed infants, because they receive the mother's antibodies through the breast milk. As the child grows, the immune system matures, but the child is still susceptible to organisms that cause the common cold, intestinal infections, and infectious diseases such as mumps and measles if not vaccinated.

The young or middle-age adult has refined defenses against infection. Normal flora, body system defenses, inflammation, and the immune response provide protection against invading microorganisms. Viruses are the most common cause of infectious illness in young or middle-age adults.

Defenses against infection may change with aging (Gantz, Tkatch, and Makris, 2000). The immune response, particularly cell-mediated immunity, declines. Older adults also undergo alterations in the structure and function of the skin, urinary tract, and lungs. For example, the skin loses its turgor and the epithelium thins. As a result, the skin is more easily abraded or torn. This increases the potential for invasion by pathogens (Table 33-4).

Nutritional Status. When protein intake is inadequate as a result of poor diet or debilitating disease, the rate of protein breakdown exceeds that of tissue synthesis (see Chapter 43). A reduction in the intake of protein and other nutrients such as carbohydrates and fats reduces the body's defenses against infection and impairs wound healing (see Chapter 47).

Clients with illnesses or problems that increase protein requirements are at further risk. These problems include traumatic injury, extensive burns, and conditions causing fever. Clients who have had surgery also require increased protein.

The nurse assesses clients' dietary intakes and abilities to tolerate solid foods. Clients who have difficulty with swallowing, who experience alterations in digestion, or who are too confused or weak to feed themselves are at risk for inadequate dietary intake. A dietitian may be called to assist in calculating the calorie count of foods ingested. In preparation for discharge, the nurse evaluates the client's and family's understanding of nutritional needs.

Stress. The body responds to emotional or physical stress by the general adaptation syndrome (see Chapter 30). During the alarm stage, the basal metabolic rate increases as the body uses energy stores. Adrenocorticotropic hormone (ACTH) acts to increase serum glucose levels and decrease unnecessary antiinflammatory responses through the release of cortisone. If stress continues or becomes intense, elevated cortisone levels result in decreased resistance to infection. Continued stress leads to exhaustion, wherein energy stores are depleted and the body has no resistance to invading organisms. The same conditions that increase nutritional requirements, such as surgery or trauma, also increase physiological stress.

Disease Process. Clients with diseases of the immune system are at particular risk for infection. Leukemia, AIDS, lymphoma, and aplastic anemia are conditions that compromise a host by weakening defenses against infectious organisms. Clients with leukemia, for example, are unable to produce enough WBCs to ward off infection.

Victims of chronic diseases such as diabetes mellitus and multiple sclerosis are also more susceptible to infection because of general debilitation and nutritional impairment. Diseases that impair body system defenses, such as emphysema and bronchitis (which impair ciliary action and thicken mucus), cancer (which alters the immune response), and peripheral vascular disease (which reduces blood flow to injured tissues), increase susceptibility to infection. Burn clients have a very high susceptibility to infection because of the damage to skin surfaces. The greater the depth and extent of the burns, the higher the risk for infection.

Medical Therapy. Some drugs and medical therapies compromise immunity to infection. The nurse assesses the client's history to determine whether the client takes medications at home that increase infection susceptibility. A review of therapies received within the health care setting further reveals risks. Adrenal corticosteroids, prescribed for several conditions, are antiinflammatory drugs that cause

Table 33-4   Assessing the Risk of Infection in Older Adults

Component	Possible Changes With Age	Outcome
Skin	Thinner dermal and epidermal layers, decreased collagen strength, decreased skin elasticity, decreased sweat	Pressure ulcers
Peripheral nerves	Reduced sensitivity, particularly in clients with history of alcohol abuse, vitamin B_{12} deficiency, and diabetes mellitus	Pressure ulcers, clients unaware of trauma to skin leading to infection
Circulation	Congestive heart failure, calcified mitral and aortic valves	Pneumonia, bacterial endocarditis
Peripheral circulation	More elastic veins, less effective venous valves, blood pooling in lower extremities	Venous stasis ulcers
Mouth	Dehydration, loss of saliva production, functional inability to maintain oral hygiene	Parotid gland infection, peridontal disease, localized abscess, bacteremia
Gastrointestinal tract	Loss of ability to secrete stomach acid in 30% of persons over 70	Salmonella diarrhea
Pulmonary system	Increased colonization of oropharynx, impaired mucociliary clearance, decreased macrophage function, decreased cough reflex	Viral and bacterial pneumonia
Urinary tract	Prostatic hyperplasia, urethral strictures, age-related hormonal changes in vaginal wall, pelvic floor relaxation, ureterocele or cystocele, degeneration of nerves leading to neurogenic bladder, use of tricyclic antidepressants, dehydration	Asymptomatic bacteriuria, cystitis, pyelonephritis
Nutrition	Malnutrition, vitamin deficiency (vitamin A, pyridoxine, and riboflavin), protein and caloric malnutrition	Impaired immune response to infection
Drug therapy	Corticosteroid and cytotoxic drugs	Impaired immune response to infection
Nursing home residency	Exposure to nosocomial infections, including influenza, *Proteus* and *Providencia* organisms with an indwelling catheter, tuberculosis, and wound infections (Incidence of bacteremia after admission is 50%.)	Frequent serious infection, increased risk of pneumonia

Data from Gantz NM, Tkatch LS, Makris AT: Geriatric infections. In *APIC text of infection control and epidemiology,* Washington, DC, 2000, Association for Professionals in Infection Control and Epidemiology.

protein breakdown and impair the inflammatory response against bacteria and other pathogens. Cytotoxic or antineoplastic drugs attack cancer cells but cause side effects of bone marrow depression and normal cell toxicity. With bone marrow depression the body is unable to produce lymphocytes and sufficient WBCs. When normal cells become altered by antineoplastic agents, cellular defenses against infection fail. Cyclosporine and other immunosuppressant drugs, which decrease the body's immune response, are commonly taken by clients who are organ transplant recipients. The immunosuppressants prevent organ and tissue rejection, but they also increase susceptibility to infection.

Cancer clients receiving radiotherapy are also at risk for infection. The massive doses of radiation, which destroy cancerous cells, can also depress the bone marrow and destroy normal cells.

Clinical Appearance. The signs and symptoms of infection may be local or systemic. Localized infections are most common in areas of skin or mucous membrane breakdown, such as surgical and traumatic wounds, pressure ulcers, and mouth lesions. Infections also develop locally in cavities beneath the skin; an example is an abscess.

To assess an area for localized infection, the nurse first inspects the area for redness and swelling caused by inflammation. Because there may be drainage from open lesions or wounds, the nurse wears disposable gloves. Infected drainage may be yellow, green, or brown, depending on the pathogen. The nurse asks the client about pain or tenderness around the site. The client may complain of tightness and pain caused by edema. If the infected area is large enough, movement of a body part may be restricted. Gentle palpation of an infected area usually results in some degree of tenderness.

Systemic infections cause more generalized symptoms than local infection. They usually result in fever, fatigue, and malaise. Lymph nodes that drain the area of infection often become enlarged, swollen, and tender during palpation. For example, an abscess in the peritoneal cavity may cause enlargement of lymph nodes in the groin. An infection of the upper respiratory tract may cause cervical lymph node enlargement. If an infection is serious and widespread, all major lymph nodes may enlarge. Systemic infections commonly cause a loss of appetite, nausea, and vomiting.

Systemic infections may develop after treatment for localized infection has failed. The nurse should be alert for changes in the client's level of activity and responsiveness. As systemic infections develop, the client may become lethargic and complain of a loss of energy. An elevation in body temperature may lead to episodes of increased heart and respiratory rates and low blood pressure. Involvement

Table 33-5	Laboratory Tests to Screen for Infection	
Laboratory Value	**Normal (Adult) Values**	**Indication of Infection**
WBC count	5000-10,000/mm³	Increased in acute infection, decreased in certain viral or overwhelming infections
Erythrocyte sedimentation rate	Up to 15 mm/hr for men and 20 mm/hr for women	Elevated in presence of inflammatory process
Iron level	60-90 g/100 ml	Decreased in chronic infection
Cultures of urine and blood	Normally sterile, without microorganism growth	Presence of infectious microorganism growth
Cultures and gram stain of wound, sputum, and throat	No WBCs on gram stain, possible normal flora	Presence of infectious microorganism growth and WBCs on gram stain
Differential Count (Percentage of Each Type of WBC)		
Neutrophils	55%-70%	Increased in acute suppurative infection, decreased in overwhelming bacterial infection (older adult)
Lymphocytes	20%-40%	Increased in chronic bacterial and viral infection, decreased in sepsis
Monocytes	2%-8%	Increased in protozoal, rickettsial, and tuberculosis infections
Eosinophils	1%-4%	Increased in parasitic infection
Basophils	0.5%-1%	Normal during infection

of major body systems may produce specific signs. For example, a pulmonary infection may result in a productive cough with purulent sputum. A urinary tract infection may result in cloudy, foul-smelling urine.

An infection in older adults may not present with typical signs and symptoms. Often, older adults have advanced infection before it is identified. This is because of their reduced inflammatory and immune responses. Normally, older adults have increased fatigue and diminished pain sensitivity. A reduced or absent fever response may occur from chronic use of aspirin or nonsteroidal antiinflammatory drugs. Atypical symptoms such as confusion, incontinence, or agitation may be the only symptoms of an infectious illness (Gantz and others, 2000). An example is pneumonia, the main complication of influenza. As many as 20% of older adults with pneumonia do not have the typical signs and symptoms of fever, shaking, chills, and rusty productive sputum. The only symptoms may be an increased, unexplained heart rate, confusion, or generalized fatigue.

Laboratory Data. A review of laboratory test results may reveal infection (Table 33-5). Laboratory values, however, are not enough to detect infection. Other clinical signs must be assessed. Factors other than infection may alter test values. For example, trauma and physical stress can cause an elevation in the number of neutrophils. A culture result may show growth of an organism in the absence of infection.

Clients With Infection. A client with infection may have a variety of health problems. The nurse assesses ways that the infection affects the client's and family's needs. These may be physical, psychological, social, or economical. For example, a client with a chronic disease such as AIDS may experience serious psychological problems as a result of self-imposed isolation or rejection by family and friends. Clients or their families may not be able to afford the cost

of medical care. The nurse, using a case management approach, determines the client's and family's ability to adjust to the disease and the available resources needed for managing health care challenges (Grimes and Grimes, 1994).

Nursing Diagnosis

During assessment the nurse gathers objective findings, such as an open incision or a reduced caloric intake, and subjective data, such as a client's complaint of tenderness over a surgical wound site (Box 33-5). Then the nurse interprets the data carefully, looking for clusters of defining characteristics or risk factors that create a pattern suggesting a specific nursing diagnosis. The following are examples of nursing diagnoses that may apply:

- Disturbed body image
- Risk for infection
- Risk for injury
- Imbalanced nutrition: less than body requirements
- Impaired oral mucous membrane
- Risk for impaired skin integrity
- Social isolation
- Impaired tissue integrity

It may be necessary for the nurse to validate data (e.g., by inspecting the integrity of a wound more carefully). Likewise, additional data such as laboratory findings may help. The selection of appropriate nursing diagnoses depends on analyzing and organizing data correctly.

The diagnosis must have the appropriate etiological factor for the nurse to establish an appropriate and well-thought-out plan. For example, minimizing the *risk for infection related to broken skin* requires good hygiene measures and wound care. Minimizing the *risk for infection related to malnutrition* requires good nutritional support and fluid balance.

The nurse may diagnose a risk for infection or make diagnoses that result from the effects of infection on health

Nursing Diagnostic Process

Box 33-5

Assessment Activities	Defining Characteristics	Nursing Diagnosis
Check results of laboratory tests. Review current medications.	WBC count 5000/mm³	Risk for infection related to lowered immunity
	Client receiving azathioprine (Imuran), an immunosuppressant	
Identify potential sites of infection.	IV catheter in right forearm, in place for 3 days	
	Foley catheter draining amber-colored urine	

status. The nurse's success in planning appropriate nursing interventions depends on the accuracy of the diagnosis and the ability to meet the client's needs.

Planning

Goals and Outcomes. The client's care plan is based on each nursing diagnosis and related factor (see care plan). The nurse develops a plan that sets attainable outcomes so that interventions are purposeful and directed. The nurse caring for the client with the nursing diagnosis of *risk for infection related to broken skin* implements skin and wound care measures to promote healing. The expected outcomes of "reduction in wound size by 1 cm" and "absence of drainage" set targets for measuring the client's improvement. Once outcomes are met, the goal of "skin intact and without drainage" can be reached. Interventions are selected in collaboration with the client, the family, and others on the health care team. The nurse directs the care in the acute care setting and may involve the dietitian or respiratory therapist in assisting with instruction on procedures that need to be followed after discharge. Common goals of care applicable to clients with infection may include the following:

- Preventing exposure to infectious organisms
- Controlling or reducing the extent of infection
- Maintaining resistance to infection
- Educating the client and family about infection control techniques

Setting Priorities. The nurse establishes priorities for the goals of care. For example, a client has developed an open wound, suffers a debilitating disease such as cancer, and has been unable to tolerate solid foods. The priority of administering therapies that promote wound healing exceeds the goal of educating the client to assume self-care therapies at home. When the client's condition improves, the priorities will change, and client education becomes an essential intervention.

Continuity of Care. The development of a care plan includes infection prevention practices. The nurse may initiate appropriate referrals, such as a dietitian, infection-control professional, or home care nurse, to collaborate in the client's care. When care is being administered in the

home, the nurse plans to be sure the environment supports good infection-control practices. For example, if a client does not have running water yet requires wound care, even simple hand washing is difficult to achieve. The nurse will bring a waterless antimicrobial solution during visits to ensure adequate hand hygiene. Educating clients and families is also an important aspect of prevention.

Implementation

By recognizing and assessing a client's risk factors and implementing appropriate measures, the nurse can reduce the risk of infection.

Health Promotion. Through critical thinking, the nurse may prevent an infection from developing or spreading by minimizing the numbers and kinds of organisms transmitted to potential infection sites. Eliminating reservoirs of infection, controlling portals of exit and entry, and avoiding actions that transmit microorganisms prevent bacteria from finding a new site in which to grow. Proper use of sterile supplies, barrier protection, and proper hand hygiene are examples of methods that the nurse may use to control the spread of microorganisms. A final preventive measure is to strengthen a potential host's defenses against infection. Nutritional support, rest, maintenance of physiological protective mechanisms, and recommended immunizations protect a client from invasion by pathogens.

Having an infection-control conscience helps the nurse to apply good medical-surgical aseptic practices at the right time and in the right clinical situation. When a client develops an infection, the nurse continues preventive care so that health care personnel and other clients are not exposed to the infection. Clients with communicable diseases may require isolation precautions that control the environment by forming barriers against transmission of infection.

Acute Care Measures. Treatment of an infectious process includes eliminating the infectious organisms and supporting the client's defenses. To identify the causative organism, the nurse may collect specimens of body fluids or drainage from infected body sites for cultures. When the disease process or causative organism has been identified,

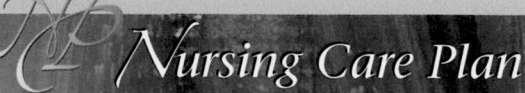

Nursing Care Plan

Risk for Infection

Assessment

Mrs. Spicer was admitted to the medical nursing unit 3 days ago with a diagnosis of lymphoma. She received her first dose of multiagent chemotherapy yesterday. Jess Ralston is the stu- dent nurse caring for Mrs. Spicer. He begins his shift of care by conducting a focused assessment.

Assessment Activities	Findings/Defining Characteristics
Reviews client's chart for laboratory data reflecting immune function.	Data show a reduction in number of white blood cells (leukopenia).
Ask client to describe appetite and review food intake for last 24 hours. Weigh client. Measure height.	Client reports she has not had an interest in eating for a couple of weeks. She has lost approximately 6 pounds. Her current weight is 125 lb, height 5'7". Her food intake yesterday consisted of a small cup of applesauce, ½ bowl of soup, some crackers, and two glasses of juice. Client states, "I get full easily and lose interest in food."
Palpate client's cervical and clavicular lymph nodes.	Lymph nodes are enlarged and painless.
Review effects of chemotherapy in drug reference.	Multi agent chemotherapy causes drug-induced pancytopenia.

Nursing Diagnosis: Risk for infection related to immunosuppression and reduced food intake.

Planning

Goal	Expected Outcomes*
	Risk Detection
Client will remain free of infection.	Client will remain afebrile.
	Client will develop no signs or symptoms of local infection (e.g., remains free of cough, cloudy or foul-smelling urine, or purulent drainage from open wound or normal body opening).
	Knowledge: Infection Control
Client will become knowledgeable of infection risks.	Client will identify routines to follow in the home that reduce transmission of microorganisms.
	Client will identify signs and symptoms to report to health care provider indicating infection.

*Outcome classification labels from: Moorhead S, Johnson M, Maas M: *Nursing Outcomes Classification (NOC)*, ed 3, St. Louis, 2004, Mosby.

Interventions†

Interventions†	Rationale
Fall Prevention	
Monitor client's body temperature routinely, inspect oral cavity for lesions, inspect urethral and vaginal orifices for drainage or discharge, inspect IV access site for drainage, and observe client for evidence of cough.	Interventions are designed to prevent and ensure early detection of infection in a client at risk (Dochterman and Bulechek, 2000).
Practice hand hygiene routinely before caring for client, between clients, and before any invasive procedures.	Rigorous hand hygiene reduces bacterial counts on the hands (Boyce and Pittet, 2002).
Teach client how to perform hand hygiene correctly.	Client can easily come in contact with infectious agents that can cause infection.
Consult with dietitian in providing a high-calorie, high-protein, low-bacteria diet. Minimize intake of salads, raw fruits and vegetables and undercooked meat, pepper, and paprika. Offer small frequent meals.	Maintaining calorie and protein intake will prevent weight loss. Foods high in bacteria should be avoided because they increase risk for gastrointestinal infection (Ignatavicius and Workman, 2002).
Infection Control	
Instruct client to report the following to physician: temperature greater than 100° F (38° C), persistent cough with or without sputum, pus or foul-smelling drainage from body site, presence of abscess, urine that is cloudy or foul smelling, or burning on urination.	Signs and symptoms are indicative of local or systemic infection.

†Intervention classification labels from Dochterman JM, Bulechek GM: *Nursing Interventions Classification (NIC)*, ed 4, St. Louis, 2004, Mosby.

Continued

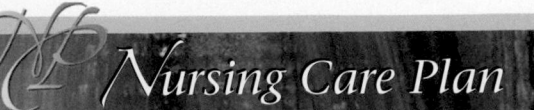

Nursing Care Plan

Risk for Infection—cont'd

Interventions†—cont'd

Infection Controls—cont'd
Teach client to follow these activities at home:
- Avoid crowds and large gatherings of people.
- Bathe daily.
- Do not share personal toilet items (toothbrush, washcloth, deodorant stick) with family.
- Take temperature twice daily.
- Do not drink water that has been standing for longer than 15 minutes.
- Do not reuse cups or glasses without washing.

†Intervention classification labels from Dochterman JM, Bulechek GM: *Nursing Interventions Classification (NIC)*, ed 4, St. Louis, 2004, Mosby.

Rationale

These measures are designed to prevent infection in those clients with impaired immune function (Ignatavicius and Workman, 2002).

Evaluation

Nursing Actions	Client Response/Finding	Achievement of Outcome
Compare client's body temperature and other physical findings with baseline data.	Client remains afebrile and denies having cough or burning on urination. No signs of drainage or discharge from body site.	Client has no active infection at this time.
Ask client to describe signs and symptoms to report to health care provider.	Client able to identify temperature range to report. Was able to describe cough. Unable to identify signs of urinary infection or local discharge.	Client has partial understanding of signs and symptoms to report. Will require additional instruction. Offer information sheet.
Ask client to explain the measures to take at home to reduce exposure to infectious agents.	Client able to discuss need to avoid sharing personal hygiene articles. Asked for a listing of other precautions and requested that husband be included in discussion.	Client has partial understanding of restrictions. Will obtain printed guidelines and include husband in discussion this evening.

the physician prescribes the treatment that is most effective for the situation. The nurse properly administers antibiotics and other treatments, watching for adverse reactions and assessing the progress of the infection.

Systemic infections require measures to prevent complications of fever (see Chapter 31). Maintaining intake of fluids prevents dehydration resulting from diaphoresis. The client's increased metabolic rate requires an adequate nutritional intake. Rest preserves energy for the healing process.

Localized infections often require measures to facilitate removal of debris to promote healing. The nurse applies principles of wound care to remove infected drainage from wound sites and support the integrity of healing wounds. Special dressings can be applied to facilitate removal of infectious drainage and promote healing of wound margins. Drainage tubes may be inserted to remove infected drainage from body cavities. The nurse uses medical and surgical aseptic techniques to manage wounds and ensure correct handling of all drainage or body fluids (see Chapter 47).

During the course of infection the nurse supports the client's body defense mechanisms. For example, if a client has infectious diarrhea, the nurse must maintain skin integrity to prevent breakdown and the entrance of microorganisms. Other routine hygiene measures such as

cleansing the oral cavity and bathing protect the skin and mucous membranes from invasion and overgrowth of microorganisms.

Asepsis. The nurse's efforts to minimize the onset and spread of infection are based on the principles of aseptic technique. **Asepsis** is the absence of pathogenic (disease-producing) microorganisms. Aseptic technique refers to practices that keep a client as free from pathogens as possible. The two types of aseptic technique are medical and surgical asepsis.

Medical asepsis, or clean technique, includes procedures used to reduce and prevent the spread of microorganisms. Hand hygiene, using clean gloves to prevent direct contact with blood or body fluids, and cleaning the environment routinely are examples of medical asepsis. Principles of medical asepsis are commonly followed in the home, as in washing hands before preparing food.

After an object becomes unsterile or unclean, it is considered contaminated. In medical asepsis an area or object is considered contaminated if it contains or is suspected of containing pathogens. For example, a used bedpan, the floor, and a used dressing are contaminated.

The nurse follows certain principles and procedures, including standard precautions to prevent infection and control its spread. During daily routine care the nurse uses basic medical aseptic techniques to break the infection chain. Because infections are readily transmissible between clients and caregivers, it may become necessary for the nurse to follow isolation precautions as appropriate.

The nurse is responsible for providing the client with a safe environment. The effectiveness of infection-control practices depends on the nurse's conscientiousness and consistency in using effective aseptic technique. It is easy to forget key procedural steps or, when hurried, to take shortcuts that break aseptic procedures. However, the nurse's failure to be meticulous will place the client at risk for an infection that can seriously impair recovery or lead to death.

Control or Elimination of Infectious Agents. Proper cleansing, disinfection, and sterilization of contaminated objects significantly reduce and often eliminate microorganisms. In health care centers a sterile processing department disinfects and sterilizes reusable supplies. However, the nurse also may be required to perform these functions. Many principles of cleaning and disinfection also apply to the home.

Cleaning. Cleaning is the removal of all soil (e.g., organic and inorganic material) from objects and surfaces (Rutala and Weber, 2002). Generally, cleaning involves use of water and mechanical action with detergents or enzymatic products. When an object comes in contact with infectious or potentially infectious material, the object is contaminated. If the object is disposable, it is usually discarded unless formal policies and procedures are in place for reprocessing the object. Reusable objects must be cleaned thoroughly before reuse and then either disinfected or sterilized according to the manufacturer's recommendations.

When cleaning equipment that is soiled by organic material such as blood, fecal matter, mucus, or pus, the nurse applies a mask and protective eyewear (or a face shield), and waterproof gloves. These barriers provide protection from infectious organisms. A brush and detergent or soap are needed for cleaning. The following steps ensure that an object is clean:

1. Rinse a contaminated object or article with cold running water to remove organic material. Hot water causes the protein in organic material to coagulate and stick to objects, making removal difficult.
2. After rinsing, wash the object with soap and warm water. Soap or detergent reduces the surface tension of water and emulsifies dirt or remaining material. Rinse the object thoroughly to remove the emulsified dirt.
3. Use a brush to remove dirt or material in grooves or seams. Friction dislodges contaminated material for easy removal. Open any hinged items for cleaning.
4. Rinse the object in warm water.
5. Dry the object and prepare it for disinfection or sterilization if indicated by the intended use of the item.
6. The brush, gloves, and sink in which the equipment is cleaned should be considered contaminated and should be cleaned and dried.

Disinfection and Sterilization. **Disinfection** describes a process that eliminates many or all microorganisms, with the exception of bacterial spores, from inanimate objects

Box 33-6   Categories for Sterilization, Disinfection, and Cleaning

Critical Items

Items that enter sterile tissue or the vascular system present a high risk of infection if the items are contaminated with microorganisms, especially bacterial spores. *Critical* items must be *sterile*. Some of these items follow:

Surgical instruments
Intravascular catheters
Urinary catheters
Needles

Semicritical Items

Items that come in contact with mucous membranes or skin that is not intact also present risks. These objects must be free of all microorganisms (except bacterial spores). *Semicritical items* must be *disinfected* or *sterilized*. Some of these items follow:

Respiratory suction tubing and catheters
Endotracheal tubes
Gastrointestinal endoscopes

Noncritical Items

Items that come in contact with intact skin but not mucous membranes must be clean. *Noncritical items* must be *disinfected*. Some of these items follow:

Bedpans
Blood pressure cuffs
Linens
Stethoscopes
Food utensils

(Rutala and Weber, 2002). This is generally accomplished by the use of a chemical disinfectant or wet pasteurization (used for respiratory therapy equipment). Examples of disinfectants are alcohols, chlorines, glutaraldehydes, and phenols. These chemicals can be caustic and toxic to tissues.

Sterilization is the complete elimination or destruction of all microorganisms, including spores. Steam under pressure, ethylene oxide (ETO) gas, hydrogen peroxide plasma, and chemicals are the most common sterilizing agents.

Whether an item is to be simply cleaned, or cleaned and disinfected or sterilized, depends on the intended use of the item. There are three categories of device classification (Box 33-6). Nurses should be familiar with agency policy and procedures for cleaning, handling, and delivering care items for eventual disinfection and sterilization. Workers especially trained in disinfection and sterilization should perform most of the procedures. Efficacy of the disinfecting or sterilizing method is influenced by the following factors:

* *Concentration of solution and duration of contact.* A weakened concentration or shortened exposure time may lessen effectiveness.
* *Type and number of pathogens.* Certain organisms are killed more easily than others by disruption. The

Table 33-6   Examples of Disinfection and Sterilization Processes

Characteristics	Examples of Use
Moist Heat	
Steam is moist heat under pressure. When exposed to high pressure, water vapor can attain temperature above boiling point to kill pathogens and spores.	Autoclave is used to sterilize surgical instruments, parenteral solutions, and surgical dressings.
Chemicals	
A number of chemical disinfectants are used in health care. These include alcohols, chlorines, formaldehyde, glutaraldehyde, hydrogen peroxide, iodophors, phenolics, and quaternary ammonium compounds. Each product performs in a unique manner and is used for a specific purpose.	Chemicals are used for disinfection of instruments and equipment such as thermometers and endoscopes. Use the appropriate facility-approved disinfectant in a safe manner (e.g., gloves, proper ventilation) for the approved purpose.
Ethylene Oxide Gas	
This gas destroys spores and microorganisms by altering cells' metabolic processes. Fumes are released within an autoclave-like chamber. Ethylene oxide gas is toxic to humans, and aeration time varies with products.	This gas sterilizes some rubber and plastic items.
Boiling Water	
Boiling is least expensive for use in home. Bacterial spores and some viruses resist boiling. It is not used in hospitals.	The items (e.g., glass baby bottles) should be boiled for at least 15 minutes.

greater the number of pathogens on an object, the longer the required disinfecting time.

- *Surface areas to treat.* All dirty surfaces and areas must be fully exposed to disinfecting and sterilizing agents.
- *Temperature of the environment.* Disinfectants tend to work best at room temperature.
- *Presence of soap.* Soap may cause certain disinfectants to be ineffective. Thorough rinsing of an object is necessary before disinfecting.
- *Presence of organic materials.* Disinfectants can become inactivated unless blood, saliva, pus, or body excretions are washed off.

Table 33-6 lists processes for disinfection and sterilization and their characteristics. Selection of the method for disinfecting or sterilizing an item depends on the intended use of the item and the nature of the item (e.g., some delicate instruments requiring sterilization cannot tolerate steam and must be processed using gas or plasma).

Control or Elimination of Reservoirs. To control or eliminate reservoir sites for infection, the nurse eliminates or controls sources of body fluids, drainage, or solutions that might harbor microorganisms. The nurse also carefully discards articles that become contaminated with infectious material (Box 33-7). The Occupational Safety and Health Act of 2001 set standards for minimizing occupational exposure to blood-borne pathogens or other potentially infectious materials (Occupational Safety and Health Administration [OSHA], 2001). All health care institutions must have guidelines for the disposal of infectious waste according to local and state regulations.

Control of Portals of Exit. The nurse follows prevention and control practices to minimize or prevent infec-

tious organisms from exiting the body. To control organisms exiting via the respiratory tract, the nurse should avoid talking directly into clients' faces or talking, sneezing, or coughing directly over surgical wounds or sterile dressing fields and wear a mask as needed. The nurse should cover the mouth or nose when sneezing or coughing. The nurse is also responsible for teaching clients to protect others when they sneeze or cough and for providing clients with disposable wipes or tissues to control the spread of microorganisms.

A nurse who has an upper respiratory tract infection and continues to work with clients should wear a mask when working closely with the client and pay special attention to hand hygiene. The same nurse should refrain from working with clients who are highly susceptible to infection (e.g., an immunosuppressed client or a neonate).

Another way of controlling the exit of microorganisms is through the careful handling of exudate (i.e., urine, feces, emesis, and blood). Contaminated fluids can easily splash while being discarded in toilets or hoppers. The nurse should always wear disposable gloves when handling exudate. Masks, gowns, and protective eyewear are worn if there is a possibility of splashing or contact with any fluids. The nurse appropriately disposes of disposable soiled items in trash bags. Laboratory specimens from all clients are handled as if they were infectious.

Control of Transmission. Effective control of infection requires a nurse to remain aware of the modes of transmission and ways to control them. In the hospital, home, or extended care facility a client should have a personal set of care items. Sharing bedpans, urinals, bath basins, and eating utensils can easily lead to transmission of infection. Thermometers, even when individually used, warrant spe-

Box 33-7   Infection Control to Reduce Reservoirs of Infection

Bathing

Use soap and water to remove drainage, dried secretions, or excess perspiration.

Dressing Changes

Change dressings that become wet and/or soiled (see Chapter 47).

Contaminated Articles

Place tissues, soiled dressings, or soiled linen in moisture-resistant bags for proper disposal.

Contaminated Needles

Engage safety features of all sharp devices and dispose in puncture-proof container. Place syringes, uncapped hypodermic needles and IV needles in puncture-proof containers, which should be located in client rooms or treatment areas so that exposed, contaminated equipment need not be carried a distance (see Chapter 34).
Do not recap needles or attempt to break them.

Bedside Unit

Keep table surfaces clean and dry.

Bottled Solutions

Do not leave bottled solutions open for prolonged periods.
Keep solutions tightly capped.
Date bottles when opened and discard according to facility policy.

Surgical Wounds

Keep drainage tubes and collection bags patent to prevent accumulation of serous fluid under the skin surface.

Drainage Bottles and Bags

Empty and dispose of drainage suction bottles according to facility policy.
Empty all drainage systems on each shift unless otherwise ordered by a physician.
Never raise a drainage system (e.g., urinary drainage bag) above the level of the site being drained unless it is clamped off.

---

cial care. Because the client's own mucus can become a source for microorganism growth, the electronic thermometer is used with a disposable sheath over the probe which is discarded after each use. Single-use chemical strip thermometers present less risk of infection than other thermometers. There has been research to suggest that use of electronic thermometers for rectal temperatures can be associated with nosocomial diarrhea (Jernigan and others, 1998). Specifically, the organism *Clostridium difficile* is able to survive on inanimate surfaces such as the thermometer probe. In institutions where nosocomial diarrhea occurs, electronic thermometers are not recommended for rectal temperatures. The same electronic thermometer should not be used for clients on contact isolation.

To prevent transmission of microorganisms through indirect contact, soiled items and equipment must be kept from touching the nurse's clothing. A common error is to carry dirty linen in the arms against the uniform. Fluid-resistant linen bags should be used, or soiled linen should be carried with hands held out from the body. Laundry hampers should be replaced before they are overflowing.

Hand Hygiene. The most important and most basic technique in preventing and controlling transmission of infections is hand hygiene. **Hand hygiene** includes using an instant alcohol hand antiseptic before and after providing client care, hand washing with soap and water when hands are visibly soiled, and performing a surgical scrub. **Hand washing** is a vigorous, brief rubbing together of all surfaces of the hands lathered in soap, followed by rinsing under a stream of water (CDC, 2002). The purpose is to remove soil and transient organisms from the hands and to reduce total microbial counts over time.

Contaminated hands are a prime cause of cross infection. For example, a nurse caring for a client who has excessive pulmonary secretions assists the client in expectorating mucus and disposes of the tissues in a bedside container. The client's roommate asks the nurse to open containers of food on the meal tray. The nurse then leaves the client's room to pour a dose of medication that is due in 5 minutes. If the nurse fails to perform hand hygiene before opening the containers of food or pouring the medication, organisms from the first client's mucus could easily be transmitted to the roommate's food or to the medication container.

The decision regarding when and what type of hand hygiene should occur depends on the following: the intensity of contact with clients or contaminated objects, the degree or amount of contamination that could occur with that contact, the susceptibility of the client or the health care worker to infection, and the procedure or activity to be performed (Larson, 1996). For example, prolonged and intense contact with a client's wound drainage would require thorough hand hygiene.

The Centers for Disease Control and Prevention (CDC) and the U.S. Public Health Service note that washing times of at least 10 to 15 seconds (Larson, 1996) will remove most transient microorganisms from the skin. If the hands are visibly soiled, more time may be needed. Routine hand washing may be performed with plain soap. Plain soap with water can physically remove a certain level of microbes, but antiseptic agents are necessary to kill or inhibit microorganisms and reduce the level still further (Larson, 1996). Skill 33-1 lists the steps for hand hygiene.

The use of alcohol-based waterless antiseptics is recommended by the CDC (2002) to improve hand hygiene

Text continued on p. 793

Research Highlight

Box 33-8

Pathogens and Artificial Fingernails

Research Focus

Female health care workers frequently have artificial or manicured nails. Researchers posed the question as to whether bacteria can reside in higher than normal numbers on artificial nail material.

Research Abstract

In two separate studies, the identity and quantity of microbial flora from health care workers (HCWs) wearing artificial nails was compared with HCWs with normal nails. In both studies, nail surfaces were swabbed and subungual (area under nails) debris was collected to obtain material for culture. In the first study, 12 HCWs who did not normally wear artificial nails wore polished artificial nails on their nondominant hand for 15 days. Identity and quantity of microflora were compared between the artificial nails and the polished normal nails of the other hand. Potential pathogens were isolated from more samples obtained from artificial nails than normal nails. Colonization of artificial nails increased over time. More organisms were found on the surface of artificial nails than normal nails.

In the second study, the flora of the nails of 30 HCWs who wore permanent acrylic artificial nails were compared with that of HCWs who had normal nails. HCWs wearing artificial nails were more likely to have a pathogen isolated than the other group.

In this study, artificial nails were more likely to harbor pathogens, especially gram-negative bacilli and yeasts, than normal nails. The longer artificial nails were worn, the more likely that a pathogen was isolated.

Evidence-Based Practice

- Nurses should not wear artificial nails when performing client care.

Reference

Hedderwick SA and others: Pathogenic organisms associated with artificial fingernails worn by healthcare workers, *Infect Control Hosp Epidemiol* 21(8):505, 2000.

Skill 33-1   *Hand* Hygiene

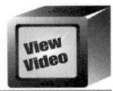

Delegation Considerations

Hand washing can be delegated to assistive personnel.
- Monitor care provider in proper method of hand hygiene.
- Instruct care provider to inform nurse if any skin irritation from soaps or antimicrobials is encountered.

Equipment

- Easy-to-reach sink with warm running water
- Antimicrobial or regular soap
- Alcohol-based waterless antiseptic
- Paper towels or air dryer
- Clean orangewood stick (optional)

Steps	Rationale
1. Inspect surface of hands for breaks or cuts in skin or cuticles. Report and cover lesions before providing client care.	Open cuts or wounds can harbor high concentrations of microorganisms. Agency policy may prevent nurses from caring for high-risk clients. If dermatitis occurs, additional interventions may be needed.
2. Inspect hands for heavy soiling.	Requires lengthier hand washing.
3. Inspect nails for length and presence of artificial acrylics.	Nails should be short and filed because most microbes on hands come from beneath the fingernails. Nails should be free of artificial applications (CDC, 2002) (Box 33-8).
4. Assess client's risk for or extent of infection (e.g., WBC count, extent of open wounds, known medical diagnosis).	Use of alcohol-based waterless antiseptic is encouraged for clients who are immunosuppressed (CDC, 2002).
5. Push wristwatch and long uniform sleeves above wrists. Avoid wearing rings. If worn, remove during procedure.	Provides complete access to fingers, hands, wrists. Wearing of rings increases number of microorganisms on hands (Garner, 1996).
6. If hands are visibly dirty or contaminated with protein-containing material, use plain soap or antimicrobial soap and water for hand washing:	
a. Stand in front of sink, keeping hands and uniform away from sink surface. (If hands touch sink during hand washing, repeat.)	Inside of sink is a contaminated area. Reaching over sink increases risk of touching edge, which is contaminated.

Steps	Rationale
b. Turn on water. Turn faucet on or push knee pedals laterally or press pedals with foot to regulate flow and temperature (see illustration).	
c. Avoid splashing water against uniform.	Microorganisms travel and grow in moisture.
d. Regulate flow of water so that temperature is warm.	Warm water removes less of the protective oils than hot water.
e. Wet hands and wrists thoroughly under running water. Keep hands and forearms lower than elbows during washing.	Hands are the most contaminated parts to be washed. Water flows from least to most contaminated area, rinsing microorganisms into the sink.
f. Apply a small amount of soap, lathering thoroughly (see illustration). Soap granules and leaflet preparations may be used.	Use of antimicrobial soaps exclusively can be drying to hands and can cause skin irritations. The decision whether to use an antimicrobial soap or alcohol-based hand antiseptic should depend on the procedure to be performed and the client's immune status.
g. Wash hands using plenty of lather and friction for at least 10 to 15 seconds. Interlace fingers and rub palms and back of hands with circular motion at least 5 times each. Keep fingertips down to facilitate removal of microorganisms.	Soap cleanses by emulsifying fat and oil and lowering surface tension. Friction and rubbing mechanically loosen and remove dirt and transient bacteria. Interlacing fingers and thumbs ensures that all surfaces are cleansed.
h. Areas under fingernails are often soiled. Clean them with fingernails of other hand and additional soap or clean orangewood stick.	Areas under nails can be highly contaminated, which will increase the risk of infection for the nurse or the client.

Critical Decision Point: Do not tear or cut skin under or around nail.

---

i. Rinse hands and wrists thoroughly, keeping hands down and elbows up (see illustration).	Rinsing mechanically washes away dirt and microorganisms.

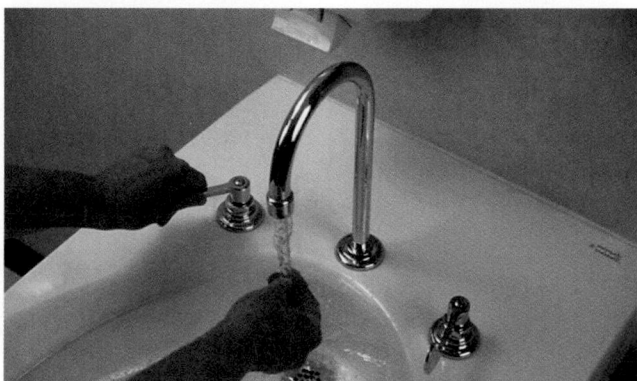

STEP **6b** Turning on water.

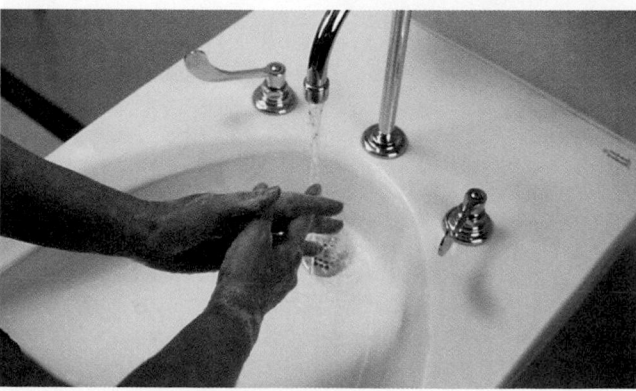

STEP **6f** Lathering hands thoroughly.

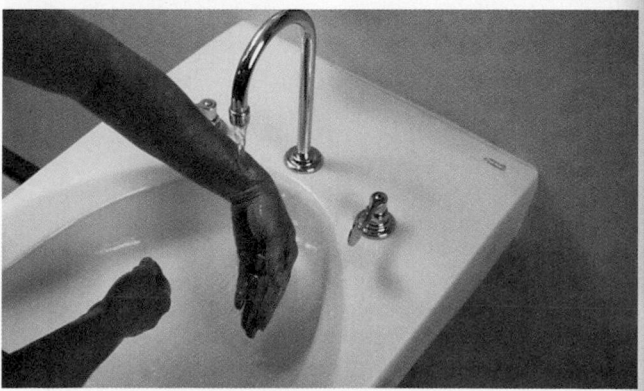

STEP **6i** Rinsing hands.

Steps	Rationale
j. *Optional:* Repeat steps a through h and extend period of washing if hands are heavily soiled.	
k. Dry hands thoroughly from fingers to wrists and forearms with paper towel, single-use cloth, or warm air dryer.	Drying from cleanest (fingertips) to least clean (forearms) area avoids contamination. Drying hands prevents chapping and roughened skin.
l. If used, discard paper towel in proper receptacle.	Prevents transfer of microorganisms.
m. Turn off water with foot or knee pedals. To turn off hand faucet, use clean, dry paper towel; avoid touching handles with hands (see illustration).	Wet towel and hands allow transfer of pathogens by capillary action.
n. If hands are dry or chapped, a small amount of lotion or barrier cream can be applied.	Use the hospital-provided container of lotion because many lotions may interfere with antimicrobial action or disintegrate gloves.
o. Inspect surfaces of hands for obvious signs of soil or other contaminants.	Determines if hand washing is adequate.
p. Inspect hands for dermatitis or cracked skin.	Indicates complications from excessive hand washing.
7. If hands are not visibly soiled, use an alcohol-based waterless antiseptic for routine decontamination of hands in all clinical situations.	
a. Apply an ample amount of product to palm of one hand (see illustration).	Enough product is needed to thoroughly cover the hands.
b. Rub hands together, covering all surfaces of hands and fingers with antiseptic (see illustration).	

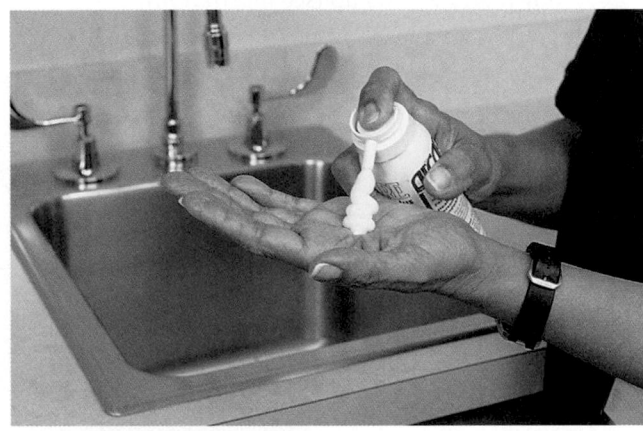

STEP **7a** Apply waterless antiseptic to hands.

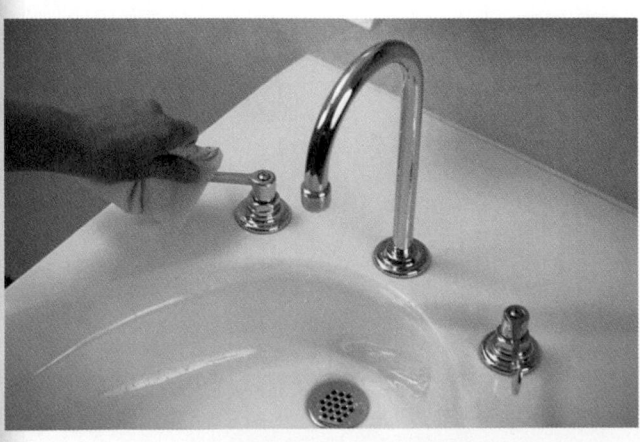

STEP **6m** Turning off faucet.

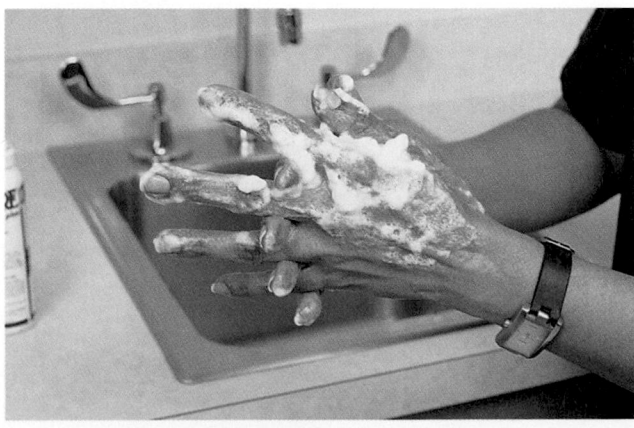

STEP **7b** Rub hands thoroughly.

Steps	Rationale
c. Rub hands together for several seconds until alcohol is dry. Allow hands to dry before applying gloves.	Drying ensures full antiseptic effect.
d. If hands are dry or chapped, a small amount of lotion or barrier cream can be applied.	Use the hospital-provided container of lotion because many lotions may interfere with antimicrobial action or disintegrate gloves.

Recording and Reporting

- It is not necessary to record or report this procedure.
- Report any dermatitis to employee health and/or infection control per agency policy.

Home Care Considerations

- Evaluate the hand-washing facilities in the home to determine the possibility of contamination, the proximity of the facilities to the client, and available supplies in the area.

- Evaluate the availability of warm running water and soap when conducting home visits and anticipate the need for alternative hand-washing products such as alcohol-based hand rubs and detergent-containing towels.
- Instruct the client and primary caregiver in proper techniques and situations for hand washing.

---

practices, protect health care worker's hands, and reduce transmission of pathogens to clients and personnel in health care settings. Alcohols have excellent germicidal activity and are more effective than either plain soap or antimicrobial soap and water. Emollients are added to alcohol-based antiseptics to prevent drying of the skin.

The CDC (2002) recommends the following:
1. Wash hands with plain soap or antimicrobial soap and water when hands are visibly dirty.
2. If hands are not visibly soiled, use an alcohol-based waterless antiseptic agent for routinely decontaminating hands in all other clinical situations:
   a. After contact with a client's intact skin (as in taking a pulse or blood pressure, or lifting a client)
   b. After contact with body fluids or excretions, mucous membranes, nonintact skin, or wound dressings as long as hands are not visibly soiled
   c. When moving from a contaminated body site to a clean body site during client care; after contact with inanimate objects (including medical equipment) in the immediate vicinity of the client
   d. Before caring for clients with severe neutropenia or other forms of severe immune suppression
   e. Before inserting indwelling urinary catheters or other invasive devices
   f. After removing gloves

The nurse instructs clients and visitors about the proper technique and times for hand hygiene. Teaching hand hygiene is particularly important if health care is to continue at home. Clients should wash their hands before eating or handling food; after handling contaminated equipment, linen, or organic material; and after elimination. Visitors are encouraged to wash their hands before eating or handling food, after coming in contact with infected clients, and after handling contaminated equipment or organic material.

Control of Portals of Entry. Many measures that control the exit of microorganisms likewise control the en-

trance of pathogens. Maintaining the integrity of skin and mucous membranes reduces the chances of microorganisms reaching a host. The client's skin should be kept well lubricated by using lotion as appropriate. Immobilized and debilitated clients are particularly susceptible to skin breakdown. Clients should not be positioned on tubes or objects that might cause breaks in the skin. Dry, wrinkle-free linen also reduces the chances of skin breakdown. Turning and positioning are needed before a client's skin becomes reddened. Frequent oral hygiene prevents drying of mucous membranes. A water-soluble ointment keeps the client's lips well lubricated.

After elimination, a woman should clean the rectum and perineum by wiping from the urinary meatus toward the rectum. Cleansing in a direction from the least to the most contaminated area helps reduce genitourinary infections. Meticulous and frequent perineal care is especially important in older adult women who wear disposable incontinent pads.

Clients, health care personnel, and even housekeepers are at risk for acquiring infections from accidental needle sticks. After administering an injection or inserting an IV catheter, the nurse should engage any safety device and carefully dispose of needles in a puncture-resistant box (see Chapter 34). A stray needle lying in bed linen or carelessly thrown into a wastebasket is a prime source for exposure to blood-borne pathogens. Hepatitis B and hepatitis C are the infections most commonly transmitted by contaminated needles (Box 33-9). A needle stick should be reported immediately. Health care agencies require the victim of a needle stick to complete an injury report and seek appropriate treatment.

Another cause for entrance of microorganisms into a host is improper handling and management of urinary catheters and drainage sets (see Chapter 44). The point of connection between a catheter and drainage tube should remain closed and intact. As long as such systems are closed, their contents are considered sterile. Outflow spigots on drainage bags should also remain closed to prevent

Box *33-9*   Hepatitis B Vaccination and Follow-Up After Exposure
Health care employers shall make available the hepatitis B vaccine and vaccination series to all employees who may have occupational exposures. Evaluation and follow-up care will be available to all employees who have been exposed. All medical evaluations and procedures, including the vaccine and vaccination series and evaluation after exposure (prophylaxis), are made available at no cost to at-risk employees. A confidential written medical evaluation will be available to employees with exposure incidents. Hepatitis B vaccinations will be made available to employees within 10 working days of assignment.

From Occupational Safety and Health Administration: Occupational Safety and Health Act of 2001, 2001, www.cdc.gov.

entrance of bacteria. Movement of the catheter at the urethra should be minimized by stabilizing the catheter with tape to reduce chances of microorganisms ascending the urethra into the bladder. Urine-measuring containers should not be shared between clients.

The nurse may care for clients with closed drainage systems that collect wound drainage, bile, or other body fluids. In each example the site from which a drainage tube exits should remain clear of excess moisture or accumulated drainage. All tubing should remain connected throughout use. Drainage receptacles should only be opened when it is necessary to discard or measure the volume of drainage.

At times the nurse obtains specimens from drainage tubes or IV tubing ports. The nurse disinfects tubes and ports by wiping the surface outward with alcohol or an iodine solution before entering the system. Temporarily placing squares of sterile gauze around the ends of an open drainage tube, such as a urinary catheter, adds further protection against bacteria. However, keeping drainage tubes closed and secure is the best practice.

A final method for reducing the entrance of microorganisms is the technique for cleansing wounds (see Chapter 47). The surgical wound itself is considered to be sterile. To prevent entrance of microorganisms into the wound, the nurse should clean outward from a wound site. When applying an antiseptic or cleaning with soap and water, the nurse wipes around the wound edge first and then cleans outward away from the wound. Clean gauze should be used for each revolution around the wound's circumference.

Protection of the Susceptible Host. A client's resistance to infection improves as the nurse protects normal body defenses against infection. The nurse intervenes to maintain the body's normal reparative processes (Box 33-10). The nurse also protects himself or herself and others through the use of isolation precautions (Box 33-11).

Isolation Precautions. The risk of transmitting nosocomial infection or infectious disease among clients is high. When a client has a suspected or known infection, health care workers become alerted and follow infection-control

Box *33-10*   Infection Control: Protecting the Susceptible Host
Protecting Normal Defense Mechanisms Regular bathing removes transient microorganisms from the skin's surface. Lubrication helps keep the skin hydrated and intact. Regular oral hygiene removes proteins in the saliva that attract microorganisms. Flossing removes tartar and plaque that can cause germ infection. Maintenance of adequate fluid intake promotes normal urine formation and a resultant outflow of urine to flush the bladder and urethral lining of microorganisms. For physically dependent or immobilized clients, the nurse encourages routine coughing and deep breathing to keep lower airways clear of mucus. The nurse encourages proper immunization of children or adult clients who become exposed to certain infectious microorganisms. Children are vaccinated for measles, mumps, rubella, chickenpox, diphtheria, and other diseases. Adults should receive tetanus-diphtheria boosters every 10 years. Influenza vaccines are recommended for health care workers. Older adults should receive pneumococcal vaccine and annual influenza vaccine. **Maintaining Healing Processes** The nurse promotes intake of adequate fluids and a well-balanced diet containing essential proteins, vitamins, carbohydrates, and fats. The nurse also uses measures to increase the client's appetite. The nurse promotes a client's comfort and sleep so that energy stores are replaced daily. The nurse assists the client in learning techniques to reduce stress.

practices. However, health care workers may not be aware that clients have infections. The majority of organisms causing nosocomial infections are found in the **colonized** body substances of clients regardless of whether a culture has confirmed infection and a diagnosis has been made (Garner, 1996). Body substances such as feces, saliva, mucus, and wound drainage always contain potentially infectious organisms.

Isolation or barrier precautions include the appropriate use of gowns, gloves, masks, eyewear, and other protective devices or clothing. Barrier protection is indicated for use with all clients because every client has the potential to transmit infection via blood and body fluids, and the risk for infection transmission can be unknown. Because of the increased attention to the prevention of blood-borne pathogens and tuberculosis, the CDC and the Occupational Safety and Health Administration (OSHA) have stressed the importance of using barrier protection (OSHA, 2001).

The CDC issued new isolation guidelines in 1996 that contain a two-tiered approach (Garner, 1996). The first and most important tier contains precautions designed to care for all clients in any setting regardless of their diagnosis or

Box 33-11 Procedural Guidelines

Caring for a Client on Isolation Precautions

Equipment
- Barrier protection determined by type of isolation
- Supplies necessary for procedures peformed in room

Delegation considerations: Care of a client in isolation can be delegated to assistive personnel (AP) when necessary procedures are within AP's competence.

1. Assess isolation indications (i.e., current laboratory test results or client's history of exposure).
2. Review agency policies and precautions necessary for the specific isolation system and consider care measures to be performed while in client's room.
3. Review nurses' notes or confer with colleagues regarding client's emotional state and adjustment to isolation.
4. Perform hand hygiene and prepare all equipment to be taken into client's room.
5. Prepare for entrance into isolation room:
   a. Apply either surgical mask or respirator around mouth and nose if needed. (Type will depend on type of isolation and facility policy.)
   b. Apply eyewear or goggles snugly around face and eyes (when needed).
   c. Apply gown, being sure it covers all outer garments. Pull sleeves down to wrist. Tie securely at neck and waist (see illustration).
   d. Apply disposable gloves (NOTE: Unpowdered, latex-free gloves should be worn if the client or the health care worker has a latex allergy.) If gloves are worn with gown, bring glove cuffs over edge of gown sleeves.

6. Enter client's room. Arrange supplies and equipment. (If equipment will be removed from room for reuse, place on clean paper towel.)
7. Explain purpose of isolation and necessary precautions to client and family. Offer opportunity to ask questions. Assess for evidence of emotional problems that may be caused by being in isolation.
8. Assess vital signs.
   a. If client is infected or colonized with a resistant organism (e.g., vancomycin-resistant enterococcus [VRE], methicillin-resistant *Staphylococcus aureus* [MRSA]), equipment remains in room. Proceed to assess vital signs by routine procedures. Avoid contact of stethoscope or blood pressure cuff with infectious material.
   b. If stethoscope is to be reused, clean diaphragm or bell with alcohol. Set aside on clean surface.
   c. Individual or disposable thermometers should be used.
9. Administer medications (see Chapter 34):
   a. Give oral medication in wrapper or cup.
   b. Dispose of wrapper or cup in plastic-lined receptacle.
   c. Administer injection.
   d. Discard syringe and uncapped needle or sheathed needle into special container.
   e. If gloves are not worn and hands contact contaminated article or body fluids, wash hands immediately.

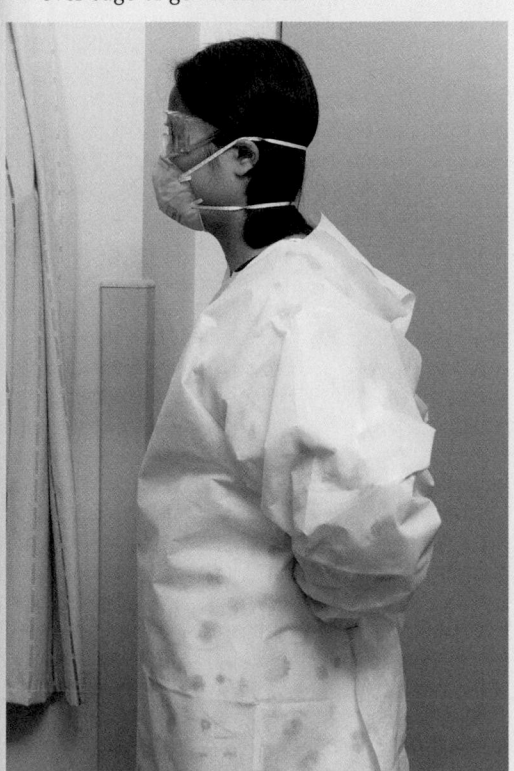

STEP **5c.**

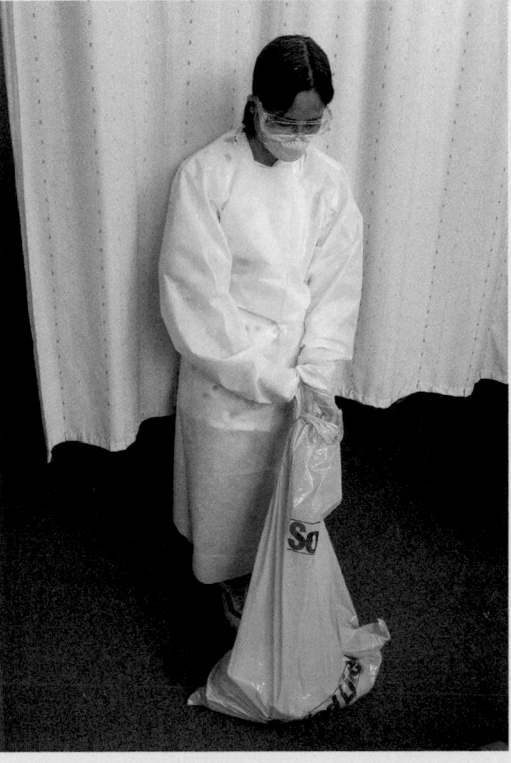

STEP **12b.**

Continued

Box 33-11 *Procedural Guidelines*

Caring for a Client on Isolation Precautions—cont'd

10. Administer hygiene, encouraging the client to discuss questions or concerns about isolation. Informal teaching can be used at this time.
    a. Avoid allowing gown to become wet.
    b. Remove linen from bed; if excessively soiled, avoid contact with gown. Place in impervious linen bag.
    c. Change gloves and wash hands if they become excessively soiled and further care is necessary.
11. Collect specimens:
    a. Place specimen containers on clean paper towel in client's bathroom.
    b. Follow procedure for collecting specimen of body fluids.
    c. Transfer specimen to container without soiling outside of container. Place container in plastic bag and place label on outside of bag or as per facility policy.
12. Dispose of linen and trash bags as they become full:
    a. Use sturdy, moisture-resistant single bags to contain soiled articles.
    b. Tie bags securely at top in knot (see illustration).
13. Resupply room as needed.

14. Leave isolation room.
    a. Remove gloves. Remove one glove by grasping cuff and pulling glove inside out over hand. Discard glove. With ungloved hand, tuck finger inside cuff of remaining glove and pull it off, inside out.
    b. Untie *top* mask string and then bottom strings, pull mask away from face and drop into trash receptacle (see illustration). (Do not touch outer surface of mask.)
    c. Untie waist and neck strings of gown. Allow gown to fall from shoulders. Remove hands from sleeves without touching outside of gown (see illustration). Hold gown inside at shoulder seams and fold inside out; discard in laundry bag.
    d. Remove eyewear or goggles.
    e. Perform hand hygiene.
    f. Explain to client when you plan to return to room. Ask whether client requires any personal care items, books, or magazines.
    g. Leave room and close door, if necessary. (Door should be closed if client is on airborne precautions.)
    h. All contaminated supplies and equipment should be disposed of in a manner that prevents spread of microorganisms to other persons (see agency policy).

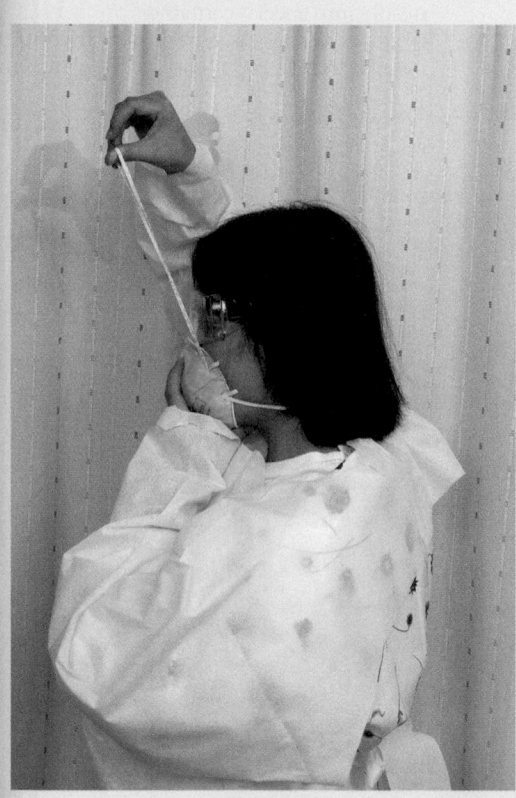

STEP **14b.**

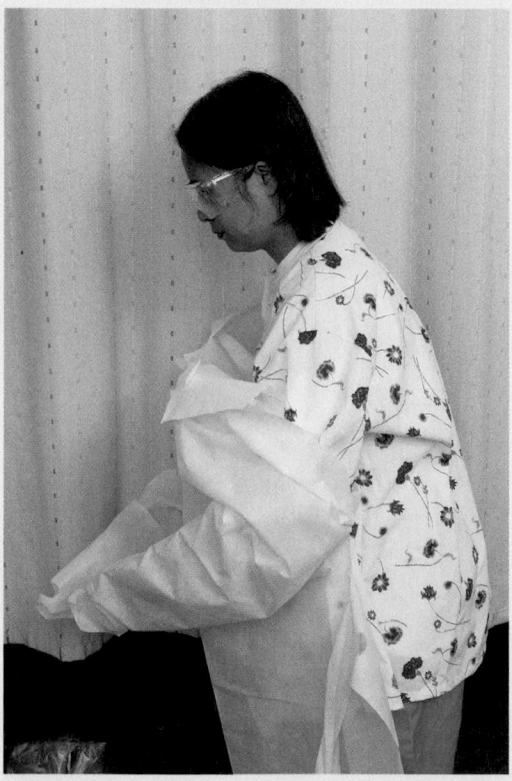

STEP **14c.**

Table 33-7	Centers for Disease Control and Prevention Isolation Guidelines

Standard Precautions (Tier One)

Standard precautions apply to blood, all body fluids, secretions, excretions (except sweat), nonintact skin, and mucous membranes.

Hands are washed between client contacts; after contact with blood, body fluids, secretions, and excretions and after contact with equipment or articles contaminated by them; and immediately after gloves are removed. (Refer to agency policy for use of an alcohol-based waterless antiseptic.)

Gloves are worn when touching blood, body fluids, secretions, excretions, nonintact skin, mucous membranes, or contaminated items. Gloves should be removed and hand hygiene performed between client care.

Masks, eye protection, or face shields are worn if client care activities may generate splashes or sprays of blood or body fluid.

Gowns are worn if soiling of clothing is likely from blood or body fluid. Perform hand hygiene after removing gown.

Client care equipment is properly cleaned and reprocessed, and single-use items are discarded.

Contaminated linen is placed in leakproof bag and handled so as to prevent skin and mucous membrane exposure.

All sharp instruments and needles are discarded in a puncture-resistant container. Safety devices must be enabled after use to prevent injury.

A private room is unnecessary unless the client's hygiene is unacceptable. Check with an infection-control professional.

Transmission Categories (Tier Two)

Category	Disease	Barrier Protection
Airborne precautions	Droplet nuclei smaller than 5 μm; measles; chickenpox (varicella); disseminated varicella zoster; pulmonary or laryngeal TB	Private room, negative-pressure airflow of at least six exchanges per hour; mask or respiratory protection device
Droplet precautions	Droplets larger than 5 μm; diphtheria (pharyngeal); rubella; streptococcal pharyngitis, pneumonia, or scarlet fever in infants and young children; pertussis; mumps; mycoplasmal pneumonia; meningococcal pneumonia or sepsis; pneumonic plague	Private room or cohort clients; mask
Contact precautions	Direct client or environmental contact; colonization or infection with multidrug-resistant organism; respiratory syncytial virus; shigella and other enteric pathogens; major wound infections; herpes simplex; scabies, varicella zoster (disseminated)	Private room or cohort clients; gloves, gowns

Modified from Garner JS: Guidelines for isolation precautions in hospitals, *Infect Control Hosp Epidemiol* 17(1):54, 1996.

presumed infectiousness. This guideline is called standard precautions. These precautions apply to (1) blood; (2) all body fluids, secretions, and excretions except sweat regardless of whether they contain blood; (3) nonintact skin; and (4) mucous membranes. Standard precautions promote hand washing and the use of gloves, masks, eye protection, or gowns, when appropriate, for client contact (Table 33-7).

The second tier uses three transmission categories: airborne, droplet, and contact precautions based on a client's diagnosed infection. These precautions are designed for specific clients with highly transmissible or epidemiologically important pathogens. For example, a client diagnosed with active tuberculosis would require the use of airborne precautions, using a special mask and ventilated room, in conjunction with standard precautions.

Users of the CDC's isolation guidelines are referred to additional CDC documents to prevent nosocomial aspergillosis and Legionnaires' disease in immunocompromised clients (CDC, 2002) and the spread of vancomycin-resistant organisms (CDC, 1995).

With the increase in numbers of reported cases of TB in the United States in the late 1980s, the CDC issued guidelines for prevention of transmission of TB in health care facilities in 1990. These and later revisions (CDC, 1994) stress the early identification and treatment of persons with known or suspected TB, facility risk assessment for TB exposures, engineering control, and proper isolation techniques. In addition, OSHA (1999) issued a mandate requiring health care facilities to follow CDC guidelines and required that health care workers be offered free TB skin tests and fitted respiratory protective devices. Airborne precautions are required for TB.

Regardless of the type of isolation system, the nurse must follow the following basic principles:
- The nurse should use thorough hand hygiene before entering and leaving the room of a client in isolation.
- Contaminated supplies and equipment should be disposed of in a manner that prevents spread of microorganisms to other persons as indicated by the mode of transmission of the organism.
- Knowledge of a disease process and the mode of infection transmission should be applied when using protective barriers.
- All persons who might be exposed during transport of a client outside the isolation room must be protected.

Psychological Implications of Isolation. When a client requires isolation in a private room, a sense of loneliness may develop because normal social relationships become disrupted. This situation can be psychologically harmful, especially for children.

As a result of the infectious process, client's body images are altered. They may feel unclean, rejected, lonely, or guilty. Infection prevention and control practices further intensify these beliefs of difference or undesirability. Isolation in a private room limits sensory contact. Unless the nurse acts to minimize feelings of psychological and physical isolation, clients' emotional states can interfere with recovery.

Before isolation measures are instituted, the client and family must understand the nature of the disease or condition, the purposes of isolation, and steps for carrying out specific precautions. If they are able to participate in maintaining infection prevention, the chances of reducing the spread of infection are increased. The client and family should be taught to perform hand hygiene and use barrier protection if appropriate. Each procedure should be demonstrated, and the client and family should be given an opportunity for practice. It is also important to explain how infectious organisms can be transmitted so that the client understands the difference between contaminated and clean objects.

The nurse also takes measures to improve the client's sensory stimulation during isolation. The room environment should be clean and pleasant. Drapes or shades should be opened, and excess supplies and equipment removed. The nurse must listen to the client's concerns or interests. If the nurse rushes through care or shows a lack of interest, the client will feel rejected and even more isolated. Mealtime is a particularly good opportunity for conversation. Providing comfort measures such as repositioning, a back massage, or a tepid sponge bath increases physical stimulation. Depending on the client's condition, the nurse should encourage the client to walk and sit up in a chair. Recreational activities such as board games or cards may be an option to keep the client mentally stimulated.

The nurse must explain to the family the client's risk for depression or loneliness. Visiting family members should be encouraged to avoid expressions or actions that convey revulsion or disgust. The nurse discusses ways to provide meaningful stimulation.

Protective Environment. Private rooms used for isolation may have negative-pressure airflow to prevent infectious particles from flowing out of the room. There are also special rooms with positive-pressure airflow that are used for highly susceptible clients, such as organ transplant recipients. On the door or wall outside the room, the nurse posts a card listing precautions for the isolation category according to agency policy. The card is a handy reference for health care personnel and visitors and alerts anyone who might enter the room accidentally that special precautions must be followed.

The isolation room or an adjoining anteroom should contain hand hygiene, bathing, and toilet facilities. Soap and antiseptic solutions are made available. Personnel and visitors perform hand hygiene before approaching the client's bedside and again before leaving the room. If toilet facilities are unavailable, there are special procedures for handling portable commodes, bedpans, or urinals. Personal protective equipment should be stored in an anteroom between the room and hallway or in a convenient location close to the point of use.

All client care rooms, including those used for isolation, contain an impervious bag for soiled or contaminated linen, as well as a trash container with plastic liners. Impervious receptacles prevent transmission of microorganisms by preventing seepage to and soiling of the outside surface. A disposable rigid container should be available in the room to discard used needles, syringes, and sharp objects.

The nurse must remain aware of infection prevention and control techniques while working with clients in protected environments. The nurse should feel comfortable performing all procedures and yet remain conscious of infection-control principles. Depending on the microorganism and the mode of transmission, the nurse must evaluate what articles or equipment may be taken into an isolation room. For example, the CDC (1995) recommends the dedicated use of articles such as stethoscopes, sphygmomanometers, or rectal thermometers in the isolation room of a client infected or colonized with vancomycin-resistant enterococci (VRE). These devices should not be used on other clients unless they are first adequately cleaned and disinfected. If after bringing any article into the room, the nurse exposes an article to infected material and then touches or removes the article, the risk of transmitting infection to other clients or personnel is increased. Box 33-11 describes the procedures commonly performed in a protective environment.

Personal Protective Equipment. Personal protective equipment (gowns, masks, protective eyewear, and gloves) should be readily available for personnel performing client care. The primary reason for gowning is to prevent soiling clothes during contact with the client. Gowns or cover-ups protect health care personnel and visitors from coming in contact with infected material and blood or body fluid. Gowns may also be required for contact precautions, depending on the expected amount of exposure to infectious material. Gowns used for barrier protection are made of a fluid-resistant material and should be changed immediately if damaged or heavily contaminated. Depending on agency policy, isolation gowns can be disposable or reusable.

Isolation gowns usually open at the back and have ties or snaps at the neck and waist to keep the gown closed and secure. Gowns should be long enough to cover all outer garments. Long sleeves with tight-fitting cuffs provide added protection. There is no special technique required for applying clean gowns as long as they are fastened securely. However, the nurse must carefully remove gowns to minimize contamination of the hands and uniform and then discard them after removal.

Full face protection (with eyes, nose, and mouth covered) should be worn when splashing or spraying of blood or body fluid into the face is anticipated. Masks should also be worn when working with a client placed on airborne or droplet precautions. The mask protects the nurse from inhaling microorganisms from a client's respiratory tract and prevents transmission of pathogens from the nurse's respiratory tract to the client. The surgical mask protects a wearer from inhaling large-particle aerosols that travel short distances (3 feet) and small-particle droplet

Box 33-12 *Procedural Guidelines*

Donning a Surgical-Type Mask

1. Find top edge of mask (usually has thin metal strip along edge). Pliable metal fits snugly against bridge of nose
2. Hold mask by top two strings or loops. Tie two top ties at top of back of head (see illustration), with ties above ears. (*Alternative:* Slip loops over each ear.)

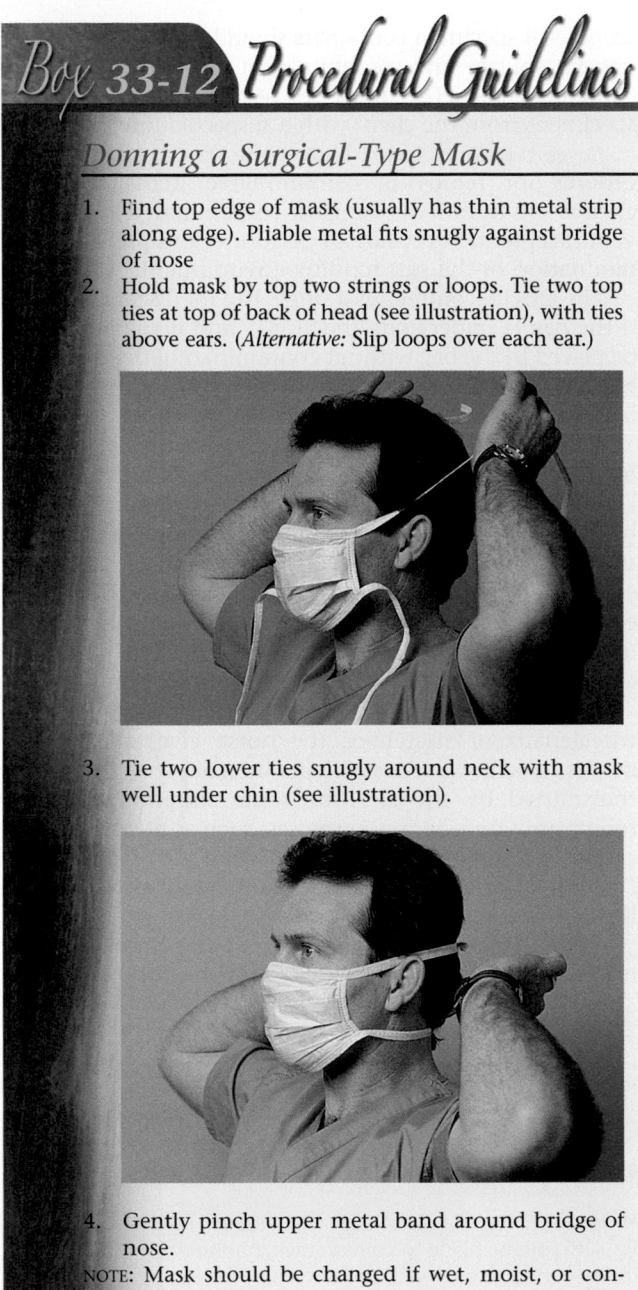

3. Tie two lower ties snugly around neck with mask well under chin (see illustration).

4. Gently pinch upper metal band around bridge of nose.
   NOTE: Mask should be changed if wet, moist, or contaminated.

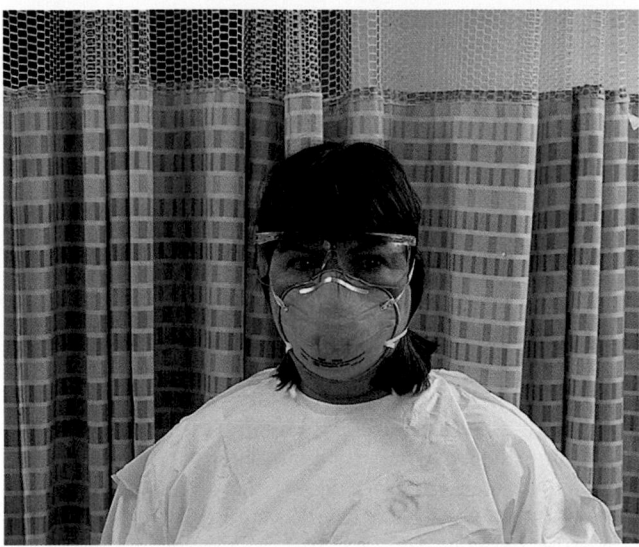

FIGURE **33–2** Nurse wearing fitted TB mask and goggles.

nuclei that remain suspended in the air and travel longer distances. At times a client who is susceptible to infection wears a mask to prevent inhalation of pathogens. Clients on droplet or airborne precautions who are transported outside of their rooms should wear masks to protect other clients and personnel. According to the CDC (Garner, 1996), masks may prevent transmission of infection by direct contact with mucous membranes. A mask discourages the wearer from touching the eyes, nose, or mouth.

A properly applied mask fits snugly over the mouth and nose so that pathogens and body fluids cannot enter or escape through the sides (Box 33-12). If a person wears glasses, the top edge of the mask fits below the glasses so that they will not cloud over as the person exhales. Talking should be kept to a minimum while wearing a

mask to reduce respiratory airflow. A mask that has become moist may not provide a barrier to microorganisms and thus may be ineffective. It should be discarded. A mask should never be reused. Clients and family members should be warned that a mask can cause a sensation of smothering. If family members become uncomfortable, they should leave the room and discard the mask.

Specially fitted respiratory protective devices or masks are required when caring for a client with known or suspected TB (Figure 33-2) (CDC, 1994; OSHA, 1994). The mask must have a higher filtration rating than the regular surgical mask and be fitted snugly to the wearer's face to prevent leakage around the sides. The nurse should be aware of agency policy regarding the type of respiratory protective device required.

Gloves help to prevent the transmission of pathogens by direct and indirect contact. The CDC (Garner, 1996) notes that clean, nonsterile gloves should be worn when touching blood, body fluid, secretions, excretions, and contaminated items. Clean gloves should be donned just before touching mucous membranes and nonintact skin. Gloves should be changed between tasks and procedures on the same client after contact with material that may contain a high concentration of microorganisms. Gloves should be removed promptly after use, before touching noncontaminated items and environmental surfaces, and before going to another client. Hand hygiene should be performed immediately to avoid transfer of microorganisms to other clients or environments. Because of allergy or sensitivity to latex gloves, facilities provide nonlatex gloves for health care staff who are allergic or sensitive to latex (see Chapter 49).

When full protective apparel is needed, the nurse first performs hand hygiene, then applies a mask and eyewear or goggle (as needed), applies a gown, and then puts on gloves. Disposable gloves are easily applied and are designed to fit either hand. The glove's thin rubber can be easily torn. The glove cuffs should be pulled up over the wrists or over the cuffs of the gown. If a break or tear is detected in a glove while providing care, the nurse should change gloves if care is not completed. If the nurse does not plan to have more contact with the client, reapplying gloves is unnecessary.

Family members visiting clients who are on a form of isolation requiring use of gloves must know when and how to apply gloves properly. The nurse demonstrates application of gloves to family members and explains the reason for use of gloves. The nurse emphasizes that it is very important to perform hand hygiene after removing gloves.

When participating in a procedure that creates droplets or splashing or spraying of blood or other body fluids, a nurse must wear protective eyewear, a mask, or a face shield (Garner, 1996). Examples of such procedures include irrigation of a large abdominal wound or insertion of an arterial catheter in which the nurse assists a physician. Eyewear may be available in the form of plastic glasses or goggles (see Figure 33-2, p. 799). The eyewear should fit snugly around the face so that fluids cannot enter between the face and the glasses.

Specimen Collection. Many laboratory studies may be required when a client is suspected of having an infectious disease. Body fluids and secretions suspected of containing infectious organisms are collected for culture and sensitivity tests. The specimen is placed in a medium that promotes growth of organisms. A laboratory technologist then identifies the microorganisms growing in the culture. Additional test results indicate antibiotics to which the organisms are resistant or sensitive. Sensitivity reports determine the antibiotics used in treatment.

The nurse obtains all culture specimens using disposable gloves and sterile equipment. Collecting fresh material from the site of infection, such as wound drainage, ensures that the specimen is not contaminated by neighboring microbes. All specimen containers should be sealed tightly to prevent spillage and contamination of the outside of the container. Box 33-13 describes techniques for collecting specimens from the client with a suspected infection.

Bagging Trash or Linen. Nurses use special bagging procedures for removing contaminated items from the client's environment. Bagging contaminated items prevents accidental exposure of personnel and prevents contamination of the surrounding environment.

The CDC recommends a single bag for discarding items if the bag is impervious and sturdy and if the article can be placed in the bag without contaminating the outside of the bag. Soiled linen should be placed in an impervious laundry bag in the client's room (OSHA, 2001).

The CDC recommends double bagging if it is impossible to prevent contamination of the bag's outer surface. Double bagging is not otherwise recommended. Studies have shown that this procedure is not necessary to control infection (Maki and others, 1986; Weinstein and others, 1989). Use of one standard-sized linen bag that is not overfilled, that is tied securely, and that is intact is adequate to prevent infection transmission. The same rule applies to trash bags.

Transporting Clients. Before transferring clients to wheelchairs or stretchers, the nurse gives them clean gowns to serve as robes. Clients infected with organisms transmitted by the airborne route should leave their rooms only for essential purposes, such as diagnostic procedures or surgery. These clients must also wear masks. Personnel transporting these clients should also wear barrier protection as needed.

At times a client being transported may drain body fluids onto a stretcher or wheelchair. When this occurs, the

---

Box 33-13   Specimen Collection Techniques*

Wound Specimen

Clean site with sterile water or saline prior to wound specimen collection. Wear gloves and use cotton-tipped swab or syringe to collect as much drainage as possible. Have clean test tube or culture tube on clean paper towel. After swabbing center of wound site, grasp collection tube by holding it with paper towel. Carefully insert swab without touching outside of tube. After securing tube's top, transfer tube into bag for transport and then perform hand hygiene.

Blood Specimen

Wearing gloves, use syringe and culture media bottles to collect up to 10 ml of blood per culture bottle (check agency policy). After prepping, perform venipuncture at two different sites to decrease likelihood of both specimens being contaminated with skin flora. Place blood culture bottles on bedside table or other surface; swab off bottle tops with alcohol. Inject appropriate amount of blood into each bottle. Remove gloves and transfer specimen into clean, labeled bag for transport. Perform hand hygiene.

Stool Specimen

Wearing gloves, use clean cup with seal top (need not be sterile) and tongue blade to collect small amount of stool, approximately the size of a walnut. Place cup on clean paper towel in client's bathroom. Using tongue blade, collect needed amount of feces from client's bedpan. Transfer feces to cup without touching cup's outside surface. Dispose of tongue blade, and place seal on cup. Transfer specimen into clean bag for transport. Remove gloves and perform hand hygiene.

Urine Specimen

Wearing gloves, use syringe and sterile cup to collect 1 to 5 ml of urine. Place cup or tube on clean towel in client's bathroom. If client has a urinary catheter, use syringe to collect specimen. Have client follow procedure to obtain a clean voided specimen (see Chapter 44) if not catheterized. Transfer urine into sterile container by injecting urine from syringe or pouring it from used collection cup. Secure top of container and transfer specimen into clean, labeled bag for transport. Remove gloves and perform hand hygiene.

From Pagana KD, Pagana TJ: *Diagnostic testing and nursing implications: a case study approach,* ed 5, St. Louis, 1998, Mosby.
*Agency policies may differ on type of containers and amount of specimen material required.

nurse must be sure to have the equipment cleaned after the client returns to the room. An extra layer of sheets may be used to cover the stretcher or seat of the wheelchair.

Personnel in diagnostic or procedural areas or the operating room should be notified that the client is on isolation precautions. The nurse explains ways that the client can help prevent transmission of infection during transport. A client on respiratory isolation is given tissues and a bag to allow proper disposal of secretions. The nurse records the type of isolation on the client's chart.

Role of the Infection-Control Professional. Many hospitals employ professionals, most of whom are nurses, who are specially trained in infection prevention and control. These individuals are responsible for advising hospital personnel regarding infection prevention and control and for monitoring infections within the hospital. Duties of an infection-control professional include the following:

- Provide staff education on infection prevention and control.
- Develop and review infection prevention and control policies and procedures.
- Recommend appropriate isolation procedures.
- Screen client records for community-acquired infections that may be reportable to the public health department.
- Consult with employee health departments concerning recommendations to prevent and control the spread of infection among personnel, such as TB testing.
- Gather statistics regarding the **epidemiology** (cause and effect) of nosocomial infections.
- Notify the public health department of incidences of communicable diseases within the facility.
- Confer with all hospital departments to investigate unusual events or clusters of infection.
- Recommend education for clients and families.
- Identify infection-control problems with equipment.
- Monitor antibiotic-resistant organisms in the institution.

An infection-control professional can be a valuable resource for assisting nurses in controlling nosocomial infections.

Infection Prevention and Control for Hospital Personnel. Health care workers are continually at risk for exposure to infectious microorganisms. The Occupational Safety and Health Act of 1991 established rules and regulations to protect employees from infectious hazards in the workplace (OSHA, 1991). The OSHA guidelines are incorporated into the policies and procedures of health care institutions and are part of regularly scheduled staff education programs.

Client Education. Often clients must learn to use infection-control practices at home (Box 33-14). Preventive technique becomes almost second nature to the nurse who practices it daily. However, the client is less aware of factors that promote the spread of infection or ways to prevent its transmission. The home environment does not always lend itself to infection prevention. Often a nurse must help a client adapt according to the resources available to maintain hygienic techniques. Generally, clients in a home care setting have a

decreased risk of infection because of decreased exposure to resistant organisms such as those found in a hospital and because of fewer invasive procedures.

After clients are at home, nurses determine their compliance with infection-control practices. The nurse educates clients about infection and techniques to prevent or control its spread. Topics the nurse can discuss in a teaching session include the following:

- Clients' susceptibility to infection
- The chain of infection, with specific reference to means of transmission
- Hygienic practices that minimize organism growth and spread, emphasizing hand washing
- Preventive health care (e.g., diet, immunizations, and exercise)
- Proper methods for handling and storage of food
- Family members who are at risk for acquiring infection
- Family members caring for such a client must be involved in the teaching plan. The nurse teaches clients and family members a commonsense approach to controlling and preventing infection.

Client Teaching   *Box 33-14*

Infection Control

Objective

- Client will assume self-care using proper infection-control techniques.

Teaching Strategies

- Instruct client about cleaning equipment using soap and water and disinfecting with an appropriate disinfectant.
- Demonstrate proper hand hygiene, explaining that it should be done before and after all treatments and when infected body fluids are contacted.
- Instruct client about the signs and symptoms of wound infection.
- For clients who receive tube feedings at home, explain the importance of preparing enough formula for only 8 hours (commercially prepared) or 4 hours (home prepared). Tell client that contaminated enteral feeding can cause infections. Rinse feeding bag and tubing with mild soap and water daily and dry.
- Instruct client to place contaminated dressings and other disposable items containing infectious body fluids in impervious plastic bags. Place needles in metal containers such as soda cans and tape the openings shut.
- Clean noticeably soiled linen separate from other laundry. Wash in water that is as hot as the fabric will tolerate. Add 1 cup of bleach to detergent. Set dryer temperature as high as fabric will allow.

Evaluation

- Ask client or family member to describe techniques used to reduce transmission of infection.
- Have client demonstrate select techniques.
- Ask client to explain the risks for infection based on the condition.

clean technique

Surgical Asepsis. **Surgical asepsis** or sterile technique requires a nurse to use different precautions from those of medical asepsis. Surgical asepsis includes procedures used to eliminate all microorganisms, including pathogens and spores, from an object or area. In surgical asepsis an area or object is considered contaminated if touched by any object that is not sterile. For example, a tear in a surgical glove exposes the outside of the glove to the skin surface, thus contaminating it. The nurse working with a sterile field or with sterile equipment must understand that the slightest break in technique results in contamination. Surgical asepsis should be used in the following situations:

- During procedures that require intentional perforation of the client's skin (e.g., insertion of IV catheters or administration of injections)
- When the skin's integrity is broken as a result of trauma surgical incision or burns
- During procedures that involve insertion of catheters or surgical instruments into sterile body cavities

Although surgical asepsis is commonly practiced in the operating room, labor and delivery area, and major diagnostic areas, the nurse may also use surgical aseptic techniques at the client's bedside. This includes, for example, inserting IV or urinary catheters, suctioning the tracheobronchial airway, and reapplying sterile dressings. A nurse in an operating room follows a series of steps to maintain sterile technique, including applying a mask, protective eyewear, and a cap; performing a surgical hand scrub; and applying a sterile gown and gloves. In contrast, a nurse performing a dressing change at a client's bedside may only perform hand hygiene and apply sterile gloves. (See following section on the principles of surgical asepsis.)

Client Preparation. Because surgical asepsis requires exact techniques, the nurse must have the client's cooperation. Therefore the nurse must prepare the client before any procedure. Certain clients may fear moving or touching objects during a sterile procedure, whereas others may even try to assist. The nurse explains how a procedure is to be performed and what the client can do to avoid contaminating sterile items, including the following:

- Avoid sudden movements of body parts covered by sterile drapes.
- Refrain from touching sterile supplies, drapes, or the nurse's gloves and gown.
- Avoid coughing, sneezing, or talking over a sterile area.

Certain sterile procedures may last an extended time. The nurse assesses the client's needs and anticipates factors that may disrupt a procedure. If a client is in pain, the nurse tries to administer analgesics no more than half an hour before a sterile procedure begins. The nurse allows the client to have elimination needs met. Often clients must assume relatively uncomfortable positions during sterile procedures. The nurse helps the client to assume the most comfortable position possible. Finally, the client's condition may result in actions or events that contaminate a sterile field; for example, a client with a respiratory infection transmits organisms by coughing or breathing. The nurse anticipates such a problem and offers the client a mask.

Principles of Surgical Asepsis. When beginning a surgically aseptic procedure, the nurse follows certain principles to ensure maintenance of asepsis. Failure to follow these principles places clients at risk for infection. The following principles are important:

1. *A sterile object remains sterile only when touched by another sterile object.* This principle guides the nurse in placement of sterile objects and how to handle them.
   a. Sterile touching sterile remains sterile; for example, sterile gloves are worn or sterile forceps are used to handle objects on a sterile field.
   b. Sterile touching clean becomes contaminated; for example, if the tip of a syringe or other sterile object touches the surface of a clean disposable glove, the object is contaminated.
   c. Sterile touching contaminated becomes contaminated; for example, when the nurse touches a sterile object with an ungloved hand, the object is contaminated.
   d. Sterile touching questionable is contaminated; for example, when a tear or break in the covering of a sterile object is found, it is discarded regardless of whether the object itself appears untouched.

2. *Only sterile objects may be placed on a sterile field.* All items are properly sterilized before use. Sterile objects are kept in clean, dry storage areas. The package or container holding a sterile object must be intact and dry. A package that is torn, punctured, wet, or open is unsterile.

3. *A sterile object or field out of the range of vision or an object held below a person's waist is contaminated.* Nurses never turn their backs on a sterile tray or leave it unattended. Contamination can occur accidentally by a dangling piece of clothing, falling hair, or an unknowing client touching a sterile object. Any object held below waist level is considered contaminated because it cannot be viewed at all times. Sterile objects should be kept in front with the hands as close together as possible.

4. *A sterile object or field becomes contaminated by prolonged exposure to air.* The nurse avoids activities that may create air currents, such as excessive movements or rearranging linen after a sterile object or field becomes exposed. When sterile packages are being opened, it is important to minimize the number of people walking into the area. Microorganisms also travel by droplet through the air. No one should talk, laugh, sneeze, or cough over a sterile field or when gathering and using sterile equipment. Microorganisms traveling through the air can fall on sterile items or fields if the nurse reaches over the work area. When opening sterile packages, the nurse holds the item or piece of equipment as close as possible to the sterile field without touching the sterile surface. Keeping movement or rearranging of sterile items to a minimum also reduces contamination by air transmission.

5. *When a sterile surface comes in contact with a wet, contaminated surface, the sterile object or field becomes contaminated by capillary action.* If moisture seeps through a sterile package's protective covering, microorganisms travel to the sterile object. When stored sterile packages become wet, the nurse discards the objects

immediately or sends the equipment for resterilization. When working with a sterile field or tray, the nurse may have to pour sterile solutions. Any spill can be a source of contamination unless the object or field rests on a sterile surface that cannot be penetrated by moisture. Urinary catheterization trays contain sterile supplies that rest in a sterile, plastic container. In this example, sterile solutions spilled within the container will not contaminate the catheter or other objects. In contrast, if a nurse places a piece of sterile gauze in its wrapper on a client's bedside table and the table surface is wet, the gauze is considered contaminated.

6. *Fluid flows in the direction of gravity.* A sterile object becomes contaminated if gravity causes a contaminated liquid to flow over the object's surface. To avoid contamination during a surgical hand scrub, the nurse holds the hands above the elbows. This allows water to flow downward without contaminating the nurse's hands and fingers. The principle of water flow by gravity is also the reason for drying from fingers to elbows with hands held up, after the scrub.

7. *The edges of a sterile field or container are considered to be contaminated.* Frequently a nurse places sterile objects on a sterile towel or drape (Figure 33-3). Because the edge of the drape touches an unsterile surface, such as a table or bed linen, a 2.5-cm (1-inch) border around the drape is considered contaminated. Objects placed on the sterile field must be inside this border. The edges of sterile containers become exposed to air after they are open and are thus contaminated. After a sterile needle is removed from its protective cap or after forceps are removed from a container, the objects must not touch the container's edge. The lip of an opened bottle of solution also becomes contaminated after it is exposed to air. When pouring a sterile liquid, the nurse first pours a small amount of solution and discards it. The solution washes away microorganisms on the bottle lip. Then the nurse pours a second time on the same side to fill a container with the desired amount of solution.

Performing Sterile Procedures. All of the equipment that will be needed should be assembled before a procedure. Thus the nurse avoids having to leave a sterile area unattended because equipment is missing. A few extra supplies should be available in case objects accidentally become contaminated. Before the sterile procedure, each step should be explained so that the client can cooperate fully. If an object becomes contaminated during the procedure, the nurse should not hesitate to discard it immediately.

Donning and Removing Caps, Masks, and Eyewear. For sterile procedures on a general nursing division, the nurse may wear a surgical mask and eyewear without a cap. Eyewear is worn as a part of standard precautions if there is a risk of fluid or blood splashing into the nurse's eyes. For sterile surgical procedures, the nurse first applies a clean cap that covers all of the hair and then the surgical mask and eyewear. A mask must fit snugly around the face and nose to prevent contamination by droplet nuclei. After a mask is worn for several hours, the area over the mouth and nose often becomes moist. Since moisture promotes the spread of microorganisms, the mask should be changed if it becomes moist.

Protective glasses or goggles should fit snugly around the forehead and face to fully protect the eyes. Eyewear needs to be worn only for procedures that create the risk of body fluids splashing into the eyes. Before removing a mask, eyewear, and cap, the nurse removes sterile gloves to prevent contamination of the hair, neck, and facial area. After untying the mask, the nurse holds it by the ties and discards it with the cap. Masks should not be worn hanging from the neck after removal. Eyewear is removed and cleaned later for reuse. After removing all protective wear, the nurse performs hand hygiene thoroughly.

Opening Sterile Packages. Sterile items such as syringes, gauze dressings, or catheters are packaged in paper or plastic containers and are impervious to microorganisms as long as they are dry and intact. Some institutions wrap reusable supplies in a double thickness of paper, linen, or muslin. These packages are permeable to steam and thus allow for steam autoclaving. Sterile items are kept in clean, enclosed storage cabinets and are separated from dirty equipment.

Sterile supplies have chemical tapes indicating that a sterilization process has taken place. The tapes change color during the sterilization process. Failure of the tapes to change color means that the item is not sterile. A sterile item should never be used if the integrity of the packaging is compromised. Health care facilities may apply the date processed and a lot number to the item after processing ("event-related expiration"), or they may apply an expiration date ("date-related expiration") to the item. With either system it is important for the nurse to check the integrity of the packaging of the item before use.

Before opening a sterile item, the nurse performs thorough hand hygiene. The nurse inspects the supplies for package integrity and sterility and assembles the supplies in the work area, such as the bedside table or treatment room, before opening packages. A bedside table or countertop provides a large, clean working area for opening items. The work area should be above waist level. Sterile supplies should not be opened in a confined space where a dirty object might fall on or strike them.

Opening a Sterile Item on a Flat Surface. Sterile packaged items must be opened without contaminating the contents. Commercially packaged items are usually designed

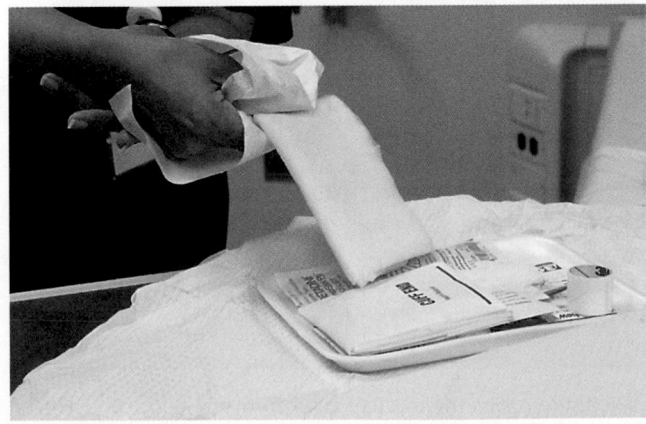

FIGURE **33–3** Placing sterile item on sterile field.

so that the nurse only has to tear away or separate the paper or plastic cover. The item is held in one hand while the wrapper is pulled away with the other (Figure 33-4). Care is then taken to keep the inner contents sterile before use. When opening items processed by the facility and packed in paper or linen, the nurse uses the following steps:

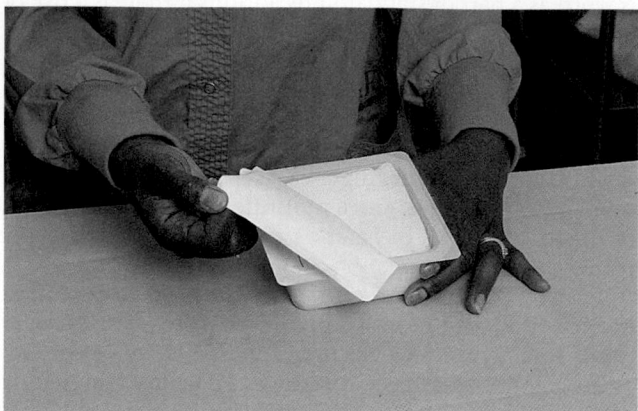

FIGURE 33-4 Nurse opens sterile package on work area above waist level.

1. Place the item flat in the center of the work surface.
2. Remove the sterilization tape or seal.
3. Grasp the outer surface of the tip of the outermost flap.
4. Open the outer flap away from the body, keeping the arm outstretched and away from the sterile field (Figure 33-5, *A*).
5. Grasp the outside surface of the first side flap.
6. Open the side flap, allowing it to lie flat on the table surface. Keep the arm to the side and not over the sterile surface (Figure 33-5, *B*). Do not allow the flaps to spring back over the sterile contents.
7. Grasp the outside surface of the second side flap and allow it to lie flat on the table surface (Figure 33-5, *C*).
8. Grasp the outside surface of the last and innermost flap.
9. Stand away from the sterile package and pull the flap back, allowing it to fall flat on the surface (Figure 33-5, *D*).
10. Use the inner surface of the package (except for the 1-inch border around the edges) as a sterile field to add additional sterile items. The 1-inch border can be grasped to maneuver the field on the table surface.

If the sterile supplies are not to be used immediately, the nurse can close the sterile package. In this case the nurse should touch only the wrapper's outside surface. To

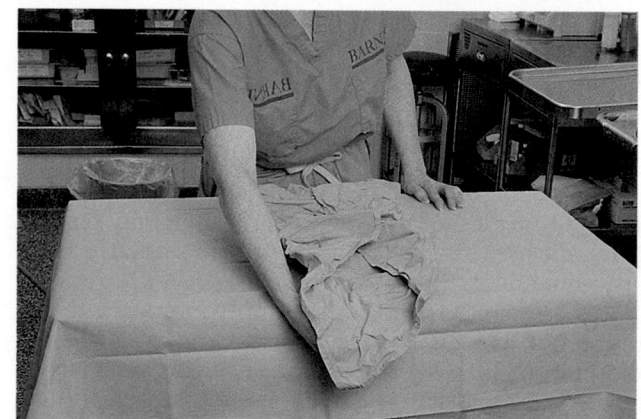
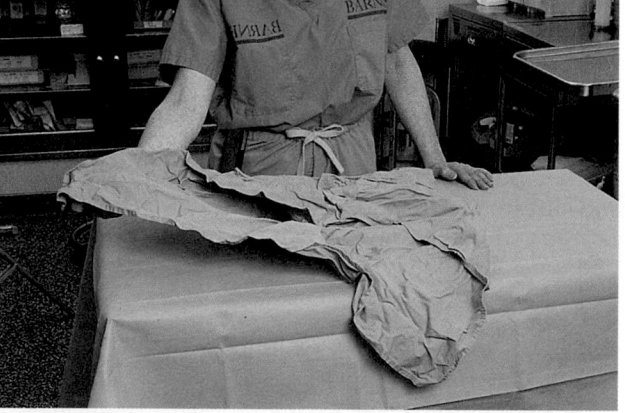
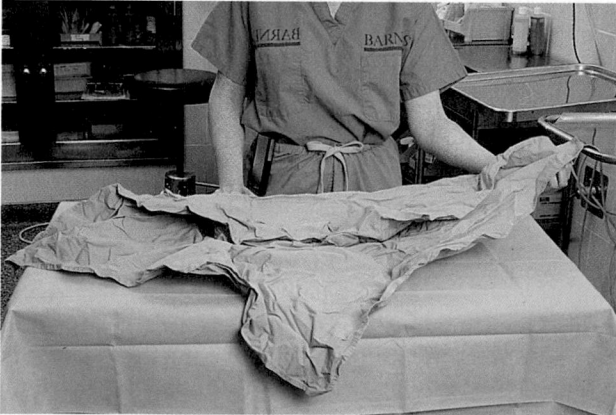
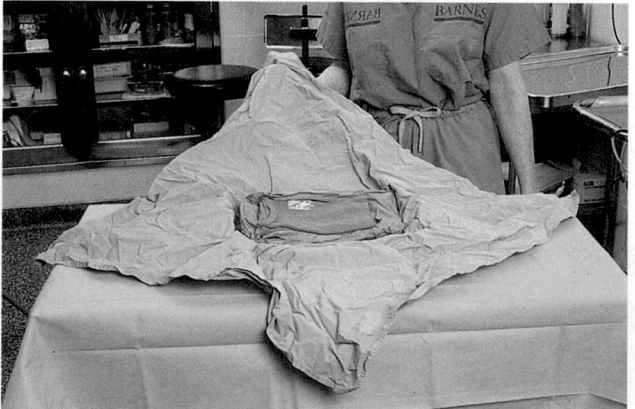

FIGURE 33-5 Opening sterile packaged items on a flat surface. **A,** The nurse opens the top flap away from the body. **B,** The nurse's arm is kept out away from the sterile field while opening a side flap. **C,** The second side flap is opened. **D,** The back flap is opened.

close a package, the order of unwrapping is reversed, and the nurse does not touch the inside contents or reach over the field.

Opening a Sterile Item While Holding It. To open a small, sterile item, the package is held in the nondominant hand while the top flap is opened and pulled away from the nurse. Using the dominant hand, the nurse carefully opens the sides and top flaps away from the enclosed sterile item in the same order previously mentioned. The nurse opens the item in a hand so that the item can be handed to a person wearing sterile gloves or transferred to a sterile field.

Preparing a Sterile Field. When performing sterile procedures, the nurse needs a sterile work area that provides room for handling and placing of sterile items. A **sterile field** is an area free of microorganisms and prepared to receive sterile items. The field may be prepared by using the inner surface of a sterile wrapper as the work surface or by using a sterile drape or dressing tray. Skill 33-2 describes preparation of a sterile field. After the surface for the field is created, the nurse adds sterile items by placing them directly on the field or by transferring them with a sterile forceps. When transferring sterile items, the nurse must carefully place objects onto the sterile field. An object that comes in contact with the 1-inch border must be discarded.

The nurse may choose to wear sterile gloves while preparing items on the field. If this is done, the nurse can touch the entire drape, but sterile items must be handed over by an assistant. The nurse's gloves cannot touch the wrappers of sterile items.

Pouring Sterile Solutions. Often the nurse must pour sterile solutions into sterile containers. A bottle containing a sterile solution is sterile on the inside and contaminated on the outside; the bottle's neck is also contaminated, but the inside of the bottle cap is considered sterile. After a cap or lid is removed, it is held in the hand or placed sterile side (inside) up on a clean surface. This means that the inside of the lid can be seen as it rests on the table surface. A bottle cap or lid should never rest on a sterile surface, even though the inside of the cap is sterile. The outer edge of the cap is unsterile and would contaminate the surface. Likewise, placing a sterile cap down on an unsterile surface increases the chances of the inside of the cap becoming contaminated.

The bottle should be held with its label in the palm of the hand to prevent the possibility of the solution wetting and fading the label. Before pouring the solution into the container, the nurse pours a small amount (1 to 2 ml) into a disposable cap or plastic-lined waste receptacle. The discarded solution cleans the lip of the bottle. The edge of the bottle is kept away from the edge or inside of the receiving container. The nurse pours the solution slowly to avoid splashing the underlying drape or field. The bottle should never be held so high above the container that even slow pouring will cause splashing. The bottle should be held outside the edge of the sterile field.

Surgical Scrub. Clients undergoing operative procedures are at an increased risk for infection. Nurses working in operating rooms perform surgical hand antisepsis to decrease and suppress the growth of skin microorganisms in case of glove tears (Association of Perioperative Nurses [AORN], 1998).

During surgical hand antisepsis, the nurse scrubs from fingertips to elbows with an antiseptic soap before each operation. The optimum duration of the surgical hand scrub is unclear, although research indicates that it may be dependent on the type of antimicrobial product (CDC, 1995). The traditional scrub time in the United States for both the initial and the subsequent scrub has been 5 minutes (Meeker and Rothrock, 1999). Larson (1996) recommends that at least 2 minutes of friction be used for surgical hand washing. The nurse should follow the agency's policy for length of scrub time. For many years, preoperative hand washing protocols required nurses to scrub with a brush. However, this practice may damage the skin and can result in increased shedding of bacteria from the hands. Scrubbing with a disposable sponge or combination sponge-brush has been shown to reduce bacterial counts on the hands as effectively as scrubbing with a brush. However, several studies suggest that neither a brush nor a sponge is necessary to reduce bacterial counts on the hands, especially when an alcohol-based product is used (CDC, 1995).

For maximum elimination of bacteria, all jewelry should be removed and the nails should be kept clean and short (AORN, 1998). Artificial nails should not be worn, because they may harbor a greater number of bacteria (CDC, 1995). Nurses who have active skin infections, open lesions or cuts, or respiratory infections should be excluded from the surgical team. Skill 33-3 describes the steps for surgical hand hygiene.

Applying Sterile Gloves. Sterile gloves are an additional barrier to bacterial transfer. There are two gloving methods: open and closed. Nurses who work on general nursing divisions use open gloving before procedures such as dressing changes or urinary catheter insertions. The closed gloving method, which is performed after nurses apply sterile gowns, is practiced in operating rooms and special treatment areas. Skills 33-4 and 33-5 review the steps of each sterile gloving technique. The proper glove size should be selected; the glove should not stretch so tightly that it can easily tear, yet it should be tight enough that objects can be picked up easily.

Donning a Sterile Gown. Nurses must wear sterile gowns when assisting at the sterile field in the operating room, delivery room, and special treatment areas so that sterile objects can be comfortably handled with less risk of contamination. The circulating nurse does not generally wear a sterile gown. The sterile gown acts as a barrier to decrease shedding of microorganisms from skin surfaces into the air and thus prevents wound contamination. Nurses caring for clients with large open wounds or assisting physicians during major invasive procedures (e.g., inserting an arterial catheter) may also wear sterile gowns.

The nurse does not apply a sterile gown until after applying a mask and surgical cap and performing surgical hand washing. The nurse picks up the gown from a sterile pack, or an assistant hands the gown to the nurse. Only a certain portion of the gown—the area from the anterior waist to, but not including, the collar and the anterior surface of the sleeves-is considered sterile. The back of the gown, the area under the arms, the collar, the area below the waist, and the underside of the sleeves are not sterile because the nurse cannot keep these areas in

Text continued on p. 816

Skill 33-2 *Preparation of a Sterile Field*

Delegation Considerations

Delegation of the preparation of a sterile field is inappropriate unless assistive personnel have received specialized training. Operating room technicians are usually trained for this skill.

Equipment

- Sterile drape
- Assorted sterile supplies

Steps	Rationale
1. Prepare sterile field just before planned procedure. Supplies are to be used immediately.	Prevents exposure of sterile field and supplies to air and contamination.
2. Select clean work surface above waist level.	Sterile object held below waist is contaminated.
3. Assemble necessary equipment.	Preparation of equipment in advance prevents break in technique.
4. Check dates or labels on supplies for sterility of equipment.	Equipment stored beyond expiration date is considered unsterile.
5. Perform hand hygiene thoroughly or use the alcohol-based hand antiseptic. *Option:* procedure may be performed with gloves.	Reduces microbial counts on skin.
6. Place pack containing sterile drape on work surface and open as described on p. 804.	Ensures sterility of packaged drape.
7. With fingertips of one hand, pick up folded top edge of sterile drape.	One-inch border around drape is unsterile and may be touched with fingers or clean gloves.
8. Gently lift drape up from its outer cover and let it unfold by itself without touching any object. Discard outer cover with your other hand.	If sterile object touches any other nonsterile object, it becomes contaminated.
9. With other hand, grasp adjacent corner of drape and hold it straight up and away from your body (see illustration).	Drape can now be properly placed while using two hands. Drape must be held away from unsterile surfaces.
10. Holding drape, first position and lay bottom half over intended work surface (see illustration).	Prevents nurse from reaching over sterile field.
11. Allow top half of drape to be placed over work surface last (see illustration).	Creates flat, sterile work surface.

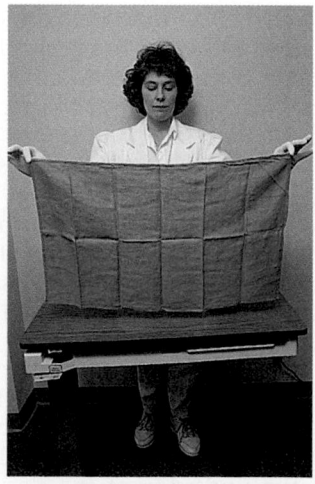

STEP **9** Hold drape straight up and away from body.

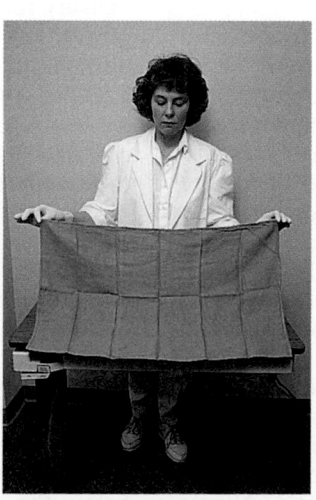

STEP **10** Lay bottom half over work surface.

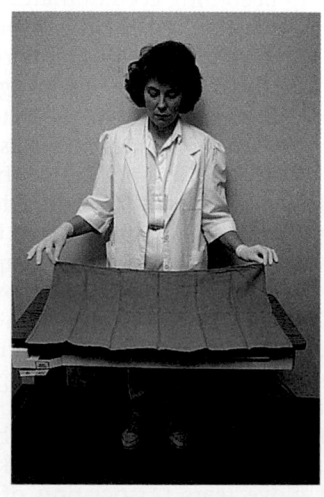

STEP **11** Place top half of drape over work surface.

Steps	Rationale
12. Grasp 1-inch border around edge to position as needed.	

Adding Sterile Items

Steps	Rationale
13. Open sterile item (following package directions) while holding outside wrapper in nondominant hand.	Frees dominant hand for unwrapping outer wrapper.
14. Carefully peel wrapper onto nondominant hand.	Item remains sterile. Inner surface of wrapper covers hand, making it sterile.
15. Being sure wrapper does not fall down on sterile field, place item onto field at angle. Do not hold arm over sterile field (see illustration).	Prevents reaching over field and contaminating its surface.
16. Dispose of outer wrapper.	Prevents accidental contamination of sterile field.
17. Perform procedure using sterile technique.	Prevents transmission of infection to client.

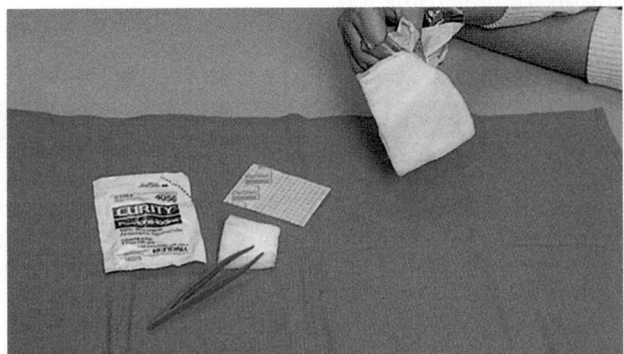

STEP **15** Adding item to sterile field.

Recording and Reporting

• It is not necessary to record or report this procedure.

Skill 33-3   *Surgical Hand Washing: Preparing for Gowning*

Delegation Considerations

The role of the scrub nurse can be delegated to a surgical technologist or licensed practical nurse.

Assistive personnel can help the registered nurse in the circulating nurse role by opening sterile supplies, setting up sterile fields, and running errands under the direction of the registered nurse.

Equipment

- Deep sink with foot or knee controls for dispensing water and soap (faucets should be high enough for hands and forearms to fit comfortably)

- Antiseptic detergent (nonirritating, broad-spectrum, fast-acting, effective in reducing skin microorganisms, and having a residual effect) (AORN, 1998)
- Surgical scrub sponge with plastic nail pick
- Alcohol-based waterless antiseptic
- Paper mask and cap or hood
- Sterile towel
- Proper scrub attire
- Protective eyewear (glasses or goggles)

Steps	Rationale
1. Consult institutional policy regarding required length of time and antiseptic to use for hand antisepsis.	Guidelines vary regarding ideal time needed and antiseptic to use for surgical scrub.
2. Be sure fingernails are short, clean, and healthy. Artificial nails should be removed. Natural nails should be less than ¼-in long.	Long nails and chipped or old polish increase number of bacteria residing on nails. Long fingernails can puncture gloves, causing contamination. Artificial nails are known to harbor gram-negative microorganisms and fungus (Hedderwick and others, 2000).

Critical Decision Point: Remove nail polish if chipped or worn longer than 4 days because it may harbor microorganisms (AORN, 1998).

Steps	Rationale
3. Inspect hands for presence of abrasions, cuts, or open lesions.	These conditions increase likelihood of more microorganisms residing on skin surfaces.
4. Apply surgical shoe covers, cap or hood, face mask, and protective eyewear.	Mask prevents escape into air of microorganisms that can contaminate hands. Other protective wear prevents exposure to blood and body fluid splashes during the procedure.
5. Surgical hand washing: a. Turn on water using knee or foot controls and adjust to comfortable temperature.	
b. Wet hands and arms under running lukewarm water and lather with detergent to 5 cm (2 inches) above elbows. (Hands need to be above elbows at all times.)	Water runs by gravity from fingertips to elbows. Hands become cleanest part of upper extremity. Keeping hands elevated allows water to flow from least to most contaminated areas. Washing a wide area reduces risk of contaminating overlying gown that the nurse later applies.
c. Rinse hands and arms thoroughly under running water. **Remember to keep hands above elbows.**	Rinsing removes transient bacteria from fingers, hands, and forearms.
d. Under running water, clean under nails of both hands with nail pick. Discard after use (see illustration).	Removes dirt and organic material that harbor large numbers of microorganisms.
e. Wet clean sponge and apply antimicrobial detergent. Scrub nails of one hand with 15 strokes. Holding sponge perpendicular, scrub palm, each side of thumb and fingers, and posterior side of hand with 10 strokes each. The arm is mentally divided into thirds, and each third is scrubbed 10 times (see illustration). Entire scrub should last 5 to 10 min. Rinse sponge and repeat sequence for other arm. A two-sponge method may be substituted. Check agency policy.	Friction loosens resident bacteria that adhere to skin surfaces. Ensures coverage of all surfaces. Scrubbing is performed from cleanest area (hands) to marginal area (upper arms).

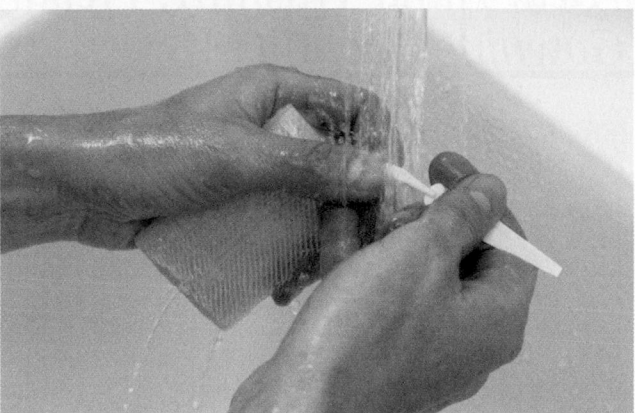

STEP **5d** Cleaning under fingernails.

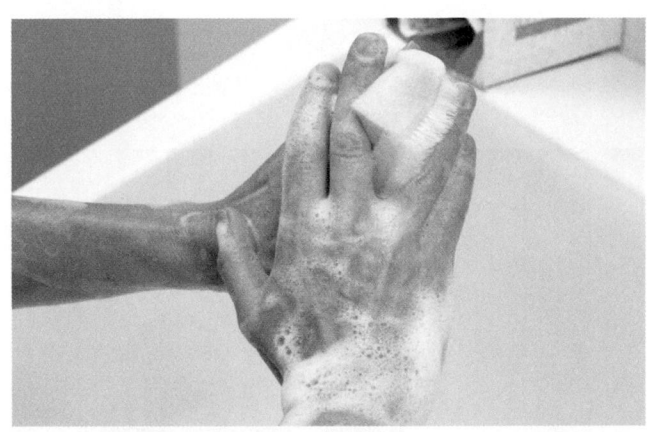

A

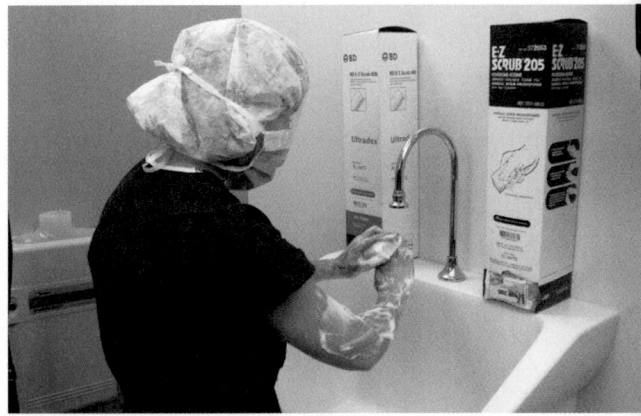

B

STEP **5e** **A,** Scrubbing side of fingers. **B,** Scrubbing forearms.

f. Discard sponge and rinse hands and arms thoroughly (see illustration). Turn off water with foot or knee control and back into room entrance with hands elevated in front of and away from the body.

After touching skin, sponge is considered contaminated. Rinsing removes resident bacteria. Prevents accidental contamination.

g. Walk up to sterile tray and lean forward slightly to pick up a sterile towel (see illustration). Dry one hand thoroughly, moving from fingers to elbow. Dry in a rotating motion. Dry from cleanest to least clean area (see illustration).

Drying prevents chapping and facilitates donning of gloves. Leaning forward prevents accidental contact of arms with scrub attire.

h. Repeat drying method for other hand by carefully reversing towel or using a new sterile towel.

Prevents accidental contamination.

i. Discard towel.

Prevents accidental contamination.

j. Proceed with sterile gowning (see Skill 33-4, p. 811).

6. **Alternate method of surgical hand hygiene using alcohol-based antiseptic:**

a. Wash hands with soap and water for 10 to 15 seconds to remove soil.

Removes dirt and organic material that harbor large numbers of microorganisms.

b. Under running water, clean under nails of both hands with nail pick. Discard after use and dry hands with a paper towel.

Skill 33-3   *S*urgical Hand Washing: Preparing
for Gowning—cont'd

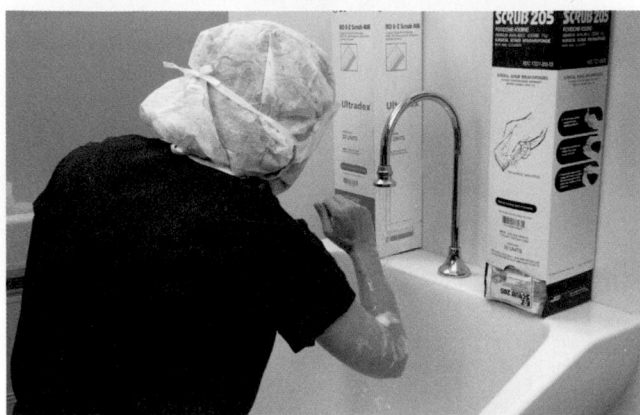

STEP **5f** Rinsing arms.

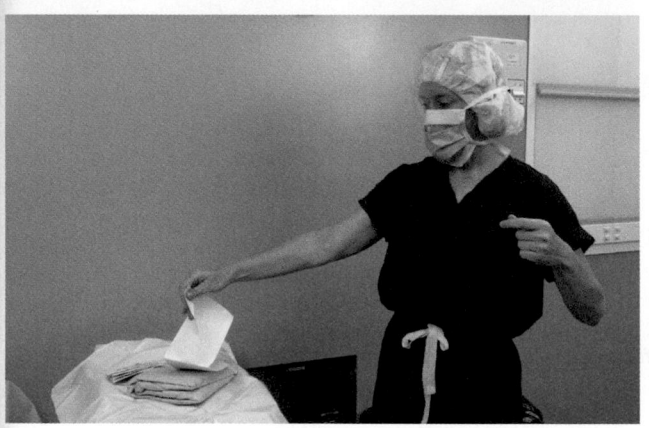

A

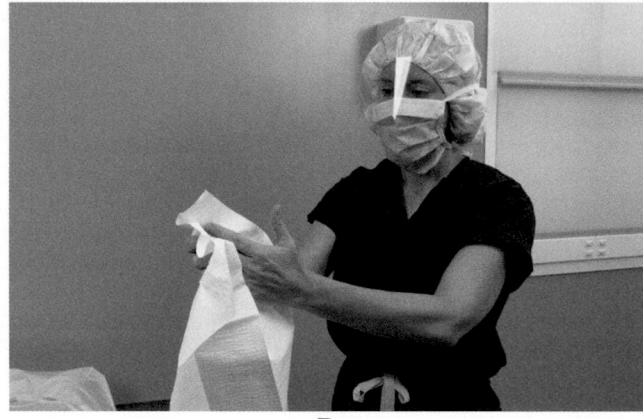

B

STEP **5g** **A,** Grasping sterile towel. **B,** Drying sequence.

STEP **6c** Application of antimicrobial agent for brushless
hand scrub. Nurse using 3M
Avagard. (Photo courtesy of
3M Health Care.)

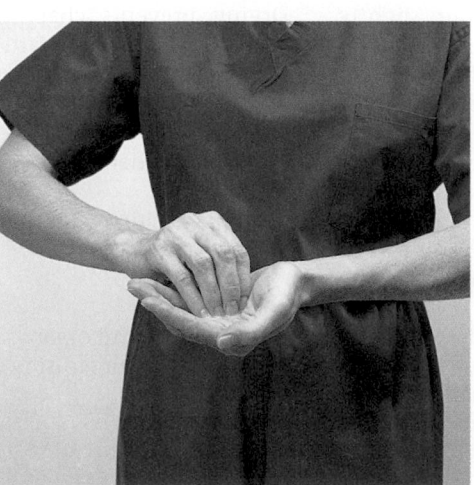

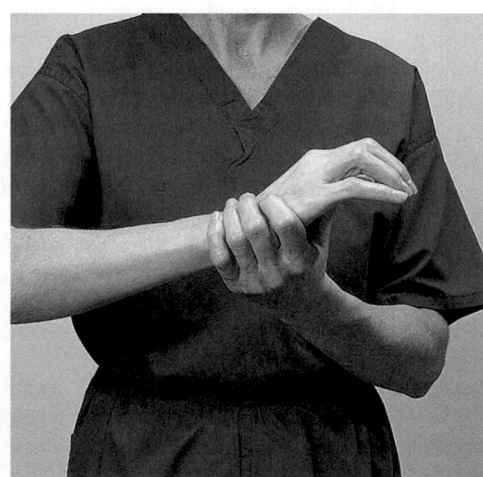

Steps	Rationale
c. Apply enough alcohol-based waterless antiseptic to one palm to cover both hands thoroughly (see illustration). Spread the antiseptic over all surfaces of the hands and fingernails. Follow product instructions for length of time to rub over hand surfaces. Allow to air-dry.	Ensures coverage of all surfaces. Air drying ensures complete antiseptis is achieved.
d. Repeat the process and allow hands to air-dry before applying sterile gloves.	

Recording and Reporting

• It is not necessary to record or report this procedure.
• Report any dermatitis to employee health or infection control per agency policy.

Skill 33-4   *A*pplying a Sterile Gown and Performing Closed Gloving

Delegation Considerations

The role of the scrub nurse can be delegated to a surgical technician.

Equipment

• Surgical cap

• Surgical mask
• Eyewear
• Foot covers
• Sterile gown (prepared by circulating nurse)

Steps	Rationale
Gowning	
1. Before entering operating room or treatment area, apply cap, face mask, and eyewear. Foot covers are also required in operating room.	Prevents hair and air droplet nuclei from contaminating sterile work areas. Eyewear protects mucous membranes of eye. Foot covers are paper or cloth and fit over work shoes.
2. Perform thorough surgical hand wash (see Skill 33-3, p. 808).	Removes transient and resident bacteria from fingers, hands, and forearms.
3. Ask circulating nurse to assist by opening sterile pack containing sterile gown (folded inside out).	Gown's outer surface remains sterile.
4. Have circulating nurse prepare glove package by peeling outer wrapper open while keeping inner contents sterile. Inner glove package is then placed on sterile field created by sterile outer wrapper.	Keeps gloves sterile and allows nurse who has scrubbed to handle sterile items.
5. Reach down to sterile gown package; lift folded gown directly upward and step back away from table.	Provides wide margin of safety, avoiding contamination of gown.
6. Holding folded gown, locate neckband. With both hands, grasp inside front of gown just below neckband.	Clean hands may touch inside of gown without contaminating outer surface.
7. Allow gown to unfold, keeping inside of gown toward body. Do not touch outside of gown with bare hands.	Outside of gown will be sterile surface.
8. With hands at shoulder level, slip both arms into armholes simultaneously (see illustration). Ask circulating nurse to bring gown over shoulders by reaching inside to arm seams and pulling gown on, leaving sleeves covering hands.	Careful application prevents contamination. Gown covers hands to prepare for closed gloving.

Applying a Sterile Gown and Performing Closed Gloving—cont'd

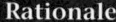

Skill 33-4

Steps	Rationale
9. Have circulating nurse securely tie back of gown at neck and waist (see illustration). (If gown is a wrap-around style, sterile flap to cover gown is not touched until the nurse has gloved.)	Gown must completely enclose underlying garments.
10. Closed Gloving	
a. With hands covered by gown sleeves, open inner sterile glove package (see illustration).	Hands remain clean. Sterile gown cuff will touch sterile glove surface.
b. With dominant hand inside gown cuff, pick up glove for nondominant hand by grasping folded cuff.	Sterile gown touches sterile glove.
c. Extend nondominant forearm with palm up and place palm of glove against palm of nondominant hand. Glove fingers will point toward elbow.	Positions glove for application over cuffed hand, keeping glove sterile.

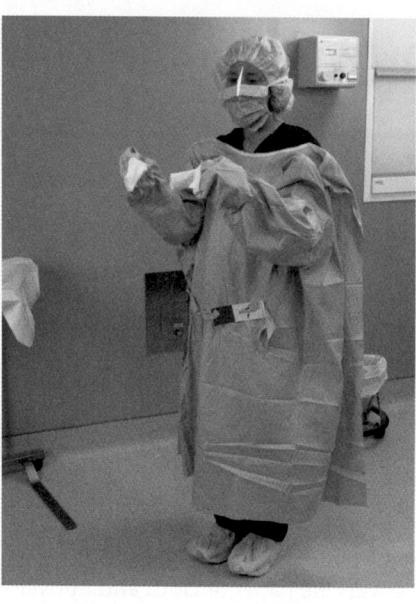

STEP **8** Placing arms in sleeves.

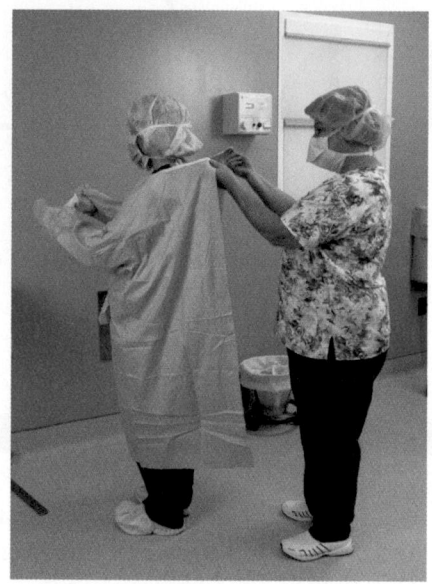

STEP **9** Circulating nurse ties scrub gown.

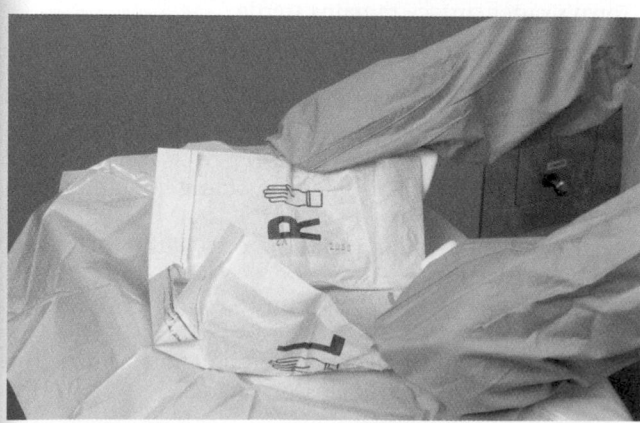

STEP **10a** Scrub nurse opens glove package.

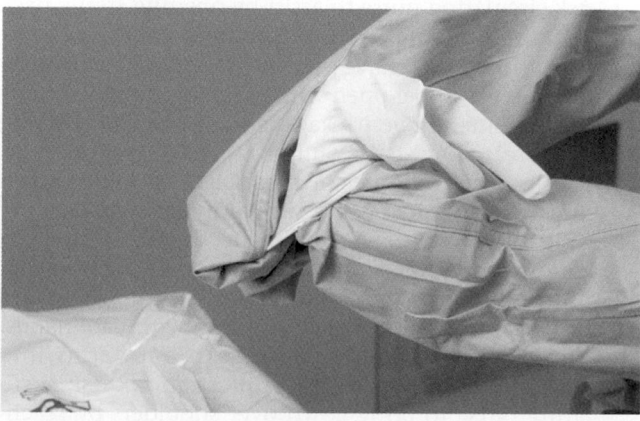

STEP **10d** Glove applied to left hand as right hand remains inside cuff.

Steps	Rationale

   d. Grasp back of glove cuff with covered dominant hand and turn glove cuff over end of nondominant hand and gown cuff (see illustration).

Seal created by glove cuff over gown prevents exit of microorganisms over operative sterile field.

   e. Grasp top of glove and underlying gown sleeve with covered dominant hand. Carefully extend fingers into glove, being sure glove's cuff covers gown's cuff.

   f. Glove dominant hand in same manner, reversing hands (see illustration). Use gloved nondominant hand to pull on glove. Keep hand inside sleeve (see illustration).

Sterile touches sterile.

   g. Be sure fingers are fully extended into both gloves.

Ensures that nurse has full dexterity while using gloved hand.

11. For wraparound sterile gowns: take gloved hand and release fastener or ties in front of gown.

Front of gown is sterile.

12. Hand tie to sterile team member who stands still (see illustration). Allowing margin of safety, turn around to the left, covering back with extended gown flap. Take back tie from team member and secure tie to gown.

Contact with team member could contaminate gown and gloves. Gown must enclose undergarments.

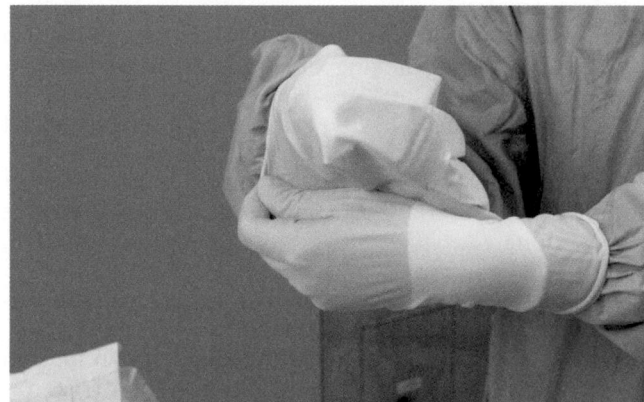
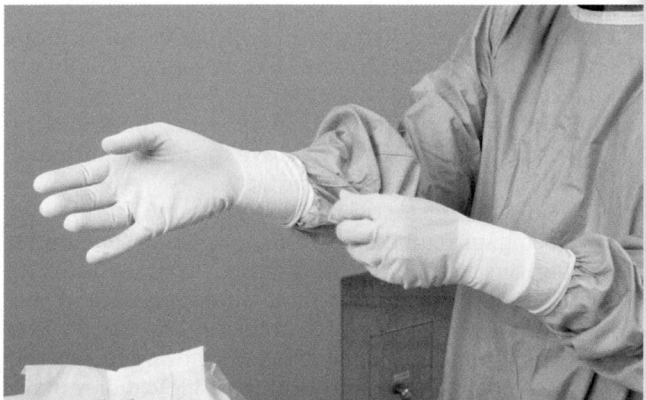

STEP **10f** Second glove applied.

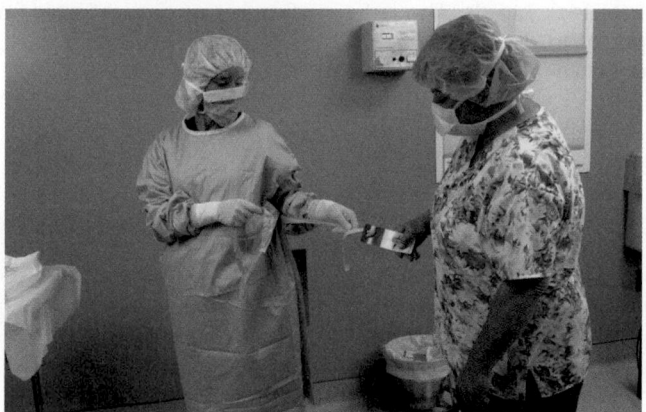

STEP **12** Handing tie to sterile team member.

Recording and Reporting

• It is not necessary to record or report this procedure.

Skill 33-5   *Open Gloving*

Delegation Considerations

Delegation of open gloving depends on whether assistive personnel have received special training and are competent to perform the sterile procedure.

Equipment

• Sterile gloves (proper size)

Steps	Rationale
1. Perform thorough hand hygiene.	Removes bacteria from skin surfaces and reduces transmission of infection.
2. Remove outer glove package wrapper by carefully separating and peeling apart sides.	Prevents inner glove package from accidentally opening and touching contaminated objects.
3. Grasp inner package and lay it on clean, flat surface just above waist level. Open package, keeping gloves on wrapper's inside surface (see illustration).	Sterile object held below waist is contaminated. Inner surface of glove package is sterile.
4. If gloves are not prepowdered, take packet of powder and apply lightly to hands over sink or wastebasket.	Powder allows gloves to slip on easily. (Some staff members do not use powder for fear of promoting growth of microorganisms.)
5. Identify right and left glove. Each glove has cuff approximately 5 cm (2 inches) wide. Glove dominant hand first.	Proper identification of gloves prevents contamination by improper fit. Gloving of dominant hand first improves dexterity.
6. With thumb and first two fingers of nondominant hand, grasp edge of cuff of glove for dominant hand. Touch only glove's inside surface.	Inner edge of cuff will lie against skin and thus is not sterile.
7. Carefully pull glove over dominant hand, leaving cuff and being sure cuff does not roll up wrist. Be sure thumb and fingers are in proper spaces (see illustration).	If glove's outer surface touches hand or wrist, then it is contaminated.
8. With gloved dominant hand, slip fingers underneath second glove's cuff (see illustration).	Cuff protects gloved fingers. Sterile touching sterile prevents glove contamination.
9. Carefully pull second glove over nondominant hand. Do not allow fingers and thumb of gloved dominant hand to touch any part of exposed nondominant hand. Keep thumb of dominant hand abducted back (see illustration).	Contact of gloved hand with exposed hand results in contamination.
10. After second glove is on, interlock hands. The cuffs usually fall down after application. Be sure to touch only sterile sides (see illustration).	Ensures smooth fit over fingers.

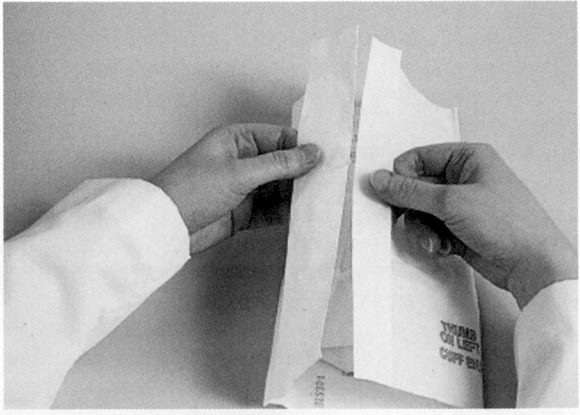

STEP **3** Opening package.

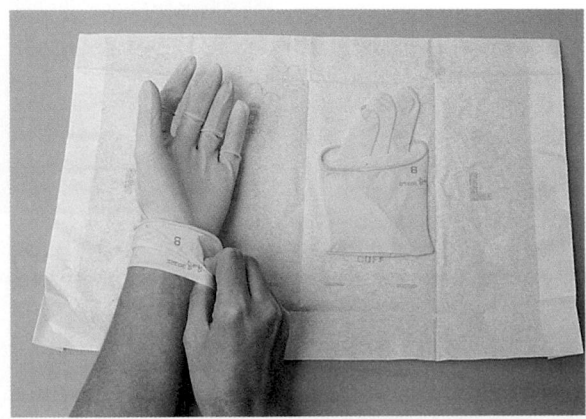

STEP **7** Pulling glove over dominant hand.

Steps	Rationale

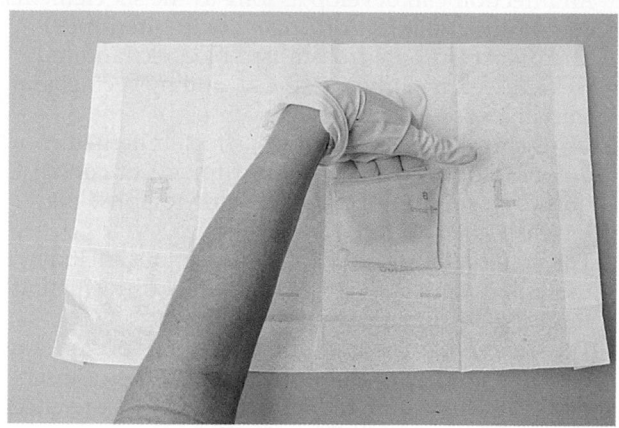

STEP **8** Slipping fingers underneath second glove's cuff.

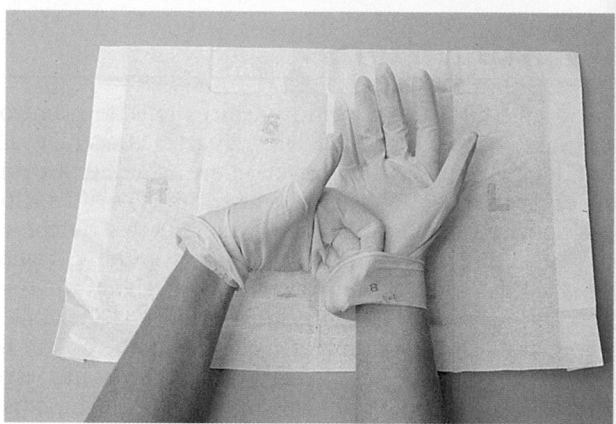

STEP **9** Pulling second glove over nondominant hand.

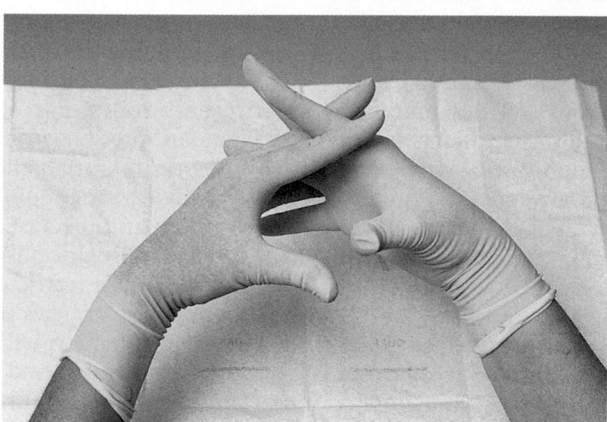

STEP **10** Hands interlocked.

Glove Disposal

11. Grasp outside of one cuff with other gloved hand; avoid touching wrist.	Minimizes contamination of underlying skin.
12. Pull glove off, turning it inside out. Discard in receptacle.	Outside of glove does not touch skin surface.
13. Take fingers of bare hand and tuck inside remaining glove cuff. Peel glove off, inside out. Discard in receptacle.	

Recording and Reporting

• It is not necessary to record or report this procedure.

constant view and ensure their sterility. Skill 33-4 reviews the steps for applying a sterile gown.

Evaluation

The success of the nurse who practices infection-control techniques is measured by determining whether the goals for reducing or preventing infection are achieved. A comparison of the client's response, such as absence of fever or development of wound drainage, with expected outcomes determines the success of nursing interventions (Figure 33-6). Similarly, a determination is made about whether interventions should be revised or eliminated. The ability to correctly assess wounds for healing and the ability to conduct a physical assessment of body systems (see Chapter 32) are important skills in evaluation. The nurse closely monitors clients, especially those at risk, for signs and symptoms of infection. For example, a client who has undergone a surgical procedure is at risk for infection at the surgical site, as well as at other invasive sites, such as the venipuncture site or central line sites. In addition, the client is at risk for a respiratory tract infection as a result of decreased mobility and for a urinary tract infection if an indwelling catheter is present. The nurse closely monitors all invasive and surgical sites for swelling, erythema, or purulent drainage. Breath sounds are monitored for changes, and sputum character is checked for purulence. Laboratory test results are reviewed for leukocytes in the urine, which may indicate a urinary tract infection. The absence of signs or symptoms of infection is the expected outcome of infection prevention and monitoring activities.

The client at risk for infection must understand the measures needed to reduce or prevent microorganism growth and spread. Providing clients or family members the opportunity to discuss infection-control measures or to demonstrate procedures will reveal their ability to comply with therapy. The nurse may determine that clients require new information or that previously instructed information needs reinforcement.

The nurse documents the client's response to therapies for infection control. A clear description of any signs and symptoms of systemic or local infection is necessary to give all nurses a baseline for comparative evaluation. The efficacy of any intervention in reducing infection must also be reported.

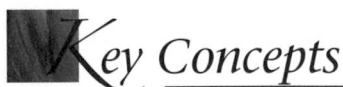

Key Concepts

- Hand hygiene is the most important technique to use in preventing and controlling transmission of infection.
- The potential for microorganisms to cause disease depends on the number of organisms, virulence, ability to enter and survive in a host, and susceptibility of the host.
- Normal body flora help to resist infection by releasing antibacterial substances and inhibiting multiplication of pathogenic microorganisms.

- The signs of local inflammation and infection are identical.
- An infection can develop as long as the six elements composing the infection chain are uninterrupted.
- Microorganisms are transmitted by direct and indirect contact, by airborne spread, and by vectors and contaminated articles.
- Increasing age, poor nutrition, stress, inherited conditions, chronic disease, and treatments or conditions that compromise the immune response may increase susceptibility to infection.
- The major sites for nosocomial infections include the urinary and respiratory tracts, bloodstream, and surgical or traumatic wounds.
- The Centers for Disease Control and Prevention now recommends use of alcohol-based waterless antiseptics as an alternative to hand washing to more effectively reduce transmission of pathogens.
- Invasive procedures, medical therapies, long hospitalization, and contact with health care personnel increase a hospitalized client's risk for acquiring a nosocomial infection.
- Isolation practices may prevent personnel and clients from acquiring infections and may prevent transmission of microorganisms to other persons.
- Standard precautions use generic barrier techniques when caring for all clients.
- Proper cleansing requires mechanical removal of all soil from an object or area.
- A client in isolation is subject to sensory deprivation because of the restricted environment.
- An infection-control professional monitors the incidence of infection within an institution and provides educational and consultative services to maintain infection prevention.
- Surgical asepsis requires more stringent techniques than medical asepsis and is directed at eliminating microorganisms.
- If the skin is broken, or if the nurse performs an invasive procedure into a body cavity normally free of microorganisms, surgical aseptic practices are followed.

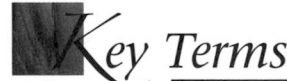

Key Terms

Aerobic, *p. 774*
Anaerobic, *p. 774*
Asepsis, *p. 786*
Bactericidal, *p. 775*
Bacteriostasis, *p. 775*
Broad-spectrum antibiotics, *p. 778*
Carriers, *p. 774*
Colonized, *p. 794*
Communicable, *p. 774*
Disinfection, *p. 787*
Edema, *p. 778*
Endogenous infection, *p. 780*
Epidemiology, *p. 801*

Exogenous infection, *p. 779*
Exudates, *p. 778*
Granulation tissue, *p. 778*
Hand hygiene, *p. 789*
Hand washing, *p. 789*
Iatrogenic infections, *p. 779*
Immunocompromised, *p. 774*
Inflammatory response, *p. 777*
Invasive, *p. 773*
Leukocytosis, *p. 778*
Localized, *p. 777*
Medical asepsis, *p. 786*
Microorganisms, *p. 773*

SEPSIS WITH NEUTROPENIA

DRG # 416
Target LOS 9 days

	DATE	DATE	DATE
Hosp day	**HOSPITAL DAY 1**	**HOSPITAL DAY 2**	**HOSPITAL DAY 3**
CONSULTS	Notify Radiation Therapy if applicable	Dr. Clements if ordered Social Service Dietician	
TESTS	CBC, SMA 18, Magnesium, Creatinine Blood cultures X 2 sites before antibiotics started Chest Xray Type and Screen	CBC Blood cultures for chills or temp>101 No more than 3 sets in 24 hours	CBC - - - - - - - - - - - - - - - -> - - - - - - - - - - - - - - - ->
SPECIMENS	U/A, c&s before antibiotics started Sputum for c&s and Gram stain if productive cough	- - - - - - - - - - - - - - - ->	- - - - - - - - - - - - - - - ->
TREATMENTS	O2 at 2L by NC if Hgb<8 Mouth care every 4 hours per protocol	- - - - - - - - - - - - - - - -> - - - - - - - - - - - - - - - ->	- - - - - - - - - - - - - - - -> - - - - - - - - - - - - - - - ->
VITAL SIGNS	Every 4 hours	- - - - - - - - - - - - - - - ->	- - - - - - - - - - - - - - - ->
I & O	Every 8 hours	- - - - - - - - - - - - - - - ->	- - - - - - - - - - - - - - - ->
DIET	Neutropenic DAT until WBC>1.5	- - - - - - - - - - - - - - - ->	- - - - - - - - - - - - - - - ->
IVs	Fluids as ordered Antibiotics as ordered	Check w/MD re: fluid changes Continue antibiotics as ordered until d/c'd	Continue until d/c'd - - - - - - - - - - - - - - - ->
MEDS	ID home meds and check with MD Check those that are ordered: ——— Tylenol gr X po temp>101 ——— Pain PRN ——— Sleeper ——— Antidiarrhea ——— Antiemetic ——— Antianxiety	Check those that are ordered: ——— Tylenol gr X po temp>101 ——— Pain PRN ——— Sleeper ——— Antidiarrhea ——— Antiemetic ——— Antianxiety	Check those that are ordered: ——— Tylenol gr X po temp>101 ——— Pain PRN ——— Sleeper ——— Antidiarrhea ——— Antiemetic ——— Antianxiety
ACTIVITY	Up as tolerated	- - - - - - - - - - - - - - - ->	- - - - - - - - - - - - - - - ->
MISC	Restrict ill visitors and staff	- - - - - - - - - - - - - - - ->	Continue until WBC>1.5
TEACHING	Instruct pt to report any: bleeding, diarrhea, N&V, pain.	Dietician to teach re: neutropenic diet. Mouth Care	Instruct re: personal hygiene
DISCHARGE PLANNING	Evaluate need for d/c planning.	Social services called if appropriate	Determine d/c destination

	Shift	Shift	Shift
Nurse signature	_____/___	_____/___	_____/___
Nurse signature	_____/___	_____/___	_____/___
Nurse signature	_____/___	_____/___	_____/___

Authored by Janie Barnett, RN; Lucy Wallace, LPN

FIGURE 33–6 First 3 days of 9-day CareMap for sepsis with neutropenia. (Courtesy Baptist Hospital, Pensacola, Fla, and The Center for Case Management, South Natick, Mass.)   *Continued*

SUMMARY
PATIENT PROBLEMS/OUTCOME CRITERIA

Sepsis w/Neutropenia   Target LOS 9 days

DATE	INITIAL	NSG DIAGNOSIS/PROBLEM	OUTCOME CRITERIA/GOAL	DATE D/C	INITIAL
		1. Activity intolerance re: disease process.	1. PT will be able to perform own hygeine care by d/c.		
		2. Imbalanced Nutrition re: less than body requirements re: anorexia, illness, dehydration.	2a Patient will be able to eat at least 1/3 of their ordered diets by d/c. 2b Patient will identify at least 3 food items that they find appealing 2c 1500cc po flds q 24 by d/c		
		3. Hyperthermia re: increase in metabolic rate and illness.	3. Pt. will be afebrile by day 5.		
		4. Potential deficient knowledge re: s/s to report neutropenic diet, personal hygiene, activity restrictions	4. Prior to d/c, the pt/s.o. will be able to demonstrate competency and/or verbalize understanding of instructions provided		

Signature   Title

_____   _____

_____   _____

_____   _____

_____   _____

_____   _____

FIGURE **33–6, cont'd** First 3 days of 9-day CareMap for sepsis with neutropenia. (Courtesy Baptist Hospital, Pensacola, Fla, and The Center for Case Management, South Natick, Mass.)

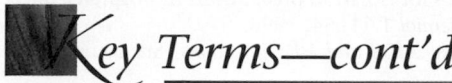

Key Terms—cont'd

Necrotic, *p. 778*	Sterile field, *p. 805*
Normal flora, *p. 778*	Sterilization, *p. 787*
Nosocomial infections, *p. 779*	Suprainfection, *p. 778*
	Surgical asepsis, *p. 802*
Pathogen, *p. 773*	Susceptibility, *p. 777*
Pathogenicity, *p. 777*	Systemic, *p. 777*
Phagocytosis, *p. 778*	Vector, *p. 776*
Purulent, *p. 778*	Virulence, *p. 774*
Sanguineous, *p. 778*	
Serous, *p. 778*	

Critical Thinking Exercises

1. Mrs. Jaycock had an indwelling urethral catheter for 1 week. The catheter has now been out for 24 hours. She complains of frequency and pain on urination. Mrs. Jaycock suggests reinsertion of the catheter because of the need to get up frequently. What can frequency or pain on urination be an indication of? Should the catheter be reinserted? Why or why not? Describe at least one appropriate assessment measure and independent nursing action for Mrs. Jaycock.

2. You are caring for Mr. Huang, who has a large, open, and draining abdominal wound. You notice another health care worker changing Mr. Huang's dressing without wearing gloves or using sterile supplies or sterile technique. When you question the health care worker regarding his or her practice, this person says, "Don't worry, the wound is already infected, and the antibiotics and draining will take care of any contaminants." How would you respond to this comment? What would your next steps be in following up on this incident?

3. Mrs. Niles is 83 years of age and lives alone. She has difficulty walking and relies on a church volunteer group to deliver lunches during the week. Her fixed income limits her ability to buy food. Last week, Mrs. Niles's 79-year-old sister died. The two sisters had been very close. As a home care nurse, explain the factors that might increase Mrs. Niles's risk for infection.

4. Mr. Vargas is admitted to the facility with a history of recent weight loss, a cough that has persisted for 2 months, and hemoptysis. His chest x-ray film shows a cavity in one lung, and his physician suspects tuberculosis. What type of isolation precautions would you use for Mr. Vargas? What protection would you use to provide care? What education would you provide for the client and his family?

Review Questions

1. If the infectious disease can be transmitted directly from one person to another, it is a:
   1. Communicable disease.
   2. Portal of entry to a host.
   3. Portal of exit from the reservoir.
   4. Susceptible host.

2. Infectious diseases such as hepatitis B or C become a reservoir for pathogens in:
   1. The urinary tract.
   2. The reproductive tract.
   3. Blood.
   4. The respiratory tract.

3. The interval when a client manifests signs and symptoms specific to a type of infection is the:
   1. Incubation period.
   2. Convalescence.
   3. Prodromal stage
   4. Illness stage.

4. The most effective way to break the chain of infection is by:
   1. Wearing gloves.
   2. Hand hygiene.
   3. Placing clients in isolation.
   4. Providing private rooms for clients.

5. After coming in contact with infected clients, and after handling contaminated equipment or organic material, visitors are encouraged to:
   1. Perform hand hygiene before eating or handling food.
   2. Leave the facility to prevent contamination of others.
   3. Wear gloves before eating or handling food.
   4. Use a private room to talk with family members.

6. A client is isolated for pulmonary tuberculosis. The nurse notes the client seems to be angry, but he knows this is a normal response to isolation. The best intervention is to:
   1. Provide a dark, quiet room to calm the client.
   2. Explain the isolation procedures and provide meaningful stimulation.
   3. Reduce the level of precautions to keep the client from becoming angry.
   4. Limit family and other caregiver visits to reduce the risk of spreading the infection.

7. A gown should be worn when:
   1. The client's hygiene is poor.
   2. The client has AIDS or hepatitis.
   3. The nurse is assisting with medication administration.
   4. Blood or body fluids may get on the nurse's clothing from a task the nurse plans to perform.

8. The nurse has redressed a client's wound and now plans to administer a medication to the client. It is important to:
   1. Remove gloves and perform hand hygiene before leaving the room.
   2. Remove gloves and perform hand hygiene before administering the medication.
   3. Leave the gloves on to administer the medication.
   4. Leave the medication on the bedside table to avoid having to remove gloves before leaving the client's room.

9. When a nurse is performing a surgical hand hygiene, he must keep hands:
   1. Above elbows.
   2. Below elbows.
   3. At a 45-degree angle.
   4. In a comfortable position.

10. To sterilize surgical instruments, parenteral solutions, and surgical dressings:
    1. Soap and water is used.
    2. Chemicals are used for disinfection.
    3. An autoclave is used.
    4. Ethylene oxide gas is used.

References

Association of Perioperative Nurses: Recommended practices for surgical hand scrubs. In *Standards and recommended practices for perioperative nursing,* Denver, 1998, The Association.

Boyce JM, Pittet D: Guideline for hand hygiene in health-care settings, *Am J Infect Control* 30(8):S1, 2002.

Centers for Disease Control and Prevention: Guideline for preventing the transmission of *Mycobacterium tuberculosis* in health-care facilities, *Federal Register* 59(208):54242, 1994.

Centers for Disease Control and Prevention, 2001

Centers for Disease Control and Prevention, Hospital Infection Control Practices Advisory Committee: Recommendations for preventing the spread of vancomycin resistance, *Am J Infect Control* 23(2):87, 1995.

Centers for Disease Control and Prevention, Hospital Infection Control Practices Advisory Committee: Draft: Guidelines for prevention of health care-associated pneumonia, 2002a, www.cdc.gov.

Centers for Disease Control and Prevention, Hospital Infection Control Practices Advisory Committee: Guideline for hand hygiene in health-care settings, 2002b, www.cdc.gov.

Dochterman JM, Bulechek GM: *Nursing interventions classification (NIC),* ed 4, St. Louis, 2004, Mosby.

Eliopoulos C: *Gerontologic nursing,* ed 5, Philadelphia, 2001, Lippincott.

Gantz NM, Tkatch LS, Makris AT: Geriatric infections. In *APIC text of infection control and epidemiology,* Washington, DC, 2000, Association for Professionals in Infection Control and Epidemiology.

Garner JS: Guidelines for isolation precautions in hospitals, *Infect Control Hosp Epidemiol* 17(1):54, 1996.

Grimes D, Grimes R: *AIDS and HIV infections,* St. Louis, 1994, Mosby.

Ignatavicius D, Workman ML: *Medical-surgical nursing: critical thinking for collaborative care,* Philadelphia, 2002, Saunders.

Jernigan JA and others: A randomized crossover study of disposable thermometers for prevention of *Clostridium difficile* and other nosocomial infections, *Infect Control Hosp Epidemiol* 19(7):494, 1998.

Keroack MA, Rosen-Kotilainen H: Microbiology/laboratory diagnostics. In *APIC infection control and applied epidemiology: principles and practice,* St. Louis, 1996, Mosby.

Larson E: APIC guideline for hand washing and hand antisepsis in health-care settings. In *APIC infection control and applied epidemiology: principles and practice,* St. Louis, 1996, Mosby.

Lueckenotte AG: *Gerontologic nursing,* ed 2, St. Louis, 2000, Mosby.

Meeker MH, Rothrock JC: *Alexander's care of the patient in surgery,* ed 11, St. Louis, 1999, Mosby.

Miller CA: Nursing care of older adults: theory and practice, ed 3, Philadelphia, 1999, Lippincott.

Moorhead S, Johnson M, and Maas M: *Nursing outcomes classification (NOC),* ed 3, St. Louis, 2004, Mosby.

Occupational Safety and Health Administration: Respiratory protection: proposed rule, *Federal Register* 59(219):58884,1994.

Occupational Safety and Health Administration: Occupational exposure to tuberculosis, *Federal Register* 64:32447, 1999.

Occupational Safety and Health Administration: Occupational Safety and Health Act of 1991: blood-borne pathogens, www.osha.gov, 1991.

Occupational Safety and Health Administration: Occupational Safety and Health Act of 2001, 2001, www.cdc.gov.

Pagana KD, Pagana TJ: *Diagnostic testing and nursing implications: a case study approach,* ed 5, St. Louis, 1998, Mosby.

Rutala W, Weber DJ: Centers for Disease Control and Prevention, Hospital Infection Control Practices Advisory Committee: Draft guideline for disinfection and sterilization in healthcare facilities, 2002, www.cdc.gov.

Research References

Hedderwick SA and others: Pathogenic organisms associated with artificial fingernails worn by healthcare workers, *Infect Control Hosp Epidemiol* 21(8):505, 2000.

Maki DG and others: Double-bagging of items from isolation rooms is unnecessary as an infection control measure: a comparative study of surface contamination with single and double-bagging, *Infect Control* 7(11):535, 1986.

Weinstein SA and others: Bacterial surface contamination of patient's linen: isolation precautions versus standard care, *Am J Infect Control* 17(5):264, 1989.

*M*edication Administration

http://evolve.elsevier.com/Potter/
fundamentals/

Media Resources

CD COMPANION

- Review Questions
- Glossary

evolve WEBSITE

- Review Questions
- Student Learning Activities
- Animations
- Video Clips
- Glossary

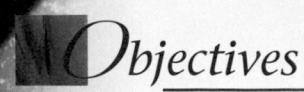

Objectives

Mastery of content in this chapter will enable the student to:

- Define the key terms listed.
- Discuss the nurse's role and responsibilities in medication administration.
- Describe the physiological mechanisms of medication action, including absorption, distribution, metabolism, and excretion of medications.
- Differentiate among different types of medication actions.
- Discuss developmental factors that influence pharmacokinetics.
- Discuss factors that influence medication actions.
- Discuss methods of educating a client about prescribed medications.
- Describe the roles of the prescriber, pharmacist, and nurse in medication administration.
- Discuss factors that commonly cause medication errors.
- Describe factors to consider when choosing routes of medication administration.
- Correctly calculate a prescribed medication dose.
- Discuss factors to include in assessing a client's needs for and response to medication therapy.
- Explain the six rights of medication administration.
- Correctly prepare and administer subcutaneous, intramuscular, and intradermal injections and intravenous medications; oral and topical skin preparations; eye, ear, and nose drops; vaginal instillations; rectal suppositories; and inhalants.

*C*lients with acute or chronic health alterations restore or maintain their health using a variety of strategies. A medication is a substance used in the diagnosis, treatment, cure, relief, or prevention of health alterations. In fact, medications are the primary treatment clients associate with restoration of health. No matter where clients receive their health care—hospitals, clinics, or home—the nurse plays an essential role in medication preparation and administration, medication teaching, and evaluating clients' responses to medications.

In the primary care setting and occasionally in the restorative care setting, the client often self-administers medications. The nurse is responsible for evaluating the effects of the medications on the client's health status, teaching clients about their medications and their side effects, ensuring adherence with the medication regimen, and evaluating client technique when the client administers medications that are not given by mouth.

In both acute care and restorative care settings, nurses spend a great deal of time administering medications to clients. The nurse also ensures that clients are adequately prepared to administer their medications when they are discharged. In the home care setting, clients usually administer their own medications.

When clients cannot administer their own medications, family members or home health care personnel may be responsible for doing so. The nurse assesses the effect the medications have in restoring or maintaining health and provides continued education to the client, family, or home care personnel on medication purpose, regimen, and side effects.

Scientific Knowledge Base

Medications administered to clients are used, almost exclusively, to prevent, diagnose, or treat disease. Because medication administration and evaluation are essential to nursing practice, nurses need to have knowledge about the actions and effects of the medications they deliver to clients. This requires an understanding of the life sciences. Moreover, to safely and accurately administer medications to clients, nurses must have an understanding of pharmacokinetics (the study of drug concentrations), growth and development, human anatomy, nutrition, and mathematics. All of the nurse's previous learning is important and is often applied to medication administration. The nursing process provides the framework for nurses to organize their thoughts and actions and is the foundation for medication administration.

Pharmacological Concepts

Drug Names. A medication may have as many as three different names. A medication's chemical name provides an exact description of the medication's composition and molecular structure. Chemical names are rarely used in clinical practice. An example of a chemical name is *N*-acetyl-para-aminophenol, which is commonly known as Tylenol. The manufacturer who first develops the medication gives the generic or nonproprietary name, with United States Adopted Name Council (USAN) approval. Acetaminophen is an example of a generic name. It is the generic name for Tylenol. The generic name becomes the official name that is listed in official publications such as the *United States Pharmacopeia* (USP). The trade name, brand name, or proprietary name is the name under which a manufacturer markets a medication. The trade name has the symbol™, at the upper right of the name, indicating that the manufacturer has trademarked the medication's name (e.g., Panadol™, Tempra™, and St. Joseph Aspirin-Free Fever Reducer for Children™).

Manufacturers have chosen names that are easy to pronounce, spell, and remember so that laypersons will recognize trade names. Many companies may produce the same medication, so similarities in trade names can be confusing. In fact, similarities in drug names is a common cause of medical errors. Hospitals and clinic pharmacies attempt to consistently dispense medications with the same trade names so nurses can become familiar with them. However, the nurse finds medications under a variety of different nomenclatures or names and must be careful to obtain the exact name and spelling for a particular medication.

Classification. Nurses learn to categorize medications with similar characteristics by their class. Medication classification indicates the effect of the medication on a body system, the symptoms the medication relieves, or the medication's desired effect. For example, clients who have type 2 diabetes (formerly called non–insulin-dependent diabetes) often take medications to lower their blood glucose level. This class of medication is called oral hypoglycemic agents. Usually each class contains more than one medication that can be prescribed for the same type of health problem. For example, there are over 12 different oral hypoglycemic agents. These medications are divided into three classifications of oral agents: first- and second-generation sulfonylureas and a miscellaneous group (McKenry and Salerno, 2003). A prescriber chooses a particular oral hypoglycemic medication based on client characteristics, cost, efficacy, dosing frequency, or prescriber experience with the medication.

One medication may also be part of more than one class. For example, aspirin is an analgesic, an antipyretic, and an antiinflammatory medication.

Medication Forms. Medications are available in a variety of forms, or preparations (Figure 34-1). The form of the medication determines its route of administration. The composition of a medication is designed to enhance its absorption and metabolism. Many medications are made in several forms such as tablets, capsules, elixirs, and suppositories. When administering a medication, the nurse must be certain to use the proper form (Table 34-1).

Medication Legislation and Standards

Federal Regulations. The role of the U.S. government in regulation of the pharmaceutical industry is to protect the health of the people by ensuring that medications are safe and effective. The first American law to regulate medications was the Pure Food and Drug Act. This law simply requires all medications to be free of impure products. Subsequent legislation (Table 34-2) has set standards related to safety, potency, and efficacy. Enforcement of medication laws rests with the Food and Drug Administration (FDA), which ensures that all medications on the market undergo vigorous testing. Medications must go through this rigorous process before they can be dispensed to the

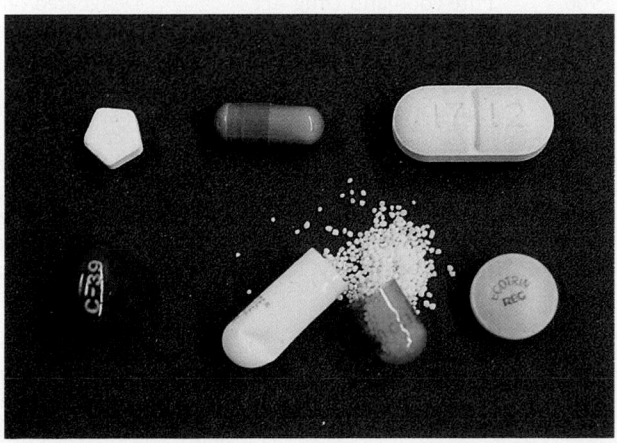

FIGURE 34-1 Forms of oral medications. *Top row:* Uniquely shaped tablet, capsule, scored tablet. *Bottom row:* Gelatin-coated liquid, extended-release capsule, enteric-coated tablet.

Table 34-1   Forms of Medication

Form	Description
Caplet	Solid dosage form for oral use; shaped like capsule and coated for ease of swallowing
Capsule	Solid dosage form for oral use; medication in powder, liquid, or oil form and encased by gelatin shell; capsule colored to aid in product identification
Elixir	Clear fluid containing water and/or alcohol; designed for oral use; usually has sweetener added
Enteric-coated tablet	Tablet for oral use coated with materials that do not dissolve in stomach; coatings dissolve in intestine, where medication is absorbed
Extract	Concentrated medication form made by removing active portion of medication from its other components (e.g., fluid extract is medication made into solution from vegetable source)
Glycerite	Solution of medication combined with glycerin for external use; contains at least 50% glycerin
Intraocular disk	A small, flexible oval consisting of two soft, outer layers and a middle layer containing medication; when moistened by ocular fluid, releases medication for up to 1 week
Liniment	Preparation usually containing alcohol, oil, or soapy emollient that is applied to skin
Lotion	Medication in liquid suspension applied externally to protect skin
Ointment (salve, cream, or unguent)	Semisolid, externally applied preparation, usually containing one or more medications
Paste	Semisolid preparation, thicker and stiffer than ointment; absorbed through skin more slowly than ointment
Pill	Solid dosage form containing one or more medications, shaped into globules, ovoids, or oblong shapes; true pills rarely used because they have been replaced by tablets
Solution	Liquid preparation that may be used orally, parenterally, or externally; can also be instilled into body organ or cavity (e.g., bladder irrigations); contains water with one or more dissolved compounds; must be sterile for parenteral use
Suppository	Solid dosage form mixed with gelatin and shaped in form of pellet for insertion into body cavity (rectum or vagina); melts when it reaches body temperature, releasing medication for absorption
Suspension	Finely divided drug particles dispersed in liquid medium; when suspension is left standing, particles settle to bottom of container; commonly oral medication and not given intravenously
Syrup	Medication dissolved in concentrated sugar solution; may contain flavoring to make medication more palatable
Tablet	Powdered dosage form compressed into hard disks or cylinders; in addition to primary medication, contains binders (adhesive to allow powder to stick together), disintegrators (to promote tablet dissolution), lubricants (for ease of manufacturing), and fillers (for convenient tablet size)
Tincture	Alcohol or water-alcohol medication solution
Transdermal disk or patch	Medication contained within semipermeable membrane disk or patch, which allows medications to be absorbed through skin slowly over long period
Troche (lozenge)	Flat, round dosage form containing medication, flavoring, sugar, and mucilage; dissolves in mouth to release medication

Table 34-2   Federal Medication Laws in the United States

Date	Title of Law	Provisions
1906	Pure Food and Drug Act	Designated official standards for medications (USP and the National Formulary); specified standards for medication labeling
1912	Sherley Amendment	Prohibited manufacturers from making fraudulent claims about medication efficacy and therapeutic effects
1914	Harrison Narcotic Act	Legally classified medications believed to be habit forming as narcotics; regulated importation, manufacture, sale, and use of narcotic substances
1938	Federal Food, Drug, and Cosmetic Act	Added the Homeopathic Pharmacopeia of the United States as a third medication standard; required that medication preparation be approved as safe by the FDA before marketing; further outlined criteria for medication labeling
1945	Amendment to the Food and Drug Act	Provided for certification of biological products used as medications (e.g., insulin, antibiotics) on batch basis; allowed for direct supervision and inspection of medication production
1952	Durham-Humphrey Amendment	Distinguished between prescription ("legend") and nonprescription medications
1962	Kefauver-Harris Amendment	Authorized FDA to supervise medication production to ensure safety and efficacy and to establish official medication names; specified greater controls on investigational medications
1970	Comprehensive Drug Abuse Prevention and Control Act (Controlled Substances Act)	Set strict controls on manufacture and distribution of controlled medication (possession of controlled substances unlawful without prescription); established government programs to promote prevention and treatment of medication dependence
1978	Drug Regulation Reform Act	Shortened the drug investigation process to release drugs sooner to the public

public. In 1993 the FDA instituted the MedWatch program. This voluntary program encourages nurses and other health care professionals to report when a medication, product, or medical event causes serious harm to a client. The MedWatch form is available to report such events (Figure 34-2).

Federal medication law has extended and refined controls on medication sales and distribution; medication testing, naming, and labeling; and the regulation of controlled substances. Official publications such as the USP and the *National Formulary* set standards for medication strength, quality, purity, packaging, safety, labeling, and dose form.

State and Local Regulation of Medication. State and local medication laws must conform to federal legislation. States can have additional controls, including control of substances not regulated by the federal government. Local governmental bodies regulate the use of alcohol and tobacco.

Health Care Institutions and Medication Laws. Health care institutions establish individual policies that must meet federal, state, and local regulations. The size of an institution, the types of services it provides, and the types of professional personnel it employs influence these policies. Institutional policies are often more restrictive than governmental controls. An institution is concerned primarily with preventing poor health outcomes resulting from medication use. For example, a common institutional policy is the automatic discontinuation of narcotics after a set number of days. Although a prescriber may reorder the narcotic, this policy helps to control unnecessarily prolonged medication therapy and requires the prescriber to review the need for this class of medication on a regular basis.

Medication Regulations and Nursing Practice. State **Nurse Practice Acts** have the most influence over nursing practice by defining the scope of a nurse's professional functions and responsibilities. In general, most state Nurse Practice Acts are purposefully broad so as not to limit the professional responsibilities of the nurse. Institutions and agencies may interpret specific actions allowed under the acts, but they cannot modify, expand, or restrict the act's intent. The primary intent of the state Nurse Practice Acts is to protect the public from unskilled, undereducated, and unlicensed personnel.

The nurse is responsible for following legal provisions when administering controlled substances or **narcotics,** which are carefully controlled through federal and state guidelines. Violations of the Controlled Substances Act are punishable by fines, imprisonment, and loss of nurse licensure. Hospitals and other health care institutions have policies for the proper storage and distribution of narcotics (Box 34-1).

Pharmacokinetics as the Basis of Medication Actions

For medications to be therapeutic, they must be taken into a client's body, must be absorbed and distributed to cells, tissues, or a specific organ, and must alter physiological functions. **Pharmacokinetics** is the study of how medications enter the body, reach their site of action, are metabolized, and exit the body. The nurse uses knowledge of pharmacokinetics when timing medication administration, selecting the route of administration, judging the client's risk for alterations in medication action, and observing the client's response.

Absorption. Absorption refers to passage of medication molecules into the blood from its site of administration. Factors that influence medication absorption are the route of administration, ability of the medication to dissolve, blood flow to the site of administration, body surface area, and lipid solubility of medication.

Route of Administration. Medications can be administered through various routes. Each route has a different rate of absorption. When medications are placed on the skin, absorption is slow due to the physical makeup of the skin. Medications placed on the mucous membranes and respiratory airways are quickly absorbed because these tissues contain many blood vessels. Because orally administered medications must pass through the gastrointestinal tract to be absorbed, the overall rate of absorption may be slowed. Intravenous (IV) **injection** produces the most rapid absorption because this route provides immediate access to the systemic circulation.

Ability of the Medication to Dissolve. The ability of an oral medication to dissolve depends largely on its form or preparation. Solutions and suspensions already in a liquid state are absorbed more readily than tablets or capsules. Acidic medications pass through the gastric mucosa rapidly. Medications that are basic are not absorbed before reaching the small intestine.

Blood Flow to the Site of Administration. When the site of administration contains a rich blood supply, medications are absorbed more rapidly. This occurs because as blood comes in contact with the site of administration, the medication is absorbed. Therefore areas that have more blood supply will experience enhanced absorption, facilitating the passage of the medication into the blood.

Body Surface Area. When a medication is in contact with a large surface area, the medication will be absorbed at a faster rate. This explains why the majority of medications are absorbed in the small intestine rather than the stomach.

Lipid Solubility of a Medication. Medications that are highly lipid soluble are absorbed more easily. They readily cross the cell membrane because it is made of a lipid layer. Another factor that may affect absorption of medication is whether or not food is in the stomach. Some oral medications are absorbed more easily when administered between meals because food can change the structure of a medication and impair its absorption. Some medications when administered together may interfere with each other so as to impair the absorption of one or both.

Safe medication administration requires knowledge of factors that may alter or impair absorption of the medications that have been prescribed. This information is

Form Approved: OMB No. 0910-0291 Expires: 4/30/96
See OMB statement on reverse

FDA Use Only
Triage unit
sequence #

MEDWATCH

THE FDA MEDICAL PRODUCTS REPORTING PROGRAM

For **VOLUNTARY** reporting
by health professionals of adverse
events and product problems

Page ____ of ____

PLEASE TYPE OR USE BLACK INK

A. Patient information

1. Patient Identifier	2. Age at time of event: ____ or Date of birth:	3. Sex ☐ female ☐ male	4. Weight ____ lbs or ____ kgs

In confidence

B. Adverse event or product problem

1. ☐ Adverse event   and/or   ☐ Product problem (e.g., defects/malfunctions)

2. Outcomes attributed to adverse event (check all that apply)

☐ death _____ (mo/day/yr)
☐ life-threatening
☐ hospitalization – initial or prolonged

☐ disability
☐ congenital anomaly
☐ required intervention to prevent permanent impairment/damage
☐ other: _____

3. Date of event (mo/day/yr)	4. Date of this report (mo/day/yr)

5. Describe event or problem

6. Relevant tests/laboratory data, including dates

7. Other relevant history, including preexisting medical conditions (e.g., allergies, race, pregnancy, smoking and alcohol use, hepatic/renal dysfunction, etc.)

C. Suspect medication(s)

1. **Name** (give labeled strength & mfr/labeler, if known)
#1
#2

2. Dose, frequency & route used #1 #2	3. Therapy dates (if unknown, give duration) from/to (or best estimate) #1 #2

4. Diagnosis for use (indication)
#1
#2

5. Event abated after use stopped or dose reduced
#1 ☐ yes ☐ no ☐ doesn't apply
#2 ☐ yes ☐ no ☐ doesn't apply

6. Lot # (if known) #1 #2	7. Exp. date (if known) #1 #2

8. Event reappeared after reintroduction
#1 ☐ yes ☐ no ☐ doesn't apply
#2 ☐ yes ☐ no ☐ doesn't apply

9. NDC # (for product problems only)
____ – ____ – ____

10. Concomitant medical products and therapy dates (exclude treatment of event)

D. Suspect medical device

1. Brand name

2. Type of device

3. Manufacturer name & address

4. Operator of device
☐ health professional
☐ lay user/patient
☐ other: _____

5. Expiration date (mo/day/yr)

6.
model # _____
catalog # _____
serial # _____
lot # _____
other #

7. If implanted, give date (mo/day/yr)

8. If explanted, give date (mo/day/yr)

9. Device available for evaluation?   (Do not send to FDA)
☐ yes   ☐ no   ☐ returned to manufacturer on _____ (mo/day/yr)

10. Concomitant medical products and therapy dates (exclude treatment of event)

E. Reporter (see confidentiality section on back)

1. Name & address	phone #

2. Health professional? ☐ yes ☐ no	3. Occupation	4. Also reported to ☐ manufacturer ☐ user facility ☐ distributor

5. If you do NOT want your identity disclosed to the manufacturer, place an " X " in this box. ☐

FDA

Mail to: MEDWATCH   *or* FAX to:
5600 Fishers Lane   1-800-FDA-0178
Rockville, MD 20852-9787

FDA Form 3500 (1/96)   **Submission of a report does not constitute an admission that medical personnel or the product caused or contributed to the event.**

FIGURE **34–2** MedWatch form, FDA form 3500 (1/96). (Courtesy FDA, MedWatch, Rockville, Md.)

ADVICE ABOUT VOLUNTARY REPORTING

Report experiences with:
- medications (drugs or biologics)
- medical devices (including in-vitro diagnostics)
- special nutritional products (dietary supplements, medical foods, infant formulas)
- other products regulated by FDA

Report SERIOUS adverse events. An event is serious when the patient outcome is:
- death
- life-threatening (real risk of dying)
- hospitalization (initial or prolonged)
- disability (significant, persistent or permanent)
- congenital anomaly
- required intervention to prevent permanent impairment or damage

Report even if:
- you're not certain the product caused the event
- you don't have all the details

Report product problems – quality, performance or safety concerns such as:
- suspected contamination
- questionable stability
- defective components
- poor packaging or labeling
- therapeutic failures

How to report:
- just fill in the sections that apply to your report
- use section C for all products except medical devices
- attach additional blank pages if needed
- use a separate form for each patient
- report either to FDA or the manufacturer (or both)

Important numbers:
- 1-800-FDA-0178   to FAX report
- 1-800-FDA-7737   to report by modem
- 1-800-FDA-1088   to report by phone or for more information
- 1-800-822-7967   for a VAERS form for vaccines

If your report involves a serious adverse event with a device and it occurred in a facility outside a doctor's office, that facility may be legally required to report to FDA and/or the manufacturer. Please notify the person in that facility who would handle such reporting.

Confidentiality: The patient's identity is held in strict confidence by FDA and protected to the fullest extent of the law. The reporter's identity, including the identity of a self-reporter, may be shared with the manufacturer unless requested otherwise. However, FDA will not disclose the reporter's identity in response to a request from the public, pursuant to the Freedom of Information Act.

The public reporting burden for this collection of information has been estimated to average 30 minutes per response, including the time for reviewing instructions, searching existing data sources, gathering and maintaining the data needed, and completing and reviewing the collection of information. Send comments regarding this burden estimate or any other aspect of this collection of information, including suggestions for reducing this burden to:

DHHS Reports Clearance Office
Paperwork Reduction Project (0910-0291)
Hubert H. Humphrey Building, Room 531-H
200 Independence Avenue, S.W.
Washington, DC 20201

"An agency may not conduct or sponsor, and a person is not required to respond to, a collection of information unless it displays a currently valid OMB control number."

Please do NOT return this form to either of these addresses.

U.S. DEPARTMENT OF HEALTH AND HUMAN SERVICES
Public Health Service • Food and Drug Administration

FDA Form 3500-back   **Please Use Address Provided Below – Just Fold In Thirds, Tape and Mail**

Department of Health and Human Services
Public Health Service
Food and Drug Administration
Rockville, MD 20857

Official Business
Penalty for Private Use $300

BUSINESS REPLY MAIL
FIRST CLASS MAIL   PERMIT NO. 946   ROCKVILLE, MD

POSTAGE WILL BE PAID BY FOOD AND DRUG ADMINISTRATION

MEDWATCH
The FDA Medical Products Reporting Program
Food and Drug Administration
5600 Fishers Lane
Rockville, MD 20852-9787

NO POSTAGE
NECESSARY
IF MAILED
IN THE
UNITED STATES
OR APO/FPO

FIGURE **34–2, cont'd**   MedWatch form, FDA form 3500 (1/96). (Courtesy FDA, MedWatch, Rockville, Md.)

Box 34–1   **Guidelines for Safe Narcotic Administration and Control**

- Store all narcotics in a locked, secure cabinet or container. (Computerized, locked cabinets are now available.)
- Nurses in charge carry a set of keys (or a special computer entry code) for the narcotics cabinet.
- During an institution's change of shift, the nurse going off duty counts all narcotics with the nurse coming on duty. Both nurses sign the narcotic record to indicate that the count is correct.
- Discrepancies in narcotic counts are reported immediately.
- A special inventory record is used each time a narcotic is dispensed and provides an accurate ongoing count of narcotics used and remaining.
- The record is used to document the client's name, date, time of medication administration, name of medication, dose, and signature of nurse dispensing the medication.
- If only one part of a premeasured dose of a controlled substance is given, a second nurse witnesses disposal of the unused portion and documents such on the record form.

---

based on an understanding of medication pharmacokinetics, the nursing history, the physical examination, and knowledge gained through daily interactions with clients. The nurse uses this knowledge to ensure that all prescribed medications are administered at the correct time. Because medications can interact with food, it may be appropriate for the nurse to administer medications before meals or after meals, with meals or on an empty stomach. Some medications interact with each other. If this occurs, the nurse ensures that they are not given at the same time. The nurse consults with and collaborates with the client's prescribers to ensure that the client achieves the therapeutic effect of all medications. Before administering any medication, the nurse should consult pharmacology books or drug references, package inserts, or pharmacists to identify medication-medication interactions or medication-nutrient interactions.

Distribution. After a medication is absorbed, it is distributed within the body to tissues and organs and ultimately to its specific site of action. The rate and extent of distribution depend on the physical and chemical properties of medications and the physiology of the person taking the medication.

Circulation. Once a medication enters the bloodstream, it is carried throughout the tissues and organs of the body. How fast it reaches the site is dependent on the vascularity of the various tissues and organs. When conditions exist that limit blood flow or intended sites of actions are poorly perfused, the distribution of a medication is inhibited. For example, clients in congestive heart failure have impaired circulation, which impairs medication delivery to the intended site of action. Therefore the efficacy of medications in these clients can be delayed or altered.

Membrane Permeability. To be distributed to an organ, a medication must pass through all of the organ's tissues and biologic membranes. Some membranes may serve as barriers to the passage of medications. For example, the blood-brain barrier allows only fat-soluble medications to pass into the brain and cerebral spinal fluid. Therefore central nervous system infections often require treatment with antibiotics injected directly into the subarachnoid space in the spinal cord. Older clients may experience adverse effects (e.g., confusion) as a result of the change in the permeability of the blood-brain barrier, with easier passage of fat-soluble medications. The placental membrane also has a nonselective barrier to medications. Fat soluble and non–fat-soluble agents may cross the placenta and produce fetal deformities, respiratory depression, and, with narcotic abuse, withdrawal symptoms.

Protein Binding. The degree to which medications bind to serum proteins such as albumin affects medication distribution. Most medications bind to this protein to some extent. When medications bind to albumin, they cannot exert any pharmacological activity. The unbound or "free" medication is the active form of the medication. Older adults have a decrease in albumin in the bloodstream, probably caused by a change in liver function. The same is true for clients with liver disease or malnutrition. Because of the potential for more medication being unbound, the older adult may be at risk for an increase in medication activity or toxicity or both.

Metabolism. After a medication reaches its site of action, it becomes metabolized into a less active or inactive form that is more easily excreted. **Biotransformation** occurs under the influence of enzymes that **detoxify,** degrade (break down), and remove biologically active chemicals. Most biotransformation occurs within the liver, although the lungs, kidneys, blood, and intestines also metabolize medications. The liver is especially important because its specialized structure oxidizes and transforms many toxic substances. The liver degrades many harmful chemicals before they become distributed to the tissues. If a decrease in liver function occurs, such as with aging or liver disease, a medication may be eliminated more slowly, resulting in an accumulation of the medication. If the organs that metabolize medications are altered, clients are at risk for medication toxicity. For example, a small sedative dose of a barbiturate may cause a client with liver disease to lapse into a hepatic coma.

Excretion. After medications are metabolized, they exit the body through the kidneys, liver, bowel, lungs, and exocrine glands. The chemical makeup of a medication determines the organ of excretion. Gaseous and volatile compounds, such as nitrous oxide and alcohol, exit through the lungs. Deep breathing and coughing (see Chapter 39) help the postoperative client to eliminate anesthetic gases more rapidly. The exocrine glands excrete lipid-soluble medications. When medications exit through sweat glands, the skin may become irritated. The nurse assists the client in good hygiene practices (see Chapter 38) to promote cleanliness and skin integrity.

If a medication is excreted through the mammary glands, there is a risk that a nursing infant will ingest the chemicals. Mothers should check on the safety of any medication used while breast-feeding.

The gastrointestinal tract is another route for medication excretion. Many medications enter the hepatic circulation to be broken down by the liver and excreted into the bile. After chemicals enter the intestines through the biliary tract, the intestines may reabsorb them. Factors that increase peristalsis (e.g., laxatives and enemas) accelerate medication excretion through the feces, whereas factors that slow peristalsis (e.g., inactivity and improper diet) may prolong a medication's effects.

The kidneys are the main organs for medication excretion. Some medications escape extensive metabolism and exit unchanged in the urine. Other medications must undergo biotransformation in the liver before being excreted by the kidney. If renal function declines, a client is at risk for medication toxicity. If the kidney cannot adequately excrete a medication, it may be necessary to reduce the dose. Maintenance of an adequate fluid intake (50 ml/kg/day) promotes proper elimination of medications for the average adult.

Types of Medication Action

Medications vary considerably in the way they act and their types of action. Factors other than characteristics of the medication also influence medication actions. A client may not respond in the same way to each successive dose of a medication. Likewise, the same medication dosage may cause very different responses in different clients. Therefore it is essential for the nurse to understand all the effects that medications can have when taken by or given to clients.

Therapeutic Effects. The **therapeutic effect** is the expected or predictable physiological response a medication causes. Each medication has a desired therapeutic effect for which it is prescribed. For example, nitroglycerin is used to reduce the cardiac workload and increase myocardial oxygen supply. A single medication may have many therapeutic effects. For example, aspirin is an analgesic, an antipyretic, an antiinflammatory, and it reduces platelet aggregation (clumping). It is important for the nurse to know for which therapeutic effect a medication is prescribed. This will allow the nurse to properly teach the client about the medication's intended effect and to accurately evaluate the medication's desired effect.

Side Effects. **Side effects** are the unintended, secondary effects a medication predictably will cause. Side effects may be harmless or injurious. If the side effects are serious enough to negate the beneficial effects of a medication's therapeutic action, the prescriber may discontinue the medication. Clients often stop taking medications because of side effects.

Adverse Effects. **Adverse effects** are generally considered severe responses to medication. For example, a client may become comatose when a drug is ingested. When adverse responses to medications occur, the prescriber must discontinue the medication immediately. Some adverse effects are unexpected effects that were not discovered during drug testing. When this situation occurs, health care providers are obligated to report the adverse effect to the FDA (see Figure 34-2, p. 826).

Toxic Effects. **Toxic effects** may develop after prolonged intake of a medication or when a medication accumulates in the blood because of impaired metabolism or excretion. Excess amounts of a medication within the body may have lethal effects, depending on the medication's action. For example, toxic levels of morphine, an opioid, may cause severe respiratory depression and death. Antidotes are available to treat specific types of medication toxicity. For example, Narcan is used to reverse the effects of opioid toxicity.

Idiosyncratic Reactions. Medications may cause unpredictable effects such as an **idiosyncratic reaction** in which a client overreacts or underreacts to a medication or has a reaction different from normal. For example, a child receiving an antihistamine (Benadryl) may become extremely agitated or excited instead of drowsy. It is not always possible to predict if a client might have an idiosyncratic response to a medication.

Allergic Reactions. Allergic reactions are another unpredictable response to a medication; they make up 5% to 10% of all medication reactions. A client can become sensitized immunologically to the initial dose of a medication. With repeated administration, the client develops an allergic response to the medication, its chemical preservatives, or a metabolite. The medication or chemical acts as an antigen, triggering the release of the body's antibodies. A client's **medication allergy** may be mild or severe. Allergic symptoms vary, depending on the individual and the medication. Among the different classes of medications, antibiotics cause a high incidence of allergic reactions. Common, mild allergy symptoms are summarized in Table 34-3. Severe or **anaphylactic reactions** are characterized by sudden constriction of bronchiolar muscles, edema of the pharynx and larynx, and severe wheezing and shortness of breath. Antihistamines, epinephrine, and bronchodilators may be used to treat anaphylactic reactions.

The client may also become severely hypotensive, necessitating emergency resuscitation measures. A client with a known history of an allergy to a medication should avoid exposure to that medication in the future. Clients might also wear an identification bracelet or medal (Figure 34-3), which alerts nurses and physicians to the allergy if the client is unconscious when receiving medical care.

Medication Interactions

When one medication modifies the action of another medication, a **medication interaction** occurs. Medication interactions are common in individuals taking several medications. A medication may potentiate or diminish the action of other medications and may alter the way in which another medication is absorbed, metabolized, or eliminated from the body. When two medications have a

Table 34-3	Mild Allergic Reactions
Symptom	**Description**
Urticaria	Raised, irregularly shaped skin eruptions with varying sizes and shapes; eruptions have reddened margins and pale centers
Rash	Small, raised vesicles that are usually reddened; often distributed over entire body
Pruritus	Itching of skin; accompanies most rashes
Rhinitis	Inflammation of mucous membranes lining nose; causes swelling and clear, watery discharge

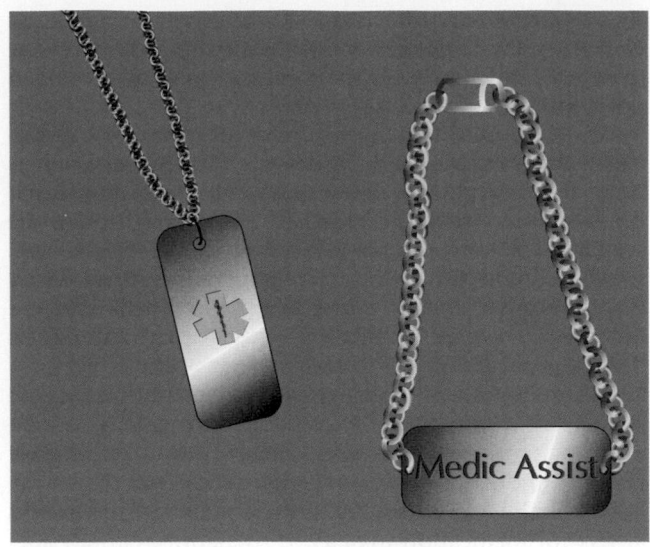

FIGURE **34-3** Identification bracelet and medal.

synergistic effect, or act synergistically, the effect of the two medications combined is greater than the effect of the medications when given separately. For example, alcohol is a central nervous system depressant that has a synergistic effect on antihistamines, antidepressants, barbiturates, and narcotic analgesics.

A medication interaction is not always undesirable. Often a prescriber combines medications to create an interaction that will have a beneficial effect on the client's condition. For example, a client with hypertension (high blood pressure) that cannot be controlled with one medication, typically receives several medications such as diuretics and vasodilators that act together to control the blood pressure.

Medication Dose Responses

After a nurse administers a medication, it undergoes absorption, distribution, metabolism, and excretion. Except when administered intravenously, medications take time to enter the bloodstream. The quantity and distribution of a medication in different body compartments change constantly. When a medication is prescribed, the goal is a constant blood level within a safe therapeutic range. Repeated doses are required to achieve a constant therapeutic **concentration** of a medication because a portion of a medication is always being excreted. The highest serum concentration (**peak** concentration) of the medication usually occurs just before the last of the medication is absorbed (McKenry and Salerno, 2003). After peaking, the serum medication concentration falls progressively. With intravenous **infusions,** the peak concentration occurs quickly, but the serum level also begins to fall immediately (Figure 34-4). The point at which the lowest amount of drug is detected in the serum is called the trough concentration. Some medications (e.g., vancomycin) are dosed based on peak and trough serum levels. The trough level is generally drawn 30 minutes before the drug is administered, and the peak level is drawn whenever the drug is expected to reach its peak concentration. The time it takes for a drug to reach its peak concentration varies depending on the medication's pharmacokinetics.

All medications have a **serum half-life,** which is the time it takes for excretion processes to lower the serum medication concentration by half. To maintain a therapeutic plateau, the client must receive regular fixed doses. For example it has been shown that pain medications are most effective when they are given "around the clock"

rather than when the client intermittently complains of pain. In this way an almost constant level of pain medication is maintained. After an initial medication dose, the client receives each successive dose when the previous dose reaches its half-life.

The client and nurse must follow regular dosage schedules and adhere to prescribed doses and dosage intervals. Some agencies set schedules for medication administration. However, the nurse can alter this schedule based on knowledge about a medication. For example, at some agencies, medications that are to be taken once a day are given at 9:00 AM. However, if the nurse knows that the medication works best when given before bedtime, the nurse administers the medication before the client goes to sleep. Table 34-4 lists common dosage schedules used in acute care settings.

When teaching clients about dosage schedules, the nurse uses language that is familiar to the client. For example, when teaching a client about medication dosing twice a day (bid), the nurse instructs the client to take a medication in the morning and again in the evening. Knowledge of the time intervals of medication action also helps the nurse to anticipate a medication's effect. With this knowledge the nurse can instruct the client when to expect a response. Table 34-5 defines common terms associated with medication actions.

Routes of Administration

The route prescribed for administering a medication depends on the medication's properties and desired effect and on the client's physical and mental condition (Table 34-6). A nurse collaborates with the prescriber in determining the best route for a client's medication, as in the following hypothetical situation:

Mr. Huels has progressively worsened physically. His temperature is 39.2° C. He complains of nausea and is unable to tolerate oral fluids. The nurse checks Mr. Huels's order, which reads, "Acetaminophen 1000 mg orally for temperature above 38.5° C." On the basis of the assessment, the nurse be-

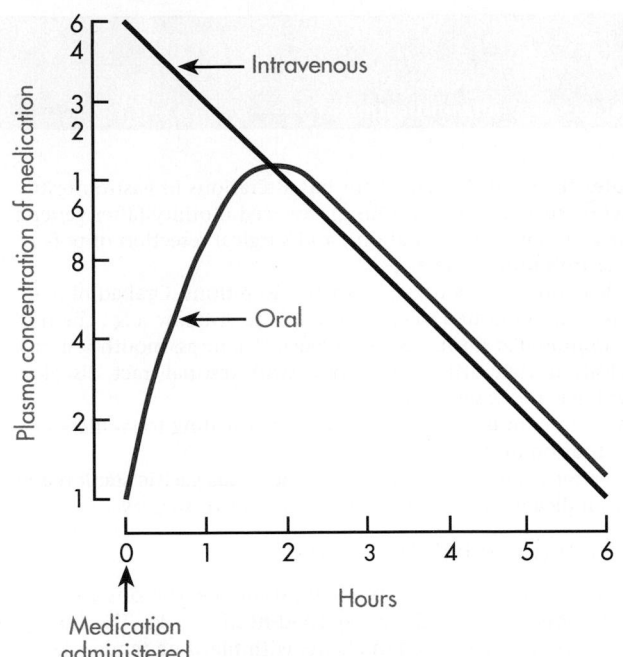

FIGURE **34–4** Curve showing therapeutic blood levels. (From Clark JF, Queener SF, Karb VB: *Pharmacological basis of nursing practice,* ed 6, St. Louis, 1998, Mosby.)

Table 34-4	Common Dosage Administration Schedules
Dosage Schedule	**Abbreviation**
Before meals	AC, ac
As desired	ad lib
Twice a day	BID, bid
Hour	H
At bedtime	
After meals	PC, pc
Whenever there is a need	prn
Every morning, every am	Qam
Every day, daily	
Every hour	Qh
Every 2 hours	q2h
Every 4 hours	q4h
Every 6 hours	q6h
Every 8 hours	q8h
4 times a day	QID, qid
Every other day	
Give immediately	STAT
3 times a day	TID, tid

Table 34-5	Terms Associated With Medication Actions
Term	**Meaning**
Onset	Time it takes after a medication is administered for it to produce a response
Peak	Time it takes for a medication to reach its highest effective concentration
Trough	Minimum blood serum concentration of medication reached just before the next scheduled dose
Duration	Time during which the medication is present in concentration great enough to produce a response
Plateau	Blood serum concentration of a medication reached and maintained after repeated fixed doses

lieves that because Mr. Huels is nauseated, he will not be able to tolerate an oral dose of acetaminophen. By consulting the physician, the nurse acquires an order for a rectal suppository instead. A rectal suppository enables the nurse to administer the appropriate medication without increasing the client's symptoms of nausea.

Oral Routes. The oral route is the easiest and the most commonly used. Medications are given by mouth and swallowed with fluid. Oral medications have a slower onset of action and a more prolonged effect than parenteral medications. Clients generally prefer the oral route.

Sublingual Administration. Some medications are designed to be readily absorbed after being placed under the tongue to dissolve (Figure 34-5). A medication given by the **sublingual** route should not be swallowed, or the desired effect will not be achieved. Nitroglycerin is commonly given by sublingual route. The client should not take a drink until the medication is completely dissolved.

Buccal Administration. Administration of a medication by the **buccal** route involves placing the solid medication in the mouth and against the mucous membranes of the cheek until the medication dissolves (Figure 34-6). Clients should be taught to alternate cheeks with each subsequent dose to avoid mucosal irritation. Clients are also warned not to chew or swallow the medication or to take any liquids with it. A buccal medication acts locally on the mucosa or systemically as it is swallowed in a person's saliva.

Parenteral Routes. Parenteral administration involves injecting a medication into body tissues. The following are the four major sites of injection:

1. **Intradermal (ID):** Injection into the dermis just under the epidermis
2. **Subcutaneous (Sub-Q):** Injection into tissues just below the dermis of the skin
3. **Intramuscular (IM):** Injection into a muscle
4. **Intravenous (IV):** Injection into a vein

Some medications are administered into body cavities other than the four types listed above. These routes of medication administration include epidural, intrathecal, intraosseous, intraperitoneal, intrapleural, and intraarterial. In some institutions, nurses may or may not be responsible for the administration of medications through these advanced techniques. Whether or not the nurse actually administers the medication by these routes, the nurse remains responsible for monitoring the integrity of the system of medication delivery, understanding the therapeutic value of the medication, and evaluating the client's response to the therapy.

Table 34-6	Factors Influencing Choice of Administration Routes
Advantages	**Disadvantages or Contraindications**

Oral, Buccal, Sublingual Routes

Routes are convenient and comfortable for client. Routes are economical. Routes are easy to administer. Medications may produce local or systemic effects. Routes rarely cause anxiety for client.	These routes are avoided when client has alterations in gastrointestinal function (e.g., nausea, vomiting), reduced motility (after general anesthesia or bowel inflammation), and surgical resection of portion of gastrointestinal tract. Some medications are destroyed by gastric secretions. Oral administration is contraindicated in clients unable to swallow (e.g., clients with neuromuscular disorders, esophageal strictures, mouth lesions). Oral medications may irritate lining of gastrointestinal tract, discolor teeth, or have unpleasant taste. Unconscious or confused client is unable or unwilling to swallow or hold medication under tongue. Oral medications cannot be given when client has gastric suction and are contraindicated in clients before some tests or surgery.

Subcutaneous (Sub-Q), Intramuscular (IM), Intravenous (IV), Intradermal (ID) Routes

Routes provide means of administration when oral medications are contraindicated. More rapid absorption occurs than with topical or oral routes. IV infusion provides medication delivery when client is critically ill or long-term therapy is required. If peripheral perfusion is poor, IV route is preferred over injections.	There is risk of introducing infection, and some medications are expensive. Clients must experience repeated needle sticks. The Sub-Q, IM, and ID routes are avoided in clients with bleeding tendencies. There is risk of tissue damage with Sub-Q injections. IM and IV routes are dangerous because of rapid absorption. These routes cause considerable anxiety in many clients, especially children.

Skin

Topical

Topical skin applications primarily provide local effect. Route is painless. Limited side effects occur.	Clients with skin abrasions are at risk for rapid medication absorption and systemic effects.

Transdermal

Transdermal applications provide prolonged systemic effects, with limited side effects.	Application leaves oily or pasty substance on skin and may soil clothing.

Mucous Membranes*

Therapeutic effects are provided by local application to involved sites. Aqueous solutions are readily absorbed and capable of causing systemic effects. Mucous membranes provide route of administration when oral medications are contraindicated.	Mucous membranes are highly sensitive to some medication concentrations. Insertion of rectal and vaginal medication often causes embarrassment. Client with ruptured eardrum cannot receive irrigations. Rectal suppositories are contraindicated if client has had rectal surgery or if active rectal bleeding is present.

Inhalation

Inhalation provides rapid relief for local respiratory problems. Route provides easy access for introduction of general anesthetic gases.	Some local agents can cause serious systemic effects.

*Includes eyes, ears, nose, vagina, rectum, and ostomy.

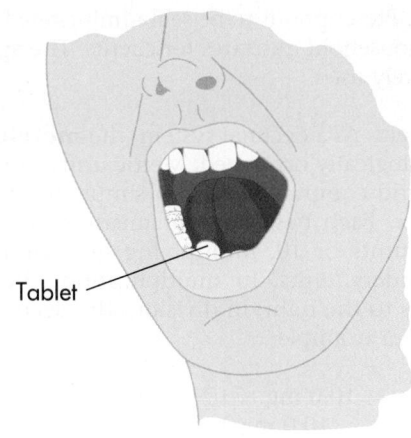

FIGURE **34–5** Sublingual administration of a tablet.

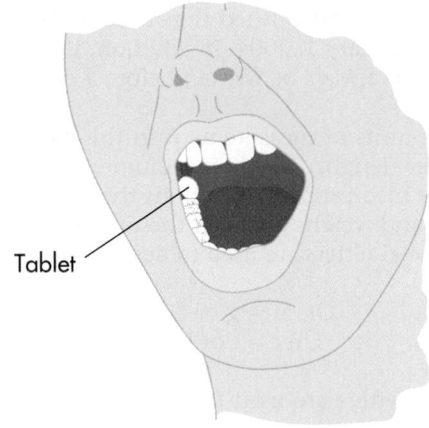

FIGURE **34–6** Buccal administration of a tablet.

Epidural. Medications are administered in the epidural space via a catheter, which has been placed by a nurse anesthetist or an anesthesiologist. This technique of medication administration is most commonly used for the administration of analgesia postoperatively (see Chapter 49). Nurses who have received extra education in the epidural route can administer medications in bolus form or by continuous infusion.

Intrathecal. Intrathecal medications are administered through a catheter that has been placed into the subarachnoid space or into one of the ventricles of the brain. Intrathecal administration is often associated with long-term medication administration through catheters that have been surgically implanted. In most institutions a physician usually injects medications into intrathecal catheters. However, specially educated nurses may also do this.

Intraosseous. This method of medication administration involves the infusion of medication directly into the bone marrow. It is most commonly used in infants and toddlers who have poor access to their intravascular space.

This method is most popular when an emergency arises and IV access is impossible. The physician inserts an intraosseous infusion needle into the bone, usually the tibia, for the administration of medication by the nurse.

Intraperitoneal. Medications are administered into the peritoneal cavity, where they are absorbed into the circulation. Chemotherapeutic agents, insulin, and antibiotics may be administered in this fashion. One method of dialysis uses the peritoneal route for the removal of fluid, electrolytes, and waste products. Nurses caring for these clients initiate and teach peritoneal dialysis management.

Intrapleural. Medications are administered through the chest wall and directly into the pleural space. This may be done through an injection or through a chest tube that has been inserted by the physician. Chemotherapeutic agents are the most common medications administered via this method. Physicians also instill medications that help resolve persistent pleural effusion. This is called pleuradesis. This technique promotes adhesion between the visceral and parietal pleura. Increasingly newer indications of this method of medication delivery are being used. One such indication is for the instillation of analgesic agents through specially designed intrapleural catheters (Clarke, 1999).

Intraarterial. This method calls for medications to be administered directly into the arteries. Intraarterial infusions are common in clients who have arterial clots. The nurse will manage a continuous infusion of clot-dissolving agents. The nurse must carefully monitor the integrity of this infusion to prevent inadvertent disconnection of the system and subsequent bleeding.

Other methods of medication administration that are usually limited to physician administration are **intracardiac,** an injection of a medication directly into cardiac tissue, and **intraarticular,** an injection of a medication into a joint.

Topical Administration. Medications applied to the skin and mucous membranes generally have local effects. The topical medication is applied to the skin by painting or spreading it over an area, applying moist dressings, soaking body parts in a solution, or giving medicated baths. Systemic effects can occur if a client's skin is thin or broken down, if the medication concentration is high, or if contact with the skin is prolonged.

Some medications (e.g., nitroglycerin, scopolamine, and estrogens) have systemic effects because they are applied topically by a **transdermal disk** or patch. The disk secures the medicated ointment to the skin. These topical applications may be applied for as little as 24 hours or as long as 7 days.

Medications can be applied to mucous membranes in a variety of ways: (1) by directly applying a liquid or ointment (e.g., eye drops, gargling, or swabbing the throat); (2) by inserting a medication into a body cavity (e.g., placing a suppository in rectum or vagina or inserting medicated packing into vagina); (3) by instilling fluid into a

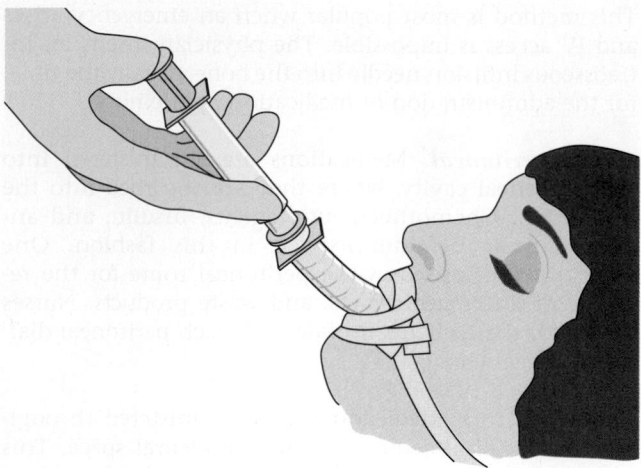

FIGURE 34–7   Medication being instilled through endotracheal tube.

body cavity (e.g., ear drops, nose drops, or bladder and rectal **instillation** [fluid is retained]); (4) by irrigating a body cavity (e.g., flushing eye, ear, vagina, bladder, or rectum with medicated fluid [fluid is not retained]); and (5) by spraying (e.g., instillation into nose and throat).

Inhalation Route. The deeper passages of the respiratory tract provide a large surface area for medication absorption. Medications can be administered through the nasal passages, oral passage, or endotracheal or tracheostomy tubes. Endotracheal tubes are inserted into the client's mouth and go to the trachea (Figure 34-7), whereas tracheostomy tubes directly enter the trachea through an incision made in the neck. Medications that are administered by the **inhalation** route are readily absorbed and work rapidly because of the rich vascular alveolar capillary network present in the pulmonary tissue. Inhaled medications may have local or systemic effects.

Intraocular Route. Intraocular medication delivery involves inserting a medication similar to a contact lens into the client's eye. The eye medication disk has two soft outer layers that have medication enclosed in them. The disk is inserted into the client's eye, much like a contact lens. The disk can remain in the client's eye for up to 1 week. Pilocarpine, a medication used to treat glaucoma, is the most common medication disk.

Systems of Medication Measurement
The proper administration of a medication depends on the nurse's ability to compute medication doses accurately and measure medications correctly. A careless mistake in placing a decimal point or adding a zero to a dose can lead to a fatal error. The nurse is responsible for checking the dose before giving a medication.

The metric, apothecary, and household systems of measurement are used in medication therapy. Most nations use the metric system as their standard of measurement. Although the U.S. Congress has not officially adopted the metric system, most health professionals in the United

States use it. Prescriptions to be self-administered are often written in household measures for clients. The apothecary system is rarely used.

Metric System. As a decimal system, the **metric system** is the most logically organized. Metric units can easily be converted and computed through simple multiplication and division. Each basic unit of measurement is organized into units of 10. Multiplying or dividing by 10 forms secondary units. In multiplication, the decimal point moves to the right; in division, the decimal moves to the left. For example:

$$10.0 \text{ mg} \times 10 = 100 \text{ mg}$$
$$10.0 \text{ mg}/10 = 1 \text{ mg}$$

When designating a metric dosage it is important to *not* have a trailing zero (e.g., 1.0 mg or 1.0 ml). The Joint Commission on Accreditation of Healthcare Organizations (2003) has established that trailing zeros cannot be used after January 1, 2004. In addition, the JCAHO requires a zero to always be written before a decimal point (e.g., 0.1 mg).

The basic units of measurement in the metric system are the meter (length), the liter (volume), and the gram (weight). For medication calculations the nurse uses only the volume and weight units. In the metric system, lowercase or capital letters are used to designate basic units:

$$\text{Gram} = \text{g or Gm}$$
$$\text{Liter} = \text{l or L}$$

Lowercase letters are used for abbreviations for other units:

$$\text{Milligram} = \text{mg}$$
$$\text{Milliliter} = \text{ml}$$

A system of Latin prefixes designates subdivision of the basic units: *deci-* (1/10 or 0.1), *centi-* (1/100 or 0.01), and *milli-* (1/1000 or 0.001). Greek prefixes designate multiples of the basic units: *deka-* (10), *hecto-* (100), and *kilo-* (1000). When writing medication doses in metric units, prescribers and nurses use fractions or multiples of a unit. Fractions should be converted to decimal form.

$$500 \text{ mg or } 0.5 \text{ g}, \textit{not } \tfrac{1}{2} \text{ g}$$
$$10 \text{ ml or } 0.01 \text{ L}, \textit{not } \tfrac{1}{100} \text{ L}$$

Household Measurements. Household units of measure are familiar to most people. The disadvantage of household measures is their inaccuracy. Household utensils such as teaspoons and cups often vary in size. Scales to measure pints or quarts are often not well calibrated. Household measures include drops, teaspoons, tablespoons, and cups for volume and pints and quarts for weight. Although pints and quarts are considered household measures, they are also used in the apothecary system.

The advantage of household measurements is their convenience and familiarity. When the accuracy of a medication dose is not critical, it is safe to use household mea-

Table 34-7	Equivalents of Measurement	
Metric	**Apothecary**	**Household**
1 ml	15-16 minims	15 drops (gtt)
4-5 ml	1 fluidram	1 teaspoon (tsp)
16 ml	4 fluidrams	1 tablespoon (tbsp)
30 ml	1 fluid ounce	2 tablespoons (tbsp)
240 ml	8 fluid ounces	1 cup (c)
480 ml (approximately 500 ml)	1 pint (pt)	1 pint (pt)
960 ml (approximately 1 L)	1 quart (qt)	1 quart (qt)
3840 ml (approximately 5 L)	1 gallon (gal)	1 gallon (gal)

Box 34-2	Common Reasons for Measurement Conversions

- Converting fluid ounces to milliliters for measurement of intake and output
- Converting body weight from pounds to kilograms and vice versa
- Converting volume equivalents to calculate IV flow rates and prepare wound irrigation solutions, enemas, or bladder irrigations

sures. For example, many over-the-counter medications can safely be measured by this method. Table 34-7 gives common equivalents of metric and household units.

Solutions. The nurse uses solutions of various concentrations for injections, **irrigations,** and infusions. A **solution** is a given mass of solid substance dissolved in a known volume of fluid or a given volume of liquid dissolved in a known volume of another fluid. When a solid is dissolved in a fluid, the concentration is in units of mass per units of volume (e.g., g/ml, g/L, mg/ml). A concentration of a solution may also be expressed as a percentage. A 10% solution, for example, is 10 g of solid dissolved in 100 ml of solution. A proportion also expresses concentrations. A 1/1000 solution represents a solution containing 1 g of solid in 1000 ml of liquid or 1 ml of liquid mixed with 1000 ml of another liquid.

Clinical Calculations

To administer medications it is essential for the nurse to have an understanding of basic arithmetic to calculate medication doses, mix solutions, and perform a variety of other activities. This skill is important because medications are not always dispensed in the unit of measure in which they are ordered. This occurs because medication companies package and bottle certain standard equivalents. For example, the prescriber may order 250 mg of a medication that is available only in grams. The nurse is responsible for converting available units of volume and weight to the desired doses. Therefore the nurse should be aware of approximate equivalents in all major measurement systems.

Medication administration is not the only function in which nurses use volume and weight conversions. Conversions are used in a variety of nursing activities (Box 34-2).

Conversions Within One System. Converting measurements within one system is relatively easy. In the metric system the nurse simply divides or multiplies. To change milligrams to grams, the nurse divides by 1000, moving the decimal 3 points to the left.

$$1000 \text{ mg} = 1 \text{ g}$$
$$350 \text{ mg} = 0.35 \text{ g}$$

To convert liters to milliliters, the nurse multiplies by 1000 or moves the decimal 3 points to the right.

$$1 \text{ L} = 1000 \text{ ml}$$
$$0.25 \text{ L} = 250 \text{ ml}$$

To convert units of measurement within the apothecary or household system, the nurse must consult an equivalent table. For example, when converting fluid ounces to quarts the nurse must first know that 32 ounces is the equivalent of 1 quart. For example, to convert 8 ounces to a quart measurement, the nurse divides 8 by 32 to get the equivalent, ¼ or 0.25 quart.

Conversion Between Systems. The nurse must frequently determine the proper dose of a medication by converting weights or volumes from one system of measurement to another. Often, metric units must be converted to equivalent household measures for use at home. To calculate medications, it is necessary to work with units in the same measurement system. Tables of equivalent measurements are available in all health care institutions. The pharmacist is also a good resource.

Before making a conversion, the nurse compares the measurement system available with that ordered. For example, the prescriber orders Robitussin 30 ml. To provide proper instruction to the client, the nurse must convert "ml" to common household measurement. To convert milliliters to tablespoons the nurse must know the equivalent or refer to a table such as Table 34-7.

Dose Calculations. There are many formulas that can be used to calculate medication doses. The following basic formula can be applied when preparing solid or liquid forms:

$$\frac{\text{Dose ordered}}{\text{Dose on hand}} \times \text{Amount on hand} = \frac{\text{Amount}}{\text{to administer}}$$

The dose ordered is the amount of medication prescribed. The dose on hand is the weight or volume of medication available in units supplied by the pharmacy; it may be expressed on the medication label as the contents of a tablet or capsule or as the amount of medication dissolved per unit volume of liquid. The amount on hand is the basic unit or quantity of the medication that contains the dose on hand. For solid medications the amount on hand may be one capsule; the amount of liquid on hand may be a milliliter or liter depending on the container. The amount to administer is the actual amount of medication the nurse will administer. The amount to administer is always expressed in the same unit as the amount on hand.

The following example illustrates how to apply the formula. The prescriber orders the client to receive morphine 2 mg IV. Thus the dose ordered is 2 mg. The medication is available in a vial containing 10 mg per milliliter. Thus the dose on hand is 10 mg in an amount on hand of 1 ml. The formula is applied as follows:

$$2 \text{ mg} / 10 \text{ mg} \times 1 \text{ ml} = \frac{\text{Volume in milliliters}}{\text{to administer}}$$

To simplify the $\frac{2}{10}$ fraction, divide numerator and denominator by 2:

$$\frac{1}{5} \times 1 \text{ ml} = \frac{1}{5} \text{ ml to administer}$$

Syringes are calibrated only in decimals. After converting the fraction $\frac{1}{5}$ to 0.2, the nurse accurately prepares the correct dose.

Another example demonstrates how the formula applies with solid dose forms. The physician orders 0.125 mg orally (PO) of digoxin. The medication is available in tablets containing 0.25 mg.

$$0.125 \text{ mg} / 0.250 \text{ mg} \times 1 \text{ tablet} = \frac{\text{Number of tablets}}{\text{to administer}}$$

The fraction $^{0.125}/_{0.250}$ equals $\frac{1}{2}$ or 0.5. Therefore,

$$0.5 \times 1 \text{ tablet} = 0.5 \text{ or } \frac{1}{2} \text{ tablet to be administered}$$

Many tablets come with scores or indentations across the center of the tablet (Figure 34-8). A scored tablet is easy to break in half for divided doses. In some institutions pharmacists are responsible for scoring tablets. The potential for giving an incorrect dose is high when the nurse estimates amounts by breaking unscored tablets. Therefore the nurse should not cut unscored tablets.

Often, liquid medications come prepared in volumes greater than 1 ml. In applying the formula, the nurse must be careful to use the correct concentration to avoid a medication error. For example, the order is "Erythromycin suspension 250 mg PO." The pharmacy delivers 100-ml bottles with the label stating, "5 ml contains 125 mg of erythromycin." Thus the appropriate concentration to use in this example to obtain the correct dose of medication is 125 mg in 5 ml.

$$250 \text{ mg} / 125 \text{ mg} \times 5 \text{ ml} = \text{Volume to administer}$$

The fraction $^{250}/_{125}$ equals 2. Therefore,

$$2 \times 5 \text{ ml} = 10 \text{ ml to administer}$$

The nurse should always double-check calculations or confer with another nurse or health care professional if an answer seems unreasonable (Table 34-8).

Pediatric Doses. Calculating children's medication doses requires caution. Children metabolize medications at different rates when compared with adults. For example, premature and newborn infants are especially vulnerable to adverse effects of medications because their liver

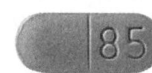

FIGURE **34-8** Scored medication tablet. (Courtesy Mosby's GenRx 1999.)

Table 34-8   Ways to Prevent Medication Administration Errors

Precaution	Rationale
Read medication labels carefully.	Many products come in similar containers, colors, and shapes.
Question administration of multiple tablets or vials for single dose.	Most doses are one or two tablets or capsules or one single-dose vial. Incorrect interpretation of order may result in excessively high dose.
Be aware of medications with similar names.	Many medication names sound alike (e.g., digoxin and digitoxin, Keflex and Keflin, Orinase and Ornade).
Check decimal point.	Some medications come in quantities that are multiples of one another (e.g., Coumadin in 2.5- and 25-mg tables, Thorazine in 30- and 300-mg spansules).
Question abrupt and excessive increases in dosages.	Most dosages are increased gradually so that physician can monitor therapeutic effect and response.
When new or unfamiliar medication is ordered, consult resource.	If prescriber is also unfamiliar with drug, there is greater risk of inaccurate dosages being ordered.
Do not administer medication ordered by nickname or unofficial abbreviation.	Many prescribers refer to commonly ordered medications by nicknames or unofficial abbreviations. If nurse or pharmacist is unfamiliar with name, wrong medication may be dispensed and administered.
Do not attempt to decipher illegible writing.	When in doubt, ask prescriber. Unless nurse questions order that is difficult to read, chance of misinterpretation is great.
Know clients with same last names. Also have clients state their full names. Check name bands carefully.	It is common to have two or more clients with same or similar last names. Special labels on Kardex or medication book can warn of potential problem.
Do not confuse equivalents.	When in a hurry, it may be easy to misread equivalents (e.g., milligram instead of milliliter).

and kidneys have not matured to full functioning levels. After the newborn period, some drugs are more quickly metabolized by the liver, which may require that the child have larger doses or more frequent administration (Hockenberry and others, 2003). Other factors that influence medication dosages in children include the difficulty in evaluating the desired effect and the hydration status of the child. In most cases, the prescriber will calculate the dose for a child before ordering the medication. However, it is the nurse's responsibility to be aware of the safe dosage range for any medication administered to a child. Therefore nurses should be aware of the formulas used to calculate pediatric doses and recheck all doses before administration. Drug package inserts or medication references often list the normal ranges for pediatric doses.

Various formulas to determine appropriate medication dosages for children exist. These formulas often take the child's age, weight, body surface area, and/or the medication amount into consideration. However, the most accurate method of calculating pediatric doses is based on a

child's body surface area (Hockenberry and others, 2003). Body surface area is estimated on the basis of the child's height and weight. A standard nomogram (e.g., the West nomogram) can be used to for estimation of a child's body surface area (Figure 34-9).

The nurse uses the formula below to calculate a pediatric dose. The formula is a ratio of the child's body surface area compared with the body surface area of an average adult (1.7 square meters, or 1.7 m²).

$$\text{Child's dose} = \frac{\text{Surface area of child}}{1.7 \text{ m}^2} \times \text{Normal adult dose}$$

For example, a prescriber orders ampicillin for a child weighing 12 kg. The normal adult dose for ampicillin is 250 mg. The West nomogram (see Figure 34-9) shows that a child weighing 12 kg has a surface area of 0.54 m². Using this information, the nurse calculates the appropriate child's dose.

$$\text{Child's dose} = 0.54 \text{m}^2 / 1.7 \text{ m}^2 \times 250 \text{ mg}$$

The m² units are canceled out.

$$\begin{aligned} \text{Child's dose} &= 0.54 / 1.7 \times 250 \text{ mg} \\ 0.54 / 1.7 &= 0.3 \\ \text{Child's dose} &= 0.3 \times 250 \text{ mg} = 75 \text{ mg} \end{aligned}$$

An alternative method to determine dosages of medications for children involves basing the amount of medication to administer (usually in mg) on how much the child weighs (usually in kg). For example, a prescriber orders 5 mg/kg to be given to a child weighing 14 kg. Using this information, the nurse calculates the appropriate dosage based on the following calculation:

$$\text{Child's dose} = 5 \text{ mg/kg} \times 14 \text{ kg} = 70 \text{ mg to be delivered}$$

*A*dministering Medications

The nurse does not have sole responsibility for medication administration. The prescriber* and pharmacist also help ensure the right medication gets to the right client. However, the nurse administering medications is accountable for knowing which medications are prescribed, their therapeutic and nontherapeutic effects, and the medications' associated nursing implications. The nurse is also responsible for knowing why the client needs the medication and determining if the client requires supervision with administration and education about the medication and its effects.

Prescriber's Role
The physician, nurse practitioner, or physician's assistant prescribes the client's medications. The prescriber writes a medication order on a form in the client's medical record, in an order book, on a legal prescription pad, by

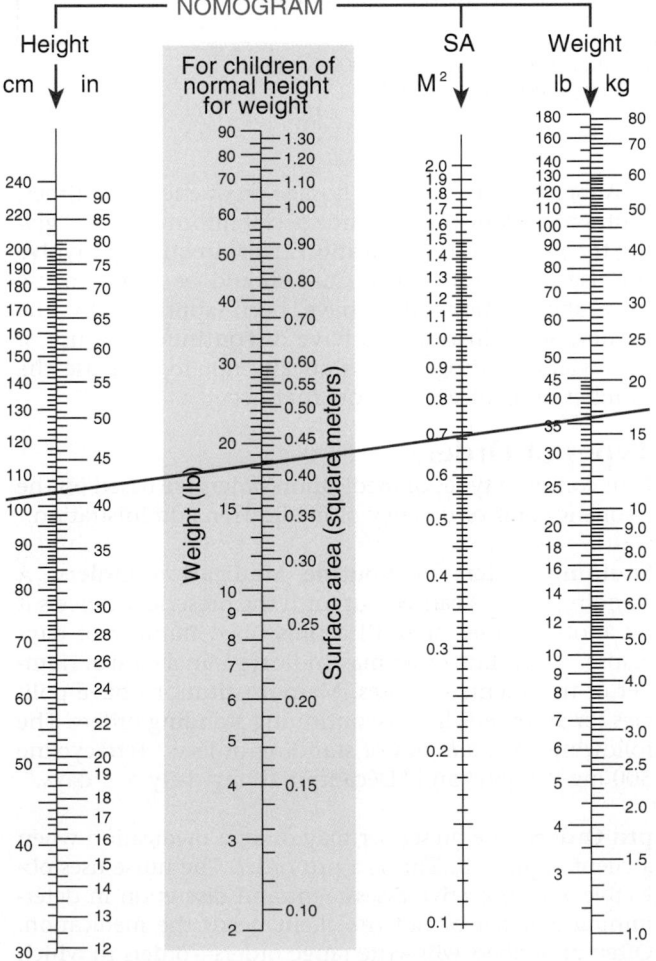

FIGURE 34–9 West nomogram for estimation of surface areas in children. A straight line is drawn between height and weight. The point where the line crosses the surface area column is the estimated body surface area. (From Behrman RE, Vaughan VC, editors: *Nelson textbook of pediatrics,* ed 13, Philadelphia, 1987, Saunders; modified from data of Boyd E, by West CD.)

---

*"Prescriber" refers to physician, advanced practice nurse, (e.g., nurse practitioner, clinical nurse specialist), or physician's assistant.

Table 34-9   Dangerous Abbreviations Used in Medication Administration

Abbreviation	Practice Problem	Preferred Term
Minimum List (Effective January 1, 2004)		
U (for unit)	Mistaken as zero, four, or cc.	Write "unit"
IU (for international unit)	Mistaken as IV or 10.	Write "international unit"
Q.D. (once daily), Q.O.D. (every other day)	Mistaken for each other.	Write "daily" and "every other day"
MS, MSO$_4$ (morphine Sulfate) MgSO$_4$	Mistaken for one another.	Write "morphine sulfate" or "magnesium sulfate"
Abbreviations To Be Considered for Minimum List by April 1, 2004		
μg	Mistaken for mg. Resulting in 1000-fold dosing overdose	Write "mcg"
H.S. (bedtime)	Mistaken for either half strength or hour of sleep. q H.S. mistaken for every hour.	Write out "half strength" or "at bedtime"
T.I.W. (for three times a week)	Mistaken for three times a day or twice weekly.	Write "three times weekly"
S.C. or S.Q. (subcutaneous)	Mistaken as SL for sublingual or "5 every."	Write "Sub-Q", subQ", or "subcutaneously"
D/C (Discharge)	Interpreted as discontinue.	Write "discharge"
cc (for cubic centimeter)	Mistaken for U (units) when poorly written.	Write "ml" for milliliters

Modified from Joint Commission for Accreditation of Healthcare Organizations: FAQs about the 2004 National Patient Safety Goals, www.jcaho.org/accredited+organizations/patient+safety, accessed 12/10/2003.

a facsimile (fax) machine, or through a computer terminal. The JCAHO (2003) requires that only medications needed to treat a client's condition are ordered. There must be a documented diagnosis, condition, or indication for use for each medication ordered.

Where allowed, a prescriber may also order a medication by talking directly to the nurse or by telephone. When medications or medical treatments are ordered over the telephone, the order is called a telephone order. If the order is given verbally to the nurse, it is called a **verbal order.** When the nurse receives a verbal or telephone order, he or she writes the complete order or enters it into a computer and then reads it back and receives confirmation from the prescriber to confirm accuracy (JCAHO, 2003). The nurse indicates the time and the name of the prescriber who gave the order and then signs the order.

Institutional policies vary regarding the personnel who can take verbal or telephone orders. Generally, nursing students cannot take these types of medication orders. Nursing students should only give newly ordered medications after the order has been written and verified by a registered nurse.

Common abbreviations may be used when writing orders (see Table 34-4, p. 831). However, the JCAHO (2003) now requires healthcare organizations to develop a "dangerous" abbreviations acronyms and symbols list. Currently, the JCAHO (2003) has issued a "minimum list" of dangerous abbreviations, acronyms, and symbols that must be included (Table 34-9). In addition, there are items the JCAHO recommends organizations add to their "do not use" list over time. The Institute of Safe Medicine Practice (ISMP) has also published a list of dangerous abbreviations (www.ismp.org, 2003).

Abbreviations indicate dosage frequencies or times, routes of administration, and special information for giving the medication. Medication errors frequently involve the use of abbreviations. Care should be taken to use only abbreviations that have been approved by the agency. Some institutions have discontinued the use of abbreviations altogether in an attempt to decrease the number of medication errors that occur.

Types of Orders

Four common types of medication orders are based on the frequency and/or urgency of medication administration.

Standing Orders or Routine Medication Orders. A standing order is carried out until the prescriber cancels it by another order or until a prescribed number of days elapse. A standing order may indicate a final date or number of treatments or doses. Many institutions have policies for automatically discontinuing standing orders. The following are examples of standing orders: "Tetracycline 500 mg PO q6h" and "Decadron 10 mg daily × 5 days."

prn Orders. The prescriber may order a medication when a client requires it. This is a prn order. The nurse uses objective and subjective assessment and discretion in determining whether or not the client needs the medication. Often prescribers will write range orders—orders in which the dose or dosing interval varies over a prescribed range depending on the client's situation. An example is "morphine sulfate 2 mg IV q 1-2 h prn for incisional pain." The JCAHO (2004) is cautioning hospitals against the use of such orders because they do pose risk for errors. The preferred order would be written "morphine sulfate 2 mg IV

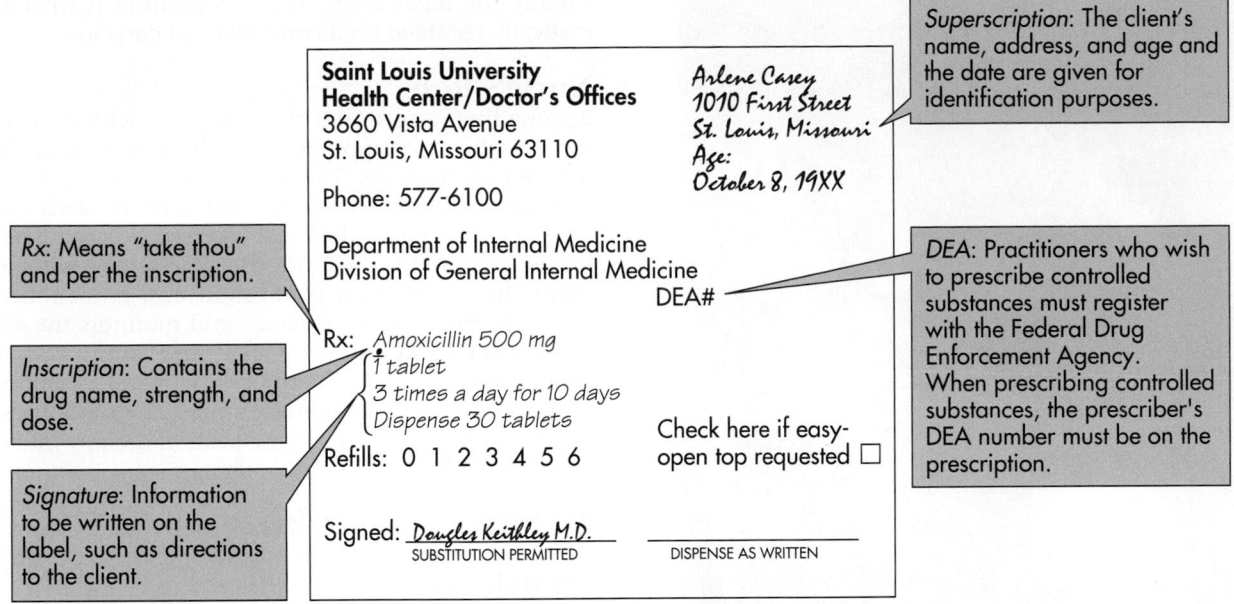

Superscription: The client's name, address, and age and the date are given for identification purposes.

Saint Louis University Health Center/Doctor's Offices
3660 Vista Avenue
St. Louis, Missouri 63110

Phone: 577-6100

Arlene Casey
1010 First Street
St. Louis, Missouri
Age:
October 8, 19XX

Rx: Means "take thou" and per the inscription.

Department of Internal Medicine
Division of General Internal Medicine
                                    DEA#

DEA: Practitioners who wish to prescribe controlled substances must register with the Federal Drug Enforcement Agency. When prescribing controlled substances, the prescriber's DEA number must be on the prescription.

Inscription: Contains the drug name, strength, and dose.

Rx: *Amoxicillin 500 mg*
     1 tablet
     3 times a day for 10 days
     Dispense 30 tablets

Refills: 0 1 2 3 4 5 6

Check here if easy-open top requested ☐

Signature: Information to be written on the label, such as directions to the client.

Signed: *Douglas Keithley M.D.*
         ‾‾‾‾‾‾‾‾‾‾‾‾‾‾‾‾‾‾‾‾‾
         SUBSTITUTION PERMITTED   DISPENSE AS WRITTEN

FIGURE **34–10** Example of a medication prescription. (Courtesy Saint Louis University Medical Center, St. Louis, Mo.)

12 hr prn for incisional pain." Nursing judgment is critical when range orders are written. The prescriber sets the minimum interval for the time of drug administration. When medications are administered, the nurse documents the assessment made and the time of medication administration. The nurse should make frequent evaluation of the effectiveness of the medication and record findings in the appropriate record.

Single (One-Time) Orders. A prescriber will often order a medication to be given only once at a specified time. This is common for preoperative medications or medications given before diagnostic examinations, for example, "Ativan 1 mg IV on call to MRI" and "Valium 10 mg PO at 0900."

STAT Orders. A STAT order signifies that a single dose of a medication is to be given immediately and only once. STAT orders are often written for emergencies when the client's condition changes suddenly. For example, "Give Apresoline 10 mg IV STAT."

Some conditions change the status of a client's medication orders. For example, surgery automatically cancels all of a client's preoperative medications (see Chapter 49). Because the client's condition changes after surgery, the prescriber must write new orders. Whenever a client is transferred to another health care agency or a different unit within a hospital or is discharged, the prescriber should review the medications and write new orders as indicated.

Prescriptions. The prescriber writes **prescriptions** for clients who are to take medications outside the hospital. The prescription includes more detailed information than a regular order because the client must understand how to take the medication and when to refill the prescription if necessary. The parts of a prescription are included in Figure 34-10.

Pharmacist's Role

The pharmacist prepares and distributes prescribed medications. Pharmacists work with nurses, physicians, and other health care providers to evaluate the efficacy of clients' medications (American Pharmaceutical Association, 2002). The pharmacist is responsible for filling prescriptions accurately and for being sure that prescriptions are valid. The pharmacist in a health care agency rarely has to mix compounds or solutions, except in the case of IV additive solutions. Most medication companies deliver medications in a form ready for use. Dispensing the correct medication, in the proper dosage and amount, with an accurate label is the pharmacist's main task. The pharmacist can also provide information about medication side effects, toxicity, interactions, and incompatibilities.

Distribution Systems

Systems for storing and distributing medications vary. Pharmacists provide the medications, but nurses distribute medications to clients. Institutions providing nursing care have a special area for stocking and dispensing medications. Special medication rooms, portable locked carts, computerized medication cabinets, and individual storage units next to clients' rooms are examples of storage areas used. Nurses must make sure that all medications are in locked containers in a room (e.g., medication room) or are under constant surveillance.

Stock Supply. With a stock system, medications are available in quantity in larger, multidose containers. This system is time consuming and costly because a nurse must dispense each medication separately for each client. This type of system of medication delivery has been associated with a high rate of medication errors and is not commonly used today.

Unit Dose. The unit-dose system uses portable carts containing a drawer with a 24-hour supply of medications for

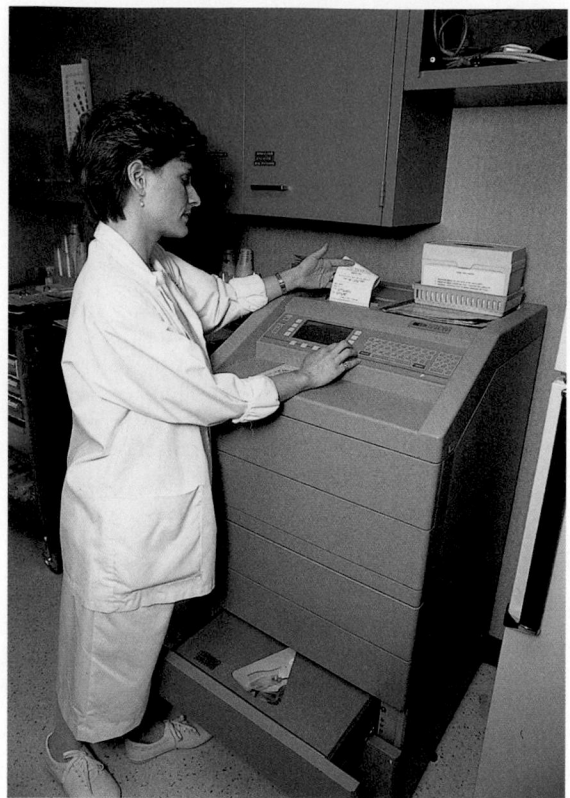

FIGURE 34-11 Nurse using automated medication dispensing system.

each client. Each drawer is labeled with the name of the client in the designated room. The unit dose is the ordered dose of medication the client receives at one time. Each tablet or capsule is wrapped in a foil or paper container. At a designated time each day the pharmacist refills the drawers in the cart with a fresh supply. The cart also contains limited amounts of prn and stock medications for special situations. Controlled substances are not kept in the individual client drawer but in a larger locker drawer in the cart. The unit-dose system is designed to reduce the number of medication errors and saves steps in dispensing medications.

Automated Medicine Dispensing Systems. Automated medication dispensing systems (AMDS) are used successfully throughout the country (Figure 34-11). The systems are designed to achieve computerized control of unit dose medication dispensing and narcotics. All procedures connected to an AMDS are controlled electronically via a client's profile. The client name and the client's drug profile must be accessed before the AMDS will dispense a medication. Each nurse has a security code allowing access to the system. The client's identification number is entered into the computer. In these systems the nurse is allowed to select the desired medication, dosage, and route from a list displayed on the computer screen. The system causes the drawer containing medication to open, records it, and charges it to the client.

Nurses may also scan bar codes to identify the client, medication (name, dosage, route), and the nurse administering the medication. This information is then automatically recorded on a computerized database.

Nurse's Role

Because the nurse spends the most time with clients, the nurse is the most appropriate health care worker to administer medications. The administration of medications to clients requires knowledge and a set of skills that is unique to the nurse. The nurse assesses the client's ability to self-administer medications, determines whether a client should receive a medication at a given time, administers medications correctly, and monitors the effects of prescribed medications. Client and family education about proper medication administration and monitoring is an integral part of the nurse's role. The nurse uses the nursing process to integrate medication therapy into care.

Critical Thinking

Knowledge

The nurse uses the knowledge learned from many disciplines when administering medications. It is this knowledge that helps the nurse understand why a particular medication has been prescribed for a client and how this medication will alter the client's physiology so as to exert a therapeutic effect. For example, in physiology the nurse learns that potassium is a major intracellular ion. When clients do not have enough potassium in their body, they may experience signs and symptoms that are associated with hypokalemia, such as muscle fatigue or weakness. Prescribed medications help to restore the client's potassium level to normal.

Knowledge about child development indicates that children often associate medication administration with a negative experience. The nurse uses principles from child development to ensure that the child cooperates with the medication experience.

Experience

The nursing student often has limited experience with medication administration as it applies to professional practice. The clinical experience provides the student with the opportunity to use the nursing process as it applies to medication administration. As the student nurse gains experiences in medication administration, psychomotor skills ("the how-to") become more refined. However, psychomotor skills represent a small part of medication administration. Client attitudes, knowledge, physical and mental status and responses can make medication administration a complex experience.

Attitudes

To administer medication safely to clients certain cognitive skills are essential. The nurse accepts full accountability and responsibility for all actions that are taken; this includes the administration of medications (Minnesota Nurses Association, 2001). When a nurse administers a medication to the client, the nurse accepts the responsibility that the medication or the nursing actions in administering it will not harm the client in any way. The nurse does not assume that the medication that is ordered for the client is the correct medication or the correct dose. The nurse could be held accountable for administering an ordered medication that is knowingly inappropriate for the client. Because of this, the nurse should be familiar with the therapeutic effect, usual dosage, laboratory interferences, and side effects of all medications that are administered. The nurse is also responsible for ensuring that clients who will self-administer medications have been properly informed about all aspects of self-administration.

Demonstrating accountability and acting responsibly in professional practice means that the nurse acknowledges when errors in professional practice occur. Most of the errors that are made by nurses are medication errors. A **medication error** is any event that could cause or lead to a client receiving inappropriate medication therapy or failing to receive appropriate medication therapy. Most medication errors occur when a nurse becomes distracted or fails to follow routine procedures such as checking dose calculations, deciphering illegible handwriting, or administering medications with which the nurse is unfamiliar (see Table 34-8, p. 836). Hospital medication delivery systems should be designed so that there is a system of checks and balances. This will help to reduce medication errors. Consider the example in Box 34-3.

Box 34-3 illustrates the crucial role that nurses play in the prevention of medication errors. The nurse is the essential link in the prevention of medication errors. Unfortunately, many medication errors are never identified. When an error occurs, it should be acknowledged immediately and reported to the appropriate hospital personnel (e.g., nurse manager and physician). Measures to counteract the effects of the error may be necessary. The nurse is also responsible for completing an incident report describing the nature of the incident. Incident reports assist administrative personnel in identifying hospital system problems that contribute to medication errors. References to incident reports should **not** be made in a client's permanent record (see Chapter 22).

Nurses administer a wide variety of medications, and new medications are constantly approved for dispensation. As a result, nurses do not always have knowledge about the medications they are asked to administer. Critical thinkers admit what they do not know and acquire the knowledge needed to safely administer unfamiliar medications. This may mean consulting more expert nurses, a pharmacist, or a medication book.

Institutional policy may place limitations on the nurse's ability to administer medications in certain units of the acute care setting. Nurses may be limited by certain medication routes or dosages. Most institutions have nursing procedure manuals that have policies that define the classes of medications nurses employed by the agency may and may not administer. The types and dosages of medications nurses may deliver can also vary from unit to unit within the same facility. For example, Dilantin, a powerful medication that is administered to treat seizures, may be administered by mouth or IV push. In large dosages, Dilantin can also affect the rhythm of the heart. Therefore some institutions place limits on how much Dilantin can be given to a client on a nursing unit that does not have the ability to monitor the client's heart rate and rhythm. Not all prescribers are aware of all of the limitations and may prescribe

Case Study　　　**Box 34-3**

The physician writes an order for a medication. The nurse receives the order and checks for completeness and appropriateness. The nurse may question the order if the written order is illegible, the dose seems unusually low or high, or the medication seems inappropriate for the client's condition. The order is sent to the pharmacy, where it is read and prepared by either a pharmacist or a pharmacy technician. If the technician prepares the medication, the pharmacist checks the technician's work. The pharmacist also verifies that the medication is the appropriate dosage and that there are no medication interactions or medication allergies. When a medication order seems inappropriate, for example, a medication order written for 2000 mg when the proper dosage calls for 200 mg, the pharmacist may ask the nurse to clarify the order from the prescriber or the pharmacist may call the prescriber directly for order clarification. When the order is appropriate, the medications are sent to the nursing unit. The nurse receives the medication and checks the administration record against what the pharmacy has sent and the prescriber ordered. Before administration, the nurse performs the six rights of medication administration. The nurse allows the client to be the final check by reviewing the name of the medication, the dosage, and why he or she is receiving the medication.

medications that cannot be given in a particular health care setting. Nurses must recognize these limitations and ensure that the prescriber is informed and that appropriate actions are taken to ensure that the client receives the mediations as prescribed and within the time prescribed in the appropriate environment.

Standards

Standards are those actions that ensure safe nursing practice. To ensure safe medication administration the nurse should be aware of a nursing standard called the six rights of medication administration. All medication errors can be linked, in some way, to an inconsistency in adhering to the six rights of medication administration. The six rights of medication administration include the following:

1. The right medication
2. The right dose
3. The right client
4. The right route
5. The right time
6. The right documentation

Right Medication. When medications are first ordered, the nurse compares the medication recording form or computer orders with the prescriber's written orders. When administering medications, the nurse compares the label of the medication container with the medication form. The nurse does this 3 times: (1) before removing the container from the drawer or shelf, (2) as the amount of medication ordered is removed from the container, and (3) before returning the container to storage. With unit-dose prepackaged medications, the nurse checks the label with the medicine form a third time even though there is no permanent container. Unit-dose medications may be checked before opening at the client's bedside.

Nurses administer only the medications they prepare. If an error occurs, the nurse who administers the medication is responsible for the error. If a client questions the medication a nurse prepares, it is important not to ignore these concerns. An alert client will know whether a medication is different from those received before. In most cases the client's medication order has been changed; however, the client's questions might reveal an error. The nurse should withhold the medication until the preparation can be rechecked against the prescriber's orders.

Clients who self-administer medications should keep them in their original labeled containers, separate from other medications, to avoid confusion. The nurse never prepares medications from unmarked containers or containers with illegible labels. If a client refuses a medication, the nurse should discard it rather than return it to the original container. Unit-dose packaged medications can be saved if they are unopened.

Right Dose. The unit-dose system is designed to minimize errors. When a medication must be prepared from a larger volume or strength than needed or when the prescriber orders a system of measurement different from what the pharmacist supplies, the chance of error increases. When performing medication calculations or conversions, the nurse should have another qualified nurse check the calculated doses.

After calculating doses, the nurse prepares the medication using standard measurement devices. Graduated cups, syringes, and scaled droppers can be used to measure medications accurately. At home, clients should use kitchen measuring spoons rather than teaspoons and tablespoons, which vary in volume.

When it is necessary to break a scored tablet, the break should be even. A scored tablet may be cut in half by using a knife-edge or a cutting device. Tablets that do not break evenly are discarded. The two halves are given in successive doses if the second half is repackaged and labeled.

Often a nurse prepares a tablet by crushing it so that it can be mixed in food. The crushing device should always be cleaned completely before the tablet is crushed. Remnants of previously crushed medications may increase a medication's concentration or result in the client receiving a portion of an unprescribed medication. Crushed medications should be mixed with very small amounts of food or liquid. The client's favorite foods or liquids should not be used because a medication may alter their taste and decrease the client's desire for them.

> *Safety Alert.* Not all medications can be crushed. Some medications, such as time-released or extended-release capsules, have special coatings to prevent the medication from being absorbed too quickly. Refer to a medication manual or some other reference before crushing a medication to ensure that the medication can be safely crushed.

Right Client. Medication errors often occur because one client gets a drug intended for another client. An important step in administering medications safely is being sure the medication is given to the right client. It is difficult to remember every client's name and face. To identify

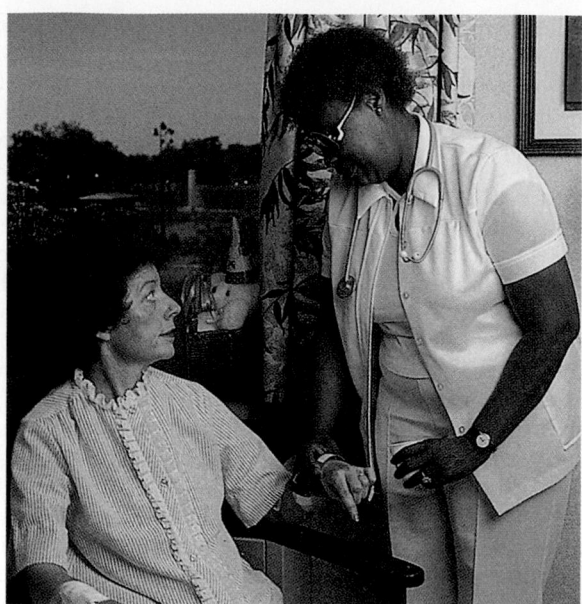

FIGURE **34–12**   Before administering any medications, the nurse checks the client's identification and allergy bracelet.

a client correctly, the nurse checks the medication administration form against the client's identification bracelet and asks the client to state his or her name to ensure the client's identification bracelet has the correct information (Figure 34-12).

If an identification bracelet becomes smudged or illegible, or is missing, the nurse must acquire a new one for the client. When asking the client's name, the nurse should not merely speak the name and assume that the client's response indicates that he or she is the right person. Instead, the nurse asks the client to state his or her full name. To avoid making the client feel uneasy, the nurse simply states that the question is routine for giving a medication.

Right Route. If a prescriber's order does not designate a route of administration, the nurse consults the prescriber. Likewise, if the specified route is not the recommended route, the nurse should alert the prescriber immediately.

When the nurse administers injections, precautions are necessary to ensure that the medications are given correctly. It is also important to prepare injections only from preparations designed for parenteral use. The injection of a liquid designed for oral use can produce local complications, such as a sterile abscess or fatal systemic effects. Medication companies label parenteral medications for "injectable use only."

Right Time. The nurse must know why a medication is ordered for certain times of the day and whether the time schedule can be altered. For example, two medications are ordered, one q8h (every 8 hours) and the other tid (3 times a day). Both medications are to be given 3 times within a 24-hour period. The prescriber intends the q8h medication to be given around the clock to maintain therapeutic blood levels of the medication. In contrast, the tid medication is given during the waking hours. Each institution has a recommended time schedule for medications ordered at frequent intervals. The nurse may alter these recommended times if necessary or appropriate.

The prescriber often gives specific instructions about when to administer a medication. A preoperative medication to be given on call means that the nurse is to administer the medication when the operating room notifies the nursing unit. A medication ordered pc (after meals) is to be given within half an hour after a meal, when the client has a full stomach. A STAT medication is to be given immediately.

Medications that must act at certain times are given priority. For example, insulin should be given at a precise interval before a meal. Antibiotics should be given on time around the clock to maintain therapeutic blood levels. All routinely ordered medications should be given within 60 minutes of the times ordered (30 minutes before or after the prescribed time) (CMS, 2003).

Some medications require the nurse's clinical judgment in determining the proper time for administration. A prn sleeping medication should be administered when the client is prepared for bed or at a time appropriate for maximum benefit. A nurse also uses judgment when administering prn analgesics. For example, the nurse may need to obtain a STAT order from the prescriber if the client requires a medication before the prn interval has elapsed.

At home a client may have to take several medications throughout the day. The nurse helps to plan schedules based on preferred medication intervals, the medication's pharmacokinetics, and the client's daily schedule. For clients who have difficulty remembering when to take medications, the nurse can make a chart that lists the times when each medication is to be taken or can prepare a special container to hold each timed dose.

Right Documentation. This right has been added to the traditional five rights of medication administration by several authors to enhance medication safety (Aschenbrenner, Cleveland, and Venable, 2002). Medication errors may result from inaccurate documentation. Therefore it is essential that nurses ensure the appropriate documentation exists before giving medications. Documentation is an important part in safe medication administration. The documentation for the medication should clearly reflect the client's name, the name of the ordered medication, the time the medication was administered, and the medication's dosage, route, and frequency. If any of these pieces of information are missing, the nurse must contact the prescriber to verify the order. After the nurse administers the medication, the medication administration record (MAR) is completed per agency policy to verify that the medication was given as ordered. Accurate documentation serves as a way for health care providers to communicate with each other.

Professional standards influence the activities of medication administration. The American Nurses Association's (ANA's) *Standards of Nursing Practice* (see Chapters 1 and 22), based on the nursing process, also apply to the activity of medication administration. Other professional nursing standards, such as what nurses can expect from pre-

---

> **Box 34-4   Nurses' Six Rights for Safe Medication Administration**
>
> 1. The right to a complete and clearly written order
> 2. The right to have the correct drug route and dose dispensed
> 3. The right to have access to information
> 4. The right to have policies on medication administration
> 5. The right to administer medications safely and to identify problems in the system
> 6. The right to stop, think, and be vigilant when administering medications

From Cook MC: Nurses' six rights for safe medication administration, *Massachusetts Nurse* 69(6):8, 1999.

---

scribers or employers in order to implement the six rights of safe medication administration, may apply (Box 34-4).

Maintaining Clients' Rights. In accordance with *The Patient Care Partnership* and because of the potential risks related to medication administration, a client has the following rights:

- To be informed of the medication's name, purpose, action, and potential undesired effects
- To refuse a medication regardless of the consequences
- To have qualified nurses or physicians assess a medication history, including allergies
- To be properly advised of the experimental nature of medication therapy and to give written consent for its use
- To receive labeled medications safely without discomfort in accordance with the six rights of medication administration
- To receive appropriate supportive therapy in relation to medication therapy
- To not receive unnecessary medications

The nurse must be aware of these rights and handle all inquiries by clients and families courteously and professionally. A nurse should not become defensive if a client refuses medication therapy. The nurse must have the necessary knowledge and skill to satisfy the responsibilities of safe and effective medication administration.

Nursing Process and Medication Administration

Assessment

To determine the need for and potential response to medication therapy, the nurse assesses many factors.

History. Before administering medications, the nurse obtains or reviews the client's medical history. A client's medical history may provide indications or contraindications for medication therapy. Disease or illness may place clients at risk for adverse medication effects. For example, if a client has a gastric ulcer, compounds containing aspirin will increase the likelihood of bleeding. Long-term health problems such as diabetes or arthritis, which require medications, suggest to the nurse the type of medications a client is taking. A client's surgical history may indicate use of medications. For example, after a thyroidectomy a client may require hormone replacement.

History of Allergies. If the client has a history of allergies to medication, the nurse informs other members of the health care team. Food allergies should also be carefully documented because many medications have ingredients also found in food sources. One example is shellfish. If clients are allergic to shellfish, the client may be sensitive to any product containing iodine such as betadine or dyes used in radiological testing. Another example is dye used in food products (e.g., candy or soda). In a hospital, clients may wear identification bands listing medications to which they are allergic. All allergies should be noted on the nurse's admission notes, medication records, and physician's history.

Medication Data. The nurse assesses information about each medication that the client takes, including length of time the medication has been taken, the current dosage, and whether or not the client has experienced adverse effects from the medication. In addition, the nurse reviews medication data, including action, purpose, normal dosages, routes, side effects, and nursing implications for administration and monitoring. Common questions to ask include the following: Is the smallest possible dose ordered (a question pertinent to older adults)? Can a certain medication interact with other medications being used? Are there special instructions for administering the medication? Often, several resources must be consulted to gather needed information. Pharmacology textbooks, nursing journals, PDR, medication package inserts, and the pharmacist are valuable resources. Helpful medication references can also be downloaded to personal handheld computers. The nurse is responsible for knowing as much as possible about each medication given. Many nursing students prepare or purchase cards containing medication data to use as a quick resource.

Diet History. A diet history reveals normal eating patterns and food preferences. The nurse can then plan the dosage schedule more effectively and advise the client in avoiding foods, such as grapefruit juice, that may interact with medications.

Client's Perceptual or Coordination Problems. For a client with perceptual fine motor or coordination limitations, self-administration may be difficult. For example, a client with arthritis may have difficulty manipulating a syringe. The nurse must assess the client's ability to prepare doses and take medications correctly. If the client is unable to self-administer medications, the nurse may need to assess whether family or friends will be available to assist.

Client's Current Condition. The ongoing physical or mental status of a client may affect whether a medication is given or how it is administered. *The nurse should assess a client carefully before giving any medication.* For example, the nurse checks blood pressure before giving an antihy-

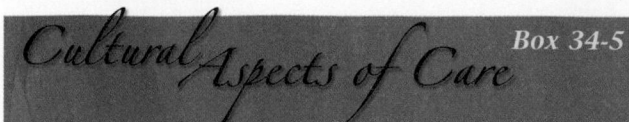

Box 34-5

Health beliefs vary by culture. These beliefs often influence how clients manage and respond to drug therapy. Significant differences in values, beliefs, and attitudes may affect a client's compliance with drug therapy. For example, cultures attach different symbolic meanings to medications and drug therapy. Herbal remedies and alternative therapies are common in various cultures and ethnic groups and may interfere with prescribed medications. In addition, there is often a marked difference in health beliefs between health providers and clients, which further affects a client's compliance with medical therapy. Demographic changes in both age and race are factors that currently affect nursing practice in medication administration. In addition to the psychosocial aspect of medication therapy, pharmacological research has shown that different ethnic and racial groups experience differences in drug response, metabolism, and side effects.

Implications for Practice

- Carefully assess cultural beliefs, attitudes, and values when administering and teaching clients about their medications.
- Conflicts between medications and cultural beliefs need to be resolved to achieve optimal client outcomes.
- When assessing medication history, nurses should investigate if the client practices any alternative therapies or is taking any herbal preparations.
- Consider cultural influences on drug response, metabolism, and side effects if a client is not responding to drug therapy as expected. A change in the client's medication may be warranted.

Data from Andrews MM, Boyle JS: *Transcultural concepts in nursing care,* ed 4, Philadelphia, 2003, Lippincott; and McKenry LM, Salerno E: *Mosby's pharmacology in nursing revised and updated,* ed 21, St. Louis, 2003, Mosby.

pertensive. A client who is nauseated may be unable to swallow a tablet. Assessment findings also serve as a baseline in evaluating the effects of medication therapy.

Client's Attitude About Medication Use. The client's attitude about medications may reveal a level of medication dependence or drug avoidance. Clients may not express their feelings about taking a particular medication, particularly if dependence is a problem. The nurse should observe the client's behavior for evidence of medication dependence or avoidance. The nurse should also be aware that the client's cultural beliefs about Western medicine could interfere with medication compliance (see Box 34-5 and Chapter 8).

Client's Knowledge and Understanding of Medication Therapy. The client's knowledge and understanding of medication therapy influence the willingness or ability to follow a medication regimen. Unless a client understands a medication's purpose, the importance of regular dosage schedules and proper administration methods, and the possible side effects, compliance is unlikely. When assessing knowledge of a medication, the nurse asks: What is it for? How is it taken? When is it taken? What side effects have there been? Has the client ever stopped taking doses? Is there anything else the client does not understand and would like to know about the medication? When the client has a history of poor compliance, the nurse should also review resources available for purchase of medications.

Client's Learning Needs. By assessing the client's level of knowledge about a medication and the resources available to take medications regularly, the nurse determines the need for instruction (see Chapter 24). It may be necessary for the nurse to explain the action and purpose of the medication, expected side effects, correct administration techniques, and ways to help the client to remember the medication regimen. If a client has been placed on a newly prescribed medication, instruction may need to be more involved.

Nursing Diagnosis

Assessment provides data about the client's condition, ability to self-administer medications, and medication use patterns, which can be used to determine actual or potential problems with medication therapy. Certain data are defining characteristics, which when clustered together reveal nursing diagnoses. For example, *noncompliance related to a medication regimen* may be indicated when a client admits not taking prescribed medications correctly, or by evidence that a medication has not reversed symptoms as expected. The following is a list of nursing diagnoses that may be used during the administration of medications:

- Anxiety
- Health maintenance, ineffective
- Health-seeking behaviors
- Deficient knowledge (medications)
- Noncompliance (medications)
- Disturbed visual sensory perception
- Impaired swallowing
- Effective therapeutic regimen management
- Ineffective therapeutic regimen management

Once the diagnosis is selected, the nurse identifies the related factor, which drives the selection of nursing interventions. For example, the related factors of inadequate resources versus lack of knowledge require different interventions. If the client's noncompliance is related to inadequate finances, the nurse will collaborate with family members, social workers, or community agencies to help a client receive necessary medications. If the related factor is lack of knowledge, the nurse will implement an extensive teaching plan and follow-up.

Planning

The nurse organizes care activities to ensure the safe administration of medications. Hurrying to give clients medications can lead to errors. It is important for the nurse to minimize distractions or interruptions when preparing and administering medications.

Goals and Outcomes. Setting goals and related outcomes will help the nurse plan to use wisely time during med-

ication administration. For example, the nurse might establish the following goal and related outcomes for a client with newly diagnosed type 2 diabetes:

Goal: The client will safely administer all ordered medications before discharge.
Outcomes:
- The client will verbalize understanding of desired effects and adverse effects of medications.
- The client will state signs, symptoms, and treatment of hypoglycemia.
- The client will establish a daily routine that will coordinate timing of medication with mealtimes.

Setting Priorities. The nurse prioritizes care when administering medications. The nurse uses information gathered from the client's assessment in determining which medications should be given first and if it is appropriate to administer prn medications. For example, if a client is in pain, it is important that the nurse provide pain medication as soon as possible. If the client is experiencing an elevated blood pressure, the blood pressure medications should be administered before other medications. The nurse also prioritizes when providing client education about medications. The most important information about the medications should be provided first. For example, if an oral hypoglycemic medication causes hypoglycemia as a side effect, the client must be able to identify and treat the hypoglycemia before taking the medication independently.

Continuity of Care. It is important to collaborate with the client's family or friends when instruction is given whenever possible. Family members will often reinforce the importance of medication regimens in the home setting. When clients are hospitalized, it is important for the nurse to not postpone instruction until the day of discharge. In order for the client to understand medications and self-administration guidelines, there must be time for questions and discussion. Early planning is critical.

In the community, the nurse ensures that the client knows where and how to obtain medications. The nurse also ensures that clients know how to read medication labels. Whether a client attempts self-administration or the nurse assumes responsibility for administering medications, the following goals and expected outcomes must be met: (1) the client and family understand medication therapy, (2) the client gains therapeutic effect of the prescribed medications without discomfort or complications, (3) the client has no complications related to the route of administration, and (4) the client safely self-administers medications.

Implementation

Health Promotion. The nurse, in promoting or maintaining the client's health, identifies factors that may improve or diminish well-being. Health beliefs, personal motivations, socioeconomic factors, and habits (e.g., smoking) can influence the client's compliance with the medication regimen.

Teaching the client and family about the benefit of a medication and the knowledge needed to take it correctly can promote adherence to the regimen and foster independence. Integrating the client's health beliefs and cultural practices into the treatment plan can assist the nurse in establishing a schedule or routine with the client. The nurse may make referrals to community resources if the client is unable to afford or obtain necessary medications.

Client and Family Teaching. Unless a client is properly informed about medications, he or she may take the medications incorrectly or not at all. The nurse provides information about the purpose of medications and their actions and effects. Many health care institutions offer easy-to-read leaflets on specific types of medications. A client must know how to take a medication properly and the effects if he or she fails to do so. For example, after receiving a prescription for an antibiotic, a client must understand the importance of taking the full prescription. Failure to do this can lead to a worsening of the condition and the development of bacteria resistant to the medication.

Nurses teach proper self-administration of medications to clients for all routes. For example, the nurse teaches a client how to accurately measure a liquid medication. Special education must be provided to clients who depend on daily injections. The client learns to prepare and administer an injection correctly using aseptic technique. Family members or friends should be taught to give injections in case the client becomes ill or physically unable to handle a syringe. Nurses can provide specially designed equipment such as syringes with enlarged calibrated scales for easier reading or Braille-labeled medication vials for clients with visual alterations.

Clients must be aware of the symptoms of medication side effects or toxicity. For example, clients taking anticoagulants learn to notify their primary care providers immediately when signs of bleeding or bruising develop. Family members or friends should be informed of medication side effects such as changes in behavior because they are often the first persons to recognize such effects. Clients are better able to cope with problems caused by medications if they understand how and when to act. All clients should learn the basic guidelines for medication safety. These guidelines ensure the proper use and storage of medications in the home (Box 34-6).

Acute Care. Clients are often hospitalized to receive expert nursing observation and documentation of responses to medications. When a nurse receives a medication order, several nursing interventions are essential for safe and effective medication administration.

Receiving Medication Orders. A medication order is required for any medication to be administered by a nurse. Before any other interventions, the nurse ensures that the medication order contains all of the elements in Box 34-7. If the medication order is incomplete, the nurse should inform the prescriber and ensure completeness before carrying out any medication order. Some medication orders can be given verbally or by telephone by the prescriber to the nurse. A verbal order is a medication or treatment order received by the nurse in the presence of the prescriber. Verbal orders are entered into the client's medical record by the registered nurse and transcribed the same way as if

---

Client Teaching   Box 34-6

Safe Medication Administration

Objective

- Client will correctly administer subcutaneous insulin

Teaching Strategies

- Instruct client in how to determine that insulin is not out of date.
- Instruct client to keep medication in its original labeled container.
- Instruct client to keep insulin refrigerated.
- Instruct client in how to rotate insulin injection sites.
- Instruct client in how to determine the amount of insulin based on the results of home capillary glucose monitoring.
- Demonstrate to client how to prepare a single insulin preparation.
- Demonstrate to client how to administer subcutaneous insulin injection.
- Instruct client in how to keep a daily log book for insulin injections, including results of home capillary glucose monitoring, type and amount of insulin given, expiration date on insulin vial, time of insulin injection, injection site used.

Evaluation

- Ask client to describe procedure used at home for determining the correct dose of insulin needed and injection site.
- Observe client preparing insulin dose based on results of capillary glucose monitoring.
- Observe client selecting injection site.
- Observe client self-administering insulin injection.
- Review client log book for insulin injections.

---

the prescriber wrote the order himself or herself. Telephone orders are medication or treatment orders given to the nurse by the prescriber, generally after the nurse updates the prescriber about a change in the client's condition. The nurse follows institutional policy regarding the receiving, recording, and transcription of verbal and telephone orders. Generally the prescriber must sign verbal and telephone orders within 24 hours. *Student nurses are prohibited from receiving verbal and telephone orders.*

Correct Transcription and Communication of Orders. The nurse or a designated unit secretary writes the prescriber's complete order on the appropriate medication form, the MAR. The transcribed order includes the client's name, room, and bed number; and medication name, dose, frequency, and route of administration. Each time a medication dose is prepared, the nurse refers to the medication form. With the unit-dose system, only one transcription is necessary, limiting the opportunity for errors. When transcribing orders, the nurse should be sure that names, dosages, and symbols are legible. The nurse rewrites any smudged or illegible transcriptions.

Some institutions have prescribed order entry. The prescriber is able to enter an order directly into the com-

Box **34-7**   Components of Medication Orders

A medication order is incomplete unless it has the following parts:

- **Client's full name:** The client's full name distinguishes the client from other persons with the same last name. In the acute care setting, clients may also be assigned special identification numbers (e.g., medical record number) to help distinguish clients with the same names. This number may be included on the order form.
- **Date that the order is written:** The day, month, year, and time must be included. Designating the time that an order is written helps clarify when certain orders are to stop automatically. If an incident occurs involving a medication error, it is easier to document what happened when this information is available.
- **Medication name:** The prescriber will order a generic or trade-name medication. Correct spelling is essential in preventing confusion with medications with similar spelling.
- **Dose:** The amount or strength of the medication is included.
- **Route of administration:** The prescriber uses accepted abbreviations for medication routes. Accuracy is important because some medications are administered by more than one route.
- **Time and frequency of administration:** The nurse needs to know when to initiate medication therapy. Orders for multiple doses establish a routine schedule for medication administration.
- **Signature of physician, nurse practitioner, or physician assistant:** Signature makes the order a legal request.

puter, preventing the need for transcription of orders. Computer interfaces transfer the order to the MAR, the pharmacy record, and automated dispensing system. The computer printout may be used as the MAR, recording which medications are given to the client (Figure 34-13).

A registered nurse checks all transcribed orders against the original order for accuracy and thoroughness. If an order seems incorrect or inappropriate, the nurse consults the prescriber. The nurse who gives the wrong medication or an incorrect dose is legally responsible for the error.

Accurate Dose Calculation and Measurement. When measuring liquid medications, the nurse uses standard measuring containers. The procedure for medication measurement is systematic to lessen the chance of error. The nurse calculates each dose when preparing the medication, pays close attention to the process of calculation, and avoids interference from other nursing activities.

Correct Administration. For safe administration, the nurse uses aseptic technique and proper procedures when handling and giving medications. For example, certain medications require the nurse to perform assessments (e.g., assessing heart rate before giving antidysrhythmic medications). The nurse must monitor when a client is receiving the first dose of a medication new to the client (JCAHO, 2003). The nurse documents the client's response on the appropriate record form (see agency policy.)

Recording Medication Administration. After administering a medication, the nurse records it immediately on the appropriate record form (see Figure 34-13, p. 848). The nurse **never** charts a medication before administering it. Recording immediately after administration prevents errors.

The recording of a medication includes the name of the medication, dose, route, and exact time of administration. Often the medication forms are prepared, and the nurse need only record the time. Agency policies may also require that the nurse record the location of an injection.

If a client refuses a medication or is undergoing tests or procedures that result in a missed dose, the nurse explains the reason the medication was not given in the nurse's notes. Some agencies require the nurse to circle the prescribed administration time on the medication record when a dose is missed.

Restorative Care. Because of the numerous types of restorative care settings, medication administration activities vary. Clients with functional limitations may require the nurse to fully administer all medications. In the home care setting, clients usually administer their own medications. Regardless of the type of medication activity, the nurse remains responsible for instructing clients and families in medication action, administration, and side effects. The nurse is also responsible for monitoring compliance with medication and determines the effectiveness of medications that have been prescribed.

Special Considerations for Administering Medications to Specific Age-Groups. A client's developmental level is a factor in the way nurses administer medications. Knowledge of a client's developmental needs helps the nurse to anticipate responses to medication therapy.

Infants and Children. Children vary in age, weight, surface area, and the ability to absorb, metabolize, and excrete medications. Children's medication doses are lower than those of adults, so special caution is needed when preparing medications for them. Medications are usually not prepared and packaged in standardized dose ranges for children. Preparing an ordered dose from an available amount requires careful calculation (see pp. 836-837).

The child's parents are often valuable resources for determining the best way to give the child medication. Sometimes it is less traumatic for the child if a parent gives the medication and the nurse supervises.

All children require special psychological preparation before receiving medications. Supportive care is needed if a child is expected to cooperate. The nurse explains the procedure to a child, using short words and simple language appropriate to the child's level of comprehension. Long explanations may increase a child's anxiety, especially for painful procedures such as an injection. The young child who refuses to cooperate or resists consistently despite explanation and encouragement may require physical coercion. If so, it is carried out quickly and carefully (Hockenberry and others, 2003). If it is possible to involve the child, the nurse may have greater success giving a medication (Cromling, 2002). For example, saying "It's time to take your tablet now. Do you want it with wa-

Room: 3700-03

Patient: PDM, Pharmacy
Birth: 11/30/79   Admit: 01/01/00
MRN: 2000403   Acct: 900015
A Doctor: Jim Smith

Age: 20 y Ht: 5 ft 2 in   Wt: 125.2 lbs
Metric: Ht: 1 m 57 cm Wt: 56.79 kg

Saint Francis Medical Center

MEDICATION ADMINISTRATION RECORD

Date: 01/18/00 – 01/19/00

ADEs/Nondrug allergies: Latex – Zosyn – Amoxicillin –
Insulins – Darvocet – Lugols soln. – Antihi +

Medication	0800	0900	1000	1100	1200	1300	1400	1500	1600	1700	1800	1900	2000	2100	2200	2300	2400	0100	0200	0300	0400	0500	0600	0700
P00014 Bacitracin ointment / AKA: Bacitracin ointment / Dose: Apply STRGH: 30 gm/tube / TID Topical: Right lower leg / For external use only / Testing			RL 10																					
P00029 Insulin/human regular / AKA: Humulin R Dose: 15 units / Strgh: 1 ml = 100 units AC Sub-Q	RL 0730																							
P00030 Fexofenadine 60 mg/psuedo 120 mg / AKA: Allegra–D Sr Tab / Dose: 1 tab STRGH: 60/120/tab / BID Oral / Auto Sub: 1 Allegra–D Tab bid / For Claritin–D 12 hr and 24 hr / Per P&T Comm			RL 10																					
P00036 Aspirin / AKA: Aspirin 325 mg Tab / Dose: 2 tab 650 mg STRGH: 325 mg/tab / Q3–4h Oral / Testing						RL 1315																		
P00039 Haloperidol tablet / AKA: Haldol 0.5 mg tab / Dose: 1 mg STRGH: 1 mg/tab / QHS Oral																								
P00035 Zolpidem / AKA: Ambien 5 mg tab / Dose: 5 mg STRGH: 5/tab / QHS PRN Oral / MR × 1 / Testing																								

Circle = Dose not given
Initials = Dose given   Page: 01 (continued)
Deltoid = R.D., L.D.
Vastus Lateralis = R.V.L., L.V.L.
Lower Abdominal = R.L.A., L.L.A.
Anterior Gluteal = R.A.G., L.A.G.
Posterior Gluteal = R.P.G., L.P.G.

Initials and signature	Initials and signature	Initials and signature
Rita Lassater RL		
Initials and signature	Initials and signature	Initials and signature
Initials and signature	Initials and signature	Initials and signature

FIGURE **34–13** Example of medication administration record (MAR). (Courtesy OSF Saint Francis Medical Center, Peoria, Ill.)

Box **34-8**   **Tips for Administering Medications to Children**

Oral Medications

- Liquid forms are safer to swallow to avoid aspiration.
- Use droppers for administering liquids to infants; straws may help older children swallow pills.
- Juice, a soft drink, or a frozen juice bar is offered after a medication is swallowed.
- Carbonated beverages poured over finely crushed ice reduce nausea.
- When mixing medications with palatable flavorings such as syrup or honey, the nurse uses only a small amount. The child may refuse to take all of a larger mixture. The nurse avoids mixing a medication with foods or liquids that the child is taking well because the child may in turn refuse them.
- A plastic, disposable syringe is the most accurate device for preparing liquid doses, especially those less than 10 ml. (Cups, teaspoons, and droppers are inaccurate.)
- When administering liquid medications, a spoon, plastic cup, or oral syringe (without needle) is useful.

Injections

- Caution is used when selecting IM injection sites because infants and small children have underdeveloped muscles.
- Children can be unpredictable and uncooperative. Someone should be available to restrain a child if needed.
- The nurse always awakens a sleeping child before giving an injection.
- Distracting the child with conversation, bubbles, or a toy may reduce pain perception.
- The nurse gives the injection quickly and does not fight with the child.
- If time allows, the nurse uses a eutectic mixture of local anesthetics (EMLA) cream.

Focus on *Older Adults*   *Box* **34-9**

- Simplify the drug therapy plan whenever possible (McKenry and Salerno, 2003).
- Keep instructions clear and simple and provide written material in large print (Maas and others, 2001).
- Assess functional status to determine if client will require assistance in taking medications (McKenry and Salerno, 2003).
- Have client drink a little fluid *before* taking oral medications to ease swallowing, and encourage the client to drink at least 5 to 6 ounces of fluid after taking medications (Ebersole and Hess, 1998).
- Older adults may have a greater sensitivity to drugs, especially those that act on the central nervous system. Therefore carefully monitor clients' responses to medications and anticipate dosage adjustments as needed (McKenry and Salerno, 2003).
- If the client has difficulty swallowing a capsule or tablet:
  - Ask the physician to substitute a liquid medication if possible (Ebersole and Hess, 1998).
  - Have the client sit up straight and tuck the chin to decrease risk of aspiration (McKenry and Salerno, 2003).
- Teach alternatives to medications, such as proper diet instead of vitamins and exercise instead of laxatives (Ebersole and Hess, 1998).
- Review medication history, including over-the-counter medications, on a frequent basis (Maas and others, 2001).

---

ter or juice?" allows a child to make a choice. The child should not be given the option of not taking a medication. After a medication is given, the nurse praises the child and may even offer a simple reward such as a star or token. Depending on the route of administration, tips exist for effective medication administration for children (Box 34-8).

Older Adults. Older adults also require special consideration during medication administration (Box 34-9). In addition to physiological changes of aging (Figure 34-14), behavioral and economic factors influence an older person's use of medications. Ebersole and Hess (1998) describe five behavioral patterns of medication use characteristic of the older client.

Polypharmacy. **Polypharmacy** means that the client is taking many medications, prescribed or not, in an attempt to treat several disorders simultaneously. Some of the medications taken may have similar effects (Mass and others, 2001). When this occurs, there is a high risk of medication interactions with other medications and with foods that the client may eat. There is also an increased risk of the client having an adverse reaction to the medications.

Self-Prescribing of Medications. A variety of symptoms can be experienced by older adult clients (e.g., pain, con-

stipation, insomnia, and indigestion). All these symptoms are amenable to over-the-counter (OTC) medications. Older adults often attempt to seek relief from the problems by using over-the-counter preparations, folk medicines, and herbs.

Over-the-Counter Medications. It is known that OTC medications are used by 75% of older adults to relieve symptoms. Many of these OTC preparations have ingredients that, when used inappropriately, may cause undesirable side effects or adverse reactions or may be contraindicated in the client's condition.

Misuse of Medications. Forms of misuse by older adults include overuse, underuse, erratic use, and contraindicated use.

Noncompliance. Noncompliance is defined as a deliberate misuse of medication. Of older adults, 75% intentionally do not adhere to their medication regimen either by not taking the medication at all or by altering the dose. Noncompliance generally occurs either because of drug ineffectiveness, uncomfortable side effects, or the prohibitive cost of the medicine.

Evaluation

The nurse monitors a client's response to medications on an ongoing basis. This requires that the nurse know the therapeutic action and common side effects of each medication. A change in a client's condition can be physiologically related to health status or may result from medications or both. The nurse must be alert for reactions in a client taking several medications. The goal of safe and

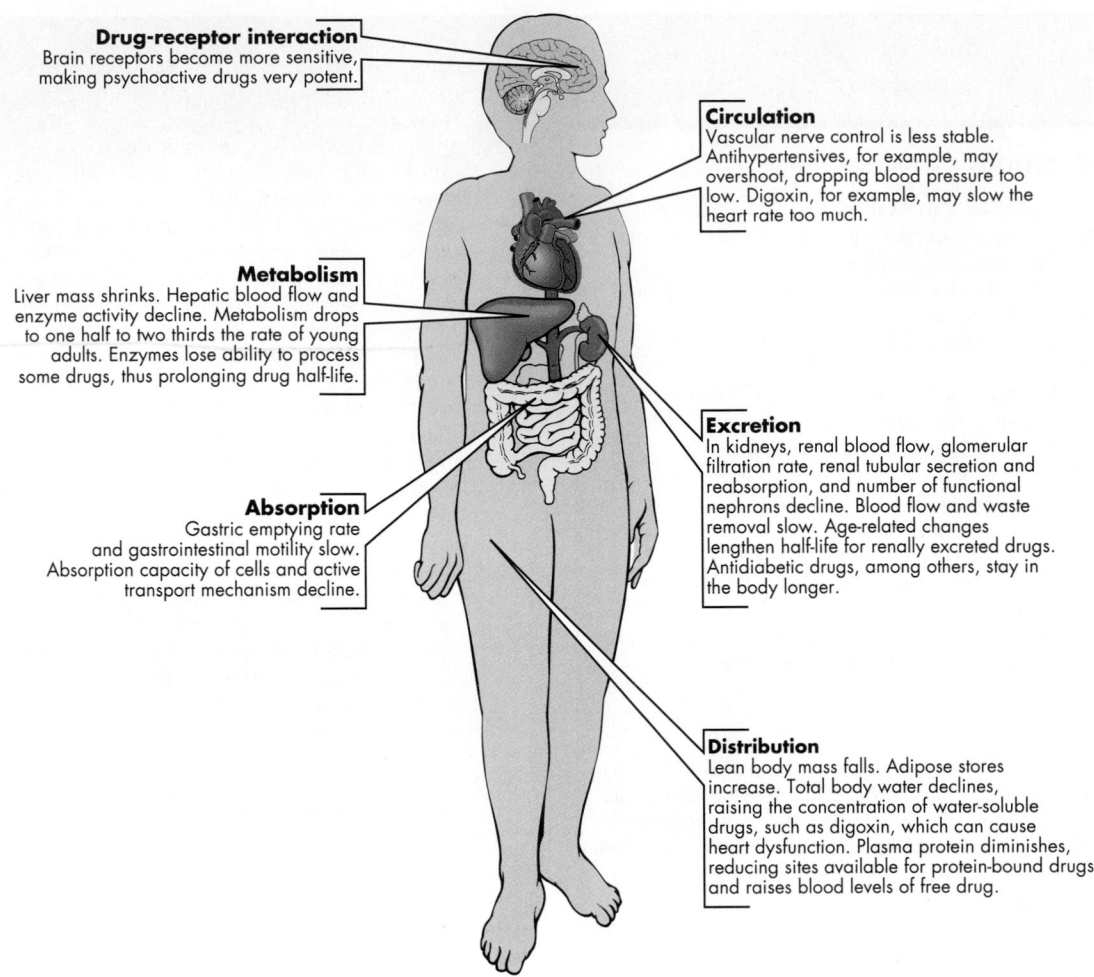

Drug-receptor interaction
Brain receptors become more sensitive, making psychoactive drugs very potent.

Circulation
Vascular nerve control is less stable. Antihypertensives, for example, may overshoot, dropping blood pressure too low. Digoxin, for example, may slow the heart rate too much.

Metabolism
Liver mass shrinks. Hepatic blood flow and enzyme activity decline. Metabolism drops to one half to two thirds the rate of young adults. Enzymes lose ability to process some drugs, thus prolonging drug half-life.

Excretion
In kidneys, renal blood flow, glomerular filtration rate, renal tubular secretion and reabsorption, and number of functional nephrons decline. Blood flow and waste removal slow. Age-related changes lengthen half-life for renally excreted drugs. Antidiabetic drugs, among others, stay in the body longer.

Absorption
Gastric emptying rate and gastrointestinal motility slow. Absorption capacity of cells and active transport mechanism decline.

Distribution
Lean body mass falls. Adipose stores increase. Total body water declines, raising the concentration of water-soluble drugs, such as digoxin, which can cause heart dysfunction. Plasma protein diminishes, reducing sites available for protein-bound drugs and raises blood levels of free drug.

FIGURE **34–14**   Aging body and drug use. (From Lewis SM and others: *Medical-surgical nursing,* ed 5, St. Louis, 2000, Mosby.)

effective medication administration involves a careful evaluation of technique and the client's response to therapy and ability to assume responsibility for self-care.

To evaluate the effectiveness of nursing interventions when meeting established goals of care, the nurse uses evaluative measures to identify if client outcomes were met. Many different evaluation measures can be used in the context of medication administration: direct observation of behavior or response, rating scales and checklists, and oral questioning. The type of measurement used varies with the action being evaluated, the reading skill and knowledge level of the client, and the client's cognitive and psychomotor ability. The most common type of measurement that the nurse uses is a physiological measure. Examples of physiological measure are blood pressure, heart rate, and visual acuity. Client statements can also be used as evaluative measures. Table 34-10 contains examples of goals, expected outcomes, and corresponding evaluative measures.

Medication Administration

Medication administration is an essential part of nursing practice, which requires a sound knowledge base in order for medications to be administered safely. Nurses must be prepared to administer medications using a variety of

routes. The following sections will explain the steps involved in administering medications using various routes.

Oral Administration

The easiest and most desirable way to administer medications is by mouth (Skill 34-1). Clients usually are able to ingest or self-administer oral medications with a minimum of problems. Most tablets and capsules should be swallowed and administered with approximately 60 to 100 ml of fluid (as allowed). There may, however, be situations that contraindicate the client's receiving medications by mouth.

The primary contraindications for giving oral medications include the presence of gastrointestinal (GI) alterations, the inability of a client to swallow food or fluids, and the use of gastric suction. An important precaution to take when administering any oral preparation is to protect clients from aspiration. Aspiration occurs when food, fluid, or medication intended for gastrointestinal administration inadvertently is administered into the respiratory tract. The nurse protects the client from aspiration by assessing the client's ability to manage oral medications. Box 34-10 provides techniques the nurse can use to protect the client from aspirating. Properly positioning the client is also essential in preventing aspiration. The nurse positions the client in a seated position when administering oral medications, if not contraindicated by

Text continued on p. 855

Table *34-10*	**Example Evaluation for Client Goals**	
Goal	**Expected Outcomes**	**Evaluative Measure With Example**
Client and family understand medication therapy.	Client and family describe information about medication, dosage, schedule, purpose, and adverse effects.	Written measurement: Have client write out medication schedule for a 24-hour period. Oral questioning: Ask client to describe purpose, dosage, and adverse effects of each prescribed medication.
	Client and family identify situations that require medical intervention.	Oral questioning: Have family describe what to do when a client has adverse effects from a medication.
	Client and family demonstrate appropriate administration technique.	Direct observation: Have client demonstrate filling of an insulin syringe and self-injection.
Client safely self-administers medications.	Client follows prescribed treatment regimen.	Anecdotal notes: Have family keep log of client's compliance with therapy for 1 week.
	Client performs administration techniques correctly.	Direct observation: For example, observe client instill eye drops.
	Client identifies available resources for obtaining necessary medication.	Oral questioning: Ask family to identify how to contact local pharmacy, or community clinic for necessary medications.

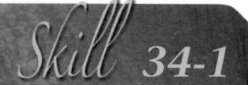 *34-1* /*A*dministering Oral Medications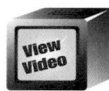

Delegation Considerations

Administering oral medications should not be delegated to assistive personnel (AP). The nurse must instruct AP about potential side effects of medications and to report their occurrence to the nurse.

Equipment

- Medication cart or tray
- Disposable medication cups
- Glass of water, juice, or preferred liquid
- Drinking straw
- Pill-crushing or pillating device (optional)
- Paper towels
- MAR or computer printout

Steps	**Rationale**
1. Assess for any contraindications to client receiving oral medication: Is client suffering from nausea/vomiting? Is client diagnosed as having bowel inflammation or reduced peristalsis? Has client had recent gastrointestinal (GI) surgery? Does client have gastric suction? Check the client's swallow, cough, and gag reflexes.	Alterations in GI function interfere with medication distribution, absorption, and excretion. Clients with GI suction might not receive benefit from the medication because it may be suctioned from the GI tract before it can be absorbed.
2. Assess client's medical history, history of allergies, medication history, and diet history. Client's food and drug allergies should be listed on *each* page of the MAR and should be prominently displayed on the client's medical record. This information may also be on an identification arm band.	These factors can influence how certain medications act. Information also reflects client's need for medications.
3. Gather physical examination and laboratory data that may influence medication administration.	Physical examination or laboratory data may contraindicate medication administration.

Critical Decision Point: If there are any contraindications to the client receiving oral medications, or if in doubt of the client's ability to swallow oral medications, temporarily withhold medication and inform prescriber.

4. Assess client's knowledge regarding health and medication use.	Determines client's need for medication education. Also assists in identifying client's adherence to medication therapy at home. Assessment may reveal medication use problems such as medication tolerance. This occurs when a client desires more and more medication to achieve the desired effect. Other medication use problems are noncompliance, abuse, addiction, or dependence.

Skill **34-1**   *Administering Oral Medications—cont'd*

Steps	Rationale
5. Assess client's preferences for fluids.	Offering fluids during medication administration increases client's fluid intake. Fluids ease swallowing and facilitate absorption from the GI tract. Fluid restrictions must be maintained when applicable.
6. Check accuracy and completeness of each MAR or computer printout with prescriber's written medication order. Check client's name, medication name and dose, route of administration, time for administration, and indication for medication.	The order sheet is the most reliable source and only legal record of medications client is to receive.
7. Prepare medications:	
a. Perform hand hygiene.	Reduces transfer of microorganisms.
b. If medication cart is used, move it outside client's room.	Organization of equipment saves time and reduces error.
c. Unlock medicine drawer or cart.	Medications are safeguarded when locked in cabinet or cart.
d. Prepare medication for one client at a time. Keep all pages of MARs or computer printouts for one client together.	Prevents preparation error. Reading labels and comparing it with transcribed order reduces error.
e. Select correct medication from stock supply or unit-dose drawer. Compare label of medication with MAR or computer printout (see illustration). Check expiration date on all medication labels.	Double-checking reduces risk of error.
f. Calculate medication dose as necessary. Double-check calculation.	Maintains clean technique required of medication administration. Tablets that are prescored can be split to ensure accurate dose is given to client.
g. To prepare tablets or capsules from a floor stock bottle, pour required number into bottle cap and transfer medication to medication cap. Do not touch medication with fingers. Extra tablets or capsules may be returned to bottle.	

Critical Decision Point: Medications that need to be broken to administer half the dose can be broken, using a gloved hand, or cut with a pill-splitting device. Tablets that are to be broken in half must be prescored. Prescored tablets are identified by a manufactured line that transverses the center of the tablet.

h. To prepare unit-dose tablets or capsules, place packaged tablet or capsule directly into medicine cup. (Do not remove wrapper; see illustration.)	Wrapper maintains cleanliness of medications and identifies medication name and dose.

Critical Decision Point: If preparing narcotics, check narcotic record for previous drug count and compare with supply available and uphold controlled substance laws.

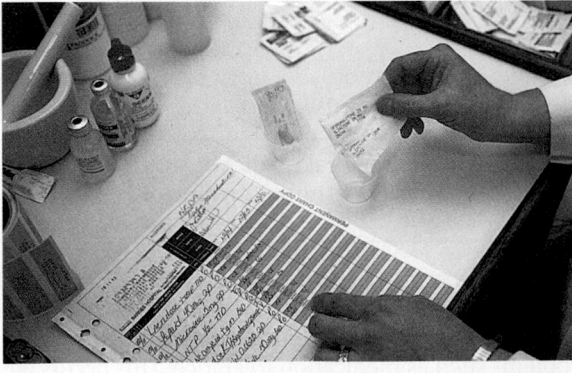

STEP **7e** The nurse verifies each medication with the MAR.

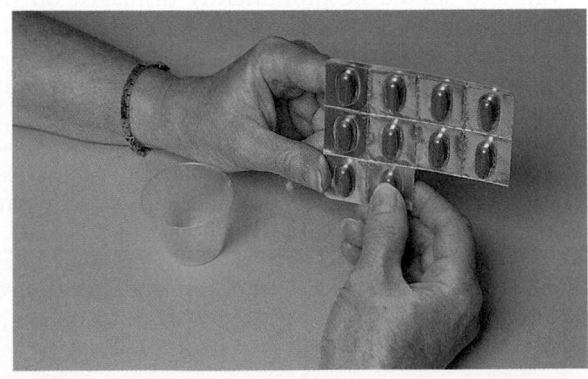

STEP **7h**   Place tablet into medicine cup without removing wrapper.

Steps   **Rationale**

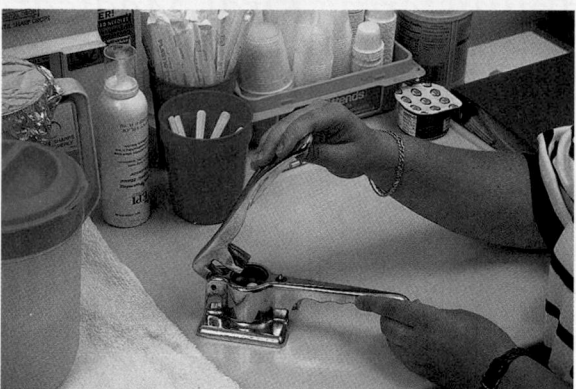

STEP **7j** Pill-crushing device used to crush pills when necessary.

i. All tablets or capsules to be given to client at same time may be placed in one medicine cup except for those requiring preadministration assessments (e.g., pulse rate or blood pressure).

Keeping medications that require preadministration assessments separate from others makes it easier for the nurse to withhold medications as necessary.

Critical Decision Point: Not all medications can be crushed (e.g., capsules, enteric-coated drugs). Consult with pharmacist when in doubt. Choking or aspiration of particles of medication or applesauce can also occur.

---

j. If the client has difficulty swallowing, and liquid medications are not an option, use pill-crushing device such as a mortar and pestle to grind pills (see illustration). If a pill-crushing device is not available, place tablet between two medication cups and grind with a blunt instrument. Mix ground tablet in small amount of soft food (custard or applesauce).

Large tablets can be difficult to swallow. Ground tablet mixed with palatable soft food is usually easier to swallow.

k. To prepare liquids:
   (1) Gently shake container. If medication is in a unit-dose container with correct amount to administer, no further preparation is needed. If medication is in a multidose bottle remove bottle cap from container and place cap upside down.

Shaking container ensures medication is mixed before administration. Placing cap of bottle upside down prevents contamination of inside of cap.

   (2) Hold multidose bottle with label against palm of hand while pouring.

Spilled liquid will not soil or fade label.

   (3) Hold medication cup at eye level and fill to desired level on scale (see illustration). Scale should be even with fluid level at its surface or base of meniscus, not edges. Draw up volumes of less than 10 ml in syringe without needle (see illustration).

Ensures accuracy of measurement.

   (4) Discard any excess liquid into sink. Wipe lip and neck of bottle with paper towel.

Prevents contamination of bottle's contents and prevents bottle cap from sticking.

l. Compare MAR or computer printout with prepared medication and container.

Reading label second time reduces error.

m. Return stock containers or unused unit-dose medications to shelf or drawer and read label again.

Third check of label reduces administration errors.

n. Do not leave medications unattended.

Nurse is responsible for safekeeping of drugs.

8. Administering medications:
   a. Take medications to client at correct time.

Medications are administered within 30 minutes before or after prescribed time to ensure intended therapeutic effect. STAT or single-order medications should be given at time ordered.

Skill 34-1   *Administering Oral Medications—cont'd*

Steps	Rationale

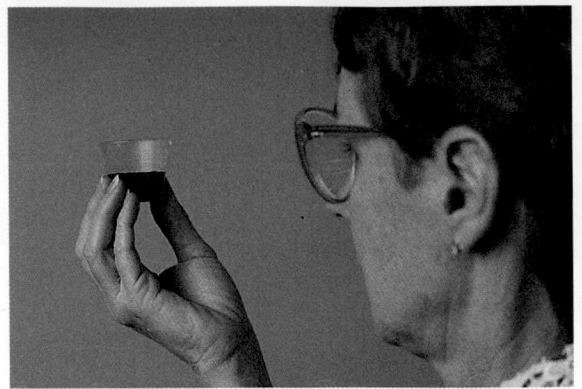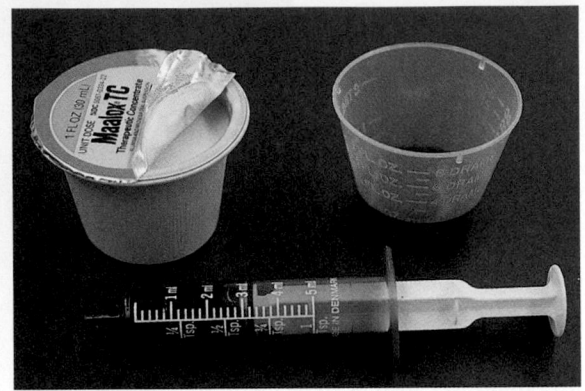

STEP **7k(3) A,** Pour the desired volume of liquid so that base of meniscus is level with line on scale. **B,** Use needleless syringe to draw up volumes less than 10 ml.

b. Identify client by comparing name on MAR or computer printout with name on client's identification bracelet. Ask client to state name.

Identification bracelets are made at time of client's admission and are most reliable source of identification.

Critical Decision Point: Client identification bracelets that are missing, illegible, or faded must be replaced.

---

c. Explain purpose of each medication and its action to client. Allow client to ask any questions about drugs.

Client has right to be informed, and client's understanding of purpose of each medication improves compliance with medication therapy.

d. Assist client to sitting or side-lying position if sitting is contraindicated.

Sitting position prevents aspiration during swallowing (Galvan, 2001).

e. Administer medications:

(1) **For tablets:** Client may wish to hold solid medications in hand or cup before placing in mouth.

Client can become familiar with medications by seeing each drug.

(2) Offer water or juice to help client swallow medications. Give cold carbonated water if available and not contraindicated.

Choice of fluid promotes client's comfort and can improve fluid intake. Carbonated water helps passage of tablet through esophagus.

(3) **For sublingual-administered medications:** Have client place medication under tongue and allow it to dissolve completely (see Figure 34-5, p. 833). Caution client against swallowing tablet.

Medication is absorbed through blood vessels of undersurface of tongue. If swallowed, medication is destroyed by gastric juices or so rapidly detoxified by liver that therapeutic blood levels are not attained.

(4) **For buccal medications:** Have client place medication in mouth against mucous membranes of the cheek until it dissolves (see Figure 34-6, p. 833). Avoid administering liquids until buccal medication has dissolved.

Buccal medications act locally on mucosa or systemically as they are swallowed in saliva.

(5) **For powdered medications:** Mix with liquids at bedside and give to client to drink.

When prepared in advance, powdered medications may thicken and even harden, making swallowing difficult.

(6) Caution client against chewing or swallowing lozenges.

Medication acts through slow absorption through oral mucosa, not gastric mucosa.

(7) Give effervescent powders and tablets immediately after dissolving.

Effervescence improves unpleasant taste of medication and often relieves GI problems.

f. If client is unable to hold medications, place medication cup to the lips and gently introduce each drug into the mouth, one at a time. Do not rush.

Administering single tablet or capsule eases swallowing and decreases risk of aspiration.

Steps	Rationale
g. If tablet or capsule falls to the floor, discard it and repeat preparation.	Medication is contaminated when it touches floor.
h. Stay until client has completely swallowed each medication. Ask client to open mouth if uncertain whether medication has been swallowed.	Nurse is responsible for ensuring that client receives ordered dosage. If left unattended, client may not take dose or may save medications, causing risk to health.
i. For highly acidic medications (e.g., aspirin), offer client nonfat snack (e.g., crackers) if not contraindicated by client's condition.	Reduces gastric irritation.
j. Assist client in returning to comfortable position.	Maintains client's comfort.
k. Dispose of soiled supplies and perform hand hygiene.	Reduces transmission of microorganisms.
9. Evaluate client's response to medications at times that correlate with the medication's onset, peak, and duration.	Evaluates medication's therapeutic benefit and can detect onset of side effects or allergic reactions.
10. Ask client or family member to identify medication name and explain purpose, action, dosage schedule, and potential side effects of drug.	Determines level of knowledge gained by client and family.

Unexpected Outcomes and Related Interventions

- Client exhibits adverse effects (side effect, toxic effect, allergic reaction).
  - Symptoms such as urticaria, rash, pruritus, rhinitis, and wheezing may indicate allergic reaction.
  - Always notify prescriber and pharmacy when the client exhibits adverse effects. Withhold further doses.
- Client refuses medication.
  - Explore reasons why client does not want medication.
  - Educate if misunderstandings of medication therapy are apparent.
  - Do not force client to take medication; clients have the right to refuse treatment.
  - If client continues to refuse medication despite educational attempts, record why the drug was withheld on client's chart and notify prescriber.

Recording and Reporting

- Record administration of oral medications on MAR, using nurse's initials or signature.
- Record the reason any drug is withheld and follow agency's policy for proper recording.

Home Care Considerations

- Instruct clients on all aspects of medication administration, including dosage, desired effect, when to take medications, anticipated side effects, and whether to take medication with or without food, to ensure safe medication administration at home.

a client's condition. Appropriate personnel (e.g., speech therapist) should evaluate clients who have difficulty swallowing before oral medications are given.

For clients with nasogastric feeding tubes, liquid medications are preferred, but some tablets can be crushed and capsules opened to mix in a solution for administration (Box 34-11).

Topical Medication Applications

Topical medications are medications that are applied locally, most often to intact skin. They can be in the form of lotions, pastes, or ointments (see Table 34-1, p. 824). They can also be applied to mucous membranes.

Skin Applications. Because many locally applied medications such as lotions, pastes, and ointments can create systemic and local effects, the nurse should apply these medications using gloves and applicators. Sterile technique is used if the client has an open wound.

Skin encrustation and dead tissues harbor microorganisms and block contact of medications with the tissues to be treated. Simply applying new medications over previously applied medications does little to prevent infection or offer therapeutic benefit. Before applying medications, the nurse cleans the skin thoroughly by washing the area gently with soap and water, soaking an involved site, or locally debriding tissue.

When applying ointments or pastes, the nurse spreads the medication evenly over the involved surface and covers the area well without applying an overly thick layer. Opaque ointments prevent visualization of underlying skin. Prescribers may order a gauze dressing to be applied over the medication to prevent soiling of clothes and wiping away of the medication. Each type of medication, whether an ointment, lotion, powder, or other type, should be applied a specific way to ensure proper penetration and absorption. The nurse applies lotions and creams by smearing them lightly onto the skin's surface; rubbing

---

Box 34-10   Protecting the Client From Aspiration

- Determine the client's ability to swallow.
- Assess the client's cough.
- Determine the presence of a gag reflex.
- Prepare oral medications in the form that is easiest to swallow.
- Allow the client to self-administer medications if possible.
- If the client has unilateral weakness, place the medication in the stronger side of the mouth.
- Administer pills one at a time, ensuring that each medication is properly swallowed before the next one is introduced.
- Thicken regular liquids or offer fruit nectars if the client cannot tolerate thin liquids.
- Avoid straws because they decrease the control the client has over volume intake, which increases the risk of aspiration.
- Have client hold and drink from cup if possible.
- Time medications to coincide with mealtimes or when the client is well rested and awake if possible.
- Administer medications using another route if risk of aspiration is severe.

Modified from Galvan TJ: Dysphagia: going down and staying down, *Am J Nurs* 101(1):37, 2001.

may cause irritation. A liniment is applied by rubbing it gently but firmly into the skin. A powder is dusted lightly to cover the affected area with a thin layer. During any application the nurse should assess the skin thoroughly. To record administration, the area applied, name of medication, and condition of skin should be noted.

Nasal Instillation. Clients with nasal sinus alterations may receive medications by spray, drops, or tampons (Skill 34-2). The most commonly administered form of nasal instillation is decongestant spray or drops, used to relieve symptoms of sinus congestion and colds. Clients must be cautioned to avoid abuse of medications because overuse can lead to a rebound effect in which the nasal congestion worsens. When excess decongestant solution is swallowed, serious systemic effects may also develop, especially in children. Saline drops are safer as a decongestant for children than nasal preparations that contain sympathomimetics (e.g., Afrin or Neo-Synephrine).

It is easier to have the client self-administer sprays, because the client can control the spray and inhale as it enters the nasal passages. For clients who use nasal sprays repeatedly, the nurse checks the nares for irritation. Nasal drops are effective in treating sinus infections. The nurse positions clients to permit the medication to reach the affected sinus.

Severe nosebleeds are usually treated with packing or nasal tampons, which are treated with epinephrine, to reduce blood flow. Usually a physician or advanced practice clinician places nasal tampons.

Eye Instillation. Common medications used by clients are eye drops and ointments, including over-the-counter preparations such as artificial tears and vasoconstrictors (e.g., Visine and Murine). However, many

---

Box 34-11   Procedural Guidelines

Giving Medications Through a Nasogastric Tube, Intestinal Tube, Gastrostomy Tube, or Small-Bore Feeding Tube

- Investigate and use alternative routes of medication administration if possible (e.g., transdermal, rectal).
- Avoid complicated medication regimens that frequently interrupt enteral feedings.
- Avoid giving elixirs or medications with a pH of less than 4.
- Verify that the medication is compatible with the enteral feeding before administration. If the medication is incompatible with the feeding, stop the feeding 1 to 2 hours before medication is given, and restart the feeding 1 to 2 hours after the medication is given. **Never** add medications directly to the tube feeding.
- Verify tube placement before administering medications (see Chapters 43 and 45).
- Administer medications in a liquid form (suspension, elixir, or solution) when possible to prevent tube obstruction.
- Before crushing tablets, be sure they can be crushed. Buccal, sublingual, enteric-coated, or sustained-released medications cannot be crushed. Read medication labels carefully before crushing a tablet or opening a capsule.
- Dissolve crushed tablets, gelatin capsules, and powders in 15 to 30 ml of warm water. Dissolve and administer each medication separately, flushing between 1 and 30 ml of water between each medication. Irrigate the tube after all medication is given. Unless contraindicated, the total amount of liquid volume administered to the client for each medication may range from 60 to 150 ml of water.
- Do not use pigtail vent for irrigation or instillation of fluid.
- Do not give whole or undissolved medications through the feeding tube.
- Continually evaluate the client's response to medication therapy. If the desired effect is not achieved, a different medication or route of administration may be indicated because of problems with the drug bioavailability when given the enteral route.

Modified from Bryson E: Drug administration via a nasogastric tube, *Nurs Times* 97(16):51, 2002; and Gilbar PJ: A guide to enteral drug administration in palliative care, *J Pain Symptom Manage* 17(3):197, 1999.

clients receive prescribed **ophthalmic** medications for eye conditions, such as glaucoma, and after cataract extraction. A large percentage of clients receiving eye medications are older adults. Age-related problems, including poor vision, hand tremors, and difficulty grasping or manipulating containers, affect the ease with which the older adult can self-administer eye medications. The nurse instructs clients and family members about the proper techniques for administering eye medications (Skill 34-3). The nurse may determine the

Text continued on p. 862

Skill 34-2 *Administering Nasal Instillations*

Delegation Considerations

Administration of nasal drops and ointments should not be delegated to assistive personnel (AP). The nurse must instruct AP about potential side effects of medications and to report their occurrence to the nurse.

Equipment

- Prepared medication with clean dropper or spray container
- Facial tissue
- Small pillow (optional)
- Washcloth (optional)
- Disposable gloves (optional, only if client has extensive nasal drainage)
- MAR or computer printout
- Penlight (to inspect nares; if ointment is to be applied to a specific lesion inside the nares)

Steps	Rationale
1. For nasal drops, determine which sinus is affected by referring to medical record.	Affects client's position during drug instillation.
2. Assess client's history of hypertension, heart disease, diabetes mellitus, and hyperthyroidism.	These conditions can contraindicate use of decongestants that stimulate central nervous system (CNS). Side effects of transient hypertension, tachycardia, palpitations, and headache may occur.
3. Review physician's order, including client's name, medication name, dosage, route, time of administration and indication.	
4. Determine whether client has any known allergies to nasal instillations	
5. Identify client; compare name on MAR with client's ID bracelet. Ask client to state name.	Ensures that correct client receives medication.
6. Perform hand hygiene. Using a penlight, inspect condition of nose and sinuses. Palpate sinuses for tenderness.	Prevents infection. Provides baseline to monitor effects of medication. Presence of discharge interferes with medication absorption.
7. Assess client's knowledge regarding use of nasal instillations and technique for instillation and willingness to learn self-administration.	May necessitate health teaching regarding use of medications. Motivation influences teaching approach.
8. Explain procedure to client regarding positioning and sensations to expect, such as burning or stinging of mucosa or choking sensation as medication trickles into throat.	Helps client anticipate experience of procedure to reduce anxiety.
9. Arrange supplies and medications at bedside. Apply gloves if client has nasal drainage.	Reduces transmission of microorganisms, ensures smooth, orderly procedure, and prevents exposure to body fluids (NIOSH, 1999).
10. Instruct client to clear or blow nose gently unless contraindicated (e.g., risk of increased intracranial pressure or nosebleeds).	Removes mucus and secretions that can block distribution of medication.
11. Administer nasal drops:	
a. Assist client to supine position.	Position provides access to nasal passages.
b. Position head properly:	
(1) For access to posterior pharynx, tilt client's head backward.	
(2) For access to ethmoid or sphenoid sinus, tilt head back over edge of bed or place small pillow under client's shoulder and tilt head back (see illustration).	
(3) For access to frontal and maxillary sinus, tilt head back over edge of bed or pillow with head turned toward side to be treated (see illustration).	Position allows medication to drain into affected sinus.
c. Support client's head with nondominant hand.	Prevents straining of neck muscles.
d. Instruct client to breathe through mouth.	Mouth breathing reduces chance of aspirating nasal drops into trachea and lungs.

Skill 34-2 Administering Nasal Instillations—cont'd

Steps	Rationale

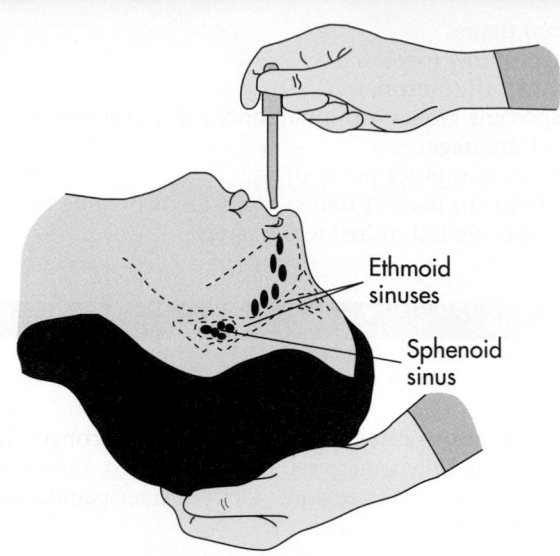

STEP **11b(2)** Position for instilling nose drops into ethmoid or sphenoid sinus.

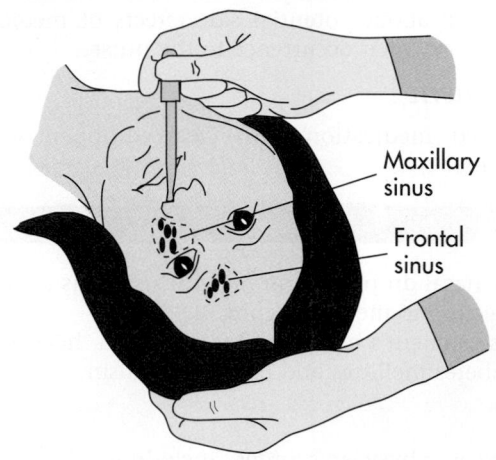

STEP **11b(3)** Position for instilling nose drops into frontal and maxillary sinus.

e. Hold dropper 1 cm (½ in) above nares and instill prescribed number of drops toward midline of ethmoid bone.	Avoids contamination of dropper. Instilling toward ethmoid bone facilitates distribution of medication over nasal mucosa.
f. Have client remain in supine position 5 min.	Prevents premature loss of medication through nares.
g. Offer facial tissue to blot runny nose, but caution client against blowing nose for several minutes.	Allows maximal amount of medication to be absorbed.
12. Assist client to a comfortable position after medication is absorbed.	Restores comfort.
13. Dispose of soiled supplies in proper container and perform hand hygiene.	Maintains neat, orderly environment. Reduces spread of microorganisms.
14. Observe client for onset of side effects 15 to 30 min after administration.	Drugs absorbed through mucosa can cause systemic reaction.
15. Ask if client is able to breathe through nose after decongestant administration. May be necessary to have client occlude one nostril at a time and breathe deeply.	Determines effectiveness of decongestant medication.
16. Reinspect condition of nasal passages between the instillations.	Condition of mucosa reveals response to medication.
17. Ask client to review risks of overuse of decongestants and methods for administration.	Feedback ensures that client can self-administer medications properly.
18. Have client demonstrate self-medication.	Feedback demonstrates learning.

Unexpected Outcomes and Related Interventions

- Client begins wheezing or displays other signs of allergic reaction to drug.
  - Follow institutional policy or guidelines for appropriate response to allergic reactions.
  - Notify client's health care provider immediately.
- Client is unable to breathe easily through nasal passages. Mucosa appears swollen, and congestion is unrelieved.
  - Client may be experiencing rebound effect. Stop medication use and notify prescriber.
- Nasal mucosa remains inflamed and tender with discharge from nares.
  - Inflammatory or infectious process remains. May need to consider alternative therapy.
- Client complains of sinus headache. Sinuses remain congested.
  - May need to consider alternative therapy.
- Client is unable to explain technique and risks of drug therapy.
  - Further explanation is required.
- Client is unable to self-administer medication.
  - Reinstruction is necessary.

Recording and Reporting

- Record medication name, concentration, number of drops, nostril into which medication was instilled, and time of administration on MAR.
- Record client's response in nurses' notes.
- Report any unusual systemic effects to nurse in charge or physician.

Home Care Considerations

- Caution clients against overuse of nasal spray decongestants at home because they can cause rebound effect, worsening mucosal swelling.
- Nasal applicators should be rinsed after each use.
- Clients should discard over-the-counter nasal sprays or nose drops after one illness because the bottles can become easily contaminated with bacteria after use.
- Each family member should have a different dropper or spray applicator.

Skill 34-3   *Administering Ophthalmic Medications*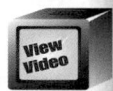

Delegation Considerations

Administration of eye drops and ointments should not be delegated to assistive personnel (AP). The nurse should instruct AP about potential side effects of medications and to report their occurrence to the nurse.

Equipment

- Medication bottle with sterile eye dropper or ointment tube or medicated intraocular disk
- Cotton ball or tissue
- Washbasin filled with warm water and washcloth if eyes have crust or drainage
- Eye patch and tape (optional)
- Clean gloves
- MAR or computer printout

Steps	Rationale
1. Review prescriber's medication order for number of drops (if a liquid) and eye (right = O.D.; left = O.S.; both = O.U.) to receive medication.	Ensures correct administration of medication.
2. Identify client. Compare name on MAR with client ID band. Ask client to state name.	Ensures that correct client receives medication.
3. Assess condition of external eye structures. (May also be done just before drug instillation.)	Provides baseline to later determine if local response to medications occurs. Also indicates need to clean eye before medication application.
4. Determine whether client has any known allergies to eye medications. Also ask if client has allergy to latex.	Protects client from risk of allergic medication response. If client has latex allergy, use nonlatex gloves.
5. Determine whether client has any symptoms of visual alterations.	Certain eye medications act to either lessen or increase these symptoms. Nurse must be able to recognize change in client's condition after drop is administered.
6. Assess client's level of consciousness and ability to follow directions.	If client becomes restless or combative during procedure, a greater risk of accidental eye injury exists.
7. Assess client's knowledge regarding medication therapy and desire to self-administer medication.	Client's level of understanding may indicate need for health teaching. Motivation influences teaching approach.

Skill 34-3 *Administering Ophthalmic Medications—cont'd*

Steps	Rationale
8. Assess client's ability to manipulate and hold dropper.	Reflects client's ability to learn to self-administer medication.
9. Explain procedure to client.	Relieves anxiety about medication being instilled into eye.
10. Perform hand hygiene and arrange supplies at bedside; apply disposable gloves.	Reduces transmission of microorganisms, ensures a smooth, orderly procedure, and follows Centers for Disease Control and Prevention (CDC) recommendations to prevent accidental exposure to body fluids (NIOSH, 1999).
11. Ask client to lie supine or sit back in chair with head slightly hyperextended.	Position provides easy access to eye for medication instillation and minimizes drainage of medication through tear duct.

Critical Decision Point: Do not hyperextend the neck of a client with cervical spine injury.

---

12. If crusts or drainage are present along eyelid margins or inner canthus, gently wash away. Soak any crusts that are dried and difficult to remove by applying damp washcloth or cotton ball over eye for a few minutes. Always wipe clean from inner to outer canthus.	Crusts or drainage harbors microorganisms. Soaking allows easy removal and prevents pressure from being applied directly over eye. Cleansing from inner to outer canthus avoids entrance of microorganism into lacrimal duct.
13. Hold cotton ball or clean tissue in nondominant hand on client's cheekbone just below lower eyelid.	Cotton or tissue absorbs medication that escapes eye.
14. With tissue or cotton resting below lower lid, gently press downward with thumb or forefinger against bony orbit.	Technique exposes lower conjunctival sac. Retraction against bony orbit prevents pressure and trauma to eyeball and prevents fingers from touching eye.
15. Ask client to look at ceiling and explain steps to client.	Action retracts sensitive cornea up and away from conjunctival sac and reduces stimulation of blink reflex.
A. Instill eye drops:	
(1) With dominant hand resting on client's forehead, hold filled medication eye dropper or ophthalmic solution approximately 1 to 2 cm (½ to ¾ in) above conjunctival sac (see illustration).	Helps prevent accidental contact of eye dropper with eye structures, thus reducing risk of injury to eye and transfer of infection to dropper (McConnell, 2001). Ophthalmic medications are sterile.
(2) Drop prescribed number of medication drops into conjunctival sac.	Conjunctival sac normally holds 1 or 2 drops. Provides even distribution of medication across eye.
(3) If client blinks or closes eye or if drops land on outer lid margins, repeat procedure.	Therapeutic effect of drug is obtained only when drops enter conjunctival sac.
(4) After instilling drops, ask client to close eye gently.	Helps to distribute medication. Squinting or squeezing of eyelids forces medication from conjunctival sac.

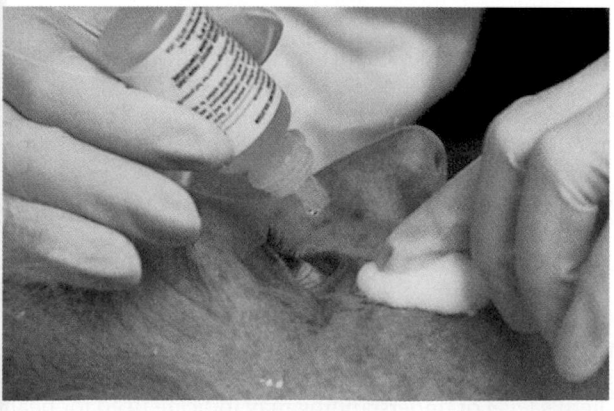

STEP **15A(1)** Hold eye dropper above conjunctival sac.

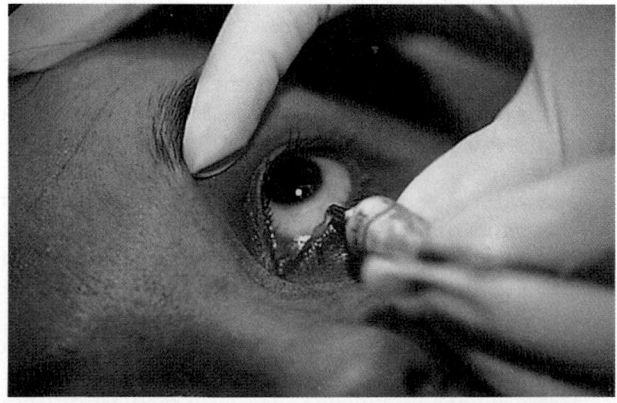

STEP **15B(1)** Apply ointment along lower eyelid.

Steps	Rationale
(5) When administering medications that cause systemic effects, apply gentle pressure with your finger and clean tissue on the client's nasolacrimal duct for 30 to 60 seconds.	Prevents overflow of medication into nasal and pharyngeal passages. Prevents absorption into systemic circulation (McConnell, 2001).
B. Instill eye ointment:	
(1) Holding ointment applicator above lower lid margin, apply thin stream of ointment evenly along inner edge of lower eyelid on conjunctiva (see illustration) from the inner canthus to outer canthus.	Distributes medication evenly across eye and lid margin.
(2) Have client close eye and rub lid lightly in circular motion with cotton ball, if rubbing is not contraindicated.	Further distributes medication without traumatizing eye.
C. Intraocular disk	
(1) Application:	
a. Open package containing the disk. Gently press fingertip against the disk so that it adheres to finger. Position the convex side of the disk on fingertip (see illustration).	Allows nurse to inspect disk for damage or deformity.
b. With other hand, gently pull the client's lower eyelid away from the eye. Ask client to look up.	Prepares conjunctival sac for receiving medicated disk.
c. Place the disk in the conjunctival sac, so that it floats on the sclera between the iris and lower eyelid (see illustration).	Ensures delivery of medication.
d. Pull the client's lower eyelid out and over the disk (see illustration).	Ensures accurate medication delivery.

Critical Decision Point: You should not be able to see the disk at this time. Repeat step 15C(1)d if you can see the disk.

---

(2) Removal:	
a. Perform hand hygiene and apply gloves.	Prevents transfer of microorganisms and follows CDC recommendations for prevention of accidental exposure to body fluids (NIOSH, 1999).
b. Explain procedure to client.	Relieves anxiety about manipulation of disk in eye.
c. Gently pull on the client's lower eyelid.	Exposes intraocular disk.
d. Using forefinger and thumb of opposite hand, pinch the disk and lift it out of the client's eye (see illustration).	

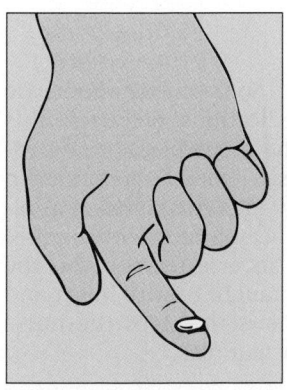

STEP **15C(1)a** Gently position the convex side of the disk against fingertips.

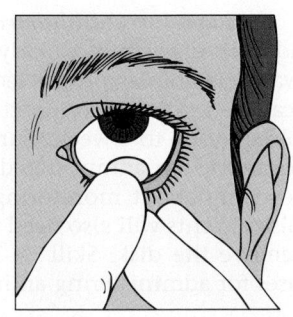

STEP **15C(1)c** Place disk in the conjunctival sac between the iris and lower eyelid.

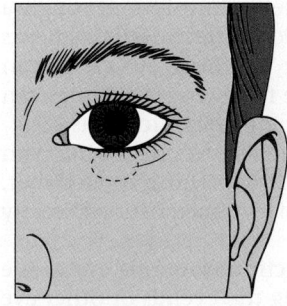

STEP **15C(1)d** Gently pull lower eyelid over the disk.

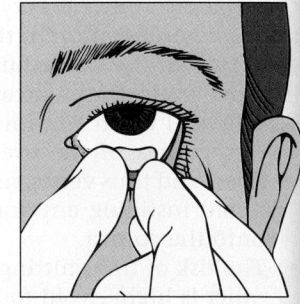

STEP **15C(2)d** Carefully pinch the disk to remove it from client's eye

Skill 34-3   *Administering Ophthalmic Medications—cont'd*

Steps	Rationale
16. If excess medication is on eyelid, gently wipe it from inner to outer canthus.	Promotes comfort and prevents trauma to eye.
17. If client had eye patch, apply clean one by placing it over affected eye so entire eye is covered. Tape securely without applying pressure to eye.	Clean eye patch reduces chance of infection.

Critical Decision Point: If client receives more than one eye medication to the same eye at the same time, wait at least 5 minutes before administering the next medication to avoid interaction between medications (Patient's Library, 2000).

Steps	Rationale
18. Remove gloves, dispose of soiled supplies in proper receptacle, and perform hand hygiene.	Maintains neat environment at bedside and reduces transmission of microorganisms.
19. Note client's response to instillation; ask if any discomfort was felt.	Determines if procedure was performed correctly and safely.
20. Observe response to medication by assessing visual changes and noting any side effects.	Evaluates effects of medication.
21. Ask client to discuss medication's purpose, action, side effects, and technique of administration.	Determines client's level of understanding.
22. Have client demonstrate self-administration of next dose.	Provides feedback regarding competency with skill.

Unexpected Outcomes and Related Interventions

- Client cannot instill drops without supervision.
  - Reinforce teaching and allow client to self-administer drops as much as possible to enhance confidence.
  - If client cannot self-administer drops, teach others, such as family members, to instill drops into the client's eye.
- Client displays signs of allergic reaction (e.g., tearing, reddened sclera) or systemic response (e.g., bradycardia) to medication.
  - Hold medication and speak with prescriber.
  - Follow institutional policy or guidelines for reporting of adverse or allergic reaction to medications.

Recording and Reporting

- Record medication, concentration, number of drops, time of administration, and eye (left, right, or both) that received medication on MAR.
- Record appearance of eye in nurses' notes.

Home Care Considerations

- Clients with chronic health care problems should consult with their health care provider before using over-the-counter eye medication.
- When using eye drops at home, clients should not share medications with other family members because risk of infection transmission is high.

client and family's ability to self-administer through a return demonstration of the procedure. Showing clients each step of the procedure for instilling eye drops can improve their compliance. The following principles can be followed when administering eye medications:

- The cornea of the eye is richly supplied with pain fibers and thus very sensitive to anything applied to it. Avoid instilling any form of eye medication directly onto the cornea.
- The risk of transmitting infection from one eye to the other is high. Avoid touching the eyelids or other eye structures with eye droppers or ointment tubes.
- Use eye medication only for the client's affected eye. Never allow a client to use another client's eye medications.

Intraocular Administration. Some medications are administered intraocularly. Medications delivered this way resemble a contact lens. The nurse places the medication into the conjunctival sac where it remains in place for up to 1 week. Currently medications such as pilocarpine are administered this way. The client requires teaching about monitoring for adverse reactions to the disk. Clients will also need to be taught how to insert and remove the disk. Skill 34-3 reviews the steps the nurse uses for administering an intraocular disk.

Ear Instillation. Internal ear structures are very sensitive to temperature extremes. Failure to instill ear drops or irrigating fluid at room temperature may cause vertigo, dizziness, or nausea. Although the structures of the outer

Box 34-12 *Procedural Guidelines*

For Administering Ear Medications

Ear Drops

1. Have client assume side-lying position (if not contraindicated by client's condition) with ear to be treated facing up, or client may sit in chair or at the bedside.
2. Perform hand hygiene. Apply gloves if drainage is present.
3. Straighten ear canal by pulling auricle down and back (children) or upward and outward (adult).

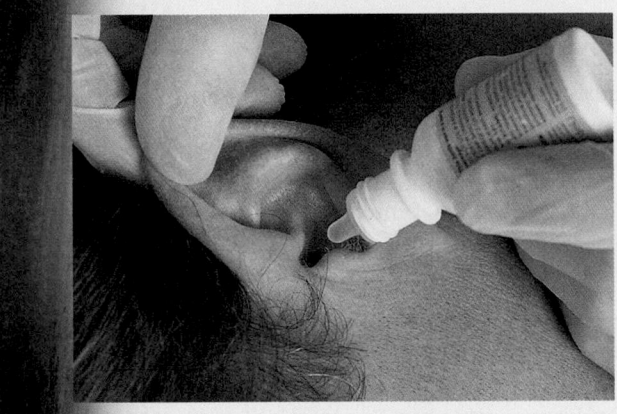

STEP **4** Placing ear drop in ear.

4. Instill prescribed drops holding dropper 1 cm (½ in) above ear canal (see illustration).
5. Ask client to remain in side-lying position 2 to 3 min. Apply gentle massage or pressure to tragus of ear with finger unless contraindicated due to pain.
6. At times the prescriber orders insertion of portion of cotton ball into outermost part of canal. Do not press cotton into canal. Remove cotton after 15 min.

Ear Irrigations

1. Assess the tympanic membrane or review medical record for history of eardrum perforation, which would contraindicate ear irrigation.
2. Assist client in assuming sitting or lying position with head tilted or turned toward affected ear. Place towel under client's head and shoulder and have client hold basin under affected ear.
3. Perform hand hygiene. Apply gloves if drainage is present.
4. Fill irrigating syringe with solution (approximately 50 ml).
5. Gently grasp auricle and straighten ear canal by pulling it down and back (children) or upward and outward (adult).
6. Slowly instill irrigating solution by holding tip of syringe 1 cm (½ in) above opening of ear canal. Allow fluid to drain out during instillation. Continue until canal is cleansed or all solution is used.

---

ear are not sterile, sterile drops and solutions are used in case the eardrum is ruptured. The entrance of nonsterile solutions into middle ear structures could result in infection. With ear drainage, the nurse should assess to be sure the client does not have a ruptured eardrum. A nurse should never occlude the ear canal with the dropper or irrigating syringe. Forcing medication into an occluded ear canal creates pressure that may injure the eardrum. Box 34-12 reviews guidelines for administering ear drops.

External ear structures of children differ from those of adults. When instilling drops or irrigating solutions, the nurse must straighten the ear canal. In infants and young children the nurse straightens the cartilaginous canal by grasping the auricle of the ear and pulling it gently down and backward. In adults the ear canal is longer and composed of underlying bone and is straightened by pulling the auricle upward and outward. Failure to straighten the canal properly may prevent medicinal solutions from reaching the deeper external ear structures.

Vaginal Instillation. Vaginal medications are available as suppositories, foam, jellies, or creams. Suppositories come individually packaged in foil wrappers and may be stored in the refrigerator to prevent the solid, oval-shaped suppositories from melting. After a suppository is inserted into the vaginal cavity, body temperature causes it to melt and be distributed and absorbed. Foam, jellies, and creams are administered with an applicator inserter (Skill

34-4). A suppository is given with a gloved hand in accordance with body substance isolation (see Chapter 33). Clients often prefer administering their own vaginal medications and should be given privacy. After instillation of the medication, a client may wish to wear a perineal pad to collect drainage. Because vaginal medications are often given to treat infection, discharge may be foul smelling. Aseptic technique should be followed, and the client should be offered frequent opportunities to maintain perineal hygiene (see Chapter 38).

Rectal Instillation. Rectal suppositories are thinner and more bullet shaped than vaginal suppositories. The rounded end prevents anal trauma during insertion. Rectal suppositories contain medications that exert local effects such as promoting defecation or systemic effects such as reducing nausea. Rectal suppositories are often stored in the refrigerator until administered.

During administration, the nurse must place the suppository past the internal anal sphincter and against the rectal mucosa (Skill 34-5). Otherwise the suppository may be expelled before it can dissolve and be absorbed into the mucosa. With practice a nurse learns to recognize the sensation of the sphincter relaxing around the finger. The suppository should not be forced into a mass of fecal material. It may be necessary to clear the rectum with a small cleansing enema before a suppository can be inserted.

Text continued on p. 867

Skill 34-4   *Administering Vaginal Medications*

Delegation Considerations

Administering medications by the vaginal route should not be delegated to assistive personnel (AP). The nurse should instruct AP about the following:

- To report any new or increased vaginal discharge or bleeding
- Potential side effects of medications and to report their occurrence to the nurse

Equipment

- Vaginal creams, foam, jelly, or suppositories, or irrigating solutions with applicator (if required)
- Clean gloves
- Towels and/or washcloth
- Perineal pad
- Drape or sheet
- Water-soluble lubricating jelly
- MAR or computer printout

Steps	Rationale
1. Review physician's order, including client's name, medication name, form (cream or suppository), route, dosage, time of administration, and drug indication.	Ensures safe and correct administration of medication.
2. Review client's history of allergies, including latex.	Protects client from risk of allergic medication response.
3. Perform hand hygiene.	Reduces transfer of microorganisms.

Critical Decision Point: Rectal and vaginal suppositories may be stored near one another in the refrigerator. Vaginal suppositories are larger and more oval.

4. Identify client; compare name on MAR with identification bracelet, and ask client's name.	Ensures that correct client receives medication.
5. Inspect condition of external genitalia and vaginal canal (see Chapter 32). (May perform just before insertion.)	Findings provide baseline to monitor effect of medication.
6. Assess client's ability to manipulate applicator or suppository and to position self to insert medication.	Mobility restriction indicates level of assistance required from nurse.
7. Explain procedure to client. Be specific if client plans to self-administer medication.	Promotes understanding. Will enable client to self-administer medication if physically able.
8. Arrange supplies at bedside.	Ensures smooth procedure.
9. Close room curtain or door.	Provides privacy.
10. Assist client to lie in dorsal recumbent position.	Provides easy access to and good exposure of vaginal canal. Also allows suppository to dissolve without escaping through orifice.
11. Keep abdomen and lower extremities draped.	Minimizes client embarrassment.
12. Apply clean gloves.	Prevents transmission of microorganisms and follows CDC recommendations to prevent accidental exposure to body fluids (NIOSH, 1999).
13. Ensure vaginal orifice is well illuminated by room light or gooseneck lamp. Cleanse area with towel or washcloth if necessary.	Proper insertion requires visualization of external genitalia.
14. Insert suppository with gloved hand:	
a. Remove suppository from foil wrapper and apply liberal amount of sterile water-based lubricating jelly to smooth or rounded end. Lubricate gloved index finger of dominant hand.	Lubrication reduces friction against mucosal surfaces during insertion.
b. With nondominant gloved hand, gently retract labial folds.	Exposes vaginal orifice.
c. Insert rounded end of suppository along posterior wall of vaginal canal entire length of finger (7.5 to 10 cm or 3 to 4 in) (see illustration).	Proper placement ensures equal distribution of medication along walls of vaginal cavity.
d. Withdraw finger and wipe away remaining lubricant from around orifice and labia.	Maintains comfort.
15. Apply cream or foam:	
a. Fill cream or foam applicator following package directions.	Dose is prescribed by volume in applicator.

Steps	Rationale

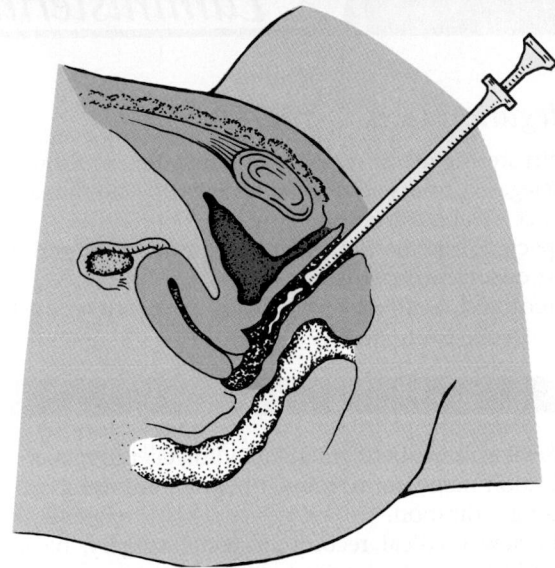

STEP **14c**   Insertion of suppository into the vaginal canal.   STEP **15c**   Instillation of medication in vaginal canal.

Steps	Rationale
b. With nondominant gloved hand, gently retract labial folds.	Exposes vaginal orifice.
c. With dominant gloved hand, insert applicator approximately 5 to 7.5 cm (2 to 3 in). Push applicator plunger to deposit medication into vagina (see illustration).	Allows equal distribution of medication along vaginal walls.
d. Withdraw applicator and place on paper towel. Wipe off residual cream from labia or vaginal orifice.	Residual cream on applicator may contain microorganisms.
16. Dispose of supplies, remove gloves, and perform hand hygiene.	Maintains neat environment and reduces transfer of microorganisms.
17. Instruct client to remain on back for at least 10 min.	Medication will be distributed and absorbed evenly throughout vaginal cavity and not be lost through orifice.
18. If applicator is used, wearing gloves, wash with soap and warm water, rinse, and store for future use.	Vaginal cavity is not sterile. Soap and water assist in removal of bacteria and residual cream. Gloves prevent transfer of microorganisms.
19. Offer client perineal pad when she resumes ambulation.	Prevents vaginal discharge from spreading to clothing.
20. Inspect appearance of discharge of vaginal canal and condition of external genitalia between applications.	Evaluates whether vaginal medication effectively reduced irritation or inflammation of tissues.

Unexpected Outcomes and Related Interventions

- Client cannot self-administer medication without supervision.
  - Reinforce teaching and allow client to self-administer medication as much as possible to enhance confidence.
  - If client is unable to administer medication, teach significant other medication administration.
- Client displays signs of allergic reaction (e.g., redness, itching) to medication.
  - Hold medication and speak with prescriber
  - Follow institutional policy or guidelines for reporting of adverse or allergic reaction to medications.

Recording and Reporting

- Record medication name, dose, route, and time of administration on MAR.
- Record character of discharge on nurses' notes.

Home Care Considerations

- Clients should perform regular perineal hygiene when receiving vaginal medications.
- Clients should be instructed to take all of the medication as prescribed, for the prescribed amount of time, to ensure effectiveness of the treatment.
- Women who have a vaginal yeast infection should abstain from sexual intercourse until treatment is completed and the infection is resolved.

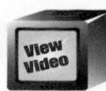

Skill 34-5   *Administering Rectal Suppositories*

Delegation Considerations

Administering medications by the rectal route should not be delegated to assistive personnel (AP). The nurse must instruct AP about the following:
- Expected fecal discharge or bowel movement and to report occurrence to the nurse
- Potential side effects of medications and to report their occurrence to the nurse

Equipment

- Rectal suppository
- Water-soluble lubricating jelly
- Clean gloves
- Drape or sheet
- Tissue
- MAR or computer printout

Steps	Rationale
1. Review prescriber's order, including client's name, medication name, form, route, time of administration, and drug indication.	Ensures safe and correct administration of medication.
2. Review medical record for rectal surgery, bleeding, and history of allergies.	Conditions contraindicate use of suppository. Prevents allergic response to medication.
3. Perform hand hygiene.	Reduces transfer of microorganisms.
4. Apply disposable gloves.	Prevents contact with infected fecal material, following CDC guidelines for body substance isolation (NIOSH, 1999).
5. Identify client; check name on MAR with client's identification bracelet and ask client's name.	Ensures that correct client receives medication.
6. Explain procedure. Be specific if client wishes to self-administer medication.	Promotes understanding and cooperation. Will enable client to self-administer medication if physically able.
7. Arrange supplies at bedside.	Ensures smooth procedure.
8. Close room curtain or door.	Maintains privacy and minimizes embarrassment.
9. Assist client in assuming Sims' position. Keep client draped with only anal area exposed.	Exposes anus and helps client relax external anal sphincter. Maintains privacy and facilitates relaxation.
10. Examine condition of anus externally and palpate rectal walls as needed (see Chapter 32). Dispose of gloves in proper receptacle if soiled.	Determines presence of active rectal bleeding. Palpation determines whether rectum is filled with feces, which may interfere with suppository placement. Reduces transmission of infection.

Critical Decision Point: Generally, rectal suppository is contraindicated in the presence of active rectal bleeding. Unless suppository is for constipation, placing medication in a rectum filled with feces may be poorly absorbed or prematurely expelled with defecation.

---

11. Apply disposable gloves (if previous gloves were discarded).	Prevents transmission of microorganisms and follows CDC guidelines to prevent accidental exposure to body substances (NIOSH, 1999).
12. Remove suppository from wrapper and lubricate rounded end (see illustration) with sterile water-soluble lubricating jelly. Lubricate index finger of dominant hand with a water-soluble lubricant.	Lubrication reduces friction as suppository enters rectal canal.

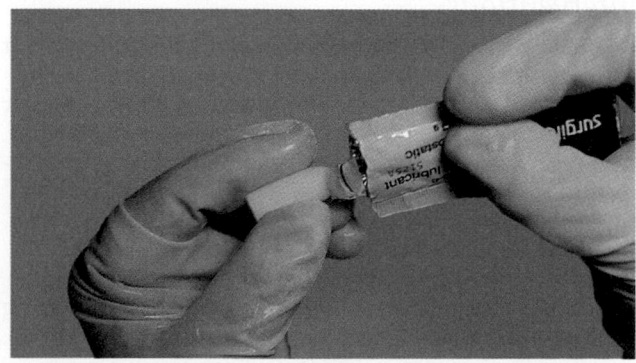

STEP **12** Remove suppository from wrapper.

Steps	Rationale
13. Ask client to take slow deep breaths through mouth and relax anal sphincter.	Forcing suppository through constricted sphincter causes pain.
14. Retract buttocks with nondominant hand. Insert suppository gently through anus, past internal sphincter and against rectal wall, 10 cm (4 in) in adults, 5 cm (2 in) in children and infants. May need to apply gentle pressure to hold buttocks together momentarily.	Suppository must be placed against rectal mucosa for eventual absorption and therapeutic action.
15. Withdraw finger and wipe anal area with tissue.	Provides comfort.
16. Discard gloves in appropriate receptacle.	Reduces transfer of microorganisms.
17. Ask client to remain flat or on side for 5 min.	Prevents expulsion of suppository.
18. If suppository contains laxative or fecal softener, place call light within reach.	Provides client with sense of control over elimination. Allows client to obtain assistance to bedpan or toilet.
19. Perform hand hygiene.	Prevents transfer of microorganisms.
20. Observe for effects of suppository (e.g., bowel movement, relief of nausea) at times that correlate with the medication's onset, peak, and duration.	Evaluates effectiveness of medication and relief of client's symptoms.

Unexpected Outcomes and Related Interventions

- Suppository falls out shortly after administration.
  - Reinsert suppository if possible.
- Client refuses medication.
  - Explore reasons why client does not want medication and clarify misunderstandings about medication.
  - Do not force client to take medication.
  - If client refuses to take medication despite educational efforts, record why drug was held in client's chart and notify prescriber.

Recording and Reporting

- Record administration of medication on MAR according to institutional policy.
- Report occurrence of rectal bleeding to physician.

Home Care Considerations

- Long-term use of laxatives often results in poor bowel tone and may result in dependency. Clients should be advised not to overuse laxatives, and they should be instructed on use of nonpharmacological measures, such as increasing fiber and fluid intake, to promote healthy bowel elimination.
- Some clients are not able to self-administer rectal medications. In this case, a family member or significant other will need to learn how to give the medication and will need to be available to administer the medication as scheduled.

Administering Medications by Inhalation

Medications administered with handheld inhalers are dispersed through an aerosol spray, mist, or powder that penetrates lung airways. The alveolocapillary network absorbs medications rapidly. **Metered-dose inhalers (MDIs)** and dry powder inhalers (DPIs) are usually used to produce local effects such as bronchodilatation. However, some medications can create serious systemic side effects.

Clients who receive medications by inhalation frequently suffer chronic respiratory disease such as chronic asthma, emphysema, or bronchitis. Medications given by inhalation provide these clients with control of airway obstruction. Because these clients depend on inhaled medications for disease control, they must learn about them and ways to administer them safely (Skill 34-6).

A metered-dose inhaler delivers a measured dose of medication with each push of a canister. Approximately 5 to 10 pounds of pressure must be used to activate the aerosol. This is important for the nurse to know because hand strength diminishes with age and from the effects of chronic respiratory disease. The nurse evaluates whether clients have enough hand strength to use the MDI appropriately. A spacer may be used with the MDI. The spacer allows the particles of medication to slow down and break into smaller pieces, which improves the drug's absorption in the client's airway. Spacers are especially helpful when the client has difficulty coordinating the steps involved in self-administering inhaled medications (Togger, 2001).

DPIs are becoming more widely available. They hold dry, powdered medication and create an aerosol when the client inhales through a reservoir that contains a dose of the medication. DPIs require less manual dexterity, and because the device is activated with the client's breath, there is no need to coordinate puffs with inhalation, as when using an MDI. They also do not require a spacer.

Text continued on p. 871

Skill 34-6 *Using Metered-Dose or Dry Powder Inhalers*

Delegation Considerations

Administering MDI or DPI and supervising clients who self-administer them should not be delegated to assistive personnel (AP). The nurse must instruct AP about the following:
- The need to report to the nurse any change in client's respiratory status or increased coughing
- Potential side effects of medications and to report their occurrence to the nurse

Equipment

- MDI or PDI
- Spacer (optional with MDI)
- Facial tissues (optional)
- Washbasin or sink with warm water
- Paper towel
- MAR or computer printout

Steps	Rationale
1. Review prescriber's order, including client's name, medication name, number of inhalations, and drug indication.	Ensures safe and correct administration of medication.
2. Identify client; compare name on MAR with client's ID bracelet, and ask client's name.	Ensures that correct client receives medication.
3. Assess client's ability to hold, manipulate, and depress canister and inhaler.	Any impairment of grasp or coordination interferes with client's ability to use MDI or DPI correctly.
4. Assess client's readiness to learn: client asks questions about medication, disease, or complications; requests education in use of inhaler; is mentally alert; participates in own care.	Affects client's ability to understand explanations and actively participate in teaching process.
5. Assess client's ability to learn: client should not be fatigued, in pain, or in respiratory distress; assess level of understanding of technical vocabulary terms.	Mental or physical limitations affect client's ability to learn and methods nurse uses for instruction.
6. Assess client's knowledge and understanding of disease and purpose and action of prescribed medications.	Knowledge of disease is essential for client to realistically understand use of inhaler.
7. Determine medication schedule and number of inhalations prescribed for each dose.	Influences explanations nurse provides for use of inhaler.
8. If previously instructed in self-administration of inhaled medicine, assess client's technique in using an inhaler.	Nurse's instruction may require only simple reinforcement, depending on client's level of dexterity.
9. Instruct client in comfortable environment by sitting in chair in hospital room or sitting at kitchen table in home.	Client will be more likely to remain receptive of nurse's explanations.
10. Provide adequate time for teaching session.	Prevents interruptions. Instruction should occur when client is receptive.
11. Perform hand hygiene and arrange equipment needed.	Reduces transfer of microorganisms and saves time.
12. Allow client opportunity to manipulate inhaler, canister, and spacer device. Explain and demonstrate how canister fits into inhaler.	Client must be familiar with how to use equipment.

Critical Decision Point: If client is using an MDI with or without a spacer and the inhaler is new or has not been used for several days, push a "test spray" into the air (MayoClinic.com, 2000). This does not need to be done for a DPI.

Steps	Rationale
13. Explain what metered dose is, and warn client about overuse of inhaler, including medication side effects.	Client must not arbitrarily administer excessive inhalations because of risk of serious side effects. If medication is given in recommended doses, side effects are uncommon.
14. Explain steps for administering inhaled dose of medication of MDI (demonstrate steps when possible): a. Insert MDI canister into the holder. b. Remove mouthpiece cover from inhaler. c. Shake inhaler vigorously 5 or 6 times.	Use of simple, step-by-step explanations allows client to ask questions at any point during procedure. Ensures fine particles are aerosolized.

Steps	Rationale
d. Have client take a deep breath and exhale.	Empties lungs and prepares the client's airway to receive the medication (Togger, 2001).
e. Instruct the client to position the inhaler in one of two ways.	
(1) Close mouth around MDI with opening toward back of throat (see illustration).	
(2) Position the device 2 to 4 cm (1-2 inches) in front of the mouth (see illustration).	Directs aerosol spray toward airway. Positioning the mouthpiece in front of mouth is considered the best way to deliver the medication.
f. With the inhaler properly positioned, have client hold inhaler with thumb at the mouthpiece and the index finger and middle finger at the top. This is called a three-point or lateral hand position.	MDIs work best when clients use a three-point or lateral hand position to activate canisters.
g. Instruct client to tilt head back slightly, inhale slowly and deeply through mouth for 3 to 5 seconds while depressing canister fully.	Medication is distributed to airways during inhalation. Inhalation through mouth rather than nose draws medication more effectively into airways.
h. Hold breath for approximately 10 seconds.	Allows tiny drops of aerosol spray to reach deeper branches of airways (National Heart, Lung and Blood Institute, 1995).
i. Remove MDI from mouth and exhale through pursed lips.	Keeps small airways open during exhalation.
15. Explain steps to administer MDI using a spacer such as an Aerochamber (demonstrate when possible):	
a. Remove mouthpiece cover from MDI and mouthpiece of spacer. Inspect spacer for foreign objects and ensure valve is intact if spacer has one (National Heart, Lung and Blood Institute, 1995).	Inhaler fits into end of spacer.
b. Insert MDI into end of spacer.	Spacer traps medication released from the MDI; the client then inhales the drug from the device. These devices break up and slow down the medication particles, enhancing the amount of medication received by client (Togger, 2001).
c. Shake inhaler vigorously 5 or 6 times.	Ensures fine particles are aerosolized.
d. Have client exhale completely before closing mouth around mouthpiece of the spacer. Avoid covering small exhalation slots with the lips (see illustration).	Empties lungs and prepares them for the medication (National Heart, Lung and Blood Institute, 1995).

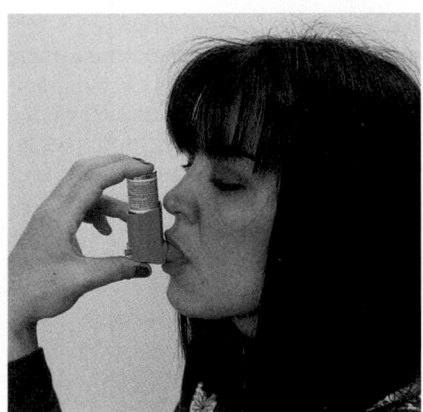

STEP **14e(1)** The client opens lips and places inhaler in mouth with opening toward back of throat.

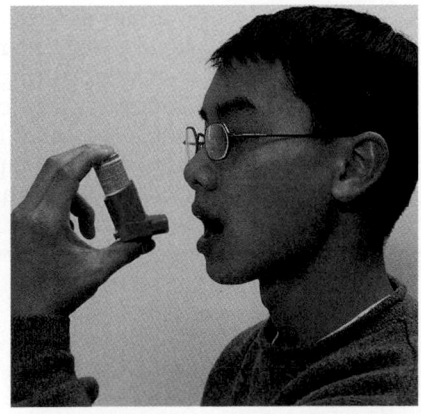

STEP **14e(2)** The client positions the mouthpiece 1 to 2 inches away from the mouth. This is considered the best way to deliver the medication.

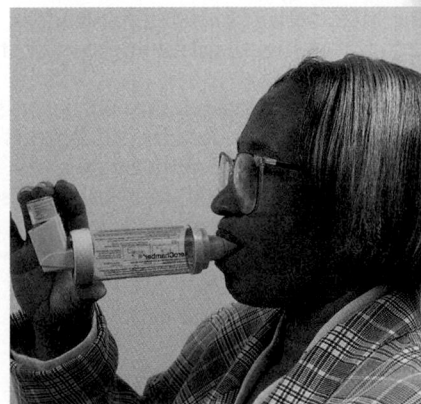

STEP **15d** Have the client place mouthpiece in mouth and close lips, being careful to keep exhalation slots exposed.

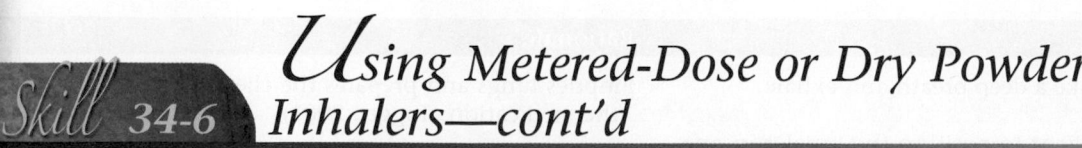

Using Metered-Dose *or Dry Powder* Inhalers—cont'd

Skill 34-6

Steps	Rationale
e. Have client depress medication canister, spraying one puff into spacer.	Emits spray that allows finer particles to be inhaled. Large droplets are retained in spacer.
f. Instruct client to inhale deeply and slowly through the mouth for 3 to 5 seconds.	Maximizes amount of medication that enters the lung.
g. Have client hold breath for 10 seconds.	Ensures full medication distribution.
h. Remove MDI and spacer before exhaling.	Allows client to exhale normally.
16. Explain steps to administer DPI (demonstrate when possible):	
a. Remove cover from mouthpiece. Do not shake the DPI (Epstein and others, 2001).	
b. Hold inhaler upright and turn wheel to the right and then to the left until a click is heard.	Primes inhaler, ensuring medication will be delivered to client (Epstein and others, 2001).
c. Exhale away from inhaler prior to inhalation.	Prevents loss of powder.
d. Position mouthpiece between the lips.	Prevents medication from escaping through mouth.
e. Inhale deeply and forcefully through the mouth.	Creates aerosol (Togger, 2001).
f. Hold breath for 5 to 10 seconds.	Ensures full medication distribution.
17. Instruct client to wait at least 20 to 30 seconds between inhalations of the same medication and 2 to 5 min between inhalations or as ordered by prescriber.	Medications must be inhaled sequentially. First inhalation opens airways and reduces inflammation. Second or third inhalation penetrates deeper airways.
18. Instruct client against repeating inhalations before next scheduled dose.	Medications are prescribed at intervals during day to provide constant drug levels and minimize side effects. Beta-adrenergic MDIs are used either on an "as needed" basis or regularly every 4 to 6 hr.
19. Explain that client may feel gagging sensation in throat caused by droplets of medication on pharynx or tongue.	Results when inhalant is sprayed and inhaled incorrectly.
20. Instruct client in cleaning inhaler:	
a. Once a day, inhaler and cap should be rinsed in warm running water. Inhaler must be completely dry before using.	Accumulation of spray around mouthpiece can interfere with proper distribution during use.
b. Twice a week, the L-shaped plastic mouthpiece should be washed with mild dishwashing soap and warm water. Rinse and dry well before putting canister back inside mouthpiece (National Heart, Lung and Blood Institute, 1995).	Removes residual medication. Inhalers holding cromolyn or nedocromil should not be placed in water (National Heart, Lung, and Blood Institute, 1995).
21. Ask if client has any questions.	Clarifies misconceptions or misunderstanding.
22. Have client explain and demonstrate steps in use of inhaler.	Return demonstration provides feedback for measuring client's learning.
23. Ask client to explain medication schedule.	Improves likelihood of compliance with therapy.
24. Ask client to describe side effects of medication and criteria for calling prescriber.	Will allow client to recognize signs of overuse and need to seek medical support when medications are ineffective.
25. After medication instillation, assess client's respirations and auscultate lungs.	Determines status of breathing pattern and adequacy of ventilation.

Unexpected Outcomes and Related Interventions

- Client needs a bronchodilator more than every 4 hours.
  - May indicate respiratory problems; reassessment of type of medication and delivery methods needed; notify health care provider if respiratory status does not improve.
- Client experiences cardiac dysrhythmias, especially if receiving beta-adrenergics
  - If client experiences symptoms with the dysrhythmias (e.g., light-headedness, syncope), withhold all further doses of medication and discuss with prescriber.
- Client is not able to self-administer medication properly.
  - Alternative delivery routes or methods of medication administration may need to be explored.

- Client experiences paroxysms of coughing.
  - Aerosolized particles irritate posterior pharynx. Notify prescriber; may need to reassess type of medication or delivery method.

Recording and Reporting

- Document in nurse's notes what skills were taught and client's ability to perform skills.
- Record time when client used MDI or DPI and the amount of puffs.
- Report any undesirable effects from medication.

Home Care Considerations

- Remind clients to carry their prescribed inhalers to use emergently in case of an acute asthma attack.

However, the medication inside the DPI may clump if the client is in a humid climate, and some clients cannot inspire fast enough to administer the entire dose of the medication (Togger, 2001). Skill 34-6 describes the steps required to administer medication through MDIs and DPIs.

One important aspect of client teaching is to help the client determine when the MDI or DPI is empty and needs to be replaced. Floating the MDI to determine how much medication is left is no longer recommended because extra propellant may cause buoyancy even if no medication is remaining. To calculate the number of days a canister will last, the nurse helps the client determine how many doses the canister contains and how many puffs per day are inhaled daily. Then, the number of doses in the canister is divided by the number of puffs taken daily. Some DPIs have mechanisms that indicate how many doses are left. These mechanisms are not foolproof, but they can help the client predict when the medication needs to be refilled (Togger, 2001).

Administering Medications by Irrigations

Medications may be used to irrigate or wash out a body cavity and are delivered through a stream of solution. Irrigations most commonly use sterile water, saline, or antiseptic solutions on the eye, ear, throat, vagina, and urinary tract. If there is a break in the skin or mucosa, the nurse uses aseptic technique. When the cavity to be irrigated is not sterile, as in the case of the ear canal (see Box 34-12, p. 863) or vagina, clean technique is used. In health care settings, however, sterile solutions are usually used. Irrigations can cleanse an area, instill a medication, or apply hot or cold to injured tissue.

Administering Parenteral Medications

Parenteral administration of medications is the administration of medications by injection. When medications are administered this way, it is an invasive procedure that must be performed using aseptic techniques (Box 34-13).

> **Box 34-13   Preventing Infection During an Injection**
>
> - To prevent contamination of solution, draw medication from ampule quickly. Do not allow it to stand open.
> - To prevent needle contamination, avoid letting needle touch contaminated surface (e.g., outer edges of ampule or vial, outer surface of needle cap, nurse's hands, countertop, table surface).
> - To prevent syringe contamination, avoid touching length of plunger or inner part of barrel. Keep tip of syringe covered with cap or needle.
> - To prepare skin, wash skin soiled with dirt, drainage, or feces with soap and water and dry. Use friction and a circular motion while cleaning with an antiseptic swab. Swab from center of site, and move outward in a 2-inch radius.

After a needle pierces the skin, there is risk of infection. Each type of injection requires certain skills to ensure that the medication reaches the proper location. The effects of a parenterally administered medication can develop rapidly, depending on the rate of medication absorption. The nurse closely observes the client's response.

Equipment. A variety of syringes and needles are available, each designed to deliver a certain volume of a medication to a specific type of tissue. The nurse uses judgment when determining the syringe or needle that will be most effective.

Syringes. Syringes consist of a cylindrical barrel with a tip designed to fit the hub of a hypodermic needle and a close-fitting plunger. Syringes, in general, are classified as being Luer-Lok or non–Luer-Lok. This nomenclature is based on the design of the syringe's tip. Luer-Lok syringes (Figure 34-15, *A*) require special needles, which are twisted onto the tip and lock themselves in place. This design prevents the inadvertent removal of the needle. Non–Luer-Lok syringes (Figure 34-15, *B-D*) require needles

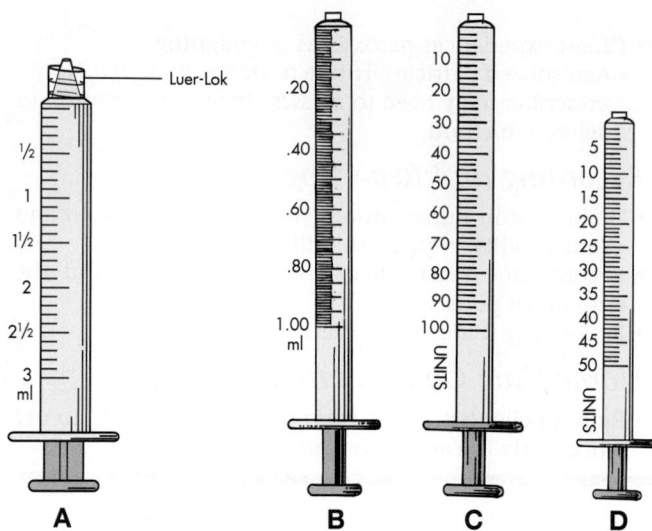

FIGURE **34–15** Types of syringes. **A,** Luer-Lok syringe marked in 0.1 (tenths). **B,** Tuberculin syringe marked in 0.01 (hundredths) for doses of less than 1 ml. **C,** Insulin syringe marked in units (100). **D,** Insulin syringe marked in units (50).

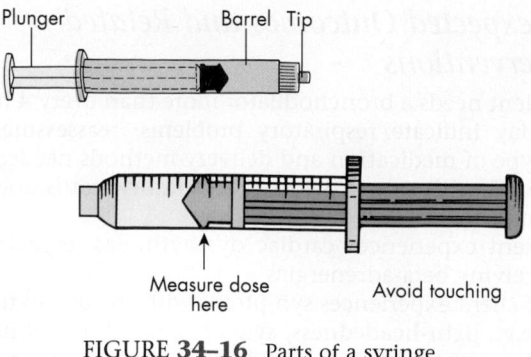

FIGURE **34–16**   Parts of a syringe.

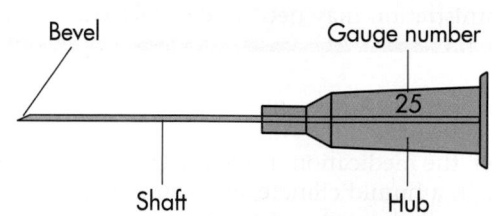

FIGURE **34–17**   Parts of the needle.

that slip onto the tip. In the clinical setting, all syringes now have safety devices to prevent needle-stick injury. The illustrations in this section are used to demonstrate different syringes, needles, and parts of the syringe.

The nurse fills a syringe by aspiration, pulling the plunger outward while the needle tip remains immersed in the prepared solution. The nurse may handle the outside of the syringe barrel and the handle of the plunger. To maintain sterility, the nurse avoids letting any unsterile object touch the tip or inside of the barrel, the hub, the shaft of the plunger, or the needle (Figure 34-16).

Syringes come in a number of sizes, from 0.5 to 60 ml. A 2- to 3-ml syringe is usually adequate for a sub-Q or IM injection. A larger volume creates discomfort. The nurse uses large syringes to administer certain intravenous medications, add medications to intravenous solutions, and irrigate wounds or drainage tubes. Syringes may come prepackaged with a needle attached. However, the nurse may change needle sizes. The hypodermic has two scales along the barrel; one is divided into minims and the other into tenths of a milliliter.

Insulin syringes (see Figure 34-15, *C* and *D*) are available in sizes that hold 0.3 to 1 ml and are calibrated in units. Each milliliter of solution contains 100 units of insulin. Insulin syringes that hold 0.3 ml are known as low-dose syringes (30 units per 0.3 ml). Most insulin syringes are U-100s (100 units per 1 ml).

The tuberculin syringe (see Figure 34-15, *B*) has a long, thin barrel with a preattached thin needle. The syringe is calibrated in sixteenths of a minim and hundredths of a milliliter and has a capacity of 1 ml. The nurse uses a tuberculin syringe to prepare small amounts of medications. A tuberculin syringe is also useful when preparing small precise doses for infants or young children.

Needles. Needles come packaged in individual sheaths to allow flexibility in choosing the right needle for a

client. Some needles are preattached to standard-sized syringes. Most needles are made of stainless steel and are disposable.

The needle has three parts: the hub, which fits onto the tip of a syringe; the shaft, which connects to the hub; and the bevel, or slanted tip (see Figure 34-17). The tip of a needle or the bevel is always slanted. The bevel creates a narrow slit when injected into tissue. This slit quickly closes when the needle is removed to prevent leakage of medication, blood, or serum. A short beveled tip is best for intravenous injections because it is not easily occluded against the inside of a blood vessel wall. Long beveled tips are sharper and narrower, which minimizes discomfort when entering tissue used for subcutaneous or intramuscular injections.

Needles vary in length from ¼ to 3 inches (Figure 34-18). The nurse chooses the needle length according to the client's size and weight and the type of tissue into which the medication is to be injected. A child or slender adult generally requires a shorter needle. The nurse uses longer needles (1 to 1½ inches) for intramuscular injections and a shorter needle (⅜ to ⅝ inch) for subcutaneous injections.

Needle diameter is measured by gauge. As the gauge becomes smaller, the needle diameter becomes larger (see Figure 34-18). The selection of a gauge depends on the viscosity of fluid to be injected or infused. An intramuscular injection usually requires an 18- to 27-gauge needle, depending on the viscosity of the medication (Nicoll and Hesby, 2002). Subcutaneous injections require smaller-diameter needles such as a 25-gauge needle. A 26-gauge needle is used for an intradermal injection.

Disposable Injection Units. Disposable, single-dose, prefilled syringes are available for some medications. The nurse must be careful to check the medication and con-

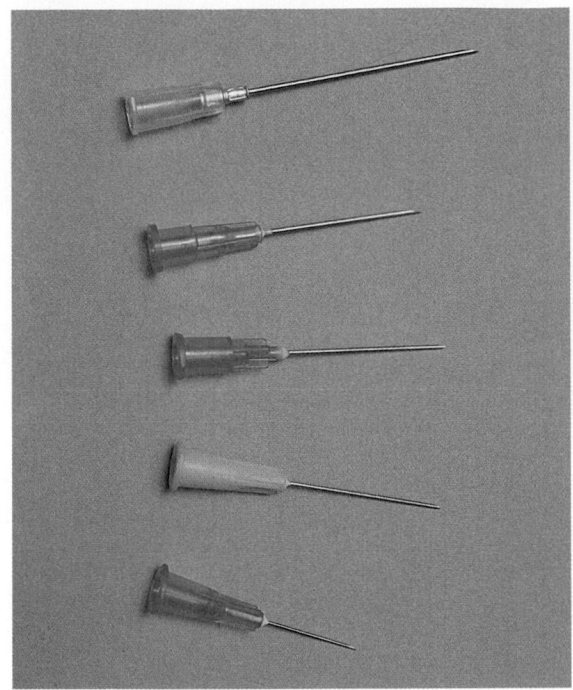

FIGURE **34–18**   Needles. *Top to bottom:* 19 gauge, 1½-inch length; 20 gauge, 1-inch length; 21 gauge, 1-inch length; 23 gauge, 1-inch length; and 25 gauge, ⅝-inch length.

centration because all prefilled syringes appear very similar. With these syringes the nurse does not have to prepare medication doses, except perhaps to expel portions of unneeded medications.

The Tubex and Carpuject injection systems include reusable plastic mechanisms that hold prefilled, disposable, sterile cartridge-needle units (Figure 34-19). The nurse slips the cartridge into the syringe, secures it (following package directions), and checks for air bubbles in the syringe. The nurse advances the plunger to expel excess medication as in a regular syringe. A new type of injection system involves screwing a plungerlike device into the end of a prefilled vial containing a needle. After the medication is given, the entire unit is disposed of in a receptacle. This design reduces the risk of needle-stick injuries.

Preparing an Injection From an Ampule. Ampules contain single doses of medication in a liquid. Ampules are available in several sizes, from 1 ml to 10 ml or more (Figure 34-20, *A*). An ampule is made of glass with a constricted neck that must be snapped off to allow access to the medication. A colored ring around the neck indicates where the ampule is prescored to be broken easily. Aspiration of the medication into a syringe (Skill 34-7) is completed with a filter needle to prevent small glass fragments from entering the syringe (Koschel, 2001).

Preparing an Injection From a Vial. A vial is a single-dose or multidose container with a rubber seal at the top (see Figure 34-20, *B*). A metal cap protects the seal until it is ready for use. Vials contain liquid or dry forms of medications. Medications that are unstable in solution are

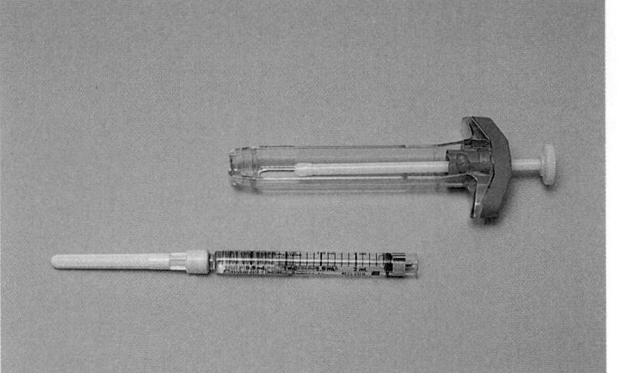

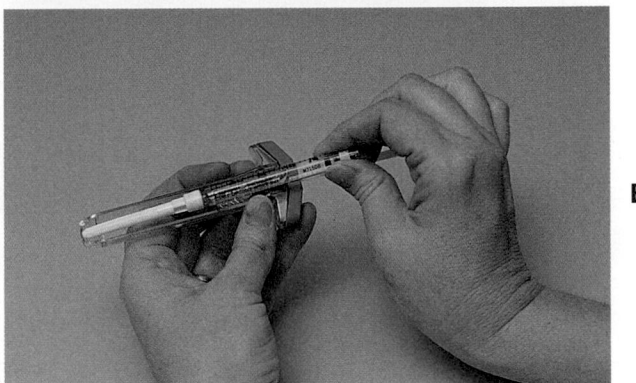

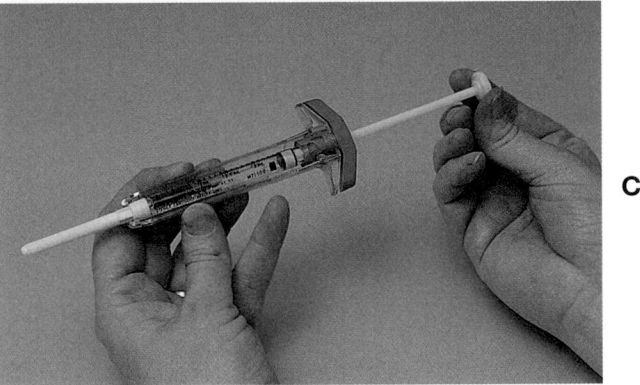

FIGURE **34–19** **A,** Carpuject syringe and prefilled sterile cartridge with needle. **B,** Assembling the Carpuject. **C,** Cartridge locks at needle end; plunger screws into opposite end.

packaged dry. The vial label specifies the solvent or diluent used to dissolve the medication and the amount of diluent needed to prepare a desired medication concentration. Normal saline and sterile distilled water are solutions commonly used to dissolve medications.

Unlike the ampule, the vial is a closed system, and air must be injected into it to permit easy withdrawal of the solution. Failure to inject air when withdrawing creates a vacuum within the vial that makes withdrawal difficult (see Skill 34-7, p. 875).

To prepare a powdered medication, the nurse draws up the amount of diluent or solvent recommended on the vial's label. The nurse injects the diluent into the vial in the same manner as injecting air into the vial. Most powdered medications dissolve easily, but it may be necessary

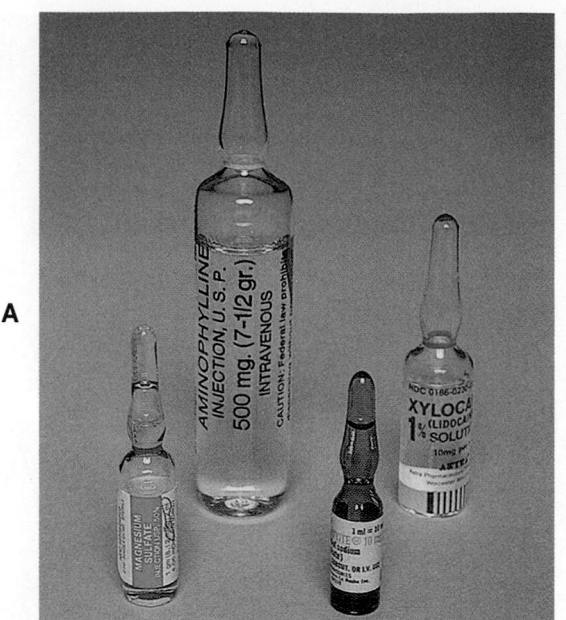 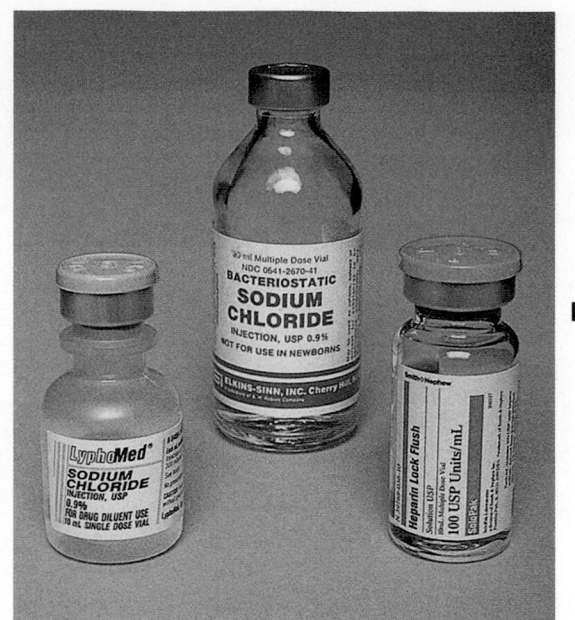

FIGURE **34–20** **A,** Medication in ampules. **B,** Medication in vials.

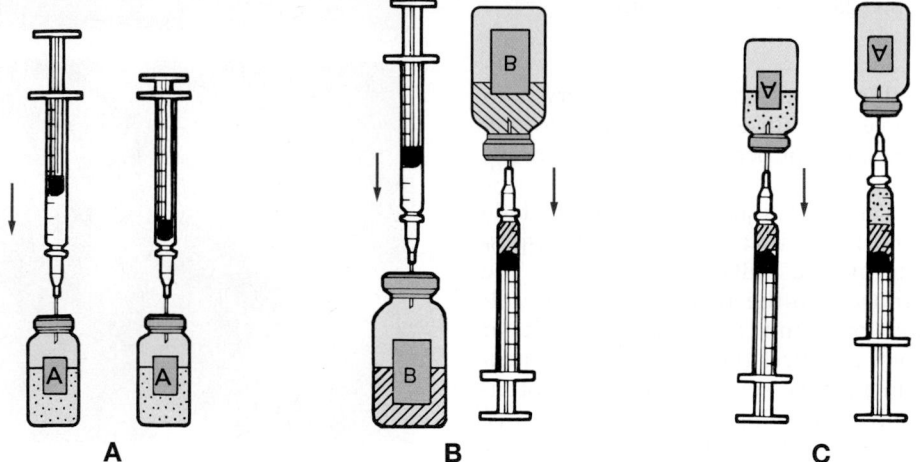

FIGURE **34–21** **A,** Injecting air into vial A. **B,** Injecting air into vial B and withdrawing dose. **C,** Withdrawing medication from vial A; medications are now mixed.

to withdraw the needle to mix the contents thoroughly. Gently rolling the vial between the hands will dissolve the powdered medication. The needle is reinserted to draw up the dissolved medication. After mixing multidose vials, the nurse makes a label that includes the date and time of mixing and the concentration of medication per milliliter. Multidose vials may require refrigeration after the contents are reconstituted.

Mixing Medications. If two medications are compatible, it is possible to mix them in one injection if the total dose is within accepted limits so that a client will not have to receive more than one injection at a time. Most nursing units have charts that list common compatible medica-

tions. If there is any uncertainty about medication compatibilities, a pharmacist should be consulted.

Mixing Medications From Two Vials. The nurse applies these principles when mixing medications from two vials:

1. Do not contaminate one medication with another.
2. Ensure the final dose is accurate.
3. Maintain aseptic technique.

Only one syringe is needed to mix medications from two vials (Figure 34-21). The nurse takes a syringe with a needle attached and aspirates the volume of air equivalent to the first medication's dose (vial A). The nurse injects the air into vial A, making sure the needle does not

Text continued on p. 879

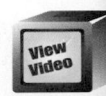

Skill 34-7 Preparing Injections

Delegation Considerations

Preparing injections from ampules and vials should not be delegated to assistive personnel.

Equipment

- **Medication in an ampule**
  - Syringe, needle, and filter needle
  - Small gauze pad or unopened alcohol swab
- **Medication in a vial**
  - Syringe

- Needles:
  - Blunt tip vial access cannula (if needleless system used)
  - Filter needle (if indicated)
  - Needle for drawing up medication (if needed) and needle for injection
- Small gauze pad or alcohol swab
- Diluent (e.g., normal saline or sterile water) (if indicated)
- **Both**
  - MAR or computer printout

Steps	Rationale
1. Check client's name and medication order, including medication name, dose, route of administration, time of administration, and drug indication.	Ensures correct administration of medication.
2. Review pertinent information related to medication, including action, purpose, side effects, and nursing implications.	Allows nurse to administer medication properly and to monitor client's response.
3. Assess client's body build, muscle size, and weight.	Determines type and size of syringe and needles for injection.
4. Perform hand hygiene and assemble supplies.	Reduces transmission of microorganisms and saves nurse's time.
5. Check medication order against MAR and check date of expiration for medication vial or ampule.	Ensures correct medication and dose are prepared. Medication potency may increase or decrease when outdated.
6. Prepare medication.	
A. **Ampule preparation**	
(1) Tap top of ampule lightly and quickly with finger until fluid moves from neck of ampule (see illustration).	Dislodges any fluid that collects above neck of ampule. All solution moves into lower chamber.
(2) Place small gauze pad or unopened alcohol swab around neck of ampule (see illustration).	Placing pad around neck of ampule protects nurse's fingers from trauma as glass tip is broken off.
(3) Snap neck of ampule quickly and firmly away from hands (see illustration).	Protects nurse's fingers and face from shattering glass.

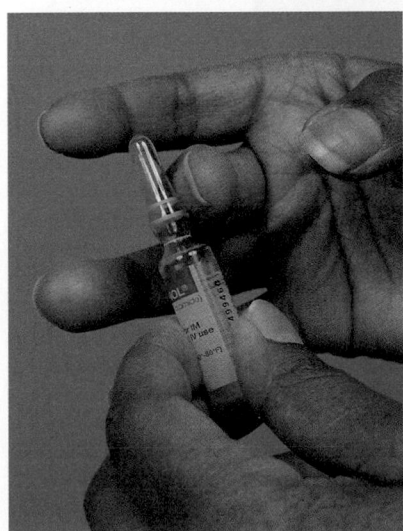

STEP **6A(1)** Tapping ampule moves fluid down neck.

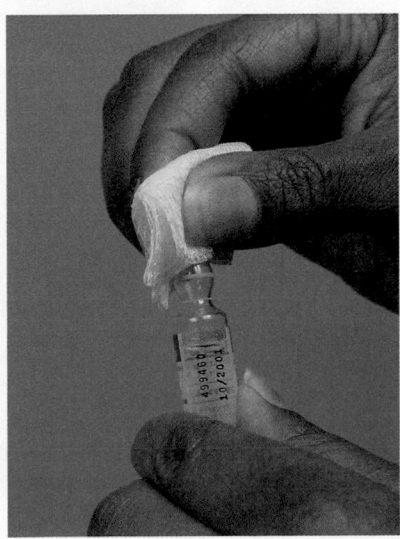

STEP **6A(2)** Gauze pad placed around neck of ampule.

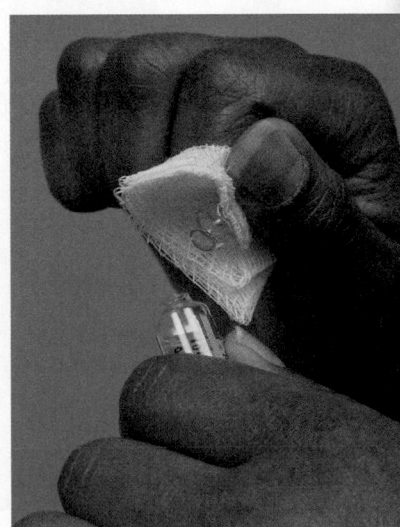

STEP **6A(3)** Snapping neck away from hands.

Skill 34-7 *Preparing Injections—cont'd*

Steps	Rationale
(4) Draw up medication quickly, using filter needle long enough to reach bottom of ampule.	System is open to airborne contaminants. Needle must be long enough to access medication for preparation. Filter needles are used to filter out any fragments of glass (Nicoll and Hesby, 2002).
(5) Hold ampule upside down, or set it on a flat surface. Insert filter needle into center of ampule opening. Do not allow needle tip or shaft to touch rim of ampule.	Broken rim of ampule is considered contaminated. When ampule is inverted, solution does dribble out if needle tip or shaft touches rim of ampule.
(6) Aspirate medication into syringe by gently pulling back on plunger (see illustration).	Withdrawal of plunger creates negative pressure within syringe barrel, which pulls fluid into syringe.
(7) Keep needle tip under surface of liquid. Tip ampule to bring all fluid within reach of the needle.	Prevents aspiration of air bubbles.
(8) If air bubbles are aspirated, do not expel air into ampule.	Air pressure may force fluid out of ampule and medication will be lost.
(9) To expel excess air bubbles, remove needle from ampule. Hold syringe with needle pointing up. Tap side of syringe to cause bubbles to rise toward needle. Draw back slightly on plunger, and then push plunger upward to eject air. Do not eject fluid.	Withdrawing plunger too far will remove it from barrel. Holding syringe vertically allows fluid to settle in bottom of barrel. Pulling back on plunger allows fluid within needle to enter barrel so fluid is not expelled. Air at top of barrel and within needle is then expelled.
(10) If syringe contains excess fluid, use sink for disposal. Hold syringe vertically with needle tip up and slanted slightly toward sink. Slowly eject excess fluid into sink. Recheck fluid level in syringe by holding it vertically.	Medication is safely dispersed into sink. Position of needle allows medication to be expelled without flowing down needle shaft. Rechecking fluid level ensures proper dose.
(11) Cover needle with its safety sheath or cap. Replace filter needle with needle for injection.	Prevents contamination of needle. Filter needles cannot be used for injection.

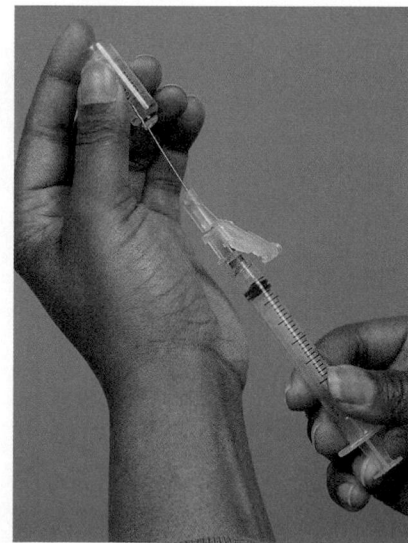

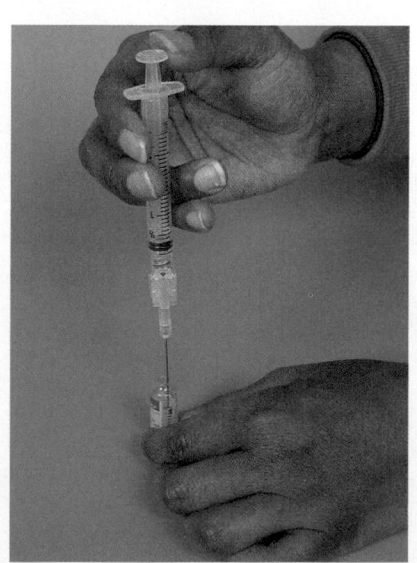

STEP **6A(6)** **A,** Medication aspirated with ampule inverted. **B,** Medication aspirated with ampule on flat surface.

Steps	Rationale

B. Vial containing a solution

(1) Remove cap covering top of unused vial to expose sterile rubber seal, keeping rubber seal sterile. If a multidose vial has been used before, cap is already removed. Firmly and briskly wipe surface of rubber seal with alcohol swab and allow it to dry.

Vial comes packaged with seal that cannot be replaced after cap removal. Not all drug manufacturers guarantee that caps of unused vials are sterile. Therefore seals must be swabbed with alcohol before preparing medication. Allowing alcohol to dry prevents needle from being coated with alcohol and mixing with medication.

(2) Pick up syringe and remove needle cap or cap covering needleless vial access device (see illustration). Pull back on plunger to draw amount of air into syringe equivalent to volume of medication to be aspirated from vial.

Air must first be injected into vial to prevent buildup of negative pressure in vial when aspirating medication.

Critical Decision Point: Some medications and some institutions require that a filter needle be used when preparing medications from a vial. Check agency policy to determine if use of filter needle is indicated (Nicoll and Hesby, 2002).

---

(3) With vial on flat surface, insert tip of needle with beveled tip entering first through center of rubber seal (see illustration). Apply pressure to tip of needle during insertion.

Center of seal is thinner and easier to penetrate. Injecting beveled tip first and using firm pressure prevent coring of rubber seal, which could enter vial or needle.

(4) Inject air into the vial's airspace, holding on to plunger. Hold plunger with firm pressure; plunger may be forced backward by air pressure within the vial.

Air must be injected before aspirating fluid. Injecting into vial's airspace prevents formation of bubbles and inaccuracy in dose.

(5) Invert vial while keeping firm hold on syringe and plunger (see illustration). Hold vial between thumb and middle fingers of nondominant hand. Grasp end of syringe barrel and plunger with thumb and forefinger of dominant hand to counteract pressure in vial.

Inverting vial allows fluid to settle in lower half of container. Position of hands prevents forceful movement of plunger and permits easy manipulation of syringe.

(6) Keep tip of needle below fluid level.

Prevents aspiration of air.

(7) Allow air pressure from the vial to fill syringe gradually with medication. If necessary, pull back slightly on plunger to obtain correct amount of solution.

Positive pressure within vial forces fluid into syringe (unless vial has been used several times).

(8) When desired volume has been obtained, position needle into vial's airspace; tap side of syringe barrel carefully to dislodge any air bubbles. Eject any air remaining at top of syringe into vial.

Forcefully striking barrel while needle is inserted in vial may bend needle. Accumulation of air displaces medication and causes dose errors.

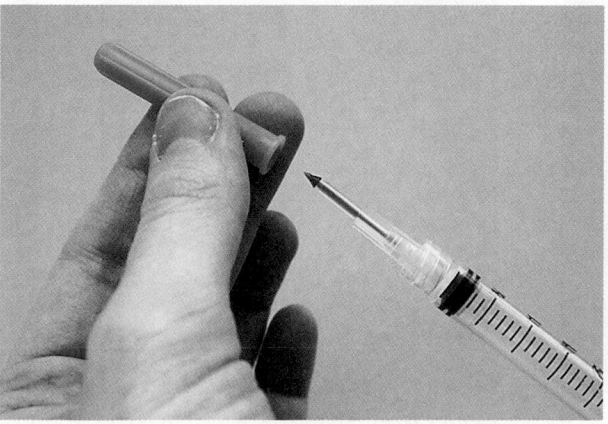

STEP 6B(2) Syringe with needleless adapter.

Skill **34-7**   *Preparing Injections—cont'd*

Steps	Rationale
(9) Remove needle from vial by pulling back on barrel of syringe.	Accidentally pulling plunger rather than barrel causes plunger to separate from barrel, resulting in loss of medication.
(10) Hold syringe at eye level, at 90-degree angle, to ensure correct volume and absence of air bubbles. Remove any remaining air by tapping barrel to dislodge any air bubbles (see illustration). Draw back slightly on plunger; then push plunger upward to eject air. Do not eject fluid. Recheck volume of medication.	Holding syringe vertically allows fluid to settle in bottom of barrel. Pulling back on plunger allows fluid within needle to enter barrel so fluid is not expelled. Air at top of barrel and within needle is then expelled.
(11) If medication is to be injected into client's tissue, change needle to appropriate gauge and length according to route of medication.	Inserting needle through a rubber stopper may dull beveled tip. New needle is sharper. Because no fluid is along shaft, needle will not track medication through tissues.
(12) For multidose vial, make label that includes date of mixing, concentration of medication per milliliter, and nurse's initials.	Ensures that future doses will be prepared correctly. Some medications must be discarded after certain number of days after mixing of vial.

C. **Vial containing a powder (reconstituting medications)**

(1) Remove cap covering vial of powdered medication and cap covering vial of proper diluent. Firmly swab both seals with alcohol swab and allow to dry.	Not all drug manufacturers guarantee that caps of unused vials are sterile. Therefore, seals must be swabbed with alcohol before preparing medication. Allowing alcohol to dry prevents needle from being coated with alcohol and mixing with medication.
(2) Draw up diluent into syringe following steps 5B(2) through 5B(10).	Prepares diluent for injection into vial containing powdered medication.
(3) Insert tip of needle through center of rubber seal of vial of powdered medication. Inject diluent into vial. Remove needle.	Diluent begins to dissolve and reconstitute medication.

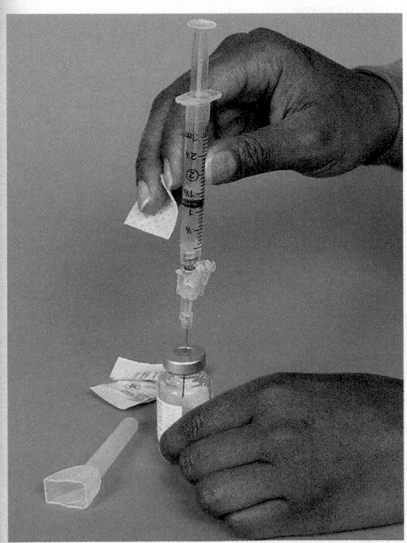

STEP **6B(3)**   Insert adapter through center of vial diaphragm (with vial flat on table).

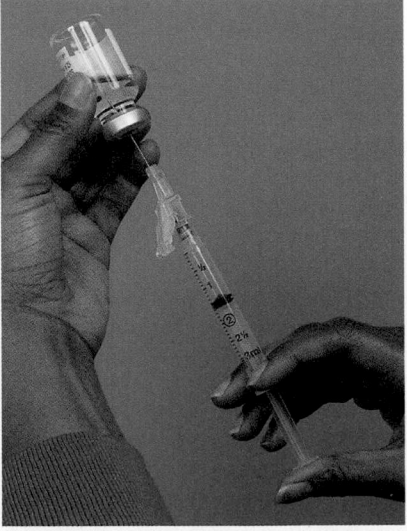

STEP **6B(5)**   Withdraw fluid with vial inverted.

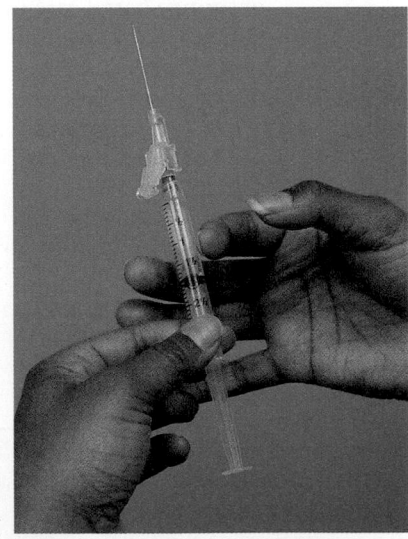

STEP **6B(10)**   Hold syringe upright, tap barrel to dislodge air bubbles.

Steps	Rationale
(4) Mix medication thoroughly. Roll in palms. Do not shake.	Ensures proper dispersal of medication throughout solution. Shaking produces bubbles.
(5) Reconstituted medication in vial is ready to be drawn into new syringe. Read label carefully to determine dose after reconstitution.	Once diluent has been added, concentration of medication (mg/ml) determines dose to be given.
(6) Prepare medication in syringe following steps 5B(2) through 5B(12).	

Critical Decision Point: Some institutions may require prepared parenteral medications to be verified for accuracy by another nurse. Check agency policy.

7. Dispose of soiled supplies. Place broken ampule and/or used vials and used needle in puncture-proof and leak-proof container. Clean work area and perform hand hygiene.	Proper disposal of glass and needle prevents accidental injury to staff. Controls transmission of infection.

Unexpected Outcomes and Related Interventions

- Air bubbles remain in syringe.
  - Expel air from syringe, and add medication to syringe until correct dose is prepared.
- Incorrect dose is prepared.
  - Discard prepared dose and prepare corrected new dose.

touch the solution. The nurse withdraws the needle, aspirates air equivalent to the second medication's dose (vial B), and then injects the volume of air into vial B. The nurse immediately withdraws the medication from vial B into the syringe. The nurse then inserts the needle back into vial A, being careful not to push the plunger and expel the medication within the syringe into the vial. The nurse withdraws the desired amount of medication from vial A into the syringe. After withdrawing the necessary amount, the nurse withdraws the needle and applies a new needle.

Mixing Medications From One Vial and One Ampule. When mixing medication from both a vial and ampule, the nurse prepares medication from the vial first and then, using the same syringe and filter needle, withdraws medication from the ampule. The medications are prepared in this order because it is not necessary to add air to withdraw medication from an ampule.

Insulin Preparation. Insulin is the hormone used to treat diabetes. It must be administered by injection because it is a protein and therefore would be broken down and destroyed in the gastrointestinal tract. Most clients with diabetes requiring insulin learn to self-administer injections. In the United States, the medication is available in 100 units or 500 units per milliliter of solution. U-500 insulin is 5 times as strong as U-100 insulin. Therefore it is ordered for clients who are very resistant to insulin, decreasing the number of units that must be administered.

When preparing insulin, a 100-unit insulin syringe is used. If the client is to receive 100-unit insulin, the nurse

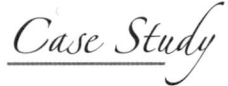
           Box 34-14

Mr. Dodds has severe insulin resistance and requires an unusually high regular insulin dosage to control his blood glucose levels. Therefore the physician has ordered that he begin taking 20 units of U-500 insulin. The nurse goes through the following medication calculation steps to determine how much insulin to prepare in the U-100 syringe:

- U-500 insulin is 5 times as strong as U-100 insulin.
- Therefore the amount of U-500 insulin should be divided by 5.
- Dosage of U-500 insulin/5 = amount of insulin to draw into U-100 syringe.
- 20 units of U-500 insulin/5 = 4 units of insulin to draw into U-100 syringe.

simply places the ordered number of units in the syringe. However, when 500-unit insulin is ordered, a medication calculation must be performed to correctly prepare the insulin (Box 34-14).

Insulin is classified by rate of action, including rapid, short, intermediate, and long acting. Each type has a different onset, peak, and duration of action (Table 34-11). Some insulins come in a stable premixed solution (e.g., 70/30 insulin is 70% NPH and 30% regular). Clients receiving these insulins avoid the need to mix insulins.

A client with diabetes may require more than one type of insulin. For example, by receiving a short-acting (regular) and an intermediate-acting (NPH) insulin, a client

Table 34-11	A Comparison of Insulin Preparations				
Type	Onset	Peak	Duration	Color	Route
Rapid-acting (Insulin lispro, insulin aspart)	15 min	1 hour	2-4 hours	Clear	Sub-Q
Short-acting (Regular)	30 min	2-4 hours	6-8 hours	Clear	IV or Sub-Q
Intermediate-acting (NPH, Lente)	1-2½ hours	6-12 hours	18 hours	Cloudy	Sub-Q
Long-acting (Ultralente)	4-8 hours	None	24-36 hours	Cloudy	Sub-Q
Long-acting (Insulin glargine)	1 hour	None	24 hours	Clear	Sub-Q*

Modified from Strowig S: Insulin therapy, *RN* 64(9):38, 2001.
***Cannot** be mixed with other insulins.

Box 34-15	Example of Sliding Scale Insulin Order

Give regular insulin Sub-Q:
2 units for glucose 150 to 200
4 units for glucose 201 to 250
6 units for glucose 251 to 300
For glucose greater than 300, call physician

---

receives more sustained control of blood glucose levels over 24 hours. Only regular insulin can be given intravenously.

Insulin is ordered by a specific dose at select times or by a sliding scale. A sliding scale dictates a certain dose based on the client's blood glucose level (Box 34-15). Usually, rapid or short-acting insulins are used for sliding scales. If more than one type of insulin is required to manage the client's diabetes, the nurse can mix two different types of insulin into one syringe if they are compatible (Box 34-16) using the steps demonstrated in Figure 34-21, p. 874. This minimizes the discomfort to the client associated with multiple injections.

Before withdrawing insulin from a vial, the nurse should rotate the vial at least 1 minute between both hands. This resuspends the modified insulin preparations and helps to warm the medication. The nurse should not shake insulin vials. Shaking causes bubbles to form, which take up space and alters the dose.

Administering Injections

Each injection route differs based on the type of tissues the medication enters. The characteristics of the tissues influence the rate of medication absorption and thus the onset of medication action. Before injecting a medication, the nurse should know the volume of the medication to administer, the medication's characteristics and viscosity, and the location of anatomical structures underlying injection sites (Skill 34-8).

If a nurse does not administer injections correctly, negative client outcomes result. Failure to select an injection site in relation to anatomical landmarks can result in nerve or bone damage during needle insertion. Inability to maintain stability of the needle and syringe

---

Box 34-16	*Procedural Guidelines*

Mixing Two Kinds of Insulin in One Syringe

- Lente insulins (Semilente, Lente, Ultralente) may be mixed with each other, in any ratio.
- Because Lente insulin binds with regular insulin, mixing of regular and Lente insulin is not recommended except for clients already adequately controlled on such a mixture.
- Insulin glargine (Lantus) **cannot** be mixed with other insulins.
- Insulin should not be mixed with any other medications unless approved by the prescriber.

To prepare insulin from two vials, the nurse or client follows these steps:

1. With an insulin syringe and needle, inject air, equal to the dose of insulin to be withdrawn, into the vial of intermediate- or long-acting (cloudy) insulin. Do not touch the tip of the needle to the solution.
2. Remove the syringe from the vial of cloudy insulin.
3. With the same syringe, inject air, equal to the dose of insulin to be withdrawn, into the vial of rapid- or short-acting insulin (clear vial). Then withdraw the correct dose into the syringe.
4. Remove the syringe from the clear insulin vial after carefully removing air bubbles in the syringe to ensure correct dose.
5. Return to the vial of intermediate- or long-acting (cloudy) insulin, and withdraw the correct dose.
6. Administer mixture of insulins within 5 minutes of preparing it. Rapid- or short-acting insulin can bind with intermediate- or long-acting insulin, thus reducing the action of the faster-acting insulin.

Modified from Strowig S: Insulin therapy, *RN* 64(9):38, 2001.

---

unit could result in pain for the client and possibly tissue damage. If the nurse fails to aspirate the syringe before injecting an intramuscular medication, the medication may accidentally be injected directly into an artery or vein. Injecting too large a volume of medication for the site selected causes extreme pain and may result in local tissue damage.

Text continued on p. 886

Skill 34-8   *Administering Injections*

Delegation Considerations

Administering injections should not be delegated to assistive personnel (AP). The nurse should instruct AP about the following:

- Potential medication side effects and to report their occurrence to the nurse
- Any impact of medication on client's vital signs or level of consciousness (e.g., sedation)

Equipment

- Proper size syringe and needle:
  - *Sub-Q:* Syringe (1 to 3 ml) and needle (27 to 25 gauge, ⅜ to ⅝ in)
  - *IM:* Syringe 2 to 3 ml for adult, 0.5 to 1 ml for infants and small children.
- Needle, length corresponding to site of injection and age of client according to following guidelines (Nicoll and Hesby, 2002):
  - *Children:* ⅝ to 1¼ inch (based on size of child)
  - *Vastus lateralis (adults):* 1 to 1½ inch
  - *Deltoid (adults):* 1 to 1½ inch
  - *Ventrogluteal (adults):* 1½ inch
  - *ID:* 1-ml tuberculin syringe with preattached 26- or 27-gauge needle
- Small gauze pad and/or alcohol swab
- Vial or ampule of medication or skin test solution
- Disposable gloves
- MAR or computer printout

Steps	Rationale
For All Injections	
1. Review prescriber's medication order for client's name, medication name, dose, time, route of administration, and drug indications.	Ensures safe and correct administration of medication.
2. Assess client's history of allergies and know substances client is allergic to and normal allergic reaction.	Certain substances have similar compositions; nurse should not administer any substance to which client is known to be allergic.
3. Check date of expiration for medication.	Drug potency may increase or decrease when outdated.
4. Observe verbal and nonverbal responses toward receiving injection.	Injections can be painful. Clients may have anxiety, which can increase pain.
5. Assess for contraindications.	
A. For subcutaneous injections Assess for factors such as circulatory shock or reduced local tissue perfusion. Assess adequacy of client's adipose tissue.	Reduced tissue perfusion interferes with medication absorption and distribution. Physiological changes of aging or client illness may influence the amount of subcutaneous tissue a client possesses. This influences methods for administering injections.
B. For intramuscular injections Assess for factors such as muscle atrophy, reduced blood flow, or circulatory shock.	Atrophied muscle absorbs medication poorly. Factors interfering with blood flow to muscles impair medication absorption.

Critical Decision Point: Because of documented adverse effects of IM injections, other routes of medication administration are safer. Verify that IM injection is necessary and explore alternative medication routes if possible (Rodger and King, 2000; Nicoll and Hesby, 2002).

6. Aseptically prepare correct medication dose from ampule or vial (see Skill 34-7, p. 875). Check carefully. Be sure all air is expelled.	Ensures that medication is sterile. Preparation techniques differ for ampule and vial.
7. Perform hand hygiene. Identify client; check identification bracelet with MAR and ask client's name.	Ensures correct client receives ordered medication.
8. Explain steps of procedure and tell client injection will cause a slight burning or sting.	Helps minimize client's anxiety.
9. Close room curtain or door.	Provides privacy.
10. Apply disposable gloves.	Reduces transfer of microorganisms.
11. Keep sheet or gown draped over body parts not requiring exposure.	Respects dignity of client while area to be injected is exposed.

Skill 34-8 *Administering Injections—cont'd*

Steps	Rationale
12. Select appropriate injection site. Inspect skin surface over sites for bruises, inflammation, or edema.	Injection sites should be free of abnormalities that may interfere with medication absorption. Site used repeatedly can become hardened from lipohypertrophy (increased growth in fatty tissue). Do not use an area that is bruised or has signs associated with infection.
a. *Sub-Q:* Palpate sites for masses or tenderness. Avoid these areas. For daily insulin, rotate site daily. Be sure needle is correct size by grasping skinfold at site with thumb and forefinger. Measure fold from top to bottom. Needle should be one-half length.	Sub-Q injections can be inadvertently given in the muscle, especially in the abdomen and thigh sites. Appropriate size of needle ensures that medication will be injected in the subcutaneous tissue.
b. *IM:* Note integrity and size of muscle and palpate for tenderness or hardness. Avoid these areas. If injections are given frequently, rotate sites.	The ventrogluteal site is the preferred site for children older than 7 months and adults unless there are contraindications to this site. In infants younger than 7 months, the vastus lateralis should be used (Rodger and King, 2000; Nicoll and Hesby, 2002).
c. *ID:* Note lesions or discolorations of forearm. Select site three to four fingerwidths below antecubital space and a handwidth above wrist. If forearm cannot be used, inspect the upper back. If necessary, sites for Sub-Q injections may be used (Workman, 1999).	An ID site should be clear so that results of skin test can be seen and interpreted correctly.
13. Assist client to comfortable position:	
a. *Sub-Q:* Have client relax arm, leg, or abdomen, depending on site chosen for injection.	Relaxation of site minimizes discomfort.
b. *IM:* Have client lie flat, on side, or prone, depending on site chosen.	Reduces strain on muscle and minimizes discomfort of injections.
c. *ID:* Have client extend elbow and support it and forearm on flat surface.	Stabilizes injection site for easiest accessibility.
d. Talk with client about subject of interest.	Distraction reduces anxiety.

Critical Decision Point: Ensure that client's position is not contraindicated by medical condition.

Steps	Rationale
14. Relocate site using anatomical landmarks.	Injection into correct anatomical site prevents injury to nerves, bones, and blood vessels.
15. Cleanse site with an antiseptic swab. Apply swab at center of the site and rotate outward in a circular direction for about 5 cm (2 inches) (see illustration).	Mechanical action of swab removes secretions containing microorganisms.

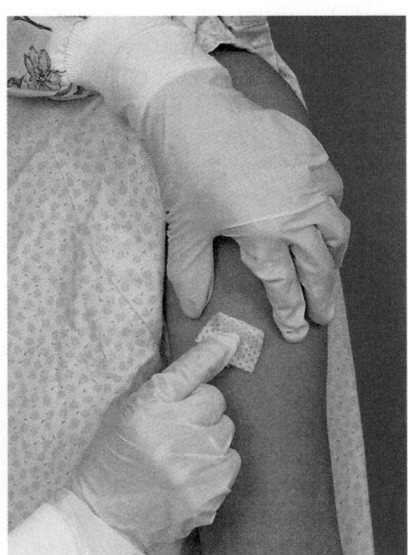

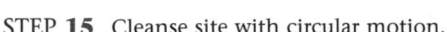
STEP **15** Cleanse site with circular motion.

Steps	Rationale
16. Hold swab or gauze between third and fourth fingers of nondominant hand.	Gauze or swab remains readily accessible when needle is withdrawn.
17. Remove needle cap or sheath from needle by pulling it straight off.	Preventing needle from touching sides of cap prevents contamination.
18. Hold syringe between thumb and forefinger of dominant hand	
a. *Sub-Q:* Hold as dart, palm down or hold syringe across tops of fingertips (see illustration).	Quick, smooth injection requires proper manipulation of syringe parts.
b. *IM:* Hold as dart, palm down.	
c. *ID:* Hold bevel of needle pointing up.	With bevel up, medication is less likely to be deposited into tissues below dermis.
19. Administer injection:	
A. Subcutaneous	
(1) For average-size client, spread skin tightly across injection site or pinch skin with nondominant hand.	Needle penetrates tight skin easier than loose skin. Pinching skin elevates subcutaneous tissue and may desensitize area.
(2) Inject needle quickly and firmly at 45- to 90-degree angle. Then release skin, if pinched.	Quick, firm insertion minimizes discomfort. (Injecting medication into compressed tissue irritates nerve fibers.)
(3) For obese client, pinch skin at site and inject needle at 90-degree angle below tissue fold.	Obese clients have fatty layer of tissue above subcutaneous layer.

Critical Decision Point: Piercing a blood vessel during a Sub-Q injection is very rare, so aspiration is not necessary when administering Sub-Q injections (Peragallo-Dittko, 1997; McConnell, 2000; American Diabetes Association, 2001)

---

(4) Inject medication slowly (see illustration).	Minimizes discomfort. Injecting heparin over 30 seconds may create less bruising (Chan, 2001).
B. Intramuscular	
(1) Position nondominant hand at proper anatomical landmarks and pull skin down to administer in a Z-track.	Z-track creates zigzag path through tissues that seals needle track to avoid tracking of medication. Z-track should be used for all IM injections (Nicoll and Hesby, 2002).
(2) If client's muscle mass is small, grasp body of muscle between thumb and fingers.	Ensures that medication reaches muscle mass (Hockenberry and others, 2003).

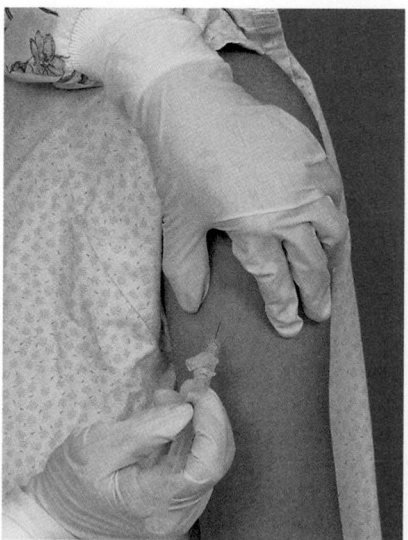

STEP **18A** Hold syringe as if grasping a dart.

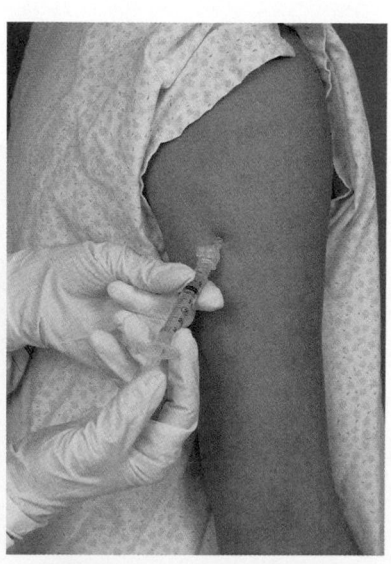

STEP **19A(4)** Inject medication slowly.

Skill 34-8   *Administering Injections—cont'd*

Steps	Rationale
(3) Insert needle quickly at 90-degree angle into muscle. After needle pierces skin, grasp lower end of syringe barrel with nondominant hand to stabilize syringe. Continue to hold skin tightly with nondominant hand. Move dominant hand to end of plunger. Do not move syringe.	Smooth manipulation of syringe reduces discomfort from needle movement. skin must remain pulled until after drug is injected to ensure Z-track administration.
(4) Pull back on plunger 5 to 10 seconds If no blood appears, inject medicine slowly, at a rate of 10 sec/ml.	Slow injection rate reduces pain and tissue trauma (Nicoll and Hesby, 2002).

Critical Decision Point: If blood appears in syringe, remove needle and dispose of medication and syringe properly. Prepare another dose of medication for injection.

(5) Wait 10 seconds Then smoothly and steadily withdraw needle and release skin. Apply gentle pressure with dry gauze if desired.	Allows time for medication to absorb into muscle before removing syringe. Some advocate use of dry gauze to minimize client discomfort (Nicoll and Hesby, 2002).
C. Intradermal	
(1) With nondominant hand, stretch skin over site with forefinger or thumb.	Needle pierces tight skin more easily.
(2) With needle almost against client's skin, insert it slowly with bevel up at a 5- to 15-degree angle until resistance is felt. Then advance needle through epidermis to approximately 3 mm (⅛ inch) below skin surface. Needle tip can be seen through skin.	Ensures needle tip is in dermis.
(3) Inject medication slowly. Normally, resistance is felt. If not, needle is too deep; remove and begin again.	Slow injection minimizes discomfort at site. Dermal layer is tight and does not expand easily when solution is injected.
(4) While injecting medication, notice that small bleb approximately 6 mm (¼ inch) in diameter (resembling mosquito bite) appears on skin's surface (see illustration).	Bleb indicates medication is deposited in dermis.
20. Withdraw needle while applying alcohol swab or gauze gently over site.	Support of tissue around injection site minimizes discomfort during needle withdrawal. Dry gauze may minimize client discomfort associated with alcohol on nonintact skin.

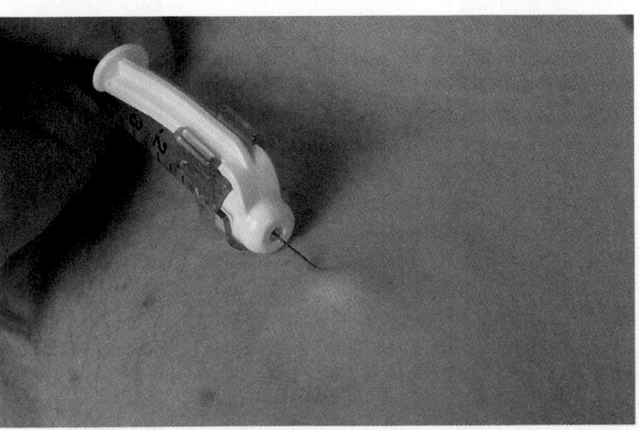

STEP **19C(4)** Injection creates a small bleb.

Steps	Rationale
21. Apply gentle pressure. Do not massage site. Apply bandage if needed.	Massage may cause underlying tissue damage. Massage of ID site may disperse medication into underlying tissue layers and alter test results.
22. Assist client to comfortable position.	Gives client sense of well-being.
23. Discard uncapped needle or needle enclosed in safety shield and attached syringe into puncture and leakproof receptacle. When nurse is unable to leave client's bedside, a one-handed technique can be used to recap a needle.	Prevents injury to client and health care personnel. Recapping needles increases risk of needle-stick injury (NIOSH, 1999).
24. Remove disposable gloves and perform hand hygiene.	Reduces transmission of microorganisms.
25. Stay with client 3 to 5 min and observe for any allergic reactions.	Severe anaphylactic reaction is characterized by dyspnea, wheezing, and circulatory collapse.
26. Return to room and ask if client feels any acute pain, burning, numbness, or tingling at injection site.	Continued discomfort may indicate injury to underlying bones or nerves.
27. Inspect site, noting any bruising or induration.	Bruising or induration indicates complication associated with injection. Document findings and notify health care provider. Provide warm compress to site.
28. Observe client's response to medication at times that correlate with the medication's onset, peak, and duration.	IM medications are rapidly absorbed. Adverse effects of parenteral medications may develop rapidly. Nurse's observations determine efficacy of medication action.
29. Ask client to explain purpose and effects of medication.	Evaluates client's understanding of information taught.
30. *For ID injections,* use skin pencil and draw circle around perimeter of injection site. Read site within 48 to 72 hr of injection.	Pencil mark makes site easy to find. Site must be read at various intervals to determine test results. Refer to manufacturer's directions to determine when to read the test's results.

Unexpected Outcomes and Related Interventions

- Raised, reddened, or hard zone (induration) forms around ID test site.
  - Notify client's health care provider.
  - Document sensitivity to injected allergen or positive test if tuberculin skin testing was completed.
- Hypertrophy of skin develops from repeated Sub-Q injections.
  - Do not use this site for future injections.
  - Instruct client not to use site for 6 months.
- Client develops signs and symptoms of allergy or side effects.
  - Follow institutional policy or guidelines for appropriate response to adverse drug reactions.
  - Notify client's health care provider immediately.
- Client complains of localized pain, numbness, tingling, or burning at injection site.
  - Potential injury to nerve or tissues may have occurred.
  - Assess injection site.
  - Document findings.
  - Notify client's health care provider.

Recording and Reporting

- Chart medication dose, route, site, time, and date given in medication record.
- Report any undesirable effects from medication to nurse in charge or physician.
- Record client's response to medications in nurses' notes.

Home Care Considerations

- Assess the client's readiness to learn before instructing on self-injections. Some clients are hesitant to administer injections to themselves, so relieve any anxiety before teaching this skill to a client.
- Some clients prefer to reuse their syringes to save costs. This practice is safe and practical if the needle is not contaminated during the preparation and administration of the injection. Needles should be recapped immediately after use.
- Clients can often purchase or obtain sharps boxes for home use. If this is not feasible, a hard plastic bottle that cannot be seen through (e.g., a fabric softener bottle or detergent bottle) may be used to safely store syringes after use. Disposal of needles used in the home varies among communities. Check with local authorities to verify how to dispose of needles.

Many clients, particularly children, fear injections. Clients with serious or chronic illness often are given several injections daily. The nurse may be able to minimize the client's discomfort in the following ways:

- Use a sharp-beveled needle in the smallest suitable length and gauge.
- Position the client as comfortably as possible to reduce muscular tension.
- Select the proper injection site, using anatomical landmarks.
- Divert the client's attention from the injection through conversation.
- Insert the needle quickly and smoothly to minimize tissue pulling.
- Hold the syringe steady while the needle remains in tissues.
- Inject the medication slowly and steadily.

Subcutaneous Injections. Subcutaneous injections involve placing medications into the loose connective tissue under the dermis (see Skill 34-8, p. 881). Because subcutaneous tissue is not as richly supplied with blood as the muscles, medication absorption is somewhat slower than with intramuscular injections. However, medications are absorbed completely if the client's circulatory status is normal. Because subcutaneous tissue contains pain receptors, the client may experience some discomfort.

The best subcutaneous injection sites include the outer posterior aspect of the upper arms, the abdomen from below the costal margins to the iliac crests, and the anterior aspects of the thighs (Figure 34-22). The site most frequently recommended for heparin injections is the abdomen (Figure 34-23). Other sites include the scapular areas of the upper back and the upper ventral or dorsal gluteal areas. The injection site chosen should be free of skin lesions, bony prominences, and large underlying muscles or nerves.

Clients with diabetes should practice intrasite rotation of insulin injections. Use of the same part of the body for a sequence of injections provides more consistency in the absorption of the insulin. For example, if the morning insulin is injected into the client's arm, then a subsequent injection should also be given in the arm. The injections are to be given at least an inch away from the previous site. No injection site should be used again for at least 1 month.

Only small doses (0.5 to 1 ml) of water-soluble medications should be given subcutaneously because the tissue is sensitive to irritating solutions and large volumes of medications. Collection of medications within the tissues can cause sterile abscesses, which appear as hardened, painful lumps under the skin.

A client's body weight indicates the depth of the subcutaneous layer. Therefore the nurse must choose the needle length and angle of insertion based on weight. Generally a 25-gauge ⅝-inch needle inserted at a 45-degree angle (Figure 34-23) or a ½-inch needle inserted at a 90-degree angle deposits medications into the subcutaneous tissue of a normal-size client. A child may require only a ½-inch needle. If the client is obese, the nurse often pinches the tissue and uses a needle long enough to insert through fatty tissue at the base of the skinfold. The preferred needle length is one half the width of the skinfold. With this method, the angle of insertion may be between 45 and 90 degrees. Thin clients may have insufficient tissue for subcutaneous injections. The upper abdomen is the best site for injection with this client.

Insulin syringes generally come with 26- to 29-gauge needles. To ensure the insulin reaches the subcutaneous tissue, the nurse follows this rule: If 2 inches of tissue can be grasped, the needle should be inserted at a 90-degree angle; if 1 inch of tissue can be grasped, the needle should be inserted at a 45-degree angle.

Intramuscular Injections. The intramuscular route provides faster medication absorption than the subcuta-

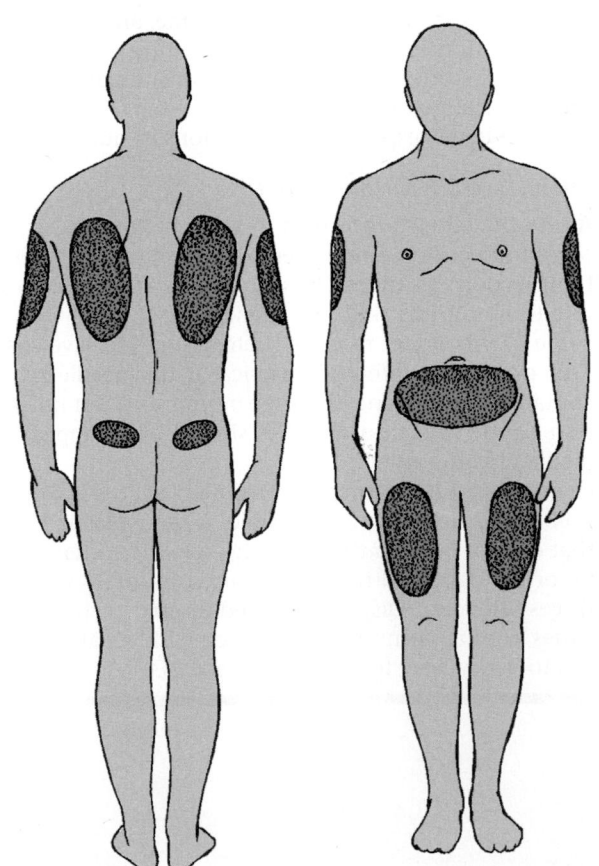

FIGURE **34–22** Sites recommended for subcutaneous injections.

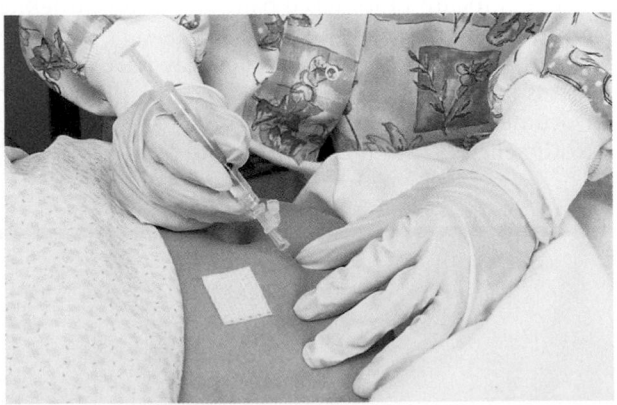

FIGURE **34–23** Giving Sub-Q heparin in the abdomen.

neous because of a muscle's greater vascularity. However, IM injections are associated with many risks. Therefore, whenever administering a medication by the IM route, the nurse must first verify that the injection is justified (Nicoll and Hesby, 2002).

The nurse uses a longer and heavier-gauge needle to pass through subcutaneous tissue and penetrate deep muscle tissue (see Skill 34-8, p. 881). Weight and the amount of adipose tissue can influence needle size selection. For example, an obese client may require a needle 3 inches long, and a thin client may only require a ½- to 1-inch needle.

The angle of insertion for an intramuscular injection is 90 degrees (see Figure 34-24). Muscle is less sensitive to irritating and viscous medications. A normal, well-developed client can tolerate 3 ml of medication into a larger muscle without severe muscle discomfort. A larger volume of medication is unlikely to be absorbed properly. Children, older adults, and thin clients can tolerate only 2 ml of an intramuscular injection. Hockenberry and others (2003) recommend giving no more than 1 ml to small children and older infants.

The nurse assesses the integrity of a muscle before giving an injection. The muscle should be free of tenderness. Repeated injections in the same muscle can cause severe discomfort. With the client relaxed, the nurse can palpate the muscle to rule out any hardened lesions. The nurse can minimize discomfort during an injection by helping the client assume a position that will help reduce muscle strain. Other interventions, such as distraction and applying pressure to the IM site may be used to decrease pain during an IM injection (Box 34-17).

Research Highlight

Box 34-17

Reducing Pain During Intramuscular Injections

Research Focus

Intramuscular injections are often associated with pain. Touch and massage has been used to decrease perceptions of pain. Further research is necessary to determine if the application of pressure at an injection site will decrease the client's perception of pain.

Research Abstract

The purpose of this study was to determine if the application of pressure at an intramuscular injection site would reduce the client's experience of pain. This study used an experimental design with intrasubject comparison. The 74 participants were Chinese students who were participating in an immunization program. Each participant received the hepatitis A vaccine and the hepatitis B vaccine, one in each arm. Pressure was applied to one arm for 10 seconds before the injection and was not applied to the other arm. The arm that received the pressure was determined randomly. After each injection, the participants ranked their pain on a Cantonese 0 to 10 pain scale. A pressure-sensing device measured the amount of pressure exerted. Females in this study reported higher levels of pain for all injections when compared with males. However, male and female participants both reported significantly less pain when they received a pressure of about 200 mm Hg for 10 seconds before the immunization.

Evidence-Based Practice

- Applying pressure at the site of an IM injection may reduce the pain experienced by the client.
- The findings of this study support the gate-control theory of the physiology of pain.
- The gender difference in the report of pain supports that men and women experience and report pain differently.
- Further research is needed to support these results with other client populations, medication types, and injection sites.

Reference

Chung J, Ng WMY, Wong TKS: An experimental study on the use of manual pressure to reduce pain in intramuscular injections, *J Clin Nurs* 11(4):457, 2002.

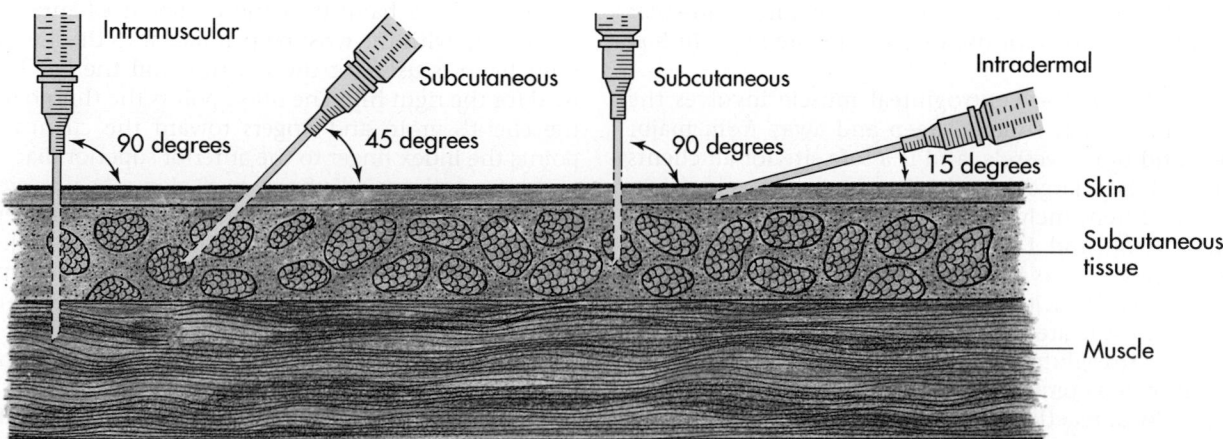

FIGURE **34-24** Comparison of angles of insertion for intramuscular (90 degrees), subcutaneous 90 degrees), and intradermal (15 degrees) injections.

Box 34-18   Characteristics of Intramuscular Sites and Indications for Usage

Vastus Lateralis

- Lacks major nerves and blood vessels
- Rapid drug absorption
- Preferred site for infants (less than 12 months) receiving immunizations
- May also be used in older children and toddlers receiving immunizations

Ventrogluteal

- A deep site, situated away from major nerves and blood vessels
- Less chance of contamination in incontinent clients or infants
- Easily identified by any prominent bony landmark
- Preferred site for medications (e.g., antibiotics) that are larger in volume, more viscous, and irritating for adults, children, and infants

Deltoid

- Easily accessible but muscle not well developed in most clients
- Used for small amounts of medications
- Not used in infants or children with underdeveloped muscles
- Potential for injury to radial and ulnar nerves or brachial artery
- May be used for immunizations for toddlers, older children, and adults
- Recommended site for hepatitis B vaccine and rabies injections

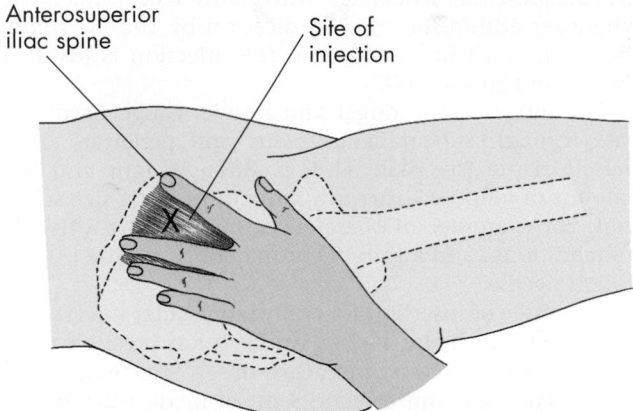

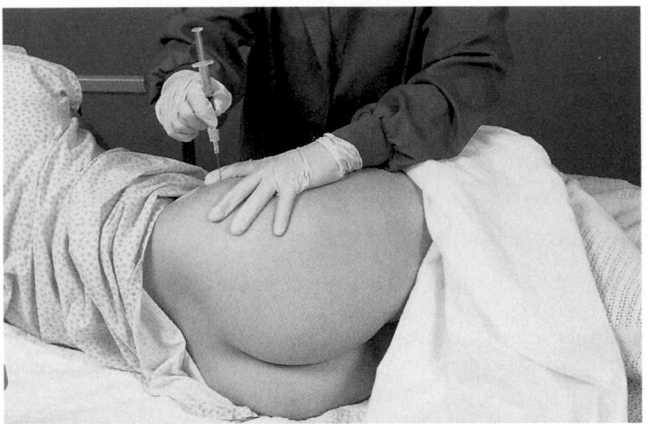

FIGURE 34–25 **A,** Landmarks for ventrogluteal site. **B,** Giving IM injection in ventrogluteal muscle.

Sites. When selecting an intramuscular site, the nurse considers the following: Is the area free of infection or necrosis? Are there local areas of bruising or abrasions? What is the location of underlying bones, nerves, and major blood vessels? What volume of medication is to be administered? Each site has certain advantages and disadvantages. The characteristics of each intramuscular site and indications for use of each site are listed in Box 34-18.

Ventrogluteal. The ventrogluteal muscle involves the gluteus medius, is situated deep and away from major nerves and blood vessels, and is a safe site for all clients because it is a large muscle that is well developed in young children, including those who do not walk, and adults (Nicoll and Hesby, 2002). Research has shown that injuries such as fibrosis, nerve damage, abscess, tissue necrosis, muscle contraction, gangrene, and pain have been associated with all the common IM sites except the ventrogluteal site. Actually, the only published case study of a complication at the ventrogluteal site reported a local reaction to the medication, which is not a complication associated with the site itself (Nicoll and Hesby, 2002).

Safety Alert. Research that has investigated complications associated with IM injection sites indicates that the ventrogluteal site is the preferred site for most injections given to adults and children over 7 months (Hockenberry and others, 2003; Nicoll and Hesby, 2002).

The nurse locates the ventrogluteal muscle by placing the heel of the hand over the greater trochanter of the client's hip with the wrist perpendicular to the femur. The right hand is used for the left hip, and the left hand is used for the right hip. The nurse points the thumb toward the client's groin and fingers toward the client's head, points the index finger to the anterior superior iliac spine, and extends the middle finger back along the iliac crest toward the buttock. The index finger, the middle finger, and the iliac crest form a V-shaped triangle, and the injection site is the center of the triangle (Figure 34-25, *A* and *B*). The client may lie on his or her side or back. Flexing of the knee and hip helps the client relax this muscle.

Vastus Lateralis. The vastus lateralis muscle is another injection site. The muscle is thick and well developed, is located on the anterior lateral aspect of the thigh, and extends in an adult from a handbreadth above the knee to a handbreadth below the greater trochanter of the femur

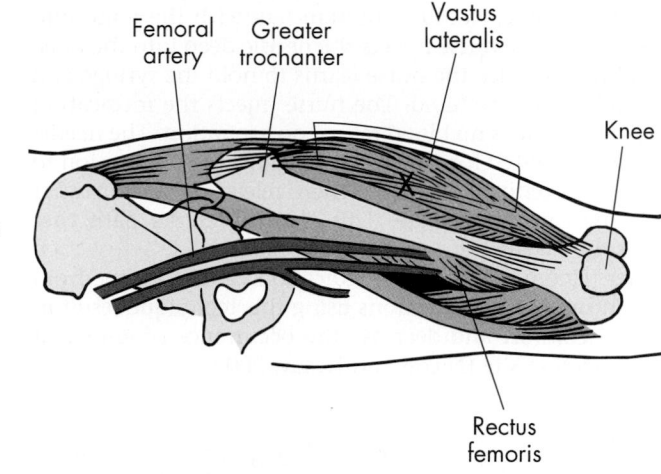

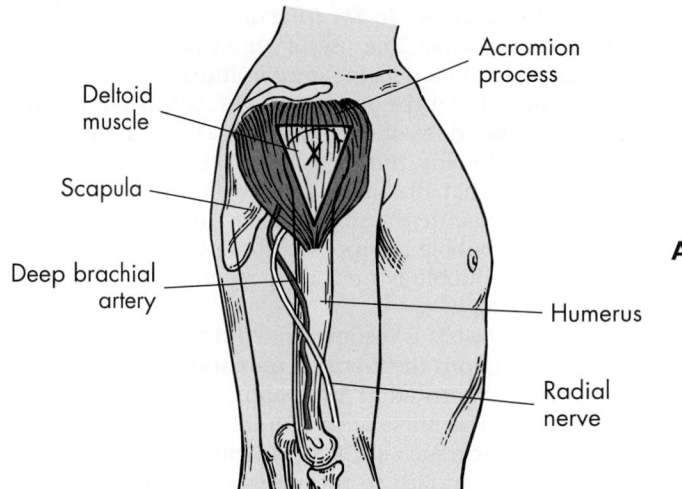

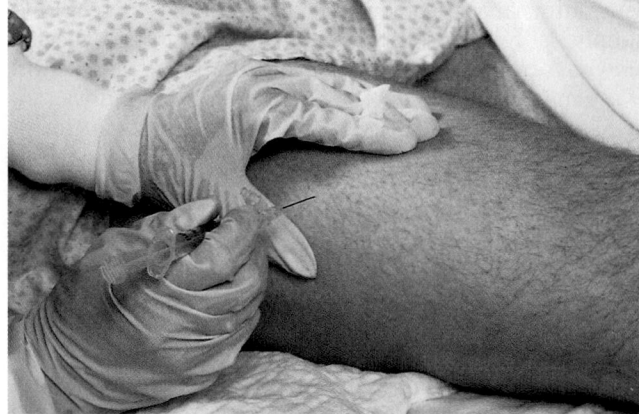

FIGURE **34–26 A,** Landmarks for vastus lateralis site. **B,** Giving IM injection in vastus lateralis muscle.

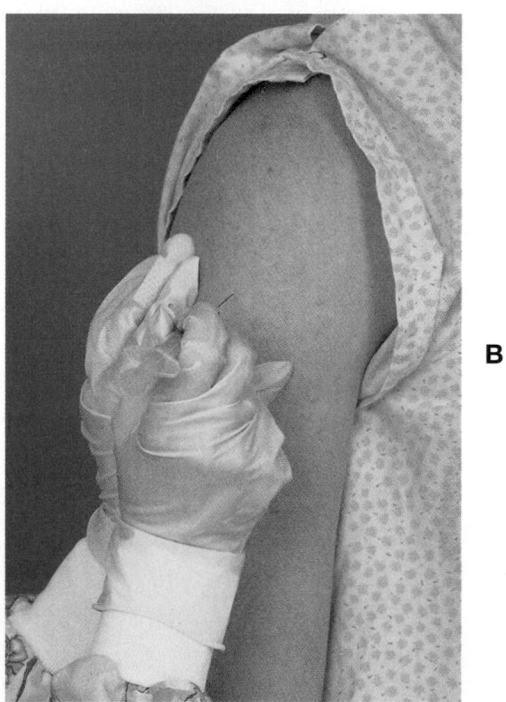

FIGURE **34–27 A,** Landmarks for deltoid site. **B,** Giving IM injection in deltoid muscle.

(Figure 34-25). The middle third of the muscle is the suggested site for injection. The width of the muscle usually extends from the midline of the thigh to the midline of the thigh's outer side. With young children or cachectic clients, it helps to grasp the body of the muscle during injection to be sure that the medication is deposited in muscle tissue. To help relax the muscle, the nurse asks the client to lie flat with the knee slightly flexed or in a sitting position.

Dorsogluteal. The dorsogluteal muscle has been a traditional site for intramuscular injections. However, studies have demonstrated that the exact location of the sciatic nerve varies from one person to another. If a needle hits a sciatic nerve, the client may experience permanent or partial paralysis of the involved leg. Therefore this site should **not** be used. (Beyea and Nicoll, 1995; Rodger and King, 2000.)

Deltoid. Although the deltoid site is easily accessible, the muscle is not well developed in many adults. There is a potential for injury when using this site because the axillary, radial, brachial, and ulnar nerves and brachial artery lie within the upper arm along the humerus (Figure 34-27, *A*). The nurse should use this site only for small medication volumes, when giving immunizations, or when other sites are inaccessible because of dressings or casts (Nicoll and Hesby, 2002).

To locate the deltoid muscle, the nurse fully exposes the client's upper arm and shoulder. A tight-fitting sleeve should not be rolled up. The nurse has the client relax the arm at the side and flex the elbow. The client may sit, stand, or lie down (Figure 34-27, *B*). The nurse palpates the lower edge of the acromion process, which forms the base of a triangle in line with the midpoint of the lateral aspect of the upper arm. The injection site is in the center of the triangle, about 3 to 5 cm (1 to 2 inches) below the acromion process (Nicoll and Hesby, 2002). The nurse may also locate the site by placing four fingers across the deltoid muscle, with the top finger along the acromion process. The injection site is then three fingerwidths below the acromion process.

Special Techniques in IM Injections

Air-Lock Technique. The use of an air bubble is a topic that draws heated debate among nurses. Historically, nurses believed that the air bubble was required to ensure that the correct dose of medication was prepared in the syringe. Additionally, nurses were told that the air bubble would ensure that the medication would remain in the muscle. However, neither of these two arguments for the use of the air bubble is supported today. Therefore drawing up an air bubble is no longer recommended (Nicoll and Hesby, 2002).

Z-Track Method. It is recommended that when administering IM injections the **z-track method** be used to minimize local skin irritation by sealing the medication in muscle tissue. The nurse selects an IM site, preferably in a large, deep muscle such as the ventrogluteal muscle. A new needle must be applied to the syringe after preparing the medication so that no solution remains on the outside needle shaft. After preparing the site with an antiseptic swab, the nurse pulls the overlying skin and subcutaneous tissues approximately 2.5 to 3.5 cm (1 to 1½ inches) later-

ally to the side. Holding the skin taut with the nondominant hand, the nurse injects the needle deep into the muscle. With practice the nurse learns to hold the syringe and aspirate with one hand. The nurse injects the medication slowly if there is no blood return on aspiration. The needle remains inserted for 10 seconds to allow the medication to disperse evenly. The nurse then releases the skin after withdrawing the needle. This leaves a zigzag path that seals the needle track where tissue planes slide across each other (Figure 34-28). The medication cannot escape from the muscle tissue. Injections using this technique result in less discomfort and decrease the occurrence of lesions at the injection site (Nicoll and Hesby, 2002).

Intradermal Injections. The nurse typically gives intradermal injections for skin testing (e.g., tuberculin screening and allergy tests). Because these medications are potent, they are injected into the dermis, where blood supply is reduced and medication absorption occurs slowly. A client may have a severe anaphylactic reaction if the medications enter the circulation too rapidly.

Skin testing requires that the nurse be able to clearly see the injection sites for changes in color and tissue integrity. Intradermal sites should be lightly pigmented,

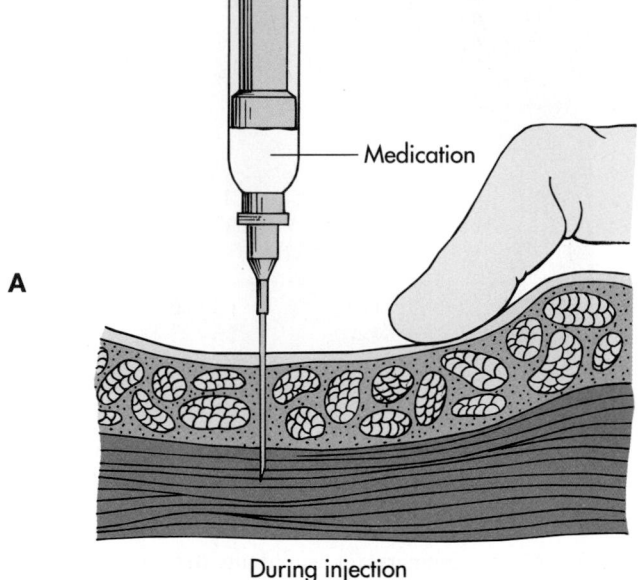

During injection

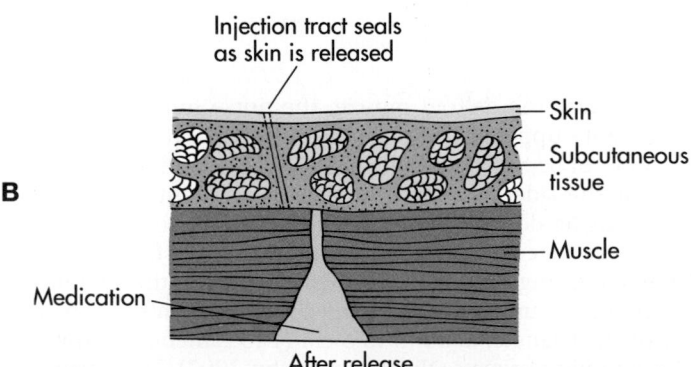

After release

FIGURE **34–28 A,** Pulling on overlying skin during IM injection moves tissue to prevent later tracking. **B,** The Z-track left after injection prevents the deposit of medication through sensitive tissue.

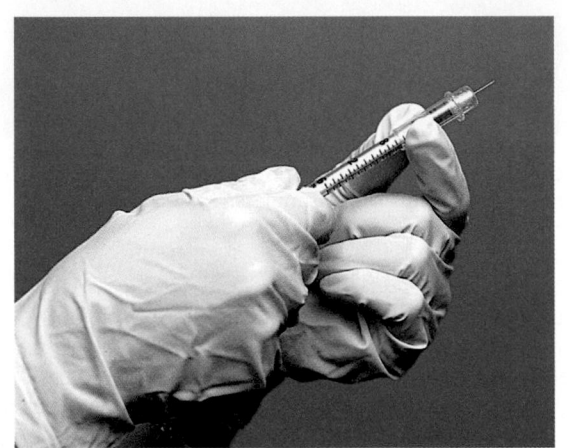

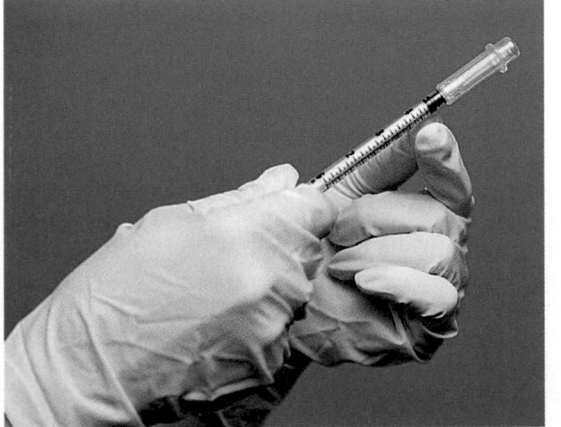

FIGURE **34–29** Needle with plastic guard to prevent needle sticks. **A,** Position of guard before injection. **B,** After injection the guard locks in place, covering the needle.

free of lesions, and relatively hairless. The inner forearm and upper back are ideal locations.

The nurse uses a tuberculin or small hypodermic syringe for skin testing. The angle of insertion for an intradermal injection is 5 to 15 degrees (see Figure 34-24, p. 887) and the bevel of the needle is pointed up. As the nurse injects the medication, a small bleb resembling a mosquito bite should appear on the skin's surface (see Skill 34-8, p. 881). If a bleb does not appear or if the site bleeds after needle withdrawal, there is a good chance the medication entered subcutaneous tissues. In this case, test results will not be valid.

Safety in Administering Medications by Injection

Needleless Devices. Between 600,000 and 1 million accidental needle sticks and sharps injuries occur annually in health care settings (American Nurses Association, 1999). These injuries commonly occur when needles are recapped, IV lines and needles are mishandled, or needles are left at a client's bedside. The risk of exposure of health care workers to blood-borne pathogens has led to the development of "needleless devices" or special needle safety devices.

Special syringes are designed with a sheath or guard that covers the needle after it is withdrawn from the skin (Figure 34-29). The needle is immediately covered, eliminating the chance for a needle-stick injury. The syringe and sheath are disposed of together in a receptacle. "Needleless" devices should be used whenever possible to reduce the risk to health care workers of needle sticks and sharps injuries (OSHA, 2001).

Needles and other instruments considered "sharps" are always disposed of into clearly marked, appropriate containers (Figure 34-30). Containers should be puncture proof and leakproof. A needle should never be forced by anyone into a full needle disposable receptacle. Used needles and syringes are never placed in any wastebasket, in the nurse's pocket, on a client's meal tray, or at the client's bedside. Box 34-19 summarizes recommendations for the prevention of needle-stick injuries.

One-Handed Needle Recapping Technique. In administering injections it may be necessary, for client safety reasons, to recap a contaminated needle. For example, the nurse may be assisting with emergency measures at the bedside and cannot reach a disposable container. If a commercially made recapping device is not available, then the nurse should use the one-handed needle recapping technique that is described in Box 34-20.

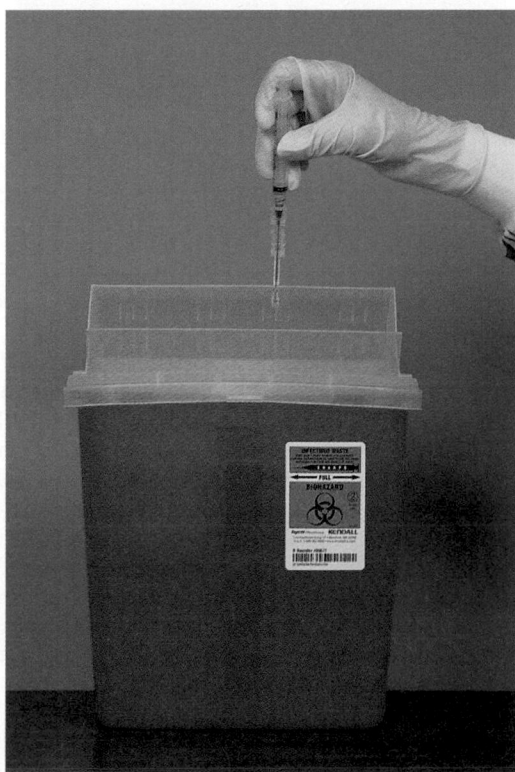

FIGURE **34–30** Sharps disposal using only one hand.

Box *34-19* **Recommendations for the Prevention of Needle-Stick Injuries**

- Avoid using needles when effective needless systems or Sharps With Engineered Sharps Injury Protections (SESIP) safety devices are available.
- Do not recap any needle.
- Plan safe handling and disposal of needles before beginning the procedure.
- Immediately dispose of needles, needleless systems, and SESIP into puncture-proof and leak-proof sharps disposal containers.
- Maintain an exposure control plan (ECP) that includes the following:
    - Assessment and implementation of innovations in procedures and technological developments to reduce risks of exposure to contaminated sharps
    - Documentation of consideration and use of appropriate, commercially available, and effective safer devices
    - Selection of devices that do not jeopardize client or employee safety or are determined to be medically inadvisable
    - Documentation of input from employees in ECP as to methods to reduce exposure
    - Annual reexamination of ECP
- Maintain a sharps injury log that includes the following:
    - Type and brand of device involved in the incident
    - Location of the incident (e.g., department or work area)
    - Description of the incident
    - Maintains privacy of the employees who have had sharps injuries

Data from Occupational Safety and Health Administration (OSHA): Occupational exposure to bloodborne pathogens: needlestick and other sharp injuries—final rule, *Federal Register,* CFR 29, part 1910(66:5317), January 18, 2001; and National Institute for Occupational Safety and Health (NIOSH): NIOSH alert preventing needle-stick injuries in health care settings, NIOSH Publications Dissemination, DHHS (NIOSH) Publication No. 2000-108, November, 1999.

Box 34-20 **Procedural Guidelines**

One-Handed Needle Recapping Technique

Needles should never be recapped. **This procedure should be used only when a sharps disposal box is unavailable and the nurse cannot leave the client's room.** Needle-stick injuries place the health care worker at risk for blood-borne pathogens. After using a needle, the health care worker should dispose of the sharp in the nearest designated container.

1. Before giving the injection, place the needle cover on a solid, immovable object such as the rim of a bedside table. The open end of the cap should face the nurse and be within reach of the nurse's dominant, or injection, hand.
2. Give the injection.
3. Place the tip of the needle at the entrance of the cap. *Gently* slide the needle into the needle cover (see illustrations).
4. Once the needle is inside the cover, use the object's resistance to completely cover the needle (see illustration).
5. Dispose of the needle at the first opportunity.
6. Perform hand hygiene.

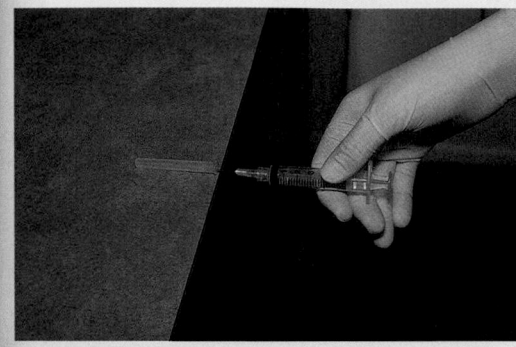

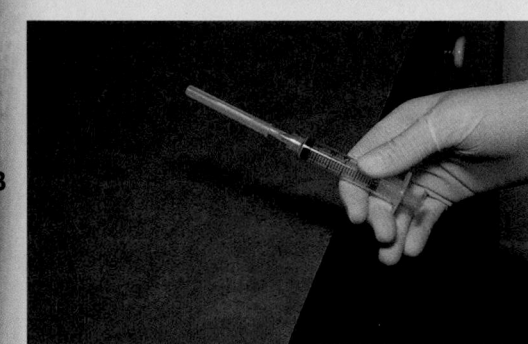

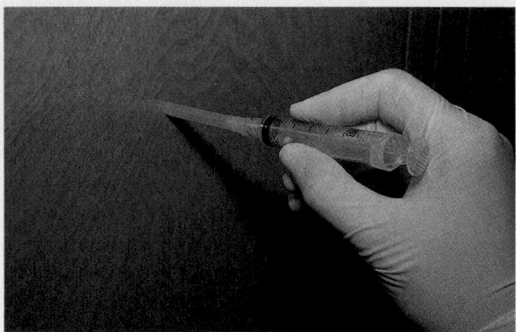

STEP 3 **A,** Place needle tip at entrance of the cap. **B,** Slide needle into the cover.

STEP 4 Place needle cover against resistance to secure.

Intravenous Administration. The nurse administers medications intravenously by the following methods:
1. As mixtures within large volumes of IV fluids
2. By injection of a bolus, or small volume, of medication through an existing intravenous infusion line or intermittent venous access (heparin or saline lock)
3. By "piggyback" infusion of a solution containing the prescribed medication and a small volume of IV fluid through an existing IV line.

In all three methods the client has either an existing IV infusion line or an IV access site such as an intermittent infusion (sometimes called a heparin or saline lock). In most institutions, policies and procedures list persons who may give IV medications and the situations in which they may be given. These policies are based on the medication, capability and availability of staff, and type of monitoring equipment available.

Chapter 40 describes the technique for performing venipuncture and establishing continuous IV fluid infusions. Medication administration is only one reason for supplying IV fluids. Intravenous fluid therapy is used primarily for fluid replacement in clients unable to take oral fluids and as a means of supplying electrolytes and nutrients.

When using any method of IV medication administration, the nurse must observe clients closely for symptoms of adverse reactions. After a medication enters the bloodstream, it begins to act immediately, and there is no way to stop its action. Thus the nurse takes special care to avoid errors in dose calculation and preparation. The nurse should double-check the six rights of safe medication administration and know the desired action and side effects. If the medication has an antidote, it must be available during administration. When administering potent medications, the nurse assesses vital signs before, during, and after infusion.

Administering medications by the IV route has advantages. Often the nurse uses the IV route in emergencies when a fast-acting medication must be delivered quickly. The IV route is also best when it is necessary to establish constant therapeutic blood levels. Some medications are highly alkaline and irritating to muscle and subcutaneous tissue. These medications cause less discomfort when given intravenously.

Safety Alert. Because IV medications are immediately available to the bloodstream once they are administered, the nurse must verify the prescribed rate of administration so that the medication is given over the appropriate amount of time. Clients may experience severe adverse reactions if IV medications are administered too quickly. Verify the rate of administration with a drug reference or a pharmacist before giving any IV medication.

Large-Volume Infusions. Of the three methods of administering IV medications, mixing medications in large volumes of fluids is the safest and easiest. Medications are diluted in large volumes (500 ml or 1000 ml) of compatible IV fluids such as normal saline or lactated Ringer's solution (Skill 34-9). In most institutions the pharmacist adds medications to the primary container of IV solution to ensure asepsis. Because the medication is not in a concentrated form, the risk of side effects or fatal reactions is minimal when infused over the prescribed time frame. Vitamins and potassium chloride are two types of medications commonly added to IV fluids. However, there is a danger with continuous infusion: if the IV fluid is infused too rapidly, the client may suffer circulatory fluid overload.

Intravenous Bolus. An IV bolus involves introducing a concentrated dose of a medication directly into the systemic circulation (Skill 34-10). Because a bolus requires only a small amount of fluid to deliver the medication, it is an advantage when the amount of fluid the client can take is restricted. The IV bolus, or "push," is the most dangerous method for administering medications because there is no time to correct errors. In addition, a bolus may cause direct irritation to the lining of blood vessels. Therefore some have added three additional "rights" to administering IV push medications: the right dilution or flush, the right speed, and the right monitoring (Zurlinden, 2002).

Before administering a bolus the nurse confirms placement of the IV line. This involves obtaining a blood return through the IV catheter or needle. The inability to obtain a blood return suggests that the needle or catheter is in the client's tissues or resting against the vein wall. A medication should never be given intravenously if the insertion site appears puffy or edematous or the IV fluid cannot flow at the proper rate. Accidental injection of a medication into the tissues around a vein can cause pain, sloughing of tissues, and abscesses, depending on the medication's composition.

The rate of administration of an IV bolus medication is usually determined by the amount of medication that can be given each minute. The nurse should look up each medication to determine the recommended concentration and rate of administration. The purpose for which a medication is prescribed and any potential adverse effects related to the rate or route of administration must be considered when a nurse gives a medication IV push.

Volume-Controlled Infusions. Another way of administering IV medications is through small amounts (50 to 100 ml) of compatible IV fluids. The fluid is within a secondary fluid container separate from the primary fluid bag. The container connects directly to the primary IV

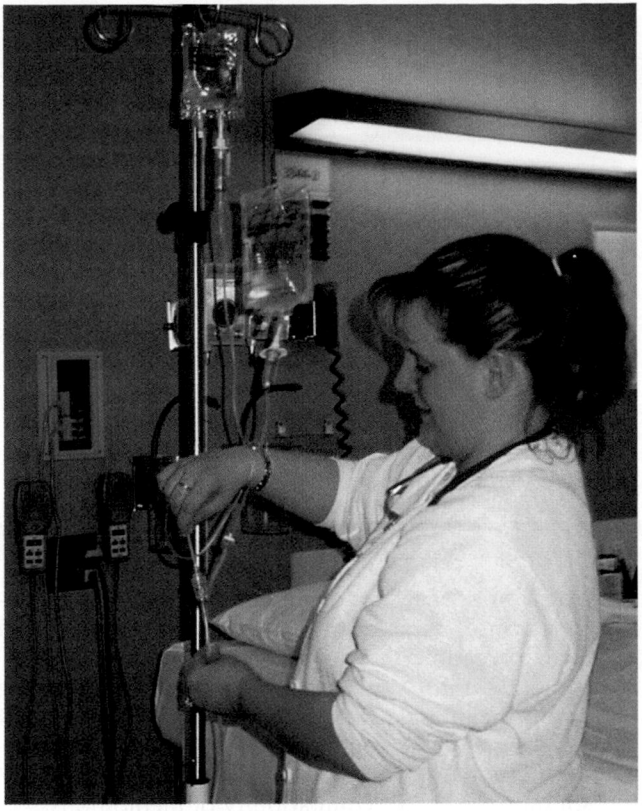

FIGURE **34–31**   Piggyback setup.

line or to separate tubing that inserts into the primary line. Three types of containers are volume control administration sets (e.g., Volutrol or Pediatrol), piggyback and/or tandem set, and miniinfusors. Using volume-controlled infusions has several advantages:

- It reduces risk of rapid-dose infusion by IV push. Medications are diluted and infused over longer time intervals (e.g., 30 to 60 minutes).
- It allows for administration of medications (e.g., antibiotics) that are stable for a limited time in solution.
- It allows for control of IV fluid intake.

Piggyback. A piggyback is a small (25 to 250 ml) IV bag or bottle connected to short tubing lines that connects to the *upper* Y-port of a primary infusion line or to an intermittent venous access (Figure 34-31). The piggyback tubing is a microdrip or macrodrip system (see Chapter 40). The set is called a piggyback because the small bag or bottle is set higher than the primary infusion bag or bottle. In the piggyback setup the main line does not infuse when the piggybacked medication is infusing. The port of the primary IV line contains a back-check valve that automatically stops flow of the primary infusion once the piggyback infusion flows. After the piggyback solution infuses and the solution within the tubing falls below the level of the primary infusion drip chamber, the back-check valve opens and the primary infusion again flows.

Tandem. A tandem setup is a small (25 to 100 ml) IV bag or bottle connected to a short tubing line to the *lower* Y-port of a primary infusion line or to an intermittent venous access. The tandem set is placed at the same height

Text continued on p. 900

Adding Medications to Intravenous Fluid Containers

Skill 34-9

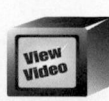

Delegation Considerations

Adding medications to IV fluid containers should not be delegated to assistive personnel. (In some institutions the pharmacist may add medications to primary containers of IV solutions to ensure asepsis.)

Equipment

- Vial or ampule of prescribed medication
- Syringe of appropriate size (5 to 20 ml)
- Sterile needle (1 to 1½ in, 19 to 21 gauge) with special filters (optional)
- Correct diluent if indicated (e.g., sterile water, normal saline)
- Sterile IV fluid container (bag or bottle, 25 to 1000 ml in volume)
- Alcohol or antiseptic swab
- Label to attach to IV bag or bottle
- MAR or computer printout

Steps	Rationale
1. Check prescriber's order to determine type of IV solution to use, name of medication, dosage, route, and drug indication.	Client's overall physical condition dictates type of IV solution used. Ensures safe and accurate medication administration.
2. Collect information necessary to administer drug safely, including action, purpose, side effects, normal dose, time of peak onset, and nursing implications.	Allows nurse to give medication safely and to monitor client's response to therapy.
3. When more than one medication is to be added to IV solution, assess for compatibility of medications.	Medications often are incompatible when mixed together. Chemical reactions that occur result in clouding or crystallization of IV fluids. Check hospital policy for approved medication compatibility list.
4. Assess client's systemic fluid balance, as reflected by skin hydration and turgor, body weight, pulse, and blood pressure.	Danger of continuous IV infusions is that fluids may infuse too rapidly, causing circulatory overload (Hockenberry and others, 2003).
5. Assess client's history of medication allergies.	IV administration of medications causes rapid effects. Allergic response can be immediate.
6. Perform hand hygiene.	Reduces transfer of microorganisms.
7. Assess IV insertion site for signs of infiltration or phlebitis (see Chapter 40).	An intact, properly functioning site ensures medication is given safely.
8. Assemble supplies in medication room.	Ensures procedure will be orderly, with less likelihood of contaminating supplies.
9. Prepare prescribed medication from vial or ampule (see Skill 34-7, p. 875).	Ensures accurate delivery of medication.
10. Identify client by reading identification band and asking name. Compare with MAR or medication order.	Ensures correct client receives medication.
11. Assess client's understanding of purpose of medication therapy.	May reveal need for education.
12. Add medication to new container (usually done in medication room or at medication cart):	
a. *Solution in a bag:* Locate medication injection port on plastic IV solution bag. Port has small rubber stopper at end. Do not select port for the IV tubing insertion or air vent.	Medication injection port is self-sealing to prevent introduction of microorganisms after repeated use.
b. *Solution in a bottle:* Locate injection site on IV solution bottle, which is often covered by a metal or plastic cap.	Accidental injection of medication through main tubing port or air vent can alter pressure within bottle and cause fluid leaks through air vent. Cap seals bottle to maintain its sterility.
c. Wipe off port or injection site with alcohol or antiseptic swab (see illustration).	Reduces risk of introducing microorganisms into bag during needle insertion.
d. Remove needle cap or sheath from syringe and insert needle of syringe or needleless device through center of injection port or site; inject medication (see illustration).	Injection of needle into sides of port may produce leak and lead to fluid contamination.

Steps	Rationale

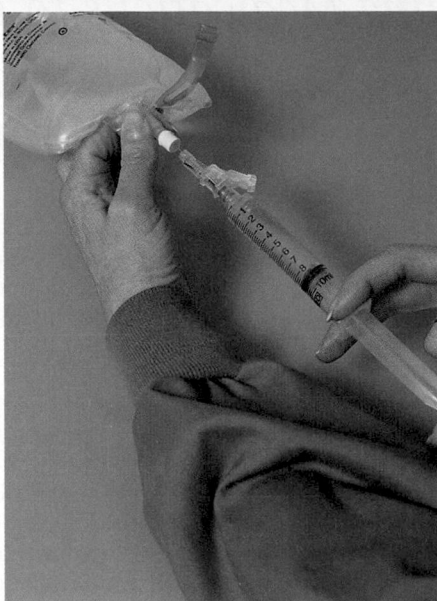

STEP **12c** Cleanse injection port with anti-septic swab.

STEP **12d** Inject medication through port.

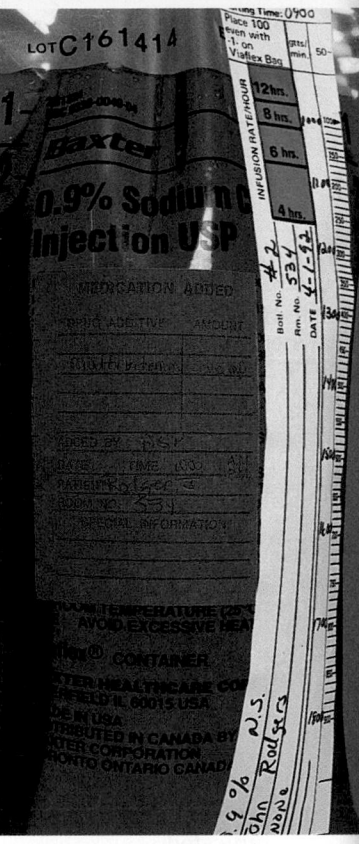

STEP **12g** Affix label to IV bag.

e. Withdraw syringe from bag or bottle.	Open tubing port in bottle provides direct route for microorganisms to enter solution. Bags have self-sealing port.
f. Mix medication and IV solution by holding bag or bottle and turning it gently end to end.	Allows even distribution of medication.
g. Complete medication label with name and dose of medication, date, time, and nurse's initials. Apply it to bottle or bag. *Optional (check agency policy): Apply a flow strip that identifies the time the solution was hung and intervals indicating fluid levels (see illustration).* Spike bag or bottle with IV tubing.	Label can be easily read during infusion of solution. Informs nurses and physicians of contents of bag or bottle.

Critical Decision Point: Do not use felt-tip markers to draw on flow strip. The ink can penetrate the plastic and leak into the IV solution.

---

13. Bring assembled items to client's bedside.	Ensures correct client receives ordered medication.
14. Prepare client by explaining that medication is to be given through existing IV line or one to be started. Explain that no discomfort should be felt during medication infusion. Encourage client to report symptoms of discomfort.	Most IV medications do not cause discomfort when diluted. However, potassium chloride can be irritating. Pain at insertion site may be early indication of infiltration.
15. Regulate infusion at ordered rate.	Prevents rapid infusion of fluid.

Critical Decision Point: Some medications (e.g., potassium chloride) can cause serious adverse reactions, including fatal cardiac dysrhythmias. These medications should be infused on an IV pump. Check institutional guidelines or policies indicating which IV medications require administration on an IV pump.

Adding Medications to Intravenous Fluid Containers—cont'd

Skill 34-9

Steps	Rationale

16. Add medication to existing container:

Critical Decision Point: Because there is no way to know exactly how much IV fluid is in an existing hanging IV container, there is no way to determine the exact concentration of the medication in the IV solution. Therefore it is recommended that medications be added to new IV fluid containers whenever possible.

---

a. Prepare vented IV bottle or plastic bag:	
(1) Check volume of solution remaining in bottle or bag.	Proper minimal volume (see drug insert) is needed to dilute medication adequately.
(2) Close off IV infusion clamp.	Prevents medication from directly entering circulation as it is injected into bag or bottle.
(3) Wipe off medication port with an alcohol or antiseptic swab.	Mechanically removes microorganisms that could enter container during needle insertion.
(4) Insert syringe needle or needleless device through injection port and inject medication.	Injection port is self-sealing and prevents fluid leaks.
(5) Withdraw syringe from bag or bottle.	
(6) Lower bag or bottle from IV pole and gently mix. Rehang bag.	Ensures medication is evenly distributed.
b. Complete medication label and apply it to bag or bottle.	Informs nurses and physicians of contents of bag or bottle.
c. Regulate infusion to desired rate. Use IV pump if indicated.	Prevents rapid infusion of fluid.
17. Properly dispose of equipment and supplies. Do not cap needle of syringe. Specially sheathed needles are discarded as a unit with needle covered.	Proper disposal of needle prevents injury to nurse and client. Capping of needles increases risk of needle-stick injuries.
18. Perform hand hygiene.	Reduces transmission of microorganisms.
19. Observe client for signs or symptoms of medication reaction.	IV medications can cause rapid effects.
20. Observe for signs and symptoms of fluid volume excess.	Rapid uncontrolled infusion can cause circulatory overload.
21. Periodically return to client's room to assess IV insertion site and rate of infusion.	Over time IV site may become infiltrated or needle malpositioned. Flow rate may change according to client's position or volume left in container.
22. Observe for signs or symptoms of IV infiltration.	Infiltrated medications can injure tissue.

Unexpected Outcomes and Related Interventions

- Client has adverse or allergic reaction to medication.
  - Follow institutional policy or guidelines for appropriate response and reporting of adverse drug reactions.
  - Notify client's health care provider immediately.
- Client develops signs of fluid volume overload (e.g., abnormal breath sounds, shortness of breath, intake greater than output).
  - Circulatory regulation may be compromised.
  - Stop IV infusion.
  - Notify client's health care provider immediately.
- IV site becomes swollen, warm, reddened, and tender to touch (see Chapter 40).
  - Indicates phlebitis.
  - Stop IV infusion and discontinue IV.
  - Treat IV site as indicated by institutional policy.

  - Insert new IV site if continuation of IV therapy is indicated.
- IV site becomes cool, pale, and swollen (see Chapter 40).
  - Indicates signs of infiltration.
  - Some IV medications are extremely harmful to subcutaneous tissue.
  - Provide IV extravasation care (e.g., inject phentolamine [Regitine] around the IV infiltration site) as indicated by institutional policy, or use a medication reference manual or consult a pharmacist to determine appropriate follow-up care.

Recording and Reporting

- Record solution and medication added to parenteral fluid on appropriate form.
- Report any adverse effects to client's health care provider, and document adverse effects according to institutional policy.

*A*dministering Medications by Intravenous Bolus

Skill **34-10**

Delegation Considerations

Administering medications by intravenous bolus should not be delegated to assistive personnel (AP). The nurse should instruct AP to do the following:

- Report any unexpected drug reactions to the nurse.
- Report discomfort at infusion site as soon as possible.
- Obtain any required vital signs and report these findings to the nurse.

Equipment

- Watch with second hand
- MAR or computer printout
- Disposable gloves
- Antiseptic swab

- **IV push (existing line)**
  - Medication in vial or ampule
  - Syringe for medication preparation
  - Needleless device or sterile needle (21 to 25 gauge)
- **IV push (IV lock)**
  - Medication in vial or ampule
  - Syringe for medication preparation
  - Vial of appropriate flush solution (saline most common, but heparin may also be used; if heparin is used, most common concentration is 10 to 100 units; check agency policy)
  - Needleless device or sterile needle (21 to 25 gauge)

Steps	Rationale
1. Check the prescriber's order for name of medication to be administered, dosage, route, and drug indication.	Ensures safe and accurate medication administration.

Critical Decision Point: Some IV medications can only be pushed safely when the client is being continuously monitored for dysrhythmias, blood pressure changes, or other adverse effects. Therefore some medications can only be pushed in specific areas within a health care agency. Confirm institutional guidelines regarding requirements for special monitoring and verify these requirements are available before giving medication (Zurlinden, 2002).

Steps	Rationale
2. Perform hand hygiene. Assess IV or saline (heparin) lock insertion site for signs of infiltration or phlebitis (see Chapter 40).	Confirming the placement of the IV catheter and the integrity of the surrounding tissue ensures that the medication is administered safely.
3. If medication is to be pushed into an IV line, assess the patency of the line by noting infusion rate.	The IV line must be patent, and fluids must infuse easily for medication to reach venous circulation effectively.
4. Prepare ordered medication from vial or ampule (see Skill 34-7, p. 875).	

Critical Decision Point: Some IV medications require dilution before administration. Verify with agency policy. If a small amount of medication is given (e.g., less than 1 ml), dilute medication in 5 to 10 ml of normal saline or sterile water so that the medication does not collect in the "dead spaces" (e.g., Y-site injection port, IV cap) of the IV delivery system.

Steps	Rationale
5. Perform hand hygiene. Apply gloves.	Reduces transmission of infection. During IV bolus administration, risk of blood exposure is low. However, nurse may manipulate IV dressing or expose site while completing other activities. Gloves reduce exposure (NIOSH, 1999).
6. Check client's identification by looking at identification bracelet and asking name.	Ensures that medication is administered to correct client.
7. Administer medication by IV push (existing line):	
a. Select injection port of IV tubing closest to client. Whenever possible, injection port should accept a needleless syringe. Use IV filter if required by medication reference or agency policy.	The Occupational Safety and Health Administration (OSHA) and CDC strongly recommend that all IV injection sites be needleless to prevent needle-stick injuries (NIOSH, 1999).
b. Clean off injection port with antiseptic swab. Allow to dry.	Prevents introduction of microorganisms during needle insertion.

Administering Medications by Intravenous Bolus—cont'd

Skill 34-10

Steps	Rationale
c. Connect syringe to IV line. Insert needleless tip or small-gauge needle of syringe containing prepared drug through center of injection port.	Prevents damage to port's diaphragm and subsequent leakage.
d. Occlude IV line by pinching tubing just above injection port. Pull back gently on syringe's plunger to aspirate blood return.	Final check that medication is being delivered into the bloodstream.

Critical Decision Point: In some cases, especially with a smaller gauge IV needle, blood return may not be aspirated, even if IV is patent. If IV site does not show signs of infiltration, and IV fluid is infusing without difficulty, proceed with IV push.

e. Release tubing and inject medication within amount of time recommended by institutional policy, pharmacist, or medication reference manual. Use watch to time administration (see illustration). Intravenous line may be pinched while pushing medication and released when not pushing medication (see illustration). Allow IV fluids to infuse when not pushing medication.	Ensures safe medication infusion. Rapid injection of IV medication can prove fatal.

Critical Decision Point: If IV medication is incompatible with IV fluids, stop the IV fluids, clamp the IV line, flush with 10 ml of normal saline or sterile water, give the IV bolus over the appropriate amount of time, flush with another 10 ml of normal saline or sterile water at the same rate as the medication was administered, and then restart the IV fluids at the prescribed rate. If IV that is currently hanging is a medication (e.g., rantidine), disconnect IV and administer IV push as outlined in step 8 to avoid giving a sudden bolus of the medication in the existing IV line to the client and to avoid creating potential risks associated with IV incompatibilities. Some IV medications and fluids cannot be stopped. Verify institutional policy regarding the temporary stopping of IV fluids or continuous IV medications. If unable to stop IV infusion, start a new IV site (see Chapter 40) and administer medication using the IV lock method.

f. After injecting medication, release tubing, withdraw syringe, and recheck fluid infusion rate.	Injection of bolus may alter rate of fluid infusion. Rapid fluid infusion can cause circulatory overload.

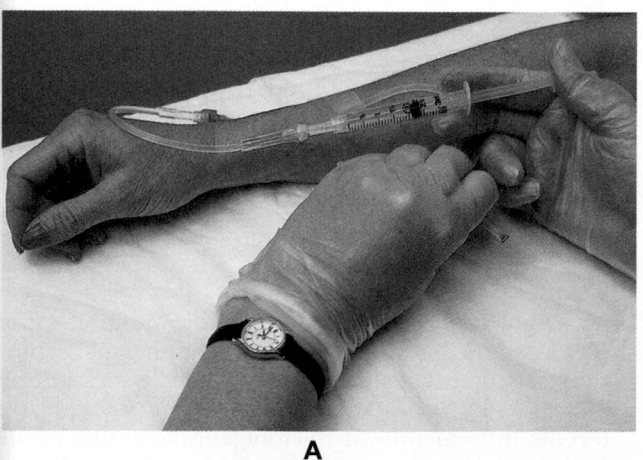 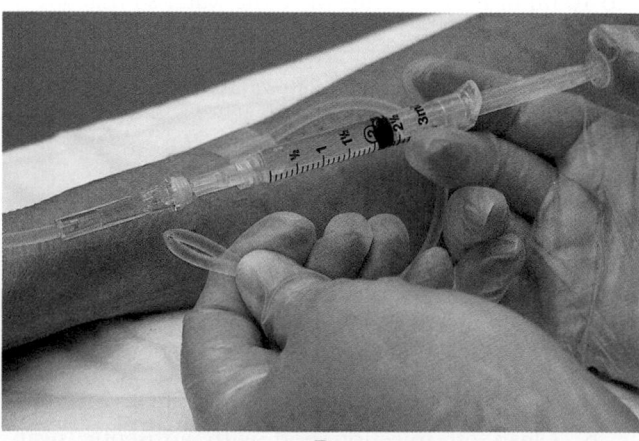

A	B

STEP **7e A,** Timing IV push medication. **B,** Intravenous line pinched off for medication infusion (optional).

Steps	**Rationale**

8. Administering medications by IV push (IV lock or a needleless system)
　　A. Prepare flush solutions according to agency policy
　　　　(1) Saline flush method (preferred method):

• Prepare two syringes with 2 to 3 ml of normal saline (0.9%) in syringe.	Normal saline has been found to be effective in keeping IV locks patent and is compatible with a wide range of medications.

　　　　(2) Heparin flush method (traditional method):
　　　　　　• Prepare one syringe with ordered amount of heparin flush solution.
　　　　　　• Prepare two syringes with 2 to 3 ml of normal saline.
　　B. Administer medication:

(1) Clean lock's injection port with antiseptic swab.	Prevents introduction of microorganisms during needle insertion.
(2) Insert syringe containing normal saline into injection port of IV lock (see illustration).	
(3) Pull back gently on syringe plunger and look for blood return.	Determines whether IV needle or catheter is positioned in vein.

Critical Decision Point: At times a saline (or heparin) lock will not yield a blood return even though the lock is patent. If IV site does not show signs of infiltration, proceed with IV push.

---

(4) Flush IV lock with 1 ml saline by pushing slowly on plunger.	Clears IV lock of blood.

Critical Decision Point: Observe closely the area of skin above the IV catheter. Note any puffiness or swelling as the IV lock is flushed, which could indicate infiltration into the vein, requiring removal of the catheter.

---

(5) Remove saline-filled syringe.	
(6) Clean lock's injection port with antiseptic swab.	Prevents transmission of infection.
(7) Insert syringe containing prepared medication into injection port of IV lock.	
(8) Inject medication within amount of time recommended by institutional policy, pharmacist, or medication reference manual. Use a watch to time administration.	Rapid injection of IV medication can result in death (Zurlinden, 2002).
(9) After administering bolus, withdraw syringe.	
(10) Clean lock's injection port with antiseptic swab.	Prevents transmission of microorganisms.

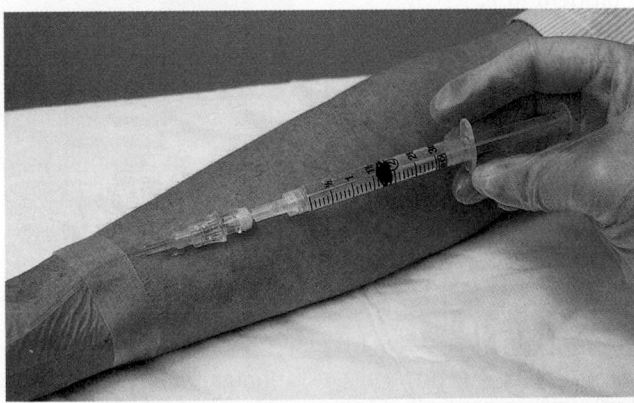

STEP **8B(2)** Syringe inserted into injection port.

Skill 34-10 *A*dministering Medications by Intravenous Bolus—cont'd

Steps	Rationale
(11) Attach syringe with normal saline and inject normal saline flush at the same rate the medication was delivered.	Irrigation with saline prevents occlusion of IV access device and ensures all medication is delivered. Flushing IV site at same rate as medication ensures that any medication remaining within IV needle is delivered at the correct rate.
(12) *Heparin flush option:* Insert needle of syringe containing heparin through diaphragm. Inject heparin slowly, and remove syringe.	Maintains patency of needle by inhibiting clot formation.
9. Dispose of uncapped needles and syringes in puncture-proof and leak-proof container.	Reduces accidental needle sticks.
10. Remove and dispose of gloves. Perform hand hygiene.	Reduces the transmission of microorganisms.
11. Observe client closely for adverse reaction as drug is administered and for several minutes thereafter.	IV medications act rapidly.

Unexpected Outcomes and Related Interventions

- Client develops adverse reaction to medication.
  - Stop delivering medication immediately and follow institutional policy or guidelines for appropriate response and reporting of adverse drug reactions.
  - Notify client's health care provider of adverse effects immediately.

- Intravenous site becomes puffy.
  - Immediately discontinue administration of injection and discontinue site.
  - Follow institutional guidelines on appropriate extravasation care.

Recording and Reporting

- Record medication, dose, time, and route on appropriate form.
- Report any adverse reactions immediately to health care provider because they could be life threatening. Client's response may indicate need for additional medical therapy.

as the primary infusion bag or bottle. In the tandem setup the tandem and the main line infuse simultaneously. The nurse must monitor the tandem setup closely. If the tandem setup is not immediately clamped when the medication is infused, the IV solution from the primary line will back up into the tandem line.

Volume-Control Administration. Volume-control administration (Volutrol, Buretrol, Pediatrol) sets are small (50 to 150 ml) containers that attach just below the primary infusion bag or bottle. The set is attached and filled in a manner similar to that used with a regular IV infusion. However, the priming filling of the set is different, depending on the type of filter (floating valve or membrane) within the set. Follow package directions for priming sets (see Chapter 40).

Miniinfusion Pump. The miniinfusion pump is battery operated and allows medications to be given in very small amounts of fluid (5 to 60 ml) within controlled infusion times using standard syringes (Skill 34-11).

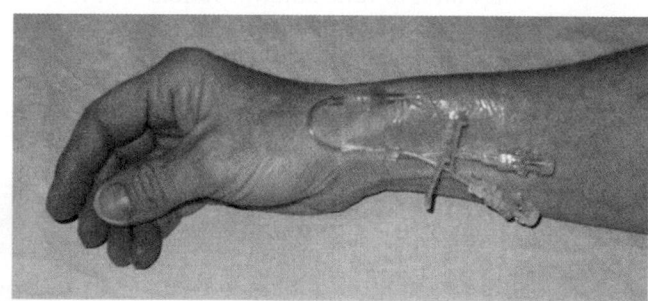

FIGURE **34–32**   Intermittent lock covered with a rubber diaphragm

Intermittent Venous Access. An intermittent venous access (commonly called a heparin lock or saline lock) is an IV catheter with a small chamber covered by a rubber diaphragm or a specially designed cap (Figure 34-32). Special rubber-seal injection caps accept needle safety devices and can be inserted into most IV catheters (see Chapter 40).

Text continued on p. 906

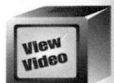

Administering Intravenous Medications by Piggyback, Intermittent Intravenous Infusion Sets, and Miniinfusion Pumps

Skill 34-11

Delegation Considerations

Administering medications by IV fluid by piggyback, intermittent intravenous infusion sets, and miniinfusion pumps should not be delegated to assistive personnel (AP). The nurse must instruct AP to report the following:
- Any unexpected drug reactions
- Discomfort at infusion site as soon as possible.

Equipment

- Antiseptic swab
- IV pole
- MAR or computer printout
- Medication label

- **Piggyback, Tandem, or Miniinfusion Pump**
  - Medication prepared in 5- to 150-ml labeled infusion bag or syringe
  - Short microdrip or macrodrip tubing set for piggyback (may have needleless system attachment)
  - Needleless device or stopcocks if available
  - Needles (21 or 23 gauge, only if stopcocks or other needleless methods are not available)
  - Miniinfusion pump
  - Adhesive tape (optional)
- **Volume-Control Administration Set**
  - Volutrol or Buretrol
  - Infusion tubing (may have needleless system attachment)
  - Syringe (1 to 20 ml)
  - Vial or ampule of ordered medication

Steps	Rationale
1. Check prescriber's order to determine type of IV solution to be used, name of medication, dose, route, time of administration, and drug indication.	Client's overall physical condition dictates type of IV solution used. Ensures safe and accurate medication administration.
2. Collect information necessary to administer medication safely, including action, purpose, side effects, normal dose, time of peak onset, and nursing implications.	Allows nurse to give medication safely and to monitor client's response to therapy.
3. Assess compatibility of drug with existing IV solution.	Drugs that are incompatible with IV solutions may result in clouding or crystallization of solution in IV tubing, which may harm the client.

Critical Decision Point: Never administer IV medications through tubing that is infusing blood, blood products, or parenteral nutrition solutions.

4. Assess patency of client's existing IV infusion line by noting infusion rate of main IV line.	IV line must be patent and fluids must infuse easily for medication to reach venous circulation effectively.

Critical Decision Point: If the client's IV site is saline locked, cleanse the port with alcohol and assess the patency of the IV line by flushing it with 2 to 3 ml of sterile normal saline. Attach appropriate IV tubing to the saline lock, and administer the medication via piggyback, tandem, miniinfusion, or volume-control administration set. When the infusion is completed, disconnect the tubing, cleanse the port with alcohol, and flush the IV line with 2 to 3 ml sterile normal saline. Maintain sterility of IV tubing between intermittent infusions.

5. Perform hand hyiene. Assess IV insertion site for signs of infiltration or phlebitis: redness, pallor, swelling, tenderness on palpation.	Confirmation of placement of IV needle or catheter and integrity of surrounding tissues ensures medication is administered safely.
6. Assess client's history of medication allergies.	Effects of medications can develop rapidly after IV infusion. Nurse should be aware of clients at risk.
7. Assess client's understanding of purpose of medication therapy.	May reveal need for education.
8. Assemble supplies at bedside. Prepare client by informing client that medication will be given through IV equipment.	Medication preparation usually is not required. Nurse may assemble infusion tubing and bag of medication in medication room or client's room. Allows client to understand procedure and minimizes anxiety.

*A*dministering Intravenous Medications by Piggyback, Intermittent Intravenous Infusion Sets, and Miniinfusion Pumps—cont'd

Skill 34-11

Steps	Rationale
9. Perform hand hygiene.	Reduces transmission of infection.
10. Check client's identification by looking at identification bracelet and asking client's name.	Ensures medication is administered to correct client.
11. Explain purpose of medication and side effects to client and explain that medication is to be given through existing IV line. Encourage client to report symptoms of discomfort at site.	Keeps client informed of planned therapies. Clients who can verbalize pain at the IV site can help detect IV infiltrations early, lessening damage to surrounding tissues.
12. Administer infusion:	
A. Piggyback or tandem infusion	
(1) Connect infusion tubing to medication bag (see Chapter 40). Allow solution to fill tubing by opening regulator flow clamp. Once tubing is full, close clamp and cap end of tubing.	Infusion tubing should be filled with solution and free of air bubbles to prevent air embolus.
(2) Hang piggyback medication bag above level of primary fluid bag. (Hook may be used to lower main bag.) Hang tandem infusion at same level as primary fluid bag.	Height of fluid bag affects rate of flow to client.
(3) Connect tubing of piggyback or tandem infusion to appropriate connector on primary infusion line:	
(a) *Stopcock:* Wipe off stopcock port with alcohol swab and connect tubing. Turn stopcock to open position.	Stopcock eliminates need for needle.
(b) *Needleless system:* Wipe off needleless port, and insert tip of piggyback or tandem infusion tubing (see illustrations).	The CDC strongly recommends needleless connections to prevent accidental needle-stick injuries (NIOSH, 1999). Establishes route for IV medication to enter main IV line.
(c) *Tubing port:* Connect sterile needle to end of piggyback or tandem infusion tubing, remove cap, cleanse injection port on main IV line, and insert needle through center of port. Secure by taping connection.	Prevents introduction of microorganisms during needle insertion.

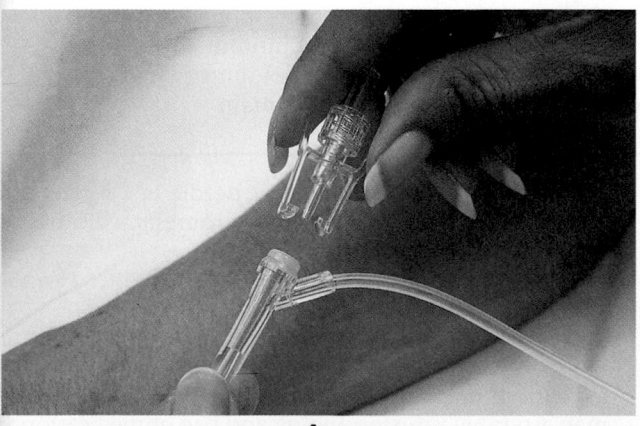
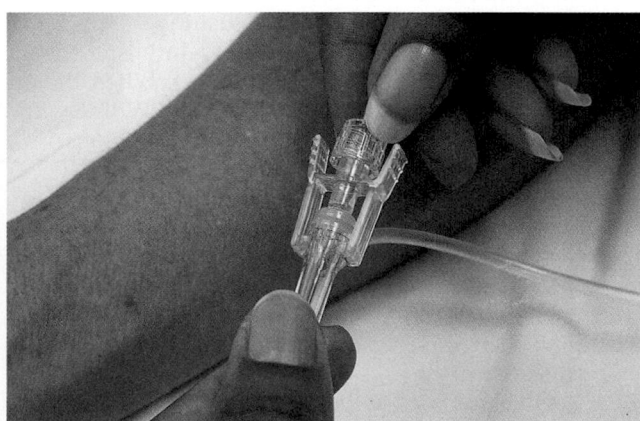

A	B

STEP **12A(3)(b)**   **A,** Needleless lever lock cannula system. **B,** Blunt-ended cannula inserts into port and locks.

Steps	Rationale
(4) Regulate flow rate of medication solution by adjusting regulator clamp. (Infusion times vary. Refer to medication reference or institutional policy for safe flow rate.)	Provides slow, intermittent infusion of medication and maintains therapeutic blood levels.
(5) After medication has infused, check flow regulator on primary infusion. The primary infusion should automatically begin to flow after the piggyback or tandem solution is empty.	Back-check valve on piggyback stops flow of the primary infusion until second medication infuses. The tandem and primary infusions flow together until the tandem set empties. Checking flow rate ensures proper administration of IV fluids.
(6) Regulate main infusion line to desired rate, if necessary.	Infusion of piggyback may interfere with the main line infusion rate.
(7) Leave IV piggyback bag and tubing in place for future medication administration or discard in appropriate containers.	Establishment of secondary line produces route for microorganisms to enter main line. Repeated changes in tubing increase risk of infection transmission (check agency policy).

B. Volume-control administration set (e.g., Volutrol)

(1) Assemble supplies in medication room.	Controls risk of contaminating IV solution.
(2) Prepare medication from vial or ampule (see Skill 34-7, p. 875).	Ensures medication is sterile.
(3) Fill Volutrol with desired amount of fluid (50 to 100 ml) by opening clamp between Volutrol and main IV bag (see illustration).	Small volume of fluid dilutes IV medication and reduces risk of too-rapid infusion.
(4) Close clamp and check to be sure clamp on air vent of Volutrol chamber is open.	Prevents additional leakage of fluid into Volutrol. Air vent allows fluid in Volutrol to exit at regulated rate.
(5) Clean injection port on top of Volutrol with antiseptic swab.	Prevents introduction of microorganisms during needle insertion.
(6) Remove needle cap or sheath and insert syringe needle through port, then inject medication (see illustrations). Gently rotate Volutrol between hands.	Rotating mixes medication with solution in Volutrol to ensure equal distribution.

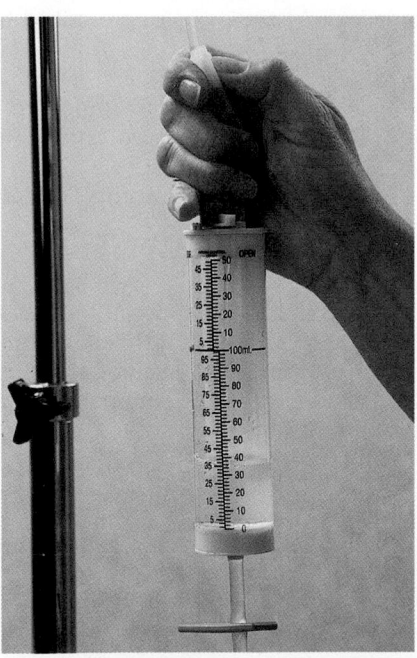

STEP **12B(3)** Filling volume-control administration device.

*A*dministering Intravenous Medications by Piggyback, Intermittent Intravenous Infusion Sets, and Miniinfusion Pumps—cont'd

Skill 34-11

Steps	Rationale

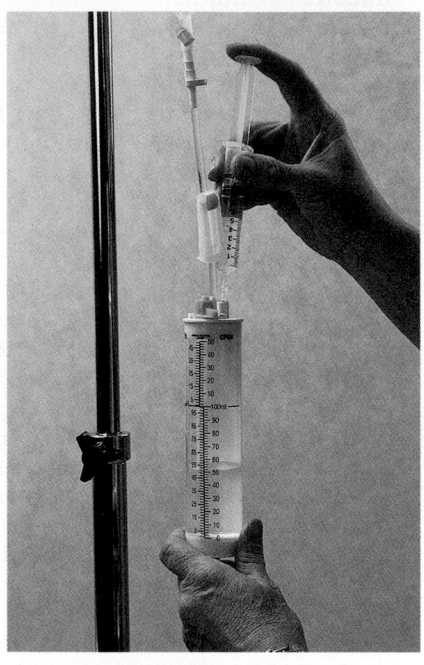 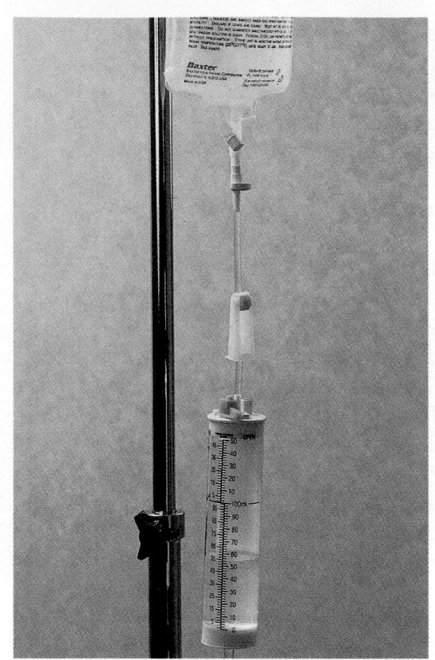

STEP **12B(6)** **A,** Medication injected into device. **B,** Prepared device.

Steps	Rationale
(7) Regulate IV infusion rate to allow medication to infuse in time recommended by institutional policy, a pharmacist, or a medication reference manual.	For optimal therapeutic effect, medication should infuse in prescribed time interval.
(8) Label Volutrol with name of medication, dosage, total volume including diluent, and time of administration.	Alerts nurses to medication being infused. Prevents other medications from being added to Volutrol.
(9) Dispose of uncapped needle or needle enclosed in safety shield and syringe in proper container.	Prevents accidental needle sticks.
C. Miniinfusion administration	
(1) Connect prefilled syringe to miniinfusion tubing.	Special tubing designed to fit syringe delivers medication to main IV line.
(2) Carefully apply pressure to syringe plunger, allowing tubing to fill with medication.	Ensures that tubing is free of air bubbles to prevent air embolus.
(3) Place syringe into miniinfusor pump (follow product directions). Be sure syringe is secure (see illustration).	
(4) Connect miniinfusion tubing to main IV line.	
(a) *Stopcock:* Wipe off stopcock port with alcohol swab and connect tubing. Turn stopcock to open position.	Stopcock reduces risk of needle-stick injuries.

Steps	Rationale

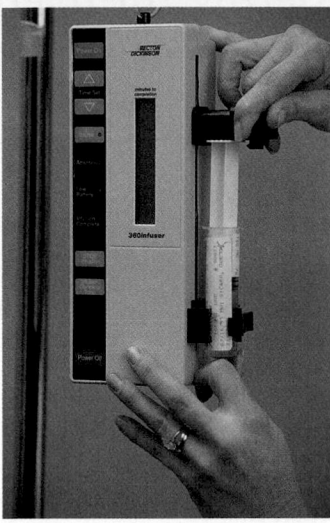

STEP **12C(3)**   Securing syringe into miniinfusor.

(b) *Needleless system:* Wipe off needleless port and insert tip of miniinfusor tubing.	Needleless system reduces risk of needle-stick injuries.
(c) *Tubing port:* Connect sterile needle to miniinfusion tubing, remove cap, cleanse injection port on main IV line, and insert needle through center of port. Consider placing tape where IV tubing enters port to secure connection.	Cleansing reduces transmission of microorganisms.
(5) Explain purpose of medication and side effects to client and explain that medication is to be given through existing IV line. Ask client to report symptoms of discomfort at site.	Informs client of planned therapies.
(6) Hang infusion pump with syringe on IV pole alongside main IV bag. Set pump to deliver medication within time recommended by institutional policy, pharmacist, or medication reference manual. Press button on pump to begin infusion. *Optional:* Set alarm.	Pump automatically delivers medication at safe, constant rate based on volume in syringe. (Alarm is used if medication is delivered into heparin/saline lock.)
(7) After medication has infused, check flow regulator on primary infusion. The infusion should automatically begin to flow once the pump stops. Regulate main infusion line to desired rate as needed. (NOTE: If stopcock is used, turn off miniinfusion line.)	Maintains patency of primary IV line.
13. Observe client for signs of adverse reactions.	IV medications act rapidly.
14. During infusion, periodically check infusion rate and condition of IV site.	IV must remain patent for proper medication administration. Development of infiltration necessitates discontinuing infusion.
15. Ask client to explain purpose and side effects of medication.	Evaluates client's understanding of instruction.

*A*dministering Intravenous Medications by Piggyback, Intermittent Intravenous Infusion *Skill* 34-11 Sets, and Miniinfusion Pumps—cont'd

Unexpected Outcomes and Related Interventions

- Client develops adverse drug reaction.
  - Stop medication infusion immediately.
  - Follow institutional policy or guidelines for appropriate response and reporting of adverse drug reactions.
  - Notify client's health care provider of adverse effects immediately.
- Medication does not infuse over desired period.
  - Determine reason (e.g., improper calculation of flow rate, malpositioning of IV needle at insertion site, or infiltration).
  - Take corrective action as indicated.
- IV site becomes swollen, warm, reddened, and tender to touch (see Chapter 40).
  - Indicates phlebitis.
  - Stop IV infusion.
  - Discontinue IV.
  - Treat IV site as indicated by institutional policy.
  - Insert new IV site if continuation of therapy is indicated.

- IV site becomes cool, pale, and swollen (see Chapter 40).
  - Indicates signs of infiltration.
  - Some IV medications are extremely harmful to subcutaneous tissue.
  - Provide IV extravasation care (e.g., injecting phentolamine [Regitine] around IV infiltration site) as indicated by institutional policy or use a medication reference or consult a pharmacist to determine appropriate follow-up care.

Recording and Reporting

- Record medication, dose, route, and time administered on MAR or computer printout.
- Record volume of fluid in medication bag or Volutrol on intake and output form.
- Report any adverse reactions to nurse in charge or physician.

Home Care Considerations

- Teach client and caregiver to dispose of needles and contaminated equipment in puncture-proof containers, (e.g., coffee can)
- Instruct family about community resources to obtain supplies.

Advantages to intermittent venous access include the following:

- Cost savings resulting from the omission of continuous IV therapy
- Convenience to the nurse by eliminating constant monitoring of flow rates
- Increased mobility, safety, and comfort for the client

Before administering an IV bolus or piggyback medication, the nurse must assess the patency and placement of the IV site. After the medication has been administered through an intermittent venous access, the access must be flushed with a solution to keep it patent. Generally, normal saline is an effective flush solution for peripheral catheters. Some institutions require the use of heparin. Nurses must verify and follow the institution's policies regarding the care and maintenance of the IV site.

Administration of Intravenous Therapy in the Home. Sometimes clients may be discharged from an acute care setting and continue to receive intravenous therapy in the home setting. Medications such as antibiotics, chemotherapy, total parenteral nutrition, pain medications, and blood transfusions may be given in the home. Most clients who have home intravenous therapy will have a central venous catheter inserted before discharge (see Chapter 40). In addition, clients who need to

receive intravenous therapy in the home have home care nurses who assist in the management of the intravenous therapy.

However, clients and their families need to be carefully assessed as to their ability to manage this therapy at home. Instruction on intravenous care management must be provided while the client is still in the hospital. Clients and families need to be taught how to recognize problems and what to do when these problems occur. It is important for the family to recognize signs of infection and complications and to know that when these occur the home care nurse or physician must be notified. In addition, clients and their families need information regarding maintenance of intravenous administration equipment, including the infusion pump.

*K*ey Concepts

- Learning medication classifications improves understanding of nursing implications for administering medications with similar characteristics.
- Federal medication legislation regulates the production, distribution, prescription, and administration of medications.

- All controlled substances are handled according to strict procedures that account for each medication.
- The nurse applies understanding of the physiology of medication action when timing administration, selecting routes, initiating actions to promote medication efficacy, and observing responses to medications.
- The older adult's body undergoes structural and functional changes that alter medication actions and influence the manner in which nurses provide medication therapy.
- Children's medication doses are computed on the basis of body surface area or weight.
- Medications given parenterally are absorbed more quickly than medications administered by other routes.
- Each medication order should include the client's name, the order date, the medication name, dosage, route, time of administration, drug indication, and the prescriber's signature.
- A medication history reveals allergies, medications a client is taking, and the client's compliance with therapy.
- The nursing process should be used when administering medication.
- The six rights of medication administration ensure accurate preparation and administration of medication doses.
- The six rights of medications administration are the right medication, right dose, right client, right route, right time, and right documentation.
- Nurses administer only medications they prepare, and prepared medications are never left unattended.
- Medications should be charted immediately after administration.
- A nurse uses clinical judgment in determining the best time to administer prn medications.
- The nurse reports a medication error immediately.
- When preparing medications, the nurse checks the medication container label against the medication administration record or computer printout 3 times.
- The Z-track method for intramuscular injections protects subcutaneous tissues from irritating parenteral fluids.
- Failure to select injection sites by anatomical landmarks may lead to tissue, bone, or nerve damage.

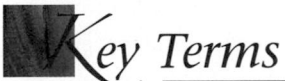

Key Terms

Absorption, *p. 825*	Instillation, *p. 834*
Adverse effects, *p. 829*	Intraarticular, *p. 833*
Anaphylactic reactions, *p. 829*	Intracardiac, *p. 833*
Biotransformation, *p. 828*	Intradermal (ID), *p. 831*
Buccal, *p. 831*	Intramuscular (IM), *p. 831*
Concentration, *p. 830*	Intraocular, *p. 834*
Detoxify, *p. 828*	Intravenous (IV), *p. 831*
Idiosyncratic reaction, *p. 829*	Irrigations, *p. 835*
Infusions, *p. 830*	Medication allergy, *p. 829*
Inhalation, *p. 834*	Medication error, *p. 841*
Injection, *p. 825*	Medication interaction, *p. 829*

Key Terms—cont'd

Metered-dose inhalers (MDIs), *p. 867*	Serum half-life, *p. 830*
Metric system, *p. 834*	Side effects, *p. 829*
Narcotics, *p. 825*	Solution, *p. 835*
Nurse Practice Acts, *p. 825*	Subcutaneous (Sub-Q), *p. 831*
Ophthalmic, *p. 856*	Sublingual, *p. 831*
Parenteral administration, *p. 831*	Synergistic effect, *p. 830*
Peak, *p. 830*	Therapeutic effects, *p. 829*
Pharmacokinetics, *p. 825*	Toxic effects, *p. 829*
Polypharmacy, *p. 849*	Transdermal disk, *p. 833*
Prescriptions, *p. 834*	Verbal order, *p. 838*
	Z-track method, *p. 890*

Critical Thinking Exercises

1. Mrs. O'Toole, a 69-year-old woman, has recently experienced a stroke. She is experiencing right-sided weakness. The neurological clinical nurse specialist wrote orders to start oral medications today. What steps should the nurse take to ensure that it is safe for this client to receive her oral medications? What should the nurse do if the client is unable to swallow?
2. Marissa is a 25-year-old who just delivered a healthy infant. She is to receive RhoGAM 300 mcg IM today. What size needle and which injection site and technique should the nurse use when administering this medication?
3. Jack, a 70-year-old retired farmer, has been experiencing new respiratory difficulties. His physician has ordered for him to start using an albuterol inhaler with a spacer. What steps will the nurse take to ensure that he can self-administer his MDI?
4. The nurse receives an order to give Lasix 40 mg IV push. The nurse has never given this medication while working on this unit. What steps should the nurse take before administering the Lasix?

Review Questions

1. Which of the following rights has been added to the traditional five rights of medication administration:
   1. Right documentation.
   2. Right route.
   3. Right medication.
   4. Right time.

2. The nurse is having difficulty reading a physician's order for a medication. The nurse knows the physician is very busy and does not like to be called. The nurse should:
   1. Call a pharmacist to interpret the order.
   2. Call the physician to have the order clarified.
   3. Consult the unit manager to help interpret the order.
   4. Ask the unit secretary to interpret the physician's handwriting.

3. The client has an order for 2 tablespoons of Milk of Magnesia. The nurse converts this dose to the metric system and would give the client:
   1. 2 ml.
   2. 5 ml.
   3. 16 ml.
   4. 30 ml.

4. Most medication errors occur when the nurse:
   1. Fails to follow routine procedures.
   2. Is responsible for administering numerous medications.
   3. Is caring for too many clients.
   4. Is administering unfamiliar medications.

5. A client is to receive cephalexin (Keflex) 500 mg PO. The pharmacy has sent 250 mg tablets. The nurse should give:
   1. ½ tablet.
   2. 1 tablet.
   3. 1½ tablets.
   4. 2 tablets.

6. The primary intent of the state Nurse Practice Act is to:
   1. Protect the public from unskilled, undereducated, and unlicensed personnel.
   2. Protect the nurse from client abuse.
   3. Determine the nurse's salary.
   4. Prevent poor health outcomes resulting from medication use.

7. The nurse is responsible for following legal provisions when administering controlled substances or narcotics. Failure to do so may result in:
   1. Fines, imprisonment, and loss of nurse licensure.
   2. Loss of employment.
   3. Medication errors.
   4. Poor health outcomes resulting from narcotic use.

8. Pharmacokinetics is the study of how medications:
   1. Are derived from plants.
   2. Enter the body, reach their site of action, are metabolized, and exit the body.
   3. Are used for certain disease processes.
   4. Are manufactured and distributed to pharmaceutical companies.

9. Official publications such as the following, set standards for medication strength, quality, purity, packaging, safety, labeling, and dose form.
   1. *Physicians Reference Guide.*
   2. *Nurse's Drug Guide.*
   3. MedWatch program.
   4. *USP* and the *National Formulary.*

10. Enforcement of medication laws rests with the:
    1. Food and Drug Administration (FDA).
    2. Nurse or physician dispensing and prescribing medications.
    3. MedWatch program.
    4. Health care institutions.

References

American Diabetes Association: Position statement: insulin administration, *Diabetes Care* 24(11):1984, 2001.

American Nurses Association: *Nursing facts about needlestick injuries,* 1999, http://www.nursingworld.org/readroom/fsneedle.htm

American Pharmaceutical Association: The pharmacy profession: transitioning from prescription provider to health care manager, 2002, http://www.pharmacyandyou.org/about/pharmcarefacts.html.

Andrews MM, Boyle JS: *Transcultural concepts in nursing care,* ed 4, Philadelphia, 2003, Lippincott.

Aschenbrenner DS, Cleveland LW, Venable SJ: *Drug therapy in nursing,* Philadelphia, 2002, Lippincott.

Bryson E: Drug administration via a nasogastric tube, *Nurs Times* 97(16):51, 2001.

Centers for Medicare and Medicaid Services: Clarifying policies related to the responsibilities of medicare-partner hospitals in the treatment of individuals with emergency conditions, update 10/2003. CMS-1063-F, USH HHS, Baltimore, Md, www.cms.hhs.gov.

Clarke K: Effective pain relief with intrapleural analgesia, *Nurs Times,* 95(12):49, 1999.

Cook MC: Nurses' six rights for safe medication administration, *Massachusetts Nurse* 69(6):8, 1999.

Cromling T: Giving meds to children needn't be a hassle, *RN* 65(3):28hf1, 2002.

Ebersole P, Hess P: *Toward healthy aging: human needs and nursing response,* ed 5, St. Louis, 1998, Mosby.

Galvan TJ: Dysphagia: going down and staying down, *Am J Nurs* 101(1):37, 2001.

Gilbar PJ: A guide to enteral drug administration in palliative care, *J Pain Symptom Manage* 17 (3):197, 1999.

Hockenberry MJ and others: *Wong's nursing care of infants and children,* ed 7, St. Louis, 2003, Mosby.

Institute of Safe Medicine Practices: ISMP list of error-prone abbreviations, symbols, and dose designations, 8(24), November 27, 2003. www.ismp.org, 2003.

Joint Commission on Accreditation of Healthcare Organizations: 2004 National patient safety goals-FAQs, 2004. www.jcaho.org/accredited+organizations.

Koschel MJ: Filter needles: question of practice, *Am J Nurs* 101(1):75, 2001.

Maas ML and others: *Nursing care of older adults: diagnoses, outcomes, and interventions,* St. Louis, 2001, Mosby.

MayoClinic.com: Asthma Center, 2000, www.mayoclinic.com/invoke.cfm?objectid=E05029A1-9E99-427BBE47BA91B7-BD70B5.

McConnell EA: Administering subcutaneous heparin, *Nursing* 30(6):17, 2000.

McConnell EA: Clinical do's and don'ts: instilling eyedrops, *Nursing* 31(9):17, 2001.

McKenry LM, Salerno E: *Mosby's pharmacology in nursing revised and updated,* ed 21, St. Louis, 2003, Mosby.

Minnesota Nurses Association: Position statement: Commission on Nursing Practice—Role of the registered nurse in safe administration of medications, *Minnesota Nursing Accent* 73(9):4, 2001.

National Heart, Lung, and Blood Institute: *Nurses: partners in asthma care,* NIH Publication No. 95-3308, October 1995, www.nhlbi.nih.gov/health/prof/lung/index.htm.

National Institute for Occupational Safety and Health (NIOSH): NIOSH alert preventing needle-stick injuries in health care settings, NIOSH Publications Dissemination, DHHS (NIOSH) Publication No. 2000-108, November, 1999.

Occupational Safety and Health Administration (OSHA): Occupational exposure to bloodborne pathogens: needlestick and other sharp injuries—final rule, *Federal Register,* CFR 29, part 1910(66:5317), January 18, 2001.

Patient's Library: Using eye drops, *RN* 63(4):230, 2000.

Peragallo-Dittko V: Research for practice: rethinking subcutaneous injection technique, *Am J Nurs* 97(5):71, 1997.

Strowig S: Insulin therapy, *RN* 64(9):38, 2001.

Togger D: Metered dose inhalers, *Am J Nurs* 101(10):26, 2001.

Workman B: Safe injection techniques, *Nurs Stand* 13(39):47, 1999.

Zurlinden J: Double check IV push, *Nurs Spectr* 15(25IL):16, 2002.

*R*esearch References

Beyea SC, Nicholl LH: Administration of medicines via the intramuscular route: an integrative review of the literature and research based protocol for the procedure *Appl Nurs Res* 8(1): 23, 1995.

Chan H: Effects of injection duration on site-pain intensity and bruising associated with subcutaneous heparin, *J Adv Nurs* 35(6):882, 2001.

Chung J, Ng WMY, Wong TKS: An experimental study on the use of manual pressure to reduce pain in intramuscular injections, *J Clin Nurs* 11(4):457, 2002.

Epstein S and others: Patient handling of a dry-powder inhaler in clinical practice, *Chest* 120(5):1480, 2001.

Nicoll LH, Hesby A: Intramuscular injection: an integrative research review and guideline for evidence-based practice, *Appl Nurs Res* 16(2):149, 2002.

Rodger MA, King, L: Drawing up and administering intramuscular injections: a review of the literature, *J Adv Nurs* 31(3):574, 2000.

35

Complementary and Alternative Therapies

Media Resources

http://evolve.elsevier.com/Potter/
fundamentals/

CD COMPANION

- Review Questions
- Glossary

evolve WEBSITE

- Review Questions
- Student Learning Activities
- Glossary

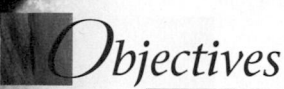

Objectives

Mastery of content in this chapter will enable the student to:

- Define the key terms listed.
- Differentiate between complementary and alternative therapies.
- Describe the clinical applications of relaxation therapies.
- Discuss the relaxation response and its effect on somatic ailments.
- Identify the principles and effectiveness of imagery, meditation, and breathwork.
- Describe the purpose and principles of biofeedback.
- Describe the methods of and the psychophysiological responses to therapeutic touch.
- Explain the scope of practice of chiropractic therapy.
- Discuss the principles and applications of acupuncture.
- Describe safe and unsafe herbal therapies.

The general health of North American people has steadily improved over the course of the last century as evidenced by lower mortality rates and increased life expectancies. Changes in science and medicine have provided the knowledge and technology to successfully alter the course of many illnesses. Despite the success of **allopathic medicine** (traditional Western medicine), many conditions such as arthritis, chronic back pain, gastrointestinal problems, allergies, headache, and insomnia have been difficult to treat, and more clients are exploring alternative methods to relieve their symptom distress. It is estimated that up to 75% of clients seek care from their primary care practitioners for stress, pain, and health conditions for which there are no known causes or cures (Fontaine, 2000). While allopathic medicine is quite effective in treating numerous physical ailments (e.g., bacterial infections, structural abnormalities, and acute emergencies), it is in general less effective in preventing disease, decreasing stress-induced illnesses, managing chronic disease, and caring for the emotional and spiritual needs of individuals.

The number of clients seeking unconventional treatments has risen considerably. In part this increase is due to (1) the perception that the treatments offered by the medical profession do not provide relief for a variety of common illnesses, (2) the increasing interest of clients in becoming more educated about their health and the need to take a more active role in their treatment, (3) the increased number of articles in journals such as *Annals of Behavioral Medicine, Alternative Therapies in Health and Medicine,* the *Journal of Alternative and Complementary Medicine,* and *Holistic Nursing,* and (4) the attraction to a holistic approach to health care that incorporates the mind, body, and spirit (Fontaine, 2000; Pelletier, 2000).

Complementary or Alternative Medicine Therapies in Health Care

Unconventional therapies are frequently referred to as either complementary or alternative medicine (CAM) therapies. **Complementary therapies** are those therapies used in addition to conventional treatment recommended by the person's health care provider. As the name implies, complementary therapies complement the conventional treatment. Many of the complementary therapies, such as acupuncture, contain diagnostic and therapeutic methods specific to their field, whereas others, such as guided imagery and breathwork, are generally easily learned and applied. Complementary therapies also include relaxation; exercise; massage (Figure 35-1); reflexology; prayer; biofeedback; hypnotherapy; shamanism; creative therapies, including art, music, or dance therapy (Figure 35-2); acupuncture and Chinese medicine; Ayurveda medicine; meditation; chiropractic therapy; osteopathy; herbalism; and homeopathy (Fontaine, 2000; Pelletier, 2000).

Alternative therapies, on the other hand, may include the same interventions as complementary therapies but frequently become the primary treatment that replaces allopathic medical care. Both complementary and alternative therapies vary in the degree to which they are compatible with allopathic medicine. For example, chiropractic and Feldenkrais (gentle body-movement therapy) practitioners frequently use diagnostic terminology and methods similar to those utilized by allopathic practitioners. They base interventions on conventional pathophysiology, anatomy, and kinesiology but at the same time, explore mind-body connections that may cause or contribute to the physiological condition. Some alternative therapies are not supported by scientific data, such as use of shark cartilage and coffee enemas, and must be regarded with caution. Even some of the more well-established therapies have only been rigorously tested on small or otherwise limited populations. This is mostly because funding for such research is limited. Types of complementary and alternative therapies are presented in Table 35-1.

Between one third and one half of the population in the United States uses one or more forms of CAM (Fontaine, 2000). Furthermore, data from a recent survey of U.S. citizens suggest a 47.3% increase in the number of visits to alternative medicine practitioners. This exceeds the number of visits to allopathic practitioners (Eisenberg and others, 1998). Because of this increased interest and use of CAM, many institutions, including some mainstream medical schools, have established training programs that incorporate CAM philosophy and content into the curriculum. As of July 1998, 100 educational programs or courses in complementary and alternative medicine were available for physicians at 65 universities in the United States (Pelletier, 2000). **Integrative medical programs** are being developed that allow health care consumers the opportunity to be treated by a team of providers consisting of both allopathic and complemen-

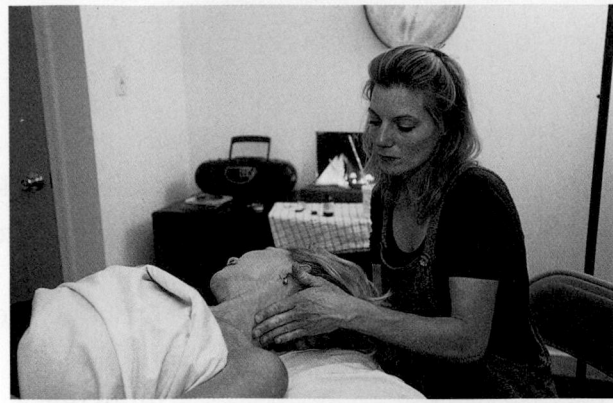

FIGURE **35–1** Massage therapy can be effectively used to relieve tension.

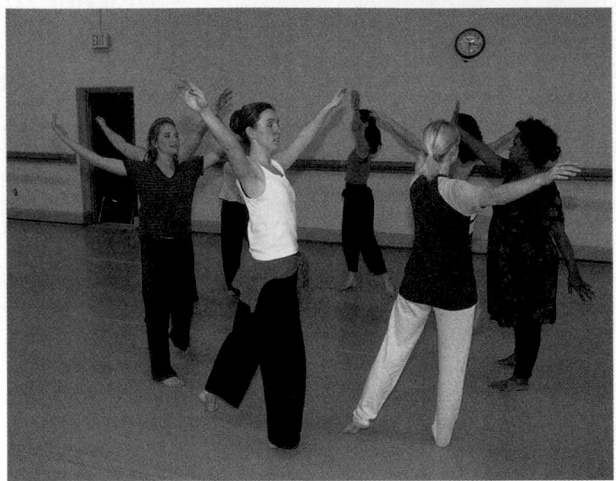

FIGURE **35–2** Young adults participating in dance therapy.

tary practitioners. Furthermore, an increasing number of insurance companies are now covering costs for certain types of CAM therapies such as herbal therapy, biofeedback, chiropractic medicine, megavitamin therapy, and acupuncture (Pelletier, 2000). However, this increase in insurance coverage is not proportionate to the increased use of CAM therapy. Many clients continue to pay out-of-pocket for a number of these therapies. Demographically, persons seeking CAM therapies typically include those who are professional, well educated, and from a higher socioeconomic standing.

The interest in CAM is also evident in the increased number of articles about it in respected medical journals and the development of several journals that specifically focus on complementary and alternative medicine. The Office of Alternative Medicine was established in 1992 as a part of the National Institutes of Health and then elevated to the status of the National Center for Complementary and Alternative Medicine (NCCAM) in 1998. The goals of this office are to facilitate the evaluation of alternative medical treatment modalities, specifically acting as a clearinghouse to disseminate information to the public, media, and professionals and funding, support-

Table 35-1	Complementary and Alternative Therapies
Types	**Definitions**

Alternative Medical Systems

Acupuncture	A traditional Chinese method of producing analgesia or altering the function of a body system by inserting thin needles along a series of lines or channels, called meridians. Direct needle manipulation of energetic meridians influences deeper internal organs.
Ayurveda	Traditional Hindu system of medicine practiced in India since the first century AD. Combination of remedies such as herbs, purgative, and rubbing oils used in treating disease.
Homeopathic medicine	System of medical treatments based on the theory that certain diseases can be cured by giving small doses of substances that in a healthy person would produce symptoms like those of the disease. Prescribed substances called remedies are made from naturally occurring plant, animal, or mineral substances.
Latin American practices	*Curanderismo* medical system, which includes a humoral model for classifying food, activity, drugs, and illnesses and a series of folk illnesses.
Native American practices	Therapies include sweating and purging, herbal remedies, and shamanic healing (healer makes contact with spirits to ask their direction in bringing healing to people).
Naturopathic medicine	System of therapeutics based on natural foods, light, warmth, massage, fresh air, regular exercise, and avoidance of medications. Recognition of inherent healing ability of the body. Treatments integrate traditional natural therapies with modern diagnostic science; includes botanical (plant) medicine.
Traditional Chinese (Oriental) medicine	Set of systematic techniques and methods including acupuncture, herbal medicines, massage, acupressure, moxibustion (use of heat from burning herbs), Qigong (balancing energy flow through body movement), and oriental massage. Fundamental concepts embedded in Taoism, Confucianism, and Buddhism.

Biologically Based Therapies

The "Zone"	Dietary program that requires eating protein, carbohydrate, and fat in a 30:40:30 ratio: 30% of calories from protein, 40% from carbohydrate, and 30% from fat. Used to balance insulin and other hormones for optimal health.
Macrobiotic diet	Predominantly a vegan diet (no animal products except fish). Initially used in the management of a variety of cancers. Emphasis placed on whole cereal grains, vegetables, and unprocessed foods.
Orthomolecular medicine (megavitamin)	Increased intake of nutrients such as vitamin C and beta-carotene. Diet used in treatment of cancer, schizophrenia, and certain chronic diseases such as hypercholesterolemia and coronary artery disease.
European phytomedicines	Products developed under strict quality control in sophisticated pharmaceutical factories, packaged professionally in tablets or capsules. Examples of well-studied herbal medicines include gingko biloba, milk thistle, and bilberry. Herbs have a wide variety of uses.
Traditional Chinese herbal remedies	Over 50,000 medicinal plant species, many of which have been studied extensively. Herbs considered the backbone of medicine.
Ayurvedic herbs	Traditional Hindu system of herbs used for over 2000 years.

Manipulative and Body-Based Methods

Acupressure	Therapeutic technique of applying digital pressure in a specified way on designated points on the body to relieve pain, produce analgesia, or regulate a body function.
Chiropractic medicine	System of therapy that involves manipulation of the spinal column and may also include physiotherapy and diet therapy.
Feldenkrais method	Alternative therapy based on establishment of good self-image through awareness and correction of body movements. Technique integrates the understanding of the physics of the body's movement patterns with an awareness of the way people learn to move, behave, and interact.
Tai chi	Technique that incorporates breath, movement, and meditation to cleanse, strengthen, and circulate vital life energy and blood. Therapy used to stimulate immune system and maintain external and internal balance.
Massage therapy	Manipulation of soft tissue through stroking, rubbing, or kneading to increase circulation, improve muscle tone, and relaxation.
Simple touch	Touching the client in appropriate and gentle ways to make connection, display acceptance, and give appreciation.

Continued

Table 35-1	Complementary and Alternative Therapies—cont'd
Types	**Definitions**
Mind-Body Interventions	
Art therapy	Use of art to reconcile emotional conflicts, foster self-awareness, and express clients' unspoken and frequently unconscious concerns about their disease.
Biofeedback	A process providing a person with visual or auditory information about autonomic physiological functions of the body, such as muscle tension, skin temperature, and brain wave activity, through the use of instruments.
Dance therapy	Intimate and powerful medium for therapy because it is a direct expression of the mind and body. Therapy used to treat persons with social, emotional, cognitive, or physical problems.
Breathwork	Using any of a variety of breathing patterns to relax, invigorate, or open emotional channels.
Guided imagery	Therapeutic technique used to treat pathological conditions by concentrating on an image or series of images.
Hypnotherapy	Induction of trance states and therapeutic suggestion for treatment of paralysis, headaches, joint pains, addictions, pain control, and phobias.
Meditation	Self-directed practice for relaxing the body and calming the mind using focused rhythmic breathing.
Music therapy	Use of music to address physical, psychological, cognitive, and social needs of individuals with disabilities and illnesses. Therapy used to improve physical movement for people with impaired movement, improve communication in people with communication disorders, develop emotional expression for people with mental health problems, evoke memories for persons with memory impairment, and distract people who are in pain or having painful treatments or chemotherapy.
Prayer therapies	Variety of techniques used in multiple cultures that incorporate caring, compassion, love, or empathy with the target of prayer.
Psychotherapy	Treatment of emotional and mental disorders by psychological techniques.
Yoga	Discipline that focuses on the body's musculature, posture, breathing mechanisms, and consciousness. Goal of yoga is attainment of physical and mental well-being through mastery of body achieved through exercise, holding of postures, proper breathing, and meditation.
Energy Therapies	
Reiki therapy	Therapy derived from ancient Buddhist practices in which practitioner places hands on or above a body area and transfers "universal life energy" to the client. This energy provides strength, harmony, and balance to treat health disturbances.
Therapeutic Touch	Treatment involving direction of a practitioner's balanced energies in an intentional manner toward those of a client. Involves laying of practitioner's hands on or close to a client's body.

ing, coordinating, and conducting research and research training in the area of alternative medicine. NCCAM has organized complementary and alternative therapies into 5 categories which researchers find useful (Box 35-1). Some of these complementary and alternative therapies are presented in Table 35-1. CAM is also reflected in the holistic health model (see Chapter 1).

Holistic nursing regards and treats the mind-body-spirit of the client. Nurses use holistic nursing interventions such as relaxation therapy, guided imagery, music therapy, simple touch, massage, and prayer (Box 35-2). Such interventions affect the whole person (mind-body-spirit) and are effective, economical, noninvasive, nonpharmacological complements to medical care. Holistic interventions can be used to augment standard treatments, to replace interventions that are ineffective or debilitating, and to promote or maintain health (Dossey, Keegan, and Guzzetta, 2000). The American Holistic Nursing Association maintains Standards of Holistic Nursing Practice that define and

establish the scope of holistic practice and describe the level of care expected from a holistic nurse (American Holistic Nurses' Association, 1998).

This chapter will discuss several types of complementary and alternative medicine therapies. The therapies are organized into two types. The first are nursing-accessible therapies. These are therapies that a nurse can begin to learn and apply in client care. The second type includes training-specific therapies, such as chiropractic therapy or acupressure, that a nurse cannot perform without additional training and/or certification. A description, clinical applications, and limitations of each therapy will be presented.

Nursing-Accessible Therapies

Some CAM therapies and techniques are general in nature and use natural processes (breathing, thinking and concentration, simple touch, movement, etc.) to help people

Box 35-1   NCCAM Categoreies of CAM Therapies

1. Alternative Medical Systems

Alternative medical systems are built upon complete systems of theory and practice. Often, these systems have evolved apart from and earlier than the conventional medical approach used in the United States. Examples of alternative medical systems that have developed in Western cultures include homeopathic medicine and naturopathic medicine. Examples of systems that have developed in non-Western cultures include traditional Chinese medicine and Ayurveda (a system from India).

2. Mind-Body Interventions

Mind-body medicine uses a variety of techniques designed to enhance the mind's capacity to affect bodily function and symptoms. Some techniques that were considered CAM in the past have become mainstream (for example, patient support groups and cognitive-behavioral therapy). Other mind-body techniques are still considered CAM, including meditation, prayer, mental healing, and therapies that use creative outlets such as art, music, or dance.

3. Biologically Based Therapies

Biologically based therapies in CAM use substances found in nature, such as herbs, foods, and vitamins. Some examples include dietary supplements, herbal products, and the use of other so-called natural but as yet scientifically unproven therapies (for example, using shark cartilage to treat cancer). Some uses of dietary supplements have been incorporated into conventional medicine. For example, scientists have found that folic acid prevents certain birth defects, and a regimen of vitamins and zinc can slow the progression of an eye disease called age-related macular degeneration (AMD).

4. Manipulative and Body-Based Methods

Manipulative and body-based methods in CAM are based on manipulation and/or movement of one or more parts of the body. Some examples include chiropractic or osteopathic manipulation, and massage.

5. Energy Therapies

Energy therapies involve the use of energy fields. They are of two types:
- **Biofield therapies** are intended to affect energy fields that purportedly surround and penetrate the human body. The existence of such fields has not yet been scientifically proven. Some forms of energy therapy manipulate biofields by applying pressure and/or manipulating the body by placing the hands in, or through, these fields. Examples include qi gong, Reiki, and Therapeutic Touch.
- **Bioelectromagnetic-based therapies** involve the unconventional use of electromagnetic fields, such as pulsed fields, magnetic fields, or alternating current or direct current fields.

From National Center for Complementary and Alternative Medicine: What is complementary and alternative medicine?, NCCAM publication no. D156, 2002, http://altmed.od.nih.gov/health/whatiscam/#11.

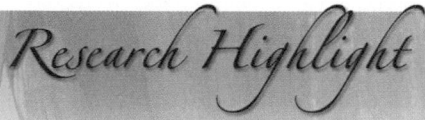
Research Highlight

Box 35-2

Use of Prayer

Research Focus

People use prayer to cope with distressing symptoms, anxiety-provoking medical procedures, and the illness experience in general. Yet no research has explored the lived experience of using prayer to cope with illness. Some research suggests that prayer is highly valued by those who use it, but there is minimal empirical knowledge about clients' prayer experiences and perspectives that nurses can use to support their clients.

Research Abstract

Because prayer appears to be a significant coping strategy for persons with cancer, this study sought to describe the experience of prayer among persons with cancer. Specific aims directed the researchers to (1) obtain descriptions of cancer clients' prayer from semistructured interviews; (2) analyze and present these descriptions using qualitative methods; (3) identify why, when, and how clients pray, as well as what they pray about and the outcomes expected; and (4) propose implications for cancer practice based on these clients' descriptions of prayer. Thirty persons with diagnosed cancer were interviewed in depth about why, when, and how they prayed, as well as what they prayed for and the outcomes expected. Findings detail how people with cancer used prayer to ease the physical, emotional, and spiritual distresses of illness. A range of approaches to prayer and topics for prayer was observed, often determined by illness circumstances.

Evidence-Based Practice

- Nurses who provide holistic care need to recognize that prayer is a valued and frequently used coping strategy for many cancer patients.
- Clinicians can facilitate coping by recognizing and facilitating client's use of prayer.
- Clients are likely to pray at times of symptom distress, emotional distress, and during diagnostic and therapeutic processes. At such times, nurses can help by fostering a condition and environment conducive to prayer.
- Although there are commonalities in prayer experiences, it typically is unique to individuals. Therefore nursing strategies for facilitating prayer must be designed with sensitivity to the uniqueness of each client.
- The nurse can help the client to relax, offer spiritual reading material, place the client with a view of nature, offer a notebook for journaling, or guard the client's room from intruders.

Reference

Taylor EJ, Outlaw FH: Use of prayer among persons with cancer, *Holist Nurs Pract* 16(3):46, 2002.

feel better and cope with chronic conditions. Nurses can learn these kinds of techniques with minimum preparation, and many of these procedures can be used with clients as independent nursing practice (Dossey and others, 2000). Adequate assessment and the client's permission are prerequisite for implementation. Also remember that some CAM therapies may alter physiological responses such that physician-prescribed therapies, such as drug doses, may need to be changed.

These therapies are designed to teach individuals ways in which to change their behavior to alter physical responses to stress and improve symptoms such as muscle tension, gastrointestinal discomfort, pain, or sleep disturbances. One of the principles of these therapies is that the individual becomes actively involved in the treatment. Individuals achieve better responses if they practice the techniques or exercises daily. A major principle is that the individual commits to implementing and maintaining the therapy until a desired outcome is achieved.

Relaxation Therapy

People are exposed to stressful situations in everyday life that evoke the **stress response** (see Chapter 30). The biochemical functions of the major organ systems are modulated by the mind. Thoughts and feelings influence the production of chemicals (i.e., neurotransmitters, neurohormones, and peptides) that circulate throughout the body and convey messages via cells to various systems within the body. The stress response is a good example of the way in which systems cooperate to protect an individual from harm (see Chapter 30). Physiologically, the cascade of changes associated with the stress response appears as increased heart and respiratory rates, tightened muscles, increased metabolic rate, and a general sense of foreboding, fear, nervousness, irritability, and negative mood. Other physiological responses include elevated blood pressure, dilated pupils, stronger cardiac contractions, and increased levels of blood glucose, serum cholesterol, circulating free fatty acids, and triglycerides. Although these responses prepare a person for short-term stress, the effects on the body of long-term stress can include structural damage and chronic illness such as angina, tension headaches, cardiac arrhythmias, pain, ulcers, and atrophy of the immune system organs (Dossey and others, 2000).

Relaxation is the state of generalized decreased cognitive, physiological, and/or behavioral arousal. Relaxation is also defined as arousal reduction. The process of relaxation elongates the muscle fibers, reduces the neural impulses sent to the brain, and thus decreases the activity of the brain as well as other body systems. The relaxation response is characterized by decreased heart and respiratory rates, blood pressure, oxygen consumption, and increased alpha brain activity and peripheral skin temperature. The relaxation response can be obtained through a variety of techniques that incorporate a repetitive mental focus and the adoption of a calm, peaceful attitude (Benson, 1975). Client teaching strategies for relaxation are listed in Box 35-3.

Relaxation helps individuals develop cognitive skills for reducing the negative ways in which they respond to situations within their environment. The cognitive skills include focusing (the ability to identify, differentiate, maintain attention on, and return attention to simple stimuli for an extended period), passivity (the ability to stop unnecessary goal-directed and analytic activity), and receptivity (the ability to tolerate and accept experiences that may be uncertain, unfamiliar, or paradoxical). The long-term goal of relaxation therapy is for the person to continually monitor himself or herself for indicators of tension and to consciously let go and release the tension contained in various body parts.

Progressive relaxation training teaches the individual how to effectively rest and reduce tension in the body. The person learns to detect subtle localized sensations of muscle tension in one muscle group (e.g., the forearm muscle). In addition, the individual learns to differentiate between high-intensity tension (strong fist clenching) and very subtle tension (Dossey and others, 2000). This activity is then practiced using different muscle groups. One active progressive relaxation technique involves the use of slow, deep abdominal breathing while tightening and relaxing an ordered succession of muscle groups. When guiding a client, the nurse may elect to begin with the muscles in the face, followed by those in the arms, hands, abdomen, legs, and feet.

Passive relaxation involves teaching the individual to relax individual muscle groups passively (i.e., without actively contracting the muscles). One passive relaxation technique incorporates slow, abdominal breathing exercises in addition to the person imagining warmth and relaxation flowing through specific muscle groups while letting go of muscle tension during expiration. Passive relaxation is useful for persons for whom the effort and energy expenditure of active muscle contracting leads to discomfort or exhaustion.

Clinical Applications of Relaxation Therapy. Relaxation techniques are effective in lowering heart rate and blood pressure, decreasing muscle tension, improving well-being, and reducing symptom distress in persons experiencing a variety of situations (e.g., complications from medical treatment or disease or grieving the loss of a significant other) (Jacobs, 2001). The type of relaxation intervention should be matched to the individual's functional status, the energy expenditure of the relaxation technique, and the motivation of the individual for frequent practice.

Relaxation, alone or in combination with deep breathing, imagery, yoga (Figure 35-3, p. 918), and music has been shown to reduce pain (Astin and others, 2002; Good and others, 2001); improve chronic fatigue syndrome (Deale and others, 2001); control hypertension (Yung, French, and Leung, 2001); improve preterm labor outcomes (Janke, 1999); contribute significantly to cancer palliative care (Ernst, 2001); and increase survival following cardiac arrest (Cowan, Pike, and Budzynski, 2001). However, more well-controlled studies are needed to validate and support the effects of relaxation therapy. For example, other variables or activities that may also lead to reduced physiological activity and pain level should be controlled in studies to determine if an individual's improved response is due to the relaxation therapy alone. Such variables may include a healthy support network, a positive attitude including humor, and other behavioral therapies such as yoga and tai chi.

Box 35-3

Client Teaching

Relaxation

Objective

- The client will demonstrate decreased anxiety, tension, and other manifestations of the stress response as a result of the relaxation intervention.

Teaching Strategies

Meditation and Rhythmic Breathing (Eliciting the Relaxation Response)

1. Provide a quiet environment.
2. Help the client get comfortable while seated or lying on back. Have client remain as still as possible and encourage to move only if necessary to remain comfortable.
3. Instruct the client to close eyes and to hold a receptive attitude—"There is nothing more important for me to do for the next 15 minutes" or "What will be, will be."
4. Instruct client to breathe in and out slowly and deeply using the abdominal muscles, keeping the chest still.
5. At the beginning of every out-breath, have client repeat the number "one" silently in his or her mind. Continue for period of meditation.
6. Explain that when the mind wanders, bring it back to counting the out-breath without judgment.
7. Have client practice for 5, 10, 15, or 20 minutes per session. Practice daily for at least one session.

Progressive Relaxation

1. Follow steps 1, 2, 3, and 4 of meditation and rhythmic breathing.
2. Once the client is breathing slowly and comfortably, instruct client to tighten and relax an ordered succession of muscle groups, tensing them and then relaxing them, while feeling each part relax.
3. Instruct client to tense and then relax the calves, knees, and so on.

Relaxation by Sensory Pacing

1. Follow steps 1, 2, 3, and 4 of meditation and rhythmic breathing.
2. Instruct client to slowly repeat and finish either in a low voice or to self each of the following sentences:
   Now I am aware of seeing . . .
   Now I am aware of feeling . . .
   Now I am aware of hearing . . .
   Instruct client to repeat and complete each sentence 4 times, then 3 times, then twice, and finally once.

Relaxation by Color Exchange

1. Follow steps 1, 2, 3, and 4 of meditation and rhythmic breathing.
2. Instruct client to notice any tension, tightness, aches, or pains in the body and to give that sensation the first color that comes to mind.
3. Instruct client to breathe in pure white light from the universe and send the light to the tense or painful place in the body, letting the white light surround the color of the discomfort.
4. Instruct client to exhale the color of the discomfort and let the white light take its place.
5. Instruct client to continue breathing in the white light and exhaling the color of the discomfort, allowing the white light to fill the entire body and bring about a sense of peace, well-being, and energy.

Modified Autogenic Relaxation

1. Follow steps 1, 2, 3, and 4 of meditation and rhythmic breathing.
2. Instruct client to repeat each of the following phrases to self 4 times, saying the first part of the phrases while breathing in for 2 to 3 seconds, holding the breath for 2 to 3 seconds, then saying the last part of the phrases while breathing out for 2 to 3 seconds:

Breathing In	Breathing Out
I am	relaxed.
My arm and legs	are heavy and warm.
My heartbeat	is calm and regular.
My breathing	is free and easy.
My abdomen	is loose and warm.
My forehead	is cool.
My mind	is quiet and still.

Relaxing With Music

1. Provide client with a tape recorder and headset.
2. Ask client to select a favorite cassette of slow, quiet music.
3. Instruct client to get into a comfortable position (either sitting or lying down but with arms and legs uncrossed) and to close eyes and listen to the music through the headset.
4. Instruct client to imagine floating or drifting with the music while listening.

Evaluation

- Assess client's vital signs, particularly respiratory pattern.
- Ask client to describe level of tension or uneasiness felt.
- Observe client for presence of behaviors that display anxiety.

Relaxation is a valuable technique because it enables individuals to exert some control over their lives. Persons may experience a decreased feeling of helplessness and a more positive psychological state overall, which helps them to have a less negative view of their situation.

Limitations of Relaxation Therapy. Individuals undergoing relaxation training have reported fearing loss of control, feeling like they are floating, and experiencing relaxation-induced anxiety related to these feelings. During relaxation training, individuals learn to differentiate between low and high levels of muscle tension. During the first months of training sessions, when the person is learning how to focus on body sensations and tensions, there are reports of increased sensitivity in detecting muscle tension. Usually these feelings are minor and resolve as the person continues with the relaxation training. However, nurses must be aware that on occasion some relaxation techniques may result in continued intensification of symptoms or the development of altogether new symptoms (Dossey and others, 2000).

An important consideration when choosing the type of relaxation technique is the physiological and psychological status of the individual. Clients with advanced

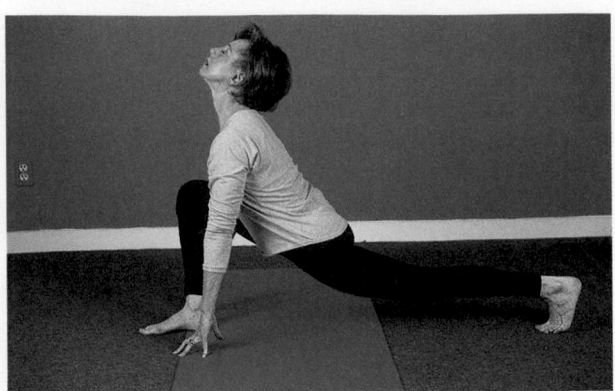

FIGURE **35–3** Yoga is a discipline that focuses on muscles, posture, breathing, and consciousness.

Box *35-4* **Indications for Meditation**

Anxiety or tension states	Irritability
Chronic bereavement	Low self-esteem or
Chronic fatigue syndrome	self-blame
Chronic pain	Mild depression
Drug abuse (alcohol or	Psychophysiological
tobacco)	disorders
Hypertension	Sleep disorders

---

disease such as cancer may seek relaxation training to reduce their stress response. However, techniques such as active progressive relaxation training require a moderate expenditure of energy, which can amplify a person's existing fatigue and limit the person's ability to complete individual relaxation sessions and practice. Therefore, active progressive relaxation would not be appropriate for clients with advanced disease or those who have decreased energy reserves. Passive relaxation or guided imagery is more appropriate for these individuals.

Meditation and Breathing

Meditation is any activity that limits stimulus input by directing attention to a single unchanging or repetitive stimulus (Pelletier, 2000). It is a general term for a wide range of practices that involve relaxing the body and stilling the mind. The root word, *meditari,* means to consider, or one can say, to pay attention to something. Dr. Herbert Benson wrote the book *The Relaxation Response* (1975), which drew the attention of Western health care practitioners to physical and psychological benefits of relaxation. As Benson pointed out, the components of relaxation are quite simple: (1) a quiet space, (2) a comfortable position, (3) a receptive attitude, and (4) a focus of attention. He described meditation as a process that anyone can use to calm down, cope with stress, and, for those with spiritual inclinations, feel as one with God or the universe. Meditation requires no change in belief system and is compatible with most religious practices. It can be practiced individually or in groups and is easy to learn. Practicing meditation does not require a teacher; many people learn the process from books or audiotapes, and it is easy to teach (Fontaine, 2000). Most meditation techniques involve slow, relaxed, deep, usually abdominal, breathing (see Box 35-3, p. 917). Meditation evokes a restful state, lowers oxygen consumption, reduces respiratory and heart rates, and generates reports of reduced anxiety.

Clinical Applications of Meditation. There are many indications for meditation (Box 35-4). There is some evidence that meditation improves stress-related illnesses and breathing patterns in asthmatics, lowers blood pressure in hypertensive clients (King, Carr, and D'Cruz, 2002;

Lee and others, 2000) and blood glucose levels in diabetics, decreases episodes of angina pectoris (Cunningham, Brown, and Kaski, 2000), and lowers cholesterol in hypercholesterolemic clients. It has also been used to reduce anxiety (Speca and others, 2000), sleep-onset insomnia, stuttering, the symptoms of irritable bowel syndrome (Keefer and Blanchard, 2001, 2002; Shannahoff-Khalsa, 2002), and even the incidence of dental caries by lowering salivary bacteria (Pelletier, 2000). Meditation has also increased productivity, improved mood, increased sense of identity, and lowered irritability (Dossey and others, 2000).

Considerations for the appropriateness of meditation include the degree of self-discipline of the person. Meditation can be easily learned and does not require memorization or particular procedures. It actually requires less self-discipline than most other behavioral therapies. Another consideration involves the self-reinforcing properties that meditation offers. Meditation can induce a peaceful, drifting mental state that is unusually pleasurable and provides an incentive for individuals to continue.

Limitations of Meditation. Although meditation has demonstrated improvement in a variety of physiological and psychological ailments, it may be contraindicated in some people. For example, a person who has a strong fear of losing control may perceive meditation as a form of mind control and thus may be resistant to learning the technique. Some individuals may also be hypersensitive to meditation and require a much shorter session than the average 15- to 20-minute session.

Meditation may also augment the effects of certain drugs. For example, individuals taking antihypertensive medications or thyroid-regulating, antidepressant, or antianxiety medications should be monitored. Prolonged practice of meditation techniques may lead to the reduced need for certain medications such as antihypertensive medications. Whatever the case, individuals learning meditation should be monitored closely for physiological changes with respect to their medications. Adjustment of the medication may be needed (Pelletier, 2000).

Imagery

Imagery or visualization techniques use the conscious mind to create mental images to stimulate physical changes in the body, improve perceived well-being, and/or enhance self-awareness. Frequently imagery is combined with some form of relaxation training to facilitate the effect of the re-

Box 35-5

Client Teaching

Creative Visualization

Objective

- The client will demonstrate skills in creative visualization.

Teaching Strategies

1. Set goals that can be accomplished, because confidence and increased self-esteem are achieved through success.
2. The created image must be clear. Although it may be difficult to develop a visual image, if the goals of the imagery are viewed with clear thoughts and in the present tense, the individual may be more successful in creating an effective image.
3. Frequently visualize the image. This visualization should be done during relaxing states as well as throughout the day, but particularly before bedtime or upon wakening, when the person's mind usually is more relaxed.
4. While focusing on the image, repeat encouraging statements, such as positive affirmations. Alleviate any doubts about one's ability to achieve one's goals.

Evaluation

- Observe client behaviors for presence of anxiety.
- Ask client to describe if the visualization experience was helpful.
- Have client report if positive self-dialogue is used with visualization.
- The client reports using images of desired health habits, feelings, and desires for healing.
- The client reports increased coping with daily stressors.

laxation technique. Imagery can be self-directed, in which individuals create their own mental images, or it can be guided, during which a practitioner leads an individual through a particular scenario (Dossey and others, 2000). For example, the client may be directed to begin slow, abdominal breathing while focusing on the rhythm of breathing. The client is then instructed to visualize ocean waves coming to shore with each inspiration, then receding with each expiration. Next the client is instructed to take notice of the smells, sounds, and temperatures that he or she is experiencing. As the imagery session progresses, the client may be instructed to visualize warmth entering the body during inspiration and tension leaving the body during expiration. Imagery scenarios should be individualized for each client and/or left up to the client to develop.

Imagery can evoke powerful psychophysiological responses such as alterations in immune function (Fontaine, 2000). Many imagery techniques involve visual imagery, but they can also include the auditory, proprioceptive, gustatory, and olfactory senses. An example of this involves visualizing a lemon being sliced in half and squeezing the lemon juice under the tongue. This visualization has been observed to produce increased salivation as effectively as the actual event. People typically respond to their environment according to the way they perceive it, as well as

by their own visualizations and expectancies. Therefore individuals can learn to regulate themselves by selecting appropriate visualizations and expectations (Dossey and others, 2000).

Creative visualization is one form of self-directed imagery that is based on the principle of mind-body connectivity (i.e., every mental image leads to physical or emotional changes) (Gawain, 2002). Client teaching strategies for creative visualization are listed in Box 35-5.

Clinical Applications of Imagery. Imagery has applications in a number of client populations. Imagery has been used to visualize cancer cells being destroyed by cells of the immune system, control or relieve pain, and achieve calmness and serenity. It has also been used in the treatment of chronic conditions such as asthma, hypertension, functional urinary disorders, menstrual and premenstrual syndromes, gastrointestinal disorders such as irritable bowel syndrome and ulcerative colitis, and rheumatoid arthritis (Dossey and others, 2000).

Limitations of Imagery. Imagery, for the most part, is a behavioral intervention that has few side effects. However, it is probably one of the least clearly defined interventions and can range from being highly structured to consisting of spontaneous daydreams by the individual (Pelletier, 2000).

Training-Specific Therapies

Training-specific therapies are CAM treatments that may be administered by nurses but only after completing a specific course of study and training. A nurse must have a certification, degree, or license beyond the RN to administer most of these therapies. Several training-specific therapies are recognized as being very effective and are recommended by Western health care practitioners (e.g., biofeedback and therapeutic touch). But many have not been studied in a systematic way to establish their effectiveness. Many of these unproven techniques are very popular in our society and used by many persons from other cultures who live in the United States. Many have positive effects, but some have negative effects too. Some of these may also have harmful results when used in conjunction with standard Western medical therapies. Therefore the nurse should acquire at least a passing knowledge of such treatments and be aware of possible harmful interactions.

Biofeedback

Biofeedback techniques are frequently used in addition to relaxation interventions to assist individuals in learning how to control specific autonomic nervous system responses. **Biofeedback** is a group of therapeutic procedures that use electronic or electromechanical instruments to measure, process, and provide information to persons about their neuromuscular and autonomic nervous system activity (Figure 35-4). The information, or feedback, is given in physical, physiological, auditory and/or visual feedback signals. For example, clients may

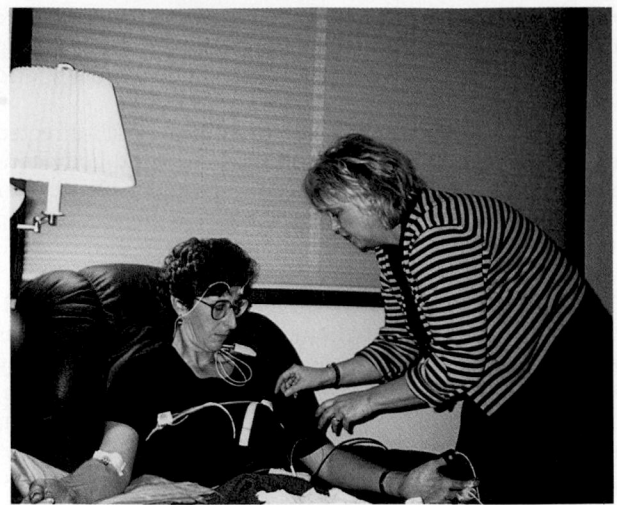

FIGURE **35–4**   Biofeedback monitoring. Electrodes are placed on the frontalis and trapezius muscles and the fingers of the left hand. Pneumograph measurements are also made.

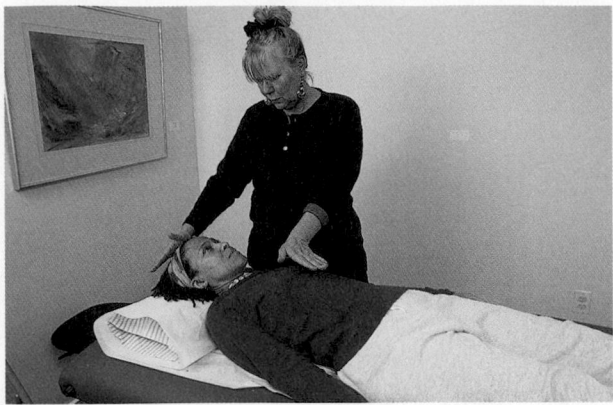

FIGURE **35–5**   In therapeutic touch the practitioner directs the practitioner's own interpersonal energy to help or heal another.

hear a sound if their pulse rate or blood pressure increases out of their therapeutic zone. Practitioners help persons develop greater awareness and resulting voluntary control over their physiological responses, of which they are otherwise unaware (Pelletier, 2000).

Biofeedback is considered an effective addition to more traditional relaxation programs because it can immediately demonstrate to clients their ability to control some physiological responses. It can also help individuals to focus on and monitor specific body parts. By providing immediate feedback in terms of what stress relaxation behaviors work most effectively, it helps the client control physiological functions that are most difficult to control. Eventually the client will be able to notice positive physiological changes without the need for instrument feedback. Finally, biofeedback demonstrates to the client the relationship between thoughts, feelings, and physiological responses.

Clinical Applications of Biofeedback. Biofeedback in a variety of forms has application in a number of situations. Biofeedback has been successful in treating migraine headaches (Sarafino and Goehring, 2000; Scharff, Marcus, and Masek, 2002), phantom limb pain (Belleggia and Birbaumer, 2001), abdominal pain, temporomandibular pain (Crider and Glaros, 1999), urinary incontinence (Abdelghany and others, 2001), hypertension (Nakao and others, 1999), and some anxiety disorders (Moore, 2000).

One of the most critical components of any behavioral program is adherence to the treatment regimen. Clients who are compliant with appointments, practice times, and goal setting and basically take responsibility for their treatment tend to be the most successful.

Limitations of Biofeedback. Although biofeedback has demonstrated effectiveness in a number of client populations, there are several precautions. During relaxation therapy and/or biofeedback sessions repressed emotions or feelings may be uncovered that clients cannot cope with by themselves. For this reason, it is recommended

that practitioners who offer biofeedback should either be trained in more traditional psychological methods or have qualified professionals available for referral.

Therapeutic Touch

Therapeutic touch (Krieger, 1979) is a training-specific therapy that was developed by a nurse. Although the philosophical and religious assumptions of therapeutic touch are different from those of other Eastern healing modalities, therapeutic touch is similar in that it involves trained health care professionals who attempt to direct their own balanced energies in an intentional and motivated manner toward those of the client.

Therapeutic touch (TT) is a natural human potential that consists of placing the practitioner's hands either on or close to the body of a person (Figure 35-5). The process of therapeutic touch involves the practitioner scanning the body of the client and diagnosing areas of accumulated tensions. The practitioner then attempts to redirect these energies to bring the person back into energy balance similar to that of the practitioner (Krieger, 1975, 1979). TT consists of five phases: centering, assessment, unruffling, treatment, and evaluation. Centering is the process whereby the practitioner becomes aware and fully present during the entire treatment. The next phase involves the assessment of the client, in which the practitioner moves his or her hands (roughly 2 to 6 inches from the body) in a rhythmic and symmetrical movement from the head to the toes. During this phase the practitioner notices the quality of **energy flow** and detects accumulations of energy. The physiological indicators of energy imbalance are perceived as feelings of congestion, pressure, warmth, coolness, blockage, pulling or drawing, or static or tingling (Krieger, 1975). During the third phase, the practitioner unruffles the energy flow or facilitates the symmetrical and rhythmical flow of energy through the body. This technique is accomplished by long downward strokes over the energy field located over the entire body. During the actual treatment the practitioner directs and balances the energy, attempting to rebalance the energy flow. This rebalancing of energy is achieved either by the practitioner touching the body or maintaining the hands in a position a few inches away from the body. The final phase consists of an evaluation of the client and a reassessment of the energy field. If a rebalance has occurred, the practitioner detects a more symmetrical, freely flowing energy field and greater well-being (Krieger, 1979).

Clinical Applications of Therapeutic Touch. Some of the earliest studies found that TT was able to increase hemoglobin (Hb) levels in several clients (Krieger, 1975, 1979). Other studies have found that TT was effective in reducing anxiety levels in hospitalized clients with cardiovascular disease, reducing headache pain, and improving mood in bereaved adults (Krieger, 1975, 1979). Several research review articles support the effectiveness of TT and call for the support of further research (Peters, 1999; Winstead-Fry and Kijek, 1999). Completed research has shown that TT can improve outcomes in postpartum women (Kiernan, 2002), reduce pain and shorten hospital stay following abdominal surgery (Smyth, 2001), help treat drug addiction (Hagemaster, 2000), and reduce or eliminate phantom limb pain (Leskowitz, 2000).

Limitations of Therapeutic Touch. Although some studies have demonstrated that therapeutic touch produced positive outcomes, others have not. Suggestions for this lack of response include an absence of eye and facial contact during the therapeutic session and too brief of a session. Therapeutic touch may be contraindicated in certain client populations. For example, persons who are sensitive to human interaction and touch (e.g., those who have been physically abused or have psychiatric disorders) may misinterpret the intent of the treatment and may feel threatened and anxious by the treatment. Other clients who are sensitive to energy repatterning may also need to avoid therapeutic touch. These include premature infants, newborns, children, pregnant women, older or debilitated people, or those in critical, unstable conditions (Fontaine, 2000).

Chiropractic Therapy

Chiropractic therapy, a manual healing art, was developed in 1895 in Iowa. Of the independently practicing health professions, it is the third largest in the Western world (Pelletier, 2000). Chiropractors graduate from well-established preparatory programs similar to medical schools. The central tenet of the chiropractic profession is spinal manipulation directed at certain joints by practitioners using their hands or an instrument. Manipulation is defined as the forceful passive movement of a joint beyond its active limit of motion. Chiropractic therapy is considered a holistic therapy that does not typically use drugs or surgery.

Spinal manipulation received an endorsement from the U.S. Department of Health and Human Service's Agency for Health Care Policy and Research in 1994. The agency developed guidelines that concluded "spinal manual therapy provides relief of symptomatic discomfort as well as functional improvement." The basic principles of chiropractic therapy incorporate the idea that human beings have an innate healing potential, and the goal of this healing profession is to access this potential. Chiropractic therapy promotes both a natural diet and

regular exercise as critical components for the body to function properly (Fontaine, 2000).

Clinical Applications of Chiropractic Therapy. The basic goals of chiropractic therapy focus on restoring the structural and functional imbalances that may result in pain. It is believed that structure and function coexist with one another and that alterations or distortions in structure can ultimately lead to abnormalities in function. One of the major structural distortions that chiropractors treat is vertebral subluxation, in which the motion of the joints is decreased due to slight changes in the position of the articulating bones and subjective symptoms such as pain. A more severe form of subluxation, called fixation, exists when joint motion is restricted. Chiropractic interventions are used to treat not only musculoskeletal abnormalities, but headaches, dysmenorrhea, blood pressure, vertigo, tinnitus, and visual disorders (Pelletier, 2000).

Limitations of Chiropractic Therapy. Several diseases or joint conditions should not be treated with manipulation. If a malignancy is suspected or determined through diagnostic testing, the client should be referred to a medical physician for further evaluation and treatment. Bone and joint infections also require pharmaceutical or surgical intervention, and the structural integrity of the bone may be compromised if excessive force is used. Contraindications for chiropractic therapy include acute myelopathy, fractures, dislocations, rheumatoid arthritis, and osteoporosis.

Traditional Chinese Medicine

Traditional Chinese medicine (TCM) comprises several healing modalities, including herbs, acupuncture, moxibustion, diet, exercise, and meditation. TCM is several thousand years old and has its roots in Taoism. There are several major concepts that constitute Chinese medicine. The most important of these is the concept of **yin and yang,** which represent opposing, yet complementary phenomena that exist in a state of dynamic equilibrium. Examples are night/day, hot/cold, and shady/sunny. Yin represents shade, cold, and inhibition, whereas yang represents fire, light, and excitement. Yin also represents the inner part of the body, specifically the viscera, liver, heart, spleen, lung, and kidney, whereas yang represents the outer part, specifically the bowels, stomach, and bladder. When there is an imbalance in these two paired opposites, then it is thought that disease occurs (Fontaine, 2000).

Qi (pronounced *chi*) is defined as the vital energy of the human body. Disease is classified into three major categories: external causes, internal causes, and neither internal nor external causes (Table 35-2). Regardless of the cause, it is thought that yin and yang go out of balance, thus altering the movement of *qi*. The body consists of several forms of this energy that directly influence physiological functions of the body and help to maintain homeostasis.

Channels of energy run in regular patterns through the body and over its surface. These channels, called **meridians,** are like rivers flowing through the body. An obstruction in the movement of these energy rivers is like a dam

Table 35-2	Three Causes of Disease According to Traditional Chinese Medicine
Cause of Disease	**Influences**
External causes, or "the six evils"	Wind, cold, fire, damp, summer heat, dryness
Internal causes, or internal damage by seven effects	Joy, anger, anxiety, thought, sorrow, fear, fright
Nonexternal, noninternal causes	Dietary irregularities, excessive sexual activity, taxation fatigue, trauma, parasites

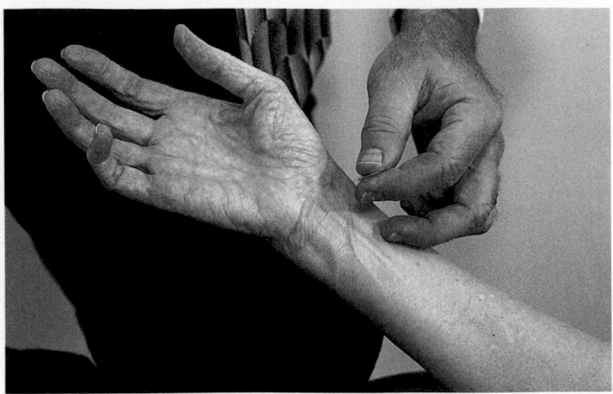

FIGURE **35–6**   Acupuncture.

that backs up the flow in one part of the body and restricts it in others. Any obstruction and blockages or deficiencies of energy would eventually lead to disease. Evaluations have been done to identify and systematize the meridians or channels through which *qi* flows. Twelve primary and eight secondary or extra channels have been identified. Located along the channels are **acupoints,** or holes through which *qi* can be influenced by the insertion of needles, a process known as **acupuncture.**

Another important component of Chinese medicine involves five elements. The five elements consist of earth, metal, water, wood, and fire. Various health phenomena are organized according to these phases and interact with each other. In Chinese medicine outward manifestations are reflective of the internal environment. There are two primary areas that are assessed in Chinese medicine: the tongue and several pulses. The color, shape, and coating of the tongue are reflective of the general condition of the internal organs. The pulses provide information about the condition and balance of *qi,* blood, ying and yang, and the internal organs (Fontaine, 2000).

Acupuncture

Acupuncture is a method of stimulating certain points (acupoints) on the body by the insertion of special needles to modify the perception of pain, normalize physiological functions, or treat or prevent disease (Figure 35-6). Acupuncture is used to regulate the flow of *qi.* According to Chinese traditional medicine, acupuncture needles unblock the obstruction of energy and reestablish the flow of *qi* through the meridians, thereby stimulating and activating the body's self-healing mechanism. Effects of needles may be enhanced by application of heat or weak electrical currents to the needles (Fontaine, 2000).

Clinical Applications of Acupuncture. Acupuncture is the primary treatment modality used by physicians of Chinese medicine. Many allopathic physicians and health care professionals are also being trained and certified in acupuncture. Many states now have regulations and licensure requirements to practice as an acupuncturist.

The most common problems for which acupuncture is used include low back pain, myofascial pain, simple and migraine headaches, sciatica, shoulder pain, tennis elbow, osteoarthritis, whiplash, and musculoskeletal sprains. Other problems that have been successfully treated in-

clude sinusitis, gastrointestinal disorders, perimenstrual symptoms, neurological disorders, chronic pulmonary diseases (including asthma), hypertension, smoking and other addictions, and clinical depression (Pelletier, 2000).

Limitations of Acupuncture. Acupuncture is considered a safe therapy when the practitioner has been appropriately trained and uses sterilized needles. Although complications have been noted, they are rare if appropriate steps are taken to ensure the safety of the equipment and the client. These complications include infections resulting from inadequately sterilized needles or those that are left in place for an extended length of time, broken needles, puncture of an internal organ, bleeding, fainting, seizures, miscarriage, and posttreatment drowsiness.

Acupuncture should be used with caution in pregnant clients and those who have a history of seizures, are carriers of hepatitis, or are infected with human immunodeficiency virus (HIV). Treatment is contraindicated in persons who have bleeding disorders, thrombocytopenia, or skin infections. The semipermanent needles should not be used with persons who have valvular heart disease because of the increased risk of infection. Electroacupuncture should be avoided in persons with a pacemaker and those who have cardiac arrhythmias, epilepsy, or are pregnant (Fontaine, 2000).

Herbal Therapies

It is estimated that approximately 25,000 plant species are used medicinally throughout the world. It is the oldest form of medicine known to man, and archeological evidence suggests that herbal remedies were used 60,000 years ago by Neanderthals. Use of **herbal therapy** gained widespread popularity in many countries as early as 3000 BC but began to decline with the development of modern scientific medicine in the early eighteenth century. However, because approximately 80% of the world's population lives in developing countries, herbal medicine constitutes a prominent part of health care in these countries. Furthermore, resurgence in interest has developed in countries whose health care is dominated by allopathic medicine. The increase in herbal medicine has occurred because of a growing concern by the general public about the complications and limitations of modern scientific medicine and consumer interest in "natural" foods (Fontaine, 2000).

The federal Food, Drug, and Cosmetic Act mandates that all drugs have to be proven safe and effective before being sold to the public. Because herbal medicines have not undergone the same rigorous research as have pharmaceuticals, the majority have not received approval for use as drugs. For this reason many herbal medicines are sold as foods or food supplements in health food stores and through private companies. The Dietary Supplement Health and Education Act passed in 1994 now allows herbs to be sold as dietary supplements as long as there are no health claims written on their labels.

Herbal substances used in Chinese medicine are taken from plants, animals, or minerals, whereas those used in Western herbal medicine are prepared primarily from plant materials. The active ingredients are "packaged" in tinctures or extracts, elixirs, syrups, capsules, pills, tablets, lozenges, powders, ointments or creams, drops, and suppositories. Many people tend to think that because herbs are natural plants they will not cause harm or side effects but this is not always true. Some herbal substances contain powerful chemicals and, as with any other medication, should be examined for interaction and compatibility with other prescribed or unprescribed substances. Many herbs are also sold with claims that they can "cure" certain ailments, such as pau d'arco for curing cancer, when their efficacy has not been determined through clinical trials. Herbs are generally classified as beneficial, harmful, or neutral, in which case they have no effects on the specific ailment.

The philosophy of herbal therapy is different from that of conventional drug therapy. The goal of herbal therapy is to restore balance within the individual by facilitating the person's self-healing ability. Drug therapy, on the other hand, is aimed at the treatment of specific diseases or symptoms. Herbal therapy is also prescribed on an individual basis with unique herbal concoctions tailored for each person (Kuhn and Winston, 2001).

Clinical Applications of Herbal Therapy. A number of herbs have been determined to be safe and effective for a variety of conditions (Table 35-3). Milk thistle, for example, has been observed to be effective in treating a number of liver and gallbladder conditions. It is thought to protect the liver through its antioxidant properties and by facilitating regeneration of liver cells. St. John's Wort has effectiveness as a mild antidepressant and mild sedative. Hypericin and pseudohypericin, major constituents of the drug, have also been shown to have potent action against viruses. Clinical trials investigating the effectiveness of St. John's wort against acquired immunodeficiency syndrome have begun (Kuhn and Winston, 2001; Skidmore-Roth, 2001).

Limitations of Herbal Therapy. Although herbal medicine has shown to provide beneficial effects for a variety of conditions, a number of problems may exist. When herbal medicines are developed, concentrations of the active ingredients have been found to vary considerably. Contamination with other herbs or chemicals, including pesticides and heavy metals, may also occur. Not all companies follow strict quality control and manufacturing guidelines, which set standards for acceptable levels of pesticides, residual solvents, bacterial levels, and heavy metals. For this reason, herbal medicine should be purchased only from reputable manufacturers. In addition, labels on herbal products should contain the scientific name of the botanical, the name and address of the actual manufacturer, a batch or lot number, the date of manufacture, and the expiration date. Some herbs have also been found to contain very toxic products and can cause cancer. Comfrey, for example, has been used for its wound-healing properties. However, various species of comfrey contain certain pyrrolizidine alkaloids that are highly carcinogenic. Comfrey has been shown to produce liver cancer in small animals. For this reason comfrey should not be used internally and, as a poultice, only on intact skin (Kuhn and Winston, 2001). Other unsafe herbs are listed in Table 35-4.

Despite the increased use of herbal products, there has not been a parallel increase in reports of toxicity. Nonetheless, herbal products should be used with caution in pregnant women, nursing mothers, infants or young children, or older adults with liver or cardiovascular disease (Fontaine, 2000).

Nursing Role in Complementary and Alternative Therapies

The interest in CAM therapies has increased significantly in the past 15 years. The majority of people using and seeking information about complementary and alternative therapies are well educated and have a strong desire to actively participate in the decision making about their health care. This increased interest comes not only from health care consumers, but also allopathic physicians who have increasing concerns that current Western medicine is not meeting the needs of their clients. Many allopathic physicians do not refer their clients for CAM therapies because they are not familiar with the therapies and have had little, if any, education and training in complementary and alternative medicine. Many physicians have reservations about CAM therapies because they have not been appropriately tested in clinical trials in which other factors that may influence the outcomes are strictly controlled.

In North America and the United Kingdom many professional groups are exploring the use of CAM and facilitating and monitoring research being conducted in this area. Proposals put forth by several of the these groups include assessing the need of the public for CAM therapies, incorporating CAM educational components in the curriculum for all health care programs, providing appropriate information to the public, and encouraging and facilitating communication between CAM practitioners and allopathic physicians so each can be open to the other's approaches and values. For example, if CAM therapies are to be accepted and incorporated into Western medicine as a more integrative medical approach, practitioners of

Table 35-3	Safe or Effective Herbs Determined by Non-U.S. Regulatory Authorities	
Common Name	**Effects**	**Examples of Uses**
Aloe	Antiinflammatory	Minor burns
	Acceleration of wound healing	Wound healing
	Alkalinization of digestive juices	Gastrointestinal disorders
Cat's claw	Stimulant of immune system	Cancer
	Antioxidant	Gastrointestinal disorders
	Antiinflammatory	Hypertension
	Lowering of blood pressure	Infections
Chamomile	Antiinflammatory	Inflammatory diseases of gastrointestinal and upper respiratory tracts
	Antispasmodic	
	Antiinfective	Inflammation of skin and mucous membranes
		Gastrointestinal spasms
Dong quai	Antispasmodic	Menstrual cramps
	Vasodilation	Premenstrual syndrome
	Balancing effects of estrogen	Menstrual irregularities
	Mild sedative effect	Hot flashes
		Vaginal dryness
Echinacea	Stimulant of immune system	Upper respiratory tract infections
	Antiinflammatory	Allergic rhinitis
	Antibacterial	Wound healing
Feverfew	Antiinflammatory	Arthritis
	Inhibition of serotonin and prostaglandins	
	Vasodilator	
Garlic	Lowering of lipids	Elevated cholesterol levels
	Inhibition of platelet aggregation	Hypertension
	Antibacterial	Diabetes
Ginger	Antiemetic	Nausea and vomiting
		Motion sickness
Gingko biloba	Memory improvement	Alzheimer's disease
	Increasing blood flow	Dementia
	Antioxidant	Eye disease
	Increased metabolism efficiency	Heart disease
		Poor circulation
		Varicose veins
		Anxiety
		Age-related diseases
Ginseng	Increased physical endurance	Fatigue
	Balancing of body	Headaches
	Resistance to stress	Decreased libido
Hawthorn	Increased oxygen utilization by heart	Angina
	Lowering of cholesterol	Coronary artery disease
	Peripheral vasodilator	
Milk thistle	Stimulation of production of new liver cells	Liver disease
	Protection of liver from damage	
St. John's wort (hypericum)	Inhibition of monoamine oxidase (MAO) and serotonin reuptake	Mild to moderate depression
		Wound healing
	Antiviral	Viral infections
	Antibacterial	*Warning:* Avoid foods containing tyramine, such as aged cheese, red wine
Saw palmetto	Prevention of conversion of testosterone to dihydrotestosterone (needed for prostate cell multiplication)	Benign prostatic hyperplasia
		Urinary problems
Valerian	Minor tranquilizer	Sleep disorders
	Central nervous system depression	Restlessness

Table 35-4   Unsafe Herbs

Common Name	Effects	Comments
Borage	Diuretic Antidiarrheal	Contains toxic pyrrolizidine alkaloids
Calamus	Fever Digestive aid	Contains varying amounts of carcinogenic *cis*-isoasarone Indian-type most toxic North American–type nontoxic
Chaparral	Anticancer	No proven efficacy May induce severe liver toxicity
Coltsfoot	Antitussive Demulcent	Contains carcinogenic pyrrolizidine alkaloids
Comfrey	Wound healing	May induce venoocclusive disease
Ephedra *(ma huang)*	Central nervous system stimulant Anorectic Bronchodilator Cardiac stimulation	Unsafe for people with hypertension, diabetes, or thyroid disease Avoid consumption with caffeine
Germander	Anorectic	Causes hepatotoxicity
Life root	Menstrual flow stimulant	Hepatotoxic
Pokeroot	Antirheumatic Anticancer	May be fatal in children
Sassafras	Stimulant Antispasmodic Antirheumatic	Volatile oil Contains carcinogenic safrole

CAM should realize the advantages of their therapies' being researched more rigorously. On the other hand, allopathic physicians and more conventional practitioners should also begin to understand the benefits of therapies that encourage active participation by their clients in preventing illness or managing chronic illness rather than relying solely on surgery or drugs (Pelletier, 2000).

Integrative medicine, a health care strategy that is gaining popularity, involves a multiple-practitioner treatment group in which a client seeks care simultaneously from more than one type of practitioner. The clients are given the option to choose the kind of practitioner they feel would benefit their particular health problem. Clients who may benefit from these groups are those who have chronic health problems that have historically been difficult to treat using traditional allopathic medicine, such as fibromyalgia or chronic fatigue syndrome. This represents a pluralistic and truly complementary health care system in which both alternative and allopathic practitioners work side-by-side to improve the well-being of their clients. Although this is not reality in the majority of settings, this approach of open communication and practice between allopathic and alternative practitioners could potentially benefit a large number of clients.

The integrative medicine approach is consistent with the holistic approach nurses are taught to practice. Nurses have the potential for becoming essential participants in this type of health care philosophy. Many nurses already practice the use of touch (Box 35-6). Nurses should be knowledgeable of CAM therapies to make appropriate recommendations to allopathic primary care providers about which therapies may be useful for clients. Nurses should also provide advice to clients regarding when to seek conventional therapy or CAM therapy. For example, if a client complains of right lower abdominal pain, nausea, and vomiting, the nurse should be suspicious of ap-

Focus on Older Adults   **Box 35-6**

- Touch is a primal need, as necessary as food, growth, or shelter. Touch can be thought of as a nutrient transmitted through the skin. "Skin hunger" has been described as a form of malnutrition that has reached epidemic proportions in the United States, especially among older adults (Fontaine, 2000).
- Older adults need touch as much as or more than any other age-group. However, skin hunger or poverty of touch is often acute among older adults. It is an unfortunate coincidence that older adults often have fewer family members or friends to touch them at a time when simple touch could be an enhanced form of communication when other senses may be reduced (Dossey, Keegan, and Guzzetta, 2000).
- Simple touch helps older adult clients feel more connected to and accepted by those around them and to their environment. Self-esteem and sense of worth are enhanced.
- A nurse who reacts adversely to the skin changes of older people may find it difficult to touch an older client. The nurse's reluctance may then communicate a negative message to the older adult (Dossey and others, 2000).
- A holistic nursing approach to care of older adults should also include the caregivers, who often experience poor health or have neglected their own health, encounter their own psychosocial issues as they relate to the caregiving experience, feel the effects of multiple stressors, or feel spiritual distress (Eliopoulos, 2001).

pendicitis and recommend that the client be assessed by an allopathic physician. However, if the client has a chronic gastrointestinal disorder and has been diagnosed with irritable bowel syndrome, the client may benefit from relaxation and herbal therapy. Nurses need to be aware of their state Nurse Practice Acts with regard to complementary therapies and practice only within the scope of these laws.

Nurses work very closely with their clients and are in the unique position of becoming familiar with the client's religious and cultural viewpoints. Nurses may be able to determine which CAM therapies would be more appropriately aligned with these beliefs and offer recommendations accordingly.

Client interest and participation in CAM therapies is increasing. Therefore it is important for nurses to be knowledgeable of the multiple CAM therapies available and the use of these therapies by their clients. It is also important for nurses to keep abreast of the current research being done in this area to provide accurate information, not only to the clients, but to other health care professionals.

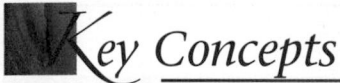

ey Concepts

- Alternative and complementary therapies can be the same, depending on whether the therapy is a primary treatment or treatment in addition to the Western medicine treatment.
- Integrative medical programs utilize a multidisciplinary (both allopathic and complementary) treatment approach providing holistic care to clients.
- The stress response is an adaptive response allowing individuals to react to stressful situations.
- A chronic stress response may be maladaptive, leading to chronic muscle tension, mood changes, and immune changes.
- Relaxation is a beneficial state characterized by lowered pulse rates, respiratory rates, blood pressure, and muscle tension and improved mood states.
- CAM therapies require commitment and regular involvement by the client to be most effective and have prolonged beneficial outcomes.
- CAM therapies should be appropriately chosen according to the person's functional status, belief or religious perspectives, access to health care, and insurance coverage.
- Some CAM therapies may alter physiological responses such that routine medication doses may need changing.
- Imagery is usually visual but can also involve the auditory, proprioceptive, gustatory, and olfactory senses.
- Many complementary and alternative therapies lack a scientific basis but are thought to be effective based on observed positive outcomes in a number of clients.

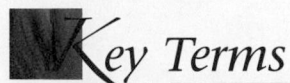

ey Terms

ritical Thinking Exercises

Client Profile: Margaret is a 76-year-old Catholic woman who has been diagnosed with a slow-growing renal tumor. She has been scheduled for surgery in 2 weeks. She is afraid of both the surgical procedure and the outcome. Is it cancer? Will the surgery result in a disability? Following surgery she becomes depressed.

1. What specific nursing-accessible CAM interventions can the nurse offer Margaret to prepare for the surgery and reduce her anxiety?
2. What CAM therapies may be appropriate to help her deal with her depression?

eview Questions

1. Despite the success of allopathic medicine (traditional Western medicine), many clients with conditions such as the following find relief in complementary therapies:
   1. Heart disease and pancreatitis.
   2. Ulcers and hepatitis.
   3. Chronic back pain and arthritis.
   4. Lupus and diabetes.

2. Many of the complementary therapies, such as acupuncture, contain diagnostic and therapeutic methods specific to their field, whereas others, such as the following, are more easily learned and applied.
   1. Massage therapy.
   2. Chinese medicine.
   3. Shamanism.
   4. Breathwork and imagery.

3. It is estimated that half of U.S. citizens use a CAM practitioner and that these visits:
   1. Exceed the visits to allopathics.
   2. Are equal to visits to allopathics.
   3. Are slightly less than visits to allopathics.
   4. Are double those visits to allopathics.

4. Holistic nursing regards and treats the:
   1. Mind, body, and spirit of the client.
   2. Disease, spirit, and family.
   3. Desires and emotions of the client.
   4. Muscles, nerves, and spine disorders.

5. When the nurse utilizes CAM, adequate assessment and the client's:
   1. Permission are a prerequisite for implementation.
   2. Physician must give approval for implementation.
   3. Family must give permission.
   4. Total understanding of CAM must be documented.

6. One of the principles of CAM therapies is that the individual becomes:
   1. Actively involved in the treatment.
   2. A total believer in what is being taught.
   3. Submissive to the practitioner.
   4. Less competent in his or her own care.

7. The stress response is a good example of the way in which systems:
   1. React the same way for all individuals.
   2. Cooperate to protect an individual from harm.
   3. Fail and cause illness and disease.
   4. Cause structural damage to the body.

8. Client's medications should be monitored carefully because meditation may augment the effects of certain drugs such as:
   1. Antihypertensive and thyroid-regulating medications.
   2. Insulin and vitamins.
   3. Prednisone.
   4. Cough syrups and aspirin.

9. Biofeedback techniques are frequently used in addition to relaxation interventions to assist individuals:
   1. To eat less food.
   2. In learning how to control specific autonomic nervous system responses.
   3. To control diabetes.
   4. With AIDS to live longer.

10. Therapeutic touch is a training-specific therapy that was developed by a (an):
    1. Physician.
    2. Nurse.
    3. Physical therapist.
    4. Ancient Scandinavian culture.

References

Benson H: *The relaxation response,* New York, 1975, Avon.

Dossey B, Keegan L, Guzzetta C: *Holistic Nursing: a handbook for practice,* ed 3, Gaithersburg, Md, 2000, Aspen.

Eisenberg D and others: Trends in alternative medicine use in the United States, 1990-1997, *JAMA* 280:1569, 1998.

Eliopoulos C: *Gerontologic nursing,* ed 5, Philadelphia, 2001, Lippincott Williams & Wilkins.

Enst E: Complementary therapies in palliative cancer care, *Cancer* 91(11):2181, 2001.

Fontaine K: *Healing practices: alternative therapies for nursing,* Upper Saddle River, NJ, 2000, Prentice Hall.

Gawain S: *Creative visualization (25th anniversary edition),* New York, 2002, New World Library.

Jacobs J: Clinical applications of the relaxation response and mind-body interventions, *J Altern Complement Med* 7 (Suppl 1): S93, 2001.

Krieger D: Therapeutic touch: the imprimatur of nursing, *Am J Nurs* 75:784, 1975.

Krieger D: Searching for evidence of physiological change, *Am J Nurs* 79:660, 1979.

Kuhn M, Winston D: *Herbal therapy and supplements: a scientific and traditional approach,* New York, 2001, Lippincott, Williams & Wilkins.

Pelletier K: *The best alternative medicine: what works? What does not?* New York, 2000, Simon & Schuster.

Skidmore-Roth L: *Handbook of herbs and supplements,* St. Louis, 2003, Mosby.

Research References

Abdelghany S and others: Biofeedback and electrical stimulation therapy for treating urinary incontinence and voiding dysfunction: one center's experience, *Urol Nurs* 21(6):401, 2001.

American Holistic Nurses' Association: *Standards of holistic nursing practice,* Flagstaff, Ariz, 1998, The Association.

Astin J and others: Psychological interventions for rheumatoid arthritis: a meta-analysis of randomized controlled trials, *Arthritis Rheum* 47(3):291, 2002.

Belleggia G, Birbaumer N: Treatment of phantom limb pain with combined EMG and thermal biofeedback: a case report, *Appl Psychophysiol Biofeedback* 26(2):141, 2001

Cowan M, Pike K, Budzynski H: Psychosocial nursing therapy following sudden cardiac arrest: impact on two-year survival, *Nurs Res* 50(2):68, 2001.

Crider A, Glaros A: A meta-analysis of EMG biofeedback treatment of temporomandibular disorders, *J Orofac Pain* 13(1):29, 1999.

Cunningham C, Brown S, Kaski, J: Effects of transcendental meditation on symptoms and electrocardiographic changes in patients with cardiac syndrome X, *Am J Cardiol* 85(5):653, 2000.

Deale A and others: Long-term outcome of cognitive behavior therapy versus relaxation therapy for chronic fatigue syndrome: a five-year follow-up study, *Am J Psychiatry* 158(12):2038, 2001.

Good M and others: Relaxation and music to reduce postsurgical pain, *J Adv Nurs* 33(2):208, 2001.

Hagemaster J: Use of therapeutic touch in treatment of drug addictions, *Holist Nurs Pract* 14(3):14, 2000.

Janke J: The effect of relaxation therapy on preterm labor outcomes, *J Obstet Gynecol Neonatal Nurs* 28(3):255, 1999.

Keefer L, Blanchard E: The effects of relaxation response meditation on the symptoms of irritable bowel syndrome, *Behav Res Ther* 39(7):801, 2001.

Keefer L, Blanchard E: A one-year follow-up of relaxation response meditation as a treatment for irritable bowel syndrome, *Behav Res Ther* 40(5):541, 2002.

Kiernan J: The experience of Therapeutic Touch in the lives of five postpartum women, *MCN Am J Matern Child Nurs* 27(1):47, 2002.

King M, Carr T, D'Cruz C: Transcendental meditation, hypertension and heart disease, *Aust Fam Physician* 31(2):164, 2002.

Lee M and others: Effect of Qi-training on blood pressure, heart rate and respiration rate, *Clin Physiol* 20(3):173, 2000.

Leskowitz E: Phantom limb pain treated with therapeutic touch: a case report, *Arch Phys Med Rehabil* 81(4):522, 2000.

Moore N: A review of EEG biofeedback treatment of anxiety disorders, *Clin Electroencephalogr* 31(1):1-6, 2000.

Nakao M and others: Blood pressure biofeedback treatment, organ damage and sympathetic activity in mild hypertension, *Psychother Psychosom* 68(6):341, 1999.

National Center for Complementary and Alternative Medicine: What is complementary and alternative medicine?, NCCAM publication no. D156, 2002, http://altmed.od.nih.gov/health/whatiscam/#11.

Peters R: The effectiveness of therapeutic touch: a meta-analytic review, *Nurs Sci Q* 12(1):52, 1999.

Sarafino E, Goehring P: Age comparisons in acquiring biofeedback control and success in reducing headache pain, *Ann Behav Med* 22(1):10, 2000.

Scharff L, Marcus D, Masek, B: A controlled study of minimal contact controlled biofeedback treatment in children with migraine, *J Pediatr Psychol* 27(2):109, 2002.

Shannahoff-Khalsa D: Complementary healthcare practices: stress management for gastrointestinal disorders—the use of kundalini yoga meditation techniques, *Gastroenterol Nurs* 25(3):126, 2002.

Smyth P: Therapeutic touch for a patient after a Whipple procedure, *Crit Care Nurs Clin North Am* 13(3):357, 2001.

Speca M and others: A randomized, wait-list controlled clinical trial: the effect of a mindfulness meditation-based stress reduction program on mood and symptoms of stress in cancer outpatients, *Psychosom Med* 62(5):613, 2000.

Taylor EJ, Outlaw FH: Use of prayer among persons with cancer, *Holist Nurs Pract* 16(3):46, 2002.

Winstead-Fry P, Kijek J: An integrative review and meta-analysis of therapeutic touch research, *Altern Ther Health Med* 5(6):58, 1999.

Yung P, French P, Leung B: Relaxation training as complementary therapy for mild hypertension control and the implications of evidence-based medicine, *Complement Ther Nurs Midwifery* 7(2):59, 2001.

36

Activity and Exercise

Media Resources

http://evolve.elsevier.com/Potter/
fundamentals/

 CD COMPANION

- Review Questions
- Glossary

evolve WEBSITE

- Review Questions
- Student Learning Activities
- Concept Map Exercise
- Critical Thinking Exercise
- Glossary

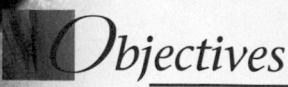

Objectives

Mastery of content in this chapter will enable the student to:

- Define the key terms listed.
- Describe the role of the musculoskeletal and nervous systems in the regulation of movement.
- Discuss physiological and pathological influences on body alignment and joint mobility.
- Describe how to maintain and use proper body mechanics.
- Describe how exercise and activity benefit physiological and psychological functioning.
- Describe the benefits of implementing an exercise program for the purpose of health promotion.
- Describe the benefits of implementing exercise and activity during the acute, restorative, and continuing care of clients.
- Describe important factors to consider when planning an exercise program for clients across the life span and for those with specific chronic illnesses.
- Assess clients for impaired mobility and activity intolerance.
- Formulate nursing diagnoses for clients experiencing problems with impaired mobility and activity intolerance.
- Write a nursing care plan for a client with impaired mobility and activity intolerance.
- Describe the interventions for maintaining activity tolerance and mobility during the acute, restorative, and continuing care of clients.
- Evaluate the nursing care plan for maintaining activity and exercise for clients across the life span and with specific chronic illnesses.

The actions of walking, turning, lifting, and carrying are essential components in the provision of nursing care. Such activities require muscle exertion by the nurse. To reduce the risk of injury to the client or nurse, the nurse must know and practice proper **body mechanics.** This includes knowledge of the actions of various muscle groups, understanding of the factors involved in the coordination of body movement, and familiarity with the integrated functioning of the skeletal, muscular, and nervous systems.

In addition, nurses must promote activity and **exercise** because of the beneficial impact on wellness, prevention of illness, and restoration of optimal functioning. A program of regular physical activity and exercise has the potential to enhance all aspects of a client's biopsychosocial and spiritual model of health (Box 36-1). This chapter provides the student with knowledge of exercise and activity as it relates to health promotion, the acute phase of illness, and the restorative and continuing care of clients. Nursing strategies are included to help plan an individualized exercise and activity program for a variety of clients with specific disease entities and needs.

Box 36-1   The Gift of Exercise

The other day I was looking for a gift to give to a friend. This friend is very important to me and I want her to be around for a long time; I want her to live a long and healthy life. I thought how great it would be if I could give her a gift that would improve the quality of her life.

So I sat down and made a list of what I would look for in this special gift:
It would help her to be stronger, firmer, leaner, more flexible, and energetic.
It would help lower her risk of dying from heart disease, help lower blood pressure and improve lipid profile, control blood glucose level, fight obesity, and help her to age more gracefully.
It would help improve immune function, concentration and task performance, and the quality of sleep.
It would help reduce stress, improve mood, enhance self-esteem, and increase optimism and confidence.
It would help to increase self-awareness and control over choices in her life.
It would be fun but also challenging.
It would allow for socialization but also time alone, depending on her needs.
It would come in all different modes and styles and adapt to various environments and weather conditions.
Finally, it would have a good *Consumer Reports* rating, supported by scientific data from reputable sources.

After completing my list, I realized that the only gift that meets all the criteria is the gift of exercise. Have a happy and healthy life, my friend.

From Huddleston JS: Exercise. In Edelman CL, Mandle CL editors: *Health promotion throughout the lifespan*, ed 5, St. Louis, 2002, Mosby.

Scientific Knowledge Base

Activity and exercise are important to all individuals' well-being. The nurse is able to provide a more individualized approach to care by knowing the physiology and regulation of body mechanics, exercise, and activity.

Overview of Body Mechanics, Exercise, and Activity

The coordinated efforts of the musculoskeletal and nervous systems to maintain balance, **posture,** and body alignment during lifting, bending, moving, and performing **activities of daily living (ADLs)** provide the foundation for body mechanics. The proper implementation of these activities reduces the risk of injury to the musculoskeletal system and facilitates body movements, allowing physical mobility without muscle strain and excessive use of muscle energy.

Body Alignment. Body alignment refers to the relationship of one body part to another body part along a horizontal or vertical line. Correct alignment reduces the strain on musculoskeletal structures, maintains adequate **muscle tone,** and contributes to balance.

Body Balance. Body balance is achieved when a relatively low **center of gravity** is balanced over a wide, stable base of support and a vertical line falls from the center of gravity through the base of support. The base of support is the foundation. When the vertical line from the center of gravity does not fall through the base of support, the body loses balance. Body balance is also enhanced by proper posture, or the body position that most favors function, requires the least muscular work to maintain, and places the least strain on muscles, ligaments, and bones (Thibodeau and Patton, 2002).

The nurse uses balance to maintain proper body alignment and posture by using two simple techniques. First, the base of support can easily be widened by separating the feet to a comfortable distance. Second, balance is increased by bringing the center of gravity closer to the base of support. This is achieved by bending the knees and flexing the hips until the person is squatting and still maintaining proper back alignment by keeping the trunk erect. The nervous system is responsible for muscle tone and regulates and coordinates the amount of pull exerted by the individual muscles (Thibodeau and Patton, 2002).

Coordinated Body Movement. Coordinated body movement is a result of weight, center of gravity, and balance. Weight is the force exerted on a body by gravity. When an object is lifted, the lifter must overcome the object's weight and be aware of its center of gravity. In symmetrical objects the center of gravity is located at the exact center of the object. The force of weight is always directed downward. An object that is unbalanced has its center of gravity away from the midline and falls without support. Because people are not geometrically perfect, their centers of gravity are usually at 55% to 57% of standing height and are located in the midline. Like unbalanced objects, clients who fail to maintain a balance with their center of gravity are unsteady, which places them at risk for falling. Nurses must be able to identify such clients and intervene in such a way that safety is maintained.

Friction. **Friction** is a force that occurs in a direction to oppose movement. As the nurse turns, transfers, or moves a client up in bed, friction must be overcome. A nurse can reduce friction by following some basic principles. The greater the surface area of the object to be moved, the greater the friction. If a client is unable to assist in moving up in bed, the client's arms should be placed across the chest. This decreases surface area and reduces friction.

A passive or immobilized client produces greater friction to movement (see Chapter 46). Thus when possible, the nurse should use some of the client's strength and mobility when lifting, transferring, or moving the client up in bed. This can be done by explaining the procedure and telling the client when to move. For instance, friction is decreased if the client can bend his or her knees as the nurse assists him or her in moving up in the bed.

Friction can also be reduced by lifting rather than pushing a client. Lifting has an upward component and decreases the pressure between the client and the bed or the chair. The use of a lift sheet reduces friction because the client is more easily moved along the bed's surface.

Exercise and Activity. Exercise is physical activity for the purpose of conditioning the body, improving health, and maintaining fitness, or it may be used as a therapeutic measure. The exercise program chosen and developed for a client depends heavily on the individual's **activity tolerance,** or the kind and amount of exercise or activity that the person is able to perform. Physiological, emotional, and developmental factors influence the client's activity tolerance.

A program of regular physical activity and exercise promotes physical and psychological health. An active lifestyle is important for maintaining and promoting health; it is also an essential treatment modality for chronic illnesses (Flood and Constance, 2002; Konradi and Anglin, 2001). Regular physical activity and exercise enhances functioning of all body systems, including cardiopulmonary functioning (endurance), musculoskeletal fitness (flexibility and bone integrity), weight control and maintenance (body image), and psychological well-being (Burbank and others, 2002; Huddleston, 2002).

The best program of physical activity includes a combination of exercises that produce different physiological and psychological benefits. Isotonic, isometric, and resistive isometric are three categories of exercise classified according to the type of muscle contraction involved. Isotonic exercises cause muscle contraction and change in muscle length **(isotonic contraction).** Examples of isotonic exercises are walking, swimming, dance aerobics, jogging, bicycling, and moving arms and legs with light resistance. The benefits of isotonic exercises are increased circulation and respiratory functioning; increased osteoblastic activity (activity by bone-forming cells), thus combating osteoporosis; and increased muscle tone, mass, and strength.

Isometric exercises involve tightening or tensing of muscles without moving body parts **(isometric contraction).** Examples of isometric exercises are quadriceps set exercises and contraction of the gluteal muscles. This form of exercise is ideal for clients who are unable to tolerate an increase in activity that is expected during isotonic exercises. Isometric exercises are easily accomplished by an immobilized client in bed. The benefits are increased muscle mass, tone, and strength, thus decreasing the potential for muscle wasting; increased circulation to the involved body part; and increased osteoblastic activity.

Isometric exercises may also be resistive. Resistive isometric exercises are those in which the individual contracts the muscle while pushing against a stationary object or resisting the movement of an object (Hoeman, 2002). A gradual increase in the amount of resistance and length of time that the muscle contraction is held will increase muscle strength and endurance. Examples of resistive isometric exercises are push-ups, pushing against a **footboard** to move up in bed, and hip lifting. In hip lifting, the client, who is in a sitting position, pushes with the hands against a surface such as the seat of a chair and raises the hips. Resistive isometric exercises help to promote muscle strength and provide sufficient stress against bone to promote osteoblastic activity.

Regulation of Movement

Coordinated body movement involves the integrated functioning of the skeletal, muscular, and nervous systems. Because these three systems cooperate so closely in mechanical support of the body, they are often considered as a single functional unit.

Skeletal System. Bones perform five functions in the body: support, protection, movement, mineral storage, and hematopoiesis (blood cell formation). In the discussion of body mechanics two of these functions—support and movement—are most important (see Chapter 46). In support, bones serve as the framework and contribute to the shape, alignment, and positioning of the body parts. In movement, bones together with their joints constitute levers for muscle attachment. As muscles contract and shorten, they pull on bones, producing joint movement (Thibodeau and Patton, 2002).

Joints. An articulation, or **joint,** is the connection between bones. Each joint is classified according to its structure and degree of mobility. On the basis of connective structures, joints are classified as fibrous, cartilaginous, or synovial (Huether and McCance, 2000). **Fibrous joints** fit closely together and are fixed, permitting little, if any, movement such as the syndesmosis between the tibia and fibula. **Cartilaginous joints** have little movement but are elastic and use cartilage to unite separate body surfaces such as the synchondrosis that attaches the ribs to the costal cartilage. **Synovial joints,** or true joints, are freely moveable and are the most mobile, numerous, and anatomically complex of the body's joints, such as the hinge type at the elbow.

Ligaments, Tendons, and Cartilage. Ligaments, tendons, and cartilage are structures that support the skeletal system (see Chapter 46). **Ligaments** are white, shiny, flexible bands of fibrous tissue that bind joints and connect bones and cartilage. Ligaments are elastic and aid joint flexibility and support. **Tendons** are white, glistening, fibrous bands of tissue that connect muscle to bone. **Cartilage** is nonvascular, supporting connective tissue with the flexibility of a firm, plastic material. The gristle-like nature of cartilage permits it to sustain weight and serve as a shock absorber between articulating bones.

Skeletal Muscle. When we walk, talk, run, breathe, or participate in physical activity, we do so by the contraction of skeletal muscles. There are over 600 skeletal muscles in the body. In addition to facilitating movement, these muscles determine the form and contour of our bodies. Most of our muscles span at least one joint and attach to both articulating bones. When contraction occurs, one bone is fixed while the other moves. The origin is the point of attachment that remains still; the insertion is the point that moves when the muscle contracts (Thibodeau and Patton, 2002).

Muscles Concerned With Movement. The muscles of movement are located near the skeletal region, where movement is caused by a lever system (Thibodeau and Patton, 2002). The lever system makes the work of moving a weight or load easier. It occurs when specific bones, such as the humerus, ulna, and radius, and the associated joints, such as the elbow, act as a lever. Thus the force applied to one end of the bone to lift a weight at another point tends to rotate the bone in the direction opposite that of the applied force. Muscles that attach to bones of leverage provide the necessary strength to move the object.

Muscles Concerned With Posture. Gravity pulls on parts of the body all the time; the only way the body can be held in position is for muscles to exert pull on bones in the opposite direction. Muscles accomplish this counterforce by maintaining a low level of sustained contraction. Poor posture places more work on muscles to counteract the force of gravity. This leads to fatigue and can eventually interfere with bodily functions and cause deformities.

Muscle Groups. The antagonistic, synergistic, and antigravity muscle groups are coordinated by the nervous system and maintain posture and initiate movement. **Antagonistic muscles** bring about movement at the joint. During movement the active mover muscle contracts while its antagonist relaxes. For example, during flexion of the arm the active mover, the biceps brachii, contracts and its antagonist, the triceps brachii, relaxes. During extension of the arm the active mover, now the triceps brachii, contracts and the new antagonist, the biceps brachii, relaxes.

Synergistic muscles contract to accomplish the same movement. When the arm is flexed, the strength of the contraction of the biceps brachii is increased by contraction of the synergistic muscle, the brachialis. Thus with synergistic muscle activity there are now two active movers—the biceps brachii and the brachialis—which contract while the antagonistic muscle, the triceps brachii, relaxes.

Antigravity muscles are involved with joint stabilization. These muscles continuously oppose the effect of gravity on the body and permit a person to maintain an upright or sitting posture. In an adult the antigravity muscles are the extensors of the leg, the gluteus maximus, the quadriceps femoris, the soleus muscles, and the muscles of the back.

Skeletal muscles support posture and carry out voluntary movement. The muscles are attached to the skeleton by tendons, which provide strength and permit motion. The movement of the extremities is voluntary and requires coordination from the nervous system.

Nervous System. Movement and posture are regulated by the nervous system. The major voluntary motor area, located in the cerebral cortex, is the precentral gyrus, or motor strip. A majority of motor fibers descend from the motor strip and cross at the level of the medulla. Thus the motor fibers from the right motor strip initiate voluntary movement for the left side of the body, and motor fibers from the left motor strip initiate voluntary movement for the right side of the body.

Transmission of the impulse from the nervous system to the musculoskeletal system is an electrochemical event and requires a neurotransmitter. Basically, neurotransmitters are chemicals (e.g., acetylcholine) that transfer the electric impulse from the nerve across the myoneural junction to stimulate the muscle, causing movement.

Movement can be impaired by disorders that alter neurotransmitter production as in Parkinson's disease, transfer from the neurotransmitter to the muscle as in myasthenia gravis, or activation of muscle activity as in multiple sclerosis (Huether and McCance, 2000).

Proprioception. **Proprioception** is the awareness of the position of the body and its parts (Huether and McCance, 2000). Proprioception is monitored by proprioceptors located on nerve endings in muscles, tendons, and joints. Posture is regulated by the nervous system and requires coordination of proprioception and balance. As a person carries out ADLs, proprioceptors monitor muscle activity and body position. For example, the proprioceptors on the soles of the feet contribute to correct posture while standing or walking. In standing, pressure is continuous on the bottom of the feet. The proprioceptors monitor the pressure, communicating this information through the nervous system to the antigravity muscles. The standing person remains upright until deciding to change position. As a person walks, the proprioceptors on the bottom of the feet monitor pressure changes. Thus when the bottom of the moving foot comes in contact with the walking surface, the individual automatically moves the stationary foot forward. The proprioceptors allow people to walk without having to watch their feet.

Balance. When standing, running, lifting, or performing ADLs, a person must have adequate balance. Balance is controlled by the nervous system, specifically by the cerebellum and the inner ear. The major function of the cerebellum is to coordinate all voluntary movement, particularly highly skilled movements, such as those required in skiing.

Within the inner ear are the semicircular canals, three fluid-filled structures that assist in maintaining balance. Fluid within the canals has a certain inertia, and when the head is suddenly rotated in one direction, the fluid remains stationary for a moment, whereas the canal turns with the head. This allows a person to change position suddenly without losing balance.

Principles of Body Mechanics

Using principles of body mechanics during routine activities also prevents injury (Box 36-2). The nurse teaches colleagues and clients' families to lift, transfer, or position clients properly. A nurse who is teaching a client's family to transfer the client from bed to chair can increase and reinforce the family's knowledge by consistently demonstrating proper body mechanics.

Whether the nurse is moving an immobilized client, assisting a client from the bed to the chair, or teaching a client to carry out ADLs efficiently, knowledge of basic principles of body mechanics is crucial. The nurse also incorporates knowledge of physiological and pathological influences on body alignment and mobility.

Pathological Influences on Body Mechanics. Many pathological conditions affect body alignment and mobility. These conditions include congenital defects; disorders of bones, joints, and muscles, central nervous system damage, and musculoskeletal trauma.

Congenital Defects. Congenital abnormalities affect the efficiency of the musculoskeletal system in regard to alignment, balance, and appearance. Osteogenesis imper-

Box *36-2*   **Principles of Body Mechanics**

The wider the base of support, the greater the stability of the nurse.

The lower the center of gravity, the greater the stability of the nurse.

The equilibrium of an object is maintained as long as the line of gravity passes through its base of support.

Facing the direction of movement prevents abnormal twisting of the spine.

Dividing balanced activity between arms and legs reduces the risk of back injury.

Leverage, rolling, turning, or pivoting requires less work than lifting.

When friction is reduced between the object to be moved and the surface on which it is moved, less force is required to move it.

Reducing the force of work reduces the risk of injury.

Maintaining good body mechanics reduces fatigue of the muscle groups.

Alternating periods of rest and activity helps to reduce fatigue.

fecta is an inherited disorder that affects bone. Bones are porous, short, bowed, and deformed; as a result, children experience curvature of the spine and shortness of stature (Wong and Hockenberry-Eaton, 2001). Scoliosis is a structural curvature of the spine associated with vertebral rotation. Muscles, ligaments, and other soft tissues become shortened. Balance and mobility are affected in proportion to the severity of abnormal spinal curvatures (Wong and Hockenberry-Eaton, 2001).

Disorders of Bones, Joints, and Muscles. Osteoporosis is a well-known and well-publicized disorder of aging in which the density or mass of bone is reduced. The bone remains biochemically normal but has difficulty maintaining integrity and support. The cause is uncertain, and theories vary from hormonal imbalances to insufficient intake of nutrients (Huether and McCance, 2000; Lewis and others, 2000).

Osteomalacia is an uncommon metabolic disease characterized by inadequate and delayed mineralization, resulting in compact and spongy bone (Lewis and others, 2000). Mineral calcification and deposition do not occur. Replaced bone consists of soft material rather than rigid bone.

Joint mobility can be altered by inflammatory and noninflammatory joint diseases and by articular disruption. Inflammatory joint disease (e.g., arthritis) is characterized by inflammation or destruction of the synovial membrane and articular cartilage, and by systemic signs of inflammation. Noninflammatory diseases have none of these characteristics, and the synovial fluid is normal (Huether and McCance, 2000). Joint degeneration, which can occur with inflammatory and noninflammatory disease, is marked by changes in articular cartilage combined with overgrowth of bone at the articular ends. Degenerative changes commonly affect weight-bearing joints.

Articular disruption may be as mild as a sprain or as severe as dislocation. Articular disruption involves trauma to the articular capsules, such as a tear in a sprain or a separation in a dislocation. Articular disruption usually results from trauma but can also be congenital, as with developmental dysplasia of the hip (Wong and Hockenberry-Eaton, 2001).

Central Nervous System Damage. Damage to any component of the central nervous system that regulates voluntary movement results in impaired body alignment and mobility. For example, the motor strip in the cerebrum can be damaged by trauma from a head injury. The amount of voluntary motor impairment is directly related to the amount of destruction of the motor strip. A client with a right-sided cerebral hemorrhage and damage to the right motor strip may have left-sided **hemiplegia.** However, a client with a right-sided head injury may only have cerebral edema (but not destruction) of the motor strip. With extensive physical therapy, voluntary movement gradually returns to the left side.

Musculoskeletal Trauma. Musculoskeletal trauma can result in bruises, contusions, sprains, and fractures. A fracture is a disruption of bone tissue continuity. Fractures most commonly result from direct external trauma. They can also occur because of some deformity of the bone, as with pathological fractures of osteoporosis (see Chapter 46).

Safety Alert. The first 6 to 12 hours is the most crucial period of time for treating soft tissue injuries (Lewis and others, 2000). Basic treatment of soft tissue injuries is summarized by the acronym *ICES:*

I – Ice: Reduces pain threshold; should not be applied for longer than 30 minutes at a time.

C – Compression: A wet elastic wrap should be applied to hold ice in place and provide compression.

E – Elevate: The injured part should be held several inches above the heart to facilitate venous return and reduce swelling.

S – Support: Usual treatment is immobilization either by application of a brace or cast.

*N*ursing Knowledge Base

This section is concerned with knowledge from areas of nursing practice that enable the nurse to meet the holistic needs of the client. Developmental changes, behavioral aspects, family and social support, cultural and ethnic origin, and environmental issues are important aspects of an individual and must be incorporated into the plan of care whether the client is seeking health promotion, acute care, or restorative and continuing care.

Developmental Changes

Throughout the life span the body's appearance and functioning undergo change. The greatest change and impact on the maturational process is observed in childhood and old age.

Infants Through School-Age Children. The newborn infant's spine is flexed and lacks the anteroposterior curves of the adult. The first spinal curve occurs when the infant extends the neck from the prone position. As growth and stability increase, the thoracic spine straightens, and the lumbar spinal curve appears, which allows sitting and standing.

The toddler's posture is awkward because of the slight swayback and protruding abdomen. As the child walks, the legs and feet are usually far apart and the feet are slightly everted. Toward the end of toddlerhood, posture appears less awkward, curves in the cervical and lumbar vertebrae are accentuated, and foot eversion disappears.

By the third year the body is slimmer, taller, and better balanced. Abdominal protrusion is decreased, the feet are not as far apart, and the arms and legs have increased in length. The child appears more coordinated. From the third year through the beginning of adolescence, the musculoskeletal system continues to grow and develop (see Chapter 11).

Adolescence. The period of adolescence is usually initiated by a tremendous growth spurt. Growth is frequently uneven. As a result, the adolescent may appear awkward and uncoordinated. Adolescent girls usually grow and develop earlier than boys. Hips widen, and fat is deposited in the upper arms, thighs, and buttocks. The adolescent boy's changes in shape are usually a result of long-bone growth and increased muscle mass (see Chapter 11).

Young to Middle Adults. An adult who has correct posture and body alignment feels good, looks good, and generally appears self-confident. The healthy adult also has the necessary musculoskeletal development and coordination to carry out ADLs (see Chapter 12). Normal changes in posture and body alignment in adulthood occur mainly in pregnant women. These changes result from the body's adaptive response to weight gain and the growing fetus. The center of gravity shifts toward the anterior. The pregnant woman leans back and is slightly swaybacked. She may complain of back pain.

Older Adults. A progressive loss of total bone mass occurs with the older adult. Some of the possible causes of this loss include physical inactivity, hormonal changes, and increased osteoclastic activity (activity by cells responsible for bone tissue absorption). The effect of bone loss is weaker bones, causing vertebrae to be softer and long shaft bones to be less resistant to bending.

In addition, older adults may walk more slowly and appear less coordinated. They may also take smaller steps, keeping their feet closer together, which decreases the base of support. Thus body balance is unstable, and they are at greater risk for falls and injuries (see Chapter 13).

> ***Safety Alert.*** Falls and the resulting injuries are among the most debilitating medical problems that prevent the older adult from remaining independent. Regular exercise that includes strengthening, flexibility, and balance can help prevent falls in the older adult (Burbank and others, 2002; Connelly, 2000; Huddleston, 2002; Resnick, 1999).

Box *36-3*   General Guidelines for Initiating and Maintaining an Exercise Program

The client will most likely initiate and maintain an exercise program if the individual:

Perceives a net benefit

Chooses an enjoyable activity

Feels competent doing the activity

Feels safe doing the activity

Can easily access the activity on a regular basis

Can fit the activity into the daily schedule

Feels that the activity does not generate financial or social costs that he or she is unwilling to bear

Experiences a minimum of negative consequences such as injury, loss of time, negative peer pressure, and problems with self-identity

Is able to successfully address issues of competing time demands

Recognizes the need to balance the use of labor-saving devices and sedentary activities with activities that involve a higher level of physical exertion

Data from National Institutes of Health Consensus Development Panel on Physical Activity and Cardiovascular Health: Physical activity and cardiovascular health, *JAMA* 276(3):241, 1996; and Schlicht J and others: Build self-efficacy to promote exercise adherence, *ACSM's Health Fitness Journal* 3(6):27, 1999.

Behavioral Aspects

Clients are more likely to incorporate an exercise program into their daily lives if this is supported and assisted by family and friends, nurses, physicians, and other members of the health care team. The nurse should take into consideration the client's knowledge of exercise and activity, barriers to a program of exercise and physical activity, and current exercise habits. Clients are more open to developing an exercise program if they are at the stage of readiness to change their behavior (Prochaska, Norcross, and DiClemente, 1994). Information on the benefits of regular exercise may be helpful to the client who is not at the stage of readiness to act. Clients' decisions to change behavior and include a daily exercise routine in their lives may occur gradually with repeated information that is individualized to their needs and lifestyle (Box 36-3). Once the client has reached the stage of readiness, the nurse must develop in collaboration with the client an exercise program that is customized to fit his or her needs; the nurse then provides continued follow-up support and assistance until the exercise program becomes a daily routine.

Environmental Issues

Work Site. A common barrier for many clients is the lack of time that is needed to engage in a daily exercise program. Work sites have the potential to help their employees overcome the obstacle of time constraints by offering opportunities, reminders, and rewards for those committed to physical fitness (National Institutes of Health [NIH], 1996). Reminders such as signs could be used to encourage employees to use the stairs instead of elevators. Rewards such as free parking or discounted parking fees could be given to employees who park in distant lots and walk (NIH, 1996).

Schools. It has become increasingly clear that children are becoming less active with the result being an increase in childhood obesity (U.S. Department of Health and Human Services [USDHHS], 2000). Children and adolescents spend a great deal of their time in school. However, the number of students involved in daily school physical education decreased from 42% in 1991 to 32% in 1997 (USDHHS, 2000). Schools can be an excellent facilitator of physical fitness and exercise. Strategies for physical activity incorporated early into a child's daily routine could provide a foundation for lifetime commitment to exercise and physical fitness. The NIH Consensus Development Panel (1996) recommends that all schools provide physical activity programs that are appropriate for children of all skill levels and not limited to competitive sports or physical education classes, that appeal to both girls and boys, as well as to children from diverse backgrounds, and that are offered on a daily basis.

Community. The community's support of physical fitness can be instrumental in promoting the health of its members. Examples of community involvement to promote physical fitness are the provision of walking trails and track facilities in community parks and physical fitness classes offered by trained professionals in exercise and physical fitness. This may be a difficult task because of cost restraints. However, success in implementing physical fitness programs is dependent on a collaborative effort from public health agencies, parks and recreational associations, state and local government agencies, health care agencies, and the members of the community.

Cultural and Ethnic Influences

Exercise and physical fitness is beneficial to all people. When developing a physical fitness program for culturally diverse populations, the nurse must consider what motivates and what is deemed appropriate and enjoyable. The nurse must also have knowledge of what specific disease entities are associated with different cultural and ethnic origins (Box 36-4).

Family and Social Support

Social support can be used as a motivational tool to encourage and promote exercise and physical fitness. The client can engage a friend or significant other to participate in a "buddy system" whereby they walk together each day at a specified time. This companionship provides for socialization and increases the enjoyment for some clients and thus develops a lifelong commitment to physical fitness. Parents can support their children in sports and physical activity by providing encouragement, praise, and transportation (Prochaska, Rodgers, and Sallis, 2002). In addition, parents can include their children in family outings that include such activities as bicycling or a basketball game in the neighborhood schoolyard.

Critical Thinking

Successful critical thinking requires a synthesis of knowledge, experience, information gathered from clients, critical thinking attitudes, and intellectual and professional standards. Client's conditions are always changing. Clinical judgments require the nurse to anticipate the information necessary, analyze the data, and make decisions regarding client care.

To understand activity tolerance and physical fitness and the impact on the client, the nurse must integrate knowledge from nursing and other disciplines, previous experiences, and information gathered from clients. As the nurse begins the process of problem solving for client care, a variety of concepts must be considered and woven together to provide the best outcome for the client. Knowledge of the musculoskeletal system and health alterations that create problems for the client in the area of activity, exercise, and body mechanics, lays the foundation for planning and decision making. The use of professional standards, such as those developed by the American College of Sports Medicine (ACSM, 1998) and the American Diabetes Association (2002), provides valuable guidelines for exercise and physical fitness. The nurse's experiences and critical thinking attitude affect

---

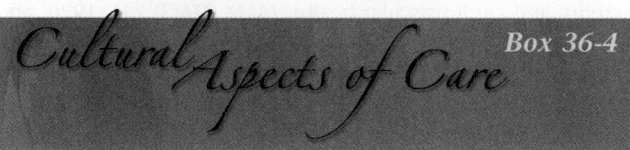
Cultural Aspects of Care **Box 36-4**

Epidemiological studies of ethnic groups indicate that physical inactivity is one of the risk factors associated with non–insulin dependent diabetes (NIDDM). In the United States, NIDDM is more prevalent in blacks and the Native American population. Physical activity has been identified as having an important role in the prevention and treatment of NIDDM, yet blacks and Native Americans have a disproportionate number of poor, unemployed, and disadvantaged individuals who lack access to the health care system.

Implications for Practice

- Physical inactivity is a modifiable risk factor for the development of NIDDM. Prevention and treatment programs need to focus heavily upon exercise and be tailored to the activity tolerance of the individual client.
- Promotion of physical activity should be supported through formal programs in schools, churches, and government agencies within black and Native American communities.
- Incorporate motivational factors into the exercise program such as providing a healthy snack or meal for the participants and furnishing each client with a log to monitor weight loss and blood glucose levels.
- Development of an exercise/prevention program should remove potential barriers such as transportation and cost to facilitate commitment to the program.

Data from Huddleston JS: Exercise. In Edelman CL, Mandle CI editors: *Health promotion throughout the lifespan*, ed 5, St. Louis, 2002, Mosby; and Lee ET and others: Incidence of diabetes in American Indians of three geographic areas, *Diabetes Care* 25: 49, 2002; Rimmer JH and others: Feasibility of a health promotion intervention for a group of predominantly African American women with type 2 diabetes, *Diabetic Educ* 28(4):571, 2002.

the problem-solving approach with clients and must be reevaluated with each new client.

Any acquired or congenital condition that affects the structure of the musculoskeletal or nervous system impairs to some degree activity, body alignment, or joint mobility. The impairment can be temporary, such as casting of an extremity, or permanent, as in contractures. For clients with limited **range of motion (ROM)** or mobility, the nursing care plan should include interventions that maintain the present level of alignment and joint mobility and increase the level of motor function.

The nurse must remember that clients may have the capacity for recovery in spite of the loss of some physical function. Restoration of functioning begins early in the care of clients experiencing disruption in their ability to perform self-care. Encouragement, support, commitment, and perseverance are important attitudes in critical thinking for these clients.

When intervening with clients experiencing problems with body mechanics and who may depend on the nurse for assistance with positioning, turning, or ambulation, perseverance is one attitude the nurse must possess. Hourly responsibility for turning often becomes repetitive, and the nurse may lose sight of its importance. Perseverance is especially important in the delegation of these activities to unlicensed health care providers or family members. Making certain that the task is performed and is performed correctly is an essential nursing function.

Another attitude for the nurse to demonstrate is one of creativity. Because problems with activity and mobility are often prolonged, the more creative the nurse's approach for improving activity tolerance and mobility skills, the greater the chance of success. This is especially important with children. Children enjoy receiving rewards for any accomplishment. When a child makes strides toward greater mobility, the nurse can make it a game by giving the child stickers in pretty colors to symbolize successes.

Nursing Process

Assessment

Assessment of body alignment and posture can be carried out with the client standing, sitting, or lying down. Through assessment the nurse will be able to determine normal physiological changes in growth and development; deviations related to poor posture, trauma, muscle damage, or nerve dysfunction; and any learning needs of clients. In addition, during assessment the nurse can provide opportunities for clients to observe their posture and obtain important information about other factors that contribute to poor alignment, such as inactivity, fatigue, malnutrition, and psychological problems. During assessment (Figure 36-1) the nurse must consider all of the elements that build toward making appropriate nursing diagnoses.

The first step in assessing body alignment is to put the client at ease so that unnatural or rigid positions are not assumed. When assessing body alignment of an immobi-

lized or unconscious client, pillows and positioning supports should be removed from the bed if not contraindicated, and the client placed in the supine position.

Standing. Assessment for the standing client includes the following: the head is erect and midline; body parts are symmetrical; the spine should be straight with normal curvatures (cervical concave, thoracic convex, lumbar concave); the abdomen is comfortably tucked; the knees should be in a straight line between the hips and ankles and slightly flexed; the feet should be flat on the floor and pointed directly forward and slightly apart to maintain a wide base of support; and the arms should hang comfortably at the sides (Figure 36-2). The client's center of gravity is in the midline, and the line of gravity is from the middle of the forehead to a midpoint between the feet. Laterally, the line of gravity runs vertically from the middle of the skull to the posterior third of the foot (Wilson and Giddens, 2001).

Sitting. Assessment of the client in the sitting position includes the following: the head is erect, and the neck and vertebral column are in straight alignment; the body weight is distributed on the buttocks and thighs; the thighs are parallel and in a horizontal plane (be careful to avoid pressure on the popliteal nerve and blood supply); the feet are supported on the floor; and the forearms are supported on the armrest, in the lap, or on a table in front of the chair.

Assessment of alignment in the sitting position is particularly important for the client with muscle weakness, muscle paralysis, or nerve damage. A client with these alterations has diminished sensation in affected areas and is unable to perceive pressure or decreased circulation. Proper sitting alignment reduces the risk of musculoskeletal system damage in such a client.

Recumbent Position. Assessment of the client in the recumbent position requires that the client be placed in the lateral position with all but one pillow and all positioning supports removed from the bed. The vertebrae should be in straight alignment without observable curves. This assessment provides baseline data concerning the client's body alignment.

Conditions that create a risk of damage to the musculoskeletal system when lying down include impaired mobility (e.g., traction), decreased sensation (e.g., **hemiparesis** from a stroke), impaired circulation (e.g., diabetes), and lack of voluntary muscle control (e.g., spinal cord injuries).

When a client is unable to change position voluntarily, the nurse assesses the position of body parts while the client is lying down. The vertebrae should be in straight alignment without any observable curves. The extremities should be in alignment and not crossed over one another. The head and neck should be aligned without excessive flexion or extension.

Mobility. Assessment of mobility enables the nurse to determine the client's coordination and balance while walking, the ability to carry out ADLs, and the ability to participate in an exercise program. The assessment of **mobility** has three components: range of motion, **gait,** and exercise.

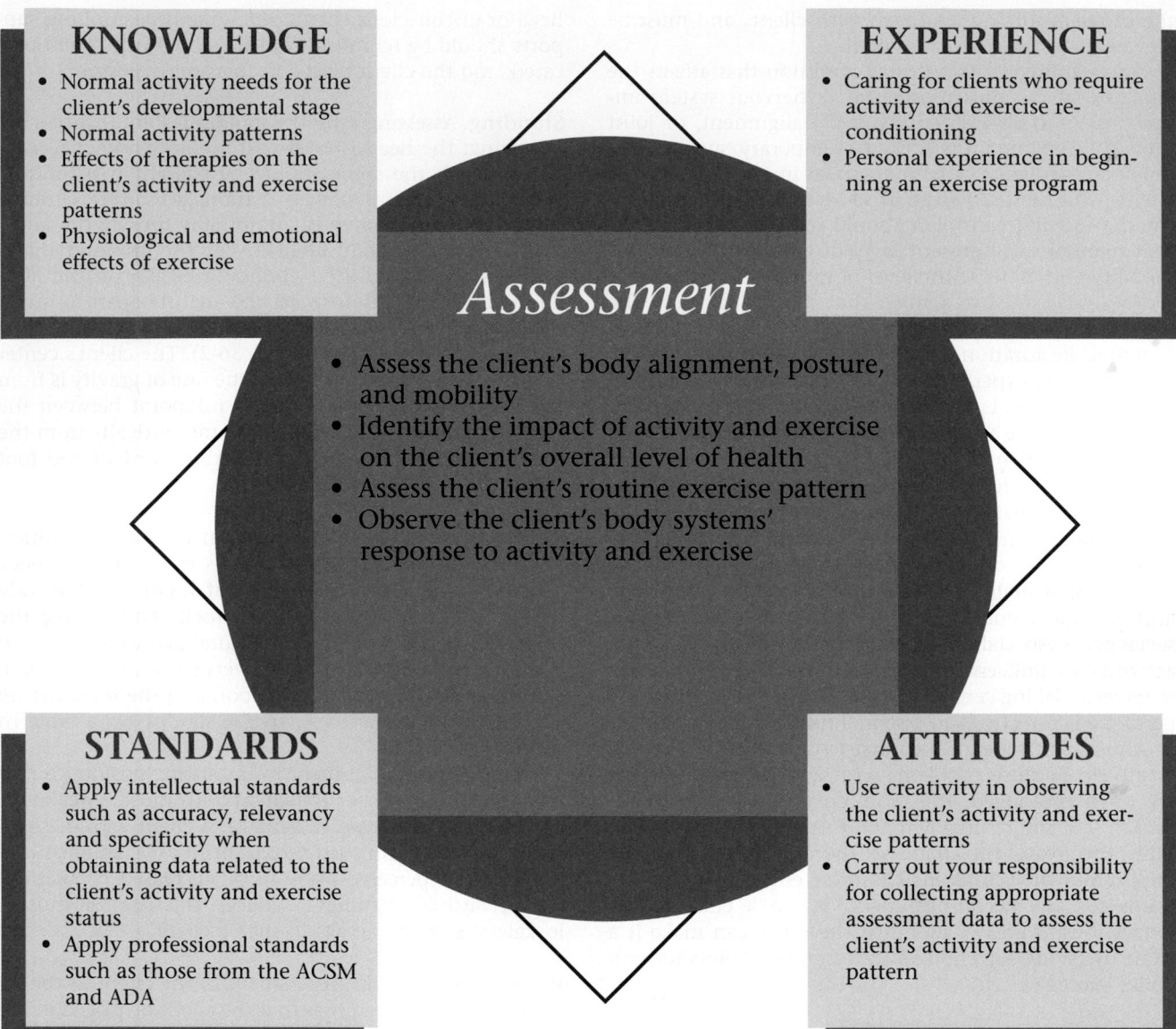

KNOWLEDGE

- Normal activity needs for the client's developmental stage
- Normal activity patterns
- Effects of therapies on the client's activity and exercise patterns
- Physiological and emotional effects of exercise

EXPERIENCE

- Caring for clients who require activity and exercise re-conditioning
- Personal experience in beginning an exercise program

Assessment

- Assess the client's body alignment, posture, and mobility
- Identify the impact of activity and exercise on the client's overall level of health
- Assess the client's routine exercise pattern
- Observe the client's body systems' response to activity and exercise

STANDARDS

- Apply intellectual standards such as accuracy, relevancy and specificity when obtaining data related to the client's activity and exercise status
- Apply professional standards such as those from the ACSM and ADA

ATTITUDES

- Use creativity in observing the client's activity and exercise patterns
- Carry out your responsibility for collecting appropriate assessment data to assess the client's activity and exercise pattern

FIGURE **36–1** Critical thinking model for activity and exercise assessment.

Range of Motion. Assessing ROM is one of the first assessment techniques used to determine the degree of damage or injury to a joint (see Chapter 32). The nurse assesses ROM to collect data to answer questions about joint stiffness, swelling, pain, limited movement, and unequal movement. Limited range of motion may indicate inflammation such as arthritis, fluid in the joint, altered nerve supply, or contractures. Increased mobility (beyond normal) of a joint may indicate connective tissue disorders, ligament tears, or possible joint fractures.

Gait. Gait is the manner or style of walking, including rhythm, cadence, and speed. Assessing gait allows the nurse to draw conclusions about balance, posture, and the ability to walk without assistance. The nurse should note conformity; a regular, smooth rhythm; symmetry in the length of leg swing; smooth swaying related to the gait

phase; and a smooth, symmetrical arm swing (Wilson and Giddens, 2001).

Exercise. Exercise is physical activity for conditioning the body, improving health, maintaining fitness, or providing therapy for correcting a deformity or restoring the overall body to a maximal state of health. When a person exercises, physiological changes occur in body systems (Box 36-5). The nurse determines how much the client regularly exercises. What type of exercise does the client prefer? How many times per week? How long does the client exercise at any given time?

Activity Tolerance. Activity tolerance is the kind and amount of exercise or activity a person is able to perform. Assessment of activity tolerance is necessary when planning physical activity for health promotion and for clients

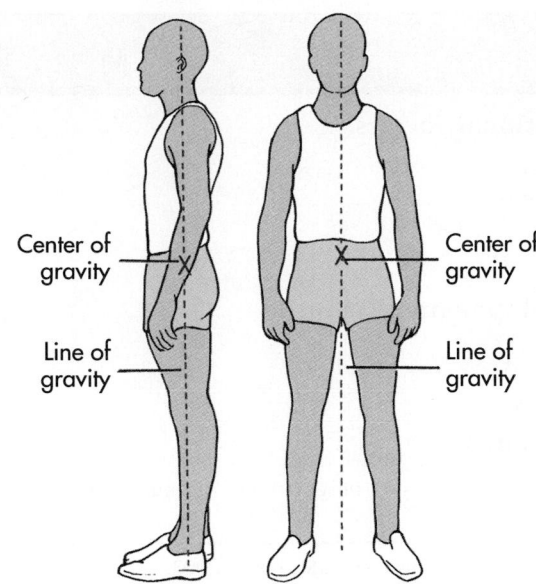

FIGURE **36–2** Correct body alignment when standing.

Box **36-5**	**Effects of Exercise**

Cardiovascular System

Increased cardiac output
Improved myocardial contraction, thereby strengthening cardiac muscle
Decreased resting heart rate
Improved venous return

Pulmonary System

Increased respiratory rate and depth followed by a quicker return to resting state
Improved alveolar ventilation
Decreased work of breathing
Improved diaphragmatic excursion

Metabolic System

Increased basal metabolic rate
Increased use of glucose and fatty acids
Increased triglyceride breakdown
Increased gastric motility
Increased production of body heat

Musculoskeletal System

Improved muscle tone
Increased joint mobility
Improved muscle tolerance to physical exercise
Possible increase in muscle mass
Reduced bone loss

Activity Tolerance

Improved tolerance
Decreased fatigue

Psychosocial Factors

Improved tolerance to stress
Reports of "feeling better"
Reports of decrease in illness (e.g., colds, influenza)

Data from Huether SE, McCance KL: *Understanding pathophysiology,* St. Louis, 2000, Mosby; and Hoeman SP: *Rehabilitation nursing: process, application, and outcomes,* ed 3, St. Louis, 2002, Mosby.

---

with acute or chronic illness. This assessment provides the nurse with baseline data about the client's activity patterns and assists in determining which factors (physical, psychological, or motivational) are affecting activity tolerance. Box 36-6 lists factors affecting activity tolerance.

Client Expectations. In assessing the client's expectations concerning activity and exercise, the nurse will first need insight into the client's perception of what is normal or acceptable in regard to physical fitness. For example, one of the factors affecting physical activity is freedom from pain. If exercising is painful or tiresome to the client, compliance and commitment to the desired interventions may be lacking. Clients may be content with their present physical activity and fitness and may not perceive a need for improvement. Unless there is a real threat to health maintenance, forcing the client to accept the nurse's perspective is a breach of standards of care.

Nursing Diagnosis

Assessment of the client's activity tolerance, physical fitness, body alignment, and joint mobility provides related clusters of data or defining characteristics that lead the nurse to identify nursing diagnoses. The nurse must be accurate identifying diagnoses. For example, a client who reports being tired or weakened could be potentially diagnosed as having activity intolerance or fatigue. Further review of assessed defining characteristics (e.g., abnormal heart rate or dyspnea) can lead to the definitive diagnosis (activity intolerance).

When activity and exercise are problems for a client, nursing diagnoses often focus on the individual's ability to move. The diagnostic label should direct nursing interventions. This requires the correct selection of the related factors. For example, activity intolerance related to excess weight gain and lack of cardiovascular fitness will require very different interventions if the related factor is prolonged bed rest. Box 36-7 provides an example of how the diagnostic process leads to accurate diagnosis selection. The following are examples of nursing diagnoses related to activity and exercise:

- Activity intolerance
- Disturbed body image
- Ineffective coping
- Impaired gas exchange
- Risk for injury
- Impaired physical mobility
- Imbalanced nutrition: more than body requirements
- Acute or chronic pain
- Impaired skin integrity

Box 36-6   **Factors Influencing Activity Tolerance**

Physiological Factors

Skeletal abnormalities
Muscular impairments
Endocrine or metabolic illnesses (e.g., diabetes mellitus or thyroid disease)
Hypoxemia
Decreased cardiac function
Decreased endurance
Impaired physical stability
Pain
Sleep pattern disturbance
Prior exercise patterns
Infectious processes and fever

Emotional Factors

Anxiety
Depression
Chemical addictions
Motivation

Developmental Factors

Age
Sex

Pregnancy

Physical growth and development of muscle and skeletal support

---

Modified from Phipps WJ and others: *Medical-surgical nursing: health and illness perspectives,* ed 7, St. Louis, 2003, Mosby.

Nursing Diagnostic Process   *Box* 36-7

Assessment Activities	**Defining Characteristics**	**Nursing Diagnosis**
Observe client's gait.	Shuffled gait Uncoordinated gait Client reports slower walking speed	Impaired physical mobility related to decreased muscle strength and control
Observe client performing tasks such as feeding, dressing, or recreational activities.	Uncoordinated movements Limited fine motor coordination	
Measure range of joint motion.	Reduced joint motion in lower and/or upper extremities Stiffness in joints	

Planning

During planning the nurse again synthesizes information from multiple resources (Figure 36-3). Critical thinking ensures that the client's plan of care integrates all that the nurse knows about the individual, as well as key critical thinking elements. Professional standards are especially important to consider when the nurse develops a plan of care. These standards often establish scientifically proven guidelines for selecting effective nursing interventions.

Concept maps are a new tool to assist in the planning of care. Figure 36-4 shows the relationship between a client's medical diagnosis of congestive heart failure and the identified nursing diagnosis.

Goals and Outcomes. Once the nursing diagnoses have been defined, the nurse and client set goals and expected outcomes to direct interventions. The plan should include consideration of any risks for injury to the client. It should also take into consideration preexisting health concerns. It is especially important to have knowledge of the client's home environment when planning therapies to maintain or improve activity, body alignment, and mobility. The client's family should be included in the care plan. For some clients with alterations in joint mobility, family members may be the providers of care. The general goal related to exercise and activity is to improve or maintain the client's motor function and independence. The following are examples of outcomes for clients with deficits in activity and exercise (Ackley and Ladwig, 2002):

• Participates in prescribed physical activity while maintaining appropriate heart rate, blood pressure, and breathing rate
• Verbalizes an understanding of the need to gradually increase activity based on tolerance and symptoms
• Expresses understanding of balancing rest and activity

Setting Priorities. Care planning is individualized to the client, taking into consideration the client's most immediate needs. The immediacy of any problem is determined

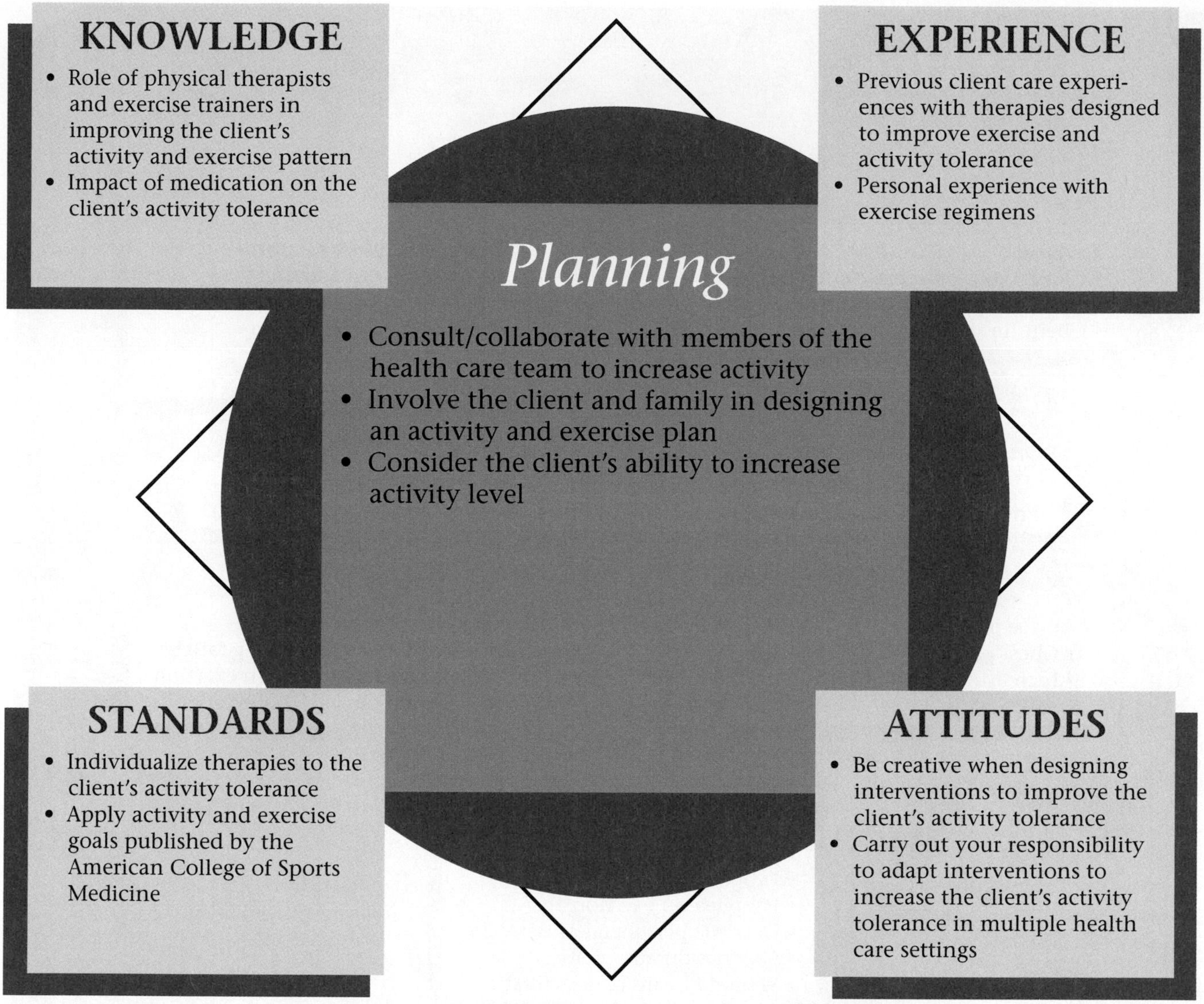

KNOWLEDGE

- Role of physical therapists and exercise trainers in improving the client's activity and exercise pattern
- Impact of medication on the client's activity tolerance

EXPERIENCE

- Previous client care experiences with therapies designed to improve exercise and activity tolerance
- Personal experience with exercise regimens

Planning

- Consult/collaborate with members of the health care team to increase activity
- Involve the client and family in designing an activity and exercise plan
- Consider the client's ability to increase activity level

STANDARDS

- Individualize therapies to the client's activity tolerance
- Apply activity and exercise goals published by the American College of Sports Medicine

ATTITUDES

- Be creative when designing interventions to improve the client's activity tolerance
- Carry out your responsibility to adapt interventions to increase the client's activity tolerance in multiple health care settings

FIGURE 36–3 Critical thinking model for activity and exercise planning.

by the effect the problem has on the client's mental and physical health. Because of the many skills associated with the care of clients with activity intolerance, improper body mechanics, and/or impaired mobility, such as turning, transferring, and positioning, it may be easy to overlook the complications associated with these health alterations. Therefore the nurse must be vigilant in monitoring the client and supervising assistive personnel in carrying out activities to prevent complications and potential injury.

Continuity of Care. Planning also involves an understanding of the client's need to maintain motor function and independence. Collaboration with other members of the health care team, for example, physical and occupational therapists, will be especially important for these clients. Long-term rehabilitation may be necessary, and discharge planning is begun when a client enters the health care system. In addition, the nurse always individualizes a plan of care directed at meeting the actual or potential needs of the client (see care plan).

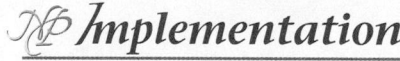 *Implementation*

Health Promotion. A sedentary lifestyle contributes to the development of health-related problems. Nurses promote health by encouraging clients to engage in a regular exercise program (Box 36-8). A holistic approach is taken to develop and implement a plan to enhance the client's overall physical fitness. The recommendations for physical activity and fitness should be discussed with the client, and a program of exercise designed in collaboration with the client (Box 36-9).

Before starting an exercise program, clients should calculate their maximum heart rate (MHR) by subtracting their current age in years from 220 and then obtain their target heart rate by taking 60% to 90% of the maximum. No matter what exercise prescription is implemented for the client, a warm-up and cool-down period must be included in the program (Huddleston, 2002). The warm-up period usually lasts about 5 to 10 minutes and may in-

Concept Map

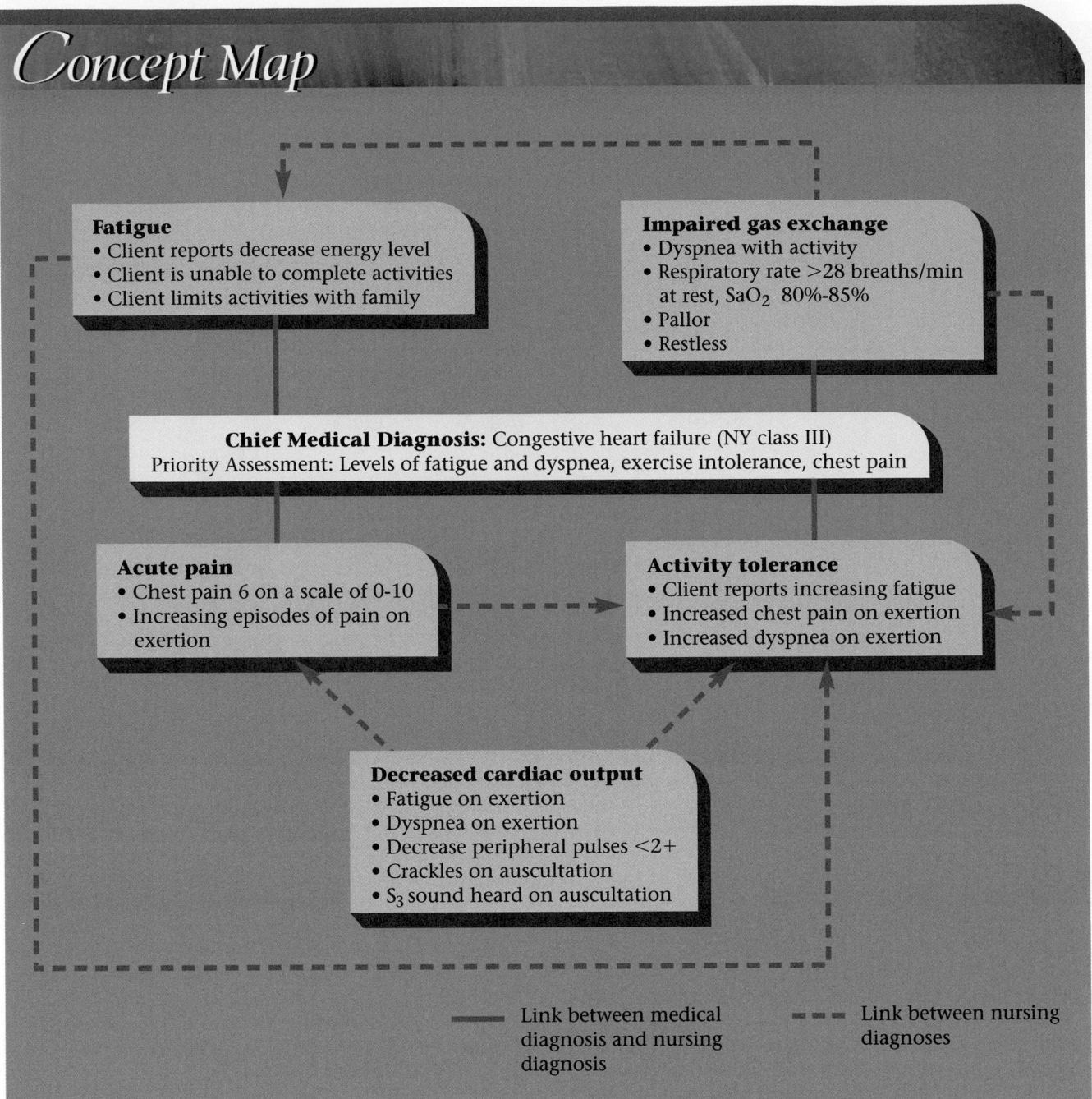

Fatigue
- Client reports decrease energy level
- Client is unable to complete activities
- Client limits activities with family

Impaired gas exchange
- Dyspnea with activity
- Respiratory rate >28 breaths/min at rest, SaO_2 80%-85%
- Pallor
- Restless

Chief Medical Diagnosis: Congestive heart failure (NY class III)
Priority Assessment: Levels of fatigue and dyspnea, exercise intolerance, chest pain

Acute pain
- Chest pain 6 on a scale of 0-10
- Increasing episodes of pain on exertion

Activity tolerance
- Client reports increasing fatigue
- Increased chest pain on exertion
- Increased dyspnea on exertion

Decreased cardiac output
- Fatigue on exertion
- Dyspnea on exertion
- Decrease peripheral pulses <2+
- Crackles on auscultation
- S_3 sound heard on auscultation

——— Link between medical diagnosis and nursing diagnosis

- - - Link between nursing diagnoses

FIGURE **36–4** Concept map for a client with congestive heart failure and decreased activity.

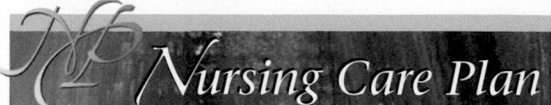

Nursing Care Plan

Activity Intolerance

Assessment

Mrs. Mary Smith is a 45-year-old housewife. She has enrolled in a cardiovascular disease prevention (CDP) program prescribed by her physician and conducted by Erich Sieple, a registered nurse.

Erich's assessment included a discussion of Mrs. Smith's current health problem, as well as a pertinent physical examination.

Assessment Activities	Findings/Defining Characteristics
Ask Mary what prompted her physician to recommend a CDP program.	She responds, "I gained 50 pounds over the past year. I become easily fatigued and lack the energy to keep up with even simple household chores. I don't want to leave the house anymore."
Ask Mary about her exercise and eating habits.	She responds, "I want to exercise but with the demands of child care and taking care of my aging parents, I just don't feel like it. I feel pulled in every direction, that increases my stress, then I want to eat, eat, and eat!"
Perform baseline assessment.	Height: 5 feet 3 inches Weight: 225 pounds (102 kg) Blood pressure: 152/90 mm Hg (at rest) Pulse: 96 beats per minute (at rest) Breathing rate: 20 breaths per minute (at rest)
Assess endurance.	Level 2-3 = moderately to substantially compromised. Erich rated Mary's endurance using the nursing outcomes classification (NOC) (Moorhead, Johnson, Maas, 2004): 1 = extremely compromised 2 = substantially compromised 3 = moderately compromised 4 = mildly compromised 5 = not compromised Blood pressure: 164/96 mm Hg (climbing 10 steps) Pulse: 120 beats per minute (climbing 10 steps) Breathing rate: 36 breaths per minute (climbing 10 steps)

Nursing Diagnosis: Activity intolerance related to excessive weight gain, inactivity, and lack of cardiovascular fitness.

Planning

Goal	Expected Outcomes*
	Health Beliefs
Client will develop a plan of exercise incorporating isotonic and isometric exercises.	Client will state the physiological and psychological effects of exercise. Client will commit to performing physical exercise at home.
	Activity Tolerance
Client's activity tolerance will improve.	Client will perform and record exercise patterns 3-4 times over the next 2 weeks. Client performed active exercise 4 times over last 2 weeks. Client's level of fatigue associated with exercise will remain the same or decrease.
	Cardiovascular Pump Effectiveness
Client's cardiopulmonary response to exercise will improve.	Client's resting diastolic blood pressure will remain below 80 mm Hg. Client's systolic blood pressure will be below 140 mm Hg. Client's resting heart rate will range between 75 and 85 beats per minute.

*Outcome classification labels from Moorhead S, Johnson M, Maas M: *Nursing outcomes classification (NOC)*, ed 3, St. Louis, 2004, Mosby.

Continued

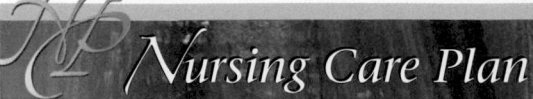

Nursing Care Plan

Activity Intolerance —cont'd

Interventions†—cont'd	Rationale
Exercise Promotion	
• Instruct client about the physiological benefits of a regular exercise program.	Physical activity and exercise protect against the development of cardiovascular disease (CVD) and decreases other risk factors associated with CVD, such as obesity, hypertension, and hyperlipidemia (Adams and others, 1999; Manson and others, 1999; Konradi and Anglin, 2001).
• Develop a progressive plan of exercise with the client, such as 2 to 3 miles of brisk walking and quadriceps, bicep, and gluteal muscle isometric exercises 3 to 4 times per week.	Cross training (combination of exercise activities) provides variety to combat boredom and increases potential for total-body conditioning (Huddleston, 2002).
• Instruct client to use an exercise log and to record the day, time, duration, and responses (pulse, feelings, shortness of breath, daily weight).	Keeping a log may increase adherence to exercise prescription (Kim, McFarland, and McLane, 1997).
• Schedule weekly meetings with the client for follow-up and review of exercise log, progress, and barriers.	Clients are more likely to increase physical activity and remain compliant with an exercise program if they are counseled by a health care professional (Huddleston, 2002).

†Intervention classification labels from Dochterman JM, Bulecheck GM: *Nursing interventions classification (NIC)*, ed 4, St. Louis, 2004, Mosby.

Evaluation

Nursing Actions	Client Response/Finding	Achievement of Outcome
Review client's exercise log at each visit.	She responds, "I make time to exercise because of this log. I hate missing a day and leaving a blank page, this represents failure. I want to succeed." Exercise log documents activity 4 times per week	Client reports enjoying exercise, as well as observing some personal benefits of exercise. The exercise log is facilitating adherence to the exercise prescription.
Record weight, blood pressure, and pulse.	Weight, 210 pounds. Resting heart rate remaining between 80 and 85 beats per minute. Blood pressure, 146/86 mm Hg.	Improved cardiovascular effects of exercise: • Heart rate is within normal range. • Blood pressure is lower but not at expected range. Monitor blood pressure as client continues to lose weight.
Ask client if exercise is helping to lower fatigue level.	She responds, "At first, finding time to exercise was hard, but once I started feeling less tired and even less stressed, it was easy to integrate exercise into my daily activities."	Achieved improved activity tolerance with exercise.

clude stretching, calisthenics, and/or the aerobic activity performed at a lower intensity. The warm-up activity prepares the body and decreases the potential for injury. The cool-down period follows the exercise routine and usually lasts about 5 to 10 minutes. The cool-down period allows the body to readjust gradually to baseline functioning and provides an opportunity to combine movement such as stretching with relaxation-enhancing mind-body awareness (Huddleston, 2002).

Many clients find it difficult to incorporate an exercise program into their daily lives because of time constraints. For these clients it is beneficial to reinforce that many ADLs can be used to accumulate the recommended 30 minutes or more per day of moderate-intensity physical activity (Box 36-10).

Other clients may benefit from a prescribed exercise and physical fitness program carefully designed to meet their needs and expectations. An exercise prescription may incorporate a combination of aerobic exercise, stretching and flexibility exercises, and resistance training. Aerobic exercise includes such activities as walking, running, bicycling, aerobic dance, jumping rope, and cross-country skiing. Recommended frequency of aerobic exercise is 3 to 5 times per week or every other day. Cross training is recommended for the client who prefers to exercise every day. For example, the client may run one day and do yoga the next day.

Stretching and flexibility exercises include active ROM that allows for stretching of all muscle groups and joints. This form of exercise is ideal for warm-up and cool-down periods. Benefits include increased flexibility, improved circulation and posture, and an opportunity for relaxation.

Resistance training increases muscle strength and endurance and is associated with improved performance of

Box 36-8 *Procedural Guidelines*

Helping Clients to Exercise

Assisting clients in exercising is an important nursing activity. The nurse is responsible for assessing the client's ability to exercise and tolerance to exercise. In addition, the nurse teaches clients and their families how to implement exercise programs. For these reasons, only selection portions of helping clients to exercise may be delegated to assistive personnel (AP). These activities may include preparing the client for exercise (e.g., shoes, clothing, hygiene needs, and obtaining preexercise and postexercise vital signs). The nurse instructs AP to do the following:

- Notify nurse of client reports of pain before, during, or after exercise.
- Notify nurse of client complaints of increased fatigue, dizziness, light-headedness when obtaining preexercise and/or postexercise vital signs.

1. Assess for any medical limitations (e.g., weight-bearing status, untreated fracture, cardiovascular disease).
2. Teach clients breathing skills to help reduce anxiety and to fully oxygenate tissues and expand lungs.
3. Asses for client's physiological and psychological limitations for learning and implementing an exercise program.
4. Assess for joint limitations and do not force a muscle or a joint during exercise.
5. Let each client move at his or her own pace.
6. Assess for proper posture, body alignment, and good body mechanics during exercise.
7. Monitor vital signs before, during, and after exercise.
8. Assess for pain, shortness of breath, or a change in vital signs. If present, stop exercise.
9. Clients should wear shoes and comfortable clothing.
10. Know what the client's mobility skills were before hospitalization.
11. Document client's progress and provide feedback as the client exercises.

Box 36-9 Recommendations for Exercise

Adults should accumulate 30 minutes or more a day of moderate-intensity (brisk) physical activity on most (or all) days of the week for a weekly total of 3 to 4 hours.

The activity does not have to be continuous; benefits can be realized with short bouts of activity (10 minutes minimum) over the course of the day.

This amount of activity will expend about 150 to 200 calories per day (the equivalent of walking 2 miles briskly) or 1000 to 1400 calories per week.

All types of activity can be applied to the daily total (e.g., raking leaves, dancing, gardening).

Lower-intensity activities should be done more often, for longer periods of time, or both. More vigorous activities should be done for shorter periods of time or less frequently.

Data from Konradi DB, Anglin LT: Moderate-intensity exercise: for our patients, for ourselves, *Orthop Nurs* 20(1):47, 2001; Pate RR and others: Physical activity and public health: a recommendation from the Centers for Disease Control and Prevention and the American College of Sports Medicine, *JAMA* 273(5):402, 1995; and Huddleston JS: Exercise. In Edelman CL, Mandle CL, editors: *Health promotion throughout the lifespan,* ed 5, St. Louis, 2002, Mosby.

Box 36-10 Incorporating Active Exercise Into Activities of Daily Living

Nodding head "yes" exercises *neck* (flexion and extension).
Shaking head "no" exercises *neck* (rotation).
Moving right ear to right shoulder exercises *neck* (lateral flexion).
Moving left ear to left shoulder exercises *neck* (lateral flexion).
Reaching to turn on overhead light exercises *shoulder* (flexion).
Reaching to bedside stand for book exercises *shoulder* (abduction).
Scratching back exercises *shoulder* (extension and internal rotation).
Rotating shoulders toward chest exercises *shoulder* (scapular protraction).
Rotating shoulders toward back exercises *shoulder* (scapular retraction).
Eating, bathing, shaving, and grooming exercise *elbow* (flexion, extension).
All activities requiring fine motor coordination, such as writing and eating, exercise *fingers* and *thumb* (flexion, extension, abduction, adduction, opposition).
Walking exercises *hip* (flexion, extension).
Rolling toes inward exercises *hip* (internal rotation).
Rolling toes outward exercises *hip* (external rotation).
Walking exercises *knee* (flexion, extension).
Walking exercises *ankle* (dorsiflexion, plantar flexion).
Pointing toe toward head of bed exercises *ankle* (dorsiflexion).
Pointing toe toward foot of bed exercises *ankle* (plantar flexion).
Walking exercises *toes* (extension).
Wiggling toes exercises *toes* (abduction, adduction).

Table 36-1	Body Mechanics for Health Care Workers
Action	**Rationale**
When planning to move a client, arrange for adequate help. Use mechanical aids if help is unavailable.	Two workers lifting together divide the workload by 50%.
Encourage client to assist as much as possible.	This promotes client's independence and strength while minimizing workload.
Keep back, neck, pelvis, and feet aligned. Avoid twisting.	Reduces risk of injury to lumbar vertebrae and muscle groups. Twisting increases risk of injury.
Flex knees; keep feet wide apart.	A broad base of support increases stability.
Position self close to client (or object being lifted).	The force is minimized. Ten pounds held at waist height close to body is equal to 100 pounds held at arms' length.
Use arms and legs (not back).	The leg muscles are stronger, larger muscles capable of greater work without injury.
Slide client toward yourself using a pull sheet.	Sliding requires less effort than lifting. Pull sheet minimizes shearing forces, which can damage client's skin.
Set (tighten) abdominal and gluteal muscles in preparation for move.	Preparing muscles for the load minimizes strain and stabilizes the trunk.
Person on a lift team with the heaviest load coordinates efforts of the lift team involved by counting to three.	Simultaneous lifting minimizes the load for any one lift.

daily activities and avoidance of injuries and disability (Pate and others, 1995). People lose about ½ pound of muscle mass per year from lack of use (Huddleston, 2002). Formal resistance training includes weight training, but the same benefits can be obtained by performing ADLs such as pushing a vacuum cleaner, raking leaves, shoveling snow, and kneading bread. Some clients may use weight training to bulk up their muscles. However, the purpose of weight training from a health perspective is to develop tone and strength and to stimulate and maintain healthy bone (Hass and others, 2000; Huddleston, 2002).

Body Mechanics. In November 2000, the U.S. Occupational Safety and Health Administration released federal ergonomic standards to prevent musculoskeletal injuries in the workplace (Occupational Safety and Health Administration, 2000). Half of all back pain is associated with manual lifting tasks (Gassett and others, 1996). The most common back injury is strain on the lumbar muscle group, which includes the muscles around the lumbar vertebrae. Injury to these areas affects the ability to bend forward, backward, and from side to side. The ability to rotate the hips and lower back is also decreased. To protect the client and the nurse, proper body mechanics must be learned and mastered (Table 36-1).

Lifting Techniques. Before lifting, the nurse should assess the weight to be lifted and what assistance, if any, is needed. If help is needed, the nurse should assess if a second person is adequate or if mechanical assistance is needed. Once the amount of needed assistance is determined, these steps are followed:

1. Tighten stomach muscles and tuck pelvis; this provides balance and protects the back.
2. Bend at the knees; this helps to maintain the nurse's center of gravity and lets the strong muscles of the legs do the lifting (Figure 36-5).
3. Keep the weight to be lifted as close to the body as possible; this places the weight in the same plane as the lifter and close to the center of gravity for balance.

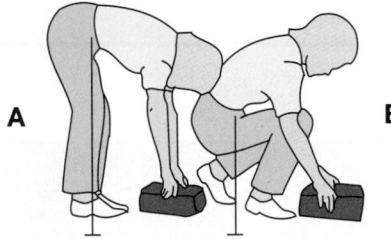

FIGURE 36–5 Incorrect **(A)** and correct **(B)** body position for lifting.

4. Maintain the trunk erect and the knees bent so that multiple muscle groups work together in a synchronized manner (Gassett and others, 1996).
5. Avoid twisting. Twisting can overload your spine and lead to serious injury.

The best height for lifting vertically is approximately 2 feet off the ground and close to the lifter's center of gravity (Gassett and others, 1996).

To reach an object overhead the nurse should do the following:

1. Use a safe, stable step stool or ladder for elevation. Avoid standing on tiptoes with the feet together. This decreases the base of support, elevates the center of gravity, and decreases balance.
2. Stand as close to the shelf as possible. This decreases the amount of time the nurse must support the weight of the object with the arms.
3. Transfer the weight of the object from the shelf to the arms and over the base of support. This maintains the nurse's base of support and aligns the weight of the object close to the nurse's center of gravity.

Acute Care. Hospitalized clients can be encouraged to do stretching and isometric exercises, active ROM exercises, and low-intensity walking, depending on their condition. The nurse is responsible for maintaining musculoskeletal function by implementing passive ROM in those clients who are unable to perform physical activity for themselves.

Musculoskeletal System. The musculoskeletal system can be maintained during the acute care of the client by encouraging the use of stretching and isometric-type exercises. Review of the client's chart and collaboration with the physician is undertaken to alert the nurse to any possible contraindications before initiating isometric exercises. An isometric exercise program is designed for the specific needs of a client. For example, an exercise program may be implemented that includes biceps and triceps isometric exercises to prepare the client for crutch walking. The nurse needs to tell the client to stop the activity if pain, fatigue, or discomfort is experienced, and reinforce this as necessary.

Generally, the muscle group is tightened (contracted) for 10 seconds and then completely relaxed for several seconds (Hoeman, 2002). Repetitions are gradually increased for each muscle group until the isometric exercise can be repeated 8 to 10 times. Clients should be instructed to perform the exercises slowly and increase repetitions as their physical condition improves. Muscle groups (quadriceps and gluteal) used for walking should be exercised isometrically 4 times per day until the client is ambulatory.

Joint Mobility. The easiest intervention to maintain or improve joint mobility for clients and one that can be coordinated with other activities is the use of ROM exercises (see Chapter 46). In active ROM exercises, the client is able to move his or her joints independently. With passive ROM exercises, the nurse moves each joint in clients who are unable to perform these exercises themselves. The use of ROM exercises enables the nurse to systematically assess and improve the client's joint mobility.

Joints that are not moved periodically can develop contractures, a permanent shortening of a muscle followed by the eventual shortening of associated ligaments and tendons. Over time, the joint may become fixed in one position and the client loses normal use of the joint. For the client who does not have voluntary motor control, passive ROM exercises are the exercises of choice.

The older adult has a decline in physical activity and changes in joints that may predispose the client to problems with mobility, and joint flexibility may be limited. The nurse can recommend approaches to help older adults use proper body mechanics and prevent injury (Box 36-11).

Mechanical devices are available to place specific joints through continuous passive ROM (CPM). These CPM machines are used postoperatively to place joints through a selective repetitive range of motion. The machine can be set to certain degrees of joint mobility with increasing joint mobility or flexion as the goal. The most common clients who use the CPM machine are those who have undergone some form of total joint replacement surgery.

Unless contraindicated, the nursing care plan should include exercising each joint through as nearly a full ROM as possible. Passive ROM exercises should be initiated as soon as the client loses the ability to move the ex-

---

Box 36-11

Focus on Older Adults

- Encourage the sedentary older client to avoid prolonged sitting, to get up and stretch. Frequent stretching decreases joint contractures.
- Be sure that the older client maintains proper body alignment when sitting to minimize joint and muscle stress.
- Teach clients how to use stronger joints or larger muscle groups. Efficient distribution of the workload decreases joint stress and pain.
- Provide resources for planned exercise programs. Weight-bearing and resistance exercise slow further bone loss and prevent fractures in the older adult with osteoporosis (Burbank and others, 2002; Phipps and others, 2003).
- Recommend tai chi, a Chinese traditional conditioning exercise. This form of exercise has resulted in reduced fear of falling and increased sense of well-being in older adults (Chewning and others, 2000).
- It is never too late to begin an exercise program (Burbank and others, 2002; Huddleston, 2002). Consult a health care provider before beginning an exercise program, particularly in the presence of heart or lung disease and other chronic illnesses.
- Exercise is extremely beneficial to older adults, but adjustments may have to be made to an exercise program for those in advanced age to prevent problems.
- When developing an exercise program for any older adult, consider not only the person's current activity level, range of motion, muscle strength and tone, and response to physical activity, but also their interests, capacities, and limitations (Eliopoulos, 2001).
- Older adults who are unable to participate in a formal exercise program can achieve the benefits of improved joint mobility and enhanced circulation by simply stretching and exaggerating movements during the performance of routine daily activities (Eliopoulos, 2001).

---

tremity or joint. Chapter 46 details ROM exercises for each area and illustrates the motion of each joint.

Walking. Joint mobility is also increased by walking. Distances walked should be measured in feet or yards instead of charting "ambulated to nurses' station and back." In the normal walking posture the head is erect; the cervical, thoracic, and lumbar vertebrae are aligned; the hips and knees have appropriate flexion; and the arms swing freely in alternation with the legs. Illness or trauma can reduce activity tolerance, resulting in the need for assistance with walking or the use of mechanical devices such as crutches, canes, or walkers.

Helping a Client to Walk. Helping a client to walk requires preparation. The nurse assesses the client's activity tolerance, strength, coordination, and balance to determine the type of assistance needed. The nurse should also assess the client's orientation and determine if there are any signs of distress. This would preclude attempts at ambulation.

The nurse evaluates the environment for safety before ambulation; this includes the removal of obstacles, a clean and dry floor, and the establishment of rest points should the client's activity tolerance become less than

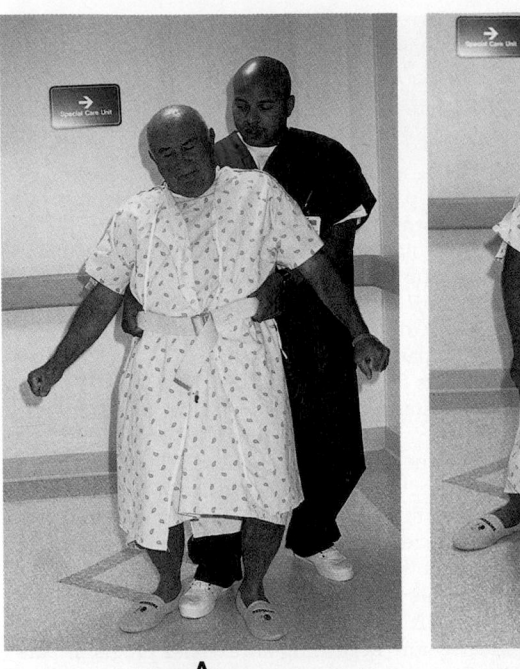
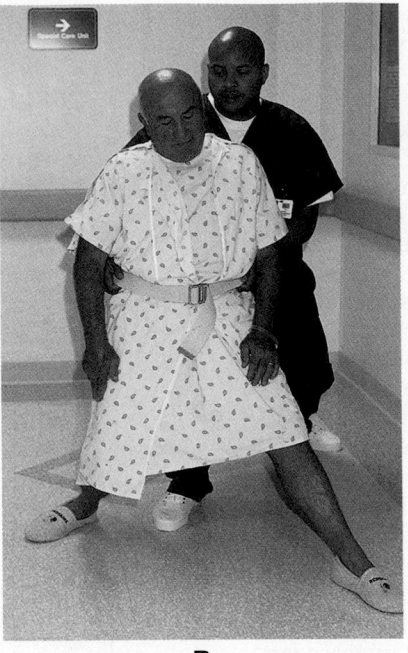
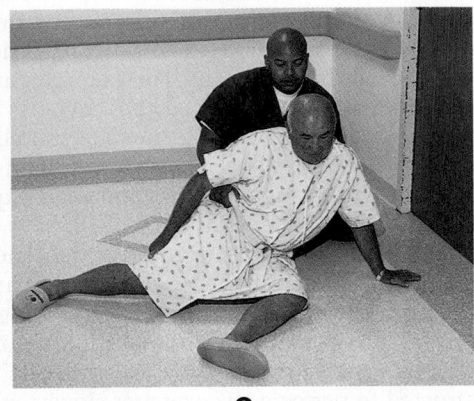

A   **B**   **C**

FIGURE **36–6 A,** Stand with feet apart to provide a broad base of support. **B,** Extend one leg and let client slide against it to the floor. **C,** Bend knees to lower body as client slides to the floor.

expected. The client should also wear supportive, non-skid shoes. Resting points should be established in the event that the client's activity tolerance is less than was estimated or the client becomes dizzy.

The client should be assisted to a position of sitting at the side of the bed and should rest for 1 to 2 minutes before standing. The longer the period of inactivity, or **immobility,** the greater are the physiological changes (see Chapter 46). Several methods are used for assisting a client with ambulation. The nurse provides support at the waist so that the client's center of gravity remains midline. This can be achieved when the nurse places both hands at the client's waist or uses a gait belt. A gait belt is a leather belt that encircles the client's waist and has handles attached for the nurse to hold while the client ambulates.

If the client has a syncopal episode or begins to fall, the nurse should assume a wide base of support with one foot in front of the other, thus supporting the client's body weight (Figure 36-6, *A*). The nurse then extends one leg and lets the client slide against the leg and gently lowers the client to the floor, protecting the client's head (Figure 36-6, *B* and *C*). Although lowering a client to the floor is not difficult, the student should practice this technique with a friend or classmate before attempting it in a clinical setting. When the client next ambulates, the nurse proceeds more slowly, monitoring for complaints of dizziness, as well as the client's blood pressure before, during, and after ambulation.

Restorative and Continuing Care. Restorative and continuing care involves implementing activity and exercise strategies to assist the client in ADLs after acute care is no longer warranted. The nurse, in collaboration with other health care professionals such as physical therapists, pro-

motes activity and exercise by teaching the use of canes, walkers, or crutches, depending on the assistive device most appropriate for the client's condition. Restorative and continuing care includes activities and exercises that restore and promote optimal functioning in clients with specific chronic illnesses, such as coronary heart disease (CHD), hypertension, chronic obstructive pulmonary disease (COPD), and diabetes mellitus.

Assistive Devices for Walking. Walkers are extremely light, moveable devices that are about waist high and made of metal tubing (Figure 36-7). They have four widely placed, sturdy legs. The client holds the handgrips on the upper bars, takes a step, moves the walker forward, and takes another step.

Canes. Canes are lightweight, easily moveable devices that are made of wood or metal. They provide less support than a walker and are less stable. A person's cane length is equal to the distance between the greater trochanter and the floor (Hoeman, 2002). Two common types of canes are the single straight-legged cane and the quad cane. The single straight-legged cane is more common and is used to support and balance a client with decreased leg strength. This cane should be kept on the stronger side of the body. For maximum support when walking, the client places the cane forward 15 to 25 cm (6 to 10 inches), keeping body weight on both legs. The weaker leg is moved forward to the cane so that body weight is divided between the cane and the stronger leg. The stronger leg is then advanced past the cane so that the weaker leg and the body weight are supported by the cane and weaker leg. During walking, the client continually repeats these three steps. The client must be taught that two points of support, such as both feet or one foot and the cane, are present at all times.

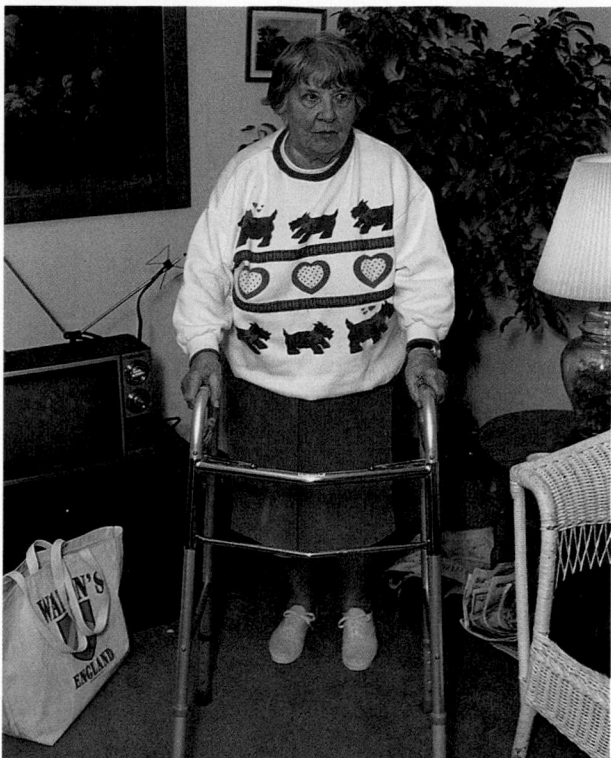

FIGURE **36–7**   Client using a walker.

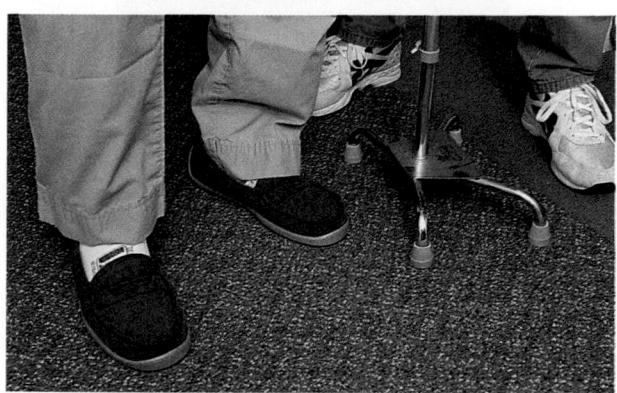

FIGURE **36–8**   Bottom of quad cane.

The quad cane provides the most support and is used when there is partial or complete leg paralysis or some hemiplegia (Figure 36-8). The same three steps that are used with the straight-legged cane are taught to the client.

Crutches. Crutches are often needed to increase mobility. The nurse begins crutch instruction with guidelines for safe use (Box 36-12). The use of crutches may be temporary, such as after ligament damage to the knee. However, crutches may be needed permanently by a client with paralysis of the lower extremities. A crutch is a wooden or metal staff. The two types of crutches are the double adjustable Lofstrand, or forearm, crutch (Figure 36-9) and the axillary wooden or metal crutch. The forearm crutch has a handgrip and a metal band that fits around the client's forearm. The metal band and the handgrip are adjusted to fit the client's height. The axillary crutch has a padded curved surface at the top, which fits under the axilla. A handgrip in the form of a crossbar is held at the level of the palms to support the body. It is important that crutches be measured for the appropriate length and that clients be taught to use their crutches safely, to achieve a stable gait, to ascend and descend stairs, and to rise from a sitting position.

Measuring for Crutches. The axillary crutch is the more common crutch used. Measurements include the client's height, the angle of elbow flexion, and the distance between the crutch pad and the axilla. When crutches are fitted, the length of the crutch should be from three to four fingerwidths from the axilla to a point 15 cm (6 inches) lateral to the client's heel (Hoeman, 2002) (Figure 36-10).

The handgrips should be positioned so that the client's body weight is not supported by the axillae. Pressure on the axillae increases risk to underlying nerves, which could result in partial paralysis of the arm. Correct position of the handgrips is determined with the client upright, supporting weight by the handgrips with the elbows slightly flexed at 30 degrees (Hoeman, 2002). Elbow flexion may be verified with a goniometer (Figure 36-11).

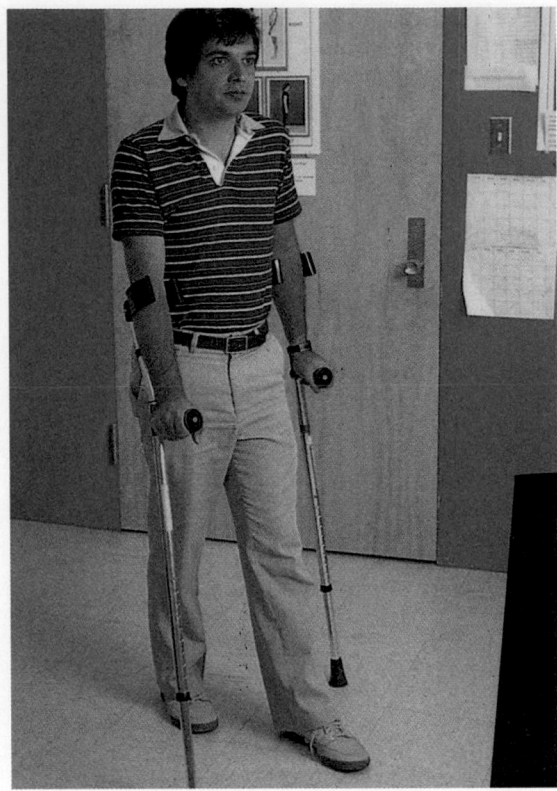

FIGURE **36–9** Double adjustable Lofstrand or forearm crutch.

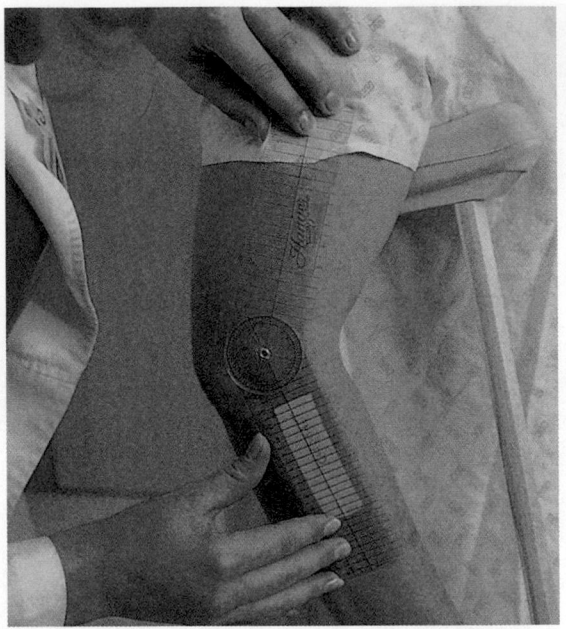

FIGURE **36–11** Using the goniometer to verify correct degree of elbow flexion for crutch use.

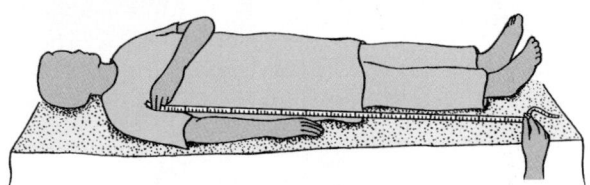

FIGURE **36–10** Measuring crutch length.

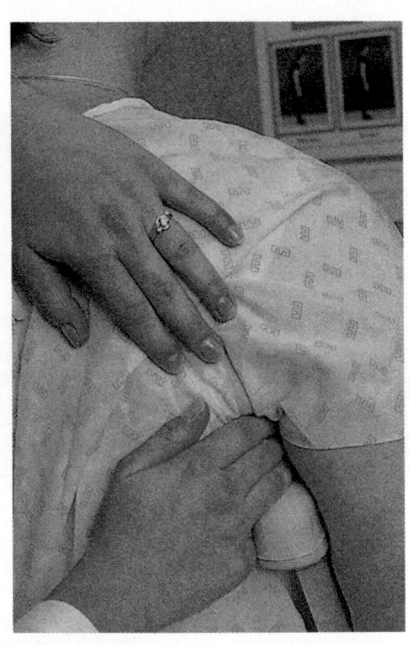

FIGURE **36–12** Verifying correct distance between crutch pads and axilla.

When the height and placement of the handgrips have been determined, the nurse should again verify that the distance between the crutch pad and the client's axilla is three to four fingerwidths (Figure 36-12).

Crutch Gait. The **crutch gait** is assumed by alternately bearing weight on one or both legs and on the crutches. The gait selected by the physician is determined by assessing the client's physical and functional abilities and the disease or injury that resulted in the need for crutches. This section summarizes the basic crutch stance and the four standard gaits: four-point alternating gait, three-point alternating gait, two-point gait, and swing-through gait.

The basic crutch stance is the tripod position, formed when the crutches are placed 15 cm (6 inches) in front of and 15 cm to the side of each foot (Figure 36-13). This position improves the client's balance by providing a wider base of support. The body alignment of the client in the tripod position includes an erect head and neck, straight vertebrae, and extended hips and knees. No weight should be borne by the axillae. The tripod position is assumed before crutch walking.

Four-point alternating, or four-point, gait gives stability to the client but requires weight bearing on both legs. Each leg is moved alternately with each opposing crutch so that three points of support are on the floor at all times (Figure 36-14).

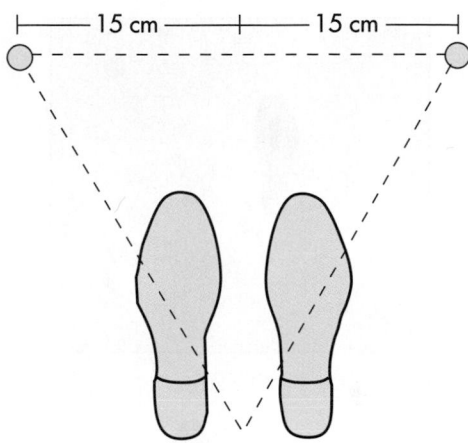

FIGURE **36–13** Tripod position, basic crutch stance.

Three-point alternating, or three-point, gait requires the client to bear all of the weight on one foot. In a three-point gait, weight is borne on both crutches and then on the uninvolved leg, and the sequence is repeated (Figure 36-15). The affected leg does not touch the ground during the early phase of the three-point gait. Gradually the client progresses to touchdown and full weight bearing on the affected leg.

The two-point gait requires at least partial weight bearing on each foot (Figure 36-16). The client moves a crutch at the same time as the opposing leg, so that the crutch movements are similar to arm motion during normal walking.

The swing-through, or swing-through gait, is frequently used by paraplegics who wear weight-supporting braces on their legs. With weight placed on the supported legs, the client places the crutches one stride in front and then swings to or through the crutches while they support the client's weight.

Crutch Walking on Stairs. When ascending stairs on crutches, the client usually uses a modified three-point gait (Figure 36-17). The client stands at the bottom of the stairs and transfers body weight to the crutches. The unaffected leg is advanced between the crutches to the stairs. The client then shifts weight from the crutches to the unaffected leg. Finally, the client aligns both crutches on the stairs. This sequence is repeated until the client reaches the top of the stairs.

To descend the stairs (Figure 36-18), a three-phase sequence is also used. The client transfers body weight to the unaffected leg. The crutches are placed on the stairs, and the client begins to transfer body weight to the crutches, moving the affected leg forward. Finally, the unaffected leg is moved to the stairs with the crutches. Again, the client repeats the sequence until reaching the bottom of the stairs.

Because in most cases clients will need to use crutches for some time, they should be adequately taught to use crutches on stairs before discharge. This instruction applies to all crutch-dependent clients, not only those who have stairs in their homes.

Sitting in a Chair With Crutches. As with crutch walking and crutch walking up and down stairs, the procedure for

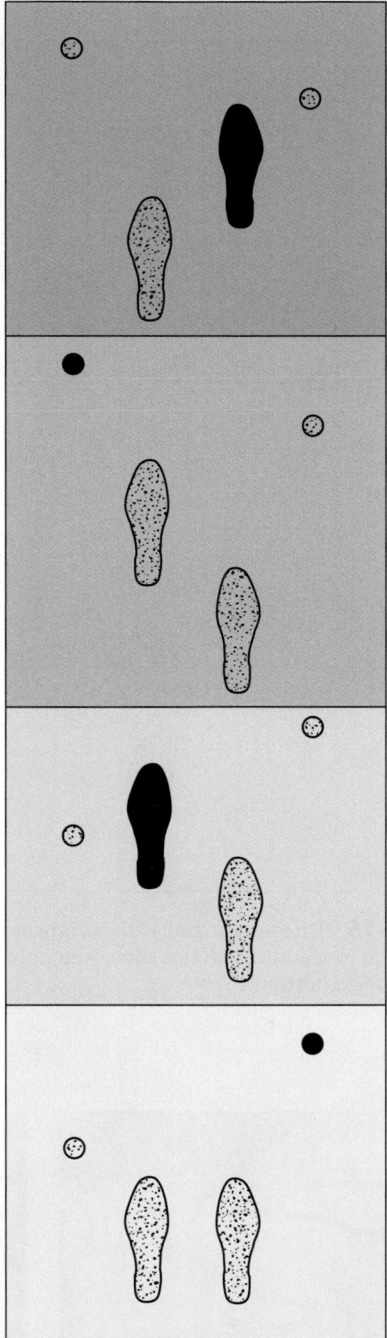

FIGURE **36–14**   Four-point alternating gait. Solid feet and crutch tips show foot and crutch tip moved in each of the four phases. (Read from bottom to top.)

sitting in a chair involves phases and requires the client to transfer weight (Figure 36-19). First, the client gets positioned at the center front of the chair with the posterior aspect of the legs touching the chair. Then the client holds both crutches in the hand opposite the affected leg. If both legs are affected, as with a paraplegic who wears weight-supporting braces, the crutches are held in the hand on the client's stronger side. With both crutches in one hand, the client supports body weight on the unaf-

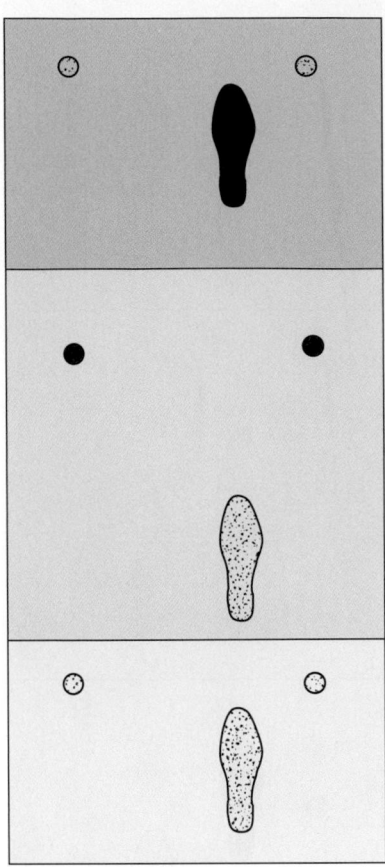

FIGURE **36–15** Three-point gait with weight borne on unaffected leg. Solid foot and crutch tips show weight bearing in each phase. (Read from bottom to top.)

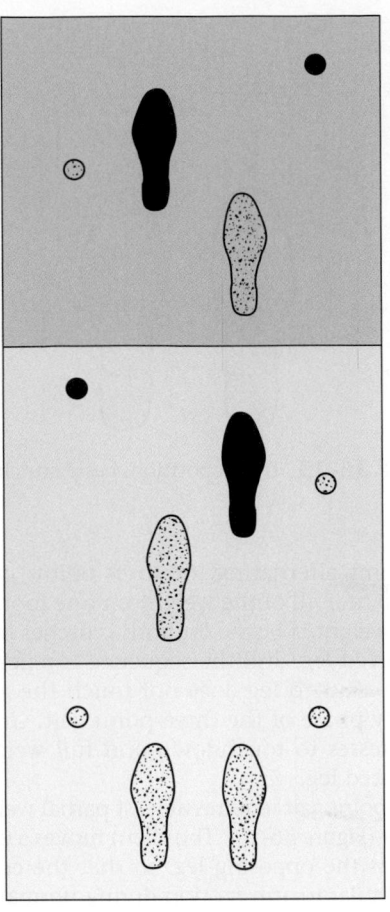

FIGURE **36–16** Two-point gait with weight born partially on each foot and each crutch advancing with opposing leg. Solid areas indicate leg and crutch tips bearing weight. (Read from bottom to top.)

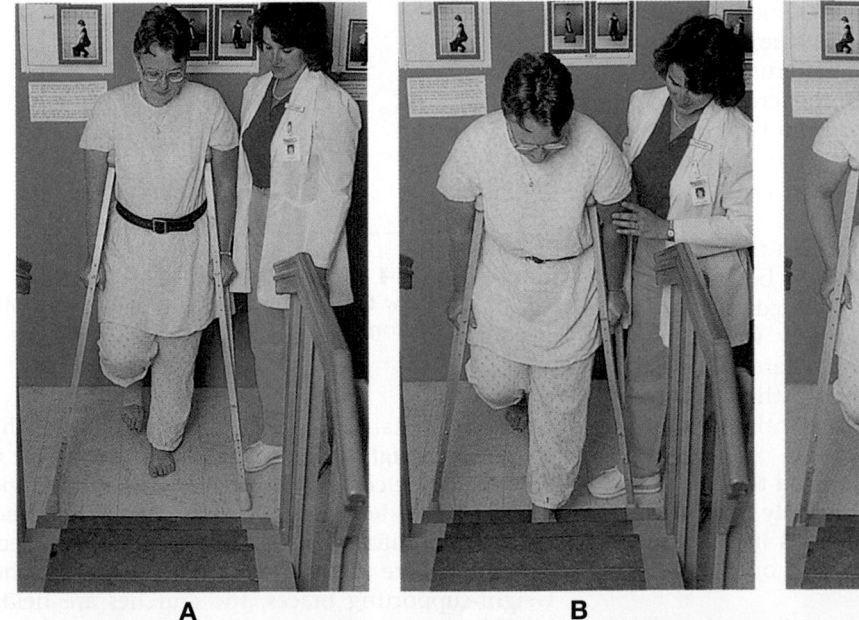

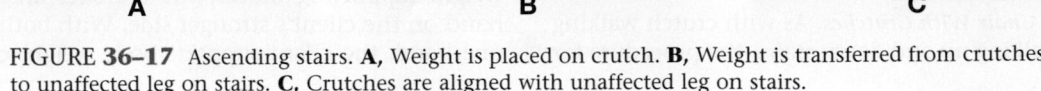

FIGURE **36-17** Ascending stairs. **A,** Weight is placed on crutch. **B,** Weight is transferred from crutches to unaffected leg on stairs. **C,** Crutches are aligned with unaffected leg on stairs.

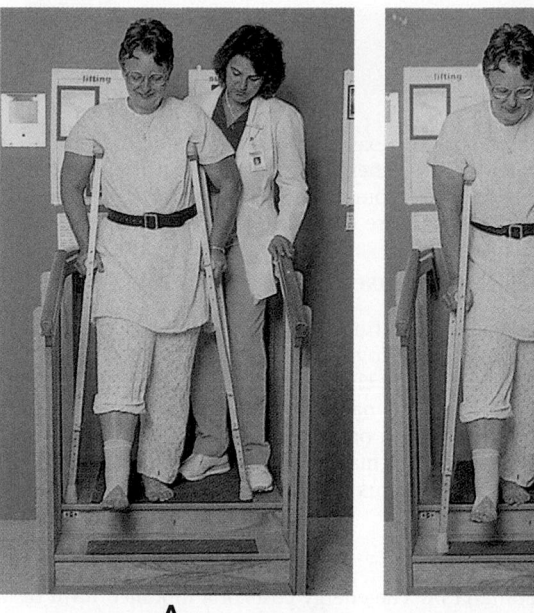
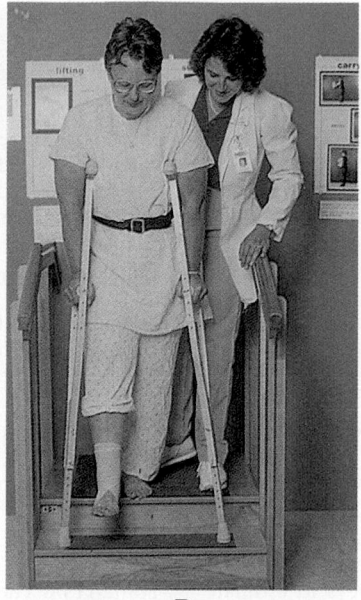
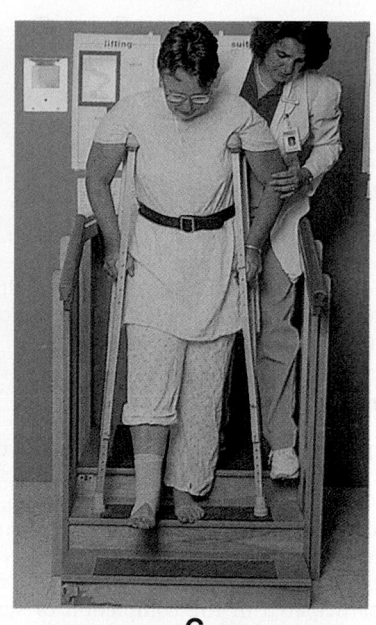

A   B   C

FIGURE 36–18 Descending stairs. **A,** Body weight is on unaffected leg. **B,** Body weight is transferred to crutches. **C,** Unaffected leg is aligned on stairs with crutches.

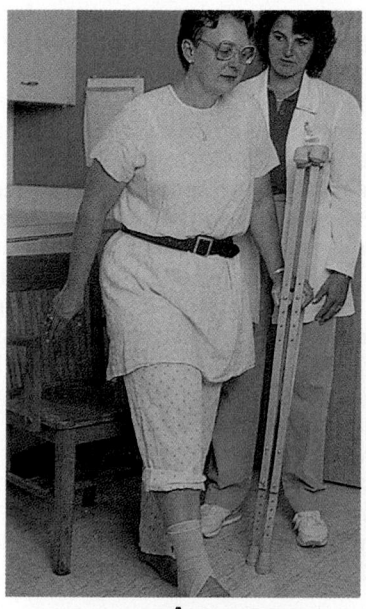
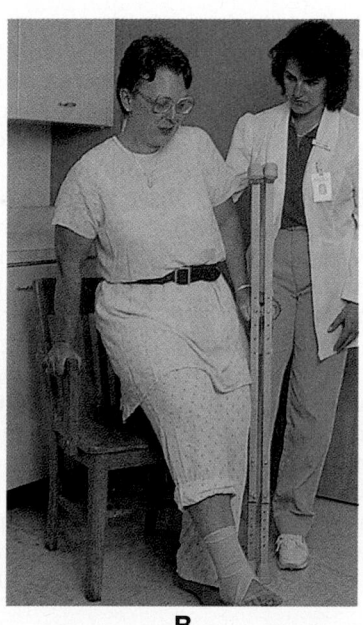
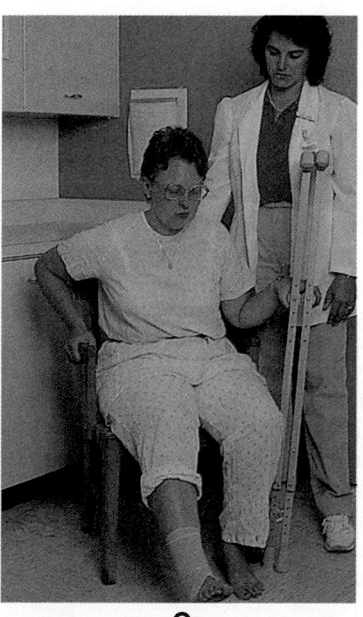

A   B   C

FIGURE 36–19 Sitting in a chair. **A,** Both crutches are held by one hand. Client transfers weight to crutches and unaffected leg. **B,** Client grasps arm of chair with free hand and begins to lower herself into chair. **C,** Client completely lowers herself into chair.

fected leg and the crutches. While still holding the crutches, the client grasps the arm of the chair with the remaining hand and lowers his or her body into the chair. To stand, the procedure is reversed, and the client, when fully erect, should assume the tripod position before beginning to walk.

Restoration of Activity and Chronic Illness. The nurse implements a plan of care designed to increase activity and exercise in clients with specific disease conditions and chronic illnesses such as CHD, hypertension, COPD, and diabetes mellitus (Box 36-13).

Coronary Heart Disease (CHD). Activity and exercise have been shown to play a role in secondary prevention or recurrence of CHD. Cardiac rehabilitation is becoming an integral part of comprehensive care of clients who have been diagnosed with CHD. Nurses are involved in many as-

Research Highlight

Box 36-13

Energy Requirements of Tai Chi

Research Focus

Developing alternative exercise strategies for clients with very low functional capacities is a challenge due to the increased risk for complications. Tai chi c'hih, a modified version of tai chi, may be an approach to health promotion in populations with chronic illness and older adults.

Research Abstract

The purpose of this study was to determine the energy cost of tai chi c'hih, which is a form of exercise consisting of a series of slow balanced movements and breathing. The objective of this study was to measure the energy costs and cardiovascular effects to assist in the planning of a safe exercise prescription for clients with very low energy reserves. Twenty-six healthy adults participated in the completion of surveys to estimate functional capacity and exercise participation, a select series of nine tai chi c'hih movements, and oxygen consumption test-

ing during the exercise program. The results of the study indicated that the energy requirements for this alternative form of exercise were comparable with low-level exercises for persons with low exercise tolerance.

Evidence-Based Practice

* Before initiating exercise, clients should consult their primary care provider.
* Encouraging clients with chronic illness to exercise has the potential to maintain and improve activity tolerance.
* Tai chi c'hih promotes feelings of relaxation and increased energy, thus making it an ideal alternative exercise prescription for clients with chronic illness.

Reference

Fontana JA: The energy costs of a modified form of tai chi exercise, *Nurs Res* 49(2):91, 2000.

---

pects of cardiac rehabilitation and may assist clients in developing a program of exercise that fits their needs and level of functioning. Increased physical activity appears to benefit individuals with myocardial infarction (MI), angina pectoris, or congestive heart failure, as well as clients who have had a coronary artery bypass graft (CABG) or percutaneous transluminal coronary angioplasty (PTCA). Clients with CHD benefit from exercise and activity in terms of reduced mortality and morbidity, improved quality of life, improved left ventricular function, increased functional capacity, and psychological well-being (NIH, 1996; Thompson and Bowman, 1998; Konradi and Anglin, 2001).

Hypertension. Exercise is instrumental in the reduction of systolic and diastolic blood pressure readings. Low- to moderate-intensity aerobic exercise (brisk walking, bicycling) appears to be the most effective in lowering blood pressure, whereas weight training and high-intensity aerobics seem to have minimal benefits (Konradi and Anglin, 2001; Huddleston, 2002).

Chronic Obstructive Pulmonary Disease. Pulmonary rehabilitation is a beneficial therapeutic tool in helping clients reach an optimal level of functioning. Some clients are fearful of participating in exercise because of the potential of worsening dyspnea (difficulty breathing). This aversion to physical activity sets up a progressive deconditioning in which minimal physical exertion results in dyspnea. Pulmonary rehabilitation provides a safe environment for monitoring the progress of clients. In addition, clients receive encouragement and support to increase activity and exercise.

Diabetes Mellitus. Along with diet, glucose monitoring, and medication, exercise is an important component

in the care of clients with diabetes mellitus. Individuals with type 1 diabetes are encouraged to exercise because it leads to improved cardiovascular fitness and psychological well-being. The nurse instructs the diabetic with type 1 diabetes about certain risks and precautions regarding exercise. Instruction should include the need for a preexercise physical examination and precautions to monitor blood glucose immediately before and after exercise. The nurse also instructs clients to avoid injecting insulin into muscles that will be active during exercise, to perform low- to moderate-intensity exercises, to carry a concentrated form of carbohydrates (sugar packets, hard candy), and to wear a medical alert bracelet. The client with type 2 diabetes who decides to participate in a regular program of exercise should include low-intensity warm-up and cool-down exercises, include aerobic exercise at 50% to 75% of maximal oxygen uptake, and exercise for 20 to 45 minutes 3 days per week (American Diabetes Association, 2002; Flood and Constance, 2002).

Evaluation

Client Care. For activity and exercise, the effectiveness of nursing interventions is measured by the success of meeting the client's expected outcomes and goals of care. The client is the only one who will know the effectiveness and benefits of activity and exercise (Figure 36-20). To evaluate the effectiveness of nursing interventions to enhance activity and exercise, comparisons are made with baseline measures that include pulse, blood pressure, strength, endurance, and psychological well-being. Actual outcomes are compared with expected outcomes to determine the client's health status and progression.

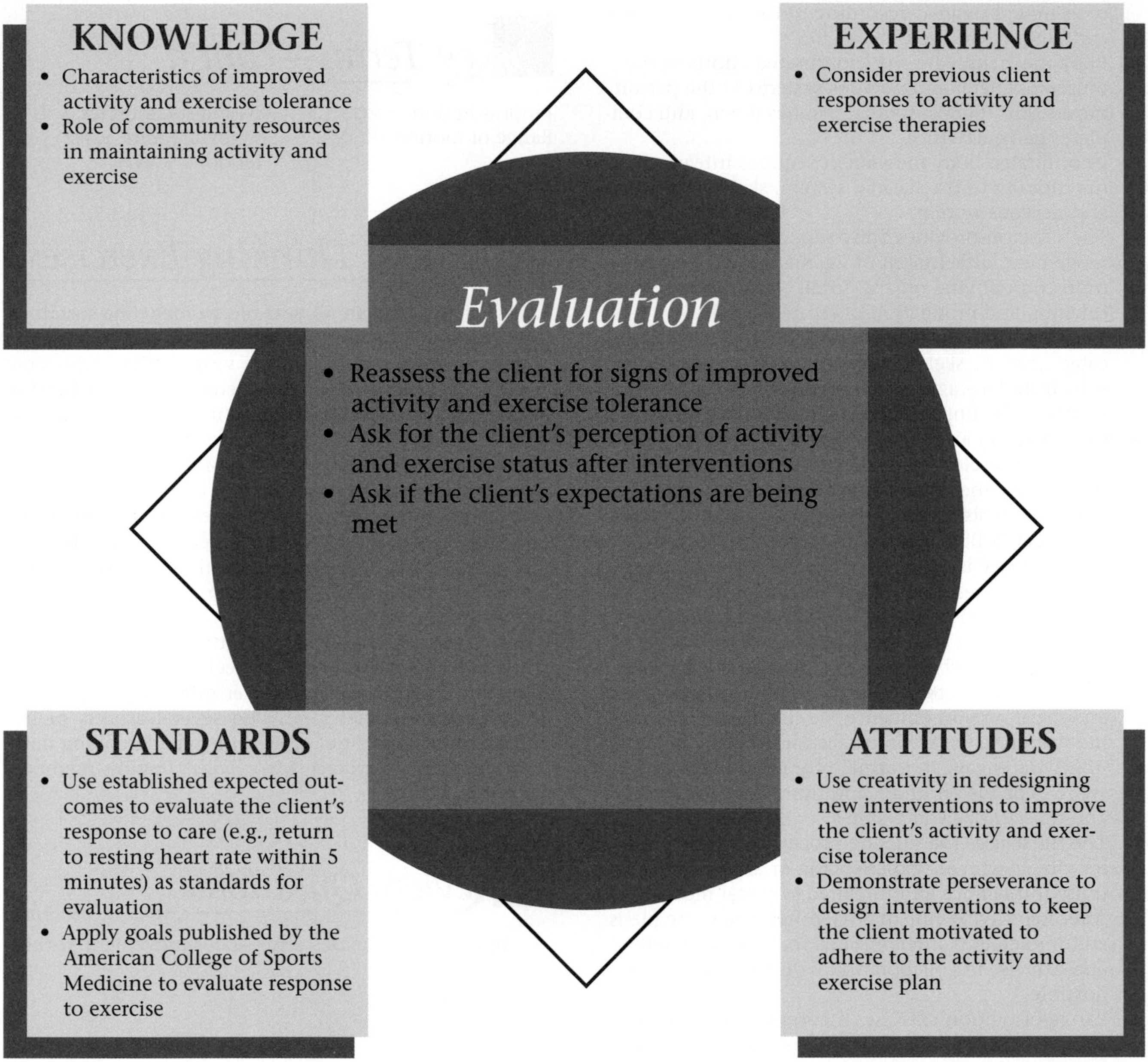

KNOWLEDGE

- Characteristics of improved activity and exercise tolerance
- Role of community resources in maintaining activity and exercise

EXPERIENCE

- Consider previous client responses to activity and exercise therapies

Evaluation

- Reassess the client for signs of improved activity and exercise tolerance
- Ask for the client's perception of activity and exercise status after interventions
- Ask if the client's expectations are being met

STANDARDS

- Use established expected outcomes to evaluate the client's response to care (e.g., return to resting heart rate within 5 minutes) as standards for evaluation
- Apply goals published by the American College of Sports Medicine to evaluate response to exercise

ATTITUDES

- Use creativity in redesigning new interventions to improve the client's activity and exercise tolerance
- Demonstrate perseverance to design interventions to keep the client motivated to adhere to the activity and exercise plan

FIGURE 36–20 Critical thinking model for activity and exercise evaluation.

Continuous evaluation allows the nurse to determine whether new or revised therapies are required and if new nursing diagnoses have developed.

Client Expectations. For the nurse to evaluate the client's perception of nursing care, the nurse must first have knowledge of the client's expectations concerning activity and exercise. What is acceptable or anticipated on the part of the nurse may be vastly different from what the client and family members anticipate or can accept. It is important for the nurse to ask the client if his or her expectations of care have been met. Working closely with the client will enable the nurse to redefine those expectations that can be realistically met within the limits of the client's conditions and treatment.

Key Concepts

- Exercise is physical activity for the purpose of conditioning the body, improving health, and maintaining fitness, or it may be used as a therapeutic measure.
- Activity tolerance is the kind and amount of exercise or work that a person is able to perform. Physiological, emotional, and developmental factors influence the client's activity tolerance.
- The best program of physical activity includes a combination of exercises that produce different physiological and psychological benefits. Isotonic, isometric, and resistive isometric are three categories

of exercise classified according to the type of muscle contraction involved.

- Body mechanics are the coordinated efforts of the musculoskeletal and nervous systems as the person moves, lifts, bends, stands, sits, lies down, and completes daily activities.
- Coordinated body movement requires integrated functioning of the skeletal system, skeletal muscles, and nervous system.
- The skeleton provides bony support structure for movement, attachment of ligaments and muscles, protection of vital organs, some of the regulation of calcium, and production of red blood cells.
- Muscles primarily associated with movement are located near the skeletal region, where movement results from leverage, which is characteristic of movements of the upper extremities.
- Coordination and regulation of muscle groups depend on muscle tone and activity of antagonistic, synergistic, and antigravity muscles.
- Balance is assisted through nervous system control in the cerebellum and inner ear function.
- Body balance is achieved when there is a wide base of support, the center of gravity falls within the base of support, and a vertical line falls from the center of gravity through the base of support.
- Developmental changes, behavioral aspects, environmental issues, cultural and ethnic origin, and family and social support influence the client's perception and motivation to engage in physical activity and exercise.
- Ability to engage in normal physical activity and exercise depends on intact and functioning nervous and musculoskeletal systems.
- The nurse uses the nursing process to provide care for clients who are experiencing or are at risk for activity intolerance and impaired physical mobility.
- After identifying nursing diagnoses, the nurse plans and implements interventions to increase activity and exercise in collaboration with the client when possible.
- Range-of-motion exercises incorporated into daily activities can include one or all of the body joints.
- Mechanical devices to promote walking include canes, walkers, and crutches.

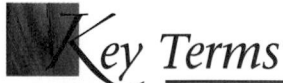

Key Terms

Activities of daily living (ADLs), *p. 931*	Friction, *p. 931*
Activity tolerance, *p. 932*	Gait, *p. 937*
Antagonistic muscles, *p. 933*	Hemiparesis, *p. 937*
Antigravity muscles, *p. 933*	Hemiplegia, *p. 934*
Body mechanics, *p. 930*	Immobility, *p. 948*
Cartilage, *p. 932*	Isometric contraction, *p. 932*
Cartilaginous joints, *p. 932*	Isotonic contraction, *p. 932*
Center of gravity, *p. 931*	Joint, *p. 932*
Crutch gait, *p. 950*	Ligaments, *p. 932*
Exercise, *p. 930*	Mobility, *p. 937*
Fibrous joints, *p. 932*	Muscle tone, *p. 931*
Footboard, *p. 932*	Posture, *p. 931*

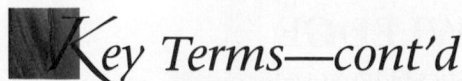

Key Terms—cont'd

Proprioception, *p. 933*	Synergistic muscles, *p. 933*
Range of motion (ROM), *p. 937*	Synovial joints, *p. 932*
	Tendons, *p. 932*

Critical Thinking Exercises

1. Ms. Moushey is an 52-year-old woman. She sustained a fracture of the left femur and must use crutches for 1 week until her follow-up visit at the orthopedic clinic. Her physician has ordered no weight bearing on the left leg. You are conducting the first home visit after her discharge from the hospital. What is the appropriate crutch gait for Ms. Moushey? List several teaching strategies that focus on crutch safety.
2. Mr. Neel has just undergone extensive abdominal surgery. What assessment parameters need to be considered before ambulation of this client? What precautions should you take before ambulating him for the first time?
3. The family of Mrs. Parks made the decision to care for her at home. She is a quadriplegic, weights 72 kg, and requires total care. You are her nurse and responsible for instructing her family on several aspects of her care. Develop a list of basic principles describing body mechanics to protect Mrs. Parks's family members from injury.

Review Questions

1. Antagonistic muscles bring about movement at the:
   1. Muscle.
   1. Joint.
   1. Ligaments.
   1. Bones.

2. Proprioception is:
   1. Awareness of the position of the body.
   2. Needed for antigravity.
   3. Located within the semicircular canals.
   4. An uncommon metabolic disease.

3. Balance is controlled by the nervous system, specifically by the:
   1. Cerebrum and pons.
   2. Cerebellum and inner ear.
   3. Eye and ear.
   4. Cerebral cortex and gyrus.

4. A client with a right-sided cerebral hemorrhage may have:
   1. Left-sided hemiplegia.
   2. Right-sided hemiplegia.
   3. Bilateral hemiplegia.
   4. Degenerative hemiplegia.

5. The greatest change in and impact on the maturational process is observed in:
   1. Infants and elders.
   2. Adults and infants.
   3. Childhood and old-age.
   4. Adults and elders.

6. The period of adolescence is usually initiated by a tremendous growth spurt. For many of these adolescents:
   1. The growth is even and smooth.
   2. The growth is uneven.
   3. Pain is felt during growth.
   4. The males will develop earlier than the females.

7. Clients are more open to developing an exercise program if they:
   1. Are at the stage of readiness to change their behavior.
   2. Ordered by the physician to begin an exercise program.
   3. Have been requested to exercise by a family member.
   4. Have been diagnosed with a chronic disease such as diabetes.

8. The result of children being less physically active outside of school has resulted in:
   1. An increase in heart disease.
   2. An increase in obesity.
   3. Improved school attendance and grades.
   4. More computer-literate children.

9. A principle of good body mechanics includes:
   1. Keeping the knees in a locked position.
   2. Maintaining a wide base of support and bending at the knees.
   3. Bending at the waist to maintain a center of gravity.
   4. Holding objects away from the body for improved leverage.

10. A client begins to fall during ambulation. To prevent injury to the client the nurse should:
    1. Call for assistance.
    2. Slide the client down the nurse's body and leg to the floor.
    3. Instruct the client to sit in the nearest chair.
    4. Allow the client to fall to prevent injury to the nurse.

*R*eferences

Ackley BJ, Ladwig GB: *Nursing diagnosis handbook: a guide to planning care,* ed 5, St. Louis, 2002, Mosby.

American Diabetes Association: Diabetes and exercise: position statement, *Diabetes Care* 25(suppl 1):S64, 2002.

Burbank PM and others: Exercise and older adults: changing behavior with the transtheoretical model, *Orthop Nurs* 21(4):51, 2002.

Dochterman JM, Bulecheck GM: *Nursing interventions classification (NIC),* ed 4, St. Louis, 2004, Mosby.

Eliopoulos C: *Gerontologic nursing,* ed 5, Philadelphia, 2001, Lippincott Williams & Wilkins.

Flood L, Constance A: Diabetes and exercise safety, *Am J Nurs* 102(6):47, 2002.

Gassett RS and others: Ergonomics and body mechanics in the work place, *Nurs Clin North Am* 274(10):861, 1996.

Hoeman SP: *Rehabilitation nursing: process, application, and outcomes,* ed 3, St. Louis, 2002, Mosby.

Huddleston JS: Exercise. In Edelman CL, Mandle CL, editors: *Health promotion throughout the lifespan,* ed 5, St. Louis, 2002, Mosby.

Huether SE, McCance KL: *Understanding pathophysiology,* ed 2, St. Louis, 2000, Mosby.

Kim MJ, McFarland GK, McLane AM: *Pocket guide to nursing diagnoses,* ed 7, St. Louis, 1997, Mosby.

Konradi DB, Anglin LT: Moderate-intensity exercise: for our patients, for ourselves, *Ortho Nurs* 20(1):47, 2001.

Lewis SM and others: *Medical-surgical nursing assessment and management of clinical problems,* ed 5, St. Louis, 2000, Mosby.

Moorhead S, Johnson M, Maas M: *Nursing outcomes classification (NOC),* ed 3, St. Louis, 2004, Mosby.

Occupational Safety and Health Administration: *Ergonomics standard regulatory text,* 2000, www.osha-slc.gov/ergonomics-standard/regulatory/regtext.html.

Phipps WJ and others: *Medical-surgical nursing: health and illness perspectives,* ed 7, St. Louis, 2003, Mosby.

Prochaska JO, Norcross JC, DiClemente CC: *Changing for good,* New York, 1994, William Morrow.

Thibodeau GA, Patton KT: *Anatomy and physiology,* ed 5, St. Louis, 2002, Mosby.

U.S. Department of Health and Human Services: *Healthy people 2010,* vols 1 and 2, Washington, DC, 2000, Centers for Disease Control and Prevention, President's Council on Physical Fitness and Sports.

Wilson SF, Giddens JF: *Health assessment for nursing practice,* ed 2, St. Louis, 2001, Mosby.

Wong DL, Hockenberry-Eaton M: *Wong's essentials of pediatric nursing,* ed 6, St. Louis, 2001, Mosby.

*R*esearch References

Adams KJ and others: Combined high-intensity strength and aerobic training in diverse phase II cardiac rehabilitation patients, *J Cardiopulm rehabil* 19:209, 1999.

American College of Sports Medicine: The recommended quantity and quality of exercise for developing and maintaining cardiorespiratory and muscular fitness, and flexibility in healthy adults, *Med Sci Sports Exerc* 30:975, 1998.

Chewning B and others: Tai chi: effects on health, *ACSM's Health Fitness J* 4:17, 2000.

Connelly DM: Resisted exercise training of institutionalized older adults for improved strength and functional mobility: a review, *Topics Geriatr Rehabil* 15(3):6, 2000.

Fontana JA: The energy costs of a modified form of tai chi exercise, *Nurs Res* 49(2):91, 2000.

Hass CJ and others: Single versus multiple sets in long-term recreational weightlifters, *Med Sci Sports Exerc* 32:235, 2000.

Lee ET and others: Incidence of diabetes in American Indians of three geographic areas, *Diabetes Care* 25:49, 2002.

Manson JE and others: A prospective study of walking as compared with vigorous exercise in the prevention of coronary disease in women, *N Engl J Med* 341:650, 1999.

National Institutes of Health Consensus Development Panel on Physical Activity and Cardiovascular Health: Physical activity and cardiovascular health, *JAMA* 276(3):241, 1996.

Pate RR and others: Physical activity and public health: a recommendation from the Centers for Disease Control and Prevention and the American College of Sports Medicine, *JAMA* 273(5):402, 1995.

Prochaska JJ, Rodgers MW, Sallis JF: Association of parent and peer support with adolescent physical activity, *Res Q Exerc Sport* 73(2):206, 2002.

Resnick B: Falls in a community older adults, *Clin Nurs Res* 8(3):251, 1999.

Rimmer JH and others: Feasibility of a health promotion intervention for a group of predominantly African American women with type 2 diabetes, *Diabetes Educ* 28(4):571, 2002.

Schlicht J and others: Build self-efficacy to promote exercise adherence, *ACSM's Health Fitness J* 3(6):27, 1999.

Thompson DR, Bowman GS: Evidence for the effectiveness of cardiac rehabilitation, *Intensive Crit Care Nurs* 14:38, 1998.

37

Client Safety

Media Resources

http://evolve.elsevier.com/Potter/
fundamentals/

CD COMPANION

- Review Questions
- Glossary

evolve WEBSITE

- Review Questions
- Student Learning Activities
- Concept Map Exercise
- Critical Thinking Exercise
- Video Clips
- Glossary

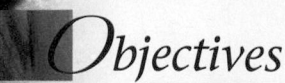

Objectives

Mastery of content in this chapter will enable the student to:

- Define the key terms listed.
- Describe how unmet basic physiological needs of oxygen, nutrition, temperature, and humidity can threaten clients' safety.
- Discuss the purpose of the National Patient Safety Goals.
- Discuss the specific risks to safety related to developmental age.
- Identify factors to assess when it becomes necessary to physically restrain a client.
- Describe the four categories of risks in a health care agency.
- Describe assessment activities designed to identify clients' physical, psychosocial, and cognitive status as it pertains to their safety status.
- Identify nursing diagnoses associated with risks to safety.
- Develop care plans for clients whose safety is threatened.
- Describe nursing interventions specific to clients' age for reducing risk of falls, fires, poisonings, and electrical hazards.
- Describe methods to evaluate interventions designed to maintain or promote safety.

*S*afety, often defined as freedom from psychological and physical injury, is a basic human need that must be met. Health care, provided in a safe manner, and a safe community environment are essential for a client's survival and well-being. The nurse, incorporating critical thinking skills when using the nursing process, is responsible for assessing the client and the environment for hazards that threaten safety, as well as planning and intervening appropriately to maintain a safe environment. By doing this, the nurse is not only a provider of safe acute, restorative, and continuing care, but also an active participant in health promotion.

Scientific Knowledge Base

Environmental Safety

A client's **environment** includes all of the many physical and psychosocial factors that influence or affect the life and survival of that client. This broad definition of environment crosses the continuum of care for settings in which the nurse and client interact (e.g., the home, community center, school, clinic, hospital, and long-term care facility). Safety in health care settings reduces the incidence of illness and injury, shortens the length of treatment and/or hospitalization, improves or maintains a client's functional status, and increases the client's sense of well-being. A safe environment affords protection to the staff as well, allowing them to function at an optimal level. A safe environment is an environment in which basic needs are met, physical hazards are reduced, transmission of pathogens is reduced, sanitation is maintained, and pollution is controlled. In addition, a safe environment is one where the threat of attack from biological, chemical, or nuclear weapons is prevented or minimized.

Basic Needs. Physiological needs, including the need for sufficient oxygen, nutrition, and optimum temperature and humidity, influence a person's safety.

Oxygen. The nurse must be aware of factors in a client's environment that decrease the amount of available oxygen. A common environmental hazard in the home is an improperly functioning heating system. A furnace that is not properly vented or a car left running inside a closed garage may introduce carbon monoxide into the environment. **Carbon monoxide** is a colorless, odorless, poisonous gas produced by the combustion of carbon or organic fuels. Carbon monoxide binds strongly with hemoglobin, preventing the formation of oxyhemoglobin and thus reducing the supply of oxygen delivered to tissues (see Chapter 39). Low concentrations can cause nausea, dizziness, headache, and fatigue. Very high concentrations can cause death (National Safety Council Fact Sheet: Carbon Monoxide, 2002). Annual inspections of heating systems, chimneys, and appliances should be done in private homes, as well as in institutions. Carbon monoxide detectors (Figure 37-1) are available for home or institutional use at a reasonable cost but should not be used as a replacement for proper use and maintenance of fuel-burning appliances.

Nutrition. Meeting nutritional needs adequately and safely requires environmental controls and knowledge. In the home the client needs a refrigerator with a freezer compartment to keep perishable foods fresh. An adequate, clean water supply is needed for drinking and to wash fresh produce and dishes. Provisions for garbage collection are necessary to maintain sanitary conditions.

Foods that are inadequately prepared or stored, or that are subject to unsanitary conditions, increase the client's risk for infections and food poisoning. Bacterial food infections result from eating food contaminated by bacteria such as *Escherichia coli* or *Salmonella, Shigella,* or *Listeria* organisms. **Food poisoning** is caused by ingestion of bacterial toxins produced in food; staphylococcal and clostridial bacteria are the most common causes. Although most food-borne diseases are bacterial, the hepatitis A virus is spread by fecal contamination of food, water, or milk (Williams, 2000).

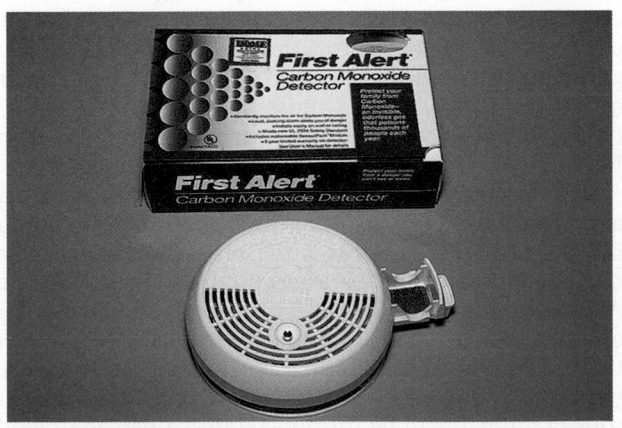

FIGURE **37-1** Carbon monoxide detector.

For illnesses caused by bacterial contamination, the onset of symptoms may be very rapid or may take a week or longer. The average incubation period for hepatitis A is 28 days (Centers for Disease Control and Prevention [CDC], 2002). Preventive measures include thorough hand washing before handling food, adequate cooking, and proper storage and refrigeration of perishable foods.

To protect consumers, commercially processed and packaged foods are subject to **Food and Drug Administration (FDA)** regulations. The FDA is a federal agency responsible for the enforcement of federal regulations regarding the manufacture, processing, and distribution of foods, drugs, and cosmetics to protect consumers against the sale of impure or dangerous substances.

Temperature and Humidity. The comfort zone for environmental temperature varies among individuals, but the usual comfort range is between 18.3° and 23.9° C (65° and 75° F). Temperature extremes that frequently occur during the winter and summer affect not only comfort and productivity, but also safety.

Exposure to severe cold for prolonged periods causes frostbite and accidental hypothermia. Frostbite occurs when a surface area of the skin freezes as a result of exposure to extremely cold temperatures. **Hypothermia** occurs when the core body temperature is 35° C (95° F) or below (see Chapter 31). Older adults, the young, clients with cardiovascular conditions, clients who have ingested drugs or alcohol in excess, and the homeless are at high risk for hypothermia (see Chapter 31).

Exposure to extreme heat can raise the core body temperature, resulting in heatstroke or heat exhaustion. Chronically ill clients, older adults, and infants are at greatest risk for injury from extreme heat. These clients should avoid extremely hot, humid environments.

The relative humidity of the air in the environment may affect the client's health and safety. **Relative humidity** is the amount of water vapor in the air compared with the maximum amount of water vapor that the air could contain at the same temperature. The comfort zone varies from person to person, but most people are comfortable when the humidity is between 60% and 70%. Increasing the environmental humidity can have therapeutic benefits for clients with upper respiratory tract infections because humidity helps to liquefy pulmonary secretions and improve breathing. It is important to follow the manufacturer's directions regarding the cleaning and maintenance of home humidifiers to reduce the contamination of the water.

Physical Hazards. Physical hazards in the environment place clients at risk for accidental injury and death. Motor vehicle accidents are the leading cause of unintentional death, followed by falls, poisonings, drownings, fires, and burns. Among older adults, most falls occur in the home; however, 10% of the falls occur in the health care facility (*Fact Book for the Year 2000*, 2001). Falls are the most common cause of hospital admissions for trauma for older clients. Among people over age 65, hip fractures result in more hospital admissions than any other injury (National Center for Injury Prevention and Control, 2000). Many physical hazards, especially those contributing to falls, can be minimized through adequate lighting, reduction of obstacles, control of bathroom hazards, and security measures.

Lighting. Adequate lighting reduces physical hazards by illuminating areas in which a person moves and works. Outside the home, there should be adequate lighting on all walkways. Outdoor lighting also helps protect the home and its inhabitants from crime. Well-lighted garages, walkways, and doorways discourage intruders from entering the premises or hiding in shadows.

Inside the house, halls, staircases, and individual rooms should be adequately lighted so that residents can safely carry out activities of daily living. Night-lights in dark halls, bathrooms, and the rooms of children and older adults help maintain safety by reducing the risk of falls. A night-light in a guest room can help orient an overnight guest who needs to get up in the middle of the night. Artificial lighting should be soft and nonglaring, because glare is a major problem for older adults (Ebersole and Hess, 2003).

Obstacles. Injuries in the home frequently result from tripping over or coming into contact with common household objects, including doormats, small rugs on the stairs and floor, wet spots on the floor, and clutter on bedside tables, closet shelves, the top of the refrigerator, and bookshelves. The risk of falls from obstacles is present for all age-groups; however, it is greatest for older adults. Falls are usually a result of a combination of intrinsic risk factors (e.g., illness, drug therapy, or alcohol use) and extrinsic or environmental factors. In some cases an obstacle or extrinsic factor may be the only cause of a fall. Intrinsic factors may be difficult to modify or eliminate, but extrinsic ones are usually not.

Bathroom Hazards. Accidents such as falls, burns, and poisoning frequently occur in the bathroom. Secure, easily seen grab bars and nonslip, colored adhesive tape on the bottom of the tub are useful in reducing falls in the bathtub. An elevated toilet seat with armrests and nonslip strips on the floor in front of the toilet are also helpful (Tideiksaar, 1989). Lowering the thermostat setting on the water heater reduces the risk of scalding. In the medicine cabinet, medications should be clearly marked and out of the reach of children. Child-resistant caps should be on all medication containers when there are children living in the home or visiting the home. Medication not in use or out-of-date should be discarded by flushing it down the toilet.

Security. Home fires are a major cause of death and injury. According to the National Fire Protection Association (*Fact Sheets: Home Fires,* 2001), there were 368,000 home fires in the United States in 2000, resulting in 3,420 deaths and 16,975 injuries. The leading cause of fire deaths is careless smoking, and most fire deaths occur between the hours of 10 PM and 6 AM. Cooking equipment and appliances, particularly stoves, are the main sources for in-home fires and fire injuries. Smoke detectors (Figure 37-2), along with carbon monoxide detectors, should be placed strategically throughout the home.

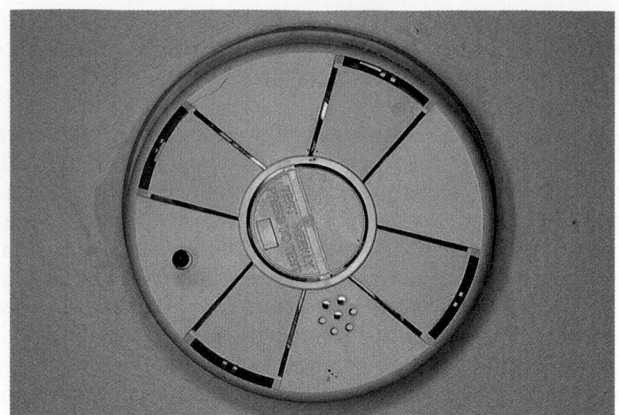

FIGURE **37–2** Smoke and fire detector.

Multipurpose fire extinguishers should be installed near the kitchen and any workshop areas.

Although lead has not been used in house paint or plumbing materials since the U.S. Consumer Product Safety Commission banned it in 1978, older homes continue to contain high lead levels. Soil and water systems may also be contaminated. Poisoning may occur from swallowing or inhaling lead. Fetuses, infants, and children are more vulnerable to lead poisoning than adults because lead is more easily absorbed into growing bodies and the tissues of small children are more sensitive to the damaging effects of lead. Exposure to excessive levels of lead can affect a child's growth or cause brain and kidney damage. Other health effects include impaired hearing, vomiting, headaches, appetite loss, and learning and behavioral problems (*Lead Poisoning Fact Sheet,* 2002).

An insecure home places the client at risk for injury or burglary. Inadequate locks on doors and windows make the home susceptible to intruders. Clients need to take precautions to secure their homes. When assessing the home for safety, the nurse guides the client to evaluate doors and windows for the presence and quality of locks. Clients should be encouraged to join block associations and work closely with law enforcement personnel to reduce crime in their neighborhoods.

Transmission of Pathogens. A **pathogen** is any microorganism capable of producing an illness. One of the most effective methods for limiting the transmission of pathogens is the medical aseptic practice of hand hygiene (see Chapter 33). Clients must be instructed in proper hand-hygiene techniques and encouraged to use them frequently in the home and hospital.

The transmission of disease from person to person can also be reduced, and in some cases prevented, by immunization. **Immunization** is the process by which resistance to an infectious disease is produced or augmented. Active immunity is acquired by injecting a small amount of attenuated (weakened) or dead organisms or modified toxins from the organism (toxoids) into the body. Passive immunity occurs when antibodies produced by other persons or animals can be introduced into a person's bloodstream for protection against a pathogen.

The human immunodeficiency virus (HIV)—the pathogen that causes acquired immunodeficiency syndrome (AIDS)—and the hepatitis B virus are transmitted through blood and other body fluids. Drug abusers frequently share syringes and needles, which increases the risk of acquiring these viruses. Safe sexual practices, including the correct use of condoms and engaging in monogamous relationships, reduce the risk for both of these diseases, as well as for other sexually transmitted diseases (STDs). Nurses use standard precautions when caring for all clients to protect themselves from contact with blood and body fluids (see Chapter 33).

At the community level, the transmission of disease is also controlled by adequate disposal of human waste through proper construction and repair of sewers and drains. Insect and rodent control (e.g., spraying for mosquitoes) is also necessary to reduce the transmission of disease.

Pollution. A healthy environment is free of pollution. A **pollutant** is a harmful chemical or waste material discharged into the water, soil, or air. People commonly think of pollution only in terms of air, land, or water pollution, but excessive noise can also be a form of pollution that presents health risks. **Air pollution** is the contamination of the atmosphere with a harmful chemical. Prolonged exposure to air pollution increases the risk of pulmonary disease. In urban areas, industrial waste and vehicle exhaust are common contributors to air pollution. In the home, school, or workplace, cigarette smoke is the primary cause of air pollution. **Land pollution** of soil can be caused by improper disposal of radioactive and bioactive waste products (e.g., dioxin).

Water pollution is the contamination of lakes, rivers, and streams, usually by industrial pollutants. Water treatment facilities filter harmful contaminants from the water, but these systems may contain flaws. If water becomes contaminated, the public should use bottled or boiled water for drinking and cooking. Flooding frequently causes damage to water treatment stations and also requires the use of bottled or boiled water.

Noise pollution occurs when the noise level in an environment becomes uncomfortable to the inhabitants of the environment. Noise levels are measured in units of sound intensity called decibels. Tolerance for noise varies from individual to individual and is influenced by health status. Irreversible hearing loss may result from constant exposure to high sound intensity. Clients working in environments with high noise levels need to wear protective devices to reduce hearing loss (Figure 37-3). Adolescents should limit their exposure to intense noise such as that found at rock concerts.

A health care facility can also be polluted by noise. The sounds of machines, people talking, intercoms, and paging systems can create increased noise levels. Even when the noise level is not high enough to affect hearing acuity, it may produce a syndrome called sensory overload. Sensory overload is a marked increase in the intensity of auditory and visual stimuli. It disrupts processing of information, and the client no longer perceives the environment in a meaningful way (see Chapter 48).

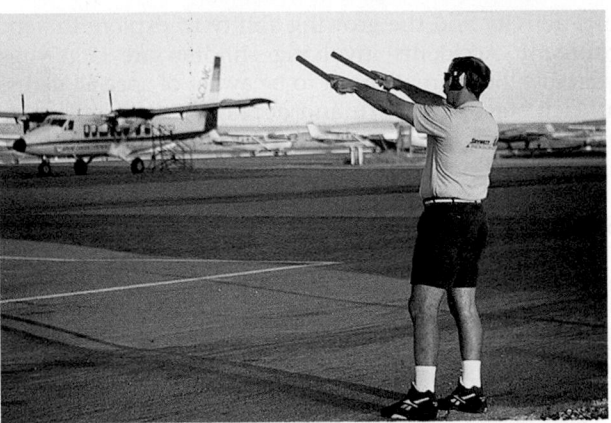

FIGURE **37-3**　Protective device to reduce hearing loss.

Terrorism. A new potential environmental health threat is the possibility of a terrorist attack. Before 1990 and the Gulf War, the possibility of the United States coming under attack from terrorists groups using biological, chemical, or nuclear weapons seemed remote. Today, however, we are concerned about an attack by an individual or small group on one of our cities, a large sporting event, or a unit of our military forces (Jones and others, 2002). **Bioterrorism,** or the use of biological agents to create fear and threat, is the most likely form of terrorist attack to occur. Health care facilities must be prepared to treat mass casualties from an attack. The answer lies in the facility's emergency management plan. Such a plan details how to respond to a terrorist attack; for example, determining the agent used, determining the time and location of the attack and the affected population, obtaining and delivering supplies, and providing treatment (Giovachino and Carey, 2001). Nurses must be prepared through education and training to be able to respond to an attack by taking the necessary steps to initiate an agency's emergency management plan.

Nursing Knowledge Base

Nurses, in addition to being knowledgeable about the environment, must be familiar with a client's developmental level; mobility, sensory, and cognitive status; lifestyle choices; and knowledge of common safety precautions. They must also be aware of the special risks to safety that are found in agency settings.

Risks at Developmental Stages

A client's developmental stage creates threats to safety as a result of lifestyle, mobility status, sensory impairments, and safety awareness.

Infant, Toddler, and Preschooler. Injuries are the leading cause of death in children over age 1 and cause more death and disabilities than do all diseases combined (Wong, 2003). The nature of the injury sustained is closely related to normal growth and development. For example, the incidence of lead poisoning is highest in late infancy and toddlerhood because of a child's increased level of oral activity and the growing ability to explore the environment. Accidents involving children are largely preventable, but parents need to be aware of specific dangers at each stage of growth and development. Accident prevention thus requires health education for parents and the removal of dangers whenever possible.

School-Age Child. When a child enters school, the environment expands to include the school, transportation to and from school, school friends, and after-school activities. Parents, teachers, and nurses must instruct the child in safe practices to follow at school or play. Using examples when discussing safe practices is an effective way to teach the school-age child.

Because school-age children are participating in more activities outside their home and neighborhood environments, they are at greater risk of injury from strangers. A child should be warned repeatedly not to accept candy, food, gifts, or rides from strangers. In addition, a child needs to know what to do if a stranger approaches. Frequently neighborhoods have a "block home" or "safe house." In these homes the owner ensures that an adult is home during the times when children are walking to and from school. If a stranger approaches a child, the child can run to that home, and the adult will protect the child and call the proper authorities. Nurses can work with school systems or neighborhoods to initiate such a system to protect children.

Sports safety is stressed in school sports, but parents and health professionals can reinforce these safety tips by insisting that children wear protective gear while participating in sports such as skateboarding and snowboarding. For example, schools provide hard batting helmets for baseball games, and parents should also provide this equipment when children are playing baseball in their own backyards.

Bicycle-related injuries, including scooters, are a major cause of death and disability among children. Children 5 to 14 years of age account for nearly one third of bicyclists killed in traffic accidents (*Injury Fact Book 2001-2002*, 2002). Bikes should be in good working order and be the proper size for the child. The child should be taught the rules of the road and cautioned not to engage in dangerous stunts or activities while bike riding. A properly fitted helmet should be worn. Because most fatalities from bicycle accidents are related to head injuries, many states are implementing laws requiring bicycle helmets (Figure 37-4).

Adolescent. As children enter adolescence, they develop greater independence and begin to develop a sense of identity and their own values. In addition, adolescents begin to separate emotionally from their families, and peers generally have a stronger influence. The struggle toward identity may cause the teenager to experience shyness, fear, and anxiety, with resulting dysfunction at home or school. In an attempt to relieve the tensions associated with physical and psychosocial changes, as well as peer pressures, adolescents may begin to act impulsively and engage in risk-taking behaviors such as smoking and using drugs. In addition to the health risks posed by nicotine and other drugs, the ingestion of drugs, in-

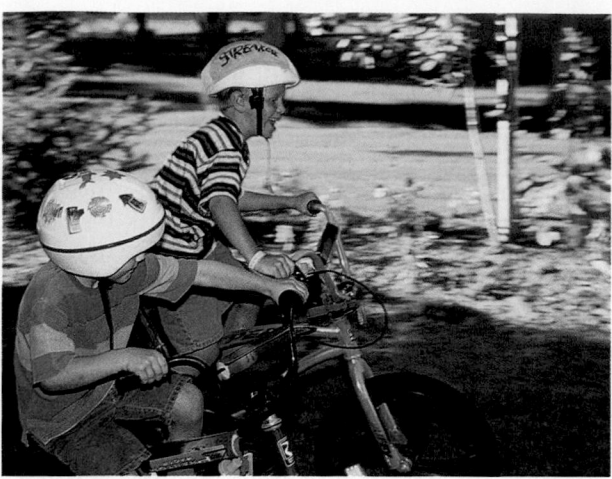

FIGURE **37-4** Proper bicycle safety equipment for school-age child.

cluding alcohol, increases the incidence of accidents such as drowning and motor vehicle accidents.

When adolescents learn to drive, their environment expands and so does their potential for injury. The risk of motor vehicle accidents is higher among teen drivers than any other age-group. Teens are more likely to speed, run red lights, ride with intoxicated drivers, and drive after using alcohol and drugs. The young driver must be taught to comply with rules and regulations regarding use of a car.

> *Safety Alert.* Reinforce to new drivers and parents of new drivers the need to consistently wear safety belts and to never ride in a car with a driver who has been drinking. Assist parents and teen in developing a plan of action if teen is with a driver who drinks at an outing.

Because adolescence is a time when mature sexual physical characteristics develop, adolescents may begin to have physical relationships with others. They need prompt, accurate instruction about abstinence and/or safe sexual practices and birth control.

Adult. The threats to an adult's safety are frequently related to lifestyle habits. For example, the client who uses alcohol excessively is at greater risk for motor vehicle accidents. The long-term smoker has a greater risk of cardiovascular or pulmonary disease as a result of the inhalation of smoke into the lungs and the effect of nicotine on the circulatory system. Likewise, the adult experiencing a high level of stress is more likely to have an accident or illness such as headaches, gastrointestinal (GI) disorders, and infections (see Chapter 30).

Older Adult. The physiological changes that occur during the aging process increase the client's risk for falls and other types of accidents such as burns and car accidents (Box 37-1). Older clients are more likely to fall in the bedroom, bathroom, and kitchen, and outside as a result of ice on walkways or obstacles in the garden. Inside falls

Physical Assessment Findings in the Older Adult That Increase the Risk of Accidents

Musculoskeletal Changes

Muscle strength and function decrease, joints become less mobile, bones are brittle due to osteoporosis, postural changes (e.g., kyphosis) are common, and range of motion is limited.

Nervous System Changes

All voluntary or automatic reflexes slow to some extent, ability to respond to multiple stimuli decreases, and sensitivity to touch is decreased.

Sensory Changes

Peripheral vision and lens accommodation decrease, lens may develop opacity (cataracts), stimuli threshold for light touch and pain increases, transmission of hot and cold impulses is delayed, and hearing is impaired as high-frequency tones become less perceptible.

Genitourinary Changes

Nocturia and occurrences of incontinence increase.

Modified from Ebersole P, Hess P: *Toward healthy aging,* ed 6, St. Louis, 2003, Mosby.

most often occur while transferring from beds, chairs, and toilets; getting into or out of bathtubs; tripping over carpet edges or doorway thresholds; slipping on wet surfaces; and descending stairs (Tideiksaar, 1989).

●●●

Unfortunately, clients throughout all developmental stages may be subject to abuse. Child abuse, domestic violence, and abuse of older adults are serious threats to safety. These topics are discussed in Chapters 11 through 13.

Individual Risk Factors

Other risk factors posing threats to safety include lifestyle, impaired mobility, sensory or communication impairment, and lack of safety awareness.

Lifestyle. Lifestyle can increase safety risks. People who drive or operate machinery while under the influence of chemical substances (drugs or alcohol), who work at inherently dangerous jobs, or who are risk takers are at greater risk of injury. In addition, people experiencing stress, anxiety, fatigue, or alcohol or drug withdrawal, or those taking prescribed medications may be more accident-prone. Because of these factors, clients may be too preoccupied to notice the source of potential accidents, such as cluttered stairs or a stop sign.

Impaired Mobility. Impaired mobility due to muscle weakness, paralysis, or poor coordination or balance is a

major factor in client falls. Immobilization predisposes the client to additional physiological and emotional hazards, which in turn can further restrict mobility and independence (see Chapter 36).

Sensory or Communication Impairment. Clients with visual, hearing, tactile, or communication impairment, such as aphasia or a language barrier, are at greater risk for injury. Such clients may not be able to perceive a potential danger or express their need for assistance (see Chapter 48).

Lack of Safety Awareness. Some clients are unaware of safety precautions, such as keeping medicine or poisons away from children or reading the expiration date on food products. A complete nursing assessment, including a home inspection, will help the nurse identify the client's level of knowledge regarding home safety so that deficiencies can be corrected with an individualized nursing care plan.

Risks in the Health Care Agency

Environmental safety pertains to the health care agency, as well as to the client's home and community. However, there are specific risks in health care agencies that must also be addressed.

A report by the Institute of Medicine (IOM) estimates that at least 44,000 to 98,000 Americans die each year as a result of medical errors, exceeding the number attributable to the eighth leading cause of death (Kohn, Corrigan and Donaldson, 1999). The most common preventable errors identified in this report include technical errors, diagnostic-related errors, failure to prevent injury, and errors in the use of a drug. One study on adverse drug events showed that 78% were due to system failures such as lack of knowledge about a drug, lack of information about a client, failure to follow established procedures, transcription errors, faulty drug identification and checking, faulty dose checking, inadequate monitoring, preparation errors, drug stocking and delivery problems, and lack of standardization (Agency for Healthcare Research and Quality [AHRQ], 2000). It is essential that nurses and health care facilities build safety into processes of care and take a systems approach when taking on efforts to reduce medical errors.

Various forms of chemicals used in health care settings are a source of an environmental risk. Chemicals such as mercury (see Chapter 31) and those found in some medications, anesthetic gases, cleaning solutions, and disinfectants can be potentially toxic if ingested or inhaled. Material Safety Data Sheets (MSDs) are available to provide detailed information about the chemical, any health hazards imposed, precautions for safe handling and use, and steps to take in case the material is released or spilled.

Specific risks to a client's safety within the health care environment also include falls, client-inherent accidents, procedure-related accidents, and equipment-related accidents. The nurse must assess for these four potential problem areas and, considering the developmental level of the client, take steps to prevent or minimize accidents.

An accident necessitates the filing of an incident report, a confidential document that completely describes any client accident occurring on the premises of a health care agency (see Chapter 22). The report documents the accident, client assessment, and interventions carried out for the client. In addition to completing the incident report, the nurse must objectively document the incident in the client's medical record. Because this is a confidential document, completion of the incident report should not be mentioned in the medical record because this eliminates the health care agency's protective clause.

Falls. Falls account for up to 90% of all reported incidents in hospitals. The risk for falling is significantly higher in older clients. In addition to age, a history of previous falls, gait disturbance, balance and mobility problems, postural hypotension, sensory impairment, urinary and bladder dysfunction, and certain medical diagnostic categories (e.g., cancer and cardiovascular, neurological, and cerebrovascular diseases) increase the risk. One of the more common factors precipitating a fall is a client's attempt to get out of bed to toilet. Drug use and drug interactions are also implicated in falls. Hip fractures are among the most serious fall-related injuries. Half of older adults who suffer a hip fracture never regain their previous level of functioning, and many are unable to live independently after the injury (*Injury Fact Book 2001-2002*, 2002). Falls that result in injuries can extend a client's length of stay in the health care environment, placing them at an even greater risk for other complications.

Client-Inherent Accidents. Client-inherent accidents are accidents (other than falls) where the client is the primary reason for the accident. Examples of client-inherent accidents are self-inflicted cuts, injuries, and burns; ingestion or injection of foreign substances; self-mutilation or fire setting; and pinching fingers in drawers or doors.

A client-inherent accident may occur as a result of a seizure. A **seizure** is a hyperexcitation and disorderly discharge of neurons in the brain leading to a sudden, violent, involuntary series of muscle contractions that may be paroxysmal and episodic, as in a seizure disorder, or transient and acute, such as following a head injury. A generalized tonic-clonic, or grand mal, seizure lasts approximately 2 minutes (no longer than 5) and is characterized by a cry, loss of consciousness with falling, tonicity (rigidity), clonicity (jerking), and incontinence (Beare and Meyers, 1998). During a fall, or as a result of muscle jerking, musculoskeletal injuries can occur. Before a convulsive episode, a few clients may report an aura, which serves as a warning or sense that a seizure is about to occur. An **aura** may be a bright light, smell, or taste. During the seizure activity the client may have shallow breathing, cyanosis, and possibly loss of bladder and bowel control. Following the seizure there is a postictal phase during which the client may have amnesia or confusion and may fall into a deep sleep.

Continuous seizures that last 15 minutes or a series of seizures over a 20- to 30-minute period in which the client does not regain consciousness between attacks is status epilepticus. This condition is a medical emergency

and requires intensive monitoring and treatment. It is important that the nurse observe the client carefully before, during, and after the seizure so that the episode can be documented accurately (Beare and Meyers, 1998).

Procedure-Related Accidents. Procedure-related accidents occur during therapy. They include medication and fluid administration errors, improper application of external devices, and accidents related to improper performance of procedures (e.g., Foley catheter insertion).

The nurse can prevent many procedure-related accidents. For example, strictly following the procedure for administering medications will prevent medication errors (see Chapter 34). Proper administration of intravenous (IV) fluids prevents fluid overload or deficit (see Chapter 40). The potential for infection is reduced when surgical asepsis is used for sterile dressing changes or any invasive procedure, such as insertion of a Foley catheter. Finally, correct use of body mechanics and transfer techniques reduces the risk of injuries when moving and lifting clients (see Chapter 46).

Equipment-Related Accidents. Equipment-related accidents result from the malfunction, disrepair, or misuse of equipment or from an electrical hazard. For example, too-rapid infusion of IV fluids may result from a dysfunctional IV pump. The JCAHO (2004) now requires that all general use and patient-controlled analgesic pumps have free-flow protection devices. To avoid accidents, the nurse should not operate monitoring or therapy equipment without instruction. A checklist should be used to assess potential electrical hazards to reduce the risk of electrical fires, electrocution, or injury from faulty equipment. In health care settings, clinical engineering staff makes regular safety checks of equipment.

Critical Thinking

Successful critical thinking requires a synthesis of knowledge, experience, information gathered from clients, critical thinking attitudes, and intellectual and professional standards. Clinical judgments require the nurse to anticipate necessary information, analyze the data, and make decisions regarding client care. Critical thinking is an ongoing process. During assessment (Figure 37-5) the nurse must consider all critical thinking elements, as well as information about the specific client, to make appropriate nursing diagnoses.

In the case of safety the nurse integrates knowledge from nursing and other scientific disciplines, previous experiences in caring for clients who had an injury or were at risk, critical thinking attitudes such as perseverance, and any standards of practice that are applicable. For example, the American Nurses Association (ANA) standards for nursing practice address the nurse's responsibility in maintaining client safety. The Joint Commission for Accreditation of Healthcare Organizations (JCAHO) also provides standards for safety (e.g., in the administration of medications, use of restraints, and use of medical devices). The nurse refers to all of this information and ex-

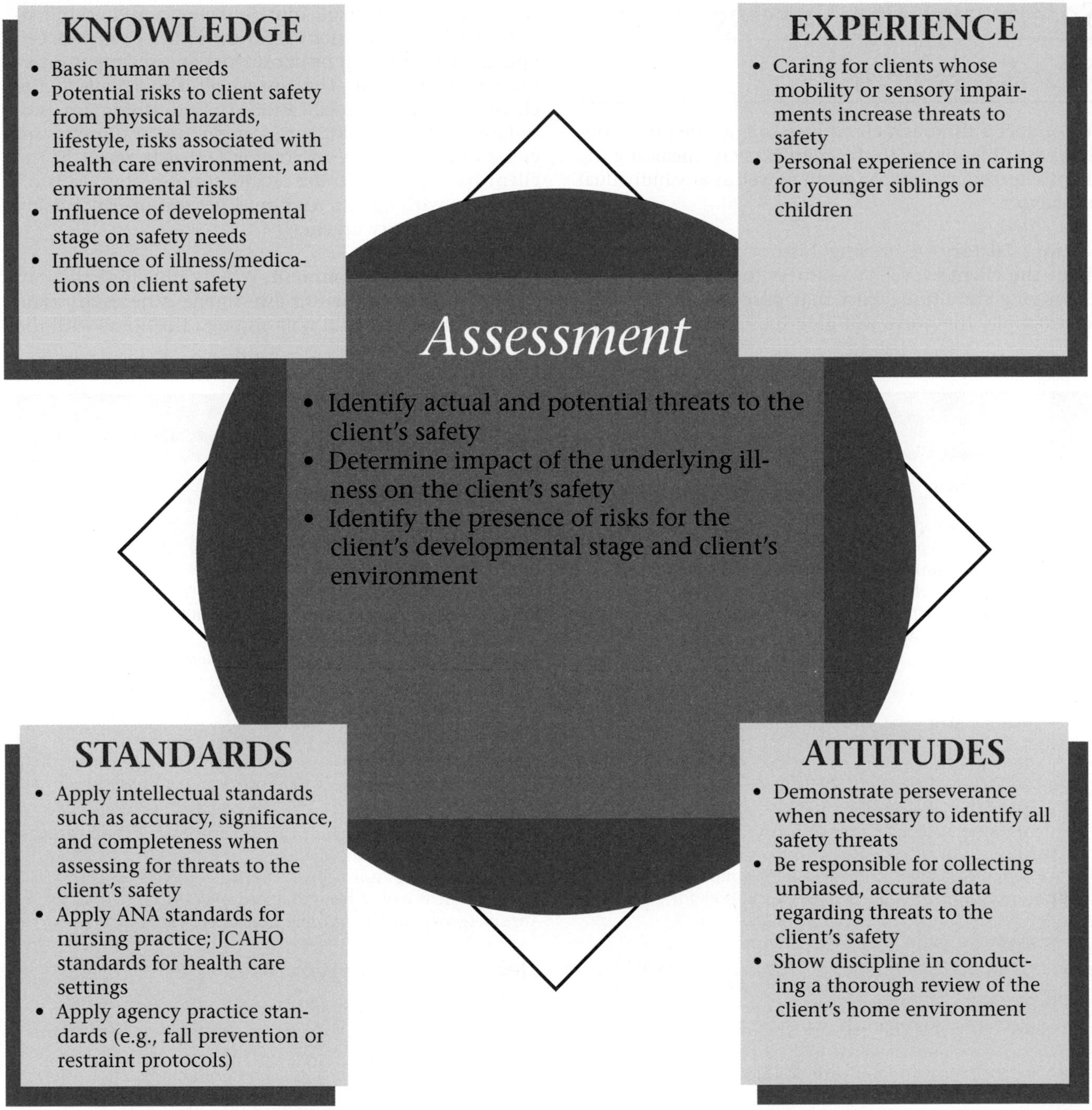

KNOWLEDGE

- Basic human needs
- Potential risks to client safety from physical hazards, lifestyle, risks associated with health care environment, and environmental risks
- Influence of developmental stage on safety needs
- Influence of illness/medications on client safety

EXPERIENCE

- Caring for clients whose mobility or sensory impairments increase threats to safety
- Personal experience in caring for younger siblings or children

Assessment

- Identify actual and potential threats to the client's safety
- Determine impact of the underlying illness on the client's safety
- Identify the presence of risks for the client's developmental stage and client's environment

STANDARDS

- Apply intellectual standards such as accuracy, significance, and completeness when assessing for threats to the client's safety
- Apply ANA standards for nursing practice; JCAHO standards for health care settings
- Apply agency practice standards (e.g., fall prevention or restraint protocols)

ATTITUDES

- Demonstrate perseverance when necessary to identify all safety threats
- Be responsible for collecting unbiased, accurate data regarding threats to the client's safety
- Show discipline in conducting a thorough review of the client's home environment

FIGURE **37–5**   Critical thinking model for safety assessment.

perience as he or she conducts a detailed assessment of a specific client. For example, while assessing a specific client's home environment, the nurse will consider knowledge regarding typical locations within the home where dangers commonly exist. If a client has a visual im-pairment, the nurse will apply previous experiences in caring for clients with visual changes to anticipate how to thoroughly assess the client's needs. Critical thinking di-rects the nurse to anticipate what needs to be assessed and how to make conclusions about available data.

Safety and the Nursing Process

NP Assessment

To conduct a thorough client assessment, the nurse considers possible threats to the client's safety, including the client's immediate environment, as well as any individual risk factors.

Nursing History. A nursing history will include data about the client's level of wellness to determine if any underlying conditions exist that pose threats to safety. For example, the nurse will give special attention to as-sessing the client's gait, muscle strength and coordina-tion, balance, and vision. A review of the client's devel-opmental status must be considered as assessment infor-mation is analyzed. The nurse will also review if the client is taking any medications or undergoing any pro-cedures that pose risks. For example, use of diuretics in-creases the frequency of voiding and may result in the client having to use toilet facilities more often. Falls of-ten occur with clients who must get out of bed quickly because of urinary urgency.

Client's Home Environment. When caring for a client in the home, a home hazard assessment is necessary (Box 37-2). The nurse should walk through the home with the

---

Box 37-2   Home Hazard Assessment

Home Exterior

Are sidewalks uneven?
Are steps in good repair?
Is ice and snow removal adequate?
Do steps have securely fastened handrails?
Is there adequate lighting?
Is outdoor furniture sturdy?

Home Interior

Do all rooms, stairways, and halls have adequate, nonglare lighting?
Are night-lights available?
Are area rugs secured?
Are wooden floors nonslippery?
Are floors where water accumulates covered by nonslip floor mats?
Is furniture placed appropriately to permit mobility?
Is furniture sturdy enough to provide support for getting up and down?
Are temperature and humidity within normal range?
Are there any steps or thresholds that may pose a hazard?
Are step edges clearly marked with colored tape?
Are handrails available and secure?
In homes with young children, are window guards and electri-cal outlet covers installed?
Can all doors and windows with security gates and locks be opened from the inside without a key?

Kitchen

Are hand-washing facilities available?
Is the pilot light on for the gas stove?
Are the stovetop and oven clean?
Are the dials on the stove readable?
Are storage areas within easy reach?
Are fluids such as cleaners and bleach in original containers and stored properly?
In homes with young children, are safety locks on cabinets and corner counter protectors installed?
Is the water temperature within normal range?
Are there clean areas for food storage and preparation?
Is refrigeration adequate? Are the refrigerator and freezer tem-peratures correct?

Bathroom

Are hand-washing facilities available?
Are there skidproof strips or surfaces in the tub or shower?
Are bath mats secured?
Does the client need grab bars near the bathtub and toilet?
Does the client need an elevated toilet seat?
Is the medicine cabinet well lighted?
Are medications in their original containers?
Are medication containers child resistant if children live in the home or visit?
Is ipecac syrup available in households with small children?
Have outdated medications been discarded?

Bedroom

Are beds of adequate height to allow getting on and off easily?
Is day and night lighting adequate?
Are floor coverings nonskid?
Does the client have a telephone nearby?
Are emergency numbers visible near the telephone?

Electrical and Fire Hazards

Are smoke and carbon monoxide detectors installed?
Are the batteries for all detectors tested every month and changed twice a year?
Have furnaces, chimneys, and stoves been checked for proper ventilation?
Are extension cords in good condition and used appropriately?
Are appliances in good working order?
Are electrical appliances located away from water sources?
Is there a multipurpose fire extinguisher near the cooking area, and does client understand how to use it?
Are combustible items such as oil-based paints, gasoline, and oily rags being stored in a garage and/or basement?
Are electrical outlets overloaded?
Are flashlights available?
Is there a first aid kit available to the adult members of the household?
Does everyone in the family have easy access to emergency phone numbers?

Modified from Tideiksaar R: Home safe home: practical tips for fall-proofing, *Geriatr Nurs* 11(6):280, 1989; and Ebersole P, Hess P: *Toward healthy aging,* ed 6, St. Louis, 2003, Mosby.

client and discuss how the client normally conducts daily activities. Key areas to inspect are the bathroom, kitchen, and areas with stairs. For example, when assessing adequacy of lighting, the nurse inspects areas where the client moves and works, such as outside walkways, steps, interior halls, and doorways. Getting a sense of the client's routines helps the nurse recognize hazards that are not as obvious.

Assessment for risks of food infections or poisoning encompass obtaining a detailed dietary assessment for the past week; conducting an examination of GI and central nervous system (CNS) function; observing for a fever; and analyzing the results of cultures of feces and vomitus. Suspected food and water sources are also studied. The nurse should also assess the client's hand-washing practices. It is useful for the nurse to ask clients when they routinely wash their hands. This can then prompt a helpful discussion about the purpose and importance of hand washing.

Assessment of the environmental comfort of a client's home should include a review of when the client normally has heating and cooling systems serviced. Does the client have a functional furnace or space heater? Does the home have air conditioning or fans? Clients who use space heaters must be informed of the risk for fires.

When clients live in older homes, the nurse should encourage inspections for the presence of lead in paint, dust, or soil. Because lead can also come from the solder or plumbing fixtures in a home, water from each faucet should also be tested. Local health offices can assist a homeowner in locating a trained lead inspector who will take samples from various locations and have them analyzed at a laboratory for content of lead.

Health Care Environment. When the client is cared for within a health care facility, the nurse must determine if any hazards exist in the immediate care environment. Does the placement of equipment or furniture pose barriers when the client attempts to ambulate? Does positioning of the client's bed allow the client to reach items on a bedside table or stand? Does the client need assistance with ambulation? The nurse also collaborates with clinical engineering staff to make sure that equipment has been assessed to ensure proper function and condition.

Risk for Falls. Assessment of a client's fall risk factors is essential in determining specific needs and developing targeted interventions to prevent falls. The nurse begins by asking clients if they have had a history of falls. A fall assessment tool (Table 37-1) can help the nurse assess for potential risks before accidents and injuries result. The illustrated tool has weighted risk factors. A client's risk of falling increases dramatically as the number of risk factors increases. Initial and daily assessment of fall risk is important in identifying clients who are at risk of falling. In many cases family members can be important resources in assessing a client's fall risk. Families often are able to report on the client's level of confusion and ability to ambulate.

Risk for Medical Errors. Nurses must also be alert to factors within their own environment that create conditions in which medical errors are more likely to occur. Studies have shown that overwork and fatigue have been shown to cause a significant decrease in alertness and concentration, leading to errors (Leonard and others, 1998). It is important for nurses to be aware of these factors and to

---

Table 37-1   **Fall Assessment Tool**

Directions: Circle the score for the risk factor that corresponds to the patient. The tool should be administered on admission to the facility or agency and again at specified intervals and when warranted by changes in health status. Scores of 15 and higher indicate high risk, and preventive measures should be implemented.

Client Factors	Date Admit	Initial Score	Date	Reassessed Score
History of falls		15		15
Confusion		5		5
Age (over 65)		5		5
Impaired judgment		5		5
Sensory deficit		5		5
Unable to ambulate independently		5		5
Decreased level of cooperation		5		5
Increased anxiety/emotional liability		5		5
Incontinence/urgency		5		5
Cardiovascular/respiratory disease affecting perfusion and oxygenation		5		5
Medications affecting blood pressure or level of consciousness		5		5
Postural hypotension with dizziness		5		5
Environmental Factors				
First week on unit/facility/services, etc.		5		5
Attached equipment (e.g., IV pole, chest tubes, appliances, oxygen, tubing, etc.)		5		5

Modified from Farmer B: *Try this: best practices in nursing care to older adults,* New York, 2000, The Hartford Institute for Geriatric Nursing, New York University.

include checks and balances when working under stressful conditions. For example, to reduce the potential for a medical error, it is essential for the nurse to check the client's identification bracelet before beginning any procedure or administering a medication (see Chapter 34).

In January 2003 the JCAHO established National Patient Safety Goals in an effort to reduce the risk of medical errors. These evidence-based recommendations require health care facilities to focus their attention on a series of specific actions. Data on the achievement of the goals will be made public each year. New goals are announced each year in July. The National Patient Safety Goals for 2004 include: improving the accuracy of patient identification; improving the effectiveness of communication among caregivers; improving the safety after using high-alert medications; eliminating wrong site, wrong client, wrong procedure surgery; improving the safety of using infusion pumps; improving the effectiveness of clinical alarm systems; and reducing risk of nosocomial infections (JCAHO 2004).

Bioterrorist Attacks. Although the occurrence of a bioterrorist attack has been limited to the anthrax deaths following September 11, 2001, the threat is very real. Nurses must be prepared to make accurate and timely assessments in any type of setting. If an attack occurs, it will most likely involve the use of biological agents such as anthrax, botulism, smallpox, or bubonic plague. A bioterrorist attack would likely resemble a natural outbreak initially, but nurses must recognize that the microorganisms used may have been modified for increased virulence or may have resistance to antibiotics or vaccines (Jones and others, 2002). Biological attacks may be either overt (announced) or covert (unannounced). Overt attacks require rapid assessment of their true occurrence, followed by an appropriate response. Covert attacks become obvious only after victims present for medical care, after the incubation period has passed and clinical signs begin to appear (Jones and others, 2002). In both cases it is essential for nurses to recognize and know high-risk syndromes (Box 37-3). Acutely ill clients representing the earliest cases after a covert attack will seek care in emergency departments. Less ill clients at the onset of an illness may seek care in primary care settings.

There are basic epidemiological principles to assess whether a client's presentation of symptoms is typical of an endemic disease or is an unusual event that should raise concern. Features that should alert nurses to the possibility of a bioterrorism-related outbreak include the following (English and Malone, 1999):

- A rapidly increasing incidence of a disease (e.g., within hours or days) in a normally healthy population
- An unusual increase in the number of people seeking care, especially with fever, respiratory, or gastrointestinal complaints
- An endemic disease rapidly emerging at an uncharacteristic time or in an unusual pattern

---

Box 37-3   Biological Agent Syndromes

1. **Anthrax** (acute infectious disease caused by *Bacillus anthracis*, a spore-forming, gram-positive bacillus). Humans become infected through skin contact, ingestion, or inhalation. Person-to-person transmission of inhalational disease does not occur. Direct exposure to vesicle secretions of skin anthrax may result in secondary cutaneous infection.
   Clinical Features: Pulmonary: flulike symptoms, possible brief interim improvement, within 2 to 4 days, abrupt onset of respiratory failure and hemodynamic collapse. Gram-positive bacilli on blood culture rests. *Cutaneous:* local skin involvement, common on the head, forearms, or hands; localized itching followed by a papular lesion that turns vesicular and within 2 to 6 days become a depressed black eschar. *Gastrointestinal:* abdominal pain, nausea, vomiting, and fever after eating contaminated food (usually meat); bloody diarrhea, hematemesis; gram-positive bacilli on blood culture. Symptoms begin within 1 day to 8 weeks (average 5 days) depending on exposure route and amount of agent.
2. **Botulism** (caused by *Clostridium botulinum,* an anaerobic gram-positive bacillus that produces a potent neurotoxin). Food-borne botulism is the most common form. An airborne form of botulism is also possible.
   Clinical Features: Food-borne botulism causes abdominal cramping, diarrhea, and other gastrointestinal symptoms. Both food-borne and inhalation botulism cause responsive client with absence of fever; drooping eyelids, weakened jaw clench, difficulty swallowing or speaking; blurred vision and double vision; symmetric paralysis of arms first, followed by respiratory muscles, then legs; respiratory dysfunction from respiratory muscle paralysis; no sensory deficits. Neurological symptoms of food-borne botulism begin 12 to 36 hours after ingestion and 24 to 72 hours after inhalation. The disease is not transmitted from person to person.
3. **Plague** (an acute bacterial disease caused by the gram-negative bacillus *Yersinia pestis*). A bioterrorism-related outbreak may be expected to be airborne.
   Clinical Features: Fever, cough, chest pain, hemoptysis, mucopurulent or watery sputum with gram-negative rods in a Gram stain test. X-ray film shows bronchopneumonia. Person-to-person transmission is possible via large aerosol droplets. Symptoms usually appear within 1 to 3 days.
4. **Smallpox** (an acute viral illness caused by the variola virus). Disease has the potential to cause severe morbidity in a nonimmune population, and it can be transmitted via the airborne route. A single case of smallpox is a public health emergency.
   Clinical Features: Symptoms similar to other acute viral illnesses, such as the flu. Skin lesions appear, quickly progressing from macules to papules to vesicles. Other symptoms include 2 to 4 days of fever and myalgia; rash most prominent on face and extremities (including palms and soles); rash scabs over in 1 to 2 weeks. Smallpox is transmitted by large and small respiratory droplets. Patient-to-patient transmission is likely from airborne and droplet exposure, and by contact with skin lesions or secretions. Symptoms begin in 7 to 17 days (average 12 days).

Modified from English J, Malone JD: *Bioterrorism readiness plan: a template for healthcare facilities,* April 13, 1999, APIC Bioterrorism Task Force and CDC Hospital Infections Program Bioterrorism Working Group.

- Lower attack rates among clients who had been indoors, in areas with filtered or closed ventilation, compared with people who had been outdoors
- Clusters of clients arriving from a single locale
- Large numbers of rapidly fatal cases
- Any client presenting with a disease that is relatively uncommon and has bioterrorism potential

Nurses must be able to recognize a biological casualty and to carry out their roles and responsibilities quickly and efficiently. Timely communication is critical for alerting both the medical and general community at large to a bioterrorist attack. Health care agencies' emergency plans will outline the predetermined departments and locations to contact in the event of an attack.

Client Expectations. Clients generally expect to be safe in their home and in the health care setting. However, there are times when a client's view of what is safe does not agree with that of the nurse. For this reason, any assessment must include the client's understanding of his or her perception of risk factors. This will be important later as the nurse attempts to make changes in the client's environment. Clients usually do not purposefully put themselves in jeopardy. When clients are uninformed or inexperienced, threats to their safety can occur. Clients must always be consulted on ways to reduce hazards in their environment.

Nursing Diagnosis

After completing an assessment of the client's safety status, the nurse reviews any clusters of data to determine if there are patterns suggesting that safety is threatened. Identification of defining characteristics from the data guide the nurse in identifying appropriate nursing diagnoses. The diagnostic process requires accurate recognition of defining characteristics, as well as the related factors (Box 37-4).

The related factor becomes the basis for selecting nursing therapies. For example, *risk for injury related to impaired mobility* and *risk for injury related to barriers in the home environment* require different nursing interventions. The client with altered mobility may require ambulatory aids and physical therapy. When the related factor is barriers in the home, the nurse intervenes to recommend changes

that will create a safer environment. At times, as in the example in Box 37-4, multiple related factors may apply. Examples of nursing diagnoses that may apply for clients whose safety is threatened include the following:

- Risk for imbalanced body temperature
- Impaired home maintenance
- Risk for injury
- Deficient knowledge
- Risk for poisoning
- Disturbed sensory/perception
- Risk for suffocation
- Disturbed thought processes
- Risk for trauma

Planning

During planning, the nurse critically synthesizes information from multiple sources (Figure 37-6). Critical thinking ensures that the client's plan of care integrates all that the nurse has learned about the client, as well as the key critical thinking elements. For example, the nurse will reflect on knowledge regarding the services other disciplines (e.g., occupational therapy) can provide in helping clients return to their home environments safely. The nurse will also reflect on any previous experience whereby a client benefited from safety interventions. Such experience helps the nurse adapt approaches with a new client. Applying critical thinking attitudes such as creativity helps the nurse and client collaborate in planning interventions that are relevant and most useful, particularly when changes are made in the home environment.

Goals and Outcomes. Planning and goal setting need to be done in collaboration with the client, family, and other members of the health care team (see care plan). The client who is an active participant in reducing threats to safety will be more alert to potential hazards. Goals and outcomes must be measurable and realistic, with consideration of the resources available to the client. The overall goal for a client with a threat to safety is remaining free from injury. The following are examples of expected outcomes that focus on the client's need for safety:

- Modifiable hazards will be reduced in the home environment by 100% within 1 month.

Nursing Diagnostic Process

Box 37-4

Assessment Activities	Defining Characteristics	Nursing Diagnosis
Observe client's mobility and body alignment.	Uncoordinated gait Poor posture	Risk for injury related to impaired mobility, decreased vision, poorly lighted home, and cluttered environment
Ask client about visual acuity.	Reports difficulty seeing at night Reports "tripping" over rugs and furniture	
Complete a home hazard appraisal.	Poorly lighted home Rooms filled with small items Excessive amount of furniture for size of room Rugs not secure	

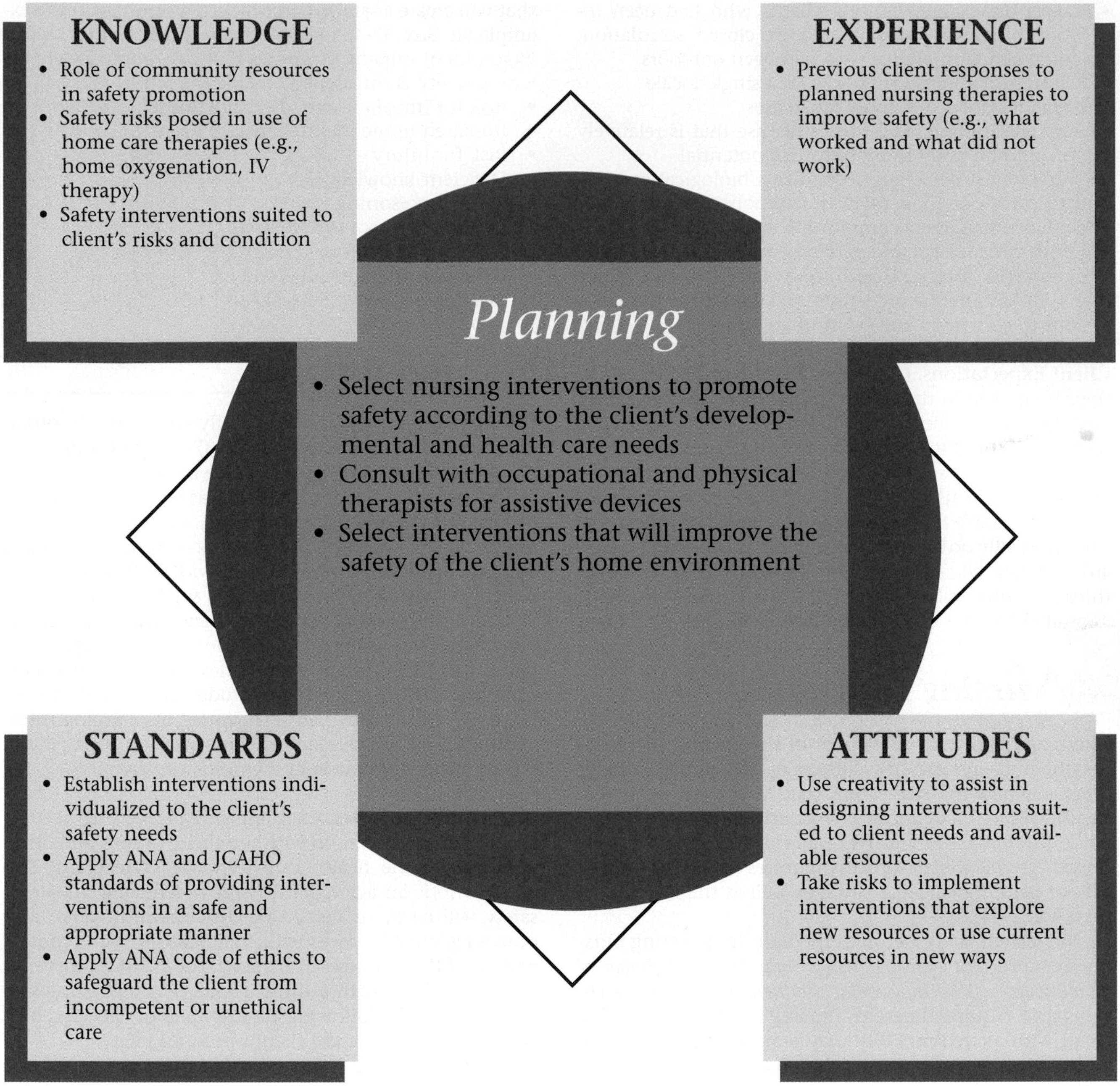

KNOWLEDGE

- Role of community resources in safety promotion
- Safety risks posed in use of home care therapies (e.g., home oxygenation, IV therapy)
- Safety interventions suited to client's risks and condition

EXPERIENCE

- Previous client responses to planned nursing therapies to improve safety (e.g., what worked and what did not work)

Planning

- Select nursing interventions to promote safety according to the client's developmental and health care needs
- Consult with occupational and physical therapists for assistive devices
- Select interventions that will improve the safety of the client's home environment

STANDARDS

- Establish interventions individualized to the client's safety needs
- Apply ANA and JCAHO standards of providing interventions in a safe and appropriate manner
- Apply ANA code of ethics to safeguard the client from incompetent or unethical care

ATTITUDES

- Use creativity to assist in designing interventions suited to client needs and available resources
- Take risks to implement interventions that explore new resources or use current resources in new ways

FIGURE **37–6** Critical thinking model for safety planning.

- Client does not suffer a fall or injury
- Client identifies risks associated with visual impairment

Setting Priorities. Nursing interventions are prioritized to provide safe and efficient care. For example, the client described in the concept map (Figure 37-7) has several nursing diagnoses. The client's mobility problem is an obvious priority because of its influence on skin integrity and risks for falls. The nurse plans individualized interventions based on the severity of risk factors and the client's developmental stage, level of health, lifestyle, and culture (Box 37-5). Planning also involves an understanding of the client's need to maintain independence within physical and cognitive capabilities. The nurse and

client collaborate to establish ways of maintaining the client's active involvement within the home and health care environment. Education of the client and family is also an important intervention to reduce safety risks over the long term.

Continuity of Care. Clients need to learn how to identify and select resources within their community that enhance safety (e.g., neighborhood block homes, local police departments, and neighbors willing to check on a client's well-being). Collaboration with the client and family and other disciplines such as social work and occupational and physical therapy may become an important part of the nurse's plan of care. For example, a hospitalized client may need to go to a rehabilitation facility to gain strength

Concept Map

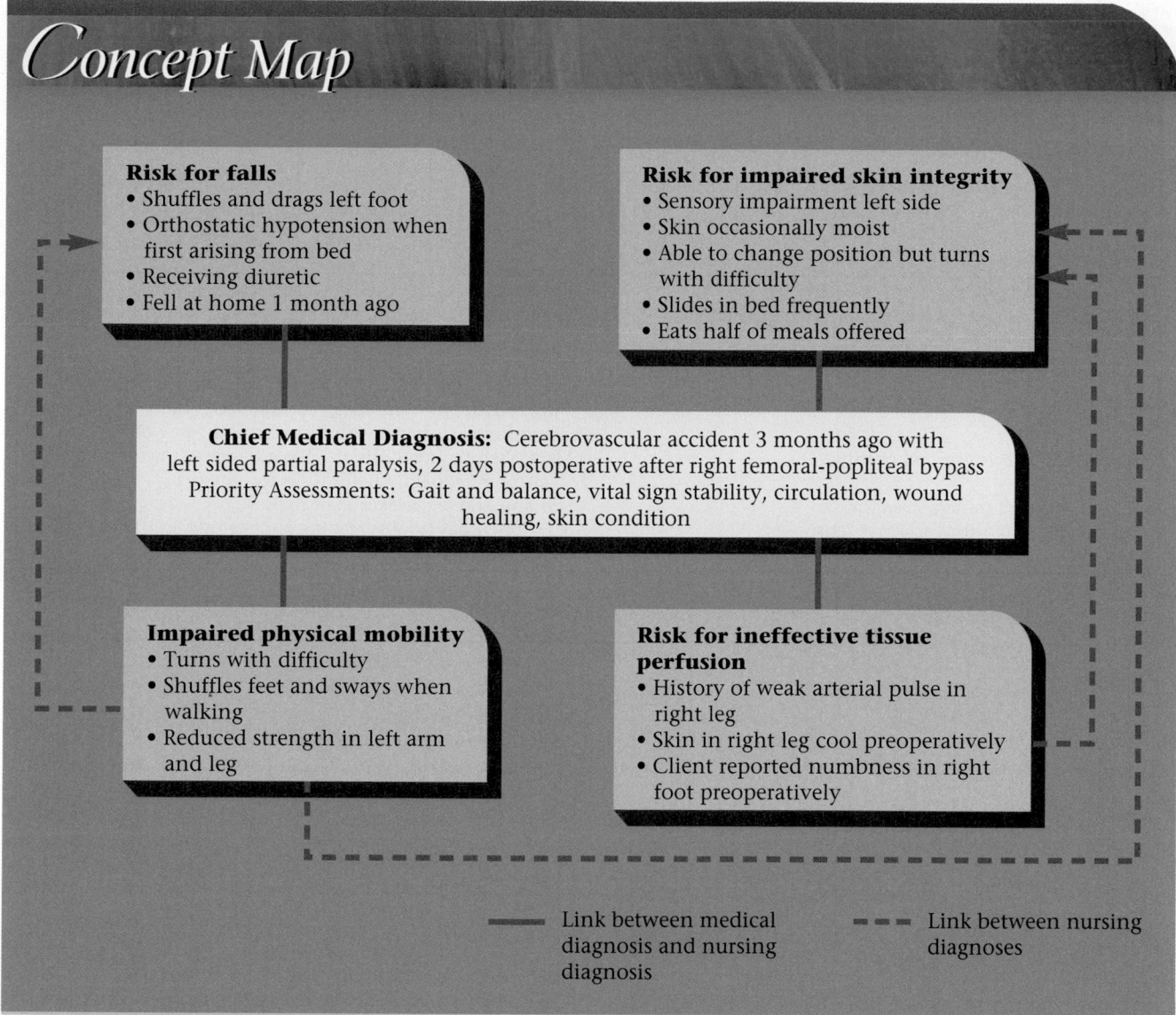

Risk for falls
- Shuffles and drags left foot
- Orthostatic hypotension when first arising from bed
- Receiving diuretic
- Fell at home 1 month ago

Risk for impaired skin integrity
- Sensory impairment left side
- Skin occasionally moist
- Able to change position but turns with difficulty
- Slides in bed frequently
- Eats half of meals offered

Chief Medical Diagnosis: Cerebrovascular accident 3 months ago with left sided partial paralysis, 2 days postoperative after right femoral-popliteal bypass
Priority Assessments: Gait and balance, vital sign stability, circulation, wound healing, skin condition

Impaired physical mobility
- Turns with difficulty
- Shuffles feet and sways when walking
- Reduced strength in left arm and leg

Risk for ineffective tissue perfusion
- History of weak arterial pulse in right leg
- Skin in right leg cool preoperatively
- Client reported numbness in right foot preoperatively

—— Link between medical diagnosis and nursing diagnosis

- - - Link between nursing diagnoses

FIGURE 37–7 Concept map for a client with a cerebrovascular accident 3 months ago with left-sided paralysis, 2 days postoperative after right femoral-popliteal bypass.

and endurance before being discharged home. The nurse must be sure the client and family understand the need for resources and are willing to make changes that will promote their safety.

Implementation

Nursing interventions are directed toward maintaining the client's safety in all types of settings. Nursing measures for providing a safe environment include health promotion, developmental interventions, and environmental interventions.

Health Promotion. To promote an individual's health, it is necessary for the individual to be in a safe environment and to practice a lifestyle that minimizes risk of injury. Edelman and Mandle (1998) describe passive and active strategies aimed at health promotion. Passive strategies

are implemented through public health and government legislative interventions (e.g., sanitation and clean water laws) (see Chapter 3). Active strategies are those in which the individual is actively involved through changes in lifestyle (e.g., wearing seat belts or installing outdoor lighting) and participation in wellness programs.

The nurse participates by supporting legislation and working in community-based settings. Because environmental and community values have the greatest influence on health promotion, community and home health nurses can assess and recommend safety measures in the home, school, neighborhood, and workplace.

Developmental Interventions

Infant, Toddler, and Preschooler. Infants, toddlers, and preschoolers depend on adults to protect them from injury. Growing children are curious and completely trusting of their environment and do not perceive themselves to be in danger. Nurses are frequently in a position to ed-

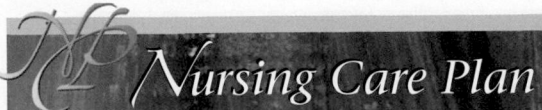

Nursing Care Plan

Risk for Injury

Assessment

Mr. Key, a visiting nurse, is seeing Ms. Cohen, an 85-year-old woman, at her home. The client has been recovering from a mild stroke affecting her left side. Ms. Cohen lives alone but receives regular assistance from her daughter and son, who both live within 10 miles. Mr. Key's assessment included a discussion of Ms. Cohen's health problem and how the stroke has affected her, as well as a pertinent physical examination.

Assessment Activities	Findings/Defining Characteristics
Ask Ms. Cohen how the stroke has affected her mobility.	She responds, "I bump into things, and I'm afraid I'm going to fall."
Conduct a home hazard assessment.	Cabinets in kitchen are in disarray and full of breakable items that could fall out. Throw rugs are on floors; bathroom lighting is poor (40-watt bulbs); bathtub lacks safety strips or grab bars; home cluttered with furniture and small objects.
Observe Ms. Cohen's gait and posture.	Ms. Cohen has kyphosis and has a hesitant, uncoordinated gait. She frequently holds walls for support.
Assess Ms. Cohen's muscle strength.	Left arm and leg weaker than right.
Assess visual acuity with corrective lenses.	Ms. Cohen has trouble reading and seeing familiar objects at a distance while wearing current glasses.

Nursing Diagnosis: Risk for injury related to impaired mobility, decreased visual acuity, and physical environmental hazards.

Planning

Goal	Expected Outcomes*
	Risk Control
Home will be free of hazards within 1 month.	Modifiable hazards in kitchen and hallway will be reduced in the home within 1 week. Revisions to bathroom completed in 1 month.
	Knowledge: Personal Safety
Client and family will be knowledgeable of potential hazards for Ms. Cohen's age-group within 1 week.	Client and daughter will identify risks and the steps to avoid them in the home at the conclusion of a teaching session next week.
	Safety Behavior: Fall Prevention
Ms. Cohen will express greater sense of feeling safe from falls in 1 month.	Ms. Cohen will report improved vision with the aid of new eyeglasses.
Client will be free of injury within 2 weeks.	Client will be able to safely ambulate throughout the home and perform personal care activities within 2 weeks.

*Outcome labels from Moorhead S, Johnson M, Maas M: *Nursing outcomes classification (NOC)*, ed 3, St. Louis, 2004, Mosby.

Interventions†	Rationale
Fall Prevention	
• Review findings from home hazard assessment with client and daughter.	Fall risks for homebound older adults include visual disturbances, unsteady gait, and postural changes (Lueckenotte, 2000). Evaluation of home hazards will highlight extrinsic factors that may lead to falls (Tideiksaar, 1989).
• Establish a list of priorities to modify, and have Ms. Cohen's son assist in installing bathroom safety devices.	Modification of environment reduces fall risk.
• Install lighting (75-watt bulbs, nonglare) throughout the home. Have son install blinds over kitchen windows.	With aging, the pupil loses the ability to adjust to light, causing sensitivity to glare. Glare can make it difficult to clearly see a walking path (Lueckenotte, 2000).
• Discuss with client and daughter the normal changes of aging, effects of recent stroke, associated risks for injury, and how to reduce risks.	Education regarding hazards can reduce fear of falling (American Geriatrics Society, 2001).

Continued

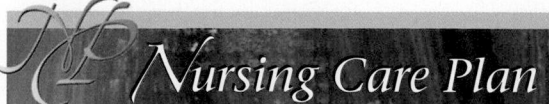

Nursing Care Plan

Risk for Injury—cont'd

Interventions†—cont'd

Fall Prevention

- Encourage daughter to schedule vision testing for new prescription within 2 to 4 weeks.
- Refer to a physical therapist to assess need for assistive devices for kyphosis, left-sided weakness, and gait.

Rationale

Improved visual acuity reduces incidence of falls (Ebersole and Hess, 2001).

Exercise often improves gait, balance, and flexibility. Modifying gait problems by increasing lower extremity strength reduces fall risk (Schoenfelder, 2000).

†Intervention classification labels from Dochterman JM, Bulechek GM: *Nursing interventions classification (NIC)*, ed 4, St. Louis, 2004, Mosby.

Evaluation

Nursing Actions	Client Response/Finding	Achievement of Outcome
Ask client and family to identify risks.	Ms. Cohen and daughter able to identify risks during a walk through the home and expressed a greater sense of safety as a result of changes made.	Client and daughter are more knowledgeable of potential hazards.
Observe environment for elimination of hazards.	Throw rugs have been removed. Lighting has increased to 75 watts except in bathroom and bedroom.	Environmental hazards have been partially reduced.
Reassess Ms. Cohen's visual acuity.	Ms. Cohen has new glasses and says she can read better, as well as see distant objects more clearly.	Ms. Cohen's vision has improved, enabling her to ambulate more safely.
Observe Ms. Cohen's gait and posture.	Ms. Cohen's gait remains hesitant and uncoordinated; she reports that her daughter has not had time to take her to the physical therapist.	Outcome of safe ambulation has not been totally achieved; continue to encourage Ms. Cohen and daughter to go to physical therapy appointment.

ucate parents or guardians about reducing risks of injuries for young children (see Chapter 11). Nurses working in prenatal and postpartum settings can easily incorporate safety into the care plan of the childbearing family. Community health nurses can assess the home and show parents how to promote safety in their homes (Table 37-2). Educate parents that children under 5 are also more susceptible to diseases such as measles, mumps, and chickenpox. Immunizations, given before the age of 2 and at recommended intervals, can protect a child from life-threatening diseases.

School-Age Child. School-age children increasingly explore their environment (see Chapter 11). They have friends outside their immediate neighborhood, and they become more active in school, church, and community activities. The school-age child needs specific teaching regarding safety in school and at play. See Table 37-2, p. 978, for nursing interventions to help guide the parent in providing for the safety of the school-age child.

Adolescent. Risks to the safety of adolescents involve many factors outside the home environment, particularly their almost constant involvement with members of their peer group (see Chapter 11). Adults serve as role models for adolescents and, through providing examples, setting expectations, and providing education, can help adolescents minimize risks to their safety. This age-group has a high incidence of suicide because of feelings of decreased self-worth and hopelessness. The nurse must be aware of the risks posed at this time and be prepared to teach adolescents and their parents measures to prevent accidents and injury.

Adult. Risks to young and middle-age adults frequently result from lifestyle factors such as child rearing, high stress levels, inadequate nutrition, use of firearms, excessive alcohol intake, and substance abuse (see Chapter 12). In this fast-paced society there also appears to be more expression of anger, which can quickly precipitate accidents (e.g., "road rage"). Adults need to have the opportunity to discuss the choices they have made in their lifestyle and the types of threats to safety that exist. Given information about threats to their well-being, adults may make necessary modifications in lifestyle practices. Useful resources are stress management centers (see Chapter 30), employee assistance programs, and health promotion activities, which can be found in many communities and hospitals. In addition, neighborhood centers, community clinics, and outpatient clinics are equipped to assist adults in modifying lifestyle habits (e.g., smoking, overeating, lack of exercise, and alcoholism) that present risks to health.

Older Adult. Nursing interventions for older adults are designed to reduce the risk of falls and other accidents and to compensate for the physiological changes of aging (Box 37-6, p. 979). Most injuries to older adults involve falls, automobile accidents, and those related to burns or

Box 37-5

Cultural Aspects of Care

Cultural phenomena affecting health and safety include personal space, social organizations, communication, and environmental control. While conducting a home assessment for risks to safety, nurses must realize that they have entered the client's territory and that the client's attitude toward his or her residence and belongings must be appreciated. For example, clients from Western Europe and the British Isles are considered aloof and distant in terms of space. It may be very difficult for them to have an outsider in their home who is suggesting changes with regard to their personal belongings to reduce physical hazards. It is particularly difficult to determine a client's attitude toward his or her home environment when another language is spoken.

Another culturally sensitive issue is the client's sense of environmental control. The nurse must be aware of health beliefs and practices that will affect the outcome of interventions. For example, reliance on family and religious organizations, as opposed to community resources, may affect the client's compliance with nursing interventions and referrals.

Nurses and health care providers need to learn to ask questions sensitively and show respect for different cultural beliefs. Adapting to different cultural beliefs and practices requires flexibility and a respect for others' viewpoints. Respect for the belief systems of others and the effects of those beliefs on the client's well-being are critically important to competent care. Nurses must have the ability and knowledge to communicate and to understand health behaviors influenced by culture.

Implications for Practice

- Resistance to change long-standing habits can interfere with a cultural group's acceptance of injury prevention practices. Include family members who have a strong influence, such as a dominant male or older woman, when providing safety education.
- Evaluate the use of traditional ethnic remedies or foods that contain lead because they can increase a client's risk for lead poisoning.
- Living in rural areas and in manufactured housing places the client at greater risk for fire-related injuries and death. Stress the importance of having working smoke detectors and a multipurpose fire extinguisher.
- Assess the client's smoking and drinking habits. Residential fire deaths can be attributed to the use of cigarettes and alcohol.
- Clients who live in poverty and have low educational levels are at greater risk for injury and disease. Assist the client and family in identifying community resources such as the local health office or clinic.
- Be aware of family patterns and how the client and family interact with each other. Family disruption and weak intergenerational ties can increase a client's risk for injury due to violent behavior.

---

fires (*Injury Fact Book 2001-2002,* 2002). Advancing age and the concurrent physiological changes in vision, hearing, mobility, reflexes, circulation, and the ability to make quick judgments all predispose older adults to falls (see Chapter 13). When a client is hospitalized, confusion, multiple medical problems, sedating medications, generalized weakness, postural instability, and an unfamiliar environment are major contributors to falling (Ebersole and Hess, 2001). Certain disease states common to older adults, such as arthritis or cerebrovascular accidents, increase chances of injury.

Older adults are more likely to have automobile accidents because of three specific physiological changes. First, changes in visual acuity, depth perception, and poor peripheral vision prevent the client from quickly observing situations in which an accident is likely to occur. Second, decreased hearing acuity alters the older client's ability to hear emergency vehicle sirens or car and truck horns. Third, because of decreased nervous system response, older adults may be unable to react as quickly as they once could to avoid an accident (Ebersole and Hess, 2001). A decline in these skills may account for the most common types of accidents, including right-of-way and turning accidents. The nurse can educate clients regarding safe driving tips (e.g., driving shorter distances or only in daylight, using side and rearview mirrors carefully, and looking behind them toward their "blind spot" before changing lanes). If hearing is a problem, the client might try to keep a window rolled down while driving or

reduce the volume of the radio or CD or cassette player. Eventually, counseling may be necessary to help clients make the decision of when to stop driving. At that time the nurse should help locate resources in the community that provide transportation.

Burns and scalds are also more apt to occur with older people because they may forget and leave hot water running or become confused when turning the dials on a stove or other heating appliance. Nursing measures for preventing burns are designed to minimize the risk from impaired vision. Hot water faucets and dials can be color coded to make it easier for the adult to know what has been turned on. Recommending a reduction in temperature of the water heater can also be very beneficial.

Older adults love to walk. Pedestrian accidents can be reduced for older adults and for all other age-groups by persuading people to wear reflectors on garments when walking at night; to stand on the sidewalk and not in the street when waiting to cross a street; to always cross at corners and not in the middle of the block (particularly if the street is a major one); to cross with the traffic light and not against it; and to look left, right, and left again before entering the street or crosswalk.

Environmental Interventions. Nursing interventions directed at eliminating environmental threats include general preventive measures such as meeting basic needs, reducing physical hazards, and reducing pathogen transmission.

Table 37-2 Interventions to Promote Safety for Children and Adolescents

Intervention	Rationale
Infants and Toddlers	
Have infants sleep on their backs or sides. Teach parents the mnemonic "back to sleep."	Sleeping on the stomach with the mouth and nose in close proximity to the mattress is associated with sudden infant death syndrome (SIDS) (Hauk and others, 2003).
Do not fill cribs with pillows, large stuffed toys, or comforters. Sheets should fit snugly.	Infants may become entwined in sheets and other bedding and suffocate.
Pacifiers should not be attached to string or ribbon and placed around a child's neck.	Choking may occur.
All instructions for preparing and storing formula must be followed.	Proper formula preparation and storage prevents contamination. A formula may come in a concentrated form, or it may already be diluted and ready to use. Following directions ensures proper concentration of the formula. Undiluted formula can cause fluid and electrolyte disturbances; very diluted formula will not provide sufficient nutrients.
Use large, soft toys without small parts, such as buttons.	Small parts can become dislodged, and choking and aspiration may occur.
Playpens with mesh sides should not be left with a side down; spaces between crib slats should be less than 2⅜ inches (6 cm) apart.	A child's head may become wedged in the lowered mesh side or in between crib slats, and asphyxiation may occur.
Never leave crib sides down or leave babies unattended on changing tables or in infant seats, walkers, swings, strollers, or high chairs.	Infants and toddlers can roll or move and fall from changing tables or out of accessories such as infant seats or walkers.
Discontinue using accessories such as infant seats, walkers, and swings when the child becomes too active, physically too big, and/or according to the manufacturer's directions.	When physically active or too big, the child can fall out of or tip over these accessories and suffer an injury.
Never leave a child alone in the bathroom, tub, or near any water source (e.g., pool).	Accidental drowning may occur.
Baby-proof the home; remove small or sharp objects and toxic or poisonous substances, including plants; install safety locks on floor-level cabinets.	Babies explore their world with their hands and mouth. Choking and poisoning may occur.
Remove plastic bags from the cleaners or grocery store from the home.	Suffocation may occur if plastic covers the nose and mouth.
Electrical outlets should have covers (Figure 37-8).	Crawling babies may insert objects into outlets and experience an electrical shock.
Window guards should be on all windows.	This prevents children from falling out of windows.
Install keyless locks (e.g., deadbolts) on doors above a child's reach, even when they are standing on a chair.	This prevents a toddler from leaving the house and wandering off. Death from exposure, car accidents, and drowning may occur. Keyless locks allow for rapid exit in case of fire.
Children weighing less than 80 pounds or under 8 years of age should always be in an age/weight-appropriate car seat that has been installed according to the manufacturer's instructions (Figure 37-9). This includes car seats and booster seats. In cars with a passenger air bag, children under 12 should be in the back seat. All passengers should have seat belts on.	In case of a sudden stop or crash, an unrestrained child may suffer severe head injuries and death.

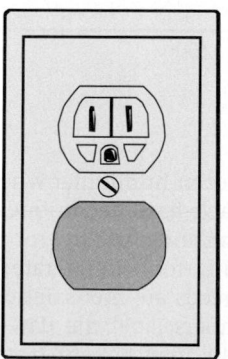

FIGURE **37-8** Safety covers for electrical outlets.

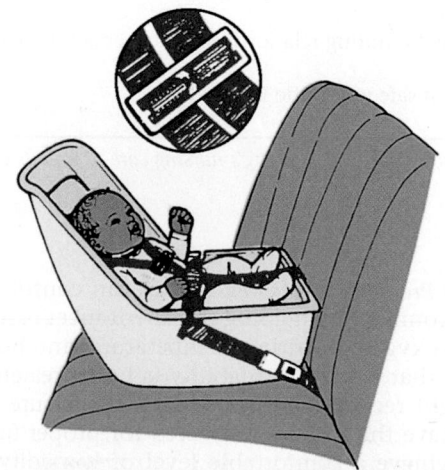

FIGURE **37-9** Infant car seat.

Continued

Table 37-2 Interventions to Promote Safety for Children and Adolescents—cont'd

Intervention	Rationale
Infants and Toddlers—*cont'd*	
Caregivers should learn cardiopulmonary resuscitation (CPR) and the Heimlich maneuver.	Caregivers should be prepared to intervene in acute emergencies, such as choking.
Preschoolers	
Teach children to swim at an early age, but always provide supervision near water.	Learning to swim is a useful skill that may someday save a child's life. However, all children need constant supervision near water.
Teach children how to cross streets and walk in parking lots. Instruct them to never run out after a ball or toy.	Pedestrian accidents involving young children are common.
Teach children not to talk to, go with, or accept any item from a stranger.	This reduces the risk of injury and stranger abduction.
Teach children basic physical safety rules, such as proper use of safety scissors, never running with an object in their mouth or hand, and never attempting to use the stove or oven unassisted.	Risk of injury is lowered if children are taught basic safety procedures.
Teach children not to eat items found in the street or grass.	Poisoning may occur.
Remove doors from unused refrigerators and freezers. Instruct children not to play or hide in a car trunk or unused appliances.	If a child cannot freely exit from appliances and car trunks, asphyxiation may occur.
School-Age Children	
Teach children the safe use of equipment for play and work.	The child needs to learn the safe, appropriate use of implements to avoid injury.
Teach children proper bicycle safety, including use of helmet and rules of the road.	This may reduce injuries from falling off a bike or being hit by a car.
Teach children proper techniques for specific sports, as well as the need to wear proper safety gear (e.g., eyewear, mouth guards).	Using proper sports techniques, correct equipment, and protective gear prevents injuries.
Teach children not to operate electrical equipment while unsupervised.	If an electrical mishap were to occur, no one would be available to help.
Children should never have access to firearms or other weapons. All firearms should be kept in locked cabinets.	Children are often fascinated by firearms and weapons and may attempt to play with them.
Adolescents	
Encourage enrollment in driver's education classes.	Many injuries in this age-group are related to motor vehicle accidents.
Provide information about the effects of using alcohol and drugs.	Adolescents are prone to risk-taking behaviors and are subject to peer pressures.
Provide sex education, emphasizing safe sex practices, including abstinence.	Many adolescents begin sexual relationships. Pregnancy and sexually transmitted diseases may result.
Refer adolescents to community and school-sponsored activities.	The adolescent needs to socialize with peers, yet needs some supervision.
Encourage mentoring relationships between adults and adolescents.	Adolescents are in need of role models after whom they can pattern their behavior.
Teach them safe use of the Internet.	Avoids overuse and possible exposure to inappropriate websites.

Modified from Wong DL: *Wong's nursing care of infants and children,* ed 7, St. Louis, 2003, Mosby.

General Preventive Measures. Nurses can contribute to a safer environment by helping the client meet basic needs related to oxygen, nutrition, temperature, and humidity. To ensure that oxygen availability is not threatened, the nurse might recommend that the client be sure to periodically have the furnace inspected for proper functioning. To achieve a comfortable level of humidity in the home, the client might attach a humidifier to the furnace or, in the case of clients who have upper respiratory tract infections, use a room humidifier where the client sleeps. The nurse can teach basic techniques for food handling (e.g., hand washing and checking for spoilage) and preparation (e.g., keeping food refrigerated before serving) so that nutritional needs are met safely. It is also helpful to have family members label the date when leftovers are saved. Older adults may benefit from Meals on Wheels services. These services provide fresh nutritious meals to older adults who have difficulty preparing their own

Focus on Older Adults   **Box 37-6**

- The older adult experiences alterations in vision and hearing. The nurse should encourage yearly vision and hearing examinations and frequent cleansing of glasses and hearing aids as a means of preventing falls and burns.
- Older adults may have slowed reaction time. Teach clients safety tips for avoiding automobile accidents. Driving may need to be restricted to daylight hours or suspended.
- Range of motion, flexibility, and strength are decreased. The nurse should encourage supervised exercise classes for older adults and teach them to seek assistance with household tasks as needed. Safety features, such as grab bars in the bathroom, may be needed.
- Reflexes are slowed, and the ability to respond to multiple stimuli is reduced. The nurse should provide adequate, meaningful stimuli but prevent sensory overload.
- Nocturia and incontinence are more frequent in older adults. The nurse should institute a regular toileting schedule for the client. A recommended frequency is every 3 hours. Diuretics should be given in the morning. Assistance should be provided, along with adequate lighting, to clients who need to go to the bathroom at night.
- Memory may be impaired. Clients should use medication organizers, which can be purchased at any drugstore at a very reasonable cost. These dispensers can be filled once a week with the proper medications to be taken at a specific time during the day.
- The family plays a significant role in the care of older adults. It is estimated that more than 8 million older adults living at home need and get some form of help from family and friends (Ebersole and Hess, 2001). Encourage the family to allow the older adult to remain as independent as possible and provide help only for those things that are especially stressful or depleted.
- The high prevalence of chronic conditions in older adults results in the use of a high number of prescription and over-the-counter medications. Coupled with age-related changes in pharmacokinetics, there is a greater risk of serious adverse effects. Medications typically prescribed for older adults include anticholinergics, diuretics, anxiolytic and hypnotic agents, antidepressants, antihypertensives, vasodilators, analgesics, and laxatives, all of which may themselves pose risks or may interact to increase the risk for falls. The nurse should review the client's drug profile to ensure that any of the above noted drugs are used cautiously and assess the client regularly for any adverse effects that may increase fall risk.

food. Client education for older adults or clients who enjoy outdoor activities should include ways to prevent and treat frostbite, hypothermia, heatstroke, and heat exhaustion (see Chapter 31).

Adequate lighting and security measures in and around the home, including the use of night-lights, exterior lighting, and locks on windows and doors, enable clients to reduce the risk of injury from crime. The local police department and community organizations often have safety classes available for residents to learn how to take precautions to minimize the chance of becoming involved in a crime. For example, some useful tips include always parking the car near a bright light or busy public area, carrying a whistle attached to the car keys, keeping car doors locked while driving, and always paying attention while driving to notice if anyone starts to follow the car.

To prevent the transmission of pathogens, nurses can teach aseptic practices. Medical asepsis, which includes hand hygiene and environmental cleanliness, reduces the transfer of organisms (see Chapter 33). Clients and family members need to learn thorough hand hygiene (hand washing or use of hand rub) and when to use it (e.g., before and after caring for a family member, before food preparation, before preparing a medication for a family member, and after contacting any body fluids). When clients require dressing changes or the use of syringes and needles, families should be shown how to properly dispose of contaminated items in the home. Most communities have regulations for the disposal of biohazardous waste.

Acute Care. There are a number of specific safety measures applicable to clients in the acute care environment. The nurse takes measures to help clients avoid falls, injuries from use of restraints and side rails, fires, poisoning, and electrical hazards. Special precautions are necessary to prevent injury in clients susceptible to having seizures. Radiation injuries are also a specific safety concern. Finally, the nurse must be prepared to respond to the emergency of a bioterrorist attack.

Falls. Modifications in the home and health care environment can easily reduce the risk of falls (Table 37-3). A heavy or debilitated client in a bed or wheelchair or on a toilet should be properly supported and secured. Side rails may be necessary unless a client is able to freely and easily ambulate independently. Safety bars on toilets, locks on beds and wheelchairs, and call lights are additional safety features found in health care settings (Figures 37-10 and 37-11). Excess furniture and equipment should be removed, and a weakened client should wear rubber-soled shoes or slippers for walking or transferring. When clients use assistive aids such as canes, crutches, or walkers, it is important to routinely check the condition of rubber tips and the integrity of the aid.

To reduce the risk of injury in the home, all obstacles should be removed from halls and other heavily traveled areas. Necessary objects such as clocks, glasses, tissues, or medications should remain on bedside tables within reach of the client but out of the reach of children. Care should also be taken to ensure that end tables are secure and have stable, straight legs. Nonessential items should be placed in drawers to eliminate clutter. If small area rugs are used, they should be secured with a nonslip pad or skid-resistant adhesive strips. Any carpeting on the stairs should be secured with carpet tacks.

Because falls cannot always be prevented, client-specific modifications may be necessary to reduce the risk of injury related to a fall. Research has shown that the use of an external hip protector can considerably reduce the risk of hip fractures among ambulatory older adults (Box 37-7).

Table 37-3   Measures to Prevent Falls by Older Adults

Measure	Rationale
Stairs	
Install treads with uniform depth of 9 inches (22.5 cm) and 9-inch risers (vertical face of steps).	If stairs are of uniform size, older adults do not have to continually adjust vision.
Install uniform-textured or plain-colored surfaces on each tread, and mark edge of tread with contrasting color.	Uniform textures or color help to decrease vertigo. Marking edge of tread provides obvious visual clue to end of stair.
Ensure proper lighting of each tread. Block sun or lightbulb glare with translucent shades or screen, or use lower-wattage or nonglare bulbs.	Older adults' vision is unable to adjust quickly to changes in lighting.
Ensure adequate head room so that users do not have to duck to negotiate stairs.	Sudden changes in head position may result in dizziness.
Remove protruding objects from staircase walls.	Decreased peripheral vision may prevent client from seeing object.
Maintain outdoor walkways and stairs in good condition and free of holes, cracks, and splinters.	Decreased visual acuity can prevent client from seeing any structural defect.
Handrails	
Install smooth but slip-resistant handrail at least 2 inches (5 cm) from wall.	Two-inch distance allows client to grasp handrail firmly for support.
Secure handrail firmly so that user's weight is supported, especially at bottom and top of stairway.	Older adults have greatest risk of falling at top and bottom of stairs, because center of gravity is being shifted and balance is unstable.
Install grab rails in bathroom near toilet and tub.	This enables client to have support while rising from sitting to standing position.
Floors	
Ensure that clients wear properly fitting shoes or slippers with nonskid surface.	Reduces chances of slipping.
Secure all carpeting, mats, and tile; place nonskid backing under small rugs.	Sudden slip may cause dizziness and inability to regain balance.
Place bath mats or nonskid strips on bathtub or shower stall floors.	Wet surfaces increase the risk of falling.
Secure electrical cords against baseboards.	Prevents tripping.
Maintain proper illumination in areas both inside and outside where the client moves and walks.	Reduces the risk of falling due to eyestrain.
Health Care Facility	
Orientation	
Place disoriented clients in room near nurses' station.	Provides for more frequent observation by nursing staff.
Maintain close supervision of confused clients.	Confused clients often attempt to wander out of bed or room.
Show the client how to use the call light at the bedside and in bathroom, and place within easy reach.	Location and use of the call light is essential to client safety.
Place bedside tables and over-bed tables close to client.	Prevents client from searching or overreaching for items such as eyeglasses, dentures, hearing aid, or telephone.
Remove clutter from bedside tables, hallways, bathrooms, and grooming areas.	Eliminates potential hazards and promotes client independence.
Leave one side rail up and one down on the side where the oriented and ambulatory client gets out of bed.	Client can use the side rail for support when getting in and out of bed and to position self once in bed.
Transport	
Lock beds and wheelchairs when transferring a client from a bed to a wheelchair or back to bed.	Provides stability and support during transfer.
Place side rails in the up position, and secure safety straps around the client on a stretcher.	Prevents the client from rolling off the stretcher.

Restraints. A physical **restraint** is a mechanical or physical device that is used to immobilize a client or extremity, restricts the freedom of movement or normal access to a person's body, and is not a usual part of treatment plans indicated by the person's condition or symptoms (Zusman, 2001). The optimal goal for all clients is a restraint-free environment; however, clients who are at risk for injury from wandering, falls, and disruptive or agitated behavior may need restraints temporarily.

Whenever a client is restrained, there is a natural tendency for the client to try to remove the restraint. When this occurs, client injury is common. Restrained clients can

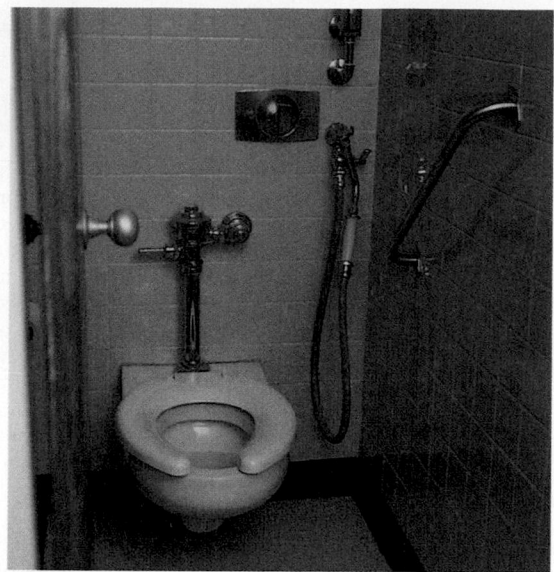

FIGURE **37–10** Safety bars around toilets and showers

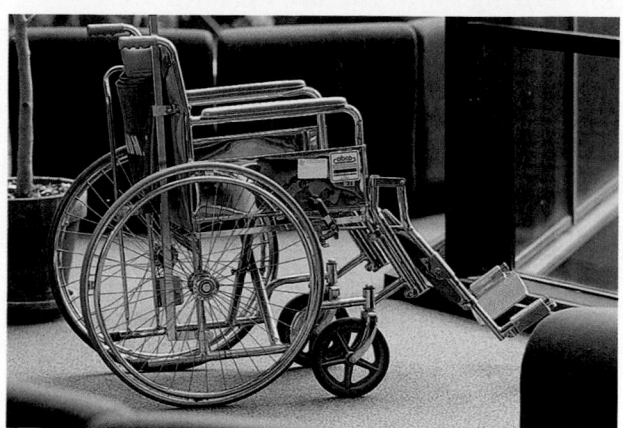

FIGURE **37–11** Safety locks on wheelchairs.

easily become entangled in a restraint device in attempts to get out of the device. In some cases, death has resulted due to strangulation or asphyxiation. As a result, nursing homes and many health care facilities have banned the use of the jacket (vest) restraint because of this risk. This text will discuss proper use of the vest restraint because if it becomes necessary for a nurse to apply a vest restraint, it must be done safely. The use of any restraint is also associated with serious complications, including pressure ulcers, constipation, pneumonia, urinary and fecal incontinence, and urinary retention (see Chapter 46). Contractures, nerve damage, and circulatory impairment are also potential hazards. In addition, restrained clients can experience a loss of self-esteem, humiliation, fear, and anger.

> *Safety Alert.* Routine assessment of a client in restraint is critical to prevent injury. Because of the risk of injury from restraints, regulatory agencies such as the JCAHO and the Centers for Medicaid and Medicare Services (CMS) enforce standards for the safe use of restraints and define clients' rights and choices regarding their use. Under these guidelines, reasons for use of a physical restraint are to be clearly stated. The use of restraints must be part of the client's medical treatment, all less restrictive interventions must be tried first, other disciplines must be consulted, and supporting documentation must be provided (CMS, 2001).

The impetus is for health care organizations to move to a restraint-free environment. Restraints do not prevent falls or injury. In fact, it has been shown that clients incur less severe injuries if left unrestrained (Capezuti and others, 1998; Strumpf and others, 1998). Research has shown that a multidisciplinary approach that conducts individualized assessments and develops structured treatment plans can reduce the number of restraints used. It is imperative that nurses try alternative measures instead of restraints (Box 37-8). The University of Iowa Gerontological Nursing Interventions

Research Center has developed a restraint use algorithm (Figure 37-12). The algorithm provides evidenced-based guidelines for how to determine if a restraint is appropriate and what interventions might be employed.

The use of restraints involves a psychological adjustment for the client and family. If restraints must be used, the nurse assists family members and clients by explaining their purpose, expected care while the client is restrained, precautions taken to avoid injury, and that the restraint is temporary and protective. Informed consent from family members may also be required before using restraints, as is the case in long-term care settings.

For legal purposes, the nurse must know agency-specific policy and procedures for appropriate use and monitoring of restraints. The use of a restraint must be clinically justified and be a part of the client's prescribed medical treatment and plan of care. A physician's order is required, based on a face-to-face assessment of the client. The order must state the type of restraint, location, and specific client behaviors for which restraints are to be used and must have a limited time frame. These orders should be renewed within a specific time frame according to the agency's policy. Restraints are not to be ordered prn (as needed). Assessment of clients who are restrained must be ongoing. Proper documentation, including the behaviors that necessitated the application of restraints, the procedure used in restraining, the condition of the body part restrained (e.g., circulation to hand), and the evaluation of the client response, is essential. Restraints must be periodically removed, and the nurse must assess the client to determine if the restraints continue to be needed.

Skill 37-1 includes guidelines for the proper use and application of restraints. Use of restraints must meet the following objectives:
- Reduce the risk of client injury from falls.
- Prevent interruption of therapy such as traction, IV infusions, nasogastric (NG) tube feeding, or Foley catheterization.

Text continued on p. 990

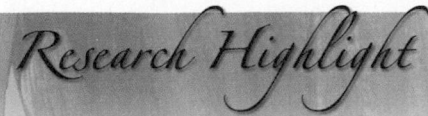

Box 37-7

Preventing Hip Fractures From Falls

Research Focus

Hip fractures in older adults are a major cause of disability, functional impairment, and death. Frequency of hip fractures is expected to increase because the number and age of older adults is also increasing. Nurses play a key role in the prevention of falls, as well as injuries related to falls.

Research Abstract

This article describes a study investigating the effect of an anatomically designed external hip protector in the prevention of hip fractures among older adults. The hip protector is shaped to cover the proximal femur and designed to shunt the energy of an impact away from the hip to the soft tissues surrounding the hip. Two protectors are worn with the use of a stretchy undergarment containing a pocket on each side for placement of the protector. In this study 1801 ambulatory, but frail, older adults (1409 women and 392 men) with a mean age of 82 years were randomly assigned (in a 1:2 ratio) either to a group that wore a hip protector or to a control group that did not wear a hip protector; 643 subjects entered the hip protector group, whereas 1148 subjects entered the control group. All fractures, including pelvic, leg, and arm fractures, were recorded until the end of the first full month (2 years later) after 62 hip fractures had occurred in the control group. The risk of fracture in the two groups was compared. In the hip protector group the risk of fracture was also analyzed according to whether the protector had been worn at the time of the fall.

A total of 1404 falls occurred in the hip protector group. Of those falls, 74% (1034) occurred while subjects wore the hip protector. The results showed that 13 subjects in the hip protector group had a hip fracture, as compared with 67 subjects in the control group. In the hip protector group 4 of those subjects were wearing the hip protector, whereas 9 subjects did not wear their hip protector. In the hip protector group 2 subjects had pelvic fractures, as compared with 12 subjects in the control group. The risk of other fractures was similar in the two groups. The results of this trial indicate that the risk of hip fracture among ambulatory older adults can be reduced by more than 80% if the protector is worn at the time of a fall.

Evidenced-Based Practice

- Identify clients who are at high risk for hip fractures (previous fall or fracture, impaired balance or mobility, use of a walking aid, cognitive impairment, impaired vision, poor nutrition, disease or medication known to predispose a person to a fall and/or fracture).
- Utilize hip protectors on those clients who are at high risk for hip fractures.
- Provide frequent reminders to the client and family about the importance of fall prevention strategies and ways to reduce the risk of injury.

Reference

Kannus P and others: Prevention of hip fracture in elderly people with use of a hip protector, *N Engl J Med* 343:1506, 2000.

Box 37-8   **Alternatives to Restraints**

- Orient clients and families to surroundings; explain all procedures and treatments to them.
- Encourage family and friends to stay, or use trained sitters for clients who need continuous supervision.
- Assign confused or disoriented clients to rooms near the nurses' station. Observe these clients frequently. Institute reality orientation measures (e.g., frequent reminders of person, time, and place; use of environmental aids such as clocks or calendars [see Chapter 48]).
- Provide appropriate visual and auditory stimuli (e.g., family pictures, clock, radio).
- Eliminate bothersome treatments as soon as possible. For example, discontinue tube feedings and begin oral feedings as quickly as allowed by the client's condition.

- Use relaxation techniques (e.g., music suited to client's taste, massage).
- Institute exercise and ambulation schedules as allowed by the client's condition.
- Provide scheduled toileting, especially during peak fall times such as 6 to 8 AM and 4 to 6 PM.
- Consult with physical and occupational therapists to enhance clients' abilities to carry out activities of daily living.
- Evaluate all medications clients are receiving to determine if the medication is having the desired therapeutic effect.
- Conduct ongoing assessment and evaluation of clients' care and their ongoing response to care.

Data from Stolley J: Freeing your patients from restraints, *Am J Nurs* 95(2): 27, 1995; Quinn CA: The advanced practice nurse and changing perspectives on physical restraint, *Clin Nurs Spec* 10(5): 223, 1996.

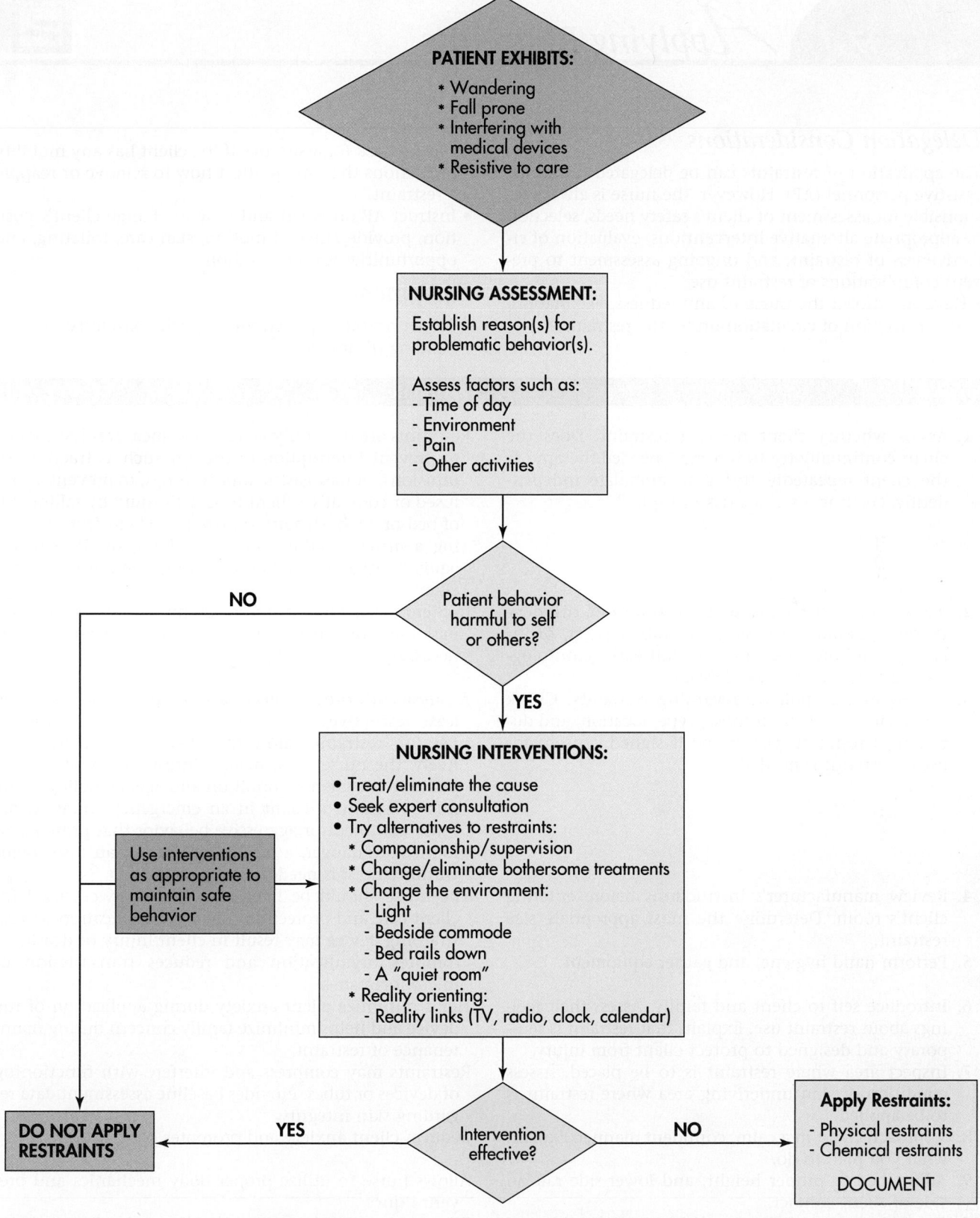

FIGURE **37–12** Restraint use algorithm. (Developed from "Restraints"—a research-based protocol by L. Ledford, MA, ARNP and J. Mentals, MS, RNCS, GNP. Copyright 1998, University of Iowa Gerontological Nursing Interventions Research Center.)

Skill 37-1   *Applying Restraints*

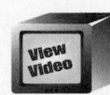

Delegation Considerations

The application of restraints can be delegated to trained assistive personnel (AP). However, the nurse is always responsible for assessment of client's safety needs, selection of appropriate alternative interventions, evaluation of effectiveness of restraint, and ongoing assessment to prevent complications of restraint use.

• Have AP inform the nurse of any redness, excoriation, or constriction of circulation under the restraint.

• Have AP ask for assistance if the client has any mobility restrictions that might affect how to remove or reapply a restraint.

• Instruct AP on when and how to change client's position, provide range of motion, skin care, toileting, and opportunities for socialization.

Equipment

• Proper restraint: jacket, mitten, belt, extremity
• Padding (if needed)

Steps	Rationale
1. Assess whether client needs a restraint. Does the client continually try to interrupt needed therapy? Is the client repeatedly trying to ambulate independently, creating a serious risk of injury?	Restraints are used only when other measures have failed to prevent interruption of therapy such as traction, IV infusions, or nasogastric tube feedings; to prevent a confused or combative client from self-injury by falling out of bed or a wheelchair; to prevent a client from removing a urinary catheter, surgical drain, or life support equipment; and to reduce risk of injury to others by the client.
2. Assess client's behavior, such as confusion, disorientation, agitation, restlessness, combativeness, or inability to follow directions. Consult with gerontological nurse specialist if available.	If client's behavior continues despite attempts to eliminate cause of behavior, use of physical restraint may be necessary.
3. Review agency policies regarding restraints. Check physician's order for purpose, type, location, and duration of restraint. Determine if signed consent for use of restraint is needed.	A physician's order is necessary to apply restraints. The least restrictive type of restraint should be ordered. Because restraints limit the client's ability to move freely, the nurse must make clinical judgments appropriate to the client's condition and agency policy. If the nurse restrains a client in an emergency situation because of violent or aggressive behavior that presents an immediate danger, a face-to-face physician assessment within 1 hour is needed (CMS, 2001).
4. Review manufacturer's instructions before entering client's room. Determine the most appropriate size restraint.	The nurse should be familiar with all devices used for client care and protection. Incorrect application of a restraining device may result in client injury or death.
5. Perform hand hygiene, and gather equipment.	Promotes organization and reduces transmission of microorganisms.
6. Introduce self to client and family. Assess their feelings about restraint use. Explain that restraint is temporary and designed to protect client from injury.	Helps minimize client anxiety during application of the device and helps minimize family concern during maintenance of restraint.
7. Inspect area where restraint is to be placed. Assess condition of skin underlying area where restraint is to be applied.	Restraints may compress and interfere with functioning of devices or tubes. Provides baseline assessment data regarding skin integrity.
8. Approach client in a calm, confident manner. Explain what you plan to do.	Reduces client anxiety and promotes cooperation.
9. Adjust bed to proper height, and lower side rail on side of client contact.	Allows nurse to utilize proper body mechanics and prevent injury.
10. Provide privacy. Make sure client is comfortable and in proper body alignment. Drape client as needed.	Privacy prevents lowering of self-esteem. Proper body alignment promotes comfort, prevents contractures and neurovascular injury.
11. Pad skin and bony prominences (if necessary) before applying restraints.	Padding reduces friction and pressure on skin and underlying tissue.

Steps	Rationale
12. Apply appropriate size restraint, making sure it is not over an IV line or other device (e.g., dialysis shunt).	IV lines and other therapeutic devices may become occluded.
A. **Jacket (vest or Posey) restraint:** Front and back of garment should be labeled as such. Apply over clothing or hospital gown (see illustration). Place client's hands through armholes or sleeves, and secure according to manufacturer's directions. Place straps at client's hips.	Restrains client while lying or reclining in bed and while sitting in chair or wheelchair. Proper application prevents suffocation or choking. Clothing or gown prevents friction against skin.

Critical Decision Point: Check agency policy. Some health care facilities no longer use vest restraints because they have been known to cause death due to strangulation.

B. **Belt restraint:** Device that secures client to bed or stretcher. Apply over clothes or gown. Remove wrinkles from front and back of restraint while placing it around client's waist. Bring ties through slots in belt. Avoid placing belt across the chest or too tightly across the abdomen (see illustration).	Restrains center of gravity and prevents client from rolling off stretcher or sitting up while on stretcher or from falling out of bed. Tight application may interfere with ventilation.

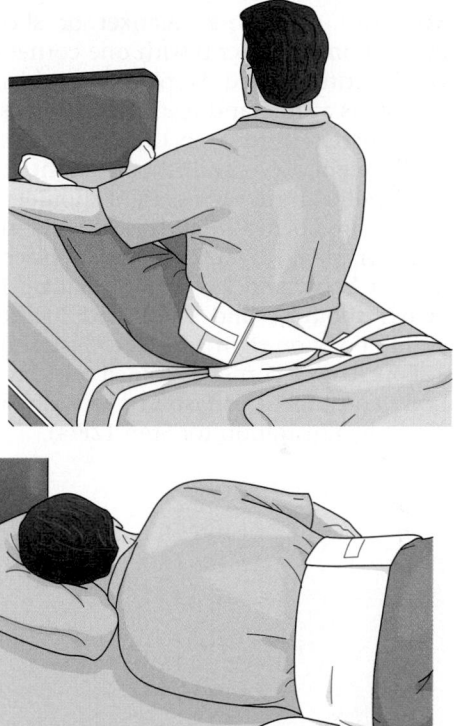

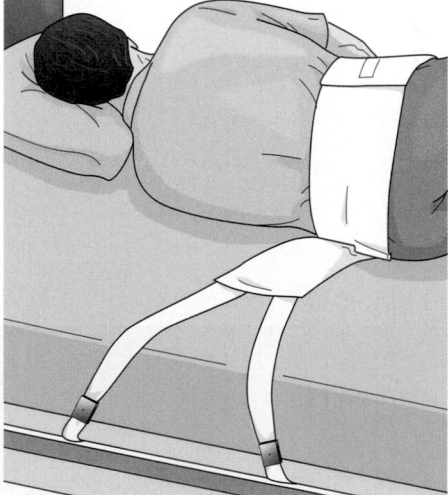

Warning: When a patient is in a restrictive (restraint or self-release) product in bed or on a stretcher or gurney, all side rails MUST be in the UP position. Side rail covers and/or gap protectors must be used when necessary to keep the patient's entire body on the mattress and to eliminate entrapment hazards.

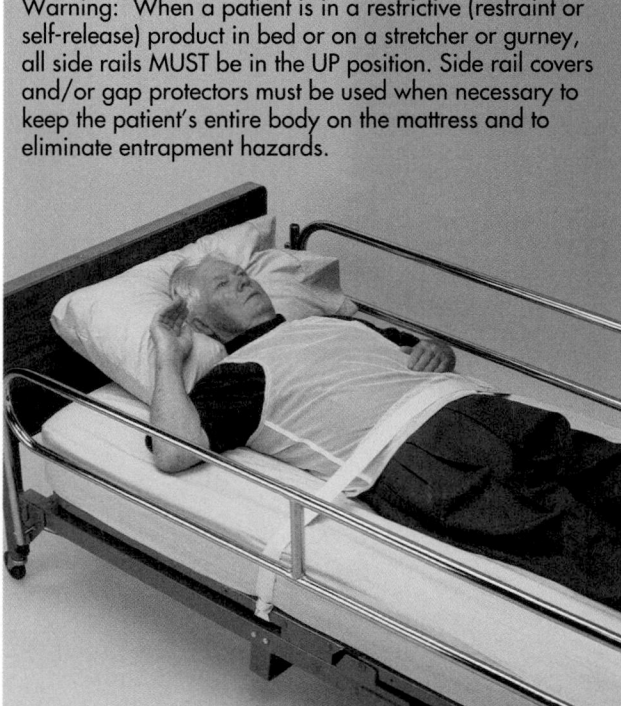

STEP **12A** Vest restraint securely attached to bed frame. (Courtesy JT Posey Co, Arcadia, Calif.)

STEP **12B** Belt restraint tied to the bed frame and to an area that does not cause the restraint to tighten when the side rail is raised or lowered. (From Sorrentino SA: *Mosby's textbook for nursing assistants*, ed 5, St. Louis, 2000, Mosby.)

Skill **37-1**   *Applying Restraints—cont'd*

Steps	Rationale
C. Extremity (ankle or wrist) restraint: Restraint designed to immobilize one or all extremities. Commercially available limb restraints are composed of sheepskin or foam padding (see illustration). Limb restraint is wrapped around wrist or ankle with soft part toward skin and secured snugly in place by Velcro straps.	Maintains immobilization of extremity to protect client from injury from fall or accidental removal of therapeutic device (e.g., IV tube or Foley catheter). Tight application may interfere with circulation.
D. Mitten restraint: Thumbless mitten device to restrain client's hands (see illustration). Place hand in mitten, being sure end is brought all the way up over the wrist.	Prevents clients from dislodging invasive equipment, removing dressings, or scratching, yet allows greater movement than a wrist restraint.
E. Elbow restraint: Piece of fabric with slots in which tongue blades are placed so that elbow joint remains rigid (see illustration).	Commonly used with infants and children to prevent elbow flexion (e.g., when an IV line is in place).
F. Mummy restraint: Blanket or sheet that is opened on bed or crib with one corner folded toward center. Child is placed on blanket with shoulders at fold and feet toward opposite corner (see illustration for Step 12F-1). With child's right arm straight down against body, right side of blanket is pulled firmly across right shoulder and chest and secured beneath left side of body (see illustration for Step 12F-2). Left arm is placed straight against body, and left side of blanket is brought across shoulder and chest and locked beneath child's body on right side (see illustration for Step 12F-3). Lower corner is folded and brought over body and tucked or fastened securely with safety pins (see illustration for Step 12F-4).	Maintains short-term restraint of small child or infant for examination or treatment involving head and neck. Effectively controls movement of torso and extremities.

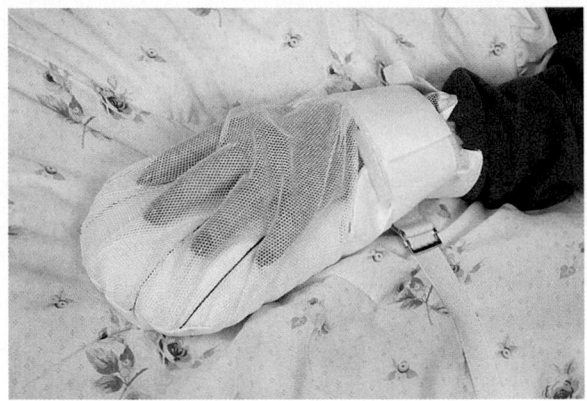

STEP **12D** Mitten restraint.

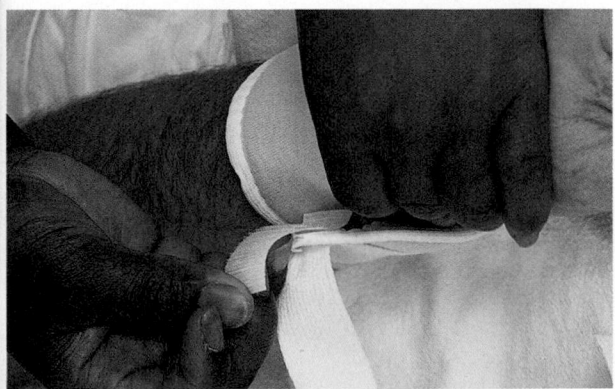

STEP **12C** Extremity restraint being applied to wrist.

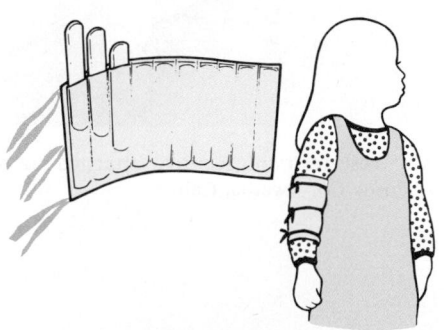

STEP **12E** Elbow restraint.

Steps	Rationale

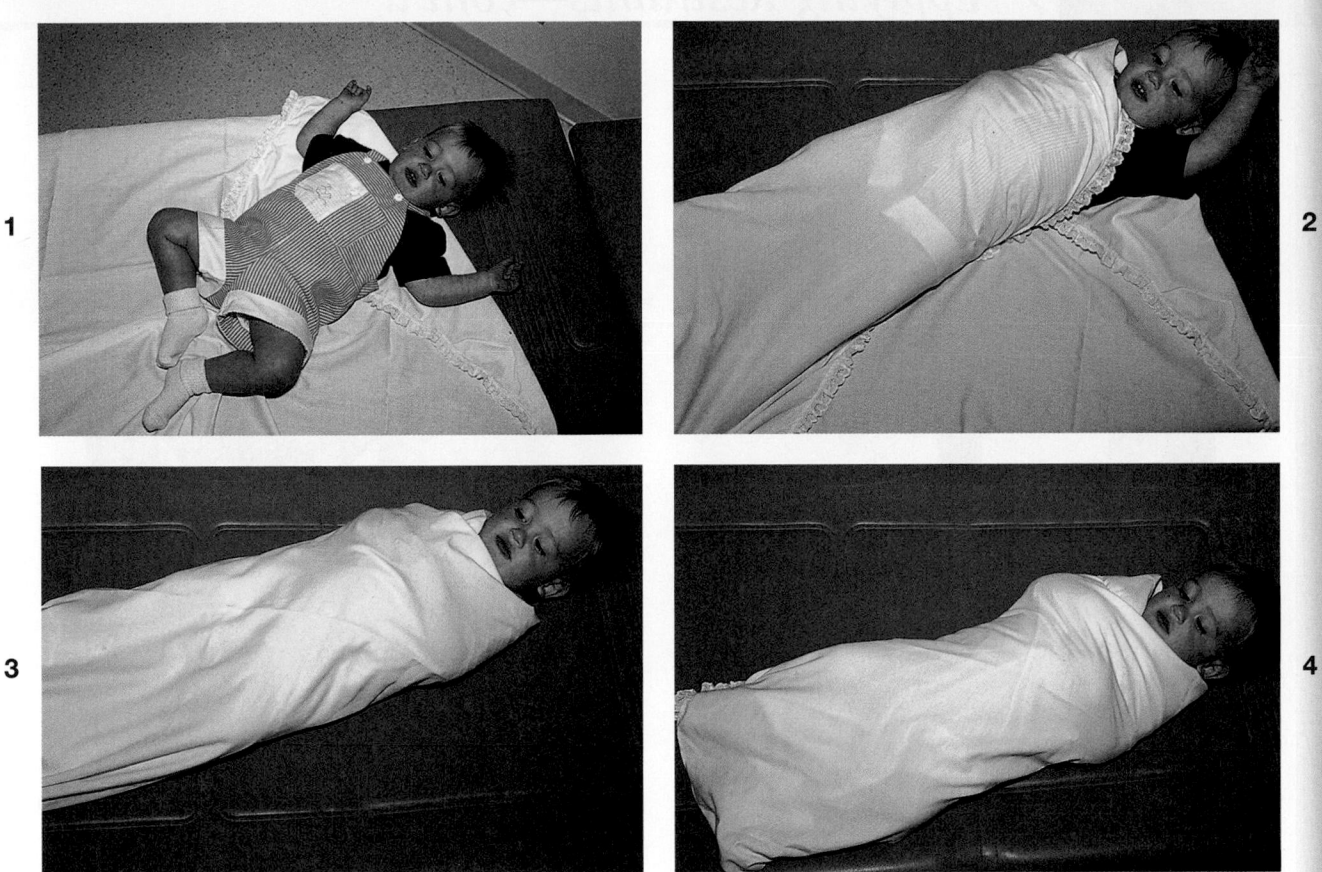

STEP **12F** Mummy restraint.

Steps	Rationale
13. Attach restraints to bed frame, which moves when the head of bed is raised or lowered (see illustration).	Client may be injured if restraint is secured to side rail and it is lowered.

Critical Decision Point: Do not attach end of restraint to side rails.

14. When a jacket restraint is used on a client in a wheel-chair, it should be secured by placing ties under armrests and securing at the back of chair (see illustration).	Prevents client from sliding restraint ties up the back of the chair.

Critical Decision Point: If ties are not under armrests, clients may be able to slide ties up the back of the chair and free themselves.

15. Secure restraints with a quick-release tie (see illustration). Do not tie in a knot.	Allows for quick release in an emergency.
16. Insert two fingers under the secured restraint (see illustration).	A tight restraint may cause constriction and impede circulation. Checking for constriction prevents neurovascular injury.
17. Proper placement of restraint, skin integrity, pulses, temperature, color and sensation of the restrained body part should be assessed at least every hour or according to agency policy.	Frequent assessment prevents complications, such as suffocation, skin breakdown, and impaired circulation.

Skill 37-1 *Applying Restraints—cont'd*

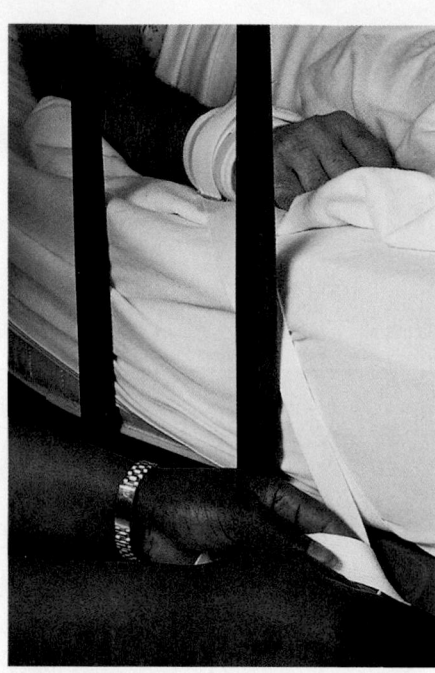

STEP **13**　Tie restraint strap to bed frame.

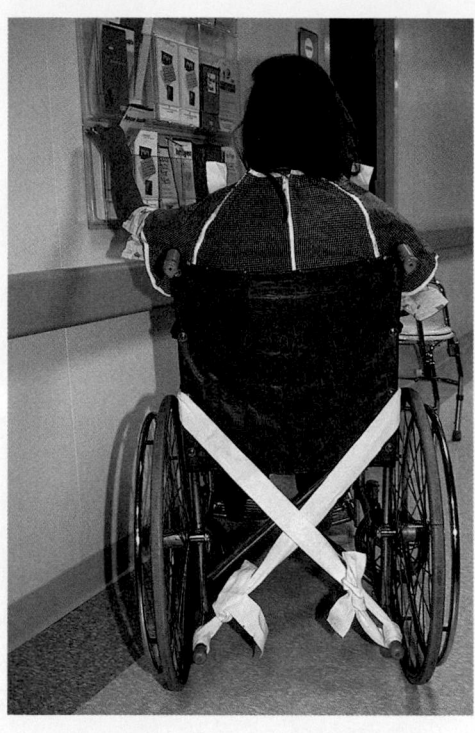

STEP **14**　Straps of vest restraint secured at back of chair.

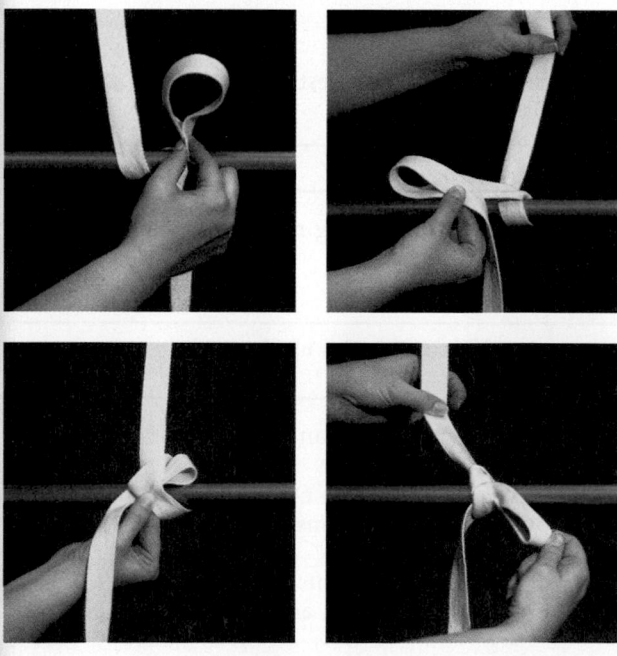

STEP **15**　The Posey quick-release tie. (Courtesy JT Posey Co, Arcadia, Calif.)

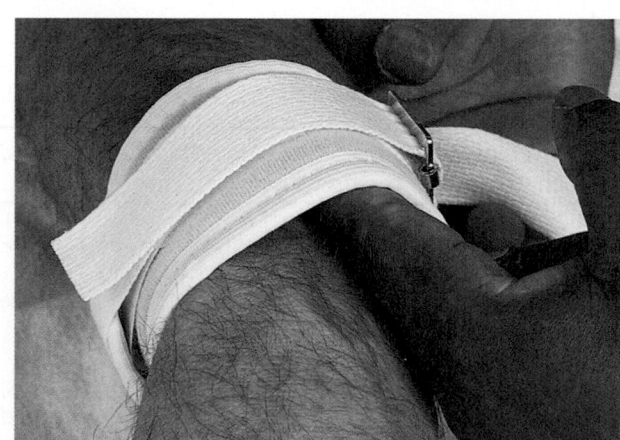

STEP **16**　Place two fingers under restraint to check tightness.

Steps	Rationale
18. Restraints should be removed at least every 2 hours (JCAHO, 2002). If client is violent and noncompliant, remove one restraint at a time and/or have staff assistance while removing restraints. Client should not be left unattended at this time.	Provides opportunity to change client's position and perform full range of motion (ROM), toileting, and exercise and to provide food or fluids.
19. Secure call light or intercom system within reach.	Allows client, family, or caregiver to obtain assistance quickly.
20. Leave bed or chair with wheels locked. Bed should be in lowest position.	Locked wheels prevent bed or chair from moving if client attempts to get out. If client falls when bed is in lowest position, the chances of injury are reduced.
21. Perform hand hygiene.	Reduces transmission of microorganisms.
22. Inspect client for any injury, including all hazards of immobility, while restraints are in use.	Client should be free of injury and not exhibit any signs of immobility complications.
23. Observe IV catheters, urinary catheters, and drainage tubes to ensure that they are positioned correctly and that therapy remains uninterrupted.	Reinsertion can be uncomfortable and can increase risk of infection or interrupt therapy.
24. Reassess client's need for continued use of restraint at least every 24 hours (for medical or surgical reason) with the intent of discontinuing restraint at the earliest possible time (JCAHO, 2002) (see agency-specific policy).	Use of restraints should be seen as a temporary measure and discontinued as soon as possible (Strumpf and others, 1998).
25. Provide appropriate sensory stimulation and reorient client as needed.	Use of restraints can further increase disorientation.

Recording and Reporting

- Record behaviors that place client at risk for injury.
- Describe restraint alternatives attempted and client's response.
- Record client's and/or family's understanding of and consent to restraint application.
- Record type and location of restraint and time applied.
- Record time of assessments and releases.
- Document client's behavior after application of restraint.
- Document specific assessments related to orientation, oxygenation, skin integrity, circulation, and positioning.
- Describe client's response when restraints were removed.

Unexpected Outcomes and Related Interventions

1. Client has signs of impaired skin integrity.
   a. Assess skin, and provide appropriate therapy.
   b. Notify the physician, and reassess the need for continued use of the restraint
   c. Ensure correct application of restraint. Pad skin under a restraint, and remove restraint more frequently.
2. Client has altered neurovascular status to an extremity (cyanosis, pallor, coldness of the skin, or complaints of tingling, pain, or numbness).
   a. Remove restraint immediately, stay with the client, and notify the physician. Protect extremity from further injury (e.g., pressure from tubing or encumbrance, positioning).

3. Client has increased confusion, disorientation, or agitation.
   a. Identify reason for change in behavior, and attempt to eliminate cause.
   b. Attempt a restraint alternative.
4. Client escapes from the restraint device and suffers a fall or injury.
   a. Attend to client's immediate physical needs, and inform physician.
   b. Reassess type of restraint used, correct application, and if alternatives can be used.

Home Care Considerations

- Plan care with family. If possible, use of an Ambularm may free client from physical restraints.
- Instruct family (or other caregiver) in use of alternatives to restraints (see Box 37-8).
- A physical restraint is a device that requires a physician order. It should not be sent home with family unless the device is needed to protect client from injury. If physical restraints are necessary, the family (or other caregiver) must be instructed in proper application, care needed while in restraints, and complications to look for. Also inform caregiver whom to contact if any abnormal findings occur.
- A client who needs to be restrained in bed should have a hospital bed and will require constant supervision in the home.

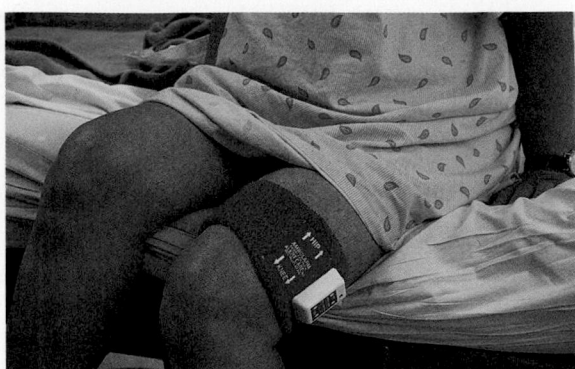

FIGURE **37–13** Client wearing an Ambularm device.

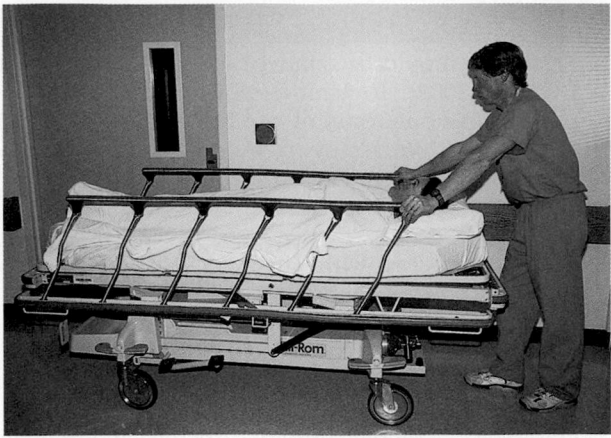

FIGURE **37–15** Side rails in the *up* position on a stretcher.

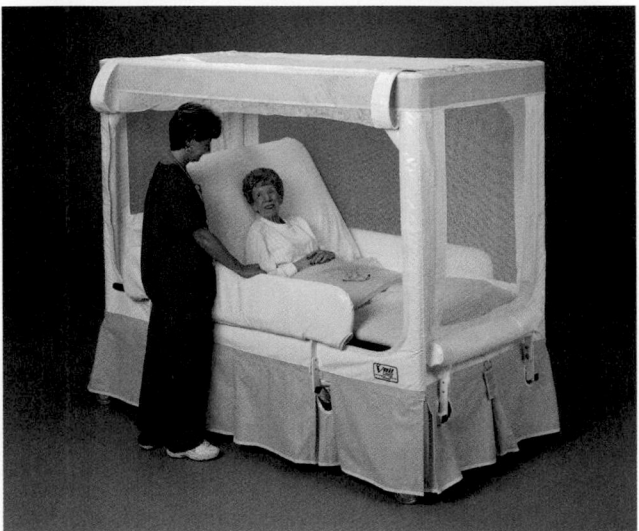

FIGURE **37–14** The Vail Enclosed Bed. (Courtesy Vail Products, Inc., Toledo, Ohio.)

• Prevent the confused or combative client from removing life support equipment.
• Reduce the risk of injury to others by the client.

In keeping with current trends toward health promotion, improved assessment techniques and modifications of the environment are offered as alternatives to restraints. A device known as the **Ambularm** is worn on the leg and signals when the leg is in a dependent position, such as over the side rail or on the floor (Figure 37-13). The device is used for clients who climb out of bed unassisted and are in danger of falling. There are also devices that can be placed on clients' mattresses or attached to the client's nightgown or chair that sound an alarm when triggered. The devices allow a zone of free movement. When the safe zone is exceeded, an alarm sounds. The alarm can be designed to signal at the central nurses' station so that staff are alerted quickly when a client is up and out of bed. There are also alarms that can be placed on doors to alert staff or family members when a confused or disoriented client, prone to wandering, opens a door.

Another alternative to a restraint is the Vail Enclosed Bed (Figure 37-14). The bed is a soft-sided, self-contained enclosed bed that is much less restrictive than chemical or physical restraints. It allows for freedom of movement and thus reduces the side effects caused by physical restraints such as pressure ulcers and loss of dignity. The padded upper frame of the bed is covered by a vinyl top and the nylon-net canopy surrounds the mattress and completely encloses the client in the bed. Zippers on the four sides of the enclosure provide access to the client. The Vail Enclosed Bed works well for clients who are restless and unpredictable, cognitively impaired, and at risk for injury if they were to fall or get out of bed, such as clients on anticoagulant therapy at risk for intracranial bleed. The bed may also be a safer alternative to side rails.

Side Rails. Side rails may help to increase a client's mobility and/or stability when in bed or when moving from bed to chair. Side rails also help prevent the unconscious client from falling out of bed or from a stretcher (Figure 37-15). A full set of raised side rails is considered a restraint if they restrict a client's freedom of voluntary movement in and out of bed (CMS, 2001). The use of side rails alone for a disoriented client may cause more confusion and further injury. A confused client who is determined to get out of bed attempts to climb over the side rail or climbs out at the foot of the bed. Either attempt usually results in a fall or injury. Nursing interventions to reduce a client's confusion should first focus on the cause of the confusion. Frequently nurses mistake a client's attempt to explore his or her environment or to self-toilet as confusion. A thorough assessment is essential. Whenever side rails are used, the bed should be maintained in the lowest position possible.

Safety Alert. Side rails have the potential to cause entrapment of the head and body, especially in older adult clients who are confused and restless. Entrapment has resulted in death, due to asphyxiation, and injuries, such as fractures and lacerations (Capezuti, 2000). To prevent this hazard, assess for excessive gaps and openings between the bed frame and mattress and utilize side rail netting, protective padding, and/or antiskid mats to prevent the mattress from being pushed to one side.

Box 37-9	Fire Intervention Guidelines for Nurses Working in Health Care Agencies

Keep the phone number for reporting fires visible on the telephone at all times.

Know the agency's fire drill and evacuation plan.

Know the location of all fire alarms, exits, extinguishers, and oxygen shut-off.

Use the mnemonic RACE to set priorities in case of fire:

R Rescue and remove all clients in immediate danger.

A Activate the alarm. Always do this before attempting to extinguish even a minor fire.

C Confine the fire by closing doors and windows and turning off oxygen and electrical equipment.

E Extinguish the fire using an extinguisher (see Box 37-10).

Fires. A fire is always possible in the home or hospital. Accidental home fires typically result from smoking in bed, placing cigarettes in trashcans, grease fires, or electrical fires resulting from faulty wiring or appliances. Institutional fires typically result from an electrical or anesthetic-related fire. Although smoking is usually not allowed in the hospital setting, smoking-related fires continue to pose a significant risk due to unauthorized smoking in bed.

The interventions described here are directed toward fires occurring in health care agencies, but the same principles apply for fires in the home (Box 37-9). Homes should be equipped with smoke and fire alarms. It is important to have a plan of action in the event of fire, including a route of exit and identification of a location where family members will meet. All clients, even young children, should be familiar with the phrase "stop, drop and roll," which describes the actions to be followed when a client's clothing and skin are burning.

If a fire occurs in a health care agency, the nurse protects clients from immediate injury, reports the exact location of the fire, and contains the fire and extinguishes it if possible. All personnel are mobilized to evacuate clients. Clients who are close to the fire, regardless of its size, are at risk of injury and should be moved to another area. If a client is receiving oxygen but not life support, the nurse discontinues the oxygen, which is combustible and can fuel an existing fire. If the client is on life support, the nurse may need to maintain the client's respiratory status manually with an Ambu-bag (see Chapter 39) until the client is moved away from the fire. Ambulatory clients can be directed to walk by themselves to a safe area and in some cases may be able to assist in moving clients in wheelchairs. Bedridden clients are generally moved from the scene of a fire by a stretcher, their bed, or a wheelchair. If none of these methods is appropriate, clients must be carried from the area. If a client must be carried, the nurse should be careful not to overextend physical limits for lifting because injury to the nurse can result in further injury to the client. If fire department personnel are on the scene, they can help evacuate the clients.

Client Teaching	Box 37-10

Correct Use of a Fire Extinguisher in the Home

Objectives

- Client will correctly place the extinguisher in the home.
- Client will describe when it is appropriate to use a home fire extinguisher.
- Client will demonstrate the correct technique when using a fire extinguisher.
- Client will state when fire extinguishers need to be replaced.

Teaching Strategies

- Discuss correct location of the extinguisher. It is recommended that one be placed on each level of the home, near an exit, in clear view, away from stoves and heating appliances, and above the reach of small children. Keep a fire extinguisher in the kitchen, near the furnace, and in the garage. The instructions should be read when the extinguisher is purchased and kept available for periodic review.
- Describe the steps to take before using the extinguisher. Attempt to fight the fire only when all occupants have left the home, the fire department has been called, the fire is confined to a small area, there is an exit route readily available, the extinguisher is the right type for the fire (see discussion in text below for a description of the types of extinguishers), and the client knows how to use the extinguisher.
- Instruct the client to memorize the mnemonic PASS: *P*ull the pin to unlock handle, *A*im low at the base of the fire, *S*queeze the handles, and *S*weep the unit from side to side (see Figure 37-16, p. 992).

Evaluation

- Client can correctly place an extinguisher in the home.
- Client correctly lists the steps to take before attempting to use an extinguisher.
- Client demonstrates correct use of the extinguisher while reciting the instructions with the mnemonic PASS.

Modified from *Home fire prevention and preparedness fact sheet*, Itasca, Ill, 2002, National Safety Council.

After a fire has been reported and clients are out of danger, nurses and other personnel must take measures to contain or put out the fire, such as closing doors and windows, placing wet towels along the base of doors, turning off oxygen and electrical equipment, and using a fire extinguisher. Fire extinguishers are categorized as type A, used for ordinary combustibles (e.g., wood, cloth, paper, and many plastic items); type B, used for flammable liquids (e.g., gasoline, grease, paint, and anesthetic gas); and type C, used for electrical equipment. The correct use of an extinguisher is discussed in Box 37-10 and demonstrated in Figure 37-16.

The best intervention is to prevent fires. Nursing measures include complying with the agency's smoking policies and keeping combustible materials away from heat sources. Some agencies have fire doors that are held open by magnets and close automatically when a fire alarm

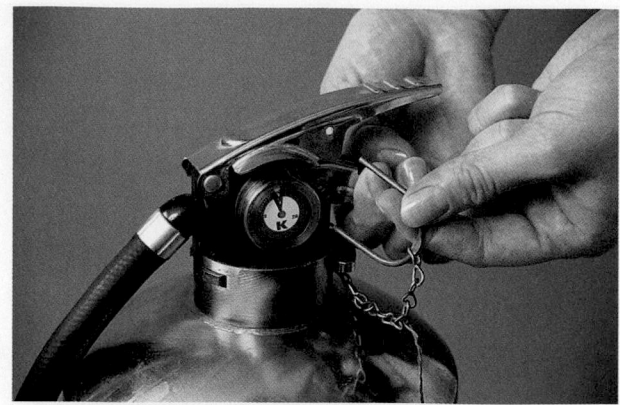

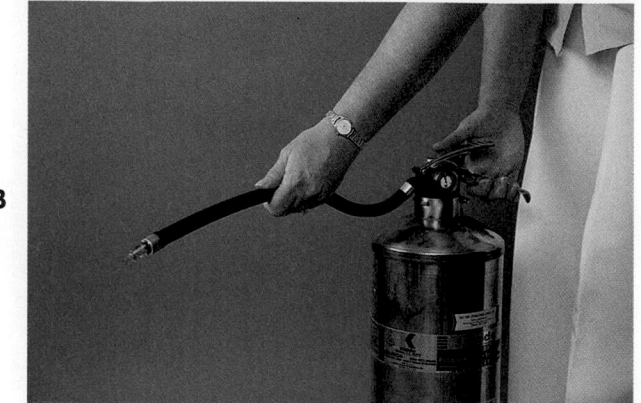

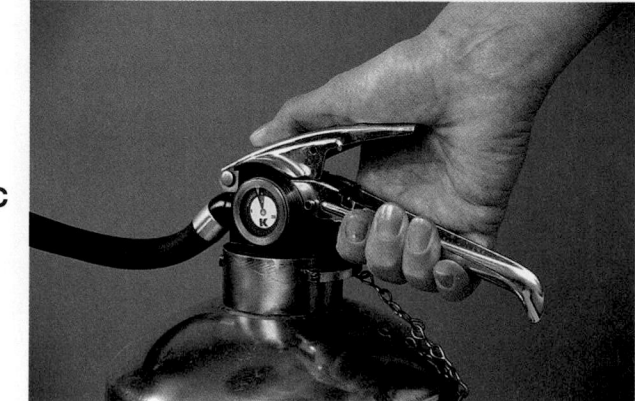

FIGURE **37–16** **A,** *P*ull the pin. **B,** *A*im at the base of the fire. **C,** *S*queeze the handles. *S*weep from side to side to coat the area evenly. (Modified from Sorrentino SA: *Mosby's assisting with patient care,* St. Louis, 1999, Mosby.)

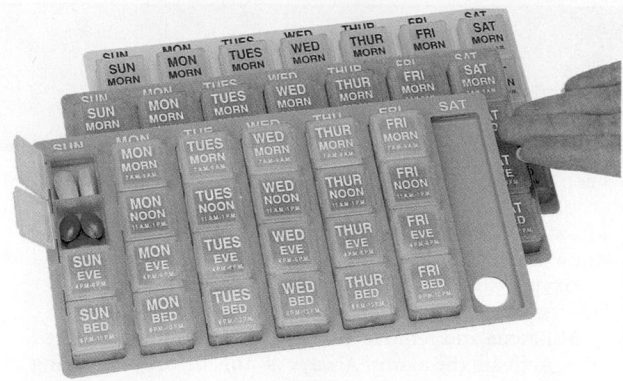

FIGURE **37–17**   One-Day-At-A-Time medicine organizer. (Courtesy Apothecary Products, Inc., Burnsville, Minnesota.)

sounds. It is important to keep equipment away from these doors.

Poisoning. A **poison** is any substance that impairs health or destroys life when ingested, inhaled, or otherwise absorbed by the body. Specific antidotes or treatments are available for only some types of poisons. The capacity of body tissue to recover from the poison determines the reversibility of the effect. Poisons can impair the respiratory, circulatory, central nervous, hepatic, GI, and renal systems of the body.

The toddler, preschooler, young school-age child, and older adult must be protected from accidental poisoning. Using child-resistant caps, placing medications and cleaning fluids and powders out of the reach of children, leaving potentially poisonous materials in original containers, and removing poisonous plants from the home prevent accidental ingestion of poisonous materials. Poisoning can also result from swallowing miniature button or disk batteries commonly found in games, cameras, calculators, and watches. In older adults, diminished eyesight and impaired memory may result in accidental ingestion of poisonous substances or in accidental overdose of prescribed medications. To prevent medication errors on the part of clients in the home, the nurse should recommend the use of medication organizers that are filled once a week by the client and/or family. These organizers have the day and time on each box, so the client knows when and what to take at any given time (Figure 37-17). This is particularly useful for clients who may forget whether they have taken their medications.

Guidelines for intervening in accidental poisoning should be adhered to. The Poison Control Center phone number should be visible on the telephone in homes with young children. In all cases of suspected poisoning, this number should be called immediately (Box 37-11).

Electrical Hazards. Electrical equipment must be maintained in good working order and should be grounded. The third (longer) prong in an electrical plug is the ground. Theoretically, the ground prong carries any stray electrical current back to the ground, hence its name. The other two prongs carry the power to the piece of electrical equipment. Improperly grounded or malfunctioning electrical equipment increases the risk of electrical injury and fire. Educating both the client and the family can reduce the risk for electrical hazards in the home environment (Box 37-12).

If a client receives an electrical shock in a health care setting, the nurse should immediately determine whether the client has a pulse. If the client has no pulse, cardiopulmonary resuscitation (CPR) should be initiated and emergency personnel should be notified (see Chapter

Box 37-11 Procedural Guidelines

Interventions in Accidental Poisoning

1. Assess for airway patency, breathing, and circulation (ABCs) in all clients in whom accidental poisoning is suspected.
2. Remove any visible materials from areas such as the mouth and eyes to terminate exposure.
3. Identify the type and amount of substance ingested, if possible. This may help to determine the antidote.
4. Call the Poison Control Center before attempting any interventions. The universal phone number for poison control is (800) 222-1222.
5. If directed by a physician, give oral fluids to assist vomiting.
6. If directed, save vomitus for laboratory analysis, which may assist with further treatment.
7. Position the victim with the head to the side to prevent aspiration of vomitus, and assist in keeping the airway open.
8. Never induce vomiting in an unconscious victim or in a client experiencing convulsions, because aspiration may occur.
9. Never induce vomiting if any of the following substances have been ingested: lye, household cleaners, hair care products, grease or petroleum products, or furniture polish. Vomiting may increase internal burns.
10. If instructed to take the victim to the emergency department, call an ambulance. Emergency equipment may be needed en route.
11. In the case of convulsions, cessation of breathing or unconsciousness, call 911.
12. Do not administer syrup of ipecac to induce vomiting. It has not been proven effective in preventing poisoning (AAP, 2004).

American Academy of Pediatrics: News release—don't treat swallowed poison with syrup of ipecac, www.aap.org/advocacy/releases/novpoison.htm. Accessed Feb 27, 2004.

---

39). If the client has a pulse and remains alert and oriented, the nurse should quickly obtain vital signs and assess the skin for signs of thermal injury. The client's physician must be notified. If an electrical shock occurs in the home, the nurse follows the same procedure but has the client go to the emergency department and then notifies the client's physician.

Seizures. Clients who have experienced some form of neurological injury or metabolic disturbance are at risk for a seizure. A seizure involves a hyperexcitation of neurons in the brain leading to a sudden, violent, involuntary series of contractions of a group of muscles. The client often loses consciousness. **Seizure precautions** encompass all nursing interventions to protect the client from traumatic injury, positioning for adequate ventilation and drainage of oral secretions, and providing privacy and support following the seizure (Skill 37-2).

During a seizure a client's jaw muscles can become tense. It has been found that significant injury to the client's oral cavity is rare, even during the most violent seizures. Injury may instead occur from a caregiver forcing an object into the client's mouth and from the teeth biting down on a hard object. Soft objects may break in the mouth during a seizure and be aspirated. Therefore the Epilepsy Foundation of America, in its recommendations for seizure first aid, includes avoiding the insertion of objects into the mouth (Seizure Recognition and Observation, 1992). The exception is in the case of **status epilepticus,** a medical emergency whereby a person has continual seizures without interruption. An adequate airway is maintained with an oral airway. Clients experiencing a seizure are never restrained but are placed on seizure precautions and need to be adequately protected from traumatic injury.

Client Teaching 　　　　　*Box 37-12*

Prevention of Electrical Hazards

Objective

- Client will recognize electrical hazards in the home and eliminate them.

Teaching Strategies

- Discuss grounding appliances and other equipment.
- Provide examples of common hazards: frayed cords, damaged equipment, and overloaded outlets.
- Discuss guidelines to prevent electrical shocks:
  - Use extension cords only when necessary, and use electrical tape to secure the cord to the floor where it will not be stepped on.
  - Do not run wires under carpeting.
  - Grasp the plug, not the cord, when unplugging items.
  - Keep electrical items away from water.
  - Do not operate unfamiliar equipment.
  - Disconnect items before cleaning.

Evaluation

- Have client list electrical hazards existing in the home.
- Review steps the client will take to eliminate these hazards.
- Check the home after the client has had an opportunity to eliminate hazards.

Skill 37-2   *Seizure Precautions*

Delegation Considerations

Assessment of a client's need for seizure precautions cannot be delegated. If a seizure occurs, the nurse must constantly assess the client's airway patency, adequacy of breathing, and circulatory status. Clinical judgments must be made quickly. Setting up seizure precautions and protecting clients at risk for seizures may be delegated to assistive personnel (AP).

- Have AP protect at-risk clients from falls by assisting with ambulation and transfer.

- Caution AP against any attempt to restrain client's extremities during an actual seizure.

Equipment

- Oral airway
- Padding for side rails and headboard
- Suction machine, oral suction equipment
- Clean disposable gloves

Steps	Rationale
1. Assess seizure history, noting frequency of seizures, presence of aura, and sequence of events, if known. Assess for medical and surgical conditions that may lead to seizures or exacerbate existing seizure condition. Assess medication history.	This enables the nurse to anticipate onset of seizure activity. Seizure medications must be taken as prescribed and not stopped suddenly, because this may precipitate seizure activity.
2. Inspect client's environment for potential safety hazards if risk for seizure exists: bedside stand or table, IV pole or other medical equipment.	Prevents client from sustaining injury by striking head or body on furniture or equipment.
3. Perform hand hygiene and prepare bed with padded side rails and headboard, bed in low position, and client positioned in side-lying position when possible (see illustration).	Minimizes risks associated with seizure activity.
4. For clients with a history of seizures, an airway (see illustration), suction apparatus, clean gloves, and pillows should be visible in the hospital setting for immediate use.	This ensures prompt, organized intervention.
5. When a seizure begins, position client safely. If client is standing or sitting, guide client to floor and protect head by cradling in nurse's lap or placing a pillow under head. Clear surrounding area of furniture. If client is in bed, raise side rails, add padding, and put bed in low position.	Protects client from traumatic injury, especially head injury.

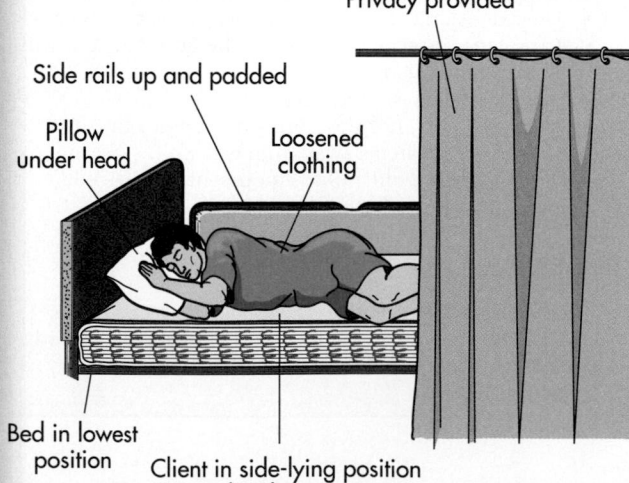

STEP **3**   Provide client privacy. Put bed in lowest position with side rails up and padded. Position client in side-lying position, with pillow under head and loosened clothing.

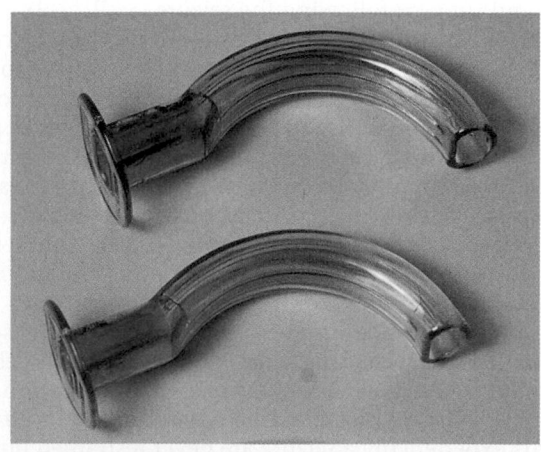

STEP **4**   Oral airways.

Steps	Rationale
6. Provide privacy.	Embarrassment is common after a seizure, especially if others witnessed the seizure.
7. If possible, turn client on side, with head flexed slightly forward.	Prevents tongue and dentures from blocking the airway and promotes drainage of secretions, thus reducing risk of aspiration.
8. Do not restrain client. Loosen clothing.	Prevents musculoskeletal injury.
9. Do not put anything into the client's mouth such as fingers, tongue depressor, or medicine.	

Critical Decision Point: Putting something in the client's mouth could result in injury to the jaw, tongue, or teeth and cause stimulation of the gag reflex, causing vomiting, aspiration, and respiratory distress (National Institute of Neurological Disorders and Stroke, 2001).

10. Stay with client, observing the sequence and timing of seizure activity.	Continued observation is necessary to ensure adequate ventilation during and following seizure activity. Accurate, specific observations will assist in documentation, diagnosis, and treatment of the seizure disorder.
11. After the seizure is over, explain what happened and answer client's questions. Foster an atmosphere of acceptance and respect.	Informing clients of the type of seizure activity experienced will assist them in participating knowledgeably in their care.
12. Following seizure, perform hand hygiene and assist client to position of comfort in bed with padded side rails up and bed in low position. Place call light within reach, and provide a quiet, nonstimulating environment.	Provides for continued safety. Clients are often confused and sleepy following a seizure.

Status Epilepticus

13. For a client experiencing status epilepticus, put on clean gloves and insert an oral airway (see illustration for Step 4) when the jaw is relaxed between seizure activity. Hold airway with curved side up, insert downward until airway reaches back of throat, then rotate and follow natural curve of the tongue. Do not place fingers near or in client's mouth.	Prevents transmission of infection. Client is in continual seizure state and requires oral airway to ensure airway patency. Client may inadvertently bite nurse's fingers during a seizure if caution is not used.
14. Access oxygen and suction equipment. Prepare for IV insertion.	Intensive monitoring and treatment are required for this medical emergency.
15. Use pillows/pads to protect client from injuring self.	Traumatic injury will be avoided.

Recording and Reporting

- Record the timing of seizure activity and sequence of events. Record presence of aura (if any), level of consciousness, posture, color, movements of extremities, incontinence, and patterns of sleep following the seizure.
- Document client's response and expected or unexpected outcomes.
- Report to physician immediately as seizure begins. Status epilepticus is an emergency situation requiring immediate medical management.

Unexpected Outcomes and Related Interventions

1. Client suffers traumatic injury.
   a. Continue to protect client from further injury.
   b. Notify the physician immediately.
   c. Ensure environment is free of safety hazards.
2. Client verbalizes feelings of embarrassment and humiliation.
   a. Offer support, and allow client to verbalize feelings.
   b. Encourage client and family to participate in decision making and planning care.

Home Care Considerations

- Communicate with client and family to identify precipitating factors.
- Teach family to care for the client during a seizure.
- Client's home should be assessed for environmental hazards in light of seizure condition.
- Provide family with guidelines to detect status epilepticus.
- Until a seizure condition is well controlled (usually for at least 1 year), the client should not take a tub bath or engage in activities such as swimming unless a knowledgeable family member is present. Driving may also be restricted during this time.
- Client should wear a medical alert bracelet or tag and have an ID card noting the presence of a seizure disorder and listing the medications taken.
- Referral to a support group or the Epilepsy Foundation may help to improve client's self-esteem and coping ability.

Radiation. Radiation is a health hazard in the health care setting and the community. Radiation and radioactive materials are used in the diagnosis and treatment of clients. Hospitals have strict guidelines on the care of clients who are receiving radiation and radioactive materials. The nurse must be familiar with established agency protocols. To reduce the nurse's exposure to radiation, time spent near the source should be limited, the distance from the source should be as great as possible, and shielding devices such as lead aprons should be used. Staff working near radiation will wear devices that can track the accumulative exposure to radiation.

The community may be at risk for radiation exposure because of incorrect disposal and transportation of radioactive waste products. Community health agencies and the Environmental Protection Agency (EPA) have established specific, strict guidelines for the disposal of radioactive waste. If a radioactive leak occurs, these agencies institute measures to prevent exposure of surrounding neighborhoods, to clean up radioactive leaks as quickly as possible, and to ensure that injured parties receive prompt medical care.

Bioterrorist Attack. Should a bioterrorist attack occur, nurses working in hospital settings must be prepared to respond and care for a sudden influx of clients. The JCAHO (2001) requires hospitals to have an emergency management plan that addresses four phases:

- *Mitigation*—Assessment process to determine hazard vulnerability for the hospital's service area. This includes an identification of the kinds of emergency situations that are most likely to occur and their probable impact.
- *Preparedness*—Steps taken to increase a hospital's ability to manage the effects of an attack. Hospital preparedness includes creating an inventory of resources (staff to supplies) that may be needed. This includes establishing agreements with product vendors and

other health care facilities to provide increased resources in the event of an attack. In addition, preparedness includes establishing primary and backup communications systems, training staff, and conducting organization-wide drills.

- *Response*—Steps taken by staff in the event of an attack. A formal response includes reporting to predetermined locations, using specific triage strategies to identify the most acutely ill, and management activities such as issuing warnings and notifications to the community. Decontamination procedures and disease reporting are also part of a hospital's response plan.
- *Recovery*—Steps taken to restore essential services and resume normal agency operations. This phase begins almost as soon as the response phase.

All hospitals must test their emergency plans twice a year. This includes implementation of planned drills. Communication is a key to any emergency management plan. If a bioterrorist attack occurs, nursing staff must know what happened, how many clients to expect, and when clients will begin to arrive so they can prepare both themselves and their facility (Steinhauer and Bauer, 2002).

Infection control practices are critical in the event of a biological attack. All clients symptomatic with suspected or confirmed bioterrorism-related illnesses must be managed using standard precautions (see Chapter 33). For certain diseases, such as smallpox or pneumonic plague, additional precautions may be needed, such as airborne or contact isolation precautions. Although most infections associated with biological agents cannot be transmitted from client to client, in general the transport and movement of clients should be limited to movement that is essential for treatment and care. An important aspect of care for clients who have a bioterrorism-related illness is postexposure management. Table 37-4 summarizes the steps to take to manage exposure to anthrax, botulism, plague, and smallpox.

Table 37-4	Postexposure Management of Bioterrorist-Related Illnesses
Illness	**Decontamination/Exposure Management**
Anthrax	In settings where threat of gross exposure exists, instruct clients to remove contaminated clothing and store in labeled, plastic bags. Handle clothing minimally to avoid agitation. Instruct clients to shower thoroughly with soap and water. Use standard precautions, and wear appropriate protective barriers when handling contaminated clothing or other items. Recommended postexposure prophylaxis includes the administration of oral fluoroquinolones (e.g., ciprofloxacin, levofloxacin, and ofloxacin).
Botulism	Even a single case of botulism should immediately raise concerns of an outbreak associated with contaminated food. The aim is to locate contaminated food and identify other persons who may have been exposed. Decontamination is not required because clients are not at risk for skin exposure or reaerosolization.
Plague	Risk for reaerosolization from contaminated clothing of exposed persons is low. In the case of gross exposure, instruct clients to remove contaminated clothing and store in labeled, plastic bags. Handle clothing minimally to avoid agitation. Instruct clients to shower thoroughly with soap and water. Use standard precautions, and wear appropriate protective barriers when handling contaminated clothing or other items. Postexposure prophylaxis is recommended for clients and health care workers. The antimicrobial agent of choice is doxycycline or ciprofloxacin.
Smallpox	Client decontamination after exposure to smallpox is not indicated. Items potentially contaminated by infectious lesions should be handled using contact isolation precautions. Postexposure immunization with smallpox vaccine is available and effective.

Modified from English J, Malone JD: *Bioterrorism readiness plan: a template for healthcare facilities,* April 13, 1999, APIC Bioterrorism Task Force and CDC Hospital Infections Program Bioterrorism Working Group.

NP Evaluation

Client Care. The components of critical thinking are applied to the evaluation step of the nursing process (Figure 37-18). The actual care delivered by the health care team is evaluated based on the expected outcomes. If the client's goals have been met, the nursing interventions can be considered effective and appropriate. If not, the nurse determines whether new risks to the client have developed or whether previous risks remain. The client and family need to participate to find permanent ways to reduce risks to safety. The nurse continually assesses the client's and family's need for additional support services such as home care, physical therapy, counseling, and further teaching.

Client Expectations. When the nurse has developed a good relationship with a client and the client feels safe and secure in their relationship, as well as in the environment, the client will most likely demonstrate less anxiety and verbalize satisfaction with the surroundings. The nurse must determine, however, if client expectations have been met. Is the client satisfied with any changes made to the environment? Does the client believe that his or her safety is ensured? If client expectations have not been met, the nurse must reassess not only the client and the environment but also the client's expressed desires.

•••

A safe environment is essential to promoting, maintaining, and restoring health. Incorporating critical thinking skills in the application of the nursing process, the nurse assesses the client and the environment to determine risk factors for injury; clusters risk factors; formulates a nursing diagnosis; and plans specific interven-

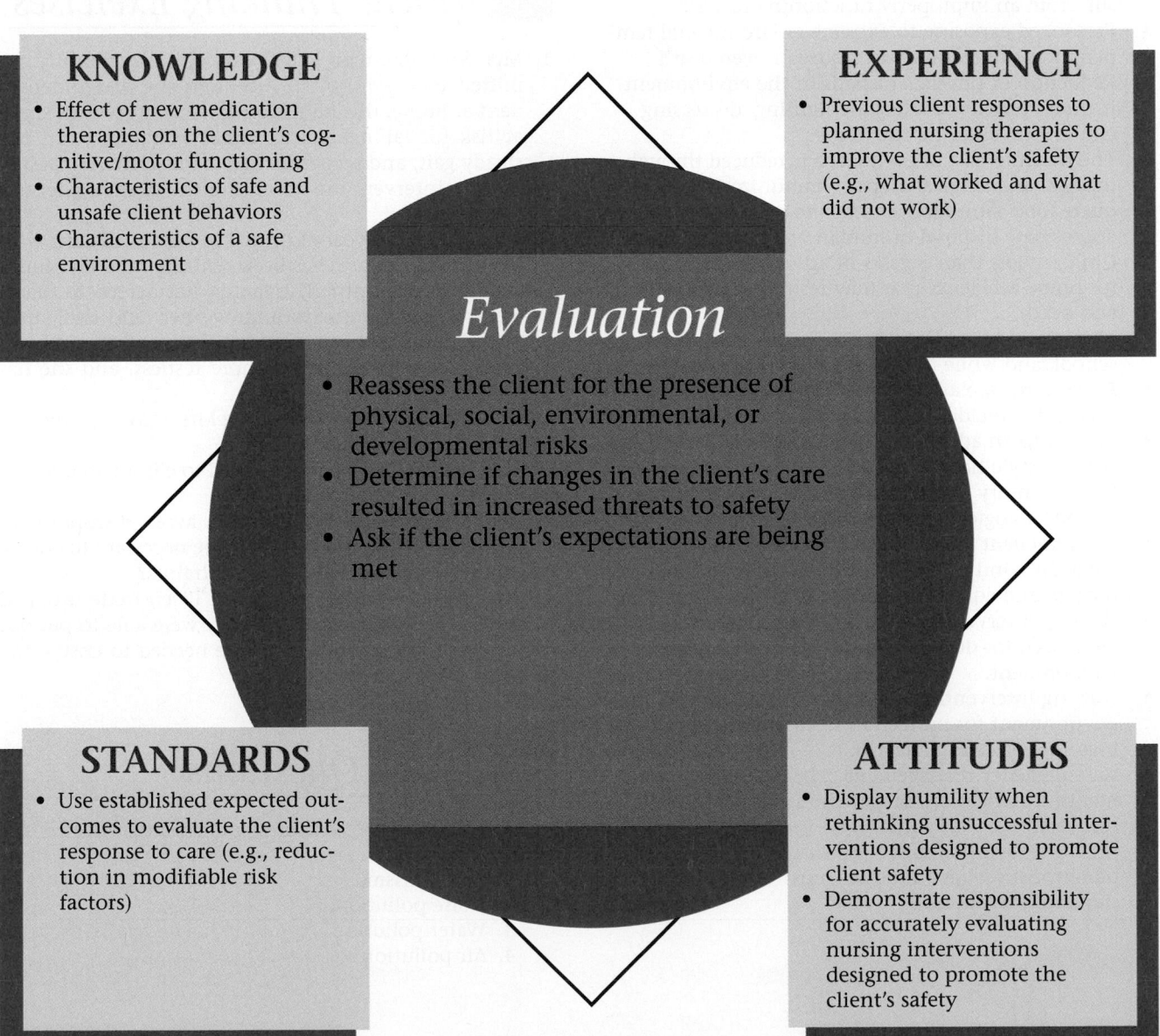

KNOWLEDGE
- Effect of new medication therapies on the client's cognitive/motor functioning
- Characteristics of safe and unsafe client behaviors
- Characteristics of a safe environment

EXPERIENCE
- Previous client responses to planned nursing therapies to improve the client's safety (e.g., what worked and what did not work)

Evaluation
- Reassess the client for the presence of physical, social, environmental, or developmental risks
- Determine if changes in the client's care resulted in increased threats to safety
- Ask if the client's expectations are being met

STANDARDS
- Use established expected outcomes to evaluate the client's response to care (e.g., reduction in modifiable risk factors)

ATTITUDES
- Display humility when rethinking unsuccessful interventions designed to promote client safety
- Demonstrate responsibility for accurately evaluating nursing interventions designed to promote the client's safety

FIGURE 37–18   Critical thinking model for safety evaluation.

tions, including client education. The expected outcomes include a safe physical environment, a client whose expectations have been met, a client who is knowledgeable about safety factors and precautions, and a client free of injury.

Key Concepts

- In the community a safe environment is one in which basic needs are achievable, physical hazards are reduced, transmission of pathogens is reduced, pollution is controlled, and sanitation is maintained.
- In a health care agency a safe environment is one that minimizes falls, client-inherent accidents, procedure-inherent accidents, and equipment-related accidents.
- A factor that reduces atmospheric oxygen is the presence of high carbon monoxide levels, which may result from an improperly functioning furnace.
- Prolonged exposure to extreme environmental temperatures can cause client injury or even death.
- Reduction of physical hazards in the environment includes providing adequate lighting, decreasing clutter, and securing the home.
- The transmission of pathogens is reduced through medical and surgical asepsis, immunization, adequate food sanitation, insect and rodent control, and appropriate disposal of human waste.
- Children less than 5 years of age are at greatest risk for home accidents that may result in severe injury and death.
- The school-age child is at risk for injury at home, at school, and while traveling to and from school.
- Adolescents are at risk for injury from automobile accidents, suicide, and substance abuse.
- Threats to an adult's safety are frequently associated with lifestyle habits.
- Risks of injury for older clients are directly related to the physiological changes of the aging process.
- Risks to client safety within a health care agency include falls and other client-inherent, procedure-related, and equipment-related accidents.
- Nursing interventions for promoting safety are individualized for developmental stage, lifestyle, and environment.
- Nursing interventions are developed to modify the environment for protection from falls, fires, poisonings, and electrical hazards.
- An emergency management plan includes the elements of mitigation, preparedness, response, and recovery.
- All clients symptomatic with suspected or confirmed bioterrorism-related illnesses must be managed using standard precautions.

Key Terms

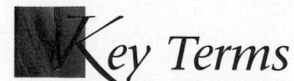

Air pollution, *p. 963*
Ambularm, *p. 990*
Aura, *p. 966*
Bioterrorism, *p. 963*
Carbon monoxide, *p. 961*
Environment, *p. 960*
Food and Drug Administration (FDA), *p. 961*
Food poisoning, *p. 961*
Hypothermia, *p. 961*
Immunization, *p. 962*

Land pollution, *p. 963*
Noise pollution, *p. 963*
Pathogen, *p. 962*
Poison, *p. 992*
Pollutant, *p. 963*
Relative humidity, *p. 961*
Restraint, *p. 980*
Seizure, *p. 966*
Seizure precautions, *p. 993*
Status epilepticus, *p. 993*
Water pollution, *p. 963*

Critical Thinking Exercises

1. Mrs. Santiago, who is 88 years old, was recently admitted to the hospital. Although she was independent at home, the admission assessment reveals she is at risk for falling due to urinary frequency, an unsteady gait, and recent mental status changes. Design specific interventions to ensure the client's safety in the hospital.
2. Mrs. Carr, a 76-year-old nursing home resident with Alzheimer's disease, has been refusing food and fluids for the past month. The family has agreed to placement of an NG tube to improve her fluid and nutritional status. Shortly after the first tube feeding was started, Mrs. Carr became more restless, and she has been picking at the tube.
   a. What might be precipitating Mrs. Carr's behavior of picking at the tube?
   b. What approaches can be used to eliminate interference with the treatment?
   c. If a restraint is necessary to avoid disruption of therapy, what interventions are necessary to ensure the client's safety while in restraints?
3. A family member reports that a lit cigarette dropped on the client's mattress, but they were able to put out the small fire. What actions are needed to ensure the safety of this client?

Review Questions

1. A new potential environmental health threat is the possibility of:
   1. Bioterrorism.
   2. Noise pollution.
   3. Water pollution.
   4. Air pollution.

2. The physiological changes that occur during the aging process increase the older client's risk for:
   1. Falls and burns.
   2. Poisoning.
   3. Alcoholism.
   4. Medication errors.

3. Unfortunately, clients throughout all developmental stages may be subject to:
   1. Alcoholism.
   2. Illiteracy.
   3. Abuse.
   4. Alzheimer's disease.

4. When teaching parents about accidental poisoning in children, the nurse would instruct them to:
   1. Give oral fluids.
   2. Induce vomiting.
   3. Call the poison control center.
   4. Drive the child to the emergency department.

5. Adolescents are at a greater risk for injury from:
   1. Poisoning and child abduction.
   2. Automobile accidents, suicide, and substance abuse.
   3. Home accidents.
   4. Physiological changes of aging.

6. While conducting a home assessment for risks to safety, nurses must realize that they have entered the client's territory and that the:
   1. Client's attitude toward his or her residence and belongings must be appreciated.
   2. The nurse is in charge, and the client must follow directions.
   3. The client must follow the physician and nurse safety recommendations.
   4. The client has no involvement in planning safety regimens.

7. A culturally sensitive issue is the client's sense of environmental control. The nurse realizes this means:
   1. Health beliefs and practices that will affect the outcome of interventions.
   2. The clients will not follow any recommendations from the nurse.
   3. The clients will want outside agency help in care.
   4. The clients will allow the nurse to plan all care.

8. The older adult experiences alterations in vision and hearing; therefore the nurse:
   1. Should encourage the client not to drive a car.
   2. Should inform the client to not attend any outside social functions.
   3. Should inform the client to give up reading because it irritates the eyes further.
   4. Should encourage yearly vision and hearing examinations.

9. During the night shift a client is found wandering the hospital halls looking for a bathroom. The nurse's initial intervention would be to:
   1. Insert a urinary catheter.
   2. Assign a staff member to stay with the client.
   3. Ask the physician to order a vest restraint.
   4. Provide scheduled toileting during the night shift.

10. The high prevalence of chronic conditions in older adults results in the increased use of:
    1. Alcohol to help with pain control.
    2. Ancillary services.
    3. High number of prescription and over-the-counter medications.
    4. Durable medical equipment

*R*eferences

American Academy of Pediatrics: News Release: *Don't treat swallowed poison with syrup of ipecac,* www.aap.org/advocacy/releases/novpoison.htm.

American Academy of Pediatrics Task Force on Infant Sleep Positioning and SIDS: Positioning and SIDS, *Pediatrics* 89:1120, 1992.

American Geriatrics Society Panel on Falls Prevention: Guideline for the prevention of falls in older persons, *J Am Geriatr Soc* 49(5):664, 2001.

Beare P, Meyers J: *Adult health nursing,* ed 3, St. Louis, 1998, Mosby.

Centers for Disease Control and Prevention: Prevention of hepatitis A through active or passive immunization: recommendations of the advisory committee on immunization practices (ACIP), *MMWR Morbid Mort Wkly Rep* 48(RR-12): 1-37. National Center for Infectious Disease, Division of Viral Hepatitis, U.S. Department of Health and Human Services, Atlanta, Ga, 2002.

Centers for Medicare and Medicaid Services: *Conditions of participation for hospitals,* 42 CFR 482.13, U.S. Department of Health and Human Services, Baltimore, Md, revised October 1, 2001.

Dochterman JM, Bulechek GM: *Nursing interventions classification (NIC),* ed 3, St. Louis, 2000, Mosby.

Ebersole P, Hess P: *Geriatric nursing and healthy aging,* St. Louis, 2001, Mosby.

Ebersole P, Hess P: *Toward healthy aging,* ed 6, St. Louis, 2003, Mosby.

Edelman CL, Mandle CL: *Health promotion throughout the lifespan,* ed 4, St. Louis, 1998, Mosby.

English J, Malone JD: *Bioterrorism readiness plan: a template for healthcare facilities,* April 13, 1999, APIC Bioterrorism Task Force and CDC Hospital Infections Program Bioterrorism Working Group.

Fact book for the year 2000, Atlanta, Ga, 2000, National Center for Injury Prevention and Control, Centers for Disease Control and Prevention.

Fact sheet: carbon monoxide, Itasca, Ill, 2002, National Safety Council.

Fact sheets: home fires, Quincy, Mass, 2001, National Fire Protection Association, http://www.nfpa.org/research/nfpafactsheets.

Farmer B: *Try this: best practices in nursing care to older adults,* New York, 2000, The Hartford Institute for Geriatric Nursing, New York University.

Giovachino M, Carey N: Modeling the consequences of bioterrorism response, *Mil Med* 166(11):925, 2001.

Giger JN, Davidhizar RE: *Transcultural nursing intervention,* ed 3, St. Louis, 1999, Mosby.

Hauck C and others: The contribution of prone sleeping position to racial disparity in SIDS: the Chicago Infant Mortality Study, *Pediatrics* 110(4): 772-780.

Home fire protection and preparedness fact sheet, Itasca, Ill, 2002, National Safety Council.

Injury Fact Book 2001-2002, Atlanta, Ga, 2002, National Center for Injury Prevention and Control, Centers for Disease Control and Prevention.

Joint Commission on Accreditation of Healthcare Organizations: *Comprehensive accreditation manual for hospitals: the official handbook,* Oakbrook Terrace, 2002, The Commission.

Joint Commission Resources, Joint Commission on Accreditation of Healthcare Organizations. Using JCAHO standards as a starting point to prepare for an emergency, *Jt Comm Perspect* 21(12):4, 2001.

Jones J and others: Future challenges in preparing for and responding to bioterrorism events, *Emerg Med Clin North Am* 20(2):501, 2002.

Kohn LT, Corrigan JM, Donaldson MS, editors: *To err is human: building a safer health system,* Washington, DC, 1999, Institute of Medicine, National Academy Press, Committee on Quality of Healthcare in America.

Lead poisoning fact sheet, Itasca, Ill, 2002, National Safety Council, nsc.org/library/facts/lead.htm.

Lueckenotte AG: *Gerontologic nursing,* St. Louis, 2000, Mosby.

Moorhead S, Johnson M, Maas, M: *Nursing outcomes classification (NOC),* ed 3, St. Louis, 2004, Mosby.

Reducing errors in healthcare: translating research into practice, AHRQ Pub No. 00-PO58, Rockville, Md, 2000, Agency for Healthcare Research and Quality.

Seizure recognition and observation: a guide for allied health professionals, ed 2, Baltimore, Md, 1992, Epilepsy Foundation of America.

Seizures and epilepsy: hope through research, Bethesda, Md, 2001, National Institute of Neurological Disorders and Stroke, National Institutes of Health.

Sorrentino SA: *Mosby's assisting with patient care,* St. Louis, 1999, Mosby.

Sorrentino SA: *Mosby's textbook for nursing assistants,* ed 5, St. Louis, 2000, Mosby.

Steinhauer R, Bauer J: The emergency management plan, *RN,* 65(6):40, 2002.

Strumpf N and others: *Restraint free care: individualized approaches for frail elders,* New York, 1998, Springer.

Williams SR: *Basic nutrition and diet therapy,* ed 11, St. Louis, 2000, Mosby.

Wong DL: *Wong's nursing care of infants and children,* ed 7, St. Louis, 2003, Mosby.

Zusman J: *Restraint and seclusion: understanding the JCAHO standards and federal regulations,* ed 3, Marblehead, Mass, 2001, Opus Communications.

*R*esearch References

Capezuti E: Preventing falls and injuries while reducing siderail use, *Ann Long-Term Care* 8(6):57, 2000.

Capezuti E and others: The relationship between physical restraint removal and falls and injuries among nursing home residents, *J Gerontol A Biol Sci Med Sci* 53A:M47, 1998.

Kannus P and others: Prevention of hip fracture in elderly people with use of a hip protector, *N Engl J Med* 343:1506, 2000.

Leonard C and others: The effect of fatigue, sleep deprivation and onerous working hours on the physical wellbeing of pre-registration house officers, *Ir J Med Sci* 167(1):22, 1998.

Quinn CA: The advanced practice nurse and changing perspectives on physical restraint, *Clin Nurs Spec* 10(5):223, 1996.

Schoenfelder DP: A fall prevention program for elderly individuals: exercise in long-term care settings, *J Gerontol Nurs* 26(3):43, 2000.

Tideiksaar R: Home safe home: practical tips for fall-proofing, *Geriatr Nurs* 11(6):280, 1989.

38

Hygiene

Media Resources

http://evolve.elsevier.com/Potter/fundamentals/

 CD COMPANION

- Review Questions
- Glossary

evolve WEBSITE

- Review Questions
- Student Learning Activities
- Concept Map Exercise
- Critical Thinking Exercise
- Video Clips
- Glossary

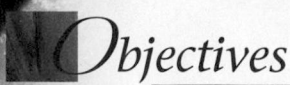

Objectives

Mastery of content in this chapter will enable the student to:

- Define the key terms listed.
- Describe factors that influence personal hygiene practices.
- Discuss the role critical thinking plays in the provision of hygienic care.
- Conduct a comprehensive assessment of a client's total hygiene needs.
- Discuss conditions that place clients at risk for impaired skin integrity.
- Discuss factors that influence the condition of the nails and feet.
- Explain the importance of foot care for the diabetic client.
- Discuss conditions that place clients at risk for impaired oral mucous membranes.
- List common hair and scalp problems and their related interventions.
- Describe how hygiene care for the older adult client may differ from that for the younger client.
- Discuss the different approaches used in maintaining a client's comfort during hygiene care.
- Successfully perform hygiene procedures for the care of the skin, perineum, feet and nails, mouth, eyes, ears, and nose.

*P*ersonal hygiene affects an individual's comfort, safety, and well-being. Well people are capable of meeting their own hygiene needs. Ill or physically challenged people may require various levels of assistance. A variety of personal, social, and cultural factors influence hygiene practices. In agency or home care settings the nurse determines a client's ability to perform self-care and provides hygienic care according to the client's needs and preferences. In addition in the home setting, the nurse assists in helping the client and family adapt hygiene techniques and approaches.

Because hygienic care requires close contact with the client, the nurse uses communication skills (see Chapter 23) to promote a caring therapeutic relationship and to use the time with the client for teaching and counseling. The nurse can integrate other nursing activities during hygiene care, including client assessment and interventions such as range-of-motion exercises, application of dressings, or inspection and care of intravenous sites. During hygiene care the nurse tries to preserve as much of the client's independence as possible, ensure privacy, convey respect, and foster the client's physical comfort.

Scientific Knowledge Base

Proper hygienic care requires an understanding of the anatomy and physiology of the integument, oral cavity, and the eyes, ears, and nose. The skin and mucosa cells exchange oxygen, nutrients, and fluids with underlying blood vessels. The cells require adequate nutrition, hydration, and circulation to resist injury and disease. Good hygiene techniques promote the normal structure and function of body tissues.

In addition, the nurse must apply knowledge of pathophysiology to provide good preventive hygienic care. The nurse learns to recognize those disease states that create changes in the integument, oral cavity, and sensory organs. For example, diabetes mellitus results in chronic vascular changes that impair healing of the skin and mucosa. In the early stages of acquired immunodeficiency syndrome (AIDS), fungal infections of the oral cavity are common. As a result of a stroke, paralysis of the trigeminal nerve eliminates the blink reflex, causing risk of corneal drying. In the presence of conditions such as these, the nurse adapts hygiene practices to anticipate client needs and minimize any injurious effects. When the nurse integrates knowledge of anatomy, physiology, and pathophysiology during hygiene care, there is the opportunity for timely recognition of abnormalities and initiation of appropriate actions to prevent further injury to sensitive tissues.

The Skin

The skin is an active organ with the functions of protection, secretion, excretion, temperature regulation, and sensation (Table 38-1). The skin has three primary layers: epidermis, dermis, and subcutaneous. The **epidermis** (outer layer) is composed of several thin layers of cells undergoing different stages of maturation. It shields underlying tissue against water loss and injury and prevents entry of disease-producing microorganisms. The innermost layer of the epidermis generates new cells to replace the dead cells that are continuously shed from the skin's outer surface. Bacteria commonly reside on the outer epidermis. These resident bacteria are normal flora (see Chapter 33) that do not cause disease but instead inhibit the multiplication of disease-causing microorganisms.

The **dermis** is a thicker skin layer containing bundles of collagen and elastic fibers to support the epidermis. Nerve fibers, blood vessels, sweat glands, sebaceous glands, and hair follicles course through the dermal layers. Sebaceous glands secrete sebum, an oily, odorous fluid, into the hair follicles.

The subcutaneous tissue layer contains blood vessels, nerves, lymph, and loose connective tissue filled with fat cells. The fatty tissue is a heat insulator for the body. Subcutaneous tissue also supports upper skin layers to withstand stresses and pressure without injury. Very little subcutaneous tissue underlies the oral mucosa.

The skin often reflects a change in physical condition by alterations in color, thickness, texture, turgor, temperature, and hydration (see Chapter 32). As long as the skin remains intact and healthy, its physiological function remains optimal.

Table 38-1	Function of the Skin and Implications for Care
Function/Description	**Implications for Care**
Protection	
Epidermis is relatively impermeable layer that prevents entrance of microorganisms. Although microorganisms reside on skin surface and in hair follicles, relative dryness of skin's surface inhibits bacterial growth. Sebum removes bacteria from hair follicles. Acidic pH of skin further retards bacterial growth.	Weakening of epidermis occurs by scraping or stripping its surface (e.g., use of dry razors, tape removal, or improper turning or positioning techniques). Excessive dryness causes cracks and breaks in skin and mucosa that allow bacteria to enter. Emollients soften skin and prevent moisture loss, soaking of skin improves moisture retention, and hydration of mucosa prevents dryness. However, constant exposure of skin to moisture causes maceration or softening, which interrupts dermal integrity and promotes ulcer formation and bacterial growth. Bed linen and clothing should be kept dry. Misuse of soap, detergents, cosmetics, deodorant, and depilatories can cause chemical irritation. Alkaline soaps neutralize the protective acid condition of skin. Cleansing of skin removes excess oil, sweat, dead skin cells, and dirt that can promote bacterial growth.
Sensation	
Skin contains sensory organs for touch, pain, heat, cold, and pressure.	Friction should be minimized to avoid loss of stratum corneum, which can result in development of pressure ulcers. Smoothing linen removes sources of mechanical irritation. Removing rings from fingers prevents nurse from accidentally injuring client's skin. Bath water should not be excessively hot or cold.
Temperature Regulation	
Body temperature is controlled by radiation, evaporation, conduction, and convection.	Factors that interfere with heat loss can alter temperature control. Wet bed linen or gowns interfere with convection and conduction. Excess blankets or bed coverings can interfere with heat loss through radiation and conduction. Coverings can promote heat conservation.
Excretion and Secretion	
Sweat promotes heat loss by evaporation. Sebum lubricates skin and hair.	Perspiration and oil can harbor microorganisms. Bathing removes excess body secretions, although if excessive it can cause drying of skin.

The Feet, Hands, and Nails

The feet, hands, and nails often require special attention to prevent infection. Any injury or deformity to the foot, including any growths or injuries to the overlying skin, can be painful and thus interfere with a client's normal ability to walk and bear weight. The hand, in contrast to the foot, is constructed largely for manipulation rather than support.

A wide range of dexterity exists in the hand because of the wide range of movement between the thumb and fingers. Any condition that interferes with movement of the hand (e.g., superficial or deep pain or joint inflammation) can impair a client's self-help abilities.

The nails are epithelial tissues that grow from the root of the nail bed, located in the skin at the nail groove, hidden by the fold of skin called the **cuticle.** The visible part of the nail is the nail body. It has a crescent-shaped white area known as the **lunula.** Under the nail lies a layer of epithelium called the nail bed (Figure 38-1). A normal healthy nail is transparent, smooth, and convex, with a pink nail bed and translucent white tip. Disease can cause changes in the shape, thickness, and curvature of the nail (see Chapter 32).

The Oral Cavity

The oral cavity is lined with mucous membranes continuous with the skin. The oral or buccal cavity consists of the lips surrounding the opening of the mouth, the cheeks running along the sidewalls of the cavity, the tongue and its muscles, and the hard and soft palate. The oral mucosa is normally light pink and moist. The floor of the mouth and the undersurface of the tongue are richly supplied with blood vessels. Any type of ulceration or trauma can

result in significant bleeding. There are three pairs of salivary glands that secrete about 1 L of saliva a day. The **buccal glands** found in the mucosa lining the cheeks and mouth maintain the hygiene and comfort of oral tissues. Salivary secretion in the mouth can be impaired through the effects of medications, exposure to radiation, and mouth breathing.

The teeth are the organs of chewing, or **mastication.** They are designed to cut, tear, and grind ingested food so it can be mixed with saliva and swallowed. A normal tooth consists of the crown, neck, and root (Figure 38-2). The periodontal membrane lies just below the gum margins, surrounds a tooth, and holds it firmly in place. Healthy teeth appear white, smooth, shiny, and properly aligned.

Difficulty in chewing can develop when surrounding gum tissues become inflamed or infected or when teeth are lost or become loosened. Regular oral hygiene is necessary to maintain the integrity of tooth surfaces and to prevent **gingivitis,** or gum inflammation.

The Hair

Hair growth, distribution, and pattern can indicate a person's general health status. Hormonal changes, emotional and physical stress, aging, infection, and certain illnesses can affect hair characteristics. The hair shaft itself is inert and cannot be directly affected by physiological factors. However, changes in its color or condition are caused by hormonal and nutrient deficiencies of the hair follicle (Figure 38-3).

The Eyes, Ears, and Nose

When nurses provide hygienic care, the eyes, ears, and nose require careful attention. Chapter 32 describes the

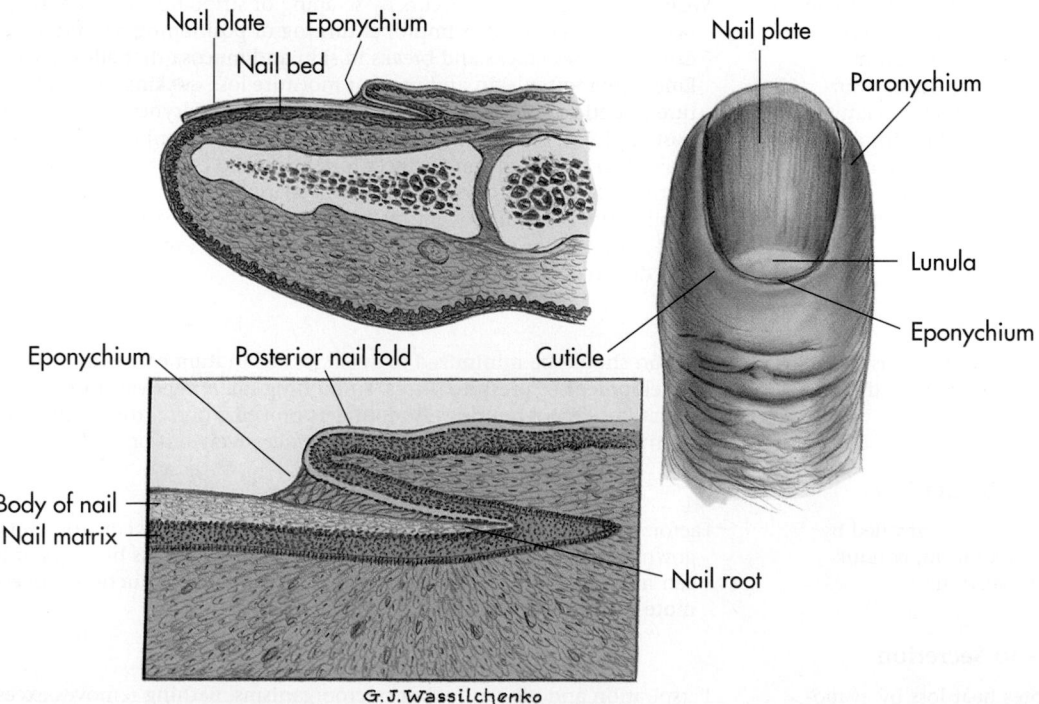

G. J. Wassilchenko

FIGURE **38–1** Anatomic structure of a normal nail. (From Thompson and others: *Clinical nursing,* ed 4, St. Louis, 1997, Mosby.)

structure and function of these organs. Cleansing of the sensitive sensory tissues should be done in a way that prevents injury and discomfort for the client, such as using care not to get soap in the client's eyes. In addition, the time a nurse spends with a client during hygiene provides

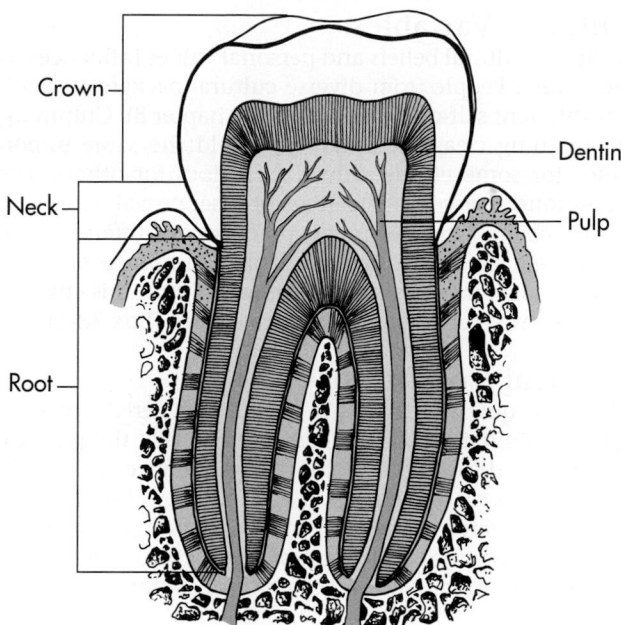

FIGURE **38–2** A normal tooth.

an excellent opportunity to ask if there have been any changes in vision, hearing, or sense of smell.

*N*ursing Knowledge Base

A client's personal preferences for hygiene are influenced by a number of factors. No two individuals perform hygiene in the same manner, and it is important that the nurse individualize the client's care based on knowing about the client's unique hygiene practices and preferences.

Hygiene care is never routine; the care requires intimate contact with the client and communication skills to promote the therapeutic relationship. In addition, during this care the nurse can learn about the client's health promotion practices and needs, emotional needs, and health care education needs.

Social Practices

Social groups influence hygiene preferences and practices, including the type of hygienic products used and the nature and frequency of personal care. During childhood, hygiene is influenced by family customs. This may include, for example, the frequency of bathing, the time of day bathing is performed, and the type of oral hygiene practiced. As children enter their adolescent years, personal hygiene may be influenced by peer group behavior. Young girls, for example, may become more interested in their personal appearance and begin to wear makeup. During

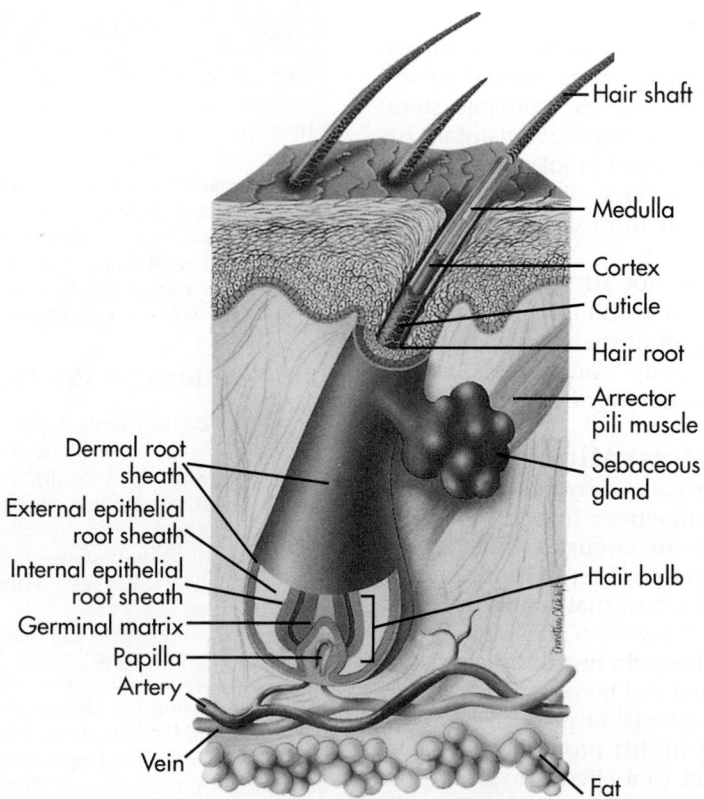

FIGURE **38–3**   Hair follicle, relationship of a follicle and related structures to the epidermal and dermal layers of the skin. (From Thibodeau GA, Patton KT: *Anatomy and physiology,* ed 5, St. Louis, 2003, Mosby.)

the adult years, involvement with friends and work groups shape the expectations people have about their personal appearance. Older adults' hygiene practices may change because of living conditions and available resources.

Personal Preferences

Each client has individual desires and preferences about when to bathe, shave, and perform hair care. Clients select different products according to personal preferences, needs, and financial resources. These desires should assist the nurse in delivering individualized care for the client. In addition, the nurse should also assist the client in developing new hygiene practices when indicated by an illness or condition.

Body Image

A client's general appearance may reflect the importance hygiene holds for that person. Body image is a person's subjective concept of his or her physical appearance (see Chapter 26). These images can change frequently. When clients undergo surgery, illness, or a change in functional status, body image can change dramatically. For this reason, the nurse will take extra effort to promote the client's hygienic comfort and appearance.

Body image affects the way in which hygiene is maintained. If a client is neatly groomed, the nurse considers the details of grooming when planning care and consults the client before making decisions about how hygienic care is to be provided. Clients who appear unkempt or uninterested in hygiene may require education about the importance of hygiene.

Socioeconomic Status

A person's economic resources influence the type and extent of hygiene practices used. The nurse should be sensitive in considering that the client's economic status may influence his or her ability to regularly maintain hygiene. When clients have the added problem of a lack of socioeconomic resources, it becomes difficult to participate and take a responsible role in health promotion activities such as basic hygiene.

When basic care items are not affordable, the nurse will work to find alternatives. It is also important to learn if use of these products is a part of the social habits practiced by the client's social group. For example, not all clients may choose to use deodorant or cosmetics.

Health Beliefs and Motivation

Knowledge about the importance of hygiene and its implications for well-being influences hygiene practices. However, knowledge alone is not enough. The client also must be motivated to maintain self-care. Health motivation is a generalized state of intent that results in behaviors to maintain or improve health (Champion, 1984). Motivation is part of an individual's health beliefs or attitudes that influence health-related behaviors.

Studies have shown that clients' health beliefs predict the likelihood of assuming health promotion behavior (Champion, 1984). In regard to a client's hygiene practices it is important for the nurse to know if a client, for example, perceives being at risk for dental disease, perceives dental disease to be serious, perceives brushing and flossing to be effective in reducing risk, and perceives any negative implications from following recommended hygiene practices. When a client recognizes there is a risk and reasonable action can be taken with no negative consequence, he or she will be more receptive to the nurse's counseling and teaching efforts.

Cultural Variables

A client's cultural beliefs and personal values influence hygiene care. People from diverse cultural backgrounds follow different self-care practices (see Chapter 8). Culturally, maintaining cleanliness may not hold the same importance for some ethnic groups as it does for others. The nurse must not convey feelings of disapproval when caring for clients whose hygienic practices are different from the nurse's. In North America it is common to bathe or shower daily, whereas in some other cultures it is customary to completely bathe only once a week (Box 38-1).

Physical Condition

The nurse quickly learns that clients with certain types of physical limitations or disabilities often lack the physical energy and dexterity to perform hygienic care. A client in traction or a cast or who has an intravenous line or other device connected to the body will need assistance with hygiene. Illnesses that cause pain may limit the dexterity and range of motion needed to perform certain measures.

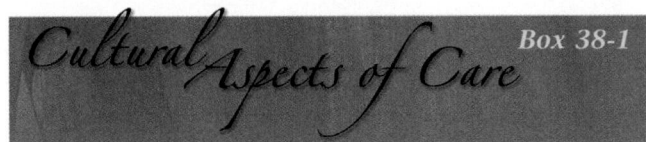

Box 38-1

Cultural Aspects of Care

Identifying changes in skin color and determining if these changes are normal reactive hyperemia or abnormal reactive hyperemia is important in evaluating clients' risks for pressure ulcers (see Chapter 47). When client's natural skin contains more melanin, it becomes more difficult to determine abnormal reactive hyperemia or cyanosis. There are normal hyperpigmentation areas, such a Mongolian spots that are seen on the sacrum of African, Native American, and Asian clients. These areas should not be confused with skin color changes such as abnormal reactive hyperemia or cyanosis.

Implications for Practice

- For dark-skin clients, know the individual's baseline skin tone by asking the client or family to point out an area of normal skin color for that individual client.
- Frequently assess for changes in baseline skin tone and skin temperature over pressure areas.
- Use natural light sources when possible because fluorescent light sources casts a bluish hue on darkly pigmented skin tones.
- Examine body sites with least melanin for underlying skin color identification.

Data from Gaskin FC: Detection of cyanosis in the person with dark skin, *J Black Nurs Assoc* 1:52, 1986; Bennet MA: Report of the Task Force on the Implications for Darkly Pigmented Intact Skin in the Prediction and Prevention of Pressure Ulcers, *Adv Wound Care* 8(6):34, 1995; and Henderson CT and others: Draft definition of stage I pressure ulcers: inclusion of persons with darkly pigmented skin, *Adv Wound Care* 10(5):16, 1997.

Clients still under the effects of sedation will not have the mental clarity or coordination to perform self-care. Chronic illnesses, such as cardiac disease, cancer, neurological disorders, and certain psychiatric conditions may exhaust or incapacitate a client. A weakened grasp resulting from arthritis, stroke, or muscular disorders can prevent a client from using a toothbrush, washcloth, or comb.

Critical Thinking

Successful critical thinking requires synthesis of knowledge, experience, information gathered from clients, critical thinking attitudes, and intellectual and professional

standards. Clinical judgments require the nurse to anticipate the information necessary to analyze data, and make decisions regarding client care. A client's condition is always changing, requiring ongoing critical thinking. During assessment, the nurse must consider all elements that build toward making appropriate nursing diagnoses (Figure 38-4).

Because hygienic care is so important for a client to feel comfortable, refreshed, and renewed, the nurse avoids making hygiene care a simple routine. Instead, the nurse integrates knowledge from nursing and other disciplines, previous experiences, and information gathered from clients. In addition, the use of critical thinking attitudes, such as curiosity and humility is needed in order to

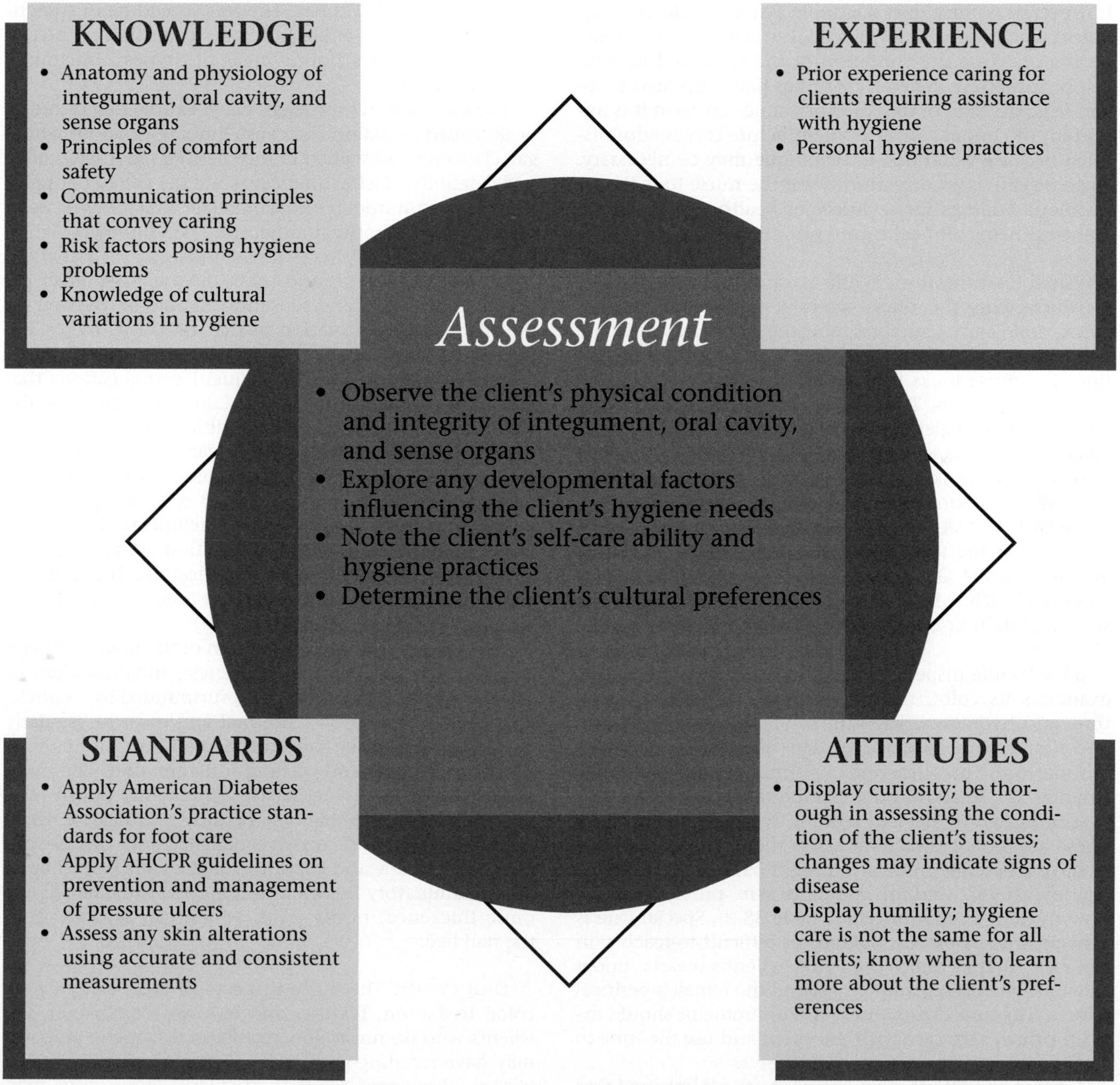

KNOWLEDGE

- Anatomy and physiology of integument, oral cavity, and sense organs
- Principles of comfort and safety
- Communication principles that convey caring
- Risk factors posing hygiene problems
- Knowledge of cultural variations in hygiene

EXPERIENCE

- Prior experience caring for clients requiring assistance with hygiene
- Personal hygiene practices

Assessment

- Observe the client's physical condition and integrity of integument, oral cavity, and sense organs
- Explore any developmental factors influencing the client's hygiene needs
- Note the client's self-care ability and hygiene practices
- Determine the client's cultural preferences

STANDARDS

- Apply American Diabetes Association's practice standards for foot care
- Apply AHCPR guidelines on prevention and management of pressure ulcers
- Assess any skin alterations using accurate and consistent measurements

ATTITUDES

- Display curiosity; be thorough in assessing the condition of the client's tissues; changes may indicate signs of disease
- Display humility; hygiene care is not the same for all clients; know when to learn more about the client's preferences

FIGURE 38–4   Critical thinking model for hygiene assessment.

design a plan of care to meet the client's hygiene needs. The nurse uses professional standards, such as those from the American Diabetes Association and skin care practices developed by the Agency for Health Care Policy and Research (AHCPR, 1992), which is now the Agency for Healthcare Quality and Research (AHRQ), when planning care to meet the client's hygiene needs.

Nursing Process

Assessment

Nursing assessment is an ongoing process. The nurse may not assess all body regions before administering hygiene; however, the nurse does routinely assess the client's condition whenever care to the client is given. For example, during oral care the condition of the teeth and mucosa can be inspected. When a client has had a repeated problem (e.g., dry skin or inflamed oral mucosa), then it is important to conduct an assessment before care is administered because variations in technique may be necessary. Hygiene care is an opportunity for the nurse to make assessment findings for a variety of health care problems and thus helps set health care priorities.

Physical Examination. While assisting a client with personal hygiene, the nurse carefully assesses the integument, oral cavity structures, and the eyes, ears, and nose (see Chapter 32). Using the skills of inspection and palpation, the nurse looks for alterations in the integrity and function of tissues. The assessment also reveals the type and extent of hygienic care required. Special attention is given to the characteristics most influenced by hygiene measures. Is the skin intact, especially over bony prominences? Is the skin dry from too much bathing? Are there calluses of the feet that may benefit from soaking? Is there a coating of the tongue that requires frequent brushing and hydration? Over time, the nurse's assessment provides the baseline for determining whether hygienic measures maintain or improve the client's condition.

Skin. While inspecting the skin, the nurse thoroughly examines its color, texture, thickness, turgor, temperature, and hydration. The skin should be smooth, warm, and supple with good turgor. The nurse pays special attention to the presence and condition of any lesions (see Chapter 32). In addition, it is important to assess for dryness indicated by flaking, redness, scaling, and cracking. These are tools available to assess the degrees of dryness to have a baseline in determining if bathing is beneficial (Handy, 1996). Certain common skin problems affect how hygiene is administered (Table 38-2). Special care is also given to assess less obvious or difficult-to-reach skin surfaces, such as under the female client's breasts, under the male client's scrotum, or around the female's perineal tissues. The nurse who observes skin problems should explain proper skin care with the client and use the time to instruct on specific hygiene techniques.

Certain conditions place clients at risk for impaired skin integrity (Box 38-2). Nurses must be particularly alert when assessing clients with reduced sensation, vascular insufficiency, and immobility. Be sure to assess both extremities and assist in turning a client so that a skin surface can be fully viewed. The development of pressure ulcers is a common complication that can extend hospital stays and threaten the well-being of the long-term care client. When caring for clients with darkly pigmented skin, be aware of unique assessment techniques and skin characteristics unique to highly pigmented skin (Box 38-3).

Feet and Nails. Assessment of the feet involves a thorough examination of all skin surfaces, including areas between the toes and over the soles of the feet. The heels, soles, and sides of the feet are prone to irritation from poorly fitting shoes. In addition, the nurse inspects the shape and size of toes and shape of the foot. The toes are normally straight and flat. The feet should be in straight alignment with the ankle and tibia. Inspection of the feet for lesions includes noting areas of dryness, inflammation, or cracking.

The nurse assesses the client's gait. Painful foot disorders or decreased sensation can cause limping or an unnatural gait. The nurse asks whether the client has foot discomfort and determines factors that aggravate the pain. Foot problems may result from bone or muscular alterations or wearing poor fitting footwear rather than skin disorders.

Clients with peripheral vascular disease, such as those with diabetes mellitus and other diseases that affect peripheral circulation and sensation, should be assessed for the adequacy of circulation to the feet (see Chapter 32). Inspection and daily foot care can prevent the development of foot ulcers and subsequent complications that may lead to amputation (Neil, 2002). Palpation of the dorsalis pedis and posterior tibial pulses indicates whether adequate blood flow is reaching peripheral tissues. Edema and changes in skin color, texture, and temperature can indicate if the client requires special hygienic care. Persons with diabetes mellitus should also be checked for **neuropathy,** degeneration of the peripheral nerves characterized by a loss of sensation. The nurse assesses the client's sensation to light touch, pinprick, and temperature (see Chapter 32).

The nurse inspects the condition of the fingernails and toenails, looking for lesions, dryness, inflammation, or cracking (Table 38-3). The nail is surrounded by a cuticle, which slowly grows over the nail and must be regularly pushed back. The skin around the nail beds and cuticles should be smooth and without inflammation. The nurse should ask women whether they frequently polish their nails and use polish remover, because chemicals in these products can cause excessive nail dryness. Disease can change the shape and curvature of the nails (see Chapter 32). Inflammatory lesions and fungus of the nail bed can cause thickened, horny nails, which can separate from the nail bed.

Oral Cavity. The nurse inspects all areas carefully for color, hydration, texture, and lesions (see Chapter 32). Clients who do not follow regular oral hygiene practices may have receding gum tissue, inflamed gums, a coated tongue, discolored teeth (particularly along gum margins), dental caries, missing teeth, and **halitosis** (bad

Table 38-2   Common Skin Problems

Characteristics	Implications	Interventions
Dry Skin		
Flaky, rough texture on exposed areas such as hands, arms, legs, or face	Skin may become infected if epidermal layer is allowed to crack.	Have client bathe less frequently and rinse body of all soap because residue left on skin can cause irritation and breakdown. Add moisture to air through use of humidifier. Increase fluid intake when skin is dry. Use moisturizing cream to aid healing. (Cream forms protective barrier and helps maintain fluid within skin.) Use cream such as Eucerin. Use creams to clean skin that is dry or allergic to soaps and detergents.
Acne		
Inflammatory, papulopustular skin eruption, usually involving bacterial breakdown of sebum; appears on face, neck, shoulders, and back	Infected material within pustule can spread if area is squeezed or picked. Permanent scarring can result.	Wash hair and skin thoroughly each day with hot water and soap to remove oil. Use cosmetics sparingly because oily cosmetics or creams accumulate in pores and tend to make condition worse. Implement dietary restrictions, if necessary. (Foods that aggravate condition should be eliminated from diet.) Inform client that exposure to ultraviolet rays, either from sunshine or heat lamp, may help control acne. (Caution should be used to prevent burning of skin.) Use prescribed topical antibiotics for severe forms of acne.
Skin Rashes		
Skin eruption that may result from overexposure to sun or moisture or from allergic reaction (may be flat or raised, localized or systemic, pruritic or nonpruritic)	If skin is continually scratched, inflammation and infection may occur. Rashes can also cause discomfort.	Wash area thoroughly and apply antiseptic spray or lotion to prevent further itching and aid in healing process. Apply warm or cold soaks to relieve inflammation, if indicated.
Contact Dermatitis		
Inflammation of skin characterized by abrupt onset with erythema, pruritus, pain, and appearance of scaly oozing lesions (seen on face, neck, hands, forearms, and genitalia)	Dermatitis is often difficult to eliminate because person is usually in continual contact with substance causing skin reaction. Substance may be hard to identify.	Avoid causative agents (e.g., cleansers and soaps).
Abrasion		
Scraping or rubbing away of epidermis that may result in localized bleeding and later weeping of serous fluid	Infection occurs easily because of loss of protective skin layer.	Be careful not to scratch client with jewelry or fingernails. Wash abrasions with mild soap and water; dry thoroughly and gently. Observe dressing or bandage for retained moisture because it could increase risk of infection.

breath). Localized pain and infection are common symptoms of a gum disease and certain tooth disorders.

Clients in acute care settings require complete oral assessment. Identification of risks for infection and other conditions identify the type and frequency of oral care. Proper oral care has been shown to reduce pneumonia in nursing home residents because it reduces the bacterial count in oral secretions, which may be aspirated, causing a bacterial infection (Research update, 2002). It is especially important to examine the oral cavity of clients re-

ceiving radiation or chemotherapy. Both treatments can cause reduction in the amount of saliva, and, as a result, there is drying and inflammation of the oral mucosal tissues. The nurse's assessment serves as a basis for preventive care for clients as they undergo treatment.

Hair. Before performing hair care, the nurse assesses the condition of the hair and scalp. Normally the hair is clean, shiny, and untangled, and the scalp is clear of lesions. The hair of black-skinned clients is usually thicker,

---

Box 38-2   **Risk Factors for Skin Impairment**

Immobilization

When restricted from moving freely, dependent body parts are exposed to pressure, reducing circulation to affected body parts. The nurse should know which clients require assistance to turn and change positions.

Reduced Sensation

Clients with paralysis, circulatory insufficiency, or local nerve damage are unable to sense an injury to the skin. During a bath assess the status of sensory nerve function by checking for pain, tactile sensation, and temperature sensation.

Nutrition and Hydration Alterations

Clients with limited caloric and protein intake can develop thinner, less elastic skin, with loss of subcutaneous tissue. This can result in impaired or delayed wound healing.

Secretions and Excretions on the Skin

Moisture on the skin's surface serves as a medium for bacterial growth and can cause irritation, soften epidermal cells, and lead to skin maceration. Presence of perspiration, urine, watery fecal material, and wound drainage on the skin can result in breakdown and infection.

Vascular Insufficiency

Inadequate arterial supply to tissues and impaired venous return decrease circulation to the extremities. Inadequate blood flow can cause ischemia and breakdown. Risk of infection also exists because delivery of nutrients, oxygen, and white blood cells to injured tissues is inadequate.

External Devices

An external device applied to or around the skin exerts pressure or friction on the skin. The nurse assesses all surfaces exposed to casts, cloth restraints, bandages and dressings, tubing, or orthopedic braces.

Box 38-3   **Skin Assessment for the Client With Darkly Pigmented Intact Skin**

- Assess localized skin color changes.
  - Any of the following may occur:
    - Color darker than surrounding skin, purplish, bluish, eggplant
    - Taut
    - Shiny
    - Induration
- Assess for edema (nonpitting, swelling).
- Importance of lighting for skin assessment:
  - Use natural or halogen light.
  - Avoid fluorescent lamps, which can give the skin a bluish tone.
- Assess skin temperature.
  - Initially area of skin impairment may feel warmer than surrounding skin.
  - Subsequently area of skin impairment may feel cooler than surrounding skin.
  - Use the back of your hand and fingers and, if client's condition permits, do not use gloves when doing this assessment.

Data from Bennet MA: Report of the Task Force on the Implications for Darkly Pigmented Intact Skin in the Prediction and Prevention of Pressure Ulcers, *Adv Wound Care* 8(6):34, 1995.

---

drier, and curlier than that of lighter skinned clients. Table 38-4 summarizes hair and scalp problems the nurse may identify. In the community health and home care settings it is particularly important to inspect the hair for lice so that appropriate hygienic treatment can be provided. If pediculosis capitis (head lice) is suspected, the nurse guards against self-infestations by hand washing and use of gloves or tongue blades to inspect the client's hair. The loss of hair **(alopecia)** can result from the effects of chemotherapy medications, hormonal changes, or improper hair care practices. Clients at risk for scalp problems are those who have experienced head trauma and those who practice poor hygiene.

Eyes, Ears, and Nose. The nurse's examination assesses the condition and function of the eyes, ears, and nose (see Chapter 32). Normally the eyes are free of infection and irritation. The sclerae are visible anteriorly as the white portion of the eye. The conjunctivae (the lining of the eyelids) are clear, pink, and without inflammation. The eyelid margins are in close approximation with the eyeball, and the lashes are turned outward. The lid margins are without inflammation, drainage, or lesions. The eyebrows should be symmetrical.

Another important aspect of an eye examination is to determine if the client wears contact lenses. This is especially significant for clients who enter hospitals or other agencies unresponsive or in a confused state. To determine if a contact lens is present, stand to the side of the client's eye and observe the cornea for the presence of a soft or rigid lens. It is also important to observe the sclera to detect the presence of a contact lens that may have shifted off the client's cornea. An undetected lens can cause severe corneal injury when left in place too long.

Assessment of the external ear structures includes inspection of the auricle, external ear canal, and tympanic membrane. Use of an otoscope is necessary (see Chapter 32). While performing hygienic measures, the nurse is most concerned with noting the presence of accumulated **cerumen** or drainage in the ear canal, local inflammation, or tenderness on palpation or the client's report of pain (see Chapter 32).

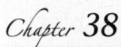

Table 38-3   Common Foot and Nail Problems

Characteristics	Implications	Interventions
Callus Thickened portion of epidermis consists of mass of horny, keratotic cells. Callus is usually flat, painless, and found on undersurface of foot or on palm of hand. Problem is caused by local friction or pressure.	Condition may cause discomfort when wearing tight shoes.	Nurse advises client to wear gloves when using tools or objects that may create friction on palmar surfaces. Soft-sole shoes with insoles are recommended. Nurse soaks callus in warm water and Epsom salts to soften cell layers. Applications of creams or lotions can reduce reformation. Encourage client to see podiatrist.
Corns Keratosis is caused by friction and pressure from ill-fitting or loose shoes. It is seen mainly on or between toes, over bony prominence. Corn is usually cone shaped, round, and raised. Soft corns are macerated.	Conical shape compresses underlying dermis, making it thin and tender. Pain is aggravated when tight shoes are worn. Tissue can become attached to bone if allowed to grow. Client may suffer alteration in gait resulting from pain.	Surgical removal may be necessary, depending on severity of pain and size of corn. Nurse avoids use of oval corn pads, which increase pressure on toes and reduce circulation. Warm water soaks can soften corns before gentle rubbing with a callus file or pumice stone (consult with physician). Wider and softer shoes are suggested.
Plantar Warts Fungating lesion appears on sole of foot and is caused by papilloma virus.	Warts may be contagious. They are painful and make walking difficult.	Treatment ordered by physician may include applications of salicylic acid, electrodesiccation (burning with electrical spark), or freezing with solid carbon dioxide.
Athlete's Foot (Tinea Pedis) Athlete's foot is fungal infection of foot; scaliness and cracking of skin occurs between toes and on soles of feet. Small blister containing fluid may appear. Problem is apparently induced by wearing of constricting footwear.	Athlete's foot can spread to other body parts, especially hands. It is contagious and frequently recurs.	Feet should be well ventilated. Drying feet well after bathing and applying powder help prevent infection. Wearing of clean socks or stockings reduces incidence. Physician may order application of griseofulvin, miconazole, or tolnaftate.
Ingrown Nails Toenail or fingernail grows inward into soft tissue around nail. Ingrown nail often results from improper nail trimming.	Ingrown nails can cause localized pain when pressure is applied.	Treatment is frequent hot soaks in antiseptic solution and removal of portion of nail that has grown into skin. Instruct client on proper nail-trimming techniques and refer to podiatrist.
Ram's Horn Nails Ram's horn nails are unusually long curved nails.	Attempt by nurse to cut nails may result in damage to nail bed with risk of infection.	Nurse refers client to podiatrist.
Paronychia Inflammation of tissue surrounding nail occurs after hangnail or other injury. It occurs in people who frequently have their hands in water and is common in diabetic clients.	Area can become infected.	Treatment is hot compresses or soaks and local application of antibiotic ointments. Paronychia can be prevented by careful manicuring.
Foot Odors Foot odors are the result of excess perspiration promoting microorganism growth.	Condition may cause discomfort because of excess perspiration.	Frequent washing, use of foot deodorants and powders, and wearing clean footwear prevent or reduce problem.

Table 38-4 Hair and Scalp Problems

Characteristics		Interventions
Dandruff		
Scaling of scalp is accompanied by itching. In severe cases, dandruff is found on eyebrows.	Dandruff causes person embarrassment. If dandruff enters eyes, conjunctivitis may develop.	Shampoo regularly with medicated shampoo. In severe cases, obtain physician's advice.
Ticks		
Small, gray-brown parasites burrow into skin and suck blood.	Ticks transmit several diseases to people. Most common are Rocky Mountain spotted fever, tularemia, and Lyme disease.	Do not pull ticks from skin because sucking apparatus remains and may become infected. Suffocate tick by placing a drop of oil or ether on tick or covering it with petrolatum to ease removal.
Pediculosis (Lice)		
Tiny, grayish-white parasite insects infest mammals.		
Pediculosis Capitis (Head Lice)		
Parasite is found on scalp attached to hair strands. Eggs look like oval particles, similar to dandruff. Bites or pustules may be observed behind ears and at hairline.	Head lice are difficult to remove and may spread to furniture and other people if not treated.	Check entire scalp. Use medicated shampoo for eliminating lice; **Caution against use of products containing Lindane, because the ingredient is toxic and known to cause adverse reactions** (National Pediculosis Association, 2001); repeat treatment 12 to 24 hours later. Manual removal is best option when treatment has failed. Vacuum infested areas of home.
Pediculosis Corporis (Body Lice)		
Parasites tend to cling to clothing, so they may not be easily seen. Body lice suck blood and lay eggs on clothing and furniture.	Client itches constantly. Scratches seen on skin may become infected. Hemorrhagic spots may appear on skin where lice are sucking blood.	Bathe or shower thoroughly. After skin is dried, apply recommended pediculocid lotion. After 12-24 hr, take another bath or shower. Bag infested clothing or linen until laundered in hot water. Vacuum rooms thoroughly and throw away bag after completion.
Pediculosis Pubis (Crab Lice)		
Parasites are found in pubic hair. Crab lice are grayish white with red legs.	Lice may spread through bed linen, clothing, or furniture or between persons via sexual contact.	Shave hair off affected area. Cleanse as for body lice. If lice were sexually transmitted, notify partner.
Hair Loss (Alopecia)		
Alopecia occurs in all races. Balding patches are seen in periphery of hair line. Hair becomes brittle and broken. Condition is caused by use of hair curlers, hair picks, tight braiding, and use of hot comb.	Patches of uneven hair growth and loss alter client's appearance.	Stop hair-care practices that damage hair.

The nurse inspects the nares for signs of inflammation, discharge, lesions, edema, and deformity (see Chapter 32). The nasal mucosa is normally pink and clear and has little or no discharge. A clear, watery discharge may be the result of allergies. If clients have any form of tubing exiting the nose (e.g., nasogastric), the nurse should look at the nares surfaces that come in contact with the tubing for tissue sloughing, localized tenderness, inflammation, and bleeding.

Developmental Changes. The normal process of aging influences the condition of body tissues and structures and thus the manner in which hygienic measures are performed. Chapter 48 addresses the changes in hearing, vision, and olfaction across the life span as a result of growth and development.

Skin. The neonate's skin is relatively immature at birth. The epidermis and dermis are loosely bound together, and the skin is very thin. Friction against the skin layers can cause bruising. The nurse must handle the neonate carefully during bathing. Any break in the skin can easily lead to infection.

A toddler's skin layers are more tightly bound together. Thus the child has a greater resistance to infection and skin irritation. However, because of the child's more active play and the absence of established hygienic habits, greater attention is needed from parents and caregivers to provide thorough hygiene and to begin teaching good hygiene habits.

During adolescence the growth and maturation of the integument increases. In girls, estrogen secretion causes the skin to become soft, smooth, and thicker, with increased vascularity. In boys, male hormones produce an increased thickness of the skin with some darkening in color. Sebaceous glands become more active, predisposing adolescents to **acne. Eccrine** and **apocrine** sweat glands become fully functional during puberty. Adolescents usually begin to use antiperspirants. More frequent bathing and shampooing also become necessary to reduce body odors and eliminate oily hair. Sweating is usually more pronounced in boys.

The condition of the adult's skin depends on hygienic practices and exposure to environmental irritants. Normally the skin is elastic, well hydrated, firm, and smooth. When an adult practices frequent bathing or is exposed to an environment with low humidity, the skin can become very dry and flaky.

As we age, the skin loses its resiliency and moisture, and sebaceous and sweat glands become less active. The epithelium thins and elastic collagen fibers shrink, making the skin fragile and subject to bruising and breaking. These changes warrant caution when turning and repositioning older adults (Lueckenotte, 2000). Typically the older person's skin is dry and wrinkled. Daily bathing as well as bathing with water that is too hot or soap that is harsh may cause the skin to become excessively dry.

Feet and Nails. During standing, the foot provides body support and absorbs shock. With aging, the feet begin to show signs of wear and tear. This may occur earlier if a person has failed to wear comfortable, supportive footwear. The cushioning layer of fat on the soles of the feet becomes thin.

Chronic foot problems are a common part of poor foot care, improper fit of footwear, aging, or systemic disease. Older adults often have dry feet because of a decrease in sebaceous gland secretion, dehydration of epidermal cells, and poor condition of footwear. Fissures that result in itching frequently develop (Bryant and Beinlich, 1999). One of the most common problems for older adults is foot pain (Lueckenotte, 2000). Painful feet can be the result of congenital deformities, weak structure, injuries, and diseases such as diabetes, rheumatoid arthritis, or osteoarthritis. Arthritis is generally the cause for changes in the feet after age 55. Additional common

problems of the feet include hammer and claw toes (flexion contractures); bunions, corns, and calluses; loss of sensation; and pathological nail conditions (Boyer, 2001).

Fungal infections occur under toenails, causing dirty yellow streaks or total discoloration. The nails can also become opaque, scaly, and hypertrophied. If foot or nail problems stay unresolved, the client can easily become disabled. The nurse applies knowledge of typical changes in the feet and nails when anticipating the type of hygiene a client will require.

The Mouth. At approximately 6 to 8 months of age, infants begin teething (Wong, 1999). The first permanent (secondary) teeth erupt at about 6 years of age (Wong, 1999). From adolescence, when all of the permanent teeth are in place, through middle adulthood, the teeth and gums remain healthy if a person follows good eating patterns and good dental care. Avoidance of fermentable carbohydrates and sticky sweets are central to keeping the teeth free of **caries.** Regular brushing and flossing helps to prevent caries and periodontal disease.

As a person grows older there are numerous factors that can result in poor oral care. These include age-related changes of the mouth, chronic disease such as diabetes, physical disabilities involving hand grasp or strength affecting the ability to perform oral care, lack of attention to oral care, and prescribed medications that have oral side effects. Aging teeth become brittle, drier, and darker in color. Teeth become uneven, jagged, and fractured, gums lose vascularity and tissue elasticity, which can cause dentures to fit poorly. Often older adults are **edentulous** and wear complete or partial dentures. It is important for the nurse to learn if older adults wear dentures and the condition of underlying supportive gum tissue.

Hair. Throughout life, changes in the growth, distribution, and condition of the hair influence the hygiene that a person requires. As males reach adolescence, shaving becomes a part of routine grooming. Young girls who reach puberty may begin to shave their legs and axillae. With aging, as scalp hair becomes thinner and drier shampooing is usually performed less frequently.

Although much of the hygiene care focuses preventing infection, injury, and maintaining function, the nurse must be aware of developmental changes and risks to these special sensory organs. While the structure of the eyes do not have marked developmental changes, altered visual acuity can occur at several points during the aging process; for example, when children start school or when clients reach middle age there may be changes in visual acuity. In addition, as clients age they are at risk for changes in visual clarity, such as those that occur with glaucoma, and visual field losses, such as those that may occur with macular degeneration or glaucoma.

Structures of the ears do not change as the client ages; however, changes in hearing acuity or balance may occur with aging. In the young child changes in hearing acuity may result from foreign objects being placed in the ear; this may be a temporary change and is resolved once the object is removed. Changes may also result from repeated ear infections or exposure to loud music, especially when the child listens to loud music while wearing headphones.

Older adults may have changes in the structure and function of the small bones in the inner ear that affect changes in hearing acuity. Aging may result in increased cerumen production, which can also impede hearing acuity. In addition, there may be age-related changes in the movement of fluid through the semicircular canals and the client may experience positional dizziness or some balance problem. While changes in the sense of smell can occur at any time, it seems to be more frequent in the older adult population. It is important to remember that changes in the sense of smell may also affect taste and the client's appetite.

New and acute changes in the structure and function of the eyes, ears, and nose must be fully assessed and evaluated. Timely evaluation of these changes may identify other illnesses or verify that they are age related.

Use of Sensory Aids. For clients who wear eyeglasses, contact lenses, artificial eyes, or hearing aids the nurse assesses client's knowledge and methods used for care and has the client describe his or her typical approach used in routine care (Box 38-4). The nurse compares information gathered from the client with what the nurse knows is the proper care technique. Any differences in client practice with standard practice may indicate a need for client education.

Box 38-4   Assessing a Client's Use of Sensory Aids

Eyeglasses

Purpose for wearing glasses (e.g., reading, distance, or both)
Methods used to clean glasses
Presence of symptoms (e.g., blurred vision, photophobia, headaches, irritation)

Contact Lenses

Type of lens worn
Frequency and duration of time lenses are worn (including sleep time)
Presence of symptoms (e.g., burning, excess tearing, redness, irritation, swelling, sensitivity to light)
Techniques used by the client to cleanse, store, insert, and remove lenses
Use of eye drops or ointments
Use of emergency identification bracelet or card that warns others to remove client's lenses in case of emergency

Artificial Eye

Method used to insert and remove eye
Method for cleansing eye
Presence of symptoms (e.g., drainage, inflammation, pain involving the orbit)

Hearing Aid

Type of aid worn
Methods used to cleanse aid
Client's ability to change battery and adjust hearing aid volume

---

Self-Care Ability. Clients with physical or cognitive impairments need assistance with all or some aspects of personal hygiene. Assessment of the client's physical and cognitive status determines specifically what aspects of hygiene care can be performed independently, those that require some assistance, and those that require total assistance.

The nurse's assessment must include measurement of a client's muscle strength, flexibility and dexterity, balance, coordination, and activity tolerance necessary in performing activities such as bathing, brushing teeth, and bending over to inspect the feet (Figure 38-5). The degree of assistance needed by a client during hygienic care may also depend on vision, the ability to sit without support, hand grasp strength, the range of motion in the client's extremities, or the presence of equipment, such as an intravenous (IV) line, dressings, or traction. Painful conditions of the upper extremities pose special problems. The nurse can assess self-care ability by asking clients to perform activities such as tooth brushing or combing the hair. Observe the client carefully and note not only if the activity is performed correctly, but if the client is able to be thorough and complete the task.

When clients have self-care limitations, part of the nurse's assessment becomes determining if family or friends are available to assist. Assisting with hygiene measures can at times be unpleasant. The nurse's assessment should include how the family assists, how often is this assistance provided, and what are their feelings about be-

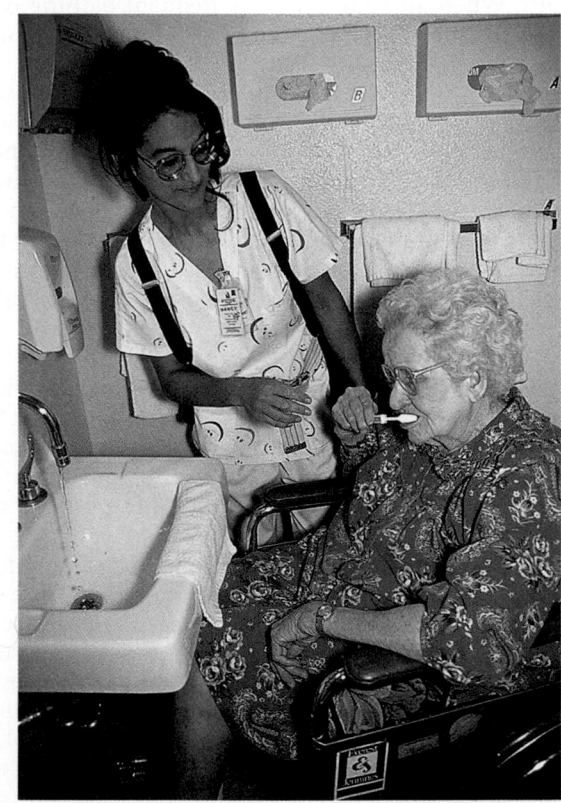

FIGURE 38-5 The nurse observes client brushing teeth. During such observations the nurse can determine how much assistance the client may need.

ing caregivers. In addition, the nurse also assesses the home environment and its influence on the client's hygiene practices. Are there barriers in the home that may affect the client's self-care abilities? Water faucets that are too tight to easily adjust, bathtubs with high sides, and a bathroom too small to fit a chair in front of a sink are a few examples.

Hygiene Practices. Assessment of hygiene practices reveals the client's preferences for how to perform grooming. For example, a client may choose to groom the hair in a certain style or choose to trim nails in a certain way. When a client has a physical disability, special precautions may be needed to perform grooming without injury. Asking the client to assist or teach the nurse how to perform preferred grooming practices gives the client a greater sense of independence and helps the nurse avoid causing the client any discomfort or injury.

Cultural Factors. A client's cultural background is an influential factor when determining hygiene needs. Culture plays a role not only in hygiene practices and preferences but also in sensitivity to personal space (see Chapter 8). For example, some Chinese-Americans may view tasks associated with closeness and touch as being offensive or impolite, whereas Vietnamese-Americans may feel very uneasy during a back rub. The nurse should ask a client what will make him or her feel most comfortable during a bath. Perhaps the client would prefer only a partial instead of a full bath from the nurse, with a family member completing the bathing of more private body parts. The client may also defer part of hygiene. If in the nurse's judgment, hygiene is critical to prevent developing or worsening problems, such as skin breakdown, the nurse must take the time to understand the client's concerns and then offer an explanation that will help the client accept the nurse's intervention.

Clients at Risk for Hygiene Problems. There are clients who present risks that require more attentive and rigorous hygienic care (Table 38-5). These risks result from side effects of medications, a lack of knowledge, an inability to perform hygiene, or a physical condition that potentially injures the skin, integument, or other structures. An immobilized client who has a fever, for example, will require more frequent bathing to minimize perspiration on the skin, and more frequent turning and positioning to reduce the chance of skin breakdown.

The nurse anticipates whether a client is predisposed to such risks and follows through with a complete assessment. For example, if a client is receiving chemotherapy, there is the risk of the medication destroying normal flora in the mouth, allowing for the overgrowth of opportunistic bacteria. Therefore the oral examination should be more thorough and detailed with the nurse examining all surfaces of the tongue and mucosa. If a client is diaphoretic, the nurse will give special attention to body areas, such as a woman's breasts and perineal area, to check where moisture may collect and irritate skin surfaces. The nurse anticipates problems created by these risks so as to provide appropriate preventive care. The nurse's assessment will include a review of the client's medical and sur-

gical history, medications, and the specific risk factors the client is likely to have.

Special Considerations in Hygiene Assessment. Depending on the type of hygiene a nurse plans to provide, there are focused assessments that are important to conduct. Before giving foot care, the nurse assesses the type of footwear worn by a client. Children or young adults who frequently fail to wear socks may have excess perspiration that promotes fungal growth. Tight or poorly fitting shoes, socks, garters, or knee-high nylon stockings may cause skin irritation and interfere with circulation to the feet. The nurse also assesses whether clients wear clean footwear daily because repeated use of soiled footwear can lead to infection. If the client has diabetes mellitus or other peripheral vascular disease, it is extremely important that correct footwear be worn. Extra wide and extra deep shoes will accommodate bunions or hammer toes. Cushioned inner soles help redistribute pressure on the metatarsal head. Rocker-bottom shoes help with ambulation (Strauss, Hart, and Winant, 1998).

A client's eating patterns are important to assess before oral care. The presence of any problems may help the nurse to locate abnormalities. The nurse asks a client if any problems are noted with chewing, denture fit, or swallowing. A client may have changed the type of food in the diet as a result of chewing difficulties. The presence of an ulcer or irritation may impair chewing and cause a client to avoid eating. This is common in an older adult with poorly fitting dentures.

Client Expectations. As is the case in any nursing assessment, it is important to know what a client expects from nursing care. In regard to hygienic care, the client may simply expect to have hygiene preferences and practices applied in the health care setting. The nurse can learn a client's expectations by asking questions such as, "To make you most comfortable and feel at home, how can I best perform your bath and personal care?" or "How can we help you care for your teeth, nails, and hair, now that you are back home?"

Learning a client's expectations and applying them in practice is important in establishing a caring relationship. Truly individualizing hygienic care shows the nurse's respect for the client's needs. As the nurse learns what the client expects, this information can be incorporated into goal development (see Planning).

Nursing Diagnosis

The nurse's assessment will reveal the condition of the skin, oral cavity, and other tissues, as well as the client's need for and ability to meet personal hygiene needs. The nurse reviews all data gathered, considers previous clients cared for, reviews knowledge pertaining to preexisting conditions, and then looks for clusters of data suggesting a problem trend. For example, an older adult with degenerative arthritis presents to the home care nurse with pain in the joints, weakness, and mobility limitations in the dominant hand, and a generally unkempt appearance. Closer review of assessment data reveals defining charac-

Table 38-5	Risk Factors for Hygiene Problems
Risks	**Hygiene Implications**

Oral Problems

Risks	Hygiene Implications
Clients who are unable to use upper extremities due to paralysis, weakness, or restriction (e.g., cast or dressing)	Client lacks upper extremity strength or dexterity needed to brush teeth (Lewis and others, 2000).
Dehydration, inability to take fluids or food by mouth (NPO)	Causes excess drying and fragility of mucosa; increases accumulation of secretions on tongue and gums.
Presence of nasogastric or oxygen tubes; mouth breathers	Causes drying of mucosa.
Chemotherapeutic drugs	Drugs kill rapidly multiplying cells, including normal cells lining oral cavity. Ulcers and inflammation can develop.
Lozenges, cough drops, antacids, and chewable vitamins over-the-counter (OTC)	Medications contain large amounts of sugar. Repeated use increases sugar or acid content in mouth.
Radiation therapy to head and neck	Reduces salivary flow and lowers pH of saliva; can lead to stomatitis and tooth decay (Lewis and others, 2000).
Oral surgery, trauma to mouth, placement of oral airway	Cause trauma to oral cavity with swelling, ulcerations, inflammation and bleeding.
Immunosuppression; alters blood clotting	Predisposes to inflammation and bleeding gums.
Diabetes mellitus	Prone to dryness of mouth, gingivitis, periodontal disease, and loss of teeth.

Skin Problems

Risks	Hygiene Implications
Immobilization	Dependent body parts are exposed to pressure from underlying surfaces. The inability to turn or change position increases risk for pressure ulcers.
Reduced sensation due to stroke, spinal cord injury, diabetes, local nerve damage	Client does not receive normal transmission of nerve impulses when excessive heat or cold, pressure, friction, or chemical irritants are applied to skin.
Limited protein or caloric intake and reduced hydration (e.g., fever, burns, gastrointestinal alterations, poorly fitting dentures)	Limited caloric and protein intake predispose to impaired tissue synthesis. Skin becomes thinner, less elastic, and smoother with a loss of subcutaneous tissue. Poor wound healing may result. Reduced hydration impairs skin turgor.
Excessive secretions or excretions on the skin from perspiration, urine, watery fecal material, and wound drainage	Moisture is a medium for bacterial growth and can cause local skin irritation, softening of epidermal cells, and skin maceration.
Presence of external devices (e.g., casts, restraint, bandage, dressing)	Device can exert pressure or friction against skin's surface.
Vascular insufficiency	Arterial blood supply to tissues is inadequate, or venous return is impaired, causing decreased circulation to extremities. Tissue ischemia and breakdown may occur. Risk for infection is high.

Foot Problems

Risks	Hygiene Implications
Client unable to bend over or has reduced visual acuity	Client is unable to fully visualize entire surface of each foot, impairing ability to adequately assess condition of skin and nails.

Eye Care Problems

Risks	Hygiene Implications
Reduced dexterity and hand coordination	Physical limitations create inability to safely insert or remove contact lenses.

teristics of an inability to wash body parts and difficulty turning and regulating a water faucet. The nursing diagnosis of *bathing/hygiene self-care deficit* is supported and becomes part of the nurse's plan of care. The nurse's accurate selection of nursing diagnoses requires critical thinking to identify actual or potential health problems. Assessment activities must be thorough in revealing all appropriate defining characteristics so that an accurate diagnosis can be made (Box 38-5).

Whether a client has an actual alteration (e.g., impaired tissue integrity) or is at risk (e.g., risk for infection) determines the focus of nursing interventions. The client with an actual alteration will require extensive hygienic

care, often more thorough than what routine hygiene might involve. For example, if the client has skin breakdown, the nurse must initiate care more frequently to keep existing skin surfaces clean and dry and to eliminate factors such as moisture or drainage that can worsen the condition of the skin. The nurse would also provide care to promote healing of injured skin surfaces (see Chapter 47). If the client is at risk for a problem, the nurse will institute preventive measures. In the case of risk for impaired oral mucous membranes, the nurse will keep the mucosa well hydrated, minimize foods irritating to tissues, and provide cleansing that soothes and reduces tissue inflammation.

Nursing Diagnostic Process   Box 38-5

Assessment Activities	Defining Characteristics	Nursing Diagnosis
Observe client attempt to bathe self either in bed or at bathroom sink. (NOTE: Be sure positioning does not restrict potential movement.)	Unable to wash body or body parts	Self-care deficit, bathing/hygiene related to upper extremity weakness and generalized fatigue
Assess client's upper extremity strength, range of motion, and coordination.	Restricted upper extremity range of motion and strength	
Ask client about level of fatigue after bathing.	Coordination adequate	
Obtain vital signs after bathing.	Complains of fatigue and needs to rest after bathing	
	Pulse elevated from 90 to 110 beats per minute, BP stable, respirations elevated from 16 to 22 breaths per minute	

The identification of related factors guides the nurse in the selection of nursing interventions. *Impaired oral mucous membrane related to malnutrition* and a diagnosis of *impaired oral mucous membrane related to chemical trauma* require very different interventions. When malnutrition is a causal factor, the nurse will obviously confer with a dietitian for appropriate dietary supplements and incorporate client education into the plan. When mucosa are injured as a result of chemical trauma from chemotherapy, techniques for cleansing and hydrating inflamed tissues and eliminating sources of irritation will be the focus of nursing care. Although there are many possible nursing diagnoses that apply to clients in need of hygienic care, the following lists selects a few of the more common nursing diagnoses associated with hygiene problems:

- Impaired dentition
- Fatigue
- Ineffective health maintenance
- Risk for infection
- Deficient knowledge about hygiene practices
- Impaired physical mobility
- Impaired oral mucous membrane
- Self-care deficit, bathing/hygiene, dressing/grooming, toileting
- Chronic low self-esteem
- Risk for impaired skin integrity
- Ineffective tissue perfusion

Planning

During planning the nurse synthesizes information from multiple resources (Figure 38-6). Critical thinking ensures that the client's plan of care integrates all that the nurse knows about the individual client and key critical thinking elements.

There are situations when clients have multiple nursing diagnoses. The concept map (Figure 38-7) shows graphically how numerous nursing diagnoses can be interrelated.

Previous experience with other clients can be very useful in knowing how to adapt hygiene techniques for special needs. Professional standards are especially important to consider when the nurse develops a plan of care. These standards often establish evidence-based guidelines for care. For example, the American Diabetes Association's clinical practice recommendations for 1999 offer valuable guidelines for preventive foot care in diabetic clients (Pinzur, Slovenkai, and Trepman, 1999).

Goals and Outcomes. The nurse and client partner together to identify goals and expected outcomes and develop an individualized plan of care based on the client's nursing diagnoses (see care plan). Goals are established with the client's self-care abilities and resources in mind and focus on maintaining or improving the condition of the skin and mucosa, oral mucosa, or dental hygiene, for example. Outcomes should be measurable and achievable within client limitations. The nurse works further with the client to then select hygiene measures that are appropriate and realistic.

When providing for client hygiene, nurses care for a variety of clients with different self-care abilities and needs. For example, the nurse and a client, who has one-sided paralysis following a cerebral vascular accident, might develop the following goal: "Client's musculoskeletal system remains free of breakdown or contractures." A series of realistic individualized expected outcomes would then be established to assist the client in meeting this goal. These outcomes may include the following:

- Client's skin is clean, dry, and intact without signs of inflammation.
- Clients skin remains elastic and well hydrated.
- Client's range of joint motion remains within normal limits on both affected and unaffected side.
- Client tolerated bathing without excessive fatigue.

Setting Priorities. The client's condition influences the plan for delivering hygiene. A seriously ill client usually needs a daily bath because body secretions accumulate. An older client at home may require a visit from a home care aide to assist with a tub bath. Clients who are normally inactive during the day and have skin that tends to be dry may need to bathe only twice a week. The nurse must plan for necessary assistance for clients who are

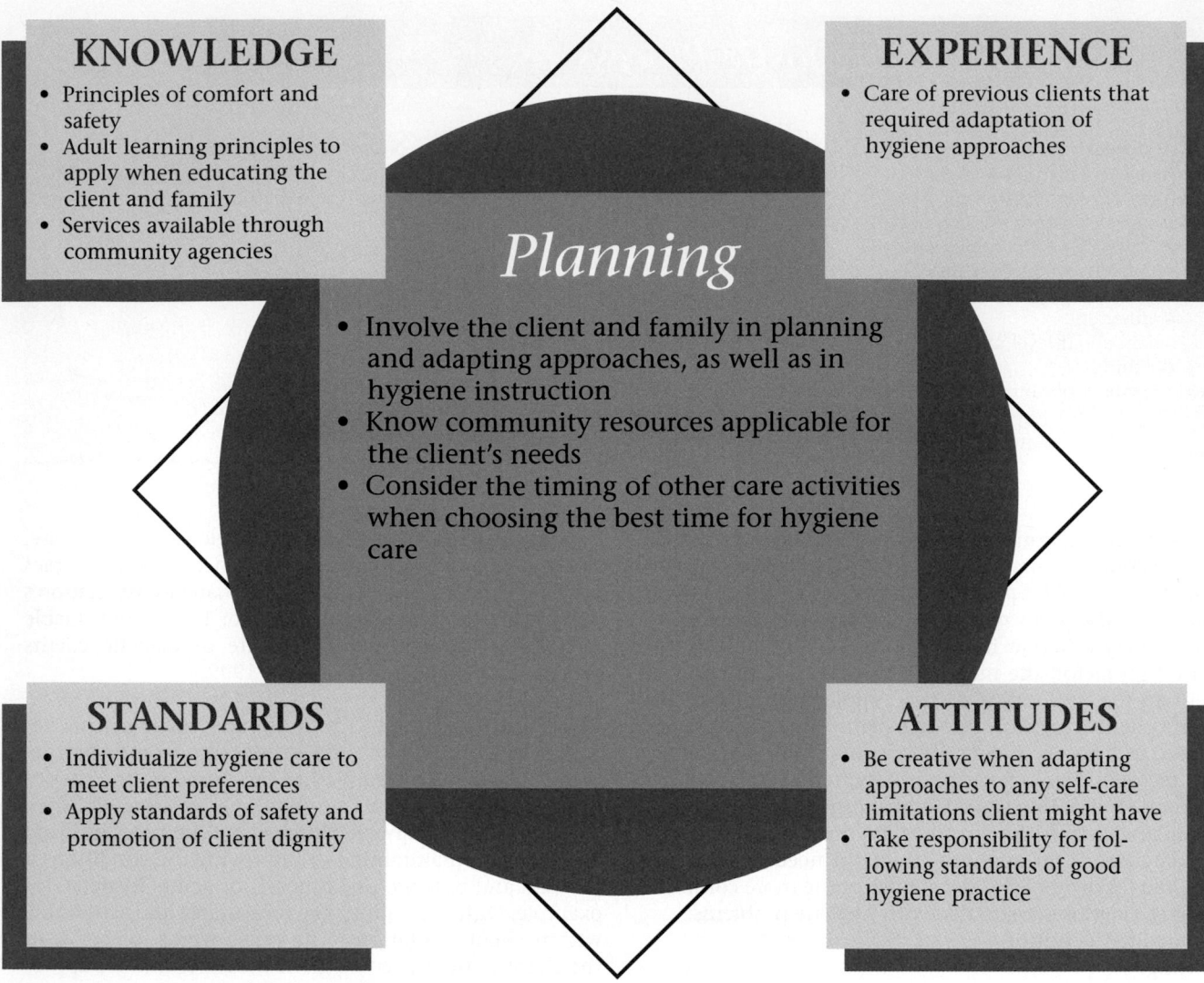

KNOWLEDGE

- Principles of comfort and safety
- Adult learning principles to apply when educating the client and family
- Services available through community agencies

EXPERIENCE

- Care of previous clients that required adaptation of hygiene approaches

Planning

- Involve the client and family in planning and adapting approaches, as well as in hygiene instruction
- Know community resources applicable for the client's needs
- Consider the timing of other care activities when choosing the best time for hygiene care

STANDARDS

- Individualize hygiene care to meet client preferences
- Apply standards of safety and promotion of client dignity

ATTITUDES

- Be creative when adapting approaches to any self-care limitations client might have
- Take responsibility for following standards of good hygiene practice

FIGURE **38–6** Critical thinking model for hygiene planning.

weakened or possess poor coordination. For example, a partially paralyzed client who has had difficulty getting out of a tub should have a tub chair, handrails, or extra personnel available for help.

Timing is also important in planning hygiene. Being interrupted in the middle of a bath to go to an x-ray examination can frustrate and embarrass a client. Following extensive diagnostic tests (e.g., a stress test), it may be best to delay hygiene and allow a client to rest.

Continuity of Care. It is important to plan for care throughout the stay in a hospital, discharge to a rehabilitation facility, and home. When a client needs assistance as a result of a self-care limitation, the family becomes a valuable resource to the nurse. Family members can usually assist with hygiene measures but may need guidance in adapting techniques to fit client limitations. Be aware of equipment and procedures used in the agency so that the client and family are knowledgeable about the care, have the skill needed to provide the care, and have access to necessary equipment. In addition, various community

resources may be needed. For example, the nurse involved in the care of a homeless client may need to be aware of the location of clothing distribution centers for basic hygiene supplies or a shelter where bathing facilities are available. Frequently the nurse will consult with social workers or staff in local area churches and schools to be sure clients have the resources they need to maintain hygiene.

Implementation

Providing hygiene is a very basic part of a client's care. The nurse learns to use caring practices that help to alleviate the client's anxiety and promote comfort and relaxation while performing each hygiene measure. For example, while giving a client a bath and changing a gown, the nurse uses a gentle approach in turning and repositioning. Using a soft, gentle voice while conversing with the client helps to relieve any fears or concerns. For clients suffering symptoms such as pain or nausea, administer-

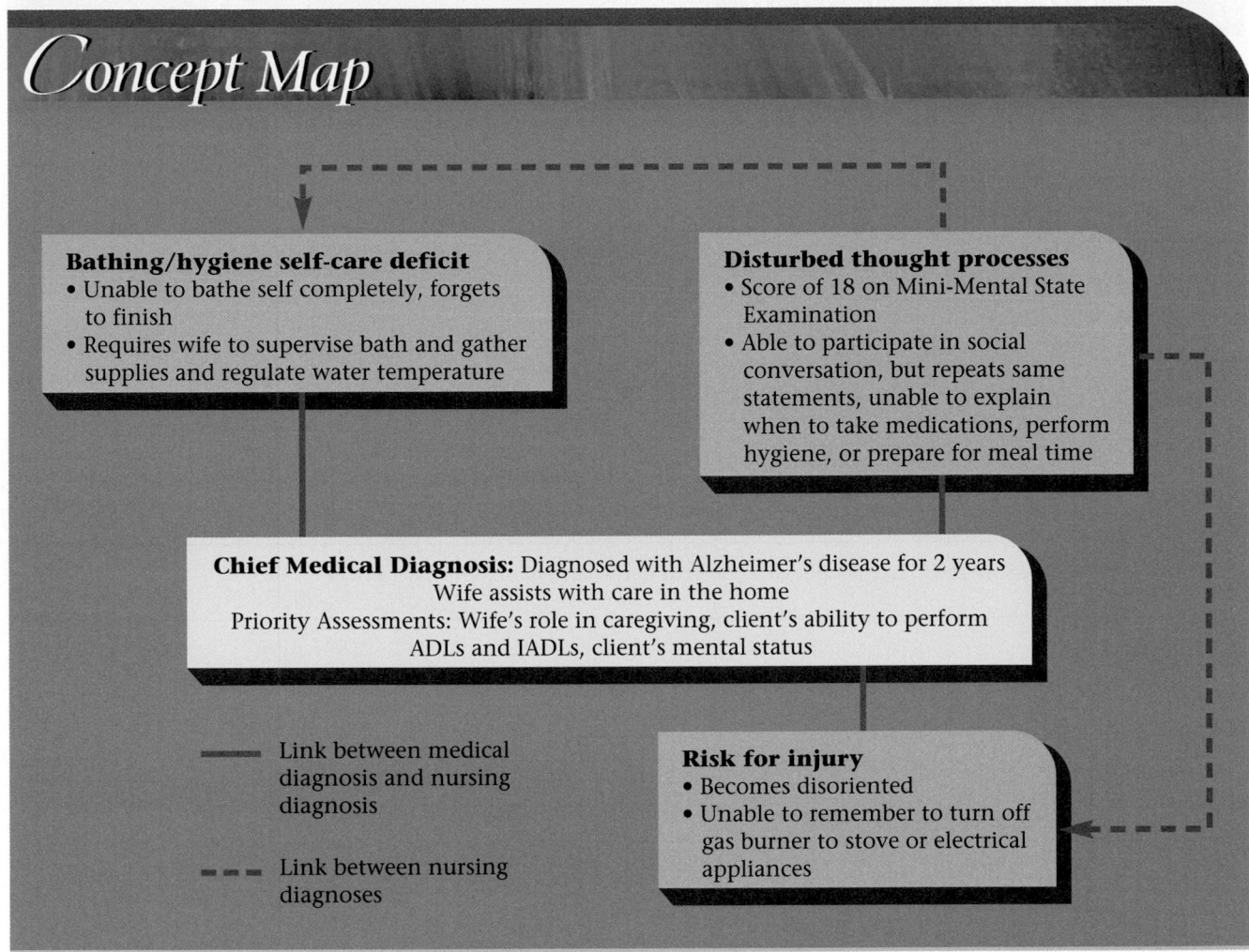

FIGURE **38–7** Concept map for client with hygiene needs.

ing symptom relief therapies before hygiene will better prepare the client for any procedure.

Another important part of implementation is assisting and preparing clients so that they are able to administer their own hygiene. This includes educating clients on proper hygienic techniques and connecting clients with the community resources necessary to enable them to perform hygienic care. The same clients at risk for hygiene problems are the ones in greatest need of understanding their risks, knowing the implications, and then having the information they need to make choices about when and how hygiene is performed.

Health Promotion. In primary health care settings, nurses educate and counsel clients and families on proper hygiene techniques. A new mother will need assistance in learning how to bathe her newborn infant. An older adult will need to become informed on the importance of regular ear care to avoid any hearing deficits resulting from accumulated cerumen. The hygiene skills described throughout this chapter provide standards for excellent

physical care. When assisting clients, the nurse tries to maintain these standards and incorporate adaptations as needed to the client's lifestyle, living arrangements, and preferences. Tips to help the nurse in educating clients about hygiene include the following:

- Make any instruction relevant. After assessing a client's knowledge, motivations, and health beliefs, provide information that relates to the client's situation and will be most useful in resolving the client's problem. For example, when offering foot care instruction to a client with diabetes mellitus, explain how the circulation to the feet can be impaired and how that poses a risk for poor healing and infection, especially when the skin becomes cut or broken.
- Adapt instruction of any techniques to the client's personal bathing facilities. Not all clients will have the ideal situation that exists in a health care setting (e.g., easily accessible shower or a bedside table to place over a bed). Use what facilities or equipment the client has so that personal care items are easy to reach, the client's safety is ensured, and the client feels comfort-

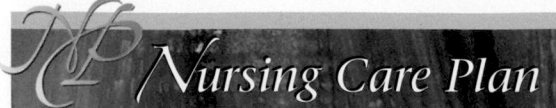

Nursing Care Plan

Hygiene

Assessment

Mrs. Wyatt is a 77-year-old who has had diabetes mellitus for 20 years. She was recently hospitalized for an acute exacerbation of the disease. The nurse, Jeannette, makes the initial home visit for Mrs. Wyatt. Jeannette's assessment reveals Mrs.

Wyatt has an unbalanced gait and appears to limp. Mrs. Wyatt continues to be very independent in making decisions about her care. She tells Jeannette, "It is important for me to be able to care for myself."

Assessment Activities	Findings/Defining Characteristics
Ask Mrs. Wyatt about the comfort of her shoes.	Mrs. Wyatt complains that in the winter her shoes feel tight with socks so she eliminates wearing any type of sock.
Observe Mrs. Wyatt's feet.	Mrs. Wyatt has bilateral heel blisters.
	Her toenails are long, tissue surrounding nail is peeling, and the nails are dirty. There is tissue inflammation between left great and second toes.
Palpate lower extremities.	Popliteal pulses are within normal limits. Dorsalis pedis pulses are weak. Feet are pale and cool to touch.
	Capillary refill time of great toe is increased in left foot at >2 seconds.
Ask Mrs. Wyatt about routine foot and nail care.	She cannot describe any specific foot care practice.

Nursing Diagnosis: Ineffective peripheral tissue perfusion related to improper diabetic foot care and nail hygiene practices.

Planning

Goal	Expected Outcomes*
	Skin Integrity
Skin integrity in both feet will improve within 1 month	Blisters will heal within 2 weeks.
	Tissue inflammation on left toes will resolve within 10 days.
	Tissue Perfusion: Peripheral
Client will have improved peripheral circulation to both feet.	Within 3 months, feet will be warm to touch, capillary refill brisk.
	Deficient Knowledge: Treatment Regimen
Client will be able to complete diabetic foot care regimen within 1 month.	Client is able to accurately inspect tissue integrity of feet and toenails within 1 month.
	Client describes correct preventive diabetic foot care practices.
	Client has improved diabetic foot care and nail hygiene within 2 weeks.

*Outcome classification labels from Moorhead S, Johnson M, Maas M: *Nursing outcomes classification (NOC)*, ed 3, St. Louis, 2004, Mosby.

Interventions†

Skin Surveillance

Review with client how to assess feet for breaks in skin, friction from shoes, and how to avoid foot injury.

Instruct client to observe feet for reddened areas, abrasions, blisters, and swollen areas immediately after removing shoes.

Rationale

Injury to the diabetic foot from improper nail care, friction from poorly fitting shoes, and minor injuries to the foot increase the client's risk for infection, impaired mobility, and amputation (Strauss, Hart, and Winant, 1998).

Improperly fitting shoes produce friction, redness, and swelling. Observation for these conditions immediately after removing shoes promotes timely identification of early foot problems (Bryant and Beinlich, 1999).

†Intervention classification labels from Dochterman JM, Bulecheck GM: *Nursing interventions classification (NIC)*, ed 4, St. Louis, 2004, Mosby.

Continued

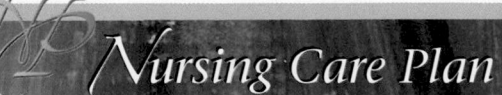

Nursing Care Plan

Hygiene—cont'd

Interventions†—cont'd	Rationale
Skin Care	
Show client how to clean and apply moisturizers and other skin care products to feet daily.	Proper foot care practices include daily cleaning and moisturizing the feet (Boyer, 2001).
Demonstrate to client how to apply moleskin over blistered areas.	Moleskin preparations are useful in avoiding pressure and friction. Avoiding pressure and friction then allows the area to heal.
Explain that client should see a podiatrist every 4 to 6 weeks for toenail care.	Regular nail care, callus removal, and inspection of feet by a professional reduces the risk for peripheral tissue injury and subsequent immobility and morbidity (Green, Aliabaide, and Green 2002).
Refer client to orthotic footwear specialist.	Orthotic footwear specialist can evaluate client's walk patterns and create footwear individualized to client's walk, weight, and other individual needs. Specialized footwear can reduce the risk of impaired skin integrity of the feet.

†Intervention classification labels from Dochterman JM, Bulecheck GM: *Nursing interventions classification (NIC)*, ed 4, St. Louis, 2004, Mosby.

Evaluation

Nursing Actions	Client Response/Finding	Achievement of Outcome
Observe client's feet.	Blisters are healed.	Resolution of foot blisters has been achieved.
	Inflammation between toes on left foot has resolved.	Resolution of tissue inflammation has occurred, and no new foot injury is observed.
	Toenails are clean and properly trimmed, and no cracks around nail tissue are observed.	Mrs. Wyatt has improved diabetic foot and nail hygiene.
Palpate lower extremities.	Pulses are equal bilaterally, capillary refill is still sluggish.	Tissue perfusion to feet has not improved.
Ask client about frequency of foot inspection.	Mrs. Wyatt states she observes her feet daily after removing her shoes and immediately before bed.	Mrs. Wyatt inspects feet daily; because no new foot injuries are observed, Mrs. Wyatt appears to have achieved this outcome.
Observe client's foot care practice.	Mrs. Wyatt correctly washed and moisturized feet but was not wearing socks with her shoes. She states that she does not consistently wear socks.	Mrs. Wyatt is able to perform diabetic foot hygiene practice but is not consistent in preventive practice.
Ask client about podiatrist appointment.	Mrs. Wyatt has been to the podiatrist twice and will be returning every 6 weeks for toenail trimming and care.	Mrs. Wyatt has improved diabetic foot and nail hygiene practice.

able in performing hygiene. For example, a young mother may have more room and feel that bathing an infant will be safer if she uses her kitchen sink and counter rather than her bathroom sink.

- Be sure to teach the client steps to take to avoid injury. Almost any hygienic procedure can pose risks (e.g., cutting a nail too close to the skin, failing to adjust the water temperature of the bath, or using tap water for contact lens care). Any instruction must clearly outline safety risks.
- Reinforce infection-control practices. Damage to the skin, mucosa, eyes, or other tissues create an immediate risk for infection. Be sure the client understands the relationship between healthy and intact skin and

tissues, hand hygiene practices, and the prevention of infection.

The *Healthy People 2010* initiative (see Chapter 6) includes recommendations to improve the dental health of the population of the United States. The goals for oral health are to decrease tooth loss caused by tooth decay or periodontal disease for people ages 35 to 44; reduce the number of older adults who have lost their natural teeth; reduce the prevalence of gingivitis; and reduce destructive periodontal disease among individuals ages 35 to 44 (Gadbury-Amyot and others, 2002).

Acute and Restorative Care. Nursing knowledge and skills needed for performing hygiene care are consistent

---

Box 38-6   **Hygiene Care Schedule in Acute and Long-Term Care Settings**

Early Morning Care

Nursing personnel on the night shift may provide basic hygiene to clients getting ready for breakfast, scheduled tests, or early morning surgery. "AM care" includes offering a bedpan or urinal if the client is not ambulatory, washing the client's hands and face, and assisting with oral care.

Routine Morning Care

In care performed after breakfast, the nurse assists by offering a bedpan or urinal to clients confined to bed; providing a bath or shower; providing perineal care; providing oral, foot, nail, and hair care; giving a back rub; changing the client's gown or pajamas; changing the bed linens; and straightening the client's bedside unit and room. This is often referred to as "complete AM care."

Afternoon Care

Hospitalized clients often undergo many exhausting diagnostic tests or procedures in the morning. In rehabilitation centers, clients may participate in physical therapy during the morning. Afternoon hygiene care includes washing the hands and face, assisting with oral care, offering a bedpan or urinal, and straightening bed linen.

Evening, or Hour-Before-Sleep, Care

Before bedtime the nurse offers personal hygiene care that helps a client relax to promote sleep. "PM care" may include changing soiled bed linens, gowns, or pajamas; assisting the client in washing the face and hands; providing oral hygiene; giving a back massage; and offering the bedpan or urinal to nonambulatory clients. Some clients may enjoy a beverage such as juice.

---

across all health care settings where acute care and restorative care are provided. In addition, some of the skills in this section are applicable in areas of health promotion.

In health care settings where clients receive direct nursing care, nurses provide a variety of hygiene measures (Box 38-6). Times may change because of factors affecting the nurse's organization or scheduling of care such as client preferences, planned diagnostic and treatment procedures, the client's need for more hygiene, or the nurse's work assignment. In extended care facilities and nursing homes, the schedule for hygiene may be less frequent.

Bathing and Skin Care. Bathing and skin care are a part of total hygiene. The extent of a client's bath and the methods used for bathing depend on the client's physical abilities, health problems, and the degree of hygiene required. If a client is physically dependent or cognitively impaired, the nurse increases skin assessment and provides skin care directed toward reducing the risk for skin breakdown. When bathing cognitively impaired clients there are special needs and challenges that the nurse must consider (Box 38-7). These clients can easily become afraid, use physical and verbal aggressive behaviors to avoid bathing, and may also display self-injurious behaviors (Hall and Buckwalter, 2001).

A **complete bed bath** is for clients who are totally dependent and require total hygiene care (Skill 38-1). It is an activity that can be exhausting for a client, even if the nurse provides all of the care. Turning during a complete bed bath and receiving back care have been shown to increase oxygen consumption in healthy men and women (Verderber and Gallagher, 1994). The nurse must anticipate and assess whether clients are physically able to tolerate a complete bath. Measuring heart rate before, during, and after the bath provides a measure of the client's physical tolerance. A **partial bed bath** involves bathing only body parts that would cause discomfort or odor if left unbathed. This includes perineal care. Aging or dependent clients in need of only partial hygiene or self-sufficient bedridden clients unable to reach all body

Evidence-Based Practice Guideline   *Box 38-7*

Bathing Persons With Dementia

Individualized and flexible client-centered
- Obtain bathing history: what works, what doesn't work. Identify client's preferences
- Determine method that is least distressing to the client, e.g., letting them soak their feet in the bathtub
- Minimize the time the client is unclothed

Use distraction and negotiation instead of demands
- Minimize noise in bathing area
- Be sure bathing environment is warm
- Set priorities as to which body parts need bathing and which can be "skipped"
- Use as few staff as possible
- If client fears water, colored water or bubble bath may help

Reward client after bathing
- Praise and rewards should be realistic
- Rewards should always be given

Modified from Hall, G.R., Buckwalter K.C. (1995). Evidence-Based protocol: Bathing persons with Dementia. In M.G. Titler (Series Ed.), Series on Evidence-Based Practice for Older Adults. Iowa City, IA. The University of Iowa College of Nursing Gerontological Nursing Interventions Research Center, Research Dissemination Core. For more information, http://www.nursing.uiowa.edu/center/gnirc/disseminatecore.htm

parts receive partial bed baths. Nurses assess carefully to determine that clients can sufficiently bathe other body parts on their own.

When administering either a complete or partial bath, it is important for the nurse to assess the condition of the skin in determining if soap is necessary or if the client requires daily bathing. Clients with excessively dry skin are predisposed to skin impairment. The nurse may decide to skip a bath for a day or bathe only badly soiled areas. Use of soaps that contain emollients is another option. Lubricating the skin with lotion can also help reduce dryness.

Text continued on p. 1030

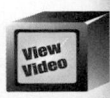

Skill 38-1 *Bathing a Client*

Delegation Considerations

Skills of bathing may be delegated to assistive personnel (AP).

- Instruct AP on the importance of not massaging reddened skin areas.
- Clarify the early signs of impaired skin integrity for select clients and their situation.
- Have AP report changes in the client's skin to the nurse.

Equipment

- Two washcloths
- Two bath towels
- Bath blanket
- Soap and soap dish
- Toiletry items (deodorant, powder, lotion, cologne)
- Clean hospital gown or client's own pajamas or gown
- Laundry bag
- Disposable gloves (when risk for contacting body fluids)

Steps	Rationale
1. Assess client's tolerance for activity, discomfort level, cognitive ability, and musculoskeletal function.	Determines client's ability to perform self-care and level of assistance required from nurse. Also determines type of bath to administer (e.g., tub bath or partial bed bath).

Critical Decision Point: Clients whose level of independence and mobility change frequently may require more or less assistance during bathing.

Steps	Rationale
2. Assess client's bathing preferences: frequency and time of day preferred for bathing, type of hygiene products, and other factors related to client preferences.	Client participates in plan of care. Promotes client's comfort and provides opportunity to include cultural or personal hygiene preferences in hygiene care.
3. Ask if client has noticed any problems or unusual marks on skin.	Provides information to direct physical assessment of skin during bathing.
4. Review orders for specific precautions concerning client's movement or positioning.	Prevents accidental injury to client during bathing activities. Determines level of assistance required by client.
5. Explain procedure, and ask client for suggestions on how to prepare supplies. If partial bath, ask how much of bath client wishes to complete.	Promotes client's cooperation and participation.
6. Adjust room temperature and ventilation, close room doors and windows, and draw room divider curtain.	Warm room that is free of drafts prevents rapid loss of body heat during bathing. Privacy ensures client's mental and physical comfort.
7. Prepare equipment and supplies.	Avoids interrupting procedure or leaving client unattended to retrieve missing equipment.
8. Offer client bedpan or urinal. Provide towel and washcloth.	Client will feel more comfortable after voiding. Prevents interruption of bath.
9. Perform hand hygiene. If client's skin is soiled with drainage or body secretions, apply disposable gloves. Ensure client is not allergic to latex.	Reduces transmission of microorganisms.
10. Bathe client.	
A. Complete or partial bed bath	
(1) If raised, lower side rail closest to you, and assist client in assuming comfortable position, maintaining body alignment. Bring client toward side closest to nurse. Place hospital bed at appropriate level.	Aids nurse's access to client. Maintains client's comfort throughout procedure. Nurse does not have to reach across bed, thus minimizing strain on back muscles. Raising the height of the bed to appropriate position for the nurse facilitates proper body mechanics.
(2) Loosen top covers at foot of bed. Place bath blanket over top sheet. Fold and remove top sheet from under blanket. If possible, have client hold bath blanket while withdrawing sheet. *Optional:* Use top sheet when bath blanket is not available.	Removal of top linens prevents them from becoming soiled or moist during bath. Blanket provides warmth and privacy.
(3) If top sheet is to be reused, fold it for replacement later. If not, dispose in laundry bag, taking care not to allow linen to contact uniform.	Proper disposal prevents transmission of microorganisms.

Skill 38-1   *Bathing a Client—cont'd*

Steps	Rationale
(4) Remove client's gown or pajamas. If an extremity is injured or has reduced mobility, begin removal from *unaffected* side. If client has intravenous (IV) tube, remove gown from arm *without* IV first; then lower IV container or remove from pump and slide gown covering affected arm over tubing and container. Rehang IV container and check flow rate (see illustrations) or reset pump rate. Do not disconnect tubing.	Provides full exposure of body parts during bathing. Undressing unaffected side first allows easier manipulation of gown over body part with reduced range of motion (ROM).

Critical Decision Point: If available, be sure that clients with an IV or upper extremity injury have a gown with snap or tie sleeves. Thus there is easy access to upper extremities during hygiene.

Critical Decision Point: When an IV pump is used, it may be appropriate to manually adjust the IV flow rate to a keep vein open (KVO) flow and remove the IV tubing from the pump (check agency policy). When the bath is complete, the nurse resets the pump to the prescribed IV flow rate (see Chapter 40).

A

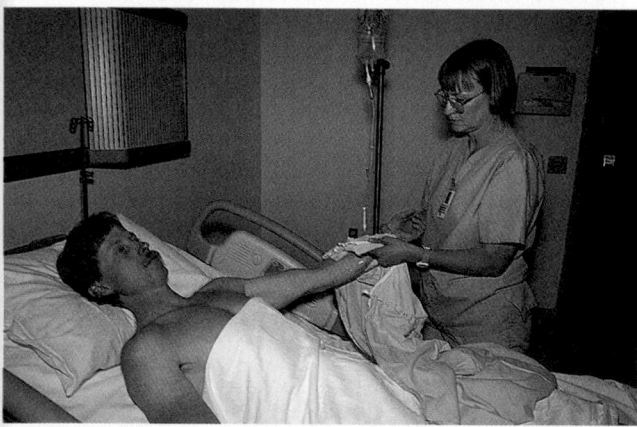

B

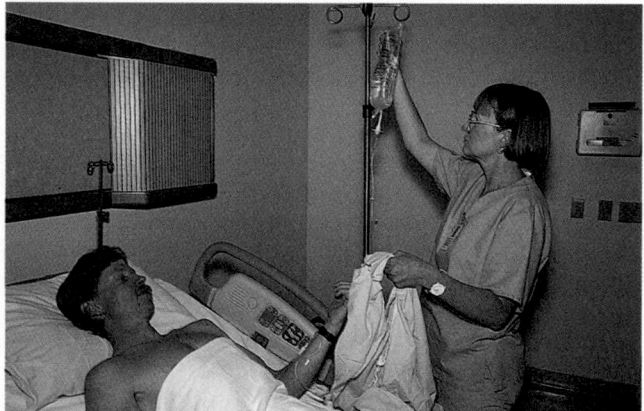

C

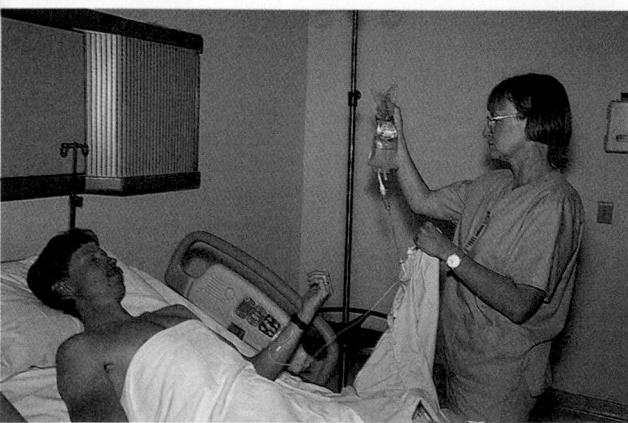

D

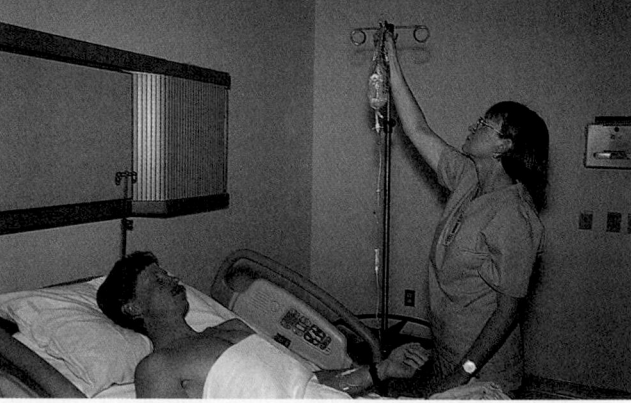

STEP **10 A(4)** **A,** Remove client's gown. **B,** Remove IV from pole. **C,** Slide IV tubing through arm of client's gown. **D,** Rehang IV bag.

Steps	**Rationale**
(5) Pull side rail up. Fill washbasin two thirds full, with warm water. Have client place fingers in water to test temperature tolerance. Place plastic container of bath lotion in bath water to warm, if desired.	Raising side rail maintains client's safety as nurse leaves bedside. Warm water promotes comfort, relaxes muscles, and prevents unnecessary chilling. Testing temperature prevents accidental burns. Bath water warms lotion for application to client's skin.
(6) Remove pillow if allowed, and raise head of bed 30 to 45 degrees. Place bath towel under client's head. Place second bath towel over client's chest.	Removal of pillow makes it easier to wash client's ears and neck. Placement of towels prevents soiling of bed linen and bath blanket.
(7) Immerse washcloth in water and wring thoroughly. If desired, fold washcloth around fingers of nurse's hand to form mitt (see illustration).	Mitt retains water and heat better than loosely held washcloth; keeps cold edges from brushing against client and prevents splashing.
(8) Wash client's eyes with plain warm water. Inquire if client is wearing contact lenses. Use different section of mitt for each eye. Move mitt from inner to outer canthus (see illustration). Soak any crusts on eyelid for 2 to 3 min with damp cloth before attempting removal. Dry eye thoroughly but gently.	Soap irritates eyes. Use of separate sections of mitt reduces infection transmission. Bathing eye from inner to outer canthus prevents secretions from entering nasolacrimal duct. Pressure can cause internal injury.
(9) Ask if client prefers to use soap on face. Wash, rinse, and dry well forehead, cheeks, nose, neck, and ears. (Men may wish to shave at this point or after bath.)	Soap tends to dry face, which is exposed to air more than other body parts.
(10) Remove bath blanket from client's arm that is closest to nurse. Place bath towel lengthwise under arm.	Prevents soiling of bed.
(11) Bathe arm with soap and water using long, firm strokes from distal to proximal areas (fingers to axilla). Raise and support arm as needed while thoroughly washing axilla (see illustration).	Soap lowers surface tension and facilitates removal of debris and bacteria when friction is applied during washing. Long, firm strokes stimulate circulation. Movement of arm exposes axilla and exercises joint's normal ROM.

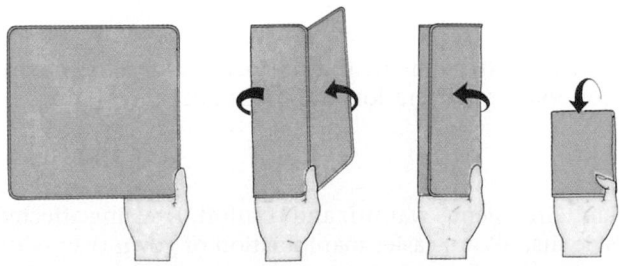

STEP **10A(7)** Steps for folding washcloth to form a mitt.

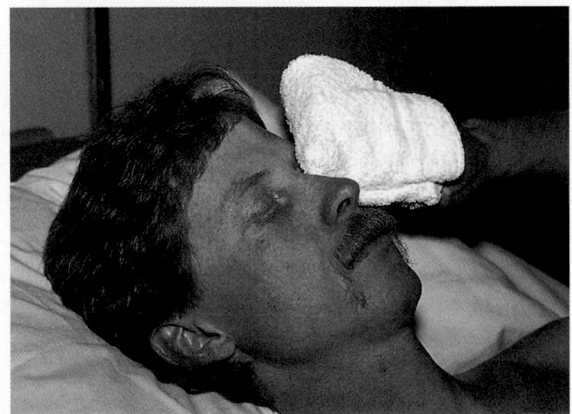

STEP **10A(8)** Wash eye from inner to outer canthus.

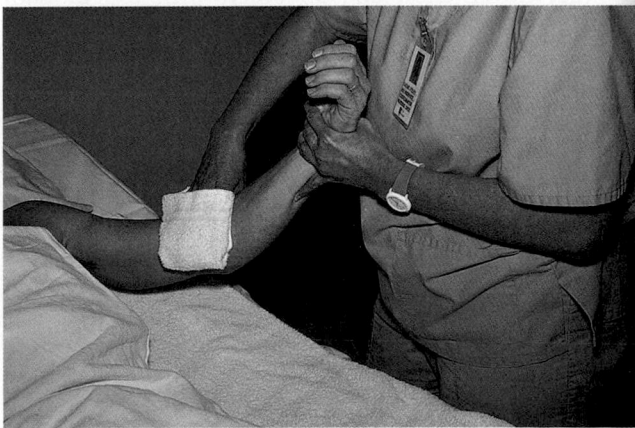

STEP **10A(11)** Washing from fingers to axilla.

Skill 38-1   *Bathing a Client—cont'd*

Steps	Rationale
(12) Rinse and dry arm and axilla thoroughly. If client uses deodorant or talcum powder, apply it.	Alkaline residue from soap discourages growth of normal skin bacteria (Barnes, 1987). Excess moisture causes skin maceration or softening. Deodorant controls body odor.
(13) Fold bath towel in half, and lay it on bed beside client. Place basin on towel. Immerse client's hand in water. Allow hand to soak for 3 to 5 min before washing hand and fingernails (see Skill 38-3). Remove basin and dry hand well.	Soaking softens cuticles and calluses of hand, loosens debris beneath nails, and enhances feeling of cleanliness. Thorough drying removes moisture from between fingers. NOTE: Do not soak if client is diabetic.
(14) Raise side rail, and move to other side of bed. Lower side rail, and repeat steps 10 through 13 for other arm.	
(15) Check temperature of bath water, and change water if necessary.	Warm water maintains client's comfort.

Critical Decision Point: If a client is at risk for falls, be sure two side rails are up before obtaining fresh water or other supplies. Remember, side rails cannot be used as a restraint.

Steps	Rationale
(16) Cover client's chest with bath towel, and fold bath blanket down to umbilicus. With one hand, lift edge of towel away from chest. With washcloth or mitted hand, bathe chest using long, firm strokes. Take special care to wash skinfolds under female client's breasts. It may be necessary to lift breast upward while bathing underneath it. Keep client's chest covered between wash and rinse periods. Dry well.	Draping prevents unnecessary exposure of body parts. Towel maintains warmth and privacy. Secretions and dirt collect easily in areas of tight skinfolds. Skinfolds are susceptible to excoriation if breasts are pendulous.
(17) Place bath towel lengthwise over chest and abdomen. (Two towels may be needed.) Fold blanket down to just above pubic region.	Prevents chilling and exposure of body parts.
(18) With one hand, lift bath towel. With mitted hand, bathe abdomen, giving special attention to bathing umbilicus and abdominal folds. Stroke from side to side. Keep abdomen covered between washing and rinsing. Dry well.	Moisture and sediment that collect in skinfolds predispose skin to maceration and irritation.
(19) Apply clean gown or pajama top. If one extremity is injured or immobilized, always dress affected side first. This step may be omitted until completion of bath; gown should not become soiled during remainder of bath.	Maintains client's warmth and comfort. Dressing affected side first allows easier manipulation of gown over body part with reduced ROM.
(20) Cover chest and abdomen with top of bath blanket. Expose near leg by folding blanket toward midline. Be sure other leg and perineum are draped.	Prevents unnecessary exposure.
(21) Bend client's leg at knee by positioning nurse's arm under leg. While grasping client's heel, elevate leg from mattress slightly, and slide bath towel lengthwise under leg. Ask client to hold foot still. Place bath basin on towel on bed, and secure its position next to foot to be washed.	Towel prevents soiling of bed linen. Support of joint and extremity during lifting prevents strain on musculoskeletal structures. Sudden movement by client could spill bath water. (Omit this step if client is unable to hold leg in basin.)
(22) With one hand supporting lower leg, raise it and slide basin under lifted foot. Make sure foot is firmly placed on bottom of basin. Allow foot to soak while washing leg. If client is unable to hold leg, do not immerse; simply wash with washcloth (see illustration).	Proper positioning of foot prevents pressure being applied from edge of basin against calf. Soaking softens calluses and rough skin.

Steps	Rationale
(23) Unless contraindicated, use long, firm strokes in washing from ankle to knee and from knee to thigh. Dry well.	Promotes venous return.

Critical Decision Point: Clients with history of deep vein thromboses or hypercoagulation disorders should not have their lower extremities washed with long firm strokes.

(24) Cleanse foot, making sure to bathe between toes. Clean and clip nails as per physician orders (see Skill 38-3). Dry well. If skin is dry, apply lotion.	Secretions and moisture may be present between toes. Lotion helps retain moisture and soften skin.

Critical Decision Point: Do not massage any reddened area on client's skin because massaging causes breaks in the skin's surface capillaries and increased risk of skin breakdown (AHCPR, 1992).

(25) Raise side rail, and move to other side of the bed. Lower side rail, and repeat steps 20 through 24 for other leg and foot.	
(26) Cover client with bath blanket, raise side rail for client's safety, and change bath water.	Decreased bath water temperature can cause chilling. Clean water reduces microorganism transmission.
(27) Lower side rail. Assist client in assuming prone or side-lying position (as applicable). Place towel lengthwise along client's side.	Exposes back and buttocks for bathing.
(28) Keep client draped by sliding bath blanket over shoulders and thighs. Wash, rinse, and dry back from neck to buttocks using long, firm strokes (see illustration). Pay special attention to folds of buttocks and anus. Give a back rub (see Chapter 42). Change bath water.	Maintains warmth, and prevents unnecessary exposure. Skinfolds near buttocks and anus may contain fecal secretions that harbor microorganisms. Changing water prevents transfer of microorganisms from anal area to genitalia.
(29) Apply disposable gloves if not done previously.	Prevents contact with microorganisms in body secretions.
(30) Assist client in assuming side-lying or supine position. Cover chest and upper extremities with towel and lower extremities with bath blanket. Expose only genitalia. (If client can wash, covering entire body with bath blanket may be preferable.) Provide perineal care (see Skill 38-2). Pay special attention to skinfolds. Apply water-repellent ointment to area exposed to moisture.	Maintains client's privacy. Clients capable of performing partial bath usually prefer to wash their own genitalia. Water-repellent ointments (e.g., A & D, Pericare) protect skin from moisture.
(31) Dispose of gloves in receptacle.	Prevents transmission of infection.
(32) Apply additional body lotion or oil as desired.	Moisturizing lotion prevents dry, chapped skin.

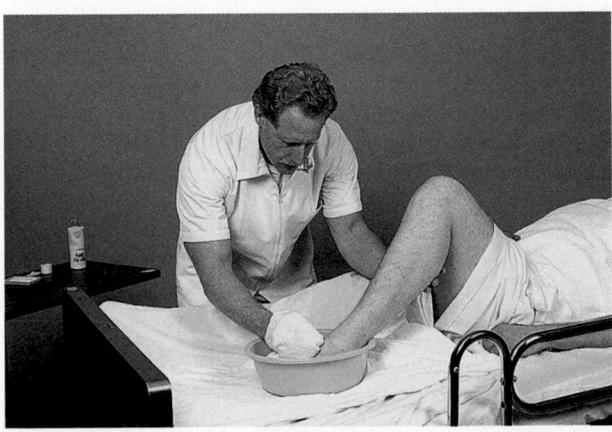

STEP 10A(22) Supporting client's leg and foot in water basin.

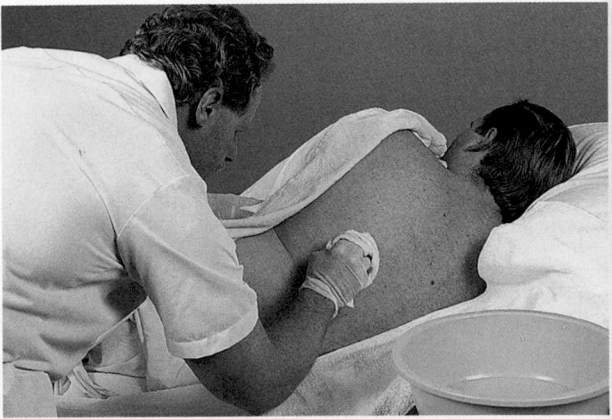

STEP 10A(28) Washing client's back.

Skill 38-1 *Bathing a Client—cont'd*

Steps	Rationale
(33) Assist client in dressing. Comb client's hair. Women may want to apply makeup.	Promotes client's body image.
(34) Make client's bed (see Skill 38-6).	Provides clean environment.
(35) Remove soiled linen, and place in dirty-linen bag. Clean and replace bathing equipment. Replace call light and personal possessions. Leave room as clean and comfortable as possible.	Prevents transmission of infection. Clean environment promotes client's comfort. Keeping call light and articles of care within reach promotes client's safety.
(36) Perform hand hygiene.	Reduces transmission of microorganisms.
B. Tub or whirlpool bath or shower; verify with agency policy if a physician's order is needed.	
(1) Consider client's condition, and review orders for precautions concerning client's movement or positioning.	Prevents accidental injury to client during bathing.
(2) Check tub or shower for cleanliness. Use cleaning techniques outlined in agency policy. Place rubber mat on tub or shower bottom. Place disposable bath mat or towel on floor in front of tub or shower.	Cleaning prevents transmission of microorganisms. Mats prevent slipping and falling.
(3) Collect all hygienic aids, toiletry items, and linens requested by client. Place within easy reach of tub or shower.	Placing items close at hand prevents possible falls when client reaches for equipment.
(4) Assist client to bathroom if necessary. Have client wear robe and slippers to bathroom.	Assistance prevents accidental falls. Wearing robe and slippers prevents chilling.
(5) Demonstrate how to use call signal for assistance.	Bathrooms are equipped with signaling devices in case client feels faint or weak or needs immediate assistance. Clients prefer privacy during bath if safety is not jeopardized.
(6) Place "occupied" sign on bathroom door.	Maintains client's privacy.
(7) Provide shower seat or tub chair if needed (see illustration). Fill bathtub halfway with warm water. If sensation is normal, ask client to test water, and adjust temperature if water is too warm. Explain which faucet controls hot water. If client is taking shower, turn shower on, and adjust water temperature before client enters shower stall.	Adjusting water temperature prevents accidental burns. Older adults and clients with neurological alterations (e.g., spinal cord injury) are at high risk for burns as a result of reduced sensation. Use of assistive devices facilitates bathing and minimizes physical exertion.

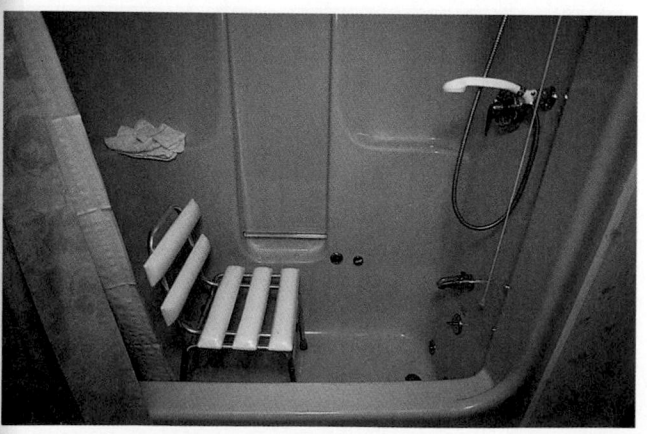

STEP **10B(7)** Shower seat for client safety.

Steps	Rationale
(8) Instruct client to use safety bars when getting in and out of tub or shower. Caution client against use of bath oil in tub water.	Prevents slipping and falling. Oil causes tub surfaces to become slippery.
(9) Instruct client not to remain in tub longer than 20 min. Check on client every 5 min.	Prolonged exposure to warm water may cause vasodilation and pooling of blood, leading to light-headedness or dizziness.
(10) Return to bathroom when client signals, and knock before entering.	Provides privacy.
(11) For client who is unsteady, drain tub of water before client attempts to get out of it. Place bath towel over client's shoulders. Assist client in getting out of tub as needed, and assist with drying. If client is weak or unstable, have assistive personnel assist.	Prevents accidental falls. Client may become chilled as water drains.

Critical Decision Point: Weak or unstable clients need extra assistance in getting out of a tub. Planning for additional personnel is essential before attempting to assist the client from tub.

Steps	Rationale
(12) Assist client as needed in donning clean gown or pajamas, slippers, and robe. (In home setting, client may don regular clothing.)	Maintains warmth to prevent chilling.
(13) Assist client to room and comfortable position in bed or chair.	Maintains relaxation gained from bathing.
(14) Clean tub or shower according to agency policy. Whirlpool baths may require special cleansing. Remove soiled linen and place in dirty-linen bag. Discard disposable equipment in proper receptacle. Place "unoccupied" sign on bathroom door. Return supplies to storage area.	Prevents transmission of infection through soiled linen and moisture.
(15) Perform hand hygiene.	Reduces transfer of microorganisms.
11. Observe skin, paying particular attention to areas that were previously soiled, reddened, or showed early signs of breakdown.	Techniques used during bathing should leave skin clean and clear.
12. Observe ROM during bath.	Measures joint mobility.
13. Ask client to rate level of comfort.	Evaluates success of bath in promoting client's comfort.

Unexpected Outcomes and Related Interventions

1. Areas of excessive dryness, rashes, irritation, or pressure ulcer appear on skin.
   a. Review agency skin care policy regarding special cleansing and moisturizing products.
   b. Limit frequency of complete baths.
   c. Complete pressure ulcer assessment (see Chapter 47).
   d. Obtain special bed surface if client is at risk for skin breakdown.
2. Client becomes excessively fatigued and unable to cooperate or participate in bathing.
   a. Reschedule bathing to a time when client is more rested.
   b. Clients with cardiopulmonary conditions and breathing difficulties require pillow or elevated head of bed during bathing.
   c. Notify physician about changes in client's fatigue level.
   d. Schedule rest periods.
3. Client seems unusually restless or complains of discomfort.
   a. Consider analgesia before bathing.
   b. Schedule rest periods before bathing.

Recording and Reporting

- Record condition of skin and any significant findings (e.g., reddened areas, bruises, nevi, or joint or muscle pain).
- Report evidence of alterations in skin integrity, break in suture line, or increased wound secretions to nurse in charge or physician.
- Record procedure and amount of assistance, client participation.

Home Care Considerations

- Assess client's tub and shower area for the need for safety devices (e.g., grab bars).
- Assess client for the need for assistive bathing devices (e.g., shower chair, handheld shower).

The tub bath or shower can be used to give a more thorough bath than a bed bath. Safety is of primary concern because the surface of a tub or shower stall is slippery. In some settings a physician's order for a shower or tub bath is necessary. In some agencies, showers are equipped with a chair for clients with weakness or poor balance. Both tubs and showers should be equipped with grab bars for clients to hold on to during entry and exit and maneuvering. Clients vary in how much help they will need. Regardless of the type of bath the client receives, the nurse should use the following guidelines:

- *Provide privacy.* Close the door, or pull room curtains around the bathing area. While bathing the client, expose only the areas being bathed.
- *Maintain safety.* Keep side rails up while away from the client's bedside. (This is critical for dependent and unconscious clients.) NOTE: When side rails are used as a restraint, a physician's order is needed. Place the call light in the client's reach if leaving the room temporarily.
- *Maintain warmth.* The room should be kept warm because the client is partially uncovered and may easily be chilled. Wet skin causes an excess loss of heat through convection. Control drafts, and keep windows closed. Keep client covered, only exposing the body part being washed during the bath.
- *Promote independence.* Encourage the client to participate in as much of the bathing activities as possible. Offer assistance when needed.
- *Anticipate needs.* Bring a new set of clothing and hygiene products to the bedside or bathroom.

Bag Baths. An innovative approach to the traditional bed bath was developed because of nurses' concern for clients who are predisposed to dry skin and the risk for infection. When washbasins are not cleaned and dried completely after use, there is the risk of contamination by gram-negative organisms. Successive uses of the basin may cause the client's skin to harbor more gram-negative organisms. The "bag bath" is a specially prepared package containing 10 washcloths that are premoistened in a mixture of water and a nonrinsable cleanser. A bag is warmed in a microwave before use, and then the nurse uses a different cloth for each part of the client's body. In this technique the skin is allowed to air dry, since towel drying removes the emollient that is left behind after the water/cleanser solution evaporates. Staff who have used the bag bath report shorter bathing times and client and nurse satisfaction (Skewes, 1994).

Perineal Care. **Perineal care** is usually part of the complete bed bath (Skill 38-2). Clients most in need of perineal care are those at greatest risk for acquiring an infection (e.g., uncircumcised males, clients who have indwelling urinary catheters, or clients who are recovering from rectal or genital surgery or childbirth). In addition, women who are having a menstrual period will require good perineal care. A client able to perform self-care should be allowed to do so. Nurses can become embarrassed about providing perineal care, particularly to clients of the opposite sex. Similarly, the client usually feels embarrassed. This should not cause the nurse to overlook the client's hygiene needs. When staffing levels permit, it may help to have a nurse of the opposite sex present in the room when providing perineal care. A professional, dignified, and sensitive approach can reduce embarrassment and put the client at ease.

If a client performs self-care, various problems such as vaginal and urethral discharge, skin irritation, and unpleasant odors may go unnoticed. The nurse must be alert for complaints of burning during urination or localized soreness, excoriation, or pain in the perineum. The nurse also inspects the client's bed linen for signs of discharge. Clients most at risk for skin breakdown in the perineal area are those with urinary or fecal incontinence, rectal and perineal surgical dressings, indwelling urinary catheters, and the morbidly obese.

Back Rub. A back rub or back massage usually follows the client's bath. It promotes relaxation, relieves muscular tension, and stimulates skin circulation. Labyak and Metzger (1997) evaluated the efficacy of massage and its effects on the physiological measures of relaxation. Their analysis showed that the long, slow, gliding strokes (**effleurage**) of a massage are associated with a reduction in heart rate and respiratory rate. Males seem to achieve greater reductions in systolic and diastolic blood pressure during back rub than females. Because effleurage causes an immediate rise in blood pressure and heart rate in clients who have had coronary artery bypass surgery, the researchers do not recommend the therapy for those clients within the first 48 hours of their surgery. Clients generally report that they are more comfortable following a back rub and find the experience pleasant, regardless of the length of the massage. However, a back rub of 3 minutes' duration can actually enhance client comfort and relaxation and thus be very therapeutic (Labyak and Metzger, 1997).

When providing a back rub, the nurse can enhance relaxation by reducing any noise and ensuring the client is comfortable. It is important to ask whether a client would like a back rub, or if the client prefers gentle instead of heavy massage, because some individuals dislike physical contact. The nurse should consult the medical record for any contraindications to a massage (e.g., fractured ribs, burns of the skin, and heart surgery).

Foot and Nail Care. Foot and nail care should be incorporated into a person's regular hygiene routine. Routine care involves soaking to soften cuticles and layers of horny cells, thorough cleansing, drying, and proper nail trimming. The exception involves clients with diabetes mellitus who do not soak their nails due to the risk of infection. When the nurse administers care, the client may remain in bed or sit in a chair (Skill 38-3). In some settings or with specific clients, such as a person with diabetes mellitus, a physician's order is needed to trim a client's toenails. Before implementing this procedure, check agency policy to determine if a physician's order is needed.

The nurse takes time during the procedure to teach the client and family proper techniques for cleaning and nail trimming. Measures to prevent infection and promote good circulation should be stressed. Clients learn to pro-

Text continued on p. 1038

Skill 38-2   Perineal Care

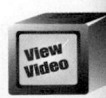
View Video

Delegation Considerations

Skills of perineal care can be delegated to assistive personnel (AP).

- Inform AP when client has physical restrictions that will affect proper way to position for procedure
- Provide information about proper positioning of indwelling catheter during perineal care.
- Instruct AP to inform nurse if any perineal drainage, excoriation, or rash is observed.

Equipment

- Washbasin
- Soap dish with soap
- Two or three washcloths
- Bath towel
- Bath blanket
- Waterproof pad or bedpan
- Toilet tissue or diaper wipes
- Disposable gloves

Additional supplies are needed when pericare is given other than during a bath:

- Cotton balls or swabs
- A solution bottle or container filled with warm water or prescribed rinsing solution
- Waterproof bag

Steps	Rationale
1. Identify clients at risk for developing infection of genitalia, urinary tract, or reproductive tract (e.g., uncircumcised male, presence of indwelling catheter, fecal incontinence).	Secretions that accumulate on surface of skin surrounding female and male genitalia act as reservoir for infection. Tissues traumatized by surgery or by presence of foreign object provide route for introduction of infectious organisms.
2. Assess client's cognitive and musculoskeletal function.	Determines client's ability to perform self-care and determines level of assistance required from nurse.
3. Apply disposable gloves and assess genitalia for signs of inflammation, skin breakdown, or infection (see Chapter 32). Discard gloves. Perform hand hygiene.	Reduces infection. Determines extent of perineal care required by client.

Critical Decision Point: Assessment of genitalia may be deferred until perineal care is administered.

Steps	Rationale
4. Assess client's knowledge of importance of perineal hygiene.	Clients at risk for infection in perineal area may be unaware of importance of cleanliness. Reflects client's need for education.
5. Explain procedure and its purpose to client.	Helps minimize anxiety during procedure that is often embarrassing to nurse and client.
6. Prepare necessary equipment and supplies.	Used when administering a bed bath.
7. Pull curtain around client's bed, or close room door. Assemble supplies at bedside.	Maintains client's privacy and ensures orderly procedure.
8. Raise bed to comfortable working position. If raised, lower side rail, and assist client in assuming side-lying position, placing towel lengthwise along client's side and keeping client covered with bath blanket or top sheet.	Facilitates good body mechanics. Provides easy access to genitalia.
9. Apply disposable gloves.	Eliminates transmission of microorganisms.
10. If fecal material is present, enclose in a fold of underpad or toilet tissue, and remove with disposable wipes or tissue. Cleanse buttocks and anus, washing front to back (see illustration). Cleanse, rinse, and dry area thoroughly. If needed, place an absorbent pad under client's buttocks. Remove and discard underpad, and replace with clean one.	Cleansing reduces transmission of microorganisms from anus to urethra or genitalia.
11. Change gloves when they are soiled. Perform hand hygiene.	

Skill 38-2   *Perineal Care—cont'd*

Steps	Rationale

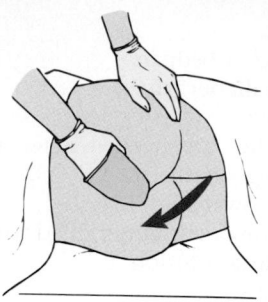

STEP **10** Cleanse buttocks from front to back.

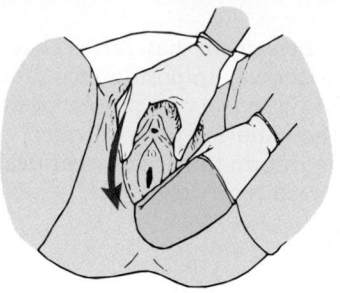

STEP **15A(5)** Cleanse from perineum to rectum (front to back).

12. Fold top bed linen down toward foot of bed, and raise client's gown above genital area. Prepare bed linen to protect client's privacy.

   Exposes perineal area for easy accessibility.

   a. "Diamond" drape client by placing bath blanket with one corner between client's legs, one corner pointing toward each side of bed, and one corner over client's chest. Tuck side corners around client's legs and under hips.

   Prevents unnecessary exposure of body parts and maintains client's warmth and comfort during procedure.

13. Raise side rail. Fill washbasin with warm water.

   Prevents client from falling. Proper water temperature prevents burns to perineum.

14. Place washbasin and toilet tissue on overbed table. Place washcloths in basin.

   Equipment placed within nurse's reach prevents accidental spills.

15. Provide perineal care.

   A. Female perineal care

   (1) Assist client to dorsal recumbent position.

   Provides easy access to genitalia.

   (2) Lower side rail, and help client flex knees and spread legs. Note restrictions or limitations in client's positioning.

   Provides full exposure of female genitalia. Minimize degree of abduction in female if position causes pain because of arthritis or reduced joint mobility.

   (3) Fold lower corner of bath blanket up between client's legs onto abdomen. Wash and dry client's upper thighs.

   Minimizes transmission of microorganisms. Keeping client draped until procedure begins minimizes anxiety. Buildup of perineal secretions can soil surrounding skin surfaces.

   (4) Wash labia majora. Use nondominant hand to gently retract labia from thigh; with dominant hand, wash carefully in skinfolds. Wipe in direction from perineum to rectum (front to back). Repeat on opposite side using separate section of washcloth. Rinse and dry area thoroughly.

   Skinfolds may contain body secretions that harbor microorganisms. Wiping from perineum to rectum (front to back) reduces chance of transmitting fecal organisms to urinary meatus.

   (5) Separate labia with nondominant hand to expose urethral meatus and vaginal orifice. With dominant hand, wash downward from pubic area toward rectum in one smooth stroke (see illustration). Use separate section of cloth for each stroke. Cleanse thoroughly around labia minora, clitoris, and vaginal orifice.

   Cleansing method reduces transfer of microorganisms to urinary meatus. (For menstruating women or clients with indwelling urinary catheters, cleanse with cotton balls.)

   (6) If client uses bedpan, pour warm water over perineal area. Dry perineal area thoroughly, using front-to-back method.

   Rinsing removes soap and microorganisms more effectively than wiping. Retained moisture harbors microorganisms.

   (7) Fold lower corner of bath blanket back between client's legs and over perineum. Ask client to lower legs and assume comfortable position.

Steps	**Rationale**

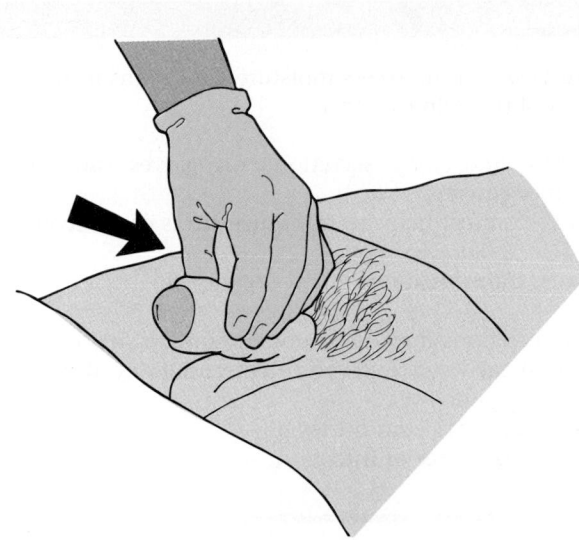

STEP **15B(3)**   Retract foreskin.

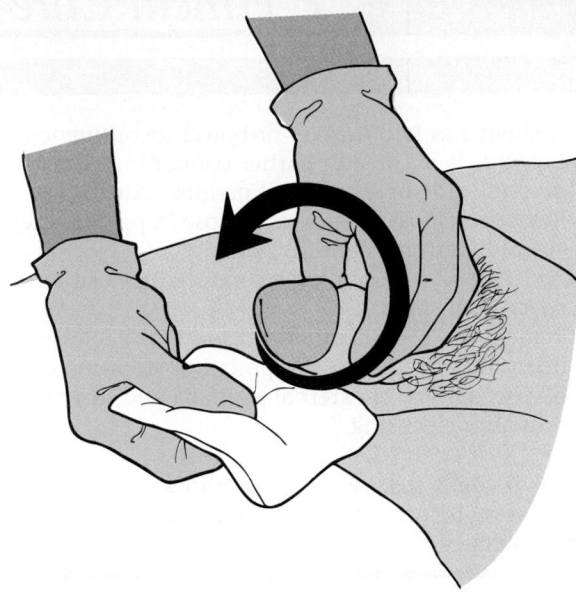

STEP **15B(4)**   Use circular motion to cleanse tip of penis.

B. **Male perineal care**

(1) Lower side rails, and assist client to supine position. Note restriction in mobility.

Provides full exposure of male genitalia.

(2) Fold lower corner of bath blanket up between client's legs and onto abdomen. Wash and dry client's upper thighs.

Minimizes transmission of microorganisms. Keeping client draped until procedure begins minimizes anxiety. Buildup of perineal secretions can soil surrounding skin surfaces.

(3) Gently raise penis, and place bath towel underneath. Gently grasp shaft of penis. If client is uncircumcised, retract foreskin (see illustration). If client has an erection, defer procedure until later.

Towel prevents moisture from collecting in inguinal area. Gentle but firm handling reduces chance of client having an erection. Secretions capable of harboring microorganisms collect underneath foreskin.

(4) Wash tip of penis at urethral meatus first. Using circular motion, cleanse from meatus outward (see illustration). Discard washcloth, and repeat with clean cloth until penis is clean. Rinse and dry gently.

Direction of cleansing moves from area of least contamination to area of most contamination, preventing microorganisms from entering urethra.

(5) Return foreskin to its natural position.

Tightening of foreskin around shaft of penis can cause local edema and discomfort.

Critical Decision Point: After administering male perineal care, make sure the foreskin is in its natural position. This is extremely important in those clients with decreased sensation in their lower extremities.

(6) Wash shaft of penis with gentle but firm downward strokes. Pay special attention to underlying surface of penis. Rinse and dry penis thoroughly. Instruct client to spread legs apart slightly.

Vigorous massage of penis can lead to erection, which can embarrass client and nurse. Underlying surface of penis may have greater accumulation of secretions. Abduction of legs provides easier access to scrotal tissues.

(7) Gently cleanse scrotum. Lift it carefully, and wash underlying skinfolds. Rinse and dry.

Pressure on scrotal tissues can be painful to client. Secretions collect between skinfolds.

(8) Fold bath blanket back over client's perineum, and assist client in turning to side-lying position.

Draping promotes comfort and minimizes client's anxiety. Side-lying position provides access to anal area.

Skill 38-2   *Perineal Care—cont'd*

Steps	Rationale
16. If client has had urinary or bowel incontinence, apply thin layer of skin barrier containing petrolatum or zinc oxide over anal and perineal skin.	Protects skin from excess moisture and toxins from urine or stool (Makelbust, 1991).
17. Remove disposable gloves, dispose in proper receptacle, and perform hand hygiene.	Moisture and body secretions on gloves can harbor microorganisms.
18. Assist client in assuming a comfortable position, and cover with sheet.	Client's comfort helps to minimize stress of procedure.
19. Remove bath blanket, and dispose of all soiled bed linen. Return unused equipment to storage area.	Reduces transmission of microorganisms.
20. Inspect surface of external genitalia and surrounding skin after cleansing.	Thick secretions may cover underlying skin lesions or areas of breakdown. Evaluation determines need for additional hygiene.
21. Ask if client feels sense of cleanliness.	Evaluates client's comfort level.
22. Observe for abnormal drainage or discharge from genitalia.	Evaluates presence of infection.

Unexpected Outcomes and Related Interventions

1. Skin and genitalia may be inflamed, with localized tenderness, swelling, and presence of foul-smelling discharge.
   a. Bathe area frequently to keep clean and dry.
   b. Obtain order for sitz bath.
   c. Apply protective barrier.
   d. Notify physician and apply prescribed antibacterial or antifungal ointment/cream.
2. Client expresses discomfort.
   a. Increase frequency of perineal care.
   b. Assess perineum for signs of irritation or discharge.
3. Client unable to perform perineal care correctly.
   a. Review perineal care.
   b. Position client and have client observe cleansing procedure.

Recording and Reporting

- Record procedure and presence of any abnormal findings (e.g., character and amount of discharge or condition of genitalia).
- Record appearance of suture line, if present.
- Report any break in suture line or presence of abnormalities to nurse in charge or physician.

Home Care Considerations

- Instruct caregivers to daily assess client's perineal area for signs of infection and skin breakdown.

Skill 38-3 Performing Nail and Foot Care

Delegation Considerations

The skill of nail and foot care of the nondiabetic client can be delegated to assistive personnel (AP). If the client is diabetic, this skill should not be delegated.
- Instruct AP that if client's nails need clipping this must be performed by the nurse.
- Instruct AP on any special considerations for client positioning.

Equipment

- Washbasin
- Emesis basin
- Washcloth
- Bath or face towel
- Nail clippers
- Orange stick
- Emery board or nail file
- Body lotion
- Disposable bath mat
- Paper towels
- Disposable gloves

Steps	Rationale
1. Inspect all surfaces of fingers, toes, feet, and nails. Pay particular attention to areas of dryness, inflammation, or cracking. Also inspect areas between toes, heels, and soles of feet.	Integrity of feet and nails determines frequency and level of hygiene required. Heels, soles, and sides of feet are prone to irritation from ill-fitting shoes.

Critical Decision Point: Client with peripheral vascular diseases, diabetes mellitus, older adults, and clients whose immune system is suppressed may require nail care from a specialist to reduce the risk of infection.

Steps	Rationale
2. Assess color and temperature of toes, feet, and fingers. Assess capillary refill of nails. Palpate radial and ulnar pulse of each hand and dorsalis pedis pulse of foot; note character of pulses (see Chapter 32).	Assesses adequacy of blood flow to extremities. Circulatory alterations may change integrity of nails and increase client's chance of localized infection when break in skin integrity occurs (Bryant and Beinlich, 1999).
3. Observe client's walking gait. Have client walk down hall or walk straight line (if able).	Structural as well as painful disorders of feet can cause limping or unnatural gait. These disorders may be the result of impaired circulation, improper fitting shoes, or structural foot abnormalities (e.g., bunions) (Bryant and Beinlich, 1999).
4. Ask female clients about whether they use nail polish and polish remover frequently.	Chemicals in these products can cause excessive dryness.
5. Assess type of footwear worn by clients: Are socks worn? Are shoes tight or ill fitting? Are garters or knee-high nylons worn? Is footwear clean?	Types of shoes and footwear may predispose client to foot and nail problems (e.g., infection, areas of friction, ulcerations). These conditions decrease mobility and increase the risk for amputation in the diabetic client (Pinzur, Slovenkai, and Trepman, 1999).
6. Identify client's risk for foot or nail problems:	Certain conditions increase likelihood of foot or nail problems.
a. Older adult	Poor vision, lack of coordination, or inability to bend over contributes to difficulty in performing foot and nail care. Normal physiological changes of aging also result in nail and foot problems (Lueckenotte, 2000).
b. Diabetes mellitus	Vascular changes associated with diabetes mellitus reduce blood flow to peripheral tissues. Break in skin integrity places diabetic at high risk for skin infection. Meticulous foot assessment reduces the diabetic client's risk of debilitating foot problems (Green, Aliabaide, and Green, 2002; Neil, 2002).
c. Heart failure, renal disease	Both conditions can increase tissue edema, particularly in dependent areas (e.g., feet). Edema reduces blood flow to neighboring tissues.

Skill 38-3   *Performing* Nail and Foot Care—*cont'd*

Steps	Rationale
d. Cerebrovascular accident (stroke)	Presence of residual foot or leg weakness or paralysis results in altered walking patterns. Altered gait pattern causes increased friction and pressure on feet.
7. Assess type of home remedies client uses for existing foot problems:	Certain preparations or applications may cause more injury to soft tissue than initial foot problem (Neil, 2002).
a. Over-the-counter liquid preparations to remove corns	Liquid preparations can cause burns and ulcerations.
b. Cutting of corns or calluses with razor blade or scissors	Cutting of corns or calluses may result in infection caused by break in skin integrity. The diabetic client or any client with decreased peripheral circulation has an increased risk for infection secondary to a break in skin integrity (Green, Aliabaide, and Green, 2002).
c. Use of oval corn pads	Oval pads may exert pressure on toes, thereby decreasing circulation to surrounding tissues.
d. Application of adhesive tape	Skin of older adult is thin and delicate and prone to tearing when adhesive tape is removed.
8. Assess client's ability to care for nails or feet: visual alterations, fatigue, musculoskeletal weakness.	Determines client's ability to perform self-care and degree of assistance required from nurse (Neil, 2002).
9. Assess client's knowledge of foot and nail care practices.	Determines client's need for health teaching.
10. Explain procedure to client, including fact that proper soaking requires several minutes.	Client must be willing to place fingers and feet in basins for 10 to 20 min. Client may become anxious or fatigued.

Critical Decision Point: Diabetic clients do not soak hands and feet. Soaking increases risk of infection in diabetic due to maceration of the skin.

Steps	Rationale
11. Obtain physician's order for cutting nails if agency policy requires it.	Client's skin may be accidentally cut. Certain clients are more at risk for infection, depending on their medical condition.
12. Perform hand hygiene. Arrange equipment on overbed table.	Easy access to equipment prevents delays.
13. Pull curtain around bed or close room door (if desired).	Maintaining client's privacy reduces anxiety.
14. Assist ambulatory client to sit in bedside chair. Help bed-bound client to supine position with head of bed elevated. Place disposable bath mat on floor under client's feet or place towel on mattress.	Sitting in chair facilitates immersing feet in basin. Bath mat protects feet from exposure to soil or debris.
15. Fill washbasin with warm water. Test water temperature.	Warm water softens nails and thickened epidermal cells, reduces inflammation of skin, and promotes local circulation. Proper water temperature prevents burns.
16. Place basin on bath mat or towel, and help client place feet in basin. Place call light within client's reach.	Clients with muscular weakness or tremors may have difficulty positioning feet. Client's safety is maintained.
17. Adjust overbed table to low position, and place it over client's lap. (Client may sit in chair or lie in bed.)	Easy access prevents accidental spills.
18. Fill emesis basin with warm water, and place basin on paper towels on overbed table.	Warm water softens nails and thickened epidermal cells.
19. Instruct client to place fingers in emesis basin and place arms in comfortable position.	Prolonged positioning can cause discomfort unless normal anatomical alignment is maintained.
20. Allow client's feet and fingernails to soak for 10 to 20 min. Rewarm after 10 min.	Softening of corns, calluses, and cuticles ensures easy removal of dead cells and easy manipulation of cuticle.
21. Clean gently under fingernails with orange stick or wooden end of cotton-tipped swab while fingers are immersed (see illustration). Remove emesis basin, and dry fingers thoroughly.	Orange stick removes debris under nails that harbors microorganisms. Thorough drying impedes fungal growth and prevents maceration of tissues.
22. Using nail clippers, clip fingernails straight across and even with tops of fingers (see illustration). Shape nails with emery board or file. If client has circulatory problems, do not cut nail; file the nail only.	Cutting straight across prevents splitting of nail margins and formation of sharp nail spikes that can irritate lateral nail margins. Filing prevents cutting nail too close to nail bed.

Steps	Rationale

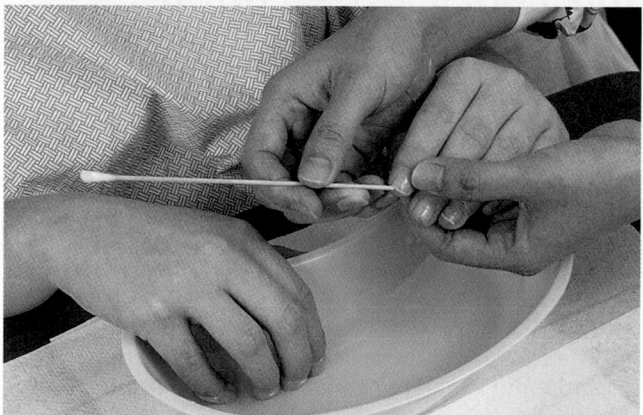

STEP 21 Clean fingernails with end of cotton-tipped swab or an orange stick.

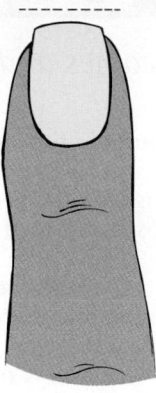

STEP 22 Using nail clippers, trim nails straight across.

Steps	Rationale
23. Push cuticle back gently with orange stick.	Reduces incidence of inflamed cuticles.
24. Move overbed table away from client.	Provides easier access to feet.
25. Put on disposable gloves, and scrub callused areas of feet with washcloth.	Gloves prevent transmission of fungal infection. Friction removes dead skin layers.
26. Clean gently under nails with orange stick. Remove feet from basin, and dry thoroughly.	Removal of debris and excess moisture reduces chances of infection.
27. Clean and trim toenails using procedures in steps 22 and 23. Do not file corners of toenails.	Shaping corners of toenails may damage tissues.
28. Apply lotion to feet and hands, and assist client back to bed and into comfortable position.	Lotion lubricates dry skin by helping to retain moisture.
29. Remove disposable gloves, and place in receptacle. Clean and return equipment and supplies to proper place. Dispose of soiled linen in hamper. Perform hand hygiene.	Reduces transmission of infection.
30. Inspect nails and surrounding skin surfaces after soaking and nail trimming.	Evaluates condition of skin and nails. Allows nurse to note any remaining rough nail edges.
31. Ask client to explain or demonstrate nail care.	Evaluates client's level of learning techniques.
32. Observe client's walk after toenail care.	Evaluates level of comfort and mobility achieved.
33. Record procedure and observations (e.g., breaks in skin, inflammation, ulcerations).	Documents procedure, client's response, and presence of abnormalities requiring additional therapy.
34. Report any breaks in skin or ulcerations to nurse in charge or physician.	These abnormalities can seriously increase client's risk of infection and must be carefully observed.

Skill 38-3   Performing Nail and Foot Care—cont'd

Unexpected Outcomes and Related Interventions

1. Cuticles and surrounding tissues may be inflamed and tender to touch.
   a. Repeated soakings may be needed to relieve inflammation and loosen layers of cells from calluses or corns.
   b. Diabetic client or client with peripheral vascular disease may require referral to a podiatrist.
   c. Evaluate need for antifungal cream.
2. Localized areas of tenderness occur on feet with calluses or corns at point of friction.
   a. Change in footwear may be needed.
   b. Refer to a podiatrist.
3. Ulcer appears between toes or other pressure areas in foot.
   a. Notify physician.
   b. Refer to a podiatrist.
   c. Increase frequency of foot assessment and hygiene.

Recording and Reporting

- Record procedure and observations (e.g., breaks in skin, inflammation, ulcerations).
- Report any breaks in skin or ulcerations to nurse in charge or physician. These are serious in client with peripheral vascular disease and illnesses in which client's circulation is impaired. Special foot care treatments may be needed.

Home Care Considerations

- If the client is diabetic or has decreased peripheral circulation, alternative therapies or foot soaking should only be done after consulting with a physician.
- Alternative therapies: moleskin applied to areas of feet that are under friction is less likely to cause pressure than corn pads; spot adhesive bandages can guard against friction, but they do not have padding to protect against pressure; wrapping small pieces of lamb's wool around toes reduces irritation of soft corns between toes.
- If client is ambulatory, instruct to soak feet in bathtub. When client's mobility is limited, a large basin or pan can be used.

Box 38-8   Signs of Peripheral Neuropathy or Vascular Insufficiency

Peripheral Neuropathy

Muscle wasting of lower extremities
Absence of deep tendon reflexes
Foot deformities
Infections
Abnormal gait
Decreased or absent vibratory sensation

Vascular Insufficiency

Decreased hair growth on legs and feet
Absent or decreased pulses
Infection in the foot
Poor wound healing
Thickened nails
Shiny appearance of the skin
Blanching of the skin on elevation

Data from American Diabetes Association: Position statement on preventive foot care in people with diabetes: clinical practice recommendations 1999, *Diabetes Care* 22(suppl 1), 1999; Pinzur MS, Slovenkai MP, Trepman E: Guidelines for diabetic foot care, The Diabetes Committee of the American Orthopaedic Foot and Ankle Society, *Foot Ankle Int* 20:695, 1999; and Neil JA: Assessing foot care knowledge in a rural population with diabetes, *Ostomy Wound Manage* 48(1):50, 2002.

tect the feet from injury, keep the feet clean and dry, and wear footwear that fits properly. The nurse instructs clients on the proper way to inspect all surfaces of the feet and hands for lesions, dryness, or signs of infection. It is important for clients to know the appearance of any abnormalities and the importance of reporting these conditions to their caregiver (Boyer, 2001).

A client with diabetes mellitus or peripheral vascular disease is at risk for foot and nail problems as a result of poor peripheral blood supply to the feet (Box 38-8). In addition, sensation in the feet can be reduced. These clients are especially at risk for the development of chronic foot ulcers. These lesions typically heal very slowly and once present are difficult to treat. Over time, circulation can become compromised enough to cause ischemia and sloughing of tissue. Although ongoing foot care can help prevent toe amputation, studies show that many clients have not learned proper care (Bryant and Beinlich, 1999) (Box 38-9). The American Diabetes Association (ADA) (1999) identifies the following risk conditions as associated with an increased risk of amputation: peripheral neuropathy; altered biomechanics; evidence of increased pressure from callus, erythema, or hemorrhage under a callus; limited joint mobility, bony deformity, or severe nail pathological condition; peripheral vascular disease; a history of ulcers or amputation (Pinzur, Slovenkai, and Trepman, 1999).

The nurse observes for changes that would indicate peripheral neuropathy or vascular insufficiency (see Box 38-8). The client must be given information to understand how circulation directly affects the health and integrity of tissues. The nurse advises clients to use the fol-

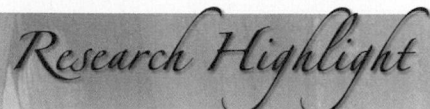

Box 38-9

Foot Care Practices of Rural Adults

Research Focus

Foot injuries are debilitating and painful; however, to the diabetic population foot injuries, even minor injuries, can result in long-term disability or even death. When clients are taught and implement proper foot care practices, the risk for developing foot ulcers and the subsequent complications are greatly reduced.

Research Abstract

The purpose of this study was to determine knowledge about foot care practices in a sample of adults (N = 61) who had either type 1 or type 2 diabetes mellitus. These adults all lived in an impoverished rural area that had little access to health care, and going barefoot and wading in local streams were normal activities. Thirty-seven of the adults were ulcer free, whereas the remaining adults had a foot ulcer present. Factors surveyed included foot inspection, foot cleaning, nail care, and use of proper footwear. The scores of both groups were low, and it appeared to the investigators that the foot care practices for both groups were the same. These two groups of clients were inconsistent in preventive foot care practices, but the lowest scores ranged in foot inspection and wearing proper footwear. The in-

vestigators concluded that ongoing assessment and use of preventive practices was necessary to reduce the risk of foot ulcers in this risk population. In addition, the assessment of these practices at point of client contact either in the home or clinic environment was essential in increasing the client's adherence to foot care practice protocols.

Evidence-Based Practice

- Use of an assessment designed to evaluate foot care practices helps to increase client's awareness of potential disease-related complications.
- Each point of client contact is an effective method to reinforce foot care practices.
- When possible, conducting an assessment of foot care practices in the client's home environment can assist the nurse in determining true foot care practices and correcting any client misconceptions at that time.

Reference

Neil JA: Assessing foot care knowledge in a rural population with diabetes, *Ostomy Wound Manage* 48(1):50, 2002.

---

lowing guidelines in a routine foot and nail care program (ADA, 1999; Pinzur, Slovenkai, and Trepman, 1999):

- Inspect the feet daily, including the tops and soles of the feet, the heels, and the areas between the toes. Use a mirror to help inspect the feet thoroughly or ask a family member to check daily.
- All clients with diabetes mellitus should receive a thorough foot examination at least once a year. People with one or more high-risk foot conditions should be evaluated more frequently. People with neuropathy should have a visual inspection of their feet at every visit with a health care professional (ADA, 1999).
- Wash the feet daily using lukewarm water; **do not soak.** Clients with reduced sensation may want to use a bath thermometer at home to test water temperature. Thoroughly pat the feet dry, and dry well between toes.
- Do not cut corns or calluses or use commercial removers. Consult a physician or podiatrist.
- If the feet perspire, apply an unscented foot powder. Wear shoes with porous uppers.
- If dryness is noted along the feet or between the toes, apply lanolin, baby oil, or even corn oil, and rub gently into the skin.
- File the toenails straight across and square; do not use scissors or clippers. Consult a podiatrist as needed.
- Do not use over-the-counter preparations to treat athlete's foot or ingrown toenails. Consult a physician or podiatrist.
- Avoid wearing elastic stockings, knee-high hose, or constricting garters. Do not cross the legs while sitting. Both impair circulation to the lower extremities.

- Wear clean socks or stockings daily. Change socks twice a day if feet perspire heavily. Socks should be dry and free of holes or darns that might cause pressure.
- Do not walk barefoot.
- Wear properly fitted shoes. The soles of shoes should be flexible and nonslipping. Small amounts of lamb's wool can be used between toes that rub or overlap. Shoes should be sturdy, closed in, and not restrictive to the feet. Clients with increased plantar pressure (e.g., erythema or callus) should use footwear that cushions and redistributes pressure. Clients with bony deformity (e.g., bunion or Charcot's joint) may need extra wide or extra deep shoes with cushioned insoles.
- Do not wear new shoes for an extended time. Wear them for short periods over several days to break them in.
- Exercise regularly to improve circulation to the lower extremities. Walk slowly and elevate, rotate, flex, and extend the feet at the ankles. Dangle the feet over the side of the bed 1 minute, and then extend both legs and hold them parallel to the bed while lying supine for 1 minute, and, finally, rest 1 minute.
- Avoid applying hot-water bottles or heating pads to the feet; use extra coverings instead.
- Minor cuts should be washed immediately and dried thoroughly. Use only mild antiseptics (e.g., Neosporin ointment). Avoid iodine or Mercurochrome. Contact a physician to treat cuts or lacerations.

Generally, any client who requires regular, thorough foot care should have a family member who is able to provide care during times when the client is incapacitated. Clients with visual difficulties, physical constraints preventing movement, or cognitive problems that impair their ability to assess the condition of the feet will need family assistance (ADA, 1999).

Oral Hygiene. Oral hygiene helps to maintain the healthy state of the mouth, teeth, gums, and lips (Ring, 2002). Brushing cleans the teeth of food particles, plaque, and bacteria. It also massages the gums and relieves discomfort resulting from unpleasant odors and tastes. Flossing further helps remove plaque and tartar from between teeth to reduce gum inflammation and infection. Complete oral hygiene enhances well-being and comfort and stimulates the appetite. Clients also benefit from a proper diet, which excludes foods promoting plaque formation and tooth decay and promotes healthy periodontal structures (Hornick, 2002). Plaque-forming foods include carbonated beverages, breads, and starches. In addition, oral hygiene immediately following a meal further reduces plaque. The nurse assists clients in maintaining good oral hygiene by teaching the importance of correct techniques and a routine daily schedule.

Clients of all ages should be advised to have a dental checkup at least every 6 months. Education about common gum and tooth disorders and methods of prevention can motivate clients to follow good oral hygiene practices. The nurse also assists in performing hygiene for weakened or disabled clients. When clients have variations in oral mucosal integrity, the nurse adapts hygiene techniques to ensure thorough and effective care (Box 38-10).

Focus on **Older Adults**   **Box 38-10**

- Many older adults are edentulous (without teeth), and the teeth that are present are often diseased or decayed (Lueckenotte, 2000).
- The periodontal membrane weakens, making it more prone to infection; periodontal disease can predispose the older adult to systemic infection.
- The presence of chronic illnesses (e.g., diabetes mellitus, renal insufficiency, and cardiovascular diseases) increases the older adult's risk for periodontal disease (Bush and Donley, 2002).
- Dentures or partial plates may not fit properly, causing pain and discomfort, which can in turn affect digestive processes, enjoyment of food, and nutritional status.
- Weaker jaw muscles and a shrinkage of the bony structure of the mouth may increase the work of chewing and lead to increased fatigue when eating (Lueckenotte, 2000).
- Dry mouth can be caused by an age-related decline in saliva secretion, as well as by medications that are frequently used by older adults (e.g., antihypertensives, diuretics, antiinflammatories, and antidepressants) (Eliopoulos, 2001).
- Poor nutritional status in some older adults can increase the risk for and severity of dental problems (e.g., caries, periodontal disease, receding gums, and tooth degeneration) (Hornick, 2002).
- Financial limitations and the belief that dentures eliminate the need for routine dental care are reasons why older adults do not seek dental care (Eliopoulos, 2001).

Data from Eliopoulos C: *Gerontologic nursing*, ed 5, Philadelphia, 2001, Lippincott Williams & Wilkins.

Brushing and Flossing. Thorough tooth brushing at least 4 times a day (after meals and at bedtime) is basic to an effective oral hygiene program. A toothbrush should have a straight handle and brush small enough to reach all areas of the mouth. An even, rounded brushing surface with soft, multitufted, nylon bristles is best. Rounded soft bristles stimulate the gums without causing abrasion and bleeding. Older adult clients with reduced dexterity and grip may require an enlarged handle with an easier grip or an electric toothbrush (Felder and others, 1994). One simple way to devise an enlarged brush handle is to pierce a soft rubber ball and push the brush handle through or glue a short piece of plastic tubing around the handle. Clients should know to obtain a new toothbrush every 3 months or following a cold or strep throat to minimize growth of microorganisms on the brush surfaces.

All tooth surfaces should be brushed thoroughly using a fluoride toothpaste. Commercially made foam rubber toothbrushes are useful for clients with sensitive gums. However, swabbing fails to cleanse teeth adequately because plaque accumulates around the base of the teeth. Foam rubber swabs should be used in moderation. Electric toothbrushes can be used, but the nurse working in an agency setting should check for electrical hazards. Lemon-glycerin sponges should not be used because they dry mucous membranes and erode teeth enamel. Moi-Stin is a salivary supplement that improves moisture and texture of the tongue and mucosa (Poland, 1987).

When teaching clients about mouth care, the nurse should recommend they do not share toothbrushes with family members or drink directly from a bottle of mouthwash. Cross contamination occurs easily. The use of disclosure tablets or drops to stain the plaque that collects at the gum line can be useful for showing clients how effectively they brush. Many clients can perform their own oral care and should be encouraged to do so. The nurse observes the client to be sure proper techniques are used.

Clients will experience conditions that threaten the integrity of oral mucosa. For example, mucosal changes associated with aging, use of chemotherapeutic drugs, or dehydration require the nurse to adapt oral hygiene approaches. More frequent mouth care and use of antiinfective agents are examples of ways the nurse will revise approaches to meet client needs. Unconscious clients and those with artificial airways (e.g., endotracheal or tracheal tubes) need more frequent and specialized oral hygiene. These clients have an increased risk of aspiration and subsequently aspiration pneumonia, and they also have more problems with dry and inflamed oral mucosa.

The amount of assistance needed by the client when brushing the teeth may vary. When assisting with or providing oral hygiene, the nurse determines the amount of assistance needed, as well as individual oral hygiene preferences (Skill 38-4).

Flossing. Dental flossing removes plaque and tartar between teeth. Flossing involves inserting waxed or unwaxed dental floss between all tooth surfaces, one at a time. The seesaw motion used to pull floss between teeth removes plaque and tartar from tooth enamel. To prevent bleeding, clients who are receiving chemotherapy or radiation or are on anticoagulant therapy should use unwaxed floss and avoid vigorous flossing near the gum

Skill 38-4 | *Providing Oral Hygiene*

Delegation Considerations

Skills of brushing teeth can be delegated to assistive personnel (AP).

- Instruct AP how to adapt procedure for a client who is at risk of aspiration. These clients include those with impaired level of consciousness, impaired swallowing, or those who are confused.
- Instruct AP to immediately report to the nurse excessive client coughing or choking during or after oral hygiene
- Instruct AP to report any bleeding of oral mucosa or gums, client report of pain, or lesions to the nurse.

Equipment

- Soft-bristled toothbrush
- Nonabrasive fluoride toothpaste or dentifrice
- Dental floss
- Water glass with cool water
- Normal saline or an essential oil antiseptic mouthwash (*optional;* follow client's preference)
- Emesis basin
- Tongue blade
- Face towel
- Paper towels
- Disposable gloves

Steps	Rationale
1. Perform hand hygiene and apply disposable gloves.	Reduces transmission of microorganisms.
2. Inspect integrity of lips, teeth, buccal mucosa, gums, palate, and tongue (see Chapter 32).	Determines status of client's oral cavity and extent of need for oral hygiene.
3. Identify presence of common oral problems:	Helps determine type of hygiene client requires and information client requires for self-care.
a. Dental caries—chalky white discoloration of tooth or presence of brown or black discoloration	
b. Gingivitis—inflammation of gums	
c. Periodontitis—receding gum lines, inflammation, gaps between teeth	Receding gums occur with aging, and as a result older clients require meticulous oral hygiene (Walton, Miller, and Tordecilla, 2002).
d. Halitosis—bad breath	
e. Cheilosis—cracking of lips	
f. Stomatitis—inflammation of the mouth	Clients receiving immunosuppressive chemotherapy (e.g., cancer chemotherapy, anti-rejection medication post organ transplant) or those clients with suppressed immune function are at risk for stomatitis (Fulton, Middleton, and McPhail, 2002).
4. Remove gloves and perform hand hygiene.	Prevents spread of microorganisms.
5. Assess risk for oral hygiene problems (see Table 38-5, p. 1016).	Certain conditions increase likelihood of impaired oral cavity integrity and need for preventive care.
6. Assess client's risk for aspiration: impaired swallowing, reduced gag reflex.	Accumulation of secretions and dentifrice can increase client's risk for aspiration due to reduced ability to control oral secretions.
7. Determine client's oral hygiene practices:	Allows nurse to identify errors in technique, deficiencies in preventive oral hygiene, and client's level of knowledge regarding dental care.
a. Frequency of toothbrushing and flossing	
b. Type of toothpaste or dentifrice used	
c. Last dental visit	
d. Frequency of dental visits	
e. Type of mouthwash or moistening preparation	Lemon-glycerin preparations can be detrimental. Glycerin is an astringent that dries and shrinks mucous membranes and gums. Lemon exhausts salivary reflex and can erode tooth enamel (Poland, 1987). Mouthwash provides pleasant aftertaste but can dry mucosa after extended use if it has an alcohol base.
8. Assess client's ability to grasp and manipulate toothbrush. (For older adult try 30-sec toothbrush assessment.)	Toothbrush test useful in assessing dexterity and strength.
9. Prepare equipment at bedside.	Determines level of assistance required.

Skill 38-4   *Providing Oral Hygiene—cont'd*

Steps	Rationale
10. Explain procedure to client and discuss preferences regarding use of hygiene aids.	Some clients feel uncomfortable about having the nurse care for their basic needs. Client involvement with procedure minimizes anxiety.
11. Place paper towels on overbed table, and arrange other equipment within easy reach.	
12. Raise bed to comfortable working position. Raise head of bed (if allowed) and lower side rail. Move client, or help client move closer. Side-lying position can be used.	Raising bed and positioning client prevent nurse from straining muscles. Semi-Fowler's position helps prevent client from choking or aspirating.
13. Place towel over client's chest.	
14. Apply gloves.	Prevents contact with microorganisms or blood in saliva.
15. Apply toothpaste to brush, holding brush over emesis basin. Pour small amount of water over toothpaste.	Moisture aids in distribution of toothpaste over tooth surfaces.
16. Client may assist by brushing. Hold toothbrush bristles at 45-degree angle to gum line (see illustration). Be sure tips of bristles rest against and penetrate under gum line. Brush inner and outer surfaces of upper and lower teeth by brushing from gum to crown of each tooth. Clean biting surfaces of teeth by holding top of bristles parallel with teeth and brushing gently back and forth (see illustration). Brush sides of teeth by moving bristles back and forth (see illustration).	Angle allows brush to reach all tooth surfaces and to clean under gum line where plaque and tartar accumulate. Back-and-forth motion dislodges food particles caught between teeth and along chewing surfaces.
17. Have client hold brush at 45-degree angle and lightly brush over surface and sides of tongue (see illustration). Avoid initiating gag reflex.	Microorganisms collect and grow on tongue's surface and contribute to bad breath. Gagging may cause aspiration of toothpaste.
18. Allow client to rinse mouth thoroughly by taking several sips of water, swishing water across all tooth surfaces, and spitting into emesis basin.	Irrigation removes food particles.
19. Allow client to gargle to rinse mouth with mouthwash as desired.	Mouthwash leaves a pleasant taste in mouth but can dry mucosa after extended use if it has an alcohol base. An essential oil antiseptic mouthwash can be effective in reducing plaque and gingivitis (Bauroth and other, 2003).
20. Assist in wiping client's mouth.	Promotes sense of comfort.
21. Allow client to floss.	Reduces tartar on tooth surfaces.
22. Allow client to rinse mouth thoroughly with cool water and spit into emesis basin. Assist in wiping client's mouth.	Irrigation removes plaque and tartar from oral cavity.

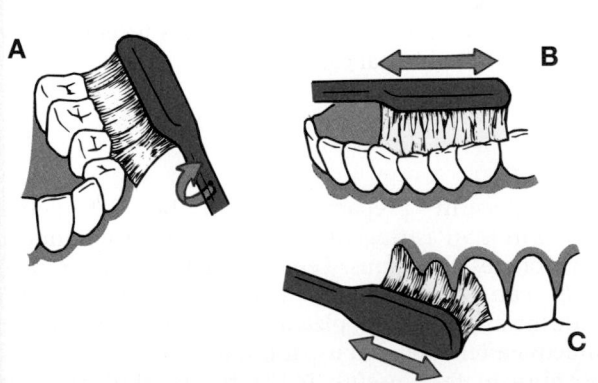

STEP **16**   Direction for toothbrush placement. **A,** A forty-five degree angle brushes gum line. **B,** Parallel position brushes biting surfaces. **C,** Lateral position brushes sides of teeth.

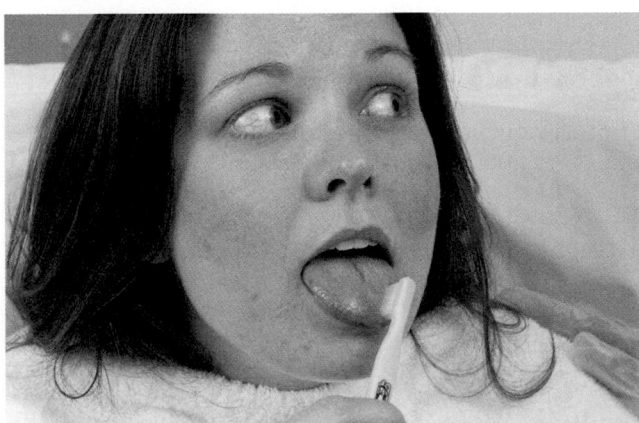

STEP **17**   Assisting client with brushing.

Steps	Rationale
23. Assist client to comfortable position, remove emesis basin and bedside table, raise side rail, and lower bed to original position.	Provides for client comfort and safety.
24. Wipe off overbed table, discard soiled linen and paper towels in appropriate containers, remove soiled gloves, and return equipment to proper place.	Proper disposal of soiled equipment prevents spread of infection.
25. Perform hand hygiene.	Reduces transmission of microorganisms.
26. Ask client if any area of oral cavity feels uncomfortable or irritated.	Pain indicates more chronic problem.
27. Apply gloves and inspect condition of oral cavity.	Determines effectiveness of hygiene and rinsing.
28. Ask client to describe proper hygiene techniques.	Evaluates client's learning.
29. Observe client brushing.	Evaluates client's ability to use correct technique.

Unexpected Outcomes and Related Interventions

1. Oral mucosa is dry and inflamed.
   a. Increase frequency of oral hygiene.
   b. Increase client's hydration.
   c. Apply protectant to client's lips.
2. Gum margins are retracted from teeth, with localized areas of inflammation. Bleeding occurs around gum margins.
   a. Determine if client has underlying bleeding tendency (e.g., anti-coagulant therapy).
   b. Report findings to physician.
   c. Use soft-bristled toothbrush.
   d. Increase frequency or oral hygiene.
3. Teeth show signs of dental caries.
   a. Refer client to dentist.
   b. Teach client oral hygiene.

Recording and Reporting

- Record procedure on flow sheet. Note condition of oral cavity in nurses' notes.
- Report bleeding or presence of lesions to nurse in charge or physician.

Home Care Considerations

- Teach client and caregiver to assess oral cavity daily to determine any effects of medications on the oral cavity (e.g., reddened, inflamed gums).

line. If toothpaste is applied to the teeth before flossing, fluoride can come in direct contact with tooth surfaces, aiding in cavity prevention. Flossing once a day is sufficient. Because it is important to clean all teeth surfaces thoroughly, the nurse should not rush to complete flossing. Placing a mirror in front of the client will help the nurse to demonstrate the proper method for holding the floss and cleaning between the teeth. Flossing a client's teeth is not realistic, nor appropriate in all care settings. However, flossing may be done more frequently in extended and rehabilitation care settings.

Clients With Special Needs. Some clients require special oral hygiene methods because of their level of dependence on the nurse or the presence of oral mucosa problems. Unconscious clients are susceptible to drying of mucous-thickened salivary secretions because they are unable to eat or drink, frequently breathe through the mouth, and often receive oxygen therapy. The unconscious client also cannot swallow salivary secretions that accumulate in the mouth. These secretions often contain gram-negative bacteria that can cause pneumonia if aspirated into the lungs. While providing hygiene to an unconscious client, the nurse must protect the client from choking and aspiration. To reduce the risk of aspiration and subsequent pneumonia, the safest technique is to have two nurses provide the care. The nurse may delegate assistive personnel to participate. One nurse does the actual cleaning, and the other removes secretions with suction equipment. While cleansing the oral cavity, the nurse should never use fingers to hold the client's mouth open. A human bite is highly contaminated. It may be necessary to perform mouth care at least every 2 hours. The nurse explains the steps of mouth care and the sensations the client will feel. The nurse also tells the client when the procedure is completed (Skill 38-5).

Clients who receive chemotherapy, radiation, or nasogastric tube intubation, or who have an infection of the mouth can suffer from **stomatitis.** Inflammation of the oral mucosa can cause oral burning, pain, and change in food tolerance. Gentle brushing and flossing are important in preventing bleeding of the gums. Clients should be advised to avoid alcohol and commercial mouthwash and to stop smoking. Normal saline rinses (approximately 30 ml) upon awaking in the morning, after each meal, and at bedtime can effectively clean the oral cavity. The rinses can be increased to every 2 hours if necessary. The physician may order a mild oral analgesic for pain control.

Performing Mouth Care for an Unconscious or Debilitated Client

Skill 38-5

Delegation Considerations

The skill of brushing teeth of an unconscious or debilitated client can be delegated to assistive personnel (AP). RN must first assess client for gag reflex and inform AP about proper way to position clients for mouth care.

- AP must be able to safely use oral suctioning for clearing oral secretions (see Chapter 39).
- Instruct AP to report to the nurse any bleeding of mucosa or gums, painful reaction by client, or excessive coughing or choking.

Equipment

- Antiinfective solution (e.g., commercial diluted hydrogen peroxide solution) that loosens crusts
- Small soft-bristled toothbrush
- Sponge toothette or tongue blade wrapped in single layer of gauze
- Padded tongue blade
- Face towel
- Paper towels
- Emesis basin
- Water glass with cool water
- Water-soluble lip lubricant
- Small-bulb syringe (optional)
- Suction machine equipment (optional)
- Disposable gloves (three pair)

Steps	Rationale
1. Perform hand hygiene. Apply disposable gloves.	Reduces transmission of microorganisms. Gloves prevent contact with microorganisms in blood or saliva.
2. Assess client's risk for oral hygiene problems (see Table 38-5, p. 1016).	Impaired levels of consciousness increases the likelihood of alterations in integrity of oral cavity structures and may require more frequent care. Proper oral care is shown to reduce the risk of pneumonia (Research update, 2002).
3. Test for presence of gag reflex by placing tongue blade on back half of client's tongue.	Reveals whether client is at risk for aspiration.

Critical Decision Point: Clients with impaired gag reflex require oral care as well. The nurse determines the type of suction apparatus needed at the bedside to protect the client's airway against aspiration.

Steps	Rationale
4. Inspect condition of oral cavity (see Chapter 32).	Determines condition of oral cavity and need for hygiene.
5. Remove gloves. Perform hand hygiene.	Prevents spread of infection.
6. Explain procedure to client.	Allows debilitated client to anticipate procedure without anxiety. Unconscious client may retain ability to hear.
7. Apply disposable gloves.	Reduces transfer of microorganisms.
8. Place paper towels on overbed table and arrange equipment. If needed, turn on suction machine, and connect tubing to suction catheter.	Prevents soiling of table top. Equipment prepared in advance ensures smooth, safe procedure.
9. Pull curtain around bed, or close room door.	Provides privacy.
10. Raise bed to the appropriate height for nurse; lower head of bed and then lower side rail.	Use of good body mechanics with bed in elevated position reduces the risk of injury to the nurse.
11. Position client on side (Sims' position) with head turned well toward dependent side. Move client close to side of bed. Then raise side rail.	Turning the client's head to the side allows secretions to drain from mouth instead of collecting in back of pharynx. Prevents aspiration. Moving the client close to the side of the bed facilitates proper body mechanics as the nurse performs this skill.
12. Place towel under client's head and emesis basin under chin.	Prevents soiling of bed linen.
13. Carefully separate upper and lower teeth with padded tongue blade by inserting blade, quickly but gently, between back molars. Insert when client is relaxed, if possible. Do not use force (see illustration).	Prevents client from biting down on nurse's fingers and provides access to oral cavity.

Steps	Rationale

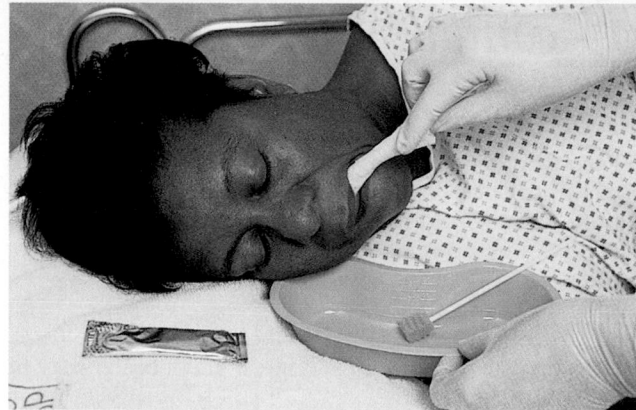

STEP **13** Separate upper and lower teeth with padded tongue blade.

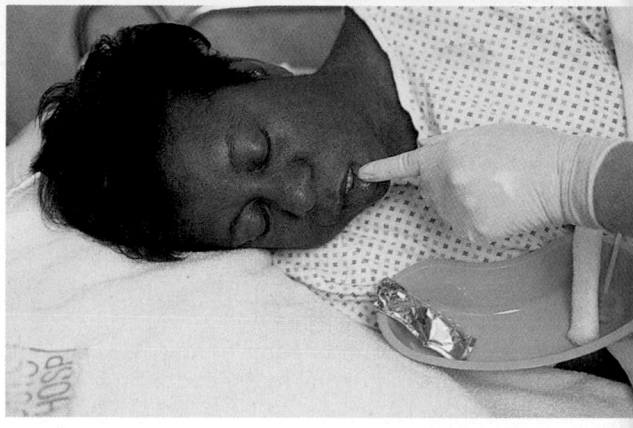

STEP **16** Application of water-soluble moisturizer to lips.

Critical Decision Point: Never use fingers to separate client's teeth.

---

14. Clean mouth using brush or sponge toothettes moistened with commercial hydrogen peroxide solution. Clean chewing and inner tooth surfaces first. Clean outer tooth surfaces. Swab roof of mouth, gums, and inside cheeks. Gently swab or brush tongue but avoid stimulating gag reflex (if present). Moisten clean swab or toothette with water to rinse. (Bulb syringe may also be used to rinse.) Repeat rinse several times.

Brushing action removes food particles between teeth and along chewing surfaces. Swabbing helps remove secretions and crusts from mucosa and moistens mucosa. Repeated rinsing removes peroxide that can be irritating to mucosa.

15. Suction secretions as they accumulate, if necessary.

Suction removes secretions and fluid that can collect in posterior pharynx.

16. Apply thin layer of water-soluble jelly to lips (see illustration).

Lubricates lips to prevent drying and cracking.

17. Inform client that procedure is completed.

Provides meaningful stimulation to unconscious or less responsive client.

18. Reposition client comfortably, raise side rail as appropriate or as ordered, and return bed to original position.

Maintains client's comfort and safety. Raising all four side rails may be considered a restraint, and a physician's order is needed.

19. Clean equipment and return to its proper place. Place soiled linen in proper receptacle.

Proper disposal of soiled equipment prevents spread of infection.

20. Remove and discard gloves. Perform hand hygiene.

Reduces transmission of microorganisms.

21. Apply clean gloves, and inspect oral cavity.

Determines efficacy of cleansing. Once thick secretions are removed, underlying inflammation or lesions may be revealed.

22. Ask debilitated client if mouth feels clean.

Evaluates level of comfort.

23. Assess client's respirations on an ongoing basis.

Ensures early recognition of aspiration.

Skill 38-5   ## *P*erforming Mouth Care for an Unconscious or Debilitated Client—cont'd

Unexpected Outcomes and Related Interventions

1. Secretions or crusts remain on oral mucosa, tongue, or gums.
   a. Increase frequency of oral hygiene.
   b. A pediatric-size toothbrush may provide better hygiene (Fitch and others, 1999).
2. Localized inflammation of gums or mucosa is present.
   a. Increase frequency of oral hygiene with a soft-bristled toothbrush.
   b. Apply moisturizing gel on oral mucosa (Fitch and others, 1999).
   c. Chemotherapy and radiation can cause stomatitis. Antiseptic mouthwashes provide relief, promote oral hygiene, and improve healing (Fulton, Middleton, and McPhail, 2002).
3. Client aspirated secretions.
   a. Suction oral airway.
   b. Perform tracheal bronchial suctioning.
   c. Notify physician.

Recording and Reporting

- Record procedure, including pertinent observations (e.g., presence of bleeding gums, dry mucosa, ulcerations, crusts on tongue).
- Report any unusual findings to nurse in charge or physician.

Home Care Considerations

- Irrigate cavity with bulb syringe; a gravy baster may be substituted.
- Mouth care should be given at least twice a day. Caregivers can get nonprescription oral care solutions (e.g., carbamide peroxide solutions) at most pharmacies.
- Have caregivers demonstrate positioning client to prevent aspiration.

Clients with diabetes mellitus frequently have periodontal disease. Visits to the dentist are needed every 3 to 4 months. All tissues should be handled gently with a minimum of trauma. Clients should learn to follow rigid cleansing schedules, at least 4 times a day.

Denture Care. Clients should be encouraged to clean their dentures on a regular basis to avoid gingival infection and irritation. When clients become disabled, the nurse or family caregiver can assume responsibility for denture care (Box 38-11). Dentures are the client's personal property and need to be handled with care because they can be easily broken. Dentures must be removed at night to give the gums a rest and prevent bacterial buildup. To prevent warping, dentures should be kept covered in water when they are not worn, and they should always be stored in an enclosed, labeled cup with the cup placed in the client's bedside stand. Discourage clients from removing their dentures and placing them on a napkin or tissue because they could be easily thrown away.

Hair and Scalp Care. A person's appearance and feeling of well-being often depend on the way the hair looks and feels. Illness or disability may prevent a client from maintaining daily hair care. An immobilized client's hair soon becomes tangled. Dressings may leave sticky blood or antiseptic solutions on the hair. In the clinic and home care setting, nurses will encounter clients who have head lice. Proper hair care is important to the client's body image. Brushing, combing, and shampooing are basic hygiene measures for all clients.

Brushing and Combing. Frequent brushing helps to keep hair clean and distributes oil evenly along hair shafts. Combing prevents hair from tangling. The client should be encouraged to maintain routine hair care. However, clients with limited mobility or weakness and those who are confused require help. Clients in a hospital or extended care facility appreciate the opportunity to have their hair brushed and combed before being seen by others.

When caring for clients from different cultures, it is important to learn as much as possible from them or their family about preferred hair care practices. For example, the hair of African-Americans tends to be quite dry. Special lanolin conditioners may be used for conditioning. Cultural preferences will also affect how hair is combed and styled.

Long hair can easily become matted after a client is confined to bed, even for a short period. When lacerations or incisions involve the scalp, blood and topical medications can also cause tangling. Frequent brushing and combing keep long hair neatly groomed. Braiding can help to avoid repeated tangles; however, braids should be unbraided periodically and hair combed to ensure good hygiene. Braids made too tightly can lead to bald patches. The nurse obtains permission from the client before braiding his or her hair.

To brush hair the nurse parts the hair into two sections and separates each into two more sections. It is easier to brush smaller sections of hair. Brushing from the scalp toward the hair ends minimizes pulling. Moistening the hair with water or alcohol frees tangles for easier combing. The nurse never cuts a client's hair without written consent.

Box *38-11* *Procedural Guidelines*

Care of Dentures

Equipment: Soft-bristled toothbrush or denture toothbrush, denture cleaning agent or toothpaste, denture adhesive (optional), glass of water, emesis basin or sink, washcloth, disposable gloves, denture cup (if dentures are to be stored after cleaning).

Delegation Considerations: The skill denture care can be delegated to assistive personnel (AP). The nurse intructs AP to:

- Inform the nurse if cracks are found in the dentures.
- Inform the nurse if the client complains of oral discomfort.

1. Ask client if dentures fit and if there is any gum or mucous membrane tenderness or irritation.
2. Ask client about preferences for denture care and products used. If client is unable to care for own dentures, the nurse must provide this care Clean dentures for client during routine mouth care.
3. Fill emesis basin with tepid water, or if using sink, place washcloth in bottom of sink and fill sink with an inch of water.
4. Remove dentures: If client is unable to do this independently, perform hand hygiene and apply gloves, grasp upper plate at front with thumb and index finger wrapped in gauze, and pull downward. Gently lift lower denture from jaw, and rotate one side downward to remove from client's mouth. Place dentures in emesis basin or sink.
5. Apply cleaning agent to brush and brush surfaces of dentures (see illustration). Hold dentures close to water. Hold brush horizontally, and use back-and-forth motion to cleanse biting surfaces. Use short strokes from top of denture to biting surfaces to clean outer and inner teeth surfaces. Hold brush vertically, and use short strokes to clean inner tooth

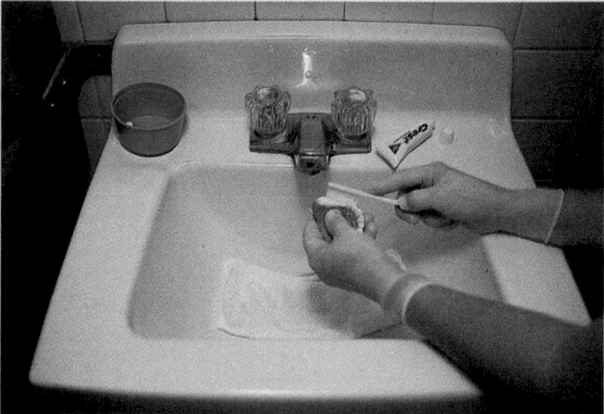

STEP **5** Brushing dentures.

surfaces. Hold brush horizontally, and use back-and-forth motion to clean undersurface of dentures.
6. Rinse thoroughly in tepid water.
7. Some clients use an adhesive to seal dentures in place. Apply a thin layer to undersurface before inserting.
8. If client needs assistance with insertion of dentures, moisten upper denture and press firmly to seal it in place. Then insert moistened lower denture. Ask if dentures feel comfortable.
9. Some clients prefer to have their dentures stored to give the gums a rest and to reduce risk of infection. Keeping dentures moist will prevent warping and facilitate easier insertion. Store in a secure place to prevent loss.
10. Remove and discard gloves and perform hand hygiene.

Clients who develop head lice require special considerations in the way combing is performed. The lice are small, about the size of a sesame seed. Bright light or natural sunlight is necessary for the lice to be seen. Thorough combing is recommended and may be more effective than use of pediculicidal shampoos, which are often toxic and ineffective against resistant lice. Follow these steps:

- Apply disposable gown and gloves.
- Use a grooming comb or hairbrush to remove tangles.
- Divide the client's hair in sections and fasten off hair that is not being combed.
- Comb out from the scalp to the end of the hair (special combs are available in drug stores).
- Dip the comb in a cup of water or use a paper towel to remove lice between each passing.
- After combing, look through the hair carefully for attached lice.
- Live lice may be caught with a tweezers or comb.
- Move to next section of hair after combing thoroughly.
- Instruct family to clean the comb with an old toothbrush and dental floss and boil the comb (if possible). The ideal would be to discard the comb after each use, but some client's financial situations may prevent the purchase of multiple combs.

- Instruct family to comb and screen for lice daily.
- Instruct family to contain client's clothes and to wash in hot water.
- Instruct family to vacuum the home and client's room, and to immediately empty vacuum bag or bagless collection device.
- Instruct caregivers on how to prevent transmission of lice:
  - Do not share any bed linens.
  - Avoid placing bare hand on client's head.
  - Immediately wash hands after providing hair care.
  - Contain all hair care products.

If a pediculicidal shampoo is ordered, instruct the client and caregiver on proper use of shampoo. These shampoos have neurological side effects. The very young and very old have increased susceptibility to the toxic effects of seizure, dizziness, headache, paresthesia, and death. This type of medication should never be used on clients infected with HIV, those with neurological conditions, the neonate, or clients who weigh less than 110 pounds (Zurlinden, 2003). As with any medication preparation, it is important to review and understand pertinent information. Most side effects associated with pediculicidal shampoos occurred due to applying too much med-

Box 38-12 Procedural Guidelines

Shampooing Hair of Bed-Bound Client

Equipment: Bath towels, washcloths, shampoo and hair conditioner (optional), water pitcher, plastic shampoo trough, washbasin, bath blanket, waterproof pad, clean comb and brush, hair dryer *(optional)*, disposable gloves *(optional)*

Delegation Considerations: The skill of shampooing hair can be delegated to assistive personnel (AP). The nurse instructs AP:

- Of any precautions needed in positioning the client.
- To inform the nurse if the client reports neck pain.
- To inform the nurse of any new skin lesions.

1. Before washing client's hair, determine that there are no contraindications to this procedure. Certain medical conditions, such as head and neck injuries, spinal cord injuries, and arthritis, could place the client at risk for injury during shampooing because of positioning and manipulation of client's head and neck.
2. Apply gloves if needed. Inspect the hair and scalp before initiating the procedure. This determines the presence of any conditions that may require the use of special shampoos or treatments (e.g., for dandruff or the removal of dried blood).
3. Place waterproof pad under client's shoulders, neck, and head (see illustration). Position client supine, with head and shoulders at top edge of bed. Place plastic trough under client's head and washbasin at end of trough. Be sure trough spout extends beyond edge of mattress.

4. Place rolled towel under client's neck and bath towel over client's shoulders.
5. Brush and comb client's hair.
6. Obtain warm water.
7. Offer client the option of holding face towel or washcloth over eyes.
8. Slowly pour water from water pitcher over hair until it is completely wet (see illustration). If hair contains matted blood, don gloves, apply peroxide to dissolve clots, and then rinse hair with saline. Apply small amount of shampoo.
9. Work up lather with both hands. Start at hairline, and work toward back of neck. Lift head slightly with one hand to wash back of head. Shampoo sides of head. Massage scalp by applying pressure with fingertips.
10. Rinse hair with water. Make sure water drains into basin. Repeat rinsing until hair is free of soap.
11. Apply conditioner or cream rinse if requested, and rinse hair thoroughly.
12. Wrap client's head in bath towel. Dry client's face with cloth used to protect eyes. Dry off any moisture along neck or shoulders.
13. Dry client's hair and scalp. Use second towel if first becomes saturated.
14. Comb hair to remove tangles, and dry with dryer if desired.
15. Apply oil preparation or conditioning product to hair, if desired by client.
16. Assist client to comfortable position, and complete styling of hair.

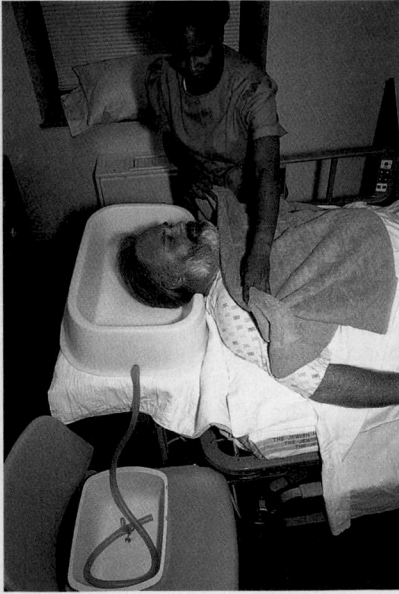

STEP **3**   Pad under shoulders, neck, and head.

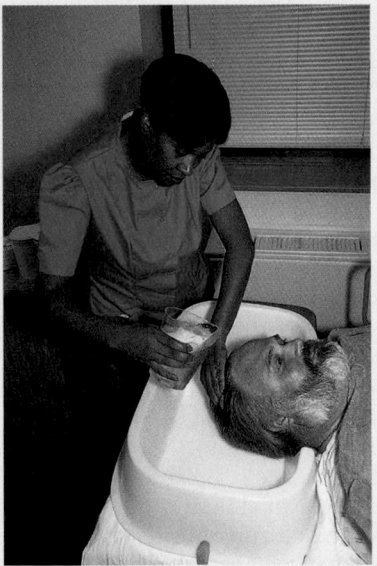

STEP **8**   Pouring water over hair.

icated shampoo, leaving the shampoo in place too long, or repeated shampooing too soon. Many clients were overtreated because they incorrectly believed that continued itching meant that lice survived the initial treatment. They did not know that itching was a common side effect of the shampoo (Zurlinden, 2003).

Shampooing. Frequency of shampooing depends on a person's daily routines and the condition of the hair. The nurse should remind clients in hospitals or extended care facilities that staying in bed, excess perspiration, or treatments that leave blood or solutions in the hair may require more frequent shampooing. For clients at home, the nurse is challenged to find ways the client can shampoo the hair without causing injury.

If the client is able to take a shower or bath, the hair can usually be shampooed without difficulty. A shower or tub chair may be used for the ambulatory, weight-bearing client who becomes tired or faint. Handheld shower nozzles allow clients to easily wash the hair in the tub or shower. Clients allowed to sit in a chair may choose to be shampooed in front of a sink or over a washbasin. However, bending is limited or contraindicated in certain conditions (e.g., eye surgery or neck injury). In these situations the nurse needs to teach the client the degree of bending allowed.

If a client is unable to sit but can be moved, the nurse may transfer the client to a stretcher for transportation to a sink or shower equipped with a handheld nozzle. Long-term care facilities are commonly equipped with this option. Caution is again needed when the client's head and neck are positioned, particularly in clients with any form of head or neck injury.

If the client is unable to sit in a chair or be transferred to a stretcher, shampooing must be done with the client in bed (Box 38-12). A special shampoo trough can be positioned under the client's head to catch water and suds. After shampooing, clients like having their hair styled and dried. Most health care centers have portable hair dryers. Dry shampoos that reduce the need to wet the client's hair are also available but are not highly effective. These dry shampoo preparations vary, and the application procedures, listed on the container, should be followed exactly. In most agencies a physician's order is necessary for shampooing the dependent client.

Shaving. Shaving facial hair can be done after the bath or shampoo. Women may prefer to shave their legs or axillae while bathing. When assisting a client, the nurse should take care to avoid cutting the client with a razor blade. Clients prone to bleeding (e.g., those receiving anticoagulants or high doses of aspirin or those with low platelet counts) must use an electric razor. Before using an electric razor, the nurse should check for frayed cords or other electrical hazards. Electric razors should be used on only one client because of infection-control considerations.

When a razor blade is used for shaving, the skin must be softened to prevent pulling, scraping, or cuts. For example, placing a warm washcloth over the male client's face for a few seconds, followed by application of shaving cream or a lathering of mild soap, softens the skin. If the

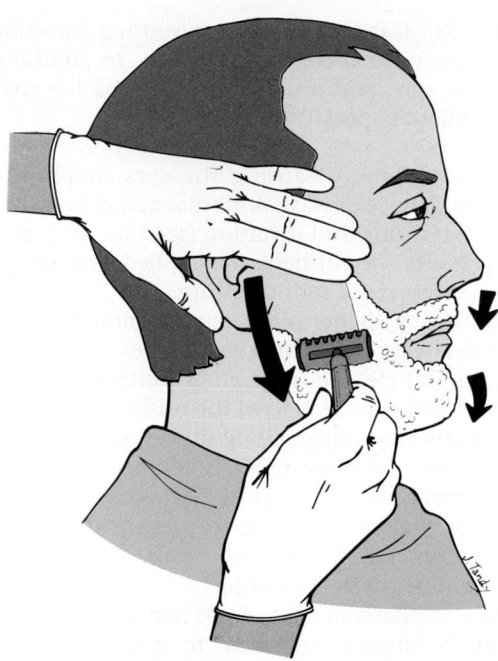

FIGURE **38–8** Shave in the direction of hair growth. Use longer strokes on the larger areas of the face. Use short strokes around the chin and lips. (From Sorrentino SA: *Assisting with patient care,* St. Louis, 1999, Mosby.)

client is unable to shave, the nurse may perform the shave. To avoid causing discomfort or razor cuts, the nurse gently pulls the skin taut and uses short, firm razor strokes in the direction the hair grows (Figure 38-8). Short downward strokes work best to remove hair over the upper lip. A client usually can explain to the nurse the best way to move the razor across the skin. In the case of African-Americans, facial hair tends to be curly and can become ingrown unless shaved close to the skin.

Mustache and Beard Care. Clients with mustaches or beards require daily grooming. Keeping these areas clean is important because food particles and mucus can easily collect in the hair. If the client is unable to carry out self-care, the nurse should do so at the client's request. Beards can be gently combed out. A shaggy or unkempt mustache or beard can be trimmed. Shaving off a mustache or beard cannot be performed without the client's consent.

Hair and Scalp Care. To best promote and restore hair and scalp health, clients should be instructed to keep hair clean, combed, and brushed regularly. Clients may also need to know how to check for and remove parasites, such as lice (see Table 38-4, p. 1012). The nurse should tell clients they need to notify their primary caregiver of changes in the texture and distribution of hair, which may indicate a serious systemic problem.

Care of the Eyes, Ears, and Nose. Special attention is given to cleansing the eyes, ears, and nose during a routine bath and when drainage or discharge accumulate. This aspect of hygiene not only makes the client more comfortable but also improves sensory reception

(Chapter 48). Care focuses on preventing infection and maintaining normal sensory function. In addition, care of the eyes, ears, and nose requires approaches that consider the client's special needs.

Basic Eye Care. Cleansing the eyes simply involves washing with a clean washcloth moistened in water. Soap may cause burning and irritation (see Skill 38-1, p. 1023). Direct pressure should never be applied over the eyeball because it may cause serious injury.

Unconscious clients often require more frequent eye care. When cleansing the client's eyes, obtain a clean washcloth and cleanse from inner canthus to outer canthus. Use a different section of the washcloth for each eye.

Secretions may collect along the lid margins and inner canthus when the blink reflex is absent or when the eye does not totally close. It may be necessary to place an eye patch over the involved eye to prevent corneal drying and irritation. Lubricating eye drops may be given according to the physician's orders.

Eyeglasses. Glasses are made of hardened glass or plastic that is impact resistant to prevent shattering. Nevertheless, because of the cost, the nurse should be careful when cleaning glasses and should protect them from breakage or other damage when they are not worn. Glasses should be put in a case in a drawer of the bedside table when not in use.

Cool water is sufficient for cleaning glass lenses. A soft cloth is best for drying to prevent scratching the lens. Paper towels can scratch a lens. Plastic lenses in particular are scratched easily, and special cleansing solutions and drying tissues are available. Use whatever the client's eye care specialist recommends.

Contact Lenses. A contact lens is a small, round, transparent, and sometimes colored disk that fits directly over the cornea of the eye. Contact lenses are designed specifically to correct refractive errors of the eye or abnormalities in the cornea's shape. They are relatively easy to apply and remove.

Contact lenses are available as daily wear, extended wear, and disposable. In terms of a client's hygiene care it is important to know that all lenses must be removed periodically to prevent ocular infection and corneal ulcers or abrasions. Common infectious agents are *Pseudomonas aeruginosa* and staphylococci. Client education must include a discussion of proper lens care techniques (Box 38-13).

Daily-wear lenses should be removed overnight for cleaning and disinfection and should not be worn for more than 10 to 14 hours daily (Cohen and Krachmer, 1992). It is recommended that all extended-wear lenses be worn no longer than 6 consecutive nights without cleaning and disinfecting (Johnson & Johnson Vision Products, 1994).

Disposable lenses are available for daily wear and extended wear and are usually replaced every 1 to 2 weeks. Pain, tearing, discomfort, and redness of the conjunctivae may be symptoms of lens overwear. Persistence of symptoms even after lens removal is abnormal, however, and may indicate serious ocular damage.

As contact lenses are worn, they accumulate secretions and foreign matter. This material deteriorates and then irritates the eye, causing distorted vision and risk for infection. Once removed, contact lenses should be cleaned and thoroughly disinfected. Clients should be cautioned to never use saliva, homemade saline, or tap water when

---

Client Teaching

Box 38-13

Contact Lens Care

Objectives

- Client will be able to identify warning signs of corneal irritation and eye infection.
- Client will be able to clean and care for contact lenses correctly.

Teaching Strategies

- Encourage client to see a vision care specialist (**ophthalmologist** or **optometrist**) regularly: every 3 to 5 years before age 40, every 2 years after age 40, and yearly after age 65.
- Plastic lenses scratch easily. Special cleaning solutions and drying tissues are recommended.
- Never use fingernail on lens to remove dirt or debris that does not loosen during washing.
- Follow recommendations of lens manufacturer or eye care practitioner when cleaning and disinfecting lenses.
- Encourage client to remember the mnemonic RSVP: *R*edness, *S*ensitivity, *V*ision problems, and *P*ain. If one of these problems occurs, remove contact lenses immediately. If problems continue, contact vision care specialist (Lewis and others, 2000).

- Lenses become very slippery once cleaning solution is applied.
- If lens is dropped on a hard surface, moisten finger with cleaning or wetting solution and gently touch lens to pick it up. Then clean, rinse, and disinfect lens.
- Lens should be kept moist or wet when not worn.
- Use fresh solution daily when storing and disinfecting lenses.
- Do not wipe lens with tissue or towel.
- Thoroughly wash and rinse lens storage case on a daily basis. Clean periodically with soap or liquid detergent; rinse thoroughly with warm water and air dry.
- To avoid mix-up, always start with the same lens when removing or inserting lenses.
- Disposable or planned replacement lenses should be thrown away after prescribed wearing period.

Evaluation

- Have client identify warning signs of corneal irritation and eye infection.
- Ask client to describe methods of contact lens care that can lead to infection.
- Ask client to describe techniques to use in cleaning and storing contact lenses.

cleaning lenses as these solutions may contain microorganisms that can cause serious infection.

Artificial Eyes. Clients with artificial eyes have had an **enucleation** of an entire eyeball as a result of tumor growth, severe infection, or eye trauma. Some artificial eyes are permanently implanted. Others can be removed for routine cleaning. Clients with artificial eyes usually prefer to care for their own eyes. The nurse should respect the client's wishes and help by assembling needed equipment.

Clients may at times require assistance in prosthesis removal and cleansing. To remove an artificial eye, the nurse retracts the lower eyelid and exerts slight pressure just below the eye (Figure 38-9). This action causes the artificial eye to rise from the socket because the suction holding the eye in place has been broken. The nurse may also use a small, rubber bulb syringe or medicine dropper bulb to create a suction effect. The suction created by placing the bulb tip directly over the eye and squeezing lifts the eye from the socket.

The artificial eye is usually made of glass or plastic. Warm normal saline cleanses the prosthesis effectively. The nurse also cleanses the edges of the eye socket and surrounding tissues with soft gauze moistened in saline or clean tap water. Signs of infection should be reported immediately because bacteria can spread to the neighboring eye, underlying sinuses, or even underlying brain tissue. To reinsert the eye, the nurse retracts the upper and lower lids and gently slips the eye into the socket, fitting it neatly

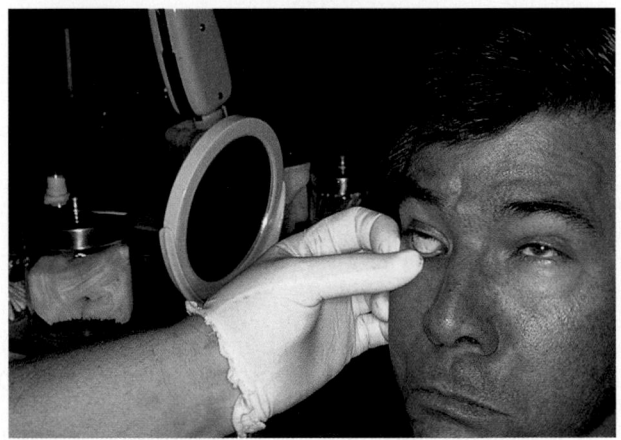

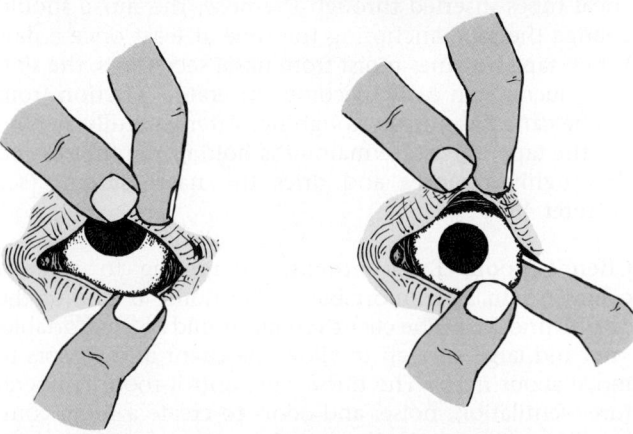

FIGURE **38–9** Removal of prosthetic eye.

under the upper eyelid. An artificial eye may be stored in a labeled container filled with tap water or saline.

Ear Care. Routine ear care involves cleansing the ear with the end of a moistened washcloth, rotated gently into the ear canal. When cerumen is visible, gentle, downward retraction at the entrance of the ear canal may cause the wax to loosen and slip out. The nurse warns clients never to use sharp objects such as bobby pins or paper clips to remove ear wax. The use of such objects can traumatize the ear canal and rupture the tympanic membrane. Use of cotton-tipped applicators should also be avoided because they can cause ear wax to become impacted within the canal.

Children and older adults commonly have impacted cerumen. Excessive or impacted cerumen can usually be removed only by irrigation, which usually requires a physician's order. If a client has a history of a perforated eardrum or if perforation is discovered during assessment, the procedure is contraindicated. Before irrigation first instill three drops of glycerin at bedtime to soften the wax, and three drops of hydrogen peroxide twice a day to loosen the wax. Then the instillation of approximately 250 ml of warm water (37° C, or 98.6° F) into the ear canal mechanically washes away loosened wax. Cold or hot water causes nausea or vomiting.

The client may sit or lie on his or her side with the affected ear up. The nurse places a small curved basin under the affected ear to catch the irrigating solution. A Water Pik (set on No. 2 setting) or a bulb irrigating syringe can be used to irrigate the ear canal. The tip of the syringe or Water Pik should not occlude the canal to avoid exerting pressure against the tympanic membrane. Gentle irrigation directed at the top of the canal loosens the cerumen from the sides of the canal. After the canal is clear, the nurse wipes off any moisture from the ear and inspects the canal for remaining cerumen.

Hearing Aid Care. Hearing aids are instruments made up of miniature parts working together as a system to amplify sound in a controlled manner. The aid receives normal low-intensity sound inputs and delivers them to the client's ear as louder outputs. The new class of hearing aids can reduce background noise interference. Computer chips placed in the aids allow for fine adjustments to the specific client's hearing needs. Hearing aids are used by both hard-of-hearing (slight or moderate hearing loss) and deaf persons (severe or prolonged hearing loss).

There are three popular types of hearing aids. An in-the-canal (ITC) aid is the newest, smallest, and least visible and fits entirely in the ear canal. It has cosmetic appeal, is easy to manipulate and place in the ear, does not interfere with wearing eyeglasses or using the telephone, and can be worn during most physical exercise. However, it requires adequate ear diameter and depth for proper fit. It does not accommodate progressive hearing loss, and it requires manual dexterity to operate, insert, remove, and change batteries. Also, cerumen tends to plug this model more than the others.

An in-the-ear (ITE, or intraaural) aid (Figure 38-10, *A*) fits into the external auditory canal and allows for more fine tuning. It is more powerful and stronger and therefore is useful for a wider range of hearing loss than the

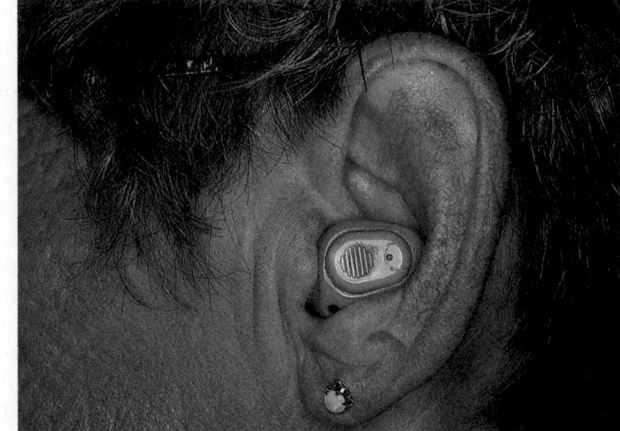

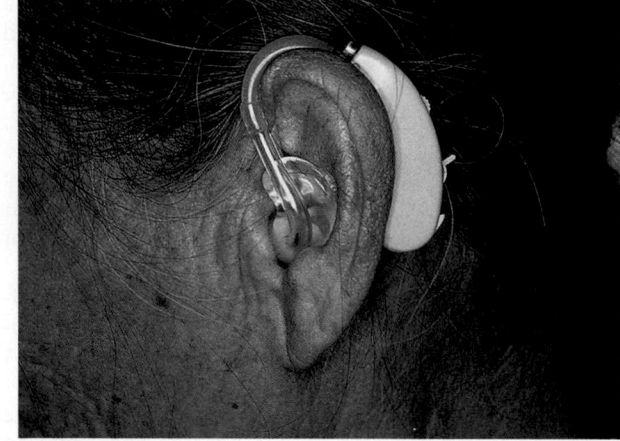

FIGURE **38–10** Two common types of hearing aids. **A,** In the ear. **B,** Behind the ear.

<table>
<tr><td colspan="2">

Box **38-14**   **Care and Use of Hearing Aids**

</td></tr>
</table>

Box **38-14**   **Care and Use of Hearing Aids**

- Initially wear a hearing aid 15 to 20 minutes; then gradually increase time until 10 to 12 hours.
- Once inserted, turn the aid slowly to one-third to one-half volume.
- A whistling sound indicates incorrect ear mold insertion, improper fit of aid, and buildup of earwax or fluid.
- Adjust volume to a comfortable level for talking at a distance of 1 yard.
- Do not wear aid under heat lamps; a hair dryer; or in very wet, cold weather.
- Batteries last 1 week with daily wearing of 10 to 12 hours.
- Remove or disconnect battery when not in use.
- Replace ear molds every 2 or 3 years.
- Routinely check battery compartment: Is it clean? Are batteries inserted properly? Is compartment shut all the way?
- Dials on hearing aid should be clean and easy to rotate, creating no static during adjusting.
- Keep aid clean.
  - See manufacturer's instructions, but aids are usually cleaned with a soft cloth.
  - Avoid use of hairspray and perfume while wearing hearing aids, the residue from the spray can cause aid to become oily and greasy.
  - Do not submerse in water.
- Routinely check cord or tubing (depending on type of aid) for cracking, fraying, and poor connections.
- Routine follow-up with audiologist is recommended to evaluate effectiveness of current aid.
- Newer computerized hearing aids can have frequencies easily adjusted.

Data from Ebersole P, Hess P: *Toward healthy aging,* ed 5, St. Louis, 2000, Mosby; Lueckenotte AG: *Gerontologic nursing,* ed 2, St. Louis, 2000, Mosby; and National Institute on Deafness and Other Communication Disorders (NIDCD): *Hearing aids,* Pub No. 99-4340, Bethesda, Md, 2001, National Institutes of Health, www.nidcd.nih.gov/health/hearing/hearingaid.asp.

ITC aid. It is easy to position and adjust and does not interfere with eyeglass wearing. It is, however, more noticeable than the ITC aid and is not recommended for persons with moisture or skin problems in the ear canal.

A behind-the-ear (BTE, or postaural) aid (Figure 38-10, *B*) hooks around and behind the ear and is connected by a short, clear, hollow plastic tube to an ear mold inserted into the external auditory canal. It allows for fine tuning. It is the largest of the three aids and is useful for clients with rapidly progressive hearing loss or manual dexterity difficulties or those who find partial ear occlusion intolerable. Disadvantages are that it is more visible and may interfere with wearing eyeglasses and using a phone, and it is more difficult to keep in place during physical exercise. Box 38-14 reviews client education guidelines for the care and cleaning of a hearing aid.

Nasal Care. The client can usually remove secretions from the nose by gently blowing into a soft tissue. The nurse cautions the client against harsh blowing that creates pressure capable of injuring the eardrum, nasal mucosa, and even sensitive eye structures. Bleeding from the nares is a sign of harsh blowing.

If the client is unable to remove nasal secretions, the nurse assists by using a wet washcloth or a cotton-tipped applicator moistened in water or saline. The applicator should never be inserted beyond the length of the cotton tip. Excessive nasal secretions can also be removed by gentle suctioning.

When clients have nasogastric, feeding, or endotracheal tubes inserted through the nose, the nurse should change the tape anchoring the tube at least once a day. When tape becomes moist from nasal secretions, the skin and mucosa can easily become macerated. Friction from a tube can cause tissue sloughing. After carefully removing the tape, the nurse maintains hold of the tubing and thoroughly cleanses and dries the nasal surface (see Chapter 43).

Client's Room Environment. Attempting to make a client's room as comfortable as the home is one of the nurse's priorities. The client's room should be comfortable, safe, and large enough to allow the client and visitors to move about freely. The nurse can control room temperature, ventilation, noise, and odors to create a more comfortable environment. Keeping the room neat and orderly also contributes to the client's sense of well-being.

Maintaining Comfort. The nature of what constitutes a comfortable environment depends on the client's age, severity of illness, and level of normal daily activity. Depending on the client's age and physical condition, the room temperature should be maintained between 20° and 23° C (68° and 74° F). Infants, older adults, and the acutely ill may need a warmer room. However, certain ill clients benefit from cooler room temperatures to lower the body's metabolic demands.

A good ventilation system keeps stale air and odors from lingering in the room. The nurse must protect the acutely ill, infants, and older adults from drafts by ensuring they are adequately dressed and covered with a light-weight blanket.

Good ventilation also reduces lingering odors caused by draining wounds, vomitus, bowel movements, and unemptied urinals. Room deodorizers can help remove many unpleasant odors but should be used with discretion in consideration of the client's possible embarrassment. Nurses should always empty and rinse bedpans or urinals promptly. Thorough hygiene measures are the best way to control body or breath odors. Most health care institutions now prohibit smoking. Before using room deodorizers the nurse should determine that the client is not allergic to or sensitive to the deodorizer itself.

Ill clients seem to be more sensitive to common hospital noises (e.g., intravenous pump alarms, suction apparatus, or stretchers exiting an elevator). Until the client is familiar with hospital noises, the nurse should try to control the noise level. This can also help the client gain necessary sleep (see Chapter 41). The nurse also explains the source of any unfamiliar noise to the client and family members.

Proper lighting is necessary for everyone's safety and comfort. A brightly lit room is usually stimulating, but a darkened room is best for rest and sleep. Room lighting can be adjusted by closing or opening drapes, regulating overbed and floor lights, and closing or opening room doors. When entering a client's room at night, refrain from abruptly turning on an overhead light unless necessary.

Room Equipment. Although there may be variation across health care settings, a typical hospital room contains the following basic pieces of furniture: overbed table, bedside stand, chairs, lamp, and bed (Figure 38-11). Long-term care and rehabilitation facilities may have similar equipment. The overbed table rolls on wheels and can be adjusted to various heights over the bed or a chair. The table provides ideal working space for the nurse performing procedures. It also provides a surface on which to place meal trays, toiletry items, and objects frequently used by the client. The bedpan and urinal should not be placed on the overbed table. The bedside stand is used to store the client's personal possessions and hygiene equipment. The telephone, water pitcher, and drinking cup are commonly found on top of the bedside stand.

Most hospital rooms contain an armless straight-backed chair or an upholstered lounge chair with arms. Straight-backed chairs are convenient when temporarily transferring the client from the bed, such as during bed making. Lounge chairs tend to be more comfortable when a client is willing and able to sit for an extended period.

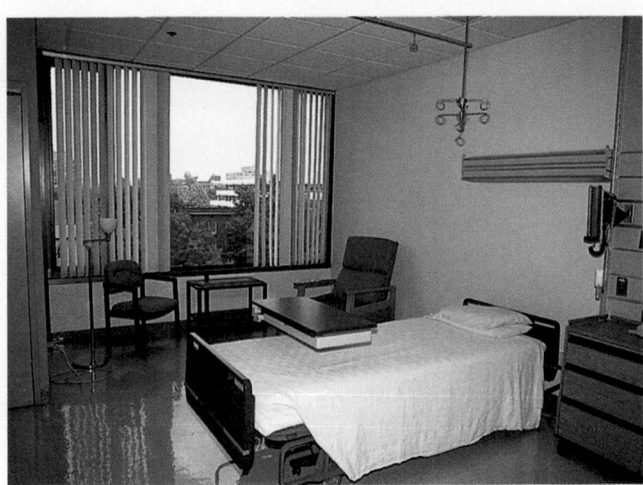

FIGURE **38-11** Typical hospital room.

Each room usually has an overbed light and a floor or table lamp. Moveable lights that extend over the bed from the wall should be positioned for easy reach but moved aside when not in use. Additional portable lighting is used to provide extra light during bedside procedures.

Other equipment usually found in a client's room includes a call light, a television set, a wall-mounted blood pressure gauge, oxygen and vacuum wall outlets, and personal care items. Special equipment designed for comfort or positioning clients includes footboards and foot boots (Figure 38-12), special mattresses (see Chapter 47), and bed boards. Whenever using comfort and positioning equipment, check agency policy and manufacturer's directions before application.

Beds. Seriously ill clients may remain in bed for a long time. Because a bed is the piece of equipment used most by a hospitalized client, it should be designed for comfort, safety, and adaptability for changing positions.

The typical hospital bed has a firm mattress on a metal frame that can be raised and lowered horizontally. More and more hospitals are converting the standard hospital bed to one in which the mattress surface can be electronically adjusted for client comfort. Different bed positions are used to promote client comfort, minimize symptoms, promote lung expansion, and to improve access during certain procedures (Table 38-6).

The position of a bed is usually changed by electrical controls incorporated into the client's call light and in a panel on the side or foot of the bed (Figure 38-13). It is important for the nurse to become familiar with use of the bed controls. Ease in raising and lowering a bed and in changing position of the head and foot eliminates undue musculoskeletal strain on the nurse. Nurses should instruct clients on the proper use of controls and caution them against raising the bed to a position that might cause harm.

Beds contain safety features such as locks on the wheels or casters. Wheels should be locked when the bed is stationary to prevent accidental movement. Side rails protect clients from accidental falls. The headboard can be removed from most beds. This is important when the

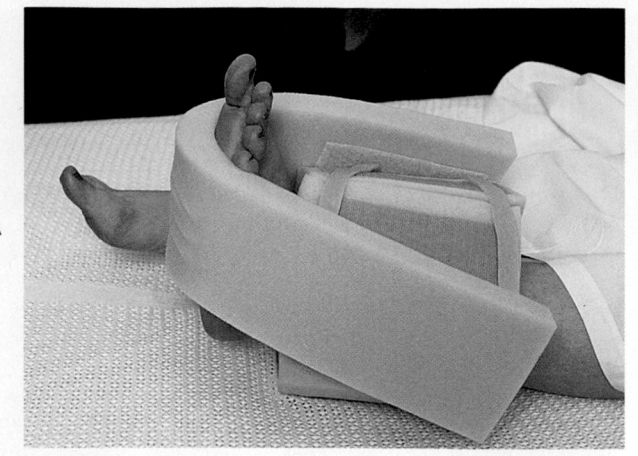 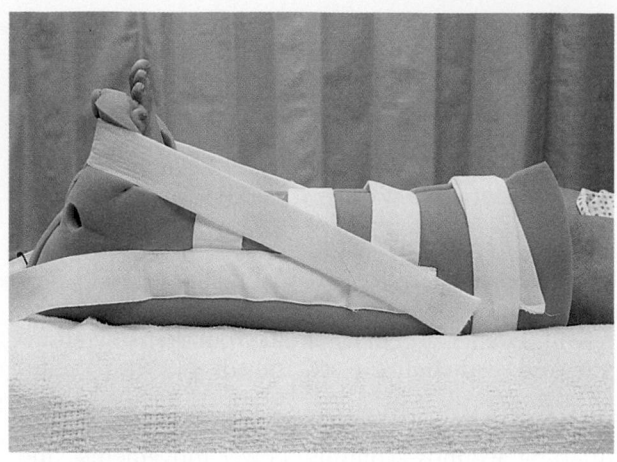

A   B

FIGURE **38–12**   **A,** Foot boot. **B,** Foot boot with lower leg extension.

Table **38-6**   **Common Bed Positions**

Position	Description	Uses
Fowler's	Head of bed raised to angle of 45 degrees or more; semisitting position; foot of bed may also be raised at knee	Is preferred while client eats Is used during nasogastric tube insertion and nasotracheal suction Promotes lung expansion
Semi-Fowler's	Head of bed raised approximately 30 degrees; inclination less than Fowler's position; foot of bed may also be raised at knee	Promotes lung expansion Used when clients receive gastric feedings to reduce regurgitation and risk of aspiration
Trendelenburg's	Entire bed frame tilted with head of bed down	Is used for postural drainage Facilitates venous return in clients with poor peripheral perfusion
Reverse Trendelenburg's	Entire bed frame tilted with foot of bed down	Is used infrequently Promotes gastric emptying Prevents esophageal reflux
Flat	Entire bed frame horizontally parallel with floor	Is used for clients with vertebral injuries and in cervical traction Is used for clients who are hypotensive Is generally preferred by clients for sleeping

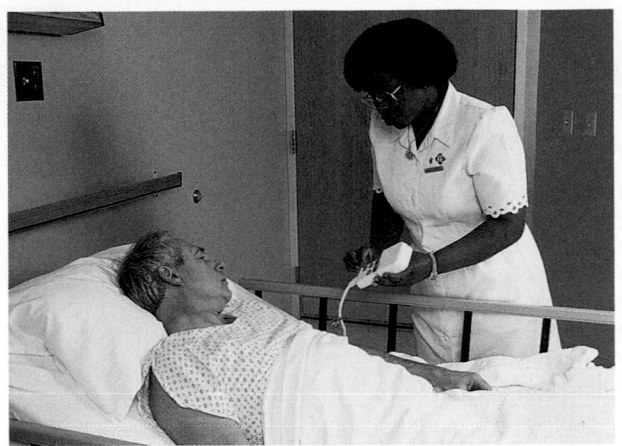

FIGURE **38–13** Nurse instructing client in use of call light and bed controls.

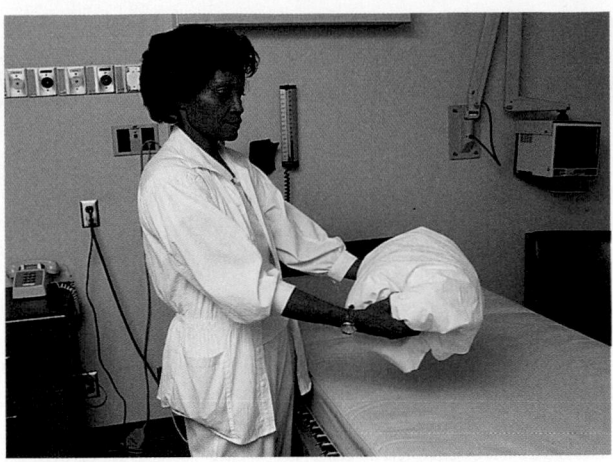

FIGURE **38–14** Holding linen away from the uniform prevents contact with microorganisms.

medical team must have easy access to the head, such as during cardiopulmonary resuscitation.

Bed Making. A client's bed should be kept clean and comfortable. This requires frequent inspections to be sure linen is clean, dry, and free of wrinkles. When clients are diaphoretic, have draining wounds, or are incontinent, the nurse should check frequently for soiled linen.

The nurse usually makes a bed in the morning after the client's bath or while the client is bathing in a shower, sitting in a chair eating, or out of the room for procedures or tests. Throughout the day the nurse straightens linen that becomes loose or wrinkled. The bed linen should also be checked for food particles after meals and for wetness or soiling. Linen that becomes soiled or wet should be changed.

When changing bed linen, the nurse follows principles of medical asepsis by keeping soiled linen away from the uniform (Figure 38-14). Soiled linen is placed in special linen bags before discarding in a hamper. To avoid air currents, which can spread microorganisms, the nurse never shakes the linen. To avoid transmitting infection, the nurse should not place soiled linen on the floor. If clean linen touches the floor, it is immediately discarded.

During bed making, the nurse uses proper body mechanics (see Chapter 36). The bed should always be raised to the appropriate height before changing linen so that the nurse does not have to bend or stretch over the mattress. The nurse also moves back and forth to opposite sides of the bed while applying new linen. Body mechanics is also important when turning or repositioning the client in bed.

When clients are confined to bed, the nurse organizes bed-making activities to conserve time and energy (Skill 38-6). The client's privacy, comfort, and safety are all important when making a bed. Using side rails to aid positioning and turning, keeping call lights within the client's reach, and maintaining the proper bed position help promote comfort and safety. After making a bed, the nurse always returns it to the lowest horizontal position to prevent accidental falls should the client get in and out of the bed alone.

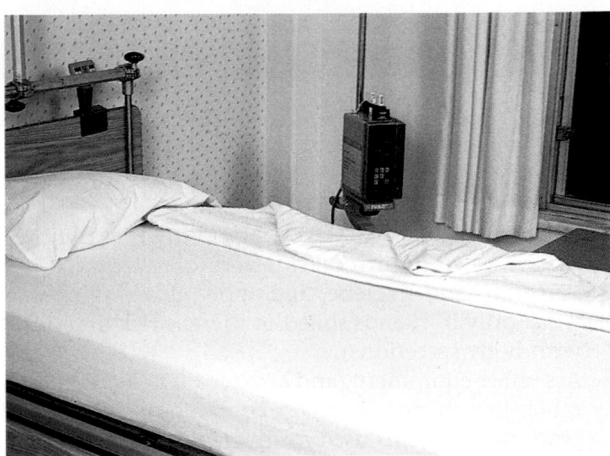

FIGURE **38–15** Surgical or recovery bed.

When possible the nurse should make the bed while it is unoccupied (Box 38-15). The nurse uses judgment in regard to when is the best time to have the client sit up in a chair while the bed is made. When making an unoccupied bed, the nurse follows the same basic principles as for occupied bed making.

An unoccupied bed can be open or closed. In an open bed, the top covers are folded back so that a client can easily get into bed. In a closed bed, the top sheet, blanket, and bedspread are drawn up to the head of the mattress and under the pillows. A closed bed is prepared in a hospital room before a new client is admitted to that room. A surgical, recovery, or postoperative bed is a modified version of the open bed. The top bed linen is arranged for easy transfer of the client from a stretcher to the bed. The top sheets and spread are not tucked or mitered at the corners. Instead, the top sheets are folded to one side or folded to the bottom third of the bed (Figure 38-15). This makes it easier to transfer the client into the bed.

Linens. In any health care agency, it is important to have an adequate supply of linen to care appropriately for

Text continued on p. 1061

Skill 38-6   *Making an Occupied Bed*

Delegation Considerations

The skill of making an occupied bed can be delegated to assistive personnel (AP).
- Before delegating this skill, review any precautions or activity restrictions for the client.
- Be sure assistive personnel know what to do if wound drainage, dressing material, drainage tubes, or IV tubing becomes dislodged or is found in the linens.
- Instruct the care provider in what to do if client becomes fatigued.

Equipment (Figure 38-16)

- Linen bag(s)
- Mattress pad (needs to be changed only when soiled)
- Bottom sheet (flat or fitted)
- Drawsheet
- Top sheet
- Blanket
- Bedspread
- Waterproof pads and/or bath blankets (optional)
- Pillowcases
- Bedside chair or table
- Disposable gloves (optional)
- Towel
- Disinfectant

Steps	Rationale
1. Assess potential for client incontinence or for excess drainage on bed linen.	Determines need for protective waterproof pads or extra bath blankets on bed.
2. Check chart for orders or specific precautions concerning movement and positioning.	Ensures client safety and use of proper body mechanics.
3. Explain procedure to the client, noting that the client will be asked to turn on side and roll over linen.	Minimizes anxiety and promotes cooperation.
4. Perform hand hygiene, and apply gloves (gloves are worn only if linen is soiled or there is risk for contact with body secretions).	Reduces transmission of microorganisms.
5. Assemble equipment, and arrange on bedside chair or table. Remove unnecessary equipment such as a dietary tray or items used for hygiene.	Assembling all equipment provides for smooth procedure and assists in increasing client's comfort. Placing linen on clean surface minimizes spread of infection.
6. Draw room curtain around bed or close door.	Maintains client's privacy.
7. Adjust bed height to comfortable working position. Lower any raised side rail on one side of bed. Remove call light.	Minimizes strain on back. It is easier to remove and apply linen evenly to bed in flat position. Provides easy access to bed and linen.
8. Loosen top linen at foot of bed.	Makes linen easier to remove.

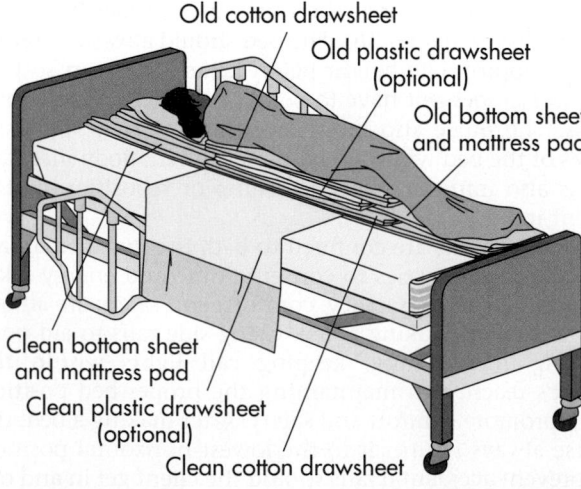

FIGURE **38–16**   Equipment for making occupied bed

Steps	Rationale
9. Remove bedspread and blanket separately. If spread and blanket are soiled, place them in linen bag. Keep soiled linen away from uniform.	Reduces transmission of microorganisms.
10. If blanket and spread are to be reused, fold them by bringing the top and bottom edges together. Fold farthest side over onto nearer bottom edge. Bring top and bottom edges together again. Place folded linen over back of chair.	Folding method facilitates replacement and minimizes wrinkles.
11. Cover client with bath blanket in the following manner: unfold bath blanket over top sheet. Ask client to hold top edge of bath blanket. If client is unable to help, tuck top of bath blanket under shoulder. Grasp top sheet under bath blanket at client's shoulders and bring sheet down to foot of bed. Remove sheet and discard in linen bag.	Bath blanket provides warmth and keeps body parts covered during linen removal.
12. With assistance from another nurse, slide mattress toward head of bed.	If mattress slides toward foot of bed when head of bed is raised, it is difficult to tuck in linen. In addition, it is uncomfortable for the client because the client's feet may be pressed against or hang over the foot of the bed.
13. Position client on the far side of the bed, turned onto side and facing away from you. Be sure side rail in front of client is up. Adjust pillow under client's head.	Turning client onto side provides space for placement of clean linen. Side rail ensures client's safety from forward falls from the bed surface and helps client in moving.
14. Loosen bottom linens, moving from head to foot. With seam side down (facing the mattress), fanfold bottom sheet and drawsheet toward client—first drawsheet, then bottom sheet. Tuck edges of linen just under buttocks, back, and shoulders. Do not fanfold mattress pad if it is to be reused (see illustration).	Prepares for removal of all bottom linen simultaneously. Provides maximum work space for placing clean linen. Later, when client turns to other side, soiled linen can be removed easily.
15. Wipe off any moisture on exposed mattress with towel and appropriate disinfectant.	Reduces transmission of microorganisms.
16. Apply clean linen to exposed half of bed: a. Place clean mattress pad on bed by folding it lengthwise with center crease in middle of bed. Fanfold top layer over mattress. (If pad is reused, simply smooth out any wrinkles.)	Applying linen over bed in successive layers minimizes energy and time used in bed making.
b. Unfold bottom sheet lengthwise so that center crease is situated lengthwise along center of bed. Fanfold sheet's top layer toward center of bed alongside the client. Smooth bottom layer of sheet over mattress, and bring edge over closest side of mattress. Pull fitted sheet smoothly over mattress ends. Allow edge of flat unfitted sheet to hang about 25 cm (10 in) over mattress edge. Lower hem of bottom flat sheet should lie seam down and even with bottom edge of mattress (see illustration).	Proper positioning of linen on one side ensures that adequate linen will be available to cover opposite side of bed. Keeping seam edges down eliminates irritation to client's skin.

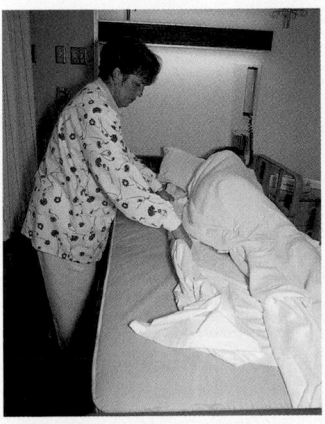

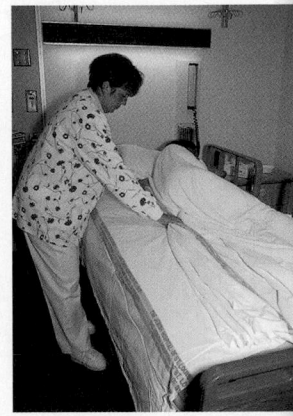

STEP **14**   Old linen tucked under client.

STEP **16b**   Clean linen applied to bed.

Skill 38-6   *Making an Occupied Bed—cont'd*

Steps	Rationale
17. Miter bottom flat sheet at head of bed:	
a. Face head of bed diagonally. Place hand away from head of bed under top corner of mattress, near mattress edge, and lift.	Ensures secure flat sheet will not loosen easily.
b. With other hand, tuck top edge of bottom sheet smoothly under mattress so that side edges of sheet above and below mattress would meet if brought together.	
c. Face side of bed and pick up top edge of sheet at approximately 45 cm (18 in) from top of mattress (see illustration).	
d. Lift sheet, and lay it on top of mattress to form a neat triangular fold, with lower base of triangle even with mattress side edge (see illustration).	
e. Tuck lower edge of sheet, which is hanging free below the mattress, under mattress. Tuck with palms down, without pulling triangular fold (see illustration).	
f. Hold portion of sheet covering side of mattress in place with one hand. With the other hand, pick up top of triangular linen fold and bring it down over side of mattress (see illustrations). Tuck this portion under mattress (see illustration).	Mitered corner cannot be loosened easily even if client moves frequently in bed.
18. Tuck remaining portion of sheet under mattress, moving toward foot of bed. Keep linen smooth.	Folds of linen are source of irritation.
19. *(Optional)* Open drawsheet so that it unfolds in half. Lay centerfold along middle of bed lengthwise, and position sheet so that it will be under the client's buttocks and torso (see illustration). Fanfold top layer toward client, with edge along client's back. Smooth bottom layer out over mattress, and tuck excess edge under mattress (keep palms down).	Drawsheet is used to lift and reposition client. Placement under client's torso distributes most of client's body weight over sheet.
20. Place waterproof pad over drawsheet, with centerfold against client's side. Fanfold top layer toward client.	Protects bed linen from being soiled.

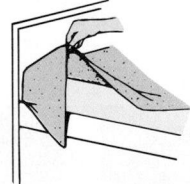

STEP **17c**   Top edge of sheet picked up.

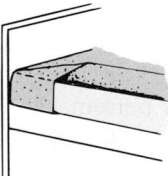

STEP **17e**   Lower edge of sheet tucked under mattress.

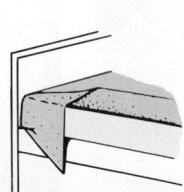

STEP **17d**   Sheet on top of mattress in a triangular fold.

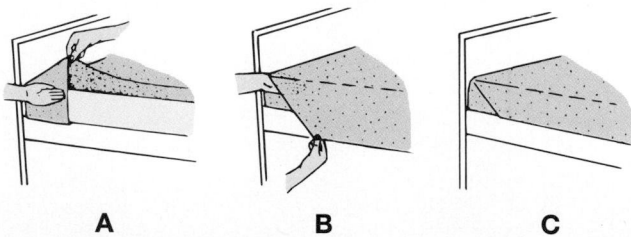

A   **B**   **C**

STEP **17f**   **A** and **B,** Triangular fold placed over side of mattress. **C,** Linen tucked under mattress.

Steps	Rationale

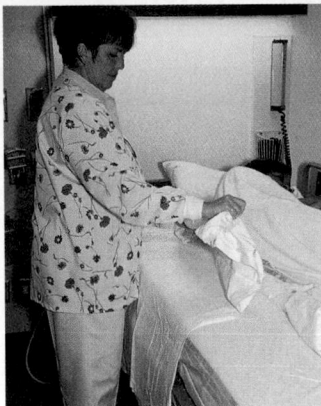

STEP **19**   Optional draw sheet.

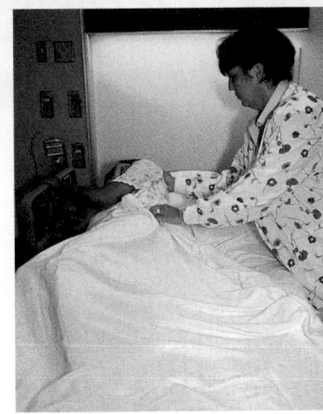

STEP **22**   Assisting client to roll over folds of linen.

Steps	Rationale
21. Have client roll slowly toward you, over the layers of linen. Raise side rail on working side, and go to other side of bed.	Positions client for removal and placement of linens. Maintains client's safety and body alignment during turning.
22. Lower side rail. Assist client in positioning on other side, over folds of linen. Loosen edges of soiled linen from under mattress (see illustration).	Exposes opposite side of bed for removal of soiled linen and placement of clean linen. Makes linen easier to remove.
23. Remove soiled linen by folding it into a bundle or square, with soiled side turned in. Discard in linen bag. If necessary, wipe mattress with antiseptic solution, and dry mattress surface before applying new linen.	Reduces transmission of microorganisms.
24. Pull clean, fanfold linen smoothly over edge of mattress from head to foot of bed.	Smooth linen will not irritate client's skin.
25. Assist client in rolling back into supine position. Reposition pillow.	Maintains client's comfort.
26. Pull fitted sheet smoothly over mattress ends. Miter top corner of bottom sheet (see step 17). When tucking corner, be sure that sheet is smooth and free of wrinkles.	Wrinkles and folds can cause irritation to skin.
27. Facing side of bed, grasp remaining edge of bottom flat sheet. Lean back; keep back straight; and pull while tucking excess linen under mattress. Proceed from head to foot of bed. (Avoid lifting mattress during tucking to ensure fit.)	Proper use of body mechanics while tucking linen prevents injury.
28. Smooth fanfolded drawsheet out over bottom sheet. Grasp edge of sheet with palms down; lean back; and tuck sheet under mattress. Tuck from middle to top and then to bottom.	Tucking first at top or bottom may pull sheet sideways, causing poor fit.
29. Place top sheet over client with centerfold lengthwise down middle of bed. Open sheet from head to foot, and unfold over client.	Sheet should be equally distributed over bed by correctly positioning centerfold.
30. Ask client to hold clean top sheet, or tuck sheet around client's shoulders. Remove bath blanket and discard in linen bag.	Sheet prevents exposure of body parts. Having client hold sheet encourages client participation in care.
31. Place blanket on bed, unfolding it so that crease runs lengthwise along middle of bed. Unfold blanket to cover client. Top edge should be parallel with edge of top sheet and 15 to 20 cm (6 to 8 in) from top sheet's edge.	Blanket should be placed to cover client completely and provide adequate warmth.
32. Place spread over bed according to step 31. Be sure that top edge of spread extends about 2.5 cm (1 in) above blanket's edge. Tuck top edge of spread over and under top edge of blanket.	Gives bed neat appearance and provides extra warmth.

Skill 38-6   *Making an Occupied Bed—cont'd*

Steps   **Rationale**

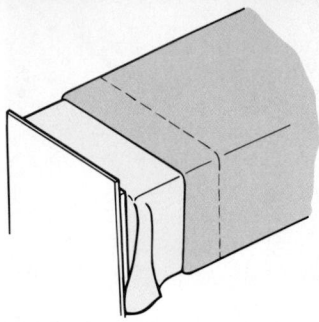

STEP **34**   Optional toe pleat.

33. Make cuff by turning edge of top sheet down over top edge of blanket and spread.

Protect client's face from rubbing against blanket or spread.

34. Standing on one side at foot of bed, lift mattress corner slightly with one hand and tuck linens under mattress. Top sheet and blanket are tucked under together. Be sure that linens are loose enough to allow movement of client's feet. Making a horizontal toe pleat is an option (see illustration).

Makes neat-appearing bed. Pressure ulcers can develop on client's toes and heels from feet rubbing against tight-fitting bed sheets.

35. Make modified mitered corner with top sheet, blanket, and spread (see illustration in Box 38-15, p. 1062):
    a. Pick up side edge of top sheet, blanket, and spread approximately 45 cm (18 in) from foot of mattress. Lift linen to form triangular fold, and lay it on bed.
    b. Tuck lower edge of sheet, which is hanging free below mattress, under mattress. Do not pull triangular fold.
    c. Pick up triangular fold, and bring it down over mattress while holding linen in place along side of mattress. Do not tuck tip of triangle.

Ensures top covers will not loosen easily.

Secures top linen but keeps even edge of blanket and top sheet draped over mattress.

36. Raise side rail. Make other side of bed; spread sheet, blanket, and bedspread out evenly. Fold top edge of spread over blanket and make cuff with top sheet (see step 33); make modified mitered corner at foot of bed (see step 35).

Side rail protects client from accidental falls.

37. Change pillowcase:
    a. Have client raise head. While supporting neck with one hand, remove pillow. Allow client to lower head.
    b. Remove soiled case by grasping pillow at open end with one hand and pulling case back over pillow with the other hand. Discard case in linen bag.
    c. Grasp clean pillowcase at center of closed end. Gather case, turning it inside out over the hand holding it. With the same hand, pick up middle of one end of the pillow. Pull pillowcase down over pillow with the other hand.
    d. Be sure pillow corners fit evenly into corners of pillowcase. Place pillow under client's head.

Support of neck muscles prevents injury during flexion and extension of neck.

Pillows slide out easily, thus minimizing contact with soiled linen.

Eases sliding of pillowcase over pillow.

Poorly fitting case constricts fluffing and expansion of pillow and interferes with client comfort.

38. Place call light within client's reach, and return bed to comfortable position.

Ensures client safety and comfort.

Steps	Rationale
39. Open room curtains, and rearrange furniture. Place personal items within easy reach on over-bed table or bedside stand. Return bed to a comfortable height.	Promotes sense of well-being.
40. Discard dirty linen in hamper or chute and perform hand hygiene.	Prevents transmission of microorganisms.
41. Ask if client feels comfortable.	Ensures bed linens are clean and smooth.
42. Inspect skin for areas of irritation.	Folds in linen can cause pressure on skin.
43. Observe client for signs of fatigue, dyspnea, pain, or discomfort.	Provides you with data about client's level of activity tolerance and ability to participate in other procedures.

Unexpected Outcomes and Related Interventions

1. Client feels discomfort from linen fold.
   a. Tighten sheets.
   b. Change client's position frequently.
2. Client's skin shows signs of breakdown.
   a. Institute skin care measures to reduce risk of pressure ulcer (see Chapter 34).
   b. Change client's position frequently.

Recording and Reporting

• Making an occupied bed need not be recorded.

---

clients. Many agencies have what are called "nurse servers" either within or just outside a client's room where a daily supply of linen is stored. Because of the importance of cost control in health care, it is important to not bring excess linen into a client's room. Once the linen is brought into a client's room, if unused, it must be discarded for laundering. This can increase an agency's costs. Excess linen lying around a client's room creates clutter and obstacles for client care activities.

Before bed making, it is important to collect necessary bed linens and the client's personal items. In this way the nurse will have all equipment accessible to prepare the bed and room. Linens are pressed and folded to prevent the spread of microorganisms and to make bed making easier. When fitted sheets are not available, flat sheets usually are pressed with a center crease to be placed down the center of the bed. The linens unfold easily to the sides, with creases often fitting over the mattress edge. A complete linen change is not always necessary. The nurse may reuse the mattress pad, sheet, blanket, and bedspread for the same client if they are not wet or soiled.

Disposal of linen must be done to minimize the spread of infection (see Chapter 33). Agency policies provide guidelines for the proper way to bag and dispose of soiled linen. After a client is discharged, all bed linen is sent to the laundry, the mattress and bed are cleansed by housekeeping staff, and new bed linen is applied.

Evaluation

Client Care. Evaluation of hygiene measures occurs both during and after each particular skill. For example, as the nurse bathes a client, close inspection of the skin reveals if drainage or other soiling is effectively removed from the skin's surface. Once the bath is completed the nurse will ask if the client's comfort and relaxation have improved. When evaluating for the effectiveness of hygiene measures, the nurse observes for changes in the client's behavior. Does the client assume a more relaxed position? Is the client free of body odor? Is the client able to fall asleep? Does the client's facial expression convey a sense of comfort?

Frequently it takes time for hygienic care to result in an improvement in the client's condition. The presence of oral lesions, a scalp infestation, or skin excoriation will often require repeated measures and a combination of nursing interventions. The nurse will evaluate for improvement in the client's condition over time and determine if existing therapies are effective.

Throughout evaluation the nurse considers the goals of care and evaluates whether expected outcomes are achieved. A critical thinking approach ensures that the nurse considers all factors when evaluating the client's care (Figure 38-17). The nurse's knowledge base and experience provide important perspectives when the nurse analyzes observations made about a client. For example, if the nurse has seen how dehydration of the oral mucosa clears with repeated hygiene, this helps in recognizing when another client's progress is slow. The standards for evaluation are the expected outcomes established in the planning stage of the client's care. If outcomes are not met, the care plan may need to be revised. The nurse continues to apply critical thinking attitudes when considering all evaluation findings.

Client Expectations. The final portion of the evaluation considers whether or not the client's expectations

Box 38-15 *Procedural Guidelines*

Making an Unoccupied Bed

Equipment: Linen bag, mattress pad (change only when soiled), bottom sheet (flat or fitted), drawsheet (optional), top sheet, blanket, bedspread, waterproof pads (optional), pillowcases, bedside chair or table, disposable gloves (if linen is soiled), washcloth, and antiseptic cleanser.

Delegation Considerations: The skill of making an unoccupied bed can be delegated to assistive personnel.

1. Determine if client has been incontinent or if excess drainage is on linen. Gloves will be necessary.
2. Assess activity orders or restrictions in mobility in planning if client can get out of bed for procedure. Assist to bedside chair or recliner.
3. Lower side rails on both sides of bed and raise bed to comfortable working position.
4. Remove soiled linen and place in laundry bag. Avoid shaking or fanning linen.
5. Reposition mattress and wipe off any moisture using a washcloth moistened in antiseptic solution. Dry thoroughly.
6. Apply all bottom linen on one side of bed before moving to opposite side.
7. Be sure fitted sheet is placed smoothly over mattress. To apply a flat unfitted sheet, allow about 25 cm (10 in) to hang over mattress edge. Lower hem of sheet should lie seam down, even with bottom edge of mattress. Pull remaining top portion of sheet over top edge of mattress.
8. While standing at head of bed, miter top corner of bottom sheet (see Skill 38-6, step 20).
9. Tuck remaining portion of unfitted sheet under mattress.
10. *Optional:* Apply drawsheet, laying center fold along middle of bed lengthwise. Smooth drawsheet over mattress and tuck excess edge under mattress, keeping palms down.
11. Move to opposite side of bed and spread bottom sheet smoothly over edge of mattress from head to foot of bed.
12. Apply fitted sheet smoothly over each mattress corner. For an unfitted sheet, miter top corner of bottom sheet (see step 8) making sure corner is taut.
13. Grasp remaining edge of unfitted bottom sheet and tuck tightly under mattress while moving from head to foot of bed. Smooth folded drawsheet over

bottom sheet and tuck under mattress, first at middle, then at top, and then at bottom.

14. If needed, apply waterproof pad over bottom sheet or drawsheet.
15. Place top sheet over bed with vertical center fold lengthwise down middle of bed. Open sheet out from head to foot, being sure top edge of sheet is even with top edge of mattress.
16. Make horizontal toe pleat: stand at foot of bed and fanfold in sheet 5 to 10 cm (2 to 4 in) across bed. Pull sheet up from bottom to make fold approximately 15 cm (6 in) from bottom edge of mattress (see Skill 38-6, step 38).
17. Tuck in remaining portion of sheet under foot of mattress. Then place blanket over bed with top edge parallel to top edge of sheet and 15 to 20 cm (6 to 8 in) down from edge of sheet. (*Optional:* Apply additional spread over bed.)
18. Make cuff by turning edge of top sheet down over top edge of blanket and spread.
19. Standing on one side at foot of bed, lift mattress corner slightly with one hand, and with other hand tuck top sheet, blanket, and spread under mattress. Be sure toe pleats are not pulled out.
20. Make modified mitered corner with top sheet, blanket, and spread. After triangular fold is made, do not tuck tip of triangle (see illustration).
21. Go to other side of bed. Spread sheet, blanket, and spread out evenly. Make cuff with top sheet and blanket. Make modified corner at foot of bed.
22. Apply clean pillowcase.
23. Place call light within client's reach on bed rail or pillow and return bed to height allowing for client transfer. Assist client to bed.
24. Arrange client's room. Remove and discard supplies. Perform hand hygiene.

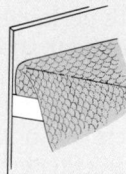

STEP **20** Modified mitered corner.

---

were met through hygienic care. The nurse might ask: Do you feel your bath and back rub helped to make you comfortable? Are there ways you feel we can do a better job with your foot care? What further measures do you think are necessary to keep your mouth clean and refreshed?

The client's expectations are important guidelines in determining client satisfaction. The nurse must feel comfortable in addressing the client's concerns and expectations. A caring approach can help in facilitating discussion of these issues.

Key Concepts

- The nurse determines a client's ability to perform self-care and provides hygienic care according to the client's needs and preferences.
- During hygiene, the nurse integrates other activities such as physical assessment, wound care, and range-of-motion exercises.

KNOWLEDGE

- Characteristics of intact and healthy skin, mucosa, nails, hair, and sense organs
- Recognition that time is necessary for integument and other structures to heal

EXPERIENCE

- Prior experience evaluating client responses to hygiene care

Evaluation

- Reassess condition of the client's integument, nails, oral cavity, and sense organs
- Determine if the client's comfort level improves
- Ask the client to demonstrate hygiene self-care skills
- Ask the client if expectations are being met

STANDARDS

- Use established expected outcomes to evaluate the client's response to care (e.g., improved skin integrity, hydration of mucosa) as standards for evaluation
- Measure all characteristics such as size of lesions, degree of edema with accuracy and preciseness

ATTITUDES

- Act with discipline; be very thorough in examining the condition of the client's tissues for improvement

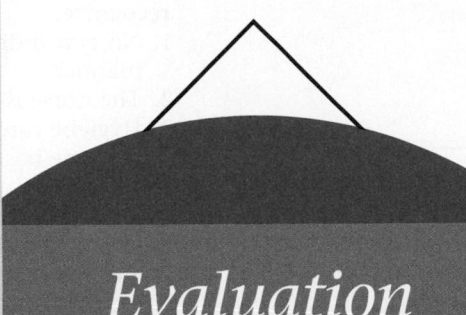
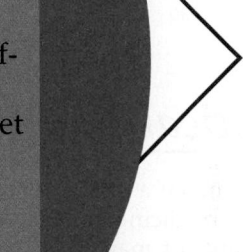
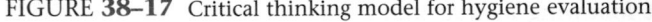

FIGURE 38–17 Critical thinking model for hygiene evaluation.

- While providing daily hygiene needs, the nurse uses teaching and communication skills in developing a caring relationship with the client.
- Various personal, sociocultural, economic, and developmental factors influence clients' hygiene practices.
- Clients' health beliefs predict the likelihood of assuming health promotion behavior, such as the maintenance of good hygiene.
- The nurse may not assess all body regions before administering hygiene; however, the nurse does routinely assess the client's condition whenever care is given.
- Clients with reduced sensation, vascular insufficiency, and immobility are at greater risk for impaired skin integrity.

- The nurse assesses a client's physical and cognitive ability to perform basic hygiene measures, including muscle strength, flexibility and dexterity, balance, coordination, activity tolerance, and ability to attend.
- For clients suffering symptoms such as pain or nausea, administering symptom relief therapies before hygiene will better prepare the client for any procedure.
- Clients with diabetes mellitus require special nail and foot care.
- When administering oral care to unconscious clients, the nurse takes measures to prevent aspiration.
- The client's room should be comfortable, safe, and large enough to allow the client and visitors to move about freely.

- Evaluation of hygiene care is based on the client's sense of comfort, relaxation, well-being, and understanding of hygiene techniques.

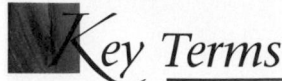ey Terms

Acne, *p. 1013*	Enucleation, *p. 1051*
Alopecia, *p. 1010*	Epidermis, *p. 1003*
Apocrine, *p. 1013*	Gingivitis, *p. 1004*
Buccal glands, *p. 1004*	Halitosis, *p. 1008*
Caries, *p. 1013*	Lunula, *p. 1004*
Cerumen, *p. 1010*	Mastication, *p. 1004*
Complete bed bath, *p. 1022*	Neuropathy, *p. 1008*
Cuticle, *p. 1004*	Ophthalmologist, *p. 1050*
Dermis, *p. 1003*	Optometrist, *p. 1050*
Eccrine, *p. 1013*	Partial bed bath, *p. 1022*
Edentulous, *p. 1013*	Perineal care, *p. 1030*
Effleurage, *p. 1030*	Stomatitis, *p. 1043*

Critical Thinking Exercises

1. Mrs. Truman is a 62-year-old woman being seen in the internal medicine clinic during her follow-up appointment for management of her diabetes mellitus. During the nurse's conversation with Mrs. Truman, the client says, "You know, last week I found a sore on my left foot; I didn't even know it was there." What type of assessment should the nurse conduct for Mrs. Truman, and what recommendations are needed for Mrs. Truman's foot care regimen?

2. Mr. Golf suffered abdominal trauma in a motorcycle accident. Abdominal surgery resulted in an ileostomy, which is leaking liquid fecal material on his skin. In addition, his has a postoperative infection, is diaphoretic and has a high fever, and has a nasogastric tube in place. What factors must you consider when providing hygiene care? Include rationales for assessments and interventions.

3. Peter Nixon is an 18-year-old admitted to the neurosurgical intensive care unit following a head injury. Peter is currently unconscious, responsive only to painful stimulus. What assessment is critical for the nurse to perform before providing oral hygiene?

Review Questions

1. Hygienic care requires close contact with the client; the nurse initially uses which of the following to promote a caring therapeutic relationship.
   1. Communication skills.
   2. Therapeutic touch.
   3. Assessment skills.
   4. Fundamental skills.

2. A client's personal preferences for hygiene are influenced by a number of factors. The nurse must recognize:
   1. No two individuals perform hygiene in the same manner.
   2. The nurse is in charge of the care.
   3. Hygiene care is a routine procedure.
   4. Hygiene has no influence on client outcomes.

3. A person's body image is which of these concepts of his or her physical appearance:
   1. Subjective.
   2. Objective.
   3. Social
   4. Developmental.

4. The *Healthy People 2010* initiative included recommendations to improve:
   1. American diet adding more carbohydrates.
   2. Dental health.
   3. Medication management in the elderly.
   4. Skin care in the elderly.

5. Clients most in need of perineal care are those at greatest risk of:
   1. Acquiring an infection.
   2. Death.
   3. Needing to be institutionalized.
   4. Falling.

6. In addition to bathing, the following intervention may best promote client comfort:
   1. Back rub.
   2. Books on tape.
   3. Snacks.
   4. Postural drainage.

7. Clients will experience conditions that threaten the integrity of oral mucosa; therefore:
   1. Less oral hygiene is needed.
   2. More frequent mouth care is needed.
   3. No mouth care should be performed.
   4. No antiinfective agents should be used.

8. The priority when providing oral hygiene to an unconscious client is to:
   1. Prevent aspiration.
   2. Prevent mouth odor.
   3. Prevent dental caries.
   4. Prevent mouth ulcerations.

9. Depending on the client's age and physical condition, the room temperature should be maintained between:
   1. 68° and 74° F.
   2. 75° and 77° F.
   3. 78° and 80° F.
   4. 65° and 70° F.

10. The method for trimming nails is to:
1. Cut the nail in a curve.
2. File the nail straight across.
3. Call a foot specialist.
4. Cut the nails to the cuticles.

References

Agency for Health Care Policy and Research: *Pressure ulcers in adults: prediction and prevention,* Pub Nos. 92-0047, 92-0050, Rockville, Md, 1992, U.S. Department of Health and Human Services, Public Health Service.

American Diabetes Association: Position statement on preventive foot care in people with diabetes: clinical practice recommendations 1999, *Diabetes Care* 22(suppl 1), 1999.

Bennet MA: Report of the Task Force on the Implications for Darkly Pigmented Intact Skin in the Prediction and Prevention of Pressure Ulcers, *Adv Wound Care* 8(6):34, 1995.

Bryant JL, Beinlich NR: Foot care: focus on the elderly, *Orthoped Nurs* 18(6): 53-60.

Bush BC, Donley TG: A model for dental hygiene education concerning the relationship between periodontal health and systemic health, *Education for Health* 15(1):19, 2002.

Champion VL: Instrument development for health belief model constructs, *Adv Nurs Sci* 6(3):73, 1984.

Cohen E, Krachmer J: Red eyes and contact lenses, *Patient Care* 26(9):143, 1992.

Dochterman JM, Bulecheck GM: *Nursing interventions classification (NIC),* ed 4, St. Louis, 2004, Mosby.

Ebersole P, Hess P: *Toward healthy aging,* ed 5, St. Louis, 2000, Mosby.

Eliopoulos C: *Gerontologic nursing,* ed 5, Philadelphia, 2001, Lippincott Williams & Wilkins.

Felder R and others: Dexterity testing as a prediction of oral care ability, *J Am Geriatr* 42(10):1081, 1994.

Fulton JS, Middleton GJ, McPhail JT: Management of oral complications, *Semin Oncol Nurs* 18:28, 2002.

Gaskin FC: Detection of cyanosis in the person with dark skin, *J Black Nurs Assoc* 1:52, 1986.

Green MF, Aliabaide Z, Green BT: Diabetic foot: evaluation and management, *South Med J* 95(1):95, 2002.

Henderson CT and others: Draft definition of stage I pressure ulcers: inclusion of persons with darkly pigmented skin, *Adv Wound Care* 10(5):16, 1997.

Johnson & Johnson Vision Products: *Your guide to healthy contact lens wear,* New Brunswick, NJ, 1994, Johnson & Johnson.

Labyak SE, Metzger BL: The effects of effleurage backrub on the physiological components of relaxation: a meta-analysis, *Nurs Res* 46:59, 1997.

Lewis SL and others: *Medical surgical nursing: assessment and management of clinical problems,* ed 5, St. Louis, 2000, Mosby.

Lueckenotte AG: *Gerontologic nursing,* ed 2, St. Louis, 2000, Mosby.

Moorhead S, Johnson M, Maas M: *Nursing outcomes classification (NOC),* ed 3, St. Louis, 2004, Mosby.

National Institute on Deafness and Other Communication Disorders (NIDCD): *Hearing aids,* Pub No. 99-4340, Bethesda, Md, 2001, National Institutes of Health, www.nidcd.nih.gov/health/hearing/hearingaid.asp.

Poland JM: Comparing Moi-Stin to lemon glycerin swabs, *Am J Nurs* 87:422, 1987.

Research update: oral care prevents pneumonia in nursing homes, *Aust Nurs J* 9(11):18, 2002.

Skewes SM: No more bed baths! *RN* 57:34, 1994.

Verderber A, Gallagher KJ: Effects of bathing, passive range-of-motion exercises, and turning on oxygen consumption in health men and women, *Am J Crit Care* 3:374, 1994.

Walton JC, Miller J, Tordecilla: Elder oral assessment and care, *ORL Head Neck Nurs* 202:12, 2002.

Wong DL: *Wong and Whaley's clinical manual of pediatric nursing,* ed 5, St. Louis, 1999, Mosby.

Zurlinden J: Drug news: new warnings for Lindane Shampoo and Lotion, *Nursing Spectrum—Midwestern Edition* 40(6):10, 2003.

Research References

Bauroth K and others: The efficacy of an essential oil antiseptic mouthwash vs. dental flossing in controlling interproximal gingivitis: a comparative study, *J Am Dental Assoc* 134(3):359-365, 2003.

Boyer L: News from NNGF: home care nurse's thoughts on dry skin and foot care in the older person, *World Council of Enterostomal Therapists Journal* 21(1):9, 2001. Bryant J L, Beinlich NR: Foot care: focus on the elderly, *Orthop Nurs* 18(6):53, 1999.

Gadbury-Amyot CC and others: Prioritization of the National Dental Hygiene Research Agenda, *J Dent Hyg* 76(2):157, 2002.

Hall GR, Buckwalter KC: Evidence-based protocol bathing persons with dementia. In Titler MG, series editor: Series on evidence-based practice for older adults, Iowa City, Ia, 1995, The University of Iowa Gerontological Nursing Interventions Research Center, Research Dissemination Core, revised 2001.

Handy M: A pilot study of the diagnosis and treatment of impaired skin integrity: dry skin in older persons. *Nurs Diagn* 1(2):57-63, 1996.

Hornick B: Diet and nutrition implications for oral health, *J Dent Hyg* 76(1):67, 2002.

Neil JA: Assessing foot care knowledge in a rural population with diabetes, *Ostomy Wound Manage* 48(1):50, 2002.

Pinzur MS, Slovenkai MP, Trepman E: Guidelines for diabetic foot care, The Diabetes Committee of the American Orthopaedic Foot and Ankle Society, *Foot Ankle Int* 20:695, 1999.

Ring T: Trends in dental hygiene education, *Access* 16(7):16, 2002.

Strauss MB, Hart JD, Winant DM: Preventive foot care: a user-friendly system for patients and physicians, *Postgrad Med* 103(5):233, 1998.

Oxygenation

Media Resources

 CD COMPANION

- Review Questions
- Glossary

evolve WEBSITE

- Review Questions
- Student Learning Activities
- Animations
- Concept Map Exercise
- Critical Thinking Exercise
- Video Clips
- Glossary

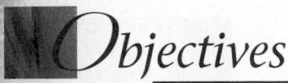

Objectives

Mastery of content in this chapter will enable the student to:

- Define the key terms listed.

- Describe the structure and function of the cardiopulmonary system.

- Identify the physiological processes of cardiac output, myocardial blood flow, and coronary artery circulation.

- Diagram the electrical conduction system of the heart.

- Describe the relationship of cardiac output, preload, afterload, contractility, and heart rate.

- Identify the physiological processes involved in ventilation, perfusion, and exchange of respiratory gases.

- Describe the neural and chemical regulation of respiration.

- Describe the impact of a client's level of health, age, lifestyle, and environment on tissue oxygenation.

- Identify and describe clinical outcomes as a result of disturbances in conduction, altered cardiac output, impaired valvular function, myocardial ischemia, and impaired tissue perfusion.

- Identify and describe clinical outcomes of hyperventilation, hypoventilation, and hypoxemia.

- Identify nursing care interventions in the primary care, acute care, and restorative and continuing care settings that promote oxygenation.

Scientific Knowledge Base

Oxygen is required to sustain life. The cardiac and respiratory systems function to supply the body's oxygen demands. Blood is oxygenated through the mechanisms of ventilation, perfusion, and transport of respiratory gases. Neural and chemical regulators control the rate and depth of respiration in response to changing tissue oxygen demands.

Cardiovascular Physiology

Cardiopulmonary physiology involves delivery of deoxygenated blood, (blood high in carbon dioxide and low in oxygen), to the right side of the heart and to the pulmonary circulation and oxygenated blood from the lungs to the left side of the heart and the tissues. The cardiac system delivers oxygen, nutrients, and other substances to the tissues and removes the waste products of cellular metabolism through the cardiac pump, the circulatory vascular system, and the integration of other systems (e.g., respiratory, digestive, and renal) (McCance and Huether, 2001).

Structure and Function. The right ventricle pumps blood through the pulmonary circulation. The left ventricle pumps blood to the systemic circulation

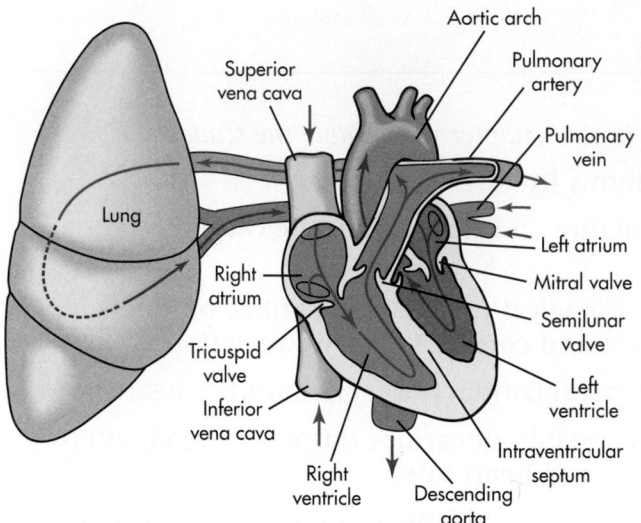

FIGURE **39–1** Schematic representation of blood flow through the heart. Arrows indicate direction of flow. (From Lewis SM and others: *Medical-surgical nursing: assessment and management of clinical problems,* ed 5, St. Louis, 2000, Mosby.)

Box 39-1   **Coronary Arteries**

Right Coronary Artery

Right Atrium, Anterior Right Ventricle
Supplies
- Posterior aspect of septum (90% of population)
- Posterior papillary muscle
- Sinus and atrioventricular nodes (80% to 90% of population)
- Inferior aspect of left ventricle

Left Coronary Arteries

Left Anterior Descending (LAD) Artery
Supplies
- Anterior left ventricular wall
- Anterior interventricular septum (septal branches supply conduction system, bundle of His, and bundle branches)
- Anterior papillary muscle
- Left ventricular apex

Circumflex Artery

Supplies
- Left atrium
- Posterior surfaces of left ventricle
- Posterior aspects of septum

(Figure 39-1). The circulatory system exchanges respiratory gases, nutrients, and waste products between the blood and the tissues.

Myocardial Pump. The pumping action of the heart is essential to maintaining oxygen delivery. Coronary artery disease (CAD) and cardiomyopathic (enlarged heart) conditions result in a diminished stroke volume—the volume of blood ejected from the ventricles, and decreased pump effectiveness. Hemorrhage and dehydration decrease pump effectiveness by decreasing the amount of blood ejected from the ventricles thereby reducing circulating blood volume. The four chambers of the heart fill with blood during diastole and empty during systole.

The myocardial fibers have contractile properties that enable them to stretch during filling. In a healthy heart this stretch is proportionally related to the strength of contraction. As the myocardium stretches, the strength of the subsequent contraction increases; this is known as the Frank-Starling (Starling's) law of the heart. In the diseased heart, Starling's law does not apply because the stretch of the myocardium is beyond the heart's physiological limits. The subsequent contractile response results in insufficient ventricular ejection (volume), and blood begins to "back up" in the pulmonary (left heart failure) or systemic circulation (right heart failure).

Myocardial Blood Flow. To maintain adequate blood flow to the pulmonary and systemic circulation, myocardial blood flow must supply sufficient oxygen and nutrients to the myocardium itself. Blood flow through the heart is unidirectional. There are four heart valves that ensure this forward blood flow (see Figure 39-1). During ventricular diastole the atrioventricular (mitral and tricuspid) valves open and blood flows from the higher-pressure atria into the relaxed ventricles. This represents

S_1, or the first heart sound. After ventricular filling, the systolic phase begins.

During the systolic phase semilunar (aortic and pulmonic) valves open and blood flows from the ventricles into the aorta and pulmonary artery. Closure of aortic and pulmonic valves represents S_2, or the second heart sound. Clients with valvular disease may have backflow or regurgitation of blood through the incompetent valve, causing a murmur that is heard on auscultation (see Chapter 32).

Coronary Artery Circulation. Blood in the atria and ventricles does not supply oxygen and nutrients to the myocardium itself. The coronary circulation is the branch of the systemic circulation that supplies the myocardium with oxygen and nutrients and removes waste. The coronary arteries fill during ventricular diastole (McCance and Huether, 2001). The right and left coronary arteries arise from the aorta just above and behind the aortic valve through openings called the coronary ostia (coronary openings). The left coronary artery, the most abundant blood supply, feeds the left ventricular myocardium, which is more muscular and does most of the heart's work (Box 39-1).

Systemic Circulation. The arteries and veins of the systemic circulation deliver nutrients and oxygen to and remove waste from the tissues. Oxygenated blood flows from the left ventricle by way of the aorta and into large systemic arteries. These arteries branch into smaller arteries, into arterioles, and finally into the smallest vessels, the capillaries. At the capillary level the exchange of respiratory gases, nutrients, and wastes occurs, and the tissues are oxygenated. The waste products exit the capillary network by way of the venules that join to form veins. These veins form larger veins, which carry deoxygenated blood to the right side of the heart, where it is returned to pulmonary circulation.

Blood Flow Regulation. The amount of blood ejected from the left ventricle each minute is the **cardiac output.** The normal cardiac output is 4 to 6 L/min in the healthy 150-pound (68-kg) adult at rest. The circulating volume of blood changes according to the oxygen and metabolic needs of the body. For example, during exercise, pregnancy, and fever, the cardiac output increases, but during sleep it decreases. Cardiac output is represented by the following formula:

$$\text{Cardiac output (CO)} = \text{Stroke volume (SV)} \times \text{Heart rate (HR)}$$

Cardiac output in the older adult may be affected by increased arterial wall tension and moderate myocardial hypertrophy due to an increased systolic blood pressure.

Cardiac index (CI) is the adequacy of the cardiac output for an individual. It takes into account the body surface area (BSA) of the client. The CI is determined by dividing the cardiac output by the BSA. The normal range is 2.5 to 4 L/min/m³. Both cardiac output and the CI are measured with invasive pulmonary artery catheters.

Stroke volume is the amount of blood ejected from the left ventricle with each contraction. It can be affected by the amount of blood in the left ventricle at the end of diastole (preload), the resistance to left ventricular ejection (afterload), and myocardial contractility.

Preload is essentially the end-diastolic volume. The ventricles stretch when filling with blood. The more stretch on the ventricular muscle, the greater the contraction and the greater the stroke volume (Starling's law). In clinical situations the preload and subsequent stroke volume can be manipulated by changing the amount of circulating blood volume. For example, in the client with hemorrhagic shock, fluid therapy and replacement of blood increases volume, thus increasing the preload and cardiac output. If volume is not replaced, preload decreases, the cardiac output decreases, and ultimately the venous return to the right atrium decreases, further decreasing preload and cardiac output.

Afterload is the resistance to left ventricular ejection: the work the heart must overcome to fully eject blood from the left ventricle. The diastolic aortic pressure is a good clinical measure of afterload. In a client with an acute hypertensive crisis, the afterload is increased, increasing the cardiac workload. Afterload in this situation can be manipulated by decreasing systemic blood pressure.

The measurement and monitoring of these cardiopulmonary hemodynamics is usually performed in critical care units. Some step-down or special care units may also have the capability to measure and monitor hemodynamics.

Myocardial contractility also affects stroke volume and cardiac output. Poor contraction decreases the amount of blood ejected by the ventricles during each contraction. Drugs that can increase the force of myocardial contraction include digitalis preparations, epinephrine, and sym-

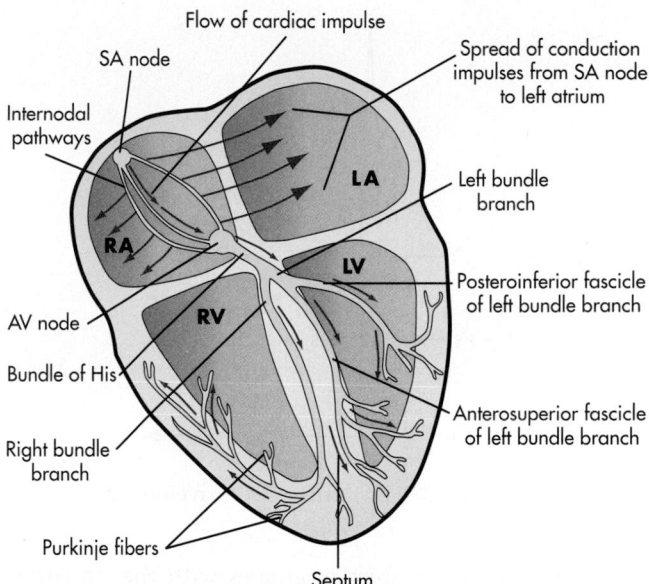

FIGURE 39–2 Conduction system of the heart. *LA,* Left atrium; *LV,* left ventricle; *RA,* right atrium; *RV,* right ventricle; *SA,* sinoatrial; *AV,* atrioventricular. (From Lewis SM and others: *Medical-surgical nursing: assessment and management of clinical problems,* ed 5, St. Louis, 2000, Mosby.)

pathomimetic drugs (drugs that mimic the effects of the sympathetic nervous system). Injury to the myocardial muscle, such as an acute myocardial infarction (AMI) can cause a decrease in myocardial contractility. The myocardium of the older adult is more rigid and slower in recovering its contractility (Lueckenotte, 2000).

Heart rate affects blood flow because of the interaction between rate and diastolic filling time. With a sustained heart rate greater than 160 beats per minute, diastolic filling time decreases, decreasing stroke volume and cardiac output. The heart rate of the older adult is slow to increase under stress. The stroke volume may increase to increase the cardiac output and blood pressure (Lueckenotte, 2000).

Conduction System. The rhythmic relaxation and contraction of the atria and ventricles depend on continuous, organized transmission of electrical impulses. These impulses are generated and transmitted by way of the cardiac conduction system (Figure 39-2).

The heart's conduction system generates the necessary action potentials that conduct the impulses required to initiate the electrical chain of events resulting in the heartbeat. The autonomic nervous system influences the rate of impulse generation, as well as the speed of transmission through the conductive pathway and the strength of atrial and ventricular contractions. Sympathetic nerve fibers, which increase the rate of impulse generation and the speed of impulse transmission, innervate all parts of the atria and ventricles. The parasympathetic fibers originating from the vagus nerve decrease the rate and also innervate all parts of the atria and ventricles, as well as the sinoatrial and atrioventricular nodes (McCance and Huether, 2001).

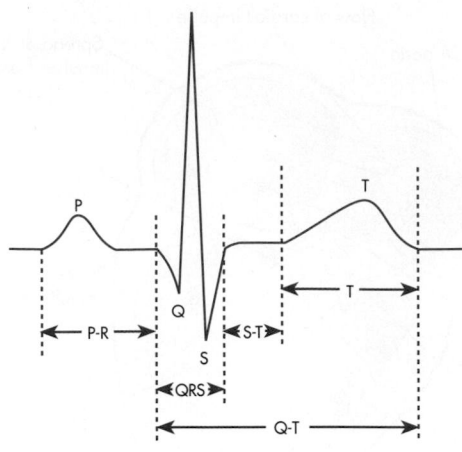

FIGURE **39–3**   Normal ECG waveform.

The conduction system originates with the sinoatrial (SA) node, the "pacemaker" of the heart. The SA node is in the right atrium next to the entrance of the superior vena cava (McCance and Huether, 2001). Impulses are initiated at the SA node at an intrinsic rate of 60 to 100 beats per minute. The resting adult rate is approximately 75 beats per minute.

The electrical impulses are then transmitted through the atria along intraatrial pathways to the atrioventricular (AV) node. The AV node mediates impulses between the atria and the ventricles. The intrinsic rate of the normal AV node is 40 to 60 beats per minute. The AV node assists atrial emptying by delaying the impulse before transmitting it through the bundle of His and the ventricular Purkinje network. The intrinsic rate of the bundle of His and the ventricular Purkinje network is 20 to 40 beats per minute.

An **electrocardiogram (ECG)** reflects the electrical activity of the conduction system. An ECG monitors the regularity and path of the electrical impulse through the conduction system; however, it does not reflect muscular work of the heart. The normal sequence on the ECG is called **normal sinus rhythm (NSR)** (Figure 39-3).

NSR implies that the impulse originates at the SA node and follows the normal sequence through the conduction system. The P wave represents the electrical conduction through both atria. Atrial contraction follows the P wave. The PR interval represents the impulse travel time through the AV node, through the bundle of His, and to the Purkinje fibers. The normal length for the PR interval is 0.12 to 0.20 second. An increase in the time, 0.20 second, indicates that there is a block in the impulse transmission though the AV node, whereas a decrease, 0.12 second, indicates the initiation of the electrical impulse from a source other than the SA node.

The QRS complex indicates that the electrical impulse has traveled through the ventricles. Normal QRS duration is 0.06 to 0.12 second. An increase in QRS duration indicates a delay in conduction time through the ventricles. Ventricular contraction usually follows the QRS complex.

The QT interval represents the time needed for ventricular depolarization and repolarization. The normal QT interval is 0.12 to 0.42 second. Changes in electrolyte values, such as hypocalcemia, or therapy with drugs such as disopyramide, amiodarone, and theophylline (Theo-Dur) can increase the QT interval. Shortening of the QT interval occurs with digitalis therapy, hyperkalemia, and hypercalcemia.

Respiratory Physiology

Most cells in the body obtain their energy from chemical reactions involving oxygen and the elimination of carbon dioxide. The exchange of respiratory gases occurs between environmental air and the blood (Figure 39-4). There are three steps in the process of oxygenation: ventilation, perfusion, and diffusion (McCance and Huether, 2001).

Structure and Function. Conditions or diseases that change the structure and function of the lung can alter respiration. The respiratory muscles, pleural space, lungs, and alveoli (Figure 39-5) are essential for ventilation, perfusion, and exchange of respiratory gases. Gases are moved into and out of the lungs through pressure changes. Intrapleural pressure is negative or less than atmospheric pressure, which is 760 mm Hg at sea level. For air to flow into the lungs, intrapleural pressure must become more negative, setting up a pressure gradient between the atmosphere and the alveoli. The diaphragm and external intercostals muscles contract to create a negative pleural pressure and increase the size of the thorax for inspiration. Relaxation of the diaphragm and contraction of the internal intercostals muscles allows air from the lung to escape. The coordination of the respiratory muscles is essential for effective respiration and gas exchange. The lung transfers oxygen from the atmosphere into the alveoli, where the oxygen is exchanged for carbon dioxide. The alveoli transfer oxygen and carbon dioxide to and from the blood through the alveolar membrane.

Ventilation is the process of moving gases into and out of the lungs. Ventilation requires coordination of the muscular and elastic properties of the lung and thorax, as well as intact innervation. The major inspiratory muscle of respiration is the diaphragm. It is innervated by the phrenic nerve, which exits the spinal cord at the fourth cervical vertebra. Perfusion relates the ability of the cardiovascular system to pump oxygenated blood to the tissues and return de-oxygenated blood to the lungs. Last, diffusion is responsible for moving the molecules from one area to another. For the exchange of respiratory gases to occur, the organs, nerves, and muscles of respiration must be intact and the central nervous system able to regulate the respiratory cycle.

Work of Breathing. Breathing is the effort required for expanding and contracting the lungs. In the healthy individual, breathing is quiet and accomplished with minimal effort. The amount of energy expended on breathing depends on the rate and depth of breathing, the ease in which the lungs can be expanded (compliance), and airway resistance (Jevon and Evans, 2001).

Inspiration is an active process, stimulated by chemical receptors in the aorta. **Expiration** is a passive process that depends on the elastic recoil properties of the lungs, requiring little or no muscle work. Elastic recoil

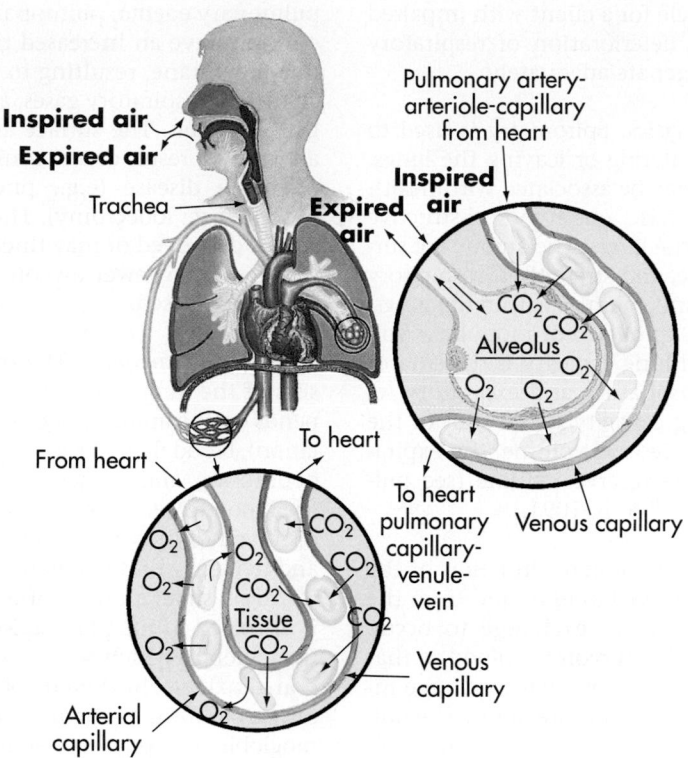

FIGURE **39–4** Structures of the pulmonary system. The circle denotes the alveoli. (From Thompson J and others: *Mosby's manual of clinical nursing,* ed 3, St. Louis, 1993, Mosby.)

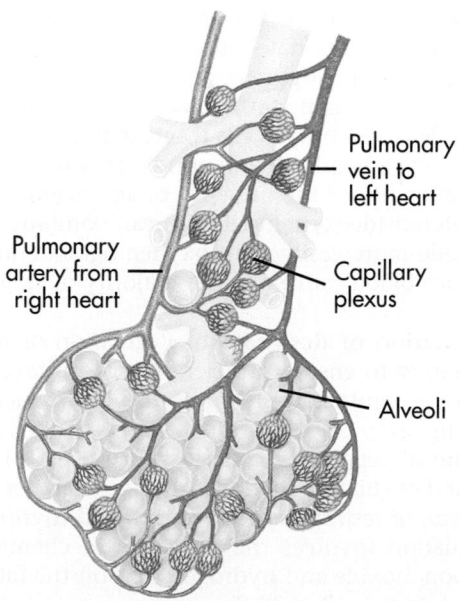

FIGURE **39–5** Alveoli at the terminal end of the lower airway. (From Thompson J and others: *Mosby's manual of clinical nursing,* ed 3, St. Louis, 1993, Mosby.)

is produced by elastic fibers in lung tissue and by surface tension in the fluid film lining the alveoli. Surfactant is a chemical produced in the lungs that maintains the surface tension of the alveoli and keeps them from collapsing. Clients with advanced chronic obstructive pul-

monary disease (COPD) lose the elastic recoil of the lungs and thorax. As a result, the client's work of breathing is increased. In addition, clients with certain pulmonary diseases can have decreased surfactant production and in turn may develop atelectasis.

Accessory muscles of respiration can increase lung volume during inspiration. Clients with COPD, especially emphysema, frequently use these muscles to increase lung volume. Prolonged use of the accessory muscles of respiration does not promote effective ventilation and causes fatigue. During assessment the nurse may observe elevation of the client's clavicles during inspiration.

Compliance is the ability of the lungs to distend or to expand in response to increased intraalveolar pressure. Compliance is decreased in diseases such as pulmonary edema, interstitial and pleural fibrosis, and congenital or traumatic structural abnormalities such as kyphosis or fractured ribs.

Airway resistance is the pressure difference between the mouth and the alveoli in relation to the rate of flow of inspired gas. Airway resistance can be increased by an airway obstruction, small airway disease (such as asthma), and tracheal edema. When resistance is increased, the amount of air traveling through the anatomical airways is decreased.

Decreased lung compliance, increased airway resistance, active expiration, or the use of accessory muscles increases the work of breathing, resulting in increased energy expenditure. To meet this expenditure, the body increases its metabolic rate, and the need for oxygen, as well as for the elimination of carbon dioxide, increases.

This sequence is a vicious cycle for a client with impaired ventilation, causing further deterioration of respiratory status and the ability to oxygenate adequately.

Lung Volumes and Capacities. Spirometry is used to measure the volume of air entering or leaving the lungs. Variations in lung volumes may be associated with health states such as pregnancy, exercise, obesity, or obstructive and restrictive conditions of the lungs. The amount of surfactant, degree of compliance, and strength of respiratory muscles can affect pressures and volumes within the lungs.

Lung capacities are made up of two or more lung volumes. For example, the total lung capacity is the sum of the tidal volume and the inspiratory and expiratory reserve volume. The total lung capacity is the sum of the tidal volume, the inspiratory reserve volume, the expiratory reserve volume, and the reserve volume (see pulmonary function tests, Table 39-9, p. 1091.)

Pulmonary Circulation. The primary function of the pulmonary circulation is to move blood to and from the alveolocapillary membrane for gas exchange to occur. The pulmonary circulation is a reservoir for blood so that the lung can increase its blood volume without large increases in pulmonary artery or venous pressures. The pulmonary circulation also acts as a filter, removing small thrombi before they can reach vital organs.

The pulmonary circulation begins at the pulmonary artery, which receives poorly oxygenated mixed venous blood from the right ventricle. Blood flow through this system depends on the pumping ability of the right ventricle, which has an output of approximately 4 to 6 L/min. The flow continues from the pulmonary artery through the pulmonary arterioles to the pulmonary capillaries, where blood comes in contact with the alveolocapillary membrane and the exchange of respiratory gases occurs. The oxygen-rich blood then circulates through the pulmonary venules and pulmonary veins, returning to the left atrium.

Pressure and resistance within the pulmonary circulatory system is lower than that within the systemic circulatory system. The walls of the pulmonary vessels are thinner and contain less smooth muscle. The lung accepts the total cardiac output from the right ventricle and, except in cases of alveolar hypoxia or cor pulmonale, does not direct blood flow from one region to another.

Respiratory Gas Exchange. Respiratory gases are exchanged in the alveoli and the capillaries of the body tissues. Oxygen is transferred from the lungs to the blood, and carbon dioxide is transferred from the blood to the alveoli to be exhaled as a waste product. At the tissue level, oxygen is transferred from the blood to tissues, and carbon dioxide is transferred from tissues to the blood to return to the alveoli and be exhaled. This transfer is dependent on the process of diffusion.

As mentioned, **diffusion** is the movement of molecules from an area of higher concentration to an area of lower concentration. Diffusion of respiratory gases occurs at the alveolocapillary membrane, and the rate of diffusion can be affected by the thickness of the membrane. Increased thickness of the membrane impedes diffusion because gases take longer to transfer across. Clients with

pulmonary edema, pulmonary infiltrates, or a pulmonary effusion have an increased thickness of the alveolocapillary membrane, resulting in slowed diffusion, slowed exchange of respiratory gases, and impaired delivery of oxygen to tissues. The surface area of the membrane can be altered as a result of a chronic disease (e.g., emphysema), an acute disease (e.g., pneumothorax), or a surgical process (e.g., lobectomy). The alveolocapillary membrane can be destroyed or may thicken, changing the rate of diffusion. When fewer alveoli are functioning, the surface area is decreased.

Oxygen Transport. The oxygen transport system consists of the lungs and cardiovascular system. Delivery depends on the amount of oxygen entering the lungs (ventilation), blood flow to the lungs and tissues (perfusion), rate of diffusion, and oxygen-carrying capacity. The capacity of the blood to carry oxygen is influenced by the amount of dissolved oxygen in the plasma, amount of hemoglobin, and tendency of hemoglobin to bind with oxygen. Only a relatively small amount of required oxygen, less than 1%, is dissolved in the plasma. Most oxygen is transported by hemoglobin, which serves as a carrier for oxygen and carbon dioxide. The hemoglobin molecule combines with oxygen to form oxyhemoglobin. The formation of oxyhemoglobin is easily reversible, allowing hemoglobin and oxygen to dissociate, which frees oxygen to enter tissues.

Carbon Dioxide Transport. Carbon dioxide diffuses into red blood cells and is rapidly hydrated into carbonic acid (H_2CO_3) because of the presence of carbonic anhydrase. The carbonic acid then dissociates into hydrogen (H^+) and bicarbonate (HCO_3^-) ions. The hydrogen ion is buffered by hemoglobin, and the HCO_3^- diffuses into the plasma (see Chapter 40). In addition, some of the carbon dioxide in red blood cells reacts with amino acid groups, forming carbamino compounds. This reaction can occur rapidly without the presence of an enzyme. Reduced hemoglobin (deoxyhemoglobin) can combine with carbon dioxide more easily than oxyhemoglobin, and therefore venous blood transports the majority of carbon dioxide.

Regulation of Respiration. Regulation of respiration is necessary to ensure sufficient oxygen intake and carbon dioxide elimination to meet the body's demands (e.g., during exercise, infection, or pregnancy). Neural and chemical regulators control the process of respiration. Neural regulation includes the central nervous system control of respiratory rate, depth, and rhythm. Chemical regulation involves the influence of chemicals such as carbon dioxide and hydrogen ions on the rate and depth of respiration (Box 39-2).

Factors Affecting Oxygenation

Adequacy of circulation, ventilation, perfusion, and transport of respiratory gases to the tissues is influenced by four types of factors: (1) physiological, (2) developmental, (3) lifestyle, and (4) environmental. Developmental, lifestyle, and environmental factors will be presented in a later section.

Physiological Factors. Any condition that affects cardiopulmonary functioning directly affects the body's

Box 39-2   Physiological Processes of Oxygenation

Neural Regulation

Maintains rhythm and depth of respiration and balance between inspiration and expiration.

Cerebral Cortex

Voluntary control of respiration delivers impulses to the respiratory motor neurons by way of the spinal cord; accommodates speaking, eating, and swimming.

Medulla Oblongata

Automatic control of respiration occurs continuously.

Chemical Regulation

Maintains appropriate rate and depth of respirations based on changes in the blood's carbon dioxide (CO_2), oxygen (O_2), and hydrogen ion (H^+) concentration.

Chemoreceptors

Located in the medulla, aortic body, and carotid body. Changes in chemical content of O_2, CO_2, and H^+ stimulate chemoreceptors, which in turn stimulate neural regulators to adjust the rate and depth of ventilation to maintain normal arterial blood gas levels. Chemical regulation can occur during physical exercise and in some illnesses. It is a short-term adaptive mechanism.

---

ability to meet oxygen demands. The general classifications of cardiac disorders include disturbances in conduction, impaired valvular function, myocardial hypoxia, cardiomyopathic conditions, and peripheral tissue hypoxia. Respiratory disorders include hyperventilation, hypoventilation, and hypoxia.

Other physiological processes affecting a client's oxygenation include alterations that affect the oxygen-carrying capacity of blood, such as the anemias; increases in the body's metabolic demands, such as pregnancy or fever and infection; and alterations that affect the client's chest wall movement or the central nervous system (Table 39-1).

Decreased Oxygen-Carrying Capacity. Hemoglobin carries 99% of the oxygen to tissues (Lewis and others, 2000). Anemia and inhalation of toxic substances decreases the oxygen-carrying capacity of blood by reducing the amount of available hemoglobin to transport oxygen. Anemia, a lower than normal hemoglobin level, is a result of decreased hemoglobin production, increased red blood cell destruction, and/or blood loss. Clients will have complaints of fatigue, decreased activity tolerance, and increased breathlessness, as well as pallor (especially seen in the conjunctiva of the eye) and an increased heart rate.

Carbon monoxide is the most common toxic inhalant that decreases the oxygen-carrying capacity of blood. The affinity for hemoglobin to bind with carbon monoxide is greater than 200 times its affinity to bind with oxygen, creating a functional anemia. Because of the bond's strength, carbon monoxide is not easily dissociated from hemoglobin, making the hemoglobin unavailable for oxygen transport.

Decreased Inspired Oxygen Concentration. When the concentration of inspired oxygen declines, the oxygen-carrying capacity of the blood is decreased. Decreases in the fraction of inspired oxygen concentration (FiO_2) can be caused by an upper or lower airway obstruction limiting delivery of inspired oxygen to alveoli; decreased environmental oxygen, such as at high altitudes; or decreased inspiration as a result of an incorrect oxygen concentration setting on respiratory therapy equipment.

Hypovolemia. Conditions such as shock and severe dehydration resulting from extracellular fluid loss and reduced circulating blood volume cause **hypovolemia.** With a significant fluid loss, the body tries to adapt by increasing the heart rate and peripheral vasoconstriction to increase the volume of blood returned to the heart and, in turn, increase the cardiac output.

Increased Metabolic Rate. Increased metabolic activity causes increased oxygen demand. When body systems are unable to meet this increased demand, the level of oxygenation declines. An increased metabolic rate is a normal physiological response to pregnancy, wound healing, and exercise because the body is building tissue. Most people can meet the increased oxygen demand and do not display signs of oxygen deprivation. Fever increases the tissues' need for oxygen, and as a result, carbon dioxide production also increases. If the febrile state persists, the metabolic rate remains high and the body begins to break down protein stores, resulting in muscle wasting and decreased muscle mass. Respiratory muscles such as the diaphragm and intercostal muscles are also wasted. The body attempts to adapt to the increased carbon dioxide levels by increasing the rate and depth of respiration. The client's work of breathing increases, and the client will eventually display signs and symptoms of hypoxemia. Those clients with pulmonary diseases are at greater risk for hypoxemia and hypercapnia. Assessment findings include an increased rate and depth of respiration, use of the accessory muscles of respiration, pursed-lip breathing, and decreased activity tolerance.

Conditions Affecting Chest Wall Movement. Any condition that reduces chest wall movement can result in decreased ventilation. If the diaphragm cannot fully descend with breathing, the volume of inspired air decreases and less oxygen is delivered to the alveoli and subsequently to tissues.

Pregnancy. As the fetus grows during pregnancy, the greater size of the uterus pushes abdominal contents upward against the diaphragm. In the last trimester of pregnancy the inspiratory capacity declines, resulting in dyspnea on exertion and increased fatigue.

Obesity. Obesity is increasing in the United States population. Twenty percent of the U.S. population is morbidly obese. Morbidly obese clients have reduced lung volumes from the heavy lower thorax and abdomen, particularly

Table 39-1   Physiological Processes Affecting Oxygenation

Process	Effect on Oxygenation
Anemia	Decreases oxygen-carrying capacity of blood
Toxic inhalant	Decreases oxygen-carrying capacity of blood
Airway obstruction	Limits delivery of inspired oxygen to alveoli
High altitude	Atmospheric oxygen concentration is lower and inspiratory oxygen concentration decreases
Fever	Increases metabolic rate and tissue oxygen demand
Decreased chest wall motion (e.g., from musculoskeletal impairments)	Prevents lowering of diaphragm and reduces anteroposterior diameter of thorax on inspiration, reducing volume of air inspired

when in the recumbent and supine positions. Morbidly obese clients have a reduction in compliance as a result of encroachment of the abdomen into the chest, increased work of breathing, and decreased lung volumes, and they may have fatigue and carbon dioxide retention. In some clients an obesity-hypoventilation syndrome develops in which oxygenation is decreased and carbon dioxide is retained, resulting in daytime sleepiness. Morbidly obese clients may also develop obstructive sleep apnea, characterized by excessive daytime somnolence and loud snoring and apneic periods during sleep. The obese client is also susceptible to pneumonia after an upper respiratory tract infection because the lungs cannot fully expand and pulmonary secretions are not mobilized in the lower lobes.

Musculoskeletal Abnormalities. Musculoskeletal impairments in the thoracic region reduce oxygenation. Such impairments may result from abnormal structural configurations, trauma, muscular diseases, and diseases of the central nervous system. Abnormal structural configurations impairing oxygenation include those that affect the rib cage, such as pectus excavatum, and those that affect the vertebral column, such as kyphosis, lordosis, or scoliosis.

Trauma. The person with multiple rib fractures can develop a flail chest, a condition in which fractures cause instability in part of the chest wall. The unstable chest wall allows the lung underlying the injured area to contract on inspiration and bulge on expiration, resulting in hypoxia. Chest wall or upper abdominal incisions may also decrease chest wall movement as the client uses shallow respirations to minimize chest wall movement to avoid pain. Excessive or high doses of narcotic analgesics may depress the respiratory center, further decreasing respiratory rate and chest wall expansion.

Neuromuscular Diseases. Diseases such as muscular dystrophy affect oxygenation of tissues by decreasing the client's ability to expand and contract the chest wall. Ventilation is impaired, and atelectasis, hypercapnia, and hypoxemia can occur. Myasthenia gravis, Guillain-Barré syndrome, and poliomyelitis affect respiratory functioning and result in hypoventilation. Myasthenia gravis interferes with normal transmission of impulses from nerves to muscles, involving the whole body, including muscles of respiration. Guillain-Barré syndrome and poliomyelitis cause inflammation and paralysis of muscle groups. Guillain-Barré syndrome usually results in an ascending pattern of

paralysis. Respiratory muscles become paralyzed as paralysis ascends to the thoracic region. Poliomyelitis may lead to general or local paralysis. Both may reverse, but poliomyelitis usually results in more residual paralysis.

Central Nervous System Alterations. Diseases or trauma involving the medulla oblongata and spinal cord may result in impaired respiration. When the medulla oblongata is affected, neural regulation of respiration is damaged and abnormal breathing patterns may develop. If the phrenic nerve is damaged, the diaphragm may not descend, thus reducing inspiratory lung volumes and causing hypoxemia. Cervical trauma at C3 to C5 can result in paralysis of the phrenic nerve. Spinal cord trauma below the fifth cervical vertebra usually leaves the phrenic nerve intact but damages nerves that innervate the intercostal muscles, preventing anteroposterior chest expansion.

Influences of Chronic Disease. Oxygenation can be decreased as a direct consequence of chronic disease. It can also be decreased as a secondary effect, as with anemia. The physiological response to chronic hypoxemia is the development of a secondary polycythemia. This adaptive response is the body's attempt to increase the amount of circulating hemoglobin to increase the available oxygen-binding sites.

Alterations in Cardiac Functioning

Illnesses and conditions that affect cardiac rhythm, strength of contraction, blood flow through the chambers, myocardial blood flow, and peripheral circulation cause alterations in cardiac functioning. Older adults experience alterations in cardiac function due to calcification of the conduction pathways, thicker and stiffer heart valves due to lipid accumulation and fibrosis, and a decrease in the number of pacemaker cells in the SA node (Lueckenotte 2000).

Disturbances in Conduction. Some disturbances in conduction are a result of electrical impulses that do not originate from the SA node. These rhythm disturbances are called **dysrhythmias,** meaning a deviation from the normal sinus heart rhythm (Table 39-2). Dysrhythmias may occur as a primary conduction disturbance; as a response to ischemia, valvular abnormality, anxiety, or drug toxicity; as a result of caffeine, alcohol, or tobacco use; or as a complication of acid-base or electrolyte imbalance (see Chapter 40).

Table 39-2	Common Basic Cardiac Dysrhythmias
Rhythm Characteristics and Etiology	**Clinical Significance and Management**

Sinus Tachycardia

Regular rhythm, rate 100-180 beats/min (higher in infants), normal P wave, normal QRS complex

Rate increase may be normal response to exercise, emotion, or stressors such as pain, fever, pump failure, hyperthyroidism, and certain drugs (e.g., caffeine, nitrates, epinephrine, nicotine)

Client with damaged heart may not be able to sustain increased myocardial oxygen consumption by increased heart rate

Correct underlying factors; discontinue drugs producing the side effect

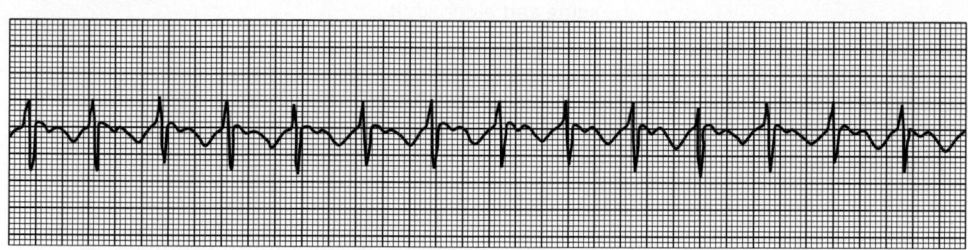

Sinus Bradycardia

Regular rhythm, rate less than 60 beats/min, normal P wave, normal PR interval, normal QRS complex

Rate decrease may be normal response to sleep or in well-conditioned athlete; abnormal drops in rate may be caused by diminished blood flow to SA node, vagal stimulation, hypothyroidism, increased intracranial pressure, or pharmacological agents (e.g., digoxin, propranolol, quinidine, procainamide)

No clinical significance unless associated with signs and symptoms of reduced cardiac output such as dizziness or syncope or presence of chest pain

Bradycardia with hypotension and decreased cardiac output is treated with atropine; a pacemaker may be required

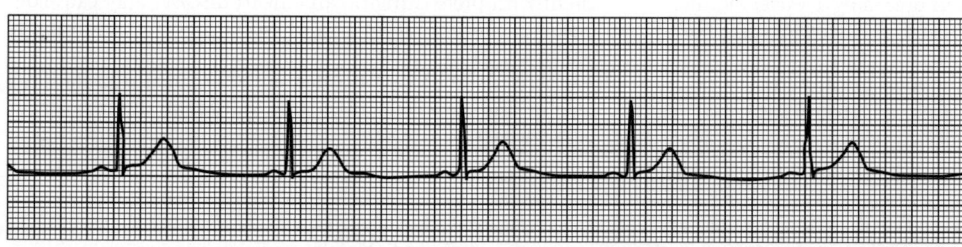

Sinus Dysrhythmia

Sinus rhythm with cyclic variation; slows during inspiration and increases with expiration; rate of 60-100 beats/min; normal P wave; normal PR interval; normal QRS complex

Caused by vagal impulses; occurs commonly in children, young adults, and older adults; usually disappears as heart rate increases

No clinical significance unless dizziness occurs with decreased rate

No management indicated unless heart rate decreases and symptoms occur

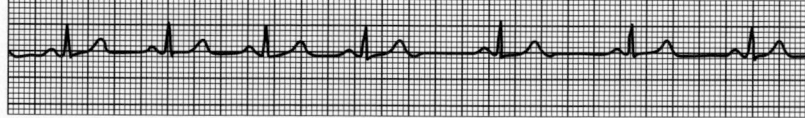

Modified from Canobbio MM: *Cardiovascular disorders,* St. Louis, 1990, Mosby.

PSVT management: Vagal stimulation such as carotid sinus massage or Valsalva maneuver to decrease ventricular response with medication to block AV conduction; adenosine 6 mg IV over 1-3 seconds; adenosine 12 mg IV over 1-3 seconds; assess complex width; narrow-check blood pressure, normal verapamil 2.5-5 mg IV; if blood pressure low or unstable, proceed to synchronized cardioversion; wide complex, lidocaine 1-1.5 mg/kg IV push, procainamide 20-30 mg/min; synchronized cardioversion if resistant to drug therapy (ECC, 1992).

Sinus bradycardia management: Correct underlying causes. If symptomatic (e.g., hypotension, chest pain, decreased level of consciousness, shortness of breath), administer atropine 0.04 mg/kg IV; transcutaneous pacing if available; dopamine 5-20 mcg/kg/min; epinephrine 2-10 mcg/min; temporary transvenous pacemaker if resistant to drug therapy (ECC, 1992).

Continued

Table 39-2   Common Basic Cardiac Dysrhythmias—cont'd

Rhythm Characteristics and Etiology	Clinical Significance and Management

Atrial Fibrillation (A-fib)

Chaotic, irregular atrial activity resulting in an irregular ventricular response. No identifiable P waves. Irregular ventricular response resulting in an irregular cardiac rate and rhythm. The rate is determined by the conduction of the multiple atrial impulses across the AV node.

Caused by aging, calcification of the SA node, or changes in myocardial blood supply

There is a loss of the atrial kick (portion of the cardiac output squeezed in the ventricles with a coordinated atrial contraction), pooling of blood in the atria, and development of microemboli. The client may complain of fatigue, a fluttering in the chest or shortness of breath if the ventricular response is rapid. Commonly occurring dysrhythmia in the aging and older adult

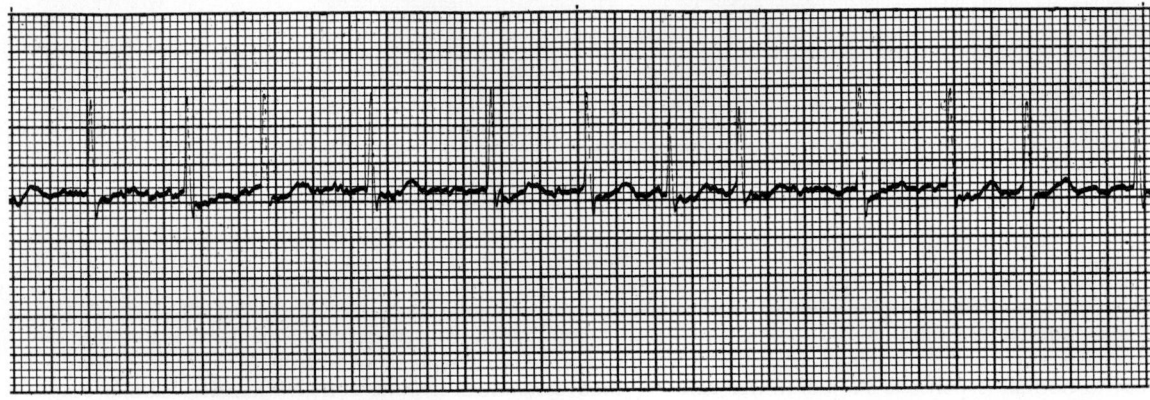

Paroxysmal Supraventricular Tachycardia (PSVT)

Sudden, rapid onset of tachycardia with stimulus originating above AV node; regular rhythm; rate 150-250 beats/min; P wave uniform, possibly buried in preceding T wave; PR interval variable, often difficult to measure; normal QRS complex

May begin and end spontaneously or be precipitated by excitement, fatigue, caffeine, smoking, or alcohol use

Usually no significant impairment; client complains of palpitations and shortness of breath; if persistent or occurring in client with preexisting organic heart disease, may cause decrease in cardiac output and/or blood pressure, resulting in pump failure or shock

Treatment includes Valsalva maneuver or vagal stimulation by carotid sinus massage, adenosine, diltiazem, digitalis, or beta-adrenergic blockers

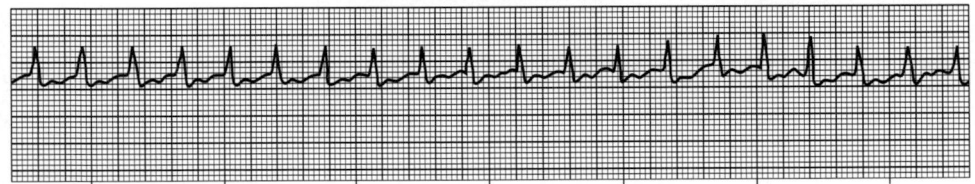

Modified from Canobbio MM: *Cardiovascular disorders,* St. Louis, 1990, Mosby.
PSVT management: Vagal stimulation such as carotid sinus massage or Valsalva maneuver to decrease ventricular response with medication to block AV conduction; adenosine 6 mg IV over 1-3 seconds; adenosine 12 mg IV over 1-3 seconds; assess complex width; narrow—check blood pressure, normal verapamil 2.5-5 mg IV; if blood pressure low or unstable, proceed to synchronized cardioversion; wide complex, lidocaine 1-1.5 mg/kg IV push, procainamide 20-30 mg/min; synchronized cardioversion if resistant to drug therapy (ECC, 1992). Sinus bradycardia management: Correct underlying causes. If symptomatic (e.g., hypotension, chest pain, decreased level of consciousness, shortness of breath), administer atropine 0.04 mg/kg IV; transcutaneous pacing if available; dopamine 5-20 mcg/kg/min; epinephrine 2-10 mcg/min; temporary transvenous pacemaker if resistant to drug therapy (ECC, 1992).

Table 39-2	Common Basic Cardiac Dysrhythmias—cont'd
Rhythm Characteristics and Etiology	**Clinical Significance and Management**

Premature Ventricular Contractions (PVCs)

Irregular rhythm with ectopic beats followed by full compensatory pause; rate normal or increased rate, P wave absent in ectopic beat; PR interval absent; QRS complex widened and distorted; T wave in opposition to R wave

Caused by changes in the normal pacemaker of the heart such as decrease in blood flow, ischemia, or embolus

PVCs occurring more than 6/min, in pairs, or with multiple configurations indicates increased ventricular irritability

Treat underlying cause such as myocardial infarction, hypoxia, hypocalcemia, or acidosis

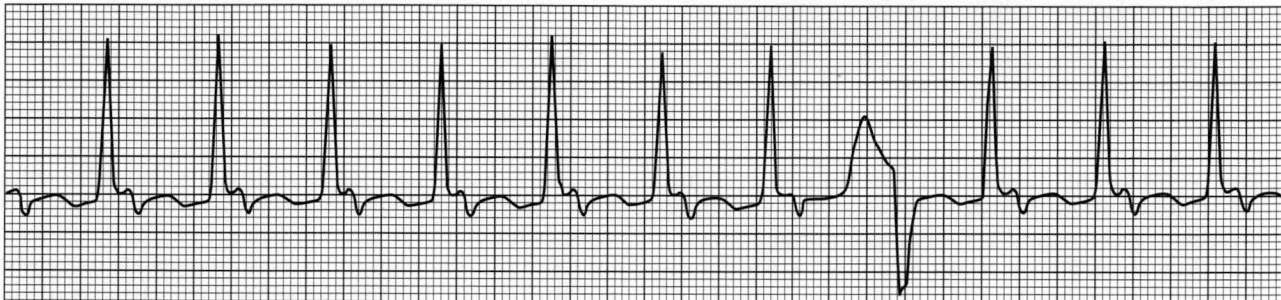

Ventricular Tachycardia

Rhythm slightly irregular, rate 100-200 beats/min, P wave absent, PR interval absent, QRS complex wide and bizarre, >0.12 second

Caused by changes in the normal pacemaker of the heart such as decrease in blood flow, ischemia, or embolus

Results in a decreased cardiac output due to decreased ventricular filling time; may lead to severe hypotension, and loss of pulse and consciousness

If refractory to defibrillation, amiodarone 300 mg IV followed by an additional 150 mg IV in 3-5 minutes (AHA, 2000)

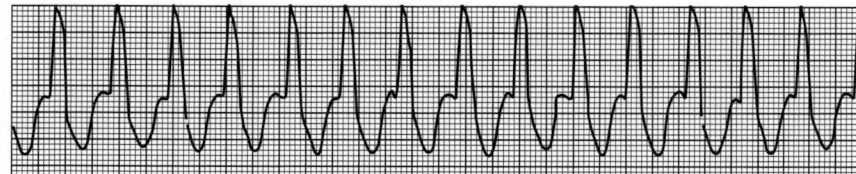

Ventricular Fibrillation

Uncoordinated electrical activity. No identifiable P, QRS, or T wave

Causes include sudden cardiac death, electrical shock, acute myocardial infarction, drowning, or trauma

Acute loss of pulse and respiration. Immediate defibrillation after assessment of ABCs of CPR. Availability of automated external defibrillator (AED) is recommended in public and/or private places where large numbers of people gather or where people who are at high risk for heart attack live (AHA, 2003) (Box 39-3)

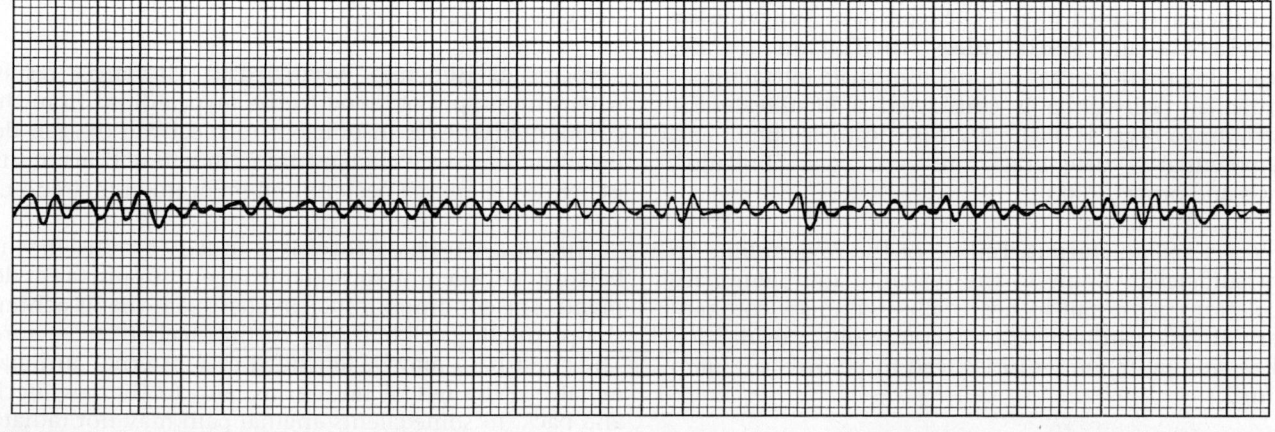

Dysrhythmias are classified by cardiac response and site of impulse origin. Cardiac response can be either tachycardiac (greater than 100 beats per minute), bradycardiac (less than 60 beats per minute), a premature (early) beat, or a blocked (delayed or absent) beat. Tachydysrhythmias and bradydysrhythmias can lower cardiac output and blood pressure. Tachydysrhythmias reduce cardiac output by decreasing diastolic filling time. Bradydysrhythmias lower cardiac output because of the decreased heart rate.

Atrial fibrillation is a commonly occurring dysrhythmia seen in older adults. The electrical impulse in the atria is chaotic and originates from multiple sites. The rhythm is irregular due to the multiple pacemaker sites and the unpredictable conduction to the ventricles. The QRS complex is normal; however, it occurs at irregular intervals. Atrial fibrillation is often described as an irregularly irregular rhythm.

Abnormal impulses originating above the ventricles are referred to as supraventricular dysrhythmias. The abnormality on the waveform is the configuration and placement of the P wave. Ventricular conduction usually remains normal, and a normal QRS complex is observed.

Ventricular dysrhythmias represent an ectopic site of impulse formation within the ventricles. It is ectopic in that the impulse originates in the ventricle, not the SA node. The configuration of the QRS complex is usually widened and bizarre. P waves may or may not be present; often they are buried in the QRS complex. **Ventricular tachycardia** and **ventricular fibrillation** are life-threatening rhythms that require immediate intervention. Ventricular tachycardia is considered a life-threatening dysrhythmia because of the decreased cardiac output and the potential to deteriorate into ventricular fibrillation (Lewis and others, 2000).

Altered Cardiac Output. Failure of the myocardium to eject sufficient volume to the systemic and pulmonary circulations can result in heart failure. Primary coronary artery disease, cardiomyopathic conditions, valvular disorders, and pulmonary disease lead to myocardial pump failure.

Left-Sided Heart Failure. Left-sided heart failure is an abnormal condition characterized by impaired function-

ing of the left ventricle due to elevated pressures and pulmonary congestion. If left ventricular failure is significant, the amount of blood ejected from the left ventricle drops greatly, resulting in decreased cardiac output. Assessment findings may include decreased activity tolerance, breathlessness, dizziness, and confusion as a result of tissue hypoxia from the diminished cardiac output. As the left ventricle continues to fail, blood begins to pool in the pulmonary circulation, causing pulmonary congestion. Clinical findings include crackles on auscultation, hypoxia, shortness of breath on exertion and often at rest, cough, and paroxysmal nocturnal dyspnea.

Right-Sided Heart Failure. Right-sided heart failure results from impaired functioning of the right ventricle characterized by venous congestion in the systemic circulation. Right-sided heart failure more commonly results from pulmonary disease or as a result of long-term left-sided failure. The primary pathological factor in right-sided failure is elevated pulmonary vascular resistance (PVR). As the PVR continues to rise, the right ventricle must generate more work, and the oxygen demand of the heart increases. As the failure continues, the amount of blood ejected from the right ventricle declines, and blood begins to "back up" in the systemic circulation. Clinically the client has weight gain, distended neck veins, hepatomegaly and splenomegaly, and dependent peripheral edema.

Impaired Valvular Function. Valvular heart disease is an acquired or congenital disorder of a cardiac valve characterized by stenosis and obstructed blood flow or valvular degeneration and regurgitation of blood. When stenosis occurs in the semilunar valves (aortic and pulmonic valves), the adjacent ventricles must work harder to move the ventricular volume beyond the stenotic valve. Over time the stenosis can cause the ventricle to hypertrophy (enlarge), and if the condition is untreated, left- or right-sided heart failure can occur. If stenosis occurs in the atrioventricular valves (mitral and tricuspid valves), the atrial pressure rises, causing the atria to hypertrophy. When regurgitation occurs, there is a backflow of blood into an adjacent chamber. For example, in mitral regurgitation the mitral leaflets do not close completely. When the ventricles contract, blood escapes back into the atria, causing a murmur, or "whooshing" sound (see Chapter 32).

Myocardial Ischemia. **Myocardial ischemia** results when the supply of blood to the myocardium from the coronary arteries is insufficient to meet the oxygen demands of the organ. Two common manifestations of this ischemia are angina pectoris and myocardial infarction.

Angina. **Angina pectoris** is usually a transient imbalance between myocardial oxygen supply and demand. The condition results in chest pain that is aching, sharp, tingling, or burning, or that feels like pressure. The chest pain may be left sided or substernal and may radiate to the left or both arms, and to the jaw, neck, and back. In some clients anginal pain may not radiate. The pain can last from 1 to 15 minutes. Clients report that pain is often precipitated by activities that increase myocardial oxygen demand (e.g., exercise, anxiety, or stress). The pain is usually relieved with rest and coronary vasodilators, the most common being a nitroglycerin preparation.

Myocardial Infarction. **Myocardial infarction (MI)** results from sudden decreases in coronary blood flow or an increase in myocardial oxygen demand without adequate coronary perfusion. Infarction occurs because of ischemia (which is reversible) and necrosis (which is not reversible) of myocardial tissue.

Chest pain associated with myocardial infarction in men is usually described as crushing, squeezing, or stabbing. The pain may be retrosternal and left precordial, and it may radiate down the left arm to the neck, jaws, teeth, epigastric area, and back. The pain occurs at rest or exertion, lasts more than 30 minutes, and is unrelieved by rest, position change, or sublingual nitroglycerin administration.

Current research indicates that there is a significant difference between men and women in relation to coronary artery disease. It is known that women do not present the same type of symptoms as men (Anderson and Kessenich, 2001). The most common initial symptom in women is angina. Women may also present with complaints of epigastric pain, radiation through to the back and into the jaw. Women tend to have fewer Q waves and ST segment changes with chest pain when compared with men. The initial signs and symptoms in women may be more atypical, including epigastric pain, shortness of breath, variant angina, and vasospasm (Denke, 2001).

Acute Coronary Syndrome. Acute coronary syndrome (ACS) includes unstable angina, non-ST segment elevation MI, and ST-segment elevation MI. There is an imbalance in the oxygen supply and demand to the myocardium. Causes include nonocclusive thrombus on preexisting plaque, coronary vasospasm, arterial narrowing from atherosclerosis, inflammation or infection, and secondary unstable angina from anemia, fever, or hypoxemia (Granger and Miller, 2001). Symptoms may not be constant and may present atypically. Clients with classic AMI symptoms are more easily identified. Intermediate risk factors for ACS include male gender, age greater than 70 years with diabetes mellitus, extracardiac vascular disease, fixed Q waves, and previous abnormal ST segment and T wave changes (Granger and Miller, 2001).

Alterations in Respiratory Functioning

Illnesses and conditions that affect ventilation or oxygen transport cause alterations in respiratory functioning. The three primary alterations are hyperventilation, hypoventilation, and hypoxia.

The goal of ventilation is to produce a normal arterial carbon dioxide tension ($PaCO_2$) between 35 and 45 mm Hg and maintain a normal arterial oxygen tension (PaO_2) between 95 and 100 mm Hg. Hyperventilation and hypoventilation refer to alveolar ventilation and not to the client's respiratory rate. Arterial oxygen levels can be monitored using a noninvasive oxygen saturation monitor. The normal range is 95% to 100%. Hypoxia refers to a decrease in the amount of arterial oxygen.

Hyperventilation. **Hyperventilation** is a state of ventilation in excess of that required to eliminate the normal venous carbon dioxide produced by cellular metabolism. Anxiety, infections, drugs, or an acid-base imbalance can induce hyperventilation, as well as hypoxia associated with pulmonary embolus or shock. Acute anxiety can lead to hyperventilation and may cause loss of consciousness from excess carbon dioxide exhalation. Fever can cause hyperventilation. As a client's body temperature increases, there is an increase in the metabolic rate, thereby increasing carbon dioxide production. The clinical response is an increased rate and depth of respiration.

Hyperventilation may also be chemically induced. Salicylate (aspirin) poisoning causes excessive stimulation of the respiratory center as the body's attempt to compensate for excess carbon dioxide. Amphetamines also increase ventilation by raising carbon dioxide production. Hyperventilation can also occur as the body tries to compensate for metabolic acidosis by producing a respiratory alkalosis. For example, the diabetic client who has gone into diabetic ketoacidosis is producing large amounts of metabolic acids. The respiratory system tries to correct the acid-base balance by overbreathing. Ventilation increases to reduce the amount of carbon dioxide available to form carbonic acid (see Chapter 40). Hemoglobin does not release oxygen to tissues as readily, and tissue hypoxia results. As symptoms worsen, the client may become more agitated, which further increases the respiratory rate and can result in respiratory alkalosis.

Hypoventilation. **Hypoventilation** occurs when alveolar ventilation is inadequate to meet the body's oxygen demand or to eliminate sufficient carbon dioxide. As alveolar ventilation decreases, $PaCO_2$ is elevated. Severe atelectasis can produce hypoventilation. **Atelectasis** is a collapse of the alveoli that prevents normal respiratory exchange of oxygen and carbon dioxide. As alveoli collapse, less of the lung can be ventilated and hypoventilation occurs.

In clients with COPD, the inappropriate administration of excessive oxygen can result in hypoventilation. These clients have adapted to a high carbon dioxide level, and their carbon dioxide–sensitive chemoreceptors are essentially not functioning. Their stimulus to breathe is a decreased PaO_2. If excessive oxygen is administered, the oxygen requirement is satisfied and the stimulus to breathe is negated. High concentrations of oxygen (e.g., greater than 24% to 28% [1 to 3 L/min]) prevent the PaO_2 from falling and obliterate the stimulus to breathe, resulting in hypoventilation. The excessive retention of carbon dioxide may lead to respiratory arrest.

Signs and symptoms of hypoventilation include mental status changes, dysrhythmias, and potential cardiac arrest. Treatment requires improving tissue oxygenation, restoring ventilatory function, treating the underlying cause of the hypoventilation, and achieving acid-base balance. If untreated, the client's status can rapidly decline, leading to convulsions, unconsciousness, and death.

Hypoxia. **Hypoxia** is inadequate tissue oxygenation at the cellular level. This can result from a deficiency in oxygen delivery or oxygen utilization at the cellular level.

Hypoxia can be caused by (1) a decreased hemoglobin level and lowered oxygen-carrying capacity of the blood; (2) a diminished concentration of inspired oxygen, which may occur at high altitudes; (3) the inability of the tissues to extract oxygen from the blood, as with cyanide poisoning; (4) decreased diffusion of oxygen from the alveoli to the blood, as in pneumonia; (5) poor tissue perfusion with oxygenated blood, as with shock; and (6) impaired ventilation, as with multiple rib fractures or chest trauma.

The clinical signs and symptoms of hypoxia include apprehension, restlessness, inability to concentrate, declining level of consciousness, dizziness, and behavioral changes. The client with hypoxia is unable to lie down and appears fatigued and agitated. Vital sign changes include an increased pulse rate and increased rate and depth of respiration. The client with a narcotic overdose, such as a heroin overdose, may display signs of hypoventilation. During early stages of hypoxia the blood pressure is elevated unless the condition is caused by shock. As the hypoxia worsens, the respiratory rate may decline as a result of respiratory muscle fatigue.

Cyanosis, blue discoloration of the skin and mucous membranes caused by the presence of desaturated hemoglobin in capillaries, is a late sign of hypoxia. The presence or absence of cyanosis is not a reliable measure of oxygenation status. Central cyanosis, observed in the tongue, soft palate, and conjunctiva of the eye, where blood flow is high, indicates hypoxemia. Peripheral cyanosis, seen in the extremities, nail beds, and earlobes, is often a result of vasoconstriction and stagnant blood flow. Hypoxia is a life-threatening condition. Untreated, it can produce cardiac dysrhythmias that result in death. Hypoxia is managed by administration of oxygen and treatment of the underlying cause, such as airway obstruction.

Nursing Knowledge Base

Developmental Factors
The developmental stage of the client and the normal aging process can affect tissue oxygenation.

Infants and Toddlers. Infants and toddlers are at risk for upper respiratory tract infections as a result of frequent exposure to other children and exposure to secondhand smoke. In addition, during the teething process some infants develop nasal congestion, which encourages bacterial growth and increases the potential for respiratory tract infection. Upper respiratory tract infections are usually not dangerous, and infants or toddlers recover with little difficulty.

School-Age Children and Adolescents. School-age children and adolescents are exposed to respiratory infections and respiratory risk factors such as secondhand smoke and cigarette smoking. A healthy child usually does not have adverse pulmonary effects from respiratory infections. A person who starts smoking in adolescence and continues to smoke into middle age, however, has an increased risk for cardiopulmonary disease and lung cancer.

Focus on Older Adults   **Box 39-4**

- The tuberculin skin test is an unreliable indicator of tuberculosis in older clients. They frequently display false-positive or false-negative skin test reactions.
  - Older clients are at an increased risk for reactivation of dormant organisms that have been present for decades as a result of age-related changes in the immune system.
  - The standard 5-TU Mantoux test is given and repeated or repeated with the 250-TU strength to create a booster effect.
  - If the older client has a positive reaction, a complete history is necessary to determine any risk factors.
- Older adults have more atypical signs and symptoms of coronary artery disease (Lueckenotte, 2000).
  - The incidence of atrial fibrillation increases with age and is the leading contributing factor for stroke in the older adult (Lueckenotte, 2000).
- Mental status changes are often the first signs of respiratory problems and may include forgetfulness and irritability.
- Older adults may not complain of dyspnea until it affects the activities of daily living that are important to them.
- Changes in the older adult's cough mechanism may lead to retention of pulmonary secretions, airway plugging, and atelectasis if cough suppressants are not used with caution.

Young and Middle-Age Adults. Young and middle-age adults are exposed to multiple cardiopulmonary risk factors: an unhealthy diet, lack of exercise, stress, over-the-counter and prescription drugs not used as intended, illegal drugs, and smoking. Reducing these modifiable factors may decrease the client's risk for cardiac or pulmonary diseases. This is also the time when lifelong habits and lifestyles are established. It is important to help these clients make good choices and informed decisions about the rest of their lives and their health care practices.

Older Adults. The cardiac and respiratory systems undergo changes throughout the aging process (Box 39-4). The changes are associated with calcification of the heart valves, SA node, and costal cartilages. The arterial system develops atherosclerotic plaques. Osteoporosis leads to changes in the size and shape of the thorax.

The trachea and large bronchi become enlarged from calcification of the airways. The alveoli enlarge, decreasing the surface area available for gas exchange. The number of functional cilia is reduced, causing a decrease in the effectiveness of the cough mechanism, putting the older adult at increased risk for respiratory infections (Lueckenotte, 2000). Ventilation and transfer of respiratory gases decline with age, because the lungs are unable to expand fully, leading to lower oxygenation levels.

Lifestyle Risk Factors
Lifestyle modifications that influence cardiopulmonary functioning are frequently difficult because a client is being asked to change a habit or behavior that may be enjoyed, such as cigarette smoking or eating certain foods;

- Maintain ideal body weight.
- Eat a low-fat, low-salt, calorie-appropriate diet.
- Engage in regular aerobic exercise of 1 hour daily.
- Use a filter mask when exposed to occupational hazards.
- Use stress reduction techniques.
- Reduce exposure to secondary infections.
- Be smoke free.
  - Avoid secondhand smoke and other pollutants.
- Have annual visits with health care provider.
  - Monitor blood pressure.
  - Monitor cholesterol and triglyceride levels.
  - Get an annual influenza vaccine if at risk for the development of influenza.
  - Get a pneumococcal vaccine if appropriate.

*Target population: young to older adults.

however, these changes can be achieved with encouragement, support, and time (Box 39-5). Risk factor modification is important, including smoking cessation, weight reduction, a low-cholesterol and low-sodium diet, management of hypertension, and moderate exercise. Although it may be more difficult to get older adults to change long-term behavior, assisting older adults to healthy behaviors can slow or halt the progression of their cardiopulmonary disease (Lueckenotte, 2000).

Nutrition. Nutrition affects cardiopulmonary function in several ways. Severe obesity decreases lung expansion, and the increased body weight increases oxygen demands to meet metabolic needs. The malnourished client may experience respiratory muscle wasting, resulting in decreased muscle strength and respiratory excursion. Cough efficiency is reduced secondary to respiratory muscle weakness, putting the client at risk for retention of pulmonary secretions. Diets high in fat increase cholesterol and atherogenesis in the coronary arteries.

Clients who are morbidly obese and/or malnourished are at risk for anemia. Diets high in carbohydrates may play a role in increasing the carbon dioxide load for clients with carbon dioxide retention. As carbohydrates are metabolized, an increased load of carbon dioxide is created and excreted via the lungs.

Dietary restriction of sodium has been shown to be beneficial in reducing antihypertensive medication requirements and may cause left ventricular hypertrophy to regress (Joint National Committee [JNC], 2003). Diets high in potassium may prevent hypertension and help improve control in clients with hypertension. A 2000-calorie diet high in fiber, potassium, calcium, and magnesium; made up of fruits, vegetables, and low-fat dairy foods; and low in saturated and total fat is recommended to help prevent and reduce the effects of hypertension (JNC, 2003).

Exercise. Exercise increases the body's metabolic activity and oxygen demand. The rate and depth of respiration

increase, enabling the person to inhale more oxygen and exhale excess carbon dioxide. A physical exercise program has many benefits (see Chapter 36). People who exercise for 1 hour daily have a lower pulse rate, blood pressure, decreased cholesterol level, increased blood flow, and greater oxygen extraction by working muscles. Fully conditioned people can increase oxygen consumption by 10% to 20% because of increased cardiac output and increased efficiency of the myocardial muscle (JNC, 2003).

Smoking Cessation. Cigarette smoking is associated with a number of diseases, including heart disease, chronic obstructive lung disease, and lung cancer. Cigarette smoking can worsen peripheral vascular and coronary artery diseases (JNC, 1997). Inhaled nicotine causes vasoconstriction of peripheral and coronary blood vessels, increasing blood pressure and decreasing blood flow to peripheral vessels. The risk of lung cancer is 10 times greater for a person who smokes than for a nonsmoker. Exposure to secondhand smoke increases the risk of lung cancer and cardiovascular disease in the nonsmoker (American Heart Association [AHA], 2001).

The number of female smokers has increased substantially over the past 30 years, resulting in a tenfold increase in the number of women diagnosed with lung cancer. Only recently has the rate of increase among women begun to slow (American Cancer Society [ACS], 2004). The 5-year survival rate for all clients with lung cancer is only 14%, regardless of the diagnosis (ACS, 2004). Frequently lung cancer is diagnosed only when it has reached an advanced stage. If lung cancer is detected when the disease is still localized, the survival rate is 49%. Only 15% of lung cancers are diagnosed when the disease is still localized (ACS, 2004). Women who take birth control pills and smoke cigarettes are at increased risk for cardiovascular problems such as thrombophlebitis and pulmonary emboli.

Substance Abuse. Excessive use of alcohol and other drugs can impair tissue oxygenation in two ways. First, the person who chronically abuses substances often has a poor nutritional intake. With the resultant decrease in intake of iron-rich foods, hemoglobin production declines. Second, excessive use of alcohol and certain other drugs can depress the respiratory center, reducing the rate and depth of respiration and the amount of inhaled oxygen. Substance abuse by either smoking or inhaling, such as crack cocaine or inhaling fumes from paint or glue cans, causes direct injury to lung tissue that can lead to permanent lung damage and impaired oxygenation.

Stress Reduction. A continuous state of stress or severe anxiety increases the body's metabolic rate and the oxygen demand. The body responds to anxiety and other stresses with an increased rate and depth of respiration. Most people can adapt, but some, particularly those with chronic illnesses or acute life-threatening illnesses such as a myocardial infarction, cannot tolerate the oxygen demands associated with anxiety (see Chapter 30).

Environmental Factors
The environment can also influence oxygenation. The incidence of pulmonary disease is higher in smoggy, urban

areas than in rural areas. In addition, the client's workplace may increase the risk for pulmonary disease. Occupational pollutants include asbestos, talcum powder, dust, and airborne fibers. For example, farm workers in dry regions of the southwestern United States are at risk for coccidioidomycosis, a fungal disease caused by inhalation of spores of the airborne bacterium *Coccidioides immitis*. Asbestosis is an occupational lung disease that develops after exposure to asbestos. The lung in asbestosis is characterized by diffuse interstitial fibrosis, creating a restrictive lung disease. It can also cause pleural mesotheliomas and pleural plaques. Clients at risk for developing asbestosis include those working with textiles, fireproofing, or milling, or in the production of paints, plastics, or some prefabricated construction. Clients exposed to asbestos who also smoke are at increased risk of developing lung cancer.

Critical Thinking

Successful critical thinking requires a synthesis of knowledge, experience, information gathered from clients, critical thinking attitudes, and intellectual and professional standards. Clinical judgments require the nurse to anticipate the information necessary, analyze the data, and make decisions regarding the client's care. During assessment the nurse must consider all elements that build toward making an appropriate nursing diagnosis (Figure 39-6).

To understand the oxygen demands of a client and the ability of the client's body to meet those demands, the nurse integrates knowledge from nursing and other disciplines, previous experiences, and information gathered from clients. The use of professional standards, such as those developed by the Agency for Healthcare Research and Quality (AHRQ) (formerly the Agency for Health Care Policy and Research [AHCPR]), the Respiratory Nursing Society (RNS), the American Heart Association (AHA), the American Lung Association (ALA), the American Thoracic Society (ATS), and the American Nurses Association (ANA), provide valuable guidelines for care and management of clients with altered oxygenation.

Nursing Process

Assessment

The nursing assessment of a client's cardiopulmonary functioning includes an in-depth history of the client's normal and present cardiopulmonary function, past impairments in circulatory or respiratory functioning, and measures that the client uses to optimize oxygenation. The history should include a review of drug, food, and other allergies, such as pet dander, mold, and environmental triggers.

Physical examination of the client's cardiopulmonary status reveals the extent of existing signs and symptoms.

A review of laboratory and diagnostic test results provides valuable data on respiratory and ventilatory parameters.

Nursing History. The nursing history should focus on the client's ability to meet oxygen needs. The nursing history for cardiac function includes pain and characteristics of pain, dyspnea, fatigue, peripheral circulation, cardiac risk factors (see p. 1080), and the presence of past or concurrent cardiac conditions. The nursing history for respiratory function includes the presence of a cough, shortness of breath, wheezing, pain, environmental exposures, frequency of respiratory tract infections, pulmonary risk factors, past respiratory problems, current medication use, and smoking history or secondhand smoke exposure.

Pain. The presence of chest pain needs to be thoroughly evaluated with regard to location, duration, radiation, and frequency. Cardiac pain does not occur with respiratory variations and is most often on the left side of the chest and radiates to the left arm in men. Chest pain in women is much less definitive and may be a sensation of choking, breathlessness, or pain that radiates through to the back. Pericardial pain resulting from an inflammation of the pericardial sac is usually nonradiating and may occur with inspiration.

Pleuritic chest pain is peripheral and may radiate to the scapular regions. It is worsened by inspiratory maneuvers, such as coughing, yawning, and sighing. Pleuritic pain is often caused from an inflammation or infection in the pleural space and is described as knifelike, lasting from a minute to hours and always in association with inspiration.

Musculoskeletal pain may be present following exercise, rib trauma, and prolonged coughing episodes. This pain is also aggravated by inspiratory movements and may easily be confused with pleuritic chest pain.

Fatigue. Fatigue is a subjective sensation in which the client reports a loss of endurance. Fatigue in the client with cardiopulmonary alterations is often an early sign of a worsening of the chronic underlying process. To provide an objective measure of fatigue, the client may be asked to rate the fatigue on a scale of 0 to 10, with 10 being the worst level of fatigue and 0 representing no fatigue.

Smoking. It is important to determine clients' direct and secondary exposure to tobacco. Ask the client about any history of smoking; include the number of years smoked and the number of packages smoked per day. This is recorded as pack-year history. For example, if a client smoked two packs a day for 20 years, the client would have a 40 pack-year history (packages per day × years smoked).

It is also important to determine if the client is exposed to secondhand smoke from family or co-workers. Exposure to tobacco increases the client's risk for chronic lung or cardiac diseases.

Dyspnea. **Dyspnea** is a clinical sign of hypoxia and manifests as breathlessness. It is the subjective sensation of difficult or uncomfortable breathing (Box 39-6). Dyspnea is shortness of breath associated with exercise or excitement, but in some clients dyspnea may be present without any relation to activity or exercise. Dyspnea is associated with many conditions, such as pulmonary diseases, cardiovascular diseases, neuromuscular conditions, and ane-

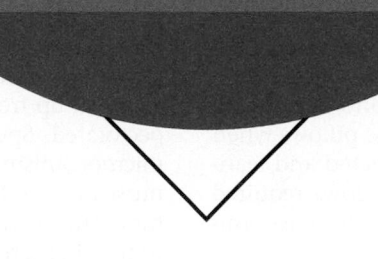

KNOWLEDGE

- Cardiac and respiratory anatomy and physiology
- Cardiopulmonary pathophysiology
- Clinical signs and symptoms of altered oxygenation
- Developmental factors affecting oxygenation
- Impact of lifestyle
- Environmental impact

EXPERIENCE

- Caring for clients with impaired oxygenation, activity intolerance, and respiratory infections
- Observations of changes in client respiratory patterns made during poor air quality days
- Personal experience with how a change in altitudes or physical conditioning affects respiratory patterns
- Personal experience with respiratory infections or cardiopulmonary alterations

Assessment

- Identify recurring and present signs and symptoms associated with the client's impaired oxygenation
- Determine the presence of risk factors that apply to the client
- Ask the client about use of medication
- Determine the client's normal and current activity status
- Determine the client's tolerance to activity

STANDARDS

- Apply intellectual standards of clarity, precision, specificity, and accuracy when obtaining a health history for the client with cardiopulmonary alterations

ATTITUDES

- Carry out the responsibility of obtaining correct information about the client
- Display confidence while assessing extent of client's respiratory alterations

FIGURE **39–6** Critical thinking model for oxygenation assessment.

mia. In addition, dyspnea may occur in the pregnant woman in the final months of pregnancy. Last, environmental factors, such as pollution, cold air, and smoking, may also cause or worsen dyspnea.

Dyspnea can be associated with clinical signs such as exaggerated respiratory effort, use of the accessory muscles of respiration, nasal flaring, and marked increases in the rate and depth of respirations (Jevon and Evans, 2001). The use of a visual analog scale (VAS) can help clients to make an objective assessment of their dyspnea. The visual analog scale is a 100-mm vertical line with end points of 0 and 10. Zero is equated with no dyspnea and 10 is equated

Research Highlight

Box 39-6

The Efficacy of Exercise Training in Clients With COPD

Research Focus

Clients with dyspnea often have a difficult time controlling their breathing. Assisting clients with dyspnea self-management may improve their quality of life. Knowing what interventions are helpful will be beneficial in developing a plan of care.

Research Abstract

The purpose of this study was to determine (1) whether exercise training adds benefit to dyspnea self-management and (2) if there is a response to supervised exercise training sessions in dyspnea, exercise performance, and health-related quality of life. Method: Subjects with COPD, age 58 to 74, with a forced expiratory volume at 1 second (FEV_1) ranging from 30.8% to 58.8% of predicted were randomized into three groups, in which one group had dyspnea self-management and supervised exercise training. Dyspnea self-management included individualized education about dyspnea management strategies, a home-walking prescription, and daily logs. Outcomes were measured at baseline and at every 2-month interval as part of a 1-year longitudinal randomized clinical trial using the Chronic Respiratory Questionnaire (CRQ), Shortness of Breath Questionnaire, and Baseline/Transitional Dyspnea Index. Outcomes measured included dyspnea during laboratory exercise and with activities of daily living, exercise performance and endurance testing, a 6-minute walk, and a quality of life survey (SF-36). Results: The group supervised which had exercise training had a significantly greater improvement in dyspnea management than the group that had no exercise training.

Evidence-Based Practice

- Supervised exercise (rehabilitation) programs improve dyspnea management for clients with COPD.
- Simply providing dyspnea self-management techniques information does not have a significant impact on clients' ability to manage their dyspnea.
- A prescription for exercise is not an effective tool in helping clients with COPD learn to manage their dyspnea.
- Individualized programs for dyspnea self-management lead to better management of the client's dyspnea and improvement in quality of life.

Reference

Stulbarg MS and others: Exercise training improves outcomes of a dyspnea self-management program, *J Cardiopulm Rehabil* 22(2):109, 2002.

---

with the worst breathlessness the client has experienced. Studies have validated the use of the visual analog scale to evaluate a client's dyspnea in the clinical setting. The nurse can evaluate the effectiveness of nursing interventions by monitoring the client's assessment of their dyspnea.

The nursing history of dyspnea includes the circumstances under which it occurred, such as with exertion, stress, or respiratory tract infection. The nurse also determines whether the client's perception of dyspnea affects the ability to lie flat. **Orthopnea** is an abnormal condition in which the person must use multiple pillows when lying down or must sit with the arms elevated and leaning forward to breathe. The number of pillows required for sleeping, such as two- or three-pillow orthopnea, usually quantifies the presence of orthopnea.

Cough. Cough is a sudden, audible expulsion of air from the lungs. The person breathes in, the glottis is partially closed, and the accessory muscles of expiration contract to expel the air forcibly. Coughing is a protective reflex to clear the trachea, bronchi, and lungs of irritants and secretions. The carina, the point of bifurcation of the right and left mainstem bronchus, is the most sensitive area for cough production. A cough is difficult to evaluate, and almost everyone has periods of coughing. Clients with a chronic cough tend to deny, underestimate, or minimize their coughing, often because they are so accustomed to it that they are unaware of how frequently it occurs.

Coughing is classified according to the time when the client most frequently coughs. Clients with chronic sinusitis may cough only in the early morning or immediately after rising from sleep. This clears the airway of mucus resulting from sinus drainage. Clients with chronic bronchitis generally produce sputum all day, although greater amounts are produced after rising from a semirecumbent or flat position. This is a result of the dependent accumulation of sputum in the airways and is associated with reduced mobility (see Chapter 36). Once the nurse determines that the client has a cough, it must be identified as productive or nonproductive and its frequency must be assessed. A productive cough results in sputum production, material coughed up from the lungs that may be swallowed or expectorated. Sputum contains mucus, cellular debris, and microorganisms, and it may contain pus or blood. The nurse must collect data about the type and quantity of sputum. The client is instructed to try to produce some sputum, being careful not to simply clear the throat to produce a sample of saliva. The nurse then inspects it for color, consistency, odor, and amount (Box 39-7).

If **hemoptysis** (bloody sputum) is reported, the nurse determines if it is associated with coughing and bleeding from the upper respiratory tract, from sinus drainage, or from the gastrointestinal tract **(hematemesis).** In addition, the hemoptysis should be described according to amount, color, and duration and whether it is mixed with sputum. When the client reports bloody or blood-tinged sputum, diagnostic tests, such as examination of sputum specimens, chest x-ray examinations, **bronchoscopy,** and other x-ray studies, should be performed.

Wheezing. **Wheezing** is characterized by a high-pitched musical sound caused by high-velocity movement of air through a narrowed airway. Wheezing may be associated with asthma, acute bronchitis, or pneumonia.

Box 39-7　Sputum Characteristics

Color

- Clear
- White
- Yellow
- Green
- Brown
- Red
- Streaked with blood

Changes in Color

- Same color throughout the day
- Clearing with coughing
- Progressively darker

Odor

- None
- Foul

Quantity

- Same as usual
- Increased
- Decreased

Consistency

- Frothy
- Watery
- Tenacious, thick

Presence of Blood

- Occasional
- Early morning
- Bright or dark red
- Blood tinged

Wheezing can occur on inspiration, expiration, or both. The nurse should determine any precipitating factors, such as respiratory infection, allergens, exercise, or stress.

Environmental or Geographical Exposures. Environmental exposure to many inhaled substances is closely linked with respiratory disease. The nurse should investigate exposures in the client's home and workplace. The most common environmental exposures in the home are cigarette smoke, carbon monoxide, and radon. The nurse should determine whether a client who is a nonsmoker is passively exposed to smoke.

Carbon monoxide poisoning can result from a blocked furnace flue or fireplace. The client may have vague complaints of general malaise, flulike symptoms, and excessive sleepiness. Clients are particularly at risk in the late fall when they turn the heat on or begin to use the fireplace again. Radon gas, a radioactive substance, enters homes through the ground. When homes are underventilated, this gas is not able to escape into the atmosphere and becomes trapped in the home.

An employment history is obtained to assess exposure to substances such as asbestos, coal, cotton fibers, fumes, or chemical inhalants. This is particularly important with middle-age and older adults, who may have worked in places without regulations to protect workers from carcinogens, such as asbestos.

Exposure to pathogens may occur during travel. Schistosomiasis can be acquired in Asia, Africa, the Caribbean, and South America. This is infection of a human with a species of fluke found in fresh water that has been contaminated by human feces. Coccidioidomycosis is a fungal disease caused by inhalation of *C. immitis,* a windborne spore carried on dust particles.

Respiratory Infections. A nursing history should contain information about the client's frequency and dura-

tion of respiratory tract infections. Although everyone occasionally experiences a cold, for some people it can result in bronchitis or pneumonia. On average, clients will have four colds per year. The nurse should determine if the client has had a pneumococcal or flu vaccine in the past and should also ask about any known exposure to tuberculosis and the results of the tuberculin skin test.

The client's risk for human immunodeficiency virus (HIV) infection is determined. Clients with a history of intravenous (IV) drug use and multiple unprotected sexual partners are at risk of developing HIV infection. Clients may not display any symptoms of HIV infection until they present with *Pneumocystis carinii* (PCP) or *Mycoplasma* pneumonia. Presentation with PCP or *Mycoplasma* pneumonia indicates a significant depression of the client's immune system and progression to acquired immunodeficiency syndrome (AIDS).

Allergies. When obtaining a history regarding the client's respiratory system it is important to inquire about airborne allergens. The client's allergic response may be watery eyes, sneezing, runny nose, or respiratory symptoms, such as cough or wheezing. When obtaining information ask the client specific questions about the type of allergens, response to these allergens, and successful and unsuccessful relief measures. In addition, determine what impact environmental air quality and secondhand smoke exposure has on the client's allergy and symptoms.

Safe nursing practice also includes obtaining information about food, drug, or insect sting allergies. These data are usually obtained on initial history and physical. However, the nurse should always double-check this information with the client, especially when obtaining information about respiratory allergens.

Health Risks. The nurse must also investigate familial risk factors, such as a family history of lung cancer or cardiovascular disease. Documentation should include which blood relatives have had the disease and their present level of health or age at time of death. Other family risk factors include the presence of infectious diseases, particularly tuberculosis. The nurse should determine who in the client's household has been infected and the status of treatment.

Medications. Another component of the nursing history should describe medications the client is using. These include prescribed, over-the-counter, folk medicine, herbal medicines, alternative therapies, and illicit drugs and substances. Such medications may have adverse effects by themselves or because of interactions with other drugs. A person using a prescribed bronchodilator drug, for example, may decide that using an over-the-counter inhalant as well will be beneficial. Many of these contain ephedrine or *ma huang,* a natural ephedrine, which acts like epinephrine. This product may react with the prescribed medication by potentiating or decreasing the effect of the prescribed medication. Clients taking warfarin (Coumadin) for blood thinning will prolong the prothrombin time (PT)/ international normalized ratio (INR) results if they are taking gingko biloba, garlic, or ginseng with the anitcoagulant. The drug interaction could precipitate a life-threatening bleed.

When clients are prescribed drugs for which toxic levels can be monitored by blood analyses, the nurse needs to review these laboratory values. Common drugs that can be monitored include theophylline (theophylline levels), digitalis preparations (digitalis levels), anticoagulants such as warfarin (Coumadin) (INR level), and phenobarbital (phenobarbital levels). Toxic effects of these medications can impair cardiopulmonary functioning.

It is important to determine if a client uses illicit drugs. Illicit drugs, particularly parenterally administered narcotics, which are often diluted with talcum powder, can cause pulmonary disorders resulting from the irritant effect of the powder on lung tissues.

As with all medication, the nurse assesses the client's knowledge and ability to use the six rights of medication administration (see Chapter 34). Of particular importance is the nurse's assessment of the client's understanding of potential side effects of the medications. Clients should be able to recognize adverse reactions and be aware of the dangers in combining prescribed medications with over-the-counter drugs.

Physical Examination. The physical examination performed to assess the client's level of tissue oxygenation includes evaluation of the cardiopulmonary system (Chapter 32). Special consideration should be given when assessing the older adult client because there are changes that occur with the aging process (Table 39-3). These changes may result in changes in the client's activity tolerance, level of fatigue, or transient changes in vital signs and may not be associated with a specific cardiopulmonary disease.

Inspection. Using inspection techniques, the nurse performs a head-to-toe observation of the client for skin and mucous membrane color, general appearance, level of consciousness, adequacy of systemic circulation, breathing patterns, and chest wall movement (Table 39-4). Any abnormalities should be investigated during palpation, percussion, and auscultation.

Inspection includes observations of the nails for clubbing. Clubbed nails, obliteration of the normal angle between the base of the nail and the skin, are seen in clients with prolonged oxygen deficiency, endocarditis, and congenital heart defects.

Table 39-3   Assessment Findings in the Aging Cardiopulmonary System

Function	Pathophysiological Change	Key Clinical Findings
Heart		
Muscle contraction	Thickening of the ventricular wall, increased collagen and decreased elastin in the heart muscle	Decreased cardiac output Diminished cardiac reserve
Blood flow	Heart valves become thicker and stiffer, more often in the mitral and aortic valves	Systolic ejection murmur
Conduction system	The SA node becomes fibrotic from calcification; the number of pacemaker cells in the SA node decreases	Increased PR, QRS, and Q-T intervals, decreased amplitude of the QRS complex
Arterial vessel compliance	Vessels become calcified, loss of arterial distensibility, decreased elastin in the vessel walls, more tortuous vessels	Hypertension, with an increase in systolic blood pressure Fluctuation in blood pressure
Lungs		
Breathing mechanics	Decreased chest wall compliance, loss of elastic recoil	Prolonged exhalation phase
	Decreased respiratory muscle mass/strength	Decreased vital capacity
Oxygenation	Increased ventilation/perfusion mismatch	Decreased PaO_2
	Decreased alveolar surface area	Decreased cardiac output
	Decreased carbon dioxide diffusion capacity	Slightly increased $PaCO_2$
Breathing control/breathing pattern	Decreased responsiveness of central and peripheral chemoreceptors to hypoxemia and hypercapnia	Increased respiratory rate Decreased tidal volume
Lung defense mechanisms	Decreased number of cilia	Decreased airway clearance
	Decreased IgA production and humoral and cellular immunity	Diminished cough reflex
Sleep and breathing	Decreased respiratory drive	Increased risk of aspiration and infection
	Decreased tone of upper airway muscles	Increased risk of arterial oxygen desaturation Snoring, obstructive sleep apnea

Observe the chest wall movement for retraction, sinking in of soft tissues of the chest between the intercostal spaces. Also observe for paradoxical breathing, asynchronous breathing, and the client's breathing pattern (Table 39-5). In paradoxical breathing the chest wall contracts during inspiration and expands during exhalation. Infants can experience sternal and substernal chest wall retractions with only a slight inspiratory effort due the pliability of the chest wall. Note the anteroposterior diameter of the chest wall. Conditions such as emphysema, advancing age, and COPD can cause the chest to assume a rounded shape.

Palpation. Palpation of the chest provides assessment data in several areas. It documents the type and amount of thoracic excursion, elicits any areas of tenderness, and can identify tactile fremitus, thrills, heaves, and the cardiac point of maximal impulse (PMI). Palpation also allows the nurse to feel for abnormal masses or lumps in the axilla and breast tissue. Palpation of the extremities provides data about the peripheral circulation, the pres-

ence and quality of peripheral pulses, skin temperature, color, and capillary refill (see Chapter 32).

Palpation should also include the feet and legs to assess the presence or absence of peripheral edema. Clients with alterations in their cardiac function, such as those with congestive heart failure or hypertension, often have pedal or lower extremity edema. Edema is graded from 1+ to 4+, depending on the depth of visible indentation after firm application of a finger (Chapter 32).

Palpation of the pulses in the neck and extremities is performed to assess arterial blood flow (see Chapter 32). A scale of 0 (absent pulse) to 3+ (full, bounding pulse) is used to describe what is palpated. The normal pulse is graded at 2+, and a weak, thready pulse is graded as 1+.

Percussion. Percussion allows the nurse to detect the presence of abnormal fluid or air in the lungs. It is also used to determine diaphragmatic excursion (see Chapter 32).

Auscultation. Auscultation enables the nurse to identify normal and abnormal heart and lung sounds (see

Table 39-4   Inspection of Cardiopulmonary Status

Abnormality	Cause
Eyes	
Xanthelasma (yellow lipid lesions on eyelids)	Hyperlipidemia
Corneal arcus (whitish opaque ring around junction of cornea and sclera)	Hyperlipidemia in young to middle adults, normal finding in older adults with arcus senilis
Pale conjunctivae	Anemia
Cyanotic conjunctivae	Hypoxemia
Petechiae on conjunctivae	Fat embolus or bacterial endocarditis
Mouth and Lips	
Cyanotic mucous membranes	Decreased oxygenation (hypoxia)
Pursed-lip breathing	Associated with chronic lung disease
Neck Veins	
Distention	Associated with right-sided heart failure
Nose	
Flaring nares	Air hunger, dyspnea
Chest	
Retractions	Increased work of breathing, dyspnea
Asymmetry	Chest wall injury
Skin	
Peripheral cyanosis	Vasoconstriction and diminished blood flow
Central cyanosis	Hypoxemia
Decreased skin turgor	Dehydration (normal finding in older adults as a result of decreased skin elasticity)
Dependent edema	Associated with right- and left-sided heart failure
Periorbital edema	Associated with kidney disease
Fingertips and Nail Beds	
Cyanosis	Decreased cardiac output or hypoxia
Splinter hemorrhages	Bacterial endocarditis
Clubbing	Chronic hypoxemia

From Potter PA, Weilitz PB: *Health assessment, pocket guide series,* St. Louis, 2003, Mosby.

Table 39-5	Assessment of Breathing Pattern
Pattern and Rate (Breaths per Minute)	**Clinical Significance**
Eupnea (16-20) 	Normal rate in the adult
Tachypnea (>35) 	Can result from anxiety or response to pain or fever, respiratory failure, anxiety, shortness of breath, or a respiratory infection. May lead to respiratory alkalosis, paresthesia, tetany, and confusion
Bradypnea (<10) 	Results from sleep, respiratory depression, drug overdose, or central nervous system (CNS) lesion
Apnea (Absence of respiration >15 seconds) 	May be intermittent, such as in sleep apnea, or prolonged, as in a respiratory arrest
Kussmaul's respirations (Usually >35, may be slow or normal) 	Tachypnea pattern associated with metabolic imbalance such as diabetic ketoacidosis, metabolic acidosis, or renal failure

Chapter 32). Auscultation of the cardiovascular system should include assessment for normal S_1 and S_2 sounds, the presence of abnormal S_3 and S_4 sounds (gallops), and murmurs or rubs. The examiner must identify the location, radiation, intensity, pitch, and quality of a murmur. Auscultation is also used to identify a bruit over the carotid arteries, abdominal aorta, and femoral arteries.

Auscultation of lung sounds involves listening for movement of air throughout all lung fields: anterior, posterior, and lateral. Adventitious breath sounds occur with collapse of a lung segment, fluid in a lung segment, or narrowing or obstruction of an airway. Auscultation also evaluates the client's response to interventions for improving the respiratory status.

Diagnostic Tests. There are a variety of diagnostic tests to monitor cardiopulmonary functioning. Some of these tests can be obtained through screening, simple blood specimens, x-ray films, or other noninvasive means. One such screening mechanism is tuberculosis (TB) skin testing (Box 39-8). This is a simple test, which is usually required for health care workers, restaurant employees, students entering schools, teachers and other school employees, and in residents of long-term care facilities (Centers for Disease Control and Prevention [CDC], 2002).

In contrast, invasive diagnostic tests, such as a thoracentesis, are quite painful. Tables 39-6 through 39-9 summarize diagnostic testing used in the assessment and evaluation of the client with cardiopulmonary alterations. When reviewing results of pulmonary function

Box 39-8	**Tuberculosis Skin Testing**

- Skin testing is used to determine the presence of *Mycobaterium* tuberculosis.
- The antigen is injected intradermally (see Chapter 34). Afterward, the injection site may be circled, and the client is instructed not to wash it off.
- Tuberculin skin tests are read at 72 hours.
- *Positive results:* A palpable, elevated, hardened area around the injection site, caused by edema and inflammation from the antigen-antibody reaction, measured in millimeters.
- Reddened flat areas are ***not*** positive reactions and are not measured.
- TB testing in older adults is less reliable (see Box 39-4, p. 1080).

studies, the nurse must learn that there are expected variations in clients of different cultures. These changes are due to structural variations in chest wall size in these clients (Box 39-9).

Whether a diagnostic procedure is painful depends on the client's tolerance for pain (see Chapter 42). The nurse can reduce the client's anxiety by explaining the procedure and telling the client what to expect. The client must understand the importance of following instructions, such as holding the breath as requested and of not coughing during the procedure. After any procedure the

Table 39-6   Cardiopulmonary Diagnostic Blood Studies

Test and Normal Values	Interpretation
Complete Blood Count (CBC)	
Normal values for a CBC vary with age and gender	A CBC determines the number and type of red and white blood cells per cubic millimeter of blood.
Cardiac Enzymes	
MB-CK 10-13 units/L; a serial MB-CK with 50% increase between two samples 4 hours apart, or a single MB-CK elevation twofold is diagnostic for an acute myocardial infarction	Cardiac enzymes are used to diagnose acute myocardial infarcts.
Plasma Cardiac Troponin I	
<0.3 mg/ml	Value elevates within 12 hours of a cardiac event and remains elevated for 10-14 days.
Plasma Cardiac Troponin T	
<0.2 mg/ml	
Serum Electrolytes	
Potassium (K$^+$) 3.5-5 mmol/L	Clients on diuretic therapy are at risk for hypokalemia (low potassium). Clients receiving angiotensin-converting enzyme (ACE) inhibitors are at risk for hyperkalemia (elevated potassium).
Cholesterol	
Fasting cholesterol ≤200 mg/100 ml	Contributing factors include sedentary lifestyle with intake of saturated fatty acids, familial hypercholesterolemia.
LDL cholesterol (bad cholesterol) ≤130 mg/100 ml	High LDL cholesterol (hypercholesterolemia) is caused by excessive intake of saturated fatty acids, dietary cholesterol intake, and obesity. Familial hypercholesterolemia and hyperlipidemia are also contributing factors, as well as hypothyroidism, nephrotic syndrome, and diabetes mellitus.
HDL cholesterol (good cholesterol) >40 mg/100 ml	Low HDL cholesterol is caused by factors such as cigarette smoking, obesity, lack of regular exercise, beta-adrenergic blocking agents, genetic disorders of HDL metabolism, hypertriglyceridemia, and type 2 diabetes.
Triglycerides ≤130 mg/100 ml	Obesity, excessive alcohol intake, diabetes mellitus, beta-adrenergic blocking agents, and familial hypertriglyceridemia cause hypertriglyceridemia.

Table 39-7   Cardiac Function Diagnostic Tests

Test	Significance
12-Lead electrocardiogram (ECG)	Graphic recording of the electrical activity of the heart used to detect abnormal electrical activity and the electrical position of the heart. The ECG includes 12 leads: I, II, III, AVR, AVL, AVF, V$_{1-6}$. Provides a 360-degree view of the heart.
Holter monitor	Portable ECG worn by the client. The test produces a continuous ECG tracing over a period of time. Clients keep a diary of activity, noting when they experience rapid heartbeats or dizziness. Evaluation of the ECG recording along with the diary provides information about the heart's electrical activity during activities of daily living.
ECG exercise stress test	ECG is monitored while the client walks on a treadmill at a specified speed and duration of time. Used to evaluate the cardiac response to physical stress. The test is not a valuable tool for evaluation of cardiac response in women due to an increased false-positive finding.
Thallium stress test	An ECG stress test with the addition of talliuym-201 injected IV. Determines coronary blood flow changes with increased activity.
Electrophysiological study (EPS)	Invasive measure of intracardiac electrical pathways. Provides more specific information about difficult-to-treat dysrhythmias. Assess adequacy of antidysrhythmic medication.
Echocardiography	Noninvasive measure of heart structure and heart wall motion. Graphically demonstrates overall cardiac performance.
Scintigraphy	Radionuclide angiography. Used to evaluate cardiac structure, myocardial perfusion and contractility.
Cardiac catheterization and angiography	Used to visualize cardiac chambers, valves, the great vessels, and coronary arteries. Pressures and volumes within the four chambers of the heart are also measured.

Measurement and Normal Values	Interpretation
Pulmonary Function Tests	
Basic ventilation studies (see Table 39-9, p. 1091). Pulmonary functions are variable by ethnic group (see Box 39-9, p. 1091).	Determines the ability of the lungs to efficiently exchange oxygen and carbon dioxide. Used to differentiate pulmonary obstructive from restrictive disease.
Peak Expiratory Flow Rate (PEFR)	
The point of highest flow during maximal expiration. Normal is based on age and body weight.	The PEFR reflects changes in large airway sizes and is an excellent predictor of overall airway resistance in the client with asthma. Daily measurement is used for early detection of asthma exacerbations.
Arterial Blood Gas	
pH 7.35-7.45 $PaCO_2$ 35-45 mm Hg PaO_2 80-100 mm Hg SaO_2 95-100%	Measures the hydrogen ion concentration (pH), partial pressure of carbon dioxide, partial pressure of oxygen, oxygen concentration.
Oximetry	
SpO_2 98%-100%	Accuracy is directly related to the perfusion of the probe area, a systolic blood pressure >90 mm Hg, and the hemoglobin level. Decreased levels correlate well with arterial oxygen levels and are used to trend oxygenation over time.
Chest X-Ray Examination	
Clear with normal bony structures	Usually posteroanterior and lateral films are taken to adequately visualize all of the lung fields. A radiograph of the thorax is used to observe the lung fields for fluid (e.g., pneumonia), masses (i.e., lung cancer), fractures, pneumothoraxes, and other abnormal processes (i.e., tuberculosis).
Bronchoscopy	
Normal airways without masses, pus, or foreign bodies	Visual examination of the tracheobronchial tree through a narrow, flexible fiberoptic bronchoscope. Performed to obtain fluid, sputum, or biopsy samples; remove mucous plugs or foreign bodies.
Lung Scan	
Normal lung structure with masses	Used to identify abnormal masses by size and location. Identification of masses is used in planning therapy and treatments.
Thoracentesis	
Thoracentesis is a surgical perforation of the chest wall and pleural space with a needle to aspirate fluid for diagnostic or therapeutic purposes or to remove a specimen for biopsy. The procedure is performed using aseptic technique and local anesthetic. The client usually sits upright with the anterior thorax supported by pillows or an over-bed table.	Specimen of plural fluid is obtained for cytological examination. The results may indicate an infection or neoplastic disease. Identification of infection or a type of cancer is important in determining a plan of care.
Throat Cultures	
Normal: Clear	Obtained by swabbing the oropharynx and tonsillar regions with a sterile swab to determine the presence of pathogenic microorganisms. Positive results are used to determine the correct antibiotic for treatment based on the organism cultured.
Sputum Specimens	
Normal: Negative Sputum culture and sensitivity (C and S) Sputum for AFB Sputum for cytology	Obtained to identify a specific microorganism, organism growing in the sputum. Identifies drug resistance and sensitivities. Used to screen for the presence of acid-fast bacillus (AFB) for detection of TB by early morning specimens on 3 consecutive days. Obtained to identify abnormal lung cancer. Differentiates type of cancer cells (small cell, oat cell, large cell).

Table 39-9   Pulmonary Function Measurements

Measurement	Normal Range	Clinical Significance
Tidal Volume (V$_t$)		
Volume of air (ml) inhaled or exhaled per breath	5-10 ml/kg	Decreased in restrictive lung disease and older client
Residual Volume (RV)		
Volume of air (ml) left in lungs after a maximal exhalation	1000-1200 ml	Increased in clients with COPD and older clients due to decreased respiratory muscle mass, strength, elastic recoil, and chest wall compliance
Functional Residual Capacity (FRC)		
Volume of air (ml) left in lungs after a normal exhalation	2000-2400 ml	Increased in clients with COPD and older clients due to decreased respiratory muscle mass, strength, elastic recoil, and chest wall compliance
Vital Capacity (VC)		
Volume of air (ml) exhaled after a maximal inhalation	4500-4800 ml	Decreased in pulmonary edema, atelectasis, and changes associated with aging
Total Lung Capacity (TLC)		
Total volume of air (ml) in lungs following a maximal inhalation	5000-6000 ml	Decreased in restrictive lung disease; increased in obstructive lung disease

Cultural Aspects of Care   Box 39-9

Pulmonary functions vary between cultures as a result of the variation in chest size. Whites have the largest chest volumes, followed by African-Americans, Asian-Americans, and Native Americans. The variations in the chest size affect the forced expiratory volume (FEV$_1$), forced vital capacity (FVC), and the FEV$_1$/FVC ratio.

	FEV$_1$ (L)	FVC (L)	FEV$_1$/FVC (%)
White	3.22	4.3	74.4
African-American	2.85	3.7	76.7
Asian-American	2.53	3.27	77.0
Native American	2.53	3.27	77.0

Modified from Lueckenotte AG: *Gerontologic nursing*, ed 2, St. Louis, 2000, Mosby.

nurse monitors the client for signs of changes in cardiopulmonary functioning, sudden shortness of breath, pain, oxygen desaturation, and anxiety.

Client Expectations. The nurse asks clients what they expect from the encounter and what their priority is for management of their health. Identifying expectations involves clients in the decision-making process and allows them to participate in their care and know what will happen to them. For example, planning a smoking cessation or weight reduction program for a client who is not ready for the change will be frustrating for both the client and the nurse. Short-term realistic goals are established that build to a larger goal. For example, reducing the fat in the

client's diet may start out with replacing food such as whole milk with 2% milk and gradually introducing skim milk. A sudden change from whole to skim milk will most likely fail, because the change is too much. A plan for adding exercise to the client's lifestyle may start with a commitment to exercise once a week for 20 minutes, or the client may commit to a weight reduction plan of 5 pounds per month.

It is important to remember that the goals and expectations of the nurse may not always coincide with those of the client. By addressing the client's concerns and expectations, the nurse will establish a relationship that can address other health care goals and expected outcomes. Knowing clients' mind-set and respecting their wishes will go a long way in helping clients to make significant lifestyle changes to benefit their health.

Nursing Diagnosis

Clients with an altered level of oxygenation can have nursing diagnoses that are primarily from a cardiovascular or pulmonary origin. Each nursing diagnosis is based on specific defining characteristics and the related etiology (Box 39-10). The nurse uses the information gathered in the nursing assessment to identify and cluster the defining characteristics. The clustered defining characteristics support the nursing diagnosis.

Nursing diagnoses appropriate for the client with alterations in oxygenation include, but are not limited to, the following:

- Activity intolerance
- Risk for activity intolerance
- Ineffective airway clearance

Nursing Diagnostic Process

Box 39-10

Assessment Activities	Defining Characteristics	Nursing Diagnosis
Ask client or family about client's mood, attentiveness, memory, and activity level.	Confusion Decreased activity Fatigue Irritability Restlessness Sleepiness	Impaired gas exchange related to decreased lung expansion
Observe client's respirations.	Dyspnea Impaired gas exchange related to collapsed alveoli Nasal flaring Tachypnea Use of accessory muscles	
Inspect skin and mucous membranes.	Diaphoresis Pallor Moist skin Abnormal lung sounds may be present	
Auscultate chest.	Decreased respiratory excursion Distant lung sounds	

- Anxiety
- Ineffective breathing pattern
- Decreased cardiac output
- Impaired comfort
- Impaired verbal communication
- Ineffective individual coping
- Fatigue
- Fear
- Risk for imbalanced fluid volume
- Impaired gas exchange
- Ineffective health maintenance
- Risk for infection
- Deficient (specify) knowledge
- Risk for impaired skin integrity
- Disturbed sleep pattern
- Ineffective tissue perfusion
- Impaired spontaneous ventilation

Planning

During planning the nurse again synthesizes information from multiple sources (Figure 39-7). Critical thinking ensures that the client's plan of care integrates all that the nurse knows about the individual, as well as key critical thinking elements. Professional standards are especially important to consider when the nurse develops a plan of care. These standards often establish scientifically proven guidelines for selecting effective nursing interventions.

Goals and Outcomes. The nurse develops an individualized plan of care for each nursing diagnosis (see care plan). The nurse and client set realistic expectations for care. Goals are to be individualized and realistic with measurable outcomes.

Clients with impaired oxygenation require a nursing care plan directed toward meeting the actual or potential oxygenation needs of the client. Individual outcomes are derived from client-centered needs. For example, the goal of maintaining a patent airway can be evaluated by specific outcomes for the client. These might include the following expected outcomes:

- Client's lungs are clear to auscultation.
- Client achieves maintenance and promotion of bilateral lung expansion.
- Client coughs productively.
- Tissue oxygenation (SaO_2) is maintained or improved.

Often a client with cardiopulmonary disease has multiple nursing diagnoses (Figure 39-8). In this case the nurse identifies when goals or outcomes apply to more than one diagnosis. The presence of multiple diagnoses also makes priority setting a critical activity.

Setting Priorities. The client's level of health, age, lifestyle, and environmental risks affect the level of tissue oxygenation. Clients with severe impairments in oxygenation frequently require nursing interventions in multiple areas. The nurse must consider what is the most important goal to reach in the limited amount of time the client is seen in the hospital or primary care setting. For example, in an acute care setting maintaining a patent airway has a higher priority than improving the client's exercise tolerance. The need for a patent airway is an immediate need, whereas as the client's level of oxygen improves the tolerance to activity will improve. In a second example, when caring for a client who has an abdominal incision, pain control may have a greater priority than coughing and deep breathing. Again, in this situation controlling the client's pain ultimately will facilitate coughing and deep breathing.

However, in a community-based or primary setting, the priority may focus on smoking cessation, exercise, and/or diet modifications. Both the client and nurse need to be focused on the same goal and expected outcomes to be successful. In addition to being individualized, each goal should be realistic and attainable for the client.

KNOWLEDGE

- Role of other health care professionals in caring for the client with impaired oxygenation
- Role of community support groups in assisting the client to manage cardiopulmonary disease
- Knowledge of effects of pulmonary interventions

EXPERIENCE

- Previous client responses to planned nursing therapies for impaired oxygenation

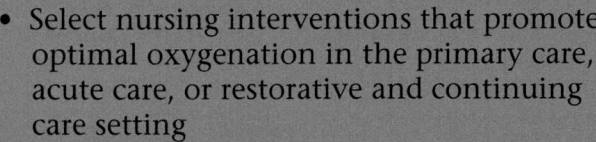

Planning

- Select nursing interventions that promote optimal oxygenation in the primary care, acute care, or restorative and continuing care setting
- Consult with other health care professionals as needed
- Involve the client and family in designing the plan of care

STANDARDS

- Individualize therapies to client's needs
- Apply established pulmonary and cardiac rehabilitation guidelines
- Apply established nursing care guidelines for care of the client with cardiopulmonary disease (e.g., protocols, care paths)

ATTITUDES

- Display confidence when selecting interventions
- Use creativity when developing home care strategies for the client's disease management
- Demonstrate responsibility and accountability when delegating care for client

FIGURE 39–7 Critical thinking model for oxygenation planning.

Continuity of Care. The time a nurse gets to spend with the client in any setting is limited. Therefore the nurse must rely on collaboration with family members, colleagues, and other specialists to accomplish the goals and outcomes that have been determined. Some clients may need to improve their exercise and activity tolerance; for some clients their continuity of care may involve enrolling in a community-based cardiopulmonary rehabilitation program. Another client may have the same health care need but is unable to leave the home, and home physical therapy is needed.

Collaboration with physical therapists, nutritionists, and community-based nurses may be valuable for a client with congestive heart failure or chronic lung conditions. These professionals work with the client and the community to optimize resources to assist the client in at-

taining the highest level of wellness. In addition, professionals can help to identify community resources and support systems for both the client and family in preventing and managing symptoms related to cardiopulmonary diseases.

Implementation

Nursing interventions for promoting and maintaining adequate oxygenation include independent nursing actions such as health promotion and prevention behaviors, positioning, and coughing techniques. Interdependent or dependent interventions include oxygen therapy, lung inflation techniques, hydration, medication administration, and chest physiotherapy.

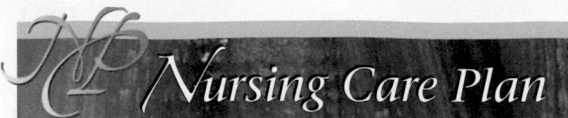

Nursing Care Plan

Respiratory Alterations

Assessment

Mr. Edwards, an older adult with a history of COPD, comes to the primary care office with complaints of continued cough-ing. He continues to smoke 2 to 3 cigarettes a day, an improvement from his previous 10 to 15 per day.

Assessment Activities	Findings/Defining Characteristics
Ask Mr. Edwards how long he has had this cough.	He replies, "I have a morning cough every day, but this cough is different. It started about a week ago."
Ask Mr. Edwards what is different about this cough.	He replies, "My ribs are getting sore. I can't cough up anything, my mouth is dry, and I have become more fatigued over the past week."
Observe Mr. Edwards's skin and mucous membranes.	His skin and mucous membranes are dry.
Auscultate lung fields.	Abnormal lung sounds in the upper lobes. The lower lobes are clear.
Ask Mr. Edwards how many glasses of water he drinks daily.	Over last week has drank 2-3 glasses a day.
Ask Mr. Edwards to produce a sputum sample.	He is unable to produce a sputum sample for evaluation.

Nursing Diagnosis: Ineffective airway clearance related to retained secretions and reduced fluid intake.

Planning

Goal	Expected Outcomes*
	Respiratory Status: Airway Patency
Client will be able to effectively clear secretions.	Lung sounds will be normal in 48 hours.
	Sputum will be thin, white, and watery.
	Respiratory rate will be within 20 to 24 breaths per minute in 48 hours.
	Client will be able to clear airway by coughing.
Client will increase oral hydration to 1000 ml of water every 24 hours.	Oral mucous membranes will be pink and moist.
	Client will verbalize that his mouth is not dry.
	Client will notice an increase in ease of sputum production.
	Client will report that his sputum is thin, white, and watery.

*Outcome classification labels from Moorhead S, Johnson M, Maas M: *Nursing outcomes classification (NOC),* ed 3, St. Louis, 2004, Mosby.

Interventions†

Airway Management

Rationale

Interventions†	Rationale
• Increase fluids to 1000 ml in 24 hours if not contraindicated by cardiovascular disease (Lewis and others, 2000).	Fluids help to liquefy secretions and promote ease of removal (Snow and others, 2001). Fluids will relieve oral mucosa and skin dryness.
• Have client deep breathe and cough every 2 hours 4 to 5 times (Lewis and others, 2000).	Retained secretions predisposes client to atelectasis and pneumonia (Day and others, 2002).
• Teach client effective cough techniques.	Coughing techniques will help to clear the airway effectively and decrease fatigue from ineffective coughing (Snow and others, 2001).
• Consider chest physiotherapy (CPT) if there is evidence of infiltrates on chest x-ray film.	Standards for CPT include sputum production greater than 30 ml/day or infiltrates on chest x-ray film

†Intervention classification labels from Dochterman JM, Bulechek GM: *Nursing interventions classification (NIC),* ed 4, St. Louis, 2004, Mosby.

Evaluation

Nursing Actions	Client Response/Finding	Achievement of Outcome
Ask Mr. Edwards if he can deep breathe and cough.	Mr. Edwards reports, "It is easier to cough up my secretions now."	Client is able to clear airway by coughing.
Assess the chest for adventitious lung sounds.	Mr. Edwards reports that he has not heard any wheezing or rattling in his chest.	Lungs clear to auscultation in all fields.
Assess respiratory rate.	No use of accessory muscles of respiration. Normal breathing pattern and respiratory rate.	Respiratory rate is between 20 and 24 breaths per minute.
Assess client's level of hydration.	Mucous membranes are moist. Mr. Edwards reports, that "My mouth isn't so dry anymore."	Oral mucous membranes are pink and moist.
Observe appearance of sputum.	Sputum is thin, white, and watery.	Sputum is thin, white, and watery.

Concept Map

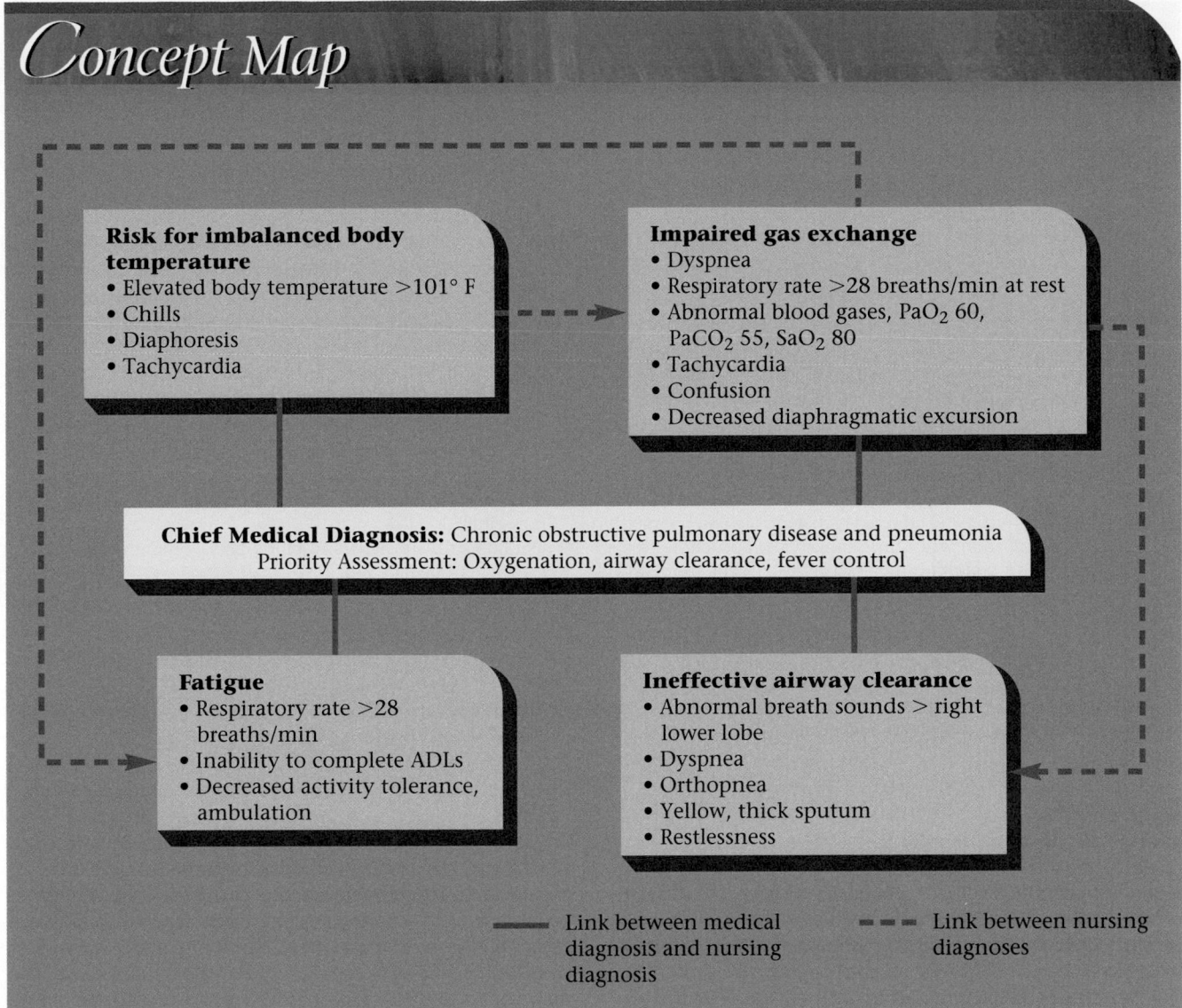

Risk for imbalanced body temperature
- Elevated body temperature >101° F
- Chills
- Diaphoresis
- Tachycardia

Impaired gas exchange
- Dyspnea
- Respiratory rate >28 breaths/min at rest
- Abnormal blood gases, PaO_2 60, $PaCO_2$ 55, SaO_2 80
- Tachycardia
- Confusion
- Decreased diaphragmatic excursion

Chief Medical Diagnosis: Chronic obstructive pulmonary disease and pneumonia
Priority Assessment: Oxygenation, airway clearance, fever control

Fatigue
- Respiratory rate >28 breaths/min
- Inability to complete ADLs
- Decreased activity tolerance, ambulation

Ineffective airway clearance
- Abnormal breath sounds > right lower lobe
- Dyspnea
- Orthopnea
- Yellow, thick sputum
- Restlessness

——— Link between medical diagnosis and nursing diagnosis

– – – Link between nursing diagnoses

FIGURE **39–8** Concept map for a client with chronic obstructive pulmonary disease and pneumonia.

Health Promotion. Maintaining the client's optimal level of health is important in reducing the number and/or severity of respiratory symptoms. Prevention of respiratory infections is foremost in maintaining optimal health. Providing cardiopulmonary-related health information (Box 39-11) is an important nursing responsibility.

Vaccinations. Annual influenza vaccines are recommended for older clients and clients with chronic illnesses. This includes clients older than 65 years of age; clients of any age with chronic disease of the heart, lung, or kidneys; clients with diabetes; and clients with immunosuppression or severe forms of anemia. The vaccine is also recommended for people in close or frequent contact with anyone in the high-risk groups. The vaccine has been shown to be 70% to 90% effective in healthy young adults (Zimmerman and Ball, 2001). The vaccine is most effective in reducing the severity of ill-

ness and the risk of serious complications and death. Studies have shown a 70% reduction in the number of older adults requiring hospitalization for pneumonia and an 85% reduction in mortality for those not in nursing homes (CDC, 2002).

Influenza in the United States occurs from November until April. The incidence is usually very low until December and peaks between January and March. Vaccines should be given between September and mid-November. It takes about 1 to 2 weeks after vaccination for antibody development and protection that lasts for approximately 6 months in most adults (CDC, 2002).

The value of vaccination of immunocompromised clients is not completely understood. HIV-positive clients may receive the flu vaccine; however, they may require a second vaccine to gain protection. Persons who should not be vaccinated include those with a known hypersensitivity to eggs or other components of the vaccine and

Client Teaching

Box 39-11

Cardiovascular Disease

Objectives

- Client will be able to verbalize risk factors associated with cardiovascular disease.
- Client will be able to demonstrate health promotion behaviors.

Teaching Strategies

- Teach risk factors that cannot be changed and those that can, such as smoking, alcohol intake, high blood pressure, and blood cholesterol levels.
- Educate the client about other risk factors for cardiovascular disease, such as diabetes, obesity, physical inactivity, stress, and oral contraceptives.
- Educate the client about the importance of regular blood pressure monitoring and adherence to a medication regimen.
- Educate client about the importance of blood cholesterol monitoring and maintaining a fasting total cholesterol and triglyceride level less than 200 mg/100 ml.
- Educate the client about low-fat, low-salt, and calorie-appropriate diets. Provide sample menus.
- Discuss strategies for stress reduction, such as realistic goal setting, relaxation techniques, exercise, proper diet, and rest.

- Educate client about the benefits of exercising for 1 hour daily to help reduce weight and help lower blood pressure.
- Set realistic goals with the client for follow-up for blood pressure monitoring.
- Determine the cultural, religious, or economic issues that may interfere with client's ability to complete the plan of care.
- Determine age-related issues that may prevent client from achieving the goals.

Evaluation

- Have client verbalize his or her risk factors for cardiovascular disease.
- Ask client to verbalize what he or she will do to achieve some balance in his or her life and reduce stress.
- Client can list his or her medications, use, and dosage and reports that he or she has been taking the medication as prescribed.
- Obtain client's weight and blood pressure and measure for presence of pedal edema.
- Monitor the serum cholesterol (total, high- and low-density lipids) and triglyceride levels.
- Client returns for follow-up as scheduled.

Modified from Canobbio MM: *Mosby's handbook of patient teaching,* St. Louis, 2000, Mosby.

---

adults with an acute febrile illness. The vaccines are formulated annually based on worldwide surveillance data.

Pneumococcal vaccine is recommended for clients at increased risk of developing pneumonia, those with chronic illnesses or immunosuppression (such as HIV/AIDS), those living in special environments such as nursing homes or the American Indian population, and clients over the age of 65. HIV-positive clients can also receive the pneumococcal vaccination. Revaccination has been recommended for clients at 65 years of age (CDC, 2002).

Both the influenza vaccine and pneumococcal vaccine can be used in pregnant women after the first trimester. However, in all cases it is important to consult the client's obstetrician before administering either vaccine.

Healthy Lifestyle Behavior. Identification and elimination of risk factors for cardiopulmonary disease is an important part of primary care. Clients are encouraged to eat a healthy low-fat, high-fiber diet; monitor their cholesterol, triglyceride, high-density lipoprotein (HDL), and low-density lipoprotein (LDL) levels; reduce stress; exercise; and maintain a body weight in proportion to their height.

Elimination of cigarettes and other tobacco, reduction of pollutants, monitoring of air quality, and adequate hydration are additional healthy behaviors. Clients should be encouraged to examine their habits and make changes to achieve their goals.

Exercise is a key factor in promoting and maintaining a healthy heart and lungs. Clients should be encouraged

to exercise 3 to 4 times a week for 20 to 30 minutes. Aerobic exercise is necessary to improve lung function, strengthen muscles, and achieve the desired outcome. Walking is one of the most efficient ways to achieve a good aerobic workout. Many shopping malls have programs that allow people to enter the mall before the shops open and use the enclosed area for walking. Some even have measured the distances to help clients plan their activity and measure their progress. Clients should be taught how to take their pulse and pace themselves. It is better to walk 15 minutes every day than to walk to exhaustion to achieve a goal. Clients should plan a time interval and walk for the designated time. Gradually they will notice that the distance increases as their endurance and fitness improve.

Clients with cardiopulmonary alterations need to minimize their risk for infection, especially during the winter months. Clients are taught to avoid large, crowded places, keep their mouth and nose covered, and be sure to dress warmly, including a scarf, hat, and gloves. This is especially important during the peak of the influenza season.

Clients with known cardiac disease and those with multiple risk factors should be cautioned to avoid exertion in cold weather. Shoveling snow is especially risky and has been known to precipitate a cardiac event in many clients. Other activities such as hanging holiday lights and decorations in the extreme cold can precipitate chest pain and bronchospasm. Clients are advised to avoid alcohol, because it blunts the respiratory drive when used in excess and may contribute to exposure to the cold by making the client feel warm when the client is really not protected.

Clients should also be taught to plan for the hot summer months. Activities should be limited to early in the day or late in the evening, when temperatures are lower. Care should be taken to maintain adequate hydration and sodium intake, especially in those clients who are taking diuretics. Caffeinated and alcoholic beverages should be limited or avoided completely, because they act as diuretics and can contribute to dehydration.

Environmental Pollutants. Avoiding exposure to secondhand smoke is essential to maintaining optimal cardiopulmonary function. Most businesses and restaurants now ban smoking or have separate areas designated as smoking areas. If clients are exposed to secondhand smoke in their home environments, counseling and support may be necessary to assist the smoker in successful smoking cessation or alterations in behavior patterns, such as smoking outside.

Exposure to chemicals and pollutants in the work environment must also be considered. Clients such as farmers, painters, carpenters, and others benefit from the use of particulate filter masks to reduce inhalation of particles.

Acute Care. Clients with acute pulmonary illnesses require nursing interventions directed toward halting the pathological process, as with a respiratory tract infection, shortening the duration and severity of the illness, such as hospitalization with pneumonia, and preventing complications from the illness or treatments, such as nosocomial infection resulting from invasive procedures.

Dyspnea Management. Dyspnea is difficult to quantify and to treat. Treatment modalities need to be individualized for each client, and more than one therapy is usually implemented. The underlying process that causes or worsens dyspnea must be treated and stabilized initially, and then four additional therapies—pharmacological measures, oxygen therapy, physical techniques, and psychosocial techniques—are implemented. Pharmacological agents may include bronchodilators, steroids, mucolytics, and low-dose antianxiety medications. Oxygen therapy can reduce dyspnea associated with exercise. Physical techniques, such as cardiopulmonary reconditioning through exercise, breathing techniques, and cough control, can help to reduce dyspnea. Relaxation techniques, biofeedback, and meditation are physiological measures that can lessen the sensation of dyspnea.

Airway Maintenance. The airway is patent when the trachea, bronchi, and large airways are free from obstructions. Airway maintenance requires adequate hydration to prevent thick, tenacious secretions. Proper coughing techniques remove secretions and keep the airway open. A variety of interventions, such as suctioning, chest physiotherapy, and nebulizer therapy, assist the client in managing alterations in airway clearance.

Mobilization of Pulmonary Secretions. The ability of a client to mobilize pulmonary secretions may make the difference between a short-term illness and a long recovery involving complications. Nursing interventions that promote mobilization of pulmonary secretions assist the client in achieving and maintaining a clear airway and help promote lung expansion and gas exchange.

Humidification. **Humidification** is the process of adding water to gas. Temperature is the most important factor affecting the amount of water vapor a gas can hold. The percentage of water in the gas in relation to its capacity for water is the relative humidity. Air or oxygen with a high relative humidity keeps the airways moist and helps loosen and mobilize pulmonary secretions. Humidification is necessary for clients receiving oxygen therapy at greater than 4 L/min. Bubbling oxygen through water can add humidity to the oxygen delivered to the upper airways, as with a nasal catheter, nasal cannula, or face mask. The humidity tent is used for infants and children with illnesses such as croup and tracheitis to liquefy secretions and help reduce fever. The nebulizer at the top of the humidity tent must remain filled with water to prevent nonhumidified air or oxygen from entering the tent. Air in the humidity tent can become cool and fall below 20° C (68° F), causing the child to become chilled. The nurse monitors the child's body temperature, as well as respiratory status. Children in humidity tents require frequent changes of clothing and bed linen to remain warm and dry.

Nebulization. **Nebulization** is a process of adding moisture or medications to inspired air by mixing particles of varying sizes with the air. A nebulizer uses the aerosol principle to suspend a maximum number of water drops or particles of the desired size in inspired air. The moisture added to the respiratory system through nebulization improves clearance of pulmonary secretions. Nebulization is often used for administration of bronchodilators and mucolytic agents.

When the thin layer of fluid that supports the mucous layer over the cilia is allowed to dry, the cilia are damaged and cannot adequately clear the airway. Humidification through nebulization enhances mucociliary clearance, the body's natural mechanism for removing mucus and cellular debris from the respiratory tract.

The major types of nebulizers are the jet-aerosol nebulizer and the ultrasonic nebulizer. A jet-aerosol nebulizer uses gas under pressure, and the ultrasonic nebulizer uses high-frequency vibrations to break up the water or medication into fine drops or particles. When inspired with air or administered oxygen, the drops of particles are then deposited throughout the tracheobronchial tree.

Chest Physiotherapy. **Chest physiotherapy (CPT)** is a group of therapies used in combination to mobilize pulmonary secretions. These therapies include postural drainage, chest percussion, and vibration. Chest physiotherapy should be followed by productive coughing and suctioning of the client who has a decreased ability to cough. Chest physiotherapy is recommended for clients who produce greater than 30 ml of sputum per day or have evidence of atelectasis by chest x-ray examination. This procedure can be safely used with infants and young children; however, conditions and diseases unique to children may at times contraindicate this procedure. Chest physiotherapy is used for a select group of clients. Box 39-12 describes the guidelines to determine if CPT is indicated for the client.

Guidelines for Chest Physiotherapy

Nursing care and selection of chest physiotherapy (CPT) skills are based on specific assessment findings. The following guidelines help the nurse in physical assessment and subsequent decision making:

- Know the client's normal range of vital signs. Conditions such as atelectasis and pneumonia requiring CPT can affect vital signs. The degree of change is related to the level of hypoxia, overall cardiopulmonary status, and tolerance to activity.
- Know the client's medications. Certain medications, particularly diuretics and antihypertensives, cause fluid and hemodynamic changes. These may decrease the client's tolerance to the positional changes of postural drainage. Steroid medications increase the client's risk of pathological rib fractures and often contraindicate rib shaking.
- Know the client's medical history. Certain conditions such as increased intracranial pressure, spinal cord injuries, and abdominal aneurysm resection contraindicate the positional changes of postural drainage. Thoracic trauma or surgery may also contraindicate percussion, vibration, and rib shaking.
- Know the client's level of cognitive function. Participation in controlled coughing techniques requires the client to follow instructions. Congenital or acquired cognitive limitations may alter the client's ability to learn and participate in these techniques.
- Be aware of the client's exercise tolerance. CPT maneuvers are fatiguing. When the client is not used to physical activity, initial tolerance to the maneuvers may be decreased. However, with gradual increases in activity and planned CPT, client tolerance for the procedure improves.

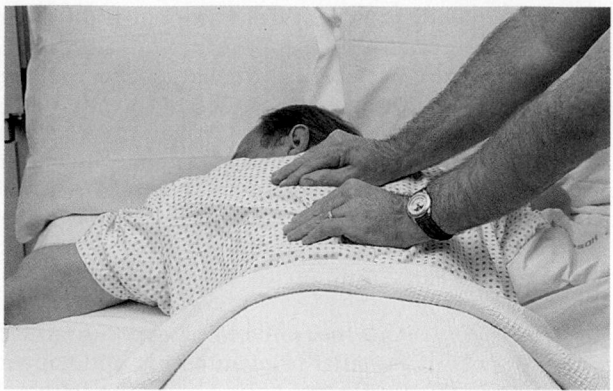

FIGURE **39-9** Hand position for chest wall percussion during physiotherapy.

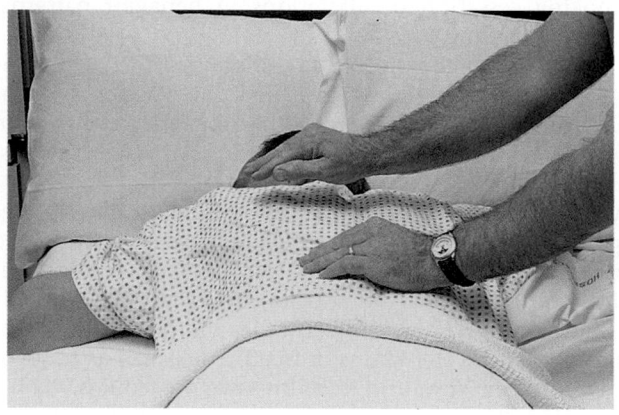

FIGURE **39-10** Chest wall percussion, alternating hand clapping against the client's chest wall.

Chest percussion involves striking the chest wall over the area being drained. The hand is positioned so that the fingers and thumb touch and the hands are cupped (Figure 39-9). Percussion on the surface of the chest wall sends waves of varying amplitude and frequency through the chest, changing the consistency and location of the sputum. Chest percussion is performed by striking the chest wall alternately with cupped hands (Figure 39-10). Percussion is performed over a single layer of clothing, not over buttons, snaps, or zippers. The single layer of clothing prevents slapping the client's skin. Thicker or multiple layers of material dampen the vibrations.

Percussion is contraindicated in clients with bleeding disorders, osteoporosis, or fractured ribs. Caution should be taken to percuss the lung fields and not the scapular regions, or trauma may occur to the skin and underlying musculoskeletal structures.

Vibration is a fine, shaking pressure applied to the chest wall only during exhalation. This technique is thought to increase the velocity and turbulence of exhaled air, facilitating secretion removal. Vibration increases the exhalation of trapped air and may shake mucus loose and induce a cough.

Postural drainage is the use of positioning techniques that draw secretions from specific segments of the lungs and bronchi into the trachea. Coughing or suc-

tioning normally removes secretions from the trachea. The procedure for postural drainage can include most lung segments (Table 39-10). Because clients may not require postural drainage of all lung segments, the procedure is based on clinical assessment findings. For example, clients with left lower lobe atelectasis may require postural drainage of only the affected region, whereas a child with cystic fibrosis may require postural drainage of all lung segments.

Suctioning Techniques. When a client is unable to clear respiratory tract secretions with coughing, the nurse must use suctioning to clear the airways. The suctioning techniques include oropharyngeal and nasopharyngeal suctioning, orotracheal and nasotracheal suctioning, and suctioning an artificial airway.

These techniques are based on common principles. Because the oropharynx and trachea are considered sterile, sterile technique is used for suctioning. The mouth is considered clean, and therefore the suctioning of oral secretions should be performed after suctioning of the oropharynx and trachea. Each type of suctioning requires the use of a rounded-tipped catheter with a number of side holes at the distal end of the catheter. Frequency of

Table 39-10	Positions for Postural Drainage
Lung Segment	**Position of Client**
Adult	
Bilateral	High-Fowler's position
Apical segments Right upper lobe—anterior segment	Supine with head of bed elevated 15 to 30 degrees
Left upper lobe—anterior segment	Supine with head elevated
Right upper lobe—posterior segment	Side lying with right side of chest elevated on pillows
Left upper lobe—posterior segment	Side lying with left side of chest elevated on pillows
Right middle lobe—anterior segment	Three-fourths supine position with dependent lung in Trendelenburg's position
Right middle lobe—posterior segment	Prone with thorax and abdomen elevated
Both lower lobes—anterior segments	Supine in Trendelenburg's position

Continued

Table 39-10   **Positions for Postural Drainage—cont'd**

Lung Segment	Position of Client
Adult—cont'd	
Left lower lobe—lateral segment	Left lateral in Trendelenburg's position.
Right lower lobe—lateral segment	Right side-lying in Trendelenburg's position.
Right lower lobe—posterior segment	Prone in Trendelenburg's position with abdomen and thorax elevated.
Both lower lobes—posterior segments	Prone in Trendelenburg's position with abdomen and thorax elevated.
Child	
Bilateral—apical segments	Sitting on nurse's lap, leaning slightly forward, flexed over pillow
Bilateral—middle anterior segments	Sitting on nurse's lap, leaning against nurse
Bilateral lobes— anterior segments	Lying supine on nurse's lap, back supported with pillow

suctioning is determined by client assessment and need. If secretions are identified by inspection or auscultation techniques, suctioning is required. Sputum is not produced continuously or every 1 or 2 hours but occurs as a response to a pathological condition. Therefore there is no rationale for routine suctioning of all clients every 1 to 2 hours. In addition, suctioning reduces the amount of the available dead space in the oropharynx and trachea, often resulting in significant desaturation of the client. The nurse must be careful to monitor the client to ensure adequate oxygenation. Too-frequent suctioning can put the client at risk for development of hypoxemia, hypotension, arrhythmias, and possible trauma to the mucosa of the lungs (Day and others, 2002).

Oropharyngeal and Nasopharyngeal Suctioning. The oropharynx extends behind the mouth from the soft palate above the level of the hyoid bone and contains the tonsils. The nasopharynx is located behind the nose and extends to the level of the soft palate. Oropharyngeal or nasopharyngeal suctioning is used when the client is able to cough effectively but is unable to clear secretions by expectorating or swallowing. The suction procedure is used after the client has coughed (Skill 39-1). As the amount of pulmonary secretions is reduced and the client is less fatigued, the client may be able to expectorate or swallow the mucus and suctioning is no longer required.

Orotracheal and Nasotracheal Suctioning. Orotracheal or nasotracheal suctioning is necessary when the client with pulmonary secretions is unable to manage secretions by coughing and does not have an artificial airway present (see Skill 39-1). A catheter is passed through the mouth or nose into the trachea. The nose is the preferred route because stimulation of the gag reflex is minimal. The procedure is similar to nasopharyngeal suctioning, but the

Text continued on p. 1108

Skill 39-1 *Suctioning*

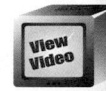

Delegation Considerations

This skill may be delegated to assistive personnel (AP) in special situations. When the client is assessed by the nurse to be stable, the skill of performing suctioning of an established tracheostomy can be delegated to an AP when the client has a permanent tracheostomy tube or is receiving home mechanical ventilation. Before delegating this skill the nurse must do the following:

- Discuss with care provider any unique modifications of the skill, such as the need to re-apply any supplemental oxygen equipment following the procedure
- Instruct the AP to report any change in client's respiratory status, secretion color or volume, or unresolved coughing or gagging
- Instruct the AP to report any change in client's color, vital signs, or complaints to pain

Equipment

- Appropriate-size suction catheter (smallest diameter that will remove secretions effectively) or Yankauer catheter (oral suction)
- Nasal or oral airway (if indicated)
- Two sterile gloves or one sterile and one clean disposable glove, or one disposable (refer to technique)
- Clean towel or paper drape
- Portable or wall suction
- Mask or face shield
- 30-ml sterile saline ampules
- Connecting tube (6 feet)

Equipment that will be needed if not using closed-suction catheter:

- Small Y adapter (if catheter does not have a suction-control port)
- Water-soluble lubricant
- Sterile basin
- Sterile normal saline solution or water (about 100 ml)

Steps	Rationale
1. Assess signs and symptoms of upper and lower airway obstruction requiring nasotracheal or orotracheal suctioning, including respiratory rate or adventitious sounds, nasal secretions, drooling, gastric secretions, or vomitus in mouth.	Physical signs and symptoms result from pooling of secretions in upper and lower airways.
2. Assess signs and symptoms associated with hypoxia and hypercapnia: apprehension, anxiety, decreased ability to concentrate, lethargy, decreased level of consciousness (especially acute), increased fatigue, dizziness, behavioral changes (especially irritability), increased pulse rate or rate of breathing, decreased depth of breathing, elevated blood pressure, cardiac dysrhythmias, pallor, cyanosis, and dyspnea.	Physical signs and symptoms resulting from decreased oxygen to tissues indicate need for suctioning.

Skill 39-1   *Suctioning—cont'd*

Steps	Rationale
3. Determine factors that normally influence upper or lower airway functioning.	
a. Fluid status	Fluid overload may increase amount of secretions. Dehydration promotes thicker secretions.
b. Lack of humidity	The environment influences secretion formation and gas exchange, necessitating airway suctioning when client cannot clear secretions effectively.
c. Infection	Clients with respiratory infections are prone to increased secretions that are thicker and sometimes more difficult to expectorate.
d. Anatomy	Abnormal anatomy can impair normal drainage of secretions. For example, nasal swelling, a deviated septum, or facial fractures may impair nasal drainage. Tumors in or around the lower airway may impair secretion removal by occluding or externally compressing the lumen of the airway.
4. Assess client's understanding of procedure.	Reveals need for client instruction and also encourages cooperation.
5. Obtain physician's order if indicated by agency policy.	Some institutions require a physician's order for tracheal suctioning.
6. Explain to client how procedure will help clear airway and relieve breathing problems and that temporary coughing, sneezing, gagging, or shortness of breath is normal. Encourage client to cough out secretions. Practice coughing, if able. Splint surgical incisions, if necessary.	Encourages cooperation and minimizes risks, anxiety, and pain.
7. Explain importance of and encourage coughing during procedure.	Facilitates secretion removal and may reduce frequency and duration of future suctioning.
8. Help client to assume position comfortable for nurse and client (usually semi-Fowler's or sitting upright with head hyperextended, unless contraindicated).	Reduces stimulation of gag reflex, promotes client comfort and secretion drainage, and prevents aspiration. Position lessens strain on nurse's back. Hyperextension facilitates insertion of catheter into trachea.
9. Place pulse oximeter on client's finger. Take reading and leave pulse oximeter in place.	Provides baseline SpO_2 to determine client's response to suctioning.
10. Place towel across client's chest.	Reduces transmission of microorganisms by protecting gown from secretions.
11. Perform hand hygiene.	Reduces transmission of microorganisms.
12. Preparation for all types of suctioning.	
A. Open suction kit or catheter with use of aseptic technique. If sterile drape is available, place it across client's chest or on the over-bed table. Do not allow the suction catheter to touch any nonsterile surfaces.	Prepares catheter and prevents transmission of microorganisms. Provides sterile surface on which to lay suction catheter between passes, if needed.
B. Unwrap or open sterile basin and place on bedside table. Fill basin or cup with approximately 100 ml of sterile normal saline solution or water (see illustration).	Unwrap or open sterile cup/basin. Place on bedside table.
C. Connect one end of connecting tubing to suction machine. Place other end in convenient location near client. Check that equipment is functioning properly by suctioning a small amount of water from basin.	
D. Turn on suction device. Set regulator to appropriate negative pressure: wall suction, 80 to 120 mm Hg; portable suction, 7 to 15 mm Hg for adults.	Elevated pressure settings increase risk of trauma to mucosa and can induce greater hypoxia (Brooks and others, 2001).

Steps	Rationale

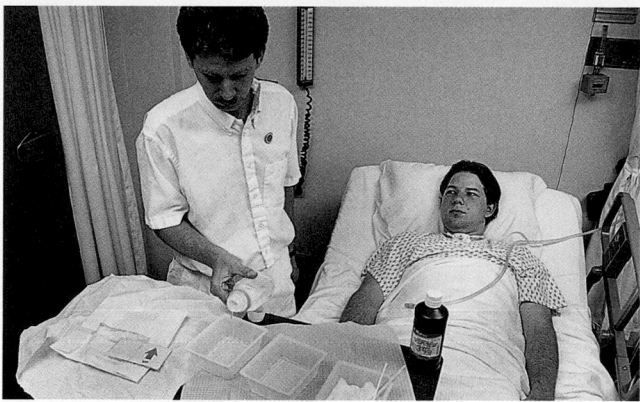

STEP **12B** Pouring sterile saline into basin.

13. Suction Airway.
    A. Oropharyngeal Suctioning.
(1) Apply clean disposable glove to dominant hand.	Suction of oral cavity does not require sterile glove use.
(2) Consider applying mask or face shield.	Suction may cause splashing of body fluids.
(3) Attach suction catheter to connecting tubing. Remove oxygen mask if present.	
(4) Insert catheter into client's mouth. With suction applied, move catheter around mouth, including pharynx and gum line, until secretions are cleared.	If catheter does not have a suction control to apply intermittent suction, take care not to allow suction tip to invaginate oral mucosal surfaces with continuous suction (St. John, 1999).
(5) Encourage client to cough, and repeat suctioning if needed. Replace oxygen mask if used.	Coughing moves secretions from lower to upper airways into mouth.
(6) Suction water from basin through catheter until catheter is cleared of secretions.	Clearing secretions before they dry reduces probability of transmission of microorganisms and enhances delivery of preset suction pressures.
(7) Place catheter in a clean, dry area for reuse with suction turned off or within client's reach, with suction on, if client is capable of suctioning self.	Facilitates prompt removal of airway secretions when suctioning is needed in the future.

    B. Nasopharyngeal and Nasotracheal Suctioning.
(1) If indicated, increase supplemental oxygen therapy to 100% or as ordered by physician. Encourage client's deep breathing.	Preoxygenation and deep breathing assist in reducing suction-induced hypoxemia (Day and others, 2002). Preoxygenation should be used with caution in oxygen-sensitive clients, such as those with chronic heart and lung conditions and those with pneumonia.

Critical Decision Point: Following the suction procedure, the client's oxygen must be readjusted as ordered by physician after procedure to avoid increased risk of oxygen toxicity and absorption atelectasis from prolonged administration of high concentrations of oxygen and increased carbon dioxide retention in clients with chronic obstructive lung diseases (Day and others, 2002).

---

(2) Open lubricant. Squeeze small amount onto open sterile catheter package without touching package.	Prepares lubricant while maintaining sterility. Water-soluble lubricant is used to avoid lipoid aspiration pneumonia. Excessive lubricant can occlude catheter.
(3) Apply sterile glove to each hand, or apply nonsterile glove to nondominant hand and sterile glove to dominant hand.	Reduces transmission of microorganisms and allows nurse to maintain sterility of suction catheter.

Critical Decision Point: In selected settings, such as the home or long-term care facility, or with clients with an established tracheostomy who do not have an airway infection a clean technique is used.

Skill **39-1**   *Suctioning—cont'd*

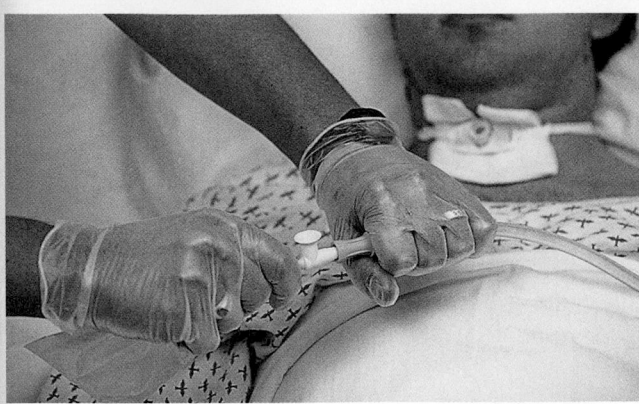

STEP **13B(4)** Attaching catheter to suction.

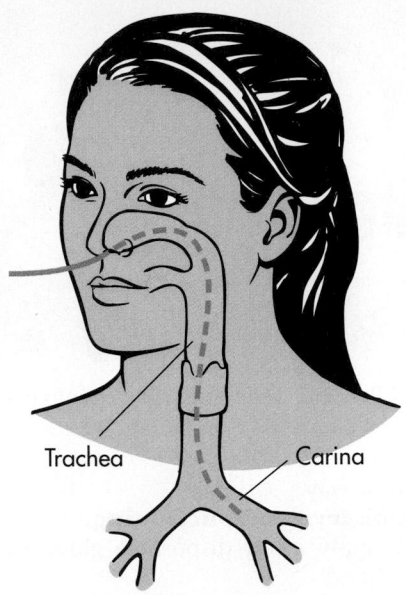

Trachea   Carina

STEP **13B(9)** Distance of insertion of nasotracheal catheter.

(4) Pick up suction catheter with dominant hand without touching nonsterile surfaces. Pick up connecting tubing with nondominant hand. Secure catheter to tubing (see illustration).	Maintains catheter sterility. Connects catheter to suction.
(5) Check that the equipment is functioning properly by suctioning small amount of normal saline solution from basin.	Ensures equipment function; lubricates catheter and tubing.
(6) Lightly coat distal 6 to 8 cm (2 to 3 inches) of catheter with water-soluble lubricant.	Lubricates catheter for easier insertion.
(7) Remove oxygen delivery device, if applicable, with nondominant hand. **Without applying suction** and using dominant thumb and forefinger, gently insert catheter into naris during inhalation.	Application of suction pressure while introducing catheter into nasopharyngeal tissues increases risk of damage to mucosa. When advanced into trachea, suction could damage mucosa and increase risk of hypoxia. Proper placement ensures removal of pharyngeal secretions.
(8) *Nasopharyngeal:* Follow natural course of naris; slightly slant catheter downward and advance to back of pharynx. In adults insert catheter about 16 cm; in older children, 8 to 12 cm (3 to 5 inches); in infants and young children, 4 to 8 cm (2 to 3 inches). Rule of thumb is to insert catheter distance from tip of nose (or mouth) to base of earlobe.	
(a) Apply intermittent suction for up to 10 to 15 seconds by placing and releasing nondominant thumb over catheter vent. Slowly withdraw catheter while rotating it back and forth between thumb and forefinger.	Intermittent suction safely removes pharyngeal secretions.

Steps	Rationale
(9) *Nasotracheal:* Follow natural course of naris and advance catheter slightly slanted and downward to just above entrance into trachea. Allow client to take a breath. Quickly insert catheter about 16 to 20 cm (6 to 8 inches in adult) into trachea (see illustration). Client will begin to cough. NOTE: In older children advance 14 to 20 cm (5½ to 8 inches); in young children and infants, 8 to 14 cm (3 to 5½ inches).	Ensures catheter will be inserted into trachea with minimum stress to client.

Critical Decision Point: Insert catheter during client inhalation, especially if inserting catheter into trachea because epiglottis is open. **Do not insert during swallowing** or catheter will most likely enter esophagus. **Never** apply suction during insertion. Client should cough. If client gags or becomes nauseated, catheter is most likely in esophagus and must be removed.

(a) *Positioning option for nasotracheal suctioning:* In some instances turning client's head to right helps nurse suction left mainstem bronchus; turning head to left helps nurse suction right mainstem bronchus. If resistance is felt after insertion of catheter for maximum recommended distance, catheter has probably hit carina. Pull catheter back 1 cm before applying suction.	

Critical Decision Point: Use nasal approach and perform tracheal suctioning before pharyngeal suctioning whenever possible. The mouth and pharynx contain more bacteria than the trachea does. If copious oral secretions are present before beginning the procedure, suction mouth with oral suction device.

(b) Apply intermittent suction for up to 10 to 15 seconds by placing and releasing nondominant thumb over vent of catheter and slowly withdrawing catheter while rotating it back and forth between dominant thumb and forefinger (see illustration). Encourage client to cough. Replace oxygen device, if applicable.	Intermittent suction and rotation of catheter prevent injury to mucosa. If catheter "grabs" mucosa, remove thumb to release suction. Suctioning longer than 10 seconds can cause cardiopulmonary compromise, usually from hypoxemia or vagal overload.

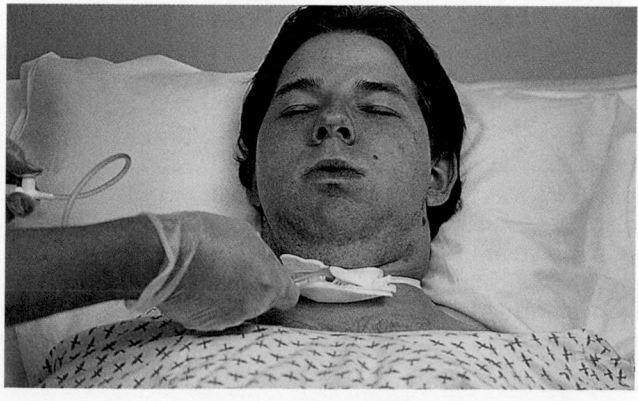

STEP **13B(9)(b)**   Suctioning tracheostomy.

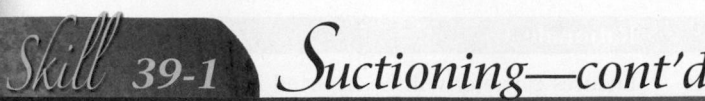

Skill 39-1   *Suctioning—cont'd*

Steps	Rationale

Critical Decision Point: If ordered to monitor client's vital signs and oxygen saturation during procedure, note if there is a 20 beats per minute change (either increase or decrease) or if pulse oximetry falls below 90% or 5% from baseline (Akgul and Akyolcu, 2002).

Steps	Rationale
(10) Rinse catheter and connecting tubing with normal saline or water until cleared.	Removes secretions from catheter. Secretions that remain in suction catheter or connecting tubing decrease suctioning efficiency.
(11) Assess for need to repeat suctioning procedure. Allow adequate time between suction passes for ventilation and oxygenation. Ask client to deep breathe and cough.	Observe for alterations in cardiopulmonary status. Suctioning can induce hypoxemia, dysrhythmias, laryngospasm, and bronchospasm. Deep breathing reventilates and reoxygenates alveoli. Repeated passes clear the airway of excessive secretions but can also remove oxygen and may induce laryngospasm.
C. Performing Artificial Airway Suctioning	
(1) Apply face shield.	Reduces transmission of microorganisms.
(2) Prepare proper suction catheter.	Suction catheter's outer diameter should not exceed one half of internal diameter of the endotracheal tube (ET) or tracheostomy tube (St. John, 1999).
(3) Apply one sterile glove to each hand, or apply nonsterile glove to nondominant hand and sterile glove to dominant hand.	Reduces transmission of microorganisms and allows nurse to maintain sterility of suction catheter.
(4) Pick up suction catheter with dominant hand without touching nonsterile surfaces. Pick up connecting tubing with nondominant hand. Secure catheter to tubing.	Maintains catheter sterility. Establishes suction.
(5) Check that equipment is functioning properly by suctioning small amount of saline from basin.	Ensures equipment function; lubricates catheter and tubing.
(6) Hyperinflate and/or hyperoxygenate client before suctioning, using manual resuscitation Ambu-bag connected to oxygen source or sigh mechanism on mechanical ventilator. Some mechanical ventilators have a button that when pushed delivers 100% oxygen for a few minutes and then resets to the previous value.	Hyperinflation decreases the risk for atelectasis caused by negative pressure of suctioning (St. John, 1999). Preoxygenation converts large proportion of resident lung gas to 100% oxygen to offset amount used in metabolic consumption while ventilator or oxygenation is interrupted, as well as to offset volume lost during suction procedure (Wood, 1998; Day and others 2002).
(7) If client is receiving mechanical ventilation, open swivel adapter or if necessary remove oxygen or humidity delivery device with nondominant hand.	Exposes artificial airway.
(8) Without applying suction, gently but quickly insert catheter using dominant thumb and forefinger into artificial airway (best to time catheter insertion with inspiration) until resistance is met or client coughs; then pull back 1 cm (½ inch).	Application of suction pressure while introducing catheter into trachea increases risk of damage to tracheal mucosa, as well as increased hypoxia related to removal of entrained oxygen present in airways. Pulling back stimulates cough and removes catheter from mucosal wall so that catheter is not resting against tracheal mucosa during suctioning.

Critical Decision Point: If unable to insert catheter past the end of the ET tube, the catheter is probably caught in the Murphy eye (i.e., side hole at the distal end of the ET tube that allows for collateral air flow in the event of main stem intubation. If this happens, rotate the catheter to reposition it away from the Murphy eye, or withdraw it slightly and reinsert with the next inhalation. Usually the catheter meets resistance at the carina. One indication that the catheter is at the carina is acute onset of coughing because the carina contains many cough receptors. The catheter should be pulled back.

Steps	Rationale
(9) Apply intermittent suction by placing and releasing nondominant thumb over vent of catheter; slowly withdraw catheter while rotating it back and forth between dominant thumb and forefinger. Encourage client to cough. Watch for respiratory distress.	Intermittent suction and rotation of catheter prevent injury to tracheal mucosal lining. If catheter "grabs" mucosa, remove thumb to release suction.

Critical Decision Point: If client develops respiratory distress during the suction procedure, immediately withdraw catheter and supply additional oxygen and breaths as needed. Oxygen can be administered directly through the catheter in an emergency. Disconnect suction and attach oxygen at prescribed flow rate through the catheter.

(10) If client is receiving mechanical ventilation, close swivel adapter or replace oxygen delivery device.	Reestablishes the artificial airway.
(11) Encourage client to deep breathe, if able. Some clients respond well to several manual breaths from the mechanical ventilator or Ambu-bag.	Reoxygenates and reexpands alveoli. Suctioning can cause hypoxemia and atelectasis.
(12) Rinse catheter and connecting tubing with normal saline until clear. Use continuous suction.	Removes catheter secretions. Secretions left in tubing decrease suction and provide environment for microorganism growth. Secretions left in connecting tube decrease suctioning efficiency.
(13) Assess client's cardiopulmonary status for secretion clearance and complications. Repeat steps 13C(6) through (12) once or twice more to clear secretions. Allow adequate time (at least 1 full minute) between suction passes for ventilation and reoxygenation. Perform nasopharyngeal and oropharyngeal suctioning (steps 13A, 13B). After nasopharyngeal and oropharyngeal suctioning is performed, catheter is contaminated; do not reinsert into ET or tracheostomy tube.	Suctioning can induce dysrhythmias, hypoxia, and bronchospasm and impair cerebral circulation or adversely affect hemodynamics (Kerr and others, 1999; Akgul and Akyolcu, 2002). Repeated passes with suction catheter clear airway of excessive secretions and promote improved oxygenation (Wood, 1998). Upper airway is considered "clean" and lower airway is considered "sterile." Therefore the same catheter can be used to suction from sterile to clean areas, but not from clean to sterile areas.

14. Complete procedure.

A. Disconnect catheter from connecting tubing. Roll catheter around fingers of dominant hand. Pull glove off inside out so that catheter remains in glove. Pull off other glove over first glove in same way to contain contaminants. Discard into appropriate receptacle. Turn off suction device.	Reduces transmission of microorganisms. Clean equipment should not be touched with contaminated gloves.
B. Remove towel and place in laundry or remove drape and discard in appropriate receptacle.	
C. Reposition client as indicated by condition. Nurse may need to reapply clean gloves for client's personal care (e.g., oral hygiene).	Proper positioning based on client's condition promotes comfort, encourages secretion drainage, and reduces risk of aspiration.
D. If indicated, readjust oxygen to original level because client's blood oxygen level should have been returned to baseline.	
E. Discard remainder of normal saline into appropriate receptacle. If basin is disposable, discard into appropriate receptacle. If basin is reusable, rinse and place in soiled utility room.	Solution is contaminated.
F. Remove and discard face shield, and perform hand hygiene.	Reduces transmission of microorganisms.
G. Place unopened suction kit on suction machine table or at head of bed according to institution preference.	Provides for immediate access of suction catheter and equipment in the event of an emergency or for the next suctioning procedure.

Skill 39-1 *Suctioning—cont'd*

Steps	Rationale
15. Compare client's vital signs and O$_2$ saturation before and after suctioning.	Identifies physiological effects of suction procedure to restore airway patency.
16. Ask client if breathing is easier and if congestion is decreased.	Provides subjective confirmation that airway obstruction is relieved with suctioning procedure.
17. Observe airway secretions.	Provides data to document presence or absence of respiratory tract infection.

Unexpected Outcomes and Related Interventions

1. Worsening respiratory status
   a. Limit length of suctioning.
   b. Determine need for more frequent suctioning, possibly of shorter duration.
   c. Notify physician.
2. Return of bloody secretions
   a. Determine amount of suction pressure used. May need to be decreased.
   b. Evaluate suctioning frequency.
   c. Provide more frequent oral hygiene.
3. Unable to pass suction catheter through first naris attempted
   a. Try other naris or oral route.
   b. Insert nasal airway, especially if suctioning through client naris frequently.
   c. Guide catheter along naris floor to avoid turbinates.
   d. If obstruction is mucus, apply suction to relieve obstruction, but do not apply suction to mucosa. If obstruction is thought to be a blood clot, consult physician.
   e. Increase lubrication of catheter.
4. Paroxysms of coughing
   a. Administer supplemental oxygen.
   b. Allow client to rest between passes of suction catheter.
   c. Consult physician regarding need for inhaled bronchodilators or topical anesthetics.
5. No secretions obtained
   a. Evaluate client's fluid status.
   b. Assess for signs of infection.
   c. Determine need for chest physiotherapy.
   d. Assess adequacy of humidification on oxygen delivery device.

Recording and Reporting

- Record the amount, consistency, color, and odor of secretions and client's response to procedure; document client's presuctioning and postsuctioning cardiopulmonary status.

Home Care Considerations

- It is necessary to adhere to best practices for infection control while weighing cost-effectiveness in the presence of a chronic situation. If the client has an established tracheostomy or requires long-term nasotracheal suctioning and infection is not present, clean suction technique is appropriate.
- Instruct client and family how to practice infection-control measures when emptying the secretion jar.

catheter tip is moved farther into the client's trachea. The entire procedure from catheter passage to its removal should be done quickly, lasting no longer than 15 seconds. Unless in respiratory distress, the client should be allowed to rest between passes of the catheter. If the client is using supplemental oxygen, the oxygen cannula or mask should be replaced during rest periods.

Tracheal Suctioning. Tracheal suctioning is accomplished through an artificial airway such as an endotracheal tube or tracheostomy tube. The suction catheter should be no greater than one half the size of the internal diameter of the artificial airway. Secretion removal should be as atraumatic as possible. To avoid trauma to the mucosa of the lung, suction pressure should never be applied while inserting the catheter and suction pressure should be maintained between 120 and 180 mm Hg.

Suction is applied intermittently as the catheter is withdrawn. Rotating the catheter will enhance removal of secretions that have adhered to the sides of the endotracheal tube. The nurse should wear a mask and goggles and may need to wear a barrier gown to prevent splashes with body fluids.

The two current methods of suctioning are the open and closed methods. Open suctioning involves a sterile catheter that is opened at the time of suctioning. The nurse wears sterile gloves to perform the suction procedure. Closed suctioning involves a multiple-use suction catheter that is encased in a plastic sheath (Figure 39-11). Closed suctioning is most often used on clients who require mechanical ventilation to support their respiratory efforts, because it permits continuous delivery of oxygen while suction is performed, thus reducing the risk of oxy-

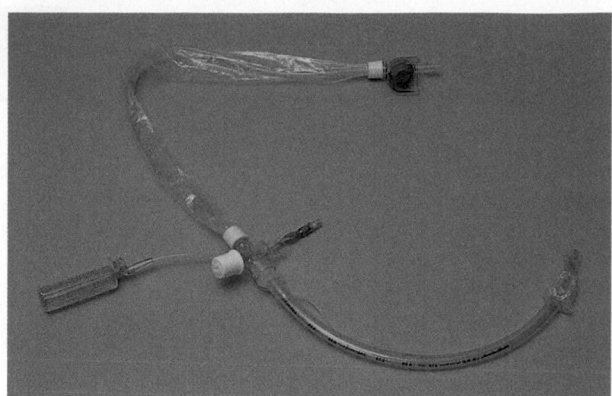

FIGURE **39–11** Ballard tracheal care, closed suction.

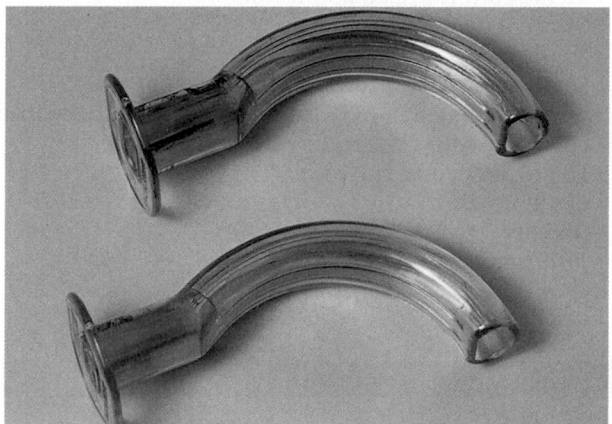

FIGURE **39–12** Artificial oral airways.

gen desaturation. Although sterile gloves are not used in this procedure, nonsterile gloves are recommended to prevent contact with splashes from body fluids.

Artificial Airways. An artificial airway is indicated for clients with decreased level of consciousness or airway obstruction and to aide in removal of tracheobronchial secretions.

Oral Airway. The oral airway, the simplest type of artificial airway, prevents obstruction of the trachea by displacement of the tongue into the oropharynx (Figure 39-12). The oral airway extends from the teeth to the oropharynx, maintaining the tongue in the normal position. The correct-size airway must be used. Proper oral airway size is determined by measuring the distance from the corner of the mouth to the angle of the jaw just below the ear. The length is equal to the distance from the flange of the airway to the tip. If the airway is too small, the tongue is not held in the anterior portion of the mouth; if the airway is too large, it may force the tongue toward the epiglottis and obstruct the airway.

The nurse inserts the airway by turning the curve of the airway toward the cheek and placing it over the tongue. When the airway is in the oropharynx, the nurse turns it so that the opening points downward. Correctly placed, the airway moves the tongue forward away from the oropharynx and the flange, the flat portion of the airway, rests against the client's teeth. Incorrect insertion merely forces the tongue back into the oropharynx.

Endotracheal and Tracheal Airway. The presence of an artificial airway places the client at high risk for infection and airway injury. Sterile technique is used in caring for and maintaining an artificial airway to prevent nosocomial infections. Artificial airways need be maintained in the correct position to prevent airway damage (Skill 39-2).

Endotracheal tubes (ETs) are used as short-term artificial airways to administer mechanical ventilation, relieve upper airway obstruction, protect against aspiration, or clear secretions. ET tubes are generally removed within 14 days; however, they may be used for a longer period of time if the client is showing progress toward weaning from mechanical ventilation and extubation.

If the client requires long-term assistance from an artificial airway, a tracheostomy is considered. A surgical incision is made into the trachea, and a short artificial airway (a tracheostomy tube) is inserted.

Maintenance and Promotion of Lung Expansion. Nursing interventions to maintain or promote lung expansion include noninvasive techniques. These include positioning, procedures using equipment such as incentive spirometry, and invasive procedures such as management of a chest tube.

Positioning. In the healthy, completely mobile person, adequate ventilation and oxygenation are maintained by frequent position changes during daily activities. However, when a person's illness or injury restricts mobility, there is an increased risk for respiratory impairment. Frequent changes of position are simple and cost-effective methods for reducing the risks of stasis of pulmonary secretions and decreased chest wall expansion.

The most effective position for client with cardiopulmonary diseases is the 45-degree semi-Fowler's position, using gravity to assist in lung expansion and reduce pressure from the abdomen on the diaphragm. When the client uses this position, the nurse needs to ensure that the client does not slide down in bed, which could reduce lung expansion. A client with unilateral lung disease, such as pneumothorax, atelectasis, pneumonia, thoracotomy, and multiple trauma affecting one lung, should be positioned with the "good lung down." This promotes better perfusion of the healthy lung, improving oxygenation. In the presence of pulmonary abscess or hemorrhage, the client should be placed with the affected lung down to prevent drainage toward the healthy lung.

Incentive Spirometry. **Incentive spirometry** is a method of encouraging voluntary deep breathing by providing visual feedback to clients about inspiratory volume. Incentive spirometry is used to promote deep breathing and to prevent or treat atelectasis in the postoperative client. Studies have shown no respiratory benefit to postoperative incentive spirometry when compared with deep breathing and early ambulation (Fujimoto and others, 2002; Stulberg, 2002).

Flow-oriented incentive spirometers consist of one or more plastic chambers that contain freely moving colored balls. The client inhales slowly and with an even flow to

Text continued on p. 1117

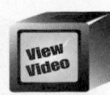

Skill 39-2 Care of an Artificial Airway

Delegation Considerations

This skill should not be routinely delegated to assistive personnel (AP). It is the responsibility of the nurse to perform endotracheal care. In some setting, clients who have well-established tracheostomy tubes may have the care delegated to AP. It is the responsibility of the nurse to assess and ensure that proper artificial airway care is provided. In addition, AP may perform other aspects of the client's care. The nurse should instruct AP about the following:

- To report to nurse any changes in client's respiratory status, level of consciousness, confusion, pain
- Emergency procedures in case the tracheostomy tube inadvertently becomes dislodged when ties are changed
- Expected drainage from tracheostomy

Equipment

- Endotracheal tube care
  - Towel
  - ET and oropharyngeal suction equipment
  - 1 to 1½-inch adhesive or waterproof tape (not paper tape) or commercial ET holder (follow manufacturer's instructions for securing)
  - Two pairs of nonsterile gloves
  - Adhesive remover swab or acetone on a cotton ball
  - Mouth care supplies (e.g., toothbrush, toothpaste, mouth swabs)
  - Face cleanser (e.g., wet washcloth, towel, soap, shaving supplies)
  - Clean 2 × 2 gauze
  - Tincture of benzoin or liquid adhesive
  - Face shield (if indicated)
- Tracheostomy care
  - Towel
  - Tracheostomy suction supplies
  - Sterile tracheostomy care kit, if available, or three sterile 4 × 4 gauze pads
  - Sterile cotton-tipped applicators
  - Sterile tracheostomy dressing
  - Sterile basin
  - Small sterile brush (or disposable cannula)
  - Tracheostomy ties (e.g., twill tape, manufactured tracheostomy ties, Velcro tracheostomy ties)
  - Hydrogen peroxide
  - Normal saline (NS)
  - Scissors
  - Two sterile gloves
  - Face shield, if indicated

Steps	Rationale
1. Perform pulmonary assessment.	
a. Auscultate lung sounds.	Provides baseline information.
b. Assess condition and potency of airway and surrounding tissues.	Indicates if additional skin care to irritated areas is needed. Identifies potential pressure areas.
c. Note type and size of tube, movement of tube, cuff size.	Movement of tube predisposes client to tracheal trauma or tube dislodgement and may indicate the need for another size airway. Cuff size indicates the amount of air needed to properly inflate cuff. An underinflated cuff increases client's risk for aspiration.
2. Explain procedure to client and family.	Reinforces information given to client and family and provides opportunity to ask additional questions
3. Position client. Clients usually prefer to be lying down. A client with a long-term well-established tracheostomy may be seated.	Provides access to site and facilitates completion of the procedure.
4. Place towel across client's chest.	Reduces transmission of microorganisms and protects linens and bedclothes.
5. Perform hand hygiene.	Reduces transmission of microorganisms.
6. Perform airway care.	
A. **Endotracheal Tube Care**	
(1) Observe for signs and symptoms of need to perform care of the artificial airway:	A client with an artificial airway is at increased risk due to an inability or difficulty controlling secretions and due to pressure points of the artificial airway.
(a) Soiled or loose tape	
(b) Pressure sores on nares, lip, or corner of mouth	
(c) Unstable tube	
(d) Excessive secretions	

Steps	Rationale
(2) Identify factors that increase risk of complications from ET tubes: (a) Type and size of tube (b) Movement of tube up and down trachea (c) Cuff size (d) Duration of placement	Tube moving up and down trachea disposes client to tracheal trauma or dislodgement. Cuff underinflation may allow aspiration, whereas overinflation may cause ischemia or necrosis of tracheal tissue. Longer duration increases risk of lower airway complications such as pneumonia.
(3) Suction endotracheal tube (see Skill 37-1, p. 1101).	Removes secretions. Diminishes client's need to cough during procedure.

Critical Decision Point: An oral airway should be immediately accessible in the event that the client bites down and obstructs the ET tube.

Steps	Rationale
(a) Instruct client not to bite or move ET tube with tongue or pull on tubing; removal of tape can be uncomfortable.	Prepares client for procedure and what to expect.
(b) Leave Yankauer suction catheter connected to suction source.	Prepares for oropharyngeal suctioning.
(4) Prepare tape. Cut piece of tape long enough to go completely around client's head from naris to naris plus 15 cm (6 inches): (a) Adult, about 30 to 60 cm (1 to 2 feet). (b) Lay adhesive side up on bedside table. (c) Cut and lay 8 to 16 cm (3 to 6 inches) of tape, adhesive side down, in center of long strip to prevent tape from sticking to hair.	Adhesive tape must be placed around head from cheek to cheek below ears. Avoid over ears as this may result in a pressure sore.
(5) Have an assistant apply a pair of gloves and hold ET tube firmly so that tube does not move.	Reduces transmission of microorganisms. Maintains proper tube position and prevents accidental extubation.
(a) Carefully remove tape from ET tube and client's face. If tape is difficult to remove, moisten with water or adhesive tape remover. Discard tape in appropriate receptacle if nearby. If not, place soiled tape on bedside table or on distant end of towel.	Provides nurse with access to skin under tape for assessment and hygiene. Reduces transmission of microorganisms.
(b) Use adhesive remover swab to remove excess adhesive left on face after tape removal.	Promotes hygiene. Retained adhesive can cause damage to skin and prevent poor adhesion of new tape.
(c) Remove oral airway or bite block if present.	Provides access and complete observation of client's oral cavity.
(d) Clean mouth, gums, and teeth opposite ET tube with mouthwash solution and 4 × 4 gauze, sponge-tipped applicators, or saline swabs. Brush teeth as indicated. If necessary, administer oropharyngeal suctioning with Yankauer catheter.	Provides oral hygiene and allows for observation of any pressure ulcers.
(e) Note "cm" ET tube marking at lips or gums. With help of assistant, move ET tube to opposite side or center of mouth. Do not change tube depth.	Prevents pressure sore formation at sides of client's mouth. Ensures correct position of tube and allows for quick visual of displaced tube.
(f) Repeat oral cleaning as in step (d) on opposite side of mouth.	Removes secretions from mouth and oropharynx.
(g) Clean face and neck with soapy washcloth; rinse and dry. Shave male client as necessary.	Moisture and beard growth prevent adhesive tape adherence.
(h) Use tincture of benzoin swab or pour small amount of tincture of benzoin on clean 2 × 2 gauze and dot on upper lip (oral ET tube) or across nose (nasal ET tube) and cheeks to ear. Allow tincture to dry completely.	Protects and makes skin more receptive to tape.

Skill 39-2 · *Care of an Artificial Airway—cont'd*

Steps	Rationale
(i) Slip tape under client's head and neck, adhesive side up. Take care not to twist tape or catch hair. Do not allow tape to stick to itself. It helps to stick tape gently to tongue blade, which serves as a guide as tape is passed behind the client's head. Center tape so that double-faced tape extends around back of neck from ear to ear.	Positions tape to secure ET tube in proper position.
(j) On one side of face, secure tape from ear to naris (nasal ET tube) or edge of mouth (oral ET tube). Tear remaining tape in half lengthwise, forming two pieces that are ½- to ¾-inch wide. Secure bottom half of tape across upper lip (oral ET tube) or across top of nose (nasal ET tube) (see illustration, *A*). Wrap top half of tape around tube (see illustration, *B*).	Secures tape to face. Using top tape to wrap prevents downward drag on ET tube.
(k) Gently pull other side of tape firmly to pick up slack and secure to remaining side of face (see illustration). Assistant can release hold when tube is secure. Nurse may want assistant to help reinsert oral airway.	Secures tape to face and tube. ET tube should be at same depth at the lips. Check earlier assessment for verification of tube depth in centimeters.
(l) Clean oral airway in warm soapy water and rinse well. Hydrogen peroxide can aid in removal of crusted secretions. Shake excess water from oral airway.	Promotes hygiene. Reduces transmission of microorganisms.
(m) For unconscious client, reinsert oral airway without pushing tongue into oropharynx.	Prevents client from biting ET tube and allows access for oropharyngeal suctioning. An oral airway in a conscious, cooperative client may cause excessive gagging and pressure ulcers to the mouth and tongue.

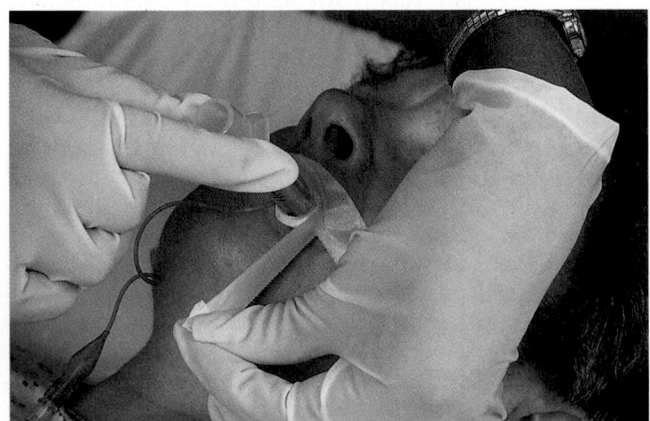

A   **B**

STEP **6A(5)(j)**   **A,** Securing bottom half of tape across client's upper lip. **B,** Securing top half of tape around tube.

Steps	Rationale

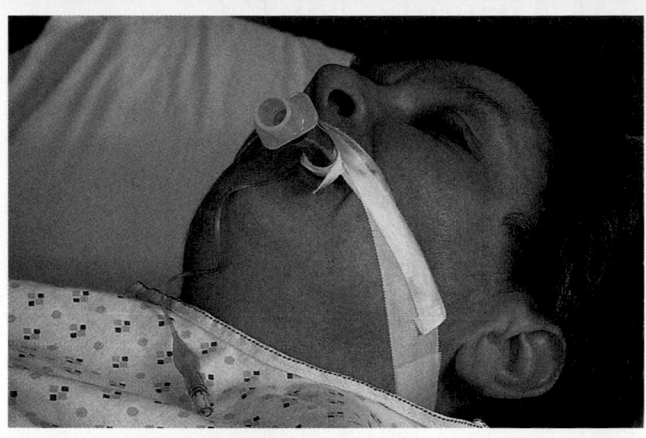

STEP **6A(5)(k)**   Tape securing ET tube.

B. **Tracheostomy Care**

(1) Observe for signs and symptoms of need to perform tracheostomy care:
    (a) Soiled/loose ties or dressing
    (b) Nonstable tube
    (c) Excessive secretions.

A client with a tracheostomy tube is at increased risk due to loss of natural airway protection of the upper airway.

(2) Suction tracheostomy (see Skill 39-1, p. 1101). Before removing gloves, remove soiled tracheostomy dressing and discard in glove with coiled catheter.

Removes secretions so as not to occlude outer cannula while inner cannula is removed. Reduces need for client to cough. Prevents aspiration of retained secretions. Disposal method contains microorganisms.

(3) Prepare equipment.
    (a) Open two packages of cotton-tipped swabs and pour NS on one package and hydrogen peroxide on the other.
    (b) Open sterile tracheostomy package.
    (c) Unwrap sterile basin and pour about 2 cm (¾ inch) of hydrogen peroxide into it.
    (d) Open small sterile brush package and place aseptically into sterile basin.
    (e) If using large roll of twill tape, cut appropriate length of tape and lay aside in dry area. Do not recap hydrogen peroxide and NS.

Preparation and organization of equipment allows the nurse to complete tracheostomy care procedure efficiently and then re-connect client to oxygen source in a timely manner.

(4) Apply gloves. Keep dominant hand sterile throughout procedure.

Reduces transmission of microorganisms.

(5) Remove oxygen source. Apply oxygen source loosely over tracheostomy if client desaturates during procedure.

Helps reduce amount of desaturation.

Critical Decision Point: It is important to stabilize the tracheostomy tube at all times during tracheostomy care to prevent injury and unnecessary discomfort.

---

(6) If a ***nondisposable inner cannula*** is used:
    (a) While touching only the outer aspect of the tube, remove the inner cannula with nondominant hand. Drop inner cannula into hydrogen peroxide basin.

Removes inner cannula for cleaning. Hydrogen peroxide loosens secretions from inner cannula.

    (b) Place tracheostomy collar or T tube and ventilator oxygen source over or near outer cannula. (NOTE: T tube and ventilator oxygen devices cannot be attached to all outer cannulas when inner cannula is removed.)

Maintains supply of oxygen to client.

Skill **39-2**   *Care of an Artificial Airway—cont'd*

Steps	Rationale

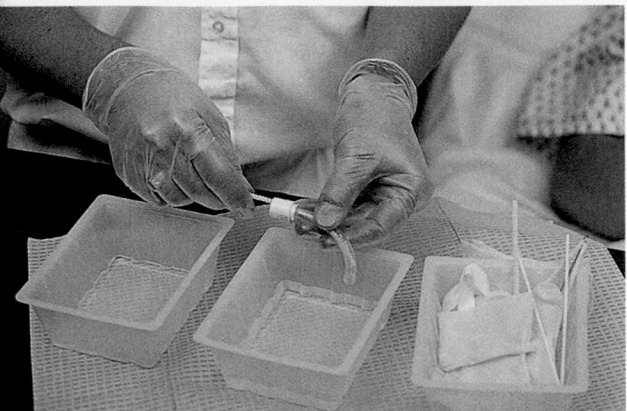

STEP **6B(6)(c)** Cleaning the tracheostomy inner cannula.

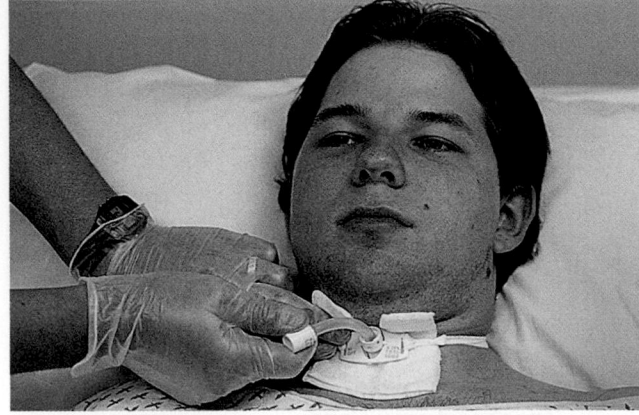

STEP **6B(6)(e)** Reinserting the inner cannula.

Steps	Rationale
(c) To prevent oxygen desaturation in affected clients, quickly pick up inner cannula and use small brush to remove secretions inside and outside cannula (see illustration).	Tracheostomy brush provides mechanical force to remove thick or dried secretions.
(d) Hold inner cannula over basin and rinse with NS, using nondominant hand to pour.	Removes secretions and hydrogen peroxide from inner cannula.
(e) Replace inner cannula and secure "locking" mechanism (see illustration). Reapply ventilator or oxygen sources.	
(7) If a ***disposable inner cannula*** is used:	
(a) Remove cannula from manufacturer's packaging.	
(b) While touching only the outer aspect of the tube, withdraw inner cannula and replace with new cannula. Lock into position.	
(c) Dispose of contaminated cannula in appropriate receptacle and apply oxygen source.	Prevents unnecessary oxygen desaturation.
(8) Using hydrogen peroxide–prepared cotton-tipped swabs and 4 × 4 gauze, clean exposed outer cannula surfaces and stoma under faceplate, extending 5 to 10 cm (2 to 4 inches) in all directions from stoma (see illustration). Clean in circular motion from stoma site outward, using dominant hand to handle sterile supplies.	Aseptically removes secretions from stoma site.
(9) Using NS-prepared cotton-tipped swabs and 4 × 4 gauze, rinse hydrogen peroxide from tracheostomy tube and skin surfaces.	Rinses hydrogen peroxide from surfaces, preventing possible irritation.
(10) Using dry 4 × 4 gauze, pat lightly at skin and exposed outer cannula surfaces.	Dry surfaces prohibit formation of moist environment from growth of microorganisms and skin excoriation.

Steps	**Rationale**

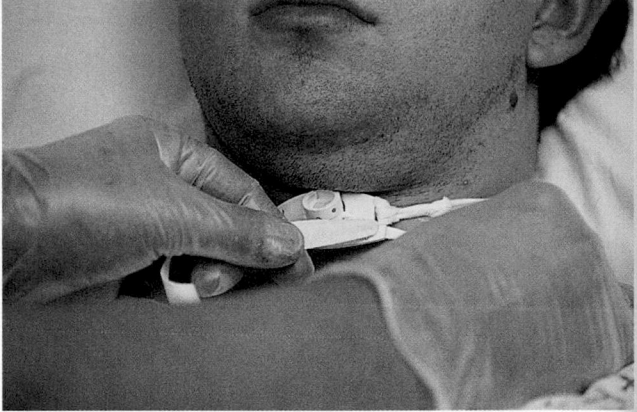

STEP **6B(8)** Cleansing around stoma.

STEP **6B(11)(b)** Replacing tracheostomy ties when an assistant is not available. Do not remove old tracheostomy ties until new ones are secure.

(11) Instruct assistant, if available, to hold tracheostomy tube securely in place while ties are cut.	Promotes hygiene, reduces transmission of microorganisms, and secures tracheostomy tube.

Critical Decision Point: Assistant must not release hold on tracheostomy tube until new ties are firmly tied to reduce risk of accidental extubation. If no assistant is present, do not cut old ties until new ties are in place and securely tied. (Follow manufacturer's guidelines for Velcro ties.)

(a) Cut length of twill tape long enough to go around client's neck two times, about 60 to 75 cm (24 to 30 inches) for an adult. Cut ends on a diagonal.	Cutting ends of tie on a diagonal aids in inserting tie through eyelet.

Critical Decision Point: Secure tracheostomy ties with one-finger slack. For accidental extubation, call for assistance and manually ventilate client with Ambu-bag, if necessary. Tracheostomy obturator should be kept at bedside with a fresh tracheostomy to facilitate reinsertion of the outer cannula, if dislodged. An additional tracheostomy tube of the same size and shape should be kept on hand for emergency replacement. If another tracheostomy tube is not available, insert a size 6 ET to keep airway open until physician arrives.

(b) Insert one end of tie through faceplate eyelet and pull ends even (see illustration).	
(c) Slide both ends of tie behind head and around neck to other eyelet, and insert one tie through second eyelet.	
(d) Pull snugly.	Secures tracheostomy tube in place.
(e) Tie ends securely in double square knot, allowing space for only one finger in tie.	One-finger slack prevents ties from being too tight when tracheostomy dressing is in place.
(f) Insert fresh tracheostomy dressing under clean ties and faceplate (see illustration).	Absorbs drainage. Dressing prevents pressure on clavicle heads.
(g) Position client comfortably and assess respiratory status.	Promotes comfort. Some clients may require post–tracheostomy care suctioning.
7. Replace any oxygen delivery devices.	Maintains oxygen therapy.
8. Remove and discard gloves. Perform hand hygiene.	
9. Compare respiratory assessments before and after procedure.	Identifies any changes in presence and quality of breath sounds after procedure.
10. Observe depth and position of tubes.	Verifies that position of tube is correct.

Skill 39-2   *Care of an Artificial Airway—cont'd*

Steps	Rationale

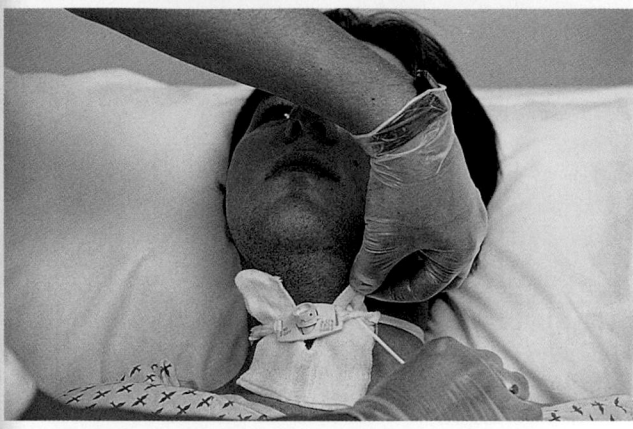

STEP **6B(11)(f)**   Applying tracheostomy dressing.

11. Assess security of tape or commercial ET or trach tube holder by tugging at tube.

Artificial airway should not move. Client may cough.

12. Assess skin around mouth and oral mucosa (ET tube) and tracheostomy stoma for drainage, pressure, and signs of irritation.

Skin breakdown and/or irritation should not be present.

Unexpected Outcomes and Related Interventions

1. Accidental extubation occurs.
   a. Call for assistance.
   b. Maintain patent airway: replace old tracheostomy tube with new tube.
   c. Observe vital signs and signs of respiratory distress.
2. Breath sounds are not equal bilaterally with an ET tube in place.
   a. Evaluate ET tube for proper depth. If incorrect, arrange for ET tube to be repositioned as allowed by institution.
   b. Obtain order for chest x-ray study to verify placement if applicable.
3. Hard, reddened areas with or without excessive or foul-smelling secretions are observed.
   a. Indicates infection. Notify physician.
   b. Increase frequency of tube care.
   c. Remove inner cannula, if applicable, for cleaning and suctioning.
4. Tube is not secure, and artificial airway moves in or out or is coughed out by client.
   a. Assess client's respiratory status and observe for the presence of mucus plugs.
   b. Adjust or apply new ties.

5. Breakdown, pressure areas, or stomatitis (tracheostomy tube) are observed.
   a. Increase frequency of tube care.
   b. Make sure skin areas are clean and dry.

Recording and Reporting

- Record respiratory assessments before and after care.
- Record ET tube care: depth of ET tube, frequency and extent of care, client tolerance, and any complications related to presence of the tube.
- Record tracheostomy care: type and size of tracheostomy tube, frequency and extent of care, client tolerance, and any complications related to presence of the tube.

Home Care Considerations (Tracheostomy Only)

   a. Instruct caregivers how to obtain supplies.
   b. Instruct caregivers on signs and symptoms of respiratory distress, tube dysfunction, respiratory and stoma infections.

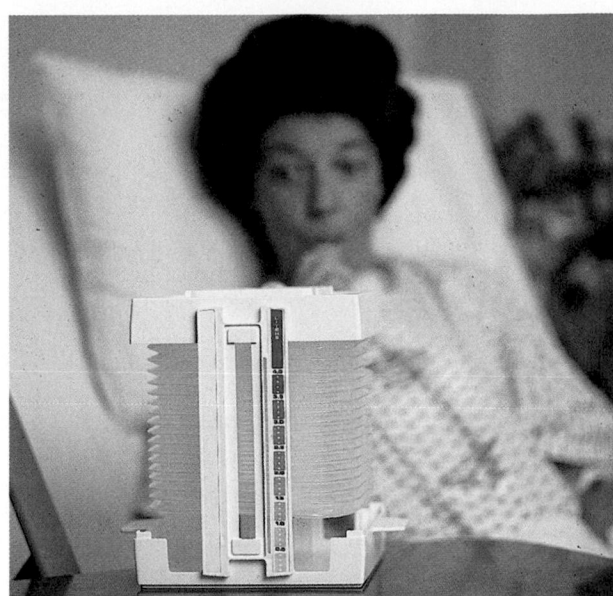

FIGURE **39-13** Volume-oriented spirometer.

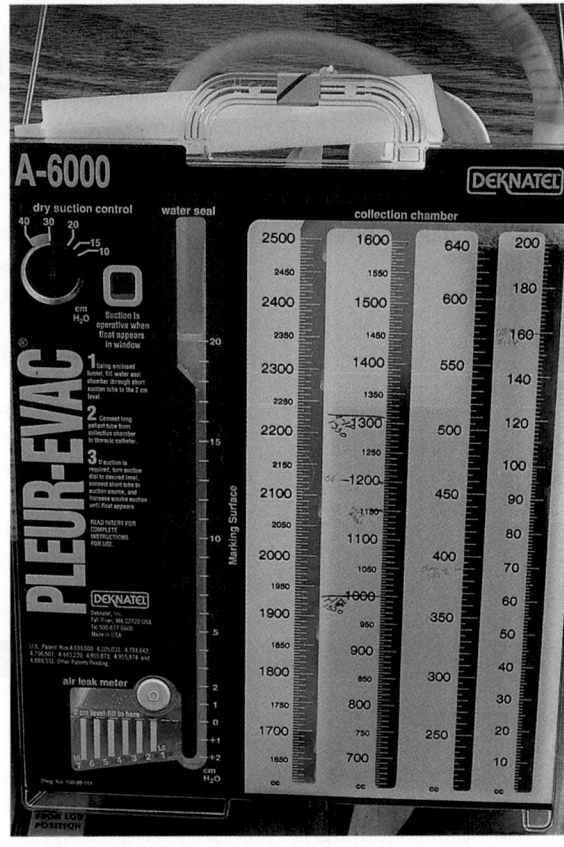

FIGURE **39-14** Disposable, commercial chest drainage system.

elevate the balls and to keep them floating as long as possible to ensure a maximally sustained inhalation.

Volume-oriented incentive spirometry devices have a bellows that is raised to a predetermined volume by an inhaled breath (Figure 39-13). An achievement light or counter is used to provide feedback. Some devices are constructed so that the light will not turn on unless the bellows is held at a minimum desired volume for a specified period to enhance lung expansion.

Incentive spirometry encourages clients to breathe to their normal inspiratory capacities. A postoperative inspiratory capacity one half to three fourths of the preoperative volume is acceptable because of postoperative pain. Administration of pain medications before incentive spirometry will help the client achieve deep breathing by reducing pain and splinting (see Chapter 49).

Chest Tubes. Chest tubes are inserted to remove air and fluids from the pleural space, to prevent air or fluid from reentering the pleural space, and to reestablish normal intrapleural and intrapulmonic pressures. A **chest tube** is a catheter inserted through the thorax to remove fluid or air. There are a variety of chest tubes on the market. In addition to the usual disposable waterless system, the traditional reusable glass three-bottle systems may still be used. The newest system available is the mobile chest drain. Regardless of the system used, the principles of client management are the same (Carroll, 2002). Chest tubes are commonly used after chest surgery and chest trauma and for pneumothorax or hemothorax to promote lung reexpansion (Skill 39-3).

A **pneumothorax** is a collection of air in the pleural space. The loss of negative intrapleural pressure causes the lung to collapse. There are a variety of mechanisms for a pneumothorax. It may occur spontaneously or as a result of chest trauma, such as a stabbing or the chest striking the steering wheel in an automobile accident. A pneumothorax may result from the rupture of an em-

physematous bleb on the surface of the lung (a large bulla resulting from the destruction caused by emphysema) or from an invasive procedure, such as insertion of a subclavian IV line.

A client with a pneumothorax usually feels pain as atmospheric air irritates the parietal pleura. The pain may be sharp and pleuritic. Dyspnea is common and worsens as the size of the pneumothorax increases.

A **hemothorax** is an accumulation of blood and fluid in the pleural cavity between the parietal and visceral pleurae, usually as a result of trauma. It produces a counterpressure and prevents the lung from full expansion. A hemothorax can also be caused by rupture of small blood vessels from inflammatory processes, such as pneumonia or tuberculosis. In addition to pain and dyspnea, signs and symptoms of shock can develop if blood loss is severe.

A disposable system, such as a Thora-Sene III or Pleur-Evac chest drainage system (DeKnatel), is a one-piece molded plastic unit that provides for a single- or multiple-chamber closed drainage system (Figure 39-14). The disposable units appear to be the system of choice because they are cost-effective and some facilitate autotransfusion, a common practice in open-heart surgeries. Knowledge of the basics of chest tube management and troubleshooting maneuvers reduces the client's risk of complications.

The simplest closed drainage system is the use of a single chamber. The chamber serves as a collector and a water seal. During normal respiration the fluid will ascend

Skill **39-3**   *Care of Clients With Chest Tubes*

Delegation Considerations

This skill should not be delegated to assistive personnel (AP). However, an AP may be assisting with other aspects of the client's care and should be informed of the following:

- Proper positioning of the client with chest tubes to facilitate chest tube drainage and optimal function of the system
- How to ambulate and transfer client with chest drainage
- Appropriate setup of drainage equipment for the type of system to be used
- To inform the nurse of any changes in vital signs, chest pain, or sudden shortness of breath, or excessive bubbling in water-seal chamber
- To notify the nurse immediately if there is disconnection of system, change in type and amount of drainage, sudden bleeding, or sudden cessation of bubbling.

Equipment

- Disposable chest drainage system (see Figure 39-14, p. 1117)
- Suction source and setup (wall canister or portable)
- Nonsterile gloves
- 2-inch tape
- Sterile gauze sponges
- Two shodded hemostats

Steps	Rationale
1. Perform hand hygiene and assess client	Signs and symptoms should reflect improvement in respiratory distress and chest pain after insertion of chest tube. Notify physician immediately.
a. *Pulmonary status:* Assess for: respiratory distress, chest pain, breath sounds over affected lung area, and stable vital signs (see Chapter 31). Signs and symptoms of increased respiratory distress and/or chest pain are decreased breath sounds over the affected and nonaffected lungs, marked cyanosis, asymmetrical chest movements, presence of subcutaneous emphysema around tube insertion site or neck, hypotension, and tachycardia (Carroll, 2002).	
b. Vital signs	Changes in pulse and blood pressure may indicate infection, respiratory distress, pain.
c. Pain: If possible, ask client to rate level of comfort on a scale of 0 to 10.	Chest tubes can be painful and interfere with client's mobility, coughing and deep breathing, and rehabilitation.
2. Observe:	
a. Chest tube dressing and site surrounding tube insertion.	Ensures that dressing is intact and occlusive seal remains, without air or fluid leaks and that area surrounding insertion site is free of drainage or skin irritation (Carroll, 2002).
b. Tubing for kinks, dependent loops, or clots.	Maintains a patent, freely draining system, preventing fluid accumulation in chest cavity. The presence of kinks, dependent loops, or clotted drainage increases the client's risk for infection, atelectasis, and tension pneumothorax (Allibone, 2003).
c. Chest drainage system, which should be upright and below level of tube insertion.	Facilitates drainage; system must be in this position to function properly.

3. Provide two shodded hemostats or approved clamps for each chest tube, attached to top of client's bed with adhesive tape. Chest tubes are only clamped under specific circumstances per physician order or nursing policy and procedure:
  a. To assess air leak
  b. To quickly empty or change disposable systems; performed by a nurse who has received education in the procedure
	Shodded hemostats have a covering to prevent hemostat from penetrating chest tube once changed. The use of these shodded hemostats or other clamp prevent air from reentering the pleural space (Allibone, 2003).

Steps	Rationale

c. If there is an accidental disconnection of drainage tubing from the drainage collection device or damage to the device

d. To assess if client is ready to have chest tube removed (which is done by physician's order); monitor the client for recurrent pneumothorax

4. Position client. — Permits optimal drainage of fluid and/or air.

   A. Semi-Fowler's position to evacuate air (pneumothorax) — Air rises to highest point in chest. Pneumothorax tubes are usually placed on anterior aspect at midclavicular line, second or third intercostal space.

   B. High-Fowler's position to drain fluid (hemothorax, effusion) — Permits optimal drainage of fluid. Posterior tubes are placed on midaxillary line, eighth or ninth intercostal space.

5. Maintain tube connection between chest and drainage tubes intact and taped. — Secures chest tube to drainage system and reduces risk of air leak causing breaks in airtight system.

   a. Water-sealed vent must be without occlusion. — Permits displaced air to pass into atmosphere.

   b. Suction-control chamber vent must be without occlusion when suction is used. — Provides safety factor of releasing excess negative pressure into atmosphere. Too little suction prevents lung reexpansion and increases client risk for infection, atelectasis, and tension pneumothorax. Too much suction damages the lung tissue and perpetuates existing air leaks (Allibone, 2003).

6. Avoid excess tubing; the tubing should be laid horizontally across the client bed or chair before dropping vertically into the drainage bottle. If the client is in a chair and the tubing is coiled, the tubing should be lifted every 15 minutes to promote drainage. — The length of tubing should be tailored to each client to avoid excessive coiling or loop formation. Coiled, looped, or clotted tubing impedes chest tube drainage (Allibone, 2003).

7. Adjust tubing to hang in straight line from top of mattress to drainage chamber. If chest tube is draining fluid, indicate time (e.g., 0900) that drainage was begun on drainage bottle's adhesive tape or on write-on surface of disposable commercial system. — Provides a baseline for continuous assessment of type and quality of drainage.

8. Strip or milk chest tube only if indicated (this means compressing the tube to encourage clots to pass through the tube). — Stripping may cause complications because it creates excessive negative intrapleural pressure (over -100 cm H_2O pressure). Milking causes less of a pressure change.

   a. Stripping—compression along length of the tubing beginning at client and continuing until drainage unit is reached

   b. Milking—compressing and releasing the tube sequentially

---

Critical Decision Point: Check your institutional policy before stripping or milking chest tubes. This practice is being discontinued at most institutions because it is believed that stripping the tube greatly increases intrapleural pressure, which could damage the pleural tissue and cause or worsen an existing pneumothorax. However, even though the literature is contradictory, stripping or milking may be done in selected clients (e.g., fresh postoperative thoracic surgery, chest trauma) because the presence of clotted drainage causes decreased reexpansion and increases risk of tension pneumothorax (Allibone, 2003), and the benefits or stripping or milking outweigh the risks.

---

9. Perform hand hygiene. — Reduces transmission of infection.

10. Evaluate:

   a. Chest tube dressing. — Appearance of drainage may be due to tube occlusion, causing drainage to exit around tube.

Critical Decision Point: Check the dressing carefully because it must remain occlusive. It can come loose from the skin, although this may not be readily apparent.

---

   b. Tubing should be free of kinks and dependent loops. — Straight and coiled drainage tube positions are optimal for pleural drainage. However, when a dependent loop is unavoidable, periodic lifting and drainage of the tube will promote pleural drainage.

 **39-3** *Care of Clients With Chest Tubes—cont'd*

Steps	Rationale
c. The chest drainage system should be upright and below level of tube insertion. Note presence of clots or debris in tubing.	System must be in the upright position to function and facilitate proper drainage.
d. Water seal for fluctuations with client's inspiration and expiration.	
(1) Waterless system: diagnostic indicator for fluctuations with client's inspirations and expirations	In the non–mechanically ventilated client, fluid should rise in the water seal or diagnostic indicator with inspiration and fall with expiration. The opposite occurs in the client who is mechanically ventilated. This indicates the system is properly functioning.
(2) Water-seal system: bubbling in the water-seal chamber	When system is initially connected to client, bubbles are expected from the chamber. These are from air that was present in the system and in client's intrapleural space. After a short time, the bubbling stops. Fluid will continue to fluctuate in the water seal on inspiration and expiration until the lung is reexpanded or the system becomes occluded.
e. Waterless system: Bubbling is diagnostic indicator.	Indicates proper functioning of the system.
f. Type and amount of fluid drainage: Nurse should note color and amount of drainage, client's vital signs, and skin color. What is the normal amount of drainage?	
(1) *In the adult:* less than 50 to 200 ml/hr immediately after surgery in a mediastinal chest tube; approximately 500 ml in first 24 hours.	Dark-red drainage is expected only in the postoperative period, turning serous with time.
(2) Between 100 and 300 ml of fluid may drain in pleural chest tube in an adult during first 3 hours after insertion. This rate will decrease after 2 hours; 500 to 1000 ml can be expected in first 24 hours. Drainage is grossly bloody during first several hours after surgery and then changes to serous. Remember that a sudden gush of drainage may be retained blood and not active bleeding. This increase in drainage can result from client position changes.	Reexpansion of lungs forces drainage into the tube. Coughing can also cause large gushes of drainage or air. Excessive amounts and/or continued presence of frank, bloody drainage the first several hours of surgery should be reported to the physician, along with client's vital signs and respiratory status.

Critical Decision Point: If drainage suddenly increases or if there is more than 100 ml/hr of blood drainage (except for the first 3 hours postoperative) the nurse should inform the physician (Allibone, 2003).

Steps	Rationale
g. Water-sealed system: bubbling in the suction-control chamber (when suction is being used).	Suction-control chamber has constant, gentle bubbling. Tubing to suction source should be free of obstruction, and suction source should be turned on to appropriate setting.
h. Waterless system: The suction control (float ball) indicates the amount of suction the client's intrapleural space is receiving.	The suction float ball dictates the amount of suction in the system. The float ball allows no more suction than dictated by its setting. If the suction source is set too low, the suction float ball cannot reach the prescribed setting. In this case the suction must be increased for the float ball to reach the prescribed setting.
i. Auscultate lungs and observe for symmetry.	Breath sounds should be equal. Decreased breath sounds on the affected side may indicate that air or fluid has reaccumulated in the pleural space. Percuss the area. A hollow sound indicates retained air, a dull/flat sound may indicate the presence of fluid (Carroll, 2002).
j. Ask client to evaluate pain on a level of 0 to 10.	May indicate the need for medication for pain.

Steps	Rationale

Unexpected Outcomes and Related Interventions

1. Continuous bubbling is seen in water-sealed chamber, indicating that leak is between client and water seal.
   a. Tighten loose connections between client and water seal.
   b. Cross-clamp chest tube close to client's chest. If bubbling stops, air leak is inside client's thorax or at chest tube insertion site. Unclamp tube, and notify physician immediately. Reinforce chest dressing. Leaving chest tube clamped causes a tension pneumothorax and mediastinal shift.
   c. Gradually move clamps down drainage tubing away from client and toward drainage chamber, moving one clamp at a time. When bubbling stops, leak is in section of tubing or connection distal to the clamp. Replace tubing or secure connection and release clamp.
2. Leak is in drainage system.
   a. Change drainage system.
3. Tension pneumothorax is present.
   a. Determine that chest tubes are not clamped, kinked, or occluded. Obstructed chest tubes trap air in intrapleural space when air leak originates within client.
   b. Notify physician immediately.
   c. Prepare immediately for another chest tube insertion; obtain a flutter (Heimlich) valve or large-gauge needle for short-term emergency release of air in intrapleural space; have emergency equipment (e.g., oxygen, code cart) near client.

4. Dependent loops of drainage tubing have trapped fluid.
   a. Drain tubing contents into drainage bottle. Coil excess tubing onto mattress, and secure in place or place in a straight line down the length of the bed.

Recording and Reporting

a. Record in nurse's notes patency of chest; presence, type, and amount of drainage; presence of fluctuations; client's vital signs; chest dressing status; amount of suction and/or water seal; and level of comfort.

Home Care Considerations

a. Client with chronic conditions (e.g., uncomplicated pneumothorax, effusions, empyema) that require a chest tube may be discharged home with smaller mobile chest drains. These systems do not have a suction-control chamber and use a mechanical one-way valve instead of a water-seal chamber (Carroll, 2002).
b. Instruct client how to ambulate and remain active with a home chest tube drainage system
c. Provide client with information as to when to contact health care professionals regarding changes in drainage system (e.g., chest pain, breathlessness, change in drainage).

---

with inspiration and descend with expiration. A single chamber is used for smaller amounts of drainage, such as an empyema—a collection of infected fluid or pus in the pleural space.

The use of two chambers permits the liquid to flow into the collection chamber as air flows into the water-sealed chamber. Fluctuations in the water-seal tube are still anticipated. Use of two chambers allows for more accurate measurement of chest drainage and is used when larger amounts of drainage are expected.

When a volume of air or fluid needs to be evacuated with controlled suction, all three chambers are used. The suction control is marked with cm readings to adjust the amount of suction. Usually 15 to 20 cm of water is used for adults. This means that the chamber is filled with sterile water to the 15- or 20-cm water level. Children require less pressure.

Special Considerations. Clamping a chest tube is contraindicated when the client is ambulating or being transported. The nurse should instead handle the chest drainage unit carefully and maintain the drainage device below the client's chest. If the tubing disconnects from the drainage unit, the nurse should instruct the client to exhale as much as possible and to cough. This maneuver rids the pleural space of as much air as possible. The nurse needs to cleanse the tips of the tubing and reconnect them quickly. If the drainage unit is broken, the end of the chest tube can be quickly submerged in a container of sterile water to reestablish the seal. Clamping the chest tube may result in a tension pneumothorax. Air pressure builds in the pleural space, collapsing the lung and creating a life-threatening event.

Removal of chest tubes requires client preparation. Clients report sensations during chest tube removal. The most frequent sensations include burning, pain, and a pulling sensation.

Maintenance and Promotion of Oxygenation. Promotion of lung expansion, mobilization of secretions, and maintenance of a patent airway assists the client in meeting oxygenation needs. Some clients, however, also require oxygen therapy to keep a healthy level of tissue oxygenation.

Oxygen Therapy. Oxygen therapy is cheap, widely available, and used in a variety of settings to relieve or prevent tissue hypoxia (Thomson and others, 2002). The goal of oxygen therapy is to prevent or relieve hypoxia. Any client with impaired tissue oxygenation can benefit from controlled oxygen administration. Oxygen is not a substitute for other treatment, however, and should be used only when indicated. Oxygen should be treated as a drug. It has dangerous side effects, such as atelectasis or oxygen toxicity (Thomson, 2002). As with any drug, the dosage or concentration of oxygen should be continuously monitored. The nurse should routinely check the physician's orders to verify that the client is receiving the prescribed oxygen concentration. The six rights of medication administration also pertain to oxygen administration (see Chapter 34).

Safety Precautions. Oxygen is a highly combustible gas. Although it will not spontaneously burn or cause an explosion, it can easily cause a fire to ignite in a client's room if it contacts a spark from an open flame or electrical equipment. With increasing use of home oxygen therapy, clients and health care professionals must be aware of the dangers of combustion.

> *Safety Alert.* Oxygen in high concentrations has a great combustion potential and readily fuels fire.

The nurse should promote safety by using the following measures:

- "No smoking" signs should be placed on the client's room door and over the bed. The client, visitors and roommates, and all personnel should be informed that smoking is not permitted in areas where oxygen is in use.
- Determine that all electrical equipment in the room is functioning correctly and is properly grounded (see Chapter 37). An electrical spark in the presence of oxygen can result in a serious fire.
- Locate the closest fire extinguisher.
- Know the fire procedures and the route for evacuation of the area.
- Check the oxygen level of portable tanks before transporting a client to ensure that there is enough oxygen in the tank.

Supply of Oxygen. Oxygen is supplied to the client's bedside either by oxygen tanks or through a permanent wall-piped system. Oxygen tanks are transported on wide-based carriers that allow the tank to be placed upright at the bedside. Regulators are used to control the amount of oxygen delivered. One common type is an upright flowmeter with a flow adjustment valve at the top. A second type is a cylinder indicator with a flow adjustment handle. In the home setting, oxygen therapy is also supplied in a variety of methods, including refillable cylinders (Cuvelier and others, 2002).

In the hospital or home, oxygen tanks are delivered with the regulator in place. In the hospital the respiratory care department usually connects the regulator to the oxygen source. Home care vendors are usually responsible for connecting the oxygen tank to the regulator for home use.

Methods of Oxygen Delivery. Oxygen can be delivered to the client by nasal cannula, nasal catheter, face mask, or mechanical ventilator.

Nasal Cannula. A **nasal cannula** is a simple, comfortable device used for oxygen delivery (Skill 39-4). The two cannulas, about 1.5 cm (½ inch) long, protrude

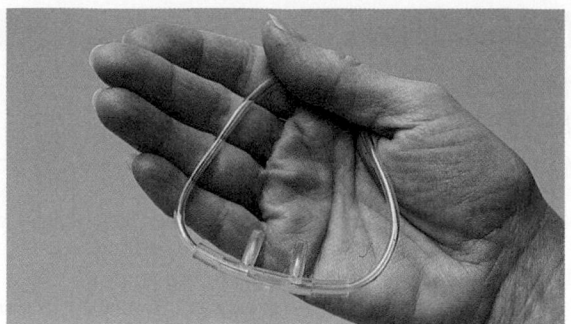

FIGURE **39–15** Nasal cannula.

Table 39-11	Approximate FiO₂ With Different Oxygen Delivery Devices	
Oxygen Delivery Device	Required liter flow (L/min)	Approximate Percent Oxygen
Nasal cannula	1-2	24-28
	3-4	32-36
	5-6	40-44
Simple face mask	5-6	40
	6-7	50
	7-8	60
Venturi mask	2	24
	3	28
	4	30
	6	35
	8	40
	10	50
	14	55

from the center of a disposable tube and are inserted into the nares (Figure 39-15). Oxygen is delivered via the cannulas with a flow rate of up to 6 L/min. Flow rates greater than 4 L/min are not often used because of the drying effect on the mucosa and the relatively little increase in delivered oxygen concentration. The nurse must know what flow rate produces a given percentage of inspired oxygen concentration (FiO_2) (Table 39-11). The nurse must also be alert for skin breakdown over the ears and in the nares from too tight an application of the nasal cannula.

Transtracheal Oxygen. Transtracheal oxygen (TTO) is a method of oxygen delivery for clients with chronic lung diseases in which a small, IV-size catheter is inserted directly into the trachea through a surgical tract in the lower neck. Oxygen is delivered directly into the trachea. The advantages of TTO are (1) no oxygen is lost to the atmosphere; (2) clients achieve adequate oxygenation at lower flow rates; (3) oxygen delivery is more efficient and less expensive, (4) there are fewer side effects, such as drying of the nasal mucosa; and (5) clients are more likely to use oxygen because of increased mobility, comfort, and cosmetic improvement.

Once the tracheal stoma is healed, the client is taught to remove and irrigate the catheter with normal saline at

Skill 39-4 — *Applying a Nasal Cannula or Oxygen Mask*

Delegation Considerations

This skill cannot be delegated to assistive personnel (AP). The nurse is responsible for assessing the client and providing safe and accurate oxygen therapy including adjustment of oxygen flow rate and evaluation of client response. The nurse should instruct AP about the following:
• Correct placement and adjustment of delivery device
• The type of equipment and the oxygen flow rate
• Unexpected outcomes associated with the oxygen delivery device (e.g., increased rate of breathing, decreased level of consciousness, increased confusion, pain) and the need to inform the nurse if any occur

Equipment

• Nasal cannula or oxygen mask
• Oxygen tubing
• Humidifier, if indicated
• Sterile water for humidification, if indicated
• Oxygen source
• Oxygen flowmeter
• Appropriate room signs

Steps	Rationale
1. Inspect client for signs and symptoms associated with hypoxia and presence of airway secretions.	Left untreated, hypoxia can produce cardiac dysrhythmias and death. Presence of airway secretions decreases effectiveness of oxygen delivery.

Critical Decision Point: Clients with sudden changes in their vital signs, level of consciousness, or behavior may be experiencing profound hypoxia. Clients who demonstrate subtle changes over time may have worsening of a chronic or existing condition or a new medical condition (Jevon and Evans, 2001).

Steps	Rationale
2. Explain to client and family what procedure entails and purpose of oxygen therapy.	Decreases client's anxiety, which reduces oxygen consumption and increases client cooperation.
3. Perform hand hygiene.	Reduces transmission of infection.
4. Attach nasal cannula to oxygen tubing, and attach to humidified oxygen source adjusted to prescribed flow rate (see illustration).	Prevents drying of nasal and oral mucous membranes and airway secretions.

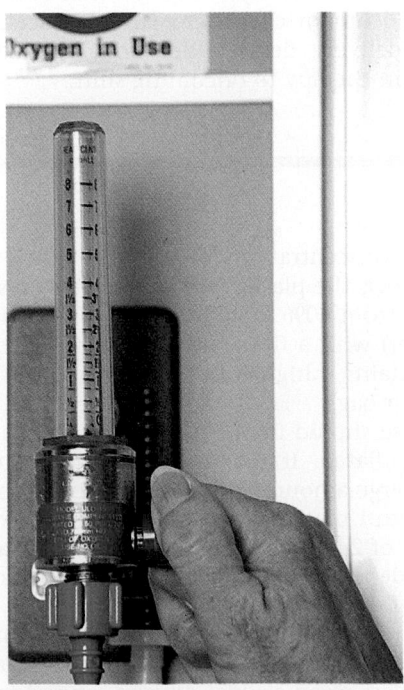

STEP **4** Adjusting flowmeter to prescribed oxygen flow rate.

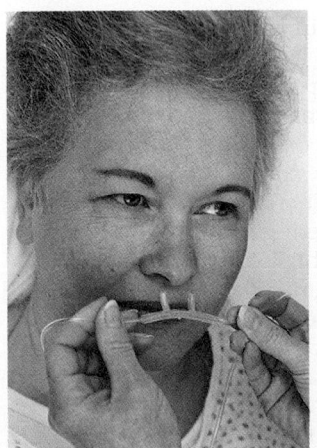 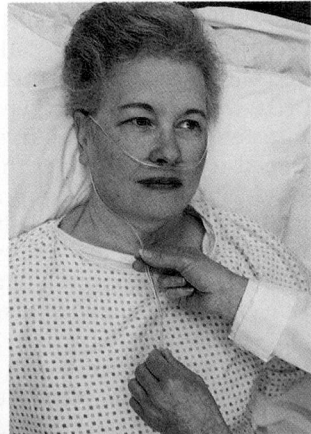

STEP **5** Applying nasal cannula and adjusting fit to client comfort.

Applying a Nasal Cannula or Oxygen Mask—cont'd

Skill 39-4

Steps	Rationale
5. Place tips of cannula into client's nares, and adjust elastic headband or plastic slide until cannula fits snugly and comfortably (see illustration).	Directs flow of oxygen into client's upper respiratory tract. Client is more likely to keep cannula in place if it fits comfortably.
6. Maintain sufficient slack on oxygen tubing and secure to client's clothes.	Allows client to turn head without dislodging cannula and reduces pressure on tips of nares.
7. Check cannula every 8 hours. Keep humidification jar filled at all times.	Ensures patency of cannula and oxygen flow. Prevents inhalation of dehumidified oxygen.
8. Observe client's nares and superior surface of both ears for skin breakdown.	Oxygen therapy can cause drying of nasal mucosa. Pressure on ears from cannula tubing or elastic can cause skin irritation.
9. Check oxygen flow rate and physician's orders every 8 hours.	Ensures delivery of prescribed oxygen flow rate and patency of cannula.
10. Perform hand hygiene.	Reduces transmission of microorganisms.
11. Inspect client for relief of symptoms associated with hypoxia.	Indicates that hypoxia is corrected or reduced.

Unexpected Outcomes and Related Interventions

1. Worsening respiratory status
   a. Check that oxygen delivery device is patent, not kinked, and attached to the oxygen flowmeter.
   b. Check oxygen level set on flowmeter; determine if delivered amount is consistent with physician order.
   c. If not using wall oxygen, determine if the oxygen source contains enough oxygen to deliver the prescribed oxygen amount.
   d. Notify physician.
2. Dry nasal and upper airway mucosa
   a. If oxygen flow rate is greater than 4 L/min, determine the need for humidification.
   b. Assess the client's fluid status and increase fluids if appropriate.
   c. Provide frequent oral care.
   d. Obtain physician order for use of sterile nasal saline intermittently.
4. Skin breakdown over the ears
   a. Adjust tightness of elastic strap to looser level.
   b. Use good hygiene and skin care around the ears.
   c. Use soft, woven 4 × 4s as nonabrasive pad between elastic and ears.
   d. Reposition elastic strap frequently.

Recording and Reporting

- Record oxygen delivery device and liter flow in medical record; document client and family education; report oxygen delivery device, liter flow, and response to changes in therapy to oncoming shift.

least 3 times a day to maintain a patent catheter. The final oxygen flow rate, usually less than 4 L/min, is delivered through an 8 Fr catheter through the mature tract.

Oxygen Masks. An oxygen mask is a device used to administer oxygen, humidity, or heated humidity. It is shaped to fit snugly over the mouth and nose and is secured in place with a strap. There are two primary types of oxygen masks: those delivering low concentrations of oxygen and those delivering high concentrations.

The simple face mask (Figure 39-16) is used for short-term oxygen therapy. It fits loosely and delivers oxygen concentrations from 30% to 60%. The mask is contraindicated for clients with carbon dioxide retention because retention can be worsened.

A plastic face mask with a reservoir bag (Figure 39-17) and a Venturi mask (Figure 39-18) are capable of delivering higher concentrations of oxygen. When used as a nonrebreather, the plastic face mask with a reservoir bag can deliver from 80% to 90% oxygen (70% when used as a rebreather) with a flow rate of 10 L/min. This oxygen mask maintains a high-concentration oxygen supply in the reservoir bag.

The nurse should frequently inspect the bag to make sure it is inflated. If it is deflated, the client may be breathing large amounts of exhaled carbon dioxide.

The Venturi mask can be used to deliver oxygen concentrations of 24% to 55% with oxygen flow rates of 2 to 14 L/min, depending on which flow-control meter is selected (see Table 39-11, p. 1122).

Home Oxygen Therapy. Indications for home oxygen therapy include an arterial partial pressure (PaO_2) of 55 mm Hg or less or an arterial oxygen saturation (SaO_2) of

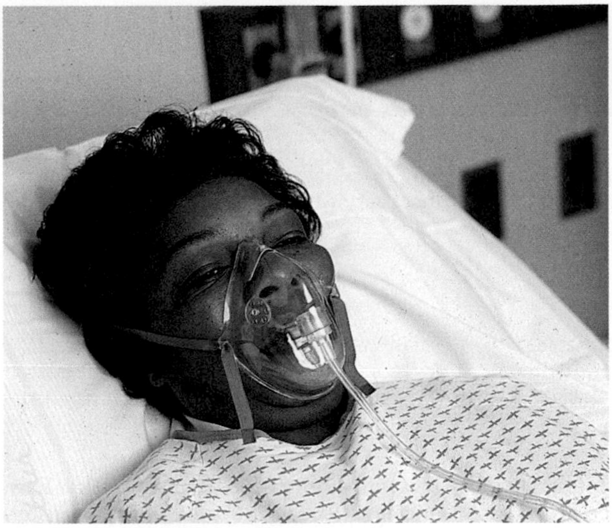

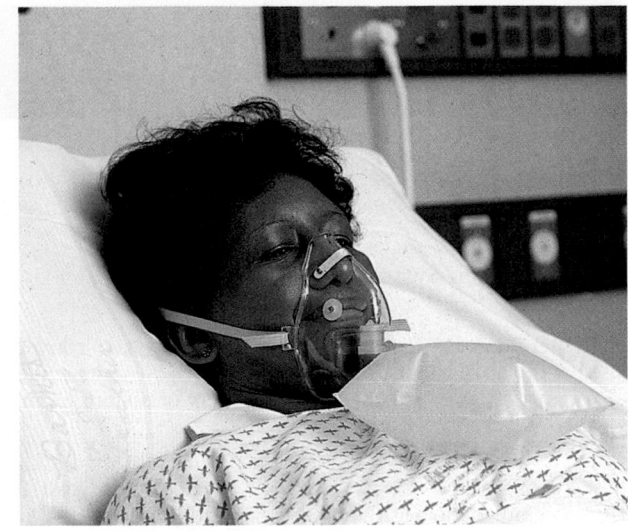

FIGURE **39–16** Simple face mask.

FIGURE **39–17** Plastic face mask with reservoir bag.

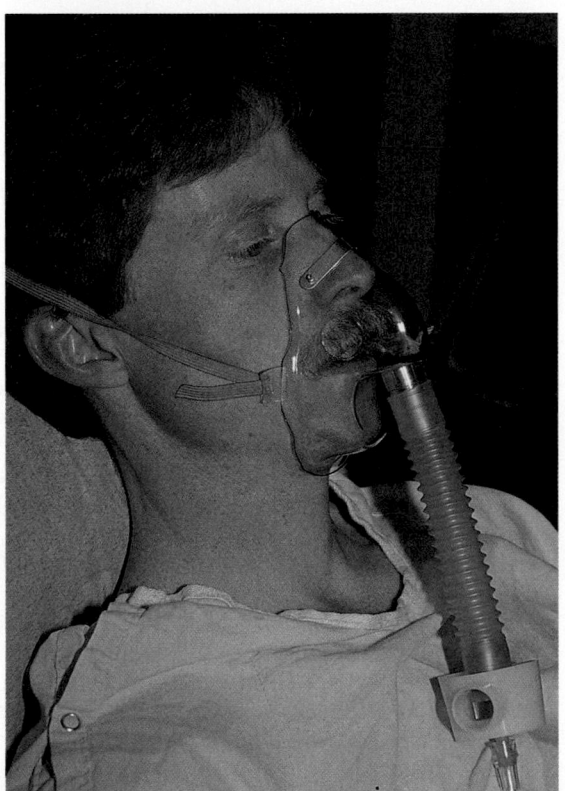

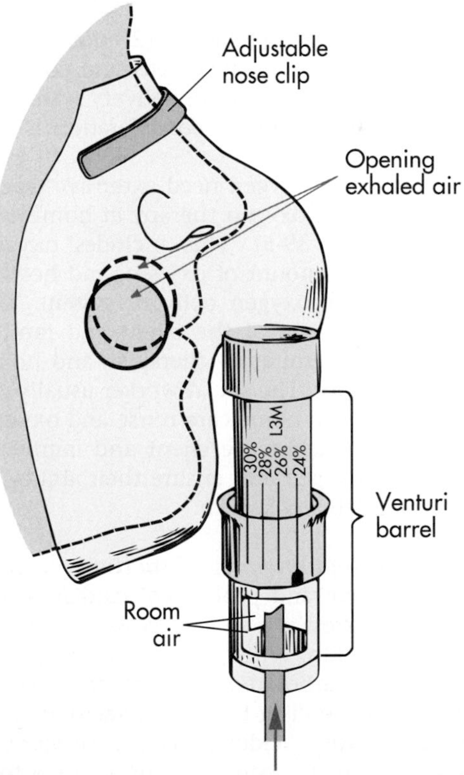

Adjustable nose clip

Opening exhaled air

Venturi barrel

Room air

FIGURE **39–18** Venturi mask

88% or less on room air at rest, on exertion, or with exercise. Clients with a PaO_2 from 56 to 59 mm Hg may also receive oxygen if there is also evidence of cor pulmonale, pulmonary hypertension, erythrocytosis, central nervous system dysfunction, impaired mental status, or increasing hypoxemia with exertion.

Home oxygen therapy has beneficial effect with clients with chronic cardiopulmonary diseases (Snow and others, 2001). This therapy improves clients' exercise tolerance and fatigue levels and in some situations assists in the management of dyspnea (Fujimoto and others, 2002). When home oxygen is required, it is usually delivered by nasal cannula. When a client has a permanent tracheostomy, however, a T tube or tracheostomy collar is necessary. Three types of oxygen are used: compressed oxygen, liquid oxygen, and oxygen concentrators. The

Table 39-12	Home Oxygen Systems	
Primary Use	**Advantages**	**Disadvantages**
Compressed Gas Cylinders		
Intermittent therapy Used for exercise or sleep only	100% oxygen, relatively inexpensive, no loss of gas during storage, relatively portable, delivery of up to 15 L/min	Bulky, possibly unsightly, frequent refilling necessary with continuous use
Liquid Oxygen Systems (Figure 39-19)		
High liter flows Used with active clients	100% oxygen, conveniently portable, portable units refilled at home, delivery of up to 6 L/min	Usually weekly delivery necessary for refill, evaporates if not used, potential for frostbite at connections and if liquid is spilled
Oxygen Concentrators		
Moderate liter flows Homebound clients with limited mobility inside or outside home	Fixed monthly cost, minimal interruption of household by supplier, no refills of "main tank," most units with delivery of up to 4 or 5 L/min	Oxygen concentration decreases as liter flow increases (usually 85% to 90%), power supply needed, electric bill increase, second system needed for portability, usually E tank gas cylinders

advantages and disadvantages (Table 39-12) of each type are assessed, along with the client's needs and community resources, before placing a certain delivery system in the home. In the home the major consideration is the oxygen delivery source.

Clients requiring home oxygen need extensive teaching to be able to continue oxygen therapy at home efficiently and safely (Skill 39-5). This includes oxygen safety, regulation of the amount of oxygen, and how to use the prescribed home oxygen delivery system. The nurse coordinates the efforts of the client and family, home care nurse, home respiratory therapist, and home oxygen equipment vendor. The social worker usually assists with arranging for the home care nurse and oxygen vendor. The nurse must assist the client and family in learning about home oxygen and ensure their ability to maintain the oxygen delivery system.

Restoration of Cardiopulmonary Functioning. If a client's hypoxia is severe and prolonged, cardiac arrest may result. A cardiac arrest is a sudden cessation of cardiac output and circulation. When this occurs, oxygen is not delivered to tissues, carbon dioxide is not transported from tissues, tissue metabolism becomes anaerobic, and metabolic and respiratory acidosis occurs. Permanent heart, brain, and other tissue damage occur within 4 to 6 minutes.

Cardiopulmonary Resuscitation. Cardiac arrest is characterized by an absence of pulse and respiration. If the nurse determines that the client has cardiac arrest, **cardiopulmonary resuscitation (CPR)** must be initiated. CPR is a basic emergency procedure of artificial respiration and manual external cardiac massage. Most nursing students are required to have successfully completed a CPR course before their clinical experiences.

The "ABCs" of cardiopulmonary resuscitation are to establish an **A**irway, initiate **B**reathing, and maintain **C**irculation. When an airway cannot be established, the nurse must reassess proper head position and assess for airway obstruction. There is no clinical benefit to cardiac compressions if an airway cannot be established. The purpose of CPR is to circulate oxygenated blood to the brain to prevent permanent tissue damage (AHA, 2001).

Restorative and Continuing Care. Restorative and continuing care may emphasize cardiopulmonary reconditioning as a structured rehabilitation program. **Cardiopulmonary rehabilitation** is actively helping the client to achieve and maintain an optimal level of health through controlled physical exercise, nutrition counseling, relaxation and stress management techniques, prescribed medications and oxygen, and compliance. As physical reconditioning occurs, the client's complaints of dyspnea, chest pain, fatigue, and activity intolerance should decrease. The client's anxiety, depression, or somatic concerns also often decrease. The client and the rehabilitation team define goals of rehabilitation.

Hydration. Maintenance of adequate systemic hydration keeps mucociliary clearance normal. In clients with adequate hydration, pulmonary secretions are thin, white, watery, and easily removable with minimal coughing. Excessive coughing to clear thick, tenacious secretions is fatiguing and energy depleting. The best way to maintain thin secretions is to provide a fluid intake of 1500 to 2000 ml/day unless contraindicated by cardiac status. The color, consistency, and ease of secretion expectoration can determine adequacy of hydration.

Coughing Techniques. Coughing is effective for maintaining a patent airway. Coughing permits the client to remove secretions from both the upper and lower airways. The normal series of events in the cough mechanism are deep inhalation, closure of the glottis, active contraction of the expiratory muscles, and glottis opening. Deep inhalation increases the lung volume and airway diameter,

Skill 39-5 | *U*sing Home Liquid Oxygen Equipment

Delegation Considerations

This skill should not be delegated to assistive personnel (AP). However, once the client is stable on home oxygen therapy, AP may perform certain aspects of care. The nurse is responsible for assessing the client, checking the device setup, and providing safe and accurate oxygen therapy. The nurse should instruct AP about the following:

- Unique needs of the client (e.g., amount of assistance in applying home nasal cannula or mask) and any assistance needed in filling liquid canisters
- The type of equipment the client should have in the home and the oxygen flow rate

- Unexpected outcomes associated with the oxygen delivery device (e.g., increased rate of breathing, decreased level of consciousness, increased confusion, pain) and the need to inform the nurse if any occur

Equipment

- Nasal cannula equipment (see Skill 39-4, p. 1123)
- Primary and portable liquid oxygen source for ambulation (see Figure 39-19, p. 1129)

Steps	Rationale
1. Assess: **a.** Client for need for home oxygen therapy.	Candidates for home oxygen have a PaO_2 ≤55 mm Hg or oxygen saturation of 88% on room air, or PaO_2 of 55 to 59 mm Hg or oxygen saturation of 86% to 89% with evidence of right heart failure, cor pulmonale, or polycythemia.
b. Client or family's ability to use oxygen equipment properly, or for appropriate use of oxygen equipment in home setting.	Physical or cognitive impairments may require instructing family members or significant others on how to operate home oxygen equipment.
c. Client's and family's ability to observe for signs and symptoms of hypoxia: apprehension, anxiety, decreased ability to concentrate, decreased level of consciousness, increased fatigue, dizziness, behavioral changes, increased pulse, increased respiratory rate, pallor, or cyanosis of the mucous membranes.	Hypoxia can occur at home despite use of oxygen therapy. It can be caused by worsening of client's physical condition or another underlying condition, such as a change in the respiratory status.
2. Explain procedure to client and family.	Reinforces information given to client and family; allows opportunity to ask questions.
3. Perform hand hygiene.	Reduces transmission of infection.
4. Demonstrate steps for preparation and completion of oxygen therapy.	Teaches psychomotor skill and enables client to ask questions.

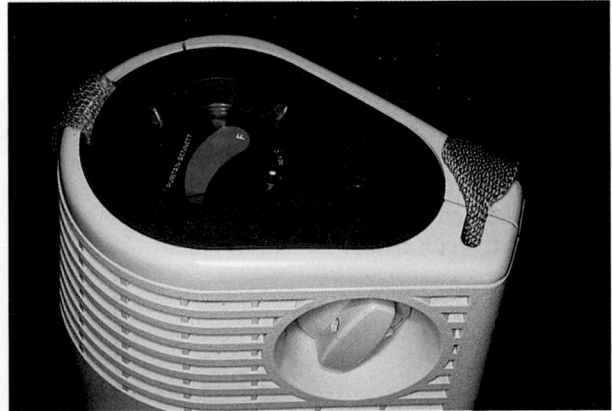
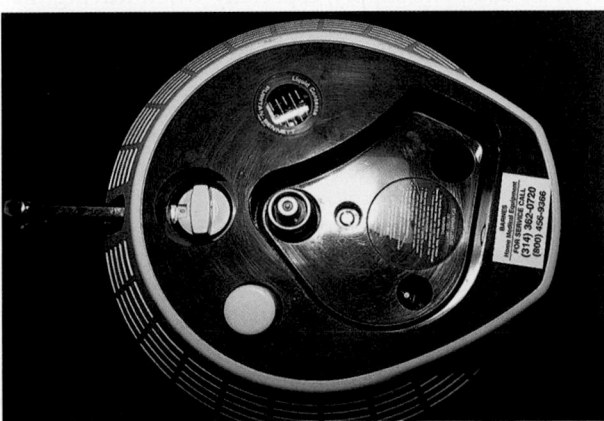

STEP **5B** Oxygen level is verified by the gauges on top of the canisters.

Skill 39-5   *Using Home Liquid Oxygen Equipment—cont'd*

Steps   **Rationale**

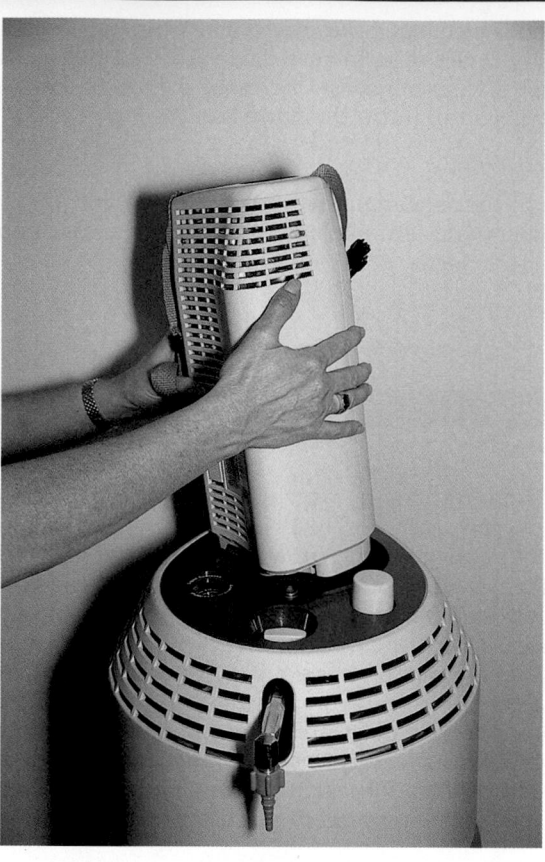

STEP **5C** Refilling portable oxygen delivery system.

5. Prepare primary and portable oxygen.

   a. Place primary oxygen source in clutter-free environment.

Primary oxygen source replaces compressed oxygen cylinders.

Critical Decision Point: Check oxygen levels in the primary and portable sources to ensure that there is an adequate supply, especially when leaving the home.

---

   b. Check oxygen levels of both sources by reading gauge on top (see illustrations).
   c. Refill portable source by placing on top of primary source and pressing down firmly. Check oxygen gauge to determine fullness of portable source (see illustration).
   d. Select prescribed rate.
   e. Connect nasal cannula and oxygen tubing to oxygen source.
   f. Perform hand hygiene.
6. Have client and family perform each step with guidance from the nurse.

Ensures adequate amount of oxygen available for use and timely refills of primary source.
Provides secure connection and prevents leakage of oxygen into room. If not seated securely, the cold liquid oxygen will leak out, creating a snowlike precipitate.

Ensures delivery of prescribed amount of oxygen.
Connects oxygen source to delivery method.

Allows nurse to correct for errors in technique and discuss their implications.

Unexpected Outcomes and Related Interventions

1. Client reports no oxygen flow.
   a. Check tank pressure gauge. If level of oxygen is low, refill tank if portable, or provide alternate source of oxygen, such as concentrator or H cylinder.
   b. Notify home oxygen supplier of need for refill.
   c. Reassure client and family.
2. Unable to fill portable liquid oxygen from main source.
   a. Check to see that portable tank is connected correctly.
   b. Determine if valve is frozen.
   c. Contact home oxygen supplier for service visit.
   d. Provide alternate oxygen source if necessary.

Recording and Reporting

- Record the client's and family's ability to safely use the home oxygen equipment; report the type of home oxygen equipment to be used, the client's and family's understanding of how to use the equipment, knowledge of safety guidelines and unexpected outcomes, and ability to return demonstrate proper use of the oxygen delivery device.

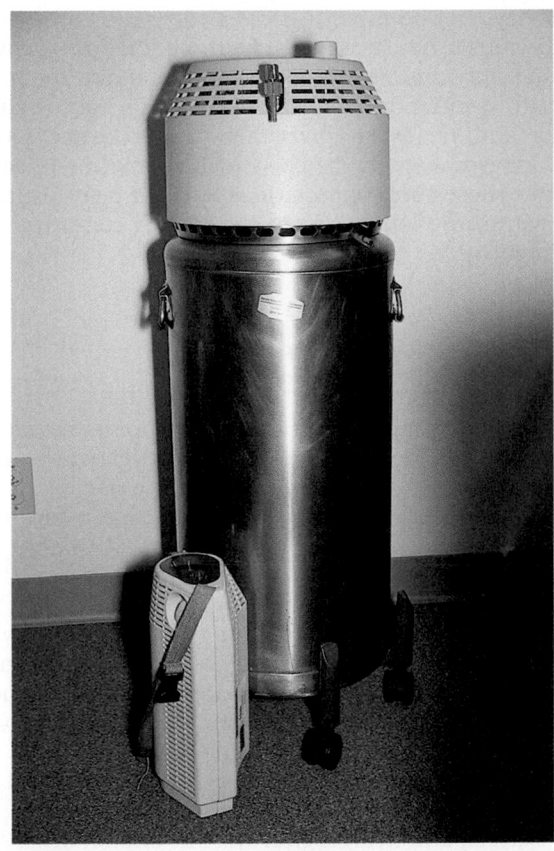

FIGURE **39–19** Primary and portable liquid oxygen source for ambulation.

allowing the air to pass through partially obstructing mucous plugs or other foreign matter. Contraction of the expiratory muscles against the closed glottis causes a high intrathoracic pressure to develop. When the glottis opens, a large flow of air is expelled at a high speed, providing momentum for mucus to move to the upper airways, where it can be expectorated or swallowed.

The effectiveness of coughing is evaluated by sputum expectoration, the client's report of swallowed sputum, or clearing of adventitious sounds by auscultation. Clients with chronic pulmonary diseases, upper respiratory tract infections, and lower respiratory tract infections should be encouraged to deep breathe and cough at least every 2 hours while awake. Clients with a large amount of sputum should be encouraged to cough every hour while awake and every 2 to 3 hours while asleep until the acute phase of mucus production has ended. Coughing techniques include deep breathing and coughing for the postoperative client, cascade, huff, and quad coughing.

With the *cascade cough,* the client takes a slow, deep breath and holds it for 2 seconds while contracting expiratory muscles. Then the client opens the mouth and performs a series of coughs throughout exhalation, thereby coughing at progressively lowered lung volumes. This technique promotes airway clearance and a patent airway in clients with large volumes of sputum.

The *huff cough* stimulates a natural cough reflex and is generally effective only for clearing central airways. While exhaling, the client opens the glottis by saying the word *huff.* With practice the client inhales more air and may be able to progress to the cascade cough.

The *quad cough* technique is used for clients without abdominal muscle control, such as those with spinal cord injuries. While the client breathes out with a maximal expiratory effort, the client or nurse pushes inward and upward on the abdominal muscles toward the diaphragm, causing the cough.

Respiratory Muscle Training. Respiratory muscle training improves muscle strength and endurance, resulting in improved activity tolerance. Respiratory muscle training may prevent respiratory failure in clients with COPD.

One method for respiratory muscle training is the incentive spirometer resistive breathing device (ISRBD). Resistive breathing is achieved by placing a resistive breathing device into a volume-dependent incentive spirometer. Muscle training is achieved when the client uses the ISRBD on a scheduled routine (e.g., twice a day for 15 minutes or 4 times a day for 15 minutes).

Breathing Exercises. Breathing exercises include techniques to improve ventilation and oxygenation. The three basic techniques are deep breathing and coughing exercises, pursed-lip breathing, and diaphragmatic breathing. Deep breathing and coughing exercises are routine interventions for postoperative clients (see Chapter 49).

Pursed-Lip Breathing. **Pursed-lip breathing** involves deep inspiration and prolonged expiration through pursed lips to prevent alveolar collapse. While sitting up, the client is instructed to take a deep breath and to exhale slowly through pursed lips, as if blowing through a straw. The nurse can also have the client blow through a straw into a glass of water to learn the technique. Clients need to gain control of the exhalation phase so that it is longer than inhalation. The client is usually able to perfect this technique by counting the inhalation time and gradually increasing the count during exhalation. In studies using pulse oximetry as a feedback tool, clients have been able to demonstrate an increase in their arterial oxygen saturation during pursed-lip breathing.

Diaphragmatic Breathing. **Diaphragmatic breathing** is more difficult and requires the client to relax intercostal and accessory respiratory muscles while taking deep inspirations. The client concentrates on expanding the diaphragm during controlled inspiration, and is taught to place one hand flat below the breastbone above the waist and the other hand 2 to 3 cm below the first hand. The client is asked to inhale while the lower hand moves outward during inspiration. The client observes for inward movement as the diaphragm ascends. These exercises are initially taught with the client in the supine position and then practiced while the client sits and stands. The exercise is often used with the pursed-lip breathing technique.

Diaphragmatic breathing is also useful for clients with pulmonary disease, for postoperative clients, and for women in labor to promote relaxation and provide pain control. The exercise improves efficiency of breathing by decreasing air trapping and reducing the work of breathing.

Evaluation

Nursing interventions and therapies are evaluated by comparing the client's progress with the goals and expected outcomes of the nursing care plan. Client care evaluates the actual care given to the client by the health care team based on the expected outcomes (Figure 39-20). Client expectations evaluate the care from the client's perspective.

Client Care. The client is the only one who can evaluate his or her degree of breathlessness. The client should be asked to rate his or her breathlessness on a scale of 1 to 10, with 1 being no shortness of breath and 10 being severe shortness of breath. Evaluation of arterial blood gas levels, pulmonary function tests, vital signs, ECG tracings, and physical assessment data provide the nurse with objective measurement of the success of therapies and treatments. Outcomes are compared with expected outcomes to determine the client's health status. Continuous evaluation allows the nurse to determine whether new or revised therapies are required and if new nursing diagnoses have developed and require a new plan of care.

When nursing measures directed to improve oxygenation are unsuccessful, the nurse must immediately modify the nursing care plan. The nurse should not hesitate to notify the physician about a client's deteriorating oxygenation status. Prompt notification can avoid an emergency situation or even the need for CPR. Continuous evaluation allows the nurse to determine whether new or revised therapies are required and if new nursing diagnoses have developed and require a new plan of care.

Client Expectations. If the nurse has successfully developed a good relationship with a client, the client will be more willing to share his or her satisfaction. It is important for the nurse to ask the client if his or her expectations of care have been met. For example, the nurse can ask the client, "Do you feel like you will be able to use the breathing techniques we have practiced at home?" If the client states that he or she does not think this will work at home, then the client's expectations for care management have not been met.

The nurse should ask the client whether all of his or her questions and needs have been met. If not, the nurse needs to spend more time understanding what the client wants and needs to meet his or her expectations. Working closely with the client will enable the nurse to redefine those client expectations that can be realistically met within the limitations of the client's condition and treatment.

Key Concepts

- The primary function of the heart is to deliver deoxygenated blood to the lungs for oxygenation and to deliver oxygen and nutrients to the tissues.
- Preload, afterload, contractility, and heart rate alter cardiac output.
- Cardiac dysrhythmias are classified by cardiac activity and site of impulse origin.
- The primary function of the lungs is to transfer oxygen from the atmosphere into the alveoli and to transfer carbon dioxide out of the body as a waste product.
- Ventilation is the process of providing adequate oxygenation from the alveoli to the blood.
- Compliance, or the ability of the lungs to expand and contract, depends on the function of musculoskeletal and neurological systems and on other physiological factors.
- The process of inspiration (active process) and expiration (passive process) is caused by changes in intrapleural and intraalveolar pressures and lung volumes.
- Respiration is controlled by the central nervous system and by chemicals within the blood.
- Decreased hemoglobin levels alter the client's ability to transport oxygen.
- Impaired chest wall movement reduces the level of tissue oxygenation.
- Hyperventilation is a respiratory rate greater than that required to maintain normal levels of carbon dioxide.

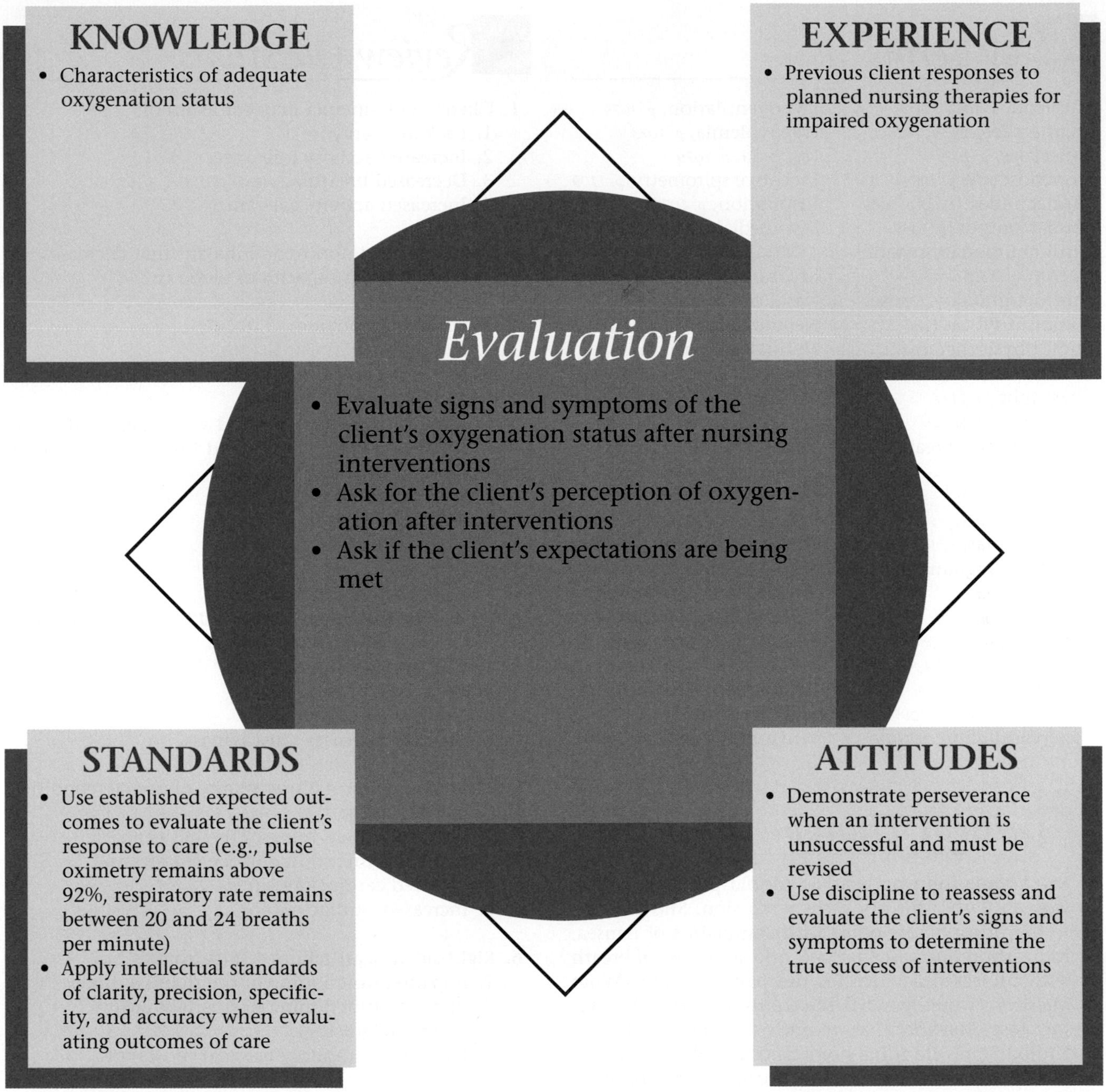

KNOWLEDGE

• Characteristics of adequate oxygenation status

EXPERIENCE

• Previous client responses to planned nursing therapies for impaired oxygenation

Evaluation

• Evaluate signs and symptoms of the client's oxygenation status after nursing interventions
• Ask for the client's perception of oxygenation after interventions
• Ask if the client's expectations are being met

STANDARDS

• Use established expected outcomes to evaluate the client's response to care (e.g., pulse oximetry remains above 92%, respiratory rate remains between 20 and 24 breaths per minute)
• Apply intellectual standards of clarity, precision, specificity, and accuracy when evaluating outcomes of care

ATTITUDES

• Demonstrate perseverance when an intervention is unsuccessful and must be revised
• Use discipline to reassess and evaluate the client's signs and symptoms to determine the true success of interventions

FIGURE **39-20** Critical thinking model for oxygenation evaluation.

• Hypoventilation causes carbon dioxide retention.
• Hypoxia occurs if the amount of oxygen delivered to tissues is too low.
• The nursing history and assessment includes information about the client's cough, dyspnea, fatigue, wheezing, chest pain, environmental exposures, respiratory infection, cardiopulmonary risk factors, and use of medications.
• Diagnostic and laboratory tests may be needed to complete the database for a client with decreased oxygenation.
• Breathing exercises improve ventilation, oxygenation, and sensations of dyspnea.

• Nebulization delivers small drops of water or particles of medication to the airways.
• Chest physiotherapy includes postural drainage, percussion, and vibration to mobilize pulmonary secretions.
• Coughing and suctioning techniques are used to maintain a patent airway.
• Oxygen therapy is used to improve levels of tissue oxygenation and is delivered by a nasal cannula, nasal catheter, or oxygen mask.

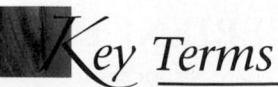

Key Terms

Afterload, *p. 1064*
Angina pectoris, *p. 1078*
Atelectasis, *p. 1079*
Bronchoscopy, *p. 1084*
Cardiac index (CI), *p. 1069*
Cardiac output, *p. 1069*
Cardiopulmonary rehabilitation, *p. 1126*
Cardiopulmonary resuscitation (CPR), *p. 1126*
Chest physiotherapy (CPT), *p. 1097*
Chest tube, *p. 1117*
Cyanosis, *p. 1080*
Diaphragmatic breathing, *p. 1130*
Diffusion, *p. 1072*
Dyspnea, *p. 1082*
Dysrhythmias, *p. 1074*
Electrocardiogram (ECG), *p. 1070*
Expiration, *p. 1070*
Hematemesis, *p. 1084*
Hemoptysis, *p. 1084*
Hemothorax, *p. 1117*
Humidification, *p. 1097*
Hyperventilation, *p. 1079*

Hypoventilation, *p. 1079*
Hypovolemia, *p. 1073*
Hypoxia, *p. 1079*
Incentive spirometry, *p. 1109*
Inspiration, *p. 1070*
Myocardial infarction (MI), *p. 1079*
Myocardial ischemia, *p. 1078*
Nasal cannula, *p. 1122*
Nebulization, *p. 1097*
Normal sinus rhythm (NSR), *p. 1070*
Orthopnea, *p. 1084*
Peak expiratory flow rate (PEFR), *p. 1090*
Pneumothorax, *p. 1117*
Postural drainage, *p. 1098*
Preload, *p. 1069*
Pursed-lip breathing, *p. 1130*
Stroke volume, *p. 1069*
Thoracentesis, *p. 1090*
Ventilation, *p. 1070*
Ventricular fibrillation, *p. 1078*
Ventricular tachycardia, *p. 1078*
Wheezing, *p. 1084*

Critical Thinking Exercises

1. Ms. Wanda Johnson is a 56-year-old postmenopausal woman with a history of hypertension. She presents to her primary care office with complaints of nausea, indigestion, increased fatigue, and shortness of breath with increased activity for the past 16 hours. What questions would you ask Ms. Johnson in the history?
2. Mr. Jose Martinez has recently immigrated to the United States from his homeland of Cuba to join his family. He comes to the clinic because he has been increasingly fatigued, has a persistent cough, has been losing weight, and awakens at night with sweats. What questions would be important to ask when completing the health history?
3. Mrs. Amanda Miller, age 45, has been admitted to the hospital with community-acquired pneumonia. She has a productive cough, fever, chills, crackles and wheezes on auscultation of her chest, and a heart rate of 104 beats per minute. What nursing diagnosis would you consider for this client? What nursing interventions would be appropriate for Mrs. Miller? What health promotion interventions need to be initiated before discharge from the hospital?
4. Mr. Chen Lee, age 72, has been having chest pain, shortness of breath, and pain down his left arm for about 2 hours. He comes to the emergency department because the pain has been getting worse over the past hour. What nursing interventions would you initiate?

Review Questions

1. Clients with anemia may complain of:
   1. Lack of energy.
   2. Increased activity tolerance.
   3. Decreased breathlessness.
   4. Increased activity tolerance.

2. The most common toxic inhalant that decreases the oxygen-carrying capacity of blood is:
   1. Carbon dioxide.
   2. Carbon monoxide.
   3. Nitrogen.
   4. Mustard gas.

3. Conditions such as shock and severe dehydration resulting from extracellular fluid loss and reduced circulating blood volume cause:
   1. Hypovolemia.
   2. Hypervolemia.
   3. Uncontrolled bleeding.
   4. Hypoxia.

4. Fever increases the tissues' need for oxygen, and as a result:
   1. Carbon dioxide decreases.
   2. Carbon dioxide increases.
   3. Cyanosis occurs.
   4. There is increases muscle mass.

5. Left-sided heart failure is an abnormal condition characterized by:
   1. Impaired functioning of the left ventricle.
   2. Impaired functioning of the left atrium.
   3. Lowered cardiac pressures.
   4. Increased cardiac output.

6. Right-sided heart failure results from:
   1. Impaired functioning of the right ventricle.
   2. Impaired functioning of the right atrium.
   3. Severe weight loss.
   4. Lowered pulmonary vascular resistance.

7. Cyanosis, the blue discoloration of the skin and mucous membranes caused by the presence of desaturated hemoglobin in capillaries, is a (an):
   1. Early sign of hypoxia.
   2. Late sign of hypoxia.
   3. Reliable measure of oxygenation status.
   4. Non–life threatening event.

8. A person who starts smoking in adolescence and continues to smoke into middle age:
   1. Has an increased risk for cardiopulmonary disease and lung cancer.
   2. Has an increased risk for obesity and diabetes.
   3. Has an increased risk for stress–related illnesses.
   4. Has an increased risk for alcoholism.

9. A simple and cost-effective method for reducing the risks of stasis of pulmonary secretions and decreased chest wall expansion is:
   1. Oxygen humidification.
   2. Chest physiotherapy.
   3. Frequent change of position.
   4. Antiinfectives.

10. The most effective position for client with cardiopulmonary diseases is the:
    1. Supine position.
    2. Prone position.
    3. High Fowler's.
    4. 45-degree semi-Fowlers.

References

Allibone L: Nursing management of chest drains, *Nurs Stand* 17(22):45, 2003.

American Cancer Society: *Cancer prevention and early detection facts and figures 2004,* Atlanta, 2004, The Society, www.career.org.

American Heart Association in collaboration with the international liaison committee on resuscitation: Guidelines 2000 for cardiopulmonary resuscitation and emergency cardiovascular care. VI. Advanced cardiovascular life support, *Circulation* 102(8 suppl):I-86, 2000.

American Heart Association: *CPR and AEDs,* 2003, www.AHA.org.

Anderson J, Kessenich CR: Women and coronary heart disease, *Nurse Pract* 26(8), 2001.

Canobbio MM: *Cardiovascular disorders,* St. Louis, 1990, Mosby.

Canobbio MM: *Mosby's handbook of patient teaching,* St. Louis, 2000, Mosby.

Carroll P: A guide to mobile chest drains, *RN* 65(5):56, 2002.

Centers for Disease Control and Prevention: Notice to readers: recommended adult immunization schedule—United States, 2002-2003, *MMWR Morb Mortal Wkly Rep* 51(40):904, 2002.

Dochterman JM, Bulechek GM: *Nursing interventions classification (NIC),* ed 4, St. Louis, 2004, Mosby.

Fujimoto K and others: Benefits of oxygen on exercise performance and pulmonary homodynamic in patients with COPD mild hypoxemia, *Chest* 122(2): 457, 2002.

Granger BB, Miller CM: Acute coronary syndrome: putting the new guidelines to work, *Nursing* 31(11):36, 2001.

Jevon P, Evans B: Assessment of a breathless patient, *Nurs Stand* 15(16):48, 2001.

Lewis SM and others: *Medical-surgical nursing: assessment and management of clinical problems,* ed 5, St. Louis, 2000, Mosby.

Lueckenotte AG: *Gerontologic nursing,* ed 2, St. Louis, 2000, Mosby.

McCance KL, Huether SE: *Pathophysiology: the biologic basis for disease in adults and children,* ed 4, St. Louis, 2001, Mosby.

Moorhead S, Johnson M, Maas M: *Nursing outcomes classification (NOC),* ed 3, St. Louis, 2004, Mosby.

Potter PA, Weilitz PB: *Health assessment pocket guide series,* ed 5, St. Louis, 2003, Mosby.

St. John RE: Airway management, *Crit Care Nurse* 19(4):79, 1999.

Stulberg MS and others: Exercise training improves outcomes of a dyspnea self-management program, *J Cardiopulm Rehabil* 22(2):109, 2002.

Thomson A and others: Oxygen therapy in acute medical care: the potential dangers of hyperoxia need to be recognised, *Br Med J* 324(7351):1406, 2002.

Zimmerman RK, Ball JA: Adult vaccination, *Prim Care* 28(4), 2001.

Research References

Akgul S, Akyolcu N: Effects of normal saline on endotracheal suctioning, *J Clin Nurs* 11(6): 826, 2002.

Cuvelier A and others: Refillable oxygen cylinders may be an alternative for ambulatory oxygen therapy in COPD, *Chest* 122(2):451, 2002.

Day T and others: Tracheal suctioning: an exploration of nurses' knowledge and competence in acute and high dependency ward areas, *J Adv Nurs* 39(1):35, 2002.

Denke MA: Primary prevention of heart disease in women, *Curr Artheroscler Rep* 3(2):136, 2001.

Joint National Committee on Prevention, Detection, Evaluation and Treatment of High Blood Pressure: The sixth report of the Joint National Committee on Prevention, Detection, Evaluation and Treatment of High Blood Pressure (JNC VII), Bethesda, Md, 2003, US Deparment of Health and Human Services, National Heart, Lung, and Blood Institute. www.nhlbi.nih.gov/guidelines/hypertension/express.pdf.

Kerr ME and others: Effect of endotracheal suctioning on cerebral oxygen in traumatic brain injured patients, *Crit Care Med* 27(2):2776, 1999.

Snow V and others: The evidence base for management of acute exacerbations of COPD: clinical practice guideline, part 1, *Chest* 119(4):1185, 2001.

Wood CJ: Endotracheal suctioning: a literature review, *Intensive Care Nurse* 14(930):124, 1998.

Fluid, Electrolyte, and Acid-Base Balances

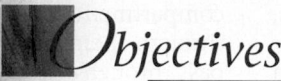

Objectives

Mastery of content in this chapter will enable the student to:

- Define the key terms listed.
- Describe the distribution, composition, movement, and regulation of body fluids.
- Describe the regulation and movement of major electrolytes.
- Describe the processes involved in acid-base balance.
- Describe common disturbances in fluid, electrolyte, and acid-base balances.
- Identify the variables affecting normal fluid, electrolyte, and acid-base balances.
- Discuss the clinical assessment for a client for fluid, electrolyte, and acid-base balances.
- Describe laboratory studies associated with fluid, electrolyte, and acid-base imbalances.
- List and discuss nursing interventions for clients with fluid, electrolyte, and acid-base imbalances.
- Discuss purpose and procedure for initiation and maintenance of intravenous therapy.
- Calculate intravenous flow rate.
- Measure and record fluid intake and output.
- Demonstrate how to change intravenous solutions, tubing, and dressings and how to discontinue an infusion.
- Discuss the complications of intravenous therapy.
- Discuss the procedure for administering a blood transfusion and nursing actions for a transfusion reaction.

*F*luid, electrolyte, and acid-base balances within the body are necessary to maintain health and function in all body systems. These balances are maintained by the intake and output of water and electrolytes and regulation by the renal and pulmonary systems. Imbalances may result from many factors, including illnesses, altered fluid intake, or prolonged episodes of vomiting or diarrhea. Acid-base balance is necessary for many physiological processes, and imbalances can alter respiration, metabolism, and the function of the central nervous system. Knowledge and understanding of the mechanisms that contribute to fluid, electrolyte, and acid-base imbalances are essential (Phipps and others, 2003).

Scientific Knowledge Base

Water is the largest single component of the body; 60% of the average adult's weight is fluid. A healthy, mobile, well-oriented adult can usually maintain normal fluid, electrolyte, and acid-base balances because of the body's adaptive physiological mechanisms.

Distribution of Body Fluids

Body fluids are distributed in two distinct compartments, one containing **intracellular fluids** and the other **extracellular fluids** (Table 40-1). Intracellular fluid (ICF) comprises all fluid within body cells. In adults, approximately 40% of body weight is ICF (Phipps and others, 2003).

Extracellular fluid (ECF) is all the fluid outside a cell, which is divided into three smaller compartments: **interstitial fluid, intravascular fluid** and transcellular fluids. Interstitial fluid, which contains lymph, is the fluid between the cells and outside the blood vessels, whereas intravascular fluid is blood plasma. Transcellular fluid consists of cerebrospinal, pleural, peritoneal, and synovial fluids (McCance and Huether, 2002). Extracellular fluid makes up about 20% of the total body weight.

Composition of Body Fluids

As water moves through the compartments of the body, it contains substances that are sometimes called minerals or salts but are technically known as **electrolytes** (Christensen and Kockrow, 2003). An electrolyte is an element or compound that, when melted or dissolved in water or another solvent, separates into **ions** and is able to carry an electrical current. Positively charged electrolytes are **cations** (e.g., sodium [Na^+], potassium [K^+], calcium [Ca^{2+}]). Negatively charged electrolytes are **anions** (e.g., chloride [Cl^-], bicarbonate [HCO_3^-], sulfate [SO_4^-]).

Electrolytes are vital to many body functions. The value **milliequivalents per liter (mEq/L)** represents the number of grams of the specific electrolyte **(solute)** dissolved in a liter of plasma **(solution).** The solution in which a solute is dissolved is called a **solvent** (Speakman and Weldy, 2002).

Minerals, which are ingested as compounds, are constituents of all body tissues and fluids and are important in maintaining physiological processes. Minerals also act as catalysts in nerve response, muscle contraction, and metabolism of nutrients in foods. In addition, they regulate electrolyte balance and hormone production and strengthen skeletal structures. Examples of minerals are iron and zinc.

Movement of Body Fluids

Fluids and electrolytes constantly shift from compartment to compartment to facilitate body processes such as tissue oxygenation, acid-base balance, and urine forma-

tion. Because cell membranes separating the body fluid compartments are selectively permeable, water can pass through them easily. However, most ions and molecules pass through them more slowly. Fluids and solutes move across these membranes by four processes: osmosis, diffusion, filtration, and active transport.

Osmosis. **Osmosis** involves the movement of a pure solvent, such as water, through a semipermeable membrane from an area of lesser solute concentration to an area of greater solute concentration in an attempt to equalize concentrations on both sides of the membrane (Figure 40-1). The membrane is permeable to the solvent, but it is impermeable to the solute. The rate of osmosis depends on the concentration of the solutes in the solution, the temperature of the solution, the electrical charges of the solutes, and the differences between the osmotic pressures exerted by the solutions. The concentration of a solution is measured in **osmols,** which reflect the amount of a substance in solution in the form of molecules, ions, or both. For example, boiling a hot dog is an example of osmosis. The concentration of molecules inside the hot dog is greater than in water. The water passes through the hot dog skin, a semipermeable membrane, in an attempt to equalize the number of molecules on both sides of the membrane. Finally, when the hot dog can no longer hold anymore water, the skin ruptures (Christensen and Kockrow, 2003).

Osmotic pressure is the drawing power for water and depends on the number of molecules in solution. A solution with a high solute concentration has a high osmotic pressure and draws water into itself. If the concentration of the solute is greater on one side of the semipermeable membrane, the rate of osmosis is quicker, and a more rapid transfer of solvent across the membrane occurs. This continues until an equilibrium is reached. The osmotic pressure of a solution is called its osmolarity, which is expressed in osmols, or milliosmols per kilogram (mOsm/kg) of the solution. The normal serum osmolarity is 280 to 295 mOsm/kg. **Osmolarity** is the measure used to evaluate serum and urine in clinical practice. Changes

Table 40-1	Electrolyte Distribution in Body Fluid
Electrolytes	**Extracellular (mEq/L)**
Sodium (Na^+)	135-145
Potassium (K^+)	3.5-5.0
Calcium (Ca^{2+})	4.5-5.5
Bicarbonate (HCO_3^-)	22-26 (arterial) 24-30 (venous)
Chloride (Cl^-)	90-110
Magnesium (Mg^{2+})	1.5-2.5
Phosphate (PO_4^{3-})	1.7-4.6

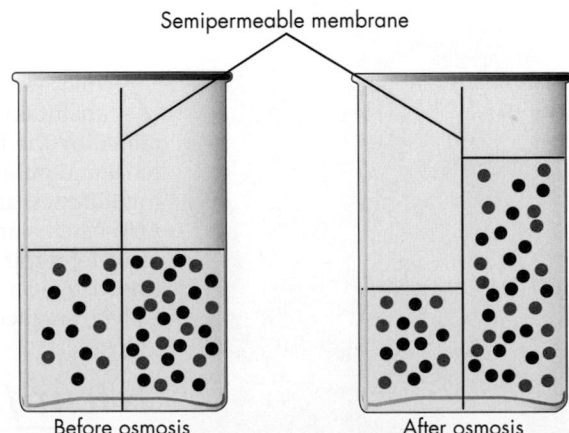

FIGURE 40-1 Osmosis through a semipermeable membrane. (From Lewis SM, Collier IC, Heitkemper M: *Medical-surgical nursing: assessment and management of clinical problems*, ed 4, St. Louis, 2002, Mosby.)

in extracellular osmolarity may result in changes in both ECF and ICF volume.

Solutions are classified as **hypertonic, isotonic,** or **hypotonic.** A solution with the same osmolarity as blood plasma is called isotonic. A hypertonic solution (a solution of higher osmotic pressure), such as 3% sodium chloride, pulls fluid from cells causing them to shrink; an isotonic solution (a solution of same osmotic pressure), such as 0.9% sodium chloride, expands the body's fluid volume without causing a fluid shift from one compartment to another; and a hypotonic solution (a solution of lower osmotic pressure), such as 0.45% sodium chloride, moves fluid into the cells, causing them to enlarge. Each of these actions occurs through osmosis.

The osmotic pressure of the blood is affected by plasma proteins, especially albumin, a serum protein naturally produced by the body. Albumin exerts **colloid osmotic** or **oncotic pressure,** which tends to keep fluid in the intravascular compartment by pulling water from the interstitial space back into the capillaries (Speakman and Weldy, 2002).

Diffusion. Diffusion is the movement of a solute (gas or substance) in a solution across a semipermeable membrane from an area of higher concentration to an area of lower concentration (Figure 40-2). The result is an even distribution of the solute in a solution. For example, when you pour a small amount of cream into a cup of black coffee, the cream left unmixed will diffuse through the whole cup of coffee (Speakman and Weldy, 2002). A physiological example is the movement of oxygen and carbon dioxide between the alveoli and blood vessels in the lungs. The difference between the two concentrations is known as a **concentration gradient.**

Filtration. Filtration is the process by which water and diffusible substances move together in response to fluid pressure, moving from an area of higher pressure to one of lower pressure. This process is active in capillary beds, where **hydrostatic pressure** differences determine the movement of water (Figure 40-3). When there is increased hydrostatic pressure on the venous side of the capillary bed, as occurs in congestive heart failure (CHF), the normal movement of water from the interstitial space into the intravascular space by filtration is reversed, resulting in an accumulation of excess fluid in the interstitial space, known as **edema.**

Active Transport. Unlike diffusion, osmosis, and filtration, **active transport** requires metabolic activity and expenditure of energy to move materials across cell membranes. This allows cells to admit larger molecules than they would otherwise be able to admit or to move molecules from areas of lesser concentration to areas of greater concentration "uphill" (Figure 40-4). Examples of active transport are the sodium and potassium pump. Sodium is pumped out of the cell and potassium is pumped in, against the concentration gradient. This process makes it possible to keep a higher concentration of potassium in the ICF and a higher concentration of sodium in the ECF.

Active transport is enhanced by carrier molecules within a cell that bind themselves to incoming molecules. For example, glucose is able to enter cells after it binds with the transport vehicle insulin. Active transport is the mechanism by which cells absorb glucose and other substances to carry out metabolic activities.

Regulation of Body Fluids

Body fluids are regulated by fluid intake, hormonal controls, and fluid output. This physiological balance is termed **homeostasis** (Heitz and Horne, 2001). In health,

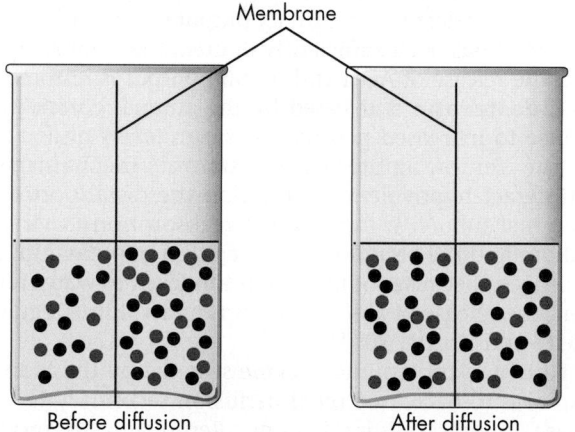

Membrane

Before diffusion   After diffusion

FIGURE **40-2** Diffusion across a semipermeable membrane. (From Lewis SM, Collier IC, Heitkemper M: *Medical-surgical nursing: assessment and management of clinical problems,* ed 4, St. Louis, 2002, Mosby.)

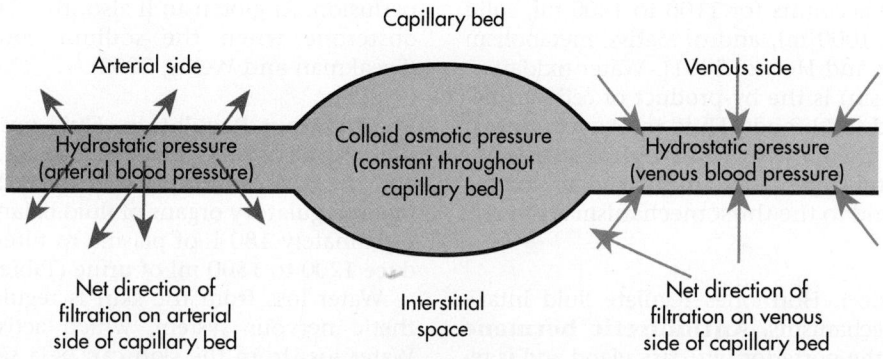

Capillary bed

Arterial side   Venous side

Hydrostatic pressure (arterial blood pressure)   Colloid osmotic pressure (constant throughout capillary bed)   Hydrostatic pressure (venous blood pressure)

Net direction of filtration on arterial side of capillary bed   Interstitial space   Net direction of filtration on venous side of capillary bed

FIGURE **40-3** An example of filtration and hydrostatic pressure.

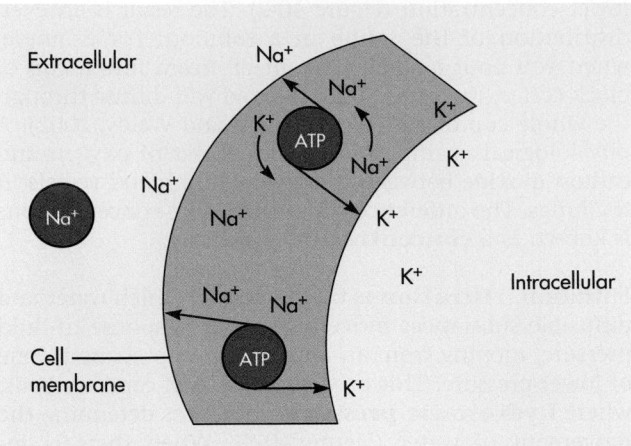

FIGURE **40–4** The sodium-potassium pump. As sodium diffuses into the cell and potassium out of the cell, active transport delivers sodium back to the extracellular compartment and potassium to the intracellular compartment. (From Lewis SM, Collier IC, Heitkemper M: *Medical-surgical nursing: assessment and management of clinical problems,* ed 4, St. Louis, 2002, Mosby.)

the body is able to respond to disturbances in fluids and electrolytes to prevent and repair damage.

Fluid Intake. Fluid intake is regulated primarily through the thirst mechanism. The thirst-control center is located within the hypothalamus in the brain. Thirst is the conscious desire for water and is one of the major factors that determines fluid intake (Speakman and Weldy, 2002). The **osmoreceptors** continually monitor the serum osmotic pressure, and when osmolality increases, the hypothalamus is stimulated. Eating potato chips is an example; the salt on the chips increases the osmotic pressure of the body fluids and stimulates the thirst mechanism (Phipps and others, 2003). Increased plasma osmolality can occur with any condition that interferes with the oral ingestion of fluids, or it can occur with the intake of hypertonic fluids. The hypothalamus will also be stimulated when excess fluid is lost and **hypovolemia** occurs, as in excessive vomiting and hemorrhage. In addition, the stimulation of the renin- angiotensin-aldosterone mechanism, potassium depletion, psychological factors, and oropharyngeal dryness initiate the sensation of thirst (Figure 40-5).

The average adult's intake is about 2200 to 2700 ml per day; oral intake accounts for 1100 to 1400 ml, solid foods about 800 to 1000 ml, and oxidative metabolism 300 ml daily (Heitz and Horne, 2001). Water oxidation (oxidative metabolism) is the by-product of cellular metabolism of ingested solid foods. Fluid intake requires an alert state. Infants, clients with neurological or psychological problems, and some older adults who are unable to perceive or respond to the thirst mechanism are at risk for **dehydration.**

Hormonal Regulation. Hormones regulate fluid intake through various mechanisms. **Antidiuretic hormone (ADH)** is stored in the posterior pituitary gland and is released in response to changes in blood osmolarity. The os-

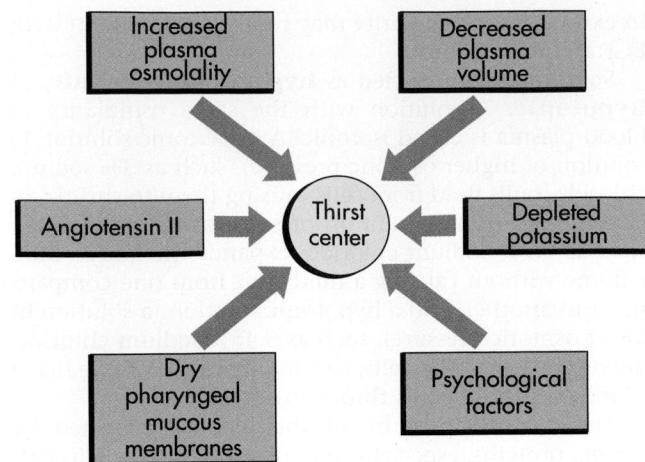

FIGURE **40–5** Stimuli affecting the thirst mechanism.

moreceptors in the hypothalamus are stimulated when there is an increase in the osmolarity to release the hormone ADH. The ADH works directly on the renal tubules and collecting ducts to make them more permeable to water. This in turn causes water to return to the systemic circulation, which dilutes the blood and decreases its osmolarity. As the body attempts to compensate, the client will experience a decrease in urinary output temporarily. When the blood has been sufficiently diluted, the osmoreceptors stop the release of ADH and urinary output is restored.

Aldosterone is released by the adrenal cortex in response to increased plasma potassium levels or as a part of the renin-angiotensin-aldosterone mechanism to counteract hypovolemia. It acts on the distal portion of the renal tubule to increase the reabsorption (saving) of sodium and the secretion and excretion of potassium and hydrogen. Because sodium retention leads to water retention, the release of aldosterone acts as a volume regulator (Heitz and Horne, 2001).

Renin, a proteolytic enzyme secreted by the kidneys, responds to decreased renal perfusion secondary to a decrease in extracellular volume. Renin acts to produce **angiotensin** I, which causes some vasoconstriction. However, angiotensin I almost immediately becomes reduced by an enzyme that converts angiotension I into angiotensin II. Angiotensin II then causes massive selective vasoconstriction of many blood vessels and relocates and increases the blood flow to the kidney, improving renal perfusion. Angiotensin II also stimulates the release of aldosterone when the sodium concentration is low (Speakman and Weldy, 2002).

Fluid Output Regulation. Fluid output occurs through four organs of water loss: the kidneys, the skin, the lungs, and the gastrointestinal (GI) tract. The kidneys are the major regulatory organs of fluid balance. They receive approximately 180 L of plasma to filter each day and produce 1200 to 1500 ml of urine (Table 40-2).

Water loss from the skin is regulated by the sympathetic nervous system, which activates sweat glands. Water loss from the skin can be a sensible or insensible loss. An average of 500 to 600 ml of sensible and insensi-

Table 40-2		Adult Average Daily Fluid Gains and Losses	
Fluid Gains	**(ml)**	**Fluid Losses**	**(ml)**
Oral fluids	1100-1400	Kidneys	1200-1500
Solid foods	800-1000	Skin	500-600
Metabolism	300	Lungs	400
		Gastrointestinal	100-200
TOTAL GAINS	2200-2700	TOTAL LOSSES	2200-2700

ble fluid is lost via the skin each day (Heitz and Horne, 2001). **Insensible water loss** is continuous and is not perceived by the person but can increase significantly with fever or burns (Heitz and Horne, 2001). **Sensible water loss** occurs through excess perspiration and can be perceived by the client or by the nurse through inspection. The amount of sensible perspiration is directly related to the stimulation of the sweat glands.

The lungs expire about 400 ml of water daily. This insensible water loss may increase in response to changes in respiratory rate and depth. In addition, devices for giving oxygen can increase insensible water loss from the lungs.

The GI tract plays a vital role in fluid regulation. Approximately 3 to 6 L of isotonic fluid is moved into the gastrointestinal tract and then returns again to the extracellular fluid. Under normal conditions, the average adult loses only 100 to 200 ml of the 3 to 6 L each day through feces. However, in the presence of a disease process, for example, diarrhea, the GI tract may become a site of a large amount of fluid loss. This loss may have a significant impact on maintaining normal fluid regulation.

Regulation of Electrolytes

Cations. Major cations within the body fluids include sodium (Na^+), potassium (K^+), calcium (Ca^{2+}), and magnesium (Mg^{2+}). Cations interchange when one cation leaves the cell and is replaced by another. This occurs because cells tend to maintain electrical neutrality.

Sodium Regulation. Sodium is the most abundant cation (90%) in ECF. Sodium ions are the major contributors to maintaining water balance through their effect on serum osmolality, nerve impulse transmission, regulation of acid-base balance, and participation in cellular chemical reactions (McCance and Huether, 2002). Sodium is regulated by dietary intake and aldosterone secretion. The normal extracellular sodium concentration is 135 to 145 mEq/L.

Potassium Regulation. Potassium is the major electrolyte and principle cation in the intracellular compartment (Phipps and others, 2003). It regulates many metabolic activities and is necessary for glycogen deposits in the liver and skeletal muscle, transmission and conduction of nerve impulses, normal cardiac conduction, and skeletal and smooth muscle contraction (McCance and Huether, 2002). A relatively small amount (approximately 2%) of potassium is located within the ECF (Heitz and Horne, 2001). The normal range for serum potassium

concentrations is 3.5 to 5 mEq/L. Potassium is regulated by dietary intake and renal excretion. The body conserves potassium poorly, so any condition that increases urine output decreases the serum potassium concentration.

Calcium Regulation. Calcium is stored in bone, plasma, and body cells. Ninety-nine percent of calcium is located in bone, and only 1% is located in ECF. Approximately 50% of calcium in the plasma is bound to protein, primarily albumin, and 40% is free ionized calcium. The remaining small percentage is combined with nonprotein anions such as phosphate, citrate, and carbonate (Heitz and Horne, 2001). Normal serum ionized calcium is 4.5 to 5.5 mEq/L. Normal total calcium is 8.5 to 10.5 mg/100 ml. Calcium is necessary for bone and teeth formation, blood clotting, hormone secretion, cell membrane integrity, cardiac conduction, transmission of nerve impulses, and muscle contraction.

Magnesium Regulation. Magnesium is essential for enzyme activities, neurochemical activities, and cardiac and skeletal muscle excitability. Plasma concentrations of magnesium range from 1.5 to 2.5 mEq/L. Serum magnesium is regulated by dietary intake, renal mechanisms, and actions of the parathyroid hormone (PTH). About 50% to 60% of body magnesium is contained within the bone, and only 1% is contained within the ECF compartment; the rest is located inside the cell (Phipps and others, 2003).

Anions. The three major anions of body fluids are chloride (Cl^-), bicarbonate (HCO_3^-), and phosphate (PO_4^{3-}) ions.

Chloride Regulation. Chloride is the major anion in ECF. The transport of chloride follows sodium. Normal concentrations of chloride range from 90 to 110 mEq/L. Serum chloride is regulated by dietary intake and the kidneys. A person with normal renal function who has a high chloride intake will excrete a higher amount of urine chloride.

Bicarbonate Regulation. Bicarbonate is the major chemical base buffer within the body. The bicarbonate ion is found in ECF and ICF. The bicarbonate ion is an essential component of the carbonic acid-bicarbonate buffering system essential to acid-base balance. The kidneys regulate bicarbonate. Normal arterial bicarbonate levels range between 22 and 26 mEq/L; venous bicarbonate is measured as carbon dioxide content, and the normal value is 24 to 30 mEq/L.

Phosphorus-Phosphate Regulation. Nearly all the phosphorus in the body exists in the form of phosphate (PO_4^{3-}), and the terms phosphorus and phosphate often are used interchangeably (Heitz and Horne, 2001). Phosphate is a buffer anion found primarily in ICF, with a small amount found in ECF. It assists in acid-base regulation. Phosphate and calcium help to develop and maintain bones and teeth. Calcium and phosphate are inversely proportional; if one rises, the other falls. Phosphate also promotes normal neuromuscular action and participates in carbohydrate metabolism. Phosphate is normally absorbed through the GI tract. It is regulated by dietary intake, renal excretion, intestinal absorption, and PTH. The normal serum level is 1.7 to 4.6 mg/100 ml.

Regulation of Acid-Base Balance

For optimal functioning of the cells, metabolic processes maintain a steady balance between acids and bases. Arterial pH is inversely proportioned to the hydrogen ion (H^+) concentration (i.e., the greater the concentration, the more acidic the solution and the lower the pH; the lower the concentration, the more alkaline the solution and the higher the pH). The pH is also a reflection of the balance between carbon dioxide (CO_2), which is regulated by the lungs, and bicarbonate (HCO_3^-), a base regulated by the kidneys (Heitz and Horne, 2001). Acid-base balance exists when the net rate at which the body produces acids or bases equals the rate at which acids or bases are excreted. This balance results in a stable concentration of hydrogen ions in body fluids that is expressed as the pH value. Normal hydrogen ion level is necessary to maintain cell membrane integrity and the speed of cellular enzymatic actions. The pH is a scale for measuring the acidity or alkalinity of a fluid. A pH value of 7 is neutral, below 7 is acid, and above 7 is alkaline. Normal values in arterial blood range from 7.35 to 7.45. The three general types of acid-base regulators in the body are chemical, biological, and physiological buffering systems. A **buffer** is a substance or a group of substances that can absorb or release H^+ to correct an acid-base imbalance.

Chemical Regulation. The largest chemical buffer in ECF is the carbonic acid and bicarbonate buffer system (Figure 40-6). This system can be expressed as the following:

$$CO_2 + H_2O \leftrightarrow H_2CO_3 \leftrightarrow H^+ + HCO_3^-$$

Carbon dioxide + Water ↔ Carbonic acid ↔ Hydrogen ion + Bicarbonate

The carbonic acid–bicarbonate buffer system is the first buffering system to react to change in the pH of ECF, and it reacts within seconds. The previous equation demonstrates how hydrogen ions (H^+) and carbon dioxide (CO_2) concentrations are directly related to each other. Whenever carbon dioxide increases, there is an increase in hydrogen ions produced, and whenever hydrogen ions are produced, there is more carbon dioxide produced (Ignatavicius and Workman, 2002). Remember, the excretion of carbon dioxide resulting from metabolism is controlled primarily by the lungs, and the excretion of hydrogen and bicarbonate ions is controlled by the kidneys.

Biological Regulation. Biological buffering occurs when hydrogen ions are absorbed or released by cells. Biological buffering occurs after chemical buffering and takes 2 to 4 hours. The hydrogen ion has a positive charge and must be exchanged with another positively charged ion, frequently potassium (K^+). In conditions with excess acid, a hydrogen ion enters the cell and a potassium ion leaves the cell and enters the ECF, thus causing an elevated serum potassium. An example is the release of fatty acids that occurs with diabetic ketoacidosis and starvation. A second biological buffer is the hemoglobin-oxyhemoglobin system. Carbon dioxide diffuses into the RBC and forms carbonic acid. The carbonic acid dissociates into hydrogen and bicarbonate ions. The hydrogen ions attach to hemoglobin, and the bicarbonate ion becomes available for buffering by exchanging with extracellular chloride (Metheney, 2000).

Another biological buffer is the chloride shift within RBCs. When blood is oxygenated in the lungs, bicarbonate diffuses into the cells and chloride travels from the hemoglobin to the plasma to maintain electrical neutrality. The reverse occurs when carbon dioxide moves into the red cells in tissue capillary beds. This process is referred to as the chloride shift and is a reciprocal exchange between these anions (Groer, 2000).

Physiological Regulation. The two physiological buffers in the body are the lungs and the kidneys. The lungs adapt rapidly to an acid-base imbalance; they act to return the pH to normal before the action of the biological buffers. Ordinarily, increased levels of hydrogen ions and carbon dioxide provide the stimulus for respiration. When the concentration of hydrogen ions is altered, the lungs react to correct the imbalance by altering the rate and depth of respiration. For example, when metabolic acidosis is present, respirations are increased, resulting in a greater amount of carbon dioxide being exhaled, which results in a decrease in the acidic level; when metabolic alkalosis is present, the lungs retain carbon dioxide by decreasing the respirations, thereby increasing the acidic level (Phipps and others, 2003).

The kidneys take from a few hours to several days to regulate acid-base imbalance. They reabsorb bicarbonate in cases of acid excess and excrete it in cases of acid deficit. In addition, the kidneys use a phosphate ion (PO_4^{3-}) to excrete hydrogen ions by forming phosphoric acid (H_3PO_4); sulfuric acid (H_2SO_4) may also be excreted. Finally, the kidneys use the ammonia mechanism to regulate acid-base balance. In this mechanism certain amino acids are chemically changed within the renal tubules into ammonia, which in the presence of hydrogen ions forms ammo-

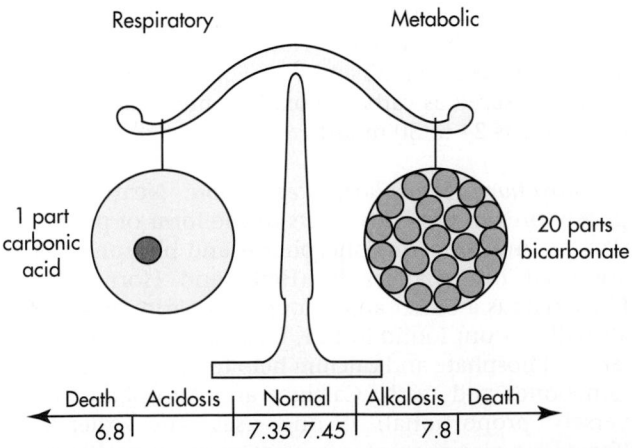

FIGURE **40–6** Carbonic acid–bicarbonate ratio and pH.

nium and is excreted in the urine, hence releasing hydrogen ions from the body (Phipps and others, 2003).

Disturbances in Electrolyte, Fluid, and Acid-Base Balances

Disturbances in electrolyte, fluid, or acid-base balances seldom occur alone and can disrupt normal body processes. When there is a loss of body fluids because of burns, illnesses, or trauma, the client is also at risk for electrolyte imbalances (Table 40-3). In addition, some untreated electrolyte imbalances (e.g., potassium loss) result in acid-base disturbances.

Electrolyte Imbalances

Sodium Imbalances. Hyponatremia is a lower-than-normal concentration of sodium in the blood (serum), which can occur with a net sodium loss or net water excess (see Table 40-3). It occurs frequently in seriously ill clients. Clinical indicators and treatment depend on the cause of hyponatremia and whether it is associated with a normal, decreased, or increased ECF volume (Heitz and Horne, 2001). The usual situation is a loss of sodium

without a loss of fluid, and results in a decrease in the osmolality of ECF. The body initially adapts by reducing water excretion and thus sodium excretion occurs in order to maintain serum osmolality at near normal levels. As the sodium loss continues, the body continues to preserve the blood and interstitial (tissue) volume. As a result, the sodium in ECF becomes diluted.

Hypernatremia is a greater-than-normal concentration of sodium in ECF that can be caused by excess water loss or an overall sodium excess (see Table 40-3). When the cause of hypernatremia is an increased aldosterone secretion, sodium is retained and potassium is excreted. When hypernatremia occurs, the body attempts to conserve as much water as possible through renal reabsorption.

Potassium Imbalances. Hypokalemia is one of the most common electrolyte imbalances, in which an inadequate amount of potassium circulates in ECF (see Table 40-3). When severe, hypokalemia can affect cardiac conduction and function. Because the normal amount of serum potassium is so small, there is little tolerance for fluctuations. The most common cause of hypokalemia is

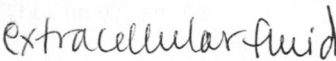

extracellular fluid

Table 40-3 Electrolyte Imbalances	
Causes	**Signs and Symptoms**
Hyponatremia	
Kidney disease resulting in salt wasting Adrenal insufficiency GI losses Increased sweating Use of diuretics, especially when combined with low-sodium diet Psychogenic polydipsia Syndrome of inappropriate ADH (SIADH)	*Physical examination:* apprehension, personality change, postural hypotension, postural dizziness, abdominal cramping, nausea and vomiting, diarrhea, tachycardia, convulsions and coma, and fingerprints remaining on sternum after palpation *Laboratory findings:* serum sodium level **below** 135 mEq/L, serum osmolality 280 mOsm/kg, and urine specific gravity **below** 1.010 (if not caused by SIADH)
Hypernatremia	
Ingestion of large amounts of concentrated salt solutions Iatrogenic administration of hypertonic saline solution parenterally Excess aldosterone secretion Diabetes insipidus Increased sensible and insensible water loss Water deprivation	*Physical examination:* thirst, dry and flushed skin, dry and sticky tongue and mucous membranes, fever, agitation, convulsions, restlessness, and irritability *Laboratory findings:* serum sodium levels **above** 145 mEq/L, serum osmolality 295 mOsm/kg, and urine specific gravity 1.030 (if not caused by diabetes insipidus)
Hypokalemia	
Use of potassium-wasting diuretics Diarrhea, vomiting, or other GI losses Alkalosis Excess aldosterone secretion Polyuria Extreme sweating Excessive use of potassium-free intravenous (IV) solutions Treatment of diabetic ketoacidosis with insulin	*Physical examination:* weakness and fatigue, decreased muscle tone, intestinal distention, decreased bowel sounds, ventricular dysrhythmias, paresthesias and weak, irregular pulse *Laboratory findings:* serum potassium level **below** 3.5 mEq/L and electrocardiogram (ECG) abnormalities (e.g., ventricular dysrhythmias)*

*Data from Heitz UE and Horne MM: *Mosby's pocket guide series: fluid, electrolyte, and acid-base balance,* ed 4, St. Louis, 2001, Mosby.

Table 40-3	Electrolyte Imbalances—cont'd
Causes	**Signs and Symptoms**

Hyperkalemia

Renal failure
Fluid volume deficit
Massive cellular damage such as from burns and trauma
Iatrogenic administration of large amounts of potassium
   intravenously
Adrenal insufficiency
Acidosis, especially diabetic ketoacidosis
Rapid infusion of stored blood
Use of potassium-sparing diuretics

Physical examination: anxiety, dysrhythmias, paresthesia, weakness, abdominal cramps, and diarrhea

Laboratory findings: serum potassium level **above** 5.0 mEq/L and ECG abnormalities (bradycardia, heart block, dysrhythmias); eventually QRS pattern widens and cardiac arrest occurs*

Hypocalcemia

Rapid administration of blood transfusions containing citrate
Hypoalbuminemia
Hypoparathyroidism
Vitamin D deficiency
Pancreatitis
Alkalosis

Physical examination: numbness and tingling of fingers and circumoral region, hyperactive reflexes, positive Trousseau's sign (carpopedal spasm with hypoxia), positive Chvostek's sign (contraction of facial muscles when facial nerve is tapped), tetany, muscle cramps, and pathological fractures (chronic hypocalcemia)

Laboratory findings: serum calcium level **below** 4.5 mEq/L or 8.5 mg/100 ml and ECG abnormalities

Hypercalcemia

Hyperparathyroidism
Osteometastasis
Paget's disease
Osteoporosis
Prolonged immobilization
Acidosis

Physical examination: anorexia, nausea and vomiting, weakness, lethargy, low back pain (from kidney stones), decreased level of consciousness, personality changes, and cardiac arrest

Laboratory findings: serum calcium level **above** 5.5 mEq/L or 10.5 mg/100 ml; x-ray examination showing generalized osteoporosis, widespread bone cavitation, radiopaque urinary stones; and elevated blood urea nitrogen (BUN) level 25 mg/100 ml and elevated creatinine level 1.5 mg/100 ml caused by fluid volume deficit (FVD) or renal damage caused by urolithiasis; ECG abnormalities

Hypomagnesemia

Inadequate intake: malnutrition and alcoholism
Inadequate absorption: diarrhea, vomiting, nasogastric
   drainage, fistulas; diseases of small intestine
Excessive loss resulting from thiazide diuretics
Aldosterone excess
Polyuria

Physical examination: muscular tremors, hyperactive deep tendon reflexes, confusion and disorientation, dysrhythmias, and positive Chvostek's sign and Trousseau's sign

Laboratory findings: serum magnesium level **below** 1.5 mEq/L

Hypermagnesemia

Renal failure
Excess oral or parenteral intake of magnesium

Physical examination: physical findings that are more frequent in acute elevations in magnesium levels: hypoactive deep tendon reflexes, decreased depth and rate of respirations, hypotension, and flushing

Laboratory findings: serum magnesium level **above** 2.5 mEq/L

*Data from Heitz UE and Horne MM: *Mosby's pocket guide series: fluid, electrolyte, and acid-base balance,* ed 4, St. Louis, 2001, Mosby.

the use of potassium-wasting diuretics such as thiazide and loop diuretics.

Hyperkalemia is a greater-than-normal amount of potassium in the blood. Severe hyperkalemia produces marked cardiac conduction abnormalities (see Table 40-3). The primary cause of hyperkalemia is renal failure, because any decrease in renal function diminishes the amount of potassium the kidney can excrete. Elevations in potassium may also be seen in crushing injuries where cells are broken and potassium is released from with the cells.

Calcium Imbalances. Hypocalcemia represents a drop in serum and/or ionized calcium. It can result from several illnesses, some of which directly affect the thyroid and parathyroid glands (see Table 40-3, p. 1141). Another cause is renal insufficiency (in which the kidneys' inability to excrete phosphorus causes the phosphorus level to rise and the calcium level to decline) or prolonged bed rest. Signs and symptoms can be related to a diminished function of the neuromuscular, cardiac, and renal systems.

Hypercalcemia is an increase in the total serum concentration of calcium and/or ionized calcium. Hypercalcemia is frequently a symptom of an underlying disease resulting in excess bone reabsorption with release of calcium.

Magnesium Imbalances. Disturbances in magnesium levels are summarized in Table 40-3. Symptoms are the result of changes in neuromuscular excitability. Hypomagnesemia, a drop in serum magnesium, occurs with malnutrition and with malabsorption disorders, and signs and symptoms are directly related to the neuromuscular system. Hypermagnesemia is an increase in serum magnesium levels. It depresses skeletal muscles and nerve function. The depression of acetylcholine leads to a sedative effect, which can lead to bradycardia, ECG changes, cardiac arrhythmias, and decreased respiratory rate and depth (Phipps and others, 2003).

Chloride Imbalances. Hypochloremia occurs when the serum chloride level falls below normal. Vomiting or prolonged and excessive nasogastric or fistula drainage can result in hypochloremia because of the loss of hydrochloric acid. The use of loop and thiazide diuretics also results in increased chloride loss as sodium is excreted. When serum chloride levels fall, metabolic alkalosis results as the body adapts by increasing reabsorption of the bicarbonate ion to maintain electrical neutrality.

Hyperchloremia occurs when the serum chloride level rises above normal, which usually occurs when the serum bicarbonate value falls or sodium level rises. Hypochloremia and hyperchloremia rarely occur as single disease processes but are commonly associated with acid-base imbalance. There is no single set of symptoms associated with these two alterations.

Fluid Disturbances. The basic types of fluid imbalances are isotonic and osmolar. Isotonic deficit and excess exist when water and electrolytes are gained or lost in equal proportions. In contrast, osmolar imbalances are losses or excesses of only water so that the concentration (osmolality) of the serum is affected. Table 40-4 lists the causes and symptoms of common disturbances.

Acid-Base Balance. Arterial blood gas (ABG) analysis is the best way to evaluate acid-base balance. Measurement of ABGs involves analysis of six components. Deviation from a normal value will indicate that the client is experiencing an acid-base imbalance. These six components are pH, $PaCO_2$, PaO_2, oxygen saturation, base excess, and HCO_3^-.

pH. pH measures hydrogen ion (H^+) concentration in the body fluids. Even a slight change can be potentially life threatening. An increase in concentration of H^+ makes a solution more acidic; a decrease makes the solution more alkaline. Normal pH value is 7.35 to 7.45 (acidic is 7.35, and alkalotic is 7.45).

PaCO₂. $PaCO_2$ is the partial pressure of carbon dioxide in arterial blood and is a reflection of the depth of pulmonary ventilation. The normal range is 35 to 45 mm Hg. When the $PaCO_2$ is less than 35 mm Hg, it is an indication that hyperventilation has occurred. As rate and depth of respiration increase, more carbon dioxide is exhaled and the carbon dioxide concentration decreases. When the $PaCO_2$ is more than 45 mm Hg, hypoventilation has occurred. As rate and depth of respiration decrease, less carbon dioxide is exhaled and more is retained, increasing the concentration of carbon dioxide.

PaO₂. PaO_2 is the partial pressure of oxygen in arterial blood. It has no primary role in acid-base regulation if it is within normal limits. A PaO_2 less than 60 mm Hg can lead to anaerobic metabolism, resulting in lactic acid production and metabolic acidosis. There is a normal decline in PaO_2 in older adults. Hypoxemia also may cause hyperventilation, resulting in respiratory alkalosis (Heitz and Horne, 2001). Normal range is 80 to 100 mm Hg.

Oxygen Saturation. Saturation is the point at which hemoglobin is saturated by oxygen (O_2). When a client is hypoxic and uses up readily available oxygen, the reserve oxygen (oxygen attached to hemoglobin) is drawn upon to provide oxygen to the tissues (Ignatavicius and Workman, 2002). Oxygen can be affected by changes in temperature, pH, and $PaCO_2$. When the PaO_2 falls below 60 mm Hg, there is a large drop in saturation (Heitz and Horne, 2001). Normal range is 95% to 99%.

Base Excess. Base excess is the amount of blood buffer (hemoglobin and bicarbonate) that exists. A high value indicates alkalosis and can result from the ingestion of large amounts of sodium bicarbonate solutions (some antacids), citrate excess with rapid blood transfusions, or intravenous infusion of sodium bicarbonate to correct ketoacidosis. A low value indicates acidosis and is usually the result of the elimination of too many bicarbonate ions. An example is diarrhea, where the increased intestinal motility that accompanies diarrhea forces the bicarbonate-containing fluid to be lost instead of being absorbed (Ignatavicius and Workman, 2002). The normal range is ±2.

Bicarbonate. Serum bicarbonate (HCO_3^-) is the major renal component of acid-base balance and is excreted and reproduced by the kidneys to maintain a normal acid-base environment. It is the principal buffer of the extracellular fluids of the body, and once bicarbonate is in the ECF, it is maintained at a concentration of 20 times that of the fluid concentration of carbonic acid (Ignatavicius and Workman, 2002). The normal range is 22 to 26 mEq/L. Less than 22 mEq/L usually indicates metabolic acidosis, more than 26 mEq/L indicates metabolic alkalosis.

Table 40-4   Fluid Disturbances

Causes	Signs and Symptoms
Isotonic Imbalances	
Fluid Volume Deficit (FVD)—Water and Electrolytes Lost in Equal or Isotonic Proportions	
Losses from the GI system, such as from diarrhea, vomiting, or drainage from fistulas or tubes Loss of plasma or whole blood, such as with burns or hemorrhage Excessive perspiration Fever Decreased oral intake of fluids Use of diuretics	*Physical examination:* postural hypotension, tachycardia, dry mucous membranes, poor skin turgor, thirst, confusion, rapid weight loss, slow vein filling, lethargy, oliguria, weak pulse *Laboratory findings:* urine specific gravity greater than 1.030, increased hematocrit level, and increased BUN level (hemoconcentration)
Fluid Volume Excess (FVE)—Water and Sodium Retained in Isotonic Proportions	
Congestive heart failure Renal failure Cirrhosis of the liver Increased serum aldosterone and steroid levels Excessive sodium intake or administration	*Physical examination:* rapid weight gain, edema (especially in dependent areas), hypertension, polyuria (if renal mechanisms are normal), neck vein distention, increased venous pressure, crackles in lungs *Laboratory findings:* decreased hematocrit level and decreased BUN level **below** 10 mg/100 ml (hemodilution)
Osmolar Imbalances	
Hyperosmolar Imbalance—Dehydration	
Diabetes insipidus Interruption of neurologically driven thirst drive Diabetic ketoacidosis Osmotic diuresis Administration of hypertonic parenteral fluids or tube feeding formulas	*Physical examination:* dry and sticky mucous membranes, flushed and dry skin, thirst, elevated body temperature, irritability, convulsions, coma *Laboratory findings:* increased serum sodium level **above** 145 mEq/L and increased serum osmolality **above** 295 mOsm/kg
Hypoosmolar Imbalance—Water Excess	
SIADH Excess water intake	*Physical examination:* decreased level of consciousness, convulsions, coma *Laboratory findings:* decreased serum sodium level **below** 135 mEq/L and decreased serum osmolality **below** 280 mOsm/kg

Types of Acid-Base Imbalances. The four primary types of acid-base imbalance are respiratory acidosis, respiratory alkalosis, metabolic acidosis, and metabolic alkalosis (Table 40-5).

Respiratory Acidosis. **Respiratory acidosis** is marked by an increased arterial carbon dioxide concentration ($PaCO_2$), excess carbonic acid (H_2CO_3), and an increased hydrogen ion concentration (decreased pH). With respiratory acidosis, the cerebrospinal fluid and brain cells become acidic, causing neurological changes. Hypoxemia occurs because of respiratory depression, resulting in further neurological impairment. Electrolyte changes such as hyperkalemia and hypercalcemia may accompany the acidosis.

Respiratory Alkalosis. **Respiratory alkalosis** is marked by decreased $PaCO_2$ and increased pH. Like respiratory acidosis, respiratory alkalosis can begin outside the respiratory system (e.g., anxiety with hyperventilation)

or within the respiratory system (e.g., initial phase of an asthma attack).

Metabolic Acidosis. **Metabolic acidosis** results because of the high acid content of the blood, which also causes a loss of sodium bicarbonate, the alkaline half of the carbonate buffer system (Speakman and Weldy, 2002). In an attempt to identify the cause of the metabolic acidosis, an analysis of serum electrolytes to detect an anion gap may be helpful. An **anion gap** reflects unmeasurable anions present in plasma and is calculated by subtracting the sum of chloride and bicarbonate from the amount of plasma sodium concentration (Table 40-6) (Heitz and Horne, 2001).

Metabolic Alkalosis. **Metabolic alkalosis** is marked by the heavy loss of acid from the body or by increased levels of bicarbonate. The most common causes are vomiting and gastric suction. Other causes include the overcorrection of metabolic acidosis, potassium deficiency,

Table **40-5** Acid-Base Imbalances	
Causes	**Signs and Symptoms**

Respiratory Acidosis

Hypoventilation Resulting
From Primary Respiratory Problems

Atelectasis (obstruction of small airways often caused by retained mucus)
Pneumonia
Cystic fibrosis
Respiratory failure
Airway obstruction
Chest wall injury

Physical examination: confusion, dizziness, lethargy, headache, ventricular dysrhythmias, warm and flushed skin, muscular twitching, convulsions, and coma

Laboratory findings: arterial blood gas alterations: pH **below** 7.35, partial pressure of carbon dioxide in arterial blood ($PaCO_2$) **above** 45 mm Hg, arterial partial pressure of oxygen (PaO_2) **less than** 80 mm Hg, and bicarbonate level normal (if uncompensated) or **above** 26 mEq/L (if compensated)

Hypoventilation Resulting
From Factors Outside of the Respiratory System

Drug overdose with a respiratory depressant
Paralysis of respiratory muscles caused by various neurological alterations
Head injury
Obesity

Respiratory Alkalosis

Hyperventilation Resulting
From Primary Respiratory Problems

Asthma
Pneumonia
Inappropriate mechanical ventilator settings

Physical examination: dizziness, confusion, dysrhythmias, tachypnea, numbness and tingling of extremities, convulsions, and coma

Laboratory findings: arterial blood gas alterations: pH **above** 7.45, $PaCO_2$ 35 mm Hg, PaO_2 normal, and bicarbonate level normal (if short lived or uncompensated) or **below** 22 mEq/L (if compensated)

Hyperventilation Resulting
From Factors Outside of the Respiratory System

Anxiety
Hypermetabolic states (fever, exercise)
Disorders of the central nervous system (head injuries, infections)
Salicylate overdose

Metabolic Acidosis

High Anion Gap

Starvation
Diabetic ketoacidosis
Renal failure
Lactic acidosis from heavy exercise
Use of drugs (methanol, ethanol, formic acid, paraldehyde, aspirin)

Physical examination: headache, lethargy, confusion, dysrhythmias, tachypnea with deep respirations, abdominal cramps, and flushed skin

Laboratory findings: arterial blood gas alterations: pH **below** 7.35, $PaCO_2$ normal (if uncompensated) or **below** 35 mm Hg (if compensated), PaO_2 normal or increased (with rapid, deep respirations), bicarbonate level **below** 22 mEq/L, and oxygen saturation normal

Normal Anion Gap

Renal tubular acidosis
Diarrhea

Metabolic Alkalosis

Excessive vomiting
Prolonged gastric suctioning
Hypokalemia or hypercalcemia
Excess aldosterone
Use of drugs (steroids, sodium bicarbonate, diuretics)

Physical examination: dizziness; dysrhythmias; numbness and tingling of fingers, toes, and circumoral region; muscle cramps; tetany

Laboratory findings: arterial blood gas alterations: pH **above** 7.45, $PaCO_2$ normal (if uncompensated) or **above** 45 mm Hg (if compensated), PaO_2 normal, and bicarbonate level above 26 mEq/L

Table 40-6	Anion Gap	
Anion Gap Type	**Values**	**Causes**
Normal anion gap	12 ($\pm$2) mEq/L	Diarrhea, renal tubular acidosis, or pancreatic fistula causing a direct loss of HCO_3^-; addition of chloride-containing acids
Increased anion gap	>14 mEq/L	Lactic acidosis, uremia, diabetic ketoacidosis (DKA), or salicylate and methanol toxicity, resulting in accumulation of nonvolatile acids with decrease in HCO_3^-

From Heitz UE and Horne MM: *Mosby's pocket guide series: fluid, electrolyte, and acid-base balance,* ed 4, St. Louis, 2001, Mosby.

Box 40-1	Risk Factors for Fluid, Electrolyte, and Acid-Base Imbalances

Age

Very young
Very old

Chronic Diseases

Cancer
Cardiovascular disease, such as congestive heart failure
Endocrine disease, such as Cushing's disease and diabetes mellitus
Malnutrition
Chronic obstructive pulmonary disease
Renal disease, such as progressive renal failure
Changes in level of consciousness

Trauma

Crush injuries
Head injuries
Burns

Therapies

Diuretics
Steroids
Intravenous (IV) therapy
Total parenteral nutrition (TPN)

Gastrointestinal Losses

Gastroenteritis
Nasogastric suctioning
Fistulas

---

hyperaldosteronism, and the use of thiazide therapy that causes an increase of renal excreted acid (Phipps and others, 2003).

Nursing Knowledge Base

Fluid and electrolyte imbalances may affect anyone regardless of age, sex, color, or religious beliefs. Infants, severely ill adults, disoriented or immobile clients, and older adults are frequently at greater risk because of their inability to respond independently to the early warnings of an impending problem. Over time, the body's adaptive compensatory mechanisms can no longer maintain fluid and electrolyte or acid-base balance adequately, and the client's health becomes compromised. The severity and long-term effects on the client's health will influence a client's ability to return to a state of optimal functioning. Prolonged or severe compromises may lead to irreversible chronic health problems that not only may change the lifestyle of the client but also may have an impact on the

caregiver(s), guardians, parents, families, and/or friends (Box 40-1).

Critical Thinking

Successful critical thinking requires a synthesis of knowledge, experience, information gathered from clients, critical thinking attitudes, and intellectual and professional standards. Clinical judgments require the nurse to anticipate the information necessary, to analyze the data, and to make decisions regarding client care. Client's conditions are always changing. During assessment (Figure 40-7) the nurse must consider all critical thinking elements, as well as data about the specific client, to make appropriate nursing diagnoses.

In the case of fluid, electrolyte, and acid-base balance, the nurse must integrate knowledge of physiology, pathophysiology, and pharmacology, as well as previous experiences and information gathered from clients. Critical analysis of data enables the nurse to understand how fluid, electrolyte, and acid-base imbalances affect the client and family. In addition, the use of critical thinking attitudes such as discipline and integrity is needed to correctly identify diagnoses and then plan successful interventions. The use of professional standards, such as those developed by the clinical laboratory for electrolyte values, provides valuable guidelines for comprehensive assessment.

Nursing Process

Assessment

The nurse understands the importance of fluid, electrolyte, and acid-base balances to homeostasis dynamics. By gathering assessment data through a history and physical examination and using critical thinking skills, the nurse will identify clients at risk and then identify all appropriate nursing diagnoses.

Nursing History. The nursing assessment begins with a client history, which is designed to reveal any risk factors or preexisting conditions that may cause or contribute to a disturbance of fluid, electrolyte, and acid-base balances. The nurse will explore with the client any factors that may cause a disturbance and integrate the information

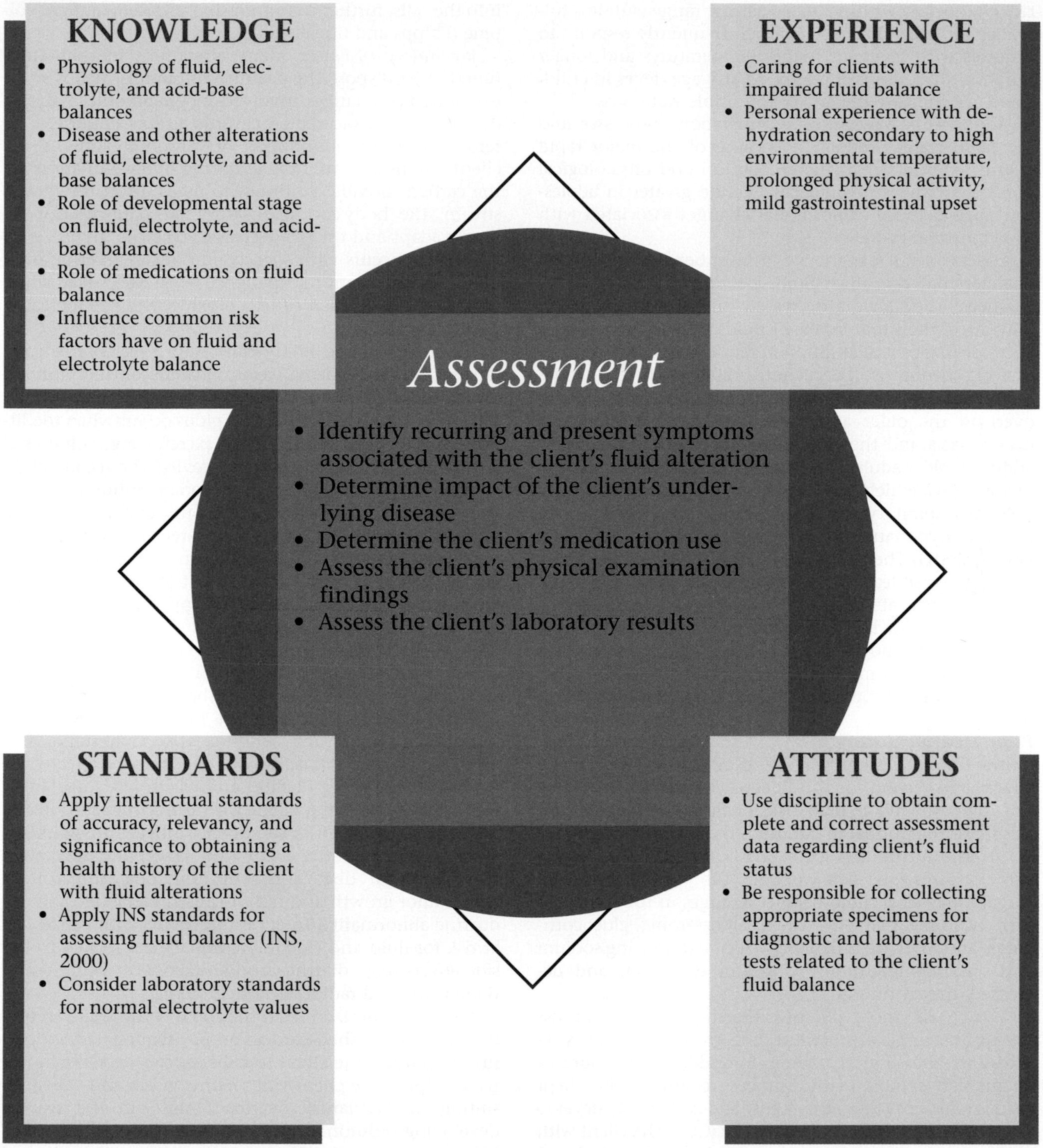

KNOWLEDGE

- Physiology of fluid, electrolyte, and acid-base balances
- Disease and other alterations of fluid, electrolyte, and acid-base balances
- Role of developmental stage on fluid, electrolyte, and acid-base balances
- Role of medications on fluid balance
- Influence common risk factors have on fluid and electrolyte balance

EXPERIENCE

- Caring for clients with impaired fluid balance
- Personal experience with dehydration secondary to high environmental temperature, prolonged physical activity, mild gastrointestinal upset

Assessment

- Identify recurring and present symptoms associated with the client's fluid alteration
- Determine impact of the client's underlying disease
- Determine the client's medication use
- Assess the client's physical examination findings
- Assess the client's laboratory results

STANDARDS

- Apply intellectual standards of accuracy, relevancy, and significance to obtaining a health history of the client with fluid alterations
- Apply INS standards for assessing fluid balance (INS, 2000)
- Consider laboratory standards for normal electrolyte values

ATTITUDES

- Use discipline to obtain complete and correct assessment data regarding client's fluid status
- Be responsible for collecting appropriate specimens for diagnostic and laboratory tests related to the client's fluid balance

FIGURE 40–7 Critical thinking model for fluid, electrolyte, and acid-base balances assessment.

with knowledge of fluid volume regulation, electrolyte concentration, and acid-base regulation.

Age. The nurse first considers the client's age. An infant's proportion of total body water (70% to 80% total body weight) is greater that that of children or adults. Infants are not protected from fluid loss because they in-

gest and excrete a relatively greater daily water volume than adults (Heitz and Horne, 2001). Therefore they are at a greater risk for **fluid volume deficits (FVDs)** and hyperosmolar imbalance because body water loss is proportionately greater per kilogram of weight.

Children ages 2 through 12 have less stable regulatory responses to imbalance, and in childhood illnesses they tend to operate within a more narrow range with less tolerance for large changes. Children frequently respond to illnesses with fevers of higher temperatures and longer duration than those of adults. At any age, fever in childhood can increase the rate of insensible water loss.

Adolescents have increased metabolic processes and increased water production because of the major rapid changes that occur in the anatomical and physiological process. Changes in fluid balance are greater in adolescent girls because of hormonal changes associated with the menstrual cycle.

Older adults experience a number of age-related changes that can affect fluid, electrolyte, and acid-base balances. They have a decreased thirst sensation which may affect their oral intake of fluids. The kidneys have a decrease in glomerular filtration rate and in the number of filtering nephrons (Lueckenotte, 2000). These changes can mean that in the presence of sodium depletion or overload the older adult may be unable to maintain homeostasis and the imbalance is instead worsened. In addition, older adults are at risk for decreased excretion of medications, which can lead to imbalances causing metabolic or respiratory acidosis, FVD, and hyperosmolar imbalance, hyponatremia, and hypernatremia (Heitz and Horne, 2001). The changes in lung function that accompany aging can lead to respiratory acidosis and the inability to compensate for metabolic acidosis. Therefore the older adult who has any condition that involves renal function, fluid and electrolyte balance, or plasma volume and osmolality is more likely to experience more serious consequences (Phipps and others, 2003).

Prior Medical History

Acute Illness. Recent surgery, head and chest trauma, shock, and second- or third-degree burns are conditions that place clients at high risk for fluid, electrolyte, and acid-base alterations. In addition, the client continues to be at risk during the acute phase until the underlying process is resolved. For example, the stress response of surgery may cause fluid-balance changes in the second to fifth postoperative day, when aldosterone, glucocorticoids, and ADH are increasingly secreted, causing sodium and chloride retention, potassium excretion, and decreased urinary output.

Surgery. The more extensive the surgery and fluid loss during the surgical procedure, the greater the body's response to the surgical trauma. In addition, after surgery clients can exhibit many acid-base changes. The client who is reluctant to breathe deeply and cough may develop respiratory acidosis due to retained $PaCO_2$. The client with nasogastric suction may develop metabolic alkalosis due to the loss of gastric acid, fluids, and electrolytes.

Burns. The greater the body surface burned, the greater the fluid loss. The burned client loses body fluids by one of five routes. First, plasma leaves the intravascular space and becomes trapped edema. This is also called the plasma-to-interstitial fluid shift. It is accompanied by a loss of serum proteins. Second, plasma and interstitial fluids are lost as burn exudate. Third, water vapor and heat are lost in proportion to the amount of skin that is burned away. Fourth, blood leaks from damaged capillaries, adding to the intravascular fluid volume loss. Last, sodium and water shift

into the cells, further compromising extracellular fluid volume (Phipps and others, 2003).

Respiratory Disorders. Many alterations in respiratory function predispose the client to respiratory acidosis. For example, the changes involved in pneumonia, sedative overdose, and exacerbated chronic airflow limitation interfere with the elimination of carbon dioxide as the client retains carbon dioxide during hypoventilation. As the carbon dioxide continues to build up in the bloodstream, the body's compensatory mechanisms can no longer adapt and the pH decreases. Likewise, hyperventilation that occurs with such conditions as fever or anxiety causes the client to experience respiratory alkalosis by blowing off too much carbon dioxide with the increased respiratory rate.

Head Injury. Head injury can result in cerebral edema. Occasionally this edema creates pressure on the pituitary gland, and as a result, ADH secretion is changed. Two alterations can occur. Diabetes insipidus occurs when too little ADH is secreted and the client excretes large volumes of diluted urine with a low specific gravity. The second alteration is the syndrome of inappropriate antidiuretic hormone (SIADH), in which there is continued inappropriate secretion of ADH. This results in water intoxication characterized by fluid volume expansion and hyponatremia, and hypotonicity of fluids as a result of high urine osmolality and low serum osmolality (Phipps and others, 2003).

Chronic Illness. Chronic disease (e.g., cancer, CHF, or renal disease) comprises a variety of conditions that can create fluid, electrolyte, and acid-base imbalances. In the presence of chronic disease the nurse must review the normal course of such conditions to understand how fluid, electrolyte, and acid-base status may be affected.

Cancer. The types of fluid and electrolyte imbalances that are observed in a client with cancer depend on the type and progression of the cancer. All electrolyte imbalances can occur in the client with cancer and are caused by anatomical distortion and functional impairment from tumor growth and tumor-caused metabolic and endocrine abnormality. In addition, clients with cancer are at risk for fluid and electrolyte imbalances related to the side effects (e.g., diarrhea and anorexia) of their chemotherapeutic and radiological treatments.

Cardiovascular Disease. In the client with cardiovascular disease a diminished cardiac output reduces kidney perfusion, causing the client to experience a decrease in urinary output. The client will retain sodium and water, resulting in circulatory overload, and run the risk of developing pulmonary edema. Fluid and electrolyte imbalances associated with heart disease can be controlled for a time with medications and fluid and sodium restrictions. The goal of fluid reduction is to decrease the workload of the left ventricle by reducing the excess circulating fluid volume.

Renal Disorders. Kidney disease alters fluid and electrolyte balance by the abnormal retention of sodium, chloride, potassium, and water in the extracellular compartment. The plasma levels of metabolic waste products such as blood urea nitrogen (BUN) and creatinine are elevated because the kidneys are unable to filter and excrete the waste products of cellular metabolism. This elevation is toxic to cellular processes. Metabolic acidosis results when hydrogen ions are retained due to decreased renal function. Because of the renal disorder, the usual renal compensatory mechanisms such as bicarbonate reabsorption are not available, so the body's ability to restore normal acid-base balance is limited.

The severity of fluid and electrolyte imbalance is proportional to the degree of renal failure. Occasionally, acute renal failure–induced shock or a decrease in extracellular fluid may be reversible. Although chronic renal failure is progressive, the client may be treated successfully with dietary control of protein and salt intake, diuretic medications, and fluid restrictions.

Gastrointestinal Disturbances. Gastroenteritis and nasogastric suctioning result in a loss of fluid, potassium, and chloride ions. Hydrogen ions are also lost, causing a disturbance in acid-base balance. Timely education of infant and child caregivers is necessary to prevent dehydration when the infant or child is experiencing diarrhea. Gastrointestinal fistulas can also result in a loss of potassium, resulting in an increased risk for hypokalemia. The loss of potassium increases the risk for acid-base disturbances as well.

Regardless of the presence of any disease process, the nurse must determine how long the client has suffered from that disease and the type of treatment currently being administered. In addition to chronic health problems, the nurse determines if the client has a history of new-onset acute illnesses such as diarrhea, vomiting, colostomy, nasogastric suctioning, or intestinal drainage. Any condition that results in the loss of GI fluids predisposes the client to dehydration and a variety of electrolyte disturbances.

Environmental Factors. The nurse should also include certain environmental factors in the nursing history. Clients who have participated in vigorous exercise or who have become exposed to temperature extremes may have clinical signs of fluid and electrolyte alterations. Exposure to environmental temperatures exceeding 28° to 30° C (82.4° to 86° F) results in excessive sweating with weight loss. A body weight loss over 7% decreases the ability of the cooling mechanism to conserve water. Loss of fluid from sweating varies and can reach a maximal rate of 2 L/hr (Ignatavicius and Workman, 2002). Inadequate fluid replacement can lead to fluid volume disturbances.

Diet. A client's current dietary history is an important component of nursing assessment. Dietary intake of fluids, salt, potassium, calcium, magnesium, and necessary carbohydrates, fats, and protein helps maintain normal fluid, electrolyte, and acid-base status. Recent changes in appetite or the ability to chew and swallow can affect nutritional status and fluid hydration. When nutritional intake is inadequate, the body tries to preserve its protein stores by breaking down glycogen and fat stores. When excess free fatty acids are released, metabolic acidosis can occur because the liver converts free fatty acids to ketone, a strong acid. However, after those resources are depleted, the body begins to destroy protein stores. When serum protein levels drop below normal, hypoalbuminemia results. In hypoalbuminemia the serum colloid osmotic pressure is de-

Box 40-2	**Medications That Cause Fluid, Electrolyte, and Acid-Base Disturbances**

Diuretics—metabolic alkalosis, hyperkalemia, and hypokalemia
Steroids—metabolic alkalosis
Potassium supplements—GI disturbances, including intestinal and gastric ulcers and diarrhea
Respiratory center depressants such as opioid analgesics—decreased rate and depth of respirations, resulting in respiratory acidosis
Antibiotics—nephrotoxicity (e.g., vancomycin, methicillin, aminoglycosides); hyperkalemia and/or hypernatremia (e.g., azlocillin, carbenicillin, piperacillin, ticarcillin, Unasyn)*
Calcium carbonate (Tums)—mild metabolic alkalosis with nausea and vomiting*
Magnesium hydroxide (Milk of Magnesia)—hypokalemia*

*Data from McKenry LM, Salerno E: *Mosby's pharmacology in nursing,* ed 21, St. Louis, 2003, Mosby.

creased, and fluid shifts from the circulating blood volume and enters the interstitial fluid space in the peritoneal cavity. In addition, dieting can lead to acidosis, because rapid water loss can lead to osmolar fluid imbalance.

Lifestyle. Lifestyle factors should also be included in the nurse's history. If a client already has preexisting medical risks, such as a history of smoking or alcohol consumption, they can further impair the client's ability to adapt to fluid, electrolyte, and acid-base alterations. For example, the consistent use of alcohol and tobacco use can ultimately cause respiratory depression, which can result in respiratory acidosis and alteration in maintaining adequate fluid and electrolyte balance.

Medication. A final category to include in the nurse's assessment is a history of medication use (Box 40-2). If the assessment reveals a medication that is likely to cause an electrolyte or acid-base disorder, the nurse will also closely examine laboratory values. In addition, the nurse will assess the client's knowledge of side effects and adherence to medication schedules and the client's knowledge of the potential side effects of over-the-counter medications on fluid, electrolyte, and acid-base balances (Phipps and others, 2003).

Physical Assessment. A thorough examination is necessary, because fluid and electrolyte imbalances or acid-base disturbances can affect all body systems. While examining each system, the nurse carefully considers the signs and symptoms to expect as a result of any imbalance. For example, an examination of the oral cavity will likely reveal signs of dehydration if the nurse suspects the client is experiencing a fluid loss. Table 40-7 summarizes possible physical findings for clients with fluid, electrolyte, and acid-base imbalances.

Measuring Fluid Intake and Output. Measuring and recording all liquid intake and output (I&O) during a 24-hour period is an important part of the client's assessment

Table 40-7   Physical and Behavioral Nursing Assessment for Fluid, Electrolyte, and Acid-Base Imbalances

Assessment	Imbalance
Weight Changes	
2%-5% loss	Mild FVD*
5%-10% loss	Moderate FVD*
10%-15% loss	Severe FVD*
15%-20% loss	Death*
2% gain	Mild fluid volume excess (FVE)
5% gain	Moderate FVE
8% gain	Severe FVE
Head	
History:	
Headache	FVD,* metabolic or respiratory acidosis, metabolic alkalosis
Dizziness	FVD,* respiratory acidosis or alkalosis, hyponatremia
Observation:	
Irritability	Metabolic or respiratory alkalosis, hyperosmolar imbalance, hypernatremia, hypokalemia
Lethargy	FVD,* metabolic acidosis or alkalosis, respiratory acidosis, hypercalcemia
Confusion, disorientation	FVD,* hypomagnesemia, metabolic acidosis, hypokalemia
Eyes	
Inspection:	
Sunken, dry conjunctivae, decreased or absent tearing	FVD
Periorbital edema, papilledema	FVE
History:	
Blurred vision	FVE
Throat and Mouth	
Inspection:	
Sticky, dry mucous membranes, dry cracked lips, decreased salivation	FVD, hypernatremia
Longitudinal tongue furrows	
Cardiovascular System	
Inspection:	
Flat neck veins	FVD
Distended neck veins	FVE
Slow venous filling	FVD*
Palpation:	
Edema (dependent body parts: back, sacrum, legs)	FVE*
Dysrhythmias (also noted as ECG changes)	Metabolic acidosis, respiratory alkalosis and acidosis, potassium imbalance, hypomagnesemia
Increased pulse rate	Metabolic alkalosis, respiratory acidosis, hyponatremia, FVD, hypomagnesemia
Decreased pulse rate	Metabolic alkalosis, hypokalemia
Weak pulse	FVD, hypokalemia
Decreased capillary filling	FVD
Bounding pulse	FVE
Auscultation:	
Blood pressure low or without orthostatic changes	FVD, hyponatremia, hyperkalemia, hypermagnesemia
Third heart sound	FVE
Hypertension	FVE

Table 40-7	Physical and Behavioral Nursing Assessment for Fluid, Electrolyte, and Acid-Base Imbalances—cont'd
Assessment	**Imbalance**

Respiratory System

Inspection:	
Increased rate	FVE, respiratory alkalosis, metabolic acidosis
Dyspnea	FVE
Auscultation:	
Crackles	FVE

Gastrointestinal System

History:	
Anorexia	Metabolic acidosis
Abdominal cramps	Metabolic acidosis
Inspection:	
Sunken abdomen	FVD
Distended abdomen	Third-space syndrome
Vomiting	FVD, hypercalcemia, hyponatremia, hypochloremia, metabolic alkalosis
Diarrhea	Hyponatremia, metabolic acidosis
Auscultation:	
Hyperperistalsis with diarrhea, or hypoperistalsis	FVD, hypokalemia

Renal System

Inspection:	
Oliguria or anuria	FVD, FVE
Diuresis (if kidneys are normal)	FVE
Increased urine specific gravity	FVD

Neuromuscular System

Inspection:	
Numbness, tingling	Metabolic alkalosis, hypocalcemia, potassium imbalances
Muscle cramps, tetany	Hypocalcemia, metabolic or respiratory alkalosis
Coma	Hyperosmolar or hypoosmolar imbalances, hyponatremia
Tremors	Respiratory acidosis, hypomagnesemia
Palpation:	
Hypotonicity	Hypokalemia, hypercalcemia*
Hypertonicity	Hypocalcemia, hypomagnesemia, metabolic alkalosis
Percussion:	
Decreased or absent deep tendon reflexes	Hypercalcemia, hypermagnesemia
Increased or hyperactive deep tendon reflexes	Hypocalcemia, hypomagnesemia

Skin

Body temperature:	
Increased	Hypernatremia, hyperosmolar imbalance, metabolic acidosis
Decreased	FVD
Inspection:	
Dry, flushed	FVD, hypernatremia, metabolic acidosis
Palpation:	
Inelastic skin turgor, cold, clammy skin	FVD

*Data from Heitz UE and Horne MM: *Mosby's pocket guide series: fluid, electrolyte, and acid base balance,* ed 4, St. Louis, 2001, Mosby.

database for fluid and electrolyte balance. Recognition of trends in the I&O is important (e.g., a gradually decreasing urine output can indicate that the body is trying to adapt to an FVD or hyperosmolar fluid imbalance). Accurate I&O measurements can identify both clients at risk for and clients who are experiencing fluid, electrolyte, and acid-base disturbances.

For clients in health care settings, I&O measurement is a nursing intervention routinely used for clients following a procedure, clients who are febrile, clients with restricted fluids, or clients who receive diuretic or intravenous (IV) therapy. The nurse also measures I&O for clients with chronic cardiopulmonary or renal illnesses and clients whose health status has deteriorated or has become unstable.

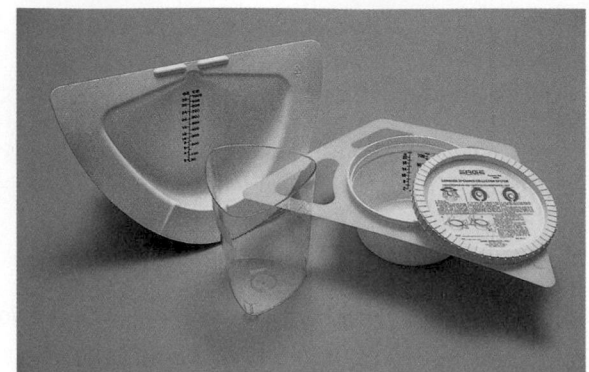

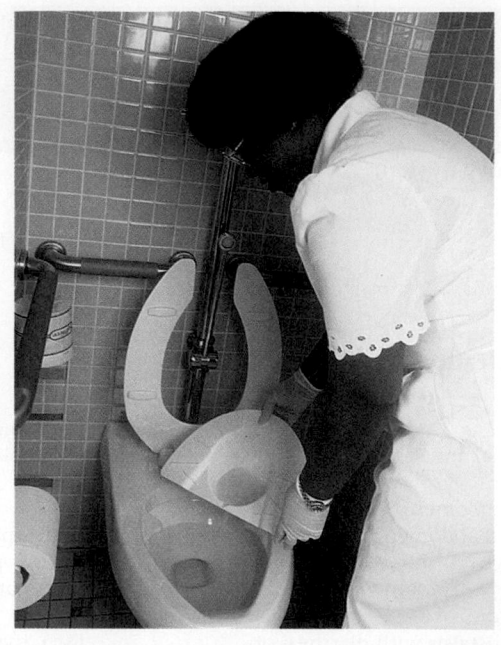

A

B

FIGURE **40–8 A,** Graduated measuring containers. Clockwise from far left: "hat" receptacle, specipan, and graduated measuring container. **B,** Emptying collected urine.

Intake includes all liquids taken by mouth, (e.g., gelatin, ice cream, soup, juice, and water), through nasogastric or jejunostomy feeding tubes (see Chapter 43), IV fluids (including both large-volume and intermittent IVs), and blood or its components. Occasionally, clients receive a specific amount of a liquid medication every 1 to 2 hours. A client receiving tube feedings may receive numerous liquid medications, and water may be used to flush the tube for the medications. Over a 24-hour period, these liquids can amount to significant intake and should always be recorded on the I&O record. Output includes urine, diarrhea, vomitus, gastric suction, and drainage from postsurgical wounds or other tubes (see Chapter 49).

Ambulatory clients are instructed to save their urine in a calibrated insert, which attaches to the rim of the toilet bowl (Figure 40-8). When a client has an indwelling Foley catheter, drainage tube, or suction, output is recorded (e.g., at the end of each nursing shift or every hour) as the client's condition requires. Cooperation from the client and family is essential with I&O measurements. It is important for the client to have good vision and motor skills to ensure accuracy. The nurse teaches the client and family the purpose of the measurements and either to notify the nurse to empty any container with voided fluid or how to measure and empty the container themselves.

In the hospital, forms for recording I&O are attached to the bedside chart or room door (see Figure 40-9). The 24-hour total is calculated as directed by agency policy. The nurse who still retains responsibility may delegate I&O recording to assistive personnel with competent skills in measurement and calculation with accuracy, not estimation, and timeliness.

Recording I&O is essential for obtaining an accurate database. This information helps maintain an ongoing evaluation of the client's hydration status to prevent severe imbalances.

Laboratory Studies. The nurse reviews laboratory tests to obtain further objective data about fluid, electrolyte, and acid-base balances. These tests include serum and urinary electrolyte levels, hematocrit, blood creatinine level, BUN levels, urine specific gravity, and ABG readings (Box 40-3, p. 1154). Serum electrolyte levels are measured to determine the hydration status, the electrolyte concentration of the blood plasma, and acid-base balance. The frequency with which these electrolyte levels are measured depends on the severity of the client's illness. Serum electrolyte tests are routinely performed on any client entering a hospital to screen for alterations and to serve as a baseline for future comparisons.

Client Expectations. Often a fluid, electrolyte, or acid-base disturbance is so serious or acute that the client's condition prevents a review of his or her expectations. However, if a client is alert enough to discuss care with the nurse, a review of expectations may reveal short-term needs (e.g., provision of comfort from nausea) or long-term needs (e.g., understanding how to prevent alterations from occurring in the future). The client must be able to understand the implications of fluid, electrolyte, or acid-base changes to be able to express expectations of care. The client's trust in the nurse is strengthened through the nurse's competent response to sudden changes in the client's condition.

Nursing Diagnosis

When caring for clients with suspected fluid, electrolyte, and acid-base imbalances, it is particularly important that the nurse be skilled in using critical thinking to formulate nursing diagnoses. The assessment data that establish the risk for or the actual presence of a nursing diagnosis in these areas may be subtle, and patterns and trends emerge

Intake and Output Summary

Patient Label	P.O. Intake	Tube Feedings	Hyperalimentation	I.V. Primary	I.V.P.B.	Blood/Blood Products	Other:	Urine	Emesis	G.I. Suction	Drainage	Other: *Chest tube*
Date: *6–10–XX*												
2200–0600	120				50			325			50	75
0600–1400	800							700			75	50
1400–2200	650				50			500			30	50
24Hr. Subtotal	1570				100			1525			155	175
Total Intake/Output	1570/100							1525/330				
Date:												
2200–0600												
0600–1400												
1400–2200												
24Hr. Subtotal												
Total Intake/Output												
Date:												
2200–0600												
0600–1400												
1400–2200												
24Hr. Subtotal												
Total Intake/Output												
Date:												
2200–0600												
0600–1400												
1400–2200												
24Hr. Subtotal												
Total Intake/ Output												
Date:												
2200–0600												
0600–1400												
1400–2200												
24Hr. Subtotal												
Total Intake/Output												
Date:												
2200–0600												
0600–1400												
1400–2200												
24Hr. Subtotals												
Total Intake/Output												
Date:												
2200–0600												
0600–1400												
1400–2200												
24Hr. Subtotals												
Total Intake/Output												

FIGURE **40–9** Twenty-four-hour intake and output record. (Courtesy St. Mary's Health Center, St. Louis, Mo.)

Box 40-3 Laboratory Data for Fluid, Electrolyte, and Acid-Base Imbalances

Fluid and Electrolytes

Altered concentrations of sodium, potassium, magnesium, calcium, phosphates, chloride, and bicarbonate (venous CO_2 contentions)

Increase in hematocrit, BUN, sodium, and osmolality in serum (related to loss of ECF fluid orr gain of solutes)

Decrease in hematocrit, BUN, sodium, and osmolality in serum (related to gain of ECF fluid or loss of solutes)

Concentrated urine demonstrated by urine specific gravity >1.030

Dilute urine demonstrated by a specific gravity <1.012

Metabolic Alkalosis

pH >7.45
$PaCO_2$ normal or >45 mm Hg if lungs are compensating
PaO_2 normal
O_2 saturation (SaO_2) normal
HCO_3^- >26 mEq/L
K^+ <3.5 mEq/L

Metabolic Acidosis

pH <7.35
$PaCO_2$ normal or <35 mm Hg if lungs are compensating

Metabolic Acidosis—continued

PaO_2 normal
SaO_2 normal
HCO_3^- <22 mEq/L
K^+ >5.3 mEq/L
K^+ <3.5 mEq/L

Respiratory Alkalosis

pH >7.45
$PaCO_2$ <35 mm Hg
PaO_2 normal
SaO_2 normal
HCO_3^- normal
K^+ <3.5 mEq/L

Respiratory Acidosis

pH <7.35
$PaCO_2$ >45 mm Hg
PaO_2 normal or <80 mm Hg, depending on cause of acidosis
SaO_2 normal or <95%, depending on cause of acidosis
HCO_3^- normal if early respiratory acidosis or >26 mEq/L if kidneys are compensating
K^+ >5.3 mEq/L

Nursing Diagnostic Process   Box 40-4

Assessment Activities	Defining Characteristics	Nursing Diagnosis
Assess blood pressure and pulse.	Client is hypotensive with increased heart rate.	Deficient fluid volume related to loss of gastrointestinal fluids via vomiting
Obtain daily weight measurements.	Client experiences sudden weight loss.	
Observe volume of urine output related to intake and specific gravity.	Decreased volume of output in comparison to intake; increased urine specific gravity is present.	
Palpate skin turgor.	Inelastic skin turgor noted.	
Ask if client is thirsty or weak.	Client verbalizes thirst and weakness.	
Inspect mucous membranes for degree of moisture.	Dry mucous membranes are noted.	
Observe for abnormal losses of fluids.	Client is vomiting.	
Assess client's tolerance to changing from lying to sitting position.	Client complains of dizziness when changing position.	

only when the nurse consciously assesses for them. The nurse must keep in mind that many body systems may be involved. Clustering of defining characteristics will lead the nurse to selection of the appropriate diagnoses. For example, the nursing diagnosis *deficient fluid volume* is developed in Box 40-4.

An important part of formulating nursing diagnoses is identifying the relevant causative or related factor. The nursing interventions that are chosen must treat or modify the related factor for the diagnosis to be resolved. *Deficient fluid volume related to loss of gastrointestinal fluids*

via vomiting will require therapies different to a degree from therapies needed for *deficient fluid volume related to elevated body temperature.*

Possible nursing diagnoses for clients with fluid, electrolyte, and acid-base alterations may include the following:
- Risk for imbalanced body temperature
- Ineffective breathing pattern
- Decreased cardiac output
- Deficient fluid volume
- Risk for deficient fluid volume
- Excess fluid volume

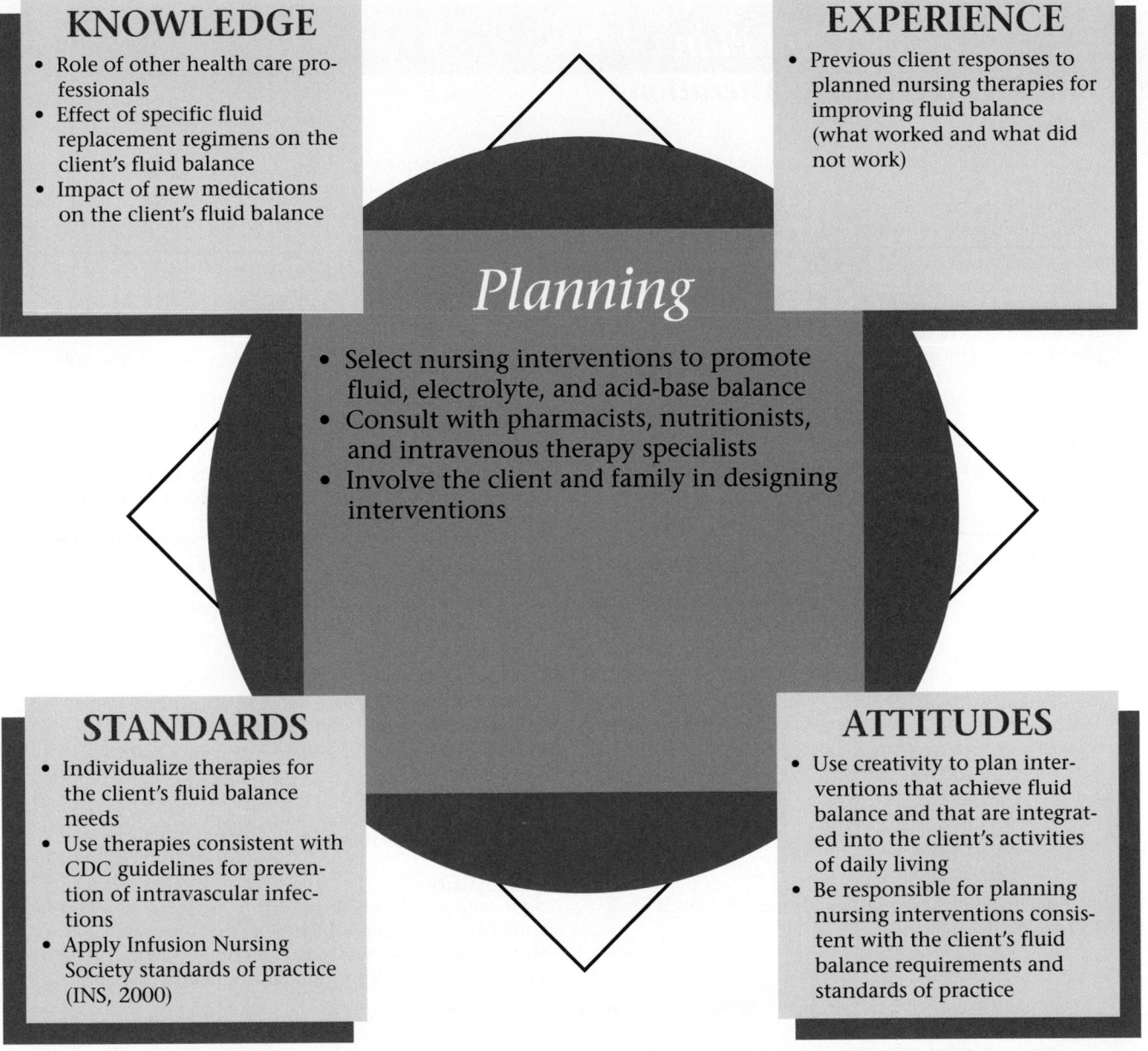

KNOWLEDGE

- Role of other health care professionals
- Effect of specific fluid replacement regimens on the client's fluid balance
- Impact of new medications on the client's fluid balance

EXPERIENCE

- Previous client responses to planned nursing therapies for improving fluid balance (what worked and what did not work)

Planning

- Select nursing interventions to promote fluid, electrolyte, and acid-base balance
- Consult with pharmacists, nutritionists, and intravenous therapy specialists
- Involve the client and family in designing interventions

STANDARDS

- Individualize therapies for the client's fluid balance needs
- Use therapies consistent with CDC guidelines for prevention of intravascular infections
- Apply Infusion Nursing Society standards of practice (INS, 2000)

ATTITUDES

- Use creativity to plan interventions that achieve fluid balance and that are integrated into the client's activities of daily living
- Be responsible for planning nursing interventions consistent with the client's fluid balance requirements and standards of practice

FIGURE **40-10** Critical thinking model for fluid, electrolyte, and acid-base balances planning.

- Impaired gas exchange
- Deficient knowledge regarding disease management
- Impaired mobility
- Impaired oral mucous membrane
- Impaired skin integrity
- Risk for impaired skin integrity
- Ineffective therapeutic regimen management
- Impaired tissue integrity
- Ineffective tissue perfusion

Planning

During the planning process the nurse uses critical thinking to synthesize information from multiple resources (Figure 40-10) and to ensure that the client's plan of care integrates both the nurse's scientific and nursing knowl-edge, as well as all the knowledge the nurse has gathered about the individual client.

Goals and Outcomes. The nurse develops an individual plan of care for each of the nursing diagnoses (see care plan). The nurse and client set expectations for care that are individualized and realistic with measurable outcomes. For example, the following related outcomes might be established for the goal "The client will restore hydration status at discharge":

- The client will be free of complications associated with the IV device throughout the duration of IV therapy.
- The client will demonstrate fluid balance by moist, mucous membranes, balanced I&O measurements, and stable daily weights within 48 hours.
- The client will have serum electrolytes within the normal range within 48 hours.

Nursing Care Plan

Fluid and Electrolyte Alterations

Assessment

Mrs. Hilda Bottomley is a 72-year-old seen by her physician this morning with complaints of flulike symptoms and difficulty breathing. She admits that she has not felt like eating and drinking much lately. After an outpatient chest x-ray examina-tion, Mrs. Bottomley has been admitted for respiratory toileting and IV antibiotic and fluid therapy. The physician orders O_2 at 4 L/min with humidification, respiratory treatments, fluids by mouth and IV, pulse oximetry, and activity with assistance.

Assessment Activities	Findings/Defining Characteristics
Ask Mrs. Bottomley to describe when her respiratory discomfort began and what accompanying signs and symptoms she may have experienced.	She states that she became congested about 2 weeks ago and now she is coughing up mucus, has chills, feels weak, is not interested in eating, and aches all over.
Observe her pulmonary secretions.	Mrs. Bottomley coughed up thick and yellowish-greenish sputum.
Assess Mrs. Bottomley's vital signs.	Mrs. Bottomley's temperature is 36.7° C (101° F), her respiratory rate is 28 breaths per minute, and rhonchi breath sounds are present. Other vital signs are within normal limits.
Evaluate her arterial blood gas values and review her chest x-ray report.	Mrs. Bottomley's arterial blood gas results indicate a mild respiratory acidosis and the chest x-ray film revealed a left lower lobe pneumonia.

Nursing Diagnosis: Ineffective airway clearance related to increased mucus in response to airway infection and manifested by mild respiratory acidosis; risk for deficient fluid volume related to reduced fluid intake.

Planning

Goal	Expected Outcomes*
	Electrolyte and Acid/Base Balance
Client's airway will be free from secretions with normal ABG levels by discharge.	ABG levels will be within normal limits in 24 hours.
	Respiratory rate will be within normal limits with activity in 24 hours.
	Temperature will be within normal limits in 24 hours.
	Breath sounds will be clear on auscultation.
	Mucus will become thin and clear in 48 hours.
	Fluid Balance
Client's fluid volume will remain within normal limits throughout hospital stay.	Urine output will equal intake of approximately 1500 ml.
	Daily weights will not vary ±2 pounds.
	Mucous membranes will remain moist.
	Vital signs will remain within normal limits.

*Outcome classification labels from Moorhead S, Johnson M, Maas M: *Nursing outcomes classification (NOC)*, ed 3, St. Louis, 2004, Mosby.

Interventions†	Rationale
Airway Maintenance	
• Schedule coughing and deep breathing exercises every 2 hours while awake.	Cough control exercises and deep breathing promote pulmonary secretion clearance (Woods, 2002).
• Administer chest physiotherapy every 4 hours while awake to affected regions of the lung.	Chest physiotherapy, breathing exercises, cough techniques, along with ambulating the client, are effective in promoting airway clearance (Woods, 2002).
• Ambulate client once every 8 hours and encourage client to get out of bed into chair often.	Mobility promotes air exchange and position change prevents settling of secretions in lung tissue.
Fluid Management	
• Provide client with an additional 16 ounces of noncaffeinated oral fluids every 8 hours.	Increased fluid intake helps to liquefy pulmonary secretions and in turn facilitate productive coughing (Woods, 2002).

†Intervention classification labels from Dochterman JM, Bulechek GM: *Nursing interventions classification (NIC)*, ed 4, St. Louis, 2004, Mosby.

Nursing Care Plan

Fluid and Electrolyte Alterations—cont'd

Evaluation

Nursing Actions	Client Response/Finding	Achievement of Outcome
Monitor ABG levels, vital signs, I&O, daily weight and O₂ saturation levels. Assess mucous membranes.	She is able to walk down the hall without respiratory discomfort. Mrs. Bottomley states she is drinking more fluids. She no longer experiences chills and a fever.	Mrs. Bottomley's arterial blood gas levels have returned to normal values. Vital signs, and O₂ saturation are within normal range. Her I&O measurements are negative for fluid loss or excess. Daily weight remained stable. Mucous membranes are moist.
Auscultate breath sounds.	Mrs. Bottomley denies any discomfort with breathing in or out.	Mrs. Bottomley's breath sounds are clear bilaterally on inspiration and expiration.
Evaluate effectiveness of coughing and deep breathing exercises.	Mrs. Bottomley demonstrated three deep breaths followed by coughing and said she no longer coughs up sputum.	Mrs. Bottomley is free of sputum production.
Identify methods to provide for adequate rest.	Mrs. Bottomley says she takes naps between her morning and afternoon treatments.	Mrs. Bottomley schedules her activities throughout the day and rests in bed before her respiratory therapy.

Setting Priorities. The client's clinical condition will determine which of the diagnoses takes the greatest priority. Many nursing diagnoses in the area of fluid, electrolyte, and acid-base balances are of highest priority, because the consequences for the client can be serious or even life threatening. For example, in the concept map (Figure 40-11) for the client with gastroenteritis and dehydration, the occurrence of nausea and diarrhea have created a serious problem of deficient fluid volume. In this situation, the nurse must intervene to help resolve the client's nausea and diarrhea. If these priorities are unmet, the client's fluid imbalance will likely worsen.

Consultation with the client's physician may assist in setting realistic time frames for the goals of care, particularly when the client's physiological status is unstable. During planning the nurse collaborates as much as possible with the client and family and other members of the interdisciplinary health care team such as IV therapy and pharmacy. The family can be particularly helpful in identifying subtle changes in a client's behavior associated with any imbalances (e.g., anxiety, confusion, or irritability). The nurse also incorporates client preferences and resources into the plan of care.

Continuity of Care. For those clients with acute disturbances, discharge planning must begin early. In the hospital the nurse anticipates the needs of the client and family and collaborates with the other members of the health care team to ensure that care can continue in the home or long-term care setting with few disruptions. For example, for the client who is discharged on IV therapy the nurse must determine the knowledge and skills of the family member or friend who is to assume caregiving responsibilities and make a referral to home IV therapy as soon as possible. The nurse also collaborates closely with other members of the health care team, such as the physician, dietician, and pharmacist. The di-

etitian can be a valuable resource in recommending food sources to either increase or reduce intake of certain electrolytes. Chapter 43 describes various therapeutic diets (e.g., low sodium). The pharmacist can assist the nurse and physician in identifying medications or combinations of medications likely to cause electrolyte or acid-base disturbances. Furthermore, the pharmacist can offer information regarding client education on side effects to anticipate for those drugs prescribed to the client. The physician will direct the treatment of any fluid, electrolyte, or acid-base alteration.

Implementation

Health Promotion. Health promotion activities in the area of fluid, electrolyte, and acid-base imbalances focus primarily on client teaching. Clients and caregivers need to recognize risk factors for these imbalances and implement appropriate preventive measures. For example, parents of infants need to understand that GI losses can quickly lead to serious imbalances; therefore when vomiting or diarrhea occur in the infant, the parent needs to recognize the risk and promptly seek health care to restore normal balance. Even the healthy adult is at risk for developing imbalances when subjected to elevated environmental temperatures. Nurses need to advise them to supplement the fluid loss from perspiration by increasing oral fluids such as water, maintaining adequate environmental ventilation, and refraining from excessive activity during this period of time.

Sometimes it is difficult to separate the effects of age-related changes from changes associated with disease processes. For an example, any older adult who has a chronic condition involving renal or respiratory function is more likely to suffer serious consequences when an acute disease process occurs (Phipps and others, 2003).

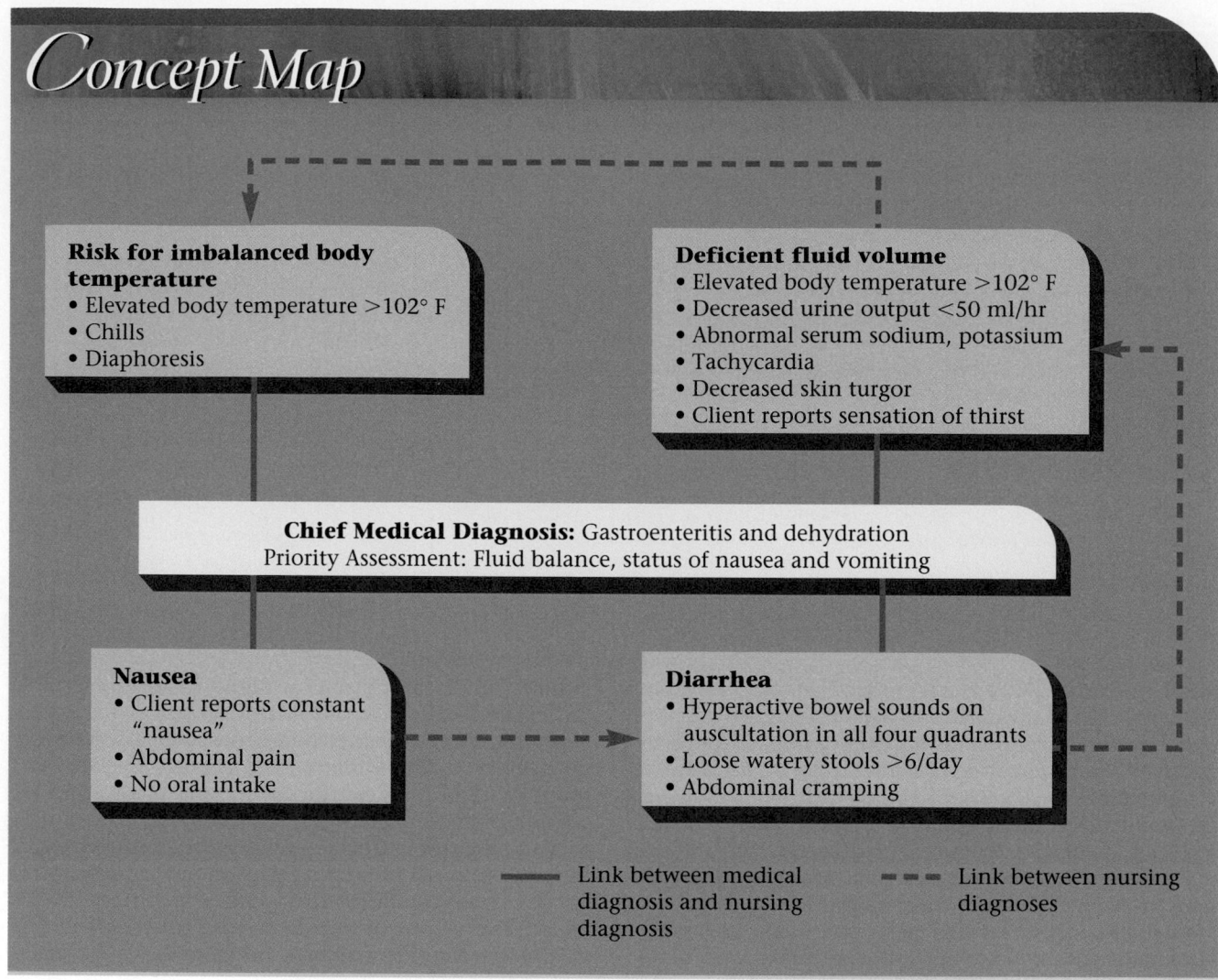

FIGURE **40–11** Concept map for a client with gastroenteritis and dehydration.

All clients with a chronic health alteration are at risk for developing changes in their fluid, electrolyte, and acid-base balances. They need to understand their own risk factors and the measures to be taken to avoid imbalances. For example, clients with renal failure must avoid excess intake of fluid, sodium, potassium, and phosphorus. Through diet education these clients learn the types of foods to avoid and the suitable volume of fluid they are permitted daily (see Chapter 43). Clients with chronic health diseases need to be made aware of early signs and symptoms of fluid, electrolyte, and acid-base imbalances. A client with heart disease should be instructed to obtain an accurate body weight each day at the approximate same time and to inform the physician of significant changes of weight from one day to another. Increase in weight, shortness of breath, orthopnea, and dependent edema are all associated with fluid retention.

Acute Care. Although fluid, electrolyte, and/or acid-base imbalance can occur in all settings, changes in the acute care delivery system place more demanding expectations on the nurse. Today the nurse must manage the client's complex medical care in a shorter span of time while being expected to perform more difficult technological skills.

Daily Weights and Intake and Output Measurement. When implementing specific measures to increase or decrease fluid, two nursing interventions are necessary: daily weight and I&O measurements. Clients with fluid and electrolyte alterations should be weighed daily. Daily weights are the single most important indicator of fluid status (Heitz and Horne, 2001). Weight should be determined at the same time each day with the same scale after the client voids. The scale should be calibrated each day or routinely. The client should wear the same clothes or clothes that weigh the same; if a bed scale is used, the same number of sheets should be used on the scale with each weighing.

I&O records provide additional information about fluid balance (see section on assessment). I&O measurements, when examined for trends, can indicate whether excess fluid volume is excreted in the form of urine or whether excretion of fluids through the kidneys has diminished. The I&O is not as accurate as daily weights in

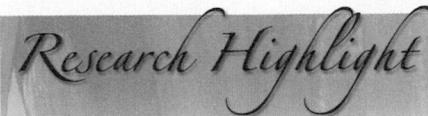

Measuring Intake and Output

Research Focus

Continuous fluid intake and output (I&O) measurement is a traditional practice for nurses to monitor the client's cardiovascular and renal function. Validation of this standard of care as an effective determination of fluid balance is questioned.

Research Abstract

The purpose of this study was to determine whether I&O measurements and daily weights revealed redundant information and, if so, which of the two practices was least efficient and could be deleted. A chart audit of clients in three nursing units was conducted to evaluate the efficiency and effectiveness of assessing the client's fluid balance using both a 24-hour I&O and daily weight measurements. Clients were selected who had a physician's order for both I&O and daily weights, the client was treated under this order for at least 48 hours, and the record was complete. The nursing team examined 48-hour records of daily weight and I&O for 73 patients meeting the criteria and correlated the two. Analyses illustrated the unreliability of weight and fluid balance measurements for determining day-to-day changes in true weight variation. Daily weights

alone provide more reliable fluid balance than cumulative I&O measurements. A reduction in personnel resources and costs are realized with elimination of labor-intensive interventions.

Evidenced-Based Practice

- Multiple sources of inaccuracy contribute to unreliable fluid measurements such as inadvertent omission recording, inaccurate measurement, insensible fluid loss, and required multiple recording.
- Sources of error with daily client weights are limited to accuracy of scale and user competency.
- Nursing time and resource expenditure are conserved with only daily weight measurements for evaluating fluid balance.
- Limit the use of combined I&O and daily weights to circumstances where reliability can be ensured.
- Cumulative I&O is best applied for short-term fluid monitoring and for clients in whom acute changes in fluid balance are critical.

Reference

Wise L and others: Evaluating the reliability and utility of cumulative intake and output, *J Nurs Care Qual* 14(3):37, 2000.

Box 40-5

---

assessing daily fluid balance unless it has been measured strictly and precisely (Box 40-5).

Enteral Replacement of Fluids. Oral replacement of fluids and electrolytes is appropriate as long as the client is not so physiologically unstable that oral fluids cannot be replaced rapidly. Oral replacement of fluids is contraindicated when the client is vomiting, has a mechanical obstruction of the GI tract, is at risk for aspiration, or has impaired swallowing. Clients unable to tolerate solid foods may still be able to ingest fluids. The nurse should employ strategies to encourage fluid intake such as offering small sips of fluid frequently, popsicles, and ice chips.

When replacing fluids by mouth in a client with a fluid deficit, it is wise to choose fluids with adequate calories and electrolyte content (e.g., fruit juices, gelatin, and replacements such as Pedialyte and Gastrolyte). However, it is important to remember that liquids containing lactose, caffeine, or low-sodium content may not be appropriate when the client has diarrhea.

A feeding tube may be appropriate when the client's GI tract is healthy but the client cannot ingest fluids (e.g., after oral surgery or with impaired swallowing). Fluids can also be replaced through a gastrostomy or jejunostomy feeding tube, or they can be administered via a small-bore nasogastric feeding tube.

Restriction of Fluids. Clients who retain fluids and have **fluid volume excess (FVE)** require restricted fluid intake. Fluid restriction is often difficult for clients, particularly if they take drugs that dry the oral mucous membranes or if they breathe through the mouth and experience the sensation of thirst. The nurse should explain the reason fluids are restricted. In addition, the client needs to know the amount of fluid permitted orally and should understand that ice chips, gelatin, and ice cream are considered fluid. The client should help to decide the amount of fluid with each meal, between meals, before bed, and with medications. Frequently clients on fluid restriction can swallow a number of pills with as little as 1 ounce (30 ml) of liquid.

A good rule of thumb for fluid restrictions is to allow half of the allotted total oral fluids between 7 AM and 3 PM, the period when clients usually are more active, receive two meals, and take most of their oral medications. Clients on fluid restriction require mouth care frequently to moisten mucous membranes, decrease the chance of mucosal drying and cracking, and maintain comfort (see Chapter 38).

Parenteral Replacement of Fluids and Electrolytes. Fluid and electrolytes may be replaced through infusion directly into the blood rather than via the digestive system. Parenteral replacement includes total parenteral nutrition (TPN), IV fluid and electrolyte therapy **(crystalloids),** and blood and blood component **(colloids)** administration.

With increasing risk to health care workers for transmission of the human immunodeficiency virus (HIV), the cause of acquired immunodeficiency syndrome (AIDS), hepatitis B virus (HBV), and other infectious diseases, standard precautions must be practiced when administering parenteral fluids (see Chapter 33).

Vascular Access Devices. **Vascular access devices** (VADs) are catheters, cannulas, or infusion ports designed for repeated access to the vascular system. Peripherally placed catheters are designed for short-term use (e.g., fluid restoration postoperative and short-term antibiotic administration). Devices such as central line catheters, peripherally inserted catheters, and implanted parts are more effective than peripherally placed catheters for administering medications and solutions that are irritating to veins and for the delivery of long-term IV therapy. Increased use of central venous catheters and implanted infusion ports (Figure 40-12) requires nurses to be educated in the care of these devices.

Total Parenteral Nutrition. **Total parenteral nutrition** is a nutritionally adequate hypertonic solution consisting of glucose and other nutrients and electrolytes given through an indwelling or central IV catheter which may be inserted peripherally or percutaneously, implanted, or tunneled. Chapter 43 reviews principles and guidelines for TPN administration, which is used as an intervention in severe cases of malnutrition.

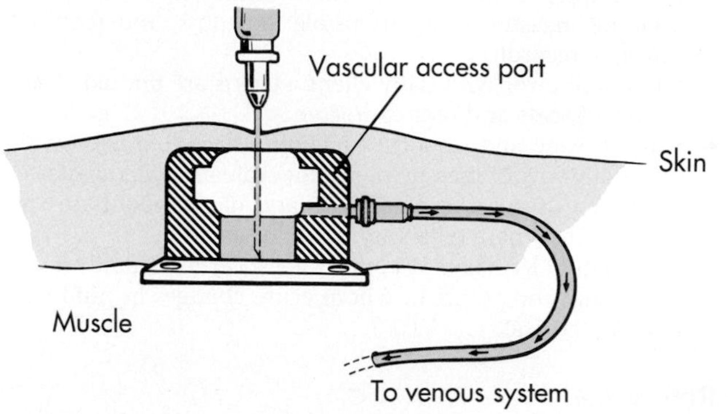

Intravenous Therapy (Crystalloids). The goal of IV fluid administration is to correct or prevent fluid and electrolyte disturbances. It allows for direct access to the vascular system, permitting the infusion of continuous fluids over a period of time. Intravenous fluid therapy must be continuously regulated because of continual changes in the client's fluid and electrolyte balance.

When IV fluid administration is required, the nurse must know the correct ordered solution, the equipment needed, the procedures required to initiate an infusion, how to regulate the infusion rate and maintain the system, how to identify and correct problems, and how to discontinue the infusion if necessary.

Administration of Intravenous Therapy

Types of Solutions. Many prepared IV solutions are available for use (Table 40-8). Intravenous solutions fall into the following categories: isotonic, hypotonic, and hypertonic. Isotonic solutions are those that have the same effective osmolality as body fluids. Hypotonic solutions are those

FIGURE 40–12 Example of an implantable vascular access device.

Table 40-8　Intravenous Solutions

Solution	Concentration	Other Names
Dextrose in Water Solutions		
Dextrose 5% in water*	Isotonic	D_5W
Dextrose 10% in water	Hypertonic	$D_{10}W$
Saline Solutions		
0.45% sodium chloride (half normal saline)	Hypotonic	½ NS 0.45% NS
0.9% sodium chloride† (normal saline)	Isotonic	NS 0.9% NS 0.9% NaCl
3%-5% sodium chloride	Hypertonic	3%-5% NS 3%-5% NaCl
Dextrose in Saline Solutions		
Dextrose 5% in 0.9% sodium chloride	Hypertonic	$D_5$0.9% NaCl $D_5$0.9% NS D_5NS
Dextrose 5% in 0.45% NaCl sodium chloride	Hypertonic	$D_5$0.45% NaCl $D_5$0.45% NS D_5½ NS
Multiple Electrolyte Solutions		
Lactated Ringer's‡	Isotonic	LR
Dextrose 5% in lactated Ringer's	Hypertonic	D_5LR

*Dextrose is quickly metabolized, leaving free water to be distributed evenly in all fluid compartments (Heitz and Horne, 2001).

†Although it is isotonic because the total concentration of electrolytes equals plasma concentration, it contains 154 mEq of both sodium and chloride, which is a higher concentration of these electrolytes than is found in the plasma, which can cause FVE (Metheny, 2000).

‡Contains sodium, potassium, calcium, chloride, and lactate.

that have an effective osmolality less than body fluids. Hypertonic solutions are those that have an effective osmolality greater than body fluids (Heitz and Horne, 2001).

In general, isotonic fluids are used most commonly for extracellular volume replacement (e.g., FVD after prolonged vomiting). The decision to use a hypotonic or hypertonic solution is based on the specific fluid and electrolyte imbalance. For example, the client with a hypertonic fluid imbalance will generally receive a hypotonic IV to dilute the ECF and rehydrate the cells. All IV fluids should be given carefully, especially hypertonic solutions, because these pull fluid into the vascular space by osmosis, resulting in an increased vascular volume that can lead to pulmonary edema, particularly in clients with heart or renal failure. Certain additives, most commonly vitamins and potassium chloride (KCl), are frequently added to IV solutions.

> **Safety Alert.** *Under no circumstances should potassium chloride (KCl) be given IV push. A direct IV infusion of KCl may be fatal.* If an IV is to have additives added, a physician's order must be obtained that includes the required additives, for example, Bottle 1: 1000 ml D$_5$½ NS with 20 mEq KCl at 125 ml/hr.

Clients with normal renal function who are receiving nothing by mouth should have potassium added to IV solutions. The body cannot conserve potassium, and even when the serum level falls, the kidneys continue to excrete potassium. If there is no potassium intake orally or parenterally, hypokalemia can develop quickly. Conversely, the nurse should verify that the client has adequate urine output before administering an IV solution containing potassium, because hyperkalemia can quickly develop.

Equipment. Correct selection and preparation of IV equipment assists in safe and quick placement of an IV line. Because fluids are instilled into the bloodstream, sterile technique is necessary; the nurse must therefore have all equipment organized and at the bedside. The nurse who must leave the bedside to obtain another piece of equipment will need to start the procedure over again. Intravenous equipment includes needles or catheters, tourniquet, gloves, dressings, solution containers, various types of tubing, and IV pumps or volume control devices. Injectable medications such as antibiotics may be added to a small IV solution bag and "piggybacked" into the primary line or as a primary intermittent infusion to be administered over a 30- to 60-minute period (see Chapter 34). The type and amount of solution depend on the medication added and the client's physiological status. Different types of tubing are used to administer medications or IV fluids. A solution given rapidly needs to be infused with macrodrip tubing, which delivers large drops (standard drop size is 10 or 15 gtt/ml depending on the manufacturer) so that the prescribed rate can be maintained. In contrast, microdrip tubing provides a standard drop size of 60 gtt/ml. Microdrip tubing is used to allow precise regulation of IV fluids even at slow rates. In addition, clients may require IV extension tubing to increase mobility, decrease manipulation and potential contamination at insertion site, or to facilitate changes in position.

> **Safety Alert.** Intravenous pumps or volume control devices are vital with children, with clients with renal or cardiac failure, with medications that require precise rates or with critically ill clients to ensure prescribed rate and prevent uncontrolled fluid administration. However, in many agencies, these devices are used routinely in most clients.

Initiating the Intravenous Line. After the equipment is collected at the bedside, the nurse prepares to place the IV line by assessing the client for a venipuncture site (Skill 40-1). Common IV puncture sites include the hand and the arm (Figure 40-13). The use of the foot for an IV site is common with children but is avoided in the adult because of the danger of thrombophlebitis (INS, 2000).

Text continued on p. 1174

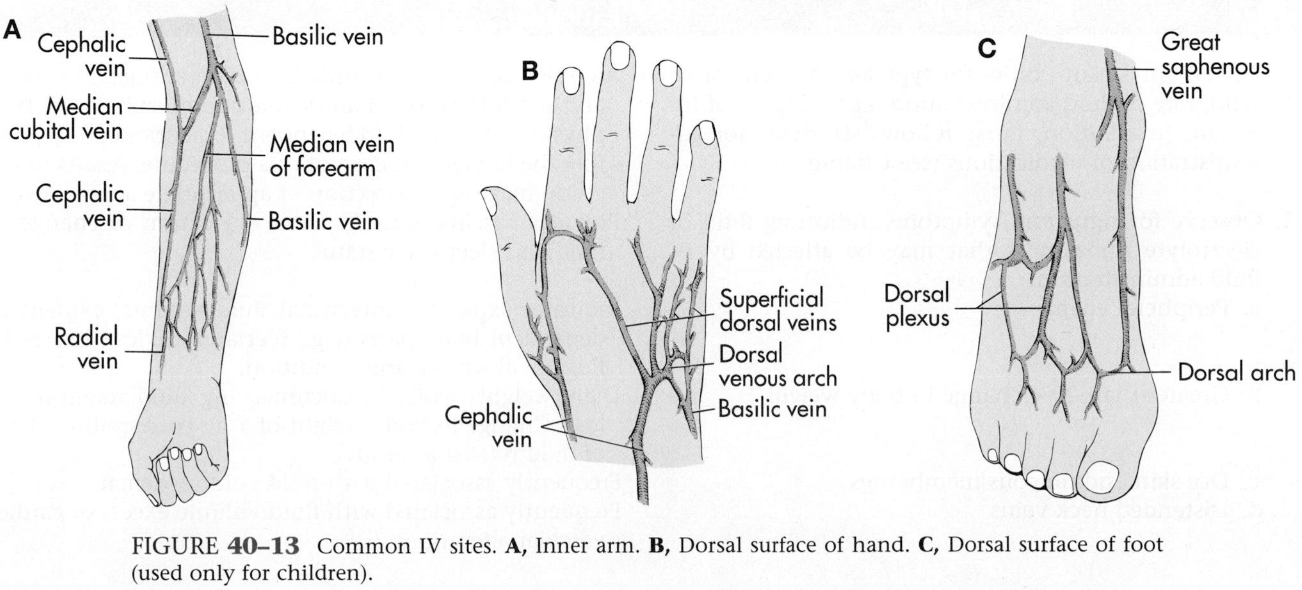

FIGURE **40–13** Common IV sites. **A,** Inner arm. **B,** Dorsal surface of hand. **C,** Dorsal surface of foot (used only for children).

Skill 40-1   *Initiating a Peripheral Intravenous Infusion*

Delegation Considerations

The skill of initiating intravenous (IV) therapy should not be delegated to assistive personnel (AP). In many states this skill is included within the scope of practice for licensed practical (vocational) nurses (LPN/LVN). Other aspects of the client's care may be delegated to AP. The nurse should instruct AP about the following:

- To inform the nurse if the client complains of burning, bleeding, swelling, or coolness at the catheter insertion site
- The prescribed flow rate and to report if rate has slowed or increased
- To inform the nurse if the IV dressing becomes wet
- To inform the nurse if the volume of fluid in the IV bag is low

Equipment

- Correct IV solution (with time tape attached)
- Proper catheter for venipuncture (gauge will vary with client's body size and reason for IV fluid administration). In an adult a 22-gauge catheter is appropriate for fluid maintenance (Ellenberger, 1999)
- IV start kit (if available): may contain a sterile drape to place under the client's arm, tourniquet, cleansing and antiseptic preparations, dressings, and a small roll of sterile tape
- Local anesthetic (optional)
- **For IV fluid infusion**
  - Administration set (choice depends on type of solution and rate of administration; infants and children, clients with cardiac and renal disease, and certain medications require microdrip tubing, which provides 60 gtt/ml)
  - 0.22 μm filter (if required by agency policy or if particulate matter is likely; size appropriate to type of solution)

- Extension tubing (used when a longer IV line is necessary or to avoid manipulation of the catheter insertion site with frequent tubing changes)
- Antiseptic swabs or sticks (chlorhexidine, povidone-iodine, alcohol)
- Disposable gloves
- Tourniquet (Determine type of tourniquet based on client assessment, e.g., blood pressure cuff [older adult], rubber band [infants]. Tourniquets can be a source of contamination; use a single-use product.)
- Arm board and protective cover, if needed (used to maintain wrist or elbow joint position when over-the-needle catheter [ONC] is placed close to or over a joint; will help prevent infiltration of IV and mechanical phlebitis)
- Nonallergenic tape and sterile tape (for use under the dressing)
- Towel (to place under client's hand or arm)
- IV pole, rolling or ceiling mounted
- Special client gown with snaps at shoulder seams (makes removal with IV tubing easier), if available
- Needle disposal container (also called sharps container)
- IV site protection device (optional)
- **For heparin or normal saline lock**
  - Injection cap (also called IV plug, adapter, hep-lok)
  - IV loop or short piece of extension tubing, if necessary
  - 1 to 3 ml of sterile normal saline or heparin flush solution (10 to 100 units/ml as ordered or per agency protocol)
  - Syringes and 25-gauge needles
- **Gauze dressing only**
  - 2 × 2 or 4 × 4 sterile gauze sponge
- **Transparent dressing only**
  - Transparent dressing

Steps	Rationale
1. Review physician's order for type and amount of IV fluid, rate of fluid administration, and purpose of infusion. In addition, nurse follows six rights for administration of medications (see Chapter 34).	An order requesting the initiation of a peripheral IV access and administration of an IV solution must be made by a physician/Licensed Independent Practitioner (LIP) before the implementation of this procedure. Assists in decision making for selection of appropriate access device.
2. Observe for signs and symptoms indicating fluid or electrolyte imbalances that may be affected by IV fluid administration.	Provides baseline data for later evaluation of change in fluid and electrolyte status.
a. Peripheral edema	Indicates expanded interstitial fluid volume, evident in dependent body parts (e.g., feet and ankles). Excess IV fluids will worsen this condition.
b. Greater than 20% change in body weight	Daily weights assist in documenting fluid retention or loss. Change in body weight of 1 kg corresponds to 1 L of fluid retention or loss.
c. Dry skin and mucous membranes	Frequently associated with fluid volume deficit.
d. Distended neck veins	Frequently associated with fluid volume excess or cardiovascular alterations.

Steps	Rationale
e. Blood pressure changes	Elevations in blood pressure (BP) may indicate volume excess, and decreased pressure may indicate fluid volume deficit. These changes can be more sudden and pronounced in those clients with underlying cardiopulmonary disease.
f. Irregular pulse rhythm; tachycardia	Rate and rhythm change can occur with changes in intravascular volume, as well as changes in potassium, calcium, and/or magnesium.
g. Auscultation of abnormal lung sounds	With fluid volume excess, the cardiovascular system is unable to compensate for this excess and fluid builds up in the lungs, creating abnormal lung sounds.
h. Decreased skin turgor	With decreased fluid volume, the skin when pinched remains in that state for several seconds. This is called "tenting."

Critical Decision Point: Changes in skin turgor are a less reliable indicator for older adult clients due to the natural loss in skin elasticity caused by the normal aging process (Lueckenotte, 2000).

i. Thirst	Symptomatic of fluid volume deficit. Very young, confused, and severely debilitated clients may not be able to indicate their thirst.
j. Anorexia, nausea, and vomiting	May be present with fluid volume excess or deficit. These symptoms may also be present with the client's underlying disease.
k. Decreased urine output	During dehydration, the kidneys attempt to restore fluid balance by reducing urine production.
l. Behavioral changes	May occur with fluid volume deficit and acid-base imbalance. In addition, behavioral changes may be due to fever, the underlying condition, or preexisting disease.
3. Assess client's previous or perceived experience with IV therapy and arm placement preference.	Determines level of emotional support and instruction necessary. If hypersensitive to venipunctures, a local anesthetic may be indicated. Anesthetic cream needs to be applied for duration of 60 minutes. Transdermal anesthetic may be administered before venipuncture.
4. Determine if client is to undergo any planned surgeries or is to receive blood infusion later.	Allows nurse to place an adequate-size catheter (i.e., 18 or 16 gauge for surgery) and avoids placement in an area that will interfere with medical procedures.
5. Assess laboratory data and client's history of allergies.	May reveal information that affects insertion of devices, such as fluid volume deficit, anemia, or allergy to iodine, adhesive, or latex.
6. Assess for the following risk factors: child or older adult, presence of heart failure or renal failure, or low platelet count.	Persons at extremes in age develop fluid imbalances more rapidly because they have proportionately larger ECF volume; persons with heart failure may require fluid restriction and cannot adapt to sudden increases in vascular volume, and persons with renal failure cannot eliminate excess ECF. A low platelet count predisposes clients to bleeding at IV site.
7. Prepare client and family by explaining the procedure, its purpose, and what is expected of client.	Decreases anxiety and promotes cooperation.
8. Perform hand hygiene.	Reduces transmission of microorganisms.
9. Assist client to comfortable sitting or supine position.	Enables client to extend arm.
10. Organize equipment on clean clutter-free bedside stand or over-bed table.	Reduces risk of contamination and accidents.
11. Change client's gown to the more easily removed gown with snaps at the shoulder, if available.	Use of a special IV gown facilitates safe removal of the gown.
12. Open sterile packages using sterile aseptic technique.	Maintains sterility of equipment and reduces spread of microorganisms.

Skill **40-1**   *Initiating a Peripheral Intravenous Infusion—cont'd*

Steps	Rationale
13. Check IV solution, using six rights of drug administration (see Chapter 34). Make sure prescribed additives, such as potassium and vitamins, have been added. Check solution for color, clarity, and expiration date. Check bag for leaks, which is best if done before reaching the bedside.	IV solutions are medications and should be carefully checked to reduce risk of error. Solutions that are discolored, contain particles, or are expired are not to be used. (Some solutions may have slight discoloration [e.g., be pink-tinged] and still be suitable for use.) Leaky bags present an opportunity for infection and must not be used.
14. Open infusion set, maintaining sterility of both ends of tubing. Many sets allow for priming of tubing without removal of end cap.	Prevents bacteria from entering infusion equipment and bloodstream.
15. Place roller clamp about 2 to 5 cm (1 to 2 in) below drip chamber and move roller clamp to "off" position (see illustrations).	Close proximity of roller clamp to drip chamber allows more accurate regulation of flow rate. Moving clamp to "off" prevents accidental spillage of fluid.
16. Remove protective sheath over IV tubing port on plastic IV solution bag (see illustration). For bottled IV solution, remove metal cap and metal and rubber disks beneath cap. Use caution not to touch exposed opening.	Provides access for insertion of infusion tubing into solution.
17. Insert infusion set into fluid bag or bottle by removing protector cap from tubing insertion spike (keeping spike sterile), and inserting spike into opening of IV bag (see illustration). Cleanse rubber stopper on glass bottled solution with antiseptic, and insert spike into black rubber stopper of IV bottle. Hang solution container on IV pole at a minimum height of 35 inches (90 cm) above planned insertion site.	Prevents contamination of solution from contaminated insertion spike. Container heights of 36 to 48 inches are usually sufficient to overcome venous pressure and other resistance from tubing and catheter.
18. Compress drip chamber and release, allowing it to fill one-third to one-half full (see illustration). Open clamp and prime infusion tubing by filling with IV solution.	Creates vacuum effects; fluid enters drip chamber to prevent air from entering tubing.

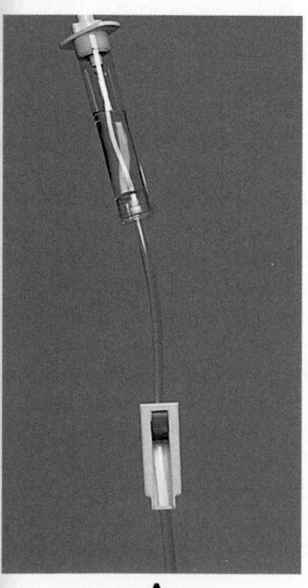
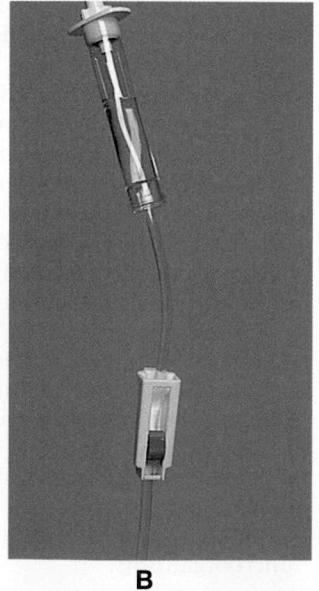

STEP **15** **A,** Roller clamp in open position. **B,** Roller clamp in closed position.

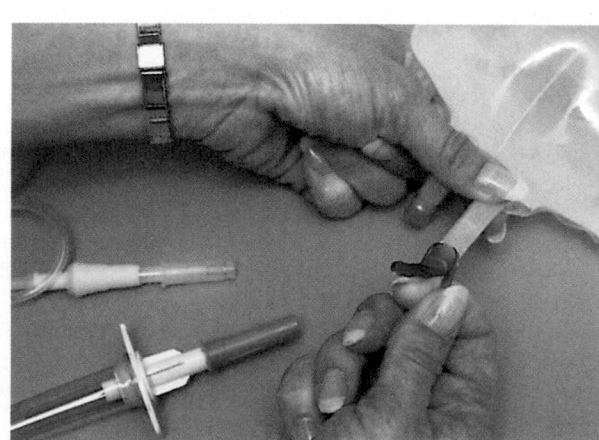

STEP **16** Removing protective sheath from IV bag port.

Steps	Rationale

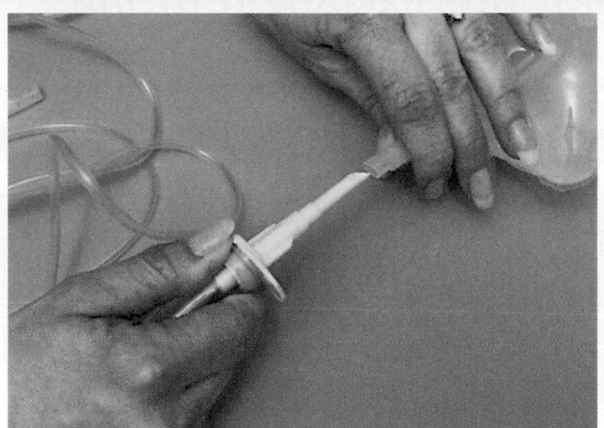

STEP **17** Inserting spike into IV bag.

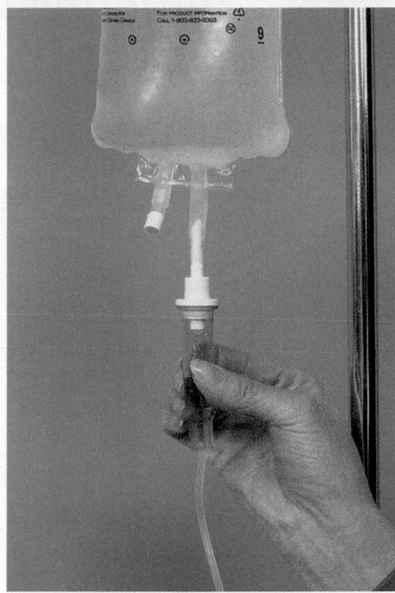

STEP **18** Squeezing drip chamber to fill with fluid.

19. Remove tubing protector cap (some tubing can be primed without removal) and slowly release roller clamp to allow fluid to travel from drip chamber through tubing to needle adapter. Return roller clamp to "off" position after tubing is primed (filled with IV fluid).

Slow fill of tubing decreases turbulence and chance of bubble formation. Removes air from tubing and permits tubing to fill with solution. Closing the clamp prevents accidental loss of fluid.

20. Be certain tubing is clear of air and air bubbles. To remove small air bubbles, firmly tap IV tubing where air bubbles are located. Check entire length of tubing to ensure that all air bubbles are removed (see illustration).

Large air bubbles can act as emboli. Air bubbles may contribute to anxiety related to IV therapy.

Critical Decision Point: Extra extension tubing may be added to IV tubing to allow for more length, which will enable the client to move more freely while still keeping the IV line stable. But remember, adding extensions increases risk for infection.

---

21. Replace tubing cap protector on end of tubing.

Maintains system sterility.

22. Optional: Prepare heparin or normal saline lock for infusion. If a loop or short extension tubing is needed, use sterile technique to connect the IV plug to the loop or short extension tubing. Inject 1 to 3 ml normal saline through the plug and through the loop or short extension tubing.

Removes air to prevent introduction into the vein. Do the same with the saline plug.

23. Apply disposable gloves. Eye protection and mask may be worn (see agency policy) if splash or spray of blood is possible. NOTE: Gloves can be left off to locate vein but must be applied before preparing site.

Reduces transmission of microorganisms. Decreases exposure to HIV, hepatitis, and other blood-borne organisms (INS, 2000).

24. Identify accessible vein for IV placement. Apply tourniquet 4 to 6 in (10 to 15 cm) above the proposed insertion site (see illustration). Position tourniquet so that ends are away from proposed venipuncture site. Check for presence of radial pulse. OPTION: Apply blood pressure cuff instead of tourniquet. Inflate to a level just below client's normal diastolic pressure. Maintain inflation at that pressure until venipuncture is completed.

Tourniquet should be tight enough to impede venous return but *not* occlude arterial flow.

Skill 40-1   *Initiating a Peripheral Intravenous Infusion—cont'd*

Steps	Rationale

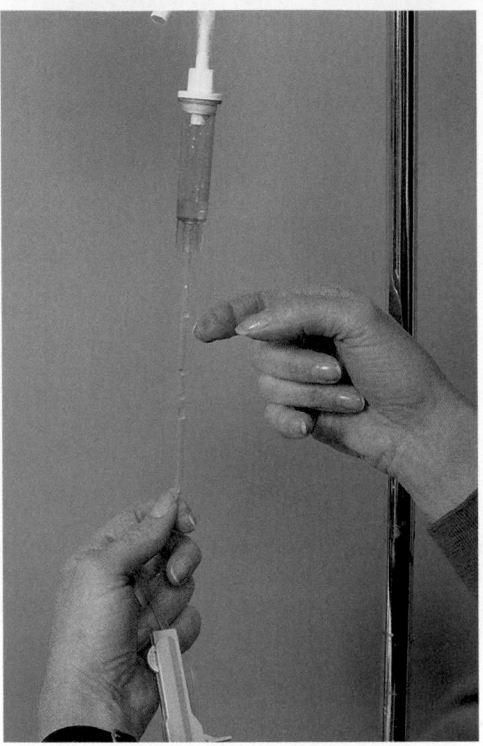

STEP **20**   Removing air bubbles from tubing.

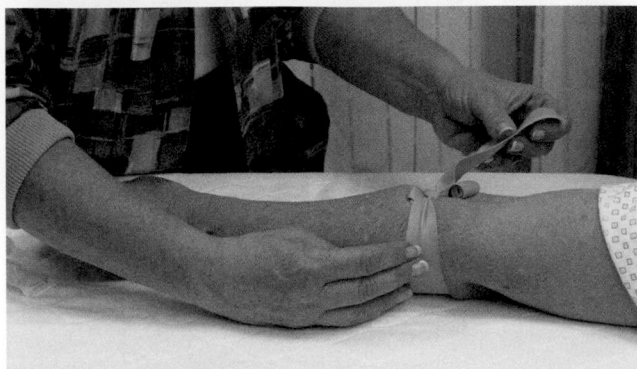

STEP **24**   Apply tourniquet.

25. Select the vein. Common IV sites for the adult include cephalic, basilic, and median cubital veins (see Figure 40-13, p. 1161).

a. Use the most distal site in the nondominant arm, if possible.

    Venipuncture should be performed distal to proximal, which increases the availability of other sites for future IV therapy.

b. Avoid areas that are painful to palpation.

    May indicate inflamed vein.

c. Select a vein large enough for catheter placement.

    Prevents interruption of venous flow while allowing adequate blood flow around the catheter.

d. Choose a site that will not interfere with client's activities of daily living (ADLs) or planned procedures.

e. Use the fingertips to palpate the vein by pressing downward and noting the resilient, soft, bouncy feeling as the pressure is released (see illustration).

    Fingertips are more sensitive and are better to assess vein condition.

f. Promote venous distention by instructing the client to open and close the fist several times, lowering the client's arm in a dependent position, rubbing or stroking the client's arm from distal to proximal below proposed site.

    These activities increase blood flow to the area of insertion. When these techniques are properly used, they foster venous dilation and access to the vein.

Critical Decision Point: Avoid vigorous rubbing and multiple tapping of client's veins. These techniques may cause injury to the vein, such as a hematoma, or cause venous constriction.

Steps	Rationale

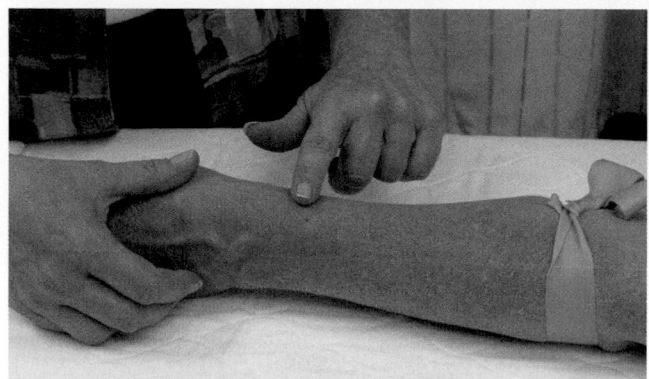

STEP **25E** Palpate vein for resilience.

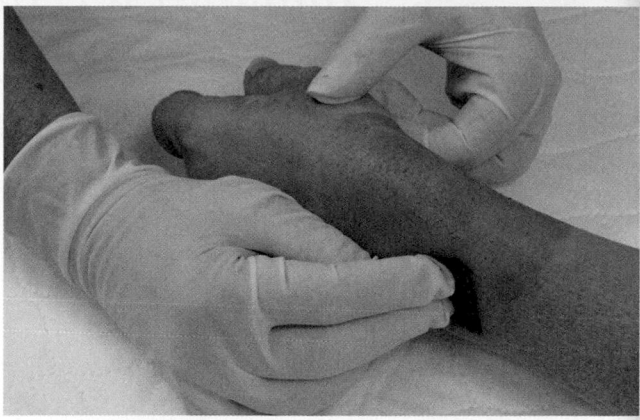

STEP **27** Cleanse site chosen for insertion.

g. Avoid sites distal to previous venipuncture site, sclerosed or hardened cordlike veins, infiltrated site or phlebotic vessels, bruised areas, and areas of venous valves or bifurcation. Avoid veins in antecubital fossa and ventral surface of the wrist.

h. Avoid fragile dorsal veins in older adult clients and vessels in an extremity with compromised circulation (e.g., in cases of mastectomy, dialysis graft, or paralysis).

26. Release tourniquet temporarily and carefully. Clip arm hair with scissors (if necessary). Do not shave area.

27. (If area of insertion appears to need cleansing, use soap and water first.) Cleanse insertion site using firm, circular motion (center to outward) in concentric circles 2 to 3 inches from insertion site. Use antiseptic prep as a single agent or in combination. Refrain from touching the cleansed site. Allow the site to dry for at least 2 minutes (see illustration). If skin is touched after cleansing, repeat cleansing procedure.

28. Reapply tourniquet or BP cuff.

Such sites increase the risk of infiltration of newly placed IV line and excessive vessel damage.

Veins in the antecubital fossa are used for blood draws and placement in this area limits mobility. Inner wrist contains numerous tendons that could be damaged.

Venous alterations can increase risk of complications (e.g., infiltration and decreased catheter dwell time).

Hair impedes venipuncture and adherence of dressing. Shaving can cause microabrasions and predispose client to infection.

Chlorhexidine is the antiseptic cleansing agent of choice (Centers for Disease Control and Prevention, 2002). Povidone-iodine is a topical antiinfective that reduces skin surface bacteria; 70% alcohol is another antiseptic cleansing agent. Povidone-iodine must dry to be effective in reducing microbial counts (Millam and others, 2000). Air-drying prevents chemical reactions between agents and allows time for maximum microbicidal activity of agents (INS, 2000). Touching the cleansed area would introduce organisms from nurse's hand to the site.

Critical Decision Point: Do not use povidone-iodine if the client is allergic to iodine; use an alternate cleansing agent.

---

29. Perform venipuncture. Anchor vein by placing thumb over vein beneath insertion site and by stretching the skin against the direction of insertion 5 to 7.5 cm (2 to 3 inches) distal to the site (see illustration). Warn client of a sharp stick. Puncture skin and vein, holding catheter at 10- to 30-degree angle with the bevel pointed upwards.

A. **Butterfly needle:** Hold needle at 10- to 30-degree angle with bevel up slightly distal to actual site of venipuncture.

B. **Needleless ONC safety device:** Insert ONC (see illustration) with bevel up at 10- to 30-degree angle slightly distal to actual site of venipuncture in the direction of the vein.

The vascular access device (VAD) selected should be the smallest gauge and shortest length that will accommodate the therapy (INS, 2000).

Places needle parallel to vein. When vein is punctured, risk of puncturing posterior vein wall is reduced.

Superficial veins require a smaller angle; deeper veins require a greater angle.

The Needlestick Safety and Prevention Act effective April 2001 requires use of needle safety devices (Saladow, 2002).

Skill 40-1 — *Initiating a Peripheral Intravenous Infusion—cont'd*

Steps	Rationale

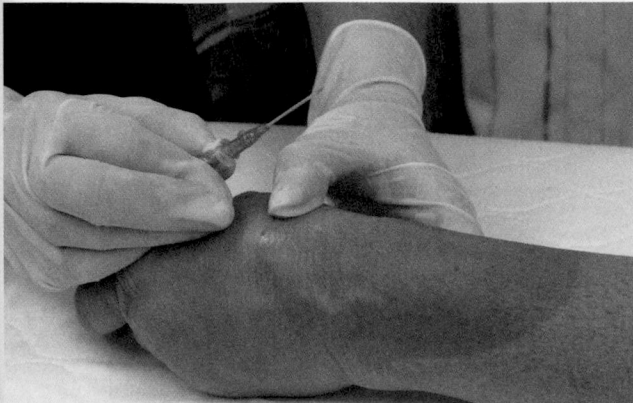

STEP **29** Stabilize vein below insertion site with skin taut.

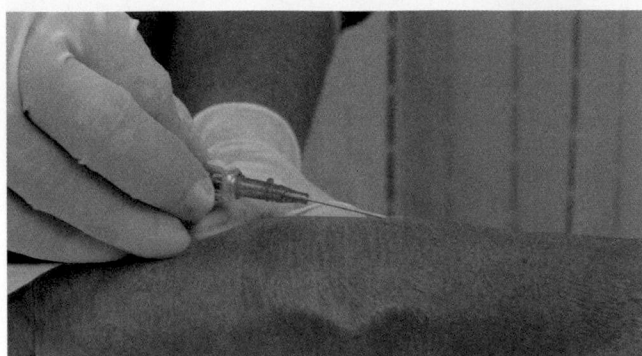

STEP **29B** Puncture skin with catheter at 10- to 30-degree angle. Catheter enters vein.

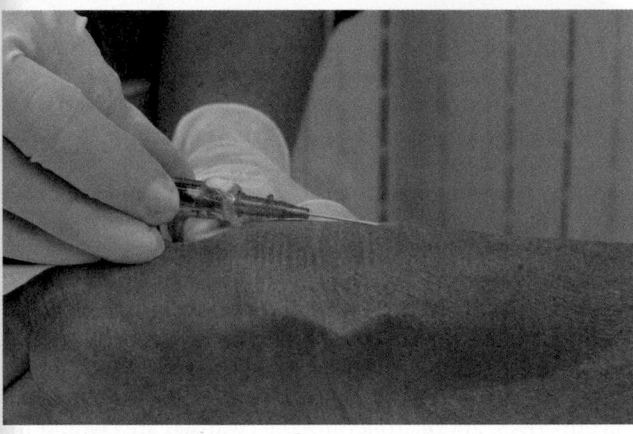

A

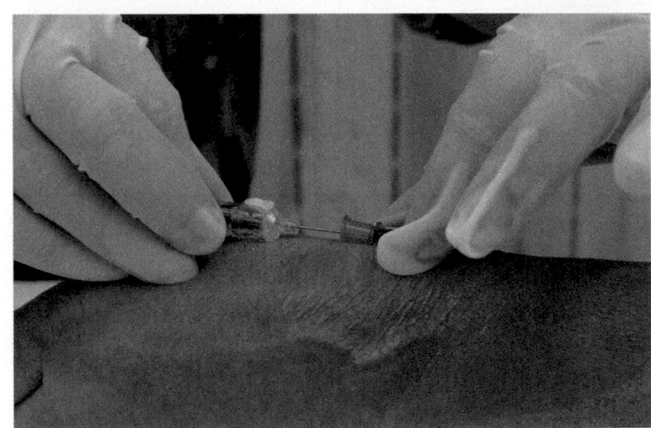

B

STEP **30** **A,** Blood return in flashback chamber, catheter lowered flush with skin. **B,** Advance catheter into vein; use safety device push-tab.

Critical Decision Point: No more than two attempts at inserting an IV should be made by a single nurse (INS, 2000).

---

30. Look for blood return through tubing of butterfly needle or flashback chamber of ONC, indicating that needle has entered vein (see illustration). Lower catheter/needle until almost flush with skin. Advance butterfly needle until hub rests at venipuncture site. Advance ONC catheter ¼ inch into vein and then loosen stylet. Advance catheter off the stylet into vein until hub rests at venipuncture site (see illustration). Do not reinsert the stylet once it is loosened. (Advance the safety device by using push-off tab to thread the catheter.)

Increased venous pressure from tourniquet increases backflow of blood into catheter or tubing.

Lowering the angle and advancing the cannula slightly allows for full penetration of vein wall, placement of catheter within vein's inner lumen, and easy advancement of catheter off stylet.

Threading catheter up to hub reduces the risk of introduction of infectious organisms along the catheter length. Reinsertion of the stylet can cause catheter damage and potential catheter embolization.

Steps	Rationale

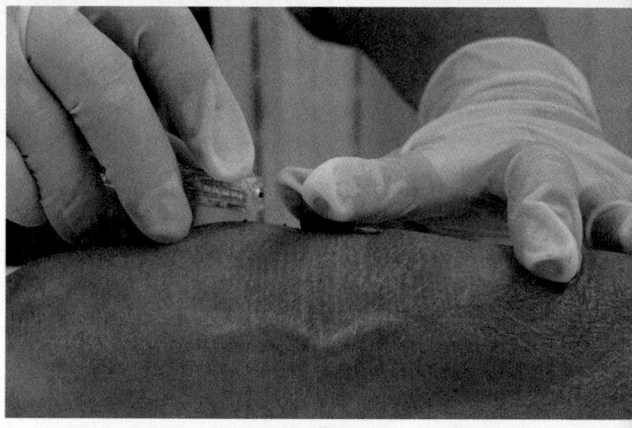

A   **B**

STEP **31 A,** Apply pressure above insertion site with index finger of nondominant hand. **B,** Retract the stylet by pushing safety tab.

31. Stabilize the catheter. Apply gentle, but firm, pressure with the index finger of nondominant hand 1¼ inches (3 cm) above insertion site (see illustration, *A*). Release tourniquet or BP cuff with dominant hand and retract stylet from ONC (see illustration, *B*). Do not recap the stylet. For a safety device, slide the catheter off the stylet while gliding the protective guard over the stylet. A click indicates the device is locked over the stylet.	Permits venous flow, reduces backflow of blood, and prevents accidental withdrawal or dislodgment.
32. Quickly connect adapter of primed fluid administration set (see illustration) or heparin lock to hub of ONC or butterfly tubing. Be sure connection is secure. Do not touch point of entry of adapter.	Prompt connection of infusion set maintains patency of vein. Maintains sterility.
33. Release roller clamp slowly to begin infusion at a rate to maintain patency of IV line.	Permits venous flow and prevents clotting of vein and obstruction of flow of IV solution.
a. *Intermittent infusion:* Continue to stabilize catheter with nondominant hand and attach injection cap of adapter. Insert prefilled flush solution into injection cap. Flush slowly (see illustration). Maintain thumb pressure on syringe during withdrawal or close clamp on extension tubing of injection cap while still flushing last 0.2 to 0.4 ml of flush solution.	Positive pressure in the catheter prevents reflux of blood into the catheter lumen (Phillips, 2001).

Critical Decision Point: Be sure to calculate rate so as not to infuse IV solution too rapidly or too slowly.

---

34. Tape or secure catheter.	
A. **If applying transparent dressing,** secure catheter with nondominant hand while preparing to apply dressing.	
B. **If applying a gauze dressing**	
(1) Tape the IV catheter. Place narrow piece (½ in wide) of sterile tape under hub of catheter with adhesive side up (see illustration, *A*) and criss-cross tape over hub to form a chevron (see illustration, *B*).	Securing the catheter and tubing prevents movement and tension on the device, reducing mechanical irritation and possible phlebitis or infection. Tape placed underneath the dressing should be sterile; nonsterile tape is a potential source of pathogenic bacteria.

Initiating a Peripheral Intravenous Infusion—cont'd

Steps	Rationale

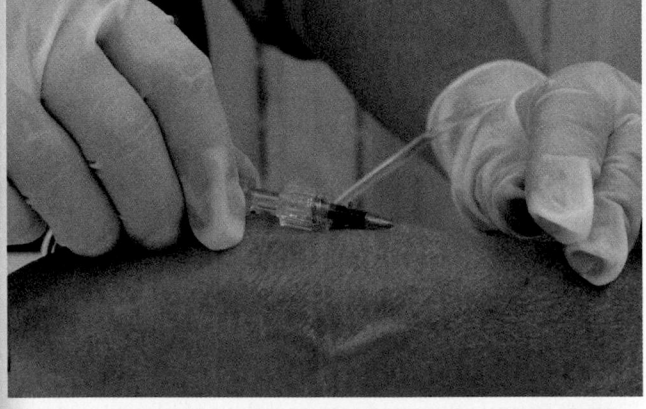

STEP **32** Connect end of IV tubing to catheter tubing. Secure connector.

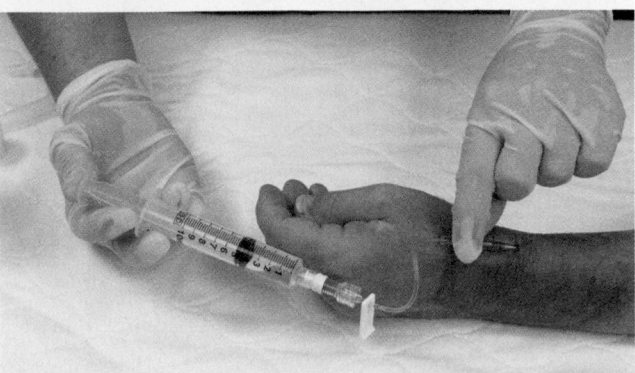

STEP **33A** Flush injection cap slowly.

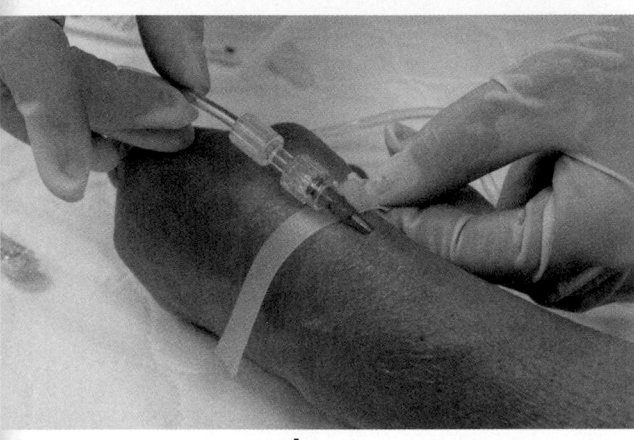

A

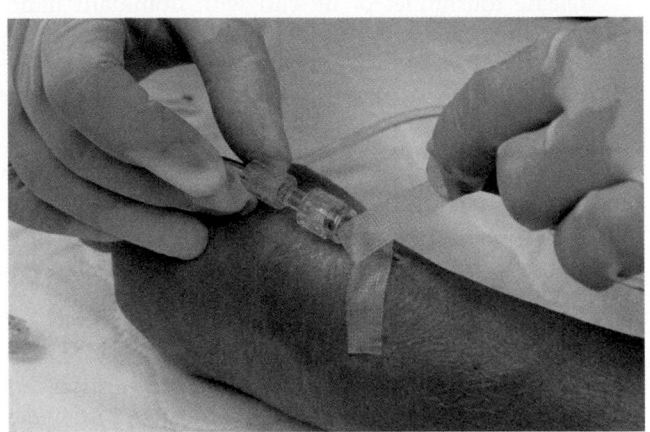

B

STEP **34B(1)** **A,** Place tape under catheter hub. **B,** Cross-cross ends of tape over hub.

(2) Place tape only on the catheter, *never* over the insertion site. Secure the site to allow easy visual inspection and early recognition of infiltration and phlebitis. Avoid applying tape around the extremity.

   Taping around extremity could result in a "tourniquet effect" and impede venous return.

35. Apply sterile dressing over site.
  A. **Transparent dressing**
    (1) Carefully remove adherent backing. Apply one edge of dressing and then gently smooth remaining dressing over site, leaving end of catheter hub uncovered (see illustration). Refer to manufacturer's directions.

   Transparent dressings are occlusive to moisture and microorganisms.
   Transparent dressings allow continuous inspection of the IV site, are more comfortable, and permit clients to bathe and shower without saturating the dressing (Phillips, 2001).

    (2) Take a 1-inch piece of tape, and place it from end of hub of the catheter to insertion site, over transparent dressing (see illustration).

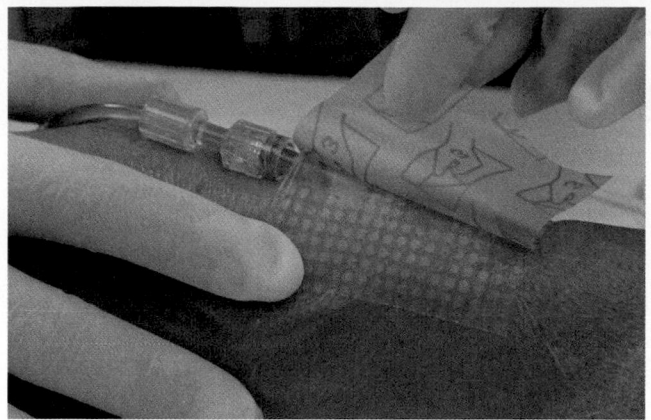

STEP **35A(1)** Apply transparent dressing.

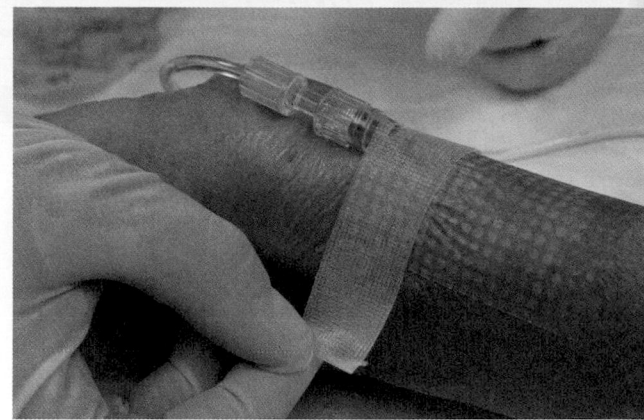

STEP **35A(2)** Place tape over transparent dressing.

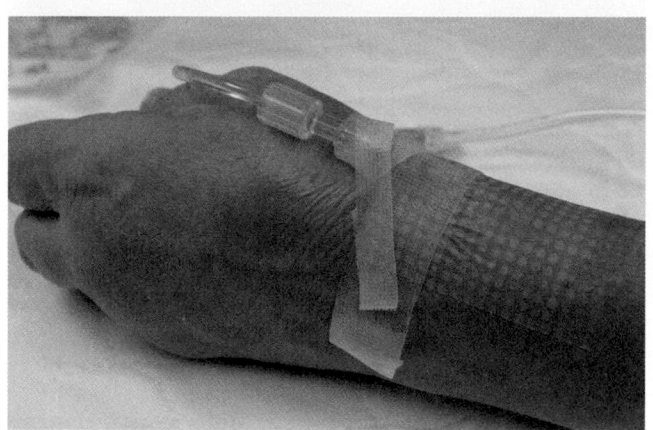

STEP **35A(3)** Apply chevron over tape.

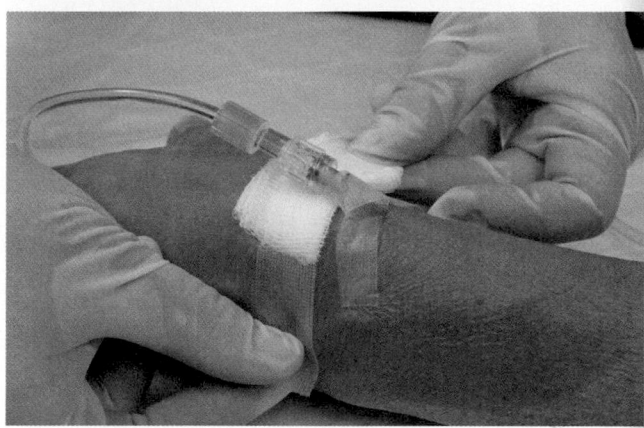

STEP **35B(1)** Fold 2 × 2 gauze in half, cover with 1-inch tape, and place under catheter hub.

(3) Then apply chevron and place only over tape, not the transparent dressing (see illustration).

B. Sterile gauze dressing

(1) Fold a 2 × 2 gauze in half and cover with a 1-in-wide piece of sterile tape extending about an inch from each side. Place it under the tubing/catheter hub junction (see illustration).

(2) Place a 2 × 2 gauze pad over venipuncture site and catheter hub. Secure all edges with tape. Do not cover connection between IV tubing and catheter hub (see illustration).

(3) Curl a loop of tubing alongside the arm and place a second piece of tape directly over the padded 2 × 2, securing tubing in two places.

Tape on top of tape makes it easier to access hub/tubing junction. Securing loop of tubing reduces risk of dislodging catheter from accidental pull.

Gauze is less expensive than transparent dressing and may also be useful if there is bleeding or excessive moisture at the site.

Initiating a Peripheral Intravenous Infusion—cont'd

Steps	Rationale

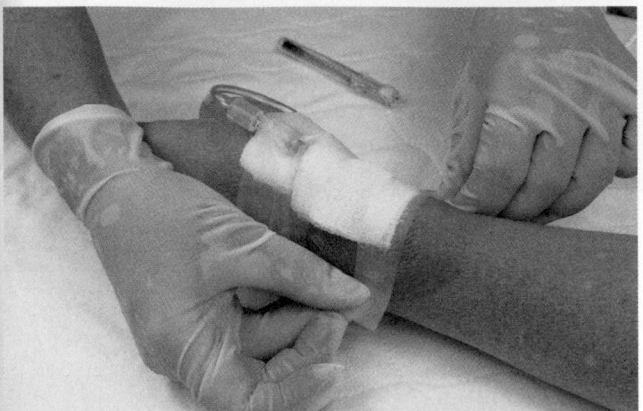

STEP **35B(2)** Apply 2 × 2 gauze.

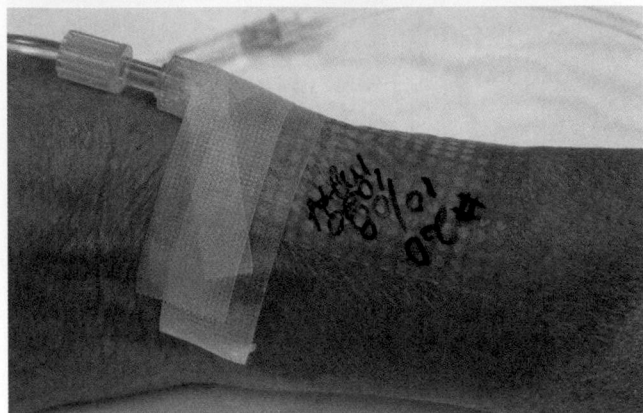

STEP **37** Dressing labeled with date and time.

36. For *IV fluid administration* adjust flow rate to correct drops per minute (see Skill 40-2) or connect to electronic infusion device (EID).

Maintains correct rate of flow for IV solution. Flow can fluctuate, so it must be checked at intervals.

   A. **Heparin lock.** Flush with 1 to 3 ml of heparin flush solution (10 to 100 units/ml) at prescribed frequency or agency policy.

Maintains patency of IV catheter.

   B. **Saline lock.** Flush with 1 to 3 ml of sterile normal saline at prescribed frequency or agency policy.

Maintains patency of IV catheter.

37. Label dressing with date, time, gauge size and length of catheter, and nurse's initials (see illustration).

Allows for easy recognition of type of device and time interval for site rotation. INS standard for site rotation of peripheral IV access device is every 72 hours (INS, 2000).

38. Dispose of used needles in appropriate sharps container. Discard supplies. Remove gloves and perform hand hygiene.

Reduces transmission of microorganisms and protects staff from injury.

39. Observe client every hour to determine if fluid is infusing correctly.

   a. Check if correct amount of solution is infused as prescribed by looking at time tape.

Correct administration of fluid volume prevents fluid imbalance.

   b. Count flow rate or check rate on infusion pump.

Accurate monitoring of rate furthers ensures correct volume administration.

   c. Check patency of IV catheter or needle.

   d. Observe client for signs of discomfort.

   e. Inspect insertion site for absence of phlebitis (Table 40-9), infiltration (Table 40-10), or inflammation.

Provides continuous evaluation of type and amount of fluid delivered to client. Hourly inspection prevents accidental fluid overload or inadequate infusion rate and identifies early incidence of vein inflammation or tissue damage.

40. Observe client every hour to determine response to therapy (i.e., measure vital signs, conduct postprocedure assessments).

IV fluids and additives are given to maintain or restore fluid and electrolyte balance. They can also cause unexpected effects, which can be serious.

Steps	Rationale

Table 40-9	Phlebitis Scale
Grade	**Clinical Criteria**
0	No clinical symptoms
1	Erythema at access site with or without pain
2	Pain at access site with erythema and/or edema
3	Pain at access site with erythema and/or edema
	Streak formation
	Palpable venous cord
4	Pain at access site with erythema and/or edema
	Streak formation
	Palpable venous cord >1 inch in length
	Purulent drainage

From Infusion Nurses Society: Infusion nursing standards of practice, *J Intraven Nurs* 23(6S): S56, 2000.

Table 40-10	Infiltration Scale
Grade	**Clinical Criteria**
0	No symptoms
	Skin blanched
	Edema, 1 inch in any direction
	Cool to touch
	With or without pain
1	Skin blanched
	Edema 1-6 inches in any direction
	Cool to touch
	With or without pain
3	Skin blanched, translucent
	Gross edema >6 inches in any direction
	Cool to touch
	Mild-moderate pain
	Possible numbness
4	Skin blanched, translucent
	Skin tight, leaking
	Skin discolored, bruised, swollen
	Gross edema >6 inches in any direction
	Deep pitting tissue edema
	Circulatory impairment
	Moderate to severe pain
	Infiltration of any amount of blood product, irritant, or vesicant

From Infusion Nurses Society: Infusion nursing standards of practice, 23(6S): S57, 2000.

Unexpected Outcomes and Related Interventions

1. Fluid volume deficit (FVD) as manifested by decreased urine output, dry mucous membranes, hypotension, tachycardia.
   - Notify physician; may require readjustment of infusion rate.
2. Fluid volume excess (FVE) as manifested by crackles in the lungs, shortness of breath, edema.
   - Reduce IV flow rate if symptoms appear, and notify physician.
3. Electrolyte imbalances as manifested by abnormal serum electrolyte levels, changes in mental status, and alterations in neuromuscular function, changes in vital signs, and other manifestations.
   - Notify physician. Additives in IV or type of IV fluid may be adjusted.
4. Infiltration as indicated by swelling and possible pitting edema, pallor, coolness, pain at insertion site, and possible decrease in flow rate.
   - Stop infusion and discontinue IV. Elevate affected extremity. Restart new IV if continued therapy is necessary.
5. Phlebitis is indicated by pain, increased skin temperature, erythema along path of vein.
   - Stop infusion and discontinue IV. Restart new IV if continued therapy is necessary.
   - Place moist warm compress over area of phlebitis.

6. Bleeding occurs at venipuncture site.
   - Bleeding from vein is usually slow, continuous seepage. Common in clients who have received heparin or have a bleeding disorder or if the IV site is over bend in arm/hand.
   - If bleeding occurs around venipuncture site and catheter is within vein, gauze dressing may be applied over site. Eventually, IV may need to be discontinued.
   - Blood on the dressing can result when the administration set becomes disconnected from the catheter's hub. When blood appears on the dressing, verify that the system is intact and change the dressing.

Recording and Reporting

- Record in nurses' notes number of attempts for insertion, type of fluid, insertion site by vessel, flow rate, size and type of catheter or needle, and when infusion was begun. A special parenteral therapy flow sheet may be used.
- Record client's response to IV fluid, amount infused, and integrity and patency of system every 4 hours or according to agency policy.
- Report the following to oncoming nursing staff: type of fluid, flow rate, status of venipuncture site, amount of fluid remaining in present solution, expected time to hang next IV bag or bottle, and any side effects.

Skill 40-1 *Initiating a Peripheral Intravenous Infusion—cont'd*

Home Care Considerations

- Teach caregiver to apply pressure with sterile gauze if catheter falls out and, if client is on anticoagulant therapy, to tape several pieces of sterile gauze in place for at least 20 min with pressure or until bleeding stops.
- Teach client and caregiver to perform tub bath without getting IV tubing wet and to unplug pump first if one is used. For showering, the client must protect the IV site and dressing from getting wet by covering completely with plastic.

- Teach client and family to monitor I&O using measuring devices.
- Teach client and family to dispose of any open and sheathed needles into sharps container. All sharps containers must be stored in safe area away from children.

Box 40-6

Focus on Older Adults

- Use the smallest gauge catheter or needle possible (e.g., 24 to 26 gauge). This is less traumatizing to the vein and allows better blood flow to provide increased hemodilution of the IV fluids or medications.
- Consider the client's need for independence, mobility, and limitations when selecting the site for the IV catheter.
- Impaired skin integrity leads to susceptibility of tearing, difficulty detecting complications, and venous sclerosis.
- Avoid veins that are easily bumped because there is less subcutaneous support tissue.
- If the client has fragile skin and veins, use minimal or no tourniquet pressure.
- After tourniquet is applied, venous pressure rises rapidly, the vein is overstretched, and puncture with even a thin needle can rupture the wall of vein (Chukhraev and Grekov, 2000).
- Place tourniquet, if used, over the client's sleeve to decrease shearing of fragile skin.

- With loss of supportive tissue, veins tend to lie more superficially; lower insertion angle for venipuncture to 5 to 15 degrees (INS, 2000).
- If the client has lost subcutaneous tissue, the veins lose stability and will roll away from the needle. To stabilize the vein, apply traction to the skin below the projected insertion site.
- Secure the device well with minimal tape or specialized products for protection.
- Nutritional deficiencies promote fluid to migrate into tissues surrounding vessels, making IV access more difficult.
- Multiple medication usage (e.g., anticoagulants, antibiotics, and steroids) increases the likelihood of fragile, transparent skin that bruises and bleeds easily.
- Dehydration related to a lower percentage of body weight as water, diminished thirst mechanism, and social factors of bladder control contribute to difficult IV access (Toth, 2002).

The nurse assessing the client for potential venipuncture sites for IV infusion should consider conditions and contraindications that exclude certain sites. Because the very young and older adults have fragile veins, the nurse should avoid sites easily moved or bumped such as the dorsal surface of the hand (Box 40-6). Venipuncture is contraindicated in a site that has signs of infection, infiltration, or thrombosis. An infected site is red, tender, swollen, and possibly warm to the touch. Exudate may be present. An infected site is not used because of the danger of introducing bacteria from the skin surface into the bloodstream. Avoid using an extremity with a vascular (dialysis) graft/fistula or on the side of a mastectomy. Place IVs at the most distal point when possible. Using a distal site first allows for the use of proximal sites later if the client would need a venipuncture site change.

A **venipuncture** is a technique in which a vein is punctured through the skin by a sharp rigid stylet (e.g., butterfly needle or metal needle), a partially covered plastic catheter (over-the-needle catheter [ONC]), or a needle attached to a syringe. Catheters placed into a central vein such as the subclavian vein and superior vena cava are used to deliver large volumes of fluids and TPN or to administer irritating medications. Peripherally inserted central catheters may be placed by nurses; however, some central line catheters require insertion by physicians. Nurses are responsible for maintaining both of them. When veins are fragile or collapse, venipuncture may become extremely difficult, but it may be a life-saving measure as well. For these difficult clients, venipuncture should be performed by an experienced practitioner. The general purposes of venipuncture are to collect a blood specimen, to instill a medication, to start an IV infusion, or to inject a radiopaque or radioactive tracer for special examinations. Skill 40-1 describes venipuncture for IV fluid infusion.

Regulating the Infusion Flow Rate. After the IV infusion is secured and the line is patent, the nurse must regulate the rate of infusion according to the prescriber's orders (Skill 40-2). An infusion rate that is too slow can lead to further cardiovascular and circulatory collapse in a critically ill

Text continued on p. 1179

Skill 40-2   *R*egulating Intravenous Flow Rate

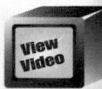

Delegation Considerations

The skill of regulating IV therapy should not be delegated to assistive personnel (AP). In many states this skill is included within the scope of practice for licensed practical (vocational) nurses (LPN/LVN). The nurse should instruct AP about the following;

- To inform nurse if client complains of burning, bleeding, swelling, coolness at the catheter insertion site
- The prescribed flow rate and to report if rate has slowed or increased

- To notify nurse if the alarm on an electronic infusion device (EID) sounds
- To inform the nurse if the volume of fluid in the IV bag is low

Equipment

- Watch with second hand
- Paper and pencil or calculator
- IV electronic infusion controller/pump (optional)
- Volume control device (optional)
- Time indicator tape

Steps	Rationale
1. Check client's medical record for correct solution, additives, and time of infusion. Usual order includes solution for 24 hours, usually divided into 2 or 3 L. Occasionally, IV order contains only 1 L to keep vein open (KVO). Order also indicates time over which each liter is to infuse.	Six rights of drug administration ensure correct fluids are given to correct client.
2. Perform hand hygiene. Observe for patency of IV line and needle or catheter:	For fluid to infuse at proper rate, IV line and needle must be free of kinks, knots, and clots.
a. Open drip regulator and observe for rapid flow of fluid from solution into drip chamber, then close drip regulator to prescribed rate.	Rapid flow of fluid into drip chamber indicates patency of IV line. Closing drip chamber to prescribed rate prevents fluid overload.
3. Check client's knowledge of how positioning of the IV site affects flow rate.	Fosters client participation in maintaining most effective position of arm with IV equipment.
4. Verify with client how venipuncture site feels (e.g., determine if there is pain or burning).	Pain or burning may be early indication of phlebitis. Includes client in decision making.
5. Have paper and pencil or calculator to calculate flow rate or use calculator.	The beginning student is unfamiliar with IV fluid rates and should use mathematical calculations to obtain correct rate.
6. Know calibration (drop factor) in drops per milliliter (gtt/ml) of infusion set: **A. Microdrip:** 60 gtt/ml **B. Macrodrip:** 15 gtt/ml or 10 gtt/ml depending upon manufacturer (will state on package)	Microdrip tubing, also called pediatric tubing, universally delivers 60 gtt/ml, and is used when small or very precise volumes are to be infused. However, there are different commercial parenteral administration sets for macrodrip tubing. Macrodrip tubing should be used when large quantities or fast rates are necessary.

Critical Decision Point: Know which company's infusion set your agency uses.

7. Calculate flow rate (hourly volume) of prescribed infusion. Flow rate ml/hr = total infusion (volume in ml)/hours of infusion (time to be infused) Example: $\dfrac{1000\ ml}{8\ hr} = \dfrac{125\ ml}{1\ hr}$	Once hourly rate has been determined, these formulas give correct flow rate.
8. Read physician's orders and follow six rights for correct solution and proper additives.	IV fluids are medications; following six rights decreases chance of medication error.

Skill 40-2   *Regulating Intravenous Flow Rate—cont'd*

Steps	Rationale
9. IV fluids are usually ordered for 24-hour period, indicating how long each liter of fluid should run; for example, IV order for client is: Bottle 1: 1000 ml D_5W with 20 mEq KCl to run 8 hr Bottle 2: 1000 ml D_5W with 20 mEq KCl to run 8 hr Bottle 3: 1000 ml D_5W with 20 mEq KCl to run 8 hr Total 24-hour IV intake: 3000 ml	Determines volume of fluid that should infuse hourly.
10. Place adhesive or fluid indicator tape on IV bottle or bag next to volume markings (see illustration).	Time taping IV bag gives nurse visual cue as to whether fluids are being administered over correct period of time. Time tapes may be required for all IV infusions, including those on therapies infused via electronic infusion devices. Check agency policy.

Critical Decision Point: Do not use felt-tip pens or permanent markers on IV bags, because ink could contaminate the solution (Millam and others, 2000).

---

11. After hourly flow rate has been determined, calculate minute rate based on drop factor of infusion set. Microdrip infusion set has a drop factor of 60 gtt/ml. Regular drip or macrodrip infusion set used in this example has drop factor of 15 gtt/ml. Use the following formula: $\dfrac{gtt\ factor}{60} \times \dfrac{flow\ rate}{1} = $ Drop rate Calculate minute flow rates for 120 ml/hr via 15 gtt/ml drop factor: $15/60 \times \dfrac{120}{1} = 30$ gtt/min via 60 gtt/ml (microdrip) drop factor: $60/60 \times \dfrac{120}{1} = 120$ gtt/ml.	Allows nurse to calculate minute flow rate based on this formula: Total volume × Drop factor/infusion time in minutes When using microdrip, ml/hr always equals gtt/min.

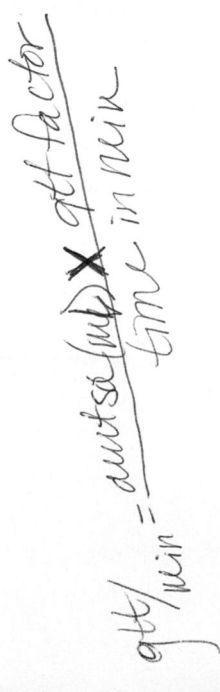

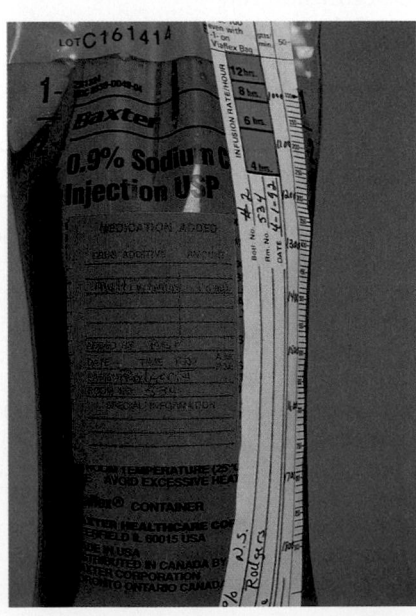

STEP **11** IV fluid bag with time tape.

Steps	Rationale
12. Establish flow rate by counting drops in drip chamber for 1 min by watch, then adjust roller clamp to increase or decrease rate of infusion (see illustration).	Determines if fluids are administered too slowly or too fast.
13. Follow this procedure for infusion controller or pump:	
a. Place electronic eye on half-filled drip chamber below origin of drop and above fluid level in chamber, or consult manufacturer's directions for setup of the infusion (see illustration). If a controller is used, ensure that IV bag is 36 in above the IV site.	The electronic eye counts the number of drops flowing from administration set to ensure that proper rate infuses. IV controller works by gravity.
b. IV infusion tubing is placed within ridges of control box in direction of flow (i.e., portion of tubing nearest IV bag at top and portion of tubing nearest client at bottom) or consult manufacturer's directions for use of pump (see illustration). Some devices require securing tubing through "air in line" alarm system. Close control chamber door. Turn on pump. Required drops per minute or volume per hour and volume to be infused are selected. Open rate control clamp and press start button.	Infusion pumps move fluid by compressing and milking IV tubing, thus propelling fluid through tubing. Rate control clamp should be open completely while infusion controller or pump is in use.

Critical Decision Point: Special infusion tubing is required for some pumps (check manufacturer's directions).

---

c. Monitor infusion rates and IV site for complications according to agency policy.	Infusion controllers or pumps are not infallible and do not replace frequent, accurate nursing assessments. Infusion pumps may continue to infuse IV fluids after an infiltration has begun. All EIDs must have free-flow protector device.
d. Assess patency and integrity of system when alarm sounds.	Alarm indicates that electronic eye has not noted precise number of drops from drip chamber, or there is an empty solution bag or bottle, or flow obstruction (e.g., kink in tubing, closed drip regulator, infiltrated or clotted needle, and/or air in the tubing).

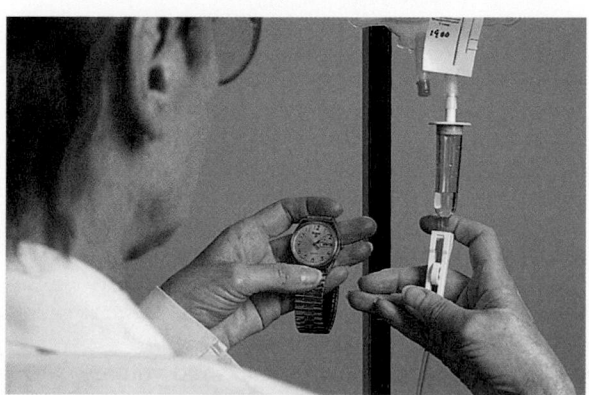

STEP **12** Counting IV drip rate.

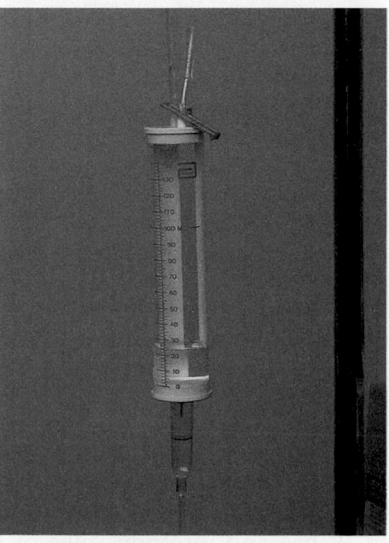

STEP **13a** Place electronic eye above fluid level in drip chamber.

Skill 40-2 *Regulating Intravenous Flow Rate—cont'd*

Steps   **Rationale**

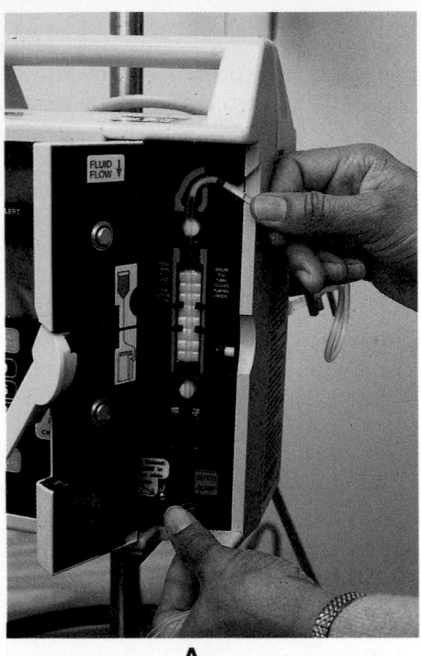

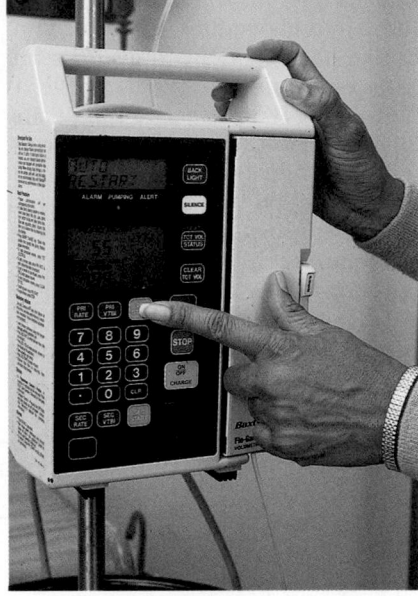

A   **B**

STEP **13b** **A,** Place infusing tubing within ridges of pump. **B,** Press start button to begin infusion.

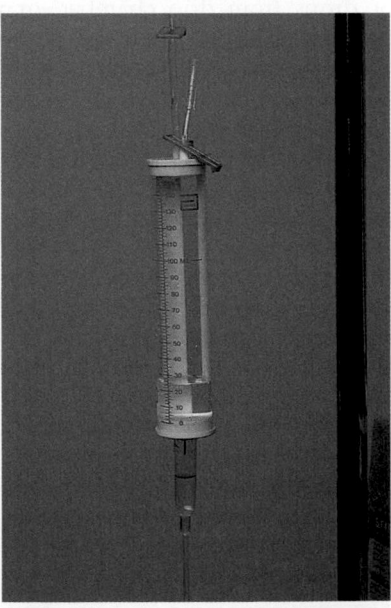

STEP **14a** Volume control device.

14. Follow this procedure for volume control device:
    a. Place volume control device (see illustration) be-   Reduces risk of sudden increase in fluid volume.
       tween IV bag and insertion spike of infusion set
       using sterile technique.

Steps	Rationale
b. Place 2 hours' fluid allotment into chamber device.	Prevents IV line from running dry if nurse does not return in exactly 60 min. In addition, if there is accidental increase in flow rate, client receives at most only a 2-hr allotment of fluid.
c. Assess system at least hourly; add fluid to volume control device. Regulate flow rate.	Maintains patency of system.
15. Observe client for signs of overhydration or dehydration to determine response to therapy and restoration of fluid and electrolyte balance.	Signs and symptoms of dehydration or overhydration warrant changing rate of fluid infused.
16. Evaluate infusion site for signs of infiltration, inflammation, clot in catheter, kink or knot in infusion tubing.	Prevents decrease or cessation of flow rate.

Unexpected Outcomes and Related Interventions

1. Sudden infusion of large volume of solution occurs with client having symptoms of dyspnea, crackles in the lung, and increased urine output, indicating fluid overload.
   - Slow infusion to KVO rate, and notify physician immediately. New IV orders will be required. Client may require diuretics.
2. IV fluid bag runs empty with subsequent loss of IV line patency.
   - IV will be restarted.
3. The IV infusion is slower than ordered.
   - Check client for positional change that might affect rate, height of IV bag, kinking of tubing.
   - An infiltration may be developing at IV site. Check condition of site.
   - If volume infused is deficient, consult physician for new order to provide necessary fluid volume.

Recording and Reporting

- Record name of solution, rate of infusion, drops/min, and ml/hr in nurses' notes or flow sheet every 4 hours or according to agency policy.

- Immediately record in nurses' notes or flow sheet any new IV fluid rates.
- Document use of any EID or controlling device and number on that device.
- At change of shift or when leaving on break, report rate of infusion to nurse in charge or next nurse assigned to care for client.

Home Care Considerations

- Ensure that client is able and willing to operate the EID (if applicable) and administer IV therapy or that there is a reliable caregiver or nursing support personnel at home to provide this IV therapy care.
- Teach client and primary caregiver to time drops per minute using watch with second hand.
- Ensure that electric outlets are functioning properly, are grounded, and infusion device has back-up power, if required by type of infusate.

---

client who has FVD or hyperosmolar imbalance or who is in shock. An IV that is running too slowly can also become clotted off more easily. An infusion rate that is too rapid can result in FVE. The nurse calculates the infusion rate to prevent too-slow or too-rapid administration of the IV fluids. Numerous methods are used to ensure an accurate hourly infusion rate for IV therapy. Fluids that run by gravity are adjusted through use of a flow control/regulator clamp. Fluids infused by an electronic infusion device or rate controller are regulated by a mechanical mechanism set at the prescribed rate. Regardless of the device in use, the client requires close monitoring to verify the correct infusion of the IV solution and to detect the occurrence of any complication. Electronic **infusion pumps** are necessary when administering low hourly volumes (e.g., 5 ml/hr or less or 20 ml/hr) and for clients who are at risk for volume overload such as neonatal, pediatric, and geriatric clients. In addition, when infusing high volumes of IV fluids (more than 150 ml/hr) to clients with impaired renal clearance, older adults, or pediatric clients, or when infusing drugs or IV fluids that require specific hourly volumes, electronic infusion devices permit accurate infusion. Electronic infusion pumps deliver the infusion via positive pressure. A rate controller used on gravity infusions regulates the infusion, but unlike the electronic pump, is affected by many mechanical and client factors. Recent advances in infusion technology have resulted in a variety of devices available for use to ensure accurate delivery.

Many devices have operating and programming capabilities that allow for single- and multiple-solution infusions at different rates. A variety of detectors and alarms respond to air in IV lines, completion of infusion, high and low pressure, low battery power, occlusion, and the inability to deliver at a preset rate.

> *Safety Alert.* An anti–free flow safeguard (preventing bolus infusion in the event of machine malfunction) is an important element of an electronic infusion device and is required. Manufacturer's recommendations for specific device features should always be checked.

Patency of the IV needle or catheter means that there are no clots at the tip of the needle or catheter and that the catheter or needle tip is not against the vein wall. A blocked catheter or needle can affect the rate of infusion of the IV fluids. IV flow rates can also be affected by the patency of the IV needle or catheter, infiltration, a knot or kink in the tubing, the height of the solution, a restrictive IV dressing and the position of the client's extremity. One way that the nurse may assess patency is by lowering the IV bag below the level of the IV insertion site and observing for a blood return, however, this method does not confirm patency. If no blood return occurs and fluid does not flow easily from the drip chamber when the roller clamp is opened, the nurse should assess potential causes: a too-tight IV dressing may be impeding the flow, a clot may be occluding the cannula of the IV catheter, or the catheter tip may be occluded against the wall of the vein. The tubing and area around the insertion site should be inspected for anything that could obstruct the flow of IV fluids. A knot or kink in the tubing can decrease the flow rate. Occasionally the tubing is kinked under a dressing, which requires the nurse to remove the dressing to locate the problem. The flow rate frequently resumes after the tubing is straightened. The client may also occlude the tubing by lying or sitting on it. The height of the IV bag can also affect flow rates. Raising the bag usually increases the rate because of increased hydrostatic pressure.

The position of the extremity, particularly at the wrist or elbow, can decrease flow rates. Occasionally the use of an arm board helps to keep the joint extended (Figure 40-14). The arm board also provides some protection to the IV site and tubing. Sometimes it is more comfortable for the client to have an infusion started in a new location rather than relying upon a site that causes problems. However, before discontinuing the infusion hampered by an extremity position, the nurse should start the infusion in another site to verify that the client has other accessible veins.

Children, older adults, clients with severe head trauma, and clients susceptible to volume overload must be protected from sudden increases in infusion volumes. The nurse needs to understand that when certain IV controller devices are opened, the IV fluid will infuse rapidly. If this is not controlled, an excessive amount of solution can infuse. Sudden increases can occur accidentally. For example, a restless client may loosen the roller clamp with a sudden movement and increase the flow rate, or the flow rate may be accidentally increased if the client ambulates. A sudden increase in IV infusion rate causes a rapid increase in vascular volume, which can make the client critically ill or even cause death. Volume control

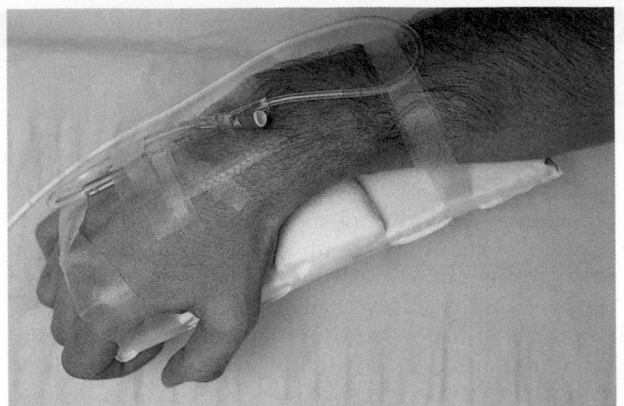

FIGURE **40–14**   IV arm board and cover.

devices, such as a Volutrol burette, can prevent sudden excessive increases in the volume of IV solution infused.

Maintaining the System. After the IV line is in place and the flow rate is regulated, the nurse must maintain the system. The nurse keeps in mind agency policy regarding the maintenance of IV lines. Line maintenance is achieved by (1) keeping the system sterile; (2) changing solutions, tubing, and site dressings; and (3) assisting the client with self-care activities so as to not disrupt the system.

The nurse plays an important role in maintaining the integrity of an IV to prevent infection from developing. Figure 40-15 demonstrates the potential sites for contamination of an intravascular device. The client's microflora and contamination by insertion are initially controlled for in the procedure for IV insertion. However, the other factors are controlled through conscientious use of infection-control principles. This begins with the use of thorough hand hygiene before and after the nurse handles any component of the IV system.

The integrity of the IV system must always be maintained. The nurse never disconnects tubing because it becomes tangled or because it might be more convenient in positioning or moving a client or applying a gown. If a client needs more room to maneuver, extension tubing can be added to an IV line. However, the use of extension tubing should be kept to a minimum, as each connection of tubing provides opportunity for contamination. Stopcocks for connecting more than one solution to a single IV site are sources of contamination and should be avoided (Centers for Disease Control and Prevention [CDC], 2002). Whenever an IV line is disconnected from a stopcock, the port should be plugged with a sterile cap. Do not allow a port to remain exposed to air for contamination. A new administration set should be exchanged with the subsequent fluid change. Intravenous tubing also contains injection ports through which adapters can be inserted for medication injections. An injection port must be cleaned thoroughly with 70% alcohol or povidone-iodine solution before accessing the system (Infusion Nurses Society [INS], 2000).

Clients receiving IV therapy over several days will require changing of solutions. It is important for the nurse to organize tasks so that this can be done in plenty of time before the solution empties and possibly becomes clotted.

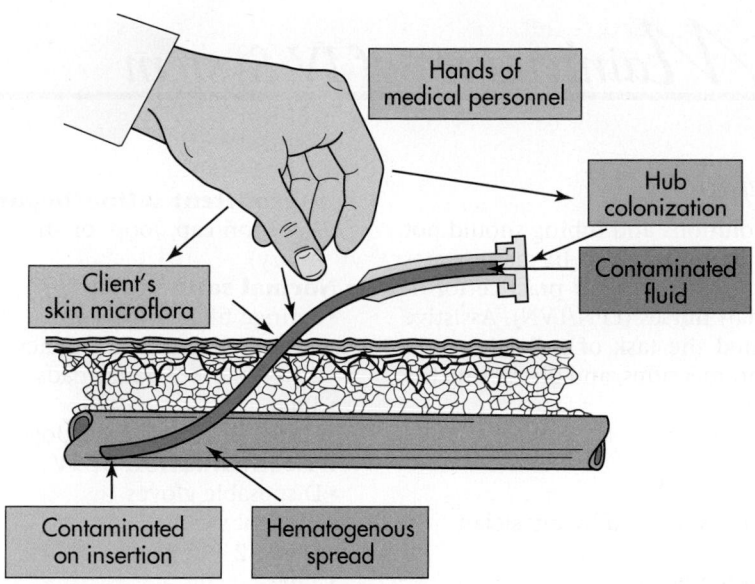

FIGURE **40–15** Potential sites for contamination of an intravascular device.

The Centers for Disease Control and Prevention (CDC) (2002) has no recommendation for the hang time of IV fluids. Skill 40-3 reviews steps for changing IV solutions.

Intravenous tubing administration sets can remain sterile for 72 hours (CDC, 2002). The CDC (2002) recommends changing tubing no more frequently than every 72 hours. The INS (2000) recommends 72-hour intervals for continuous tubing changes, adding that 48-hour tubing changes should be considered if the rate of catheter-related infection and phlebitis in an agency exceeds 5%. The exception is tubing containing blood, TPN, blood products, and lipid emulsions, which are more likely to promote bacterial growth. Agency policy may require more frequent tubing changes (e.g., every 24 hours). Whenever possible, schedule tubing changes when it is time to hang a new container to promote aseptic technique. To prevent entry of bacteria into the bloodstream, sterility must be maintained during tubing and solution changes.

The dressings over IV sites are applied to reduce the entrance of bacteria into the insertion site. The two forms of dressings are transparent and gauze. Transparent dressings reliably secure the IV device, allow continuous visual inspection of the IV site, become less easily soiled or moistened, and require less frequent changes than standard gauze (CDC, 2002). Either form of dressing must be changed when the IV device is removed or replaced or when the dressing becomes damp, loosened, or soiled (INS, 2000). Agency policy may require IV dressings to be routinely changed within a certain time frame (e.g., 48 to 72 hours) (Skill 40-4).

To prevent the accidental disruption of an IV system, the nurse may need to assist the client with hygiene, comfort measures, meals, and ambulation. Because a client with an infusion in the arm finds it difficult to meet hygiene needs, the nurse should help with bathing and changing gowns. It helps to use a gown specifically made with snaps along the top sleeve seam to facilitate changing the gown without disturbing the venipuncture

site. Regular gowns are changed by following these six steps for maximum arm mobility and speed:
1. Remove the sleeve of the gown from the arm without the IV, maintaining the client's privacy.
2. Remove the sleeve of the gown from the arm with the IV.
3. Remove the IV solution container from its stand and pass it and the tubing through the sleeve. (If this involves removing the tubing from an IV electronic infusion device, use the roller clamp to slow the infusion to prevent the accidental infusion of a large volume of solution or medication).
4. Place the IV solution container and tubing through the sleeve of the clean gown and hang it on its stand. (If the IV is connected to a electronic infusion device, reassemble and open the roller clamp. Turn the pump on.)
5. Place the arm with the IV through the gown sleeve.
6. Place the arm without the IV through the gown sleeve. (Breaking the integrity of an IV line to change a gown leads to contamination.)

There are now protective devices designed to prevent accidental dislodgement of an IV catheter (Figure 40-16, p. 1189). The device fits comfortably around a client's hand or arm and provides a plastic shield to cover the IV device.

The client with an arm or a hand infusion is able to walk, unless contraindicated. A rolling IV pole (a standard IV pole with wheels) is needed. The nurse helps the client get out of bed and places the pole next to the involved arm. The client is instructed to hold on to the pole with the involved hand and to push it while walking. The nurse should assess the equipment to make sure that the IV bag is at the proper height, that there is no tension on the tubing, and that the flow rate is correct. The nurse should instruct the client to report any blood in the tubing, a stoppage in the flow, or increased discomfort. Intravenous medications, especially antibiotics and potassium, can cause discomfort and burning sensations at the IV site. While discomfort may be relieved by repositioning the extremity, the source of discomfort must always be

Text continued on p. 1189

Skill 40-3   *Maintenance of IV System*

Delegation Considerations

The skill of changing IV solutions and tubing should not be delegated to assistive personnel (AP). In many states this skill is included within the scope of practice for licensed practical (vocational) nurses (LPN/LVN). Assistive personnel may be delegated the task of collecting supplies, assisting with comfort measures, and distracting the client during the procedure.

Equipment

• **IV infusion**
  ▪ Bottle/bag of IV solution as ordered by physician
  ▪ Time tape
  ▪ Infusion tubing and tubing label
  ▪ Filter (size appropriate to solution) and extension tubing (if necessary)

• **Intermittent saline/heparin lock**
  ▪ Injection cap, loop, or short extension tubing (if necessary)
• **Normal saline flush**
  ▪ Syringe filled with normal saline or heparin flush solution (check agency policy)
  ▪ 2 sterile 2 × 2 gauze pads
  ▪ Tape
  ▪ Disposable nonsterile gloves
• **Discontinuation of IV**
  ▪ Disposable gloves
  ▪ Alcohol swabs
  ▪ Sterile 2 × 2 gauze
  ▪ Tape

Steps	Rationale
Changing IV Solution	
1. Check physician's orders.	Ensures that correct solution will be used. IV therapy requires the six rights of medication administration.
2. If order is written for keep vein open (KVO) or to keep open (TKO), contact physician/LIP for clarification of the rate of the infusion. Note date and time when solution was last changed.	Orders for KVO do not provide complete information and can result in fluid overload or deficit and electrolyte imbalance. A KVO order should contain a specific infusion rate (INS, 2000). Refer to agency policy. IV tubing and solution should be changed at the same time.
3. Determine the compatibility of all IV fluids and additives by consulting appropriate literature or the pharmacy.	Incompatibilities may lead to precipitate formation and can cause physical, chemical, and therapeutic client changes. Precipitation may occlude patency of catheter.
4. Determine client's understanding of need for continued IV therapy.	Reveals need for client instruction.
5. Assess patency of current IV access site.	If patency is occluded, a new IV access site may be needed. Notify physician.
6. Have next solution prepared and accessible at least 1 hr before needed. Check that solution is correct and properly labeled. Check solution expiration date and for presence of precipitate and discoloration.	Adequate planning reduces risk of clot formation in vein caused by empty IV bag. Checking prevents medication error.
7. Prepare to change solution when less than 50 ml of fluid remains in bottle or bag or when a new type of solution is ordered.	Prevents air from entering tubing and vein from clotting from lack of flow.
8. Prepare client and family by explaining the procedure, its purpose, and what is expected of client.	Decreases anxiety and promotes cooperation.
9. Be sure drip chamber is at least half full.	Provides fluid to vein while bag is changed.
10. Perform hand hygiene.	Reduces transmission of microorganisms.
11. Prepare new solution for changing. If using plastic bag, remove protective cover from IV tubing port. If using glass bottle, remove metal cap and metal and rubber disks.	Permits quick, smooth, and organized change from old to new solution.
12. Move roller clamp to stop flow rate.	Prevents solution remaining in drip chamber from emptying while changing solutions.
13. Remove old IV fluid container from IV pole.	Brings work to nurse's eye level.
14. Quickly remove spike from old solution bag or bottle and, without touching tip, insert spike into new bag or bottle.	Reduces risk of solution in drip chamber running dry and maintains sterility.

Critical Decision Point: If spike is contaminated, a new IV tubing set is required.

Steps	Rationale

15. Hang new bag or bottle of solution on IV pole.

Gravity assists with delivery of fluid into drip chamber.

16. Check for air in tubing. If bubbles form, they can be removed by closing the roller clamp, stretching the tubing downward, and tapping the tubing with the finger (the bubbles rise in the fluid to the drip chamber, see illustration). For larger amounts of air, swab injection port below the air with alcohol and allow to dry. Connect a syringe to this port and aspirate the air into the syringe. Reduce air in tubing by priming slowly instead of allowing a wide-open flow.

Reduces risk of air embolus. Use of an air-eliminating filter also reduces this risk.

17. Make sure drip chamber is one-third to one-half full. If the drip chamber is too full, pinch off tubing below the drip chamber, invert the container, squeeze the drip chamber (see illustration), hang up the bottle, and release the tubing.

Reduces risk of air entering tubing.

18. Regulate flow to prescribed rate.

Maintains measures to restore fluid balance and deliver IV fluid as ordered.

19. Mark time on label tape and place on bag. Do not use felt-tip pens or permanent markers on IV bags.

Ink from markers may leach through polyvinyl chloride containers.

20. Observe client for signs of overhydration or dehydration to determine response to IV fluid therapy.

Provides ongoing evaluation of client's fluid and electrolyte status.

21. Observe IV system for patency and development of complications (e.g., infiltration or phlebitis).

Provides ongoing evaluation of IV system.

Changing IV Tubing

22. Determine when new infusion set is needed:

   a. Agency policy will indicate frequency of routine change for IV administration sets and heparin/saline flush tubing.

The CDC (2002) and INS (2000) recommend changing tubing for primary infusions no more frequently than 72-hour intervals or whenever tubing has been compromised.

   b. Puncture of infusion tubing requires immediate change.

Punctured tubing results in fluid leakage and bacterial contamination.

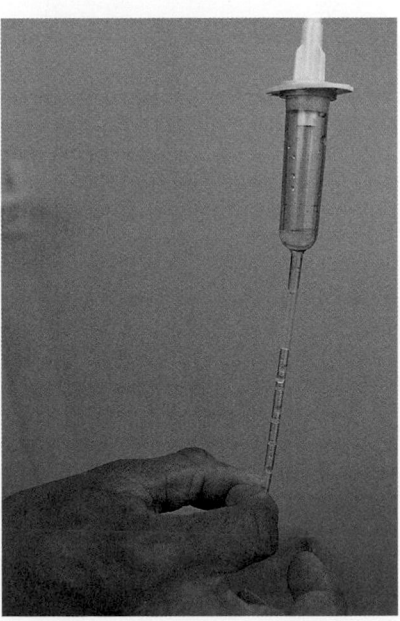

STEP **16** Tap tubing to cause air bubbles to rise up to drip chamber.

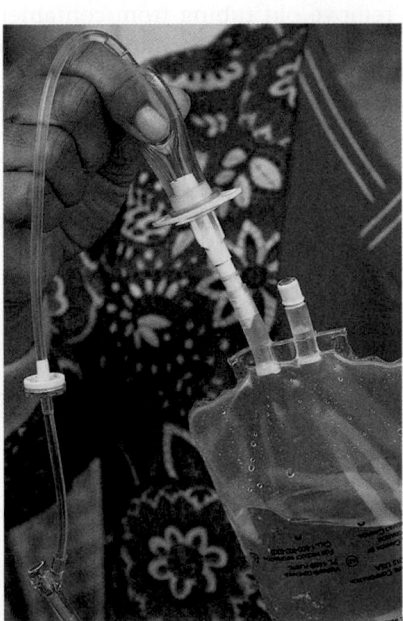

STEP **17** Squeeze drip chamber to remove a portion of fluid. Be sure to leave chamber one-third to one-half full.

Steps	Rationale
c. Contamination of tubing requires immediate change.	Contamination of tubing allows entry of bacteria into client's bloodstream.
d. Occlusions in existing tubing. Such occlusions can occur after infusion of packed red cells, whole blood, albumin, or other blood components.	Whole blood or blood component product can occlude or partially occlude tubing, because viscous solutions adhere to walls of tubing and decrease the size of the lumen.
23. Prepare client and family by explaining the procedure, its purpose, and what is expected of client.	Decreases anxiety, promotes cooperation, and prevents sudden movement of extremity, which could dislodge IV needle or catheter.
24. Perform hand hygiene.	Reduces transmission of microorganisms.
25. Open new infusion set, keeping protective coverings over infusion spike and distal adapter. Secure all junctions with Luer-loks, clasping devices, or threaded devices.	Provides nurse with ready access to new infusion set and maintains sterility of infusion set.
26. Apply nonsterile, disposable gloves.	Reduces risk of exposure to HIV, hepatitis, and other blood-borne bacteria.
27. If needle or catheter hub is not visible, remove IV dressing while maintaining stability of catheter. If transparent dressing has to be removed, place small piece of sterile tape across hub temporarily to anchor catheter during disconnection. Do not remove tape securing needle or catheter to skin with gauze dressing.	Needle hub must be accessible to provide smooth transition when removing old and inserting new tubing.
28. For IV continuous infusion:	
a. Move roller clamp on new IV tubing to "off" position.	Prevents spillage of solution after bag or bottle is spiked.
b. Slow rate of infusion by regulating drip rate on old tubing. Be sure rate is at KVO rate.	Prevents complete infusion of solution that remains in tubing, which can increase risk of occlusion of IV catheter or needle.
c. Compress and fill drip chamber of old tubing.	Provides surplus of fluid in drip chamber so there is enough fluid to maintain IV patency while changing tubing.
d. Remove IV container from pole, invert container and remove old tubing from container. Carefully hold container while hanging or taping drip chamber on IV pole 36 inches above IV site.	Fluid in drip chamber will run slowly to keep catheter patent.
e. Place insertion spike of new tubing into old solution bag opening and hang solution bag on IV pole.	Permits flow of fluid from solution into new infusion tubing.
f. Compress and release drip chamber on new tubing; fill drip chamber one-third to one-half full.	Allows drip chamber to fill and promotes rapid, smooth flow of solution through new tubing.
g. Slowly open roller clamp, remove protective cap from needle adapter (if necessary), and flush new tubing with solution. Replace cap.	Removes air from tubing and replaces it with fluid.
h. Turn roller clamp on old tubing to "off" position.	Prevents spillage of fluid as tubing is removed from needle hub.
29. For saline/heparin lock:	
a. If a loop or short extension tubing is needed because of an awkward IV site placement, use sterile technique to connect the new injection cap to the loop or tubing.	
b. Swab injection cap with alcohol, povidone-iodine or chlorhexidine. Insert syringe with 1 to 3 ml saline or heparin flush solution and inject through the injection cap into the loop or short extension tubing (see illustration).	Removes air to prevent introduction into the vein.

Steps	Rationale

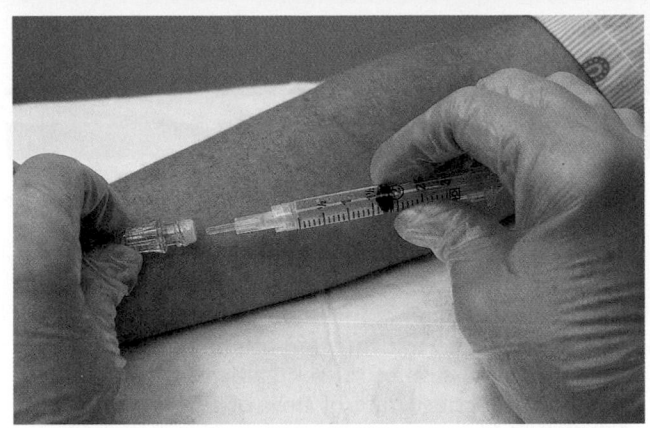

A

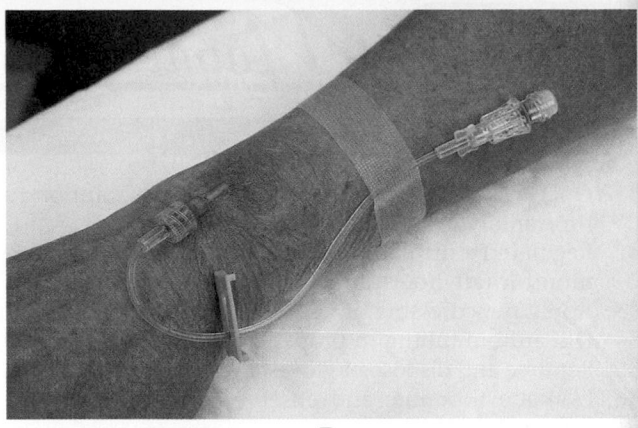

B

STEP **29B** Inject saline into injection cap **(A)** connected to saline lock extension tube **(B).**

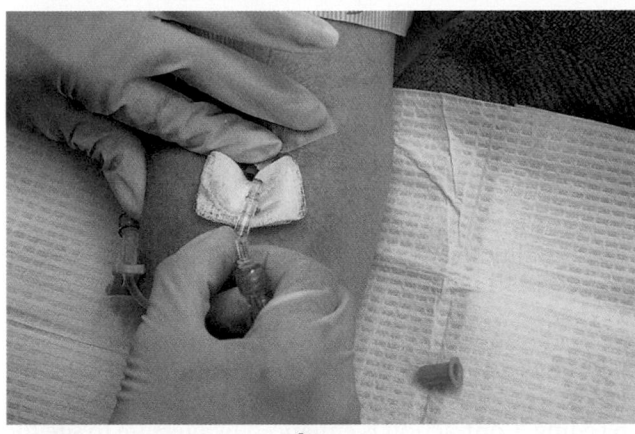

A

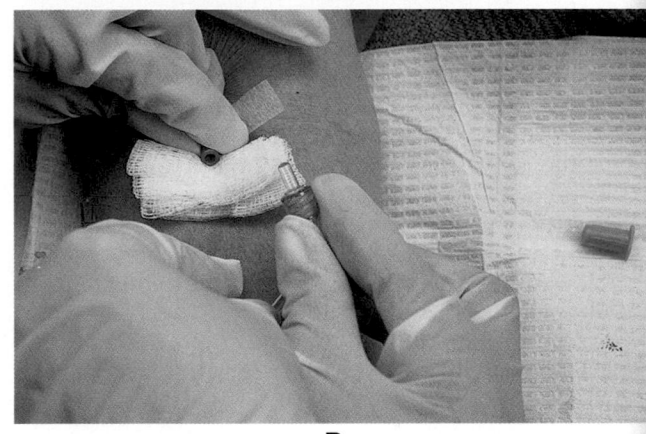

B

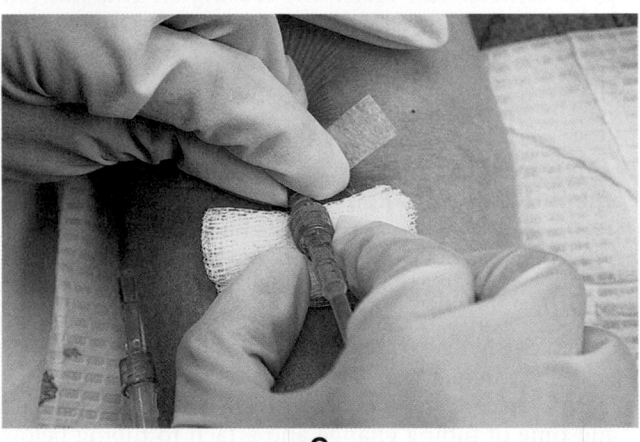

C

STEP **30 A,** Maintain stability of catheter hub while removing old tubing. **B,** Connect new infusion tubing. **C,** Be sure connection at hub is secure.

30. Stabilize hub of catheter and apply pressure over vein just above catheter tip at least 1½ inches above insertion site. Gently disconnect old tubing from catheter hub (see illustration). Maintain stability of hub and quickly insert adapter of new tubing or saline/heparin lock into hub (see illustrations).

Prevents accidental displacement of catheter or needle.

Prevents clot formation in catheter or needle and backflow of blood.

Skill **40-3**   *Maintenance of IV System—cont'd*

Steps	Rationale
31. Open roller clamp on new tubing. Allow solution to run rapidly for 30 to 60 seconds.	Permits IV solution to enter catheter to prevent catheter occlusion.
32. Regulate IV drip according to physician's orders and monitor rate hourly.	Maintains infusion flow at prescribed rate.
33. Apply new dressing, if needed.	Reduces risk of bacterial infection from skin.
34. Discard old tubing in proper container.	Reduces accidental transmission of microorganisms.
35. Remove and dispose of gloves. Perform hand hygiene.	Reduces transmission of microorganisms.
36. Evaluate flow rate and observe connection site for leakage	Maintains prescribed rate of flow of IV fluid and determines if fit is secure.

Discontinuing Peripheral IV Access

Steps	Rationale
37. Check physician's order for discontinuation of IV.	Order is required for discontinuation of fluids/medication.
38. Explain procedure to client. Explain that affected extremity must be held still and how long procedure will take.	Minimizes client's anxiety and discomfort.
39. Perform hand hygiene and apply disposable gloves.	Reduces trasmission of microorganisms.
40. Turn IV tubing roller clamp to "off" position. Remove tape securing tubing.	
41. Remove IV site dressing and tape while stabilizing catheter.	Movement of catheter will cause discomfort.
42. With dry gauze or alcohol swab held over site, apply light pressure and withdraw the catheter, using a slow steady movement, keeping the hub parallel to the skin.	Changing the angle of the catheter inside the vein could cause additional vein irritation, increasing the risk of postinfusion phlebitis.
43. Apply pressure to the site for 2 to 3 minutes, using the dry, sterile gauze pad. Secure with tape.	Dry pad causes less irritation to the puncture site. Subcutaneous hematoma is common complication. When needle is removed, vein wall contracts to stop bleeding. Contraction is enhanced by pressure to site for at least 2 to 3 minutes (Chukhraev and Grekov, 2000).
44. Inspect the catheter for intactness, noting tip integrity and length.	Tips of catheter can break off, causing an embolus, an emergency situation. Notify physician if tip is broken.
45. Discard used supplies.	
46. Remove and discard gloves, and perform hand hygiene.	
47. Instruct client to report any redness, pain, drainage, or swelling that may occur after catheter removal.	Postinfusion phlebitis may occur within 48 to 96 hours after catheter removal.

Unexpected Outcomes and Related Interventions

1. Flow rate is incorrect; client receives too little or too much fluid.
   - Readjust infusion rate to ordered rate; evaluate client for adverse effects; notify physician.
2. Flow of IV fluid is decreased or absent.
   - Assess IV infusion system for patency.
   - Recalibrate drip rate on new tubing.
   - Assess IV site for infiltration.

Recording and Reporting

- Record changing of tubing and solution on client's record. A special parenteral therapy flow sheet may be used.
- Place a piece of tape or preprinted label with the date and time of tubing change and attach to tubing below the level of drip chamber.

Home Care Considerations

- Emphasize to client and family the importance of changing solutions when IV tubing still contains fluid.

Skill 40-4   Changing a Peripheral Intravenous Dressing

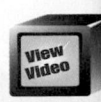

Delegation Considerations

The skill of changing a peripheral IV dressing should not be delegated to assistive personnel (AP). In many states, this skill is included within the scope of practice for licensed practical (vocational) nurses. Assistive personnel may be delegated the task of collecting supplies, assisting with comfort measures, and distracting the client during the procedure.

Equipment

- Antiseptic swab stick (chlorhexidine, povidone-iodine, and/or 70% alcohol)
- Alcohol swab stick
- Adhesive remover (if needed)
- Strips of nonallergenic sterile tape for use underneath the dressing
- Disposable gloves
- Arm board or housing device (if needed)
- For gauze dressing
  - Sterile 2 × 2 gauze pad
  OR
  - Sterile 4 × 4 gauze pad
- For transparent dressing
  - Sterile transparent dressing

Steps	Rationale
1. Determine when dressing was last changed. Many institutions require nurse to write date and time on dressing and date the device was first placed.	Provides information regarding length of time present dressing has been in place. In addition, nurse is able to plan for dressing change. CDC recommends that, whenever possible, peripheral IV dressings be scheduled when IV system is changed.
2. Perform hand hygiene. Observe present dressing for moisture and intactness.	Moisture is a medium for bacterial growth and renders dressing contaminated.
3. Observe IV system for proper functioning or complications: kinks in infusion tubing or IV catheter. Palpate the catheter site through the intact dressing for inflammation or subjective complaints of pain or burning.	Unexplained decrease in flow rate requires the nurse to investigate placement and patency of the IV catheter. Pain can be associated with both phlebitis and infiltration.
4. Inspect exposed catheter site for swelling or blanching.	Indicates fluid infusing into surrounding tissues. Will require removal of IV catheter.
5. Assess client's understanding of need for continued IV infusion.	Determines need for client instruction.
6. Explain procedure and purpose to client and family. Explain that affected extremity must be held still and how long procedure will take.	Decreases anxiety, promotes cooperation, and gives client time frame around which personal activities can be planned.
7. Apply disposable gloves.	Reduces transmission of microorganisms.
8. Remove tape, gauze, and/or transparent dressing from old dressing one layer at a time, leaving tape (if present) that secures IV catheter in place. Be cautious if catheter tubing becomes tangled between two layers of dressing. When removing transparent dressing, hold catheter hub and tubing with nondominant hand.	Prevents accidental displacement of catheter or needle.
9. Observe insertion site for signs and/or symptoms of infection, namely redness, swelling, and exudate. If present, remove catheter and insert a new IV in another site.	
10. If infiltration, phlebitis, or clot occurs or if ordered by physician, stop infusion and discontinue IV. Restart new IV if continued therapy is necessary. Place moist warm compress over area of phlebitis (see Tables 40-9, 40-10, p. 1173).	
11. If IV is infusing properly, gently remove any tape securing catheter. Stabilize needle or catheter with one hand. Use adhesive remover to cleanse skin and remove adhesive residue, if needed.	Exposes venipuncture site. Stabilization prevents accidental displacement of catheter or needle. Adhesive residue decreases ability of new dressing to adhere tightly to skin.
12. Stabilize catheter at all times with one finger over catheter until tape or dressing is replaced.	Prevents decannulation from vein.

Changing a Peripheral Intravenous Dressing—cont'd

Skill **40-4**

Steps	Rationale

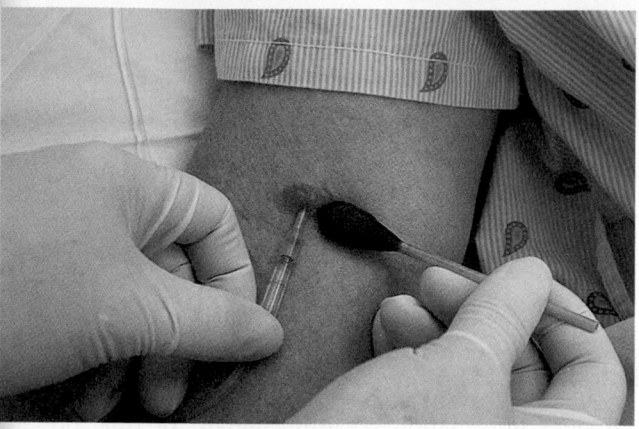

STEP **13** Cleanse peripheral insertion site.

13. Using circular motion, cleanse peripheral IV insertion site with antiseptic swab starting at insertion site and working outward creating concentric circles (see illustration). Allow swab solution to air dry completely.

Circular motion prevents cross contamination from skin bacteria near venipuncture site. Antiseptics may include chlorhexidine, povidone-iodine, and alcohol. CDC recommends 2% chlorhexidine-based solution. Povidone-iodine is a topical antiinfective that reduces skin surface bacteria; the solution must be dry to be effective in reducing microbial counts (CDC, 2002). If antiseptic agents are used in combination, allow each to dry separately.

Critical Decision Point: Do not tape over connection of access tubing or port to IV catheter.

---

14. Apply new transparent or gauze dressing (See Skill 40-1).
15. Remove and discard gloves.
16. Anchor IV tubing with additional pieces of tape. When using transparent polyurethane dressing, minimize the tape placed over dressing.
17. Place insertion date (if known), date and time of dressing change, size and gauge of catheter, and initials of nurse directly on dressing.

    Apply arm board and/or commercial housing device if site is affected by joint motion.
18. Discard used equipment and perform hand hygiene.
19. Observe functioning and patency of IV system in response to changing dressing.
20. Monitor client's body temperature.

Ensures protection of IV site and reduces chance of infection.

Prevents accidental displacement of IV needle or catheter or separation of IV tubing from needle adapter.

Documents dressing change.

Reduces transmission of microorganisms.
Validates that IV is patent and functioning correctly.

Elevated temperature indicates an infection that may be associated with bacterial contamination of the venipuncture site.

Unexpected Outcomes and Related Interventions

1. IV catheter is infiltrated, as evidenced by decreased flow rate or edema, pallor, or decreased temperature around insertion site.
   - Stop infusion and discontinue IV. Restart new IV in other extremity if continued therapy is necessary. Elevate affected extremity.
2. Phlebitis is present, as evidenced by erythema and tenderness along vein pathway.
   - Stop infusion and discontinue IV. Restart new IV in other extremity if continued therapy is necessary.
   - Apply warm moist compress to area of phlebitis.
3. IV catheter or needle is accidentally removed.
   - Restart IV if continued therapy is needed.

4. Client has an elevated temperature.
   - Notify physician. IV may be removed and restarted. Client will be evaluated for source of infection.
5. Insertion site is red and/or edematous and/or painful and/or has presence of exudates, indicating infection at venipuncture site.
   - IV is discontinued. Antibiotic therapy may begin.
   - Apply warm moist compress to area of inflammation.

Recording and Reporting

- Record appearance of IV site, type of dressing, and status of IV fluid infusion.
- A special parenteral fluid flow sheet may be used for recording.

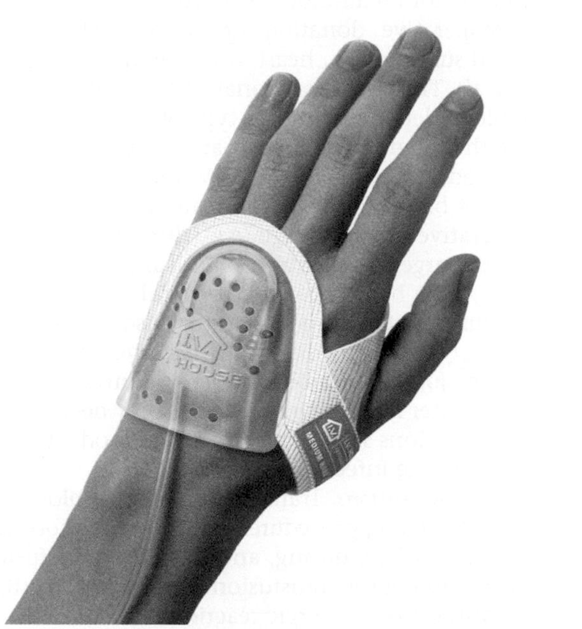

FIGURE **40–16** IV House Protective Device (Courtesy IV House, St. Louis, MO).

carefully evaluated, and may necessitate starting a new IV line in a larger vein.

Complications of Intravenous Therapy. An **infiltration** occurs when IV fluids enter the surrounding space around the venipuncture site. This is manifested as swelling (from increased tissue fluid) and pallor and coolness (caused by decreased circulation) around the venipuncture site. Fluid may be flowing through the IV line at a decreased rate or may have stopped flowing. Pain may also be present and usually results from edema and increases proportionately as the infiltration continues.

When infiltration occurs, the infusion must be discontinued and, if IV therapy is still necessary, a new cannula is inserted into a vein in another extremity. To reduce discomfort, the nurse raises the extremity, which promotes venous drainage. To help decrease the edema, the nurse wraps the extremity in a warm, moist towel for 20 minutes while

keeping it elevated on a pillow. This promotes venous return, increases circulation, and reduces pain and edema.

Phlebitis is inflammation of the vein. Selected risk factors for phlebitis include the type of catheter material, chemical irritation of additives and drugs given intravenously (e.g., antibiotics), and the anatomical position of the catheter. Signs and symptoms may include pain, edema, **erythema,** and increased skin temperature over the vein, and, in some instances, redness traveling along the path of the vein (INS, 2000). Dehydration may also be a contributing factor because of the increase in blood viscosity.

When phlebitis develops, the IV line must be discontinued and a new line inserted in another vein. Warm, moist heat on the site of phlebitis can offer some relief to the client (see Chapter 47). Phlebitis can be dangerous, because blood clots (thrombophlebitis) can occur and in some cases may result in emboli. This may result in permanent damage to veins as well as resulting in extended agency care. Phlebitis may be prevented by the routine removal and rotation of IV sites. The CDC recommends replacing peripheral venous catheters and rotating sites at least every 72 to 96 hours (CDC, 2002).

Fluid volume excess occurs when the client has received a too-rapid administration of IV solutions. The assessment findings include shortness of breath, crackles in the lungs, and tachycardia. The nurse should slow the rate of infusion, notify the physician, raise the head of the bed, and monitor vital signs.

Bleeding can occur around the venipuncture site during the infusion or through the catheter needle or tubing if these become inadvertently disconnected. Bleeding is common in clients who have received heparin or who have a bleeding disorder (e.g., leukemia or thrombocytopenia). If bleeding occurs around the venipuncture site and the catheter is within the vein, a pressure dressing may be applied over the site to control the bleeding. Bleeding from a vein is usually a slow, continuous seepage and is not serious.

Discontinuing Intravenous Infusions. Discontinuing an infusion is necessary after the prescribed amount of fluid has been infused, when an infiltration occurs, if phlebitis

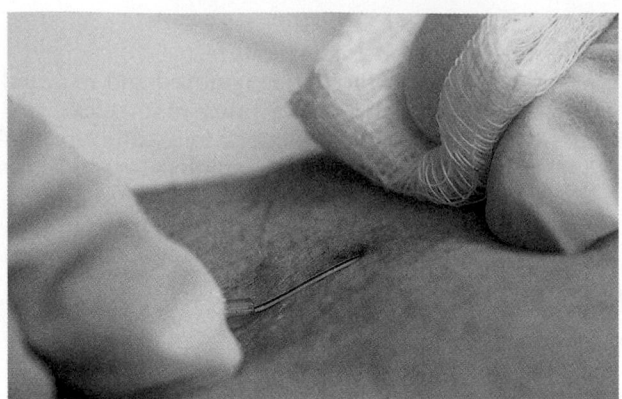

FIGURE **40–17** IV catheter is removed slowly, keeping catheter parallel to vein.

is present, or if the infusion catheter or needle develops a clot at its tip. The nurse discontinuing an infusion first applies disposable gloves and then removes the tape and dressing in the same manner as for the daily infusion dressing changes. The nurse then moves the roller clamp to the "off"/closed position to prevent spillage of IV fluid. The site may be cleansed with antiseptic solution(s) before removal. Allow each solution to dry completely. Check agency policy. The nurse places a sterile 2 × 2 gauze pad over the venipuncture site and, using the other hand, with a slow, steady movement withdraws the cannula by pulling straight back away from the puncture site (Figure 40-17). The catheter should be inspected for intactness and integrity. If necessary, alcohol or soap and water can be used to remove dried blood or other drainage from around the site. The nurse elevates the extremity and applies pressure to the site for 1 to 2 minutes to control bleeding and prevent hematoma formation. Clients who have received heparin require longer pressure because of the action of heparin on blood-clotting mechanisms. If needed, the nurse applies a bandage over a sterile cotton ball or applies a larger sterile dressing over the venipuncture site. The nurse records the amount of fluid infused and the time of the discontinuation as well as the appearance of the insertion site.

Blood Replacement (Colloids). Blood replacement or transfusion is the IV administration of whole blood or a component such as plasma, packed red blood cells (RBCs), or platelets. The objectives for blood transfusions include (1) to increase circulating blood volume after surgery, trauma, or hemorrhage; (2) to increase the number of RBCs and to maintain hemoglobin levels in clients with severe anemia; and (3) to provide selected cellular components as replacement therapy (e.g., clotting factors, platelets, albumin).

Blood Groups and Types. The most important grouping for transfusion purposes is the ABO system, which includes A, B, O, and AB blood types. The determination of blood groups is based on the presence or absence of A and B red cell antigens. Individuals with A antigens, B antigens, or no antigens belong to groups A, B, and O, re-

spectively. The person with A and B antigens has AB blood. Individuals with type A blood naturally produce anti-B antibodies in their plasma. Similarly, type B individuals naturally produce anti-A antibodies. A type O individual has neither type A nor type B antigen and thus is considered a universal blood donor. A type AB individual produces neither antibody, which is why a type AB individual, can be a universal recipient and receive any type of blood. If blood that is mismatched with the client's blood is transfused, a **transfusion reaction** occurs. The transfusion reaction is an antigen-antibody reaction and can range from a mild response to severe anaphylactic shock, which can be life threatening.

Another consideration when matching for blood transfusions is the Rh factor, which is an antigenic substance in the erythrocytes of most people. A person with the factor is Rh positive, and a person without it is Rh negative.

Autologous Transfusion. **Autologous transfusion** or autotransfusion is the collection of a client's own blood. The blood for an autologous transfusion can be obtained by preoperative donation up to 5 weeks before the planned surgery (e.g., heart, orthopedic, plastic, or gynecological). The client can donate 1 to 5 units of his or her own blood depending on the type of surgery and the ability of the client to maintain an acceptable hematocrit. The blood will be tested for HIV and HBV. Another way to collect blood for an autologous transfusion is during perioperative blood salvage (e.g., during vascular and orthopedic surgery, organ transplant surgery, and traumatic injuries). The blood that has been salvaged is then reinfused during the surgery. Blood can also be salvaged postoperatively from mediastinal and chest-tube drainage and after joint and spinal surgery. Autologous transfusions are safer for the client because they decrease the risk of complications such as mismatched blood and exposure to blood-borne infectious agents.

Blood Transfusions. Transfusing blood or blood components is a nursing procedure. The nurse is responsible for assessment before, during, and after the transfusion and for regulation of the transfusion. Assessment is critical because of the risk of allergic reactions.

If the client has an IV line in place, the nurse should assess the venipuncture site for signs of infection or infiltration. The nurse should also determine the gauge of the IV catheter. A large catheter such as an 18 gauge or 19 gauge is preferred because blood is thicker and stickier than IV fluids, although smaller gauge sizes will accommodate transfusions. The nurse should determine that the IV catheter is patent and functioning properly. The tubing for blood administration has an in-line filter (Figure 40-18). The tubing should be filled with 0.9% normal saline to prevent **hemolysis,** or breakdown of RBCs.

Pretransfusion assessment also includes obtaining information from the client. The nurse asks whether the client knows the reason for the blood transfusion and whether the client has ever had a previous transfusion or transfusion reaction. A client who has had a transfusion reaction is usually at no greater risk for a reaction with a subsequent transfusion. However, the client may be anxious about the transfusion, requiring nursing intervention. Before giving a transfusion, the nurse explains the proce-

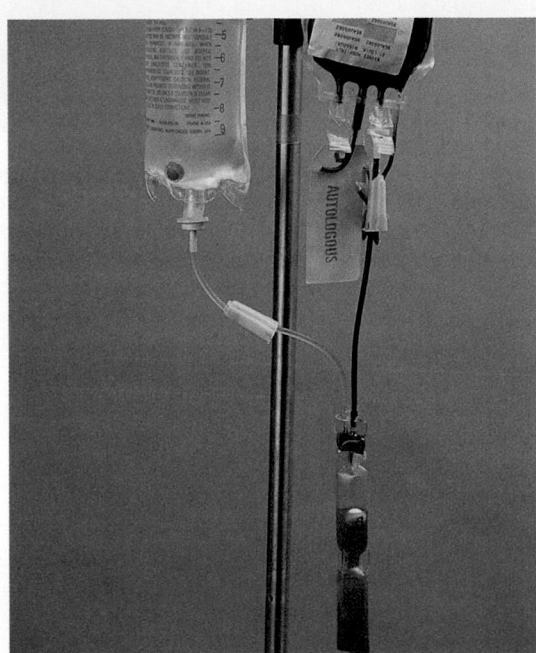

FIGURE **40–18** Tubing for blood administration has an in-line filter.

Cultural Aspects of Care   *Box 40-7*

When a client's natural skin contains more melanin, it becomes more difficult to determine color changes. Early assessment for IV complications such as phlebitis and infiltration may not be easily detected.
Clients within certain cultural backgrounds have fear related to the donor process for blood.
Clients with certain religious or personal beliefs may abstain from receiving blood transfusions and/or medications.

Implications for Practice

- Use light palpation to assess for tenderness associated with phlebitis.
- Use light palpation to assess for edema and coolness associated with infiltration.
- Assess clients individually to determine their acceptance or abstinence toward therapeutic regimens.
- Appreciate clients' choice related to their therapy.
- Although some clients will abstain from receiving whole blood or packed red blood cells, there are other blood products or alternatives that they will accept.

Modified from Rudnicke C: Transfusion alternatives, *J Infus Nurs* 26(3):29, 2003.

dure and instructs the client to report any side effects (e.g., chills, dizziness, or fever) once the transfusion begins. The nurse also checks to be sure the client has signed an informed consent. Clients with certain cultural backgrounds may abstain from blood transfusions (Box 40-7).

Because of the danger of transfusion reactions, it is very important to use specific precautions in administering blood or blood products. The nurse must obtain the client's baseline vital signs before the transfusion begins. This data will allow the nurse to determine when changes in vital signs occur, which can indicate that a transfusion reaction is developing. To ensure that the right client receives the correct type of blood or blood product, a thorough procedure is used to check the identity of the blood products, the client, and the compatibility of the blood and the client. The nurse, although not involved in the blood labeling process, is responsible for determining that the blood delivered to the client corresponds to the client's blood type listed in the medical record. Two registered nurses or one registered nurse and a licensed practical nurse (see agency policy) must together check the label on the blood product against the client's identification number, blood group, and complete name. If even a minor discrepancy exists, the blood should not be given and the blood bank should be notified immediately.

Initiation of a transfusion begins slowly to allow for the early detection of a transfusion reaction. The nurse maintains the infusion rate, monitors for side effects, assesses vital signs, and promptly records all findings. The nurse usually stays with the client during the first 15 minutes, the time when a reaction is most likely to occur. The nurse will continue to monitor the client and obtain vital signs periodically during the transfusion as directed by agency policy. If a transfusion reaction is anticipated or

suspected, the nurse will obtain vital signs more frequently (Table 40-11).

The rate of transfusion is usually specified in the physician's orders. Ideally a unit of whole blood or packed RBCs is transfused in 2 hours. This time can be lengthened to 4 hours if the client is at risk for FVE. Beyond 4 hours there is a risk of the blood becoming contaminated.

When clients have a severe blood loss such as with hemorrhage, they may receive rapid transfusions through a central venous catheter. A blood-warming device is often necessary, because the tip of the central venous catheter lies in the superior vena cava, above the right atrium. Rapid administration of cold blood can result in cardiac dysrhythmia (Otto, 2001).

Transfusion Reactions. A transfusion reaction is a systemic response by the body to incompatible blood. Causes include red cell incompatibility or allergic sensitivity to the components of the transfused blood or to the potassium or citrate preservative in the blood. Blood transfusion can also result in the transmission of infectious disease. Several types of acute reactions can result from blood transfusions (see Table 40-9, p. 1192).

A second category of reactions includes diseases transmitted by infected blood donors who are asymptomatic. Diseases transmitted through transfusions are malaria, hepatitis, and AIDS. Because all units of blood collected must undergo serological testing and screening for HIV and HBV, the risk of acquiring blood-borne infections from blood transfusions is reduced.

Circulatory overload is a risk when a client receives massive whole blood or packed RBC transfusions for massive hemorrhagic shock or when a client with normal

Table 40-11   **Acute Transfusion Reactions**

Reaction	Cause	Clinical Manifestations	Management	Prevention
Acute hemolytic	Infusion of ABO-incompatible whole blood, RBCs, or components containing 10 ml or more of RBCs. Antibodies in the recipient's plasma attach to antigens on transfused RBCs, causing RBC destruction	Chills, fever, low back pain, flushing, tachycardia, tachypnea, hypotension, vascular collapse, hemoglobinuria, hemoglobinemia, bleeding, acute renal failure, shock, cardiac arrest, death	Stop transfusion. Treat shock, if present. Draw blood samples for serological testing slowly to avoid hemolysis from the procedure. Send urine specimen to the laboratory. Maintain BP with IV colloid solutions. Give diuretics as prescribed to maintain urine flow. Insert indwelling catheter or measure voided amounts to monitor hourly urine output. Dialysis may be required if renal failure occurs. Do not transfuse additional RBC-containing components until transfusion service has provided newly crossmatched units.	Meticulously verify and document client identification from sample collection to component infusion.
Febrile, nonhemolytic (most common)	Sensitization to donor white blood cells, platelets, or plasma proteins	Sudden chills and fever (rise in temperature of greater than 1° C), headache, flushing, anxiety, muscle pain	Give antipyretics as prescribed—avoid aspirin in thrombocytopenic patients. **Safety Alert. Do not restart transfusion.**	Consider leukocyte-poor blood products (filtered, washed, or frozen).
Mild allergic	Sensitivity to foreign plasma proteins	Flushing, itching, urticaria (hives)	Give antihistamine as directed. If symptoms are mild and transient, transfusion may be restarted slowly. **Safety Alert. Do not restart transfusion if fever or pulmonary symptoms develop.**	Treat prophylactically with antihistamines.
Anaphylactic	Infusion of IgA proteins to IgA-deficient recipient who has developed IgA antibody	Anxiety, urticaria, wheezing, progressing to cyanosis, shock, possible cardiac arrest	Initiate CPR, if indicated. Have epinephrine ready for injection (0.4 ml of a 1:1000 solution subcutaneously or 0.1 ml of 1:1000 solution diluted to 10 ml with saline for IV use). **Safety Alert. Do not restart transfusion.**	Transfuse extensively washed RBC products, from which all plasma has been removed. Alternately, use blood from IgA-deficient donor.
Circulatory overload	Fluid administered faster than the circulation can accommodate	Cough, dyspnea, pulmonary congestion (rales), headache, hypertension, tachycardia, distended neck veins	Place client upright with feet in dependent position. Administer prescribed diuretics, oxygen, morphine. Phlebotomy may be indicated.	Adjust transfusion volume and flow rate based on client size and clinical status. Have transfusion service divide unit into smaller aliquots for better spacing of fluid input.
Sepsis	Transfusion of contaminated blood components	Rapid onset of chills, high fever, vomiting, diarrhea, and marked hypotension and shock	Obtain culture of client's blood and send bag with remaining blood to transfusion service for further study. Treat septicemia as directed—antibiotics, IV fluids, vasopressors, steroids.	Collect, process, store, and transfuse blood products according to blood banking standards and infuse within 4 hours of starting time.

Data from Young J: Transfusion reaction, *Nursing* 30(12):33, 2000; and Vengelen-Tyler V, editor: *AABB technical manual,* ed 13, Bethesda, Md, 1999, AABB.

ABO, Blood group consisting of groups A, AB, B, and O; *RBCs,* red blood cells; *BP,* blood pressure; *IV,* intravenous; *IgA,* immunoglobulin A; *CPR,* cardiopulmonary resuscitation.

blood volume receives blood. Clients particularly at risk for circulatory overload are older adults and those with cardiopulmonary diseases.

Blood transfusion reactions are life threatening, but prompt nursing intervention can maintain the client's physiological stability.

> **Safety Alert.** If a blood reaction is suspected, the nurse *stops the transfusion immediately.*

- The nurse keeps the IV line open by "piggybacking" 0.9% normal saline directly into the IV line and running the saline.
- The nurse should not turn off the blood and simply turn on the 0.9% normal saline that is connected to the Y-tubing infusion set. This would cause blood remaining in the Y-tubing to infuse into the client. Even a small amount of mismatched blood can cause a major reaction.
- The nurse has the physician notified immediately.
- The nurse remains with the client, observing signs and symptoms and monitoring vital signs as often as every 5 minutes.
- The nurse prepares to administer emergency drugs such as antihistamines, vasopressors, fluids, and steroids as per physician order or protocol.
- The nurse prepares to perform cardiopulmonary resuscitation.
- The nurse obtains a urine specimen and sends it to the laboratory to determine presence of hemoglobin as a result of RBC hemolysis.
- The blood container, tubing, attached labels, and transfusion record are saved and returned to the laboratory.

Interventions for Acid-Base Imbalances. Nursing interventions to promote acid-base balance support prescribed medical therapies and are aimed at reversing the acid-base imbalance that exists. Such imbalances can be life threatening and require rapid correction. The nurse must maintain a functional IV line and frequently check the physician's orders for new medications or fluids. Prescribed drugs, such as insulin or sodium bicarbonate, and fluid and electrolyte replacement should be given promptly. Chapter 39 reviews appropriate therapies for clients with respiratory acidosis.

The nurse also monitors clients closely for changes in acid-base balance. Clients with acid-base disturbances usually require repeated ABG analysis. This procedure provides arterial blood samples for analysis of hydrogen ion concentration.

Arterial Blood Gases. Determination of ABG levels requires the removal of a sample of blood from an artery to assess the client's acid-base status and the adequacy of ventilation and oxygenation. Arterial blood is drawn from a peripheral artery (usually the radial) or from an arterial line inserted by a physician. In some agencies, nurses are responsible for radial artery punctures. Beginning nursing students do not draw arterial samples but frequently assist in the sampling process and care for the client after the procedure. After the specimen is obtained, care is taken to prevent air from entering the syringe because this will affect the blood gas analysis. To re-

duce metabolism of cells, the syringe is submerged in crushed ice and transported immediately to the laboratory. The nurse applies pressure to the puncture site for at least 5 minutes to reduce the risk of hematoma formation. The nurse might also reassess the radial pulse after pressure has been removed.

Restorative Care. After experiencing acute alterations in fluid, electrolyte, or acid-base balance, clients often require ongoing maintenance to prevent a recurrence of health alterations. Older adults and the chronically ill require special considerations to prevent complications from developing (see Box 40-6, p. 1174).

Home Intravenous Therapy. Intravenous therapy is often continued in the home setting for clients who are discharged from the hospital and have not completed their prescribed treatment. The presence of a family member at home is preferred who can be available if the client suddenly cannot manage the IV or if a problem develops. A home IV therapy nurse will work closely with the client to ensure that a sterile IV system is maintained and that complications can be avoided or recognized promptly. Box 40-8 summarizes client education guidelines for home IV therapy.

Nutritional Support. Most clients who have had electrolyte disorders or metabolic acid-base disturbances require ongoing nutritional support. Depending on the type of disorder, fluid or food intake may be encouraged or restricted (see Chapter 43).

Medication Safety. Numerous drugs contain components or create potential side effects that can alter fluid and electrolyte balance. Clients with chronic disease who are receiving multiple medications and those with renal or liver disorders are at significant risk for alterations to develop. Once clients return to a restorative care setting, whether in the home, long-term care, or a nursing home, drug safety becomes very important. Client and family education is essential to provide information on knowing what is contained in a drug and what side effects to observe for. The nurse should review all medications with clients and encourage them to consult with their local pharmacist, especially if they try a new over-the-counter medication.

Evaluation

Client Care. The evaluation of a client's clinical status is especially important if an acute fluid and electrolyte or acid-base disturbance exists. The client's condition can change very quickly, and the nurse must be able to recognize the signs and symptoms of impending problems. To do this well, the nurse integrates what he or she knows about the health alterations, the effects of medications and fluids, and the client's presenting clinical status (Figure 40-19).

The nurse will perform evaluative measures and determine if changes have occurred from the last client as-

Client Teaching

Home Intravenous Therapy

Objective

- The client and caregiver will demonstrate understanding and competence with IV therapy for safe delivery in the home setting.

Teaching Strategies

- Explain to client and caregiver the importance of IV therapy in maintaining hydration and access for the delivery of medications.
- Emphasize the risks involved when the IV system is not kept sterile.
- Be sure the client and/or caregiver is able to manipulate the required equipment.
- Instruct client or caregiver in how to change IV solutions, tubing, and dressing when they become soiled or dislodged. (NOTE: The home care nurse may be able to visit frequently enough to perform scheduled tubing and dressing changes.)

- Instruct client and caregiver about signs and symptoms of infiltration, phlebitis, and infection and to notify the home care nurse immediately.
- Instruct client and caregiver to notify the home care nurse if the infusion slows or stops or if blood is seen in the tubing.
- Teach client with caregiver's assistance how to ambulate, perform hygiene, and participate in other activities of daily living without dislodging or disconnecting catheter and tubing.

Evaluation

- Ask client and caregiver why it is necessary to maintain hydration and IV access for the delivery of medications.
- Ask client and caregiver what to do if IV stops.
- Ask the client and caregiver to describe signs and symptoms of complications and the action they should take.
- Observe the client or caregiver changing the IV container, tubing, and dressing.
- Observe the client ambulate and participate in activities of daily living to see how he or she protects and manipulates the IV catheter and apparatus.

---

sessment. For example, if the nurse's assessment of a client's hypokalemia is showing signs of improvement, the physical signs and symptoms of hypokalemia should begin to disappear or lessen in intensity. The client's heart rhythm becomes more regular and normal bowel function returns.

For clients with less acute alterations, evaluation likely occurs over a longer period of time. In this situation the nurse's evaluation may be focused more on behavioral changes (e.g., the client's ability to follow dietary restrictions and medication schedules). The family's ability to anticipate alterations and prevent problems from recurring is also an important element of evaluation.

The client's level of progress determines whether the nurse needs to continue or revise the plan of care. If goals are not met as a result of the failure to meet expected outcomes, the nurse may need to consult with a physician and discuss additional methods such as increasing the frequency of an intervention (e.g., provide more fluids to a dehydrated client), introducing a new therapy (e.g., initiate insertion of an IV), or discontinuing a particular therapy. Once outcomes have been met, the nurse can resolve the nursing diagnosis and focus on other priorities.

Client Expectations. The nurse routinely reviews with the client his or her success in meeting the client's expectations of care. "Tell me if I have helped you feel more comfortable" is a question that the nurse might raise if the client's expectations revolve around comfort and symptom management. If the client's concerns involve having a better understanding of a chronic problem, the nurse's evaluation might focus on the client's satisfaction with educational offerings. Often the client's level of satisfaction with care also depends on the nurse's success in

involving family and friends. If the client has concerns about returning home or to a different care setting, it will be important to evaluate if the client feels prepared for the transition from acute care.

Key Concepts

- Body fluids are distributed in ECF and ICF compartments.
- Body fluids are composed of electrolytes, minerals, cells, and water.
- Body fluids are regulated through fluid intake, output, and hormonal regulation.
- Volume disturbances include isotonic and osmolar deficits and excesses.
- Electrolytes are regulated by dietary intake and hormonal controls.
- Acid-base imbalances are buffered by chemical, biological, and physiological buffering, especially the lungs and kidneys.
- Chronic and serious illnesses increase the risk of fluid, electrolyte, and acid-base imbalances.
- Clients who are very young or very old are at greater risk for fluid, electrolyte, and acid-base imbalances.
- Assessment for fluid, electrolyte, and acid-base alterations includes the nursing history, physical and behavioral assessment, measurements of I&O, daily weights, and specific laboratory data.
- Osmolar imbalances and FVD can be corrected by enteral or parenteral administration of fluid.
- Common complications of IV therapy include infiltration, phlebitis, infection, FVE, and bleeding at the infusion site.

KNOWLEDGE

- Characteristics of normal fluid and electrolyte balances
- Characteristics of normal acid-base balance
- Pathophysiologic effects on fluid, electrolyte, and acid-base balances
- Effects of nursing interventions on fluid and electrolyte balance

EXPERIENCE

- Previous client responses to planned nursing therapies for improving fluid balance (what worked and what did not work)

Evaluation

- Reassess signs and symptoms of the client's fluid and/or acid-base balances
- Ask the client for perceptions of fluid balance after interventions
- Ask if the client's expectations are being met

STANDARDS

- Use established expected outcomes to evaluate the client's response to care (e.g., mucous membranes will be moist, BP remains at 10% of baseline)

ATTITUDES

- Display integrity when identifying those interventions that were not successful
- Be independent when redesigning successful hospital-based interventions for the home care setting

FIGURE **40–19** Critical thinking model for fluid, electrolyte, and acid-base balances evaluation.

- Blood transfusions are given to replace fluid volume loss from hemorrhage, treat anemia, or replace coagulation factors.
- Blood transfusions can be donor, autologous, or obtained through perioperative salvage.
- Administration of blood or blood products requires the nurse to follow a specific procedure to identify transfusion reactions quickly.
- In addition to transfusion reactions, the risks of transfusion also include hyperkalemia, hypocalcemia, FVE, and infection.
- Treatment for electrolyte disturbances include dietary and pharmacological interventions.
- The body's chemical buffering system responds first to acid-base abnormalities.

- The goals of therapy for acid-base imbalances are to treat the underlying illness and to restore the arterial pH to normal.

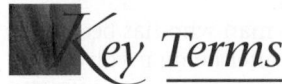 *ey Terms*

Active transport, *p. 1137*
Aldosterone, *p. 1138*
Angiotensin, *p. 1138*
Anion gap, *p. 1144*
Anions, *p. 1136*
Antidiuretic hormone (ADH), *p. 1138*

Arterial blood gas (ABG), *p. 1143*
Autologous transfusion, *p. 1190*
Buffer, *p. 1140*
Cations, *p. 1136*

Key Terms—cont'd

Colloid osmotic pressure, *p. 1137*	Intravascular fluid, *p. 1136*
Colloids, *p. 1159*	Ions, *p. 1136*
Concentration gradient, *p. 1137*	Isotonic, *p. 1137*
Crystalloids, *p. 1159*	Metabolic acidosis, *p. 1144*
Dehydration, *p. 1138*	Metabolic alkalosis, *p. 1144*
Diffusion, *p. 1137*	Milliequivalents per liter (mEq/L), *p. 1136*
Edema, *p. 1137*	Oncotic pressure, *p. 1137*
Electrolytes, *p. 1136*	Osmolarity, *p. 1136*
Erythema, *p. 1189*	Osmols, *p. 1136*
Extracellular fluids, *p. 1136*	Osmoreceptors, *p. 1138*
Filtration, *p. 1137*	Osmosis, *p. 1136*
Fluid volume deficit (FVD), *p. 1147*	Osmotic pressure, *p. 1136*
Fluid volume excess (FVE), *p. 1159*	Phlebitis, *p. 1189*
	Renin, *p. 1138*
Hemolysis, *p. 1190*	Respiratory acidosis, *p. 1144*
Homeostasis, *p. 1137*	Respiratory alkalosis, *p. 1144*
Hydrostatic pressure, *p. 1137*	Sensible water loss, *p. 1139*
Hypertonic, *p. 1137*	Solute, *p. 1136*
Hypotonic, *p. 1137*	Solution, *p. 1136*
Hypovolemia, *p. 1138*	Solvent, *p. 1136*
Infiltration, *p. 1189*	Total parenteral nutrition, *p. 1160*
Infusion pumps, *p. 1179*	Transfusion reaction, *p. 1190*
Insensible water loss, *p. 1139*	Vascular access devices, *p. 1159*
Interstitial fluid, *p. 1136*	Venipuncture, *p. 1174*
Intracellular fluids, *p. 1136*	

Critical Thinking Exercises

1. Mrs. Emanuele is an 81-year-old admitted to the hospital with a 3-day history of vomiting and diarrhea. She has had only ice chips since the first episode of vomiting and is now complaining of malaise, cramping muscles, and a temperature of 101° F. Which laboratory findings would you expect to be abnormal based on her complaints? What interventions would you expect the physician to order?
2. Caroline has just received a new client on her unit who is to receive 1 unit of RBCs within the next hour. What nursing actions are necessary before administering blood? What are the signs and symptoms of a transfusion reaction? Can Caroline delegate the administration of blood to a licensed practical nurse or a nursing assistant on her team?
3. Bob is caring for a 52-year-old man who has been seen in the emergency department after being involved in a motor vehicle accident. He is complaining of difficulty breathing and a respiratory rate of 40 breaths per minute. Bob's client is transferred to the intensive care unit, intubated, and placed on a ventilator. After the client leaves, a nursing student asks Bob to interpret his client's last ABG results: pH, 7.30; PaO₂, 70; PaCO₂, 50; HCO₃, 24. What interpretation will Bob give to the student nurse? What is the relationship between the ABG results and the client being intubated and ventilated?

4. Jane is the nurse caring for Betty, a 59-year-old who has just had a total knee replacement. The physician has ordered Ancef 1 g in 50 ml to run over 30 minutes IV piggyback tid. Betty has a continuous infusion of Ringer's lactate at 75 ml/hr in the left forearm. What type of tubing will Jane use to administer the IV piggyback medication? Calculate the drops per minute of the piggyback using both microtubing (60 drops/ml) and macrotubing (15 drops/ml).
5. John Patrick, a 24-year-old tennis professional, was admitted to the clinic with a temperature of 105° F. He has a history of playing in a 5-hour tennis match in 100° F heat. His coach brought him to the clinic because he was weak and lethargic. What assessment findings would the nurse expect to find? What interventions would be necessary? Describe a teaching plan for John upon discharge.

Review Questions

1. One of the most common electrolyte imbalances is:
   1. Hypokalemia.
   2. Hyperkalemia.
   3. Hyponatremia.
   4. Hypocalcemia.

2. The client most at risk for fluid volume deficits (FVDs) is a (an):
   1. Elder adult.
   2. Adult.
   3. Child.
   4. Infant.

3. One reason older adults experience fluid and electrolyte imbalance and acid-base imbalances, is they:
   1. Eat poor-quality food.
   2. Have a decreased thirst sensation.
   3. Have more stress response.
   4. Have an overly active thirst response.

4. Output recorded on an Intake and Output record (I&O) includes:
   1. Urine, vomitus, diarrhea, and drainage from wounds.
   2. Diarrhea, gastric suction, and drainage from wounds.
   3. Medications, juices, and water.
   4. Urine, diarrhea, vomitus, gastric suction, and drainage from wounds or tubes.

5. Health promotion activities in the area of fluid and electrolyte imbalances focuses primarily on:
   1. Client teaching.
   2. Dietary intake.
   3. Medication regimen.
   4. Physician involvement in care.

6. Total parenteral nutrition (TPN) is delivered by which of the following methods?
   1. Mouth and rectum.
   2. Mouth and intravenous.
   3. Indwelling or central IV catheter.
   4. Via a nasogastric tube.

7. As a safety alert the nurse is aware the following medication is never given directly intravenously:
   1. Potassium chloride (KCl).
   2. Lasix.
   3. Dextrose.
   4. Calcium gluconate.

8. Many factors are initially controlled for in the IV insertion procedure. This nurse understands this begins with:
   1. Hand hygiene.
   2. Checking sterility of supplies.
   3. Ensuring the six rights of medication administration.
   4. Carefully checking the order for the IV therapy.

9. Indications of IV fluid infiltration include:
   1. Phlebitis and coolness.
   2. Edema and erythema.
   3. Pallor and coolness
   4. Pain and erythema.

10. The Centers for Disease Control (CDC) recommends that replacing peripheral venous catheters and rotating sites should occur at least every:
    1. 72 to 96 hours.
    2. 48 to 72 hours.
    3. 24 to 48 hours.
    4. 48 hours.

*R*eferences

Centers for Disease Control and Prevention: Guidelines for the prevention of intravascular catheter-related infections, *MMWR Morb Mortal Wkly Rep* 51(RR-10), 2002.

Christensen B, Kockrow E: *Foundations of nursing,* ed 4, St. Louis, 2003, Mosby.

Dochterman JM, Bulechek GM: *Nursing interventions classification (NIC),* ed 4, St. Louis, 2004, Mosby.

Ellenberger A: Starting an IV line, *Nursing* 99(3):56, 1999.

Groer MW: *Advanced pathophysiology: application to clinical practice,* St. Louis, 2000, Mosby.

Heitz UE, Horne MM: *Mosby's pocket guide series: fluid, electrolyte, and acid-base balance,* ed 4, St. Louis, 2001, Mosby.

Ignatavicius D, Workman MJ: *Medical-surgical nursing,* ed 4, Philadelphia, 2002, WB Saunders.

Infusion Nurses Society: Infusion nursing standards of practice, *J Intraven Nurs* 23(6S)51, 2000.

Lewis SM and others: *Medical-surgical nursing: assessment and management of clinical problems,* ed 6, St. Louis, 2002, Mosby.

Lueckenotte A: *Gerontologic nursing,* ed 2, St. Louis, 2000, Mosby.

McCance KL, Huether SE: *Pathophysiology: the biologic basis for disease in adults and children,* ed 4, St. Louis, 2002, Mosby.

McKenry LM, Salerno E: *Mosby's pharmacology in nursing,* ed 21, St. Louis, 2003, Mosby.

Metheney NM: *Fluid and electrolyte balance: nursing considerations,* ed 4, Philadelphia, 2000, JB Lippincott.

Millam DA and others: On the road to successful IV starts, *Nursing* 30(4):34, 2000.

Moorhead S, Johnson M, Maas M: *Nursing outcomes classification (NOC),* ed 3, St. Louis, 2004, Mosby.

Otto SE: *Pocket guide to intravenous therapy,* ed 4, St. Louis, 2001, Mosby.

Phillips D: *Manual of IV therapeutics,* ed 3, Philadelphia, 2001, FA Davis.

Phipps and others: *Medical-surgical nursing: health and illness perspectives,* ed 7, St. Louis, 2003, Mosby.

Rudnicke C: Transfusion alternatives, *J Infus Nurs* 26(3):29, 2003.

Speakman ES, Weldy NJ: *Body fluids and electrolytes: a programmed presentation,* ed 8, St. Louis, 2002, Mosby.

Vengelen-Tyler V, editor: AABB *Technical manual,* ed 13, Bethesda, Md, 1999, AABB.

Woods AW: Pneumonia, *Nursing* 32(11):56, 2000.

Young, J: Transfusion reaction, *Nursing* 30(12):33, 2000.

*R*esearch References

Chukhraev AM, Grekov IG: Local complications of nursing interventions on peripheral veins, *J Infus Nurs* 23(3), 167, 2000.

Saladow J: The use of vascular access devices with needle safety features, *JVAD* 7(3):41, 2002.

Toth L: Monitoring infusion therapy in patients residing in long-term care facilities, *JVAD* 7(1): 34-38, 2002.

Wise L and others: Evaluating the reliability and utility of cumulative intake and output, *J Nurs Care Qual* 14(3):37, 2000.

41

_S_leep

http://evolve.elsevier.com/Potter/fundamentals/

Media Resources

CD COMPANION

- Review Questions
- Glossary

evolve WEBSITE

- Review Questions
- Student Learning Activities
- Concept Map Exercise
- Critical Thinking Exercise
- Glossary

Objectives

Mastery of content in this chapter will enable the student to:

- Define the key terms listed.
- Compare the characteristics of rest and sleep.
- Explain the effect the 24-hour sleep-wake cycle has on biological function.
- Discuss mechanisms that regulate sleep.
- Describe the stages of a normal sleep cycle.
- Explain the functions of sleep.
- Compare and contrast the sleep requirements of different age-groups.
- Identify factors that normally promote and disrupt sleep.
- Discuss characteristics of common sleep disorders.
- Conduct a sleep history for a client.
- Identify nursing diagnoses appropriate for clients with sleep alterations.
- Identify nursing interventions designed to promote normal sleep cycles for clients of all ages.
- Describe ways to evaluate sleep therapies.

*P*roper rest and sleep are as important to good health as good nutrition and adequate exercise. Individuals need different amounts of sleep and rest. Physical and emotional health depends on the ability to fulfill these basic human needs. Without proper amounts of rest and sleep, the ability to concentrate, make judgments, and participate in daily activities decreases and irritability increases.

Identifying and treating clients' sleep pattern disturbances is an important goal for a nurse. To help clients, a nurse must understand the nature of sleep, the factors influencing it, and clients' sleep habits. Clients require an individualized approach based on their personal habits and pattern of sleep, as well as the particular problem influencing sleep. Nursing interventions can be effective in resolving short- and long-term sleep disturbances.

One theory about the function of sleep is that it is associated with healing and restoration (McCance and Huether, 2002). Achieving the best possible sleep quality is important for the promotion of good health as well as the recovery from illness. Nurses care for clients who often have preexisting sleep disturbances and for clients who develop sleep problems as a result of illness or hospitalization. Sometimes clients seek health care because they have a sleep problem that may have gone unnoticed for many years. Ill clients often require more sleep and rest than healthy clients. However, the nature of illness may prevent clients from gaining adequate rest and sleep. The institutional environment of a hospital or long-term care facility and the activities of health care personnel make sleep difficult.

Scientific Knowledge Base

Physiology of Sleep

Sleep is a cyclical physiological process that alternates with longer periods of wakefulness. The sleep-wake cycle influences and regulates physiological function and behavioral responses.

Circadian Rhythms. People experience cyclical rhythms as part of their everyday life. The most familiar rhythm is the 24-hour, day-night cycle known as the diurnal or **circadian rhythm** (derived from Latin: *circa,* "about," and *dies,* "day"). A woman's menstrual cycle is an infradian rhythm, one that occurs in a cycle longer than 24 hours. Biological cycles lasting less than 24 hours are called ultradian rhythms. Circadian rhythms influence the pattern of major biological and behavioral functions. The fluctuation and predictability of body temperature, heart rate, blood pressure, hormone secretion, sensory acuity, and mood depend on the maintenance of the 24-hour circadian cycle.

Circadian rhythms, including daily sleep-wake cycles, are affected by light and temperature and external factors such as social activities and work routines. All persons have **biological clocks** that synchronize their sleep cycles. Some people can fall asleep at 8 PM, whereas others go to bed at midnight or early in the morning. Different people also function best at different times of the day.

Hospitals or extended care facilities usually do not adapt care to an individual's sleep-wake cycle preferences. Typical routines cause interruptions in sleep or prevent clients from falling asleep at their usual time. If a person's sleep-wake cycle is altered significantly, a poor quality of sleep can result. Reversals in the sleep-wake cycle such as falling asleep during the day (or vice versa for people who work nights) can indicate a serious illness. Anxiety, restlessness, irritability, and impaired judgment are common symptoms of disturbances in the sleep cycle.

The biological rhythm of sleep frequently becomes synchronized with other body functions. Changes in body temperature, for example, correlate with sleep patterns. Normally, body temperature peaks in the afternoon, decreases gradually, and then drops sharply after a person falls asleep. When the sleep-wake cycle becomes disrupted (e.g., by working rotating shifts), other physiological functions may change as well. For example, the person may experience a decreased appetite and lose weight (National Sleep Foundation, 2001). Failure to maintain the individual's usual sleep-wake cycle can adversely influence the client's overall health.

Sleep Regulation. Sleep involves a sequence of physiological states maintained by highly integrated central nervous system (CNS) activity that is associated with changes in the peripheral nervous, endocrine, cardiovascular, respiratory, and muscular systems (McCance and Huether, 2002). Each sequence can be identified by specific physiological responses and patterns of brain activity. Instruments such as the electroencephalogram (EEG), which measures electrical activity in the cerebral cortex, the electromyogram (EMG), which measure muscle tone,

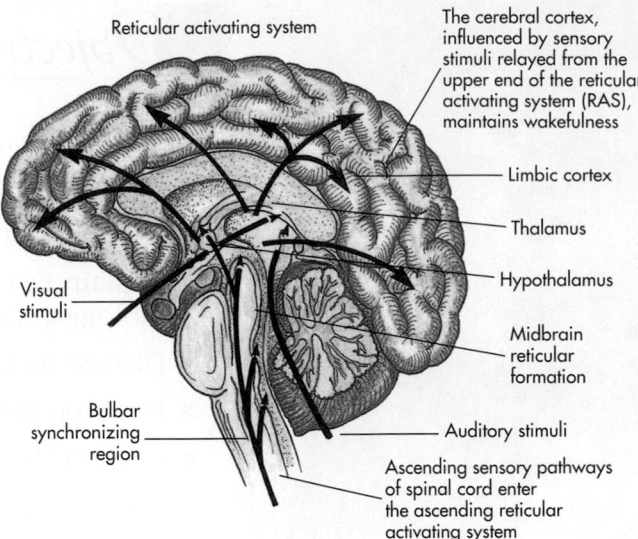

FIGURE 41-1 RAS and BSR control sensory input, intermittently activating and suppressing the brain's higher centers to control sleep and wakefulness.

and the electrooculogram (EOG), which measures eye movements, provide information about some structural physiological aspects of sleep.

Current theory indicates sleep is thought to be an active inhibitory process. Therefore, the control and regulation of sleep may depend on the interrelationship between two cerebral mechanisms that intermittently activate and suppress the brain's higher centers to control sleep and wakefulness (Zachary, 2000). One mechanism causes wakefulness, whereas the other causes sleep. The ascending reticular activating system (RAS) located in the upper brain stem is believed to contain special cells that maintain alertness and wakefulness. The RAS receives visual, auditory, pain, and tactile sensory stimuli. Activity from the cerebral cortex (e.g., emotions or thought processes) also stimulates the RAS. Wakefulness results from neurons in the RAS that release catecholamines such as norepinephrine (Chokroverty, 2000).

Sleep may be produced by the release of serotonin from specialized cells in the raphe sleep system of the pons and medulla. This area of the brain is also called the bulbar synchronizing region (BSR). Whether a person remains awake or falls asleep depends on a balance of impulses received from higher centers (e.g., thoughts), peripheral sensory receptors (e.g., sound or light stimuli), and the limbic system (emotions) (Figure 41-1).

As people try to fall asleep, they close their eyes and assume relaxed positions. Stimuli to the RAS decline. If the room is dark and quiet, activation of the RAS further declines. At some point the BSR takes over, causing sleep.

Stages of Sleep. EEG, EMG, and EOG electrical signals show that different brain-wave, muscle, and eye activity are associated with different stages of sleep (Zachary, 2000). Normal sleep involves two phases: **nonrapid eye movement (NREM) sleep** and **rapid eye movement (REM) sleep** (Box 41-1). During NREM a sleeper pro-

---

Box **41-1**   **Stages of the Sleep Cycle**

Stage 1: NREM

Includes lightest level of sleep.
Stage lasts a few minutes.
Decreased physiological activity begins with gradual fall in vital signs and metabolism.
Person is easily aroused by sensory stimuli such as noise.
Awakened, person feels as though daydreaming has occurred.

Stage 2: NREM

Period of sound sleep.
Relaxation progresses.
Arousal remains relatively easy.
Stage lasts 10 to 20 minutes.
Body functions continue to slow.

Stage 3: NREM

Involves initial stages of deep sleep.
Sleeper is difficult to arouse and rarely moves.
Muscles are completely relaxed.
Vital signs decline but remain regular.
Stage lasts 15 to 30 minutes.

Stage 4: NREM

Deepest stage of sleep.
Very difficult to arouse sleeper.
If sleep loss has occurred, sleeper will spend considerable portion of night in this stage.
Vital signs are significantly lower than during waking hours.
Stage lasts approximately 15 to 30 minutes.
Sleepwalking and enuresis may occur.

REM Sleep

Vivid, full-color dreaming may occur.
Less vivid dreaming may occur in other stages.
Stage usually begins about 90 minutes after sleep has begun.
Typified by autonomic response of rapidly moving eyes, fluctuating heart and respiratory rates, and increased or fluctuating blood pressure.
Loss of skeletal muscle tone occurs.
Gastric secretions increase.
Very difficult to arouse sleeper.
Duration of REM sleep increases with each cycle and averages 20 minutes.

---

gresses through four stages during a typical 90-minute sleep cycle. The quality of sleep from stage 1 through stage 4 becomes increasingly deep. Lighter sleep is characteristic of stages 1 and 2, and a person is more easily arousable. Stages 3 and 4 involve a deeper sleep, called slow-wave sleep, from which a person is more difficult to arouse. Rapid eye movement sleep is the phase at the end of each sleep cycle. Different factors may promote or interfere with various stages of the sleep cycle. The nurse chooses therapies that foster sleep or attempts to eliminate factors that can disrupt it.

Sleep Cycle. The normal sleep pattern for an adult begins with a presleep period during which the person is aware only of a gradually developing sleepiness. This period normally lasts 10 to 30 minutes, but if a person has difficulty falling asleep, it may last an hour or more.

Once asleep, the person usually passes through four to six complete sleep cycles per night, each consisting of four stages of NREM sleep and a period of REM sleep (McCance and Huether, 2002). The cyclical pattern usually progresses from stage 1 through stage 4 of NREM, followed by a reversal from stage 4 to 3 to 2, ending with a period of REM sleep (Figure 41-2). A person usually reaches REM sleep about 90 minutes into the sleep cycle.

With each successive cycle, stages 3 and 4 shorten, and the period of REM lengthens. REM sleep may last up to 60 minutes during the last sleep cycle. Not all people progress consistently through the stages of sleep. For example, a sleeper may fluctuate for short intervals between NREM stages 2, 3, and 4 before entering REM stage. The amount of time spent in each stage varies over the life span. Newborns and children spend more time in deep

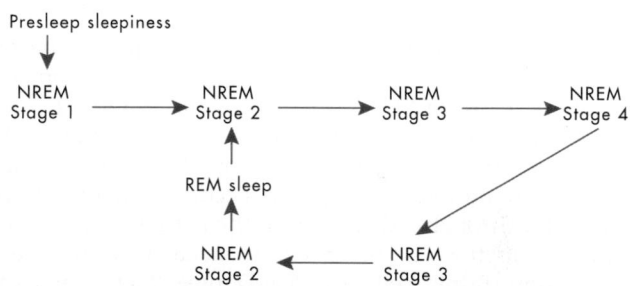

FIGURE **41–2** The stages of the adult sleep cycle.

sleep. With aging, sleep becomes more fragmented and more time is spent in lighter stages (National Sleep Foundation, 2003). Shifts from stage to stage tend to accompany body movements, and shifts to light sleep or wakefulness tend to occur suddenly, whereas shifts to deep sleep tend to be gradual (Zachary, 2000). The number of sleep cycles depends on the total amount of time that the client spends sleeping.

Functions of Sleep

The purpose of sleep remains unclear. Sleep is believed to contribute to physiological and psychological restoration (McCance and Huether, 2002). NREM sleep contributes to body tissue restoration (Chokroverty, 2000). During NREM sleep, biological functions slow. A healthy adult's normal heart rate throughout the day averages 70 to 80 beats per minute or less if the individual is in excellent physical condition. However, during sleep the heart rate falls to 60 beats per minute or less. This means that the heart beats 10 to 20 fewer times in each minute during sleep or 60 to 120 fewer times in each hour. Clearly, restful sleep may be beneficial in preserving cardiac function. Other biological functions decreased during sleep are respirations, blood pressure, and muscle tone (McCance and Huether, 2002).

Sleep appears to be needed to routinely restore biological processes. During deep slow-wave (NREM stage 4) sleep, the body releases human growth hormone for the repair and renewal of epithelial and specialized cells such as brain cells (Jones, 2000; McCance and Huether, 2002). Protein synthesis and cell division for renewal of tissues such as the skin, bone marrow, gastric mucosa, or brain occur during rest and sleep. NREM sleep may be especially important in children, who experience more stage 4 sleep.

Another theory about the purpose of sleep is that the body conserves energy during sleep. The skeletal muscles relax progressively, and the absence of muscular contraction preserves chemical energy for cellular processes. Lowering of the basal metabolic rate further conserves the body's energy supply (Chokroverty, 2000).

REM sleep is needed for brain tissue restoration and appears to be important for cognitive restoration (Chokroverty, 2000). REM sleep is associated with changes in cerebral blood flow, increased cortical activity, increased oxygen consumption, and epinephrine release. This association may assist with memory storage and learning. During sleep, the brain filters stored information about the day's activities.

The benefits of sleep on behavior often go unnoticed until a person develops a problem resulting from sleep deprivation. A loss of REM sleep can lead to feelings of confusion and suspicion. Various body functions (e.g., mood, motor performance, memory, and equilibrium) can be altered when prolonged sleep loss occurs (National Sleep Foundation, 2002b). Alterations in the natural and cellular immune function also occur with moderate to severe sleep deprivation (Brink, Kelly, and Rae-Dupree, 2000). Some of the more recent industrial accidents, such as the nuclear accident in Chernobyl, have been attributed to human error associated with sleep deprivation. Traffic, home, and work-related accidents caused by falling asleep have been estimated to cost billions of dollars a year in the United States (Mahowald, 2000; National Sleep Foundation, 2002b). Because of concern over an increased incidence of automobile accidents, some states in the United States have implemented guidelines regulating the driving privileges of people with disorders that cause excessive sleepiness (Pakola, Dinges, and Pack, 1995).

Dreams. Although dreams occur during both NREM and REM sleep, the dreams of REM sleep are more vivid and elaborate and are believed to be functionally important to learning, memory processing, and adaptation to stress (Pagel, 2000). REM dreams may progress in content throughout the night from dreams about current events to emotional dreams of childhood or the past. Personality can influence the quality of dreams; for example, a creative person may have elaborate and complex dreams, and a depressed person may dream of helplessness.

Most people dream about immediate concerns such as an argument with a spouse, plans for a wedding, or worries over work. Sometimes a person is unaware of fears represented in bizarre dreams. Clinical psychologists often try to analyze the symbolic nature of dreams as part of a client's psychotherapy. Objects in dreams hold symbolic significance. For example, an apple may represent a forbidden object, or a lion may symbolize rage, water often has a sexual meaning. The ability to describe a dream and interpret its significance may help resolve personal concerns or fears.

Another theory suggests that dreams erase certain fantasies or nonsensical memories. Because most dreams are forgotten, many people have little dream recall and do not believe they dream at all. To remember a dream, a person must consciously think about it on awakening. People who recall dreams vividly usually awake just after a period of REM sleep.

Physical Illness

Any illness that causes pain, physical discomfort (e.g., difficulty breathing), or mood problems, such as anxiety or depression, can result in sleep problems. Persons with such alterations may have trouble falling or staying asleep. Illnesses also may force clients to sleep in positions to which they are unaccustomed. For example, assuming an awkward position when an arm or leg has been immobilized in traction can interfere with sleep.

Respiratory disease often interferes with sleep. Clients with chronic lung disease such as emphysema are short of breath and frequently cannot sleep without two or three pillows to raise their heads. Asthma, bronchitis, and allergic rhinitis alter the rhythm of breathing and disturb sleep. A person with a common cold has nasal congestion, sinus drainage, and a sore throat, which impair breathing and the ability to relax.

A connection between heart disease, sleep, and sleep disorders exists. Sleep-related breathing disorders have been linked to increased incidence of high blood pressure and risk of heart diseases and stroke (American Academy of Sleep Medicine, 2002). Hypertension often causes early morning awakening and fatigue. Hypothyroidism decreases stage 4 sleep, whereas hyperthyroidism causes persons to take more time to fall asleep. Last, an increased risk of sudden cardiac death in the first hours after wakening has been identified.

Nocturia, or urination during the night, disrupts sleep and the sleep cycle. This condition is most common in older people with reduced bladder tone or persons with cardiac disease, diabetes, urethritis, or prostatic disease. After a person awakens repeatedly to urinate, returning to sleep may be difficult.

Older adults often experience restless legs syndrome (RLS), which occurs before sleep onset. People experience recurrent, rhythmical movements of the feet and legs. An itching sensation is felt deep in the muscles. Relief comes only from moving the legs, which prevents relaxation and subsequent sleep. Depending on how severely sleep is disrupted, RLS may be a relatively benign condition. Primary restless legs syndrome is a central nervous disorder. Secondary RLS has been found to be associated with lower levels of iron, pregnancy, and uremia (National Heart, Lung, and Blood Institute, 2000). In contrast, people who have severe leg cramps during the night may have a problem with arterial circulation.

Persons with peptic ulcer disease often awaken in the middle of the night. Research results demonstrating a relationship between gastric acid secretion and stages of sleep are conflicting. One consistent finding is that persons with duodenal ulcers fail to suppress acid secretion in the first 2 hours of sleep (Orr, 2000).

Sleep Disorders

Sleep disorders are conditions that, if untreated, generally cause disturbed nighttime sleep that results in one of three problems: insomnia, abnormal movements or sensation during sleep or when awakening at night, or excessive daytime sleepiness (Aldrich and Naylor, 2000). Many adults in the United States have significant sleep debt from inadequacies in either the quantity or quality of their nighttime sleep and experience **hypersomnolence** on a daily basis (National Sleep Foundation, 2002b).

Sleep disorders have been classified into four major categories (American Sleep Disorders Association, 1997) (Box 41-2). The **dyssomnias** are primary disorders that have their origin in different body systems and are subdivided into three major groups: intrinsic, extrinsic, and circadian rhythm disorders. The intrinsic sleep disorders include disorders of initiating and maintaining sleep, that is, various forms of insomnia and disorders of excessive sleepiness such as narcolepsy and obstructive sleep apnea. Extrinsic sleep disorders develop from external factors, which if removed, lead to resolution of the sleep disorder. The circadian rhythm sleep disorders arise from a misalignment between the timing of sleep and what is desired by the individual or is a societal norm. The **parasomnias** are undesirable behaviors that occur predominantly during sleep: arousal disorders, partial arousals, or disorders during transitions in the sleep cycle or from sleep to wakefulness. Many medical and psychiatric sleep disorders are associated with sleep and wake disturbances. These sleep disturbances are divided into those associated with psychiatric, neurological, or other medical specialty

---

Box *41-2*   Classification of Sleep Disorders

Dyssomnias

Intrinsic Sleep Disorders
Psychophysiological insomnia
Narcolepsy
Periodic limb movement disorder
Sleep apnea syndromes

Extrinsic Sleep Disorders
Inadequate sleep hygiene
Insufficient sleep syndrome
Hypnotic-dependent sleep disorders
Alcohol-dependent sleep disorders

Circadian Rhythm Sleep Disorders
Time-zone change (jet lag) syndrome
Shift-work sleep disorder
Delayed sleep phase syndrome

Parasomnias

Arousal Disorders
Sleepwalking
Sleep terrors

Sleep-Wake Transition Disorders
Sleeptalking
Sleep starts
Nocturnal leg cramps

Parasomnias Usually Associated With REM Sleep
Nightmares
REM sleep behavior disorder
Sleep paralysis

Parasomnias—cont'd

Other Parasomnias
Sleep bruxism (teeth grinding)
Sleep enuresis (bed-wetting)
Sudden infant death syndrome

Sleep Disorders Associated With Medical-Psychiatric Disorders

Associated With Psychiatric Disorders
Mood disorders
Anxiety disorders
Psychoses
Alcoholism

Associated With Neurological Disorders
Dementia
Parkinsonism
Central degenerative disorders

Associated With Other Medical Disorders
Nocturnal cardiac ischemia
Chronic obstructive pulmonary disease
Peptic ulcer disease

Proposed Sleep Disorders

Menstruation-associated sleep disorders
Sleep choking syndrome
Pregnancy-associated sleep disorders

Modified from American Sleep Disorders Association, Diagnostic Classification Steering Committee: International classification of sleep disorders, 1997. In Thorpy M: Classification of sleep disorders. In Kryger M and others, editors, *Principles and practice of sleep medicine,* ed 3, Philadelphia, 2000, WB Saunders.

disorders. The proposed sleep disorders are newly described disturbances for which inadequate information currently exists to substantiate their existence.

Sleep laboratory studies such as a nighttime **polysomnogram** (PSG), the Multiple Sleep Latency Test (MSLT), and actigraphy are often used to diagnose a sleep disorder (Mahowald, 2000). A polysomnogram involves the use of EEG, EMG, and EOG to monitor stages of sleep and wakefulness during nighttime sleep. The MSLT provides objective information about sleepiness and selected aspects of sleep structure by measuring eye movements, muscle-tone changes, and brain electrical activity during at least four napping opportunities spread throughout the day. Sleep-onset REM episodes are also noted because this abnormality is associated with several sleep disorders. The MSLT takes 8 to 10 hours to complete. The actigraph is worn on the wrist and measures the sleep-wake patterns of clients over an extended period of time (Attarian, 2000). Actigraphy data provides information on sleep time, sleep efficiency, number and duration of awakenings, and levels of activity and rest (Redecker, 2000).

Insomnia. **Insomnia** is a symptom experienced by clients who have chronic difficulty falling asleep, frequent awakenings from sleep, and/or a short sleep or nonrestorative sleep (Zorick and Walsh, 2000). It is the most common sleep-related complaint (Attarian, 2000). The insomniac complains of excessive daytime sleepiness, as well as insufficient quantity and quality of sleep. Frequently, however, the client gets more sleep than is realized. Insomnia may signal an underlying physical or psychological disorder. Insomnia occurs more frequently in women and is women's most common sleep problem (National Sleep Foundation, 2001).

People may experience transient insomnia as a result of situational stresses such as family, work, or school problems; jet lag; illness; or loss of a loved one. Insomnia may recur, but between episodes the client is able to sleep well. However, a temporary case of insomnia due to a stressful situation can lead to chronic difficulty in obtaining sufficient sleep, perhaps due to the worry and anxiety that develops about obtaining adequate sleep.

Insomnia is often associated with poor **sleep hygiene,** or habits and practices the client uses that are associated with sleep. If the condition continues, the fear of not being able to sleep can be enough to cause wakefulness. During the day, persons with chronic insomnia may feel sleepy, fatigued, depressed, and anxious.

Because there are many causes of insomnia, management involves several approaches (Attarian, 2000). As appropriate, it is important to treat underlying emotional or medical problems that may be causing this nighttime sleep problem. Treatment can also be symptomatic, including improved sleep hygiene measures, biofeedback, cognitive techniques, and relaxation techniques. When insomnia develops secondary to inappropriate health behaviors, treatment is directed at changing these behaviors. For example, in drug-dependence insomnia the client is unable to fall asleep because of excessive use of hypnotic medications. This client usually benefits from a gradual withdrawal of the hypnotics.

Sleep Apnea. **Sleep apnea** is a disorder characterized by the lack of airflow through the nose and mouth for periods of 10 seconds or longer during sleep. There are three types of sleep apnea: central, obstructive, and mixed apnea, which has both a central and an obstructive component.

The most common form is obstructive sleep apnea (OSA). It is estimated that 18 million people in the United States meet the diagnostic criteria for OSA (National Sleep Foundation, 2002a). OSA occurs when muscles or structures of the oral cavity or throat relax during sleep. The upper airway becomes partially or completely blocked, and nasal airflow is diminished (hypopnea) or stopped (apnea) for as long as 30 seconds (Basin and Guilleminault, 2000; Dobbin and Strollo, 2002). The person still attempts to breathe because chest and abdominal movement continue, which often results in loud snoring and snorting sounds. When breathing is partially or completely diminished, each successive diaphragmatic movement becomes stronger until the obstruction is relieved. Structural abnormalities such as a deviated septum, nasal polyps, certain jaw configurations, or enlarged tonsils predispose a client to obstructive apnea. The effort to breathe during sleep results in arousals from deep sleep often to the stage 2 cycle. In severe cases, hundreds of hypopnea/apnea episodes can occur every hour, resulting in severe interference with deep sleep.

Excessive daytime sleepiness (EDS) is the most common complaint of people with OSA. Persons with severe OSA may report taking daytime naps and experiencing a disruption in their daily activities because of sleepiness (National Sleep Foundation, 2002a). Feelings of sleepiness are usually most intense upon awakening from, or right before going to, sleep, and about 12 hours after the midsleep period. EDS often results in impaired waking function, poor work or school performance, accidents while driving or using equipment, and behavioral or emotional problems.

Middle-age men are thought to be more frequently affected by OSA, particularly when they are obese (Elliott, 2001). However, obstructive sleep apnea is also seen in postmenopausal women as well as younger women and children (Mahowald, 2000). Obstructive apnea causes a serious decline in arterial oxygen saturation level. Clients are at risk for cardiac dysrhythmias, right heart failure, pulmonary hypertension, angina attacks, stroke, and hypertension. Sleep apnea has been shown to contribute to high blood pressure and increased risk for heart attack and stroke (National Sleep Foundation, 2002a).

Surgery and anesthesia disrupt normal sleep patterns in clients. Postoperatively, these clients may reach deep levels of REM sleep. This deep sleep causes muscle relaxation that can lead to obstructive sleep apnea (Cullen, 2001). Clients with OSA who are given opioid analgesics after surgery have an increased risk of developing airway obstruction because normal arousal mechanisms that occur with obstruction are suppressed (Cullen, 2001).

Central sleep apnea (CSA) involves dysfunction in the brain's respiratory control center. The impulse to breathe temporarily fails, and nasal airflow and chest wall movement cease. The oxygen saturation of the blood falls. The condition is seen in clients with brain stem injury, muscular dystrophy, and encephalitis and people who breathe normally during the day. Less than 10% of sleep apnea is predominantly central in origin. People with CSA tend to awaken during sleep and therefore complain of insomnia and excessive daytime sleepiness. Mild and intermittent snoring is also present.

The client with sleep apnea is often significantly deprived of deep sleep. In addition to complaints of excessive daytime sleepiness, sleep attacks, fatigue, morning headaches, and decreased sex drive are common (White, 2000). Treatment includes therapy for underlying cardiac or respiratory complications and emotional problems that arise as a result of the symptoms of this disorder. Sleep hygiene and a weight-loss program may help. One of the most effective therapies is use of a nasal continuous positive airway pressure (CPAP) device at night, which requires a client to wear a mask over the nose. Room air is delivered through the mask at a high pressure. The air pressure prevents airway collapse. The CPAP device is portable and effective particularly for obstructive apnea. In cases of severe sleep apnea the tonsils, uvula, or portions of the soft palate may be surgically removed. Success with surgical procedures is variable.

Narcolepsy. **Narcolepsy** is a dysfunction of mechanisms that regulate the sleep and wake states. Excessive daytime sleepiness is the most common complaint associated with this disorder. During the day a person may suddenly feel an overwhelming wave of sleepiness and fall asleep; REM sleep can occur within 15 minutes of falling asleep. **Cataplexy,** or sudden muscle weakness during intense emotions such as anger, sadness, or laughter, may occur at any time during the day. If the cataplectic attack is severe, the client may lose voluntary muscle control and fall to the floor. A person with narcolepsy may have vivid dreams that occur as the person is falling asleep that are difficult to distinguish from reality (called hypnagogic hallucinations). Sleep paralysis, or the feeling of being unable to move or talk just before waking or falling asleep, is another symptom (Cohen, Nehring, and Cloninger, 1996). Some studies show a genetic link for narcolepsy (Mahowald, 2000).

A significant problem for the person with narcolepsy is that the individual falls asleep uncontrollably at inappropriate times. Unless this disorder is understood, a sleep attack can easily be mistaken for laziness, lack of interest in activities, or drunkenness. Typically, the symptoms first begin to arise in adolescence and may be confused with the excessive daytime sleepiness that is thought to commonly occur in teens. Narcoleptics are treated with stimulants that may only partially increase wakefulness and reduce sleep attacks, and antidepressant medications that suppress cataplexy and the other REM-related symptoms. Brief daytime naps no longer than 20 minutes may help reduce subjective feelings of sleepiness. The newest drug for treating narcolepsy is a wakefulness-promoting agent, modafinil. Modafinil has little or no potential for abuse (Zordis, 2001). Other management methods that have been reported as helpful are following a regular exercise program, eating light meals high in protein, practicing deep breathing, chewing gum, and taking vitamins (Cohen, Nehring, and Cloninger, 1996). Factors that in-

crease a narcoleptic client's drowsiness should be avoided (e.g., alcohol, heavy meals, exhausting activities, long-distance driving, long periods of sitting, hot stuffy rooms).

Sleep Deprivation. **Sleep deprivation** is a problem many clients experience as a result of the dyssomnia. Causes may include illness (e.g., fever, difficulty breathing, or pain), emotional stress, medications, environmental disturbances (e.g., frequent nursing care), and variability in the timing of sleep due to shift work. Physicians and nurses may be particularly prone to sleep deprivation due to long work schedules and rotating shifts.

Hospitalization, especially in intensive care units, makes clients particularly vulnerable to the extrinsic and circadian sleep disorders (Redeker, 2000). Sleep deprivation involves decreases in the quantity and quality of sleep and inconsistency in the timing of sleep. When sleep becomes interrupted or fragmented, changes in the normal sequencing of the sleep cycles occur. A cumulative sleep deprivation develops.

A person's response to sleep deprivation is highly variable. Clients may experience a variety of physiological and psychological symptoms (Box 41-3). The severity of symptoms is often related to the duration of sleep deprivation. The most effective treatment for sleep deprivation is elimination or correction of factors that disrupt the sleep pattern. Nurses can play an important role in identifying treatable sleep deprivation problems.

Parasomnias. The parasomnias are sleep problems that are more common in children than in adults. Sudden infant death syndrome (SIDS) is hypothesized to be related to apnea, hypoxia, and cardiac arrhythmias caused by abnormalities in the autonomic nervous system that are manifested during sleep (Gillis, 2000). Currently, the American Academy of Pediatrics (2000) recommends

---

Box 41-3   Sleep Deprivation Symptoms

Physiological Symptoms

Ptosis, blurred vision
Fine motor clumsiness
Decreased reflexes
Slowed response time
Decreased reasoning and judgment
Decreased auditory and visual alertness
Cardiac arrhythmias

Psychological Symptoms

Confusion and disorientation
Increased sensitivity to pain
Irritable, withdrawn, apathetic
Excessive sleepiness
Agitation
Hyperactivity
Decreased motivation

that apparently healthy infants should be placed in the supine position during sleep because of an association between the prone position and the occurrence of SIDS.

Parasomnias that occur among older children include somnambulism (sleepwalking), night terrors, nightmares, nocturnal enuresis (bed-wetting), body rocking, and tooth grinding (bruxism) (D'Cruz and Vaughn, 2001). When adults have these problems, it may indicate more serious disorders. Specific treatment for these disorders varies. However, in all cases it is important to support clients and maintain their safety. For example, sleepwalkers are unaware of their surroundings and are slow to react. Thus the risk of falls is great. A nurse should not startle sleepwalkers but instead gently awaken them and lead them back to bed.

*N*ursing Knowledge Base

Sleep and Rest

When people are at **rest** they usually feel mentally relaxed, free from anxiety, and physically calm. Rest does not imply inactivity, although everyone often thinks of it as settling down in a comfortable chair or lying in bed. When people are at rest they are in a state of mental, physical, and spiritual activity that leaves them feeling refreshed, rejuvenated, and ready to resume the activities of the day (Mornhinweg and Voignier, 1996). People have their own habits for obtaining rest and can find ways to adjust to new environments or conditions that affect the ability to rest. Rest may be gained from reading a book, practicing a relaxation exercise, listening to music, taking a long walk, or sitting quietly (Mornhinweg and Voignier, 1996).

Nurses frequently care for clients on bed rest in a variety of health care settings. This treatment confines clients to bed to reduce physical and psychological demands on the body. However, these people do not necessarily feel rested. They still may have emotional worries that prevent complete relaxation. For example, concern over physical limitations or a fear of being unable to return to their usual lifestyle may cause such clients to feel stressed and unable to relax.

Sleep is a recurrent, altered state of consciousness that occurs for sustained periods. When people obtain proper sleep, they feel that their energy has been restored. Some sleep experts believe that these feelings of energy restoration imply that sleep provides time for the repair and recovery of body systems for the next period of wakefulness.

The usual rest and sleep patterns of persons entering a hospital or other health care facility can easily be affected by illness or unfamiliar health care routines. The extent of change in usual sleep and rest patterns depends on the client's physiological and psychological states and the physical environment, such as background noise and the work patterns of caregivers. The nurse must always be aware of the client's need for rest. A lack of rest for long periods can cause illness or worsening of existing illness. The nurse can help clients learn the importance of rest and ways to promote it at home or in the health care environment.

Normal Sleep Requirements and Patterns

Sleep duration and quality vary among persons of all age-groups. One person may feel adequately rested with 4 hours of sleep, whereas another requires 10 hours.

Neonates. The neonate up to the age of 3 months averages about 16 hours of sleep a day. The sleep cycle is generally 40 to 50 minutes with wakening occurring after one to two sleep cycles (Renaud, 1996). For the first week the neonate sleeps almost constantly. Approximately 50% of this sleep is REM sleep, which stimulates the higher brain centers. This is thought to be essential for development because the neonate is not awake long enough for significant external stimulation.

Infants. Infants usually develop a nighttime pattern of sleep by 3 months of age. The infant may take several naps during the day but usually sleeps an average of 8 to 10 hours during the night for a total daily sleep time of 15 hours. About 30% of sleep time is spent in the REM cycle. Awakening commonly occurs early in the morning, although it is not unusual for an infant to awaken during the night. If awakening during the night becomes routine, the problem may be with diet because hunger frequently awakens the child. Compared with older children, active (REM) sleep makes up a larger proportion of sleep.

Toddlers. By the age of 2, children usually sleep through the night and take daily naps. Total sleep averages 12 hours a day. After 3 years of age, children often give up daytime naps (Hockenberry and others, 2003). It is common for toddlers to awaken during the night. The percentage of REM sleep continues to fall. During this period the toddler may be unwilling to go to bed at night. This unwillingness may be due to a need for autonomy or a fear of separation from their parents.

Preschoolers. On average a preschooler sleeps about 12 hours a night (about 20% is REM). By the age of 5, the preschooler rarely takes daytime naps except in cultures where a siesta is the custom (Wong and others, 2003). The preschooler usually has difficulty relaxing or quieting down after long, active days. A preschooler also has problems with bedtime fears, waking during the night, or nightmares. Parents are most successful in getting a preschooler to bed by establishing a consistent ritual that includes some quiet time activity before bedtime. Partial wakening followed by normal return to sleep may be seen (Hockenberry and others, 2003). In the waking period, the child may exhibit brief crying, walking around, unintelligible speech, sleepwalking or bed-wetting. Partial wakening can also occur in school-age children.

School-Age Children. The amount of sleep needed during the school years is individualized because of varying states of activity and levels of health. A 6-year-old averages 11 to 12 hours of sleep nightly, whereas an 11-year-old sleeps about 9 to 10 hours (Hockenberry and others, 2003). The 6- or 7-year-old can usually be persuaded to go to bed by encouraging quiet activities. The older child often resists sleeping because of an unawareness of fatigue or a need to be independent. A school-age child will be tired the following day if allowed to stay up later than usual. An older child may seek a later bedtime as a symbol of dominance over a younger child. Parents are usually successful in getting the older child to bed by using a firm, consistent approach. The older school-age child may be allowed to go to bed later, but such a privilege may be dependent on the child going to bed promptly without complaints.

Adolescents. Typically, teenagers get about 7½ hours of sleep per night. At a time when sleep needs actually increase, the typical adolescent is subject to a number of changes that often reduce the time spent sleeping (Dahl and Carskadon, 1995). Usually parents are no longer involved in setting a specific bedtime. School demands, after-school social activities, and part-time jobs may result in compressed time available for sleep. Teens go to bed later and rise earlier during the high school years. Because of lifestyle demands that shorten the time available for sleep and probable physiological need, teens often experience EDS. Performance in school, vulnerability to accidents, behavior and mood problems, and increased use of alcohol can be the result of EDS due to insufficient sleep (Mitler and others, 2000).

Young Adults. Most young adults average 6 to 8½ hours of sleep a night, but this can vary. Young adults rarely take regular naps. Approximately 20% of sleep time is spent in REM sleep, which remains consistent throughout life. Healthy young adults require adequate sleep to participate in the busy activities that fill their days. However, it is common for lifestyle demands to interrupt usual sleep patterns. The stresses of jobs, family relationships, and social activities may lead to insomnia (i.e., difficulties initiating and/or maintaining sleep) and the use of medication for sleep. Long-term use of such medications can disrupt sleep patterns and make the insomnia problem worse. Daytime sleepiness contributes to an increased number of accidents, decreased productivity, and interpersonal problems in this age-group. Pregnancy increases the need for sleep and rest. Insomnia is a common problem during the third trimester of pregnancy (Mindell and Jacobsen, 2000).

Middle Adults. During middle adulthood the total time spent sleeping at night begins to decline. The amount of stage 4 sleep begins to fall, a decline that continues with advancing age. Sleep disturbances are often initially diagnosed among people in this age range even when the symptoms of a disorder have been present for several years. Insomnia is particularly common, probably because of the changes and stresses of middle age. Sleep disturbances can be caused by anxiety, depression, or certain physical ailments. Women experiencing menopausal symptoms often experience insomnia. Members of this age-group may rely on herbal supplements or sleeping medications.

Older Adults. Complaints of sleeping difficulties increase with age. More than 80% of adults 65 years or older report problems with sleep (Schneider, 2002). Episodes of REM sleep tend to shorten. There is a progressive decrease in stages 3 and 4 NREM sleep; some older adults have almost no stage 4, or deep sleep. An older adult awakens more often during the night, and it may take more time for an older adult to fall asleep.

Variability in the sleep behaviors of older adults is common. Complaints about difficulties with nighttime sleep frequently occur among older adults, often resulting from the presence of another chronic illness. For example, an older adult with arthritis may have difficulty sleeping because of painful joints. The tendency to nap seems to increase progressively with age. The increase in daytime napping may occur because of the frequent awakenings experienced at night. The changes in an older person's sleep pattern may be due to changes in the CNS that affect the regulation of sleep. Sensory impairment, which is common with aging, may reduce an older person's sensitivity to time cues that maintain circadian rhythms.

Factors Affecting Sleep
A number of factors affect the quantity and quality of sleep. Often a single factor may not be the only cause for a sleep problem. Physiological, psychological, and environmental factors can alter the quality and quantity of sleep.

Drugs and Substances. Sleepiness, insomnia, and fatigue often result as a direct effect of commonly prescribed medications (Box 41-4). These medications alter sleep and impair daytime alertness, which can be problematic for individuals (McKenry and Salerno, 2003; Schweitzer, 2000). Medications prescribed for sleep may cause more problems than benefits. Older adults often take a variety of drugs to control or treat chronic illness, and the combined effects of several drugs can seriously disrupt sleep. One substance that may promote sleep is L-tryptophan, a natural protein found in foods such as milk, cheese, and meats.

Lifestyle. A person's daily routine may influence sleep patterns. An individual working a rotating shift (e.g., 2 weeks of days followed by a week of nights) often has difficulty adjusting to the altered sleep schedule. The body's internal clock might be set at 11 PM, but the work schedule forces sleep at 9 AM instead. The individual may be able to sleep only 3 or 4 hours because the body's clock perceives that it is time to be awake and active. Difficulties with maintaining alertness during work time can result in decreased and even hazardous performance. After several weeks of working a night shift a person's biological clock usually does adjust. Other alterations in routines that can disrupt sleep patterns include performing unaccustomed heavy work, engaging in late-night social activities, and changing evening mealtime.

Usual Sleep Patterns. In the past century the amount of sleep obtained nightly by U.S. citizens has decreased over 20% (National Sleep Foundation, 2003), indicating that many Americans are sleep deprived and experience excessive sleepiness during the day. Sleepiness becomes pathological when it occurs at times when individuals need or want to be awake. People who experience tem-

---

Box 41-4   **Drugs and Their Effect on Sleep**

Hypnotics

Interfere with reaching deeper sleep stages
Provide only temporary (1 week) increase in quantity of sleep
Eventually cause "hangover" during day; excess drowsiness, confusion, decreased energy
May worsen sleep apnea in older adults

Diuretics

Nighttime awakenings caused by nocturia

Antidepressants and Stimulants

Suppress REM sleep
Decrease total sleep time

Alcohol

Speeds onset of sleep
Reduces REM sleep
Awakens person during night and causes difficulty returning to sleep

Caffeine

Prevents person from falling asleep
May cause person to awaken during night
Interferes with REM sleep

Beta-Adrenergic Blockers

Cause nightmares
Cause insomnia
Cause awakening from sleep

Benzodiazepines

Alter REM sleep
Increase sleep time
Increase daytime sleepiness

Narcotics

Suppress REM sleep
Cause increased daytime drowsiness

Anticonvulsants

Decrease REM sleep time
May cause daytime drowsiness

---

porary sleep deprivation as a result of an active social evening or lengthened work schedule usually feel sleepy the next day. However, they may be able to overcome these feelings even though they have difficulty performing tasks and remaining attentive. Chronic lack of sleep is much more serious than temporary sleep deprivation and can cause serious alterations in the ability to perform daily functions. Sleepiness tends to be most difficult to overcome during sedentary tasks. For example, single-vehicle accidents related to a driver falling asleep at the wheel occur most often between 2 AM and 6 AM due to the sleepiness that can occur when people are awake during what is their normal period of sleep (National Sleep Foundation, 2003).

Emotional Stress. Worry over personal problems or situations can disrupt sleep. Emotional stress causes a person to be tense and often leads to frustration when sleep does not come. Stress may also cause a person to try too hard to fall asleep, to awaken frequently during the sleep cycle, or to oversleep. Continued stress may cause poor sleep habits.

Older clients frequently experience losses that lead to emotional stress such as retirement, physical impairment, or the death of a loved one. Older adults and other individuals who experience depressive mood problems often experience delays in falling asleep, earlier appearance of REM sleep, frequent awakening, increased total bed time, feelings of sleeping poorly, and early awakening (Beck-Little and Weinrich, 1998).

Environment. The physical environment in which a person sleeps has a significant influence on the ability to fall and remain sleep. Good ventilation is essential for restful sleep. The size, firmness, and position of the bed can affect the quality of sleep. If a person usually sleeps with another individual, sleeping alone can cause wakefulness. On the other hand, sleeping with a restless or snoring bed partner can disrupt sleep.

Sound also influences sleep. The level of noise needed to awaken people depends on the stage of sleep (Webster and Thompson, 1986). Low noises are more likely to arouse a person from stage 1 sleep, whereas louder noises awaken people in stage 3 or 4 sleep. Some persons require silence to fall asleep, whereas others prefer background noise such as soft music or television.

In hospitals and other in-patient facilities, noise creates a problem for clients. Noise in hospitals is usually new or strange. Thus clients are prone to awaken. This problem is greatest the first night of hospitalization, when clients often experience increased total wake time, increased awakenings, and decreased REM sleep and total sleep time. The level of noise in hospitals can be very loud. Normal conversation measures about 50 decibels. People-induced noises (e.g., nursing activities) are sources of increased sound levels. Intensive care units are sources for high noise levels (Box 41-5). Close proximity of clients, noise from confused and ill clients, the ringing of alarm systems and telephones, and disturbances caused by emergencies make the environment unpleasant.

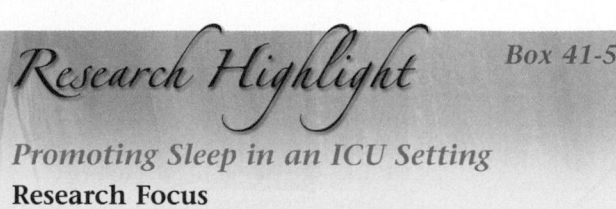

Box 41-5

Promoting Sleep in an ICU Setting

Research Focus

Noise combined with other environmental factors in intensive care units disrupts normal sleep-wake patterns in clients. This disruption leads to sleep deprivation that is associated with poor client outcomes. Nursing interventions to promote sleep in these clients need to be tested. Little research focusing on the effect of specific nursing interventions is available.

Research Abstract

The purpose of this study was to examine the effect that a "quiet time" protocol to reduce noise and light stimulation had on sleep in clients in a neuroscience critical care unit. The protocol reduced noise and environmental stimuli by limiting visitors, turning down lights, closing blinds, and turning off television. The study also evaluated whether a "quiet time" in the ICU unit was feasible. One hundred twenty-one clients in the treatment group received the "quiet time" protocol. One hundred eighteen clients in the control group received the usual care conditions. Data collection included 1446 observations on the clients in the control group and 1529 observations on the clients in the treatment group. Trained RN observers collected data on clients' sleeping behavior 8 times each day. Measurement of light and noise were taken at the same time. The results showed that significantly more clients were observed to be asleep during the period in which the "quiet time" protocol was implemented. Light and sound levels were also significantly reduced during the protocol implementation. Implementing the "quiet time" protocol did present a challenge to the nursing staff in the ICU setting because it was difficult for the nurses to organize care to provide the uninterrupted 2-hour rest period and it was difficult to control noise from ventilators, monitor alarms, and other equipment.

Evidence-Based Practice

- Implementing a "quiet time" protocol on ICU units is a low-cost nursing intervention.
- Reduction of environmental stimuli can help promote needed rest and sleep in clients in an ICU.
- Use of "quiet time" protocols can improve sleep in acutely ill clients.

Reference

Olson DM and others: Quiet time: a nursing intervention to promote sleep in neurocritical care units, *Am J Crit Care* 10(2):74, 2001.

Light levels may affect the ability to fall asleep. Some clients may prefer a dark room, whereas others, such as children or older adults, may prefer keeping a soft light on during sleep. Clients also may have trouble sleeping based on the temperature of a room. A room that is too warm or too cold often causes a client to become restless.

Exercise and Fatigue. A person who is moderately fatigued usually achieves restful sleep, especially if the fatigue is the result of enjoyable work or exercise. Exercising 2 hours or more before bedtime allows the body to cool down and maintains a state of fatigue that promotes relaxation. However, excess fatigue resulting from exhausting or stressful work can make falling asleep difficult. This can be a common problem for grade school children and adolescents.

Food and Caloric Intake. Following good eating habits is important for proper health, including sleep. Eating a large, heavy, and/or spicy meal at night may result in indigestion that interferes with sleep. Caffeine and alcohol consumed in the evening have insomnia-producing effects. A drastic reduction or avoidance of these substances is an important strategy that people can use to improve sleep. Food allergies may cause insomnia. In infants, a milk allergy requiring that breast milk or a no-milk formula be used may cause nighttime waking and crying or colic. Besides milk, other foods that often result in an insomnia-producing allergy among both children and adults include corn, wheat, nuts, chocolate, eggs, seafood, red and yellow food dyes, and yeast (Hauri and Linde, 1990). Restoration of normal sleep may take up to 2 weeks when the particular food that is causing the difficulty has been eliminated from the diet.

Weight loss or gain influences sleep patterns. When a person gains weight, sleep periods become longer with fewer interruptions. Weight loss can cause short and fragmented sleep. Certain sleep disorders may be the result of the semistarvation diets popular in a weight-conscious society.

Critical Thinking

Successful critical thinking requires a synthesis of knowledge, including information gathered from clients, experience, critical thinking attitudes, and intellectual and professional standards. Clinical judgments require the nurse to anticipate the information necessary, analyze the data, and make decisions regarding client care. The nurse must adapt critical thinking to the changing needs of the client. During assessment (Figure 41-3), the nurse must consider all elements that build toward making appropriate nursing diagnoses.

In the case of sleep, the nurse integrates knowledge from nursing and disciplines such as pharmacology and psychology. Personal experience with a sleep problem, as well as experience with clients, prepares a nurse to know effective forms of sleep therapies. The use of critical thinking attitudes such as perseverance, confidence, and discipline are needed to complete a comprehensive assessment and to develop a plan of care to provide successful management of the sleep problem. The use of professional standards, such as the *Standards of Clinical Nursing Practice* (American Nurses Association, 1998) and the "Nursing Standard-of-Practice Protocol: Sleep Disturbances in Elderly Patients" (Foreman and Wykle, 1995), provide valuable guidelines for the nurse to assess and address the needs of clients with sleep disorders. The standard-of-practice protocol was developed for hospital nurses to use to prevent or manage sleep problems in older hospitalized adults. The project was

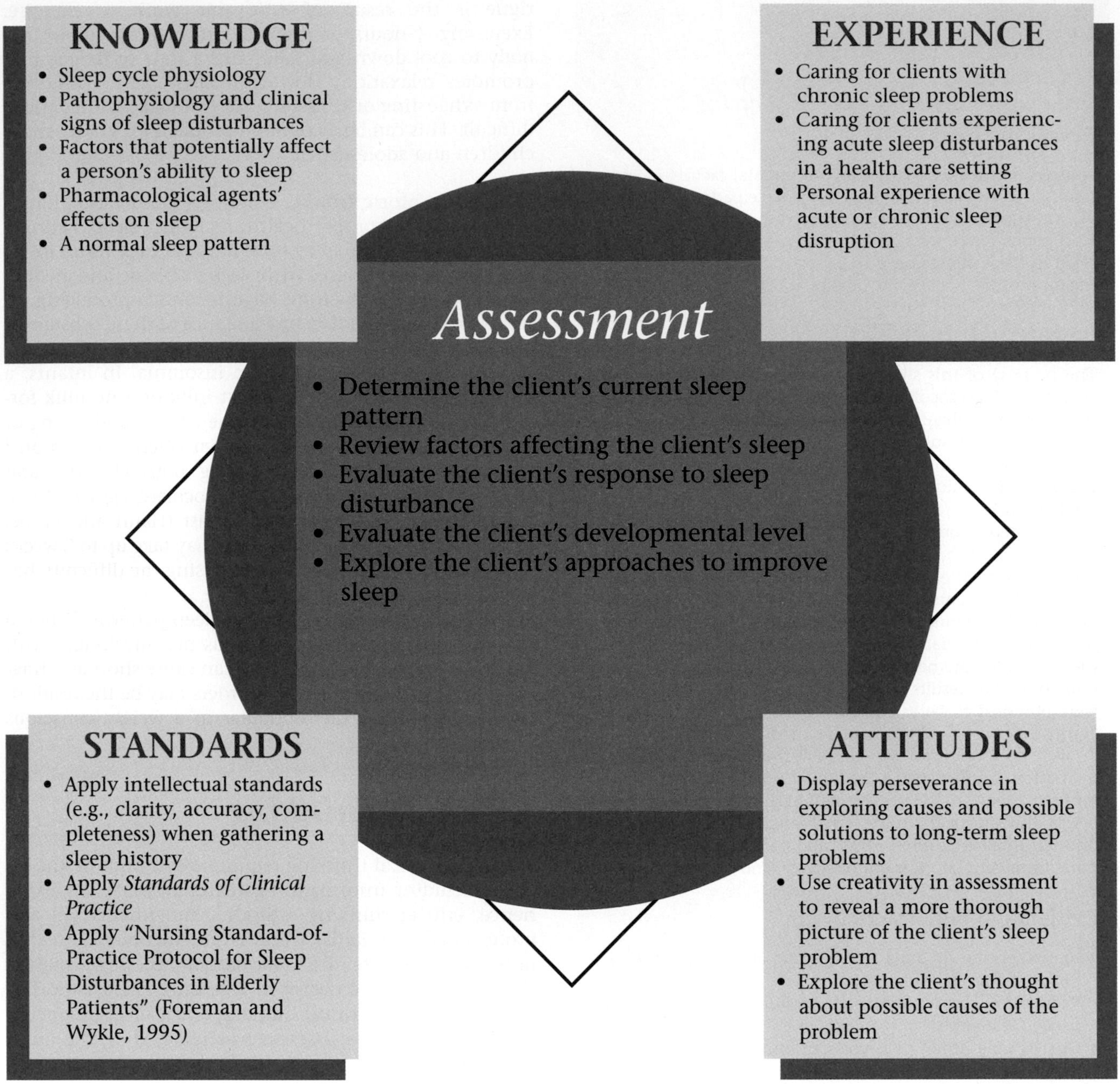

KNOWLEDGE

- Sleep cycle physiology
- Pathophysiology and clinical signs of sleep disturbances
- Factors that potentially affect a person's ability to sleep
- Pharmacological agents' effects on sleep
- A normal sleep pattern

EXPERIENCE

- Caring for clients with chronic sleep problems
- Caring for clients experiencing acute sleep disturbances in a health care setting
- Personal experience with acute or chronic sleep disruption

Assessment

- Determine the client's current sleep pattern
- Review factors affecting the client's sleep
- Evaluate the client's response to sleep disturbance
- Evaluate the client's developmental level
- Explore the client's approaches to improve sleep

STANDARDS

- Apply intellectual standards (e.g., clarity, accuracy, completeness) when gathering a sleep history
- Apply *Standards of Clinical Practice*
- Apply "Nursing Standard-of-Practice Protocol for Sleep Disturbances in Elderly Patients" (Foreman and Wykle, 1995)

ATTITUDES

- Display perseverance in exploring causes and possible solutions to long-term sleep problems
- Use creativity in assessment to reveal a more thorough picture of the client's sleep problem
- Explore the client's thought about possible causes of the problem

FIGURE **41–3** Critical thinking model for sleep assessment.

part of the John A. Hartford Foundation's Nurses Improving Care of Hospitalized Elderly (NICHE) Project (Foreman and Wykle, 1995).

Nursing Process

Assessment

The nurse assesses clients' sleep patterns by using the nursing history to gather information about factors that usually influence sleep. If the client perceives that sleep is adequate, the nursing history can be brief. Sleep is a

subjective experience. Only the client can report whether or not it is sufficient and restful. If the client is satisfied with the quantity and quality of sleep received, it may be considered normal. If a client admits to or the nurse suspects a sleep problem, a more detailed history is needed.

Sleep Assessment. Most persons can provide a reasonably accurate estimate of their sleep patterns, particularly if any changes have occurred. Assessment is aimed at understanding the characteristics of any sleep problem and the client's usual sleep habits so that ways for promoting sleep can be incorporated into nursing care. For example, if the nursing history reveals that a client always reads before falling asleep, it makes sense to offer reading material at bedtime.

Sources for Sleep Assessment. Usually clients are the best resource for describing sleep problems and the extent to which problems represent a change from their usual sleep and waking patterns. Often the client knows the cause for sleep problems, such as a noisy environment or worry over a relationship.

In addition, bed partners can provide information on the client's sleep patterns that may reveal the nature of certain sleep disorders. For example, partners of clients with sleep apnea often complain that the client's snoring disturbs their sleep. Often the partners must sleep in different beds or rooms to obtain adequate sleep. The nurse should ask bed partners whether the clients have pauses of breathing during sleep and how frequently the apneic attacks occur. Some partners mention becoming fearful when clients apparently stop breathing for periods during sleep.

When caring for children, the nurse seeks information about sleep patterns from parents because they are usually a good source of information about how their child is having trouble sleeping. However, older children can usually explain their sleep problem. Some parents may not realize that there is a wide variability in the sleeping patterns of infants. Hunger, excessive warmth, and separation anxiety are factors that may contribute to an infant's difficulty with going to sleep or frequent awakenings during the night. Older children often are able to relate fears or worries that inhibit their ability to fall asleep. If children frequently awaken in the middle of bad dreams, parents can identify the problem but perhaps do not understand the meanings of the dreams. Parents can also describe the typical behavior patterns that foster or impair sleep. For example, excessive stimulation from active play or visiting friends may predictably impair sleep. With chronic sleep problems, parents can relate the duration of the problem, its progression, and children's responses. Parents of infants may need to keep a 24-hour log of their infant's waking and sleeping behavior for several days to determine what may be causing the problem. The infant's eating pattern and sleeping environment also need to be described because these may influence sleeping behavior.

Tools for Assessment of Sleep. Subjective reports of sleep have been shown to be reliable and valid measures of sleep (Libman and others, 2000). There are several subjective sleep assessment tools that are easy and quick to administer.

One effective, brief method for assessing sleep quality is the use of a visual analog scale (Closs, 1988). The nurse draws a straight horizontal line 100 mm (4 inches) long. Opposing statements such as "best night's sleep" and "worst night's sleep" are at opposite ends of the line. Clients are asked to place a mark on the horizontal line at the point corresponding to their perceptions of the previous night's sleep. The distances of the mark along the line can be measured in millimeters and offers a numerical value for satisfaction with sleep. The scale can be repeatedly administered to show change over time. Such a scale is useful to assess an individual client, not to com-

pare clients. The Richards-Campbell Sleep Questionnaire, a five-item visual analog scale, has been developed to measure sleep in critically ill clients (Richards, O'Sullivan, and Phillips, 2000).

Another brief subjective method to assess sleep is a 0 to 10 sleep rating scale similar to the concept of the 0 to 10 pain scale (Richards, 1996). Individuals should separately rate their quantity and quality of sleep on the scale. Instruct clients to indicate with a number between 0 and 10 their sleep quantity then their quality of sleep with 0 being the worst sleep and 10 being the best sleep. Additional paper-and-pencil tools are available, such as the St. Mary's Hospital Sleep Questionnaire, the Baekeland-Hoy Sleep Log, the Pittsburgh Sleep Quality Index, the Epworth Sleepiness Scale, and the Verran-Snyder-Halpern Sleep Scale (Elliott, 2001; Leigh and others, 1988; Richardson, 1997; Smyth, 1999, 2002).

Sleep History. When a client reports having adequate sleep, a sleep history can be brief. A determination of usual bedtime, normal bedtime rituals, preferred environment for sleeping, and what time the client usually rises gives the nurse information for planning care conducive to sleep. When suspecting a sleep problem, the nurse assesses the quality and characteristics of sleep in greater depth. For example, the nurse asks the client to describe the sleep problem; including recent changes in sleep pattern and sleep symptoms experienced during waking hours; use of sleep and other prescribed or over-the-counter medications; the pattern of dietary intake and amount of substances that influence sleep; and recent life events that have affected the client's mental and emotional status.

Description of Sleeping Problems. When a client has a sleep problem, the nursing history must be detailed so that therapeutic care can be provided. Open-ended questions help a client to describe a problem more fully. A general description of the problem followed by more focused questions usually reveals specific characteristics that can be used in planning therapies.

To begin, the nurse needs to understand the nature of the sleep problem, its signs and symptoms, its onset and duration, its severity, any predisposing factors or causes, and the overall effect on the client. Assessment questions might include the following:

- *Nature of the problem:* Tell me what type of problem you have with your sleep. Tell me why you think your sleep is inadequate. Describe for me a recent typical night's sleep. How is this sleep different from what you are used to?
- *Signs and symptoms:* Do you have difficulty falling asleep, staying asleep, or waking up? Have you been told that you snore loudly? Do you have headaches when awakening? Does your child awaken from nightmares?
- *Onset and duration:* When did you notice the problem? How long has this problem lasted?
- *Severity:* How long does it take you to fall asleep? How often during the week do you have trouble falling asleep? Tell me how many hours of sleep a night you got this week; compare that to what is usual for you.

What do you do when you awaken during the night or too early in the morning?

- *Predisposing factors:* Tell me what you do just before going to bed. Have you recently had any changes at work or at home? How is your mood, and have you noticed any changes recently? What medications or recreational drugs do you take on a regular basis? Are you taking any new prescription or over-the-counter medications? How long have you been taking medications? Do you eat food (e.g., spicy or greasy foods) or drink substances (e.g., alcohol or caffeinated beverages) that could be interfering with your sleep? Do you have a physical illness that might be interfering with your sleep? Does anyone in your family have a history of sleep problems?

- *Effect on client:* How has the loss of sleep affected you? (Ask a spouse or friend: Have you noticed any changes in behavior since the sleep problem started?) Do you feel excessively sleepy, irritable, or have trouble concentrating during waking hours? Do you have trouble staying awake or have you fallen asleep at inappropriate times, for example, while driving, sitting quietly in a meeting, or watching TV?

Proper questioning helps the nurse determine the type of sleep disturbance and the nature of the problem. Box 41-6 gives examples of additional questions for the nurse to ask the client when specific sleep disorders are suspected. The questions assist in selecting specific sleep therapies and the best time for implementation.

As an adjunct to the sleep history, a client and bed partner may be asked to keep a sleep-wake log for 1 to 4 weeks (Attarian, 2000; Beck-Little and Weinrich, 1998). The sleep-wake log is completed daily to provide information on day-to-day variations in sleep-wake patterns over extended periods. Entries in the log often include 24-hour information about various waking and sleeping health behaviors such as physical activities, mealtimes, type and amount of intake (alcohol and caffeine), time and length of daytime naps, evening and bedtime routines, the time the client tries to fall asleep, nighttime awakenings, and the time of morning awakening. A partner can help record the estimated times the client falls asleep or awakens. Although the log is helpful, the client must be motivated to participate in its completion. Ordinarily it is not used with acutely ill clients who have short hospital stays.

Usual Sleep Pattern. Normal sleep is difficult to define because individuals vary in the quantity and quality of sleep that they perceive as adequate for them. It is important, however, to have clients describe their usual sleep pattern to determine the significance of the changes being created by a sleep disorder. Knowing a client's usual, preferred sleep pattern allows a nurse to try to match sleeping conditions in a health care setting with those in the home. To determine the client's sleep pattern the nurse asks the following questions:

1. What time do you usually get in bed each night?
2. What time do you usually fall asleep? Do you do anything special to help you fall asleep?
3. How many times do you awaken at night? Why?
4. What time do you typically wake up in the morning?

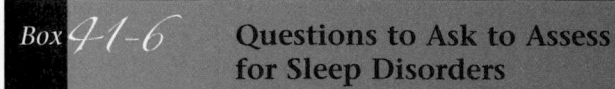

Box 41-6   Questions to Ask to Assess for Sleep Disorders

Insomnia

How easily do you fall asleep?
Do you fall asleep and have difficulty staying asleep? How many times do you awaken?
Do you awaken early from sleep?
What time do you awaken for good? What causes you to awaken early?
What do you do to prepare for sleep? To improve your sleep?
What do you think about as you try to fall asleep?
How often do you have trouble sleeping?

Sleep Apnea

Do you snore loudly?
Has anyone ever told you that you often stop breathing for short periods during sleep? (Spouse or bed partner/roommate may report this).
Do you experience headaches after awakening?
Do you have difficulty staying awake during the day?
Does anyone else in your family snore loudly or stop breathing during sleep?

Narcolepsy

Are you tired during the day?
Do you fall asleep at inopportune times? (Friends or relatives may report this.)
Do you have episodes of losing muscle control or falling to the floor?
Have you ever had the feeling of being unable to move or talk just before falling asleep?
Do you have vivid lifelike dreams when going to sleep or waking up?

5. What time do you get out of bed for good once you have awakened?
6. What is the average number of hours you sleep each night?

The nurse compares these data with the predominant pattern usually found for other clients of the same age. Based on this comparison, the nurse begins to assess for identifiable patterns such as insomnia.

Clients with sleep problems may show patterns drastically different from their usual one, or the change may be relatively minor. Hospitalized clients usually need or want more sleep as a result of illness. However, some may require less sleep because they are less active. Clients who are ill may think that it is important to try to sleep more than what is usual for them, eventually making sleeping difficult.

Physical and Psychological Illness. The nurse determines whether the client has any preexisting health problems that might interfere with sleep. A history of psychiatric problems may also make a difference. For example, a bipolar or manic-depressive client sleeps more when depressed than when manic. A depressed client often experiences an inadequate amount of sleep that is fragmented. Chronic diseases such as chronic obstructive pulmonary disease and painful disorders such as arthritis interfere with sleep. The nurse also assesses the client's medication history, including a description of over-the-counter and prescribed drugs. If a client takes medications to aid sleep, the nurse gathers information about the type and amount of medication that is being used. The nurse may also assess daily caffeine intake.

If the client has recently undergone surgery, the nurse can expect the client to experience some disturbance in sleep. Clients may awaken frequently during the first night after surgery and receive little deep or REM sleep. Depending on the type of surgery, it may take several days for a normal sleep cycle to return.

Current Life Events. The nurse learns whether the client is experiencing any changes in lifestyle that may be disrupting sleep. A person's occupation may offer a clue to the nature of the sleep problem. Changes in job responsibilities, rotating shifts, or long hours can contribute to a sleep disturbance. Questions about social activities, recent travel, or mealtime schedules help clarify the sleep assessment.

Emotional and Mental Status. If a client is anxious, excitable, or angry, mental preoccupations can seriously disrupt sleep. The client may be experiencing emotional stress related to illness or situational crises such as loss of job or a loved one. Thus the client's emotions may affect the ability to sleep. Clients with psychiatric disorders may need mild sedation for adequate rest. The nurse assesses the effectiveness of the medication and its effect on daytime function.

Bedtime Routines. The nurse asks what the client does to prepare for sleep. For example, the client may drink a glass of milk, take a sleeping pill, eat a snack, or watch television. The nurse assesses habits that are beneficial compared with those that have been found to disturb sleep. Not all clients are alike. Watching television may promote sleep for one person, whereas another individual may be stimulated to stay awake while watching TV. Sometimes pointing out that a particular habit may be interfering with sleep can help clients to find ways to change or eliminate habits that may be disrupting sleep.

The nurse should pay special attention to a child's bedtime rituals. The parents can report whether it is necessary, for example, to read the child a bedtime story, rock the child to sleep, or engage in quiet play. Some young children need a special blanket or stuffed animal when going to sleep.

Bedtime Environment. The nurse asks the client to describe preferred bedroom conditions. The bedroom may be dark or light, and the door to the room may be open or closed. The client may listen to the radio or watch television, or prefer a quiet environment. The nurse also asks if the client prefers a soft or firm mattress. In addition, a child may require the company of a parent to fall asleep. The nurse may learn that changes in the home or institutional environment may be necessary to promote sleep. In a health care environment there may be environmental distractions that can interfere with sleep such as a roommate's television, an electronic monitor in the hallway, a noisy nurses' station, or another client who cries out at night. The nurse identifies factors that can be reduced or controlled.

Behaviors of Sleep Deprivation. Some clients may be unaware of how their sleep problems are affecting their behavior. The nurse observes for behaviors such as irritability, disorientation (similar to a drunken state), frequent yawning, and slurred speech. If sleep deprivation has lasted a long time, psychotic behavior such as delusions and paranoia may develop. For example, a client may report seeing strange objects or colors in the room. The client may act afraid when the nurse enters the room.

Clients hospitalized in intensive care units (ICUs) for extended time may show the "ICU syndrome" of sleep deprivation (Dines-Kalinowski, 2002). Constant environmental stimuli within the ICU, such as strange noises from equipment, the frequent monitoring and care given by nurses, and ever-present lights, confuse clients. Repeated environmental stimuli and the client's poor physical status lead to sleep deprivation (Olson and others, 2001).

Client Expectations. A poor night's sleep for a client often starts a vicious cycle of anticipatory anxiety, with fear that sleep will again be disturbed as the client tries harder and harder to sleep (Attarian, 2000). The nurse must use a skilled and caring approach to assess the client's sleep needs. A caring nurse is one perceived to tailor care to the individual's needs. The nurse should always ask clients what they expect regarding sleep. This includes asking clients what interventions they currently use and how successful the interventions are. The nurse also asks clients what other interventions to promote sleep they prefer and how they might be implemented. It is important to understand clients' expectations regarding their sleep pattern. When clients ask the nurse for assistance because of sleep disturbances, they typically expect the nurse to respond promptly to assist them in improving their quantity and quality of sleep.

Nursing Diagnosis

The nurse reviews assessment data looking for clusters of data that include defining characteristics for a sleep pattern disturbance. If a sleep pattern disturbance is identified, the nurse specifies the condition. By specifying the nature of a sleep disturbance, the nurse can design more effective interventions. For example, the nurse will choose different therapies for clients with insomnia who are unable to fall asleep than for those with sleep apnea. Box 41-7 demonstrates how to use nursing assessment activities to identify and cluster defining characteristics to make an accurate nursing diagnosis.

Assessment should also identify the related factor or probable cause of the sleep disturbance, such as a noisy environment, a high intake of caffeinated beverages in the evening, or stress involving a marital relationship. These causes become the focus of interventions for mini-

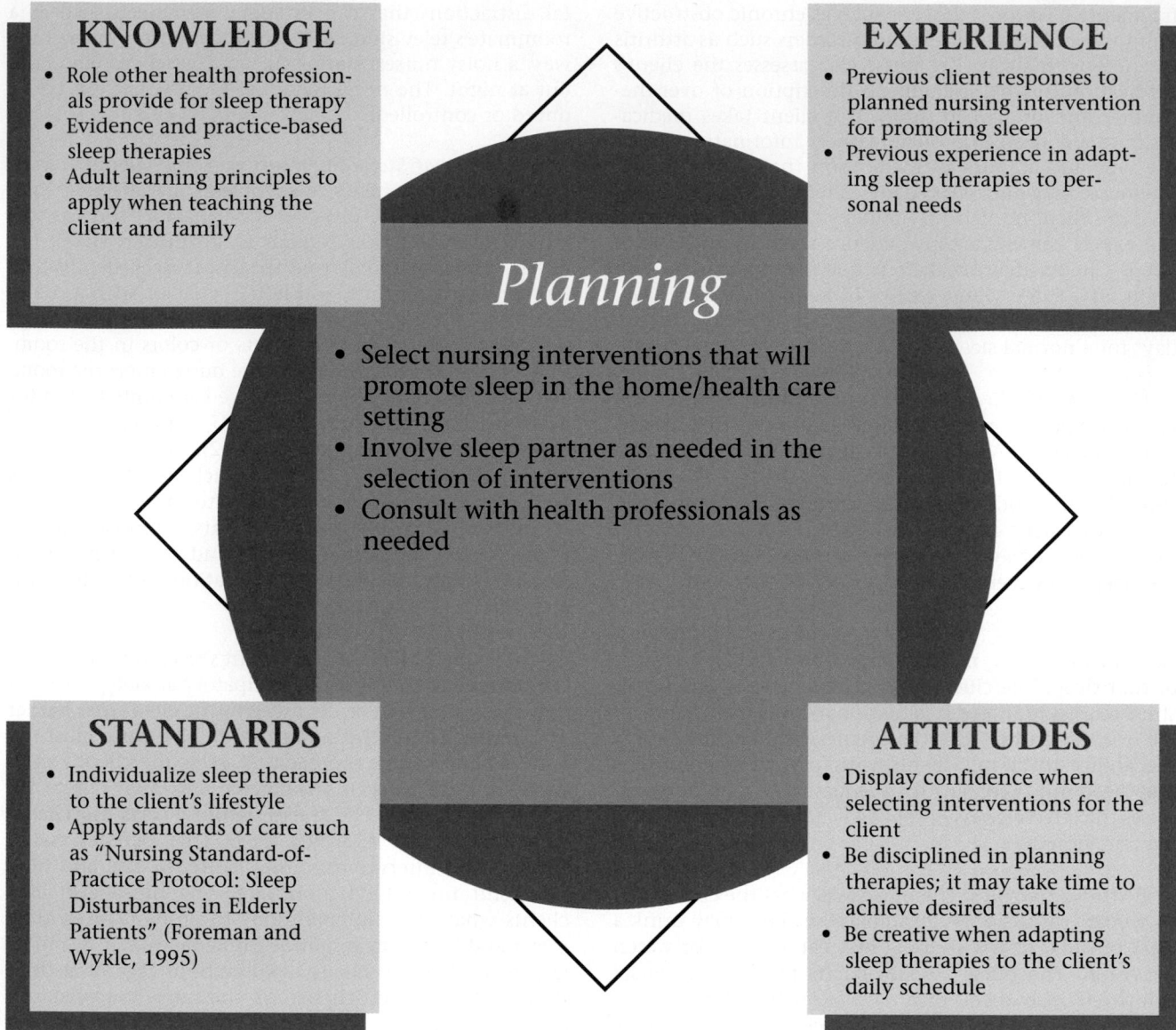

FIGURE **41–4** Critical thinking model for sleep planning.

mizing or eliminating the problem. For example, if a client is experiencing insomnia as a result of a noisy health care environment, the nurse could offer some basic recommendations for helping sleep such as controlling the noise of hospital equipment, reducing interruptions, or keeping doors closed. If the insomnia is related to worry over a threatened marital separation, the nurse's actions involve introduction of coping strategies and creation of an environment for sleep. If the probable cause or related factors are incorrectly defined, the client may not benefit from care.

Sleep problems may affect clients in other ways. For example, a nurse may find that a client with sleep apnea has problems with a spouse who is tired and frustrated over the client's snoring. In addition, the spouse is concerned that the client is breathing improperly and thus is

in danger. The nursing diagnosis of *compromised family coping* indicates that the nurse must provide support to the client and spouse so that they can understand sleep apnea and obtain the medical treatment needed. Nursing diagnoses for clients with sleep problems may include the following:

- Anxiety
- Ineffective breathing pattern
- Acute confusion
- Compromised family coping
- Ineffective coping
- Fatigue
- Ineffective protection
- Disturbed sensory perception
- Sleep deprivation
- Disturbed sleep pattern

Nursing Diagnostic Process

Box *41-7*

Assessment Activities	Defining Characteristics	Nursing Diagnosis
Ask client to explain nature of sleep problem.	Client reports difficulty in falling asleep, taking up to an hour. Client reports awakening two to three times nightly, with difficulty returning to sleep.	Disturbed sleep pattern
Observe client's behavior and ask bed partner if behavior changes have been noted.	Client admits to not feeling well rested. Spouse describes episodes of client being lethargic and irritable.	
Determine if client has had recent lifestyle changes.	Spouse reports client recently lost job, has concern over finding new position.	

Planning

Goals and Outcomes. During planning the nurse again synthesizes information from multiple resources in order to develop an individualized plan of care (Figure 41-4) (see care plan). Professional standards are especially important to consider in developing a care plan. These standards often offer scientifically proven guidelines for effective nursing interventions. For example, the "Nursing Standard-of-Practice Protocol: Sleep Disturbances in Elderly Patients" (Foreman and Wykle, 1995) recommends individualized nursing interventions that maintain and support an older adult's normal sleep pattern and bedtime ritual. It is important for a plan of care for sleep promotion to include strategies appropriate to the client's sleep routines, living environment, and lifestyle.

As care is planned for the client with sleep disturbances, creation of a concept map is another method for developing holistic client-centered care (Figure 41-5). The nurse creates the map after identifying relevant nursing diagnoses from the assessment database. In this example, the nursing diagnoses are linked to the client's medical diagnosis of depression following the death of the spouse. The concept map shows the relationships between the nursing diagnoses: *dysfunctional grieving, disturbed sleep pattern, and impaired social interaction*. This approach to planning care assists the nurse in recognizing relationships between interventions that are planned. For this client, interventions and successful outcomes for one nursing diagnosis can affect the resolution of another nursing diagnosis.

When developing goals and outcomes, it is important for the nurse and client to collaborate. As a result, realistic goals and measurable outcomes will more likely be set. An effective plan includes outcomes established over a realistic time frame that focus on the goal of improving the quantity and quality of sleep in the home. Often family members can be very helpful in contributing to the plan. A sleep promotion plan may require many weeks to accomplish. An example of a goal with client outcomes includes:

Goal: The client will control environmental sources disrupting sleep within 1 month.

Outcomes:
- Client will identify factors in the immediate home environment that disrupt sleep in 2 weeks.
- Client will report having a discussion with family members about environmental barriers to sleep in 2 weeks.
- Client will report changes made in the bedroom to promote sleep within 4 weeks.
- Client will report having fewer than two awakenings per night within 4 weeks.

Setting Priorities. Working with the client, the nurse establishes the priority outcomes and interventions for the client. Frequently sleep disturbances are the result of other health problems. For example, when physical symptoms are interfering with sleep, management of the symptoms will be the nurse's priority. Once symptoms are relieved, the nurse can then focus on sleep therapies. Clients are a helpful resource in determining which interventions hold priority. For example, once clients understand the factors that disrupt sleep, they can make choices in the types of changes they would like to make in their lifestyle or sleeping environment.

Continuity of Care. The nurse partners closely with the client and significant others to ensure that any therapies, such as a change in the sleep schedule or changes to the bedroom environment, are realistic and achievable. In a health care setting the nurse plans treatments or routines so that the client will be able to rest. For example, in the intensive care unit, nurses check available electronic monitors to track trends in vital signs without awakening a client each hour. Other staff members should be aware of the care plan so that they can cluster activities at certain times to reduce awakenings. In a nursing home the focus of the plan may involve better planning of rest periods around the activities of the other residents. Often the schedule of one roommate may not coincide with that of another.

The nature of the sleep disturbance determines whether referrals to additional health care providers are necessary. For example, if a sleep problem is related to a situational crisis or emotional problem, the nurse may refer the client to a psychiatric clinical nurse specialist or clinical psychologist for counseling. When chronic insomnia is the problem, a medical referral or referral to a sleep center may be

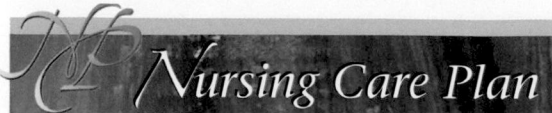

Nursing Care Plan

Disturbed Sleep Pattern

Assessment

Julie Arnold, a 42-year-old attorney, is the first client of the morning at the neighborhood health clinic where you work. When you ask her how she is doing, she tells you she is having difficulty sleeping. Julie is married and has two school-age chil-dren. Julie's assessment includes a thorough sleep history and a discussion of how the sleep problem has affected her life. A physical examination is also completed.

Assessment Activities	Findings/Defining Characteristics
Ask Julie to explain the nature of her sleep problem.	Julie explains that she wakes up once or twice a night. She states, "I feel tired when I wake up, and I have trouble concentrating at work in the afternoon." She also reports that she has less patience with her children at home.
Ask Julie if there have been any recent changes in her life.	Julie says she is feeling pressured at work to complete an important case that she started on 2 weeks ago. She also reports that due to her heavy work schedule, she has stopped her routine of walking 1 to 2 miles daily.
Ask Julie to describe her bedtime routine.	Julie responds that she is going to bed between 12 AM and 1 AM, which is 2 hours later than her usual bedtime. It takes her an hour to fall asleep. She says she used to get 7 to 8 hours of sleep a night and now it is more like 5 to 6 hours. She drinks 2 to 3 cups of coffee after dinner while she is working on her case before bedtime. Julie reports drinking a glass of wine just before bedtime to help relax because she has been having trouble falling asleep.
Assess Julie for signs of sleep problems.	During the examination, the nurse notes Julie has dark circles under her eyes, she shifts her position in the chair multiple times, and yawns frequently.

Nursing Diagnosis: Disturbed sleep pattern related to psychological stress from job pressures.

Planning

Goal	Expected Outcomes*
	Sleep
Client will achieve an improved sense of adequate sleep within 2 weeks.	Client will report waking up less frequently during the night and feeling rested within 2 weeks.
	Client will verbalize adherence to a regular bedtime routine within 1 week.
Client will achieve a more normal sleep pattern within 2 weeks.	Client will fall asleep within 30 minutes of going to bed within 2 weeks.
	Client will report sleeping 7 hours nightly within 2 weeks.

*Outcomes classification label from Moorhead S, Johnson M, and Maas M: *Nursing outcomes classification (NOC)*, ed 3, St. Louis, 2004, Mosby.

Interventions†

Sleep Enhancement

Interventions†	Rationale
Encourage client to establish a bedtime routine and a regular sleep pattern.	Maintaining a consistent schedule helps induce sleep (Schneider, 2002).
Instruct client to limit caffeine, nicotine, and alcohol before bedtime.	Caffeine and nicotine are stimulants and cause difficulty in falling asleep. Alcohol lightens and fragments sleep (Kwentus, 2000).
Assist client in identifying ways to eliminate stressful concerns about work before bedtime (e.g., taking time before actual sleep time to read a light novel).	Excess worry and intense activities before bedtime may stimulate client and prevent sleep (Elliott, 2001).
Adjust environment, have client control noise, temperature, and light in the bedroom.	This develops an environment conducive to sleep (Kwentus, 2000).

†Intervention classification labels from Dochterman JM, Bulechek GM, editors: *Nursing interventions classification (NIC)*, ed 4, St. Louis, 2004, Mosby.

Continued

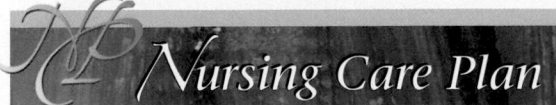

Nursing Care Plan

Disturbed Sleep Pattern—cont'd

Interventions†—cont'd	Rationale
Exercise Promotion Encourage client to reinstitute walking routinely during the day, but not 2 to 3 hours before bedtime.	Exercise can increase activity levels and the need for sleep. Exercise just before bedtime is a stimulant that prevents sleep (Elliott, 2001).
Simple Relaxation Therapy Instruct client on how to perform muscle relaxation before bedtime.	Relaxation therapy can help reduce anxiety, which interferes with sleep (Elliott, 2001).

†Intervention classification labels from Dochterman JM, Bulechek GM, editors: *Nursing interventions classification (NIC)*, ed 4, St. Louis, 2004, Mosby.

Evaluation

Nursing Actions	Client Response/Finding	Achievement of Outcome
Ask Julie if she is able to fall asleep and stay asleep.	Julie responds, "It usually takes me 15 to 20 minutes to fall asleep, and I woke up once for only two nights last week."	Julies reports she falls asleep within 30 minutes and wakes up less frequently during the night.
Ask Julie to describe her waking behaviors at work and home during the day.	Julie responds that she has completed her case at work and feels less pressure. She has restarted her walking routine. She reports that she is better able to cope with her children and that she is able to concentrate at work.	Julie reports feeling more rested.
Observe Julie's waking nonverbal expressions and behavior.	Julie sits in the chair without shifting position. She does not yawn during the conversation. The dark circles under her eyes are almost gone.	Julies reports she is sleeping an average of 7 hours a night.

---

beneficial. If the nurse works in an in-patient setting and the client is to receive a referral for continued care after discharge, offering information about the sleep problem will be useful to the home care nurse. The success of sleep therapy depends on an approach that fits the client's lifestyle and the nature of the sleep disorder.

Implementation

Nursing interventions designed to improve the quality of a person's rest and sleep are largely focused on health promotion. Clients need adequate sleep and rest to maintain active and productive lifestyles. During times of illness, rest and sleep promotion is important for recovery. Nursing care in an acute care, restorative care, or continuing care setting differs from that provided in a client's home. The primary differences are in the environment and the nurse's ability to support normal rest and sleep habits. The client's age also influences the types of therapies that are most effective. Box 41-8 provides principles for promoting sleep in older clients. Despite the cause or related factors for sleep problems, the nurse performs specific interventions that promote normal sleep patterns.

Health Promotion. In community health and home settings the nurse helps clients develop behaviors conducive to rest and relaxation. This may include suggesting changes in the environment or certain lifestyle habits. To develop good sleep habits at home, clients and their bed partners should learn techniques that promote sleep and conditions that interfere with sleep (Zarcone, 2000) (Box 41-9). Parents should also learn how to promote good sleep habits for their children. Clients benefit most from instructions based on information about their homes and lifestyles such as what type of activities will promote sleep in a third-shift worker or how the home environment can be made more conducive to sleep. Similarly, they will more likely apply information that is useful and valued.

Environmental Controls. All clients require a sleeping environment with a comfortable room temperature and proper ventilation, minimal sources of noise, a comfortable bed, and proper lighting (Dochterman and Bulechek, 2004). Infants sleep best when the room temperature is 64.4° to 69.8° F (18° to 21° C) at night. Cribs should be positioned away from open windows or drafts. The infant is covered with a light, warm blanket. Children and adults vary more in regard to comfortable room temperature. Some prefer to sleep without covers. Older adults often require extra blankets or covers.

Distracting noise needs to be eliminated so that the bedroom is as quiet as possible. In the home the television, telephone, or the intermittent chiming of a clock

Concept Map

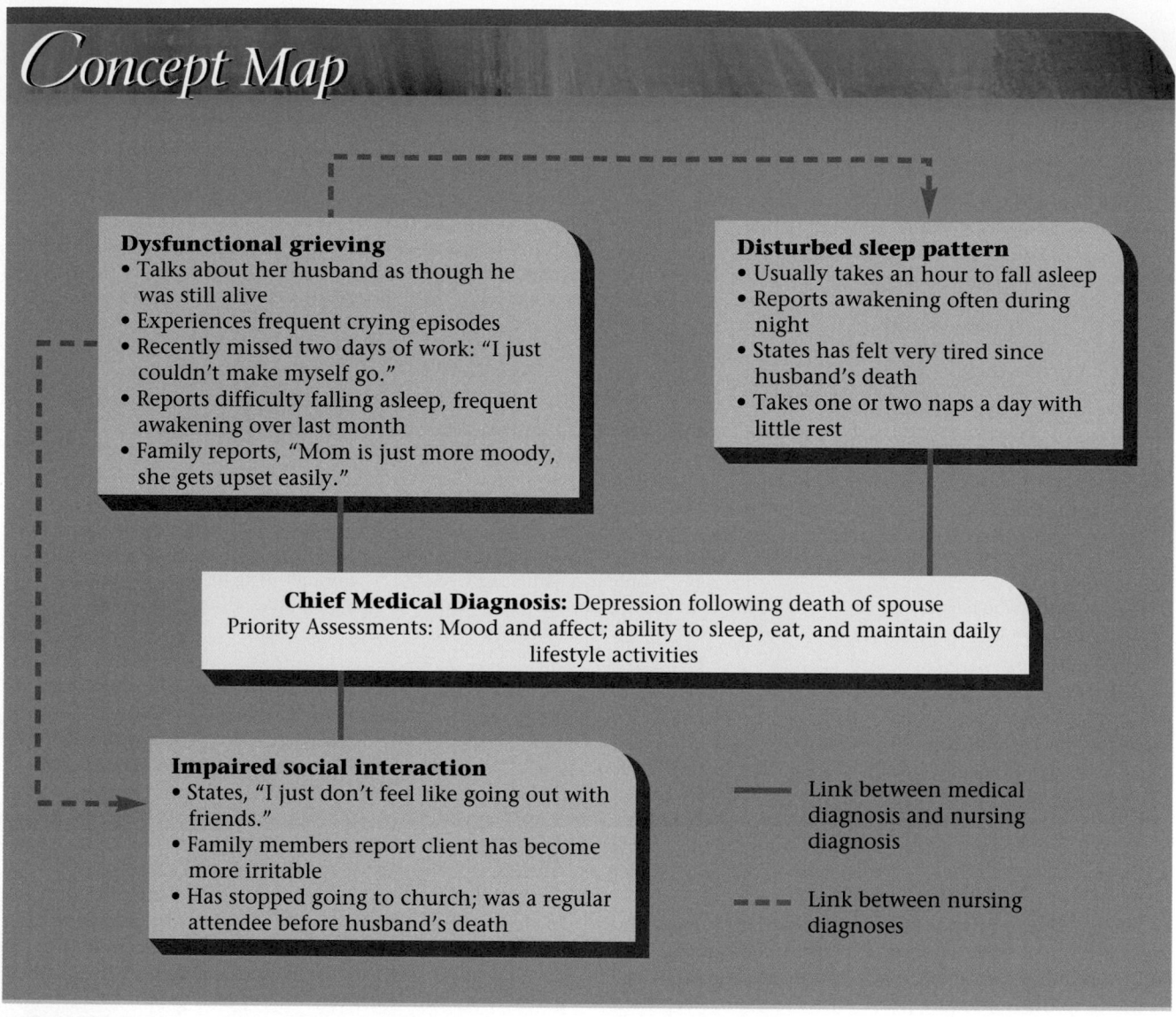

Dysfunctional grieving
- Talks about her husband as though he was still alive
- Experiences frequent crying episodes
- Recently missed two days of work: "I just couldn't make myself go."
- Reports difficulty falling asleep, frequent awakening over last month
- Family reports, "Mom is just more moody, she gets upset easily."

Disturbed sleep pattern
- Usually takes an hour to fall asleep
- Reports awakening often during night
- States has felt very tired since husband's death
- Takes one or two naps a day with little rest

Chief Medical Diagnosis: Depression following death of spouse
Priority Assessments: Mood and affect; ability to sleep, eat, and maintain daily lifestyle activities

Impaired social interaction
- States, "I just don't feel like going out with friends."
- Family members report client has become more irritable
- Has stopped going to church; was a regular attendee before husband's death

—— Link between medical diagnosis and nursing diagnosis

- - - Link between nursing diagnoses

FIGURE **41–5** Concept map for client with depression following death of spouse.

may disrupt a client's sleep. The family becomes an important part of the nurse's approach, especially if there are several family members, all with different schedules for going to sleep. At home it may require the cooperation of several people living with the client to reduce noise. It is also important to remember that some clients are used to sleeping with familiar inside noises, such as the hum of a fan. Commercial products that produce a soothing noise such as ocean waves or rainfall may be purchased and used to create a soothing environment for sleep.

A bed and mattress should provide support and comfortable firmness. Bed boards can be placed under mattresses to add support. Sometimes extra pillows are important to help a person position comfortably in bed. The position of the bed in the room may also make a difference for some clients.

Infants' beds must be safe. To reduce the chance of suffocation, pillows, stuffed toys, or the ends of loose blankets should not be placed in cribs. Loose-fitting plastic mattress covers should not be used because infants might pull them over their faces and suffocate. Infants are usually placed on their back to prevent suffocation or on their sides to prevent aspiration of stomach contents.

For any client prone to confusion or falls, safety is critical. In the home a small night-light might assist the client in orienting to the room environment before arising to go to the bathroom. Beds set lower to the floor may lessen the chance of a person falling when first standing. Clutter and throw rugs should always be removed from the path a client uses to walk from the bed to the bathroom. If a client needs assistance in ambulating from a bed to the bathroom, a small bell at the bedside can be used to call family members.

Clients vary in regard to the amount of light that they prefer at night. Infants and older adults sleep best in softly lit rooms. Light should not shine directly on their eyes. Small table lamps prevent total darkness. For older adults this reduces the chance of confusion and prevents

Promoting Sleep

Sleep-Wake Pattern

- Maintain a regular bedtime and wake-up schedule (Kwentus, 2000).
- Eliminate naps unless they are a routine part of the schedule.
- If naps are used, limit to 20 minutes or less twice a day.
- Go to bed when sleepy.
- Use warm bath and relaxation techniques to promote sleep (Schneider, 2002).
- If unable to sleep in 15 to 30 minutes, get out of bed.

Environment

- Sleep where you sleep best.
- Keep noise to minimum; use soft music to mask noise if necessary.
- Use night-light and keep path to bathroom free of obstacles.
- Set room temperature to preference; use socks to promote warmth.

Medications

- Use sedatives and hypnotics as last resort and then only short-term if absolutely necessary (Lueckenotte, 2000).
- Adjust medications being taken for other conditions and assess for drug interactions that may cause insomnia or excessive daytime sleepiness (EDS).

Diet

- Limit alcohol, caffeine, and nicotine in late afternoon and evening (Lueckenotte, 2000).
- Consume carbohydrates or milk as a light snack before bedtime (Foreman and Wykle, 1995).
- Decrease fluids 2 to 4 hours before sleep (Lueckenotte, 2000).

Physiological/Illness Factors

- Elevate head of bed and provide extra pillows as preferred.
- Use analgesics 30 minutes before bed to ease aches and pains (Foreman and Wykle, 1995).
- Use therapeutics to control symptoms of chronic conditions as prescribed (Beck-Little and Weinrich, 1998).

Sleep Hygiene Habits

Objective

- Client will follow proper sleep hygiene habits at home.

Teaching Strategies

- Instruct client to try to exercise daily, preferably in morning or afternoon, and to avoid vigorous exercise in the evening within 2 hours of bedtime.
- Caution client against sleeping long hours during weekends or holidays to prevent disturbance of normal sleep-wake cycle.
- Explain that if possible, the bedroom should not be used for intensive studying, snacking, TV watching, or other nonsleep activity, besides sex.
- Explain that client should try to avoid worrisome thinking when going to bed and should use relaxation exercises.
- Advise to get out of bed and do some quiet activity until feeling sleepy enough to go back to bed if client does not fall asleep within 30 minutes of going to bed.
- Recommend client limit caffeine to morning coffee and limit alcohol intake (more than 1 to 2 drinks a day can interrupt sleep cycle).
- Ask client to examine environment: keep room dark, well ventilated, quiet, and at a comfortable temperature. Instruct that use of earplugs and eyeshades may be helpful.
- Instruct client to avoid heavy meals for 3 hours before bedtime; a light snack may help.

Evaluation

- Have client complete sleep-wake log for 1 week, and compare it with previous sleep-wake log.
- Ask client to periodically complete visual analog or sleep rating scale for perceptions of quality of sleep.

falls en route to the bathroom. If streetlights shine through windows or when clients nap during the day, heavy shades, drapes, or slatted blinds are helpful.

Promoting Bedtime Routines. Bedtime routines relax clients in preparation for sleep (Dochterman and Bulechek, 2004). It is always important for persons to go to sleep when they feel fatigued or sleepy. Going to bed while fully awake and thinking about other things can cause insomnia and interfere with the bed as a stimulus for sleep.

Newborns and infants sleep through so much of the day that a specific routine is hardly necessary. However, quieting activities, such as holding them snugly in blankets, singing or talking softly, and gentle rocking, help infants fall asleep.

A bedtime routine (e.g., same hour for bedtime, snack or quiet activity) used consistently helps young children avoid delaying sleep. Toddlers and preschoolers may be too excited and full of energy to go to bed. Patterns of preparing for bedtime need to be reinforced. Reading stories, allowing children to sit in a parent's lap while listening to music, or listening to a prayer are routines that can be associated with preparing for bed. Quiet activities such as coloring and reading work well with school-age children.

Adults need to avoid excessive mental stimulation just before bedtime. Reading a light novel, watching an enjoyable television program, or listening to music helps a person relax. Relaxation exercises can be useful at bedtime. Slow, deep breathing for 1 or 2 minutes induces calm (see Chapter 42). Relaxation of muscles alleviates tension and prepares the body for rest (Elliott, 2001). Guided imagery and praying may also promote sleep.

At home a client should not try to finish office work or resolve family problems before bedtime. The bedroom should not be used as a place to work and should always be associated with sleep. Working toward a consistent time for sleep and wakening helps most clients gain a healthy sleep pattern and strengthens the rhythm of the sleep-wake cycle.

Promoting Comfort. People fall asleep only after feeling comfortable and relaxed (Dochterman and Bulechek, 2004). Minor irritants can keep clients awake. Soft cotton nightclothes keep infants or small children warm and comfortable. Clients should be instructed to wear loose-fitting nightwear. An extra blanket may be all that is needed to prevent a person from feeling chilled and being unable to fall asleep. Clients should void before retiring so they are not kept awake by a full bladder.

Establishing Periods of Rest and Sleep. In the home it may help to encourage clients to stay physically active during the day so that they are more likely to sleep at night. Increasing daytime activity lessens problems with falling asleep. Rigorous exercise should always be planned at least several hours before bedtime.

In the home setting the nurse frequently cares for clients with chronic debilitating disease. The nursing care plan might include having clients set aside afternoons for rest to promote optimal health. The nurse helps adjust medication schedules, instructs clients to regularly void before rest periods, and suggests unplugging the telephone so that rest periods are uninterrupted.

Stress Reduction. The inability to sleep because of emotional stress can also make a person feel irritable and tense. When clients feel emotionally upset, they should be encouraged to try not to force sleep. Otherwise, insomnia frequently develops, and soon bedtime is associated with the inability to relax. A client who has difficulty falling asleep can be helped by getting up and pursuing a relaxing activity, such as sewing or reading, rather than staying in bed and thinking about sleep.

Preschoolers have bedtime fears (fear of the dark or strange noises), awaken during the night, or have nightmares. After nightmares, the parent should enter the child's room immediately and talk to them briefly about fears to provide a cooling-down period. One approach is to comfort children and leave them in their own beds so that their fears are not used as excuses to delay bedtime. Keeping a light on in the room may also help. Cultural tradition may cause families to approach sleep practices differently (Box 41-10). The nurse should respect those that differ from traditional recommendations.

Bedtime Snacks. Some persons enjoy bedtime snacks, whereas others cannot sleep after eating. A dairy product snack such as warm milk or cocoa that contains L-tryptophan may be helpful in promoting sleep. A full meal before bedtime can often cause gastrointestinal upset and interfere with the ability to fall asleep.

Nurses should encourage clients to try to refrain from drinking or ingesting caffeine before bedtime. Coffee, tea, cola, and chocolate act as stimulants, causing a person to stay awake or awaken throughout the night. Alcohol can interrupt sleep cycles and reduce the amount of deep

---

Box 41-10

Cultural Aspects of Care

Practices and patterns of sleep and rest vary among cultures. Sleep patterns are a component of the cultural practices related to the use of space and interaction distances. Traditionally experts recommend having infants and children sleep in their own beds. Co-sleeping, in which children are allowed to sleep with parents or siblings, is a more common practice among African-American, Hispanic, Middle Eastern, Eastern Europe, Asian, and American Samoan families. The type of bed for a child may also vary. Some Native American tribes use a cradle board for infants, whereas American Samoan infants sleep on a pandanus mat covered with a blanket. These approaches lessen the child's anxiety and create a strong sense of security.

Implications for Practice

- Assess thoroughly the sleep practices and preferred bedroom environment of clients from different cultures.
- Ask clients and their families how the hospital environment can be adapted to accommodate their cultural preferences.

Data from Andrews MM, Boyle JS: *Transcultural concepts in nursing care*, ed 4, Philadelphia, 2003, Lippincott; Giger JN, Davidhizar RE: *Transcultural nursing: assessment and intervention*, ed 3, St. Louis, 1999, Mosby; and Lozoff B: Culture and family: influences on childhood sleep practices and problems. In Ferber R, Kryger M, editors: *Principles and practice of sleep medicine in the child*, Philadelphia, 1995, WB Saunders.

---

sleep. Coffee, tea, colas, and alcohol act as diuretics and may cause a person to awaken in the night to void (Foreman and Wykle, 1995).

Infants require special measures to minimize nighttime awakenings for feeding. It is common for children to have a need for middle-of-the-night bottle- or breast-feeding. Hockenberry and others (2003) recommend offering the last feeding as late as possible. Infants should not be given bottles in bed.

Pharmacological Approaches. Melatonin is a neurohormone produced in the brain that helps control circadian rhythms and promote sleep (Cheng and Umland, 2000). It is a popular nutritional supplement to aid sleep. The recommended dosage is 0.3 to 1 mg taken 2 hours before bedtime. Older adults who have decreased levels of melatonin may find melatonin more beneficial as a sleep aid (Elliott, 2001). There are several other herbal products that are shown to assist in sleep. Valerian is effective in mild insomnia. It effects release of neurotransmitters and produces very mild sedation (Cheng and Umland, 2000; Elliott, 2001). Kava is recommended to help promote sleep in clients who have sleep problems related to anxiety. Chamomile, passionflower, lemon balm, and lavender are other herbal products that have mild sedative effects (Elliott, 2001). Clients should be cautioned about the dosage and use of herbal compounds because the Food and Drug Administration (FDA) does not regulate them (Cheng and Umland, 2000). Herbal compounds may create interactions with prescribed medication, and concurrent use should be avoided (Merritt and others, 2000) (see Chapter 35).

The use of nonprescription sleeping medications is not advisable. Clients should learn the risks of such drugs. Over the long term, these drugs can lead to further sleep disruption even when they initially seemed to be effective. Older adults should be cautioned about using over-the-counter antihistamines because of their long duration of action that can cause confusion, constipation, urinary retention, and increased risk of falls (Cheng and Umland, 2000). The nurse can help clients use behavioral and proper sleep hygiene measures to establish sleep patterns that do not require the use of drugs.

Acute Care. Clients in an acute care setting have their normal rest and sleep routine disrupted, which generally leads to sleep problems. In this setting the nursing interventions focus on controlling factors in the environment that disrupt sleep, relieving physiological or psychological disruptions to sleep, and providing for uninterrupted rest and sleep periods for the client. The "Nursing Standard-of-Practice Protocol: Sleep Disturbances in the Elderly" practice guidelines are based on the principle that an effective strategy must be individualized based on client needs and that sleep medications should be considered a last-resort intervention (Foreman and Wykle, 1995).

Environmental Controls. In a hospital the nurse can control the environment in several ways. Nurses should close the curtains between clients in semiprivate rooms. Lights on a hospital nursing unit can be dimmed at night. One of the biggest problems for clients in the hospital is noise. Important ways to reduce noise are to conduct conversations and reports in a private area away from client rooms and to keep necessary conversations to a minimum, especially at night (Foreman and Wykle, 1995). Additional ways to control noise in the hospital can be found in Box 41-11.

Promoting Comfort. Compared with beds at home, hospital beds are often harder and of a different height, length, or width. Keeping beds clean and dry and in a comfortable position may help clients relax. Some clients suffer painful illnesses requiring special comfort measures such as application of dry or moist heat, use of supportive dressings or splints, and proper positioning before retiring (Figure 41-6).

Establishing Periods of Rest and Sleep. In a hospital or extended care setting it is difficult to provide clients with the time needed to rest and sleep. However, the nurse plans care to avoid awakening clients for nonessential tasks. The nurse can help by scheduling assessments, treatments, procedures, and routines for times when clients are awake. For example, if a client's physical condition has been stable, the nurse should avoid awakening the client to check vital signs. Allowing clients to determine the timing and methods of delivery of basic care measures can promote rest. Baths and routine hygiene measures should not be given during the night for nurs-

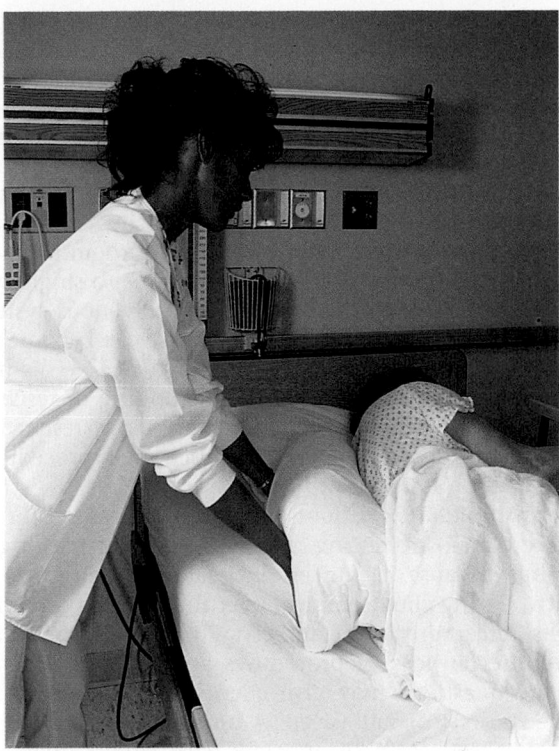

FIGURE **41-6** Positioning client for sleep.

Box 41-11	Control of Noise in the Hospital

Close doors to client's room when possible.
Keep doors to work areas on unit closed when in use.
Reduce volume of nearby telephone and paging equipment.
Wear rubber-soled shoes. Avoid clogs.
Turn off bedside oxygen and other equipment that is not in use.
Turn down alarms and beeps on bedside monitoring equipment.
Turn off room TV and radio unless client prefers soft music.
Avoid abrupt loud noise such as flushing a toilet or moving a bed.
Keep necessary conversations at low levels, particularly at night.
Conduct conversations and reports in a private area away from client rooms.

ing convenience. Blood should be drawn at a time when the client is awake. Unless maintaining a drug's therapeutic blood level is essential, medications should be given during waking hours. The nurse should work with the radiology department and other support services to schedule diagnostic studies and therapies at intervals that allow clients time for rest. Attempts should be made to provide the client with 2 to 3 hours of uninterrupted sleep during the night (Foreman and Wykle, 1995).

When the client's condition demands more frequent monitoring, the nurse can plan activities to allow extended rest periods. The nurse can instruct assistive personnel on the coordination of client care to reduce client disturbances. This means planning activities so that instead of a nurse or other personnel returning to the room every few minutes, the client may have up to an hour or more to rest quietly. For example, if a client needs frequent dressing changes, is receiving intravenous therapy, and has drainage tubes from several sites, the nurse should not make a separate trip into the room to check each problem. Instead the nurse should use a single visit to change the dressing, regulate the intravenous system, and empty the drainage tubes. The nurse can become the client's advocate for promoting optimal sleep. This may mean becoming a gatekeeper by postponing or rescheduling visits by family, asking consultants to reschedule visits, or questioning the frequency of certain procedures.

Stress Reduction. Clients who are hospitalized for extensive diagnostic testing may have difficulty resting or sleeping because of uncertainty about their state of health. Giving clients control over their health care minimizes uncertainty and anxiety. Providing information about the purpose of procedures and routines and answering questions may give clients the peace of mind needed to rest or fall asleep. A nurse on the night shift should take time to sit and talk with clients unable to sleep. This helps the nurse determine the factors keeping clients awake. Back rubs can also be used to help clients relax more thoroughly. If a sedative is indicated, the nurse confers with the physician to be sure that the lowest dosage is used initially. Discontinuing a sedative as soon as possible prevents a dependence that can seriously disrupt the normal sleep cycle. Older adults' metabolism of drugs is slowed, making them more vulnerable to the side effects of sedatives, hypnotics, antianxiety drugs, or analgesics.

Restorative or Continuing Care. The nursing interventions that are implemented in the acute care setting can also be used in the restorative or continuing care environment. Controlling the environment, especially noise, establishing periods of rest and sleep, and promoting comfort are important considerations. Nursing interventions related to stress reduction and controlling physiological disturbances are also implemented in these settings. Helping a client achieve restful sleep in this environment may take a period of time.

Promoting Comfort. Providing for personal hygiene improves a client's sense of comfort. A warm bath or shower before bedtime can be relaxing. Clients restricted to bed should be offered the opportunity to void and wash their face and hands. Toothbrushing and care of dentures also help to prepare the client for sleep. Position the client to support dependent body parts and protect pressure points. The nurse can offer a massage to aid in muscle relaxation just before the client goes to sleep (Foreman and Wykle, 1995) (see Chapter 42).

Controlling Physiological Disturbances. For clients with physical illness, the nurse can help control symptoms that disrupt sleep. For example, a client with res-

piratory abnormalities should sleep with two pillows or in a semisitting position to ease the effort to breathe. The client may benefit from taking prescribed bronchodilators before sleep to prevent airway obstruction. A client with a hiatal hernia also needs special care. After meals the client may experience a burning sensation as a result of gastric reflux. To prevent sleep disturbances, the client should eat a small meal several hours before bedtime and sleep in a semisitting position. Clients with pain, nausea, or other recurrent symptoms should receive any symptom-relieving medication timed so that the drug takes effect at bedtime. The nurse should remove or change any irritants against the client's skin such as moist dressings or drainage tubes.

Pharmacological Approaches. The liberal use of drugs to manage insomnia is quite common in American culture. Central nervous system stimulants such as amphetamines, caffeine, nicotine, terbutaline, theophylline, and pemoline should be used sparingly and under medical management (McKenry and Salerno, 2003). In addition, withdrawal from CNS depressants such as alcohol, barbiturates, tricyclic antidepressants (amitriptyline, imipramine, and doxepin), and triazolam can cause insomnia and must be managed carefully.

Medications that are used to induce sleep are called **hypnotics. Sedatives** are medications that produce a calming or soothing effect (McKenry and Salerno, 2003). Hypnotics and sedatives as sleep medications can help if used correctly. A client who takes sleep medications should know about their proper use, as well as the risks and possible side effects. However, long-term use of antianxiety, sedative, or hypnotic agents can disrupt sleep and lead to more serious problems. One group of drugs considered to be relatively safe is the benzodiazepines (Table 41-1). The benzodiazepines cause relaxation, antianxiety, and hypnotic effects by facilitating the action of neurons in the CNS that suppress responsiveness to stimulation, thereby decreasing levels of arousal (Mendelson, 2000). These medications do not cause general CNS depression as sedatives or hypnotics do. Physicians prescribe this group of drugs because antianxiety effects occur at safe, nontoxic doses.

The benzodiazepines are used cautiously with children under 12 years of age and are contraindicated in infants less than 6 months. Pregnant clients should avoid benzodiazepines because their use is associated with risk of congenital anomalies. Nursing mothers should not receive the drugs because they are excreted in breast milk. Short-acting benzodiazepines such as oxazepam or lorazepam are usually recommended. Initial doses should be small, and increments are added gradually, based on client response, for a limited period of time. Nurses should warn clients not to take more than the prescribed dose, especially if the medication seems to become less effective after initial use. If older clients who were recently continent, ambulatory, and alert become incontinent, confused, and/or demonstrate impaired mobility, the use of benzodiazepines should be considered as a possible cause.

Regular use of any sleep medication can lead to tolerance and withdrawal. Rebound insomnia can occur after stopping the medication. Immediately administering a

Table 41-1	Pharmacology of Antiinsomnia Agents			
Generic Name	Trade Name	Onset of Action (in Minutes)	Oral Dosage* (mg)	Indications
Alprazolam	Xanax	15-60	0.25-0.5 (3 times/day)	Anxiety
Diazepam	Valium	15-45	5-10 at bedtime	Sleep disorder
Flurazepam	Dalmane Apo-Flurazepam	15-45	15-30 at bedtime	Sleep disorder
Lorazepam	Ativan Apo-Lorazepam	15-60	2-4 at bedtime	Anxiety, sleep disorder
Oxazepam	Serax Zapex	45-90	10-30 (3-4 times/day)	Anxiety
Temazepam	Restoril	25-27	15-30 at bedtime	Sleep disorder
Triazolam	Halcion	15-30	0.125-0.25, give 1-1½ hr before bedtime	Sleep disorder
Zolpidem	Ambien	15-45	5-10 at bedtime	Sleep disorder

*Dosage may be reduced in older adult clients.

sleeping medication when a hospitalized client complains of being unable to sleep may be doing the client more harm than good. Alternative approaches to promote sleep must be considered. Routine monitoring of client response to sleeping medications is important.

Evaluation

Client Care. With regard to problems with sleep, the client is the source for evaluating outcomes. Each client has a unique need for sleep and rest. The client is the only who will know if sleep problems are improved and which interventions or therapies are most successful in promoting sleep (Figure 41-7). To evaluate the effectiveness of nursing interventions, the nurse makes comparisons with baseline sleep assessment data to evaluate if sleep has improved.

The nurse determines whether expected outcomes have been met. Evaluative measures may be used shortly after a therapy has been tried (e.g., observing whether a client falls asleep after reducing noise and darkening a room). Other evaluative measures may be used after a client awakens from sleep (e.g., asking a client to describe the number of awakenings during the previous night). The client and bed partner can usually provide accurate evaluative information. Over longer periods, the nurse may use assessment tools such as the visual analog scale or sleep rating scale to determine whether sleep has progressively improved or changed.

The nurse also assesses the level of understanding that clients or family members gain after receiving instruction on sleep habits. Compliance with these practices may best be measured during a home visit, when the environment can be observed. When expected outcomes are not met, the nurse revises the nursing measures or expected outcomes based on the client's needs or preferences.

Client Expectations. If the nurse has successfully developed a good relationship with a client and has developed a therapeutic plan of care, subtle behaviors often indicate the level of the client's satisfaction. The nurse may note the absence of signs of sleep problems, such as lethargy, frequent yawning or position changes, in the client. It is important for the nurse to ask the client if his or her sleep needs have been met. For example, ask the client, "Are you feeling more rested?" or "Can you tell me if you feel we have done all we can to help improve your sleep?" If the client's expectations have not been met, the nurse needs to spend more time trying to understand the client's needs and preferences. Working closely with the client and bed partner will enable the nurse to redefine those expectations that can be realistically met within the limits of the client's condition and treatment. The nurse is effective in promoting rest and sleep if the client's goals and expectations are met.

Key Concepts

- Sleep is believed to provide physiological and psychological restoration.
- The 24-hour sleep-wake cycle is a circadian rhythm that influences physiological function and behavior.
- The control and regulation of sleep depends on a balance between regulators within the central nervous system.
- During a typical night's sleep a person passes through four to six complete sleep cycles. Each sleep cycle contains three NREM stages of sleep and a period of REM sleep.
- Neonates, infants, children, and adolescents require more sleep than adults.
- The most common type of sleep disorder is insomnia, which is characterized by the inability to fall asleep, remain asleep during the night, or go back to sleep after awakening earlier than is desired.
- The hectic pace of a person's lifestyle, emotional and psychological stress, and alcohol ingestion can disrupt the sleep pattern.
- Only a client can report whether sleep is restful.
- If a client's sleep is adequate, the nurse assesses the client's usual bedtime, normal bedtime ritual, the preferred environment for sleeping, and usual preferred rising time.

KNOWLEDGE

- Characteristics of desirable sleep pattern
- Behaviors reflecting adequate sleep

EXPERIENCE

- Previous client responses to planned nursing interventions for promoting sleep
- Previous experience in adapting sleep therapies to personal needs

Evaluation

- Evaluate signs and symptoms of the client's sleep disturbance
- Review the client's sleep pattern
- Ask the client's sleep partner to report the client's response to sleep therapies
- Ask client if expectations of care are being met

STANDARDS

- Use established expected outcomes to evaluate the client's response to care (e.g., improved duration of sleep, fewer awakenings)

ATTITUDES

- Demonstrate humility if an intervention is unsuccessful; rethink your approach
- Display perseverance in staying with a plan or in trying new approaches in the case of chronic sleep problems

FIGURE **41–7** Critical thinking model for sleep evaluation.

- When a client has a sleep problem, the nurse conducts a complete sleep history. Diagnosing sleep problems depends on identifying factors that impair sleep.
- When planning interventions to promote sleep, the nurse should consider the usual characteristics of the client's home environment and normal lifestyle.
- A regular bedtime routine of relaxing activities prepares a person physically and mentally for sleep.
- An environment with a darkened room, reduced noise, comfortable bed, and good ventilation promotes sleep.
- One of the most important nursing interventions for promoting sleep in the hospitalized client is establishing periods for uninterrupted sleep and rest.
- Noise is one of the most common causes of sleep disturbances in the hospitalized client. The nurse should implement noise-reducing interventions to promote sleep.
- Pain or other disease symptom control is essential to promote the ability to sleep.

- Long-term use of sleeping pills may lead to difficulty in initiating and maintaining sleep.

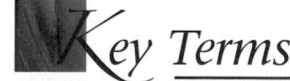 *ey Terms*

Biological clocks, *p. 1200*
Cataplexy, *p. 1205*
Circadian rhythm, *p. 1200*
Dyssomnias, *p. 1203*
Excessive daytime sleepiness (EDS), *p. 1204*
Hypersomnolence, *p. 1203*
Hypnotics, *p. 1222*
Insomnia, *p. 1204*
Narcolepsy, *p. 1205*
Nocturia, *p. 1202*
Nonrapid eye movement (NREM) sleep, *p. 1200*

Parasomnias, *p. 1203*
Polysomnogram, *p. 1204*
Rapid eye movement (REM) sleep, *p. 1200*
Rest, *p. 1206*
Sedatives, *p. 1222*
Sleep, *p. 1200*
Sleep apnea, *p. 1204*
Sleep deprivation, *p. 1205*
Sleep hygiene, *p. 1204*

Critical Thinking Exercises

1. Mr. Collins, age 45, comes to the doctor for a checkup. He tells you that he feels like he is not getting enough sleep and that his wife says he snores loudly. What assessment data should you gather from Mr. Collins?

2. You are doing a presentation to a preschool parents group on the topic of sleep and rest. What information should you provide to parents to help promote sleep in preschool and school-age children?

3. Mrs. Augustine is a 75-year-old who recently moved into a nursing home. She says she has not been sleeping well since moving. Develop a plan of care to promote sleep for Mrs. Augustine.

Review Questions

1. When assessing a client for obstructive sleep apnea (OSA), the nurse understands the most common symptom is:
   1. Headache.
   2. Early wakening.
   3. Impaired reasoning.
   4. Excessive daytime sleepiness.

2. One priority nursing intervention to promote sleep for a hospitalized client is to:
   1. Turn television on low to late-night programming.
   2. Avoid awakening client for nonessential tasks.
   3. Give prescribed sleeping medications at dinner.
   4. Have client follow hospital routines.

3. The use of nonprescription sleeping medications is not advisable because these medications can:
   1. Lead to further sleep disruption even when they initially seemed to be effective.
   2. Be expensive and difficult to obtain.
   3. Cause severe depression and anxiety.
   4. Cause headaches and nausea.

4. If a client is using herbal compounds such as valerian for sleep, the nurse should caution the client that these compounds may:
   1. Interfere with prescribed mediations.
   2. Cause diarrhea and anxiety.
   3. Not be used indefinitely.
   4. Produce severe insomnia.

5. The nurse understands that the most vivid dreaming occurs during:
   1. REM sleep.
   2. Stage 1 NREM sleep.
   3. Stage 4 NREM sleep.
   4. Transition period from NREM to REM sleep.

6. A client taking a beta-adrenergic blocker for hypertension can experience interference with sleep patterns such as:
   1. Nocturia.
   2. Increased daytime sleepiness.
   3. Increased awakening from sleep.
   4. Increased difficulty falling asleep.

7. The care plan for improving sleep in an older person may include:
   1. A nap during the day to make up for lost sleep.
   2. Exercise in the evening to increase fatigue.
   3. Allowing the client to sleep as late as possible.
   4. Decreasing fluids 2 to 4 hours before sleep.

8. Currently the American academy of Pediatrics recommends that healthy infants be placed in a side-lying or supine position during sleep to decrease the incidence of:
   1. Falls.
   2. Vomiting.
   3. Cradle cap.
   4. Sudden infant death syndrome (SIDS).

9. Narcolepsy can be best explained as:
   1. A sudden muscle weakness during exercise.
   2. Stopping breathing for short intervals during sleep.
   3. Frequent awakenings during the night.
   4. An overwhelming wave of sleepiness and falling asleep.

10. A nursing measure to promote sleep in school-age children is to:
    1. Make sure the room is dark and quiet.
    2. Encourage evening exercise.
    3. Encourage television viewing.
    4. Encourage quiet activities prior to bed time.

References

Aldrich MS, Naylor MW: Approach to the patient with disordered sleep. In Kryger MH, Roth T, Dement WC, editors: *Principles and practice of sleep medicine,* ed 3, Philadelphia, 2000, WB Saunders.

American Academy of Pediatrics Task Force on Infant Sleep Position and Sudden Infant Death Syndrome: Changing concepts of sudden infant death syndrome: implications for infant sleeping environment and sleep position, *Pediatrics* 105(3):650, 2000.

American Academy of Sleep Medicine: *Sleep and heart disease,* Westchester, Ill, 2002, The Academy.

American Nurses Association: *Standards of clinical nursing practice,* ed 2, Washington, DC, 1998, American Nurses Publishing, American Nurses Foundation/American Nurses Association.

American Sleep Disorders Association, Diagnostic Classification Steering Committee: International classification of sleep disorders, 1997. In Thorpy M: Classification of sleep disorders. In Kryger M and others, editors: *Principles and practice of sleep medicine,* ed 3, Philadelphia, 2000, WB Saunders.

Andrews MM, Boyle JS: *Transcultural concepts in nursing care,* 4e, Philadelphia, 2003, Lippincott.

Attarian HP: Helping patients who say they cannot sleep: practical ways to evaluate and treat insomnia, *Postgrad Med* 107(3):127, 2000.

Basin AG, Guilleminault C: Clinical features and evaluation of obstructive apnea. In Kryger MH, Roth T, Dement WC, editors, *Principles and practice of sleep medicine,* ed 3, Philadelphia, 2000, WB Saunders.

Beck-Little R, Weinrich SP: Assessment and management of sleep disorders in the elderly, *J Gerontol Nurs* 24(4):14, 1998.

Brink S, Kelly K, Rae-Dupree J: Sleepless society, *U.S. News & World Report* 129(15), electronic version, 2000.

Cheng C, Umland E: New and old drugs to treat insomnia, *Patient Care* 34(11):34, 2000.

Chokroverty S: *Clinical companion to sleep disorders in medicine,* ed 2, Boston, 2000, Butterworth Heineman.

Closs SJ: Assessment of sleep in hospital patients: a review of methods, *J Adv Nurs* 13:501, 1988.

Cohen FL, Nehring WM, Cloninger L: Symptom description and management in narcolepsy, *Holist Nurs Pract* 10(4):44, 1996.

Cullen DF: Obstructive sleep apnea and postoperative analgesia—a potentially dangerous combination, *J Clin Anesth* 13:83, 2001.

Dahl RE, Carskadon MA: Sleep and its disorders in adolescence. In Ferber E, Kryger M, editors: *Principles and practice of sleep medicine in the child,* Philadelphia, 1995, WB Saunders.

D'Cruz OF, Vaughn BV: Parasomnias: an update, *Semin Pediatr Neurol* 8(4):251, 2001.

Dines-Kalinowski CM: Promoting sleep in the ICU, *Nursing* 32(2):326, 2002.

Dobbin KR, Strollo PJ: Obstructive sleep apnea: recognition and management considerations for the aged patient, *AACN Clin Issues* 13(1):103, 2002.

Dochterman JM, Bulechek GM, editors: *Nursing interventions classification (NIC),* ed 4, St. Louis, 2004, Mosby.

Elliott AC: Primary care assessment and management of sleep disorders, *J Am Acad Nurse Pract* 13(9):409, 2001.

Foreman MD, Wykle M: Nursing standard-of-practice protocol: sleep disturbances in elderly patients, *Geriatr Nurs* 16(3):238, 1995.

Giger JN, Davidhizar RE: *Transcultural nursing: assessment and intervention,* ed 3, St. Louis, 1999, Mosby.

Gillis AM: Cardiac arrhythmias. In Kryger MH, Roth T, Dement WC, editors: *Principles and practice of sleep medicine,* ed 3, Philadelphia, 2000, WB Saunders.

Hauri P, Linde S: *No more sleepless nights,* New York, 1990, Wiley.

Jones B: Basic mechanisms of sleep-wake states. In Kryger MH, Roth T, Dement WC, editors: *Principles and practice of sleep medicine,* ed 3, Philadelphia, 2000, WB Saunders.

Kwentus JA: Sleep problems, *Clin Geriatrics,* 8(9):64, 2000.

Leigh TJ and others: Factor analysis of the St. Mary's Hospital Sleep Questionnaire, *Sleep* 11(5):448, 1988.

Lozoff B: Culture and family: influences on childhood sleep practices and problems. In Ferber R, Kryger M, editors: *Principles and practice of sleep medicine in the child,* Philadelphia, 1995, WB Saunders.

Lueckenotte AG: *Gerontologic nursing,* ed 2, St. Louis, 2000, Mosby.

Mahowald MW: What is causing excessive daytime sleepiness? Evaluation to distinguish sleep deprivation from sleep disorders, *Postgrad Med* 107(3):108, 2000.

McCance KL, Huether SE: *Pathophysiology: the biologic basis for disease in adults and children,* ed 4, St. Louis, 2002, Mosby.

McKenry LM, Salerno E: *Mosby's pharmacology in nursing,* ed 21, St. Louis, 2003, Mosby.

Mendelson WB: Hypnotics: basic mechanisms and pharmacology. In Kryger MH, Roth T, Dement WC, editors: *Principles and practice of sleep medicine,* ed 3, Philadelphia, 2000, WB Saunders.

Merritt SL and others: Herbal remedies: efficacy in controlling sleepiness and promoting sleep, *Nurse Pract Forum* 11(2):87, 2000.

Mitler H and others: Sleep medicine, public policy and public health. In Kryger MH, Roth T, Dement WC, editors: *Principles and practice of sleep medicine,* ed 3, Philadelphia, 2000, WB Saunders.

Moorhead S, Johnson M, Maas M: *Nursing outcomes classification (NOC),* ed 3, St. Louis, 2004, Mosby.

Mornhinweg GC, Voignier RR: Rest, *Holist Nurs Pract* 10(4):54, 1996.

National Heart, Lung, and Blood Institute Working Group on Restless Leg Syndrome: Restless leg syndrome: detection and management in primary care, *Am Fam Physician* 61(1):108, 2000.

National Sleep Foundation: *Sleep strategies for shiftworkers,* Washington, DC, 2001, The Foundation.

National Sleep Foundation: *Sleep apnea,* Washington, DC, 2002a, The Foundation.

National Sleep Foundation: *The ABCs of ZZZs,* Washington, DC, 2002b, The Foundation.

National Sleep Foundation: *The nature of sleep,* http://www.sleepfoundation.org/publications/nos.html#1, 2003.

Orr WC: Gastrointestinal physiology. In Kryger MH, Roth T, Dement WC, editors: *Principles and practice of sleep medicine,* ed 3, Philadelphia, 2000, WB Saunders.

Pagel JF: Nightmares and disorders of dreaming, *Am Fam Physician* 61(7):2037, 2000.

Pakola SJ, Dinges, DF, Pack AI: Driving and sleepiness: review of regulations and guidelines for commercial and noncommercial drivers with sleep apnea and narcolepsy, *Sleep* 18(9):787, 1995.

Renaud MT: Neonatal sleep patterns: implications for nursing, *Holist Nurs Pract* 10(4):27, 1996.

Richards KC: Sleep promotion, *Crit Care Nurs Clin North Am* 8(1):39, 1996.

Richardson SJ: A comparison of tools for assessment of sleep pattern disturbance in critically ill adults, *Dimens Crit Care Nurs* 16(5):226, 1997.

Schneider DL: Insomnia: safe and effective therapy for sleep problems in the older patient, *Geriatrics* 57(5):24, 2002.

Schweitzer PK: Drugs that disturb sleep and wakefulness. In Kryger MH, Roth T, Dement WC, editors: *Principles and practice of sleep medicine,* ed 3, Philadelphia, 2000, WB Saunders.

Smyth C: Try this: The Pittsburgh Sleep Quality Index (PSQI), *Clin Nurse Spec* 14(3):139, 1999.

Smyth C: The Pittsburgh Sleep Quality Index, *Geriatr Nurs* 23(1):56, 2002.

Webster RA, Thompson DR: Sleep in the hospital, *J Adv Nurs* 11:447, 1986.

White DP: Central sleep apnea. In Kryger MH, Roth T, Dement WC, editors: *Principles and practice of sleep medicine,* ed 3, Philadelphia, 2000, WB Saunders.

Wong DL and others: *Whaley and Wong's nursing care of infants and children,* ed 7, St. Louis, 2003, Mosby.

Zachary M: Understanding changes in brain waves during sleep, *AARC Times* 24(8):40, 2000.

Zarcone VP: Sleep hygiene. In Kryger MH, Roth T, Dement WC, editors: *Principles and practice of sleep medicine,* ed 3, Philadelphia, 2000, WB Saunders.

Zordis JD: Narcolepsy: Recognition is key to proper management, *RT J Respir Care Pract* 14(2):33, 2001.

Zorick F, Walsh J: Evaluation and management of insomnia: an overview. In Kryger MH, Roth T, Dement WC, editors: *Principles and practice of sleep medicine,* ed 3, Philadelphia, 2000, WB Saunders.

*R*esearch References

Libman E and others: Sleep questionnaire versus sleep diary: which measure is better? *Int J Rehabil Health* 5(3):205, 2000.

Mindell JA, Jacobson BJ: Sleep disturbances during pregnancy, *J Obstet Gynecol Neonatal Nurs* 29(6):590, 2000.

Olson DM and others: Quiet time: a nursing intervention to promote sleep in neurocritical care units, *Am J Crit Care* 10(2):74, 2001.

Redeker N: Sleep in acute care settings: an integrative review, *Image J Nurs Sch* 32(1):31, 2000.

Richards KC, O'Sullivan PS, Phillips RL: Measurement of sleep in critically ill patients, *J Nurs Meas* 8(2):131, 2000.

42

Comfort

Media Resources

http://evolve.elsevier.com/Potter/
fundamentals/

CD COMPANION

- Review Questions
- Glossary

evolve WEBSITE

- Review Questions
- Student Learning Activities
- Concept Map Exercise
- Critical Thinking Exercise
- Glossary

Objectives

Mastery of content in this chapter will enable the student to:

- Define the key terms listed.
- Discuss common misconceptions about pain.
- Describe the physiology of pain.
- Identify components of the pain experience.
- Explain how the physiology of pain relates to selecting interventions for pain relief.
- Describe the components of pain assessment.
- Perform an assessment of a client experiencing pain.
- Explain how cultural factors influence the pain experience.
- Describe the appropriate nursing diagnoses, outcomes, and interventions for a client with pain.
- Describe guidelines for selecting and individualizing pain interventions.
- Explain the various pharmacological approaches to treating pain.
- Describe applications for use of nonpharmacological pain interventions.
- Discuss nursing implications for administering analgesics.
- Identify barriers to effective pain management.
- Evaluate a client's response to pain interventions.

Everyone has experienced some type or degree of **pain.** It is the most common reason why people seek health care. Despite being one of the most commonly occurring symptoms in the medical world, pain is one of the least understood. A person in pain feels distress or suffering and seeks relief. The nurse uses a variety of interventions to bring relief or to restore comfort. However, the nurse cannot see or feel the client's pain. Pain is subjective; no two persons experience pain in the same way, and no two painful events create identical responses or feelings in a person. The International Association for the Study of Pain (IASP, 1979) defined pain as "an unpleasant, subjective sensory and emotional experience associated with actual or potential tissue damage, or described in terms of such damage." Thus, physical pain can cause psychological pain and visa versa.

Nurses care for clients in many settings and situations in which interventions are provided to promote comfort. Comfort is a concept central to the art of nursing. As Donahue (1989) summarized, "Through comfort and comfort measures . . . nurses provide strength, hope, solace, support, encouragement, and assistance." A variety of nursing theorists refer to comfort as a basic client need for which nursing care is delivered. The concept of comfort is as subjective as that of pain. Each individual has physiological, social, spiritual, psychological, and cultural characteristics that influence how comfort is interpreted and experienced.

The context of comfort is the umbrella under which pain and pain management options are viewed. Since the experience of pain is dynamic, the nurse has a responsibility to understand the pain experience. The nurse, client, family, and members of the health care team must collaborate to find the most effective approach to pain control. According to McCaffery (1979), "Pain is whatever the experiencing person says it is, existing whenever he says it does." Providing pain relief is considered a basic human right and is incorporated into the Pain Care Bill of Rights (American Pain Foundation, 2001). Furthermore, the American Bar Association (2000) declared pain relief a basic legal right. Nurses are ethically and legally responsible for managing pain and relieving suffering. Effective pain management not only reduces physical discomfort, but also improves quality of life and promotes earlier mobilization and return to work, resulting in fewer hospital/clinic visits, shortened hospital stays, and reduced health care costs.

Scientific Knowledge Base

Recorded history allows us to see that pain has been an integral component of the human experience. Traditionally pain has been viewed simply as a symptom of an illness or condition. However, pain itself is now considered to be a separate disease.

Nature of Pain

Pain is much more than a physical sensation caused by a specific stimulus. The pain experience is complex, involving physical, emotional and cognitive components. Pain is subjective and highly individualized. The stimulus for pain can be physical and/or mental in nature. Pain is exhausting and demands a person's energy. It can interfere with personal relationships and influence the meaning of life (Davis, 2002). Pain cannot be objectively measured, such as with a blood test. Only the client knows whether pain is present and what the experience is like. It is not the responsibility of clients to prove that they are in pain; it is the nurse's responsibility to accept patients' report of pain (American Pain Society [APS], 1999).

Physiology of Pain

There are four processes of nociceptive (normal) pain: transduction, transmission, perception, and modulation (McCaffery and Pasero, 1999). A client in pain cannot discriminate among the processes. However, understanding each process helps the nurse recognize factors that can cause pain, symptoms that accompany pain, and the rationale and actions of select therapies.

Pain is usually caused by thermal, chemical, or mechanical stimuli. The energy of these stimuli is converted to electrical energy. This energy conversion is known as **transduction.** Transduction begins in the periphery when a pain-producing stimulus sends an impulse across a peripheral pain nerve fiber **(nociceptor),** initiating an action potential. Once transduction is complete, **transmission** of the pain impulse begins.

> **Box 42-1**   **Neurophysiology of Pain: Neuroregulators**
>
> ### Neurotransmitters (Excitatory)
>
> **Substance P**
> Found in the pain neurons of the dorsal horn (excitatory peptide)
> Needed to transmit pain impulses from the periphery to higher brain centers
> Causes vasodilation and edema
>
> **Serotonin**
> Released from the brain stem and dorsal horn to inhibit pain transmission
>
> **Prostaglandins**
> Generated from the breakdown of phospholipids in cell membranes
> Believed to increase sensitivity to pain
>
> ### Neuromodulators (Inhibitory)
>
> **Endorphins and Dynorphins**
> They are the body's natural supply of morphinelike substances
> Activated by stress and pain
> Located within the brain, spinal cord, and gastrointestinal tract
> Cause analgesia when they attach to opiate receptors in the brain
> Present in higher levels in people who have less pain than others with a similar injury
>
> **Bradykinin**
> Released from plasma that leaks from surrounding blood vessels at the site of tissue injury
> Binds to receptors on peripheral nerves, increasing pain stimuli
> Binds to cells that cause the chain reaction producing prostaglandins

All cellular damage caused by thermal, mechanical, or chemical stimuli results in the release of excitatory **neurotransmitters** such as **prostaglandins,** bradykinin, potassium, histamine, and substance P (Box 42-1). These pain-sensitizing substances surround the pain fibers in the extracellular fluid, creating the spread of the pain message and causing an inflammatory response (Paice, 1994). The pain fiber enters the spinal cord and travels one of several routes until ending within the gray matter of the spinal cord. Within the dorsal horn, substance P is released, causing a synaptic transmission from the afferent (sensory) peripheral nerve to spinothalamic tract nerves (Wall and Melzack, 1999) (Figure 42-1).

Nerve impulses resulting from the painful stimulus travel along afferent (sensory) peripheral nerve fibers. Two types of peripheral nerve fibers conduct painful stimuli: the fast, myelinated A-delta fibers and the very small, slow, unmyelinated C fibers. The A fibers send sharp, localized, and distinct sensations that localize the source of the pain and detect its intensity. The C fibers relay impulses that are poorly localized, burning, and persistent (Wall and Melzack, 1999). For example, after stepping on a nail, a person initially feels a sharp, localized pain, which is a result of A-fiber transmission. Within a few seconds, the pain becomes more diffuse and widespread, until the whole foot aches because of C-fiber innervation.

Transmission of the pain stimulus continues along the afferent nerve fibers until they end in the dorsal horn of the spinal cord. Pain stimuli continue to travel through nerve fibers in the spinothalamic tracts that cross to the opposite side of the spinal cord. Pain impulses then travel up the spinal cord. Figure 42-2 shows the normal pain reception pathway. After the pain impulse ascends the spinal cord, information is transmitted quickly by the thalamus to higher centers in the brain, including

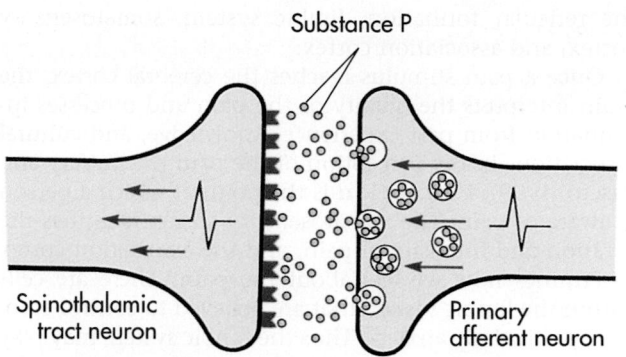

FIGURE **42–1** Substance P and other neurotransmitters are released from primary afferent fibers that terminate in the dorsal horn of the spinal cord. (From Paice JA: Unraveling the mystery of pain, *Oncol Nurs Forum* 18[5]:843, 1991.)

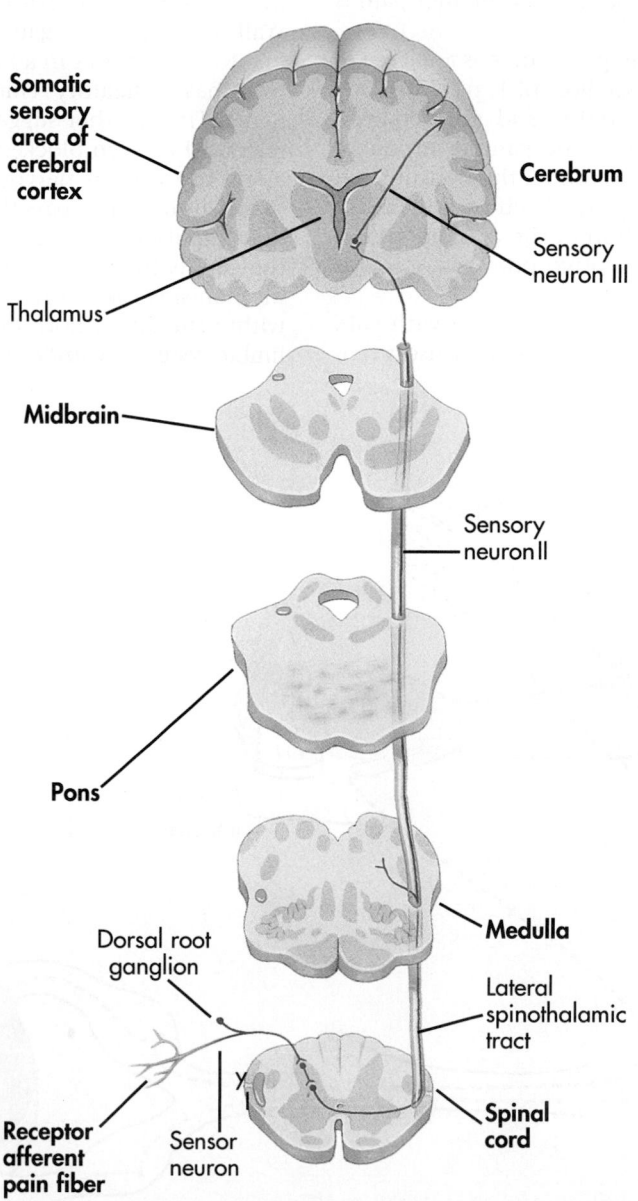

FIGURE **42–2** Spinothalamic pathway that conducts pain stimuli to the brain.

the reticular formation, limbic system, somatosensory cortex, and association cortex.

Once a pain stimulus reaches the cerebral cortex, the brain interprets the quality of the pain and processes information from past experience, knowledge, and cultural associations in the perception of the pain (McCaffery and Pasero, 1999). **Perception** is the point at which a person is aware of pain. The somatosensory cortex identifies the location and intensity of pain, and the association cortex determines how we feel about the pain. There are cells within the limbic system that are believed to control emotion, particularly anxiety. Thus the limbic system may play an active role in processing the emotional reaction to pain.

As a person becomes aware of pain, a complex reaction unfolds. Psychological and cognitive factors interact with neurophysiological ones in the perception of pain. Perception gives awareness and meaning to pain so that a person can then react. The reaction to pain is the physiological and behavioral responses that occur after pain is perceived.

Once the brain perceives the pain, there is a release of inhibitory neurotransmitters (see Box 42-1, p. 1230) such as endogenous opioids (endorphins and enkephalins), serotonin (5HT), norepinephrine, and gamma aminobutyric acid (GABA), which work to hinder the transmission of pain and help produce an analgesic effect (McCaffery and Pasero, 1999). This inhibition of the pain impulse is the fourth phase of the nociceptive process known as **modulation.**

A protective reflex response may also occur with pain reception (Figure 42-3). A-delta fibers send sensory impulses to the spinal cord, where they synapse with spinal motor neurons. The motor impulses travel via a reflex arc along efferent (motor) nerve fibers back to a peripheral muscle near the site of stimulation; thus bypassing the brain. Contraction of the muscle leads to a protective withdrawal from the source of pain. For example, when a person accidentally touches a hot iron, a burning sensation is felt, but the hand also reflexively withdraws from the iron's surface. When superficial fibers in the skin are stimulated, a person moves away from the pain source. If internal tissues such as muscle or mucous membranes become stimulated, tightening and guarding of muscles occur. This reflex is usually absent, below the injury, in clients with spinal cord injuries. However, spinal cord injured clients can still experience pain (Siddall, Yezierski, and Loeser, 2000).

Gate-Control Theory of Pain. Researchers know that there is no specific pain center in the nervous system. Wall and Malzack's gate-control theory (1965) was the first to suggest that in addition to the physical sensation, pain has obligatory emotional and cognitive components. They further suggested that pain impulses can be regulated or even blocked by gating mechanisms located along the central nervous system. The theory suggests that pain impulses pass through when a gate is open and that impulses are blocked when a gate is closed. Closing the gate is the basis for pain-relief interventions. Gating mechanisms can be found in substantia gelatinosa cells within the dorsal horn of the spinal cord, thalamus, and limbic system. By understanding what can influence these

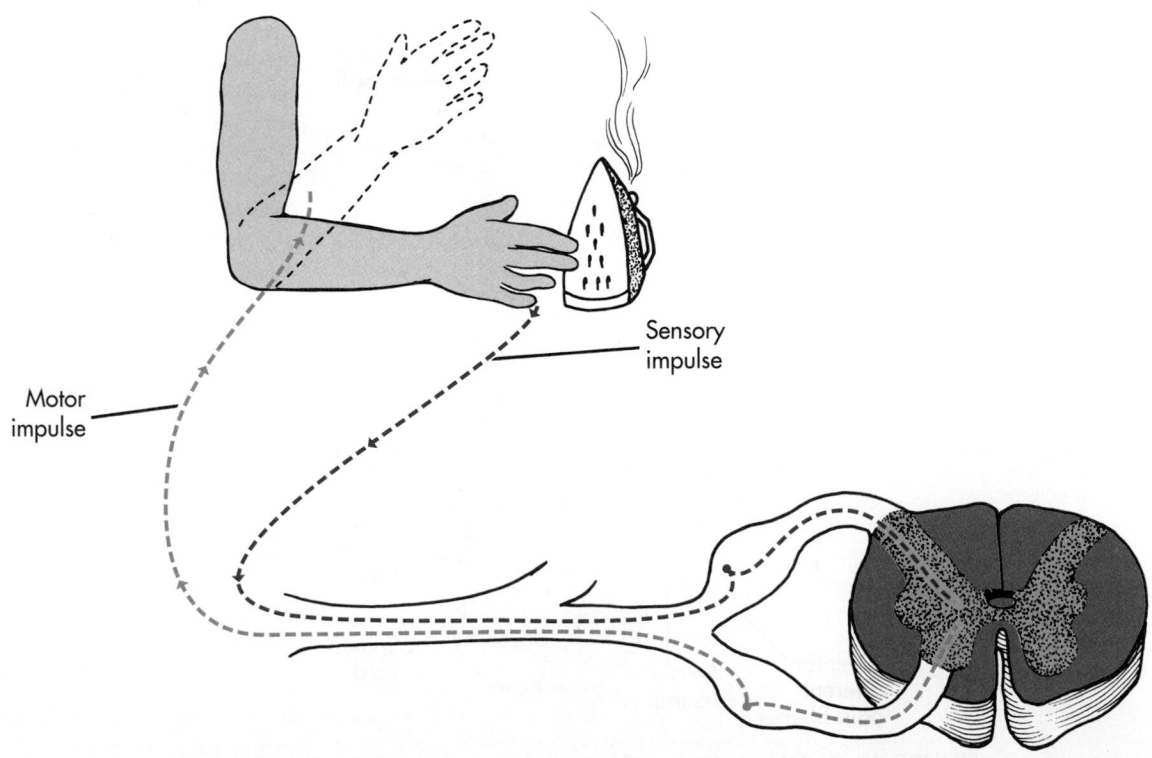

Motor impulse

Sensory impulse

FIGURE **42–3** Protective reflex to pain stimulus.

gates (physiology, emotional and cognitive processes), nurses can gain a useful conceptual framework for pain management. For example, stress, exercise, and other factors increase the release of endorphins, raising an individual's **pain threshold** (the point at which a person feels pain). Because the amount of circulating substances vary with every individual, the response to pain will be different. Recently N-methyl-D-aspartate (NMDA) receptors have been implicated in the pain experience (Helmy and Bali, 2001).

Physiological Responses. As pain impulses ascend the spinal cord toward the brain stem and thalamus, the autonomic nervous system becomes stimulated as part of the stress response. Pain of low to moderate intensity and superficial pain elicit the fight-or-flight reaction of the general adaptation syndrome (see Chapter 30). Stimulation of the sympathetic branch of the autonomic nervous system results in physiological responses (Table 42-1). If the pain is continuous, severe, or deep, typically involving the visceral organs (e.g., with a myocardial infarction or colic from gallbladder or renal stones), the parasympathetic nervous system goes into action. Sustained physiological responses to pain could cause serious harm to an individual. Except in cases of severe traumatic pain, which may send a person into shock, most people reach a level of adaptation in which physical signs return to normal. Thus clients in pain will *not* always have changes in their vital signs.

Behavioral Responses. Once pain is experienced, there begins a cycle of events that if left untreated or unrelieved can significantly alter the quality of a person's life. Pain can have a dominating nature, interfering with the ability to relate and care for oneself. This component of pain

reaction helps to explain why the management of pain can be such a challenge.

Pain threatens physical and psychological well-being. Clients may choose not to report pain if they believe their pain would inconvenience others or signal loss of self-control. Some clients will endure severe pain without assistance. Often a nurse must encourage such a client to accept pain-relieving measures so that activity or nutritional intake is not seriously curtailed. In contrast, other clients may seek relief before pain occurs having learned that pain is easier to prevent than to treat. For example, a client may request an aspirin in anticipation of a headache. The client's ability to tolerate pain significantly influences the nurse's perceptions of the degree of the discomfort. Clients deemed to have a low **pain tolerance** (level of pain a person is willing to put up with) may be perceived as whiners. The nurse teaches clients the importance of reporting their pain.

Typical body movements and facial expressions that indicate pain include clenching the teeth, holding the painful part, bent posture, and grimaces. A client may cry or moan, be restless, or make frequent requests of the nurse. The nurse soon learns to recognize patterns of behavior that reflect pain. This becomes especially important in clients who are unable to report their pain such as the cognitively impaired. However, lack of pain expression does not necessarily mean that the client is not experiencing pain (McCaffery and Pasero, 1999).

Types of Pain
Pain may be categorized by duration or pathology. Acute and chronic pain are categorized by duration.

Acute Pain. Everyone experiences some level of acute pain during their lifetime. **Acute pain** is protective, has

Table 42-1	Physiological Reactions to Pain
Response	**Cause or Effect**
Sympathetic Stimulation*	
Dilation of bronchial tubes and increased respiratory rate	Provides increased oxygen intake
Increased heart rate	Provides increased oxygen transport
Peripheral vasoconstriction (pallor, elevation in blood pressure)	Elevates blood pressure with shift of blood supply from periphery and viscera to skeletal muscles and brain
Increased blood glucose level	Provides additional energy
Diaphoresis	Controls body temperature during stress
Increased muscle tension	Prepares muscles for action
Dilation of pupils	Affords better vision
Decreased gastrointestinal motility	Frees energy for more immediate activity
Parasympathetic Stimulation†	
Pallor	Causes blood supply to shift away from periphery
Muscle tension	Results from fatigue
Decreased heart rate and blood pressure	Results from vagal stimulation
Rapid, irregular breathing	Causes body defenses to fail under prolonged stress of pain

*Pain of low to moderate intensity and superficial pain.
†Severe or deep pain.

an identifiable cause, is of short duration (usually less than 6 months), and has limited tissue damage and emotional response. Acute pain eventually resolves with or without treatment after a damaged area heals. Because acute pain has a predictable ending (healing) and an identifiable cause, this usually results in a willingness by health team members to treat acute pain aggressively. It is important to realize that unrelieved acute pain can progress to chronic pain.

Acute pain can seriously threaten a client's recovery by resulting in prolonged hospitalization, increased risks of complications from immobility (see Chapter 36), and delayed rehabilitation. There cannot be physical or psychological progress as long as acute pain persists, because the client focuses all energy on pain relief. The nurse's efforts at teaching and motivating the client toward self-care will often be hampered until the pain is successfully managed. Complete pain elimination may not be achievable, but reducing pain to an acceptable level is realistic. Thus a primary nursing goal should be to provide pain relief that allows clients to participate in their recovery.

Chronic Pain. One of the most important differences between chronic pain and acute pain is that chronic pain is not considered protective and thus serves no purpose. **Chronic pain** lasts longer than anticipated, may *not* have an identifiable cause, and leads to great personal suffering. Chronic pain may be noncancerous (nonmalignant) or cancerous. Examples of chronic noncancer pain include arthritis, low back pain, myofascial pain, headache, and peripheral neuropathy (McCaffery and Pasero, 1999). Chronic noncancer pains are usually non–life threatening. An injured area may have healed long ago, yet the pain is ongoing and may not respond to treatment.

The possible unknown cause of noncancer pain, combined with the unrelenting pain and uncertainty of its duration frustrates the client, frequently leading to psychological depression and perhaps suicide. Chronic noncancer pain is a major cause of psychological and physical disability, leading to problems such as loss of a job, inability to perform simple daily activities, sexual dysfunction, and social isolation from family and friends.

The person with chronic noncancer pain often does not show overt symptoms and does not adapt to the pain; rather, the person seems to suffer more with time because of physical and mental exhaustion. Chronic noncancer pain creates the insecurity of never knowing how one will feel from day to day. Symptoms of chronic noncancer pain include fatigue, insomnia, anorexia, weight loss, apathy, hopelessness, and anger.

Health care workers are usually less willing to treat chronic noncancer pain with opioids, although a recent policy statement on the use of opioids for noncancer pain was released by the American Pain Society (APS) (2002). The American Society of Anesthesiologists (1997) developed Practice Guidelines for Chronic Pain Management, which includes the use of opioids. Often a person with chronic noncancer pain who "doctor shops" is labeled a drug seeker, when they are actually seeking a pain relief. This is known as **pseudoaddiction.** Nurses should discourage the client from having multiple health care providers for treating pain and refer them to pain experts. Pain centers offer a holistic approach to chronic pain us-ing nonpharmacological as well as pharmacological strategies for pain management. Caring for the client with chronic noncancer pain can be challenging. The nurse should emphasize that the pain can successfully be managed, although not necessarily cured, via a comprehensive approach.

Cancer Pain. Not all clients with cancer will experience pain. But for those who do, the Agency for Healthcare Research and Quality (AHRQ), formerly the Agency for Health Care Policy and Research (AHCPR), reports that up to 90% can have their pain managed with relatively simple means (Jacox and others, 1994). Pain in a client with cancer pain may be acute and/or chronic. The pain may also be nociceptive and/or neuropathic. Cancer pain may be due to tumor progression and its related pathological process, invasive procedures, toxicities of treatment, infection, and physical limitations. It can be sensed at the actual site of the tumor or distant to the site, which is called referred pain. A new report of pain by a client with existing pain needs to be investigated. Although the need for treatment of cancer pain has become more visible, the issue of undertreatment continues. In a study conducted in a hospice setting, of those clients with pain, only 42% stated they had pain-relief scores of 5 or less on a scale of 1 to 10 (1 being no relief and 10 being complete relief) (McMillan, 1996).

Pain by Inferred Pathology Process. Identifying the cause of pain is the first step in successfully treating pain. Nociceptive or normal pain is subdivided into somatic (musculoskeletal) and visceral (internal organ) pain. Neuropathic pain arises from abnormal or damaged pain nerves (Table 42-2). Each of these pathological processes has distinct pain characteristics that will be discussed under pain assessment.

Idiopathic Pain. Because not all pain has an identifiable cause, a third category is necessary: idiopathic pain. **Idiopathic pain** is chronic pain in the absence of an identifiable physical or psychological cause or pain perceived as excessive for the extent of organic pathological condition. An example of idiopathic pain is complex regional pain syndrome (CRPS), previously known as reflex sympathetic dystrophy (RSD) and causalgia. The cause is unknown. It is hoped that future technology will identify the cause or causes, thus leading to a more effective treatment.

*N*ursing Knowledge Base

In *Notes on Nursing: What It Is and What It Is Not,* Florence Nightingale (reprint, 1969) states that ". . . pain . . . perpetuates and intensifies itself." Thus nurses have a long history of dealing with the effect of pain on clients. Traditionally, pain was considered a symptom of a disease or condition. If the condition was successfully treated, the pain would cease. Pain is now considered a comorbid medical condition needing treatment. Knowing that pain affects every aspect of a client's life, pain management is one of the most researched concepts in nursing. Through nursing research of pain mechanisms and interventions

Table 42-2 **Classification of Pain by Inferred Pathology**	
Nociceptive Pain	**Neuropathic Pain**

I. *Nociceptive pain:* Normal processing of stimuli that damages normal tissues or has the potential to do so if prolonged; usually responsive to nonopioids and/or opioids.
 	
A. Somatic pain: Arises from bone, joint, muscle, skin, or connective tissue. It is usually aching or throbbing in quality and is well localized.
 	
B. Visceral pain: Arises from visceral organs, such as the gastrointestinal tract and pancreas. This may be subdivided:
  1. Tumor involvement of the organ capsule that causes aching and fairly well localized pain.
  2. Obstruction of hollow viscus, which causes intermittent cramping and poorly localized pain.
	II. *Neuropathic pain:* Abnormal processing of sensory input by the peripheral or central nervous system; treatment usually includes adjuvant analgesics.
	
	A. Centrally generated pain
	  1. Deafferentation pain: Injury to either the peripheral or central nervous system. *Examples:* Phantom pain may reflect injury to the peripheral nervous system; burning pain below the level of a spinal cord lesion reflects injury to the central nervous system.
	  2. Sympathetically maintained pain: Associated with dysregulation of the autonomic nervous system. *Examples:* pain associated with reflex sympathetic dystrophy/causalgia (complex regional pain syndrome, type I, type II).
	
	B. Peripherally generated pain
	  1. Painful polyneuropathies: Pain is felt along the distribution of many peripheral nerves. *Examples:* diabetic neuropathy, alcohol-nutritional neuropathy, and those associated with Guillain-Barré syndrome.
	  2. Painful mononeuropathies. Usually associated with a known peripheral nerve injury, and pain is felt at least partly along the distribution of the damaged nerve. *Examples:* nerve root compression, nerve entrapment, trigeminal neuralgia.

Modified from McCaffery M, Pasero C: *Pain: clinical manual,* ed 2, St. Louis, 1999, Mosby; data from Max MB, Portenoy RK: Methodological challenges for clinical trials of cancer pain treatments. In Chapman CR, Foley KM, editors: *Current and emerging issues in cancer pain: research and practice,* New York, 1993, Raven Press; and Portenoy RK: Neuropathic pain. In Portenoy RK, Kanner RM, editors: *Pain management: theory and practice,* Philadelphia, 1996, FA Davis.

to reduce pain, nursing knowledge of pain management will continue to grow. In this section factors that influence pain are explored.

Knowledge, Attitudes, and Beliefs

Health care personnel often have attitudes regarding clients in pain. Unless clients have objective signs of pain, a nurse may not believe that they are uncomfortable. These attitudes about pain are caused in part by the traditional medical model of illness. This model suggests that physical problems result from physical causes. Thus pain is viewed as a physical response to organic dysfunction. When no obvious source of pain can be found (e.g., the client with chronic low back pain or neuropathies), nurses, as well as physicians, may stereotype pain sufferers as complainers or difficult clients.

McCaffery and others (2000) studied the attitudes of nurses regarding pain management and found that the nurse's personal opinion about the client's report of pain affected the pain assessment and titration of opioid doses. In a study by Zalon (1993), the greater the client's pain intensity, the worse the nurse's estimation of the pain. Nurses need to be aware of their own biases when managing pain.

The extent to which nurses make assumptions about clients in pain seriously limits their ability to offer pain relief. Unfortunately, all people are influenced by biases based on their culture, education, and experience. Too of-

Box 42-2   **Common Biases and Misconceptions About Pain**
The following statements are *false:* Drug abusers and alcoholics overreact to discomforts. Clients with minor illnesses have less pain than those with severe physical alteration. Administering analgesics regularly will lead to drug addiction. The amount of tissue damage in an injury can accurately indicate pain intensity. Health care personnel are the best authorities on the nature of a client's pain. Psychogenic pain is not real. Chronic pain is psychological. Clients should expect to have pain in a hospital. Clients who cannot speak do not feel pain.

ten, nurses allow misconceptions about pain (Box 42-2) to affect their willingness to intervene. Many nurses even avoid acknowledging a client's pain because of their own fear and denial. Nurses may not believe a client's report of pain if they do not "look" like they are in pain. Nurses are entitled to their personal beliefs; however, they must *accept* the client's report of pain and act according to professional guidelines, standards, position statements, policies and procedures, and evidence-based research findings.

To help a client gain comfort or relief, the nurse must view the experience through the client's eyes. Pain is tiring and demands energy from the person experiencing it. It interferes with relationships and the individual's ability to maintain self-care. Acknowledging personal prejudices or misconceptions helps the nurse address the client's problem more professionally. The nurse who becomes an active, knowledgeable observer of a client in pain will make a more objective analysis of the pain experience. The client makes the diagnosis that pain is present, and the nurse works to apply techniques and skills that ultimately give relief.

Factors Influencing Pain

Pain is complex, involving physiological, social, spiritual, psychological, and cultural influences. Thus each individual's pain experience is different. The nurse considers all factors that affect the client in pain. This is necessary to ensure a holistic approach to the assessment and care of the client in pain.

Physiological Factors

Age. Age is an important variable that influences pain, particularly in infants and older adults. Developmental differences found among these age-groups influence how children and older adults react to pain. Young children have difficulty understanding pain and the procedures nurses administer that may cause pain. Young children who have not developed full vocabularies also have difficulty verbally describing and expressing pain to parents or caregivers. Cognitively, toddlers and preschoolers are unable to recall explanations about pain or associate pain with experiences that can occur in various situations. With these developmental considerations in mind, the nurse must adapt approaches for assessing a child's pain (including what to ask and the behaviors to observe for) and how to prepare a child for a painful medical procedure (Table 42-3).

It is important to remember that pain is not an inevitable part of aging. However, because of the aging process, there is a greater likelihood of an older adult developing a pathological condition, which is accompanied by pain (Herr, 2002a; Kelly, 2003). Once an older client suffers pain, there can be serious impairment of functional status. Mobility, activities of daily living (ADLs), social activities outside the home, and activity tolerance can all be reduced. The presence of pain in an older adult requires aggressive assessment, diagnosis, and management (Box 42-3).

The ability of older clients to interpret pain can be complicated by the presence of multiple diseases with vague symptoms that may affect similar parts of the body. When there is more than one source of pain, a nurse must make detailed assessments (Herr, 2002b). The manifestations of different diseases can cause an atypical presentation of painful conditions. In other words, different diseases can cause similar symptoms. For example, chest pain does not always indicate a heart attack; it may be a symptom of arthritis of the spine or of an abdominal disorder. Not all older adults experience cognitive impairment. However, when an older adult experiences confusion, recalling pain experiences and providing detailed explanations is difficult. It is important to recognize that there are misconceptions about pain management in the very young and in older adults that need to be addressed before nurses can adequately intervene in a client's pain (Miaskowski and Levine, 2000) (Table 42-4).

Fatigue. Fatigue heightens the perception of pain. The sense of exhaustion intensifies pain and decreases coping abilities. This can be a common problem with any person

Table 42-3	Pain in Infants
Misconception	**Correction**
Infants are incapable of feeling pain.	Infants have the anatomical and functional requirements for pain processing by mid to late gestation.
Infants are less sensitive to pain than older children and adults.	Term neonates have the same sensitivity to pain as older infants and children. Preterm neonates may have a greater sensitivity to pain than term neonates or older children.
Infants are incapable of expressing pain.	Although infants cannot verbalize pain, they respond with behavioral cues and physiological indicators that can be observed by others.
Infants must learn about pain from previous painful experiences.	Pain requires no prior experience; it need not be learned from earlier painful experience. Pain is present with the first insult.
Pain cannot be accurately assessed in infants.	Behavioral cues (i.e., facial expressions, cry, body movements) and physiological indicators of pain can be reliably and validly assessed either alone or in combination. The most valid approach is facial expression (Craig, 1998). A composite pain measure can also be used (Stevens, 1998).
Infants are incapable of remembering pain.	Early exposure to noxious stimuli may have an effect on the infant's future responses to painful events (Grunau and others, 1994; Taddio and others, 1997).
Analgesics and anesthetics cannot be safely given to infants and neonates because of their immature capacity to metabolize and eliminate drugs and their sensitivity to opioid-induced respiratory depression.	Infants older than 1 month of age metabolize drugs in the same manner as older infants and children. Careful selection of the agent, dosage, administration route and time, and frequent monitoring for desired and undesired effects, and drug titration and weaning can minimize the adverse effects of opioids and nonopioids for pain management in neonates (Stevens, 1998).

Modified from McCaffery M, Pasero C: *Pain: clinical manual*, ed 2, St. Louis, 1999, Mosby.

Box 42-3

Focus on Older Adults

- With aging there is a decrease in muscle mass, an increase in body fat, and a decrease in percentage body water. This results in an increased concentration of water-soluble drugs such as morphine. Also, the volume of distribution for fat-soluble drugs such as fentanyl increases (Popp and Portenoy, 1996).
- Older adults frequently eat poorly, resulting in low serum albumin levels. Many drugs are highly protein bound. In the presence of low serum albumin, more free drug (active form) is available, thus increasing the risk for side and/or toxic effects (Lehn, 2001).

- Decline of liver and renal function is a natural occurrence with aging. This results in reduced metabolism and excretion of drugs. Hence, older adults often experience a greater peak effect and longer duration of analgesics (Kelly, 2003).
- Age-related changes in the skin such as thinning and loss of elasticity could affect the absorption rate of topical analgesics.

Table 42-4   Pain in Older Adults

Misconception	Correction
Pain is a natural outcome of growing old.	It is true that older adults are at greater risk (as much as twofold) than younger adults for many painful conditions; however, pain is not an inevitable result of aging.
Pain perception, or sensitivity, decreases with age.	This assumption is unsafe. Although there is evidence that emotional suffering specifically related to pain may be less in older than in younger clients, no scientific basis exists for the assertion that a decrease in perception of pain occurs with age or that age dulls sensitivity to pain.
If the older client does not report pain, he or she does not have pain.	Older clients commonly underreport pain. Reasons include expecting to have pain with increasing age; not wanting to alarm loved ones; being fearful of losing their independence; not wanting to distract, anger, or bother caregivers; and believing caregivers know they have pain and are doing all that can be done to relieve it. The absence of a report of pain does not mean the absence of pain.
If an older client appears to be occupied, asleep, or otherwise distracted from pain, he or she does not have pain.	Older clients often believe it is unacceptable to show pain and have learned to use a variety of ways to cope with it instead (e.g., many clients use distraction successfully for short periods of time). Sleeping may be a coping strategy or it may indicate exhaustion, not pain relief. Assumptions about the presence or absence of pain cannot be made solely on the basis of a client's behavior.
The potential side effects of opioids make them too dangerous to use to relieve pain in older adults.	Opioids may be used safely in older adults. Although the opioid-naive older adult may be more sensitive to opioids, this does not justify withholding the use of them in the management of pain in this population. The key to use of opioids in the older adult is to "start low and go slow." Potentially dangerous opioid-induced side effects can be prevented with slow titration; regular, frequent monitoring and assessment of the client's response; and adjustment of dose and interval between doses when side effects are detected. If necessary, clinically significant respiratory depression can be reversed by an opioid antagonist drug.
Clients with Alzheimer's disease and others cognitive impairments do not feel pain, and their reports of pain are most likely invalid.	No evidence exists that cognitively impaired older adults experience less pain or that their reports of pain are less valid than those of individuals with intact cognitive function. It is probable that clients with dementia or other deficits of cognition suffer significant unrelieved pain and discomfort. Assessment of pain in these clients is challenging but possible. The best approach is to accept the client's report of pain and treat the pain as it would be treated in an individual with intact cognitive function.
Older clients report more pain as they age.	Even though older clients experience a higher incidence of painful conditions, such as arthritis, osteoporosis, peripheral vascular disease, and cancer, than younger clients, studies have shown that they underreport pain. Many older adult clients grew up valuing the ability to "grin and bear it," and, unfortunately, have been heavily influenced by the "Just Say No" to drugs campaign.

Modified from McCaffery M, Pasero C: *Pain: clinical manual,* St. Louis, 1999, Mosby; data from Butler RN, Gastel B: Care of the aged: perspectives on pain and discomfort. In Turk DC, Melzack R, editors: *The handbook of pain assessment,* New York, 1992, Guilford Press; Harkins SW, Price DD: Are there special needs for pain assessment in the elderly? *APS Bull* 3:1, January/February 1993; Harkins SW and others: Geriatric pain. In Wall PD, Melzack R, editors: *Textbook of pain,* London, 1999, Churchill Livingstone; and American Geriatrics Society: the management of persistent pain in older persons, *J Am Geriatr Soc* 50(S6):205, 2002.

experiencing a long-term illness or who has fatigue as a result of treatment. If fatigue occurs along with sleeplessness, the perception of pain may be even greater. Pain is often experienced less after a restful sleep than at the end of a long day.

Genes. Recently research on animal models suggests that genetic information passed on by parents might increase or decrease the person's sensitivity to pain. What was historically described as pain threshold or pain tolerance may, in fact, be determined by genetic makeup. In addition, exposure to pain at a young age may increase sensitivity to pain (Ruda and others, 2000).

Neurological Function. A client's neurological function can easily influence the pain experience. Any factor that interrupts or influences normal pain reception or perception affects the client's awareness and response to pain. For example, a client who has a spinal cord injury; peripheral neuropathy, as in the case of diabetes mellitus; or a neurological disease, such as multiple sclerosis, experiences altered pain sensation. Certain pharmacological agents influence pain perception and response. Analgesics, sedatives, and anesthetics depress functions of the central nervous system. It is important for the nurse to conduct a neurological assessment (see Chapter 32) of a client at risk for being insensitive to pain. This client could suffer injury easily and thus requires preventive nursing care.

Social Factors
Attention. The degree to which a client focuses attention on pain can influence pain perception. Increased attention has been associated with increased pain, whereas distraction has been associated with a diminished pain response (Carroll and Seers, 1998). This concept is one that nurses apply in various pain-relief interventions such as relaxation, guided imagery, and massage. By focusing a client's attention and concentration on other stimuli, the nurse places pain on the periphery of awareness.

Previous Experience. Each person learns from painful experiences. Previous experience does not mean that a person will accept pain more easily in the future. If a person has had frequent episodes of pain without relief or has had bouts of severe pain, anxiety or even fear may recur. In contrast, if a person has had repeated experiences with the same type of pain but the pain has been successfully relieved, it becomes easier to interpret the pain sensation. As a result, the client is better prepared to take necessary actions to relieve the pain.

When a client has had no experience with pain, the first perception of it can impair the ability to cope. For example, after abdominal surgery, it is common for a client to experience severe incisional pain for several days. Unless the client is aware of this, the onset of pain may be viewed as a serious complication. Rather than participate actively in postoperative breathing exercises (see Chapter 49), the client may lie immobile in bed and maintain shallow breathing because of fear that something has gone wrong. The nurse should prepare the client with a clear explanation of the type of pain that will be experienced and methods to reduce it.

Family and Social Support. People in pain often depend on family members or close friends for support, assistance, or protection. Although pain still exists, the presence of a loved one can minimize loneliness and fear. An absence of family or friends can often make the pain experience more stressful. The presence of parents is especially important for children experiencing pain.

Spiritual Factors. Spirituality is a concept that stretches beyond religion and includes an active searching for meaning to situations in which one finds oneself. Spiritual questions may include, "Why has this happened to me?" "Why now?" "What will become of me?" "Why am I suffering?" Spiritual pain goes beyond what we can see. "Why has God done this to me?" "Have I not lived an honest life?" "Is this suffering teaching me something?" Other spiritual concerns include loss of independence and becoming a burden to family (Otis-Green and others, 2002). It is important for the nurse to convey to the client that he or she matters. Requesting a clergy consult for a client with chronic pain is a recommended strategy. Recall that pain is an experience that has physical *and* emotional components. Thus, providing interventions designed to treat both aspects is essential for optimum pain management.

Psychological Factors
Anxiety. The degree and quality of pain perceived by a client are related to the meaning of pain. The relationship between pain and anxiety is complex. Anxiety often increases the perception of pain, but pain may also cause feelings of anxiety. It is difficult to separate the two sensations. Wall and Melzack (1999) reported that painful stimuli activate the portion of the limbic system believed to control emotion, particularly anxiety. The limbic system may process the emotional reaction to pain, aggravating or relieving it.

Critically ill or injured clients, who often perceive a lack of control over their environment and care, may have high anxiety levels. This anxiety, if it has gone unnoticed in the high-tech environment of an intensive care unit (ICU), can lead to serious pain management problems. The challenge is to relieve the pain in a client who is anxious in any setting. Although pharmacological and nonpharmacological approaches to the management of anxiety are appropriate, anxiolytic medications should not be a substitute for analgesia.

Coping Style. The experience of pain can be lonely. When clients experience pain in health care settings such as hospitals, the loneliness can be unbearable. Coping style influences the ability to deal with pain. Persons with internal loci of control perceive themselves as having personal control over their environments and the outcome of events, such as pain (Gil, 1990). In contrast, persons with external loci of control perceive other factors in their environments, such as nurses, as being responsible for the outcome of events. This concept is applied in the use of patient-controlled analgesia (PCA). Clients who are able to self-administer small doses of intravenous (IV) pain medication during an acute episode successfully achieve pain control more quickly than those who rely on nurses to administer intermittent doses of pain medications.

Pain may cause partial or total disability. Clients often find various ways to cope with the physical and psychological effects of pain. It is important to understand a client's coping resources during a painful experience. These resources, such as communicating with a supportive family, exercise, or singing, can be used in the nurse's plan of care to support the client and offer a degree of pain relief.

Cultural Factors

Meaning of Pain. The meaning that a person associates with pain affects the experience of pain and how one adapts to it. This can be closely associated with the person's cultural background. A person will perceive pain differently if it suggests a threat, loss, punishment, or challenge. For example, a woman in labor will perceive pain differently than a woman with a history of cancer who is experiencing a new pain and fearing recurrence. The degree and quality of pain perceived by a client are related to the meaning of pain.

Ethnicity. Cultural beliefs and values affect how individuals deal with pain. Individuals learn what is expected and accepted by their culture, including how to react to pain (Lasch, 2000; Steefel, 2002). Health care providers of-ten assume that their ways and beliefs are equal to those of others. Thus they try to presume how clients will respond to pain. There are different meanings and attitudes associated with pain across various cultural groups. An understanding of the cultural meaning of pain helps the nurse to design culturally sensitive care for people with pain.

How people express pain is another cultural trait. Some cultures believe it is natural to be demonstrative about pain. Others tend to be more introverted. In addition, it is also important to know to what extent a member of a particular culture has assimilated into American society. For example, if several generations of a Hispanic client's family have lived in the United States, the influence of the Spanish culture may be limited. In contrast, a client who has recently come to the United States and who embraces the cultural norms of his or her ethnic group may have very different attitudes than an Anglo-Saxon American.

Knowing that cultural differences exist is not enough in the treatment of pain. Nurses must explore the impact of those differences and include cultural patterns and beliefs into the plan of care (Box 42-4). The nurse, the client, and the family must work together to facilitate communication about the assessment and management of pain. Finding a common assessment tool and communicating that tool to other health care providers is imperative.

Cultural Aspects of Care   Box 42-4

Culture models our responses, behaviors, and attitudes about pain. Culturally acquired patterns of pain responses may influence the neurophysiological processing of pain information as well as psychological, behavioral, and verbal response to pain. A client's meaning of pain may influence how much pain can be tolerated and endured. Response to pain may be limited by language used to describe or report pain. The degree of pain expression does not necessarily correlate with pain intensity. Preferences for pain coping strategies are usually determined by culture; thus nontraditional interventions to manage pain need to be explored with the client. How people view pain will influence teaching strategies appropriate for learning.

Implications for Practice

- Be aware of perceived causal factors of pain (fate, lifestyle, punishment, witchcraft).
- Emotional responses to pain (overt, stoic) vary between and within cultures.
- Words used to express pain vary among cultures (hurt, ache, discomfort).
- Personal and social meaning of pain and past pain experiences affect pain perception.
- Definitions of pain change the perception of pain intensity.
- Feelings about pain direct treatment.
- Health care provider beliefs and expectations regarding pain expression sway pain management strategies.
- Therapeutic goals of pain management are influenced by cultural beliefs.

Data from Lasch K: Culture, pain, and culturally sensitive pain care, *Pain Manag Nurs* 1(3):S16, 2000; Steefel L: Treat pain in any culture, *Nurs Spectr* 6(5):8, 2002; Ramer L and others: Multimeasure pain assessment in an ethnically diverse group of patients with cancer, *J Transcult Nurs* 10(2):94, 1999.

Critical Thinking

Successful critical thinking requires a synthesis of knowledge, experience, information gathered from clients, critical thinking attitudes, and intellectual and professional standards. Clinical judgments require that the nurse anticipate what information is needed, analyze the data, and make decisions regarding client care. A client's condition or situation is always changing. During assessment the nurse must consider all critical thinking elements that build toward making appropriate nursing diagnoses.

In the case of comfort, knowledge of pain physiology and the many factors that influence pain place the nurse in a better situation to anticipate ways to manage a client's pain. Previous experience in caring for clients with pain sharpens the nurse's assessment skills and ability to choose effective therapies. Critical thinking attitudes and intellectual standards ensure the aggressive assessment, creative planning, and diligent evaluation that are needed on the part of the nurse for the client to obtain an acceptable level of comfort. Successful pain management does not necessarily mean pain elimination, but rather attainment of a mutually agreed upon pain relief goal that allows clients to control their pain instead of the pain controlling them.

Nursing Process and Pain

Nurses need to approach pain management systematically to understand a client's pain and to provide appropriate intervention. Successful management of pain depends on establishing a relationship of trust between the health care provider, client, and family. Pain management extends beyond pain relief, encompassing the client's quality of life and ability to work productively, to enjoy recreation, and to function normally in the family and society (Jacox and others, 1994).

NP Assessment

Nurses care for clients with pain on a daily basis. Therefore it is necessary to monitor pain on a consistent basis along with temperature, pulse, respirations, and blood pressure. In some institutions pain is treated as the fifth vital sign.

Establishing a nursing diagnosis, deciding on appropriate interventions, and evaluating the client's response (outcomes) to the interventions are contingent on the fundamental activity of a factual, timely, accurate pain assessment (Figure 42-4). The core of this complex activity is the exploration of the pain experience through the eyes of the client. A variety of tools are available to assist the nurse in

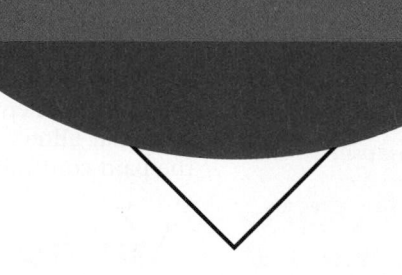

KNOWLEDGE
- Physiology of pain
- Factors that potentially increase or decrease responses to pain
- Pathophysiology of conditions causing pain
- Awareness of biases affecting pain assessment and treatment
- Cultural variations in how pain is expressed
- Knowledge of nonverbal communication

EXPERIENCE
- Caring for clients with acute, chronic, and cancer pain
- Caring for clients who experienced pain as a result of a health care therapy
- Personal experience with pain

Assessment
- Determine the client's perspective of pain including history of pain; its meaning; and physical, emotional, and social effects
- Measure objectively the characteristics of the client's pain
- Review potential factors affecting the client's pain

STANDARDS
- Refer to AHCPR guidelines for acute pain management
- Apply intellectual standards (e.g., clarity, specificity, accuracy, and completeness when gathering assessment)
- Apply relevance when letting the client explore the pain experience

ATTITUDES
- Persevere in exploring causes and possible solutions for chronic pain
- Display confidence when assessing pain to relieve the client's anxiety
- Display integrity and fairness to prevent prejudice from affecting assessment

FIGURE **42–4** Critical thinking model for comfort assessment.

assessing the client's pain. However, the goal in using these tools is not to identify how much pain the client can tolerate, rather it is to identify how much pain can exist without interfering with client function.

AHRQ has established specific guidelines for assessing clients with acute and cancer pain. The focus is on planning successful pain management interventions before pain is experienced. Because it involves a collaborative approach, the AHRQ pain treatment flow chart (Figure 42-5) offers a useful conceptual approach to the control of acute pain. Clients must understand that informed reporting of pain is valuable and necessary if the health care team is to manage pain effectively.

When assessing pain, the nurse must be sensitive to the client's level of discomfort. In addition, the nurse must ask the client at what level will the discomfort not interfere with his or her functional ability. For example, the nurse caring for a client with pain should ask, "What is an acceptable level of pain for you?" The client might answer that a level 2 pain (on a scale of 0 to 10, with 0 being no pain and 10 being worse pain imaginable) is acceptable. The nurse then focuses efforts on getting the pain decreased to at least that level. If pain is acute or severe, it is unlikely that the client can provide a detailed description of the entire experience. During an episode of acute pain the nurse primarily assesses the location, severity, and quality of the pain. A more thorough pain assessment can occur when the client has been made more comfortable (Kim, 2002).

For clients with chronic pain, assessment may best be focused on affective, cognitive, and behavioral dimensions of the pain experience and on its history and context (Lawler, 1997). In the case of chronic noncancer pain, assessment should include the level of function, because it may not be possible to achieve complete pain relief. In the home care setting, family members may become the assessors of pain. Using the *ABC*s of pain management is an effective way to manage pain (Box 42-5).

The nurse should be aware of possible errors in pain assessment (Box 42-6). Using the right tools and methods can help to avoid errors and to ensure that the right pain interventions are chosen. Failure of clinicians to assess a client's pain, accept the findings, and treat the report of pain is a common cause of unrelieved pain and suffering (McCaffery and Pasero, 1999).

Client's Expression of Pain. A client's self-report of pain is the single most reliable indicator of the existence and

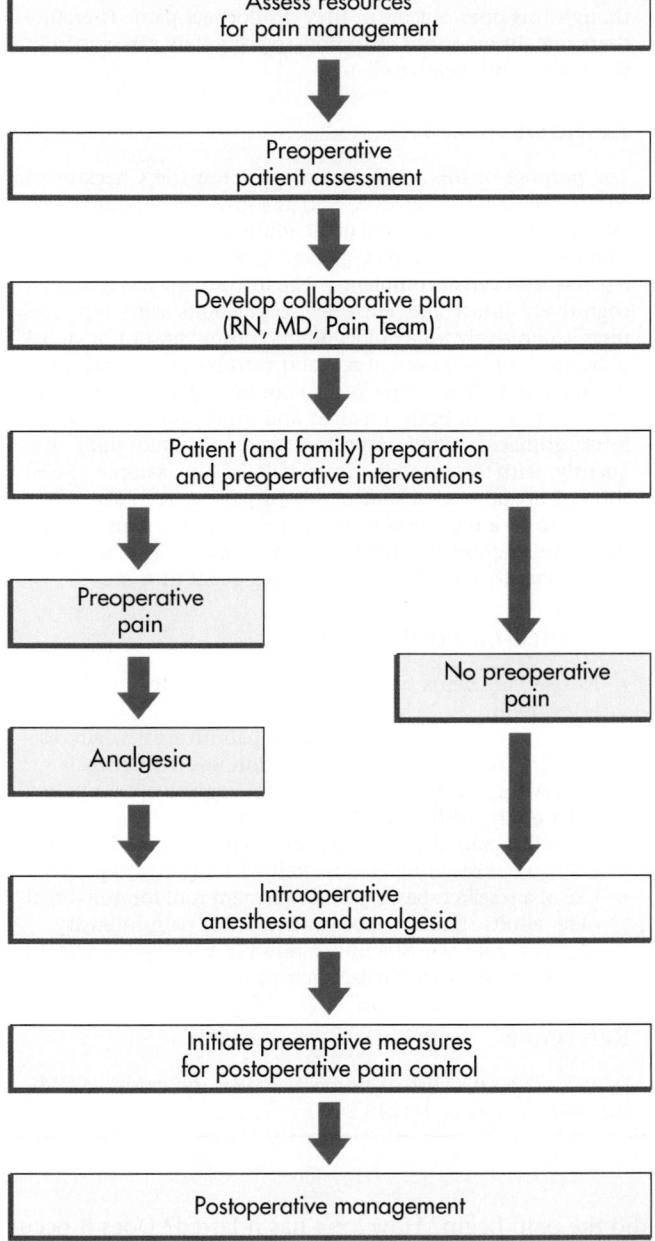

FIGURE **42–5** Pain treatment flow chart: preoperative and intraoperative phases. (From Agency for Health Care Policy and Research, Acute Pain Management Guideline Panel: *Acute pain management: operative or medical procedures and trauma,* Clinical Practice Guideline, AHCPR Pub No. 92-0032, Rockville, Md, 1992, Agency for Health Care Policy and Research, Public Health Service, U.S. Department of Health and Human Services.) (From Jacox A and others: *Management of cancer pain,* Clinical Practice Guideline No. 9, AHCPR Publication No. 94-0592, Rockville, Md, 1994, Agency for Health Care Policy and Research, Public Health Service, U.S. Department of Health and Human Services.)

Box *42-5* **Routine Clinical Approach to Pain Assessment and Management: *ABCDE***

A *Ask about pain regularly. Assess pain systematically.*
B *Believe the client and family in their report of pain and what relieves it.*
C *Choose pain control options appropriate for the client, family, and setting.*
D *Deliver interventions in a timely, logical, and coordinated fashion.*
E *Empower clients and their families. Enable them to control their course to the greatest extent possible.*

From Jacox A and others: *Management of cancer pain,* Clinical Practice Guideline No. 9, AHCPR Publication No. 94-0592, Rockville, Md, 1994, Agency for Health Care Policy and Research, Public Health Service, U.S. Department of Health and Human Services.

Box 42-6 Possible Sources for Error in Pain Assessment

- Bias, which causes nurses to consistently overestimate or underestimate the pain that clients experience
- Vague or unclear assessment questions, which lead to unreliable assessment data
- Use of pain assessment tools that have not been proven reliable and valid with identical clients (a reliable assessment tool focuses only on pain cues that provide a reliable measure of relevant clinical changes)
- Clients who do not always provide complete, pertinent, and accurate pain information
- Cognitively impaired older clients who are unable to use pain scales

---

intensity of pain and any related discomfort (AHCPR, 1992; APS, 1999). Pain is individualistic. Many clients fail to report or discuss discomfort; at the same time, many nurses believe that clients will report pain if they have it. In addition, if clients sense that the nurse doubts that pain exists, they will share little information about their pain experience or will minimize their report. It is imperative that the nurse set the stage for the relationship that allows for open communication about pain. Simple measures such as sitting when talking to clients about pain lets clients know that the nurse has the time and the interest to assess their pain.

Clients unable to communicate effectively often require special attention during assessment. Children, persons who are developmentally delayed, clients who are psychotic, the critically ill, clients with dementia, and clients who do not speak English all require different approaches. Feldt (2000) has designed a tool for use with cognitively impaired clients that focuses on behaviors (Box 42-7).

Cognitively impaired clients might require simple assessment approaches involving close observation of behavior changes, especially with movement. A critically ill client who may have a clouded sensorium or the presence of nasogastric tubes or artificial airways may require the nurse to ask specific directive questions that the client can answer with a nod of the head or by writing out a response. If the client speaks a different language, pain assessment will be difficult. A family member or interpreter may be necessary to describe the client's feelings and sensations. Assessment tools such as the visual analog scale (VAS) have been translated into several languages to aid the nurse when an interpreter or family is not present (McCaffery and Pasero, 1999).

Characteristics of Pain. Assessment of common characteristics of pain helps the nurse form an understanding of the type of pain, its pattern, and types of interventions that may bring relief. Use of instruments to quantify the extent and degree of pain depends on a client being sufficiently cognitively alert to be able to understand a nurse's instructions.

Onset and Duration. The nurse asks questions to determine the onset, duration, and sequence of pain. When

---

Research Highlight *Box 42-7*

Nonverbal Pain Indicators

Research Focus

Assessing pain in a nonverbal client is difficult. Nurses encounter many clients who are unable to express their pain, although this does not mean they do not feel pain. Therefore there remain questions as to how to accurately assess pain in the noncommunicative client.

Research Abstract

The purpose of this study was to pilot test the Checklist of Nonverbal Pain Indicators (CNPI) as a measure of pain behaviors in cognitively impaired older adults. Nonverbal behaviors studied were vocalizations, grimaces, bracing, rubbing, restlessness, and verbal complaints. The instrument was tested on cognitively intact and impaired older adults with hip fractures. Cognitively intact older adults showed fewer nonverbal indications of pain both at rest and with movement than did the impaired clients. The most common observed pain behavior, at rest, in both impaired and unimpaired clients was facial grimaces. CNPI indicators were observed more frequently with movement. Over half of the sample (56%) showed no nonverbal indications of pain at rest. The CNPI proved to be a reliable and simple tool to assess pain in postoperative cognitively impaired older adults. The tool was more accurate in assessing pain during client movement.

Evidence-Based Practice

- Nonverbal clients require focused, around-the-clock pain assessment.
- Impaired clients may forget about painful areas when resting, thus requesting pain medication less frequently.
- Observing for pain behaviors in cognitively impaired older adults with activity is essential.
- Assessing pain at rest in cognitively impaired older adults may give misleading cues to staff with regards to pain.
- Use of a research-based pain assessment tool for nonverbal older adults should improve accuracy of pain intensity.
- Accurate pain assessment can result in better pain relief in clients unable to verbalize their pain.

Reference

Feldt K: The checklist of nonverbal pain indicators (CNPI), *Pain Manag Nursing* 1(1):13,2000.

---

did the pain begin? How long has it lasted? Does it occur at the same time each day? How often does it recur?

Certain types of headaches can be characterized by the time of day when they occur. The onset of sudden and severe pain is easier to assess than is gradual, mild discomfort. An understanding of the time cycle of pain helps the nurse to know when to intervene before the pain occurs or worsens.

Location. To assess pain location, the nurse asks the client to tell or to point to all areas of discomfort. Do not assume that pain will always occur in the same location.

Table 42-5   Classification of Pain by Location

Location	Characteristics	Examples of Causes
Superficial or Cutaneous		
Pain resulting from stimulation of skin	Pain is of short duration and is localized. It usually is a sharp sensation.	Needle stick; small cut or laceration
Deep or Visceral		
Pain resulting from stimulation of internal organs	Pain is diffuse and may radiate in several directions. Duration varies but it usually lasts longer than superficial pain. Pain may be sharp, dull, or unique to organ involved.	Crushing sensation (e.g., angina pectoris); burning sensation (e.g., gastric ulcer)
Referred		
Common phenomenon in visceral pain because many organs themselves have no pain receptors; entrance of sensory neurons from affected organ into same spinal cord segment as neurons from areas where pain is felt; perception of pain is in unaffected areas	Pain is felt in part of body separate from source of pain and may assume any characteristic.	Myocardial infarction, which may cause referred pain to jaw, left arm, and left shoulder; kidney stones, which may refer pain to groin
Radiating		
Sensation of pain extending from initial site of injury to another body part	Pain feels as though it travels down or along body part. It may be intermittent or constant.	Low back pain from ruptured intravertebral disk accompanied by pain radiating down leg from sciatic nerve irritation

When describing pain location, the nurse uses anatomical landmarks and descriptive terminology. The statement "The pain is localized in the upper right abdominal quadrant" is more specific than "The client states the pain is in the abdomen." Pain, classified by location, may be superficial or cutaneous, deep or visceral, referred, or radiating (Table 42-5).

Intensity. One of the most subjective, and therefore most useful, characteristics for the reporting of pain may be its severity, or intensity. Clients are often asked to describe pain as mild, moderate, or severe. However, the meaning of these terms differs for the nurse and client. This type of information is also difficult to verify over time.

Descriptive scales are a more objective means of measuring pain intensity (Figure 42-6). When scales are used to rate pain, a 10-cm (4-inch) baseline is recommended (AHCPR, 1992). A verbal descriptor scale (VDS) consists of a line with three- to five-word descriptors equally spaced along the line. The descriptors are ranked from "no pain" to "unbearable pain." The nurse shows the client the scale and asks the client to choose the current intensity of pain. The nurse also asks what rating to give the average pain and the worse pain over the past 24 hours. The VDS enables a client to choose a category for describing pain. A numerical rating scale (NRS) may be used instead of word descriptors. In this case clients rate pain on a scale of 0 to 10. A report of 0 to 3 indicates mild pain, 4 to 6 moderate pain, and 7 to 10 severe pain. The scales work best when assessing pain intensity before and after therapeutic interventions.

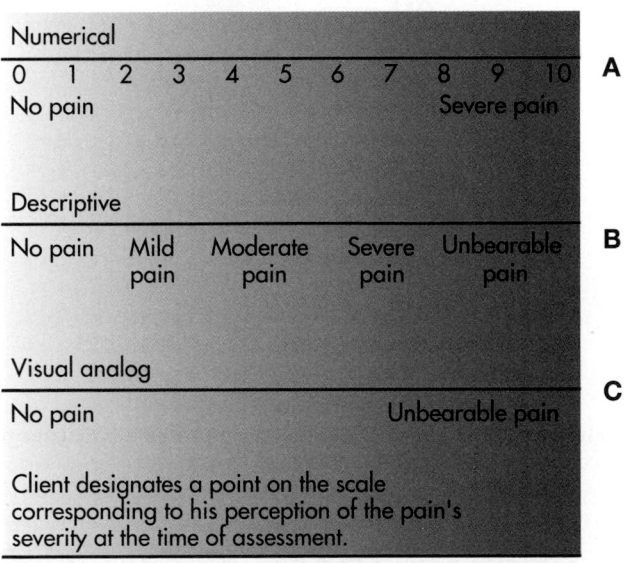

FIGURE 42-6 Sample pain scales. **A,** Numerical. **B,** Verbal descriptive. **C,** Visual analog.

The VAS does not have labeled subdivisions. It consists of a straight line, representing a continuum of intensity, and has verbal descriptors at each end. This scale gives the client total freedom in identifying the severity of pain. The VAS may not be as practical for daily use as an NRS (McCaffery and Pasero, 1999). Although the pain scale chosen varies among individuals, once selected it should be used consistently.

Assessing pain intensity in children requires special techniques. Children's verbal statements are most important (Hockenberry and others, 2003). Young children may not know what the word *pain* means, and therefore assessment may require the nurse to use words such as *owie, boo-boo,* or *hurt.* There are some unique tools available to measure pain intensity in children. Beyer and others (1992) have developed the "Oucher," which consists of two separate scales: a 0 to 100 scale on the left for older children

and a six-picture photographic scale on the right for younger children (Figure 42-7). Photographs of the face of a child (in increasing levels of discomfort) are designed to cue children into understanding what pain is and its severity. A child merely points to the selection, thus simplifying the task of describing the pain. New ethnic versions of the tool have also been developed. Wong and Baker (1988) developed the FACES scale to assess pain in children (Figure 42-8). The scale consists of six cartoon faces ranging from a smiling face ("no hurt") to increasingly less happy faces, to a final sad, tearful face ("hurts worse"). Children as young as 3 years of age can use the scale. There are also a variety of tools for assessing pain in neonates, infants, and nonverbal toddlers such as the Premature Infant Pain Profile (PIPP) and the Newborn Infant Pain Scale (NIP).

A pain scale should be designed so that it is easy to use and is not time consuming for the client to complete. If the client can read and understand the scale, the description of pain should be more accurate. Descriptive scales are useful not only in assessing the severity of pain, but also in evaluating changes in a client's condition. The nurse can use the scales after an intervention or when symptoms become aggravated to evaluate whether the pain has decreased or increased. Although different clients might prefer different pain scales, it is important for the nurse to select and consistently use the same scale on a specific client. A pain scale cannot be used to compare the pain of one client to that of another client. A rating of 7 or more on a 0 to 10 scale requires immediate attention.

Quality. Another subjective characteristic of pain is its quality. Because there is no common or specific pain vocabulary in general use, the words a client may choose to describe pain are varied. Clients of American descent often use *hurt* and *ache* to describe their pain, reserving the word *pain* for severe discomfort. The nurse uses words other than *pain* to obtain an accurate report. For example, the nurse might say, "Tell me what your discomfort feels like." The client may describe the pain as crushing, throbbing, sharp, or dull. Although a list of descriptive terms is available, it is more accurate to have clients describe the pain in their own words whenever possible.

There is some consistency in the way people describe certain types of pain. The pain associated with a myocardial infarction is often described as crushing or viselike, whereas the pain of a surgical incision is often described as dull, aching, and throbbing, indicating nociceptive

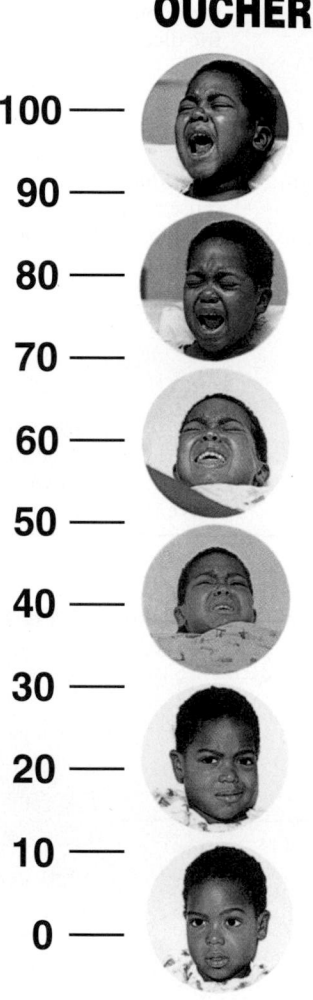

OUCHER.

100 —
90 —
80 —
70 —
60 —
50 —
40 —
30 —
20 —
10 —
0 —

FIGURE **42–7** African-American version of the Oucher pain scale. (Copyright Denyes Villarrael, 1990.)

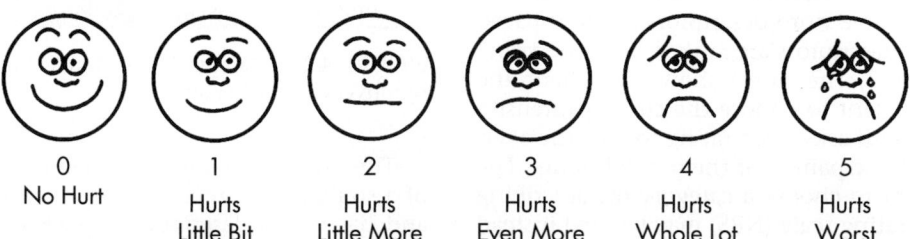

0	1	2	3	4	5
No Hurt	Hurts Little Bit	Hurts Little More	Hurts Even More	Hurts Whole Lot	Hurts Worst

Brief word instructions: Point to each face using the words to describe the pain intensity. Ask the child to choose face that best describes own pain and record the appropriate number.

FIGURE **42–8** Wong-Baker FACES Pain Rating Scale. (From Hockenberry MJ and others: *Wong's nursing care of infants and children,* ed 7, St. Louis, 2003, Mosby.)

pain. Neuropathic pain is usually described as burning, shooting, or electric-like (Portenoy, 1996). When the client's descriptions fit the pattern forming in the nurse's assessment, a clearer analysis can be made of the nature and type of pain. This will lead to more appropriate pain management because nociceptive and neuropathic pain are treated differently.

Pain Pattern. Various factors affect the pattern of pain. It helps to assess specific events or conditions that precipitate or aggravate pain. The nurse asks the client to describe activities that cause pain, such as physical movement, coffee ingestion, or urination. The nurse may also ask the client to demonstrate actions that cause a painful response, such as coughing or turning a certain way. In the example of a ruptured intravertebral disk, the low back pain and radiation down the leg is usually aggravated by bending over or lifting objects. Swallowing and talking typically aggravate the pain of pharyngitis. Asking the client if there is a particular time of day the pain is worse, or if the pain is intermittent, constant, or a combination helps the nurse to plan interventions to prevent pain from occurring or worsening.

Relief Measures. It is useful to know whether a client has an effective way of relieving pain, such as changing position, using ritualistic behavior (pacing, rocking, rubbing), eating, meditation, prayer, or applying heat or cold to the painful site. The client's methods often work best for the nurse, too. Clients gain comfort from knowing that the nurse is willing to try their relief measures. Clients also gain a sense of control over the pain instead of the pain controlling them (Haythornthwaite and others, 1998). Assessment of relieving factors should also include identification of practitioners (e.g., internist, orthopedist, acupuncturist, chiropractor, or dentist) whose services the client has used.

Contributing Symptoms. There are some symptoms (depression, anxiety, fatigue, sedation, anorexia, sleep disruption, spiritual distress, guilt) that may cause worsening of pain. The nurse needs to assess for these associated symptoms and evaluate their effects on the client's pain perception. Reporting and treating contributing symptoms contributes to successful pain management.

Effects of Pain on the Client. Pain is a stressful event that can alter a person's lifestyle and affect psychological well-being. In the case of cancer and chronic noncancer pain, it can cause suffering, loss of control, and impaired quality of life throughout the client's course of care. By recognizing the effects pain has on clients, the nurse can better identify the nature and existence of pain.

When a client has acute pain, the nurse should assess vital signs, conduct a focused physical examination, and observe for nonverbal responses to pain. At the initial onset of acute pain, the heart and respiratory rate and blood pressure increase. However, the body adapts quickly to acute pain and the vital signs return to within normal range quickly. The nurse should not confuse signs and symptoms of pain with other pathological changes. Changes in vital signs are more often indicative of problems other than pain. For example, a client who is highly

anxious also has elevated heart and respiratory rates. The nurse performs a physical and neurological assessment based on the client's pain history. The painful area should be examined to see if palpation or manipulation of the site increases pain (Jacox and others, 1994). During a general overview, the nurse looks for cues indicating pain (e.g., posturing or guarding a painful area). If pain is unrelieved, the nurse looks for signs of physical exhaustion.

Behavioral Effects. When a client has pain, the nurse assesses verbalization, vocal response, facial and body movements, and social interaction. A verbal report of pain is a vital part of assessment. The nurse must be willing to listen and understand. Many clients cannot verbalize discomfort because of the inability to communicate. An infant or a client who is unconscious, disoriented or confused, or aphasic, or who speaks a foreign language is unable to explain the pain experience. In these cases it is especially important for the nurse to be alert for behaviors that indicate pain (Box 42-8).

Groaning, grunting, and crying are examples of vocalizations used to express pain. Certain vocalizations may be involuntary and may occur without warning when acute pain occurs. For some clients, vocalizations are culturally acceptable ways to communicate and do not necessarily indicate a higher severity of pain or reduced pain tolerance.

Subtle facial expressions or body movements often reveal more about the character of pain than does precise questioning. For example, the client may grimace or begin to toss and turn at regular intervals. The amount of restlessness or protective movement may increase as the assessment progresses. Some nonverbal expressions characterize sources of pain. The client with chest pain often grabs or holds the chest. A child or adult with severe abdominal pain often assumes a fetal position. The nonverbal expression of pain may support or contradict other information about pain. If a woman in labor reports that her labor pains are occurring more frequently, and if she

---

Box 42-8   Behavioral Indicators of Effects of Pain

Vocalizations

Moaning
Crying
Gasping
Grunting

Facial Expressions

Grimace
Clenched teeth
Wrinkled forehead
Tightly closed or widely opened eyes or mouth
Lip biting

Body Movement

Restlessness
Immobilization
Muscle tension
Increased hand and finger movements
Pacing activities
Rhythmic or rubbing motions
Protective movement of body parts

Social Interaction

Avoidance of conversation
Focus only on activities for pain relief
Avoidance of social contacts
Reduced attention span

begins to massage her abdomen more frequently, her report is confirmed. If a client complains of severe abdominal pain but continues to grasp the chest, a more detailed assessment may be necessary.

The nature of a person's pain causes the person to attend to the discomfort and fight it or give in to the discomfort and withdraw socially. The extent to which a client interacts with the environment can provide a clue for the nurse about the intensity or nature of the pain. Severe pain can seriously hamper a person's lifestyle.

Influence on Activities of Daily Living. Clients who live with daily pain are less able to participate in routine activities, which can lead to physical deconditioning. Assessment of these changes reveals the extent of the client's disability and adjustments necessary to help clients participate in self-care. The primary goal of the nurse should be to improve client function.

The nurse asks whether pain interferes with sleep. There may be initial difficulty falling asleep. Sleeping pills or other medications may be needed to induce sleep. The pain may awaken the client during the night and create difficulty in falling back to sleep (see Chapter 41).

Depending on the location of the pain, the client may have difficulty performing normal hygiene measures. The nurse determines whether the client can perform hygiene and dressing/grooming activities independently. The pain may restrict mobility to the point that the client is no longer able to bathe in a bathtub. The client may have problems performing other activities of daily living. For example, clients with severe arthritis may find it painful to grasp eating utensils or lower themselves to a toilet seat. The nurse assesses the client's need for assistance with self-care activities and collaborates with members of the health care team (e.g., physical therapy and occupational therapy). The nurse also considers the need for family members or friends to assist the client with basic hygiene.

Pain can impair the ability to maintain normal sexual relations. Conditions such as arthritis, degenerative diseases of the hip, and chronic back pain make it difficult for a person to assume usual positions during intercourse. Prolonged use of opioids for cancer pain is known to affect sexual function and libido in men and women (Jacox and others, 1994). The nurse should assess the extent to which pain has affected sexual activity. It also helps to learn whether a client is physically unable to participate or if the desire for sexual intercourse has been reduced by the pain.

The ability of people to work can be seriously threatened by pain. The more physical activity required in a job, the greater the risk of discomfort when the pain is associated with musculoskeletal and certain visceral alterations. Pain related to emotional stress is probably increased in individuals whose jobs involve tension-laden decision making. The nurse assesses the work that clients do and their abilities to function in regular jobs. The daily chores of homemakers are assessed in the same manner as the duties involved in jobs outside the home. The nurse assesses whether it is necessary for clients to stop activity occasionally because of pain. Often the nurse can help clients select ways of minimizing or controlling the pain so that they can remain productive.

It is also important to include an assessment of the effect of pain on social activities. The pain may be so debilitating that the client becomes too exhausted to socialize. The nurse identifies the client's normal social activities, the extent to which they have been disrupted, and the client's wish to participate.

Client Expectations. A national survey states that the public views pain as a "part of life" and would rather bear it than take action to relieve it (Bostrom, 1997). Clients who seek treatment with pain as a major symptom may have experienced this pain for many hours or days before seeking health care assistance. They may expect and even accept a certain amount of pain while being hospitalized. Asking the client the comfort level that is acceptable to him or her is an initial step in encouraging the client to regain control. Assessing previous pain experiences and what interventions were effective at home provides a foundation on which the nurse can build. Clients expect that nurses will believe their reports of pain and be prompt in meeting their pain needs.

Nursing Diagnosis

The development of an accurate nursing diagnosis for a client in pain results from thorough data collection and analysis (Box 42-9). A nurse must not diagnose pain simply because it is presumed that a client will be uncomfortable. Careful assessment will or will not indicate pain as a (potential) problem. An accurate diagnosis is made only after a complete assessment has been performed. In the example of the diagnosis of pain, the nurse may assess the client's withdrawal from communication, grimacing, and moaning, as well as the client's verbalization of discomfort. In contrast, the diagnosis of anxiety may be made by observing a client's facial tension and appearance, poor eye contact, restlessness, and verbalizations of feeling scared. The two diagnoses have similar defining characteristics. The nurse sorts out patterns of data to identify pain as the correct diagnosis.

The nursing diagnosis should focus on the specific nature of the pain to help the nurse identify the most useful types of interventions for alleviating pain and minimizing its effect on the client's lifestyle and function. *Acute pain related to physical trauma* versus *acute pain related to natural childbirth processes* require very different nursing interventions. Accurate identification of related factors ensures that appropriate nursing interventions will be chosen.

The nurse may make diagnoses other than that of *acute* or *chronic pain*. The extent to which pain affects a client's lifestyle and general state of health determines whether other nursing diagnoses are relevant. For example, the nurse's assessment may reveal that a client suffers from pain of the hands and shoulders as a result of crippling arthritis that the client has had for over 3 years. As a result, the client is unable to remove or fasten necessary items of clothing. The nursing diagnoses for this client would be that of *self-care deficit: dressing/grooming* and *chronic pain*. The diagnosis of *self-care deficit* would lead the nurse to involve members of the health care team to provide the client with assistive devices for performing

Nursing Diagnostic Process

Box *42-9*

Assessment Activities	Defining Characteristics	Nursing Diagnosis
Have client describe pain intensity. Assess onset and location of pain. Observe client behaviors.	Pain is constant; 5 out of 10 Present for 7 months in lower lumbar area Grimaces and grunts with movement, rubs flanks frequently; reduced movement	Chronic pain related to chronic physical disability
Assess effect of pain on activities of daily living (ADLs). Review medical history.	Appetite poor; gets little sleep; difficulty dressing Previous trauma; previous exposure to opioids	

self-care. Examples of other diagnoses that may be applicable to clients at risk for experiencing pain include the following:

- Anxiety
- Ineffective coping
- Fatigue
- Fear
- Hopelessness
- Impaired physical mobility
- Imbalanced nutrition: less than body requirements
- Acute pain
- Chronic pain
- Powerlessness
- Ineffective role performance
- Self-care deficit
- Chronic low self-esteem
- Situational low self-esteem
- Risk for situational low self-esteem
- Sexual dysfunction
- Disturbed sleep pattern
- Impaired social interaction
- Spiritual distress

Planning

During planning the nurse synthesizes information from multiple resources. Critical thinking ensures that the client's plan of care integrates all that the nurse knows about the individual client, as well as key critical thinking elements (Figure 42-9, p. 1248). Professional standards are especially important to consider when the nurse develops a plan of care (see care plan, p. 1249). These standards often establish scientifically proven guidelines for selecting effective nursing interventions. Professional standards of care regarding pain management are available as agency policies or through professional organizations such as the American Society of Pain Management Nurses.

Another effective method for planning care is a concept map. Clients who are in pain may frequently have interrelated problems. As one problem gets worse, other aspects of the client's level of health also change. The concept map assists the nurse in relating how the nursing diagnoses are interrelated with each other and linked to the client's medical diagnosis. Using the example here, as care is planned

for the client with rheumatoid arthritis, the nurse notes the relationships between *acute pain, impaired physical mobility, self-care, and fatigue* (Figure 42-10, p. 1251). Identifying these relationships assists the nursing in developing a holistic and client-centered plan of care.

Goals and Outcomes. Goals of pain management permit the client to function to the best possible extent. This requires that the nurse and client first identify what the pain has prevented the client from doing. Then a mutually acceptable level of pain that will allow return of function is decided. An indication of plan success is determined through attainment of goals and outcomes. For example, in the case of the goal of "the client will achieve a satisfactory level of pain relief within 24 hours," the following are possible outcomes:

- Reporting that pain is a 3 or less on a scale of 0 to 10, or does not interfere with ADLs
- Identifying factors that intensify pain and modifying behavior accordingly
- Using pain relief measures safely

Setting Priorities. Together the nurse and client discuss realistic expectations for an individualized plan of care. Planned interventions must be appropriate for the nature and type of pain. For example, pain related to acute incisional pain usually responds to analgesics, whereas pain related to early labor contractions can often be reduced with relaxation exercises. An intervention that works for one client will not work for all. When developing a plan of care, the nurse selects priorities based on the client's level of pain and its effect of the client's condition. For severe pain it is important to provide relief as soon as possible. A pain intensity of 7 or greater out of 10 requires the nurse's immediate attention.

Analgesics can provide relatively rapid relief and lessen the chance of pain worsening. After a client gains some relief from the pain, the nurse plans other interventions such as relaxation or the application of cold to enhance the effect of analgesics.

Continuity of Care. A comprehensive plan includes a variety of resources for pain control. Resources available include nurse specialists, doctors of pharmacology (PharmDs), physical therapists, occupational therapists, and clergy. An oncology nurse specialist is very familiar with the pharmaco-

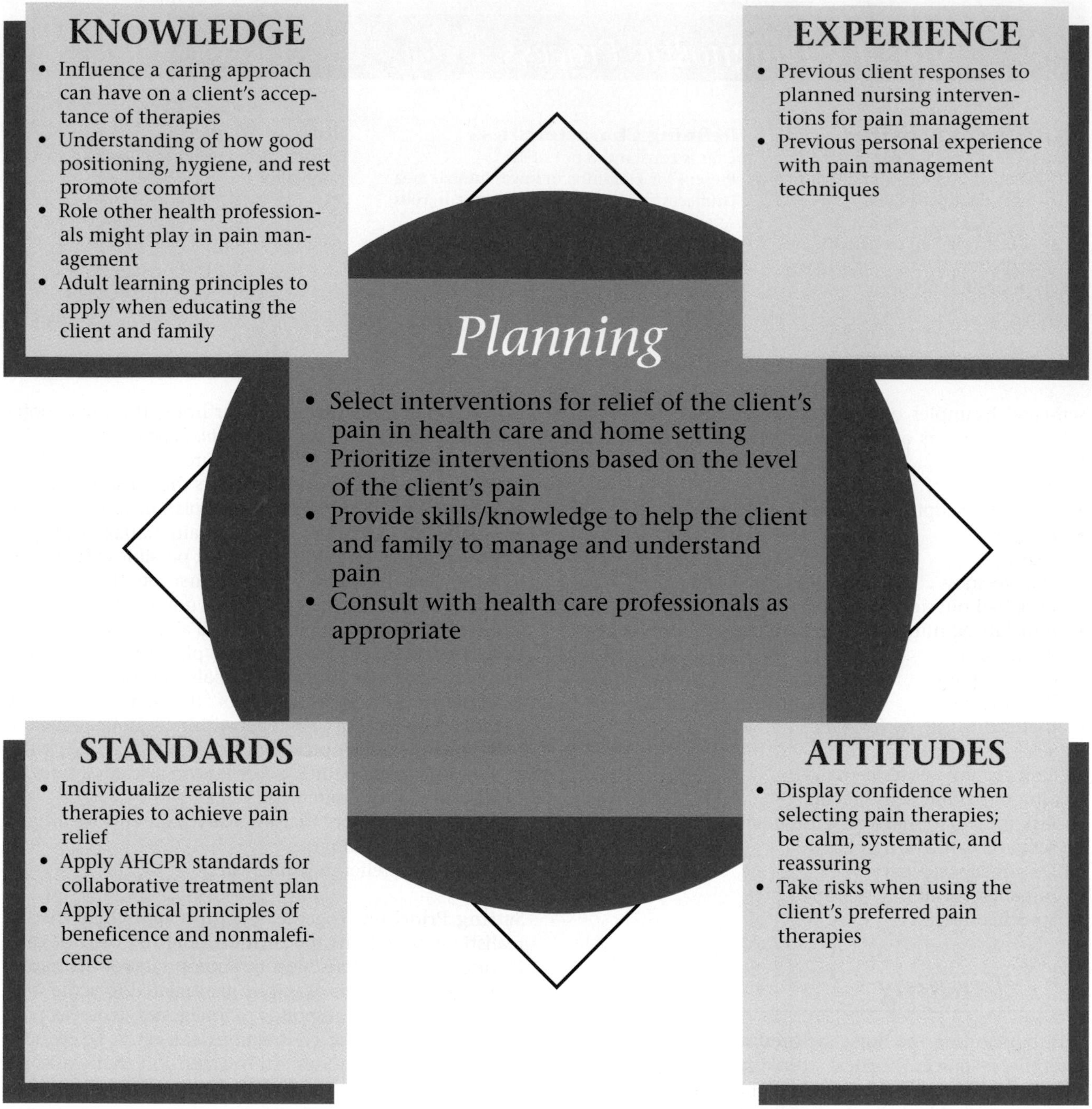

KNOWLEDGE

- Influence a caring approach can have on a client's acceptance of therapies
- Understanding of how good positioning, hygiene, and rest promote comfort
- Role other health professionals might play in pain management
- Adult learning principles to apply when educating the client and family

EXPERIENCE

- Previous client responses to planned nursing interventions for pain management
- Previous personal experience with pain management techniques

Planning

- Select interventions for relief of the client's pain in health care and home setting
- Prioritize interventions based on the level of the client's pain
- Provide skills/knowledge to help the client and family to manage and understand pain
- Consult with health care professionals as appropriate

STANDARDS

- Individualize realistic pain therapies to achieve pain relief
- Apply AHCPR standards for collaborative treatment plan
- Apply ethical principles of beneficence and nonmaleficence

ATTITUDES

- Display confidence when selecting pain therapies; be calm, systematic, and reassuring
- Take risks when using the client's preferred pain therapies

FIGURE **42–9** Critical thinking model for comfort planning.

logical and nonpharmacological interventions that are most effective for chronic noncancer and cancer pain. Doctors of pharmacology are knowledgeable about pharmacological treatments of pain. Physical therapists can plan exercises that strengthen muscle groups and lessen pain in affected areas. Occupational therapists may devise splints to support painful body parts. Clergy members can help clients resolve spiritual pain. It is important to involve the family in the plan of care because they may need to administer care in the home after discharge. If the pain management plan is not successful in achieving the identified pain relief goal, the nurse should talk with the physi-

cian about changing the plan. Pain expert consultation might be necessary.

Implementation

The nature of the pain and the extent to which it affects a person's well-being determine the choice of pain-relief interventions. Pain therapy requires an individualized approach, perhaps more so than any other client problem. The nurse, client, and oftentimes the family must be partners in using pain-control measures. Nurses administer

Nursing Care Plan

Impaired Comfort

Assessment

Mrs. Mays was diagnosed with a cancerous tumor in her left lung 8 months ago. After treatment she was taking oral analgesics on a prn basis. However, she is now admitted to the hospital with uncontrollable chest pain and possible pneumonia. Her husband is with her. A PCA of morphine 0.5 mg demand dose with a 10-minute lockout is begun.

Assessment Activities	Findings/Defining Characteristics
Ask Mrs. Mays what she did at home to control her pain.	Her pain escalated from a 3 to a 10 so she doubled her medication and went to bed, but this did not help.
Ask Mrs. Mays what her pain intensity is now.	On a scale of 0 to 10, she reports a 9.
Ask Mrs. Mays what her pain has prevented her from doing.	She responds that she is unable to complete her own hygiene activities or sleep well.
Observe Mrs. Mays's nonverbal behavior.	She is restless, unable to stay focused, and remains very still during the history taking.
Ask Mrs. Mays her pain intensity goal (out of 10).	She says that a pain intensity of 5 out of 10 would help her function better right now. A goal of 3 would be preferred.

Nursing Diagnosis: Acute pain related to a biological injuring agent (tumor).

Planning

Goal	Expected Outcomes*
	Pain Control
Client will obtain an acceptable level of comfort before discharge.	Client will report pain at stated goal or below.
Husband will assist in restoring Mrs. Mays to a pain-free state.	Husband will provide slow-stroke massage to Mrs. Mays before bedtime.
Client will actively participate in ADLs.	**Pain: Disruptive Effects**
	Mrs. Mays will report sleeping for 5 to 6 hours without interruption from pain.
	She will complete her own hygiene with minimal assistance.
	She will walk the hallway with her husband every 4 hours for 15 minutes.
	Medication Response
Mrs. Mays will not experience unmanageable opioid side effects.	Mrs. Mays will report having a normal bowel movement every other day.

*Outcome classification labels from Moorhead S, Johnson M, Maas S: *Nursing outcomes classification (NOC)*, ed 3, St. Louis, 2004, Mosby.

Interventions†	Rationale
Pain Management	
• Begin PCA at ordered dose. Explain to client and spouse how to use the PCA. Emphasize the importance of only the client pushing the button, not the husband.	Client is experiencing an acute episode of her cancer pain. A report of 7 (or more) out of 10 requires immediate-release opioid. Discouraging the husband from pushing the button will minimize potential toxic effects of the opioid because client must be awake to perceive the pain and push the button (Reiff and Nizolek, 2001).
• Monitor IV PCA morphine use. Explain to client and spouse the action of the medication; potential side effects, and the importance of reporting if the pain is not relieved.	Pain is easier to prevent than to treat. Side effects are usually transient, except for constipation. Calculating 24-hour dose of opioid helps determine appropriate oral dose (McCaffery and Pasero, 1999).
• Have client select nonpharmacological interventions that have relieved pain in the past (e.g., distraction, music, simple relaxation therapy).	Personal control allows a client to shape immediate circumstances through own actions. (Salerno and Willens, 1996). Nonpharmacological interventions augment pharmacological strategies, but should not be used in place of analgesics (McCaffery and Pasero, 1999).
• Teach spouse how to perform slow-stroke back massage.	Slow-stroke back massage is easy to do, takes a brief time, and has been shown to induce relaxation (Meek, 1993).

†Intervention classification labels from Dochterman JM, Bulechek GM: *Nursing interventions classification (NIC)*, ed 4, St. Louis, 2004, Mosby.

Continued

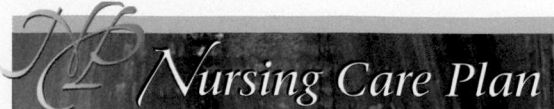

Nursing Care Plan

Impaired Comfort—cont'd

Evaluation

Nursing Actions	Client Response/Finding	Achievement of Outcome
Ask Mrs. Mays if she attained her pain relief goal most of the time.	She responds, "My pain usually runs around a 3, which is my goal, except when I start walking."	Mrs. Mays reports an acceptable level of comfort on a scale of 0 to 10. Instruct her to push her button before ambulating.
Observe Mrs. Mays performing ADLs, walking, and ability to sleep.	She is dressed for breakfast, walking the hallway every 4 hours with her husband. The night nurse's notes indicate she slept through the night.	Ability to perform ADLs and sleep has improved. Continue to monitor.
Ask Mr. Mays if he was able to give his wife a back rub.	He reported that she did not want a back rub but preferred to have her feet rubbed, which he was happy to do. "She said it made her feel more relaxed."	Nonpharmacological intervention successful, but needs changing from back rub to foot rub in the nursing care plan.
Ask Mrs. Mays when was the last time she had a bowel movement and its consistency.	She has not had a bowel movement in 3 days (since starting the morphine PCA).	Assess her abdomen for bowel sounds and distention. Consult with physician about starting a stimulant laxative once intestinal obstruction is ruled out (McCaffery and Pasero, 1999).

and monitor interventions ordered by physicians for pain relief and independently use pain-relief measures that complement those prescribed by a physician. Client remedies are often most successful, especially when the client has already had experience with pain. Generally, the least invasive or safest therapy should be tried first. If there is doubt about a nursing therapy, the nurse should consult with a physician.

Health Promotion. Clients are better prepared to handle almost any situation when they understand it. The experience of pain is no exception. However, clients with moderate to severe pain may not be able to participate in the decision-making process until the pain is controlled to an acceptable level. Once this is accomplished, teaching may begin.

Teaching clients about the pain experience reduces anxiety and helps clients achieve a sense of control. For example, clients entering a clinic or hospital for the first time may know that tests will be performed but do not understand them. As a result, they may be anxious about the experience. Fears are enhanced if friends have had unpleasant experiences in similar circumstances. Fear increases the perception of painful stimuli.

During the anticipatory phase of a pain experience, the nurse needs to teach clients about the procedures and associated discomfort. Explaining the procedure in a confident tone conveys a sense that the nurse will care for the client correctly. When clients receive instruction about an upcoming painful experience, they often perceive the actual experience as less unpleasant.

Because comfort affects a person's physical and mental functioning, holistic health approaches are becoming important interventions for maintaining a person's wellness. Holistic health is an ongoing state of wellness that involves taking care of the physical self, expressing emotions appropriately and effectively, using the mind constructively, being creatively involved with others, and becoming aware of higher levels of consciousness (American Holistic Health Association, 1999). The use of holistic health approaches assumes a person's own capacity for healing and returns responsibility for health back to the individual (Edelman and Mandle, 1998). The concept of holistic health parallels the values nursing has always had in maintaining the integrity of the whole person.

Holistic health is more than just self-care. It also is a process of personal inquiry. Individuals learn to look at the emotional meaning of any health problems they might have and the significance of the problem in light of their purpose in life (Edelman and Mandle, 1998). A person becomes consciously aware of the relationship between emotional health and physical health. The role of clients is to participate actively in their own well-being. Common holistic health approaches include wellness education, regular exercise, rest, attention to good hygiene practices and nutrition, and management of interpersonal relationships. When a person develops pain or other symptoms of discomfort, there are nonpharmacological as well as pharmacological strategies the nurse can offer. Several of the nonpharmacological interventions do not need an order, but are nurse initiated.

Nonpharmacological Pain-Relief Interventions. There are a number of nonpharmacological interventions that might lessen pain and that can be used in combination with pharmacological measures (Titler and Rakel, 2001). Nonpharmacological interventions include cognitive-behavioral and physical approaches. The goals of cognitive-behavioral interventions are to change clients' perceptions of pain, to alter pain behavior, and to provide clients

Concept Map

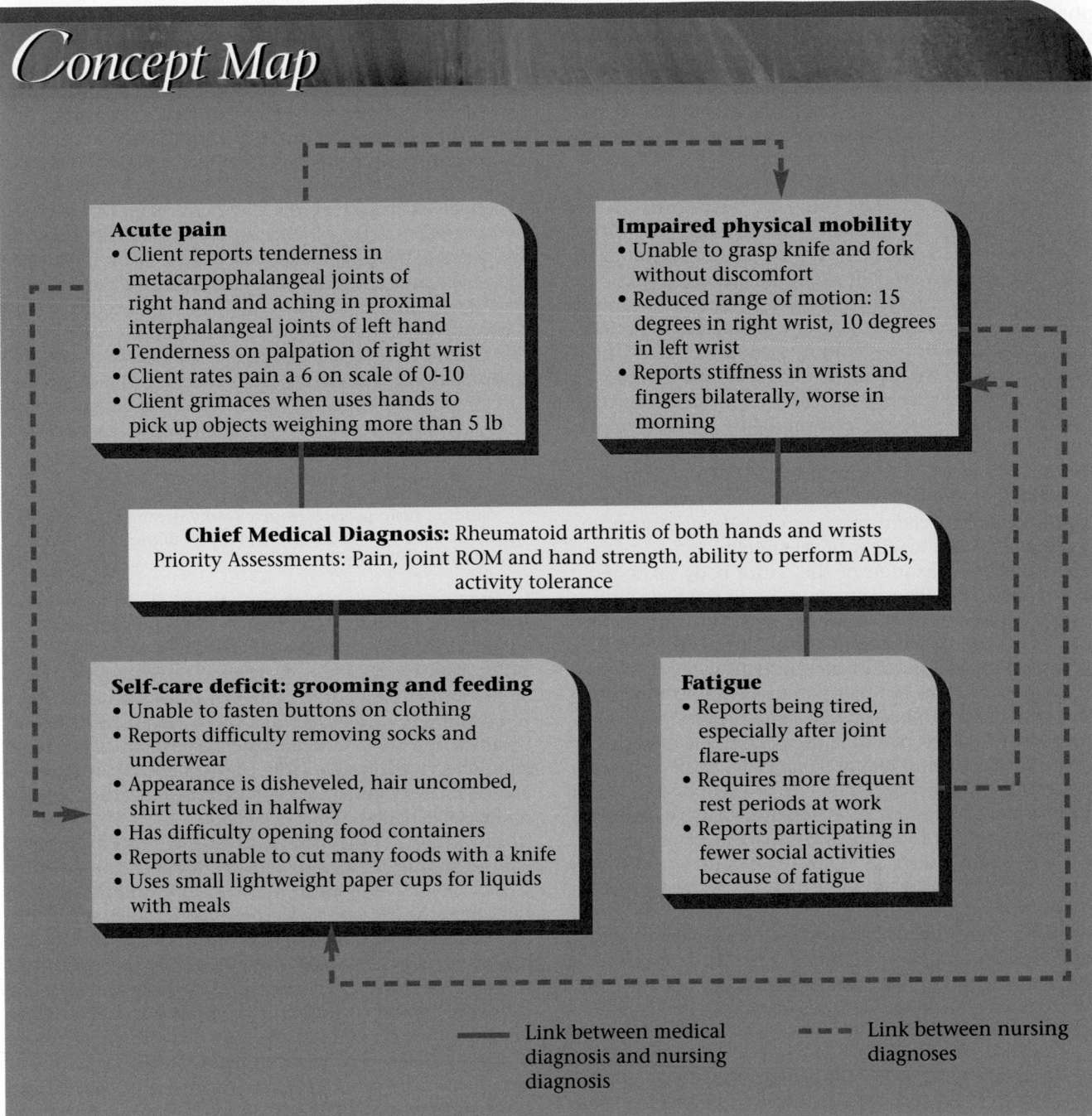

Acute pain
- Client reports tenderness in metacarpophalangeal joints of right hand and aching in proximal interphalangeal joints of left hand
- Tenderness on palpation of right wrist
- Client rates pain a 6 on scale of 0-10
- Client grimaces when uses hands to pick up objects weighing more than 5 lb

Impaired physical mobility
- Unable to grasp knife and fork without discomfort
- Reduced range of motion: 15 degrees in right wrist, 10 degrees in left wrist
- Reports stiffness in wrists and fingers bilaterally, worse in morning

Chief Medical Diagnosis: Rheumatoid arthritis of both hands and wrists
Priority Assessments: Pain, joint ROM and hand strength, ability to perform ADLs, activity tolerance

Self-care deficit: grooming and feeding
- Unable to fasten buttons on clothing
- Reports difficulty removing socks and underwear
- Appearance is disheveled, hair uncombed, shirt tucked in halfway
- Has difficulty opening food containers
- Reports unable to cut many foods with a knife
- Uses small lightweight paper cups for liquids with meals

Fatigue
- Reports being tired, especially after joint flare-ups
- Requires more frequent rest periods at work
- Reports participating in fewer social activities because of fatigue

—— Link between medical diagnosis and nursing diagnosis

--- Link between nursing diagnoses

FIGURE **42–10** Concept map for client with pain related to rheumatoid arthritis.

with a greater sense of control. Relaxation and guided imagery are examples. Physical agents have the goal of providing comfort, correcting physical dysfunction, altering physiological responses, and reducing fears associated with pain-related immobility. The AHCPR guidelines for acute pain management (1992) cite nonpharmacological interventions to be appropriate for clients who meet the following criteria:
- Find such interventions appealing
- Express anxiety or fear
- May benefit from avoiding or reducing drug therapy

- Are likely to experience and need to cope with a prolonged interval of postoperative pain
- Have incomplete pain relief after use of pharmacological interventions

Relaxation and Guided Imagery. Clients can alter affective-motivational and cognitive pain perception through relaxation and guided imagery. **Relaxation** is mental and physical freedom from tension or stress. Relaxation techniques provide individuals with self-control when discomfort or pain occurs, reversing the physical and emotional stress of pain. Relaxation techniques can be used at any phase of health or illness Clients who use relaxation techniques successfully experience several physiological and behavioral changes such as decreased pulse, blood pressure, and respirations; heightened global awareness; decreased oxygen consumption; a sense of peace; and decreased muscle tension and metabolic rate. Relaxation techniques include meditation, yoga, Zen, guided imagery, and progressive relaxation exercises (see Chapter 35).

For effective relaxation, the individual's participation and cooperation are needed. Relaxation techniques are taught only when the client is not in acute discomfort because the inability to concentrate makes the exercise ineffective. The nurse explains the technique in detail and describes common sensations the client may experience (e.g., a decrease in temperature or numbness of a body part). The client should use these sensations as feedback.

The nurse is a coach, guiding the client slowly through steps of the exercise. The environment should be free of noises or other irritating stimuli. The client may sit in a comfortable chair or lie in bed (Box 42-10). A light sheet or blanket for warmth often helps the client feel more comfortable. The client may use guided imagery and relaxation exercises together or separately.

Progressive relaxation of the entire body takes about 15 minutes. The client pays attention to the body, noting areas of tension. Tense areas are replaced with warmth and relaxation. Some clients relax better with their eyes closed. Soft background music can help.

Progressive relaxation exercise involves a combination of controlled breathing exercises and a series of contractions and relaxation of muscle groups. The client begins by breathing slowly and diaphragmatically, allowing the abdomen to rise slowly and the chest to expand fully. When the client establishes a regular breathing pattern, the nurse coaches the client to locate any area of muscular tension, to think about how it feels, to tense muscles fully, and then completely to relax them. This creates the sensation of removing all discomfort and stress. Gradually the client can relax the muscles without first tensing them. When full relaxation is achieved, pain perception is lowered and anxiety toward the pain experience becomes minimal. Chapter 35 offers several relaxation exercise approaches.

Box 42-10   Body Positions for Relaxation

Sitting

Sit with entire back resting against back of chair.
Place feet flat on floor.
Keep legs separated.
Hang arms at the side or rest on chair arms.
Keep head aligned with spine.

Lying

Keep legs separated with toes pointed slightly outward.
Rest arms at sides without touching sides of body.
Keep head aligned with spine.
Use thin, small pillow under head.

If a client becomes agitated or uncomfortable, the nurse stops the exercise. If the client seems to have difficulty relaxing any part of the body, the nurse slows the progression of the exercise and concentrates on the tensed body part. The client must also know from the beginning that the exercise can be stopped at any time. With practice the client can soon perform relaxation exercises independently (Aspen Reference Group, 1999).

In **guided imagery** the client creates an image in the mind, concentrates on that image, and gradually becomes less aware of pain. The nurse coaches the client in forming the image and concentrating on the sensory experience. Initially the nurse asks the client to think of a pleasant scene or experience that promotes the use of all the senses. The client describes the image and the nurse records it so that it can be used during later exercises. The nurse uses specific information given by the client and does not make changes in the client's image. The following is an example of a portion of a guided imagery exercise:

> Imagine yourself lying on a cool bed of grass with the sounds of rushing water from a nearby stream. It's a balmy day. You turn to see a patch of blue wildflowers in bloom and can smell their fragrance.

The nurse sits closely enough to the client to be heard but is not intrusive. The nurse's calm, soft voice helps the client focus more completely on the suggested image. While relaxing, the client focuses on the image, and it becomes unnecessary for the nurse to speak continuously. If the client shows signs of agitation, restlessness, or discomfort, the nurse should stop the exercise and begin later when the client is more at ease. The client may use guided imagery and relaxation exercises together or separately (see Chapter 35).

Distraction. The reticular activating system inhibits painful stimuli if a person receives sufficient or excessive sensory input. With meaningful sensory stimuli, a person can ignore or become unaware of pain. Pleasurable stimuli cause the release of endorphins. Persons who are bored or in isolation have only their pain to think about and thus perceive it more acutely. Distraction directs a client's attention to something else and thus can reduce the awareness of pain and even increase tolerance. There is one disadvantage. If it works, health care personnel or family may question the existence or severity of the pain. Distraction may work best for short, intense pain lasting a few minutes, such as during an invasive procedure or while waiting for an analgesic to work. The nurse assesses activities enjoyed by the client that may act as distractions. These might include singing, praying, describing photos or pictures aloud, listening to music, and playing games. Most distractions can be used in a hospital, home, or long-term care facility.

Music. One effective distraction is music, which decreases physiological pain, stress, and anxiety by diverting the person's attention away from the pain and creating a relaxation response. The nurse can use music creatively in many clinical situations. Clients generally prefer to perform (play an instrument or sing a song) or listen to music. All forms of music are used in music therapy. It is important to let the client select the type of music he or she prefers. Popular music does not usually produce a deep level of relaxation because it is short with a steady beat and words. Music produces an altered state of consciousness through sound, silence, space, and time. It must be listened to for at least 15 minutes to be therapeutic. The use of earphones helps clients to concentrate on music while also avoiding annoying other clients or staff. In an acute care setting, listening to music can be highly effective in reducing a client's postoperative pain. The nurse assists clients by creating a relaxing setting so music can be listened to uninterrupted. If pain becomes acute, the nurse suggests increasing the volume of music until the pain subsides.

A special group of clients have been found to benefit significantly from individualized or preferred music. Clients with Alzheimer's disease or related disorders (ADRD) often experience agitation and disruptive behavior. When this same group of clients experiences pain, the level of agitation can worsen. Research has shown that music may be used as a method of communicating with this population even in advanced stages of dementia when the person is unable to understand verbal language

---

Evidence-Based Practice Guideline

Box 42-11

Individualized Music

- Determine if client is able to hear a normal speaking voice at a distance of 1½ feet. Impaired hearing may distort sound, which may be source of irritation.
- Assess client's personal music preference.
  - Ask client how important a role music played in his or her life.
  - Ask if client played a musical instrument.
  - Ask if client enjoys singing and dancing.
  - Ask client to identify three most favorite types of music (e.g., Country and western, folk, blues, jazz, rock and roll, ethnic).
  - Ask client which of the following is their favorite form of music: vocal, instrumental, or both.
  - Ask client to identify songs that make him or her happy.
  - Have client identify specific artists or performers he or she enjoys listening to.
  - Have client identify specific albums, tapes, CDs he or she has at home.
- If client is unable to provide information due to cognitive impairment, interview a family member who is knowledgeable about the client's music preference.
- Play the music selections:
  - Use an audio cassette player or CD player that functions properly.
  - Plan each music intervention session to last about 30 minutes, in a location where client is comfortable or spends most of time.
  - Set volume at an appropriate level.
  - Headphones may be an option; however, they can be uncomfortable or confusing to persons with dementia.

Modified from Gerdner L: *Individualized music: evidence-based protocol,* 2001, The University of Iowa Gerontological Nursing Interventions Research Center, Research Dissemination Core. Iowa City, Ia. In M.G. Titler (Series Ed.), Series on Evidence-Based Practice for Older Adults. Iowa City, IA. The University of Iowa College of Nursing Gerontological Nursing Interventions Research Center, Research Dissemination Core. For more information, http:// www.nursing.uiowa.edu/center/gnirc/disseminatecore.htm.

---

and has decreased ability to interpret environmental stimuli (Gerdner, 2001). Box 42-11 provides an evidenced-based protocol for use of music with ADRD clients.

Biofeedback. **Biofeedback** is a behavioral therapy that involves giving individuals information about physiological responses (e.g., blood pressure or tension) and ways to exercise voluntary control over those responses (McGrady and others, 1994). The therapy is used to produce deep relaxation and is especially effective for muscle tension and migraine headaches. When headaches are treated, electrodes are attached externally over each temple. The electrodes measure skin tension in microvolts. A polygraph machine visibly records the tension level for the client to see. The client learns to achieve optimal relaxation using feedback from the polygraph while lowering the actual level of tension experienced. The therapy takes several weeks to learn. Chapter 35 describes the benefits and limitations of biofeedback.

Cutaneous Stimulation. **Cutaneous stimulation** is the stimulation of the skin to relieve pain. A massage, warm bath, ice bag, and transcutaneous electrical nerve stimulation (TENS) are simple ways to reduce pain perception. The specific way in which cutaneous stimulation works is unclear. One suggestion is that it causes release of endorphins, thus blocking the transmission of painful stimuli. The gate-control theory suggests that cutaneous stimulation activates larger, faster-transmitting A-beta sensory nerve fibers. This decreases pain transmission through small-diameter A-delta and C fibers. Synaptic gates close to the transmission of pain impulses. In a review by O'Mathuna (2000), touch and massage influenced autonomic nervous system activity. When a person perceives touch to be relaxing, the relaxation response is elicited.

An advantage to cutaneous stimulation is that the measures can be used in the home, giving clients and families some control over pain symptoms and treatment. The proper use of cutaneous stimulation can reduce pain perception and help to reduce muscle tension that might otherwise increase pain. When using cutaneous stimulation methods, the nurse eliminates sources of environmental noise, helps the client to assume a comfortable position, and explains the purpose of the therapy. Cutaneous stimulation should not be used directly on sensitive skin areas (e.g., burns, bruises, skin rashes, inflammation, and underlying bone fractures).

Massages have been used by nurses as a safe and effective way to produce physical and mental relaxation, reduce pain, and enhance the effectiveness of pain medications for many years (Figure 42-11). Massaging the back and shoulders or the hands and feet for 3 to 5 minutes can help relax muscles and promote sleep and comfort (Grealish and others, 2000). Massages communicate caring and can easily be taught to family members or other health care personnel (Box 42-12, p. 1255).

Cold and heat applications (see Chapter 47) relieve pain and promote healing. The selection of heat versus cold interventions varies with clients' conditions. For example, moist heat can help relieve the pain from a tension headache, and cold applications can reduce the acute pain from inflamed joints. When using any form of heat or cold application, the nurse instructs the client to avoid injury to the skin by checking the temperature and avoiding

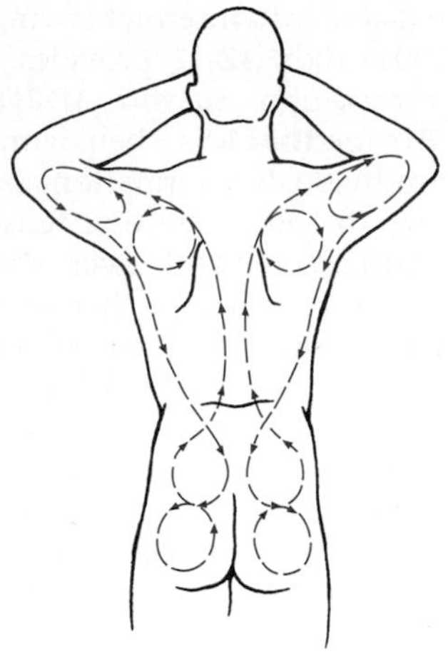

FIGURE **42–11** Back massage pattern.

direct application of the cold or hot surface to the skin. Especially at risk are clients with spinal cord or other neurological injury, older adults, and confused clients.

Ice massage and application of cold packs are two types of cold therapy that are particularly effective for pain relief. Ice massage involves the use of a large ice cube or a small paper cup filled with water and frozen (water rises out of the cup as it freezes to create a smooth surface of ice for massage). The massage is simple. A nurse or the client can apply the ice with firm pressure to the skin, followed by a slow, steady, circular massage over the area. Cold may be applied near the pain site, on the opposite side of the body corresponding to the pain site, or on a site located between the brain and the pain site. It takes 5 to 10 minutes to apply cold. Each client responds differently to the site of application that is most effective. Application near the actual site of pain tends to work best. A client feels cold, burning, and aching sensations and numbness. When numbness occurs, the ice should be removed. Cold is particularly effective for tooth or mouth pain when ice is placed on the web of the hand between the thumb and index finger. This point on the hand is an **acupressure** point that apparently influences nerve pathways to the face and head. Cold applications are also effective before invasive needle punctures.

Heat application might be more effective for some clients. Heating pads or hot water bottles may be used, but clients should be taught not to lay on the heating element because burning could occur. Commercial pillows that can be warmed in the microwave and that contour to the body are also available.

Another form of cutaneous stimulation, sometimes called counterstimulation, is **transcutaneous electrical nerve stimulation (TENS),** involving stimulation of the skin with a mild electrical current passed through external electrodes (Slucka, 2001). The therapy requires a physician's order. The TENS unit consists of a battery-powered transmitter, lead wires, and electrodes. The electrodes are placed directly over or near the site of pain. Hair or skin preparations should be removed before attaching the electrodes. When a client feels pain, the transmitter is turned on and a buzzing or tingling sensation is created. The client may adjust the intensity and quality of skin stimulation. The tingling sensation can be applied until pain relief occurs. TENS is effective for postsurgical pain control and reduction of pain caused by postoperative procedures.

Herbals. Although herbals have not been sufficiently studied to recommend for pain relief, many clients self-medicate using herbals. Herbals could have an interaction with prescribed analgesics, thus the nurse asks the client to report all substances taken to relieve pain (see Chapter 35).

Reducing Pain Perception. One simple way to promote comfort is by removing or preventing painful stimuli (Box 42-13, p. 1256). This is especially important for clients who are immobilized or unable to sense discomfort. Pain can also be prevented by anticipating painful events. For example, a client who is allowed to become constipated may suffer from distention and abdominal cramping. The nurse actively intervenes to ensure that the normal elimination process continues. Before performing procedures, the nurse considers the client's condition, aspects of the procedure that may be uncomfortable, and techniques to avoid causing pain. For example, in a client with severe arthritic knee pain, the nurse knows that any extreme flexion of the knee causes much pain. Before walking the client to the bathroom, the nurse makes sure that an elevated toilet seat is available. The client can then be seated and can rise with minimal discomfort. It takes only simple consideration of the client's comfort and a little extra time to avoid pain-producing situations.

Acute Care

Acute Pain Management. Nurses care for clients who have acute pain due to invasive procedures (e.g., surgery or endoscopy) or trauma. The AHCPR (1992) has established a pain treatment flow chart (Figure 42-12, p. 1257) for the aggressive treatment of postoperative pain and pain from medical procedures and trauma. The systematic approach ensures quick response on the part of caregivers to client discomfort. The key to success is ongoing evaluation of interventions: Is relief obtained? Are there any unacceptable side effects from the medications? It is the responsibility of the health care team to collaborate to find the combination of therapy that works best for a client.

Pharmacological Pain-Relief Interventions. There are several pharmacological agents that provide pain relief and require a physician's order to administer. The nurse's judgment in the use and management of these medications helps ensure the best pain relief possible. The ideal analgesic has yet to be developed.

Analgesics. **Analgesics** are the most common method of pain relief. Although analgesics can effectively relieve pain, nurses and physicians still tend to undertreat clients because of incorrect drug information, concerns about addiction, anxiety over errors in using opioid analgesics, and administration of less medication than was ordered. It is necessary for nurses to understand the drugs available for pain relief and their pharmacological effects.

There are three types of analgesics: (1) nonsteroidal anti-inflammatory drugs (NSAIDs) and nonopioids, (2) **opioids** (traditionally called narcotics), and (3) **adjuvants.**

Box 42-12 Procedural Guidelines

Massage

Equipment: Bath towel, moisturizing lotion, bath towel or blanket
1. Assist client to assume comfortable position.
2. Dim room lights and/or turn on soft music according to client preference.
3. Perform hand hygiene. Warm lotion in hands or place container in warm water.
4. Adjust or remove client's bed clothing.
5. Place small amount of lotion in hands.

Delegation considerations: It is the nurse's responsibility to assess for any possible contraindication or client response to massage. The skill of administering a massage may be delegated to assistive personnel (AP). Before delegation the nurse must:
- Instruct AP as to which body parts to massage.
- Instruct AP on the importance of not massaging reddened skin areas.
- Clarify the early signs of impaired skin integrity for select clients and their situation and instruct AP to report changes in the client's skin to the nurse.

Critical Decision Point

Clients who have had neck or spinal trauma and/or surgery should not have back or neck massage without order by their physician.

6. Massage each body part at least 10 minutes.
   a. *Back:* Beginning a sacral area massage on a circular motion (see Figure 42-11) while moving upward form buttocks to shoulders. Use a firm smooth stroke over the scapula. Continue in one smooth stroke to upper arms and laterally along sides of back down to iliac crests. Use long, gliding strokes along muscles of spine. Knead any muscles that feel tense or tight. Knead skin by gently grasping tissue between thumb and fingers (see illustrations). Knead upward along one side of the spine from buttocks to shoulders around nape of neck. Knead or stroke downward toward sacrum. Repeat along other side of the back.
   b. *Neck:* Support the neck at the hairline with one hand and massage up with a gliding stroke. Knead muscles on one side. Switch hands to support neck and knead other side. Stretch the neck slightly, with one hand at the top and the other at the bottom.
   c. *Arms:* Use a gliding stroke to massage from the client's wrist or forearm. With thumb and forefinger of both hands, knead muscles from forearm to shoulder. Continue kneading biceps, deltoid, and tricep muscles. Finish with gliding strokes from the wrists to the shoulder.
   d. *Hands:* Slowly open the client's palm; glide fingers over the palmar surface. Use thumbs to apply friction to the palm and move thumbs in a circular motion; stretch the palm outward. Massage each finger using a corkscrew-like motion from base of finger to the tip. Gently knead each muscle in the client's fingers. Glide hands smoothly from fingertips to wrists. Repeat for other hand.
   e. *Feet:* Gently massage the top and bottom of each foot. Using gliding motion, massage from heel to toe. Gently massage the dorsal surface of the foot and each toe Repeat for other foot.

Critical Decision Point

Do not massage client's legs or calf muscle.

7. Wipe excess lotion off client's back, neck, or extremity. If necessary retie gown or assist with pajamas and assist client to comfortable position.
8. Ask client about level of comfort. Note any areas of muscle pain or tension.

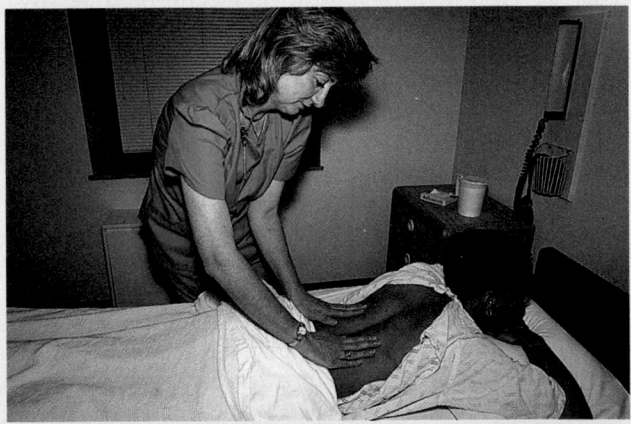
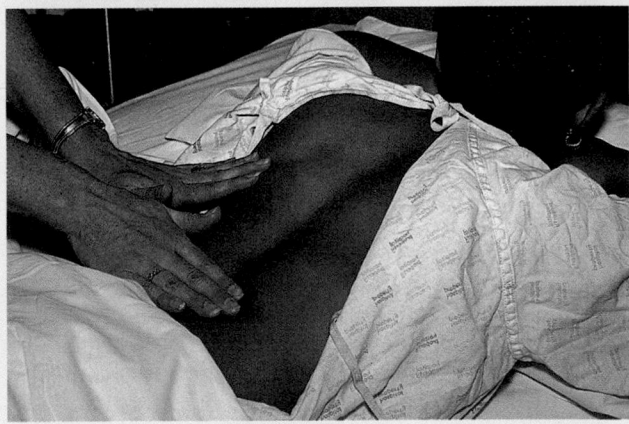

STEP **6a**

Box 42-13   **Controlling Painful Stimuli in the Client's Environment**

Tighten and smooth wrinkled bed linen.

Position tubing on which client is lying.

Loosen constricting bandages (unless specifically applied as a pressure dressing).

Change wet dressings and linens.

Position client in anatomical alignment.

Check temperature of hot or cold applications, including bathwater.

Lift client in bed—do not pull.

Position client correctly on bedpan.

Avoid exposing skin or mucous membranes to irritants (e.g., urine, stool, wound drainage).

Prevent urinary retention by keeping Foley catheters patent and free flowing.

Prevent constipation with fluids, diet, and exercise.

NSAIDs generally provide relief for mild to moderate acute intermittent pain, such as the pain associated with a headache. Treatment of mild to moderate postoperative pain should begin with an NSAID unless contraindicated (AHCPR, 1992). Although the exact mechanism of action is unknown, NSAIDs are believed to act by inhibiting the synthesis of prostaglandins (Halverson, 1999) thus inhibiting the cellular responses during inflammation. Most NSAIDs act on peripheral nerve receptors to reduce transmission and reception of pain stimuli. Unlike opioids, NSAIDs do not depress the central nervous system, nor do they interfere with bowel or bladder function (AHCPR, 1992). Chronic NSAID use in the older client, though, is associated with more frequent adverse effects (gastrointestinal bleeding and renal insufficiency) and should be avoided. Mild to moderate musculoskeletal pain in older adults is effectively managed with the nonopioid acetaminophen (American Geriatrics Society [AGS], 2002).

Opioid or opioid-like analgesics are generally prescribed for moderate to severe acute pain, such as postoperative pain. They may also be ordered for chronic noncancer and cancer pain. They act on the central nervous system to produce a combination of depressing and stimulating effects. These analgesics, when given orally or by injection, act on higher centers of the brain and spinal cord by binding with opiate receptors to modify perception of pain. One of the risks of opioid and opioid-like analgesics is the potential for depression of vital nervous system functions. Opiates depress the respiratory center within the brain stem. However, this is rare (Wheeler and others, 2002). Respiratory depression is only clinically significant if there is a decrease in the rate *and* depth of respirations from the client's baseline assessment (McCaffery and Pasero, 1999). Clients who are breathing deeply rarely have clinical respiratory depression. It is important to note that sedation *always* occurs before respiratory depression. Thus the nurse should closely monitor opioid-naive clients receiving opioids for sedation (Pasero and McCaffery, 2002).

Clients can also experience side effects such as nausea, vomiting, constipation, and altered mental processes. Except for constipation, these side effects usually stop once the client has been receiving the opioid around-the-clock (ATC) for 4 to 7 days. One way to maximize pain relief while minimizing drug toxicity is to administer the medication on a regular ATC basis rather than on an as-needed (prn) basis. The American Pain Society (1999) and AHCPR (1992) state that if pain is anticipated for the majority of the day ATC administration should be considered.

Opioids are effective in the older adult population. Although there is controversy about the use of opioids for chronic noncancer pain in all age-groups, the American Geriatrics Society (AGS) (2002) does feel that opioids are probably not used enough with older persons. The AGS suggests a "start low" (dose) and "go slow" (upward dose titration) philosophy. In addition, several professional organizations have developed position statements advocating the use of opioids for noncancer pain after careful client assessment.

The proper use of analgesics requires careful assessment and critical thinking in the application of pharmacological principles and logic (Box 42-14, p. 1258). A person's response to an analgesic is highly individualized. An NSAID may be as or more effective than an opioid for some clients if the pain is due to inflammation. An orally administered analgesic usually has a longer duration of action than an injectable form. Nurses must stay familiar with comparative doses of different analgesics. In addition, nurses must know the route of administration most effective for a client so that controlled, sustained pain relief is achieved.

The nurse should always know the comparative potencies of analgesics in oral and injectable form. If nurses on succeeding shifts choose different routes for the same doses, the client will not receive the same level of analgesia, and pain control will be poor. Nurses must provide controlled, sustained pain relief. Equianalgesic charts are available on most nursing units or by contacting pharmacy staff. The charts convert parenteral forms to oral forms, and gives equivalent doses of different opioids (e.g., morphine to hydromorphone).

Adjuvants are drugs with analgesic properties that were not originally developed to relieve pain. Tricyclic antidepressants and anticonvulsants are used to successfully treat neuropathic pain (Collins and others, 2000). Corticosteroids are used to relieve pain associated with inflammation and bone metastasis. Other adjuvants are bisphosphonates and calcitonin given for bone pain (Jacox and others, 1994). Additional adjuvants are also available.

Although sedatives, antianxiety agents, and muscle relaxants may be ordered with opioids to enhance pain control or relieve other symptoms associated with pain, they have *no* analgesic effect. However, they can cause drowsiness and impairment of coordination, judgment, and mental alertness and contribute to respiratory depression. It is important for the nurse to avoid attributing these side effects to the opioid. A thorough reassessment must be conducted.

Patient-Controlled Analgesia. Clients benefit from having control over pain therapy. When clients depend on nurses for prn analgesia, an erratic cycle of alternating

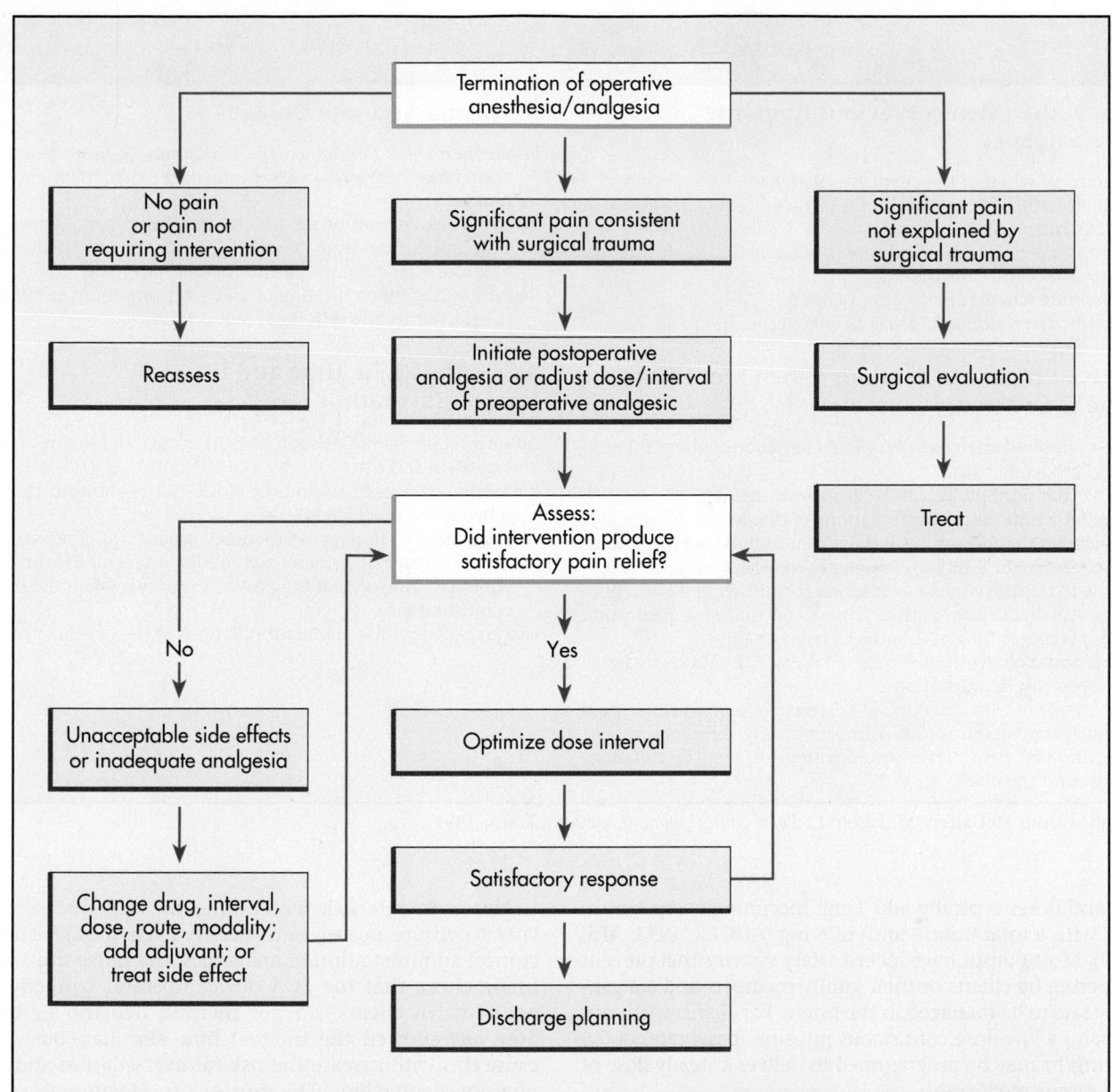

FIGURE **42-12** Pain treatment flow chart: postoperative phase. (From Agency for Health Care Policy and Research, Acute Pain Management Guideline Panel: *Acute pain management: operative or medical procedures and trauma,* Clinical Practice Guideline, AHCPR Pub No. 92-0032, Rockville, Md, 1992, Agency for Health Care Policy and Research, Public Health Service, U.S. Department of Health and Human Services.)

pain and analgesia often occurs. The client feels pain and asks for medication, but the nurse must first assess the client and then prepare the medication. Within an hour, analgesia finally occurs, but pain relief may last only 30 minutes. Then, gradually, the client again feels discomfort, and the cycle begins again. The client is constantly going in and out of analagesic therapeutic range.

A drug delivery system called **patient-controlled analgesia (PCA)** is a safe method for postoperative and cancer pain management that most clients prefer. It is a drug delivery system that allows clients to self-administer opioids (morphine, hydromorphone, fentanyl) with minimal risk of overdose. The goal is to maintain a constant plasma level of analgesic so that the problems of prn dosing are avoided. Systemic PCA usually involves IV drug administration, but it can also be given subcutaneously. PCAs are portable infusion pumps (usually computerized), containing a chamber for a syringe (Figure 42-13, p. 1259) or bag that delivers a small, preset dose of medication. To receive a demand dose, the client pushes a button attached to the PCA device. The system is designed to deliver no more than a specified number of doses either every hour or every 4 hours (depending on the pump) to avoid overdoses. A typical PCA prescription relies on a series of "loading" doses (e.g., 3 to 5 mg of morphine) repeated every 5 minutes until initial postoperative pain diminishes. On-

---

Box 42-14   Nursing Principles for Administering Analgesics

Know the Client's Previous Response to Analgesics

Determine whether the client has allergies.
Know whether client is at risk for using opioids (e.g., history of obstructive sleep apnea).
Identify previous doses and routes of analgesic administration to avoid undertreatment.
Determine whether relief was obtained.
Ask whether a nonopioid was as effective as an opioid.

Select Proper Medications When More Than One Is Ordered

Use nonopioid analgesics or opioid combination drugs for mild to moderate pain.
Know that nonopioids can be given with opioids.
In older adults, avoid combinations of opioids.
Remember that morphine and hydromorphone are the opioids of choice for long-term management of severe pain.
Know that intravenous medications act quicker and can relieve severe, acute pain within 1 hour and that oral medication may take as long as 2 hours to relieve pain.
Understand that intramuscular analgesics should be avoided, especially in older adults.
Use an opioid with a nonopioid analgesic for severe pain because such combinations treat pain peripherally and centrally.
For chronic pain, give sustained-release oral formulations around the clock.

Know the Accurate Dosage

Recall that 4 g is considered the maximum 24-hour dose for acetaminophen and acetylsalicylic acid (ASA); 3200 mg for ibuprofen.
Adjust doses, as appropriate, for children and older clients.
Bear in mind that large doses of opioids are acceptable in opioid-tolerant clients, but not opioid-naive clients.
Recognize that when titrating opioids, it is important to titrate to effect or to uncontrollable side effects.

Assess the Right Time and Interval for Administration

Administer analgesics as soon as pain occurs and before it increases in severity.
Remember that an around-the-clock (ATC) administration schedule is usually best.
Give analgesics before pain-producing procedures or activities.
Know the average duration of action for a drug and the time of administration so that the peak effect occurs when the pain is most intense.
Use extended-release opioid formulations to treat chronic pain.

Modified from McCaffery M, Pasero C: *Pain: clinical manual,* ed 2, St. Louis, 1999.

---

demand doses typically add 1 mg morphine every 6 minutes, with a total hourly limit of 6 mg (AHCPR, 1992; APS, 1999). Most pumps have locked safety systems that prevent tampering by clients or their family members and are generally safe to be managed in the home. For clients with cancer pain, a low-dose continuous infusion (basal rate) of 0.5 to 1 mg/hr may be programmed to deliver a steady dose of continuous medication.

> *Safety Alert.* PCA basal doses are *not* recommended for opioid-naive clients following surgery because of the possibility for respiratory depression.

There are many benefits to PCA use. The client gains control over pain, and pain relief does not depend on nurse availability. Clients can also access medication when they need it. This can decrease anxiety and lead to decreased medication use. Small doses of medications are delivered at short intervals, stabilizing serum drug concentrations for sustained pain relief. Client preparation and teaching is critical to the safe and effective use of PCA devices (Box 42-15). Clients must be able to understand the use of the equipment and be physically able to locate and press the button to deliver the dose. Family members must be instructed not to "hit the button" for the client, as this could cause toxic effects (Reiff and Nizolek, 2001). Nurse-controlled analgesia may be implemented in lieu of the client, with physician approval, after assessing the client.

Nurses must check the IV line and PCA device regularly to ensure proper functioning. Even though clients control administration of analgesics, the nurse must routinely check that the PCA device operates correctly. In opioid-naive clients, do not increase demand or basal dose *and* shorten the interval time simultaneously because this will increase the risk for oversedation and respiratory depression. The nurse also documents drug dosages and tracks any waste of medications according to agency policy (Pasero, 2003)

Local Analgesic Infusion Pump. Following orthopedic surgery, to avoid systemic effects of oral analgesics, an application of a local anesthetic may be appropriate. A catheter from the wound placed during surgery is connected to a pump containing a local anesthetic (Marcaine). The pump may be set as a demand or continuous mode. The device is usually left in place for 48 hours. The client is taught how to discontinue the pump at home and to bring the catheter to the next physician visit. Oral analgesics may still be needed by the client, but the total dose is often reduced (Pasero, 2000). Safe use of the pump in surgeries other than orthopedic has not yet been established.

Topical Analgesics and Anesthetics. A topical anesthetic often used on children is EMLA (eutectic mixture of local anesthetics). This anesthetic disk or cream (thickly applied) is placed on the skin 15 minutes before local anesthetic infiltration or minor procedures (e.g., IV start).

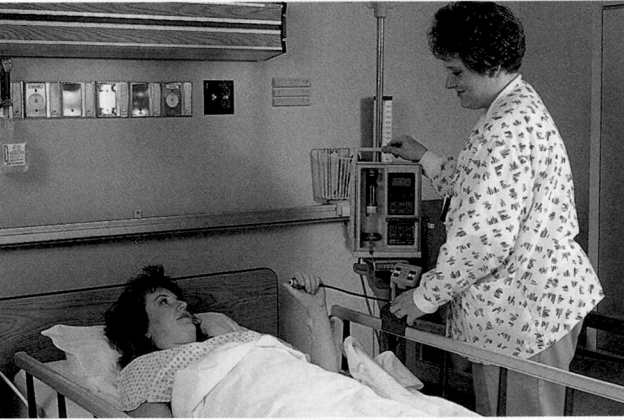

FIGURE 42–13 **A,** PCA pump with syringe chamber. **B,** Patient learns to use PCA pump.

EMLA should not be placed around eyes, the tympanic membrane, or over large skin surfaces. The lidoderm patch is a topical analgesic effective for cutaneous neuropathic pain. Three patches are placed on and around the pain site using a 12-hour on, 12-hour off schedule to avoid lidocaine toxicity

Local and Regional Anesthetics. **Local anesthesia** is the infiltration of a local anesthetic medication to induce loss of sensation to a localized body part. Physicians use local anesthesia during brief surgical procedures such as removal of a skin lesion or suturing a wound. Local anesthetics can be applied topically on skin and mucous membranes or injected subcutaneously or intradermally to anesthetize a body part. The drugs produce temporary loss of sensation by inhibiting nerve conduction. Local anesthetics can also block motor and autonomic functions depending on the amount used and the location and depth of an injection. Smaller sensory nerve fibers are more sensitive to local anesthetics than are large motor fibers. As a result, the client loses sensation before losing motor function, and conversely, motor activity returns before sensation.

Local anesthetics can cause side effects, depending on their absorption into the circulation. Itching or burning of the skin or a localized rash is common after topical applications. Application to vascular mucous membranes increases the chance of systemic effects, such as a change in heart rate. Injection of anesthetics increases the risk of systemic side effects, depending on the amount of drug used and the area injected. Each produces a different level of anesthesia as a result of the amount of anesthetic used and location of the spinal nerve affected.

Regional anesthesia is the injection of a local anesthetic to block a group of sensory nerve fibers. Tissues are anesthetized layer by layer, as the surgeon or anesthesia provider introduces the agent into deeper structures of the body. Kinds of regional anesthesia include epidural anesthesia, pudendal blocks, and spinal anesthesia. **Epidural analgesia** is now commonly used for the treatment of acute postoperative pain, labor and delivery pain, and chronic pain, especially that associated with cancer (Cox, 2001). It permits control or reduction of severe pain without the more serious sedative effects of parenteral or oral narcotics. However, intraspinal morphine can produce the same side effects of nausea, mental clouding, and sedation, because it is absorbed via the cerebrospinal fluid into the circulation of the epidural vascular plexus. Epidural analgesia can be short or long term, depending on the client's condition and life expectancy. Short-term therapy is used for pain after intrathoracic, abdominal, and orthopedic surgery. Long-term therapy is used for intractable pain in the lower part of the body, particularly when it is bilateral (DuPen and Williams, 1992).

Epidural analgesia is administered into the spinal **epidural space** (Figure 42-14). The physician inserts a blunt-tip needle into the level of the vertebral interspace nearest to the area requiring analgesia. When the needle reaches the space, solutions may be freely injected and small catheters may be passed into it. Once a catheter is advanced into the epidural space and the needle is removed, the remainder of the catheter is secured with a dressing and taped along the back of the client (Figure 42-15). If the catheter is only temporary, it is connected to tubing positioned along the spine and over the client's shoulder. The end of the catheter can then be placed on the client's chest for the nurse's access. Epidural analgesia may be anesthesiology or nurse controlled, depending on agency policy. Clients may also be given control of the demand dose, known as patient-controlled epidural analgesia (PCEA).

Nursing Implications. The nurse provides emotional support to clients receiving local or regional anesthesia by explaining insertion or application sites and warning clients that they will temporarily lose sensory function. In the case of regional anesthesia the nurse must explain when motor and autonomic function are expected to be temporarily lost. It is common for clients to fear paralysis because epidural and spinal injections come close to the spinal cord. Autonomic function (bowel and bladder control) may also be temporarily lost. To reassure the client, the nurse explains the sensations to be experienced. Injection can be painful unless the physician first numbs the injection site. The nurse prepares clients for such discomfort. Before a client receives an anesthetic, the nurse

checks for allergies. To monitor systemic effects, the nurse assesses blood pressure and pulse. Spinal anesthesia may also cause respiratory changes.

After administration of a local anesthetic, the nurse protects the client from injury until full sensory and motor function return. Until a local anesthetic is absorbed and metabolized, the client must be careful in using an anesthetized body part. Clients can easily injure themselves without knowing it. For example, after an injection into a joint, the nurse warns the client to avoid using the joint until function returns. For clients with topical anesthesia, the nurse avoids applying heat or cold to numb areas. After spinal anesthesia the client stays in bed until sensory and motor function return. The nurse assists the client during the first attempt at getting out of bed.

When managing epidural infusions, the catheter is connected to an epidural infusion pump, a port, or reservoir or is capped off for bolus injections. To reduce the risk of accidental epidural injection of drugs intended for IV use, the catheter should be clearly labeled "epidural catheter." Continuous infusions must be administered through electronic infusion devices for proper control. Because of the catheter location, strict surgical asepsis is needed to prevent a serious and potentially fatal infection. Physicians are notified immediately of any signs or symptoms of infection or pain at the insertion site. Thorough nursing care is needed during hygiene procedures to keep the catheter system clean and dry.

The nursing implications for managing epidural analgesia are numerous (Table 42-6). Supplemental doses of opioids or sedative/hypnotics are avoided because of possible additive central nervous system adverse effects.

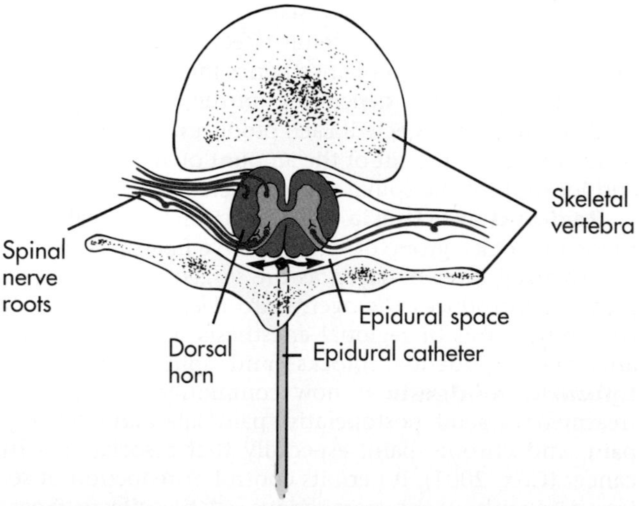

FIGURE **42–14** Anatomical drawing of epidural space.

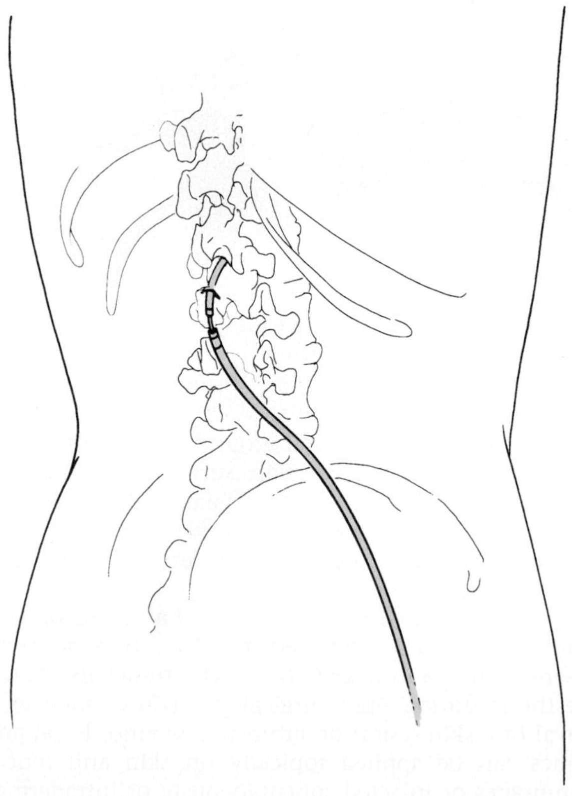

FIGURE **42–15** Epidural catheter taped in place.

Monitoring of medications' effects differs, depending on whether infusions are intermittent or continuous. Complications of epidural opioid use include nausea and vomiting, urinary retention, constipation, respiratory depression, and **pruritus** (Cox, 2001). When clients are receiving epidural analgesia, monitoring occurs as often as every 15 minutes, including assessment of respiratory rate, respiratory effort, and skin color. Once stabilized, monitoring can move to every hour (refer to agency policy).

The client must receive thorough education about epidural analgesia in terms of the action of the medication and its advantages and disadvantages. Clients should know about the potential for side effects and should be instructed to notify a health care provider if they develop. If the client requires long-term epidural use, a permanent catheter may be tunneled through the skin and exit at the client's side. A client on long-term therapy can be taught to safely administer infusions in the home with minimal ongoing intervention by the nurse.

Surgical Interventions for Pain Relief. When a client's pain persists despite medical treatment, surgical interventions may give relief. Neurosurgical treatment is appropriate for clients in whom more conservative treatment is neither tolerated nor effective (Jacox and others, 1994). The risks include new pain symptoms from nerve damage or nerve division, recurrence of pain, and postoperative neurological impairment. Surgery involves resection of either peripheral nerve roots or pain pathways in the spinothalamic tract. For example, a **dorsal rhizotomy** involves surgically cutting the dorsal (posterior) nerve roots as they enter the spinal cord. It is effective for relieving localized acute pain in the area supplied by the nerve root and deep visceral pain. The client loses sensation of pain but retains full motor function. A **chordotomy** is more extensive and involves resection of the spinothalamic tract. The procedure is used to treat unrelieved pain. The risks of the procedure are great because permanent paralysis may result from edema of the spinal cord or accidental resection of motor nerves. After the procedure, the client has a permanent loss of pain and temperature sensation in the affected areas.

When nurses care for these clients, they need to be aware of the area of resection to assess for paresthesia, change in temperature sensation, and loss of motor function. When performed correctly, these procedures can relieve persistent pain without causing serious neurological deficits. Additional invasive pain-relieving procedures available for intractable pain include spinal cord stimulators, and vertebroplasty.

Procedure Pain Management. The Thunder Project II (Puntillo and others, 2001) identified several procedures in critical care clients that cause pain:
- Turning
- Wound drain removal
- Tracheal suctioning
- Femoral catheter removal
- Placement of central line
- Changing of nonburn wound dressings

Premedicating clients before painful procedures allows clients to cooperate more fully and reduces the experience of pain. This is also true for clients with abdominal pain who present in the emergency department. APS (1999) recommends medicating the client in pain *before* an extensive physical examination and diagnostic procedures to attain more accurate data.

Chronic Noncancer and Cancer Pain Management. Cancer pain can be chronic or acute. The AHCPR released clinical practice guidelines for the management of cancer pain (Jacox and others, 1994). The guidelines are designed to treat cancer pain in a more comprehensive and aggressive manner. Similarly, they provide clients and families more options for pain relief. Figure 42-16 is a flow chart depicting cancer pain management from assessment to various treatment options. The best choice of treatment often changes as the client's condition and the characteristics of pain change. Nonpharmacological interventions, as well as pharmacological interventions, can be used together.

Various medications and routes of administration can provide relief for clients with cancer pain. There are relatively new oral analgesics with fewer side effects. Long-

Table 42-6	Nursing Care for Clients With Epidural Infusions
Goal	**Actions**
Prevent catheter displacement.	Secure catheter (if not connected to implanted reservoir) carefully to outside skin.
Maintain catheter function.	Check external dressing around catheter site for dampness or discharge. (Leak of cerebrospinal fluid may develop.)
	Use transparent dressing to secure catheter and to aid inspection.
	Inspect catheter for breaks.
Prevent infection.	Use strict aseptic technique when caring for catheter (see Chapter 33).
	Do not routinely change dressing over site.
	Change infusion tubing every 24 hours.
Monitor for respiratory depression.	Monitor vital signs, especially respirations, per policy.
	Pulse oximetry and apnea monitoring may be used.
Prevent undesirable complications.	Assess for pruritus (itching) and nausea and vomiting.
	Administer antiemetics as ordered.
Maintain urinary and bowel function.	Monitor intake and output.
	Assess for bladder and bowel distention.
	Assess for discomfort, frequency, and urgency.

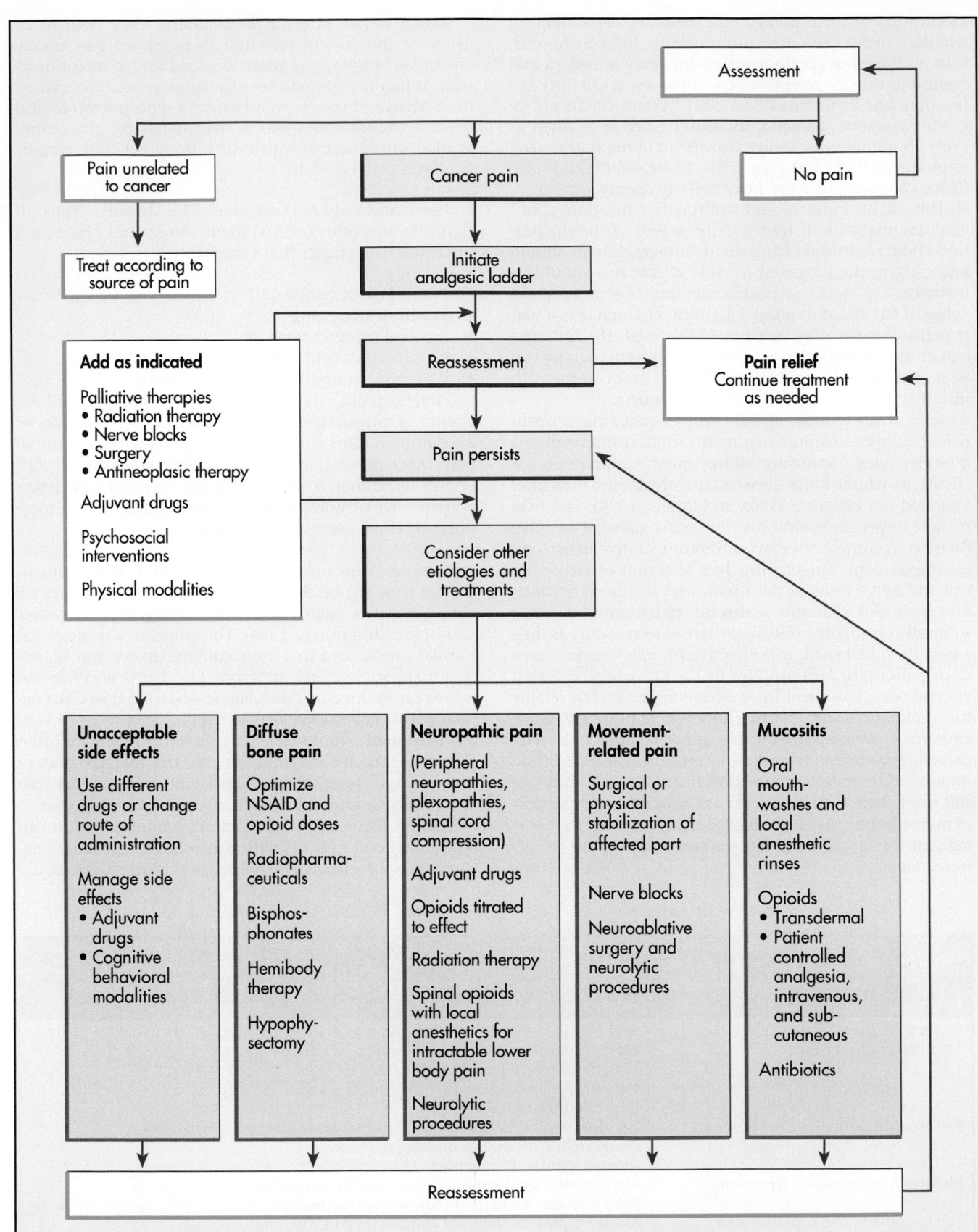

FIGURE **42–16** Flow chart: continuing pain management in patients with cancer. (From Jacox A and others: *Management of cancer pain*, Clinical Practice Guideline No. 9, AHCPR Pub No. 94-0592, Rockville, Md, 1994, Agency for Health Care Policy and Research, Public Health Service, U.S. Department of Health and Human Services.)

acting or controlled-release medications have been very successful in managing cancer pain as well as noncancer pain. These controlled-released medications (e.g., MS Contin, Roxanol SR, and OxyContin) can provide pain relief for 6 to 12 hours. Although most noncancer and cancer pain can be managed by using oral medications, there are times when other routes are needed. Epidural analgesia and intrathecal infusions (administration of opioids via catheters placed within the brain's ventricles) have been highly effective with select clients.

Estimates of addiction in clients with chronic pain range from 1% to 24% (Passik, Kirsh, and Portenoy, 2002). It has been demonstrated that clients with persistent pain requiring prolonged opioid administration can develop an opioid tolerance. As a result, clients require higher doses of opioids to attain pain relief. The higher opioid dose is not lethal because clients also develop a tolerance to respiratory depression.

For clients with chronic pain it is necessary to give required analgesics on a regular basis. Prescribing analgesics on a prn basis for chronic pain is ineffective and causes more suffering. The client with chronic pain must take an analgesic regularly, even when the pain subsides. Regular administration maintains therapeutic drug blood levels for ongoing pain control.

Administering analgesics to treat chronic noncancer and cancer pain requires applying principles different from those used to treat acute pain. The World Health Organization (1990) recommends a three-step approach to managing cancer pain (Figure 42-17). Therapy begins with using NSAIDs and/or adjuvants and progresses to strong opioids if pain persists. However, when a client with cancer first experiences pain, it is best to begin with a higher dosage than will be needed for continued pain relief. The physician can slowly decrease the dosage to the amount needed, thus providing the client with immediate pain relief. There is aggressive treatment of the side effects of analgesia, such as nausea and constipation, so that analgesia can be continued. Clients can become tolerant to the side effects of nausea but not to the constipating effects of analgesics. Clients should

have prescribed stimulant laxatives, not simple stool softeners, routinely administered both to prevent and to treat constipation.

Transdermal drug systems administer fentanyl at predetermined doses for up to 48 to 72 hours. Fentanyl is about 100 times more potent than morphine.

Safety Alert. Fentanyl should **only** be used in clients who are opioid tolerant.

The transdermal route is useful when clients are unable to take drugs orally. Clients find these systems easy to use, and they allow for continuous opioid administration without needles or pumps. Self-adhesive patches release the medication slowly over time, achieving effective analgesia. Caution is needed in administering transdermal patches to adult clients who weigh less than 100 pounds (too little subcutaneous tissue for absorption) or who are hyperthermic. Hyperthermia causes more rapid drug absorption. The patch should not ever be cut and should be disposed of down the toilet, witnessed by two nurses.

A transmucosal fentanyl "unit" has been developed to treat **breakthrough pain** (Box 42-16) in opioid-tolerant clients. It is placed in the client's mouth and swabbed over the inside of the cheeks and lower gums. The unit needs to be left intact and not chewed, but allowed to dissolve and absorb over a 15-minute period. No more than two units should be used per breakthrough pain episode. If pain is not relieved, the physician should be notified.

Analgesics may be given rectally when clients have nausea and vomiting or are fasting before or after surgery (Jacox and others, 1994). This route is contraindicated if clients have diarrhea or if cancerous lesions involve the anus or rectum. Morphine, hydromorphone, and oxymorphone are available in suppositories.

Another way to treat severe cancer pain in the home or acute care setting is with continuous infusions or a basal rate on a PCA device. This provides improved, uniform pain control with fewer peaks and valleys in plasma concentration, more effective drug action, and lower drug dosages overall. Candidates for continuous infusions include clients with severe pain for whom oral and injectable medications provide minimal relief, clients with severe nausea and vomiting, and clients unable to swallow oral medications. The intramuscular route should not be used for controlling cancer pain because the injection itself is painful and there is inconsistent, erratic absorption of the drug.

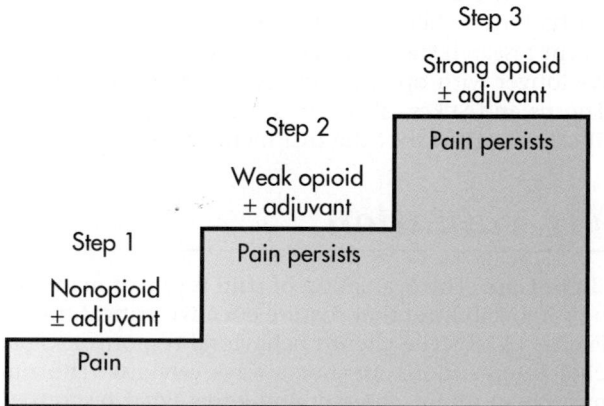

FIGURE **42-17** WHO analgesic ladder is a three-step approach to using drugs in cancer pain management. ± *adjuvant,* With or without adjuvant medications. (From World Health Organization: *Cancer pain relief and palliative care: report of a WHO expert committee,* WHO Tech Rep Series No. 804, Geneva, 1990, The Organization.)

Box 42-16   Types of Breakthrough Pain: Pain That Extends Beyond Treated Steady Chronic Pain

Incident pain: Pain that is predictable and elicited by specific behaviors
End-of-dose failure pain: Pain that occurs toward the end of the usual dosing interval of a regularly scheduled analgesic
Spontaneous pain: Pain that is unpredictable and not associated with any activity or event

When a client is first given continuous-drip morphine sulfate, it is essential that the IV access be patent and that the IV site be without complications (see Chapter 40). A central line catheter such as a Groshong or Hickman catheter, an implanted venous access port, or a peripherally inserted central catheter is usually best suited for long-term IV infusion. When IV access is poor, the subcutaneous route with a concentrated dose is possible. When infusions begin, the client continues to be monitored. Clients who are placed on continuous analgesic infusions are not usually opioid naive, and thus respiratory depression is rare.

In the home, clients may use ambulatory infusion pumps. State-of-the-art ambulatory pumps are small devices, often no larger than a deck of cards, that contain a 1- to 30-day supply of medication. The pumps are lightweight and allow free movement. The pump is battery powered and worn in a pouch attached to a belt or harness. The bag of medication and IV fluid fits inside the pump.

Although the pumps are programmed by physicians, pharmacists, or nurses, clients or families must be highly motivated to care for the pump properly. The client must show the capacity to learn the procedures and to assume responsibility for proper pump operation (Bernstein and others, 1993). In addition, it is important that the client have the physical capabilities to make adjustments to the pump (e.g., change batteries). The client and family learn to manage the pump, to observe for side effects, and to maintain function of the central venous catheter. Because the client is initially managed with opioids in the hospital before going home, the risk of side effects is not as great unless the client or family member increases the dosage. A home care nurse makes routine visits to ensure that the client manages the pump correctly. The IV fluid bag and tubing are changed routinely by the nurse. This maintains the sterility of the system.

Barriers to Effective Pain Management. Barriers to effective pain management can be complex, involving the client, health care provider, and health care system (Box 42-17). A deep-seated and often inappropriate concern shared by health care providers and clients is the fear of addiction when long-term opioid use is prescribed to manage pain. There is a difference between **physical dependence, addiction,** and **drug tolerance** (Box 42-18). The nurse needs to provide clarification of the differences to clients and other health care providers. Experiencing a physical dependency does not imply addiction, and drug tolerance in and of itself does not constitute addiction. That is not to say that addiction does not occur or that true addicts should not be treated for pain. The nurse monitors for addiction while also providing adequate pain management for all clients, including addicts (Newshan, 2000).

Placebos are "sugar pills" with no active ingredient, but they can produce positive or negative responses in 30% to 50% of people who take them (Thompson, 2000). The use of placebos to treat pain is discouraged by many professional organizations. It is considered unethical and deceitful to administer placebos (Tucker, 2001). This jeopardizes the trust between clients and health care providers.

If a placebo is ordered, the nurse must question the order and ask, "Why?" Many health care agencies have policies that limit the use of placebos to research only.

Restorative and Continuing Care

Pain Clinics, Palliative Care, and Hospices. During the last decade, health professionals have recognized pain as a significant health problem (A Controlled Trial to Improve Care, 1995). With an increased awareness of the multiple problems that pain can cause for clients, programs have been designed for pain management. Pain clinics may offer several options. A comprehensive pain center can treat persons on an inpatient or outpatient basis. Staff members representing all health care disciplines, such as nursing, medicine, physical therapy, pastoral care, and dietetics, work with clients to find the most effective pain-relief measures. A comprehensive clinic can provide not only diverse therapy but also research into new treatments and training for professionals.

Many hospitals are developing palliative care teams to assist clients and their family members to successfully manage their diseases (Ferrell and Coyle, 2001). Learning to live life fully with an incurable condition is the goal of palliative care (see Chapter 29). It is essential that clients and their family members be given ongoing assistance in managing their pain at home (Schumacher and others, 2002).

Hospices are programs for care of clients at the end of life. The term *hospice* comes from the Latin word *hospes,* which means "a place to rest." Often, hospice programs are affiliated with hospitals. The programs help terminally ill clients continue to live at home in comfort and privacy with the help of a hospice health care team. Pain control is a priority for hospices. Clients receive the proper dosage and form of analgesics that provide pain relief. Under the guidance of hospice nurses, families learn to monitor clients' symptoms and become the primary caregivers. A hospice client may become hospitalized in the event of a brief, acute care crisis or family problem.

Hospice programs help nurses overcome their fears of contributing to a client's death when administering large doses of opioids. The American Nurses Association (ANA) supports aggressive treatment of pain and suffering even if it hastens a client's death (ANA Code of Ethics, 2002). Recent research suggests that dying clients suffer less and live longer with opioid administration at the end of life (Thorns and Sykes, 2000). It is the client's disease that is killing the client, not the treatment of pain.

Evaluation

Client Care. The evaluation of pain is one of many nursing responsibilities that require effective critical thinking (Figure 42-18). The client's behavioral responses to pain-relief interventions are not always obvious. The nurse must be an intent observer and know what responses to anticipate on the basis of the type of pain, the intervention, the timing of the interventions, the physiological nature of the injury or disease, and the client's previous responses. The nurse evaluates psychological as well as physiological responses to pain.

Box 42-17   Barriers to Effective Pain Management

Client Barriers

Fear of addiction
Worry about side effects
Fear of tolerance (won't be there when I need it)
Take too many pills already
Fear of injections
Concern about not being a "good" client
Don't want to worry family and friends
May need more tests
Need to suffer to be cured
Pain is for past indiscretions
Inadequate education
Reluctance to discuss pain
Pain is inevitable
Pain is part of aging
Fear of disease progression
Physicians and nurses are doing all that they can
Just forget to take analgesics
Weak in character
Fear of distracting physicians from treating illness
Physicians have more important or ill clients to see
Suffering in silence is noble and expected

Health Care Provider Barriers

Inadequate pain assessment
Concern with addiction
Opiophobia, fear of opioids

Health Care Provider Barriers—cont'd

Fear of legal repercussions
No visible cause of pain
Clients must learn to live with pain
Reluctance to deal with side effects of analgesics
Not believing client's report of pain
Fear of giving a dose that will kill the client
Physician time constraints
Inadequate reimbursement
Belief that opioids may "mask" symptoms
Belief that pain is part of aging
Overestimation of rates of respiratory depression

Health Care System Barriers

Concern with creating "addicts"
Ability to fill prescriptions
Absolute dollar restriction on amount reimbursed for prescriptions
Mail order pharmacy restrictions
Nurse practitioners and physician assistants not used efficiently
Extensive documentation requirements
Poor pain policies and procedures regarding pain management
Lack of money
Inadequate access to pain clinics
Poor understanding of economic impact of unrelieved pain

Box 42-18   Definitions Related to the Use of Opioids in Pain Treatment

Approved by the Boards of Directors of the American Academy of Pain Medicine, The American Pain Society, and the American Society of Addiction Medicine, February 2001.

Physical Dependence

A state of adaptation that is manifested by a drug class specific withdrawal syndrome that can be produced by abrupt cessation, rapid dose reduction, decreasing blood level of the drug, and/or administration of an antagonist.

Drug Tolerance

A state of adaptation in which exposure to a drug induces changes that result in a diminution of one or more of the drug's effects over time.

Addiction

A primary, chronic, neurobiologic disease, with genetic, psychosocial, and environmental factors influencing its development and manifestations. It is characterized by behaviors that include one or more of the following: impaired control over drug use, compulsive use, continued use despite harm, and craving.

Pseudoaddiction

Client behaviors (drug seeking) that may occur when pain is undertreated.

Pseudotolerance

Need to increase opioid dose for reasons other than opioid tolerance: progression of disease, onset of new disorder, increased physical activity, lack of adherence, change in opioid formulation, drug-drug interaction, drug-food interaction (Wall and Malzack, 1999).

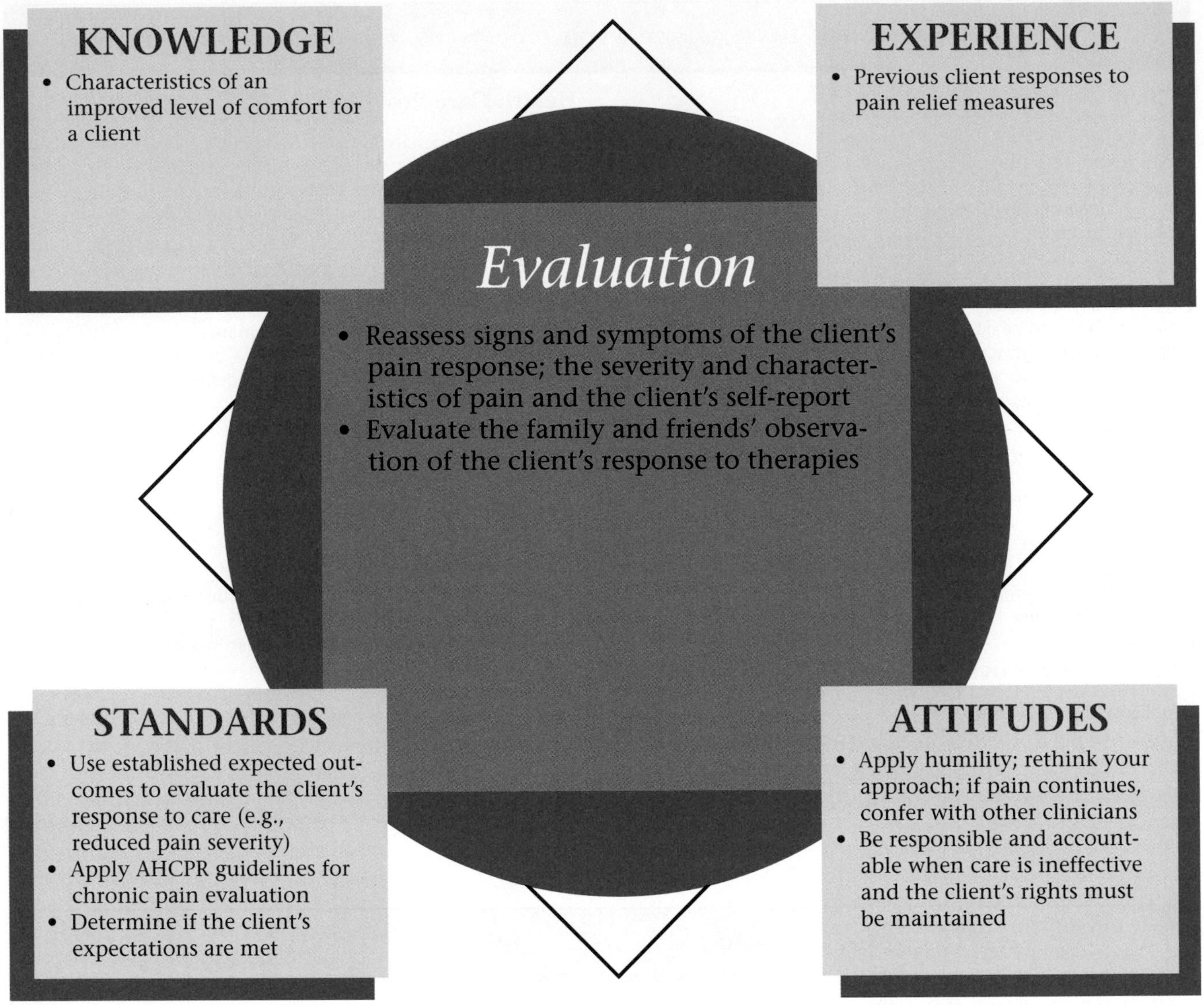

KNOWLEDGE
- Characteristics of an improved level of comfort for a client

EXPERIENCE
- Previous client responses to pain relief measures

Evaluation
- Reassess signs and symptoms of the client's pain response; the severity and characteristics of pain and the client's self-report
- Evaluate the family and friends' observation of the client's response to therapies

STANDARDS
- Use established expected outcomes to evaluate the client's response to care (e.g., reduced pain severity)
- Apply AHCPR guidelines for chronic pain evaluation
- Determine if the client's expectations are met

ATTITUDES
- Apply humility; rethink your approach; if pain continues, confer with other clinicians
- Be responsible and accountable when care is ineffective and the client's rights must be maintained

FIGURE **42–18** Critical thinking model for comfort evaluation.

If the nurse assesses that a client continues to have discomfort after an intervention, it may be necessary to try a different approach. For example, if an analgesic provides only partial relief, the nurse may add relaxation exercises or guided-imagery exercises. The nurse may also consult with the physician about increasing the dosage, decreasing the interval between doses, or trying different analgesics.

The nurse evaluates the client's perceptions of the effectiveness of interventions. The client may help decide the best times to attempt a treatment. In essence, the client is the best judge of whether an intervention works. The nurse also evaluates tolerance to therapy and the overall relief obtained. For example, if a nurse administers an analgesic, side effects from the medication and the client's reported pain relief must be assessed. Similarly, af-

ter turning a client, the nurse should return to determine whether the client is tolerating the new position and whether pain has subsided. If an intervention aggravates discomfort, the nurse stops it immediately and seeks an alternative. Time and patience are necessary to maximize the effectiveness of pain management. The nurse evaluates the entire pain experience to determine interventions that are most effective and times that they should be administered.

Client Expectations. The client, if able, is the best resource for evaluating the effectiveness of pain-relief measures. The nurse must continually assess whether the character of the client's pain changes and whether individual interventions are effective. The family often

Modified from McCaffery M, Pasero C: *Pain: clinical manual,* St. Louis, 1999, Mosby.

Box 42-19 Nurse-Physician Pain Communication

1. Identify physician by name.
2. Give your name.
3. State the general nature of the call.
4. Identify the client by name and diagnosis.
5. State the pain management goal: rating and activities.
6. Summarize the current pain rating and effect of pain on activities.
7. List the current analgesic doses and relevant side effects.
8. Identify nonpharmacological strategies used.
9. Suggest a solution (on the basis of a clinical practice guideline, if possible).

is another valuable resource, particularly in the case of the client with cancer who may not be able to express discomfort during the latter stages of terminal illness. The nurse is successful in treating pain when the client's expectations of pain relief are met. The nurse uses evaluative criteria in determining the outcome of pain-relief interventions.

Effective communication of a client's assessment of pain and his or her response to intervention is facilitated by accurate and thorough documentation. This communication needs to transpire from nurse to nurse, shift to shift, and nurse to other health care providers. It is the professional responsibility of the nurse caring for the client to report what has been effective for managing the client's pain. The client is not responsible for ensuring that this information is accurately transmitted. A variety of tools such as a pain flow sheet or diary will help centralize information about pain management. The client expects the nurse to be sensitive to his or her pain and to be diligent in attempts to manage that pain. Effectively communicating with physicians (Box 42-19) will assist the nurse in achieving optimal pain relief for clients.

Key Concepts

- Pain is a purely subjective physical and psychosocial experience.
- A nurse's misconceptions about pain often result in doubt about the degree of the client's suffering and unwillingness to provide relief.
- Knowledge of the nociceptive pain processes of the pain experience—transmission, transduction, perception, and modulation—provides the nurse with guidelines for determining pain-relief measures.
- An interaction of psychological and cognitive factors affects pain perception.
- A person's cultural background influences the meaning of pain and how it is expressed.
- It is common for older clients not to report pain.
- Clients who are in chronic pain are unlikely to show behavioral changes.
- The difference between acute and chronic pain involves the concept of harm. Acute pain is protective, thus preventing harm; chronic pain is no longer protective.
- The nurse does not collect an in-depth pain history when the client is experiencing severe discomfort.
- Pain can cause physical signs and symptoms similar to the signs and symptoms of other diseases.
- Clients waiting to undergo invasive tests may gain some pain relief by anticipatory guidance.
- The nurse individualizes pain interventions by collaborating closely with the client, using assessment findings, and trying a variety of interventions.
- Eliminating sources of painful stimuli is a basic nursing measure for promoting comfort.
- Using a regular schedule for analgesic administration is more effective than an as-needed schedule in controlling pain.
- A patient-controlled analgesic device gives clients pain control with low risk of overdose.
- While caring for a client who receives local anesthesia, the nurse protects the client from injury.
- Nursing implications for administering epidural analgesia include preventing infection and monitoring closely for respiratory depression.
- The goal of pain management is to anticipate and prevent pain rather than treat it.
- Evaluation of the client's pain interventions requires consideration of the changing character of pain, the client's response to interventions, and the client's perceptions of a therapy's effectiveness.

Key Terms

Acupressure, *p. 1254*
Acute pain, *p. 1233*
Addiction, *p. 1214*
Adjuvants, *p. 1254*
Analgesics, *p. 1254*
Biofeedback, *p. 1253*
Breakthrough pain, *p. 1263*
Chordotomy, *p. 1261*
Chronic pain, *p. 1234*
Cutaneous stimulation, *p. 1253*
Dorsal rhizotomy, *p. 1261*
Drug tolerance, *p. 1264*
Epidural anesthesia, *p. 1250*
Epidural space, *p. 1260*
Guided imagery, *p. 1252*
Idiopathic pain, *p. 1234*
Local anesthesia, *p. 1259*
Modulation, *p. 1231*
Neurotransmitters, *p. 1230*
Nociceptor, *p. 1230*

Opioids, *p. 1254*
Pain, *p. 1229*
Pain threshold, *p. 1233*
Pain tolerance, *p. 1233*
Patient-controlled analgesia (PCA), *p. 1257*
Perception, *p. 1231*
Physical dependence, *p. 1264*
Placebos, *p. 1264*
Prostaglandins, *p. 1230*
Pruritus, *p. 1261*
Pseudoaddiction, *p. 1234*
Pseudotolerance, *p. 1265*
Regional anesthesia, *p. 1259*
Relaxation, *p. 1251*
Transcutaneous electrical nerve stimulation (TENS), *p. 1254*
Transduction, *p. 1230*
Transmission, *p. 1230*

Critical Thinking Exercises

1. John is a 32-year-old construction worker who sustained an injury to the lumbar region of his back during a fall approximately 8 months ago. John is 6 feet tall and weighs 280 pounds. He continues to report pain intensity as a 5 (on a scale of 0 to 10), increasing with activity; he has limited flexibility and is unable to return to work. He has recently been admitted for treatment at a comprehensive pain clinic. What interventions might the health care team employ?

2. Alexis is a 3-year-old admitted to the pediatric unit for a third-degree burn to her right lower extremity. What tools might be useful when assessing this child's pain?

3. You are caring for an unconscious client who was involved in an automobile accident and sustained multiple injuries. The client has several lacerations, wounds, and surgical incisions, as well as multiple lines and tubes. What measures might you take to promote the client's comfort?

4. Mary Beth Jones, a 55-year-old woman with metastatic breast cancer to the bone, has been receiving IV morphine sulfate (MSO_4) for a week for severe back and leg pain. Her frequently increased infusion of MSO_4 is not reducing her pain to an acceptable level, and she is becoming increasingly sedated. What other pharmacological interventions might be considered?

5. Ms. Wilkins, 65 years old, returns from surgery following a small bowel resection. The physician orders a 25-mcg fentanyl patch applied to help manage the postoperative pain. Ms. Wilkins received one dose of morphine 4 mg IV push in the recovery room 1 hour ago, which relieved her pain. What actions would be appropriate for you to take at this time?

Review Questions

1. The following organization declared pain relief a basic legal right:
   1. State Boards of Nursing.
   2. American Bar Association.
   3. American Nurses Association.
   4. National League for Nursing.

2. Pain is viewed as a:
   1. Separate disease.
   2. Symptom of an illness.
   3. Symptom of a condition.
   4. Objective finding.

3. This type of pain lasts longer than anticipated, may not have an identifiable cause, and leads to great personal suffering:
   1. Cancer pain.
   2. Chronic pain.
   3. Acute pain.
   4. Idiopathic pain.

4. One of the reasons many nurses avoid acknowledging a client's pain is:
   1. Inadequate pain management skills.
   2. Insufficient time to respond to the client.
   3. Fear that the intervention may cause addiction.
   4. Inability to manage their increased client load.

5. Cognitively this age-group is unable to recall explanations about pain or associate pain with experiences that can occur in various situations:
   1. Preschoolers.
   2. Adolescents.
   3. Young adults.
   4. Elderly.

6. An 82-year-old man with Alzheimer's disease is restless and moaning. The client's daughter states the client did not sleep well most of the night. The nurse's first response would be to:
   1. Recommend giving the client sleeping medication.
   2. Obtain a psychiatric evaluation.
   3. Administer pain medication as ordered.
   4. Assess and document physical and behavioral data.

7. The client requested medication for her abdominal incision pain, which she rates as 5 (scale of 0 to 10, with 10 the worse pain). One hour after administration of her pain medication, she was able to walk in the hall for 10 minutes and rated her pain as a 7. This indicated that the dosage of pain was:
   1. Adequate.
   2. Excessive.
   3. Insufficient.
   4. Unnecessary.

8. Approximately 30 minutes after administering a complementary treatment such as heat therapy or back massage, the nurse should:
   1. Turn and reposition the client.
   2. Document the pain assessment data.
   3. Evaluate the effectiveness of the treatment.
   4. Administer the prescribed medication.

9. A preventive approach for acute pain relief means that analgesic medications are given:
   1. Before the pain is experienced.
   2. With complementary therapies.
   3. Before the pain becomes severe.
   4. When the pain tolerance level is exceeded.

10. One of the reasons that patient-controlled analgesia (PCA) pumps are frequently used for postoperative pain management is to:
    1. Increase client satisfaction.
    2. Decrease the frequency of client complaints.
    3. Control client use of narcotics and reduce the chance of addiction.
    4. Encourage the use of pain medications before the client experiences severe pain.

References

Agency for Health Care Policy and Research, Acute Pain Management Guideline Panel: *Acute pain management: operative or medical procedures and trauma,* Clinical Practice Guideline, AHCPR Pub No. 92-0032, Rockville, Md, 1992, Agency for Health Care Policy and Research, Public Health Service, U.S. Department of Health and Human Services.

American Bar Association: *Commission on legal problems of the elderly: report to the house of delegates,* 2000, http://www.abanet.org.

American Geriatrics Society: The management of persistent pain in older persons, *J Am Geriatr Soc* 50(S6):205, 2002.

American Holistic Health Association: *Wellness from within: the first step,* Anaheim, Calif, 1999, The Association.

American Nurses Association: *Code of ethics with interpretive statements,* Washington, DC, 2002, The Association.

American Pain Foundation: *Pain care bill of rights,* 2001, http://www.painfoundation.org/www.painfoundation.org.

American Pain Society: *Principles of analgesic use in the treatment of acute and cancer pain,* ed 4, Glenview, Ill, 1999, The Society.

American Pain Society: *The use of opioids for the treatment of chronic pain,* Glenview, Ill, 2002, The Society, http://www.ampainsoc.org/advocacy/opioids.htm.

American Society of Anesthesiologists: Practice guidelines for chronic pain management, *Anesthesiology* 86:995, 1997.

Aspen Reference Group/Health Science: *Pain management patient education manual,* Gaithersburg, Md, 1999, Aspen Publication.

Bernstein LH and others: Portable medicine pumps in primary care, *Patient Care* 27:91, 1993.

Butler RN, Gastel B: Care of the aged: perspectives on pain and discomfort. In Turk DC, Melzack R, editors: *The handbook of pain assessment,* New York, 1992, Guilford Press.

Carroll D, Seers K: Relaxation for the relief of chronic pain: a systematic review, *J Adv Nurs* 27(3):1, 1998.

Collins S and others: Antidepressants and anticonvulsants for diabetic neuropathy and postherpetic neuralgia: a quantitative systematic review, *J Pain Symptom Manage* 206:449, 2000.

Cox F: Clinical care of patients with epidural infusions, *Prof Nurse* 16(10):1429, 2001.

Craig KD: The facila display of pain in infants and children. In Finley GA, McGrath PJ editors: Measurement of pain in infants and children, *Prog Pain Res Manage* 10:103, 1998.

Dochterman JM, Bulechek GM: *Nursing interventions classifications (NIC),* ed 4, St. Louis, 2004, Mosby.

Donahue P: *Nursing: the finest art,* St. Louis, 1989, Mosby.

DuPen SL, Williams AR: Management of patients receiving combined epidural morphine and bupivacine for the treatment of cancer pain. *J Pain Sympton Manage* 7(2):125, 1992.

Edelman CL, Mandle CL: *Health promotion throughout the lifespan,* ed 4, St. Louis, 1998, Mosby.

Feldt K: Improving assessment and treatment of pain in cognitively impaired nursing home residents, *Ann Long-Term Care* 8(9):36, 2000.

Ferrell B, Coyle N: *Textbook of palliative nursing,* London, 2001, Oxford Press.

Gil K: Psychologic aspects of acute pain, *Anesthesiol Rep* 2(2):246, 1990.

Halverson P: Nonsteroidal anti-inflammatory drugs: benefits, risks, and COX-2 selectivity, *Orthop Nurs* 18(6):21, 1999.

Harkins SW, Price DD: Are there special needs for pain assessment in the elderly? *APS Bull* 3:1, January/February 1993.

Harkins SW and others: Geriatric pain. In Wall PD, Melzack R, editors: *Textbook of pain,* London, 1999, Churchill Livingstone.

Herr K: Chronic pain: challenges and assessment strategies, *J Gerontol Nurs* 28(1):20, 2002a.

Herr K: Chronic pain in the older patient: management strategies, *J Gerontol Nurs* 28(2):28, 2002b.

Hockenberry MJ and others: *Wong's nursing care of infants and children,* ed 7, St. Louis, 2003, Mosby.

International Association for the Study of Pain, Subcommittee on Taxonomy: Pain terms: a list with definitions and notes on usage, *Pain* 6:249, 1979.

Jacox A and others: *Management of cancer pain,* Clinical Practice Guideline No. 9, AHCPR Pub No. 94-0592, Rockville, Md, 1994, Agency for Health Care Policy and Research, Public Health Service, U.S. Department of Health and Human Services.

Kelly A: *Geriatric pain assessment: self-directed learning module,* Pensacola, Fla, 2003, American Society of Pain Management Nurses (ASPMN).

Lasch K: Culture, pain, and culturally sensitive pain care, *Pain Manag Nurs* 1(3):S16, 2000.

Lawler K: Pain assessment, *Professional Nurse Study Supplement* 13(1):S5, 1997.

Lehn R: *Pharmacology for nursing care,* ed 4, Philadelphia, 2001, WB Saunders.

Max MB, Portenoy RK: Methodological challenges for clinical trials of cancer pain treatments. In Chapman CR, Foley KM, editors: *Current and emerging issues in cancer pain: research and practice,* New York, 1993, Raven Press

McCaffery M: *Nursing management of the patient with pain,* ed 2, Philadelphia, 1979, Lippincott.

McCaffery M, Pasero C: *Pain: clinical manual,* ed 2, St. Louis, 1999, Mosby.

McMillan SC: Pain and pain relief experienced by hospice patients with cancer, *Cancer Nurs* 19:298, 1996.

Melzack R, Wall PD: Pain mechanisms: a new theory, *Science* 150:971, 1965.

Miaskowski C: The impact of age on a patient's perception of pain and ways it can be managed, *Pain Manag Nurs* 1(3):2, 2000.

Moorhead S, Johnson M, Maas S: *Nursing outcomes classification (NOC),* ed 3, St. Louis, 2004, Mosby.

Newshan G: Pain management in the addicted patient: practical considerations, *Nurs Outlook* 48(2):81, 2000.

Nightingale F: *Notes on nursing: what it is and what it is not,* New York, 1969, Dover.

O'Mathuna D: Evidence-based practice and reviews of therapeutic touch, *J Nurs Scholarsh* 32(3): 279, 2000.

Otis-Green S and others: An integrated psychosocial model for cancer pain management, *Cancer Pract* 10(S1):58, 2002.

Paice JA: Unraveling the mystery of pain, *Oncol Nurs Forum* 18(5):843, 1991.

Paice JA: *The physiology and pharmacologic management of pain: physiology of pain: unraveling the mystery,* Baltimore, 1994, Williams & Wilkins.

Pasero C: Continuous local anesthetics, *Am J Nurs* 100(8):22, 2000.

Pasero C: *Intravenous patient-controlled analgesia for acute pain management: self-directed learning module,* Pensacola, Fla, 2003, American Society of Pain Management Nurses (ASPMN).

Pasero C, McCaffery M: Monitoring sedation, *Am J Nurs* 102(2):67, 2002.

Passik S, Kirsh K, Portenoy R: Substance abuse issues in palliative care. In Berger A, Portenoy R., Weissman D, editors: *Principles and practice of palliative care and supportive oncology,* Philadelphia, 2003, Lippincott Williams & Wilkins.

Popp B, Portenoy R: Management of chronic pain in the elderly: pharmacology of opioids and other analgesics. In Ferrell BA, Ferrell BR, editors: *Pain in the elderly,* Seattle, 1996, IASP Press.

Portenoy RK: Neuropathic pain. In Portenoy RK, Kanner RM, editors: *Pain management: theory and practice,* Philadelphia, 1996, FA Davis.

Reiff P, Nizolek, M: Troubleshooting tips for PCA, *RN* 64(4):33, 2001.

Rodriquez D: Pain measurement in the elderly: a review, *Pain Manag Nurs* 2(2):38, 2001.

Salerno E, Willens JS: *Pain management handbook: an interdisciplinary approach.* St. Louis, 1996, Mosby.

Siddall P, Yezierski R, Loeser J: Pain following spinal cord injury: clinical features, prevalence, and taxonomy, *IASP Technical Corner from IASP Newsletter,* 2000, http://www.iasp-pain.org/TC00-3.html.

Slucka K: The basic science mechanisms of TENS and clinical applications, *APS Bulletin* 11(2):10, 2001.

Steefel L: Treat pain in any culture, *Nurs Spectr* 6(5):8, 2002.

Thompson W: Placebos: a review of the placebo response, *Am J Gastroenterol* 95(7):1637, 2000.

Titler M, Rakel B: Nonpharmacological treatment of pain, *Crit Care Nurs Clin North Am* 13(2):221, 2001.

Tucker K: Deceptive placebo administration, *Am J Nurs* 101(8):55, 2001.

Wall P, Melzack R: *Textbook of pain,* ed 4, London, 1999, Churchill Livingstone.

Wong DL, Baker CM: Pain in children: comparison of assessment scales, *Okla Nurse* 33(1):8, 1988.

World Health Organization: *Cancer pain relief and palliative care, report of a WHO expert committee,* WHO Tech Rep Series No. 804, Geneva, 1990, The Organization.

*R*esearch References

A controlled trial to improve care for seriously ill hospitalized patients: the study to understand prognoses and preferences for outcomes and risks of treatments (SUPPORT): *JAMA* 274(20):1591, 1995.

Beyer JE and others: The creation, validation, and continuing development of the Oucher: a measure of pain intensity in children, *J Pediatr Nurs* 7(5):335, 1992.

Bostrom M: Summary of the Mayday fund survey: public attitudes about pain and analgesics, *J Pain Symptom Manage* 13(3):166, 1997.

Davis G: Barriers to managing chronic pain of older adults with arthritis, *J Nurs Scholarsh* 34(2):121, 2002.

Feldt K.: The checklist of nonverbal pain indicators (CNPI), *Pain Manag Nurs* 1(1):13, 2000.

Gerdner L. *Evidence-based protocol: individualized music,* revised 2001, The University of Iowa Gerontological Nursing Interventions Research Center, Research Dissemination Core, Iowa City, Ia.

Grealish L and others: Foot massage: a nursing intervention to modify the distressing symptoms of pain and nausea in patients hospitalized with cancer, *Cancer Nurs* 23(3):237, 2000.

Grunau RVE and others: Early pain experience, child and family factors, as precursors of somatization: a prospective study of extremely premature and full-term children, *Pain* 56:353, 1994.

Haythornthwaite J and others: Pain coping strategies predict perceived control over pain, *Pain* 77(1):33, 1998.

Helmy S, Bali A: The effect of preemptive use of the NMDA receptor antagonist dextromethorphan on postoperative analgesic requirements, *Anesth Analg* 92:739, 2001.

Kim MK: Analgesia for children with acute abdominal pain, *Acad Emerg Med* 9(4):281, 2002.

McCaffery M and others: Nurses' personal opinion about patients' pain and their effect of recorded assessments and titration of opioid doses, *Pain Manag Nurs* 1(3):79, 2000.

McGrady A and others: Effect of biofeedback-assisted relaxation on migraine headache and changes in cerebral blood flow velocity in the middle cerebral artery, *Headache* 34(7):424, 1994.

Meek SS: Effects of slow-stroke back massage on relaxation in hospice clients, *Image J Nurs Sch* 25(1):17, 1993.

Miaskowski C, Levine D: Does opioid analgesia show a gender preference for females, *Pain Forum* 8:34, 2000.

Puntillo K and others: Patients' perceptions and responses to procedural pain: results from Thunder Project II, *Am J Crit Care* 10(4):238, 2001.

Ramer L and others: Multimeasure pain assessment in an ethnically diverse group of patients with cancer, *J Transcult Nurs* 10(2):94, 1999.

Ruda R and others: Altered nociceptive neuronal circuits after neonatal peripheral inflammation, *Science* 289(5479):628, 2000.

Schumacher K and others: Putting cancer pain management regimens into practice at home, *J Pain Symptom Manage* 23(5):369, 2002.

Stevens B: Composite measures of pain. In Finley GA, McGrath PJ editors: Measurement of pain in infants and children, *Prog Pain Res Manage* 10:161, 1998.

Taddio A and others: Neonatal circumcision and pain response during routine vaccination 4 to 6 months later, *Lancet* 349:599, 1997.

Thorns A, Sykes N: Opioid use in last week of life and implications for end-of-life decision-making, *Lancet* 356(9927):398, 2000.

Wheeler M and others: Adverse events associated with postoperative opioid analgesia: a systemic review, *J Pain* 3(3):159, 2002.

Zalon ML: Nurses' assessment of post operative patients' pain, *Pain* 54(3):329, 1993.

43

$\mathcal{N}$utrition

Media Resources

http://evolve.elsevier.com/Potter/fundamentals/

 CD COMPANION

- Review Questions
- Glossary

evolve WEBSITE

- Review Questions
- Student Learning Activities
- Animations
- Concept Map Exercise
- Critical Thinking Exercise
- Video Clips
- Glossary

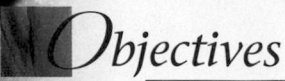

Objectives

Mastery of content in this chapter will enable the student to:

- Define the key terms listed.
- Explain the importance of each of the five food groups for good nutrition.
- Explain the importance of a balance between energy intake and energy requirements.
- List the end products of carbohydrate, protein, and fat metabolism.
- Explain the significance of saturated, unsaturated, and polyunsaturated fats.
- Describe the food guide pyramid and the healthy eating index and discuss their value in planning meals for good nutrition.
- Explain dietary reference intakes.
- List seven dietary guidelines for health promotion.
- Explain the variance in nutritional requirements throughout growth and development.
- Discuss the major methods of nutritional assessment.
- Identify three major nutritional problems and describe clients at risk.
- State the goals of enteral and parenteral nutrition.
- Describe the procedure for initiating and maintaining tube feedings.
- Describe the methods to avoid complications of tube feedings.
- Describe the methods to avoid complications of parenteral nutrition.
- Discuss medical nutrition therapy in relation to three medical conditions.
- Discuss diet counseling and client teaching in relation to client expectations.

Food provides sustenance and also holds symbolic meaning. The giving or taking of food is part of ceremonies, social gatherings, holiday traditions, religious events, the celebration of birth, and the mourning of death. The difficulty of the decision to withdraw food in a terminal illness, even in the form of intravenous (IV) nutrients, is a testament to the symbolic power of food and feeding.

Florence Nightingale understood the importance of nutrition, stressing the nurse's role in the science and art of feeding during the mid-1800s (Dossey, 1999). Since then, the nurse's role in nutrition and diet therapy has changed. Medical nutrition therapy (MNT) is now recognized as a disease-specific treatment modality when clients are at risk for malnutrition (American Academy of

Family Physicians, 1997). In some illnesses, such as type 1 diabetes mellitus or mild hypertension, diet therapy may be the major treatment for disease control (American Heart Association, 2000; American Diabetes Association, 2002). Other conditions, such as inflammatory bowel disease, may require specialized nutrition support such as enteral nutrition (EN) or parenteral nutrition (PN). Standards now exist that clearly designate the standard of care for promotion of optimal nutrition in all health care clients (American Cancer Society, 1997).

Scientific Knowledge Base

Nutrients: The Biochemical Units of Nutrition

The body requires fuel to provide energy for cellular metabolism and repair, organ function, growth, and body movement. An individual's energy requirements are influenced by several factors. The energy requirement of a person at rest is called the **basal metabolic rate (BMR).** This is the energy needed to maintain life-sustaining activities (breathing, circulation, heart rate, and temperature) for a specific period of time. Factors such as age, body mass, gender, fever, starvation, menstruation, illness, injury, infection, activity level, or thyroid function affect energy requirements. The **resting energy expenditure (REE)** is a measurement that accounts for BMR plus energy to digest meals and perform mild activity. Resting energy expenditure is a baseline of energy requirement that accounts for approximately 60% to 75% of our daily needs. Factors that affect metabolism include illness, pregnancy, lactation, and activity level. In hospitals, energy requirements may be estimated by measuring oxygen consumption, carbon dioxide production, and nitrogen excretion by means of a metabolic chart.

In general, when energy requirements are completely met by kilocalorie (kcal) intake in food, weight does not change. When the kilocalories ingested exceed energy demands, a person gains weight. If the kilocalories ingested fail to meet energy requirements, a person loses weight.

Nutrients are the elements necessary for body processes and function. Energy needs are met from a variety of nutrients: carbohydrates, proteins, fats, water, vitamins, and minerals. Water is a vital body component that acts as a solvent for metabolic processes. Vitamins and minerals do not provide energy but are essential to metabolic processes, including acid-base balance.

Foods are sometimes described according to their **nutrient density,** the proportion of essential nutrients to the number of kilocalories. High-nutrient-density foods, such as fruits and vegetables, provide a large number of nutrients in relationship to kilocalories. Low-nutrient-density foods, such as alcohol or sugar, are high in kilocalories but are nutrient poor.

Carbohydrates. Carbohydrates are the main source of energy in the diet. Each gram of carbohydrate produces 4 kcal and serves as the main source of fuel (glucose) for the brain, skeletal muscles during exercise, erythrocyte and leukocyte production, and cell function of the renal medulla. Carbohydrates are obtained primarily from plant foods, except for lactose (milk sugar). Carbohydrates are classified according to their carbohydrate units, or **saccharides.**

Monosaccharides such as glucose (dextrose) or fructose cannot be broken down into a more basic carbohydrate unit. Disaccharides such as sucrose, lactose, and maltose are composed of two monosaccharides and water. Both monosaccharides and disaccharides are classified as **simple carbohydrates** and are found primarily in sugars. Polysaccharides such as glycogen are composed of many carbohydrate units and are classified as complex carbohydrates. They are insoluble in water and are digested to varying degrees. Starches are polysaccharides.

Some polysaccharides cannot be digested because humans do not have enzymes capable of breaking them down. **Fiber** has received attention as a dietary factor in disease prevention and treatment and prevention of diarrhea in tube-fed clients. Insoluble fibers are not digestible and include cellulose, hemicellulose, and lignin. Soluble fibers include pectin, guar gum, and mucilage.

Proteins. Although proteins may provide a source of energy (4 kcal/g), they are essential for synthesis (building) of body tissue in growth, maintenance, and repair. Collagen, hormones, enzymes, immune cells, DNA, and RNA are all composed of protein. In addition, blood clotting, fluid regulation, and acid-base balance require proteins. Nutrients and many pharmacological substances are transported in the blood by proteins.

The simplest form of protein is the amino acid. **Essential amino acids** are those that the body cannot synthesize but must have provided in the diet. Others can be synthesized and are classified as **nonessential amino acids. Amino acids** can be linked together. Albumin and insulin are simple proteins because they contain only amino acids or their derivatives. The combination of a simple protein with a nonprotein substance produces a complex protein, such as lipoprotein, formed by a combination of a lipid and a simple protein.

A complete protein contains all essential amino acids in sufficient quantity to support growth and maintain nitrogen balance. Ingestion of proteins is not primary for meeting energy needs but is most important for continued positive nitrogen balance. Complete proteins are also referred to as high-quality proteins. Incomplete proteins lack one or more of the nine essential amino acids and include cereals, legumes (beans, peas), and vegetables. **Complementary proteins** are pairs of incomplete proteins that when combined supply the total amount of protein provided by complete protein sources.

Nitrogen balance is achieved when the intake and output of nitrogen are equal. When the intake of nitrogen exceeds the output, the body is in positive nitrogen balance, which is required for growth, normal pregnancy, maintenance of lean muscle mass and vital organs, and wound healing. The nitrogen retained by the body is used for building, repair, and replacement of body tissues. Negative nitrogen balance occurs when the body loses more nitrogen than the body gains, for example, with infection, sepsis, burns, fever, starvation, head injury, and trauma. The increased nitrogen loss is the result of body-tissue destruction or loss of nitrogen-containing body fluids. Nutrition during this period must provide nutrients to put clients into positive balance for healing.

Protein can be used to provide energy, but because of protein's essential role in growth, maintenance, and repair, adequate kilocalories should be provided in the diet from nonprotein sources. Protein is spared as an energy source when there is sufficient carbohydrate in the diet to meet the energy needs of the body.

Fats. Fats **(lipids)** are the most caloric dense nutrient because they provide 9 kcal/g. Fats are composed of triglycerides and fatty acids. **Triglycerides** circulate in the blood and are made up of three fatty acids attached to a glycerol. **Fatty acids** are composed of chains of carbon and hydrogen atoms with an acid group on one end of the chain and a methyl group at the other. Fatty acids can be **saturated,** in which each carbon in the chain has two attached hydrogen atoms, or **unsaturated,** in which an unequal number of hydrogen atoms are attached and the carbon atoms attach to each other with a double bond. **Monounsaturated** fatty acids have one double bond, whereas **polyunsaturated** fatty acids have two or more double carbon bonds. The various types of fatty acids have significance for health and the incidence of disease and are referred to in dietary guidelines.

Fatty acids are also classified as essential or nonessential. Linoleic acid, an unsaturated fatty acid, is the only essential fatty acid in humans. Linolenic acid and arachidonic acid (also unsaturated fatty acids) are important for metabolic processes but can be manufactured by the body when linoleic acid is available. Deficiency occurs when fat intake falls below 10% of daily nutrition. Most animal fats have high proportions of saturated fatty acids, whereas vegetable fats have higher amounts of unsaturated and polyunsaturated fatty acids (Figure 43-1).

Water. Water is a critical component of the body because cell function depends on a fluid environment. Water composes 60% to 70% of total body weight. The percent of total body water is greater for lean people than obese people because muscle contains more water than any other tissue except blood. Infants have the greatest percentage of total body water, and older people have the least. When deprived of water, a person cannot survive for more than a few days.

Fluid needs are met by ingesting liquids and solid foods high in water content, such as fresh fruits and vegetables. Water is also produced during digestion when food is oxidized. In a healthy individual, fluid intake from all sources equals fluid output through elimination, respiration, and sweating (see Chapters 40 and 44). An ill person can have an increased need for fluid (e.g., with

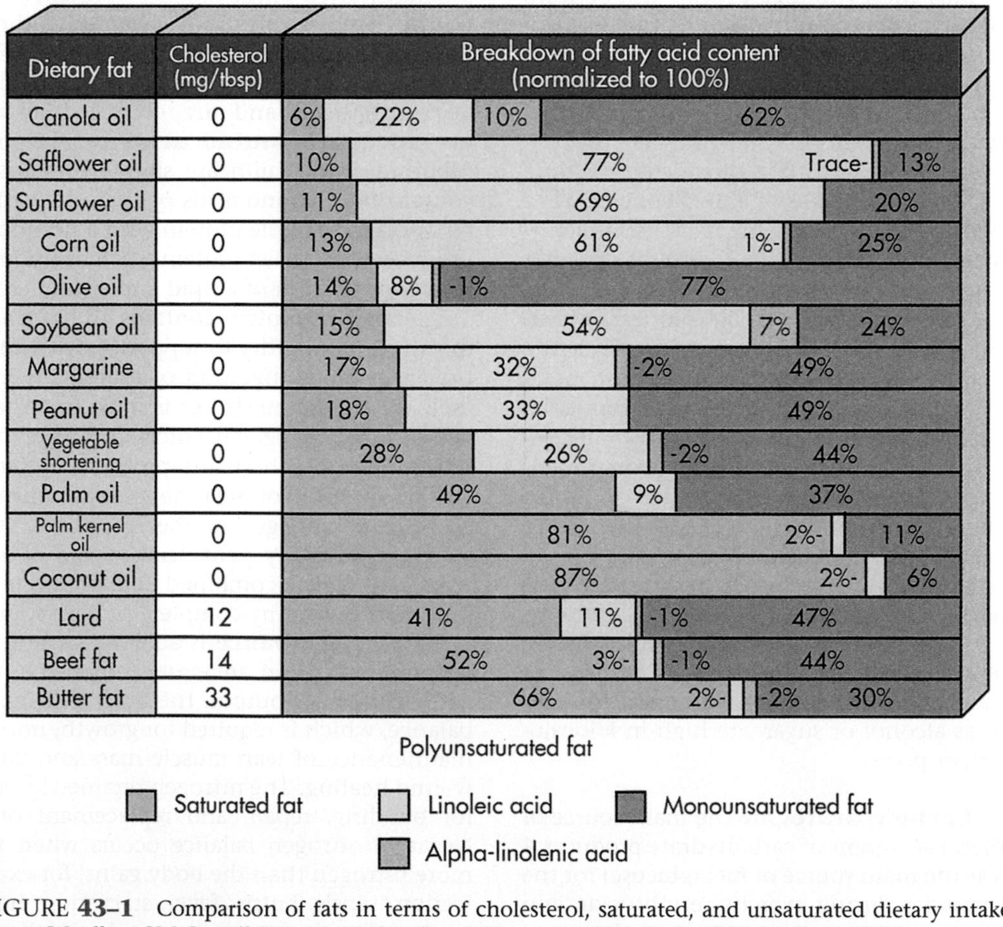

Dietary fat	Cholesterol (mg/tbsp)	Breakdown of fatty acid content (normalized to 100%)
Canola oil	0	6% / 22% / 10% / 62%
Safflower oil	0	10% / 77% / Trace- / 13%
Sunflower oil	0	11% / 69% / 20%
Corn oil	0	13% / 61% / 1%- / 25%
Olive oil	0	14% / 8% / -1% / 77%
Soybean oil	0	15% / 54% / 7% / 24%
Margarine	0	17% / 32% / -2% / 49%
Peanut oil	0	18% / 33% / 49%
Vegetable shortening	0	28% / 26% / -2% / 44%
Palm oil	0	49% / 9% / 37%
Palm kernel oil	0	81% / 2%- / 11%
Coconut oil	0	87% / 2%- / 6%
Lard	12	41% / 11% / -1% / 47%
Beef fat	14	52% / 3%- / -1% / 44%
Butter fat	33	66% / 2%- / -2% / 30%

Polyunsaturated fat

■ Saturated fat   □ Linoleic acid   ■ Monounsaturated fat

■ Alpha-linolenic acid

FIGURE **43–1** Comparison of fats in terms of cholesterol, saturated, and unsaturated dietary intake. (From Wardlaw GM, Insell PM: *Perspectives in nutrition,* ed 2, New York, 1993, McGraw-Hill.)

fever or gastrointestinal losses). By contrast, an ill person can also have a decreased ability to excrete fluid (e.g., with cardiopulmonary or renal disease), which may lead to the need to restrict fluid intake.

Vitamins. Vitamins are organic substances present in small amounts in foods that are essential to normal metabolism. The body is unable to synthesize vitamins in the required amounts and depends on dietary intake. Vitamin content is usually highest in fresh foods that are used quickly after minimal exposure to heat, air, or water. Vitamins are classified as fat soluble and water soluble.

Fat-Soluble Vitamins. The **fat-soluble vitamins** (A, D, E, and K) can be stored in the body. With the exception of vitamin D, these vitamins are provided through dietary intake. **Hypervitaminosis** of fat-soluble vitamins can result from megadoses (intentional or unintentional) of supplemental vitamins, excessive amounts in fortified food, and large intake of fish oils.

Certain vitamins are currently of considerable interest in their role as antioxidants that neutralize substances called free radicals, which are thought to produce oxidative damage to body cells and tissues. It is believe that oxidative damage increases a person's risk for various cancers. These vitamins include beta-carotene and vitamins A, C, and E (Williams, 2001).

Water-Soluble Vitamins. The **water-soluble vitamins** are vitamin C and B complex (which consists of eight vitamins). Water-soluble vitamins cannot be stored in the body and must be provided in the daily food intake. Although water-soluble vitamins are not stored, toxicity may still occur. Vitamins are chemicals used as catalysts in biochemical reactions. When there is enough of any specific vitamin to meet the catalytic demands, the rest of the vitamin supply acts as a free chemical and may be toxic to the body.

Minerals. Minerals are inorganic elements essential to the body as catalysts in biochemical reactions. Minerals are classified as **macrominerals** when the daily requirement is 100 mg or more and microminerals or trace elements when less than 100 mg is needed daily. Selenium is a **trace element** that also has antioxidant properties. Silicon, vanadium, nickel, tin, cadmium, arsenic, aluminum, and boron may play an unidentified role in nutrition. Toxic effects of arsenic, aluminum, and cadmium are documented.

Anatomy and Physiology of the Digestive System

Digestion. Digestion of food consists of mechanical breakdown that results from chewing, churning, and mixing with fluid, as well as chemical reactions by which food is reduced to its simplest form. Each part of the gastrointestinal (GI) system has an important digestive or absorptive function (Figure 43-2) . Enzymes are an essential component of the chemistry of digestion. **Enzymes** are the proteinlike substances that act as catalysts to speed up chemical reactions.

Most enzymes have one specific function. Each enzyme functions best at a specific pH. The secretions of the GI tract have vastly different pH levels. For example, saliva is relatively neutral, gastric juice is highly acidic, and the secretions of the small intestine are alkaline. For example, the enzyme amylase in the saliva breaks down starches into sugars.

The mechanical, chemical, and hormonal activities of digestion are interdependent. Enzyme activity depends on the mechanical breakdown of food to increase its surface area for chemical action. Hormones regulate the flow of digestive secretions needed for enzyme supply. The secretion of digestive juices and the motility of the GI tract are also regulated by physical, chemical, and hormonal factors, because they are bound to psychological, emotional, and nervous system alterations. Gastrointestinal tract action is increased by nerve stimulation from the parasympathetic nervous system (e.g., the vagus nerve).

Digestion begins in the mouth, where chewing mechanically breaks down food. The food is mixed with saliva, which contains ptyalin (salivary amylase), an enzyme that acts on cooked starch to begin its conversion to maltose. The longer food is chewed, the more starch digestion occurs in the mouth. Proteins and fats are broken down physically but remain unchanged chemically because enzymes in the mouth do not react with these nutrients. Chewing reduces food particles to a size suitable for swallowing, and saliva provides lubrication to further ease swallowing of the food. The epiglottis is a flap of skin that closes over the trachea as a person swallows to prevent aspiration. Swallowed food enters the esophagus and is moved along by wavelike muscular contractions **(peristalsis)** to the base of the esophagus, above the cardiac sphincter. Pressure from a bolus of food at the cardiac sphincter causes it to relax, allowing the food to enter the fundus, or uppermost portion, of the stomach. Difficulty swallowing is referred to as **dysphagia.**

In the stomach, pepsinogen is secreted by chief cells and then activated by hydrochloric acid (HCl) to pepsin, a protein-splitting enzyme. The stomach's pyloric glands secrete gastrin, a hormone that triggers parietal cells to secrete HCl. Parietal cells secrete HCl as well as intrinsic factor (IF), which is necessary for absorption of vitamin B_{12} in the ileum. Gastric lipase and amylase are produced to begin fat and starch digestion, respectively. The lining of the stomach is protected from autodigestion by a thick layer of mucus. Alcohol and aspirin are two substances directly absorbed through the lining of the stomach. The stomach acts as a reservoir where food remains for approximately 3 hr, with a range of 1 to 7 hr.

Food leaves the antrum, or distal stomach, via the pyloric sphincter and enters the duodenum. Food has now become an acidic, liquefied mass called **chyme.** Chyme flows into the duodenum and is quickly mixed with bile, intestinal juices, and pancreatic secretions. Secretin and cholecystokinin (CCK) are hormones secreted by the small intestine mucosa. Secretin activates release of bicarbonate from the pancreas, raising the pH of chyme. Cholecystokinin inhibits further gastrin secretion and initiates release of additional digestive enzymes from the pancreas and gallbladder.

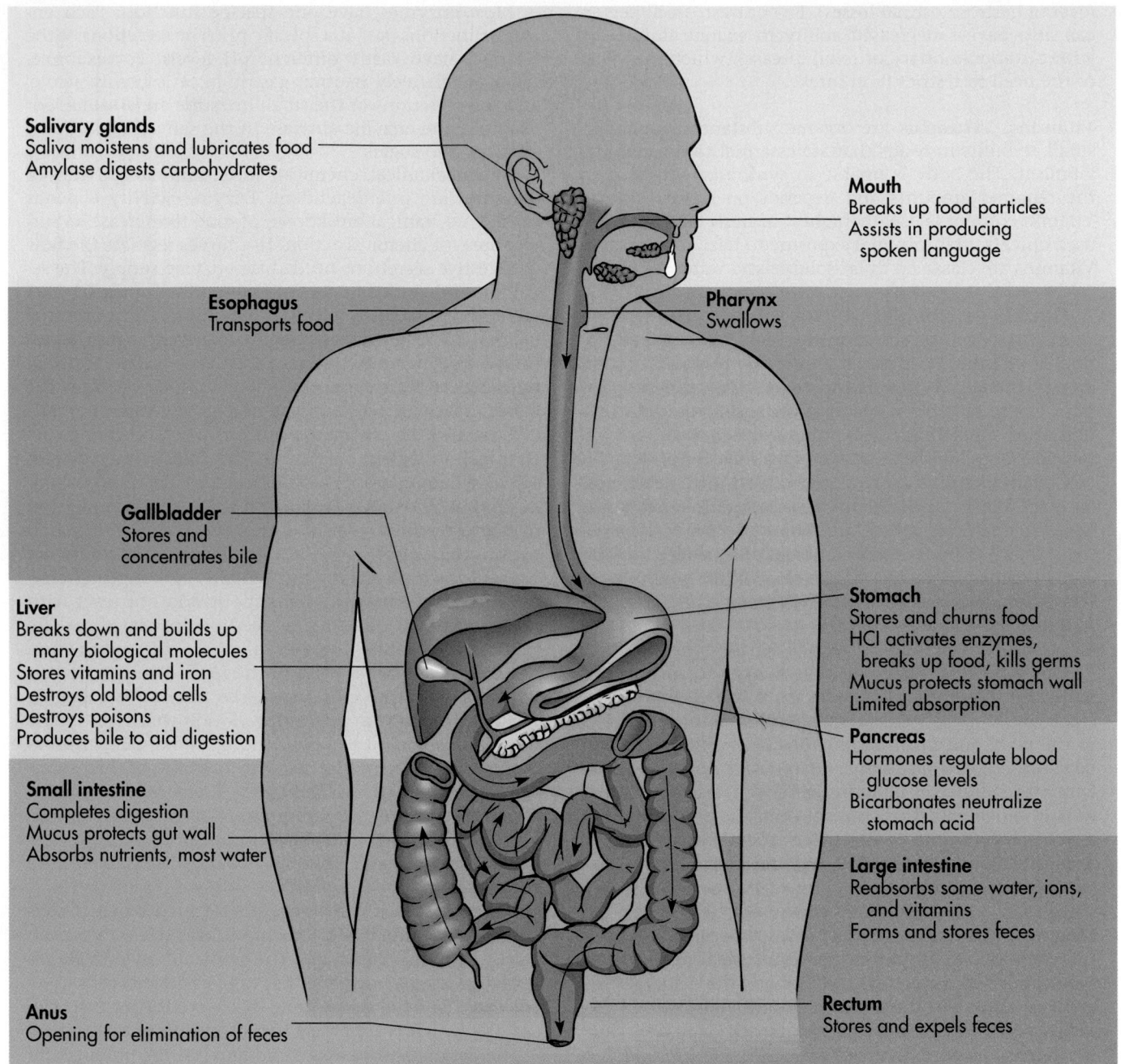

Salivary glands
Saliva moistens and lubricates food
Amylase digests carbohydrates

Mouth
Breaks up food particles
Assists in producing
spoken language

Esophagus
Transports food

Pharynx
Swallows

Gallbladder
Stores and
concentrates bile

Stomach
Stores and churns food
HCl activates enzymes,
breaks up food, kills germs
Mucus protects stomach wall
Limited absorption

Liver
Breaks down and builds up
many biological molecules
Stores vitamins and iron
Destroys old blood cells
Destroys poisons
Produces bile to aid digestion

Pancreas
Hormones regulate blood
glucose levels
Bicarbonates neutralize
stomach acid

Small intestine
Completes digestion
Mucus protects gut wall
Absorbs nutrients, most water

Large intestine
Reabsorbs some water, ions,
and vitamins
Forms and stores feces

Anus
Opening for elimination of feces

Rectum
Stores and expels feces

FIGURE **43–2** Summary of digestive system anatomy/organ function. (From Rolin Graphics.)

Bile is manufactured in the liver and stored in the gallbladder. Bile acts as a detergent, because it emulsifies fat to permit enzyme action while suspending fatty acids in solution. Pancreatic secretions contain six enzymes: amylase to digest starch; lipase to break down emulsified fats; and trypsin, elastase, chymotrypsin, and carboxypeptidase to break down proteins.

Peristalsis continues in the small intestine, mixing the secretions with the chyme. The mixture becomes increasingly alkaline, inhibiting the action of the gastric enzymes and promoting the action of the duodenal secretions. Epithelial cells in the small intestinal villi secrete enzymes to facilitate digestion. These include sucrase, lac-

tase, maltase, lipase, and peptidase. The major portion of digestion occurs in the small intestine, producing glucose, fructose, and galactose from carbohydrates; amino acids and dipeptides from proteins; and fatty acids, glycerides, and glycerol from lipids. Approximately 5 hours are required to pass food through the small intestine via peristalsis.

Absorption. The small intestine is the primary absorption site for nutrients. It is lined with fingerlike projections called villi, which increase the surface area available for absorption. Nutrients are absorbed by means of passive diffusion, osmosis, active transport, and pinocytosis.

Table 43-1	Intestinal Absorption of Major Nutrients			
Nutrient	**From**	**Absorption Method**	**Control Agent/Cofactor**	**Route**
Carbohydrate*	Monosaccharides (glucose and galactose)	Competitive	—	Blood
		Selective	—	Blood
		Active transport (via sodium pump)	Sodium	Blood
Fat†	Fatty acids	Fatty acid-bile complex (micelles)	Bile	Lymph
	Glycerides (mono, di)		—	Lymph
	Triglycerides (few) (neutral fat)	Pinocytosis	—	Lymph
Protein	Amino acids	Selective	—	Blood
	Dipeptides (some)	Carrier transport systems	Pyridoxine (pyridoxal phosphate)	Blood
	Whole protein (rare)	Pinocytosis	—	Blood
Minerals	Sodium	Active transport via sodium pump	—	Blood
	Calcium	Active transport	Vitamin D	Blood
	Iron	Active transport	Ferritin mechanism (as transferritin)	Blood
Vitamins‡	B$_{12}$	Carrier transport	IF	Blood
	A	Bile complex	Bile	Blood
	K	Bile complex	Bile	From large intestine to blood
Water§	H$_2$O	Osmosis	—	Blood, lymph, interstitial fluid

Modified from Williams SR: *Basic nutrition and diet therapy,* ed 11, St. Louis, 2001, Mosby.
*Carbohydrates, protein, minerals, and water-soluble vitamins are absorbed by villus capillaries within the small intestine, processed within the liver, and released via the portal vein circulatory means.
†Fatty acids are absorbed into the lymphatic circulatory system via lacteal ducts at the center of each microvilli found within the small intestine.
‡Exceptions to vitamin absorption are listed (i.e., B$_{12}$, A, and K). Vitamins A and K are fat soluble and are transported via bile to the blood. Vitamin B$_{12}$ is water soluble, but requires specialized transport factor for absorption.
§Water is reabsorbed in the large intestine through capillaries to the blood, also flows to the lymphatic system by absorption via large intestinal lymphatic ducts, and serves as a source of interstitial fluid per osmosis.

Table 43-1 describes the means and route of absorption of major nutrients.

The main source of water absorption is via the intestine. Approximately 8.5 L of GI secretions and 1.5 L of oral intake, totaling 10 L of fluid, must be managed daily within the GI tract. The small intestine reabsorbs 9.5 L, and approximately 0.4 L is reabsorbed in the colon. The remaining 0.1 L is eliminated in feces. In addition to water, electrolytes and minerals are absorbed, and bacteria in the colon synthesize vitamin K and some B complex vitamins. Finally, feces are formed in the colon for elimination.

Metabolism and Storage of Nutrients. Metabolism refers to all the biochemical reactions within the cells of the body. Metabolic processes can be anabolic (building) or catabolic (breaking down). **Anabolism** is the building of more complex biochemical substances by synthesis of nutrients. Anabolism occurs when lean muscle is added through diet and exercise. Amino acids are anabolized into tissues, hormones, and enzymes. **Catabolism** is the breakdown of biochemical substances into simpler substances. Starvation is an example of catabolism, when wasting of body tissues occurs. Normal metabolism and anabolism are physiologically possible when the body is in positive nitrogen balance, whereas catabolism occurs during physiological states of negative nitrogen balance.

Nutrients absorbed in the intestines, including water, are transported through the circulatory system to body tissues. Through the chemical changes of metabolism, nutrients are converted into a number of substances required by the body. Carbohydrates, protein, and fat undergo metabolism to produce chemical energy and to maintain a balance between anabolism and catabolism. To carry out the body's work, the chemical energy produced by metabolism is converted to other types of energy by different tissues. Muscle contraction involves mechanical energy, nervous system function involves electrical energy, and the mechanisms of heat production involve thermal energy. All of these forms of energy originate in metabolism.

Some of the nutrients required by the body are stored in tissues. The body's major form of reserve energy is fat, stored as adipose tissue. Protein is stored in muscle mass. When the body's energy requirements exceed the energy supplied by ingested nutrients, stored energy is used. Monoglycerides from the digested portion of fats can be converted to glucose by gluconeogenesis. Amino acids can also be converted to fat and stored or catabolized into energy via gluconeogenesis. All body cells except red blood cells and neurons can oxidize fatty acids into **ketones** for energy in the absence of dietary carbohydrates (glucose). Glycogen, synthesized from glucose, provides energy during brief periods of fasting. Glycogen is stored in small reserves in liver and muscle tissue. For example, blood glucose levels are maintained by this mechanism as we sleep. Nutrient metabolism consists of three main processes:

1. Catabolism of glycogen into glucose, carbon dioxide, and water **(glycogenolysis)**
2. Anabolism of glucose into glycogen for storage **(glycogenesis)**
3. Catabolism of amino acids and glycerol into glucose for energy **(gluconeogenesis)**

Elimination. Chyme is moved by peristaltic action through the ileocecal valve into the large intestine, where it becomes feces (see Chapter 45). As feces moves toward the rectum, water is absorbed in the mucosa. The longer the material stays in the large intestine, the more water is absorbed, causing the feces to become firmer. Exercise and fiber stimulate peristalsis, and water maintains consistency. Feces contains cellulose and similar indigestible substances, sloughed epithelial cells from the GI tract, digestive secretions, water, and microbes.

Dietary Guidelines

Dietary Reference Intakes. In 1997 the Food and Nutrition Board of the National Institute of Medicine/ National Academy of Sciences, in partnership with Health Canada, initiated **dietary reference intakes (DRIs).** The Food and Nutrition Board (1997) of the National Academy of Sciences published DRIs in response to the increased public use of nutritional supplements. The DRIs broaden the base of information on nutrients, vitamins and minerals. These DRIs present evidenced-based criteria for minimum to maximum amounts of vitamins and nutrients to avoid deficiencies or toxicities. In as much as this evidence is continually evolving, clinicians should consult with current resources, such as web pages and evidenced-based literature, when determining a client's specific nutrition needs or supplementation. This new format presents a range of acceptable intake in place of absolute values.

As research has expanded the scientific body of nutrition knowledge, absolute values are no longer sufficient. Studies addressing the reduction of risk of chronic diseases such as cardiovascular disease, cancer, and osteoporosis have launched a need for expanded nutrient information.

Food Guidelines. The *Food Guide Pyramid,* (U.S. Department of Agriculture, 1996) was designed as a basic guide for buying food and meal preparations (Figure 43-3). This basic system provides for diets ranging from 1600 to 2800 kcal/day (USDA, 1996). Additional foods to round out meals and meet energy requirements can be selected from enriched cereals, complex carbohydrates, and additional grains. To further augment the food pyramid, the U.S. Department of Agriculture (USDA) and the U.S. Department of Health and Human Services (USDHHS) have published the 2000 Dietary Guidelines for Americans and provide average daily consumption guidelines for the five food groups: grains, vegetables, fruits, dairy products, and meats (Box 43-1).

Daily Values. **Daily values** for food labels were created by the Food and Drug Administration (FDA) in response

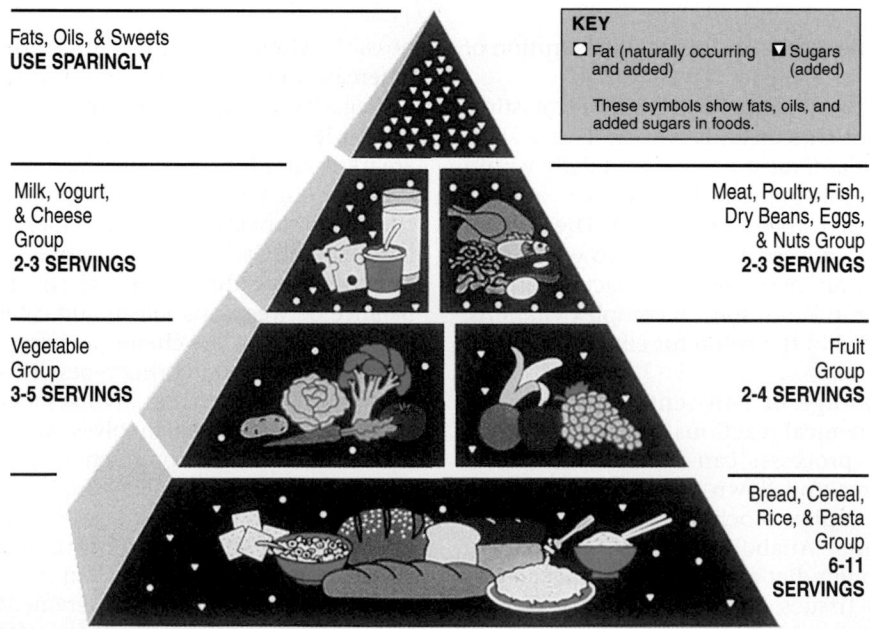

FIGURE **43–3**   U.S. food guide pyramid. (From U.S. Department of Agriculture: *USDA's food guide pyramid,* USDA Human Nutrition Information Service Pub No. 249, Washington, DC, 1996, U.S. Government Printing Office.)

to the 1990 Nutrition Labeling and Education Act (NLEA). The FDA first established two sets of reference values. The referenced daily intakes (RDI) are the first set, comprising protein, vitamins, and minerals based upon the RDA. The daily reference values (DRV) make up the second set and consist of nutrients such as total fat, saturated fat, cholesterol, carbohydrates, fiber, sodium, and potassium. Combined, both sets make up the daily values used on food labels (FDA, 1995). Daily values did not replace RDAs but provided a separate, more understandable format for the public. Daily values are based on percentages of 2000 kcal/day (Figure 43-4).

Healthy People 2010. In 1997 the USDHHS and the Public Health Service (PHS) began a consensus process, establishing nutritional goals and objectives for *Healthy People 2010: National Health Promotion and Disease Prevention Objectives. Healthy People 2010* is the United States' contribution to the World Health Organization's (WHO's) "Health for All" strategy. The report defines national goals to be met to increase the proportion of Americans who live long, healthy lives (Box 43-2). *Healthy People 2010* continues the objectives initiated in *Healthy People 2000*. All nutrition-related objectives include baseline data, from which progress is measured. The challenge remains to motivate consumers to put these dietary recommendations into practice. Many objectives of *Healthy People 2010* show positive indicators, including decreasing fat consumption and death rates from coronary heart disease. An increase in overall life expectancy has also occurred; however, obesity remains problematic. Health professionals can play a key role in promoting healthy dietary practices.

Nursing Knowledge Base

Nutrition During Human Growth and Development

Infants Through School-Age. Infancy is marked by rapid growth and high protein, vitamin, mineral, and energy requirements. The average birth weight of an American baby is 3.2 to 3.4 kg (7 to 7½ pounds). The infant usually doubles birth weight at 4 to 5 months and triples it at 1 year. An energy intake of approximately 108 kcal/kg of body weight is needed in the first half of infancy and 98 kcal/kg in the second half (USDA, 2000). Commercial formulas and human breast milk both provide approximately 20 kcal/oz. A full-term newborn is able to digest and absorb simple carbohydrates, proteins, and a moderate amount of emulsified fat. Infants need about 100 to 150 ml/kg/day of fluid because a large portion of total body weight is water.

Breast-Feeding. The American Academy of Pediatrics (1997a) strongly recommends breast-feeding. There are multiple benefits of breast-feeding to both infant and mother. These benefits include, but are not limited to, reducing food allergy risks; convenient, always correct temperature, available, and fresh; economical, because it is less expensive than formula; and increased time for mother and infant interaction (Grodner, Anderson, and DeYoung, 2000).

Formula. Infant formulas are designed to contain the approximate nutrient composition of human milk. Protein in the formula is typically supplied as whey, soy, cow's milk base, casein hydrolysate, or elemental amino acids. The American Academy of Pediatrics (1997b) has set standards for the level of nutrients in infant formulas. The addition of nucleotides to infant formula is a new area of research, intending to more closely parallel human milk and boost immune function (Pickering and others, 1998).

Regular cow's milk should not be used for infant formula during the first year of life. It may cause gastrointestinal bleeding and is too concentrated for the infant's kidneys to manage. The American Academy of Pediatrics (1994) issued a policy statement citing research supporting a possible relationship between cow's milk given in the first year of life and later development of type 1 diabetes mellitus. Honey and corn syrup are potential sources of botulism toxin and should not be used in the infant's diet. The toxin can be fatal in children under 1 year of age (Williams, 2001).

Introduction to Solid Food. Breast milk or formula provides sufficient nutrition for the first 4 to 6 months of life. The development of fine motor skills of the hand and fin-

---

Box 43-1   2000 Dietary Guidelines: ABCs for Good Health

Aim for fitness.
- Aim for a healthy weight.
- Choose sensible portion sizes.
- Be physically active each day.

Build a healthy base.
- Let the pyramid guide food selections.
- Choose a diet with plenty of grains, vegetables, fruits, dairy, and meat/protein sources.

- Maintain food safety.
  - Cook meats completely.
  - Keep food fresh.
  - Discard questionable food; when in doubt, throw it out.

Choose sensibly.
- Choose a diet low in fat, saturated fat, and cholesterol.
- Use sugar in moderation.
- Use salt and sodium in moderation.
- Drink alcoholic beverages in moderation, if at all.

Data from U.S. Department of Agriculture and U.S. Department of Health and Human Services: *Nutrition and your health: dietary guidelines for Americans*, ed 5, USDA/DHHS Home and Garden Bulletin No. 232, Washington, DC, 2000, U.S. Government Printing Office, www.usda.gov/cnpp/Pubs/DG2000/Index.html.

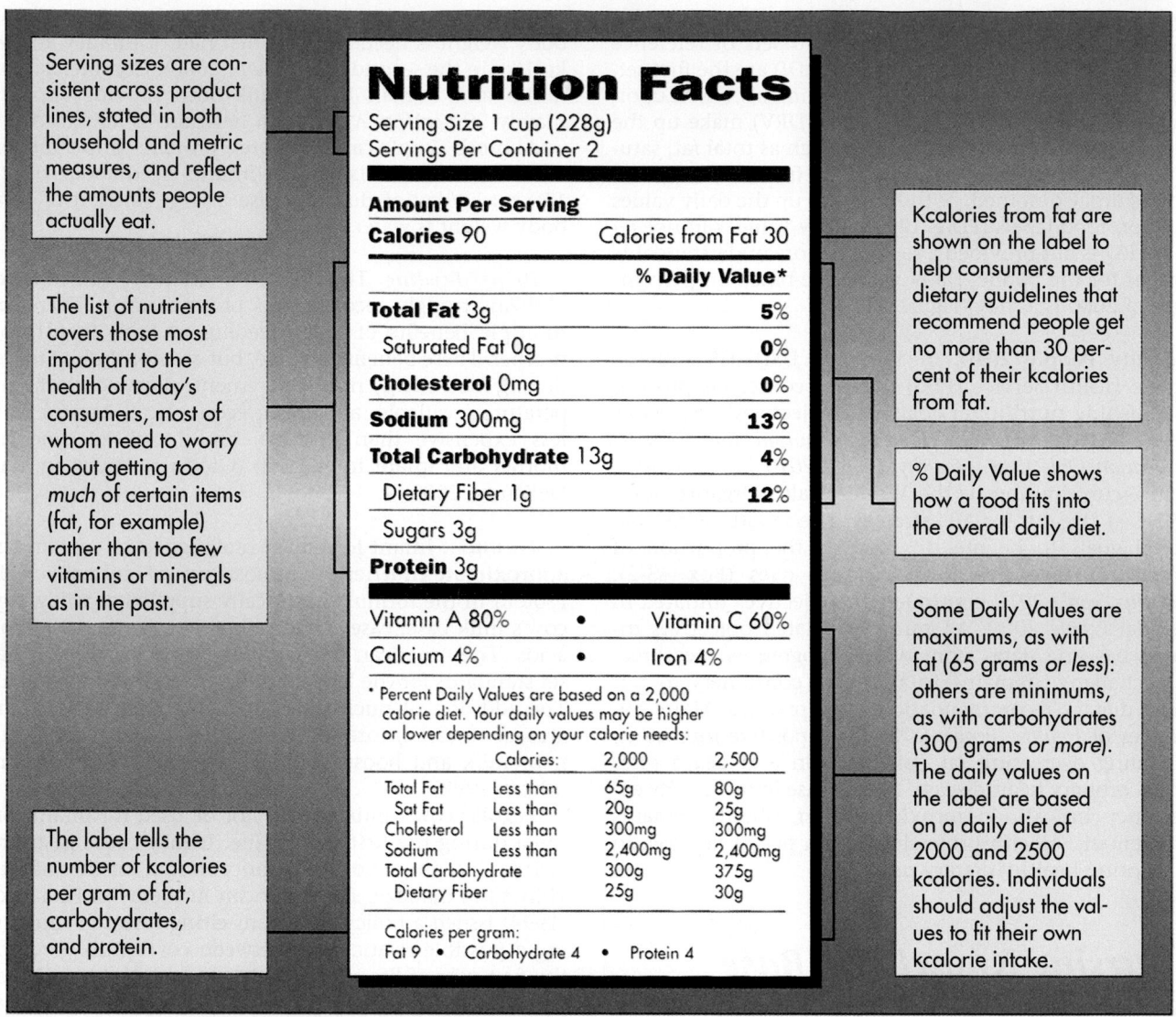

FIGURE **43–4**   FDA daily values for food labels. (From Food and Drug Administration: *Daily values for food labels,* Washington DC, 1995, U.S. Government Printing Office.)

Box *43-2*   **Nutrition Objectives for *Healthy People 2010***

Healthy weight
Reduction of obesity in adults
Reduction of obesity in children (6 to 11) and adolescents (12 to 19)
Decrease in growth retardation to <30% daily intake
Decrease in fat intake to <30% daily intake
Vegetable and fruit intake of five daily servings in 75% of people
Grain products intake of six daily servings in 80% of people
Calcium DRI met in 90% of people
Sodium daily intake no more than 2400 mg in 65% of people
Reduction of prevalence of iron deficiency in children and childbearing women

Reduction of prevalence of anemia in pregnant women to <23%
Nutrient-dense meals and snacks at school for children and adolescents
Nutrition education required in elementary schools
Nutrition education required in middle/junior high schools
Nutrition education required in senior high schools
Work-site nutrition education and weight management programs
Nutrition assessment and individualized planning at primary care sites
Nutritional education and counseling services for diabetics at primary care sites
Increase in prevalence of food security to 94% of households

Data from U.S. Department of Health and Human Services: *Healthy people 2010,* 2002, www.health.gov./healthypeople.

gers parallels the infant's interest in food and self-feeding. Iron-fortified cereals are typically the first semisolid food to be introduced.

The addition of foods to an infant's diet should be governed by the infant's nutrient needs, physical readiness to handle different forms of foods, and the need to detect and control allergic reactions. New foods should be introduced one at a time, approximately 4 to 7 days apart to identify allergies. It is best to introduce new foods before milk or other foods to avoid satiety (Wong, 2001).

The growth rate slows during toddler years (1 to 3). The toddler needs fewer kilocalories but an increased amount of protein in relation to body weight; consequently appetite may decrease at 18 months of age. Toddlers exhibit strong food preferences and become picky eaters. Small frequent meals consisting of breakfast, lunch, and dinner with three interspersed high-nutrient-density snacks may improve nutritional intake (Wong, 2001). Calcium and phosphorus are important for healthy bone growth.

Toddlers who consume more than 24 ounces of milk daily in lieu of other foods may develop milk anemia, because milk is a poor source of iron. Whole milk should be used until the toddler reaches 2 years of age to help ensure adequate intake of fatty acids necessary for brain and neurological development. Certain foods such as hot dogs, candy, nuts, grapes, raw vegetables, and popcorn have been implicated in choking deaths and should be avoided. Preschoolers' (3 to 5 years) dietary requirements are similar to toddlers. They consume slightly more than toddlers, and nutrient density is more important than quantity.

School-age children, 6 to 12 years old, grow at a slower and steadier rate, with a gradual decline in energy requirements per unit of body weight. Despite better appetites and more varied food intake, school-age children's diets should be carefully assessed for adequate protein and vitamins A and C. School-age children frequently fail to eat a proper breakfast and have unsupervised intake at school. High fat, sugar, and salt can result from too-liberal intake of snack foods. Kennedy-Caldwell (1998) notes that children are spending more time away from home, as do parents, further compounding this modern-day problem. Over the last 3 years there has been a consistent increase in sedentary activity level and increase in childhood obesity (USDHHS, 2002).

Adolescents. During adolescence, physiological age is a better guide to nutritional needs than chronological age. Energy needs increase to meet greater metabolic demands of growth. Daily requirement of protein also increases. Calcium is essential for the rapid bone growth of adolescence, and girls need a continuous source of iron to replace menstrual losses. Boys also need adequate iron for muscle development. Iodine supports increased thyroid activity, and use of iodized table salt ensures availability. B complex vitamins are needed to support heightened metabolic activity.

The adolescent's diet is influenced by many factors other than nutritional needs, including concern about body image and appearance, desire for independence, and fad diets. Nutritional deficiencies may occur in ado-

lescent girls as a result of dieting and use of oral contraceptives. The adolescent boy's diet may be inadequate in total kilocalories, protein, iron, folic acid, B vitamins, and iodine. Snacks provide approximately 25% of the teenager's total dietary intake. Fast food is common and adds extra salt, fat, and kilocalories. Skipping meals or eating meals with wrong choices of snacks contributes to nutrient deficiency and obesity (Wong, 2001).

Fortified foods (nutrients added) are important sources of vitamins and minerals. Snack food from the dairy and fruit and vegetable groups are good choices. To counter obesity, increasing physical activity is often more important than curbing intake. The onset of eating disorders such as **anorexia nervosa** or **bulimia nervosa** is often during adolescence. Recognition of eating disorders is essential for early intervention (Box 43-3).

Sports and regular moderate-to-intense exercise necessitate dietary modification to meet increased energy needs for adolescents. Carbohydrates, both simple and complex, should be the main source of energy, providing 55% to 60% of total daily kilocalories. Protein needs are increased to 1.0 to 1.5 g/kg/day. Fat needs are not increased. Adequate hydration is very important for all athletes. Water should be ingested before and after exercise

---

Box *43-3*   **Potential Assessment for Eating Disorders**

Anorexia Nervosa

A. Refusal to maintain body weight over a minimal normal weight for age and height, e.g., weight loss leading to maintenance of body weight less than 85% of IBW; or failure to make expected weight gain during period of growth, leading to body weight less than 85% of that expected.

B. Intense fear of gaining weight or becoming fat, although underweight.

C. Disturbance in the way in which one's body weight, size, or shape is experienced, e.g., the person claims to "feel fat" even when emaciated, believes that one area of the body is "too fat" even when obviously underweight.

D. In females, absence of at least 3 consecutive menstrual cycles when otherwise expected to occur (primary or secondary amenorrhea). (A woman is considered to have amenorrhea if her periods occur only following hormone, e.g., estrogen, administration.)

Bulimia Nervosa

A. Recurrent episodes of binge eating (rapid-consumption of a large amount of food in a discrete period of time).

B. A feeling of lack of control over eating behavior during the eating binges.

C. The person regularly engages in either self-induced vomiting, use of laxatives or diuretics, strict dieting or fasting, or vigorous exercise in order to prevent weight gain.

D. A minimum average of 2 binge eating episodes a week for at least 3 months.

Reprinted with permission from American Psychiatric Association: *Diagnostic and statistical manual of mental disorders,* ed 4-revised, Washington, DC, Copyright 1994, American Psychiatric Association.

to prevent dehydration, especially in hot, humid environments. Vitamin and mineral supplements are not required, but intake of iron-rich foods is required to prevent anemia.

Parents often have more influence on the adolescent diet than they believe. Effective strategies include limiting the amount of unhealthy food choices kept at home and enhancing the appearance and taste of healthy foods. Making healthy food choices more convenient and available and working to change social norms of what foods are "cool" are also ways to promote optimal nutritional health in adolescents (Neumark-Sztainer and others, 1999)

Pregnancy occurring within 4 years of menarche may place mother and fetus at risk because of anatomical and physiological immaturity. Malnutrition at the time of conception increases risk to the adolescent and her fetus. Most teenage girls do not want to gain weight. Counseling related to nutritional needs of pregnancy may be difficult, and suggestions are better tolerated than rigid directions. The diet of pregnant adolescents is often deficient in calcium, iron, and vitamins A and C. Prenatal vitamin and mineral supplements are recommended.

Young and Middle Adults. The demands for most nutrients are reduced as the growth period ends. Mature adults need nutrients for energy, maintenance, and repair. Energy needs usually decline over the years. Obesity may become a problem due to decreased physical exercise, dining out more often, and increased ability to afford more luxury foods. Adult women who use oral contraceptives may need extra vitamins. Iron and calcium intake continues to be important.

Maintaining good oral health is significant throughout adulthood. Poor oral hygiene and periodontal disease are potential risk factors for systemic diseases such as bacteremia, endocarditis, cardiopulmonary disease, diabetes mellitus, and adverse outcomes in pregnancy (Hornick, 2002).

Pregnancy. Poor nutrition during pregnancy can cause low birth weight in infants and decreased chances of survival. Generally the fetus's needs are met at the expense of the mother. However, if nutrient sources are not available, both suffer. The nutritional status of the mother at the time of conception is important. Significant aspects of fetal growth and development often occur before pregnancy is even suspected. The energy requirements of pregnancy are related to the mother's body weight and activity. The quality of nutrition during pregnancy is important, and food intake in the first trimester should include balanced portions of essential nutrients with emphasis on quality. Protein intake throughout pregnancy is increased. Calcium intake is especially critical in the third trimester, when fetal bones are mineralized. Iron may be supplemented to provide for increased maternal blood volume, for fetal blood storage, and for blood loss during delivery.

Folic acid intake is particularly important for DNA synthesis and the growth of red blood cells. Inadequate intake may lead to fetal neural tube defects, anencephaly, or maternal megaloblastic anemia (Daly and others, 1997). It is now recommended that women planning future pregnancies discuss preconception folic acid supple-

ments. In 1998 the FDA began requiring that grain products be fortified with folic acid. Prenatal care usually includes vitamin and mineral supplementation to ensure daily intakes; however, pregnant women should not take additional supplements beyond prescribed amounts.

Lactation. The lactating woman needs 500 kcal/day above the usual allowance because the production of milk increases energy requirements. Protein requirements for lactation exceed the protein requirement during pregnancy. The need for calcium remains the same as during pregnancy. There is an increased need for vitamins A and C. Daily intake of water-soluble vitamins (B and C) is needed to ensure adequate levels in breast milk. Fluid intake should be adequate but need not be excessive. Caffeine, alcohol, and drugs are excreted in breast milk and should be avoided. Tobacco use can decrease milk production (Food and Nutrition Board, 1992).

Older Adults. Adults 65 years and older have a decreased need for energy as metabolic rate slows with age. However, vitamin and mineral requirements remain unchanged from middle adulthood. Numerous factors influence the nutritional status of the older adult. Income is significant because living on a fixed income may reduce the amount of money available to buy food (Box 43-4). Health is another important influence. The older adult may be on a therapeutic diet or have difficulty eating because of physical symptoms, lack of teeth, or dentures or be at risk for drug-nutrient interactions (Table 43-2). Thirst sensation may diminish, leading to inadequate fluid intake or dehy-

---

Focus on **Older Adults**   Box 43-4

Factors Affecting Nutritional Status

- Age-related gastrointestinal changes that affect digestion of food and maintenance of nutrition include changes in the teeth and gums, reduced saliva production, atrophy of oral mucosal epithelial cells, increased taste threshold, decreased thirst sensation, reduced gag reflex, and decreased esophageal and colonic peristalsis.
- Presence of comorbidities increases risk of poor nutrition (Millen and others, 2001).
- Malnutrition in older adults has multiple causes, such as income, educational level, physical functional level to meet activities of daily living (ADLs), loss, dependency, loneliness, and transportation (Chen and others, 2001).
- Nutrition knowledge: Reading food labels, nutrient value of foods.
- Adverse effects of medications such as anorexia, xerostomia, early satiety, and impaired smell and taste perception.
- Factors affecting nutrient needs: Calcium, vitamin D, or phosphorus for basic metabolic demand (BMD). B_{12} may not be synthesized because of lack of intrinsic factor in terminal ileum, decreased lean muscle mass, lower basic energy expenditure (BEE) (Lueckenotte, 2000; Chen and others, 2001).
- Cognitive impairments related to delirium, dementia, and depression.

Table 43-2   Sample of Drug-Nutrient Interactions*

Drug	Effect
Analgesic/Narcotic	
Acetaminophen	Decreased drug absorption with food; overdose associated with liver failure
Aspirin	Absorbed directly through stomach; decreased drug absorption with food; decreased folic acid, vitamins C and K, and iron absorption
Opiates	Decreased peristalsis; constipation
Antacid	
Aluminum hydroxide	Decreased phosphate absorption
Sodium bicarbonate	Decreased folic acid absorption
Antiarrhythmic	
Amiodarone	Taste alteration
Digitalis	Anorexia, decreased renal clearance in older persons
Propranolol	Increased drug absorption with food
Antiarthritic	
Methotrexate	Decreased drug absorption with food, decreased folic acid
Penicillamine	Taste alteration
Antibiotic	
Amoxicillin, doxycycline, penicillin	Decreased drug absorption with food
Ampicillin	Taste alteration, decreased drug absorption with food
Cephalosporin	Decreased vitamin K
Clarithromycin	Taste alteration
Gentamicin	Anorexia, decreased renal excretion in older persons
Metronidazole	Anorexia
Neomycin	Decreased fat, nitrogen, vitamin B_{12}, lactose, sucrose, sodium, potassium, iron, calcium
Rifampin	Decreased vitamin B_6, niacin, vitamin D
Tetracycline	Decreased drug absorption with milk and antacids, decreased nutrient absorption of calcium, riboflavin, vitamin C due to binding
Trimethoprim/sulfamethoxazole	Decreased folic acid
Anticoagulant	
Coumarin	Acts as antagonist to vitamin K
Anticonvulsant	
Carbamazepine	Increased drug absorption with food
Phenobarbital	Decreased drug absorption with food, decreased vitamin D
Phenytoin	Decreased calcium absorption; decreased vitamins D and K and folic acid; taste alteration; decreased drug absorption with food
Primidone	Decreased calcium absorption, increased metabolism of vitamins D and K
Antidepressant	
Amitriptyline	Appetite stimulant
Clomipramine	Taste alteration, appetite stimulant
Fluoxetine (selective serotonin reuptake inhibitors [SSRIs])	Taste alteration, anorexia
Antifungal	
Amphotericin B	Anorexia
Griseofulvin	Taste alteration, enhanced absorption with food
Antihistamine	
Astemizole	Increased appetite, decreased drug absorption with food
Cyproheptadine	Increased appetite

*Not intended to be an exhaustive or all-inclusive list. Always check pharmacology references before administering medications.

Continued

Table 43-2 Sample of Drug-Nutrient Interactions*—cont'd

Drug	Effect
Antihypertensive	
Captopril	Taste alteration, anorexia
Hydralazine	Enhanced drug absorption with food, decreased vitamin B_6
Labetalol	Taste alteration (weight gain for all beta-blockers)
Methyldopa	Decreased vitamin B_{12}, folic acid, iron
Antiinflammatory	
All steroids	Increased appetite and weight, increased folic acid, decreased calcium (osteoporosis with long-term use), promotes gluconeogenesis of protein
Indomethacin	Decreased iron absorption
Salicylazosulfapyridine (Azulfidine)	Decreased folic acid
Antiparkinson	
Levodopa	Taste alteration, decreased vitamin B_6 and drug absorption with food
Antipsychotic	
Chlorpromazine	Increased appetite
Thiothixene	Decreased riboflavin, increased need
Bronchodilator	
Albuterol sulfate	Appetite stimulant
Theophylline	Anorexia
Cholesterol Lowering	
Cholestyramine	Decreased fat-soluble vitamins (A, D, E, K); vitamin B_{12}; iron
Diuretic	
Furosemide	Decreased drug absorption with food
Spironolactone	Increased drug absorption with food
Thiazides	Decreased magnesium, zinc, and potassium
Triamterene	Decreased folic acid
Estrogen/Progestin	
Oral contraceptive hormone replacement therapy (HRT)	Decreased vitamin B_6, B_{12}, folic acid, zinc; increased transferrin as above
Laxative	
Mineral oil	Decreased absorption of fat-soluble vitamins (A, D, E, K), carotene
Phenolphthalein	Decreased calcium, potassium, vitamin D
Muscle Relaxant	
Baclofen	Taste alteration
Dantrolene	Taste alteration, anorexia
Platelet Aggregate Inhibitor	
Dipyridamole	Decreased drug absorption with food
Potassium Replacement	
Potassium chloride	Decreased vitamin B_{12}
Stimulant	
Dextroamphetamine	Taste alteration, anorexia
Methylphenidate	Anorexia, decreased weight, decreased growth
Tranquilizer	
Benzodiazepines	Increased appetite

*Not intended to be an exhaustive or all-inclusive list. Always check pharmacology references before administering medications.

dration (see Chapter 40). Some symptoms of dehydration in older adults may include confusion, weakness, hot dry skin, furrowed tongue, rapid pulse, and high urinary sodium. Meats may be avoided because of cost or because they are difficult to chew. Cream soups and meat-based vegetable soups are nutrient-dense sources of protein. Cheese, eggs, and peanut butter are also useful high-protein alternatives. Milk continues to be an important food for older women (and men) who need adequate calcium to protect against osteoporosis (a decrease of bone mass density). Research has shown that older men lag behind women in developing osteoporosis by approximately a decade. However, screening and treatment are also necessary for older men, as well as older women (Atkinson and Ward, 2001; Ybarra, Ade, and Romeo, 1996). The diet of older adults should contain choices from all food groups and may require a vitamin and mineral supplement.

The USDHHS's Administration on Aging (AOA) now requires states to provide nutritional screening services to older adult clients who benefit from home-delivered or congregate meal services. Reports of findings are sent to AOA. An estimated 2.5 million community-dwelling older adults suffer from food inadequacies within any 6-month period, and 40% to 50% of this group have a moderate-to-high risk of malnutrition. A public-private partnership with the USDHHS and General Mills was recently formed to provide breakfast as a second meal to older homebound adults in a Morning Meals on Wheels program (USDHHS, 1997).

> **Safety Alert.** Homebound older adults with chronic illness have additional nutritional risks. Frequently this group lives alone with little or no social resources to assisting in obtaining or preparing nutritionally sound meals. Increased nutritional screening during regular medical provider visits may result in more timely recognition of potential nutritional deficiencies and subsequent treatment of these deficiencies (Millen and others, 2001; Todorovic, 2001).

Alternative Food Patterns

Long before recommended allowances and guidelines were issued, many people followed special patterns of food intake based on religion (Table 43-3), cultural background (Box 43-5), ethics, health beliefs, personal preference, or concern for the efficient use of land to produce food. Such special diets are not necessarily more or less nutritious than diets based on the food pyramid or other nutritional guidelines, because good nutrition depends on a balanced intake of all required nutrients. Nurses will care for clients who practice a variety of food intake patterns.

Vegetarian Diet. A common alternative dietary pattern is the vegetarian diet. **Vegetarianism** is the consumption of a diet consisting predominantly of plant foods. Vegetarians may be ovolactovegetarian (avoid meat, fish, and poultry but eat eggs and milk), lactovegetarians (drink milk but avoid eggs), or vegans (consume only plant foods). Vegan, Zen macrobiotic (eat primarily brown rice, other grains, and herb teas), and fruitarian (eat only fruit, nuts, honey, and olive oil) diets are nutrient poor and can result in malnutrition. Knowledge related to complementary use of complete and incomplete proteins is necessary. Children who follow a vegetarian diet are especially at risk for protein and vitamin deficiencies, such as vitamin B_{12}.

Critical Thinking

Successful critical thinking requires a synthesis of knowledge, experience, information collected from clients, critical thinking attitudes, and intellectual and professional standards. Clinical judgments require the nurse to anticipate the required information, analyze the data, and make decisions regarding client care. Critical thinking is a dynamic process. During assessment (Figure 43-5, p. 1287) the nurse must consider all elements that build toward making appropriate nursing diagnoses.

Table **43-3**	**Religious Dietary Restrictions**					
Islam	**Christianity**	**Hinduism**	**Judaism**		**Church of Jesus Christ of Latter-Day Saints (Mormons)**	**Seventh-Day Adventists Church**
Pork	Minimal or	All meats	Pork		Alcohol	Pork
Alcohol	no alcohol		Predatory fowl		Tobacco	Shellfish
Caffeine	Holy day		Shellfish (eat only fish with		Caffeine	Alcohol
Ramadan fasting	observances		scales)			Vegetarian
sunrise to sun-	may restrict		Rare meats			diet
set for month	meat		Blood (blood sausage, etc.)			encouraged
Ritualized meth-			Mixing of milk or dairy			
ods of animal			products with meat dishes			
slaughter re-			Must adhere to kosher food			
quired for meat			preparation methods			
ingestion			24 hr of fasting on Yom			
			Kippur, a day of atonement			
			No leavened bread eaten			
			during Passover (8 days)			
			No cooking on the Sabbath			
			(Saturday)			

Cultural Aspects of Care   Box 43-5

Nutrition

The incidence of lactose intolerance around the world occurs from high to low in the following ethnic or racial groups: Asian-Pacific, African and African-American, Native American, Mexican-American, Middle Eastern, followed by whites. This condition affects nutrient absorption, and calcium deficiency results. Calcium is necessary for maintaining bone mass density.

The theory of hot and cold foods predominates in many cultures. The origin appears to be from Hippocratic beliefs concerning health and the four humors. Arabs were keepers of this knowledge during the Dark Ages and later influenced the Spanish to adopt this belief system in the later Middle Ages. The foundation of the theory is keeping harmony with nature by balancing "cold," "hot," "wet," and "dry." Some cultures believe hot is warmth, strength, and reassurance, whereas cold is menacing and weak. Classification has nothing to do with spiciness but is a symbolic representation of temperature.

Implications for Practice

- Lactose and other food intolerances unique to specific cultures may necessitate diet adaptation to meet nutrient, mineral, and vitamin daily intake requirements.
- When clients use hot and cold foods as part of their cultural health practices, dietary modifications may be needed for hospitalized clients or those clients in extended care facilities. For example, a client may wish to have an increase in hot foods (e.g., rice, grain cereals, alcohol, beef, lamb, chili peppers, chocolate, cheese, temperate zone fruits, eggs, peas, goat's milk, cornhusks, oils, onions, pork, radishes, and tamales). By contrast, cold foods encompass beans, citrus fruits, tropical fruits, dairy products, most vegetables, honey, raisins, chicken, fish, and goat.
- Hot or cold foods are not the result of spices or ingredients. Rather, foods can be made hot or cold through methods of preparation. A blending of hot and cold balances food.
- Some specific conditions may require hot foods. Menstruation, cancer, pneumonia, earache, colds, paralysis, headache, and rheumatism are cold illnesses requiring hot foods.
- Other conditions, such as pregnancy, fever, infections, diarrhea, rashes, ulcers, liver problems, constipation, kidney problems, and sore throats are believed to be hot conditions requiring cold foods.

Modified from Giger JN, Davidhizar RE: *Transcultural nursing: assessment and intervention,* ed 2, St. Louis, 1995, Mosby.

In the case of nutrition, the nurse must integrate knowledge from nursing and other disciplines, previous experiences, and information gathered from clients and families regarding customary food preferences, as well as recent dietary history. The use of professional standards, such as the DRIs, the USDA's food guide pyramid, dietary guidelines, and *Healthy People 2010* objectives provide guidelines for assessing and maintaining clients' nutritional status. Other professional standards by the American Heart Association (2000), the American Diabetic Association (ADA) (2002), The American Cancer Society (1997), and the American Society for Parenteral and Enteral Nutrition (ASPEN) (2001) are available. These standards are evidence based and are regularly updated for optimal client care.

Nursing Process and Nutrition

Nurses are in an excellent position to recognize signs of poor nutrition and to take steps to initiate change. Close contact with clients and their families enables nurses to make observations about physical status, food intake, weight changes, and response to therapy.

Assessment

Early recognition of malnourished or at-risk clients has a strong positive influence on both short- and long-term health outcomes (Evans-Stoner, 1997; ASPEN, 2001). Studies have identified 40% to 55% of adult hospitalized clients as being either malnourished or at risk for malnutrition and have also found a relationship between malnutrition and adverse outcomes, including mortality. Nutrition assessment forms used to identify clients in need or at risk are useful. Hennessy and Orr (1996), Kovacevich and others (1997), and Costello and Todd-Magel (1997) are sources of useable forms. Assessment of nutritional status is essential due to the common need of all human beings for nutrients, energy, and fluids. Nutrition assessment centers on five major areas: anthropometry, laboratory tests, dietary and health history, clinical observation, and client expectations.

The Nutrition Screening Initiative is a multidisciplinary effort begun in 1991 to assess for warning signs of malnutrition in older adults. A three-tiered approach was designed for the nutritional assessment of older adults. Ten key risk factors are shown in the checklist to determine nutritional health (Figure 43-6), which serves as the first tier (Nutrition Screening Initiative, 1998; USDA, 2000).

Anthropometry. **Anthropometry** is a measurement system of the size and makeup of the body. Height and weight should be obtained for each client on hospital admission or entry into any health care setting. If possible, the client should be weighed at the same time each day, on the same scale, and with the same clothing or linen. Rapid weight gain usually reflects fluid shifts. One pint or 500 ml of fluid equals 1 pound. Height and weight can be compared to standards for height-weight relationships. Recent weight changes should be documented. For example, for a client with renal failure or congestive heart failure a weight increase of 2 pounds is significant, as it may indicate that the client has retained a liter (1000 ml) of fluid.

Anthropometric measurements that aid in identifying nutritional problems include the ratio of height to wrist circumference, mid-upper arm circumference (MAC), triceps skin fold (TSF), and mid-upper arm muscle circumference (MAMC). Significant variation may result unless

KNOWLEDGE

- Normal nutrition parameters
- Anatomy and physiology of gastrointestinal system
- Cultural influences on nutrition
- Developmental factors affecting nutrition
- Effects of medications on nutrition

EXPERIENCE

- Caring for clients with altered nutrition
- Observation of nutritional practices of friends and family
- Personal assessment of nutritional practices

Assessment

- Identify the signs and symptoms associated with altered nutrition
- Gather data from clients regarding nutritional practices
- Determine client's nutritional energy needs (REE × activity or illness factor)
- Obtain client's dietary history

STANDARDS

- Apply intellectual standards of accuracy, completeness, and significance when obtaining a health history for clients with altered nutrition
- Compare gathered data with established nutritional standards, (e.g., dietary reference intake, food pyramid, *Healthy People 2010,* and healthy eating index)

ATTITUDES

- Be open minded about the client's nutritional practices when obtaining nutritional assessment
- Display confidence when collecting data related to culture, socioeconomic status, physical functioning, dietary restrictions, and personal preferences as necessary to a complete nutritional assessment

FIGURE **43–5**   Critical thinking model for nutrition assessment.

the examiner is skilled and has proper equipment. Values for MAC, TSF, and MAMC are compared to standards and calculated as a percentage of the standard. Changes in values for an individual over time are of greater significance than isolated measurements (Williams, 2001).

Body Mass Index. **Body mass index (BMI)** measures weight corrected for height and serves as an alternative to traditional height-weight relationships. Calculation of BMI is achieved by dividing the client's weight in kilograms by height in meters squared: Weight (kg) divided by Height² (m²).

A BMI of greater than 25 defines the upper boundaries of healthy weight, and places a client at higher medical risk of respiratory disease, tuberculosis, digestive disease, and some cancers. By contrast, a BMI of greater than 35 places a client at higher medical risk of coronary heart disease, some cancers, diabetes mellitus, and hypertension (Grodner, Anderson, and DeYoung, 2000; USDA, 2000).

Ideal Body Weight. An **ideal body weight (IBW)** provides an estimate of what a person should weigh. This can be calculated using the body mass index as a reference guide. BMI between 25 and 30 indicates overweight,

The Warning Signs of poor nutritional health are often overlooked. Use this checklist to find out if you or someone you know is at nutritional risk.

DETERMINE YOUR NUTRITIONAL HEALTH

Read the statements below. Circle the number in the yes column for those that apply. For each yes answer, score the number in the box. Total the nutritional score.

	YES
I have an illness or condition that made me change the kind and/or amount of food I eat.	2
I eat fewer than 2 meals per day.	3
I eat few fruits or vegetables, or milk products.	2
I have 3 or more drinks of beer, liquor or wine almost every day.	2
I have tooth or mouth problems that make it hard for me to eat.	2
I don't always have enough money to buy the food I need.	4
I eat alone most of the time.	1
I take 3 or more different prescribed or over-the-counter drugs a day.	1
Without wanting to, I have lost or gained 10 pounds in the last 6 months.	2
I am not always physically able to shop, cook and/or feed myself.	2
TOTAL	

Total Your Nutritional Score. If it's –

0–2   Good! Recheck your nutritional score in 6 months.

3–5   You are at moderate nutritional risk. See what can be done to improve your eating habits and lifestyle. Your office on aging, senior nutrition program, senior citizens center or health department can help. Recheck your nutritional score in 3 months.

6 or more   You are at high nutritional risk. Bring this checklist the next time you see your doctor, dietitian or other qualified health or social service professional. Talk with them about any problems you may have. Ask for help to improve your nutritional health.

These materials developed and distributed by the Nutritional Screening Initiative, a project of:

AMERICAN ACADEMY
OF FAMILY PHYSICIANS

THE AMERICAN
DIETETIC ASSOCIATION

NATIONAL COUNCIL
ON THE AGING

Remember that warning signs suggest risk, but do not represent diagnosis of any condition.

FIGURE **43–6** Nutrition screening tool for older adults. (Reprinted with permission from the Nutrition Screening Initiative, 1998, a project of the American Academy of Family Physicians, the American Dietetic Association, and the National Council of the Aging, Inc. and funded in part by a grant from Ross Products Division, Abbott Laboratories, Inc.)

and a BMI greater than 30 defines obesity (USDA, 2000). If height cannot be measured with the client standing, position the client lying flat in bed as straight as possible, arms folded on the client's chest, and measure the client lengthwise.

Laboratory and Biochemical Tests. No single laboratory or biochemical test is diagnostic for malnutrition. Factors that may alter test results include fluid balance, liver function, kidney function, and the presence of disease. Common laboratory tests used to study nutritional status include measures of plasma proteins such as albumin, transferrin, prealbumin, retinol binding protein, total iron-binding capacity, and hemoglobin. After feeding, the response time for changes in these proteins ranges from hours to weeks. The metabolic half-life of albumin is 21 days, transferrin is 8 days, prealbumin is 2 days, and retinol binding protein is 12 hours. This range demonstrates why albumin level, for example, is not an accurate short-term indicator of serum protein status (Pagana and Pagana, 1999).

Furthermore, serum albumin levels are affected by the following factors: hydration; hemorrhage; renal or hepatic disease; high-output drainage of wounds, drains, burns, or the gut; steroid administration; exogenous albumin infusions; age; and trauma, burns, stress, or surgery. In summary, albumin level is a better indicator for chronic illnesses, whereas prealbumin level is preferred for acute conditions.

Nitrogen balance is important to establish serum protein status (see the discussion of protein in this chapter). Nitrogen intake is calculated by dividing 6.25 into the total grams of protein ingested in a day (24 hours). The output of nitrogen is established through laboratory analysis of a 24-hour urinary urea nitrogen (UUN). For clients with diarrhea or fistula drainage, a further addition of 2 to 4 g of nitrogen output is estimated. Nitrogen balance is found by subtracting the nitrogen output from the nitrogen intake. A positive (more nitrogen is taken in than is put out) 2- to 3-g nitrogen balance is ideal for anabolism. By contrast, negative (more nitrogen is put out than is taken in) nitrogen balance is present when cata-

Table 43-4	Obtaining a Dietary History
Components of a Dietary History	**Areas to Assess and /or Questions to Ask**
Diet	
• Number of meals per day	• How many meals do you eat? Are these scheduled meals or snacks?
• Food preferences	• What type of food do you like?
• Food preparation practices	• Who prepares the food?
• Food purchasing practices	• Who purchases the food?
Unpleasant symptoms	
• Indigestion, heartburn, gas	• What foods cause indigestion, gas, or heartburn? Does this occur each time you have the food?
• Relief practices	• What relieves the symptoms?
Allergies	• Are you allergic to any foods?
	• Get specific listing of foods and allergic response (e.g., hives, itching, anaphylaxis).
	• Determine what is done to treat allergies (e.g., EpiPen, oral antihistamines).
Taste	• Have you noticed any changes in taste?
	• Did these changes occur with medications or following an illness?
Chewing and swallowing	• Does the client wear dentures? Are the dentures comfortable?
	• Assess the condition of the client's teeth.
	• Does the client experience mouth pain or sores (e.g., cold sore, canker sores).
	• Do you have difficulty swallowing?
	• Do you cough or gag when you swallow?
Appetite	• Have you had a change in appetite?
	• Have you noticed a change in weight?
	• Was this change an anticipated change (e.g., client was on a weight reduction diet)?
Elimination patterns	• Frequency of bowel movements.
	• Diarrhea associated with meals or specific foods.
	• Constipation.
Use of medications	• What medications do you take?
	• Do you take any over-the-counter medications that your doctor does not prescribe?
	• Do you take any nutritional or herbal supplements?

bolic states exist, seen in either starvation or physiological stress.

Dietary History and Health History. In addition to the general nursing history, the nurse obtains a more specific diet history to assess the client's actual or potential needs (Table 43-4). The diet history focuses on the client's habitual intake of foods and liquids, as well as information about preferences, allergies, and other relevant areas, such as the client's ability to obtain food. The nurse gathers information about the client's illness/activity level to determine energy needs and compares food intake. Nursing assessment of nutrition includes health status; age; cultural background (see Box 43-5, p. 1286); religious food patterns (see Table 43-3, p. 1285); socioeconomic status; personal food preferences; psychological factors; use of alcohol or illegal drugs; use of vitamin, mineral, or herbal supplements; prescription or over-the-counter (OTC) drugs (see Table 43-2); and the client's general nutrition knowledge (Evans-Stoner, 1997).

In outpatient settings, a 3- to 7-day food diary may be kept by the client. This allows the nurse to calculate nutritional intake and to compare it with DRIs to see if dietary habits are adequate. Food-frequency questionnaires may be used to establish patterns over time.

Clinical Observation. Clinical observations can be among the most important aspects of a nutritional as-

sessment. As in other kinds of nursing assessment, the nurse observes the client for signs of nutritional alterations. Because improper nutrition affects all body systems, clues to malnutrition may be observed during physical assessment (see Chapter 32). When the general physical assessment of body systems is complete, the nurse can recheck pertinent areas to evaluate the client's nutritional status. The clinical signs of nutritional status (Table 43-5) provide guidelines for observation during physical assessment.

The nurse must also assess the client's risk of aspiration. Clients at high risk for aspiration are those clients with decreased level of alertness, decreased gag and/or cough reflexes, and clients who have difficulty managing saliva and may or may not have a wet gurgly voice. The nurse should assess for adequate swallowing (see Chapter 32) before giving food or medications (see Chapter 34). To check adequacy of the client's swallow, place fingers at the level of the client's throat at the level of the larynx, and then ask client to swallow. The nurse should be able to palpate the movement of the larynx. Clients with risk of aspiration will need specialized assistance with feeding.

Client Expectations. Clients rely on health care professionals to identify problems of which they may not be aware. Most nutritional problems tend to develop insidiously over weeks and months, not overnight (ADA, 2002). Weigley (1995) found several specific nutrition

Table 43-5	Clinical Signs of Nutritional Status	
Body Area	**Signs of Good Nutrition**	**Signs of Poor Nutrition**
General appearance	Alert: responsive	Listless, apathetic, cachexia, cachectic appearance
Weight	Weight normal for height, age, body build	Obesity (usually 10% above IBW) or underweight appearance (special concern for underweight)
Posture	Erect posture; straight arms and legs	Sagging shoulders; sunken chest; humped back
Muscles	Well-developed, firm muscles; good tone; some fat under skin	Flaccid appearance, poor tone, underdeveloped tone; tenderness; edema; wasted appearance; inability to walk properly
Nervous system control	Good attention span; lack of irritability or restlessness; normal reflexes; psychological stability	Inattention; irritability; confusion; burning and tingling of hands and feet (paresthesia); loss of position and vibratory sense; weakness and tenderness of muscles (may result in inability to walk); decrease or loss of ankle and knee reflexes; absent vibratory sense
Gastrointestinal function	Good appetite and digestion; normal regular elimination; no palpable organs or masses	Anorexia; indigestion; constipation or diarrhea; liver or spleen enlargement
Cardiovascular function	Normal heart rate and rhythm; lack of murmurs; normal blood pressure for age	Rapid heart rate (above 100 beats/min), enlarged heart; abnormal rhythm; elevated blood pressure
General vitality	Endurance; energy, good sleep habits; vigorous appearance	Easily fatigued; lack of energy; falling asleep easily, tired and apathetic appearance
Hair	Shiny, lustrous appearance; firmness; strands not easily plucked, healthy scalp	Stringy, dull, brittle, dry, thin, and sparse, depigmented appearance; strands that can be easily plucked
Skin (general)	Smooth and slightly moist skin with good color	Rough, dry, scaly, pale, pigmented, irritated appearance; bruises; petechiae; subcutaneous fat loss
Face and neck	Uniform color; smooth, pink, healthy appearance; lack of swelling	Greasy, discolored, scaly, swollen appearance; dark skin over cheeks and under eyes; lumpiness or flakiness of skin around nose and mouth
Lips	Smoothness; good color; moist (not chapped or swollen) appearance	Dry, scaly, swollen appearance; redness and swelling (cheilosis); angular lesions at corners of mouth; fissures or scars (stomatitis)
Mouth, oral membranes	Reddish pink mucous membranes in oral cavity	Swollen, boggy oral mucous membranes
Gums	Good pink color; healthy and red appearance; lack of swelling or bleeding	Spongy gums that bleed easily; marginal redness, inflammation; receding gums
Tongue	Good pink or deep reddish color; lack of swelling; smoothness, presence of surface papillae; lack of lesions	Swelling, scarlet and raw appearance; magenta color, beefiness (glossitis); hyperemic and hypertrophic papillae; atrophic papillae
Teeth	Lack of cavities and pain; bright, straight appearance; lack of crowding; well-shaped jaw; clean appearance with no discoloration	Unfilled caries; absent teeth; worn surfaces; mottled (fluorosis), malpositioned appearance
Eyes	Bright, clear, shiny appearance; lack of sores at corner of membranes; eyelids; moist and healthy pink color; prominent blood vessels or lack of mound of tissue or sclera; lack of fatigue circles beneath eyes	Pale eye membranes (pale conjunctivas); redness of membrane (conjunctival injection); dryness; signs of infection; Bitot's spots, redness and fissuring of eyelid corners (angular palpebritis); dryness of eye membrane (conjunctival xerosis); dull appearance of cornea (corneal xerosis); soft cornea (keratomalacia)
Neck (glands)	Lack of enlargement	Thyroid enlargement
Nails	Firm, pink appearance	Spoon shape (koilonychia); brittleness; ridges
Legs, feet	Lack of tenderness, weakness, or swelling; good color	Edema; tender calf; tingling; weakness
Skeleton	Lack of malformations	Bowlegs; knock-knees; chest deformity at diaphragm; prominent scapulae and ribs

From Williams SR: *Basic nutrition and diet therapy*, ed 11, St. Louis, 2001, Mosby.

tasks that were performed least by nurses. These tasks included development of nutrition plans, reference to diet manuals and research literature, use of nutritional materials in teaching, and use of resources to learn about clients' cultural food habits. A firm knowledge base is important to meet client expectations.

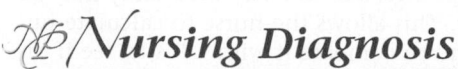

Nursing Diagnosis

Assessment enables the nurse to determine existence of actual or potential nutrition problems (Box 43-6). Knowledge of normal nutrition parameters, anatomy and physiology of the GI system, and cultural, developmen-

Nursing Diagnostic Process

Box *43-6*

Assessment Activities	Defining Characteristics	Nursing Diagnosis
BMI	BMI=37	Imbalanced nutrition: more than body requirements
Obtain height and weight	52-year-old man	
	Height: 5 feet 11 inches	
	Weight: 270 pounds (122.7 kg)	
Obtain 24-hour food history	Lack of satiety	
	High fat and carbohydrate intake, 3 to 4 beers/day	
Fluid	Fluid intake is coke, beer, and juice, all high caloric	
Physical assessment	Short of breath on walking	
	Large abdomen	
	Blood pressure: 125/85 mm Hg	
	Pulse: 102 beats per minute	
	Respirations: 32 breaths per minute	
Laboratory values	Cholesterol and triglycerides elevated. All others within normal limits (WNL).	
Medication	None	
Social	Wife and family eat out or have large family dinners 2 times a week.	

tal, pharmacological, and dietary guidelines is necessary for complete assessment. A problem may occur when overall intake is significantly decreased or increased or when one or more nutrients are not ingested, completely digested, or completely absorbed. Specific nursing diagnoses are related to the actual nutrition problem (e.g., inadequate intake) but may also involve problems that place the client at risk for nutritional deficiencies, such as oral trauma, severe burns, or infections. There are also clinical situations in which clients have multiple related problems. The concept map in Figure 43-7 shows the relationship of nursing diagnoses in a client with myasthenia gravis.

The nursing diagnostic statement is based on defining characteristics present in the assessment database. In addition, the suspected health problem related to the nursing diagnosis is stated. The following are examples of nursing diagnoses that apply to clients with nutritional problems:

- Risk for aspiration in enteral nutrition therapy
- Constipation
- Diarrhea
- Deficient fluid volumes
- Excess fluid volume
- Health maintenance, ineffective
- Health-seeking behaviors (nutrition)
- Risk for infection
- Deficient knowledge (nutrition)
- Ineffective management of therapeutic regimen, individuals
- Imbalanced nutrition: less than body requirements
- Imbalanced nutrition: more than body requirements
- Risk for imbalanced nutrition: more than body requirements
- Feeding self-care deficit

Planning

Planning to maintain optimal nutritional status requires a higher level of care than simply correction of nutritional problems. Synthesis of client information from multiple sources is necessary to devise an individualized approach of care that is relevant to the client's needs (Figure 43-8). Critical thinking application is the best way to ensure that all data sources are considered in developing a client's plan of care. The identification of clients at risk for nutritional problems should result in a care plan that will prevent or minimize nutritional problems (see care plan). Referring to professional standards for nutrition is especially important during this step, because published standards are based on scientific findings.

Goals and Outcomes. Goals and outcomes and priorities of care reflect the client's physiological, therapeutic, and individualized needs. Nutritional education and counseling are important for clients on regular diets to prevent disease and promote health. Clients on therapeutic diets must understand the implications of the diet and how the diet assists in controlling their illness. For example, clients with congestive heart failure who follow a low-sodium diet in conjunction with medication therapy and a prescribed exercise program show improvement in their functional activities (Hunt and others, 2001).

Individualized client planning cannot be overemphasized. For example, obese clients will usually respond better to obtainable goals of smaller weight loss accomplished in a series over time than to one large overwhelming goal (Foster and others, 1997). Mutually planned goals negotiated between the client, dietitian, and nurse will ensure success. For this type of client an overall goal might be

Concept Map

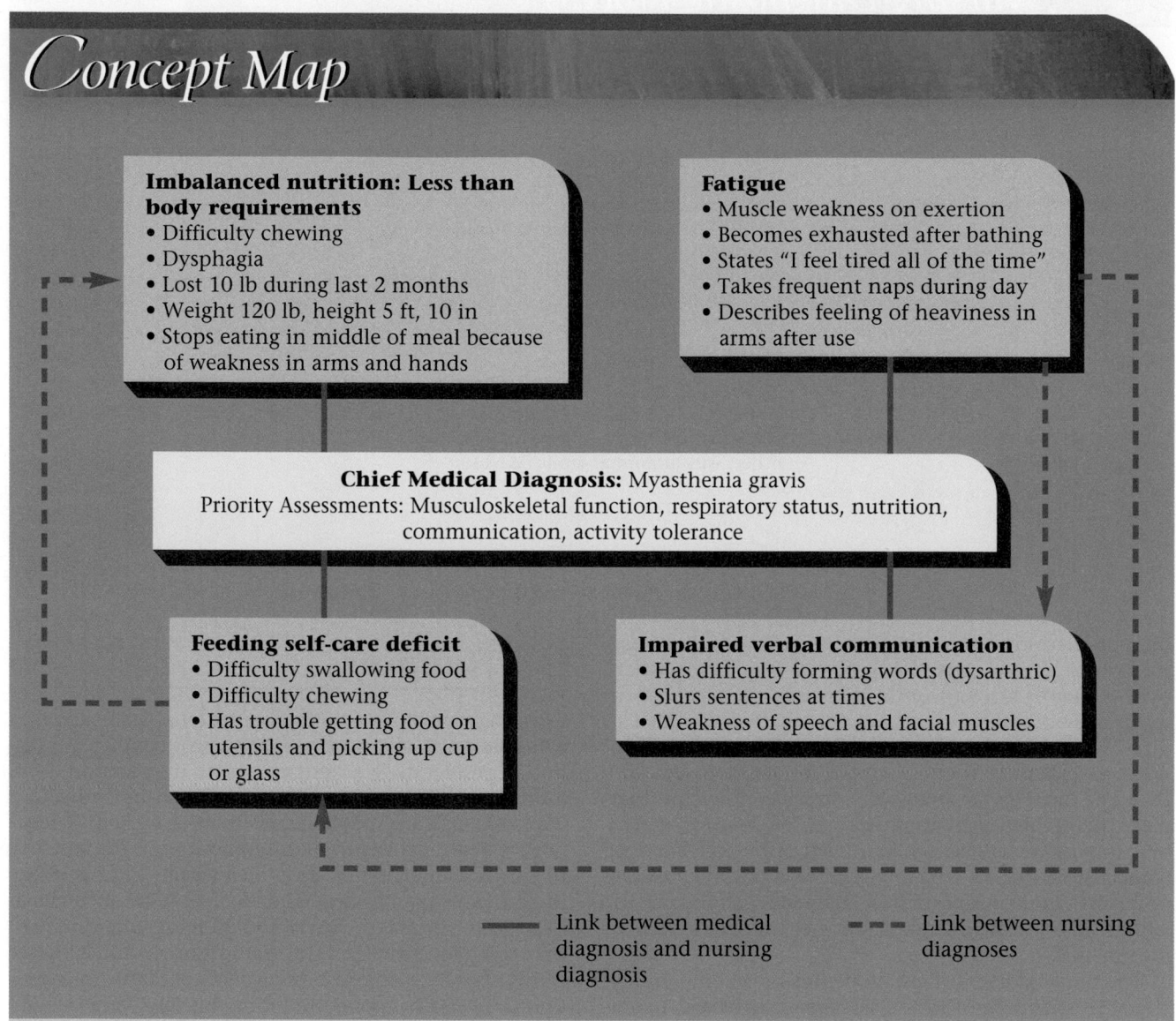

Imbalanced nutrition: Less than body requirements
- Difficulty chewing
- Dysphagia
- Lost 10 lb during last 2 months
- Weight 120 lb, height 5 ft, 10 in
- Stops eating in middle of meal because of weakness in arms and hands

Fatigue
- Muscle weakness on exertion
- Becomes exhausted after bathing
- States "I feel tired all of the time"
- Takes frequent naps during day
- Describes feeling of heaviness in arms after use

Chief Medical Diagnosis: Myasthenia gravis
Priority Assessments: Musculoskeletal function, respiratory status, nutrition, communication, activity tolerance

Feeding self-care deficit
- Difficulty swallowing food
- Difficulty chewing
- Has trouble getting food on utensils and picking up cup or glass

Impaired verbal communication
- Has difficulty forming words (dysarthric)
- Slurs sentences at times
- Weakness of speech and facial muscles

—— Link between medical diagnosis and nursing diagnosis

--- Link between nursing diagnoses

FIGURE **43–7**   Concept map for client with myasthenia gravis.

"Client will achieve appropriate BMI height-weight range or within 10% of IBW." The following outcomes assist in achievement of the goal:
- Client's daily nutritional intake meets the minimal DRIs.
- Client's daily fat nutritional fat intake is less than 30%.
- Client removes sugared beverages from diet.
- Client refrains from eating between meals and after dinner.
- Client loses at least ½ to 1 pound per week.

Meeting nutritional goals requires multidisciplinary input. Knowledge of each discipline's role in provision of nutrition support is necessary to maximize nutritional outcomes. For example, collaboration with a reg-

istered dietitian ensures appropriate nutrition treatment plans. Calorie counts are frequently ordered, and assistance is necessary in obtaining accurate data. A good plan of care requires accurate exchange of information between disciplines.

Setting Priorities. The identification of clients at risk for nutritional problems results in timely interventions to prevent or minimize nutritional problems. Although changes in the client's weight may be gradual, a priority is to improve nutritional intake.

During acute illness or surgery, the intake of food is often altered in the perioperative period. The priority of care may be to provide optimal preoperative nutrition support in clients with malnutrition. The priority for the

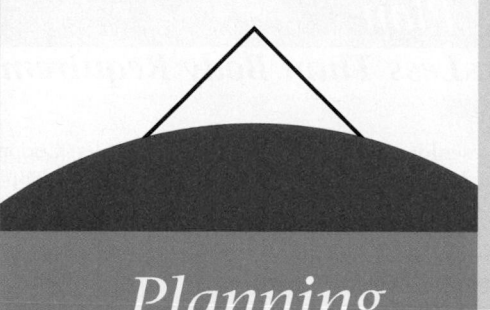

KNOWLEDGE

- Role of dietitians/nutrition-ists in caring for clients with altered nutrition
- Impact of community support groups/resources in assisting clients to manage nutrition
- Impact of bad diets on clients' nutritional status

EXPERIENCE

- Previous client responses to nursing interventions for altered nutrition
- Personal experiences with dietary change strategies (what worked and what did not)

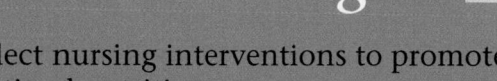

Planning

- Select nursing interventions to promote optimal nutrition
- Select nursing interventions consistent with therapeutic diets
- Consult with other health care professionals (e.g., dieticians, nutritionists, physicians, pharmacists, and physical and occupational therapists) to adopt interventions that reflect the client's needs
- Involve family when designing interventions

STANDARDS

- Individualize therapy according to client needs
- Select therapies consistent with established standards of normal nutrition (e.g., USDA, FDA, WHO, HWC)
- Select therapies consistent with established standards for therapeutic diets (e.g., AHA, ADA, ASREP)

ATTITUDES

- Display confidence in selecting interventions
- Creatively adapt interventions for the client's physical limitations, culture, personal preferences, budget, and home care needs

FIGURE 43–8 Critical thinking model for nutrition evaluation.

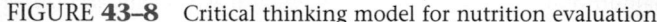

resumption of food intake postoperatively is dependent upon the return of bowel function, the extent of the surgical procedure, and the presence of any complications (see Chapter 49).

In another example, when clients have had oral and throat surgery they must chew and swallow food in the presence of excision sites, sutures, or otherwise manipulated tissue. The priority of care may be to first provide comfort and pain control. Then the nurse can address nutritional priorities and plan care to maintain nutrition and not cause pain or injury to the healing tissues.

The client and family need to collaborate with the nurse in the planning of care and setting of priorities. This is important because food purchase and preparation may involve the family and the plan of care may not suc-

ceed without their commitment to, involvement in, and understanding of the nutritional priorities.

Continuity of Care. The continuity of care extends beyond the hospital setting, and it is important that discharge planning extend the nutritional interventions as clients return to their home or extended care facilities. Client nutritional needs often extend beyond the acute, hospital setting. Enteral tube feedings can be administered into the stomach or intestines via a tube inserted through the nose or a percutaneous access (see Skill 43-2, p. 1305 and Skill 43-3, p. 1309). These enteral feedings often supplement the client's oral nutritional intake in the home or rehabilitation setting. In these extended settings, the dietitian monitors the client's nutritional status and intake and

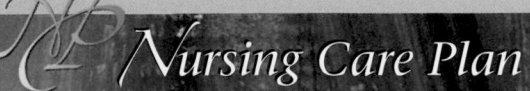

Nursing Care Plan

Imbalanced Nutrition: Less Than Body Requirements

Assessment

Ms. Maria Diaz, a nurse practitioner in a senior citizens' center is seeing Mrs. Cooper, who is 68 years old and has a history of congestive heart failure. Recently Mrs. Cooper noticed a weight loss (15%). Three months have passed since Mrs. Cooper had been started on sertraline for depression related to the loss of her husband 6 months ago. This was an initial episode of de-

pression. Mrs. Cooper had also been referred for counseling 3 months ago for help with grief and depression through a local senior service agency. When Maria inquired as to her financial situation, Mrs. Cooper responded that it was tight living on a small pension and Social Security, but she was able to manage.

Assessment Activities	Findings/Defining Characteristics
Ask Mrs. Cooper about her food intake during the last 2 days.	She responds that she drinks some juice in the morning and two or three cups of coffee. In addition, she may have a sandwich in the late afternoon. "I'm just not interested in food. It has no taste."
Ask Mrs. Cooper about social interaction.	Mrs. Cooper complains of loneliness and said she does not get out much, although her psychologist recommended more socializing. Her friends at church call her to come back to meetings, but she is just not ready. She says she tires easily.
Weigh client and assess posture.	Her weight is 20% below her IBW, and she had a low BMI of 17. This weight loss had occurred in 6 months' time, down 24 pounds. Stooped posture
Observe Mrs. Cooper for signs of poor nutrition.	Dull, thinning hair Dry scaling skin Pale conjunctivae and mucous membranes
Palpate muscles and extremities.	2+ bilateral pitting ankle edema Generalized poor muscle tone

Nursing Diagnosis: Imbalanced nutrition: less than body requirements related to a decreased ability to ingest food as a result of depression.

Planning

Goals	Expected Outcomes*
	Weight Control
Client will progressively gain weight.	Client will gain 1 to 2 pounds per month until goal of 130 pounds is reached.
	Nutritional Status: Nutrient Intake
Client will consume adequate nourishment each day.	Client will ingest 1900 kcal/day, including 50 g of protein per day.
Client will exhibit no signs of malnutrition.	Physical assessment and laboratory values will be within normal limits.

*Outcome classification labels from Moorhead S, Johnson M, Maas M: *Nursing outcomes classification (NOC)*, ed 3, St. Louis, 2004, Mosby.

Interventions†	Rationale
Nutritional Counseling	
• Coordinate plan of care with physician, psychologist, client, and dietitian.	Successful nutrition care planning is a multidisciplinary approach throughout the continuum of care (Chen and others, 2001).
• Individualize menu plans.	Individualized meal planning is more useful to the client.
• Frequent small meals.	Frequent small meals offset early satiety.
• Review food pyramid.	USDA (1996) and *Healthy People 2010* recommendations for food selections provide optimal nutrition (USDA, 2002).

†Intervention classification labels from Dochterman JM, Bulechek GM: *Nursing interventions classification (NIC)*, ed 4, St. Louis, 2004, Mosby.

Continued

Nursing Care Plan

Risk for Injury—cont'd

Interventions†—cont'd

Nutritional Monitoring

- Monitor client monthly for weight gain, anemia, serum albumin level, and total lymphocyte count (TLC).

- Perform physical assessment of hair, eyes, mouth, skin, and muscle tone.

Nutritional Management

- Encourage client to eat small meals and to increase dietary intake and to help off set anorexia secondary to sertraline.

- Encourage fluid intake.

- Encourage fiber intake.
- Consult with client about referral for congregate meals (lunch at senior center) 5 times per week.

Rationale

Weight gain should be slow and progressive. Serum albumin of 4.0 g/100 ml and TLC 1500/mm³ are within normal limits (Grodner, Anderson, and DeYoung, 2000).
Provides progressive monitoring for improved nutritional status

Sertraline is an SSRI medication, which caused diminished taste and anorexia. Frequent small meals helps to reduce anorexia-associated weight loss.
Older adults need eight 8-ounce glasses per day of fluid from beverage and food sources. Concentrating intake in morning and early afternoon is acceptable to prevent nocturia (Lueckenotte, 2000).
Adequate fluid, fiber, and exercise deter constipation.
Congregate meal participation would encourage good nutrition and promote socialization with peers (Millen and others, 2001).

†Intervention classification labels from Dochterman JM, Bulechek GM: *Nursing interventions classification (NIC)*, ed 4, St. Louis, 2004, Mosby.

Evaluation

Nursing Actions	Client Response/Finding	Achievement of Outcome
Ask Mrs. Cooper to review her diet for the last 2 to 3 days.	Client responds that she ate her main meal at the senior center, has fruit and grain-fiber for breakfast, and in the evening either has soup or a sandwich with fruit.	Mrs. Cooper is selecting more nutritionally rich foods, consistent with current guidelines.
Observe client's appearance.	Skin is less pale, hair appears to be in better condition and styled. Ankle edema is present, but less than 1+.	Mrs. Cooper has improved physical parameters of nutrition, still needs follow-up.
Weigh client.	Weight gain of 4 pounds in 4 weeks.	Weight gain is steady; client is still below ideal body weight.
Ask client about appetite and energy level.	Mrs. Cooper responds that on days she eats at the senior center her appetite seems better and she "wants to do more things." She notes that weekends are very lonely.	Weekday support for nutritional status appears effective, needs to increase client's activity status and nutritional intake during weekends.

---

makes recommendations for changes, based primarily upon data documented in the client's chart. Dietitians are expert in choice of enteral formulas and dietary modifications required for specific disease states.

When parenteral nutrition (PN), a solution consisting of glucose, amino acids, lipids, minerals, electrolytes, trace elements, and vitamins, is needed, it is given through an indwelling peripheral or central venous catheter (see Chapter 40). The pharmacist is expert in drug-nutrient interactions and mixture of total parenteral nutrition (TPN).

When clients require continuing care in the restorative care setting, occupational therapists work with clients and families to identify assistive devices. Devices such as utensils with large handles and plates with elevated sides assist a client with self-feeding. A speech therapist can as-

sist a client with swallowing exercises and techniques to reduce the risk of aspiration. Home therapists can also help clients maintain function in the home setting by rearranging food preparation areas in an effort to maximize the client's functional capacity.

Implementation

Ill or debilitated clients often have poor appetites **(anorexia).** The ketosis that accompanies starvation is an appetite suppressant, and surgical procedures and trauma cause pain. Deficiencies in certain vitamins and minerals can cause anorexia. Nurses can help clients to understand the factors that cause anorexia and use cre-

Table 43-6	Metabolic Responses to Severe Stress	
Ebb Phase (onset)	**Flow Phase (36-48 hours post injury)**
Decreased oxygen consumption	Increased oxygen consumption
Normal or increased cardiac output	Increased cardiac output
Hypothermia	Increased nitrogen excretion
Decreased insulin levels	Elevated insulin levels
Hyperglycemia	Hyperglycemia
Hypovolemia	
Hypotension	Normal lactate
Increased lactate	
Normal free fatty acids	Increased free fatty acids
Increased cortisol	Decreased cortisol
	Hyperthermia
	Increased gluconeogenesis

From Grodner M, Anderson S, DeYoung S: *Foundations and clinical applications of nutrition: a nursing approach,* ed 2, St. Louis, 2000, Mosby.

ative approaches to stimulate appetite. During hospitalizations diagnostic testing disrupts many mealtimes or requires nothing by mouth (NPO) status before tests. Clients worried about families, finances, employment, or illnesses are often not able to eat an adequate diet. Both physiological stress due to illness and emotional stress influence dietary need and intake (Table 43-6). Medications may interfere with taste, cause nausea, interfere with absorption, or affect metabolism (see Table 43-2, p. 1283).

Health Promotion. Nurses are in a key position to educate clients about good nutrition habits. Incorporating knowledge of nutrition into lifestyle serves as prevention against the development of many diseases. Outpatient and community-based settings may be optimal locations for nursing assessment of nutritional practices and status. Early identification of potential or actual problems is the best way to avoid more serious problems. Similarly, in other health care settings, clients with nutritional problems such as obesity may require assistance in menu planning and compliance strategies. The nurse's role as educator often includes educating families and providing information about community resources. A means, such as telephone numbers, of contacting a dietitian or nurse for follow-up questions should always be part of counseling.

Meal planning must take into account the family's budget and different preferences of family members. Specific foods are chosen on the basis of the dietary prescription and food groups. For families on limited budgets, substitutes can be used. For example, bean or cheese dishes can often replace meat in a meal, and evaporated milk or dry skim milk can be used for cooking. The method of preparation may also be modified when it is necessary to minimize certain substances. Baking rather than frying reduces fat intake, and lemon juice or spices can be used to add flavor to low-sodium diets.

Planning menus a week in advance has several benefits. It helps ensure good nutrition or compliance with a specific diet and helps the family stay within the allotted budget. Menus may in turn be checked by a nurse or dietitian for content. Often a simple tip can be of value in meal planning, such as advice to avoid grocery shopping when hungry, which can lead to spontaneous purchases of more expensive or less nutritional foods that are not included in meal plans. The USDA (2000) provides sample weekly meal planning services for a range of sample budgets accessible on the USDA website.

Safety Alert. Food safety is also an important public health issue. Food-borne bacteria can occur from improper food cleansing, preparation, or poor hygiene practices of food workers. Health care professionals not only need to be aware of the factors related to food safety but should also provide client education to reduce the risks for food-borne illnesses (Table 43-7, Box 43-7).

Acute Care. The nutritional care of acutely ill clients requires the nurse to consider a variety of factors that influence nutritional intake. Ill or debilitated clients frequently have poor appetites. In addition, diagnostic testing and procedures in the acute care setting is another disruptive influence on intake. Frequently as preparation for or immediately following a diagnostic procedure the client is NPO. The mealtimes in a health care setting are interrupted, or the client is too fatigued or may be too uncomfortable to eat. It is important that the nurse continuously assess the client's nutritional status and adopt interventions that promote normal intake, digestion, and metabolism of nutrients. Clients who are NPO and receive only standard IV fluids for more than 4 to 7 days are at nutritional risk.

Advancing Diets. Acute and chronic conditions affect the client's immune system and in turn can affect the client's nutritional status. Clients who have conditions, such as human immunodeficiency virus (HIV) infections or cancers, or treatments, such as cancer chemotherapy or post–organ transplant chemotherapy, may have a decreased immune function. As a result, these clients may require nutritional supplements or diets that are higher in selected nutrients. Table 43-8 gives an overview of the immune system, the malnutrition impact, and what nutrients are beneficial. In addition, clients who are ill, who have had surgical procedures, or who were NPO for a period of time have specialized dietary needs. They may have a gradual progression of dietary intake or need therapeutic diets to manage their illness. Box 43-8 lists the diets commonly used in health care settings.

Promoting Appetite. Providing an environment conducive to nutritional intake includes keeping the client's environment free of odors, providing oral hygiene as needed to remove unpleasant tastes, and maintaining client comfort. In addition, certain medications can affect dietary intake and nutrient use. For example, medications such as insulin, glucocorticoids, and thyroid hormones affect metabolism. Other medications, such as antifungal

Table *43-7* Food Safety

Food-Borne Disease	Organism	Food Source	Symptoms*
Botulism	*C. botulinum*	Improperly home-canned foods, smoked and salted fish, ham, sausage, shellfish	Symptoms are varied from mild discomfort to death in 24 hours, initially nausea and dizziness, progressing to motor (respiratory) paralysis
Escherichia coli	*Escherichia coli* 0157:H7	Undercooked meat (ground beef)	Severe cramps, nausea, vomiting, diarrhea (may be bloody), renal failure. Appears 1-8 days after eating, lasts 1-7 days
Listeriosis	*Listeria* *L. monocytogenes*	Soft cheese, meat (hot dogs, pate, lunch meats), unpasteurized milk, poultry, seafood	Severe diarrhea, fever, headache, pneumonia, meningitis, endocarditis. Appears 3-21 days after infection
Perfringens enteritis	*Clostridium* *C. perfringens*	Cooked meats, meat dishes held at room or warm temperature	Mild diarrhea, vomiting. Appears 8-24 hours after eating, lasts 1-2 days
Salmonellosis	*Salmonella* *S. typhi* *S. paratyphi*	Milk, custards, egg dishes, salad dressings, sandwich fillings, polluted shellfish	Mild to severe diarrhea, cramps, vomiting. Appears 12 to 24 hours after ingestion, lasts 1-7 days
Shigellosis	*Shigella* *S. dysenteriae*	Milk, milk products, seafood, salads	Mild diarrhea to fatal dysentery. Appears 7-36 hours after ingestion; lasts 3-14 days.
Staphylococcus	*Staphylococcus* *S. aureus*	Custards, cream fillings, processed meats, ham, cheese, ice cream, potato salad, sauces, casseroles	Severe abdominal cramps, pain, vomiting, diarrhea, perspiration, headache, fever, prostration. Appears 1-6 hours after ingestion, lasts 1-2 days

From Williams SR: *Basic nutrition and diet therapy,* ed 11, St. Louis, 2001, Mosby.
*Symptoms are generally most severe for youngest and oldest age-groups.

Client Teaching

Box 43-7

Food Safety

Objectives

- Client will be able to verbalize measures to protect from food-borne illness.
- Client will understand the primary types of illness and how they are transmitted.
- Client will not experience food-borne illness.

Teaching Strategies

- Explain that food safety has become an important public health issue in recent years. Populations particularly at risk are older and younger persons, as well as immunosuppressed individuals.
- Instruct clients on the following:
  - Wash hands with hot, soapy water before touching or eating food.
  - Cook meat, poultry, fish, and eggs until they are well done.
- Wash fresh fruits and vegetables thoroughly.
- Do not eat raw meats or unpasteurized milk.
- Do not buy or consume food that has passed the expiration date.
- Keep foods properly refrigerated at 40° F and frozen at 0° F.
- Wash dishes and cutting boards with hot soapy water.
- Do not save leftovers for more than 2 days in refrigerator.
- Wash dishrags, towels, and sponges regularly, or use paper towels.
- Clean the inside of refrigerator and microwave regularly to prevent microbial growth.

Evaluation

- Ask client to verbalize measures to prevent food-borne illnesses.
- Observe the client at home for safe practices, if making home visit.

Modified from Keithley JK, Swanson B: Minimizing HIV/AIDS malnutrition, *Medsurg Nurs* 7(5):256, 1998.

---

agents, can affect taste. Some of the psychotropic medications affect appetite, cause nausea, and may also alter taste. Sometimes the nurse and dietitian can help the client to select foods that can reduce the altered taste sensations or nausea. In other situations the medication may need to be changed. Assessing clients for the need for pharmacological agents to stimulate appetite such as cyproheptadine (Periactin), megestrol (Megace), or dron-

abinol (Marinol) or to manage symptoms that interfere with nutrition may require physician consultation.

Assisting Clients With Feeding. When clients need assistance with eating, it important to protect the client's safety, independence, and dignity. The nurse should assess the client's risk of aspiration. Clients at high risk for aspiration are those clients with decreased level of alert-

Table 43-8   **Nutrition and the Immune System**

Immune/Physiological Component	Malnutrition Effect	Vital Nutrient
Antibodies	Decreased amount	Protein, vitamins A, C, B_{12}, B_6, folic acid, thiamin, biotin, riboflavin, niacin
GI tract	Translocation of bacteria to systemic bodily areas	Arginine, glutamine, omega-3 fatty acids
Granulocytes and macrocytes	Longer time for phagocytosis kill time and lymphocyte activation	Protein, vitamins A, C, B_{12}, B_6, folic acid, thiamin, riboflavin, niacin, zinc, iron
Mucus	Flat microvilli in GI tract, decreased antibody secretion	Vitamins B_{12}, B_6, C, biotin
Skin	Integrity compromised, density reduced, wound healing slowed	Protein, vitamins A, B_{12}, C, niacin, copper, zinc
T-lymphocytes	Depressed T-cell distribution	Protein, arginine, iron, zinc, omega-3 fatty acids, vitamins A, B_{12}, B_6, folic acid, thiamin, riboflavin, niacin, pantothenic acid

Total Lymphocyte Count (TLC)

TLC = % lymphocytes $\times$ WBC count $\div$ 100*

Modified from Grodner M, Anderson S, DeYoung S: *Foundations and clinical applications of nutrition: a nursing approach,* ed 2, St. Louis, 2000, Mosby.

*Results <2000 cells/mm^3 suggest impaired immunocompetence; results <1500 cells/mm^3 are associated with greater morbidity and mortality.

Box 43-8   **Diet Progression and Therapeutic Diets**

Clear Liquid

Broth, bouillon, coffee, tea, carbonated beverages, clear fruit juices, gelatin, Popsicles

Full Liquid

As above with addition of smooth-textured dairy products, custards, refined cooked cereals, vegetable juice, pureed vegetables, all fruit juices

Pureed

All of above with addition of scrambled eggs, pureed meats, vegetables, fruits, mashed potatoes and gravy

Mechanical Soft

All of above with addition of ground or finely diced meats, flaked fish, cottage cheese, cheese, rice, potatoes, pancakes, light breads, cooked vegetables, cooked or canned fruits, bananas, soups, peanut butter

Soft/Low Residue

Addition of low-fiber, easily digested foods, such as pastas, casseroles, moist tender meats, and canned cooked fruits and vegetables. Desserts, cakes, and cookies without nuts or coconut

High Fiber

Addition of fresh uncooked fruits, steamed vegetables, bran, oatmeal, and dried fruits

Low Sodium

4 g (no added salt), 2 g, 1 g, or 500 mg sodium diets. These diets vary from no added salt to severe sodium restriction (500 mg sodium diet) that requires selective food purchases.

Low Cholesterol

300 mg/day cholesterol, in keeping with AHA guidelines for serum lipid reduction

Diabetic

Recommended food exchanges by the American Diabetic Association. Usually the caloric recommendations are around 1800 calories. The exchange diet results in a balanced intake of carbohydrates, fats, and proteins. The total calories may vary to accommodate the client's metabolic demands, which may be affected by an exercise program, pregnancy, or in some situations another illness.

Regular

No restrictions, unless specified

ness, decreased gag and/or cough reflexes, and clients who have difficulty managing saliva (see assessment section of this chapter).

Clients at risk for aspiration need more assistance with feeding and swallowing. The client should be positioned in an upright, seated position. If the client has unilateral weakness, teach the client and caregiver to place food in the stronger side of the mouth. Thicker fluids are easier to swallow, and the client should not use a straw (Galvin, 2001). In addition, the rate of feeding is slower, and more frequent chewing and swallowing assessments throughout the meal are needed. In some cases, a speech therapist needs to evaluate the client's ability to swallow and this therapist is valuable in teaching the client how to swallow safely.

Clients with visual deficits also need special assistance. For example, clients with decreased vision may be able to independently feed themselves if adequate information is given. Identify the food location on the plate as if it were a clock (e.g., meat at 9 o'clock and vegetable at 3 o'clock). Tell the client where the beverages are located in relation to the plate. Be sure other care providers set the meal tray and plate in the same manner. Clients with impaired vision, as well as those clients with decreased motor skill, may be more independent during mealtimes with the use of large-handled adaptive utensils. These are easier to grip and manipulate.

Provide opportunities for clients to direct the order in which they want to eat the food items, as well as the speed at which they wish to eat. Determine the client's food preferences, and, unless contraindicated, try to have these items included on the client's dietary tray. If the client requests the food to be warmer or cooler, try to meet this need. These seem like small items, but they may go a long way in maintaining some of the client's sense of independence.

Clients need to protect their clothes and bedding with napkins or towels, and these items should not be referred to as a "bib." Likewise, mealtime is usually a social activity; instruct other nurses or care providers to converse and engage the client in a conversation. Mealtime is an excellent opportunity for client education. The nurse can instruct the client about any therapeutic diets, medications, energy conservation measures, or adaptive devices to assist the client in independently feeding.

Enteral Tube Feeding. **Enteral nutrition (EN)** refers to nutrients given via the GI tract. Enteral nutrition is the preferred method of meeting nutritional needs if the client's GI tract is functioning by providing physiological, safe, and economical nutritional support. Enterally fed clients receive formula via nasogastric, jejunal, or gastric tubes. Gastric feedings may be given to clients with a low risk of aspiration; however, if there is a risk of aspiration, jejunal feeding is preferred. Box 43-9 lists indications for tube feeding. In addition, enteral tube feedings are easily given in the home setting by either the nurse or the family. The nurse inserts the enteral tube, and verification of tube placement by x-ray examination must occur before the client receives the first enteral feeding (Skill 43-1).

Text continued on p. 1304

Box *43-9* Indications for Enteral and Parenteral Nutrition

Enteral Nutrition	**Parenteral Nutrition**
Cancer Head and neck Upper GI Critical illness/trauma	**Nonfunctional GI Tract** Massive small bowel resection/GI surgery Paralytic ileus Intestinal obstruction Trauma to abdomen, head, or neck Severe malabsorption Intolerance to enteral feeding (established by trial) Chemotherapy, radiation therapy, bone marrow transplantation
Neurological and Muscular Disorders Brain neoplasm Cerebrovascular accident Dementia Myopathy Parkinson's disease	
Gastrointestinal Disorders Enterocutaneous fistula Inflammatory bowel disease Mild pancreatitis	**Extended Bowel Rest** Enterocutaneous fistula Inflammatory bowel disease exacerbation Severe diarrhea Moderate to severe pancreatitis
Respiratory Failure With Prolonged Intubation **Inadequate Oral Intake** Continuous feedings Supine positioning Cerebral vascular accident Local trauma Anorexia nervosa Difficulty chewing, swallowing Severe depression	**Preoperative TPN** Preoperative bowel rest Treatment for comorbid severe malnutrition in clients with nonfunctional GI tracts Severely catabolic clients when GI tract nonusable for >4 to 5 days

View Video

Inserting a Small-Bore Nasoenteric Tube for Enteral Feedings

Skill 43-1

Delegation Considerations

This skill requires problem solving and knowledge application unique to a professional nurse. For this reason, delegation of this skill to assistive personnel is inappropriate.

Equipment

- Nasogastric or nasointestinal tube (8 to 12 Fr) with guide wire or stylet
- Stethoscope
- 60-ml or larger Luer-Lok or catheter-tip syringe
- Hypoallergenic tape and tincture of benzoin or tube fixation device

- pH indicator strip (scale 0.0 to 14.0)
- Glass of water and straw
- Emesis basin
- Safety pin
- Rubber band
- Towel
- Facial tissues
- Clean gloves
- Suction equipment in case of aspiration
- Penlight to check placement in nasopharynx
- Tongue blade

Steps	Rationale
1. Assess client for the need for enteral tube feeding: NPO or insufficient intake for more than 5 days, functional GI tract, unable to ingest sufficient nutrients.	Identifying clients who need tube feedings before they become nutritionally depleted may help to prevent complications related to malnutrition.
2. Perform hand hygiene. Assess patency of nares. Have client close each nostril alternately and breathe. Examine each naris for patency and skin breakdown.	Evaluates nares for patency. Nares may be obstructed or irritated, or septal defect may be present.
3. Assess for gag reflex. Place tongue blade in client's mouth, touching uvula to induce a gag response.	Identifies ability to swallow and determines if there is a risk for aspiration.

Critical Decision Point: Clients with impaired level of consciousness may also have impaired gag reflex, and their risk of aspiration is increased during this type of procedure and subsequent tube feedings.

4. Review client's medical history for nasal problems (e.g., nosebleeds, oral facial surgery; past history of aspiration, or anticoagulation therapy).	Nasoenteric tubes are contraindicated in clients with recent nasal surgery, facial traumas, nosebleeds, and receiving anticoagulation. This includes clients with surgical procedures requiring a transphenoid approach used to remove pituitary tumors, because there is a risk for improper tube placement (Metheny, 2002).
5. Review physician's order for type of tube and enteral feeding schedule.	Procedure and tube feedings require a physician's order.
6. Auscultate abdomen for bowel sounds	Absence of bowel sounds may indicate decreased or absent peristalsis and increased risk for aspiration and/or abdominal distention.
7. Perform hand hygiene.	Reduces transfer of microorganisms.
8. Explain procedure to client and how to communicate during intubation by raising index finger to indicate gagging or discomfort.	Reduces anxiety and helps client to assist in insertion.
9. Stand on same side of bed as naris for insertion, and assist client to high-Fowler's position unless contraindicated. Place pillow behind head and shoulders.	Allows easier manipulation of tube. Fowler's position reduces risk of aspiration and promotes effective swallowing.
10. Place bath towel over chest. Keep facial tissues within reach.	Prevents soiling of gown. Insertion of tube may produce tearing.
11. Determine length of tube to be inserted and mark with tape:	Length approximates distance from nose to stomach in 98% of clients. For duodenal or jejunal placement, an additional 20 to 30 cm is required.
a. Traditional method: measure distance from tip of nose to earlobe to xiphoid process of sternum (see illustration).	

Steps	Rationale

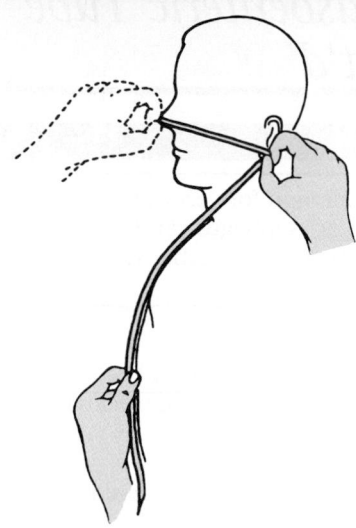

STEP **11a**   Determine length of tube to be inserted.

12. Prepare nasogastric or nasointestinal tube for intubation:

a. Plastic tubes should not be iced.

Tubes will become stiff and inflexible, causing trauma to mucous membranes.

b. Inject 10 ml of water from 30-ml or larger Luer-Lok or catheter-tip syringe into the tube.

Aids in guide wire or stylet insertion.

c. Make certain that guide wire is securely positioned against weighted tip and that both Luer-Lok connections are snugly fitted together.

Promotes smooth passage of tube into GI tract. Improperly positioned stylet can induce serious trauma.

13. Cut tape 10 cm (4 inches) long or prepare tube fixation device.

To be used to anchor tubing following insertion.

14. Put on clean gloves.

Reduces transmission of microorganisms.

15. Dip tube with surface lubricant into glass of water.

Activates lubricant to facilitate passage of tube into naris to GI tract.

16. Insert tube through nostril to back of throat (posterior nasopharynx). Aim back and down toward ear.

Natural contour facilitates passage of tube into GI tract and reduces gagging by client.

17. Have client flex head toward chest after tube has passed through nasopharynx.

Closes off glottis and reduces risk of tube entering trachea.

Critical Decision Point: Encourage client to swallow by giving small sips of water or ice chips when possible. Advance tube as client swallows. Rotate tube 180 degrees while inserting.

---

18. Emphasize need to mouth breathe and swallow during the procedure.

Helps facilitate passage of tube and alleviates client's fears during the procedure.

19. When tip of tube reaches the carina (about 25 cm [10 inches] in an adult), stop, hold end of tube near ear and listen for air exchange from the distal portion of the tube.

If air is heard, the tube could be in the respiratory tract; remove tube and start over. This step should never be used for tube verification (Metheny and Titler, 2001).

20. Advance tube each time client swallows until desired length has been passed.

Reduces discomfort and trauma to client.

Critical Decision Point: Do not force tube. If resistance is met or client starts to cough, choke, or become cyanotic, stop advancing the tube and pull tube back.

---

21. Check for position of tube in back of throat with penlight and tongue blade.

Tube may be coiled, kinked, or entering trachea.

22. Perform measures to verify placement of tube (see Box 43-10, p. 1312):

Skill 43-1 | *Inserting a Small-Bore Nasoenteric Tube for Enteral Feedings—cont'd*

Steps	Rationale

Critical Decision Point: Auscultation is no longer considered a reliable method for verification of tube placement because a tube inadvertently placed in the lungs, pharynx, or esophagus can transmit a sound similar to that of air entering the stomach (Metheny and others, 1990b; Metheny, Titler, 2001; Chang and others, 1982).

Steps	Rationale
23. After gastric aspirates are obtained, anchor tube to nose and avoid pressure on nares. Mark exit site with indelible ink. Select one of the following options.	A properly secured tube allows the client more mobility and prevents trauma to nasal mucosa.
a. Apply tape	
(1) Apply tincture of benzoin or other skin adhesive on tip of client's nose and tube and allow it to become "tacky."	Helps tape adhere better. Protects skin.
(2) Remove gloves and split one end of tape lengthwise 5 cm (2 inches).	
(3) Place the intact end of tape over bridge of client's nose. Wrap each of the 5-cm strips around tube as it exits nose (see illustration).	Securing tape to nares prevents tissue necrosis.
b. Apply tube fixation device using shaped adhesive patch.	Secures tube and reduces friction on naris.
(1) Apply wide end of patch to bridge of nose (see illustration).	
(2) Slip connector around tube as it exits nose (see illustration).	
24. Fasten end of nasogastric tube to client's gown by looping rubber band around tube in slipknot. Pin rubber band to gown (see illustration).	Reduces traction on the naris if tube moves.
25. For intestinal placement, position client on right side when possible until radiological confirmation of correct placement has been verified. Remove gloves, perform hand hygiene, and assist client to a comfortable position.	Promotes passage of the tube into the small intestine (duodenum or jejunum).

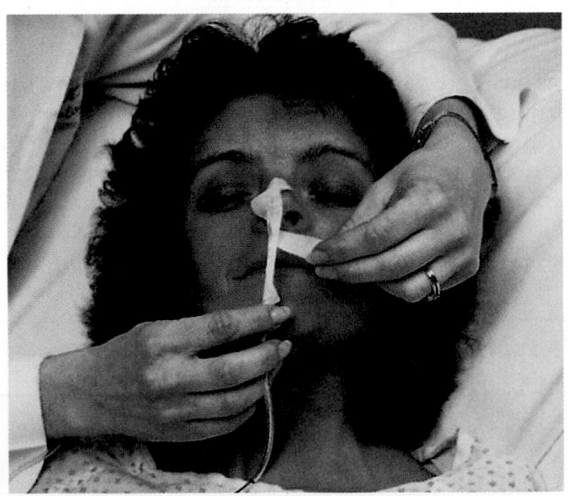

STEP **23a(3)**   Wrapping tape to anchor nasoenteral tube.

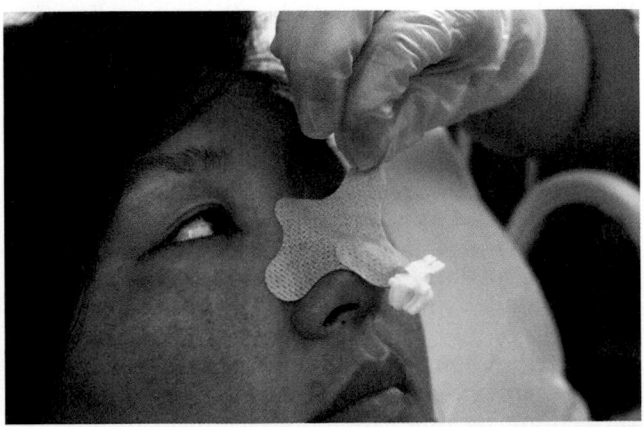

STEP **23b(1)**   Applying patch to bridge of nose.

Steps	Rationale

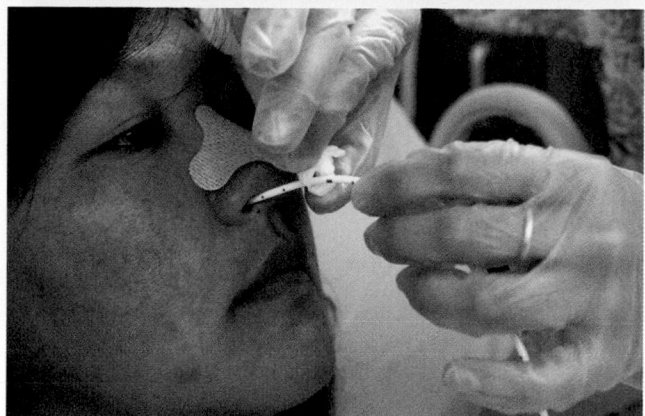

STEP **23b(2)** Slip connector around feeding tube.

STEP **24** Fastening feeding tube to client's gown.

Critical Decision Point: Leave guide wire or stylet in place until correct position is ensured by x-ray film. Never attempt to reinsert partially or fully removed guide wire or stylet while feeding tube is in place.

---

26. Obtain x-ray film of abdomen.	Placement of tube is verified by x-ray examination (Metheny and others, 1988; Metheny and Titler, 2001).
27. Apply clean gloves, and administer oral hygiene (see Chapter 38). Cleanse tubing at nostril.	Promotes client comfort and integrity of oral mucous membranes.
28. Remove gloves, dispose of equipment, and perform hand hygiene.	Reduces transmission of microorganisms.
29. Inspect naris and oropharynx for any irritation after insertion.	If insertion was difficult, irritation of naris or oropharynx may have occurred.
30. Ask if client feels comfortable.	Evaluates client's level of comfort.
31. Observe client for any difficulty breathing, coughing, or gagging.	Malposition of the tube may cause these symptoms.
32. Auscultate lung sounds.	Abnormal lung sounds can be an early sign of aspiration.

Unexpected Outcomes and Related Interventions

1. Aspiration of stomach contents into the respiratory tract (immediate response), evidenced by coughing, dyspnea, cyanosis, auscultation of crackles or wheezes
   a. Position client on side.
   b. Suction nasotracheally and oral tracheally.
   c. Consult physician immediately to order chest x-ray examination.
2. Aspiration of stomach contents into respiratory tract (delayed response), evidenced by dyspnea, fever, auscultation of crackles or wheezes
   a. Consult physician to obtain order for chest x-ray film.
   b. Prepare for possible initiation of antibiotics.
3. Displacement of feeding tube to another site (e.g., from duodenum to stomach, mark at exit site if tube is moved); may occur when client coughs or vomits
   a. Aspirate GI contents and measure pH (Metheny and Titler, 2001).

   b. Remove displaced tube and insert and verify placement of new tube.
   c. If there is a question of aspiration, obtain chest x-ray film.
4. Clogging of feeding tube
   a. Aspirate gastric contents to assess patency of tube.
   b. Irrigate tube.
5. Irritation of naris or nasal mucosa
   a. Provide hygiene and remove and replace tape.
   b. Consider removing tube and inserting into other naris (physician order required).

Recording and Reporting

• Record and report type and size of tube placed, location of distal tip of tube, client's tolerance of procedure, pH value, and confirmation of tube position by x-ray examination.

Enteral formulas are usually one of four types. Polymeric (1.0 to 2.0 kcal/ml) include milk-based blenderized foods prepared by hospital dietary staff or in the client home. The polymeric classification also includes commercially prepared whole nutrient formulas. For this type of formula to be effective, the client's gastrointestinal tract must be able to absorb whole nutrients. The second type, modular formulas (3.8 to 4.0 kcal/ml), are single macronutrient (e.g., protein, glucose, polymers, or lipids) preparations and are not nutritionally complete. This type of formula is added to other foods for meeting the client's individual nutritional needs. The third type, elemental (1.0 to 3.0 kcal/ml) formulas, contain predigested nutrients that are easier for a partially dysfunctional gastrointestinal tract to absorb. The last type are the specialty (1.0 to 2.0 kcal/ml) formulas that are designed to meet specific nutritional needs in certain illness (e.g., liver failure, pulmonary disease, or HIV infection).

Tube feedings are typically started at full strength at slow rates (see Skill 43-2, Box 43-12, p. 1308). The hourly rate is increased every 12 to 24 hours if no signs of intolerance appear (nausea, cramping, vomiting, diarrhea). Studies have demonstrated a beneficial effect of enteral feedings compared with parenteral nutrition. Feeding by the enteral route may reduce sepsis, blunt the hypermetabolic response to trauma, and maintain intestinal structure and function (Guenter, Ericson, and Jones, 1997; ASPEN, 2002). Enteral nutrition has been used successfully within 24 to 48 hours after surgery or trauma to provide fluids, electrolytes, and nutritional support. Gastric ileus may prevent nasogastric feedings, whereas nasointestinal or jejunal tubes allow successful postpyloric feeding, where formula is placed directly into the small intestine or jejunum or beyond the pyloric sphincter of the stomach (ASPEN, 2002).

A serious complication associated with enteral feedings is aspiration of formula into the tracheobronchial tree. Aspiration of enteral formula into the lungs irritates the bronchial mucosa, resulting in decreased blood supply to affected pulmonary tissue (Metheny and others, 2002). This then leads to necrotizing infection, pneumonia, and potential abscess formation. The high glucose content of a feeding serves as a bacterial medium for growth, promoting infection. Adult respiratory distress syndrome (ARDS) is also an outcome frequently associated with pulmonary aspiration. Some of the common conditions that increase the risk of aspiration include coughing, nasotracheal suctioning, an artificial airway, decreased level of consciousness, and lying flat.

Enteral Access Tubes. When the client is unable to ingest food but is still able to digest and absorb nutrients, enteral tube feeding is indicated. Feeding tubes can be inserted through the nose (nasogastric or nasointestinal), surgically (gastrostomy or jejunostomy), or endoscopically (percutaneous endoscopic gastrostomy or jejunostomy [PEG or PEJ]). If EN therapy is for less than 4 weeks total, nasogastric or nasojejunal feeding tubes may be used. Surgical or endoscopically placed tubes are preferred for long-term feeding (more than 4 weeks) to reduce the discomfort of a nasal tube and to provide a more secure, reliable access (Bowers, 1996). Clients with gastroparesis (decreased or absent innervation to the stomach

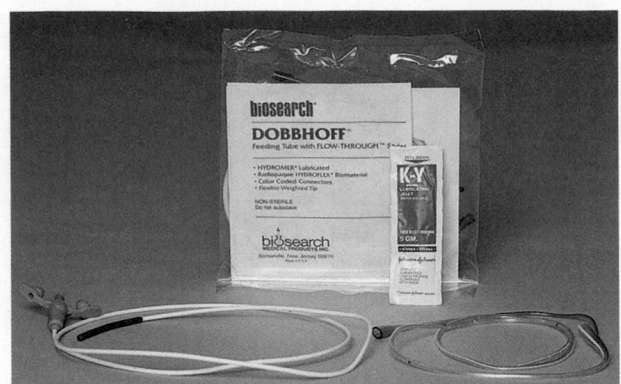

FIGURE **43–9**   Enteral tubes, small bore.

that results in delayed gastric emptying) or esophageal reflux, or with a history of aspiration pneumonia are some types of clients that require placement of tubes beyond the stomach into the intestine (Edwards and Metheny, 2000; Metheny and others, 2002).

Nursing research has investigated the problems associated with nasoenteric tube placement, type of feeding instilled, rate of feeding, and complications associated with tube feeding. Small-bore feeding tubes create less discomfort for the client and are currently most often used (Figure 43-9). For the adult, most of these tubes are 8 to 12 Fr and 36 to 43 inches long. A stylet is often used during insertion of a small-bore tube to stiffen it. The stylet is removed when the correct position of the feeding tube is confirmed. Skills 43-2 and 43-3 describe the procedure for initiating nasogastric and gastrostomy and jejunostomy enteral feedings.

Historically, feeding tube placement was checked by injecting air through the tube while auscultating the stomach for a gurgling or bubbling sound, or asking the client to speak (Metheny and others, 1998b). These methods have a high degree of inaccuracy. Rombeau and Rolandelli (1997) report that clients have been able to speak despite placement of feeding tubes in the lung. Auscultation has repeatedly been shown to be ineffective in detecting tubes accidentally placed in the lung; further, it is not effective in distinguishing between gastric and intestinal placement for stationary feeding tubes (Metheny and others, 1997, 1999). Thus the nurse must suspect tube displacement in clients at risk and use meticulous assessment skills. Metheny and others (1998a) reported several cases in which nasoenteral feeding tube displacement in the lung went undetected by auscultation.

At present, the most reliable method for verification of placement of small-bore feeding tubes is x-ray examination (Box 43-11). The measurement of pH of secretions withdrawn from the feeding tube may help to differentiate the location of the tube (Box 43-12). For accurate pH measurements, 30 ml of air is injected into the tube before measurement. Flushing the tube with air clears out formula, medications, or flush solutions. Only 5 to 10 ml of gastric fluid is needed for pH testing. A client who takes acid-inhibitor medications will usually have an acidic pH value ranging from 4.0 (after 4 hours of fasting) to 6.0 (with continuous EN infusion). By contrast, intestinal

Text continued on p. 1311

Skill 43-2   *Administering Enteral Feedings via Nasoenteric Tubes*

View Video

Delegation Considerations

Administration of enteral tube feeding via nasogenteric tube is a procedure that can be delegated to assistive personnel (AP) after the tube placement is verified by the nurse. The nurse is also responsible for client assessment.

- Ensure that the client is sitting upright in a chair or in bed, and instruct assistive personnel to infuse the feeding slowly.
- Assistive personnel should be instructed to report any difficulty infusing the feeding or any discomfort voiced by the client.

Equipment

- Disposable feeding bag and tubing or ready-to-hang system
- 30-ml or larger Luer-lok or catheter-tip syringe
- Stethoscope
- pH indicator strip (scale 0.0 to 14.0)
- Infusion pump (required for intestinal feedings): use pump designed for tube feedings
- Prescribed enteral feedings
- Gloves
- Equipment to obtain blood glucose by finger stick

Steps	Rationale
1. Assess client's need for enteral tube feedings: impaired swallowing, decreased level of consciousness, head or neck surgery, facial trauma, surgeries of upper alimentary canal.	Identify clients who need tube feedings before they become nutritionally depleted.
2. Evaluate client's nutritional status (see Table 43-5). Obtain baseline weight and laboratory values. Assess client for fluid volume excess or deficit, electrolyte abnormalities, and metabolic abnormalities such as hyperglycemia.	Enteral feedings are to restore or maintain a client's nutritional status. Provides objective data to measure effectiveness of feedings.
3. Verify physician's order for formula, rate, route, and frequency. Laboratory data and bedside assessments, such as finger-stick blood glucose measurement, are also ordered by the physician.	Tube feedings, laboratory tests, and bedside tests must be ordered by physician.
4. Explain procedure to client.	Well-informed client is more cooperative and at ease.
5. Perform hand hygiene.	Reduces transmission of microorganisms.
6. Auscultate for bowel sounds before feeding.	Absent bowel sounds may indicate decreased ability of GI tract to digest or absorb nutrients.
7. Prepare feeding container to administer formula: a. Check expiration date on formula and integrity of container.	Tube feedings administered within the designated shelf life from a container without cracks or breaks reduces the client's risk of obtaining tube-feeding-borne GI infections. In addition, a container without cracks or breaks prevents leakage of tube feeding.
b. Have tube feeding at room temperature.	Cold formula may cause gastric cramping and discomfort because the liquid is not warmed by mouth and esophagus.
c. Connect tubing to container as needed or prepare ready-to-hang container.	Tubing must be free of contamination to prevent bacterial growth.
d. Shake formula container well, and fill container with formula (see illustration). Open stopcock on tubing and fill with formula to remove air. Hang on intravenous (IV) pole.	Filling the tubing with formula prevents excess air from entering GI tract.
8. For intermittent feeding have syringe ready and be sure formula is at room temperature	Cold formula may cause gastric cramping.
9. Place client in high-Fowler's position, or elevate head of bed 30 degrees.	Elevated head helps prevent aspiration.
10. Verify tube placement (see Box 43-11, p. 1312): Consider together the results from pH testing and the aspirate's appearance.	On occasion, color alone may differentiate gastric from intestinal placement. Because most intestinal aspirates are stained by bile to a distinct yellow color, and most gastric aspirates are not, the difference can often distinguish sites (Metheny and others, 1999). The pH aspirate offers valuable data as well in tracking advancement of a feeding tube (Metheny and Titler, 2001).

Skill 43-2   *Administering Enteral Feedings via Nasoenteric Tubes—cont'd*

Steps	Rationale

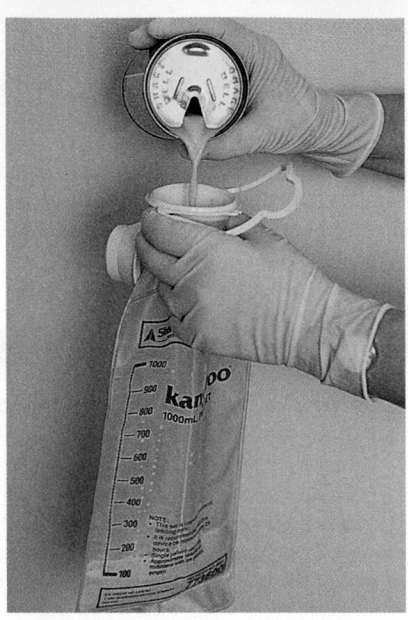

STEP **7d**   Pour formula into feeding container.

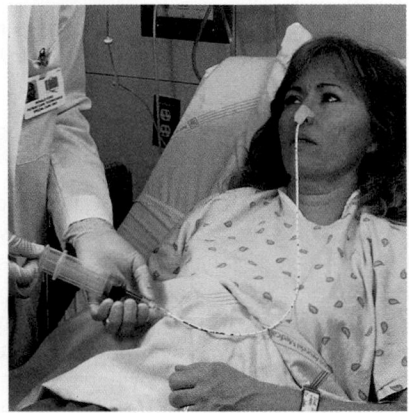

STEP **11b**   Check for gastric residual (small-bore tube).

Critical Decision Point: Auscultation is no longer considered a reliable method for verification of placement of tube because a tube inadvertently placed in lungs, pharynx, or esophagus can transmit sound similar to that of air entering stomach (Chang and others, 1982; Metheny and others, 1990a, 1990b).

Steps	Rationale

11. Check for gastric residual.
   a. Draw up 30 ml of air with syringe. Connect to end of feeding tube. Flush tube with air.
   b. Pull back evenly to aspirate gastric contents (see illustration).
   c. Return aspirated contents to stomach unless the volume exceeds 100 ml (check agency policy).
	Residual volume indicates if gastric emptying is delayed. Delayed gastric emptying may be reflected if 100 ml or more remain in the client's stomach (McClave and others, 1999). Return of aspirate prevents fluid and electrolyte imbalance.

12. Flush tubing with 30 ml water.	Ensures tube is clear and patent.

13. Initiate feeding:
  A. Syringe or intermittent feeding
    (1) Pinch proximal end of the feeding tube.
	Prevents air from entering client's stomach.

(2) Remove plunger from syringe and attach barrel of syringe to end of tube.
    (3) Fill syringe with measured amount of formula (see illustration). Release tube and hold syringe high enough to allow it to empty gradually by gravity, refill; repeat until prescribed amount has been delivered to the client.
    (4) If feeding bag is used, hang feeding bag on an IV pole (see illustration). Fill bag with prescribed amount of formula, and allow bag to empty gradually over at least 30 min.
	Gradual emptying of tube feeding by gravity from syringe or feeding bag reduces risk of abdominal discomfort, vomiting, or diarrhea induced by bolus or too-rapid infusion of tube feedings.

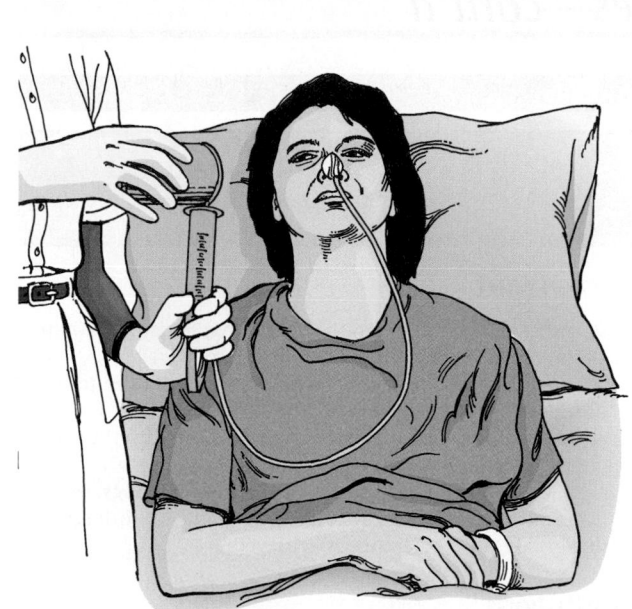

STEP **13A(3)**   Fill syringe with formula.

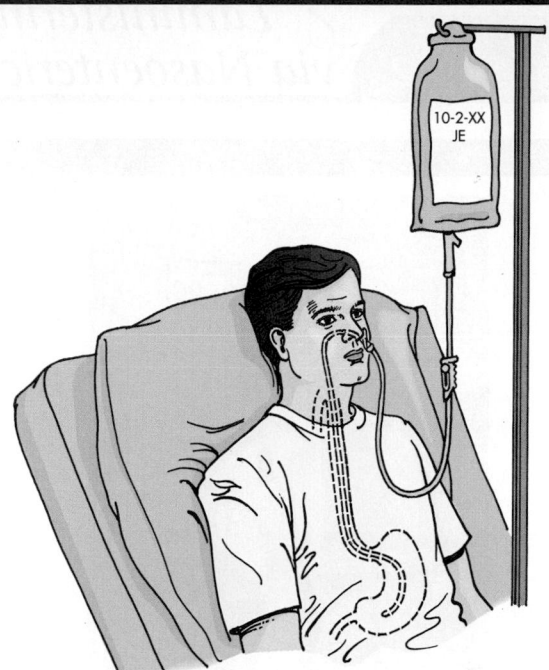

STEP **13A(4)**   Administer feeding.

B. Continuous-drip method
  (1) Hang feeding bag and tubing on IV pole.
  (2) Connect distal end of tubing to the proximal end of the feeding tube.
  (3) Connect tubing through infusion pump and set rate (see illustration).
14. Advance tube feeding gradually (Box 43-10, p. 1308).

Continuous feeding method is designed to deliver prescribed hourly rate of feeding. This method reduces risk of abdominal discomfort. Clients who receive continuous drip feedings should have residuals checked every 4 hr and tube placement verified.

Tube feedings should be advanced gradually to prevent diarrhea and gastric intolerance to formula.

Critical Decision Point: Tube feedings should be infused by feeding pumps and not by an intravenous (IV) pump.

---

15. Following intermittent infusion or at end of continuous infusion, flush nasoenteral tubing with 30 ml of water. Repeat every 4 to 6 hr. Remove gloves or perform hand hygiene.

Maintains patency of feeding tube and provides client with a source of water to help maintain fluid and electrolyte balance.

Critical Decision Point: It may be necessary to consult with a dietitian to recommend a total free water requirement per day. This avoids the potential of fluid overload.

---

16. When tube feedings are not being administered, cap or clamp the proximal end of the feeding tube.
17. Rinse bag and tubing with warm water whenever feedings are interrupted.
18. Change bag and tubing every 24 hr.

19. Measure amount of aspirate (residual) every 8 to 12 hr.
20. Monitor finger-stick blood glucose every 6 hr until maximum administration rate is reached and maintained for 24 hr.
21. Monitor intake and output every 8 hr and do 24-hr totals.

Prevents air from entering stomach between feedings.

Rinsing bag and tubing with warm water clears old tube feedings and reduces bacterial growth.
Reduces client's exposure to bacterial growth occurring in bag and tubing.
Evaluates tolerance of tube feeding.
Alerts nurse to client's tolerance of glucose.

Intake and output are indications of fluid balance or fluid volume excess or deficit.

*A*dministering Enteral Feedings via Nasoenteric Tubes—cont'd

Skill 43-2

Steps	Rationale

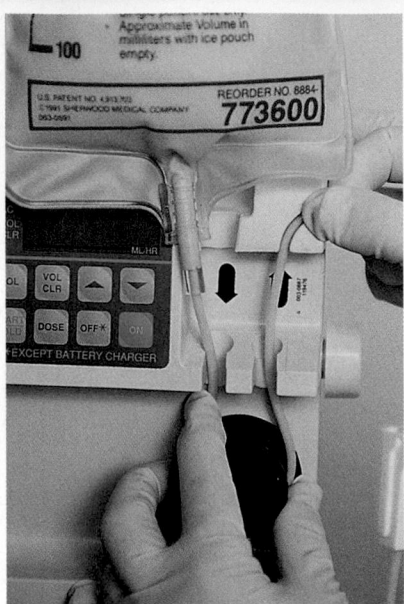

STEP **13B(3)**　Connect tubing through infusion pump.

Box 43-10　Advancing the Rate of Tube Feeding

Intermittent

1. Start formula at full strength for isotonic formulas (300 to 400 mOsm) or at ordered concentration.
2. Infuse bolus of formula over at least 20 to 30 minutes via syringe or feeding container.
3. Begin feedings with no more than 150 to 250 ml at one time. Increase by 50 ml per feeding per day to achieve needed volume and calories in six to eight feedings. (NOTE: Concentrated formulas at full strength may be infused at slower rate until tolerance is achieved.)

Continuous

1. Start formula at full strength for isotonic formulas (300 to 400 mOsm) or at ordered concentration. Usually hypertonic formulas are also started at full strength but at a slower rate.
2. Begin infusion rate at designated rate.
3. Advance rate slowly (e.g., 10 to 20 ml/hr per day) to target rate if tolerated (tolerance indicated by absence of nausea and diarrhea, and low gastric residuals).

22. Weigh client daily until maximum administration rate is reached and maintained for 24 hr; then weigh client 3 times per week.
23. Observe return of normal laboratory values.

Weight gain is indicator of improved nutritional status; however, sudden gain of more than 2 lb in 24 hr usually indicates fluid retention.

Improving laboratory values (e.g., albumin, transferrin, and prealbumin) indicate an improved nutritional status.

Unexpected Outcomes and Related Interventions (in addition to those in Skill 43-1)

1. Gastric residual exceeds 100 ml (see agency policy).
   a. Hold feeding.
   b. Notify physician.
   c. Maintain client in semi-Fowler's or at least have head of bed elevated 30 degrees.
   d. Recheck residual in 1 hour.
2. Client develops diarrhea 3 times or more in 24 hr.
   a. Notify physician.
   b. Confer with dietitian.
   c. Institute skin care measures.
   d. Consider change in antibiotics, only for clients receiving antibiotics.
3. Client develops nausea and vomiting.
   a. Notify physician.
   b. Check patency of tube.

   c. Aspirate for residual.
   d. Auscultate for bowel sounds.

Recording and Reporting

- Record amount and type of feeding. Client's response to tube feeding, patency of tube, and any side effects.
- Report client's tolerance and adverse effects.

Home Care Considerations

- Teach client or primary caregiver how to determine correct placement of feeding tube.
- Inform client or primary caregiver of signs associated with pulmonary aspiration, delayed gastric emptying.
- Reinforce signs and symptoms associated with feeding tube complications and when to call physician.

Administering Enteral Feedings via Gastrostomy or Jejunostomy Tube

Skill 43-3

Delegation Considerations

Administration of enteral tube feeding via a gastrostomy or jejunostomy tube or a jejunal tube is a procedure that can be delegated to assistive personnel (AP) after tube placement is verified by the nurse.

- Ensure that the client is sitting upright in a chair or in bed and instruct the assistive personnel to infuse the feeding slowly.
- Assistive personnel should be instructed to report any difficulty infusing the feeding or any discomfort voiced by the client.

Equipment

- Disposable feeding container or ready-to-hang bag
- 30-ml or larger Luer-Lok or catheter-tip syringe
- Formula
- Infusion pump: Use pump designed for tube feedings
- pH indicator strips (scale 0.0 to 14.0)
- Stethoscope
- Clean gloves
- Equipment to obtain blood glucose by finger stick

Steps	Rationale
1. Assess client's need for enteral tube feedings (see Skill 43-1, p. 1300 and Skill 43-2, p. 1305): impaired swallowing, decreased level of consciousness, surgeries of upper alimentary tract, need for long-term enteral nutrition.	Identifies clients who need tube feedings before they become nutritionally depleted. Enteral feeding preserves the function and mass of the gut, promotes wound healing, diminishes hypermetabolism in burn injuries, and may decrease infection in critically ill clients (Zaloga, 1994).
2. Auscultate for bowel sounds before feeding. Consult physician if bowel sounds are absent.	Absence of bowel sounds may indicate decreased or absent peristalsis and increased risk of aspiration or abdominal distention.
3. Obtain baseline weight and laboratory values.	Enteral feedings are to restore or maintain nutritional status. Provides objective data to measure effectiveness of feedings.
4. Verify physician's order for formula, rate, route, and frequency.	Tube feedings must be ordered by physician.
5. Perform hand hygiene.	Reduces transmission of microorganisms.
6. Assess gastrostomy/jejunostomy site for breakdown, irritation, or drainage.	Infection, pressure from tube, or drainage of gastric secretions can cause skin breakdown.
7. Explain procedure to client.	Well-informed client is more cooperative and feels more at ease.
8. Prepare feeding container to administer formula: a. Have tube feeding at room temperature.	Cold formula may cause gastric cramping and discomfort because the liquid is not warmed by mouth and esophagus.
b. Connect tubing to container as needed, or prepare ready-to-hang bag.	Tubing must be free of contamination to prevent bacterial growth.
c. Shake formula well. Fill container and tubing with formula.	Placement of formula through tubing prevents excess air from entering gastrointestinal tract.
9. For intermittent feeding have syringe ready and be sure formula is at room temperature.	Cold formula may cause gastric cramping.
10. Elevate head of bed 30 to 45 degrees.	Elevating client's head helps prevent chance of aspiration.
11. Apply gloves and verify tube placement: A. **Gastrostomy tube:** Attach syringe and aspirate gastric secretions; observe their appearance and check pH. Return aspirated contents to stomach unless the volume exceeds 100 ml. If the volume is greater than 100 ml on several consecutive occasions, hold feeding and notify physician (McClave and others, 1999).	Fluid from gastric tube of client who has fasted for at least 4 hr usually has a pH of 1 to 4, especially when client is not receiving a gastric-acid inhibitor. Continuous administration of tube feedings may elevate pH (Metheny and Titler 2001). Gastric residual determines if gastric emptying is delayed. Delayed gastric emptying may be indicated by 100 ml or more remaining in client's stomach from previous feeding (McClave and others, 1999).

Skill 43-3   *Administering Enteral Feedings via Gastrostomy or Jejunostomy Tube—cont'd*

Steps	Rationale
B. Jejunostomy tube: Aspirate intestinal secretions, observe their appearance and check pH.	Presence of intestinal fluid indicates that the end of the tube is in the small intestine (i.e., duodenum or jejunum). Generally the intestinal residual is very small (10 ml or less). If fluid tests acidic on pH test, looks like gastric fluid, or the residual volume is large (more than 10 ml), displacement of the tube into the stomach may have occurred.
12. Flush with 30 ml of water.	
13. Initiate feedings:	Usually gastrostomy and jejunostomy feedings are given continuously to ensure proper absorption. However, initial feedings may be given by bolus to assess client's tolerance to formula. See Box 43-10, p. 1308, for guidelines to advance enteral feedings.
A. Syringe feedings (1) Pinch proximal end of gastrostomy/jejunostomy tube.	Prevents excessive air from entering the client's stomach or leaking of gastric contents.
(2) Remove plunger and attach barrel of syringe to end of tube, then fill syringe with formula.	
(3) Release tube, and elevate syringe. Allow syringe to empty gradually by gravity. Refill until prescribed amount has been delivered to client.	Gradual administration of tube feedings by gravity reduces the risk of diarrhea induced by bolus tube feedings.
B. Continuous drip method	Continuous-feeding method is designed to deliver a prescribed hourly rate of feeding. This method reduces the risk of diarrhea. Clients who receive continuous-drip feedings should have residuals checked every 8 to 12 hr.
(1) Verify that volume in container is sufficient for length of feeding (4 to 8 hr, check manufacturers recommendations).	
(2) Hang container on IV pole, and clear tubing of air.	Allows for gravity flow of formula. Prevents accumulation of air in the client's stomach.
(3) Thread tubing into pump according to manufacturer's directions.	
(4) Connect tubing to end of gastrostomy/jejunostomy tube.	
(5) Begin infusion at prescribed rate.	
14. Administer water via feeding tube as ordered with or between feedings.	Provides client with source of water to help maintain fluid and electrolyte balance.
15. Flush tube with 30 ml of water every 4 to 6 hr and before and after administering medications via feeding tube.	Maintains patency of tube and provides client with some free water. Small jejunal tubes are very prone to clogging and are difficult to replace (Simon and Fink, 1999).
16. When tube feedings are not being administered, cap or clamp the proximal end of the gastrostomy/jejunostomy tube.	Prevents excess air from entering the gastrointestinal tract between feedings and prevents leakage of gastric contents.
17. Rinse container and tubing with warm water after all intermittent feedings.	Clears feeding from tubing and reduces bacterial growth in container and tubing.
18. Assess skin around tube exit site. The skin around the tube should be cleansed daily with warm water and mild soap. Tubing exit site is left open to air. If a dressing is needed because of drainage, assess drainage and change dressing as needed.	Report any drainage, redness, swelling, or displacement of the tube to the physician. Leakage of gastric drainage may cause skin irritation. Skin around feeding tube should be cleansed daily with warm water and mild soap. When needed, a small precut gauze dressing may be applied to exit site.
19. Dispose of supplies, and perform hand hygiene.	Prevents transmission of microorganisms.
20. Evaluate client's tolerance to tube feeding. Measure the amount of aspirate (residual) every 8 to 12 hr.	Evaluates tolerance of tube feeding.

Steps	Rationale
21. Monitor finger-stick blood glucose every 6 hr until maximum administration rate is reached and maintained for 24 hr.	Alerts nurse to client's tolerance of glucose.
22. Monitor intake and output every 24 hr.	Intake and output are indications of fluid balance or fluid volume excess.
23. Weigh client daily until maximum administration rate is reached and maintained for 24 hr; then weigh client 3 times per week.	Weight gain is indicator of improved nutritional status; however, a sudden gain of more than 2 lb in 24 hr usually indicates fluid retention.
24. Observe return of normal laboratory values.	Improving laboratory values (albumin, transferrin, prealbumin) indicate an improved nutritional status.
25. Inspect stoma site for signs of impaired skin integrity.	Enteral tubes can cause pressure and excoriation at the stoma site. In addition, gastric secretions also cause irritation to client's skin.

Unexpected Outcomes and Related Interventions (in addition to Skill 43-2)

1. Client aspirates formula when gastric emptying is delayed or formula is administered too rapidly and produces vomiting.
   a. Position client in side-lying position.
   b. Suction airway.
   c. Notify physician.
   d. Obtain chest x-ray film.
2. Skin around gastrostomy/jejunostomy site breaks down.
   a. Institute skin care practices.
   b. Use pressure relief measures around tube.
   c. Provide appropriate wound care (see Chapter 47).

Recording and Reporting

- Record amount and type of feeding and client's response to tube feeding, patency of tube, and any side effects.
- Report to oncoming nursing staff: type of feeding, status of feeding tube, client's tolerance, and adverse effects.

Home Care Considerations

- Teach client or primary caregiver how to determine correct placement of feeding tube.
- Inform client or primary caregiver of signs associated with pulmonary aspiration, delayed gastric emptying.
- Reinforce signs and symptoms associated with feeding tube complications and when to call physician.

---

spirate has a pH of 7.8 to 8.0. More precise indicators are needed to help differentiate the source of tube feeding aspirate (Metheny and others, 2000).

The addition of blue food coloring to enteral formula to assist with the detection of formula aspirated into the lung, presumably by staining the tracheobronchial secretions is now questioned and should not be used. The FDA issued a public health advisory reporting an association between use of Blue No. 1 food coloring and client deaths (USFDA, 2003). Research has determined that the absence of blue-stained tracheobronchial secretions does not rule out pulmonary aspiration (Davis and others, 1995; Metheny, Aud, and Wuderlich, 1999).

Major complications of enteral nutrition are outlined in Table 43-9. Of special note, severely malnourished clients are at risk for electrolyte disturbances from refeeding syndrome as cations such as potassium, magnesium, and phosphate move intracellularly during EN or PN therapy.

Parenteral Nutrition. **Parenteral nutrition (PN)** is a form of specialized nutrition support in which nutrients are provided intravenously. Safe administration of this form of nutrition depends on appropriate assessment of nutrition needs, meticulous management of the central venous catheter (CVC), and careful monitoring to prevent or treat metabolic complications. Parenteral nutrition is administered in a variety of settings, including the client's home. Regardless of the setting, the nurse adheres to the same principles of asepsis and infusion management to ensure safe nutrition support.

Clients who are unable to digest or absorb enteral nutrition benefit from PN. Clients in highly stressed physiological states such as sepsis, head injury, or burns are candidates for PN therapy (see Box 43-9, p. 1299).

Clinical and laboratory monitoring by a multidisciplinary team is required throughout PN therapy. The need for continued PN is consistently reevaluated. The goal to move toward use of the GI tract is constant (ASPEN, 2002). Disuse of the GI tract has been associated with villus atrophy and generalized cell shrinkage. Translocation of bacteria from the local gut to systemic regions has been noted in relation to GI cell shrinkage, resulting in gram-negative septicemia.

Lipid emulsions provide supplemental kilocalories and prevent essential fatty acid deficiencies. These emulsions can be administered through a separate peripheral line, through the central line by Y-connector tubing (see

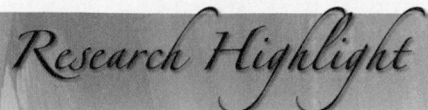

Research Highlight

Box 43-11

Accuracy in Determining Placement of Feeding Tubes

Research Focus

Two possible adverse outcomes of enteral nutrition are accidental placement of a nasoenteric feeding tube into the lung and pulmonary aspiration of gastric contents.

Research Abstract

No one knows the precise incidence of accidental tube misplacements into the lung, but estimates of close to 5% have been cited; clients at highest risk are those with a decreased level of consciousness (LOC), confusion, uncooperativeness, agitation, presence of an endotracheal tube, recent extubation, and poor gag reflex. A feeding tube accidentally inserted into the lung may end in the tracheobronchial tree or perforate into the pleural space. In either event, efforts are made to detect the misplacement before the introduction of tube feedings because inadvertent infusion of formula into the lung promotes tissue consolidation, pneumonia, and respiratory failure. The most accurate method for checking feeding tube placement is x-ray examination; the most effective nonradiological methods include aspirating fluid from the feeding tube and measuring its pH and describing its appearance. Although observing for respiratory distress is helpful in alert clients (especially when firm large-diameter tubes are used), it is of little benefit in those who have a decreased LOC and when small-bore tubes are used. Risk factors for pulmonary aspiration in tube-fed clients include feeding into the stomach when gastric atony is present (resulting in high gastric residual volumes), poor gag reflexes, mechanical ventilation, and flat positioning in bed. Bedside methods used to detect pulmonary aspiration are not well defined.

Evidence-Based Practice

- X-ray verification of feeding tube placement is the most reliable method available to confirm correct feeding tube location and is required in most acute care facilities when small-bore tubes are initially inserted.
- When the x-ray method is not feasible, the next best method involves testing the feeding tube aspirate's pH and observing its appearance. A properly obtained pH of 0 to 4 is a good indication of gastric placement; a pH of 6 or higher could indicate placement in the lung, intestine, or even the stomach when gastric pH is unusually high. Intestinal fluid is usually bile-stained (dark golden yellow); in contrast, gastric fluid is usually grassy green, off-white to tan, or clear and colorless.
- The auscultatory method should not be used to determine tube location.
- If the dye method is used to detect aspiration of enteral feedings, the dye should be sterile to reduce the risk of pulmonary infection in the event of aspiration.

References

Metheny N, Aud M, Ignatavicius D: Detection of improperly placed feeding tubes, *J Healthc Risk Manage* 18(3):37, 1998; Metheny NA, Aud MA, Wunderlich RJ: A survey of bedside methods used to detect pulmonary aspiration of enteral formula in intubated tube-fed patients, *Am J Crit Care* 8(3):160, 1999; and Metheny N, Titler M: Assessing placement of feeding tubes, *Am J Nurs* 101(5):36, 2001.

Chapter 40), or as an admixture to the PN solution. The addition of lipid emulsion to the PN solution is called a 3-in-1 admixture and is given over a 24-hour period. The admixture should not be used if oil droplets are observed or if an oil or creamy layer is observed on the surface of the admixture. This observation indicates that the emulsion has broken into large lipid droplets that can cause fat emboli if administered. Lipid emulsions are white and opaque; thus care should be taken to avoid confusing enteral formula with parenteral lipids.

Initiating PN. Clients with short-term nutritional needs often receive intravenous solutions of less than 10% dextrose via a peripheral vein in combination with amino acids and lipids. Peripheral solutions are not as caloricly dense as TPN solutions and therefore are usually temporary. Parenteral nutrition with greater than 10% dextrose requires a CVC that is placed into a high-flow central vein such as the superior vena cava by a physician under sterile conditions (see Chapter 40). Nurses who have special training insert peripherally inserted central catheters (PICCs) that are started in a vein of the forearm and threaded into the subclavian or superior vena cava vein.

After catheter placement, the catheter is flushed with saline or heparin until the position is radiographically confirmed. The physician sutures the CVC catheter in place and covers the site with a sterile dressing. A PICC is usually stabilized with sterile strips of tape and a sterile dressing. A chest x-ray examination identifies any complications.

Before beginning any parenteral nutrition infusion, verify the physician's order and inspect the solution for particulate matter or a break in the lipid emulsion. An infusion pump is always used. An initial rate of 40 to 60 ml/hr is recommended. The rate is gradually increased until the client's complete nutrition needs are supplied. Clients receiving PN at home frequently administer the entire daily solution over 12 hours at night. This allows the client to disconnect from the infusion each morning, flush the central line, and have independent mobility during the day.

Preventing Complications. Complications of PN include mechanical complications from insertion of the CVC, infection, and metabolic alterations (Table 43-10). Pneumothorax results from a puncture insult to the pulmonary system and results in accumulation of air in the pleural cavity with subsequent collapse of the lung and impaired breathing. Pneumothorax is usually accompanied

Box 43-12 Procedural Guidelines

Obtaining GI Aspirate for pH Measurement, Large- and Small-Bore Feeding Tubes: Intermittent and Continuous Feeding

Equipment: Cone tipped or asepto syringe, pH test paper (scale of 1 to 11), paper towel, small medication cup, disposable gloves.

Delegation Considerations: The skill of measuring pH in GI aspirate should not be delegated to assistive personnel.

1. Perform measures to verify placement of tube:
   a. For intermittently fed clients, test placement immediately before feeding (usually a period of at least 4 hours will have elapsed since previous feeding). More frequent checking has been associated with increased clogging of small-bore tubes. To avoid clogging, flush tube with 30 ml water after aspirating for the residual volume (Edwards and Metheny, 2000).
   b. For continuously tube-fed clients, check agency policy. If the client is tolerating the feedings without incident and other indicators of correct location are present (the mark on the tube at the exit site has remained in its original position and the most recent x-ray films confirm tube's correct position), it is reasonable to continue feedings. **If risk of tube displacement is high and the tube has moved, consider the need for an x-ray film to verify placement** (Metheny and Titler, 2001). Plan pH testing at times when feeding may be withheld (e.g., during diagnostic testing, chest physical therapy, or to avoid medication interaction).
   c. Wait at least 1 hour after medication administration by tube or mouth.
      Perform hand hygiene.
2. Apply disposable gloves.
3. Draw up 30 ml of air into syringe, then attach to end of feeding tube. Flush tube with 30 ml of air before attempting to aspirate fluid. It will likely be more difficult to aspirate fluid from the small intestine than from the stomach. Repositioning the client from side to side may be helpful. More than one bolus of air through the tube may be needed in some cases. Burst of air aids in aspirating fluid more easily (Metheny and others, 1993b).
4. Draw back on syringe and obtain 5 to 10 ml of gastric aspirate. Observe appearance of aspirate (see illustration Step 4A).

   Gently mix aspirate in syringe. Then expel a few drops into a clean medicine cup. Dip the pH strip into the fluid or apply a few drops of the fluid to the strip (see illustration Step 4B). Compare the color of the strip with the color on the chart provided by the manufacturer (Metheny and others, 1998b).
   a. Gastric fluid from client who has fasted for at least 4 hours usually has pH range of 1 to 4 (Metheny and others, 1998a).
   b. Fluid from nasointestinal tube of fasting client usually has pH greater than 6 (Metheny and others, 1989).

   c. Client with continuous tube feeding may have pH of 5 or higher.
   d. pH of pleural fluid from tracheobronchial tree is generally greater than 6.
5. Remove gloves and discard supplies. Perform hand hygiene.

Critical Decision Point

If after repeated attempts, it is not possible to aspirate fluid from a tube that was originally established by x-ray examination to be in desired position, and (a) there are no risk factors for tube dislocation, (b) tube has remained in original taped position, and (c) client is not experiencing difficulty, assume tube is correctly placed (Metheny and others, 1993a).

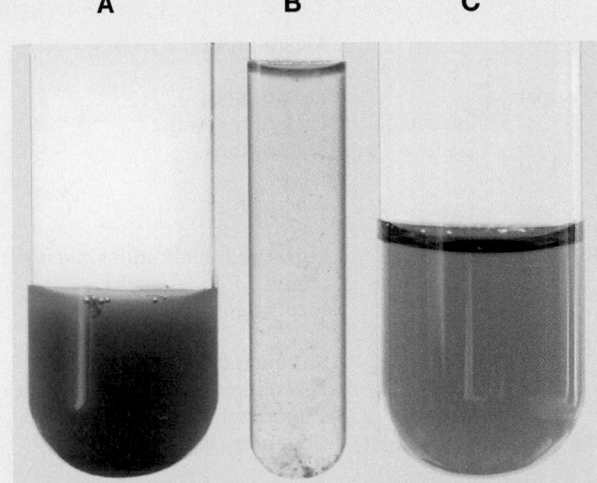

STEP **4A**   Gastrointestinal contents. **A,** Stomach. **B,** Stomach. **C,** Intestinal (Courtesy Dr. Normal Metheny, Professor, St. Louis University School of Nursing.)

STEP **4B**   Comparing pH strip with color chart.

Table 43-9	Enteral Tube Feeding Complications	
Problem	**Possible Cause**	**Intervention***
Pulmonary aspiration	Regurgitation of formula	Verify tube placement.
	Feeding tube displaced	Reposition tube and verify tube placement.
	Client in supine position	Elevate head of bed 30 to 45 degrees during feedings and for 2 hours afterwards.
	Deficient gag reflex	Reassess for return of normal gag reflex, until then place client on aspiration precautions and place client in supine position.
	Gastroesophageal reflux disease (GERD)	Verify tube placement.
	Delayed gastric emptying	(See delayed gastric emptying below.)
Diarrhea	Hyperosmolar formula or medications	Deliver formula continuously, lower rate, dilute, or change to isotonic EN.
	Allergy to elixir ingredients (sorbitol)	Liquid medications are often sweetened with sorbitol, consider as possible cause.
	Malnutrition/hypoalbuminemia	Albumin 2.5 g/100 ml lessens oncotic pressure equilibrium.
	Antibiotic therapy	Antibiotics may destroy normal intestinal flora; physician may change medication; treat symptoms with antidiarrhea agents.
	Bacterial contamination	Do not hang formula longer than 4-8 hours in bag, wash bag out well when refilling, change tube feeding bags q24h, and use aseptic practices. Check expiration dates.
	Malabsorption	Check for pancreatic insufficiency; use low-fat, lactose-free formula, and continuous feedings.
Constipation	Lack of fiber	Select a formula containing fiber.
	Lack of free water	Add water as needed as flushes.*
	Medications	Evaluate side effects; suggest stool softener or bulk-forming laxative.
	Inactivity	Monitor client's ability to ambulate; collaborate with physician for activity order or physical therapy.
Tube occlusion	Pulverized medications given per tube	Irrigate with 30 ml water before and after each medication per tube.*
	Insufficient tube irrigation	Dilute crushed medications if not liquid.
		Avoid crushed medications, if liquid available.
	Sedimentation of formula	Shake cans well before administering (read label).
	Reaction of incompatible medications or formula	Read pharmacological information on compatibility of drugs and formula.
Tube displacement	Coughing, vomiting	Replace tube and confirm placement before restarting tube feeding.
	Not taped securely	With placement verification, check that tape is secure (nasoenteric).
Abdominal cramping, nausea/vomiting	High osmolality of formula	Suggest an isotonic formula, or dilute current formula.
	Rapid increase in rate/volume	
	Delayed gastric emptying	Lower rate of delivery to increase tolerance.
	Lactose intolerance	Suggest use of lactose-free formula.
	Intestinal obstruction	Stop feeding with GI obstruction.
	High-fat formula used	Use greater proportion of carbohydrate.
	Cold formula used	Warm formula to room temperature.
Delayed gastric emptying	Diabetic gastroparesis	Consult with physician regarding medication for increasing gastric motility.
	Prematurity	
	Serious illnesses	Check for residual (see agency policy).
	Inactivity	Consult physician regarding advancing tube to intestinal placement.
		Monitor medications and pathological conditions that may affect GI motility.
Serum electrolyte imbalance	Excess GI losses	Monitor serum electrolyte levels daily.
	Dehydration	Provide free water as per dietitian recommendation
	Cirrhosis	Know of links with specific pathological condition.
	Renal insufficiency	
	Congestive heart failure, edema	
	Diabetes mellitus	

*Check first for fluid-restricted conditions that would affect volume of water given.

Table 43-9 Enteral Tube Feeding Complications—cont'd

Problem	Possible Cause	Intervention*
Increased respiratory quotient	Overfeeding of carbohydrates	Balance kilocalorie needs provided from fat, protein, and carbohydrate with greater proportion of fat in formula (to decrease CO_2 production).
Fluid overload	Refeeding syndrome in malnutrition	Restrict fluids if necessary and use either a specialized formula or a diluted enteral formula at first.
	Excess free water or diluted (hypotonic) formula	Monitor levels of serum proteins and electrolytes.
		Use a more concentrated formula with fluid volume excess without risk of refeeding syndrome.
Hyperosmolar dehydration	Hypertonic formula with insufficient free water	Slow rate of delivery, dilute, or change to isotonic formula.

*Check first for fluid-restricted conditions that would affect volume of water given.

Table 43-10 Complications of Parenteral Nutrition (PN)

Problem	Signs/Symptoms	Intervention
Air embolism	Tachypnea, apnea, wheezing, hypotension, cyanosis	Turn client to left lateral decubitus position, instruct client to perform Valsalva maneuver, and lower head of bed. Cap open end of catheter or tape perforation in catheter wall. Administer oxygen; notify physician. Maintain integrity of closed system to prevent air emboli, and have client perform Valsalva maneuver when changing cap.
Catheter occlusion	No flow or sluggish flow through the catheter	Temporarily stop infusion and flush with saline or heparin. If effort to flush is unsuccessful, attempt to aspirate a clot; if still unsuccessful, follow protocol for use of thrombolytic agent (e.g., urokinase).
Catheter sepsis	Fever, chills, glucose intolerance, positive blood culture	To prevent, change catheter site dressing if it becomes wet or contaminated, use aseptic technique when changing dressing or handling IV tubing, catheter caps, or PN containers. Do not hang a single container of PN for more than 24 hours, or lipids more than 12 hours; use an in-line 0.22-μm filter to remove bacteria.*
Electrolyte imbalance	Monitor Na, Ca, K, Cl, PO_4, Mg, and CO_2 levels	See Chapter 40 for signs of deficiency/toxicity. Check TPN for supplemental electrolyte levels. Notify physician of imbalances.
Hypercapnia	Increased oxygen consumption, increased CO_2, respiratory quotient >1.0, minute ventilation	To prevent; ventilator-dependent clients are at risk; monitor parameters; provide 30% to 60% of energy requirements as fat per physician's order.
Hypoglycemia	Diaphoresis, shakiness, confusion, loss of consciousness	To prevent; do not abruptly discontinue TPN but taper rate down to within 10% of infusion rate 1 to 2 hours before stopping. If hyperglycemia is suspected, test blood glucose, administer IV bolus of dextrose per physician order if necessary.
Hyperglycemia	Thirst, headache, lethargy, increased urination	Monitor blood glucose level daily until stable, then as ordered or prn. TPN is initiated slowly and tapered up to maximal infusion rate. Additional insulin may be required during therapy if problem persists (or if client has diabetes mellitus).
Hyperglycemic hyperosmolar nonketotic dehydration/ coma (HHNC)	Hyperglycemia (>500 mg%/dl), glycosuria, serum osmolarity >350 mOsm/L, confusion, azotemia, headache, severe signs of dehydration (see Chapter 40) hypernatremia, metabolic acidosis, convulsions, coma	To prevent, monitor blood glucose, BUN, serum osmolarity, glucose in urine, and fluid losses; administer insulin as ordered; replace fluids as needed; maintain consistent infusion rate; and provide 30% of daily energy needs as fat. Clients at risk are hypermetabolic, receiving steroids, older adults, diabetic, have impaired renal or pancreatic function, or are septic.
Pneumothorax	Severe dyspnea, cyanosis, x-ray confirmation	Complication that occurs upon catheter insertion, may evolve slowly afterwards. Monitor for first 24 hours for pulmonary distress.
Thrombosis of central vein	Unilateral edema of neck, shoulder, and arm, pain	Repeated or traumatic catheter insertions place clients at risk; notify physician.

*With 3-in-1-admixture TPN, filtration is not possible due to large lipid molecules.

by symptoms of sudden sharp chest pain, dyspnea, and coughing. In relation to PN, pneumothorax most often occurs during CVC placement.

Air embolus can occur during insertion of the catheter or when changing the tubing or cap. Having the client perform a Valsalva maneuver (holding the breath and "bearing down") while assuming a left lateral decubitus position can prevent air embolus. The increased venous pressure created by the maneuver prevents air from entering the bloodstream during catheter insertion.

To avoid infection, the infusion tubing should be changed every 24 hours with lipids and every 48 hours when lipids are not infused. During CVC dressing changes, sterile mask and gloves are always used and insertion sites should be assessed for signs and symptoms of infection (see Chapter 40).

The PN solution contains most of the major electrolytes, vitamins, and minerals. Supplemental vitamin K must be given as ordered throughout therapy. Vitamin K can be synthesized by microflora found in the jejunum and ileum with normal use of the GI tract; however, because PN circumvents GI use, exogenous vitamin K must be administered.

Electrolyte and mineral imbalances may occur. Administration of concentrated glucose is accompanied by increases in endogenous insulin production, which causes cations (potassium, magnesium, and phosphorus) to move intracellularly. In malnourished or cachectic clients the resulting low serum (extracellular) levels of electrolytes and edema may cause cardiac dysrhythmias, congestive heart failure, respiratory distress, convulsions, coma, or death. This has been called refeeding syndrome.

Too-rapid administration of hypertonic dextrose can result in an osmotic diuresis and dehydration (see Chapter 40). If an infusion falls behind schedule, the nurse should not increase the rate in an attempt to catch up. Sudden discontinuation of the solution can cause hypoglycemia. Usually, 5% to 10% dextrose is infused when PN solution is suddenly discontinued. Diabetic clients are more at risk.

The goal is to move clients from PN to EN and/or oral feeding. Once clients are meeting one third to one half of their kilocalorie needs per day, PN is usually decreased to half the original volume. EN feedings should then be increased to meet needs. When 75% of daily energy needs are consistently met with tube feeding, PN may be discontinued. Clients who make the transition from PN to oral feedings typically have early satiety and decreased appetite. Parenteral nutrition should be gradually decreased in response to increased oral intake. If oral intake is inadequate, small frequent meals may prove helpful. Calorie/protein counts are recommended when clients begin taking soft foods. When 75% of needs are being met by reliable dietary intake, PN therapy may be discontinued.

Restorative and Continuing Care. Clients discharged from a hospital with diet prescriptions often need dietary education to plan meals that meet specific therapeutic requirements. Restorative care includes both immediate postsurgical care and routine medical care and therefore includes hospitalized and home care clients. The following sections address nutritional interventions for some common disease states.

Medical Nutrition Therapy. Optimal nutrition is important in health and illness, but the specific dietary intake pattern that results in optimal nutrition must be modified for clients with particular diseases. **Medical nutrition therapy (MNT)** is the use of specific nutritional therapies to treat an illness, injury, or condition. Medical nutrition therapy may be necessary to assist the body's ability to metabolize certain nutrients, correct nutritional deficiencies related to the disease, and eliminate foods that may exacerbate disease symptoms. Sheils, Rubin, and Stapleton (1999) examined the cost savings generated by MNT and found specific savings associated with diabetes and cardiovascular disease and an overall decrease in physician office visits of 23.5%. This section provides a summary of MNT for a variety of diseases.

Gastrointestinal Diseases. Peptic ulcers are controlled with regular meals and medications such as cimetidine. Cimetidine is one of a class of drugs that are histamine receptor antagonists that block secretion of hydrochloric acid. *Helicobacter pylori* was first identified by Marshall and Warren in 1984 and is a bacteria that causes peptic ulcers. This is confirmed by laboratory tests and treated with antibiotics. Stress and overproduction of gastric HCl also contribute to peptic ulcer disease. Clients are encouraged to avoid foods that increase stomach acidity, such as caffeine, decaffeinated coffee, frequent milk intake, citric acid juices, and certain seasonings (hot chili peppers, chili powder, black pepper). Smoking, alcohol, and aspirin are also discouraged.

Inflammatory bowel disease includes Crohn's disease and idiopathic ulcerative colitis. Treatment of acute inflammatory bowel disease may include elemental diets (formula with the nutrients in their simplest form ready for absorption) or parenteral nutrition when symptoms such as diarrhea and weight loss are prevalent. In the chronic stage of the disease a regular highly nourishing diet is appropriate. Vitamins and iron supplements may be required to correct or prevent anemia. Irritable bowel syndrome is managed by increasing fiber, reducing fat, avoiding large meals, and avoiding lactose or sorbitol-containing foods for susceptible individuals.

The treatment of **malabsorption** syndromes, such as celiac disease, includes a gluten-free diet. Gluten is present in wheat, rye, barley, and oats. Short-bowel syndrome results from extensive resection of bowel after which clients suffer from malabsorption due to lack of intestinal surface area. These clients may require lifetime feeding with either elemental enteral formulas or parenteral nutrition.

Diverticulitis is a condition that results from an inflammation of diverticula, which are abnormal but common pouchlike herniations that occur in the bowel lining. This conditions is nutritionally treated with a moderate- or low-residue diet until the infection subsides. Afterward, a high-fiber diet is generally prescribed for chronic diverticula problems.

Diabetes Mellitus. Type 1 diabetes mellitus (DM) requires both insulin and dietary restrictions for optimal control, beginning with diagnosis (ADA, 2002). By contrast, type 2 diabetes mellitus may initially be controlled solely by exercise and diet therapy. If these measures prove ineffective, it is common to add oral medications. Insulin injections may follow if type 2 diabetes worsens or fails to respond to these initial interventions. In both cases the diet is individualized according to the client's age, build, weight, and activity level. Fats are moderately controlled (30% or less), and complex carbohydrates make up the majority (50% to 60%) of the diet, rather than simple carbohydrates. Protein comprises 10% to 20% of daily intake. Foods that contain soluble fiber are recommended, with a daily intake of 40 g of fiber. Foods for dietary planning are classified into two exchange groups: the carbohydrate group and the meat and meat substitute group. Foods from within the same group can be exchanged, but it is not recommended to exchange a carbohydrate food for a meat item. Each item has about the same nutrient value as other foods in the group (for more information, see ADA, 2002, and www.diabetes.org). The goal of treatment is normal glycemic levels, and hemoglobin A_{Ic} level of less than 7%, with resultant minimization of complications of ophthalmic, vascular, renal, and neuropathic damage (Lipkin, 1999). Nurses also need to be aware of signs and symptoms of hypoglycemia and hyperglycemia.

Cardiovascular Diseases. The American Heart Association's (AHA's) dietary guidelines are intended to reduce risk factors for the development of coronary artery disease (AHA, 2000, and www.americanheart.org). Dietary therapy following an acute myocardial infarction includes initial reduction in kilocalories, soft-textured foods, and amounts of fat, sodium, and cholesterol that conform to AHA recommendations. Magnesium, folic acid, and vitamin B_6 appear to be important for primary prevention of coronary heart disease. Increases in folic acid are associated with a decrease in homocysteine, which is associated with greater risk of coronary artery disease (Rimm and others, 1998).

Nutritional therapy for hypertension includes kilocalorie reduction to promote weight loss as appropriate, decreased sodium intake, and potassium-rich foods if potassium-wasting diuretics are part of the treatment.

Cancer and Cancer Treatment. Malignant cells compete with normal cells for nutrients, increasing the metabolic needs of the client. Most cancer treatments cause nutritional problems. Clients with cancer typically complain of anorexia and taste distortions. Malnutrition in cancer is associated with increased morbidity and mortality. Enhanced nutritional status may improve the client's quality of life.

Radiation therapy is intended to destroy rapidly dividing malignant cells; however, other normal rapidly dividing cells, such as the epithelial lining of the GI tract, are often affected. Radiation therapy can cause anorexia, stomatitis, severe diarrhea, strictures of the intestine, and pain. Radiation treatment of the head and neck region can cause taste and smell disturbances, decreased salivation, and dysphagia. Nutrition management of the client with cancer focuses on maximizing intake of nutrients and fluids. The nurse should use creative approaches to manage alterations in taste and smell. For example, clients with altered taste may prefer chilled foods or foods that are highly spiced.

Human Immunodeficiency Virus. HIV-infected clients typically experience body wasting and severe weight loss. The wasting can be related to anorexia, stomatitis, oral thrush infection, nausea, or recurrent vomiting, all resulting in inadequate intake. Factors associated with weight loss and malnutrition are severe diarrhea, GI malabsorption, and altered metabolism of nutrients. Systemic infection results in hypermetabolism from cytokine elevation. Often the medications taken to treat HIV infection cause side effects that alter nutritional status.

Restorative care of acquired immunodeficiency syndrome (AIDS) malnutrition focuses upon maximizing kilocalories and nutrients. Each cause of nutritional depletion should be diagnosed and addressed in the care plan. Individually tailored nutrition support should progress in stages from oral, to enteral, and lastly to parenteral. Good hand hygiene and food safety are essential because of the client's reduced resistance to infection. For example, minimization of exposure to *Cryptosporidium* in drinking water, lakes, or swimming pools is important. Low-fat diets and small, frequent, nutrient-dense meals may be better tolerated (Keithley and Swanson, 1998).

Evaluation

Care plans should reflect achievable goals and outcomes. Nurses need to evaluate outcomes of nursing actions and be alert for signs that goals are being met. Adequate time should be allowed to test each nursing approach to a problem. Multidisciplinary collaboration remains essential in provision of nutrition support.

Client Care. Effectiveness of nutritional interventions is best measured by meeting the client's expected outcomes and goals of care (Figure 43-10). Nutrition therapy does not always produce rapid results. Ongoing comparisons may be made with baseline measures of weight, serum albumin or prealbumin, and protein and kilocalorie intake. EN therapy is frequently interrupted. Medications may produce unwanted side effects. If gradual weight gain is not observed, or if weight loss continues, the dietary EN prescription may need to be increased. Changes in condition may also indicate a need to change the nutritional plan of care. Multidisciplinary members of the health care team should be consulted in an effort to better individualize the client's plan of care. The client should be an active participant whenever possible. In the end, the client's ability to incorporate dietary changes into his or her lifestyle with the least amount of stress or disruption will ensure that outcome measures are successfully met.

Client Expectations. Clients expect competent and accurate care. If ongoing nutritional therapies are not resulting in successful outcomes, clients expect nurses to recognize this fact and alter the plan of care accordingly. Expectations held by nurses may differ from those held by clients. For example, Young, Minnick, and Marcantonio (1996) found discrepancies among nursing staff, nursing managers, and clients regarding health care values. Successful interventions and outcomes depend on recognition of this concept in addition to nursing knowledge and skill. Working closely with the client will enable the nurse to redefine those expectations that can be realistically met within the limits of the client's conditions and treatment.

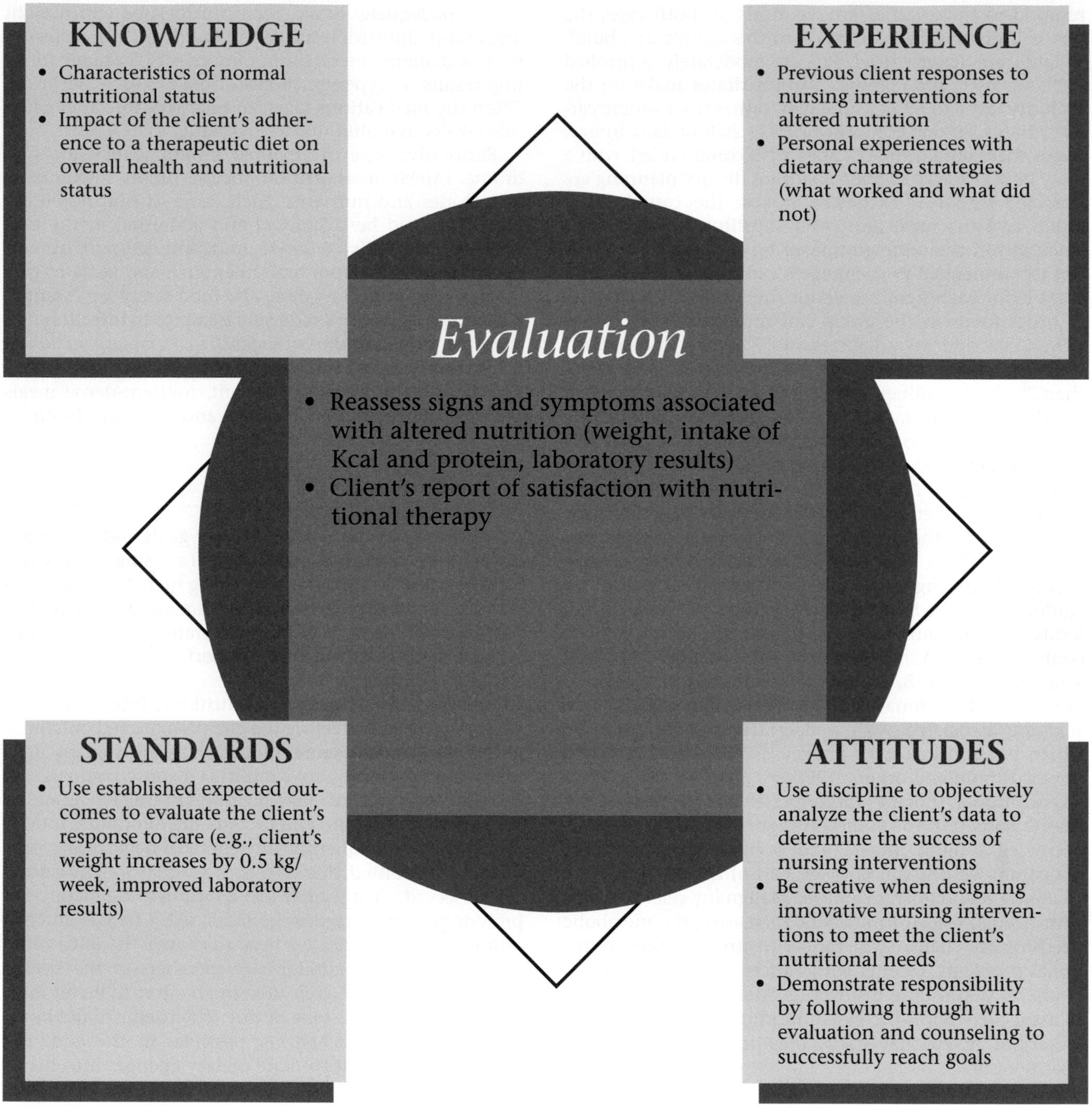

KNOWLEDGE

- Characteristics of normal nutritional status
- Impact of the client's adherence to a therapeutic diet on overall health and nutritional status

EXPERIENCE

- Previous client responses to nursing interventions for altered nutrition
- Personal experiences with dietary change strategies (what worked and what did not)

Evaluation

- Reassess signs and symptoms associated with altered nutrition (weight, intake of Kcal and protein, laboratory results)
- Client's report of satisfaction with nutritional therapy

STANDARDS

- Use established expected outcomes to evaluate the client's response to care (e.g., client's weight increases by 0.5 kg/week, improved laboratory results)

ATTITUDES

- Use discipline to objectively analyze the client's data to determine the success of nursing interventions
- Be creative when designing innovative nursing interventions to meet the client's nutritional needs
- Demonstrate responsibility by following through with evaluation and counseling to successfully reach goals

FIGURE **43–10**   Critical thinking model for nutrition evaluation.

Key Concepts

- Ingestion of a diet balanced with carbohydrates, fats, proteins, vitamin, and minerals provides the essential nutrients to carry out the body's normal physiological functioning throughout the life span.
- Through digestion, food is broken down into its simplest form for absorption. Digestion and absorption occur mainly in the small intestine.
- Dietary reference intakes provide a range of values that address the needs of both groups (estimated average requirement) and individuals (adequate intakes, recommended dietary allowances, and tolerable upper intake level).
- Guidelines for dietary change advocate reduced fat, saturated fat, sodium, refined sugar, and cholesterol and increased intake of complex carbohydrates and fiber.
- Because improper nutrition can affect all body systems, nutritional assessment includes a review of total physical assessment.
- Multidisciplinary collaboration is essential to optimal nutrition.

- Tube feedings can be used for clients who are unable to ingest food but are able to digest and absorb food.
- Enteral nutrition may protect intestinal structure and function and enhance immunity.
- Total parenteral nutrition supplies essential nutrients in appropriate amounts to support life through the introduction of a concentrated nutrient solution into the superior vena cava near the right atrium of the heart.
- Medical nutrition therapy is a recognized treatment modality for both acute and chronic disease states.
- Special diets alter the composition, texture, digestibility, and residue of foods to suit the client's particular needs.

Key Terms

Amino acids, *p. 1273*
Anabolism, *p. 1277*
Anorexia, *p. 1295*
Anorexia nervosa, *p. 1281*
Anthropometry, *p. 1286*
Basal metabolic rate (BMR), *p. 1273*
Body mass index (BMI), *p. 1287*
Bulimia nervosa, *p. 1281*
Carbohydrates, *p. 1273*
Catabolism, *p. 1277*
Chyme, *p. 1275*
Complementary proteins, *p. 1273*
Daily values, *p. 1278*
Dietary reference intakes (DRIs), *p. 1278*
Dysphagia, *p. 1275*
Enteral nutrition (EN), *p. 1299*
Enzymes, *p. 1275*
Essential amino acids, *p. 1273*
Fat-soluble vitamins, *p. 1275*
Fatty acids, *p. 1274*
Fiber, *p. 1273*
Gluconeogenesis, *p. 1278*
Glycogenesis, *p. 1278*
Glycogenolysis, *p. 1278*
Hypervitaminosis, *p. 1275*
Ideal body weight (IBW), *p. 1287*
Ketones, *p. 1278*
Lipid emulsions, *p. 1311*

Lipids, *p. 1274*
Macrominerals, *p. 1275*
Malabsorption, *p. 1316*
Medical nutrition therapy (MNT), *p. 1316*
Metabolism, *p. 1277*
Minerals, *p. 1275*
Monounsaturated (fatty acids), *p. 1274*
Nitrogen balance, *p. 1273*
Nonessential amino acids, *p. 1273*
Nutrient density, *p. 1273*
Nutrients, *p. 1311*
Parenteral nutrition (PN), *p. 1311*
Peristalsis, *p. 1275*
Polyunsaturated (fatty acids), *p. 1274*
Resting energy expenditure (REE), *p. 1273*
Saccharides, *p. 1273*
Saturated (fatty acids), *p. 1274*
Simple carbohydrates, *p. 1273*
Trace element, *p. 1275*
Triglycerides, *p. 1274*
Unsaturated (fatty acids), *p. 1274*
Vegetarianism, *p. 1285*
Vitamins, *p. 1275*
Water-soluble vitamins, *p. 1275*

Critical Thinking Exercises

1. Jean, age 35, has just had surgery for a bowel obstruction. Her medical history includes Crohn's disease. Before this exacerbation, 3 months ago, Jean's weight was 123 pounds (55.8 kg). Admission weight was 115 pounds (52.2 kg); 3 days after surgery she now weighs 108 pounds (49.0 kg). Her height is 5 feet, 5 inches (165 cm). Reported laboratory values are white blood cell count, 8.3; % lymphocytes 13; albumin, 2.3 g/dl. What is Jean's BMI? What is her percent weight loss? What is her total lymphocyte count? Jean remains NPO with nasogastric suction; what intervention(s) would you discuss with her physician?

2. Darrin Thomas, 86, was admitted for a viral infection. He has had a recent weight loss of 6 pounds in the week before admission. He has lost an additional 4 pounds during the week of hospitalization. His appetite is poor; he has frequent nausea and vomiting. His abdomen is soft, nontender, and cancer free, and bowel sounds are present. Enteral feedings will be initiated.
   a. What type of tube should be selected?
   b. How will the tube placement be verified?
   c. Describe the type of feeding and initiation of feedings.
   d. What complications should be assessed?

3. Roberta is being treated for breast cancer with chemotherapy as adjunct to a lumpectomy. She has maintained a positive attitude as well as possible but is concerned about the side effects of the medication. Roberta has bleeding gums, stomatitis, nausea, and diarrhea. As a result she has no desire to eat. She is 85% of her usual body weight at present. How could you assist Roberta in improving her nutritional status?

Review Questions

1. The nutrient that provides the body's most preferred energy source is:
   1. Fat.
   2. Protein.
   3. Vitamin.
   4. Carbohydrate.

2. The nutrient that is preferred to repair tissue is:
   1. Fat.
   2. Protein.
   3. Vitamin.
   4. Carbohydrate.

3. Positive nitrogen balance would occur in:
   1. Infection.
   2. Starvation.
   3. Burn injury.
   4. Pregnancy.

4. Water composes 60% to 70% of
   1. Total body weight.
   2. Digested food.
   3. Carbohydrates.
   4. Water-soluble vitamins.

5. When feeding tubes are first positioned, verification is done by:
   1. Auscultation.
   2. X-ray confirmation.
   3. pH testing of gastric contents.
   4. Confirmation of distal mark on feeding tube.

6. Parenteral nutrition is used when the client is:
   1. NPO.
   2. Critically ill.
   3. Recovering from abdominal surgery.
   4. Experiencing a condition resulting in gastrointestinal dysfunction.

7. The bacteria that causes peptic ulcers is:
   1. *Micrococcus.*
   2. *Helicobacter pylori.*
   3. *Staphyloccocus.*
   4. *Corynebacteria.*

8. Inflammatory bowel disease include(s):
   1. Crohn's disease and idiopathic ulcerative colitis.
   2. Celiac disease.
   3. Peptic ulcers.
   4. Diverticulitis.

9. Nutritional therapy for hypertension includes:
   1. A moderate or low-residue diet.
   2. Reduction in kilocalories, soft-textured foods, and amounts of fat, sodium, and cholesterol.
   3. Kilocalorie reduction to promote weight loss as appropriate, decreased sodium intake, and potassium-rich foods if potassium-wasting diuretics are part of the treatment.
   4. A high-fiber diet.

10. Homebound elderly have an increased risk of:
    1. Diverticulitis.
    2. Poor nutrition.
    3. Food intolerances.
    4. Peptic ulcers.

References

American Academy of Family Physicians: *A position paper on disease state management,* (November 7, 1997), http://www.aafp.org/family/managed/disease.

American Academy of Pediatrics: Infant feeding practices and their possible relationship to the etiology of diabetes mellitus (RE9430), *Pediatrics* 94(5):752, 1994.

American Academy of Pediatrics: Breastfeeding recommendations, *Pediatrics* 100(6):1035, 1997a.

American Academy of Pediatrics: Pediatrician's responsibility for infant nutrition, *Pediatrics* 99(5):749, 1997b.

American Cancer Society: American Cancer Society Guidelines on Diet and Cancer, 1997, http://www.cancer.org.

American Diabetic Association: Evidenced-based nutrition principles: recommendations for the treatment and prevention of diabetes related complications, *Diabetic Care* 25(suppl 1):S50, 2002, http://www.diabetes.org.

American Heart Association: AHA scientific position: "Dietary guidelines for healthy American adults," *Circulation* 102:2284, 2000, http://www.americanheart.org.

American Psychiatric Association: *Diagnostic and statistical manual of mental disorders,* ed 4-revised, Washington, DC, 1994, The Association.

American Society for Parenteral and Enteral Nutrition: Standards of practice, nutrition support nurse, *Nutr Clin Pract* 16(1):56, 2001.

American Society for Parenteral and Enteral Nutrition: Guidelines for the use of parenteral and enteral nutrition in adult and pediatric patients, *J Parenter Enteral Nutr* 26(1):1SA, 2002.

Bowers S: Tubes: a nurse's guide to enteral feeding devices, *Medsurg Nurs* 5(5):313, 1996.

Chen CC and others: A concept analysis of malnutrition in the elderly, *J Adv Nurs* 36(1):131, 2001.

Costello MC, Todd-Magel C: Bridging the gap: hospital to home nutrition support, *Medsurg Nurs* 6(6):328, 1997.

Davis AE and others: Preventing feeding-associated aspiration, *Medsurg Nurs* 4(2):111, 1995.

Dochterman JM, Bulechek GM: *Nursing interventions classification (NIC),* ed 4, St. Louis, 2004, Mosby.

Dossey B: *Florence Nightingale: mystic, visionary, and healer,* Philadelphia, 1999, Springhouse.

Edwards S, Metheny N: Measurement of gastric residual volume: state of the science, *Medsurg Nurs* 9(3):125, 2000.

Evans-Stoner N: Nutritional assessment: a practical approach, *Nurs Clin North Am* 32(4):637, 1997.

Food and Nutrition Board: *Nutrition during pregnancy and lactation: an implementation guide,* Washington, DC, 1992, National Academy Press.

Food and Nutrition Board: *Dietary reference intakes for calcium, phosphorus, magnesium, vitamin D, and fluoride,* Washington, DC, 1997, National Academy Press.

Galvin TJ: Dysphagia: going down and staying down, *Am J Nurs* 101(1):37, 2001.

Giger JN, Davidhizar RE: *Transcultural nursing: assessment and intervention,* ed 2, St. Louis, 1995, Mosby.

Grodner M, Anderson S, DeYoung S: *Foundations and clinical applications of nutrition: a nursing approach,* ed 2, St. Louis, 2000, Mosby.

Guenter P, Ericson M, Jones S: Enteral nutrition therapy, *Nurs Clin North Am,* 32(4):651, 1997.

Hennessy KA, Orr ME: *Nutrition support core curriculum,* ed 3, Silver Spring, Md, 1996, American Society of Parenteral and Enteral Nutrition.

Hornick B: Diet and nutrition implications for oral health, *J Dent Hyg* 76(1):67, 2002.

Moorhead S, Johnson M, Maas M: *Nursing outcomes classification (NOC),* ed 3, St. Louis, 2004, Mosby.

Keithley K, Swanson B: Minimizing HIV/AIDS malnutrition, *Medsurg Nurs* 7(5):256, 1998.

Kennedy-Caldwell CM: Childhood nutrition, *Annu Rev Nurs Res* 16:3, 1998.

Lueckenotte AG: *Gerontolologic nursing,* ed 2, St. Louis, 2000, Mosby.

Nutrition Labeling and Education Act, PL 100-535, 104 Stat 2353, 21 USC §301 (1990).

Nutrition Screening Initiative: A project of the American Academy of Family Physicians, the American Dietetic Association, and the National Council of the Aging, Inc and funded in part by a grant from Ross Products Division, Abbott Laboratories, 1998.

Pagana KD, Pagana TJ: *Mosby's diagnostic and laboratory test reference,* ed 4, St. Louis, 1999, Mosby.

Rombeau JL, Rolandelli RH, editors: *Enteral feeding and tube feeding,* Philadelphia, 1997, WB Saunders.

Todorovic V: Detecting and managing nutrition of older people in the community, *Br J Community Nurs* 6(2):54, 2001.

U.S. Department of Agriculture: *Healthy eating index,* Washington, DC, October 1995, U.S. Department of Agriculture.

U.S. Department of Agriculture: *USDA's food guide pyramid,* USDA Human Nutrition Information Service Pub No. 249, Washington, DC, 1996, U.S. Government Printing Office.

U.S. Department of Health and Human Services: *Morning Meals on Wheels program initiative announced,* March 19, 1997, http://www.hhs.gov.

U.S. Department of Agriculture and U.S. Department of Health and Human Services: *Nutrition and your health: dietary guidelines for Americans,* ed 5, USDA/DHHS Home and Garden Bulletin No. 232, Washington, DC, 2000, U.S. Government Printing Office, http://www.usda.gov/cnpp/pubs.

U.S. Department of Health and Human Services: *Healthy people 2010,* 2002, http://www.health.gov/healthypeople.

U.S. Food and Drug Administration: *FDA Public Health Advisory: reports of blue discoloration and death in patients receiving enteral feedings tinted with the dye FD&C Blue No. 1,* Washington, DC, 2003, U.S. Food and Drug Administration, pp. 1-3.

Weigley ES: Nutrition-related activities of entry level nurses, *Nurse Educ* 20:3, 1995.

Williams SR: *Basic nutrition and diet therapy,* ed 11, St. Louis, 2001, Mosby.

Wong DL: *Whaley & Wong's essentials of pediatric nursing,* ed 6, St. Louis, 2001, Mosby.

Ybarra J, Ade R, Romeo JH: Osteoporosis in men: a review, *Nurs Clin North Am* 31(4):805, 1996.

Young WB, Minnick AF, Marcantonio R: How wide is the gap in defining quality care? Comparison of patient and nurse perceptions of important aspects of patient care, *J Nurs Adm* 26(2):15, 1996.

Zaloga G: Frontiers in critical care nutrition, *New Horizons* 2(2):121, 1994.

Research References

Atkinson SA, Ward WE: The role of nutrition in the prevention and treatment of adult osteoporosis, *Can Med Assoc J* 105(11):1511, 2001.

Chang J and others: Inadvertent endobronchial intubation with nasogastric tube, *Arch Otolaryngol* 108:528, 1982.

Daly S and others: Minimum effective dose of folic acid for food fortification to prevent neural tube defects, *Lancet* 347:657, 1997.

Foster GD and others: What is a reasonable weight loss? Patient expectations of obesity treatment, *J Consult Clin Psychol* 65(1):79, 1997.

Hunt S and others: ACC/AHA guidelines for the evaluation and treatment of chronic heart failure in the adult: executive summary—ACC/AHA practice guidelines, *Circulation* 104:2996, 2001.

Kovacevich DS and others: Nutrition risk classification: a reproducible and valid tool for nurses, *Nutr Clin Pract* 12(1):20, 1997.

Lipkin E: New strategies for the treatment of type 2 diabetes, *J Am Diet Assoc* 99(3):329, 1999.

McClave SA and others: Enteral tube feeding in the intensive care unit: factors impeding adequate delivery, *Crit Care Med* 27(7):1252, 1999.

Metheny NA: Inadvertent intracranial nasogastric tube placement, *Am J Nurs* 102(8):25, 2002.

Metheny N, Titler, M: Assessing placement of feeding tubes, *Am J Nurs* 101(5):36, 2001.

Metheny N, Aud M, Ignatavicius D: Detection of improperly placed feeding tubes, *J Healthc Risk Manage* 18(3):37, 1998a.

Metheny N, Aud MA, Wunderlich RJ: A survey of bedside methods used to detect pulmonary aspiration of enteral formula in intubated tube-fed patients, *Am J Crit Care* 8(3):160, 1999.

Metheny N and others: Measures to test placement of nasogastric and nasointestinal feeding tubes: a review, *Nurse Res* 37:324, 1988.

Metheny N and others: Effectiveness of pH measurement in predicting feeding tube placement, *Nurse Res* 38(5):262, 1989.

Metheny N and others: Detection of inadvertent respiratory placement of small-bore feeding tubes: a report of 10 cases, *Heart Lung* 19(6):631, 1990a.

Metheny N and others: Effectiveness of the auscultatory method in predicting feeding tube location, *Nurse Res* 39(5):262, 1990b.

Metheny N and others: Effectiveness of pH measurements in predicting feeding tube placement: an update, *Nurs Res* 42(6):324, 1993a.

Metheny N and others: How to aspirate fluid from small bore feeding tubes, *Am J Nurs* 93(5):86, 1993b.

Metheny N and others: Visual characteristics of aspirates from feeding tubes as a method for predicting tube location, *Nurs Res* 43:282, 1994.

Metheny N and others: pH and concentrations of pepsin and trypsin in feeding tube aspirates as predictors of tube placement, *J Parenter Enteral Nutr* 21(5):279, 1997.

Metheny N and others: pH, color, and feeding tubes, *RN* 61(1):277, 1998a.

Metheny N and others: Testing feeding tube placement: auscultation vs. pH method, *Am J Nurs* 98:37, 1998b.

Metheny N and others: pH and concentrations of bilirubin in feeding tube aspirates as predictors of tube placement, *Nurs Res* 48(4):189, 1999.

Metheny N and others: Development of a reliable and valid bedside test for bilirubin and its utilization for improving prediction of feeding tube location, *Nurs Res* 49(6):202, 2000.

Metheny N and others: Pepsin as a marker for pulmonary aspiration, *Am J Crit Care* 11(2):150, 2002.

Millen BE and others: Nutritional risk in an urban homebound older population: the nutrition and healthy aging project, *J Nutr Health Aging* 5(4):269, 2001.

Neumark-Sztainer D and others: Factors influencing food choices of adolescents: findings from focus-group discussions with adolescents, *J Am Diet Assoc* 99(8):929, 1999.

Pickering LK and others: Modulation of the immune system by human milk and infant formula containing nucleotides, *Pediatrics* 101:242, 1998.

Rimm EB and others: Folate and vitamin B_6 from diet and supplements in relation to risk of coronary heart disease among women, *JAMA* 279(5):359, 1998.

Sheils JF, Rubin R, Stapleton DC: The estimated costs and savings of medical nutrition therapy: the Medicare population, *J Am Diet Assoc* 99(4):428, 1999.

Simon T, Fink AS: Current management of endoscopic feeding tube dysfunction, *Surg Endosc* 13:403, 1999.

$\mathcal{U}$rinary Elimination

44

Media Resources

http://evolve.elsevier.com/Potter/
fundamentals/

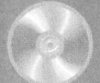 **CD COMPANION**

- Review Questions
- Glossary

evolve WEBSITE

- Review Questions
- Student Learning Activities
- Animations
- Concept Map Exercise
- Critical Thinking Exercise
- Video Clips
- Glossary

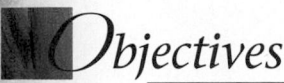bjectives

Mastery of content in this chapter will enable the student to:

- Define the key terms listed.
- Describe the process of urination.
- Identify factors that commonly influence urinary elimination.
- Compare and contrast common alterations in urinary elimination.
- Obtain a nursing history for a client with urinary elimination problems.
- Identify nursing diagnoses appropriate for clients with alterations in urinary elimination.
- Obtain urine specimens.
- Describe characteristics of normal and abnormal urine.
- Describe the nursing implications of common diagnostic tests of the urinary system.
- Discuss nursing measures to promote normal micturition and reduce episodes of incontinence.
- Insert a urinary catheter.
- Discuss nursing measures to reduce urinary tract infection.
- Irrigate a urinary catheter.
- Identify two modalities of renal replacement therapy.

*N*ormal elimination of urinary wastes is a basic function most people take for granted. When the urinary system fails to function properly, virtually all organ systems will be eventually affected. Clients with alterations in urinary elimination may also suffer emotionally from body image changes. The nurse provides understanding and a sensitivity to all clients' needs. The nurse must understand the reasons for urinary elimination problems and find acceptable solutions.

Scientific Knowledge Base

Urinary elimination depends on the function of the kidneys, ureters, bladder, and urethra. Kidneys remove wastes from the blood to form urine. Ureters transport urine from the kidneys to the bladder. The bladder holds urine until the urge to urinate develops. Urine leaves the body through the urethra. All organs of the urinary system must be intact and functional for successful removal of urinary wastes (Figure 44-1).

Kidneys
The kidneys lie on either side of the vertebral column behind the peritoneum and against deep muscles of the back. The kidneys extend from the twelfth thoracic to the third lumbar vertebrae. Normally, the left kidney is higher than the right because of the anatomical position of the liver.

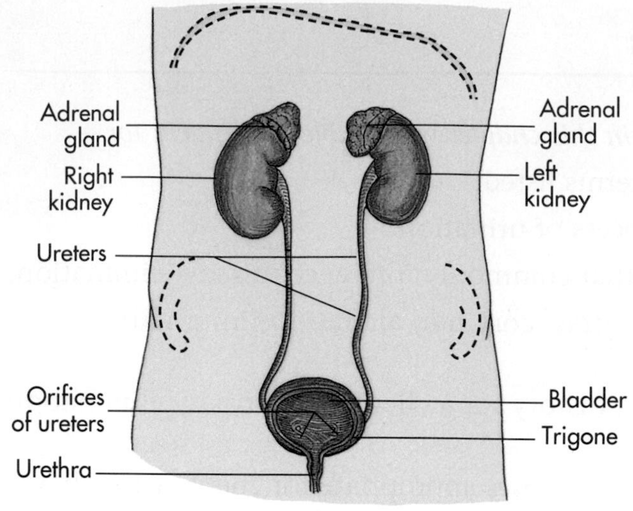

FIGURE **44–1** Organs of the urinary system.

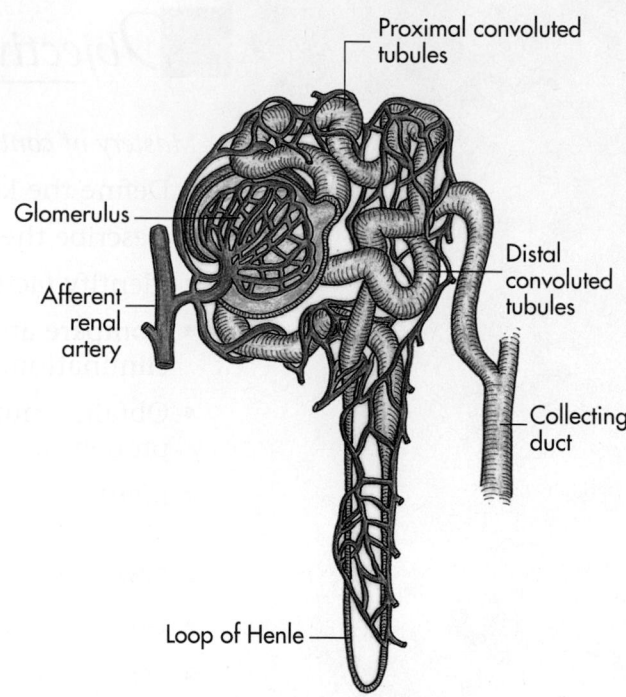

FIGURE **44–2** Renal nephron.

Waste products of metabolism that collect in the blood are filtered in the kidneys. Blood reaches each kidney by a renal (kidney) artery that branches from the abdominal aorta. Approximately 20% to 25% of the cardiac output circulates each minute through the kidneys. The **nephron,** the functional unit of the kidney, forms the urine. The nephron is composed of the glomerulus, Bowman's capsule, proximal convoluted tubule, loop of Henle, distal tubule, and collecting duct (Figure 44-2).

A cluster of blood vessels forms the capillary network of the glomerulus, which is the initial site of filtration of the blood and the beginning of urine formation. The glomerular capillaries permit filtration of water, glucose, amino acids, urea, creatinine, and major electrolytes into Bowman's capsule. Large proteins and blood cells do not normally filter through the glomerulus. The presence of large proteins in the urine **(proteinuria)** is a sign of glomerular injury. The glomerulus filters approximately 125 ml of filtrate per minute.

Not all the glomerular filtrate is excreted as urine. About 99% of the filtrate is reabsorbed into the plasma, with the remaining 1% excreted as urine (McCance and Huether, 2002). The kidneys play a key role in fluid and electrolyte balance (see Chapter 40). Although output does depend on intake, the normal adult urine output is 1500 to 1600 ml/day. An output of less than 30 ml/hr may indicate renal alterations. The kidneys also produce several substances vital to production of red blood cells (RBCs), blood pressure regulation, and bone mineralization.

The kidneys are responsible for maintaining a normal RBC volume by producing **erythropoietin.** Erythropoietin functions within the bone marrow to stimulate red blood cell production and maturation and prolongs the life of mature RBCs (McCance and Huether, 2002). Clients with chronic alterations in kidney function cannot produce sufficient quantities of this hormone; therefore they are prone to anemia.

Renin is another hormone produced by the kidneys. Its major role is the regulation of blood flow in times of renal ischemia (decreased blood supply). Renin is released from juxtaglomerular cells (Figure 44-3). The kid-

neys also produce prostaglandin E_2 and prostacyclin, which are important in maintaining renal blood flow through vasodilation.

Renin functions as an enzyme to convert angiotensinogen (a substance synthesized by the liver) into angiotensin I. Angiotensin I is converted to angiotensin II in the lungs. Angiotensin II causes vasoconstriction and stimulates aldosterone release from the adrenal cortex. Aldosterone causes retention of water, which increases blood volume. Both of these mechanisms increase arterial blood pressure and renal blood flow (McCance and Huether, 2002).

The kidneys also play a role in calcium and phosphate regulation by producing a substance that converts vitamin D into its active form. Clients with chronic alterations in kidney function do not make sufficient amounts of the active vitamin D. They are prone to develop renal bone disease resulting from the demineralization of bone caused by impaired calcium absorption.

Ureters

Urine enters the renal pelvis from the collecting ducts and travels to the bladder through ureters. The ureters are tubular structures that enter the urinary bladder in the pelvic cavity at the ureterovesical junction. Urine draining from the ureters to the bladder is usually sterile.

Three layers of tissue form the wall of the ureter. The inner layer is a mucous membrane continuous with the lining of the renal pelvis and urinary bladder. The middle layer consists of smooth muscle fibers that transport urine by peristaltic waves. An outer layer of fibrous connective tissue supports the ureters.

Peristaltic waves cause the urine to enter the bladder in spurts rather than steadily. The ureters enter obliquely through the posterior bladder wall. This arrangement normally prevents the reflux of urine from the bladder into

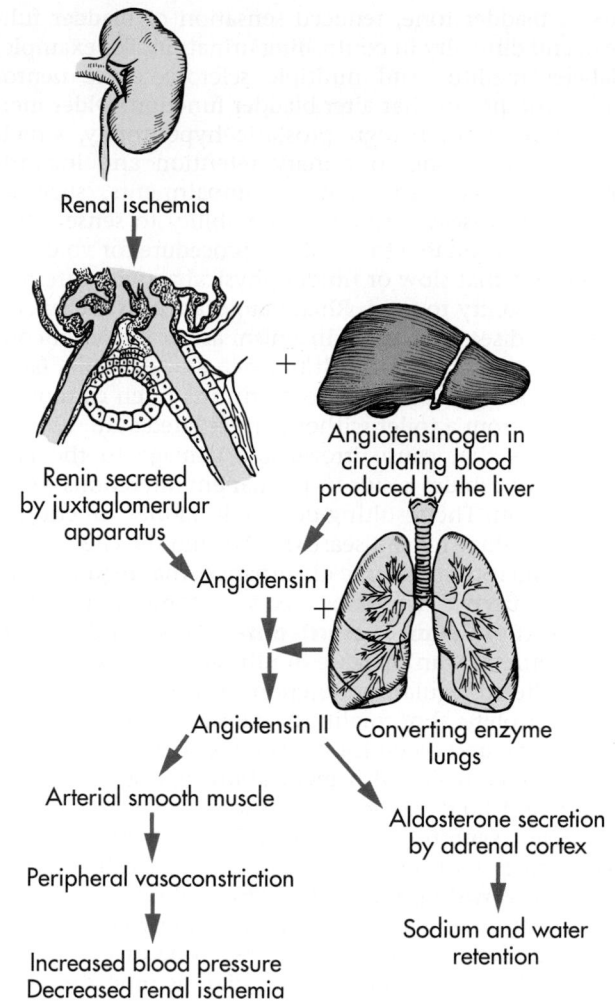

FIGURE **44-3** Physiological effects of renin-angiotensin mechanism.

the ureters during the act of **micturition** by the compression of the ureter at the ureterovesical junction (the juncture of the ureters with the bladder). An obstruction within a ureter, such as a kidney stone **(renal calculus),** results in strong peristaltic waves that attempt to move the obstruction into the bladder. These strong peristaltic waves result in pain often referred to as renal colic.

Bladder

The urinary bladder is a hollow, distensible, muscular organ that stores and excretes urine. When empty, the bladder lies in the pelvic cavity behind the symphysis pubis. In men the bladder lies against the anterior wall of the rectum and in women it rests against the anterior walls of the uterus and vagina.

The bladder expands as it becomes filled with urine. Pressure within the bladder is usually low, even when partly full, a factor that protects against infection. When the bladder is full, it expands and extends above the symphysis pubis. A greatly distended bladder may reach the umbilicus. In a pregnant woman the developing fetus pushes against the bladder, reducing the bladder's capacity and causing a feeling of fullness. This effect is more likely to occur in the first and third trimester.

The trigone (a smooth triangular area on the inner surface of the bladder) is at the base of the bladder. An opening exists at each of the trigone's three angles. Two are for the ureters, and one is for the urethra.

The wall of the bladder has four layers: the inner mucous coat, a submucous coat of connective tissue, a muscular coat, and an outer serous coat. The muscular layer has bundles of muscle fibers that form the detrusor muscle. The internal urethral sphincter, made of a ringlike band of muscle, is at the base of the bladder where it joins the urethra. The sphincter prevents escape of urine from the bladder and is under voluntary control.

Urethra

Urine travels from the bladder through the urethra and passes outside of the body through the urethral meatus. Normally the turbulent flow of urine through the urethra washes it free of bacteria. Mucous membrane lines the urethra, and urethral glands secrete mucus into the urethral canal. Thick layers of smooth muscle surround the urethra. In addition, the urethra descends through a layer of skeletal muscles called the pelvic floor muscles. When these muscles are contracted, it is possible to prevent urine flow through the urethra (McCance and Huether, 2002).

In women the urethra is approximately 4 to 6.5 cm (1½ to 2½ inches) long. The external urethral sphincter, located about halfway down the urethra, permits voluntary flow of urine. The short length of the urethra predisposes women and girls to infection. Bacteria can easily enter the urethra from the perineal area. In men the urethra, which is both a urinary canal and a passageway for cells and secretions from reproductive organs, is about 20 cm (8 inches) long. The male urethra has three sections: the prostatic urethra, the membranous urethra, and the penile urethra.

Act of Urination

Several brain structures influence bladder function, including the cerebral cortex, thalamus, hypothalamus, and brain stem. Together they suppress contraction of the bladder's detrusor muscle until a person wishes to urinate or void. Once voiding occurs, the response is a contraction of the bladder and coordinated relaxation of pelvic floor muscles.

The bladder normally holds as much as 600 ml of urine. However, the desire to urinate can be sensed when the bladder contains a smaller amount of urine (150 to 200 ml in an adult and 50 to 100 ml in a child). As the volume increases, the bladder walls stretch, sending sensory impulses to the micturition center in the sacral spinal cord. Impulses from the micturition center stimulate the detrusor muscle to contract. The internal urethral sphincter relaxes; urine enters the urethra, although voiding does not yet occur. As the bladder contracts, nerve impulses to the midbrain and cerebral cortex make a person conscious of the need to urinate. Older children and adults can respond to or ignore this urge, thus making urination under voluntary control. If the person chooses not to void, the external urinary sphincter remains contracted, and the micturition reflex is inhibited. However, when a person is ready to void, the external sphincter relaxes, the micturition reflex stimulates the detrusor muscle to contract, and efficient emptying of the bladder occurs.

If the urge to void has been ignored repeatedly, the bladder capacity may be reached and the resulting pressure on the sphincter may make continued voluntary control impossible.

Damage to the spinal cord above the sacral region causes loss of voluntary control of urination, but the micturition reflex pathway may remain intact, allowing urination to occur reflexively. This condition is called a **reflex bladder.** If bladder emptying is hindered by chronic obstruction such as prostate enlargement, over time the micturition reflex becomes nonfunctional and severe urinary retention occurs.

Factors Influencing Urination. Many factors influence the volume and quality of urine and the client's ability to urinate. Some pathophysiological conditions may be acute and reversible (urinary tract infection), whereas others may be chronic and irreversible (slow, progressive development of renal dysfunction). Diseases that slow or hinder physical activity interfere with the ability to void. Sociocultural factors and psychological factors may influence the client's expectation of the degree of privacy and location for attending to urinary needs. Muscle tone of the abdominal and pelvic floor muscles impairs urination. Fluid balance directly affects the quantity of urine produced. Surgical and diagnostic procedures affect urine and urination in several ways. Medications may interfere with both the production and characteristics of urine and affect the act of urination. Problems related to the act of urination may be the result of cognitive, functional, or physical means resulting in incontinence, retention, or infection.

Disease Conditions. Disease processes that affect urine elimination may affect renal function (changes in urine volume or quality), the act of urine elimination, or both. Those conditions that affect urine volume and quality are generally categorized as prerenal, renal, or postrenal in origin.

Prerenal alterations decrease circulating blood flow to and through the kidneys with resulting decreased blood flow to renal tissue. In other words, the alterations occur before the urinary system. The decrease in renal blood flow leads to **oliguria** (diminished capacity to form urine) or, less commonly, **anuria** (inability to produce urine). Selected causes include dehydration, hemorrhage, and congestive heart failure.

Renal alterations result from factors that cause injury directly to the glomeruli or renal tubule, interfering with their normal filtering, reabsorptive, and secretory functions. Selected causes include transfusion reactions, diseases of the glomeruli, and systemic diseases such as diabetes mellitus.

Postrenal alterations result from obstruction to the flow of urine in the urinary collecting system caused by calculi, blood clots, or tumors anywhere from the calyces (drainage structures within the kidney) to the urethral meatus. Urine is formed by the urinary system but cannot be eliminated by normal means.

Several diseases can affect the ability to micturate. Any lesion of peripheral nerves leading to the bladder causes loss of bladder tone, reduced sensation of bladder fullness, and difficulty in controlling urination. For example, diabetes mellitus and multiple sclerosis cause neuropathic conditions that alter bladder function. Older men may suffer from benign prostatic hypertrophy, which makes them prone to urinary retention and incontinence. Clients with cognitive impairments, such as Alzhiemer's disease, may lose the ability to sense a full bladder or be unable to recall the procedure for voiding.

Diseases that slow or hinder physical activity interfere with the ability to void. Rheumatoid arthritis, degenerative joint disease, and Parkinsonism are examples of conditions that make it difficult to reach and use toilet facilities. A client with rheumatoid arthritis often cannot sit on or rise from a toilet without an elevated seat.

Diseases that cause irreversible damage to the glomerulus or tubules result in permanent alterations in renal function. The resulting decline in kidney function is called end-stage renal disease (ESRD), and the client manifests numerous metabolic disturbances that require treatment for survival. The associated symptoms occur as a result of the **uremic syndrome.** This syndrome is characterized by an increase in nitrogenous wastes in the blood, altered regulatory functions (causing marked fluid and electrolyte abnormalities), nausea, vomiting, headache, coma, and convulsions. The problem may be managed conservatively with medications and a regimen of dietary and fluid restrictions. However, as worsening of the uremic symptoms becomes evident, more aggressive treatment is indicated (Box 44-1). These treatments are known as **renal replacement therapies.**

Dialysis and organ transplantation are two methods of renal replacement. Dialysis may take one of two forms, peritoneal or hemodialysis. Both dialysis modalities can be applied for a short or long time, but they require specialized equipment and nurses with specific training.

Peritoneal dialysis is an indirect method of cleansing the blood of waste products using osmosis and diffusion. The peritoneum functions as a semipermeable membrane. Excess fluid and waste products are readily removed from the bloodstream when a sterile electrolyte solution (dialysate) is instilled into the peritoneal cavity by gravity via a surgically placed catheter. The dialysate is left in the cavity for a prescribed time interval and then is drained out by gravity, taking accumulated wastes and excess fluid and electrolytes with it.

Hemodialysis uses a machine equipped with a semipermeable filtering membrane (artificial kidney) that removes accumulated waste products and excess fluids

---

Box 44-1   Indications for Dialysis

Renal failure that can no longer be controlled by conservative management (i.e., dietary modifications and administration of medications to correct electrolyte abnormalities)
Worsening of uremic syndrome associated with ESRD (i.e., nausea, vomiting, neurological changes, pericarditis)
Severe electrolyte and/or fluid abnormalities that cannot be controlled by simpler measures (e.g., hyperkalemia, pulmonary edema)

from the blood. In the dialysis machine, dialysate fluid is pumped through one side of the filter membrane (artificial kidney) while the client's blood passes through the other side. The processes of diffusion, osmosis, and ultrafiltration cleanse the client's blood, and it is returned through a specially placed vascular access device (Gore-Tex graft, arteriovenous fistula, or hemodialysis catheter).

Organ transplantation is the replacement of the client's diseased kidneys with a healthy one from a living or cadaver donor of compatible blood and tissue type. The new organ is surgically implanted into the abdomen. Special medications (immunosuppressives) are administered for life to prevent the body from rejecting the transplanted organ. Unlike the other treatments, successful organ transplantation offers the client the potential for restoration of normal kidney function.

Sociocultural Factors. The degree of privacy needed for urination varies with cultural norms. North Americans expect toilet facilities to be private, whereas some European cultures accept communal toilet facilities. Social expectations (e.g., school recesses) influence the time of urination.

The nurse's approach to a client's elimination needs must consider cultural, social, and gender habits. If a client prefers privacy, the nurse tries to prevent interruptions as the client voids. A client with less need for privacy should be treated with understanding and acceptance. Place clients in a position of comfort. Men generally urinate best in a standing position, whereas women generally sit on a toilet. In some cultures the client would squat over a receptacle rather than sit on one. Culture dictates when and where it is appropriate to urinate. Culture determines whether it is proper for a male to care for the urinary needs of a female (see Chapter 8).

Psychological Factors. Anxiety and emotional stress may cause a sense of urgency and increased frequency of urination. Anxiety may prevent a person from being able to urinate completely; as a result, the urge to void may return shortly after voiding. Emotional tension makes it difficult to relax abdominal and perineal muscles. If the external urethral sphincter is not completely relaxed, voiding may be incomplete, and urine is retained in the bladder. Attempting to void in a public restroom may result in a temporary inability to void. Privacy and adequate time to urinate are usually important to most people. Some people need distractions (e.g., reading) to relax.

Muscle Tone. Weak abdominal and pelvic floor muscles impair bladder contraction and control of the external urethral sphincter. Poor control of micturition can result from muscle wasting caused by prolonged immobility, stretching of muscles during childbirth, menopausal muscle atrophy, or traumatic damage to muscles. Continuous drainage of urine through an indwelling catheter causes loss of bladder tone and/or damage to urethral sphincters. When a catheter is removed, the client may have difficulty regaining urinary control.

Fluid Balance. The kidneys maintain a sensitive balance between retention and excretion of fluids (see Chapter 40). If fluids and the concentration of electrolytes and solutes are in equilibrium, an increase in fluid intake causes an increase in urine production. Ingested fluids increase the body's circulating plasma and thus increase the volume of urine excreted.

This amount varies with food and fluid intake. The volume of urine formed at night is about half that formed during the day because both intake and metabolism decline. Nocturia can be a sign of renal alteration. In a healthy person, the intake of water in food and fluids balances the output of water in urine, feces, and insensible losses in perspiration and respiration. An excessive output of urine is known as **polyuria.** A urine output that is decreased despite normal intake is called oliguria. Oliguria may occur when fluid losses through other means is increased (perspiration, diarrhea, or vomiting) or may occur with kidney disease.

Ingestion of certain fluids directly affects urine production and excretion. Coffee, tea, cocoa, and cola drinks that contain caffeine promote increased urine formation **(diuresis).** Alcohol inhibits the release of antidiuretic hormone (ADH), also resulting in increased water loss in urine. Foods that contain a high fluid content, such as fruits and vegetables, may also increase urine production.

Febrile conditions affect urine production. The client who becomes diaphoretic loses a large amount of fluids through insensible water loss, which decreases urine production. However, the increased body metabolism associated with fever increases accumulation of body wastes. Although urine volume may be reduced, it is highly concentrated.

Surgical Procedures. The stress of surgery initially triggers the general adaptation syndrome (see Chapter 30). The surgical client is often in an altered state of fluid balance before surgery due to the disease process or preoperative fasting, which aggravates the reduction in urine output. The stress response releases an increased amount of ADH, which increases water reabsorption. Stress also elevates the level of aldosterone, causing retention of sodium and water. Both of these substances reduce urine output in an effort to maintain circulatory fluid volume.

Anesthetics and narcotic analgesics may alter the glomerular filtration rate, reducing urine output. These pharmacological agents also impair sensory and motor impulses traveling between the bladder, spinal cord, and brain. Clients recovering from anesthesia and deep analgesia are often unable to sense bladder fullness and are unable to initiate or inhibit micturition. Spinal anesthetics, in particular, create the risk of urinary retention because of an inability to sense the need to void and a possible inability of the bladder muscles and sphincters to respond (Lewis, Heitkemper, and Dirksen, 2000).

Surgery of lower abdominal and pelvic structures can impair urination because of local trauma to surrounding tissues. The edema and inflammation may obstruct the flow of urine from the kidneys to the bladder or from the bladder or urethra, interfere with relaxation of pelvic and sphincter muscles, or cause discomfort during voiding. After returning from surgery involving the ureters, bladder, and urethra, clients routinely have urinary catheters.

The surgical formation of a **urinary diversion** temporarily or permanently bypasses the bladder and urethra as the exit routes for urine. Permanent urinary diversions may be needed in the client with cancer of the bladder. The client with a urinary diversion has a **stoma** (artificial opening) on the abdomen to drain urine.

Medications. Diuretics prevent reabsorption of water and certain electrolytes to increase urine output. Urinary retention may be caused by use of anticholinergics (e.g., atropine), antihistamines (e.g., Sudafed), or antihypertensives (e.g., Aldomet). Some medications change the color of urine. Phenazopyridine (Pyridium) colors the urine a bright orange to rust; amitriptyline causes a green or blue discoloration, whereas levodopa may discolor the urine to brown or black. Cancer chemotherapy drugs may also color the urine and be toxic to the kidneys or the bladder. Clients with alterations in kidney function require dosage adjustments in medications excreted by the kidneys.

Diagnostic Examination. Examination of the urinary system can influence micturition. Procedures such as an intravenous pyelogram may require that the client limit fluids before the test. A restriction in fluid intake commonly lowers urine output. A laxative used to cleanse the bowel may limit fluid available for urine production. Diagnostic examinations (e.g., cystoscopy) that involve direct visualization of urinary structures may cause localized edema of the urethral passageway and spasm of the bladder sphincter. The client often has urinary retention after such a procedure and may pass red or pink urine because of trauma to the urethral or bladder mucosa.

Alterations in Urinary Elimination. Most clients with urinary problems have disturbances in the act of micturition that involve a failure to store urine or a failure to empty urine. These disturbances result from impaired bladder function, obstruction to urine outflow, or inability to voluntarily control micturition. Some clients may have permanent or temporary changes in the normal pathway of urinary excretion. The client with a urinary diversion has special problems because urine drains to the outside through a stoma.

Urinary Retention. **Urinary retention** is the marked accumulation of urine in the bladder as a result of the inability of the bladder to empty. Normally urine production slowly fills the bladder and prevents activation of stretch receptors until it distends to a certain level of stretch. The micturition reflex occurs, and the bladder empties. In urinary retention the bladder becomes unable to respond to the micturition reflex and thus unable to empty. Urine continues to collect in the bladder, stretching its walls and causing feelings of pressure, discomfort, tenderness over the symphysis pubis, restlessness, and diaphoresis (sweating).

As retention progresses, retention with overflow may develop. Pressure in the bladder builds to a point where the external urethral sphincter is unable to hold back urine. The sphincter temporarily opens to allow a small volume of urine (25 to 60 ml) to escape. As urine exits, the bladder pressure falls enough to allow the sphincter to regain control and close. With retention overflow the

client voids small amounts of urine 2 or 3 times an hour with no real relief of discomfort. The nurse should be aware of the volume and frequency of voiding to assess this condition in the client. The nurse should assess the abdomen for evidence of bladder distention.

In acute retention key signs are bladder distention and absence of urine output over several hours. The client under the influence of anesthetics or analgesics may feel only pressure, but the alert client has severe pain as the bladder distends beyond its normal capacity. In severe urinary retention the bladder may hold as much as 2000 to 3000 ml of urine. Retention occurs as a result of urethral obstruction, surgical or childbirth trauma, alterations in motor and sensory innervation of the bladder, medication side effects, or anxiety.

Urinary Tract Infections. Urinary tract infections (UTIs) are responsible for more than 7 million physician visits a year and are the most common hospital-acquired (nosocomial) infections in the United States, accounting for 40% of the total (Foxman, 2002). Many cases result from catheterization or surgical manipulation. Although several different microorganisms may cause UTIs, *Escherichia coli* remains the most common causative pathogen, responsible for 80% of uncomplicated infections. Bacteria in the urine **(bacteriuria)** may lead to the spread of organisms into the kidneys and bloodstream, leading to **urosepsis** (O'Donnell and Hofmann, 2002). Microorganisms most commonly enter the urinary tract through the ascending urethral route. Bacteria inhabit the distal urethra, external genitalia, and vagina in women. Organisms enter the urethral meatus easily and travel up the inner mucosal lining to the bladder. Women are more susceptible to infection because of the proximity of the anus to the urethral meatus and because of the short urethra. In men, prostatic secretions that contain an antibacterial substance and the length of the urethra reduce the susceptibility to UTIs. Older adults and clients with progressive underlying disease or decreased immunity are also at increased risk.

In a healthy person with good bladder function, organisms are flushed out during voiding. Residual urine in the bladder becomes more alkaline and is an ideal site for microorganism growth. Any interference with the free flow of urine can cause infection. A kinked, obstructed, or clamped catheter and any condition resulting in urinary retention increase the risk of a bladder infection.

Poor perineal hygiene is a common cause of UTIs in women. Inadequate hand washing, failure to wipe from front to back after voiding or defecating, and frequent sexual intercourse predispose women to infection.

Clients with lower UTIs have pain or burning during urination **(dysuria)** as urine flows over inflamed tissues. Fever, chills, nausea, vomiting, and malaise may develop as the infection worsens. An irritated bladder **(cystitis)** causes a frequent and urgent sensation of the need to void. Irritation to bladder and urethral mucosa results in blood-tinged urine **(hematuria).** The urine appears concentrated and cloudy because of the presence of white blood cells (WBCs) or bacteria. If infection spreads to the upper urinary tract (kidneys—**pyelonephritis**), flank pain, tenderness, fever, and chills are common.

One of the most common causes of infection is the introduction of instruments into the urinary tract. For example, the introduction of a catheter through the urethra provides a direct route for microorganisms. With an indwelling bladder catheter, bacteria ascend along the outside of the catheter on the urethral wall or travel up the catheter's lumen. Local irritation to the urethra or bladder predisposes tissues to bacterial invasion.

Urinary Incontinence. **Urinary incontinence (UI)** is the involuntary loss of urine that is sufficient to be a problem (Lee, Phanumus, and Fields, 2000). It may be temporary or permanent. Leakage of urine may be continuous or intermittent. Urinary incontinence can be identified as functional, overflow, reflex, stress, or urge. Some clients may have a mixed form of incontinence that has features of stress and urge incontinence. Table 44-5 in a later section of this chapter describes the types of UI, their symptoms, and nursing interventions.

Incontinence should not be associated only with older adults. It may develop in people of every age, although it is more common in older adults (Neuman, Palmer, 2003). It is estimated that 15% to 30% of adult women experience UI. It is present in as many as 50% of nursing home residents and in 15% to 56% of homebound elders (Lee, Phanumus, and Fields, 2000; Neuman and Palmer, 2003). Incontinence can impair body image and often leads to a loss of independence. Clothing may become wet with urine, and the accompanying odor adds to embarrassment. As a result, clients with this problem often avoid social activities. Clients often fail to discuss this condition with physicians or nurses, and as a result urinary incontinence is underreported and undertreated. Resources for information about continence care and treatment may be found at Access to Continence Care & Treatment (http://wellnessweb.com/INCONT/acct/contents.htm).

Older adults may have special problems with incontinence because of physical limitations and environmental barriers. Older persons with restricted mobility have greater chances of being incontinent because of their inability to reach toilet facilities in time. Low-set chairs and beds raised well above the floor may be obstacles for older adults who must get up to reach a toilet. Older clients often lack the energy to walk very far at one time. The toilet may be too far away for clients with urge incontinence. Older clients who have difficulty undoing buttons or manipulating zippers face another obstacle.

Continued episodes of incontinence create the potential for skin breakdown. The character of urine changes when allowed to remain in contact with skin and may cause skin breakdown. The immobilized client who has frequent incontinence is especially at risk for pressure ulcers (see Chapter 46). Additional information about urinary elimination issues may be located at the websites for The American Geriatrics Society (http://www.americangeriatrics.org) or the American Urogynecologic Society (http://augs.org).

Urinary Diversions. A urinary stoma to divert the flow of urine from the kidneys directly to the abdominal surface is created for several reasons (e.g., cancer of the blad-

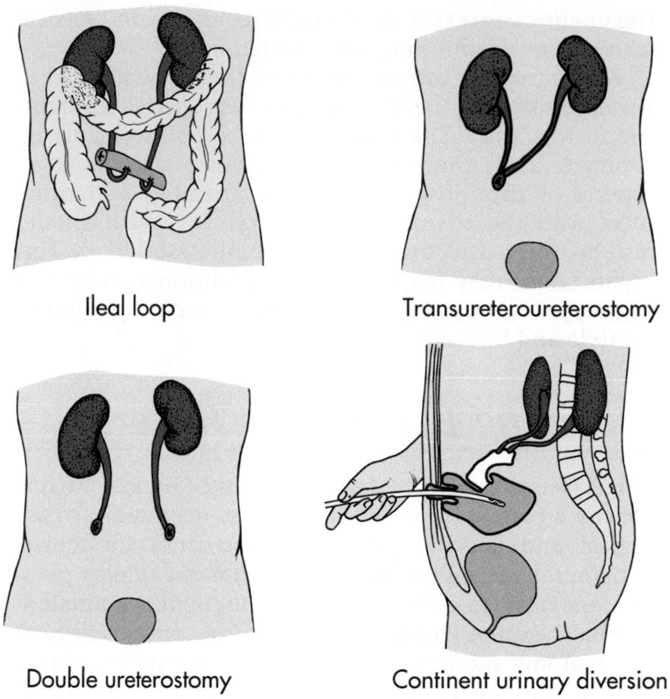

FIGURE **44-4** Types of urinary diversions.

der, trauma, radiation injury to the bladder, fistulas, and chronic cystitis). Such a urinary diversion may be temporary or permanent. Figure 44-4 illustrates several approaches to urinary diversion.

The ileal loop or conduit involves separating a loop of intestinal ileum with its blood supply intact. The ureters are implanted into the isolated segment of ileum. The remaining ileum is reconnected to the rest of the digestive tract. The ileal segment can then be used as a conduit for continuous urine drainage or fashioned into a continent reservoir (McCance and Huether, 2002). The continent pouch is constructed to provide urinary storage in a leakproof pouch. The portion of the ileum connected to the abdominal wall acts as a continent nipple, requiring intermittent catheterization for emptying. The disadvantage of either an ileal conduit or reservoir is that if urine outflow becomes obstructed, irreversible damage to the kidneys can occur secondary to chronic infections or hydronephrosis.

A **ureterostomy** involves bringing the end of one or both ureters to the abdominal surface. To avoid the need for two collecting devices, a transureteroureterostomy connects the ureters and brings one out through the abdominal wall. In some cases a tube may need to be placed directly into the renal pelvis to provide urinary drainage. This procedure is called a **nephrostomy.**

The client with an incontinent urinary diversion must wear a stomal pouch continuously because there is no sphincter control for regulation of urine flow. Local irritation and skin breakdown occur when urine comes in contact with the skin for long periods.

A urinary diversion poses threats to a client's body image. The client must learn to manage the diversion, and those who do not have a continent urinary diversion must wear an artificial device to collect urine. However, the client can wear normal clothing, engage in physical activity, travel, and have sexual relations.

A client with a urinary diversion should be referred to the enterostomal therapist (a nurse with specialized training in this area). The therapist can be an invaluable resource to assist the client with matters pertaining to all aspects of care. The enterostomal therapist will often meet with the client before surgery. The client should also be referred to the United Ostomy Association. This organization may help in providing information regarding support groups to enhance coping and adaptation to lifestyle and body-image changes.

Nursing Knowledge Base

Urinary elimination is a basic function of humans that is usually a private process. Many clients may need physiological and psychological assistance from the nurse. Whether the client has an actual or potential urinary problem, the nurse must be sensitive to the client's elimination needs. The nurse will need knowledge of concepts beyond the anatomy and physiology of the urinary system to give appropriate care. Other concepts that must be understood are infection control, hygiene measures, growth and development, and psychosocial influences.

Infection Control and Hygiene

The urinary tract is usually considered sterile. The nurse must use infection-control principles to help prevent the development and spread of urinary tract infections, as well as to treat existing infections (see Chapter 33). Many UTIs are caused by *E. coli*, common bacteria found in feces. Infection can occur in any location of the urinary tract from the urethra to the kidneys. Hospital-acquired UTIs are often related to poor hand hygiene, improper catheter care, or faulty catheterization technique (Kunin, 2001).

Knowledge of both medical and surgical asepsis must be applied meticulously when providing care involving the urinary tract or external genitalia (see Chapter 33). Any invasive procedure of the urinary tract such as catheterization requires sterile technique. Procedures such as perineal care or examination of the genitalia require medical asepsis.

Growth and Development

Growth and development factors determine the client's ability to control the act of urination during the life span. Infants and young children cannot effectively concentrate urine. Their urine appears light yellow or clear. In relation to their small body size, infants and children excrete large volumes of urine. For example, a 6-month-old infant who weighs 6 to 8 kg (13 to 18 pounds) excretes 400 to 500 ml of urine daily.

As the neurological system matures, a toddler of 2 to 3 years is able to associate the sensations of bladder filling and urination. A child must be able to recognize the feeling of bladder fullness, to hold urine for 1 to 2 hours, and to communicate the sense of urgency to an adult. Many toddlers may then be able to control the external sphincter, and toilet training will begin. The young child needs parents' understanding, patience, and consistency. A child may not gain full control of micturition until age 4 or 5. Daytime control of micturition is easier to accomplish than nighttime control and occurs earlier in the child's development, usually by 2 years of age. Occasional daytime accidents or nocturnal enuresis may continue until age 5 (see Chapter 11).

The adult normally voids 1500 to 1600 ml of urine daily. The kidney concentrates urine, producing a normal, amber-colored urine. A person does not normally wake to void during sleep because of reduction of renal blood flow during rest and the kidney's ability to concentrate urine.

Aging may impair micturition. In the male, prostate enlargement may begin during the 40s and continue throughout life, resulting in urinary frequency and possible urinary retention. In the female, childbearing and/or hormonal changes of menopause may cause changes that lead to urinary difficulties. During a pregnancy urinary frequency is common, and susceptibility to urinary tract infection is increased. Temporary or permanent changes that result from repeated deliveries or hormonal changes might result in decreased perineal muscle tone, leading to urgency and stress incontinence (see Chapter 13). The changes in the urethral mucosa associated with loss of estrogen during and after menopause also contribute to increased susceptibility to infection (McCance and Huether, 2002).

Problems of mobility sometimes make it difficult for the older adult to reach a toilet in time. An older person may be too weak to rise from a toilet seat without assistance. The older adult with chronic neurological disease such as parkinsonism or cerebrovascular accident may have difficulty standing or walking to the toilet. Advancing age also causes changes that may result in voiding problems.

Changes in kidney and bladder function also occur with aging. The kidney's ability to concentrate urine declines. The older adult often experiences **nocturia** (excessive urination at night). The bladder loses muscle tone and capacity to hold urine, resulting in increased **urinary frequency.** Because the bladder cannot contract as effectively, an older person often retains urine in the bladder after voiding **(residual urine).** These changes increase the risk for bacterial growth and development of urinary tract infections (UTIs).

Psychosocial Considerations

The nurse must consider that urinary elimination problems may result in alterations of self-concept and sexuality. Culture may influence the choice of appropriate nursing interventions. In some cultures, the embarrassment related to urinary elimination problems is so great that many clients, especially women, refuse to seek treatment (Gray, 2003). Self-concept, which includes body image, self-esteem, roles, and identity, develops over a life span. Gender influences positioning for urination: males stand, whereas females sit. In addition, gender differences also affect risk factors associated with urinary alterations. Men are at risk for urinary incontinence and have greater psychological distress related to UI (Gray, 2003). Although women are at greater risk for urinary tract infections, men have a greater risk for infection-related renal disease.

Critical Thinking

Successful critical thinking requires a synthesis of knowledge, experience, information gathered from clients, critical thinking attitudes, and intellectual and professional standards. Clinical judgments require the nurse to collect necessary information, analyze the data, and anticipate and make decisions regarding client care.

During assessment the nurse must consider all elements that build toward making appropriate nursing diagnoses. In the case of urinary elimination, the nurse must integrate knowledge from nursing and other disciplines, previous experiences, and information gathered from clients to understand the process of urinary elimination and the impact on the client and family. As a result, the nurse is able to identify the unique impact of these problems on the client and family.

In addition, the use of critical thinking attitudes such as perseverance is needed to find a plan of care to provide successful management of urinary elimination problems. Professional standards provide valuable directions for management.

When planning and implementing care for the client with alterations in urinary elimination, the nurse also uses standards developed by professional organizations such as the Agency for Healthcare Policy and Research (AHCPR), the American Nurses Association (ANA), and the United Ostomy Association as a guide for individualized client care.

Nursing Process and Alterations in Urinary Function

Assessment

To identify a urinary elimination problem and gather data for a care plan, the nurse uses scientific and nursing knowledge, obtains information by a nursing history, performs a physical assessment, assesses the client's urine, and reviews information from diagnostic tests and examinations. The nurse uses critical thinking to synthesize this information as assessment proceeds (Figure 44-5). Adequate assessment should result in the formulation of nursing diagnoses appropriate for alterations in urinary elimination. When assessing for problems with urinary elimination, the nurse must be aware of the impact of the client's culture and language in the assessment process (Box 44-2).

Nursing History. The nursing history includes a review of the client's elimination patterns and symptoms of urinary alterations and an assessment of other factors that may be affecting the ability to urinate normally.

Pattern of Urination. The nurse asks the client about daily voiding patterns, including frequency and times of day, normal volume at each voiding, and any recent changes. Frequency varies among individuals and varies with intake and other types of fluid losses. The common

times for urination are on awakening, after meals, and before bedtime. Most people void an average of 5 or more times a day. The client who voids frequently during the night may have renal disease or prostate enlargement. Information about the pattern of urination establishes a baseline for comparison.

Symptoms of Urinary Alterations. Certain symptoms specific to urinary alterations may occur in more than one type of disorder. During assessment the nurse asks the client about any symptoms related to urination (Table 44-1). The nurse also assesses whether the client is aware of conditions or factors that precipitate or aggravate symptoms. Likewise, it is important that the nurse determine what the client does when any of these symptoms occur.

Factors Affecting Urination. The nurse summarizes factors in the client's history that normally affect urination such as age, environmental factors, medication history, psychological factors, muscle tone, fluid balance, current surgical or diagnostic procedures, and presence of disease conditions. The nurse should be alert to individual needs related to normal changes of aging that predispose older adults to certain elimination problems (Box 44-3). The name, amount, and frequency of each prescription and over-the-counter medication should be noted as part of the history. Another factor to consider is the bowel elimination pattern. Constipation may often interfere with normal urine elimination. Environmental barriers in the home or health care setting are also evaluated. Such aids as elevated toilet seats, grab bars, or a portable commode may be needed. Limitations such as visual or physical impairments are assessed.

The nurse assesses for the presence of an indwelling catheter. A client recovering from major surgery or suffering critical illness or disability often has an indwelling catheter to aid urinary drainage and provide a measurement of urine output. The presence of a catheter places a client at risk for infection, catheter blockage, or skin care problems (Getliffe, 2003). A client's physical condition affects the frequency with which the nurse monitors fluid balance through regular intake and output (I&O) measurements (see Chapter 40). Clients with a urinary diversion may need special assistance to maintain adequate urine elimination and skin care integrity.

Physical Assessment. A physical examination (see Chapter 32) provides the nurse with data to determine the presence and severity of urinary elimination problems. The primary structures reviewed include the skin and mucosal membranes, kidneys, bladder, and urethral meatus.

Skin and Mucosal Membranes. The nurse assesses the condition of the skin and mucosal membranes. Problems with urinary elimination are often associated with fluid and electrolyte disturbances. By assessing skin turgor and the oral mucosa the nurse assesses the client's hydration status. Urinary incontinence increases the risk of skin breakdown.

Kidneys. If the kidneys become infected or inflamed, flank pain typically develops. The nurse assesses for flank

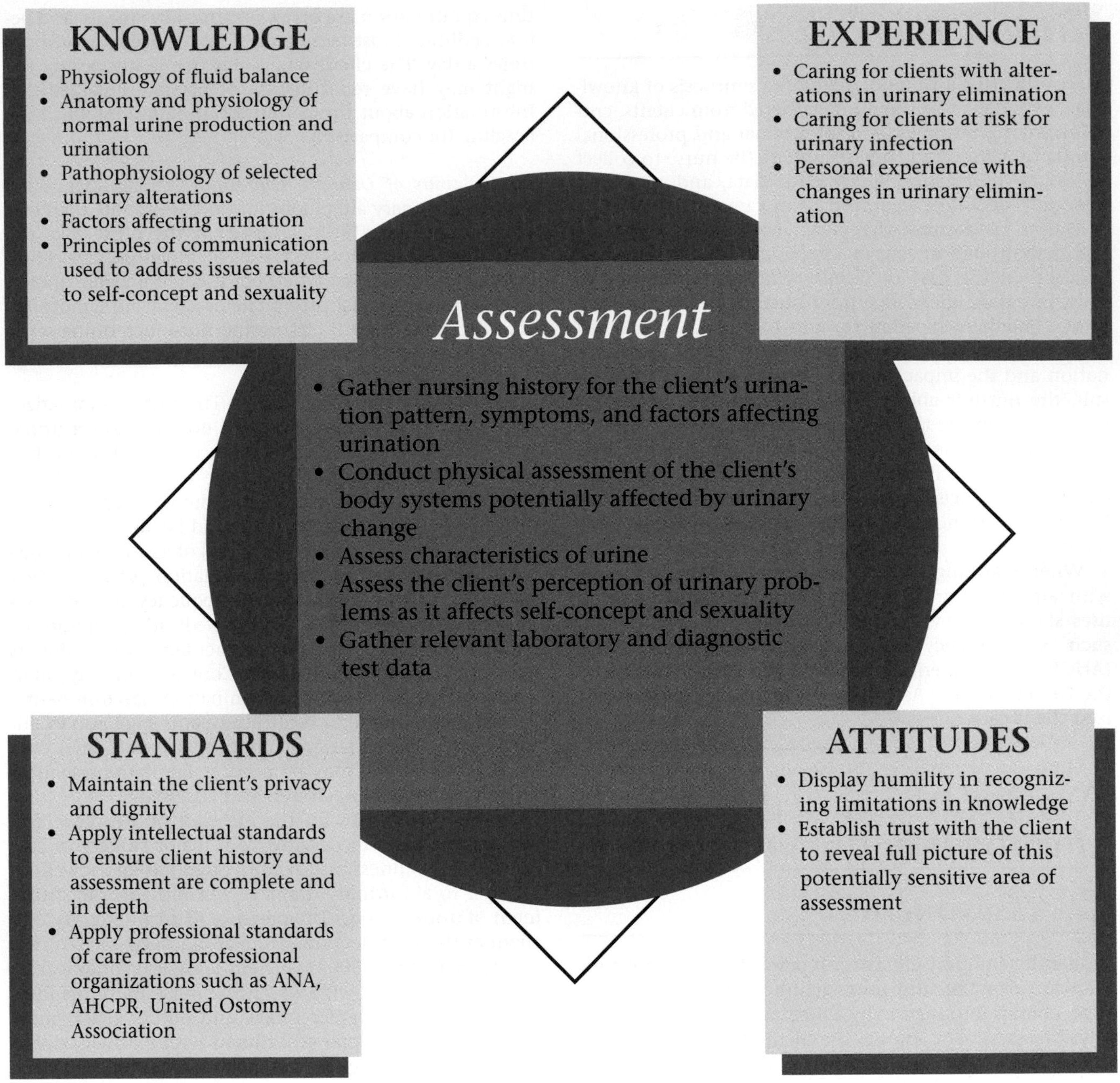

KNOWLEDGE

- Physiology of fluid balance
- Anatomy and physiology of normal urine production and urination
- Pathophysiology of selected urinary alterations
- Factors affecting urination
- Principles of communication used to address issues related to self-concept and sexuality

EXPERIENCE

- Caring for clients with alterations in urinary elimination
- Caring for clients at risk for urinary infection
- Personal experience with changes in urinary elimination

Assessment

- Gather nursing history for the client's urination pattern, symptoms, and factors affecting urination
- Conduct physical assessment of the client's body systems potentially affected by urinary change
- Assess characteristics of urine
- Assess the client's perception of urinary problems as it affects self-concept and sexuality
- Gather relevant laboratory and diagnostic test data

STANDARDS

- Maintain the client's privacy and dignity
- Apply intellectual standards to ensure client history and assessment are complete and in depth
- Apply professional standards of care from professional organizations such as ANA, AHCPR, United Ostomy Association

ATTITUDES

- Display humility in recognizing limitations in knowledge
- Establish trust with the client to reveal full picture of this potentially sensitive area of assessment

FIGURE **44–5** Critical thinking model for urinary elimination assessment.

tenderness early in the disease by percussing the costovertebral angle (the angle formed by the spine and the twelfth rib). Auscultation is also performed to detect the presence of a renal artery bruit (sound resulting from turbulent blood flow through a narrowed artery).

Nurses with advanced examination skills learn to palpate the kidneys during abdominal examination. The kidneys' position, shape, and size can reveal problems such as tumors.

Bladder. In adults the bladder rests below the symphysis pubis and cannot be examined by the nurse. When distended, the bladder rises above the symphysis pubis at the midline of the abdomen and may extend to just be-

low the umbilicus. On inspection the nurse may note a swelling or convex curvature of the lower abdomen. The nurse lightly palpates the lower abdomen. The partially filled bladder normally feels smooth and rounded. As the nurse applies light pressure to the bladder, the client may feel the urge to urinate, tenderness, or even pain. Percussion of a full bladder yields a dull percussion note.

Urethral Meatus. The nurse assesses the urinary **meatus** to note the presence of discharge, inflammation, and lesions. To examine the female, a dorsal recumbent position provides full exposure of the genitalia. While wearing clean gloves, the nurse retracts the labial folds to see the urethral meatus. Normally the

Cultural Aspects of Care

Box 44-2

Urine elimination is usually a personal activity that is not shared with others. When clients have needs related to urine elimination, the nurse must be aware of the intrusive nature of intervention. In addition, other characteristics of the client, such as culture, may also affect the nurse's care. Nurses cannot be knowledgeable about every culture's impact on client care, but it is important to be open to and respect practices different from one's own.

Implications for Practice

- If language differences are causing miscommunication, it may be necessary to use a bicultural medical translator initially. Learn at least a few important words in the client's language to allow for future interchanges.

- In some cultures a female nurse is required for a female client when a physical examination is to be done or questions or procedures are of an intimate nature.
- Cultures view disease differently. It is important to understand how the culture views the cause and treatment of the condition and how traditional Western medicine may or may not fit with that understanding.
- Cultures allow for varying involvement of client's families in the client's care. This source of strength is important to the health of the client, and family must be included in the plan of care.
- Cultural influences may affect the willingness of the client to seek care.

Data from Leonard BJ, Plotnikoff GA: Awareness: the heart of cultural competence. *AACN Clin Issues* 11(1):51, 2000; and Gray ML: Gender, race, and culture in research on UI, *Am J Nurs* 103(3 suppl):20, 2003.

Table **44-1**	Common Types of Urinary Alterations	
Symptoms	**Description**	**Causes or Associated Factors**
Urgency	Feeling of need to void immediately	Full bladder, bladder irritation or inflammation from infection, incompetent urethral sphincter, psychological stress
Dysuria	Painful or difficult urination	Bladder inflammation, trauma or inflammation of urethral sphincter
Frequency	Voiding at frequent intervals (<2 hr)	Increased fluid intake, bladder inflammation, increased pressure on bladder (pregnancy, psychological stress)
Hesitancy	Difficulty initiating urination	Prostate enlargement, anxiety, urethral edema
Polyuria	Voiding large amounts of urine	Excess fluid intake, diabetes mellitus or insipidus, use of diuretics, postobstructive diuresis
Oliguria	Diminished urinary output relative to intake (usually 400 ml/24 hr)	Dehydration, renal failure, UTI, increased ADH secretion, congestive heart failure
Nocturia	Urination, particularly excessive or frequent, at night	Excessive fluid intake before bed (especially coffee or alcohol), renal disease, aging process, prostate enlargement
Dribbling	Leakage of urine despite voluntary control of urination	Stress incontinence, overflow from urinary retention
Incontinence	Involuntary loss of urine	Multiple factors: unstable urethra, loss of pelvic muscle tone, estrogen depletion, fecal impaction, neurological impairment
Hematuria	Blood in the urine	Neoplasms of the kidney or bladder, glomerular disease, infection of kidney or bladder, trauma to urinary structures, calculi, bleeding disorders
Retention	Accumulation of urine in the bladder, with inability of bladder to empty fully	Urethral obstruction, bladder inflammation, decreased sensory activity, neurogenic bladder, prostate enlargement, postanesthesia effects, side effects of medications (e.g., anticholinergics, antidepressants)
Residual urine	Volume of urine remaining after voiding (>100 ml)	Inflammation or irritation of bladder mucosa from infection, neurogenic bladder, prostate enlargement, trauma, or inflammation of urethra

meatus is pink and appears as a small slitlike opening below the clitoris and above the vaginal orifice. There is normally no discharge from the meatus. If present, specimens of urethral discharge should be obtained before the client voids.

Women with vaginal infections are susceptible to UTIs because the vaginal discharge may travel easily to the ure-

thral meatus. Older women commonly have vaginitis as a result of hormonal deficiencies. The nurse inspects the vaginal orifice carefully for signs of inflammation and describes any drainage.

A man's urethral meatus is normally a small opening at the tip of the penis. The nurse inspects the meatus for discharge, inflammation, and lesions. It may be necessary

- High-quality nursing care is essential in care of the older adult. When older adults become dependent on others for personal care, maintenance of their urinary health falls into the domain of nursing practice (Dowd, Kolbaca, and Steiner, 2000).
- Dilute urine discourages bacterial growth, so older adults should be encouraged to increase their fluid intake to at least six to eight glasses a day, unless medically contraindicated (Gray and Krissovich, 2003).
- Fluids, such as cranberry juice, that promote an acidic urine should be made available as part of the client's fluid intake, because an acidic urine also inhibits bacterial growth (Gray, 2002).
- Restricting fluid intake does not decrease urinary incontinence severity or frequency. However, transient restriction, 2 hours before sleep, combined with nocturnal toileting diminished the severity of UI (Gray and Krissovich, 2003).
- Indwelling catheters should not be used routinely in older adults or if used, for no longer than 3 days. The risk of infection increases dramatically for catheterized clients (Kunin, 2001).
- The nurse should note that incontinence is not a normal part of aging, and efforts should be made to assess incontinence and provide interventions to promote return to continence (Thompson and Smith, 2002).

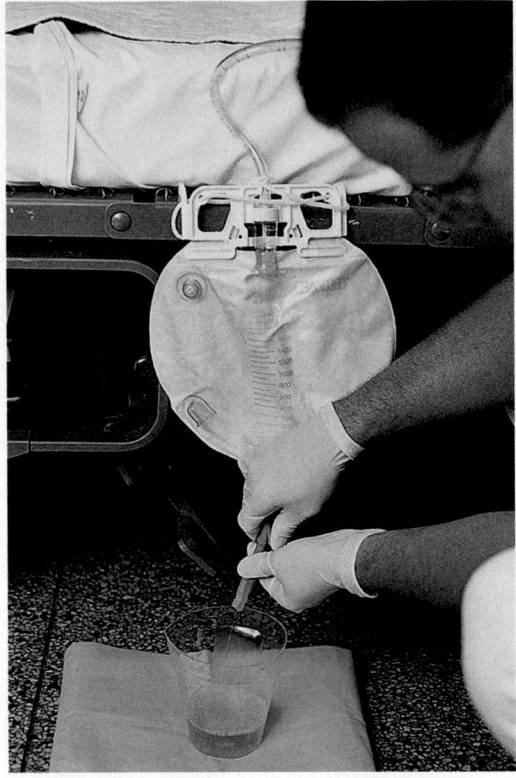

FIGURE **44-6** Urine drainage bag.

to retract the foreskin in uncircumcised men to see the meatus. Clean gloves should be worn when retracting the foreskin.

Assessment of Urine. Assessment of urine involves measuring the client's fluid intake and urine output and observing characteristics of the client's urine.

Intake and Output. The nurse assesses the client's average daily fluid intake. If an accurate measurement of fluid intake is needed from the client who is at home, the nurse may ask the client to show a commonly used glass or cup on which the intake estimate is based.

In a health care setting the nurse measures a client's fluid intake either when the physician orders I&O measurements or when nursing judgment warrants a more precise measurement (see Chapter 40). A change in urine volume is a significant indicator of fluid alterations or kidney disease. While caring for the client, the nurse assesses volume by measuring (with plastic receptacles, bedpans, or urinals) urinary output with each voiding. Special receptacles (urimeters) attach between indwelling catheters and drainage bags and are a convenient means of accurately measuring urine volume. A urimeter holds 100 to 200 ml of urine. After measuring urine from a urimeter, the nurse can drain the cylinder into the urinary drainage bag or into a receptacle for disposal. Urimeters are indicated when precise hourly measurements of urine are needed.

When urine from a drainage bag is measured, the use of a separate plastic graduated measuring receptacle obtains a more precise measurement of urine output (Figure 44-6). Each client should have a graduated receptacle for his or her exclusive use to prevent potential cross contamination.

The nurse reports any extreme increase or decrease in volume. An hourly output of less than 30 ml for more than 2 hours is cause for concern. Similarly, consistently high volumes of urine (polyuria), over 2000 to 2500 ml daily, should be reported to a physician.

Characteristics of Urine. The nurse inspects the client's urine for color, clarity, and odor.

Color. Normal urine ranges from a pale, straw color to amber, depending on its concentration. Urine is usually more concentrated in the morning or with fluid volume deficits. As the person drinks more fluids, urine becomes less concentrated.

Bleeding from the kidneys or ureters causes urine to become dark red; bleeding from the bladder or urethra causes a bright red urine. Various medications and foods also change urine color. For example, Pyridium, a urinary analgesic, colors the urine bright orange. Eating beets, rhubarb, or blackberries may cause red urine. Special dyes used in intravenous diagnostic studies eventually discolor urine. Dark amber urine may be the result of high concentrations of bilirubin caused by liver dysfunction. The nurse documents and reports any abnormal color or sediment, especially if the cause is unknown.

Clarity. Normal urine appears transparent at voiding. Urine that stands several minutes in a container becomes cloudy. Freshly voided urine in clients with renal disease

Table 44-2	Urine Testing
Collection Type/Use of Specimen	**Nursing Considerations**
Random (routine urinalysis)	Can be collected during normal voiding, from an indwelling catheter or urinary diversion collection bag. Collected in a clean specimen cup.
Clean-voided or midstream (culture and sensitivity)	See Skill 44-1. Collected in a sterile specimen cup.
Sterile specimen (culture and sensitivity)	If the client has an indwelling catheter, a sterile specimen can be collected using aseptic technique through the special port (Figure 44-7) found on the side of the catheter. The nurse clamps the tubing below the port, allowing fresh, uncontaminated urine to collect in the tube. After the nurse wipes the port with an antimicrobial swab, a sterile syringe needle is inserted and at least 3 to 5 ml of urine is withdrawn. Using sterile aseptic technique, the nurse transfers the urine to a sterile container (see Chapter 33).
Timed urine specimens (for measuring levels of adrenocortical steroids or hormones, creatinine clearance, or protein quantity tests)	Time required may be 2-, 12-, or 24-hour collections. The timed period begins after the client urinates and ends with a final voiding at the end of the time period. The client voids into a clean receptacle, and the urine is transferred to the special collection container, which may contain special preservatives. Each specimen must be free of feces and toilet tissue. Missed specimens make the whole collection inaccurate. Check with agency policy and the laboratory for specific instructions.

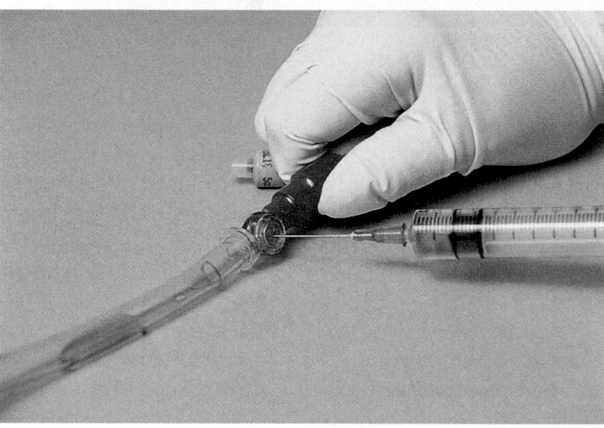

FIGURE 44-7 Urine specimen collection: aspiration from a collection port in drainage tubing of an indwelling catheter.

may appear cloudy or foamy because of high protein concentrations. Urine also appears thick and cloudy as a result of bacteria.

Odor. Urine has a characteristic odor. The more concentrated the urine, the stronger the odor. Stagnant urine has an ammonia odor, which is common in clients who are repeatedly incontinent. A sweet or fruity odor occurs from acetone or acetoacetic acid (by-products of incomplete fat metabolism) seen with diabetes mellitus or starvation.

Urine Testing. The nurse often collects urine specimens for laboratory testing. The type of test determines the method of collection. All specimens are labeled with the client's name, date, and time of collection. Specimens should be transported to the laboratory in a timely fashion to ensure accuracy of test results. Agency infection-control policies require the adherence to standard precautions by all personnel during specimen handling (see Chapter 33).

Specimen Collection. The nurse collects random, clean-voided or midstream, sterile, and timed specimens (Table 44-2).

Urine Collection in Children. Specimen collection from infants and children is often difficult. Adolescents and school-age children are usually able to cooperate, although they may be embarrassed. Preschool children and toddlers have difficulty voiding on request. Offering a young child fluids 30 minutes before requesting a specimen may help. The nurse must use terms for urination that the child can understand. A young child may be reluctant to void in unfamiliar receptacles. A potty chair or specimen hat placed under the toilet seat is usually effective. The nurse must use special collection devices for infants or toddlers who are not toilet trained. Clear plastic, single-use bags with self-adhering material can be attached over the child's urethral meatus. Specimens should not be obtained by squeezing urine from the diaper material because the results may be inaccurate.

Text continued on p. 1339

Collecting Midstream (Clean-Voided) Urine Specimen

Skill 44-1

Delegation Considerations

Collecting midstream (clean-voided) urine specimen may be delegated to assistive personnel (AP). If appropriate, an alert client who is physically able may be instructed to collect the specimen. It is the nurse's responsibility to ensure that this specimen is obtained correctly and in a timely manner. Be aware of agency policy regarding specimen collection.

Instruct AP to do the following:
- Inform the nurse when the specimen was obtained
- Inform the nurse if client is unable to initiate a stream or has pain or burning on urination
- Inform the nurse if the collected specimen is dark, bloody, or cloudy, is odorous, or contains mucus

Equipment

- Soap or cleansing solution, washcloth, and towel
- Commercial kit for clean-voided specimen or individual supplies as listed
  - Sterile cotton balls or sterile 2 × 2 or 4× 4 gauze pads
  - Antiseptic solution (e.g., providone-iodine); check for client allergy, if allergic provide an alternative
  - Sterile water
- Sterile specimen collection cup or jar
- Sterile and nonsterile gloves
- Bedpan, bedside commode, or specimen hat
- Completed specimen label

Steps	Rationale
1. Assess voiding status of client.	
a. When client last voided	May indicate bladder fullness.
b. Level of awareness or developmental stage	Reveals client's ability to cooperate during procedure.
c. Mobility, balance, and physical limitations	Determines level of assistance in acquiring specimen.
2. Assess client's understanding of purpose of test and method of collection.	Information allows you to clarify misunderstandings and promotes client cooperation.
3. Explain procedure to client:	
a. Reason midstream specimen is needed	Helps client understand the procedure.
b. Ways client and family can assist	
c. Ways to obtain specimen free of feces	Feces change characteristics of urine and may cause abnormal values.
4. Provide fluids to drink ½ hour before collection unless contraindicated (i.e., fluid restriction) if client does not feel urge to void.	Improves likelihood of client being able to void.
5. Provide privacy for client by closing door or bed curtain.	Privacy allows client to relax and produce specimen more quickly.
6. Give client or family members soap, washcloth, and towel to cleanse perineal area.	Client may prefer to wash own perineal area.
7. Perform hand hygiene and apply nonsterile gloves and assist nonambulatory clients with perineal care. Assist female client onto bedpan.	Prevents transmission of microorganisms to nurse, provides easy access to perineal area to collect specimen.
8. Change gloves if necessary.	Reduces transfer of infection.
9. Using surgical asepsis, open sterile kit (see illustration) or prepare sterile supplies. Apply sterile gloves after opening sterile specimen cup, placing cap with sterile inside surface up, and do not touch inside of container or cap (see Chapter 33).	Sterile technique is essential to maintain sterility of equipment and specimen. Sterile gloves prevent the transmission of microorganisms to the specimen from the nurse or from the client to the nurse. Contaminated specimen is most frequent reason for inaccurate reporting of urine cultures and sensitivities.
10. Pour antiseptic solution over cotton balls or gauze pads unless kit contains prepared gauze pads in antiseptic solution.	Cotton balls or gauze pads will be used to further cleanse the perineum.
11. Assist or allow client to independently cleanse perineum and collect specimen:	
A. Female	
(1) Spread labia with thumb and forefinger of nondominant hand.	Provides access to urethral meatus.
(2) Cleanse area with cotton ball or gauze, moving from front (above urethral orifice) to back (toward anus) (see illustration).	Cleanse from area of least contamination to area of greatest contamination to decrease bacterial levels.

Steps	Rationale

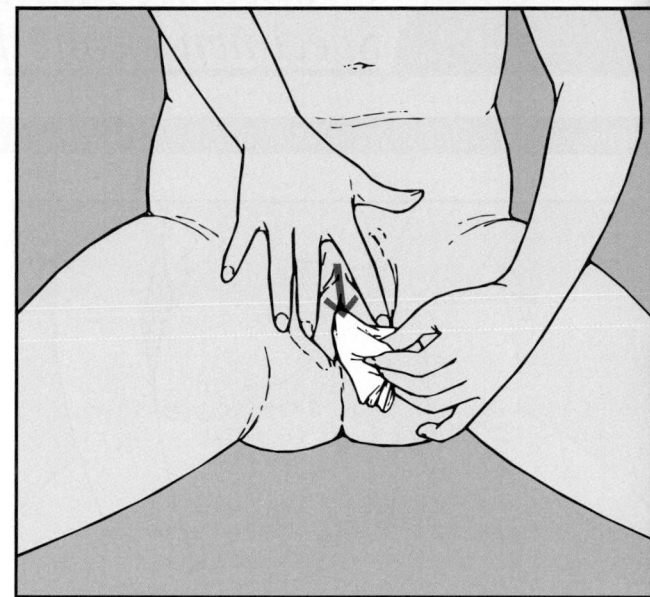

STEP **9**   Commercial midstream urine collection kit.

STEP **11A(2)**   Cleansing technique (female).

(3) If agency policy indicates, rinse area with sterile water, and dry with dry cotton ball or gauze.

> Prevents contamination of specimen with antiseptic solution.

(4) While continuing to hold labia apart, client should initiate stream and after stream is achieved, pass container into stream and collect 30 to 60 ml (see illustration).

> Initial stream flushes out microorganisms that accumulate at urethral meatus and prevents transfer into specimen.

B. Male

(1) Hold penis with one hand, and using circular motion and antiseptic swab, cleanse end of penis, moving from center to outside (see illustration). In uncircumcised men, the foreskin should be retracted before cleansing.

> Cleanse from area of least contamination to area of greatest contamination to decrease bacterial levels.

(2) If agency procedure indicates, rinse area with sterile water, and dry with cotton or gauze.

> Prevents contamination of specimen with antiseptic solution.

(3) After client has initiated urine stream, pass specimen collection container into stream, and collect 30 to 60 ml (see illustration).

> Initial stream flushes out microorganisms that accumulate at urethral meatus and prevents transfer into specimen.

12. Remove specimen container before flow of urine stops and before releasing labia or penis. Client finishes voiding in bedpan or toilet. If foreskin was retracted for specimen collection, it must be replaced over the glans.

> Prevents contamination of specimen with skin flora. If foreskin not replaced, swelling and constriction may occur, causing pain and possible obstruction to urine flow.

13. Replace cap securely on specimen container (touch outside only).

> Retains sterility of inside of container and prevents spillage of urine.

14. Cleanse any urine from exterior surface of container, and place in a plastic specimen bag.

> Prevents transfer of microorganisms to others.

15. Remove bedpan (if applicable), and assist client to comfortable position.

> Promotes relaxing environment.

16. Label specimen, and attach laboratory requisition.

> Prevents inaccurate identification that could lead to errors in diagnosis or treatment.

*C*ollecting Midstream (Clean-Voided) Urine Specimen—cont'd

Skill 44-1

Steps	Rationale

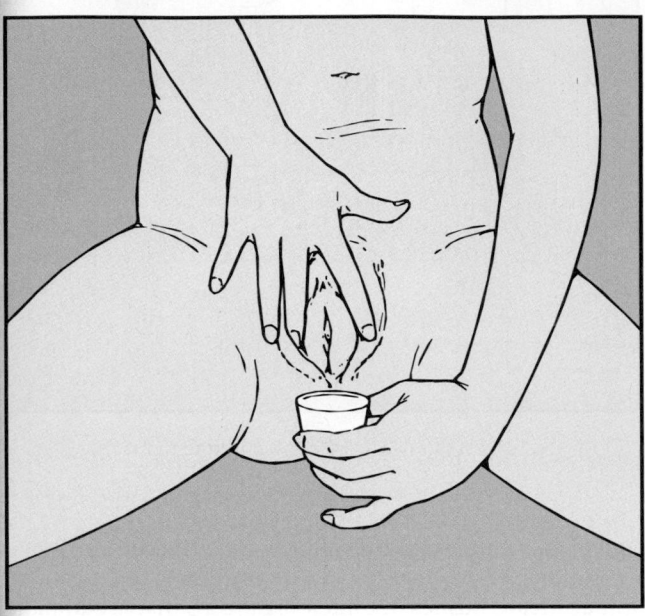

STEP **11A(4)** Specimen collection (female).

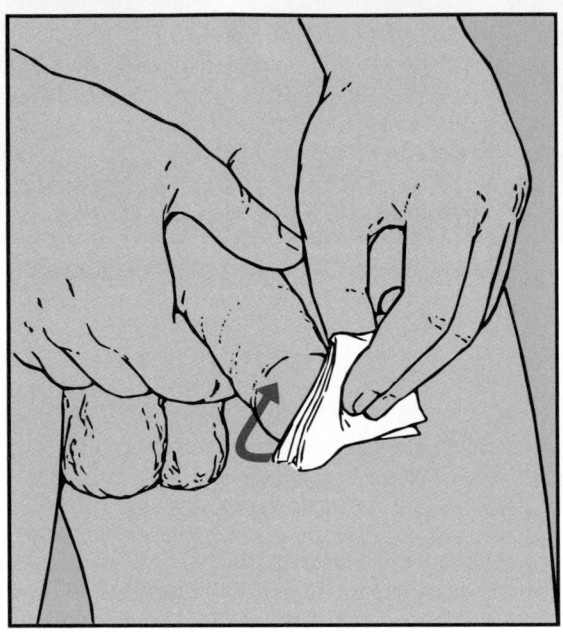

STEP **11B(1)** Cleansing technique (male).

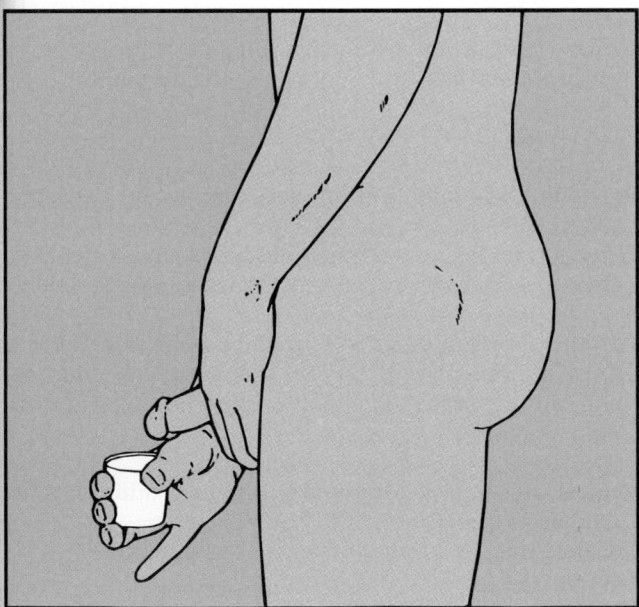

STEP **11B(3)** Specimen collection (male).

Critical Decision Point: If client is menstruating, indicate information on laboratory requisition.

17. Remove gloves, dispose in proper receptacle, and perform hand hygiene.	Reduces transmission of infection.
18. Transport specimen to laboratory within 15 minutes or refrigerate immediately.	Bacteria grow quickly in urine, and specimen should be analyzed immediately to obtain correct results.

Unexpected Outcomes and Related Interventions

1. Urine specimen is contaminated with feces or toilet paper.
   a. Repeat instruction to client or assist client in obtaining specimen.
   b. Obtain a new specimen.
   c. Consider using a straight catheterization to obtain specimen.
2. Specimen is accidentally discarded.
   a. Repeat specimen collection.

Recording and Reporting

- Record date and time urine specimen was obtained in nurses' notes.
- Notify physician of any significant abnormalities.

Home Care Considerations

- If client is to collect specimen as outpatient, proper instruction for collection needs to be given.
- Appropriate equipment will need to be given to client and family.
- Information on storing specimen until time for delivery to doctor's office or hospital laboratory needs to be given.

Table 44-3 Routine Urinalysis	
Measurement and Normal Value	**Interpretation**
pH (4.6-8.0) average 6.0	pH helps indicate acid-base balance. Urine that stands for several hours becomes alkaline. An acid pH helps protect against bacterial growth.
Protein (none or up to 8 mg/100 ml)	Normally protein is not present in urine. It is seen in renal disease because damage to glomeruli or tubules allows protein to enter urine.
Glucose (none)	Diabetic clients have glucose in urine as a result of inability of tubules to reabsorb high glucose concentrations (>180 mg/100 ml). Ingestion of high concentrations of glucose may cause some glucose to appear in urine of healthy persons.
Ketones (none)	Clients whose diabetes mellitus is poorly controlled experience breakdown of fatty acids. End products of fat metabolism are ketones. Clients with dehydration, starvation, or excessive aspirin usage also may have **ketonuria.**
Blood (up to 2 RBCs)	Damage to glomeruli or tubules may allow RBCs to enter the urine. Trauma, disease, or surgery of the lower urinary tract also may cause blood to be present. In women, blood in a routine urine specimen may be contaminated with menstrual fluid.
Specific gravity (1.010-1.025)	Specific gravity measures concentration of particles in urine. High specific gravity reflects concentrated urine, and low specific gravity reflects diluted urine. Dehydration, reduced renal blood flow, and increased ADH secretion elevate specific gravity. Overhydration, early renal disease, and inadequate ADH secretion reduce specific gravity.
Microscopic Examination	
WBCs (0-4 per low-power field)	Greater numbers may indicate urinary tract infection.
Bacteria (none)	Bacteria indicate urinary tract infection. (Client may or may not have symptoms.)
Casts (none)	Casts are cylindrical bodies whose shapes take on likeness of objects within the renal tubule. Types include hyaline, WBCs, RBCs, granular cells, and epithelial cells. Their presence is always an abnormal finding and indicates renal alterations.

Modified from Pagana KD, Pagana TJ: *Mosby's manual of diagnostic and laboratory tests,* ed 2, St. Louis, 2002, Mosby.

Common Urine Tests

Urinalysis. The laboratory performs a **urinalysis** on a specimen obtained by any of the previously described methods. Table 44-3 lists normal values for a urinalysis. The specimen should be examined as soon as possible, preferably within 2 hours. It should be the first voided specimen in the morning to ensure a uniform concentration of constituents. For a quick screening the nurse can perform certain portions of the urinalysis with special reagent strips. The nurse dips the strips into the urine and then observes for a color change in the time interval designated on the package (Figure 44-8).

Specific Gravity. The **specific gravity** is the weight or degree of concentration of a substance compared with an equal volume of water. A urine specimen is poured into a special clean, dry cylinder. The weighted urinometer is suspended in the cylinder of urine. The concentration of dissolved substances in the urine aids in determination of a client's fluid balance. This measurement is always done as part of a complete urinalysis. The nurse in a critical care unit may be responsible for doing periodic measurement of specific gravity of urine as part of complete client assessment for specific clients.

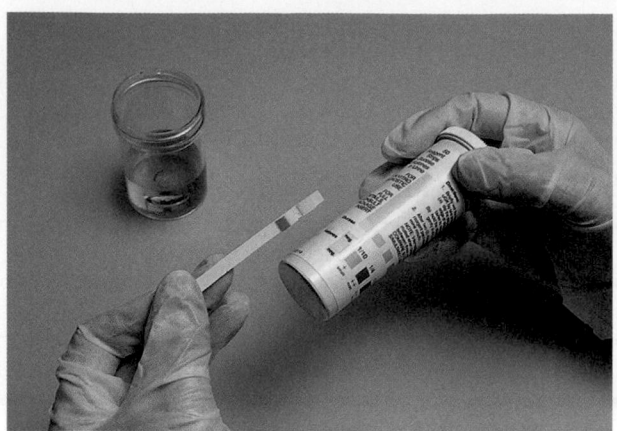

FIGURE **44–8** Checking results of a chemical reagent strip dipped in urine.

If questions regarding the accuracy of specific gravity measurements arise, a urine osmolality test should be obtained. Although both tests measure urine concentration, the osmolality test is more accurate because it measures the total number of particles in a solution (see Chapter 40).

Urine Culture. A urine culture requires a sterile or clean-voided sample of urine. It takes approximately 24 to 48 hours before the laboratory can report findings of bacterial growth. While awaiting results, a broad-spectrum antibiotic may be ordered as soon as a culture has been obtained. The test for sensitivity determines which specific antibiotics are effective. The results (sensitivities) of a urine culture may indicate a change in choice of medication.

Diagnostic Examinations. The urinary system is one of the few organ systems amenable to accurate diagnostic study by several radiographic techniques. The two approaches for visualization of urinary structures, direct and indirect techniques, can be quite simple or very complex, requiring extensive nursing intervention. These procedures are further subdivided into invasive or noninvasive categories (Table 44-4).

Many of the nursing responsibilities related to diagnostic examinations of the urinary tract are common to many of the studies. The common responsibilities before the study include the following:
- Obtaining a signed consent (if agency policy)
- Assessing client for history of shellfish (iodine) allergy, which predicts allergy to the dye used in specific studies (intravenous pyelogram [IVP] and renal arteriogram)
- Administering bowel cleansing medications (check agency policy)
- Ensuring client receives appropriate pretest diet (clear liquids) or nothing by mouth (NPO), as needed

Common postprocedure interventions may include the following:
- Assessing intake and output
- Observing characteristics of urine (color, clarity, presence of blood)

Client Expectations. Clients are dependent on their caregivers to recognize and meet their needs. Nurses need to use a skilled and caring approach, to be creative in using a variety of assessment techniques, and to serve as a client advocate. A caring nurse will meet the client's needs in a way that is acceptable and individualized for the client and family situation. The client having needs related to urinary function expects that the nurse will be respectful of privacy needs and sensitive to the impact of urinary impairments on sexuality and self-concept. The nurse should always include the client in the plan of care and develop goals that are mutually acceptable. Cultural practices and personal preferences should be considered. Clients expect that assistance from the nurse will be prompt. Once children and adults have achieved continence, urinary incontinence is often a source of embarrassment and shame.

Nursing Diagnosis

A thorough assessment of the client's urinary elimination function reveals patterns of data that allow the nurse to make relevant and accurate nursing diagnoses. The nurse thinks critically by reflecting on knowledge of previous clients, applying knowledge of urinary function and the effects of disorders, reviewing defining characteristics identified, and then making a specific diagnosis. The diagnosis may focus on a specific urinary elimination alteration or an associated problem such as *impaired skin integrity related to urinary incontinence.* Identification of defining characteristics leads the nurse to select an appropriate diagnosis. Specifying related factors for each diagnosis allows selection of individualized nursing interventions (Ackley and Ludwig, 2002). One sample of diagnostic reasoning is found in Box 44-4. Some nursing diagnoses common to clients with urine elimination alterations include the following:
- Disturbed body image
- Urinary incontinence (functional, reflex, stress, urge)
- Pain (acute, chronic)
- Risk for infection
- Self-care deficit, toileting
- Impaired skin integrity
- Impaired urinary elimination
- Urinary retention

Planning

During planning, the nurse integrates the knowledge from assessment and the knowledge related to resources and available therapies to develop an individualized plan of care (see care plan). The client's needs should be matched with clinical and professional standards recommended in the literature (Figure 44-10). Building a relationship of trust with the client is important because the implementation of care involves interaction of a very personal nature.

Goals and Outcomes. The plan of care for urinary elimination alterations must include realistic and individualized goals along with relevant outcomes. The nurse and the client must collaborate in setting goals and outcomes and ultimately in choosing nursing interventions. A general goal might be normal urinary elimination, but the individual goal may differ depending on the problem. The

Table 44-4	Diagnostic Examinations	
Name of Procedure	**Purpose and Method of Procedure**	**Special Nursing Considerations**
Noninvasive Procedures		
Abdominal roentgenogram (plain film; kidney, ureter, bladder [KUB], or flat plate)	To determine the size, shape, symmetry, and location of the kidneys.	No special preparation or precautions.
Computerized axial tomography (CT) scan (Figure 44-9)	A computerized x-ray procedure used to obtain detailed images of structures within a selected plane of the body. The computer reconstructs cross-sectional image and thus allows the physician to view pathologic conditions such as tumors, obstructions.	Bowel cleansing as per agency or physician preference. Assess for shellfish (iodine) allergy if a CT with contrast is ordered. Prepare client for the procedure (e.g., client will be placed into a large machine, need to lie still, feelings of claustrophobia in some clients).
Intravenous pyelogram (IVP)	To view the collecting ducts and renal pelvis and outline the ureters, bladder, and urethra using dye that is excreted through the urine. A special intravenous injection that converts to a dye in urine will be injected intravenously.	Bowel cleansing will be completed as per agency or physician preference. Only clear liquids are permitted until after test completed. Assess client for shellfish (iodine) allergy before test. After test, fluid intake is encouraged to dilute and flush dye from client. Observe for late symptoms of allergy (rash, etc.).
Renal (kidney) scan	To determine renal blood flow, anatomical structure of the kidneys, and excretory function using a radioisotope.	Usually no bowel cleansing needed, but check agency policy. After test, only precaution is rinsing bedpan or urinal after use and flushing the urine, as urine will contain a minute amount of radioisotope. Rinse fluid carefully using a double flush.
Ultrasound Renal	To identify gross renal structures and structural abnormalities in the kidney using high-frequency, inaudible sound waves.	No bowel cleansing needed.
Bladder	To identify structural abnormalities of bladder or lower urinary tract. May also be used to estimate the volume of urine in the bladder either prevoiding or postvoiding.	If needed, client may be asked to drink fluids before the test to cause bladder distention for better results. No special care necessary after either study.
Invasive Procedures		
Endoscopy	Use of an endoscope (cystoscope) will allow for direct visualization, specimen collection, and/or treatment of the interior of the bladder and urethra. Surgery on the male prostate may also be accomplished using an endoscope. Although this procedure may be accomplished using local anesthesia, it is more commonly performed using general anesthesia or conscious sedation to avoid unnecessary anxiety and trauma for the client.	Signed consent is obtained. If ordered, a bowel cleansing will be completed. Follow agency policy for preoperative preparation and checklist (see Chapter 49). After client's return, assess the vital signs, the characteristics of urine, monitor intake and output (I&O), encourage fluids, and observe for fever, dysuria, and pain in suprapubic region.

Continued

Table 44-4	Diagnostic Examinations—cont'd	
Name of Procedure	**Purpose and Method of Procedure**	**Special Nursing Considerations**
Invasive Procedures—cont'd		
Arteriogram (angiography)	This procedure is used primarily to visualize the renal arteries and/or their branches to detect narrowing or occlusion. A catheter is placed in one of the femoral arteries and introduced up to the level of the renal arteries. Radiopaque contrast is injected through the catheter while x-ray images are taken in rapid succession.	Signed consent is obtained. Assess for shellfish (iodine) allergy. Follow agency preprocedure checklist. After the procedure, the nurse must monitor vital signs frequently until stable, bed rest is maintained for prescribed time interval, fluids are encouraged to flush the contrast from the system. The nurse will also monitor the affected extremity for neuro-circulatory function (pulse, skin temperature, sensation, and movement), as well as observe catheter site for bleeding, swelling, increased tenderness, or hematoma formation. Physician must be notified immediately of any post procedure abnormality.
Urodynamic testing (cystometrogram)	This procedure determines bladder muscle function. This procedure is indicated to evaluate causes of urinary incontinence. A catheter is inserted, the urine drained, and either carbon dioxide gas or sterile saline is used to fill the bladder. Pressure readings are taken and compared with the client's reported sensations.	The nurse explains the need for the client to report all sensations during the test. After the test the nurse assesses the client for sensations of sweating, pain, nausea, bladder fullness, or a strong urge to void.

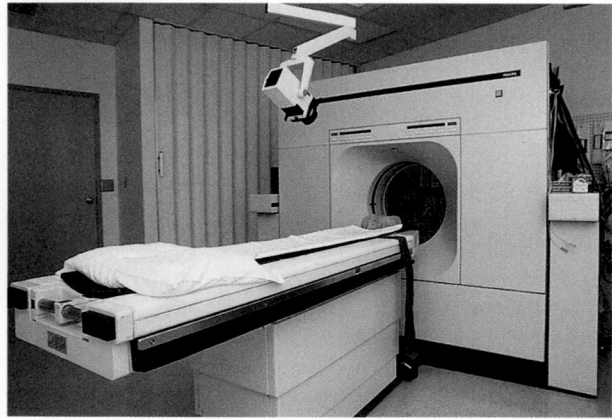

FIGURE **44-9** CT equipment. (From Brundage DJ: *Renal disorders,* St. Louis, 1992, Mosby.)

goals may be short term or long term. For example, urinary retention following surgery may require the short-term goal "Client will have normal voiding with complete bladder emptying within 24 hours." Relevant expected outcomes for this goal may include the following:
- Client will void within 8 hours.
- Urinary output of 300 ml or greater will occur with each voiding.
- Client's bladder is not distended to palpation.
- Client will not continually feel an urge to void.

Conversely, the client with stress incontinence may have a long-term goal that is dependent on weeks of pelvic floor muscle exercise to achieve urinary control: "Client will achieve full urinary continence within 8 weeks after start of exercise program (Kegel)." Goals must be reasonably achievable for the client situation and be relevant to the client's own situation.

Setting Priorities. Urinary elimination is a personal and intimate activity. The nurse must establish a relationship with the client that allows discussion and intervention. While the nurse is collaborating with the client, the client's priorities will become apparent to the nurse and the client should develop an understanding of all the goals.

In the case when a client has multiple nursing diagnoses (Figure 44-11), it becomes important for the nurse to recognize the primary health problem and its influence on other problems. In the example of the client with chronic confusion, the resultant incontinence creates several risks. Focusing on the management of incontinence will help to resolve more than one nursing diagnosis. Although physical care needs may appear to have higher priority, the psychological needs related to self-esteem or sexuality may be of higher priority for the client. Attention to the client's perceived needs may be the most satisfactory and successful approach to accomplishing all the goals. Reinforcement of good health habits that are already followed improves compliance with the care plan.

Nursing Diagnostic Process

Box 44-4

Assessment Activities	Defining Characteristics	Nursing Diagnosis
Have client describe situations that accompany urine leakage.	Client states that she "loses a little urine" whenever she sneezes, coughs, or laughs.	Stress urinary incontinence related to decreased pelvic muscle tone and urethral sphincter trauma
	Client states she has been having problems for the past year.	
Observe client behavior.	Client is wearing a menstrual minipad continuously.	
	Client is reluctant to interact with others and tries not to cough or laugh.	
Review medical history.	Client is postmenopausal after three vaginal births.	

Continuity of Care. The plan incorporates health promotion activities and therapeutic interventions for clients. Preventive interventions may be required for clients at risk for urinary problems. It is important in the nursing process to consider the client's home environment and normal elimination routines when planning therapies. In planning the care for some clients, consultation with other health care professionals and the client's family may be needed. For example, the physical therapist can design an exercise plan to increase strength and endurance so the client will be able to ambulate to the bathroom. The need for home care services should be explored and appropriate referrals made. The family may need to alter the home environment to make it easier and safer for the client to use the bathroom.

Implementation

Implementation is the action phase of the nursing process. The nurse will carry out the independent and collaborative behaviors needed to assist the client in achieving the desired outcomes and goals. The independent activities are those in which nurses use their own judgment. An example of this is teaching self-care activities to the client. Collaborative activities are those prescribed by the physician and carried out by the nurse, such as medication administration.

Health Promotion. The focus of health promotion is to assist the client in understanding and participating in self-care practices that will preserve and protect healthy urinary system function. This focus can be achieved using several means.

Client Education. Success of therapies aimed at eliminating or minimizing urinary elimination problems depends in part on successful client education. Box 44-5 describes an example of nursing education related to one area of urinary elimination needs. Although many clients may need to learn about all aspects of urinary elimination, the nurse first focuses the teaching on the client's specific elimination problems. For example, clients who

practice poor hygiene benefit most from learning about normal sterility of the urinary tract and ways to prevent infection. Clients also learn the significance of symptoms of urinary alterations so that early preventive health care can be initiated.

The nurse can easily incorporate teaching when giving nursing care. For example, if the nurse is attempting to increase the client's fluid intake, a good time to discuss the benefits is while giving fluids with medications or meals. The nurse may be more successful in teaching about perineal hygiene while giving a bath or performing catheter care.

Promoting Normal Micturition. Maintaining normal urinary elimination will help to prevent many urination problems. Many nursing measures have been designed to promote normal voiding in clients at risk for urination difficulties and in clients with established urination problems. The nurse can initiate many of these measures independently.

Stimulating Micturition Reflex. The client's ability to void depends on feeling the urge to urinate, being able to control the urethral sphincter, and being able to relax during voiding. The nurse can help a client learn to relax and stimulate the reflex to void by assuming the normal position for voiding. A woman is better able to void in a squatting or sitting position. If the client is unable to use toilet facilities, the nurse positions the client in a squatting position on a bedpan (see Chapter 45) or bedside commode. A man voids more easily in the standing position. If the man cannot reach toilet facilities, he may stand at the bedside and void into a urinal (a metal or plastic receptacle for urine) (Figure 44-12). At times it may be necessary for one or more nurses to assist a man in standing.

Other measures that promote relaxation and the ability to void include sensory stimuli. The sound of running water helps many clients void through the power of suggestion. Stroking the inner aspect of the thigh may stimulate sensory nerves and promote the micturition reflex. The nurse can also pour warm water over the client's perineum and create the sensation to urinate. If urine output is to be measured, the nurse must first measure the volume of water to be poured over the perineal area.

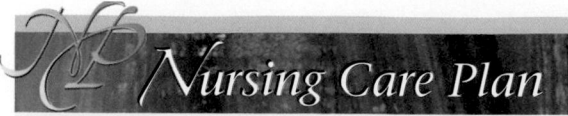

Nursing Care Plan

Functional Urinary Incontinence

Assessment

Mrs. Kay, the home care nurse, is seeing Mrs. Grayson, a 75-year-old widow at her home. Mrs. Grayson has type 2 diabetes mellitus and arthritis and was referred by her physician because of urinary incontinence. She lives alone, but her daughter lives less than a 10-minute drive away. Mrs. Kay's assessment included a discussion of Mrs. Grayson's current health problems with emphasis on the more recent urinary concerns.

Assessment Activities	**Findings/Defining Characteristics**
Ask Mrs. Grayson about the effects of her arthritis on her mobility.	She responds, "It is hard for me to get up once I'm down. Even when I'm up, I have such pain I have trouble walking."
Observe Mrs. Grayson's gait and ability to get up and down.	You observe that she has difficulty standing to an upright position. She limps on the right side. Mrs. Grayson grimaces as she walks.
Ask Mrs. Grayson about any other effects that her difficulty in walking have had.	Mrs. Grayson begins to cry and states, "You can see the plastic cover on my chair. I'm so embarrassed, sometimes I can't get out of the chair fast enough and I lose my water. I've been wearing those diapers lately."

Nursing Diagnosis: Functional incontinence related to impaired mobility.

Planning

Goal	Expected Outcomes*
	Urinary Continence
Client will have reduced episodes of incontinence within 1 week.	Client will report less frequent episodes of incontinence following initiation of a pattern of timed voiding.
	Independent Toileting
Client will ambulate with less discomfort within 1 week.	Client will demonstrate ability to walk comfortably with a steady gait to bathroom within 1 week.

*Outcome classification labels from Moorhead S, Johnson M, Maas M: *Nursing outcomes classification (NOC),* ed 3, St. Louis, 2004, Mosby.

Interventions†

Urinary Incontinence Care
- Have client complete a 3-day 24-hr log of urination.

- Establish interval for toileting to anticipate need for voiding based on bladder log data. Interval may vary from 1½ to 4 hours.

- Work with client to establish a reasonable, manageable voiding program using environmental cues to minimize or eliminate incontinence episodes.

- Consult with physician to prescribe an alternative antiarthritic.

Rationale

The bladder log provides objective verification of urine elimination pattern and patterns of urine leakage and provides a baseline for evaluation of effectiveness of management plans (Lyons and Specht, 2001; Wyman, 2003).
Bladder log also demonstrates pattern of voiding that may indicate more serious urinary problems related to urinary tract infections or other renal diseases (Lewis, Heitkemper, and Dirksen, 2000).
Timed voiding (habit training) will empty the bladder before the usual stimuli (bladder stretch) and avoid association with inability to get to bathroom facilities in time (Lyons and Specht, 2001; Wyman, 2003).
Uncontrolled incontinence can lead to institutionalization of older adults who prefer to remain in their own homes and contributes to increased illness (urinary tract infections, skin breakdown) (Gray, 2003).
Reduction in joint pain will increase mobility.

†Intervention classification label from Dochterman JM, Bulechek GM: *Nursing interventions classification (NIC),* ed 4, St. Louis, 2004, Mosby.

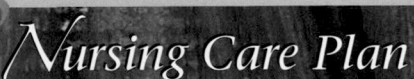

Nursing Care Plan
Functional Urinary Incontinence—cont'd

Evaluation

Nursing Actions	Client Response/Finding	Achievement of Outcome
Ask Mrs. Grayson about degree of continence since starting timed voiding.	She responds, "I'm dry most of the time now."	Mrs. Grayson reports partial success with bladder control. She is satisfied that with time her success will be complete.
Observe Mrs. Grayson's gait and ability to get up and down.	Mrs. Grayson is taking a new arthritis medication. You observe improved ambulation and ease of getting up and down.	Mrs. Grayson reports improved ambulation and increased comfort.

Maintaining Elimination Habits. Many clients follow routines to promote normal voiding. In a hospital or long-term care facility the nurse's routines may conflict with those of clients. Integrating clients' habits into the care plan fosters normal voiding and will assist in preventing problems related to urination.

Maintaining Adequate Fluid Intake. A simple method of promoting normal micturition is maintaining good fluid intake. A client with normal renal function who does not have heart or kidney disease should drink 2000 to 2500 ml of fluid daily. However, an average daily intake of 1200 to 1500 ml of fluids is usually adequate unless the client has a history of urinary tract infection.

When fluid intake is increased, the excreted urine flushes out solutes or particles that may collect in the urinary system. Because a client may be unwilling to drink 2500 ml of water daily, the nurse should encourage fluids that the client prefers. Many vegetables and fruits also have a high fluid content. At home it may help to set a schedule for drinking fluids (e.g., with meals or medications). To minimize nocturia, fluids should be avoided 2 hours before bedtime.

Promoting Complete Bladder Emptying. Under normal conditions, a small amount of the client's urine remains in the bladder after voiding (residual urine) because urinary sphincters close. Thus persons normally remain continent and dry. Urinary incontinence may occur because pressure in the bladder is too great or because the sphincters are too weak. Urinary retention occurs from a strong or contracted sphincter or a weak detrusor muscle that prevents normal bladder emptying.

Measures that promote micturition may help clients with incontinence or retention. Additional measures are used to promote and control bladder emptying so clients gain a sense of elimination control (Table 44-5).

Preventing Infection. One of the most important considerations for a client with urinary alterations is the need to prevent infection of the urinary system. Good perineal hygiene that includes cleansing the urethral meatus after each voiding or bowel movement is essential. A daily fluid intake of 2000 to 2500 ml dilutes urine, promotes regular micturition, and flushes the urethra of microorganisms.

Acidifying Urine. Urine is normally acidic and tends to inhibit growth of microorganisms. Meats, eggs, whole-grain breads, cranberries, and prunes increase urine acidity. Cranberry juice has been shown to lower urine pH and decrease bacterial adherence to the bladder wall (Gray, 2002). High doses of ascorbic acid may also be used to lower the pH.

Acute Care

Maintaining Elimination Habits. Clients usually require time to void. Requesting a urine specimen on demand does not contribute to relaxation and normal voiding habits. Clients should be given at least 30 minutes to provide a specimen. The nurse knows that clients normally void upon awakening or before meals, and offers the opportunity to use toilet facilities then. Also important is the need to respond to clients' urges to urinate. Delay in assisting clients to the bathroom may interfere with normal micturition and contribute to incontinence.

> **Safety Alert.** Many falls in the older adult are related to the urge to urinate. Anticipate the need and provide for scheduled bathroom visits. Make sure the pathway is clear of any barriers between the bed and the facilities.

Privacy is essential for normal voiding. If the client cannot reach the bathroom, the nurse makes sure that the bedside curtain is closed. The debilitated client at home may prefer using a bedside commode screened by a partition or room divider. Young children are often unable to void in the presence of persons other than their parents.

When possible, the nurse should encourage the continued use of special measures that the client uses to void. The client may be able to relax and void more easily while reading or listening to music. Having a cup or glass of fluids may also promote urination.

Medications. Drug therapy given alone or with other therapies can help problems of incontinence or retention. The bladder is innervated by the parasympathetic nervous system. Local bladder irritants such as calculi or infection may cause uncontrolled bladder contractions. Drugs that depress the neurotransmitter acetylcholine, which stimulates the bladder, reduce incontinence caused by bladder

KNOWLEDGE

- Importance of caring in maintenance of the client's self-esteem
- Role other health professionals might provide in the care of the client with urinary elimination alterations
- Adult learning principles to apply when educating the client and family
- Services of community-based resources
- Nursing interventions effective in maintaining normal urinary elimination

EXPERIENCE

- Previous client responses to planned nursing interventions to promote urinary elimination

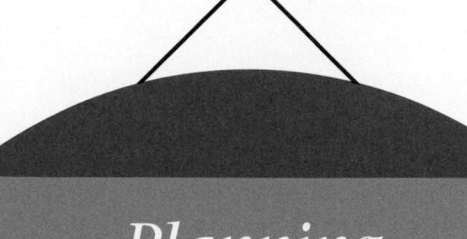

Planning

- Reinforce adherence to good hygiene practices
- Select interventions that promote normal physiology of micturition
- Involve the family in learning knowledge and skills for the client's care in the home
- Refer the client to appropriate health care professionals and/or community agencies

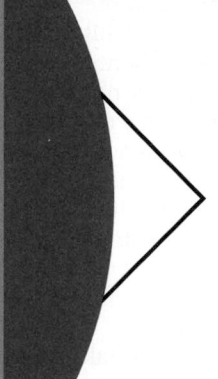

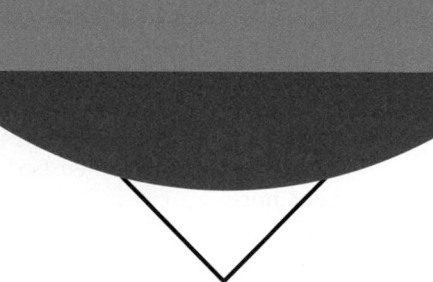

STANDARDS

- Individualize interventions to adapt to a normal urination pattern
- Apply standards of care from the agency and professional organizations such as ANA, AHCPR, and United Ostomy Association in planning care

ATTITUDES

- Use risk taking and creativity in trying alternatives in care (e.g., skin care, ostomy management)

FIGURE **44–10** Critical thinking model for urinary elimination planning.

Concept Map

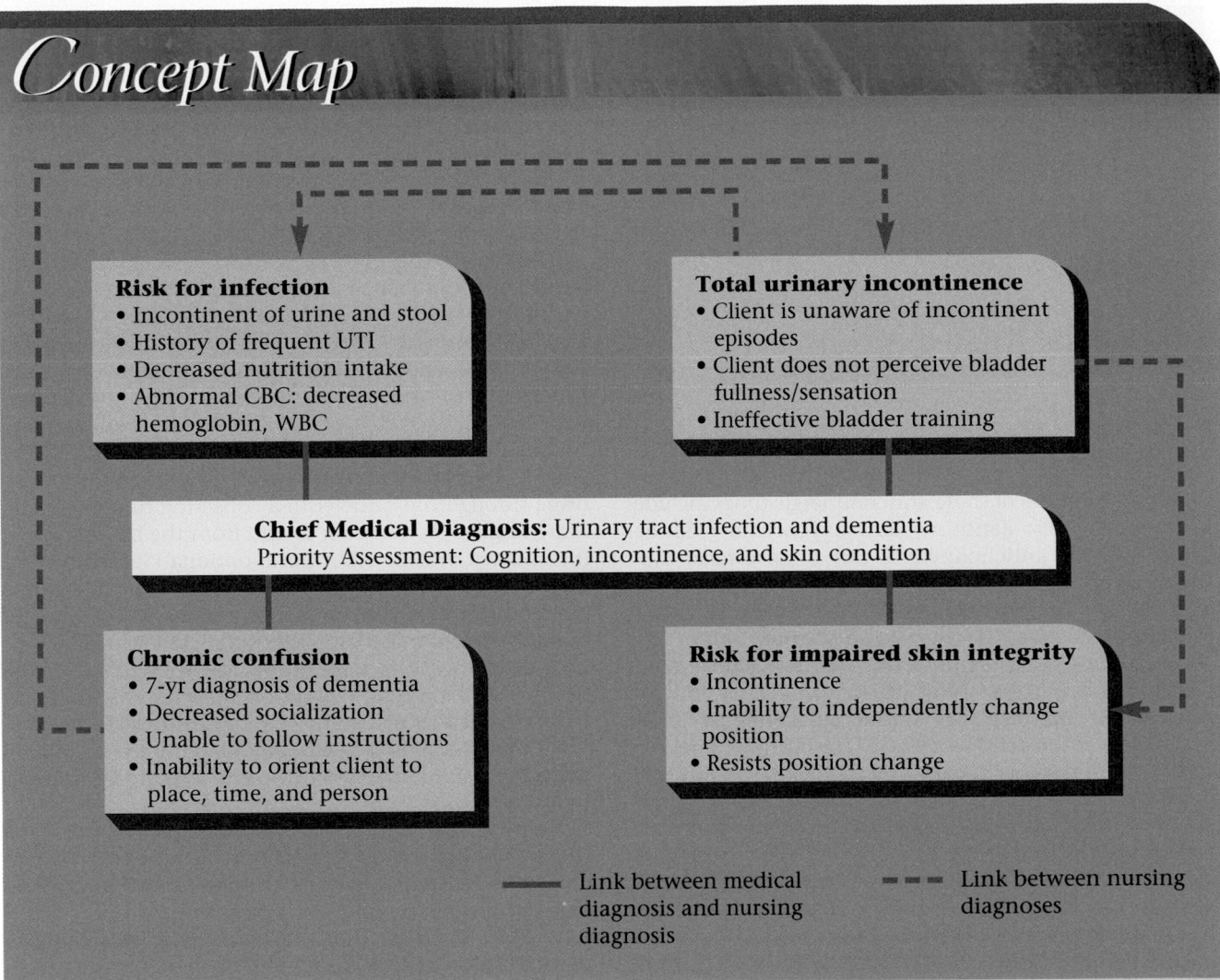

Risk for infection
- Incontinent of urine and stool
- History of frequent UTI
- Decreased nutrition intake
- Abnormal CBC: decreased hemoglobin, WBC

Total urinary incontinence
- Client is unaware of incontinent episodes
- Client does not perceive bladder fullness/sensation
- Ineffective bladder training

Chief Medical Diagnosis: Urinary tract infection and dementia
Priority Assessment: Cognition, incontinence, and skin condition

Chronic confusion
- 7-yr diagnosis of dementia
- Decreased socialization
- Unable to follow instructions
- Inability to orient client to place, time, and person

Risk for impaired skin integrity
- Incontinence
- Inability to independently change position
- Resists position change

—— Link between medical diagnosis and nursing diagnosis

- - - Link between nursing diagnoses

FIGURE **44–11** Concept map for client with urinary tract infection and dementia.

Client Teaching

Box 44-5

Urinary Elimination Problems Related to Urinary Sphincter Dysfunction

Objectives

- Client will achieve continence through increased sphincter control.

Teaching Strategies

- Have client attempt to tighten urinary sphincter during urination to feel the sensations associated with urinary sphincter contraction.
- Teach client progressive use of pelvic floor exercises (PFEs).
- Provide written instructions.
- Have client sit or stand without tensing muscles of legs, buttocks, or abdomen.

- Have client contract and relax circumvaginal muscles and urinary and anal sphincters for 3 to 4 seconds and repeat in quick succession.
- Have client repeat these cycles for 25 to 30 times 3 times a day for 6 months.
- Teach and monitor use of a voiding record.

Evaluation

- Ask client and caregiver about voiding record to identify changes in patterns of urinary elimination.
- Ask client and caregiver about degree of satisfaction related to control achieved in urinary elimination.
- Ask client and caregiver about selection and usage of incontinence control devices.

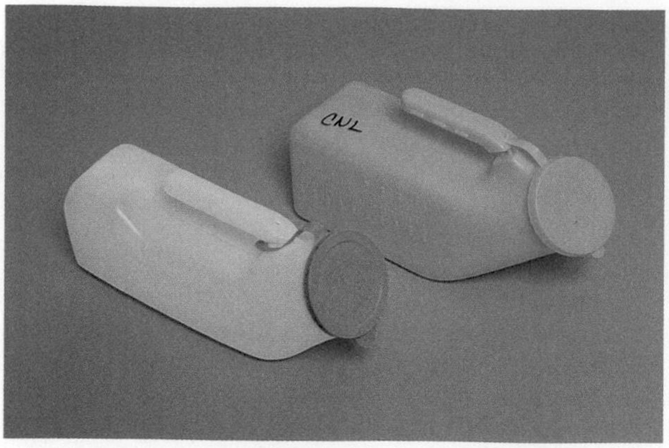

FIGURE **44-12** Types of male urinals.

irritation. Examples of these anticholinergic drugs include propantheline (Pro-Banthine) and oxybutynin chloride (Ditropan). The anticholinergics can cause cardiac dysrhythmias and should be used with caution in clients with heart disease. Anticholinergics may also cause constipation and a dry mouth (McKenry and Salerno, 2003).

When the bladder empties, the detrusor muscle contracts in response to parasympathetic stimulation. Incomplete bladder emptying results from impaired innervation or weakness of the detrusor muscle. The client experiences retention and possible overflow incontinence. Cholinergic drugs increase contraction of the bladder and improve emptying. Bethanechol (Urecholine) stimulates parasympathetic nerves to increase bladder wall contraction and relax the sphincter. Bethanechol can be given by subcutaneous or oral routes. Cholinergic drugs may cause diarrhea as a side effect (McKenry and Salerno, 2003).

The dribbling or overflow incontinence seen in men with prostatic enlargement can be treated with an alpha$_1$-adrenergic blocker, such as terazosin (Hytrin). Terazosin is given orally and relaxes prostatic smooth muscle, thus relieving obstructive symptoms. This drug may cause hypotension because it is also used in treatment of hypertension (McKenry and Salerno, 2003).

> *Safety Alert.* Medications that cause transient hypotension also increase the client's risk of fall or injury. Instruct clients taking these medications to plan their nighttime toileting and to get out of bed slowly.

Catheterization. **Catheterization** of the bladder involves introducing a rubber or plastic tube through the urethra and into the bladder. The catheter provides a continuous flow of urine in clients unable to control micturition or those with obstructions. It also provides a means of assessing urine output in hemodynamically unstable clients. Because bladder catheterization carries the risk of UTI, blockage, and trauma to the urethra, it is preferable to rely on other measures for either specimen collection or management of incontinence (Getliffe, 2003).

Types of Catheterization. Intermittent and indwelling retention catheterizations are the two forms of catheter insertion. With the intermittent technique a straight single-

use catheter (Figure 44-13, *A*) is introduced long enough to drain the bladder (5 to 10 minutes). When the bladder is empty, the nurse immediately withdraws the catheter. Intermittent catheterization can be repeated as necessary, but repeated use increases the risks of trauma and infection. An indwelling or Foley catheter (Figure 44-13, *B*) remains in place for a longer period until a client is able to void completely and voluntarily or as long as accurate measurements are needed (Box 44-6).

The straight single-use catheter has a single lumen with a small opening about 1.3 cm ($^1/_2$ inch) from the tip. Urine drains from the tip, through the lumen, and to a receptacle. An indwelling Foley catheter has a small inflatable balloon that encircles the catheter just above the tip. When inflated, the balloon rests against the bladder outlet to anchor the catheter in place. The indwelling retention catheter may have two or three lumens within the body of the catheter (Figure 44-13, *B*). One lumen drains urine through the catheter to a collecting tube. A second lumen carries sterile water to and from the balloon when it is inflated or deflated. A third (optional) lumen may be used to instill fluids or medications into the bladder. It is easy to determine the number of lumens by the number of drainage and injection ports at the catheter's end.

A second type of intermittent catheter has a curved tip. A Coudé catheter is used on male clients who may have enlarged prostates that partly obstruct the urethra. The Coudé catheter is less traumatic during insertion because it is stiffer and easier to control than the straight-tip catheter.

Catheters come in many diameters to fit the size of a client's urethral canal. Suggestions on how to make appropriate decisions regarding catheter selection are provided in Box 44-7.

Catheter Insertion. Urethral catheterization requires a physician's order. The nurse must use strict aseptic technique (see Chapter 33). Organizing equipment before the procedure prevents interruptions. The steps for inserting indwelling and single-use straight catheters are basically the same. The difference lies in the procedure taken to inflate the indwelling catheter balloon and secure the catheter. Skill 44-2 lists steps for performing female and male urethral catheterization.

Closed Drainage Systems. After inserting an indwelling catheter, the nurse maintains a closed urinary drainage system to minimize the risk of infection. Urinary drainage bags are plastic and can hold about 1000 to 1500 ml of urine. The bag should hang on the bed frame or wheelchair without touching the floor. Never hang the bag on the bed rail because it can be accidentally raised above the level of the bladder.

When the client ambulates, the nurse or client carries the bag below the client's waist. The drainage bag should never be raised above the level of the client's bladder. Urine in the bag and tubing can become a medium for bacteria, and infection is likely to develop if urine flows back into the bladder.

Most drainage bags contain an antireflux valve to prevent urine in the bag from reentering the drainage tubing and contaminating the client's bladder. A spigot at the base of the bag provides a means for emptying the bag. The spigot should always be clamped, except during emp-

Table 44-5	Urinary Incontinence and Treatment Options	
Description/Causes	**Symptoms**	**Interventions**
Functional		
Involuntary, unpredictable passage of urine in a client with intact urinary and nervous system Change in environment: sensory, cognitive, or mobility deficits	Urge to void that causes loss of urine before reaching appropriate receptacle. The client with cognitive changes may have forgotten what to do.	Habit training Environmental alterations Scheduled toileting Condom catheter (men) Protective undergarments
Overflow		
Voluntary or involuntary loss of a small amount of urine (20-30 ml) from an overdistended bladder Hypotonic or underactive detrusor secondary to drugs, fecal impaction, diabetes, spinal cord injury; men—prostate enlargement; women—severe uterine prolapse	Symptoms may vary from dribbling of a few drops of urine to larger amounts with urgency and frequency.	Intermittent catheterization Surgery Indwelling or condom catheter Credé's method
Reflex		
Involuntary loss of urine occurring at somewhat predictable intervals; large or small volume Spinal cord dysfunction (either inhibition of cerebral awareness or impairment of the reflex arc)	Unawareness of bladder filling, lack of urge to void, uninhibited bladder spasm contraction	Anticholinergic medications Surgery Intermittent catheterization Indwelling or condom catheter Estrogen replacement Credé's method
Stress		
Leakage of small volumes of urine caused by sudden increase in intraabdominal pressure Coughing, laughing, sneezing, or lifting with a full bladder; obesity; full uterus in third trimester; incompetent bladder outlet; weak pelvic musculature	Loss of urine with increased intraabdominal pressure, urinary urgency and frequency	Pelvic floor exercises (Kegel) Surgery Artificial sphincter Biofeedback Scheduled toileting Electrical stimulation Lifestyle modifications (e.g., weight reduction, smoking cessation)
Urge		
Involuntary passage of urine after a strong sense of urgency to void Decreased bladder capacity; irritation of bladder stretch receptors; alcohol or caffeine ingestion; increased fluid intake; infection	Urinary urgency, often with frequency (more often than every 2 hours); bladder spasm or contraction; voiding in either small amounts (<100 ml) or large amounts (>500 ml)	Anticholinergic medications Bladder retraining Scheduled toileting Treatment of UTI or vaginitis Biofeedback Electrical stimulation Lifestyle modifications (e.g., selected dietary and fluid modifications)

Data from Ackley BJ, Ludwig GB: *Nursing diagnosis handbook: a guide to planning care,* St. Louis, 1997, Mosby; Wyman JF: Treatment of urinary incontinence in men and older women, *Am J Nurs* 103(3 suppl): 26, 2003.

tying, and tucked into the protective pouch on the side of the bag (see agency policy). To keep the drainage system patent the nurse checks for kinks or bends in the tubing, avoids positioning the client on the drainage tubing, and observes for clots or sediment that may occlude the collecting tubing.

Routine Catheter Care. Clients with indwelling catheters have a number of special care needs. Nursing measures are directed at preventing infection and maintaining unobstructed flow of urine through the catheter drainage system

Perineal Hygiene. Buildup of secretions or encrustation at the catheter insertion site is a source of irritation and potential infection. Nurses provide perineal hygiene (see Chapter 38) at least twice daily or as needed for a client with a retention catheter. Soap and water are effective in reducing the number of organisms around the urethra. The nurse must not accidentally advance the catheter up into the bladder during cleansing or risk introducing bacteria.

Catheter Care. In addition to routine perineal hygiene, many institutions recommend that clients with catheters

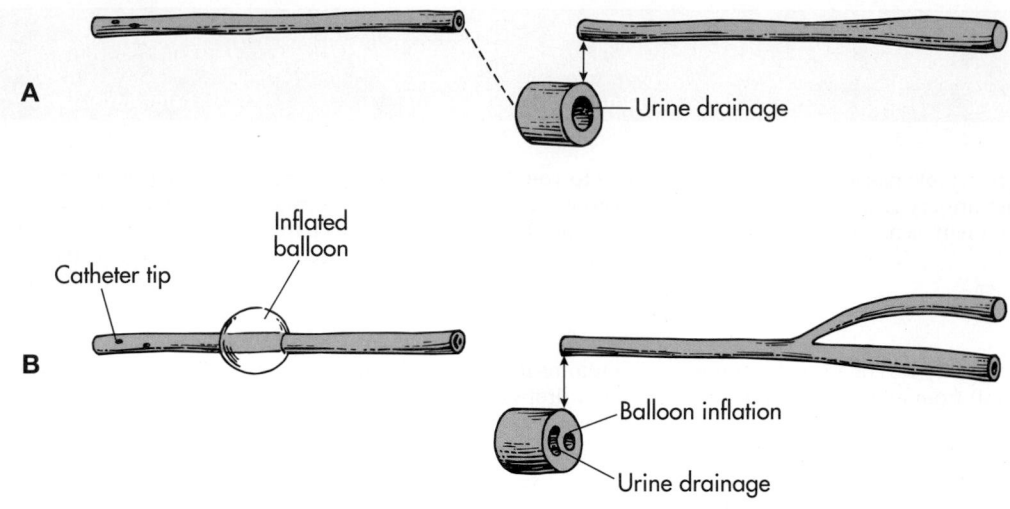

FIGURE **44–13** Types of urinary catheters. **A,** Straight catheter. **B,** Indwelling (Foley).

<table>
<tr><td>

Box **44-6**   **Indications for Catheterization**

Intermittent Catheterization

Relief of discomfort of bladder distention, provision of decompression
Obtaining sterile urine specimen
Assessment of residual urine after urination
Long-term management of clients with spinal cord injuries, neuromuscular degeneration, or incompetent bladders

Short-Term Indwelling Catheterization

Obstruction to urine outflow (e.g., prostate enlargement)
Surgical repair of bladder, urethra, and surrounding structures
Prevention of urethral obstruction from blood clots
Measurement of urinary output in critically ill clients
Continuous or intermittent bladder irrigations

Long-Term Indwelling Catheterization

Severe urinary retention with recurrent episodes of UTI
Skin rashes, ulcers, or wounds irritated by contact with urine
Terminal illness when bed linen changes are painful for client

</td><td>

Box **44-7**   **Guidelines for Appropriate Catheter Selection**

- The catheter size should be determined by the size of the client's urethral canal. When the French system is used, the larger the gauge number, the larger the catheter size. Generally, children require an 8 to 10 Fr, women require a 14 to 16 Fr, whereas men require a 16 to 18 Fr (Lewis, Heitkemper, and Dirksen, 2000). To prevent trauma, the smallest effective catheter size is preferred.
- The expected time required for the catheterization will determine the catheter material selection.
- Plastic catheters are suitable only for intermittent use due to their inflexibility.
- Latex and rubber catheters are recommended for use up to 3 weeks. Be aware of allergies to either of these materials.
- Pure silicon or Teflon catheters are best suited for long-term use (2 to 3 months) because they cause less encrustation at the urethral meatus.
- Balloon size is also important in selecting an indwelling catheter. Balloon sizes range from 3 ml (pediatric) to large postoperative volumes (75 ml). In adults, the 5-ml and 30-ml sizes are the most common: The 5-ml size allows for optimal drainage, whereas the 30-ml size is used after prostatectomies to provide hemostasis of the prostatic bed (Lewis, Heitkemper, and Dirksen, 2000).
- Only sterile water should be used to inflate the balloon because saline may crystallize, resulting in incomplete deflation of the balloon at the time of removal.
- If leakage should occur around the catheter, a change in lumen size or use of antispasmodic medication may be warranted.

</td></tr>
</table>

receive special care 3 times a day and after defecation or bowel incontinence to help minimize discomfort and infection (Skill 44-3).

Fluid Intake. All clients with catheters should have a daily intake of 2000 to 2500 ml if permitted. This can be met through oral intake or intravenous infusion. A high fluid intake produces a large volume of urine that flushes the bladder and keeps catheter tubing free of sediment.

Preventing Infection. Maintaining a closed urinary drainage system is important in infection control. A break in the system can lead to introduction of microorganisms. Sites at risk are the site of catheter insertion, the

drainage bag, the spigot, the tube junction, and the junction of the tube and the bag (Figure 44-14).

In addition, the nurse monitors the patency of the system to prevent pooling of urine within the tubing. Urine in the drainage bag is an excellent medium for microorganism growth. Bacteria can travel up drainage tubing to

Text continued on p. 1361

Skill 44-2 *Inserting a Straight or an Indwelling Catheter*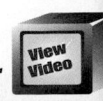

Delegation Considerations

Catheterization is not usually delegated to assistive personnel (AP). However, in some settings, agency policy may permit this skill to be delegated to AP who have been properly instructed.

- AP routinely assist with positioning the client and maintaining client privacy and comfort, empty urine from the collection bag, and provide perineal care.
- Instruct AP to report client discomfort or fever to the nurse.
- Instruct AP to report abnormal color, odor, and amount of urine in drainage bag to the nurse.

Equipment

- Catheterization kit containing the following sterile items:
  - Gloves (extra pair optional)
  - Drapes, one fenestrated
- Lubricant
- Antiseptic cleansing solution
- Cotton balls
- Forceps
- Prefilled syringe with sterile water to inflate the balloon of indwelling catheter
- Catheter of correct size and type for procedure (i.e., intermittent or indwelling)
- Sterile drainage tubing with collection bag and multipurpose tube holder or tape, safety pin, and elastic band for securing tubing to bed if client is bed bound (for indwelling catheter)
- Receptacle or basin (usually bottom of catheterization tray)
- Specimen container
- Blanket

Steps	Rationale
1. Assess status of client:	
a. Ask client when last voided, or check I&O flow sheet, or palpate bladder.	Determine time of last voiding or potential for bladder fullness.
b. Level of awareness or developmental stage.	Reveals the client's ability to cooperate and level of explanation needed.
c. Mobility and physical limitations of client.	Affect way the nurse positions client.
d. Client's gender and age.	Determines catheter size: 8 to 10 Fr is generally used for children, 14 to 16 Fr is indicated for women, 12 Fr may be considered for young girls, and 16 to 18 Fr is used for male clients unless larger size is ordered by physician.
e. Distended bladder.	Causes pain. Can indicate need to insert catheter if client is unable to void independently.
f. Perform hand hygiene. Inspect perineum for erythema, drainage, and odor.	Reduces infection. Determines condition of the perineum.
g. Any pathological condition that may impair passage of catheter (e.g., enlarged prostate in men).	Obstruction prevents passage of catheter through urethra into the bladder. May require use of coude catheter.
h. Allergies.	Procedure risks exposure to antiseptic, tape, latex, and lubricant. Betadine allergies are common; if the client is unaware of allergy, ask if allergic to shellfish.
2. Review client's medical record, including physician's order and nurses' notes.	Determines purpose of inserting catheter: preparation for surgery, urinary irrigations, collection of sterile specimens, or measurement of residual urine. Assess for previous catheterization, including catheter size, response of client, and time of last catheterization.
3. Assess client's knowledge of the purpose for catheterization.	Reveals need for client instruction.
4. Explain procedure to client.	Promotes cooperation.
5. Arrange for extra nursing personnel to assist as necessary.	Client may be unable to assume positioning for procedure.
6. Perform hand hygiene.	Reduces transmission of microorganisms.
7. Close curtain or door.	Offers privacy, reduces embarrassment, and aids in relaxation during procedure.
8. Raise bed to appropriate working height.	Promotes use of proper body mechanics.
9. Facing client, stand on left side of bed if right-handed (on right side of bed if left-handed). Clear the bedside table and arrange equipment.	Successful catheter insertion requires nurse to assume comfortable position with all equipment easily accessible.
10. Raise side rail on opposite side of bed, and put side rail down on working side.	Promotes client safety.

Inserting a Straight or an Indwelling Catheter—cont'd

Steps	Rationale
11. Place waterproof pad under client.	
12. Position client.	Prevents soiling of bed linen.
A. Female client	Provides good visualization of perineal structures.
(1) Assist to dorsal recumbent position (supine with knees flexed). Ask client to relax thighs so the hips can be externally rotated.	Legs may be supported with pillows to reduce muscle tension and promote comfort.
(2) Position female client in side-lying (Sims') position with upper leg flexed at hip if unable to assume dorsal recumbent position. If this position is used, nurse must take extra precautions to cover rectal area with drape to reduce chance of cross contamination.	This alternate position is used if client cannot abduct leg at hip joint (e.g., if client has arthritic joints). Also, this position may be more comfortable for client. Support client with pillows if necessary to maintain position.
B. Male client	
(1) Assist to supine position with thighs slightly abducted.	Comfortable position for client that aids in visualization.
13. Drape client.	
A. Female client (see illustration)	
(1) Drape with bath blanket. Place blanket diamond fashion over client, with one corner at client's midsection, side corners over each thigh and abdomen, and last corner over perineum.	
B. Male client (see illustration)	
(1) Drape upper trunk with bath blanket, and cover lower extremities with bed sheets, exposing only genitalia.	

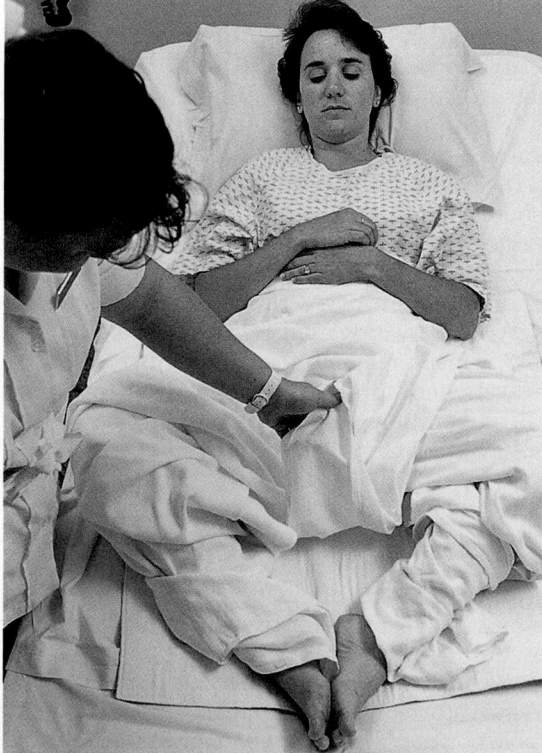

STEP **13A** Draping technique (female).

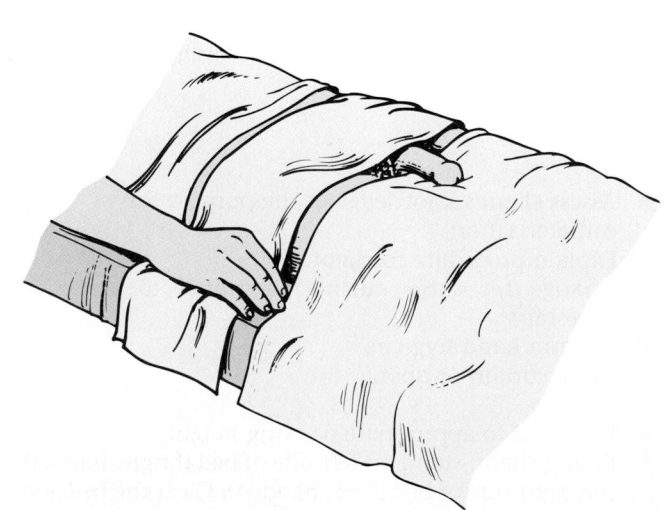

STEP **13B** Draping technique (male).

Steps	Rationale
14. Wearing disposable gloves, wash perineal area with soap and water as needed; dry thoroughly. Remove and discard gloves; perform hand hygiene.	Avoids unnecessary exposure of body parts and maintains client's comfort.
15. Position lamp to illuminate perineal area. (When using flashlight have an assistant hold it.)	Reduces microorganisms near urethral meatus and allows further opportunity to visualize perineum and landmarks.
16. Open package containing drainage system; place drainage bag over edge of bottom bed frame, and bring drainage tube up between side rails and mattress.	Permits accurate identification and good visualization of urethral meatus. Prepare system for eventual connection with catheter.

Critical Decision Point: This step is necessary only when an indwelling catheter is to be inserted and drainage system is not part of the catheterization kit.

---

17. Open catheterization kit according to directions, keeping bottom of container sterile.	Prevents transmission of microorganisms from table or work area to sterile supplies. The materials in the kit are arranged in sequence of use.
18. Place plastic bag that contained kit within reach of work area to use as a waterproof bag to dispose of used supplies.	
19. Apply sterile gloves (see Chapter 33).	Allows nurse to handle sterile supplies without contamination.

Critical Decision Point: If underpad is first item in kit, place pad plastic side down under client, touching only the edges so as to maintain sterility. Then apply sterile gloves.

---

20. Organize supplies on sterile field. Open inner sterile package containing catheter. Pour sterile antiseptic solution into correct compartment containing sterile cotton balls. Open packet containing lubricant. Remove specimen container (lid should be placed loosely on top) and prefilled syringe from collection compartment of tray, and set them aside on sterile field.	Maintains principles of surgical asepsis and organizes work area.
21. Before inserting indwelling catheter, test balloon by injecting fluid from prefilled syringe into balloon port (see illustration).	Checks integrity of balloon. Do not use the catheter if the balloon does not inflate or leaks.
22. Lubricate 2.5 to 5 cm (1 to 2 inches) of catheter for women and 12.5 to 17.7 cm (5 to 7 inches) for men.	

Critical Decision Point: Some catheters will have a plastic sheath over the catheter that must be removed before lubrication. In some cases the physician may order the use of a lubricant containing a local anesthetic.

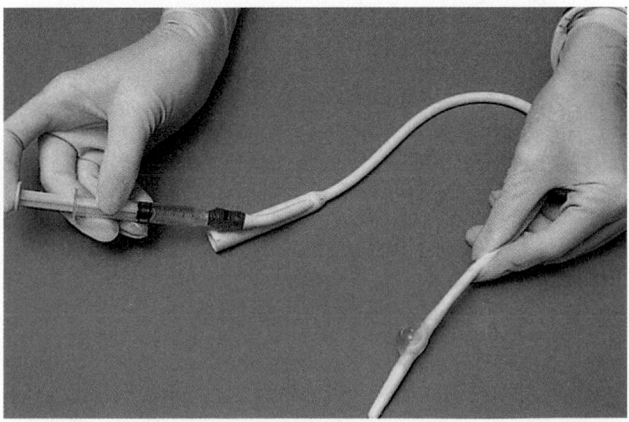

STEP **21** Checking balloon (indwelling catheter).

Inserting a Straight or an Indwelling Catheter—cont'd

Skill 44-2

Steps	Rationale

23. Apply sterile drape:

  A. Female client

    (1) Allow top edge of drape to form a cuff over both gloved hands. Place drape down on bed between client's thighs. Slip cuffed edge just under buttocks, taking care not to touch contaminated surface with gloves. — Outer surface of drape covering hands remains sterile. Sterile drape against sterile gloves is sterile.

    (2) Pick up fenestrated sterile drape, and allow it to unfold without touching an unsterile object. Apply drape over perineum, exposing labia, and being sure not to touch contaminated surface. — Maintains sterility of work surface.

  B. Male client

    (1) Two methods are used for draping depending on preference. *First method:* Apply drape over thighs and under penis without completely opening fenestrated drape. *Second method:* Apply drape over thighs just below penis. Pick up fenestrated sterile drape, allow it to unfold, and drape it over penis with fenestrated slit resting over penis. — Maintains sterility of work surface.

24. Place sterile tray and contents on sterile drape. Open specimen container. — Provides easy access to supplies during catheter insertion. Maintains aseptic technique during procedure.

25. Cleanse urethral meatus:

  A. Female client

    (1) With nondominant hand, carefully retract labia to fully expose urethral meatus. Maintain position of nondominant hand throughout procedure. — Full visualization of urethral meatus is provided. Full retraction prevents contamination of urethral meatus during cleansing.

    (2) Using forceps in sterile dominant hand, pick up cotton ball saturated with antiseptic solution and clean perineal area, wiping from front to back from clitoris toward anus. Using a new cotton ball for each area, wipe along the far labial fold, near labial fold, and directly over center of urethral meatus (see illustration). — Cleansing reduces number of microorganism at urethral meatus.
Use of a single cotton ball for each wipe prevents transfer of microorganisms. Cleansing proceeds from area of least contamination to that of most contamination. Dominant hand remains sterile.

STEP **25A(2)** Cleansing technique (female).

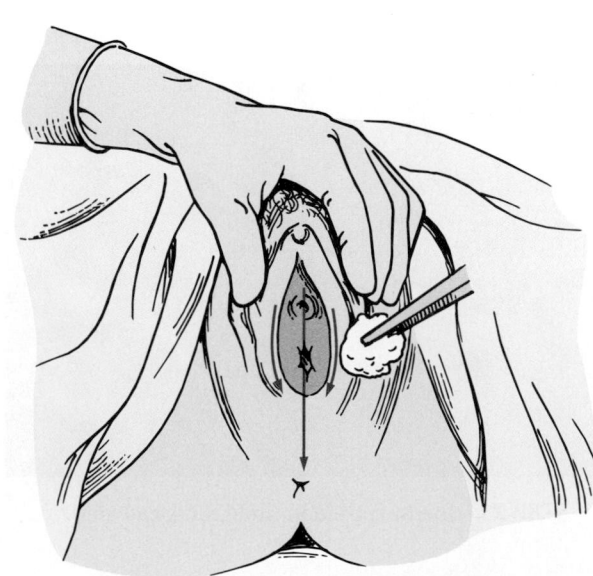

Steps	Rationale

Critical Decision Point: Closure of labia during cleansing requires that the cleansing procedure be repeated because the area has become contaminated.

B. Male client
    (1) If client is not circumcised, retract foreskin with nondominant hand. Grasp penis at shaft just below glans. Retract urethral meatus between thumb and forefinger. Maintain nondominant hand in this position throughout procedure.

Accidental release of foreskin or dropping of penis during cleansing requires process to be repeated because area has become contaminated.

    (2) With dominant hand, pick up cotton ball with forceps and clean penis. Move in a circular motion from urethral meatus down to base of glans. Repeat cleansing three more times, using a clean cotton ball each time (see illustration).

Reduces number of microorganisms at urethral meatus and moves from area of least to most contamination. Dominant hand remains sterile.

Critical Decision Point: If foreskin does not remain retracted during insertion, then the cleansing process must be repeated because the area has become contaminated.

26. Pick up catheter with gloved dominant hand 7.5 to 10 cm (3 to 4 inches) from catheter tip. Hold end of catheter loosely coiled in palm of dominant hand. (Optional: May grasp catheter with forceps.)
27. Insert catheter:

A. Female client
    (1) Ask client to bear down gently as if to void, and slowly insert catheter through urethral meatus (see illustration).

Relaxation of external sphincter aids in insertion of catheter.

    (2) Advance catheter a total of 5 to 7.5 cm (2 to 3 inches) in adult or until urine flows out of catheter's end. When urine appears, advance catheter another 2.5 to 5 cm (1 to 2 inches). Do not force against resistance.

Female urethra is short. Appearance of urine indicates that catheter tip is in bladder or lower urethra. Advancement of catheter ensures bladder placement.

    (3) Release labia, and hold catheter securely with nondominant hand. Slowly inflate balloon if retention catheter is used (see illustrations) (see step 30).

Bladder or sphincter contraction may cause accidental expulsion of catheter.

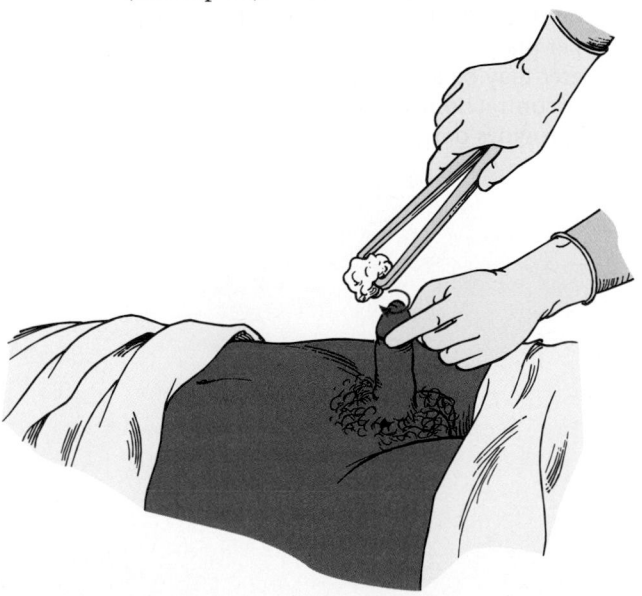

STEP **25B(2)** Cleansing technique (male).

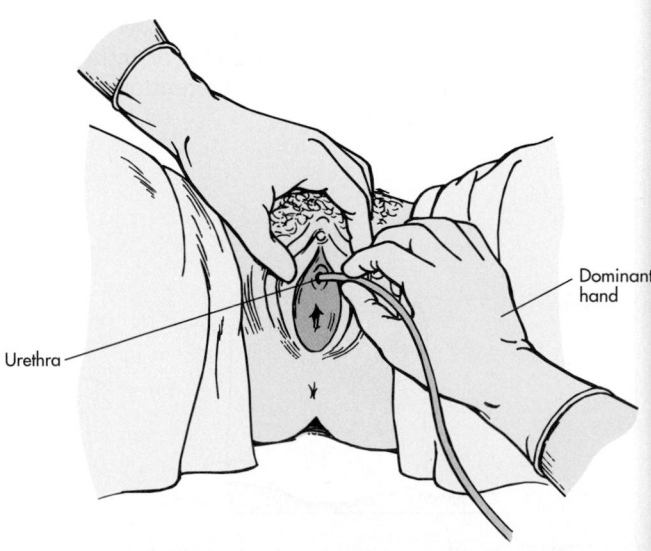

STEP **27A(1)** Inserting the catheter.

Skill 44-2   *Inserting a Straight or an Indwelling Catheter—cont'd*

Steps	Rationale

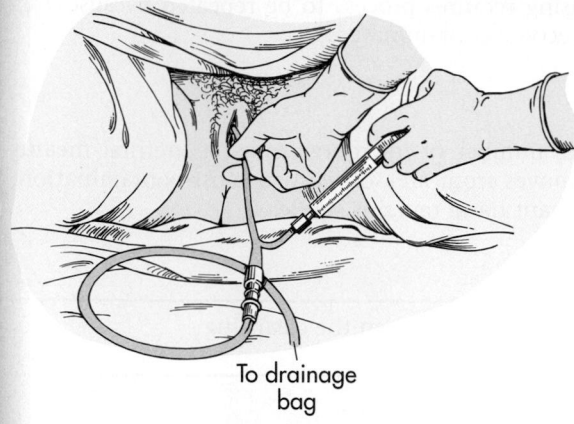

STEP 27A(3) Inflating the balloon (indwelling catheter).

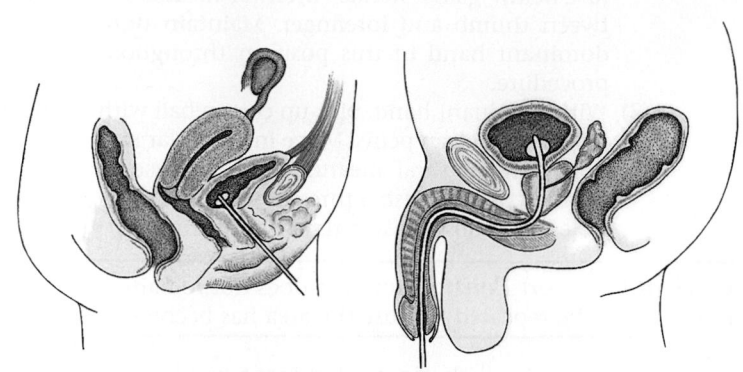

STEP 27A(3) Placement of inflated balloon in bladder.

Critical Decision Point: If no urine appears, check if catheter is in vagina. If misplaced, leave catheter in vagina as landmark indicating where not to insert, and insert another.

B. Male client

  (1) Lift penis to position perpendicular to client's body and apply light traction (see illustration).

     Straightens urethral canal to ease catheter insertion.

  (2) Ask client to bear down as if to void, and slowly insert catheter through urethral meatus.

     Relaxation of external sphincter aids in insertion of catheter.

  (3) Advance catheter 17 to 22.5 cm (7 to 9 inches) in adult or until urine flows out catheter's end. If resistance is felt, withdraw catheter; do not force it through urethra. When urine appears, advance catheter another 2.5 to 5 cm (1 to 2 inches). **Do not use force to insert a catheter.**

     The adult male urethra is long. It is normal to meet resistance at the prostatic sphincter. When resistance is met, nurse should hold catheter firmly against sphincter without forcing catheter. After a few seconds, the sphincter relaxes, and the catheter is advanced. Appearance of urine indicates catheter tip is in bladder or urethra. Further advancement of catheter ensures proper placement.

  (4) Lower penis and hold catheter securely in nondominant hand. Place end of catheter in urine tray. Inflate balloon if retention catheter is used (see step 30).

     Catheter may be accidentally expelled by bladder or urethral contraction. Collection of urine prevents soiling and provides output measurement.

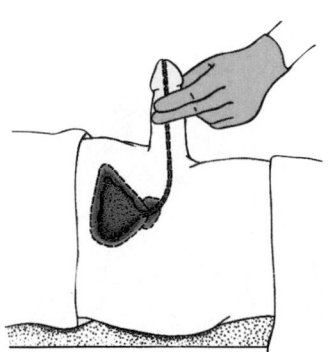

STEP 27B(1) Position penis perpendicular to body for catheter insertion.

Steps	Rationale
(5) Reduce (or reposition) the foreskin.	Paraphimosis (retraction and constriction of the foreskin behind the glans penis) secondary to catheterization may occur if foreskin is not reduced.
28. Collect urine specimen as needed. Fill specimen cup or jar to desired level (20 to 30 ml) by holding end of catheter in dominant hand over cup.	Allows sterile specimen to be obtained for culture analysis.
29. Allow bladder to empty fully (about 800 to 1000 ml) unless institution policy restricts maximal volume of urine to drain with each catheterization. Check institution policy before beginning catheterization. If a restriction is in place, the range is often 800 to 1000 ml.	As always the nurse should monitor the client's condition, and if the vital signs change or bleeding occurs, temporarily stop the flow of urine and continue when the client's condition warrants. Retained urine may serve as a reservoir for growth of microorganisms.

Critical Decision Point: If a straight, single-use catheter was inserted, withdraw it slowly, but smoothly until it is removed.

30. Inflate balloon fully per manufacturer's recommendation and then release catheter with nondominant hand and pull gently.	Inflation of balloon anchors catheter tip in place above the bladder outlet to prevent removal of the catheter. Note size of balloon on catheter. Most commonly a 5-ml balloon is used, but a 300-ml balloon may be ordered in some cases. A prefilled syringe may be included with the kit. Use only the amount included. Do not overinflate the balloon.

Critical Decision Point: If resistance to inflation is noted or client complains of pain, the balloon may not be entirely in the bladder. Stop inflation, aspirate the fluid injected into the balloon and advance the catheter a little more before attempting to inflate the balloon again.

31. Attach end of retention catheter to collecting tube of drainage system. Drainage bag must be below level of bladder; attach bag to bed frame, do not place bag on side rails of bed (see illustration).	
32. Anchor catheter:	
A. Female client	
(1) Secure catheter tubing to inner thigh with strip of nonallergenic tape (or multipurpose tube holders with a Velcro strap). Allow for slack so movement of thigh does not create tension on catheter (see illustration).	Anchoring catheter to inner thigh reduces pressure on urethra, thus reducing possibility of tissue injury.

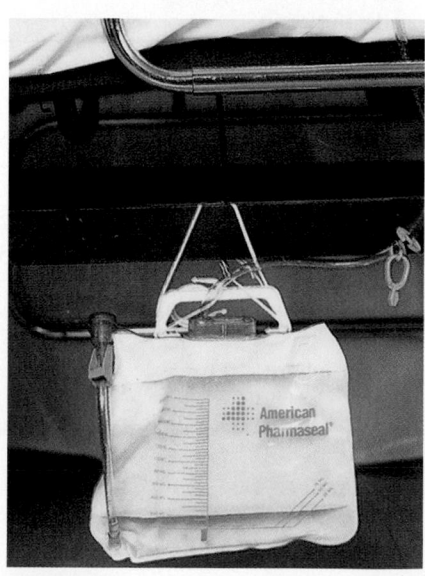

STEP **31** Attach drainage to lower bed frame.

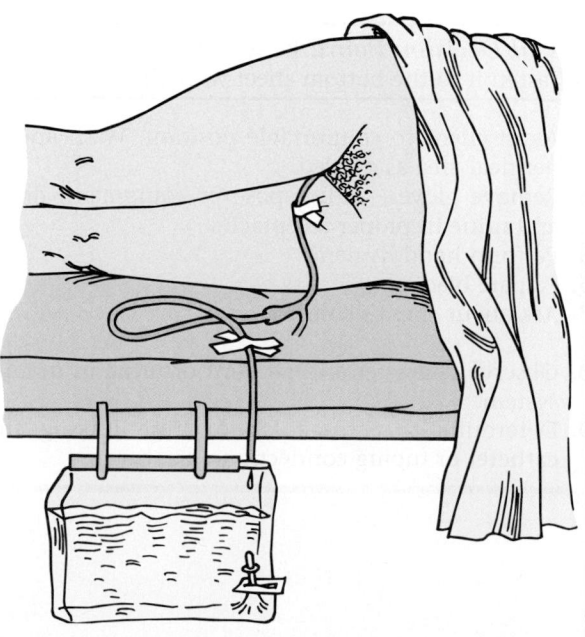

STEP **32A(1)** Tape catheter to inner thigh (female) and coil extra tubing on bed and attach to sheet.

*I*nserting a Straight or Indwelling Catheter—cont'd

Skill 44-2

Steps	Rationale

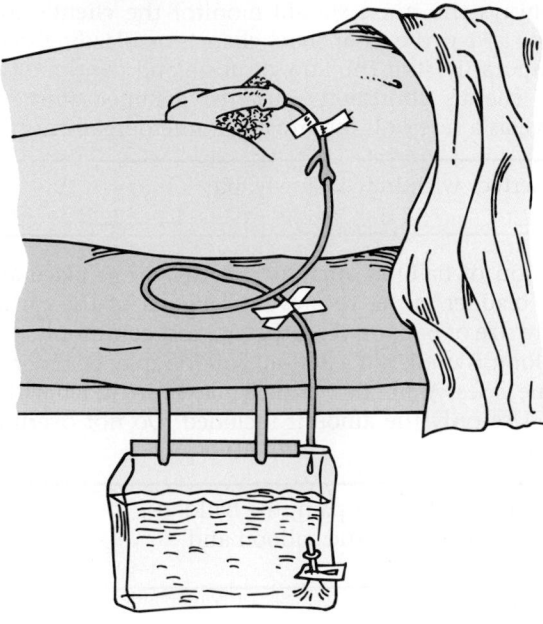

STEP 32B(1) Tape catheter to lower abdomen (male) and coil extra tubing on bed and attach to sheet.

Steps	Rationale
B. Male client (1) Secure catheter tubing to top of thigh or lower abdomen (with penis directed toward chest). Allow slack in catheter so movement does not create tension on catheter (see illustration).	Anchoring catheter to lower abdomen reduces pressure on urethra at junction of penis and scrotum, thus reducing possibility of tissue injury.

Critical Decision Point: Be sure there are no obstructions in tubing. Coil excess tubing on bed and fasten it to the bottom sheet with clip from kit or use rubber band and safety pin.

Steps	Rationale
33. Assist client to comfortable position. Wash and dry perineal area as needed.	Maintains comfort and security.
34. Remove gloves, and dispose of equipment, drapes, and urine in proper receptacles.	Reduces transmission of microorganisms.
35. Perform hand hygiene.	Reduces transmission of microorganisms.
36. Palpate bladder.	Determines if distention is relieved.
37. Ask about client's comfort.	Determines if client's sensation of discomfort or fullness has been relieved.
38. Observe character and amount of urine in drainage system.	Determines if urine is flowing adequately.
39. Determine that there is no urine leaking from catheter or tubing connections.	Prevents injury to client's skin.

Unexpected Outcomes and Related Interventions

1. Urethral or perineal irritation is present.
   a. Observe for catheter leaking, replace if necessary.
   b. Assess that indwelling catheter is anchored properly.
   c. Perform perineal hygiene and catheter more frequently.
2. Client has fever and/or odor is present, or client experiences small frequent voidings, burning or bleeding on voiding.
   a. Obtain clean voided urine specimen.
   b. Notify physician.
3. Client experiences urinary retention and is unable to void after catheter is removed.
   a. Provide adequate fluid intake and ensure client privacy.
   b. If client unable to void 6 to 8 hours following catheter removal, notify physician.

Recording and Reporting

- Report and record type and size of catheter inserted, amount of fluid used to inflate the balloon, characteristics of urine, amount of urine, reasons for catheterization, specimen collection if appropriate, and client's response to procedure and teaching concepts.
- Initiate I&O record.
- If catheter is definitely in bladder and no urine is produced within an hour, absence of urine should be immediately reported to physician.

Home Care Considerations

- Clients who are at home may use a leg bag during the day and switch to a large-volume bag at night so sleep can be uninterrupted.
- Clients may catheterize themselves at home using a clean technique.

Skill 44-3 *Indwelling Catheter Care*

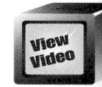
View Video

Delegation Considerations

Perineal care is often part of routine hygiene care that is delegated to assistive personnel (AP). Proper assessment and care of the perineal area will need professional clinical judgment.

If client has had trauma or surgical procedures that involve the perineal area, this care should not be delegated.

- Instruct AP to report client discomfort, perineal pain, perineal discharge, and/or odor to the nurse.

Equipment

- Catheter care kit or individual supplies
  - Nonsterile gloves
  - Cotton balls or large swabs
  - Clean washcloth and towel
  - Warm water and soap
  - Antibiotic ointment (if agency policy)
- Bath blanket
- Waterproof absorbent pad

Steps	Rationale
1. Assess for episode of bowel incontinence or client discomfort or provide care as per agency routine as part of hygiene measures (see Chapter 38).	Accumulation of secretions or feces causes irritation to perineal tissues and acts as a source of bacterial growth.
2. Explain procedure to client. Offer opportunity to perform self-care to able client.	Reduces anxiety and promotes cooperation. Embarrassment may motivate client to perform own hygiene.
3. Close door or bedside curtain.	Maintains client privacy.
4. Perform hand hygiene.	Reduces transmission of infection.
5. Position client:	
A. **Female**	
(1) Dorsal recumbent position	Ensures easy access to perineal tissues.
B. **Male**	
(1) Supine or Fowler's position	
6. Place waterproof pad under client.	Protects bed linens from soiling.
7. Drape bath blanket on client so that only perineal area is exposed.	Prevents unnecessary exposure of body parts.
8. Apply gloves.	

Skill 44-3   *I*ndwelling Catheter Care

Steps	Rationale
9. Remove anchor device to free catheter tubing.	
10. With nondominant hand:	
A. Female	
(1) Gently retract labia to fully expose urethral meatus and catheter insertion site, maintaining position of hand throughout procedure.	Provides full visualization of urethral meatus. Full retraction prevents contamination of meatus during cleansing.
B. Male	
(1) Retract foreskin if not circumscribed, and hold penis at shaft just below glans, maintaining position throughout procedure.	Accidental closure of labia or dropping of penis during cleansing requires procedure to be repeated.
11. Assess urethral meatus and surrounding tissue for inflammation, swelling, and discharge. Note amount, color, odor, and consistency of discharge. Ask client if any burning or discomfort is felt.	Determines presence of local infection and status of hygiene.
12. Cleanse perineal tissue:	
A. Female	
(1) Use clean cloth, soap, and water. Cleanse around urethral meatus and catheter. Cleaning from pubis toward anus, clean labia minora. Use a clean side of cloth for each wipe. Finally clean around anus. Dry each area well.	Reduces the number of microorganisms at urethral meatus. Use of clean cloth prevents transfer of microorganisms.
B. Male	
(1) While spreading urethral meatus, cleanse around catheter first, and then wipe in circular motion around meatus and glans.	Cleansing moves from area of least to most contamination.
13. Reassess urethral meatus for discharge.	Determines if cleansing is complete.
14. With towel, soap, and water, wipe in a circular motion along length of catheter for 10 cm (4 inches).	Reduces presence of secretions or drainage on exterior of catheter surface.
15. Apply an antibiotic ointment at urethral meatus and along 2.5 cm (1 inch) of catheter if ordered by physician or part of agency policy.	Further reduces growth of microorganisms at insertion site.
16. In male client reduce (or reposition) the foreskin.	
17. Place client in a safe, comfortable position.	Promotes comfort.
18. Dispose of contaminated supplies, remove gloves, and perform hand hygiene.	Prevents spread of infection.

Unexpected Outcomes and Related Interventions

1. Urethral discharge
   a. Increase frequency of indwelling catheter care.
   b. Apply topical antibiotic ointment per agency policy.
   c. Notify physician.
2. Accidental catheter dislodgement
   a. Notify physician.
   b. Assess for urethral trauma.
   c. Monitor urine output.

Recording and Reporting

- Report and record presence and characteristics of drainage, condition of perineal tissue, and any discomfort reported by client.
- If infection is suspected, report findings to physician.

Home Care Considerations

- If client is discharged with indwelling catheter, the client and family should be taught catheter care and signs and symptoms to report to nurse or physician.

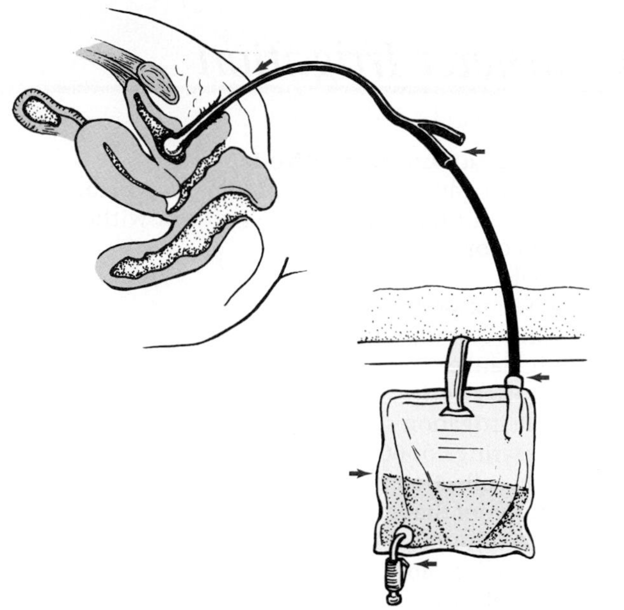

FIGURE **44–14** Potential sites for introduction of infectious organisms into a urinary drainage system.

Box 44-8 Tips for Preventing Infection in Catheterized Clients

Follow good hand-hygiene techniques (see Chapter 33).
Do not allow the spigot on the drainage system to touch a contaminated surface.
Only use sterile technique to collect specimens from a closed drainage system.
If the drainage tube becomes disconnected, do not touch the ends of the catheter or tubing. Wipe the end of the tubing and catheter with an antimicrobial solution before reconnecting.
Ensure that each client has a separate receptacle for measuring urine to prevent cross contamination.
Prevent pooling of urine in the tubing and reflux of urine into the bladder.
Avoid raising the drainage bag above the level of the bladder.
If it becomes necessary to raise the bag during transfer of the client to a bed or stretcher, clamp the tubing or empty the tubing contents to the drainage bag first.
Provide for drainage of urine from the tubing to the bag by positioning the tubing.
Before exercise or ambulation drain all urine from the tubing into the drainage bag.
Avoid prolonged kinking or clamping of the tubing.
Empty the drainage bag at least every 8 hours. If large outputs are noted, empty more frequently.
Encourage fluid intake (if not contraindicated). Inclusion of cranberry juice has been shown to decrease the adherence of bacteria to the bladder wall and to catheter lumen (Gray, 2002).
Remove the catheter as soon as clinically warranted (Kunin, 2001).
Tape or secure the catheter appropriately for the client (see Skill 44-2, p. 1351).
Perform routine perineal hygiene per agency policy and after defecation or bowel incontinence (see Skill 44-3, p. 1359).

grow in pools of urine. If this urine flows back into the client's bladder, an infection will likely develop (Kunin, 2001). Suggestions for ways to prevent infections in catheterized clients are provided in Box 44-8.

Catheter Irrigations and Instillations. To maintain the patency of indwelling urinary catheters, it sometimes becomes necessary to irrigate or flush a catheter. Blood, pus, or sediment can collect within tubing and result in bladder distention and the buildup of stagnant urine. Instillation of a sterile solution ordered by the physician clears the tubing of accumulated material. For clients with bladder infections, a physician may order antiseptic or antibiotic bladder irrigations to wash out the bladder or treat local infection. In both irrigations, sterile aseptic technique is followed.

Before performing an irrigation, the nurse assesses the catheter for blockage. If the amount of urine in the drainage bag is less than the client's intake or less than the output during the previous shift, blockage can be expected. If urine does not drain freely, the nurse may milk the tubing. Milking is done by gently squeezing then releasing the drainage tube starting from the client to the drainage bag so a clot or sediment will not be forced back into the catheter.

Maintenance of a closed system is recommended during intermittent irrigations or instillations. This technique is effective for irrigating a partially blocked catheter or for bladder instillations. A single intermittent irrigation is safer and less likely to introduce infections into the urinary tract than repeated irrigations. There are two additional methods for catheter irrigation. One is a closed bladder irrigation system (Skill 44-4). This system provides for frequent intermittent irrigations or continuous irrigation without disruption of the sterile catheter system through use of a three-way catheter. This method is used most often in clients who have had genitourinary surgery and are at risk for blood clots and mucus fragments occluding the catheter. The other system involves opening the closed drainage system to instill bladder irrigations (see Skill 44-4). This technique poses greater risk for causing infection. However, it may be needed when catheters become blocked and it is undesirable to change the catheter (e.g., after recent bladder or prostate surgery).

Removal of Indwelling Catheter. When removing an indwelling catheter, the nurse promotes normal bladder function and prevents trauma to the urethra.

To remove a catheter the nurse requires a clean, disposable towel; a trash receptacle; and a sterile syringe the same size as the volume of solution within the catheter's inflated balloon. Disposable gloves are also recommended. The end of each catheter contains a label that denotes the volume of solution (5 to 30 ml) within the balloon.

The nurse positions the client in the same position as during catheterization. Some institutions recommend collecting a sterile urine specimen at this time or sending the catheter tip for culture and sensitivity tests. After removing the tape, the nurse places the towel between a female client's thighs or over a male client's thighs. The nurse inserts the syringe into the injection port. Most ports are

Text continued on p. 1365

Skill 44-4   *Closed and Open Catheter Irrigation*

Delegation Considerations

Although closed catheter irrigation carries less risk of infection, neither closed nor open catheter irrigation are usually delegated to assistive personnel (AP). Catheter irrigation is usually done in clients with complications such as urinary tract infections or postsurgically after prostatectomy.

- AP may assist with other aspects of client care, such as positioning and measuring intake and output.
- Instruct AP to report complaints of pain, discomfort, or fever to the nurse.
- Instruct AP to report the presence of clots in the output or a change in output to the nurse.

Equipment

- **Closed intermittent method**
  - Sterile irrigation solution at room temperature
  - Sterile graduated container
  - Sterile 30- to 50-ml syringe
  - Sterile 19- to 22-gauge 1-inch needle
  - Antiseptic swab
  - Clamp for catheter or tubing
  - Bath blanket

- **Closed continuous method**
  - Sterile irrigation solution at room temperature
  - Irrigation tubing and clamp (with or without Y connector)
  - IV pole
  - Antiseptic swab
  - Y connector (optional)
  - Bath blanket
- **Open method**
  - Sterile irrigation set with tray
  - Bulb syringe or 60-ml piston-type syringe
  - Sterile collection basin
  - Waterproof drape
  - Sterile solution container
  - Antiseptic swabs
  - Sterile gloves
  - Sterile correct irrigation solution at room temperature
  - Tape or elastic band to resecure catheter
  - Bath blanket

Steps	Rationale
1. Assess physician's order for type of irrigation and irrigation solution to use.	Ensures proper selection of equipment.
2. Assess color of urine and presence of mucus or sediment.	Determines if client is bleeding, has infection, or is sloughing tissue.

3. Determine type of catheter in place:
  a. Triple lumen (one lumen to inflate balloon, one to instill irrigation solution, one to allow outflow of urine).
  b. Double lumen (one lumen to inflate balloon, one to allow outflow of urine).
	Indicates method for irrigation.

4. Determine patency of drainage tubing.	Ensures that drainage tubing is not kinked, clamped incorrectly, or looped.
5. Assess amount of urine in drainage bag (may want to empty drainage bag before irrigation).	If not empty, will need to subtract urine volume from amount drained to determine if all irrigant returned.
6. Explain procedure and purpose to client.	Helps client relax and cooperate during procedure.
7. Perform hand hygiene and apply clean gloves for closed methods.	Prevents transmission of microorganisms.
8. Provide privacy by pulling bed curtains closed. Fold back covers so that catheter is exposed. Cover client's upper torso with bath blanket.	Promotes client comfort.
9. Assess lower abdomen for bladder distention.	Detects whether catheter is malfunctioning or blocking urinary drainage.
10. Position client in dorsal recumbent or supine position.	Promotes client comfort and provides easy access to catheter. Promotes flow of irrigating solution into bladder.

11. Closed intermittent irrigation:
  a. Prepare prescribed sterile solution in sterile graduated cup.
  b. Draw sterile solution into syringe using aseptic technique.
	Ensures that irrigating fluid remains sterile.

Steps	**Rationale**

Critical Decision Point: Avoid cold solution as irrigant because it may result in bladder spasm and discomfort.

c. Clamp indwelling retention catheter just below soft injection port.	Occlusion of catheter provides resistance against which irrigant can be forcefully instilled into catheter.
d. Cleanse injection port with antiseptic swab (same port used for specimen collection).	Reduces transmission of infection.
e. Insert needle of syringe through port at 30-degree angle towards bladder.	Ensures that needle tip enters lumen of catheter and flow is directed into bladder.
f. Slowly inject fluid into catheter and bladder.	Slow, continuous pressure dislodges clots and sediment without traumatizing bladder wall.

Critical Decision Point: If catheter does not irrigate easily, the tip may be incorrectly placed in the urethra and not in the bladder. Use slow pressure when injecting fluid. Too much pressure may traumatize the urethal or bladder wall.

g. Withdraw syringe, remove clamp, and allow solution to drain into drainage bag. If ordered by physician, keep clamped to allow solution to remain in bladder for short time (20-30 min).	Allows drainage by gravity.

Critical Decision Point: If solution is to remain in bladder, do not forget to unclamp tubing at the end of the instillation period.

12. Closed continuous irrigation (see illustration):	
a. Using aseptic technique, insert tip of sterile irrigation tubing into bag of sterile irrigating solution.	Prevents entrance of microorganisms.
b. Close clamp on tubing and hang bag of solution on IV pole.	

STEP **12** Closed continuous bladder irrigation.

Skill 44-4   *Closed and Open Catheter Irrigation—cont'd*

Steps	Rationale
c. Open clamp and allow solution to flow through tubing, keeping end of tubing sterile. Close clamp.	Removes air from tubing.
d. Wipe off irrigation port of triple lumen catheter, or attach sterile Y connector to double lumen catheter and then attach to irrigation tubing.	Third lumen or Y connector provides means for irrigation solution to enter bladder. System must remain sterile.
e. Be sure that drainage bag and tubing are securely connected to drainage port of triple lumen catheter or other arm of Y connector.	Ensures that urine and irrigation solution will drain from bladder.
f. For intermittent flow, clamp tubing on drainage system, open clamp on irrigation tubing, and allow prescribed amount of fluid to enter bladder (100 ml is normal for adults). Close irrigation clamp, and then open drainage tubing clamp. (Optional: Leave clamp closed for 20-30 min if ordered. See previous Critical Decision Point.)	Fluid instills through catheter into bladder, flushing system. Fluid drains out after irrigation is completed.
g. For continuous drainage, calculate drip rate and adjust clamp on irrigation tubing accordingly. Be sure that clamp on drainage tubing is open, and check volume of drainage in drainage bag. Make sure drainage tubing is patent, and avoid kinks.	Ensures continuous, even irrigation of catheter system. Prevents accumulation of solution in bladder, which may cause bladder distention and possible injury.
13. Open irrigation (when double lumen catheter is in place):	
a. Open sterile irrigation tray, establish sterile field, pour required volume of sterile solution into sterile container, and replace cap on large container of solution.	Adheres to principles of surgical asepsis (see Chapter 33).
b. Apply sterile gloves.	Reduces transmission of infection.
c. Position sterile waterproof drape under catheter.	Prevents soiling of bed linens.
d. Aspirate 30 ml of solution into sterile irrigating syringe.	Prepares irrigant for instillation into catheter.
e. Move sterile collection close to client's thighs.	Prevents soiling of bed linen and prohibits reaching over sterile field.
f. Disconnect catheter from drainage tubing, allowing urine from catheter to flow into collection basin. Allow urine in tubing to flow into drainage bag. Cover end of tubing with sterile protective cap. Position tubing in a safe place.	Maintains sterility of inner aspect of catheter and drainage tubing and reduces potential of introducing pathogens into bladder.
g. Insert tip of syringe into catheter lumen, and gently instill solution.	Gentle instillation reduces incidence of bladder spasm but clears catheter of obstruction.

Critical Decision Point: If resistance is noted, do not force the irrigation.

Steps	Rationale
h. Withdraw syringe, lower catheter, and allow solution to drain into basin. Repeat instillation until prescribed solution has been used or until drainage is clear (will depend on purpose of irrigation).	Allows drainage to flow by gravity. Provides for adequate flushing of catheter.
i. If solution does not return, have client turn onto side facing you. If changing position does not help, reinsert syringe and gently aspirate solution.	Change of position may move catheter tip in bladder, increasing likelihood that fluid instilled will flow out.
j. After irrigation is complete, remove protector cap from tubing, cleanse end with alcohol swab (or recommended agency solution), and reestablish drainage system.	Reduces entrance of microorganisms into system.
14. Reanchor catheter to client with tape or elastic tube holder.	Prevents trauma to urethral tissue.
15. Assist client to comfortable position.	Promotes relaxation and rest.

Steps	Rationale
16. Lower bed to lowest position. Put side rails up if appropriate.	Promotes client safety.
17. Dispose of contaminated supplies, remove gloves, and perform hand hygiene.	Prevents spread of infection.
18. Calculate fluid used to irrigate bladder and catheter and subtract from total output.	Determines accurate urinary output.
19. Assess characteristics of output: viscosity, color, and presence of matter (e.g., sediment, clots, blood).	Evaluates results of irrigation.

Unexpected Outcomes and Related Interventions

1. Irrigating solution does not return or is not flowing a prescribed rate, which may indicate possible occlusion of catheter.
   a. Examine tubing for kinks, clots, or urine sediment.
   b. Notify physician if irrigant is retained, client complains of pain, or bladder is distended.
2. Cloudy or foul urine, fever
   a. Monitor fever.
   b. Notify physician.
   c. Obtain sterile urine specimen if ordered by physician.
3. Increase in bladder spasms; may indicate occlusion of catheter with foreign object (e.g., blood clot)
   a. Notify physician.
   b. May be instructed to perform intermittent irrigations until clots clear.

Recording and Reporting

- Record type and amount of irrigation solution used, amount returned as drainage, and the character of drainage.
- Record and report any findings such as complaints of bladder spasms, inability to instill fluid into bladder, and/or presence of blood clots.

Home Care Considerations

- If client is discharged with indwelling catheter and requires bladder irrigations, either the client and or the family must be properly instructed.
- In the home it is most likely that open irrigation will be required. Because this method carries the highest risk of contamination, the nurse must assess the level of understanding of surgical asepsis by the client and family.

self-sealing and require that only the tip of the syringe be inserted. The nurse slowly withdraws all of the solution to deflate the balloon totally. If a portion of the solution remains, the partially inflated balloon will traumatize the urethral canal as the catheter is removed. After deflation the nurse explains that the client may feel a burning sensation as the catheter is withdrawn. The nurse then pulls the catheter out smoothly and slowly.

It is normal for the client to experience some dysuria, especially if the catheter has been in place several days or weeks. Until the bladder regains full tone, the client may also experience frequency of urination or urinary retention.

The nurse assesses the client's urinary function by noting the first voiding after catheter removal and documenting the time and amount of voiding for the next 24 hours. If amounts are small, frequent assessment of bladder distention is necessary. If 8 hours has elapsed without voiding or the client experiences discomfort, it may become necessary to reinsert the catheter.

Alternatives to Urethral Catheterization. To avoid the risks associated with catheters inserted through the urethra, there are two alternatives for urinary drainage.

Suprapubic Catheterization. Suprapubic catheterization involves surgical placement of a catheter through the abdominal wall above the symphysis pubis and into the urinary bladder. The physician performs the procedure under local or general anesthesia. The catheter is anchored in place with sutures, a commercially prepared body seal, or both. Urine drains into a urinary drainage bag. Maintenance of the tubing and drainage bag is the same as for an indwelling catheter. The suprapubic catheter is relatively painless and reduces the incidence of infection commonly seen with retention catheters. Women who have undergone a vaginal hysterectomy may also benefit temporarily from the insertion of a suprapubic catheter after surgery.

Sediment, clots, or the abdominal wall itself can block the suprapubic catheter. Adequate fluid intake will help to minimize risk of blockage by sediment or infection due to stagnation. The suprapubic catheter must remain patent at all times. Nurses must monitor the client's I&O carefully, monitor the appearance of urine, and observe for signs of infection (e.g., fever and chills). The nurse also administers skin care around the insertion site.

Condom Catheter. The second alternative to catheterization is the condom catheter (Box 44-9), which may be suitable for incontinent or comatose men who still have complete and spontaneous bladder emptying. The condom is a soft, pliable, rubber sheath that slips over the penis. It may be worn at night only or continuously, depending on the client's needs. There are three general methods of securing the condom catheter. One method uses a strip of elastic tape or rubber that encircles the top of the condom to secure it in place. Another type uses a self-adhesive condom sheath. The third method uses an inflatable ring within the condom to secure placement. Care must be taken to ensure that whatever type or size is used, blood supply to the penis is not impaired. Standard adhesive tape should never be used to secure a condom catheter because it does not expand with change in penis size and is painful to remove.

The end of the condom is attached to plastic drainage tubing that can be attached to the side of the bed or strapped to the client's leg. The condom catheter itself poses little risk of infection. Infections usually result from buildup of secretions around the urethra, trauma to the urethral meatus, or buildup of pressure in the outflow tubing.

If the condom catheter is made of opaque material, the nurse should remove the condom catheter daily to check for skin irritation. Some new condom catheters are more transparent, and the skin may be observed through them more easily. With each catheter change the nurse cleans the urethral meatus and penis thoroughly. The drainage tubing must be checked often for patency.

Box 44-9 *Procedural Guidelines*

Condom Catheter

Equipment: Condom catheter (may come with self-adhesive or elastic adhesive), collection bag, basin with warm water, towel and washcloth, clean gloves, scissors.
Delegation Considerations: The skill of applying a condom catheter can be delegated to assistive personnel. The RN is responsible for assessing the condition of the penis over time. The RN informs the staff member to notify the RN of signs of skin irritation or swelling of tissues.

1. Check physician's order.
2. Perform hand hygiene.
3. Assess urinary elimination patterns, client's ability to voluntarily urinate, and continence.
4. Assess mental status of client so appropriate teaching related to condom care can be implemented.
5. Assess condition of penis and scrotum.
6. Assess client's knowledge of the purpose for the condom catheter.
7. Explain procedure to client.
8. Raise bed to working height and raise far upper side rail.
9. Using sheet, drape client so only genitals are exposed.
10. Prepare condom catheter and drainage system (see manufacturer's directions).
11. Apply gloves and provide perineal care.
    a. If needed, clip hair at base of penile shaft.
12. Apply skin prep to penile shaft and allow to dry.
13. Holding penis in nondominant hand, apply condom by rolling smoothly onto penis. NOTE: Leave a 2.5- to 5-cm (1- to 2-inch) space between tip of penis and end of catheter (see illustration).
14. Secure condom catheter:
    a. If using elastic adhesive, wrap the strip of adhesive over the condom to secure it in place by using a spiral technique (see illustration). NOTE: Adhesive tape must never be used.
    b. For self-adhesive catheter, follow manufacturer's directions.
15. Attach catheter to drainage bag and attach drainage bag to lower bed frame.
16. Make client comfortable.
17. Observe urinary drainage, drainage tube patency, condition of penis, and tape placement.

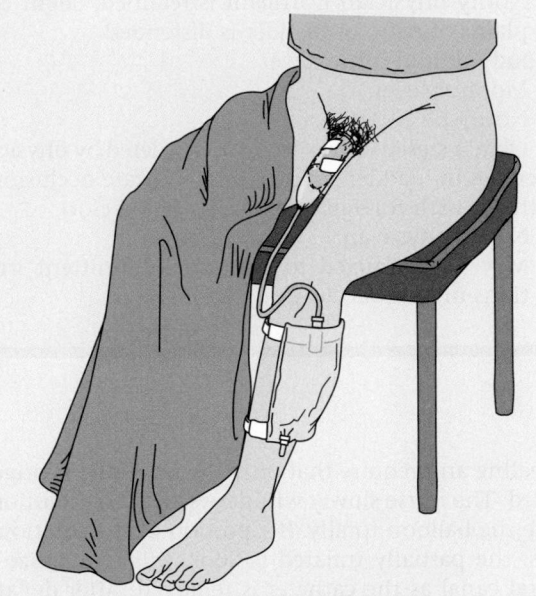

STEP **13**   Distance between end of penis and tip of catheter.

Tape

STEP **14a**   Elastic tape is applied in spiral fashion to secure the condom catheter to the penis.

For a man with a retracted penis, maintaining a conventional condom catheter may prove difficult. Special devices are available to help alleviate this problem (Figure 44-15). Manufacturer's guidelines for product application should be consulted.

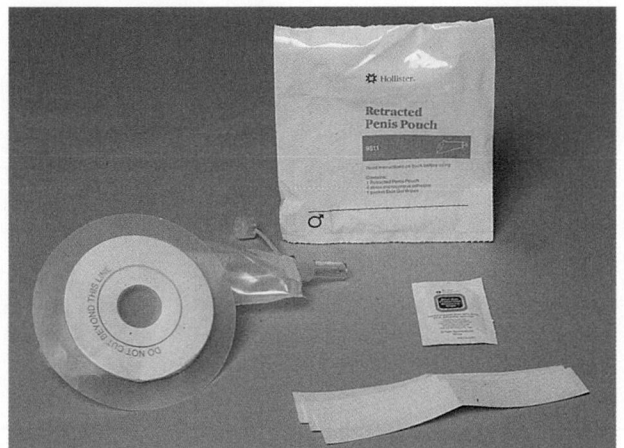

FIGURE **44–15**   Retracted penis pouch external urinary device.

There are no collection devices for women as effective as the condom catheter is for men, so frequently the only incontinent devices used are pads and protective clothing. To maintain dignity, pads and protective clothing should not be referred to as adult diapers and should be changed frequently to control odor. These devices should be only used temporarily to minimize or prevent episodes of incontinence while treatment is ongoing. Clients should be monitored frequently and good skin care given to prevent irritation caused by urine.

Restorative Care. The client may regain normal urinary voiding function through special activities such as bladder retraining, habit training, or cognitive therapy (Box 44-10). If either of those activities is not possible, then self-catheterization may restore a measure of control to the client.

Strengthening Pelvic Floor Muscles. Clients who have difficulty starting or stopping the urine stream may benefit from **pelvic floor exercises (PFEs).** Pelvic floor exercises, also known as Kegel exercises, improve the strength of pelvic floor muscles and consist of repetitive contractions of muscle groups (Thompson and Smith,

---

Research Highlight

Box 44-10

Cognitive Measures for Bladder Control

Research Focus

Alterations in urine elimination often include urinary leakage and/or frequency that cause discomfort for clients. Skin breakdown is a common condition resulting from consistent exposure of the skin to urine. Falls may occur secondary to clients' need to use toilet facilities. Because these urinary problems are often manageable by cognitive strategies, research has been done to determine the best methods to use.

Research Abstract

The purpose of this study was to determine if the introduction of an audiotape with reinforcing cognitive strategies would be successful in enhancing the comfort and quality of life for clients with urinary incontinence and/or frequency. Dowd and others investigated the use of cognitive strategies with two groups of adults with a history of incontinence and/or frequency. Thirty-one women and nine men entered into the study and were randomly assigned to the treatment group or the control group. Both groups received education about bladder health and recorded incontinence and/or frequency episodes in the voiding diary, but only the treatment group listened to an audiotape that contained relaxation, music, and cognitive strategies. The verbal side of the tape contained instructions for relaxation followed by cognitive strategy statements. These statements focused on concepts of self and on specific aspects of bladder management. Statements such as, "I am not alone; many other men and women have loss of urine and are okay" were designed to enhance social comfort. The statements ". . . being physically fit is important" and "I often tighten and relax the muscles that control my urine flow"

were designed to enhance physical comfort. Other statements reinforced concepts such as the effect of fluids on output and how to manage urge to void. Music was on the second side of the tape. Comfort was measured at four intervals during the study using the Urinary Incontinence and Frequency Comfort Questionnaire. The results demonstrated that self-report of increased comfort and decreased urinary episodes were significant, with the treatment group having better results. In addition, after the control group was given the audiotape treatment their levels of comfort and episodes of incontinence and or frequency approximated the levels of the original treatment group.

Evidence-Based Practice

- Incontinence and/or frequency are experienced by adults of all ages, educational levels, economic status, and health status.
- Many adults wrongly believe that urinary incontinence and/or frequency are an expected part of the aging process.
- Clients who take an active part in their management of bladder control have improved self-esteem and decreased physical complications such as skin breakdown.
- Nurses can support the use of this inexpensive nonpharmacological intervention to enhance comfort in community-based and selected institutionalized older adults.

Reference

Dowd T, Kolcaba K, Steiner R: Using cognitive strategies to enhance bladder control and comfort. *Holist Nurs Pract* 14(2):91, 2000.

2002). These exercises have demonstrated effectiveness in treating stress incontinence, overactive bladders, and mixed cause of urinary incontinence (Sampselle, 2003). A client begins these exercises during voiding to learn the technique. They are then practiced at nonvoiding times. Improvement is usually gradual. Clients should be alert and motivated to perform the exercises. The client must continue to use these exercises to maintain effectiveness (see Box 44-5, p. 1347). These exercises are noninvasive and carry a low risk of adverse effects.

Bladder Retraining. The goal of bladder retraining is to gradually increase the interval between voidings and to decrease voiding frequency during both waking and sleeping hours (Sampselle, 2003). Ultimately the overall goal of this retraining is to restore a normal pattern of voiding. For bladder retraining to be successful, clients must be alert and physically able to follow a training program. The program includes education, scheduled voiding, and positive reinforcement.

The nurse first assesses the client's current pattern of urination. This information allows the nurse to plan a program that often takes 2 weeks or more to learn. Although the program may be started in the hospital or rehabilitation unit, it may need to be continued in an extended care facility or at home. If the client has an underlying UTI, this should be treated at the same time. The following measures may help the incontinent client gain control over urination and are part of restorative and rehabilitative care:

- Learning exercises to strengthen the pelvic floor
- Initiating a toileting schedule on awakening, at least every 2 hours during the day and evening, before getting into bed, and every 4 hours at night (individualizing time frame as needed)
- Using methods to initiate voiding (e.g., running water and stroking the inner thigh)
- Using methods to relax to aid complete bladder emptying (e.g., reading and deep breathing)
- Never ignoring the urge to void (if problem involves infrequent voidings that result in retention)
- Minimizing tea, coffee, other caffeine drinks, and alcohol
- Taking prescribed diuretic medication or fluids that increase diuresis (such as tea or coffee) early in the morning
- Progressively lengthening or shortening periods between voiding as appropriate for control of specific cause of incontinence
- Offering protective undergarments to contain urine and reduce the client's embarrassment (not diapers)
- Following a weight-control program if obesity is a problem
- Providing positive reinforcement when continence is maintained

These guidelines help the client to establish a routine for voiding and control factors that might increase the number of incontinent episodes.

Habit Training. A client with functional incontinence may benefit from habit training, which helps clients improve voluntary control over urination. A flexible toileting schedule based on the client's pattern is established.

Evidence-Based Practice Guideline   Box 44-11

Prompted Voiding for Persons With Urinary Incontinence

- Apply prompted voiding protocol (Lyons, Specht, 2001).
- Approach person at scheduled prompted voiding times.
  - Wait 5 seconds for individual to self-initiate request (SIR) to toilet.
- Ask person if he or she is wet or dry.
  - Physically assess person to determine continence status.
  - Provide feedback. Praise if client is dry, no comment if client is wet.
- Prompt individual to toilet.
  - Offer assistance with toileting.
- Provide feedback.
- Inform individual of next scheduled prompted voiding session.
- Encourage individual to self-initiate requests to toilet.
- Record result of prompted voiding session.

Modified from Lyons S.S., Specht J.K.P. (1999). *Evidence-based protocol: Prompted voiding for persons with urinary incontinence.* In M.G. Titler (Series Ed.), Series on Evidence-Based Practice for Older Adults. Iowa City, IA. The University of Iowa College of Nursing Gerontological Nursing Interventions Research Center, Research Dissemination Core. For more information, http:// www.nursing.uiowa.edu/center/gnirc/disseminatecore.htm.

The nurse helps the client to the bathroom before incontinent episodes occur. Fluids and medications are timed to prevent interference with the toileting schedule. Clients with moderate or severe mental or physical dysfunction can benefit. When combined with positive reinforcement to reward successful voiding, this approach is also called prompted voiding (Box 44-11).

Self-Catheterization. Some clients with chronic disorders such as spinal cord injury learn to perform self-catheterization. The client must be able to physically manipulate equipment and assume a position for successful catheterization. The nurse teaches the client the structures of the urinary tract, clean versus sterile technique, the importance of adequate fluid intake, and the frequency of self-catheterization. Generally, the goal is to have clients perform self-catheterization every 6 to 8 hours, but the schedule should be individualized.

Maintenance of Skin Integrity. The normal acidity of urine is irritating to skin. Urine allowed to remain in contact with the skin becomes alkaline, causing encrustations or precipitates to collect on the skin, fostering breakdown. Continuous exposure of the perineal area or skin around an ostomy leads to gradual maceration and excoriation (see Chapter 47). Washing with mild soap and warm water is the best way to remove urine from skin. Body lotion keeps skin moisturized and petroleum-based ointments provide a barrier to the urine. Clients who wet their clothing should receive partial baths and dry clothing after voiding.

When the skin becomes irritated or inflamed, the physician may prescribe a cream or spray containing steroids (e.g., Kenalog) to reduce inflammation. If fungal growth develops, the antifungal drug nystatin (Mycostatin), available in cream or powder, is effective.

Promotion of Comfort. Clients with urinary alterations become uncomfortable as a result of the symptoms of urinary problems. Frequent or unpredictable voiding, dysuria, and painful distention are sources of discomfort.

The incontinent client gains comfort from having clean, dry clothing. When stress incontinence is the problem, a protective pad offers protection against soiling. Wet clothing adheres to the skin and can cause rubbing and irritation.

Urinary analgesics that act on the urethral and bladder mucosa relieve dysuria (e.g., phenazopyridine [Pyridium]). This drug may be combined with sulfonamide antibiotics in preparations such as Azo-Gantanol and Azo-Gantrisin. Clients taking drugs with phenazopyridine should be aware that their urine will be orange. They must drink large amounts of fluids to prevent toxicity from the sulfonamides and to maintain optimal flow through the urinary system (McKenry and Salerno, 2003).

If the client has local discomfort from an inflamed urethra, a warm sitz bath may provide pain relief. The warm water soothes inflamed tissues near the urethral meatus by improving blood supply. The client is often relaxed after a sitz bath, so voiding occurs easily. Pain of distention cannot be relieved unless the client is able to empty the bladder. Interventions that stimulate micturition or intermittent catheterization may be the only sources of pain relief.

Evaluation

Client Care. The client is the best source of evaluation of outcomes and responses to nursing care (Figure 44-16). However, the nurse will also evaluate the effectiveness of nursing interventions through comparisons with baseline data. The nurse evaluates for change in the client's voiding pattern, presence of urinary tract alteration, and physical condition. Outcomes are compared with expected outcomes to determine the client's health status. Continuous evaluation allows the nurse to determine whether new or revised therapies are required or if any new nursing diagnoses have developed.

Client Expectations. If the nurse has developed a trust relationship with a client, indications of the client's degree of satisfaction with his or her care are evident. The client may smile or nod in appreciation. However, the nurse needs to confirm whether the client's expectations have been met to full satisfaction. The nurse may need to ask specifically about the client's degree of urinary control and comfort. If just asked "How are you feeling today?" the client may reply with a noncommittal "OK." However, the nurse needs specific information about how well an intervention has met the need in order to continue or revise the plan of care. The nurse can also assist the client in redefining unrealistic client goals when impairment in function is not likely to be altered as completely as the client might like.

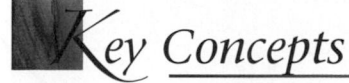

Key Concepts

- The act of micturition or voiding is influenced by voluntary control from higher brain centers and involuntary control from the spinal cord.
- Symptoms common to urinary disturbances include urgency, dysuria, polyuria, oliguria, and difficulty in starting the urinary stream.
- When collected properly, a clean-voided urine specimen does not contain bacteria from the urethral meatus.
- Methods of promoting the micturition reflex assist clients in sensing the urge to urinate and controlling urethral sphincter relaxation.
- An increased fluid intake results in increased diluted urine formation that reduces the risk of urinary tract infections.
- An indwelling urinary catheter remains in the bladder for an extended period, making the risk of infection greater than with intermittent catheterization.
- Catheter irrigation becomes necessary when the catheter becomes occluded with sediment or blood clots.
- A catheter drainage system should be a closed system positioned to allow free drainage of urine by gravity.
- Incontinence is classified as functional, overflow, stress, urge, or total. Each type has specific nursing interventions.
- Specific guidelines for catheter selection should be followed so that the catheter does not cause harm.

Key Terms

Anuria, *p. 1326*
Bacteriuria, *p. 1328*
Catheterization, *p. 1348*
Cystitis, *p. 1328*
Diuresis, *p. 1327*
Dysuria, *p. 1328*
Erythropoietin, *p. 1324*
Hematuria, *p. 1328*
Ketonuria, *p. 1339*
Meatus, *p. 1332*
Micturition, *p. 1325*
Nephron, *p. 1324*
Nephrostomy, *p. 1329*
Nocturia, *p. 1330*
Oliguria, *p. 1326*
Pelvic floor exercises
　(PFEs) (Kegel exercises),
　p. 1367
Polyuria, *p. 1327*

Proteinuria, *p. 1324*
Pyelonephritis, *p. 1328*
Reflex bladder, *p. 1326*
Renal calculus, *p. 1325*
Renal replacement
　therapies, *p. 1326*
Renin, *p. 1324*
Residual urine, *p. 1330*
Specific gravity, *p. 1339*
Stoma, *p. 1328*
Uremic syndrome, *p. 1326*
Ureterostomy, *p. 1329*
Urinalysis, *p. 1339*
Urinary diversion, *p. 1327*
Urinary frequency, *p. 1330*
Urinary incontinence (UI),
　p. 1329
Urinary retention, *p. 1328*
Urosepsis, *p. 1328*

KNOWLEDGE

- Clinical signs of normal micturition
- Characteristics of normal urine
- Behaviors that demonstrate learning

EXPERIENCE

- Previous client responses to planned nursing interventions to promote urinary elimination

Evaluation

- Reassess the client's urination pattern and signs and symptoms of alterations
- Inspect the character of the client's urine
- Have the client and family demonstrate any self-care skills
- Have the client discuss feelings regarding any permanent changes in elimination
- Ask client if expectations are being met

STANDARDS

- Use expected outcomes established in client's plan of care
- Use established expected outcomes from professional organizations such as ANA and AHCPR to evaluate the client's response to care

ATTITUDES

- Be accountable and responsible for onset of any complications related to care
- Demonstrate perseverance when necessary because some interventions (e.g., pelvic floor exercises) may take weeks to months to effect any change
- Adapt and revise approaches if interventions are ineffective

FIGURE **44–16** Critical thinking model for urinary elimination evaluation.

Critical Thinking Exercises

1. Mrs. Rodriquez is a 77-year-old woman who has had problems with urgency for the past 2 years. The episodes are becoming increasingly frequent. She has been attempting to deal with the problem by using an absorbent pad in her underwear but she feels as though everyone knows her problem. The embarrassment of having an odor often keeps her at home. She has given up attending daily mass at church.
   a. How can the nurse help her regain control of her urinary elimination?
   b. What are the actual nursing diagnoses that apply to Mrs. Rodriquez?
   c. For one diagnosis give one goal/outcome and two nursing interventions.
2. Mrs. Brownell is a 37-year-old woman who has been admitted with back pain radiating down into her groin. She has also noticed blood in her urine for a week, but she was hoping it would go away. She is to undergo an IVP in 4 hours.
   a. What is the purpose of the IVP?
   b. What nursing care is needed before she goes to the x-ray department?
   c. Give at least two nursing responsibilities for care of the client who has undergone an IVP.
3. Mrs. Fenton is a 70-year-old woman with physical limitations related to rheumatoid arthritis. Her daughter, with whom she lives, has brought her to her family practitioner's office. You are the family nurse practitioner in the practice. As you assess Mrs. Fenton, you ask her how she is coping. Mrs. Fenton begins to answer but the starts to cry. "I know when I have to go to the bathroom, but I often don't make it in time." The daughter asks you for suggestions on how to manage, as she noticed that her mother's perineal skin is reddened and sore. What assessments does the nurse need to complete before planning interventions for Mrs. Fenton's care?

Review Questions

1. The normal adult urine output is.
   1. 1000 ml/day.
   2. 1500 to 1600 ml/day.
   3. 3000 to 3200 ml/day.
   4. 4000 ml/day.

2. Renal alterations result from factors that cause injury directly to the glomeruli or renal tubule, interfering with their normal filtering, reabsorptive, and secretory functions. Selected causes include:
   1. Transfusion reactions.
   2. Dehydration.
   3. Hemorrhage.
   4. Congestive heart failure.

3. Postrenal alterations result from obstruction to the flow of urine in the urinary collecting system caused by:
   1. Dehydration.
   2. Blood clots
   3. Hemorrhage.
   4. Diabetes mellitus.

4. The most common hospital-acquired (nosocomial) infections are:
   1. Urethral.
   2. Bladder.
   3. Kidney.
   4. Urinary tract.

5. Hospital-acquired UTIs are often related to poor hand washing and:
   1. Urinary drainage bags.
   2. Poor perineal hygiene.
   3. Improper catheter care.
   4. Poor urinary output.

6. The urine appears concentrated and cloudy because of the presence of white blood cells or
   1. Bacteria.
   2. Urinary drainage bags.
   3. Blood clots.
   4. Poor perineal hygiene.

7. Some medications change the color of urine. Pyridium colors the urine:
   1. Blue.
   2. Bright orange to rust.
   3. Yellow.
   4. Brown.

8. To minimize nocturia, clients should avoid fluids:
   1. 4 hours before bedtime.
   2. After lunch.
   3. 2 hours before bedtime.
   4. In the late afternoon.

9. Maintaining a Foley catheter drainage bag in the dependent position prevents:
   1. Urinary reflux.
   2. Urinary retention.
   3. Reflex incontinence.
   4. Urinary incontinence.

10. When applying a condom catheter, it is important to secure the catheter in the penile shaft in such a manner that the catheter is:
    1. Tight and draining well.
    2. Dependent and draining well.
    3. Secured with adhesive tape applied in a circular pattern.
    4. Snug and secure, but does not cause constriction to blood flow.

References

Ackley BJ, Ludwig GB: *Nursing diagnosis handbook: a guide to planning care,* St. Louis, 2002, Mosby.

Dochterman JM, Bulechek GM: *Nursing interventions classification (NIC),* ed 4, St. Louis, 2004, Mosby.

Lee SY, Phanumus D, Fields SD: Urinary incontinence: a primary care guide to managing acute and chronic symptoms in older adults, *Geriatrics* 55(11):65, 2000.

Leonard BJ, Plotnikoff GA: Awareness: the heart of cultural competence, *AACN Clin Issues* 11(1):51, 2000.

Lewis SM, Heitkemper MM, Dirksen SR : *Medical-surgical nursing,* ed 5, St. Louis, 2000, Mosby.

McCance KL, Huether SE: *Pathophysiology: the biological basis for disease in adults and children,* ed 4, St. Louis, 2002, Mosby.

McKenry LM, Salerno E: *Mosby's pharmacology in nursing,* ed 21, St. Louis, 2003, Mosby.

Moorhead S, Johnson M, Maas M: *Nursing outcomes classification (NOC),* ed 3, St. Louis, 2004, Mosby.

Pagana KD, Pagana TJ: *Mosby's manual of diagnostic and laboratory tests,* ed 2, St. Louis, 2002, Mosby.

Thompson DL, Smith DA: Continence nursing: a whole person approach, *Holist Nurs Pract* 16(2):14, 2002.

Research References

Dowd T, Kolcaba K, Steiner R: Using cognitive strategies to enhance bladder control and comfort, *Holist Nurs Pract* 14(2):91, 2000.

Foxman B: Epidemiology of urinary tract infections: incidence, morbidity, and economic costs, *Am J Med* 113(1A):5S, 2002.

Getliffe K: Managing recurrent urinary catheter blockage: problems, promises, and practicalities, *J Wound Ostomy Continence Nurs* 30(3):146, 2003.

Gray M: Are cranberry juice or cranberry products effective in the prevention or management of urinary tract infection? *J Wound Ostomy Continence Nurs* 29(3):122, 2002.

Gray M, Krissovich M: Does fluid intake influence the risk for urinary incontinence, urinary tract infection, and bladder cancer? *J Wound Ostomy Continence Nurs* 30(3):126, 2003.

Gray ML: Gender, race, and culture in research on UI. *Am J Nurs* 103(3 suppl):20, 2003.

Kunin CM: Nosocomial urinary tract infections and the indwelling catheter, *Chest* 120(1):10, 2001.

Lyons SS, Specht JKP: *Prompted voiding for persons with urinary incontinence: evidence-based protocol,* The University of Iowa, Gerontological Nursing Interventions research Center, Research Dissemination Core, revised 2001.

Neuman DK, Palmer MH: State of the science on urinary incontinence: executive summary, *Am J Nurs* 103(3 suppl):4, 2003.

O'Donnell JA, Hofmann MT: Urinary tract infections: how to manage nursing home patients with or without chronic catheterization, *Geriatrics* 57(5):45, 2002.

Sampselle CM: Behavioral interventions in young and middle-age women, *Am J Nurs* 103(3 suppl):9, 2003.

Wyman JF: Treatment of urinary incontinence in men and older women, *Am J Nurs* 103(3 suppl):26, 2003.

45

*B*owel Elimination

Media Resources

http://evolve.elsevier.com/Potter/
fundamentals/

CD COMPANION

- Review Questions
- Glossary

evolve WEBSITE

- Review Questions
- Student Learning Activities
- Animations
- Concept Map Exercise
- Critical Thinking Exercise
- Video Clips
- Glossary

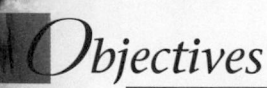

Mastery of content in this chapter will enable the student to:

- Define the key terms listed.
- Discuss the role of gastrointestinal organs in digestion and elimination.
- Describe three functions of the large intestine.
- Explain the physiological aspects of normal defecation.
- Discuss psychological and physiological factors that influence the elimination process.
- Describe common physiological alterations in elimination.
- Assess a client's elimination pattern.
- List nursing diagnoses related to alterations in elimination.
- Describe nursing implications for common diagnostic examinations of the gastrointestinal tract.
- List nursing measures that promote normal elimination.
- List nursing measures included in bowel training.
- Discuss nursing care measures required for clients with a bowel diversion.
- Utilize critical thinking in the provision of care to clients with alterations in bowel elimination.

Regular elimination of bowel waste products is essential for normal body functioning. Alterations in elimination are often early signs or symptoms of problems within either the gastrointestinal or another body system. Because bowel function depends on the balance of several factors, elimination patterns and habits vary among individuals.

To manage the elimination problems of clients, the nurse must understand normal elimination and factors that promote, impede, or cause alterations in elimination. Supportive nursing care respects the client's privacy and emotional needs. Measures designed to promote normal elimination should also minimize discomfort for the client.

Scientific Knowledge Base

The gastrointestinal (GI) tract is a series of hollow mucous membrane–lined muscular organs. The purposes of these organs are to absorb fluid and nutrients, prepare food for absorption and use by the body's cells, and provide for temporary storage of feces (Figure 45-1). The volume of fluids absorbed by the GI tract is high, making fluid and electrolyte balance a key function of the GI system. In addition to ingested fluids and foods, the GI tract also receives secretions from the gallbladder and pancreas.

Mouth
The mouth mechanically and chemically breaks down nutrients into usable size and form. The teeth **masticate** food, breaking it down into a size suitable for swallowing. Saliva, produced by the salivary glands in the mouth,

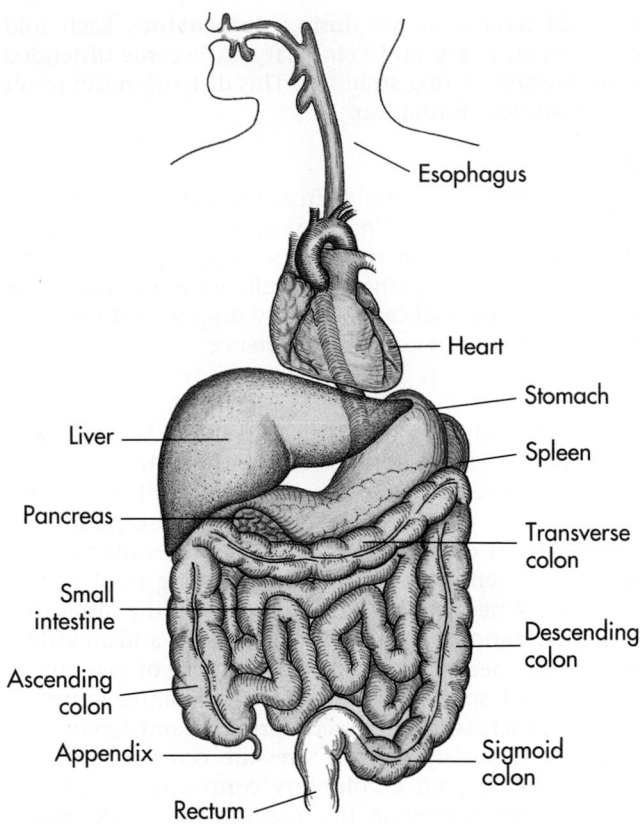

FIGURE 45-1   Organs of the gastrointestinal tract (with the heart as a reference point).

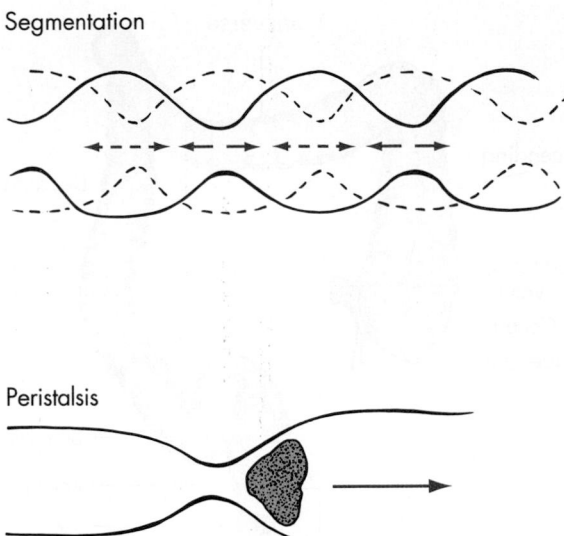

FIGURE 45-2   Segmented and peristaltic waves.

dilules and softens the food in the mouth for easier swallowing. Digestion begins in the mouth and ends in the small intestine.

Esophagus

As food enters the upper esophagus, it passes through the upper esophageal sphincter, a circular muscle that prevents air from entering the esophagus and food from refluxing into the throat. The **bolus** of food travels down the esophagus and is pushed along by **peristalsis,** which propels food through the length of the GI tract.

The food moves down the esophagus and reaches the cardiac or lower esophageal sphincter, which lies between the esophagus and the upper end of the stomach. The sphincter is not a muscle but a physiological pressure difference that prevents reflux of stomach contents back into the esophagus.

Stomach

The stomach performs three tasks, including the storage of the swallowed food and liquid; the mixing of food, liquid, and digestive juices; and the emptying of its contents into the small intestine. The stomach produces and secretes hydrochloric acid (HCl), mucus, the enzyme pepsin, and intrinsic factor. Pepsin and HCl facilitate the digestion of protein. Mucus protects the stomach mucosa from acidity and enzyme activity. The intrinsic factor is essential in the absorption of vitamin B_{12}.

Small Intestine

Movement within the small intestine, occurring by both **segmentation** and peristalsis (Figure 45-2), facilitates both digestion and absorption. **Chyme** mixes with digestive juices (e.g., bile and amylase). Reabsorption in the small intestine is so efficient that by the time the chyme reaches the end of the small intestine, it is pastelike in consistency. The small intestine is divided into three sections: the duodenum, the jejunum, and the ileum.

The duodenum is approximately 2 feet long and continues to process the chyme from the stomach. The second section, the jejunum, is approximately 9 feet long and has the primary function of absorption of carbohydrates and proteins. The ileum, which is approximately 12 feet long, specializes in the absorption of water, fats, and bile salts. Most nutrients and electrolytes are absorbed in the small intestine, specifically by the duodenum and jejunum. The ileum absorbs certain vitamins, iron, and bile salts.

If small intestine function is impaired, the digestive process is greatly altered. For example, conditions such as inflammation, surgical resection, or obstruction can disrupt peristalsis, reduce the area of absorption, or block the passage of chyme. Electrolyte and nutrient deficiencies then develop.

Large Intestine

The lower GI tract is called the *large intestine* (colon) because it is larger in diameter than the small intestine. However, its length (1.5 to 1.8 m [5 to 6 feet]) is much shorter. The large intestine is divided into the cecum, colon, and rectum (Figure 45-3). The large intestine is the primary organ of bowel elimination.

Chyme enters the large intestine by waves of peristalsis through the ileocecal valve, a circular muscle layer that prevents regurgitation. The colon is divided into the ascending, transverse, descending, and sigmoid colons. The colon's muscular tissue allows it to accommodate

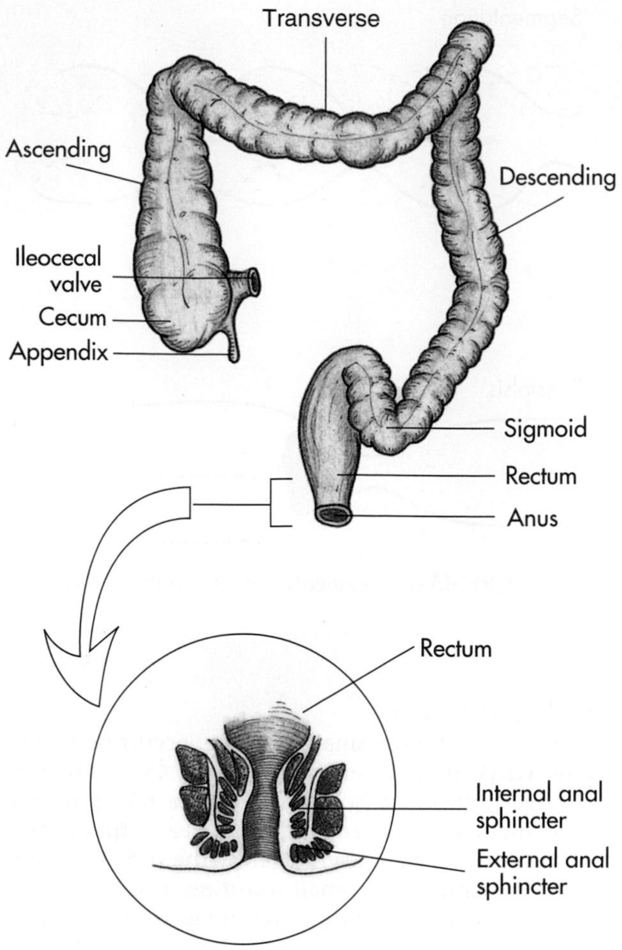

FIGURE **45–3**   Divisions of the large intestine.

and eliminate large quantities of waste and gas (flatus). The colon has three functions: absorption, secretion, and elimination. A volume of water and significant amounts of sodium and chloride are absorbed by the colon daily (Doughty, 2000b). The amount of water absorbed from chyme depends on the speed at which colonic contents move. Chyme is normally a soft, formed mass. If peristalsis is abnormally fast, there is less time for water to be absorbed and the stool will be watery. If peristaltic contractions slow down, water continues to be absorbed and a hard mass of stool forms, resulting in constipation.

The secretory function of the colon aids in electrolyte balance. Bicarbonate is secreted in exchange for chloride. About 4 to 9 mEq of potassium is also excreted daily. Serious alterations in colon function (e.g., diarrhea) can cause severe electrolyte disturbances.

Slow peristaltic contractions move contents through the colon. Intestinal content is the main stimulus for contraction. Mass peristalsis pushes undigested food toward the rectum. These mass movements occur only three or four times daily, with the strongest during the hour after mealtime.

The rectum is the final portion of the large intestine. Normally the rectum is empty of waste products (feces) until just before defecation. The rectum contains vertical and transverse folds of tissue that may help to temporar-

ily hold fecal contents during **defecation.** Each fold contains an artery and vein that can become distended from pressure during straining. This distention can result in hemorrhoid formation.

Anus
Feces and flatus are expelled from the rectum through the anal canal and anus. Contraction and relaxation of the internal and external sphincters, innervated by sympathetic and parasympathetic stimuli, aid in the control of defecation. The anal canal is richly supplied with sensory nerves that help to control continence.

Defecation
The physiological factors critical to bowel function and defecation include normal GI tract function, sensory awareness of rectal distention and rectal contents, voluntary sphincter control, and adequate rectal capacity and compliance (Doughty, 2000a). Normal defecation begins with movement in the left colon, moving stool toward the anus. When stool reaches the rectum, the distention causes relaxation of the internal sphincter, and an awareness of the need to defecate. At the time of defecation, the external sphincter relaxes and abdominal muscles contract, increasing intrarectal pressure and forcing the stool out (Doughty, 2000a). Pressure can be exerted to expel feces through a voluntary contraction of the abdominal muscles while maintaining forced expiration against a closed airway. This is termed the **Valsalva maneuver.** This will assist in stool passage. Clients with cardiovascular disease, glaucoma, increased intracranial pressure, or a new surgical wound can be placed at further risk, such as cardiac irregularities and elevated blood pressure, with this maneuver and should be cautioned to avoid straining to pass the stool. Normal defecation is painless, resulting in passage of soft, formed stool.

Nursing Knowledge Base

Factors Affecting Bowel Elimination
Many factors influence the process of bowel elimination. Knowledge of these factors enables the nurse to anticipate measures required to maintain a normal elimination pattern.

Age. Developmental changes that affect elimination occur throughout life. An infant has a small stomach capacity and less secretion of digestive enzymes. Some foods such as complex starches are tolerated poorly. Food passes quickly through an infant's intestinal tract because of rapid peristalsis. The infant is unable to control defecation because of a lack of neuromuscular development. This development usually does not take place until 2 to 3 years of age.

Systemic changes in the function of digestion and absorption of nutrients result from changes in older clients' cardiovascular and neurological systems, rather than their gastrointestinal system. For example, arteriosclerosis may cause decreased splanchnic and mesenteric blood flow, thus decreasing absorption from the small intestine (Lueckneotte, 2000). In addition, there is a decrease in

Table **45-1**	Normal Age-Related Changes in the Gastrointestinal Tract	
Portion of GI Tract	**Functional or Physiological Change**	**Causes**
Mouth	Decreased chewing and decreased salivation, including oral dryness	Degeneration of cells, medications.
Esophagus	Reduced motility, especially in lower third	Degeneration of neural cells.
Stomach	Decrease in:	
	Acid secretions	Degeneration of gastric mucosa. Alkaline gastric medium contributes to malabsorption of iron. Although digestive enzymes are decreased, enough remain available for digestion.
	Motor activity	Delayed gastric emptying causing fewer hunger contractions.
	Mucosal thickness	Loss of parietal cells also leads to loss of intrinsic factor, which is needed for vitamin B_{12} absorption.
Small intestine	Decreased nutrient absorption	Fewer absorbing cells.
Large intestine	Increase in pouches on the weakened intestinal wall called diverticulosis	Weakened musculature. Absorption not significantly affected.
	Constipation	Decreased peristalsis.
	Missed defecation signal. Increasing risk for fecal incontinence	Duller nerve sensations.
Liver	Size decreased	Reduced storage capacity and ability to synthesize protein and metabolize medications.

Data from Lueckenotte AG: *Gerontologic Nursing,* ed 2, St. Louis, 2000, Mosby.

peristalsis, and esophageal emptying slows. Older adults often experience changes in the GI system that impair digestion and elimination (Table 45-1).

Older adults also loose muscle tone in the perineal floor and anal sphincter. Although the integrity of the external sphincter may remain intact, older adults may have difficulty controlling bowel evacuation and are at risk for incontinence. In addition, there is a slowing of nerve impulses to the anal region and some individuals become less aware of the need to defecate and as a result develop irregular bowel movements and are at risk for constipation.

Diet. The food that a person eats influences elimination. Regular daily food intake helps maintain a regular pattern of peristalsis in the colon. **Fiber,** the undigestible residue in the diet, provides the bulk of fecal material. Bulk-forming foods, such as grains, fruits, and vegetables, absorb fluids and increase stool mass. The bowel walls are stretched, creating peristalsis and initiating the defecation reflex. By stimulating peristalsis, bulk foods pass quickly through the intestines, keeping the stool soft. Ingestion of a high-fiber diet improves the likelihood of a normal elimination pattern if other factors are normal. Fiber intake can help resolve constipation, and further research has documented the use of supplemental dietary fiber to reduce bowel incontinence (Bliss and others, 2001).

Gas-producing foods such as onions, cauliflower, and beans also stimulate peristalsis. The gas formed distends intestinal walls and increases colon motility. Some spicy foods can increase peristalsis but can also cause indigestion and watery stools.

Some foods, such as milk and milk products, are difficult or impossible for some people to digest. This is caused by a **lactose intolerance,** which may have a genetic link. Lactose, a simple form of sugar found in milk, is normally broken down by the enzyme lactase. Intolerance to lactose-containing foods may result in diarrhea, gaseous distention, and cramping (Mishkin, 1997).

Fluid Intake. An inadequate fluid intake or disturbances resulting in fluid loss (such as vomiting) affect the character of feces. Fluid liquefies intestinal contents, easing its passage through the colon. Reduced fluid intake slows passage of food through the intestine and can result in hardening of stool contents. Unless there is a medical contraindication, an adult should drink six to eight glasses (1400 to 2000 ml) of noncaffeinated fluid daily. An increase in fluid intake with the use of fruit juices softens stool and increases peristalsis. Older adults are at risk of insufficient intake of fluids and are thus predisposed to constipation (Selma, Beizer, and Highbee, 1997). In addition, an increased ingestion of milk or milk products may slow peristalsis in some persons and cause constipation (Anti and others, 1998).

Physical Activity. Physical activity promotes peristalsis, whereas immobilization depresses peristalsis. Early ambulation as illness begins to resolve or as soon as possible after surgery is encouraged to promote maintenance of peristalsis and normal elimination. Maintaining tone of skeletal muscles used during defecation is important. Weakened abdominal and pelvic floor muscles impair the ability to increase intraabdominal pressure and to control the external sphincter. Muscle tone may be weakened or lost as a result of long-term illness or neurological disease that impairs nerve transmission. As a result of these changes in the abdominal and pelvic floor muscles, there is an increased risk for constipation.

Psychological Factors. The function of almost all body systems can be impaired by prolonged emotional stress (see Chapter 30). If an individual becomes anxious, afraid, or angry, the stress response is initiated, which allows the body to restore defenses. The digestive process is accelerated, and peristalsis is increased. Side effects of increased peristalsis are diarrhea and gaseous distention. If a person becomes depressed, the autonomic nervous system slows impulses and peristalsis can decrease, resulting in constipation. A number of diseases of the GI tract are believed to be associated with stress. These include ulcerative **colitis,** certain gastric and duodenal ulcers, and **Crohn's disease.**

Personal Habits. Personal elimination habits influence bowel function. Most people benefit from being able to use their own toilet facilities at a time that is most effective and convenient for them. A busy work schedule may prevent the individual from responding appropriately to the urge to defecate, disrupting regular habits and causing possible alterations such as constipation. A person should recognize the best time for elimination. The gastrocolic reflex is frequently stimulated to cause defecation after meals.

Chronically ill and hospitalized clients may not be able to maintain privacy during defecation. In a hospital or extended care setting, bathroom facilities are often shared with a roommate whose hygienic habits might be quite different. In addition, a chronic illness may limit a client's balance, activity tolerance, or physical activity and requires the use of a bedpan or bedside commode. The sights, sounds, and odors associated with sharing toilet facilities or using bedpans are often embarrassing. Embarrassment prompts clients to ignore the urge to defecate, which can begin a vicious cycle of constipation and discomfort.

Position During Defecation. Squatting is the normal position during defecation. Modern toilets are designed to facilitate this posture, allowing the person to lean forward, exert intraabdominal pressure, and contract the thigh muscles. For the client immobilized in bed, defecation is often difficult. In a supine position it is impossible to contract the muscles used during defecation. If the client's condition permits, raise the head of the bed; this

assists the client to a more normal sitting position on a bedpan, enhancing the ability to defecate.

Pain. Normally the act of defecation is painless. However, a number of conditions, including hemorrhoids, rectal surgery, rectal fistulas, and abdominal surgery, can result in discomfort. In these instances the client often suppresses the urge to defecate to avoid pain, and constipation may develop.

Pregnancy. As pregnancy advances, the size of the fetus increases and pressure is exerted on the rectum. A temporary obstruction created by the fetus impairs passage of feces. Slowing of peristalsis during the third trimester often leads to constipation. A pregnant woman's frequent straining during defecation or delivery can result in formation of permanent hemorrhoids.

Surgery and Anesthesia. General anesthetic agents used during surgery cause temporary cessation of peristalsis (see Chapter 49). Inhaled anesthetic agents block parasympathetic impulses to the intestinal musculature. The anesthetic's action slows or stops peristaltic waves. The client who receives local or regional anesthesia is less at risk for elimination alterations because bowel activity may be affected minimally or not at all.

Any surgery that involves direct manipulation of the bowel temporarily stops peristalsis. This condition, called **paralytic ileus,** usually lasts about 24 to 48 hours. If the client remains inactive or is unable to eat after surgery, return of normal bowel function may be further delayed.

Medications. Medication may have certain expected actions on the bowel; for example, there are medications to promote defecation or control diarrhea. In addition, medications prescribed for acute and chronic conditions may have secondary effects on the client's bowel elimination patterns (Table 45-2).

Laxatives and **cathartics** soften the stool and promote peristalsis. Although similar, laxatives are milder in

Table 45-2	Medications and the Gastrointestinal System
Medications	**Action**
Dicyclomine HCl (Bentyl)	Suppresses peristalsis and can decrease gastric emptying.
Narcotic analgesics	Slow peristalsis and segmental contractions, often resulting in constipation (McKenry and Salerno, 2001).
Anticholinergic drugs, such as atropine or glycopyrrolate (Robinul)	Inhibit gastric acid secretion and depress GI motility (McKenry and Salerno, 2001). Although useful in treating hyperactive bowel disorders, anticholinergics can cause constipation.
Antibiotics	May produce diarrhea by disrupting the normal bacterial flora in the GI tract. If the diarrhea and associated abdominal cramping become severe, the client might need to change medications (Bartlett, 2002).
Nonsteroidal antiinflammatory drugs	Promote gastrointestinal irritation that can range from dyspepsia to life-threatening hemorrhage (Cooke, 1996).
Aspirin	A prostaglandin inhibitor, it can interfere with the formation and production of protective mucus and can predispose clients to gastritis.
Histamine$_2$ (H$_2$) antagonists	Suppress the secretion of hydrochloric acid and may interfere with the digestion of some foods.
Iron	Can cause discoloration of the stool (black) and lead to constipation (McKenry and Salerno, 2001).

action than cathartics. When used correctly, laxatives and cathartics safely maintain normal elimination patterns. However, chronic use of cathartics causes the large intestine to lose muscle tone and become less responsive to stimulation by laxatives. Laxative overuse can also cause serious diarrhea that can lead to dehydration and electrolyte depletion. Mineral oil, a common laxative, decreases fat-soluble vitamin absorption. Laxatives can influence the efficacy of other medications by altering the transit time (i.e., the time the medication remains in the GI tract and is available for absorption).

Diagnostic Tests. Diagnostic examinations involving visualization of GI structures often require that portions of the bowel be empty of contents. The client usually receives a prescribed bowel preparation (e.g., medications, cathartics, and/or enemas) before the test. In addition, the client is not allowed to eat or drink after midnight of the day preceding examinations such as a colonoscopy, **endoscopy**, or other testing that requires visualization of the lower GI tract. Following the diagnostic procedure, there may be changes in elimination, such as increased gas or loose stools, until the client resumes a normal eating pattern.

Common Bowel Elimination Problems

The nurse might care for clients who have or are at risk for elimination problems because of emotional stress (anxiety or depression), physiological changes in the GI tract such as surgical alteration of intestinal structures, inflammatory diseases, prescribed therapy, or disorders impairing defecation.

Constipation. **Constipation** is a symptom, not a disease (Box 45-1). The signs of constipation vary among clients, but they usually include infrequent bowel move-

---

Box 45-1   Common Causes of Constipation

- Irregular bowel habits and ignoring the urge to defecate.
- Chronic illnesses (e.g., Parkinson's disease, multiple sclerosis, rheumatoid arthritis, chronic bowel diseases, depression, eating disorders) (Annells and Koch, 2002; Richmond, 2003).
- Low-fiber diet high in animal fats (e.g., meats, dairy products, eggs) and refined sugars (rich desserts). Also, low fluid intake slows peristalsis (Bliss and others, 2001).
- Situational stress (e.g., illness of a family member, death of a loved one, divorce) (Dosh, 2002).
- Lengthy bed rest or lack of regular exercise.
- Heavy laxative use causes loss of normal defecation reflex. In addition, the lower colon is completely emptied, requiring time to refill with bulk (Annells and Koch, 2002).
- Older adults experience slowed peristalsis, loss of abdominal muscle elasticity, and reduced intestinal mucus secretion. Older adults often eat low-fiber foods.
- Neurological conditions that block nerve impulses to the colon (e.g., spinal cord injury, tumor).
- Organic illnesses such as hypothyroidism, hypocalcemia, or hypokalemia (Richmond, 2003).

---

ments, difficult evacuation of feces, inability to defecate at will, and hard feces (Dosh, 2002). Straining during defecation is an associated sign. When intestinal motility slows, the fecal mass becomes exposed over time to the intestinal walls and most of the fecal water content is absorbed. Little water is left to soften and lubricate the stool. Passage of a dry, hard stool may cause rectal pain.

Constipation can be a significant hazard to health. Straining during defecation may cause problems to the client with recent abdominal, gynecological, or rectal surgery. The effort to pass a stool can cause sutures to separate, reopening the wound. In addition, clients with histories of cardiovascular disease, diseases causing elevated intraocular pressure (glaucoma), and increased intracranial pressure should prevent constipation and avoid using the Valsalva maneuver (see Chapter 31). Exhaling through the mouth during straining avoids a Valsalva maneuver (Stewart, 1998). Clients may have constipation from certain medications that they are taking. Some medications that cause constipation include aspirin, antihistamines, diuretics, tranquilizers, hypnotics, antacids with aluminum or calcium, and drugs used to control Parkinson's disease.

Impaction. Fecal **impaction** results from unrelieved constipation. It is a collection of hardened feces, wedged in the rectum, that cannot be expelled. In cases of severe impaction, the mass can extend up into the sigmoid colon. Clients who are debilitated, confused, or unconscious are most at risk for impaction. They are too weak or unaware of the need to defecate, or they may be dehydrated so that the stool becomes too hard and dry to pass.

An obvious sign of impaction is the inability to pass a stool for several days, despite the repeated urge to defecate. When a continuous oozing of diarrhea stool develops, impaction should be suspected. The liquid portion of feces located higher in the colon seeps around the impacted mass. Loss of appetite (anorexia), nausea and/or vomiting, abdominal distention and cramping, and rectal pain may accompany the condition. The nurse who suspects an impaction can gently perform a digital examination of the rectum and palpate for the impacted mass.

Diarrhea. **Diarrhea** is an increase in the number of stools and the passage of liquid, unformed feces. It is associated with disorders affecting digestion, absorption, and secretion in the GI tract. Intestinal contents pass through the small and large intestine too quickly to allow the usual absorption of fluid and nutrients. Irritation within the colon can result in an increased mucus secretion. As a result, feces become watery and the client may be unable to control the urge to defecate.

Excess loss of colonic fluid can result in serious fluid and electrolyte or acid-base imbalances. Infants and older adults are particularly susceptible to associated complications (see Chapter 40). Because repeated passage of diarrhea stools also exposes the skin of the perineum and buttocks to irritating intestinal contents, meticulous skin care and containment of fecal drainage is needed to prevent skin breakdown (see Chapter 38).

Many conditions cause diarrhea. Antibiotic use via any route of administration may alter the normal flora in the gastrointestinal tract (Bartlett, 2002). Clients receiving enteral nutrition are also at risk for diarrhea, which may be due to the GI response to the nutritional components, frequency, or volume of the enteral feeding (Eisenberg, 2002). Food allergies and intolerances increase peristalsis and cause diarrhea. Diseases, surgeries, or diagnostic testing of the lower gastrointestinal tract can also cause diarrhea. The aims of treatment are to remove precipitating conditions and to slow peristalsis.

In addition, communicable food-borne pathogens can cause diarrhea. The risk of food-borne illnesses can be greatly reduced by simple hand washing following the use of the bathroom, before and after preparing foods, and cleaning and storing fresh produce and meats. When diarrhea is the result of a food-borne virus, the goal is usually to rid the system of the pathogen, rather than to slow peristalsis.

Incontinence. Fecal **incontinence** is the inability to control passage of feces and gas from the anus. Incontinence can harm a client's body image (see Chapter 26). In many situations the client is mentally alert but physically unable to avoid defecation. The embarrassment of soiling clothes can lead to social isolation. Physical conditions that impair anal sphincter function or control can cause incontinence. Incontinence can occur in a variety of settings. Conditions that create frequent, loose, large-volume, watery stools also predispose to incontinence (Box 45-2).

Flatulence. As gas accumulates in the lumen of the intestines, the bowel wall stretches and distends **(flatulence).** It is a common cause of abdominal fullness, pain, and cramping. Normally, intestinal gas escapes through the mouth (belching) or the anus (passing of flatus). However, if there is a reduction in intestinal motility resulting from opiates, general anesthetics, abdominal surgery, or immobilization, flatulence can become severe enough to cause abdominal distention and severe sharp pain.

Hemorrhoids. **Hemorrhoids** are dilated, engorged veins in the lining of the rectum. They are either external or internal. External hemorrhoids are clearly visible as protrusions of skin. If the underlying vein is hardened, there can be a purplish discoloration (thrombosis). This causes increased pain and may need to be excised. Internal hemorrhoids have an outer mucous membrane. Increased venous pressure from straining at defecation, pregnancy, heart failure, and chronic liver disease can cause hemorrhoids.

Bowel Diversions

Certain diseases cause conditions that prevent normal passage of feces through the rectum. The treatment for these disorders may result in the need for a temporary or permanent artificial opening **(stoma)** in the abdominal wall. Surgical openings may be created in the ileum **(ileostomy)** or colon **(colostomy)** with the ends of the intestine brought through the abdominal wall to create the stoma.

The standard bowel diversion creates a stoma, or the client has reconstructive bowel surgery that uses the native sphincter for bowel continence. The reconstructive surgery includes a continent stoma procedure, or the

Research Highlight   *Box 45-2*

Factors Associated With Fecal Incontinence

Research Focus

Identifying causes for fecal incontinence of clients in acute care settings is difficult. Nurses care for many clients who are incontinent. This condition is embarrassing for the client. However, it also increases the client's risk of complications secondary to incontinence, such as impaired skin integrity or prolonged hospital stays.

Research Abstract

The purpose of this study was to determine the presence of fecal incontinence in hospitalized clients who were acutely ill and to determine if there was a relationship between fecal incontinence and stool consistency, and between two well-known nosocomial or iatrogenic causes of diarrhea: *Clostridium difficile* and enteral tube feedings. Data from 152 clients were collected on fecal incontinence, stool frequency and consistency, presence of tube feedings and medications, severity of illness, and nutritional information. Rectal swabs and stool specimens were obtained weekly and cultured for nosocomial infections.

Evidence-Based Practice

- The presence of diarrhea was more frequently associated with incontinence.
- Clients who were incontinent of loose, watery diarrhea had little or no warning before the incontinence episode.
- Diarrhea is present without a positive stool culture.
- Controlling the diarrhea is beneficial because as the stool becomes more formed the frequency of incontinence declines.
- When clients have organism-related diarrheas, as with *C. difficile,* treatments to slow intestinal transit should be avoided.

Reference

Bliss DZ and others: Fecal incontinence in hospitalized patients who are acutely ill, *Nurs Res* 49(2):101, 2000.

ileoanal pouch anastomosis, which is described later (Colwell and others, 2001).

Ostomies. The location of the ostomy determines the consistency of stool. An ileostomy bypasses the entire large intestine. As a result, stools are frequent and liquid. The same is true for a colostomy of the ascending colon. A colostomy of the transverse colon generally results in a more solid, formed stool. The sigmoid colostomy emits near-normal stool. The location of a colostomy is determined by the client's medical problem and general condition. There are three types of colostomy construction: loop colostomy, end colostomy, and double-barrel colostomy.

Loop Colostomy. A loop colostomy is usually performed in a medical emergency when closure of the colostomy is anticipated. These are usually temporary large stomas constructed in the transverse colon (Figure 45-4, *A-D*). The surgeon pulls a loop of bowel onto the abdomen (Figure 45-4, *E*). An external supporting device such as a plastic rod, bridge (Figure 45-4, *C* and *D*), or rubber catheter is temporarily placed under the bowel loop to keep it from slipping back (Figure 45-4, *A*). The surgeon then opens the bowel and sutures it to the skin of the abdomen (Figure 45-4, *F*). A communicating wall remains between the proximal and distal bowel. The loop ostomy has two openings through the one stoma (Figure 44-5, *D* and *G*). The proximal end drains stool, whereas the distal portion drains mucus. Within 7 to 10 days the external supporting device is removed.

End Colostomy. The end colostomy consists of one stoma formed from the proximal end of the bowel with the distal portion of the GI tract either removed or sewn closed (called Hartmann's pouch) and left in the abdominal cavity. For many clients, end colostomies are a result of surgical treatment of colorectal cancer. In such cases the rectum might also be removed. Clients with diverticulitis who are treated surgically often have a temporary end colostomy with a Hartmann's pouch (Figure 45-5).

Double-Barrel Colostomy. Unlike the loop colostomy, the bowel is surgically severed in a double-barrel colostomy (Figure 45-6, *A*), and the two ends are brought out onto the abdomen (Figure 45-6, *B*). The double-barrel colostomy consists of two distinct stomas: the proximal functioning stoma and the distal nonfunctioning stoma.

Alternative Procedures

Ileoanal Pouch Anastomosis. The ileoanal pouch anastomosis is a new surgical procedure that may be used in clients who need to have a colectomy for treatment of ulcerative colitis or familial **polyps.** In this procedure the colon is removed, a pouch is created from the end of the small intestine, and the pouch is attached to the client's anus (Figure 45-7).This pouch provides for the collection of waste material, which is similar to the rectum. The client is continent of stool because stool is evacuated via the anus. When the ileal pouch is created, the client has a temporary ileostomy to allow the anastomosis to heal.

Kock Continent Ileostomy. The Kock continent ileostomy is created using the client's small intestine to create a pouch (Figure 45-8). This procedure is occasionally used in the treatment of ulcerative colitis. The pouch has a continent stoma, a nipple type of valve that is drained with an external catheter, which is placed intermittently in the stoma. The client empties the pouch several times a day. The stoma is covered with a protective dressing or stoma cap (Colwell and others, 2001).

Psychological Considerations. A stoma can cause serious body image changes, particularly if it is permanent. A study reported by Walsh and others (1995) measured the perception of body image in clients who had a stoma. Clients who had a long-standing history of chronic bowel disease such as Crohn's disease or ulcerative colitis had improved quality of life, but a lower body image. Conversely, clients who needed an ostomy because of cancer had a higher body image but a reduced quality of life. Clients often perceive a stoma as invasive and disfiguring. However, a well-placed stoma should not interfere with the client's activities and can be concealed with clothing (Banks and Razor, 2003). However, even though clothing may conceal the ostomy, the client feels different. Many clients have difficulty maintaining or initiating normal sexual relations (see Chapter 27). An important factor in the client's reactions is the character of fecal secretions and the ability to control them. Foul odors, spillage, or leakage of liquid stools and inability to regulate bowel movements give the client a loss of self-esteem.

Critical Thinking

Successful critical thinking requires a synthesis of knowledge, experience, information gathered from clients, critical thinking attitudes, and intellectual and professional standards. Clinical judgments require the nurse to anticipate the information necessary, analyze the data, and make decisions regarding client care. During assessment (Figure 45-9) the nurse must consider all critical thinking elements that build toward making appropriate diagnoses.

In the case of bowel elimination, the nurse must integrate the knowledge from nursing and other disciplines to better understand the client's response to bowel elimination interruptions. Often clients respond to disruptions in bowel elimination with fright and embarrassment. Sensitivity on the part of the nurse is essential. For clients with significant interruptions such as a bowel diversion, the nurse will find the inclusion of information from an enterostomal specialist an important part of the care plan.

Nursing Process and Bowel Elimination

Assessment

Assessment for bowel elimination patterns and abnormalities includes a nursing history, a physical assessment of the abdomen, inspection of fecal characteristics, and a review of relevant test results. In addition, the nurse needs to determine the client's medical history pattern and types of fluid and food intake, chewing ability, medications, and recent illnesses and/or stressors.

Nursing History. The nursing history provides a review of the client's usual bowel pattern and habits. What a client describes as normal or abnormal may be different from factors and conditions that tend to promote normal elimination. Identifying normal and abnormal patterns, habits, and the client's perception of normal and abnormal in regard to bowel elimination allows the nurse to determine the client's problems. Much of the nursing history can be organized around the factors that affect elimination (Norton and Chelvanayagam, 2000):

- *Determination of the usual elimination pattern:* Frequency and time of day are included. The accurate assessment of a client's current bowel elimination pattern may be

Text continued on p. 1385

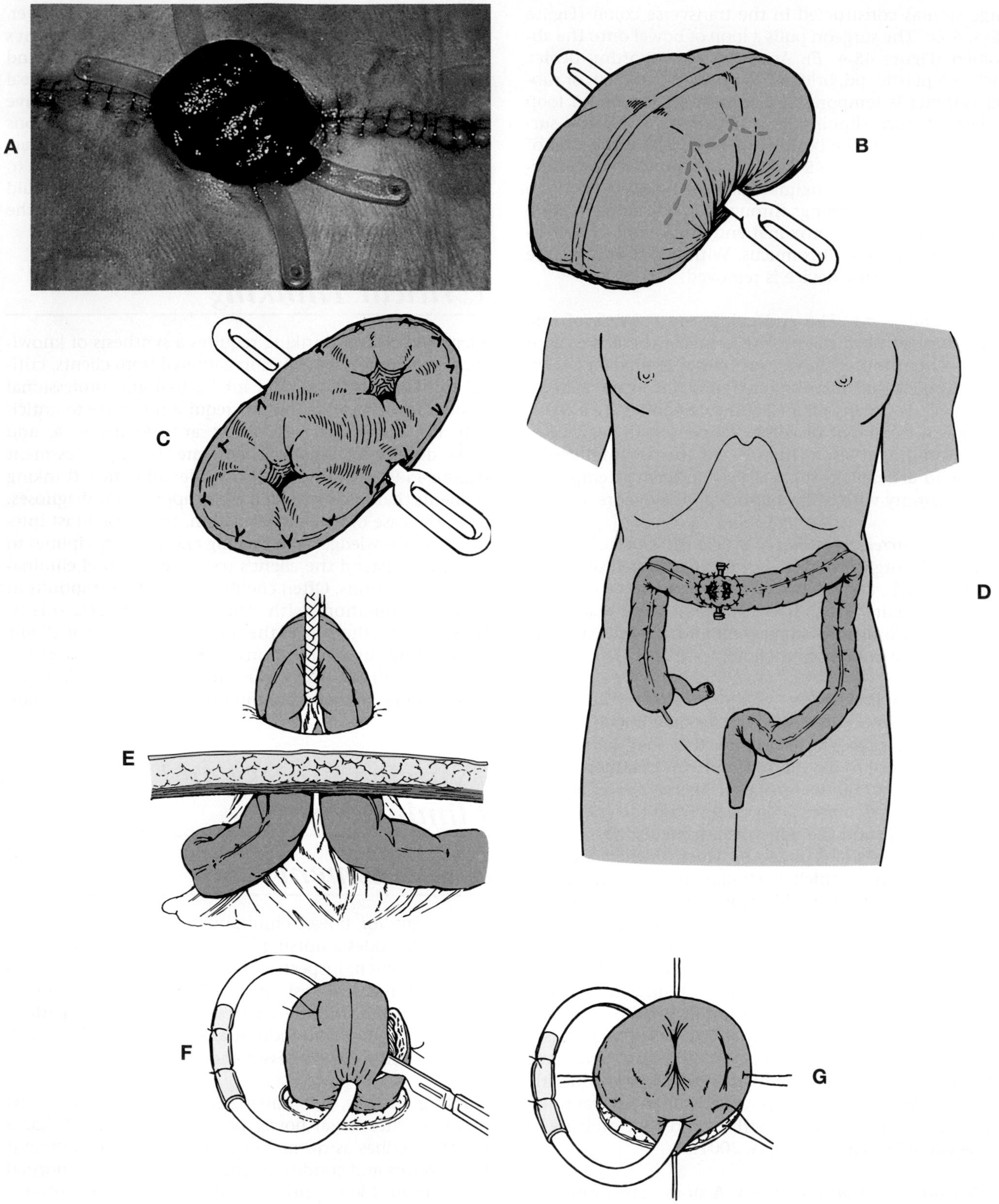

FIGURE **45–4 A,** Transverse loop colostomy supported with a flexible red rubber catheter. **A, B,** Abdominal view of loop colostomy in transverse colon. **C,** Loop colostomy construction is much the same as construction of loop ileostomy. Stoma is created with longitudinal incision through sacculations in colon. **D,** Loop colostomy matured. **E,** Loop ostomy construction, loop of bowel exteriorized. **F,** Support device placed to maintain position of bowel on abdominal surface. Distal bowel of ileum is incised, mesentery. Stitch placed to designate proximal bowel. **G,** Loop ileostomy matured with protruding functional limb. (**A,** Permission to use and/or reproduce this copyrighted photo has been granted by the owner, Hollister, Incorporated; **B** to **G** From Hampton BG, Bryant RA: *Ostomies and continent diversions: nursing management,* St. Louis, 1992, Mosby.)

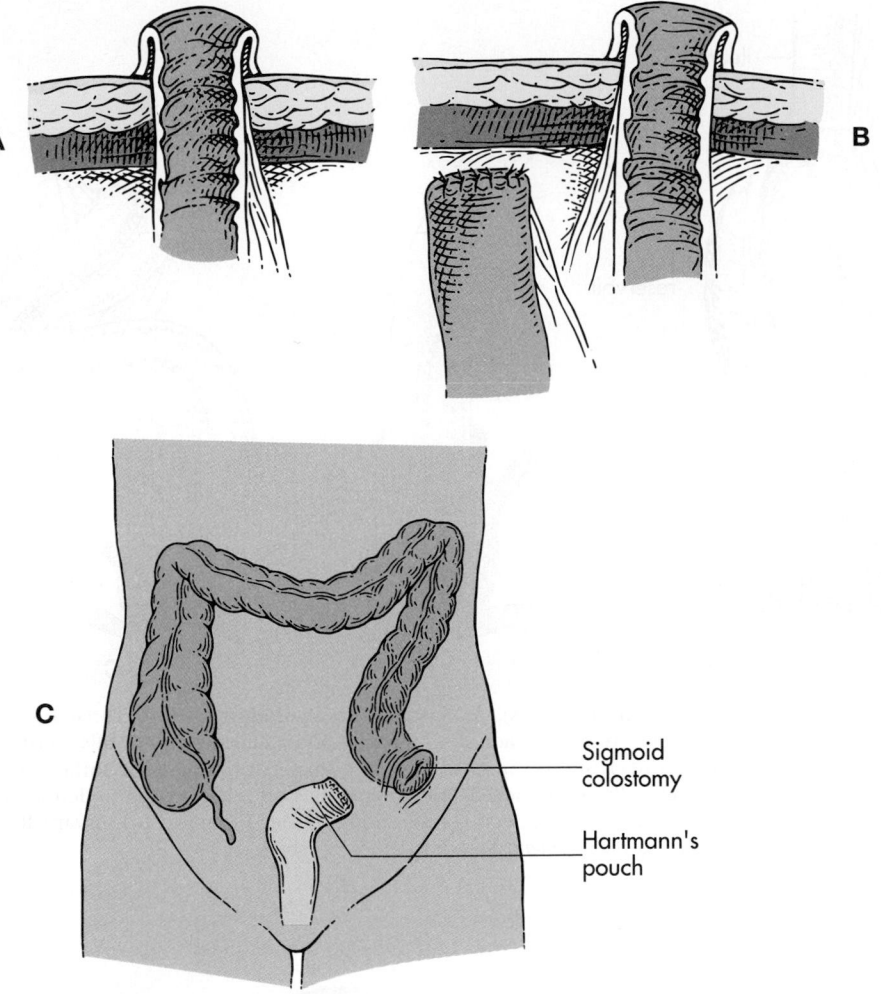

FIGURE **45-5** End colostomy. **A,** Cross-sectional view of end stoma. **B,** Cross-sectional view of end stoma with distal bowel oversewn and secured to anterior peritoneum at stoma site. **C,** Sigmoid colostomy. Distal bowel is oversewn and left in place to create Hartmann's pouch. (From Hampton BG, Bryant RA: *Ostomies and continent diversions: nursing management,* St. Louis, 1992, Mosby.)

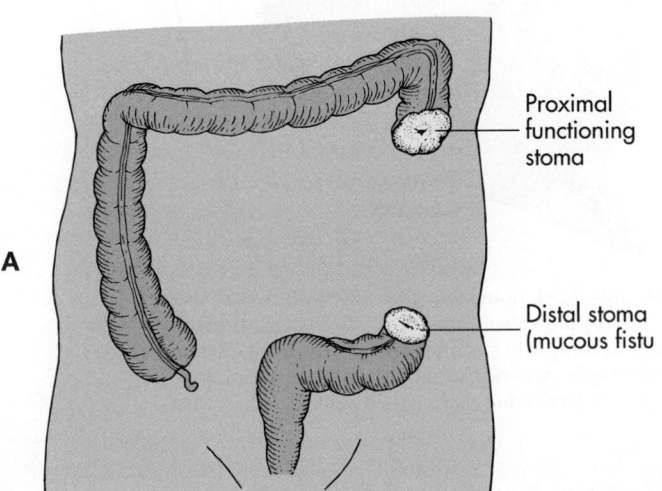

FIGURE **45-6** Double-barrel colostomy. **A,** Double-barrel colostomy in the descending colon. **B,** Cross-sectional view of double-barrel stoma. (From Hampton BG, Bryant RA: *Ostomies and continent diversions: nursing management,* St. Louis, 1992, Mosby.)

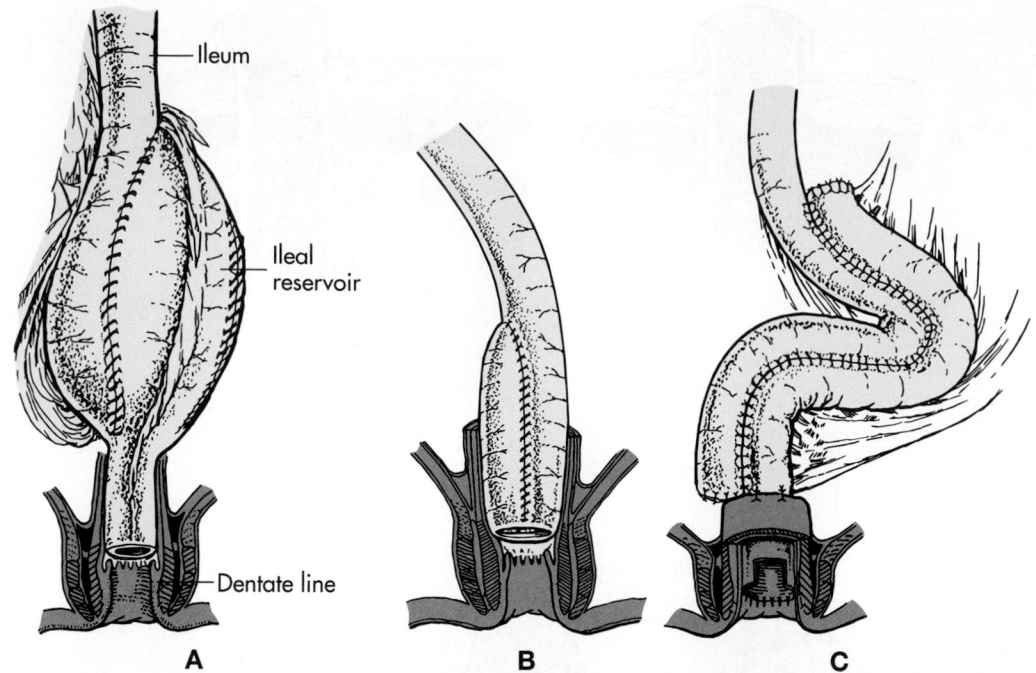

FIGURE **45–7**   Ileaoanal reservoirs (IARs). **A,** S-shaped configuration for IAR. Three 10-cm limbs of ileum are used, antimesenteric surface of each limb opened, and adjacent bowel walls anastomosed. **B,** J-shaped configuration for IAR. Distal ileum is aligned in J shape; antimesenteric surface of J shape is opened, and adjacent bowel walls anastomosed. Side-to-end anastomosis of bowel to dentate line is evident. **C,** Lateral or side-by-side ileoanal pouch configuration. (From Hampton BG, Bryant RA: *Ostomies and continent diversions: nursing management,* St. Louis, 1992, Mosby.)

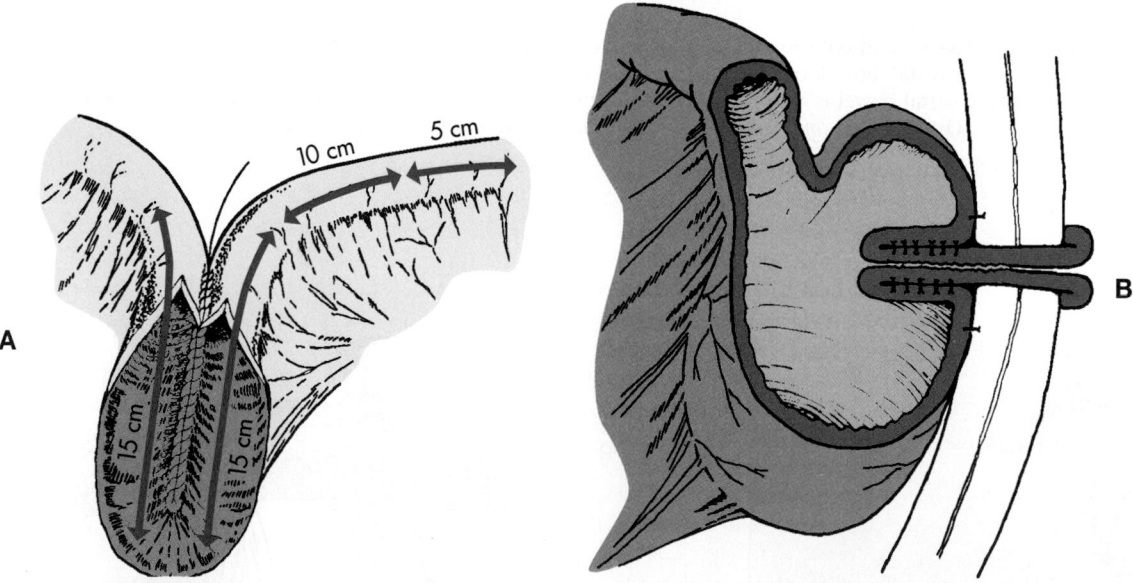

FIGURE **45–8**   Construction of Kock continent ileostomy—Kock pouch. **A,** Two 15-cm limbs are used to create pouch, and one 15-cm limb is used to fashion a nipple valve and stoma. **B,** Distal limb is intussuscepted into reservoir to create one-way valve and accomplish continence. Sutures or staples, or both, are placed to stabilize and maintain intussuscepted nipple. Anterior surface of reservoir is anchored to anterior peritoneal wall. (From Hampton BG, Bryant RA: *Ostomies and continent diversions: nursing management,* St. Louis, 1992, Mosby.)

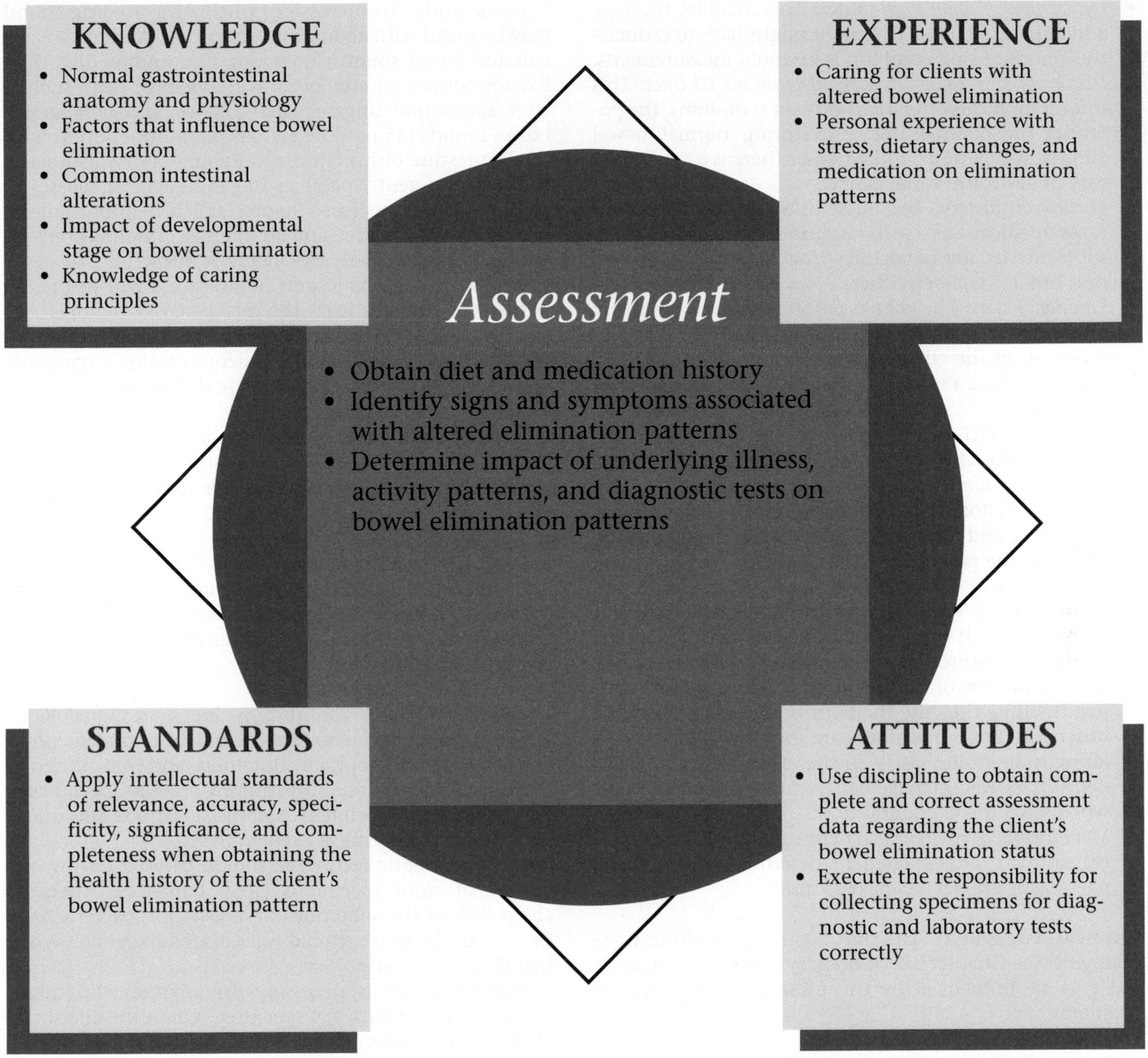

KNOWLEDGE

- Normal gastrointestinal anatomy and physiology
- Factors that influence bowel elimination
- Common intestinal alterations
- Impact of developmental stage on bowel elimination
- Knowledge of caring principles

EXPERIENCE

- Caring for clients with altered bowel elimination
- Personal experience with stress, dietary changes, and medication on elimination patterns

Assessment

- Obtain diet and medication history
- Identify signs and symptoms associated with altered elimination patterns
- Determine impact of underlying illness, activity patterns, and diagnostic tests on bowel elimination patterns

STANDARDS

- Apply intellectual standards of relevance, accuracy, specificity, significance, and completeness when obtaining the health history of the client's bowel elimination pattern

ATTITUDES

- Use discipline to obtain complete and correct assessment data regarding the client's bowel elimination status
- Execute the responsibility for collecting specimens for diagnostic and laboratory tests correctly

FIGURE 45-9 Critical thinking model for elimination assessment.

assisted by having the client or caregiver complete a bowel elimination diary.
- *Client's description of usual stool characteristics:* Determines whether the stool is normally watery or formed, soft or hard, the typical color, and the presence of blood. Ask the client to describe the usual shape of the stool and the number of stools per day.
- *Identification of routines followed to promote normal elimination:* Examples are drinking hot liquids, eating specific foods, or taking time to defecate during a certain part of the day.
- *Assessment of the use of artificial aids at home:* The nurse assesses whether the client uses enemas, laxatives, or bulk-forming food additives before having a bowel movement. Ask how often client used them.

- *Presence and status of bowel diversions:* If the client has an ostomy, the nurse assesses frequency of fecal drainage, character of feces, appearance and condition of the stoma (color, swelling, and irritation), type of fecal collection device used, and methods used to maintain the ostomy's function.
- *Changes in appetite:* Also include changes in eating patterns and a change in weight (amount of loss or gain). If a change of weight is present, the nurse should inquire if the weight change was planned, such as weight loss with a diet.
- *Diet history:* The nurse determines the client's dietary preferences for a day. The nurse determines the intake of fruits, vegetables, cereals, and breads and also if meals are regular or irregular.

- *Description of daily fluid intake:* This includes the type and amount of fluid. The client might have to estimate the amount using common household measurements.
- *History of surgery or illnesses affecting the GI tract:* This information can often help explain symptoms, the potential for maintaining or restoring normal bowel elimination pattern, and whether there is a family history of gastrointestinal cancer.
- *Medication history:* The nurse asks whether the client takes medications (such as laxatives, antacids, iron supplements, and analgesics) that might alter defecation or fecal characteristics.
- *Emotional state:* The client's emotions can significantly alter frequency of defecation. During assessment, observation of the client's emotions, tone of voice, and mannerisms can reveal significant behaviors that indicate stress.
- *History of exercise:* The nurse asks the client to specifically describe the type and amount of daily exercise.
- *History of pain or discomfort:* Ask the client whether there is a history of abdominal or anal pain. The type, frequency, and location of pain may help identify the source of the problem.
- *Social history:* Clients have many different living arrangements. Where clients live may affect their toileting habits. If the client is sharing living quarters, how many bathrooms are there? Do clients have their own bathroom, or do they need to share and thus adjust the time they use the bathroom to accommodate others? If clients live alone, are they capable of ambulating to the toilet safely? If the client is not independent in bowel management, the nurse determines who assists the client and how.
- *Mobility and dexterity:* The client's mobility and dexterity need to be evaluated to determine if the client needs assistive devices or personnel.

Physical Assessment. The nurse conducts a physical assessment (see Chapter 32) of body systems and functions likely to be influenced by the presence of elimination problems.

Mouth. The nurse inspects the client's teeth, tongue, and gums. Poor dentition or poorly fitting dentures influence the ability to chew (see Chapter 43). Sores in the mouth can make eating not only difficult, but also painful.

Abdomen. The nurse inspects all four abdominal quadrants for contour, shape, symmetry, and skin color. Inspection also includes noting masses, peristaltic waves, scars, venous patterns, stomas, and lesions. Normally, peristaltic waves are not visible. However, observable peristalsis can be a sign of intestinal obstruction.

Abdominal distention appears as an overall outward protuberance of the abdomen. Intestinal gas, large tumors, or fluid in the peritoneal cavity may cause distention. A distended abdomen feels tight, like a drum, and the skin appears taut, as if stretched.

The nurse auscultates the abdomen with the stethoscope to assess bowel sounds in each quadrant (see Chapter 32). Normal bowel sounds occur every 5 to 15 seconds and last a second to several seconds. While auscultating, the nurse notes the character and frequency of bowel sounds. An increase in pitch or a tinkling sound may be heard with abdominal distention. Absent (no auscultated bowel sounds) or hypoactive sounds (less than five sounds per minute) occur with paralytic ileus, such as after abdominal surgery. High-pitched and hyperactive bowel sounds (35 or more sounds per minute) occur with small intestine obstruction and inflammatory disorders.

The nurse gently palpates the abdomen for masses or areas of tenderness (see Chapter 32). It is important for the client to relax. Tensing abdominal muscles interferes with palpating underlying organs or masses.

Percussion detects lesions, fluid, or gas within the abdomen. Familiarity with the five percussion notes (see Chapter 32) also permits identification of underlying abdominal structures. Gas or flatulence creates a tympanic note. Masses, tumors, and fluid are dull to percussion.

Rectum. The nurse inspects the area around the anus for lesions, discolorations, inflammation, and hemorrhoids. Abnormalities should be carefully recorded (see Chapter 32).

Laboratory Tests. Laboratory and diagnostic examinations yield useful information concerning elimination problems (Table 45-3). Laboratory analysis of fecal contents can detect pathological conditions such as tumors, bleeding, and infection.

Fecal Specimens. The nurse is directly responsible for ensuring that specimens are accurately obtained, properly labeled in appropriate containers, and transported to the laboratory on time. Institutions provide special containers for fecal specimens. Some tests require specimens to be placed in chemical preservatives.

Medical aseptic technique should be used during collection of stool specimens (see Chapter 33). Because about 25% of the solid portion of a stool is bacteria from the colon, the nurse should wear disposable gloves when handling specimens.

Hand hygiene is necessary for anyone who might come in contact with the specimen. Often the client can obtain the specimen if properly instructed. The nurse explains that feces cannot be mixed with urine or water. For this reason the client must defecate into a clean, dry bedpan or special container placed under the toilet seat.

Tests performed by the laboratory for occult (microscopic) blood in the stool and stool cultures require only a small sample. The nurse collects about an inch of formed stool or 15 to 30 ml of liquid diarrhea stool. Tests for measuring the output of fecal fat require a 3- to 5-day collection of stool. All fecal material must be saved throughout the test period.

After obtaining a specimen, the nurse labels and tightly seals the container and completes laboratory requisition forms. The nurse then records specimen collections in the client's medical record. It is important to avoid delays in sending specimens to the laboratory. Some tests such as measurement for ova and parasites require the stool to be warm. When stool specimens are allowed to stand at room temperature, bacteriological changes that alter test results can occur.

A common laboratory test that can be done at home or at the client's bedside is **fecal occult blood testing**

Table 45-3	Laboratory and Diagnostic Tests for Bowel Function
Measurement and Normal Values	**Interpretation**
Laboratory tests	
• Total bilirubin: 0.1-1.0 mg/dl	• Increased in hepatobiliary diseases, obstructions in bile duct, certain anemias, and following transfusion reactions.
• Alkaline phosphatase: 30-85 ImU/ml	• Elevated in obstructive hepatobiliary diseases, hepatobiliary carcinomas, bone tumors, healing fractures.
• Amylase: 56-190 international units/L	• Elevated in abnormalities of the pancreas, such as inflammation or tumors, cholecystitis, necrotic bowel, and diabetic ketoacidosis.
• Carcinoembryonic antigen: (CEA): <5 ng/ml	• Elevated in the presence of cancer or inflammation of the GI tract or hepatobiliary organs.
Direct visualization	
• Endoscopy	• Routine examination, such as a colonoscopy is routine for people after 50 year of age. Normally the GI tract should be free of polyps, tumors, inflammation, ulcers, hernias, obstruction, and ulcerations. If a lesion such as a polyp is identified, the physician removes the growth or a portion of the growth and sends it to pathology for analysis. If bleeding is present, the physician may attempt to coagulate the source. In some cases the identification of an abnormality may indicate the need for follow-up surgery for the client.
Indirect visualization	
• X-ray film with contrast medium	• The x-ray film may identify the presence of abnormalities in the GI tract. A series of x-ray films may be completed to allow for indirect visualization of the entire tract. The presence of tumors, ulcerations, inflammation, or other abnormalities may indicate the need for further diagnostic testing and medical or surgical intervention.

From Pagana KD, Pagana TJ: *Mosby's diagnostic and laboratory test reference*, ed 5, St. Louis, 2001, Mosby.

(FOBT), or guaiac test, which measures microscopic amounts of blood in feces (Box 45-3). It is useful as a diagnostic screening test for colon cancer (Box 45-4). One positive result does not confirm GI bleedings. The test should be repeated at least 3 times while the client refrains from ingesting foods and medications that can cause false-positive results. For example, red meat, poultry, fish, and some raw vegetables are food sources and vitamin C, aspirin, and nonsteroidal antiinflammatory drugs are medications that can cause false-positive results (Ransohoff and Lang, 1997). Clients who are receiving anticoagulants or who have a bleeding disorder or a GI disorder known to cause bleeding (e.g., intestinal tumors, bowel inflammation, or ulcerations) should be regularly screened for fecal occult blood.

Fecal Characteristics. Inspection of fecal characteristics (Table 45-4) reveals information about the nature of elimination alterations. Several factors can influence each characteristic. A key to assessment is knowing whether there have been any recent changes. The client can best provide this information during the nursing history.

Diagnostic Examinations. A variety of radiological and diagnostic tests are used with the client experiencing altered bowel elimination (Box 45-5). Visualization of GI structures may be by direct or indirect approach. Many facilities employ the use of conscious sedation during these procedures. Midazolam (Versed) is often the sedative drug of choice with possible augmentation with meperidine (Demerol) or morphine. It is essential for the nurse to understand the safety precautions involved concerning the use of this form of anesthesia. In many institutions special training is required. A crash cart must be present at the bedside, and the client must be monitored continuously with pulse oximetry and frequent vital signs, usually every 15 minutes during and immediately following the procedure (check agency policy).

Client Expectations. Clients expect the nurse to be able to answer all of their questions regarding diagnostic tests and the preparation for those tests. Clients will be concerned about discomfort and exposure of their more personal areas. Fear of loss of control over bowel elimination is especially worrisome. Clients will need reassurance that their needs will be met and that the nurse will be supportive. Constipation is more of a problem as people age (Abyad and Mourad, 1996). Some older clients who may fail to recognize their elimination needs will need the nurse to monitor elimination patterns so that negative consequences will not occur. It is important for the nurse to remember that the client brings to any situation an individual perception of what is "right" for them. In the area of bowel elimination the client will expect a knowledgeable nurse who can teach them methods of promoting and maintaining a normal bowel elimination pattern. Clients of different cultures may also have various expectations as well (Box 45-6).

Nursing Diagnosis

The nurse's assessment of the client's bowel function reveals data that may indicate an actual or potential elimination problem or a problem resulting from elimination alterations. The concept map (Figure 45-10) shows how the nursing diagnosis of constipation is related to three

Box 45-3 *Procedural Guidelines*

Measuring Fecal Occult Blood

Equipment: Hemoccult test paper, Hemoccult developer, and wooden applicator (see illustration below).

Delegation Considerations: This skill can be delegated to assistive personnel. The nurse assesses significance of findings.

1. Explain purpose of the test and ways client can assist. Client can collect own specimen if possible.
2. Perform hand hygiene.
3. Apply, clean disposable gloves.
4. Use tip of wooden applicator (see figure for step 1) to obtain a small portion of a stool specimen. Be sure that specimen is free of tissue paper.
5. Perform Hemoccult slide test.
   a. Open flap of slide and, using the wooden applicator, thinly smear stool in the first box of the guaiac paper. Apply a second fecal specimen from a different portion of the stool to the slide's second box (see illustration).
   b. Close slide cover and turn the packet over to the reverse side (see illustration). Open cardboard flap and apply two drops of developing solution on each box of guaiac paper. A blue color indicates a positive guaiac, or presence of fecal occult blood.
   c. Assess color of the guaiac paper after 30 to 60 seconds.
   d. Dispose of test slide in proper receptacle.

6. Wrap wooden applicator in paper towel, remove gloves, and discard in proper receptacle.
7. Perform hand hygiene
8. Record results of test, note any unusual fecal characteristics.

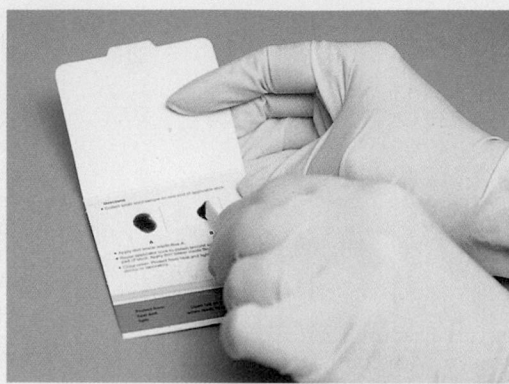

STEP **5a**   Application of fecal specimen on guaiac paper.

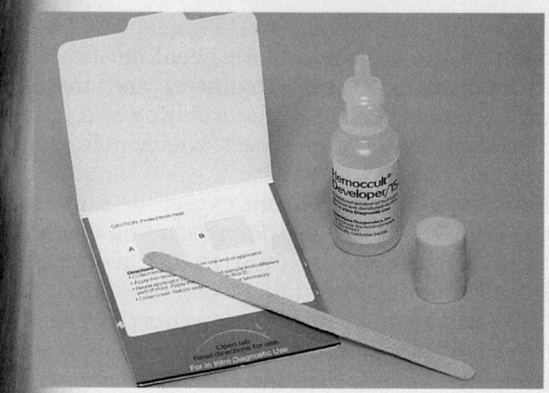

Equipment for performing fecal occult blood testing.

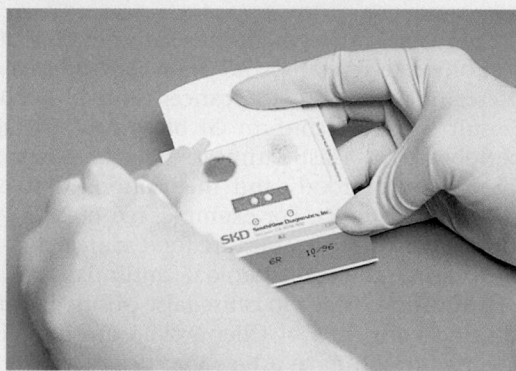

STEP **5b**   Application of Hemoccult developing solution on the guaic paper on the reverse side of the test kit.

Box 45-4   **Screening for Colon Cancer**

Risk Factors

- Age: over 50 years of age
- Family history: colon polyps or colorectal cancer
- History of inflammatory bowel disease (colitis, Crohn's disease)
- Personal history of polyps
- Diet: high intake of animal fats and low fiber intake
- Obesity and inactivity

Warning Signs

- Change in bowel habits
- Rectal bleeding
- Sensation of incomplete bowel evacuation

Screening Tests

- Digital rectal examination every year after age 40
- Fecal occult blood test every year after age 50
- Direct visualization of colon at age 50, and every 3 to 5 years thereafter. Colonoscopy is the preferred method of visualization.

From American Cancer Society: *Colon and rectal cancer: 2003, 2003,* Atlanta, 2003, The Society, www.cancer.org.

Table 45-4 **Fecal Characteristics**

Characteristic	Normal	Abnormal	Abnormal Cause
Color	Infant: yellow; adult: brown	White or clay	Absence of bile
		Black or tarry (melena)	Iron ingestion or upper GI bleeding
		Red	Lower GI bleeding, hemorrhoids
		Pale with fat	Malabsorption of fat
		Translucent mucus	Spastic constipation, colitis, excessive straining
		Bloody mucus	Blood in feces, inflammation, infection
Odor	Pungent; affected by food type	Noxious change	Blood in feces or infection
Consistency	Soft, formed	Liquid	Diarrhea, reduced absorption
		Hard	Constipation
Frequency	*Varies:* Infant 4 to 6 times daily (breast-fed) or 1 to 3 times daily (bottle-fed); adult daily or 2 to 3 times a week	Infant more than 6 times daily or less than once every 1-2 days; adult more than 3 times a day or less than once a week	Hypomotility or hypermotility
Amount	150 g per day (adult)		
Shape	Resembles diameter of rectum	Narrow, pencil shaped	Obstruction, rapid peristalsis
Constituents	Undigested food, dead bacteria, fat, bile pigment, cells lining intestinal mucosa, water	Blood, pus, foreign bodies, mucus, worms	Internal bleeding, infection, swallowed objects, irritation, inflammation
		Excess fat	Malabsorption syndrome, enteritis, pancreatic disease, surgical resection of intestine

Box 45-5 **Radiologic and Diagnostic Tests**

Plain Film of Abdomen/Kidneys, Ureter, Bladder

A simple x-ray film of the abdomen requiring no preparation.

Upper GI/Barium Swallow

An x-ray examination using an opaque contrast medium (barium) to examine the structure and motility of the upper GI tract, including pharynx, esophagus, and stomach.
Client must be allowed nothing by mouth (NPO) after midnight the night before the examination.
Client must remove all jewelry or other metallic objects.
After the test, client must increase fluids to facilitate passage of barium.

Upper Endoscopy

An endoscopic examination of the upper GI tract allowing more direct visualization through a lighted fiber-optic tube that contains a lens, forceps, and brushes for biopsy.
Preparation is similar to that of the upper GI.
Light sedation is required.

Barium Enema

An x-ray examination using an opaque contrast medium to examine the lower GI tract.
Preparation includes NPO after midnight, a bowel prep such as magnesium citrate, and in some instances enemas to empty out any remaining stool particles.

Ultrasound

A technique that uses high-frequency sound waves to echo off body organs, creating a picture.
Preparation depends on the organ to be visualized and may include NPO or no prep.

Colonoscopy

An endoscopic examination of the entire colon with the use of colonoscopy inserted into the rectum.
Preparation is similar to that of barium enema: clear liquids the day before and then some form of bowel cleanser, such as GoLytely. Enemas until clear may also be ordered. Light sedation is required.

Flexible Sigmoidoscopy

An examination of the interior of the sigmoid colon through the use of a flexible or rigid lighted tube.
Preparation is similar to that of a barium enema or colonoscopy.
Light sedation is required.

Computerized Tomography Scan

An x-ray examination of the body from many angles utilizing a scanner analyzed by a computer.
Preparation may be NPO, or nothing may be required.
The client must be informed of the need to lie very still. If claustrophobia is a problem, light sedation may be utilized.

Magnetic Resonance Imaging

A noninvasive examination that uses magnet and radio waves to produce a picture of the inside of the body.
Preparation is NPO 4 to 6 hours before examination.
No metallic objects are allowed in the room, including metal objects on clothes.

Enteroclysis

Introduction of contrast material to jejunum, allowing entire small intestine to be studied.
Preparation is 24 hours of clear liquid diet and colon cleansing, such as a GoLytely or enemas until clear.

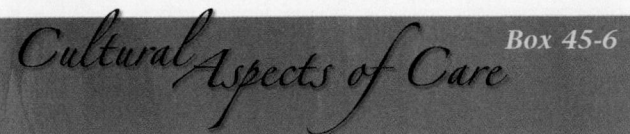

Box 45-6

Colorectal cancer is one of the most frequently occurring cancers among older adult African-Americans. Although the use of fecal occult blood testing (FOBT) to detect colorectal cancer early has decreased mortality rates in the general population, the mortality rate in African-Americans has increased. This may be because older adult African-Americans are least likely to participate in early detection and therefore when they are diagnosed their cancers are at an advanced stage.

Implications for Care

- Increasing the participation in FOBT by older adult African-Americans is a national nursing priority and must be part of African-American clients' primary prevention screening activities.
- Health care services targeting the African-American population need to have African-American health care providers for health promotion screening activities.
- Providing educational opportunities regarding the need for FOBT in the community can increase participation in colorectal cancer screening.

Modified from Powe BD: Fatalism among elderly African Americans: effects on colorectal cancer screening, *Cancer Nurs* 18(5):385, 1995.

other diagnoses. In this example a client with cancer has developed constipation as a result of activity intolerance and imbalanced nutrition. Both of those conditions were a result of the client's pain. Examples of diagnoses that may apply to clients with elimination problems include the following:

- Bowel incontinence
- Constipation
- Risk for constipation
- Perceived constipation
- Diarrhea

Associated problems, such as body-image changes or skin breakdown, require interventions unrelated to bowel function impairment. However, in some instances the nurse must direct as much attention to the elimination problem as to the associated problem.

The nurse's ability to identify the correct diagnosis depends not only on the thoroughness of assessment but also on recognition of defining characteristics and factors that can impair elimination (Box 45-7). The nurse determines the client's risk and institutes measures to ensure maintenance of normal bowel function.

Planning

During the planning of care the nurse synthesizes information from multiple resources (Figure 45-11). Critical thinking ensures that the plan of care integrates all the nurse knows about the client and the clinical problem. The nurse relies on professional standards. The guidelines on incontinence (see Chapter 44) can assist the nurse in protecting the client's skin, promoting continence, and reducing the embarrassment associated with incontinence. In addition, the Agency for Health Care Policy and Research (AHCPR), now the Agency for Health Care Research and Quality (AHCRQ), guidelines on reduction of pressure ulcers also assist in developing care for clients with bowel incontinence (see Chapter 47).

Goals and Outcomes. The nurse and the client establish goals and outcomes by incorporating the client's elimination habits or routines as much as possible and reinforcing those routines that promote health. In addition, preexisting health concerns are also considered. For example, if the client is at risk for the worsening of heart failure, an outcome of increased fluid intake must be tailored to the client's cardiac function and ability to safely handle the increased fluid. In another example, if the client's bowel habits caused the elimination problem, the nurse helps the client learn new ones. The overall goal of returning the client to a normal bowel elimination pattern may include the following outcomes:

- Client sets regular defecation habits.
- Client is able to list proper fluid and food intake needed to achieve bowel elimination.
- Client implements a regular exercise program.
- Client reports daily passage of soft, formed brown stool.
- Client does not report any discomfort associated with defecation.

Setting Priorities. Defecation patterns vary among individuals. For this reason, the nurse and client must work together closely to plan effective interventions (see care plan). What may be a realistic time frame to establish a normal defecation pattern for one client might be very different for another. In the client with a new ostomy resulting from newly diagnosed cancer the priority of coping with cancer and its treatment may need to precede the client's need to independently manage the bowel diversion. In addition, when a bowel diversion is necessary, coping with the changes in body image may become a high priority for both the client and family.

Continuity of Care. When clients are disabled or debilitated by illness, it is necessary to include the family in the plan of care. Often family members have the same ineffective elimination habits as the client. Thus client and family teaching is an important part of the care plan. Other health team members such as dietitians and enterostomal therapist (ET) nurses can be valuable resources. When clients require surgical intervention, a critical pathway may be used to coordinate the activities of the multidisciplinary health care team.

The client with alterations in bowel elimination will require intervention from many members of the health care team. Certain tasks, such as assisting clients onto the bedpan or bedside commode, are appropriate to delegate to assistive personnel. It will be important for the nurse to remind the assistant to report any abnormal findings or difficulties encountered during the elimination process. Many of the diagnostic tests for evaluation of the gastrointestinal system will be performed by nonnursing personnel. The nurse must maintain ongoing communi-

Concept Map

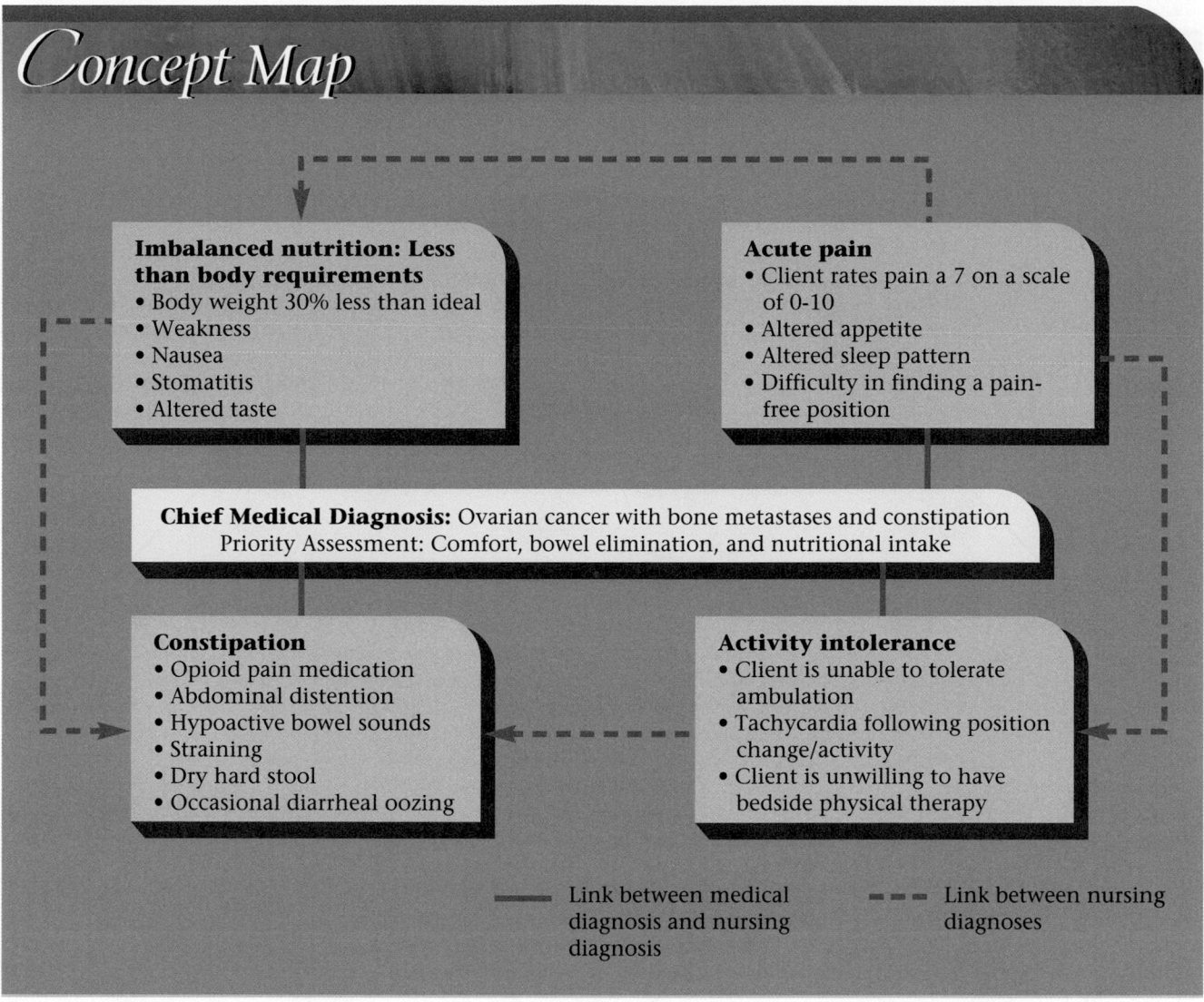

Imbalanced nutrition: Less than body requirements
- Body weight 30% less than ideal
- Weakness
- Nausea
- Stomatitis
- Altered taste

Acute pain
- Client rates pain a 7 on a scale of 0-10
- Altered appetite
- Altered sleep pattern
- Difficulty in finding a pain-free position

Chief Medical Diagnosis: Ovarian cancer with bone metastases and constipation
Priority Assessment: Comfort, bowel elimination, and nutritional intake

Constipation
- Opioid pain medication
- Abdominal distention
- Hypoactive bowel sounds
- Straining
- Dry hard stool
- Occasional diarrheal oozing

Activity intolerance
- Client is unable to tolerate ambulation
- Tachycardia following position change/activity
- Client is unwilling to have bedside physical therapy

——— Link between medical diagnosis and nursing diagnosis

- - - Link between nursing diagnoses

FIGURE **45–10** Concept map for client with ovarian cancer with bone metastases and constipation.

Nursing Diagnostic Process

Box **45-7**

Assessment Activities	Defining Characteristics	Nursing Diagnosis
Ask client to describe recent food intake.		
Auscultate bowel sounds.	Bowel sounds will be hyperactive and may be audible without a stethoscope.	Diarrhea related to food-borne pathogen, changes in diet, and alteration in gastrointestinal functioning
Assess frequency of stools.	Frequency is an early indication of increased risk for fluid and electrolyte imbalance, which is further indicated by muscle cramps.	
Assess hydration status.	Loss of skin turgor and dry mucous membranes indicate fluid deficit.	
Have clients describe pain, cramping, or any associated factors.	Pain is colicky in nature and spasmodic.	
Evaluate perianal area for redness and irritation.	Frequent stools lead to breakdown of perianal tissues.	

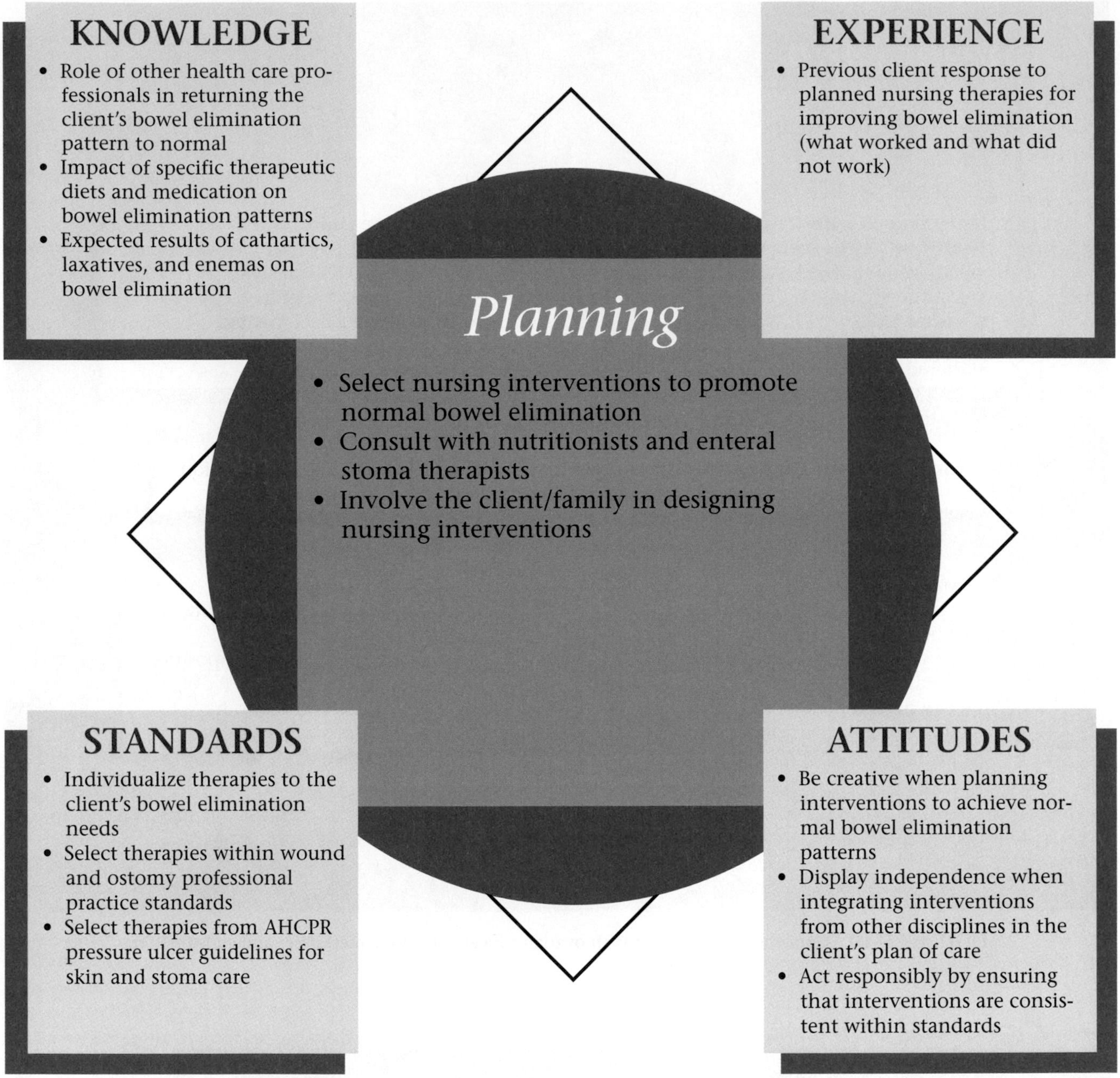

KNOWLEDGE

- Role of other health care professionals in returning the client's bowel elimination pattern to normal
- Impact of specific therapeutic diets and medication on bowel elimination patterns
- Expected results of cathartics, laxatives, and enemas on bowel elimination

EXPERIENCE

- Previous client response to planned nursing therapies for improving bowel elimination (what worked and what did not work)

Planning

- Select nursing interventions to promote normal bowel elimination
- Consult with nutritionists and enteral stoma therapists
- Involve the client/family in designing nursing interventions

STANDARDS

- Individualize therapies to the client's bowel elimination needs
- Select therapies within wound and ostomy professional practice standards
- Select therapies from AHCPR pressure ulcer guidelines for skin and stoma care

ATTITUDES

- Be creative when planning interventions to achieve normal bowel elimination patterns
- Display independence when integrating interventions from other disciplines in the client's plan of care
- Act responsibly by ensuring that interventions are consistent within standards

FIGURE **45–11**   Critical thinking model for elimination planning.

cation with these caregivers to ensure that the client's needs, wants, and concerns are addressed.

₦₽Implementation

Success of the nurse's interventions depends on improving the clients and family members' understanding of bowel elimination. In the home, hospital, or long-term care facility, clients capable of learning can be taught effective bowel habits.

The nurse should teach the client and family about proper diet, adequate fluid intake, and factors that stimulate or slow peristalsis, such as emotional stress. This of-

ten can best be done during the client's mealtime. The client should also learn the importance of establishing regular bowel routines and regular exercise and taking appropriate measures when elimination problems develop.

Health Promotion. One of the most important habits a nurse can teach regarding bowel habits is to take time for defecation. To establish regular bowel habits, a client must know when the urge to defecate normally occurs. The nurse advises the client to begin establishing a routine during a time when defecation is most likely to occur, usually an hour after a meal. Many evidenced-based interventions are available to reduce the risk of constipation (Box 45-8). If a client is restricted to bed or requires

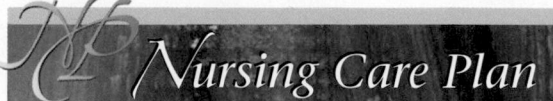

Nursing Care Plan
Bowel Elimination Alterations

Assessment

Javier is visiting Larry at his home on one of the local cattle ranches. Larry lives 20 miles from town. He is 22 years old and had surgery 6 days ago for repair of a badly broken right leg. Larry also tells Javier that he "just doesn't feel good."

Assessment Activities	Findings/Defining Characteristics
Ask Larry about his recent bowel elimination patterns over the last 5 days.	Larry tells Javier that he has not had a bowel movement since he left the hospital 4 days ago, and that he feels like his abdomen is tight and sore.
Review client's medication.	Client has been prescribed Lortabs for pain. Larry says he is taking one tablet every 6 hours, up to three a day.
Review dietary intake over last day.	Larry has eaten eggs, bacon, and toast and had soup for lunch. For supper Larry had chicken, rice and corn. He drinks about six cups of coffee each day, no water but will drink a Coke.
Ask about any nausea or vomiting.	Client has not felt nauseated.
Auscultate client's abdomen.	Decreased bowel sounds are auscultated throughout all four abdominal quadrants.
Palpate abdomen.	While Javier is palpating Larry's abdomen, Larry tells Javier, "It really hurts." On palpation, left lower quadrant is tender and firm.

Nursing Diagnosis: Constipation related to opiate-containing pain medication and decreased fiber intake.

Planning

Goals	Expected Outcomes*
	Bowel Elimination
Client will establish normal defecation.	Client will drink at least 1500 ml of fluid over the next 8 hours.
Client will voice relief from constipation.	Client will report passage of soft, formed stool without straining in next 24 hours.
Client will identify measures that will prevent constipation.	**Nutritional Status: Food and Fluid Intake** Client will increase the fiber content of his diet. Client will increase exercise.

*Outcome classification labels from Moorhead S, Johnson M, Maas M: *Nursing outcomes classification (NOC)*, ed 3, St. Louis, 2004, Mosby.

Interventions†

Constipation/Impaction Management
- Encourage fluid intake of appropriate fluids, fruit juice, water.
- Encourage activity within the limits of client's mobility regimen.
- Add bran flakes or bran to the diet.
- Provide laxative or stool softeners as ordered.
- Provide privacy.

Rationale

Adequate fluid intake is necessary to prevent hard, dry stool.

Even minimal activity (such as leg lifts) increases peristalsis.

The number of bowel movements are increased with bran (Bliss and others, 2001).
Medications can soften the stool and prevent straining (McKenry and Salerno, 2001).
Clients should feel relaxed when moving bowels (Stewart, 1998).

†Intervention classification label from Dochterman JM, Bulechek GM: *Nursing interventions classification (NIC)*, ed 4, St. Louis, 2004, Mosby.

Continued

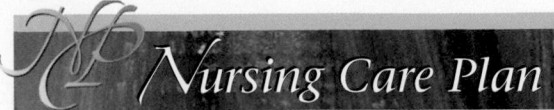

Nursing Care Plan

Bowel Elimination Alterations—cont'd

Evaluation

Nursing Actions	Client Response/Finding	Achievement of Outcome
Ask client to identify foods high in fiber.	Client able to state appropriate foods. Review of 24-hour diet diary shows client is selecting high-fiber, low-fat foods.	Larry is making excellent progress in introducing high-fiber and low-fat foods into his diet.
Ask client to plan menus to increase fiber.	Review of 24-hour diet diary showed meals plans with high fiber content. Client reviewed shopping list with bran, oat, and fruit products.	Larry is knowledgeable about fiber content and purchases food that is high in fiber.
Ask client about increased activity.	Client states that he has not changed his activity pattern.	Client has not increased activity pattern and needs to continue to work on this activity.
Observe client's subsequent stool for characteristics such as consistency and color.	Stools are now every 24 to 48 hours. Larry does not "feel regular." Abdomen is soft and nondistended. Stools are formed and hard, and client does report straining.	Client has not achieved passage of regular, formed stool.

Evidence-Based Practice Guideline

Box 45-8

Management of Constipation

- Fluid intake of at least 1.5 L/day is recommended. Preferred fluid is water because it is sodium and calorie free. Client may benefit from one to two glasses of fruit juice as well.
- Coffee, tea, and alcohol should be avoided due to their diuretic properties.
- High-fiber diet (25 to 30 g/day) reduces constipation; as fiber passes though the colon, it acts as a sponge. As a result, bulkier and softer stools develop. In addition, the waste moves through the body more easily and results in more regular bowel movements. **High-fiber diet is not recommended for individuals who are immobile or who do not consume at least 1.5 L of fluid per day.**
- Most beneficial means to prevent constipation is a combination of insoluble and soluble fiber (e.g. bran, fruits, and vegetables).
- Physical activity in combination with adequate fluid intake and high-fiber diet is beneficial in the management of constipation. For those who are fully mobile, walking once or twice a day for 15 to 20 minutes is sufficient.
- For individuals who are unable to walk, chair or bed exercises such as pelvic tilt, low trunk rotation, and single leg lifts are recommended.
- Laxatives should be used with caution, and a stepwise progression of laxatives is recommended: first bulk-forming laxatives, followed by stool softeners, osmotics, stimulants, suppositories, and enemas as a last resort.

Modified from Hinrichs, M., Huseboe, J. (1998). *Evidence-based protocol: management of constipation.* In M.G. Titler (Series Ed.), Series on Evidence-Based Practice for Older Adults. Iowa City, IA. The University of Iowa College of Nursing Gerontological Nursing Interventions Research Center, Research Dissemination Core. For more information, http://www.nursing.uiowa.edu/ center/gnirc/disseminatecore.htm.

assistance in ambulating, the nurse should offer a bedpan or help the client reach the bathroom in a timely manner.

Many clients have established routines for defecation. In a hospital or long-term care facility, the nurse should make certain that treatment routines do not interfere with the client's routine. It is important to provide privacy. When clients forced to use a bedpan share rooms with other persons, the nurse should pull the curtain around the area so that clients can relax, knowing that interruptions will not occur. The call light should always be placed within the client's reach. Bathroom doors should be closed, although the nurse may stand close in case the client needs assistance.

Promotion of Normal Defecation. To help clients evacuate bowel contents normally and without discomfort, a number of interventions can stimulate the defecation reflex, affect the character of feces, or increase peristalsis.

Sitting Position. The nurse might need to assist clients who have difficulty sitting because of muscular weakness and mobility problems. Regular toilets are too low for clients unable to lower themselves to a sitting position because of joint- or muscle-wasting diseases. Clients can purchase elevated toilet seats for the home. With such a seat, less effort is needed to sit or stand.

Positioning on Bedpan. Clients restricted to bed must use bedpans for defecation. Women use bedpans to pass both urine and feces, whereas men use bedpans only for defecation. Sitting on a bedpan can be extremely uncomfortable. The nurse should help position clients comfortably. Two types of bedpans are available (Figure 45-12). The regular bedpan, made of metal or hard plastic, has a curved smooth upper end and a sharp-edged lower end and is about 5 cm (2 inches) deep. A fracture pan, designed for clients with body or leg casts, has a shallow upper end about 1.3 cm (½ inch) deep. The upper end of the

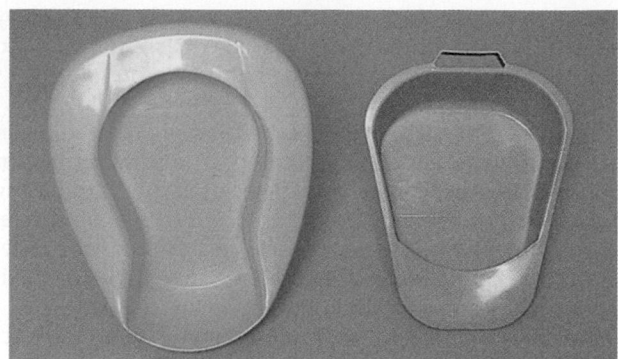

FIGURE **45–12** Types of bedpans. *From left,* regular bedpan and fracture bedpan.

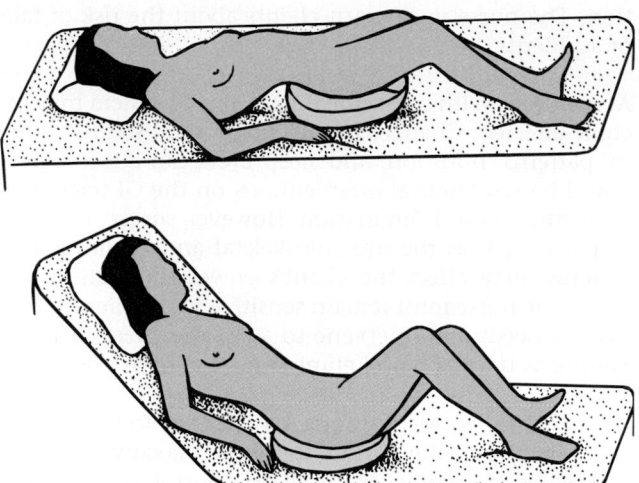

FIGURE **45–13** Positions on a bedpan. *Top,* Improper positioning of client. *Bottom,* Proper position reduces client's back strain.

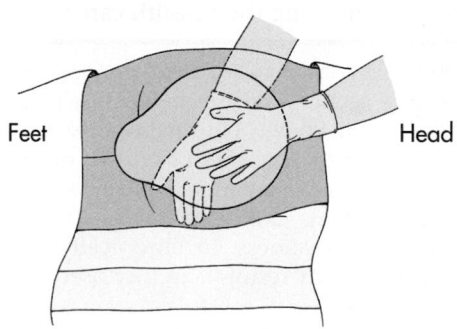

FIGURE **45–14** Positioning an immobilized client on a bedpan.

pan fits under the buttocks toward the sacrum, with the lower end just under the upper thighs. The pan should be high enough so that feces enter the pan. A metal bedpan should be warmed with water first, then dried.

When positioning a client, it is important to prevent muscle strain and discomfort. A nurse should never try to lift a client onto a bedpan. A client should also never be placed on a bedpan and then left with the bed flat unless activity restrictions demand it. If the bed is flat, the hips remain hyperextended.

Figure 45-13 shows proper and improper positions on bedpans. The best method for bedpan placement is to first be sure the client is positioned high in bed. The nurse then raises the client's head about 30 degrees, to prevent hyperextension of the back and to provide support to the upper torso. The client then raises the hips by bending the knees and lifting the hips upward. The nurse places a hand palm up under the client's sacrum, resting the elbow on the mattress and using it as a lever to help in lifting, while slipping the pan under the client. Clients who have had abdominal surgery are hesitant to exert strain on suture lines and may have difficulty positioning on a pan. Gloves should always be worn by the nurse when handling a bedpan.

If the client is immobile or it is unsafe to allow the client to exert such effort, the client remains flat and rolls onto the bedpan by using the following steps:

1. Lower the head of the bed flat and assist the client in rolling onto one side, backside toward you.
2. Apply a little powder to back and buttocks to prevent skin from sticking to the pan
3. Place the bedpan firmly against the buttocks, down into the mattress with the open rim toward the client's feet (Figure 45-14).
4. Keeping one hand against the bedpan, place the other around the client's far hip. Ask the client to roll back onto the pan, flat in bed. Do not shove the pan under the client.
5. With the client positioned comfortably, raise the head of the bed 30 degrees.
6. Place a rolled towel or small pillow under the lumbar curve of the client's back for added comfort.
7. Raise the knee gatch or ask the client to bend the knees to assume a squatting position. Do not raise the knee gatch if contraindicated.

Privacy. The nurse should maintain the client's privacy during bowel elimination. This is especially important for a client using a bedpan. The call light and a supply of toilet paper should be within easy reach. When the client finishes, the nurse responds to the call signal immediately and removes the pan. The client might require assistance with wiping. To remove the pan the nurse asks the client to roll off to the side or raise the hips. The nurse holds the pan steady to avoid spilling. The nurse should avoid pulling or shoving the pan from under the client's hips because this can pull the client's skin and cause tissue injury such as shearing (see Chapter 47). After the pan is removed, the nurse, while wearing gloves, cleans the anal and perineal areas.

After assessing the stool, the nurse should immediately empty the bedpan's contents into the toilet or in a special receptacle in the utility room. A spray faucet attached to most toilets allows the nurse to rinse the bedpan thoroughly. The client uses the same bedpan each time. The nurse should chart the characteristics of the feces.

The nurse should offer the bedpan often. Clients may accidentally soil bedclothes if forced to wait. Many clients try to avoid using a bedpan because it is embarrassing and uncomfortable. They may try to get to the bathroom even though their conditions prohibit ambulation. The nurse must warn clients about the risk of falls or accidents.

Acute Care. With any acute illness, the GI system may become affected. Changes in the client's fluid status, mobility patterns, nutrition, and sleep cycle can affect regular bowel habits. Surgical interventions on the GI tract obviously affect bowel elimination. However, surgery on other systems, such as the musculoskeletal and cardiovascular systems, may affect the client's bowel elimination patterns. The nurse must remain sensitive to the client's elimination needs and intervene to assist the client in maintaining as normal bowel elimination habits as possible.

Medications. Medications may be used to initiate and facilitate bowel elimination. Cathartics, laxatives, and occasionally an enema are used to control constipation, whereas antidiarrheal preparations assist the client in resolving diarrhea. All of these medications are available over-the-counter; stronger preparations are available through prescriptions. Clients must be cautioned not to use these over-the-counter medications on a prolonged basis without consulting their health care provider.

> *Safety Alert.* Excessive use of laxatives, enemas, and/or bulk forming agents increase the client's risk for diarrhea and abnormal bowel elimination. Excessive use of these agents destroys the client's normal defecation reflex. In addition, the client may develop altered absorption of nutrients, fluid and electrolyte imbalances, and generalized weakness. In chronically ill or older adult clients this may result in an increased risk for falls and other injuries.

Cathartics and Laxatives. Often a client is unable to defecate normally because of pain, constipation, or impaction. Cathartics and laxatives have the short-term action of emptying the bowel. They are also used in bowel evacuation for clients undergoing GI tests and abdominal surgery. Although the terms cathartic and laxative are often used interchangeably, cathartics have a stronger effect on the intestines. Five types of laxatives and cathartics are available (Table 45-5).

Cathartics and laxatives are available in oral, tablet, and powder suppository dosage forms (see Chapter 34). Although the oral route is most commonly used, cathartics that come prepared as suppositories are more effective because of their stimulant effect on the rectal mucosa. Cathartic suppositories such as bisacodyl (Dulcolax) can act within 30 minutes. Older adults often get a strong sudden urge to defecate with Dulcolax.

Antidiarrheal Agents. For clients with diarrhea, frequent passage of liquid stools becomes a problem. Many clients will use over-the-counter agents, such as Imodium, to relieve common diarrhea. However, the most effective antidiarrheal agents are prescriptive opiates such as codeine phosphate, opium tincture (paregoric), and diphenoxylate (Lomotil). Antidiarrheal opiate agents decrease intestinal muscle tone to slow passage of feces. Opiates inhibit peristaltic waves that move feces forward, but they also increase segmental contractions that mix intestinal contents. As a result, more water is absorbed by the intestinal walls. Antidiarrheal agents should be used with caution because opiates are habit forming.

Enemas. An **enema** is the instillation of a solution into the rectum and sigmoid colon. The primary reason for an enema is to promote defecation by stimulating peristalsis. The volume of fluid instilled breaks up the fecal mass, stretches the rectal wall, and initiates the defecation reflex. Enemas are also given as a vehicle for medications that exert a local effect on rectal mucosa.

The most common use for an enema is temporary relief of constipation. Other indications include removing impacted feces; emptying the bowel before diagnostic tests, surgery, or childbirth; and beginning a program of bowel training.

Cleansing Enemas. Cleansing enemas promote the complete evacuation of feces from the colon. They act by stimulating peristalsis through the infusion of a large volume of solution or through local irritation of the colon's mucosa. Cleansing enemas include tap water, normal saline, soapsuds solution, and low-volume hypertonic saline. Each solution exerts a different osmotic effect (see Chapter 40), influencing the movement of fluids between the colon and interstitial spaces beyond the intestinal wall. Infants and children should receive only normal saline because they are at risk for fluid imbalance.

Tap Water. Tap water is hypotonic and exerts a lower osmotic pressure than fluid in interstitial spaces. After infusion into the colon, tap water escapes from the bowel lumen into interstitial spaces. The net movement of water is low. The infused volume stimulates defecation before large amounts of water leave the bowel. Tap water enemas should not be repeated because water toxicity or circulatory overload can develop if large amounts of water are absorbed.

Normal Saline. Physiologically normal saline is the safest solution to use because it exerts the same osmotic pressure as fluids in interstitial spaces surrounding the bowel. The volume of infused saline stimulates peristalsis. Giving saline enemas does not create the danger of excess fluid absorption.

Hypertonic Solutions. Hypertonic solutions infused into the bowel exert osmotic pressure that pulls fluids out of interstitial spaces. The colon fills with fluid, and the resultant distention promotes defecation. Clients unable to tolerate large volumes of fluid benefit most from this type of enema, which is, by design, low volume. Contraindications for this type of enema are clients who are dehydrated and young infants. A hypertonic solution of 120 to 180 ml (4 to 6 oz) is usually effective. The commercially prepared Fleets Enema is the most commonly used.

Soapsuds. Soapsuds may be added to tap water or saline to create the effect of intestinal irritation to stimulate peristalsis. Only pure castile soap is safe, and it comes in a liquid form included in most soapsuds enema kits. Harsh soaps or detergents can cause serious bowel inflammation.

A physician may order a high or low cleansing enema. The terms *high* and *low* refer to the height from which, and hence the pressure with which, the fluid is delivered. High enemas are given to cleanse the entire colon. After the enema is infused, the client is asked to turn from the

Table 45-5   Common Types of Laxatives and Cathartics

Agent/Brand Name	Action	Indications	Risks
Bulk Forming			
Methylcellulose (Cologel, Hydrolose) Psyllium (Metamucil, Naturacil)	High-fiber content absorbs water and increases solid intestinal bulk. Agents stretch intestinal wall to stimulate peristalsis.	Agents are least irritating, most natural, and safest cathartics. Agents are drugs of choice for chronic constipation (e.g., pregnancy, low-residue diet). Agents may also be used to relieve mild, watery diarrhea.	Agents can cause obstruction if not mixed with at least 240 ml of water or juice and swallowed quickly. Caution is used with bulk-forming laxatives that also contain stimulants. Agents are not used in clients for whom large fluid intake is contraindicated.
Emollient or Wetting			
Docusate sodium (Colace, Disonate) Docusate calcium (Surfak) Docusate potassium (Dialose)	Stool softeners are detergents that lower surface tension of feces, allowing water and fat to penetrate. They may increase secretion of water by intestine.	Agents are used for short-term therapy to relieve straining on defecation (e.g., hemorrhoids, perianal surgery, pregnancy, recovery from myocardial infarction).	Agents are of little value for treatment of chronic constipation.
Saline			
Magnesium citrate or citrate of magnesia (Citroma) Magnesium hydroxide (Milk of Magnesia) Sodium phosphate (Fleet Phospho-Soda, Fleet Enema)	Agents contain salt preparation not absorbed by intestines. Osmotic effect increases pressure in bowel to act as stimulant for peristalsis. Agents may also lubricate feces.	Agents are used only for acute emptying of bowel (e.g., endoscopic examination, suspected poisoning, acute constipation).	Agents are not used in long-term management of constipation. Agents are not used in clients with kidney dysfunction (toxic buildup of magnesium). Phosphate salts are not used for clients on fluid restriction.
Stimulant Cathartics			
Bisacodyl (Dulcolax) Castor oil (Neoloid, Purge) Casanthranol (Dialose Plus, Peri-Colace) Danthron (Modane Bulk) Phenolphthalein (Doxidan, Correctol, Ex-Lax)	Agents irritate intestinal mucosa to increase motility. Agents decrease absorption in small bowel and colon. Phenolphthalein and danthron may cause pink or red urine.	Agents may be used to prepare bowel for diagnostic procedures.	Agents may cause severe cramping. Agents are not for long-term use. Chronic use may cause fluid and electrolyte imbalances. Agents are avoided during pregnancy and lactation.
Lubricants			
Mineral oil (Haley's M-O, Petrogalar Plain)	Agents coat fecal contents, allowing easier passage of stool. Agents reduce water absorption in colon.	Agents are used to prevent straining on defecation (e.g., hemorrhoids, perianal surgery).	Agents decrease absorption of fat-soluble vitamins (A, D, E, and K). Agents can cause dangerous form of pneumonia if aspirated into lungs. Mineral oil when taken with emollients can increase risk for fat emboli.

left lateral to the dorsal recumbent, over to the right lateral position. The position change ensures that fluid reaches the large intestine. A low enema cleanses only the rectum and sigmoid colon.

Oil Retention. Oil-retention enemas lubricate the rectum and colon. The feces absorb the oil and become softer and easier to pass. To enhance action of the oil, the client retains the enema for several hours if possible.

Other Types of Enemas. Carminative enemas provide relief from gaseous distention. They improve the ability to pass flatus. An example of a carminative enema is MGW solution, which contains 30 ml of magnesium, 60 ml of glycerin, and 90 ml of water.

Medicated enemas contain drugs. An example is sodium polystyrene sulfonate (Kayexalate), used to treat clients with dangerously high serum potassium levels. This drug contains a resin that exchanges sodium ions for potassium ions in the large intestine. Another medicated enema is neomycin solution, an antibiotic used to reduce bacteria in the colon before bowel surgery.

Enema Administration. The nurse administers enemas in commercially packaged, disposable units or with reusable equipment prepared before use. Sterile technique is unnecessary because the colon normally contains bacteria. However, the nurse wears gloves to prevent the transmission of fecal microorganisms.

The nurse should explain the procedure, including the position to assume, precautions to take to avoid discomfort, and the length of time necessary to retain the solution before defecation. If the client is to receive the enema at home, the nurse explains the procedure to a family member.

Often the physician orders "enemas till clear." This means that the enema is repeated until the client passes fluid that is clear and contains no fecal material. It may be necessary to give as many as three enemas, but the nurse should caution the client against using more than three. Excess enema use seriously depletes fluids and electrolytes. If the enema fails to return a clear solution after three times (check agency policy) or if the client seems to not be tolerating the rigors of repeated enemas, the physician should be notified.

Giving an enema to a client who is unable to contract the external sphincter can pose difficulties. The nurse gives the enema with the client positioned on the bedpan. Giving the enema with the client sitting on the toilet is unsafe because the curved rectal tubing can abrade the rectal wall. Skill 45-1 outlines the steps for an enema administration.

Digital Removal of Stool. For clients with an impaction, the fecal mass may be too large to be passed voluntarily. If enemas fail, the nurse must break up the fecal mass with the fingers and remove it in sections. The procedure can be very uncomfortable for the client. Excess rectal manipulation may cause irritation to the mucosa, bleeding, and stimulation of the vagus nerve, which results in a reflex slowing of the heart rate. Because of the procedure's potential complications, a physician's order is necessary for the nurse to remove a fecal impaction (Box 45-9).

Box 45-9 *Procedural Guidelines*

Digital Removal of Stool

Equipment: Disposable gloves, lubricant, bedpan, towel, washcloth, soap and water, and bedpan.
Delegation considerations: The procedure of digital removal of stool should not be delegated to assistive personnel.

1. Explain the procedure to the client.
2. Take baseline vital signs before the procedure. Help the client lie on the left side with knees flexed and back toward you.
3. Drape the trunk and lower extremities with a bath blanket and place a waterproof pad under the buttocks. Keep a bedpan next to the client.
4. Apply disposable gloves and lubricate the index finger of your dominant hand with lubricating jelly.
5. Gently insert the gloved index finger into the rectum and advance the finger slowly along the rectal wall toward the umbilicus.
6. Gently loosen the fecal mass by massaging around it. Work the finger into the hardened mass.
7. Work the feces downward toward the end of the rectum. Remove small pieces at a time and discard into bedpan.
8. Reassess the client's vital signs and look for signs of fatigue. Stop the procedure if the heart rate drops significantly or the rhythm changes.
9. Continue to remove feces and allow the client to rest at intervals.
10. After completion, wash and dry the buttocks and anal area.
11. Remove bedpan and dispose of feces. Remove gloves by turning them inside out, then discard.
12. Assist client to toilet or clean bedpan if urge to defecate develops.
13. Perform hand hygiene. Record results of removal of impaction by describing fecal characteristics.
14. Follow procedure with enemas or cathartics as ordered by physician.
15. Reassess client's vital signs and level of comfort.

Inserting and Maintaining a Nasogastric Tube. A client's condition or situation may warrant special interventions to decompress the GI tract. Such conditions include surgery (see Chapter 49), infections of the GI tract, trauma to the GI tract, and conditions in which peristalsis is absent.

A nasogastric (NG) tube is a pliable tube that is inserted through the client's nasopharynx into the stomach. The tube has a hollow lumen that allows removal of gastric secretions and introduction of solutions into the stomach. Nasogastric intubation has several purposes (Table 45-6).

The Levin and Salem sump tubes are the most common for stomach decompression. The Levin tube is a single-lumen tube with holes near the tip. It may be connected to a drainage bag or to an intermittent suction device to drain stomach secretions.

Text continued on p. 1402

Skill 45-1   *Administering a Cleansing Enema*

Delegation Considerations

The skill of administering an enema can be delegated to assistive personnel (AP). It is the nurse's responsibility to assess client for specific considerations such as need for alternative positioning, comfort, and stable vital signs before procedure. In addition, it is the nurse's responsibility to determine client's response to the enema.

- Inform and assist caregiver in proper way to position clients who have mobility restrictions, such as those clients with arthritis or severe fatigue.
- Instruct AP how to position clients who also have therapeutic equipment present, such as drains, intravenous catheters, or traction.
- Instruct AP in the specific signs and symptoms of client not tolerating the procedure and when it must be stopped. For example, these signs and symptoms may include abdominal pain more than a pressure sensation, abdominal cramping, abdominal distention, or rectal bleeding.

Equipment

- Disposable gloves
- Water-soluble lubricant
- Waterproof, absorbent pads
- Bath blanket
- Toilet tissue
- Bedpan, bedside commode, or access to toilet
- Washbasin, washcloths, towel, and soap
- Intravenous (IV) pole
- Enema bag administration
  - Enema container
  - Tubing and clamp (if not already attached to container)
  - Appropriate size rectal tube:
    - *Adult:* 22 to 30 Fr
    - *Child:* 12 to 18 Fr
  - Correct volume of warmed solution:
    - *Adult:* 750 to 1000 ml
    - *Child:*
      150 to 250 ml, infant
      250 to 350 ml, toddler
      300 to 500 ml, school-age child
      500 to 750 ml, adolescent
  - Prepackaged enema
- Prepackaged enema container with rectal tip

Steps	Rationale
1. Assess status of client: last bowel movement, normal bowel patterns, hemorrhoids, mobility, external sphincter control, and abdominal pain.	Determines factors indicating need for enema and influencing the type of enema used.
2. Assess for presence of increased intracranial pressure, glaucoma, or recent rectal or prostate surgery.	Conditions contraindicate use of enemas.
3. Check client's medical record to clarify the rationale for the enema.	Determines purpose of enema administration: preparation for special procedure or relief of constipation.
4. Review physician's order for enema.	Order by physician is required. Determines number and type of enema to be given.
5. Determine client's level of understanding of purpose of enema.	Allows nurse to plan for appropriate teaching measures.
6. Perform hand hygiene. Collect appropriate equipment.	Reduces transmission of microorganisms.
7. Correctly identify client and explain procedure.	Information promotes client cooperation and reduces anxiety.
8. Assemble enema bag with appropriate solution and rectal tube.	
9. Apply gloves.	Reduces transmission of microorganisms.
10. Provide privacy by closing curtains around bed or closing door.	Reduces embarrassment for client.
11. Raise bed to appropriate working height for nurse: raise side rail on client's left.	Promotes good body mechanics and client safety.
12. Assist client into left side-lying (Sims') position with right knee flexed. Children may also be placed in dorsal recumbent position.	Allows enema solution to flow downward by gravity along natural curve of sigmoid colon and rectum, thus improving retention of solution.

Critical Decision Point: If client is suspected of having poor sphincter control, position in dorsal recumbent position on bedpan. Client will have difficulty retaining enema solution.

13. Place waterproof pad under hips and buttocks.	Prevents soiling of linen.

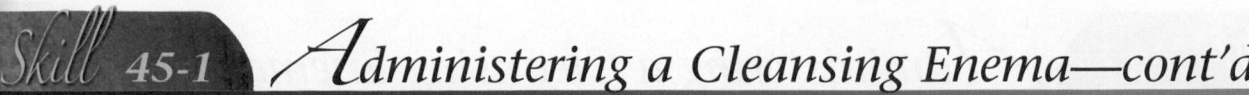

Skill 45-1 *Administering a Cleansing Enema—cont'd*

Steps	Rationale
14. Cover client with bath blanket, exposing only rectal area, clearly visualizing anus.	Provides warmth, reduces exposure of body parts, and allows client to feel more relaxed and comfortable.
15. Place bedpan or commode in easily accessible position. If client will be expelling contents in toilet, ensure that toilet is free. (If client will be getting up to bathroom to expel enema, place client's slippers and bathrobe in easily accessible position.)	Used in case client is unable to retain enema solution.
16. Administer enema:	
A. Enema bag	
(1) Add warmed solution to enema bag: warm tap water as it flows from faucet, place saline container in basin of hot water before adding saline to enema bag, check temperature of solution by pouring small amount of solution over inner wrist.	Hot water can burn intestinal mucosa. Cold water can cause abdominal cramping and is difficult to retain.
(2) Raise container, release clamp, and allow solution to flow long enough to fill tubing.	Removes air from tubing.
(3) Reclamp tubing.	Prevents further loss of solution.
(4) Lubricate 6 to 8 cm (2½ to 3 inches) of tip of rectal tube with lubricating jelly.	Allows smooth insertion of rectal tube without risk of irritation or trauma to mucosa.
(5) Gently separate buttocks and locate anus. Instruct client to relax by breathing out slowly through mouth.	Breathing out promotes relaxation of external anal sphincter.

(6) Insert tip of rectal tube slowly by pointing tip in direction of client's umbilicus (see illustration). Length of insertion varies:
   Adult: 7.5 to 10 cm (3 to 4 inches)
   Child: 5 to 7.5 cm (2 to 3 inches)
   Infant: 2.5 to 3.75 cm (1 to 1½ inches)
	Careful insertion prevents trauma to rectal mucosa from accidental lodging of tube against rectal wall. Insertion beyond proper limit can cause bowel perforation.

Critical Decision Point: If tube does not pass easily, do not force. Consider allowing a small amount of fluid to infuse and then try reinserting tube slowly.

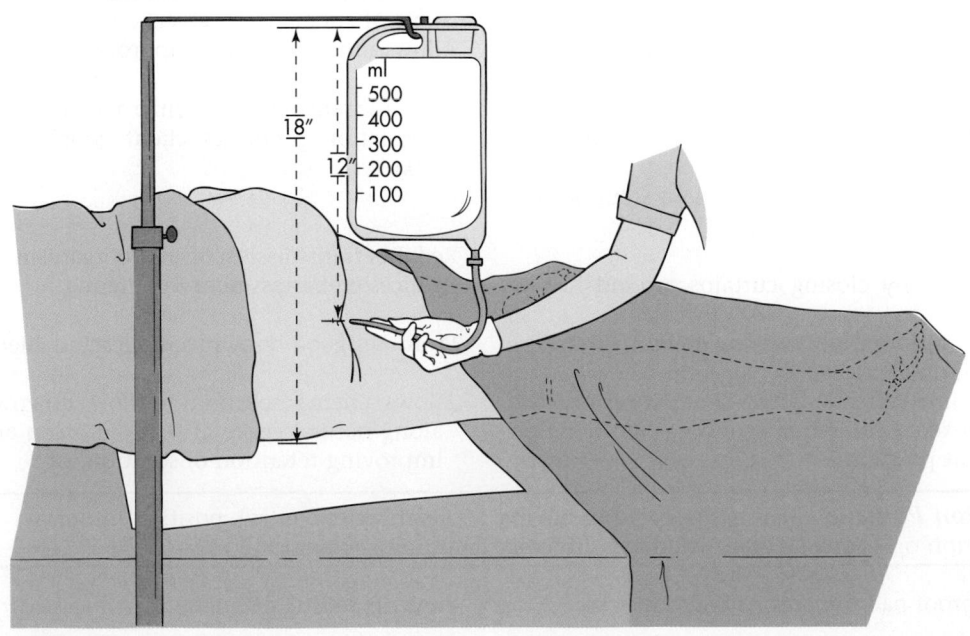

STEP **16A(6)**   Insertion of a rectal tube into rectum

Steps	Rationale
(7) Hold tubing in rectum constantly until end of fluid instillation.	Bowel contraction can cause expulsion of rectal tube.
(8) Open regulating clamp and allow solution to enter slowly with container at client's hip level.	Rapid instillation can stimulate evacuation of rectal tube.
(9) Raise height of enema container slowly to appropriate level above anus: 30 to 45 cm (12 to 18 inches) for high enema, 30 cm (12 inches) for regular enema, 7.5 cm (3 inches) for low enema (see illustration for step 16A[6]). Instillation time varies with the volume of solution administered.	Allows for continuous, slow instillation of solution. Raising container too high causes rapid instillation and possible painful distention of colon. High pressure can cause rupture of bowel in infant.
(10) Lower container or clamp tubing if client complains of cramping or if fluid escapes around rectal tube.	Temporary cessation of instillation prevents cramping, which may prevent client from retaining all fluid, altering effectiveness of enema.
(11) Clamp tubing after all solution is instilled.	Prevents entrance of air into rectum.
B. **Prepackaged disposable container**	
(1) Remove plastic cap from rectal tip. Tip is already lubricated, but more jelly can be applied as needed.	Lubrication provides for smooth insertion of rectal tube without causing rectal irritation or trauma.
(2) Gently separate buttocks and locate rectum. Instruct client to relax by breathing out slowly through mouth.	Breathing out promotes relaxation of external rectal sphincter.
(3) Insert tip of bottle gently into rectum: *Adult:* 7.5 to 10 cm (3 to 4 inches) *Child:* 5 to 7.5 cm (2 to 3 inches) *Infant:* 2.5 to 3.75 cm (1 to 1½ inch)	Gentle insertion prevents trauma to rectal mucosa.
(4) Squeeze bottle until all of solution has entered rectum and colon. Instruct client to retain solution until the urge to defecate occurs, usually 2 to 5 minutes.	Hypertonic solutions require only small volumes to stimulate defecation.
17. Place layers of toilet tissue around tube at anus and gently withdraw rectal tube.	Provides client's comfort and cleanliness.
18. Explain to client that feeling of distention is normal. Ask client to retain solution as long as possible while lying quietly in bed. (For infant or young child, gently hold buttocks together for a few minutes.)	Solution distends bowel. Length of retention varies with type of enema and client's ability to contract rectal sphincter. Longer retention promotes more effective stimulation of peristalsis and defecation.
19. Discard enema container and tubing in proper receptacle or rinse out thoroughly with warm soap and water if container is to be reused.	Reduces transmission and growth of microorganisms.
20. Assist client to bathroom or help to position client on bedpan.	Normal squatting position promotes defecation.
21. Observe character of feces and solution (caution client against flushing toilet before inspection).	Determines efficacy of enema.

Critical Decision Point: When enemas are ordered "until clear," observe contents of solution passed. Return is "clear" when no solid fecal material exists, but solution may be colored.

22. Assist client as needed to wash anal area with warm soap and water (if nurse administers perineal care, use gloves).	Fecal contents can irritate skin. Hygiene promotes client's comfort.
23. Remove and discard gloves and perform hand hygiene.	Reduces transmission of microorganisms.
24. Inspect color, consistency, amount of stool, and fluid passed.	Determines if stool is evacuated or fluid is retained. Note abnormalities such as presence of blood or mucus.
25. Assess condition of abdomen; cramping, rigidity, or distention can indicate a serious problem.	Determines if distention is relieved. Excess volume can distend or perforate the bowel.

Skill 45-1   *Administering a Cleansing Enema—cont'd*

Unexpected Outcomes and Related Interventions

1. Abdomen becomes rigid and distended.
   a. Stop enema if fluid is still being instilled.
   b. Notify physician and obtain vital signs.
2. Abdominal pain or cramping develops.
   a. Slow rate of instillation.
3. Bleeding occurs.
   a. Stop enema administration
   b. Notify physician and obtain vital signs.

Recording and Reporting

- Record type and volume of enema given and characteristics of results.
- Report failure of client to defecate to physician.

Home Care Considerations

- For clients who require enemas for bowel preparation at home, instruct family not to exceed recommended fluid volume levels or number of enemas. Encourage family about the need for slow administration of warmed fluid.
- Instruct family about the negative side effects of tap water enemas.

Table 45-6	Purposes of Nasogastric Intubation	
Purpose	**Description**	**Type of Tube**
Decompression	Removal of secretions and gaseous substances from gastrointestinal tract; prevention or relief of abdominal distention	Salem sump, Levin, Miller-Abbott
Feeding (gavage) (see Chapter 43)	Instillation of liquid nutritional supplements or feedings into stomach for clients unable to swallow fluid	Duo, Dobhoff, Levin
Compression	Internal application of pressure by means of inflated balloon to prevent internal esophageal or gastrointestinal hemorrhage	Sengstaken-Blakemore
Lavage	Irrigation of stomach in cases of active bleeding, poisoning, or gastric dilation	Levin, Ewald, Salem sump

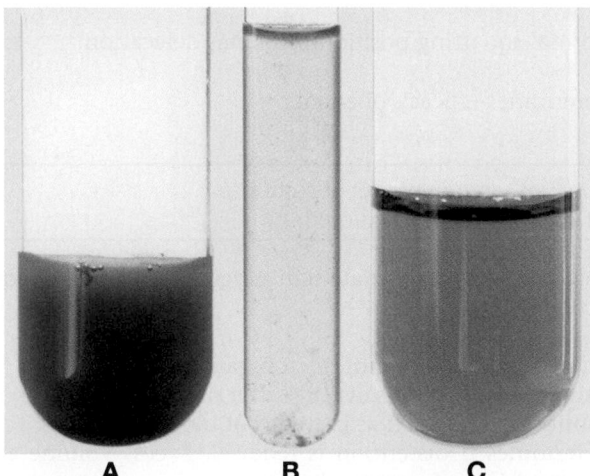

FIGURE **45–15** Gastric contents. **A,** Stomach. **B,** Stomach. **C,** Intestinal. (Courtesy Dr. Norma Metheny, St. Louis University, School of Nursing.)

The Salem sump tube is preferable for stomach decompression. The tube has two lumina: one for removal of gastric contents (Figure 45-15) and one to provide an air vent. A blue "pigtail" is the air vent that connects with the second lumen. When the sump tube's main lumen is connected to suction, the air vent permits free, continuous drainage of secretions. The air vent should never be clamped off, connected to suction, or used for irrigation.

Nasogastric tube insertion (Skill 45-2) does not require sterile technique. The nurse simply uses clean technique. The procedure is uncomfortable. The client experiences a burning sensation as the tube passes through the sensitive nasal mucosa. When the tube reaches the back of the pharynx, the client may begin to gag. The nurse must help the client relax to make tube insertion easier. Some institutions allow xylocaine jelly to be used when inserting the tube as it increases client comfort during the procedure.

One of the greatest problems in caring for a client with an NG tube is maintaining comfort. The tube is a constant irritation to nasal mucosa. The nurse must assess the condition of the nares and mucosa for inflammation and **excoriation.** The tape used to anchor the tube

Text continued on p. 1409

Skill 45-2   *Inserting and Maintaining a Nasogastric Tube*   View Video

Delegation Considerations

The skill of inserting and maintaining the nasogastric (NG) tube should not be delegated to assistive personnel (AP). The nurse is responsible for the proper function and drainage of the nasogastric tube, all relevant assessments, and determining the client's level of comfort. The nurse may instruct AP to do the following:

- Measure and record the drainage
- Provide oral and nasal hygiene
- Perform selected comfort measures

Equipment

- No. 14 or no. 16 Fr NG tube (smaller-lumen catheters are not used for decompression in adults because they must be able to remove thick secretions)
- Water-soluble lubricating jelly
- pH test strips (measure gastric aspirate acidity)

- Tongue blade
- Flashlight
- Emesis basin
- Asepto bulb or catheter-tipped syringe
- 1-inch (2.5-cm) wide hypoallergenic tape (3-4 inches long) or commercial fixation device
- Safety pin and rubber band
- Clamp, drainage bag, or suction machine or pressure gauge if wall suction is to be used
- Towel
- Glass of water with straw
- Facial tissues
- Normal saline
- Tincture of benzoin (optional)
- Suction equipment
- Disposable gloves

Steps	Rationale
1. Perform hand hygiene. Inspect condition of client's nasal and oral cavity.	Baseline condition of nasal and oral cavity determines need for special nursing measures for oral hygiene after tube placement.
2. Ask if client has had history of nasal surgery and note if deviated nasal septum is present.	Nurse should insert tube into uninvolved nasal passage. Procedure may be contraindicated if surgery is recent.
3. Palpate client's abdomen for distention, pain, and rigidity. Auscultate for bowel sounds.	Baseline determination of level of abdominal distention later serves as comparison once tube is inserted.
4. Assess client's level of consciousness and ability to follow instructions.	Determines client's ability to assist in procedure.

Critical Decision Point: If client is confused, disoriented, or unable to follow commands, obtain assistance from another staff member to insert the tube.

Steps	Rationale
5. Check medical record for physician's order, type of NG tube to be placed, and whether tube is to be attached to suction or drainage bag.	Procedure requires physician's order. Adequate decompression depends on NG suction.
6. Perform hand hygiene. Prepare equipment at the bedside. Cut a piece of tape about 4 inches (10 cm) long and split one end in half to form a V, or have NG tube fixator device available.	Reduces transmission of infection. Ensures well-organized procedure. Tape or fixator device will be used to hold the tube in place after insertions.
7. Identify client and explain procedure.	Identification prevents error of placing tube in wrong client. Explanation gains client's cooperation and lessens possibility that client will remove tube.
8. Apply disposable gloves.	Reduces transmission of microorganisms.
9. Position client in high-Fowler's position with pillows behind head and shoulders. Raise bed to a horizontal level comfortable for the nurse.	Promotes client's ability to swallow during procedure. Good body mechanics prevent injury to nurse or client.
10. Place bath towel over client's chest; give facial tissues to client. Place emesis basin within reach.	Prevents soiling of client's gown. Tube insertion through nasal passages may cause tearing and coughing with increased salivation.
11. Pull curtain around the bed or close room door.	Provides privacy.
12. Stand on client's right side if right-handed, left side if left-handed.	Allows easiest manipulation of tubing.
13. Instruct client to relax and breathe normally while occluding one naris. Then repeat this action for other naris. Select nostril with greater air flow.	Tube passes more easily through naris that is more patent.

*I*nserting and Maintaining a Nasogastric Tube—cont'd

Skill 45-2

Steps	Rationale

14. Measure distance to insert tube:
   a. Measure distance from tip of nose to earlobe to xiphoid process (see illustration).
   b. First mark 50-cm point on tube, then do traditional measurement. Tube insertion should be to midway point between 50 cm (20 inches) and traditional mark.
	Approximates distance from naris to stomach. tube should extend from naris to stomach; distance varies with each client.

15. Mark length of tube to be inserted with small piece of tape placed so it can easily be removed.	Marks length of tube to be inserted from nares to stomach.
16. Curve 10 to 15 cm (4 to 6 inches) of end of tube tightly around index finger, then release.	Curving tube tip aids insertion and decreases stiffness of tube.
17. Lubricate 7.5 to 10 cm (3 to 4 inches) of end of tube with water-soluble lubricating jelly.	Minimizes friction against nasal mucosa and aids insertion of tube.
18. Alert client that procedure is to begin.	Decreases client anxiety and increases client cooperation.
19. Initially instruct client to extend neck back against pillow; insert tube gently and slowly through nares with curved end pointing downward (see illustration).	Facilitates initial passage of tube through naris and maintains clear airway for open naris.
20. Insert tube slowly through naris with curved end pointing downward. Continue to insert tube along floor of nasal passage aiming down toward client's ear. If resistance is met, apply gentle downward pressure to advance tube. (Do not force past resistance).	Minimizes discomfort of tube rubbing against upper nasal turbinates. Resistance is caused by posterior nasopharynx. Downward pressure helps tube curl around corner of nasopharynx.
21. If resistance is met, try to rotate the tube and see if it advances. If still resistant, withdraw tube, allow client to rest, relubricate tube, and insert into other naris.	Forcing against resistance can cause trauma to mucosa. Helps relieve client's anxiety.

Critical Decision Point: If unable to insert tube in either naris, stop procedure and notify physician.

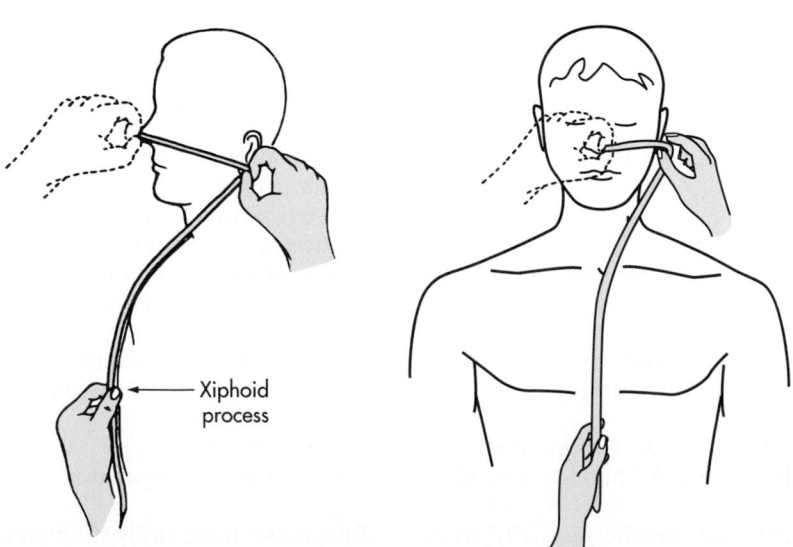

STEP **14a**   Technique for measuring distance to insert NG tube.

Steps	Rationale
22. Continue insertion of tube until just past nasopharynx by gently rotating tube toward opposite naris.	Helps prevent coiling of tube in oropharynx.
a. Stop tube advancement, allow client to relax, and provide tissues.	Relieves client's anxiety; tearing is natural response to mucosal irritation, and excessive salivation may occur because of oral stimulation.
b. Explain to client that next step requires that client swallow. Give client glass of water unless contraindicated.	Sipping of water aids passage of NG tube into esophagus.
23. With tube just above oropharynx, instruct client to flex head forward, take a small sip of water, and swallow. Advance tube 2.5 to 5 cm (1 to 2 inches) with each swallow of water. If client is not allowed fluids, instruct to dry swallow or suck air through straw.	Flexed position closes off upper airway to trachea and opens esophagus. Swallowing closes epiglottis over trachea and helps move the tube into the esophagus. Swallowing water reduces gagging or choking. Water can be removed later from stomach by suction.
24. If client begins to cough, gag, or choke, withdraw tube slightly (do not remove the tube) and stop tube advancement. Instruct client to breathe easily and take sips of water.	Tube may be displaced into larynx and produce coughing. Swallowing water closes epiglottis over trachea and helps move the tube into the esophagus. Risk for aspiration increases if vomiting occurs.

Critical Decision Point: If vomiting occurs, assist client in clearing airway; oral suctioning may be needed. Do not proceed until airway is cleared.

Steps	Rationale
25. If client continues to gag and cough or complains that tube feels as though it is coiling in the back of throat, check back of oropharynx using tongue blade. If tube has coiled, withdraw it until the tip is back in the oropharynx. Then reinsert with client swallowing.	Tube may coil around itself in the back of the throat and stimulate the gag reflex.
26. Continue to advance tube with swallowing until tape or mark is reached. Temporarily anchor tube to client's cheek with a piece of tape until tube placement is checked.	Tip of tube must be well within stomach for adequate decompression. Tube should be anchored before placement if verified.
27. Verify tube placement. Check agency policy for preferred methods for checking NG tube placement.	
a. Ask client to talk.	Inability to speak can indicate that tube is through client's vocal cords into the lungs.
b. Inspect posterior pharynx for presence of coiled tube.	Tube is pliable and can coil up in back of pharynx instead of advancing into esophagus.
c. Aspirate gently back on syringe to obtain gastric contents, observing color.	Gastric contents are usually cloudy and green, but may be off-white, tan, bloody, or brown in color. Aspiration of contents provides means to measure fluid pH and thus determine tube tip placement in gastrointestinal tract (see Figure 45-14). Other common aspirate colors include the following: duodenal placement (yellow or bile stained), esophagus (may or may not have saliva-appearing aspirate).

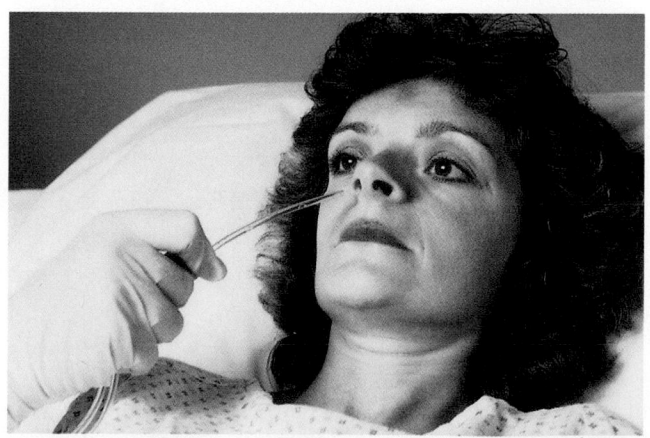

STEP **19**   Insert NG tube with curved end pointing downward.

*I*nserting and Maintaining a Nasogastric Tube—cont'd

Steps	Rationale
d. Measure pH of aspirate with color-coded pH paper with range of whole numbers 1 to 11 (see illustration).	Gastric aspirates have decidedly acidic pH values, preferably 4 or less, compared with intestinal aspirates, which are usually greater than 4, or respiratory secretions, which are usually greater than 5.5 (Metheny and others, 1993, 1994, 1998; Metheny and Titler, 2001).
e. Have ordered x-ray examination performed of chest/abdomen.	Placement of tube can be reliably verified by x-ray exam.

Critical Decision Point: Be sure to use gastric (Gastrocult) pH test and not Hemoccult test.

f. If tube is not in stomach, advance another 2.5 to 5 cm (1 to 2 inches) and repeat steps 27b, c, and d to check tube position.	Tube must be in stomach to provide decompression.
28. Anchoring tube:	
a. After tube is properly inserted and positioned, either clamp end or connect it to drainage bag or suction machine.	Drainage bag is used for gravity drainage. Intermittent suction, low suction, is most effective for decompression. Client going to the operating room often has tube clamped.
b. Tape tube to nose; avoid putting pressure on nares.	Prevents tissue necrosis. Tape anchors tube securely.
(1) Before taping tube to nose, apply small amount of tincture of benzoin to lower end of nose and allow to dry (optional). Be sure top end of tape over nose is secure.	Benzoin prevents loosening of tape if client perspires.
(2) Carefully wrap two split ends of tape around tube (see illustration).	
(3) Alternative: Apply tube fixation device using shaped adhesive patch (see illustration).	

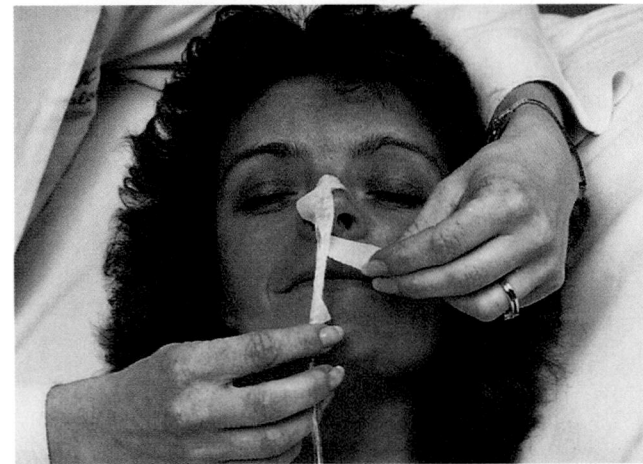

STEP **28b(2)**   Tape is crossed over and around NG tube.

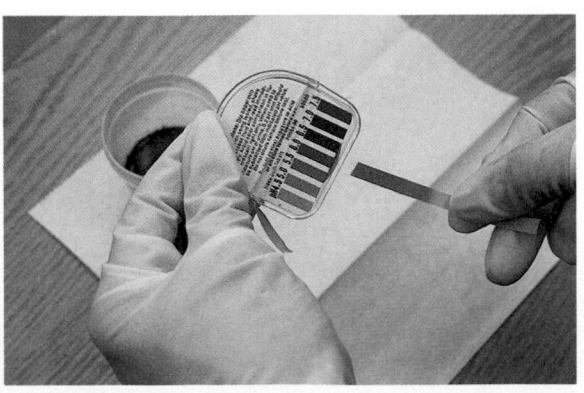

STEP **27d**   Checking pH of gastric aspirate.

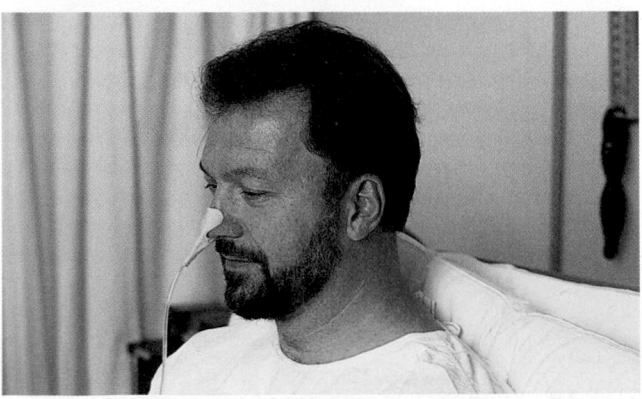

STEP **28b(3)**   Client with tube fixation device.

Steps	Rationale

c. Fasten end of NG tube to client's gown by looping rubber band around tube in slip knot. Pin rubber band to gown (provides slack for movement).

Reduces pressure on the nares if tube moves.

d. Unless physician orders otherwise, head of bed should be elevated 30 degrees.

Helps prevent esophageal reflux and minimizes irritation of tube against posterior pharynx.

e. Explain to client that sensation of tube should decrease somewhat with time.

Adaptation to continued sensory stimulus.

f. Remove gloves and wash hands.

Reduces transmission of microorganisms.

29. Once placement is confirmed:

a. Place a mark, either a red mark or tape, on the tube to indicate where the tube exists in the nose.

The mark or tube length is to be used as a guide to indicate whether displacement may have occurred.

b. Measurement of the tube length from nares to connector is an alternate method.

c. Document the tube length in the client record.

30. Tube irrigation:

a. Wash hands and apply gloves.

Reduces transmission of microorganisms.

b. Check for tube placement in stomach (see step 27). Reconnect NG tube to connecting tube.

Prevents accidental entrance of irrigating solution into lungs.

c. Draw up 30 ml of normal saline into Asepto or catheter-tipped syringe.

Use of saline minimizes loss of electrolytes from stomach fluids.

d. Clamp NG tube. Disconnect from connection tubing and lay end of connection tubing on towel.

Reduces soiling of client's gown and bed linen.

e. Insert tip of irrigating syringe into end of NG tube. Remove clamp. Hold syringe with tip pointed at floor and inject saline slowly and evenly. Do not force solution.

Position of syringe prevents introduction of air into vent tubing, which could cause gastric distention. Solution introduced under pressure can cause gastric trauma.

Critical Decision Point: Do not introduce saline through blue colored "pigtail" air vent of Salem sump tube.

---

f. If resistance occurs, check for kinks in tubing. Turn client onto left side. Repeated resistance should be reported to the physician.

Tip of tube may lie against stomach lining. Repositioning on left side may dislodge tube away from the stomach lining. Buildup of secretions will cause distention.

g. After instilling saline, immediately aspirate or pull back slowly on syringe to withdraw fluid. If amount aspirated is greater than amount instilled, record the difference as output. If amount aspirated is less than amount instilled, record the difference as intake.

Irrigation clears tubing, so stomach should remain empty. Fluid remaining in stomach is measured as intake.

h. Reconnect NG tube to drainage or suction. (If solution does not return, repeat irrigation.)

Reestablishes drainage collection; may repeat irrigation or repositioning of tube until NG tube drains properly.

i. Remove gloves and perform hand hygiene.

Reduces transmission of microorganisms.

31. Discontinuation of NG tube:

a. Verify order to discontinue NG tube.

Physician's order required for procedure.

b. Explain procedure to client and reassure that removal is less distressing than insertion.

Minimizes anxiety and increases cooperation. Tube passes out smoothly.

c. Wash hands and apply disposable gloves.

Reduces transmission of microorganisms.

d. Turn off suction and disconnect NG tube from drainage bag or suction. Remove tape from bridge of nose and unpin tube from gown.

Have tube free of connections before removal.

e. Stand on client's right side if right-handed, left side if left-handed.

Allows easiest manipulation of tube.

f. Hand the client facial tissue; place clean towel across chest. Instruct client to take and hold a deep breath.

Client may wish to blow nose after tube is removed. Towel may keep gown from getting soiled. Airway will be temporarily obstructed during tube removal.

g. Clamp or kink tubing securely and then pull tube out steadily and smoothly into towel held in other hand while client holds breath.

Clamping prevents tube contents from draining into oropharynx. Reduces trauma to mucosa and minimizes client's discomfort. Towel covers tube, which can be an unpleasant sight. Holding breath helps to prevent aspiration.

Skill 45-2   *Inserting and Maintaining a Nasogastric Tube—cont'd*

Steps	Rationale
h. Measure amount of drainage and note character of contents. Dispose of tube and drainage equipment into proper container.	Provides accurate measure of fluid output. Reduces transfer of microorganisms.
i. Clean nares and provide mouth care.	Promotes comfort.
j. Position client comfortably and explain procedure for drinking fluids, if not contraindicated.	Depends on physician's order. Sometimes clients are allowed nothing by mouth (NPO) for up to 24 hours. When fluids are allowed, the order usually begins with a small amount of ice chips each hour and increases as client is able to tolerate more.
32. Clean equipment and return to proper place. Place soiled linen in utility room or proper receptacle.	Proper disposal of equipment prevents spread of microorganisms and ensures proper exchange procedures.
33. Remove gloves and perform hand hygiene.	Reduces transmission of microorganisms.
34. Observe amount and character of contents draining from NG tube. Ask if client feels nauseated.	Determines if tube is decompressing stomach of contents.
35. Palpate client's abdomen periodically, noting any distention, pain, and rigidity and auscultate for the presence of bowel sounds. Turn off suction while auscultating.	Determines success of abdominal decompression and the return of peristalsis. The sound of the suction apparatus may be transmitted to abdomen and be misinterpreted as bowel sounds.
36. Inspect condition of nares and nose.	Evaluates onset of skin and tissue irritation.
37. Observe position of tubing.	Determines if tension is being applied to nasal structures.
38. Ask if client feels sore throat or irritation in pharynx.	Evaluates level of client's discomfort.

Unexpected Outcomes and Related Interventions

1. Client's abdomen becomes distended and/or painful.
   a. Assess patency of tube and irrigate as needed.
2. Client complains of sore throat from dry, irritated mucous membranes.
   a. Increase frequency of oral hygiene.
   b. Ask physician if client may suck on ice chips, throat lozenges.
3. Client develops irritation of skin around naris.
   a. Provide skin care to naris.
   b. Retape so tube does not press against naris.
   c. Consider switching tube to other naris.
4. Client develops signs of pulmonary aspiration: fever, shortness of breath, pulmonary congestion.
   a. Perform respiratory assessment.
   b. Notify physician.
   c. Obtain chest x-ray examination as ordered.

Recording and Reporting

- Record in nurses' notes time and type of NG tube inserted, client's tolerance of procedure, confirmation of placement, character of gastric contents, pH value, whether tube is clamped or connected to drainage device, and amount of suction applied.
- Record in nurses' notes and/or flow sheet amount and character of contents draining from NG tube every shift, unless ordered more frequently by physician.

often becomes soiled. The nurse changes it every day to lessen irritation. Frequent lubrication of the nares also minimizes excoriation. With one nares occluded, the client may breathe through the mouth. Frequent mouth care (at least every 2 hours) helps minimize dehydration. A glass of cool water for rinsing is useful, but the client who is allowed nothing by mouth (NPO) should not swallow the water. The client will frequently complain of a sore throat. An ice bag applied externally to the throat may help. Gargling with topical xylocaine jelly and/or lozenges may be used if ordered by the physician.

After the tube is inserted, the nurse must maintain its patency. If the tip of the tubing rests against the stomach wall or if the tube becomes blocked with thick secretions, regular irrigation is necessary. Flushing the tube with normal saline by way of a catheter-tipped syringe clears blockage within the tube (see Skill 45-2, p. 1403). If an NG tube continues to drain improperly after irrigation, the nurse must reposition it by advancing or withdrawing it slightly. Any change in tube position requires the nurse to verify the placement of the tube in the client's GI tract (see Skill 45-2, p. 1403).

The NG tube can cause distention. The presence of the tube causes many clients to swallow large volumes of air. Channels of gastric secretions also form along the walls of the stomach and bypass the suction holes. Turning the client regularly helps to collapse the channels and promotes emptying of stomach contents.

Continuing and Restorative Care. As the client recovers and is able to return home or to an extended care facility, regular elimination patterns must begin. When clients have a colostomy they must learn to care for the ostomy. Other clients may require bowel retraining. It is important to remember that ostomy care and bowel retraining may be initiated or take place in the acute care settings as well. However, because these are long-term care needs, these activities are usually completed in the restorative care settings.

Care of Ostomies. Clients with temporary or permanent bowel diversions have unique elimination needs. Persons with an ostomy wear a pouch or appliance to collect effluent from the stomas (Hyland, 2002). The stool discharged from an ostomy is called **effluent,** and that term will be used throughout this section. These client's must use meticulous skin care to prevent liquid stool from irritating the skin around the stoma (Box 45-10).

Irrigating a Colostomy. Although this practice is not as common as it once was, some clients may be instructed to irrigate their left-sided colostomies in order to regulate colon emptying. Other clients do not want to spend the additional 60 to 90 minutes in the bathroom every day, so they empty their pouch as necessary (Hyland, 2002). Only a colostomy can be irrigated.

Specific equipment for irrigating a colostomy should be used. An enema set should ***never*** be used to irrigate a colostomy. A special cone-tipped irrigator (Figure 45-16) is used. This device prevents bowel penetration and prevents backflow of the irrigating solution. Clients usually sit on the toilet and place an irrigating sleeve over the stoma. The

---

Box 45-10

Client Teaching

Stomal Care (Incontinent Ostomy)

Objective

- Client will demonstrate the correct procedure for stomal care.

Teaching Strategies

- Teach the client that the drainage from the stoma is very irritating to the skin and contact of the skin with the drainage should be avoided. However, when contact does occur the client should cleanse the area as soon a possible.
- Show client how to inspect the appearance of the skin and surrounding stoma. The stoma should be moist, shiny, and pink (Hyland, 2002). Bleeding should be minimal. The skin around the stoma, called the peristomal area, should be normal skin tone.
- Skin surrounding the stoma should be cleansed with mild soap and water or even plain water (Hyland, 2002). The client must also dry the area thoroughly.
- Instruct client to avoid the use of creams, ointments, or baby wipes or other moist towelettes on peristomal skin, as these agents can prevent the pouch from adhering securely on the client's skin (Hyland, 2002).
- Instruct client to report excess bleeding or prolonged oozing to the nurse or physician.
- Demonstrate to client how to select and apply a skin barrier and pouch; also instruct client regarding length of wear.
- Demonstrate to client how to empty and change the pouching system.
- Instruct client how to reduce odor and what commercial agents to use.
- Assist client in determining what ostomy supplies should be carried at all times. Provide client and family with a list of resources to obtain supplies in the community.
- Instruct the client that if a yeast infection occurs, perform thorough cleansing, followed by patting the area dry and applying a prescribed topical agent, such as triamcinolone acetonide (Kenalog) spray or nystatin (Mycostatin), to the affected region.

Evaluation

- Client will correctly state skin care procedures.
- Client will correctly perform stoma skin care procedure.

---

end of this sleeve extends into the bowl of the commode. The physician orders the amount and type of solution. For adults, the amount ranges from 500 to 700 ml of tap water. The solution is instilled slowly through the lubricated cone tip. Irrigation should take 5 to 10 minutes. The client then removes the cone tip and waits 30 to 45 minutes for the solution and feces to drain out of the irrigation sleeve. Once the drainage stops, the client applies a stoma cap or a pouch. If a client chooses to irrigate the colostomy, the time of irrigation is individualized to the client's lifestyle.

Pouching Ostomies. Ostomies require a pouch to collect fecal material. An effective pouching system protects

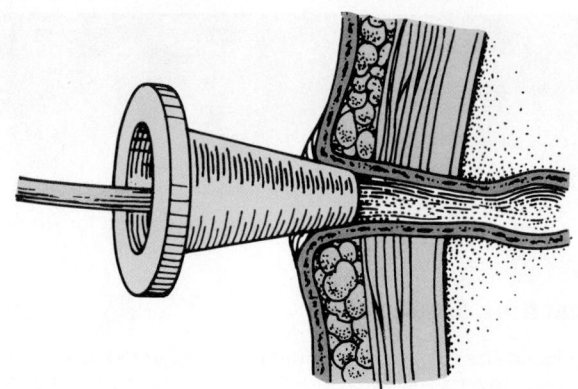

FIGURE **45–16**   Ostomy irrigation cone inserted into stoma.

the skin, contains fecal material, remains odor free, and is comfortable and inconspicuous. A person wearing a pouch should feel secure in participating in any activity.

Many pouching systems are available. To ensure that a pouch fits well and meets the client's needs, the nurse considers the location of the ostomy, type and size of the stoma, type and amount of ostomy drainage, size and contour of the abdomen, condition of the skin around the stoma, physical activities of the client, client's personal preference, age and dexterity, and cost of equipment. An **enterostomal therapist (ET)** is a nurse trained to care for ostomy clients. The staff nurse collaborates with the ET to be sure the correct pouching system is used. For example, referral to an ET nurse would be appropriate to plan the care of a client who has a high-output ostomy that requires a pouch modification.

A pouching system consists of a pouch and skin barrier. Some pouching systems, such as Squibb-ConvaTec, Hollister, Coloplast, and Smith & Nephew, are attached to the client's skin from the product's adhesive surface, whereas other pouching systems, such as VIP, are nonadhesive systems. Pouches come in one- and two-piece systems that are disposable or reusable. Some pouches have the opening precut by the manufacturer; others require the stoma opening to be custom cut by someone to the client's specific stoma size.

Skin barriers include wafers, pastes, powders, and liquid film that are applied to the skin around the stoma. Some wafer skin barriers are permanently attached to the ostomy pouch. These are called one-piece pouch systems. In a two-piece system, the pouch can be detached from the skin barrier for emptying or changing. This allows the skin barrier to remain around the client's stoma for several days, thus minimizing the chance of skin damage from too-frequent removal of the skin barrier from the peristomal skin. When using a two-piece pouching system, it is important to remember that the skin barrier and pouch must be the same corresponding size and from the same manufacturer. The pouch from one manufacturer will not fit correctly on the skin barrier from another manufacturer. The nurse must be sure to use an ostomy pouch made for collecting fecal matter (colostomy or ileostomy) and not one for collecting urine.

It is important to measure the stoma size carefully when selecting and cutting out the opening on the wafer skin barrier. A good skin barrier protects the skin, prevents irritation from repeated removal of the pouch, and is comfortable for the client to wear. Skill 45-3 describes steps for applying one type of pouch system.

Nutritional Considerations for Clients With Ostomies. Nutritional therapy is important for clients with ostomies. During the first weeks after surgery, many physicians recommend low-fiber diets, particularly for ileostomy clients because the small bowel requires time to adapt to the diversion. Low-fiber foods include bread, noodles, rice, cream cheese, eggs (not fried), strained fruit juices, lean meats, fish, and poultry. As ostomies heal, clients can eat almost any food. High-fiber foods such as fresh fruits and vegetables help ensure a more solid stool needed to achieve success at irrigation. Blockage must be avoided. The stoma's surgical construction can affect the likelihood of blockage.

Clients with an ileostomy should eat slowly and chew food completely. Drinking 10 to 12 glasses of water daily also prevents blockage. High-fiber foods that may cause problems include stringy meats, mushrooms, popcorn, fruits such as cherries, and some seafood such as shrimp and crab. Ostomy clients may benefit from avoiding foods that cause gas and odor, including broccoli, cauliflower, dried beans, and Brussels sprouts.

Bowel Training. The client with incontinence is unable to maintain bowel control. A **bowel training** program can help some clients achieve normal defecation; especially those who still have some neuromuscular control.

The training program involves setting up a daily routine. By attempting to defecate at the same time each day and using measures that promote defecation, the client gains control of bowel reflexes. The program requires time, patience, and consistency. The physician determines the client's physical readiness and ability to benefit from bowel training. A successful program includes the following:

- Assessing the normal elimination pattern and recording times when the client is incontinent
- Incorporating principles of gerontologic nursing when providing bowel retraining programs for the older adult client (Box 45-11)
- Choosing a time in the client's pattern to initiate defecation-control measures
- Giving stool softeners orally every day or a cathartic suppository at least half an hour before the selected defecation time (lower colon must be free of stool so that suppository contacts intestinal mucosa)
- Offering a hot drink (hot tea) or fruit juice (prune juice) (or whatever fluids normally stimulate peristalsis for the client) before the defecation time
- Assisting the client to the toilet at the designated time
- Avoiding medications, such as analgesics, that may increase constipation
- Providing privacy and setting a time limit for defecation (15 to 20 minutes).
- Instructing the client to lean forward at the hips while sitting on the toilet, to apply manual pressure with the hands over the abdomen, and to bear down but not strain to stimulate colon emptying

Text continued on p. 1416

Skill 45-3   Pouching an Ostomy

View Video

Delegation Considerations

The skill of pouching an ostomy, especially a newly established ostomy, should not be delegated to assistive personnel (AP). Pouching of an established ostomy can be delegated to AP. The nurse must do the following:

- Assist caregiver in selecting appropriate pouch and skin barrier.
- Inform caregiver of the signs of stomal and peristomal skin changes that should be reported to a registered professional nurse (RN).
- Have caregiver monitor and report characteristics and volume of ostomy output and report changes in volume and/or consistency to the nurse for further assessment.

Equipment (Figure 45-17)

- Clear drainable colostomy/ileostomy pouch in correct size for two-piece system or custom cut-to-fit one-piece type with attached skin barrier
- Pouch closure device, such as clamp
- Clean disposable gloves
- Deodorant specific for an ostomy collection bag
- Gauze pads and washcloths
- Towel or disposable waterproof barrier
- Basin with warm tap water
- Scissors/pen
- Adhesive remover (optional)

Steps	Rationale
1. Perform hand hygiene and auscultate for bowel sounds.	Documents presence of peristalsis.
2. Apply gloves and perform hand hygiene. Observe skin barrier and pouch for leakage and length of time in place. Depending on type of pouching system used (such as with an opaque pouch), the nurse may have to remove the pouch to fully observe the stoma. Clear pouches permit the viewing of the stoma without their removal.	May indicate need for different type of pouch or sealant.

Critical Decision Point: Intact skin barriers with no evidence of leakage do not need to be changed daily and can remain in place for 3 to 5 days (Ayello, 2000).

3. Observe stoma for color, swelling, trauma, and healing; stoma should be moist and reddish-pink. Assess type of stoma. Stomas can be flush with the skin or be a budlike protrusion on the abdomen (see illustration for a normal bud stoma).	Stoma characteristics should be one of the factors to consider when selecting an appropriate pouching system.

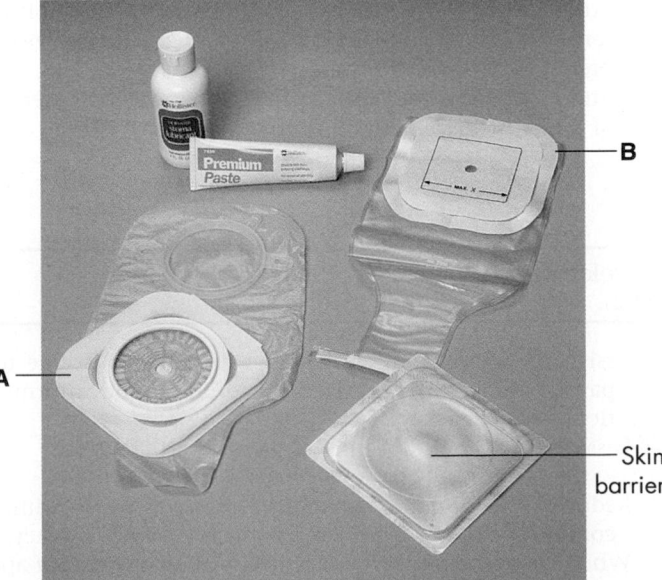

A

B

Skin barrier

FIGURE **45-17** Ostomy pouches and skin barriers. **A,** Two-piece detachable system. (NOTE: Skin barrier would need to be custom cut according to stoma size.) The pouch opening is already precut by the manufacturer to fit the size of the flange on the skin barrier. **B,** One-piece pouch with skin barrier attached. (Permission to use and/or reproduce this copyrighted photo has been granted by the owner, Hollister Incorporated.)

Skill 45-3   *Pouching an Ostomy—cont'd*

Steps	Rationale

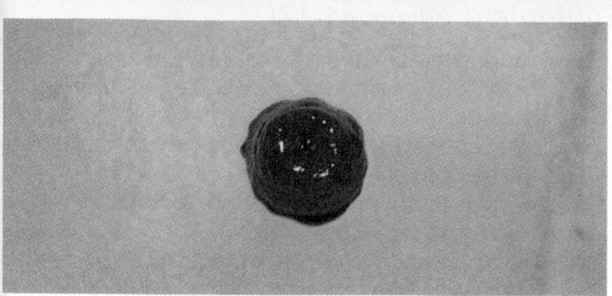

STEP **3**   Bud stoma. (Permission to use and/or reproduce this copyrighted photo has been granted by the owner, Hollister Incorporated.)

4. Measure the stoma with each pouching change. Follow pouch manufacturer's directions and measuring guide as to which pouch to use based on client's stoma size. The opening around the appliance should be no more than $\frac{1}{16}$ inch larger than the stoma (Hyland, 2002).

Determines correct size equipment, preventing trauma to stoma. Too large an opening can permit fecal drainage to ooze from under the appliance, causing skin irritation. Too small an opening can cause the appliance to cut into the stoma (Hyland, 2002).

5. Observe abdominal incision (if present).

Relationship of abdominal incision to stoma determines proper placement of pouch.

6. Observe effluent from stoma and keep a record of intake and output. Ask client about skin tenderness. Remove gloves and perform hand hygiene.

Effluent from stoma is caustic, and if it comes in contact with the sensitive peristomal skin, the risk of skin breakdown increases (Hyland, 2002).

7. Assess abdomen for best type of pouching system to use. Consider the following:
  a. Contour and peristomal plane
  b. Presence of scars, incisions
  c. Location and type of stoma

Determines pouching system selection and need for other equipment. For a stoma to have an adequate seal with an ostomy appliance, the stoma must be placed within the abdominal rectus muscle, away from abdominal creases and folds, away from the bony understructures, and surrounded by at least 2 inches of smooth surface on all sides (Banks and Razor, 2003).

8. Assess the client's self-care ability to determine the best type of pouching system to use.

Clients who have difficulty using their hands or who have limited vision may find a one-piece system or a precut pouch and skin barrier more desirable to use; others prefer being able to keep the skin barrier in place for several days, changing just the pouch, and therefore prefer the two-piece system.

9. After skin barrier and pouch removal, assess skin around stoma, noting scars, folds, skin breakdown, and peristomal suture line, if present. Keep pouch loosely attached to stoma to collect any drainage while the system is being changed.

Determines need for barrier paste to increase adherence of pouch to skin or to fill in irregularities.

Critical Decision Point: If the skin around the stoma is discolored, weeping, itchy, or sore, the client should be referred to an ostomy specialist (Hyland, 2002).

10. Determine client's emotional response and knowledge and understanding of an ostomy and its care.

Assists in determining extent to which client is able to participate in care and need for teaching and information clarification.

11. Explain procedure to client; encourage client's interaction and questions.

Lessens anxiety and promotes client's participation.

12. Perform hand hygiene. Assemble equipment and close room curtains or door.

Reduces infection transmission. Optimizes use of time; conserves client's and nurse's energy. Provides privacy.

13. Position client either standing or supine and drape. If seated, position either on or in front of the toilet.

When client is supine, fewer wrinkles allow for ease of application of pouching system; maintains client's dignity.

Steps	Rationale
14. Perform hand hygiene and apply disposable gloves.	Reduces transmission of microorganisms.
15. Place towel or disposable waterproof barrier under the client.	Protects bed linen.
16. Completely remove used pouch and skin barrier gently by pushing the skin away from the barrier. An adhesive remover may be used to facilitate removal of the skin barrier.	Reduces trauma; jerking irritates the skin and can cause tears.
17. Cleanse peristomal skin gently with warm tap water using gauze pads or clean washcloth; do not scrub the skin; dry completely by patting the skin with gauze or towel.	Avoid use of soap because it leaves a residue on the skin that interferes with pouch adhesion to the skin. Skin must be as dry as skin barrier; pouch does not adhere to wet skin. If blood appears on the gauze pad, do not be alarmed; the stoma, if rubbed, may ooze some blood from the cleaning process. The stoma's surface is a highly vascular mucous membrane. Bleeding into the pouch is abnormal.
18. Measure the stoma for correct size of pouching system needed, using the manufacturer's measuring guide (see illustration).	Ensures accuracy in determining correct pouch size needed. Stoma shrinks and does not reach usual size for 6 to 8 wk.
19. Select appropriate pouch for client based on client assessment. With a custom cut-to-fit pouch, use an ostomy guide to cut opening on the pouch $\frac{1}{16}$ inch larger than stoma before removing backing (Hyland, 2002). Prepare pouch by removing backing from barrier and adhesive (see illustration). With ileostomy, apply thin circle of barrier paste around opening in pouch; allow to dry.	The paste facilitates seal and protects skin. Size of pouch opening keeps drainage off skin and lessens risk of damage to stoma during peristalsis or activity. Pouch and skin barrier are changed whenever leaking. Can also be changed before or after tub bath or shower. Stool is alkaline and this irritates the skin; fecal bacteria can colonize on the skin and increase risk of infection. Change when client is comfortable; before a meal is better, because this avoids increased peristalsis and chance of evacuation during the pouch change.

Critical Decision Point: If client has a large volume of liquid stool from an ileostomy, consider using a "high-output" pouch that will contain the volume of effluent and reduce the frequency of pouch emptying.

20. Apply the skin barrier and pouch. If creases next to stoma occur, use barrier paste to fill in; let dry 1 to 2 min.

Critical Decision Point: If client has surgical incision near stoma, the skin barrier may have to be trimmed for fit.

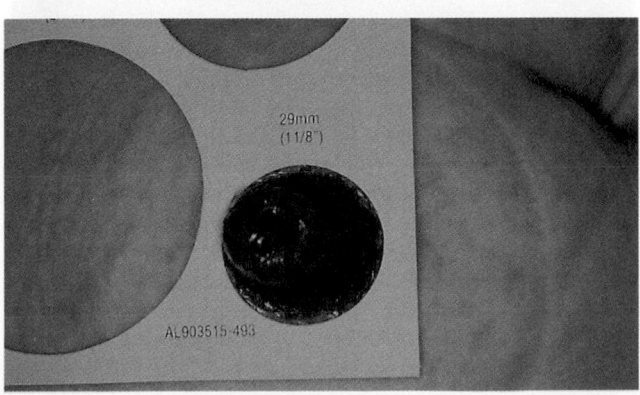

STEP **18**   Measuring a stoma.

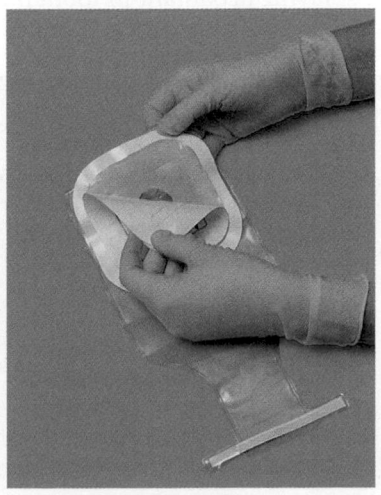

STEP **19**   Preparing an ostomy pouch.

Skill 45-3 *Pouching an Ostomy—cont'd*

Steps	Rationale

A. For one-piece pouching system
  (1) Use skin sealant wipes on skin directly under adhesive skin barrier or pouch; allow to dry. Press the adhesive backing of the pouch and/or skin barrier smoothly against the skin, starting from the bottom and working up and around the sides.
  (2) Hold pouch by barrier, center over stoma, and press down gently on barrier, bottom of pouch should point toward client's knees (see illustration).
  (3) Maintain gentle finger pressure around the barrier for 1 to 2 min.

B. For two-piece pouching system
  (1) Apply flange (barrier with adhesive) as in steps above for one-piece system (see illustration). Then snap on pouch and maintain finger pressure.   *Creates wrinkle-free, secure seal; decreases irritation from the adhesive on skin.*

C. For both pouching systems gently tug on the pouch in a downward direction.   *Determines if the pouch is securely attached.*

21. Apply nonallergic paper tape around the pectin skin barrier in a "picture frame" method. Half of the tape should be on the skin barrier and half on the client's skin. Some clients may prefer a belt attached to the pouch for extra security rather than tape.   *"Picture framing" the pectin skin barrier adds to the security of keeping the pouch system attached securely.*

Critical Decision Point: If the client chooses to wear a belt, be sure belt is not too tight by placing two fingers between belt and client's skin.

---

22. Although many ostomy pouches are odor proof, some nurses and clients like to put a small amount of ostomy deodorant into the pouch. Do not use "home remedies," such as aspirin, to control ostomy odor.   *Aspirin or other substances can harm the stoma.*

23. Fold bottom of drainable open-ended pouches up once and close using a closure device such as a clamp (or follow manufacturer's instructions for closure).   *Maintains secure seal to prevent leaking.*

24. Properly dispose of old pouch and soiled equipment. Consider spraying deodorant in room if needed.   *Lessens odors in room.*

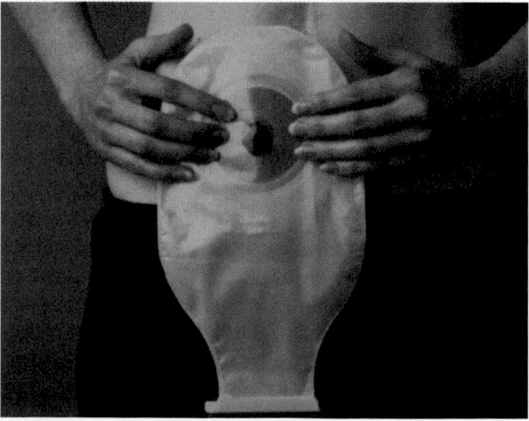

STEP **20A(2)** Applying a one-piece pouch. (Courtesy ConvaTec, Princeton NJ.)

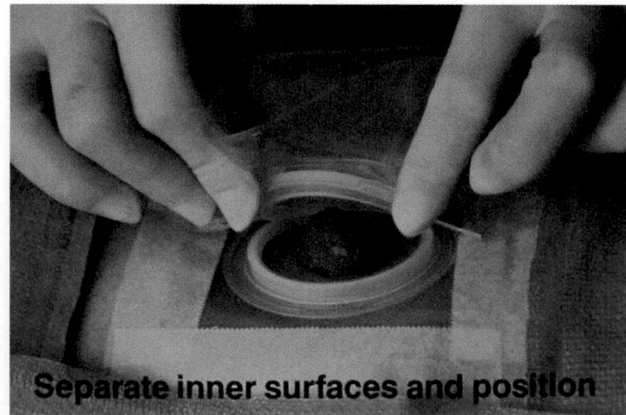

STEP **20B(1)** Application of barrier-paste flange. (Courtesy ConvaTec, Princeton NJ.)

Steps	Rationale
25. Remove gloves and perform hand hygiene.	Reduces transmission of microorganisms.
26. Change one- or two-piece pouch every 3 to 7 days unless leaking; pouch can remain in place for tub bath or shower; after bath, pat adhesive dry.	Avoids unnecessary trauma to skin from too frequent changes. Drying ensures adhesion of pouch.
27. Ask if client feels discomfort around stoma.	Determines presence of skin irritation.
28. Note appearance of stoma around skin and existing incision (if present) while pouch is removed and skin is cleansed. Reinspect condition of skin barrier and adhesive.	Determines condition of tissues and progress of healing. Determines presence of leaks.
29. Auscultate bowel sounds and observe characteristics of stool.	Determines return of peristalsis and bowel elimination.
30. Observe client's nonverbal behaviors as pouch is applied. Ask if client has any questions about pouching.	May indicate emotional response to stoma and readiness for teaching. Determines level of understanding of procedure.

Unexpected Outcomes and Related Interventions

1. Client experiences damage to peristomal skin.
   a. Assess for and report to physician for treatment:
      (1) Mechanical damage (see illustration) due to inappropriate skin care, incorrect tape removal
      (2) Chemical damage due to effluent coming into contact with peristomal skin, skin reaction to adhesive
      (3) Damage due to a fungal infection (candidiasis), usually caused from excessive skin moisture
2. Stoma becomes necrotic as manifested by purple or black color, dry instead of moist, failure to bleed, or there is tissue sloughing.
   a. Assess circulation to stoma.
   b. Observe for excessive edema or tension on bowel suture line (if present).
   c. Immediately report this finding to the physician.

Recording and Reporting

- Chart type of pouch and skin barrier applied.
- Record amount and appearance of stool, texture, condition of peristomal skin, and sutures.
- Report any of the following to the charge nurse and/or physician:
  - Abnormal appearance of stoma, suture line, peristomal skin, character of output, absence of bowel sounds
  - No flatus in 24 to 36 hours and no stool by third day
- Document abdominal distention and excessive tenderness, nature of bowel sounds.
- Record client's level of participation and need for teaching.

Home Care Considerations

- Evaluate the client's home toileting facilities. This includes presence of adequate toileting facilities, flushable toilet, and number and location of toilets.
- Caution the client that most ostomy pouches and barriers cannot be flushed down the toilet; they clog the system. Dispose of used ostomy pouch according to local sanitation regulations.

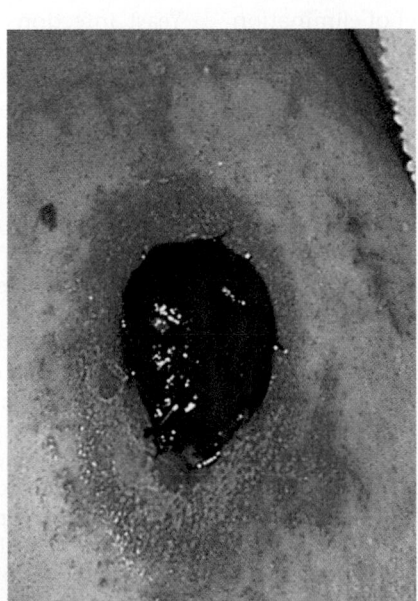

A

B

FIGURE **45–17 A,** Mechanical injury. **B,** Candidiasis. (Permission to use and/or reproduce this copyrighted photo has been granted by the owner, Hollister Incorporated.)

- The energy needs of persons over 51 years of age are considered to be less due to loss of metabolic tissue with age. Protein needs do not decrease with aging (Morrisson, 1997).
- Maintaining a well-balanced diet, high in fiber will assist in maintaining normal bowel elimination patterns (Bliss and others, 2001).
- Constipation is a common complaint in older clients. Contributing factors are impaired general health, use of medication, and decreased mobility and physical activity (Abyad and Mourad, 1996).
- If constipation is ignored, significant complications can arise. Instructing clients to establish a specific time for bowel elimination may assist in preventing constipation (Dosh, 2002).
- Clients need to feel at ease during elimination. Lack of privacy may lead the client to ignore the urge to defecate.
- Older adults are known for their concern with their elimination habits.
- Warm liquids and certain juices (prune) stimulate bowel motility.

- Not criticizing or conveying frustration if the client is unable to defecate
- Providing regular meals with adequate fluids and fiber (Bliss and others, 2001)
- Maintaining normal exercise within the client's physical ability

Maintenance of Proper Fluid and Food Intake. In choosing a diet for promoting normal elimination, the nurse should consider the frequency of defecation, characteristics of feces, and types of foods that impair or promote defecation. The client with frequent constipation or impaction requires an increased intake of high-fiber foods and more fluids. However, the client should realize that diet therapy provides only long-term relief of elimination problems and may not give immediate relief from problems such as constipation.

When diarrhea is a problem, the nurse can recommend foods with a low fiber content and discourage foods that typically cause gastric upset or abdominal cramping. Diarrhea caused by illness can be debilitating. If the client cannot tolerate foods or liquids orally, intravenous therapy (with potassium supplements) is necessary. The client returns to a normal diet slowly, often beginning with fluids. Excessively hot or cold fluids stimulate peristalsis, causing abdominal cramps and further diarrhea. As the tolerance to liquids improves, solid foods are ordered.

Promotion of Regular Exercise. A daily exercise program helps prevent elimination problems. Walking, riding a stationary bicycle, or swimming stimulates peristalsis. Clients who are sedentary at work are most in need of regular exercise.

For a client temporarily immobilized, the nurse should attempt ambulation as soon as possible. If the condition permits, the nurse assists a postoperative client in walking to a chair on the evening of the day of surgery. The client should walk farther each day.

Some clients have difficulty passing stool because of weak abdominal and pelvic floor muscles. Exercises help bedridden clients using a bedpan. The client can practice the exercises as follows:

- Lie supine; tighten the abdominal muscles as though pushing them to the floor. Hold them tight to the count of three; relax. Repeat 5 to 10 times as tolerated.
- Flex and contract the thigh muscles by raising one knee slowly toward the chest. Repeat for each leg at least 5 times and increase frequency as tolerated.

Hemorrhoids. Many clients have discomfort from alterations in elimination. Pain results when hemorrhoid tissues are directly irritated. The primary goal for the client with hemorrhoids is to have soft-formed, painless bowel movement. Proper diet, fluids, and regular exercise improve the likelihood of stools being soft. If the client becomes constipated, passage of hard stools may cause bleeding and irritation. Local heat provides temporary relief to swollen hemorrhoids. A sitz bath is the most effective means of heat application (see Chapter 47).

Maintenance of Skin Integrity. The client with diarrhea or fecal incontinence is at risk for skin breakdown when fecal contents remain on the skin. The same problem exists for the client with an ostomy that drains liquid stool. Liquid stool is usually acidic and contains digestive enzymes. Irritation from repeated wiping with toilet tissue aggravates skin breakdown. Bathing the skin after soiling helps but may result in more breakdown unless the skin is thoroughly dried.

When caring for a debilitated, incontinent client who is unable to ask for assistance, the nurse should check often for defecation. The anal areas can be protected with petrolatum, zinc oxide, or another ointment that holds moisture in the skin, preventing drying and cracking. Yeast infections of the skin can develop easily. Several powdered antifungal agents are effective against yeast. Baby powder or cornstarch should not be used because they have no medical properties and they frequently cake on the skin and become difficult to remove.

Evaluation

Client Care. The effectiveness of care depends on success in meeting the goals and expected outcomes of care. Optimally the client will be able to have regular, pain-free defecation of soft-formed stools. The client is the only one who is able to determine if the bowel elimination problems have been relieved and which therapies were the most effective (Figure 45-18). The client will also be able to demonstrate information gained regarding establishment of a normal elimination pattern. The client will be able to demonstrate any skills learned such as ostomy protocols and skin protection. The client will

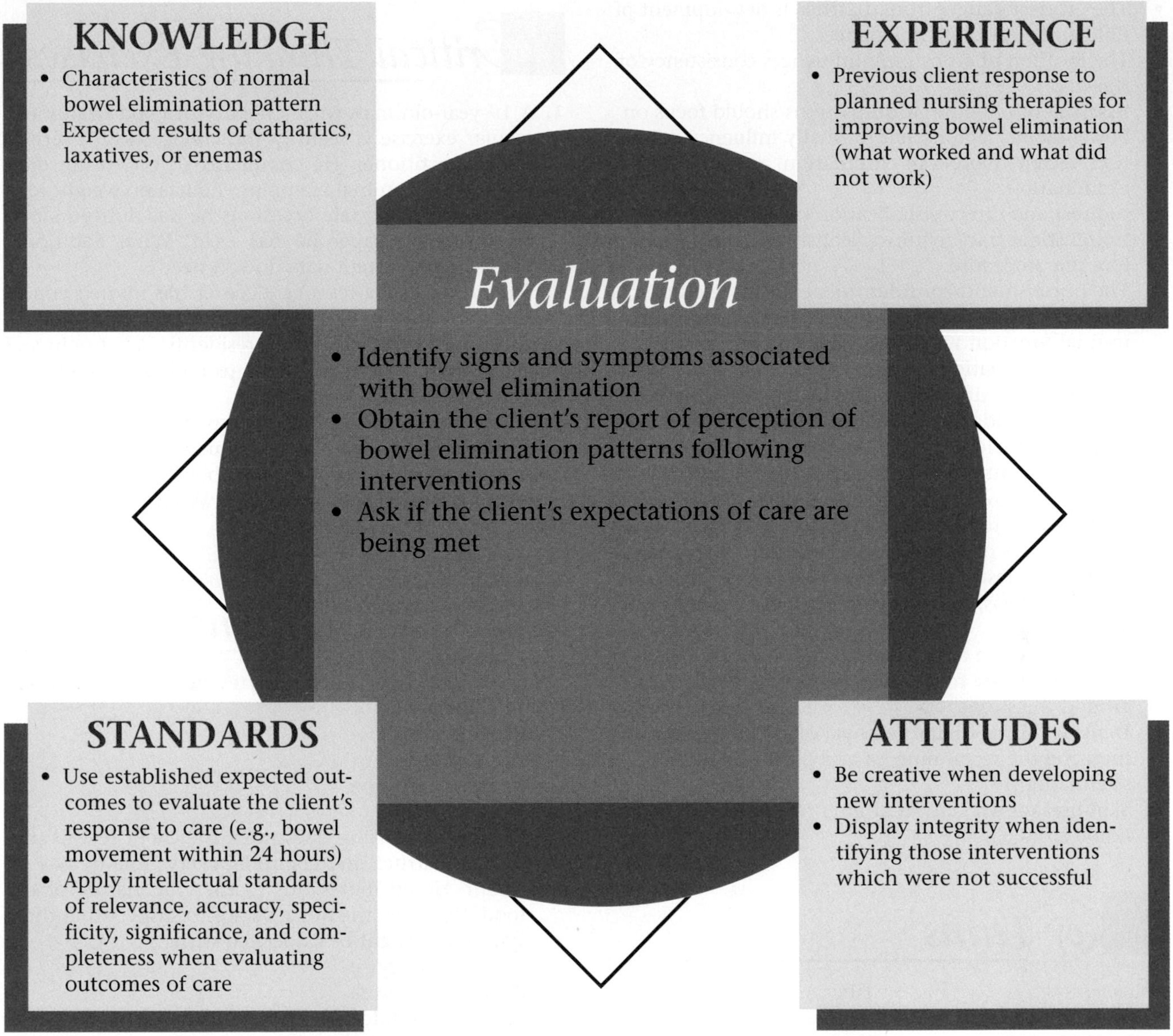

KNOWLEDGE

- Characteristics of normal bowel elimination pattern
- Expected results of cathartics, laxatives, or enemas

EXPERIENCE

- Previous client response to planned nursing therapies for improving bowel elimination (what worked and what did not work)

Evaluation

- Identify signs and symptoms associated with bowel elimination
- Obtain the client's report of perception of bowel elimination patterns following interventions
- Ask if the client's expectations of care are being met

STANDARDS

- Use established expected outcomes to evaluate the client's response to care (e.g., bowel movement within 24 hours)
- Apply intellectual standards of relevance, accuracy, specificity, significance, and completeness when evaluating outcomes of care

ATTITUDES

- Be creative when developing new interventions
- Display integrity when identifying those interventions which were not successful

FIGURE **45–18**　Critical thinking model for elimination evaluation.

be able to accomplish normal defecation by manipulating natural components of daily living such as diet, fluid intake, and exercise. The client will have minimal reliance on artificial means of defecation such as enemas and laxative use.

Client Expectations. If the nurse has been successful in establishing a therapeutic relationship with the client, the client will feel comfortable in discussing the intimate details often associated with bowel elimination. The client will not be fearful of embarrassment as the nurse assists the client with elimination needs. The client will relate a feeling of comfort and freedom from pain as elimination needs are met within the limits of the client's condition and treatment.

Key Concepts

- Mechanical breakdown of food elements, gastrointestinal motility, and selective absorption and secretion of substances by the large intestine influence the character of feces.
- Food high in fiber content and an increased fluid intake keep feces soft.
- Ongoing use of cathartics, laxatives, and enemas affects and delays normal defecation reflexes.
- Vagal stimulation, which slows the heart rate, may occur during straining while defecating, taking rectal temperatures, enemas, and digital removal of impacted stool.

- The greatest danger from diarrhea is development of fluid and electrolyte imbalance.
- The location of an ostomy influences consistency of the stool.
- Assessment of elimination patterns should focus on bowel habits, factors that normally influence defecation, recent changes in elimination, and a physical examination.
- Indirect and direct visualization of the lower gastrointestinal tract requires cleansing of the bowel before the procedure.
- The nurse should consider frequency of defecation, fecal characteristics, and effect of foods on gastrointestinal function when selecting a diet promoting normal elimination.
- Proper positioning on a bedpan allows the client to assume a position similar to squatting without experiencing muscle strain.
- Nasogastric intubation decompresses the gastric contents by removing secretions and gaseous products from the gastrointestinal tract.
- The purposes of gastric decompression are to keep the gastrointestinal tract free of secretions, reduce nausea and gas, and decrease the risk of vomiting and aspiration.
- Proper selection and use of an ostomy pouching system is necessary to prevent damage to the skin around the stoma.
- Dangers during digital removal of stool include traumatizing the rectal mucosa and promoting vagal stimulation.
- Skin breakdown can occur after repeated exposure to liquid stool.

Key Terms

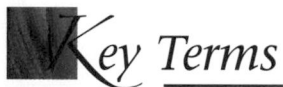

Bolus, *p. 1375*
Bowel training, *p. 1410*
Cathartics, *p. 1378*
Chyme, *p. 1375*
Colitis, *p. 1378*
Colostomy, *p. 1380*
Constipation, *p. 1379*
Crohn's disease, *p. 1378*
Defecation, *p. 1376*
Diarrhea, *p. 1379*
Effluent, *p. 1409*
Endoscopy, *p. 1379*
Enema, *p. 1396*
Enterostomal therapist
  (ET), *p. 1410*
Excoriation, *p. 1402*
Fecal occult blood testing
  (FOBT), *p. 1386*

Fiber, *p. 1377*
Flatulence, *p. 1380*
Hemorrhoids, *p. 1380*
Ileostomy, *p. 1380*
Impaction, *p. 1379*
Incontinence, *p. 1380*
Lactose intolerance, *p. 1377*
Laxatives, *p. 1378*
Masticate, *p. 1374*
Paralytic ileus, *p. 1378*
Peristalsis, *p. 1375*
Polyps, *p. 1381*
Segmentation, *p. 1375*
Stoma, *p. 1380*
Valsalva maneuver, *p. 1376*

Critical Thinking Exercises

1. A 19-year-old man with a history of good health and regular exercise is seen by the college health service nurse practitioner. He complains of increasing diarrhea and abdominal cramping; he has no weight loss. He states that on rare occasions he has noticed blood on the toilet paper he has used. What additional pieces of assessment data do you need?
2. The nursing long-term care center has invited you to come and do a presentation concerning prevention of bowel incontinence in their residents. What points of information would you want to include in your presentation?
3. A 22-year-old man is to undergo surgery for Crohn's disease. He will have a new pouching ileostomy. He and his mother need teaching about what this means for his future elimination needs. What would you tell them?

Review Questions

1. Most nutrients and electrolytes are absorbed in the:
   1. Colon.
   2. Stomach.
   3. Esophagus.
   4. Small intestine.

2. During the nursing assessment the client reveals that he has diarrhea and cramping every time he has ice cream. He attributes this to the cold nature of the food. However, the nurse begins to suspect that these symptoms might be associated with:
   1. Food allergy.
   2. Irritable bowel.
   3. Lactose intolerance.
   4. Increased peristalsis.

3. The nurse is assessing a 55-year-old client who is in the clinic for a routine physical. The nurse instructs the client to obtain fecal occult blood testing (FOBT):
   1. When there is a family history of polyps.
   2. If client reports rectal bleeding.
   3. If a palpable mass is detected on digital examination.
   4. As part of a routine examination for colon cancer.

4. These agents decrease intestinal muscle tone to slow passage of feces.
   1. Antidiarrheal opiate agents.
   2. Hypertonic.
   3. Cathartics.
   4. Laxatives

5. Diarrhea that occurs with a fecal impaction is the result of:
   1. A clear liquid diet.
   2. Irritation of the intestinal mucosa.
   3. Seepage of stool around the impaction.
   4. Inability of the client to form a stool.

6. A cleaning enema is ordered for a 55-year-old client before intestinal surgery. The maximum amount given is:
   1. 150 to 200 ml.
   2. 200 to 400 ml.
   3. 400 to 750 ml.
   4. 750 to 1000 ml.

7. During the enema the client begins to complain of pain. The nurse notes blood in the return fluid and rectal bleeding. The nurse's actions are to:
   1. Stop the instillation.
   2. Slow down the rate of instillation.
   3. Stop the instillation and obtain vital signs.
   4. Tell the client to breathe slowly and relax.

8. One of the greatest problems in caring for a client with an NG tube is:
   1. Dyhydration.
   2. Maintaining comfort.
   3. Constipation.
   4. Nutritional therapy.

9. The stool discharged from an ostomy is called:
   1. Effluent.
   2. Cathartics.
   3. Colonic fluid.
   4. Mucosa.

10. A nurse trained to care for ostomy clients is a (an):
    1. Enterostomal therapist.
    2. Nurse practitioner.
    3. Ostomy practitioner.
    4. GI therapist.

*R*eferences

Abyad A, Mourad F: Constipation: common-sense care of the older patient, *Geriatrics* 51(12):28, 1996.

American Cancer Society: *Colon and rectal cancer: 2003, 2003* Atlanta, 2003, The Society, www.cancer.org.

Annells M, Koch T: Older people seeking solutions to constipation: the laxative mire, *J Clin Nurs* 11(5):603, 2002.

Ayello EA: The ABCDs of stoma assessment and pouching, personal correspondence, 2000.

Banks N, Razor B: Preoperative stoma site assessment and marking: trained RNs can improve ostomy outcomes, *Am J Nurs* 103(3):64A, 2003.

Bliss DZ and others: Supplementation with dietary fiber improves fecal incontinence, *Nurs Res* 50(4):203, 2001.

Colwell J and others: The stare of the standard diversion, *J Wound Ostomy Continence Nurs* 28:6, 2001.

Cooke CE: Disease management: prevention of NSAID induced gastropathy, *Drug Benefit Trends* 8(3):14, 1996.

Dochterman JM, Bulechek GM: *Nursing interventions classification (NIC),* ed 4, St. Louis, 2004, Mosby.

Dosh SA: Evaluation and treatment of constipation, *J Fam Pract* 51(6):555, 2002.

Doughty D: A physiologic approach to bowel training, *J Wound Ostomy Continence Nurs* 23(1):46, 2000a.

Doughty D: *Urinary and fecal incontinence nursing,* ed 2, St. Louis, 2000b, Mosby.

Hinrichs M, Huseboe J: *Evidenced-based protocol: management of constipation,* The University of Iowa, Gerontological Nursing Interventions Research Center, Research Dissemination Core, reviewed March 2001, Iowa City, Ia.

Hyland J: Basics of ostomies, *Gastroenterol Nurs* 25(6):241, 2002.

Lueckenotte AG: *Gerontologic nursing,* ed 2, St. Louis, 2000, Mosby.

McKenry LM, Salerno E: *Pharmacology in nursing,* ed 21, St. Louis, 2001, Mosby.

Moorhead S, Johnson M, Maas M : *Nursing outcomes classification (NOC),* ed 3, St. Louis, 2004, Mosby.

Morrisson SG: Feeding the elderly population, *Nurs Clin North Am* 32(4):791, 1997.

Pagana KD, Pagana TJ: *Mosby's diagnostic and laboratory test reference,* ed 5, St. Louis, 2001, Mosby.

Powe BD: Fatalism among elderly African Americans: effects on colorectal cancer screening, *Cancer Nurs* 18(5):385, 1995.

Richmond J: Prevention of constipation through risk management, *Nurs Stand* 17(16):39, 2003.

Selma, TP, Beizer JL, Highbee MD: *Geriatric dosage handbook,* Hudson, Ohio: Lexi-Comp Inc., 1997.

Stewart KB: Helping your patient contend with constipation, *Nursing* 28(9 Hosp Nurs):32hn 22, 1998.

Walsh BA and others: Psychometric evaluation of body image and quality of life following ostomy surgery. Oral abstract presented at the Wound, Ostomy, Continence Nurses (WOCN) Society Twenty-Seventh Annual Conference, Denver, May 1995.

*R*esearch References

Annells M, Koch T: Older people seeking solutions to constipation: the laxative mire, *J Clin Nurs* 11(5):603, 2002.

Anti M and others: Water supplementation enhances the effect of high-fiber diet on stool frequency and laxative consumption in adult patients with functional constipation, *Hepatogastroenterology* 45(21):727, 1998.

Bartlett JG: Antibiotic-associated diarrhea, *N Engl J Med* 346(5):334, 2002.

Bliss DZ and others: Fecal incontinence in hospitalized patients who are acutely ill, *Nurs Res* 49(2):101, 2000.

Bliss DZ and others: Supplementation with dietary fiber improves fecal incontinence, *Nurs Res* 50(4):203, 2001.

Dosh SA: Evaluation and treatment of constipation, *J Fam Pract* 51(6):555, 2002.

Hinrichs M, Huseboe J: *Evidenced-based protocol: management of constipation,* The University of Iowa, Gerontological Nursing Interventions Research Center, Research Dissemination Core, reviewed March 2001, Iowa City, Ia.

Metheny N and others: Effectiveness of pH measurements in predicting feeding tube placement: an update, *Nurs Res* 42(6):324, 1993.

Metheny N and others: Visual characteristics of aspirates from feeding tubes as a method for predicting tube location, *Nurs Res* 43:282, 1994.

Metheny N and others: pH, color, and feeding tubes, *RN* 61(1):277, 1998.

Metheny NA, Titler MG: Assessing placement of feeding tubes, *Am J Nurs* 101(5):36, 2001.

Mishkin S: Dairy sensitivity, lactose malabsorption, and elimination diets in inflammatory bowel disease, *Am J Clin Nutr* 65(2):564, 1997.

Ransohoff DF, Lang CA: Screening for colorectal cancer with the fecal occult blood test: a background paper, Ann Intern Med 126:881, 1997.

Mobility and Immobility

Media Resources

http://evolve.elsevier.com/Potter/
fundamentals/

CD COMPANION

- Review Questions
- Glossary

evolve WEBSITE

- Review Questions
- Student Learning Activities
- Animations
- Concept Map Exercise
- Critical Thinking Exercise
- Video Clips
- Glossary

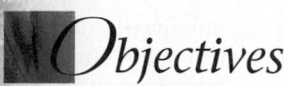

Objectives

Mastery of content in this chapter will enable the student to:

- Define the key terms listed.

- Describe the functions of the musculoskeletal (skeleton, skeletal muscles) and nervous systems in the regulation of movement.

- Discuss physiological and pathological influences on body alignment and joint mobility.

- Identify changes in physiological and psychosocial function associated with mobility and immobility.

- Assess for correct and impaired body alignment and mobility.

- State correct nursing diagnoses for impaired body alignment and mobility.

- Develop nursing care plans for clients with impaired body alignment and mobility.

- Describe essential techniques when assisting with active/passive range-of-motion (ROM) exercises, assisting a client to move up in bed, repositioning a client, assisting a client to a sitting position, transferring a client from a bed to a chair or from a bed to a stretcher, and helping a client to safely use crutches.

- Describe active/passive range-of-motion exercises.

- Describe essential techniques when helping a client to safely use crutches.

- Evaluate the nursing plan for maintaining body alignment and mobility.

Mobility serves many purposes, such as expression of an emotion with a nonverbal gesture, self-defense, satisfaction of basic needs, and performance of activities of daily living (ADLs) and recreational activities. Many functions of the body need mobility to function optimally. To maintain optimal physical mobility, the musculoskeletal and nervous systems of the body must be intact and functioning.

Clinical nursing practice related to mobility requires incorporating knowledge and skills related to body mechanics to provide competent care. *Body mechanics* is a term used to describe coordinated efforts of the musculoskeletal and nervous systems in moving and lifting the body. Knowing the movements and functions of muscles in maintaining posture and movement is vital to safe production and maintenance of motion for nurses, as well as for clients.

Scientific Knowledge Base

Physiology and Principles of Body Mechanics

Body mechanics are the coordinated efforts of the musculoskeletal and nervous systems to maintain balance, posture, and body alignment during lifting, bending, moving, and performing ADLs. Use of proper body mechanics reduces risk of injury to the musculoskeletal system, facilitates ease of body movement, and allows for more efficient use of energy.

Use of proper body mechanics is important to the safety and well-being of the nurse and of clients. The nurse uses a variety of muscle groups for each nursing activity, such as walking during nursing rounds, administering medications, lifting and transferring clients, and moving objects. The physical forces of weight and friction can influence body movement. Correctly used, these forces increase the nurse's efficiency. Incorrect use can impair the nurse's ability to lift, transfer, and position clients and cause serious injury. Knowledge of the basic structures and functions of the neuromuscular system and knowledge of physiological and pathological influences on mobility and body alignment are important to a full understanding of body mechanics (see Box 36-2, p. 934).

Alignment. The terms *body alignment* and *posture* are analogous and refer to the positioning of the joints, tendons, ligaments, and muscles while standing, sitting, and lying. Correct body alignment reduces strain on musculoskeletal structures and risk for injury, aids in maintaining adequate muscle tone, and contributes to balance and conservation of energy.

Balance. Body alignment means that the individual's center of gravity is stable and body strain is minimized. Body alignment contributes to body balance. Without balance control, the center of gravity is displaced, thus creating a risk for falls and subsequent injuries. Balance is enhanced with a wide base of support and correct body posture and when the body's center of gravity is kept low and within the base of support.

Balance is required for maintaining a static position such as sitting, for performing ADLs, and for moving freely in the community. The ability to balance can be compromised by disease, injury, pain, physical development (e.g., age), life changes (e.g., pregnancy), medications (e.g., in which dizziness is a side effect), and prolonged immobility, which may cause deconditioning. Nurses must be alert to impaired balance, because it is a major threat to physical safety. Impaired balance can also lead to a client's fear of falls and self-imposed restrictions on activity.

> *Safety Alert.* Impaired balance is a risk factor for falls among older adults. Approximately 5% of falls result in fractures, and 20% require some medical attention. Nursing interventions should be aimed at a thorough client safety assessment and implementing fall prevention strategies (Van Haastregt and others, 2000).

Gravity and Friction. Weight is the force exerted on a body by gravity. To lift safely, the lifter must overcome the weight of the object to be lifted and know its center of gravity. In symmetrical objects the center of gravity is located at the exact center of the object. Nurses do not just lift symmetrical objects, they often lift people. People are not geometrically perfect; their centers of gravity are usually at 55% to 57% of standing height and are located in the midline. The force of weight is always directed downward, which is why an unbalanced object falls. Clients or nurses who are unsteady can fall as their centers of gravity become unbalanced because of the gravitational pull of their weight. Therefore nurses are responsible for protecting clients from falling and ensuring the safety of clients and themselves (see Chapter 36).

Friction is a force that occurs in a direction to oppose movement. As the nurse turns, transfers, or moves a client up in bed, friction must be overcome. A nurse can reduce friction by following some basic principles. The greater the surface area of the object to be moved, the greater the friction. A larger object produces greater resistance to movement. To decrease surface area and reduce friction when a client is unable to assist in moving up in bed, the client's arms should be placed across the chest. This decreases surface area and reduces friction.

Whenever possible, the nurse should use some of the client's strength when lifting, transferring, or moving clients. This can be done by explaining the procedure and telling the client when and what body parts to move. The result should be a synchronized movement in which the client can participate and friction is decreased. Involving the client may have the added bonus of increasing participation in self-care, thus promoting a sense of accomplishment.

Friction can also be reduced by lifting rather than pushing a client. Lifting has an upward component and decreases the pressure between the client and the bed or chair. Placing the client on a sheet or blanket (pull sheet or lift sheet) and then pulling this sheet to move the client reduces friction because the client is more easily moved along the bed's surface.

Regulation of Movement

Coordinated body movement involves integrated functioning of the skeletal system, skeletal muscle, and nervous system. Because these three systems cooperate so closely in mechanical support of the body, they are discussed as a single functional unit.

Skeletal System. The skeleton provides attachments for muscles and ligaments and provides the leverage necessary for movement. Thus the skeleton is the body's supporting framework and comprises four types of bones: long, short, flat, and irregular. **Long bones** contribute to height (e.g., the femur, fibula, and tibia in the leg) and length (e.g., the phalanges of the fingers and toes). **Short bones** occur in clusters and, when combined with ligaments and cartilage, permit movement of the extremities. Two examples of short bones are the carpal bones in the foot and the patella in the knee. **Flat bones** provide structural contour, such as bones in the skull and the ribs in the thorax. **Irregular bones** make up the vertebral column and some bones of the skull, such as the mandible.

Bones are further characterized by firmness, rigidity, and elasticity. Firmness results from inorganic salts, such as calcium and phosphate that are laid down in the bone matrix. Firmness is related to the bone's rigidity, which is necessary to keep long bones straight, and enables bones to withstand weight bearing. In addition, bones have a degree of elasticity and skeletal flexibility that changes with age. For example, the newborn has a large amount of cartilage and is highly flexible but is unable to support weight. The toddler's bones are more pliable than those of an older person and are better able to withstand falls. Older adults, especially women, are more susceptible to bone loss (resorption) and osteoporosis.

The skeletal system has several functions. It protects vital organs (e.g., the skull around the brain; the ribs around the heart and lungs), and bones aid in calcium regulation. Bones store calcium and release it into the circulation as needed. Clients with decreased calcium regulation and metabolism are at risk for developing osteoporosis and **pathological fractures (fractures** caused by weakened bone tissue). In addition, the internal structure of bones contains bone marrow, participates in red blood cell (RBC) production, and acts as a reservoir for blood. Clients with altered bone marrow function or diminished RBC production are usually weakened and fatigue easily, which decreases their mobility and places them at risk of falling.

Joints. **Joints** are the connections between bones. Each joint is classified according to its structure and degree of mobility. There are four classifications of joints: synostotic, cartilaginous, fibrous, and synovial.

The **synostotic joint** refers to bones jointed by bones. No movement is associated with this type of joint, and the bony tissue that forms between the bones provides strength and stability. The classic example of this type of joint is the sacrum, in which vertebrae are joined (Figure 46-1, *A*).

The **cartilaginous joint,** or synchondrodial joint, has little movement but is elastic and uses cartilage to unite body surfaces. Cartilaginous joints are found when bones are exposed to constant pressure, such as the costosternal joints between the sternum and ribs (Figure 46-1, *B*).

The **fibrous joint,** or syndesmodial joint, is a joint in which two bony surfaces are united by a ligament or membrane. The fibers of ligaments are flexible and stretch, permitting a limited amount of movement. For example, the paired bones of the lower leg (tibia and fibula) are syndesmotic joints (McCance and Huether, 2002) (Figure 46-1, *C*).

The **synovial joint,** or true joint, is a freely moveable joint in which contiguous bony surfaces are covered by articular cartilage and connected by ligaments lined with a synovial membrane. Joining of the humeral radius and ulna by cartilage and ligaments forms a pivotal joint (Figure 46-1, *D*). Other types of synovial joints are the ball-and-socket joints, such as the hip joint, and the hinge joints, such as the interphalangeal joints of the fingers.

Ligaments. **Ligaments** are white, shiny, flexible bands of fibrous tissue binding joints together and connecting bones and cartilages. Ligaments are elastic and aid joint flexibility and support (Figure 46-2). In addition, some ligaments have a protective function. For example, ligaments between the vertebral bodies and the ligamentum flavum prevent damage to the spinal cord during movement of the back.

Tendons. **Tendons** are white, glistening, fibrous bands of tissue that connect muscle to bone. Tendons are strong, flexible, and inelastic, and they occur in various lengths and thicknesses. The Achilles tendon (tendo calcaneus) is the thickest and strongest tendon in the body. It begins near the middle of the posterior of the leg and attaches the gastrocnemius and soleus muscles in the calf to the calcaneal bone in the back of the foot (Figure 46-3).

Cartilage. **Cartilage** is nonvascular, supporting connective tissue located chiefly in the joints and thorax, trachea, larynx, nose, and ear. The fetus has a large amount of temporary cartilage, which is replaced by bone developed during infancy. Permanent cartilage is **unossified** (not hardened) except in advanced age and diseases such as osteoarthritis.

Joints, ligaments, tendons, and cartilage permit strength and flexibility of the skeleton. Strength enables the skeletal system to support the body. A person's flexibility is demonstrated through range of motion (ROM). However, strength and flexibility do not result entirely from these four structures. Adequate skeletal muscle is also necessary.

Skeletal Muscle. Movement of bones and joints involves active processes that must be carefully integrated to achieve coordination. Skeletal muscles, because of their ability to contract and relax, are the working elements of movement. Contractile elements of the skeletal muscle are enhanced by anatomical structure and attachment to the skeleton.

Muscles are made of fibers that contract when stimulated by an electrochemical impulse that travels from the nerve to the muscle across the neuromuscular junction. The electrochemical impulse causes the filaments (predominantly protein molecules of myosin and actin) within the fiber to slide past each other, with the filaments changing length.

Muscle contractions can be categorized by functional purpose: moving, resisting, or stabilizing body parts. In **concentric tension,** increased muscle contraction causes muscle shortening with movement resulting, such as when a client uses an overhead trapeze to pull up in bed. **Eccentric tension** helps control the speed and direction of movement. In the example of the overhead trapeze, the client should slowly lower to the bed. The lowering is controlled when the antagonistic muscles lengthen. Concentric and eccentric muscle actions are necessary for active movement and are therefore referred to as dynamic or **isotonic contraction. Isometric contraction** (static contraction) causes an increase in muscle tension or muscle work but no shortening or active movement of the muscle (e.g., instructing the client in tightening and relaxing a muscle group, as in quadriceps set exercises or pelvic floor exercises). Voluntary movement is a combination of isotonic and isometric contractions. For example, when the nurse lifts a client up in bed, the client's weight causes increased tension in the muscles of the nurse's arms until the tension (isometric) is equal to the weight to be lifted and the weight of the lower arm. When this equilibrium is reached, continued stimulation to the muscles results in muscle shortening (isotonic) and bending of the elbow (active movement), and the client is lifted off the bed.

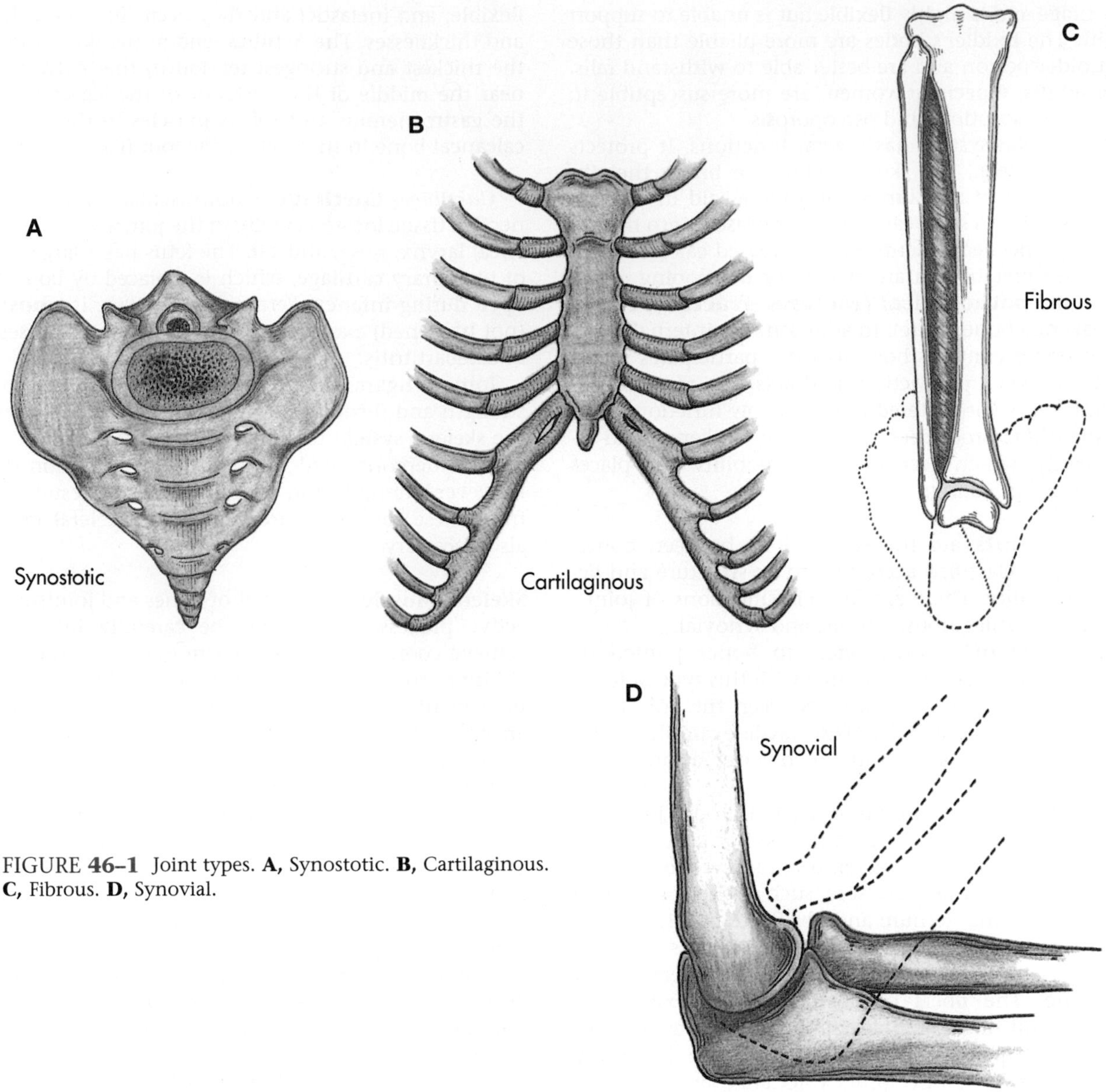

A

B

C

Fibrous

Synostotic

Cartilaginous

D

Synovial

FIGURE **46–1** Joint types. **A,** Synostotic. **B,** Cartilaginous. **C,** Fibrous. **D,** Synovial.

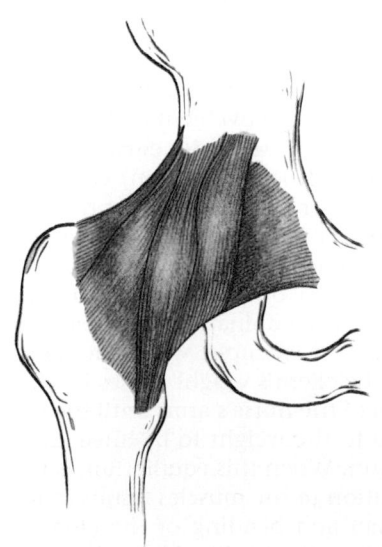

FIGURE **46–2** Ligaments of the hip joint.

Although isometric contractions do not result in muscle shortening, energy expenditure is increased. This type of muscle work is comparable to having a car in neutral with the driver continually depressing the accelerator and racing the engine. The driver is not going anywhere but expends a large amount of energy. The nurse must recognize the energy expenditure (increased respiratory rate and increased work on the heart) associated with isometric exercises because they may be contraindicated in certain clients' illnesses (e.g., myocardial infarction or chronic obstructive pulmonary disease).

Muscle Movement and Posture. Muscles that attach to bones of leverage provide necessary strength to move an object. **Leverage** is an inducing or compelling force and occurs when specific bones, such as the humerus, ulna, and radius, and the associated joint, such as the elbow, act together as a lever. Force is applied to one end of the bone to lift a weight as another point rotates the bone in the opposite direction.

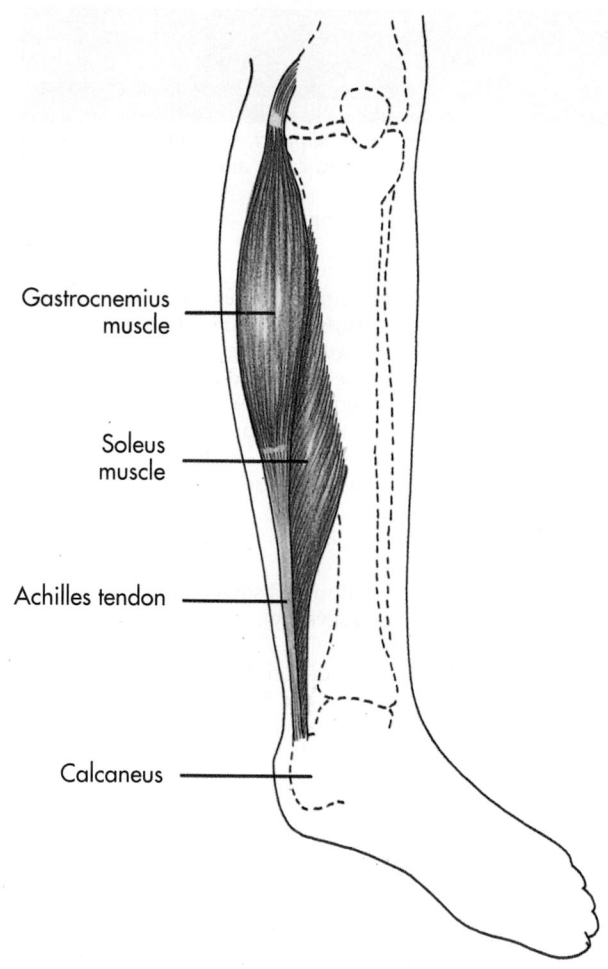

FIGURE **46-3** Tendons and muscles of the lower leg.

Gastrocnemius muscle

Soleus muscle

Achilles tendon

Calcaneus

Muscles associated primarily with maintaining posture are short and featherlike in appearance because they converge obliquely at a common tendon. Muscles of the lower extremities, trunk, neck, and back are concerned primarily with **posture** (the position of the body in relation to the surrounding space). These muscle groups work together to stabilize and support body weight standing or sitting, and they allow an individual to maintain a sitting or standing posture.

Muscle Regulation of Posture and Movement. Posture and movement can be reflections of personality, discomfort, and mood, as well as musculoskeletal function. For example, a person with a dramatic personality gestures with the hands, a person who is fatigued or depressed may slouch, and a person with abdominal pain may curl into a fetal-like position.

Posture and movement also depend on the skeleton and the shape and development of skeletal muscles. Coordination and regulation of different muscle groups depend on muscle tone and activity of antagonistic, synergistic, and antigravity muscles.

Muscle tone, or tonus, is the normal state of balanced muscle tension. Tension is achieved by alternate contraction and relaxation, without active movement, of neighboring fibers of a specific muscle group. Good muscle tone helps maintain functional positions such as sit-

ting or standing without excess muscle fatigue. Muscle tone is maintained through continual use of muscles. ADLs require muscle action and help maintain muscle tone. As a result of immobility or prolonged bed rest, activity level, activity tolerance, and muscle tone decrease.

The antagonistic, synergistic, and antigravity muscle groups are coordinated by the nervous system and work together to maintain posture and initiate movement (see Chapter 36).

Nervous System. Movement and posture are regulated by the nervous system. The precentral gyrus, or motor strip, is the major voluntary motor area and is located in the cerebral cortex. A majority of motor fibers descend from the motor strip and cross at the level of the medulla. Thus the motor fibers from the right motor strip initiate voluntary movement for the left side of the body, and motor fibers from the left motor strip initiate voluntary movement for the right side of the body.

During voluntary movement, impulses descend from the motor strip to the spinal cord. An impulse exits the spinal cord through efferent motor nerves and travels through the nerves. Through a complex process, **neurotransmitters,** or chemicals such as acetylcholine, transfer electric impulses from the nerve across the neuromuscular junction to the muscle. The neurotransmitter reaches a muscle and stimulates it, causing movement. Movement can be impaired by disorders that alter neurotransmitter production, transfer from the nerve to the muscle, or activation of muscle activity. Parkinsonism is an example of such a disorder (see Chapter 36).

Pathological Influences on Mobility
Many pathological conditions affect mobility. Although a complete description of each is beyond the scope of this chapter, an overview of four pathological influences are presented here: postural abnormalities, impaired muscle development, damage to the central nervous system, and direct trauma to the musculoskeletal system.

Postural Abnormalities. Congenital or acquired postural abnormalities affect the efficiency of the musculoskeletal system, as well as body alignment, balance, and appearance. During assessment, the nurse observes body alignment and ROM (see Chapter 36). Postural abnormalities can cause pain, impair alignment or mobility, or both. Knowledge about the characteristics, causes, and treatment of common postural abnormalities (Table 46-1) is necessary for lifting, transfer, and positioning. Some postural abnormalities may limit ROM. Nurses intervene to maintain maximum ROM in unaffected joints and then may design interventions to strengthen affected muscles and joints, improve the client's posture, and adequately use affected and unaffected muscle groups. Referral to and/or collaboration with a physical therapist may enhance the nurse's interventions for a client with a postural abnormality.

Impaired Muscle Development. Injury and disease can lead to numerous alterations in musculoskeletal function. The muscular dystrophies, for example, are a group of familial disorders that cause degeneration of skeletal muscle fibers. The most prevalent of the muscle diseases in

Table 46-1   Postural Abnormalities

Abnormality	Description	Cause	Possible Treatments*
Torticollis	Inclining of head to affected side, in which sternocleidomastoid muscle is contracted	Congenital or acquired condition	Surgery, heat, support, or immobilization, depending on cause and severity, gentle ROM
Lordosis	Exaggeration of anterior convex curve of lumbar spine	Congenital condition Temporary condition (e.g., pregnancy)	Spine-stretching exercises (based on cause)
Kyphosis	Increased convexity in curvature of thoracic spine	Congenital condition Rickets, osteoporosis Tuberculosis of spine	Spine-stretching exercises, sleeping without pillows, using bed board, bracing, spinal fusion (based on cause and severity)
Kypholordosis	Combination of kyphosis and lordosis	Congenital condition	Similar to methods used in kyphosis or lordosis (based on cause) Immobilization and surgery (based on cause and severity)
Scoliosis	Lateral "s" curvature of spine, unequal heights of hips and shoulders	Congenital condition Poliomyelitis Spastic paralysis Unequal leg length	Immobilization and surgery (based on cause and severity)
Kyphoscoliosis	Abnormal anteroposterior and lateral curvature of spine	Congenital condition Poliomyelitis Cor pulmonale	Immobilization and surgery (based on cause and severity)
Congenital hip dysplasia	Hip instability with limited abduction of hips and, occasionally, adduction contractures (head of femur does not articulate with acetabulum because of abnormal shallowness of acetabulum)	Congenital condition (more common with breech deliveries)	Maintenance of continuous abduction of thigh so that head of femur presses into center of acetabulum Abduction splints, casting, surgery
Knock-knee (genu valgum)	Legs curved inward so that knees come together as person walks	Congenital condition Rickets	Knee braces, surgery if not corrected by growth
Bowlegs (genu varum)	One or both legs bent outward at knee, which is normal until 2 to 3 years of age	Congenital condition Rickets	Slowing rate of curving if not corrected by growth With rickets, increase of vitamin D, calcium, and phosphorus intake to normal ranges
Clubfoot	95%: medial deviation and plantar flexion of foot (equinovarus) 5%: lateral deviation and dorsiflexion (calcaneovalgus)	Congenital condition	Casts, splints such as Denis-Browne splint, and surgery (based on degree and rigidity of deformity)
Footdrop	Inability to dorsiflex and invert foot because of peroneal nerve damage	Congenital condition Trauma Improper position of immobilized client	None (cannot be corrected) Prevention through physical therapy Bracing with ankle-foot orthotic (AFO)
Pigeon-toes	Internal rotation of forefoot or entire foot, common in infants	Congenital condition Habit	Growth, wearing reversed shoes

Data from McCance KL, Huether SE: *Pathophysiology: the biologic basis for disease in adults and children,* ed 4, St. Louis, 2002, Mosby.
*Severity of condition and cause will dictate treatment, which must be individualized.

childhood, the muscular dystrophies are characterized by progressive, symmetrical weakness and wasting of skeletal muscle groups, with increasing disability and deformity (McCance and Huether, 2002).

Damage to the Central Nervous System. Damage to any component of the central nervous system that regulates voluntary movement results in impaired body alignment and mobility. The motor strip in the cerebral cortex can be damaged by trauma from a head injury, ischemia from a stroke or brain attack (cerebrovascular accident [CVA]), or bacterial infection like meningitis. Motor impairment is directly related to the amount of destruction of the mo-

tor strip. For example, a person with a right-sided cerebral hemorrhage with complete necrosis will likely have destruction of the right motor strip and left-sided hemiplegia. Trauma to the spinal cord also impairs mobility. Common trauma includes transection of the spinal cord in which motor fibers are cut. A complete transection will likely result in a bilateral loss of voluntary motor control below the level of the trauma.

Direct Trauma to the Musculoskeletal System. Direct trauma to the musculoskeletal system can result in bruises, contusions, sprains, and fractures. A fracture is a disruption of bone tissue continuity. Fractures most commonly result from direct external trauma, but they can also occur as a consequence of some deformity of the bone (e.g., pathological fractures of osteoporosis, Paget's disease, or osteogenesis imperfecta). Young children are usually able to form new bone more easily than adults and, as a result, have few complications after a fracture. Treatment often includes positioning the fractured bone in proper alignment and immobilizing it to promote healing and restore function. Even this temporary immobilization can result in some **muscle atrophy,** loss of tone, and joint stiffness.

Nursing Knowledge Base

Mobility–Immobility

Fully understanding mobility requires more than an overview of body mechanics and the regulation of movement by the musculoskeletal and nervous systems. The nurse must be knowledgeable about how mobility and immobility affect the systems of the body and the psychosocial and developmental aspects of clients.

Mobility refers to a person's ability to move about freely, and **immobility** refers to the inability to move about freely. Mobility and immobility are best understood as the end points of a continuum, with many degrees of partial immobility between. Some clients move back and forth on this continuum, but for other clients, immobility is absolute and continues indefinitely. The terms *bed rest* and *impaired physical mobility* are frequently used when discussing clients on the mobility-immobility continuum.

Bed rest is an intervention that restricts clients to bed for therapeutic reasons. This intervention is most often prescribed by nurses and physicians. Bed rest has many different interpretations among health care professionals. Clients with a wide variety of conditions are placed on bed rest. The duration of bed rest depends on the illness or injury and the client's prior state of health (Box 46-1).

Impaired physical mobility is defined by the North American Nursing Diagnosis Association (NANDA) as a state in which the individual experiences or is at risk of experiencing limitation of physical movement (Ackley and Ladwig, 2002). Alterations in the level of physical mobility can result from prescribed restriction of movement in the form of bed rest, physical restriction of movement because of external devices (e.g., a cast or skeletal traction), voluntary restriction of movement, or impairment of motor or skeletal function.

The effects of muscular deconditioning associated with lack of physical activity may be apparent in a matter of days. The normal individual on bed rest loses muscle strength from baseline levels at a rate of 3% a day. Bed rest also is associated with cardiovascular, skeletal, and other organ changes. The term *disuse atrophy* has been used to describe the pathological reduction in normal size of muscle fibers after prolonged inactivity from bed rest, trauma, casting, or local nerve damage (McCance and Huether, 2002).

In a classic study, Deitrick and others (1948) found that even young healthy men put on bed rest had physiological problems. Periods of immobility or prolonged bed rest

---

Box **46-1**	General Objectives of Bed Rest

Reducing physical activity and the oxygen needs of the body

Reducing pain, including postoperative pain, and the need for large doses of analgesics

Allowing ill or debilitated clients to rest

Allowing exhausted clients the opportunity for uninterrupted rest

---

can cause major physiological, psychological, and social effects. These effects can be gradual or immediate and vary from client to client. The greater the extent and the longer the duration of immobility, the more pronounced the consequences. The client with complete mobility restrictions is continually at risk for hazardous system-wide effects.

Systemic Effects. All body systems work more efficiently with some form of movement. Exercise has been shown to have positive outcomes for all major systems of the body. Therefore when there is an alteration in mobility, each body system is at risk for impairment. The severity of the impairment depends on the client's overall health, degree and length of immobility, and age. For example, older adults with chronic illnesses develop pronounced effects of immobility more quickly than do younger clients with the same immobility problem.

Metabolic Changes. Endocrine metabolism, calcium resorption, and functioning of the gastrointestinal system are altered by changes in mobility.

The endocrine system, made up of hormone-secreting glands, helps to maintain and regulate vital functions such as (1) response to stress and injury, (2) growth and development, (3) reproduction, (4) ionic homeostasis, and (5) energy metabolism. When injury or stress occurs, the endocrine system triggers a series of responses aimed at maintaining blood pressure and preserving life. The endocrine system is important in maintaining homeostasis. Tissues and cells live in an internal environment that the endocrine system helps regulate through maintenance of sodium, potassium, water, and acid-base balance. The endocrine system also helps regulate energy metabolism. The basal metabolic rate (BMR) is increased by thyroid hormone, and energy is made available to cells through the integrated action of gastrointestinal and pancreatic hormones (McCance and Huether, 2002).

Immobility disrupts normal metabolic functioning: decreasing the metabolic rate; altering the metabolism of carbohydrates, fats, and proteins; causing fluid, electrolyte, and calcium imbalances; and causing gastrointestinal disturbances such as decreased appetite and slowing of peristalsis. However, in the presence of an infectious process, immobilized clients may have an increased BMR as a result of fever or wound healing. Fever and repair of wounds increase cellular oxygen requirements (McCance and Huether, 2002).

A deficiency in calories and protein is characteristic of clients with a decreased appetite secondary to immobility.

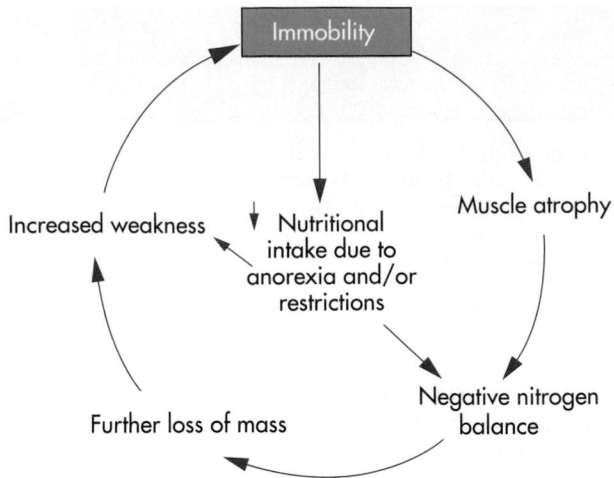

FIGURE **46–4** Factors contributing to negative nitrogen balance associated with immobility. (From Gröer MW, Shekleton ME: *Basic pathophysiology: a holistic approach,* ed 3, St. Louis, 1989, Mosby.)

Proteins are constantly being synthesized and broken down into amino acids in the body to be reformed into other proteins. Amino acids that are not used are excreted. The body can synthesize certain amino nonessential acids but depends on ingested proteins to supply the eight essential amino acids. When more nitrogen (the end product of amino acid breakdown) is excreted than is ingested in proteins, the body is said to have a **negative nitrogen balance** (Figure 46-4) and weight loss, decreased muscle mass, and weakness result from tissue catabolism (tissue breakdown). Protein loss leads to muscle loss.

Another metabolic change is calcium resorption (loss) from bones. As a result, urinary excretion of calcium increases because immobility causes the release of calcium into the circulation. Normally the kidneys can excrete the excess calcium. However, if the kidneys are unable to respond appropriately, hypercalcemia results (Maher, Salmond, and Pellino, 2002).

Impairments of gastrointestinal functioning, resulting from decreased gastrointestinal motility that develops subsequent to decreased mobility, vary. Difficulty in passing stools (constipation) is a common symptom, although diarrhea may result from a fecal impaction (accumulation of hardened feces). The nurse must be aware that this finding is not normal diarrhea, but rather liquid stool passing around the area of impaction (see Chapter 45). Left untreated, fecal impaction can result in a mechanical bowel obstruction that may partially or completely occlude the intestinal lumen, blocking normal propulsion of liquid and gas. The resulting fluid in the intestine produces distention and increases intraluminal pressure. Over time, intestinal function becomes depressed, dehydration occurs, absorption ceases, and fluid and electrolyte disturbances worsen.

Respiratory Changes. Regular aerobic exercise is known to enhance respiratory functioning. Lack of movement and exercise places clients at higher risk for respiratory complications. Postoperative and immobile clients are at high risk for developing pulmonary complications. The most common respiratory complications are **atelectasis** (collapse of alveoli) and **hypostatic pneumonia** (inflammation of the lung from stasis or pooling of secretions). Both decrease oxygenation, prolong recovery, and add to the client's discomfort (Black and others, 2001). In atelectasis a bronchiole or a bronchus becomes blocked by secretions and the distal lung tissue (alveoli) collapses as the existing air is absorbed, producing hypoventilation. The extent of atelectasis is determined by the site of the blockage. A lung lobe or a whole lung may even be collapsed. At some point in the development of these complications, there is a proportional decline in the client's ability to cough productively. Ultimately the distribution of mucus in the bronchi increases, particularly when the client is in the supine, prone, or lateral position (Figure 46-5). Mucus accumulates in the dependent regions of the airways (Figure 46-6). Because mucus is an excellent medium for bacterial growth, hypostatic pneumonia may result.

Cardiovascular Changes. The cardiovascular system is also affected by immobilization. The three major changes are orthostatic hypotension, increased cardiac workload, and thrombus formation.

Orthostatic hypotension is a drop of 20 mm Hg or more in systolic blood pressure and of 10 mm Hg in diastolic blood pressure when the client rises from a lying or sitting position to a standing position (Lance and others, 2000). In the immobilized client, decreased circulating fluid volume, pooling of blood in the lower extremities, and decreased autonomic response occur. These factors result in decreased venous return, followed by a decrease in cardiac output, which is reflected by a decline in blood pressure (McCance and Huether, 2002).

As the workload of the heart increases, its oxygen consumption does, too. The heart therefore works harder and less efficiently during periods of prolonged rest. As immobilization increases, cardiac output falls, further decreasing cardiac efficiency and increasing workload.

Clients are also at risk for thrombus formation. A **thrombus** is an accumulation of platelets, fibrin, clotting factors, and the cellular elements of the blood attached to the interior wall of a vein or artery, sometimes occluding the lumen of the vessel (Figure 46-7). There are three factors that contribute to venous thrombus formation: (1) loss of integrity of the vessel wall (e.g., injury), (2) abnormalities of blood flow (e.g., slow blood flow in calf veins associated with bed rest), and (3) alterations in blood constituents (e.g., a change in clotting factors or increased platelet activity). These three factors are sometimes referred to as Virchow's triad (McCance and Huether, 2002).

Musculoskeletal Changes. The effects of immobility on the musculoskeletal system can include permanent or temporary impairment or permanent disability. Restricted mobility may result in loss of endurance, strength, muscle mass and decreased stability and balance. Other effects of restricted mobility affecting the skeletal system are impaired calcium metabolism and impaired joint mobility.

Upright

Mucus
distribution

Supine

Effects on lumen diameter

Upright

Supine

Bronchus

Lumen change

Mucus

FIGURE **46–5** Effect of recumbency and gravity on distribution of respiratory tract and diameter of bronchiolar lumen. (From Gröer MW, Shekleton ME: *Basic pathophysiology: a holistic approach,* ed 3, St. Louis, 1989, Mosby.)

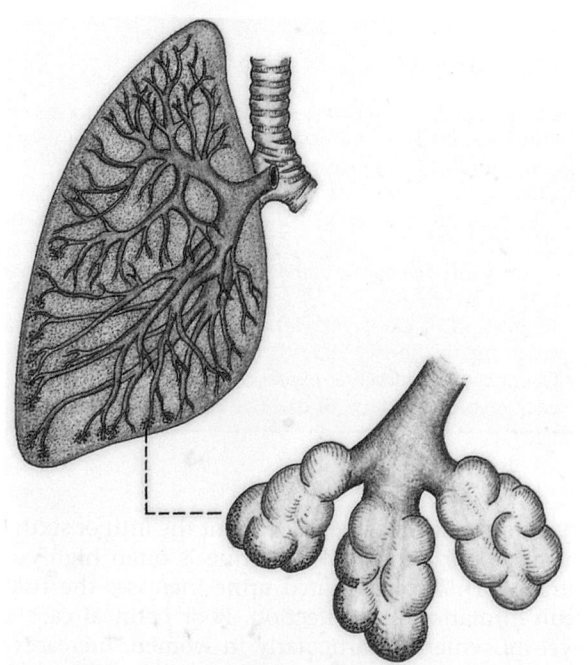

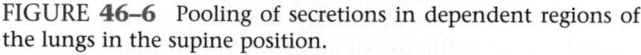

FIGURE **46–6** Pooling of secretions in dependent regions of the lungs in the supine position.

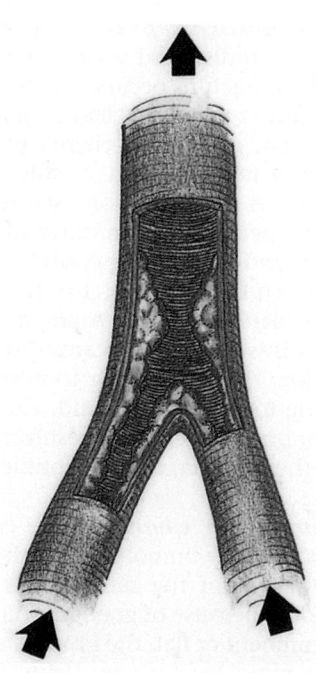

FIGURE **46–7** Thrombus formation in a vessel.

Muscle Effects. Because of protein breakdown, the client loses lean body mass, which is composed partially of muscle. The reduced muscle mass is unable to sustain activity without increased fatigue. If immobility continues and the muscles are not exercised, there is further decrease in muscle mass. Muscle weakness always occurs with immobility. Prolonged immobility often leads to muscle atrophy (or loss of muscle tissue). Therefore atrophy is widely observed in response to illness, decreased ADLs, and immobilization. Loss of endurance, decreased muscle mass and strength, and joint instability (see Skeletal Effects) put clients at risk for falls (see Chapter 37).

Skeletal Effects. Immobilization causes two skeletal changes: impaired calcium metabolism and joint abnormalities. Because immobilization results in bone resorption, the bone tissue is less dense, or is atrophied, and **disuse osteoporosis** results. When disuse osteoporosis occurs, the client is at risk for pathological fractures.

Immobilization and non–weight-bearing activities increase the rate of bone resorption. Bone resorption also causes calcium to be released in the blood, and hypercalcemia results.

Osteoporosis is a major health concern in this country. Most affected are women; 20% are men. The NOF (National Osteoporosis Foundation, 2002) reports that one out of two women will suffer the severe consequence of a pathological fracture as a result of primary osteoporosis. Although primary osteoporosis is different in origin from the osteoporosis that results from immobility, it is imperative for nurses to recognize that immobilized clients may be at high risk for accelerated bone loss if they have primary osteoporosis. Early client evaluation and consultation and referral with physicians, dietitians, and physical therapists are important interventions for preventing disability in clients with primary osteoporosis who become immobilized. For the client with osteoporosis, the goal is to maintain independence with activities of daily living. Assistive ambulatory devices, adaptive clothing, and safety bars may assist the client with maintaining independence. Client teaching should focus on limiting the severity of the disease through diet and activity (Box 46-2).

Immobility can lead to joint contractures. A **joint contracture** is an abnormal and possibly permanent condition characterized by fixation of the joint. It is caused by disuse, atrophy, and shortening of the muscle fibers. When a contracture occurs, the joint cannot obtain full ROM. Contractures may leave a joint(s) in a nonfunctional position, as seen in clients who are permanently curled in a fetal position. Resnick (2000) found that upper and lower extremity contractures significantly reduce functional performance in older adults.

One common and debilitating contracture is footdrop (Figure 46-8). When **footdrop** occurs, the foot is permanently fixed in plantar flexion. Ambulation is difficult with the foot in this position, because the client cannot dorsiflex the foot. The client with footdrop is therefore unable to lift the toes off the ground. Clients who have suffered CVAs or brain attacks with resulting left- or right-sided paralysis (hemiplegia) are susceptible to footdrop.

Urinary Elimination Changes. The client's urinary elimination is altered by immobility. In the upright position, urine flows out of the renal pelvis and into the ureters and bladder because of gravitational forces. When the client is recumbent or flat, the kidneys and the ureters move toward a more level plane. Urine formed by the kidney must enter the bladder unaided by gravity. Because the peristaltic contractions of the ureters are insufficient to overcome gravity, the renal pelvis may fill before urine enters the ureters (Figure 46-9). This condition is called **urinary stasis** and increases the risk of urinary tract infection and renal calculi (see Chapter 44). **Renal calculi** are calcium stones that lodge in the renal pelvis and pass through the ureters. Immobilized clients are at risk for calculi because of altered calcium metabolism and the resulting hypercalcemia.

As the period of immobility continues, fluid intake can diminish, and this combined with other causes, such as fever, increases the risk for dehydration. As a result, uri-

nary output may decline on or about the fifth or sixth day after immobilization and the urine is often highly concentrated. This concentrated urine increases the risk for calculi formation and infection. Poor perineal care after bowel movements, particularly in women, increases the risk of urinary tract contamination by *Escherichia coli* bacteria. Another cause of urinary tract infections in immobilized clients is the use of an indwelling urinary catheter.

Integumentary Changes. The direct effect of pressure on the skin by immobility is compounded by the changes in metabolism that accompany immobility. Any break in the skin's integrity is difficult to heal in the immobilized client. Preventing a pressure ulcer is much less expensive than treating one (Bergquist, 2001). Thus immobility is a major risk for pressure ulcers and preventive nursing interventions are imperative.

A **pressure ulcer** is an impairment of the skin as a result of prolonged ischemia (decreased blood supply to an

---

Client Teaching   Box 46-2

Clients With Osteoporosis
Objective

- Client will verbalize strategies to prevent or limit the severity of osteoporosis.

Teaching Strategies

- Instruct client and/or caregiver on common risk factors and how to modify lifestyle (e.g., smoking, caffeine, alcohol, hormone replacement as recommended by physician).
- Teach client and/or caregiver the current recommended dietary allowances for calcium and review foods high in calcium.
- Instruct clients and/or caregiver on appropriate types of weight-bearing exercises as recommended by physician or physical therapist to prevent injury or fractures.
- Teach client and/or caregiver about safety, fall prevention, and strategies to create a safe home environment.
- Instruct client and/or caregiver self-administration of appropriate medication as ordered by physician.
- Promote positive self-image in client by providing realistic yet optimistic and positive feedback about changes in appearance and mobility.

Evaluation

- Client and/or caregiver verbalize strategies to modify lifestyle such as stopping smoking, reducing caffeine or alcohol intake, or increasing dietary calcium.
- Client and/or caregiver verbalize foods high in calcium.
- Client and/or caregiver verbalize appropriate weight-bearing exercises.
- Client and/or caregiver verbalize safety strategies to prevent falls.
- Client and/or caregiver verbalize appropriate knowledge about medications.
- Client and/or caregiver express positive but realistic feedback regarding effects of disease.

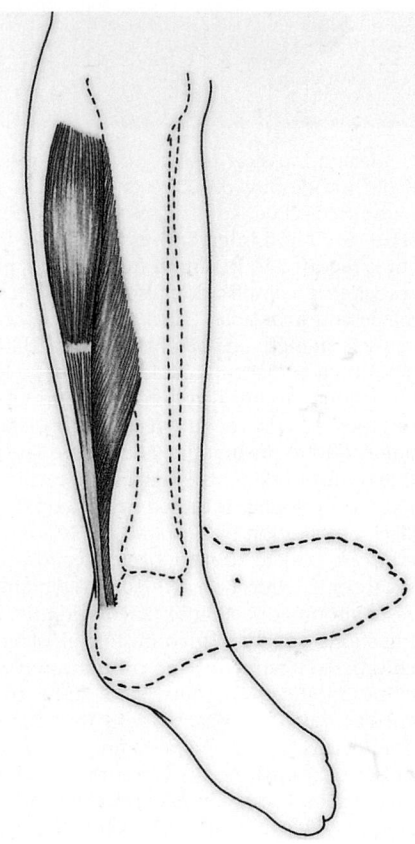

FIGURE **46–8**   Footdrop. Ankle is fixed in a plantar flexion. Normally the ankle is able to flex (*dotted line*), which eases walking.

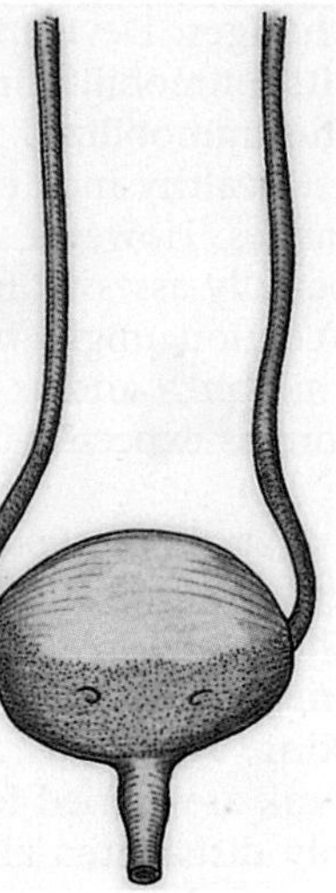

FIGURE **46–9**   Stasis of urine with reflux to ureters.

area) in tissues (see Chapter 47). The ulcer is characterized initially by inflammation and usually forms over a bony prominence. Ischemia develops when the pressure on the skin is greater than the pressure inside the small peripheral blood vessels supplying blood to the skin.

Tissue metabolism depends on the body's receipt of oxygen and nutrients from the blood supply and the elimination of metabolic wastes. Pressure affects cellular metabolism by decreasing or obliterating tissue circulation. When a client lies in bed or sits in a chair, the weight of the body is on bony prominences. The longer the pressure is applied, the longer the period of ischemia and therefore the greater the risk of skin breakdown.

> *Safety Alert:* To prevent skin breakdown, immobilized clients should be turned every 2 hours at a minimum. Defloor (2000) reports that the preferred position is a 30-degree lateral position if the client is going to remain in a position for more than 2 hours.

Psychosocial Effects. Immobilization may lead to emotional and behavioral responses, sensory alterations, and changes in coping. These changes are individualized to each client. In addition, immobilized clients may also have social and family difficulties.

Common emotional changes are depression, behavioral changes, sleep-wake disturbances, and impaired coping. The immobilized client can become depressed because of changes in role, self-concept, and other factors.

Depression is an affective disorder characterized by exaggerated feelings of sadness, melancholy, dejection, worthlessness, emptiness, and hopelessness out of proportion to reality. Depression can result from worrying about present and future levels of health, finances, and family needs. Because immobilization removes the client from a daily routine, he or she has more time to worry about disability. Worrying can quickly increase the client's depression, causing withdrawal. Assessing behavioral changes throughout restricted mobility helps the nurse to identify changes in self-concept, recognize early signs of depression, and develop nursing interventions.

Behavioral changes resulting from immobilization vary widely, depending on the client. Common behavioral changes include hostility, belligerence, giddiness, fear, and anxiety. Early in the nursing process the nurse should interview the client's family and friends about normal behavioral patterns to gain baseline data. If unexpected behaviors are observed later, the nurse can intervene to reduce the effects of immobilization on the client's behavioral patterns.

Sleep-wake alterations in the immobile client may occur from nursing care or changes in habit or environment. Disruption of normal sleeping patterns can further cause behavioral changes. Nursing interventions should be used to ensure that the client receives sufficient sleep (see Chapter 41). The client who is on bed rest and is able to change position during sleep does not require continuous physical nursing care. Unless other treatment activities are required during the night, the care plan for the physiologically stable client on bed rest should provide for uninterrupted sleep.

Long-term immobility or bed rest can affect usual coping patterns. Such a client may withdraw and become passive. The passive client allows nurses to provide care but is not interested in increasing independence or involvement in care. Early in the care of an immobilized client, the nurse should assess the client's normal coping mechanisms in order to design a nursing care plan that will allow the client to continue to use these coping abilities or will help him or her develop new ones.

Developmental Changes. Developmental changes tend to be associated with immobility in the very young and in older adults. The immobilized young or middle-age adult who has been healthy may experience few, if any, developmental changes. However, there are exceptions, and clients must be fully assessed for developmental implications. One exception might be a mother who has complications at childbirth and as a result cannot interact with the newborn as expected.

Infants, Toddlers, and Preschoolers. The newborn infant's spine is flexed and lacks the anteroposterior curves of the adult (see Chapter 11). As the baby grows, musculoskeletal development permits support of weight for standing and walking. Posture is awkward because the head and upper trunk are carried forward. Because body weight is not evenly distributed along a line of gravity, posture is off balance, and falls occur often. When the infant, toddler, or preschooler is immobilized, it is usually because of trauma or the need to correct a congenital skeletal abnormality. Prolonged immobilization can delay the child's gross motor skills, intellectual development, or musculoskeletal development. Nurses caring for immobilized children should plan activities that provide physical and psychosocial stimuli.

Adolescents. The adolescence stage is usually initiated by a tremendous growth spurt (see Chapter 11). Growth is frequently uneven. Prolonged immobilization may alter adolescent growth patterns. In addition, the adolescent may lag behind peers in gaining independence. When immobilization occurs, social isolation must be a concern for this age-group.

Adults. An adult who has correct posture and body alignment feels good, looks good, and generally appears self-confident. The healthy adult also has the necessary musculoskeletal development and coordination to carry out ADLs (see Chapter 12). When periods of prolonged immobility occur, all physiological systems are at risk. In addition, the role of the adult may change with regard to the family or social structure. The adult may lose identity associated with a job.

Older Adults. A progressive loss of total bone mass occurs with the older adult. Some of the possible causes of this loss include decreased physical activity, hormonal changes, and actual bone resorption. The effect of bone loss is weaker bones. Older adults may walk more slowly, take smaller steps, and appear less coordinated. Thus balance is impaired, and they are at greater risk for falls and injuries (see Chapter 13). The outcomes of a fall include not only possible injury, but also hospitalization, loss of independence, and psychological effects.

Older adults may experience functional status changes secondary to hospitalization and altered mobility status (Box 46-3). Immobilization of older adults may increase their physical dependence on others and accelerate functional losses. Immobilization of some older adults results from a degenerative disease, neurological trauma, or chronic illness. For some older adults, immobilization occurs gradually and progressively, whereas for others—

Box 46-3   Hazards of Hospitalization of the Older Adult

For many elders, admission to the hospital often results in functional decline despite the cure or treatment for which they were admitted. Older adults can quickly regress to a dependent state, and rapid intervention of an interdisciplinary health team is required to maintain functional capacity.

Elders experience complications from hospitalization that are explainable and avoidable. Usual aging is associated with decreased muscle strength and aerobic capacity. Placing clients on bed rest without sufficient ambulation leads to loss of mobility and functional decline. Immobility causes weakness, fatigue, and an increased risk for falls. It results in shallow breathing, which may lead to pneumonia, and inadequate turning or repositioning results in skin breakdown and pressure ulcers.

Temporary incontinence is caused by unnecessary catheterization or lack of attention by hospital staff. Catheter use and improper pericare lead to urinary tract infections. Elders are prone to nosocomial infections (infections obtained in the health care environment) because of compromised immune systems. Infections often cause confusion in older adults as well as medications, treatments, and translocation.

Hospitalization affects the nutritional status in the older adult. Limited access to fluids causes dehydration. Conversely, fluid overload occurs from improper administration of IV fluids. Treatments and medications cause fluid and electrolyte imbalances, contributing to confusion in the geriatric client. Anorexia and insufficient assistance with eating may lead to malnutrition.

Finally, multiple interruptions and noise in the environment impair sleep, causing fatigue, depression, and confusion. Any of these factors may thrust vulnerable elders into a state of irreversible functional decline.

Modified from Ebersole P, Hess P: *Geriatric nursing and healthy aging,* St. Louis, 2001, Mosby.

---

especially those who have had a stroke—immobilization is sudden. When providing nursing care for an older adult, the nurse should develop a care plan that encourages the client to perform as many self-care activities as possible, thereby maintaining the highest level of mobility. Nurses may inadvertently contribute to a client's immobility by providing unnecessary help with activities such as bathing and transferring.

Critical Thinking

Critical thinking requires the nurse to combine knowledge, experiences, client data, critical thinking attitudes, and intellectual and professional standards. Each of these sources must be weighed for its validity and applicability to the client who is facing impaired mobility. The immobile client's needs are multiple, and by integrating these sources the nurse can best judge appropriate nursing diagnoses and subsequent care.

To understand the impact of immobility on the client and family, the nurse must integrate knowledge from nursing and other disciplines, previous experiences, and information gathered from clients. In addition, the use of critical

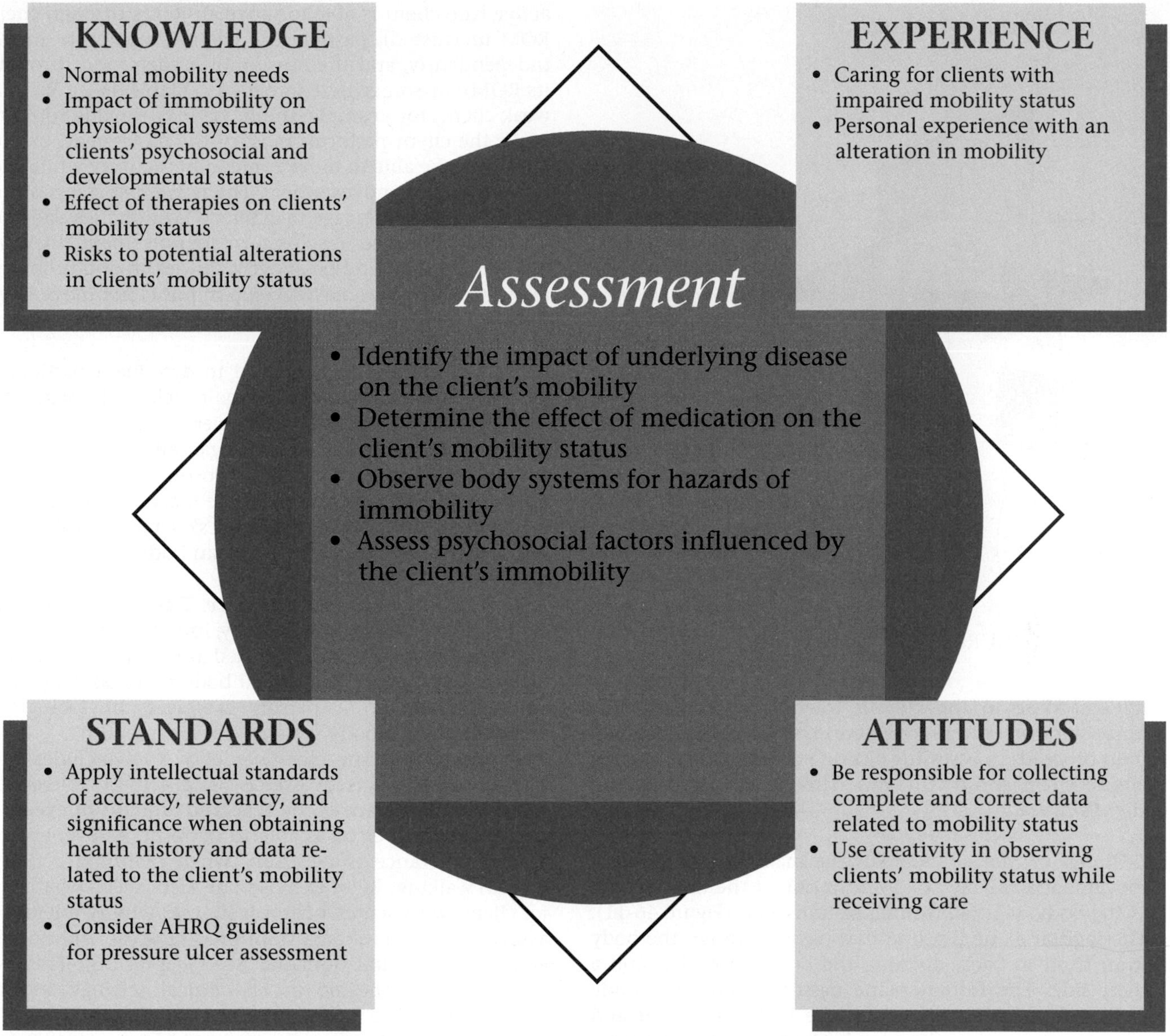

KNOWLEDGE

- Normal mobility needs
- Impact of immobility on physiological systems and clients' psychosocial and developmental status
- Effect of therapies on clients' mobility status
- Risks to potential alterations in clients' mobility status

EXPERIENCE

- Caring for clients with impaired mobility status
- Personal experience with an alteration in mobility

Assessment

- Identify the impact of underlying disease on the client's mobility
- Determine the effect of medication on the client's mobility status
- Observe body systems for hazards of immobility
- Assess psychosocial factors influenced by the client's immobility

STANDARDS

- Apply intellectual standards of accuracy, relevancy, and significance when obtaining health history and data related to the client's mobility status
- Consider AHRQ guidelines for pressure ulcer assessment

ATTITUDES

- Be responsible for collecting complete and correct data related to mobility status
- Use creativity in observing clients' mobility status while receiving care

FIGURE **46–10** Critical thinking model for immobility assessment.

thinking attitudes such as creativity is needed to devise a plan to provide successful interventions for immobility. Professional standards such as those developed by the Agency for Healthcare Research and Quality (AHRQ) and intellectual standards such as accuracy provide valuable guides for mobility management (Figure 46-10). In addition, many agencies may have standards for practice related to transferring clients and to fall and pressure sore prevention.

Nursing Process for Impaired Body Alignment and Mobility

The application of the nursing process, using a critical thinking approach enables the nurse to develop individualized care plans for clients with preexisting mobility impairments and for those who are at risk for immobility. A care plan is designed to improve the client's functional status, promote self-care, maintain psychological well-being, and reduce the hazards of immobility.

Assessment

Nursing assessment is presented in two sections: mobility and immobility. Both areas are usually assessed during the complete physical examination.

Mobility. Assessment of client mobility focuses on ROM, gait, exercise and activity tolerance, and body alignment. When unsure of the client's abilities, the nurse should begin assessment of mobility with the client in the most supportive position and move to higher levels of mobil-

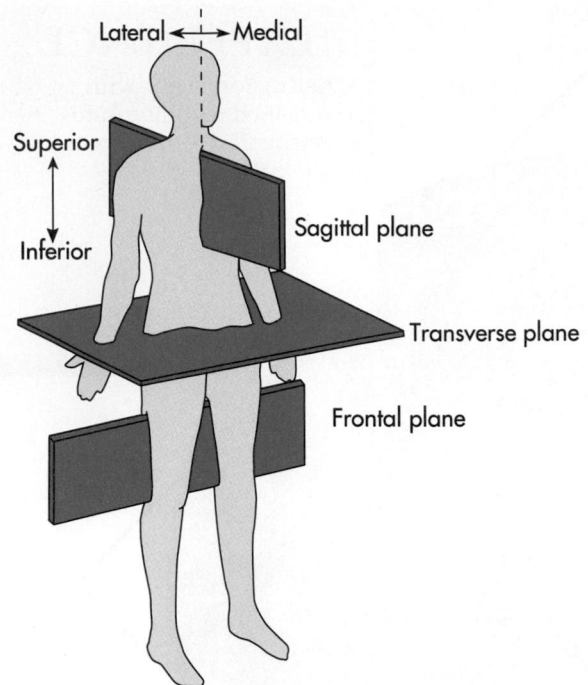

FIGURE **46–11** Planes of the body.

ity according to the client's tolerance. Generally, the nurse starts assessing movement while the client is lying, then proceeds to assessing sitting positions in bed, transfers to chair, and finally gait. This helps to protect the client's safety.

Range of Motion. **ROM** is the maximum amount of movement available at a joint in one of the three planes of the body: sagittal, frontal, or transverse (Figure 46-11). The sagittal plane is a line that passes through the body from front to back, dividing the body into a left and a right side. The frontal plane passes through the body from side to side and divides the body into front and back. The transverse plane is a horizontal line that divides the body into upper and lower portions.

Joint mobility in each of the planes is limited by ligaments, muscles, and the nature of the joint. However, some joint movements are specific to each plane. In the sagittal plane, movements are flexion and extension (e.g., fingers and elbows), dorsiflexion and plantar flexion (feet), and extension (e.g., hip). In the frontal plane, movements are abduction and adduction (e.g., arms and legs), and eversion and inversion (feet). In the transverse plane, movements are pronation and supination (hands), and internal and external rotation (hips).

When assessing ROM, the nurse asks questions about and physically examines the client for stiffness, swelling, pain, limited movement, and unequal movement. Chapter 32 describes specific techniques for measuring the degrees of motion in a joint. Assessment of ROM is important as a baseline measure to compare and evaluate whether loss in joint mobility has occurred. Clients whose mobility is restricted require ROM to reduce the hazards of immobility. Thus the nurse assesses the type of ROM exercise a client can perform. ROM exercises may be

active (the client is able to move all joints through their ROM unassisted), passive (the client is unable to move independently, and the nurse moves each joint through its ROM), or somewhere in between (Table 46-2). With a weak client, for example, the nurse may provide support while the client performs most of the movement, or the client may be able to move some joints actively while the nurse passively moves others. The nurse first assesses the client's ability to engage in active ROM exercises and the need for assistance, teaching, or reinforcement. In general, exercises should be as active as health and mobility allow. Contractures may develop in joints not moved periodically through their full ROM.

Gait. The term **gait** is used to describe a particular manner or style of walking. The gait cycle begins with the heel strike of one leg and continues to the heel strike of the other leg. Assessing a client's gait allows the nurse to draw conclusions about balance, posture, safety, and ability to walk without assistance. The mechanics of human gait involve coordination of the skeletal, neurological, and muscular systems of the human body.

Exercise and Activity Tolerance. **Exercise** is physical activity for conditioning the body, improving health, and maintaining fitness. It can be used as therapy to correct a deformity or restore the overall body to a maximal state of health. When a person exercises, physiological changes occur in body systems (see Chapter 36).

Assessment of the client's energy level includes the physiological effects of exercise and activity tolerance. **Activity tolerance** is the type and amount of exercise or work that a person is able to perform. Assessment of activity tolerance is necessary when planning activity such as walking, ROM exercises, or ADLs such as bathing for clients with acute or chronic illness. Activity tolerance assessment includes data from physiological, emotional, and developmental domains (see Chapter 36). This assessment is applicable in all clinical settings and is quickly completed by the nurse.

As activity is begun, clients should be monitored for symptoms such as dyspnea, fatigue, or chest pain and/or for a change in vital signs from baseline. The weak or debilitated client is unable to sustain activity because the greater energy needed to complete the activity creates fatigue and generalized weakness. Even seemingly simple tasks such as eating and moving in bed may need to be monitored. When decreased activity tolerance is noted, the nurse should assess the time needed by the client to recover. Decreasing recovery time may indicate improving activity tolerance.

People who are depressed, worried, or anxious are frequently unable to tolerate exercise. Depressed clients are usually not motivated to participate. Clients who are worried or anxious fatigue easily because they expend a great deal of energy in worry and anxiety. Thus they may experience physical and emotional exhaustion.

Developmental changes also affect activity tolerance. As the infant enters the toddler stage, the activity level increases and the need for sleep declines. The child entering preschool or primary grades expends mental energy in learning and may require more rest after school or

Text continued on p. 1439

Table 46-2   Range-of-Motion Exercises

Body Part	Type of Joint	Type of Movement	Range (Degrees)	Primary Muscles
Neck, cervical spine	Pivotal	*Flexion:* Bring chin to rest on chest	45	Sternocleidomastoid
		Extension: Return head to erect position	45	Trapezius
		Hyperextension: Bend head back as far as possible	10	Trapezius
		Lateral flexion: Tilt head as far as possible toward each shoulder	40-45	Sternocleidomastoid
		Rotation: Turn head as far as possible in circular movement	180	Sternocleidomastoid, trapezius
Shoulder	Ball and socket	*Flexion:* Raise arm from side position forward to position above head	180 / 45-60	Coracobrachialis, biceps brachii, deltoid, pectoralis major
		Extension: Return arm to position at side of body	180	Latissimus dorsi, teres major, triceps brachii
		Hyperextension: Move arm behind body, keeping elbow straight	45-60	Latissimus dorsi, teres major, deltoid
		Abduction: Raise arm to side to position above head with palm away from head	180	Deltoid, supraspinatus
		Adduction: Lower arm sideways and across body as far as possible	320	Pectoralis major

Continued

Table 46-2   Range-of-Motion Exercises—cont'd

Body Part	Type of Joint	Type of Movement	Range (Degrees)	Primary Muscles
Shoulder, cont'd	Ball and socket, cont'd	*Internal rotation:* With elbow flexed, rotate shoulder by moving arm until thumb is turned inward and toward back	90	Pectoralis major, latissimus dorsi, teres major, subscapularis
		External rotation: With elbow flexed, move arm until thumb is upward and lateral to head	90	Infraspinatus, teres major, deltoid
		Circumduction: Move arm in full circle (Circumduction is combination of all movements of ball-and-socket joint.)	360	Deltoid, coracobrachialis, latissimus dorsi, teres major
Elbow	Hinge	*Flexion:* Bend elbow so that lower arm moves toward its shoulder joint and hand is level with shoulder	150	Biceps brachii, brachialis, brachioradialis
		Extension: Straighten elbow by lowering hand	150	Triceps brachii
Forearm	Pivotal	*Supination:* Turn lower arm and hand so that palm is up	70-90	Supinator, biceps brachii
		Pronation: Turn lower arm so that palm is down	70-90	Pronator teres, pronator quadratus
Wrist	Condyloid	*Flexion:* Move palm toward inner aspect of forearm	80-90	Flexor carpi ulnaris, flexor carpi radialis
		Extension: Move fingers and hand posterior to midline	80-90	Extensor carpi radialis brevis, extensor carpi radialis longus, extensor carpi ulnaris
		Hyperextension: Bring dorsal surface of hand back as far as possible	80-90	Extensor carpi radialis brevis, extensor carpi radialis longus, extensor carpi ulnaris
		Abduction (radial deviation): Bend wrist laterally toward fifth finger	Up to 30	Flexor carpi radialis, extensor carpi radialis brevis, extensor carpi radialis longus
		Adduction (ulnar deviation): Bend wrist medially toward thumb	30-50	Flexor carpi ulnaris, extensor carpi ulnaris

Table 46-2	Range-of-Motion Exercises—cont'd			
Body Part	**Type of Joint**	**Type of Movement**	**Range (Degrees)**	**Primary Muscles**
Fingers	Condyloid hinge	*Flexion:* Make fist	90	Lumbricales, interosseus volaris, interosseus dorsalis
		Extension: Straighten fingers	90	Extensor digiti quinti proprius, extensor digitorum communis, extensor indicis proprius
		Hyperextension: Bend fingers back as far as possible	30-60	
		Abduction: Spread fingers apart	30	Interosseus dorsalis
		Adduction: Bring fingers together	30	Interosseus volaris
Thumb	Saddle	*Flexion:* Move thumb across palmar surface of hand	90	Flexor pollicis brevis
		Extension: Move thumb straight away from hand	90	Extensor pollicis longus, extensor pollicis brevis
		Abduction: Extend thumb laterally (usually done when placing fingers in abduction and adduction)	30	Abductor pollicis brevis
		Adduction: Move thumb back toward hand	30	Adductor pollicis obliquus, adductor pollicis transversus
		Opposition: Touch thumb to each finger of same hand		Opponeus pollicis, opponeus digiti minimi
Hip	Ball and socket	*Flexion:* Move leg forward and up	90-120	Psoas major, iliacus, sartorius
		Extension: Move back beside other leg	90-120	Gluteus maximus, semitendinosus, semimembranosus
		Hyperextension: Move leg behind body	30-50	Gluteus maximus, semitendinosus, semimembranosus

Continued

Table 4-6-2   **Range-of-Motion Exercises—cont'd**

Body Part	Type of Joint	Type of Movement	Range (Degrees)	Primary Muscles
Knee	Hinge	*Abduction:* Move leg laterally away from body	30-50	Gluteus medius, gluteus minimus
		Adduction: Move leg back toward medial position and beyond if possible	30-50	Adductor longus, adductor brevis, adductor magnus
		Internal rotation: Turn foot and leg toward other leg	90	Gluteus medius, gluteus minimus, tensor fasciae latae
		External rotation: Turn foot and leg away from other leg	90	Obturatorius internus, obturatorius externus
		Circumduction: Move leg in circle		Psoas major, gluteus maximus, gluteus medius, adductor magnus
Knee	Hinge	*Flexion:* Bring heel back toward back of thigh	120-130	Biceps femoris, semitendinosus, semimembranosus, sartorius
		Extension: Return leg to floor	120-130	Rectus femoris, vastus lateralis, vastus medialis, vastus intermedius
Ankle	Hinge	*Dorsal flexion:* Move foot so that toes are pointed upward	20-30	Tibialis anterior
		Plantar flexion: Move foot so that toes are pointed downward	45-50	Gastrocnemius, soleus

Table 46-2   Range-of-Motion Exercises—cont'd

Body Part	Type of Joint	Type of Movement	Range (Degrees)	Primary Muscles
Foot	Gliding	*Inversion:* Turn sole of foot medially	10 or less	Tibialis anterior, tibialis posterior
		Eversion: Turn sole of foot laterally	10 or less	Peroneus longus, peroneus brevis
Toes	Condyloid	*Flexion:* Curl toes downward	30-60	Flexor digitorum, lumbricalis pedis, flexor hallucis brevis
		Extension: Straighten toes	30-60	Extensor digitorum longus, extensor digitorum brevis, extensor hallucis longus
		Abduction: Spread toes apart	15 or less	Abductor hallucis, interosseus dorsalis
		Adduction: Bring toes together	15 or less	Adductor hallucis, interosseus plantaris

before strenuous play. The adolescent going through puberty may require more rest because much of the body's energy is expended for growth and hormone changes (see Chapter 41).

Changes may still occur through the adult years, but many of these changes are related to work and lifestyle choices. Pregnancy may cause fluctuations in a woman's energy tolerance; especially during the first and third trimesters, when she may have increased fatigue. Hormonal changes and fetal development use body energy, and the woman may be unable or unmotivated to carry out physical activities. During the last trimester, fetal development consumes a great deal of the mother's energy, and the size and location of the fetus may limit the ability to take a deep breath, resulting in less oxygen being available for physical activities.

As the person grows older, activity tolerance changes. Muscle mass is reduced, posture changes, and the composition of bones is altered. There are often changes in the cardiorespiratory system, such as decreased maximum heart rate and decreased lung compliance that affect the intensity of exercise. As age progresses, the older individual may still exercise but will do so at a reduced intensity. The more inactive a client is, the more pronounced these activity changes are.

Body Alignment. Assessment of body alignment can be carried out with the client standing, sitting, or lying down. This assessment has the following objectives:
- Determining normal physiological changes in body alignment resulting from growth and development for each individual client
- Identifying deviations in body alignment caused by poor posture

- Providing opportunities for clients to observe their posture
- Identifying learning needs of clients for maintaining correct body alignment
- Identifying trauma, muscle damage, or nerve dysfunction
- Obtaining information concerning other factors that contribute to poor alignment, such as fatigue, malnutrition, and psychological problems

The first step in assessing body alignment is to put clients at ease so that unnatural or rigid positions are not assumed. When the body alignment of an immobilized or unconscious client is assessed, pillows and positioning supports should be removed from the bed and the client placed in the supine position.

Standing. The nurse should focus assessment of body alignment for the standing client on the following points:
1. The head is erect and midline.
2. When observed posteriorly, the shoulders and hips are straight and parallel.
3. When observed posteriorly, the vertebral column is straight.
4. When the client is observed laterally, the head is erect and the spinal curves are aligned in a reversed S pattern. The cervical vertebrae are anteriorly convex, the thoracic vertebrae are posteriorly convex, and the lumbar vertebrae are anteriorly convex.
5. When observed laterally, the abdomen is comfortably tucked in and the knees and ankles are slightly flexed. The person appears comfortable and does not seem conscious of the flexion of knees or ankles.
6. The arms hang comfortably at the sides.
7. The feet are placed slightly apart to achieve a base of support, and the toes are pointed forward.

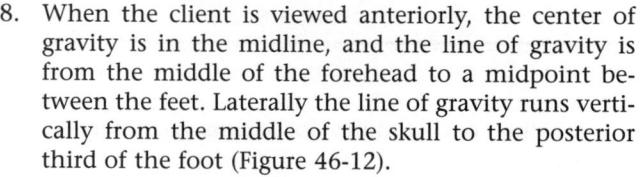

FIGURE **46–12** Correct body alignment when standing.

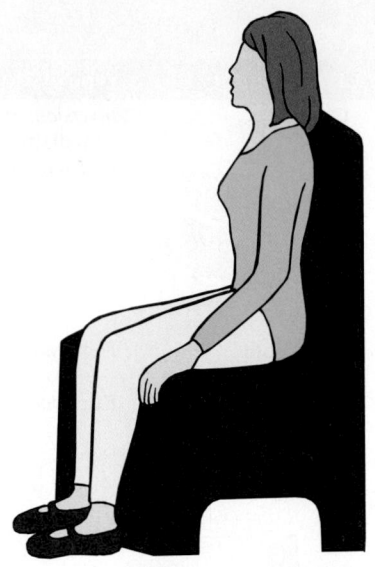

FIGURE **46–13** Correct body alignment when sitting.

8. When the client is viewed anteriorly, the center of gravity is in the midline, and the line of gravity is from the middle of the forehead to a midpoint between the feet. Laterally the line of gravity runs vertically from the middle of the skull to the posterior third of the foot (Figure 46-12).

Sitting. The nurse assesses alignment of the sitting client by the following observations:

1. The head is erect, and the neck and vertebral column are in straight alignment.
2. The body weight is evenly distributed on the buttocks and thighs.
3. The thighs are parallel and in a horizontal plane.
4. Both feet are supported on the floor (Figure 46-13). With clients of short stature, a footstool is used and the ankles are comfortably flexed.
5. A 2.5 to 5 cm (1- to 2-inch) space is maintained between the edge of the seat and the popliteal space on the posterior surface of the knee. This space ensures that there is no pressure on the popliteal artery or nerve to decrease circulation or impair nerve function.
6. The client's forearms are supported on the armrest, in the lap, or on a table in front of the chair.

It is particularly important to assess alignment when sitting if the client has muscle weakness, muscle paralysis, or nerve damage. Because of these alterations, the client has diminished sensation in the affected area and is unable to perceive pressure or decreased circulation. Proper alignment while sitting reduces the risk of musculoskeletal system damage in such a client. The client with severe respiratory disease may assume a posture of leaning on the table in front of the chair in an attempt to breathe more easily.

Lying. People who are conscious have voluntary muscle control and normal perception of pressure. As a result, they usually assume a position of comfort when lying down. Because their ROM, sensation, and circulation are within normal limits, they change positions when they perceive muscle strain and decreased circulation.

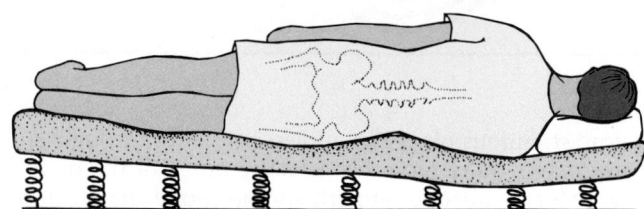

FIGURE **46–14** Correct body alignment when lying down.

Assessment of body alignment is best done with the client in the lateral position when the client is restricted to bed and not able to move well. All positioning supports should be removed from the bed except for the pillow under the head, and the body should be supported by an adequate mattress (Figure 46-14). This position allows for full view of the spine and back and will help provide other baseline body alignment data, such as whether the client can remain positioned without aid. The vertebrae should be aligned, and the position should not cause discomfort. Conditions that create a risk of damage to the musculoskeletal system when lying down include clients with impaired mobility, such as those in traction or with arthritis; clients with decreased sensation, such as those with hemiparesis (one-sided weakness) following stroke or brain attack; clients with impaired circulation, such as those with diabetes; and clients with lack of voluntary muscle control, such as those with spinal cord injuries.

Physiological Assessment. The nurse assesses the immobilized client for hazards of immobility by performing a head-to-toe physical assessment (see Chapter 32). In addition, the nursing assessment should focus on certain physiological areas, as well as the client's psychosocial and developmental dimensions. The physiological hazards of immobility that may be identified during a nursing assessment are summarized below and in Table 46-3.

Table 46-3	Physiological Hazards of Immobility	
System	**Assessment Techniques**	**Abnormal Findings**
Metabolic	Inspection	Slowed wound healing, abnormal laboratory data
	Inspection	Muscle atrophy
	Anthropometric measurements (mid-upper arm circumference, triceps skinfold measurement)	Decreased amount of subcutaneous fat
	Palpation	Generalized edema
Respiratory	Inspection	Asymmetrical chest wall movement, dyspnea, increased respiratory rate
	Auscultation	Crackles, wheezes
Cardiovascular	Auscultation	Orthostatic hypotension
	Auscultation, palpation	Increased heart rate, third heart sound, weak peripheral pulses, peripheral edema
Musculoskeletal	Inspection, palpation	Decreased ROM, erythema, increased diameter in calf or thigh
	Palpation	Joint contracture
	Inspection	Activity intolerance, muscle atrophy, joint contracture
Skin	Inspection, palpation	Break in skin integrity
Elimination	Inspection	Decreased urine output, cloudy or concentrated urine, decreased frequency of bowel movements
	Palpation	Distended bladder and abdomen
	Auscultation	Decreased bowel sounds

Metabolic System. When assessing metabolic functioning, the nurse uses **anthropometric measurements** (measures of height, weight, and skinfold thickness) to evaluate muscle atrophy (see Chapter 32). In addition, the nurse may analyze intake and output records for fluid balance. Does intake equal output? Intake and output measurements assist the nurse in determining whether a fluid imbalance exists (see Chapter 40). Dehydration and edema can increase the rate of skin breakdown in an immobilized client. Monitoring laboratory data such as electrolytes, serum protein (albumin and total protein) levels, and blood urea nitrogen (BUN) aid the nurse in determining metabolic functioning.

Assessing wound healing to evaluate alterations in the exchange of nutrients and monitoring food intake and elimination patterns will help to determine altered gastrointestinal functioning and potential metabolic problems. If an immobilized client has a wound, the rate of healing indicates how well nutrients are being delivered to tissues. Normal progression of healing indicates that metabolic needs of injured tissues are being met. Anorexia occurs commonly in immobilized clients. The client's food intake should be assessed before the meal tray is removed to determine the amount eaten. Nutritional imbalances can be avoided if the nurse assesses the client's dietary patterns and food preferences early in immobilization (see Chapter 43).

Respiratory System. A respiratory assessment should be performed at least every 2 hours for clients with restricted activity. The nurse inspects chest wall movements during the full inspiratory-expiratory cycle. If a client has an atelectatic area, chest movement may be asymmetrical. In addition, the nurse auscultates the entire lung region to identify diminished breath sounds, crackles, or wheezes. Auscultation should focus on the dependent lung fields because pulmonary secretions tend to collect in these lower regions. A complete respiratory

assessment identifies the presence of secretions and can be used to determine nursing interventions necessary for optimal respiratory function.

Cardiovascular System. Cardiovascular nursing assessment of the immobilized client includes blood pressure monitoring, evaluation of apical and peripheral pulses, and observation for signs of venous stasis (e.g., edema and poor wound healing). Although not all clients will experience orthostatic hypotension, clients should have their vital signs monitored during the first few attempts at sitting or standing.

When getting the client from a supine position into a chair, the nurse moves the client gradually. When performing this procedure, the nurse documents orthostatic changes. The nurse first obtains baseline blood pressure and pulse measurements with the client in the supine position. The nurse then assists the client to a position sitting at the side of the bed. The client should remain sitting 2 minutes before taking the blood pressure and pulse. The nurse remains with the client in a sitting position and continually monitors the client for dizziness or light-headedness. If there is no dizziness or drop in blood pressure ($\geq$20 mm Hg systolic or 10 mm Hg diastolic), the nurse assists the client to a standing position and retakes the blood pressure and pulse immediately upon standing and again after 2 minutes of standing. The nurse should monitor the client closely for dizziness throughout this procedure. The longer the period of immobility, the greater the risk of hypotension when the client stands (Lance and others, 2000).

The nurse also assesses the apical and peripheral pulses. Recumbency increases cardiac workload and results in an increased pulse rate. In some clients, particularly older adults, the heart may not tolerate the increased workload, and a form of cardiac failure may develop. A third heart sound, heard at the apex, can be an early indication of congestive heart failure. Monitoring peripheral pulses allows the nurse to evaluate the heart's ability to pump blood. The absence of a peripheral pulse in the lower extremities, particularly one that was previously present, should be documented and reported to the client's physician.

Edema may develop in clients who have had injury or whose heart is unable to handle the increased workload of bed rest. Because edema moves to dependent body regions, assessment of the immobilized client should include the sacrum, legs, and feet. If the heart is unable to tolerate the increased workload, peripheral body regions, such as the hands, feet, nose, and earlobes, will be colder than central body regions. Finally, the nurse assesses the venous system, because deep vein thrombosis (DVT) is a hazard of restricted mobility. A dislodged venous thrombus, called an **embolus,** may travel through the circulatory system to the lungs and impair circulation and oxygenation. Venous emboli that travel to the lungs may be life threatening. More than 90% of all pulmonary emboli begin in the legs or pelvis (Byrne, 2001).

To assess for a deep vein thrombosis, the nurse removes the client's elastic stockings and/or sequential compression devices (SCDs) every 8 hours and observes the calves for redness, warmth, and tenderness. Homans' sign, or calf pain on dorsiflexion of the foot, indicates a probable thrombus, but this sign is not always present (Maher, Salmond, and Pellino, 2002). Checking Homans' sign may be contraindicated in a suspected DVT as some investigators think that vigorous dorsiflexion may dislodge the thrombus. In addition, calf circumference should be measured daily. To do this, the nurse marks a point on each calf 10 cm from the midpatella. The circumference is measured each day using the mark for placement of the tape measure. Unilateral increases in calf diameter can be an early indication of thrombosis. Because DVTs can also occur in the thigh, thigh measurements should be taken daily if the client is prone to thrombosis. In many clients, DVTs can be prevented by active exercise and compression devices in conjunction with prescribed anticoagulant treatment.

Musculoskeletal System. Major musculoskeletal abnormalities that may be identified during nursing assessment include decreased muscle tone and strength, loss of muscle mass, and contractures. The anthropometric measurements described previously may indicate losses in muscle tone and muscle mass. Muscle atrophy is a common complication that arises from the lack of weight bearing found with bed rest (Takata and Yasui, 2001).

Assessment of ROM is important as a baseline against which later measurements can be compared to evaluate whether a loss in joint mobility has occurred. ROM can be measured with a goniometer (see Figure 36-10).

Disuse osteoporosis (generalized bone loss resulting from the lack of mechanical stress on bones) cannot be identified by physical assessment. However, clients on prolonged bed rest, postmenopausal women, clients taking steroids, and persons with increased serum and urine calcium levels have a greater risk for bone demineralization. The risk of disuse osteoporosis should be considered when planning nursing interventions. Not only may falls result in injury, but also falls may occur because of pathological fractures secondary to osteoporosis. Clients who are at risk for osteoporosis should have their diet assessed for calcium intake. Some clients have a lactose intolerance and need dietary teaching about alternative sources of calcium (Maher, Salmond, and Pellino, 2002).

Integumentary System. The nurse must continually assess the client's skin for breakdown and color changes such as pallor or redness. The skin should be observed when the client is turned, during hygiene measures and, when elimination needs are provided for. At a minimum, assessment should occur every 2 hours (see Chapter 47).

Elimination System. The client's elimination status should be evaluated on each shift, and total intake and output should be evaluated every 24 hours and compared over time. The nurse should determine that the client is receiving the correct amount and type of fluids orally or parenterally (see Chapter 44). Inadequate intake and output or fluid and electrolyte imbalances can increase the risk for renal system impairment, ranging from recurrent infections to kidney failure. Dehydration can also increase the risk for skin breakdown, thrombus formation, respiratory infections, and constipation.

Assessment of elimination status should also include the adequacy of dietary choices, bowel sounds, and the frequency and consistency of bowel movements (see Chapter 45). Accurate assessment enables the nurse to intervene before constipation and fecal impaction occur.

Psychosocial Assessment. Many alterations in physiological, sociocultural, and developmental functioning are related to immobility. Often, these problems are interrelated, and it is imperative that nursing care focus on all dimensions. Often the focus of immobility is on the easily visible physical problems, such as skin impairment, but the psychosocial and developmental aspects of immobility should not be overlooked (Box 46-4).

Abrupt changes in personality may have a physiological cause, such as surgery, a medication reaction, a pulmonary embolus, or an acute infection. For example, compromised older clients have confusion as their primary symptom when experiencing a pulmonary emboli or an acute urinary tract infection. Identifying confusion is an important component of the nurse's assessment. Acute confusion in older adults is not normal and should be thoroughly examined (Ludwick, 1999).

Common reactions to immobilization include boredom, feelings of isolation, depression, and anger. The nurse should observe for changes in a clients' emotional status. Examples of change that may indicate psychosocial concerns are a cooperative client who becomes less cooperative or an independent client who asks for more help than is necessary. The nurse should try to determine the reasons for such alterations. Identifying how the client usually copes with loss is vital (see Chapters 29 and 30). A change in mobility status, whether permanent or not, may cause a grief reaction. Families are a key resource for information about behavior changes.

Unexplained changes in the sleep-wake cycle must be identified and corrected. Most can be prevented or minimized, such as those occurring because of nursing activities, a noisy environment, or discomfort. They may also

Box 46-4

Research Highlight

The Meaning of Mobility

Research Focus

It is widely known that decreased mobility contributes to physical and psychological impairment. Little is known, however, about the meaning of mobility to residents and nurses in long-term care facilities. It is important for nurses to understand the phenomena of mobility in order to develop mobility strategies.

Research Abstract

The purpose of this study was to understand the perceptions regarding mobility from nurses and residents in long-term care facilities in order to develop strategies that would support mobility in the institutionalized adult. An exploratory qualitative design was used. Focus groups with residents and nursing staff were conducted in three long-term care facilities. Twenty residents and 15 nurses participated in the study. Both groups identified mobility as key to quality of life. Elders equated mobility with freedom, choice, and independence. Nurses valued mobility and associated it with freedom and autonomy. Both

nurses and residents viewed having to "wait" for assistance as a barrier to mobility. Nurses identified further obstacles such as heavy workload and lack of time. Residents focused on physical barriers such as steep ramps, crowded elevators, and negative attitudes of staff.

Evidence-Based Practice

- Mobility is central to clients' quality of life and well-being.
- Nurses play a key role in assessing and assisting clients with their mobility needs.
- Nurses focus on minimizing obstacles to mobility.
- Nurses coordinate with other health care professionals to meet client's mobility needs.
- Nurses use creative strategies to encourage mobility in elders.

Reference

Bourret E and others: The meaning of mobility for residents and staff in long-term care facilities, *J Adv Nurs* 37(4):338, 2002.

---

occur because of medications such as analgesics, sleeping pills, or cardiovascular drugs (see Chapter 41).

Because psychosocial changes usually occur gradually, the nurse should observe the client's behavior on a daily basis. If behavioral changes occur, the nurse should determine the causes and evaluate the changes as short or long term. Identifying the cause helps the nurse design appropriate nursing interventions.

Developmental Assessment. Assessment of the immobilized client should include developmental considerations to ensure that the client's needs are identified. The nurse determines whether the young child can meet developmental tasks and is progressing normally. The child's development may regress or be slowed because of immobilization. By identifying a child's overall developmental needs, the nurse can design nursing therapies to maintain normal development. The nurse may also need to assure the parents that developmental delays are usually temporary.

Immobilization of a family member changes the family's functioning. The family's response to this change may lead to problems, stress, and anxieties. Children seeing parents who are immobile may have difficulty understanding what is occurring and may have difficulty coping.

Immobility can have a significant effect on the older adult's levels of health, independence, and functional status. Nursing assessment enables the nurse to determine the older client's ability to meet needs independently and to adapt to developmental changes such as declining physical functioning and altered family and peer relationships. A decline in developmental functioning needs prompt investigation to determine why the change occurred and what can be done to return the client to an optimal level of functioning as soon as possible. Activities that reduce immobility and promote participation in ADLs are vital to

prevent functional decline (Ludwick, Dieckman, and Snelson, 1999). Assessment also includes the client's home and community to identify factors that are risks to the client's mobility and safety (see Chapter 37).

Client Expectations. Clients may have unrealistic expectations of themselves or their caregivers. They may agree with the staff and understand their limitations, or they may set their expectations of themselves too high or too low. Because clients may rely on family caregivers to provide personal care that they have not received from another since early childhood, it is vital that the caregivers take the time to learn the client's expectations.

Some clients may expect to be waited on, and other clients may want to do as much as possible. Key to understanding these expectations is the client's psychosocial reaction, knowledge about his or her condition, and developmental level. Asking clients to explain what they know about their mobility status, what questions they and their families have, and how the immobility is affecting their goals will help the nurse and other caregivers more fully appreciate and incorporate clients' expectations into care planning.

Nursing Diagnosis

An immobilized or partially immobilized client may have one or more nursing diagnoses. The two diagnoses most directly related to mobility problems are *impaired physical mobility* and *risk for disuse syndrome*. The diagnosis of *impaired physical mobility* is used for the client who has some limitation but is not completely immobile. The diagnosis of *risk for disuse syndrome* should be considered for the client who is immobile and at risk for multisystem pathophysiology because of inactivity. Beyond these diagnoses, the list of potential diagnoses is extensive, because immobility affects multiple body systems

- Activity intolerance
- Ineffective airway clearance
- Ineffective breathing pattern
- Ineffective individual coping
- Risk for disuse syndrome
- Risk for deficient fluid volume
- Impaired gas exchange
- Risk for infection
- Risk for injury
- Impaired physical mobility
- Impaired skin integrity
- Impaired risk for skin integrity
- Disturbed sleep pattern
- Social isolation
- Ineffective (peripheral) tissue perfusion
- Impaired urinary elimination

Assessment reveals clusters of data that indicate whether a client is at risk or if an actual problem exists. The clusters of data include defining characteristics that support the diagnostic label and probable cause of the diagnosis. Locating the probable cause of the diagnosis (based on assessment data) is important to planning client-centered goals and subsequent nursing interventions that will best help the client.

Impaired physical mobility related to bed rest would require slightly different interventions than *impaired physical mobility related to pain in the left shoulder.* Thus it is critical that nursing assessment activities identify and cluster defining characteristics that ultimately support the nursing diagnosis selected (Box 46-5). The diagnosis related to bed rest would require interventions aimed at keeping the client as mobile as possible and encouraging the client to do self-care and ROM in bed. The diagnosis related to pain would require the nurse to assist the client with comfort measures so that the client would then be willing and more able to move. In both situations the nurse would explain the importance of activity to healthy body functioning.

Often the physiological dimension is the major focus of nursing care for clients with impaired mobility. Thus the psychosocial and developmental dimensions are neglected. Yet all dimensions are important to health. For example, during immobilization, social interaction and stimuli are decreased. Ultimately the client may become isolated, withdrawn, and bored. Such clients may frequently use the nurse's call bell to request minor physical attention when their real need is greater socialization. Nursing diagnoses for health needs in developmental areas reflect changes from the client's normal activities. Immobility can lead to a developmental crisis if the client is unable to resolve problems and continue to mature.

Immobility may also lead to complications such as pulmonary emboli or pneumonia. If these conditions develop, the nurse will collaborate with the physician or nurse practitioner for prescribed therapy to intervene. The nurse is alert for these potential complications and works to prevent them.

Planning

During planning the nurse synthesizes information from resources such as knowledge of the role of respiratory and physical therapy, standards such as skin care guidelines from the AHRQ, protocols for clients at risk for falls, attitudes such as creativity and perseverance, and past experiences with immobilized clients (Figure 46-15). Critical thinking ensures that the client's plan of care integrates all that the nurse knows about the individual, as well as key critical thinking elements. Professional standards are especially important to consider when the nurse develops a plan of care. These standards often establish scientifically proven guidelines for selecting effective nursing interventions.

Goals and Outcomes. The nurse develops an individualized plan of care for each nursing diagnosis (see care plan). The nurse and client set realistic expectations for care. Goals are set that are individualized, realistic, and measurable. The goals focus on preventing problems or risks to body alignment and mobility. These goals are client centered and should be mutually set with client and family. A family who does too much or too little in an attempt to help the client may unknowingly impede the client's progress.

The goals and expected outcomes are developed to assist the client in achieving his or her highest level of mo-

---

Nursing Diagnostic Process   Box 46-5

Assessment Activities	Defining Characteristics	Nursing Diagnosis
Measure ROM during exercises of extremities.	Client has limited ROM with left shoulder.	Impaired physical mobility related to left shoulder pain
	Client has impaired coordination while attempting to perform ROM with left shoulder.	
Observe client use left shoulder in ADL's	Client is reluctant to attempt movement with left shoulder.	
Ask client about perception of pain.	Client complains of sharp pain in shoulder.	
Ask client about endurance and activity tolerance.	Client reports decreased muscle strength in left shoulder.	

bility. In addition, these goals may be written to reduce the hazards of immobility. For example, a client who has left-sided paralysis following a stroke may have two long-term goals. The first directed toward improved mobility may be "Client uses walker to ambulate around the home and grocery store." A parallel goal directed toward the hazards of immobility may be "Client's skin remains free of pressure." Both of these goals are essential to restoring maximal mobility for this client. Because there is impaired sensation, both the client and caregivers must be aware of the client's need to have the skin free of pressure. Expected outcomes for the second goal could include the following:

- Client's skin color and temperature return to normal baseline within 20 minutes of position change.
- Client's skin remains dry and intact

Setting Priorities. Care planning must take into consideration priority setting, so that immediate needs are attended to first. This is particularly important when clients have multiple diagnoses (Figure 46-16). The nurse plans therapies according to severity of risks to the client, and the plan is individualized according to the client's developmental stage, level of health, and lifestyle. The immediacy of any problem is determined by the effect the problem has on the client's mental and physical health.

It is especially important in priority setting to recognize that potential complications should not be overlooked. Many times actual problems such as pressure ulcers and disuse osteoporosis get addressed only after they develop. Therefore the nurse must be vigilant in monitoring the client, reinforcing prevention techniques to

KNOWLEDGE

- Benefit of mobility on body system functioning
- Role of physical, occupational, or respiratory therapists or dietitians in reducing hazards of immobility
- Effect of new medications on the client's mobility status
- Effect of mobility interventions

EXPERIENCE

- Previous client responses to planned nursing therapies for improving mobility (what worked and what did not work)

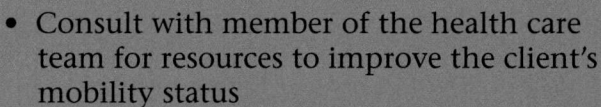

Planning

- Consult with member of the health care team for resources to improve the client's mobility status
- Identify nursing interventions designed to reduce hazards of immobility to increase mobility status
- Involve the client and family in care activities
- Determine the client's ability to increase activity level

STANDARDS

- Individualize therapies for the client's mobility needs
- Apply skin care therapies consistent with AHRQ standards
- Apply cardiopulmonary reconditioning therapies consistent with AHRQ standards
- Apply protocols for fall prevention

ATTITUDES

- Use creativity to design interventions that improve mobility
- Display perseverance to adapt interventions to multiple health care settings

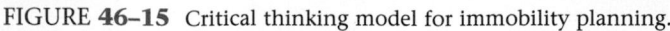

FIGURE **46-15** Critical thinking model for immobility planning.

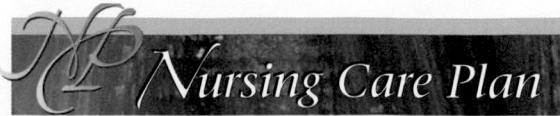

Nursing Care Plan

Immobility

Assessment

Ms. Barbara Adams, an 84-year-old client, has been admitted for rehabilitation after a total hip replacement (THR) for osteoarthritis. The wound is clean, dry, and intact. Staples will be removed in 2 days. She is not able to transfer with help from chair to bed. She states that she is "afraid of falling" and frequently refuses to get out of bed. She rates her pain as a 2 on a scale of 0 to 10. She has a history of smoking. She states that she needs pain medication to help her sleep during the night but does not need any during the day. She is to start physical therapy tomorrow.

Assessment Activities	Findings/Defining Characteristics
Assess Ms. Adams' pain level.	She rates her pain as a 2 on a scale of 0 to 10. She states that she needs pain medication at night to help her sleep, but does not need any during the day.
Assess Ms. Adams' ability to transfer.	She is not able to transfer with help from chair to bed.
Ask Ms. Adams how her surgery has affected her mobility.	She responds that she is "afraid of falling," and she frequently refuses to get out of bed.
Assess Ms. Adams' wound status.	Wound is clean, dry, and intact.

Nursing Diagnosis: Impaired mobility related to musculoskeletal impairment from surgery and a fear of falling.

Planning

Goal	Expected Outcomes*
	Tissue Integrity: Skin
Ms. Adams will be free from skin breakdown by discharge.	Client's skin will remain intact.
	Client's skin will be free of erythema.
	Tissue Perfusion: Peripheral
Ms. Adams will exhibit no evidence of DVT by discharge.	Client's calf diameters will remain within 1 cm of baseline through discharge.
	Client's lower extremity pulses will remain equal.
	Client will have no complaints of calf pain.
	Mobility Level
Ms. Adams will be able to transfer with assistance within 2 days.	Client will transfer with assistance 3 times per day within 2 days.
	Client will state fear of falling during transfer is less within 2 days.

*Outcome classification labels from Moorhead S, Johnson M, Maas M: *Nursing outcomes classification (NOC)*, ed 3, St. Louis, 2004, Mosby.

Interventions†

Circulatory Care

Interventions†	Rationale
Administer low-dose heparin as ordered.	Administration of low-dose heparin has shown reduction in risk for vein thrombosis (Nunnelee, 1997).
Apply intermittent compression stockings as ordered and remove each shift for hygiene.	Application increases venous tone, improving venous return, and reducing venous stasis (Byrne, 2001).
Reinforce antiembolic exercises while awake.	Exercises promote venous return.
Assist client out of bed slowly.	Moving slowly will decrease the likelihood of orthostatic hypotension. Moving the client slowly will also avoid the perception by the client of being rushed, which may cause the client to become fearful.

†Intervention classification labels from Dochterman JM, Bulechek GM: *Nursing interventions classification (NIC)*, ed 4, St. Louis, 2004, Mosby.

Continued

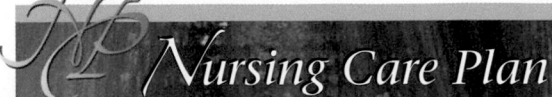

Nursing Care Plan

Immobility—cont'd

Interventions†—cont'd

Skin Surveillance

Instruct client to shift position every 1 to 1½ hours while awake.

When recumbent, place client in 30-degree lateral position.

Keep client's heels off of bed by placing a pad under the lower legs.

Positioning

Explain positioning procedure to client.
Refer to physical therapy for transfer training.
Encourage client to assist in transfer and positioning.

Rationale

Position changes should occur every 1 to 1½ hours or more frequently if needed. Reduces the risk of pressure ulcer development.

The 30-degree lateral position reduces pressure from the sacral area and reduces the risk of skin breakdown (AHRQ, 2003).
Using a thin pad under the lower legs raises the heels just enough so that a paper can slide between the heels and the bed, thereby reducing the pressure on the heels so that tissue blood flow is maintained (AHRQ, 2003).

Reduces anxiety.
Helps to strengthen muscles used in transfer.

†Intervention classification labels from Dochterman JM, Bulechek GM: *Nursing interventions classification (NIC)*, ed 4, St. Louis, 2004, Mosby.

Evaluation

Nursing Actions	Client Response/Finding	Achievement of Outcome
Ask Ms. Adams if her mobility has improved postoperatively. Observe client transfer from bed to chair.	Client is able to transfer from the chair to the bed with assistance.	Client has achieved goal of transferring with assistance.
Observe Ms. Adams's skin integrity each shift.	Client's wound remains clean, dry, and intact. No breakdown noted on extremities.	Client has achieved outcome that skin will remain intact.
Perform circulatory assessment of extremities every shift.	Client's calf diameters remain within 1 cm of baseline. No evidence of swelling, pain, redness, or warmth.	There is no evidence of a DVT.
Ask Ms. Adams to rate her fear of falling on a scale of 0 to 10.	Client rates fear of falling a 7 on a scale of 0 to 10.	Outcome of decrease in fear of falling has not been totally achieved.
	Client is getting out of bed every shift.	Continue to encourage client.

both client and other caregivers, and supervising assistive personnel in carrying out activities aimed at preventing complications of impaired mobility.

Continuity of Care. The interventions planned for the client may be done directly by the nurse or delegated to assistive personnel (AP). AP can reinforce leg exercises, use of the incentive spirometer, and coughing and deep breathing (see Chapter 39). They may turn and position clients, apply elastic stockings, and assess leg circumferences and height and weight.

Because many of the skills associated with care of the immobile client can be delegated, the nurse must be vigilant in performing routine assessments to identify any developing complications early. The nurse also informs assistive personnel when clients are at risk for immobility hazards so complications can be prevented. For example, although turning and positioning of a comatose client may be delegated, the nurse must ensure that it is done correctly and that the position is changed frequently to reduce the risk of poor alignment and future injury to the skin and musculoskeletal system. The frequency of turn-

ing is based on client assessment for risk of pressure ulcer development (see Chapter 47).

The nurse may need the help of another health team member such as a physical or occupational therapist when considering mobility needs. For example, physical therapists are a resource for planning ROM or strengthening exercises, and occupational therapists are a resource for planning ADLs that clients need to modify or relearn. Discharge planning is begun when a client enters the health care system. In anticipation of the client's discharge from an institution, a referral may be made to help the client remain mobile or regain mobility at home. Therefore consideration must be given to the client's home environment when planning therapies to maintain or improve body alignment and mobility.

Implementation

Nursing interventions related to immobility are classified into health promotion activities, acute care–based interventions, and restorative and continuing care services.

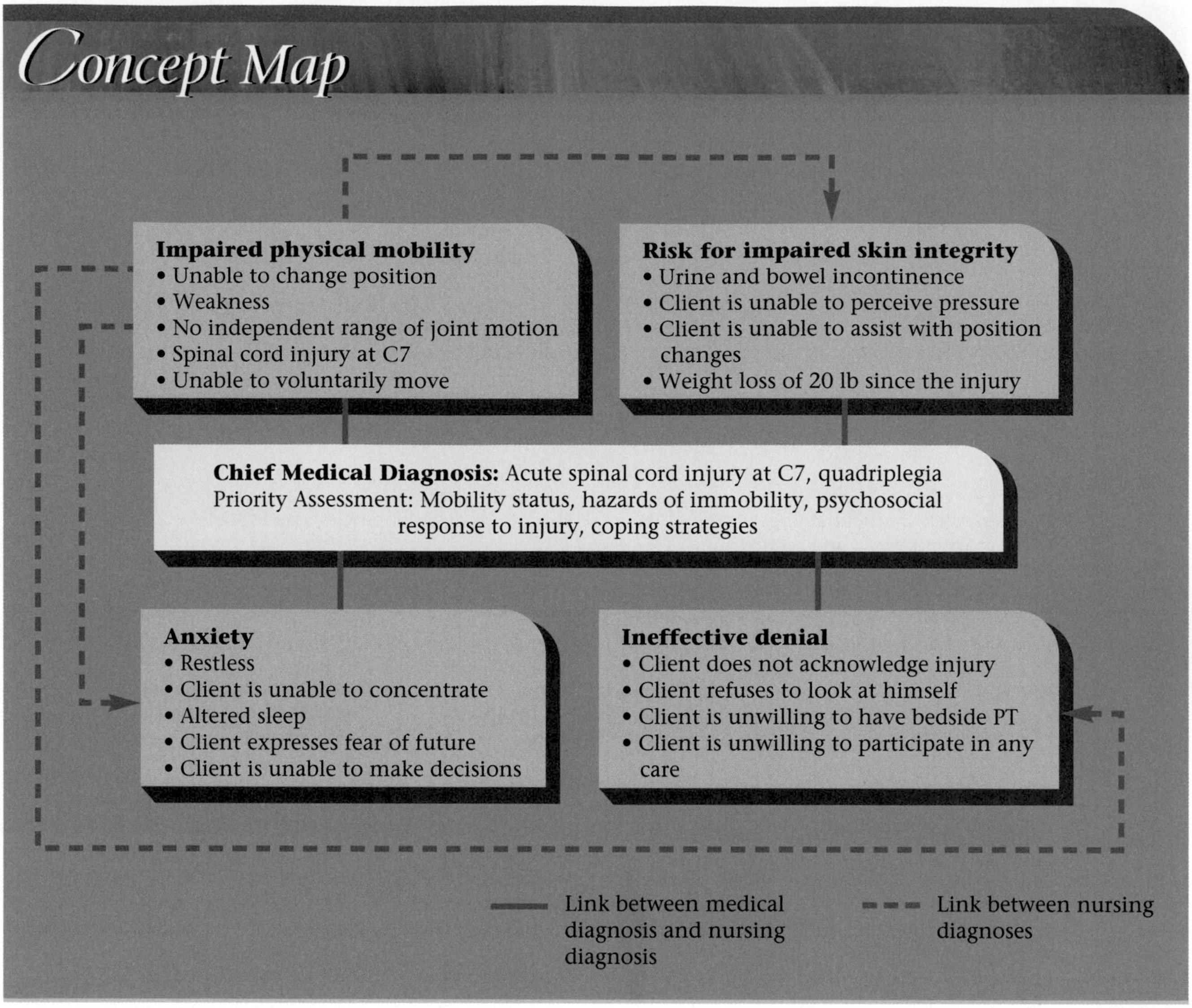

Concept Map

Impaired physical mobility
• Unable to change position
• Weakness
• No independent range of joint motion
• Spinal cord injury at C7
• Unable to voluntarily move

Risk for impaired skin integrity
• Urine and bowel incontinence
• Client is unable to perceive pressure
• Client is unable to assist with position changes
• Weight loss of 20 lb since the injury

Chief Medical Diagnosis: Acute spinal cord injury at C7, quadriplegia
Priority Assessment: Mobility status, hazards of immobility, psychosocial response to injury, coping strategies

Anxiety
• Restless
• Client is unable to concentrate
• Altered sleep
• Client expresses fear of future
• Client is unable to make decisions

Ineffective denial
• Client does not acknowledge injury
• Client refuses to look at himself
• Client is unwilling to have bedside PT
• Client is unwilling to participate in any care

——— Link between medical diagnosis and nursing diagnosis

- - - Link between nursing diagnoses

FIGURE **46–16** Concept map for client with acute spinal cord injury at C7 and quadriplegia.

Health Promotion. Health promotion activities include a variety of interventions that can be divided into education, prevention, and early detection. Examples of these health promotion activities include lifting techniques and fall prevention measures and early detection of scoliosis. In this section, lifting techniques and exercise are emphasized.

Lifting. The rate of injuries in occupational settings has increased in recent years. Back pain is the costliest job-related injury (U.S. Department of Labor, 2000). Back injuries are often the direct result of improper lifting and bending. The most common back injury is strain on the lumbar muscle group, which includes the muscles around the lumbar vertebrae. Injury to these areas affects the ability to bend forward, backward, and from side to side and limits the ability to rotate the hips and lower back.

Nurses and AP are especially at risk for injury to lumbar muscles when lifting, transferring, or positioning im-

mobilized clients. Therefore nurses need to be cognizant of good lifting techniques to protect themselves, those they supervise, and the clients being cared for. Therefore when lifting, the nurse should assess the weight to be lifted and what assistance, if any, is needed. If help is needed, the nurse should determine if a second person or mechanical assistance is needed.

Nurses should know their individual capabilities for lifting and moving clients based on their own strength and flexibility. Another consideration is the condition of the client and whether he or she can provide help while being moved. Once the amount of assistance is determined, these steps are followed:

1. Keep the weight to be lifted as close to the body as possible; this action places the object in the same plane as the lifter and close to the center of gravity for balance.
2. Bend at the knees; this helps to maintain the center of gravity and uses the stronger leg muscles to do the

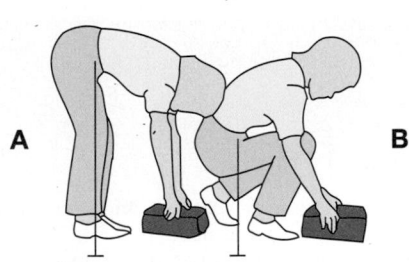

FIGURE **46–17** Incorrect **(A)** and correct **(B)** body position for lifting.

lifting (Figure 46-17). Avoid twisting. Twisting can overload the spine and lead to serious injury.

3. Tighten abdominal muscles and tuck the pelvis; this provides balance and helps protect the back.

4. Maintain the trunk erect and knees bent so that multiple groups work together in a coordinated manner (see Chapter 36).

However, it should be noted that nurse injuries are not only related to lifting. Nurses spend time in many activities bending and twisting that may also cause injury. Examples of such activities include bathing, feeding, dressing, and undressing clients (Nelson, Fragala, and Menzel, 2003).

Exercise. Although many diseases and physical problems can cause or contribute to immobility, it is important to remember that exercise programs can enhance feelings of well-being, as well as improve endurance, strength, and health. Exercise is known to reduce the risk of many health problems such as cardiovascular disease, diabetes, and osteoporosis. In the case of older adults, routine completion of ADL activities prevents contractures and improves independence (Resnick, 2000).

Exercise should be a key prescription given by nurses for health promotion of clients. Functional decline from disuse is a major concern as aging occurs. Nurses can contribute to promoting health for many types of clients by encouraging or starting managed exercise programs. Older adults can enjoy and benefit from exercise, but the chronically ill elder must overcome barriers to physical activity (Box 46-6). Other research has shown that older adults can enjoy and benefit from exercises other than traditional Western exercises such as walking or swimming (Box 46-7). Even hospitalized clients can be encouraged to do stretching, ROM, and light walking within the limits of their condition (see Chapter 36).

Acute Care. In the acute care setting, specific interventions are designed to reduce the impact of immobility on the client by reducing the hazards of immobility and by positioning and transferring clients correctly.

Immobility Hazards. Clients in acute care settings may demonstrate some problems associated with prolonged immobility, such as impaired respiratory status, orthostatic hypotension, and impaired skin integrity. For these clients, nursing interventions are designed to reduce the impact of immobility on body systems and prepare the client for the restorative phase of care.

Metabolic System. The immobilized client requires a high-protein, high-calorie diet with vitamin B and C supplements. Protein is needed to repair injured tissue and rebuild depleted protein stores. A high-calorie intake provides sufficient fuel to meet metabolic needs and to replace subcutaneous tissue. Supplementation with vitamin C is necessary to replace protein stores. Vitamin B complex is needed for skin integrity and wound healing.

If the client is unable to eat, nutrition must be provided parenterally or enterally. Enteral feedings include delivery through a nasogastric, gastrostomy, or jejunostomy tube of high-protein, high-calorie solutions with complete requirements of vitamins, minerals, and electrolytes (Chapter 43). Total parenteral nutrition refers to delivery of nutritional supplements through a central or peripheral intravenous catheter.

Respiratory System. Nursing interventions for the respiratory system are aimed at promoting expansion of the chest and lungs, preventing stasis of pulmonary secretions, maintaining a patent airway, and promoting adequate exchange of respiratory gases.

Promoting Expansion of the Chest and Lungs. Changing the position of the client at least every 2 hours allows the dependent lung regions to reexpand. Reexpansion maintains the elastic recoil property of the lungs and clears the dependent lung regions of pulmonary secretions.

The nurse encourages the client to deep breathe and cough every 1 to 2 hours. Alert clients can be taught to deep breathe or yawn every hour or to use an incentive spirometer (see Chapter 39). The nurse instructs the client to take in three deep breaths and cough with the third exhalation. This technique produces a more forceful, productive cough without excessive fatigue. These respiratory interventions will aid alveolar expansion and prevent atelectasis. Coughing reduces the stasis of pulmonary secretions. For unconscious clients with an artificial airway, the nurse can expand the chest and lungs by using an Ambu-bag (see Chapter 39).

If abdominal binders are required, they should be removed every 2 hours to allow the client to breathe deeply. Binders must be assessed for correct positioning and adjusted as necessary to prevent interference with respirations. Often clients will wear the binder only when ambulating. Specific physician instructions for the use of binders will vary.

Preventing Stasis of Pulmonary Secretions. Stagnant secretions accumulating in the bronchi and lungs may lead to growth of bacteria and subsequent development of pneumonia. Changing the client's position every 2 hours can reduce stagnation of secretions. This change rotates the dependent lung, mobilizing secretions.

The immobile client should take in a minimum of 2000 ml of fluid a day, if not contraindicated, to help keep mucociliary clearance normal. In clients free from infection and with adequate hydration, pulmonary secretions will appear thin, watery, and clear. The client can easily remove the secretions with coughing. Without adequate hydration the secretions are thick and tenacious and difficult to remove. Encouraging fluids also benefits in helping with bowel and urine elimination and aids in maintaining circulation and skin integrity.

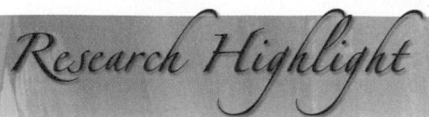

Box 46-6

Barriers to Exercise Participation

Research Focus

Exercise has been credited with increasing mobility; maintaining functional performance; decreasing the risk of cardiovascular disease, diabetes, and osteoporosis; and enhancing perceived quality of life. Elders are the most sedentary group in America despite the many benefits of exercise. Aging adults face several barriers when attempting to participate in physical activity.

Research Abstract

The purposes of this study were (1) to describe health barriers to exercise participation in older clients for a home-based walking program and (2) to explore the implications for practice. This study used self- and interviewer-administered instruments to assess potential barriers to physical activity. The 212 subjects (age 60 to 80 years old) participated in a walking program. Videotapes were used to explain the purpose of the study, and participants completed questionnaires, a health status interview, and other measures during a series of visits. Pain, fatigue, mobility, and sensory impairments were identified as primary barriers to participation in exercise.

Evidence-Based Practice

- Encourage clients to pace activities and increase speed and intensity gradually to avoid pain.
- Administer prescribed antiinflammatory medications 1 to 2 hours before starting exercise program.
- Encourage clients to balance rest and activity and get plenty of sleep.
- Advise clients to avoid caffeine and alcohol before bed.
- Teach clients to use canes or walkers to assist with walking as needed.
- Encourage clients to choose smooth and even walking surfaces.
- Advise clients not to force joints past the point of resistance or pain
- Teach clients to check legs and feet daily for redness, swelling, blisters, or broken skin.
- Teach clients to wear properly fitting shoes.
- Encourage clients to walk with a companion or group.

Reference

Cooper K and others: Health barriers to walking for exercise in elderly primary care, *Geriatr Nurs* 22(5):258, 2001.

Cultural Aspects of Care

Box 46-7

There are many activities specifically linked to culture such as: time orientation, health care practices, health promotion, nutrition, religion, family systems, and death. Less attention has been given to the impact of culture on mobility and exercise. However, cultural influences have an important role on exercise and physical activity.

In many written materials, exercise is often described based on white middle-class values. For example, not everyone has access to a tennis court or swimming pool at a local country club. Furthermore, many individuals would not feel comfortable in this environment. Certain cultures discourage involvement in organized recreational physical activities such as basketball, running, and aerobics (Johnson, 2000). Ethnic dancing is an effective activity that is more acceptable than the above organized sports activities in Western European countries (Jain, 2001). Other cultures emphasize exercise in terms of activities of daily living such as walking, gardening, and prayer/meditation. As an example, people from Bangladesh view prayer as a structured form of exercise. Muslims value participation in community activities important and consider walking to the mosque a part of their weekly exercise regime (Johnson, 2000).

Implications for Practice

- Nurses must evaluate patterns of daily living and culturally prescribed activities before suggesting specific forms of exercise to clients (Andrews and Boyle, 1999).
- Nurses must help clients plan physical activities that are culturally acceptable (Melillo and others, 2001).
- Exercise programs must be flexible and accommodate family and community responsibilities of the culture (Banks-Wallace, 2000).
- Nurses must encourage culturally specific interventions to facilitate commitment to exercise (Banks-Wallace, 2000).
- Nurses must educate clients on the importance of exercise in preserving health, and facilitate acceptance by incorporating it into socially rewarding community activities (Johnson, 2000).

Data from Andrews M, Boyle J: *Transcultural concepts in nursing care,* ed 3, Philadelphia, 1999, Lippincott; Banks-Wallace J: Staggering under the weight of responsibility: the impact of culture on physical activity among African American women, *J Multicultural Nurs Health* 6(3):24, 2000; Jain S: Cultural dance: an opportunity to encourage physical activity and health in communities, *Am J Health Education* 32(4):216, 2001; Johnson M: Perceptions of barriers to healthy physical activity among Asian communities, *Sport Education Soc* 5(1):51, 2000; and Melillo K and others: Perceptions of older Latino adults regarding physical fitness, physical activity, and exercise, *J Gerontol Nurs* 27(9):38, 2001.

Chest physiotherapy (CPT) (percussion and positioning) is an effective method for preventing pulmonary secretion stasis. CPT techniques help the client to drain secretions from specific segments of the bronchi and lungs into the trachea so that the client can cough and expel the secretions. Respiratory assessment findings identify areas of the lungs requiring CPT (see Chapter 39).

Maintaining a Patent Airway. Immobilized clients and those on bed rest are generally weakened. If weakness progresses, the cough reflex gradually becomes inefficient. The stasis of secretions in the lungs may be life threatening for an immobilized client because hypostatic pneumonia can easily develop. Dislodging and mobilizing the stagnant secretions reduce the risk of pneumonia. Assessment findings that indicate this condition include productive cough with greenish yellow sputum; fever; pain on breathing; and crackles, wheezes, and dyspnea. The nurse should actively work with the client to deep breathe and cough every 1 to 2 hours as described in promoting chest expansion.

In the immobilized client an obstructed airway is usually a result of a mucous plug. The nurse can implement several therapies, such as CPT, to reduce the risk of mucous plugs and to maintain a patent airway. Nasotracheal or orotracheal suction techniques may be used to remove secretions in the upper airways of a client who is unable to cough productively. This procedure must be performed aseptically. The nurse can also suction secretions when clients have artificial airways such as an endotracheal or tracheal tube. The nurse inserts a catheter into the artificial airway in a sterile procedure. This removes pulmonary secretions from the upper and lower airways (see Chapter 39).

Cardiovascular System. The effects of bed rest or immobilization on the cardiovascular system include orthostatic hypotension, increased cardiac workload, and thrombus formation. Nursing therapies are designed to minimize or prevent these alterations.

Reducing Orthostatic Hypotension. After bed rest, clients usually have an increased pulse rate, a decrease in pulse pressure, and a drop in blood pressure with an increase in fainting when arising to a sitting or standing position (Black, Hawks, and Keene, 2001). Interventions should be directed toward reducing or eliminating the effects of orthostatic hypotension. The nurse attempts to get the client moving as soon as the physical condition allows, even if this only involves dangling at the bedside or moving to a chair. This activity maintains muscle tone and increases venous return. Isometric exercises, those activities that involve muscle tension without muscle shortening, do not have any beneficial effect on preventing orthostatic hypotension but may improve activity tolerance. When getting an immobile client up for the first time, the nurse should usually be assisted by at least one other person. This is a precautionary step. The client will still be expected to do as much of the transfer as the condition allows.

Reducing Cardiac Workload. The nurse designs interventions to reduce cardiac workload, which is increased by immobility. A primary intervention is to discourage the client from using the Valsalva maneuver. When using this maneuver such as during straining of defecation or moving up in bed, the client holds his or her breath, which increases intrathoracic pressure. This decreases venous return and cardiac output. When the strain is released, venous return and cardiac output immediately increase and systolic blood pressure and pulse pressure rise. These pressure changes produce a reflex bradycardia and a possible decrease in blood pressure that may cause sudden cardiac death in clients with heart disease. The nurse teaches the client to breathe out while moving or being lifted up in bed.

Preventing Thrombus Formation. The most cost-effective way to address the DVT problem is through an aggressive program of prophylaxis. It begins with identification of clients at risk and continues throughout the time clients are immobile or otherwise at risk. This is clearly a collaborative role between nurses and physicians. The nurse can easily identify risk factors during an admission nursing assessment. Many interventions reduce the risk of thrombus formation in the immobilized client. Leg exercises, encouraging fluids, position changes, and teaching should begin when the client becomes immobile. Preoperative clients should be given this information before surgery (see Chapter 49). Other interventions such as medications, intermittent pneumatic compression (IPC), and sequential compression devices (SCDs) require a physician's order. Maintenance and administration of prophylaxis is a nursing role, and nurses can determine when the client is fully mobile postoperatively, decreasing the continued risk for DVT.

Heparin and low-molecular-weight heparin (LMWH) are the most widely used drugs in the prophylaxis of DVT. Standard heparin is considered the gold standard for treatment because it has been well studied and validated. Common dosage for heparin therapy is 5000 units given subcutaneously 2 hours before surgery and repeated every 8 to 12 hours until the client is fully mobile or discharged. Heparin is an anticoagulant, and it suppresses clot formation. Because of the action of this medication, the nurse must continually assess the client for signs of bleeding, such as increased bruising, guaiac-positive stools, and bleeding gums. Common dosage of Lovenox (LMWH) in the prophylaxis of DVTs is 30 to 40 mg subcutaneously 2 hours before surgery and continued throughout the postoperative period. Although the majority of clients receiving LMWH do not experience side effects, the risk remains present (Nunnelee, 1997).

SCD/IPCs consist of sleeves or stockings, made of fabric or plastic that are wrapped around the leg and secured with Velcro (Box 46-8). The sleeves are then connected to a pump that alternately inflates and deflates the stocking around the leg. A typical cycle is inflation for 10 to 15 seconds and deflation for 45 to 60 seconds. Inflation pressures average 40 mm Hg. Use of SCD/IPCs on the legs decreases venous stasis by increasing venous return through the deep veins of the legs. For optimal results, use of SCD/IPCs is begun as soon as possible and maintained until the client becomes fully ambulatory. Graded compression stockings can help prevent DVT, but clients must receive the right size, and the SCD/IPCs must be used correctly.

Elastic stockings (sometimes called thromboembolic device hose) (TED) also aid in maintaining external pressure on the muscles of the lower extremities and thus

Box 46-8 *Procedural Guidelines*

Application of Sequential Compression Stockings

Equipment: Tape measure, sequential stockings, stockinette, hygiene supplies

Delegation Considerations: The skill of applying SCSs can be delegated to assistive personnel (AP). The nurse is responsible for assessing circulation in the extremities. The nurse instructs the AP to:

- Notify nurse if client complains of pain in leg.
- Notify nurse if discoloration develops in extremities.

1. Assess client for need for sequential compression stockings
2. Obtain baseline assessment data about the status of circulation, pulse, and skin integrity on client's lower extremities before initiating sequential compression stockings.
3. Measure client for proper-size stocking by measuring around the largest part of the client's thigh. Review manufacturer's directions regarding measuring for proper fit.
4. Perform hand hygiene. Provide hygiene to lower extremities if needed.
5. Place a protective stockinette over the client's leg.
6. Wrap the stocking around the leg, starting at the ankle, with the opening over the patella (see illustration).
   a. Attach the stockings to the insufflator and verify that the intermittent pressure is between 35 and 45 mm Hg.
7. Record date and time of stocking application and stocking length and size in nurses' notes.
8. Record condition of skin and circulatory assessment.
9. Monitor skin integrity and circulation to client's lower extremities as ordered or according to manufacturer's guidelines.

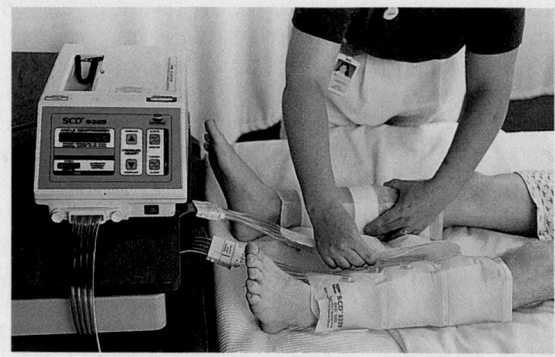

Application of sequential stocking.

---

may promote venous return (Box 46-9). When considering applying graded compression stockings, the nurse first needs to assess the client's suitability for wearing them. The stockings should not be applied if there is any local condition affecting the leg (e.g., any skin lesion, gangrenous condition, or recent vein ligation), because application may compromise circulation. The stockings must be applied properly, and they must be removed and reapplied at least twice a day. Be sure to assess circulation at the toes to ensure the hose are not too tight. In addition, the stockings should always be clean and dry, and it may be useful for the client to have two pairs.

Positioning techniques aid in reducing compression of the leg veins. Proper positioning used with other therapies (e.g., heparin or elastic stockings) aid in reducing the client's risk of thrombus formation. When positioning clients, the nurse uses caution to prevent pressure on the posterior knee and deep veins in the lower extremities. Client teaching should include avoiding crossing the legs, not sitting for prolonged periods of time, not wearing clothing that constricts the legs or waist, not putting pillows under the knees, and avoiding massaging the legs.

ROM exercises are designed to reduce the risk of contractures but may also aid in preventing thrombi. Activity causes contraction of the skeletal muscles, which in turn exerts pressure on the veins to promote venous return, thereby reducing venous stasis. Specific exercises that help prevent thrombophlebitis are ankle pumps, foot circles, and knee flexion. Ankle pumps, sometimes called calf pumps, include alternating plantar flexion and dorsiflexion. Foot circles require the client to rotate the ankle. Instructing the client to make the letters of the alphabet with their feet every 1 to 2 hours is a good exercise to teach. Knee flexion involves alternately extending and flexing the knee. These exercises are sometimes referred to as antiembolic exercises and should be done hourly while awake.

When DVT is suspected, the nurse should report it immediately. The leg should be elevated with no pressure on the thrombus. The family, client, and all health care personnel should be instructed not to massage the area because of the danger of dislodging the thrombus.

Musculoskeletal System. The immobilized client must receive some exercise to prevent excessive muscle atrophy and joint contractures. If the client is unable to move part or all of the body, the nurse must perform passive ROM exercises for all immobilized joints while bathing the client and at least 2 or 3 more times a day. If one extremity is paralyzed, the client can be taught to put each joint independently through its ROM. Clients on bed rest should have active ROM exercises incorporated into their daily schedules. Nurses can teach clients to integrate exercises during ADLs (see Box 46-11, p. 1476). Some orthopedic conditions require more frequent passive ROM exercises to restore the injured joint's function after surgery. Clients with such conditions may use automatic equipment (continuous passive motion [CPM]) for passive ROM

Box 46-9 *Procedural Guidelines*

Application of TED Hose

Equipment: Tape measure, TED hose, hygiene supplies
1. Assess the need for elastic stockings and condition of the client's skin.

Delegation Considerations: The skill of applying TED hose can be performed by assistive personnel (AP). The nurse is responsible for assessing circulation to the lower extremities. The nurse instructs the AP to:
- Notify nurse if client develops leg pain or discoloration.
2. Observe for conditions that might contraindicate use of stockings.
3. Perform hand hygiene. Provide hygiene to lower extremities if needed.
4. Use tape measure to measure client's legs to determine proper stocking size (measure according to manufacturer's directions). Elastic stockings come in two lengths: knee length and thigh length.
5. Apply stockings:
   a. Turn elastic stocking inside out up to the heel. Place one hand into sock, holding heel. Pull top of sock with the other hand inside out over foot of sock.
   b. Place client's toes into foot of elastic stocking, making sure that sock is smooth (see illustration).
   c. Slide remaining portion of sock over client's foot, being sure that the toes are covered. Make sure the foot fits into the toe and heel position of the sock (see illustration).
   d. Slide top of sock up over client's calf until sock is completely extended. Be sure sock is smooth and no ridges or wrinkles are present, particularly behind the knee (see illustration).
6. Instruct client not to roll socks partially down.
7. Record date and time of stocking application and stocking length and size in nurses' notes.
8. Record condition of skin and circulatory assessment.

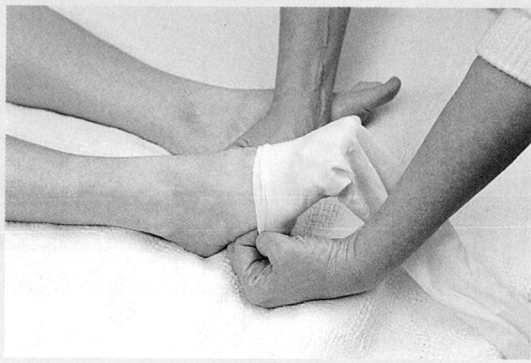

STEP **5b**

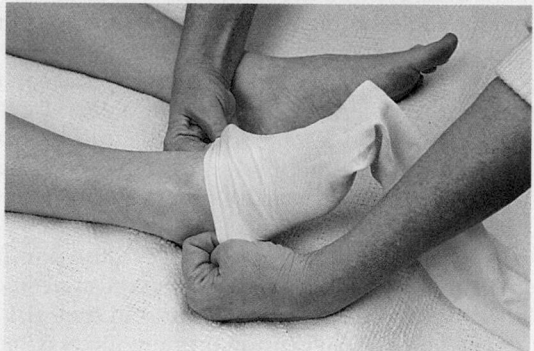

STEP **5c**

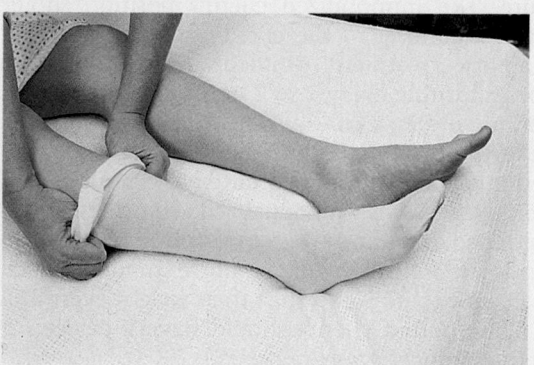

STEP **5d**

exercises (Figure 46-18). The CPM machine moves an extremity to a prescribed angle for a prescribed period. This is beneficial when the client must gradually increase the degree and duration of flexion and extension. Studies over the last 5 years have yielded varying evidence about the effectiveness of CPM in clients with total knee replacements. Short-term benefits were noted in some studies, but long-term improvement in range of motion was questionable (Maher, Salmond, and Pellino, 2002).

Active ROM exercises maintain function of the musculoskeletal system. The nurse should also plan interventions for the gradual return of mobility for clients who will be able to resume normal activity. The best nursing intervention is establishing an individualized progressive exercise program. A progressive exercise program gradually increases the client's physical activity to reverse the deconditioning associated with immobility. Progressive exercise programs are used for clients with musculoskele-

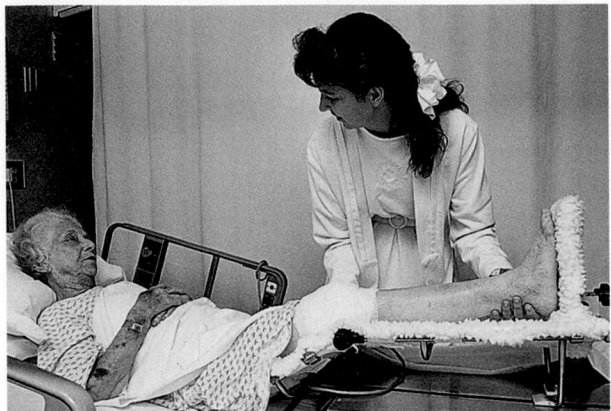

FIGURE **46–18** Continuous passive range-of-motion machine.

Modified from Ebersole P, Hess P: *Geriatric nursing and healthy aging*, St. Louis, 2001, Mosby.

tal, neurological, cardiopulmonary, renal, and other chronic diseases.

When working with older adults, the nurse must keep in mind gerontological principles that enhance the effectiveness of exercise programs and limit injuries (Box 46-10).

Teaching, referral, and interdisciplinary collaboration are important for clients with limited mobility. Depending on the setting and resources available, the nurse may want to refer the client for physical therapy. The therapist would set up the specific exercise program, and the nurse would reinforce it.

Integumentary System. The major risk to the skin from restricted mobility is the formation of pressure ulcers. Early identification of high-risk clients and their risk factors aids the nurse in preventing pressure ulcers (Chapter 17). Interventions aimed at prevention are positioning, skin care, and the use of therapeutic devices to relieve pressure. The immobilized client's position should be changed according to the client's activity level, perceptual ability, treatment protocols, and daily routines. Although turning every 1 to 2 hours is recommended for preventing ulcers, it may also be necessary to use devices for relieving pressure. The time that a client sits uninterrupted in a chair should be limited to 1 hour or less, but this time interval is individualized. The client should be repositioned frequently because uninterrupted pressure will cause skin breakdown. The nurse should teach clients who are able to do so, to shift their weight every 15 minutes. Chair-bound clients should have a device for the chair that reduces pressure (AHRQ, 2003).

Elimination System. The nursing interventions for maintaining optimal urinary functioning are directed at keeping the client well hydrated and preventing urinary stasis, calculi, and infections without causing bladder distention.

Adequate hydration (e.g., 2000 to 3000 ml of fluids per day) helps prevent renal calculi and urinary tract infections. The well-hydrated client should void large amounts of dilute urine that is approximately equal to fluid intake. If the client is incontinent, the nurse should modify the care plan to include toileting aids and a hygiene schedule so that the increased urinary output does not cause skin breakdown.

To prevent bladder distention, the nurse assesses the frequency and amount of urinary output. A client who

Box 46-10

Focus on Older Adults

- Base exercise program on individual assessment data (underlying conditions, medications, present activity level). Consult physician for specific exercise restrictions before onset of exercise program.
- Use correct body mechanics, appropriate clothing, exercise-specific shoes, and sufficient hydration.
- Perform a gradual, extended exercise warm-up (e.g.,15 minutes) to maximize flexibility and decrease muscle injury.
- Begin at low level (40% to 50% of predicted maximal heart rate), and follow gentle exercise progression.
- Avoid sudden twisting movements, rapid movements, and rapid transitions from one movement to the next.
- Avoid exercises that tax vision and balance.
- Avoid sustained isometric contractions of greater than 10 seconds.
- Avoid exercise during acute viral infections.
- Stop exercising if cardiac dysrhythmias, angina, or excessive breathlessness occurs.
- Perform cool-down until heart rate returns to resting level to decrease postural hypotension and cardiac dysrhythmias.
- Modify exercise program based on individual's responses.

continually dribbles urine and whose bladder is distended may have reflex incontinence. If the immobilized client does not have voluntary control of bladder elimination, bladder retraining may be necessary. If the client experiences bladder distention, the nurse may be required to insert a straight catheter or an indwelling Foley catheter (see Chapter 44).

The nurse must also record the frequency and consistency of bowel movements. A diet rich in fluids, fruits, vegetables, and fiber can facilitate normal peristalsis. If a client is unable to maintain regular bowel patterns, stool softeners, cathartics, or enemas may be needed (see Chapter 45).

Psychosocial Changes. Assessment can identify effects of prolonged immobilization on the client's psychosocial dimension. People who have a tendency toward depression or mood swings are at greater risk for developing psychosocial effects during bed rest or immobilization. There are many nursing interventions to meet the client's psychosocial needs.

The nurse should anticipate changes in the client's psychosocial status. The nurse can provide routine and informal socialization. Nursing activities can be planned so that the client can talk and interact with staff. If possible, the client should be placed in a room with others who are mobile and interactive. If a private room is required, staff members should be asked to visit throughout the shift to provide meaningful interaction.

The nurse also provides stimuli to maintain a clients' orientation. A daily newspaper helps the client keep track of events and time. Bedside chats at appropriate moments orient the client to nursing activities, meals, and visiting hours. Books help occupy the client when he or she is alone. The client can participate in craft activities. Radio, television, and videotapes provide stimulation and help pass the time.

Clients should also be involved in their care whenever possible. For example, the nurse should encourage the client to determine when the bed should be made. Some clients rest better during the night when fresh sheets are put on in the evening rather than in the morning. The client should provide as much self-care as possible. Hygiene and grooming articles should be kept within easy reach. Clients should be encouraged to wear their glasses or artificial teeth and to shave or apply makeup. These are activities through which people maintain their body images. Maintenance of body image can help improve the client's outlook.

In institutional health care settings, nursing care given between 10:00 PM and 7:00 AM should be scheduled to minimize interruptions of sleep. For example, the nurse may administer medications and assess vital signs at the time when the client is turned or receives special skin care.

The nurse should also observe the client's ability to cope with restricted mobility. If the nursing care plan is not improving coping patterns, a clinical nurse specialist, counselor, social worker, spiritual adviser, or other consultant may be needed. Their recommendations should be incorporated into the care plan.

Developmental Changes. Ideally, immobilized clients continue normal development. Nursing interventions can help. Nursing care should provide mental and physical stimulation, particularly for a young child. Play activities can be incorporated into the care plan. Completing puzzles, for example, helps a child to develop fine motor skills, and reading helps the child to develop cognitively. Parents can be encouraged to stay with a child who is hospitalized. An immobilized child should be placed with children of the same age who are not immobilized, unless a contagious disease is present. Nursing activities, such as dressing changes, cast care, and care of traction, can be designed to require the child's participation. The nurse must recognize significant changes from normal behavioral patterns. If these continue, the nurse should consult with a clinical nurse, counselor, or other health care professional whose specialty is children.

Restricted mobility of older clients presents unique nursing problems. Older clients who are frail or have chronic illnesses may be at increased risk for the psychosocial hazards of immobility. Maintaining a calendar and clock with a large dial, conversing about current events and family members, and encouraging visits from significant others may reduce the risk of social isolation. The nurse's spending time in the room talking and listening to the client play an important role in reducing the risk of social isolation.

Nursing care should encourage older immobilized clients to perform as many ADLs as independently as possible. Clients should continue to perform personal grooming if they did so before their mobility was restricted. This type of activity preserves the client's dignity and gives the client a sense of accomplishment.

Positioning Techniques. Clients with impaired nervous, skeletal, or muscular system functioning and increased weakness and fatigability often require help from the nurse to attain proper body alignment while in bed or sitting. Several positioning devices are available for maintaining good body alignment for clients (Table 46-4). Pillows are a positioning aid that may or may not be readily available depending on resources. Before using a pillow, the nurse should determine whether it is the proper size. A thick pillow under the client's head increases cervical flexion. A thin pillow under body prominences may be inadequate to protect skin and tissue from damage caused by pressure. When additional pillows are unavailable, or if they are an improper size, the nurse can use folded sheets, blankets, or towels as positioning aids. The 30-degree lateral position is strongly recommended in clients at risk for pressure ulcer development (see Chapter 47).

A footboard is placed perpendicular to the mattress, parallel to and touching the plantar surfaces of the client's feet. The footboard prevents footdrop by maintaining the feet in dorsiflexion. After placing it on the bed, the nurse needs to determine that it is correctly placed, with the client's feet placed firmly against the board. Another common technique is the use of high-top tennis shoes or an ankle-foot orthotic (AFO) to help maintain dorsiflexion.

A **trochanter roll** prevents external rotation of the hips when the client is in a supine position. To form a trochanter roll, a cotton bath blanket is folded lengthwise to a width that will extend from the greater trochanter of the femur to the lower border of the popliteal space. (Figure 46-19). The blanket is placed under the buttocks and then rolled counterclockwise until the thigh is in neutral position or in inward rotation. When correct alignment of the hip is achieved, the patella faces directly upward. Sandbags are sand-filled plastic tubes or bags that can be shaped to body contours. Sandbags can be used in place of or in addition to trochanter rolls. They immobilize an extremity or maintain body alignment.

Hand rolls maintain the thumb in slight adduction and in opposition to the fingers. A hand roll maintains the hand, thumb, and fingers in a functional position. The nurse evaluates the hand roll to make sure that the hand is indeed in a functional position. Hand rolls are most often used for clients whose arms are paralyzed or who are unconscious. Rolled washcloths should not be used as hand rolls, because they do not keep the thumb well abducted, especially in clients who have a spastic paralysis.

Hand-wrist splints are individually molded for the client to maintain proper alignment of the thumb (slight adduction) and the wrist (slight dorsiflexion). These splints should be used only by the client for whom the splint was made.

The **trapeze bar** is a triangular device that descends from a securely fastened overhead bar that is attached to the bed frame. It allows the client to pull with the upper extremities to raise the trunk off the bed, to assist in transfer from bed to wheelchair, or to perform upper arm exercises (see Figure 46-20). It is a useful device for helping to increase independence, maintain upper body strength, and decrease the shearing action from sliding across or up and down in bed.

Although each procedure for positioning has specific guidelines, there are some universal steps the nurse

Table 46-4 Devices Used for Proper Positioning

Devices	Uses and Descriptions
Pillows	Pillows are readily available in most health care facilities, including the home. They should be of appropriate size for the body part to be positioned. Pillows provide support, elevate body parts, and can splint incisional areas, reducing postoperative pain during activity or coughing and deep breathing.
Foot boots	Foot boots maintain feet in dorsiflexion. Boots are made of rigid plastic or heavy foam and keep the foot flexed at the proper angle. The nurse should remove the foot boots two or three times a day to assess skin integrity and joint mobility.
Trochanter rolls	Trochanter rolls prevent external rotation of legs when clients are in the supine position. To form a trochanter roll, a cotton bath blanket or a sheet is folded lengthwise to a width extending from the greater trochanter of the femur to the lower border of the popliteal space (see Figure 46-19). The blanket is placed under the buttocks and then rolled away from the client until the thigh is in the neutral position or an inward position with the patella facing upward.
Sandbags	Sandbags provide support and shape to body contours; they immobilize extremities and maintain specific body alignment. Sandbags are filled plastic tubes that can be shaped to body contours. They can be used in place of, or in addition to, trochanter rolls.
Hand rolls	Hand rolls maintain the thumb slightly adducted and in opposition to the fingers; they maintain fingers in a slightly flexed position. The nurse evaluates the position of the hand roll to make certain the hand is indeed in a functional position.
Hand-wrist splints	Hand-wrist splints are individually molded for the client to maintain proper alignment of the thumb in slight adduction and the wrist in slight dorsiflexion. These splints should be used only for the client for whom the splint was made.
Trapeze bar	The trapeze bar descends from a securely fastened overhead bar attached to the bed frame (see Figure 46-20). The trapeze allows the client to use upper extremities to raise the trunk off the bed, to assist in transfer from bed to wheelchair, or to perform upper arm strengthening exercises.
Side rails	Side rails are bars positioned along the sides of the length of the bed. They ensure client safety and are useful for increasing mobility. In addition, they provide assistance in rolling from side to side or sitting up in bed.
Bed boards	Bed boards are plywood boards placed under the entire surface area of the mattress. They are useful for increasing back support and alignment, especially with a soft mattress.
Wedge pillow	A wedge or abductor pillow is a triangular-shaped pillow made of heavy foam. It is used to maintain the legs in abduction following total hip replacement surgery.

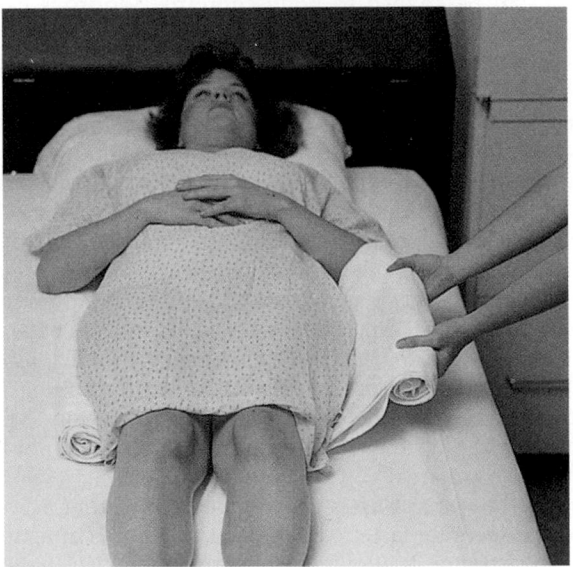

FIGURE **46–19** Trochanter roll.

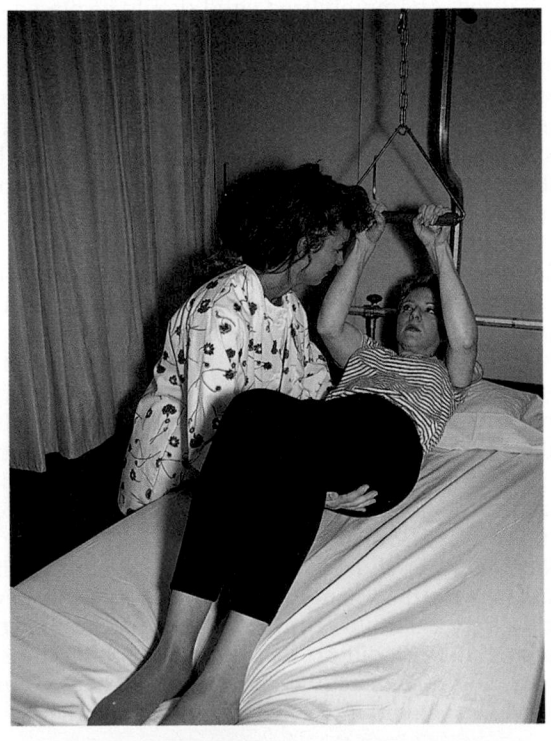

FIGURE **46–20** Client using a trapeze bar.

should follow for clients who require positioning assistance (Skill 46-1). Following the guidelines reduces the risk of injury to the musculoskeletal system when the client is sitting or lying. When joints are unsupported, their alignment is impaired. Likewise, if joints are not positioned in a slightly flexed position, their mobility is decreased. During positioning, the nurse also assesses for pressure points (see Figure 47-12, p. 1502). When actual or potential pressure areas exist, nursing interventions involve removal of the pressure, thus decreasing the risk for development of pressure ulcers and further trauma to the musculoskeletal system. In these clients the 30-degree lateral position should be used.

Supported Fowler's Position. In the supported Fowler's position, the head of the bed is elevated 45 to 60 degrees and the client's knees are slightly elevated without pressure to restrict circulation in the lower legs. The angle of head and knee elevation and the length of time that the client should remain in the supported Fowler's position are influenced by the client's illness and overall condition. Supports must permit flexion of the hips and knees and proper alignment of the normal curves in the cervical, thoracic, and lumbar vertebrae. The following are common trouble areas for the client in the supported Fowler's position:

- Increased cervical flexion because the pillow at the head is too thick and the head thrusts forward
- Extension of the knees, allowing the client to slide to the foot of the bed
- Pressure on the posterior aspect of the knees, decreasing circulation to the feet
- External rotation of the hips
- Arms hanging unsupported at the client's sides
- Unsupported feet or pressure on the heels
- Unprotected pressure points at the sacrum and heels
- Increased shearing force on the back and heels when the head of the bed is raised greater than 60 degrees

Supine Position. The supine position, involves the client resting on the back. In the supine position the relationship of body parts is essentially the same as in good standing alignment except that the body is in the horizontal plane. Pillows, trochanter rolls, and hand rolls or arm splints are used to increase comfort and reduce injury to the skin or musculoskeletal system. The mattress should be firm enough to support the cervical, thoracic, and lumbar vertebrae. Shoulders are supported, and the elbows are slightly flexed to control shoulder rotation. A foot support is used to prevent footdrop and maintain proper alignment. The following are some common trouble areas for clients in the supine position:

- Pillow at the head that is too thick, increasing cervical flexion
- Head flat on the mattress
- Shoulders unsupported and internally rotated
- Elbows extended
- Thumb not in opposition to the fingers
- Hips externally rotated
- Unsupported feet
- Unprotected pressure points at the occipital region of the head, vertebrae, coccyx, elbows, and heels

Prone Position. The client in the prone position is lying face or chest down. Often the client's head is turned to the side, but if a pillow is under the head, it should be thin enough to prevent cervical flexion or extension and maintain alignment of the lumbar spine. Placing a pillow under the lower leg permits dorsiflexion of the ankles and some knee flexion, which promotes relaxation. If a pillow is unavailable, the ankles should be in dorsiflexion over the end of the mattress. The nurse should assess for and correct any of the following potential trouble points:

- Neck hyperextension
- Hyperextension of the lumbar spine
- Plantar flexion of the ankles
- Unprotected pressure points at the chin, elbows, hips, knees, and toes

Studies show the prone position reduces risk of pressure ulcers. Areas located over the body prominences have the highest interface pressures which result in a greater likelihood of developing ulcers. Defloor (2000) found that the prone position resulted in the lowest interface pressures, reducing the risk of skin breakdown. Although the prone position is seldom used in practice, nurses should consider this as an alternative especially in clients who normally sleep in this position.

Side-Lying Position. In the side-lying (or lateral) position the client is resting on the side with the major portion of body weight on the dependent hip and shoulder. A 30-degree lateral position is recommended for clients at risk for pressure ulcers (see Chapter 47). Trunk alignment should be the same as in standing. For example, the structural curves of the spine should be maintained, the head should be supported in line with the midline of the trunk, and rotation of the spine should be avoided. The following trouble points are common in the side-lying position:

- Lateral flexion of the neck
- Spinal curves out of normal alignment
- Shoulder and hip joints internally rotated, adducted, or unsupported
- Lack of support for the feet
- Lack of protection for pressure points at the ear, shoulder, anterior iliac spine, trochanter, and ankles
- Excessive lateral flexion of the spine if the client has large hips and a pillow is not placed superior to the hips at the waist

Sims' Position. Sims' position differs from the side lying position in the distribution of the client's weight. In Sims' position the weight is placed on the anterior ilium, humerus, and clavicle. Trouble points common in Sims' position include the following:

- Lateral flexion of the neck
- Internal rotation, adduction, or lack of support to the shoulders and hips
- Lack of support for the feet
- Lack of protection for pressure points at the ilium, humerus, clavicle, knees, and ankles

Transfer Techniques. Nurses often provide care for immobilized clients whose position must be changed, who must be moved up in bed, or who must be transferred from a bed to a chair or from a bed to a stretcher. Use of proper body mechanics enables the nurse to move, lift, or transfer clients safely and also protects the nurse from injury to the musculoskeletal system. Although nurses use

Text continued on p. 1467

Skill 46-1 *Moving and Positioning Clients in Bed*

Delegation Considerations

The skills of moving and positioning clients in bed can be delegated to assistive personnel (AP). The nurse is responsible for assessing the client's level of comfort and for any hazards of immobility. It is important for the nurse to do the following:

• Instruct AP on any limitations affecting movement and positioning of client in bed.

Equipment

• Pillows
• Footboard (optional)
• High-top sneakers
• Trochanter roll
• Sandbag
• Hand rolls
• Side rails

Steps	Rationale
1. Assess client's body alignment and comfort level while client is lying down.	Provides baseline data for later comparisons. Determines ways to improve position and alignment.
2. Assess for risk factors that may contribute to complications of immobility:	Increased risk factors require client to be repositioned more frequently.
a. Paralysis: hemiparesis resulting from cerebrovascular accident (CVA); decreased sensation	Paralysis impairs movement; muscle tone changes; sensation can be affected. Because of difficulty in moving and poor awareness of involved body part, client is unable to protect and position body part for self.
b. Impaired mobility: traction or arthritis or other contributing disease processes	Traction or arthritic changes of affected extremity result in decreased ROM.
c. Impaired circulation	Decreased circulation predisposes client to pressure sores.
d. Age: very young, older adults	Premature and young infants require frequent turning because their skin is fragile. Normal physiological changes associated with aging predispose older adults to greater risks for developing complications of immobility.
e. Level of consciousness and mental status.	Comatose or semicomatose clients are unable to verbalize areas of skin pressure, increasing the risk for skin breakdown.
3. Assess client's physical ability to help with moving and positioning:	Enables nurse to use client's mobility and strength. Determines need for additional help. Ensures client and nurse safety.
a. Age	Older adult client will move more slowly with less strength.
b. Level of consciousness and mental status.	Determines need for special aids or devices. Clients with altered levels of consciousness may not understand instructions and may be unable to help.
c. Disease process	Cardiopulmonary disease may require client to have head of bed elevated.
d. Strength, coordination	Determines amount of assistance provided by client during position change.
e. ROM	Limited ROM may contraindicate certain positions.
4. Assess physician's orders. Clarify whether any positions are contraindicated because of client's condition (e.g., spinal cord injury; respiratory difficulties; certain neurological conditions; presence of incisions, drain, or tubing).	Placing client in an inappropriate position could cause injury.
5. Perform hand hygiene.	Reduces transfer of microorganisms.
6. Assess for the presence of tubes, incisions, and equipment (e.g., traction).	Will alter positioning procedure and may affect client's ability to independently change positions.
7. Assess ability and motivation of client, family members, and primary caregiver to participate in moving and positioning client in bed in anticipation of discharge to home.	Determines ability of client and caregivers to assist with positioning.
8. Raise level of bed to comfortable working height, and get extra help if needed.	Raises level of work to your center of gravity and provides for client's and your safety.

Steps	Rationale
9. Perform hand hygiene	Reduces transfer of microorganisms
10. Explain procedure to client.	Decreases anxiety and increases client cooperation.
11. Position client flat in bed if tolerated.	Repositioning from a flat position decreases friction and possible shear on client's skin.

Critical Decision Point: Before flattening bed, account for all tubing, drains, and equipment to prevent dislodgement or tipping if caught in mattress or bed frame as bed is lowered.

---

12. Position client in bed.

   A. **Move immobile client up in bed (one nurse)**

(1) Place client on back with head of bed flat. Stand on one side of bed.	Enables you to assess body alignment. Reduces gravity's pull on client's upper body.
(2) Remove pillow from under head and shoulders, and place pillow at head of bed.	Prevents striking client's head against head of bed.
(3) Begin at client's feet. Face foot of bed at 45-degree angle. Place feet apart with foot nearest head of bed behind other foot (forward-backward stance) (see illustration). Flex knees and hips as needed to bring arms level with client's legs. Shift weight from front to back leg, and slide client's legs diagonally toward head of bed.	Positioning is begun at client's legs because they are lighter and easier to move. Facing direction of movement ensures proper balance. Shifting weight reduces force needed to move load. Diagonal motion permits pull in direction of force. Flexing knees lowers your center of gravity and uses thigh muscles rather than back muscles.
(4) Move parallel to client's hips. Flex knees and hips as needed to bring arms level with client's hips.	Maintains correct body alignment. Brings you closest to object to be moved and lowers center of gravity. Uses thigh muscles rather than back muscles.
(5) Slide client's hips diagonally toward head of bed.	Aligns client's hips and feet.
(6) Move parallel to client's head and shoulders. Flex knees and hips as needed to bring arms level with client's body.	Maintains proper body alignment. Brings you closer to object to be moved. Lowers center of gravity. Uses thigh muscles rather than back muscles.
(7) Slide arm closest to head of bed under client's neck with hand reaching under and supporting client's opposite shoulder.	Supports client's head and neck, maintaining alignment and preventing injury during movement.
(8) Place other arm under client's upper back.	Supports client's body weight and reduces friction during movement.
(9) Slide client's trunk, shoulders, head, and neck diagonally toward head of bed.	Realigns client's body on one side of bed.
(10) Elevate side rail. Move to other side of bed, and lower side rail.	Protects client from falling out of bed.
(11) Repeat procedure, switching sides until client reaches desired position in bed.	

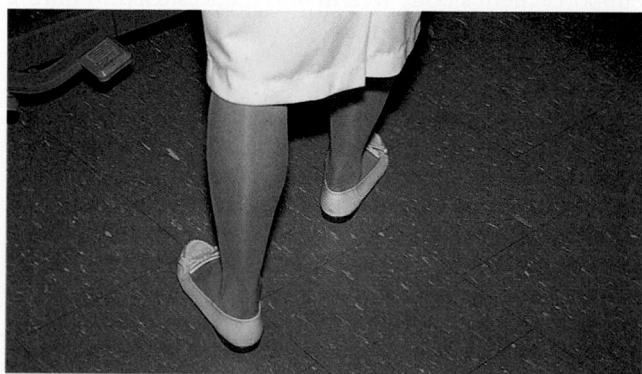

STEP **12A(3)** Position of feet: Feet placed apart in a forward to backward stance.

Skill 46-1   *Moving and Positioning Clients in Bed—cont'd*

Steps	Rationale
(12) Center client in middle of bed, moving body in same three sections.	Maintains proper body alignment. Provides ample room for turning, positioning, and other nursing activities.
B. Assist client in moving up in bed (one or two nurses)	
(1) Remove pillow from under head and shoulders, and place pillow at head of bed.	Prevents striking client's head against head of bed.
(2) Face head of bed.	Facing direction of movement prevents twisting of your body while moving client.
(a) Each nurse should have one arm under client's shoulders and one arm under client's thighs.	
(b) Alternative position: position one nurse at client's upper body. Nurse's arm nearest head of bed should be under clients' head and opposite shoulder; other arm should be under client's closest arm and shoulder. Position other nurse at client's lower torso. The nurse's arms should be under client's lower back and torso.	Prevents trauma to client's musculoskeletal system by supporting shoulder and hip joints and evenly distributing weight.
(3) Place feet apart, with foot nearest head of bed behind other foot (forward-backward stance).	Wide base of support increases balance. Stance enables you to shift body weight as client is moved up in bed, thereby reducing force needed to move load.
(4) When possible, ask client to flex knees with feet flat on bed.	Decreases friction and enables client to use leg muscles during movement.
(5) Instruct client to flex neck, tilting chin toward chest.	Prevents hyperextension of neck when moving client up in bed.
(6) Instruct client to assist moving by pushing with feet on bed surface.	Reduces friction. Increases client mobility. Decreases workload.
(7) Flex knees and hips, bringing forearms closer to level of bed.	Increases balance and strength by bringing your center of gravity closer to client. Uses thighs instead of back muscles.
(8) Instruct client to push with heels and elevate trunk while breathing out, thus moving toward head of bed on count of three.	Prepares client for move. Reinforces assistance in moving up in bed. Increases client cooperation. Breathing out avoids Valsalva maneuver.
(9) On count of three, rock and shift weight from front to back leg. At the same time client pushes with heels and elevates trunk.	Rocking enables you to improve balance and overcome inertia. Shifting your weight counteracts client's weight and reduces force needed to move load. Client's assistance reduces friction and workload.
C. Move immobile client up in bed with drawsheet or pull sheet (two nurses)	
(1) Place drawsheet or pull sheet under client by turning side to side. Have sheet extend from shoulders to thighs. Return client to supine position.	Supports client's body weight and reduces friction during movement.
(2) Position one nurse at each side of client.	Distributes weight equally between nurses.
(3) Grasp drawsheet or pull sheet firmly near the client.	
(4) Place feet apart with forward-backward stance. Flex knees and hips. Shift weight from front to back leg, and move client and drawsheet or pull sheet to desired position in bed.	Facing direction of movement ensures proper balance. Shifting weight reduces force needed to move load. Flexing knees lowers center of gravity and uses thighs instead of back muscles.
(5) Realign client in correct body alignment.	Prevents injury to musculoskeletal system.
D. Position client in supported Fowler's position (see illustration)	
(1) Elevate head of bed 45 to 60 degrees.	Increases comfort, improves ventilation, and increases client's opportunity to socialize or relax.

Steps	**Rationale**

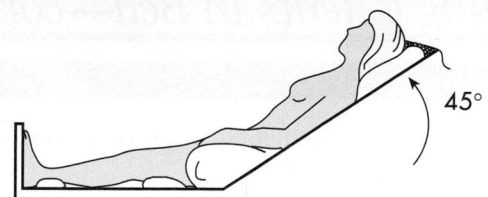

STEP **12D** Supported Fowler's position with footboard in place.

(2) Rest head against mattress or on small pillow.	Prevents flexion contractures of cervical vertebrae.
(3) Use pillows to support arms and hands if client does not have voluntary control or use of hands and arms.	Prevents shoulder dislocation from effect of downward pull of unsupported arms, promotes circulation by preventing venous pooling, and prevents flexion contractures of arms and wrists.
(4) Position pillow at lower back.	Supports lumbar vertebrae and decreases flexion of vertebrae.
(5) Place small pillow or roll under thigh.	Prevents hyperextension of knee and occlusion of popliteal artery from pressure from body weight.
(6) Place small pillow or roll under ankles.	Prevents prolonged pressure of mattress on heels.

Critical Decision Point: To keep feet in proper alignment and prevent footdrop, place footboard at bottom of client's feet.

E. Position hemiplegic client in supported Fowler's position

(1) Elevate head of bed 45 to 60 degrees.	Increases comfort, improves ventilation, and increases client's opportunity to relax.
(2) Position client in sitting position as straight as possible.	Counteracts tendency to slump toward affected side. Improves ventilation and cardiac output; decreases intracranial pressure. Improves client's ability to swallow and helps to prevent aspiration of food, liquids, and gastric secretions.
(3) Position head on small pillow with chin slightly forward. If client is totally unable to control head movement, hyperextension of the neck must be avoided.	Prevents hyperextension of neck. Too many pillows under head may cause or worsen neck flexion contracture.

Critical Decision Point: If the client has a paralyzed extremity, provide support for involved arm and hand on over-bed table in front of client. Place arm away from client's side and support elbow with pillow.
- Position *flaccid* hand in normal resting position with wrist slightly extended, arches of hand maintained, and fingers partially flexed; may use section of rubber ball cut in half; clasp client's hands together.
- Position *spastic* hand with wrist in neutral position or slightly extended; fingers should be extended with palm down or may be left in relaxed position palm up. At times it may be difficult to position spastic hands without the use of specially made splints for the client.

---

(4) Flex knees and hips by using pillow or folded blanket under knees.	Ensures proper alignment. Flexion prevents prolonged hyperextension, which could impair joint mobility.
(5) Support feet in dorsiflexion with firm pillow or footboard.	Prevents footdrop. Stimulation of ball of foot by hard surface has tendency to increase muscle tone in client with extensor spasticity of lower extremity.

F. Position client in supine position

(1) Be sure client is comfortable on back with head of bed flat.	Some clients' physical conditions will not tolerate supine position.
(2) Place small rolled towel under lumbar area of back.	Provides support for lumbar spine.

Skill **46-1**   *Moving and Positioning Clients in Bed—cont'd*

Steps	Rationale
(3) Place pillow under upper shoulders, neck, or head.	Maintains correct alignment and prevents flexion contractures of cervical vertebrae.
(4) Place trochanter rolls or sandbags parallel to lateral surface of client's thighs.	Reduces external rotation of hip.
(5) Place small pillow or roll under ankle to elevate heels (see illustration for step 11D).	Reduces pressure on heels, helping to prevent pressure sores.
(6) Place footboard or firm pillows against bottom of client's feet.	Maintains dorsiflexion and prevents footdrop.
(7) Place foot splints on client's feet.	Maintains feet in dorsiflexion. Prevents footdrop.
(8) Place pillows under pronated forearms, keeping upper arms parallel to client's body (see illustrations).	Reduces internal rotation of shoulder and prevents extension of elbows. Maintains correct body alignment.
(9) Place hand rolls in client's hands. Consider physical therapy referral for use of hand splints.	Reduces extension of fingers and abduction of thumb. Maintains thumb slightly adducted and in opposition to fingers.
G. Position hemiplegic client in supine position	
(1) Place head of bed flat.	Necessary for positioning in supine position.
(2) Place folded towel or small pillow under shoulder or affected side.	Decreases possibility of pain, joint contracture, and subluxation. Maintains mobility in muscles around shoulder to permit normal movement patterns.
(3) Keep affected arm away from body with elbow extended and palm up. (Alternative is to place arm out to side, with elbow bent and hand toward head of bed.)	Maintains mobility in arm, joints, and shoulder to permit normal movement patterns. (Alternative position counteracts limitation of ability of arm to rotate outward at shoulder [external rotation]. External rotation must be present to raise arm overhead without pain.)

Critical Decision Point: Position affected hand in one of the recommended positions for flaccid or spastic hand.

---

(4) Place folded towel under hip of involved side.	Diminishes effect of spasticity in entire leg by controlling hip position.
(5) Flex affected knee 30 degrees by supporting it on pillow or folded blanket.	Slight flexion breaks up abnormal extension pattern of leg. Extensor spasticity is most severe when client is supine.
(6) Support feet with soft pillows at right angle to leg.	Maintains foot in dorsiflexion and prevents footdrop. Pillows prevent stimulation to ball of foot by hard surface, which has tendency to increase muscle tone in client with extensor spasticity of lower extremity.

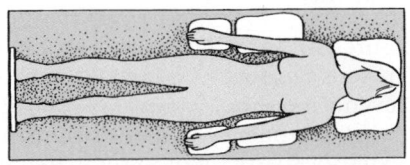
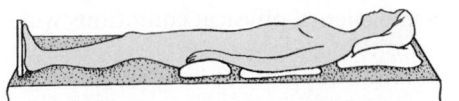
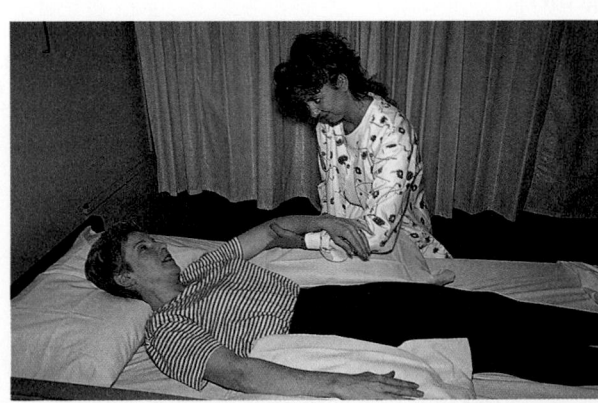

STEP **12F(8)** Supine position with pillows in place.

Steps	Rationale

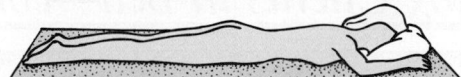

STEP **12H(2)** Prone position, head supported with pillow.

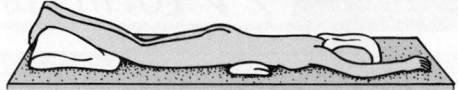

STEP **12H(3)** Prone position, pillow under client's abdomen and feet.

H. Position client in prone position	
(1) With client supine, roll client over arm positioned close to body, with elbow straight and hand under hip. Position on abdomen in center of bed.	Positions client correctly so alignment can be maintained.
(2) Turn client's head to one side and support head with small pillow (see illustration).	Reduces flexion or hyperextension of cervical vertebrae.
(3) Place small pillow under client's abdomen below level of diaphragm (see illustration).	Reduces pressure on breasts of some female clients and decreases hyperextension of lumbar vertebrae and strain on lower back.
(4) Support arms in flexed position level at shoulders.	Maintains proper body alignment. Support reduces risk of joint dislocation.
(5) Support lower legs with pillows to elevate toes (see illustration).	Prevents footdrop. Reduces external rotation of hips. Reduces mattress pressure on toes.
I. Position hemiplegic client in prone position	

Critical Decision Point: Increase frequency of position if pressure areas begin to appear, joint mobility becomes impaired or worsened, or client complains of discomfort. Consult with physical and occupational therapists as needed. Use 30-degree lateral position (see Figure 47-18, p. 1515).

---

(1) Move client toward unaffected side.	Creates room for proper client alignment in center of bed when client is rolled onto abdomen.
(2) Roll client onto side.	
(3) Place pillow on client's abdomen.	Prevents sagging of abdomen when client is rolled over; decreases hyperextension of lumbar vertebrae and strain on lower back.
(4) Roll client onto abdomen by positioning involved arm close to client's body, with elbow straight and hand under hip. Roll client carefully over arm.	Prevents injury to affected side.
(5) Turn head toward involved side.	Promotes development of neck and trunk extension, which is necessary for standing and walking.
(6) Position involved arm out to side, with elbow bent, hand toward head of bed, and fingers extended (if possible).	Counteracts limitation of arm's ability to rotate outward at shoulder (external rotation). External rotation must be present to raise arm over head without pain.

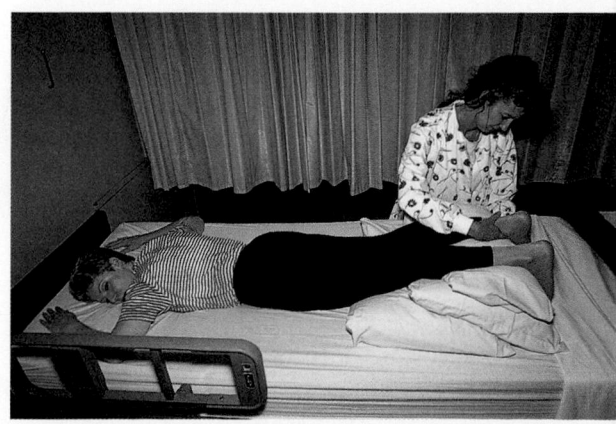

STEP **12H(5)** Prone position.

Skill 46-1   *Moving and Positioning Clients in Bed—cont'd*

Steps	Rationale
(7) Flex knees slightly by placing pillow under legs from knees to ankles.	Flexion prevents prolonged hyperextension, which could impair joint mobility.
(8) Keep feet at right angle to legs by using pillow high enough to keep toes off mattress.	Maintains feet in dorsiflexion.

J. Position client in lateral (side-lying) position

Steps	Rationale
(1) Lower head of bed completely or as low as client can tolerate.	Provides position of comfort for client and removes pressure from bony prominences on back and buttocks.
(2) Position client to side of bed.	Provides room for client to turn to side.
(3) Prepare to turn client onto side. Flex client's knee that will not be next to mattress. Place one hand on client's hip and one hand on client's shoulder.	Positioning will set up leverage for easy turning.
(4) Roll client onto side toward you.	Rolling client toward you decreases trauma to tissues. In addition, client is positioned so leverage on hip makes turning easy.
(5) Place pillow under client's head and neck.	Maintains alignment. Reduces lateral neck flexion. Decreases strain on sternocleidomastoid muscle.
(6) Bring shoulder blade forward.	Prevents client's weight from resting directly on shoulder joint.
(7) Position both arms in slightly flexed position. Upper arm is supported by pillow level with shoulder; other arm, by mattress.	Decreases internal rotation and adduction of shoulder. Supports both arms in slightly flexed position.
(8) Place tuck-back pillow behind client's back. (Make by folding pillow lengthwise. Smooth area is slightly tucked under client's back.)	Provides support to maintain client on side.
(9) Place pillow under semiflexed upper leg level at hip from groin to foot (see illustrations).	Maintains leg in correct alignment. Prevents pressure on bony prominence.
(10) Place sandbag parallel to plantar surface of dependent foot.	Maintains dorsiflexion of foot. Prevents footdrop.

K. Position client in Sims' (semiprone) position

Steps	Rationale
(1) Lower head of bed completely.	Provides for proper body alignment while client is lying down.
(2) Be sure client is comfortable in supine position.	Prepares client for position. Client is rolled partially onto abdomen.
(3) Position client in lateral position, with dependent arm straight along client's body and with client lying partially on abdomen.	

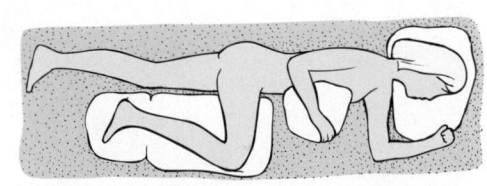

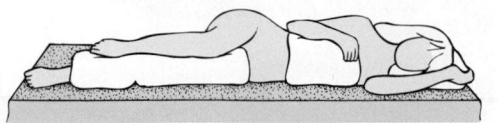

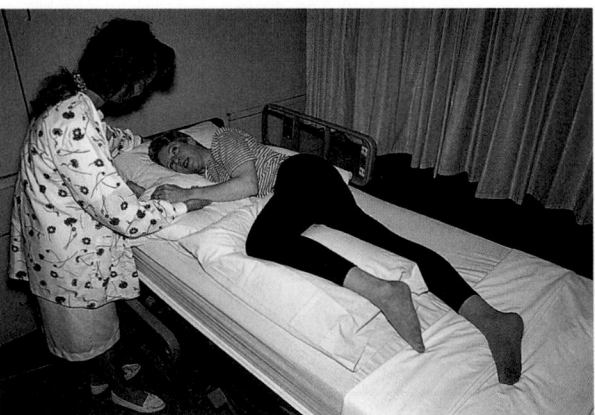

STEP **12J(9)** Side-lying position with pillows in place.

Steps	Rationale

(4) Carefully lift client's dependent shoulder and bring arm back behind cleint.

(5) Place small pillow under client's head.

(6) Place pillow under flexed upper arm, supporting arm level with shoulder. — Maintains proper alignment and prevents lateral neck flexion. Prevents internal rotation of shoulder. Maintains alignment.

(7) Place pillow under flexed upper legs, supporting leg level with hip. — Prevents internal rotation of hip and adduction of leg. Flexion prevents hyperextension of leg. Reduces mattress pressure on knees and ankles.

(8) Place sandbags parallel to plantar surface of foot (see illustration). — Maintains foot in dorsiflexion. Prevents footdrop.

L. Logrolling the client (three nurses)

Critical Decision Point: Supervise and aid assistive personnel when there is a physician's order to **logroll** a client. Clients who have suffered from spinal cord injury or are recovering from neck, back, or spinal surgery often need to keep the spinal column in straight alignment to prevent further injury.

---

(1) Place pillow between client's knees. — Prevents tension on the spinal column and adduction of the hip.

(2) Cross client's arms on chest. — Prevents injury to arms.

(3) Position two nurses on side of bed to which the client will be turned. Position third nurse on the other side of bed (see illustration). — Distributes weight equally between nurses.

(4) Fanfold or roll the drawsheet or pull sheet. — Provides strong handles in order to grip the drawsheet or pull sheet without slipping.

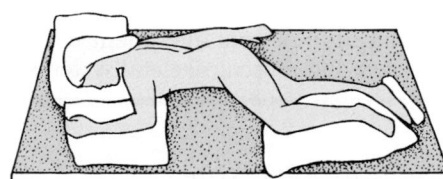

STEP **12K(8)** Sims' (semiprone) position with pillows in place.

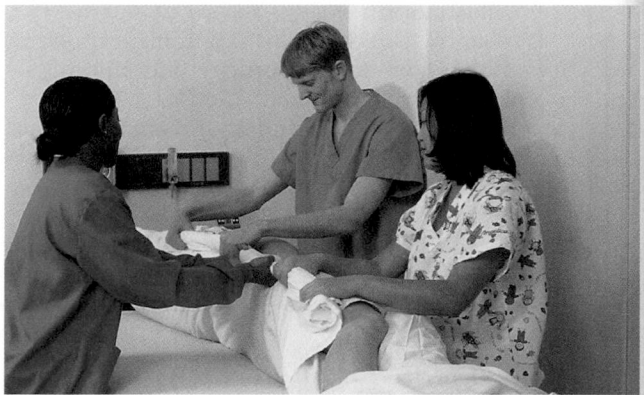

STEP **12L(5)** Move client as a unit, maintaining proper alignment.

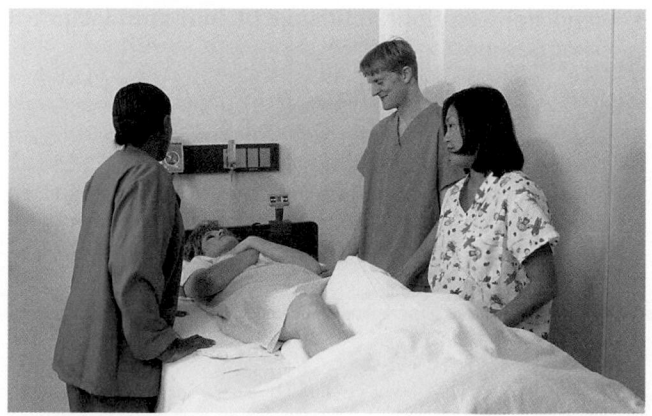

STEP **12L(3)** Position nurses on each side of client.

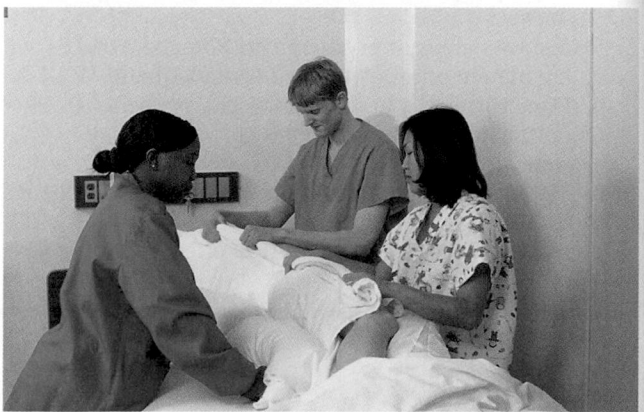

STEP **12L(6)** Place pillows along client's back for support.

Skill 46-1   *Moving and Positioning Clients in Bed—cont'd*

Steps	Rationale

STEP **12L(7)** Gently lean client as a unit against pillows.

Steps	Rationale
(5) Move the client as one unit in a smooth, continuous motion on the count of three (see illustration).	This maintains proper alignment by moving all body parts at the same time, preventing tension or twisting of the spinal column.
(6) Nurse on the opposite side of the bed places pillows along the length of the client (see illustration).	Pillows keep client aligned.
(7) Gently lean the client as a unit back towards the pillows for support (see illustration).	Ensures continued straight alignment of spinal column, preventing injury.
13. Perform hand hygiene.	Reduces transmission of microorganisms.
14. Evaluate client's level of comfort and ability to assist in position change.	Clients with reduced activity tolerance and increased levels of pain may find position changes very fatiguing and will need postposition change interventions to restore their level of comfort.
15. Following each position change evaluate client's body alignment and presence of any pressure areas.	Prompt identification of poor alignment reduces risks to the client's skin and musculoskeletal systems.

Unexpected Outcomes and Related Interventions

1. Joint contractures develop or worsen.
   a. Improper positioning results in shortening of muscles.
2. Skin shows areas of erythema and breakdown.
   a. Frequency of repositioning is inadequate.
   b. Place turning schedule above client's bed.
3. Client avoids moving.
   a. Indicates fear of pain.
   b. Medicate as ordered by a physician to ensure client's comfort before moving.
   c. Allow pain medication to take effect before proceeding.

Recording and Reporting

- Record procedure and observations (e.g., condition of skin, joint movement, client's ability to assist with positioning).
- Report observations at change of shift and document in nurses' notes.

Home Care Considerations

- Teach family the importance of body mechanics for themselves and the client.
- Teach client, family about the signs of skin breakdown and the importance of safety during positioning for clients with decreased sensation.

many transfer techniques, the following general guidelines should be followed in any transfer procedure:

- Raising the side rail on the side of the bed opposite the nurse to prevent the client from falling out of bed
- Elevating the level of the bed to a comfortable height
- Assessing the client's mobility and strength to determine what assistance the client can offer during transfer
- Determining the need for assistance from other care providers
- Explaining the procedure and describing what is expected of the client
- Assessing for correct body alignment and pressure areas after each transfer

Safety Alert: The nurse should recognize personal strength and its limits. Moving a completely immobilized client alone is difficult and dangerous. The nurse who is attempting transfer or moving techniques for the first time should request help to reduce the risk of injury to client and nurse.

Moving Clients. Clients require various levels of assistance to move up in bed, move to the side-lying position, or sit up at the side of the bed. For example, a young, healthy woman may need only a little support as she sits at the side of the bed for the first time after childbirth, whereas an older man may need help from one or more nurses to do the same task 1 day after abdominal surgery.

The nurse should always enlist the client's help to the fullest extent possible. To determine what the client is able to do alone and how many people are needed to help move the client in bed, the nurse assesses the client to determine whether the illness contradicts exertion (e.g., cardiovascular disease). Next, the nurse determines whether the client comprehends what is expected. For example, a client recently medicated for postoperative pain may be too lethargic to understand instruction; thus to ensure safety, two nurses are needed to move the client in bed. The nurse then determines the comfort level of the client. The nurse also evaluates personal strength and knowledge of the procedure. Finally, the nurse determines whether the client is too heavy or immobile for the nurse to complete the procedure alone (Nelson and others, 2003). In doubtful cases the nurse should always request assistance from another person. Skills 46-1 and 46-2 describe the steps commonly used in moving clients in bed and transferring them to a sitting position at the side of the bed.

Transferring a Client From a Bed to a Chair. Transfer of a client from a bed to a chair by one nurse requires assistance from the client and should not be attempted with a client who cannot help (see Skill 46-2, p. 1468). The nurse explains the procedure to the client before the transfer. Moving obstacles out of the way also prepares the environment. The chair is placed next to the bed with the chair back in the same plane as the head of the bed. Placement of the chair allows the nurse to pivot with the client and to transfer the client's weight quickly.

A safe transfer is the first priority. The nurse who is doubtful about personal strength or the client's ability to help should request assistance. Often a hydraulic lift can be used to transfer clients (see Skill 46-2, p. 1468). The

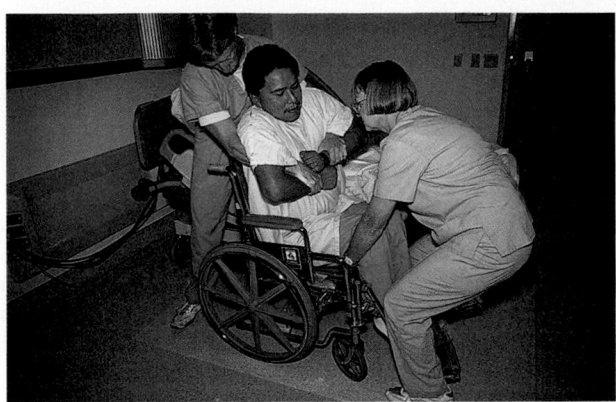

FIGURE **46–21** Transferring an immobile client from bed to wheelchair.

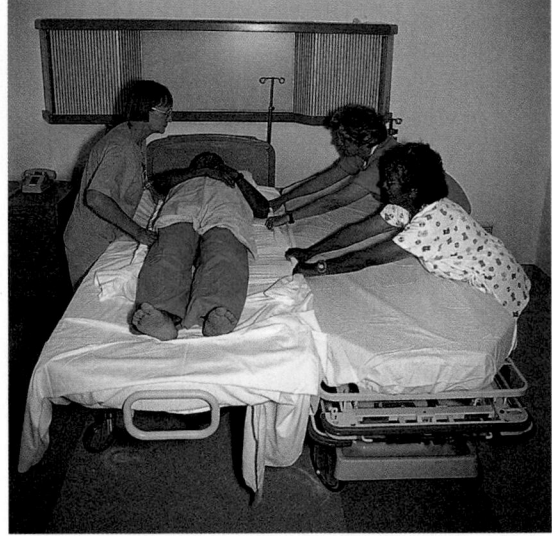

FIGURE **46–22** Use of a draw or pull sheet to transfer a client from bed to stretcher.

client should sit and dangle the feet at the side of the bed for a minute before standing. The client should then stand at the side of the bed for another minute so that the client can quickly be lowered back into it in case of dizziness or fainting. When moving an immobilized client from a bed to a wheelchair, both nurses must use proper body mechanics (Figure 46-21). If a client has an immobile lower extremity from a cast or paralysis, the transfer should be toward the unaffected leg.

Transferring a Client From a Bed to a Stretcher. An immobilized client who must be transferred from a bed to a stretcher or from a bed to another bed often requires a three-person carry (see Skill 46-2, p. 1468). This technique is best implemented when personnel who are doing the lifting are similar in height. If their centers of gravity are within the same plane, they can lift as a team. Another way to transfer a client is by using a lift sheet or a quilted transfer pad placed under the client (Figure 46-22). The lift sheet serves as a "cradle" while the client is being transferred to the stretcher. In this technique, nurses need to be

Text continued on p. 1475

Skill 46-2　*Using Safe and Effective Transfer Techniques*

Delegation Considerations

The skills of effective transfer techniques can be delegated to assistive personnel (AP). Clients who are transferred for the first time after prolonged bed rest, extensive surgery, critical illness, or spinal cord trauma usually require supervision by professional nurses. When delegating this skill the nurse should do the following:
- Instruct AP to seek assistance when moving or lifting heavy client.
- Instruct AP on any client limitations that may affect safe transfer techniques.

Equipment

- Transfer belt, sling, or lapboard (as needed), nonskid shoes, bath blankets, pillows.
- Wheelchair: Position chair at 45-degree angle to bed, lock brakes, remove footrests, lock bed brakes.
- Stretcher: Position at right angle (90 degrees) to bed, lock brakes on stretcher, lock brakes on bed.
- Mechanical/hydraulic lift: Use frame, canvas strips or chains, and hammock or canvas strips.

Steps	Rationale
1. Assess the client for the following:	Provides information relative to the client's abilities, physical status, ability to comprehend, and the number of individuals needed to provide safe transferring.
a. Muscle strength (legs and upper arms)	Immobile clients have decreased muscle strength, tone, and mass. Affects ability to bear weight or raise body.
b. Joint mobility and contracture formation	Immobility or inflammatory processes (e.g., arthritis) may lead to contracture formation and impaired joint mobility.
c. Paralysis or paresis (spastic or flaccid)	Client with central nervous system damage may have bilateral paralysis (requiring transfer by swivel bar, sliding bar, or mechanical [Hoyer] lift) or unilateral paralysis, which requires belt transfer to "best" side. Weakness (paresis) requires stabilization of knee while transferring. Flaccid arm must be supported with sling during transfer.
d. Orthostatic hypotension	Determines risk of fainting or falling during transfer. Immobile clients may have decreased ability for autonomic nervous system to equalize blood supply, resulting in drop of 15 mm Hg or more in blood pressure when rising from sitting position.
e. Activity tolerance	Determines ability of client to assist with transfer.
f. Level of comfort	Pain may reduce client's motivation and ability to be mobile. Pain relief before transfer enhances client participation.
g. Vital signs	Vital sign changes such as increased pulse and respiration may indicate activity intolerance (see Chapter 31).
2. Assess client's sensory status: a. Adequacy of central and peripheral vision b. Adequacy of hearing c. Loss of peripheral sensation	Determines influence of sensory loss on ability to make transfer. Visual field loss decreases client's ability to see in direction of transfer. Peripheral sensation loss decreases proprioception. Clients with visual and hearing losses need transfer techniques adapted to deficits. Clients with cerebrovascular accident (CVA) may lose area of visual field, which profoundly affects vision and perception.

Critical Decision Point: Clients with hemiplegia also may "neglect" one side of the body (inattention to or unawareness of one side of body or environment), which distorts perception of the visual field.

Steps	Rationale
3. Assess client's cognitive status.	Determines client's ability to follow directions and learn transfer techniques.

Critical Decision Point: Clients with head trauma or CVA may have perceptual cognitive deficits that create safety risks. If client has difficulty in comprehension, simplify instructions and maintain consistency.

Steps	Rationale
4. Assess client's level of motivation: a. Client's eagerness versus unwillingness to be mobile b. Whether client avoids activity and offers excuses	Altered psychological states reduce client's desire to engage in activity.
5. Assess previous mode of transfer (if applicable).	Determines mode of transfer and assistance required to provide continuity. Transfer belts should be used with all clients being transferred for the first time and thereafter as deemed necessary.
6. Assess client's specific risk of falling when transferred.	Certain conditions increase client's risk of falling or potential for injury. Neuromuscular deficits, motor weakness, calcium loss from long bones, cognitive and visual dysfunction, and altered balance increase risk of injury.
7. Assess special transfer equipment needed for home setting. Assess home environment for hazards.	Transfer ability at home is greatly enhanced by prior teaching of family and support persons, assessment of home for safety risks and functionality.
8. Perform hand hygiene.	Reduces transmission of microorganisms.
9. Explain procedure to client.	Increases client participation.
10. Transfer client. A. **Assist client to sitting position (bed at waist level)** (1) Place client in supine position.	Enables you to assess client's body alignment continually and to administer additional care, such as suctioning or hygiene needs.
(2) Face head of bed at a 45-degree angle, and remove pillows.	Proper positioning reduces twisting of your body when moving the client. Pillows may cause interference when the client is sitting up in bed.
(3) Place feet apart with foot nearer bed behind other foot, continuing at a 45-degree angle to the head of the bed.	Improves balance and allows transfer of body weight as client is sitting up in bed.
(4) Place hand farther from client under shoulders, supporting client's head and cervical vertebrae.	Maintains alignment of head and cervical vertebrae and allows for even lifting of client's upper trunk.
(5) Place other hand on bed surface.	Provides support and balance.
(6) Raise client to sitting position by shifting weight from front to back leg.	Improves balance, overcomes inertia, and transfers weight in direction in which client is moved.
(7) Push against bed using arm that is placed on bed surface.	Divides activity between arms and legs and protects back from stain. By bracing one hand against mattress and pushing against it as client is lifted, part of weight that would be lifted by your back muscles is transferred through your arm onto mattress.
B. **Assist client to sitting position on side of bed with bed in low position** (1) Turn client to side, facing you on side of bed on which client will be sitting (see illustration).	Decreases amount of work needed by client and you to raise client to sitting position.
(2) With client in supine position, raise head of bed 30 degrees.	Prepares client to move to side of bed and protects from falling.

*U*sing Safe and Effective Transfer Techniques—cont'd

Steps	Rationale

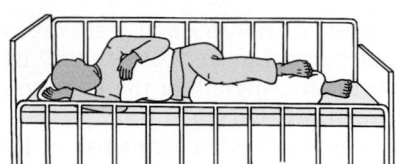

STEP **10B(1)** Side-lying position.

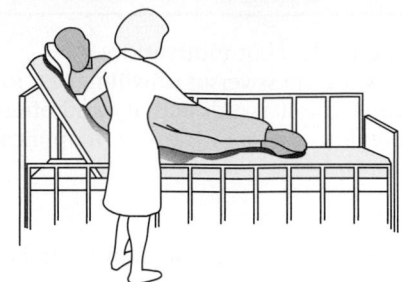

STEP **10B(6)** Nurse places arm over client's thighs.

(3) Stand opposite client's hips. Turn diagonally so you face client and far corner of foot of bed.

Places your center of gravity nearer client. Reduces twisting of your body because you are facing direction of movement.

(4) Place feet apart with foot closer to head of bed in front of other foot.

Increases balance and allows you to transfer weight as client is brought to sitting position on side of bed.

(5) Place arm nearer head of bed under client's shoulders, supporting head and neck.

Maintains alignment of head and neck as you bring client to sitting position.

(6) Place other arm over client's thighs (see illustration).

Supports hip and prevents client from falling backward during procedure.

(7) Move client's lower legs and feet over side of bed. Pivot toward rear leg, allowing client's upper legs to swing downward.

Decreases friction and resistance. Weight of client's legs when off bed allows gravity to lower legs, and weight of legs assists in pulling upper body in sitting position.

(8) At same time, shift weight to rear leg and elevate client (see illustration).

Reduces client risk for falling. Immobilized clients may experience light-headedness or dizziness when assuming a sitting position.

C. **Transferring client from bed to chair with bed in low position**

(1) Assist client to sitting position on side of bed. Have chair in position at 45-degree angle to bed.

Positions chair within easy access for transfer.

(2) Apply transfer belt or other transfer aids.

Transfer belt maintains stability of client during transfer and reduces risk of falling (Owens and others, 1999). Client's arm should be in sling if flaccid paralysis is present.

(3) Ensure that client has stable nonskid shoes. Weight-bearing or strong leg is placed forward, with weak foot back.

Nonskid soles decrease risk of slipping during transfer. Always have client wear shoes during transfer; bare feet increase risk of falls. Client will stand on stronger, or weight-bearing, leg.

(4) Spread feet apart.

Ensures balance with wide base of support.

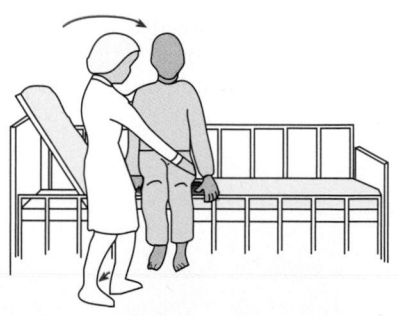

STEP **10B(8)** Nurse shifts weight to rear leg and elevates client.

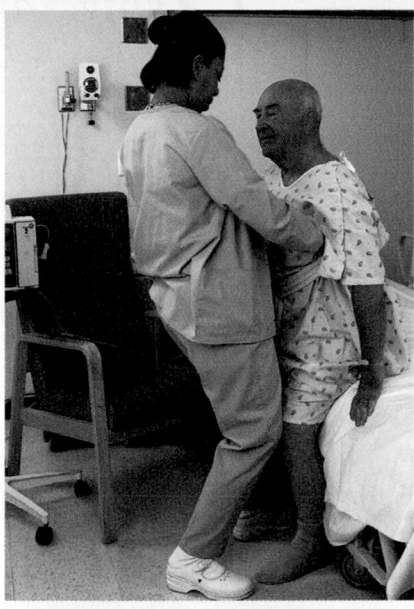

STEP **10C(5)**   Nurse flexes hips and knees, aligning knees with client's knees.

STEP **10C(7)**   Nurse rocks client to standing position.

(5) Flex hips and knees, aligning knees with client's knees (see illustration).	Flexion of knees and hips lowers the center of gravity to object to be raised; aligning knees with client's allows for stabilization of knees when client stands.
(6) Grasp transfer belt from underneath.	Transfer belt is grasped at client's side to provide movement of client at center of gravity. Clients with upper extremity paralysis or paresis should never be lifted by or under arms.

Critical Decision Point: A transfer belt or walking belt with handles should be used in place of the under-axilla technique. The under-axilla technique has been found to be physically stressful for nurses and uncomfortable for clients (Owens and others, 1999).

---

(7) Rock client up to standing position on count of three while straightening hips and legs and keeping knees slightly flexed (see illustration). Unless contraindicated, client may be instructed to use hands to push up if applicable.	Rocking motion gives client's body momentum and requires less muscular effort to lift client.
(8) Maintain stability of client's weak or paralyzed leg with knee.	Ability to stand can often be maintained in paralyzed or weak limb with support of knee to stabilize.
(9) Pivot on foot farther from chair.	Maintains support of client while allowing adequate space for client to move.
(10) Instruct client to use armrests on chair for support and ease into chair (see illustration).	Increases client stability.
(11) Flex hips and knees while lowering client into chair (see illustration).	Prevents injury to nurse from poor body mechanics.
(12) Assess client for proper alignment for sitting position. Provide support for paralyzed extremities. Lapboard or sling will support flaccid arm. Stabilize leg with bath blanket or pillow.	Prevents injury to client from poor body alignment.
(13) Praise client's progress, effort, or performance.	Continued support and encouragement provide incentive for client perseverance.

Using Safe and Effective Transfer Techniques—cont'd

Skill **46-2**

| Steps | Rationale |

STEP **10C(10)** Client uses armrests for support.

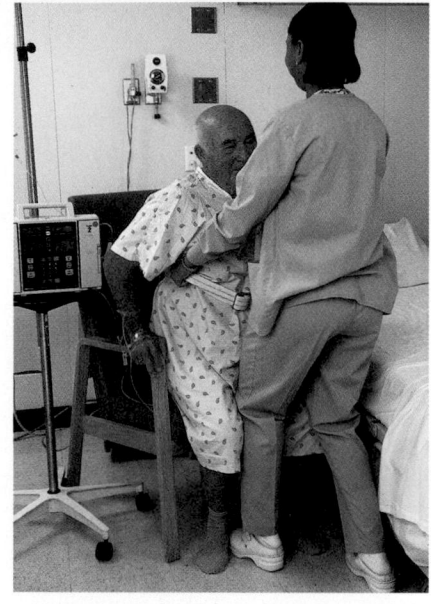

STEP **10C(11)** Nurse eases client into chair.

D. **Perform three-person carry from bed to stretcher (bed at stretcher level)**

(1) Three nurses stand side by side facing side of client's bed.

Prevents twisting of nurses' bodies. Client's alignment is maintained.

(2) Each person assumes responsibility for one of three areas: head and shoulders, hips and thighs, and ankles.

Distributes client's body weight evenly.

(3) Each person assumes wide base of support with foot closer to stretcher in front and knees slightly flexed.

Increases balance and lowers center of gravity of person lifting.

(4) Arms of lifters are placed under client's head and shoulders, hips and thighs, and ankles, with fingers securely around other side of client's body (see illustration).

Distributes client's weight over forearms of lifters.

Critical Decision Point: Verify that clients with spinal cord injuries are stabilized before transfer. The inexperienced care provider should not attempt to move the spinal cord–injured client.

---

(5) Lifters roll client toward their chests. On count of three, client is lifted and held against nurses.

Moves workload over lifters' base of support. Enables lifters to work together and safely lift client.

(6) On second count of three, nurses step back and pivot toward stretcher, moving forward if needed.

Transfers weight toward stretcher.

(7) Gently lower client onto center of stretcher by flexing knees and hips until elbows are level with edge of stretcher.

Maintains nurses' alignment during transfer.

(8) Assess client's body alignment, place safety straps across body, and raise side rails.

Reduces risk of injury from poor alignment or falling.

Steps	Rationale

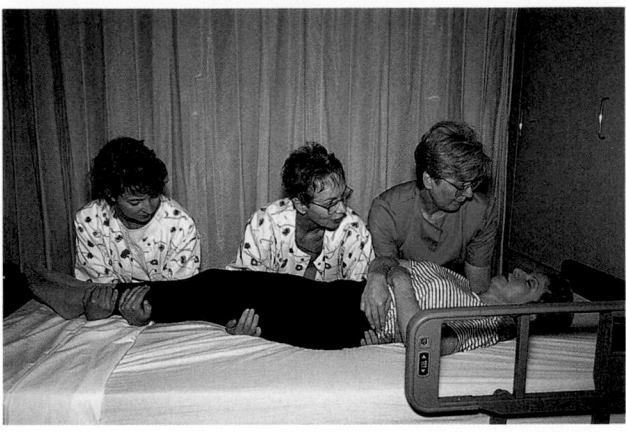

STEP **10D(4)**   Proper positioning of lifters during three-person transfer.

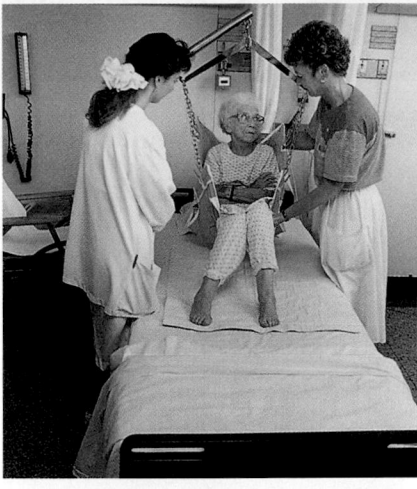

STEP **10E(17)**   Proper placement of sling under client.

E. **Use Hoyer (mechanical/hydraulic) lift to transfer client from bed to chair**

(1) Bring lift to bedside.

Ensures safe elevation of client off bed. (Before using lift, be thoroughly familiar with its operation.)

(2) Position chair near bed, and allow adequate space to maneuver lift.

Prepares environment for safe use of lift and subsequent transfer.

(3) Raise bed to high position with mattress flat. Lower side rail.

Maintains nurses' alignment during transfer.

(4) Keep bed side rail up on side opposite you.

Maintains client safety.

(5) Roll client on side away from you.

Completes positioning of client on mechanical/hydraulic sling.

(6) Place hammock or canvas strips under client to form sling. Place two canvas pieces so that lower edge fits under client's knees (wide piece), and upper edge fits under client's shoulders (narrow piece).

Two types of seat are supplied are supplied with mechanical/hydraulic lift: hammock style is better for clients who are flaccid, weak, and need support; canvas strips can be used for clients with normal muscle tone. Hooks should face away from client's skin. Place sling under client's center of gravity and greatest portion of body weight.

(7) Raise bed rail.

Maintains client safety.

(8) Go to opposite side and lower side rail.

(9) Roll client to opposite side and pull hammock (strips) through.

Completes positioning of client on mechanical/hydraulic sling.

(10) Roll client supine onto canvas seat.

Sling should extend from shoulders to knees (hammock) to support client's body weight equally.

(11) Remove client's glasses, if appropriate.

Swivel bar is close to client's head and could break eyeglasses.

(12) Place lift's horseshoe bar under side of bed (on side with chair).

Positions lift efficiently and promotes smooth transfer.

(13) Lower horizontal bar to sling level by releasing hydraulic valve. Lock valve.

Positions hydraulic lift close to client. Locking valve prevents injury to client.

(14) Attach hooks on strap (chain) to holes in sling. Short chains or straps hook to top holes of sling; longer chains hook to bottom of sling.

Secures hydraulic lift to sling.

(15) Elevate head of bed.

Positions client in sitting position.

(16) Fold client's arms over chest.

Prevents injury to paralyzed arms.

(17) Pump hydraulic handle using long, slow, even strokes until client is raised off bed (see illustration).

Positions client in sitting position.

(18) Use steering handle to pull lift from bed and maneuver to chair.

Moves client from bed to chair.

(19) Roll base around chair.

Positions lift in front of the chair in which client is to be transferred.

Skill 46-2   *U*sing Safe and Effective Transfer Techniques—cont'd

Steps	Rationale

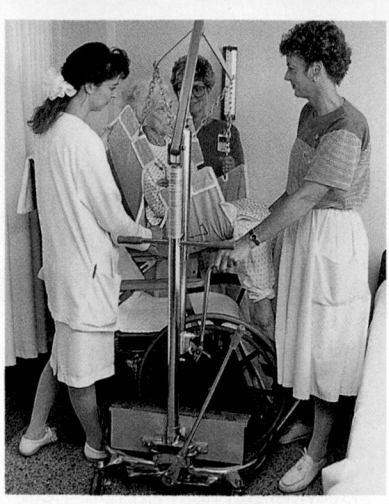

STEP **10E(20)** Use of hydraulic lift to lower client into chair.

Steps	Rationale
(20) Release check valve slowly (turn to left) and lower client into chair (see illustration).	Safely guides client into back of chair as seat descends.
(21) Close check valve as soon as client is down and straps can be released.	If valve is left open, boom may continue to lower and injure client.
(22) Remove straps and mechanical/hydraulic lift.	Prevents damage to skin and underlying tissues from canvas or hooks.
(23) Check client's sitting alignment and correct if necessary.	Prevents injury from poor posture.
11. Perform hand hygiene.	Reduces transmission of microorganisms.
12. With each transfer evaluate client's tolerance and level of fatigue and comfort.	Increased activity may result in symptoms associated with activity intolerance (e.g., increased pulse, changes in blood pressure, increased respirations, and decreased level of comfort). These clients may find transfer very fatiguing and will need posttransfer interventions to restore their level of comfort.
13. Following each transfer, evaluate client's body alignment.	Prompt identification of poor alignment reduces risks to the client's skin and musculoskeletal systems.

Unexpected Outcomes and Related Interventions

1. Client unable to comprehend and follow directions for transfer.
   a. Cognitive impairment affects learning and retention.
   b. Reassess continuity and simplicity
2. Client sustains injury on transfer.
   a. Indicates improper transfer technique was used.
   b. Evaluate incident that caused injury (e.g., assessment inadequate, change in client status, improper use of equipment).
   c. Complete incident report according to institution policy.

3. Client's level of weakness does not permit active transfer.
   a. Physical impairments require increased assistance from nursing personnel.
   b. Increase bed activity and exercise to heighten tolerance.
4. Client continues to bear weight on non–weight-bearing limb.
   a. Certain conditions (e.g., hip fractures) need to be non–weight bearing through healing process.
   b. Reassess client's understanding of weight-bearing status.

5. Client transfers well on some occasions, poorly on others.
   a. Transfers may be difficult when client is fatigued or in pain; assess before transfer (allow for a rest period before transferring, or medicate for pain if indicated).
   b. Periodic confusion may also alter performance.
6. Client is unable to stand for time required in transfer.
   a. Results from increased fatigue, orthostatic hypotension, or pain.
   b. Provide for adequate assistance during transfer.
7. Localized areas of erythema develop that do not disappear quickly.
   a. Early signs of pressure sores (see Chapter 47).

Recording and Reporting

- Record procedure, including pertinent observations: weakness, ability to follow directions, weight-bearing ability, balance, ability to pivot, number of personnel needed to assist, and amount of assistance (muscle strength) required.
- Report any unusual occurrence to nurse in charge. Report transfer ability and assistance needed to next shift or other caregivers. Report progress or remission to rehabilitation staff (physical therapist or occupational therapist).

Home Care Considerations

- Teach family members about proper body mechanics for themselves and the client.
- Provide community resources for hospital equipment that can be used in the home setting (e.g., transfer belts, mechanical lifts) to assist in safe transfer techniques.

on opposite sides of the bed and holding onto the lift sheet when transferring the client to the stretcher. The stretcher and the bed are placed side by side so that the client can be transferred quickly and easily using the lift sheet. As with all procedures, safety is the priority. Safety is increased in the three-person team if the lifters work together. Therefore one person should assume the leadership role.

Caution is used when the client has or is suspected of having spinal cord trauma. If the client must be moved, a transfer board should be placed under the client to maintain spinal alignment before transferring the client to a stretcher. The client should be prepared for the transfer and asked to help when possible (e.g., by folding the arms over the chest). The environment should be free from obstacles, and unnecessary equipment should be removed from the bed.

Restorative Care. The goal of restorative care for the client who is immobile is to maximize functional mobility and independence and reduce residual functional deficits such as impaired gait and decreased endurance. The focus in restorative care is not only on ADLs that relate to physical self-care, but also on **instrumental activities of daily living (IADLs).** IADLs are activities that are necessary to be independent in society beyond eating, grooming, transferring, and toileting and include such skills as shopping, preparing meals, banking, and taking medications.

The nurse uses many of the same interventions as described in the health promotion and acute care sections, but the emphasis is on working collaboratively with clients and their significant others and with other health care professionals. The emphasis is on facilitating the client's return to maximal functional ability in both ADLs and IADLs so that quality of life is enhanced.

Intensive specialized therapy such as occupational or physical therapy is common. The client, if in an institution, will likely go to the therapy department 2 to 3 times a day. The nurse's role is to work collaboratively with these professionals and reinforce exercises and teaching done. For example, after a complete stroke or brain attack, a client will likely receive gait training from a physical therapist, speech rehabilitation from a speech therapist, and training from an occupational therapist on food preparation or other household chores. The therapy may not be able to restore total functional health but may help the client adapt to the mobility limitations or complications.

Common restorative interventions are focused on regaining mobility. There are evidenced-based protocols that demonstrate that performing exercises to maintain or regain joint mobility and teaching the use of assistive devices for walking are common restorative nursing interventions (Box 46-11). Items frequently used to help adapt to mobility limitations include walkers, canes, wheelchairs, and assistive devices such as toilet seat extenders, reaching sticks, special silverware, and clothing with Velcro closures.

Joint Mobility. To ensure adequate joint mobility, the nurse can teach the client about ROM exercises. When the client does not have voluntary motor control, the nurse institutes passive ROM exercises. Walking also increases joint mobility. Occasionally clients need to use assistive devices such as crutches or walkers to help them walk.

Range-of-Motion Exercises. Clients with restricted mobility are unable to perform some or all ROM exercises independently. This limitation can be identified in clients in whom one extremity has limited movement or in completely immobilized clients. The nurse provides ROM exercises to maintain maximum joint mobility.

To ensure that clients routinely receive ROM exercises, the nurse should schedule them at specific times, perhaps with another nursing activity, such as during the client's bath. This enables the nurse to systematically reassesses mobility while improving the client's ROM. In addition, bathing usually requires that extremities and joints are put through complete ROM.

Unless contraindicated, the care plan should include moving the client's extremities through the fullest ROM possible. ROM exercises may be active, passive, or some-

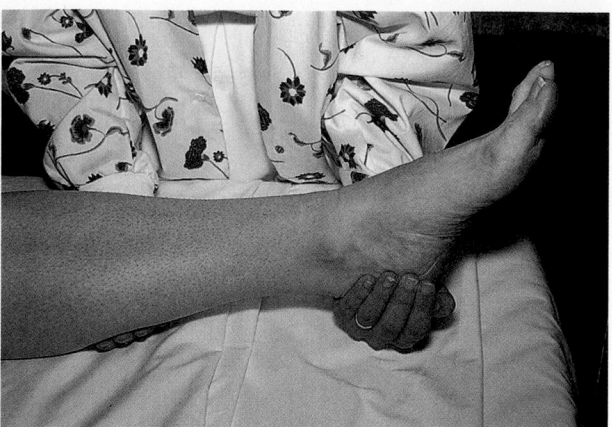

FIGURE **46–23** Using a cupped hand to support a joint.

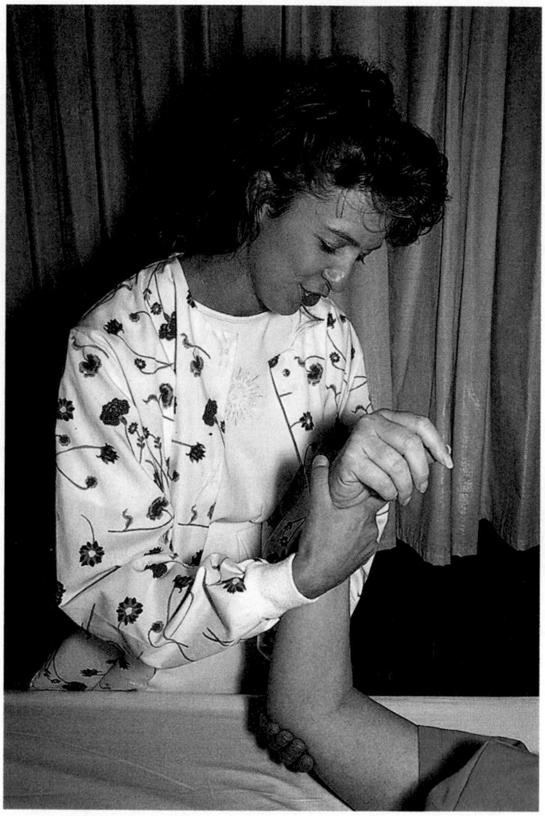

Exercise Promotion: Walking in Elders (Reinitiating Exercise in the Previously Immobile Client)

- Assist client in contemplating change in activity level.
  - Increase client's awareness of current activity.
  - Provide information about the benefits of exercise.
  - Determine any barriers to exercise.
  - Provide choices of activities.
- Assist client in preparing for an activity program.
  - Provide information about how to safely carry out the exercise (e.g., proper walking, safety considerations).
  - Assist client in strengthening exercise tolerance and activity.
  - Emphasize client's ability to become more active.
  - Provide resources for social exercise groups (e.g., older adult fitness groups, community walking programs, walking in local shopping malls).
- Assist client in establishing an activity program.
  - Provide positive, constructive feedback.
  - Increase activity as appropriate for client's mobility status.
  - Assist client in developing a long-term exercise plan.
  - Visit the client during an exercise program.
- Assist client in maintaining an activity program.
  - Recognize each success.
  - If relapse occurs, remind client that it is ok and to continue with the exercise program.
  - Maintain a supportive environment.
  - Encourage family and friends to participate in the exercise program.

Modified from Jitramontree, N. (2001). Evidence-based protocol: Exercise promotion—walking in elders—evidence-based protocol. 2001, The University of Iowa, Gerontological Nursing Interventions Research Center, Research Dissemination Core. In M.G. Titler (Series Ed.), *Series on Evidence-Based Practice for Older Adults*. Iowa City, IA. The University of Iowa College of Nursing Gerontological Nursing Interventions Research Center, Research Dissemination Core. For more information, http:// www.nursing.uiowa.edu/ center/gnirc/disseminatecore.htm.

FIGURE **46–24** Supporting the joint by holding the distal and proximal areas adjacent to the joint.

where in between. With a weak client, for example, the nurse may support an extremity while the client performs the movement, or the client may be able to move some joints actively while the nurse passively moves others. In general, exercises should be as active as health and mobility allow. Passive ROM exercises should begin as soon as the client's ability to move the extremity or joint is lost. Movements are carried out slowly and smoothly, just to the point of resistance, and should not cause pain. The nurse should never force a joint beyond its capacity. Each movement should be repeated 5 times during the session.

When performing passive ROM exercises, the nurse stands at the side of the bed closest to the joint being exercised. Passive ROM exercises are performed using a head-to-toe sequence and moving from larger to smaller joints. If an extremity is to be moved or lifted, the nurse places a cupped hand under the joint to support it (Figure 46-23), supports the joint by holding the adjacent distal and proximal areas (Figure 46-24), or supports the joint with one hand and cradles the distal portion of the extremity with the remaining arm (Figure 46-25). The fol-

lowing sections describe an overview of nursing considerations for ways to support major joints in the body. See Table 46-2, p. 1435, for detailed ROM and illustrated motion for each joint.

Neck. A flexion contracture of the neck is a serious disability because the client's neck is permanently flexed with the chin close to or actually touching the chest. Ultimately, the client's body alignment is altered, the visual field is changed, and the level of independent functioning is decreased.

Shoulder. One feature of the shoulder that sets it apart from other joints in the body is that the strongest muscle

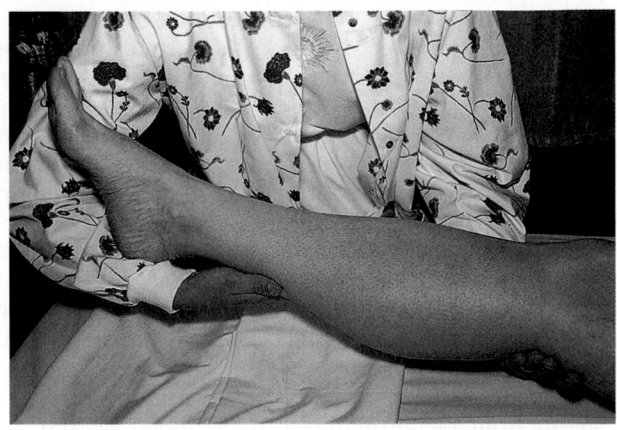

FIGURE **46–25** Cradling the distal portion of an extremity.

controlling it, the deltoid, is in complete elongation in the normal position. No other muscle exerts its full strength when in complete elongation. When caring for a client with limited shoulder mobility, the nurse may need to provide support devices for the shoulder, such as slings when the client is standing or sitting or pillows when the client is in bed. Correctly positioning the shoulder prevents pain, joint dislocation, and further changes in body alignment.

Elbow. The elbow functions optimally at an angle of about 90 degrees. An elbow fixed in full extension is disabling and limits the client's independence.

Forearm. Most functions of the hand are best carried out with the forearm in moderate pronation. When the forearm is fixed in a position of full supination, the client's use of the hand is limited.

Wrist. The primary function of the wrist is to place the hand in slight dorsiflexion, the position of functioning. Therefore full ROM is not as great a priority as maintaining the wrist in a functional position. When the wrist is fixed in even a slightly flexed position, the grasp is weakened. In the immobilized client the functional position of the wrist can be achieved by using splints.

Fingers and Thumb. The ROM in the fingers and thumb enables the client to perform ADLs and activities requiring fine motor skills, such as carpentry, needlework, drawing, and painting. The functional position of the fingers and thumb is slight flexion of the thumb in opposition to the fingers.

Hip. Because the lower extremities are concerned chiefly with locomotion and weight bearing, stability of the hip joint may be more important than its mobility. For example, if one hip has no mobility but is fixed in a neutral position and fully extended, it is possible to walk without a significant limp.

However, contractures often fix the hip in positions of deformity. Excessive abduction makes the affected leg appear too short, whereas excessive adduction makes the affected leg appear too long. In either case the client has limited locomotion and walks with an obvious limp. Internal and external rotation contractures cause an abnormal and unbalanced gait.

Knee. A primary function of the knee is stability, which is achieved by ROM, ligaments, and muscles. However, the knees cannot remain stable under weight-bearing

conditions unless there is adequate quadriceps power to maintain the knee in full extension. ROM exercises should include pulling the knee into full extension.

An immobile knee joint can result in serious disability. The degree of disability depends on the position in which the knee is stiffened. If the knee is fixed in full extension, the person must sit with the leg thrust out in front. When the knee is flexed, the person limps while walking. The greater the flexion, the greater the limp.

Ankle and Foot. Without full ROM of the ankle, there will be gait deviations. If the joint is not stable, the person will fall. If joint mobility is diminished, the nurse should maintain the joint in a position in which walking can be carried out with a forward rolling motion from the heel onto the forefoot.

When the person relaxes as in sleep or coma, the foot relaxes and assumes a position of plantar flexion. As a result, the foot may become fixed in plantar flexion (footdrop), which impairs the ability to walk. Inversion and eversion must also be avoided to allow the foot to rest flat on the floor.

Toes. Excessive flexion of the toes results in clawing. When this is a permanent deformity, the foot is unable to rest flat on the floor and the client is unable to walk properly. Flexion contractures are the most common foot deformity associated with reduced joint mobility.

Adequate ROM gives the necessary mobility to carry out ADLs and exercise and to engage in relaxing activities. In addition, adequate ROM in the lower extremities allows walking.

Walking. In the normal walking posture the head is erect; the cervical, thoracic, and lumbar vertebrae are aligned; the hips and knees have appropriate flexion; and the arms swing freely with the legs. Illness or trauma can reduce activity tolerance, so assistance in walking is required. In addition, temporary or permanent damage to the musculoskeletal and nervous systems may necessitate use of an assistive device for walking.

Helping a Client to Walk. When a client's mobility has restricted the ability to walk, the nurse must assess the client's activity tolerance, tolerance to the upright position (orthostatic hypotension), strength, presence of pain, coordination, and balance to determine the amount of assistance needed.

The nurse explains how far the client should try to walk, who is going to help, when the walk will take place, and why walking is important. In addition, the nurse and client determine how much independence the client can assume.

The nurse also checks the environment to be sure that there are no obstacles in the client's path. Chairs, over-bed tables, and wheelchairs are cleared out of the way so that the client has ample room to walk safely. Before starting, rest points should be established in case activity tolerance is less than estimated or the client becomes dizzy. For example, a chair might be placed in the hall for the client to rest if needed.

The nurse should provide support at the waist so that the client's center of gravity remains midline. This can be achieved when the nurse places both hands at the client's waist or uses a gait belt. A **gait belt** is a leather belt that encircles the waist and has handles attached for the nurse to hold. While walking, the client should not lean to one side because this alters the center of gravity, distorts balance, and increases the risk of falling.

A client who at any point appears unsteady or complains of dizziness should be returned to a nearby bed or chair. If the client faints or begins to fall, the nurse should assume a wide base of support with one foot in front of the other, thus supporting the body weight. Then the nurse should gently lower the client to the floor, protecting the head. Although lowering a client to the floor is not difficult, the student should practice this technique with a friend or classmate before attempting it in a clinical setting.

Clients with **hemiplegia** (one-sided paralysis) or **hemiparesis** (one-sided weakness) often need assistance to walk. The nurse always stands on the client's affected side and supports the client by holding one arm around the client's waist (or uses a gait belt once the client's stability is ensured) and the other arm around the inferior aspect of the client's upper arm so that the nurse's hand is under the client's axilla. Providing support by holding the client's arm is incorrect because the nurse cannot easily support the weight to lower the client to the floor if the client faints or falls. In addition, if the client falls with the nurse holding an arm, a shoulder joint may be dislocated.

A nurse who does not have a lot of strength and who is unable to ambulate a client alone should request help. The two-nurse method helps distribute the client's weight evenly. The two nurses stand on either side of the client. Each nurse's near arm is around the client's waist, and the other arm is around the inferior aspect of the client's arm so that both nurses' hands are supporting the client's axillae.

Using Assistive Devices for Walking. Clients who are recovering from a lengthy illness that required bed rest and whose mobility is impaired frequently require assistive devices to assist in ambulation. These devices include canes, walkers, crutches, and assistive personnel to teach and assist the client and family in the use of these devices. (Chapter 36).

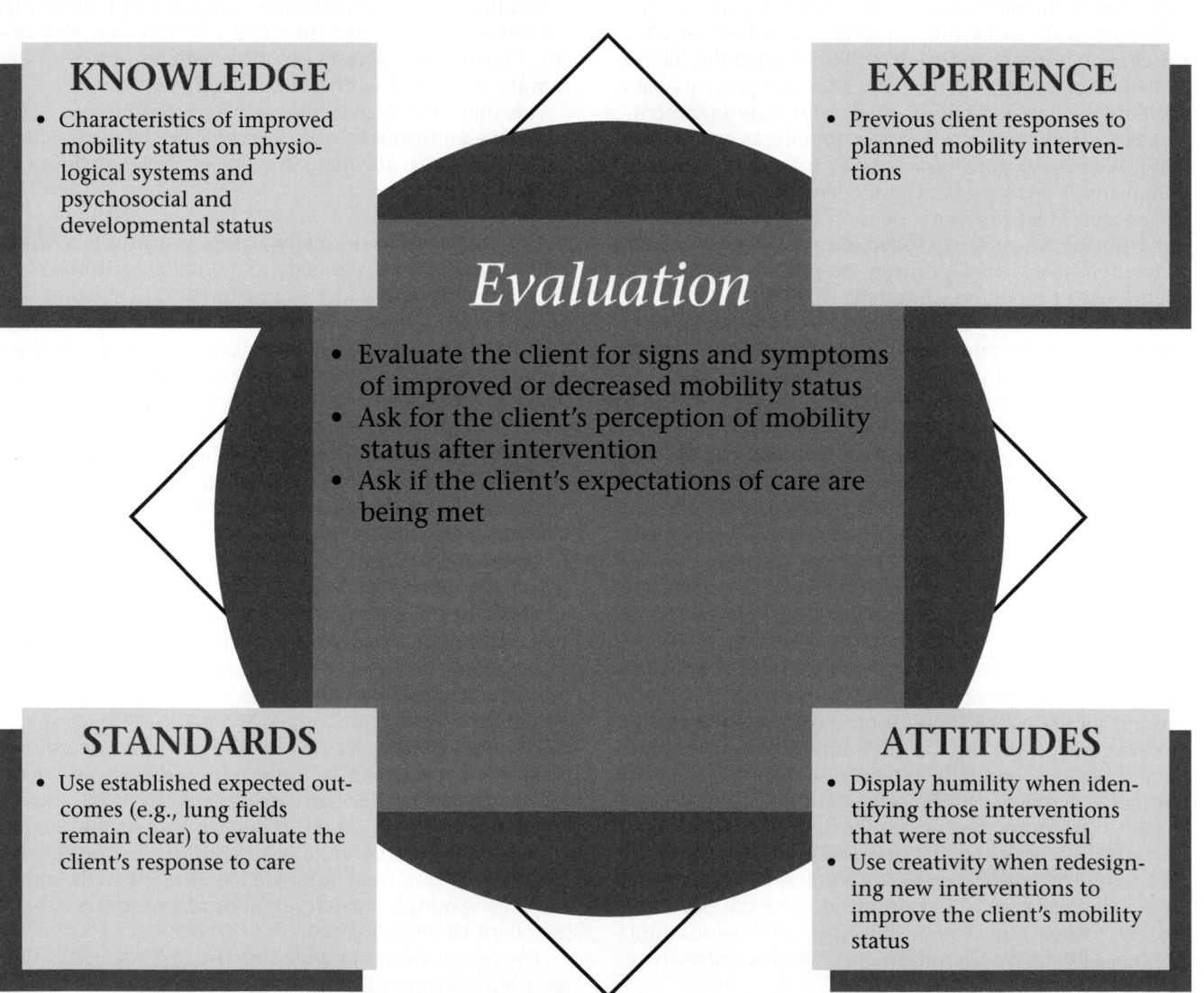

FIGURE **46–26** Critical thinking model for immobility evaluation.

ℳℰ Evaluation

Client Care. To evaluate outcomes and response to nursing care, the nurse measures the effectiveness of all interventions. The actual outcomes are compared with the outcomes selected during planning such as the client's ability to maintain or improve body alignment, joint mobility, walking, moving, or transferring, or to prevent the hazards of immobility. The nurse evaluates specific interventions designed to promote body alignment, improve mobility, and protect the client from the hazards of immobility. Client and family teaching to prevent future risks to body alignment and hazards of immobility is also evaluated (Figure 46-26). Evaluation is summative and continuous. The continuous or formative nature of evaluation allows the nurse to determine whether new or revised therapies are required and if new nursing diagnoses have developed.

Client Expectations. Movement is often taken for granted until it is lost. Lack of movement is often associated with punishment in Western society. Children are given "time-outs," teens are "grounded," and criminals are jailed. It is therefore important to recognize that immobility may lead to fear, anger, grief, withdrawal, or hostility. Whether the nurse is sensitive to these reactions and helps the client work through them or responds negatively will greatly influence clients' expectations.

Clients who are immobile and dependent on others for some or all of their needs can become overly dependent or try to do too much themselves too early. Finding the interdependent balance between independence and dependence is a difficult task. Clients will want control over their mobility that is personally satisfactory. In the client who is completely dependent on others for care, control over how and when things are done may be very important. Do clients feel they are treated with dignity? Do caregivers treat them as adults? Are they given opportunities to make meaningful choices? Clients who are dependent on others for care may see their demands as the only control they have over their life. Humility is an important attitude in critical thinking when assessing clients' expectations. Humility helps the nurse to identify modifications that may be needed in care planning.

ℳℰ Key Concepts

- Body mechanics are the coordinated efforts of the musculoskeletal and nervous systems as the person moves, lifts, bends, stands, sits, lies down, and completes daily activities.
- Coordinated body movement requires integrated functioning of the skeletal system, skeletal muscles, and nervous system.
- The skeletal system provides bony support structure for movement, attachment of ligaments and muscles, protection of vital organs, some of the regulation of calcium, and production of red blood cells.

- The nervous system provides initiation and voluntary control of movement.
- Coordination and regulation of muscle groups depend on muscle tone; activity of antagonistic, synergistic, and antigravity muscles; and neural input to muscles.
- Balance is assisted through nervous system control by the cerebellum and inner ear.
- Body alignment is the condition of joints, tendons, ligaments, and muscles in various body positions.
- Balance is achieved when there is a wide base of support, the center of gravity falls within the base of support, and a vertical line falls from the center of gravity through the base of support.
- Developmental stages influence body alignment and mobility; the greatest impact of physiological changes on the musculoskeletal system is observed in children and older adults.
- The risk of disabilities related to immobilization depends on the extent and duration of immobilization and the client's overall level of health.
- Immobility may result from illness or trauma or may be prescribed for therapeutic reasons.
- Immobility presents hazards in the physiological, psychological, and developmental dimensions.
- The nurse uses the nursing process and critical thinking synthesis to provide care for clients who are experiencing or are at risk for the adverse effects of impaired body alignment and immobility.
- After identifying nursing diagnoses, the nurse plans and implements interventions to prevent or minimize the hazards and complications of impaired body alignment and immobilization.
- Clients with impaired body alignment require nursing interventions to maintain them in the supported Fowler's, supine, prone, side-lying, and Sims' positions.
- Range-of-motion exercises include one or all of the body joints.
- Assistive devices to promote walking include canes, walkers, and crutches.

ℳℰ Key Terms

Activity tolerance, *p. 1434*
Anthropometric measurements, *p. 1441*
Atelectasis, *p. 1428*
Bed rest, *p. 1427*
Body alignment, *p. 1422*
Body mechanics, *p. 1421*
Cartilage, *p. 1423*
Cartilaginous joint, *p. 1423*
Chest physiotherapy (CPT), *p. 1451*
Concentric tension, *p. 1423*
Disuse osteoporosis, *p. 1429*
Eccentric tension, *p. 1423*
Embolus, *p. 1441*
Exercise, *p. 1434*
Fibrous joint, *p. 1423*

Flat bones, *p. 1422*
Footdrop, *p. 1430*
Fracture, *p. 1423*
Friction, *p. 1422*
Gait, *p. 1434*
Gait belt, *p. 1478*
Hemiparesis, *p. 1478*
Hemiplegia, *p. 1478*
Hypostatic pneumonia, *p. 1428*
Immobility, *p. 1427*
Instrumental activities of daily living (IADLs), *p. 1475*
Irregular bones, *p. 1422*
Isometric contraction, *p. 1423*
Isotonic contraction, *p. 1423*

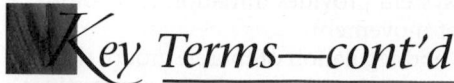

Key Terms—cont'd

Joint contracture, *p. 1430*
Joints, *p. 1423*
Leverage, *p. 1424*
Ligaments, *p. 1423*
Logroll, *p. 1465*
Long bones, *p. 1422*
Mobility, *p. 1421*
Muscle atrophy, *p. 1427*
Muscle tone, *p. 1425*
Negative nitrogen balance, *p. 1428*
Neurotransmitters, *p. 1425*
Orthostatic hypotension, *p. 1428*
Osteoporosis, *p. 1430*

Pathological fractures, *p. 1423*
Posture, *p. 1425*
Pressure ulcer, *p. 1430*
Range of motion (ROM), *p. 1434*
Renal calculi, *p. 1430*
Short bones, *p. 1422*
Synostotic joint, *p. 1423*
Synovial joint, *p. 1423*
Tendons, *p. 1423*
Thrombus, *p. 1428*
Trapeze bar, *p. 1455*
Trochanter roll, *p. 1455*
Unossified, *p. 1423*
Urinary stasis, *p. 1430*

Critical Thinking Exercises

1. You are caring for a 57-year-old man who has just had a bilateral total knee replacement for osteoarthritis. He is 2 days postoperative and beginning to transfer to a chair with help. He is 100 pounds overweight and has a history of deep vein thrombosis. He has compression stockings, continuous passive range of motion, and a heparin/saline lock. Make a list of potential nursing diagnoses.

2. When you are doing a home visit for a 75-year-old woman, the client's granddaughter runs in and says, "Did you show the nurse the sore on your leg that you got from falling yesterday?" What questions about mobility are important to ask the client? How do you begin your assessment?

3. Your clinical experience is in long-term care. You are working in assisted living. The nurse in charge of the assisted living wing asks you to help her with a program titled "Lifestyle Choices: Living Life to Its Fullest." She asks you to participate and discuss how regular exercise can improve overall health and to show how exercise can be incorporated into activities of daily living. Develop a content outline and a time frame for your presentation.

4. You are caring for a 75-year-old man who is immobilized after spinal cord trauma from a motor vehicle accident. What potential complications would you be assessing for in this geriatric client?

Review Questions

1. A physiological risk associated with prolonged immobility is:
   1. Decreased bone resorption.
   2. Decreased cardiac workload.
   3. Decreased serum calcium levels.
   4. Increased hemoglobin formation.

2. A client has been on bed rest for several days. The client stands and the nurse notes that the client's systolic pressure drops 20 mm Hg. This is referred to as:
   1. Orthostatic hypotension.
   2. Rebound hypotension.
   3. Positional hypotension.
   4. Central venous hypotension.

3. The purpose of elastic stockings after a surgical procedure is to:
   1. Prevent varicose veins.
   2. Prevent muscular atrophy.
   3. Ensure joint mobility and prevent contractures.
   4. Facilitate the return of venous blood to the heart.

4. The most important objective of bed rest for a client with bilateral pneumonia would be to:
   1. Allow the client uninterrupted sleep.
   2. Reduce the oxygen needs of the body.
   3. Decrease the need for pain medications.
   4. Prevent the client from falling due to an unsteady gait.

5. The client at greatest risk for developing adverse effects of immobility is a:
   1. 3-year-old child with a fractured femur.
   2. 48-year-old woman following a thyroidectomy.
   3. 78-year-old man in traction for a broken hip.
   4. 38-year-old woman undergoing a hysterectomy.

6. A client has been immobilized for 5 days because of extensive abdominal surgery. When getting this client out of bed for the first time a nursing diagnosis related to the safety of this client would be:
   1. Pain.
   2. Impaired skin integrity.
   3. Altered tissue perfusion.
   4. Risk for activity intolerance.

7. Heparin and low-molecular-weight heparin (LMWH) are the most widely used drugs in the prophylaxis of deep vein thrombosis (DVT). Common dosage for heparin therapy is:
   1. 5000 units given subcutaneously 2 hours before surgery and repeated every 8 to 12 hours.
   2. 500 units given subcutaneously 2 hours before surgery and repeated every 8 to 12 hours.
   3. 500 units given subcutaneously 2 hours before surgery and repeated every 8 to 12 hours.
   4. 5000 units given subcutaneously 8 hours before surgery and repeated every 2 to 4 hours.

8. This allows the client to pull with the upper extremities to raise the trunk off the bed, to assist in transfer from bed to wheelchair, or to perform upper arm exercises:
   1. Trapeze bar.
   2. Trochanter roll.
   3. Hand rolls.
   4. Footboard.

9. The client in this position is lying face or chest down:
   1. Supine.
   2. Prone.
   3. Fowler's.
   4. Lateral.

10. These activities are necessary to be independent in society and include such skills as shopping, preparing meals, banking, and taking medications:
   1. Activities of daily living (ADLs).
   2. Work activities.
   3. Instrumental activities of daily living (IADLs).
   4. Homemaker activities.

References

Ackley B, Ladwig G: *Nursing diagnosis handbook: a guide to planning care,* ed 5, St. Louis, 2002, Mosby.

Agency for Healthcare Research and Quality (AHRQ): *Pressure ulcer prevention and treatment,* http:// hstat.nlm.nih.gov/hq/ Hquest/screen/TextBrowse/t/1049658066834/s/40521.

Andrews M, Boyle, J: *Transcultural concepts in nursing care,* ed 3, Philadelphia, 1999, Lippincott.

Banks-Wallace J: Staggering under the weight of responsibility: the impact of culture on physical activity among African American women, *J Multicultural Nurs Health* 6(3):24, 2000.

Black J, Hawks J, Keene A: *Medical-surgical nursing: clinical management for positive outcomes,* ed 6, Philadelphia, 2001, Saunders.

Byrne B: Deep vein thrombosis prophylaxis: the effectiveness and implications of using below knee or thigh length graduated compression stockings, *Heart Lung* 30(4):277, 2001.

Deitrick JE and others: Effects of immobilization upon various metabolic and physiological functions of normal men, *Am J Med* 4:3, 1948.

Dochterman JM, Bulechek GM: *Nursing interventions classification (NIC),* ed 4, St. Louis, 2004, Mosby.

Ebersole P, Hess P: *Geriatric nursing and healthy aging,* St. Louis, 2001, Mosby.

Jain S: Cultural dance: an opportunity to encourage physical activity and health in communities, *Am J Health Education* 32(4):216, 2001.

Jitramontree N: *Exercise promotion: walking in elders—evidenced-based protocol,* Iowa City, Ia, 2001, The University of Iowa, Gerontological Nursing Interventions Research Center, Research Dissemination Core.

Johnson M: Perceptions of barriers to healthy physical activity among Asian communities, *Sport Education Soc* 5(1):51, 2000.

Lance R and others: Comparison of different methods of obtaining orthostatic vital signs, *Clin Nurs Res* 9(4):479, 2000.

Ludwick R, Dieckman B, and Snelson C: Assessment of the geriatric orthopaedic trauma patient, *Orthop Nurs* 18:13, 1999.

Maher A, Salmond S, Pellino T: *Orthopaedic nursing,* ed 3, Philadelphia, 2002, Saunders.

Melillo K and others: Perceptions of older Latino adults regarding physical fitness, physical activity, and exercise, *J Gerontol Nurs* 27(9):38, 2001.

Nunnelee J: Low molecular-weight heparin, *J Vasc Nurs* 15(3):94, 1997.

McCance KL, Huether SE: *Pathophysiology: the biologic basis for disease in adults and children,* ed 4, St. Louis, 2002, Mosby.

Moorhead S, Johnson M, Maas M: *Nursing outcomes classification (NOC),* ed 3, St. Louis, 2004, Mosby.

National Osteoporosis Foundation: *American's bone health: the state of osteoporosis and low bone mass in our nations,* 2002, National Osteoporosis Foundation.

Nelson A, Fragala G, Menzel N: Myths and facts about back injuries in nursing, *Am J Nurs* 103(2):32, 2003.

Nelson A and others: Safe patient handling movement, *Am J Nurs* 103(3):32, 2003.

Owens B and others: What are we teaching about lifting and transferring patients? *Res Nurs Health* 22:3, 1999.

Resnick B: Functional performance and exercise of older adults in long-term care settings, *J Gerontol Nurs* 26(3):7, 2000.

Takata S, Yasui N: Disuse osteoporosis, *J Med Invest* 48:147, 2001.

U.S. Department of Labor: Lost work time injuries and illnesses: characteristics and resulting time away from work (USDL00-115), Washington, DC, 2000, Bureau of Labor Statistics.

Research References

Banks-Wallace J: Staggering under the weight of responsibility: the impact of culture on physical activity among African American women, *J Multicultural Nurs Health* 6(3):24, 2000.

Bergquist S: Subscales, subscores, or summative score: evaluating the contribution of Braden scale items for predicting pressure ulcer risk in older adults receiving home health care, *J Wound Ostomy Continence Nurs* 28:279, 2001.

Bourret E and others: The meaning of mobility for residents and staff in long-term care facilities, *J Adv Nurs* 37(4):338, 2002.

Byrne B: Deep vein thrombosis prophylaxis: the effectiveness and implications of using below knee or thigh length graduated compression stockings, *Heart Lung* 30(4):277, 2001.

Cooper K and others: Health barriers to walking for exercise in elderly primary care, *Geriatr Nurs* 22(5):258, 2001.

Defloor T: The effect of position and mattress on interface pressure, *Appl Nurs Res* 13(1):2, 2000.

Deitrick JE and others: Effects of immobilization upon various metabolic and physiological functions of normal men, *Am J Med* 4:3, 1948.

Jain S: Cultural dance: an opportunity to encourage physical activity and health in communities, *Am J Health Education* 32(4):216, 2001.

Jitramontree N: *Exercise promotion: walking in elders—evidenced-based protocol,* Iowa City, Ia, 2001, The University of Iowa, Gerontological Nursing Interventions Research Center, Research Dissemination Core.

Johnson M: Perceptions of barriers to healthy physical activity among Asian communities, *Sport Education Soc* 5(1):51, 2000.

Lance R and others: Comparison of different methods of obtaining orthostatic vital signs, *Clin Nurs Res* 9(4):479, 2000.

Ludwick R: Clinical decision making: recognition of confusion and application of restraints, *Orthop Nurs* 18:65, 1999.

Ludwick R, Dieckman B, and Snelson C: Assessment of the geriatric orthopaedic trauma patient, *Orthop Nurs* 18:13, 1999.

Melillo K and others: Perceptions of older Latino adults regarding physical fitness, physical activity, and exercise, *J Gerontol Nurs* 27(9):38, 2001.

Nunnelee J: Low molecular-weight heparin, *J Vasc Nurs* 15(3):94, 1997.

Resnick B: Functional performance and exercise of older adults in long-term care settings, *J Gerontol Nurs* 26(3):7, 2000.

Takata S, Yasui N: Disuse osteoporosis, *J Med Invest* 48:147, 2001.

Van Haastregt J and others: Preventing falls and mobility problems in community-dwelling elders: the process of creating a new intervention, *Geriatr Nurs* 21(6):309, 2000.

47

*S*kin Integrity and Wound Care

Media Resources

http://evolve.elsevier.com/Potter/
fundamentals/

CD COMPANION

- Review Questions
- Glossary

evolve WEBSITE

- Review Questions
- Student Learning Activities
- Concept Map Exercise
- Critical Thinking Exercise
- Video Clips
- Glossary

Objectives

Mastery of content in this chapter will enable the student to:

- Define the key terms listed.
- Discuss the risks and contributing factors to pressure ulcer formation.
- List the four stages of pressure ulcers.
- Discuss normal processes of wound healing.
- Describe the differences among wounds healing by primary and secondary intention.
- Describe complications of wound healing and the usual time of occurrence.
- Explain the factors that impede or promote wound healing.
- Describe the differences between nursing care of acute and chronic wounds.
- Complete an assessment for a client with impaired skin integrity.
- List nursing diagnoses associated with impaired skin integrity.
- Develop a nursing care plan for a client with impaired skin integrity.
- List appropriate nursing interventions for a client with impaired skin integrity.
- State evaluation criteria for a client with impaired skin integrity.

The skin, the body's largest organ, composes one sixth of the total body weight (Wysocki, 2000). It is a protective barrier against disease-causing organisms, a sensory organ for pain, temperature, and touch, and can synthesize vitamin D. Injury to the skin poses risks to safety and triggers a complex healing response. It is one of the nurse's most important responsibilities to monitor skin integrity and to plan, implement, and assess interventions to maintain skin integrity. Knowing the normal healing pattern helps the nurse to recognize alterations that require intervention.

Scientific Knowledge Base

Skin

The skin has two layers: the epidermis and the dermis (Figure 47-1). These two layers are separated by a membrane, often referred to as the dermal-epidermal junction. The **epidermis,** or the top layer, has several layers. The stratum corneum is the thin, outermost layer of the epidermis. It consists of flattened, dead, keratinized cells. The cells originate from the innermost epidermal layer, commonly called the basal layer. Cells in the basal layer divide, proliferate, and migrate toward the epidermal surface. After cells reach the stratum corneum, they flatten and die. This constant movement ensures replacement of surface cells sloughed during normal desquamation. The thin stratum corneum pro-

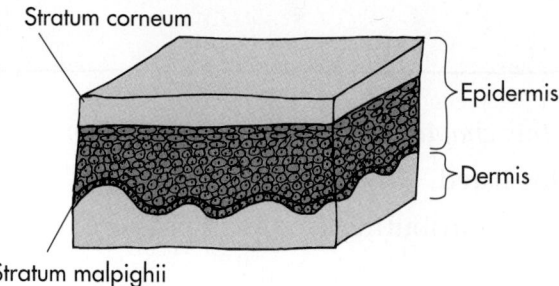

Stratum corneum

Epidermis

Dermis

Stratum malpighii

FIGURE **47–1** Layers of the integument.

tects underlying cells and tissues from dehydration and prevents entrance of certain chemical agents. The stratum corneum allows evaporation of water from the skin and permits absorption of certain topical medications.

The **dermis,** the inner layer of the skin, provides tensile strength, mechanical support, and protection to the underlying muscles, bones, and organs. It differs from the epidermis in that it contains mostly connective tissue and few skin cells. **Collagen** (a tough, fibrous protein), blood vessels, and nerves are found in the dermal layer. Fibroblasts, which are responsible for collagen formation, are the only distinctive cell type within the dermis.

Understanding skin structure helps the nurse maintain skin integrity and promote wound healing. Intact skin protects the client from chemical and mechanical injury. When the skin is injured, the epidermis functions to resurface the wound and restore the barrier against invading organisms while the dermis responds to restore the structural integrity (collagen) and the physical properties of the skin. Age can alter skin characteristics and make skin more vulnerable to damage. A summary of the normal changes in aging skin can be found in Box 47-1.

Pressure Ulcers

Pressure ulcer, pressure sore, decubitus ulcer, and *bedsore* are terms used to describe impaired skin integrity related to unrelieved, prolonged pressure. The most current terminology is **pressure ulcer** (Figure 47-2), which is consistent with the recommendations of the National Pressure Ulcer Advisory Panel (NPUAP) and the pressure ulcer guidelines panel of the Agency for Health Care Policy and Research (AHCPR) (AHCPR, 1992a). A pressure ulcer is defined as localized areas of tissue necrosis that develop when soft tissue is compressed between a bony prominence and an external surface for a prolonged period of time (NPUAP, 1995a). Any client experiencing decreased mobility, decreased sensory perception, fecal or urinary incontinence and/or poor nutrition can be at risk for pressure ulcer development.

There are many factors that contribute to the formation of a pressure ulcer. Pressure is the major cause in pressure ulcer formation. Tissues receive oxygen and nutrients and eliminate metabolic wastes via the blood. Any factor that interferes with blood flow in turn interferes with cellular metabolism and the function or life of the cells. Prolonged, intense pressure affects cellular metabolism by decreasing or obliterating blood flow, resulting in tissue ischemia and ultimately tissue death.

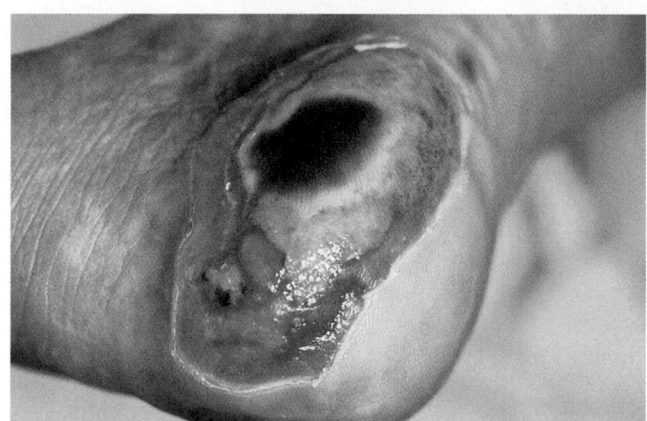

FIGURE **47–2** Pressure ulcer with tissue necrosis.

Pathogenesis of Pressure Ulcers. Pressure is the major element in the cause of pressure ulcers. Three pressure-related factors contribute to pressure ulcer development: (1) pressure intensity, (2) pressure duration, and (3) tissue tolerance.

Pressure Intensity. A classic research study identified capillary closing pressure as the minimal amount of pressure required to collapse a capillary (e.g., when the pressure exceeds the normal capillary pressure range of 16 to 32 mm Hg) (Burton and Yamada, 1951). Therefore if the pressure applied over a capillary exceeds the normal capillary pressure, the vessel is occluded, causing **tissue ischemia.** If the client has reduced sensation and cannot respond to the discomfort of the ischemia, tissue ischemia and death can occur.

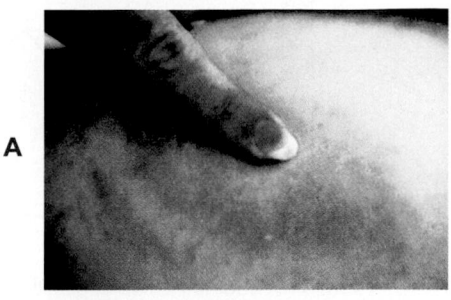

FIGURE **47–3 A,** Reactive hyperemia. **B,** Blanches with fingertip pressure. (From Pires M, Muller A: Detection and management of early tissue pressure indicators: a pictorial essay, *Progressions* 3[3]:3, 1991.)

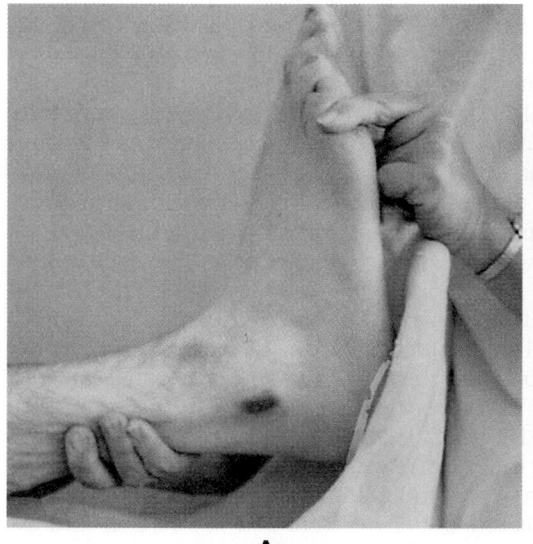
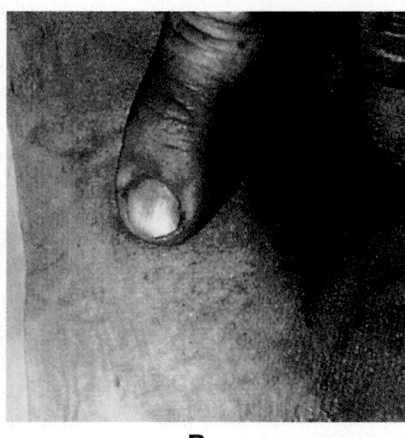
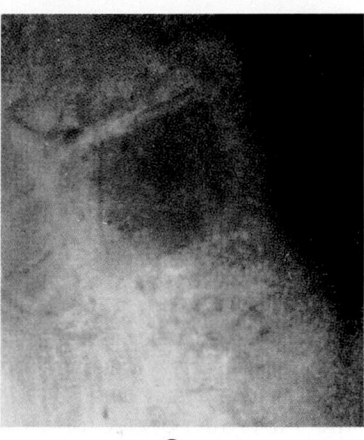

FIGURE **47–4 A,** Abnormal reactive hyperemia. **B** and **C,** In abnormal reactive hyperemia the area is much darker than the surrounding skin and does not blanch with fingertip pressure. (From Pires M, Muller A: Detection and management of early tissue pressure indicators: a pictorial essay, *Progressions* 3[3]:3, 1991.)

The clinical presentation of obstructed blood flow is demonstrated when evaluating areas of pressure. After a period of tissue ischemia, if the pressure is relieved and the blood flow returns, the skin turns red. The effect of this redness is vasodilation (blood vessel expansion), called reactive hyperemia (Figure 47-3, *A*). The area of reactive hyperemia should be evaluated by pressing a finger over the affected area. If the area blanches (turns lighter in color), (Figure 47-3, *B*) and the erythema returns when the finger is removed, the reactive hyperemia is thought to be transient and is an attempt to overcome the ischemic episode (Ratliff and Bryant, 2003). If, however, the erythemic area does not blanch (nonblanching erythema) (Figure 47-4) when finger pressure is applied, deep tissue damage should be suspected.

Blanching is seen when the normal red tones of the light-skinned client are absent. Blanching does not occur in clients with darkly pigmented skin. The Task Force on the Implications for Darkly Pigmented Intact Skin in the Prediction and Prevention of Pressure Ulcers (Bennett, 1995) defined **darkly pigmented skin** as skin that "remains unchanged (does not blanch) when pressure is applied over a bony prominence, irrespective of the client's race or ethnicity." Characteristics of intact dark skin that might alert nurses to the potential for pressure ulcers have been identified (Box 47-2).

Pressure Duration. There are two considerations with regard to the duration of pressure. Low pressures over a prolonged time period can cause tissue damage, as well as high-intensity pressure over a short period of time. Extended pressure occludes blood flow and nutrients and contributes to cell death (Pieper, 2000). Clinical implications of pressure duration include evaluating the amount of pressure (checking skin for reactive hyperemia) and determining the amount of time that a client can tolerate pressure (checking to be sure after relieving pressure that the affected area blanches).

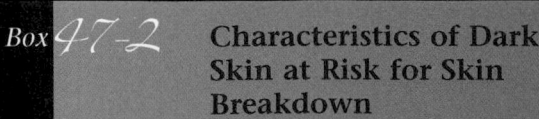

Box 47-2 Characteristics of Dark Skin at Risk for Skin Breakdown

Assessment Issues

Natural or halogen light source best for assessing skin
Fluorescent light source, to be avoided, because it casts a bluish hue, making accurate assessment difficult

Color

Appears darker than surrounding skin
May have purplish/bluish hue

Temperature

Initial warmth when compared with surrounding skin
Later coolness as tissue is devitalized

Touch	Appearance
Indurated	Taut
Edema	Shiny
Soft, boggy	Scaly

Modified from Bennett MA: Report of the Task Force on the Implications for Darkly Pigmented Intact Skin in the Prediction and Prevention of Pressure Ulcers, *Adv Wound Care* 8(6):34, 1995.

Tissue Tolerance. The ability of tissue to endure pressure depends upon the integrity of the tissue and the supporting structures. The extrinsic factors of shear, friction, and moisture affect the ability of the skin to tolerate pressure: the greater degree to which the factors of shear, friction and moisture are present, the more susceptible the skin will be to damage from pressure. The second factor related to tissue tolerance pertains to the ability of the underlying skin structures (blood vessels, collagen) to assist in redistributing pressure. Systemic factors such as poor nutrition, increased aging, and low blood pressure affect the tissue's tolerance to externally applied pressure.

Risk Factors for Pressure Ulcer Development. A variety of factors can predispose a client to pressure ulcer formation. These factors can be directly related to disease, such as decreased level of consciousness, related to the aftereffects of trauma, the presence of a cast, or secondary to an illness, such as decreased sensory input following a cerebrovascular accident.

Impaired Sensory Perception. Clients with altered sensory perception for pain and pressure are more at risk for impaired skin integrity than clients with normal sensation. Clients with intact sensory perception of pain and pressure can feel when a portion of their body senses increased, prolonged pressure or pain. In turn, when clients are alert and oriented, they can change positions or request assistance in changing positions and relieve the pressure.

Impaired Mobility. Clients unable to independently change positions are at risk for pressure ulcer develop-

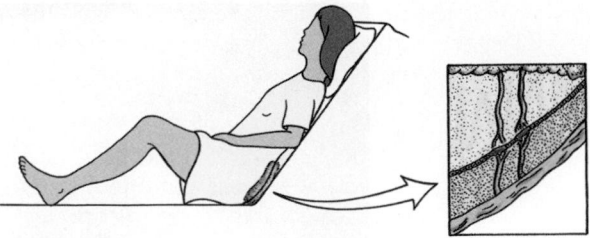

FIGURE 47-5 Diagrammatic sketch of shearing force exerted against sacral area.

ment. For example, clients with spinal cord injuries have decreased or absent motor and sensory impairment and are unable to reposition off of bony prominences.

Alteration in Level of Consciousness. Clients who are confused or disoriented, or who have changing levels of consciousness, are unable to protect themselves from pressure ulcer development. Clients who are confused or disoriented may be able to feel the pressure, but they may not be able to understand how to relieve it or communicate their discomfort. Clients in a coma cannot perceive pressure and are unable to move voluntarily to relieve pressure.

Shear. The force exerted parallel to skin resulting from both gravity pushing down on the body and resistance (friction) between the client and a surface is shear (Pieper, 2000). For example, shear force can occur when the head of the bed is elevated, and the sliding of the skeleton starts, but the skin is fixed because of friction with the bed (Figure 47-5). In addition, shear force can also occur when transferring a client from bed to stretcher and the client's skin is pulled across the bed. When shear is present, the skin and subcutaneous layers adhere to the surface of the bed, and the layers of muscle and the bones slide in the direction of body movement. The underlying tissue capillaries are stretched and angulated by the shear force. As a result, necrosis occurs deep within the tissue layers. The tissue damage occurs deep in the tissues, causing undermining at the point of pressure.

Friction. The mechanical force exerted when skin is dragged across a coarse surface such as bed linens is called **friction** (AHCPR, 1994). Unlike shearing injuries, friction injuries affect the epidermis or top layer of the skin, which is denuded as the client is repositioned. The denuded skin appears red and painful and can be referred to as a "sheet burn." A friction injury can occur in clients who are restless, in those who have uncontrollable movements, such as spastic conditions, and in those whose skin is dragged rather than lifted from the bed surface during position changes.

Moisture. The presence and duration of moisture on the skin increases the risk of ulcer formation. Moisture reduces the skin's resistance to other physical factors such as pressure and/or **shearing force.** Prolonged moisture softens skin, making it more susceptible to damage. Immobilized clients, who are unable to perform their own hygiene needs, depend on the nurse to keep the skin dry and intact. Skin moisture can originate from wound drainage, excessive perspiration, and fecal or urinary incontinence.

Classification of Pressure Ulcers

Pressure ulcers must be assessed at regular intervals using systematic parameters to evaluate wound healing, plan appropriate interventions, and evaluate progress. Assessment should include depth of tissue involvement (staging), type and approximate percentage of tissue in wound bed, wound dimensions, exudate description, and condition of surrounding skin.

An early method to classify pressure ulcers is the use of a staging system. Staging systems for pressure ulcers are based on describing the depth of tissue destroyed. Accurate staging requires knowledge of the skin layers, and a major drawback of a staging system is that an ulcer covered with necrotic tissue cannot be staged until debrided (because the necrotic tissue is covering the depth of the ulcer).

There are several different staging systems that are used clinically (AHCPR, 1994). It is important to note that the definitions are different for each of these staging systems. Therefore the same pressure ulcer could have a different stage number, depending on the staging system used.

The stages below are from the NPUAP system. In 1998 the NPUAP stage I definition was changed to reflect assessment characteristics of clients with dark skin tones. Indicators other than skin color, such as temperature, "orange peel" pore appearance, firmness or tightness, hardness, and laboratory data, may be helpful when assessing clients with dark skin (Henderson and others, 1997). Pressure ulcer staging is used to describe the pressure ulcer depth at the point of assessment. Thus once the pressure ulcer is staged, this stage endures even as the pressure ulcer heals. Pressure ulcers do not progress from a stage III to a stage I, rather a stage III ulcer demonstrating signs of healing is described as a healing stage III pressure ulcer (Cooper, 2000).

Stage I: A stage I pressure ulcer is an observable pressure-related alteration of intact skin whose indicators, as compared with an adjacent or opposite area on the body, may include changes in one or more of the following: skin temperature (warmth or coolness), tissue consistency (firm or beefy feel), and/or sensation (pain, itching). The ulcer appears as a defined area of persistent redness in lightly pigmented skin, whereas in darker skin tones the ulcer may appear with persistent red, blue, or purple hues (Figure 47-6, *A*). There are no open skin areas.

Stage II: Partial-thickness skin loss involving epidermis and/or dermis. The ulcer is superficial and presents clinically as an abrasion, blister, or shallow crater (Figure 47-6, *B*).

Stage III: Full-thickness skin loss involving damage or necrosis of subcutaneous tissue that may extend down to, but not through, underlying fascia. The ulcer presents clinically as a deep crater with or without undermining of adjacent tissue (Figure 47-6, *C*).

Stage IV: Full-thickness skin loss with extensive destruction, tissue necrosis, or damage to muscle, bone, or supporting structures (e.g., tendon and joint capsules). Undermining and sinus tracts also may be associated with stage IV pressure ulcers (Figure 47-6, *D*).

In addition, Bennett (1995) suggests that when assessing clients with darkly pigmented skin, proper lighting is important to accurately assess the skin (see Box 47-2, p. 1486). Either natural light or a halogen light is recommended. This prevents the blue tones that are produced by fluorescent light sources on darkly pigmented skin, which can interfere with accurate assessment. Additional aspects of assessing dark skin are found in Box 47-3.

The assessment of tissue type in a pressure ulcer indicates the amount (percentage) and appearance (color) of viable and nonviable tissue. Red, moist tissue is indicative of **granulation tissue,** which is progressing toward healing; yellow tissue can be characteristic of **slough** (stringy substance attached to wound bed), which is tissue that must be removed before the wound can heal; and black or brown tissue is generally **eschar** (necrotic tissue), which must be removed before healing can proceed.

Wound dimensions should include consistent measurements of depth, length, and width. These measurements can provide overall gross changes in size as an indicator of healing (Cooper, 2000). **Exudate** describes the amount, color, consistency, and odor of wound drainage. Excessive exudate can indicate the presence of a wound infection. And finally the condition of the skin surrounding the wound is evaluated for redness, warmth, maceration, or **edema** (swelling). The presence of any of these factors on the skin surrounding the wound can be indicative of wound deterioration.

Wound Classifications

A **wound** is a disruption of normal anatomical structure and function that results from pathological processes beginning internally or externally to the involved organ(s) (Lazarus and others, 1994). It is imperative for the nurse to know that *all wounds are not created equal.* Understanding the etiology of a wound is important, because the treatment for the wound varies depending on the underlying disease process. Some treatments may even be harmful to certain wounds, so the nurse should always know the complete history, including the etiology of the wound. Stotts and Cavanaugh (1999) suggest that five questions (regarding wound etiology, occurrence, chronology, aggravating and alleviating factors, and associated symptoms) be included in the nursing assessment of a wound's history

There are many ways to classify wounds. Wound classification systems describe the status of skin integrity, cause of the wound, severity or extent of tissue injury or damage, cleanliness of the wound (Table 47-1), or descriptive qualities of the wound such as color (Figure 47-7). These classifications overlap. For example, a penetrating knife wound is also an open wound, and a contused wound is a closed wound.

Wound classifications enable the nurse to understand the risks associated with a wound and implications for its care. An open wound, for example, presents a greater risk of infection than a closed wound, whereas an abrasion requires less extensive dressings than a deeply penetrating

Text continued on p. 1492

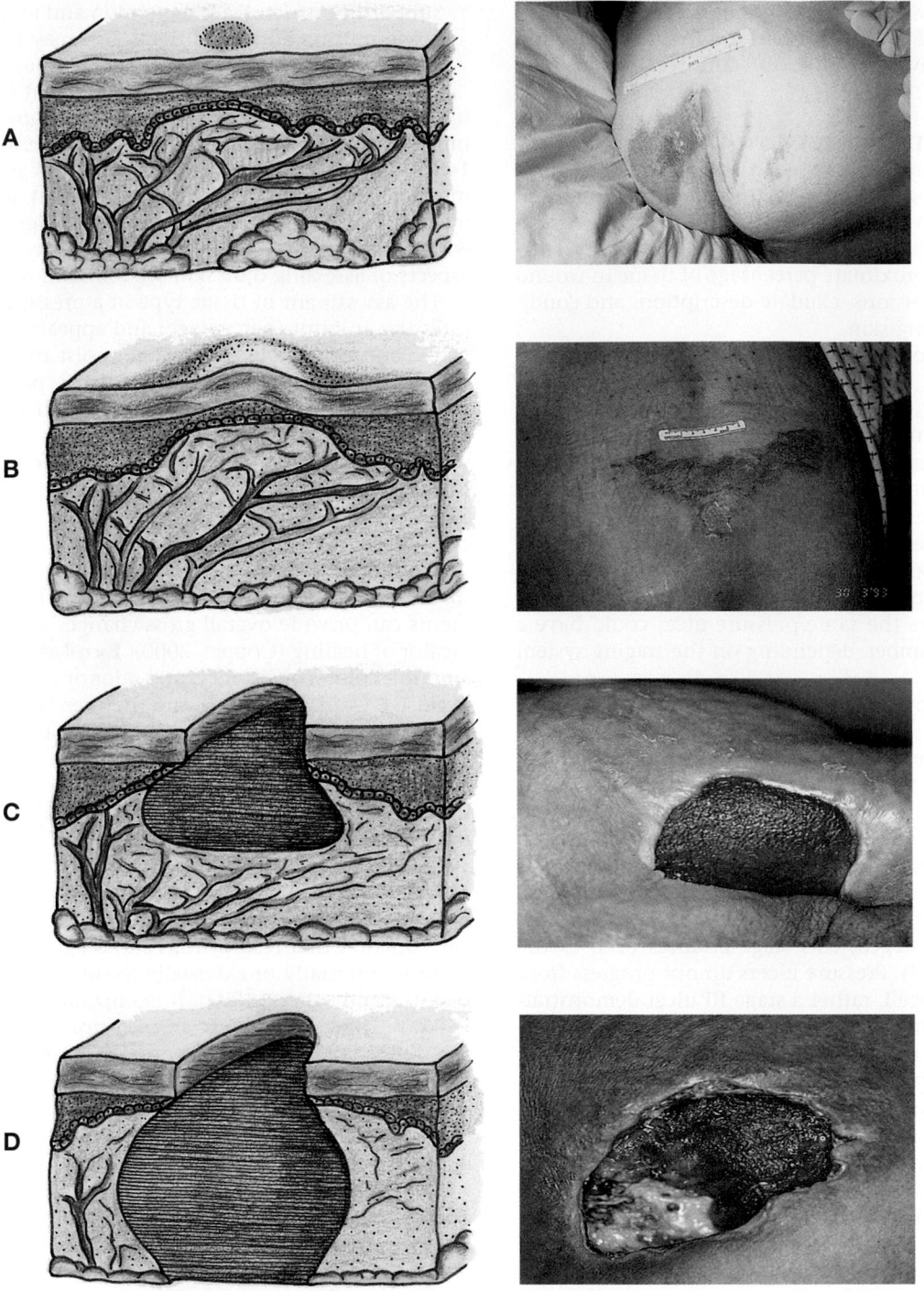

FIGURE **47–6** Diagram of stages. **A,** Stage I pressure ulcer. **B,** Stage II pressure ulcer. **C,** Stage III pressure ulcer. **D,** Stage IV pressure ulcer. (Courtesy Laurel Wiersma, RN, MSN, Clinical Nurse Specialist, Barnes-Jewish Hospital, St. Louis, Mo.)

Box 47-3

Cultural Aspects of Care

Detecting cyanosis and other changes in skin color in clients is an important clinical skill. However, this detection can become a challenge in dark-skinned clients. Cyanosis is defined as "a slightly bluish grayish slatelike or dark purple discoloration of the skin due to the presence of at least 5 grams of reduced hemoglobin in arterial blood." Color differentiation of cyanosis varies according to skin pigmentation. In dark-skinned clients, the nurse needs to know the individual's baseline skin tone. The nurse should not confuse the normal hyperpigmentation of mongolian spots that are seen on the sacrum of African, Native American, and Asian clients as cyanosis. The nurse should observe the client's skin in nonglare daylight. The Gaskin's Nursing Assessment of Skin Color (GNASC) may be a useful tool for assessment for iden-tifying changes in skin color that may increase the client's risk for pressure ulcers.

Implications for Practice

- Cyanosis is difficult but possible to detect in the dark-skinned client.
- Nurses need to be aware of situations that produce changes in skin tone.
- Examine body sites with the least melanin for underlying color identification.
- The pigmented skin should be evaluated for color-specific changes in skin tone.

Modified from Gaskin FC: Detection of cyanosis in the person with dark skin, *J Natl Black Nurses Assoc* 1:52, 1986; and Henderson CT and others: Draft definition of stage I pressure ulcers: inclusion of persons with darkly pigmented skin, *Adv Wound Care* 10(5):16, 1997.

Table 47-1   Wound Classification

Description	Causes	Implications for Healing
Status of Skin Integrity		
Open		
Wound involving a break in skin or mucous membranes	Trauma by sharp object or blow (surgical incision, venipuncture, gunshot wound)	Break in skin exposes body to invasion by microorganisms. Loss of blood and body fluids through wound occurs. Function of body part is reduced.
Closed		
Wound involving no break in skin	Part of body being struck by blunt object; twisting, straining, or deceleration force against body (bone fracture, tear of visceral organ)	Wound may predispose person to internal hemorrhage. Function of affected body part is reduced.
Acute		
Wound that proceeds through an orderly and timely reparative process that results in sustained restoration of anatomical and functional integrity	Trauma from a sharp object	Wounds are usually easily cleaned and repaired. Wound edges are clean and intact.
Chronic		
Wound that fails to proceed through an orderly and timely process to produce anatomical and functional integrity	Ulcers exposed to friction, shear, moisture, pressure	Continued exposure to pressure, friction, shear, and moisture impedes wound healing. Wound tissue may be necrotic, and drainage may be present.
Cause		
Intentional		
Wound resulting from therapy	Surgical incision; introduction of needle into body part	Incision is usually performed under aseptic technique to minimize chance of infection. Wound edges are usually smooth and clean.
Unintentional		
Wound that occurs unexpectedly	Traumatic injury (knife wound, burn)	Wound occurs under unsterile conditions. Wound edges are often jagged.

Continued

Table 47-1	Wound Classification—cont'd	
Description	**Causes**	**Implications for Healing**
Severity of Injury		
Superficial Wound that involves only epidermal layer of skin	Result of friction applied to skin surface (abrasion, first-degree burn, shearing)	Break creates risk of infection. Wound does not involve underlying injury to tissues or organs. Blood supply to area is intact.
Penetrating Wound involving break in epidermal skin layer, as well as dermis and deeper tissues or organs	Foreign object or instrument entering deep into body tissues; usually unintentional (gunshot wound, stab wound)	There is high risk of infection because foreign object is contaminated. Wound may cause internal and external hemorrhage; damage to organs causes temporary or permanent loss of function.
Perforating Penetrating wound in which foreign object enters and exits an internal organ	(See above entry.)	There is high risk of infection. Nature of injury depends on organ perforated (lung, compromised oxygenation; major vessel, hemorrhage; intestine, contamination of abdominal cavity by feces).
Cleanliness		
Clean Wound containing no pathogenic organisms	Closed surgical wound not entering gastrointestinal, respiratory, genital, or uninfected urinary tract or oropharyngeal cavity	There is low risk of infection.
Clean-Contaminated Wound made under aseptic conditions but involving body cavity that normally harbors microorganisms	Surgical wound entering gastrointestinal, respiratory, genital, or urinary tract or oropharyngeal cavity under controlled conditions	There is greater risk of infection than with clean wound.
Contaminated Wound existing under conditions in which presence of microorganisms is likely	Open, traumatic, accidental wounds; surgical wound in which break in asepsis occurred	Tissues are often not healthy and show inflammation. There is high risk of infection.
Infected Bacterial organisms present in wound site, usually above 10^5 organisms per gram of tissue	Any wound that does not properly heal and grows organisms, old traumatic wound, surgical incision into area infected (e.g., ruptured bowel)	Wound presents signs of infection (inflammation, purulent drainage, skin separation).
Colonized Wound containing microorganisms (usually multiple)	Chronic wound (vascular stasis ulcer, pressure ulcer)	Wound healing is slow, and high risk of infection exists.

Table 47-1	Wound Classification—cont'd	
Description	**Causes**	**Implications for Healing**

Descriptive Qualities

Laceration

| Tearing of tissues with irregular wound edges | Severe traumatic injury (knife wound, industrial accident involving machinery, tissues cut by broken glass) | Wound is usually created by contaminated object. Depth of wound determines other complications. |

Abrasion

| Superficial wound involving scraping or rubbing of skin's surface | Wound often resulting from fall (skinned knee or elbow); wound also resulting from dermatological procedure for removing scar tissue | Wound is painful from exposure of superficial nerves; deeper tissues are not involved. There is risk of infection from exposure to contaminated surface. |

Contusion

| Closed wound caused by a blow to body by blunt object; contusion or bruise characterized by swelling, discoloration, and pain | Bleeding in underlying tissues caused by blunt force against body part | Wound is more severe if internal organ is contused. Wound may cause temporary loss of function of body part. Localized bleeding into tissues may form hematoma (collection of blood). |

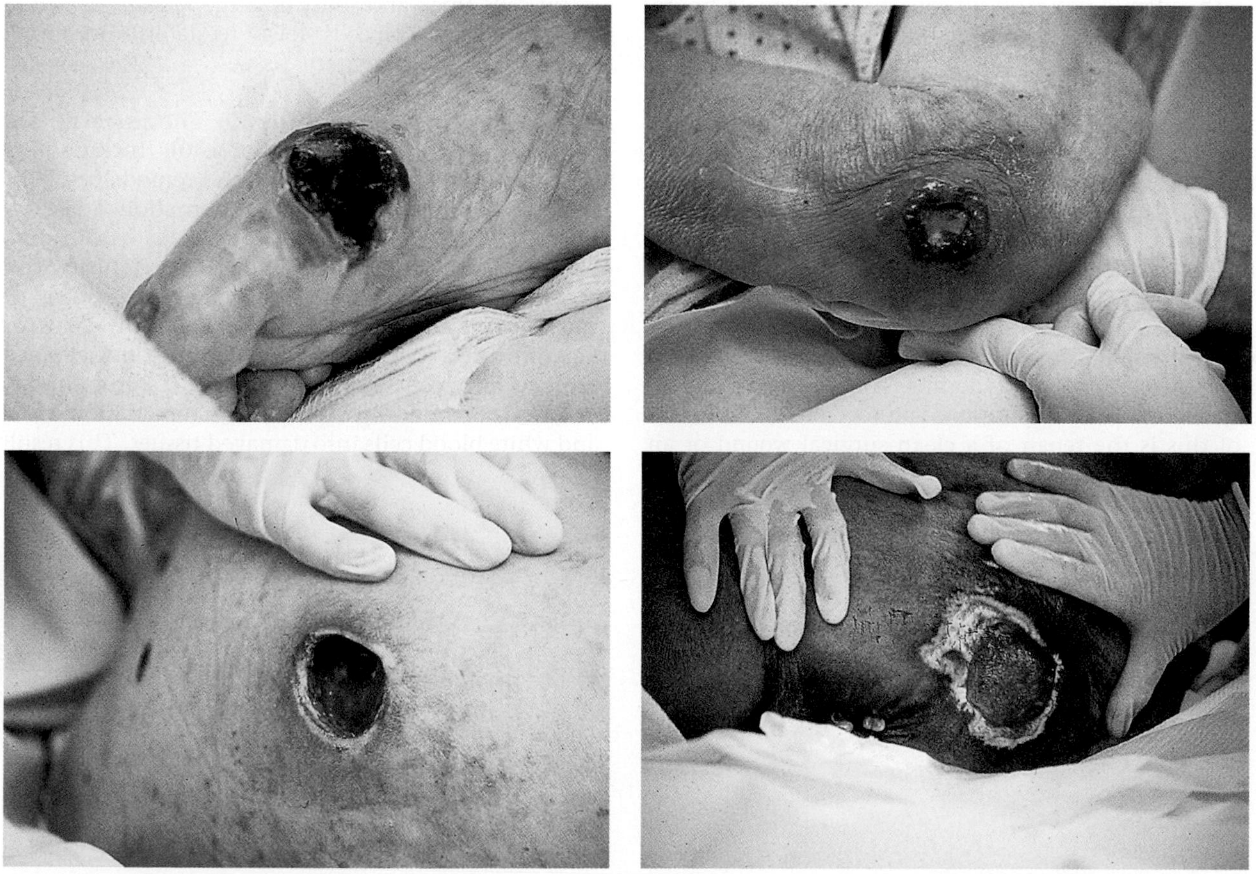

FIGURE **47–7** Wounds classified by color assessment. **A,** A "black" wound. **B,** A "yellow" wound. **C,** A "red" wound. **D,** A mixed-color wound. (Courtesy Scott Health Care—A Molnlyche Company, Philadelphia.)

wound. It is important for the nurse to understand the difference between acute and chronic wounds. Acute wounds follow the normal healing process in an orderly and timely way (Kane, 2001). Examples of acute wounds are those caused by trauma or surgery. In chronic wounds the healing trajectory is delayed, repair fails to occur, and return to normal function is slowed (Kane, 2001). Chronic wounds such as peripheral vascular venous ulcers, lower extremity arterial ulcers, neuropathic ulcers, and pressure ulcers take much longer to heal and can be a nursing challenge and client frustration.

Process of Wound Healing. Wound healing involves integrated physiological processes. The nature of healing is the same for all wounds, with variations depending on the location, severity, and extent of injury. The ability of cells and tissues to regenerate or return to normal structure by cell growth also affects healing. Cells of the liver, renal tubules, and neurons of the central nervous system typically regenerate slowly or not at all.

There are two types of wounds: those with loss of tissue and those without. A clean surgical incision is an example of a wound with little tissue loss. The surgical wound heals by **primary intention.** The skin edges are **approximated,** or closed, and the risk of infection is low. Healing occurs quickly; the inflammation (redness, warmth, edema) typically subsides in less than 24 hours, and the wound is resurfaced between day 4 and 7 (Waldrop and Doherty, 2000). In contrast, a wound involving loss of tissue, such as a burn, pressure ulcer, or severe laceration, heals by **secondary intention.** The wound is left open until it becomes filled by scar tissue. It takes longer for a wound to heal by secondary intention, and thus the chance of infection is greater. If scarring from secondary intention is severe, there may be permanent loss of tissue function (Figure 47-8).

Wound Repair. Partial-thickness wounds are shallow wounds involving loss of the epidermis (top layer) and possibly partial loss of the dermis. These wounds heal by regeneration because epidermis can regenerate. An example of this is the repair of a clean surgical wound or an abrasion. Full-thickness wounds extending into the dermis (involving both layers of tissue) heal by scar formation because deeper structures do not regenerate. Pressure ulcers are an example of full-thickness wounds.

Partial-Thickness Wound Repair. There are three components involved in the healing process of a partial-thickness wound: inflammatory response, epithelial proliferation and migration, and reestablishment of the epidermal layers.

The *inflammatory response* is triggered by tissue trauma, causing redness and swelling to the area with a moderate amount of serous exudate. This response is generally limited to the first 24 hours after wounding. The epithelial cells begin to proliferate, providing new cells to replace the lost cells. This *epithelial proliferation and migration* starts at both the wound edges and the epidermal cells lining the epidermal appendages, allowing for quick resurfacing. Epithelial cells begin to migrate across the wound bed, soon after the wound occurs. A wound left open to air can resurface within 6 to 7 days, whereas a wound that is kept moist can resurface in 4 days. The difference in the healing rate is related to the fact that epidermal cells can only migrate across a moist surface. In a dry wound, the cells must migrate down into a moist level before migration can occur (Waldrop and Doughty, 2000). New epithelium is only a few cells thick and must undergo *reestablishment of the epidermal layers.* The cells slowly reestablish normal thickness and appear as dry pink tissue.

Full-Thickness Wound Repair. The three phases involved in the healing process of a full-thickness wound are inflammatory, proliferative, and remodeling.

Inflammatory Phase. The inflammation stage is the body's reaction to wounding and begins within minutes of injury and lasts approximately 3 days. During **hemostasis,** injured blood vessels constrict, and platelets gather to stop bleeding. Clots form a **fibrin** matrix that later provide a framework for cellular repair. Damaged tissue and mast cells secrete histamine, resulting in vasodilation of surrounding capillaries and exudation of serum and white blood cells into damaged tissues. This results in

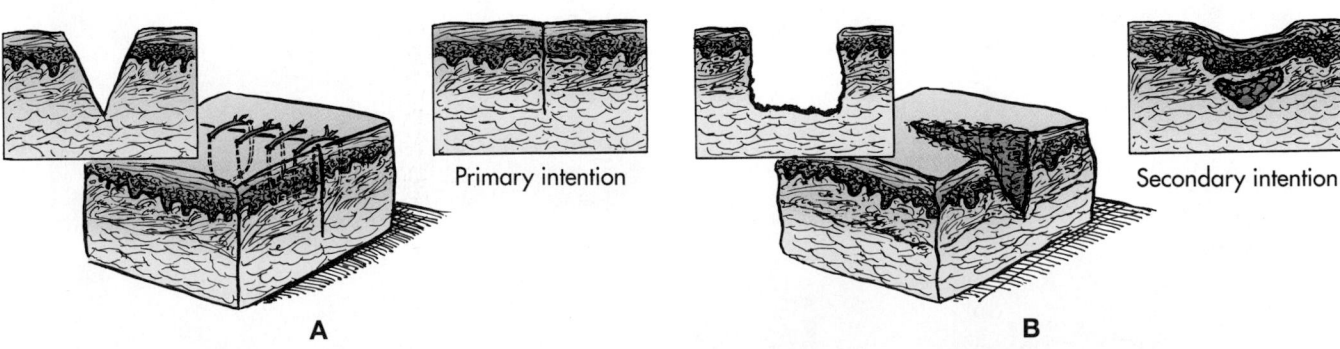

Primary intention

Secondary intention

A   **B**

FIGURE **47–8   A,** Wound healing by primary intention, such as with a surgical incision. Wound healing edges are pulled together and approximated with sutures, staples, or adhesive tapes, and healing occurs by connective tissue deposition. **B,** Wound healing by secondary intention. Wound edges are not approximated, and healing occurs by granulation tissue formation and contraction of the wound edges. (Used with permission: Bryant RA, editor: *Acute and chronic wounds: nursing management,* ed 2, St. Louis, 2000, Mosby.)

localized redness, edema, warmth, and throbbing. The inflammatory response is beneficial, and there is no value in attempting to cool the area or reduce the swelling unless the swelling occurs within a closed compartment (e.g., ankle or neck).

Leukocytes (white blood cells) reach the wound within a few hours. The primary acting white blood cell is the neutrophil, which begins to ingest bacteria and small debris. The second important leukocyte is the monocyte, which transforms into macrophages. The macrophages are the "garbage cells" that clean a wound of bacteria, dead cells, and debris by phagocytosis. Macrophages continue the process of clearing the wound of debris, release growth factors that attract **fibroblasts,** the cells that synthesize collagen (connective tissue). Collagen can be found as early as the second day and is the main component of scar tissue.

In a clean wound the inflammatory phase accomplishes control of bleeding and establishes a clean wound bed. The inflammatory phase is prolonged if too little inflammation occurs, as in debilitating disease such as cancer or after administration of steroids. Too much inflammation also prolongs healing because arriving cells compete for available nutrients. An example is a wound infection in which the increased metabolic energy requirements present in an infected wound competes for the available calorie intake.

Proliferative Phase. With the appearance of new blood vessels as reconstruction progresses, the proliferative phase begins and lasts from 3 to 24 days. The main activities during this phase are the filling of the wound with granulation tissue, contraction of the wound, and the resurfacing of the wound by **epithelialization.** Fibroblasts are present in this phase and are the cells that synthesize collagen, providing the matrix for granulation. Collagen mixes with the granulation tissue, and this matrix will support the reepithelialization. Collagen provides strength and structural integrity to a wound. During this period the wound contracts to reduce the area that requires healing. Last, the epithelial cells migrate from the wound edges to resurface. In a clean wound the proliferative phase accomplishes the following: the vascular bed is reestablished (granulation tissue), the area is filled with replacement tissue (collagen, contraction and granulation tissue), and the surface is repaired (epithelialization). Impairment of healing during this stage usually results from systemic factors such as age, **anemia,** hypoproteinemia, and zinc deficiency.

Remodeling. Maturation, the final stage of healing, may take place for more than a year, depending on the depth and extent of the wound. The collagen scar continues to reorganize and gain strength for several months. However, a healed wound usually does not have the tensile strength of the tissue it replaces. Collagen fibers undergo remodeling or reorganization before assuming their normal appearance. Usually scar tissue contains fewer pigmented cells (melanocytes) and has a lighter color than normal skin.

Complications of Wound Healing

Hemorrhage. **Hemorrhage,** or bleeding from a wound site, is normal during and immediately after the initial trauma. Hemostasis occurs within several minutes unless large blood vessels are involved or the client has poor clotting function. Hemorrhage occurring after hemostasis indicates a slipped surgical suture, a dislodged clot, infection, or erosion of a blood vessel by a foreign object (e.g., a drain). Hemorrhage may occur externally or internally. For example, if a surgical suture slips from a blood vessel, bleeding occurs internally within the tissues, and there are no visible signs of blood unless a surgical drain is present, which is inserted into tissues beneath a wound to remove fluid that collects in underlying tissues. The nurse can detect internal bleeding by looking for distention or swelling of the affected body part, a change in the type and amount of drainage from a surgical drain, or signs of hypovolemic shock. A **hematoma** is a localized collection of blood underneath the tissues. It appears as a swelling, change in color, sensation, or warmth or mass that often takes on a bluish discoloration. A hematoma near a major artery or vein is dangerous because pressure from the expanding hematoma may obstruct blood flow.

External hemorrhaging is obvious. The nurse observes dressings covering the wound for bloody drainage. If bleeding is extensive, the dressing soon becomes saturated, and frequently blood drains from under the dressing and pools beneath the client. The nurse observes all wounds closely, particularly surgical wounds, in which the risk of hemorrhage is great during the first 24 to 48 hours after surgery or injury.

Infection. Wound infection is the second most common nosocomial (hospital-related) infection (see Chapter 33). According to the Centers for Disease Control and Prevention (CDC) (2001), a wound is infected if purulent material drains from it, even if a culture is not taken or has negative results. A sample of drainage from an infected wound may not reveal bacteria due to poor culture technique or administration of antibiotics. Positive culture findings do not always indicate an infection because many wounds contain colonies of noninfective resident bacteria. In fact, all chronic dermal wounds are considered contaminated with bacteria. What differentiates contaminated wounds from infected wounds is the amount of bacteria present. It is generally agreed that wounds with more than 100,000 (10^5) organisms per gram of tissue are infected (Robson, 1997). The chances of wound infection are greater when the wound contains dead or necrotic tissue, there are foreign bodies in or near the wound, and the blood supply and local tissue defenses are reduced. Bacterial wound infection inhibits wound healing.

A contaminated or traumatic wound may show signs of infection early, within 2 to 3 days. A surgical wound infection usually does not develop until the fourth or fifth postoperative day. The client has a fever, tenderness and pain at the wound site, and an elevated white blood cell count. The edges of the wound may appear inflamed. If drainage is present, it is odorous and **purulent,** which causes a yellow, green, or brown color, depending on the causative organism (Table 47-2).

Dehiscence. When a wound fails to heal properly, the layers of skin and tissue may separate. This most commonly occurs before collagen formation (3 to 11 days af-

Table 47-2	Types of Wound Drainage
Type	**Appearance**
Serous	Clear, watery plasma
Purulent	Thick, yellow, green, tan, or brown
Serosanguineous	Pale, red, watery: mixture of clear and red fluid
Sanguineous	Bright red: indicates active bleeding

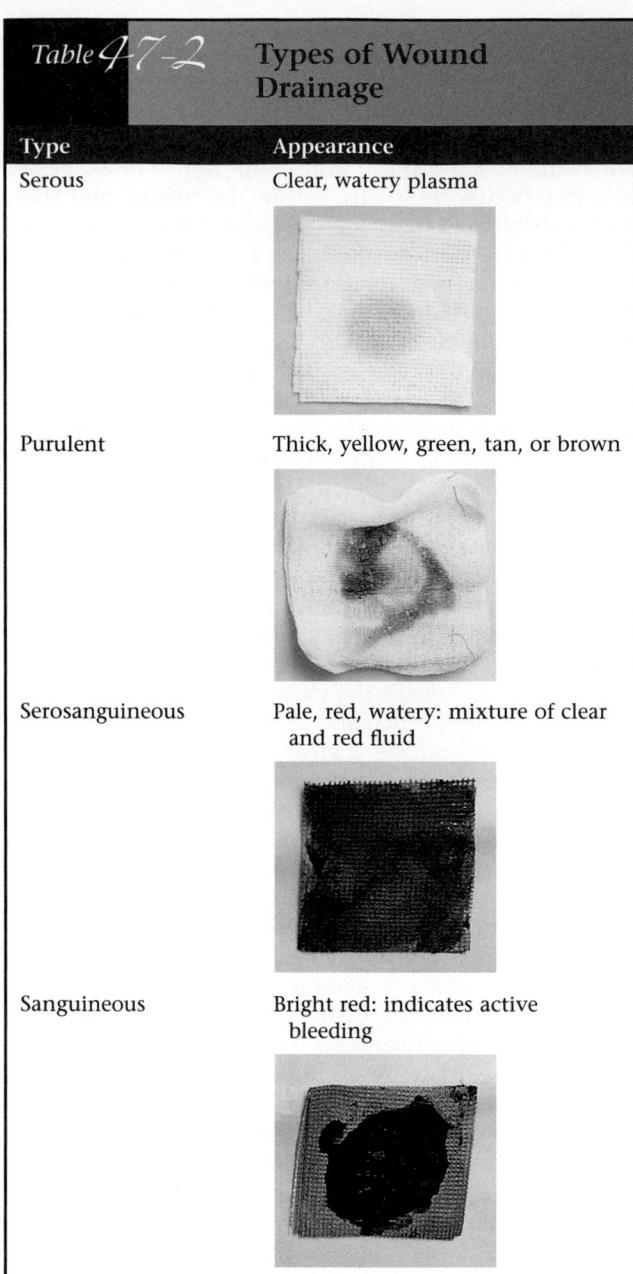

Box 47-4	Risk for Skin Breakdown From Body Fluids

Low Risk

Saliva
Serosanguineous drainage

High Risk

Gastric drainage
Pancreatic drainage

Moderate Risk

Bile
Stool
Urine
Ascetic fluid
Purulent exudate

vides a splint to the area, supporting the healing tissue when coughing increases the intraabdominal pressure.

Evisceration. With total separation of wound layers, **evisceration** (protrusion of visceral organs through a wound opening) may occur. The condition is an emergency that requires surgical repair. When evisceration occurs, the nurse places sterile towels soaked in sterile saline over the extruding tissues to reduce chances of bacterial invasion and drying of the tissues. If the organs protrude through the wound, blood supply to the tissues is compromised. The client should be allowed nothing by mouth (NPO), observed for signs and symptoms of shock, and prepared for emergency surgery.

Fistulas. A **fistula** is an abnormal passage between two organs or between an organ and the outside of the body. Most fistulas form as a result of poor wound healing or as a complication of disease, such as Crohn's disease. Trauma, infection, radiation exposure, and diseases such as cancer can prevent tissue layers from closing properly and allow the fistula tract to form. Fistulas increase the risk of infection and fluid and electrolyte imbalances from fluid loss. Chronic drainage of fluids through a fistula can also predispose a person to skin breakdown (Box 47-4).

*N*ursing Knowledge Base

Prediction and Prevention of Pressure Ulcers

A major aspect of nursing care is the maintenance of skin integrity. Consistent, planned skin care interventions are critical to ensuring high quality in care. Nurses constantly observe their clients' skin for breaks or impaired skin integrity. Impaired skin integrity occurs from prolonged pressure, irritation of the skin, or immobility, leading to the development of pressure ulcers.

A pressure ulcer is a localized area of tissue necrosis (death) that develops when soft tissue is compressed between a bony prominence and an external surface for a prolonged period (NPUAP, 1992a). Nursing care interven-

ter injury). **Dehiscence** is the partial or total separation of wound layers. A client who is a risk for poor wound healing (e.g., poor nutritional status, infection, obesity) for a local infection is at risk for dehiscence (Candido, 2002). However, obese clients have a higher risk because of the constant strain placed on their wounds and the poor healing qualities of fat tissue. Dehiscence involves abdominal surgical wounds and occurs after a sudden strain, such as coughing, vomiting, or sitting up in bed. Clients often report feeling as though something has given way. When there is an increase in serosanguineous drainage from a wound, the nurse should be alert for the potential for dehiscence. A strategy to prevent dehiscence is to utilize a folded thin blanket or pillow placed over an abdominal wound when the client is coughing. This pro-

Table 47-3		Norton Scale							
Physical Condition		**Mental Condition**		**Activity**		**Mobility**		**Continence**	
Good	4	Alert	4	Walks	4	Full	4	Good	4
Fair	3	Apathetic	3	Walks with help	3	Slightly limited	3	Occasional incontinence	3
Poor	2	Confused	2	Sits in chair	2	Very limited	2	Frequent incontinence	2
Very bad	1	Stuporous	1	Remains in bed	1	Immobile	1	Urine and fecal incontinence	1
Total		Total		Total		Total		Total	
Grand total									
A score of 14 or less indicates risk of pressure ulcer, a score of less than 12 indicates high risk.									

Agency for Health Care Policy and Research. Panel for the Prediction and Prevention of Pressure Ulcers in Adults: *Pressure ulcers in adults: prediction and prevention,* Clinical Practice Guideline No. 3. AHCPR Pub. NO 92-0047. Rockville, MD, 1992a, Agency for Health Care Policy and research, Public Health Service, U.S. Department of Health and Human Services.

tions aimed at the prevention, assessment, and treatment of pressure ulcers should be based on research (AHCPR, 1992a, 1994).

Risk Assessment. There are several instruments for assessing clients who are at high risk for developing a pressure ulcer. Clients with little risk for pressure ulcer development are spared the unnecessary and sometimes costly preventive treatments and the related risk of complications (Stotts, 1988). Prevention and treatment of pressure ulcers are major nursing priorities. The incidence of pressure ulcers in a facility or agency is an important indicator of quality of care. There is evidence that a program of prevention guided by risk assessment can simultaneously reduce the institutional incidence of pressure ulcers by as much as 60% and bring down the costs of prevention at the same time (Braden, 2001). Several assessment risk scales (Bergstrom and others, 1987; Norton, McLaren, and Exon-Smith, 1962) developed by nurses enable systematic risk assessment of clients. The Norton Scale and the Braden Scale are noted in the AHCPR guidelines (1992a) as being valid tools to use for pressure ulcer risk assessment. Each tool has a different number of risk factors (five to eight items) that are ranked by number. The client's risk assessment score is obtained by adding the individual numbers given for each risk factor. Interpretation of the meaning of the numerical score differs with each scale.

Norton Scale. The first scale reported in the literature is the Norton Scale (Norton, McLaren, and Exon-Smith, 1962) (Table 47-3). It scores five risk factors: physical condition, mental condition, activity, mobility, and incontinence. The total score ranges from 5 to 20; a lower score indicates a higher risk for pressure ulcer development (AHCPR, 1992).

Braden Scale. The Braden Scale (Table 47-4) was developed based on risk factors in a nursing home population (Bergstrom and others, 1987). The Braden Scale is composed of six subscales: sensory perception, moisture, activity, mobility, nutrition, friction and shear. The total score ranges from 6 to 23; a lower total score indicates a higher risk for pressure ulcer development (Braden and

Bergstrom, 1989). The cutoff score for onset of pressure ulcer risk with the Braden Scale in the general adult population is 18 (Ayello and Braden, 2002). For black and Latino clients with darkly pigmented skin, a cutoff score of 18 has been suggested (Lyder and others, 2001). The Braden Scale is highly reliable when used to identify clients at greatest risk for pressure ulcers (Bergstrom and others, 1987; Braden and Bergstrom, 1994; Ratliff and Bryant, 2003). The Braden Scale is the most commonly used assessment scale for pressure ulcer risk.

Prevention. The prevention of pressure ulcers is a priority in caring for clients and is not limited to clients with restrictions in mobility. Impaired skin integrity may not be a problem in healthy, immobilized individuals but is a serious and potentially devastating problem in ill or debilitated clients (AHCPR, 1992a).

Economic Consequences of Pressure Ulcers. Pressure ulcers are a continual problem in acute and restorative care settings. Prevalence refers to the "number of cases present in a population at one point in time" (AHCPR, 1994). The National Pressure Ulcer Advisory Panel estimates that pressure ulcer prevalence in acute care is 15% with incidence of 7% (Ayello and Braden, 2002). There is a lack of clarity about the prevalence of pressure ulcers among persons being cared for in the home without supervision or assistance of professionals (AHCPR, 1994). In the home care setting, prevalence rates have been reported to be 9.12%, and approximately 30% were at risk for new pressure ulcers (Ferrell and others, 2000).

When a pressure ulcer occurs, the length of stay in a hospital and the overall cost of health care increases (AHCPR, 1994). The actual cost of treatment is difficult to approximate. About 1.6 million clients each year in acute care settings develop pressure ulcers, representing a cost of $2.2 to $3.6 billion to the U.S. health care system (Pieper, 2000). Although treatment of pressure ulcers is more costly than prevention (Richardson, Gardner, and Frantz, 1998), the preventive measures themselves are expensive. Extra equipment, such as special beds and mattresses, and increased nursing time are needed to administer these measures. When an ulcer develops, mean

Table 47-4	Braden Scale for Predicting Pressure Ulcer Risk			
Patient's Name _____ Evaluator's Name _____ Date of Assessment				
Sensory Perception Ability to respond meaningfully to pressure-related discomfort	1. Completely limited Unresponsive (does not moan, flinch, or grasp) to painful stimuli due to diminished level of consciousness or sedation. OR Limited ability to feel pain over most of body surface.	2. Very limited Responds only to painful stimuli. Cannot communicate discomfort except by moaning or restlessness. OR Has a sensory impairment which limits the ability to feel pain or discomfort over $1/2$ of body.	3. Slightly limited Responds to verbal commands, but cannot always communicate discomfort or need to be turned. OR Has some sensory impairment that limits ability to feel pain or discomfort in 1 or 2 extremities.	4. No impairment Responds to verbal commands. Has no sensory deficit that would limit ability to feel or voice pain or discomfort.
Moisture Degree to which skin is exposed to moisture	1. Constantly moist Skin is kept moist almost contantly by perspiration, urine, etc. Dampness is detected every time patient is moved or turned.	2. Very moist Skin is often, but not always, moist. Linen must be changed at least once a shift.	3. Occasionally moist Skin is occasionally moist, requiring an extra linen change approximately once a day.	4. Rarely moist Skin is usually dry. Linen only requires changing at routine intervals.
Activity Degree of physical activity	1. Bedfast Confined to bed.	2. Chairfast Ability to walk severely limited or nonexistent. Cannot bear own weight and/or must be assisted into chair or wheelchair.	3. Walks occasionally Walks occasionally during day, but for very short distances, with or without assistance. Spends majority of each shift in bed or chair.	4. Walks frequently Walks outside the room at least twice a day and inside room at least once every 2 hours during waking hours.
Mobility Ability to change and control body position	1. Completely immobile Does not make even slight changes in body or extremity position without assistance.	2. Very limited Makes occasional slight changes in body or extremity position but unable to make frequent or significant changes independently.	3. Slightly limited Makes frequent though slight changes in body or extremity position independently.	4. No limitations Makes major and frequent changes in position without assistance.

Courtesy Barbara Braden and Nancy Bergstrom.

hospital costs ($37,288 versus $13,924) and length of stay (30.4 versus 12.8 days) are increased (Allman and others, 1999).

Factors Influencing Pressure Ulcer Formation and Wound Healing

Impaired skin integrity resulting in pressure ulcers is primarily the result of pressure. However, additional factors can increase the client's risk for pressure ulcer development and poor wound healing. In addition to shear force, friction, and moisture, which were previously discussed, nutrition, tissue perfusion, infection, age, and other factors influence pressure ulcer formation, as well as wound healing (Table 47-5).

Nutrition. For clients weakened or debilitated by illness, nutritional therapy is especially important. A client who has undergone surgery (see Chapter 49) and is well nourished still requires at least 1500 kcal/day for nutritional maintenance. Alternatives such as enteral feedings (see Chapter 43) and parenteral nutrition (see Chapter 40) are made available for clients unable to maintain normal food intake.

Normal wound healing requires proper nutrition (Table 47-6). Deficiencies in any of the nutrients may result in impaired or delayed healing (Stotts, 2000). Physiological processes of wound healing depend on the availability of protein, vitamins (especially A and C), and the trace minerals zinc and copper. Collagen is a protein formed from amino acids acquired by fibroblasts from protein ingested

Table **47-4**	**Braden Scale for Predicting Pressure Ulcer Risk—cont'd**

Patient's Name _____ Evaluator's Name _____ Date of Assessment

Nutrition *Usual* food intake pattern	1. Very poor Never eats a complete meal. Rarely eats more than $^1/_3$ of any food offered. Eats 2 servings or less of protein (meat or dairy products) per day. Takes fluids poorly. Does not take a liquid dietary supplement. OR Is NPO and/or maintained on clear liquids or IVs for more than 5 days.	2 Probably inadequate Rarely eats a complete meal and generally eats only about $^1/_2$ of any food offered. Protein intake includes only 3 servings of meat or dairy products per day. Occasionally will take a dietary supplement. OR Receives less than optimum amount of liquid diet or tube feeding.	3. Adequate Eats over half of most meals. Eats a total of 4 servings of protein (meat, dairy products) each day. Occasionally will refuse a meal, but will usually take a supplement if offered. OR Is on a tube feeding or total parenteral nutrition regimen that probably meets most of nutritional needs.	4. Excellent Eats most of every meal. Never refuses a meal. Usually eats a total of 4 or more servings of meat and dairy products. Occasionally eats between meals. Does not require supplementation.
Friction and Shear	1. Problem Requires moderate to maximum assistance in moving. Complete lifting without sliding against sheets is impossible. Frequently slides down in bed or chair, requiring frequent repositioning with maximum assistance. Spasticity, contractures, or agitation leads to almost constant friction.	2. Potential problem Moves feebly or requires minimum assistance. During a move skin probably slides to some extent against sheets, chair, restraints, or other devices. Maintains relatively good position in chair or bed most of the time but occasionally slides down.	3. No apparent problem Moves in bed and in chair independently and has sufficient muscle strength to lift up completely during move. Maintains good position in bed or chair at all times.	

TOTAL SCORE

Courtesy Barbara Braden and Nancy Bergstrom.

in food. Vitamin C is needed for synthesis of collagen. Vitamin A reduces the negative effects of steroids on wound healing. Trace elements are also needed; zinc is needed for epithelialization and collagen synthesis, and copper is necessary for collagen fiber linking.

Calories provide the material needed to support the cellular activity of wound healing. Protein needs are especially increased. A balanced intake of various nutrients is critical to support wound healing. A balanced diet should include protein, fat, carbohydrates, vitamin and minerals.

Albumin is a frequently measured variable used to evaluate the client's protein status. A client with a serum albumin level below 3 g/100 ml is at greater risk for pressure ulcer. In addition, low albumin levels are associated with poor wound healing (Hanan and Scheele, 1991; Pinchcofsky-Devin and Kaminski, 1989; Ratliff and Bryant, 2003). Although serum albumin levels are slow to

reflect changes in visceral proteins, they are good predictors of malnutrition in all age groups (Hanan and Scheele, 1991). Prealbumin is an excellent measure of nutritional status because it reflects not only what has been ingested but also what has been able to be absorbed, digested, and metabolized (Stotts, 2000).

Tissue Perfusion. Oxygen fuels the cellular functions essential to the healing process; therefore the ability to perfuse the tissues with adequate amounts of oxygenated blood is critical to wound healing (Waldrop and Doughty, 2000). Clients with reduced circulation, which may occur with shock or peripheral vascular diseases such as diabetes are at risk for poor tissue perfusion. Oxygen requirements depend upon the phase of wound healing; for instance, chronic tissue hypoxia is associated with impaired collagen synthesis and reduced tissue resistance to infection (see Table 47-6, p. 1499).

Table 47-5   Factors That Impair Wound Healing

Physiological Effects	Nursing Implications
Age	
Aging alters all phases of wound healing.	Instruct client on safety precautions to avoid injuries.
Vascular changes impair circulation to wound site.	Be prepared to provide wound care for longer period.
Reduced liver function alters synthesis of clotting factors.	Teach support persons in home wound care techniques.
Inflammatory response is slowed.	
Formation of antibodies and lymphocytes is reduced.	
Collagen tissue is less pliable.	
Scar tissue is less elastic.	
Malnutrition	
All phases of wound healing are impaired.	Provide balanced diet rich in protein, carbohydrates, lipids, vitamins A and C, and minerals (e.g., zinc, copper). Assess ability to chew foods; if problem noted, provide with liquid supplements.
Stress from burns or severe trauma increases nutritional requirements.	Provide adequate amounts of calories and fluid.
Obesity	
Fatty tissue lacks adequate blood supply to resist bacterial infection and deliver nutrients and cellular elements for healing.	Observe obese client for signs of wound infection and evisceration.
Impaired Oxygenation	
Low arterial oxygen tension alters synthesis of collagen and formation of epithelial cells.	Provide diet adequate in iron, Vitamin B_{12}, and folic acid. Monitor hematocrit and hemoglobin levels of clients with wounds.
If local circulating blood flow is poor, tissues fail to receive needed oxygen.	
Decreased hemoglobin in blood (anemia) reduces arterial oxygen levels in capillaries and interferes with tissue repair.	
Smoking	
Smoking reduces amount of functional hemoglobin in blood, thus decreasing tissue oxygenation.	Discourage client from smoking by explaining its effects on wound healing.
Smoking may increase platelet aggregation and cause hypercoagulability.	
Smoking interferes with normal cellular mechanisms that promote release of oxygen to tissues.	
Drugs	
Steroids reduce inflammatory response and slow collagen synthesis.	Carefully observe clients receiving these drugs because signs of inflammation may not be obvious.
Antiinflammatory drugs suppress protein synthesis, **wound contraction,** epithelialization, and inflammation.	Vitamin A can counteract effects of steroids.
Prolonged antibiotic use may increase risk of superinfection.	Caution client to use only prescribed medications.
Chemotherapeutic drugs can depress bone marrow function, lower number of leukocytes, and impair inflammatory response.	
Diabetes	
Chronic disease causes small blood vessel disease that impairs tissue perfusion.	Instruct diabetic clients to take preventive measures to avoid cuts or breaks in skin.
Diabetes causes hemoglobin to have greater affinity for oxygen, so it fails to release oxygen to tissues.	Provide preventive foot care.
Hyperglycemia alters ability of leukocytes to perform phagocytosis and also supports overgrowth of fungal and yeast infection.	Control blood sugar to reduce the physiological changes associated with diabetes.
Radiation	
Fibrosis and vascular scarring eventually develop in irradiated skin layers.	Closely observe clients who have surgery after radiation for wound complications.
Tissues become fragile and poorly oxygenated.	

Table 47-5	Factors That Impair Wound Healing—cont'd
Physiological Effects	**Nursing Implications**
Wound Stress	
Vomiting, abdominal distention, and respiratory effort may stress suture line and disrupt wound layer. Sudden, unexpected tension on incision inhibits formation of endothelial cell and collagen networks.	Control nausea with ordered antiemetics. Keep nasogastric tubes patent and draining to avoid accumulation of secretions. Instruct and help client to splint abdominal wound during coughing.

Table 47-6	Role of Selected Nutrients in Wound Healing		
Nutrient	**Role in Healing**	**Recommendations**	**Sources**
Calories	Fuel for cell energy "Protein protection"	30-35 kcal/kg/day, or enough to maintain positive nitrogen balance	
Protein	Neogenesis, collagen formation, wound remodeling	1.25-1.50 g/kg/day, or enough to maintain positive nitrogen balance	Poultry, fish, eggs, beef
Vitamin C (ascorbic acid)	Collagen synthesis, capillary wall integrity, fibroblast function	RDA = 60 mg Supplement if deficient 500 mg bid Need long time to develop clinical scurvy from vitamin C deficiency Low toxicity	Citrus fruits, tomatoes, potatoes, fortified fruit juices
Vitamin A	Epithelialization, wound closure Can reverse steroid effects on skin and delayed healing	RDA = 4000 international units Supplement if deficient 20,000 units × 10 days	Green leafy vegetables (spinach), broccoli, carrots, sweet potatoes, liver
Vitamin E	No known role in wound healing	None	Fish, oysters, liver, dark meat, eggs, legumes
Zinc	Collagen formation and protein synthesis	RDA = 12-15 mg Correct deficiencies No improvement in wound healing with supplementation unless zinc deficient Use with caution—large doses can be toxic May inhibit copper metabolism and impair immune function	Vegetables, meats, legumes
Fluid	Essential fluid environment for all cell function	30-35 ml/kg/day Increase by another 10-15 ml/kg if client is on an air-fluidized bed	Use noncaffeine, nonalcoholic fluids without sugar Water is best—6-8 glasses/day

Modified from Ayello EA, Thomas DR, Litchford MA: Nutritional aspects of wound healing, *Home Healthc Nurse* 17(11):719, 1999; and Stotts NA: Nutritional assessment and support. In Bryant RA, editor: *Acute and chronic wounds: nursing management,* ed 2, St. Louis, 2000, Mosby.

Infection. Wound infection prolongs the inflammatory phase, delays collagen synthesis, prevents epithelialization, and increases the production of proinflammatory cytokines, which may lead to additional tissue destruction (Waldrop and Doughty, 2000). Indications that a wound infection may be present include the presence of pus; change in odor, volume, or character of wound drainage; redness in the surrounding tissue; fever; or pain.

Age. Increased age affects all phases of wound healing. A decrease in the functioning of the macrophage can lead to a delayed inflammatory response, delayed collagen synthesis, and slower epithelialization.

Psychosocial Impact of Wounds. The psychosocial impact of wounds on the physiological process of healing is unknown. The client's psychological response to any wound is part of the nurse's assessment. Body image changes may impose a great stress on the client's adaptive mechanisms. In addition, body image changes influence self-concept (see Chapter 26) and sexuality (see Chapter 27). The client's personal and social resources for adaptation should also be a part of the assessment. Factors that may affect the client's perception of the wound include the presence of scars, drains (drains may be necessary for weeks or even months after certain procedures), odor from drainage, and temporary or permanent prosthetic devices.

Critical Thinking

Successful critical thinking requires a synthesis of knowledge, experience, information gathered from clients, critical thinking attitudes, and intellectual and professional standards. Clinical judgments require the nurse to anticipate the information necessary, analyze the data, and make decisions regarding client care. Critical thinking is always changing. During assessment (Figure 47-9) the

nurse must consider all elements that build toward making appropriate nursing diagnoses.

When caring for clients who have impaired skin integrity and chronic wounds, the nurse must integrate knowledge from nursing and other disciplines, previous experiences, and information gathered from clients to understand the risk to skin integrity and wound healing. Knowledge of normal musculoskeletal physiology, the pathogenesis of pressure ulcers, normal wound healing, and the pathophysiology of underlying diseases enables

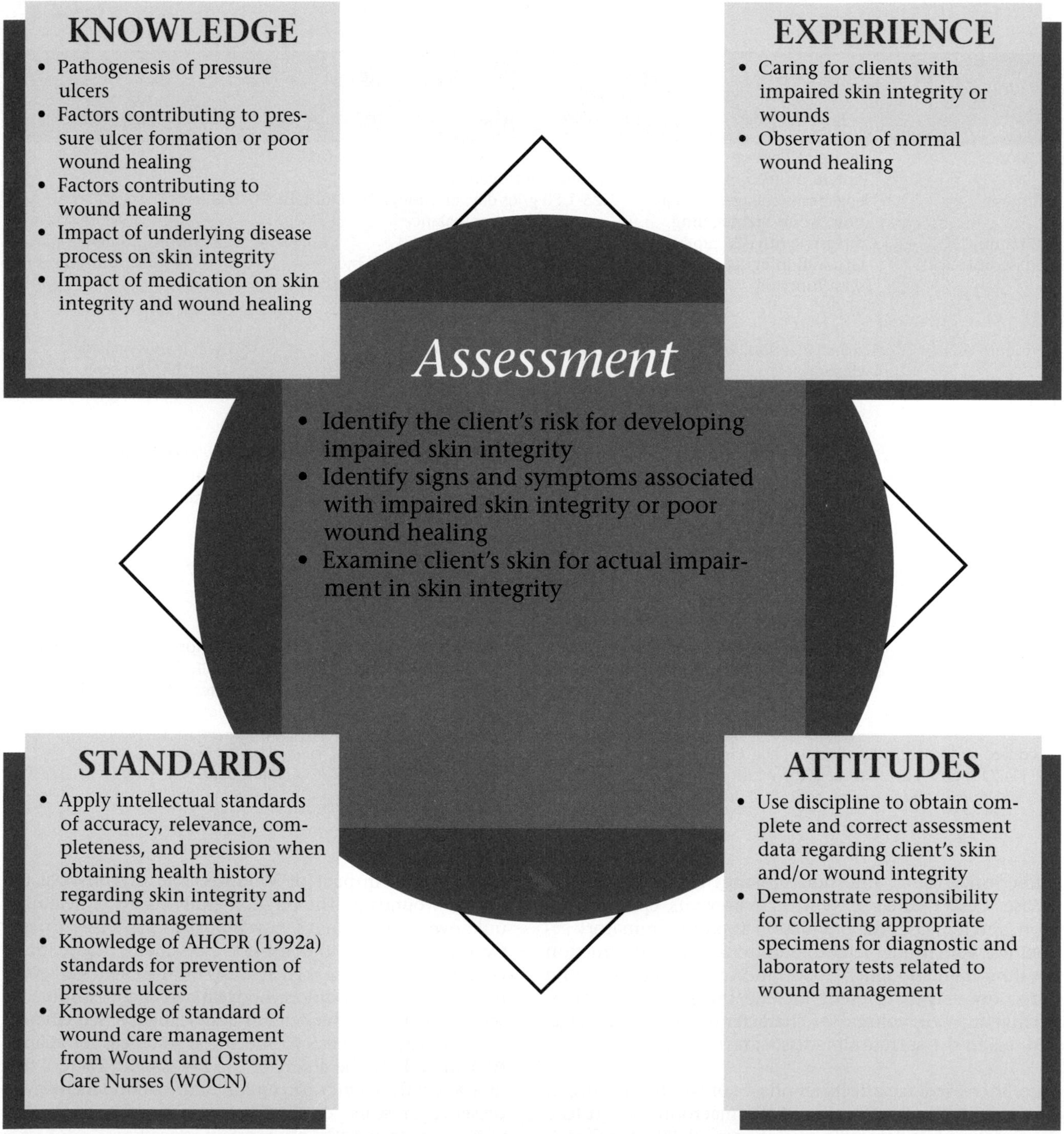

KNOWLEDGE

- Pathogenesis of pressure ulcers
- Factors contributing to pressure ulcer formation or poor wound healing
- Factors contributing to wound healing
- Impact of underlying disease process on skin integrity
- Impact of medication on skin integrity and wound healing

EXPERIENCE

- Caring for clients with impaired skin integrity or wounds
- Observation of normal wound healing

Assessment

- Identify the client's risk for developing impaired skin integrity
- Identify signs and symptoms associated with impaired skin integrity or poor wound healing
- Examine client's skin for actual impairment in skin integrity

STANDARDS

- Apply intellectual standards of accuracy, relevance, completeness, and precision when obtaining health history regarding skin integrity and wound management
- Knowledge of AHCPR (1992a) standards for prevention of pressure ulcers
- Knowledge of standard of wound care management from Wound and Ostomy Care Nurses (WOCN)

ATTITUDES

- Use discipline to obtain complete and correct assessment data regarding client's skin and/or wound integrity
- Demonstrate responsibility for collecting appropriate specimens for diagnostic and laboratory tests related to wound management

FIGURE **47-9** Critical thinking model for skin integrity and wound care assessment.

the nurse to have a scientific basis for care. The AHCPR and Wound and Ostomy Care Nurses (WOCN) have guidelines for assessment of risk for impaired skin integrity, prevention measures, and interventions to promote wound healing (AHCPR, 1992a, 1994), as well as other standards of practice, should be applied. Past experience with clients at risk for impaired skin integrity or with clients with wounds increases the experiential knowledge base from which the nurse can identify interventions. Finally, the nurse must be disciplined during assessment to obtain comprehensive and correct assessment data. Another attitude that the nurse must demonstrate is

one of creativity. Because chronic wounds are difficult to heal, the nurse must be diligent in evaluating nursing interventions and determining which interventions are effective and which need to be modified.

Nursing Process

Assessment

Baseline and continual assessment data provide critical information about the client's skin integrity and the increased risk for pressure ulcer development.

Skin. The nurse continually assesses the skin for signs of ulcer development (Box 47-5). The neurologically impaired client; the chronically ill client in long-term care; the client with diminished mental status; and the intensive care unit (ICU), oncology, hospice, or orthopedic client have increased potential for developing pressure ulcers.

Assessment for tissue pressure indicators includes visual and tactile inspection of the skin. Baseline assessment is performed to determine the client's normal skin characteristics and any actual or potential areas of breakdown. Assessment characteristics of a client's skin should be individualized, depending on the client's skin tone (Bennett, 1995; Henderson and others, 1997). Assessment characteristics of darkly pigmented skin were described earlier (see Boxes 47-2, p. 1486, and 47-3, p. 1489). The nurse pays particular attention to areas located over bony prominences, under casts, traction, splints, braces, collars, or other orthopedic devices. The frequency of pressure checks depends on the schedule of appliance application and the skin's response to the external pressure (Figure 47-10).

When hyperemia is noted, the nurse documents the location, size, and color and reassesses the area after 1 hour

---

Box 47-5 *Procedural Guidelines*

Skin Assessment

Delegation considerations: Assessment for presence of skin breakdown is a nursing responsibility and should not be delegated to assistive personnel (AP). However, it is important that the nurse instruct AP to report the following:
  a. Any changes in the client's skin to the nurse immediately
  b. Client's exposure to body fluids (e.g., urine, feces, wound drainage, gastric secretions)

1. Obtain appropriate equipment (check agency policy).
   a. Skin assessment documentation record
2. Observe pressure points. Compression of these areas for prolonged periods of time by bony prominences or external sources can cause tissue ischemia and cell death (AHCPR, 1992a).
   a. Bony prominences—heels, ankles, knees, hips, sacral area, ischial area, spinal area, shoulders, and elbows (see Figure 47-12)
   b. Cast edges, area next to nasogastric tubes, drainage tubes, or oxygen tubing
3. When reddened areas are found, gently press the area with a gloved finger to assess the ability of the tissue to blanch. Reactive hyperemia occurs when a reddened area blanches upon palpation. If the area does not blanch, suspect tissue injury.
4. Check perineal area for signs of reddened, irritated skin. Perineal skin is at high risk for skin breakdown in the client with fecal and/or urinary incontinence.
5. Observe underlying skin areas where tape, tubing, casts, or splints are in contact with skin.
6. Note previous areas of skin breakdown, check for any breaks in the skin integrity, or note nonblanching erythema in this area. Areas of previous skin breakdown do not heal to the same strength as intact noninjured skin; therefore these areas are at higher risk of skin breakdown.
7. Determine if potential or actual skin breakdown is present and institute appropriate preventative or treatment protocols.
8. Record appearance of skin under pressure.
9. Record what preventative or treatment protocols were initiated.

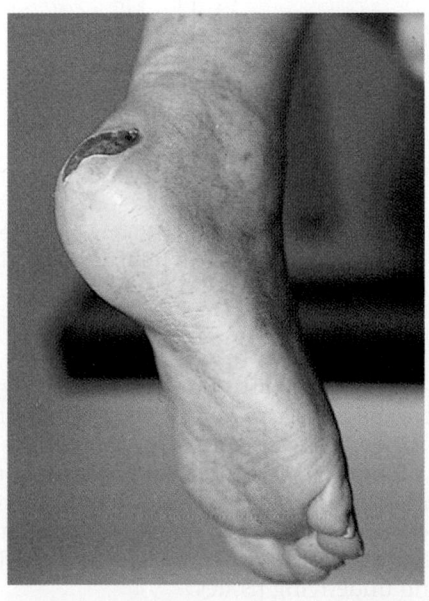

FIGURE **47–10** Formation of pressure ulcer on heel resulting from external pressure from mattress of bed.

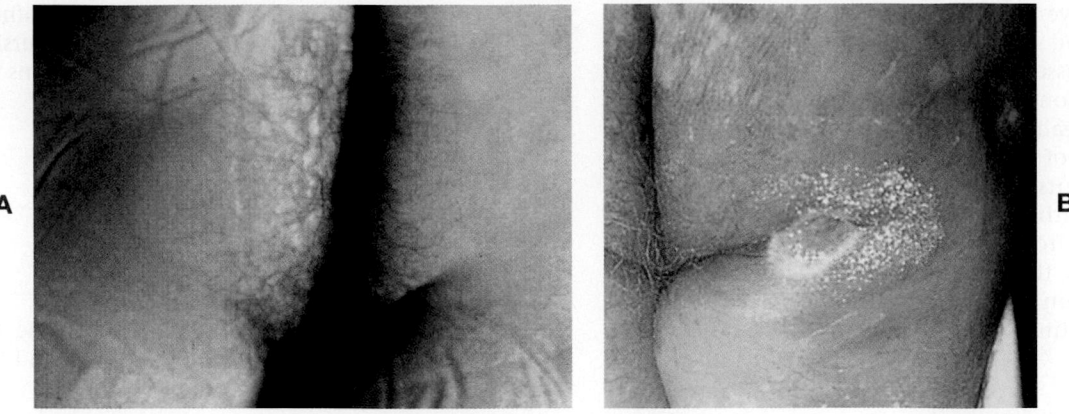

FIGURE **47–11**   **A,** Hyperemia on ischial tuberosities. **B,** Deeper stages of ulceration. (From Pires M, Muller A: Detection and management of early tissue pressure indicators: a pictorial essay, *Progressions* 3[3]:3, 1991.)

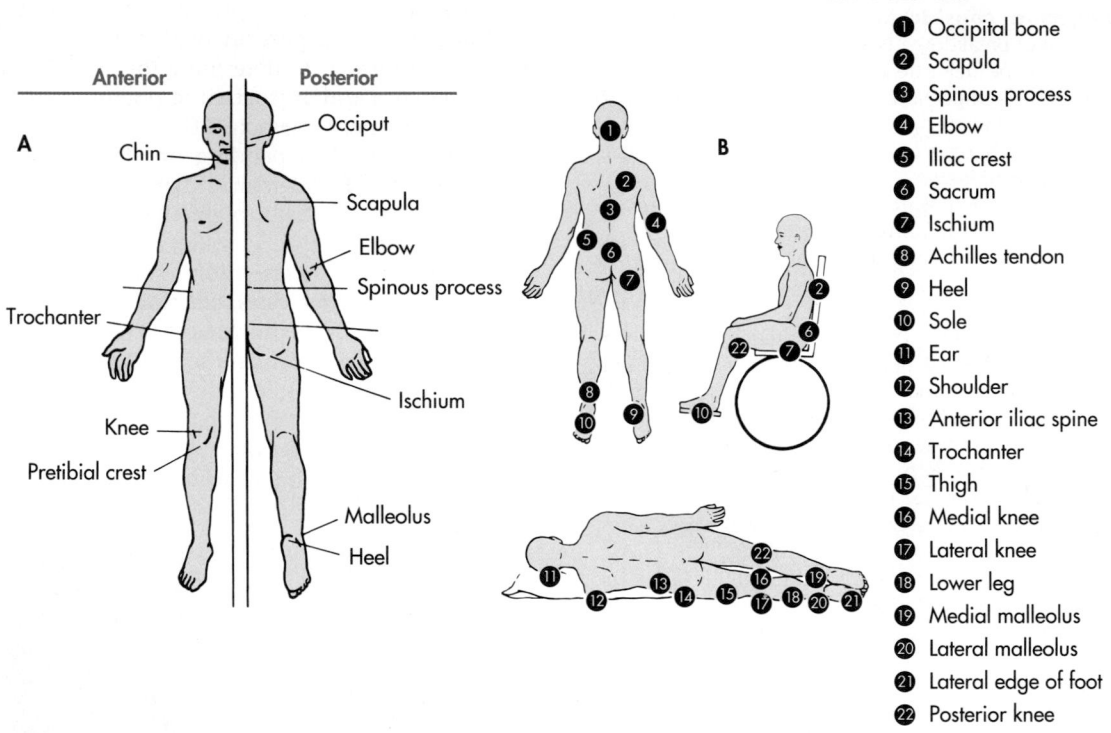

Pressure ulcer sites

❶ Occipital bone
❷ Scapula
❸ Spinous process
❹ Elbow
❺ Iliac crest
❻ Sacrum
❼ Ischium
❽ Achilles tendon
❾ Heel
❿ Sole
⓫ Ear
⓬ Shoulder
⓭ Anterior iliac spine
⓮ Trochanter
⓯ Thigh
⓰ Medial knee
⓱ Lateral knee
⓲ Lower leg
⓳ Medial malleolus
⓴ Lateral malleolus
㉑ Lateral edge of foot
㉒ Posterior knee

FIGURE **47–12**   **A,** Bony prominences most frequently underlying pressure ulcer. **B,** Pressure ulcer sites. (Modified from Trelease CC: Developing standards for wound care, *Ostomy Wound Manage* 20:46, 1988.)

(Figure 47-11, *A*). When **abnormal reactive hyperemia** is suspected, the nurse can outline the affected area with a marker to make reassessment easier. These signs are early indicators of impaired skin integrity, but damage to the underlying tissue may be more progressive (Figure 47-11, *B*). Tactile assessment enables the nurse to use palpation to acquire further data about **induration** and the damage to the skin and underlying tissues.

The nurse palpates the reddened tissue, observing for blanching with return to normal skin tones in clients with light-toned skin. In addition, the nurse palpates for induration, noting the size in millimeters or centimeters of the induration around the injured area. The nurse also uses palpation to note changes in temperature of the surrounding skin and tissues.

The nurse includes visual and tactile inspection over the body areas most frequently at risk for pressure ulcer development (Figure 47-12). When a client lies in bed or sits in a chair, body weight is heavily placed on certain bony prominences. Body surfaces subjected to the greatest weight or pressure are at greatest risk for pressure ulcer formation.

Pressure Ulcers. Because pressure ulcers have multiple etiological factors, assessment for pressure ulcer risk (Skill 47-1) includes several important factors. These include using an appropriate predictive measure and assessing the client's mobility, nutrition, presence of body fluids, and comfort level.

Predictive Measures. On admission to acute care and rehabilitation hospitals, nursing homes, home care programs, and other health care facilities, individuals should be assessed for risk of pressure ulcer development (AHCPR, 1992a). Pressure ulcer risk assessment should be done systematically (NPUAP, 1989; AHCPR, 1992a). An assessment tool, such as the Norton or Braden scales, which is designed to measure the risk for developing a pressure ulcer is recommended (see Tables 47-3, p. 1495, and 47-4, p. 1496). Interpretation of the meaning of the total numerical scores differs with each risk assessment scale. Lower numerical score on the Braden Scale or the Norton Scale indicate that a client is at high risk for skin breakdown. A benefit of the predictive instruments is to increase the nurse's early detection of clients at greatest risk for ulcer development. Once these clients are identified, appropriate interventions are instituted to maintain skin integrity. Reassessment for pressure ulcer risk should be done periodically. Once a client is identified to be at risk for developing pressure ulcers, prevention strategies should be implemented (AHCPR, 1992a; NPUAP, 1995a).

Mobility. Assessment includes documenting the level of mobility and the potential effects of impaired mobility on skin integrity. Documenting assessment of mobility should also include obtaining data regarding the quality of muscle tone and strength. For example, the nurse determines whether the client can lift weight off of the sacral area and roll the body to a side-lying position. The client may have adequate range of motion (ROM) to move independently into a more protective position. Finally, the nurse notes the client's activity tolerance (see Chapter 36).

Mobility must be assessed as part of baseline data. If the client has some degree of independence in mobility, the nurse reinforces the frequency of position changes and measures to relieve pressure. The frequency of position changes is based on ongoing skin assessment and is revised as data change. The nurse must be meticulous when assessing pressure sites.

Nutritional Status. An assessment of the client's nutritional status should be an integral part of the initial assessment data for clients at risk for impaired skin integrity and wounds (Stotts, 2000). Malnutrition is a major risk factor for pressure ulcer development (Horn and others, 2002). A loss of 5% of usual weight, weight less than 90% of ideal body weight, or a decrease of 10 pounds in a brief period are all signs of actual or potential nutritional problems (Stotts, 2000).

Body Fluids. Continual exposure of the skin to body fluids also increases the client's risk for skin breakdown and pressure ulcer formation. Some body fluids, such as saliva and serosanguineous drainage, are not a caustic to the

---

Box *47-6*   Wound History Assessment Questions

What caused the wound?
When did the wound occur? What is its location and dimensions?
When did the client receive a tetanus shot?
What happened to this wound since it occurred? What were the changes, and what caused them?
What treatments, activities, or care have slowed or helped the wound-healing process? Are there special needs for this wound to heal?
Are there associated symptoms such as pain or itching with the wound? How are they being managed, and are they effective?
What is the goal for the client, wound, and healing?

Modified from Stotts NA, Cavanaugh CE: Assessing the patient with a wound, *Home Healthc Nurse* 17(1):27, 1999.

---

skin and the risk of skin breakdown from exposure to these fluids is low. However, exposure to urine, bile, stool, acetic fluid, and purulent wound exudates carries a moderate risk for skin breakdown, especially in clients who have other risk factors, such as chronic illness or poor nutrition. Last, exposure to gastric and pancreatic drainage has the highest risk for skin breakdown. Again, it is important to prevent and reduce the client's exposure to body fluids, and when exposure occurs, meticulous hygiene and skin care must be provided.

Pain. Until recently, little has been written or researched about pain and pressure ulcers. The AHCPR (1994) has recommended that the assessment and management of pain be included in the care of clients with pressure ulcers (Krasner, 2001). Maintaining adequate pain control and client comfort increased the client's willingness and ability to increase mobility, which in turn reduces pressure ulcer risk.

Wounds. The nurse often assesses wounds under two conditions: at the time of injury before treatment and after therapy, when the wound is relatively stable. Each condition requires the nurse to make different observations and to take different actions. Regardless of the setting, it is important that the nurse initially obtain information regarding the cause and history of the wound (Box 47-6).

Emergency Setting. The nurse may see wounds in any setting, including clinic, emergency department, youth camps, or the nurse's own backyard. The type of wound determines the criteria for inspection. For example, the nurse need not inspect for signs of internal bleeding after an abrasion but should do so in the event of a puncture wound.

When a client's condition is judged to be stable because of the presence of spontaneous breathing, a clear airway, and a strong carotid pulse (see Chapter 39), the nurse inspects the wound for bleeding. An **abrasion** is superficial with little bleeding and is considered a partial-thickness

Assessment for Risk of Pressure Ulcer Development

Skill 47-1

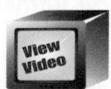

Delegation Considerations

Assessment of clients for risk of pressure ulcers should not be delegated to assistive personnel (AP). However, the AP may have other aspects of client care delegated, and the nurse should instruct AP to do the following:

- Report any changes, such as redness, blistering, abrasion, or cuts, to the client's skin to the nurse for further nursing assessment.
- Keep the client's skin dry and provide hygiene following incontinence of urine or stool or exposure to other body fluids.

- Reposition the client according to the frequency established on the nursing care plan or agency policy.
- Avoid trauma to the client's skin from tape, pressure, friction, or shear.

Equipment

- Risk assessment tool, Braden Scale (used in this skill) or Norton Scale
- Documentation record

Steps	Rationale
1. Identify at-risk individuals needing prevention and the specific factors placing them at risk.	Determines factors that increase the client's risk for developing pressure ulcers (Braden, 2001).
a. Use a validated risk assessment tool such as the Braden Scale or Norton Scale.	Ensures consistent, reliable, comparable assessments (AHCPR, 1992a; NPUAP, 1995a).
b. Assess the client upon admission to acute care, rehabilitation hospitals, nursing homes, home care programs, and other health care facilities.	Provides a baseline assessment.
c. Inspect the condition of the client's skin at least once a day (see Box 47-5, p. 1501) and examine all bony prominences, noting skin integrity. (Check agency policy for reassessment and reassess at periodic intervals.) If redness or discoloration is noted, use thumb to gently palpate area of redness. The discoloration may vary from pink to deep red.	Routine skin assessments will identify changes in client's pressure ulcer risk. Nonblanchable erythema or discoloration in the client's skin may be an early indicator of skin injury (Pieper, 2000).

Critical Decision Point: In dark-skinned clients the discoloration appears as a deepening of the normal ethnic color (see Boxes 47-2, p. 1486, and 47-3, p. 1489). Darkly pigmented skin does not always show direct changes in color (Bennett, 1995; NPUAP, 1998).

d. Observe all assistive devices, such as braces or casts, and medical equipment, such as nasogastric tubes and catheters, for pressure points.	Presence of medical equipment has the potential to cause pressure and skin breakdown to sensitive regions, such as the nares, ears, over bony prominences, and other pressure areas.
2. Determine the client's ability to respond meaningfully to pressure-related discomfort (sensory perception).	Client with completely, very, or slightly limited ability to respond to pressure-related discomfort cannot communicate discomfort, will have a limitation in the ability to feel pain, and thus will have a risk for developing pressure ulcers.
3. Assess the degree to which the client's skin is exposed to moisture.	A person whose skin is exposed to excessive moisture has an increased risk of developing skin breakdown.
4. Evaluate the client's activity level.	The client who is bedfast, chairfast, or only walks occasionally will be at risk for developing pressure areas because of the degree of physical inactivity.
a. Determine the client's ability to change and control body position (mobility).	Potential for friction and shear increases when the client is completely dependent on others for position change.
b. Determine client's preferred positions.	Weight of body will be placed on certain bony prominences, and the client may resist repositioning off these areas.

Steps	Rationale
5. Assess the client's usual food intake pattern (nutrition).	A client who never eats a complete meal or rarely eats a complete meal is at risk for pressure ulcer formation.
a. Review weight pattern and nutritional laboratory values (see Box 47-12, p. 1527).	Decreased nutrition status is linked with pressure ulcer formation and poor pressure wound healing (AHCPR, 1994).
b. Complete fluid intake assessment.	Fluid imbalance, either dehydration or edema, can increase the client's risk for pressure ulcers.
6. Evaluate the presence of friction and/or shear.	The client who has a problem in moving, requires maximum assistance in moving, or slides against sheets when moved is at an increased risk of skin damage.
7. Document the risk assessment (Cooper, 2000).	The documentation will provide a baseline for comparison of increased or decreased risk for development of pressure ulcers and allow planning of interventions.
a. As the Braden Scale scores become lower, predicted risk becomes higher.	Scores: 15 to 18, at risk 13 to 14, moderate risk 10 to 12, high risk 9 or below, very high risk
b. Link the risk assessment to preventative protocols.	Prevention protocols will target problem areas to assist in prevention of skin breakdown.
c. Institute at-risk interventions (score of 15 to 18). Consider instituting frequent turning, protection of client's heels, use of a pressure reducing support surface, and managing moisture.	Decreases the risk of skin breakdown.
d. Institute moderate risk interventions (score of 13 to 14). Consider a protocol of frequent turning, protect client's heels, provide a pressure-reducing support surface, provide foam wedges for 30-degree lateral positioning, and manage moisture, shear, and friction.	Decreases the increased risk of skin breakdown with appropriate interventions.
e. Institute high-risk interventions (score of 10 to 12). Consider a protocol that increases the frequency of turning, supplements turning with small shifts in position, facilitates maximal remobilization, protects the client's heels, provides a pressure-reducing support surface, provides foam wedges for 30-degree lateral positioning, and manages moisture, friction, and shear. If needed, institute nutritional interventions to reduce risk of pressure ulcer development.	Addresses the factors that contribute to skin breakdown and plans for interventions to address the causative factors.
f. Institute very high-risk interventions (score of 9 or below). Consider a protocol that incorporates the points for high-risk clients plus uses a pressure-relieving surface if the client has intractable pain, severe pain exacerbated by turning.	Plans interventions to decrease the effects of immobility, decreased sensory perception, moisture, friction, shear, decreased activity, and nutritional issues in a high-risk individual.
8. Provide education to client and family regarding pressure ulcer risk and prevention.	Assists clients and family to understand the interventions designed to reduce pressure ulcer risk.
9. Evaluate measures to reduce pressure ulcer development a. Observe client's skin for areas at risk.	Determines over time client's response to risk reduction interventions.
b. Observe tolerance of client for positioning.	Frequent change in position furthers reduces client's risk for pressure ulcer development.
c. Monitor the success of a toileting program or other measures to reduce the frequency of incontinence of urine or stool.	Determines timeliness of a toileting program or schedule to assist the client in meeting elimination needs.
d. Evaluate nutrition laboratory values.	Determines the success of nutritional supplements in improving nutritional status.

Skill 47-1   *Assessment for Risk of Pressure Ulcer Development—cont'd*

Unexpected Outcomes and Related Interventions

1. Skin does not blanch when firmly pressed, has purple discoloration, or has significant color change.
   a. Reassess frequency of turning schedule.
   b. Implement agency's skin care protocols.
   c. Consider support surface to reduce pressure ulcer risk.

Recording and Reporting

- Record client's risk score.
- Record appearance of skin under pressure.
- Describe position, turning intervals, pressure-relieving devices, and other prevention strategies.
- Report any need for additional consultations for the high-risk client.

Home Care Considerations

- Instruct caregiver on the use of the 30-degree lateral position. This position prolongs the time between position changes, resulting in fewer sleep interruptions for client and caregiver.
- Pressure-relief maneuvers need to be individualized for client need and home environment. Provide family with resources for hospital equipment.

---

wound. The wound may appear "weepy" because of plasma leakage from damaged capillaries. A **laceration** may bleed more profusely, depending on the wound's depth and location. For example, minor scalp lacerations tend to bleed profusely because of the rich blood supply to the scalp. Lacerations greater than 5 cm (2 inches) long or 2.5 cm (1 inch) deep can cause serious bleeding. **Puncture** wounds bleed in relation to the depth and size of the wound; for example, a nail puncture does not cause as much bleeding as a knife wound. The primary dangers of puncture wounds are internal bleeding and infection.

The nurse next inspects the wound for foreign bodies or contaminant material. Most traumatic wounds are dirty. Soil, broken glass, shreds of cloth, and foreign substances clinging to penetrating objects can become embedded in the wound.

The size of the wound is the next criterion for inspection. A deep laceration requires suturing. A large, open wound may expose bone or tissue that should be protected.

When the injury is a result of trauma from a dirty penetrating object, the nurse determines when the client last received a tetanus toxoid injection. Tetanus bacteria reside in soil and in the gut of humans and animals. A tetanus antitoxin injection is necessary if the client has not had one within 5 years.

Stable Setting. When the client's condition is stabilized (e.g., after surgery or treatment) the nurse assesses the wound to determine progress toward healing. If the wound is covered by a dressing and the physician has not ordered it changed, the nurse should not directly inspect the wound unless serious complications are suspected. In such a situation the nurse should inspect only the dressing and any external drains. If the physician prefers to change the dressing, the physician will assess the wound at least daily. When the nurse removes dressings, care is taken to avoid accidental removal or displacement of underlying drains. Because removal of dressings can be painful, it may help to give an analgesic at least 30 minutes before exposing a wound.

Wound Appearance. The nurse observes whether wound edges are closed. A surgical incision healing by primary intention should have clean, well-approximated edges. Crusts often form along the wound edges from exudate. A puncture wound is usually a small, circular wound with the edges coming together toward the center. If a wound is open, the wound edges are separated, and the nurse inspects the condition of tissue at the wound base. The nurse also looks for complications such as dehiscence and evisceration. The outer edges of a wound normally appear inflamed for the first 2 to 3 days, but this slowly disappears. Within 7 to 10 days a normally healing wound resurfaces with epithelial cells, and edges close. Table 47-7 lists assessment characteristics for abnormal wound healing in primary and secondary wounds. If infection develops, the area directly surrounding the wound becomes brightly inflamed and swollen.

Skin discoloration usually results from bruising of interstitial tissues or hematoma formation. Blood collecting beneath the skin first takes on a bluish or purplish appearance. Gradually, as the clotted blood is broken down, shades of brown and yellow appear.

Character of Wound Drainage. The nurse notes the amount, color, odor, and consistency of drainage. The amount of drainage depends on the location and extent of the wound. For example, drainage is minimal after a simple appendectomy. In contrast, wound drainage is moderate for 1 to 2 days after drainage of a large abscess.

Table 47-7	Assessment of Abnormal Healing in Primary and Secondary Intention Wounds	
Primary Wounds	**Secondary Wounds**	
Incision line poorly approximated	Pale or fragile granulation tissue, granulation tissue bed may be excessively dry or moist	
Drainage present more than 3 days after closure	Exudate present	
Inflammation decreased in first 3-5 days after injury	Necrotic or slough tissue present in wound base	
No epithelialization of wound edges by day 4	Epithelialization not continuous	
No healing ridge by day 9	Fruity, earthy, or putrid odor present	
	Presence of fistula(s), tunneling, undermining	

Modified from Stotts NA, Cavanaugh CE: Assessing the patient with a wound, *Home Healthc Nurse* 17(1):27, 1999.

If the nurse needs an accurate measurement of the amount of drainage within a dressing, the dressing can be weighed and compared with the weight of the same dressing when clean and dry. A rule of thumb is 1 g by weight of drainage equals 1 ml of volume of drainage. Another method of quantifying wound drainage would be to chart the number of dressings used and the frequency of change. An increase in the number or frequency of dressings will indicate a relative increase or decrease in wound drainage. The color and consistency of drainage vary depending on the components. Types of drainage include the following: **serous, sanguineous, serosanguineous,** and purulent (see Table 47-2, p. 1494).

If the drainage has a pungent or strong odor, an infection should be suspected. The nurse should describe the wound's appearance according to characteristics observed. An example of accurate recording follows:

> Abdominal incision is 5 cm in width, in RLQ (right lower quadrant); edges well approximated without inflammation or exudate. 1.2-cm diameter circle of serous drainage present on one 4 × 4 gauze changed every 8 hours.

Drains. The physician inserts a drain into or near a surgical wound if a large amount of drainage is expected. Some drains are sutured in place. Caution should be exercised when changing the dressing around drains that are not sutured in place to prevent accidental removal. A Penrose drain may lie under a dressing; at the time of placement a pin or clip is placed through the drain to prevent it from slipping farther into a wound (Figure 47-13). It is usually the physician's responsibility to pull or advance the drain as drainage decreases to permit healing deep within the drain site.

The nurse assesses the number of drains, drain placement, character of drainage, and condition of collecting apparatus. First the nurse observes the security of the drain and its location with respect to the wound. Next the nurse notes the character of drainage. If there is a collecting device, the nurse measures the drainage volume. Because a drainage system must be patent, the nurse looks for drainage flow through the tubing, as well as around the tubing. A sudden decrease in drainage through the tubing may indicate a blocked drain, and the physician should be notified. When a drain is connected to suction, the nurse assesses the system to be sure that the pressure ordered is being exerted. Evacuator units

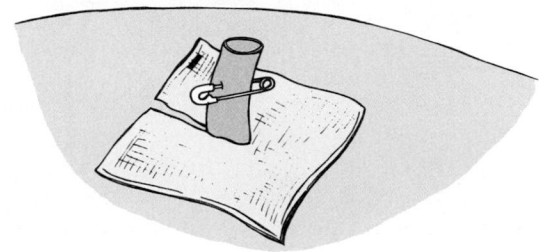

FIGURE **47–13** Penrose drain.

such as a Hemovac or Jackson-Pratt (Figure 47-14) exert a constant low pressure as long as the suction device (bladder or bag) is fully compressed. These types of drainage devices are often referred to as self-suction. When the evacuator device is unable to maintain a vacuum on its own, the nurse notifies the surgeon, who can then order a secondary vacuum system (such as wall suction). If fluid is allowed to accumulate within the tissues, wound healing will not progress at an optimal rate, and the risk of infection is increased.

Wound Closures. Surgical wounds are closed with staples, sutures, or wound closures. A frequent skin closure is the stainless-steel staple. The staple provides more strength than nylon or silk sutures and tends to cause less irritation to tissue. The nurse looks for irritation around staple or suture sites and notes whether closures are intact. The nurse may choose to count sutures when the physician has removed a portion of them. Normally for the first 2 to 3 days after surgery the skin around sutures or staples is edematous. Continued swelling may indicate that the closures are too tight. The skin can be cut by overly tight suture material, leading to wound separation. Sutures that are too tight are a common cause of wound dehiscence. Early suture removal reduces formation of defects along the suture line and minimizes chances of unattractive scar formation.

Palpation of Wound. When inspecting a wound, the nurse may observe swelling or separation of wound edges. While wearing gloves, the nurse lightly palpates wound edges, detecting localized areas of tenderness or drainage collection. The nurse gently applies the fingertips along the wound edges. If pressure causes fluid to be expressed, the nurse notes the character of the drainage.

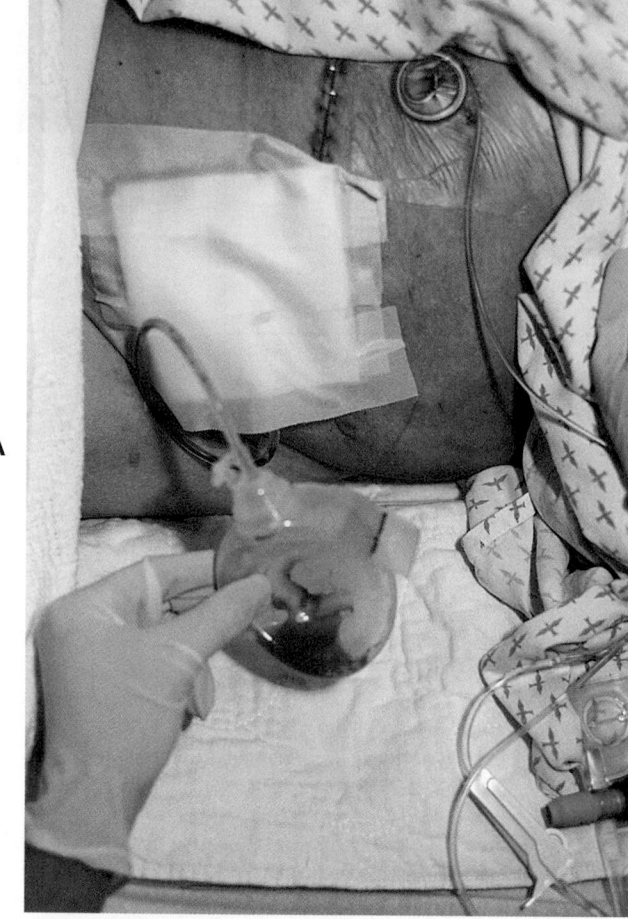

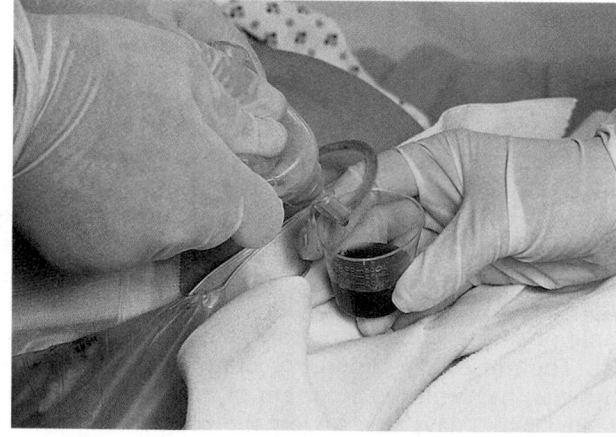

FIGURE **47–14** Jackson-Pratt drainage device. **A,** Drainage tubes and reservoir. **B,** Emptying drainage reservoir.

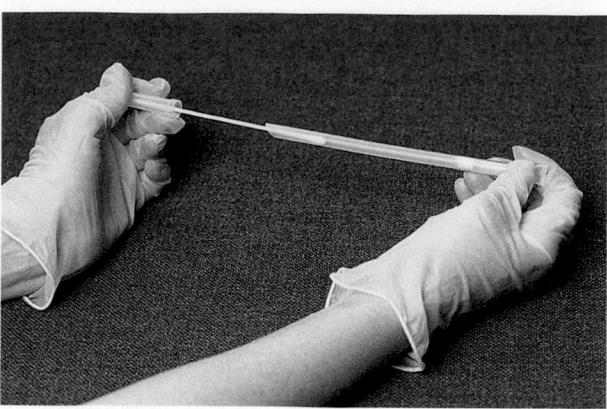

FIGURE **47–15** Wound culturette tube.

<table>
<tr><td>*Box* **47-7**</td><td>**Recommendations for Standardized Techniques for Wound Cultures***</td></tr>
</table>

Needle Aspiration Procedure

- Clean intact skin with a disinfectant solution. Allow to dry.
- Draw 0.5 ml of air into the syringe and insert the needle through intact skin adjacent to the wound.
- Apply suction by withdrawing the plunger to the 10-ml mark. Move the needle backward and forward at different angles for two to four explorations.
- Withdraw the needle from the tissue and return the plunger to the 0.5-ml mark.

Quantitative Swab Procedure

- Clean the wound surface with a nonantiseptic solution.
- Moisten the swab with normal saline.
- Rotate the swab in 1 cm² of clean tissue in the open wound. Apply pressure to the swab to elicit tissue fluid. Insert the tip of the swab is inserted into the appropriate sterile container and transport to the laboratory.

Modified from Stotts NA: Wound infection: diagnosis and management. In Bryant RA, editor: *Acute and chronic wounds: nursing management,* ed 2, St. Louis, 2000, Mosby.
*Check agency policy to determine need to obtain physician order.

It may be necessary to collect the drainage for culture. The client is normally sensitive to palpation of wound edges. Extreme tenderness may indicate infection.

Wound Cultures. If the nurse detects purulent or suspicious-looking drainage, obtaining a specimen of the drainage for culture may be necessary (see Chapter 33). The nurse never collects a wound culture sample from old drainage. Resident colonies of bacteria from the skin grow within exudate and may not be the true causative organisms of a wound infection. The nurse cleans a wound first with normal saline to remove skin flora. Aerobic organisms grow in superficial wounds exposed to the air, and anaerobic organisms tend to grow within body cavities. The nurse uses a different method of specimen collection for each type of organism (Box 47-7).

To collect an aerobic specimen, the nurse uses a sterile swab from a culturette tube (Figure 47-15). If wound edges are separated, the nurse slowly and gently inserts the tip of the swab into the wound to collect deeper secretions. The nurse needs to apply sufficient pressure with the swab

Nursing Diagnostic Process

Box 47-8

Assessment Activities	Defining Characteristics	Nursing Diagnosis
Inspect surface of skin.	Presence of wound, break in skin integrity Yellow, foul-smelling drainage from wound Edges of wound not approximated Sutures remain in place	Impaired skin integrity related to contaminated wound
Inspect wound for signs of healing.	Brown-red drainage 5 days after surgery Edges of wound not approximated	
Obtain client's temperature, heart rate, white blood cell count, and serum albumin.	Client is febrile, heart rate is 125 beats per minute, leukocyte (white blood cell) count is 12,000/mm³, serum albumin less than 3.5 mg/100 ml.	

to cause some tissue fluid to be expressed in an area the size of 1 cm^2 and collected onto the tip of the swab (Stotts, 2000). After collecting the specimen, the nurse returns the swab to the culturette tube, caps the tube, and crushes the inner ampule containing the medium for organism growth. The medium must moisten and coat the swab tip. The nurse immediately sends the labeled specimen to the laboratory for quantitative bacterial cultures rather than swab cultures (AHCPR, 1994).

If drainage from a deep body cavity has a foul odor, there is a chance of anaerobic organism growth. The nurse uses a sterile syringe tip to aspirate drainage from the inner wound. Afterward the nurse applies a sterile needle to the syringe, expels air from the syringe and needle, and places a cork over the needle to prevent entrance of air. In some institutions the nurse may inject the specimen into a special vacuum container with a culture medium.

Gram stains are often performed as well. This test often allows the physician to order appropriate treatment earlier than when only cultures are done. No additional specimens are usually required. The microbiology laboratory needs only to be notified to perform the additional test.

Client Expectations. When clients have an acute surgical or traumatic wound, the wound may heal promptly and without complications. However, when pressure ulcers or chronic wounds are present, the course of treatment is lengthy and costly. Because the client and family must be involved with wound care management, it is important to know the client's expectations. A client who has realistic goals and is informed about the length of time for wound healing is more likely to adhere to the specific therapies designed to promote wound healing and prevent further skin breakdown.

Nursing Diagnosis

Assessment reveals clusters of data that indicate whether an actual or a risk for *impaired skin integrity* exists. In addition, the assessment data may support more than one

diagnostic label. For example, a postoperative client has purulent drainage from a surgical wound and reports tenderness around the area of the wound. These data would support a nursing diagnosis of *infection* (Box 47-8). After completing an assessment of the client's wound, the nurse identifies nursing diagnoses that will direct supportive and preventive care. There are multiple nursing diagnoses associated with impaired skin integrity and wounds:

- Risk for infection
- Imbalanced nutrition: less than body requirements
- Acute or chronic pain
- Impaired physical mobility
- Impaired skin integrity
- Risk for impaired skin integrity
- Ineffective tissue perfusion
- Impaired tissue integrity

The client may be at risk for poor wound healing because of previously defined factors that impair healing. Thus even though the client's wound may appear normal, the nurse identifies nursing diagnoses, such as *impaired nutrition* or *impaired tissue perfusion*, that direct nursing care toward support of wound repair.

The nature of a wound can cause problems unrelated to wound healing. Alteration in comfort and impaired mobility are problems that have implications for the client's eventual recovery. For example, a large abdominal incision can cause enough pain to interfere with the client's ability to turn in bed effectively.

Planning

After identifying nursing diagnoses, the nurse develops a plan of care for the client who has actual or is at risk for impaired skin integrity. During planning the nurse again synthesizes information from multiple resources (Figure 47-16). Critical thinking ensures that the client's plan of care integrates all that the nurse knows about the individual, as well as key critical thinking elements. Professional standards are especially important to consider when the nurse develops a plan of care.

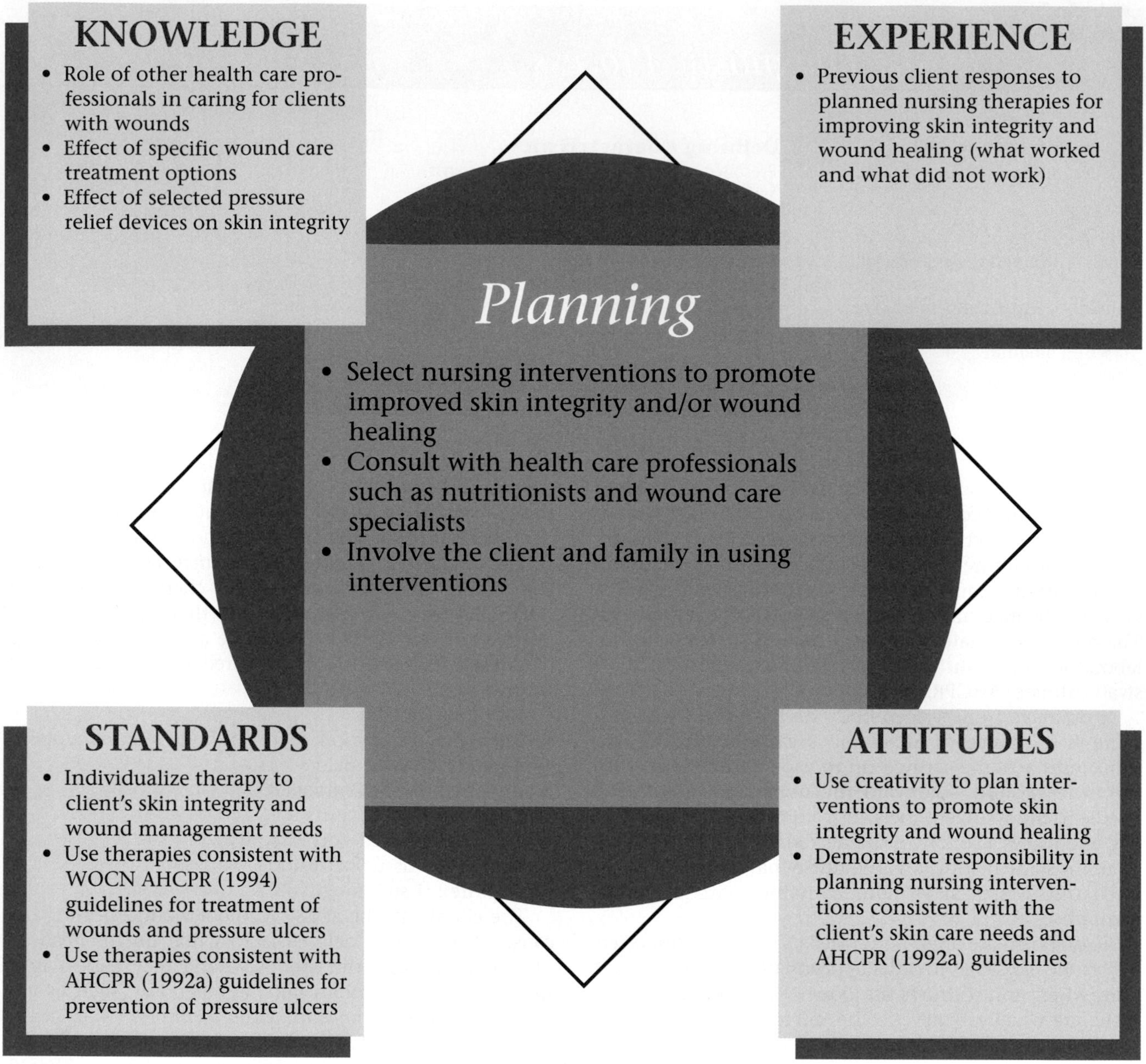

KNOWLEDGE

- Role of other health care pro-fessionals in caring for clients with wounds
- Effect of specific wound care treatment options
- Effect of selected pressure relief devices on skin integrity

EXPERIENCE

- Previous client responses to planned nursing therapies for improving skin integrity and wound healing (what worked and what did not work)

Planning

- Select nursing interventions to promote improved skin integrity and/or wound healing
- Consult with health care professionals such as nutritionists and wound care specialists
- Involve the client and family in using interventions

STANDARDS

- Individualize therapy to client's skin integrity and wound management needs
- Use therapies consistent with WOCN AHCPR (1994) guidelines for treatment of wounds and pressure ulcers
- Use therapies consistent with AHCPR (1992a) guidelines for prevention of pressure ulcers

ATTITUDES

- Use creativity to plan inter-ventions to promote skin integrity and wound healing
- Demonstrate responsibility in planning nursing interven-tions consistent with the client's skin care needs and AHCPR (1992a) guidelines

FIGURE **47–16** Critical thinking model for skin integrity and wound care planning.

Clients who have large or chronic wounds have multiple nursing care needs. For example, consider the following scenario:

A nurse is caring for Mrs. Kathy Crane. Mrs. Crane is a 65-year-old woman with a 30-year history of diabetes mellitus, for which she takes insulin. Her diabetes is poorly controlled due to her inability to adhere to a 1200-calorie diet. She is 70 pounds overweight. For the last 10 years, she has reported decreased sensation to her lower extremities. She does not practice good foot care; she cuts her own toenails and goes barefoot. She was admitted to the hospital for elective repair of an abdominal aneurysm. The surgery went well, but postoperatively Mrs. Crane had dif-

ficulty ambulating and performing coughing and deep breathing exercises. On her second postoperative day she developed a postoperative pneumonia, which required intravenous antibiotics. During the course of her pneumonia, Mrs. Crane refused to walk, she became incontinent of urine and stool, and she complained about position changes. After her position was changed, she would reposition herself on her back. Two weeks after her surgery Mrs. Crane developed a large draining sacral wound which is now 6 cm in diameter and is a stage IV pressure ulcer. In addition, she has a smaller, stage III ulcer on her left heel. Skin assessment also reveals areas of prolonged redness over pressure points, especially on the right heel and over both hips.

Concept Map

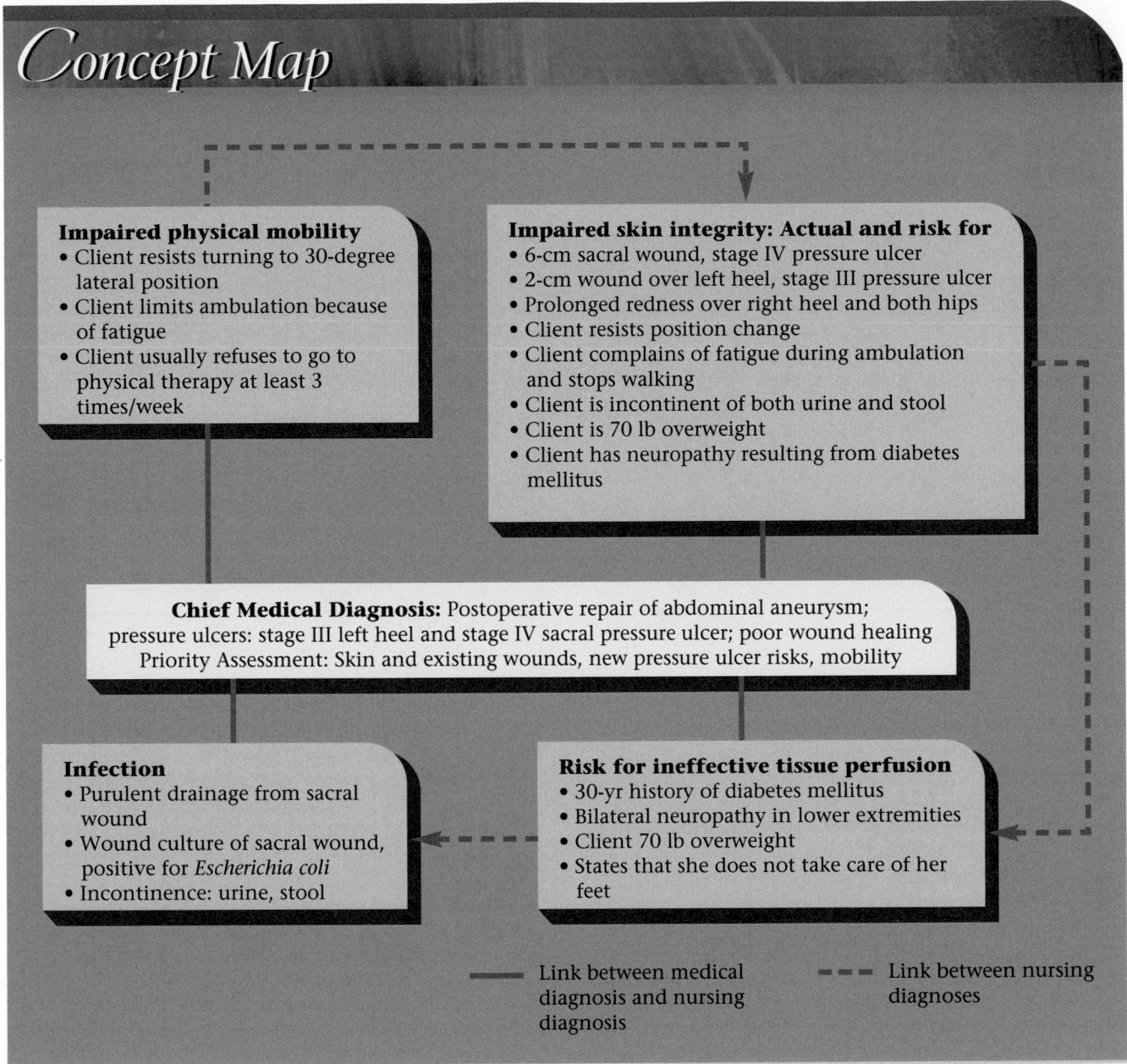

Impaired physical mobility
- Client resists turning to 30-degree lateral position
- Client limits ambulation because of fatigue
- Client usually refuses to go to physical therapy at least 3 times/week

Impaired skin integrity: Actual and risk for
- 6-cm sacral wound, stage IV pressure ulcer
- 2-cm wound over left heel, stage III pressure ulcer
- Prolonged redness over right heel and both hips
- Client resists position change
- Client complains of fatigue during ambulation and stops walking
- Client is incontinent of both urine and stool
- Client is 70 lb overweight
- Client has neuropathy resulting from diabetes mellitus

Chief Medical Diagnosis: Postoperative repair of abdominal aneurysm; pressure ulcers: stage III left heel and stage IV sacral pressure ulcer; poor wound healing
Priority Assessment: Skin and existing wounds, new pressure ulcer risks, mobility

Infection
- Purulent drainage from sacral wound
- Wound culture of sacral wound, positive for *Escherichia coli*
- Incontinence: urine, stool

Risk for ineffective tissue perfusion
- 30-yr history of diabetes mellitus
- Bilateral neuropathy in lower extremities
- Client 70 lb overweight
- States that she does not take care of her feet

——— Link between medical diagnosis and nursing diagnosis   - - - Link between nursing diagnoses

FIGURE **47–17** Concept map for client with a chronic wound.

When planning for care for Mrs. Crane, a concept map can help to individualize care for this client who may have multiple health problems and related nursing diagnoses (Figure 47-17). This map assists the nurse in using critical thinking skills to organize complex client assessment data and related nursing diagnoses with the client's chief medical diagnosis. As the nurse identifies linkages between the nursing diagnoses and the chief medical diagnosis, the concept map also links potential interventions with the client's health care needs.

Goals and Outcomes. Nursing care is based on the client's identified needs and priorities. Goals and expected outcomes are established, and from the goals the

nurse plans interventions according to the risk for pressure ulcers or the type and severity of the wound and the presence of any complications, such as infection, poor nutrition, peripheral vascular diseases, or immunosuppression, that can affect wound healing (see care plan).

A goal frequently identified when working with a client with a wound is to see wound improvement within a 2-week period. The outcomes of this goal might include the following:

- Higher percentage of granulation tissue in the wound base
- No further skin breakdown in any body location
- An increase in the caloric intake by 10%

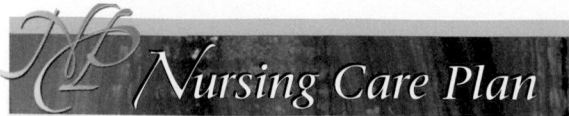

Nursing Care Plan

Skin Integrity and Wound Care

Assessment

Mrs. Stein is 3 weeks postoperative for a total hip replacement. She has developed a severe postoperative wound infection. She does not complain of discomfort in the operative site; however, she complains of a painful, burning sensation in the sacral region.

Assessment Activities	Findings/Defining Characteristics
Obtain an oral temperature.	Elevated temperature is noted.
Ask Ms. Stein how the surgical site limits her mobility.	She relates that her hip always aches and the pain is increased upon movement.
	She tells you that she prefers to keep the hip immobile to keep the pain level down.
	Position of comfort is supine, and Mrs. Stein resists position changes.
Perform a total body skin assessment, paying special attention to the sacral area.	Reactive hyperemia is noted over the sacral area; this area does not blanch upon palpation (Pieper, 2000).
	Skin over sacrum is blistered and has an abrasion (Braden, 2001).
	No other areas are noted to be open, with the exception of the surgical site.

Nursing Diagnosis: Impaired skin integrity related to pressure on the bony prominence in the sacral region.

Planning

Goal	Expected Outcomes*
	Tissue Integrity: Skin Mucous Membranes
Injury to client's skin and underlying tissue resulting from pressure on the bony prominence will be reduced within 2 to 4 weeks.	Client will have intact skin integrity in the area of non-blanching erythema.
	Mrs. Stein will maintain intact skin over other pressure points.
	Client's skin will remain clean and dry.
	Immobility Consequences: Physiological
Client's ability to tolerate position changes will improve within 2 to 4 weeks.	Reactive hyperemia will be within normal limits in all pressure points except sacral region.
	Reactive hyperemia in sacral region will have a decrease in nonblanchable pressure areas.

*Outcome classification labels from Moorhead S, Johnson M, Maas M: *Nursing outcomes classification (NOC)*, ed 3, St. Louis, 2004, Mosby.

Interventions†

Interventions†	Rationale
Pressure Management	
• Reposition client every 90 minutes. Turning interval: 120 minutes − 30 minutes hypoxia time = 90 minutes. Offer pain medication at least 20 minutes before position change.	Repositioning removes pressure and allows normal hyperemic response. Frequency of turning is based on initial assessment (Pieper, 2000; AHCPR, 1994).
• Place client on a low-air-loss overlay.	Clients with pressure ulcer development are at greater risk for new ulcers and need preventive measures to prevent ulcer progression (AHCPR, 1994; NPUAP, 1995a, 1995b).
Site Care	
• Keep area dry and clean; avoid rubbing the area.	Moisture can soften the skin and cause a break in the skin integrity. Rubbing an area of nonblanching erythema can cause further tissue damage (AHCPR, 1992a; Ratliff and Bryant, 2003).

†Intervention classification labels from Dochterman JM, Bulechek GM: *Nursing interventions classification (NIC)*, ed 4, St. Louis, 2004, Mosby.

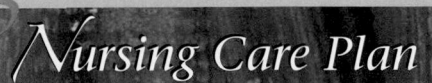

Nursing Care Plan

Skin Integrity and Wound Care—cont'd

Evaluation

Nursing Actions	Client Response/Findings	Achievement of Outcome
Perform a daily total body skin assessment. Chart results.	No new skin breakdown noted.	Client reports no other areas of pain or discomfort.
	Decreased redness at the sacral area.	Client reports decreased pain at the sacral site.
Palpate the reddened area over the sacrum	Sacral area begins to show signs of normal reactive hyperemia blanching following palpation.	Sacral region is improving; no break in epidermis.
	Other pressure points have normal reactive hyperemia and blanching.	Other pressure points remain intact.

These outcomes can be reasonable if the overall goal for the client is to heal the ulcer. The nurse plans therapies according to the severity and type of wound and the presence of any complicating conditions (e.g., infection, poor nutrition, immunosuppression, and diabetes) that may affect wound healing. Other goals of care for clients with wounds include the following: promoting wound hemostasis, preventing infection, promoting wound healing, maintaining skin integrity, gaining comfort, and health promotion.

Setting Priorities. The nursing care priorities in wound care are established based on the comprehensive client assessment and goal and established outcomes. These priorities also depend on whether the client's condition is stable or emergent. An acute wound needs immediate intervention, whereas in the presence of a chronic, stable wound, the client's hygiene needs may have a greater priority. When there is a risk for pressure ulcer development, preventive interventions, such as skin care practices, elimination of shear, and positioning, are high priorities. Promotion of wound healing is a major nursing priority, and the type of wound care administered depends on the type, size, and location of the wound, wound location, and overall treatment goals.

Other client factors to be considered when establishing priorities include client preferences, daily activities, and family factors. These factors are important regardless of the setting for health care. The priorities of care may not vary from outpatient, home, acute care, or restorative care settings.

Continuity of Care. With early discharge from the health care setting, it is important to consider the client's plan for discharge. Anticipating the client's discharge wound care needs and related equipment and resources, such as referral to a home care agency or outpatient wound care clinic, can assist not only in improving wound healing but also improve the client's level of independence. Clients and their families may need to continue the objectives of wound management after discharge (Box 47-9). The ability of the caregiver and the amount of time needed to change a particular dressing need to be considered when selecting a dressing that will be used by the client after discharge. For example, in the home setting, caregivers may choose more expensive dressing materials to reduce the frequency of dressing changes (AHCPR, 1994). The nurse and client work together to establish ways of maintaining client involvement in nursing care and to promote wound healing whether the client is in the hospital or home.

Implementation

Health Promotion. Perhaps the most effective intervention for problems with skin integrity and wound care is prevention. Prompt identification of high-risk clients and their risk factors aids in prevention of pressure ulcers.

Prevention of Pressure Ulcers. When the client is immobile, the major risk to the skin is the formation of pressure ulcers. Nursing interventions focus on prevention. The first step in prevention is to assess the client's risk factors for pressure ulcer development. The nurse plans on reducing or eliminating the identified risk factors.

Early identification of clients at risk and their risk factors aids the nurse in preventing pressure ulcers. Prevention minimizes the impact that risk factors or contributing factors may have on pressure ulcer development. Table 47-8 provides some universal preventive measures. Three major areas of nursing interventions for prevention of pressure ulcers are (1) skin care, which includes hygiene and skin care; (2) mechanical loading and support devices, which include proper positioning and the use of therapeutic surfaces; and (3) education (AHCPR, 1992a).

Topical Skin Care. The nurse must perform frequent skin assessment. This assessment should be done at a minimum on a once-a-day basis; however, high-risk clients will have more frequent skin assessments, such as at the beginning of each nursing shift. In addition, the nurse must ensure that the client's skin is clean and dry. Assessment and skin hygiene are two initial defenses for preventing skin breakdown.

When the skin is cleansed, soaps and hot water are avoided. Soaps and alcohol-based lotions cause drying

Box **47-9**   **Home Care Recommendations**

Ulcer/Wound Assessment

Assessment and documentation [of the pressure ulcer] should be carried out at least weekly, unless there is evidence of deterioration, in which case both the pressure ulcer and the client's overall management must be reassessed immediately. In the home setting, this may require the assistance of the client and family because weekly assessment by health care providers is not always feasible.

Psychosocial Assessment and Management

- Assess resources (e.g., availability and skill of caregivers, finances, equipment) of individuals being treated for pressure ulcers in the home. A successful treatment program requires adequate caregiver and equipment resources.
- Caregivers need to be evaluated for their ability to comprehend and implement the treatment requirements.
- Caregivers should also be evaluated for their level of strength and endurance.
- Economic factors should be considered, because they may limit the supply and availability of equipment, as well as opportunities to relieve caregivers.
- An approach is suggested that focuses upon the psychosocial and physical factors affecting wound care (Teare and Barrett, 2002).

Ulcer Care Dressings

- Consider caregiver time when selecting a dressing.
- In the home setting, caregivers may choose more expensive dressing materials to reduce the frequency of dressing changes.

Infection Control

- Clean dressings may also be used in the home setting.
- Clean dressings, as opposed to sterile ones, are recommended for home use until research demonstrates otherwise. This recommendation is in keeping with principles regarding nosocomial infections and with past success of clean urinary catheterization in the home setting, and it takes into account the expense of sterile dressings and the dexterity required for application. The "no-touch" technique can be used for dressing changes. This technique is a method of changing surface dressings without touching the wound or the surface of any dressing that might be in contact with the wound. Adherent dressings should be grasped by the corner and removed slowly, whereas gauze dressings can be pinched in the center and lifted off.
- Disposal of contaminated dressings in the home should be done in a manner consistent with local regulations. The Environmental Protection Agency recommends that soiled dressings be placed in securely fastened plastic bags before being added to other household trash. Local regulations vary, however, and home care agencies and clients are advised to follow procedures that are consistent with local laws.

Modified from Agency for Health Care Policy and Research, Panel for the Treatment of Pressure Ulcers in Adults: *Treatment of pressure ulcers,* Clinical Practice Guideline No. 15, AHCPR Pub No. 95-0653, Rockville, Md, 1994, Agency for Health Care Policy and Research, Public Health Service, U.S. Department of Health and Human Services.

Table **47-8**   **A Quick Guide to Pressure Ulcer Prevention**

Risk Factor	Nursing Interventions
Decreased sensory perception	Assess pressure points for signs of nonblanching reactive hyperemia.
	Provide pressure reduction or relief surface.
Moisture	Assess need for incontinence management.
	Following each incontinent episode, cleanse area with no-rinse perineal cleanser and protect skin with a moisture barrier ointment.
Friction and shear	Reposition client using a drawsheet and lifting off of surface.
	Provide a trapeze to facilitate movement.
Decreased activity/mobility	Establish and post individualized turning schedule.
	Position client at a 30-degree lateral turn and limit head elevation to 30 degrees.
Poor nutrition	Provide adequate nutritional and fluid intake; assist with intake as necessary.
	Consult dietitian for nutritional evaluation.

and leave an alkaline residue. The alkaline residue discourages the growth of normal skin bacteria, thus promoting an overgrowth of opportunistic bacteria, which can then enter an open wound (AHCPR, 1992a). There are many types of products available for skin care, and their use needs to be matched to the specific needs of the client.

After the skin is cleansed and completely dried, moisturizer should be applied to keep the epidermis well lu-

bricated but not oversaturated. Cornstarch is a dry lubricant and helps to reduce friction (AHCPR, 1992a).

Efforts should be made to control, contain, or correct incontinence, perspiration, or wound drainage (Ratliff and Bryant, 2003). Clinicians may find the AHCPR guidelines on urinary incontinence (1992b) helpful (see Chapter 44). Clients who have fecal incontinence and who are also receiving enteral tube feeding provide a man-

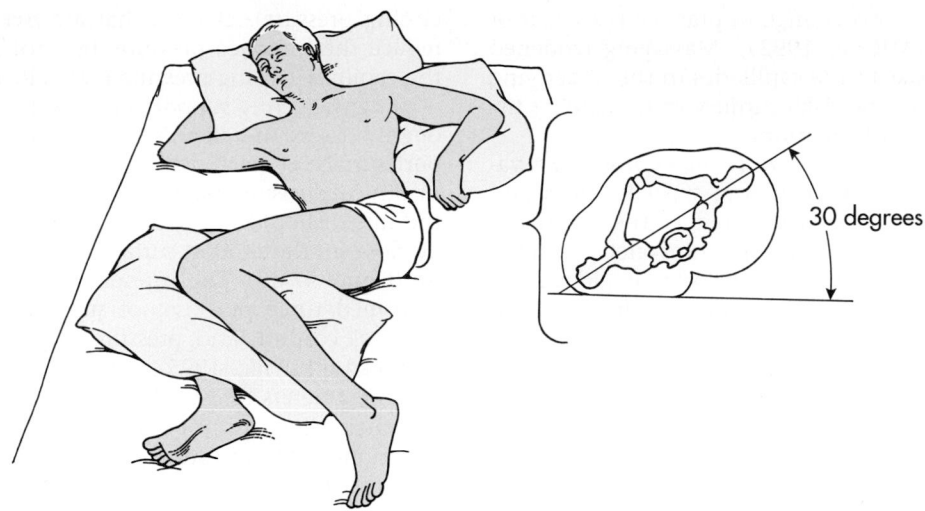

FIGURE **47–18** Thirty-degree lateral position at which pressure points are avoided. (From Pieper B and others: Pressure ulcers. In Bryant RA, editor: *Acute and chronic wounds: nursing management,* ed 2, St. Louis, 2000, Mosby.)

agement challenge. When clients have an incontinent episode, the area should be gently cleansed and dried and a thick layer of moisture barrier applied to the exposed areas. A moisture barrier protects the skin from excessive moisture and bacteria found in the urine or stool.

The expertise of an advanced practice nurse with a focus on enterostomal therapy, wound care, or management of incontinence should be used in caring for at-risk clients. Methods for controlling or containing incontinence vary. Urinary incontinence may be treated with behavioral techniques, medication, and surgery. Behavioral techniques are used to help clients learn ways to control their bladder and sphincter muscles. Two examples are bladder training and habit training, which is also called timed voiding.

Use of absorbent pads and garments should be considered only after the above measures have been tried. Although controversial, absorbent products, such as absorptive underpads and garments, may be part of the treatment plan for an incontinent client. The nurse should use only products that wick moisture away from the client's skin (AHCPR, 1992b; Ratliff and Bryant, 2003). Underpads should be used judiciously because some of these pads do not wick the drainage away from the client's skin and can cause skin damage.

Positioning. Positioning interventions are designed to reduce pressure and shearing force to the skin. Elevating the head of the bed to 30 degrees or less will decrease the chance of pressure ulcer development from shearing forces (AHCPR, 1992a). The immobilized client's position should be changed according to activity level, perceptual ability, and daily routines (Braden, 2001). Therefore a standard turning interval of 1½ to 2 hours may not prevent pressure ulcer development in some clients. The AHCPR guidelines (1992a) recommend that a written turning and positioning schedule be utilized. Clients should be repositioned at least every 2 hours. When repositioning, positioning devices should be used to protect bony prominences (AHCPR, 1992a, 1994). A 30-degree

lateral position is recommended in the AHCPR guidelines (1992a) (Figure 47-18). The 30-degree lateral position should prevent positioning directly over the bony prominence. To prevent shear and friction injuries, a sheet should be used to lift rather than drag the client when changing positions.

Safety Alert. Incorrect positioning of an immobile client can create a shearing injury. When repositioning the client, place a flat folded sheet under the client's body. Obtain assistance for repositioning and with at least one other care giver, lift the sheet up and toward the new position. Dragging the client on the sheets will place the client at high risk for shearing and friction injuries.

Clients able to sit in a chair should be limited to sitting for 2 hours or less. Again, the exact time is individualized, but the nurse should not allow the client to sit for a period longer than the recommended time that was calculated during assessment. Thus if the interval is every 1½ hours, the client should remain in a sitting position for less than 1½ hours. In the sitting position, the pressure on the ischial tuberosities is greater than in the supine position. In addition, a client at risk for skin breakdown in a sitting position should be taught to shift weight every 15 minutes (AHCPR, 1992a, Ratliff and Bryant, 2003). Shifting weight provides short-term relief on the ischial tuberosities. A client should also sit on foam, gel, or an air cushion to redistribute weight away from the ischial areas. Rigid and donut-shaped cushions are contraindicated because they reduce blood supply to the area, resulting in wider areas of ischemia (AHCPR, 1992a, 1994).

After the client is repositioned, the nurse reassesses the skin. Identifying characteristics that might indicate early signs of tissue ischemia in darkly pigmented skin can be found in Boxes 47-2 and 47-3. For clients with light-toned skin, the nurse observes for **normal reactive hyperemia** and blanching. The reddened areas should never be massaged. This change in practice is a result of nursing research (AHCPR, 1992a). Massaging reddened areas increases breaks in the capillaries in the underlying tissues and increases the risk of injury to underlying tissue and pressure ulcer formation.

Support Surfaces (Therapeutic Beds and Mattresses). A variety of support surfaces, including specialty beds and mattresses, have been designed to reduce the hazards of immobility to the skin and musculoskeletal system. However, none eliminates the need for meticulous nursing care. No single device eliminates the effects of pressure on the skin.

It is important to understand the difference between a pressure-reducing and a pressure-relieving support surface or device. A device that is **pressure relieving** relieves the interface pressure (the pressure between the body and the support surface) below 32 mm Hg (capillary closing pressure). Devices that are **pressure reducing** reduce the interface pressure, but not necessarily below the capillary closing pressure (AHCPR, 1994).

When selecting support surfaces, the nurse must thoroughly assess the client's needs. Knowledge about support surface characteristics (Table 47-9) assists the nurse in clinical decision making. In selecting a support surface, the nurse should know the client's risks, as well as the purpose for the support surface; a flow chart may be helpful (Figure 47-19). The Support Surface Consensus Panel identified three purposes of support surfaces: comfort, postural control, and pressure management (Krouskop and van Rijswijk, 1995). Furthermore, they identified nine parameters to use when evaluating support surfaces and their relationship to each of the three purposes: life expectancy, skin moisture control, skin temperature control, redistribution of pressure, product service require-

---

Table 47-9   Support Surfaces

Categories	Mechanism of Action	Indications	Examples of Manufacturers/ Product Names
Low-Air-Loss System			
Available in a full bed or as an overlay	Pressure-relief device Bed: The entire surface is a powered, inflated surface with air loss Overlay: Powered surface, constant inflation and air loss at the surface; place over the bed mattress	Prevention of skin breakdown in clients who can not be turned or have existing skin breakdown	Hill Rom/Flexicair Kinetic Concepts, Inc/First Step Select Crown Therapeutics/ Select Air Mattress
Foam			
Available as an overlay or in a full mattress	Reduces pressure and the cover (top) can reduce friction and shear Overlay: Placed on top of bed mattress Full mattress: Used in place of the usual mattress	Pressure reduction for high-risk clients	Bio Clinic/Bio Guard BG Industries/MaxiFloat
Static Air-Filled Overlays			
Available in an overlay	Interconnected air-filled cells, inflated to appropriate level Pressure relief or pressure reduction (depends on product)	High-risk clients	Crown Therapeutics/ RoHo mattress Gaymar Industries/ Sof-Care
Air-Fluidized Beds			
	Bed frame with silicone-coated beads that become fluidized when air is pumped through the beads Pressure relief, antishear, antifriction surface	For clients with burns or multiple stage III or stage IV pressure ulcers, protection of new grafts and flaps	Kinetic Concepts, Inc/FluidAir Hill Rom/Clinitron
Kinetic Therapy			
	Provides continuous passive motion, to promote mobilization of respiratory secretions; also provides low-air-loss therapy.	Clients who are at risk for or have developed atelectasis and/or pneumonia	Hill Rom/Total Care Sport Kinetic Concepts, Inc/ TriaDyne

ments, fall safety, infection control, flammability, and client-product friction (Krouskop and van Rijswijk, 1995). A summary of AHCPR recommendations (1994) regarding the use of support surfaces is found in Box 47-10. Clients and families need to be taught the reason for and proper use of the beds or mattresses (Box 47-11). Some common errors with support surfaces are placing the wrong side of the support surface toward the client, not plugging support surfaces into the electrical source, not turning on the power source for powered support surfaces, failing to do "hand checks" for some support surfaces, and improperly inflating some support surfaces.

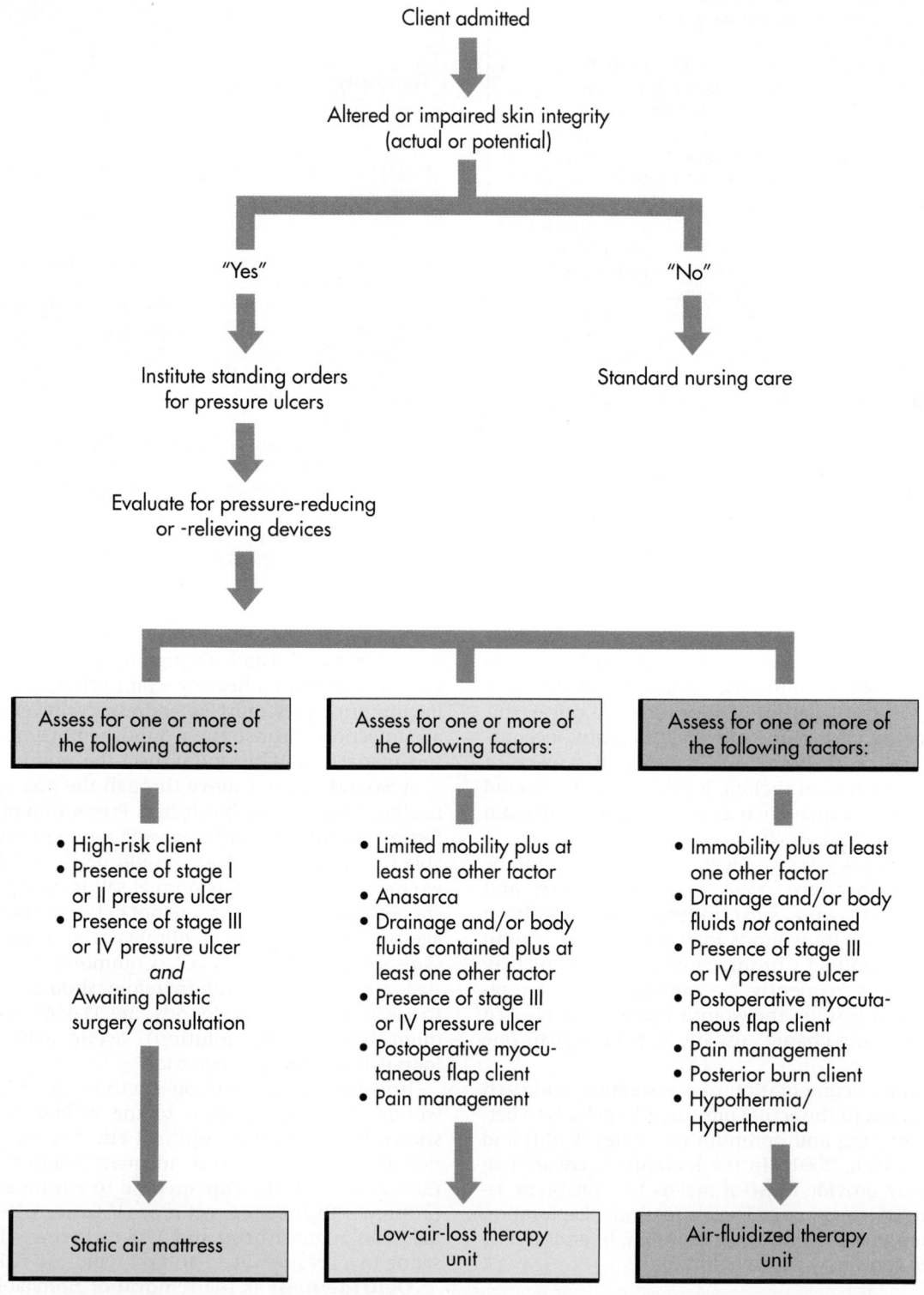

FIGURE **47–19** Flow diagram for ordering specialty beds. (From Thomas C: Specialty beds: decision-making made easy, *Ostomy Wound Manage* 23:51, 1989.)

Box *47-10*   **AHCPR Support Surface Recommendations**

- Assess all clients with existing pressure ulcers to determine their risk for developing additional pressure ulcers. If the client remains at risk, use a pressure-reducing surface.
- Use a static support surface if a client can assume a variety of positions without bearing weight on a pressure ulcer and without "bottoming out."
- Use a dynamic support surface if the client cannot assume a variety of positions without bearing weight on a pressure ulcer, if the client fully compresses the static support surface, or if the pressure ulcer does not show evidence of healing.
- If a client has large stage III or stage IV pressure ulcers on multiple turning surfaces, a low-air-loss bed or an air-fluidized bed may be indicated.
- When excess moisture on intact skin is a potential source of maceration and skin breakdown, a support surface that provides airflow can be important in drying the skin and preventing additional pressure ulcers.

Modified from Agency for Health Care Policy and Research, Panel for Treatment of Pressure Ulcers in Adults: *Treatment of pressure ulcers,* Clinical Practice Guideline No. 15, AHCPR Pub No. 95-0653, Rockville, Md, 1994, Agency for Health Care Policy and Research, Public Health Service, U.S. Department of Health and Human Services.

When used correctly, these mattresses and specialty beds assist in reducing pressure ulcers in clients at risk.

Acute Care

Management of Pressure Ulcers. Treatment of clients with pressure ulcers requires a holistic approach that uses the expertise of several multidisciplinary health care professionals (AHCPR, 1994). In addition to the nurse, this can include the physician, physical therapist, occupational therapist, nutritionist, and pharmacist. Aspects of pressure ulcer treatment include local care of the wound and supportive measures such as adequate nutrients and relief of pressure (Skill 47-2).

When treating a pressure ulcer, the wound should be reassessed for location, stage, size, tissue type and amount, exudate and surrounding skin condition (Cooper, 2000). Acute wounds may require close monitoring (every 8 hours.) Chronic wound assessment may be conducted less frequently. Depending upon the topical management system, the wound should be evaluated with every dressing change, usually not more than one time per day.

The use and documentation of a systematic approach to the assessment of the actual pressure ulcers leads to better decision making and optimum outcomes (Ratliff and Bryant, 2003; Weir, 2001). In the literature there are two tools that may provide a useful means for consistent assessment and reassessment of pressure ulcers. Exploration of the Bates-Jensen (1997) (Figure 47-20) and Ayello (1992, 1996) tools may prove helpful.

Wound Management. Maintenance of a physiologic local wound environment is the goal of effective wound

Client Teaching   Box 47-11

Therapeutic Beds and Mattresses
Objective

- Client and family will describe understanding of the purposes and basic operations of the therapeutic bed or mattress.

Teaching Strategies

- Explain to client and family the reasons for the therapeutic bed.
- Explain proper body mechanics while using the therapeutic bed.
- Educate family about the use and care of the therapeutic bed.
- Explain to client and family about additional pressure-relief measures.
- Give client and family a copy of each of the AHCPR booklets for clients on prevention and treatment of pressure ulcers.

Evaluation

- Client and family will state basic purposes for the therapeutic bed or mattress.
- Client and family will be able to describe the function of the therapeutic bed or mattress.
- Client and family will be able to demonstrate use of a therapeutic bed or mattress and other pressure-relief measures.

management (Rolstad, Ovington, and Harris, 2000). In order to maintain a healthy wound environment the following principles must be addressed: prevent and manage infection, cleanse the wound, remove nonviable tissue, manage exudate, and protect the wound.

A wound will not move through the phases of wound healing if the wound is infected. Prevention of wound infection includes wound cleansing and removal of nonviable tissue. Pressure ulcers should be cleansed only with wound cleansers such as normal saline or some commercial wound cleansers that are not cytotoxic (will not damage or kill cells, such as fibroblasts and healing tissue) (Rolstad and others, 2000). Commonly used solutions that are cytotoxic, and therefore should not be used to clean granulating wounds, are Dakin's solution (sodium hypochlorite solution), acetic acid, povidone-iodine, and hydrogen peroxide.

Irrigation is a common method of delivering the wound cleansing solution to the wound. Studies have shown that there is an optimal effective range of irrigation pressures that ensure adequate removal of bacteria (Rodeheaver, 2001). One method to ensure an irrigation pressure within the correct range is to use a 19-gauge needle or an angiocatheter and a 35-ml syringe that delivers saline to a pressure ulcer at 8 psi (Figure 47-21).

Debridement is the removal of nonviable, necrotic tissue. Removal of necrotic tissue is necessary to rid the ulcer of a source of infection, to enable visualization of

Skill **47-2**   *Treating Pressure Ulcers*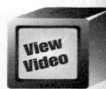

Delegation Considerations

Treatment of pressure ulcers should not be delegated to assistive personnel (AP). In some practice settings, *nonsterile* dressing application may be delegated to AP for chronic, established wounds where the protocol has been evaluated and designated by a nurse. The *assessment* of the wound remains within the scope of the nurse even if the dressing change is delegated to AP. When aspects of client care or dressing change are delegated, the nurse should instruct AP to do the following:

- Report changes in skin integrity to the nurse immediately.
- Report pain, fever, or wound drainage to the nurse immediately.
- Report any potential contamination to existing dressing (e.g., client incontinence or other bodily fluids, dressing becomes dislodged).

Equipment

- Disposable gloves (clean)
- Plastic bag for dressing disposal
- Measuring device
- Cotton-tipped applicators
- Topical cleansing agent
- Dressing of choice (see Table 47-10, p. 1534)
- Hypoallergenic tape (if needed)
- Documentation record
- Scale for assessing wound healing

Steps	Rationale
1. Assess client's level of comfort and need for pain medication.	Dressing change procedure is better tolerated if pain is controlled.
2. Determine if client has allergies to topical agents.	Topical agents may cause localized skin reactions.
3. Review order for topical agent or dressing.	Ensures that proper medication and treatment are administered.
4. Close room door or bedside curtains. Position client to allow dressing removal.	Area should be accessible for dressing change.
5. Perform hand hygiene and apply clean gloves. Remove dressing and place in plastic bag.	Reduces transmission of microorganisms and prevents accidental exposure to body fluids.
6. Assess pressure ulcer(s). All pressure ulcers should be individually assessed (see illustration).	Assessment of a pressure ulcer should be comprehensive.
a. Note color, type, and percentage of tissue present in the wound base.	The tissue type will assist in the choice of dressing. Consistent assessment will provide the basis for evaluating wound progress (Cooper, 2002).
b. Measure width and length of the ulcer(s). Width is determined by measuring the dimension from left to right, and the length is from top to bottom.	Ulcer size will change as healing progresses and therefore the longest and widest areas of the wound will change over time. Measuring the width and length by measuring consistent areas will provide a consistent measurement (Goldman and Salcido, 2002).
c. Measure depth of pressure ulcer using sterile cotton-tipped applicator or other device that will allow measurement of wound depth (see illustration).	Depth measure is important for determining wound volume. Although surface area adequately represents tissue loss in stage I and II ulcers, volume more adequately represents tissue loss in deeper stage III and IV wounds.
d. Measure depth undermining skin using a cotton-tipped applicator and gently probing under skin edges.	Undermining represents the loss of the underlying tissue (subcutaneous and muscle) to a greater extent than the skin. Undermining may indicate progressive tissue necrosis and must be accommodated with an appropriate dressing.
7. Assess the periwound skin; check for maceration, redness, denuded area.	Deterioration of the skin around a wound may indicate infection, excessive wound exudate, or skin stripping from adhesive removal (Colwell, 2003).
8. Change to sterile gloves (check agency policy).	Aseptic technique must be maintained during cleansing, and application of dressings. Refer to institutional policy regarding use of clean or sterile gloves.
9. Cleanse ulcer thoroughly with normal saline or cleansing agent. Use irrigating syringe for deep ulcers.	Removes wound debris.

Skill 47-2　　*Treating Pressure Ulcers—cont'd*

Steps	Rationale

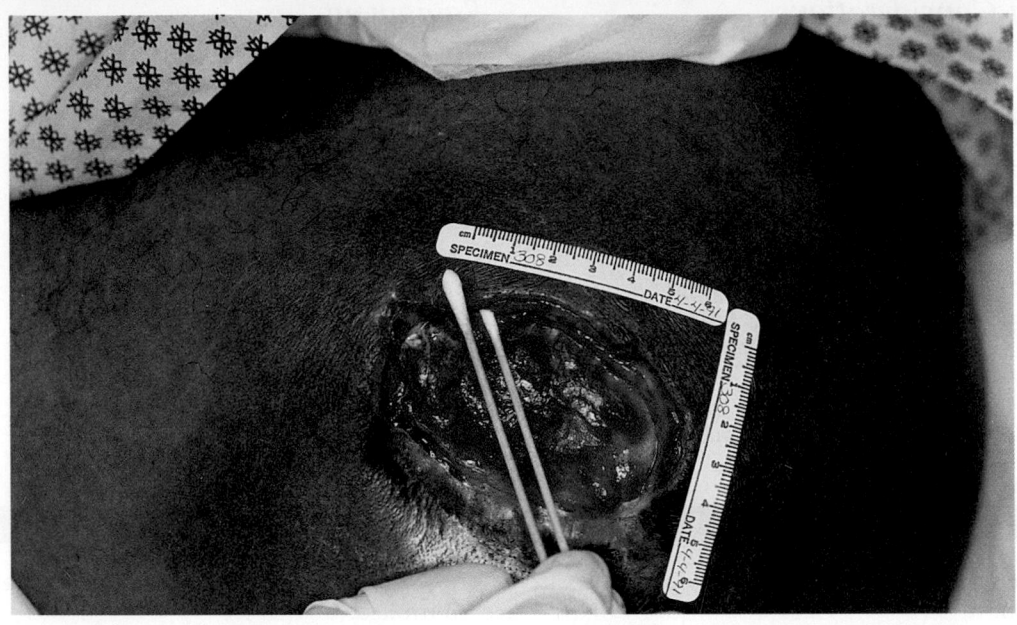

STEP **6**　Measuring wound depth (steps b, c, and d).

10. Apply topical agents, as prescribed:
　A. Enzymes
　　(1) Apply thin, even layer of ointment over necrotic areas of ulcer only. Do not apply enzyme to surrounding sk

in.

　　(2) Apply gauze dressing directly over ulcer.
　　(3) Tape securely in place.
　B. Hydrogel
　　(1) Cover surface of ulcer with hydrogel using applicator or gloved hand.
　　(2) Apply dry gauze, hydrocolloid, or transparent film dressing over wound and adhere to intact skin.
　C. Calcium alginate
　　(1) Pack wound with alginate using applicator or gloved hand.
　　(2) Apply dry gauze, foam, or hydrocolloid over alginate. Tape in place.
11. Remove gloves and dispose of soiled supplies. Perform hand hygiene.
12. Complete ulcer information required for one of the wound-healing scales per agency's protocol.

Thick layer of ointment is not necessary. Thin layer absorbs and acts more effectively. Excess medication can irritate surrounding skin (Rolstad, Ovington, and Harris, 2000). Some enzymes can cause burning, paresthesia, and dermatitis to surrounding skin. Check manufacturer's direction for frequency of application.

Protects wound. Prevents bacteria from entering wound.
Keeps dressing in place.

Provides maintenance of a moist wound environment.

Covers wound base, maintaining hydrogel wound interface.

Provides maintenance of wound moisture while absorbing excess drainage.
Holds alginate against wound surface.

Reduces transmission of microorganisms.

Allows comparison of assessments over time to determine progress toward wound healing.

Critical Decision Point: A clean pressure ulcer should show evidence of some healing within 2 to 4 weeks.

---

13. Compare subsequent ulcer measurements.

Wound-healing scales such as the PUSH or the PSST (see Figure 47-20, p. 1522) can be used to quantify and measure pressure ulcer healing.

Steps	Rationale
14. Do *not* use the pressure ulcer staging system to measure pressure ulcer healing.	System measures depth of wound, not healing (NPUAP, 1995a,b).

Unexpected Outcomes and Related Interventions

1. Skin surrounding ulcer becomes macerated.
   a. Reduce exposure of surrounding skin to topical agents and moisture.
   b. Consider the use of a liquid skin barrier on periwound skin.
2. Ulcer becomes deeper with increased drainage.
   a. Notify physician for possible change in pressure ulcer status.
   b. Obtain necessary wound cultures.
   c. Obtain additional consults (e.g., wound care specialist).

Recording and Reporting

- Record assessment of ulcer in client's record.
- Describe type of topical agent used, dressing applied, and client's response.
- Report any deterioration in ulcer appearance.

Home Care Considerations

- Cost can be a factor. Some clients have more time than financial resources. They may choose a less expensive treatment option such as dressing material, especially if there is no third-party reimbursement.
- Disposal of contaminated dressings in the home should be done in a manner consistent with local regulations (AHCPR, 1994).
- Discuss need for home pressure-relief surface or bed.

the wound bed, and to provide a clean base necessary for healing. An exception to the rule that all eschar be debrided is a dry necrotic heel pressure ulcer. According to the AHCPR guidelines (1994), "heel ulcers with dry eschar need not be debrided if they do not have edema, erythema, fluctuance, or drainage."

The method of debridement will depend on which is most appropriate to the client's condition and care goals (AHCPR, 1994). It is important to remember that during the debridement process some normal wound observations that may occur are an increase in wound exudate, odor, and size. Pain that occurs with debridement needs to be assessed and prevented or effectively managed (AHCPR, 1994).

Methods of debridement include mechanical, autolytic, chemical, and sharp/surgical. One method of mechanical debridement is the use of wet-to-dry saline gauze dressings. A moistened gauze is placed into the wound and the dressing allowed to dry thoroughly before the nurse "pulls" the gauze that has adhered to the tissue out of the pressure ulcer. This is a nonselective method of debridement because devitalized and viable tissue are both removed, and thus it is not used routinely. It should never be used in a clean, granulating wound. Other methods of mechanical debridement are wound irrigation (high-pressure irrigation and pulsatile high-pressure lavage) and whirlpool treatments (Ramundo and Wells, 2000). Whirlpool treatments are performed by physical therapists.

Autolytic debridement uses synthetic dressings over a wound to allow the eschar to be self-digested by the action of enzymes that are present in wound fluids (AHCPR, 1994). It can be accomplished by using dressings that support moisture at the wound surface. If the wound base is dry, a dressing that will add moisture is used; if there is

excessive exudate, a dressing that absorbs the excessive moisture while maintaining moisture at the wound bed is used. Some examples of dressings used are transparent film dressings and hydrocolloid dressings.

Chemical debridement can be accomplished with the use of a topical enzyme preparation, Dakin's solution, or sterile maggots. Topical enzymes induce changes in the substrate against which they are effective and result in the breakdown of necrotic tissue (Ramundo and Wells, 2000). Depending upon the type of enzyme used, the preparation either digests or dissolves the tissue. These drugs require a physician's order. Dakin's solution breaks down and loosens dead tissue in a wound. It is used by applying the solution to a gauze and packing into the wound. Sterile maggots can be used in a wound because it is thought that they ingest the dead tissue.

Surgical debridement is the removal of devitalized tissue by using a scalpel, scissors, or other sharp instrument. Physicians and, in some states, advanced practice nurses can perform surgical debridement of a pressure ulcer. Nurses should check the Nurse Practice Act for their state to see if surgical debridement is covered as a nursing function. It is the quickest method of debridement. It is usually indicated when the client has signs of cellulitis or sepsis.

A moist environment will support the movement of epithelial cells and facilitate wound closure. A wound that has excessive wound exudate (drainage) can provide an environment that may support bacterial growth, macerate the periwound skin, and slow the healing process. If excessive wound exudate is present, the nurse must evaluate the volume, consistency, and odor of the drainage to determine if signs and symptoms of infection are present.

An important factor not to be overlooked is that the wound will not heal unless the contributory factors are controlled or eliminated. Therefore it is critically important

Text continued on p. 1526

BATES-JENSEN WOUND ASSESSMENT TOOL

Instructions for use

General Guidelines:

Fill out the attached rating sheet to assess a wound's status after reading the definitions and methods of assessment described below. Evaluate once a week and and whenever a change occurs in the wound. Rate according to each item by picking the response that best describes the wound and entering that score in the item score column for the appropriate date. When you have rated the wound on all items, determine the total score by adding together the 13-item scores. The HIGHER the total score, the more severe the wound status. Plot total score on the Wound Status Continuum to determine progress.

Specific Instructions:

1. **Size:** Use ruler to measure the longest and widest aspect of the wound surface in centimeters; multiply length × width.

2. **Depth:** Pick the depth, thickness, most appropriate to the wound using these additional descriptions:
   1 = tissues damaged but no break in skin surface.
   2 = superficial, abrasion, blister or shallow crater. Even with, and/or elevated above skin surface (e.g., hyperplasia).
   3 = deep crater with or without undermining of adjacent tissue.
   4 = visualization of tissue layers not possible due to necrosis.
   5 = supporting structures include tendon, joint capsule.

3. **Edges:** Use this guide:
Indistinct, diffuse	=	unable to clearly distinguish wound outline.
Attached	=	even or flush with wound base, <u>no</u> sides or walls present; flat.
Not attached	=	sides or walls <u>are</u> present; floor or base of wound is deeper than edge.
Rolled under, thickened	=	soft to firm and flexible to touch.
Hyperkeratosis	=	callous-like tissue formation around wound and at edges.
Fibrotic, scarred	=	hard, rigid to touch.

4. **Undermining:** Assess by inserting a cotton-tipped applicator under the wound edge; advance it as far as it will go without using undue force; raise the tip of the applicator so it may be seen or felt on the surface of the skin; mark the surface with a pen; measure the distance from the mark on the skin to the edge of the wound. Continue process around the wound. Then use a transparent metric measuring guide with concentric circles divided into 4 (25%) pie-shaped quadrants to help determine percent of wound involved.

5. **Necrotic Tissue Type:** Pick the type of necrotic tissue that is <u>predominant</u> in the wound according to color, consistency, and adherence using this guide:
White/gray non-viable tissue	=	may appear prior to wound opening; skin surface is white or gray
Non-adherent, yellow slough	=	thin, mucinous substance; scattered throughout wound bed; easily separated from wound tissue
Loosely adherent, yellow slough	=	thick, stringy, clumps of debris; attached to wound tissue
Adherent, soft, black eschar	=	soggy tissue; strongly attached to tissue in center or base of wound
Firmly adherent, hard/black eschar	=	firm, crusty tissue; strongly attached to wound base <u>and</u> edges (like a hard scab)

© 2001 Barbara Bates-Jensen

FIGURE **47–20** Bates-Jensen Wound Assessment Tool (BWAT). (Based on Pressure Sore Status Tool [PSST].) (Courtesy Barbara Bates-Jensen, Reseda, Calif.)

Continued

6. **Necrotic Tissue Amount:** Use a transparent metric measuring guide with concentric circles divided into 4 (25%) pie-shaped quadrants to help determine percent of wound involved.

7. **Exudate Type:** Some dressings interact with wound drainage to produce a gel or trap liquid. Before assessing exudate type, gently cleanse wound with normal saline or water. Pick the exudate type that is <u>predominant</u> in the wound according to color and consistency, using this guide:
   Bloody   = thin, bright red
   Serosanguineous = thin, watery pale red to pink
   Serous   = thin, watery, clear
   Purulent   = thin or thick, opaque tan to yellow
   Foul purulent   = thick, opaque yellow to green with offensive odor

8. **Exudate Amount:** Use a transparent metric measuring guide with concentric circles divided into 4 (25%) pie-shaped quadrants to determine percent of dressing involved with exudate. Use this guide:
   None   = wound tissues dry
   Scant   = wound tissues moist; no measurable exudate
   Small   = wound tissues wet; moisture evenly distributed in wound; drainage involves ≤25% dressing
   Moderate = wound tissues saturated; drainage may or may not be evenly distributed in wound; drainage involves >25% to ≤75% dressing
   Large   = wound tissues bathed in fluid; drainage freely expressed; may or may not be evenly distributed in wound; drainage involves >75% of dressing

9. **Skin Color Surrounding Wound:** Assess tissues within 4 cm of wound edge. Dark-skinned persons show the colors "bright red" and "dark red" as a deepening of normal ethnic skin color or a purple hue. As healing occurs in dark-skinned persons, the new skin is pink and may never darken.

10. **Peripheral Tissue Edema and Induration:** Assess tissues within 4 cm of wound edge. Non-pitting edema appears as skin that is shiny and taut. Identify pitting edema by firmly pressing a finger down into the tissues and waiting for 5 seconds; on release of pressure, tissues fail to resume previous position and an indentation appears. Induration is abnormal firmness of tissue with margins. Assess by gently pinching the tissues. Induration results in an inability to pinch the tissues. Use a transparent metric measuring guide to determine how far edema or induration extends beyond wound.

11. **Granulation Tissue:** Granulation tissue is the growth of small blood vessels and connective tissue to fill in full-thickness wounds. Tissue is healthy when bright, beefy red, shiny, and granular with a velvety appearance. Poor vascular supply appears as pale pink or blanched to dull, dusky red color.

12. **Epithelialization:** Epithelialization is the process of epidermal resurfacing and appears as pink or red skin. In partial-thickness wounds it can occur throughout the wound bed as well as from the wound edges. In full-thickness wounds it occurs from the edges only. Use a transparent metric measuring guide with concentric circles divided into 4 (25%) pie-shaped quadrants to help determine percent of wound involved and to measure the distance the epithelial tissue extends into the wound.

© 2001 Barbara Bates-Jensen

FIGURE **47–20, cont'd** Bates-Jensen Wound Assessment Tool (BWAT). (Based on Pressure Sore Status Tool [PSST].) (Courtesy Barbara Bates-Jensen, Reseda, Calif.)

Continued

BATES-JENSEN WOUND ASSESSMENT TOOL   NAME_____

Complete the rating sheet to assess wound status. Evaluate each item by picking the response that best describes the wound and entering the score in the item score column for the appropriate date.

Location: Anatomic site. Circle, identify right **(R)** or left **(L)** and use **"X"** to mark site on body diagrams:

___ Sacrum and coccyx   ___ Lateral ankle
___ Trochanter   ___ Medial ankle
___ Ischial tuberosity   ___ Heel   Other Site ___

Shape: overall wound pattern; assess by observing perimeter and depth.

Circle and date appropriate description:

___ Irregular   ___ Linear or elongated
___ Round/oval   ___ Bowl/boat
___ Square/rectangle   ___ Butterfly   Other Shape ___

Item	Assessment	Date Score	Date Score	Date Score
1. Size	1 = Length × width <4 sq cm 2 = Length × width 4–<16 sq cm 3 = Length × width 16.1–<36 sq cm 4 = Length × width 36.1–<80 sq cm 5 = Length × width >80 sq cm			
2. Depth	1 = Non-blanchable erythema on intact skin 2 = Partial-thickness skin loss involving epidermis and/or dermis 3 = Full-thickness skin loss involving damage or necrosis of subcutaneous tissue; may extend down to but not through underlying fascia; and/or mixed partial and full thickness and/or tissue layers obscured by granulation tissue 4 = Obscured by necrosis 5 = Full-thickness skin loss with extensive destruction, tissue necrosis, or damage to muscle, bone or supporting structures			
3. Edges	1 = Indistinct, diffuse, none clearly visible 2 = Distinct, outline clearly visible, attached, even with wound base 3 = Well-defined, not attached to wound base 4 = Well-defined, not attached to base, rolled under, thickened 5 = Well-defined, fibrotic, scarred or hyperkeratotic			
4. Undermining	1 = None present 2 = Undermining <2 cm in any area 3 = Undermining 2-4 cm involving <50% wound margins 4 = Undermining 2-4 cm involving >50 % wound margins 5 = Undermining >4 cm or tunneling in any area			
5. Necrotic Tissue Type	1 = None visible 2 = White/gray non-viable tissue and/or non-adherent yellow slough 3 = Loosely adherent yellow slough 4 = Adherent, soft, black eschar 5 = Firmly adherent, hard, black eschar			
6. Necrotic Tissue Amount	1 = None visible 2 = <25% of wound bed covered 3 = 25% to 50% of wound covered 4 = >50% and <75% of wound covered 5 = 75 % to 100% of wound covered			

FIGURE **47–20, cont'd** Bates-Jensen Wound Assessment Tool (BWAT). (Based on Pressure Sore Status Tool [PSST].) (Courtesy Barbara Bates-Jensen, Reseda, Calif.)

Continued

Item	Assessment	Date Score	Date Score	Date Score
7. Exudate Type	1 = None 2 = Bloody 3 = Serosanguineous: thin, watery, pale red/pink 4 = Serous: thin, watery, clear 5 = Purulent: thin or thick, opaque, tan/yellow, with or without odor			
8. Exudate Amount	1 = None, dry wound 2 = Scant, wound moist but no observable exudate 3 = Small 4 = Moderate 5 = Large			
9. Skin Color Surrounding Wound	1 = Pink 2 = Bright red and/or blanches to touch 3 = White or grey pallor or hypopigmented 4 = Dark red or purple and/or non-blanchable 5 = Black or hyperpigmented			
10. Peripheral Tissue Edema	1 = No swelling or edema 2 = Non-pitting edema extends <4 cm around wound 3 = Non-pitting edema extends ≥4 cm around wound 4 = Pitting edema extends <4 cm around wound 5 = Crepitus and/or pitting edema extends ≥4 cm around wound			
11. Peripheral Tissue Induration	1 = None present 2 = Induration, <2 cm around wound 3 = Induration 2-4 cm extending <50% around wound 4 = Induration 2-4 cm extending ≥50% around wound 5 = Induration >4 cm in any area around wound			
12. Granulation Tissue	1 = Skin intact or partial-thickness wound 2 = Bright, beefy red; 75% to 100% of wound filled and/or tissue overgrowth 3 = Bright, beefy red; <75% and >25% of wound filled 4 = Pink, and/or dull, dusky red and/or fills ≤25% of wound 5 = No granulation tissue present			
13. Epithelialization	1 = 100% wound covered, surface intact 2 = 75% to <100% wound covered and/or epithelial tissue extends >0.5 cm into wound bed 3 = 50% to <75% wound covered and/or epithelial tissue extends to <0.5 cm into wound bed 4 = 25% to <50% wound covered 5 = <25% wound covered			
	TOTAL SCORE			
	SIGNATURE			

WOUND STATUS CONTINUUM

1	5	10 13 15	20	25	30	35	40	45	50	55	60

Tissue Health   Wound Regeneration   Wound Degeneration

Plot the total score on the Wound Status Continuum by putting an "X" on the line and the date beneath the line. Plot multiple scores with their dates to see-at-a-glance regeneration or degeneration of the wound.

© 2001 Barbara Bates-Jensen

FIGURE 47–20, cont'd Bates-Jensen Wound Assessment Tool (BWAT). (Based on Pressure Sore Status Tool [PSST].) (Courtesy Barbara Bates-Jensen, Reseda, Calif.)

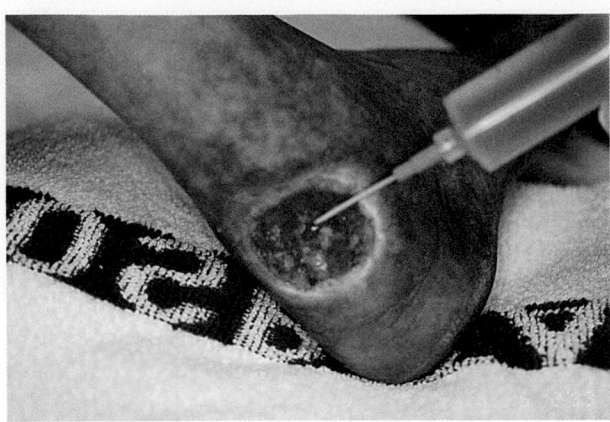

FIGURE **47-21** Wound irrigation.

that the causative factors (e.g., shear, friction, pressure, and moisture) be addressed, or it is unlikely that the wound will heal despite topical therapy (Rolstad and others, 2000).

The treatment plan will need to be altered as the ulcer heals. For example, in the management of a necrotic wound, a transparent film dressing may be used initially to autolytically debride the wound. Once the wound is cleansed of necrotic tissue, the transparent film dressing is discontinued and based upon the wound base characteristics, a new dressing may be chosen. A wound with excessive drainage will require a dressing with a high absorptive capacity. Continued reassessment is key to supporting the wound as it moves through the phases of wound healing (Colwell, 2003).

Growth Factors. It has been identified that growth factors regulate most of the key actions of cells during wound healing. As the molecular regulation of healing has been studied, the role of various growth factors is better understood. Topical growth factors have been used to regulate the healing of chronic wounds. Growth factors involved in wound healing include epidermal growth factor, platelet-derived growth factor, fibroblast growth factor, and transforming growth factor (Schultz, 2000). The nurse may be responsible for the use of this treatment modality after the physician determines that it may provide a benefit for the client's wound care. Teaching the client or significant other about the use of growth factors is also the nurse's responsibility. The nurse teaches the use of the medication, wound care, and the prevention of wound breakdown and recurrence.

Education. Education of the client and caregivers is an important nursing function (Erwin-Toth and Stenger, 2001). There are a variety of educational tools, including videotapes and written materials, that can be used by the nurse when teaching clients and caregivers/family to prevent and treat pressure ulcers. Written materials are available on a variety of topics, including dressing changes; there are also guides for measuring wounds and charts for positioning clients. AHCPR (1992a, 1994) has booklets for clients on pressure ulcer prevention and treatment that can be helpful when teaching clients and their caregivers/ family. These booklets are available in English and in Spanish. Teaching should be individualized for each client, especially with older clients.

Understanding and assessment of the experience of the client and support person are also important dimensions in the treatment of people with pressure ulcers (AHCPR, 1994). Clinicians are only just now exploring through research the caregiver's perspective of the concerns and issues faced by frail older spouses caring for their loved ones with pressure ulcers (Baharestani, 1994). Interventions should be planned to meet the identified psychosocial needs of clients and their support persons (AHCPR, 1994).

Nutritional Status. Nutritional assessment and support of the client with a wound is based upon the appreciation that nutrition is fundamental to normal cellular integrity and tissue repair (Stotts, 2000). An algorithm provided by AHCPR (1994) can be used to help clinicians meet the goals of nutritional assessment and management for clients with pressure ulcers. The AHCPR guidelines (1994) recommend that an abbreviated nutritional assessment be done every 3 months for individuals at risk for malnutrition. This includes individuals who are unable to take food by mouth or who have experienced an involuntary change in weight. Parameters for clinically significant malnutrition have been defined (AHCPR, 1994) (Box 47-12). The client's mouth and skin should be assessed for signs of nutritional deficiencies (see Chapter 43). Vitamin and mineral supplements should be given if deficiencies are confirmed or suspected. The client's hydration status, especially the amount of fluids and the weight pattern, should also be assessed (Ayello, Thomas, and Litchford, 1999).

Protein Status. Clients with a potential for or actual decreased serum albumin levels or poor protein intake need a nutritional evaluation to ensure proper caloric intake (AHCPR, 1994; Ratliff and Bryant, 2003). A client can lose as much as 50 g of protein per day from an open, weeping pressure ulcer. Although the RDA of protein for adults is 0.8 g/kg, a higher intake of protein up to 1.8 g/kg/day may be needed for healing. Increased protein intake helps rebuild epidermal tissue. Increased caloric intake helps replace subcutaneous tissue. Vitamin C promotes collagen synthesis, capillary wall integrity, fibroblast function, and immunological function.

Hemoglobin. A low hemoglobin level decreases delivery of oxygen to the tissues and leads to further ischemia. When possible, hemoglobin should be maintained at 12 g/100 ml.

First Aid for Wounds. In an emergency setting the nurse uses first aid measures for wound care. Under stable conditions the nurse uses a variety of interventions to ensure wound healing. When a client suffers a traumatic wound, first aid interventions include stabilizing cardiopulmonary function (see Chapter 39), promoting hemostasis, cleansing the wound, and protecting the wound from further injury.

Hemostasis. After assessing the type and extent of the wound, the nurse controls bleeding of a laceration by applying direct pressure on the wound with a sterile or clean dressing, such as a washcloth. After bleeding subsides, an adhesive bandage or gauze dressing taped over the laceration allows skin edges to close and a blood clot to form. If

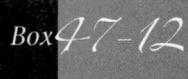

Box 47-12   AHCPR Recommendations for Nutritional Assessment and Management of Pressure Ulcers

Assessment of Clinically Significant Malnutrition

Serum albumin is less than 3.5 mg/100 ml.
Total lymphocyte count is less than 1800/mm³.
Body weight has decreased more than 15%.

Interventions

- Ensure adequate dietary intake to prevent malnutrition to the extent that this is compatible with the individual's wishes and ideal body weight.
  - Maintain serum albumin greater than 3.5 mg/100 ml.
  - Maintain total lymphocyte count greater than 1800/mm³.
- Perform an abbreviated nutritional assessment, as defined by the Nutritional Screening Initiative, at least every 3 months for individuals who are unable to take food by mouth or who experience an involuntary change in weight.
- Encourage dietary intake or supplementation if an individual with a pressure ulcer is malnourished. If dietary intake continues to be inadequate, impractical, or impossible, nutritional support (usually tube feeding) should be used to place the client into positive nitrogen balance (approximately 30 to 35 calories/kg/day and 1.25 to 1.50 g of protein/kg/day) according to the goals of care.
- Give vitamin and mineral supplements if deficiencies are confirmed or suspected.

Modified from Agency for Health Care Policy and Research, Panel for Treatment of Pressure Ulcers in Adults: *Treatment of pressure ulcers,* Clinical Practice Guideline No. 15, AHCPR Pub No. 95-0653, Rockville, Md, 1994, Agency for Health Care Policy and Research, Public Health Service, U.S. Department of Health and Human Services.

a dressing becomes saturated with blood, the nurse adds another layer of dressing, continues to apply pressure, and elevates the affected part. Further disruption of skin layers should be avoided. Serious lacerations should be sutured by a physician. Pressure dressings used during the first 24 to 48 hours after trauma help maintain hemostasis.

A puncture wound is allowed to bleed to remove dirt and other contaminants, such as saliva from a dog bite. When a penetrating object, such as a knife blade, is present, it is not removed. Removal could cause massive, uncontrolled bleeding. Except for skull injuries, the nurse may apply pressure around the penetrating object, but not on it, and the client should be transported to an emergency facility.

Cleansing. The process of cleansing a wound involves selecting both an appropriate cleansing solution and using a mechanical means of delivering that solution without causing injury to the healing wound tissue (AHCPR, 1994). Gentle cleansing of a wound removes contaminants that might serve as sources of infection. However, vigorous cleaning using a method with too much me-

chanical force can cause bleeding or further injury. For abrasions, minor lacerations, and small puncture wounds, the nurse first rinses the wound with normal saline, and lightly covers the area with a dressing. When a laceration is bleeding profusely, the nurse should only brush away surface contaminants and concentrate on hemostasis until the client can be cared for in a clinic or hospital.

Topical Agents for Cleansing Wounds. According to the AHCPR guidelines (1994), normal saline is the preferred cleansing agent. It is physiological and will not harm tissue.

Gentle cleansing with normal saline and the application of saline dressings (wet-to-wet, wet-to-damp) are often used in healing wounds and to debride wounds (wet-to-dry). The nurse uses saline to maintain the moist surface needed to promote the development and migration of epithelial tissue. Wet-to-dry saline dressings should be used only to debride wounds. They should never be used in a clean granulating wound.

Protection. Regardless of whether bleeding has stopped, the nurse protects the wound from further injury by applying sterile or clean dressings and immobilizing the body part. A light dressing applied over minor wounds prevents entrance of microorganisms.

Dressings. The more extensive the wound, the larger the dressing required. In the home a clean towel or diaper may be the best secondary dressing. A bulky dressing applied with pressure minimizes movement of underlying tissues and helps immobilize the entire body part. A bandage or cloth wrapped around a penetrating object should immobilize it adequately.

There are alternative dressings that can be used to cover and protect certain types of wounds. Examples are large wounds, wounds with drainage tubes or suction catheters in the wound, wounds that need frequent changing, and fistulas. In these wounds, pouches or special wound collection systems are used to cover the wound and collect the wound drainage. Some of these devices have a plastic door on the front of the wound pouch allowing the nurse to change the wound packing without removing the wound pouch from the skin.

The use of dressings requires an understanding of wound healing. A variety of dressing materials are commercially available. The correct dressing selection can facilitate wound healing (Currence, 2001; Rolstad and others, 2000). The dressing type will depend on the assessment of the wound and the phase of wound healing. The objectives for the wound care must be identified and the dressing choice will become clear. A wound that requires infection management will require a different set of dressings than a wound that requiring the removal of nonviable tissue.

For surgical wounds that heal by primary intention, it is common to remove dressings as soon as drainage stops. In contrast, when the nurse dresses a wound healing by secondary intention, the dressing material becomes a means for providing moisture to the wound, or assisting in debridement.

Purposes of Dressings. A dressing may serve several purposes:
- Protecting a wound from microorganism contamination
- Aiding hemostasis

- Promoting healing by absorbing drainage and debriding a wound
- Supporting or splinting the wound site
- Protecting the client from seeing the wound (if perceived as unpleasant)
- Promoting thermal insulation of the wound surface
- Providing a moist environment

When the skin becomes broken, a dressing helps reduce exposure to microorganisms. However, when wound drainage is minimal, the healing process forms a natural fibrin seal that can eliminate the need for a dressing. A dressing is always needed for wounds with extensive tissue loss.

Pressure dressings promote hemostasis. Applied with elastic bandages, a pressure dressing exerts localized downward pressure over an actual or potential bleeding site. A pressure dressing eliminates dead space in underlying tissues so that wound healing progresses normally. The nurse checks pressure dressings to be sure that they do not interfere with circulation to a body part. The nurse assesses skin color, pulses in distal extremities, the client's comfort, and changes in sensation. Pressure dressings are not routinely removed.

A primary function of a dressing on a healing wound is to absorb drainage. Most traditional surgical dressings have three layers: a contact or primary layer, an absorbent layer, and an outer protective or secondary layer. The contact dressing covers the incision and part of the adjacent skin. Fibrin, blood products, and debris adhere to the contact dressing's surface. A problem can occur if the wound drainage dries, causing the dressing to stick to the suture line. Improper removal of the dressing can cause disruption of the healing epidermal surface. If the dressing is sticking to the surgical incision, the dressing should be lightly moistened with saline solution. This will cause the dressing to become saturated, loosening it from the incisional area, allowing for no trauma to the incisional area.

The dressing technique will vary depending on the goal of the treatment plan for the wound. For example, if the goal is to maintain a moist environment for a clean granulating wound, it is important for the nurse to prevent the saline-moistened gauze dressing from drying and sticking to the healing wound. This is in direct contrast to the dressing technique that should be used if the goal of care is to mechanically debride the wound using a saline wet-to-dry dressing. When wounds require debriding, such as a necrotic wound, a wet-to-dry dressing technique can be utilized. The moist dressing (contact dressing) is placed into the wound and allowed to dry. The contact dressing debrides necrotic tissue and debris. In this case the contact dressing is allowed to dry so that it sticks to underlying tissue, and debridement occurs during removal.

Dressings applied to a draining wound require frequent changing to prevent microorganism growth and skin breakdown. Bacteria grow readily in the dark, warm, moist environment under a dressing. Skin surfaces become macerated and irritated. Periwound skin breakdown can be minimized by keeping the skin clean, dry, and reducing the use of tape.

The absorbent dressing layer serves as a reservoir for additional secretions. The wicking action of woven gauze dressings pulls excess drainage into the dressing and away from the wound.

The final outer layer of a dressing helps prevent bacteria and other external contaminants from reaching the wound surface. Usually the outer dressing is made of a thicker dressing material. Adhesives can be applied to this layer securing the dressings.

A dressing should support a moist wound environment if the wound is healing by secondary intention. A moist wound base facilitates the movement of epithelialization, thus allowing the wound to resurface as quickly as possible.

Types of Dressings. Dressings vary by type of material and mode of application (wet or dry) (Skill 47-3). They should be easy to apply, comfortable, and made of materials that promote wound healing. The AHCPR guidelines (1994) are helpful when selecting dressings based on the goal of wound treatment (Box 47-13).

Pressure ulcers require dressings. The type of dressing is usually based on the stage of the pressure ulcer and the objective of the dressing (Table 47-10). Before placing a dressing on a pressure ulcer, it is important that the nurse know the stage of the pressure ulcer, the goal of the dressing, and principles of wound care.

Gauze sponges are the oldest and most common dressing. They are absorbent and are especially useful in wounds to wick away the wound exudate. They do not interact with wound tissue and thus cause little wound irritation. Gauze is available in different textures and in squares of 4 × 4 inches or 2 × 2 inches and rolls of various

Text continued on p. 1533

| Box **47-13** | **AHCPR Dressing Recommendations** |

- Use a dressing that will keep the ulcer bed continuously moist. Wet-to-dry dressings should be used only for debridement and are not considered continuously moist saline dressings.
- Use clinical judgment to select a type of moist wound dressing suitable for the ulcer. Studies of different types of moist wound dressings showed no differences in pressure ulcer healing outcomes.
- Choose a dressing that keeps the surrounding intact (periulcer) skin dry while keeping the ulcer bed moist.
- Choose a dressing that controls exudate but does not desiccate the ulcer bed.
- Consider caregiver time when selecting a dressing.
- Eliminate wound dead space by loosely filling all cavities with dressing material. Avoid overpacking the wound.
- Monitor dressings applied near the anus, because they are difficult to keep intact.

Modified from Agency for Health Care Policy and Research, Panel for Treatment of Pressure Ulcers in Adults: *Treatment of pressure ulcers,* Clinical Practice Guideline No. 15, AHCPR Pub No. 95-0653, Rockville, Md, 1994, Agency for Health Care Policy and Research, Public Health Service, U.S. Department of Health and Human Services.

Skill 47-3 *A*pplying Dry and Wet-to-Dry Moist Dressings

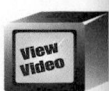

Delegation Considerations

Controversy about delegating wound care to assistive personnel (AP) exists. The care of acute new wounds and those that require sterile technique for dressing change should not be delegated to AP. In some settings, aspects of wound care such as dressing change can be delegated. This may include the changing of dressings using *clean* technique for chronic wounds. The *assessment* of the wound remains within the scope of the nurse even if the dressing change is delegated to AP. When aspects of client care or dressing change are delegated the nurse should instruct AP to do the following:

- Report pain, fever, bleeding, or wound drainage to the nurse immediately.
- Report any potential contamination to existing dressing (e.g., client incontinence or other bodily fluids, dressing becomes dislodged).

Equipment

- Sterile gloves
- Variety of gauze dressings and pads
- Irrigation kit
- Cleansing solution
- Sterile solution
- Clean, disposable gloves
- Tape, ties, or bandage as needed
- Waterproof bag
- Extra gauze dressings, or ABD pads

Steps	Rationale
1. Perform hand hygiene. Obtain information about size and location of wound to be dressed.	Reduces transmission of microorganisms. Helps nurse to plan for proper type and amount of supplies needed. Alerts nurse when assistance is needed to hold dressings in place.
2. Assess client's level of comfort.	Removal of dry dressing can be painful; client may require pain medication.
3. Review orders for dressing change procedure.	Indicates type of dressing or applications to use.
4. Explain procedure to client and instruct client not to touch wound area or sterile supplies.	Decreases anxiety. Sudden, unexpected movement on client's part could result in contamination of wound and supplies.
5. Close room or cubicle curtains and windows.	Provides privacy and reduces airborne microorganisms.
6. Position client comfortably and drape with bath blanket to expose only wound site.	Provides access to wound, yet minimizes unnecessary exposure.
7. Place disposable bag within reach of work area. Fold top of bag to make cuff (see illustration).	Ensures easy disposal of soiled dressings. Prevents soiling of bag's outer surface.
8. Apply face mask and protective eyewear, if splashing may occur, and perform hand hygiene.	Reduces transmission of pathogens to exposed tissues. Protects nurse from splashes.
9. Put on clean, disposable gloves and remove tape, bandage, or ties.	Prevents transmission of infectious organisms from soiled dressings to nurse's hands.
10. Remove tape: pull parallel to skin; pull toward dressing; remove remaining adhesive from skin.	Pulling tape toward dressing reduces stress on suture line or wound edges.
11. With gloved hand carefully remove gauze dressings one layer at a time, taking care not to dislodge drains or tubes.	Appearance of drainage may be upsetting to client. Removal of one layer at a time reduces the chance of accidental removal of underlying drains.
a. If dressing sticks on a wet-to-dry dressing, do not moisten it; instead gently free dressing and alert client of potential discomfort.	Wet-to-dry dressing should debride wound. Do not wet the dressing to remove it. It is supposed to be dry so that as it is removed from the wound, it also removes necrotic tissue from the wound.

Critical Decision Point: Never use a wet-to-dry dressing in a clean granulating wound. Use only for debridement.

Steps	Rationale
12. Observe character and amount of drainage on dressing and appearance of wound.	Provides estimate of drainage amount and assessment of wound's condition.

Applying Dry and Wet-to-Dry Moist Dressings

Skill 47-3

Steps	Rationale

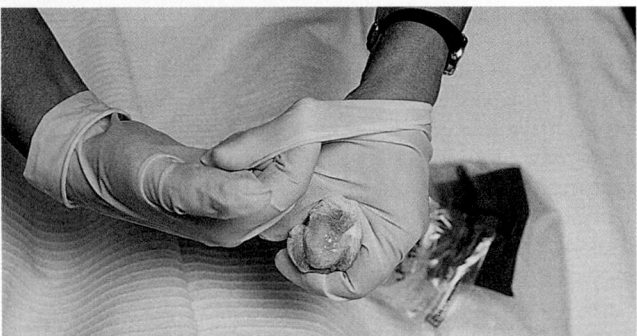

STEP **13**   Removal of disposable glove over contaminated dressing.

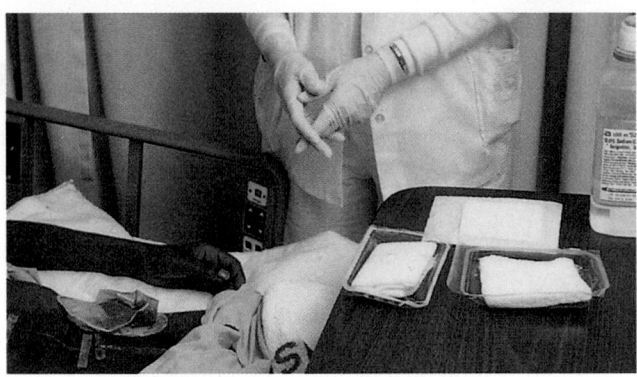

STEP **7**   Disposable waterproof bag placed near the dressing site.

STEP **14**   Sterile dressing equipment.

13. Fold dressings with drainage contained inside, and remove gloves inside out. With small dressings, remove gloves inside out over dressing (see illustration). Dispose of gloves and soiled dressings in disposable bag. Perform hand hygiene.

Reduces transmission of microorganisms. Prevents contact of nurse's hands with material on gloves.

14. Open sterile dressing tray or individually wrapped sterile supplies. Place on bedside table (see illustration).

Sterile dressings remain sterile while on or within sterile surface. Preparation of supplies prevents break in technique during dressing change.

15. Cleanse wound:
    a. Pour ordered solution into sterile irrigation container.
    b. Using syringe, gently allow solution to flow over wound.
    c. Continue until the irrigation flow is clear.
    d. Dry surrounding skin.
16. Apply dressing:
    A. Dry dressing
    (1) Apply sterile gloves.

    Allows handling of sterile supplies without contamination.

    (2) Inspect wound for appearance, drains, drainage, and integrity.

    Indicates status of wound healing.

    (3) Cleanse wound with solution:
        (a) Clean from least-contaminated area to most-contaminated area.

        Prevents contamination of previously cleaned area.

Steps	Rationale

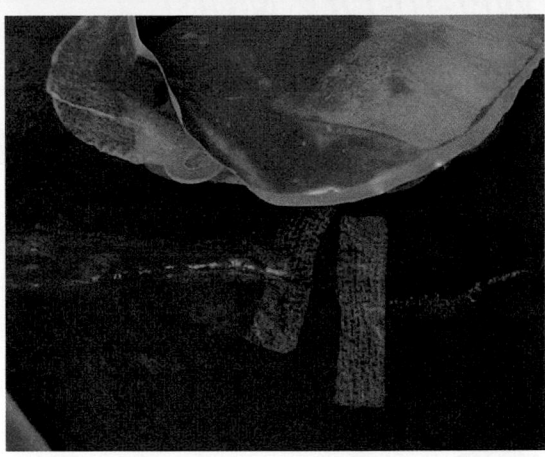

STEP **16B(3)**   Exposure of wound facilitates assessment of wound and any drainage.

Steps	Rationale
(4) Dry area. (5) Apply sterile dry dressing covering wound. (6) Apply topper dressing if indicated.	Provides protection and absorption of wound drainage. Protects wound from external environment.
B. Wet-to-dry dressing (1) Apply clean gloves. (2) Remove old dressings, discard. (3) Assess surrounding skin (see illustration). Discard gloves. (4) Apply sterile gloves. (5) Cleanse wound base with normal saline. Assess wound base.	Surrounding skin assessment provides an evaluation of wound management. Allows handling of sterile supplies without contamination. Cleansing removes wound debris for adequate assessment.
(6) Moisten gauze with prescribed solution. Wring gauze out. Unfold. (7) Apply moist fine-mesh, open-weave gauze as a single layer directly onto the wound surface. If wound is deep, gently pack dressing into wound base with sterile gloves or forceps until all wound surfaces are in contact with the gauze. If tunneling present, use a cotton-tipped applicator to place gauze into tunneled area. Be sure gauze does not touch the surrounding skin (see illustration).	Gauze should be moist to allow for absorption of wound debris. Inner gauze should be moist, not dripping wet, to absorb drainage and adhere to debris. Wound should be loosely packed to facilitate wicking of drainage into absorbent outer layer of dressing. Having inner gauze too wet (so it does not dry) is a common error in technique for this type of dressing (Barr, 1995).
(8) Cover with sterile dry gauze and topper dressing.	Topper dressing prevents strike through of wound drainage and provides a surface to tape the dressing in place.
17. Secure dressing. a. Tape: Apply nonallergenic tape to dressing.	The goal for secure a dressing is to keep the dressing in place and intact without causing damage to underlying and surrounding skin.
b. Montgomery ties (see Figure 47-26, p. 1542) (1) Expose adhesive surface of tape on end of each tie. (2) Place ties on opposites of dressing. (3) Place adhesive directly on skin or use skin barrier. (4) Secure dressing by lacing ties across it c. For dressings on an extremity, secure dressing with roller gauze or Surgiflex elastic net (see illustration).	Skin barrier (Stomahesive) protects intact skin from stretch and tension of adhesive tape.

Skill 47-3   *A*pplying Dry and Wet-to-Dry Moist Dressings—cont'd

Steps	Rationale

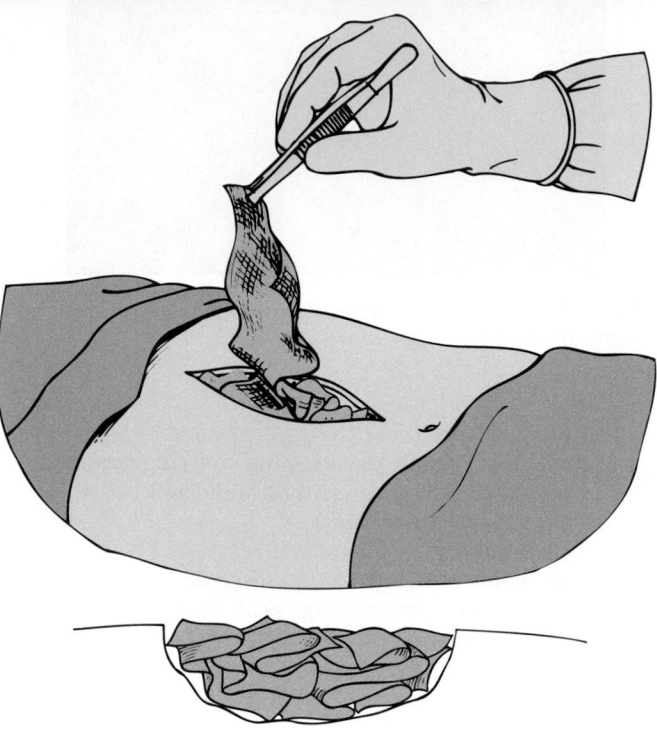

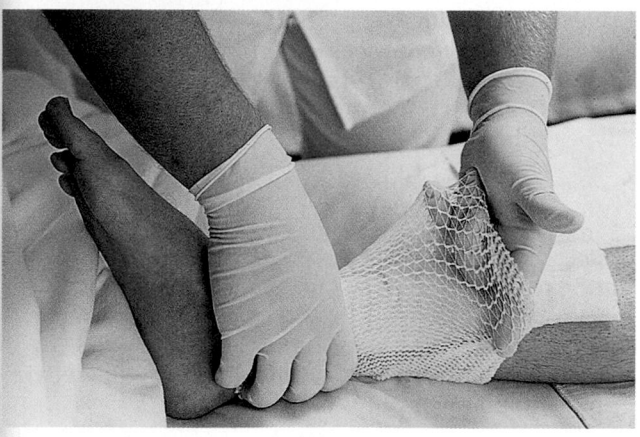

STEP **16B(7)** Packing wound with single layer of gauze.

STEP **17c**   Elastic net securing a lower extremity dressing.

18. Remove gloves and dispose of in bag. Remove any mask or eyewear.	Reduces transmission of infection.
19. Dispose of supplies and perform hand hygiene.	Reduces transmission of infection.
20. Assist client to comfortable position.	Promotes client's sense of well being. Enhances comfort.

Unexpected Outcomes and Related Interventions

1. Wound appears inflamed, tender, with or without drainage.
   a. Monitor client for signs of infection (e.g., increased temperature, white blood cell count).
   b. Obtain wound culture.
   c. Notify physician.
2. Wound drainage increases.
   a. Increase frequency of dressing changes.
   b. Notify physician, who may consider drain placement to facilitate wound drainage.
3. Wound bleeds during dressing change.
   a. Observe color. If drainage is bright red and excessive, might need to apply pressure.
   b. Inspect along dressing and underneath client to determine amount of bleeding.
   c. Obtain vital signs as needed.
   d. Notify physician.
4. Client reports a sensation that "something has given way under the dressing."
   a. Observe wound for increased drainage or separation of sutures.
   b. Protect wound. Cover with sterile moist dressing.
   c. Instruct client to lie still.
   d. Notify physician.

Recording and Reporting

- Report brisk, bright red bleeding or evidence of wound dehiscence or evisceration to physician immediately.
- Report wound and periwound tissue appearance, color, and tissue type and presence and characteristics of exudate, type and amount of dressings used, and tolerance of client to procedure.
- Record client's level of comfort.
- Write date and time dressing applied on tape in ink (not marker).

Home Care Considerations

- More expensive specialty dressings may be used, because they decrease the frequency of dressing changes.
- Clean dressings may also be used in the home setting.
- Disposal of contaminated dressings in the home should be done in a manner consistent with local regulations.

---

lengths. They can be saturated with solutions and used to cleanse and pack a wound. When used to pack a wound, the gauze is saturated with the solution (usually normal saline), wrung out, unfolded, and lightly packed into the wound. The purpose of this type of dressing is to provide moisture to the wound, yet to allow wound drainage to be wicked into the gauze pad. Unfolding the dressing allows easier wicking action.

Wet-to-dry dressings are used in treating wounds that require debridement. The nurse moistens the contact dressing layer, wrings out the excessive solution, and packs into the wound and covers with a secondary dressing. The dressing is removed once the gauze dries, and as the gauze is pulled from the wound bed, wound debris should adhere to the gauze, facilitating necrotic tissue removal.

Nonadherent gauze dressings such as Telfa are used over clean wounds with little or no drainage. Telfa gauze has a shiny, nonadherent surface that does not stick to incisions or wound openings but allows drainage to pass through to the gauze topper.

Another type of dressing is a self-adhesive, transparent film. This type of dressing traps the wound's moisture over the wound, providing a moist environment. (Figure 47-22). The transparent film dressing is ideal for small, superficial wounds such as partial-thickness wounds, or to protect high risk skin. A film dressing can also be used as a secondary dressing, as well as for autolytic debridement of small wounds. It has the following advantages:

- Adheres to undamaged skin
- Serves as a barrier to external fluids and bacteria but still allows the wound surface to "breathe," because oxygen can pass through the transparent dressing
- Promotes a moist environment that speeds epithelial cell growth
- Can be removed without damaging underlying tissues
- Permits viewing the wound
- Does not require a secondary dressing

Hydrocolloid dressings are dressings with complex formulations of colloids, elastomeric, and adhesive components. These dressings are adhesive and occlusive. The wound contact layer of this dressing forms a gel as fluid is absorbed and maintains a moist healing environment. Hydrocolloids can be used to support healing in clean granulating wounds as well as to autolytically debride necrotic wounds. These dressings come in a variety of sizes and shapes. This type of dressing has the following functions:

- It absorbs drainage through the use of exudate absorbers in the dressing.
- It maintains wound moisture.
- It slowly liquefies necrotic debris.
- It is impermeable to bacteria and other contaminants.
- It is self-adhesive and molds well.

Table 47-10   **Dressing by Ulcer Stage**

Dressing (example of two brand names)	Mechanism of Action	Comments
Stage I		
Transparent film dressing (Tegadern, Bioclusive)	Protects from friction injury	May be left in place up to 7 days if occlusive seal remains
		Allows visualization of area
Thin hydrocolloid dressing (X-Thin DuoDERM, Restore X-Thin)	Provides protection of reddened area by decreasing surface injury	Flexible dressing that can remain in place up to 7 days; translucent, allowing visualization of area
Stage II		
Hydrocolloid dressing (DuoDerm, Comfeel)	Interacts with the wound fluid to provide a moist environment	Can stay in place until the seal is broken, allowing for enhanced healing
Composite dressing (Viasorb, Alldress)	Traps wound moisture and provides surface protection	Provides absorbent, nonadherent layer over wound with occlusive cover
Hydrogel dressing (Vigilon, Saf-Gel)	Provide moisture to a clean granular wound, supporting reepithelialization	Requires a secondary dressing
Foam dressing (Lyofoam, Polymem)	Absorbs exudate and debris while maintaining moist environment*	Is absorbent and nonadherent to wound base
		May be used with topical agents
Stage III		
Polyurethane foam (Lyofoam, Polymem)	Maintains moist wound environment*	Absorbs exudates
Hydrocolloid dressing (Duoderm, Comfeel)	Interacts with the wound fluid to provide a moist environment	Can cause slough tissue to soften by autolysis
		Effective with moderate amount of wound drainage
Hydrogel dressing (Vigilon, Saf-Gel)	Provides moisture to a clean granular wound, supporting reepithelialization	May be used to soften necrotic tissue, allowing for debridement
		Available in sheet dressing that can be packed into wound
Alginate dressing (Kaltostat, AlgiSite)	Absorbs excessive moisture	Can be left in wound bed until saturated
Stage IV		
Hydrocolloid dressing (Duoderm, Comfeel)	Interacts with the wound fluid to provide a moist environment	Only indicated for a clean wound and generally used with a filler dressing
Hydrogel dressing	Provides moisture to a wound and can be used to loosen necrotic tissue	Used to fill tunneling areas
Gauze roll dressing (Intersorb, Kerlix)	Provides moisture to wound when moistened with solution; will wick drainage from wound	Should be moistened with an appropriate solution, the gauze roll wrung out, unrolled, and packed lightly into wound
		Requires a secondary dressing
		Changed when strike through is noted on secondary dressing
		Generally requires dressing changes every 8 to 12 hr

*As with *all* occlusive dressings, wounds should *not* be clinically infected.

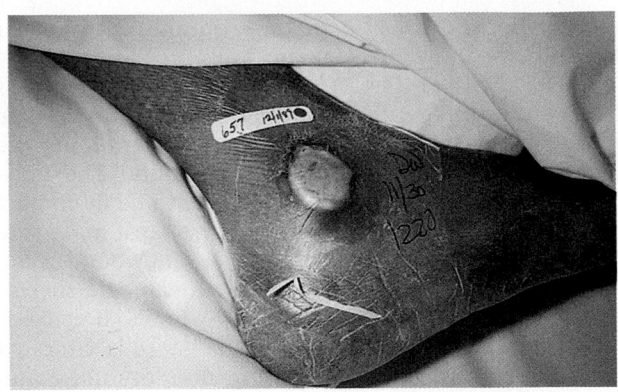

FIGURE **47–22** Transparent film dressing.

- It can be used as a preventive dressing for high-risk friction areas.
- It may be left in place for 3 to 5 days, minimizing skin trauma and disruption of healing.

This type of dressing is most useful on shallow to moderately deep dermal ulcers. A disadvantage of hydrocolloid dressings is most cannot absorb the amount of drainage from heavily draining wounds, and some are contraindicated for use in full-thickness and infected wounds. Some hydrocolloids may leave a residue in the wound bed that can be confused with pus.

Hydrogel dressings are water- or glycerin-based amorphous gel, impregnated gauze or sheet dressings. This type of dressing hydrates wounds and can absorb some but not large amounts of exudate. Hydrogel dressings are used on partial-thickness and full-thickness wounds, deep wounds with some exudate, necrotic wounds, burns, and radiation damaged skin. They are very useful in painful wounds, because they are very soothing to the client and do not adhere to the wound bed and thus cause little trauma during dressing removal. A disadvantage is that some hydrogels require a secondary dressing and care must be taken to prevent periwound maceration. Hydrogels come in a sheet dressing or in a tube where the gel can be squirted to the wound base.

Hydrogel has the following advantages:
- It is soothing and reduces pain in the wound.
- It provides a moist environment.
- It can debride the wound (by softening the necrotic tissue).
- It does not adhere to the wound base and can be easily removed.

There are many other types of dressings available. Foam dressings and alginate dressings are used in wounds with large amounts of exudate and in wounds that need packing. Foam dressings are also used around drainage tubes to absorb drainage. Calcium alginate dressings are manufactured from seaweed and come in sheet and rope form. The alginate forms a soft gel when it comes in contact with wound fluid. These highly absorbent dressings can be used on infected wounds and do not cause trauma when removed from the wound. They should not be used in dry wounds and require a secondary dressing. Several manufacturers produce composite dressings. These dress-ings combine two different dressing types into one dressing. Research is ongoing regarding what type of dressing is best for what type of wound (Cuzzell, 2002).

Changing Dressings. To prepare for changing a dressing, the nurse must know the type of dressing, the presence of underlying drains or tubing, and the type of supplies needed for wound care. Poor preparation may cause a break in aseptic technique (see Chapter 33) or accidental dislodging of a drain. The nurse's judgment in modifying a dressing change procedure is important during wound care, particularly if the character of a wound changes. Notifying the physician of any change is essential.

The physician's order for changing a dressing should indicate the dressing type, the frequency of changing, and any solutions or ointments to be applied to the wound. An order to "reinforce dressing prn" (add dressings without removing the original one) is common right after surgery, when the physician does not want accidental disruption of the suture line or bleeding. The medical or operating room record usually indicates whether drains are present and from what body cavity they drain. After the first dressing change, the nurse describes the location of drains and the type of dressing materials and solutions to use in the client's care plan. The CDC (2001) recommends the following during the dressing change procedure:
- The skin beneath the tape is also assessed.
- The nurse should perform thorough hand hygiene before and after wound care.
- Personnel should not touch an open or fresh wound directly without wearing sterile gloves (see Chapter 33).
- Dressings over closed wounds should be removed or changed when they become wet or if the client has signs or symptoms of infection and as ordered.

There is a growing body of literature about sterile versus clean dressings. The AHCPR guidelines (1994) recommend that clean dressings and gloves be used on pressure ulcers. For surgical wounds, preliminary research indicates no difference in the healing rate of wounds when clean rather than sterile dressing change technique is used (Box 47-14).

To prepare a client for a dressing change, the nurse does the following:
- Administers required analgesics so that peak effects occur during the dressing change
- Describes steps of the procedure to lessen client anxiety
- Gathers all supplies required for the dressing change
- Recognizes normal signs of healing
- Answers questions about the procedure or the wound

Often it is necessary to teach clients how to change dressings in preparation for home care. In this situation the nurse must demonstrate dressing changes to the client and family and then provide an opportunity for the client or family member to practice. Usually in this situation wound healing has progressed to the point that risks of complications such as dehiscence or evisceration are minimal. The client should be able to change a dressing independently or with assistance from a family member before discharge. The AHCPR guidelines (1994) state that "clean dressing may also be used in the home setting for pressure ulcers. Disposal of contaminated dressings in the home should be done in a manner consistent with lo-

Research Highlight   Box 47-14

Quality Care and Pressure Ulcer Risk

Research Focus

Pressure ulcers continue to present a major health care problem for hospitalized older adults. The prediction and prevention of pressure ulcers is a top priority. It is important that processes of quality care related to pressure ulcer prediction and prevention be instituted as part of the development of the plan of care to predict and prevent the incidence of pressure ulcer development.

Research Abstract

The purpose of this research was to profile and evaluate the processes of care for Medicare clients hospitalized at risk for pressure ulcer development. The study examined the quality of care delivered to older adults at risk for pressure ulcer development in hospitals throughout the United States. Medical records of 2425 clients aged 65 years and older were evaluated for use of daily skin assessment, use of pressure-reducing device, documentation of being at risk, repositioning for a minimum of 2 hours, nutritional consultation for at-risk individuals, and staging of pressure ulcer. The associations between the previously noted process of care and the occurrence of pressure ulcer development were determined. Results showed compliance with the process of care: use of daily skin assessment, 94%; use of pressure-reducing device, 7.5%; documentation of being at risk, 22.6%; repositioning for a minimum of 2 hours, 66.2%; nutritional consultation, 43.3%; stage I pressure ulcer staged, 20.2%; and stage II or greater ulcer stage, 30.9%. The authors felt that the results suggest that caregivers in U.S. hospitals have numerous opportunities to improve care related to pressure ulcer prediction and prevention.

Evidence-Based Practice

- Lack of documentation of clients at risk demonstrates the need for hospitals to increase prediction and prevention strategies. Use of a risk scale can provide triggers to plan care to decrease risk factors.
- Extended stays of over 7 days increase the risk of pressure ulcer development. Nurses must remain vigilant in the prevention of pressure ulcers in clients with longer stays.
- Use of care practices such as daily skin assessment, use of pressure-relief surfaces and objective risk assessment measures (e.g., Braden Scale) identified at risk clients and reduced evidence of pressure ulcers.
- The use of a nutritional consultation was associated with decreased incidence of pressure ulcers, suggesting a nutritional consultation may sensitize the staff that the older adult is at risk for pressure ulcer development.

Reference

Lyder CH and others: Quality of care for hospitalized Medicare patients at risk for pressure ulcers, *Arch Intern Med* 161(12): 1549, 2001.

---

cal regulations." Skill 47-3, p. 1529, outlines the steps for changing dry and wet-to-dry dressings.

Packing a Wound. The first step in packing a wound is to assess the size, depth, and shape of the wound. These wound characteristics are important in determining the size and type of dressing used to pack a wound. The dressing should be flexible and must be able to be in contact with all of the wound surface. The nurse must make sure that the type of material used to pack the wound is appropriate. There are many new dressing materials, such as alginates, that are also used to pack wounds. If gauze is the appropriate dressing material, the gauze is saturated with the ordered solution, wrung out, unfolded and lightly packed into the wound. The entire wound surface should be in contact with part of the moist gauze dressing (see Skill 47-3, p. 1529). The AHCPR guidelines (1994) recommend that wound dead space be eliminated by loosely filling all of the wound cavity with the dressing material. Dead space is "a cavity remaining in a wound" (AHCPR, 1994). It is important to remember that the wound cavity needs to be filled so that areas are not "walled off," to prevent abscesses (AHCPR, 1994).

It is important to remember that the wound should not be packed too tightly. Overpacking the wound may cause pressure on the tissue in the wound bed. The wound should be packed only until the packing material reaches the surface of the wound; there should never be so much packing material in the wound that it extends higher than the wound surface. Wound packing that overlaps onto the wound edges can cause maceration of the tissue surrounding the wound. It can also impede the proper healing and closing of the wound.

A new treatment modality for chronic wounds is vacuum-assisted closure (the brand name is Wound V.A.C.). The **Wound Vacuum Assisted Closure (Wound V.A.C.)** is a device that assists in wound closure by applying localized negative pressure to draw the edges of a wound together (Figure 47-23, *A, B*). Wound V.A.C. accelerates wound healing by promoting the formation of granulation tissue, collagen, fibroblasts, and inflammatory cells in order to completely close or improve the health of a wound in preparation for a skin graft. The use of negative pressure removes fluid from the area surrounding the wound, thus reducing local peripheral edema and improving circulation to the area (Chua and others, 2000) (Figure 47-24). In addition, after 3 to 4 days of therapy bacterial counts in the wound drop (Argenta and Morykwas, 1997; Evans and Land, 2001).

Wound V.A.C. may be used to treat acute and chronic wounds (Skill 47-4). The schedule for changing Wound V.A.C. dressings vary. An infected wound may need a dressing change every 24 hours, whereas a clean wound can be changed 3 times a week (Chua and others, 2000; Mendez-Eastman, 1998). As the wound heals, the wound base is redder and granulation tissue will line the surface of the wound. The wound has a stippled or granulated appearance. Last, the surface area of the wound may increase or decrease depending on wound location and the amount of drainage removed by the Wound V.A.C. system. As the wound heals, paler areas in the wound may develop. This indicates an increase in fibrous tissue (Mendez-Eastman, 1998).

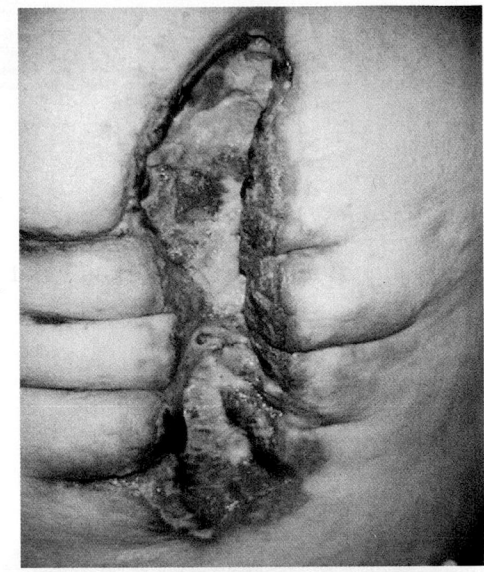

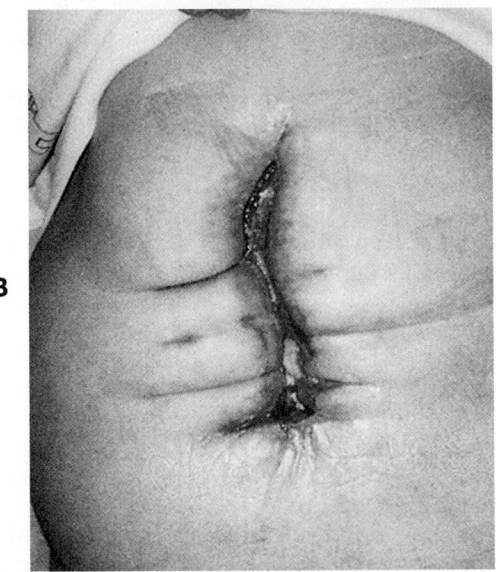

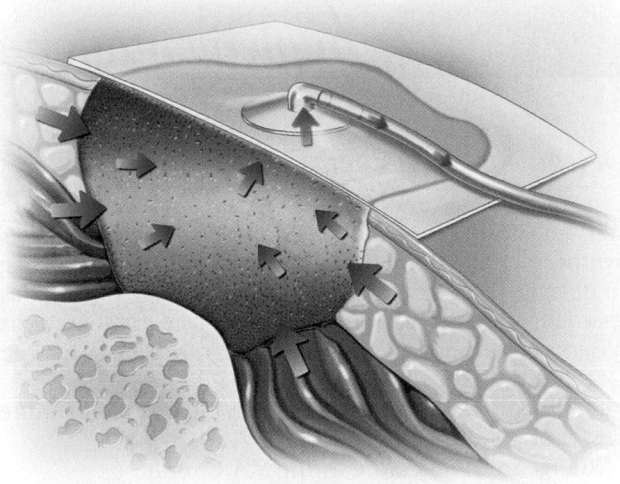

FIGURE **47–24** Wound V.A.C. system using negative pressure to remove fluid from area surrounding the wound, reducing edema and improving circulation to the area. (Courtesy Kinetic Concepts, Inc [KCI], San Antonio, Tex.)

FIGURE **47–23 A,** Dehisced wound before Wound V.A.C. therapy. **B,** Dehisced wound after Wound V.A.C. therapy. (Courtesy Kinetic Concepts, Inc [KCI], San Antonio, Tex.)

Securing Dressings. The nurse may use tape, ties, or bandages, or a secondary dressing and cloth binders to secure a dressing over a wound site. The choice of anchoring depends on the wound size and location, the presence of drainage, the frequency of dressing changes, and the client's level of activity.

The nurse most often uses strips of tape to secure dressings if the client is not allergic to tape. Nonallergenic paper and plastic tapes minimize skin reactions. Common adhesive tape adheres well to the skin's surface, whereas elastic adhesive tape compresses closely around pressure bandages and permits more movement of a body part. Skin sensitive to adhesive tape can become severely inflamed and denuded and may even slough when the tape is removed. It is important to assess skin under tape at each dressing change.

Tape is available in various widths such as ½, 1, 2, and 3 inches. The nurse chooses the size that sufficiently secures the dressing. For example, a large abdominal wound dressing must remain secure over a large area despite frequent stress from movement, respiratory effort, and possibly abdominal distention. Strips of 3-inch adhesive better stabilize such a large dressing so that it does not continually slip off. When applying tape, the nurse ensures that it adheres to several inches of skin on both sides of the dressing and that it is placed across the middle of the dressing. When securing the dressing, the nurse presses the tape gently, exerting pressure away from the wound. This way, tension occurs in both directions away from the wound, minimizing skin distortion and irritation. Tape is never applied over irritated or broken skin. Some nurses protect the skin beneath the tape with a skin sealant product.

To remove tape safely, the nurse loosens the tape ends and gently pulls the outer end parallel with the skin surface toward the wound. The nurse applies light traction to the skin away from the wound as the tape is loosened and removed. Adhesive remover can also be used to loosen the tape from the skin. The traction minimizes pulling of the skin. If tape covers an area of hair growth, the client experiences less discomfort if the nurse pulls the tape in the direction of hair growth.

To avoid repeated removal of tape from sensitive skin, the nurse can secure dressings with pairs of reusable Montgomery ties (Figure 47-26). Each section consists of a long strip; half contains an adhesive backing to apply to the skin, and the other half folds back and contains a cloth tie or a safety pin and rubber band combination to be fastened across a dressing and untied at dressing changes. A large, bulky dressing may require two or more sets of Montgomery ties. Another method to protect the surrounding skin on wounds that need frequent dressing changes is to place strips of hydrocolloid dressings on either side of the wound edges, cover the wound with a
Text continued on p. 1542

Skill 47-4   *Implementation of Vacuum Assisted Closure*

Delegation Considerations

Assessment for and placement of Wound Vacuum Assisted Closure (V.A.C.) should not be delegated to assistive personnel (AP). Other aspects of the client care may be delegated, but the nurse is responsible for wound assessment and evaluation of wound care interventions. When delegating aspects of care the nurse must instruct AP to do the following:

- Report to the nurse any change in client's temperature, level of comfort.
- Change in the pressure in the V.A.C. unit.
- Any change in the integrity of the Wound V.A.C. dressing.

Equipment

- V.A.C. unit (requires physician order) (Figure 47-25)
- V.A.C. foam dressing
- Tubing for connection between V.A.C. unit and V.A.C. dressing
- Gloves, clean and sterile
- Scissors (sterile)
- Skin prep/skin barrier
- Moist washcloth
- Plastic trash bag
- Linen bag

Steps	Rationale
1. Perform hand hygeine. Assemble supplies.	Reduces transmission of microorganisms. Organizes procedure.
2. Position client comfortably and drape to expose only wound site. Instruct client not to touch wound or sterile supplies.	Maintaining client comfort assists in completing skill smoothly. Draping provides access to wound while minimizing unnecessary exposure.
3. Place disposable waterproof bag within reach of work area with top folded to make a cuff.	Facilitates safe disposal of soiled dressings.
4. When V.A.C. is in place, push therapy on/off button. a. Keeping tube connectors with V.A.C. unit, disconnect tubes from each other to drain fluids into canister. b. Before lowering, tighten clamp on canister tube.	Deactivates therapy and allows for proper drainage of fluid in drainage tubing.
5. With dressing tube unclamped, introduce 10 to 30 ml of normal saline, if ordered, into tubing to soak underneath foam.	Facilitates loosening of foam when tissue adheres to foam (Chua and others, 2000).
6. Gently stretch transparent film horizontally and slowly pull up from the skin.	Reduces stress on suture line or wound edges and reduces irritation and discomfort.
7. Remove old V.A.C. dressing, observing appearance and drainage on dressing. Use caution to avoid tension on any drains that are present. Discard dressing and remove gloves.	Determines dressings needed for replacement. Avoids accidental removal of drains because they may or may not be sutured in place.
8. Apply sterile or clean gloves. Irrigate the wound with normal saline or other solution ordered by the physician. Gently blot to dry.	Irrigation removes wound debris.

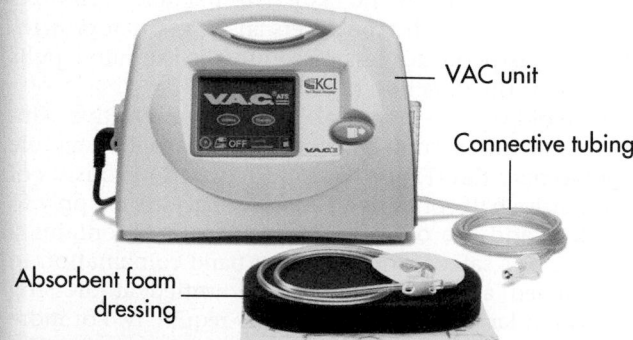

FIGURE **47–25** Wound V.A.C. unit. *Top to bottom:* V.A.C. unit itself, connective tubing to go between V.A.C. unit and V.A.C. dressing, absorbent foam dressing. (Courtesy Kinetic Concepts, Inc [KCI], San Antonio, Tex.)

Steps	Rationale

Critical Decision Point: When drainage looks purulent, or there is change in amount or color, or it has a foul odor, wound cultures should be obtained even when they are not ordered for that particular dressing change (Chua and others, 2000).

9. Measure wound as ordered: at baseline, first dressing change, weekly, and discharge from therapy. Remove and discard gloves.	Objectively documents wound healing process in response to negative pressure, wound therapy (Bannwell, Holten, and Martin, 1998).
10. Depending on the type of wound, apply sterile gloves or new clean gloves.	Fresh sterile wounds require sterile gloves. Chronic wounds may require clean technique. However, do not use the same gloves worn to remove old dressing because cross contamination may occur (Mendez-Eastman, 1998; Stotts and others, 1997).
11. Prepare V.A.C. foam. a. Select appropriate foam.	Black, polyurethane (PU) foam has larger pores and is most effective in stimulating granulation tissue and wound contraction. White, polyvinyl alcohol (PVA) soft foam is denser with smaller pores and is used when the growth of granulation tissue needs to be restricted (KCI, 1999).
b. Using sterile scissors, cut foam to wound size. Dressing must be cut to fit the size and shape of the wound including tunnels and undermined areas.	

Critical Decision Point: Clients may experience more pain with the black foam because of excessive wound contraction. For this reason they may need to be switched to the PVA soft foam.

12. Gently place foam in wound; be sure that the foam is in contact with entire wound base and margins and tunneled and undermined areas (see illustration step 12A).	Maintains negative pressure to entire wound. Edges of the foam dressing must be in direct contact with the client's skin (Broussard, Mendez-Eastman, and Frantz, 2000).
13. Apply wrinkle free transparent dressing over foam and secure tubing to the unit (see illustration step 12, B and C).	Connects the negative pressure from the V.A.C. unit to the wound foam.

Critical Decision Point: For deep wounds regularly reposition tubing to minimize pressure on wound edges. In addition, clients with restricted mobility or sensation must be repositioned frequently to prevent laying on the tubing and causing skin damage (KCI, 1999).

14. Apply skin protectant, such as skin prep or Stomahesive wafer, to skin around the wound.	Protects periwound skin from injury that may result from the occlusive dressing.
15. Apply Wound V.A.C. dressing. Secure tubing to transparent film, aligning drainage holes to ensure an occlusive seal (see illustration step 12, C). Do not apply tension to drape and tubing.	Ensures that the wound is properly covered and a negative pressure seal can be achieved (see Box 47-15, p. 1540). Excessive tension may compress foam dressing and impede wound healing. Excessive tension also produces a shear force on periwound area (KCI, 1999).
16. Secure tubing several centimeters away from the dressing.	Prevents pull on the primary dressing, which can cause leaks in the negative pressure system (Chua and others, 2000; KCI, 1999).

Implementation of Vacuum Assisted Closure—cont'd

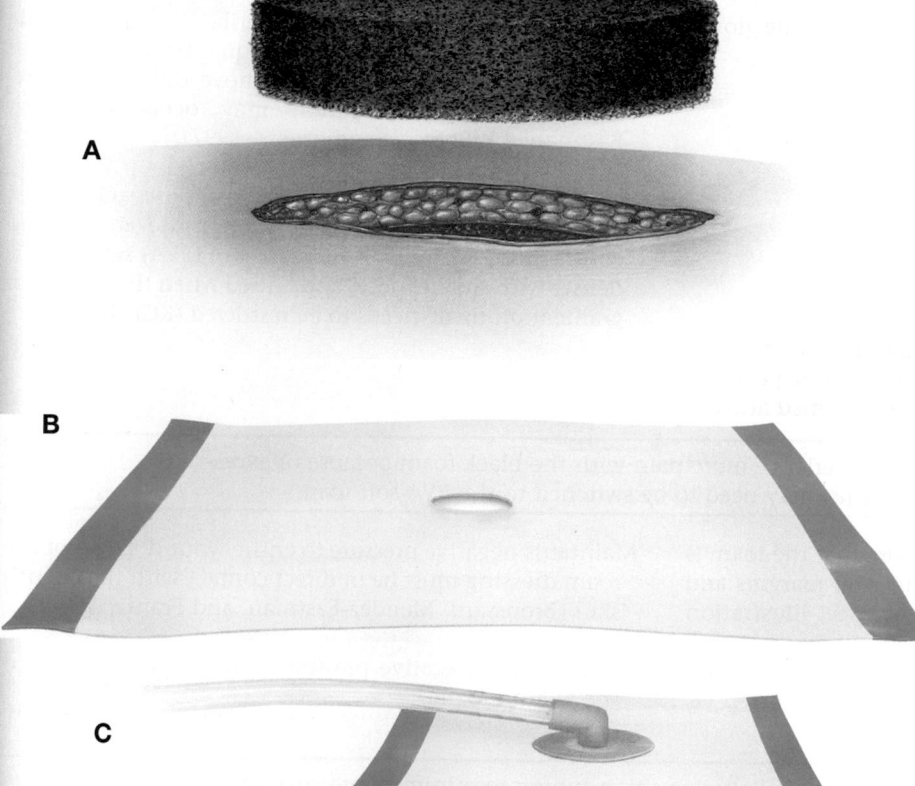

STEP **12**   Dressing application. **A,** Properly sized foam to cover wound (step 12). **B,** Wrinkle-free transparent dressing applied over foam (step 13). **C,** Secure tubing to the foam and transparent dressing unit (step 15). (Courtesy Kinetic Concepts, Inc [KCI]), San Antonio, Tex.)

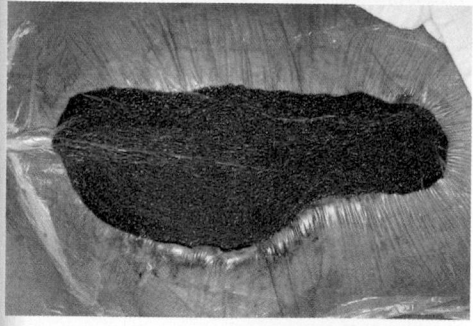

STEP **17**   Foam dressing, transparent dressing, and Wound V.A.C. tubing secured over existing wound. (Courtesy Kinetic Concepts, Inc [KCI], San Antonio, Tex.)

Box 47-15   Maintaining an Airtight Seal

To avoid wound desiccation, the wound must stay sealed once therapy is initiated. Problem seal areas include wounds around joints and near the sacrum. The following points may assist in maintaining an airtight seal:
- Shave hair around wound.
- Cut transparent film to extend 3 to 5 cm beyond wound parameter.

- Avoid wrinkles in transparent film.
- Patch leaks with transparent film.
- Use multiple small strips of transparent film to hold dressing in place before covering dressing with large piece of transparent film.
- Avoid adhesive remover because it leaves a residue that hinders film adherence.

From Chua PC and others: Vacuum-assisted wound closure, *Am J Nurs* 100(12):45, 2000.

Steps	Rationale

17. Once wound is completely covered (see illustration), connect the tubing from the dressing to the tubing from the canister and V.A.C. unit.
   a. Remove canister from sterile packaging and push into V.A.C. unit until a click is heard. NOTE: **an alarm will sound if the canister is not properly engaged.**
   b. Connect the dressing tubing to the canister tubing. Make sure both clamps are open.
   c. Place V.A.C. unit on a level surface or hang from the foot of the bed. NOTE: **The V.A.C. unit will alarm and deactivate therapy if the unit is tilted beyond 45 degrees.**
   d. Press in green-lit power button and set pressure as ordered.
	Intermittent or continuous negative pressure can be administered at 50 to 200 mm Hg, according to physician order and client comfort. The average is 125 mm Hg (Baxandall, 1996; Chua and others, 2000).

18. Discard old dressing materials; remove gloves and perform hand hygiene.	Reduces transmission of microorganisms. Negative pressure is achieved when an airtight seal is achieved.

19. Inspect Wound V.A.C. system to verify that negative pressure is achieved.
   a. Verify that display screen reads THERAPY ON.
   b. Be sure clamps are open and tubing is patent.
   c. Identify air leaks by listening with stethoscope or by moving hand around edges of wound while applying light pressure.
   d. If a leak is present, use strips of transparent film to patch areas.	

20. Compare wound with baseline wound assessment.	Provides objective documentation of wound healing.
21. Verify airtight dressing seal and proper negative pressure.	In order to achieve prescribed vacuum level, the wound must be covered with an airtight seal. This airtight seal and the negative pressure promote wound drainage, circulation, and healing.

Unexpected Outcomes and Related Interventions

1. Wound appears inflamed and tender, drainage has increased, and an odor is present.
   a. Notify physician.
   b. Obtain wound culture.
   c. Increase frequency of dressing changes.
2. Client reports increase in pain.
   a. If using black foam, switch to the PVA foam product.
   b. Client may need more analgesic support when V.A.C. is initiated.
   c. Negative pressure may need to be reduced.
3. Negative pressure seal has broken.
   a. Take preventive measures: Shave hair around wound, avoid wrinkles in transparent dressing, and avoid use of adhesive remover because it may leave residue that hinders film adherence.
   b. Reinforce with transparent dressing strips.

Recording and Reporting

- Record appearance of wound, color, characteristics of any drainage, presence of wound healing augmentation.
- Record pressure setting of Wound V.A.C.
- Record date and time of dressing change.
- Report brisk, bright bleeding, evidence of poor wound healing, and possible wound infection.

Home Care Considerations

- Wound V.A.C. can be used in the home safely. Client may need clinic visits or home care nursing visits to monitor wound healing.
- Provide resources to client for supplies for Wound V.A.C.
- Instruct family and caregiver regarding proper disposal of contaminated product.

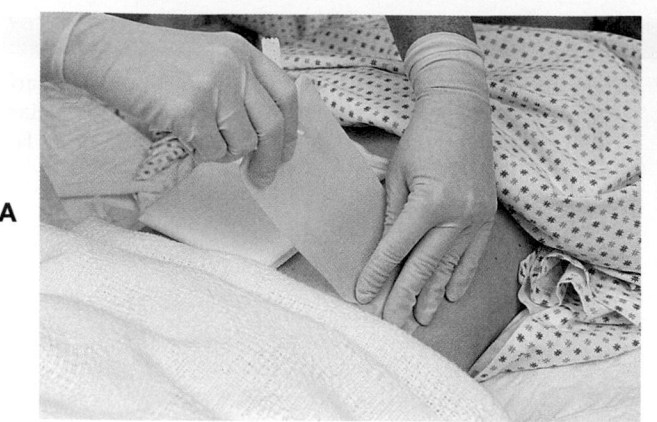
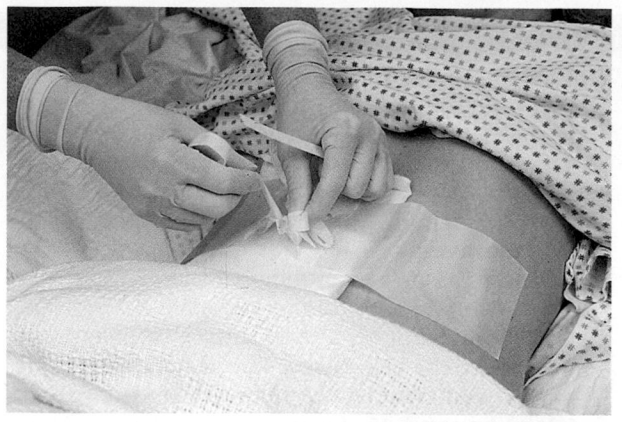

FIGURE **47–26** Montgomery ties. **A,** Each tie is placed at side of dressing. **B,** Securing ties encloses dressing.

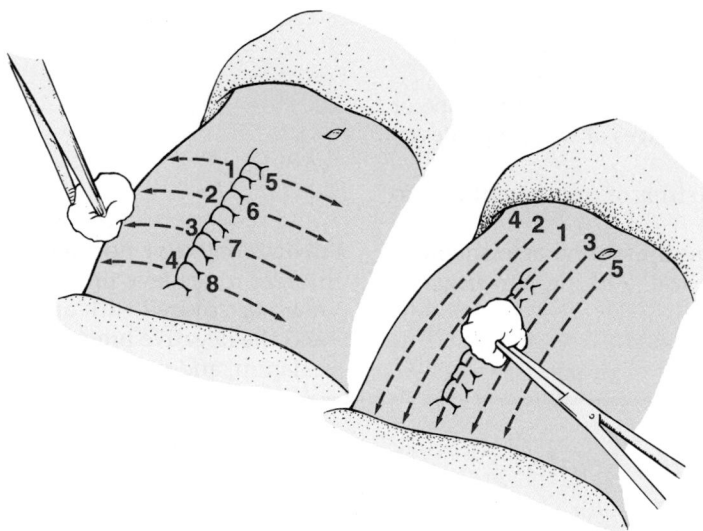

FIGURE **47–27** Methods for cleansing a wound site.

dressing, and then apply the tape to the hydrocolloid dressing. To provide even support to a wound and immobilize a body part, the nurse may apply elastic gauze or cloth bandages and binders over a dressing.

Comfort Measures. A wound can be painful, depending on the extent of tissue injury. The nurse uses several techniques to minimize discomfort during wound care. Careful removal of tape, gentle cleansing of wound edges, and careful manipulation of dressings and drains minimize stress on sensitive tissues. Careful turning and positioning also reduce strain on a wound. Administration of analgesic medications 30 to 60 minutes before dressing changes (depending on a drug's time of peak action) also reduces discomfort.

Cleansing Skin and Drain Sites. Although a moderate amount of wound exudate promotes epithelial cell growth, the physician may order cleansing of a wound or drain site if a dressing does not properly absorb drainage or if an open drain deposits drainage onto the skin. Wound cleansing requires good hand-washing and aseptic techniques (see Chapter 33). The nurse may use irrigation to remove debris.

Basic Skin Cleansing. The nurse cleanses surgical or traumatic wounds by applying noncytotoxic solutions with sterile gauze or by irrigation. The following three principles are important when cleansing an incision or the area surrounding a drain:

1. Cleanse in a direction from the least contaminated area, such as from the wound or incision to the surrounding skin (Figure 47-27) or from an isolated drain site to the surrounding skin (Figure 47-28).
2. Use gentle friction when applying solutions locally to the skin.
3. When irrigating, allow the solution to flow from the least to most contaminated area.

After applying a solution to sterile gauze, the nurse cleanses away from the wound. The nurse never uses the

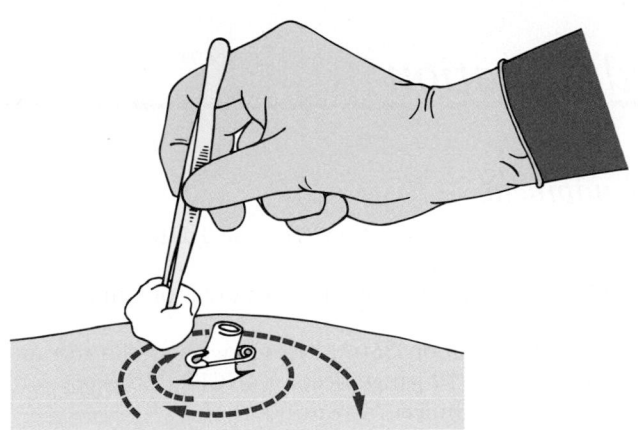

FIGURE **47–28** Cleansing a drain site.

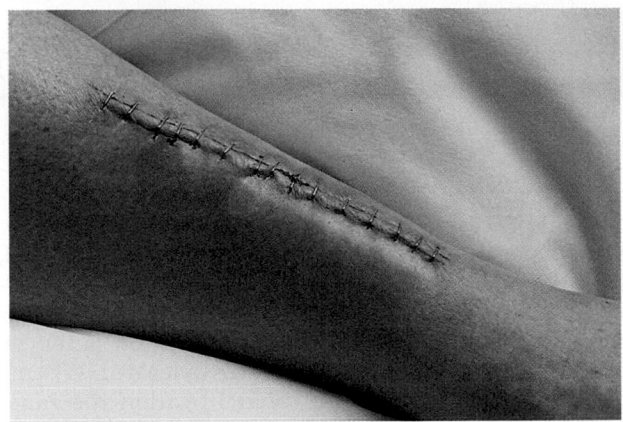

FIGURE **47–29** Incision closed with metal staples.

same piece of gauze to cleanse across an incision or wound twice.

A drain site can be contaminated because moist drainage harbors microorganisms. If a wound has a dry incisional area and a moist drain site, cleansing moves from the incisional area toward the drain. The nurse uses two separate swabs or gauze pads, one to cleanse from the top of the incision toward the drain and one to cleanse from the bottom of the incision toward the drain. To cleanse the area of an isolated drain site, the nurse cleans around the drain, moving in circular rotations outward from a point closest to the drain. In this situation the skin near the site is more contaminated than the site itself. To cleanse circular wounds, the nurse uses the same technique as in cleansing around a drain.

Irrigations. Irrigations are a special way of cleansing wounds. The nurse uses an irrigating syringe to flush the area with a constant low-pressure flow of solution. The gentle washing action of the irrigation cleanses a wound of exudate and debris. Irrigations are particularly useful for open, deep wounds involving an inaccessible body part, such as the ear canal, or when cleansing sensitive body parts, such as the conjunctival lining of the eye.

Wound Irrigations. Irrigation of an open wound requires sterile technique. The nurse uses a 35-ml syringe with a 19-gauge needle (AHCPR, 1994; Ratliff and Bryant, 2003) to deliver the solution, using an irrigation system that has a safe pressure and will not damage healing wound tissue. It is important to never occlude a wound opening with a syringe, because this results in the introduction of irrigating fluid into a closed space. The pressure of the fluid could cause tissue damage and discomfort. A wound should always be irrigated with the syringe tip over but not in the drainage site. Fluid should flow directly into the wound and not over a contaminated area before entering the wound. Skill 47-5 lists steps for wound irrigation.

Suture Care. A surgeon closes a wound by bringing the wound edges as close together as possible to reduce scar formation. Proper wound closure involves minimal trauma and tension to tissues with control of bleeding. **Sutures** are threads or metal used to sew body tissues together (Figure 47-29). The client's history of wound

healing, the site of surgery, the tissues involved, and the purpose of the sutures determine the suture material to be used. For example, if the client has had repeated surgery for an abdominal hernia, the physician might choose wire sutures to provide greater strength for wound closure. In contrast, a small laceration of the face calls for the use of very fine Dacron (polyester) sutures to minimize scar formation.

Sutures are available in a variety of materials, including silk, steel, cotton, linen, wire, nylon, and Dacron. Sutures come with or without sharp surgical needles attached. Commonly seen are steel staples, a type of outer skin closure that causes less trauma to tissues than sutures, yet provides extra strength. It is also common to see wounds closed with tape closures such as Steri-Strips applied over the wound to keep the edges closed.

Sutures are placed within tissue layers in deep wounds and superficially as the final means for wound closure. Deep sutures are usually an absorbable material that will disappear over time. Sutures are foreign bodies and thus are capable of causing local inflammation. The surgeon can minimize tissue injury by using the finest suture possible and the smallest number necessary.

Policies vary within institutions as to who may remove sutures. If it is appropriate that the nurse remove them, a physician's order is required. An order for suture removal is not written until the physician believes that the wound has closed (usually in 7 days). Special scissors with curved cutting tips or special staple removers slide under the skin closures for suture removal (Figure 47-30). The physician usually signifies the number of sutures or staples to remove. If the suture line appears to be healing in certain locations better than in others, the physician may choose to have only some sutures removed (e.g., every other one).

To remove staples, the nurse simply inserts the tips of the staple remover under each wire staple. While slowly closing the ends of the staple remover together, the nurse squeezes the center of the staple with the tips, freeing the staple from the skin.

To remove sutures, the nurse first checks the type of suturing used (Figure 47-31). With intermittent suturing, the surgeon ties each individual suture made in the skin. Continuous suturing, as the name implies, is a series of

Text continued on p. 1546

Skill 47-5   *Performing Wound Irrigation*

Delegation Considerations

The skill of wound irrigation should not be delegated to assistive personnel (AP). In the case of a chronic wound, cleansing of the wound using *clean* technique can be delegated to AP. Assessment of any wound, care of acute new wounds, and evaluation of wound irrigation is the responsibility of the nurse and is never delegated. When a wound is stable or requires clean irrigation the nurse should instruct AP to do the following:

- Report any change in wound appearance or increased wound drainage to the nurse.
- Use proper clean technique to avoid cross contamination from irrigation syringes and equipment.

Equipment

- Irrigant/cleansing solution (volume 1.2 to 2 times the estimated wound volume)
- Irrigation delivery system depending on amount of pressure desired:
    Sterile irrigation 35-ml syringe with sterile soft angiocatheter or 19-gauge needle (AHCPR, 1994) *or*
    Handheld shower or whirlpool
- Clean gloves
- Sterile gloves
- Waterproof underpad, if needed
- Dressing supplies
- Disposable waterproof bag
- Gown, if risk of spray
- Goggles, if risk of spray

Steps	Rationale
1. Assess client's level of pain. Administer prescribed analgesic 30 to 45 minutes before starting wound irrigation procedure.	Discomfort may be related directly to wound or indirectly to muscle tension or immobility. Increased comfort level permits client to move more easily and be positioned to facilitate wound irrigation.
2. Review medical record for physician's prescription for irrigation of open wound and type of solution to be used.	Open wound irrigation requires medical order, including type of solutions to use.
3. Assess recent recording of signs and symptoms related to client's open wound.	Data are used as baseline to indicate change in condition of wound (Cooper, 2000).
a. Condition of skin and wound	
b. Elevation of body temperature	May indicate response to infection.
c. Drainage from wound (amount, color)	Amount will decrease as healing takes place.
d. Odor	Strong odor indicates infectious process.
e. Consistency of drainage	Leukocytes produce thick drainage.
f. Size of wounds, including depth, length, and width	Determines stage of healing.
4. Explain procedure of wound irrigation and cleansing.	Information will reduce client's anxiety.
5. Perform hand hygiene.	Reduces transmission of microorganisms.
6. Position client comfortably to permit gravitational flow of irrigating solution through wound and into collection receptacle. Position client so that wound is vertical to collection basin.	Directing solution from top to bottom of wound and from clean to contaminated area prevents further infection. Positioning client during planning stage provides bed surfaces for later preparation of equipment.
7. Warm irrigation solution to approximate body temperature.	Warmed solution increases comfort and reduces vascular constriction response in tissues.
8. Form cuff on waterproof bag and place it near bed.	Cuffing helps to maintain large opening, thereby permitting placement of contaminated dressing without touching refuse bag itself.
9. Close room door or bed curtains.	Maintains privacy.
10. Apply gown and goggles if needed.	Protects nurse from splashes or sprays of blood and body fluids.
11. Put on clean gloves and remove soiled dressing and discard in waterproof bag. Discard gloves.	Reduces transmission of microorganisms.
12. Prepare equipment; open sterile supplies.	
13. Put on sterile gloves.	

Steps	Rationale
14. To irrigate wound with wide opening:	
a. Fill 35-ml syringe with irrigation solution.	Flushing wound helps remove debris and facilitates healing by secondary intention.
b. Attach 19-gauge needle or angiocatheter (see Figure 47-21, p. 1526).	Provides ideal pressure for cleansing and removal of debris.
c. Hold syringe tip 2.5 cm (1 inch) above upper end of wound and over area being cleansed.	Prevents syringe contamination. Careful placement of the syringe prevents unsafe pressure of the flowing solution.
d. Using continuous pressure, flush wound; repeat steps 14a, b, and c until solution draining into basin is clear.	Clear solution indicates that all debris has been removed.
15. To irrigate deep wound with very small opening:	
a. Attach soft angiocatheter to filled irrigating syringe.	Catheter permits direct flow of irrigant into wound. Expect wound to take longer to empty when opening is small.
b. Lubricate tip of catheter with irrigating solution; then gently insert tip of catheter and pull out about 1 cm (½ inch).	Removes tip from fragile inner wall of wound.
c. Using slow, continuous pressure, flush wound.	

Critical Decision Point: CAUTION: Splashing may occur during this step.

Steps	Rationale
d. Pinch off catheter just below syringe while keeping catheter in place.	Avoids contamination of sterile solution.
e. Remove and refill syringe. Reconnect to catheter and repeat until solution draining into basin is clear.	
16. To cleanse wound with handheld shower:	Useful for clients able to shower with assistance or independently. May be accomplished at home. A shower table is helpful for bed-bound or acutely ill clients.
a. With client seated comfortably in shower chair, adjust spray to gentle flow; water temperature should be warm.	
b. Cover showerhead with clean washcloth if needed.	
c. Shower for 5 to 10 minutes with showerhead 12 inches (30 cm) from wound.	

Critical Decision Point: Consider culturing a wound if it has a foul, purulent odor; inflammation surrounds the wound; a nondraining wound begins to drain; or client is febrile.

Steps	Rationale
17. Obtain cultures, if needed, after cleansing with non-bacteriostatic saline.	Routine culturing of open wounds is not recommended in the AHCPR guidelines (1994). They recommend using quantitative bacterial cultures (tissue biopsy or wound fluid by needle aspiration) rather than swab cultures, which often detect only surface bacterial contaminants.
18. Dry wound edges with gauze; dry client if shower or whirlpool is used.	Prevents maceration of surrounding tissue caused by excess moisture.
19. Apply appropriate dressing (see Skill 47-2, p. 1519 and Skill 47-3, p. 1529).	Maintains protective barrier and healing environment for wound.
20. Remove gloves and, if worn, mask, goggles, and gown.	Prevents transfer of microorganisms.
21. Dispose of equipment and soiled supplies. Perform hand hygiene.	Reduces transmission of microorganisms.
22. Assist client to comfortable position.	
23. Assess type of tissue in the wound bed.	Identifies wound-healing progress and determines type of wound cleansing needed.
24. Inspect dressing periodically.	Determines client's response to wound irrigation and need to modify plan of care.
25. Evaluate skin integrity.	Determines if extension of wound has occurred.

Skill 47-5   *Performing* Wound Irrigation—*cont'd*

Steps	Rationale
26. Observe client for signs of discomfort.	Client's pain should not increase as a result of wound irrigation.
27. Observe for presence of retained irrigant.	Retained irrigant is a medium for bacterial growth and subsequent infection.

Unexpected Outcomes and Related Interventions

1. Wound does not appear to heal.
   a. Obtain wound culture.
   b. Notify physician, who may change dressing and or irrigation frequency.
2. Wound drainage increases.
   a. Apply more absorbent gauze.
   b. Increase the frequency of irrigation.

Recording and Reporting

- Record wound irrigation and client response on progress notes.
- Immediately report any evidence of fresh bleeding, sharp increase in pain, retention of irrigant, or signs of shock to attending physician.
- At change of shift, report expected and unexpected outcomes that have actually occurred.

Home Care Considerations

- Teach client and caregiver how to make normal saline, especially if cost is an issue. Normal saline can be made by using 2 teaspoons of salt in 1 L (1 quart) of boiling water (Barr, 1995).
- Tell client and caregiver that because normal saline has no preservatives, it should be thrown out 24 to 48 hours after it is first opened or made (Barr, 1995).

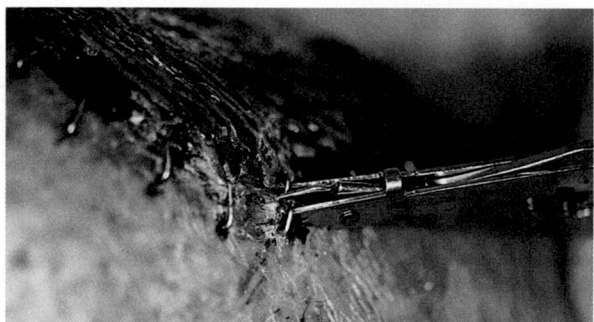

FIGURE **47–30** Staple remover.

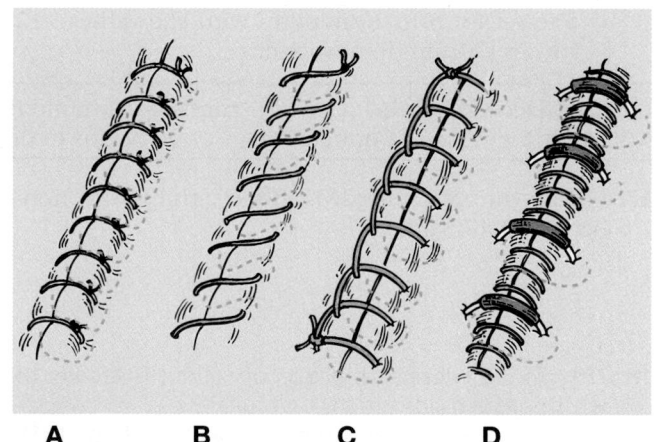

FIGURE **47–31** Examples of suturing methods. **A,** Intermittent. **B,** Continuous. **C,** Blanket continuous. **D,** Retention.

sutures with only two knots, one at the beginning and one at the end of the suture line. Retention sutures are placed more deeply than skin sutures and may or may not be removed by the nurse, depending on agency policy. The manner in which the suture crosses and penetrates the skin determines the method for removal. The most important principle in suture removal is to never pull the visible portion of a suture through underlying tissue. Sutures on the skin's surface harbor microorganisms and debris. The portion of the suture beneath the skin is sterile. Pulling the contaminated portion of the suture through tissues may

lead to infection. The nurse clips suture materials as close to the skin edge on one side as possible and pulls the suture through from the other side (Figure 47-32).

Drainage Evacuation. When drainage interferes with healing, drainage evacuation can be achieved by using either a drain alone or a drainage tube with continuous

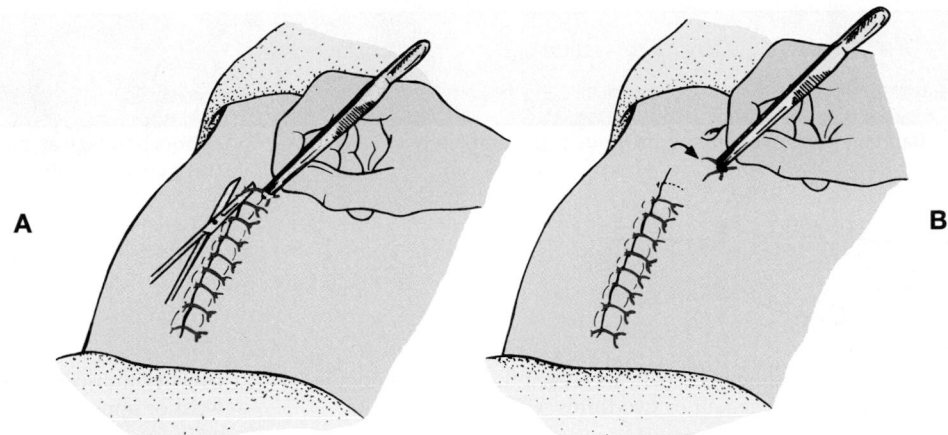

FIGURE **47–32** Removal of intermittent suture. **A,** The nurse cuts the suture as close to the skin as possible, away from the knot. **B,** The nurse removes the suture and never pulls the contaminated stitch through tissues.

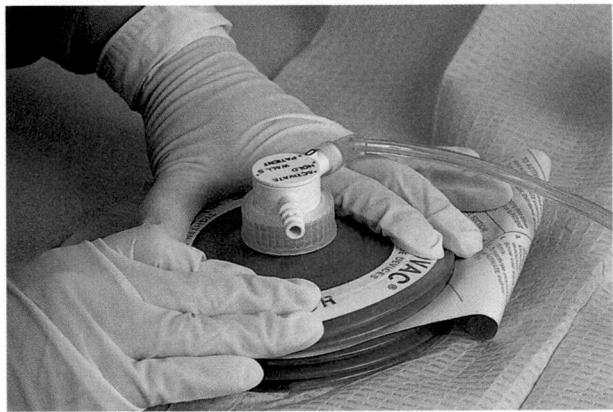

FIGURE **47–33** Setting the suction on a drainage evacuator. 1. With the drainage port open, the level on the diaphragm is raised. 2. The nurse pushes straight down on the lever to lower the diaphragm. 3. Closure of the port prevents escape of air and creates vacuum pressure.

suction. The nurse may apply special skin barriers, including hydrocolloid dressings, similar to those used with ostomies (see Chapter 45), around drain sites. The skin barriers are soft material applied to the skin with adhesive. Drainage flows on the barrier but not directly on the skin. **Drainage evacuators** (Figure 47-33) are convenient, portable units that connect to tubular drains lying within a wound bed and exert a safe, constant, low-pressure vacuum to remove and collect drainage. The nurse ensures that suction is exerted and that connection points between the evacuator and tubing are intact. The evacuator collects drainage that the nurse assesses for volume and character every shift and as needed. When the evacuator fills, the nurse measures output by emptying the contents into a graduated cylinder and immediately resets the evacuator to apply suction.

Bandages and Binders. A simple gauze dressing is often not enough to immobilize or provide support to a wound. Binders and bandages applied over or around

dressings can provide extra protection and therapeutic benefits by the following:

1. Creating pressure over a body part (e.g., an elastic pressure bandage applied over an arterial puncture site)
2. Immobilizing a body part (e.g., an elastic bandage applied around a sprained ankle)
3. Supporting a wound (e.g., an abdominal binder applied over a large abdominal incision and dressing)
4. Reducing or preventing edema (e.g., a well-supporting bra to minimize breast discomfort after delivery of a baby)
5. Securing a splint (e.g., a bandage applied around hand splints for correction of deformities)
6. Securing dressings (e.g., elastic webbing applied around leg dressings after a vein stripping)

Bandages are available in rolls of various widths and materials, including gauze, elasticized knit, elastic webbing, flannel, and muslin. Gauze bandages are lightweight and inexpensive, mold easily around contours of the body, and permit air circulation to prevent skin maceration. Elastic bandages conform well to body parts but can also be used to exert pressure.

Binders are bandages that are made of large pieces of material to fit a specific body part. Most binders are made of elastic or cotton. An abdominal binder and a breast binder are examples.

Principles for Applying Bandages and Binders. Correctly applied bandages and binders do not cause injury to underlying and nearby body parts or create discomfort for the client. For example, a chest binder must not be so tight as to restrict chest wall expansion. Before a bandage or binder is applied, the nurse's responsibilities include the following:

• Inspecting the skin for abrasions, edema, discoloration, or exposed wound edges
• Covering exposed wounds or open abrasions with a sterile dressing
• Assessing the condition of underlying dressings and changing if soiled
• Assessing the skin of underlying areas that will be distal to the bandage for signs of circulatory impairment

Table 47-11	**Types of Bandage Turns**	
Type	**Description**	**Purpose or Use**
Circular	Bandage turn overlapping previous turn completely	Anchors bandage at the first and final turn; covers small part (finger, toe)
Spiral	Bandage ascending body part, with each turn overlapping previous one by one-half or two-thirds width of bandage	Covers cylindrical body parts such as wrist or upper arm
Spiral-reverse	Turn requiring twist (reversal) of bandage halfway through each turn	Covers cone-shaped body parts such as forearm, thigh, or calf; useful with nonstretching bandages such as gauze or flannel
Figure eight	Oblique overlapping turns alternately ascending and descending over bandaged part; each turn crossing previous one to form figure eight	Covers joints; snug fit provides excellent immobilization
Recurrent	Bandage first secured with two circular turns around proximal end of body part; half turn made perpendicular up from bandage edge; body of bandage brought over distal end of body part to be covered with each turn folded back over on itself	Covers uneven body parts such as head or stump

(coolness, pallor or cyanosis, diminished or absent pulses, swelling, numbness, and tingling) to provide a means for comparing changes in circulation after bandage application

Table 47-11 outlines the principles of bandage and binder application. After a bandage is applied, the nurse assesses, documents, and immediately reports changes in circulation, skin integrity, comfort level, and body function (e.g., ventilation or movement). The nurse who applies a bandage can loosen or readjust it as necessary. The nurse should have a physician's order before loosening or removing a bandage applied by a physician. The nurse explains to the client that any bandage or binder feels relatively firm or tight. A bandage should be carefully assessed to be sure that it is properly applied and is providing therapeutic benefit, and soiled bandages should be replaced.

Binder Application. Binders are especially designed for the body part to be supported. The most common types of binders are the abdominal binder and breast binder (Skill 47-6). Breast binders, used to provide support after breast surgery or to exert pressure to reduce lactation in a woman after childbirth, are now being replaced with well-fitting bras.

Abdominal Binders. An abdominal binder supports large abdominal incisions that are vulnerable to tension or stress as the client moves or coughs (Figure 47-34). The nurse secures an abdominal binder with safety pins, Velcro strips, or metal stays.

Slings. Slings support arms with muscular sprains or fractures. A commercially manufactured sling consists of a long sleeve that extends above the elbow, with a strap that fits around the neck. In the home a large triangular piece of cloth can be used. The client may sit or lie supine during sling application (Figure 47-35). The nurse instructs the client to bend the affected arm, bringing the forearm straight across the chest. The open sling fits under the client's arm and over the chest, with the base of the triangle under the wrist and the triangle's point at the client's elbow. One end of the sling fits around the back of the client's neck. The nurse brings the other end up and over the affected arm while supporting the extremity. The nurse ties the two ends at the side of the neck so that the knot does not press against the cervical spine. The loose material at the elbow can be folded evenly around the elbow and pinned. The lower arm and hand should always be supported at a level above the elbow to prevent the formation of dependent edema.

Bandage Application. Rolls of bandage can secure or support dressings over irregularly shaped body parts. Each roll has a free outer end and a terminal end at the center of the roll. The rolled portion of the bandage is its body, and its outer surface is placed against the client's skin or dressing. Skill 47-7 describes the steps for applying an elastic bandage. The nurse may use a variety of bandage turns, depending on the body part to be bandaged.

Heat and Cold Therapy

Assessment for Temperature Tolerance. Before applying heat or cold therapies, the nurse assesses the client's physical condition for signs of potential intolerance to heat and cold. The nurse first observes the area to be treated. Alterations in skin integrity, such as abrasions, open wounds, edema, bruising, bleeding, or localized areas of inflammation, increase the client's risk of injury. Because the physician commonly orders heat and cold applications to be placed on traumatized areas, the baseline skin assessment provides a guide for evaluating skin changes that might occur during therapy.

Assessment includes identification of conditions that contraindicate heat or cold therapy. An active area of

Text continued on p. 1554

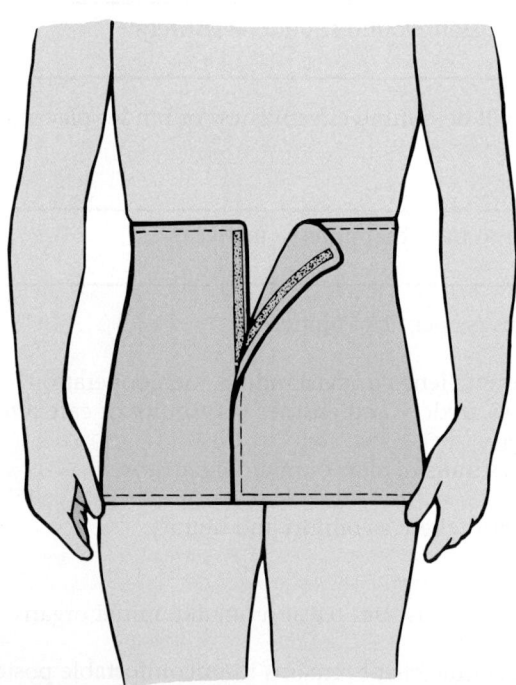

FIGURE **47–34** Securing an abdominal binder with Velcro.

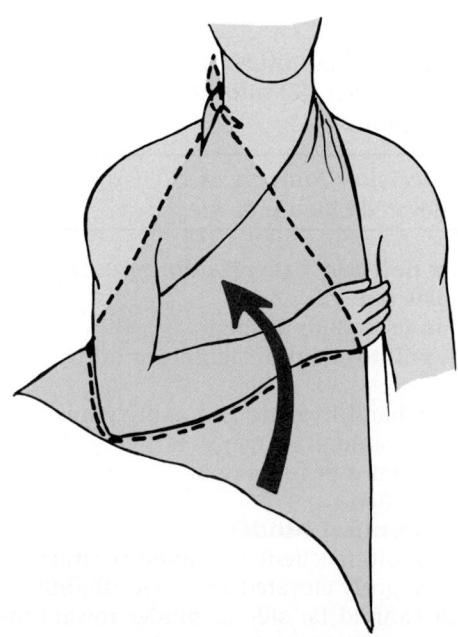

FIGURE **47–35** Application of a sling.

Skill 47-6 *Applying an Abdominal or Breast Binder*

Delegation Considerations

The skills of applying a binder (abdominal or breast) can be delegated to assistive personnel (AP). The nurse is responsible for wound assessment and the evaluation of wound care interventions. The nurse must also complete an assessment of the client's ability to breathe deeply, cough effectively, and move independently; of skin for irritation/abrasion; of incision/wound and dressing; and of comfort level before a binder or sling is applied for the first time. When delegating this skill the nurse must instruct AP to do the following:

- Immediately notify the nurse of any change in client's respiratory status.
- Report to the nurse any increase in wound drainage.
- Report to the nurses any changes in skin integrity under or adjacent to the binder.
- Remove the binder at prescribed intervals.

Equipment

- Gloves, if wound drainage is present
- Abdominal binder:
  - Correct size cloth/elastic straight binder
  - Safety pins (unless Velcro closure or metal fasteners are attached): six to eight safety pins are usually adequate for abdominal binders
- Breast binder:
  - Correct size binder
  - Safety pins (approximately 12) unless Velcro closure is attached

Steps	Rationale
1. Observe client with need for support of thorax or abdomen. Observe ability to breathe deeply and cough effectively.	Baseline assessment determines client's ability to breathe and cough. Impaired ventilation of lung can lead to alveolar atelectasis and inadequate arterial oxygenation.
2. Review medical record if medical prescription for particular binder is required and reasons for application.	Application of supportive binders may be used on nursing judgment. In some situations, physician input is required.
3. Inspect skin for actual or potential alterations in integrity. Observe for irritation, abrasion, skin surfaces that rub against each other, or allergic response to adhesive tape used to secure dressing.	Actual impairments in skin integrity can be worsened with application of a binder. Binder can cause pressure and excoriation.
4. Inspect any surgical dressing.	Dressing replacement or reinforcement precedes application of any binder.

Critical Decision Point: Dressing should be clean and dry, and incision/wound should be entirely covered by dressing.

---

5. Assess client's comfort level, using analog scale of 0 to 10 (see Chapter 42) and noting any objective signs and symptoms.	Data will determine effectiveness of binder placement.

Critical Decision Point: Expect client in moderate-to-severe pain to have diaphoresis, tachycardia, and elevated blood pressure.

---

6. Gather necessary data regarding size of client and appropriate binder.	Ensures proper fit of binder.
7. Explain procedure to client.	Promotes client's understanding and cooperation.
8. Teach skill to client or significant other.	Reduces anxiety and ensures continuity of care after discharge.
9. Perform hand hygiene and apply gloves (if likely to contact wound drainage).	Reduces transmission of microorganisms.
10. Close curtains or room door.	Maintains client's comfort and dignity.
11. Apply binder.	
A. Abdominal binder	
(1) Position client in supine position with head slightly elevated and knees slightly flexed.	Minimizes muscular tension on abdominal organs.
(2) Fanfold far side of binder toward midline of binder.	Reduces time client remains in uncomfortable position.

Steps	Rationale
(3) Instruct and help client to roll away from nurse toward raised side rail while firmly supporting abdominal incision and dressing with hands.	Reduces pain and discomfort.
(4) Place fan folded ends of binder under client.	Permits placement and centering of binder with minimal discomfort.
(5) Instruct or assist client to roll over folded ends.	
(6) Unfold and stretch ends out smoothly on far side of bed.	Maintains skin integrity and comfort.
(7) Instruct client to roll back into supine position.	Facilitates chest expansion and adequate wound support when binder is closed.
(8) Adjust binder so that supine client is centered over binder using symphysis pubis and costal margins as lower and upper landmarks.	Centers support from binder over abdominal structures, which reduces incidence of decreased lung expansion.

Critical Decision Point: Cover any exposed areas of an incision or wound with sterile dressing.

Steps	Rationale
(9) Close binder. Pull one end of binder over center of client's abdomen. While maintaining tension on that end of binder, pull opposite end of binder over center and secure with Velcro closure tabs, metal fasteners, or horizontally placed safety pins (see Figure 47-34, p. 1549).	Provides continuous wound support and comfort.
B. **Breast binder**	
(1) Assist client in placing arms through binder's armholes.	Eases binder placement process.
(2) Assist client to supine position in bed.	Supine positioning facilitates normal anatomical position of breasts; facilitates healing and comfort.
(3) Pad area under breasts if necessary.	Prevents skin contact with undersurface.
(4) Using Velcro closure tabs or horizontally placed safety pins, secure binder at nipple level first. Continue closure process above and then below nipple line until entire binder is closed.	Horizontal placement of pins may reduce risk of uneven pressure or localized irritation.
(5) Make appropriate adjustments, including individualizing fit of shoulder straps and pinning waistline darts to reduce binder size.	Maintains support to client's breasts.
(6) Instruct and observe skill development in self-care related to reapplying breast binder.	Self-care is integral aspect of discharge planning. Skin integrity and comfort level goals are ensured.
12. Assess client's comfort level.	Helps determine effectiveness of binder placement.
13. Adjust binder as necessary.	Promotes comfort and chest expansion.
14. Remove gloves and perform hand hygiene.	Prevents cross infections.
15. Observe site for skin integrity, circulation, and characteristics of the wound. (Periodically remove binder and surgical dressing to assess wound characteristics.)	Determines that binder has not resulted in complication to skin, wound, or underlying organs.
16. Assess comfort level of client, using analog scale of 0 to 10 and noting any objective signs and symptoms.	Binders should not increase discomfort.
17. Assess client's ability to ventilate properly, including deep breathing and coughing.	Identifies any impaired ventilation and potential pulmonary complications.
18. Identify client's need for assistance with activities such as hair combing, dressing, and ambulating.	Mobility of upper extremities may be limited, depending on severity and location of incision.

Skill 47-6 *Applying an Abdominal or Breast Binder—cont'd*

Unexpected Outcomes and Related Interventions

1. Client's pain increases.
   a. Remove binder and assess wound.
   b. Reapply binder using less pressure.
2. Client's respiratory rate decreases.
   a. Remove binder.
   b. Encourage client to cough and deep breathe.
   c. Reapply binder using less pressure.
3. Client develops impaired skin integrity under the binder.
   a. Remove binder.
   b. Initiate skin care measure to heal affected site.

Recording and Reporting

- Report any skin irritation to nurse at between-shift report.
- Record application of binder, condition of skin, circulation, integrity of dressing, and client's comfort level.
- Report ineffective lung expansion to physician immediately.

Home Care Considerations

- Abdominal and breast binders are washable and are placed over a line to dry.
- Instruct caregiver to avoid excessive pressure with binder application.

Skill 47-7 *Applying an Elastic Bandage*

Delegation Considerations

The application of an elastic bandage can be delegated to assistive personnel (AP). However, the nurse is responsible for wound assessment and the evaluation of the wound. In addition, the nurse is responsible for assessing for adequate circulation to the extremity distal to the elastic bandage (e.g., pulse, skin temperature, capillary refill). When delegating this skill to AP, the nurse must instruct AP about the following:

- Any restrictions that the client might have (e.g., unable to independently raise leg or independently roll over)
- To report any change in the skin color of the client's injured extremity
- To report any increases in client's pain

Equipment

- Correct width and number of bandages
- Safety pins, clips, or adhesive tape
- Disposable gloves, if wound drainage is present

Steps	Rationale
1. Perform hand hygiene and apply gloves if needed. Inspect skin for alterations in integrity as indicated by abrasions, discoloration, chafing, or edema. (Look carefully at bony prominences.)	Altered skin integrity contraindicates the use of elastic bandages.
2. Inspect surgical dressing. Remove gloves and perform hand hygiene.	Surgical dressing replacement or reinforcement precedes application of any bandage.
3. Observe adequacy of circulation (distal to bandage) by noting surface temperature, skin color, and sensation of body parts to be wrapped.	Comparison of area before and after application of bandage is necessary to ensure continued adequate circulation. Impairment of circulation may result in coolness to touch when compared with opposite side of body, cyanosis or pallor of skin, diminished or absent pulses, edema or localized pooling, and numbness or tingling of part.
4. Review medical record for specific orders related to application of elastic bandage. Note area to be covered, type of bandage required, frequency of change, and previous response to treatment.	Specific prescription may direct procedure, including factors such as extent of application (e.g., toe to knee, toe to groin) and duration of treatment.
5. Identify client's and primary caregiver's present knowledge level of skill if bandaging will be continued at home.	Ensures that planning and teaching are individualized.

Steps	Rationale
6. Explain procedure to client.	Increased knowledge promotes cooperation and reduces anxiety.
7. Teach skill to client or significant other.	Reduces anxiety and ensures continuity of care after discharge.
8. Perform hand hygiene and apply gloves if drainage is present.	Reduces transmission of microorganisms.
9. Close room door or curtains.	Maintains client's comfort and dignity.
10. Help client to assume comfortable, anatomically correct position.	Maintains alignment. Prevents musculoskeletal deformity.

Critical Decision Point: Bandages applied to lower extremities are applied before client sits or stands. Elevation of dependent extremities for 20 minutes before bandage application will enhance venous return.

11. Hold roll of elastic bandage in dominant hand and use other hand to lightly hold beginning of bandage at distal body part. Continue transferring roll to dominant hand as bandage is wrapped.	Maintains appropriate and consistent bandage tension.

Critical Decision Point: Toes or fingertips should be visible for follow-up circulatory assessment.

12. Apply bandage from distal point toward proximal boundary using variety of turns to cover various shapes of body parts (see Table 47-11, p. 1548).	Bandage is applied in manner that conforms evenly to body part and promotes venous return.
13. Unroll and very slightly stretch bandage.	Maintains uniform bandage tension.
14. Overlap turns by one-half to two-thirds width of bandage roll.	Prevents uneven bandage tension and circulatory impairment.
15. Secure first bandage with clip or tape before applying additional rolls.	
a. Apply additional rolls without leaving any uncovered skin surface. Secure last bandage applied.	Prevents wrinkling or loose ends.
16. Remove gloves if worn and perform hand hygiene	Reduces transmission of microorganisms.
17. Assess distal circulation when bandage application is complete and at least twice during 8-hour period.	Early detection and management of circulatory impairment ensures healthy neurovascular status.
a. Observe skin color for pallor or cyanosis.	
b. Palpate skin for warmth.	
c. Palpate pulses and compare bilaterally.	
d. Ask if client is aware of pain, numbness, tingling, or other discomfort.	Neurovascular changes indicate impaired venous return.
e. Observe mobility of extremity.	Determines if bandage is too tight, which restricts movement, or determines if joint immobility is attained.
18. Have client demonstrate bandage application.	Return demonstration documents learning.

Unexpected Outcomes and Related Interventions

1. Impaired circulation distal to elastic bandage
   a. Release bandage.
   b. Palpate extremity and assess pulse, temperature, and capillary refill.
   c. Reapply dressing with less pressure.
2. Break in skin under elastic bandage
   a. Remove bandage.
   b. Reapply bandage with less pressure.
3. Client unable to perform dressing change
   a. Reinstruct client on bandage application.
   b. Observe client apply bandage.

Recording and Reporting

- Document condition of wound, integrity of dressing, application of bandage, circulation, and client's comfort level.
- Report any changes in neurological or circulatory status to nurse in charge or physician.

Home Care Considerations

- Instruct client or caregiver not to make bandages too tight, which interferes with circulation.
- Elastic bandages that are used to reduce swelling are best applied to the feet in the morning, before getting out of bed.
- Always remove an elastic bandage daily and inspect skin beneath it.

bleeding should not be covered by a warm application because bleeding will continue. Warm applications are contraindicated when the client has an acute, localized inflammation such as appendicitis because the heat could cause the appendix to rupture. If a client has cardiovascular problems, it is unwise to apply heat to large portions of the body because the resulting massive vasodilation may disrupt blood supply to vital organs.

Cold is contraindicated if the site of injury is already edematous. Cold further retards circulation to the area and prevents absorption of the interstitial fluid. If the client has impaired in circulation (e.g., arteriosclerosis), cold further reduces blood supply to the affected area. Cold therapy is also contraindicated in the presence of neuropathy, because the client is unable to perceive temperature change and damage resulting from temperature extremes. One other contraindication for cold therapy is shivering. Cold applications may intensify shivering and dangerously increase body temperature.

The nurse also assesses the client's response to stimuli. Sensation to light touch, pinprick, and mild temperature variations (see Chapter 32) reveals the ability of the client to recognize when heat or cold becomes excessive. If a client has peripheral vascular disease, the nurse pays particular attention to the integrity of extremities. For example, if the physician's order is to apply a cold compress to a lower extremity, the nurse should assess circulation to the leg by assessing for capillary refill, observing skin color, and palpating skin temperatures, distal pulses, and edematous areas. If signs of circulatory inadequacy are present, the nurse should question the order.

Level of consciousness influences the ability to perceive heat, cold, and pain. If a client is confused or unresponsive, the nurse must make frequent observations of skin integrity after therapy begins.

The nurse must also assess the condition of equipment being used. Electrical equipment should be checked for cracked cords, frayed wires, damaged insulation, and exposed heating components. Equipment containing circulating fluids should not have leaks. The nurse also checks equipment for evenness of temperature distribution.

Local application of heat and cold to an injured body part can be therapeutic. Before using these therapies, however, the nurse must understand normal body responses to local temperature variations, assess the integrity of the body part, determine the client's ability to sense temperature variations, and ensure proper operation of equipment. The nurse is legally responsible for safe administration of heat and cold applications.

Bodily Responses to Heat and Cold. Exposure to heat and cold can cause systemic and local responses. Systemic responses occur through heat-loss mechanisms (sweating and vasodilation) or mechanisms promoting heat conservation (vasoconstriction and piloerection) and heat production (shivering) (see Chapter 32). Local responses to heat and cold occur through stimulation of temperature-sensitive nerve endings within the skin. This stimulation sends impulses from the periphery to the hypothalamus, which becomes aware of local temperature sensations and triggers adaptive responses for maintenance of normal body temperature. If alterations occur along temperature sensation pathways, the reception and eventual perception of stimuli will be altered.

The body can tolerate wide variations in temperature. The normal temperature of the skin's surface is 34° C (93.2° F), but temperature receptors usually adapt quickly to local temperatures between 45° and 15° C (113° and 59° F). Pain develops when local temperatures exceed this range. Excessive heat causes a burning sensation. Cold produces a numbing sensation before pain.

The body's adaptive ability creates the major problem in protecting clients from injury resulting from temperature extremes. A person initially feels an extreme change in temperature but within a short time hardly notices it. This can be dangerous because a person insensitive to heat and cold extremes can suffer serious tissue injury. The nurse must recognize clients most at risk for injuries from heat and cold applications (Table 47-12).

Local Effects of Heat and Cold. Heat and cold stimuli create different physiological responses. The choice of heat or cold therapy depends on local responses desired for wound healing.

Effects of Heat Application. Heat generally is quite therapeutic, improving blood flow to an injured part (see Table 47-13, p. 1555). If heat is applied for 1 hour or more, however, blood flow is reduced by a reflex vasoconstriction as the body attempts to control heat loss from the area. Periodic removal and reapplication of local heat restores vasodilation. Continuous exposure to heat damages epithelial cells, causing redness, localized tenderness, and even blistering.

Effects of Cold Application. The application of cold can initially diminish swelling and pain (see Table 47-13). Prolonged exposure of the skin to cold results in a reflex vasodilation. The cell's inability to receive adequate blood flow and nutrients results in tissue ischemia. The skin initially takes on a reddened appearance, followed by a bluish purple mottling with numbness and a burning type of pain. The skin's tissues can freeze from exposure to extreme cold.

Factors Influencing Heat and Cold Tolerance. The body's response to heat and cold therapies depends on the following factors:

- A person is better able to tolerate short exposure to temperature extremes.
- Certain areas of the skin are more sensitive to temperature variations. These include the neck, inner aspect of the wrist and forearm, and perineal region. The foot and palm of the hand are less sensitive.
- Exposed skin layers are more sensitive to temperature variations.
- The body responds best to minor temperature adjustments. If a body part is cool and a hot stimulus touches the skin, the response is greater than if the skin were already warm.
- A person has less tolerance to temperature changes to which a large area of the body is exposed.
- Tolerance to temperature variations changes with age. Clients who are very young and old are most sensitive to heat and cold.
- If a client's physical condition reduces the reception or perception of sensory stimuli, tolerance to temperature extremes is high, but the risk of injury is also high.

Table 47-12   Conditions That Increase Risk of Injury From Heat and Cold Application

Condition	Risk Factors
Very young clients or older clients	Thinner skin layers in children increase risk of burns. Older clients have reduced sensitivity to pain.
Open wounds, broken skin, stomas	Subcutaneous and visceral tissues are more sensitive to temperature variations. They also contain no temperature and fewer pain receptors.
Areas of edema or scar formation	Reduced sensation to temperature stimuli occurs because of thickening of skin layers from fluid buildup or scar formation.
Peripheral vascular disease (e.g., diabetes, arteriosclerosis)	Body's extremities are less sensitive to temperature and pain stimuli because of circulatory impairment and local tissue injury. Cold application further compromises blood flow.
Confusion or unconsciousness	Perception of sensory or painful stimuli is reduced.
Spinal cord injury	Alterations in nerve pathways prevent reception of sensory or painful stimuli.
Abscessed tooth of appendix	Infection is highly localized. Application of heat may cause rupture with spread of microorganisms systematically.

Table 47-13   Therapeutic Effects of Heat and Cold Applications

Physiological Response	Therapeutic Benefit	Examples of Conditions Treated
Heat		
Vasodilation	Improves blood flow to injured body part; promotes delivery of nutrients and removal of wastes; lessens venous congestion in injured tissues	Improves blood flow to injured body part; promotes delivery of nutrients and removal of wastes; lessens venous congestion in injured tissues
Reduced blood viscosity	Improves delivery of leukocytes and antibiotics to wound site	
Reduced muscle tension	Promotes muscle relaxation and reduces pain from spasm or stiffness	
Increased tissue metabolism	Increases blood flow; provides local warmth	
Increased capillary permeability	Promotes movement of waste products and nutrients	
Cold		
Vasoconstriction	Reduces blood flow to injured body part, preventing edema formation; reduces inflammation	Direct trauma (sprains, strains, fractures, muscle spasms); superficial laceration or puncture wound; minor burn; suspected malignancy in area of injury or pain; injections; arthritis and joint trauma
Local anesthesia	Reduces localized pain	
Reduced cell metabolism	Reduces oxygen needs of tissues	
Increased blood viscosity	Promotes blood coagulation at injury site	
Decreased muscle tension	Relieves pain	

- Uneven temperature distribution suggests that the equipment is functioning improperly.

Safety Alert. Before application of heat or cold therapy the client should understand its purpose, the symptoms of temperature exposure, and precautions taken to prevent injury. Box 47-16 provides methods for the safe application of heat and cold therapy.

Application of Heat and Cold Therapies. A prerequisite to using any heat or cold application is a physician's order, which should include the body site to be treated and the type, frequency, and duration of application. The nurse should consult the agency's procedure manual for correct temperatures to use.

Choice of Moist or Dry. Heat and cold applications can be administered in dry or moist forms. The type of wound or injury, the location of the body part, and the presence of drainage or inflammation are factors considered in selecting dry or moist applications. Box 47-17 summarizes advantages and disadvantages of both.

Warm, Moist Compresses. For open wounds, sterile, warm, moist compresses improve circulation, relieve edema, and promote consolidation of pus and drainage.

Box **47-16**　　　　**Safety Suggestions for Applying Heat or Cold Therapy**

Do explain to the client sensations to be felt during the procedure.

Do instruct the client to report changes in sensation or discomfort immediately.

Do provide a timer, clock, or watch so that the client can help the nurse time the application.

Do keep the call light within the client's reach.

Do refer to the institution's policy and procedure manual for safe temperatures.

Do not allow the client to adjust temperature settings.

Do not allow the client to move an application or place hands on the wound site.

Do not place the client in a position that prevents movement away from the temperature source.

Do not leave unattended a client who is unable to sense temperature changes or move from the temperature source.

Box **47-17**　　　　**Choice of Dry or Moist Applications**

Advantages

Moist Applications

Moist application reduces drying of skin and softens wound exudate.

Moist compresses conform well to body area being treated.

Moist heat penetrates deeply into tissue layers.

Warm moist heat does not promote sweating and insensible fluid loss.

Dry Applications

Dry heat has less risk of burns to skin than moist applications.

Dry application does not cause skin maceration.

Dry heat retains temperature longer because it is not influenced by evaporation.

Disadvantages

Moist Applications

Prolonged exposure can cause maceration of skin.

Moist heat will cool rapidly because of moisture evaporation.

Moist heat creates greater risk for burns to skin because moisture conducts heat.

Dry Applications

Dry heat increases body fluid loss through sweating.

Dry applications do not penetrate deep into tissues.

Dry heat causes increased drying of skin.

A compress is a piece of gauze dressing moistened in a prescribed warmed solution. A pack is a larger cloth or dressing applied to a larger body area.

Heat from warm compresses dissipates quickly. To maintain a constant temperature, the nurse must change the compress often or apply a warm aquathermic pad or waterproof heating pad over the compress. Because moisture conducts heat, any device's temperature setting should be lower for a moist compress than for a dry application. A layer of plastic wrap or a dry towel can also be used to insulate the compress and retain heat. Moist heat promotes vasodilation and evaporation of heat from the skin's surface. For this reason, a client may feel chilly. The nurse controls drafts within the room and keeps the client covered with a blanket or robe. Skill 47-8 describes the steps for applying a warm, moist compress.

Warm Soaks. Immersion of a body part in a warmed solution promotes circulation, lessens edema, increases muscle relaxation, and can provide a means to debride wounds and apply medicated solution. A soak can also be accompanied by wrapping the body part in dressings and saturating them with the warmed solution.

The nurse positions the client comfortably, places waterproof pads under the area to be treated, and heats the solution to about 40.5° to 43° C (105° to 110° F). After immersing the body part, the nurse covers the container and extremity with a towel to reduce heat loss. It is usually necessary to remove the cooled solution and add heated solution after about 10 minutes. The problem is to keep the solution at a constant temperature. The nurse never adds a hotter solution while the body part remains immersed. After any soak, the nurse dries the body part thoroughly to prevent maceration.

Sitz Baths. The client who has had rectal surgery, an episiotomy during childbirth, painful hemorrhoids, or vaginal inflammation may benefit from a **sitz bath,** a bath in which only the pelvic area is immersed in warm fluid. The client sits in a special tub or chair or in a basin that fits on the toilet seat so that the legs and feet remain out of the water. Immersing the entire body causes widespread vasodilation and nullifies the effect of local heat application to the pelvic area.

The desired temperature for a sitz bath depends on whether the purpose is to promote relaxation or to clean a wound. It may be necessary to add warm water during the procedure, which normally lasts 20 minutes, to maintain a constant temperature. Agency procedure manuals recommend safe water temperatures. A disposable sitz basin contains an attachment resembling an enema bag that allows gradual introduction of warmer water.

Applying a Warm, Moist Compress to an Open Wound

Skill 47-8

Delegation Considerations

This skill can be delegated to assistive personnel (AP). The nurse is responsible for wound assessment and evaluation of wound care interventions. When delegating this skill to AP the nurse must do the following:

- Caution caregiver to maintain proper temperature of application during duration of treatment.
- Caution caregiver to keep application in place for only the length of time specified in physician's orders.
- Have caregiver notify the nurse when treatment is complete so that an evaluation of client's response can be made.

Equipment

- Prescribed solution warmed to appropriate temperature
- Sterile gauze dressings or commercially prepared compresses
- Sterile container for solution
- Dry bath towel
- Disposable gloves
- Sterile gloves
- Waterproof pad
- Ties or tape
- Aquathermia or heating pad (optional)
- Bath blanket

Steps	Rationale
1. Refer to physician's order for type of compress, location and duration of application, desired temperature, and institutional policies regarding temperature of compress.	Ensures safe and correct application.
2. Refer to medical record to identify any systemic contraindications to heat application.	Heat causes vasodilation, which aggravates active bleeding. Heat applied to localized area of acute inflammation or tumor may cause rupture or activate cell growth.
3. Perform hand hygiene.	Reduces transmission of microorganisms.
4. Inspect condition of exposed skin and wound on which compress is to be applied.	Provides baseline to determine changes in skin during heat application.

Critical Decision Point: Very thin or damaged skin is more susceptible to injury from heat. Nonintact skin and drainage from wounds are indications to wear gloves.

Steps	Rationale
5. Assess client's extremities for sensitivity to temperature and pain by measuring light touch, pinprick, and temperature sensation.	Clients insensitive to heat or cold sensations must be monitored closely during treatment.

Critical Decision Point: Diabetic clients, victims of stroke, and clients with peripheral neuropathy are particularly at risk for thermal injury.

Steps	Rationale
6. Assemble equipment and supplies.	Organization of supplies prevents unnecessary delays in the procedure.
7. Explain steps of procedure and purpose to client. Describe sensations to be felt, such as decreasing warmth and wetness. Explain precautions to prevent burning.	Minimizes client's anxiety and promotes cooperation during the procedure.
8. Close door and bedside curtains.	Decreases drafts, thus decreasing the transmission of microorganisms. Provides for client privacy.
9. Assist client in assuming comfortable position in proper body alignment and place waterproof pad under area to be treated.	Compress remains in place for several minutes. Limited mobility in uncomfortable position causes muscular stress. Pad prevents soiling of bed linen.
10. Expose body part to be covered with compress and drape client with bath blanket.	Prevents unnecessary cooling and exposure of body part.
11. Prepare compress:	Ensures orderly procedure.
a. Pour solution into sterile container.	
b. If using portable heating source, warm solution. Commercially prepared compresses may remain under infrared lamp until just before use. Open sterile packages and drop gauze into container to become immersed in solution.	Compresses must retain warmth for therapeutic benefit.
c. Adjust temperature of aquathermia pad (if needed).	

Applying a Warm, Moist Compress to an Open Wound—cont'd

Skill 47-8

Steps	Rationale
Critical Decision Point: Temperature must be tested by applying sterile solution to nurse's forearm (without contaminating solution).	
12. Apply disposable gloves. Remove any existing dressing covering wound. Dispose of gloves and dressings in proper receptacle.	Reduces transmission of microorganisms.
13. Assess condition of wound and surrounding skin. Inflamed wound appears reddened, but surrounding skin is less red in color.	Provides baseline to determine skin changes following compress application.
Critical Decision Point: If skin surrounding wound is reddened, application may be contraindicated.	
14. Apply sterile gloves.	Allows nurse to manipulate sterile dressing and touch open wound.
15. Pick up one layer of immersed gauze, wring out any excess solution, and apply it lightly to open wound.	Excess moisture macerates skin and increases risks of burns and infection. Skin is sensitive to sudden change in temperature.
16. In a few seconds, lift edge of gauze to assess for redness.	Increased redness indicates burn.
17. If client tolerates compress, pack gauze snugly against the wound. Be sure all wound surfaces are covered by warm compress.	Packing of compress prevents rapid cooling from underlying air currents.
18. Cover moist compress with dry sterile dressing and bath towel. If necessary, pin or tie in place. Remove sterile gloves.	Dry sterile dressing will prevent transfer of microorganisms to wound via capillary action caused by moist compress. Towel insulates compress to prevent heat loss.
19. Apply aquathermia or waterproof heating pad over towel (optional). Keep it in place for desired duration of application.	Provides constant temperature to compress.
20. If an aquathermia pad is *not* used to maintain temperature of application, change warm compress using sterile technique every 5 min or as ordered during duration of therapy.	Prevents cooling and maintains therapeutic benefit of compress.
21. After prescribed time, apply disposable gloves and remove pad, towel, and compress. Reassess wound and condition of skin, and replace dry sterile dressing as ordered.	Continued exposure to moisture will macerate skin. Prevents entrance of microorganisms into wound site.
22. Assist client to preferred comfortable position.	Maintains client's comfort.
23. Dispose of equipment and soiled compress. Perform hand hygiene.	Reduces transmission of microorganisms.
24. Inspect affected area covered by compress and heating pad every 5 to 10 min.	Assists in determining effects of application.
25. Ask every 5 to 10 min if client notices any unusual burning sensation not felt before application.	It may be difficult to assess burn merely by color changes if wound is inflamed or drainage is present.
26. Have client explain and demonstrate application.	Evaluates client's understanding of and ability to perform procedure.

Unexpected Outcomes and Related Interventions

1. Client's wound remains the same.
   a. Report to physician.
   b. Evaluate the continued use of warm compress.
2. Client's skin is broken, erythematous, and warm to the touch.
   a. Verify that correct temperature of compress is maintained.
   b. Institute skin care practices.

Recording and Reporting

- Record type, location, and duration of application. Note solution and temperature.
- Describe condition of wound and skin before and after treatment, as well as client's response to therapy.
- Describe any instructions given and client's ability to explain and perform procedure.
- Report unusual findings to nurse in charge or physician.

Home Care Considerations

- When necessary, assess availability of primary caregivers to assist clients in application of compress, their understanding of purpose of procedure, and their willingness to comply with procedure and not leave client with compress in place beyond prescribed time limit.
- Assess physical environment to determine existence of adequate facilities to prepare warm compress and provide for sterile technique.

The nurse prevents overexposure of the client by draping bath blankets around the client's shoulders and thighs and controlling drafts. The client should be able to sit in the basin or tub with feet flat on the floor and without pressure on the sacrum or thighs. Because exposure of a large portion of the body to heat can cause extensive vasodilation, the nurse should assess the pulse and facial color and ask whether the client feels light-headed or nauseated.

Aquathermia (Water-Flow) Pads. A popular device in health care institutions is the **aquathermia pad,** or water-flow pad (Figure 47-36), used for treating muscle sprains and areas of mild inflammation or edema. The aquathermia unit consists of a waterproof plastic or rubber pad connected by two hoses to an electrical control unit that has a heating element and motor.

Distilled water circulates through hollowed channels within the pad to the control unit where water is heated or cooled (depending on temperature setting). Some pads have an absorbent surface to apply moist heat. The units are safer than conventional heating pads. However, the nurse should still check for equipment malfunctions. The temperature setting is fixed by inserting a plastic key into the temperature regulator. In many institutions the central supply room sets the regulators to the recommended temperature (40.5° to 43° C [105° to 110° F]). If the distilled water in the unit runs low, the nurse simply fills the reservoir two-thirds full. Plain tap water is never added, because it might leave mineral deposits in the unit.

To avoid burning the client's skin, the nurse does not place the pad directly on it. A thin towel or pillow case fits easily over the heating pad. Tape, ties, or a gauze roll holds the pad in place. Pins are never used, because they might cause a leak. The nurse checks the client's skin often for signs of burning. An application should last only 20 to 30 minutes. The nurse does not allow a client to lie

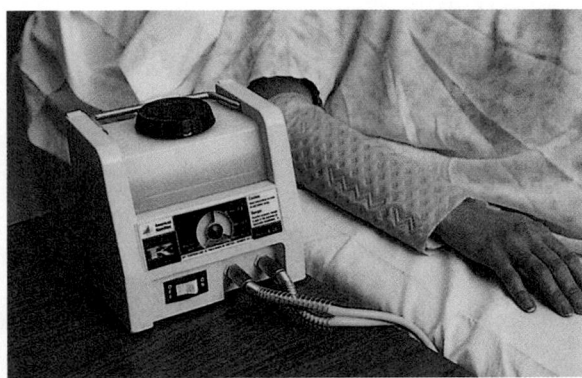

FIGURE **47–36** Aquathermia pad.

on a pad. Pressure against a mattress prevents normal heat dissipation. If the pad is to be applied to a region of the back, the client should lie prone or on one side.

Commercial Hot Packs. Commercially prepared, disposable hot packs apply warm, dry heat to an injured area. By striking, kneading, or squeezing the pack, chemicals are mixed and release heat. Package directions recommend the time for heat application.

Cold, Moist, and Dry Compresses. The procedure for applying cold, moist compresses is the same as that for warm compresses. Cold compresses should be applied for 20 minutes at a temperature of 15° C (59° F) to relieve inflammation and swelling. They may be clean or sterile.

There are commercially prepared cold packs that are similar to the disposable hot packs for dry applications. They come in various shapes and sizes to fit different body parts. When using cold compresses, the nurse observes for adverse reactions such as burning or numbness, mottling of the skin, redness, extreme paleness, and a bluish skin discoloration.

Cold Soaks. The procedure for preparing cold soaks and immersing a body part is the same as for warm soaks. The desired temperature for a 20-minute cold soak is 15° C (59° F). The nurse controls drafts and uses outer coverings to protect the client from chilling. It may be necessary to add cold water during the procedure to maintain a constant temperature.

Ice Bags or Collars. For a client who has a muscle sprain, localized hemorrhage, or hematoma or who has undergone dental surgery, an ice bag is ideal to prevent edema formation, control bleeding, and anesthetize the body part. Proper use of the bag requires the following steps:

1. Fill the bag with water, secure the cap, invert to check for leaks, and pour out the water.
2. Fill the bag two-thirds full with crushed ice so that the bag can mold easily over a body part.
3. Release any air from the bag by squeezing its sides before securing the cap, because excess air interferes with conduction of cold.
4. Wipe off excess moisture.
5. Cover the bag with a flannel cover, towel, or pillow case.

6. Apply the bag to the injury site for 30 minutes; the bag can be reapplied in an hour.

Evaluation

Client Care. Nursing interventions for reducing and treating pressure ulcers are evaluated by determining the client's response to nursing therapies and by determining whether each goal was achieved. To evaluate outcomes and responses to care, the nurse measures the effectiveness of interventions. The optimal outcomes are to prevent injury to the skin and tissues, reduce injury to the skin and underlying tissues, and restore skin integrity.

Because each client has different risk factors for impaired skin integrity, nursing interventions must be individualized. Clients with minimal mobility impairments or relatively stable health status may need only a few measures. Nursing interventions for reducing and treating pressure ulcers are evaluated by determining the client's response to nursing therapies and by determining whether each goal was achieved (Figure 47-37).

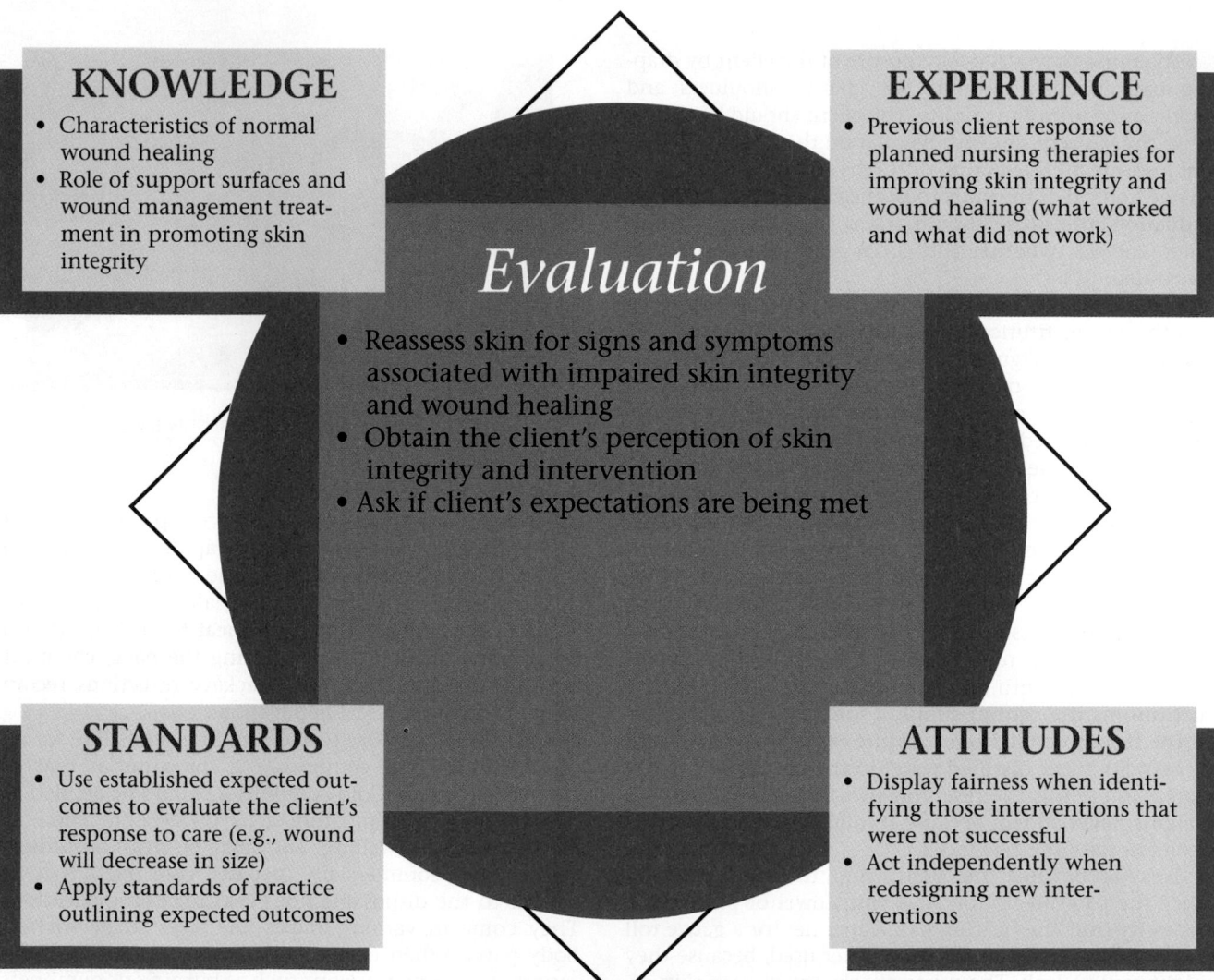

KNOWLEDGE
- Characteristics of normal wound healing
- Role of support surfaces and wound management treatment in promoting skin integrity

EXPERIENCE
- Previous client response to planned nursing therapies for improving skin integrity and wound healing (what worked and what did not work)

Evaluation
- Reassess skin for signs and symptoms associated with impaired skin integrity and wound healing
- Obtain the client's perception of skin integrity and intervention
- Ask if client's expectations are being met

STANDARDS
- Use established expected outcomes to evaluate the client's response to care (e.g., wound will decrease in size)
- Apply standards of practice outlining expected outcomes

ATTITUDES
- Display fairness when identifying those interventions that were not successful
- Act independently when redesigning new interventions

FIGURE **47–37** Critical thinking model for skin integrity and wound care evaluation.

To evaluate outcomes and responses to care, the nurse measures the effectiveness of interventions. This often occurs over an extended period of time, requiring the nurse to make careful ongoing assessments of the client with an ulcer. The nurse also evaluates specific interventions designed to promote skin integrity and to teach the client and family to reduce future threats to skin integrity.

The AHCPR panel (1992a) produced a client's guide for pressure ulcers that is short with clear illustrations. The nurse also evaluates the client's and family's need for additional support services (e.g., home care, physical therapy, and counseling) and initiates the referral process.

Finally, the nurse evaluates the need for additional referrals to other experts in pressure ulcers, such as nurses certified in wound care when indicated. Care of the client with a pressure ulcer requires a multidisciplinary team approach.

Client Expectations. The client and caregiver need to understand how to prevent or treat pressure ulcers. Helping them understand the content in the AHCPR consumer version of the prevention and treatment guidelines is helpful. Clients may enter into the wound-healing phase with unrealistic expectations with regard to the duration of care. The nurse needs to collect evaluation data about the client's perception of wound care management. Clients with chronic wounds are often cared for in their home settings and have certain expectations about their level of comfort, lifestyle, independence, and privacy. Therefore the nurse must determine from the client whether his or her expectations were respected and met.

Key Concepts

- Pressure ulcers contribute to client suffering and increase the length of stay in acute and extended care settings, as well as the overall cost of care needed to manage the wound.
- Improvement of a healing pressure ulcer can be measured by several of the newly developed healing scales; the staging systems for wound depth should not be used exclusively for this purpose.
- All clients must be evaluated for risk factors that contribute to development of impaired skin integrity.
- Alterations in mobility, sensory perception, level of consciousness, and nutrition and the presence of moisture increase the risk for pressure ulcer development.
- The risk of impaired skin integrity related to immobilization depends on the extent and duration of immobilization.
- External pressure, shearing force, and friction are contributing factors to the development of pressure ulcers.
- When the external pressure against the skin is greater than the pressure needed to keep the capillary open, blood flow decreases to the adjacent tissues.
- Meticulous assessment of the skin, and identification of risk factors are important in decreasing the opportunity for pressure ulcer development.

- Preventive skin care is aimed at controlling external pressure on bony prominences and keeping the skin clean, well lubricated and hydrated, and free of excess moisture.
- Proper positioning should reduce the effects of pressure and guard against the shearing force.
- Therapeutic beds and mattresses reduce the effects of pressure; however, selection is based on assessment data to identify the best bed for individual needs.
- Cleansing and topical agents used to treat pressure ulcers vary according to the stage of the pressure ulcer and condition of the wound bed. Assessment of the ulcer enables the nurse to select proper skin care agents.
- Nutritional interventions are directed at improving wound healing through increasing protein and calorie levels.
- Wound assessment requires a description of the appearance of the wound base, size, presence of exudate, and the periwound skin condition.
- Healing proceeds through three stages: inflammation, proliferation, and remodeling.
- When there is extensive tissue loss, a wound heals by secondary intention.
- The chances of wound infection are greater when the wound contains dead or necrotic tissue, when foreign bodies lie on or near the wound, and when the blood supply and tissue defenses are reduced.
- Principles of wound first aid include control of bleeding, cleansing, and protection.
- The layers of a dry dressing absorb drainage and prevent entrance of bacteria.
- The wet-to-dry dressing mechanically removes dead tissue and wound exudate to debride the wound.
- When cleansing wounds or drain sites, the nurse cleans from the least to most contaminated area, away from wound edges.
- A bandage or binder should be applied in a manner that does not impair circulation or irritate the skin.
- An acute sprain, closed fracture, or bruise responds best to cold applications.

Key Terms

Abnormal reactive hyperemia, *p. 1502*	Epithelialization, *p. 1493*
Abrasion, *p. 1503*	Eschar, *p. 1487*
Anemia, *p. 1493*	Evisceration, *p. 1494*
Approximated, *p. 1492*	Exudate, *p. 1487*
Aquathermia pad, *p. 1559*	Fibrin, *p. 1492*
Blanching, *p. 1485*	Fibroblasts, *p. 1493*
Collagen, *p. 1484*	Fistula, *p. 1494*
Darkly pigmented skin, *p. 1485*	Friction, *p. 1486*
	Granulation tissue, *p. 1487*
Debridement, *p. 1518*	Hematoma, *p. 1493*
Dehiscence, *p. 1494*	Hemorrhage, *p. 1493*
Dermis, *p. 1484*	Hemostasis, *p. 1492*
Drainage evacuators, *p. 1547*	Induration, *p. 1502*
Edema, *p. 1487*	Laceration, *p. 1506*
Epidermis, *p. 1483*	Normal reactive hyperemia, *p. 1515*

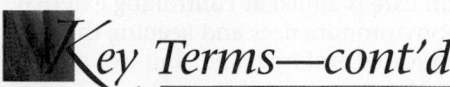

Key Terms—cont'd

Pressure reducing, *p. 1516*
Pressure relieving, *p. 1516*
Pressure ulcer, *p. 1484*
Primary intention, *p. 1492*
Puncture, *p. 1506*
Purulent, *p. 1493*
Sanguineous, *p. 1507*
Secondary intention, *p. 1492*
Serosanguineous, *p. 1507*
Serous, *p. 1507*

Shearing force, *p. 1486*
Sitz bath, *p. 1556*
Slough, *p. 1487*
Sutures, *p. 1543*
Tissue ischemia, *p. 1484*
Wound, *p. 1487*
Wound contraction, *p. 1498*
Wound Vacuum Assisted
    Closure (Wound V.A.C.),
    p. 1536

Critical Thinking Exercises

1. When removing a saline moistened dressing from a sacral pressure ulcer, you note that the gauze is dripping with beige-colored fluid. What assessments should be made and after the assessment, what should be done next? What could be the possible cause of this drainage?
2. After changing a client's position, you observe redness over the bony prominences. How should this area be assessed?
3. You have just admitted a client from a nursing home to your division. On initial assessment, you assess a stage III pressure ulcer. How do you determine the type of care and dressing to use with this particular pressure ulcer?
4. You are providing care to an older, incontinent Hispanic man who is bed-bound. How will you assess for pressure ulcers in this client? What measures can you take to prevent his skin from breaking down?

Review Questions

1. When repositioning an immobile client the nurse notices redness over a bony prominence. When the area is assessed the red spot blanches with fingertip touch, indicating:
   1. A local skin infection requiring antibiotics.
   2. This client has sensitive skin and requires special bed linen.
   3. A stage III pressure ulcer needing the appropriate dressing.
   4. Reactive hyperemia, a reaction that causes the blood vessels to dilate in the injured area.

2. This type of pressure ulcer has an observable pressure-related alteration of intact skin whose indicators, compared with an adjacent or opposite area on the body, may include changes in one or more of the following: skin temperature (warmth or coolness), tissue consistency (firm or beefy feel), and/or sensation (pain, itching).
   1. Stage I.
   2. Stage II.
   3. Stage III.
   4. Stage IV.

3. When obtaining a wound culture to determine the presence of a wound infection, the specimen should to be taken from the:
   1. Necrotic tissue.
   2. Drainage on the dressing.
   3. Wound drainage.
   4. Wound after it has first been cleansed with normal saline.

4. Postoperatively the client with a closed abdominal wound reports a sudden "pop" after coughing. When the nurse examines the surgical wound site, the sutures are open and pieces of small bowel are noted at the bottom of the now opened wound. The correct intervention would be to:
   1. Allow the area to be exposed to air until all drainage has stopped.
   2. Place several cold packs over the areas, protecting the skin around the wound.
   3. Cover the areas with sterile saline-soaked towels and immediately notify the surgical team; this is likely to indicate a wound evisceration.
   4. Cover the area with sterile gauze; place a tight binder over the areas. Ask the client to remain in bed for 30 minutes because this is a minor opening in the surgical wound and should reseal quickly.

5. Serous drainage from a wound is defined as:
   1. Fresh bleeding.
   2. Clear, watery plasma.
   3. Thick and yellow.
   4. Beige to brown and foul smelling.

6. For a client who has a muscle sprain, localized hemorrhage, or hematoma, this helps prevent edema formation, control bleeding, and anesthetize the body part:
   1. Binder.
   2. Ice bag.
   3. Ace bandage.
   4. Absorptive diaper.

7. Interventions to manage a client who is experiencing fecal and urinary incontinence include:
   1. Use of a large absorbent diaper, changing when saturated.
   2. Keeping the buttocks exposed to air at all times.
   3. Utilization of an incontinence cleanser, followed by application of a moisture barrier ointment.
   4. Frequent cleansing, application of an ointment, and covering the areas with a thick absorbent towel.

8. The best description of a hydrocolloid dressing is:
   1. A seaweed derivative that is highly absorptive.
   2. Premoistened gauze, placed over a granulating wound.
   3. A debriding enzyme that is used to remove necrotic tissue.
   4. A dressing that forms a gel that interacts with the wound surface.

9. A binder placed around a surgical client with a new abdominal wound is indicated for:
   1. Collection of wound drainage.
   2. Reduction of abdominal swelling.
   3. Reduction of stress on the abdominal incision.
   4. Stimulation of peristalsis (return of bowel function) from direct pressure.

10. Application of a warm compress is indicated:
    1. To relieve edema.
    2. For a client who is shivering.
    3. To promote healing by simulating blood flow.
    4. To protect bony prominences from pressure ulcers.

References

Agency for Health Care Policy and Research, Panel for the Prediction and Prevention of Pressure Ulcers in Adults: *Pressure ulcers in adults: prediction and prevention,* Clinical Practice Guideline No. 3, AHCPR Pub No. 92-0047, Rockville, Md, 1992a, Agency for Health Care Policy and Research, Public Health Service, U.S. Department of Health and Human Services.

Agency for Health Care Policy and Research, Panel for Urinary Incontinence Guideline: *Urinary incontinence in adults,* Clinical Practice Guideline, AHCPR Pub No. 92-0038, Rockville, Md, 1992b, Agency for Health Care Policy and Research, Public Health Service, U.S. Department of Health and Human Services.

Agency for Health Care Policy and Research, Panel for Treatment of Pressure Ulcers in Adults: *Treatment of pressure ulcers,* Clinical Practice Guideline No. 15, AHCPR Pub No. 95-0653, Rockville, Md, 1994, Agency for Health Care Policy and Research, Public Health Service, U.S. Department of Health and Human Services.

Argenta LC, Morykwas MJ: Vacuum-assisted closure: a new method for wound control and treatment: clinical experience, *Ann Plast Surg* 38(6): 563, 1997.

Ayello EA: Teaching the assessment of patients with pressure ulcers, *Decubitus* 5(7):53, 1992.

Ayello EA: Keeping pressure ulcers in check, *Nursing* 26(10):62, 1996.

Ayello EA, Braden B: How and why to do pressure ulcer risk assessment, *Adv Skin Wound Care* 15(13)125, 2002.

Ayello EA, Thomas DR, Litchford MA: Nutritional aspects of wound healing, *Home Healthc Nurse* 17(11):719, 1999.

Barr JE: Principles of wound cleansing, *Ostomy Wound Manage* 41(7A):15S, 1995.

Bates-Jensen B: The pressure sore status look a few thousand assessments later, *Adv Wound Care* 10(5):65,1997.

Baxandall T: Healing cavity wounds with negative pressure, *Nurs Stand* 11(6): 49, 1996.

Bennett MA: Report of the Task Force on the Implications for Darkly Pigmented Intact Skin in the Prediction and Prevention of Pressure Ulcers, *Adv Wound Care* 8(6):34, 1995.

Bergstrom N, Demuth PJ, Branden B: A clinical trial of the Braden scale for predicting pressure sore risk, *Nurs Clin North Am* 22(2):417, 1987.

Braden BJ: Risk assessment in pressure ulcer prevention. In Krasner DL, Rodeheaver GT, Sibbald RG, editors: *Chronic wound care: a clinical source book for healthcare professionals,* Wayne, Pa, 2001, HMP Communications.

Broussard CL, Mendez-Eastman S, Frantz, R: Adjuvant wound therapies. In Bryant RA: *Acute and chronic wounds: nursing management,* ed 2, St. Louis, 2000, Mosby.

Candido LC: Treatment of surgical wound dehiscence, *Dermatol Nurs* 14(3):187, 2002.

Centers for Disease Control and Prevention: Feeding back surveillance data to prevent hospital acquired infections, *Emerging Infect Dis* 7(2):295, 1991.

Chua PC and others: Vacuum-assisted wound closure, *Am J Nurs* 100(12): 45, 2000.

Colwell J: Skin integrity and wound care. In Potter PA, Perry AG: *Basic Nursing, Essentials for Practice,* St. Louis, 2003, Mosby.

Cooper DM: Assessment, measurement, and evaluation: their pivotal role in wound healing. In Bryant RA, editor, *Acute and chronic wounds: nursing management,* ed 2, St. Louis, 2000, Mosby.

Currence S: Product selection in the new millennium. In Krasner DL, Rodeheaver GT, Sibbald RG, editors: *Chronic wound care: a clinical source book for healthcare professionals,* Wayne, Pa, 2001, HMP Communications.

Cuzzell J: Wound assessment and evaluation: wound dressings—confusion or choice? *Dermatol Nurs* 18(6):260, 1997.

Dochterman JM, Bulechek GM: *Nursing interventions classification (NIC),* ed 4, St. Louis, 2004, Mosby.

Erwin-Toth P, Stenger B: Teaching wound care to patients, families and healthcare providers. In Krasner DL, Rodeheaver GT, Sibbald RG, editors: *Chronic wound care: a clinical source book for healthcare professionals,* Wayne, Pa, 2001, HMP Communications.

Evans L, Land L: Topical negative pressure for treating chronic wounds: a systematic review, *Br J Plast Surg* 54(3):238, 2001.

Gaskin FC: Detection of cyanosis in the person with dark skin, *J Natl Black Nurses Assoc* 1:52, 1986.

Goldman RJ, Salcido R: More than one way to measure a wound: an overview of tools and techniques, *Adv Skin Wound Care* 15(5):236, 2002.

Hanan K, Scheele L: Albumin vs. weight as a predictor of nutritional status and pressure ulcer development, *Ostomy Wound Manage* 33:22, 1991.

Henderson CT and others: Draft definition of stage I pressure ulcers: inclusion of persons with darkly pigmented skin, *Adv Wound Care* 10(5):16, 1997.

Horn SD and others: Description of the national pressure ulcer long-term care study, *J Am Geriatr Soc* 50(11):1816, 2002.

Kane DP: Chronic wound healing and chronic wound management. In Krasner DL, Rodeheaver GT, Sibbald RG, editors: *Chronic wound care: a clinical source book for healthcare professionals,* Wayne, Pa, 2001, HMP Communications.

KCI USA: The V.A.C.: vacuum assisted closure—guidelines for use, physician and caregiver reference manual. Product information, San Antonio, Tex, 1999.

Krasner D: Caring for the person experiencing chronic pain. In Krasner DL, Rodeheaver GT, Sibbald RG, editors: *Chronic wound care: a clinical source book for healthcare professionals,* Wayne, Pa, 2001, HMP Communications.

Krouskop T, van Rijswijk L: Standardizing performance-based criteria for support surfaces, *Ostomy Wound Manage* 41(1):34, 1995.

Lazarus GS and others: Definitions and guidelines for assessment of wounds and evaluation of healing, *Arch Dermatol* 130(4): 489,1994.

Mendez-Eastman S: When wounds won't heal, *RN* 61(10):20, 1998.

Moorhead S, Johnson M, and Maas M: *Nursing outcomes classification (NOC),* ed 3, St. Louis, 2004, Mosby.

National Pressure Ulcer Advisory Panel: Pressure ulcer prevalence, cost and risk assessment: consensus development conference statement, *Decubitus* 2(2):24, 1989.

National Pressure Ulcer Advisory Panel: *Pressure ulcer research: etiology, assessment, and early intervention,* Buffalo, NY, 1995a, The Panel.

National Pressure Ulcer Advisory Panel: *NPUAP proceedings of the Fourth National NPUAP Conference,* Washington, DC, February 24-25, 1995b.

National Pressure Ulcer Advisory Panel: *Position statement on stage I assessment in darkly pigmented skin,* 1998, http://www.NPUAP.org/position4/htm.

Norton D, McLaren R, Exon-Smith AN: *An investigation of geriatric nursing problems in hospital,* Edinburgh, 1962, Churchill Livingstone.

Pieper B: Mechanical forces: pressure, shear and friction. In Bryant RA, editor: *Acute and chronic wounds: nursing management,* ed 2, St. Louis, 2000, Mosby.

Pires M, Muller A: Detection and management of early tissue pressure indicators: a pictorial essay, *Progressions* 3(3):3, 1991.

Ramundo J, Wells J: Wound debridement. In Bryant RA, editor: *Acute and chronic wounds: nursing management,* ed 2, St. Louis, 2000, Mosby.

Richardson GM, Gardner S, Frantz RA: Nursing assessment: impact on type and cost of interventions to prevent pressure ulcers, *J Wound Ostomy Continence Nurs* 25(6):1273, 1998.

Robson MC: Wound infection: a failure of wound healing caused by an imbalance of bacteria, *Surg Clin North Am* 77(3):637, 1997.

Rodeheaver GT: Wound cleansing, wound irrigation, wound disinfection. In Krasner DL, Rodeheaver GT, Sibbald RG, editors: *Chronic wound care: a clinical source book for healthcare professionals,* Wayne, Pa, 2001, HMP Communications.

Rolstad BS, Ovington L, Harris A: Principles of wound management. In Bryant RA, editor: *Acute and chronic wounds: nursing management,* ed 2, St. Louis, 2000, Mosby.

Schultz G: Molecular regulation of wound healing. In Bryant RA, editor: *Acute and chronic wounds: nursing management,* ed 2, St. Louis, 2000, Mosby.

Stotts NA: Nutritional assessment and support. In Bryant RA, editor: *Acute and chronic wounds: nursing management,* ed 2, St. Louis, 2000, Mosby.

Stotts NA, Cavanaugh CE: Assessing the patient with a wound, *Home Healthc Nurse* 17(1):27, 1999.

Stotts NA and others: Sterile versus clean technique in postoperative wound care of patients with open surgical wounds: a pilot study, *J Wound Ostomy Continence Nurs* 24:10, 1997.

Teare J, Barrett C: Using a quality of life assessment in wound care, *Nurs Stand* 17(6):67, 2002.

Thomas C: Specialty beds: decision-making made easy, *Ostomy Wound Manage* 23:51, 1989.

Trelease CC: Developing standards for wound care, *Ostomy Wound Manage* 20:46, 1988.

Waldrop J, Doughty D: Wound healing physiology. In Bryant RA, editor: *Acute and chronic wounds: nursing management,* ed 2, St. Louis, 2000, Mosby.

Weir D: Pressure ulcers: assessment, classification, and management. In Krasner DL, Rodeheaver GT, Sibbald RG, editors: *Chronic wound care: a clinical source book for healthcare professionals,* Wayne, Pa, 2001, HMP Communications.

Wysocki AB: Anatomy and physiology of skin and soft tissue. In Bryant RA, editor: *Acute and chronic wounds: nursing management,* ed 2, St. Louis, 2000, Mosby.

*R*esearch References

Allman RM and others: Pressure ulcers, hospital complications, and disease severity: impact on hospital costs and length of stay, *Adv Wound Care* 12(1):22, 1999.

Baharestani MM: The lived experience of wives caring for their frail, homebound, elderly husbands with pressure ulcers, *Adv Wound Care* 7(3):40, 1994.

Banwell PE, Holten IW, Martin DL: A new concept in wound healing: the management of wounds with negative pressure therapy, *Br J Surg* 82(suppl 2):149, 1998.

Braden BJ, Bergstrom N: Clinical utility of the Braden Scale for predicting pressure sore risk, *Decubitus* 2(3):50,1989.

Braden BJ, Bergstrom N: Predictive validity of the Braden Scale for pressure sore risk in a nursing home population, *Res Nurs Health* 17(6):459, 1994.

Bergstrom N and others: The Braden Scale for predicting pressure sore risk, *Nurs Res* 36(4):205, 1987.

Burton AC, Yamada S: Relation between blood pressure and flow in the human forearm, *J Appl Physiol* 4:3291, 1951.

Ferrell BA and others: Pressure ulcers among patients admitted to home care, *J Am Geriatr Soc* 48(9):1042, 2000.

Lyder CH and others: Quality of care for hospitalized medicare patients at risk for pressure ulcers, *Arch Intern Med* 161(12):1549, 2001.

Pinchcofsky-Devin GD, Kaminski MV: Correlation of pressure sores and nutritional status, *J Am Geriatr Soc* 34(6):435, 1989.

Ratliff CR, Bryant DE. *Guidelines for the management of pressure ulcers,* Clinical Practice Guideline Series, Glenview, Ill, 2003, Wound, Ostomy and Continence Nurses Society.

Stotts NA: Predicting pressure ulcer development in surgical patients, *Heart Lung* 17(6):641, 1988.

Stotts NA and others: Sterile vs clean technique in wound care of patients with open surgical wounds in the post-op period: a pilot study, *J Wound Ostomy Continence Nurs* 24(1):10, 1997.

48

Sensory Alterations

Media Resources

http://evolve.elsevier.com/Potter/
fundamentals/

 CD COMPANION

- Review Questions
- Glossary

evolve WEBSITE

- Review Questions
- Student Learning Activities
- Animations
- Concept Map Exercise
- Critical Thinking Exercise
- Glossary

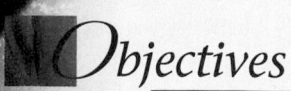

Objectives

Mastery of content in this chapter will enable the student to:

- Define the key terms listed.
- Differentiate among the processes of reception, perception, and reaction to sensory stimuli.
- Discuss the relationship of sensory function to an individual's level of wellness.
- Discuss common causes and effects of sensory alterations.
- Discuss common sensory changes that normally occur with aging.
- Identify factors to assess in determining a client's sensory status.
- Identify nursing diagnoses relevant to clients with sensory alterations.
- Develop a plan of care for clients with visual, auditory, tactile, speech, and olfactory deficits.
- List interventions for preventing sensory deprivation and controlling sensory overload.
- Describe conditions in the health care agency or client's home that can be adjusted to promote meaningful sensory stimulation.
- Discuss ways to maintain a safe environment for clients with sensory deficits.

*I*magine the world without sight, hearing, or the ability to feel objects or sense aromas around you. Human beings rely on a variety of sensory stimuli to give meaning and order to events occurring in their environment. The senses are tightly interwoven in forming the perceptual base of our world (Ebersole and Hess, 2001). Stimulation comes from many sources in and outside the body, particularly through the senses of sight (visual), hearing **(auditory),** touch **(tactile),** smell **(olfactory),** and taste **(gustatory).** The body also has a **kinesthetic** sense that enables a person to be aware of the position and movement of body parts without seeing them. **Stereognosis** is a sense that allows a person to recognize an object's size, shape, and texture. The ability to speak is not considered a sense, but it is similar in that the client may lose the ability to interact meaningfully with other human beings. Meaningful stimuli allow a person to learn about the environment and are necessary for healthy functioning and normal development. When sensory function is altered, the person's ability to relate to and function within the environment changes drastically.

Many clients seeking health care have preexisting sensory alterations. Others may develop sensory alterations as a result of medical treatment (e.g., hearing loss from antibiotic use). The environment of a health care setting (e.g., a noisy intensive care unit) can cause sensory alterations. Clients who have partial or complete loss of a major sense may have developed or may need to find alternative ways to function safely within the environment. If sensory alterations occur early in life, clients often have developmental and socialization problems because of difficulty in responding to people and the environment. A health care setting is often a place of unfamiliar sights, sounds, and smells, as well as minimal contact with family and friends. If clients feel depersonalized and are unable to receive meaningful stimuli, serious sensory alterations can develop.

The nurse must understand and help meet the needs of clients with sensory alterations, as well as recognize clients most at risk for developing sensory problems. The nurse helps clients learn to interact and react safely and effectively in their environment.

Scientific Knowledge Base

Normal Sensation

Normally the nervous system continually receives thousands of bits of information from sensory nerve organs, relays the information through appropriate channels, and integrates the information into a meaningful response. Sensory stimuli reach the sensory organs and can elicit an immediate reaction or present information to the brain to be stored for future use. The nervous system must be intact for sensory stimuli to reach appropriate brain centers and for the individual to perceive the sensation. After interpreting the significance of a sensation, the person can then react to the stimulus. Table 48-1 summarizes normal hearing and vision.

Reception, perception, and reaction are the three components of any sensory experience (see Chapter 42). Reception begins with stimulation of a nerve cell called a receptor, which is usually designed for only one type of stimulus, such as light, touch, or sound. In the case of special senses, the receptors are grouped close together or located in specialized organs (McCance and Huether, 2002), such as the taste buds of the tongue or the retina of the eye. When a nerve impulse is created, it travels along pathways to the spinal cord or directly to the brain. For example, sound waves stimulate hair cell receptors within the organ of Corti, which causes impulses to travel along the eighth cranial nerve to the acoustic area of the temporal lobe. Sensory nerve pathways usually cross over to send stimuli to opposite sides of the brain. The actual perception or awareness of unique sensations depends on the receiving region of the cerebral cortex, where specialized brain cells interpret the quality and nature of sensory stimuli. When the person becomes conscious of the stimuli and receives the information, perception takes place. Perception includes integration and interpretation of the stimuli based on the person's experiences. A person's level of consciousness influences how well stimuli are perceived and interpreted. Any factors lowering consciousness impair sensory perception. If sensation is incomplete, such as blurred vision, or if past experience is inadequate for understanding stimuli such as pain, the person may react inappropriately to the sensory stimulus.

It is impossible to react to all of the multiple stimuli entering the nervous system. The brain prevents sensory bombardment by discarding or storing sensory information. A person will usually react to stimuli that are most meaningful or significant at the time. After continued reception of the same stimulus, however, a person stops responding and the sensory experience goes unnoticed. For example, a person concentrating on reading a good book may not be aware of music in the background. This

Table 48-1	Normal Hearing and Vision
Function	**Anatomy and Physiology**
The Ear	
Transmits to the brain an accurate pattern of all sounds received from the environment, the relative intensity of these sounds, and the direction from which they originate	Two ears provide stereophonic hearing to judge sound direction.
	The external ear canal shelters the eardrum and maintains relatively constant temperature and humidity to maintain elasticity.
	The middle ear is an air-containing space between the eardrum and oval window. It contains three small bones (ossicles).
	The eardrum and ossicles transfer sound to the fluid-filled inner ear.
	Movement of the stapes in the oval window creates vibrations in the fluid that bathes the membranous labyrinth, which contains the end organs of hearing and balance.
	The union of the vestibular (balance) and cochlear (hearing) portions of the labyrinth explains the combination of hearing and balance symptoms that occur with inner ear disorders.
	Vibration of the eardrum is transmitted through the bony ossicles. Vibrations at the oval window are transmitted in perilymph within the inner ear to stimulate hair cells that send impulses along the eighth cranial nerve to the brain.
The Eye	
Transmits to the brain an accurate pattern of light reflected from solid objects in the environment and transformed into color and hue	Light rays enter the convex cornea and begin to converge.
	Fine adjustment of light rays occurs as they pass through the pupil and through the lens.
	Change in the shape of the lens focuses light on the retina.
	The retina has a pigmented layer of cells to enhance visual acuity.
	The sensory retina contains the rods and cones—photoreceptor cells sensitive to stimulation from light.
	Photoreceptor cells send electrical potentials by way of the optic nerve to the brain.

adaptability phenomenon occurs with most sensory stimuli except for those of pain.

The balance between sensory stimuli entering the brain and those actually reaching a person's conscious awareness maintains a person's well-being. If an individual attempts to react to every stimulus within the environment or if there is insufficient variety and quality of stimuli, sensory alterations will occur.

Sensory Alterations

The most common types of sensory alterations are sensory deficits, sensory deprivation, and sensory overload. When a client suffers from more than one sensory alteration, the ability to function and relate effectively within the environment is seriously impaired.

Sensory Deficits. A deficit in the normal function of sensory reception and perception is a **sensory deficit.** When senses are impaired, the sense of self is impaired. Initially a person may withdraw by avoiding communication or socialization with others in an attempt to cope with the sensory loss. It becomes difficult for the person to interact safely with the environment until new skills relying on other existing functions are learned. When a

deficit develops gradually or when considerable time has passed since the onset of an acute sensory loss, the person learns to rely on unaffected senses. Some senses may even become more acute to compensate for an alteration. For example, a blind client often develops an acute sense of hearing.

Clients with sensory deficits may change behavior in adaptive or maladaptive ways. For example, one client with a hearing impairment may turn the unaffected ear toward the speaker to hear better, whereas another client may shun other people to avoid the embarrassment of not being able to understand their speech. Box 48-1 summarizes common sensory deficits and their influence on those affected.

Sensory Deprivation. The reticular activating system in the brain stem mediates all sensory stimuli to the cerebral cortex, so even in deep sleep, clients are able to receive stimuli. Sensory stimulation must be of sufficient quality and quantity to maintain a person's awareness. The sensory deprivation that clients experience relates to the need for a comforting touch. Clients in intensive care units (ICUs) are often exposed to physical touch, but it is usually associated with technical intervention rather

---

Box 48-1   Common Sensory Deficits

Visual Deficits

Presbyopia: A gradual decline in the ability of the lens to accommodate or to focus on close objects. Individual is unable to see near objects clearly.

Cataract: Cloudy or opaque areas in part or the entire lens that interfere with passage of light through the lens. Cataracts usually develop gradually, without pain, redness, or tearing in the eye.

Dry eyes: Result when tear glands produce too few tears. Common in older adults and resulting in itching, burning, or even reduced vision.

Open-angle glaucoma: An increase in intraocular pressure caused by an obstruction to the normal flow of aqueous humor through the canal of Schlemm. Causes progressive pressure against the optic nerve, resulting in visual field loss, decreased visual acuity, and a halo effect seen around objects if untreated.

Diabetic retinopathy: Pathological changes occur in the blood vessels of the retina, resulting in decreased vision or vision loss.

Macular degeneration: Condition in which the macula (specialized portion of the retina responsible for central vision) loses its ability to function efficiently. First signs may include blurring of reading matter, distortion or loss of central vision, and distortion of vertical lines.

Hearing Deficits

Presbycusis: A common progressive hearing disorder in older adults.

Cerumen accumulation: Buildup of earwax in the external auditory canal. Cerumen, which is normally absorbed in a younger person's ear, becomes hard and collects in the canal and causes a conduction deafness.

Balance Deficit

Dizziness and disequilibrium: Common condition in older adulthood, usually resulting from vestibular dysfunction. Frequently an episode of vertigo or disequilibrium is precipitated by a change in position of the head.

Taste Deficit

Xerostomia: Decrease in salivary production that leads to thicker mucus and a dry mouth. Result of medications such as antihistamines. Can interfere with the ability to eat and leads to appetite and nutritional problems.

Neurological Deficits

Peripheral neuropathy: Disorder of the peripheral nervous system. Commonly caused by diabetes, Guillain-Barré syndrome, and neoplasms (Ebersole and Hess, 2001). Symptoms include numbness and tingling of the affected area and stumbling gait.

Stroke: Cerebrovascular accident caused by clot, hemorrhage, or emboli disrupting blood flow to the brain. Creates altered proprioception with marked incoordination and imbalance. Loss of sensation and motor function in extremities controlled by the affected area of the brain also occurs. A stroke affecting the left hemisphere of the brain results in symptoms on the right side such as difficulty with speech. A stroke on the right hemisphere will have symptoms on the left side, which may include visuospatial alterations such as loss of half of a visual field or inattention and neglect, especially to the left side.

than personal, comforting touch (Urden and others, 2002). When a person experiences an inadequate quality or quantity of stimulation, such as monotonous or meaningless stimuli, **sensory deprivation** occurs. Three types of sensory deprivation are reduced sensory input (sensory deficit from visual or hearing loss), elimination of order or meaning from input (e.g., exposure to strange environments), and restriction of the environment (e.g., bed rest or reduced environmental variation) that produces monotony and boredom (Ebersole and Hess, 2001).

There are many effects of sensory deprivation (Box 48-2). The symptoms can easily cause nurses and physicians to believe that a client is psychologically ill and confused, is suffering from severe electrolyte imbalance, or is under the influence of psychotropic drugs. Therefore the nurse must always be aware of the client's existing sensory function and the quality of stimuli within the environment.

Sensory Overload. When a person receives multiple sensory stimuli and cannot perceptually disregard or selectively ignore some stimuli, **sensory overload** occurs. Excessive sensory stimulation prevents the brain from appropriately responding to or ignoring certain stimuli. Because of the multitude of stimuli leading to overload, the person no longer perceives the environment in a way that makes sense. Overload prevents meaningful re-

sponse by the brain; the person's thoughts race, attention moves in many directions, and anxiety and restlessness occur. As a result, overload causes a state similar to that produced by sensory deprivation. However, in contrast to deprivation, overload is individualized. The amount of stimuli needed for healthy function varies with each individual. Persons may be subject to environmental overload more at one time than at another. A person's tolerance to sensory overload may vary by level of fatigue, attitude, and emotional and physical well-being.

The acutely ill client may easily fall victim to sensory overload. The client in constant pain or who undergoes frequent monitoring of vital signs or who has irritation from drainage tubes is at risk. Multiple stimuli can combine to cause overload even if the nurse offers a comforting word or provides a gentle back rub. Clients may not benefit from nursing intervention because their attention and energy are focused on more stressful stimuli. Another example is the client who is hospitalized in an ICU, where the activity is constant. Lights are always on. Sounds can be heard from monitoring equipment, staff conversations, equipment alarms, and the activities of people entering the unit. Even at night, an ICU can be very noisy.

The behavioral changes associated with sensory overload can easily be confused with mood swings or simple disorientation. The nurse must look for symptoms such as racing thoughts, scattered attention, restlessness, and anxiety. Clients in ICUs sometimes resort to constantly fingering tubes and dressings. Constant reorientation and control of excessive stimuli become an important part of the client's care.

*N*ursing Knowledge Base

Factors Affecting Sensory Function

There are multiple factors that may affect an individual's sensory function. All are conditions or situations that the nurse attempts to manage when delivering care. These factors relate to the quality and quantity of sensory stimuli. Other influences are family, environmental, and cultural factors that affect the client.

Age. Infants are unable to discriminate sensory stimuli because nerve pathways are immature. Visual changes during adulthood include presbyopia (inability to focus on near objects) and the need for glasses for reading. These changes usually occur from ages 40 to 50. Normal changes associated with aging include reduced visual fields, increased glare sensitivity, impaired night vision, reduced accommodation and depth perception, and reduced color discrimination. Hearing changes, which begin at age 30, include decreased hearing acuity, speech intelligibility, pitch discrimination, and hearing threshold. Older adults hear low-pitched sounds the best but have difficulty hearing conversation over background noise. Speech sounds are garbled, and there is a delayed reception and reaction to speech. Older adults have difficulty discriminating the consonants (*z, t, f, g*) and high-frequency sounds (s, sh, ph, k). A problem with age-related hearing loss is that some individuals who are affected may not even be aware of their deficit (Tolson,

---

Box *48-2*	**Effects of Sensory Deprivation**

Cognitive

Reduced capacity to learn
Inability to think or problem solve
Poor task performance
Disorientation
Bizarre thinking
Regression
Increased need for socialization, altered mechanisms of attention

Affective

Boredom
Restlessness
Increased anxiety
Emotional ability
Panic
Increased need for physical stimulation

Perceptual

Visual/motor coordination
Color perception
Apparent movement
Tactile accuracy
Ability to perceive size and shape
Spatial and time judgment

Modified from Ebersole P, Hess P: *Toward healthy aging; human needs and nursing response,* ed 5, St. Louis, 2001, Mosby.

1997). A serious concern for those with a hearing deficit is that they may be inappropriately labeled as confused (Maas and others, 2001).

Gustatory and olfactory changes include a decrease in the number of taste buds in later years and reduction of olfactory nerve fibers by age 50. Reduced taste discrimination and reduced sensitivity to odors are common.

Proprioceptive changes after age 60 include increased difficulty with balance, spatial orientation, and coordination. Older adults experience tactile changes, including declining sensitivity to pain, pressure, and temperature.

Persons at Risk. Older adults are a high-risk group because of normal physiological changes involving sensory organs. However, the nurse must be careful to not automatically assume that a client's sensory problem is related to advancing age. For example, adult sensorineural hearing loss can be due to exposure to excess and prolonged noise, metabolic, vascular, and other systemic alterations. A client may benefit from a referral to an audiologist or **otolaryngologist** if the assessment reveals serious hearing problems.

Individuals at risk for sensory deprivation are commonly those living in a confined environment such as a nursing home. Although most quality nursing homes or centers offer meaningful stimulation through group activities, environmental design, and mealtime gatherings, there are exceptions. The individual who is confined to a wheelchair, suffers from poor hearing and/or vision, has decreased energy, and avoids contact with others is at significant risk for sensory deprivation. If the environment creates monotony, the individual has a reduced capacity to learn and to think.

Meaningful Stimuli. Meaningful stimuli reduce the incidence of sensory deprivation. In the home, meaningful stimuli include pets, music playing on a cassette player, television, pictures of family members, and a calendar and clock. The same types of items should be present in a nursing center. In a health care setting the nurse notes whether clients have roommates or visitors. The presence of others can offer positive stimulation. However, a roommate who constantly watches television, persistently tries to talk, or continuously keeps lights on can contribute to sensory overload. A client can become disoriented in a barren environment such as in an isolation room that gives few signals for normal sensory perception. The presence or absence of meaningful stimuli influences alertness and the ability to participate in care.

Amount of Stimuli. Excessive stimuli in an environment can cause sensory overload. The frequency of observations and procedures performed in an acute care setting may be stressful. If the client is in pain, has many tubes and dressings, or is restricted by casts or traction, overstimulation can be a problem. A client's room may be near repetitive or loud noises (e.g., an elevator, stairwell, or nurses' station), which may contribute to sensory overload.

Family Factors. The amount and quality of contact with supportive family members and significant others can influence the degree of isolation the client feels. Whether a client lives alone or whether family and friends frequently visit influences client reactions. The absence of visitors during hospitalization or residency in a nursing center or extended care facility can also affect sensory status. This is a common problem in hospital intensive care settings, where visitation is often restricted. A pattern of social isolation can contribute to sensory changes. The ability to discuss fears or concerns with loved ones is an important coping mechanism for most people. Therefore the absence of meaningful conversation can cause a person to become sensorially deprived, and the nurse may not be alerted until behavioral changes occur.

Social Interaction. Clients with hearing loss tend to decrease time spent with social activities and with verbal communication (Resnick, Fries, and Verbrugge, 1997). Children with hearing deficits will be inattentive, uncooperative, or easily bored (Wong and others, 2002). Often a client becomes embarrassed by needing to continually ask another person to repeat what has been said. So instead, they initiate little communication. Clients who find their lifestyles influenced by a hearing loss experience loneliness and lowered self-esteem. Social difficulties caused by hearing loss further contribute to the feeling of loneliness.

Environmental Factors. A person's occupation can place him or her at risk for visual, hearing, and peripheral nerve alterations (Box 48-3). Individuals who are exposed to loud noises at work or who have occupations involving risk of exposure to chemicals or flying objects should be screened for hearing and visual problems. Clients who use their hands in a repetitive fashion, causing trauma to the median nerve, can develop carpal tunnel syndrome. Carpal tunnel syndrome is one of the most common industrial or work-related injuries. Occupations that involve continuous wrist movement may cause the client to develop swelling or inflammation, which creates pressure on the nerve as it passes through the narrow area in the wrist. The client experiences numbness, tingling, pain, and weakness in the hand while performing fine hand movements (Ruda, 2000).

A hospitalized client can be at risk for sensory alterations due to exposure to environmental stimuli or a change in sensory input. Clients who are immobilized because of bed rest or physical encumbrances (e.g., casts or traction) are at risk, because they are unable to experience all of the normal sensations of free movement. Another group at risk includes clients isolated in a health care setting or at home. For example, the client placed in isolation because of tuberculosis (see Chapter 33) is often restricted to a hospital room and is unable to enjoy normal interactions with visitors. A hospital environment is full of sensory stimuli. Therapeutic isolation, the sounds of electrical monitors and equipment, bright lighting, and the odors of body fluids are just some examples.

As a result of illness or hospitalization, a client is often confined to an unfamiliar and unresponsive environment. This does not mean that all hospitalized clients have sensory alterations. However, the nurse must assess more carefully those clients subjected to continued sensory stimulation (e.g., ICU settings, long-term hospitalization, or multiple therapies). The nurse assesses the

---

Box **48-3**   **Occupations and Leisure Activities That Pose Risk for Sensory Alterations**

Hearing

Factory worker
Airport worker
Rock musician
Construction worker with jackhammer
Farmer working with farm machines

Vision

Exposure to irritating gases
Welder
Exposure to high-speed machinery
Racquetball, squash, or fencing
Motorcycle riding
Power tool use

Peripheral Nerve Injury—Repetitive Motion

Computer programmer
Manicurist
Factory worker on assembly line

Peripheral Nerve Trauma

Industrial equipment
Home woodworking

Cultural Aspects of Care   *Box* **48-4**

- Whites have more hearing impairment problems than African-Americans and Asian-Americans.
- Eskimos are especially vulnerable to developing primary narrow-angle glaucoma, and it is more often seen in older adults and in women (Giger and Davidhizar, 1999).
- The percentage and acuity of glaucoma is higher in African-Americans than in whites.
- The incidence of astigmatism is higher for both African-Americans and Native Americans than for whites.
- Otitis media is more prevalent among Native Americans than among whites (Smith and Wilbur, 2000).
- Jewish Americans have a greater incidence of myopia, and it is more prevalent in boys than in girls (Lewis and others, 2000).

---

client's environment, both within the health care setting and the home, looking for factors that pose risks or that need adjustment to provide safety and more stimulation.

Cultural Factors. Certain sensory alterations occur more commonly in select ethnic groups. For example, the frequency and severity of glaucoma is higher in African-Americans as compared with whites. Other statistics have shown that the incidence of hearing impairment is greater in whites than in either African-Americans or Asian-Americans (Smith and Wilbur, 2000). Box 48-4 summarizes additional sensory alterations that can be associated with a client's cultural heritage.

Critical Thinking

Successful critical thinking requires a synthesis of knowledge and information gathered from clients, experience, critical thinking attitudes, and intellectual and professional standards. Clinical judgments require the nurse to anticipate the information necessary, analyze the data, and make decisions regarding client care. Clients' conditions are always changing. During assessment (Figure 48-1) the nurse must consider all critical thinking elements that build toward making appropriate nursing diagnoses.

In the case of sensory alterations the nurse must integrate knowledge of the pathophysiology of sensory deficits, factors that affect sensory function, and thera-

peutic communication principles. This knowledge positions the nurse to conduct appropriate assessments, anticipate what to recognize when a client describes a sensory problem and to make judgments of any abnormalities. For example, knowing the normal symptoms of a cataract helps the nurse recognize the pattern of visual changes a client with a cataract will report.

Previous experiences in caring for clients with sensory deficits enable the nurse to recognize limitations in function in each new client and how limitations might affect the client's ability to carry out daily activities. For example, after caring for a client with a hearing impairment, the nurse will be able to conduct a more effective assessment of the next client by using approaches that promote the client's ability to hear the nurse's questions.

Critical thinking attitudes and standards, when applied during assessment, ensure a thorough and accurate database from which to make decisions. For example, perseverance is needed to learn details as to how visual changes influence a client's ability to socialize. Standards of care and practice, such as those from the American Academy of Ophthalmology and the American Nurses Association (ANA) Scope and Standards of Gerontological Nursing Practice (1995), provide criteria for screening sensory problems and for establishing standards for competent, safe, effective care and practice. Using critical thinking, the nurse can conduct a thorough assessment and then plan, implement, and evaluate care that will enable the client to function safely and effectively.

Nursing Process

Assessment

When assessing clients with or at risk for sensory alterations, it is important for the nurse to consider any pathophysiology of existing deficits, as well as all of the factors influencing sensory function, to anticipate how to approach a given client's assessment. For example, if the client has a hearing disorder, the nurse will adjust his or

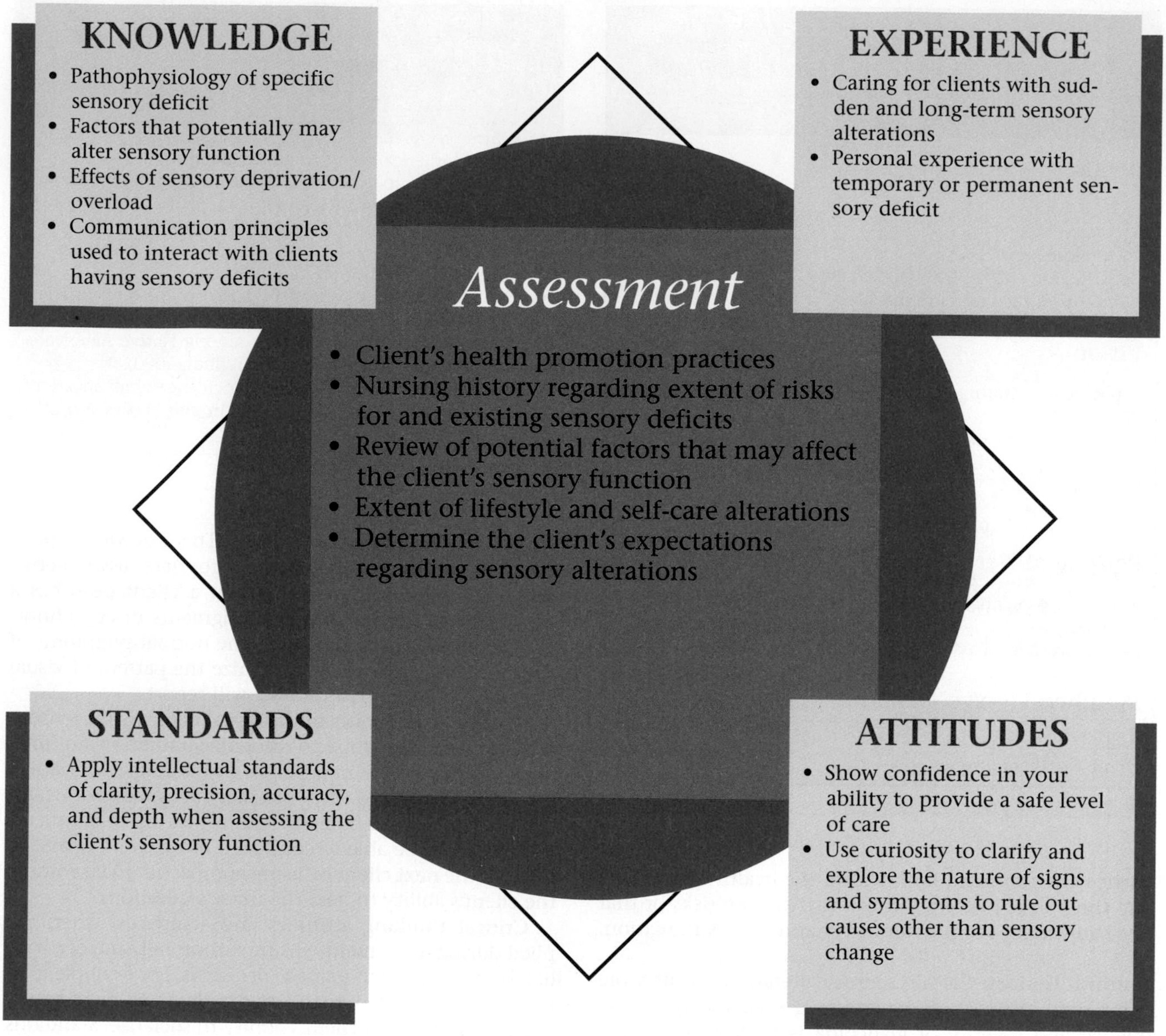

KNOWLEDGE

- Pathophysiology of specific sensory deficit
- Factors that potentially may alter sensory function
- Effects of sensory deprivation/ overload
- Communication principles used to interact with clients having sensory deficits

EXPERIENCE

- Caring for clients with sudden and long-term sensory alterations
- Personal experience with temporary or permanent sensory deficit

Assessment

- Client's health promotion practices
- Nursing history regarding extent of risks for and existing sensory deficits
- Review of potential factors that may affect the client's sensory function
- Extent of lifestyle and self-care alterations
- Determine the client's expectations regarding sensory alterations

STANDARDS

- Apply intellectual standards of clarity, precision, accuracy, and depth when assessing the client's sensory function

ATTITUDES

- Show confidence in your ability to provide a safe level of care
- Use curiosity to clarify and explore the nature of signs and symptoms to rule out causes other than sensory change

FIGURE **48–1** Critical thinking model for sensory alterations assessment.

her communication style and then focus the assessment on relevant criteria related to hearing deficits. The nurse collects a history that also assesses the client's current sensory status and the degree to which a sensory deficit affects the client's lifestyle, psychosocial adjustment, developmental status, self-care ability, and safety. The assessment must also focus on the quality and quantity of environmental stimuli.

Sensory Alterations History. The nursing history includes assessment of the nature and characteristics of sensory alterations or any problem related to an alteration. When taking the sensory alterations history, the nurse should consider the ethnic or cultural background of the client, because certain alterations are higher in some cultural groups (see Box 48-4, p. 1571). The nurse begins by asking the client to describe the sensory deficit. For example:

- Describe your hearing loss for me.
- Describe how your vision is affected.
- Explain how use of your hands has changed.
- Knowledge about the onset and duration of the sensory alteration can be helpful. The nurse begins to learn how long the client has taken measures to adjust to the alteration:
- How long have you had a visual problem?
- When did you begin to feel numbness in your hands? In your legs?
- How long have you noticed being unable to hear conversations clearly?

It is also useful to assess the client's self-rating for a sensory deficit. Lewis-Cullinan and Janken (1990) found that a client's self-rating for hearing was one of the most important defining characteristics for the nursing diagnosis of *disturbed sensory perception (auditory)*. The nurse can simply say, "Rate your hearing as excellent, good, fair, poor, or bad." Then, based on the client's self-rating, the nurse may explore more fully the client's perception of a sensory loss. This provides a more in-depth look at how the client's quality of life has been influenced. In the specific case of hearing problems, a screening tool developed by Ventry and Weinstein has been found to be effective in identifying clients needing audiological intervention. The screening version of the Hearing Handicap Inventory for the Elderly (HHIE-S) is a 5-minute, 10-item questionnaire designed to assess how a client perceives the emotional and social effects of hearing loss (Weinstein, 1994). The greater the handicapping effect from the hearing loss, the higher the scores (Demers, 2001).

A nursing history can also reveal any recent changes in a client's behavior. Frequently friends or family are the best resources for this information, because the client may be unaware of any change. The nurse asks the following:

- Has the client shown any recent mood swings (e.g., outbursts of anger, nervousness, fear, or irritability)?
- Have you noticed the client avoiding social activities?

It is important to remember that many adults are sensitive about admitting losses and may hesitate to share information.

Mental Status. Mental status assessment is an important component of any evaluation of sensory function (Box 48-5). Observation of the client during history taking, during the physical examination, and during nursing care provides valuable data for evaluation of a client's mental status. An assessment of mental status is valuable particularly if the nurse suspects sensory deprivation or overload. Observation of the client can provide data that reveal key client behaviors. The nurse will observe the client's physical appearance and behavior, measure cognitive ability, and assess the client's emotional status. The Mini Mental Status Examination (MMSE) is an example of a tool that can *formally* be used to measure disorientation, altered conceptualization and abstract thinking, and change in problem-solving abilities (see Chapter 32). For example, a client with severe sensory deprivation may not be able to carry on a conversation, remain attentive, or display recent or past memory.

Physical Assessment. To identify sensory deficits and their severity, the nurse assesses vision, hearing, olfaction, taste, and the ability to discriminate light touch, temperature, pain, and position. Chapter 32 describes assessment techniques in detail. Table 48-2 summarizes assessment techniques for identifying sensory deficits. In all examples the nurse will gather more accurate data if the examination room is private, quiet, and comfortable for the client. Finally, the nurse also relies on personal observation of the client to detect sensory alterations. Ebersole and Hess (2001) have identified some typical observations indicating hearing loss, which include the following: the client seems inattentive to others, responds with inappropriate anger when spoken to, believes people are talking about him or her, has trouble following clear directions, asks to have something repeated, has monotonous voice quality and speaks unusually loud or

---

| Box **48-5** | **Assessment of Mental Status** |

Physical Appearance and Behavior

Motor activity, posture, facial expression, hygiene

Cognitive Ability

Level of consciousness, abstract reasoning, calculation, attention, judgment
Ability to carry on conversation, ability to read, write, and copy figure
Recent and remote memory

Emotional Stability

Agitation, euphoria, irritability, hopelessness, or wide mood swings
Auditory, visual, or tactile hallucinations, illusions, delusions

---

soft, has the television unusually loud, and answers questions inappropriately.

The typical physical tests used to screen for hearing impairment rely on an examiner's whispered voice or a tuning fork. The Welch-Allyn audioscope is very effective for measuring hearing acuity. The handheld instrument includes an ear speculum that is placed within the external ear canal. The examiner can view the tympanic membrane to ensure that cerumen is not blocking the canal. A tonal sequence is initiated by pressing a button on the audioscope. The instrument is highly sensitive to detecting hearing loss.

Ability to Perform Self-Care. The nurse assesses clients' functional abilities in their home environment or health care setting, including feeding, dressing, grooming, and toileting activities. For example, the nurse assesses whether a client with altered vision can find items on a meal tray and can read directions on a prescription. The nurse also determines a visually impaired client's ability to perform daily routines such as reading bills and writing checks, differentiating money denominations, and driving a vehicle at night. If a client seems sensorially deprived, is concern shown for grooming? Does a client's loss of balance prevent rising from a toilet seat safely? Can the client with a stroke manipulate buttons or zippers for dressing? Any impairment in the ability to perform self-care has implications for planning discharge from a health care setting and in providing resources within the home.

Health Promotion Habits. It is important for the nurse to assess the daily routines clients follow to maintain sensory function. What type of eye and ear care is incorporated into daily hygiene? For those individuals who participate in sports (e.g., racquetball) or recreational activities (e.g., motorcycle riding), or who work in a setting where ear or eye injury is a possibility (e.g., chemical exposure, welding, glass or stone polishing, or constant

Table 48-2	Assessment of Sensory Function	
Assessment	**Behavior Indicating Deficit (Children)**	**Behavior Indicating Deficit (Adults)**
Vision		
Ask client to read newspaper, magazine, or lettering on menu. Measure visual acuity with Snellen chart (see Chapter 32). Assess visual fields and depth perception. Assess pupil size and accommodation to light. Ask client to identify colors on color chart or crayons.	Self-stimulation, including eye rubbing, body rocking, sniffing or smelling, arm twirling; hitching (using legs to propel while in sitting position) instead of crawling	Poor coordination, squinting, under-reaching or overreaching for objects, persistent repositioning of objects, impaired night vision, accidental falls
Hearing		
Perform conventional assessment, including ticking watch, whisper, and tuning fork (see Chapter 32). Perform audiometry. Observe client conversing with others. Compare client's ability to recognize consonants with ability to distinguish vowels. Assess client's perception of hearing ability and history of tinnitus. Inspect ear canal for hardened cerumen.	Frightened when unfamiliar people approach, no reflex or purposeful response to sounds, failure to be awakened by loud noise, slow or absent development of speech, greater response to movement than to sound, avoidance of social interaction with other children	Blank looks, decreased attention span, lack of reaction to loud noises, increased volume of speech, positioning of head toward sound, smiling and nodding of head in approval when someone speaks, use of other means of communication such as lipreading or writing, complaints of ringing in ears
Touch		
Assess client for sensitivity to light touch and temperature (see Chapter 32). Check client's ability to discriminate between sharp and full stimuli. Assess whether client can distinguish objects (coin or safety pin) in the hand with eyes closed. Ask whether client feels unusual sensations.	Inability to perform developmental tasks related to grasping objects or drawing, repeated injury from handling of harmful objects (e.g., hot stove, sharp knife)	Clumsiness, overreaction or underreaction to painful stimulus, failure to respond when touched, avoidance of touch, sensation of pins and needles, numbness
Smell		
Have client close eyes and identify several nonirritating odors (e.g., coffee, vanilla).	Difficult to assess until child is 6 or 7 years old, difficulty discriminating noxious odors	Failure to react to noxious or strong odor, increased body odor, increased sensitivity to odors
Taste		
Ask client to sample and distinguish different tastes (e.g., lemon, sugar, salt). (Have client drink or sip water and wait 1 minute between each taste.) Ask client if recent weight change has occurred.	Inability to tell whether food is salty or sweet, possible ingestion of strange-tasting things	Change in appetite, excessive use of seasoning and sugar, complaints about taste of food, weight change
Position Sense		
Perform conventional tests for balance and position sense (see Chapter 32).	Clumsiness, extraneous movement, excessive arm swinging in those with hyperactivity or learning difficulty	Poor balance and spatial orientation, shuffling gait, reduced response to brace self when falling, more precise and deliberate movements

exposure to loud noise), the nurse determines if safety glasses or hearing protective devices (HPDs) are worn. Do clients who use assistive devices such as eyeglasses, contact lenses, or hearing aids know how to provide daily care (see Chapter 38)? Are the devices used, and are they in proper working order?

The nurse also assesses the client's compliance with routine health screening. When was the last time the client had an eye examination or hearing evaluation? For adults, routine screening of visual and hearing function is imperative to detect problems early. This is especially true in the case of glaucoma, which if undetected can lead to permanent visual loss. Recommended screening guidelines are usually structured on the basis of age. When a client begins to show a hearing deficit, routine screening should be incorporated in regular examinations.

Hazards. A client with sensory alterations is at risk for injury if the living environment is unsafe. For example, a client with visual impairment cannot see potential hazards clearly. A client with proprioceptive problems may lose balance easily. The condition of the home, the rooms, and the front and back entrances can be problematic to the client with sensory alterations. Some of the more common hazards include the following:
- Uneven, cracked walkways leading to front/back door
- Doormats with slippery backing
- Extension and phone cords in the main route of walking traffic
- Loose area rugs and runners placed over carpeting
- Bathrooms without shower or tub grab bars
- Water faucets unmarked to designate hot and cold
- Bathroom floor with slippery surface
- Absence of smoke detectors in rooms
- Unlit stairways, lack of handrails.
- Cluttered floors, furniture, including footstools
- Kitchen equipment (e.g., ranges, irons, toasters) with hard-to-read settings

In the hospital environment, caregivers often forget to rearrange furniture and equipment to keep paths from the bed and chair to the bathroom and entrance clear. Walking into a client's room and looking for safety hazards can be a useful exercise:
- Is the call light within easy, safe reach?
- Are intravenous (IV) poles on wheels and easy to move?
- Are footstools in the middle of the room?
- Are suction machines, IV pumps, or drainage bags positioned so that a client can rise from a bed or chair easily?

An additional problem faced by the visually impaired is the inability to read medication labels and syringe gauges. The nurse asks the client to read a label to determine if the client can read the dosage and frequency. If a client has a hearing impairment, the nurse checks to see whether the sounds of a doorbell, telephone, smoke alarm, and alarm clock are easy to discriminate.

Communication Methods. Clients with existing sensory deficits often develop alternative ways of communicating. To interact with the client and to promote interaction with others (Figure 48-2), the nurse must understand the client's method of communication. A deaf or hearing-

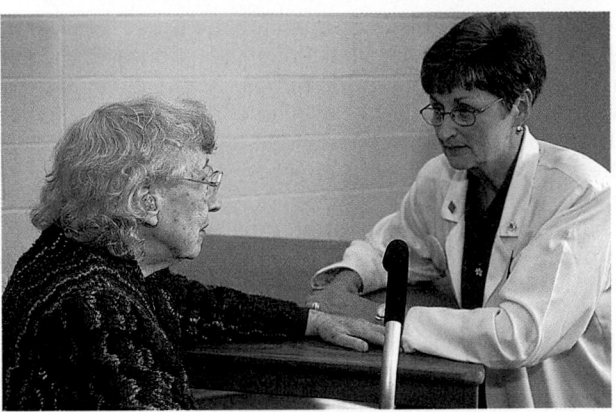

FIGURE **48–2** Nurse sits at eye level so that client with hearing impairment can communicate.

impaired client may read lips, use sign language, listen with the help of a hearing aid, or read and write notes. Vision becomes almost a primary sense for the hearing impaired.

Visually impaired clients are unable to observe facial expressions and other nonverbal behaviors that clarify the content of spoken communication. Instead, they rely on voice tones and inflections to detect the emotional tone of communication. Clients with visual deficits often learn to read Braille.

Clients with **aphasia** may be unable to produce or understand language. **Expressive aphasia,** a motor type of aphasia, is the inability to name common objects or to express simple ideas in words or writing. For example, a client may understand a question but be unable to express an answer. Sensory or **receptive aphasia** is the inability to understand written or spoken language. The client may be able to express words but is unable to understand questions or comments of others. Global aphasia is the inability to understand language or communicate orally.

The temporary or permanent loss of the ability to speak is extremely traumatic to an individual. The nurse assesses a client's alternative communication method and whether it causes anxiety in the client. Clients who have undergone laryngectomies often write notes, use communication boards or laptop computers, speak with mechanical vibrators, or use esophageal speech. Clients with endotracheal or tracheostomy tubes have a temporary loss of speech. Most use a notepad to write their questions and requests. However, the client may become incapacitated and unable to write messages. The nurse needs to determine whether the client has developed a sign language or system of symbols to communicate needs.

To understand the nature of a communication problem, the nurse must know whether a client has trouble speaking, understanding, naming, reading, or writing. Depending on the nature of the problem, the nurse selects the best way to interact with the client. For example, if the person has a visual deficit or is blind, speak normally and not from a distance and have sufficient lighting. For someone who is hearing impaired, speak clearly with a moderate rate of speech and pause to determine understanding.

Social Support. It is important for the nurse to know the client's social skills and level of satisfaction with the support given by family and friends. Is the client satisfied with the support made available from friends? Is the client able to solve problems with family members? Does the family offer the support needed when the client requires assistance as a result of a sensory loss? The long-term effects of sensory alterations can influence family dynamics and a client's willingness to remain active in society.

Use of Assistive Devices. The nurse should assess the use of assistive devices (e.g., use of a hearing aid or glasses) and the sensory effects for the client. This includes learning how often the devices are used daily, the client's or family caregiver's method for cleaning, and the client's knowledge of what to do when a problem develops. When the nurse identifies that the client has an assistive device, it is important to remember that just because the individual has the assistive device, it does not mean that it works or that the client uses it or benefits from it (McConnell, 2002).

Other Factors Affecting Perception. The nurse should remember that factors other than sensory deprivation or overload may cause impaired perception (e.g., medications or pain). The nurse assesses the client's medication history, which includes prescribed, over-the-counter medications, and herbal products. This history includes gaining information regarding the frequency, dose, method of administration, and last time these medications were taken. Some antibiotics (e.g., streptomycin, gentamicin, and tobramycin) are **ototoxic** and can permanently damage the auditory nerve; chloramphenicol can irritate the optic nerve. Narcotic analgesics, sedatives, and antidepressant medications can alter the perception of stimuli.

The nurse also conducts a thorough pain assessment (see Chapter 42) when pain is suspected to be causing perceptual problems. The nurse should also assess the use of caffeine and other remedies.

Client Expectations. Clients depend on their senses to provide them with information so as to respond or react to a specific situation or problem. Therefore clients expect caregivers to recognize and appropriately manage and adjust their environment to meet their sensory needs. This would include assisting the individual client in learning and adapting to a changed lifestyle based on the specific sensory impairment. The nurse should determine from the client exactly what the client expects to achieve and what interventions have been helpful in the past in the management of the client's limitation. The nurse should remember that clients with sensory alterations have strengthened their other senses and expect the caregivers to anticipate their needs (e.g., for safety and security).

Nursing Diagnosis

After assessment, the nurse reviews all available data and critically looks for patterns and trends suggestive of a health problem relating to sensory alterations (Box 48-6). For example, a client's advanced age, apathy, inattentiveness during conversations, and self-rating of hearing as "poor" are all defining characteristics for the nursing diagnosis of *disturbed sensory perception (auditory)*. The nurse validates findings to ensure accuracy of the diagnosis. For example, the diagnosis of *disturbed thought processes* could mistakenly be made if the nurse does not confirm the client's hearing deficit and perception of poor hearing.

The nurse determines the factor that likely causes the client's health problem. In the previous example impacted cerumen is the cause of the client's hearing alteration. The etiology or related factor of a nursing diagnosis is a condition that can be affected by nursing interventions. The etiology must be accurate; otherwise, nursing therapies will be ineffective. For a client with impacted cerumen, regular irrigations of the ear canal have the potential for improving auditory perception (Wong and others, 2002). In contrast, if the client's auditory alteration was related to hearing loss from nerve deafness, nursing interventions for alternative communication methods would be necessary.

The client may also have health care problems for which sensory alteration is the etiology, such as with the diagnosis of *risk for injury*. The nurse may also select nurs-

---

Nursing Diagnostic Process   Box 48-6

Assessment Activities	Defining Characteristics	Nursing Diagnosis
Assess client's visual acuity.	Has reduced ability to see objects clearly. Needs brighter light to read. Has trouble distinguishing edges of stairs.	Risk for injury related to visual impairment from cataract formation
Visit home setting and inspect for any hazards that may pose risks to client.	Lighting in rooms, hallways, and stairwells is very dim. Carpet in living room is old, and edges are curled up. Steps lead up to front entrance of home.	
Review medical record from clinic visit.	Client has been diagnosed as having senile cataracts in both eyes.	

ing diagnoses by recognizing the way that sensory alterations affect a client's ability to function (e.g., self-care deficit). In addition, most clients present themselves to health care professionals with multiple diagnoses (Figure 48-3). In the example of the concept map, a client with retinal detachment has the nursng diagnosis of sensory perception, which is an etiology for both risk for falls and fears. The nurse must recognize patterns of data that reveal health problems created by the client's sensory alteration. Examples of nursing diagnoses that might apply to clients with sensory alterations include the following:

- Impaired adjustment
- Impaired verbal communication
- Risk for injury
- Impaired physical mobility
- Self-care deficit, bathing/hygiene
- Self-care deficit, dressing/grooming
- Self-care deficit, toileting
- Situational low self-esteem
- Disturbed sensory perception
- Social isolation
- Disturbed thought processes

Planning

During planning the nurse again synthesizes information from multiple resources (Figure 48-4). The nurse reflects on knowledge gained from the assessment and knowledge of how sensory deficits affect normal functioning. In this way the nurse can recognize the extent of the client's deficit and know the type of interventions most likely to be helpful. The nurse also considers the role that health professionals can play in planning care and the available community resources that may be useful. The nurse's previous experience in caring for clients with sensory alterations can be invaluable. Caring for a client, for example, with a visual loss should assist the nurse in knowing how to plan nursing approaches that ensure the client's safety while maximizing the client's independence.

When applying critical thinking to planning care, professional standards can be particularly useful. These standards, in the form of clinical pathways or evidenced-based treatment protocols, often recommend scientifically proven interventions for the client's condition. For exam-

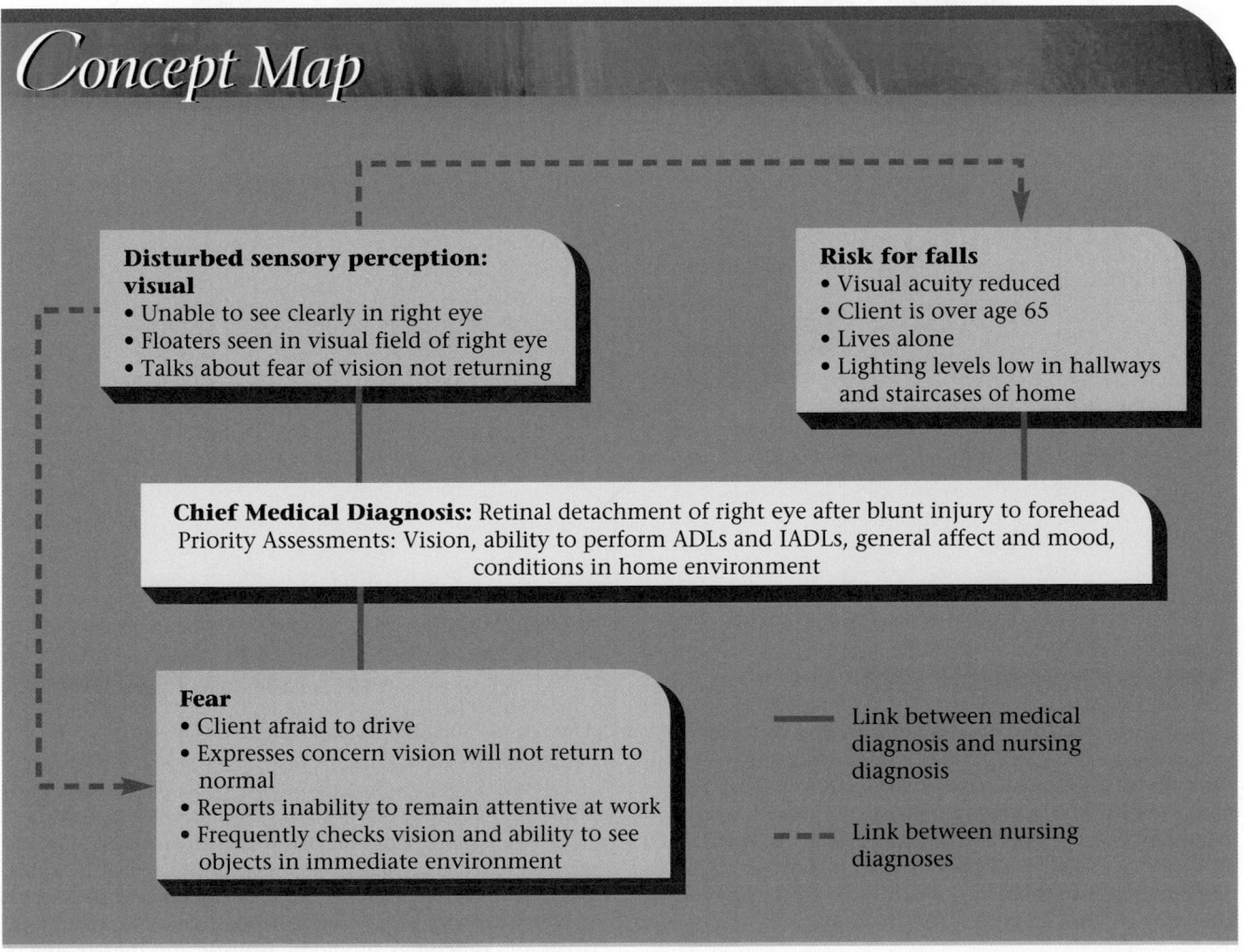

FIGURE 48-3 Concept map for client with retinal detachment of right eye after blunt injury to forehead.

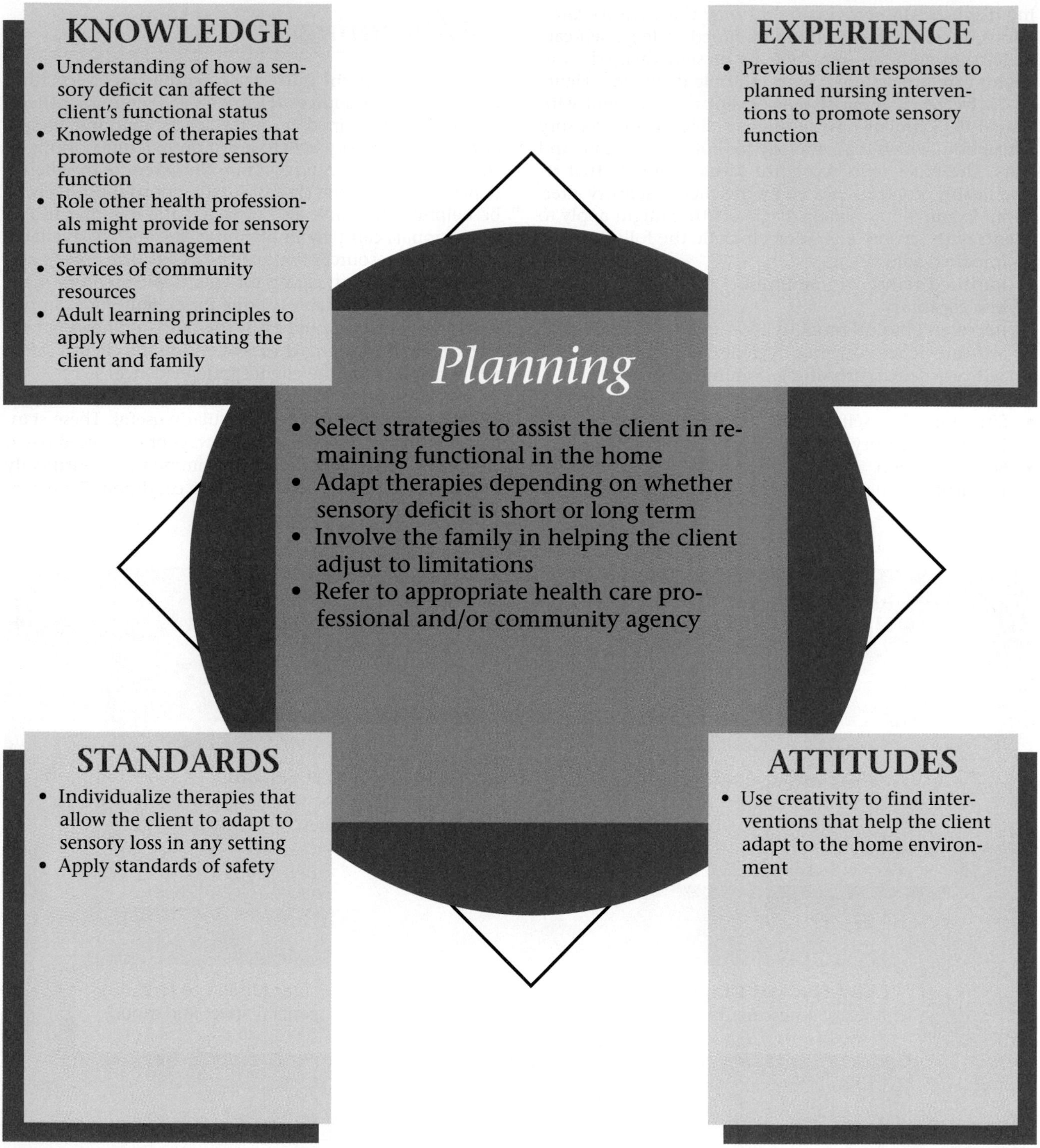

KNOWLEDGE

- Understanding of how a sensory deficit can affect the client's functional status
- Knowledge of therapies that promote or restore sensory function
- Role other health professionals might provide for sensory function management
- Services of community resources
- Adult learning principles to apply when educating the client and family

EXPERIENCE

- Previous client responses to planned nursing interventions to promote sensory function

Planning

- Select strategies to assist the client in remaining functional in the home
- Adapt therapies depending on whether sensory deficit is short or long term
- Involve the family in helping the client adjust to limitations
- Refer to appropriate health care professional and/or community agency

STANDARDS

- Individualize therapies that allow the client to adapt to sensory loss in any setting
- Apply standards of safety

ATTITUDES

- Use creativity to find interventions that help the client adapt to the home environment

FIGURE **48–4** Critical thinking model for sensory alterations planning.

ple, clients who have visual deficits and are hospitalized may be placed on a fall prevention protocol that will incorporate research-based precautions to ensure client safety.

Goals and Outcomes. During planning, the nurse develops an individualized plan of care for each nursing diagno-

sis (see care plan). The nurse and client partner together to develop a realistic plan that incorporates what the nurse knows about the client's sensory problems and the extent to which sensory function can be maintained or improved. Goals and outcomes should be realistic and measurable. A goal of care for a client with an actual or potential sensory alteration may include "The client will regain improve-

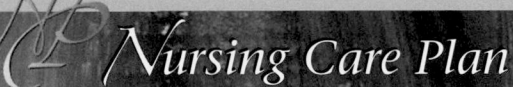

Nursing Care Plan
Disturbed Sensory Perception

Assessment

Judy Long, a 70-year-old receptionist for a college dormitory, complains to the community health nurse that lately her vision is blurred. She comments that she is having her neighbor drive her places. Judy visited an ophthalmologist, and she is scheduled for surgery in 3 weeks.

Assessment Activities	Findings/Defining Characteristics
Ask Judy to describe her vision changes.	Judy states, "My left eye seems to have a film over it that makes my vision blurred. I am having difficulty reading. I also have difficulty with night driving; the headlights are large and blurred."
Ask Judy to describe any life changes that have occurred since the change in vision.	Judy indicated that she has always worked, managed her home, and done volunteering. She says she is losing her independence because she has to have someone drive her and she is now hesitant to use stairs at home.
Assess Judy's visual acuity.	Judy cannot read the Snellen chart with the left eye.
Ask Judy the results of the visit to the ophthalmologist.	Judy states she was told she has a cataract of the left eye, and surgery is planned in 3 weeks.
Conduct a home hazard assessment.	There is clutter in the home, dim lighting, and stairs without handrails going into the house.

Nursing Diagnosis: Disturbed sensory perception related to altered sensory reception of senile cataract.

Planning

Goals	Expected Outcomes*
	Safety behavior: Home Physical Environment
Client will maintain independence in a safe home environment.	Client will verbalize changes made to protect and maintain visual acuity for indoor and outdoor activities in 2 weeks.
	A safety check of the client's home will show removal of safety hazards in 1 week.
	Client will explain plans for alternate transportation to work and social activities in 1 week.
	Sensory Function: Vision
Client will maintain existing visual function.	Client will use visual aid devices in 1 week.

*Outcome classification labels from Moorhead S, Johnson M, Maas M: *Nursing outcomes classification (NOC)*, ed 3, St. Louis, 2004, Mosby.

Interventions†	Rationale
Environmental Management	
• Instruct client to keep walking area in home and work area free of clutter, footstools, and electric cords and to avoid rearranging furniture.	Keeping the area clutter free reduces the risk of injury, and these measures help promote a safe environment (Hensel, 2000).
• Instruct client to reduce glare by wearing dark-colored sunglasses for outside and light-colored glasses for inside.	Clients have better visual acuity when they protect their eyes from bright light (Ebersole and Hess, 2001).
• Teach client to use a light over the shoulder for reading and writing.	People with cataracts see better with wider illumination (Ebersole and Hess, 2001).
• Provide magnifier for client to use to read newspaper and mail.	Devices will provide magnification to improve visual acuity.
Emotional Support	
• Encourage client to express feelings regarding loss of vision and lifestyle changes.	People who experience visual loss grieve over loss of independence (Vader, 1992).
Family Involvement	
• Confer with client on selecting a family member, friend, or community resource who can provide them with transportation until after the eye condition has been corrected.	An alternate means of transportation will foster safety (Hensel, 2000).

†Intervention classification labels from Dochterman JM, Bulechek GM: *Nursing interventions classification (NIC)*, ed 4, St. Louis, 2004, Mosby.

Continued

Nursing Care Plan

Disturbed Sensory Perception—cont'd

Evaluation

Nursing Actions	Client Response/Finding	Achievement of Outcome
Ask client to describe the changes that have made the home environment safer.	Judy responds that the family have removed the clutter and handrails have been placed at the entryway. Lighting has been placed behind her chair, and there are 100-watt lights in the living room.	Judy reports feeling safer walking the stairs and moving about in her home. The home hazards have been reduced.
During a home visit, observe the home environment for safety hazards.		
Observe client's verbal and nonverbal responses to the lifestyle adaptations.	Judy says, "I feel safer with walking in my home."	
As Judy uses magnifier, have her read a medication label.	Judy is able to read name of medication and dosage correctly.	Visual acuity has not been further compromised.
Ask if client is able to maintain a degree of independence with the environmental and lifestyle modifications.	Judy states, "I am more independent at home, and until surgery I do not mind someone driving for me."	Judy has attained some degree of independence.
Ask client to identify source of transportation.	Judy says a family member has agreed to drive her shopping and for surgery.	Judy has transportation through the weeks required for the surgical experience.

ment in hearing acuity within 2 weeks." Associated outcomes for this goal might include the following:

- The client will report using communication techniques for improved reception of messages within 2 weeks.
- The client will successfully demonstrate technique for cleansing hearing aid within 1 week.
- Client and family will be observed using proper communication skills to send and receive messages.
- Client will self-report improved hearing acuity.

Setting Priorities. Priorities of care must be set with regard to the type and extent of sensory alteration that affects a client. For example, a client who enters the emergency department after experiencing eye trauma, may have priorities of reducing anxiety and preventing further injury to the eye. In contrast, a client who is being discharged from an outpatient surgery department following cataract removal may have the priority of learning about any self-care restrictions. However, safety is always a top priority. The client can also help prioritize aspects of care. For example, the client may wish to learn ways to communicate more effectively or to participate in favorite hobbies given his or her limitation.

Some sensory alterations are short term (e.g., a client suffering sensory/perceptual alterations as a result of sensory overload in an ICU). Appropriate interventions are thus likely to be temporary (e.g., frequent reorientation or introduction of intimate and pleasant stimuli such as a back rub). Sensory alterations such as permanent visual loss require long-term goals of care for clients to adapt. However, clients who have sensory alterations at the time of entering a health care setting are usually most informed about how to adapt interventions to their lifestyles. The blind in particular need to control whatever part of their care they can. Sometimes it becomes necessary for the client to make major changes in self-care activities, communication, and socialization.

Continuity of Care. When developing a plan of care, the nurse considers all resources available to clients. The family can play a key role in providing meaningful stimulation and learning ways to help the client adjust to any limitations. The nurse may also refer the client to other health care professionals. Early referrals to occupational or speech therapists, for example, can speed a client's recovery. If a client has experienced a major loss of sensory function and is also unable to manage medical needs such as medication self-administration or dressing changes, referral to home care may be an option. There are also numerous community-based resources (e.g., local chapter of the Society for the Blind and Visually Impaired, Area on Aging, and the National Council on Independent Living Programs). The nurse may be able to arrange a volunteer to visit a client or have printed materials made available that describe ways to cope with sensory problems.

Implementation

Nursing interventions involve the client and family so that a safe, pleasant, and stimulating sensory environment can be maintained. The most effective interventions enable the client with sensory alterations to function safely with existing deficits and to continue a normal lifestyle. Learning to adjust to sensory impairments can occur at any age with the proper support and resources. The nurse uses measures to maintain a client's sensory function at the highest level possible.

Health Promotion. Good sensory function begins with prevention. Almost everyone becomes exposed to risks in the environment that may cause sensory alterations. When clients enter primary care settings, the nurse can take the opportunity to review commonsense approaches for reducing risk of sensory loss.

Screening. Nearly 12 millions Americans have some degree of visual impairment. Preventable blindness is a worldwide health issue (Smith, 2003). Therefore prevention of visual impairment begins with children and requires appropriate screening (Wong and others, 2002). There are three recommended interventions: (1) screening for rubella or syphilis in women who are considering pregnancy; (2) adequate prenatal care to prevent premature birth (with the danger of exposure of the infant to excessive oxygen); and (3) periodic screening of all children, especially newborns through preschoolers, for congenital blindness and visual impairment caused by refractive errors and **strabismus.**

Visual impairments are common during childhood. The most common visual problem is a **refractive error** such as nearsightedness. The nurse's role is one of detection and referral. Parents must know signs suggesting visual impairment (e.g., failure to react to light and reduced eye contact from the infant). The nurse instructs parents to report these signs to a physician immediately. Vision screening of school-age children and adolescents can detect problems early. The school nurse is usually responsible for vision testing.

Hearing impairment is one of the most common disabilities in the United States. It is estimated that over 28 million Americans have a hearing, speech, or language impairment (Smith and Wilbur, 2000). Children at risk include those with a family history of childhood hearing impairment, perinatal infection (rubella, herpes, cytomegalovirus), low birth weight, chronic ear infection, and Down syndrome. Nurses should advise pregnant women of the importance of early prenatal care, avoidance of ototoxic drugs, and testing for syphilis or rubella.

Children with chronic middle ear infections, a common cause of impaired hearing, should receive periodic auditory testing. Parents must be warned of the risks and should seek medical care when the child has symptoms of earache or respiratory infection.

Hearing loss from noise-induced environments was once thought to affect primarily older individuals; however, recent research has observed this in youth and young adults age 20 to 30 years old. This loss is attributed to exposure to noise at constantly high levels, such as from portable music devices, automobile music systems, concerts, and loud music in aerobics classes. This hearing impairment results in loss of sound quality. Sounds are barrel-like, and consonants are hard to hear. *Healthy People 2010* (U.S. Department of Health and Human Services, 2000) has identified goals that include the use of hearing protection devices to minimize or prevent hearing loss in children and workers. Nurses should routinely assess clients for noise exposure and participate in providing hearing conservation classes for teachers, students, and clients (Lusk, 2002; McCullagh, 2002).

In the United States, glaucoma is the second leading cause of blindness in the general population and the primary cause of blindness in African-Americans. It is important to recommend that clients between the ages of 40 and 64 have an eye examination every 2 to 4 years. Examinations should occur every 1 to 2 years if there is a family history of glaucoma or if the client is of African ancestry, has had a serious eye injury in the past, is tak-

---

Box 48-7 Tips for Preventing Eye Injury in Children

Infants and Toddlers

Avoid toys with long, pointed handles or projections.
Do not allow child to walk or run with pointed object in hand.
Keep pointed instruments and tools out of reach.

Preschoolers

Supervise use of sharp or pointed objects such as scissors.
Teach child to walk carefully when carrying pointed objects.
Keep child away from projectile activities.
Begin to teach respect for firearms and fireworks.

School-Age Children and Adolescents

Teach proper use of potentially dangerous equipment such as power tools, fireworks, and sports equipment (hockey sticks or pool cues).
Stress use of eye protection when playing ball and racquet sports, shooting, using power tools, or riding motorcycles.
Warn children not to look directly at the sun even when wearing sunglasses.
Be sure corrective lenses are made of safety glass, which is shatterproof.

---

ing steroid medications, or is over 65 years of age (Smith and Wilbur, 2000).

The guidelines for hearing screening for adults are less prescriptive. Generally, if a client works or lives in an environment where there is a high noise level, routine screening is highly recommended (Meadows, 2003). Nurses in occupational settings can assess for symptoms of tinnitus and make prompt referrals. Early detection may prevent hearing disabilities in millions of individuals (Griest and Bishop, 1998; Lusk, 2002). The most important thing for adults to understand is to not accept hearing loss as a natural part of aging. Once hearing loss becomes acknowledged by a client, it is important to have regular hearing testing. Nurses should encourage clients to follow through with recommendations for hearing aids.

Preventive Safety. Trauma is a common cause of blindness in children. Penetrating injury from propulsive objects such as firecrackers, slingshots, or rocks or from penetrating wounds from sticks, scissors, or toy weapons are just a few examples. Parents and children require counseling on ways to avoid eye trauma (Box 48-7). Safety equipment can easily be found in most sports shops and large department stores.

Adults are at risk for eye injury while playing sports and working in jobs involving exposure to chemicals or flying objects. The Occupational Safety and Health Administration has guidelines for safety in the workplace. Employers are required to have employees wear eye goggles and/or use equipment such as HPDs to reduce the risk of injury. Nurses in occupational health settings can reinforce use of protective devices.

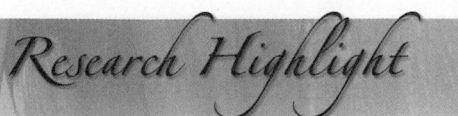

Box 48-8

Research Highlight

Farmers' Use of Hearing Protection

Research Focus

Noise-induced hearing loss (NIHL) is a consequence of exposure to high noise levels and is preventable by the appropriate use of hearing protection devices (HPDs). The focus of this research was to identify factors affecting farmers' use of HPDs. Farmers use a variety of equipment that routinely expose them to hazardous high noise levels. Nurses need to focus assessment and interventions to promote effective use of HPDs among the farming population and others. Additional research is needed to evaluate the impact of educational interventions for those exposed to high noise levels.

Research Abstract

Within the framework of Pender's Health Promotion Model, this study examined factors that influence farmers' use of HPDs. Pender's model of health-promoting behaviors shows a relationship between understanding and knowledge to explain and predict behavior. A convenience sample of 139 farmers were tested at a farm show in the Midwest. The researchers found that interpersonal support (encouragement and praise from others), situational factors, and perceived barriers were significant predictors for the reasons farmers did not use HPDs. The study showed that 17% of the farmers used HPDs with high noise levels and the majority (56%) never used HPDs. The results of the study as compared with other studies of workers' use of hearing protection showed that construction workers have more encouragement and support for the use of HPDs than the farmers, who commonly work in isolation.

Evidence-Based Practice

- Assess farmers for noise-induced hearing loss.
- Design and evaluate teaching tools to educate health care providers regarding the use of HPDs to include farmers and others exposed to high noise levels.
- Teach the value of HPDs for prevention of hearing loss to all workers, including farmers.
- Educate professionals on the necessity of family support for use of HPDs.
- Refer clients with suspected hearing impairment to a hearing clinic or to an audiologist for testing.

Reference

McCullagh M, Lusk SL, Ronis DL: Factors influencing use of hearing protection among farmers: a test of the Pender Health Promotion Model, *Nurs Res* 51:(1):33, 2002.

Box 48-9

Client Teaching

Troubleshooting Hearing Aid Malfunction

Objectives

- Family member will identify source of malfunction in hearing aid.
- Family member will demonstrate hearing aid care.

Teaching Strategies

- Show family member locations on hearing aid device where damage (e.g., cracks, fraying) is likely to occur: ear mold or case, earphone, dials, cord, and connection plugs.
- Demonstrate battery replacement: Have extra set of unused batteries available.
- Review method to check volume: turn dial to maximum gain and then check. Is voice clear?
- Consult manufacturer's directions for specific care measures for cleaning battery case and ear mold.
- Review factors to report to hearing aid laboratory: static, distortion of sound, poor volume quality.

Evaluation

- Have family member describe types of common malfunctions with hearing aid.
- Have family demonstrate battery removal and cleaning.

---

who work in physicians' offices, schools, and community clinics should reinforce the importance of early and timely immunization. When a child or an adult develops any type of health problem, caution should be used in prescribing drugs that are ototoxic.

Use of Assistive Devices. Health promotion requires appropriate use of assistive aids and good, routine hygiene measures. A client who wears corrective contact lenses, eyeglasses, or hearing aids should make sure they are kept clean, accessible, and functional (see Chapter 38). It is helpful to have a family member or friend also know how to clean an assistive aid (Box 48-9).

It is critical for contact lens wearers to frequently clean lenses (see Chapter 38) and to use the appropriate solutions for cleaning and disinfection. With the rise in use of soft contact lenses, particularly extended-wear lenses, some clients have become casual with regard to both the care and wearing time of the contacts; as a result, there has been an increase in serious corneal infections. Infrequent lens disinfection, contamination of lens storage cases and contact lens solutions, and use of homemade saline adds to a client's risk. Swimming while wearing lenses also creates a serious risk of infection.

Wearing a hearing aid no longer has to be a social stigma. There are a wide variety of aids that not only successfully enhance a person's hearing, but can also be cosmetically acceptable. Chapter 38 summarizes the types of hearing aids available and tips for proper care and use.

Preventing hearing loss requires individuals to avoid exposure to continuous high noise levels and brief loud impulse noise. HPDs should be worn by clients who must work around noise. Earplugs and earphones are useful in blocking high-decibel sounds (Box 48-8).

Another means of prevention involves regular immunization of children against diseases capable of causing hearing loss (e.g., rubella, mumps, and measles). Nurses

Smith and Wilbur (2000) identify factors that determine a person's likelihood for wearing a hearing aid: perceived need for improved hearing, attitude toward the hearing problem, and motivation to seek solutions. Acknowledging a need to improve hearing is a person's first step. The nurse can give clients useful information on the benefits of wearing a hearing aid. It is also important to have a significant other available to assist with hearing aid adjustment. Federal regulations require medical clearance from a physician before a person can be fitted with a hearing aid (Ebersole and Hess, 2001). If a client has any of the following ear conditions, a hearing aid cannot be used: visible congenital or traumatic deformity of the ear, active drainage in the last 90 days, sudden or progressive hearing loss within the last 90 days, acute or chronic dizziness, unilateral sudden hearing loss within the last 90 days, visible cerumen accumulation or a foreign body in the ear canal, pain or discomfort in the ear, or an audiometric air-bone gap of 15 decibels or greater. The nurse can detect the first seven conditions on physical examination and should refer the client to an otolaryngologist for further counseling (Ebersole and Hess, 2001).

Promoting Meaningful Stimulation. Life becomes much more enriching and satisfying when meaningful and pleasant stimuli exist within the environment. There are many ways that the nurse can help clients make adjustments to their environment so that it becomes more stimulating. This is best done when the nurse considers the normal physiological changes that accompany sensory deficits.

Vision. As a result of the normal changes of aging, the pupil's ability to adjust to light is diminished. As a result, older adults can be very sensitive to glare. The nurse can suggest ways for the client to minimize glare by selecting satin and nongloss finishes for walls and countertops in the home and choosing sheer curtains, tinted windows, or adjustable shades to reduce outdoor light. Wearing sunglasses outside obviously can reduce the glare of direct sunlight.

The ability to read is important to everyone. Therefore clients should be allowed to use their glasses whenever possible (e.g., during procedures and client instruction); it helps clients to remain oriented, maintain some control, and retain their dignity (Larsen and others, 1997). Clients with reduced visual acuity may need more than corrective lenses. A pocket magnifier can help a client read most printed material. Telescopic lens eyeglasses are smaller, easier to focus, and have a greater range. There are also books and other publications available in larger print. If a client has a legal or other important document he or she wishes to read, standard copying machines have enlarging capabilities. There are now closed-circuit television magnifying units that enlarge written characters up to 45 times (Ebersole and Hess, 2001).

With aging, a person experiences a change in color perception. Perception of the colors blue, violet, and green usually declines. Brighter colors such as red, orange, and yellow are easier to see. The nurse can offer suggestions of ways the client may decorate a room and paint hallways or stairwells so that differentiations can be made in surfaces and objects in a room.

Hearing. To maximize residual hearing function, the nurse works closely with the client to suggest ways to modify the environment. Telephones and televisions can be amplified. Alarm clocks that shake the bed or activate a flashing light are useful adaptive devices. An innovative way to enrich the lives of the hearing impaired is recorded music. Music recorded in the low-frequency sound cycles can be heard by clients with severe hearing loss.

One way to help an individual with a hearing loss is to ensure that the problem is not impacted cerumen. With aging, cerumen thickens and builds up in the ear canal. Excessive cerumen occluding the ear canal can cause a **conductive hearing loss.** Irrigation of the canal with tepid water in a 60-ml syringe (see Chapter 38) will remove cerumen. Removal of cerumen can significantly improve the client's hearing ability. Lewis-Cullinan and Janken (1990) conducted a study involving 226 older adults. They found improvement in the hearing test scores in 75% of the subjects after cerumen removal.

Taste and Smell. The nurse can easily promote the sense of taste by using measures to enhance remaining taste perception. Good oral hygiene keeps the taste buds well hydrated. Taste perception is heightened if foods are well seasoned, differently textured, and eaten separately. Flavored vinegar or lemon juice can add tartness to food. The nurse should always ask the client what foods are most taste appealing. If taste perception is improved, food intake and appetite will also improve.

Stimulation of the sense of smell with aromas such as brewing coffee, cooking garlic and baking bread can heighten taste sensation. The client should avoid blending or mixing foods, because these actions make it difficult to identify tastes. Older persons should chew food thoroughly to allow more food to contact remaining taste buds.

Smell can be improved by strengthening pleasant olfactory stimulation. A client's environment can be made more pleasant with smells such as cologne, mild room deodorizers, fragrant flowers, and sachets. The nurse also encourages clients to sniff food before eating. When the nurse assists clients with eating or sets up a meal tray in a health care setting, naming the foods may help clients imagine the aromas. The client is again an important resource. Certain aromas may actually cause clients to lose their appetites.

Removal of unpleasant odors improves the quality of a person's environment. The nurse should keep a client's room clean, empty bedpans or urinals, remove and dispose of soiled dressings, and keep bathroom doors closed.

Touch. Clients with reduced tactile sensation usually have the impairment over a limited portion of their bodies. The nurse can stimulate existing function by providing touch therapy. If the client is willing to be touched, hair brushing and combing, a back rub, and touching of the arms or shoulders are ways of increasing tactile contact. When sensation is reduced, a firm pressure may be necessary for the client to feel the nurse's hand. Turning and repositioning can also improve the quality of tactile sensation. When invasive procedures are being performed, it is important to use touch by holding the client's hands, and keeping them warm and dry.

If a client is overly sensitive to tactile stimuli **(hyperesthesia),** the nurse must minimize irritating stimuli.

Keeping bed linens loose to minimize direct contact with the client and protecting the skin from exposure to irritants are helpful measures. If the client has numbness and tingling or pain in the hands, as with carpal tunnel syndrome, special wrist splints may be worn to dorsiflex the wrist to relieve the nerve pressure. For those clients who use computers, there are special keyboards and wrist pads available to decrease the pressure on the median nerve and aid in relief of pain and promote healing.

Establishing Safe Environments. When sensory function becomes impaired, individuals become less secure, and the world around them becomes smaller. Older adults in particular find it important to feel secure about their immediate environment. This is necessary for the person to have a sense of independence. Feeling safe allows a person to function within the home. The nurse can make recommendations to assist clients in making their living environment safer without restricting their independence. During a home visit or while completing an examination in the clinic, the nurse can offer several useful suggestions for home safety. The nature of the actual or potential sensory loss determines the safety precautions taken.

Adaptations for Visual Loss. Whether a visual alteration is a result of injury, eye disease, or the changes of aging, safety becomes a factor if visual acuity, peripheral vision, adaptation to the dark, and depth perception are permanently reduced. With reduced peripheral vision a client cannot see panoramically, because the outer visual field is less discrete. This creates a special hazard for driving or walking in crowded areas. Adults with reduced adaptation to the dark require 3 times as much light to see objects as they did as young adults. With reduced depth perception a person cannot see how far away objects are located. This is a special danger when a person attempts to walk down stairs or over uneven surfaces.

> *Safety Alert:* To create a safe environment, the nurse begins by looking at the results of the home environment assessment (see Chapter 37).

Driving is a particular safety hazard for anyone with visual alterations. Reduced peripheral vision may prevent a driver from seeing a car in an adjacent lane. Reduced adaptation to the dark and a sensitivity to glare makes driving at night a significant risk. Vision is a primary consideration for safety, but there are other factors as well. In the case of older adults, decreased reaction time, reduced hearing, and decreased strength in the legs and arms may further compromise driving skills. Some safety tips the nurse can share with those who continue to drive include the following: drive in familiar areas, do not drive during rush hour, avoid interstate highways for local drives, drive defensively—use rear-view and side-view mirrors when changing lanes, avoid driving at dusk or night, go slow, but not too slow, keep the car in good working condition, and carry a portable or preprogrammed cellular phone.

The presence of visual alterations makes it difficult for a person to conduct normal activities of living within the home. Because of reduced depth perception, clients can trip on throw rugs, runners, or the edge of stairs. All flooring or carpeting should be kept in good repair. The nurse can advise the client to use low-pile carpeting. Thresholds between rooms should be level with the floor. Clutter should be removed to ensure clear pathways for walking. Furniture should be arranged so that a client can move about easily without fear of tripping or running into objects. Any stairwell should have a securely fastened banister or handrail extending the full length of the stairs.

Front and back entrances to the home, work areas, and stairwells need to be properly lighted. The nurse encourages the client to have a repairman install lights with higher wattage and wider illumination. Fluorescent lighting should be avoided. A light switch should be located at the top and bottom of stairwells. It is also important to be sure lighting on the stairs does not cast shadows. Be sure the client can clearly see the edge of each step, especially the first and last. When possible, steps inside and outside the home should be replaced with ramps.

When a client is unable to see visual contrasts, a number of interventions can be helpful. Sometimes settings on electrical appliances and equipment are only highlighted in black and white or shades of gray. Color contrasts help to distinguish settings. Colored tape, paint, or nail enamel can be used to color code appliance dials. Color can also be useful to highlight the edge of stairs. Painting the edge of stairs with bright orange paint or applying a broad strip of colored tape at the stair edge can help a person see the edges of stairs more clearly. The nurse can help the client tour the home to find opportunities for color coding. Telephones with large numbers may be helpful.

If a client is partially or totally blind, fire hazards should be removed from the home. Flammable items, such as paper and cloth, should be kept away from the stove. A client who smokes must learn to discard ashes frequently into an ashtray. Water in the bottom of an ashtray helps ensure that cigarette butts are extinguished.

An added consideration for the visually impaired is the assurance that eye medications are administered safely. For conditions such as glaucoma, clients must closely adhere to regular medication schedules. Labels on medication containers should be in large print. A friend or spouse should always be familiar with dosage schedules in case a client is unable to self-administer a medication. The visually impaired may have some difficulty manipulating eye droppers.

Adaptations for Reduced Hearing. Important environmental sounds (e.g., doorbells and alarm clocks) may best be heard if amplified or changed to a lower-pitched, buzzerlike sound. There are also sound lamps that respond with light to sounds such as doorbells, burglar alarms, smoke detectors, and babies crying. These can be purchased from hearing aid dealers, telephone companies, and appliance stores. Signaling devices allow the deaf person greater independence. Family members or anyone who calls the client regularly should learn to let the phone ring for a longer period. There are amplified receivers for telephones and telephone communications devices (TTDs) that use a computer and printer to transfer words over the telephone for the hearing impaired. Both sender and receiver must have the special device to complete a call.

Adaptations for Reduced Olfaction. A reduced sensitivity to odors means that the client may be unable to smell leaking gas, a smoldering cigarette or fire, or tainted food. The client should use smoke and carbon monoxide detectors and other alternative precautions such as checking ashtrays or placing cigarette butts in water. A client can learn to check dates on food packages and the color and texture of food. Leftovers should be kept in labeled containers with the preparation date. Pilot gas flames should be checked visually.

Adaptations for Reduced Tactile Sensation. When clients have reduced sensation in their extremities, they are at risk for injury from exposure to temperature extremes. The nurse should caution them on the use of water bottles or heating pads (see Chapter 47). The temperature setting on the home water heater should be no higher than 48.8° C (120° F). If a client also has a visual impairment, it is important to be sure that water faucets are clearly marked "hot" and "cold," or color codes (i.e., red for hot and blue for cold) can be used.

Promoting Communication. A sensory deficit can cause a person to feel isolated because of an inability to communicate with others. It is important for individuals to be able to interact with people whom they encounter. This problem can complicate a nurse's effectiveness in teaching clients information and skills. The nature of the sensory loss influences the methods and styles of communication that nurses can use (Box 48-10). Communication methods can also be taught to family members and significant others.

When beginning a conversation with a client who has a hearing deficit, it helps to reduce any background noise by turning off or lowering the volume of any TV, appliance, or radio. It is also helpful to have conversations in settings where there are better acoustics, which aid in controlling and muffling extraneous background noises. In a group setting it is better to form a semicircle in front of the client so that the client can see who is speaking next; this helps foster group involvement. The client with a hearing impairment may be able to speak normally. However, the deaf client's inability to hear self-spoken words may cause serious speech alterations. Clients may use sign language or lipreading, write with a pad and pencil, or learn to use a computer for communication. Special communication boards that contain common terms (e.g., *pain, bathroom, dizzy,* or *walk*) used in nursing care help clients express their needs.

Client instruction is one aspect of communication. There are teaching booklets available in large print for clients with visual loss. The client who is blind may require more frequent and detailed verbal descriptions of information. This is particularly true if there are no instructional booklets written in Braille. The visually im-

---

Box 48-10   Communication Methods

Clients With Aphasia

Listen to the client and wait for the client to communicate.
Do not shout or speak loudly (hearing loss is not the problem).
If the client has problems with comprehension, use simple, short questions and facial gestures to give additional clues.
Speak of things familiar and of interest to the client.
If the client has problems speaking, ask questions that require simple yes or no answers or blinking of the eyes. Offer pictures or a communication board so that the client can point.
Give the client time to understand; be calm and patient.
Do not pressure or tire the client.
Avoid patronizing and childish phrases.

Clients With an Artificial Airway

Use pictures, objects, or word cards so that the client can point.
Offer a pad and pencil or Magic Slate for the client to write messages.
Do not shout or speak loudly.
Give the client time to write messages, because these clients become easily fatigued.
Provide an artificial voice box (vibrator) for the client with a laryngectomy to use to speak words or phrases.

Clients With Hearing Impairment

Get the client's attention. Do not startle the client when entering the room. Do not approach a client from behind. Be sure the client knows you wish to speak.
Face the client and stand or sit on the same level. Be sure your face and lips are illuminated to promote lipreading. Keep hands away from mouth.
If the client wears glasses, be sure they are clean so that your gestures and face can be seen.
If the client wears a hearing aid, make sure it is in place and working.
Speak slowly and articulate clearly. Older adults may take longer to process verbal messages.
Use a normal tone of voice and inflections of speech. Refrain from speaking with something in your mouth.
When you are not understood, rephrase rather than repeat the conversation.
Use visible expressions. Speak with your hands, your face, and your eyes.
Do not shout. Loud sounds are usually higher pitched and may impede hearing by accentuating vowel sounds and concealing consonants. If it is necessary to raise your voice, speak in lower tones.
Talk toward the client's best or normal ear.
Use written information to enhance the spoken word.
Do not restrict a deaf client's hands. Never have IV lines in both of the client's hands if the preferred method of communication is sign language.
Avoid eating, chewing, or smoking while speaking.
Avoid speaking from another room or while walking away.

paired can learn by listening to audiotapes or the sound portion of a televised teaching session. Clients with hearing impairment may benefit from written instructional materials and visual teaching aids (e.g., posters and graphs). Demonstrations by the nurse are very useful. Hospitals are required to make professional interpreters available to read sign language of deaf clients.

Acute Care. When clients enter acute care settings for therapeutic management of sensory deficits or as a result of traumatic injury, the nurse uses approaches to maximize sensory function existing at the time. Safety again is an obvious priority until the client's sensory status is either stabilized or improved. For example, clients with sensory deficits have a high risk for falls in the acute care environment. It also becomes very important to know the extent of any existing sensory impairment before the acute episode of illness so that the nurse can reinforce what the client already knows about self-care or plan for more instruction before and following discharge.

Another group of clients who are at risk for developing sensory alterations while hospitalized are those in ICUs and the acutely ill. The constant activity within an ICU and the frequent monitoring of the acutely ill can easily cause clients to experience sensory overload. The nurse's main challenge becomes introducing regular, meaningful stimulation so that clients maintain a clearer perception of their immediate environment.

Orientation to the Environment. The client with recent sensory impairment requires a complete orientation to the immediate environment. Reorientation to the institutional environment may be provided by ensuring that name tags on uniforms are visible, addressing the client by name, explaining where the client is (especially if clients are transported to different areas for treatment), and using conversational cues to time or location. The tendency for clients to become confused can be reduced by offering short and simple, repeated explanations and reassurance. Family members and visitors can also help orient clients to the hospital surroundings.

A client with serious visual impairment must feel comfortable in knowing the boundaries of the immediate environment. Normally we see physical boundaries within a room. The blind or severely visually impaired must touch the boundaries or objects to gain a sense of their surroundings. The client needs to walk through a room and feel the walls to establish a sense of direction. The nurse can help by explaining objects within the room, such as furniture or equipment. It takes time for the client to absorb a room's arrangement. The client may need to reorient again, with the nurse explaining the location of key items (e.g., call light, telephone, and chair). It also helps to always approach a blind client from the front to avoid startling him or her.

It is important to keep all objects in the same position and place. After an object is moved even a short distance, it no longer exists for a blind person. Simply moving a chair aside may create a dangerous safety hazard. The nurse should ask the client if any item should be arranged to make ambulation easier. Traffic patterns should be kept clear and use of furniture with sharp edges avoided.

The client who is blind always needs extra time to perform any task. The client needs a detailed description of how to perform an activity and will move slowly to remain safe.

Bedridden clients are at risk for sensory deprivation. Normally movement gives an integrated awareness of the self through vestibular and tactile stimulation. A person's sensory perception is influenced by movement patterns. The limited movement of bed rest changes how a person interprets the environment; surroundings seem different, and objects seem to assume shapes different from normal. A person who is on bed rest requires routine stimulation through range-of-motion exercises, positioning, and participation in self-care activities (as appropriate). Comfort measures such as washing the face and hands and providing back rubs can help to improve the quality of stimulation and lessen the chance of sensory deprivation. Planning time to talk with clients is also essential. The nurse should explain unfamiliar environmental noises and sensations. A calm, unhurried approach during contact with a client gives the nurse quality time to help reorient and familiarize the client with care activities. The client who is well enough to read will benefit from a variety of reading material.

Communication. The most common language disorder following a stroke is aphasia. As a result of a disruption in blood flow to the brain, the speech center becomes damaged, altering a person's ability to either use or understand spoken words. Depending on the type of aphasia, the inability to communicate can be frustrating and frightening (see Box 48-10, p. 1585). The nurse should initially establish very basic communication and recognize that aphasia does not indicate intellectual impairment or degeneration of personality. The nurse explains situations and treatments that are pertinent to the client, because he or she may be able to understand the speaker's words (Ebersole and Hess, 2001). Because a stroke often causes partial or complete paralysis of one side of the client's body, an aphasic client may need special assistive devices. There are communication boards that have been developed for several levels of disability. Sensitive pressure switches, activated by the touch of an ear, nose, or chin, can control electronic communication boards (Ebersole and Hess, 2001). Clients who have had a stroke usually acquire referrals to speech therapists to develop appropriate rehabilitation plans.

In acute care hospitals or long-term care facilities, nurses often care for clients with artificial airways (see Chapter 39). For example, an endotracheal tube is inserted into the oropharynx and down through the vocal cords of the larynx into the upper bronchus. The placement of the tube prevents a client from speaking. In this case the nurse must use special communication methods to facilitate the client's ability to express needs (see Box 48-10, p. 1585). The client may be completely alert and able to hear and see the nurse normally. Giving the client time to convey any needs or requests is very important. Creative communication techniques (e.g., a communication board or a laptop computer) can be used to foster and strengthen the client's interactions with health care personnel, family, and friends.

Controlling Sensory Stimuli. The nurse controls excessive stimuli for clients at risk for sensory overload. Clients need time for rest and freedom from stress caused by frequent monitoring and repeated tests. The nurse can reduce sensory overload by organizing the care plan. Combining activities such as dressing changes, bathing, and vital sign measurement in one visit prevents the client from becoming overly fatigued. The client also needs scheduled time for rest and quiet. Planning for rest periods often requires cooperation from family, visitors, and health care colleagues. Coordination with laboratory and radiology departments may help minimize the number of procedures the client must undergo. The nurse may encourage a family member to sit quietly with a client or involve the client in an undemanding repetitive activity such as combing hair or brushing teeth. Helping clients to become as mobile and independent as possible within prescribed limits provides meaningful stimulation.

When clients experience sensory overload or deprivation, the resultant behavior can be difficult for family or friends to accept. The nurse encourages the family not to argue with or contradict the confused client, but to calmly explain location, identity, and time of day. Engaging the client in a normal discussion about familiar topics may assist in reorientation. Prearranging tests and procedures with departments reduces the amount of time needed for tests and examinations. Anticipating client needs such as voiding helps reduce uncomfortable stimuli.

The nurse can also try to control extraneous noise in and around the client's room. It may be necessary to ask a roommate to lower the volume on a television or to move the client to a quieter room. Equipment noise should be kept to a minimum. Bedside equipment not in use, such as suction and oxygen equipment should be turned off. The nurse also avoids abrupt loud noises, such as dropping objects or causing the over-bed table to adjust to the lowest level suddenly. Nursing staff should also try to control laughter or conversation at the nurses' station. Nurses should allow clients to close room doors.

When the client leaves an acute care setting for the home environment, nurses should communicate with colleagues in the home care setting about the interventions that helped the client adapt to sensory problems. Similarly, information describing the client's existing sensory deficits should be reported. Continuity of care is achieved when the client is required to make only minimal changes in the home setting.

Safety Measures. The client with recent visual impairment often requires help with walking. The presence of an eye patch, frequently instilled eye drops, or the swelling of eyelid structures following surgery are just a few factors that cause a client to need more assistance than usual. A sighted guide can give confidence to the visually impaired and ensure safe mobility. Ebersole and Hess (2001) list four suggestions for a sighted guide:

1. Ask the blind client if he or she wants a "sighted guide."
2. If assistance is accepted, offer an elbow or arm. Instruct the client to grasp your arm just above the elbow. If necessary, physically assist the person by guiding his or her hand to your arm or elbow (Figure 48-5).

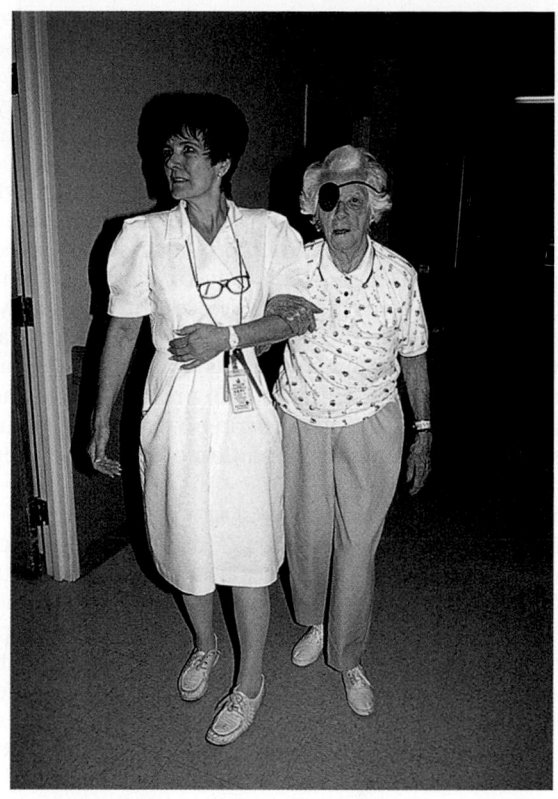

FIGURE **48–5** Nurse assists in the ambulation of a client wearing an eye patch.

3. Go one-half step ahead and slightly to the side of the blind person. The shoulder of the person should be directly behind your shoulder. If the person is frail, place the hand on your forearm.
4. Relax and walk at a comfortable pace. Warn the client when you approach doorways or narrow spaces.

While walking the client, describe the course of movement and ensure that obstacles have been removed. A client with visual impairment should never be left standing alone in an unfamiliar area. For clients who undergo eye surgery, it is important to teach family members techniques for assisting with ambulation.

A visually impaired client who spends considerable time in bed should have a call light nearby. Necessary objects should be placed in front of the client to prevent falls caused by reaching over the bedside. Side rails are also important in this regard. At night a night-light with a red bulb can help reduce falls. The red light reduces the time required for the eyes to adapt to the dark and allows the client to see well enough to function without keeping the regular light on (Matteson and McConnell, 1988).

Nurses may rely on clients in health care settings to report unusual sounds, such as a suction apparatus running improperly or an IV pump alarm. However, the client with a hearing loss may not hear such sounds and thus requires more frequent visits by the nurse. The client can also benefit from learning to use vision to discover sources of danger. The nurse should never restrict both arms of deaf or hearing-impaired clients (e.g., with restraints or IV lines), because they need their hands to communicate. The nurse should face the client when speaking, use simple sentences, and speak more slowly and in a normal volume (McConnell, 2002). It is wise to note on the intercom button and a client's chart if the client is deaf and/or blind. A client lacking the ability to speak cannot call out for assistance. Clients should have message boards or the call light close at hand.

Clients with reduced tactile sensation risk injury when their conditions confine them to bed, because they are unable to sense pressure on bony prominences or the need to change position. These clients rely on nurses for timely repositioning, moving tubes or devices the client may lie on, and turning to avoid skin breakdown. When the ability to sense temperature variations is reduced, the nurse should use extra caution in applying heat and cold therapies (see Chapter 47) and preparing bathwater. The nurse must frequently check the condition of the client's skin.

Restorative and Continuing Care

Maintaining Healthy Lifestyles. After a client has experienced a sensory loss, it becomes important to understand the implications of the loss and to make the adjustments needed to continue a normal lifestyle. Sensory impairments need not prevent a person from leading an active, rewarding life. Many of the interventions applicable to health promotion, such as adapting the home environment, can be used after a client leaves an acute care setting.

Understanding Sensory Loss. Clients who have experienced a recent loss must understand how to adapt so that their living environments can be safe and appropriately stimulating. All family members should understand the way that a client's sensory impairment affects normal daily activities. Family and friends can be more supportive when they understand sensory deficits and the types of elements that worsen or lessen sensory problems. For example, family and friends need to learn how to communicate with someone who has a hearing loss. There are resources within a community that provide information that assists clients with personal management needs. The American Foundation for the Blind, American National Red Cross, and National Association for Speech and Hearing offer resource materials and product information.

Socialization. The ability to communicate is gratifying. It tests our intellect, opens opportunities, and allows us to exchange the feelings we have about others. When interactions are hindered by sensory alterations, a person can feel ineffective and lose self-esteem. If clients feel socially unaccepted, they will perceive sensory losses as seriously impairing the quality of life.

Interacting with others can become a burden for many clients with sensory alterations. Asking people to continuously repeat what they say is both embarrassing and exhausting for a client with hearing loss. Many clients lose the motivation to engage in social situations. As a person withdraws from interaction, a deep sense of loneliness can develop. The nurse can introduce therapies to reduce loneliness, particularly for older clients (Box 48-11). In addition, family members must learn to focus on a person's ability to interact rather than on the person's disability. It should not be assumed, for example, that a person who is hard of hearing does not wish to speak. A

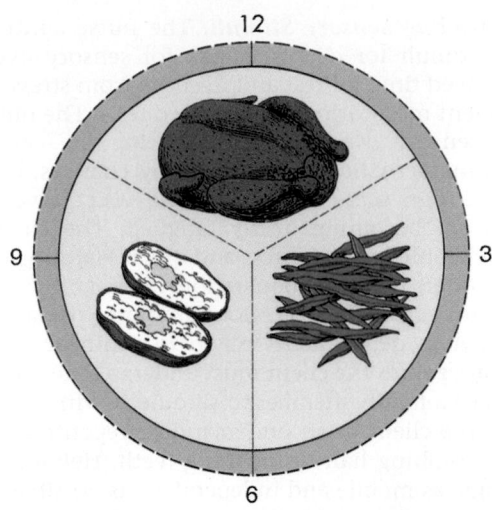

FIGURE 48-6 Location of food using clock as frame of reference.

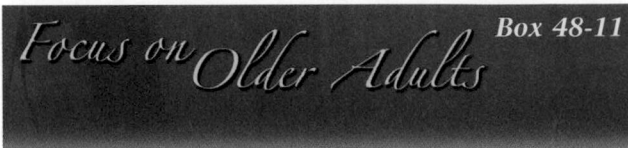

Box 48-11

Focus on Older Adults

- Spend time with a person in silence or conversation.
- Use physical contact—holding a hand, embracing a shoulder—to convey caring.
- Help recommend alterations in living arrangements if physical isolation is a factor.
- Assist older adults in keeping in contact with people important to them.
- Help obtain information about mutual help groups.
- Arrange for security escort services as needed.
- Bring a pet that is easy to care for into the home.
- Link a person with religious organizations attuned to the social needs of older adults.

blind person can still enjoy a walk through a park with a companion describing the sights around them.

Promoting Self-Care. The ability to perform self-care is essential for self-esteem. Frequently, family members and nurses believe that sensorially impaired persons require assistance, when in fact they can help themselves. There are useful guidelines to assist clients with visual or tactile impairment so that they can help themselves with daily living activities. For example, a meal tray can be set up as though food on the tray and condiments and drinks around the tray are numbers on the face of a clock (Figure 48-6). The visually impaired client can easily become oriented to the items after the nurse or family member explains each item's location.

The client with visual problems needs assistance in reaching toilet facilities safely. Safety bars should be installed near the toilet. It may be helpful to have the bar a different color than the wall for easier visibility. Towels should never be placed on safety bars, because they may interfere with a person's grasp. Toilet paper should be within easy reach. The use of colors, especially red-yellow, on drawers and other places helps promote functional independence (Swanson and Drury, 2001).

If tactile sense is diminished, the client can dress more easily with zippers or Velcro strips, pullover sweaters or blouses, and elasticized waists. If a client has partial paralysis and reduced sensation, the affected side should be dressed first. Family members responsible for selecting clothing for visually impaired clients should be encouraged to follow the client's preferences. Any sensory impairment has a significant influence on body image, and it is important for the client to feel well groomed and attractive. A client may need assistance with basic grooming such as brushing, combing, and shampooing hair. The client also may need assistance with medication selection, clothing identification, and learning to manage routine procedures such as blood pressure and glucose monitoring (Cleary, 1995). It is important to assist clients in maintaining a degree of independence and in having as much control over the management of their care and lifestyle as possible.

Clients with proprioceptive problems may lose their balance easily. Bathrooms should have nonskid surfaces in the tub and shower. Grab bars should be installed either vertically or horizontally in tubs and showers, depending on how the client is able to grasp or hold onto the bar. The nurse can instruct family members to supervise ambulation and sitting, make frequent checks to prevent falls, and caution the client against leaning forward.

Evaluation

Client Care. With regard to problems with sensory alterations, the client is the source for evaluating outcomes. The client is the only one who will know if his or her sensory abilities are improved and which specific interventions or therapies are most successful in facilitating a change in the client's performance (Figure 48-7). To evaluate the effectiveness of nursing interventions, the nurse uses critical thinking and makes comparisons with the baseline sensory assessment data to evaluate if sensory alterations have changed.

The nurse determines if the expected outcomes have been met. For example, the nurse uses evaluative data to determine whether care measures improve or at least maintain a client's ability to interact and function within the environment. The nature of a client's sensory alterations influences the way a nurse evaluates the outcome of care. For example, the nurse uses proper communication techniques with a client with a hearing deficit and then evaluates whether the client has gained the ability to hear or interact more effectively. When expected outcomes have not been achieved, there may be a need to change interventions or alter the client's environment. Family members may need to become more involved in support of the client.

If nursing care has been directed at improving sensory acuity, the nurse evaluates the integrity of the sensory organs and the client's ability to perceive stimuli. Any interventions designed to relieve problems associated with sensory alterations are evaluated on the basis of the client's ability to function normally without injury. When the nurse attempts to directly or indirectly (through education) alter the client's environment, evaluation is directed at observing whether the client makes environmental changes. When client teaching is designed to improve a client's sensory function, it is important to determine whether the client is following recommended therapies. Asking the client to explain or demonstrate self-care skills evaluates the level of learning that has occurred. It may be necessary to reinforce previous instruction if learning has not taken place.

Client Expectations. If the nurse has successfully developed a good relationship with a client and has a therapeutic plan of care, subtle behaviors often indicate the level of the client's satisfaction. The nurse may note that the client responds appropriately, such as by smiling. The nurse may observe that the client interacts more with family or with the nurse and is not asking to have information repeated. However, it is important for the nurse to ask the client if his or her sensory needs have been met. For example, the nurse may ask the client, "Can you tell me if you feel we have done all we can do to help improve your ability to hear?" If the client's expectations have not been met, then the nurse needs to spend more time understanding the client's needs and specific preferences. Working closely with the client and family will enable the nurse to redefine those expectations that can be realistically met within the limits of the client's condition and therapies. The nurse is effective when the client's goals and expectations have been met.

Key Concepts

- Sensory reception involves the stimulation of sensory nerve fibers and the transmission of impulses to higher centers within the brain.
- When sensory function is impaired, the sense of self is impaired and can affect one's ability to socialize.
- Sensory deprivation results from an inadequate quality or quantity of sensory stimuli.
- Aging results in a gradual decline of acuity in all senses.
- Clients who are older, immobilized, or confined in isolated environments are at risk for sensory alterations.
- Assessment of a client's health promotion habits helps to reveal risks for sensory impairment.
- An older adult often will not admit to a sensory loss.
- An assessment of hazards in the environment requires the nurse to tour living areas in the home and to look for conditions that increase the chances of injury such as falls.
- The plan of care for clients with sensory alterations should include participation by family members. The extent of support from family members and significant others can influence the quality of sensory experiences.
- Clients with sensory deficits develop alternative ways of communicating that rely on other senses.

KNOWLEDGE
- Characteristics of improved hearing, sight, touch, or taste
- The client's ability to recognize sensory changes

EXPERIENCE
- Previous client responses to planned nursing interventions to promote sensory function

Evaluation
- Reassess signs and symptoms of sensory alteration
- Determine the client's ability to remain functional within the home or health care environment
- Ask the client to demonstrate or explain newly learned self-care skill
- Ask client if expectations are being met

STANDARDS
- Use established expected outcomes (e.g., improved sensory acuity, creation of a safe home environment) to evaluate the client's response to care

ATTITUDES
- Think independently and consider the client's views about whether the level of care has improved his or her sensory status
- Use creativity and observe the client in the home to adequately evaluate sensory function

FIGURE **48–7** Critical thinking model for sensory alterations evaluation.

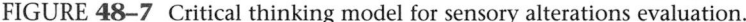

- Care of clients at risk for sensory deprivation includes introducing meaningful and pleasant stimuli for all senses.
- To prevent sensory overload, the nurse controls stimuli and orients the client to the environment.
- Clients with artificial airways can communicate effectively with communication boards, laptop computers, and written messages.

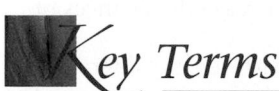

Key Terms

Aphasia, *p. 1575*
Auditory, *p. 1566*
Conductive hearing loss, *p. 1583*
Expressive aphasia, *p. 1575*

Gustatory, *p. 1566*
Hyperesthesia, *p. 1583*
Kinesthetic, *p. 1566*
Olfactory, *p. 1566*
Otolaryngologist, *p. 1570*

Ototoxic, *p. 1576*
Proprioceptive, *p. 1570*
Receptive aphasia, *p. 1575*
Refractive error, *p. 1581*
Sensory deficit, *p. 1568*

Sensory deprivation, *p. 1569*
Sensory overload, *p. 1569*
Stereognosis, *p. 1566*
Strabismus, *p. 1581*
Tactile, *p. 1566*

Critical Thinking Exercises

1. Mr. Tully is a 54-year-old farmer who is having a physical for insurance purposes. Overall, his health is good. His wife reports that over the past year he has lost interest in being involved in social gatherings, is more irritable, and often has asked her to repeat what was said. Recently, he has complained of a constant buzzing in his ears. What assessment data is needed? What specific interventions may be needed?

2. Mrs. Marfell, 79 years old, is visiting the outpatient cardiac center for a routine check-up. The nurse notices that the client needed help reading the physical forms. She also told the nurse she is having increased difficulty driving at night. What additional assessment data should the nurse gather from Mrs. Marfell?

3. You have an opportunity to speak with a group of parents and students regarding the importance of hearing protection. What information would you share with this varied age-group to promote healthy hearing?

Review Questions

1. This sense enables a person to be aware of the position and movement of body parts without seeing them:
1. Auditory.
2. Kinesthetic.
3. Tactile.
4. Gustatory.

2. A sense that allows a person to recognize an object's size, shape, and texture is:
1. Stereognosis.
2. Kinesthetic.
3. Tactile.
4. Gustatory.

3. A client who is in constant pain and undergoes frequent monitoring of vital signs is at risk for experiencing sensory:
1. Deprivation.
2. Deficits.
3. Overload.
4. Stimuli

4. Proprioceptive changes after age 60 include increased:
1. Hearing and vision impairment.
2. Difficulty with balance, spatial orientation, and coordination.
3. Hearing impairment and difficulty with balance and coordination.
4. Vision impairment and difficulty with spatial orientation.

5. For a hearing-impaired client to hear a spoken conversation, the nurse should:
1. Approach a client quietly from behind.
2. Face the client when speaking; use a louder than normal tone of voice.
3. Select a public area to have a spoken conversation.
4. Face the client when speaking; speak slower and in a normal volume.

6. When obtaining a history of the client's hearing loss, the nurse should ask:
1. How long have you been deaf?
2. Do you also have vision problems?
3. Why don't you pay attention to me while I speak?
4. How does your hearing loss compare to a year ago?

7. A realistic goal for an older adult client who drives is:
1. Drive very, very slowly all of the time.
2. Keep the car in good working condition.
3. Always drive at night to prevent sun glare.
4. Drive during rush hours when others are on the road.

8. Because hearing impairment is one of the most common disabilities among children, a nursing intervention is to teach parents, schoolteachers, and children to:
1. Avoid activities in which crowds and loud noises occur.
2. Delay childhood immunizations until hearing can be verified.
3. Take precautions when involved in activities associated with high-intensity noises.
4. Prophylactically administer antibiotics to reduce the incidence of infections.

9. A high-priority home assessment for a client with diminished olfaction is the inclusion of:
1. Low water setting.
2. Extra lighting in hallways.
3. Smoke detectors on all levels.
4. Amplified telephone receivers.

10. Sensory deficits happen when a problem with sensory reception or perception occurs. As a result clients may:
1. Withdraw socially to cope with the loss.
2. Rely solely on one sense.
3. Respond normally to stimuli.
4. Function safely within their environment.

References

American Nurses Association: *Scope and Standards of Gerontological Nursing Practice,* Washington, DC, 1995, American Nurses Association.

Cleary ME: Helping the person who is visually impaired: concerns, questions, remedies, and resources, *J Ophthalmic Nurs Technol* 14(5):205, 1995.

Dochterman JM, Bulechek GM: *Nursing interventions classification (NIC),* ed 4, St. Louis, 2004, Mosby.

Ebersole P, Hess P: *Geriatric nursing and healthy aging,* St. Louis, 2001, Mosby.

Ebersole P, Hess P: *Toward healthy aging; human needs and nursing response,* ed 5, St. Louis, 2001, Mosby.

Giger JN, Davidhizar RE: *Transcultural nursing: assessment and intervention,* ed 3, St. Louis, 1999, Mosby.

Griest SE, Bishop PM: Tinnitus as an early indicator of permanent hearing loss, *Am Assoc Occup Health Nurs J* 46(7):325, 1998.

Hensel SL: Sensory function. In Lueckenotte AG: *Gerontologic nursing,* ed 2, St. Louis, 2000, Mosby.

Larsen PD and others: Assessment and management of sensory loss in elderly patients, *AORN J* 65(2):432 1997.

Lewis SM and others, editors: *Medical-surgical nursing: assessment and management of clinical problems,* ed 5, St. Louis, 2000, Mosby.

Lusk SL: Preventing noise-induced hearing loss, *Nurs Clin North Am* 37:257, 2002.

Maas ML and others: *Nursing care of older adults, diagnoses, outcomes, & interventions,* St. Louis, 2001, Mosby.

Matteson MA, McConnell ES: *Gerontological nursing: concepts and practice,* Philadelphia, 1988, WB Saunders.

McCance KL, Huether SE: *Pathophysiology: the biologic basis for disease in adults and children,* ed 4, St. Louis, 2002, Mosby.

McConnell EA: How to converse with a hearing impaired patient, *Nursing* 32(8):20, 2002.

McCullagh M: When hearing becomes a part of healing, *Orthop Nurs* 21(4):64, 2002.

Meadows C: Assessment of the auditory system. In Phipps WJ and others: *Medical-surgical nursing health and illness perspectives,* ed 7, St. Louis, 2003, Mosby.

Moorhead S, Johnson M, Maas M: *Nursing outcomes classification (NOC),* ed 3, St. Louis, 2004, Mosby.

Resnick HE, Fries BE, Verbrugge LM: Windows to their world: the effects of sensory impairments on social engagement and activity time in nursing home residents, *J Gerontol Soc Sci* 52(3): S135, 1997.

Ruda SC: Nursing assessment: musculoskeletal system. In Lewis SM and others: *Medical-surgical nursing: assessment and management of clinical problems,* ed 5, St. Louis, 2000, Mosby.

Smith SC: Problems of the eye. In Phipps WJ and others: *Medical-surgical nursing health and illness perspectives,* ed 7, St. Louis, 2003, Mosby.

Smith SC, Wilbur ME: Vision and hearing problems. In Lewis SM and others: *Medical-surgical nursing: assessment and management of clinical problems,* ed 5, St. Louis, 2000, Mosby.

Swanson EA, Drury J: Sensory/perceptual alterations. In Maas ML and others: *Nursing care of older adults: diagnoses, outcomes and interventions,* St. Louis, 2001, Mosby.

Tolson D: Age-related hearing loss: a case for nursing intervention, *J Adv Nurs* 26(6):1150, 1997.

Urden LA and others: *Thelan's critical care nursing: diagnosis and management,* ed 4, St. Louis, 2002, Mosby.

U.S. Department of Health and Human Services: *Healthy people 2010: understanding and improving health,* Washington, DC, 2000, Jones & Bartlett Publishers.

Weinstein BE: Age-related hearing loss: how to screen for it, and when to intervene, *Geriatrics* 49(8):40, 1994.

Wong DL and others: *Maternal child nursing care,* ed 2, St. Louis, 2002, Mosby.

*R*esearch References

Demers K: Hearing screening, *J Gerontol Nurs* 27(11):8, 2001.

Lewis-Cullinan C, Janken JK: Effect of cerumen removal on the hearing ability of geriatric patients, *J Adv Nurs* 15:594, 1990.

McCullagh M, Lusk SL, Ronis DL: Factors influencing use of hearing protection among farmers: a test of the Pender Health Promotion Model, *Nurs Res* 51(1):33, 2002.

49

Care of Surgical Clients

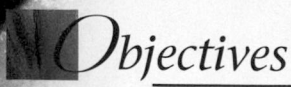

Objectives

Mastery of content in this chapter will enable the student to:

- Define the key terms listed.
- Explain the concept of perioperative nursing care.
- Differentiate between classifications of surgery and types of anesthesia.
- List factors to include in the preoperative, intraoperative, and postoperative assessment of a surgical client.
- Demonstrate postoperative exercises: diaphragmatic breathing, coughing, incentive spirometer use, turning, and leg exercises.
- Design a preoperative teaching plan
- Prepare a client for surgery.
- Explain the nurse's role in the operating room.
- Describe the rationale for nursing interventions designed to prevent postoperative complications.
- Explain the difference and similarities in caring for ambulatory surgery versus inpatient surgical clients.

Perioperative nursing care includes nursing care given before (preoperative), during (intraoperative), and after surgery (postoperative). It may take place in the hospital, in a surgical center attached to a hospital, in a free-standing surgical center, or in a physician's office. Perioperative nursing is a fast-paced, changing, and challenging field in which to work. It is based on the nurse's understanding of several important principles, including the following:

- High-quality care
- Multidisciplinary teamwork
- Effective and therapeutic communication and collaboration with the client, the client's family, and the surgical team
- Effective and efficient client assessment and intervention in all phases
- Advocacy for the client and the client's family
- Understanding of cost containment.

The nurse must practice good surgical asepsis, thoroughly document care, and emphasize client safety in all phases of care. Effective teaching and discharge planning are needed to prevent or minimize complications and ensure quality outcomes. The nursing process provides a basis for perioperative nursing, with the nurse individualizing strategies throughout the perioperative period so that the client has a smooth course from admission into the health care system through convalescence. The continuity of care is stressed in the perioperative model.

The continuing care of the surgical client has shifted from hospital-based convalescence to home-based convalescence, with the majority of responsibility shifting to the client and/or family. As the length of hospital stay decreases, the educational needs of the client undergoing a surgical procedure increases. Clients are sent home with complex medical/surgical conditions that require both education and follow-up. Proper client education is essential to ensure positive surgical outcomes (Gershenson, and others, 1999).

History of Surgical Nursing

It was not until the twentieth century that the discipline of surgery progressed as a science. Surgery gave physicians the means to treat conditions that were difficult or impossible to manage only by pure medicine. Early surgeons had little knowledge of the principles of asepsis, and anesthesia techniques were primitive and unsafe. Indeed, a surgeon's success was based on speed. The discovery of anesthesia in the 1840s revolutionized surgery. Anesthesia provided for the combination of analgesia, muscle relaxation, and amnesia, which allowed the surgical procedure time to be extended. The value of hand washing in the 1800s, along with the development of the germ theory (Pasteur), triggered the study of aseptic technique, which reduced postoperative infections and mortality.

Nursing played a major role in disease prevention, beginning with Florence Nightingale's belief that the environment was a key factor in disease prevention. Nurses working in the first operating rooms (ORs) cleaned the rooms and equipment, performed technical tasks such as obtaining supplies, and occasionally accompanied the client to the surgical ward to deliver nursing care. Massachusetts General Hospital provided the first operating room education for nurses in 1876. This trend continued into the 1900s as nursing schools included operating room experience in each nurse's clinical instruction.

During the 1970s a change occurred in nursing education. A focus on the importance of nurses acquiring a broad knowledge base resulted in less emphasis on operating room techniques. Many schools eliminated operating room experience from the curriculum. However, today many nursing schools have reinstituted clinical operating room experience.

In 1956 the **Association of Operating Room Nurses (AORN)** was formed to gain knowledge of surgical principles and explore methods to improve nursing care of surgical clients. The organization developed standards of nursing practice that outlined the scope of responsibility of the perioperative nurse. AORN was the first nursing organization to develop structure, process, and outcome standards as defined by the American Nurses Association (ANA). The standards of perioperative nursing include (1) administrative practice, (2) clinical practice, (3) professional performance, (4) quality improvement, and (5) client outcomes (AORN, 2002d). Today, AORN has changed its name to the Association of Perioperative Registered Nurses; however, AORN is still used as their acronym. The organization continues to be a driving force for the practice of perioperative nursing.

Ambulatory Surgery

A recent change in the surgery setting is the advent of **ambulatory surgery,** also referred to as outpatient surgery, short-stay surgery, or same-day surgery. Centers providing these services may be hospital based or freestanding surgicenters. Over half of all surgical procedures are conducted on an outpatient basis. These procedures include ophthalmic, gastroenterological, gynecological, eye-ear-nose-throat, orthopedic, cosmetic/restorative, and general procedures (Federated Ambulatory Surgery Association, 2002). One-day surgery in which the client is admitted the day of surgery and observed overnight (23-hour admission) has also increased in popularity.

There are distinct benefits for the client who has ambulatory surgery. Anesthetic drugs that metabolize rapidly with few aftereffects allow shorter operative times. Nurses recognize the benefit of early postoperative ambulation and encourage clients to assume an active role in recovery. Ambulatory surgery also offers cost savings by eliminating the need for hospital stays. This reduces the possibility of acquiring nosocomial infections, which occur when normal skin flora changes with hospitalization and clients become colonized with bacteria found in the hospital setting. Procedures such as tumor biopsies and gallbladder removal **(cholecystectomy)** can now be done using laparoscopic procedures. Because of the small incision, a laparoscopic cholecystectomy involves only a few hours to a 24-hour hospital stay and a recovery period of a week. By contrast, a traditional open cholecystectomy involves a large abdominal incision. Clients require a 3- to 5-day hospitalization and at least a 4-week recovery period. Thus many surgeons use laparoscopic procedures instead of traditional surgical procedures, thereby decreasing the length of surgery, hospitalization, and associated costs.

Scientific Knowledge Base

Classification of Surgery

The types of surgical procedures are classified according to seriousness, urgency, and purpose (Table 49-1). A procedure may fall into more than one classification. For example, surgical removal of a disfiguring scar is minor in seriousness, elective in urgency, and reconstructive in purpose. Frequently the classes overlap. An urgent procedure is also considered major in seriousness. The same operation may be performed for different reasons on different clients. For example, a gastrectomy may be performed as an emergency procedure to resect a bleeding ulcer or as an urgent procedure to remove a cancerous growth. The classification indicates to the nurse the level of care a client might require.

The American Society of Anesthesiologists (ASA) assigns classification based on a client's physiological condition independent of the proposed surgical procedure (Table 49-2). Intraoperative difficulties occur more frequently with clients who have a poor physical status classification (Meeker and Rothrock, 1999). ASA physical status class I and class II and also stable class III are now acceptable for ambulatory surgery. Class IV and class V require inpatient surgery.

Nursing Knowledge Base

Nursing knowledge offers important contributions for the care of the perioperative client. Nursing has made significant contributions in showing the benefit preoperative education and preparation has in promoting positive client outcomes following surgery. Structured preoperative teaching that includes the AORN standards

Table 49-1   Classification for Surgical Procedures

Type	Description	Example
Seriousness	**Seriousness**	
Major	Involves extensive reconstruction or alteration in body parts; poses great risks to well-being	Coronary artery bypass, colon resection, removal of larynx, resection of lung lobe
Minor	Involves minimal alteration in body parts; often designed to correct deformities; involves minimal risks compared with major procedures	Cataract extraction, facial plastic surgery, tooth extraction
Urgency		
Elective	Is performed on basis of client's choice; is not essential and may not be necessary for health	Bunionectomy, facial plastic surgery, hernia repair, breast reconstruction
Urgent	Is necessary for client's health, may prevent additional problems from developing (e.g., tissue destruction or impaired organ function); not necessarily emergency	Excision of cancerous tumor, removal of gallbladder for stones, vascular repair for obstructed artery (e.g., coronary artery bypass)
Emergency	Must be done immediately to save life or preserve function of body part	Repair of perforated appendix, repair of traumatic amputation, control of internal hemorrhaging
Purpose		
Diagnostic	Is surgical exploration that allows physician to confirm diagnosis; may involve removal of tissue for further diagnostic testing	Exploratory laparotomy (incision into peritoneal cavity to inspect abdominal organs), breast mass biopsy
Ablative	Is excision or removal of diseased body part	Amputation, removal of appendix, cholecystectomy
Palliative	Relieves or reduces intensity of disease symptoms; will not produce cure	Colostomy, debridement of necrotic tissue, resection of nerve roots
Reconstructive/ Restorative	Restores function or appearance to traumatized or malfunctioning tissues	Internal fixation of fractures, scar revision
Procurement for transplant	Removal of organs and/or tissues from a person pronounced brain dead for transplantation into another person	Kidney, heart, or liver transplant
Constructive	Restores function lost or reduced as result of congenital anomalies	Repair of cleft palate, closure of atrial septal defect in heart
Cosmetic	Performed to improve personal appearance	Blepharoplasty to correct eyelid deformities; rhinoplasty to reshape nose

Table 49-2   Physical Status (PS) Classification of the American Society of Anesthesiologists

Class	Description	Characteristics
PS-I	A normal healthy client	No physiological, biological, organic disturbance
PS-II	A client with a mild systemic disease	Cardiovascular (CV) disease with minimal restriction on activity
PS-III	A client with a severe systemic disease that limits activity but is not incapacitating	Hypertension (HTN), obesity, diabetes mellitus (DM)
PS-IV	A client with a severe systemic disease that is a constant threat to life	CV or pulmonary disease that limits activity; severe diabetes with systemic complications; history of myocardial infarction (MI), angina pectoris, or poorly controlled HTN
PS-V	A **moribund** client who is not expected to survive 24 hours with/without the operation	Severe cardiac, pulmonary, renal, hepatic, or endocrine dysfunction
PS-VI	A client declared brain dead whose organs are being removed for donor purpose	Clients may have a wide variety of dysfunctions that are being managed to optimize blood flow to the heart and organs (e.g., aggressive fluid replacement and blood pressure medications)
E	Emergency operation	Surgery is done as a last recourse of resuscitative effort; major multisystem or cerebral trauma, ruptured aneurysm, or large pulmonary embolus

Data from Meeker MH, Rothrock JC: *Alexander's care of the patient in surgery,* ed 11, St. Louis, 1999, Mosby; and Greenfield L and others: *Surgery: scientific principles and practice,* ed 2, Philadelphia, 1997, Lippincott-Raven.

(2002d) and return demonstration of postoperative exercises has been shown to improve outcomes such as pain severity, pulmonary function, length of stay, and clients' level of anxiety.

There is also significant evidence-based knowledge available for proper wound care interventions. Nursing research has contributed to what is known about the characteristics of wound healing and the types of applications most likely to be beneficial. Chapter 47 describes in detail a variety of interventions used to treat wounds, including surgical wounds.

Within the operating room setting, nursing knowledge has improved the standards for infection control and client safety. For example, surgical hand scrubs, which is a skill beyond the scope of this textbook, can now be performed without the use of brushes as a result of research that has shown the efficacy of alcohol-based hand antiseptics in reducing bacteria on the skin (Hobson and others, 1998; Larson and others, 1990). Evidence-based practice changes within the OR improve the quality of care for surgical clients and ultimately improve client outcomes.

Critical Thinking

Successful critical thinking requires a synthesis of knowledge, information gathered from clients, experience, critical thinking attitudes, and intellectual and professional standards. Clinical judgments require the nurse to anticipate the information necessary, analyze the data, and make decisions regarding client care. A client's condition is always changing. During assessment (Figure 49-1) the nurse must consider all of the elements that build toward making appropriate nursing diagnoses.

In the case of caring for the perioperative client, the nurse integrates knowledge from anatomy and physiology, pathophysiology, and the surgical stress response, along with previous experiences in caring for surgical clients and information gathered from an individual client, to make

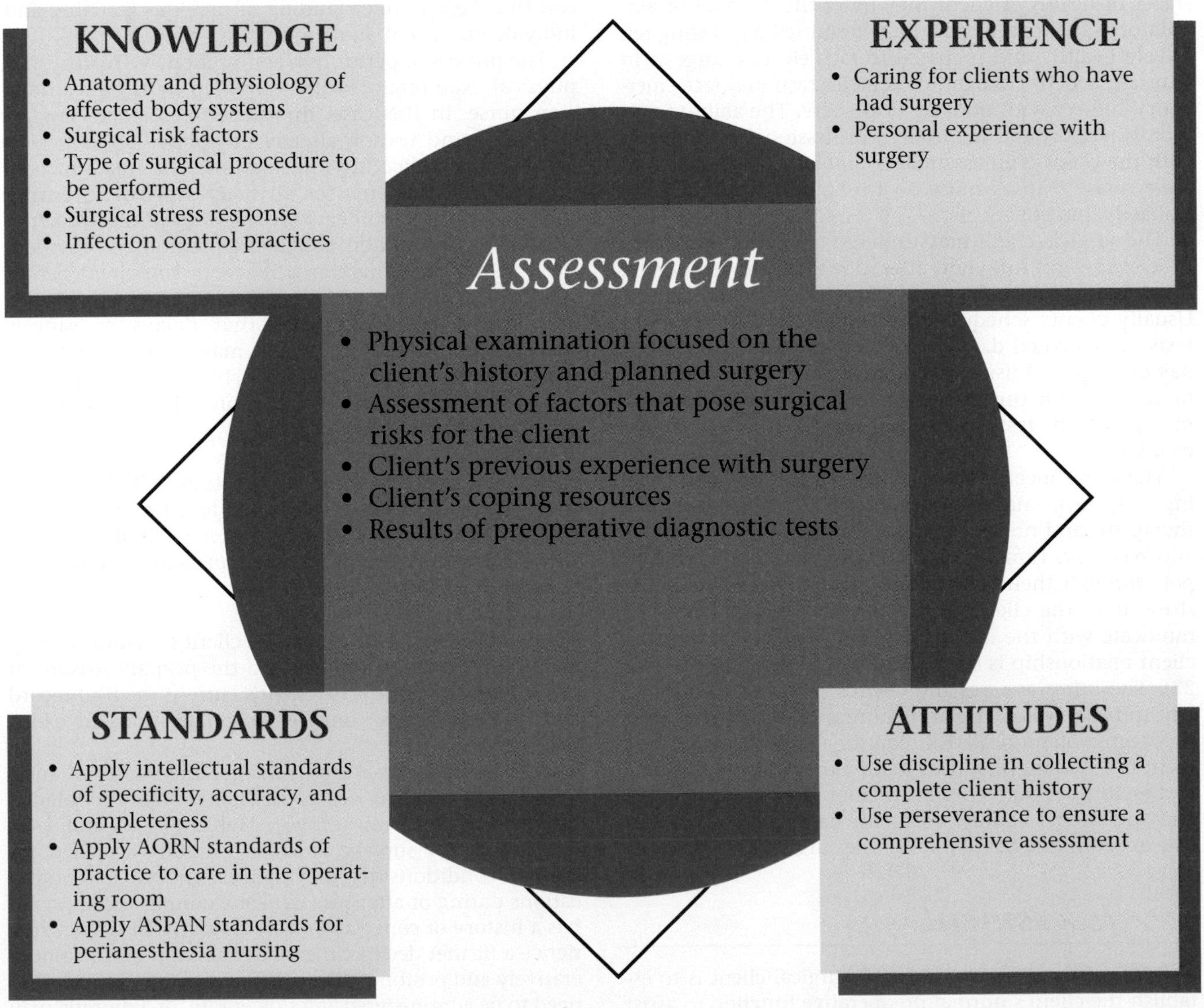

KNOWLEDGE

- Anatomy and physiology of affected body systems
- Surgical risk factors
- Type of surgical procedure to be performed
- Surgical stress response
- Infection control practices

EXPERIENCE

- Caring for clients who have had surgery
- Personal experience with surgery

Assessment

- Physical examination focused on the client's history and planned surgery
- Assessment of factors that pose surgical risks for the client
- Client's previous experience with surgery
- Client's coping resources
- Results of preoperative diagnostic tests

STANDARDS

- Apply intellectual standards of specificity, accuracy, and completeness
- Apply AORN standards of practice to care in the operating room
- Apply ASPAN standards for perianesthesia nursing

ATTITUDES

- Use discipline in collecting a complete client history
- Use perseverance to ensure a comprehensive assessment

FIGURE **49-1** Critical thinking model for surgical client assessment.

clinical decisions for the client's care. The use of critical thinking attitudes such as perseverance is needed to develop a plan of care that provides successful perioperative care (e.g., airway management, infection control, pain management, and discharge planning). The use of professional standards as developed by the Agency for Health Care Research and Quality (AHRQ), formerly known as the Agency for Health Care Policy and Research (AHCPR), AORN, and the **American Society of PeriAnesthesia Nurses (ASPAN)** provide valuable guidelines for perioperative management and evaluation of process and outcomes (www.ahcpr.gov; www.aorn.org; www.aspan.org). However, the nurse should review these guidelines within the context of new emerging evidence-based practice and agency policies.

The Nursing Process in the Preoperative Surgical Phase

Surgical clients enter the health care setting in different stages of health. A client may enter the hospital or ambulatory satellite unit on a predetermined day feeling relatively healthy and prepared to face elective surgery. In contrast, a victim of a motor vehicle crash may face emergency surgery with no time to prepare. The ability to establish rapport and maintain a professional relationship with the client is an essential component of the preoperative phase. Nurses must do this quickly, but compassionately and effectively.

The surgical client may undergo tests and procedures to confirm or rule out alterations requiring surgery. Most testing is performed before the day of surgery. Usually clients scheduled for ambulatory surgery have tests done several days before surgery. Testing done the day of surgery is usually limited to such tests as glucose monitoring for the diabetic client. Nurses must be familiar with the tests, their purpose, and how to monitor results.

The client meets many health care personnel, including surgeons, nurse anesthetists or anesthesiologists, therapists, and nurses. All play a role in the client's care and recovery. Family members attempt to provide support through their presence but face many of the same stressors as the client. The nurse must effectively communicate with the client and family because the nurse-client relationship is the foundation of care (see Chapter 23). The nurse assesses the client's physical, emotional, and spiritual well-being and cultural heritage; recognizes the degree of surgical risk; coordinates diagnostic tests; identifies nursing diagnoses and nursing interventions; and establishes outcomes in collaboration with the client and the client's family. Pertinent data and the plan of care are communicated among the surgical team.

Assessment

The aim of the assessment of the surgical client is to establish the client's normal preoperative function to assist the nurse in preventing and recognizing possible postoperative complications. Assessment of the surgical client can be extensive. Ambulatory and same-day surgical programs provide challenges in gathering a complete assessment in a limited time. A multidisciplinary team approach is essential. Clients are admitted only hours before the surgical event, so nurses must organize and verify data obtained preoperatively to implement a perioperative plan of care. This occurs not only with the ambulatory care client, but also with the client who will require a more prolonged hospital stay. It has become common practice for clients to be admitted the day of surgery, even for such major procedures as open heart surgery or craniotomy.

The majority of assessments begin before admission for surgery—in the physician's office, preadmission clinic, anesthesia clinic, or by telephone. Clients may answer a self-report inventory, a rudimentary physical examination may be completed by a surgical nurse, laboratory tests may be drawn or completed, teaching is begun, questions are answered, and paperwork is initiated. This streamlines the care required by the client on the day of surgery. Nurses in the immediate preoperative period assess the client's understanding of previous teaching and individualize client and family care.

The physician performs a comprehensive history and physical examination with follow-up by the preadmission nurse. In this case, the nurse needs to review assessments and testing already completed so as not to waste time duplicating information. The nurse focuses on key measurements for all body systems to ensure that no obvious problems are overlooked and that the client has understood education previously provided. Even though the surgeon will screen the client before scheduling surgery, preoperative assessment occasionally reveals an abnormality that delays or cancels surgery. For example, the client may have a cough and low-grade fever on admission. This may indicate the onset of infection, and the surgeon will need to be notified immediately.

Nursing History. The nurse conducts an initial interview to collect a client history similar to that described in Chapter 32. If a client is unable to relate all of the necessary information, the nurse relies on family members as resources.

Medical History. A review of the client's medical history should include past illnesses and the primary reason for seeking medical care. The client's current medical record and medical records from past hospitalizations are excellent sources of data.

Preexisting illnesses can influence the choice of anesthetic agents used, as well as the client's ability to tolerate surgery and reach full recovery (Table 49-3). Candidates for ambulatory surgery must be carefully screened for medical conditions that may increase the risk for complications during or after surgery. For example, a client who has a history of congestive heart failure (CHF) may experience a further decline in cardiac function both intraoperatively and postoperatively. Intravenous (IV) fluids may need to be administered at a slower rate, or a diuretic may need to be given after blood transfusions.

Table **49-3**	Medical Conditions That Increase the Risks of Surgery
Type of Condition	**Reason for Risk**
Bleeding disorders (thrombocytopenia, hemophilia)	Increase risk of hemorrhaging during and after surgery.
Diabetes mellitus	Increases susceptibility to infection and may impair wound healing from altered glucose metabolism and associated circulatory impairment. Stress of surgery may cause increases in blood glucose levels.
Heart disease (recent myocardial infarction, dysrhythmias, congestive heart failure) and peripheral vascular disease	Stress of surgery causes increased demands on myocardium to maintain cardiac output. General anesthetic agents depress cardiac function.
Obstructive sleep apnea	Administration of opioids increase risk of airway obstruction postoperatively. Clients will desaturate as revealed by drop in O_2 saturation by pulse oximetry.
Upper respiratory infection	Increases risk of respiratory complications during anesthesia (e.g., pneumonia and spasm of laryngeal muscles).
Liver disease	Alters metabolism and elimination of drugs administered during surgery and impairs wound healing and clotting time because of alterations in protein metabolism.
Fever	Predisposes client to fluid and electrolyte imbalances and may indicate underlying infection.
Chronic respiratory disease (emphysema, bronchitis, asthma)	Reduces client's means to compensate for acid-base alterations (see Chapter 40). Anesthetic agents reduce respiratory function, increasing risk for severe hypoventilation.
Immunological disorders (leukemia, acquired immunodeficiency syndrome [AIDS], bone marrow depression, and use of chemotherapeutic drugs or immunosuppressive agents)	Increases risk of infection and delayed wound healing after surgery.
Abuse of street drugs	Persons abusing drugs may have underlying disease (HIV/hepatitis), which affects healing.
Chronic pain	Regular use of pain medications may result in higher tolerance. Increased doses of analgesics may be required to achieve postoperative pain control.

Risk Factors. Various conditions and factors increase a person's risk in surgery. Knowledge of risk factors enables the nurse to take necessary precautions in planning care.

Age. Very young and old clients are at risk during surgery because of immature or declining physiological status. Mortality rates are higher in very young and very old surgical clients. During surgery, nurses and physicians are especially concerned with maintaining an infant's normal body temperature. The infant's shivering reflex is underdeveloped, and often wide temperature variations occur. Anesthesia adds to the risk because anesthetics can cause vasodilation and heat loss.

During surgery an infant has difficulty maintaining a normal circulatory blood volume. The total blood volume of an infant is considerably less than that of an older child or an adult. Even a small amount of blood loss can be serious. A reduced circulatory volume makes it difficult for the infant to respond to increased oxygen demands during surgery. In addition, the infant is highly susceptible to complications associated with dehydration. However, if blood or fluids are replaced too quickly, overhydration may occur. Other important and unique aspects of a child's surgical care include airway management, treatment of seizures, management of temperature alterations, identification and treatment of emergence delirium and delayed emergence from anesthesia, treatment of pain and agitation, and availability of age-appropriate emergency equipment and medications.

With advancing age, a client's physical capacity to adapt to the stress of surgery is hampered because of deterioration in certain body functions. Despite the risk, the majority of clients undergoing surgery are older adults. Table 49-4 summarizes physiological factors that place older clients at risk during surgery.

Nutrition. Normal tissue repair and resistance to infection depend on adequate nutrients. Surgery intensifies this need. After surgery a client requires at least 1500 kcal/day to maintain energy reserves. Increased protein, vitamins A and C, and zinc facilitate wound healing (see Chapters 43 and 47). A malnourished client is prone to poor tolerance to anesthesia, negative nitrogen balance, delayed blood clotting mechanisms, infection, poor wound healing, and the potential for multiple organ failure. Many hospitalized clients display some degree of malnutrition. If a client has elective surgery, attempts to correct nutritional imbalances before surgery should be made. However, if a malnourished client must undergo an emergency procedure, efforts to restore nutrients occur after surgery.

Obesity. Obesity increases surgical risk by reducing ventilatory and cardiac function. Hypertension, coronary

Table 49-4	Physiological Factors That Place the Older Adult at Risk During Surgery	
Alterations	**Risks**	**Nursing Implications**
Cardiovascular System		
Degenerative change in myocardium and valves	Reduced cardiac reserve.	Assess baseline vital signs. Recognize the longer time period required for heart rate to return to normal following stress on the heart and evaluate the occurrence of tachycardia accordingly (Eliopoulos, 2001).
Rigidity of arterial walls and reduction in sympathetic and parasympathetic innervation to heart	Alterations predispose client to postoperative hemorrhage and rise in systolic and diastolic blood pressure.	Maintain adequate fluid balance to minimize stress to the heart. Ensure blood pressure level is adequate to meet circulatory demands.
Increase in calcium and cholesterol deposits within small arteries; thickened arterial walls	Predispose client to clot formation in lower extremities.	Instruct client on techniques for performing leg exercises and proper turning. Apply elastic stockings, sequential compression devices (SCDs).
Integumentary System		
Decreased subcutaneous tissue and increased fragility of skin	Prone to pressure ulcers and skin tears.	Assess skin every 4 hours; pad all bony prominences during surgery. Turn or reposition.
Pulmonary System		
Rib cage stiffened and reduced in size	Reduced vital capacity.	Instruct client on proper technique for coughing, deep breathing, and use of spirometer. When possible, have client ambulate and sit in chair frequently.
Reduced range of movement in diaphragm	Greater residual capacity (volume of air is left in lung after normal breath) increases, reducing amount of new air brought into lungs with each inspiration.	
Stiffened lung tissue and enlarged air spaces	Alteration reduces blood oxygenation.	Obtain baseline oxygen saturation; measure as indicated throughout perioperative period.
Renal System		
Reduced blood flow to kidneys	Increased risk of shock when blood loss occurs.	For clients hospitalized before surgery, determine baseline urinary output for 24 hours.
Reduced glomerular filtration rate and excretory times	Limits ability to eliminate drugs or toxic substances.	Assess for adverse response to drugs.
Reduced bladder capacity	Voiding frequency increases, and larger amount of urine stays in bladder after voiding. Sensation of need to void may not occur until bladder is filled.	Instruct client to notify nurse immediately when sensation of bladder fullness develops. Keep call light and bedpan within easy reach. Toilet every 2 hours or more frequently if indicated.
Neurological System		
Sensory losses, including reduced tactile sense and increased pain tolerance	Decreased ability to respond to early warning signs of surgical complications.	Inspect bony prominences for signs of pressure that client may not sense. Orient client to surrounding environment. Observe for nonverbal signs of pain.
Decreased reaction time	Confusion after anesthesia	Allow adequate time to respond, process information, and perform tasks. Institute fall precautions.
Metabolic System		
Lower basal metabolic rate	Reduced total oxygen consumption.	Ensure adequate nutritional intake when diet is resumed, but avoid intake of excess calories.
Reduced number of red blood cells and hemoglobin levels	Ability to carry adequate oxygen to tissues is reduced.	Administer necessary blood products. Monitor blood test results.
Change in total amounts of body potassium and water volume	Greater risk for fluid or electrolyte imbalance occurs.	Monitor electrolyte levels and supplement as necessary.
Impaired thermoregulatory mechanisms	Cold operating rooms; exposure of body parts during procedure, IV fluids, medications.	Ensure careful, close monitoring of client temperature; provide warm blankets; monitor cardiac function; warm IV fluids.

artery disease, diabetes mellitus, and congestive heart failure are common in the **bariatric** (obese) population. Embolus, **atelectasis,** and pneumonia are also more frequent postoperative complications in the obese client. The client may have difficulty resuming normal physical activity after surgery. The obese client is susceptible to poor wound healing and wound infection because of the structure of fatty tissue, which contains a poor blood supply. This slows delivery of essential nutrients, antibodies, and enzymes needed for wound healing (see Chapter 47). It is often difficult to close the surgical wound of an obese client because of the thick adipose layer. An obese client is also at risk for **dehiscence** (opening of the suture line).

Immunocompetence. For the client with cancer, radiation therapy may be given preoperatively to reduce the size of the cancerous tumor so that it can be removed surgically. Radiation has some unavoidable effects on normal tissue, such as excess thinning of skin layers, destruction of collagen, and impaired vascularization of tissue. Ideally, the surgeon waits to perform surgery 4 to 6 weeks after completion of radiation treatments. Otherwise, the client may face serious wound-healing problems. In addition, chemotherapeutic drugs used for cancer treatment, immunosuppressive medications used to prevent rejection after organ transplantation, and steroids used to treat a variety of inflammatory conditions increase the risk for infection.

Fluid and Electrolyte Imbalance. The body responds to surgery as a form of trauma. As a result of the adrenocortical stress response, sodium and water are retained and potassium is lost within the first 2 to 5 days after surgery. Severe protein breakdown can cause a negative nitrogen balance. The severity of the stress response influences the degree of fluid and electrolyte imbalance. More extensive surgery will result in a greater stress response. A client who is hypovolemic or who has serious preoperative electrolyte alterations is at significant risk during and after surgery. For example, an excess or depletion of potassium increases the chance of dysrhythmia during or after surgery. If the client has preexisting renal, gastrointestinal, or cardiovascular abnormalities, the risk of fluid and electrolyte alterations is even greater.

Pregnancy. The perioperative plan of care must address not one, but two clients: the mother and the developing fetus. Surgery is performed on the pregnant client only on an emergent or urgent basis. All major systems of the mother are affected during pregnancy. For example, cardiac output significantly increases as does respiratory tidal volume to accommodate the increase in metabolic rate. Gastrointestinal motility decreases, hormone levels increase, and energy levels decrease with advancing pregnancy. Laboratory and hemodynamic values change. Fibrinogen levels increase, so pregnant clients are more susceptible to the development of deep vein thrombosis due to increased coagulability. Hemoglobin and hematocrit levels decrease, mostly as a result of the effects of hemodilution (increased circulating volume). The white blood cell (WBC) count is elevated when the woman is near term and postpartum without the presence of infec-

tion. General anesthesia is administered with caution because of the increased risk of fetal death and preterm labor. Psychological considerations for mother and family are essential.

Previous Surgeries. A client's past experience with surgery can influence physical and psychological responses to a procedure. The previous type of surgery, level of discomfort, extent of disability, and overall level of care provided are factors the nurse asks the client to recall. The nurse addresses any complications that the client experienced. It is also important to assess clients for motion sickness and nausea and vomiting with previous surgeries (Gan, 2002; Tramer, 2001). These factors increase the risk for aspiration. Prior anesthesia records may be a useful source of information if other previous problems occurred. This information helps the nurse anticipate the client's preoperative and postoperative needs.

Previous surgery may also influence the level of physical care required after a surgical procedure. For example, a client who has had a previous thoracotomy for resection of a lung lobe has a greater risk for postoperative pulmonary complications than a client with intact normal lungs.

Perceptions and Understanding of Surgery. The surgical experience affects not only the client, but the family unit as a whole. The nurse therefore must prepare both the client and the family for the surgical experience. Identification of a client's and family's knowledge, expectations, and perceptions allows the nurse to plan teaching and to provide individualized emotional support measures.

Each client brings fears to the surgical setting. Some are due to past hospital experiences, warnings from friends and family, or lack of knowledge. The nurse asks for a description of the client's understanding of the planned surgery and its implications. The nurse might ask questions such as "Tell me what you think will happen before and after surgery" or "Explain what you know about surgery." The nurse faces an ethical dilemma when a client is misinformed or unaware of the reason for surgery and should confer with the physician if the client has an inaccurate perception or knowledge of the surgical procedure before the client is sent to the surgical suite. The nurse also determines whether the physician explained routine preoperative and postoperative procedures. When a client is well prepared and knows what to expect, the nurse reinforces the client's knowledge and maintains accuracy and consistency.

Medication History. If a client regularly uses prescription or over-the-counter medications, the surgeon or anesthesia provider may temporarily discontinue the drugs before surgery or adjust the dosages. Certain medications have special implications for the surgical client, creating greater risks for complications (Table 49-5). The nurse instructs clients to ask the physician if usual medications should be taken the morning of surgery. Clients should also be asked if any herbal preparations are used, because many clients do not view herbs as medications and may omit them from their medication history (see Chapter

Table 49-5   **Drugs With Special Implications for the Surgical Client**

Drug Class	Effects During Surgery
Antibiotics	Antibiotics potentiate action of anesthetic agents. If taken within 2 weeks before surgery, aminoglycosides (gentamicin, tobramycin, neomycin) may cause mild respiratory depression from depressed neuromuscular transmission.
Antidysrhythmics	Antidysrhythmics can reduce cardiac contractility and impair cardiac conduction during anesthesia.
Anticoagulants	Anticoagulants alter normal clotting factors and thus increase risk of hemorrhaging. They should be discontinued at least 48 hours before surgery. Aspirin is a commonly used medication that can alter clotting mechanisms.
Anticonvulsants	Long-term use of certain anticonvulsants (e.g., phenytoin [Dilantin] and phenobarbital) can alter metabolism of anesthetic agents.
Antihypertensives	Antihypertensives interact with anesthetic agents to cause bradycardia, hypotension, and impaired circulation. They inhibit synthesis and storage of norepinephrine in sympathetic nerve endings.
Corticosteroids	With prolonged use, corticosteroids cause adrenal atrophy, which reduces the body's ability to withstand stress. Before and during surgery, dosages may be temporarily increased.
Insulin	Diabetic clients' need for insulin after surgery is altered. Stress response and intravenous (IV) administration of glucose solutions can increase dosage requirements after surgery. Decreased nutritional intake can decrease dosage requirements.
Diuretics	Diuretics potentiate electrolyte imbalances (particularly potassium) after surgery.
Nonsteroidal antiinflammatory drugs (NSAIDs)	NSAIDs inhibit platelet aggregation and may prolong bleeding time, increasing susceptibility to postoperative bleeding.
Herbal therapies: ginger, gingko, ginseng	These herbal therapies have the ability to affect platelet activity and increase susceptibility to postoperative bleeding. Ginseng may increase hypoglycemia with insulin therapy.

35). Certain herbs may interfere with the action of other medications (consult the pharmacist). For hospitalized clients, prescription drugs taken preoperatively are automatically discontinued postoperatively unless the physician reorders them.

Allergies. The nurse must assess for allergies to drugs that may be given during a phase of the surgical experience. In addition, it is also critical to assess for latex, food, and contact allergies (e.g., to tape, ointments, or solutions). A client may be too young or have too few exposures to drugs to know if he or she has allergies. The type of allergic response is very important to assess. Allergies need to be delineated from unpleasant side effects. For example, the client may state that codeine causes nausea (a side effect), or it may cause hypotension and confusion (an allergy). When asking a client about allergies, realize that the term "allergy" can be confusing for some clients. Asking a client if he or she has ever "had a problem with a medication or substance" may be another helpful approach to questioning.

It is critical that the client specifically be asked about latex allergies because a latex-free environment must be provided for clients with latex allergies. The nurse ensures that a list of the client's allergies is noted appropriately in the client's chart and/or the hospital computer system, as well as any other places designated by institutional policy, such as an allergy band.

Smoking Habits. The client who smokes is at greater risk for postoperative pulmonary complications than a client who does not. The chronic smoker already has an increased amount and thickness of mucous secretions in the lungs. General anesthetics increase airway irritation and stimulate pulmonary secretions, which are retained as a result of reduction in ciliary activity during anesthe-

sia. After surgery the client who smokes has greater difficulty clearing the airways of mucous secretions and needs emphasis on the importance of postoperative deep breathing and coughing (see Chapter 39).

Alcohol Ingestion and Substance Use and Abuse. Habitual use of alcohol and illegal drugs predisposes the client to adverse reactions to anesthetic agents. The client may also experience a cross-tolerance to anesthetic agents, necessitating higher-than-normal doses. In addition, the physician may need to increase postoperative dosages of analgesics. Clients with a history of excessive alcohol ingestion may also be malnourished, which may contribute to delayed wound healing. These clients are also at risk for liver disease, portal hypertension, and esophageal varices (predisposing the client to bleeding disorders). The client who habitually uses alcohol and is required to remain in the hospital longer than 24 hours is also at risk for acute alcohol withdrawal and its more severe form, delirium tremens (DTs).

Family Support. It is important for the nurse to determine the extent of the client's support from family members or friends. Because family is not always defined by blood relations, it is best to have the client identify his or her source of support. Surgery often results in temporary or permanent disability that requires added assistance during recovery. The client usually cannot immediately assume the same level of physical activity enjoyed before an illness. Often a client returns home with dressings to change or exercises to perform. With ambulatory surgery, clients and families assume responsibility for postoperative care. The family is an important resource for the client with physical limitations and provides the emotional support needed to motivate the client to return to a previous state of health. The family may better remember preoperative and postoperative teaching as well.

The nurse should ask if family members or friends can provide support. The client may want someone else present when the nurse provides instructions or explanations. Family presence should be encouraged when feasible, especially for clients in the ambulatory setting. Often a family member can become the client's coach, offering valuable support during the postoperative period, when the client's participation in care is vital.

Occupation. Surgery may result in physical alterations that hinder or prevent a person from returning to work. The nurse assesses the client's occupational history to anticipate the possible effects of surgery on recovery and eventual work performance. The nurse explains any restrictions before a client returns to work, such as lifting, use of the extremities, or climbing stairs. When a client is unable to return to a job, the nurse confers with a social worker and/or occupational therapist to refer the client to job-training programs or to help the client seek economic assistance.

Preoperative Pain Assessment. Surgical manipulation of tissues, treatments, and positioning on the operating room table may result in postoperative pain for the client. Pain is a very personal experience and requires an individualized plan of care. Preoperatively the nurse should conduct a comprehensive pain assessment (see Chapter 42), including the client's and family's expectations for pain management following surgery. The nurse should begin education regarding pain management as soon as possible (Barnes, 2001). Preoperative assessment should include the use of a pain instrument to rate the presence and severity of pain (see Chapter 42). Several instruments for both pediatric and adult clients have shown reliability and validity (Summers, 2001). Frequent pain assessments are necessary to alert the nurse to treat the pain and assess the adequacy (outcome) of pain interventions.

Review of Emotional Health. Surgery is psychologically stressful. The client may be anxious about the surgery and its implications. Clients often feel that they are powerless over their situation. Family members may perceive the client's surgery as a disruption of their lifestyle. Hospitalization and the recovery period at home may be lengthy. The family is usually concerned about the client returning to a normal, productive life. When the client has chronic illness, the family may be fearful that surgery may result in further disability or hopeful that it may improve their lifestyle. To understand the impact of surgery on a client's and family's emotional health, the nurse assesses the client's feelings about surgery, self-concept, body image, and coping resources.

It is often difficult to assess feelings thoroughly when ambulatory surgery is scheduled. The nurse usually has less time to establish a relationship with the client. Box 49-1 describes a study that explored the needs of ambulatory surgery clients. In some outpatient surgical programs the nurse may visit with a client in the home or on the telephone before surgery. In a hospital room the

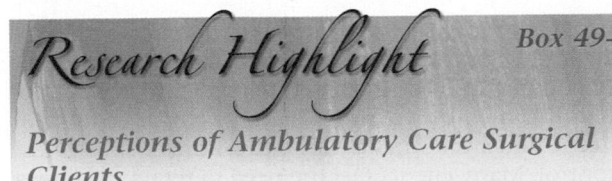

Research Highlight   Box 49-1

Perceptions of Ambulatory Care Surgical Clients

Research Focus

Over the past decade the number of ambulatory surgical procedures has continually increased. Nursing care of the ambulatory surgery client must be condensed into shorter time periods in all phases of perioperative care. Ensuring that the needs of ambulatory surgery clients are met is imperative.

Research Abstract

The purpose of this study was to explore the perceptions and views of ambulatory surgery clients. A study of 16 clients who underwent abdominal surgical procedures in an ambulatory surgery center was conducted. Data were collected by intensive semistructured interviews conducted in the surgeon's office at the time of the 1-week postoperative appointment. Topics in the interviews included client's recall of how they felt the night before surgery, experiences the day of surgery, whether the perioperative experience met their expectation, feelings regarding the discharge process, and the experience of recovering at home. The interviews were then analyzed. Three areas were identified: fear, knowing, and presence. This study supported the importance of the nurse's presence through the perioperative experience and provided the perioperative nurse with an understanding of the needs of the ambulatory surgery client.

Evidence-Based Practice

- Fear in general was expressed, and fear of anesthesia was discussed most often. Frequently, clients discuss their fears indirectly. Nurses must listen to clients for cues and provide them an opportunity to express their fears.
- Clients often had insufficient knowledge about what to expect preoperatively and postoperatively despite a good understanding of the surgical procedure itself. Education and reinforcement of the education is important throughout all phase of the perioperative experience.
- Clients wanted to know they mattered as an individual. Nurses should address clients by name and listen to individual requests and concerns. Incorporate the individual and the support system into the plan of care.
- Clients wanted to know the nurse was truly there for them both physically and emotionally.
- Connection with family or significant others is important throughout the perioperative experience.

Reference

Costa MJ: The lived perioperative experience of ambulatory surgery patients, *AORN J* 74(6):874, 2001.

nurse should choose a time for discussion after admitting procedures or diagnostic tests are completed. The nurse explains that it is normal to have fears and concerns. The client's ability to share feelings partially depends on the nurse's willingness to listen, be supportive, and clarify misconceptions.

If the client feels powerless, the nurse should attempt to determine the reason. The medical diagnosis may generate apprehension of increased dependence and loss of physical or mental function. The thought of being "put to sleep" under anesthesia may create concern about loss of control. Many clients feel the need to retain the power to make decisions about treatment. The nurse must assure clients of their right to ask questions and seek information.

A client may be angry about the need for surgery. For example, a young person may feel that it is unfair to have a disorder that typically affects older people. Surgery may occur at a time when it is inconvenient or potentially disruptive. The client may occasionally express anger by verbally attacking the nurse or physician. Being argumentative or overly demanding, refusing to cooperate, and criticizing the nurse's efforts to provide care are manifestations of anger and anxiety.

Self-Concept. Clients with a positive self-concept are more likely to approach surgical experiences appropriately. The nurse assesses self-concept by asking clients to identify personal strengths and weaknesses (see Chapter 26). Clients who are quick to criticize or scorn personal characteristics may have little self-regard or may be testing the nurse's opinion of their characters. Poor self-concept hinders the ability to adapt to the stress of surgery and aggravates feelings of guilt or inadequacy.

Body Image. Surgical removal of any diseased body part often leaves permanent disfigurement, alteration in body function, or concern over mutilation. Loss of certain body functions (e.g., with a colostomy or ureterostomy) may compound a client's fears. The nurse assesses for the body image alterations that clients perceive will result from surgery. Individuals will respond differently depending on their culture, self-concept and degree of self-esteem (see Chapter 26).

Often surgery changes the physical or psychological aspects of clients' sexuality. Excision of breast tissue, colostomies, ureterostomies, hysterectomy, or removal of prostate glands may affect clients' perceptions of their sexuality. Augustus (2002) found that African-American women delayed having a hysterectomy because of the negative sexuality connotations associated with hysterectomy. Surgery such as hernia repair or cataract extraction forces clients to temporarily refrain from sexual intercourse until they return to normal physical activity.

The nurse should encourage clients to express concerns about sexuality. The client facing even temporary sexual dysfunction requires understanding and support. Discussions about the client's sexuality should be held with the client's sexual partner so that they can gain a shared understanding of how to cope with limitations in sexual function.

Coping Resources. Assessment of feelings and self-concept helps reveal whether the client can cope with the stress of surgery. The physiological effects of stress are well documented. Activation of the endocrine system results in the release of hormones and catecholamines (epinephrine, norepinephrine), which result in increases in blood pressure, heart rate, and respiration. Platelet aggregation also occurs, along with many other physiological responses. The nurse must be aware of these responses and assist with stress management (see Chapter 30). The nurse asks the client about past stress management. If the client has had previous surgery, the nurse should determine behaviors that helped resolve any tension or nervousness. The nurse may instruct the client on relaxation exercises that can help control anxiety.

When reviewing the client's coping resources, the nurse asks the client about specific family members and friends who may provide support. Once these are identified, the nurse includes these individuals in any client teaching and interventions to manage stress and anxiety.

Culture. Culture is a system of beliefs that have developed over time and subsequently been passed on through many generations (Lipson, Dibble, and Minarik, 1996). Clients come from diverse cultural and religious backgrounds. These backgrounds affect the way each client perceives and reacts to the surgical experience. If cultural, ethnic, and religious differences are not acknowledged and planned for in the perioperative plan of care, desired surgical outcomes may not be achieved. Therefore the acquisition of knowledge regarding a client's cultural and ethnic heritage assists the nurse in caring for the perioperative client. Although it is important to recognize and plan for differences based on culture, it is also necessary to recognize that members of the

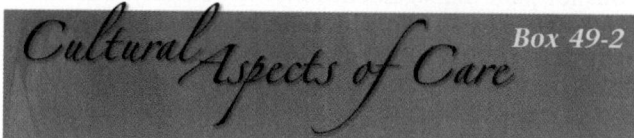

Cultural Aspects of Care   Box 49-2

Providing clients of various cultures, religious groups, and countries with individualized education and perioperative nursing care can be challenging. The use of a wide variety of resources within a health care agency, in the literature and from the Internet will help the nurse to provide culturally sensitive care.

Implications for Practice

- Preoperative assessment should include a cultural assessment with questions such as primary language spoken, feelings regarding surgery and pain, pain management, expectations, support system, and feelings toward self care with postoperative implications (e.g., Does client relate to concept of pain? Does client have feelings about gender of caregiver? Does client follow custom giving family members control over decisions?).
- Utilize professional interpreters to communicate with non–English-speaking clients.
- Utilize pictures or phrase cards with various languages to communicate and assess the non–English-speaking client, regarding pain, comfort, temperature, etc.
- Provide preoperative and postoperative educational materials in a variety of languages.

Modified from De Ruiter HP, Larsen KE: Developing a transcultural patient care web site, *J Transcult Nurs* 13(1):61, 2002; Douglas M: Pain as the fifth vital sign: will cultural variations be considered, *J Transcult Nurs* 10(4):285, 1999.

same culture are individuals and may not hold these shared beliefs. Box 49-2 highlights cultural care aspects in the perioperative period.

Client Expectations. Clients rely on their caregivers for information, comfort, pain control, adequate monitoring, and performance of interventions that ensure their safety throughout the surgical experience. This involves having a caring attitude, serving as an advocate for the client, being skilled in surgical assessment and interventions, and anticipating the client's needs throughout the perioperative period. Each plan of care must be individualized to the client, which makes it essential to understand clients' expectations. Do they expect full pain relief or simply to have their pain reduced? Do they expect to be independent immediately after surgery, or do they expect to be fully dependent on the nurse or family? These are only a few of the questions that need to be asked of the surgical client to establish a plan of care congruent with the client's needs and expectations.

Physical Examination. The nurse conducts a partial or complete physical examination, depending on the amount of time available and the client's preoperative condition. Chapter 32 describes techniques used in physical assessment. Assessment focuses on findings related to the client's medical history and on body systems that will likely be affected by the surgery. The nursing assessment should complement the surgeon's and anesthesia provider's physical examination (Barnes, 2002).

General Survey. The nurse observes the client's general appearance. Gestures and body movements may reflect weakness caused by illness. The client may appear malnourished. Height, body weight, and history of recent weight loss are important indicators of nutritional status.

Preoperative vital signs, including blood pressure while sitting and standing, provide important baseline data with which to compare alterations that occur during and after surgery. Some institutions request that blood pressure be obtained in both arms for comparison. Anxiety and fear commonly cause elevations in heart rate and blood pressure. As the effects of the anesthesia diminish after surgery, the nurse compares findings with the preoperative baseline. Preoperative assessment of vital signs is also important to rule out fluid and electrolyte abnormalities (see Chapter 40).

An elevated temperature before surgery is a cause for concern. If the client has an underlying infection, the surgeon may choose to postpone surgery until the infection has been treated. An elevated body temperature increases the risk of fluid and electrolyte imbalance after surgery.

Head and Neck. The condition of oral mucous membranes is one indicator of the level of hydration. A dehydrated client is at risk for developing serious fluid and electrolyte imbalances during surgery. Inspection of the soft palate and nasal sinuses can reveal sinus drainage indicative of respiratory or sinus infection. To rule out the possibility of local or systemic infection, the nurse palpates for cervical lymph node enlargement.

The nurse inspects the jugular veins for distention. Excess fluid within the circulatory system or failure of the heart to contract efficiently may lead to jugular vein distention and reveal a risk for cardiovascular complications during surgery.

During the examination of the oral mucosa, loose or capped teeth must be identified because they can become dislodged during endotracheal intubation. Dentures must be noted so they can be removed before surgery especially if general anesthesia is required.

Integument. The nurse carefully inspects the skin, especially over bony prominences, such as the heels, elbows, sacrum, and scapula. During surgery, a client must lie in a fixed position, often for several hours. As a result the client may have an increased risk for pressure ulcers (see Chapter 47) especially if the skin is thin and dry and has poor turgor. Chronic use of steroids also increases the client's susceptibility to skin tears. The overall condition of the skin also reveals the client's level of hydration. An older adult is at high risk for alteration in skin integrity from positioning and sliding on the operating room table, causing shear and pressure.

Thorax and Lungs. Assessment of the client's breathing pattern and chest excursion aids in assessing ventilatory capacity. A decline in ventilatory function places the client at risk for respiratory complications. For example, a client who has high abdominal surgery will have difficulty breathing deeply because of a painful abdominal incision. Auscultation of breath sounds will indicate whether the client has pulmonary congestion or narrowing of airways.

Existing atelectasis or moisture in the airways will be aggravated during surgery. Serious pulmonary congestion may cause postponement of the surgery. Certain anesthetics can cause laryngeal muscle spasm; thus if the nurse auscultates wheezing in the airways preoperatively, the client is at risk for further airway narrowing during surgery and after extubation (removal of the endotracheal tube); therefore the physician should be made aware of these findings.

Heart and Vascular System. The nurse assesses the character of the apical pulse and listens to heart sounds, assesses peripheral pulses, capillary refill, and the color and temperature of extremities. If peripheral pulses are not palpable, a Doppler instrument should be used for assessment of their presence. Acceptable capillary refill occurs in less than 2 seconds. Measurement of capillary refill and assessment of peripheral pulses are particularly important for the client having vascular surgery or for a client who may have casts or constricting bandages applied to the extremities after surgery (see Chapter 32).

Abdomen. The nurse assesses the abdomen for size, shape, symmetry, and presence of distention. Assessment of preoperative bowel sounds is useful as a baseline. The nurse should also ask whether the client has regular bowel movements and inquire about the color and consistency of stools.

Neurological Status. Preoperative assessment of neurological status is imperative for all clients receiving general anesthesia. The baseline neurological status assists with the assessment of ascent from anesthesia. During the health history and physical assessment, the nurse observes the client's level of orientation, alertness, and mood, noting whether the client answers questions appropriately and can recall recent and past events. A client who will have surgery for neurological disease (e.g., brain tumor or aneurysm) may demonstrate an impaired level of consciousness or altered behavior.

If the client is scheduled for spinal anesthesia, preoperative assessment of gross motor function and strength is important. Spinal anesthesia causes temporary paraly-

sis of the lower extremities (see Chapter 42). The nurse should be aware of a client entering surgery with weakness or impaired mobility of the lower extremities and not become alarmed when full motor function does not return as the spinal anesthetic wears off.

Diagnostic Screening. Before a client has surgery, the surgeon may order diagnostic tests to screen for preexisting abnormalities. Ordered tests are determined by the client's history and physical assessment. Table 49-6 contains common diagnostic tests performed preoperatively based on the client's medical history. Tests are also determined by the procedure itself. For procedures where blood loss is expected (e.g., hip and knee replacements),

Table 49-6   Common Diagnostic Tests Performed Preoperatively Based on Client History

History	Test
Hepatic disease	Prothrombin time, International Normalized Ratio, partial thromboplastin time (PT/INR/PTT); liver enzymes, such as serum aspartate aminotransferase (AST); alkaline phosphatase
Medications:	
Diuretics	Blood urea nitrogen (BUN), creatinine, electrolytes
Steroids	Electrolytes, glucose
Anticoagulants	PT/INR/PTT
Cardiovascular disease	BUN, creatinine, CBC, chest x-ray study, electrocardiogram (ECG)
Pulmonary disease	Complete blood count (CBC), chest x-ray study, ECG
Central nervous system disease	White blood cell (WBC) count, electrolytes, BUN, creatinine, glucose, and ECG

Table 49-7   Diagnostic Screening for Surgical Clients

Measurement and Normal Values	Interpretation
Complete blood count (CBC) *RBC:* Men: 4.7-6.1 million/mm^3 *Women:* 4.2-5.4 million/mm^3 *Hgb:* Men: 14-18 g/100 ml *Women:* 12-16 g/100 ml *Hct:* Men: 42%-52%; Women: 37%-47% *WBC:* Adults and children >2 yr: 5000-10,000/mm^3	Peripheral venous sample of blood measures red blood cells (RBCs), white blood cells (WBCs), hemoglobin (Hgb), and hematocrit (Hct). May reveal infection, low blood volume, and potential for oxygenation problems. Surgeon may order blood replacement.
Serum electrolytes *Sodium (Na):* 136-145 mEq/L *Potassium (K):* 3.5-5.0 mEq/L *Chloride (Cl):* 98-106 mEq/L *Bicarbonate (HCO$_3^-$):* 21-28 mEq/L	Peripheral venous sample of blood reveals significant fluid and electrolyte imbalances preoperatively. Attention is given to Na, K, and Cl levels. IV fluid replacement may be indicated preoperatively.
Coagulation studies *PT:* 11-12.5 seconds *INR:* 0.76-1.27 *APTT:* 30-40 seconds *Platelets:* 150,000-400,000/mm^3	Prothrombin time (PT), International Normalized Ratio (INR), activated partial thromboplastin time (APTT), and platelet counts reveal clotting ability of blood. Reveals clients at risk for bleeding tendencies and thrombus formation.
Serum creatinine *Men:* 0.6-1.2 mg/100 ml *Women:* 0.5-1.1 mg/100 ml	Ability of kidneys to excrete creatinine, by-product of muscle metabolism, assesses renal function. Elevated level can indicate renal failure.
Blood urea nitrogen (BUN) 10-20 mg/100 ml	Ability of kidneys to excrete urea and nitrogen indicates renal function. BUN becomes elevated if client is dehydrated. Preoperative IV fluid replacement may be needed.
Glucose *Fasting:* 70-105 mg/100 ml	Finger stick or peripheral blood sample. Clients may require treatment of low or high levels preoperatively and postoperatively.

Modified from Pagana KD, Pagana TJ: *Mosby's diagnostic and laboratory test reference*, ed 6, St. Louis, 2003, Mosby.

a type and crossmatch would be indicated preoperatively. The surgeon will designate the number of blood units to have available during surgery. Table 49-7 gives the purpose and normal values for the more common blood tests. If diagnostic tests reveal severe problems, the surgeon may cancel surgery until the condition stabilizes. The nurse is responsible for the preparation of clients for diagnostic studies and for coordinating completion of the tests. The nurse also reviews diagnostic results as they become available to alert physicians to findings and to assist with planning appropriate therapy.

If a client is over the age of 40 or has heart disease, the physician may order a chest x-ray examination or an electrocardiogram (ECG). The chest x-ray is an examination of the condition of the heart and lungs. An ECG measures the heart's electrical activity to determine whether the heart rate, rhythm, and other factors are normal.

Pulmonary function testing and occasionally arterial blood gas analysis may be performed on clients with preexisting lung disease. Blood glucose levels are measured preoperatively on diabetic clients.

Autologous infusions are an option for some clients who choose to donate their own blood before surgery to reduce the risk of transfusion-related infections. The donation usually must be made several weeks before the scheduled surgery. The client who does self-donation may exhibit a lower hemoglobin and hematocrit level on the day of surgery. Autotransfusion via the use of a cell-saver device in surgery may be possible if physicians are anticipating large blood loss (e.g., open heart surgery). The cell saver, although expensive, returns washed red blood cells to the client and decreases the risk of human immunodeficiency virus (HIV) infection and hepatitis B by using the client's own blood and has created positive outcomes in terms of length of client stay (Meeker and Rothrock, 1999).

Nursing Diagnosis

The nurse clusters patterns of defining characteristics gathered during assessment to identify nursing diagnoses for the surgical client (Box 49-3). The client with preexisting health problems is likely to have a variety of risk diagnoses. For example, a client with preexisting bronchitis who has abnormal breath sounds and a productive cough will be at risk for *ineffective airway clearance*. The nature of the surgery and the client's health status provide defining characteristics for a number of nursing diagnoses. For example, a client who undergoes a surgical procedure is at risk for developing infection at the surgical site, the IV site, or the bloodstream (sepsis). A diagnosis of *risk for infection* will require the nurse's attention from admission through convalescence.

The related factors for each diagnosis establish directions for nursing care that will be provided during one or all surgical phases. For example, the diagnosis of *risk for infection related to an invasive procedure* will require different interventions than if the related factors were *inadequate immune response*. Preoperative nursing diagnoses allow the nurse to take precautions and actions so that care provided during the intraoperative and postoperative phases is consistent with the client's needs.

Nursing diagnoses made preoperatively will also focus on the potential risks a client may face after surgery. Preventive care is essential so that the surgical client can be managed effectively. The following are common nursing diagnoses relevant to the surgical client:

- Ineffective airway clearance
- Risk for latex allergy response
- Anxiety
- Disturbed body image
- Risk for imbalanced body temperature
- Ineffective breathing pattern
- Ineffective coping
- Fear
- Risk for deficient fluid volume
- Risk for infection
- Risk for perioperative-positioning injury
- Deficient knowledge (specify)
- Impaired physical mobility
- Acute pain
- Powerlessness
- Impaired skin integrity
- Disturbed sleep pattern
- Delayed surgical recovery

Planning

During planning the nurse again synthesizes information from multiple resources (Figure 49-2). For example, knowledge pertaining to adult learning principles, coupled with the client's unique needs, will ensure a well-designed **preoperative teaching** plan. Critical think-

---

Nursing Diagnostic Process

Box 49-3

Assessment Activities	Defining Characteristics	Nursing Diagnosis
Ask client to describe previous surgical experiences.	Apprehension	Fear related to knowledge deficit and previous surgical experience
Ask client about preoperative education/preparation before admission.	Frightened	
Observe client's nonverbal behavior.	Identifies fear of surgery	
Assess vital signs.	Unaware of preoperative testing	
	Increased tension	
	Increased heart rate	

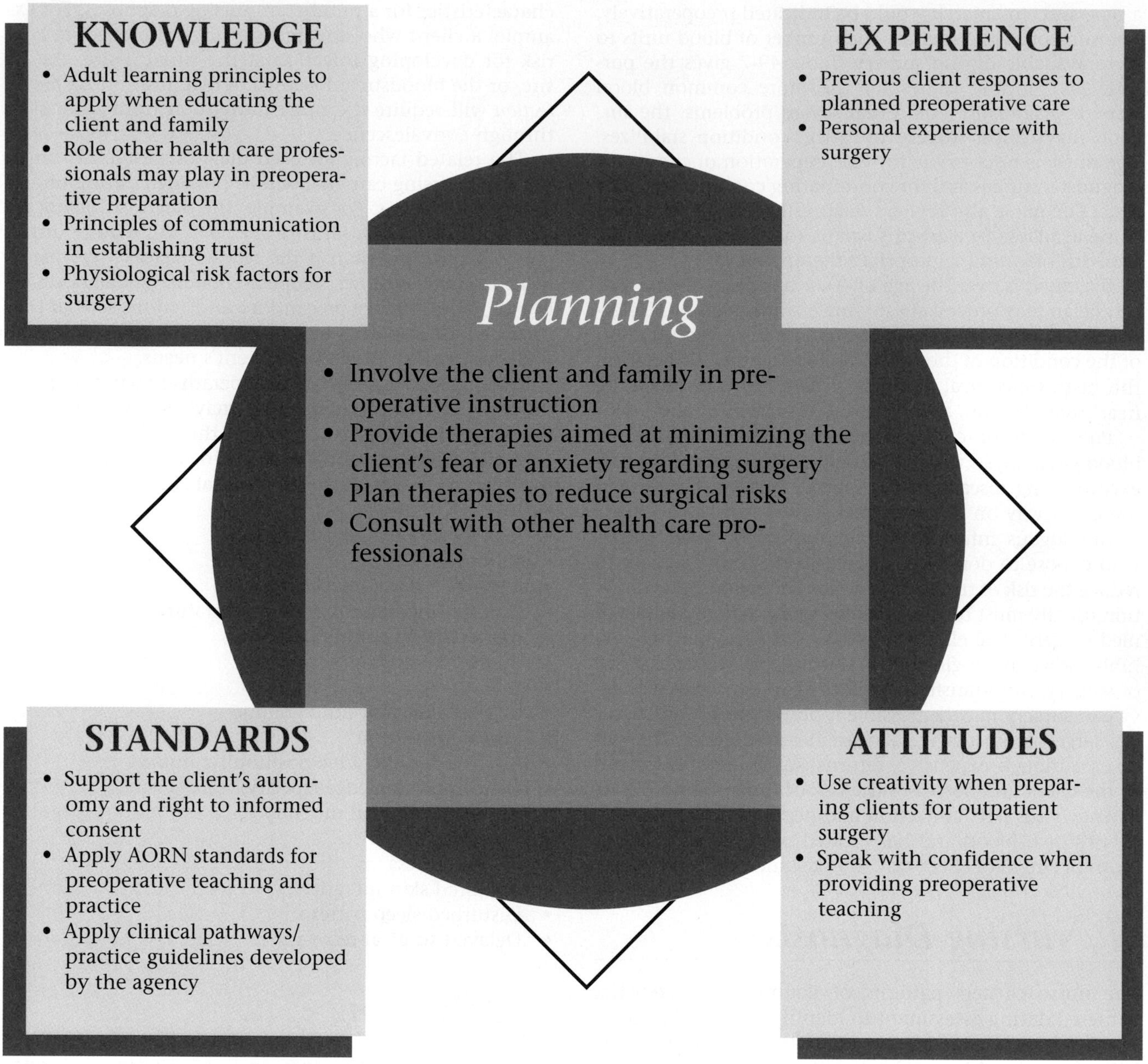

KNOWLEDGE

- Adult learning principles to apply when educating the client and family
- Role other health care professionals may play in preoperative preparation
- Principles of communication in establishing trust
- Physiological risk factors for surgery

EXPERIENCE

- Previous client responses to planned preoperative care
- Personal experience with surgery

Planning

- Involve the client and family in preoperative instruction
- Provide therapies aimed at minimizing the client's fear or anxiety regarding surgery
- Plan therapies to reduce surgical risks
- Consult with other health care professionals

STANDARDS

- Support the client's autonomy and right to informed consent
- Apply AORN standards for preoperative teaching and practice
- Apply clinical pathways/ practice guidelines developed by the agency

ATTITUDES

- Use creativity when preparing clients for outpatient surgery
- Speak with confidence when providing preoperative teaching

FIGURE **49–2** Critical thinking model for surgical client planning.

ing ensures that the client's plan of care integrates the nurse's knowledge, previous experience and established standards of care. Previous experience in caring for surgical clients helps the nurse anticipate how to approach client care (e.g., complications to prevent and anticipate and methods to reduce anxiety). Professional standards are especially important to consider when the nurse develops a plan of care. These standards often establish scientifically proven guidelines for selecting effective nursing interventions. The nurse develops an individualized plan of care for each nursing diagnosis (see care plan). The nurse and client set realistic expectations for care.

Successful planning requires the involvement of the surgical client and family in establishing the plan of care.

Early involvement of the client when developing the surgical care plan minimizes surgical risks and postoperative complications. A client informed about the surgical experience is less likely to be fearful and can prepare to participate in the postoperative recovery phase so that outcomes can be met. Diagnosis, interventions, and outcomes are established to ensure recovery or maintenance of the preoperative state.

Goals and Outcomes. The preoperative care plan is based on individualized nursing diagnoses. This plan is reviewed and modified during the intraoperative and postoperative periods. Outcomes established for each goal of care provide measurable behavioral evidence to gauge the client's progress toward meeting stated goals.

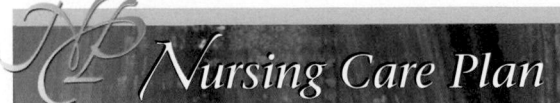

Nursing Care Plan

Perioperative Client

Assessment

Mrs. Campana is an 80-year-old client scheduled to be admitted in 5 days for elective bowel resection. Joe Marrero is the nurse in the clinic surgery service assigned to prepare Mrs. Campana for surgery. During Joe's initial discussion with Mrs. Campana, he observes her to be alert and oriented. Mrs. Campana has severely reduced visual acuity but is able to hear Joe's questions clearly.

Assessment Activities	Findings/Defining Characteristics
Ask Mrs. Campana about previous surgeries and her experience with them.	She responds, "I had surgery over 20 years ago, and I was in the hospital for 10 days."
Ask Mrs. Campana what she has been told regarding her surgery.	She states her surgeon explained the procedure with a drawing of the bowel and the location of the part to be removed.
Ask Mrs. Campana what she has been told regarding preoperative preparation and what to expect postoperatively.	She states she received information from the surgeon's office regarding medicines to stop and those she should take the morning of surgery, her diet before surgery and when to stop eating, and who to call for questions. She does not recall receiving information regarding what to expect postoperatively.
Assess Mrs. Campana's ability to read typical font type.	She is unable to read the font on the newspaper; she can read the headlines with her glasses.
Assess Mrs. Campana's family/support system for preoperative and postoperative assistance.	She states her daughter will be coming in town the day of surgery to help her after surgery.

Nursing Diagnosis: Deficient knowledge regarding preoperative and postoperative care requirements related to lack of exposure to information.

Planning

Goals	Expected Outcomes*
	Knowledge: Treatment Procedures
Client will understand the postoperative routines of surgical care by day before surgery.	Client will discuss monitoring routines following surgery by morning of surgery in the preoperative period.
	Client will be able to describe importance of postoperative exercises by morning of surgery, including turn, cough, and deep breathing, incentive spirometer, leg exercise.
	Client will be able to describe schedule for activity and nutritional management following surgery by day 1 postoperatively.
Client will participate actively in postoperative recovery activities by day 1 following surgery.	Client will successfully perform postoperative exercises by morning of surgery in the preoperative period.

Outcome classification labels from Moorhead S, Johnson M, Maas M: *Nursing outcomes classification (NOC)*, ed 3, St. Louis, 2004, Mosby.

Interventions†	Rationale
Teaching Preoperative	
• Provide client with audiotape program that explains preoperative and postoperative routines. Supply instruction booklet designed for visually impaired. Make a follow-up call to client and call the daughter to allow them the opportunity to ask questions and voice concerns. Document all phases of education provided to client in client's record, preoperative before admission, day of surgery, and postoperative.	Preadmission education can require less teaching time and better performance of exercises on admission (Rice and others, 1992). Education has a beneficial effect in reducing postoperative anxiety (Shuldham, 1999).
• On admission to hospital, demonstrate to client and daughter the performance of postoperative exercises and how to get out of bed.	Demonstration is an effective method to reinforce didactic instruction.
• Explain sensations to be expected postoperatively (e.g., incisional pain, IV, nasogastric tube, wound care).	Teaching about sensory aspects (what the client sees, feels, smells) should be structured (Shuldham, 1999).
• Give client opportunity to return demonstrate postoperative exercises before surgery.	Return demonstration measures client learning and provides opportunity to reinforce instruction.
• Correct any unrealistic expectations client or daughter may have regarding surgery.	Unrealistic expectations, when unmet, can contribute to client's anxiety. Psychological preparation for surgery reduces anxiety (Devine and Cook, 1992).

†Intervention classification labels from Dochterman JM, Bulechek GM: *Nursing interventions classification (NIC)*, ed 4, St. Louis, 2004, Mosby.

Continued

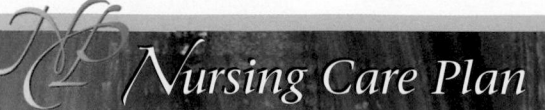

Nursing Care Plan

Perioperative Client—cont'd

Evaluation

Nursing Actions	Client Response/Finding	Achievement of Outcome
Ask client to describe typical monitoring and care activities following surgery. Document evaluation of client's understanding and demonstration of learned activities in client's record.	She is able to verbalize typical monitoring and care following surgery. She states the booklet and audiotape were both helpful.	Mrs. Campana has a good understanding of the typical postoperative course.
Observe client's demonstration of postoperative exercises.	She is able to demonstrate leg exercises and deep breathing and coughing exercises, but is having difficulty with incentive spirometer use.	Mrs. Campana is able to demonstrate most of postoperative exercises but needs further teaching and practice on incentive spirometer use.
Explore with client and daughter if they have any remaining fears or concerns.	Both Mrs. Campana and her daughter deny any fears or concerns at the present time.	Informational and psychological needs of Mrs. Campana and her daughter have been met.

The following example provides a goal of care and expected outcomes relevant for the preoperative surgical client:

- Client is able to verbalize significance of postoperative exercises.
- Client verbalizes prevention of lung congestion and pneumonia as reasons for deep breathing and coughing exercises and incentive spirometer.
- Client verbalizes promotion of blood flow to prevent leg clots as reason for postoperative leg exercises.
- Client verbalizes rationale for early ambulation as it improves lung function, assists with return of bowel function, and promotes recovery.

Setting Priorities. Using clinical judgment, the nurse prioritizes nursing diagnoses and interventions based on the assessed unique needs of each client. Clients requiring emergent surgery may experience changes in their physiological status that require the nurse to reprioritize quickly. For example, if a client's blood pressure begins to drop, hemodynamic stabilization becomes a priority over education and stress management. Generally, when the preoperative situation is more controlled, the approach to each client must be thorough and reflect an understanding of the implications of the client's age, physical and psychological health, educational level, cultural and religious practices, and stated and/or written wishes concerning advance medical directives.

Continuity of Care. For ambulatory surgery clients and clients admitted the day of their scheduled surgery, preoperative planning occurs days before admission to the hospital or surgical center. Frequently, preoperative education begins in the physician's office, continues during the scheduled preadmission testing visit, and is reinforced by the nurse the day of admission. Preoperative instruction gives the client time to think about the surgical experience, make necessary physical preparations (e.g., altering diet or discontinuing medication use), and ask

questions about postoperative procedures. The ambulatory surgical client usually returns home on the day of surgery. Thus well-planned preoperative care ensures that the client is well informed and able to be an active participant during recovery. The family or spouse can also play an active supportive role for the client.

Implementation

Preoperative nursing interventions provide the client with a complete understanding of the surgery and prepare the client physically and psychologically for surgical intervention.

Informed Consent. Surgery cannot be legally or ethically performed until a client understands the need for a procedure, the steps involved, risks, expected results, and alternative treatments. Chapter 22 discusses in detail the nurse's responsibilities for **informed consent.** It is the surgeon's responsibility to explain the procedure and obtain the informed consent. After the consent form has been completed, the nurse ensures that the form is placed in the client's medical record. The record goes to the operating room with the client.

Health Promotion. Health promotion activities during the preoperative phase focus on health maintenance, prevention of complications, and support of possible rehabilitation needs postoperatively.

Preoperative Teaching. Client education is an important aspect of the client's surgical experience. Preoperative teaching concerning a client's expected postoperative behavior, provided in a systematic and structured format with teaching and learning principles, has a positive influence on the client's recovery. Preadmission nurses may call clients up to 1 week before surgery to clarify questions and reinforce explanations. Preoperative information and instructions may include telephone calls, mailings from the physician's office or hospital, preoperative teaching guidelines and checklists, and the use of videotapes or **clinical pathways** (Figure 49-3). Lookinland and Pool (1998) found that clients who received structured education before admission had better clinical outcomes and were more satisfied. However, despite the education being provided to clients, retention of information following discharge is poor, especially in the older adult population (Bean and Waldron, 1995). Lee and others (1998) conducted postdischarge surveys of 206 clients hospitalized over a 6-week period. Results from this study indicated that continuity of care was enhanced if education was provided before, during, and after discharge. They found that half of the clients who were contacted requested additional education. Therefore it seems ideal to attempt perioperative education before admission, during the hospital stay, and after discharge. Including family members in perioperative preparation is advised. Often a family member is the coach for postoperative exercises when the client returns from surgery. If anxious relatives do not understand routine postoperative events, it is likely that their anxiety will heighten the client's fears and concerns. Perioperative preparation of family members before surgery can help to minimize anxiety and misunderstanding.

The nurse should provide clients with information about sensations typically experienced after surgery. Preparatory information helps clients anticipate the steps of a procedure and thus helps them form realistic images of the surgical experience. When events occur as predicted, clients are better able to cope and attend to the experiences. For example, in the operating room the anesthesia provider may apply ointment to clients' eyes to prevent corneal damage. Warning clients about sensations of blurred vision will reduce their anxiety on awakening from surgery. Sensations that the nurse may describe include the expected pain at the surgical site, the tightness of dressings, dryness of the mouth, or the sensation of a sore throat resulting from an endotracheal tube.

Anxiety and fear are barriers to learning, and both emotions are heightened as surgery approaches. The nurse assesses the surgical client's readiness and ability to learn. If the client is capable of and receptive to learning, the nurse presents information in a logical sequence, beginning with preoperative events and advancing to intraoperative and postoperative routines. The following standards have been established by ANA and AORN (2002d) to demonstrate client understanding of the surgical experience.

Client Cites Reasons for Preoperative Instructions and Exercises. Given a rationale for preoperative and postoperative procedures, the client is better prepared to participate in care. Every preoperative teaching program includes explanation and demonstration of postoperative exercises: diaphragmatic breathing, incentive spirometry, coughing, turning, and leg exercises. These exercises are designed to prevent postoperative complications (Skill 49-1).

If the client is measured for elastic stockings or **pneumatic compression devices,** teaching about the pur-

poses and nursing care that will be required following application is necessary (see Chapter 46).

After explaining each exercise, the nurse demonstrates it. The nurse acts as a coach, guiding the client through each exercise. For example, the nurse assesses whether the client is sitting properly and helps the client place the hands in the proper position during breathing. The nurse then allows the client time for independent practice and returns to evaluate effectiveness before surgery.

Client States the Time of Surgery. The client and family should be told the approximate time that surgery will begin. If the hospital has a busy operating room schedule, it is best to let them know how many procedures are scheduled before the client's. The surgeon usually informs the client and family of the anticipated length of surgery. Unanticipated delays may occur for many reasons. The family needs to be aware that delays occur for various reasons and does not necessarily indicate a problem.

Client States the Postoperative Unit and Location of the Family During Surgery and Recovery. The unit to which the client is admitted before surgery may be different from the postoperative unit. The family needs to know where the client will be taken after surgery. The nurse also explains where the family can wait and where the surgeon will attempt to find family members after surgery. Many institutions have implemented programs in which the circulating nurse gives periodic reports to the family in the waiting room for surgeries that are expected to be prolonged. If the client will be taken to a special unit, it helps to orient the client and family members to the unit's environment before surgery.

Client Discusses Anticipated Postoperative Monitoring and Therapies. The client and family need to know about postoperative events. If they understand the frequency of postoperative vital sign monitoring before surgery occurs, they will be less apprehensive when nurses measure vital signs. The nurse can also explain whether the client is likely to have IV lines, monitoring lines, dressings, or drainage tubes or will require ventilator support.

Client Describes Surgical Procedures and Postoperative Treatment. After the surgeon has explained the basic purpose of a surgical procedure, the client may ask the nurse additional questions to clarify misunderstandings. Preestablished teaching standards, such as those integrated in clinical pathways for preoperative and postoperative care (Figure 49-4, p. 1619), give the nurse an excellent guide for instruction. First ask what the client has been told. When the client has little or no understanding about the surgery, the physician will need to be notified to reinform the client. The nurse can augment the physician's explanations.

Client Describes Postoperative Activity Resumption. The type of surgery a client undergoes affects the speed with which normal physical activity and regular eating habits can be resumed. The nurse explains that it is normal to progress gradually in activity and eating. If the

Text continued on p. 1618

	DAY OF SURGERY— BEFORE GOING TO SURGERY	SURGICAL INTENSIVE CARE UNIT (SICU)	DAY 1 - ON PROGRESSIVE CARDIOVASCULAR UNIT (PCVU)
OBSERVATIONS & TREATMENTS	You will take your second shower with special soap before leaving home or with the nurse's help if you are in the hospital. Do not use lotions, powders, or deodorants. Put on your blood bracelet, if not already done. In the hospital, your height, weight, blood pressure, pulse, breathing rate, and temperature will be measured. You will wear a hospital gown. Give your glasses and jewelry to your family. An IV may be started in a vein in your arm.	You will come straight to the SICU after surgery. You will have several different IVs, tubes, and wires connected to various pieces of equipment. Each has a specific purpose that allows us to watch your progress closely. We will monitor your temperature, blood pressure, pulse, heart rhythm, heart function, breathing, and oxygen level. Your breathing will be controlled by a machine through a tube in your mouth until it is safe for you to breathe on your own. Tubes will drain excess fluid and blood from your chest and urine from your bladder. You may have a tube in your nose that goes into your stomach to keep it empty. You will have bandages over your incisions. Chest x-rays and blood tests will be taken as needed. Once the breathing tube is removed, you will begin your breathing exercises. We will encourage you to do a lot of deep breathing. Breathing exercises are a very important part of healing. The morning after surgery, most of the IVs, tubes, and wires will be removed and you will transfer to the PCCU.	Your blood pressure, pulse, temperature, breathing rate, and oxygen level will be checked at least every 4 hours. Your heart rhythm is constantly watched on a monitor. If you are diabetic, your blood sugar will be checked before meals and at bedtime until you go home. You will continue the breathing exercises that you started in the SICU—20 times every 2 hours. Deep breathing is very important! Some patients need other breathing treatments, which will be given by the pulmonary staff. You will be weighed every day before breakfast. Your bandages will be changed and might come off entirely today. Some drainage is normal. You will wear white elastic stockings to increase circulation and decrease swelling. They may be taken off at night while you sleep. It is important to keep your legs up on a stool (even with your hips) or up on the recliner footrest whenever you sit for more than 30 minutes.
ACTIVITY	You may be up walking until the preoperative medication is given.	After the breathing tube has been removed for a few hours, we will help you to sit on the edge of the bed. Starting the day after surgery, you will sit in the chair for meals.	You will sit in the chair for 1 hour at mealtimes. You may walk to the bathroom with help. The cardiac rehab staff will walk with you today (Step 1). The first 2 days after surgery are very busy, and your rest is very important.
DIET	You should have nothing to eat or drink.	After the breathing tube has been removed, and if you don't have any nausea, your nurse will give you clear liquids or ice chips in small amounts.	Today you will get a soft diet with small servings. It is important to eat, even if your appetite is poor. We will limit the amount of fluids that you drink to 2 quarts each day.
MEDICATIONS	One of your doctors will order a pill or shot to make you sleepy before surgery. Oxygen will be started after the medication is given.	Medications will be given to you as ordered by your doctor. Intravenous fluids and medications will be infusing as needed. You will take pain pills and other medications by mouth after the breathing tube is out.	You will be taking several different medications. Good pain control is important so you feel like doing the activity needed for recovery. Your nurse will ask you to describe your pain level on a 0-10 scale with 0 = no pain, and 10 = worst pain. It is important to take your pain medication every 3-4 hours. If you are nauseated, let your nurse know so medication can be given to help. You will have an IV in your neck or arm for medications, if needed.
EDUCATION	Preadmission patients should follow their preadmission instructions sheet. The nurses will be explaining and reinforcing information you have already heard. Please ask questions. Your family will be given directions to the waiting room. They will be notified when you have gone to the SICU.	The SICU is a busy place, and your nurse will explain noises, IVs, tubes, and equipment to you and your family. The nurses will discuss and answer any questions you or your family may have regarding your progress and plan of care. Visiting time will be discussed with you and your family. Please read the ICU visitor's brochure.	We will teach you and reinforce the following: • Proper ways to move in and out of bed • Pain control • Breathing exercises • Supporting your chest incision • 5-pound weight limit • Importance of eating • Fluid restriction You and/or your family members or visitors may attend class at 1:30 PM, Monday, Tuesday, or Wednesday each week.
GOING HOME			

FIGURE 49–3 Client instructions for a clinical pathway for coronary artery bypass graft (CABG). The first day of a 6-day pathway highlights what the client can expect the day of surgery. (Courtesy Genesis Medical Center, Davenport, Iowa.)

Skill **49-1**   *Demonstrating Postoperative Exercises*

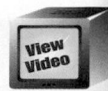

Delegation Considerations

The skill of demonstrating postoperative exercises should not be delegated to assistive personnel. However, other aspects of client care may be delegated.

- Educate AP to encourage clients to practice exercises regularly following instruction.
- Instruct AP to inform nurse if client if unwilling to perform these exercises.

Equipment

- Pillow or wrapped blanket (used to splint surgical incision during coughing)
- Incentive spirometer
- Positive expiratory pressure (PEP) device and nose clip

Steps	Rationale
1. Assess client's risk for postoperative respiratory complications. Review medical history to identify presence of chronic pulmonary conditions (e.g., emphysema, asthma), any condition that affects chest wall movement, history of smoking, and presence of reduced hemoglobin.	General anesthesia predisposes client to respiratory problems because lungs are not fully inflated during surgery; and cough reflex is suppressed, so mucus collects within airway passages. After surgery, client may have reduced lung volume and require greater efforts to cough and deep breathe; inadequate lung expansion can lead to atelectasis and pneumonia. Client is at greater risk to develop respiratory complications if other chronic lung conditions are present. Smoking damages ciliary clearance and increases mucus secretion. Reduced hemoglobin level can lead to inadequate oxygenation.
2. Assess ability to cough and deep breathe by having client take deep breath and observing movement of shoulders and chest wall. Measure chest excursion during deep breath. Ask client to cough after taking deep breath.	Reveals maximum potential for chest expansion and ability to cough forcefully; serves as baseline to measure ability to perform exercises after surgery.
3. Assess risk for postoperative thrombus formation. (Older clients, those with active cancer, and clients immobilized for more than 3 days are most at risk.) Observe for localized tenderness along the distribution of the venous system, swollen calf or thigh, calf swelling more than 3 cm compared with asymptomatic leg, pitting edema in symptomatic leg, and collateral superficial veins. If any of these signs are present, notify the physician.	Venous stasis, hypercoagulability, and vein trauma exist simultaneously for thrombus formation to occur (Lewis and others, 2000). After general anesthesia, circulation is slowed, and when rate of blood flow is slowed, there is greater tendency for clot formation. Immobilization results in decreased muscular contraction in lower extremities, which promotes venous stasis.

Critical Decision Point: A positive Homans' sign (calf pain when dorsiflexing client's foot with knee flexed) has been found to have a low specificity for deep vein thrombosis (DVT) diagnosis and often is not present or may be present when no DVT exists (Anand and others, 1998; Tick and others, 2002).

4. Assess client's ability to move independently while in bed.	Determines existence of any mobility restrictions.
5. Explain postoperative exercises to client, including importance to recovery and physiological benefits.	Information allows client to understand significance of exercises and can motivate learning. Persons tend to learn new skills when benefits can be gained.

6. Demonstrate exercises.
  A. Diaphragmatic breathing
    (1) Assist client to comfortable sitting position on side of bed or in chair or standing position.
    (2) Stand or sit facing client.
    (3) Instruct client to place palms of hands across from each other, down and along lower borders of anterior rib cage. Place tips of third fingers lightly together (see illustration). Demonstrate for client.
	Upright position facilitates diaphragmatic excursion.
	
	Allows client to observe breathing exercise.
	Position of hands allows client to feel movement of chest and abdomen as diaphragm descends and lungs expand.

Skill 49-1   *Demonstrating Postoperative Exercises—cont'd*

Steps	Rationale

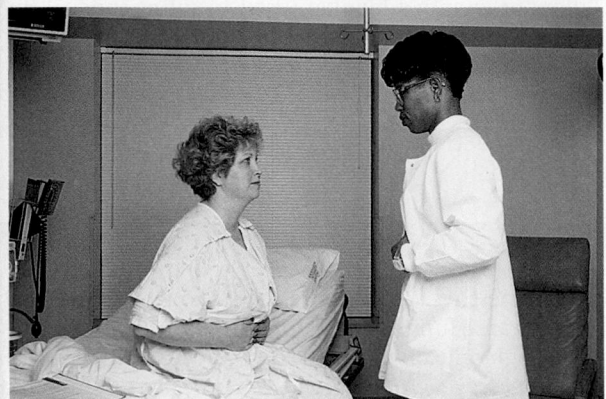

STEP **6A(3)**   Client learns how to feel proper abdominal breathing.

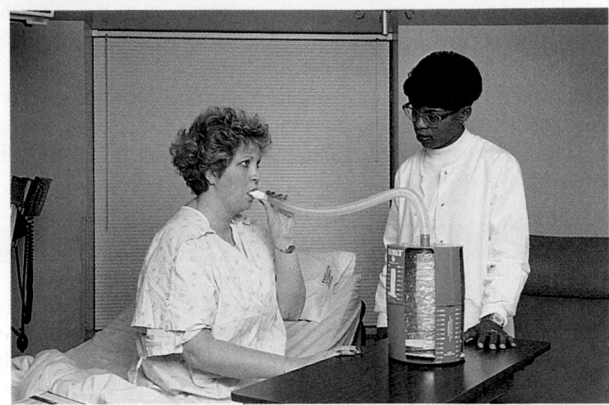

STEP **6B(4)**   Client inhales using incentive spirometer.

Steps	Rationale
(4) Have client take slow, deep breaths, inhaling through nose and push abdomen against hands. Tell client to feel middle fingers separate during inhalation. Demonstrate.	Taking slow, deep breaths prevents panting or hyperventilation. Inhaling through nose warms, humidifies, and filters air.
(5) Explain that client will feel normal downward movement of diaphragm during inspiration. Explain that abdominal organs descend and chest wall expands.	Explanation and demonstration focus on normal ventilatory movement of chest wall. Client develops understanding of how diaphragmatic breathing feels.
(6) Avoid using chest and shoulders while inhaling and instruct client in same manner.	Using auxiliary chest and shoulder muscles increases useless energy expenditure.
(7) Have client hold slow, deep breath for count of three and then slowly exhale through mouth as if blowing out a candle (pursed lips). Tell client middle fingertips will touch as chest wall contracts.	Allows for gradual expulsion of all air.
(8) Repeat breathing exercise 3 to 5 times.	Allows client to observe slow, rhythmic breathing pattern.
(9) Have client practice exercise. Instruct client to take 10 slow, deep breaths every hour while awake during postoperative period until mobile.	Repetition of exercise reinforces learning. Regular deep breathing prevents postoperative complications.

B. Incentive spirometry

Steps	Rationale
(1) Perform hand hygiene.	Reduces transmission of microorganisms.
(2) Instruct client to assume semi-Fowler's or high-Fowler's position.	Promotes optimal lung expansion during respiratory maneuver.
(3) Either set or indicate to client on the device scale, the volume level to be attained with each breath.	Establishes goal to volume level necessary for lung expansion.
(4) Demonstrate to client how to place mouthpiece of spirometer so that lips completely cover mouthpiece (see illustration).	Demonstration is reliable technique for teaching psychomotor skill and enables client to ask questions.
(5) Instruct client to inhale slowly and maintain constant flow through unit, attempting to reach goal volume. When maximal inspiration is reached, client should hold breath for 2 to 3 seconds (see illustration) and then exhale slowly. Number of breaths should not exceed 10 to 12/min each session.	Maintains maximal inspiration and reduces risk of progressive collapse of individual alveoli. Slow breath prevents or minimizes pain from sudden pressure changes in chest.
(6) Instruct client to breathe normally for short period.	Prevents hyperventilation and fatigue.

Steps	Rationale

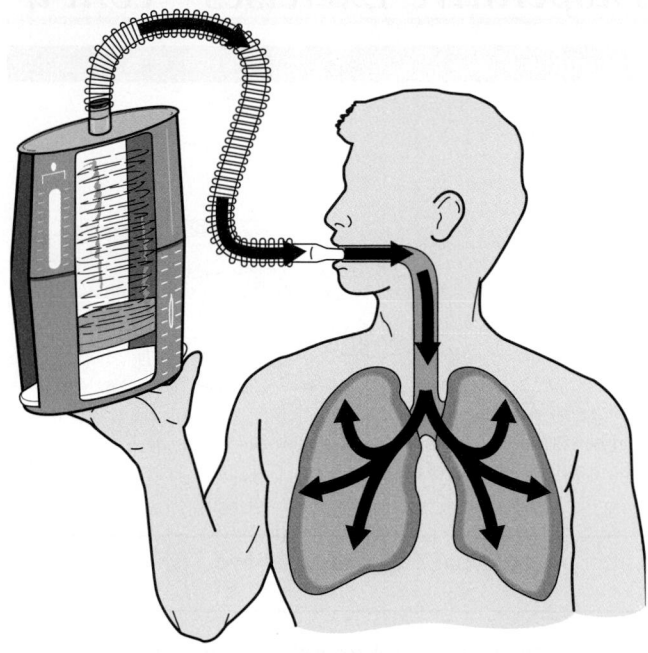

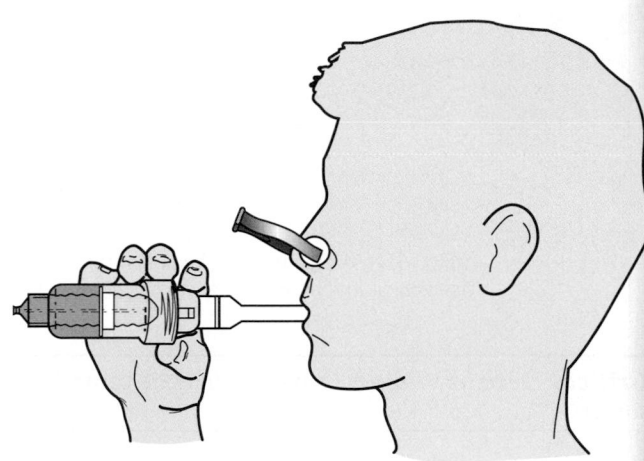

STEP **6B(5)** Incentive spirometer increase flow of air into lungs.   STEP **6C(3)** Positive expiratory pressure device.

Steps	Rationale
(7) Have client repeat maneuver until goals are achieved.	Ensures correct use of spirometer.
(8) Perform hand hygiene.	Reduces transmission of microorganisms.
C. **Positive expiratory pressure (PEP) therapy and "huff" coughing**	
(1) Perform hand hygiene.	Reduces transmission of microorganisms.
(2) Set PEP device for the setting ordered.	The higher the setting, the more effort will be required by the client. Ideally it should deliver 10 to 20 cm H_2O during passive expiration (AARC, 2002).
(3) Instruct client to assume semi-Fowler's or high-Fowler's position and place nose clip on client's nose (see illustration).	Promotes optimal lung expansion and expectoration of mucus (AARC, 2002).
(4) Have client place lips around mouthpiece. Client should take a full breath and then exhale 2 to 3 times longer than inhalation. Pattern should be repeated for 10 to 20 breaths.	Ensures that all breathing is done through the mouth and that the device is used properly.
(5) Remove device from mouth and have client take a slow, deep breath and hold for 3 seconds.	Promotes lung expansion before coughing.
(6) Instruct client to exhale in quick, short, forced exhalations or "huffs."	"Huff" coughing, or forced expiratory technique, promotes bronchial hygiene by increased expectoration of secretions.
D. **Controlled coughing**	
(1) Explain importance of maintaining upright position.	Position facilitates diaphragm excursion and enhances thorax expansion.
(2) Demonstrate coughing. Take two slow, deep breaths, inhaling through nose and exhaling through mouth.	Deep breaths expand lungs fully so that air moves behind mucus and facilitates effects of coughing.
(3) Inhale deeply third time and hold breath to count of three. Cough fully for two or three consecutive coughs without inhaling between coughs. (Tell client to push all air out of lungs.)	Consecutive coughs help remove mucus more effectively and completely than one forceful cough.

Steps	Rationale

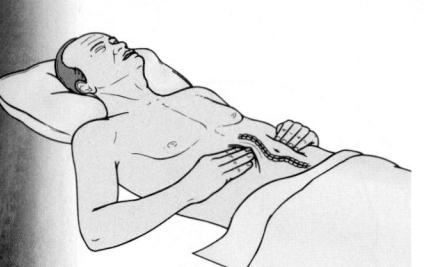 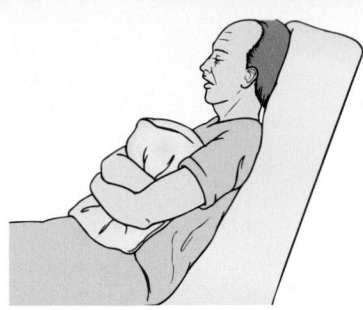 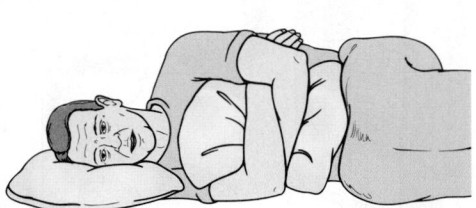

STEP **6D(5)** Techniques for splinting incision. (From Lewis S and others: *Medical-surgical nursing: assessment and management of clinical problems,* ed 5, St. Louis, 2000, Mosby.)

Critical Decision Point: Coughing may be contraindicated after brain, spinal, head, neck, or eye surgery.

---

(4) Caution client against just clearing throat instead of coughing. Explain that coughing will not cause injury to incision when done correctly.

(5) If surgical incision will be abdominal or thoracic, teach client to place one hand over incisional area and other hand on top of first. During breathing and coughing exercises, client presses gently against incisional area to splint or support it. Pillow over incision is optional (see illustration).

(6) Client continues to practice coughing exercises, splinting imaginary incision. Instruct client to cough 2 to 3 times every 2 hours while awake.

(7) Instruct client to examine sputum for consistency, odor, amount, and color changes.

E. **Turning**
(1) Instruct client to assume supine position and move to side of bed if permitted by surgery. Have client move by bending knees and pressing heels against the mattress to raise and move buttocks (see illustration). Top side rails on both sides of bed should be in up position.

(2) Instruct client to place right hand over incisional area to splint it.

(3) Instruct client to keep right leg straight and flex left knee up (see illustration). If back or vascular surgery was performed, client will need to logroll or will require assistance with turning.

Clearing throat does not remove mucus from deep in airways. Postoperative incisional pain makes it harder for the client to cough effectively.

Surgical incision cuts through muscles, tissues, and nerve endings. Deep breathing and coughing exercises place additional stress on suture line and cause discomfort. Splinting incision with hands provides firm support and reduces incisional pulling. (Some clients prefer to have pillow to place over incision.)

Value of deep coughing with splinting is stressed to effectively expectorate mucus with minimal discomfort.

Sputum consistency, odor, amount, and color changes may indicate presence of pulmonary complication, such as pneumonia.

Positioning begins on side of bed so that turning to other side will not cause client to roll toward bed's edge.

Supports and minimizes pulling on suture line during turning.

Straight leg stabilizes client's position. Flexed left leg shifts weight for easier turning.

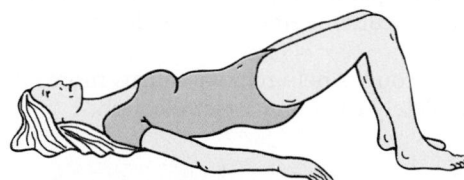 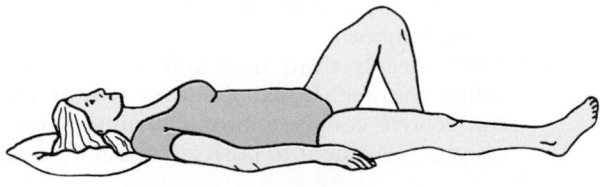

STEP **6E(1)** Buttocks lift.

STEP **6E(3)** Leg position for turning.

Steps	Rationale
(4) Have client grab right side rail with left hand, pull toward right, and roll onto right side.	Pulling toward side rail reduces effort needed for turning.
(5) Instruct client to turn every 2 hours while awake.	Reduces risk of vascular and pulmonary complications.
F. Leg exercises	
(1) Have client assume supine position in bed. Demonstrate leg exercises by performing passive range-of-motion exercises and simultaneously explaining exercise.	Provides normal anatomical position of lower extremities.
(2) Rotate each ankle in complete circle. Instruct client to draw imaginary circles with big toe (see illustration). Repeat 5 times.	Leg exercises maintain joint mobility and promote venous return to prevent thrombi.
(3) Alternate dorsiflexion and plantar flexion of both feet. Direct client to feel calf muscles contract and relax alternately (see illustrations *A* and *B*). Repeat 5 times.	Stretches and contracts gastrocnemius muscles.
(4) Perform quadriceps setting by tightening thigh and bringing knee down toward mattress, then relaxing (see illustration). Repeat 5 times.	Contracts muscles of upper legs, maintains knee mobility, and enhances venous return.
(5) Have client alternately raise each leg straight up from bed surface, keeping legs straight and then have client bend leg at hip and knee (see illustration). Repeat 5 times.	Promotes contraction and relaxation of quadricep muscles.
7. Have client practice exercises at least every 2 hours while awake. Instruct client to coordinate turning and leg exercises with diaphragmatic breathing, incentive spirometry, and coughing exercises.	Repetition of sequence reinforces learning. Establishes routine for exercises that develops habit for performance. Sequence of exercises should be leg exercises, turning, breathing, incentive spirometry, and coughing.
8. Observe client's ability to perform all five exercises independently.	Ensures that client has learned correct technique. Documents client's education and provides data for instructional follow-up.

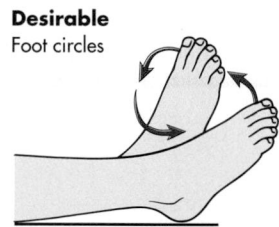

STEP **6F(2)** Foot circles. (From Lewis S and others: *Medical-surgical nursing: assessment and management of clinical problems,* ed 5, St. Louis, 2000, Mosby.)

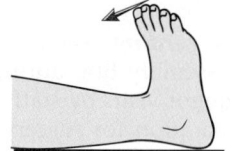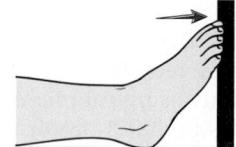

STEP **6F(3)A** Alternate dorsiflexion and plantar flexion. (From Lewis S and others: *Medical-surgical nursing: assessment and management of clinical problems,* ed 5, St. Louis, 2000, Mosby.)

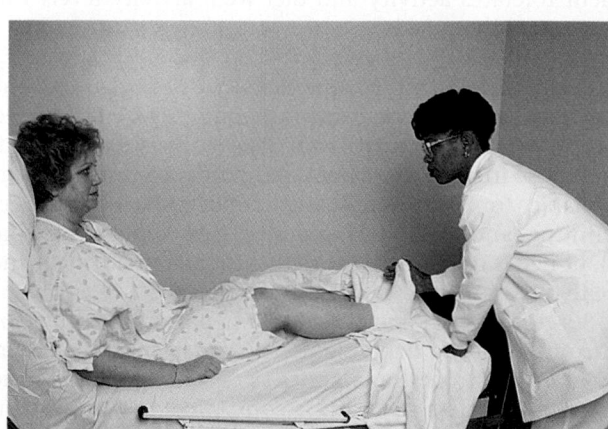

STEP **6F3B** Client pushes feet to perform plantar flexion.

Skill 49-1   *Demonstrating Postoperative Exercises—cont'd*

Steps	Rationale

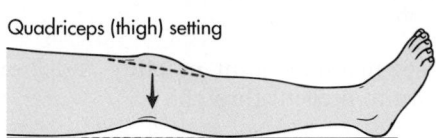

STEP **6F(4)** Quadriceps (thigh) setting. (From Lewis S and others: *Medical-surgical nursing: assessment and management of clinical problems,* ed 5, St. Louis, 2000, Mosby.)

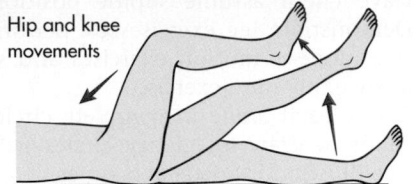

STEP **6F(5)** Hip and knee movements. (From Lewis S and others: *Medical-surgical nursing: assessment and management of clinical problems,* ed 5, St. Louis, 2000, Mosby.)

Unexpected Outcomes and Related Interventions

1. Client is unable to perform exercises correctly preoperatively.
   a. Assess for the presence of anxiety, pain, and fatigue.
   b. Teach client stress reduction techniques and/or pain management strategies.
   c. Repeat teaching using more demonstration or re-demonstration at time when family or friends are present.
2. Client is unwilling to perform exercises postoperatively because of incisional pain of thorax or abdomen (deep breathing, coughing, and turning) or because of surgery involving lower abdomen, groin, buttocks, or legs (leg exercises, turning).
   a. Instruct client to ask for pain medication 30 minutes before performing postoperative exercise or to use patient-controlled analgesia (PCA) immediately before exercising.
   b. Report to surgeon inadequate pain relief and need to change analgesic or increase dose.

Recording and Reporting

- Record exercises demonstrated and whether client can perform them independently.
- Report any problems client has in practicing exercises to nurse assigned to client on next shift for follow-up.

---

client tolerates activity and diet well, activity levels will progress more quickly.

Client Verbalizes Pain-Relief Measures. One of the surgical client's fears is pain. The family is also concerned for the client's comfort. Pain after surgery is expected. The nurse informs the client and family of interventions available for pain relief (e.g., analgesics, positioning, splinting, and relaxation exercises) (see Chapter 42). The client needs to know the schedule for analgesic drugs, the route of administration, and their effects.

Surgical clients may avoid taking pain-relief drugs for fear of becoming dependent. The nurse should encourage the client to use analgesics as needed. Explain to the client that unless the pain is controlled, it will be difficult for the client to participate in postoperative therapy. The client should be encouraged to inform nurses before the pain becomes a constant discomfort. If a client waits until pain becomes excruciating, an analgesic may not provide relief at the dose ordered. Clients who will have patient-controlled analgesia (PCA) after surgery should know how to push the button, know to push the button when beginning to feel discomfort, and

understand that use of PCA will not cause overmedication (see Chapter 42).

The client should also know the length of time that it takes for the drug to begin working. Information from preoperative pain assessment will be helpful to the nurse when teaching about pain-relief measures. Pain reporting and expectations regarding pain management based on a client's cultural beliefs are areas that need to be explored individually and systematically through research (Douglas, 1999; Ramer and others, 1999).

Client Expresses Feelings Regarding Surgery. The client may feel like part of an assembly line during the preoperative surgical phase. Frequent visits by staff, diagnostic testing, and physical preparation for surgery consume a lot of time, and the client has few opportunities to reflect on the surgical experience. The nurse recognizes the client as a unique individual. The client and family need time to express feelings about surgery. The client's level of anxiety influences the frequency of discussions. While delivering routine care, the nurse can encourage expression of concerns. The family may wish to discuss concerns without the client so that their fears will not

OPEN HEART CLINICAL PATHWAY   PROCEDURE _____
GENESIS MEDICAL CENTER, Davenport, Iowa

	PAS / Day prior to OR Date/Time	ADMISSION / Day of OR Date/Time	SICU Date Date
ASSESSMENT/ REASSESSMENT	N_____ WNL D_____ E_____ Pulm screen / protocol parameters Send old charts including cath report to PCCU Send all x-rays to OR	N_____ WNL D_____ E_____ Braden _____ Weight_____Height_____	2400_____ 2400_____ 0400_____ 0400_____ 0800_____ 0800_____ 1200_____ 1200_____ 1600_____ 1600_____ 2000_____ 2000_____ Weight _____ Notify surgeon per parameters
ACTIVITY	As Tolerated	As Tolerated	Bedrest reposition every 2 hours Dangle 5 minutes within 2 hours post extubation Up in chair post extubation, CXR / meals <u>FAST TRACK:</u> <u>Nsg</u>: Walk in place 1 minute before breakfast. Page Cardiac Rehab 15 minutes before PCCU transfer
DIET	NAS, low cholesterol then NPO midnight before surgery	NPO	NPO while intubated Open Heart Progressive Diet-ADA if diabetic
MEDICATIONS	Hold medications per physician orders	Preoperative medications per anesthesia PRN	No Atropine Central/peripheral IV (lock at transfer) Antibiotic ASA (hold if valve) Analgesic IV PRN. Add analgesic po when extubated Nitroglycerin IV, begin weaning at 0500 POD 1 Renew/start beta blockers
TESTS	PA/Lateral CXR, EKG, Comprehensive Metabolic Panel, CBC, INR, PTT, U/A, Type & Cross , 4 units RBCs PFT per protocol	Review test results and ensure availability on chart	Admission stat ABG, K+, CBC, PT/PTT, CA++, Mg, CXR 4 hour ABG, K+, CBC, CA++ \12 hour CPK 0500 ABG, CMP, CBC, & EKG 0500 daily CXR while in SICU 0500 daily INR if valve K+, ABG PRN. CBC every 4 hours PRN
TREATMENTS	DVT screen Chlorhexidine shower night before surgery	Chlorhexidine shower morning before surgery	Extubation Protocol at_____O2 Protocol PEP Therapy Protocol TEDs (Remove at hs)

INTERVENTIONS	• Discharge Planning
	• Nutritional Management
	• Preop Coordination
	• Risk Identification
	• Teaching: Preoperative
	• Teaching: Individual
	• Teaching: Procedure/ Treatment
		• Admission Care
		Discharge Planning
		• Fall Prevention
		• Infection Control
		• Nutritional Monitoring
		• Surgical Preparation
		Teaching: Individual
			• Analgesic Administration: Infection Control
			   Intraspinal • Invasive Hemodynamic
			• Autotransfusion Monitoring
			• Bleeding Precautions • Mech. Ventilation
			• Cardiac Care Weaning
			Discharge Planning • Nutritional Monitoring
			• ET Extubation • Pain Management
			Fall Prevention • Physical Restraints
			• Fl/Electrolyte Teaching :Individual
			   Management • Tube Care

TEACHING	Able to read and write ☐Y ☐N Readiness to learn barriers☐Y ☐N Other☐vision ☐hearing☐language Learns best ☐see ☐hear ☐do Initiate clinical pathway Initial Learner = Pt Method = 1:1, H/O, PAS class	Review clinical pathway Learner = Pt Method = 1:1	Review clinical pathway D___ E___ N___ D___ E___ N___ Learner = Pt. Method = 1:1
DISCHARGE PLANNING	Screen/ Notify MSS	Date_____Time_____ Transferred to OR per cart in stable condition with staff	Date_____Time_____ Transferred to PCCU per wheelchair/ambulate/bed in stable condition with staff. Day of OR 24hour I/O:_____ Transfer I/O information: Night I/O_____ Day I/O_____ Evening I/O_____
CONSULT/ OTHER	Cardiac Rehab Dietitian OR RN RT	Notify of admission Cardiologist _____ Surgeon _____ Family physician _____	Pulmonary artery line removed_____ Arterial line removed_____ Foley removed _____ MCTs removed _____ Other removed_____

Learner:		Method:
Pt = Patient	A/V	= Audio/Visual
Par = Parent	1:1	= One to One
Sp = Spouse	Demo	= Demonstrates
S.O. = Significant other	H/O	= Handouts
	P/I	= Phone Interview
	G	= Group

2

472-001   6/98   mw bn

FIGURE **49–4** Open heart clinical pathway. (Courtesy Genesis Medical Center, Davenport, Iowa.)

frighten the client and vice versa. The establishment of a trusting and therapeutic relationship with the client and family allows this to happen.

Acute Care. Acute care activities in the preoperative phase focus on interventions to physically prepare the client for surgery.

Physical Preparation. The degree of preoperative physical preparation depends on the client's health status, the surgery to be performed, and the surgeon's preferences. A seriously ill client receives more supportive care in the form of medications, IV fluid therapy, and monitoring than the client facing a minor elective procedure. The nurse explains the purpose of all procedures.

Maintenance of Normal Fluid and Electrolyte Balance. The surgical client is vulnerable to fluid and electrolyte imbalances as a result of inadequate preoperative intake or excessive fluid losses during surgery (see Chapter 40). A client traditionally took nothing by mouth (NPO) after midnight on the morning of surgery to keep the stomach empty and thus reduce the risk of vomiting and aspiration. Recommendations for preoperative fasting were published by a task force from the American Society of Anesthesiologists (ASA, 1999). Fasting from intake of a light meal or nonhuman milk for 6 or more hours, breast milk for 4 or more hours, and clear liquids for 2 to 3 hours before elective procedures requiring general anesthesia, regional anesthesia, or sedation is recommended.

Agencies vary as to the extent these guidelines have been adopted. The nurse removes fluids and solid foods from the client's bedside and posts a sign over the bed to alert hospital personnel and family members about fasting restrictions. The client may be instructed to take specific medications (e.g., anticoagulants, cardiovascular medications, and anticonvulsants, antibiotics) with a sip of water as ordered by the physician. Although the concept of preoperative fasting has changed over the past 10 years, studies demonstrate that recent guidelines have not been fully implemented and multidisciplinary improvement processes may be required (O'Callaghan, 2002; Williams, 1999).

A client who is at home the evening before surgery must understand the importance of the specific fasting period that is ordered. The nurse can allow the client to rinse the mouth with water or mouthwash and brush the teeth immediately before surgery as long as the client does not swallow water. The nurse notifies the surgeon and anesthesia provider if the client eats or drinks during the fasting period.

During surgery, normal mechanisms for controlling fluid and electrolyte balance, including respiration, digestion, circulation, and elimination, are disturbed. The surgical procedure may cause extensive losses of blood and other body fluids. The surgical stress response aggravates any fluid and electrolyte imbalance. The client's preoperative diet should include foods high in protein, with sufficient carbohydrates, fat, and vitamins. If a client cannot eat, because of gastrointestinal alterations or impairments in consciousness, an IV route for fluid replacement

is started. The physician assesses serum electrolyte levels to determine the type of IV fluids and electrolyte additives to administer. Clients with severe nutritional imbalances may require supplements with concentrated protein and glucose (see Chapter 43).

Reduction of Risk of Surgical Wound Infection. The risk of developing a surgical wound infection is determined by the amount and type of microorganisms contaminating a wound, susceptibility of the host, and the surgical wound itself. All three factors interact to cause infection. Antibiotics may be ordered in the preoperative period. A reduction in wound infection rates occurs when an antibiotic is present in sufficient concentrations at the wound site before incision (Polk and Christmas, 2000). The surgeon will order a specific time before surgery for the oral antibiotic to be taken or IV antibiotic to be administered.

The skin is a favorite site for microorganisms to grow and multiply. Without proper skin preparation, the risk of postoperative wound infection is high. Many surgeons have clients bathe or shower the evening before surgery. Some physicians may request clients to bathe or shower more than once, whereas others may have clients give special attention to cleansing the proposed operative site. This attention could include use of an antibacterial soap. Depending on the surgical procedure, a client may also shower the morning of surgery. If the surgical procedure involves the head, neck, or upper chest area, the client may also be required to shampoo the hair. Cleansing and trimming of fingernails and toenails may also be necessary.

The need for hair removal depends on the amount of hair, location of the incision, and surgical procedure planned (AORN, 2002c). Hair removal can damage and cause breaks in the client's skin, which may allow for the entry of microorganisms. If required, hair removal, preferably with a clipper or shaver, is performed as close to the time of surgery as possible. Short hospital stays are known to reduce the chance of a nosocomial infection (hospital acquired). Respiratory, urinary tract, and wound infections can all be acquired during hospitalization. This is one advantage to having ambulatory surgical procedures, because the client usually returns home when the surgery has been completed.

Prevention of Bowel and Bladder Incontinence. The client may receive a bowel preparation (e.g., a cathartic or enema) if the surgery involves the lower gastrointestinal system or lower abdominal organs. Manipulation of portions of the gastrointestinal tract during surgery results in absence of peristalsis for 24 hours and sometimes longer. Enemas and cathartics, such as GoLytely, cleanse the gastrointestinal tract to prevent intraoperative incontinence and postoperative constipation. An empty bowel reduces risk of injury to the intestines and minimizes contamination of the operative wound if a portion of the bowel is incised or opened accidentally, or if colon surgery is planned. The surgeon's order may read "give enemas until clear." This means that the nurse is to administer enemas until the enema return contains no solid fecal material (see Chapter 45). Too many enemas given over a short time, however, can cause serious fluid and electrolyte imbalances. Most agencies recommend a limit to the number of enemas (usually three) a nurse may administer successively. Potassium levels are rechecked after bowel preparation is completed.

The bladder is not prepared until the morning of surgery. The nurse instructs the client to void just before leaving for the operating room and before giving preoperative medications. An empty bladder prevents a client from being incontinent during surgery. This is important during abdominal surgery, when it may become necessary for the surgeon to manipulate the bladder. An empty bladder also makes abdominal organs more accessible during surgery. The nurse in the operating room often inserts a Foley catheter to maintain an empty bladder.

Promotion of Rest and Comfort. Rest is essential for normal healing. Anxiety about the impending surgery can easily interfere with the ability to relax or sleep. The underlying condition requiring surgery may be painful, further impairing rest.

The nurse should attempt to make the client's environment quiet and comfortable. Frequently the physician orders a sedative-hypnotic or anxiolytic agent for the night before surgery. Sedative-hypnotics (e.g., temazepam [Restoril]) affect and promote sleep. Anxiolytic agents (e.g., alprazolam [Xanax]) act on the cerebral cortex and limbic system to relieve anxiety.

An advantage to ambulatory surgery or same-day surgical admissions is that the client is able to sleep at home the night before surgery. The client is likely to get more rest in a familiar environment. The nonhospitalized client may also have medication ordered by the physician if apprehension about surgery interferes with a good night's rest.

Preparation on the Day of Surgery. The nurse completes a number of routine procedures before releasing the client for surgery.

Hygiene. Basic hygiene measures provide additional comfort before surgery. If the hospitalized client is unwilling to take a complete bath, a partial bath is refreshing and removes irritating secretions or drainage from the skin. Because the client cannot wear personal nightwear to the operating room, the nurse provides a clean hospital gown. If the client has been NPO the last several hours, the client's mouth may be very dry. The nurse may offer the client mouthwash and toothpaste, again cautioning the client not to swallow water.

Hair and Cosmetics. During surgery with the client under general anesthesia, the client's head is positioned to introduce an endotracheal tube into the airway (see Chapter 39). This procedure may involve manipulation of the client's hair and scalp. To avoid injury, the nurse asks the client to remove hairpins or clips before leaving for surgery. Hairpieces or wigs should also be removed. Long hair can be braided. The client will wear a disposable hat before entering the operating room.

During and after surgery the anesthesia provider and nurses assess skin and mucous membranes to determine the client's level of oxygenation and circulation. Therefore all makeup (lipstick, powder, blush, nail polish) should be removed to expose normal skin and nail coloring. Pulse oximetry is capable of recording accurate measurements through most nail polish colors, but removal is still considered good practice. Contact lenses, false eyelashes, and eye makeup must also be removed. The client's glasses can be given to the family immediately before the client enters the operating room.

Removal of Prostheses. It is easy for any type of prosthetic device to become lost or damaged during surgery. The client must remove all prostheses, including partial or complete dentures, artificial limbs, artificial eyes, and hearing aids. If a client has a brace or splint, the nurse checks with the physician to determine whether it should remain with the client.

For many clients it is embarrassing to remove dentures, wigs, or other devices that enhance personal appearance. Privacy should be offered as the personal items are removed. Clients may be allowed to keep personal items until they reach the preoperative area. Dentures must be placed in special containers labeled with the client's name and other identification required by the agency, for safekeeping to prevent loss or breakage. In many agencies nurses must document an inventory of all prosthetic devices or personal items and have them locked away for safekeeping according to agency policy. It is also common practice for nurses to give prostheses to family members or to keep the devices at the client's bedside. Documentation in the nursing notes, surgical checklist or per agency policy should reflect these actions.

Safeguarding Valuables. If a client has any valuables, the nurse should give them to family members or secure them for safekeeping. Many hospitals require clients to sign a release to free the institution of responsibility for lost valuables. Valuables can usually be stored and locked in a designated location. Often clients are reluctant to remove wedding rings or religious medals. A wedding band can be taped in place. However, if there is a risk that the client will experience swelling of the hand or fingers (mastectomy, hand surgery, fluid shifts), the band should be removed. Many hospitals allow clients to pin religious medals to their gowns, although the risk of loss increases. For safety, other metal items, such as for pierced areas, should also be removed. The location of valuables is documented per hospital policy.

Preparing the Bowel and Bladder. The client may require an enema or cathartic the morning of surgery to ensure that the colon is empty. If so, it should be given at least an hour before the client is scheduled to leave, allowing time for the client to defecate without rushing. The client should void before surgery. If the client is unable to void, it should be noted on the preoperative checklist. An indwelling urinary catheter may be placed if the surgery is long or the incision is in the lower abdomen.

Vital Signs. The nurse measures a final preoperative set of vital signs. The anesthesia provider uses these values as a baseline for intraoperative vital signs. If preoperative vital signs are abnormal, surgery may need to be postponed. The nurse notifies the physician of abnormalities before sending the client to surgery.

Documentation. Before the client goes to the operating room, the nurse checks the contents of the medical record to be sure that pertinent laboratory results are present. The nurse checks consent forms for accuracy of information. A preoperative checklist (Figure 49-5) provides the nurse with guidelines for ensuring completion of nursing interventions. The nurse also checks the nurse's notes to be sure that documentation of care is current. This is especially important if the hospitalized client experienced unpredicted problems the night before surgery.

Performing Special Procedures. A client's condition may warrant special interventions before surgery. The client may need IV infusions started or a nasogastric tube inserted before leaving for surgery or in the preoperative area, but this is usually done in the operating room (see Chapter 45).

Administering Preoperative Medications. The advent of ambulatory surgery has reduced the use of preoperative medications. However, the anesthesia provider or surgeon may order preanesthetic drugs ("on-call medications," "preops") to reduce the client's anxiety, the amount of general anesthesia required, the risk of nausea and vomiting and resultant aspiration, and respiratory tract secretions.

Typically the physician orders preoperative medications to be administered when the client leaves for the operating room or at an earlier prescribed time. The nurse provides all nursing care measures before giving the client preoperative medications. The consent form needs to be signed before the administration of these medications. In addition, the client should be helped to void. Because the drugs cause sedation, the client should not be allowed to leave the bed or stretcher until surgical personnel arrive to transport the client to the operating room. The client should be warned to expect drowsiness and a dry mouth.

> **Safety Alert:** Explain to the client the effects of the preoperative medications. Reinforce to the client to remain in bed or on the stretcher. The side rails should be raised and the bed or stretcher kept in the low position. The call light is placed within easy reach of the client.

Latex Sensitivity/Allergy. As the incidence and prevalence of **latex sensitivity** and allergy increases, the need for recognition of potential sources of latex is extremely critical. Federal regulations enacted in September 1998 mandate that all medical supplies contain a label notifying the consumer of the latex content (Doepke, 1998).

The operating room and postanesthesia care unit (PACU) contain innumerable products that contain latex. Some common sources include gloves, IV tubing, syringes, and rubber stoppers on bottles and vials. Latex is also present in objects that may be overlooked, including adhesive tape, disposable electrodes, endotracheal tube cuffs, protection sheets, and ventilator equipment. Those

most at risk include persons with genetic predisposition to latex allergy, children with spina bifida, clients with urogenital abnormalities or spinal cord injury (because of a long history of catheter use), clients with a history of multiple surgeries, health care professionals, and workers who manufacture rubber products (Paquet, 1998).

Signs and symptoms of a latex reaction can include local effects ranging from urticaria and flat or raised red patches to vesicular, scaling, or bleeding eruptions. Acute dermatitis may also be present. Rhinitis and/or rhinorrhea are other common reactions in both mild and severe latex reactions. Immediate hypersensitivity reactions can be life threatening, with the client exhibiting focal or generalized urticaria, edema, bronchospasm, and mucous hypersecretion, which can compromise respiratory status. Vasodilation compounded by increased capillary permeability can lead to circulatory collapse and eventual death. Because the client may be draped during surgery, any unexplained acute deterioration in a previously healthy client should be investigated for possible latex allergy (Shoup, 1998).

The American Association of Nurse Anesthetists (AANA) has developed a protocol to provide safe, competent care to the client identified as being at risk for latex allergy (AANA, 1995). A latex allergy cart should be available at all times. All of the contents must be latex free. A reference binder is kept with the cart that indicates supplies, medications, and appropriate care options for latex-sensitive clients. It is recommended that the client with a latex allergy be scheduled as the first case of the day in the operating room. The room should be thoroughly cleaned, including all equipment, and all unnecessary items removed (Doepke, 1998). The client can then be safely accommodated by using appropriate latex-free items during the perioperative period and recovery. Box 49-4 is an example of a nursing care plan for latex precautions.

Eliminating Wrong Site and Wrong Procedure Surgery. Because of errors made in the past with clients undergoing the wrong surgery or having surgery performed on the wrong site, the Joint Commission on Accreditation of Healthcare Organizations (JCAHO, 2004) has instituted guidelines for preventing such mishaps. Whenever an invasive surgical procedure is to be performed, the nurse and surgeon must be sure the site has been marked by the surgeon (see agency policy). Indelible ink is used to mark left and right distinction, multiple structures (e.g., fingers), and levels of the spine. If the client refuses a mark, the nurse notes such on the procedure checklist. The nurse also verifies the client and the procedure to be performed. In addition, once the client reaches the operating room, a "Time Out" is required. A "Time Out" is conducted just before starting the procedure. All members of the operative team must be present. During the "Time Out" the client is again identified along with the side and site.

Evaluation

Client Care. The admitting nurse and the nurse in the preoperative area will be the source for evaluating outcomes in the preoperative period (Figure 49-6). With regard to the preoperative client's plan of care, limited time

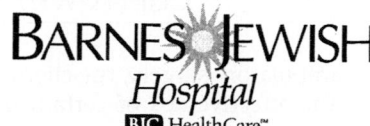

SURGICAL/PROCEDURE CHECKLIST
Complete this side for inpatients & outpatients
having any invasive procedure

Please check (✔) the appropriate box (☐) and fill in the blank(s) as needed.

ADDRESSOGRAPH

Date of Procedure: _____ Type of Procedure: _____

Off Floor Reports printed and placed in chart: ☐ Yes ☐ No ☐ N/A: _____

ITEM	Yes/Initials	NA	COMMENT	Date
Face sheet in chart				
Consent to Surgery or Other Procedure signed			☐ To be signed in treatment area.	
SPECIALTY Consent signed			☐ To be signed in treatment area. (Specify)	
Transfusion consent signed				
ID Band on				
Allergies Noted: ☐ Armband ☐ Front of Chart ☐ Medication Record				
Height & Weight documented				
Dentures, eyeglasses, contact lenses, nail polish, hairpins, prosthesis, jewelry removed				
Surgical/Procedural skin prep done				
Patient in hospital gown/pajamas				
Patient has been NPO since: _____				
Voided or catheterized				
Vital Signs taken and documented				
Patient is on Isolation			(Specify)	
History & physical in chart				
Lab work in chart (Printed Off Floor reports)				
Urinalysis in chart				
EKG in chart				
Chest X-ray (done if ordered)				
Change in condition/VS reported to:				
Valuables/Inventory checklist done				
Pre-Operative meds given:				
Addressograph plate in chart				
Patient transferred to Surgical/Procedure area in HIS				
Mode of travel: ☐ Amb ☐ W/C ☐ Stretcher ☐ Bed				
Operative Site Marked			☐ Site to be marked in holding area	
Case Cancelled				

Family contact during surgery:

Name: _____ Location: _____ Phone: _____

INITIALS	SIGNATURES	INITIALS	SIGNATURES

BJ 2-3343-465 V15 (07/03) Page 1 of 2 TAB: TREATMENT

DO NOT WRITE BELOW THIS LINE

BJ 2-3343-465

FIGURE 49–5 Preoperative checklist. (Courtesy Barnes Jewish Hospital, St. Louis.)

Box 49-4

Evidence-Based Practice Guideline

Latex Precautions

1. Survey the client care area and remove products containing latex (e.g., exam gloves, rubber sheets, or blood pressure cuff).
2. Place a latex precautions label on the client's chart and latex precautions signs on the door to the client's room and/or transport cart.
3. Use only non-latex gloves. Order an adequate supply.
4. Review supplies to be used for the client, and substitute with latex-free supplies.
5. Review medications to be administered and verify that they are latex-free. Include the following steps:
   a. Notify pharmacy of need for latex precautions.
   b. Verify that all prescribed medications are latex-free.
   c. Place a sign in area where medications (including mixing solutions) are kept, indicating that the client is on latex precautions.
   d. Use latex-free syringes.
6. Review intravenous supplies to be used and verify that they are latex-free. Include the following steps:
   a. Use latex-free solutions.
   b. Use latex-free tubing, buretrols.
   c. Use latex-free syringes, including those for patient-controlled analgesia.
   d. Use latex-free tape.
7. Verify that bedding and support garments are latex-free (e.g., mattress protectors, antiembolism stockings, and binders).
8. Verify that dressings and tape are latex-free.
9. Notify family and visitors of the use of latex precautions.
10. Routinely survey the client care area and verify latex products are not present (e.g., examination gloves, balloons).
11. Before transfer to another area or agency, notify care providers of need for latex precautions.
12. Education programs about latex allergy should be provided to health care providers, clients, and family or caregivers. This education should include the following:
    a. Definition of latex allergy
    b. Exposures to latex
    c. Latex avoidance
    d. Signs and symptoms of a reaction to latex
    e. Emergency treatment of a reaction to latex

Modified from Steelman, V.M., Titler, M.G (1997). Evidence-based protocol: latex precautions. In M.G. Titler (Series Ed.), Series on Evidence-Based Practice for Older Adults. Iowa City, IA. The University of Iowa College of Nursing Gerontological Nursing Interventions Research Center, Research Dissemination Core. For more information, http:// www.nursing.uiowa.edu/center/gnirc/disseminatecore.htm.

is available to evaluate the outcomes. The client's current status is compared with expected outcomes to determine whether new or revised interventions and/or nursing diagnoses need to be implemented.

Interventions continue during and after surgery, so that evaluation of many goals and outcomes do not occur until after surgery. For example, the nurse will not be able to evaluate the success of reducing postoperative wound infection or promoting return of normal physiological function until a few days after surgery. If the client is having ambulatory surgery, the client will return home; therefore the effectiveness of certain interventions may not be easily evaluated.

Client Expectations. It may be difficult to determine whether the client's expectations have been met regarding preoperative teaching. The nurse is evaluating the client in a "hurried" atmosphere, because there are many things that need to be accomplished in a short amount of time. The client's surgery may be an emergency, or performance of various procedures may make it difficult for the nurse to find time for evaluation. The client may feel somewhat depersonalized by the need to complete tasks. It is important that the nurse remember to attend to the personal needs (privacy, fear, anxiety) of the client, as well as the tasks at hand. The client should be given an opportunity to state whether expectations have been met. If expectations are unmet, the nurse will need to work closely with the client to redefine expectations that can be realistically met within the time limits imposed by this particular setting.

Transport to the Operating Room

Personnel in the operating room notify the nursing division or ambulatory surgery area when it is time for surgery. In many hospitals a nursing orderly or transporter brings a stretcher for transporting the client. The transporter checks the client's identification bracelet against the client's chart to be sure that the right person is going to surgery. Because the client may have received preoperative drugs, the nurses and transporter assist the client in transferring from bed to stretcher to prevent falls. The ambulatory surgery client may ambulate to the operating room if able and not medicated. Provide the family an opportunity to visit before the client is transported to the operating room. Nurses then direct the family to a waiting area. In some hospitals the family may be allowed to wait with the client in the operating room holding area until he or she is transported into the operating room.

After the client leaves the nursing division, the nurse prepares the bed and room for the client's return if the client is returning to the same nursing division. The nurse will be better prepared to care for the client after surgery if the room is readied before the client's return.

A postoperative bedside unit should include the following:

1. Sphygmomanometer, stethoscope, and thermometer
2. Emesis basin
3. Clean gown
4. Washcloth, towel, and facial tissues
5. IV pole
6. Suction equipment (if needed)
7. Oxygen equipment (if needed)
8. Extra pillows for positioning the client comfortably
9. Bed pads to protect bed linen from drainage
10. Bed raised to stretcher height with bed linens pulled back and furniture moved to accommodate the stretcher and equipment (such as IV lines)

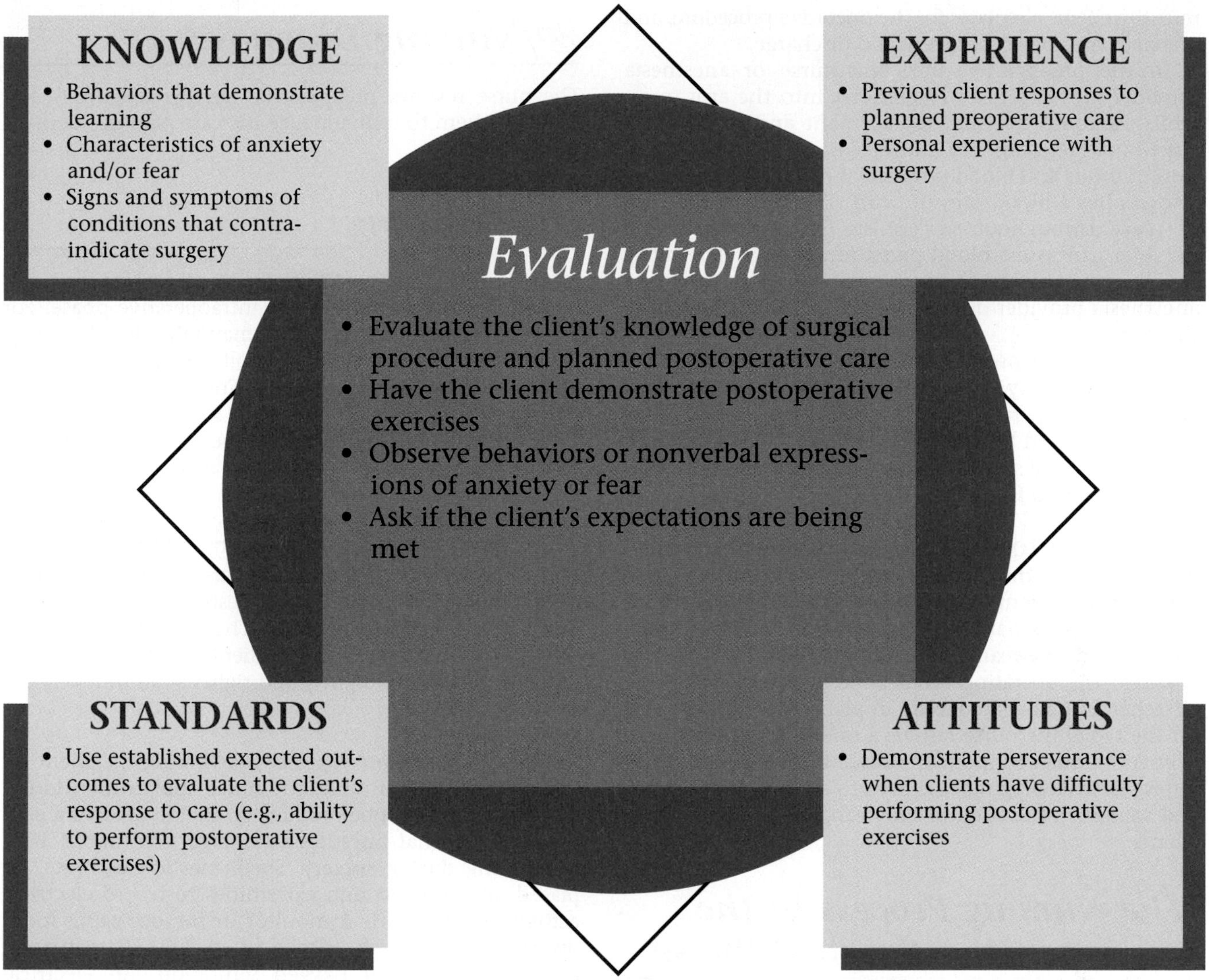

KNOWLEDGE

- Behaviors that demonstrate learning
- Characteristics of anxiety and/or fear
- Signs and symptoms of conditions that contra-indicate surgery

EXPERIENCE

- Previous client responses to planned preoperative care
- Personal experience with surgery

Evaluation

- Evaluate the client's knowledge of surgical procedure and planned postoperative care
- Have the client demonstrate postoperative exercises
- Observe behaviors or nonverbal express-ions of anxiety or fear
- Ask if the client's expectations are being met

STANDARDS

- Use established expected out-comes to evaluate the client's response to care (e.g., ability to perform postoperative exercises)

ATTITUDES

- Demonstrate perseverance when clients have difficulty performing postoperative exercises

FIGURE **49–6** Critical thinking model for surgical client evaluation.

Intraoperative Surgical Phase

Care of the client during surgery requires careful prepara-tion and knowledge of the events that occur during the surgical procedure. The nurse usually functions in one of two roles in the operating room: circulating nurse or scrub nurse. The **circulating nurse** must be an RN. Responsibilities of the circulating nurse include review of the preoperative assessment, establishing and imple-menting the intraoperative plan of care, evaluating the care, and providing for continuity of care postoperatively. The circulating nurse assists with procedures as needed such as endotracheal intubation and blood administra-tion. In addition, this nurse monitors sterile technique and a safe operating room environment, assists the sur-geon and surgical team by operating nonsterile equip-ment, provides additional supplies, verifies sponge and instrument counts and maintains accurate and complete written records.

The **scrub nurse** may be an RN, a licensed practical nurse, or a surgical technician. This nurse maintains a sterile field during the surgical procedure, assists with ap-plying sterile drapes, hands the surgeons the instruments and other sterile supplies and counts the sponges and instruments.

Preoperative (Holding) Area

In most hospitals the client enters a holding area, also known as the preanesthesia care unit or presurgical care unit (PSCU), outside the operating room. The nurse ex-plains the steps to be taken in preparing the client for surgery, verifies appropriate data has been obtained, as-sesses a client's readiness both physically and emotion-ally and reinforces teaching (Sullivan, 2000). Nurses in the holding area are members of the operating room staff and wear surgical scrub suits, hats, and footwear in ac-cordance with infection-control policies. In some ambu-latory surgical settings a perioperative primary nurse admits the client, circulates for the operative procedure, and manages the client's recovery and discharge.

In the preoperative area the nurse or anesthesia provider may insert an IV catheter into the arm to establish a route for fluid replacement and IV drugs. A large-bore (18 gauge) IV catheter is used for easy infusion of fluids and blood products if necessary. The nurse also applies a blood pressure cuff. The cuff will remain in place throughout surgery so that the anesthesia provider can assess blood pressure readings. The nurse usually reviews the preoperative checklist, and the anesthesia provider may perform a client assessment at this time.

Because of the preoperative medications, the client begins to feel drowsy. The temperature in the holding area and adjacent operating room suites is usually cool, and the client should be offered an extra blanket. Conscious sedation may be started at this time. The client's stay in the holding area is usually brief.

Admission to the Operating Room

Nurses transfer the client to the operating room via a stretcher. The client is usually still awake and will notice nurses and physicians wearing complete surgical masks, gowns, and eyewear. The staff carefully transfers the client to the operating room table, being sure that the stretcher and table are locked in place. After the client is on the table, the nurse fastens a safety strap around the client. The nurse supports the client by explaining procedures and encouraging the client to ask questions. Sights and sounds in the surgical suite can seem frightening to clients.

The Nursing Process in the Intraoperative Surgical Phase

ℵℙ*Assessment*

In the PSCU, the nurse conducts a focused preoperative assessment to verify the client is ready for surgery and to plan intraoperative care. Because clients will not be able to speak for themselves while under general anesthesia, this preoperative assessment in the operating room is important for the client's safety.

> *Safety Alert:* Verification of client name by client response compared to chart and arm band is completed. This is done before sedation. The chart is reviewed for consent forms, allergies, medical history, physical assessment findings, and test results. The nurse verifies with the client the planned surgical procedure and the surgical site before anesthesia is administered. Some agencies have the client mark the surgical site. The nurse ensures that prosthetic devices and valuables have been removed.

Review of the preoperative care plan to establish an intraoperative care plan is performed, and the nurse observes the client's psychological comfort during this assessment.

ℵℙ*Nursing Diagnosis*

The nurse reviews preoperative nursing diagnoses and modifies them to individualize the care plan in the operating room.

ℵℙ*Planning*

Goals and Outcomes. Client-centered outcomes of preoperative care extend into the intraoperative phase. For example, a goal would be to maintain skin integrity. Expected outcomes include the following:
- Client will have intact skin and show no signs of redness.
- Client will be free of burns at the grounding pad.

ℵℙ*Implementation*

A primary focus of intraoperative care is to prevent injury and complications related to anesthesia, surgery, positioning, and equipment used. The perioperative nurse serves as an advocate for the client during surgery and protects the client's dignity and rights at all times.

Acute Care
Physical Preparation. After safely securing the client on the operating room table, the nurse applies monitoring devices to the client before surgery. Clients receiving general and regional anesthesia undergo continuous ECG monitoring during surgery. Small plastic electrodes are placed on the chest and extremities to record electrical activity of the heart. A monitor in the operating room displays the heart's electrical activity. Pulse oximetry will be used to monitor oxygen saturation. An electrical cautery grounding pad is applied to the skin. **Antiembolism stockings** may be applied intraoperatively (especially for long cases) or postoperatively according to agency policy (see Chapter 46). The nurse documents device application, capillary refill, and client tolerance to procedures.

Introduction of Anesthesia. Clients undergoing surgical procedures receive one of four types of anesthesia: general, regional, local, or conscious sedation.
General Anesthesia. Modern anesthetic agents are much easier to reverse and allow the client to recover with fewer untoward effects. **General anesthesia** results in an immobile, quiet client who does not recall the surgical procedure. The client's amnesia acts as a protective measure from the unpleasant events of the procedure. An anesthesia provider gives general anesthetics by IV and inhalation routes through the three phases of anesthesia: induction, maintenance, and emergence. Surgery requiring general anesthesia involves major procedures with extensive tissue manipulation or during a procedure when analgesia, muscle relaxation, immobility, and control of the autonomic nervous system are desired.

Induction includes the administration of agents and endotracheal intubation. The maintenance phase includes positioning the client, preparation of the skin for incision, and the surgical procedure itself. Appropriate levels of anesthesia are maintained during this phase. During emergence, anesthetics are decreased and the client begins to awaken. Because of the short half-life of today's medications, emergence often occurs in the operating room.

The duration of anesthesia depends on the length of surgery. The greatest risks from general anesthesia are the side effects of anesthetic agents, including cardiovascular depression or irritability, respiratory depression, and liver and kidney damage.

Regional Anesthesia. Induction of **regional anesthesia** results in loss of sensation in an area of the body. The method of induction influences the portion of sensory pathways that are anesthetized. No loss of consciousness occurs with regional anesthesia, but the client may be sedated. The anesthesia provider gives regional anesthetics by infiltration and local application. Administration techniques include nerve blocks and spinal or epidural anesthesia, and intravenous regional anesthesia.

Risks are involved with infiltrative anesthetics, particularly in the case of spinal anesthesia. Because the level of anesthesia may rise, which means that the anesthetic agent moves upward in the spinal cord, breathing may be affected. This migration of anesthetic depends on the drug type, amount, and client position. If the level of anesthesia rises, respiratory paralysis may develop, requiring resuscitation. Elevation of the upper body prevents respiratory paralysis. The client may have a sudden fall in blood pressure, which results from extensive vasodilation caused by the anesthetic block to sympathetic vasomotor nerves and pain and motor nerve fibers. The client requires careful monitoring during and immediately after surgery.

Because the client is responsive and capable of breathing voluntarily, it is unnecessary for the anesthesia provider to use an endotracheal tube. Operating room personnel often gain a false sense of security because of the client's relative alertness. Nurses must remember that burns and other trauma can occur on the anesthetized part of the body without the client being aware of the injury. It is therefore necessary to frequently observe the position of extremities and the condition of the skin.

Local Anesthesia. **Local anesthesia** involves loss of sensation at the desired site (e.g., a growth on the skin or the cornea of the eye). The anesthetic agent (e.g., lidocaine) inhibits nerve conduction until the drug diffuses into the circulation. It may be injected locally or applied topically. The client experiences a loss in pain and touch sensation, and in motor and autonomic activities (e.g., bladder emptying). Local anesthesia is commonly used for minor procedures performed in ambulatory surgery. Physicians may infiltrate the operative area with local anesthetics to promote postoperative pain relief.

Conscious Sedation. **Conscious sedation** is routinely used for procedures that do not require complete anesthesia but rather a depressed level of consciousness. A client under conscious sedation must independently retain a patent airway and airway reflexes and be able to respond appropriately to physical and verbal stimuli (Litwack, 1999). Short-acting intravenous sedatives, such as midazolam, are given.

Advantages of conscious sedation include adequate sedation and reduction of fear and anxiety with minimal risk, amnesia, relief of pain and noxious stimuli, mood alteration, elevation of pain threshold, enhanced client cooperation, stable vital signs, and rapid recovery. A variety of diagnostic and therapeutic procedures are appropriate for conscious sedation (burn dressing changes, some cosmetic surgery, pulmonary biopsy and bronchoscopy, colonoscopy, and many others) (Litwack, 1999).

Nurses assisting with the administration of local anesthesia and conscious sedation must demonstrate competency in the care of these clients. Knowledge of anatomy, physiology, cardiac dysrhythmias, procedural complications, and pharmacological principles related to the administration of individual agents is essential. Nurses must also be able to assess, diagnose, and intervene in the event of untoward reactions and demonstrate skill in airway management and oxygen delivery. Resuscitation equipment must be readily available when local anesthesia or conscious sedation is used (AORN, 2002b).

Positioning the Client for Surgery. During general anesthesia the nursing personnel and surgeon often do not position the client until the stage of complete relaxation is achieved. The choice of position is usually determined by the surgical approach. Ideally the client's position provides good access to the operative site and sustains adequate circulatory and respiratory function. It should not impair neuromuscular structures. The client's comfort and safety must be considered.

Normal range of joint motion is maintained in an alert person by pain and pressure receptors. If a joint is extended too far, pain stimuli provide a warning that muscle and joint strain is too great. In a client who is anesthetized, normal defense mechanisms cannot guard against joint damage, muscle stretch, and strain. The muscles are so relaxed that it is relatively easy to place the client in a position the individual normally could not assume while awake. The client often remains in a given position for several hours. Although it may be necessary to place a client in an unusual position, the nurse should attempt to maintain correct alignment and protect the client from pressure, abrasion, and other injuries. Attachments to the operating room table allow protection and padding of extremities and bony prominences. Positioning should not impede normal movement of the diaphragm or interfere with circulation to body parts. If restraints are necessary, the nurse pads the area to be restrained to prevent skin trauma.

Documentation of Intraoperative Care. During the intraoperative phase the nursing staff continues the preoperative care plan. For example, strict asepsis must be followed to minimize the risk of surgical wound infection. IV fluid infusion and monitoring of urinary and nasogastric output are actions the nurse takes to maintain fluid balance. Throughout the surgical procedure the nurse keeps an accurate record of client care activities and procedures performed by operating room personnel. Documentation of intraoperative care provides useful data for the nurse who cares for the client postoperatively.

𝒩𝒫 Evaluation

Interventions implemented during the intraoperative phase are evaluated throughout the surgical procedure.

Client Care. The nurse performs intraoperative evaluation of the client. Vital signs and intake and output are continuously monitored. The client's body temperature during the procedure and on completion of the surgical procedure is measured. The skin is inspected under the grounding pad and at areas where pressure from positioning may have been exerted.

Client Expectations. For clients not undergoing general anesthesia, the nurse frequently questions them regarding pain, numbness, perceived room temperature, and overall comfort. The circulating nurse provides updates to family members in the waiting room.

Postoperative Surgical Phase

After surgery a client's care can become complex as a result of physiological changes that may occur. Clients who have undergone general anesthesia are more likely to face complications than those who have had only local anesthesia or conscious sedation. The client who requires general anesthesia usually has undergone extensive surgery as well. In contrast, an ambulatory surgical client who has had local anesthesia with no sedation and has stable vital signs may be immediately discharged. A client who has undergone regional or general anesthesia usually is transferred to the postanesthesia care unit (PACU) to be stabilized before discharge, whereas a client who has had local anesthesia may go directly to the nursing unit or back to the ambulatory surgery center.

To assess a client's postoperative condition, the nurse applies critical thinking while relying on information from the preoperative nursing assessment, knowledge regarding the surgical procedure performed, and events occurring during surgery. This information helps the nurse to detect any change and make decisions about the client's care. A variation from the client's norm may indicate the onset of surgically related complications. Along with the anesthesia provider, the circulating nurse may accompany the client to the PACU and report to the nurse to provide continuity of care.

A client's postoperative course involves two phases: the immediate recovery period and postoperative convalescence. For an ambulatory surgical client, recovery normally lasts only 1 to 2 hours, and **convalescence** occurs at home. For a hospitalized client, recovery may last a few hours, and convalescence occurs over 1 or more days depending on the extent of surgery and the client's response.

Immediate Postoperative Recovery

Before the arrival of the client in the PACU, the PACU nurse obtains data from the surgical team in the operating room regarding the client's general status and need for special equipment and nursing care. Careful planning allows the nursing staff to consider placement of clients

in the PACU. For example, clients who undergo spinal anesthesia are aware of their surroundings and may benefit from being in a quieter part of the PACU, away from clients needing frequent monitoring. The client with a serious infection such as tuberculosis should be isolated from other clients. Standard precautions for infection control (see Chapter 33) are used for all clients.

When the client is admitted to the PACU, the personnel notify the client care area of the client's arrival. This allows the nursing staff to inform family members. The nurse usually advises family members to remain in the designated waiting area so that they can be found when the surgeon arrives to explain the client's condition. *It is the surgeon's responsibility to describe the client's status, the results of surgery, and any complications that may have been encountered.* The nurse can be a valuable resource to the family if complications have arisen in the operative phase.

When the client enters the PACU (Figure 49-7), the nurse and members of the surgical team confer about the client's status. The surgical team's report includes a review of anesthetic agents administered so that the PACU nurse can anticipate how quickly a client should regain consciousness and to anticipate analgesic needs. A report on IV fluids or blood products administered during surgery alerts the nurse to the fluid and electrolyte balance. The surgeon often reports special concerns (e.g., whether the client is at risk for hemorrhaging or infection). The operating room nurse or anesthesia provider discusses whether there were complications during surgery, such as excessive blood loss or cardiac irregularities. Frequently this report takes place while PACU nurses are admitting the client. The nurse will attach the client to monitoring equipment such as the noninvasive blood pressure monitor, ECG monitor, and pulse oximeter. Clients often receive some form of oxygen in this immediate recovery period.

After reviewing events in the operating room, the PACU nurse makes a complete assessment of the client's status. The assessment should be performed rapidly and thoroughly and be targeted to the needs of the postsurgical client. The standards of care of the American Society of PeriAnesthesia Nurses (ASPAN, 2002) outline the urgent nature and components of the admission assessment. A systems approach to assessment is discussed in a later section outlining the nursing process in postopera-

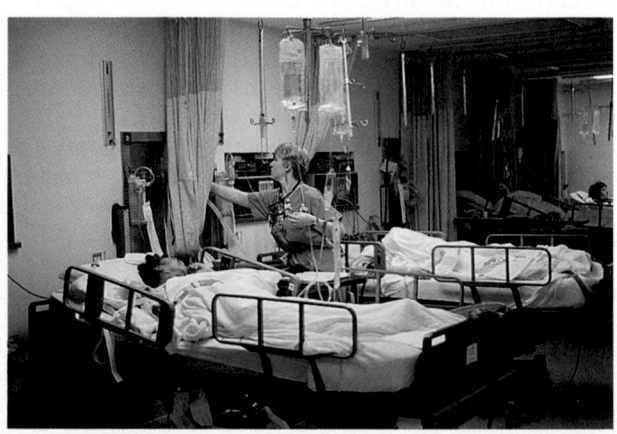

FIGURE **49–7** Postanesthesia care unit.

tive care. Nursing care in the PACU focuses on monitoring and maintaining respiratory, circulatory, and neurological status and on managing pain.

Discharge From the Postanesthesia Care Unit

The nurse evaluates readiness for discharge from the PACU on the basis of vital sign stability in comparison with the preoperative data. Other outcomes for discharge include body temperature control, good ventilatory function, orientation to surroundings, absence of complications, minimal pain and nausea, controlled wound drainage, adequate urine output, and fluid and electrolyte balance. Clients with more extensive surgery requiring anesthesia of longer duration usually recover more slowly. Many PACU staffs use an objective scoring system that helps delineate when clients may be discharged. The Aldrete score, or the **Postanesthesia Recovery Score (PARS),** is the most widely used scoring tool (Table 49-8). The client must receive a composite score of 8 to 10 before discharge from the PACU (Aldrete, 1998). If the client's condition is still poor after 2 to 3 hours, the stay lengthens or the surgeon may transfer the client to an intensive care unit (ICU).

When the client is ready to be discharged from the PACU, the nurse calls the nursing unit to report vital signs, the type of surgery and anesthesia performed, blood loss, level of consciousness, general physical con-

Table 49-8		Modified Aldrete Score								
			Admission	5 Min	15 Min	30 Min	45 Min	60 Min	Discharge
Able to move four extremities voluntarily or on command	2	Activity							
Able to move two extremities voluntarily or on command	1								
Unable to move extremities voluntarily or on command	0								
Able to breathe deeply and cough freely	2	Respiratory							
Dyspnea or limited breathing	1								
Apneic	0								
BP 20% of preanesthetic level	2	Circulation							
BP 20%-49% of preanesthetic level	1								
BP 50% of preanesthetic level	0								
Fully awake	2	Consciousness							
Arousable on calling	1								
Not responding	0								
Able to maintain O₂ saturation 92% on room air	2	O₂ saturation							
Needs O₂ inhalation to maintain O₂ saturation 90%	1								
O₂ saturation 90% even with O₂ supplement	0								
		TOTALS							

Modified from Aldrete JA, Kroulik D: A post-anesthetic recovery score, *Anesth Analg* 49:924, 1970; and Aldrete JA: Modifications to the post anesthesia score for use in ambulatory surgery, *J Perianesth Nurs* 13(3):148, 1998.
BP, Blood pressure.

dition, and presence of IV lines, drainage tubes, and dressings. The PACU nurse's report helps the nurse on the acute client care area to anticipate special client needs and obtain necessary equipment.

Personnel, which may include nurses, return the client on a stretcher. Staff members assist in safely transferring

the client to a bed (see Chapter 36). The PACU nurse, if helping to transport the client, shows the acute care nurse the recovery room record and reviews the client's condition and course of care. The PACU nurse also reviews physician orders that require attention. *Before the PACU nurse leaves the acute care area, the staff nurse assum-*

Table 49-9   Expanded Postanesthetic Recovery Score for Ambulatory Patients

Indices	Task	Score	Time in Minutes Indices						
			0	5	10	15	30	45	60
Activity	Able to move four extremities voluntarily or on command	2							
	Able to move two extremities voluntarily or on command	1							
	Unable to move extremities voluntarily or on command	0							
Respiration	Able to breathe deeply and cough freely	2							
	Dyspnea, limited breathing, or tachypnea	1							
	Apneic or on mechanical ventilator	0							
Circulation	BP 20% of preanesthetic level	2							
	BP 20%-49% of preanesthetic level	1							
	BP 50% of preanesthetic level	0							
Consciousness	Fully awake	2							
	Arousable on calling	1							
	Not responding	0							
O_2 saturation	Able to maintain O_2 saturation 92% on room air	2							
	Needs O_2 inhalation to maintain O_2 saturation 90%	1							
	O_2 saturation 90% even with O_2 supplement	0							
Dressing	Dry and clean	2							
	Wet but marked and not increasing	1							
	Growing area of wetness	0							
Pain	Pain free	2							
	Mild pain handled by oral medication	1							
	Severe pain requiring parenteral medication	0							
Ambulation	Able to stand up and walk straight*	2							
	Vertigo when erect	1							
	Dizziness when supine	0							
Fasting-feeding	Able to drink fluids	2							
	Nauseated	1							
	Nausea and vomiting	0							
Urine output	Has voided	2							
	Unable to void but comfortable	1							
	Unable to void and uncomfortable	0							
TOTALS									

Modified from Aldrete JA, Kroulik D: A post-anesthetic recovery score, *Anesth Analg* 49:924, 1970; and Aldrete JA: Modifications to the post anesthesia score for use in ambulatory surgery, *J Perianesth Nurs* 13(3):148, 1998.
NOTE: Total score must be at least 18 for client to be discharged to home.
BP, Blood pressure.
*May be substituted by Romberg's test, or picking up 12 clips in one hand.

ing care for the client takes a complete set of vital signs to compare with PACU findings. Minor vital sign variations normally occur after transporting the client.

Recovery in Ambulatory Surgery

The thoroughness and extent of postoperative recovery care depends on the ambulatory client's condition, type of surgery, and anesthesia. In some cases the client will go through both phase I (PACU) and phase II recovery. Clients in need of close monitoring are assessed and cared for in the same fashion as inpatient clients in phase I. The PARS may be used, with a score of 8 to 10 determining discharge from the PACU. After clients become stable and no longer require close monitoring, the nurse transfers them to phase II recovery

However, with new anesthetic agents and techniques, clients experience a more rapid awakening in the operating room (Apfelbaum and others, 2002; Fredman and others, 2002; Saar, 2001). Therefore many ambulatory surgery clients are able to bypass phase I. This is known as fast-tracking. Phase II recovery consists of a room equipped with medical recliner chairs, side tables, and foot rests. Kitchen facilities for preparing light snacks and beverages are usually located in the area, along with bath-

---

Client Teaching   Box 49-5

Postoperative Instructions for Ambulatory Surgical Client

Objective

- Client will verbalize resources to contact for assistance.
- Client will describe signs and symptoms of postoperative problems.
- Client will list the name and dose of medications to self-administer.
- Client will describe guidelines related to specific surgery.

Teaching Strategies

- Give instruction sheet with physician's telephone number, surgery center's number, and follow-up appointment date and time. Allow client and family to ask questions.
- Explain to family member the signs and symptoms of infection for which to observe.
- Explain name, dose, schedule, and purpose of medications. Provide drug information leaflets.
- Explain activity restrictions, diet progression, and any special wound care related to specific surgery. Provide instruction sheet with clear, focused explanations.

Evaluation

- Have client explain when and how to call physician with problems.
- Have client recite date for follow-up appointment.
- Have client and family member describe signs and symptoms of infection.
- Have client verbalize name of drug, dose, and when to take.
- Have client demonstrate proper activity/movement and wound care.

---

rooms. Aldrete (1998) has added five more areas of functional assessment for the ambulatory surgery client, which constitute the **Postanesthesia Recovery Score for Ambulatory Patients (PARSAP)** (Table 49-9). The phase II environment is designed to promote the client's and family's comfort and well-being until discharge. The nurse monitors clients but not at the same intensity as during phase I. In phase II recovery, nurses initiate postoperative teaching with clients and family members (Box 49-5).

Ambulatory surgical clients are discharged to home when they meet certain criteria. A client being monitored by the PARSAP must achieve a score of 18 or higher before being discharged. An exception may be allowed if the client was unable to walk or use extremities before surgery (Aldrete, 1998). Postoperative nausea and vomiting may occur once the client is home even if the symptoms were not present in the surgery center. Options for therapy include the prophylactic use of the drug ondansetron (an orally disintegrating tablet), transcutaneous acupoint electrical stimulation, or a transdermal scopolamine patch (Gan, 2002).

Written postoperative instructions and prescriptions are reviewed with the client and family, and the nurse ensures they verbalize understanding of these instructions. The client is discharged to a responsible adult.

Postoperative Convalescence

Inpatient clients are kept in the PACU until their condition stabilizes; they are then returned to the postoperative nursing division. Ambulatory surgery clients will return home. Nursing care focuses on returning the client to a relatively functional level of wellness as soon as possible. The speed of convalescence depends on the type or extent of surgery, risk factors, and postoperative complications.

The Nursing Process in Postoperative Care

Nursing care in the PACU focuses on monitoring and maintaining respiratory, circulatory, fluid and electrolyte, and neurological status, as well as the management of pain. Other important factors to assess include temperature control, skin and incision/wound status, and genitourinary and gastrointestinal function. These factors are not, however, unique to the PACU setting. The nurse on the acute care division continues assessment of these critical factors on a less intensive basis until the client's discharge from the acute care facility.

NP Assessment

After the assessment on the client's arrival to recovery, the nurse repeats evaluation of vital signs and other key observations at least every 15 minutes or more frequently, depending on the client's condition and unit policy. This assessment usually continues until discharge from the PACU. Vital sign monitoring on the postoperative nursing unit should initially be hourly for 4 hours and then every 4 hours. As the client's condition stabilizes, frequency of assessment will usually decrease to once a shift until discharge. Frequency of assessment should always be based on the client's current condition. *A nurse should not assume that further monitoring is unnecessary if the client appears normal during the initial assessment.* A client's condition can change rapidly, especially during the postoperative period.

The nurse thoroughly documents the assessment, including vital signs, level of consciousness, condition of dressings and drains, comfort level, IV fluid status, and urinary output measurements. Client data can be entered on flow sheets, a computerized client record, or written progress notes. The initial findings are a baseline for comparing postoperative changes.

After the assessment is completed on the acute care area and the client's immediate needs are met, the family is allowed to visit. The nurse can explain the purpose of postoperative procedures or equipment and the client's status. The family should know that the client will fall in and out of sleep for most of the rest of the day from the effects of general anesthesia and pain medication. The family should also be reminded that frequent assessments are to be expected and that loss of sensation and movement in the extremities remains for several hours if the client had spinal or epidural anesthesia.

Respiration. Certain anesthetic agents may cause respiratory depression. Thus the nurse is especially alert for shallow, slow breathing and a weak cough. The nurse assesses airway patency, respiratory rate, rhythm, depth of ventilation, symmetry of chest wall movement, breath sounds, and color of mucous membranes. If breathing is unusually shallow, placement of the hand near the client's nose or mouth allows the nurse to feel exhaled air. Pulse oximetry should reflect 92% to 100% saturation.

The client often has an oral or nasal airway (see Chapter 39) inserted in the operating room after removal of the endotracheal tube to maintain a patent airway until the client can protect his or her airway. As the client awakens, the client will spit out the airway or the nurse asks the client to spit out the airway. The ability to do so signifies the return of a normal gag reflex.

One of the nurse's greatest concerns is airway obstruction. A number of factors can contribute to obstruction, including weak pharyngeal/laryngeal muscle tone from anesthetics; secretions in the pharynx, bronchial tree, or trachea; and laryngeal or subglottic edema (Litwack, 1999). In the postanesthetic client the tongue causes the majority of airway obstructions. Ongoing assessment of airway patency is crucial. Clients are often kept in side-lying positions until airways are clear.

In the acute care area, the nurse continues to assess respiratory status and breath sounds. Older clients, smokers, and clients with a history of respiratory disease are prone to developing complications such as atelectasis or pneumonia. The client is also assessed for any signs of shortness of breath or difficulty with endurance.

Circulation. The client is at risk for cardiovascular complications resulting from actual or potential blood loss from the surgical site, side effects of anesthesia, electrolyte imbalances, and depression of normal circulatory regulating mechanisms. Careful assessment of heart rate and rhythm, along with blood pressure, reveals the client's cardiovascular status. A rhythm strip is usually obtained postoperatively, compared with preoperative ECG tracings, and mounted on the PACU record. The values are monitored at least every 15 minutes throughout the recovery phase. The nurse compares preoperative vital signs with postoperative values. If the client's blood pressure drops progressively with each check or if the heart rate changes or becomes irregular, the physician should be notified.

The nurse assesses circulatory perfusion by noting capillary refill, pulses, and the color and temperature of the nail beds and skin. If the client has had vascular surgery or has casts or constricting devices that may impair circulation, the nurse assesses peripheral pulses and capillary refill distal to the site of surgery. For example, after surgery to the femoral artery, the nurse assesses posterior tibial and dorsalis pedis pulses. The nurse also compares pulses in the affected extremity with those in the nonaffected extremity.

A common early circulatory problem is hemorrhage. Blood loss may occur externally through a drain or incision or internally. Either type of hemorrhage may result in a fall in blood pressure; elevated heart and respiratory rate; thready pulse; cool, clammy, pale skin; and restlessness. The surgeon should be notified if changes such as these are noted. The nurse maintains IV fluid infusion and may need to increase IV replacement fluids. The nurse monitors the client's vital signs every 15 minutes or more frequently until the client's condition stabilizes. Oxygen may need to be continued. Medications and volume replacement may be considered. Blood counts and coagulation studies are drawn and sent to the laboratory or measured with bedside testing methods.

The potential for cardiovascular complications remains when the client is transferred to the acute care area. The nurse continues to assess the same factors that were identified in the PACU.

Temperature Control. The operating room and recovery room environments are extremely cool. The client's anesthetically depressed level of body function results in a lowering of metabolism and fall in body temperature. When clients begin to awaken, they complain of feeling cold and uncomfortable. The length of time spent in the operating room and laminar flow rooms contributes to heat loss. Surgeries that require an open body cavity also contribute to heat loss. Older adults and pediatric clients are at higher risk for developing problems associated with hypothermia.

In rare instances **malignant hyperthermia,** a life-threatening complication of anesthesia, develops. Malignant hyperthermia causes tachypnea, tachycardia, premature ventricular contractions (PVCs), unstable blood pressure, cyanosis, skin mottling, and muscular rigidity. Despite the name, an elevated temperature occurs late. Although it is often seen during the induction phase of anesthesia, symptoms may recur 24 to 72 hours postoperatively (Karlet, 1998). Without prompt detection and treatment, it can be fatal.

Temperature is monitored closely in the acute care area. Because an elevated temperature may be the first indication of an infection, the nurse evaluates the client for a potential source of infection, including the IV site (if present), the surgical incision/wound, and the respiratory and urinary tracts. The physician must be notified, because a further evaluation, including blood, sputum and urinary cultures, will likely be needed.

Fluid and Electrolyte Balance. Because of the surgical client's risk for fluid and electrolyte abnormalities, the nurse assesses the hydration status and monitors cardiac and neurological function for signs of electrolyte alterations (see Chapter 40). Laboratory values will be monitored and compared with the client's baseline values.

An important responsibility of the nurse is maintaining patency of IV infusions. The client's only source of fluid intake immediately after surgery is through IV catheters. The nurse inspects the catheter insertion site to ensure that the catheter is properly positioned within a vein so that fluid flows freely. Accurate recording of intake and output helps assess renal and circulatory function. The nurse measures all sources of output, including urine, surgically placed drains, gastric drainage, and drainage from wounds, and notes any insensible loss from diaphoresis. The nurse should assess daily weight for the first several days after surgery and compare it with the preoperative weight. If the client has a known cardiac history such as congestive heart failure, daily weights may be continued. It is important to use a consistent scale, amount of clothing, and time of day to obtain accurate weight measurement.

Neurological Functions. In the PACU, the client is often drowsy. As anesthetic agents are metabolized, the client's reflexes return, muscle strength is regained, and a normal level of orientation returns. A client should at least be oriented to self and the hospital before discharge from the PACU. The nurse assesses pupillary and gag reflexes (see Chapter 32), hand grips, and movement of extremities. If a client has had surgery involving a portion of the neurological system, the nurse conducts a more thorough neurological assessment. For example, if the client has had low back surgery, the nurse assesses leg movement, sensation, and strength.

Clients with regional anesthesia begin to experience a return in motor function before tactile sensation returns. The nurse checks the client's sensation along **dermatomes** (segmental skin areas innervated by specific segments of the spinal cord). Knowing where anesthesia was introduced, the nurse is able to check the distribution of the spinal nerves affected (see Chapter 32). Typically, the nurse assesses the dermatome level by touching the client bilaterally and documenting where the client feels touch. The sense of touch can be tested using hand pressure or a gentle pinch of the skin. Extremity strength assessment continues to be important if spinal or epidural anesthesia has been given, although the client should remain in the PACU until sensation and voluntary movement of the lower extremities have been reestablished.

Skin Integrity and Condition of the Wound. In the PACU, the nurse assesses the condition of the client's skin, noting rashes, petechiae, abrasions, or burns. A rash may indicate a drug sensitivity or allergy. Abrasions or petechiae may result from inappropriate positioning or restraining that injures skin layers, or from a clotting disorder. Burns may indicate that an electrical cautery grounding pad was incorrectly placed on the client's skin. Burns or serious injury to the skin should be documented by an incident report (see Chapter 25). The nurse should also note if the client is complaining of any burning or pain in the eye that could indicate a corneal abrasion.

After surgery most surgical wounds are covered with a dressing that protects the wound site and collects drainage. The nurse observes the amount, color, odor, and consistency of drainage on dressings. It is most common for serosanguineous drainage immediately postoperatively. The nurse estimates the amount of drainage by noting the number of saturated gauze sponges. If drainage appears on the outer surface of a dressing, another way of assessing drainage is by drawing a circle around the outer perimeter of the drainage and dating it with the time noted. This way the nurse can easily note if drainage is increasing (see Chapter 47). However, this is not the most accurate measure of volume of fluid lost.

Many physicians prefer to change surgical dressings the first time so that they can inspect the incisional area. The nurse on the surgical nursing unit will usually have the first opportunity to view and thoroughly assess and document the status of the incision/wound. Initially it is important to note if wound edges are approximated and no active bleeding or drainage is present. Wound assessment is especially important, because it forms the baseline for continued monitoring during the client's hospital stay.

It is also important to assess the client's mobility level. If the client is unable or unwilling to turn, pressure ulcer development is a concern. The nurse should institute the use of the Braden Scale or another assessment tool to determine the client's risk of developing pressure ulcers. Preventive measures such as a turning schedule and pressure reduction devices can be instituted (see Chapter 47).

Genitourinary Function. Depending on the surgery, a client may not regain voluntary control over urinary function for 6 to 8 hours after anesthesia. An epidural or spinal anesthetic may prevent the client from feeling bladder fullness. The nurse palpates the lower abdomen just above the symphysis pubis for bladder distention. If the client has a urinary catheter, there should be a continuous flow of urine of 30 to 50 ml/hr in adults (Metheny, 2000). The nurse observes the color and odor of urine. Surgery involving portions of the urinary tract normally causes bloody urine for at least 12 to 24 hours, depending on the type of surgery. The acute care nurse will provide ongoing assessment of genitourinary function.

Gastrointestinal Function. Anesthetics slow gastrointestinal motility and may cause nausea. Normally during the immediate recovery phase, faint or absent bowel sounds are auscultated in all four quadrants. The nurse inspects the abdomen for distention that may be caused by accumulation of gas. In a client who has had abdominal surgery, distention will develop if internal bleeding occurs; however, this is a late sign of bleeding. Distention may also occur in the client who develops a **paralytic ileus** from handling of the bowel in surgery.

The acute care nurse closely monitors the client's initial oral intake for potential aspiration or the presence of nausea and vomiting. Assessment also includes checking for return of peristalsis every 4 to 8 hours. Routinely, the nurse auscultates the abdomen to detect return of normal bowel sounds; 5 to 30 loud gurgles per minute over each quadrant indicates that peristalsis has returned. High-pitched tinkling sounds accompanied by abdominal distention suggest that the bowel is not functioning properly. The nurse asks if the client is passing gas (flatus). This is an important sign indicating normal bowel function. If a nasogastric (NG) tube is in place, assess the patency of the tube (see Chapter 45) and the color and amount of any drainage.

Comfort. As clients awaken from general anesthesia, the sensation of pain becomes prominent. Pain can be perceived before full consciousness is regained. Acute incisional pain causes clients to become restless and may be responsible for temporary changes in vital signs. It is difficult for clients to begin coughing and deep breathing exercises when they experience pain. The client who had regional or local anesthesia usually does not experience pain initially, because the incisional area is still anesthetized.

Assessment of the client's discomfort and evaluation of pain-relief therapies are essential nursing functions. Pain scales are an effective method for nurses to assess postoperative pain, evaluate response to analgesics, and objectively document pain severity (see Chapter 42). Using preoperative pain assessments as a baseline, the nurse evaluates the effectiveness of interventions throughout the client's recovery.

Client Expectations. The nurse assesses the client's and family's expectations for recovery and perceived progress in the recovery and convalescence phases. Ongoing assessment of expectations regarding pain control, comfort level, dietary intake, activity level, and readiness for discharge are also performed. The nurse determines the client's and family's expectations regarding needs at home and these are incorporated into the plan of care.

Nursing Diagnosis

The nurse determines the status of problems identified from preoperative nursing diagnoses and clusters new relevant data to identify new diagnoses. Previously defined diagnoses, such as *impaired skin integrity,* may continue as a postoperative problem. The nurse may also identify new risk factors leading to identification of nursing diagnoses. For example, an older client who has undergone major abdominal surgery and who has a preexisting problem of reduced hip mobility resulting from arthritis will likely have the diagnosis of *impaired physical mobility.* The surgery itself may add risk factors for the client. The nurse also considers needs of a client's family when making diagnoses. For example, the inability of the family to cope with the client's condition requires the nurse's intervention.

Planning

Because of the critical nature of the immediate postoperative period, the plan of care in the PACU involves close monitoring of the client and frequent assessments to ensure return to stable physiological function. During the convalescent phase the nurse uses current physical assessment data and analysis of the preoperative nursing history for planning the client's care. The surgeon's postoperative orders also offer guidelines. Typical postoperative orders include the following:

* Frequency of vital sign monitoring and special assessments
* Types of IV fluids and rates of infusion
* Postoperative medications (especially those for pain and nausea)
* Resumption of preoperative medications as condition allows (some oral medications will be converted to the IV route with appropriate dose adjustment)
* Fluids and food allowed by mouth
* Level of activity that the client is allowed to resume
* Position that the client is to maintain while in bed
* Intake and output
* Laboratory tests and x-ray studies
* Special directions (e.g., surgical drains to suction, tube irrigations, dressing changes)

Goals and Outcomes. The nurse considers the effects of the stress of surgery and limitations it produces when establishing goals, expected outcomes, and interventions for the individual client. Measurable outcomes help to ensure aggressive but appropriate recovery from surgery. For example, the client at risk for impaired mobility should have specific outcomes selected that include targeted ambulation (e.g., steps to take and distance down hallway) and range of joint movement. After each outcome is met, the client will ultimately achieve the goal of independent mobility at a preoperative level or better. The nurse carefully considers all goals of care established during the preoperative surgical phase. The following is an example of a goal and expected outcomes for the postoperative period:

* Client achieves a return of normal physiological function after surgery.
* Client's vital signs return to preoperative baseline.
* Client's airway is patent and respirations are even and unlabored.
* Client's temperature returns to baseline, and he remains afebrile.
* Client's fluid and electrolyte levels remain balanced.
* Client returns to previous level of activity.

Setting Priorities. In the PACU, priorities of care include the assessment and stability of the client's airway, intervention for an impaired airway, and assessment of the client's respiratory, circulatory, and neurological status and pain control. As the client progresses, priorities should focus on advancement of client activity to return the client to preoperative functioning or better. The client will generally have multiple nursing diagnoses (Figure 49-8). The nurse may reestablish priorities several times as the status of the client's health problems change.

Concept Map

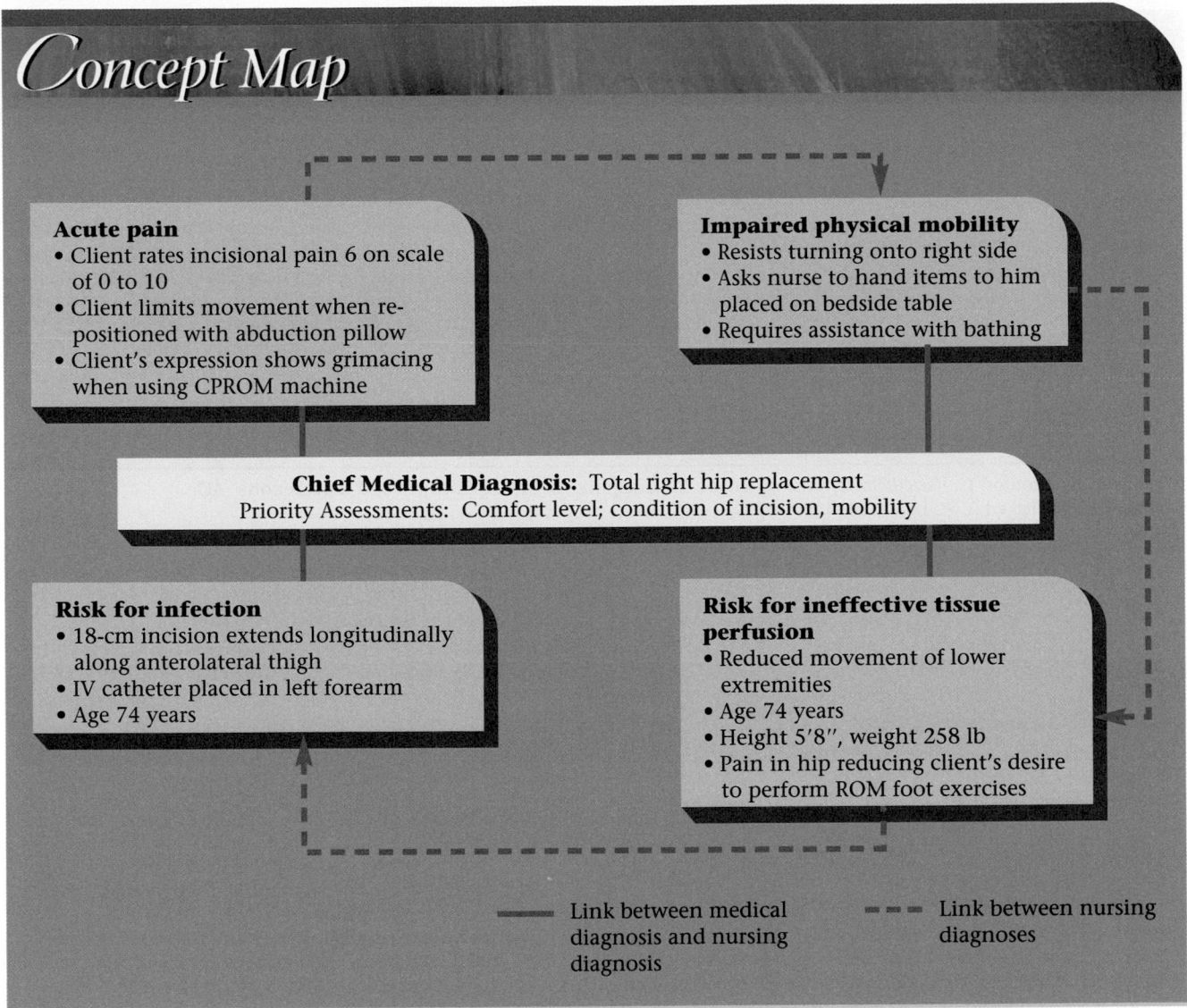

Acute pain
- Client rates incisional pain 6 on scale of 0 to 10
- Client limits movement when re-positioned with abduction pillow
- Client's expression shows grimacing when using CPROM machine

Impaired physical mobility
- Resists turning onto right side
- Asks nurse to hand items to him placed on bedside table
- Requires assistance with bathing

Chief Medical Diagnosis: Total right hip replacement
Priority Assessments: Comfort level; condition of incision, mobility

Risk for infection
- 18-cm incision extends longitudinally along anterolateral thigh
- IV catheter placed in left forearm
- Age 74 years

Risk for ineffective tissue perfusion
- Reduced movement of lower extremities
- Age 74 years
- Height 5'8", weight 258 lb
- Pain in hip reducing client's desire to perform ROM foot exercises

—— Link between medical diagnosis and nursing diagnosis

- - - Link between nursing diagnoses

FIGURE **49–8** Concept map for surgical client with total hip replacement.

Continuity of Care. In the recovery phase, the nurse collaborates on the plan of care with respiratory therapy, physical therapy, occupational therapy, dietary, social work, home health, and others to meet the multidisciplinary needs of the client. The goal of all of these disciplines is to assist the client to return to the best possible level of functioning with a smooth transition to home. The family's role in the plan of care to foster recovery is also essential.

Implementation

Health Promotion. A surgical wound, the effects of prolonged immobilization during surgery and convalescence, preoperative risks such as age (Box 49-6), and the influence of anesthesia and analgesics are the primary causes for postoperative complications. Nursing interventions in the postoperative period are directed at prevent-

ing complications so that the client returns to the highest level of functioning possible. Failure of the client to become actively involved in recovery adds to the risk of complications (Table 49-10). Virtually any body system can be affected. The nurse must consider the interrelationship of all systems and therapies provided.

Maintaining Respiratory Function. To prevent respiratory complications, the nurse begins pulmonary interventions early. The benefits of thorough preoperative teaching are realized when clients are able to participate actively. When awakening from anesthesia, the nurse may need to assist the client in maintaining a patent airway. The following measures maintain airway patency:
- Position the client on one side with the face downward and the neck slightly extended to facilitate a forward movement of the tongue and the flow of mucous secretions out of the mouth. A small folded towel supports the head. Another positioning technique to pro-

Focus on Older Adults   **Box 49-6**

- Age alone is no longer a parameter for determining the benefit one can achieve from a surgical procedure. Consequently, nurses are caring for many more surgical clients of advanced age, and are required to know the age-related factors that impact a surgical procedure (Eliopoulos, 2001).
- A smaller margin of physiologic reserve makes the older adult less able to compensate during the perioperative period for changes that can occur due to infection, hemorrhage, alterations in blood pressure, and fluid/electrolyte abnormalities.
- Older clients are at greater risk for postoperative delirium, especially those who undergo hip replacement. A rapid decline in cognitive function, fluctuations in awareness and

orientation, disturbed sleep-wake cycle, and personality and mood changes characterize the typical presentation (Lueckenotte, 2000).
- Altered and unexpected drug responses are often related to different pharmacokinetics in the older adult. Thus the nurse caring for the perioperative older client must be alert to the possibility of a high risk for adverse medication events with the administration of anesthetic agents and postoperative analgesics, especially narcotics (Lueckenotte, 2000). "Start low and go slow" should be the guiding principle when medicating older adults because of their slow drug clearance capability.

Data from Eliopoulos C: *Gerontologic nursing,* ed 5, Philadelphia, 2001, Lippincott; and Lueckenotte AG: *Gerontologic nursing,* ed 2, St. Louis, 2000, Mosby.

Table **49-10**   **Postoperative Complications**

Complication	Cause
Respiratory System	
Atelectasis: Collapse of alveoli with retained mucous secretions. Signs and symptoms include elevated respiratory rate, dyspnea, fever, crackles auscultated over involved lobes of lungs, and productive cough.	Inadequate lung expansion. Anesthesia, analgesia, and immobilized position prevent full lung expansion. There is greater risk in clients with upper abdominal surgery who have pain during inspiration and repress deep breathing.
Pneumonia: Inflammation of alveoli. It may involve one or several lobes of lung. Development in lower dependent lobes of lung is common in immobilized surgical client. Signs and symptoms include fever, chills, productive cough, chest pain, purulent mucus, and dyspnea.	Poor lung expansion with retained secretions or aspirated secretions. Common resident bacterium in respiratory tract is *Diplococcus pneumoniae,* which causes most cases of pneumonia.
Hypoxemia: Inadequate concentration of oxygen in arterial blood. Signs and symptoms include restlessness, dyspnea, high or low blood pressure, tachycardia or bradycardia, diaphoresis, and cyanosis.	Respirations are depressed by anesthetics or analgesics. Increased retention of mucus with impaired ventilation occurs because of pain or poor positioning.
Pulmonary embolism: Embolus blocking pulmonary arterial blood flow to one or more lobes of lung. Signs and symptoms include dyspnea, sudden chest pain, cyanosis, tachycardia, and drop in blood pressure.	Same factors lead to formation of thrombus or embolus. Immobilized surgical client with preexisting circulatory or coagulation disorders is at risk.
Circulatory System	
Hemorrhage: Loss of large amount of blood externally or internally in short period of time. Signs and symptoms include hypotension, weak and rapid pulse, cool and clammy skin, rapid breathing, restlessness, and reduced urine output.	Slipping of suture or dislodged clot at incisional site. Clients with coagulation disorders are at greater risk.
Hypovolemic shock: Inadequate perfusion of tissues and cells from loss of circulatory fluid volume. Signs and symptoms are same as for hemorrhage.	In surgical client, hypovolemic shock is usually caused by hemorrhage.
Thrombophlebitis: Inflammation of vein often accompanied by clot formation. Veins in legs are most commonly affected. Signs and symptoms include swelling and inflammation of involved site and aching or cramping pain. Vein feels hard, cordlike, and sensitive to touch.	Venous stasis is aggravated by prolonged sitting or immobilization. Trauma to vessel wall and hypercoagulability of blood increase risk of vessel inflammation.

Table *49-10*   Postoperative Complications—cont'd

Complication	Cause
Circulatory System—cont'd	
Thrombus: Formation of clot attached to interior wall of a vein or artery, which can occlude the vessel lumen. Symptoms include localized tenderness along distribution of the venous system, swollen calf or thigh, calf swelling >3 cm compared to asymptomatic leg, pitting edema in symptomatic leg, and collateral superficial veins, and decrease in pulse below location of thrombus (if arterial).	Venous stasis (see discussion of thrombophlebitis) and vessel trauma. Venous injury is common after surgery of legs, abdomen, pelvis, and major vessels. Clients with pelvic and abdominal cancer or traumatic injuries to the pelvis or lower extremities are at high risk for thrombus formation.
Embolus: Piece of thrombus that has dislodged and circulates in bloodstream until it lodges in another vessel, commonly lungs, heart, brain, or mesentery.	Thrombi form from increased coagulability of blood (e.g., polycythemia and use of birth control pills containing estrogen).
Gastrointestinal System	
Paralytic ileus: Nonmechanical obstruction of the bowel caused by physiological, neurogenic, or chemical imbalance associated with decreased peristalsis. Common in initial hours after abdominal surgery.	Handling of intestines during surgery can lead to loss of peristalsis for a few hours to several days.
Abdominal distention: Retention of air within intestines and abdominal cavity during gastrointestinal surgery. Signs and symptoms include increased abdominal girth, tympanic percussion over abdominal quadrants, client complaints of fullness and "gas pains."	Slowed peristalsis from anesthesia, bowel manipulation, or immobilization. During laparoscopic surgeries, influx of air for procedure causes distention.
Nausea and vomiting: Symptoms of improper gastric emptying or chemical stimulation of vomiting center. Client complains of gagging or feeling full or sick to stomach.	Abdominal distention, fear, severe pain, medications, eating or drinking before peristalsis returns, and initiation of gag reflex.
Genitourinary System	
Urinary retention: Involuntary accumulation of urine in bladder as result of loss of muscle tone. Signs and symptoms include inability to void, restlessness, and bladder distention. It appears 6-8 hours after surgery.	Effects of anesthesia and narcotic analgesics. Local manipulation of tissues surrounding bladder and edema interfere with bladder tone. Poor positioning of client impairs voiding reflexes.
Urinary tract infection: An infection of the urinary tract as a result of bacterial or yeast contamination. Signs and symptoms include dysuria, itching, abdominal pain, possible fever, cloudy urine, WBCs and leukocyte esterase positive on urinalysis.	Most frequently a result of catheterization of the bladder.
Integumentary System	
Wound infection: An invasion of deep or superficial wound tissues by pathogenic microorganisms; signs and symptoms include warm, red, and tender skin around incision; fever and chills; purulent material exiting from drains or from separated wound edges. Infection usually appears 3-6 days after surgery.	Infection is caused by poor aseptic technique or contaminated wound or surgical site before surgical exploration. For example, with a bowel perforation, the patient is at increased risk for a wound infection because of bacterial contamination from the large intestine.
Wound dehiscence: Separation of wound edges at suture line. Signs and symptoms include increased drainage and appearance of underlying tissues. This usually occurs 6-8 days after surgery.	Malnutrition, obesity, preoperative radiation to surgical site, old age, poor circulation to tissues, and unusual strain on suture line from coughing or positioning cause dehiscence.
Wound evisceration: Protrusion of internal organs and tissues through incision. Incidence usually occurs 6-8 days after surgery.	See discussion of wound dehiscence. Client with dehiscence is at risk for developing evisceration.
Skin breakdown: Result of pressure or shearing forces. Surgical clients are at increased risk if alterations in nutrition and circulation are present, resulting in edema and delayed healing.	Prolonged periods on the operating room (OR) table and in the bed postoperatively can lead to pressure breakdown. Skin breakdown results from shearing during positioning on the OR table and improper pulling of the client up in bed.
Nervous System	
Intractable pain: Pain that is not amenable to analgesics and pain-alleviating interventions.	Intractable pain may be related to the wound or dressing; anxiety, or positioning.

mote a patent airway involves the head of the bed being slightly elevated and the client's neck slightly extended, with the head turned to the side. The nurse in the PACU may need to perform a jaw thrust maneuver and/or chin lift continuously to maintain the airway in some clients. Never position the client with arms over or across the chest, because this reduces maximum chest expansion.

- The nurse suctions artificial airways and the oral cavity for mucous secretions (see Chapter 39). Care must be taken to avoid continually eliciting the gag reflex, which might cause vomiting. Before the nurse or client removes an artificial airway, the back of the airway should be suctioned so that secretions are not retained.

The following measures promote expansion of the lungs:

- Encourage diaphragmatic breathing exercises every hour while clients are awake. Maximal inspirations lasting 3 to 5 seconds open up alveoli.
- Instruct clients to use an incentive spirometer for maximum inspiration. The client should try to reach the inspiratory volume achieved preoperatively on the spirometer.
- Encourage early ambulation. Walking causes clients to assume a position that does not restrict chest wall expansion and stimulates an increased respiratory rate.
- Help clients who are restricted to bed to turn on their sides every 1 to 2 hours while awake and to sit when possible. Turning permits expansion of the lungs. Sitting causes lowering of abdominal organs, thus facilitating diaphragmatic movement and lung expansion.
- Keep the client comfortable. A client who is comfortable will be able to participate in the postoperative regimen. Assess, document, treat, and evaluate the client's pain.

The following measures promote removal of pulmonary secretions if they are present:

- Encourage coughing exercises every 2 hours while clients are awake and maintain pain control to promote a deep, productive cough. *For clients who have had eye, intracranial, or spinal surgery, coughing may be contraindicated because of the potential increase in intraocular or intracranial pressure.*
- Provide oral hygiene to facilitate expectoration of mucus. The oral mucosa becomes dry when clients are NPO or are placed on limited fluid intake.
- Initiate orotracheal or nasotracheal suction for clients who are too weak or are unable to cough (see Chapter 39).
- Administer oxygen as ordered and monitor oxygen saturation with a pulse oximeter

Preventing Circulatory Complications. Measures directed at preventing circulatory complications avert circulatory stasis. Some clients are at greater risk of venous stasis because of the nature of their surgery or medical history. The following measures promote normal venous return and circulatory blood flow:

- Encourage clients to perform leg exercises at least every hour while awake. Exercise may be contraindicated in an affected extremity involving vascular repair or realignment of fractured bones and torn cartilage.

- Apply elastic antiembolism stockings or pneumatic compression stocking as ordered by the physician (see Chapter 46). The stockings should be removed every 8 hours and left off for 1 hour. Perform a thorough assessment of the skin of the lower extremities at this time.
- Encourage early ambulation. Most clients are expected to ambulate the evening of surgery, depending on the severity of the surgery and their condition. Even if a client has an epidural catheter or PCA device, ambulation should be encouraged. The degree of activity allowed progresses as the condition improves. Before ambulation, the nurse assesses the client's vital signs. Abnormalities may contraindicate ambulation. If vital signs are at baseline, the nurse first helps the client to sit on the side of the bed. Client complaints of dizziness are a sign of postural hypotension. A recheck of blood pressure determines whether ambulation is safe. The nurse assists with ambulation by standing at the client's side and making sure that the client can walk steadily. The first few times out of bed, clients may be able to walk only a few feet. This should improve each time. Evaluate tolerance to activity by periodically assessing the pulse rate as the client ambulates.
- Avoid positioning clients in a manner that interrupts blood flow to extremities. While in bed, clients should not have pillows or rolled blankets placed under the knees. Compression of the popliteal vessels can cause thrombi. When clients sit in chairs, their legs should be elevated on footstools. A client should never be allowed to sit with one leg crossed over the other.
- Administer anticoagulant drugs as ordered. Physicians often order prophylactic doses of anticoagulants, such as heparin, for clients at greatest risk for thrombus formation. Orthopedic clients often receive aspirin, warfarin (Coumadin), or enoxaparin (Lovenox) for anticoagulation.
- Promote adequate fluid intake orally or intravenously. Adequate hydration prevents concentrated buildup of formed blood elements, such as platelets and red blood cells. When the plasma volume is low, these elements may gather and form small clots within blood vessels.

Achieving Rest and Comfort. A surgical client's pain increases as anesthesia effects diminish. The client becomes more aware of the surroundings and more perceptive of discomfort. The incisional area may be only one source of pain. Irritation from drainage tubes, tight dressings or casts, and the muscular strains caused from positioning on the operating room table can cause discomfort.

It is common to administer narcotic analgesics immediately after surgery. Initial analgesic doses are usually given by IV infusion in the PACU and titrated to client comfort. After an anesthetized client is awake and aware, PCA may be used. This is given by IV or subcutaneous infusion or via an epidural, as with fentanyl or morphine. The PCA system allows clients to administer their own IV analgesics from a specially prepared IV pump (see Chapter 42). If clients gain a sense of control over their pain, they usually have fewer postoperative problems. Gagliese and others (2000) found that both young and older adult surgical clients were able to use a PCA to attain adequate levels of pain relief. The use of subcutaneous PCA was found in one research study to result in lower pain scores and less sleep disturbance due to pain (Dawson and others, 1999). Many clients receive epidural analgesia that may be continued throughout the recovery period (see Chapter 42).

The nurse on the acute care area continues pain assessment and assessment of the effectiveness of interventions. If the client has a PCA and is using it more frequently than the amount programmed, the nurse should contact the physician to increase the amount of medication the client can receive. The PCA gives the nurse a useful monitor of the effectiveness of pain medication. As oral intake is tolerated, the nurse facilitates changing the client's pain medication from IV to oral administration. The importance of nonpharmacological interventions should not be overlooked. The nurse should assess what care routines contribute to pain and use nonpharmacological measures to treat them. An example would be to lower the head of the bed and use a pillow for incisional splinting while turning a client with recent abdominal surgery. The nurse can also use other methods of promoting pain relief, such as positioning, back rubs, distraction, or imagery. Pain can significantly slow recovery. The client becomes reluctant to cough, breathe deeply, turn, ambulate, or perform necessary exercises. The nurse assesses the client's pain thoroughly (see Chapter 42). *It should not be assumed that the pain is incisional.* When the client asks for pain medication, the nurse determines the location, intensity, and character of the pain. The nurse should provide analgesics as often as allowed, around the clock, the first 24 to 48 hours after surgery to improve pain control (AHCPR, 1992). If pain medications are not relieving discomfort, the nurse should notify the physician for additional orders after completing a thorough assessment. Recognizing potential complications of analgesics and what to do if they occur is an important role for the postoperative nurse.

Acute Care

Temperature Regulation. Temperature regulation is important in the postoperative period. Clients are often cool after surgery; the PACU nurse provides warmed blankets in the immediate postoperative period. If the temperature is 35.6° C (96° F) or below, a warming mattress or convective warming device may be used. Increasing body warmth causes the client's metabolism to rise and circulatory and respiratory functions to improve.

Shivering may not be a sign of hypothermia but rather a side effect of certain anesthetic agents. Meperidine (Demerol) may be given in small increments to decrease shivering as prescribed by the physician. Deep breathing and coughing helps to expel retained anesthetic gases.

Malignant hyperthermia is a potentially lethal condition that can occur in clients receiving general anesthesia. It should be suspected when there is unexpected tachycardia and tachypnea, jaw muscle rigidity, body rigidity of limbs, abdomen and chest, or hyperkalemia. Temperature elevation is a late sign (www.mhaus.org). The nurse will immediately administer dantrolene sodium ordered by the physician. Clients with temperature elevations should be assessed and nursing interventions planned for a possi-

ble infectious process. Postoperative interventions of deep breathing and coughing, early ambulation, prompt removal of indwelling urinary catheters and IV catheters, and aseptic care of the surgical wound will decrease the risk of postoperative infections. Clients suspected to have infections will have cultures obtained.

Maintains Neurological Function. Orientation to the environment is important in maintaining the client's mental status. The nurse reorients the client, explains that surgery is completed, and describes procedures and nursing measures. The client who was properly prepared before surgery is less likely to be anxious when nurses provide care. Any change in level of consciousness should be promptly reported to a physician.

Maintaining Fluid and Electrolyte Balance. As previously stated, an important nursing responsibility is maintaining patency of IV infusions in the postoperative period. The client's only source of fluid intake immediately after surgery is through IV catheters. The physician orders a prescribed rate for each infusion. As the client begins to take and tolerate oral fluids, the IV rate will be decreased. When an ambulatory surgical client awakens and is able to tolerate fluids by mouth without gastrointestinal upset, the IV catheter is removed. With acute care clients, when the client no longer needs a continuous IV infusion, the IV line may be saline locked to preserve the site for antibiotics or other use (see Chapter 40). The client may also receive blood products after surgery, depending on blood loss during surgery.

Promoting Normal Bowel Elimination and Adequate Nutrition. Normally a client who has had general anesthesia does not receive fluids to drink in the PACU because of bowel sluggishness, the risk of nausea and vomiting, and because of grogginess from general anesthesia. To minimize nausea, sudden movement of the client should be avoided. For clients identified to be at high risk for the development of nausea and vomiting or clients who must not vomit (e.g., eye surgery), a combination of antiemetics is recommended (Gan, 2002; Tramer, 2001). For example, the combination of ondansetron and droperidol can achieve a 90% response rate of no nausea, vomiting, or need for rescue antiemetics (Gan, 2002). If the client has a nasogastric tube, the nurse keeps it patent by regular normal saline irrigations as ordered (see Chapter 45). Occlusion of a nasogastric tube results in accumulation of gastric contents within the stomach.

The client will likely begin taking ice chips or sips of fluids when arriving on the acute care unit. If these are tolerated, a clear liquid meal will usually be ordered. Interventions for preventing gastrointestinal complications promote return of normal elimination and faster return of normal nutritional intake. It takes several days for a client who has had surgery on gastrointestinal structures (e.g., a colon resection) to resume a normal diet. Normal peristalsis may not return for 2 to 3 days. In contrast, the client whose gastrointestinal tract is unaffected directly by surgery can resume dietary intake after recovering from the effects of anesthesia. The following measures promote return of normal elimination:

- Maintain a gradual progression in dietary intake. For the first few hours after surgery a client receives only IV fluids. If bowel sounds are active and the physician orders a normal diet the first evening after surgery, first provide clear liquids, such as water, apple juice, broth, or tea, after nausea subsides. Overloading with large amounts of fluids may lead to distention and vomiting. If the client tolerates liquids without nausea, advance the diet as ordered. Clients who have had abdominal surgery are usually NPO the first 24 to 48 hours. As peristalsis returns, provide clear liquids, followed by full liquids, a light diet of solid foods, and finally a client's usual diet. Encourage intake of foods high in protein and vitamin C.
- Promote ambulation and exercise. Physical activity stimulates a return of peristalsis. The client who suffers abdominal distention and "gas pain" may obtain relief while walking.
- Maintain an adequate fluid intake. Fluids keep fecal material soft for easy passage. Fruit juices and warm liquids are especially effective.
- Promote adequate food intake by promoting the client's appetite.
  - Stimulate the client's appetite by removing sources of noxious odors and providing small servings of nonspicy foods.
  - Assist the client to a comfortable position during mealtime. The client should sit if possible to minimize pressure on the abdomen.
  - Provide desired servings of food. For example, a client may be more willing to face the first meal when servings are not large.
  - Provide frequent oral hygiene. Adequate hydration and cleansing of the oral cavity eliminate dryness and bad tastes.
- Administer fiber supplements, stool softeners, and rectal suppositories as ordered. If constipation or distention develops, the physician attempts to stimulate peristalsis with cathartics or enemas.
- Provide meals when the client is rested and free from pain. Often a client loses interest in eating if mealtime has been preceded by exhausting activities, such as ambulation, coughing and deep breathing exercises, or extensive dressing changes. When a client has pain, the associated nausea often causes a loss of appetite.

Promoting Urinary Elimination. The depressant effects of anesthetics and analgesics impair the sensation of bladder fullness. If bladder tone is reduced, the client has difficulty starting urination. However, clients should void within 8 to 12 hours after surgery. Because a full bladder can be painful and often causes restlessness in recovery, it may become necessary to insert a catheter. If the client has an indwelling urinary catheter, the goal should be to have it removed as soon as possible because of the high risk for the development of a nosocomial bladder or urinary tract infection.

Clients who undergo surgery of the urinary system frequently have an indwelling urinary catheter inserted to maintain free urinary flow until voluntary control of urination returns. The following measures promote normal urinary elimination (see Chapter 44):

- Help the client to assume normal positions during voiding. The male client may need assistance to stand to void. Bedpans make voiding difficult. A female client will have better results if she is able to use a toilet or bedside commode.
- Check the client frequently for the need to void. A surgical client restricted to bed needs assistance in handling and using bedpans or urinals. Often the client acquires a sudden feeling of bladder fullness and urgency to void and will need help quickly.
- Assess for bladder distention. If a client does not void within 8 hours of surgery or bladder distention is present, it may be necessary to insert a straight urinary catheter. A physician's order is needed. Continued difficulty in voiding may require an indwelling catheter, although the risk for a urinary tract infection increases.
- Monitor intake and output. An accepted level of urinary output is at least 1 ml/kg/hr for adults. If the urine is dark, concentrated, and low in volume, the physician should be notified. A client can easily become dehydrated as a result of fluid loss from the surgical wound. Measure intake and output for several days after surgery until normal fluid intake and urinary output are achieved.

Promoting Wound Healing. A surgical wound undergoes considerable stress during convalescence. The stress of inadequate nutrition, impaired circulation, and metabolic alterations increase the risk for delayed healing (see Chapter 47). A wound may also undergo considerable physical stress. Strain on sutures from coughing, vomiting, distention, and movement of body parts can disrupt the wound layers. The nurse protects the wound and promotes healing. A critical time for wound healing is 24 to 72 hours after surgery, after which a seal is established. If a wound becomes infected, it usually occurs 3 to 6 days after surgery. A clean surgical wound usually does not regain strength against normal stress for 15 to 20 days after surgery. The nurse uses aseptic technique during dressing changes and wound care (see Chapters 33 and 47). Surgical drains must remain patent so that accumulated secretions can escape from the wound bed. Ongoing observation of the wound identifies early signs and symptoms of infection.

Maintaining/Enhancing Self-Concept. The appearance of wounds, bulky dressings, and extruding drains and tubes threatens a client's self-concept. The effects of surgery, such as disfiguring scars, may create permanent changes in the client's body image. If surgery leads to impairment in body function, the client's role within the family can change significantly.

The nurse observes clients for alterations in self-concept. Clients may show revulsion toward their appearance by refusing to look at incisions, carefully covering dressings with bedclothes, or refusing to get out of bed because of tubes and devices. The fear of not being able to return to a functional role in their families may even cause clients to avoid participating in the care plan.

The family becomes an important part of the efforts to improve the client's self-concept. The nurse explains the client's appearance to the family and ways to avoid nonverbal expressions of revulsion or surprise. The family needs to be accepting of the client's needs and still encourage the client's independence. If the condition is permanent, the family learns to assist the client through the grieving process so that the client can reach a stage of acceptance. The following measures help to maintain the client's self-concept:

- Provide privacy during dressing changes or inspection of the wound. Keep room curtains closed around the bed, and drape the client so that only the dressing or incisional area is exposed.
- Maintain the client's hygiene. Wound drainage and antiseptic solutions from the surgical skin preparation dry on the skin's surface and cause irritation. A complete bath the first day after surgery can make the client feel renewed. When the gown becomes soiled by wound drainage, offer a clean gown and washcloth. Keep the client's hair neatly combed and offer frequent oral hygiene. Room deodorizers may be useful if the odor from drainage seems particularly troublesome to the client and family.
- Prevent drainage devices from overflowing. Typically the physician orders contents of drainage collections to be measured every 8 hours for output recording. The client sometimes becomes preoccupied with observing the gradual collection of drainage, and some drainage devices can leak contents if they become too full. Empty the devices periodically to prevent accidental spills and hampering of the client's movement.
- Maintain a pleasant environment. Self-concept is heightened by being in pleasant, comfortable surroundings. Store or remove unused supplies and keep the client's bedside orderly and clean.
- Offer opportunities for the client to discuss feelings about appearance. A client who avoids looking at an incision may need to discuss fears or concerns. A client having surgery for the first time is often more anxious than one who has had multiple surgeries. When the client chooses to look at an incision for the first time, the area should be clean. Eventually the client should be able to care for the incision site by applying simple dressings or bathing the affected area.
- Provide the family with opportunities to discuss ways to promote the client's self-concept. Encouraging independence can be difficult for a family member who has a strong desire to assist the client in any way. By knowing about the appearance of a wound or incision, family members can be supportive during dressing changes. The topic or tone of a conversation can also help family members distract a client from dwelling on fears and concerns. Family members should not avoid discussing the future. However, they need help to know when it is appropriate to discuss future plans. Then the client and family can work together to discuss realistic plans for the client's return home.

Restorative and Continuing Care. In the postoperative period, the nurse, client, and family work to prepare the client for discharge. Education regarding wound care, activity level, diet, medications, and specifics to the type of surgery is an ongoing process throughout hospitalization.

Some clients will need assistance in the postoperative period after discharge from home care, such as wound care or drain management. With ambulatory surgery clients, focused education with the limited time is essential. Including the family or support system provides a resource for the client once home (see Box 49-5, p. 1631). With both ambulatory and hospitalized surgical clients, nurses provide a wide variety of written educational materials. For example, educational materials with more pictures should be used with clients who do not speak English or have limited reading ability. All materials should be sensitive to various cultures and religions.

Evaluation

Client Care. The nurse evaluates the effectiveness of care provided to the surgical client on the basis of expected outcomes following nursing interventions. In all surgical settings the nurse consults with the client and family to gather evaluation data. The nurse can evaluate the ambulatory surgical client's outcomes via a telephone call to the client's home, asking if complications have developed and if the client understands restrictions or medications. The call is usually placed 24 hours after surgery, which allows the nurse to evaluate the progress of recovery.

In an acute care setting the evaluation of a surgical client is ongoing. If a client fails to progress as expected, the nurse revises the client's plan of care based on the priorities of the client's needs. Every effort is made to assist the client in returning to as healthy and functional a state as possible.

Part of the nurse's evaluation is determining the extent to which the client and family have learned self-care measures. A client often has to continue dressing care, follow activity restrictions, continue medication therapy, and observe for signs and symptoms of complications on returning home. A referral to home care assists clients unable to perform self-care activities. It is useful to have a home care nurse in attendance at discharge to know what a client can effectively perform.

Client Expectations. With short hospital stays and ambulatory surgery, it is especially important to evaluate client expectations early in the postoperative process. Pain relief is usually a priority in the surgical population. Asking the client if everything possible has been done to alleviate pain, including nonpharmacological measures, can determine if the client's needs have been met. Timeliness of response to the client's needs, such as scheduled times for pain medication and prompt answering of a call light, may increase satisfaction. The client usually wants to be discharged from acute care as soon as possible and when indicated by the physician. Ensuring that discharge plans are in place facilitates that process and enhances the client's satisfaction with care. A phone call to the client 24 hours after ambulatory surgery or after discharge from acute care provides reassurance and provides an opportunity for questions to assist the client to a return to the presurgical state of wellness.

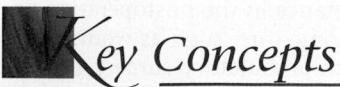

Key Concepts

- Perioperative nursing is professional nursing care provided to the surgical client before, during, and after surgery.
- Surgery is classified by level of severity, urgency, and purpose.
- The preoperative period may be several days or only a few hours long.
- Preoperative assessment of vital signs and physical findings provides an important baseline with which to compare postoperative assessment data.
- Nursing diagnoses of the surgical client may pose implications for nursing care during one or all phases of surgery.
- Primary responsibility for informed consent rests with the client's surgeon.
- Structured preoperative teaching has a positive influence on a client's postoperative recovery.
- Basic to preoperative teaching is explanation of all preoperative and postoperative routines and demonstration of postoperative exercises.
- In ambulatory surgery, nurses must use the limited time available to educate clients, assess their health status, and prepare them for surgery.
- A routine preoperative checklist is a guide for final preparation of the client before surgery.
- Many responsibilities of nurses within the operating room focus on protecting the client from potential harm.
- All medications taken before surgery are automatically discontinued after surgery unless a physician reorders the drugs.
- Family members are important in assisting clients with any physical limitations and in providing emotional support during postoperative recovery.
- Assessment of the postoperative client centers on the body systems most likely to be affected by anesthesia, immobilization, and surgical trauma.
- Accurate pain assessment and intervention are necessary for healing.

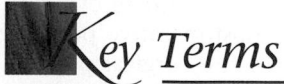

Key Terms

Ambulatory surgery, *p. 1595*
American Society of PeriAnesthesia Nurses (ASPAN), *p. 1598*
Antiembolism stockings, *p. 1626*
Association of Operating Room Nurses (AORN), *p. 1595*
Atelectasis, *p. 1601*
Bariatric, *p. 1601*
Cholecystectomy, *p. 1595*
Circulating nurse, *p. 1625*
Clinical pathways, *p. 1611*

Conscious sedation, *p. 1627*
Convalescence, *p. 1628*
Dehiscence, *p. 1601*
Dermatome, *p. 1633*
General anesthesia, *p. 1626*
Informed consent, *p. 1610*
Latex sensitivity, *p. 1622*
Local anesthesia, *p. 1627*
Malignant hyperthermia, *p. 1632*
Moribund, *p. 1596*
Paralytic ileus, *p. 1634*
Perioperative nursing, *p. 1594*

Pneumatic compression devices, *p. 1611*
Postanesthesia Recovery Score (PARS), *p. 1629*

Postanesthesia Recovery Score for Ambulatory Patients (PARSAP), *p. 1631*
Preoperative teaching, *p. 1607*
Regional anesthesia, *p. 1627*
Scrub nurse, *p. 1625*

Critical Thinking Exercises

1. Your 82-year-old client is admitted after a fall for repair of a fractured hip. What postoperative complications are seen in the older client undergoing this type of surgery?
2. Mr. B. is a 52-year-old client who will have thoracic surgery. He has a 30-year history of smoking one pack of cigarettes per day. What type of pulmonary preventive measures would you expect Mr. B to need postoperatively?
3. Mrs. C. was admitted for ambulatory surgery for an inguinal hernia repair. What discharge criteria would be used for Mrs. C., and what discharge instructions would she require?
4. Your client is scheduled for abdominal hysterectomy at 2:00 PM. Based on NPO guidelines, what fasting schedule should you implement in collaboration with the surgeon and anesthesia provider?

Review Questions

1. An obese client is at risk for poor wound healing postoperatively because:
    1. Ventilatory capacity is reduced.
    2. Fatty tissue has a poor blood supply.
    3. Risk for dehiscence is increased.
    4. Resuming normal physical activity is delayed.

2. The nurse should ask each client preoperatively for the name and dose of all prescription and over-the-counter medications taken before surgery because they:
    1. May cause allergies to develop.
    2. Are automatically ordered postoperatively.
    3. May create greater risks for complications or interact with anesthetic agents.
    4. Should be taken the morning of surgery with sips of water.

3. A client who smokes two packs of cigarettes per day is most at risk postoperatively for:
    1. Infection.
    2. Pneumonia.
    3. Hypotension.
    4. Cardiac dysrhythmias.

4. Family members should be included when the nurse teaches the client preoperative exercises to that they can:
   1. Supervise the client at home.
   2. Coach the client postoperatively.
   3. Practice with the client while waiting to be taken to the operating room.
   4. Relieve the nurse by getting the client to do exercise every 2 hours.

5. Fluid balance is best monitored by:
   1. Daily weights.
   2. Skin tugor.
   3. Capillary refill.
   4. Intake and output.

6. In the PACU the nurse notes that the client is having difficulty breathing because of an obstruction. The nurse would first:
   1. Suction the pharynx and bronchial tree.
   2. Give oxygen through a mask at 10 L/min.
   3. Position the client so that the tongue falls forward.
   4. Ask the client to use an incentive spirometer.

7. Because an older adult is at increased risk for respiratory complications after surgery, the nurse should:
   1. Ambulate every 2 hours.
   2. Monitor fluid and electrolyte status every shift.
   3. Orient the client to the surrounding environment frequently.
   4. Encourage the client to turn, deep breathe, and cough frequently.

8. A client with a prothrombin time (PT) or an activated partial thromboplastin time (APTT) greater than normal is at risk postoperatively for:
   1. Anemia.
   2. Bleeding.
   3. Infection.
   4. Cardiac dysrhythmias.

9. When the client is deep breathing and coughing it is important to have the client sitting because this position:
   1. Is more comfortable.
   2. Facilitates expansion of the thorax.
   3. Increases the client's view of the room and is more relaxing.
   4. Helps the client to splint with a pillow.

10. In the postoperative period if a client has unexpected tachycardia and tachypnea; jaw muscle rigidity; body rigidity of limbs, abdomen, and chest; or hyperkalemia, the nurse should suspect:
    1. Infection.
    2. Hypertension.
    3. Pneumonia.
    4. Malignant hyperthermia.

*R*eferences

AARC Clinical Practice Guideline: Use of positive airway pressure adjuncts to bronchial hygiene therapy, 2002, http://www.aarc.org.

Agency for Health Care Policy and Research: *Acute pain management: operative or medical procedures and trauma,* Clinical Practice Guideline, AHCPR Pub No. 92-0032, Rockville, Md, 1992, Public Health Service, U.S. Department of Health and Human Services.

Agency for Health Care Research and Quality, Acute Pain Management: *Operative or medical procedures and trauma,* Clinical Practice Guidelines No. 1, No. 92-0032: Feb, 1992, www.ahcpr.gov.

Aldrete JA: Modifications to the post anesthesia score for use in ambulatory surgery, *J Perianesth Nurs* 13(3):148, 1998.

Aldrete JA, Kroulik D: A post-anesthetic recovery score, *Anesth Analg* 49:924, 1970.

American Association of Nurse Anesthetists, Infection/Environmental Control Task Force: *Latex allergy protocol,* Park Ridge, Ill, 1995, The Association.

American Society of PeriAnesthesia Nurses: *Standards of perianesthesia nursing practice,* Cherry Hill, NJ, 2002, The Society.

American Society of PeriAnesthesia Nurses, *Standards of perianesthesia nursing practice,* 2002, www.aspan.org.

Association of Operating Room Nurses: Recommended practices for managing the patient receiving local anesthesia, *AORN J* 75(4):849, 2002a.

Association of Operating Room Nurses: Recommended practices for managing the patient receiving moderate sedation/analgesia, *AORN J* 75(3):642, 2002b.

Association of Operating Room Nurses: Recommended practices for skin preparation of patients, *AORN J* 75(1):184, 2002c.

Association of Operating Room Nurses: *Standards, recommended practices, and guidelines,* Denver, 2002d, The Association.

Association of Perioperative Registered Nurses, www.aorn.org.

Barnes S: Pain management: what do patients need to know and when do they need to know it? *J Perianesth Nurs* 16(2):107, 2001.

Barnes S: Patient preparation: the physical assessment, *J Perianesth Nurs* 17(1):46, 2002.

Bean P, Waldron K: Readmission study leads to continuum of care, *Nurs Manage* 26:65, 1995.

De Ruiter HP, Larsen KE: Developing a transcultural patient care web site, *J Transcult Nurs* 13(1):61, 2002.

Dochterman JM, Bulechek GM: *Nursing interventions classification (NIC),* ed 4, St. Louis, 2004, Mosby.

Doepke S: Identifying the risk, *Semin Perioper Nurs* 7(4):226, 1998.

Douglas M: Pain as the fifth vital sign: will cultural variations be considered, *J Transcult Nurs* 10(4): 285, 1999.

Eliopoulos C: *Gerontologic nursing,* ed 5, Philadelphia, 2001, Lippincott.

Federated Ambulatory Surgery Association: *Most common outpatient procedures,* 2002, http://www.fasa.org.

Gershenson A and others: Tilling the soil: nurturing the seeds of patient and family education, *J Nurs Care Qual* 13(6):83, 1999.

Greenfield L and others: *Surgery: scientific principles and practice,* ed 2, Philadelphia, 1997, Lippincott-Raven.

Joint Commission for Accreditation of Health Care Organizations: *Guidelines for implementing the universal protocol for preventing wrong site, wrong procedure, and wrong person surgery,* www.jcaho.org accessed 2/28/04.

Karlet MC: Malignant hyperthermia consideration for ambulatory surgery, *J Perianesth Nurs* 13(5):304, 1998.

Lewis S and others: *Medical-surgical nursing: assessment and management of clinical problems,* ed 5, St. Louis, 2000, Mosby.

Lipson J, Dibble S, Minarik P: *Culture and nursing care: a pocket guide,* San Francisco, 1996, UCSF Nursing Press.

Litwack K: *Core curriculum for perianesthesia nursing practice,* ed 4, Philadelphia, 1999, WB Saunders.

Lueckenotte AG: *Gerontologic nursing,* ed 2, St. Louis, 2000, Mosby.

Malignant Hyperthermia Association of the United States, *Managing malignant hypertension: clinical update,* online brochure, www.mhaus.org.

Meeker MH, Rothrock JC: *Alexander's care of the patient in surgery,* ed 11, St. Louis, 1999, Mosby.

Metheny NM: *Fluid and electrolyte balance: nursing considerations,* ed 4, Philadelphia, 2000, Lippincott.

Moorhead S, Johnson M, Maas M. *Nursing outcomes classification (NOC),* ed 3, St. Louis, Mosby, 2004.

Pagana KD, Pagana TJ: *Mosby's diagnostic and laboratory test reference,* ed 6, St. Louis, 2003, Mosby.

Paquet J: Latex hypersensitivity: the IgE response, *Semin Perioper Nurs* 7(4):203, 1998.

Polk HC, Christmas AB: Prophylactic antibiotics in surgery and surgical wound infections, *Am Surg* 66(2):105, 2000.

Shoup A: Why latex allergy now? *Semin Perioper Nurs* 7(4):222, 1998.

Steelman VM, Titler MG: *Evidence-based protocol: latex precautions,* Iowa City, Ia, 2001, The University of Iowa Gerontological Nursing Interventions Research Center, Research Dissemination Core.

Sullivan EE: Preoperative holding areas, *J Perianesth Nurs* 15(5):353, 2000.

*R*esearch References

American Society of Anesthesiologists Task Force on Preoperative Fasting: Practice guidelines for preoperative fasting and the use of pharmacologic agents to reduce the risk of pulmonary aspiration: application to healthy patients undergoing elective procedures, *Anesthesiology* 90(3): 896, 1999.

Anand SS and others: Does this patient have deep vein thrombosis? *JAMA* 279(14):1094, 1998.

Apfelbaum JL and others: Eliminating intensive postoperative care in same-day surgery patients using short-acting anesthetics, *Anesthesiology* 97(1): 66, 2002.

Augustus CE: Beliefs and perceptions of African American women who have had hysterectomy, *J Transcult Nurs* 13(4): 296, 2002.

Costa MJ: The lived perioperative experience of ambulatory surgery patients, *AORN J* 74(6):874, 2001.

Dawson L and others: Improving patients' postoperative sleep: a randomized control study comparing subcutaneous with intravenous patient-controlled analgesia, *J Adv Nurs* 30(4):875, 1999.

Devine EC, Cook TD: Clinical and cost saving effects of psychoeducational interventions with surgical patients: a meta-analysis, *Res Nurs Health* 9:89, 1992.

Fredman B and others: Fast-track eligibility of geriatric patients undergoing short urologic procedures, *Anesth Analg* 94:560, 2002.

Gagliese L and others: Age is not an impediment to effective use of patient-controlled analgesia by surgical patients, *Anesthesiology* 93(3):601, 2000.

Gan TJ: Postoperative nausea and vomiting—can it be eliminated? *JAMA* 287(10):1233, 2002.

Hobson DW and others: Development and evaluation of a new alcohol-based surgical hand scrub formulation with persistent antimicrobial characteristics and brushless application, *Am J Infect Control* 26:507, 1998.

Larson EL and others: Alcohol for surgical scrubbing? *Infect Control Hosp Epidemiol* 11:139, 1990.

Lee N and others: A survey of patient education postdischarge, *J Nurs Care Qual* 13(1):63, 1998.

Lookinland S, Pool M: Study on effect of methods of preoperative education in women, *AORN J* 67(1):203, 1998.

O'Callaghan N: Pre-operative fasting, *Nurs Stand* 16(36):33, 2002.

Ramer L and others: Multimeasure pain assessment in an ethnically diverse group of patients with cancer, *J Transcult Nurs* 10(2):94, 1999.

Rice VH and others: Pre-admission self-instruction effect on post-admission and post-operative indicators in CABG patients: partial replication and extension, *Res Nurs Health* 15:253, 1992.

Saar L: Use of a modified postanesthesia recovery score in phase II perianesthesia period of ambulatory surgery patients, *J Perianesth Nurs* 16(2):82, 2001.

Shuldham C: A review of the impact of pre-operative education on recovery from surgery, *Int J Nurs Stud* 36:171, 1999.

Summers S: Evidence-based practice. II. Reliability and validity of selected acute pain instruments, *J Perianesth Nurs* 16(1):35, 2001.

Tick LW and others: Practical diagnostic management of patients with clinically suspected deep vein thrombosis by clinical probability test, compression ultrasonography, and D-dimer test, *Am J Med* 113:630, 2002.

Tramer MR: A rational approach to the control of postoperative nausea and vomiting: evidence from systematic reviews. II. Recommendations for prevention and treatment, and research agenda, *Acta Anaesthesiol Scand* 45:14, 2001.

Williams JR: Pre-operative fasting: putting research into practice, *Nurs Stand* 13(39):33, 1999.

Review Question ANSWERS

For answers with rationales see answer key beginning on p. 1648.

Chapter 1
1. 1
2. 2
3. 3
4. 1
5. 1
6. 1
7. 4
8. 2
9. 2
10. 2

Chapter 2
1. 1
2. 3
3. 4
4. 3
5. 2
6. 1
7. 4
8. 4
9. 2
10. 3

Chapter 3
1. 1
2. 2
3. 3
4. 4
5. 2
6. 3
7. 3
8. 4
9. 3
10. 1

Chapter 4
1. 1
2. 4
3. 2
4. 2
5. 4
6. 4
7. 3
8. 4
9. 1
10. 1

Chapter 5
1. 1
2. 2
3. 1
4. 4
5. 1
6. 1

7. 1
8. 1
9. 4
10. 3

Chapter 6
1. 1
2. 4
3. 3
4. 2
5. 3
6. 3
7. 1
8. 3
9. 3
10. 2

Chapter 7
1. 3
2. 4
3. 4
4. 1
5. 3
6. 1
7. 3
8. 1
9. 2
10. 1

Chapter 8
1. 2
2. 2
3. 1
4. 2
5. 1
6. 1
7. 4
8. 3
9. 1
10. 4

Chapter 9
1. 3
2. 1
3. 2
4. 4
5. 1
6. 2
7. 1
8. 4
9. 2
10. 3

Chapter 10
1. 1
2. 1
3. 4
4. 3
5. 4
6. 2
7. 2
8. 1
9. 3
10. 1

Chapter 11
1. 2
2. 1
3. 3
4. 4
5. 3
6. 2
7. 1
8. 2
9. 3
10. 3

Chapter 12
1. 2
2. 1
3. 4
4. 3
5. 1
6. 2
7. 3
8. 2
9. 3
10. 4

Chapter 13
1. 4
2. 3
3. 3
4. 2
5. 1
6. 3
7. 2
8. 1
9. 4
10. 1

Chapter 14
1. 2
2. 4
3. 1
4. 2
5. 4
6. 2

7. 4
8. 3
9. 3
10. 1

Chapter 15
1. 1
2. 4
3. 1
4. 3
5. 3
6. 1
7. 1
8. 3
9. 3
10. 2

Chapter 16
1. 1
2. 3
3. 2
4. 4
5. 1
6. 2
7. 4
8. 3
9. 1
10. 2

Chapter 17
1. 1
2. 3
3. 4
4. 2
5. 1
6. 3
7. 2
8. 2
9. 1
10. 4

Chapter 18
1. 2
2. 1
3. 3
4. 3
5. 1
6. 2
7. 1
8. 2
9. 1
10. 1

Chapter 19	Chapter 24	Chapter 29	Chapter 34
1. 4	1. 3	1. 1	1. 1
2. 1	2. 2	2. 2	2. 2
3. 1	3. 3	3. 3	3. 4
4. 2	4. 4	4. 4	4. 1
5. 3	5. 3	5. 4	5. 4
6. 1	6. 1	6. 2	6. 1
7. 2	7. 3	7. 3	7. 1
8. 4	8. 1	8. 1	8. 2
9. 2	9. 2	9. 2	9. 4
10. 3	10. 4	10. 3	10. 1

Chapter 20	Chapter 25	Chapter 30	Chapter 35
1. 3	1. 1	1. 1	1. 3
2. 4	2. 4	2. 4	2. 4
3. 1	3. 1	3. 2	3. 1
4. 4	4. 3	4. 3	4. 1
5. 3	5. 1	5. 3	5. 1
6. 4	6. 3	6. 2	6. 1
7. 2	7. 2	7. 4	7. 2
8. 1	8. 2	8. 2	8. 1
9. 4	9. 1	9. 4	9. 2
10. 1	10. 4	10. 1	10. 2

Chapter 21	Chapter 26	Chapter 31	Chapter 36
1. 4	1. 2	1. 3	1. 2
2. 3	2. 2	2. 1	2. 1
3. 1	3. 4	3. 1	3. 2
4. 2	4. 3	4. 2	4. 1
5. 2	5. 1	5. 3	5. 3
6. 3	6. 4	6. 1	6. 2
7. 4	7. 3	7. 4	7. 1
8. 1	8. 1	8. 1	8. 2
9. 3	9. 3	9. 3	9. 2
10. 2	10. 1	10. 1	10. 2

Chapter 22	Chapter 27	Chapter 32	Chapter 37
1. 1	1. 4	1. 2	1. 1
2. 4	2. 2	2. 2	2. 1
3. 2	3. 4	3. 3	3. 3
4. 4	4. 1	4. 4	4. 3
5. 3	5. 1	5. 2	5. 2
6. 4	6. 3	6. 3	6. 1
7. 3	7. 1	7. 3	7. 1
8. 2	8. 2	8. 1	8. 4
9. 4	9. 2	9. 4	9. 4
10. 4	10. 1	10. 4	10. 3

Chapter 23	Chapter 28	Chapter 33	Chapter 38
1. 4	1. 3	1. 1	1. 1
2. 3	2. 2	2. 3	2. 1
3. 2	3. 4	3. 4	3. 1
4. 1	4. 1	4. 2	4. 2
5. 1	5. 4	5. 1	5. 1
6. 3	6. 1	6. 2	6. 1
7. 4	7. 1	7. 4	7. 2
8. 3	8. 4	8. 2	8. 1
9. 2	9. 2	9. 3	9. 1
10. 4	10. 1	10. 1	10. 1

Chapter 39
1. 1
2. 1
3. 1
4. 2
5. 1
6. 1
7. 2
8. 1
9. 3
10. 4

Chapter 40
1. 1
2. 4
3. 2
4. 4
5. 1
6. 3
7. 1
8. 1
9. 3
10. 1

Chapter 41
1. 4
2. 2
3. 1
4. 1
5. 1
6. 2
7. 4
8. 4
9. 4
10. 4

Chapter 42
1. 2
2. 1
3. 2
4. 3
5. 1
6. 4
7. 3
8. 3
9. 3
10. 4

Chapter 43
1. 4
2. 2
3. 4
4. 1
5. 2
6. 4
7. 3
8. 1
9. 3
10. 2

Chapter 44
1. 2
2. 1
3. 2
4. 4
5. 3
6. 1
7. 2
8. 3
9. 1
10. 4

Chapter 45
1. 4
2. 3
3. 4
4. 1
5. 3
6. 4
7. 3
8. 2
9. 1
10. 1

Chapter 46
1. 2
2. 1
3. 4
4. 2
5. 3
6. 4
7. 1
8. 1
9. 2
10. 3

Chapter 47
1. 4
2. 1
3. 4
4. 3
5. 2
6. 2
7. 3
8. 4
9. 3
10. 1

Chapter 48
1. 2
2. 2
3. 3
4. 2
5. 4
6. 4
7. 2
8. 3
9. 3
10. 1

Chapter 49
1. 2
2. 3
3. 2
4. 2
5. 1
6. 3
7. 4
8. 2
9. 2
10. 4

Review Question RATIONALES

Chapter 1

1. The correct answer is 1. *The Code of Ethics for Nurses With Interpretive Statements* provides a guide for carrying out nursing responsibilities that provide quality nursing care and provides for the ethical obligations of the profession.

2. The correct answer is 2. The founder of modern nursing, Florence Nightingale, established the first nursing philosophy based on health maintenance and restoration.

3. The correct answer is 3. Clara Barton, founder of the American Red Cross, tended soldiers on the battlefields, cleansing their wounds, meeting their basic needs, and comforting them in death.

4. The correct answer is 1. Evidence-based practice is defined as "the integration of best research evidence with clinical expertise and patient values." It involves accurate and thoughtful decision making about health care delivery for clients.

5. The correct answer is 1. The Standards of Care described in the ANA *Standards of Clinical Nursing Practice, second edition* describe a competent level of nursing care. The levels of care are demonstrated through the nursing process: assessment, diagnosis, outcome identification and planning, implementation, and evaluation.

6. The correct answer is 1. Regardless of educational preparation, the examination for RN licensure is exactly the same in every state in the United States. This provides a standardized minimum knowledge base for the client population nurses serve.

7. The correct answer is 4. Contemporary nursing requires that the nurse possess knowledge and skills for a variety of professional roles and responsibilities. In the past, the principal role of nurses was to provide care and comfort as they carried out specific nursing functions. However, changes in nursing have expanded the role to include increased emphasis on health promotion and illness prevention, as well as concern for the client as a whole.

8. The correct answer is 2. The advanced practice nurse (APN) is generally the most independent functioning nurse. An APN has a master's degree in nursing, advanced education in pharmacology and physical assessment, and certification and expertise in a specialized area of practice. The APN may work in primary, acute, or restorative care settings.

9. The correct answer is 2. In North America the major professional nursing organizations are the National League for Nursing (NLN) and American Nurses Association (ANA).

10. The correct answer is 2. As long as nurses maintain involvement in health care policy and practice, misinformed outsiders cannot attempt to impose their will on nursing and nursing practice.

Chapter 2

1. The correct answer is 1. As health care costs continued to rise out of control, regulatory and competitive approaches were created to control health care spending. Regulatory approaches included professional standards review organizations (PSROs) that functioned to review the quality, quantity, and cost of hospital care provided through Medicare.

2. The correct answer is 3. Most providers of health care (e.g., health care networks or managed care organizations) now receive capitated payments for their services. Capitation is the payment mechanism in which providers receive a fixed amount per client or enrollee of a health care plan.

3. The correct answer is 4. Managed care organizations (MCOs) provide comprehensive, preventive, and treatment services to a specific group of voluntarily enrolled persons. The *staff model* is one in which physicians are salaried employees of the MCO.

4. The correct answer is 3. Primary care is defined as the "provision of integrated, accessible health care services by clinicians who are accountable for addressing a large majority of personal health care needs, developing a sustained partnership with clients, and practicing in the context of family and community."

5. The correct answer is 2. Examples of health care services for illness prevention include blood pressure and cancer screenings, immunizations, and poison control information.

6. The correct answer is 1. A comprehensive occupational health program geared to health promotion and accident or illness prevention can increase worker productivity, decrease absenteeism, reduce use of expensive medical care, and lower disability claims. Recurring issues that nurses face are drug testing, right-to-know issues, concerns related to acquired immunodeficiency syndrome (AIDS), and exposure to environmental hazards.

7. The correct answer is 4. Churches and synagogues offer the site for parish nursing. The services might include running errands to the grocery store or pharmacy, transporting clients to a physician's office, providing respite care to family members, and being homemaker aides.

8. The correct answer is 4. Hospital emergency departments and urgent care centers, critical care units, and inpatient medical-surgical units are the sites where secondary and tertiary levels of care are provided.

9. The correct answer is 2. A skilled nursing facility (SNF) offers skilled care from a licensed nursing staff. Medicare covers stays at SNFs for 100 days but at a decreasing dollar amount after the first 20 days.

10. The correct answer is 3. The phenomenon of "knowing clients" is a measure of a nurse's experience and maturity. Knowing clients is a new concept of therapeutic decision making that comprises a nurse's understanding of a specific client and the nurse's subsequent selection of interventions. Knowing develops as a result of a nurse's experience in a specific clinical area, the time the nurse has been in practice, and the quality of relationships the nurse has formed with clients.

Chapter 3

1. The correct answer is 1. The *Healthy People Initiative* was initially created to establish health care goals for the year 2000. These goals are continually revised; for example, the overall goals of *Healthy People 2010* are to increase the life expectancy and quality of life and to eliminate health disparities.

2. The correct answer is 2. Community health nursing is a nursing approach that merges knowledge from the public health sciences with professional nursing theories to safeguard and improve the health of populations in the community.

3. The correct answer is 3. Community-based nursing involves the acute and chronic care of individuals and families that enhances their capacity for self-care and promotes autonomy in decision making.

4. The correct answer is 4. Vulnerable populations of clients are those who are more likely to develop health problems as a result of excess risks, who have limits in access to health care services, or who are dependent on others for care.

5. The correct answer is 2. Physical, emotional, and sexual abuse, as well as neglect, are major public health problems affecting older adults, women, and children.

6. The correct answer is 3. Examples of tertiary intervention include the prevention of the spread of disease.

7. The correct answer is 3. Perinatal classes, infant care, child safety, and cancer screening are just some of the health education programs in which a nurse in community practice may participate as a nurse educator.

8. The correct answer is 4. A counselor assists clients in identifying and clarifying health problems and in choosing appropriate courses of action to solve those problems. For example, a community-based nurse may work in employee assistance programs or women's shelters. In this setting a major amount of nurse client interaction is through counseling.

9. The correct answer is 3. The innovation or change must be tried on a limited basis. New ideas that can be experimented with are usually adopted more quickly. Clients trying out new technology can find out how it works in their own situation.

10. The correct answer is 1. The community can be viewed as having three components: the structure or locale, the people, and the social systems.

Chapter 4

1. The correct answer is 1. Nursing identifies its domain in a paradigm that includes four linkages: the person, health, environment/situation, and nursing.

2. The correct answer is 4. Descriptive theories are the first level of theory development. They describe phenomena, speculate on why phenomena occur, and describe the consequences of phenomena. They have the ability to explain, relate, and in some situations predict nursing phenomena.

3. The correct answer is 2. A theory is a set of concepts, definitions, relationships, and assumptions that project a systematic view of phenomena. It is developed after extensive research, which allows the researcher to have a clear perspective of all components of a phenomenon.

4. The correct answer is 2. There is a contemporary move toward nursing science- or evidence-based practice in which theories are tested and used to describe or predict client outcomes of nursing care.

5. The correct answer is 4. Knowledge from other disciplines such as the physical, social, and behavioral sciences include relevant theories that explain phenomena. An interdisciplinary theory explains a systematic view of phenomena specific to the discipline of inquiry.

6. The correct answer is 4. Health-and-wellness theoretical models are designed to help health care professionals understand the relationships between these two concepts and the client's attitudes toward health and health practices.

7. The correct answer is 3. Human growth and development is an orderly predictive process that begins with conception and continues through death. There are a variety of well-tested theoretical models that describe and predict behavior and development at various phases of the life continuum.

8. The correct answer is 4. The hierarchy of basic human needs includes five levels of priority. The most basic, or first, level includes physiological needs, such as air, water, and food.

9. The correct answer is 1. Leininger's (1991) cultural care diversity and universality theory states that care is the essence of nursing and the dominant, distinctive, and unifying feature of nursing. Human caring varies among cultures in its expressions, processes, and patterns.

10. The correct answer is 1. As an art, nursing relies on knowledge gained from practice and reflection of past experiences. As a science, nursing draws on scientifically tested knowledge that is applied in the practice setting (Kikuchi, Simmons, and Romyn, 1996). But it is the "expert nurse" who transports the art and science of nursing into the scientific realm of creative caring.

Chapter 5

1. The correct answer is 1. The conduct of nursing research has its roots with Florence Nightingale, who observed in detail the effects of nursing actions, such as the impact of nutrition and hygiene, during the Crimean War.

2. The correct answer is 2. In the 1950s there was an increase in the number of nurses with advanced degrees, and the journal *Nursing Research* was initiated.

3. The correct answer is 1. If tradition becomes so ingrained that a person does not question the practice, other, more appropriate or research-based approaches may be overlooked.

4. The correct answer is 4. The scientific method is the foundation of research. Scientific research is the most reliable and objective of all methods of gaining knowledge.

5. The correct answer is 1. The hallmark of scientific research is the experiment. In a true experimental study, the conditions under which a treatment or measure is investigated are tightly controlled.

6. The correct answer is 1. The subjects—persons selected for the comparison and experimental groups—are chosen at random from among those eligible for the study.

7. The correct answer is 1. The amount of knowledge known about the problem and the type of problem being investigated are factors that determine the methods used.

8. The correct answer is 1. Qualitative nursing research is the investigation of phenomena that are not easily quantified or categorized.

9. The correct answer is 4. ANA's position paper (1997), which describes the participation of nurses in research according to their academic preparation, does include research activities for nurses with various levels of academic preparation.

10. The correct answer is 3. Informed consent means that research subjects (1) are given full and complete information about the purpose of the study, procedures, data collection, potential harm and benefits, and alternative methods of treatment; (2) are capable of fully understanding the research and the implications of participation; (3) have the power of free choice to voluntarily consent or decline participation in the research; and (4) understand how confidentiality or anonymity is maintained.

Chapter 6

1. The correct answer is 1. When illness does occur, different attitudes about illness cause people to react in different ways to illness or the illness of a family member. Medical sociologists call the reaction to illness, illness behavior.

2. The correct answer is 4. Defining health is difficult. The World Health Organization (WHO) defines health as a "state of complete physical, mental and social well-being, not merely the absence of disease or infirmity."

3. The correct answer is 3. The health belief model addresses the relationship between a person's belief and behaviors thus: It provides a way of understanding and predicting how clients will behave in relation to their health and how they will comply with health care therapies.

4. The correct answer is 2. Nurses using the holistic nursing model recognize the natural healing abilities of the body and incorporate complementary and alternative interventions.

5. The correct answer is 3. Internal variables include a person's developmental stage, intellectual background, perception of functioning, and emotional and spiritual factors.

6. The correct answer is 3. A person's beliefs about health are shaped in part by the person's knowledge, lack of knowledge, or incorrect information about body functions and illnesses, educational background, and past experiences.

7. The correct answer is 1. Health promotion activities such as routine exercise and good nutrition help clients maintain or enhance their present levels of health.

8. The correct answer is 3. Primary prevention aimed at health promotion includes health education programs, immunization, and physical and nutritional fitness activities.

9. The correct answer is 3. Tertiary prevention occurs when a defect or disability is permanent and irreversible. It involves minimizing the effects of long-term disease or disability by interventions directed at preventing complications and deterioration.

10. The correct answer is 2. An acute illness usually has a short duration and is severe. The symptoms appear abruptly, are intense, and often subside after a relatively short period.

Chapter 7

1. The correct answer is 3. Touch is a form of relating that leads to a connection between nurse and client. However, touch can convey many messages; it must be used with discretion.

2. The correct answer is 4. To know a client means that the nurse avoids assumptions, focuses on the client, and engages in a caring relationship with the client that reveals information and cues that facilitate critical thinking and clinical judgments. Knowing the client is at the core of the process by which nurses make clinical decisions.

3. The correct answer is 4. Spiritual health is achieved when a person finds a balance between his or her own life values, goals, and belief systems and those of others. Research has shown a link between spirit, mind, and body. An individual's beliefs and expectations can and do have effects on the person's physical well-being.

4. The correct answer is 1. The family is an important resource. Success with nursing interventions often depends on the family's willingness to share information about the client and their acceptance and understanding of therapies.

5. The correct answer is 3. Strategies for creating work environments that enable nurses to demonstrate more caring behaviors include introducing greater flexibility into the work environment structure, rewarding experienced nurse mentors, improving nurse staffing, and providing nurses with autonomy over their practice.

6. The correct answer is 1. Nurses make caring a part of the philosophy and environment in the workplace by incorporating care concepts into standards of nursing care, thus establishing the guidelines for professional conduct.

7. The correct answer is 3. A nurse demonstrates caring by helping family members become active participants in a client's care.

8. The correct answer is 1. Listening is not only "taking in" what a client says, it also includes interpretation and understanding of what is said and giving back that understanding to the person talking.

9. The correct answer is 2. Presence involves a person-to-person encounter that conveys a closeness and a sense of caring that involves "being there" and "being with" clients.

10. The correct answer is 1. The study of clients' perceptions is important because health care is placing greater emphasis on client satisfaction. What clients experience in their interactions with institutional services and health care professionals, and what they think of that experience, can determine how clients use the health care system and how they can benefit from it.

Chapter 8

1. The correct answer is 2. The processes of enculturation and acculturation facilitate cultural learning. Socialization into one's primary culture as a child is known as enculturation. The process of adapting to and adopting a new culture is acculturation.

2. The correct answer is 2. Assimilation results when an individual gives up his or her ethnic identity in favor of the dominant culture.

3. The correct answer is 1. Cultural awareness is an in-depth self-examination of one's own background, recognizing biases and prejudices and assumptions about other people.

4. The correct answer is 2. Cultural competence is the process of acquiring specific knowledge, skills, and attitudes that ensure delivery of culturally congruent care.

5. The correct answer is 1. Ethnocentrism is the root of biases and prejudices comprising beliefs and attitudes associating negative permanent characteristics to people who are perceived to be different from the valued group.

6. The correct answer is 1. When action is taken on one's prejudices, discrimination occurs.

7. The correct answer is 4. The dominant value orientation in North American society is individualism and self-reliance in achieving and maintaining health. Caring approaches generally promote the client's independence and ability for self-care.

8. The correct answer is 3. Disparities in health outcomes between the rich and poor illustrate the influence of socioeconomic factors in morbidity and mortality. Social factors such as poverty and lack of universal medical insurance compromise the health status of the poor and unemployed.

9. The correct answer is 1. Nurses need not assume that pain relief is equally valued across groups. Cultural pain may be suffered by a client whose valued way of life is disregarded by practitioners.

10. The correct answer is 4. The dominant value in American society of individual autonomy and self-determination may be in direct conflict with diverse groups. Advance directives, informed consent, and consent for hospice are examples of mandates that may violate clients' values.

Chapter 9

1. The correct answer is 3. *Family durability* is the term for the intrafamilial system of support and structure that may extend beyond the walls of the household. The players may change, the parents may remarry, and the children may or may not leave home as adults, but the "family" is considered to transcend long periods and inevitable lifestyle changes.

2. The correct answer is 1. Family forms are patterns of people considered by family members to be included in the family. Alternate patterns of relationships include multiadult households, "skip-generation" families (grandparents caring for grandchildren), communal groups with children, "nonfamilies" (adults living alone), cohabiting partners, and homosexual couples.

3. The correct answer is 2. The blended family is formed when parents bring unrelated children from prior or foster parenting relationships into a new, joint living situation.

4. The correct answer is 4. Grandparents are also increasingly being called on to raise their grandchildren due to a number of societal factors: the increase in the divorce rate, dual-income families, and single parenthood. Most often it is a consequence of legal intervention when parents are deemed unfit or renounce their parental obligations.

5. The correct answer is 1. The family health system (FHS) offers a holistic perspective for nurses to examine, assess, and care for families. In this system there are five realms or processes of family life: interactive, developmental, coping, integrity, and health. The interactive processes include family relationships.

6. The correct answer is 2. Family functioning focuses on the processes used by the family to achieve its goals. These processes include communication among family members, goal setting, conflict resolution, caregiving, nurturing, and use of internal and external resources.

7. The correct answer is 1. Economic stability increases a family's access to adequate health care, creates more opportunity for education, increases sound nutrition, and decreases stress.

8. The correct answer is 4. The family is the primary social context in which health promotion and disease prevention take place. The family's beliefs, values, and practices strongly influence health-promoting behaviors of its members.

9. The correct answer is 2. When the family as client is the approach, family processes and relationships (e.g., parenting or family caregiving) are the primary focuses of nursing care.

10. The correct answer is 3. When the nurse assumes a humble position instead of coming across as an authority on the subject, this often decreases the client's defenses and makes the client more willing to listen without feeling embarrassed.

Chapter 10

1. The correct answer is 1. Growth and development are synchronous processes that are interdependent in healthy individuals. Physical growth is the quantitative, or measurable, aspect of an individual's physical measurements. Measurable growth indicators include changes in height, weight, teeth, skeletal structures, and sexual characteristics.

2. The correct answer is 1. Moral development focuses on the description of moral reasoning. It is the ability of an individual to distinguish right from wrong and to develop ethical values on which to base his or her actions.

3. The correct answer is 4. Stage 5: genital (puberty through adulthood) is Freud's final stage. This is a time of turbulence when earlier sexual urges reawaken and are directed to an individual outside the family circle. Unresolved prior conflicts surface during adolescence, making this a turbulent stage.

4. The correct answer is 3. In the stage of initiative versus guilt (3 to 6 years), children like to pretend and try out new roles. Conflicts often arise between the child's desire to explore and the limits placed on his or her behavior. These conflicts may lead to feelings of frustration and guilt. Guilt may also occur if the caregiver's responses are too punitive. Teaching impulse control and cooperative behaviors to the child can help the family avoid the risks of altered growth and development.

5. The correct answer is 4. During the stage of generativity versus self-absorption and stagnation (middle age), the ability to expand one's personal and social involvement is critical. Middle-age adults should be able to see beyond their needs and accomplishments to the needs of society. Dissatisfaction with one's place and achievements often leads to self-absorption and stagnation.

6. The correct answer is 2. Psychiatrist Roger Gould believes his research describes a sequential process that takes place between the internal life (personality) of adults and their outer world (culture, lifestyle).

7. The correct answer is 2. The fourth theme, identified in the 40s, "The die is cast," is indicative of resignation and the belief that possibilities are limited. The personality is set. Changes in career are believed to be less likely to be successful. Parents are blamed for their lack of choices. Regret is faced for mistakes made with children.

8. The correct answer is 1. During formal operations the individual's thinking moves to abstract and theoretical subjects. Thinking can venture into such subjects as achieving world peace, finding justice, and seeking meaning in life. Adolescents can organize their thoughts in their minds. They have the capacity to reason with respect to possibilities.

9. The correct answer is 3. At the preconventional level the person reflects on moral reasoning based on personal gain. These consequences can come in the form of punishment or reward.

10. The correct answer is 1. Basic to Gilligan's argument is the developmental differences in relationships and issues of dependency between women and men. Girls do not need to separate from their mothers to achieve feminine identity; it is through this attachment to their mother that their identity is formed.

Chapter 11

1. The correct answer is 2. Three risk factors have been cited as having a possible effect on prenatal development, including nutrition, stress, and mother's age.

2. The correct answer is 1. The most extreme physiological change occurs when the newborn leaves the in utero circulation and develops independent respiratory functioning. Nursing care is directed at maintaining an open airway, stabilizing and maintaining body temperature, and protecting the newborn from infection.

3. The correct answer is 3. Automobile injuries are the leading cause of death in children older than 1 year.

4. The correct answer is 4. During the preoperational thought stage (Piaget, 1952), toddlers recognize that they are separate beings from their mothers, but they are unable to assume the view of another. They use symbols to represent objects, places, and persons. This function is demonstrated when children imitate the behavior of another that they viewed earlier (e.g., pretend to shave like daddy).

5. The correct answer is 3. The play of preschool children becomes more social after the third birthday as it shifts from parallel to associative play. Most 3-year-old children are able to play with one other child in a cooperative manner in which they make something or play designated roles such as mother and baby. By age 4, children play in groups of two or three, and by 5 years the group has a temporary leader for each activity.

6. The correct answer is 2. Preschoolers average 12 hours of sleep a night and take infrequent naps.

7. The correct answer is 1. Motor development in the school-age child: 8-10 years: Can learn to floss teeth effectively and be independent in tooth care.

8. The correct answer is 2. Infections account for the majority of all childhood illnesses; respiratory infections are the most prevalent. The common cold remains the chief illness of childhood.

9. The correct answer is 3. Good communication skills are critical for adolescents in overcoming peer pressure and unhealthy behaviors. The following are some hints for communicating with adolescents: do not avoid discussing sensitive issues; asking questions about sex, drugs, and school opens the channels for further discussion; ask open-ended questions; look for the meaning behind their words or actions; be alert to clues to their emotional state; and involve other individuals and resources when necessary.

10. The correct answer is 3. Accidents remain the leading cause of death in adolescence.

Chapter 12

1. The correct answer is 2. The young adult has usually completed physical growth by the age of 20. An exception to this is the pregnant or lactating woman.

2. The correct answer is 1. The nurse's role in health promotion is to identify modifiable factors that increase support to reduce unhealthy lifestyle behaviors.

3. The correct answer is 4. When determining the amount of information that the individual needs to make decisions about the prescribed course of therapy, the nurse should consider those factors that may affect the individual's compliance with the regimen, including educational level, socioeconomic factors, and motivation and desire to learn.

4. The correct answer is 3. A current trend in some health care agencies is to provide a lay doula or support person to be present during labor to assist women who have no other source of support.

5. The correct answer is 1. Lactation, or the process of breast-feeding, offers many advantages to both the new mother and baby.

6. The correct answer is 2. Close friends and associates of the single young adult may also be viewed as the individual's "family."

7. The correct answer is 3. A family history of a disease may put a young adult at risk for developing it in the middle or older adult years. For example, a young man whose father and paternal grandfather had myocardial infarctions (heart attacks) in their 50s has a risk for a future myocardial infarction.

8. The correct answer is 2. As in all age-groups, personal hygiene habits in the young adult can be risk factors. Sharing eating utensils with a person who has a contagious illness increases the risk of illness.

9. The correct answer is 3. Health teaching and health counseling are often directed at improving health habits.

10. The correct answer is 4. Clearly, a life-threatening illness, marital transition, or job stressor increases the anxiety of the client and family. The nurse may need to use crisis intervention or stress management techniques to help the client adapt to the changes of the middle adult years.

Chapter 13

1. The correct answer is 4. Two factors contribute to the projected increase in the number of older adults: the aging of the "baby boom" generation and the growth of the population segment over age 85. The baby boomers are the large cohort of adults born between 1946 and 1964.

2. The correct answer is 3. Various theorists have attempted to describe the complex biopsychosocial process of aging. Although many theories have been developed, there is no single universally accepted theory that predicts and explains the complexities of the aging process.

3. The correct answer is 3. The three common conditions affecting cognition are delirium, depression, and dementia. Distinguishing between these three conditions is challenging, but essential.

4. The correct answer is 2. Sexuality is increasingly recognized as a factor in the care of older adults. All older adults, whether healthy or frail, need to express sexual feelings. Sexuality involves love, warmth, sharing, and touching, not just the act of intercourse.

5. The correct answer is 1. The older adult's libido does not decrease; however, frequency of sexual activity may decline. An older woman who does not understand physical changes affecting sexual activity may be concerned that her sex life is nearly over with the onset of menopause. The older man may feel the same when he discovers a change in the firmness of his erection, a decreased need for ejaculation with

each orgasm, or a longer recovery period between episodes of intercourse.

6. The correct answer is 3. Presbyopia, a progressive decline in the ability of the eyes to accommodate for close, detailed work, is common.

7. The correct answer is 2. Presbycusis affects the ability to hear high-pitched sounds and sibilant consonants such as *s, sh,* and *ch.*

8. The correct answer is 1. Taste buds atrophy and lose sensitivity. The older adult is less able to discern among salty, sweet, sour, and bitter tastes. The sense of smell is also decreased, further reducing taste. Salivary secretion is reduced.

9. The correct answer is 4. After age 55 respiratory muscle strength begins to decrease. The anteroposterior diameter of the thorax increases. Vertebral changes due to osteoporosis lead to dorsal kyphosis.

10. The correct answer is 1. Frontotemporal dementia has an insidious onset and progresses slowly. Early symptoms include poor hygiene, lack of social tact, hyperorality, and sexual disinhibition. Incontinence is an early symptom in frontotemporal dementia, although it is a late symptom in the more common Alzheimer's disease.

Chapter 14

1. The correct answer is 2. Critical thinking is an active, organized, cognitive process used to carefully examine one's thinking and the thinking of others. It involves use of the mind in forming conclusions, making decisions, drawing inferences, and reflecting.

2. The correct answer is 4. There are core critical thinking skills that, when applied to nursing, are useful in showing the complex nature of clinical decision making. Self-regulation involves self-examination and self-correction. The nurse reflects on his experiences and identifies ways he can improve his own performance.

3. The correct answer is 1. An important aspect of critical thinking is reflection, the process of purposefully thinking back or recalling a situation to discover its purpose or meaning. As a nurse it helps to think back on a client situation, to make sense of the experience, and to thus gain insight as to the meaning of the situation.

4. The correct answer is 2. Intuition is the direct understanding of particulars in a situation without conscious deliberation. It is an inner sensing that something is so. It occurs when an experienced nurse walks into a client's room, looks at the client's appearance without the benefit of a thorough assessment, and senses that the client is about to deteriorate physically.

5. The correct answer is 4. At the basic level of critical thinking a learner trusts that experts have the right answers for every problem. Thinking is concrete and based on a set of rules or principles. For example, a nurse uses an institution's procedure manual to confirm how to insert a Foley catheter.

6. The correct answer is 2. The nursing process consists of five steps: assessment, diagnosis, planning, implementation, and evaluation. The process provides a systematic approach for gathering client data, critically examining and analyzing the data, identifying the client's response to a health problem, determining priorities, establishing goals and expected outcomes of care, taking appropriate action, and then evaluating whether the action is effective.

7. The correct answer is 4. The nursing process consists of five steps: assessment, diagnosis, planning, implementation, and evaluation. The process provides a systematic approach for gathering client data, critically examining and analyzing the data, identifying the client's response to a health problem, determining priorities, establishing goals and expected outcomes of care, taking appropriate action, and then evaluating whether the action is effective.

8. The correct answer is 3. The first component of critical thinking is a nurse's specific knowledge base. This varies according to a nurse's educational experience, including basic nursing education, continuing education courses, and additional college degrees. In addition, it includes the initiative a nurse shows in reading the nursing literature so as to remain current in nursing science.

9. The correct answer is 3. A critical thinker does not customarily accept another person's ideas without question. To think independently, one questions others' ways of interpreting knowledge and looks for rational and logical answers to problems.

10. The correct answer is 1. When caring for clients, a nurse has a responsibility to correctly perform nursing care activities based upon standards of practice. Standards of practice are the minimum level of performance accepted to ensure high-quality care. For example, the nurse does not take shortcuts (e.g., failing to identify a client) when administering medications.

Chapter 15

1. The correct answer is 1. The purpose of the assessment is to establish a database about the client's perceived needs, health problems, and responses to these problems. In addition, the data reveal related experiences, health practices, goals, values, and expectations held about the health care system.

2. The correct answer is 4. While gathering data about a client, the nurse synthesizes relevant knowledge, clinical experiences, critical thinking standards and attitudes, and standards of practice simultaneously. Critical thinking thus helps the nurse to direct the assessment in a meaningful and purposeful way.

3. The correct answer is 1. An assessment should not include inferences or interpretative statements that are unsupported with data. The nurse applies intellectual standards of critical thinking to collect the level of detail necessary to fully understand a client's problems or needs.

4. The correct answer is 3. Data collection includes the gathering of subjective and objective data from or about a client. Subjective data are clients' perceptions about their health problems. Only clients can provide this kind of information.

5. The correct answer is 3. The use of good communication skills and critical thinking intellectual standards enable the nurse to collect complete, accurate, and relevant data.

6. The correct answer is 1. The first step in establishing the database is to collect subjective information by interviewing the client. An interview is an organized conversation with the client to obtain the client's health history and information about the current illness.

7. The correct answer is 1. An interview with a client includes three phases, similar to that of a therapeutic relationship: orientation, working, and termination. A successful interview requires preparation on the part of the nurse by collecting any available information about the client and then creating an environment conducive to an interview.

8. The correct answer is 3. During data clustering, the nurse organizes data and focuses attention on client functions needing support and assistance for recovery. Focused data clustering using a systems approach or functional health pattern approach assists the nurse in correctly classifying and organizing data.

9. The correct answer is 3. Closed-ended questions limit the client's answers to one or two words such as "yes" or "no" or a number or frequency of a symptom. For example, the nurse might ask, "How often does the diarrhea occur?" or "Do you have pain or cramping?" Closed-ended questions require concise answers and are used to clarify previous information or provide additional information.

10. The correct answer is 2. The use of open-ended questions prompts clients to describe a situation in more than one or two words. This technique leads to a discussion in which clients actively describe their health status. Open-ended questions give clients the chance to tell their stories and what is important to them.

Chapter 16

1. The correct answer is 1. A nursing diagnosis is a clinical judgment about individual, family, or community responses to actual and potential health problems or life processes.

2. The correct answer is 3. NANDA International's work provides a common language for the health problems nurses deal with. The organization is the leader in nursing diagnosis classification and is endorsed by the ANA as having the responsibility to do so.

3. The correct answer is 2. The use of standard formal nursing diagnostic statements serves several purposes. One of them is to help nurses to focus on the role of nursing in client care.

4. The correct answer is 4. Critical thinking is an active, organized, cognitive process used to carefully examine one's thinking and the thinking of others.

5. The correct answer is 1. *Family coping: potential for growth related to unexpected birth of twins* is a wellness nursing diagnosis. The type of nursing diagnosis describes human responses to levels of wellness in an individual, family, or community that have a readiness for enhancement.

6. The correct answer is 2. A risk nursing diagnosis describes human responses to health conditions/life processes that may develop in a vulnerable individual, family, or community. For example, a client with a spinal cord injury that limits mobility is at *risk for impaired skin integrity.*

7. The correct answer is 4. Diagnostic labels include descriptors used to give additional meaning to the diagnosis. For example, the diagnosis *impaired physical mobility* includes the descriptor *impaired* to describe the nature or change in mobility that best describes the client's response.

8. The correct answer is 3. To collect complete, relevant, and correct assessment data it may help to identify assessment activities that produce specific kinds of data. For example, using auscultation to obtain a pulse produces an objective measurement of heart rate and rhythm.

9. The correct answer is 1. The nurse determines the accuracy of data collected. For example, the nurse who auscultates abnormal lung sounds may be unsure of what is being heard through the stethoscope. Inaccurate assessment data means that data from clients are misinterpreted, inappropriate interventions may be selected, and the quality of care is jeopardized.

10. The correct answer is 2. Use of standardized nursing language such as NANDA diagnoses helps to ensure accuracy. A diagnostic statement such as "unhappy and worried about health" is not a scientifically based diagnosis, and it can lead to errors. The language needs to be more precise and appropriate, such as *ineffective individual coping related to fear of medical diagnosis.*

Chapter 17

1. The correct answer is 1. Once a nurse assesses a client's condition and identifies appropriate nursing diagnoses, a plan is developed for the client's nursing care.

2. The correct answer is 3. Planning is a category of nursing behaviors in which client-centered goals and expected outcomes are established and nursing interventions are selected. The interventions are specifically chosen to resolve the client's problem and achieve the goals and outcomes. Planning requires a nurse to use deliberate decision-making and problem-solving skills to design care for each client.

3. The correct answer is 4. Priorities are based on the urgency of the problem, the client's safety and desires, the nature of the treatment indicated, and the relationship among the diagnoses. Establishing priorities is not merely a matter of numbering the nursing diagnoses on the basis of severity or physiological importance.

4. The correct answer is 2. A client-centered goal is a specific and measurable behavior or response that reflects: a client's highest possible level of wellness and independence in function. Examples include "Client will perform self-care hygiene independently," "Client will remain free of infection," or "Client will accept body image alteration."

5. The correct answer is 1. For clients to participate in goal setting, they should be alert and have some degree of independence in completing activities of daily living, problem solving, and decision making. This is important because the nurse and client partner together in the client's care. If clients' cognitive and physical impairments are so severe that they cannot actively participate in goal setting, the nursing team acts in their behalf to develop client-centered goals.

6. The correct answer is 3. The nurse writes an expected outcome statement in measurable terms. This allows the nurse to note specifically the behavior or physiological response expected for resolution of the client's problem. For example, "Client will have less pain" is an inaccurate outcome statement because the phrase "less pain" is nonspecific. The statement "Client will report pain acuity less than 4 on a scale of 0 to 10" is accurate.

7. The correct answer is 2. As goals, outcomes, and interventions are developed, the nurse must be aware of and committed to accepted standards of practice from nursing and other disciplines in designing safe

and relevant client-centered care. In the planning of care the nurse displays attitudes such as creativity, perseverance, and humility to develop a plan of care that is individualized to the client/family needs.

8. The correct answer is 2. When establishing realistic goals, the nurse, through assessment, must know the resources of the health care facility, family, and client; the client's physiological, emotional, cognitive, and sociocultural potential; and the economic cost and resources available to reach expected outcomes in a timely manner.

9. The correct answer is 1. To initiate an intervention the nurse must be competent in three areas: (1) know the scientific rationale for the intervention, (2) possess the necessary psychomotor and interpersonal skills, and (3) be able to function within a particular setting to use the available health care resources effectively.

10. The correct answer is 4. Collaborative interventions are therapies that require the knowledge, skill, and expertise of multiple health care professionals.

Chapter 18

1. The correct answer is 2. In theory, implementation of the nursing care plan follows the planning component of the nursing process. However, in many health care settings implementation may begin directly after assessment. For example, immediate implementation is necessary when the nurse identifies urgent needs of the client in situations such as cardiac arrest or sudden death of a loved one.

2. The correct answer is 1. Indirect care interventions are treatments performed away from the client but on behalf of the client or group. Examples of indirect care include actions aimed at managing the client's environment (e.g., safety and infection control), documentation, and interdisciplinary collaboration.

3. The correct answer is 3. A standing order is a preprinted document containing orders for the conduct of routine therapies, monitoring guidelines, and/or diagnostic procedures for specific clients with identified clinical problems. The orders direct the conduct of client care in various clinical settings. Standing orders must be approved and signed by the licensed, prescribing physician or health care provider in charge of care before their implementation.

4. The correct answer is 3. When a nurse delegates aspects of a client's care to another staff member, the nurse assigning tasks is responsible for ensuring that each task is appropriately assigned and is completed according to the standard of care and that the direct care interventions are delegated to those personnel competent to provide the specific type of care.

5. The correct answer is 1. Interdisciplinary care plans represent the contributions of all disciplines caring for a client. For example, a client recovering from total hip surgery will have a care plan for the problem of impaired mobility that includes interventions from nursing, the surgeon, and physical therapy.

6. The correct answer is 2. Assessment is a continuous process that occurs each time a nurse interacts with a client. When new data are gathered and a new client need is identified, the nurse modifies the care plan.

7. The correct answer is 1. Environmental factors influence the delivery and reception of care. The surroundings in which nursing activities occur should be safe and conducive to the implementation of the therapy. Client safety is always the first concern.

8. The correct answer is 2. An out-of-date or incorrect care plan compromises the quality of nursing care, whereas review and modification enable the nurse to provide timely nursing interventions to best meet the client's needs.

9. The correct answer is 1. Goals can be achieved by providing an environment conducive to meeting such goals; adjusting care in accordance with the client's expressed or implied needs; stimulating and motivating clients, thereby enabling them to achieve self-care and independence; and encouraging clients to accept care or adhere to the treatment regimen.

10. The correct answer is 1. Because of the continual growth of health care professions and related technology, a nurse may lack the skills to perform a new procedure. When this occurs, information about the procedure is obtained from the literature and the agency's procedure book.

Chapter 19

1. The correct answer is 4. The nurse conducts evaluation measures to determine if expected outcomes are met, *not* the nursing interventions. The expected outcomes are the standards against which the nurse judges if goals have been met and thus if care is successful.

2. The correct answer is 1. Evaluation is one of the most critical phases of the nursing process because it determines the usefulness and effectiveness of nursing practice and is client driven and client centered. During evaluation the nurse decides if the previous steps of the nursing process were effective by examining the client's responses and comparing them with the behaviors or physical indicators stated in the expected outcomes.

3. The correct answer is 1. Evaluation is ongoing whenever the nurse has contact with the client. Once an intervention has been delivered, the nurse

gathers objective and subjective data from the client, family, and health care team members.

4. The correct answer is 2. The nurse must realize that evaluation is dynamic and ever changing, depending on the client's nursing diagnoses and condition. As problems change, so too may expected outcomes. A client whose health status continuously changes requires more frequent evaluation.

5. The correct answer is 3. The evaluation process, which determines the effectiveness of nursing care, includes five elements: (1) identifying evaluative criteria and standards, (2) collecting data to determine whether the criteria or standards are met, (3) interpreting and summarizing findings, (4) documenting findings and any clinical judgment, and (5) terminating, continuing, or revising the care plan.

6. The correct answer is 1. A goal specifies the expected behavior or response that indicates resolution of a nursing diagnosis or maintenance of a healthy state. It is a summary statement of what is to be accomplished when all expected outcomes have been met.

7. The correct answer is 2. Expected outcomes are the expected measurable results of the goal-oriented nursing process. A nurse-sensitive client outcome is a measurable client or family state, behavior, or perception, largely influenced by and sensitive to nursing interventions.

8. The correct answer is 4. Evaluating a client's response to nursing care requires the use of evaluative measures, which are simply the assessment skills and techniques used to collect data for evaluation. (e.g., auscultation of lung sounds, observation of a client's skill performance, discussion of the client's feelings, and inspection of the skin).

9. The correct answer is 2. The primary source of data for evaluation is the client. However, the nurse also uses the family and other caregivers.

10. The correct answer is 3. As goals are evaluated, the nurse makes adjustments to the care plan as indicated. If a goal was successfully met, that portion of the care plan is discontinued. Unmet and partially met goals require the nurse to continue intervention. After a nurse reassesses a client, nursing diagnoses may be modified or added with appropriate goals and expected outcomes, and interventions are established.

Chapter 20

1. The correct answer is 3. Functional nursing model of care is task focused, not client focused. Tasks are divided, with one nurse assuming responsibility for specific tasks, for example, hygiene and dressing changes, whereas another nurse may assume responsibility for medication administration.

2. The correct answer is 4. Primary nursing model of nursing care delivery was developed with the aim of placing RNs at the bedside and improving nursing's accountability for client outcomes and the professional relationships among staff members.

3. The correct answer is 1. Case management is a care management approach that coordinates and links health care services to clients and their families while streamlining costs and maintaining quality.

4. The correct answer is 4. Working in a decentralized structure has the potential for greater collaborative effort, increased competency of staff, and ultimately a greater sense of professional accomplishment and satisfaction.

5. The correct answer is 3. Accountability refers to individuals being answerable for their actions. It involves follow-up and a reflective analysis of one's decisions to evaluate their effectiveness.

6. The correct answer is 4. One of the manager's greatest challenges is communication with staff. The manager can use a variety of approaches to ensure that information is communicated quickly and accurately to all staff. For example, the manager can distribute biweekly or monthly newsletters of ongoing unit or health care agency activities or post minutes of committee meetings.

7. The correct answer is 2. Second-order priority needs are actual problems for which the client has requested immediate help, such as comfort measures.

8. The correct answer is 1. First-order priority needs are an immediate threat to a client's survival or safety, such as a physiological episode of obstructed airway, loss of consciousness, or a psychological episode of an anxiety attack.

9. The correct answer is 4. Assistive personnel should not be assigned sole responsibility for the care of clients. Instead, it is the professional nurse in charge of client care who decides what activities assistive personnel may perform independently and what activities must be performed by the RN and assistant in partnership. Nursing assistants have been trained to bathe clients.

10. The correct answer is 1. Quality improvement (QI) outcome indicator is a measure of the client's status after receiving care.

Chapter 21

1. The correct answer is 4. Justice refers to fairness. Health care providers agree to strive for justice in health care. The term often is used during discussions about resources. Decisions about who should receive available organs are always difficult.

2. The correct answer is 3. Maleficence refers to harm or hurt; thus nonmaleficence is the avoidance of harm or hurt. In health care ethics it is important to remember that ethical practice involves not only the will to do good, but also the equal commitment to do no harm.

3. The correct answer is 1. Beneficence refers to taking positive actions to help others. The practice of beneficence encourages the urge to do good for others. Commitment to beneficence helps to guide difficult decisions wherein the benefits of a treatment may be challenged by risks to the client's well-being or dignity.

4. The correct answer is 2. Fidelity refers to the agreement to keep promises. The standard of fidelity is an obligation to follow through with care offered to clients.

5. The correct answer is 2. The American Nurses Association (ANA) has established widely accepted codes that professional nurses attempt to follow.

6. The correct answer is 3. Nurses strengthen their ability to advocate for a client when nurses are able to identify personal values and then accurately identify the values of the client and articulate the client's point of view.

7. The correct answer is 4. A utilitarian system of ethics proposes that the value of something is determined by its usefulness.

8. The correct answer is 1. The ethic of care explores the notion of care as a central activity of human behavior. Those who write about the ethic of care advocate a more female-biased theory that is based on understanding relationships, especially personal narratives.

9. The correct answer is 3. When ethical dilemmas arise, the nurse's point of view is unique and critical. The nurse usually interacts with clients over longer time intervals than do other disciplines.

10. The correct answer is 2. Each step in the processing of an ethical dilemma resembles steps in critical thinking. The nurse begins by gathering information and moves through assessment, identification of the problem, planning, implementation, and evaluation.

Chapter 22

1. The correct answer is 1. Statutory law is created by elected legislative bodies such as state legislatures and the U.S. Congress. Examples of state statutes are the Nurse Practice Acts found in all 50 states.

2. The correct answer is 4. Nurse Practice Acts establish educational requirements for nurses, distinguish between nursing and medical practice, and generally define the scope of nursing practice.

3. The correct answer is 2. Common law is cr[...] judicial decisions made in courts when in[...] legal cases are decided. An example of com[...] is informed consent and the client's right t[...] treatment.

4. The correct answer is 4. Nurses should be sensitive to common sources of client injury, such as falls and medication errors.

5. The correct answer is 3. According to the Uniform Anatomical Gift Act, an individual who is at least 18 years of age may make an anatomical gift or organ donation (defined as a "donation of all or part of a human body to take effect upon or after death").

6. The correct answer is 4. Nurses may act as Good Samaritans by providing emergency assistance at an accident scene. Good Samaritan laws have been enacted in almost every state to encourage health care professionals to assist in emergency situations. These laws limit liability and offer legal immunity for nurses who help at the scene of an accident.

7. The correct answer is 3. There are essentially two standards for the determination of death. The cardiopulmonary standard requires irreversible cessation of circulatory and respiratory functions. The whole-brain standard requires irreversible cessation of all functions of the entire brain, including the brain stem. The reason for the development of different definitions is to facilitate recovery of organs for transplantation. Even though the client may be legally "brain dead," the client's organs may be healthy for donation to other clients.

8. The correct answer is 2. Informed consent is part of the physician-client relationship. Because nurses do not perform surgery or direct medical procedures, in most situations, obtaining clients' informed consent does not fall within the nursing duty.

9. The correct answer is 4. Malpractice or professional liability insurance is a contract between the nurse and the insurance company. Malpractice insurance provides for a defense when a nurse is sued for professional negligence or medical malpractice.

10. The correct answer is 4. The physician is responsible for directing medical treatment. Nurses are obligated to follow physician's orders unless they believe the orders are in error or would harm clients.

Chapter 23

1. The correct answer is 4. Assessment of a client's ability to communicate includes gathering data about the many contextual factors that influence communication. These include the participants' internal factors and characteristics, the nature of their relationship, the situation prompting communication, the environment, and the sociocultural elements present. Assessing these contextual factors helps the

nurse make sound decisions during the communication process.

2. The correct answer is 3. Active listening means to be attentive to what the client is saying both verbally and nonverbally. Several nonverbal skills have been identified as facilitative skills for attentive listening. S—Sit facing the client. O—Observe an open posture (i.e., keep arms and legs uncrossed). L—Lean toward the client. This posture conveys that you are involved and interested in the interaction. E—Establish and maintain intermittent eye contact.

3. The correct answer is 2. A helping relationship between nurse and client does not just happen—it is created with care and skill and is built on the client's trust in the nurse. Statements reflecting empathy are highly effective because they tell the person that the nurse heard the feeling content, as well as factual content, of the communication. It is used to establish trust.

4. The correct answer is 1. Gender is another factor that influences how we think, act, feel, and communicate. Male and female communication patterns tend to differ, which can sometimes create barriers to effective communication. Males communicate to achieve goals, establish individual status and authority, and compete for attention and power. Females communicate to build connections with others, include others, and cooperate with, respond to, show interest in, and support others.

5. The correct answer is 1. Nurses function in roles that require interaction with multiple health team members. Many elements of the nurse-client helping relationship are also applied in these collegial relationships, which are focused on accomplishing the work and goals of the clinical setting. It is especially important to involve the client and family in decisions about the plan of care to determine whether suggested methods are acceptable.

6. The correct answer is 3. Clarifying: to check whether understanding is accurate, the nurse can restate an unclear or ambiguous message to clarify the sender's meaning. Instead of restating the message, the nurse can also ask the other person to rephrase it, explain further, or give an example of what the person means.

7. The correct answer is 4. Focusing is used to center on key elements or concepts of a message. If conversation is vague or rambling or clients begin to repeat themselves, focusing is a useful technique.

8. The correct answer is 3. Giving personal opinions: when the nurse gives a personal opinion, it takes decision making away from the client. It inhibits spontaneity, stalls problem solving, and creates doubt.

9. The correct answer is 2. A tip for improved communication with older adults is to stick to one topic at a time.

10. The correct answer is 4. In the zones of personal space and touch, the personal zone (18 inches to 4 feet) includes nursing activities such as sitting at a client's bedside and taking the client's nursing history.

Chapter 24

1. The correct answer is 3. Psychomotor learning involves acquiring skills that require the integration of mental and muscular activity. Teaching a client to use a walker requires the use of the psychomotor domain. The client masters skills by manipulating equipment and practicing manual skills.

2. The correct answer is 2. If a learning ability is impaired, such as with a client in pain, the nurse should postpone teaching activities or modify teaching strategies to better meet the needs of the learner.

3. The correct answer is 3. Readiness to learn is related to the stage of grieving. Clients cannot learn when they are unwilling or unable to accept the reality of illness. However, properly timed teaching can facilitate adjustment to illness or disability. When a client is in denial or disbelief, teach in the present tense (e.g., explain what client needs to know to be discharged).

4. The correct answer is 4. The first step in forming a teaching plan is developing learning objectives. A learning objective identifies the expected outcome of a planned learning experience and helps establish priorities for learning. By developing topics for discussion that require problem solving, the freshman would be engaged in learning about nutrition.

5. The correct answer is 3. Behavioral objectives are measurable and observable and indicate how learning will be evidenced. The objective describes precise behaviors and content (e.g., the client will perform breast self-examination correctly on herself before the end of the teaching session).

6. The correct answer is 1. The telling approach is useful when limited information must be taught (e.g., preparing a client for an emergent diagnostic procedure).

7. The correct answer is 3. A nurse uses role play for teaching ideas and attitudes. During role play, people are asked to play themselves or someone else. The technique involves rehearsing a desired behavior.

8. The correct answer is 1. Older adults learn and remember effectively if the learning is paced properly and the material is relevant to the learner's needs and abilities.

9. The correct answer is 2. Generally, teaching and learning begin when a person identifies a need for knowing or acquiring an ability to do something.

10. The correct answer is 4. Demonstrations are useful methods for teaching psychomotor skills such as preparation of a syringe. The client is able to observe a skill before practicing it.

Chapter 25

1. The correct answer is 1. Accreditation agencies such as the Joint Commission on Accreditation of Healthcare Organizations (JCAHO) specify guidelines for documentation.

2. The correct answer is 4. Under the prospective payment system, hospitals are reimbursed a set dollar amount by Medicare for each diagnosis-related group (DRG).

3. The correct answer is 1. Documentation, which is anything written or printed within a client record, is a vital aspect of nursing practice. Nursing documentation must be accurate, comprehensive and flexible enough to retrieve critical data, maintain quality and continuity of care, track client outcomes, and reflect current standards.

4. The correct answer is 3. Data recorded, reported, or communicated to other health care professionals are confidential and must be protected.

5. The correct answer is 1. Clients frequently request copies of their medical records, and they have the right to read those records. Each institution has policies for controlling the manner in which records are shared. In most situations, clients are required to give written permission for release of medical information.

6. The correct answer is 3. Critical pathways are multidisciplinary care plans that include key interventions and expected outcomes within an established time frame.

7. The correct answer is 2. Acuity records provide a method of determining the hours of care and staff required for a given group of clients. A client's acuity level is based on the type and number of nursing interventions required for providing care in a 24-hour period.

8. The correct answer is 2. Ideally discharge planning begins at admission. Nurses revise the plan of care as the client's condition changes. There needs to be evidence of the involvement of the client and family members in the discharge planning process so that the client and family have the necessary information and resources to return home.

9. The correct answer is 1. An increasing number of older adults require care in long-term health care facilities. Since many individuals will live in this setting for the rest of their lives, they are referred to as residents rather than clients.

10. The correct answer is 4. A telephone order (TO) involves a physician stating a prescribed therapy over the phone to a registered nurse. A verbal order (VO) may be accepted when there is no opportunity for a physician to write the order, as in emergency situations. Clarifying for accuracy is important when a registered nurse accepts a physician's order over the telephone or verbally. The order needs to be verified by repeating it clearly and precisely. The registered nurse is responsible for writing the order on the physician's order sheet in the client's permanent record and signing it.

Chapter 26

1. The correct answer is 2. Self-concept is an individual's conceptualization about how the individual thinks about him or herself. It is a complex lifelong process that involves many factors. Mastectomy is a surgical procedure that alters the appearance and function of the body, although the changes may not be apparent to others when the individual is dressed. Although potentially undetected by others, these bodily changes have a significant impact on the individual.

2. The correct answer is 2. One of the self-concept developmental tasks of 1- to 3-year-olds is developing self through modeling, imitation, and socialization.

3. The correct answer is 4. Identity involves the internal sense of individuality, wholeness, and consistency of a person over time and in various circumstances.

4. The correct answer is 3. Body image involves attitudes related to the body, including physical appearance, structure, or function.

5. The correct answer is 1. Through the process of reinforcement-extinction, certain behaviors become common or are avoided, depending on whether they are approved and reinforced or discouraged and punished.

6. The correct answer is 4. In the process of identification, an individual internalizes the beliefs, behavior, and values of role models into a personal, unique expression of self.

7. The correct answer is 3. An individual's identity is affected by stressors throughout life, but is particularly vulnerable during adolescence, which is a time of great change.

8. The correct answer is 1. Identity confusion results when a person does not maintain a clear, consistent, and continuous consciousness of personal identity.

9. The correct answer is 3. Self-esteem: asking a client about how the client feels about himself or herself, will give the nurse information about the client's self-esteem.

10. The correct answer is 1. Increasing a client's self-awareness is achieved though establishing a trusting relationship that allows the client to openly explore thoughts and feelings.

Chapter 27

1. The correct answer is 4. The first step of gender identity development occurs as the child becomes aware of the differences of the sexes and perceives that he or she is male or female.

2. The correct answer is 2. Sexual health can be described as a person's freedom from physical and psychological impairment, the awareness of open and positive attitudes toward sexual functioning, and accurate knowledge about sexuality.

3. The correct answer is 4. Sexual dysfunction is defined as the absence of complete sexual functioning.

4. The correct answer is 1. The incidence of sexually transmitted diseases (STDs) in the United States is increasing each year. The United States has the highest rate of STDs in the industrialized world. The prevalence of STDs is a major health concern because treatment is costly and the incidence is high in minority populations of low socioeconomic attainment.

5. The correct answer is 1. Contraceptive methods that require the intervention of a health care provider include hormonal contraception, intrauterine devices (IUDs), the diaphragm, the cervical cap, and sterilization.

6. The correct answer is 3. Effectiveness rates are reported as follows: oral contraceptives, 97% to 99.9%; IUDs, 98% to 99.9%; diaphragm, 82% to 97%; and cervical cap, 82% to 95%.

7. The correct answer is 1. Sterilization is the most effective contraception method other than abstinence. It should be considered permanent. Female sterilization, or tubal ligation, involves cutting, tying, or otherwise ligating the fallopian tubes. In male sterilization, or vasectomy, the vas deferens, which carries the sperm away from the testicles, is cut and tied.

8. The correct answer is 2. Although human immunodeficiency virus (HIV) is present in the majority of body fluids, it is really a blood-borne pathogen. For transmission of HIV to occur, some exchange of body fluid, particularly blood, must occur. Primary routes of transmission include contaminated intravenous (IV) needles; anal intercourse, vaginal intercourse, and oral-genital sex; and transfusion of blood and blood products.

9. The correct answer is 2. When caring for older adults, the nurse may adjust his or her assessment approach. When the nurse gathers a sexual history from an older adult, it is important to keep in mind that older adults may have difficulty discussing intimate details with health care providers. The nurse has the responsibility to help maintain the sexuality of the aged by offering the opportunity to discuss. Often, asking questions on the topic of sexuality in a comfortable, relaxed manner facilitates older adults' discussing their sexual needs.

10. The correct answer is 1. A useful framework for guiding planning is the PLISSIT model developed by Annon (1976). In this model there are progressively more involved levels of intervention. The *P* stands for permission giving. During assessment the nurse's questions can bring up the topic of sexuality and can give the individual permission to talk about sexual concerns. *LI* stands for limited information, which involves providing basic information regarding sexuality and sexual functioning. *SS* stands for specific suggestions, whereby the nurse provides specific suggestions regarding a sexual concern or issue, or the concern expressed might be one that the nurse is not equipped to address. In this case the nurse should refer to another health care provider. The *IT* stands for intensive therapy. At this level of intervention, the nurse's role would be to refer the client to a qualified practitioner, such as a social worker or sex counselor, for individualized therapy.

Chapter 28

1. The correct answer is 3. Caring for a client's spiritual needs means caring for the whole person, accepting his or her beliefs and experiences, and helping the client with issues surrounding meaning and hope.

2. The correct answer is 2. There are individuals who either do not believe in the existence of God (atheist) or who believe that any ultimate reality is unknown or unknowable (agnostic). Agnostics believe that the existence of a God or higher power cannot be proven or disproved. This does not mean that spirituality is not an important concept for the atheist or agnostic. Atheists search for meaning in life through their work and their relationships with other individuals.

3. The correct answer is 4. Hope is a multidimensional concept that provides comfort while enduring life threats and personal challenges.

4. The correct answer is 1. Hinduism accepts modern medical science; however, the belief is that illness is caused by past sins, and the prolongation of life is discouraged.

5. The correct answer is 4. A ritual can provide the client with structure and support during difficult times. If rituals are important to the client, the nurse uses them as part of nursing intervention.

6. The correct answer is 1. The ability to establish presence is part of the art of nursing. It is not simply being in the same room with a client performing procedures or sharing technical information with a client, but presencing involves "being with" a client versus "doing for" a client. Presencing involves offering closeness with the client, physically, psychologically, and spiritually.

7. The correct answer is 1. Some sects of Hinduism are vegetarians. The belief is not to kill any living creature.

8. The correct answer is 4. Some members of the Jehovah's Witnesses may avoid food prepared with or containing blood.

9. The correct answer is 2. Members of the Mormon faith abstain from alcohol, caffeine, and tobacco.

10. The correct answer is 1. Clients who experience terminal illness or who have suffered permanent loss in body function because of a disabling disease or an injury will require the nurse's support in grieving over and coping with their loss. Supporting a client during times of grief can be strengthened by the nurse's ability to enter into a spiritual relationship with the client, whereby nurse and client come to know one another as individuals.

Chapter 29

1. The correct answer is 1. An actual loss is any loss of a person or object that can no longer be felt, heard, known, or experienced by the individual. Lost objects that have been valued by a client include any possession that is worn out, misplaced, etc.

2. The correct answer is 2. A perceived loss is any loss that is tangible and uniquely defined by the grieving client. It may be less obvious to others.

3. The correct answer is 3. Situational loss includes any sudden, unpredictable external event.

4. The correct answer is 4. During Bowlby's phase of disorganization and despair an individual may endlessly examine how and why the loss occurred.

5. The correct answer is 4. During Kübler-Ross's depression stage of dying the individual may feel overwhelmingly lonely and withdraw from interpersonal interaction.

6. The correct answer is 2. Worden's Task III is to adjust to the environment in which the deceased is missing. According to Worden, a person does not realize the full impact of a loss for at least 3 months. At this point many friends and associates stop calling, and the person is left to ponder the full impact of loneliness.

7. The correct answer is 3. Aging is frequently associated with losses such as physical changes, loss of employment, loss of social respect, loss of relationships, and *threat to a sense of fulfillment and contributions made in life.*

8. The correct answer is 1. General nursing care goals for clients with a loss include accommodating grief, accepting the reality of a loss, and renewing regular relationships.

9. The correct answer is 2. For transplantation of organs, the client must be maintained on ventilatory and circulatory support until vital organs are harvested. The family must clearly understand that the client is "brain dead," that the equipment (i.e., ventilator and vasopressor medications) is not keeping the client alive but keeping the physical body in a state so that the organs will not be damaged before harvesting.

10. The correct answer is 3. Palliative care allows clients to make more informed choices, achieve better alleviation of symptoms, and have more opportunity to work on issues of life closure.

Chapter 30

1. The correct answer is 1. The medulla oblongata controls vital functions necessary for survival. These include heart rate, blood pressure, and respiration.

2. The correct answer is 4. The general adaptation syndrome (GAS) has a three-stage reaction to stress. During the alarm reaction, rising hormone levels result in increased blood volume, blood glucose levels, epinephrine and norepinephrine amounts, heart rate, blood flow to muscles, oxygen intake, and mental alertness.

3. The correct answer is 2. Ego-defense mechanisms are indirect methods of coping with stress. Denial is avoiding emotional conflicts by refusing to consciously acknowledge anything that might cause intolerable emotional pain.

4. The correct answer is 3. Posttraumatic stress disorder (PTSD) begins with an acute stress disorder.

5. The correct answer is 3. Situational stress can arise from job changes, either one's own or that of a family member, and adjusting to chronic illness.

6. The correct answer is 2. The nurse uses the interview to determine the client's perception of stress by asking the client what is of most concern at this time.

7. The correct answer is 4. The primary modes of intervention for stress are to decrease stress-producing situations, increase resistance to stress, and learn skills that reduce physiological response to stress. A support provides emotional support benefits to a client experiencing stress.

8. The correct answer is 2. In the presence of anxiety-provoking thoughts and events, a common physiological symptom is muscle tension. Physiological tension will be diminished through a systematic approach to releasing tension in major muscle groups.

9. The correct answer is 4. Rapid changes in health care technology, diversity in the workforce, organizational restructuring, and changing work systems can place stress on nurses.

10. The correct answer is 1. A crisis creates a turning point in a person's life because it changes the direction of a person's life in some way. The precipitating event usually occurs from 1 to 2 weeks before the individual seeks help, but it may have occurred within the past 24 hours. Generally a crisis is resolved in some way within approximately 6 weeks.

Chapter 31

1. The correct answer is 3. Bradycardia is a slow heart rate, below 60 beats per minute in adults. Bradypnea is an abnormally slow rate of breathing, less than 12 breaths per minute.

2. The correct answer is 1. An inefficient contraction of the heart that fails to transmit a pulse wave to the peripheral pulse site creates a pulse deficit. To assess a pulse deficit the nurse and a colleague assess radial and apical rates simultaneously and then compare rates. The difference between the apical and radial pulse rates is the pulse deficit. Pulse deficits are frequently associated with abnormal rhythms.

3. The correct answer is 1. Careful measurement techniques ensure accurate findings. Vital signs and other physiological measurements are the basis for clinical problem solving. Vital sign assessment is an essential ingredient when nurses and physicians collaborate to determine the client's health status.

4. The correct answer is 2. Blood pressure measurements will not be accurate unless the correct size blood pressure cuff is applied appropriately. If a cuff is too small or tends to come loose, the result is a false high reading.

5. The correct answer is 3. Respirations cease for several seconds. Persistent cessation results in respiratory arrest. Any irregular respiratory pattern or periods of apnea (the cessation of respiration for several seconds) are symptoms of underlying disease in the adult and must be reported to the physician or nurse in charge.

6. The correct answer is 1. If orthostatic hypotension is assessed, the client is assisted to a lying position and the physician or nurse in charge is notified. While obtaining orthostatic measurements, the nurse observes for other symptoms of hypotension such as fainting, weakness, or light-headedness. Because the skill of orthostatic measurements re-

quires critical thinking and ongoing nursing judgment, this procedure is not delegated to unlicensed assistive personnel.

7. The correct answer is 4. When assessing the pulse, the nurse must consider the variety of factors influencing the pulse rate. A combination of these factors may cause significant changes. If the nurse detects an abnormal rate while palpating a peripheral pulse, the next step is to assess the apical rate.

8. The correct answer is 1. Conduction is the transfer of heat from one object to another with direct contact. Heat conducts through contact with solids, liquids, and gases. When the warm skin touches a cooler object, heat is lost. Conduction normally accounts for a small amount of heat loss. The nurse increases conductive heat loss when applying an ice pack or bathing a client with cool water.

9. The correct answer is 3. The pulse is the palpable bounding of blood flow noted at various points on the body. Blood flows through the body in a continuous circuit. The pulse is an indicator of circulatory status. Diseases causing poor oxygenation, such as asthma or chronic obstructive pulmonary disease (COPD), cause an increase in pulse rate.

10. The correct answer is 1. The basic techniques of inspection, palpation, and auscultation are used to determine vital signs. These skills are simple but should not be taken for granted. Careful measurement techniques ensure accurate findings. Vital signs and other physiological measurements are the basis for clinical problem solving. Vital sign assessment is an essential ingredient when nurses and physicians collaborate to determine the client's health status.

Chapter 32

1. The correct answer is 2. Inspection is a simple technique, but it is often underused. The quality of an inspection depends on the nurse's willingness to spend time doing a thorough job.

2. The correct answer is 2. The order of an abdominal examination differs slightly from previous assessments. The nurse begins with inspection and then follows with auscultation. It is important to auscultate before palpation and percussion because palpation and percussion may alter the frequency and character of bowel sounds.

3. The correct answer is 3. The nurse uses the dorsal surface of the hands/fingers to assess skin temperature.

4. The correct answer is 4. A methodical approach is used to examine the lymph nodes to avoid overlooking any single node or chain. The client relaxes with the neck flexed slightly forward and, if needed, toward the nurse. This maneuver relaxes tissues and muscles. Both sides of the neck are inspected and

palpated for comparison. During palpation the nurse faces or stands to the side of the client for easy access to all nodes. Using the pads of the middle three fingers of the hand, the nurse palpates gently in a rotary motion for superficial lymph nodes.

5. The correct answer is 2. Areas of concern when inspecting skin lesions include variegated pigmentation, irregular borders, and indistinct margins. Cancerous lesions frequently undergo changes in color and size.

6. The correct answer is 3. The movement of a body part away from the midline of the body is called abduction. Examples of joints include the legs, arms, and fingers.

7. The correct answer is 3. The nurse first inspects the shape and symmetry of the client's chest from the back and front. Normally the chest contour is symmetrical.

8. The correct answer is 1. The examiner compares lung sounds in one region on one side of the body with sounds in the same region on the opposite side. It is impossible to remember the quality of all sounds noted on one side of the body and then compare them with sounds on the other side.

9. The correct answer is 4. Interpreting abstract ideas or concepts reflects the capacity for abstract thinking. A higher level of intellectual functioning is required for an individual to explain such phrases as "A stitch in time saves nine" or "Don't count your chickens before they're hatched." The nurse notes whether the client's explanations are relevant and concrete. The client with altered mentation will likely interpret the phrase literally or merely rephrase the words.

10. The correct answer is 4. Assessment begins when the nurse first meets the client. The nurse determines the reason the client is seeking health care. Initial data from the general survey begins with a review of the client's primary health problems. The nurse makes mental notes of the client's behavior and appearance. The examination begins with a general survey that includes observation of general appearance and behavior, vital signs, and height and weight measurements. The survey provides information about characteristics of an illness, a client's hygiene and body image, emotional state, recent changes in weight, and developmental status. If abnormalities or problems are found, the affected body system is closely assessed later.

Chapter 33

1. The correct answer is 1. If the infectious disease can be transmitted directly from one person to another, it is a communicable, or contagious, disease.

2. The correct answer is 3. The blood is normally sterile, but in the case of infectious diseases such as hepatitis B or C, it becomes a reservoir for pathogens.

3. The correct answer is 4. The interval when client manifests signs and symptoms (e.g., common cold manifested by sore throat, sinus congestion, rhinitis) specific to type of infection is the illness stage.

4. The correct answer is 2. The most important and most basic technique in preventing and controlling transmission of infections is hand hygiene, which includes using an instant alcohol hand antiseptic before and after providing client care and hand washing. Hand washing is a vigorous, brief rubbing together of all surfaces of the hands lathered in soap, followed by rinsing under a stream of water.

5. The correct answer is 1. Visitors are encouraged to wash their hands before eating or handling food, after coming in contact with infected clients, and after handling contaminated equipment or organic material.

6. The correct answer is 2. Before isolation measures are instituted, the client must understand the nature of the disease or condition, the purposes of isolation, and steps for carrying out specific precautions. The nurse also takes measures to improve the client's sensory stimulation during isolation.

7. The correct answer is 4. Gowns or cover-ups protect health care personnel and visitors from coming in contact with infected material and blood or body fluid.

8. The correct answer is 2. Gloves should be removed promptly after use, before touching noncontaminated items and environmental surfaces.

9. The correct answer is 3. Autoclave is used to sterilize surgical instruments, parenteral solutions, and surgical dressings.

10. The correct answer is 1. When a nurse is doing a surgical hand washing, he or she must keep hands above elbows.

Chapter 34

1. The correct answer is 1. Right documentation has been added to the traditional five rights of medication administration to enhance medication safety. Medication errors may result from inaccurate documentation. Therefore it is essential that nurses ensure the appropriate documentation exists before giving medications.

2. The correct answer is 2. A medication order is required for any medication to be administered by a nurse. Before any other interventions, the nurse ensures that the medication order contains all of the elements. If the medication order is incomplete, the

nurse should inform the prescriber and ensure completeness before carrying out any medication order.

3. The correct answer is 4. Thirty milliliters is equivalent to 2 tablespoons. Tables of equivalent measurements are available in all health care institutions.

4. The correct answer is 1. A medication error is any event that could cause or lead to a client receiving inappropriate medication therapy or failing to receive appropriate medication therapy. Most medication errors occur when a nurse fails to follow routine procedures such as checking dose calculations, deciphering illegible handwriting, or administering medications with which the nurse is unfamiliar.

5. The correct answer is 4. This example demonstrates how the formula applies with solid dose forms. The physician orders 500 mg orally (PO) of Keflex. The medication is available in tablets containing 250 mg.

500 mg / 250 mg × 1 tablet = number of tablets to administer

The fraction 500⁄250 equals 2. Therefore

2 × 1 tablet = 2 tablets to be administered.

6. The correct answer is 1. State Nurse Practice Acts have the most influence over nursing practice by defining the scope of a nurse's professional functions and responsibilities. In general, most state Nurse Practice Acts are purposefully broad so as not to limit the professional responsibilities of the nurse. Institutions and agencies may interpret specific actions allowed under the acts, but they cannot modify, expand, or restrict the act's intent. The primary intent of the state Nurse Practice Acts is to protect the public from unskilled, undereducated, and unlicensed personnel.

7. The correct answer is 1. The nurse is responsible for following legal provisions when administering controlled substances or narcotics (medications that affect the mind and behavior), which are carefully controlled through federal and state guidelines. Violations of the Controlled Substances Act are punishable by fines, imprisonment, and loss of nurse licensure. Hospitals and other health care institutions have policies for the proper storage and distribution of narcotics.

8. The correct answer is 2. Pharmacokinetics is the study of how medications enter the body, reach their site of action, are metabolized, and exit the body. The nurse uses knowledge of pharmacokinetics when timing medication administration, selecting the route of administration, judging the client's risk for alterations in medication action, and observing the client's response.

9. The correct answer is 4. Federal medication law has extended and refined controls on medication sales and distribution; medication testing, naming, and labeling; and the regulation of controlled substances. Official publications such as the USP and the *National Formulary* set standards for medication strength, quality, purity, packaging, safety, labeling, and dose form.

10. The correct answer is 1. Enforcement of medication laws rests with the Food and Drug Administration (FDA), which ensures that all medications on the market undergo vigorous testing. Medications must go through this rigorous process before they can be dispensed to the public.

Chapter 35

1. The correct answer is 3. Despite the success of allopathic medicine (traditional Western medicine), many conditions such as arthritis, chronic back pain, gastrointestinal problems, allergies, headache, and insomnia have been difficult to treat, and more clients are exploring alternative methods to relieve their symptom distress.

2. The correct answer is 4. Many of the complementary therapies, such as acupuncture, contain diagnostic and therapeutic methods specific to their field, whereas others, such as guided imagery and breathwork, are generally easily learned and applied.

3. The correct answer is 1. Between one third and one half of the population in the United States uses one or more forms of complementary or alternative medicine (CAM). Furthermore, data from a recent survey of U.S. citizens suggest a 47.3% increase in the number of visits to alternative medicine practitioners. This exceeds the number of visits to allopathic practitioners.

4. The correct answer is 1. Holistic nursing regards and treats the mind-body-spirit of the client. Nurses use holistic nursing interventions such as relaxation therapy, guided imagery, music therapy, simple touch, massage, and prayer. Such interventions affect the whole person (mind-body-spirit) and are effective, economical, noninvasive, nonpharmacological complements to medical care.

5. The correct answer is 1. Nurses can learn CAM techniques with minimum preparation, and many of these procedures can be used with clients as independent nursing practice. Adequate assessment and the client's permission are prerequisites for implementation.

6. The correct answer is 1. One of the principles of these (CAM) therapies is that the individual becomes actively involved in the treatment. Individuals achieve better responses if they practice the techniques or exercises daily. A major principle is that the individual commits to implementing and maintaining the therapy until a desired outcome is achieved.

7. The correct answer is 2. The stress response is a good example of the way in which systems cooperate to protect an individual from harm. Although these responses prepare a person for short-term stress, the effects on the body of long-term stress can include structural damage and chronic illness such as angina, tension headaches, cardiac arrhythmias, pain, ulcers, and atrophy of the immune system organs.

8. The correct answer is 1. Meditation may augment the effects of certain drugs. For example, individuals taking antihypertensive medications or thyroid-regulating, antidepressive, or antianxiety medications should be monitored. Prolonged practice of meditation techniques may, in some instances, lead to the reduced need for certain medications such as antihypertensive medications.

9. The correct answer is 2. Biofeedback techniques are frequently used in addition to relaxation interventions to assist individuals in learning how to control specific autonomic nervous system responses.

10. The correct answer is 2. Therapeutic touch (Krieger, 1979) is a training-specific therapy that was developed by a nurse. Although the philosophical and religious assumptions of therapeutic touch are different from those of other Eastern healing modalities, therapeutic touch is similar in that it involves trained health care professionals who attempt to direct their own balanced energies in an intentional and motivated manner toward those of the client.

Chapter 36

1. The correct answer is 2. The antagonistic, synergistic, and antigravity muscle groups are coordinated by the nervous system and maintain posture and initiate movement. Antagonistic muscles bring about movement at the joint. During movement the active mover muscle contracts while its antagonist relaxes.

2. The correct answer is 1. Proprioception is the awareness of the position of the body and its parts. Proprioception is monitored by proprioceptors located on nerve endings in muscles, tendons, and joints. Posture is regulated by the nervous system and requires coordination of proprioception and balance.

3. The correct answer is 2. When standing, running, lifting, or performing activities of daily living (ADLs), a person must have adequate balance. Balance is controlled by the nervous system, specifically by the cerebellum and the inner ear. The major function of the cerebellum is to coordinate all voluntary movement, particularly highly skilled movements, such as those required in skiing.

4. The correct answer is 1. A client with a right-sided cerebral hemorrhage and damage to the right motor strip may have left-sided hemiplegia. However, a client with a right-sided head injury may only have cerebral edema (but not destruction) of the motor strip.

5. The correct answer is 3. Throughout the life span the body's appearance and functioning undergo change. The greatest change and impact on the maturational process is observed in childhood and old age.

6. The correct answer is 2. The period of adolescence is usually initiated by a tremendous growth spurt. Growth is frequently uneven. As a result, the adolescent may appear awkward and uncoordinated. Adolescent girls usually grow and develop earlier than boys. Hips widen, and fat is deposited in the upper arms, thighs, and buttocks. The adolescent boy's changes in shape are usually a result of long-bone growth and increased muscle mass.

7. The correct answer is 1. Clients are more open to developing an exercise program if they are at the stage of readiness to change their behavior. Information on the benefits of regular exercise may be helpful to the client who is not at the stage of readiness to act.

8. The correct answer is 2. It has become increasingly clear that children are becoming less active with the result being an increase in childhood obesity. Children and adolescents spend a great deal of their time in school. However, the number of students involved in daily school physical education decreased from 42% in 1991 to 32% in 1997.

9. The correct answer is 2. Bending at the knees helps to maintain the nurse's center of gravity and lets the strong muscles of the legs do the lifting.

10. The correct answer is 2. If the client has a syncopal episode or begins to fall, the nurse should assume a wide base of support with one foot in front of the other, thus supporting the client's body weight. The nurse then extends one leg and lets client slide against leg and gently lowers the client to the floor, protecting the client's head (Figure 36-5, B and C). Although lowering a client to the floor is not difficult, the student should practice this technique with a friend or classmate before attempting it in a clinical setting.

Chapter 37

1. The correct answer is 1. A new potential environmental health threat is the possibility of a terrorist attack. Before 1990 and the Gulf War, the possibility of the United States coming under attack from terrorists groups using biological, chemical, or nuclear weapons seemed remote. Today, however, we are concerned about an attack by an individual or small group on one of our cities, a large sporting event, or a unit of our military forces. Bioterrorism, or the use of biological agents to create fear and threat, is the most likely form of terrorist attack to

occur. Health care facilities must be prepared to treat mass casualties from an attack. The answer lies in the facility's emergency management plan. Such a plan details how to respond to a terrorist attack; for example, determining the agent used, determining the time and location of the attack and the affected population, obtaining and delivering supplies, and providing treatment.

2. The correct answer is 1. The physiological changes that occur during the aging process increase the older client's risk for falls and other types of accidents such as burns and car accidents. Older clients are more likely to fall in the bedroom, bathroom, and kitchen, and outside as a result of ice on walkways or obstacles in the garden. Inside falls most often occur while transferring from beds, chairs, and toilets; getting into or out of bathtubs; tripping over carpet edges or doorway thresholds; slipping on wet surfaces; and descending stairs.

3. The correct answer is 3. Unfortunately, clients throughout all developmental stages may be subject to abuse. Child abuse, domestic violence, and abuse of older adults are serious threats to safety.

4. The correct answer is 3. Guidelines for intervening in accidental poisoning should be adhered to. The Poison Control Center phone number should be visible on the telephone in homes with young children. In all cases of suspected poisoning, this number should be called immediately.

5. The correct answer is 2. Adolescents are at risk for injury from automobile accidents, suicide, and substance abuse.

6. The correct answer is 1. While conducting a home assessment for risks to safety, nurses must realize that they have entered the client's territory and that the client's attitude toward his or her residence and belongings must be appreciated.

7. The correct answer is 1. Another culturally sensitive issue is the client's sense of environmental control. The nurse must be aware of health beliefs and practices that will affect the outcome of interventions. For example, reliance on family and religious organizations, as opposed to community resources, may affect the client's compliance with nursing interventions and referrals.

8. The correct answer is 4. The older adult experiences alterations in vision and hearing. The nurse should encourage yearly vision and hearing examinations and frequent cleansing of glasses and hearing aids as a means of preventing falls and burns.

9. The correct answer is 4. Nocturia and incontinence are more frequent in older adults. The nurse should institute a regular toileting schedule for the client. A recommended frequency is every 3 hours. Diuretics should be given in the morning. Assistance should be provided, along with adequate lighting, to clients who need to go to the bathroom at night.

10. The correct answer is 3. The high prevalence of chronic conditions in older adults results in the use of a high number of prescription and over-the-counter medications. Coupled with age-related changes in pharmacokinetics, there is a greater risk of serious adverse effects.

Chapter 38

1. The correct answer is 1. Because hygienic care requires close contact with the client, the nurse uses communication skills to promote a caring therapeutic relationship and uses the time with the client for teaching and counseling. The nurse can integrate other nursing activities during hygiene care, including client assessment and interventions such as range-of-motion exercises, application of dressings, or inspection and care of intravenous sites.

2. The correct answer is 1. A client's personal preferences for hygiene are influenced by a number of factors. No two individuals perform hygiene in the same manner, and it is important that the nurse individualize the client's care based on knowing about the client's unique hygiene practices and preferences. Hygiene care is never routine.

3. The correct answer is 1. Body image is a person's subjective concept of his or her physical appearance. These images can change frequently. When clients undergo surgery, illness, or a change in functional status, body image can change dramatically. For this reason, the nurse will take extra effort to promote the client's hygienic comfort and appearance.

4. The correct answer is 2. The *Healthy People 2010* initiative included recommendations to improve the dental health of the population of the United States. The goals for oral health were to decrease tooth loss caused by tooth decay or periodontal disease for people ages 35 to 44; reduce the number of older adults who have lost their natural teeth; reduce the prevalence of gingivitis; and reduce destructive periodontal disease among individuals ages 35 to 44.

5. The correct answer is 1. Clients most in need of perineal care are those at greatest risk for acquiring an infection (e.g., uncircumcised males, clients who have indwelling urinary catheters, or clients who are recovering from rectal or genital surgery or childbirth). In addition, women who are having a menstrual period will require good perineal care.

6. The correct answer is 1. A back rub or back massage usually follows the client's bath. It promotes relaxation, relieves muscular tension, and stimulates skin circulation.

7. The correct answer is 2. Clients will experience conditions that threaten the integrity of oral mucosa. For example, mucosal changes associated with aging, use of chemotherapeutic drugs, or dehydration require the nurse to adapt oral hygiene approaches. More frequent mouth care and use of antiinfective agents are examples of ways the nurse will revise approaches to meet client needs.

8. The correct answer is 1. Unconscious clients and those with artificial airways (e.g., endotracheal or tracheal tubes) need more frequent and specialized oral hygiene. These clients have an increased risk of aspiration and subsequently aspiration pneumonia, and they also have more problems with dry and inflamed oral mucosa.

9. The correct answer is 1. Depending on the client's age and physical condition, the room temperature should be maintained between 20° and 23° C (68° and 74° F). Infants, older adults, and the acutely ill may need a warmer room. However, certain ill clients benefit from cooler room temperatures to lower the body's metabolic demands.

10. The correct answer is 1. File the toenails straight across and square; do not use scissors or clippers. Consult a podiatrist as needed.

Chapter 39

1. The correct answer is 1. Anemia, a lower than normal hemoglobin level, is a result of decreased hemoglobin production, increased red blood cell destruction, and/or blood loss. Clients will have complaints of fatigue, decreased activity tolerance, and increased breathlessness, as well as pallor (especially seen in the conjunctiva of the eye) and an increased heart rate.

2. The correct answer is 1. Carbon monoxide is the most common toxic inhalant that decreases the oxygen-carrying capacity of blood. The affinity for hemoglobin to bind with carbon monoxide is greater than 200 times its affinity to bind with oxygen, creating a functional anemia. Because of the bond's strength, carbon monoxide is not easily dissociated from hemoglobin, making the hemoglobin unavailable for oxygen transport.

3. The correct answer is 1. Conditions such as shock and severe dehydration resulting from extracellular fluid loss and reduced circulating blood volume cause hypovolemia. With a significant fluid loss, the body tries to adapt by increasing the heart rate and peripheral vasoconstriction to increase the volume of blood returned to the heart and, in turn, increase the cardiac output.

4. The correct answer is 2. Fever increases the tissues' need for oxygen, and as a result, carbon dioxide production also increases. If the febrile state persists, the metabolic rate remains high and the body begins to break down protein stores, resulting in muscle wasting and decreased muscle mass. Respiratory muscles such as the diaphragm and intercostals muscles are also wasted.

5. The correct answer is 1. Left-sided heart failure is an abnormal condition characterized by impaired functioning of the left ventricle due to elevated pressures and pulmonary congestion. If left ventricular failure is significant, the amount of blood ejected from the left ventricle drops greatly, resulting in decreased cardiac output.

6. The correct answer is 1. Right-sided heart failure results from impaired functioning of the right ventricle characterized by venous congestion in the systemic circulation. Right-sided heart failure more commonly results from pulmonary disease or as a result of long-term left-sided failure. The primary pathological factor in right-sided failure is elevated pulmonary vascular resistance (PVR). As the PVR continues to rise, the right ventricle must generate more work, and the oxygen demand of the heart increases. As the failure continues, the amount of blood ejected from the right ventricle declines, and blood begins to "back up" in the systemic circulation. Clinically the client has weight gain, distended neck veins, hepatomegaly and splenomegaly, and dependent peripheral edema.

7. The correct answer is 2. Cyanosis, the blue discoloration of the skin and mucous membranes caused by the presence of desaturated hemoglobin in capillaries, is a late sign of hypoxia. The presence or absence of cyanosis is not a reliable measure of oxygenation status.

8. The correct answer is 1. A person who starts smoking in adolescence and continues to smoke into middle age has an increased risk for cardiopulmonary disease and lung cancer.

9. The correct answer is 3. Frequent changes of position are simple and cost-effective methods for reducing the risks of stasis of pulmonary secretions and decreased chest wall expansion.

10. The correct answer is 4. The most effective position for a client with cardiopulmonary diseases is the 45-degree semi-Fowler's position, using gravity to assist in lung expansion and reduce pressure from the abdomen on the diaphragm.

Chapter 40

1. The correct answer is 1. Hypokalemia is one of the most common electrolyte imbalances, in which an inadequate amount of potassium circulates in extracellular fluid (ECF). When severe, hypokalemia can affect cardiac conduction and function. Because the normal amount of serum potassium is so small, there is little tolerance for fluctuations. The most common cause of hypokalemia is the use

of potassium-wasting diuretics such as thiazide and loop diuretics.

2. The correct answer is 4. The nurse first considers the client's age. An infant's proportion of total body water (70% to 80% total body weight) is greater than that of children or adults. Infants are not protected from fluid loss because they ingest and excrete a relatively greater daily water volume than adults. Therefore they are at a greater risk for fluid volume deficits (FVDs) and hyperosmolar imbalance because body water loss is proportionately greater per kilogram of weight.

3. The correct answer is 2. Older adults experience a number of age-related changes that can affect fluid, electrolyte, and acid-base balances. They have a decreased thirst sensation, which may affect their oral intake of fluids. The kidneys have a decrease in glomerular filtration rate and in the number of filtering nephrons. These changes can mean that in the presence of sodium depletion or overload the older adult may be unable to maintain homeostasis and the imbalance is instead worsened.

4. The correct answer is 4. For clients in health care settings, intake and output (I&O) measurement is a nursing intervention routinely used for clients following a procedure, clients who are febrile, clients with restricted fluids, or clients who receive diuretic or intravenous (IV) therapy. Output includes urine, diarrhea, vomitus, gastric suction, and drainage from postsurgical wounds or other tubes.

5. The correct answer is 1. Health promotion activities in the area of fluid, electrolyte, and acid-base imbalances focus primarily on client teaching. Clients and caregivers need to recognize risk factors for these imbalances and implement appropriate preventive measures.

6. The correct answer is 3. Total parenteral nutrition (TPN) is a nutritionally adequate hypertonic solution consisting of glucose and other nutrients and electrolytes given through an indwelling or central IV catheter, which may be inserted peripherally or percutaneously, implanted, or tunneled. TPN is used as an intervention in severe cases of malnutrition.

7. The correct answer is 1. Under no circumstances should potassium chloride (KCl) be given IV push. A direct infusion of KCl may be fatal. If an IV is to have additives added, a physician's order must be obtained that includes the required additives.

8. The correct answer is 1. The client's microflora and contamination by insertion are initially controlled for in the procedure for IV insertion. However, the other factors are controlled through conscientious use of infection-control principles. This begins with the use of thorough hand hygiene before and after the nurse handles any component of the IV system.

9. The correct answer is 3. An infiltration occurs when IV fluids enter the surrounding space around the venipuncture site. This is manifested as swelling (from increased tissue fluid) and pallor and coolness (caused by decreased circulation) around the venipuncture site.

10. The correct answer is 1. Phlebitis may be prevented by the routine removal and rotation of IV sites. The Centers for Disease Control and Prevention (CDC) recommends replacing peripheral venous catheters and rotating sites at least every 72 to 96 hours.

Chapter 41

1. The correct answer is 4. Excessive daytime sleepiness (EDS) is the most common complaint of people with obstructive sleep apnea (OSA). Persons with severe OSA may report taking daytime naps and experiencing a disruption in their daily activities because of sleepiness.

2. The correct answer is 2. In a hospital or extended care setting it is difficult to provide clients with the time needed to rest and sleep. However, the nurse plans care to avoid awakening clients for nonessential tasks. The nurse can help by scheduling assessments, treatments, procedures, and routines for times when clients are awake. For example, if a client's physical condition has been stable, the nurse should avoid awakening the client to check vital signs.

3. The correct answer is 1. The use of nonprescription sleeping medications is not advisable. Clients should learn the risks of such drugs. Over the long term, these drugs can lead to further sleep disruption even when they initially seemed to be effective. Older adults should be cautioned about using over-the-counter antihistamines because of their long duration of action that can cause confusion, constipation, urinary retention, and increased risk of falls.

4. The correct answer is 1. Clients should be cautioned about the dosage and use of herbal compounds because the Food and Drug Administration (FDA) does not regulate them. Herbal compounds may create interactions with prescribed medication, and concurrent use should be avoided.

5. The correct answer is 1. Although dreams occur during both nonrapid eye movement (NREM) and rapid eye movement (REM) sleep, the dreams of REM sleep are more vivid and elaborate and are believed to be functionally important to learning, memory processing, and adaptation to stress.

6. The correct answer is 2. Beta-adrenergic agents can cause nightmares, insomnia, and awakenings from sleep.

7. The correct answer is 4. Limiting alcohol, caffeine, and nicotine and decreasing fluids 2 to 4 hours before sleep may promote sleep for older adults.

8. The correct answer is 4. Currently, the American Academy of Pediatrics recommends that apparently healthy infants be placed in the side-lying or supine position during sleep because of an association between the prone position and the occurrence of sudden infant death syndrome (SIDS).

9. The correct answer is 4. Narcolepsy is a dysfunction of mechanisms that regulate the sleep and wake states. Excessive daytime sleepiness is the most common complaint associated with this disorder. During the day a person may suddenly feel an overwhelming wave of sleepiness and fall asleep; REM sleep can occur within 15 minutes of falling asleep.

10. The correct answer is 4. The amount of sleep needed during the school years is individualized because of varying states of activity and levels of health. A 6-year-old averages 11 to 12 hours of sleep nightly, whereas an 11-year-old sleeps about 9 to 10 hours. The 6- or 7-year-old can usually be persuaded to go to bed by encouraging quiet activities.

Chapter 42

1. The correct answer is 2. The American Bar Association declared pain relief a basic legal right.

2. The correct answer is 1. Pain itself is considered to be a separate disease.

3. The correct answer is 2. Chronic pain lasts longer than anticipated, may not have an identifiable cause, and leads to great personal suffering.

4. The correct answer is 3. One of the common biases and misconceptions about pain is that administering analgesics regularly will lead to drug addiction.

5. The correct answer is 1. Cognitively toddlers and preschoolers are unable to recall explanations about pain or associate pain with experiences that can occur in various situations.

6. The correct answer is 4. An accurate diagnosis is made only after a complete assessment has been performed. In the example of the diagnosis of pain, the nurse may assess the client's withdrawal from communication, grimacing, and moaning, as well as the client's verbalization of discomfort.

7. The correct answer is 3. Descriptive pain scales are useful not only in assessing the severity of pain, but also in evaluating changes in a client's condition. A rating of 7 or more on a 0 to 10 scale requires immediate attention. The dose was insufficient.

8. The correct answer is 3. The key to success in pain relief is ongoing evaluation of interventions. Is the pain relieved?

9. The correct answer is 3. Nurses care for clients who have acute pain due to invasive procedures (e.g., surgery, endoscopy) or trauma. A preventive measure is an aggressive treatment of postoperative pain and pain from medical procedures and trauma.

10. The correct answer is 4. A drug delivery system called patient-controlled analgesia (PCA) is a safe method for postoperative and cancer pain management that most clients prefer. The client gains control over pain, and pain relief does not depend on nurse availability. They can also access medication when they need it. This can decrease anxiety and lead to decreased medication use.

Chapter 43

1. The correct answer is 4. Carbohydrates are the main source of energy in the diet.

2. The correct answer is 2. Although proteins may provide a source of energy (4 kcal/g), they are essential for synthesis (building) of body tissue in growth, maintenance, and repair.

3. The correct answer is 4. When the intake of nitrogen exceeds the output, the body is in positive nitrogen balance, which is required for growth, normal pregnancy, maintenance of lean muscle mass and vital organs, and wound healing.

4. The correct answer is 1. Water composes 60% to 70% of total body weight.

5. The correct answer is 2. The most reliable method for verification of placement of small-bore feeding tubes is x-ray examination.

6. The correct answer is 4. Parenteral nutrition (PN) is a form of specialized nutrition support in which nutrients are provided intravenously. Clients who are unable to digest or absorb enteral nutrition or who are in highly stressed physiological states such as sepsis, head injury, or burns are candidates for PN therapy.

7. The correct answer is 3. *Helicobacter pylori* is a bacterium that causes peptic ulcers.

8. The correct answer is 1. Inflammatory bowel disease includes Crohn's disease and idiopathic ulcerative colitis.

9. The correct answer is 3. Nutritional therapy for hypertension includes kilocalorie reduction to promote weight loss as appropriate, decreased sodium intake, and potassium-rich foods if potassium-wasting diuretics are part of the treatment.

10. The correct answer is 2. Homebound older adults have an increased risk of poor nutrition.

Chapter 44

1. The correct answer is 2. The normal adult urine output is 1500 to 1600 ml/day.

2. The correct answer is 1. Renal alterations result from factors that cause injury directly to the glomeruli or renal tubule, interfering with their normal filtering, reabsorptive, and secretory functions. Selected causes include transfusion reactions, diseases of the glomeruli, and systemic diseases such as diabetes mellitus.

3. The correct answer is 2. Postrenal alterations result from obstruction to the flow of urine in the urinary collecting system caused by calculi, blood clots, or tumors anywhere from the calyces (drainage structures within the kidney) to the urethral meatus.

4. The correct answer is 4. Urinary tract infections (UTIs) are the most common hospital-acquired (nosocomial) infections in the United States.

5. The correct answer is 3. Hospital-acquired UTIs are often related to poor hand washing, improper catheter care, or faulty catheterization technique.

6. The correct answer is 1. The urine appears concentrated and cloudy because of the presence of white blood cells (WBCs) or bacteria.

7. The correct answer is 2. Some medications change the color of urine. Pyridium colors the urine a bright orange to rust.

8. The correct answer is 3. To minimize nocturia, fluids should be avoided 2 hours before bedtime.

9. The correct answer is 1. The drainage bag should never be raised above the level of the client's bladder. Urine in the bag and tubing can become a medium for bacteria, and infection is likely to develop if urine flows back into the bladder (urinary reflux).

10. The correct answer is 4. Care must be taken to ensure that whatever type or size of condom catheter is used, blood supply to the penis is not impaired.

Chapter 45

1. The correct answer is 4. Most nutrients and electrolytes are absorbed in the small intestine, specifically by the duodenum and jejunum.

2. The correct answer is 3. Intolerance to lactose-containing foods may result in diarrhea, gaseous distention, and cramping.

3. The correct answer is 4. A common laboratory test that can be done at home or at the client's bedside is the fecal occult blood test (FOBT), or guaiac test, which measures microscopic amounts of blood in feces. It is useful as a diagnostic screening test for colon cancer.

4. The correct answer is 1. Antidiarrheal opiate agents decrease intestinal muscle tone to slow passage of feces. Opiates inhibit peristaltic waves that move feces forward, but they also increase segmental contractions that mix intestinal contents.

5. The correct answer is 3. An obvious sign of fecal impaction is the inability to pass a stool for several days, despite the repeated urge to defecate. When a continuous oozing of diarrhea stool develops, impaction should be suspected.

6. The correct answer is 4. Cleansing enemas promote the complete evacuation of feces from the colon. The maximum amount given to an adult is 750 to 1000 ml.

7. The correct answer is 3. The specific signs and symptoms of a client not tolerating an enema include abdominal pain more than a pressure sensation, abdominal cramping, abdominal distention, or rectal bleeding. It must be stopped. Notify physician and obtain vital signs.

8. The correct answer is 2. One of the greatest problems in caring for a client with a nasogastric (NG) tube is maintaining comfort.

9. The correct answer is 1. The stool discharged from an ostomy is called effluent.

10. The correct answer is 1. A nurse trained to care for ostomy clients is an enterostomal therapist.

Chapter 46

1. The correct answer is 2. The effects of bed rest or immobilization on the cardiovascular system include orthostatic hypotension, increased cardiac workload, and thrombus formation.

2. The correct answer is 1. After bed rest clients usually have an increased pulse rate, a decrease in pulse pressure, and an increase in fainting in response to a tilting or an erect posture. This is referred to as orthostatic hypotension.

3. The correct answer is 4. Elastic stockings (sometimes called thromboembolic device hose) [TED]) also aid in maintaining external pressure on the muscles of the lower extremities and thus may promote venous return.

4. The correct answer is 2. In the presence of an infectious process, immobilized clients may have an increased basal metabolic rate (BMR) as a result of fever or wound healing. Fever and repair of wounds increase cellular oxygen requirements. Bed rest helps to reduce their need for oxygen.

5. The correct answer is 3. Immobility can have a significant effect on the older adult's levels of health, independence, and functional status.

6. The correct answer is 4 b. Increased activity may result in symptoms associated with activity intolerance (e.g., increased pulse, changes in blood pressure, increased respirations, and decreased level of comfort). This can jeopardize the client's safety.

7. The correct answer is 1. Heparin and low-molecular-weight heparin (LMWH) are the most widely used drugs in the prophylaxis of deep vein thrombosis (DVT). Standard heparin is considered the gold standard for treatment because it has been well studied and validated. Common dosage for heparin therapy is 5000 units given subcutaneously 2 hours before surgery and repeated every 8 to 12 hours until the client is fully mobile or discharged.

8. The correct answer is 1. The trapeze bar is a triangular device that descends from a securely fastened overhead bar that is attached to the bed frame. It allows the client to pull with the upper extremities to raise the trunk off the bed, to assist in transfer from bed to wheelchair, or to perform upper arm exercises.

9. The correct answer is 2. The client in the prone position is lying face or chest down.

10. The correct answer is 3. Instrumental activities of daily living (IADLs) are activities that are necessary to be independent in society beyond eating, grooming, transferring, and toileting and include such skills as shopping, preparing meals, banking, and taking medications.

Chapter 47

1. The correct answer is 4. After a period of tissue ischemia, if the pressure is relieved and the blood flow returns, the skin turns red. The effect of this redness is vasodilation (blood vessel expansion), called reactive hyperemia. The area of reactive hyperemia should be evaluated by pressing a finger over the affected area. If the area blanches (turns lighter in color), and the erythema returns when the finger is removed, the reactive hyperemia is thought to be transient and is an attempt to overcome the ischemic episode.

2. The correct answer is 1. A stage I pressure ulcer is an observable pressure-related alteration of intact skin whose indicators, as compared with an adjacent or opposite area on the body, may include changes in one or more of the following: skin temperature (warmth or coolness), tissue consistency (firm or beefy feel), and/or sensation (pain, itching).

3. The correct answer is 4. If the nurse detects purulent or suspicious-looking drainage, collecting a specimen for culture may be necessary. The nurse never collects a wound culture sample from old drainage. Resident colonies of bacteria from the skin grow within exudate and may not be the true causative organisms of a wound infection. The nurse cleans a wound first with normal saline to remove skin flora.

4. The correct answer is 3. When evisceration occurs, the nurse places sterile towels soaked in sterile saline over the extruding tissues to reduce chances of bacterial invasion and drying. If the organs protrude through the wound, blood supply to the tissues is compromised. The client should be allowed nothing by mouth (NPO), observed for signs and symptoms of shock, and prepared for emergency surgery.

5. The correct answer is 2. Serous drainage is clear, watery plasma.

6. The correct answer is 2. For a client who has a muscle sprain, localized hemorrhage, or hematoma or who has undergone dental surgery, an ice bag is ideal to prevent edema formation, control bleeding, and anesthetize the body part.

7. The correct answer is 3. When clients have an incontinent episode, the area should be gently cleansed and dried and a thick layer of moisture barrier applied to the exposed areas. A moisture barrier protects the skin from excessive moisture and bacteria found in the urine or stool.

8. The correct answer is 4. Hydrocolloid dressings are dressings with complex formulations of colloids, elastomeric, and adhesive components. These dressings are adhesive and occlusive. The wound contact layer of this dressing forms a gel as fluid is absorbed and maintains a moist healing environment.

9. The correct answer is 3. To provide even support to a wound and immobilize a body part, the nurse may apply elastic gauze or cloth bandages and binders over a dressing.

10. The correct answer is 1. For open wounds, sterile, warm, moist compresses improve circulation, relieve edema, and promote consolidation of pus and drainage.

Chapter 48

1. The correct answer is 2. A kinesthetic sense enables a person to be aware of the position and movement of body parts without seeing them.

2. The correct answer is 2. Stereognosis is a sense that allows a person to recognize an object's size, shape, and texture.

3. The correct answer is 3. A client who is in constant pain and undergoes frequent monitoring of vital signs is at risk for experiencing sensory overload.

4. The correct answer is 2. Proprioceptive changes after age 60 include increased difficulty with balance, spatial orientation, and coordination.

5. The correct answer is 4. For a client with hearing impairment the nurse should face the client when

speaking, use simple sentences, and speak more slowly and in a normal volume.

6. The correct answer is 4. The nursing history includes assessment of the nature and characteristics of sensory alterations or any problem related to an alteration. The nurse begins by asking the client to describe the sensory deficit. For example, "How does your hearing compare to a year ago?"

7. The correct answer is 2. For older adults: Do not drive during rush hour. Drive defensively—use rear-view and side-view mirrors when changing lanes. Avoid driving at dusk or night. Go slow, but not too slow. Keep the car in good working condition.

8. The correct answer is 3. Nurses should routinely assess children for noise exposure and participate in providing hearing conservation classes for teachers, students, and parents.

9. The correct answer is 3. Olfactory is the sense of smell. If a client cannot smell, the client might not smell smoke if there were a fire. A fire alarm would be essential.

10. The correct answer is 1. A deficit in the normal function of sensory reception and perception is a sensory deficit. When senses are impaired, the sense of self is impaired. Initially a person may withdraw by avoiding communication or socialization with others in an attempt to cope with the sensory loss.

Chapter 49

1. The correct answer is 2. The obese client is susceptible to poor wound healing and wound infection because of the structure of fatty tissue, which contains a poor blood supply. This slows delivery of essential nutrients, antibodies, and enzymes needed for wound healing.

2. The correct answer is 3. If a client regularly uses prescription or over-the-counter medications, the surgeon or anesthesia provider may temporarily discontinue the drugs before surgery or adjust the dosages. Certain medications have special implications for the surgical client, creating greater risks for complications or interacting with anesthetic agents.

3. The correct answer is 2. The client who smokes is at greater risk for postoperative pulmonary complications than a client who does not.

4. The correct answer is 2. The family is an important resource for the client with physical limitations and provides the emotional support needed to motivate the client to return to a previous state of health.

5. The correct answer is 1. Accurate recording of intake and output helps assess renal and circulatory function. The nurse should assess daily weight for the first several days after surgery and compare it with the preoperative weight to assess fluid balance.

6. The correct answer is 3. Position the client on one side with the face downward and the neck slightly extended to facilitate a forward movement of the tongue and the flow of mucous secretions out of the mouth.

7. The correct answer is 4. After surgery the client may have reduced lung volume and require greater efforts to cough and deep breathe; inadequate lung expansion can lead to atelectasis and pneumonia.

8. The correct answer is 2. Prothrombin time (PT), international normalized ratio (INR), activated partial thromboplastin time (APTT), and platelet counts reveal clotting ability of blood, which reveals clients at risk for bleeding tendencies and thrombus formation.

9. The correct answer is 2. Maintaining upright position facilitates diaphragm excursion and enhances thorax expansion.

10. The correct answer is 4. Malignant hyperthermia is a potentially lethal condition that can occur in clients receiving general anesthesia. It should be suspected when there is unexpected tachycardia and tachypnea, jaw muscle rigidity, body rigidity of limbs, abdomen, and chest, or hyperkalemia. Temperature elevation is a late sign.

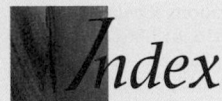

Index

A

A-delta fiber, 1230-1231
Abandonment, 418-419
Abbreviations in drug dosages, 838, 838t
Abdellah theory of nursing, 68
Abdomen, 741-746
  assessment of
    auscultation in, 743b, 743-744
    inspection in, 742-743
    nursing health history in, 741t
    palpation in, 744f, 744-746, 745f
    percussion in, 722f, 744, 744f
    physical, 1386
    positioning for, 681t
    preoperative, 1605
  landmarks of, 741-742, 742f
  of middle adult, 227t
  of older adult, 243
Abdominal binder, 1549f, 1549-1552
Abdominal cramping, enteral nutrition-related, 1314t
Abdominal distention, 742-743, 1386
  postoperative, 1637t
Abdominal radiography, 1341t
Abdominal reflex, 768t
Abducens nerve, 764t
Abduction, 758t, 759f
  of finger, 1437t
  of knee, 1438t
  of shoulder, 1435t
  of thumb, 1437t
  of toe, 1439t
  of wrist, 1436t
ABGs. See Arterial blood gases.
Ablative surgery, 1596t
Abnormal reactive hyperemia, 1502
ABO system, 1190
Abortion, 417-418, 529
Abrasion, 1009t, 1491t, 1503
Absorption
  intestinal, 1276-1277, 1277t
  of medication, 825-828
Abstinence as contraception, 526
Abstract, 83
Abstract thinking, 208, 763
Abuse
  assessment in general survey, 684b, 684-685
  child, 412, 684b
  domestic, 684b
  within family, 143
  public health laws and, 412
  sexual, 529, 684b
    clinical manifestations of, 186b
    potential signs and symptoms of, 533b
    sexual health assessment and, 533
  substance
    adolescent and, 210, 212
    assessment in general survey, 685, 685b
    community-based nursing and, 52, 54
    older adult and, 54t
    preoperative care and, 1602
    school-age child and, 202t
    skin assessment in, 690b
    surgical risks and, 1602
    young adult and, 222

Acceptance, 553
  dying and, 570
Accessory muscles of respiration, 1071
Accident
  in health care facility, 965-966
  motor vehicle
    during early childhood, 191t
    during infancy, 183b
    during school-age years, 202t
  pedestrian, 976
Accommodation, 702
Accountability, 375, 391
  critical thinking and, 270-271
  in nursing, 19
Accreditation, 477
Acculturation, 120
Acetaminophen, 823, 1283t
Achilles reflex, 768t
Achilles tendon, 1423, 1424f
Acid-base balance
  disturbances in, 1143-1146, 1145t, 1146t
  intravenous therapy for, 1193
  regulation of, 1140, 1140f
Acidification of urine, 1345
Acidosis
  metabolic, 1144, 1145t, 1154t
  respiratory, 1144, 1145t, 1148, 1154t
Acne, 1009t, 1013
Acquired immunodeficiency syndrome, 527, 775t
  adolescent and, 212
  Americans With Disabilities Act and, 408-409
  family care in, 143
  increased surgical risks and, 1599t
  nursing history of, 1085
  nutrition in, 1317
  transmission of, 963
  value of vaccinations in, 1095-1096
Acromegaly, 697
Actigraphy, 1204
Active immunity, 962
Active listening, 437
Active strategies of health promotion, 97
Active transport, 1137, 1138f
Activities of daily living, 256, 347, 931
  incorporation of exercise into, 945b
  pain and, 1246
Activity, 929-958
  acute care and, 946-948, 947b, 948f
  assistive devices for walking, 948-953, 949b, 949-953f
  behavioral aspects of, 935, 935b
  body mechanics and, 931-932
    assessment of, 937-938, 938f, 939b, 939f, 940b
    lifting techniques in, 946, 946f
    principles of, 933-934, 934b
  chronic illness and, 953-954, 954b
  critical thinking in, 936-937
  cultural and ethnic influences on, 936, 936b
  developmental changes and, 934-935
  environmental issues in, 935-936
  evaluation in, 954-955, 955f
  family and social support for, 936
  health promotion in, 941-946, 945b
  nursing diagnosis in, 939-940, 940b
  older adult and, 250
  planning in, 940-941, 941f
  postoperative, 1611-1618
  regulation of movement and, 932-933

Activity intolerance, 943-944
Activity reinforcer, 467
Activity theory, 239
Activity tolerance, 932, 938-939, 939b, 940b, 1434-1439
Actual loss, 569
Actual nursing diagnosis, 306
Acuity record, 492
Acupoints, 922
Acupressure, 913t, 1254
Acupuncture, 913t, 922, 922f
Acupuncturist, 124t
Acute care
  activity and, 946-948, 947b, 948f
  assisting client with feeding in, 1297-1299
  blood replacement in, 1190-1193, 1191b, 1191f, 1192t
  daily weights and intake and output measurement in, 1158-1159, 1159b
  dietary progression in, 1296, 1298b, 1298t
  enteral nutrition in, 1299-1311
    administration via nasoenteric tube, 1305-1308
    complications of, 1314-1315t
    determination of placement of tube, 1312b
    enteral access tubes in, 1304, 1304f
    indications for, 1299b
    insertion of nasoenteric tube for, 1300-1303
    obtaining aspirate for pH measurement, 1313
    via gastrostomy or jejunostomy tube, 1309-1311
  enteral replacement of fluids in, 1159
  family care and, 151
  grief and, 585-587
  hygiene in, 1021-1022, 1022b
  immobility and, 1449-1475
    assisting client to sitting position, 1469-1470
    cardiac workload and, 1451
    cardiovascular system and, 1451
    developmental changes and, 1455
    elimination and, 1454
    expansion of chest and lungs in, 1449
    Hoyer lift in, 1473-1474
    integumentary system and, 1454
    maintenance of patent airway in, 1451
    metabolic systemic and, 1449
    moving and positioning client in bed, 1458-1466
    musculoskeletal system and, 1452-1454, 1454b, 1454f
    positioning techniques in, 1455-1457, 1456f, 1456t
    prevention of stasis of pulmonary secretions in, 1449-1451
    psychological changes in, 1454-1455
    reduction of orthostatic hypotension in, 1451
    respiratory system and, 1449
    thrombus formation and, 1451-1452, 1452b, 1453b
    transferring client from bed to chair, 1467, 1467f, 1470-1471
    transferring client from bed to stretcher, 1467, 1467f, 1472, 1475
  infection control and, 784-786

Special Features

Client Teaching

Concept Maps

*R*esearch Highlights

Special Features—cont'd

Nursing Care Plans

Procedural Guideline

Skills